MW01195532

Lever's
Dermatopathology

Histopathology of the Skin

TWELFTH EDITION

TWELFTH EDITION

Lever's
Dermatopathology
Histopathology of the Skin

Editor-in-Chief:

David E. Elder, MB, CHB, FRCPA
Professor of Pathology and Laboratory Medicine
Hospital of the University of Pennsylvania
Philadelphia, Pennsylvania

Associate Editors:

Rosalie Elenitsas, MD
Professor of Dermatology
Director of Dermatopathology
Department of Dermatology
Hospital of the University of Pennsylvania
Philadelphia, Pennsylvania

George F. Murphy, MD
Professor of Pathology
Harvard Medical School
Boston, Massachusetts
Director, Program in Dermatopathology
Department of Pathology
Brigham and Women's Hospital
Boston, Massachusetts

Misha Rosenbach, MD
Assistant Professor of Dermatology and Internal Medicine
Associate Program Director, Dermatology Residency
Director, Dermatology Inpatient Consult Service
Director, Cutaneous Sarcoidosis Clinic
Perelman School of Medicine
University of Pennsylvania
Philadelphia, Pennsylvania

Adam I. Rubin, MD
Assistant Professor of Dermatology
Hospital of the University of Pennsylvania
The Children's Hospital of Philadelphia
Perelman School of Medicine
University of Pennsylvania
Philadelphia, Pennsylvania

John T. Seykora, MD
Professor
Section of Dermatopathology
Department of Dermatology
Hospital of the University of Pennsylvania
Philadelphia, Pennsylvania

Xiaowei Xu, MD, PhD
Associate Professor
Department of Pathology and Laboratory Medicine
University of Pennsylvania
Philadelphia, Pennsylvania

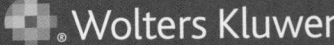

Wolters Kluwer

Philadelphia • Baltimore • New York • London
Buenos Aires • Hong Kong • Sydney • Tokyo

Acquisitions Editor: Nicole Dernoski
Senior Development Editor: Ariel S. Winter
Editorial Coordinator: Christopher Rodgers
Marketing Manager: Kirsten Watrud
Production Project Manager: Bridgett Dougherty
Manager, Graphic Arts & Design: Stephen Druding
Manufacturing Coordinator: Beth Welsh
Prepress Vendor: S4Carlisle Publishing Services

Twelfth Edition

Copyright © 2023 Wolters Kluwer.

Copyright © 2015 Wolters Kluwer. Copyright © 2009 Lippincott Williams & Wilkins, a Wolters Kluwer business. Copyright © 2004, 1997 by Lippincott Williams & Wilkins. Copyright © 1990, 1983, 1975 by JB Lippincott. All rights reserved. This book is protected by copyright. No part of this book may be reproduced or transmitted in any form or by any means, including as photocopies or scanned-in or other electronic copies, or utilized by any information storage and retrieval system without written permission from the copyright owner, except for brief quotations embodied in critical articles and reviews. Materials appearing in this book prepared by individuals as part of their official duties as U.S. government employees are not covered by the above-mentioned copyright. To request permission, please contact Wolters Kluwer at Two Commerce Square, 2001 Market Street, Philadelphia, PA 19103, via email at permissions@lww.com, or via our website at shop.lww.com (products and services). 7/2022

9 8 7 6 5 4 3 2 1

Printed in Singapore

Library of Congress Cataloging-in-Publication Data
ISBN-13: 978-1-9751-7449-1
ISBN-10: 1-975174-49-6
Library of Congress Control Number: 2022909724

This work is provided "as is," and the publisher disclaims any and all warranties, express or implied, including any warranties as to accuracy, comprehensiveness, or currency of the content of this work.

This work is no substitute for individual patient assessment based upon healthcare professionals' examination of each patient and consideration of, among other things, age, weight, gender, current or prior medical conditions, medication history, laboratory data and other factors unique to the patient. The publisher does not provide medical advice or guidance and this work is merely a reference tool. Healthcare professionals, and not the publisher, are solely responsible for the use of this work including all medical judgments and for any resulting diagnosis and treatments.

Given continuous, rapid advances in medical science and health information, independent professional verification of medical diagnoses, indications, appropriate pharmaceutical selections and dosages, and treatment options should be made and healthcare professionals should consult a variety of sources. When prescribing medication, healthcare professionals are advised to consult the product information sheet (the manufacturer's package insert) accompanying each drug to verify, among other things, conditions of use, warnings and side effects and identify any changes in dosage schedule or contraindications, particularly if the medication to be administered is new, infrequently used or has a narrow therapeutic range. To the maximum extent permitted under applicable law, no responsibility is assumed by the publisher for any injury and/or damage to persons or property, as a matter of products liability, negligence law or otherwise, or from any reference to or use by any person of this work.

shop.lww.com

MKO722

Dedication

This edition is dedicated to our families who have supported us in our endeavors leading up to this work, and to our teachers and mentors in medicine and surgery, pathology, dermatology, and dermatopathology, too numerous to name individually, whose commitment to the discovery and dissemination of knowledge, and careful tutoring at the bedside, bench, and microscope enabled this work to be accomplished. We are also grateful to those with whose care we have been in part entrusted, providing the basis for the descriptions and illustrations of conditions presented in this book.

Contributors

Khadija Aljefri, MBChB, MRCP(DERM), CCT(UK)
Consultant Dermatologist
Department of Dermatology
Dermamed Clinic
Dubai, United Arab Emirates

Emily M. Altman, MD
Associate Professor, Program Director, Vice Chair of Education
Department of Dermatology
University of New Mexico
Albuquerque, New Mexico

Raymond L. Barnhill, MD, MSc
Professor
Department of Translational Research
Institut Curie and Université de Paris UFR de Médecine
Paris, France

Trevor W. Beer, MBChB, FRCPA, FRCPath
Dermatopathologist
Clinipath Pathology
Osborne Park, Western Australia

Ryan S. Berry, MD
Staff Pathologist
Western Pathology, Inc.
San Luis Obispo, California

Steven D. Billings, MD
Professor
Department of Pathology
Cleveland Clinic Lerner College of Medicine
Cleveland, Ohio
Co-Director, Dermatopathology Section
Department of Pathology
Cleveland Clinic
Cleveland, Ohio

Scott C. Bresler, MD, PhD
Assistant Professor
Department of Pathology and Dermatology
Michigan Medicine, University of Michigan
Ann Arbor, Michigan

Eduardo Calonje, MD, DipRCpath
Lead in Dermatopathology
Honorary Reader, King's College London
Department of Dermatopathology
St John's Institute of Dermatology
St Thomas' Hospital
London, United Kingdom

Thinh Chau, MD
Resident
Department of Dermatology
Brown University
Rhode Island Hospital
Providence, Rhode Island

Lianjun Chen, MD, PhD
Associate Professor
Department of Dermatology
Hua Shan Hospital
Fu Dan University
Shanghai, China

Emily Y. Chu, MD, PhD
Associate Professor
Dermatology and Pathology and Laboratory Medicine
Perelman School of Medicine
University of Pennsylvania
Philadelphia, Pennsylvania

Mary Clark, MD, MS
Assistant Professor
Department of Pathology and Laboratory Medicine
The Geisel School of Medicine at Dartmouth
Hanover, New Hampshire
Chief
Department of Pathology and Laboratory Medicine
White River Junction VA Medical Center
White River Junction, Vermont

Caryn Cobb, BA
Medical Student
Department of Dermatology
The Warren Alpert Medical School of Brown University
Rhode Island Hospital
Providence, Rhode Island

A. Neil Crowson, MD
President of Pathology Laboratory Associates
Director of Dermatopathology
Department of Dermatology
University of Oklahoma
Tulsa, Oklahoma

Jonathan L. Curry, MD
Professor of Pathology and Translational Molecular
   Pathology
The University of Texas MD Anderson Cancer Center
Houston, Texas

William Damsky, MD, PhD
Assistant Professor
Departments of Dermatology and Pathology
Yale University
New Haven, Connecticut

Garrett T. Desman, MD
Chief of Dermatopathology Services
Optum
Lake Success, New York
Assistant Clinical Professor
Department of Pathology and Dermatology
Icahn School of Medicine at Mount Sinai
New York, New York

Lyn M. Duncan, MD
Professor of Pathology
Harvard Medical School
Boston, Massachusetts
Dermatopathologist
Department of Pathology
Massachusetts General Hospital
Boston, Massachusetts

David E. Elder, MB, CHB, FRCPA
Professor of Pathology and Laboratory Medicine
Hospital of the University of Pennsylvania
Philadelphia, Pennsylvania

Rosalie Elenitsas, MD
Professor of Dermatology, Director of
    Dermatopathology
Department of Dermatology
Hospital of the University of Pennsylvania
Philadelphia, Pennsylvania

Beverly E. Faulkner-Jones, MB, ChB, PhD
Senior Dermatopathologist and Pediatric Pathologist
Quantum Pathology, LLC
Waltham, Massachusetts

Andrew L. Folpe, MD
Professor
Department of Laboratory Medicine and Pathology
Mayo Clinic
Rochester, Minnesota

Jessica A. Forcucci, MD
Assistant Professor
Department of Pathology and Laboratory Medicine
Medical University of South Carolina
Charleston, South Carolina

Ruth K. Foreman, MD, PhD
Assistant Professor
Department of Pathology
Massachusetts General Hospital
Harvard Medical School
Boston, Massachusetts

Maxwell A. Fung, MD
Professor, Director
Department of Dermatology
University of California, Davis
Sacramento, California

Earl J. Glusac, MD
Professor of Pathology and Dermatology
Yale University School of Medicine
New Haven, Connecticut

Amrita Goyal, MD
Adjunct Assistant Professor
Department of Dermatology
University of Minnesota
Minneapolis, Minnesota

Alejandro A. Gru, MD
Associate Professor
Departments of Pathology and Dermatology
University of Virginia
Charlottesville, Virginia

Terence J. Harrist, MD
Senior Dermatopathologist
Quantum Pathology
Waltham, Massachusetts

John L. M. Hawk, BSc, MD
Emeritus Professor of Dermatological Photobiology
King's College London and St John's Institute of
    Dermatology
London, United Kingdom

Matthew L. Hedberg, MD, PhD
Instructor and Waine C. Johnson Endowed Research Fellow of
    Dermatopathology
Department of Dermatology
Perelman School of Medicine
University of Pennsylvania
Philadelphia, Pennsylvania
Instructor
Department of Dermatology
Hospital of the University of Pennsylvania
Philadelphia, Pennsylvania

Peter Heenan, MBBS, FRCPA, FRCPATH
Clinical Professor
School of Pathology and Laboratory Medicine
The University of Western Australia
Crawley, Western Australia, Australia

Edward R. Heilman, MD, FAAD, FCAP
Clinical Professor of Dermatology and Pathology
SUNY Downstate Health Sciences University
Chair Emeritus, Dermatology
Program Director, Dermatopathology Fellowship
University College of Brooklyn
Brooklyn, New York

Molly A. Hinshaw, MD, FAAD
Associate Professor of Dermatology and Pathology
Section Chief of Dermatology, Director of Dermatology Nail
    Clinic
Department of Dermatology
University of Wisconsin School of Medicine and
    Public Health
University of Wisconsin Hospital and Clinics
Madison, Wisconsin

Michael D. Ioffreda, MD
Professor
Departments of Dermatology and Pathology
Penn State College of Medicine
Penn State Health—Hershey Medical Center
Hershey, Pennsylvania

Joseph S. Kattampallil, BMBS, FRACGP, MBA, FRCPA
Anatomical Pathologist
Clinipath
Perth, Western Australia, Australia

Nigel Kirkham, MD, FRCPath
Consultant Pathologist
National Reference Laboratory
Dubai, United Arab Emirates

Christine J. Ko, MD
Professor of Dermatology and Pathology
Associate Director, Dermatopathology Laboratory
Department of Dermatology
Yale University
New Haven, Connecticut

Erica S. Kumar, MD
Physician
Department of Dermatopathology and Pathology
Pathology Laboratory Associates
Tulsa, Oklahoma
Department of Dermatology
University of Oklahoma
Oklahoma City, Oklahoma

Alvaro C. Laga, MD, MMSc
Associate Pathologist, Department of Pathology
Brigham and Women's Hospital
Harvard Medical School
Boston, Massachusetts

Christine G. Lian, MD
Associate Professor of Pathology
Brigham and Women's Hospital
Harvard Medical School
Boston, Massachusetts

B. Jack Longley, MD
Professor Emeritus
Department of Dermatology
University of Wisconsin
Madison, Wisconsin

Su Enn Low, MBChB, FRCPath
Consultant Histopathologist
Department of Histopathology
Whiston Hospital
Rainhill, United Kingdom

Cynthia Magro, MD
Professor of Pathology and Laboratory Medicine
Director of Dermatopathology
Department of Pathology
Weill Cornell Medicine
New York, New York

John C. Maize, MD
Distinguished University Professor
Medical University of South Carolina
Charleston, South Carolina

Zlatko Marušić, MD, PhD
Consultant Pathologist
Clinical Department of Pathology and Cytology
University Hospital Center—Zagreb
Zagreb, Croatia

Martin C. Mihm, Jr., MD, FACP
Associate Director, Melanoma Program
Department of Dermatology
Brigham and Women's Hospital
Boston, Massachusetts

Michael K. Miller, MD
Clinical Assistant Professor
Department of Dermatology
SUNY Downstate Medical Center
Brooklyn, New York
Active Staff
Department of Pathology
Yale New Haven Health: Greenwich Hospital
Greenwich, New York

Michael E. Ming, MD, MSCE
Associate Professor of Dermatology
School of Medicine
University of Pennsylvania
Philadelphia, Pennsylvania

Adnan Mir, MD, PhD
Assistant Professor
Department of Dermatology
Metropolitan Hospital Center and Weill Cornell Medicine
New York, New York
Dermatopathologist
Dermpath Diagnostics New York
White Plains, New York

Elizabeth A. Morgan, MD
Associate Professor
Department of Pathology
Harvard Medical School
Boston, Massachusetts
Associate Pathologist
Department of Pathology
Brigham and Women's Hospital
Boston, Massachusetts

George F. Murphy, MD
Professor of Pathology
Harvard Medical School
Boston, Massachusetts

Priyadharsini Nagarajan, MD, PhD
Associate Professor
Department of Pathology
The University of Texas MD Anderson Cancer Center
Houston, Texas

Rosalynn M. Nazarian, MD
Associate Professor
Department of Pathology
Harvard Medical School
Boston, Massachusetts
Associate Pathologist
Pathology Service, Dermatopathology Unit
Massachusetts General Hospital
Boston, Massachusetts

Cuong V. Nguyen, MD
Assistant Professor
Department of Dermatology
Northwestern University, Feinberg School of Medicine
Northwestern Memorial Hospital
Chicago, Illinois

Charles H. Palmer, MD
Staff Pathologist and Dermatopathologist (Emeritus)
Department of Pathology
Pathology Associates of Albuquerque
Presbyterian Hospital
Albuquerque, New Mexico

Rajiv M. Patel, MD
Director (Section Head) of Dermatopathology
Director, Bone and Soft Tissue Pathology Fellowship
Departments of Pathology and Dermatology
Michigan Medicine, University of Michigan
Ann Arbor, Michigan

Susan Pei, MD
Assistant Professor of Oncology
Department of Dermatology
Department of Pathology and Laboratory Medicine
Roswell Park Comprehensive Cancer Center
Buffalo, New York

Victor G. Prieto, MD, PhD
Chair
Department of Pathology
The University of Texas MD Anderson Cancer Center
Houston, Texas

Bruce D. Ragsdale, MD
Pathologist
Western Pathology, Inc.
San Luis Obispo, California

Luis Requena, MD
Professor
Department of Dermatology
Universidad Autónoma de Madrid
Madrid, Spain
Chairman
Department of Dermatology
Fundación Jiménez Diaz
Madrid, Spain

Leslie Robinson-Bostom, MD
Professor
Department of Dermatology
The Warren Alpert Medical School of Brown
    University
Providence, Rhode Island
Director, Division of Dermatopathology
Brown Dermatology
Providence, Rhode Island

Misha Rosenbach, MD
Associate Professor
Department of Dermatology
University of Pennsylvania
Philadelphia, Pennsylvania

Adam I. Rubin, MD
Associate Professor of Dermatology, Pediatrics, and Pathology
    and Laboratory Medicine
Perelman School of Medicine
University of Pennsylvania
Philadelphia, Pennsylvania

Sam Sadigh, MD
Instructor
Department of Pathology
Harvard Medical School
Boston, Massachusetts
Associate Pathologist
Department of Pathology
Brigham and Women's Hospital
Boston, Massachusetts

John T. Seykora, MD, PhD
Professor
Departments of Dermatology and Pathology
Perelman School of Medicine
University of Pennsylvania
Philadelphia, Pennsylvania

Jason S. Stratton, MD
Assistant Professor
Oklahoma University College of Medicine
Oklahoma City, Oklahoma
Anatomic and Clinical Pathologist
Pathology Laboratory Associates
Tulsa, Oklahoma

Michael T. Tetzlaff, MD
Professor
Department of Pathology and Dermatology
University of California, San Francisco
San Francisco, California

Jorge Torres-Mora, MD
Assistant Professor
Department of Laboratory Medicine and Pathology
Mayo Clinic
Rochester, Minnesota

Margaret Wat, MD, PhD
Assistant Professor
Departments of Dermatology and Pathology
University of Arizona College of Medicine—Tucson
Tucson, Arizona
Director of Dermatopathology
Departments of Dermatology and Pathology
Banner University Medical Center—Tucson
Tucson, Arizona

Michael Wilk, MD
Dermatologist and Dermatopathologist
Private Dermatohistological Laboratory
Nuernberg, Germany

Xiaowei Xu, MD, PhD
Professor
Department of Pathology and Laboratory Medicine
University of Pennsylvania
Philadelphia, Pennsylvania

Sook Jung Yun, MD, PhD
Professor and Chair
Department of Dermatology
Chonnam National University Medical School
Gwangju, South Korea
Professor
Department of Dermatology
Chonnam National University Hospital
Gwangju, South Korea

Bernhard Wilhelm Heinrich Zelger, Prof. Dr. Mag.
Associate Professor
Department of Dermatology, Venerology and Allergology
Medical University Innsbruck
Innsbruck, Austria

Preface to the Twelfth Edition

This book represents an incremental revision and update of the previous three editions, the first of which constituted a somewhat more extensive revision of the seven editions produced by Walter Lever, MD, beginning in 1949 as a 449-page volume with "221 Illustrations Including 8 Subjects in Color on 4 Plates." Thus, this will be the eleventh edition of a book that has been continuously published for more than 70 years! In this second generation of the work, the principles that made "Lever" such a success for so long continue to be applied, and are extended in this edition. These include, first and foremost, a continued organization of the book along the lines of a traditional clinicopathologic classification of cutaneous disease. This enables us to discuss lesions according to their clinical and etiologic relationships, paralleling the organization of the major clinical texts. In some other dermatopathology works, a greater emphasis has been placed on histological patterns of disease as the underpinning of the chapter organization. This has advantages in enabling beginners to develop an appropriate differential diagnosis for a given pattern of disease, but can be confusing in that etiologically and clinically disparate conditions tend to be discussed in juxtaposition to each other, and also in that polymorphous conditions need to be discussed in multiple different places.

We have taken into account the modern emphasis on pattern recognition in several ways. First, within each chapter, the conditions considered are, when appropriate, organized and discussed along pattern lines. Second, we have, as in the past, included a chapter that presents an algorithmic classification of skin diseases according to histologic pattern features. It is intended that this chapter may serve as a means of developing a differential diagnosis from an unknown slide, following which page references are provided to discuss the disorders in other areas of the book. In addition, we have prepared a companion volume "Synopsis and Atlas of Lever's Histopathology of the Skin," now in its fourth edition. This Atlas has enabled us to greatly extend the number of illustrations including a larger number of clinical images, and is organized completely on the basis of histologic patterns. Unlike some other pattern-based works, this Atlas includes neoplastic disorders among the inflammatory conditions. Thus, it becomes clear to the reader that a lichenoid actinic keratosis or in situ melanoma may share features with (and potentially be misdiagnosed as) a plaque of lichen planus or a patch of lupus. This Atlas will continue to be updated and extended to incorporate the new information in successive editions of the "Big Lever."

In another area of emphasis, we have continued the practice of providing clinical review prior to exposition of the histologic features for each group of disorders. This has been made more explicit with the addition of a specific heading "Clinical Summary" for most disease entities. In addition, we have a section entitled "Principles of Management" to serve for each disease or category of disease as a capsule summary of treatment modalities. These are becoming increasingly complex, and subject to rapid evolution and change. These innovations in our opinion will greatly enhance the value of the work, not only for pathologists and others whose primary training is not in clinical dermatology but also for dermatologists in training and, no doubt, for some who are more advanced in the field as well. We also include clinical images to enhance this distinctive aspect of the text, recognizing that the clinical morphology is the "gross pathology" of dermatopathology. Indeed, in today's environment of ubiquitous digital cameras and internet connections, we take this opportunity to encourage clinicians to submit with their biopsies not only detailed clinical differentials but also clinical images of selected cases, for the benefit of more accurate diagnosis and improved patient care.

At the other end of the spectrum of clinical science, we have continued and updated the classic work's emphasis on "histogenesis" by emphasizing underlying mechanisms of disease. The term "histogenesis," to us, includes mechanisms of development of histologic patterns of disease and might equally well be (and sometime is) labeled "pathogenesis." Because of the explosion of knowledge, molecular mechanisms of pathogenesis are presented for perhaps almost a majority of the diseases. However, it is interesting that, in most cases, these molecular mechanisms, while of explanatory interest, still have not yet supplanted traditional histopathology and immunohistology as the "gold standard" for diagnosis of most of the conditions discussed in the book.

As in the past, the book does not attempt to be a compendium of all known skin diseases. However, we have tried to make it a reference work for those skin diseases in which histopathology plays an important role in diagnosis. We are grateful for this opportunity and are excited to present another edition of this revered work to a new generation of readers. At the same time, we hope that members of earlier generations, who have used "Lever" as their primary skin pathology training and reference source, will find this new edition useful in their continuing development and in their daily practices.

David E. Elder
Philadelphia, 2022

Preface to the First Edition

This book is based on the courses of dermatopathology that I have been giving in recent years to graduate students of dermatology enrolled at Harvard Medical School and Massachusetts General Hospital. The book is written primarily for dermatologists; I hope, however, that it may be useful also to pathologists, since dermatopathology is given little consideration in most textbooks of pathology.

I have attempted to keep this book short. Emphasis has been placed on the essential histologic features. Minor details and rare aberrations from the typical histologic picture have been omitted. I have allotted more space to the cutaneous diseases in which histologic examination is of diagnostic value than to those in which the histologic picture is not characteristic. In spite of my striving for brevity I have discussed the histogenesis of several dermatoses, because knowledge of the histogenesis often is of great value for the understanding of the pathologic process.

Primarily for the benefit of pathologists who usually are not too familiar with dermatologic diseases, I have preceded the histologic discussion of each disease with a short description of the clinical features. A fairly extensive bibliography has been supplied for readers who are interested in obtaining additional information. In the selection of articles for the bibliography, preference has been given, whenever possible, to those written in English.

I wish to express my deep gratitude to Dr. Tracy B. Mallory and Dr. Benjamin Castleman of the Pathology Laboratory at the Massachusetts General Hospital for the training in pathology they have given me. It has been invaluable to me. Their teaching is reflected in this book. Furthermore, I wish to thank Mr. Richard W. St. Clair, who with great skill and patience produced all the photomicrographs in this book.

Walter F. Lever
1949

Acknowledgments

The editors acknowledge the contributions of many others to this work in its previous editions, especially those of Walter F Lever, MD, and Gundula Schaumberg-Lever, MD.

Contents

Introduction to Dermatopathologic Diagnosis

DAVID E. ELDER, ROSALIE ELENITSAS, GEORGE F. MURPHY, MISHA ROSENBACH, ADAM I. RUBIN, AND XIAOWEI XU

INTRODUCTION

Readers of this book (now in its 12th edition) have long relied on it to aid them in making accurate histopathologic diagnoses of cutaneous disease. A diagnosis is a clinical tool that assists in the process of codifying patients into disease groups that tend to share a common outcome and a common set of responses to therapy. The histopathologic diagnosis in turn is used by clinicians to aid in the management of patients. The most accurate diagnosis is the one that most closely correlates with clinical outcome and helps direct the most appropriate clinical intervention. Thus, there is a close relationship between diagnosis and prognostication. By emphasizing certain key observations that have value in identifying particular diseases, this book aids observers to make appropriate histopathologic diagnoses from skin specimens and to provide an estimate of prognosis.

Where applicable, ultrastructural, immunohistochemical, and molecular aids to diagnosis are discussed. These advances have resulted in increased specificity for many diagnoses. For example, immunofluorescence has long been used to differentiate among vesiculobullous disorders (Chapter 9). In another example, a dermal tumor composed of large nonpigmented mitotically active cells that are positive in an immunohistochemical reaction for the HMB-45 or Melan-A antigens could be a malignant melanoma, or a clear cell sarcoma. In the absence of the immunologic criteria, these diagnoses could not have been made as reliably (Chapter 28). Currently, molecular criteria are routinely utilized for diagnosis and prognosis. For example, a fusion transcript for EWS-ATF1 detected by reverse transcriptase polymerase chain reaction (RT-PCR) or by fluorescence *in situ* hybridization (FISH) can reliably distinguish between a clear cell sarcoma and a malignant melanoma involving the soft tissue, a distinction that is not always possible to make with certainty by traditional means (Chapter 28) (1). As another example, FISH testing and comparative genomic hybridization (CGH) or diagnostic gene expression profiling (GEP) or next-generation sequencing (NGS), in addition to ancillary immunohistochemical testing for markers like Ki-67, p16, HMB-45, and PRAME are all currently used to help make a more specific diagnosis in melanocytic tumors that present with conflicting criteria or with criteria whose diagnostic efficacy is uncertain (Chapter 28) (2,3).

Despite the rapid advances of molecular techniques in diagnosis and prognosis, it may seem surprising that morphology remains the basis of diagnosis for most neoplasms and many inflammatory dermatoses. Yet a histopathologic image represents a true synthesis of all of the molecular events acting in a given microscopic "scene," encompassing not only the concerted expression of genes, including oncogenes and tumor suppressor genes but also the sum total of all epigenetic effects such as gene methylation, posttranslational modification, and the spatially and temporally segregated interactions of proteins and other gene products. This level of complexity of information cannot be captured by any high-throughput molecular testing that has yet been developed. Although histopathology remains the gold standard for most dermatologic diagnoses, it must be recognized that not all specimens are amenable to a definitive "specific" histopathologic diagnosis. As reviewed by Foucar (4–6), specificity, or the "true negativity rate," is the frequency of a negative test result in individuals who actually do not have the disease of interest. Specificity studies are hard to do because they require large-scale studies of normal populations and because of the need for a "gold standard" for the disease, independent of the test under consideration. Most studies in the literature begin with data demonstrating the "sensitivity" or "true positive rate," which is a measure of the frequency of a positive test result in individuals with the disease (4). These data do not, however, indicate that a diagnostic test is perfectly reliable. For example, most melanomas are positive for the immunohistochemical marker S100 (high sensitivity). However, almost all benign melanocytic neoplasms are also positive for the same marker (low specificity). Frequent mitoses in the dermal component of the neoplasm, on the other hand, are common in bulky tumorigenic melanomas but rare in most benign melanocytic neoplasms and are therefore a useful, relatively specific but not pathognomonic marker for melanoma. Alternatively, mitotic figures are absent in most thin nontumorigenic melanomas so that their sensitivity for the diagnosis of "melanoma," overall, is low (Chapter 28).

The histopathologic features of many inflammatory dermatoses have overlapping features with each other, and only a few particular signs can be suggestive of a specific diagnosis. Even among the more readily characterized papulosquamous dermatoses, such as psoriasis or lichen planus (Chapter 7), the histopathologic picture is more typically "consistent with" rather than "diagnostic of" the clinical process. However, in patient management, the histopathology can be helpful by excluding one diagnosis out of a large differential when a specific diagnosis is not possible. For example, review of a biopsy of a psoriasiform plaque may rule out mycosis fungoides (Chapter 31) but may not be able to establish the specific diagnosis of psoriasis (Chapter 7). The obvious diagnostic limitations of histopathology extend to infectious and neoplastic processes as well, where additional testing such as special stains and/or bacterial or fungal cultures may be essential to establish a useful diagnosis. For example, the hyaline fungi of the dermatophyte group may be invisible against the backdrop of nail plate and are typically visualized only in a periodic acid–Schiff (PAS) or Grocott stain for fungus. The converse applies to noninfectious inflammatory disorders such as pyoderma gangrenosum, where infection needs to be ruled out as an etiologic possibility (Chapter 16). Similarly, in the neoplastic realm, histopathology alone may not suffice to distinguish between keratoacanthoma and squamous cell carcinoma (7) (Chapter 29) or between Spitz nevus and melanoma (8) (Chapter 28).

Some of these "difficult" diagnoses result from the existence of important data elements that are undetectable by routine histologic methods, such as sparse organisms in a granulomatous process or molecular changes in a pigmented lesion. In other instances, the data might be detectable if sought but are obscure. Many granulomatous processes can be more specifically characterized if more sensitive staining for organisms is done, as in a Grocott or acid-fast stain. If the observer does not think of infection and order the stain, the diagnosis is never made. In many other situations, however, such as the diagnosis of keratoacanthoma versus squamous cell carcinoma or of Spitz nevus versus melanoma, the available data may have been assiduously collected by the observer using complex algorithms published for these purposes, yet the diagnosis remains obscure, and agreement among observers is difficult or impossible to obtain. In such cases, there is typically a continuum of the traits that underlie diagnosis, and individual cases in the vicinity of the diagnostic cut-point are more likely to be misclassified than other cases (9). In addition, the available criteria may simply lack the discriminatory power needed to make a confident diagnosis.

In an interesting exercise published as "Tutorial on Melanocytic Lesions," a panel of six experts in pigmented lesion pathology reviewed 71 "difficult" cases (10). While agreement was substantial for many of the different categories of lesions, the categories of Spitz nevi and other variants of nevi and of nevoid melanoma were more difficult. Unanimity in diagnosis was reached in only 11 of 38 of these cases, and in 6 cases the opinions of the experts were equally divided between benign and malignant. In another category, that of six examples of "pseudomelanomas" in children, agreement on a benign diagnosis was almost unanimous, yet one of these patients had died of metastatic disease. In another study of 30 lesions selected for their difficulty, evaluation of 17 "Spitzoid" lesions yielded no clear consensus as to diagnosis; "in only one case did six or more pathologists agree on a single category, regardless of clinical outcome." In addition, some lesions that proved fatal were categorized by most observers as either Spitz nevi or atypical Spitz tumors (11). Thus, agreement on a diagnosis does not necessarily mean that the diagnosis is correct. Therefore, the best opinion that can be rendered about these lesions is that the true diagnosis is unknown and the likely behavior of these lesions is uncertain. The use of modern molecular techniques has mitigated, but not eliminated, this uncertainty (12).

Following practice in other areas of pathology where similar problems exist (13–23), such lesions, in our opinion, are best categorized as "tumors of uncertain malignant potential" (TUMPs). In these cases, we always provide a differential diagnosis, and therapy is usually tailored with the "worst-case scenario" taken into consideration. Even this latter assumption

is not without potential for controversy. However, it is not clear that therapy devised for routine cases of melanoma should be automatically applied to melanocytic tumors of uncertain malignant potential (MELTUMPs) (Chapter 28). In these "borderline" or "difficult" lesions, the clinical utility of histopathology may be aided by effective communication between the clinician and pathologist, with appropriate attention to the clinical and epidemiologic context of the lesion under study, and also by ancillary testing such as CGH, FISH, or NGS for assessment of gene amplification profiles and mutation status, which have been shown to differ between Spitz nevi and melanomas (24,25). Even when all of the clinical, histopathologic, and molecular information is at hand, a consensus diagnosis may be impossible, and there is no prospective assurance that any diagnosis is biologically "correct."

Foucar (5,6,26) has elegantly discussed the difficulties inherent in making a histopathologic diagnosis (and these considerations apply to other forms of diagnosis as well), and the issues have also been well covered by Sackett and his colleagues (27). A major reason for the difficulty in making an exact diagnosis in pathology, as in clinical medicine, is that the information required to make the diagnosis is frequently incomplete. At the most fundamental level, there may simply be no extant standard for a particular diagnosis. For example, histopathology is often taken to be a gold standard for diagnosis of a particular disease. However, if the histopathologic parameters that are considered to define this disease have been determined in a clinically defined series of cases, their independence and specificity could be called into question. A purely histopathologic study of nummular dermatitis, however complete and accurate it may be, will not glean any information that reliably distinguishes between this diagnosis and that of another spongiotic dermatitis (Chapter 7). Patches of early mycosis fungoides biopsied from patients with established plaque-stage lesions may well represent examples of "early" mycosis fungoides, yet similar histologic changes in a patient with only a solitary lesion may or may not progress to established disease (Chapter 31).

Another serious problem in histopathologic diagnosis results from the fact that specificity studies to determine the prevalence of criteria in diagnostically challenging cases are frequently not available. For example, early studies of the HMB-45 antibody determined that it had 100% specificity for melanoma cells in the dermis or deeper tissues (28). After the specificity studies were extended, however, it was recognized that this antigen is expressed not only in melanoma but also in blue nevi (29) and in other benign lesions (Chapter 28).

Foucar has pointed out that the diagnostic process is an example of complex decision-making that has intrinsic uncertainty, usually resulting from one or more of the following: (a) the large number of variables that can be evaluated in an attempt to solve the problem results in novel combinations of variables that cannot be managed consistently by problem solvers; (b) one or more key variables lack clear definition; or (c) one or more key variables is hidden from the problem solver (26). To the uncertainty inherent in these complex problems can be added (d) the uncertainty (discussed previously) of the specificity of the individual findings and (e) the uncertainty that results from deficiencies in the observer's ability to evaluate and categorize histologic findings. Even the most expert observers have inherent and often unrecognized deficiencies that result in less-than-perfect reproducibility of histopathologic observations, and thus of diagnoses (30). Furthermore, there are limitations in the ability of even the most expert observers to communicate their diagnostic acumen to others (26).

The diagnostic difficulties that result from uncertainty are compounded when there is also failure to agree on the criteria for diagnosis. In a study of inter- and intraobserver reproducibility for the diagnosis of dysplastic nevi, intraobserver reproducibility was substantial, and interobserver concordance was fair, despite differences in criteria. It was concluded that, although experienced dermatopathologists in this study used different diagnostic criteria for histopathologic dysplasia, their usage was consistent (31). In another study where observers agreed to abide by predetermined criteria, and were provided reference photomicrographs illustrative of the criteria, agreement was substantial to excellent for the histopathologic diagnosis of 112 melanocytic tumors, including typical and dysplastic nevi and melanomas. It was then concluded that, using predetermined criteria, melanocytic dysplasia can be reproducibly graded among diverse general dermatopathologists (32). It is also interesting to note that, even when reproducibility is less than what might be considered optimal, a diagnosis can still be meaningful if the association between the diagnostic observation and a biologically important result is sufficiently powerful. In a case-control study of the association of histopathologic melanocytic dysplasia with melanoma risk, a statistically significant and biologically meaningful relative risk of 3.99 was observed despite κ values for agreement among observers that were in the "poor" range (33). Presumably, the differences in criteria among observers were controlled for any given observer in the case-control format. In a subsequent evaluation of the same cases, after a discussion of criteria, the agreement rate was substantially improved, and an additional highly reproducible criterion was introduced, namely that of lesional size (34).

As discussed by Foucar, and illustrated in some of the preceding examples, differences in criteria may result from the use of different assumptions for the development of criteria (26). At the simplest level of diagnosis, an individual pathologist might establish a set of criteria that establish a diagnosis "by definition." Such a definitional diagnosis reduces uncertainty for that individual to a minimum. At a somewhat more advanced level, criteria are used that are considered likely to be acceptable to other pathologists, constituting a "consensus gold standard." At this level of diagnosis, difficulties in communicating a clear definition of the criteria among pathologists introduce uncertainty caused by lack of reproducibility, and this uncertainty increases with the number of variables under consideration and the resultant increasing subjectivity of the diagnostic exercise.

The most advanced measure of the level of diagnostic problem-solving, according to Foucar, is represented by the attempt to assign a biologically correct label, one that precisely predicts a disease's course (26). Attempts to fully resolve this more difficult level of prediction are likely in many cases, if not most, to be frustrated by the uncertainties enumerated previously, especially the existence of hidden variables—"host resistance," "virulence," "environmental effects," and so on— that are not evident to the observer of histopathology, however expert and diligent he or she may be. Efforts to improve on diagnostic efficacy at this level might, for example, pursue information at the ultrastructural or molecular level. However, the accurate and complete prediction of a particular disease outcome will always prove to be an elusive goal.

Prognostication, which describes the prediction of disease outcome, is an important biologic indicator of diagnostic efficacy. In some instances, many of them neoplasms, a histopathologic diagnosis is predictive of biologic behavior, such as the capacity for distant metastasis. Follow-up studies of outcome can serve as an appropriate gold standard for validation of diagnostic utility. Indeed, a 100% statistical probability of survival for a given neoplasm could be regarded as equivalent to a diagnosis of benignancy, illustrating a strong relationship between diagnosis and prognosis. Even when such studies are available, however, the prediction of outcome is usually in terms of statistical probabilities, which are not absolute. In addition, the course of a disease is inevitably altered by the diagnostic process; for example, excision of a melanocytic lesion that is diagnosed as a melanoma *in situ* is effective in preventing "malignant" behavior such as persistence, recurrence, continued growth, and progression to a lesion with capacity for metastasis. The information needed to accurately predict outcome in any given individual case is also frequently not available to the observer. For example, the outcome of a viral infection may depend on the presence or absence of antibodies in the patient's serum, which cannot be determined from observation of histopathologic sections. Similarly, even the most advanced and seemingly lethal primary malignant melanoma has a certain probability of survival, even after the most sophisticated prognostic models are utilized (35).

Another advanced measure of the biologic relevance of a diagnostic system is through the correlation of traditional diagnostic labels with molecular findings. In early molecular-based studies of Bastian and his colleagues (24,36–40), nevi were distinguished from melanomas, a subset of atypical Spitz nevi was distinguished from among the usual forms of this condition, the acral-lentiginous subset of melanoma was distinguished from other types, and findings traditionally associated with melanoma classification were found to relate to underlying genetic abnormalities, all through the use of CGH and/or gene-sequencing techniques to identify molecular signatures that appear to have specificity for these traditionally defined variants of melanocytic neoplasia (Chapter 28). Similarly, in a patient with a suspected infection, a PCR test for "foreign" DNA can be diagnostic of the presence of an infectious agent (Chapters 20–25). These types of correlations can be expected to increase in the future, strengthening the relationship between our present empirically-based classification schemas and the underlying biology.

Another problem that is pervasive, especially for melanocytic tumors, is a lack of agreement as to terminology, despite efforts at standardization. Generally, these standardization efforts have been limited in their scope, for example, in national guidelines for diagnosis of melanocytic lesions that tend to concentrate on malignant lesions, whereas the numerically more prevalent benign or intermediate lesions are ignored. These differences in terminology tend to be locally associated with different "schools" of pathology. In any given institution, communication between pathologists and clinicians may be quite satisfactory, because of a long history of discussion and mutual education. Difficulties may be encountered, however, when cases are shared between institutions for management or when large-scale databases are used in an attempt to evaluate the quality and efficacy of differing management approaches, for example, in terms of the outcome of different management strategies in large populations. In an extensive study of diagnostic reproducibility, it was found that agreement in the categorization of melanocytic tumors tends to be better as to the biologic implications of a diagnosis compared to the form of words used to convey it. A system called the "MPath-Dx Reporting System" has been proposed as a means of standardization of management considerations for melanocytic proliferations and melanoma. In this system, increasing degrees of presumed biologic risk are related to increasing degrees of intervention using a numeric scale (MPath 1 through MPath 5) (41,42). A similar system in breast radiology has been used to improve communication between radiologists and surgeons in patient management (43).

One inescapable source of uncertainty that impacts on diagnostic accuracy and predictive value is the nature of the tissue sample itself. For inflammatory dermatoses, it is important that the biopsy be representative of the presumed stage of lesion evolution, as it is well known that lesions have "lives" representing passages during which histomorphology may appear quite different. It is also important that the sample adequately represents tissue strata relevant to all of the processes in the clinical differential. A biopsy that does not include deep reticular dermis, for example, makes it difficult to assess for early morphea and impossible to evaluate panniculitis. It is also important to know whether the center or edge of a lesion has been sampled, as the findings may differ considerably based on location within any given lesion. For example, a biopsy in a patient with an ulcer might not even include the actual ulcer, if the goal is to exclude vasculitis or vasculopathy in the adjacent skin, whereas a biopsy from the center of the ulcer itself will usually demonstrate only a nonspecific inflammatory exudate. Generally, a biopsy from the edge of the ulcer is likely to be optimal. For neoplasms, partial samples may make it impossible to exclude more biologically significant components, and thin shave biopsies that twist and contort during processing and transect deeper dermal alterations may confound interpretation considerably. Accordingly, close interaction between clinician and dermatopathologist, both before and after a sample is obtained, is essential to enhancing diagnostic accuracy and predictive value.

It is likely that the best approximation to the goal of improving diagnostic specificity and communication will be achieved by a detailed correlation of findings at the molecular, histopathologic, and gross anatomic levels with the physical findings and clinical history, interpreted in the context of the whole patient and his or her environment, with long-term follow-up serving as the "gold standard." We emphasize the importance of clinicopathologic correlation in diagnosis, especially of inflammatory dermatoses but also in "borderline" tumors. Many diagnoses are straightforward, but when a diagnosis is difficult, clinicopathologic correlation is essential! This is often best accomplished in a multidisciplinary conference setting.

In the "real world" of clinical medicine, a histopathologic description and differential diagnosis for a difficult case are often more likely to be useful than a single "specific" diagnosis that may be correct in its own frame of reference but may be wrong or misleading without clinicopathologic correlation within the context of a particular patient. If possible, when a differential diagnosis is given, it is most helpful to the clinician to favor a particular entity to aid patient management. This is the traditional method of clinical practice, which should be aided but not supplanted by the tools of histopathology. The information in this book has been designed to assist in this clinical diagnostic process.

REFERENCES

1. Antonescu CR, Tschernyavsky SJ, Woodruff JM, Jungbluth AA, Brennan MF, Ladanyi M. Molecular diagnosis of clear cell sarcoma: detection of EWS-ATF1 and MITF-M transcripts and histopathological and ultrastructural analysis of 12 cases. *J Mol Diagn.* 2002;4:44–52.
2. Gerami P, Scolyer RA, Xu X, et al. Risk assessment for atypical spitzoid melanocytic neoplasms using FISH to identify chromosomal copy number aberrations. *Am J Surg Pathol.* 2013;37:676–684.
3. Lee JJ, Lian CG. Molecular testing for cutaneous melanoma: an update and review. *Arch Pathol Lab Med.* 2019;143(7):811–820.
4. Foucar E. Diagnostic decision-making in anatomic pathology. *Am J Clin Pathol.* 2001;116(suppl):S21–S33.
5. Foucar E. Error identification: a surgical pathology dilemma. *Am J Surg Pathol.* 1998;22:1–5.
6. Foucar E. Classification in anatomic pathology. *Am J Clin Pathol.* 2001;116(suppl):S5–S20.
7. Tisack A, Fotouhi A, Fidai C, Friedman BJ, Ozog D, Veenstra J. A clinical and biologic review of keratoacanthoma. *Br J Dermatol.* 2021;185(3):487–498.
8. Merkel EA, Mohan LS, Shi K, Panah E, Zhang B, Gerami P. Paediatric melanoma: clinical update, genetic basis, and advances in diagnosis. *Lancet Child Adolesc Health.* 2019;3(9):646–654.
9. Brenner H. How independent are multiple "independent" diagnostic classifications? *Stat Med.* 2004;15:1377–1386.
10. Cerroni L, Kerl H. Tutorial on melanocytic lesions. *Am J Dermatopathol.* 2001;23:237–241.
11. Barnhill RL, Argenyi ZB, From L, et al. Atypical Spitz nevi/tumors: lack of consensus for diagnosis, discrimination from melanoma, and prediction of outcome. *Hum Pathol.* 1999;30:513–520.
12. Raghavan SS, Peternel S, Mully TW, et al. Spitz melanoma is a distinct subset of spitzoid melanoma. *Mod Pathol.* 2020;33(6):1122–1134.
13. Lasota J, Dansonka-Mieszkowska A, Stachura T, et al. Gastrointestinal stromal tumors with internal tandem duplications in 3′ end of KIT juxtamembrane domain occur predominantly in stomach and generally seem to have a favorable course. *Mod Pathol.* 2003;16:1257–1264.
14. Lee AH, Denley HE, Pinder SE, et al. Excision biopsy findings of patients with breast needle core biopsies reported as suspicious of malignancy (B4) or lesion of uncertain malignant potential (B3). *Histopathology.* 2003;42:331–336.
15. Marion-Audibert AM, Barel C, Gouysse G, et al. Low microvessel density is an unfavorable histoprognostic factor in pancreatic endocrine tumors. *Gastroenterology.* 2003;125:1094–1104.
16. Moore SW, Satge D, Sasco AJ, Zimmermann A, Plaschkes J. The epidemiology of neonatal tumours: report of an international working group. *Pediatr Surg Int.* 2003;19:509–519.
17. Folpe AL, Fanburg-Smith JC, Miettinen M, Weiss SW. Atypical and malignant glomus tumors: analysis of 52 cases, with a proposal for the reclassification of glomus tumors. *Am J Surg Pathol.* 2001;25:1–12.
18. Medina PM, Valero Puerta JA, Perez MD. Atypical stromal hyperplasia of the prostate (stromal proliferation of uncertain malignant potential) [in Spanish]. *Arch Esp Urol.* 2000;53:722–723.
19. Nucci MR, Prasad CJ, Crum CP, Mutter GL. Mucinous endometrial epithelial proliferations: a morphologic spectrum of changes with diverse clinical significance. *Mod Pathol.* 1999;12:1137–1142.
20. Lin BT, Bonsib SM, Mierau GW, Weiss LM, Medeiros LJ. Oncocytic adrenocortical neoplasms: a report of seven cases and review of the literature. *Am J Surg Pathol.* 1998;22:603–614.
21. Menaker GM, Sanger JR. Granular cell tumor of uncertain malignant potential. *Ann Plast Surg.* 1997;38:658–660.
22. Soumakis S, Panayiotides J, Protopapa E, Kouri E, Vlachonikolis J, Delides GS. Quantitative pathology in uterine smooth muscle

tumours: the case for the standard histologic classification criteria. *Eur J Gynaecol Oncol.* 1997;18:203–207.

23. Carr NJ, Sobin LH. Unusual tumors of the appendix and pseudomyxoma peritonei. *Semin Diagn Pathol.* 1996;13:314–325.

24. Bastian BC, LeBoit PE, Pinkel D. Mutations and copy number increase of HRAS in Spitz nevi with distinctive histopathological features. *Am J Pathol.* 2000;157:967–972.

25. Zarabi SK, Azzato EM, Tu ZJ, et al. Targeted next generation sequencing (NGS) to classify melanocytic neoplasms. *J Cutan Pathol.* 2020;47(8):691–704.

26. Foucar E. Debating melanocytic tumors of the skin: does an "uncertain" diagnosis signify borderline diagnostic skill?. *Am J Dermatopathol.* 1995;17:626–634.

27. Sackett DL, Haynes RB, Tugwell P. Early diagnosis. In: Sackett DL, Haynes RB, Tugwell P, eds. *Clinical Epidemiology: A Basic Science for Clinical Medicine.* 1st ed. Little, Brown & Company; 1985:139–155.

28. Gown AM, Vogel AM, Hoak D, Gough F, McNutt MA. Monoclonal antibodies specific for melanocytic tumors distinguish subpopulations of melanocytes. *Am J Pathol.* 1986;123:195.

29. Sun J, Morton TH, Gown AM. Antibody HMB-45 identifies the cells of blue nevi. *Am J Surg Pathol.* 1990;14:748–751.

30. Farmer ER, Gonin R, Hanna MP. Discordance in the histopathologic diagnosis of melanoma and melanocytic nevi between expert pathologists. *Hum Pathol.* 1996;27:528–531.

31. Piepkorn MW, Barnhill RL, Cannon-Albright LA, et al. A multiobserver, population-based analysis of histologic dysplasia in melanocytic nevi. *J Am Acad Dermatol.* 1994;30:707–714.

32. Weinstock MA, Barnhill RL, Rhodes AR, Brodsky GL. Reliability of the histopathologic diagnosis of melanocytic dysplasia: The Dysplastic Nevus Panel. *Arch Dermatol.* 1997;133:953–958.

33. Shors AR, Kim S, White E, et al. Dysplastic naevi with moderate to severe histological dysplasia: a risk factor for melanoma. *Br J Dermatol.* 2006;155:988–993.

34. Xiong MY, Rabkin MS, Piepkorn MW, et al. Diameter of dysplastic nevi is a more robust biomarker of increased melanoma risk than degree of histologic dysplasia: a case-control study. *J Am Acad Dermatol.* 2014;71(6):1257–1258.

35. Rivers JK, McCarthy SW, Shaw HM, et al. Patients with thick melanomas surviving at least 10 years: histological, cytometric and HLA analyses. *Histopathology.* 1991;18:339–346.

36. Stephens P, Wiesner T, He J, et al. Next-generation sequencing of genomic and cDNA to identify a high frequency of kinase fusions involving ROS1, ALK, RET, NTRK1, and BRAF in Spitz tumors [ASCO meeting abstracts]. *J Clin Oncol.* 2013;31:9002.

37. Broekaert SM, Roy R, Okamoto I, et al. Genetic and morphologic features for melanoma classification. *Pigment Cell Melanoma Res.* 2010;23:763–770.

38. van Raamsdonk CD, Bezrookove V, Green G, et al. Frequent somatic mutations of GNAQ in uveal melanoma and blue naevi. *Nature.* 2009;457:599–602.

39. Curtin JA, Fridlyand J, Kageshita T, et al. Distinct sets of genetic alterations in melanoma. *N Engl J Med.* 2005;353:2135–2147.

40. Bastian BC, Olshen AB, LeBoit PE, Pinkel D. Classifying melanocytic tumors based on DNA copy number changes. *Am J Pathol.* 2003;163:1765–1770.

41. Piepkorn MW, Barnhill RL, Elder DE, et al. The MPATH-Dx reporting schema for melanocytic proliferations and melanoma. *J Am Acad Dermatol.* 2014;70(1):131–141.

42. Elmore JG, Barnhill RL, Elder DE, et al. Pathologists' diagnosis of invasive melanoma and melanocytic proliferations: observer accuracy and reproducibility study. *BMJ.* 2017;357:j2813.

43. Hamy AS, Giacchetti S, Albiter M, et al. BI-RADS categorisation of 2,708 consecutive nonpalpable breast lesions in patients referred to a dedicated breast care unit. *Eur Radiol.* 2012;22:9–17.

Biopsy Techniques

ROSALIE ELENITSAS AND MICHAEL E. MING

INTRODUCTION

Proper techniques are important for maximizing the utility of a skin biopsy. A biopsy is indicated in suspected cutaneous malignant neoplasms or inflammatory diseases and to clarify which of the diagnoses under consideration is the best fit. Appropriate communication is an important step in securing an accurate diagnosis for the patient. Biopsies submitted without a differential diagnosis, particularly biopsies of inflammatory disorders, may present challenges in interpretation for the dermatopathologist, although, of course, there are exceptions to this rule. The technique used to obtain a specimen for microscopic evaluation may have a significant impact on the ability of the dermatopathologist to arrive at the correct diagnosis. The choice of technique (punch, superficial or deep shave, ellipse) depends on many factors, including a mental review of the clinical differential diagnosis and the microscopic appearance of each disorder; the anatomic site; the morphology of the lesion, particularly its size and shape; the overall physical health of the patient; and cosmetic concerns. The treating provider must also assure that the specimen is labeled and properly submitted to the laboratory. Failure in these initial steps of the skin biopsy pathway may affect the final result (1) (Table 2-1).

Selection of the appropriate lesion to biopsy when evaluating an inflammatory disorder is crucial. In most instances,

Table 2-1

Potential Contributors to Diagnostic Error That Should Be Considered by the Clinician

Suboptimal selection of lesion to biopsy

Inappropriate biopsy technique (e.g., crushing specimen or incorrectly assessing the depth to which the biopsy should be performed)

Failure to confirm that tissue is in the bottle and within the medium

Inappropriate selection of medium to transport biopsy to lab

Insufficient medium in bottle

Failure to secure bottle lid to avoid leakage

Incorrect labeling of biopsy bottle

Incorrect labeling or demographic information on requisition form

Lack of relevant clinical information on the requisition form

histologic examination of a fully developed lesion will give more information than examination of an early or involuting lesion. However, vesiculobullous lesions, ulcers, and pustular lesions are exceptions. For their histologic examination, a very early lesion is optimal; otherwise, secondary changes such as regeneration, degeneration, scarring, or secondary infection may obscure essential features and make recognition of the primary pathologic process impossible. The ideal candidate lesion for biopsy has not been scratched or traumatized and is untouched by topical or systemic therapy, especially anti-inflammatory agents. If there are lesions in different stages of evolution, multiple biopsy specimens may be helpful. When considering diagnoses such as connective tissue nevus, anetoderma, atrophoderma, and some pigmentation disorders, the dermatopathologist may wish to compare involved and uninvolved skin. In those cases, one can perform a scalpel biopsy incorporating a portion of the lesion and adjacent normal skin or perform two separate punch biopsies.

Choosing the proper biopsy technique depends on the clinical differential diagnosis, as seen with examples in Table 2-2. Punch biopsy is the standard procedure for obtaining samples of inflammatory dermatoses, but it is often used for neoplasms as well. In most instances, a specimen obtained with a 4-mm punch biopsy is adequate for histologic study. A 3-mm punch biopsy may be preferable for small lesions or biopsies from the face or other areas where cosmesis is a concern. Either a 6-mm punch biopsy or a deep incisional biopsy using a scalpel should be performed if panniculitis is suspected, to ensure that adequate amounts of subcutaneous fat are obtained. After the skin specimen has been loosened with the biopsy punch, it should be handled very gently and, above all, should not be grasped with forceps except at the very edge. Crush artifact from forceps makes a specimen of an inflammatory process difficult to interpret, with lymphoma and leukemic infiltrates being particularly susceptible to crush. Often, a punch biopsy specimen can be squeezed gently out of its socket or carefully speared with the syringe needle that was used for injection of the local anesthetic. Sharp scissors can be used to cut through the subcutaneous fat at the base of the specimen. All punch biopsy specimens for inflammatory disease should extend to the subcutaneous fat whenever possible because, in many dermatoses, characteristic histologic features are found in the lower dermis or in the subcutaneous fat.

When performing scalp biopsies for alopecia, many laboratories prefer two specimens: one for transverse (horizontal) sectioning and the other for standard (vertical) sectioning.

Table 2-2

Selection of Biopsy Technique

Suspected Diagnosis	Biopsy Type
Neoplastic	
Actinic keratosis	Shave
Seborrheic keratosis	Shave
Verruca	Shave
Nonmelanoma skin cancer	Shave is common, but punch/ excision also options.
Mycosis fungoides	Punch; deep shave/ saucerization
Atypical nevi/suspected melanoma	Deep shave, punch, or excision (regardless of technique, clinician should try to remove entire lesion under most circumstances)
Subungual melanoma	Nail matrix shave, punch, incisional biopsy
Inflammatory	
Blistering disease*	Punch or deep shave, edge of new blister
Contact dermatitis	Punch
Allergic reactions	Punch
Lupus/dermatomyositis*	Punch
Morphea/sclerosing process	Punch
Small vessel vasculitis*	Punch
Large vessel vasculitis	Punch or ellipse
Granulomatous process	Punch
Panniculitis	Punch (6 mm or larger) or ellipse
Alopecia*	Punch, 4 mm or larger

*Also consider immunofluorescence.

Techniques utilizing only one biopsy specimen, such as the HoVert technique, allow for both horizontal (Ho) and vertical (Vert) sections for analysis (2). The punch instrument should be inserted into the skin parallel to the direction of hair growth, and the biopsy should extend well into the subcutaneous layer to be certain that the bulbs of terminal follicles are included. In scarring alopecia, it is important that a biopsy be performed in an area of erythema with visible hair shafts; a biopsy of a completely scarred area of alopecia will show only end-stage nonspecific changes. There are excellent reviews in the literature on this topic (3).

Shave biopsies may be either superficial or extend more deeply into the skin, but, in general, they should extend at least into the papillary dermis. Superficial shave biopsies should be used only for lesions in which characteristic histologic changes are expected to be present in the epidermis or the superficial dermis (e.g., seborrheic keratoses, actinic keratoses, verrucae, and basal cell carcinomas). Cosmetic results are often improved by using the superficial shave biopsy technique. A variant of the deep shave biopsy is the saucerization technique, in which the

blade is introduced at a roughly 45-degree angle. To aid in the control of the size of the tissue to be removed, some physicians score the skin before performing a shave or saucerization biopsy. Shave biopsies may hinder some diagnoses such as dermatofibrosarcoma protuberans, where the important microscopic features are in the deeper dermis. A superficial shave biopsy without adequate dermis may be suboptimal if melanoma is included in the differential diagnosis because of concerns that a melanoma might be transected at the base. A transected melanoma specimen may be more difficult to diagnose accurately, and proper assessment of tumor thickness may be hindered. If melanoma is suspected clinically, it is preferable to remove the entire lesion to a depth that ensures that the melanoma is not transected. This may be accomplished via elliptical excision, punch, or deep shave specimen (4). In addition, when biopsying atypical pigmented lesions, removal of the entire lesion may assist in diagnosis and is the preferred technique under most clinical circumstances.

Because of the thick overlying stratum corneum, a shave biopsy of acral skin may produce a superficial specimen extending only to the midepidermis or papillary dermis. This is especially important when considering a biopsy of an acral pigmented lesion; in this situation, a punch biopsy or small excision will often provide a better specimen for interpretation. With a shave biopsy, aluminum chloride is recommended for hemostasis; Monsel solution (ferric subsulfate) and electrocautery are alternatives, but they may affect the interpretation of subsequent biopsies or reexcisions, by introducing iron deposition and cautery artifacts, respectively, in the remaining tissue.

Deep incisional biopsies using a scalpel may be helpful when evaluating panniculitis or when assessing deep dermal or subcutaneous nodules.

Curettage can be a less satisfactory method of obtaining material for histologic examination because the submitted material has lost its architecture, is usually scanty and superficial, and may show crush artifact. Even if curettage is performed well, fragmentation and distortion cannot be avoided. Curettage of a melanoma that clinically was thought to be a seborrheic keratosis or basal cell carcinoma may hinder accurate diagnosis and may make assessment of microscopic features more difficult.

The biopsy specimen should be placed in a fixative immediately on removal from the patient to prevent autolysis. It should not be allowed to dry, and the dermatologist should check the specimen bottle to ensure that the tissue has not adhered to the side of the bottle or remained inside the punch. Patient information should be placed on the bottle itself, not on the lid, which could be accidentally placed on a different bottle. As fixative, 10% buffered formalin can be used in nearly all instances (see Chapter 4). However, if the specimen is mailed in cold winter climates, 10% aqueous formalin, which freezes at −11°C, may allow the formation of ice crystals in the specimen. Ice crystals cause damage and distortion in the specimen, particularly in the epithelial cells, and make adequate histologic evaluation impossible. Freezing can be prevented by adding 95% ethyl alcohol to formalin, 10% by volume. An alternative is to let the specimen stand in the formalin solution at room temperature for at least 6 hours before mailing.

Every specimen submitted for histologic diagnosis should be accompanied by detailed clinical information, including a differential diagnosis. The histopathologist's ability to render an accurate diagnosis often depends on the available clinical information, and clinicopathologic correlation is the key to providing optimal patient care. Previous biopsies at the same site, specific requests (e.g., consideration of special stains for infectious organisms), and special handling (e.g., orientation guidelines) should also be indicated on the requisition sheet sent to the laboratory with the specimen. Handling of biopsies for immunofluorescence is discussed in Chapter 4.

The quality of diagnosis can potentially be greatly enhanced by the provision of a clinical image, especially when a biopsy of a larger lesion is done. The clinical morphology represents the gross pathology, especially for inflammatory skin disease, and a clinical image can greatly facilitate interpretation. Although many diagnoses can be made in isolation, clinical correlation and discussion of difficult cases at consensus conferences, when available also add value to the diagnostic process, for the benefit of patients, clinicians, and histopathologists alike.

REFERENCES

1. Stratman EJ, Elston DM, Miller SJ. Skin biopsy. Identifying and overcoming errors in the skin biopsy pathway. *J Am Acad Dermatol.* 2016;74:19–25.
2. Nguyen JV, Hudacek K, Whitten JA, Rubin AI, Seykora JT. The HoVert technique: a novel method for the sectioning of alopecia biopsies. *J Cutan Pathol.* 2011;38(5):401–406.
3. Kolivras A, Thompson C. Primary scalp alopecia: new histopathological tools, new concepts and a practical guide to diagnosis. *J Cutan Pathol.* 2017;44:53–69.
4. Swetter SM, Tsao H, Bichakjian CK, et al. Guidelines of care for the management of primary cutaneous melanoma. *J Am Acad Dermatol.* 2019;80(1):208–250.

Histology of the Skin

CHRISTINE G. LIAN AND GEORGE F. MURPHY

OVERVIEW

An understanding of the normal histology of skin and an appreciation of our rapidly expanding knowledge of skin biology are essential to diagnostic recognition in cutaneous pathology. Many skin disorders have relatively subtle pathologic changes, either the result of biopsy during early evolutionary stages or intrinsic to a given condition. Without an awareness of what would be anticipated at a specific biopsy site normally, it may be impossible to make such diagnoses with accuracy and reproducibility. The journey to defining the normal histology of human skin is a relatively short one in terms of spatial dimensions. From an *en face* view of the skin surface, characterized by desquamating scale, furrows, and evidence of adnexal growth, to the normal ultrastructure of key organelles within underlying cellular constituents, we span a magnification range of 10^5 (1). Over this expanse, the histology of the skin is amazingly complex. Divided into two seemingly separate but functionally interdependent layers (epidermis and dermis) (Figs. 3-1 to 3-5), the skin is composed of cells with myriad functions ranging from mechanical and photoprotection, immunosurveillance, and nutrient metabolism to repair. A third layer, the subcutaneous adipose tissue, is not truly a part of the skin, but,

because of its close anatomic relationship and its tendency to respond together with the skin in many pathologic processes, it is also discussed in this chapter.

The epidermal layer is composed primarily of keratinocytes (>90%), with minority populations of Langerhans cells, melanocytes, neuroendocrine (Merkel) cells, and unmyelinated axons. In addition, the epidermis also contains specialized cuboidal epithelium that forms the spiraling acrosyringia of eccrine sweat ducts, as well as occasional cells putatively programmed for possible adnexal/glandular differentiation (e.g., Toker cells, as found in nipple epidermis in approximately 10% of individuals) (2,3). Architecturally, the epidermal layer has an undulant undersurface in two-dimensional sections, with apparent downward invaginations termed *rete* that interdigitate with underlying vascularized mesenchyme termed *dermal papillae* (not to be confused with follicular papillae of the hair bulb). In reality, three-dimensional reconstruction reveals epidermal rete to form a honeycomb of interconnected ridges, with dermal papillae representing rounded conical invaginations not dissimilar to the undersurface of an egg carton. Separated from, yet united with, the epidermis by a structurally and chemically complex basement membrane zone, the dermis consists of

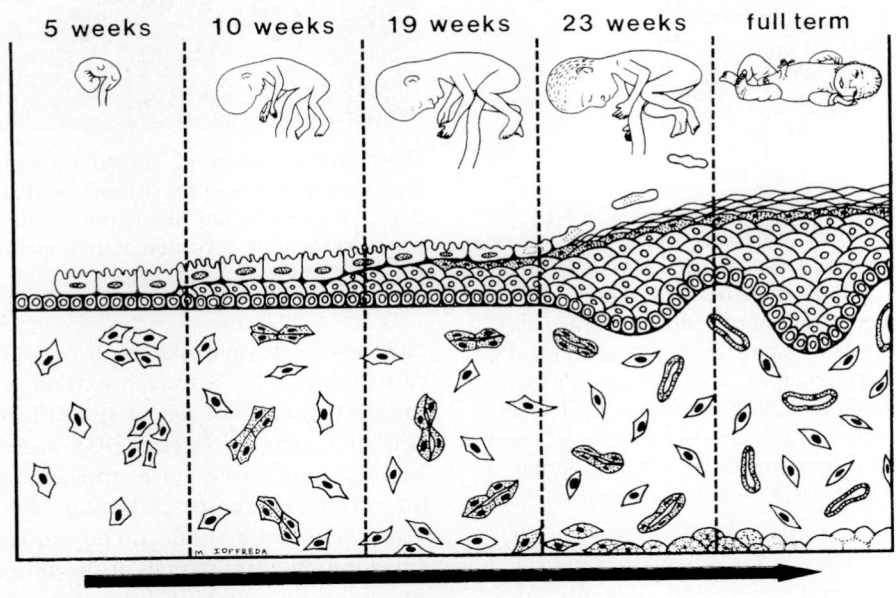

Figure 3-1 Schematic overview of embryonic development of human skin. (Courtesy of Dr. Michael Ioffreda.)

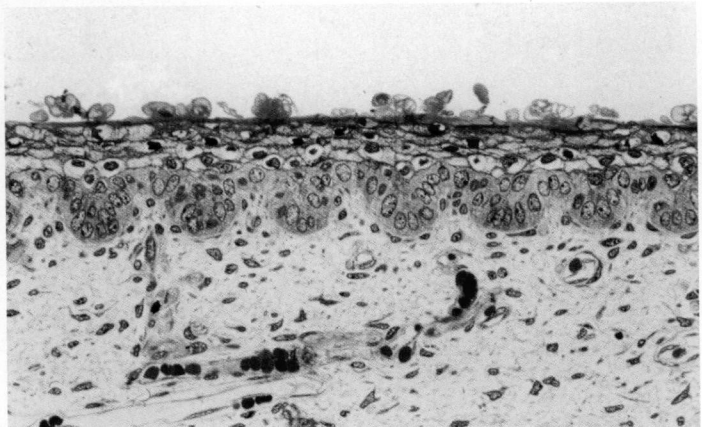

Figure 3-2 Histology of epidermis and dermis of 18-week normal human fetal skin (1-µm-thick, plastic-embedded section).

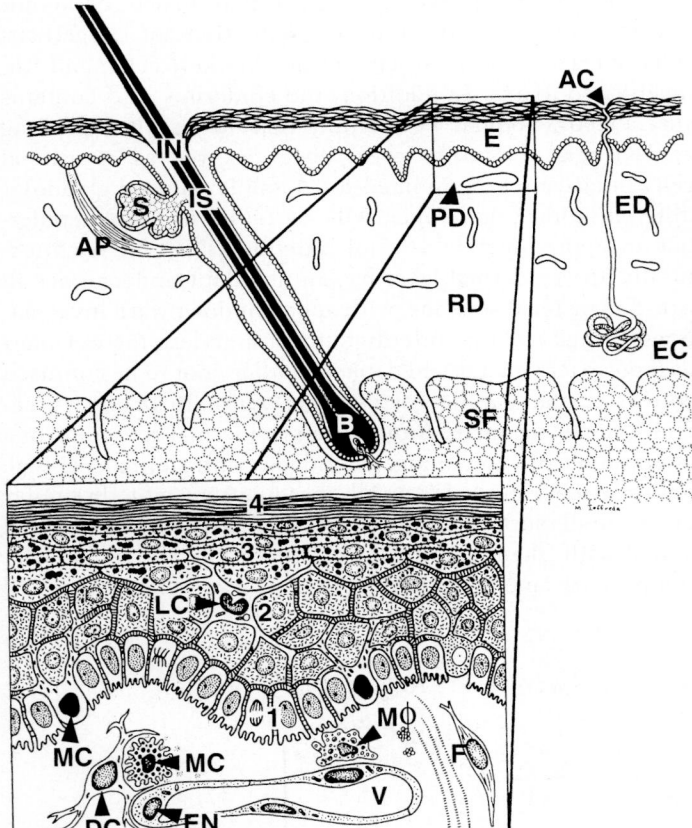

Figure 3-3 Schematic overview of the architecture and cytologic constituents of normal human skin. This projection demonstrates the cellular components of the epidermis and superficial dermis in greater detail, with epidermal strata denoted numerically. *1*, stratum basalis; *2*, stratum spinosum; *3*, stratum granulosum; *4*, stratum corneum. *AC*, eccrine acrosyringium; *AP*, arrector pili muscle; *B*, follicular bulb; *DC*, perivascular dendritic cell; *E*, epidermis; *EC*, coil of eccrine gland; *ED*, dermal eccrine duct; *EN*, endothelial cell; *F*, fibroblast; *IN*, follicular infundibulum; *IS*, follicular isthmus; *LC*, Langerhans cell; *MC*, mast cell; *Mf*, macrophage; *PD*, papillary dermis; *RD*, reticular dermis; *S*, sebaceous gland; *SF*, subcutaneous fat; *V*, vessel. (Courtesy of Dr. Michael Ioffreda.)

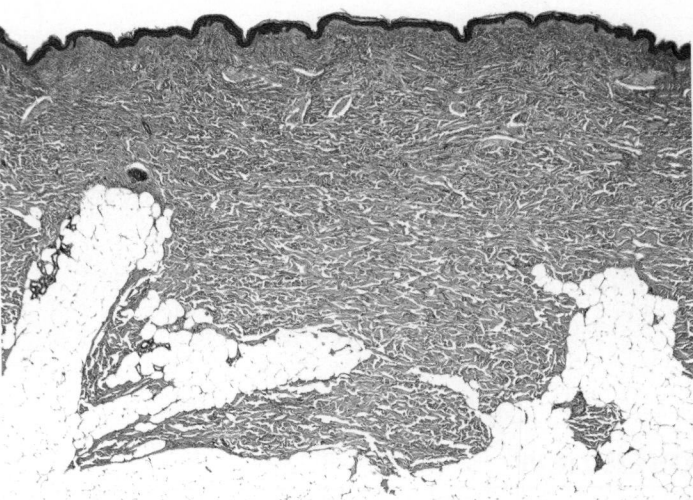

Figure 3-4 Histology of normal human skin. From **top** to **bottom:** epidermis, dermis, and upper part of the subcutaneous tissue. Note how the adipose tissue from the subcutis follows and surrounds adnexal structures within the dermis.

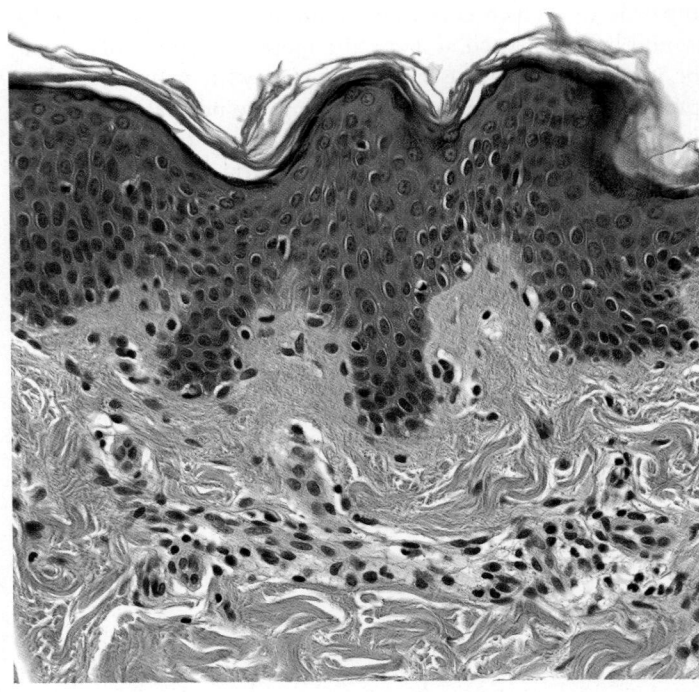

Figure 3-5 Histology of normal epidermis and superficial dermis. Note the separation of the delicate papillary dermal collagen from the underlying coarser reticular dermis by the horizontally aligned blood vessel representing a portion of the superficial vascular plexus.

endothelial and neural cells and supporting elements, fibroblasts, dendritic and nondendritic monocyte/macrophages, factor XIIIa–expressing dermal dendrocytes, and mast cells enveloped within a matrix of collagen and glycosaminoglycan (Table 3-1). Adnexae extend from the epidermis into the dermis and consist of specialized cells for hair growth, epithelial renewal (stem cells), and temperature regulation. Adnexal epithelium also appears to provide a safe haven for certain precursor cells (e.g., for melanocytes and dendritic cells) in a tissue niche sequestered from deleterious environmental influences at the skin surface. The subcutis is an underlying cushion formed by cells engorged with lipid and nourished by vessels that grow within thin intervening septae. The developmental anatomy of skin is important

Table 3-1

Structural and Staining Characteristics of Representative Skin Cells

Cell Type	Location	Characteristic Structure(s)	Immunostain(s)	Histochemical Stain(s)
Keratinocyte	Entire epidermis, adnexa	Tonofilaments, desmosomes	Cytokeratins (CKs) (see sections below)	
Melanocyte	Basal cell layer	Melanosomes	S100, MART-1/Melan-A, HMB45, MITF, SOX10	Fontana-Masson, DOPA, tyrosinase, silver nitrate
Langerhans cell	Mid epidermis	Birbeck granules	S100, CD1a, langerin	ATPase
Merkel cell	Basal layer, bulge of hair follicle	Neurosecretory granules	CK20, chromogranin, synaptophysin INSM1	Neuron-specific enolase
Fibroblast	Entire dermis	Spindle-shaped with prominent rough	Vimentin, procollagen, CD34	Masson trichrome for collagen
Dermal dendrocyte	Superficial dermis	Elongated dendrites	Factor XIIIa	
Endothelial cell	Vascular plexuses	Weibel–Palade bodies, factor VIII	CD31, CD34	
Mast cell	Perivascular space	Scroll-containing secretory granules	C-kit, tryptase	Giemsa, toluidine blue
Macrophage	Perivascular space	Lysosomes	CD68, CD163	
Eccrine/apocrine gland	Epidermis and dermis	Ducts and secretory coils containing granules	Epithelial membrane antigen (EMA), carcinoembryonic antigen (CEA)	PAS for apocrine gland
Sebaceous gland	Dermis	Lipidized epithelial cells	EMA	
Nerve fiber	Around vessels and adnexa	Neurofilaments	S100, anti-neurofilament antibodies	Bodian, osmium tetroxide

not only for understanding the basis for mature structural–functional relationships, but also in relation to certain skin tumors that recapitulate embryologic cutaneous structure.

EPIDERMIS

The epidermis comprises the following cell types:
• Keratinocytes
• Melanocytes
• Langerhans cells
• Merkel cells

Keratinocytes

Embryology

The development of *in utero* skin biopsy techniques gives practical importance to understanding the normal evolutionary histology of fetal skin. The epidermis begins as a single layer of ectodermal cells (4,5). By 5 weeks of gestational age, this has differentiated at least focally into two layers—the basal layer or stratum germinativum and the overlying periderm; by 10 weeks, an intervening layer—the stratum intermedium—develops (Fig. 3-1). Cells forming the periderm are large, bulge from the epidermal surface, and are bathed in amniotic fluid. By 19 weeks, there are several layers of intermediate cells, and the periderm has begun to flatten (Figs. 3-1 and 3-2). Keratinization is well developed by 23 weeks within the stratum intermedium in association with small keratohyalin granules. At this juncture, most of the periderm cells have shed, and the keratinizing cells

that remain beneath represent the newly formed stratum corneum (5).

By ultrastructure, the histogenesis of the epidermis involves the initial formation of immature desmosomes and early hemidesmosomes and distinct basement membrane (6 to 7 weeks of gestational age) (6,7). Anchoring filaments are observed several weeks later, and the basement membrane appears structurally mature by the end of the first trimester. The surface cells of the periderm display numerous microvilli and cytoplasmic microvesicles, increasing the area in contact with amniotic fluid and suggesting active interchange between the periderm cells and the amniotic fluid (4). Tonofilaments are sparse until 16 weeks, when dense accumulations are observed in cells of the intermediate layer as evidence of beginning keratinization (5).

Normal Microanatomy

The keratinocytes differ from the dendritic or clear cells (melanocytes and Langerhans cells) by their larger size, an ample amount of stainable cytoplasm, and the presence of intercellular bridges. As they differentiate into horny cells, the keratinocytes are arranged in four layers from bottom to top (Figs. 3-6 to 3-12):

• Basal cell layer (stratum basalis)
• Squamous cell layer (stratum spinosum)
• Granular layer (stratum granulosum)
• Horny layer (stratum corneum)

An additional layer: Stratum lucidum can be recognized on the palms and soles (see Regional Variation) (Fig. 3-7).

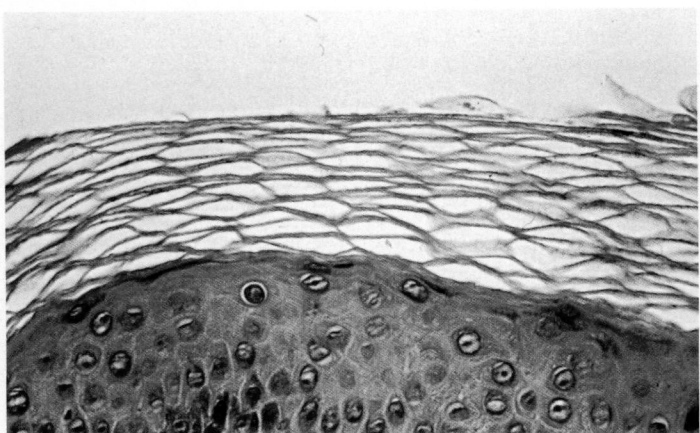

Figure 3-6 Histology of normally anucleate stratum corneum, the terminal differentiation product of underlying basal and suprabasal cells. Note the characteristic "basket-weave" architecture typical of nonacral sites.

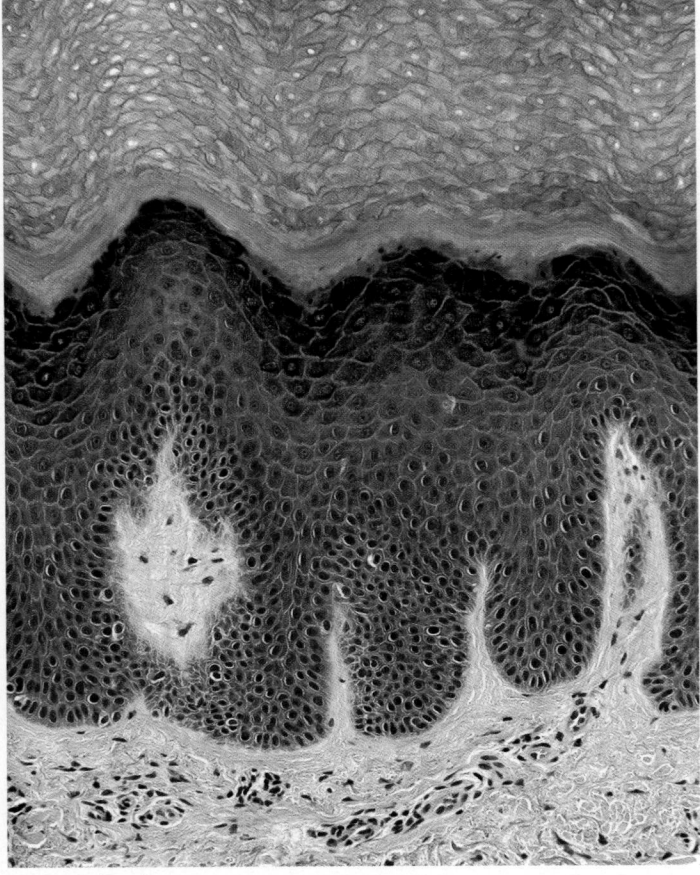

Figure 3-7 Histology of normal acral skin illustrating the thick and compact stratum corneum and the presence of a stratum lucidum (gray blue) in the lower portion of the horny layer.

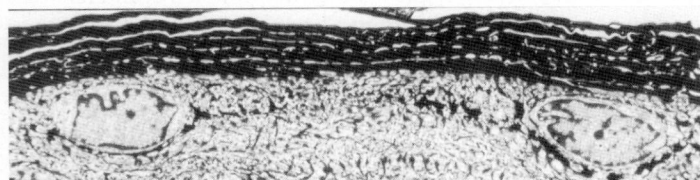

Figure 3-8 Ultrastructure of stratum corneum showing transition of intracellular tonofilaments within viable cells to anucleate stratum corneum at the epidermal surface. The darker granules directly beneath the stratum corneum represent keratohyalin granules.

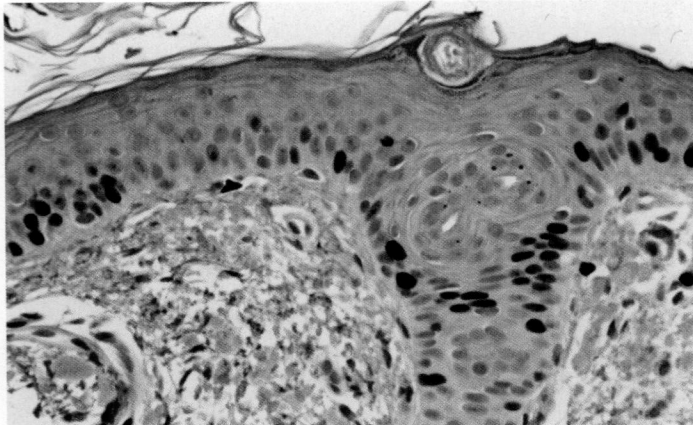

Figure 3-9 Evidence of basal cell layer replicative potential by Ki-67 immunostaining. Note the predominance of labeled cells in the basal cell layer of the epidermis and the included portion of a follicular infundibulum.

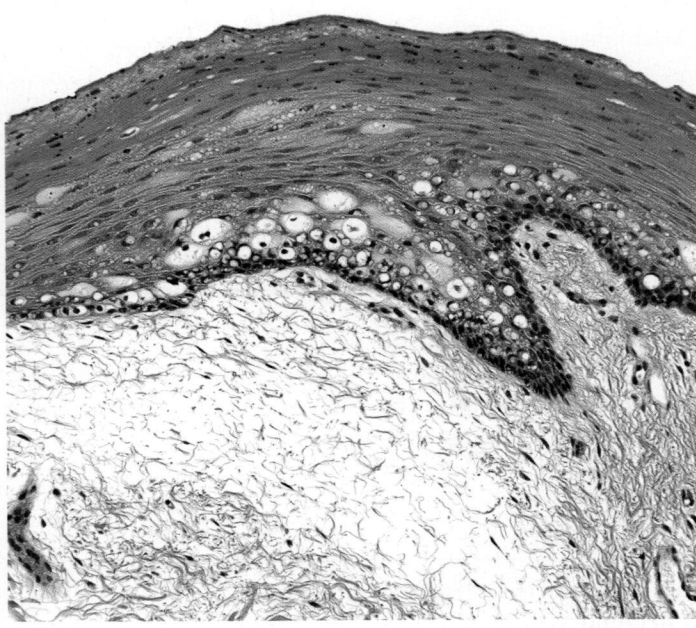

Figure 3-10 Mucosal epithelium of the oral cavity showing stratified squamous epithelium without a well-formed granular or cornified layer. Note the cytoplasmic pallor owing to glycogenation and delicate underlying connective tissue.

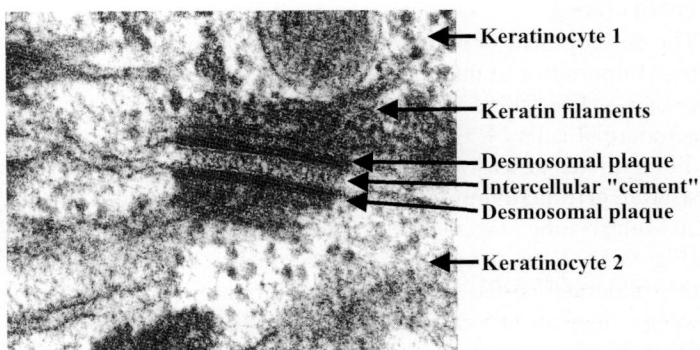

Figure 3-11 Ultrastructure of a desmosome. Note the two electrodense plaques, each located within the cytoplasm of the two keratinocytes that are connected by the desmosome.

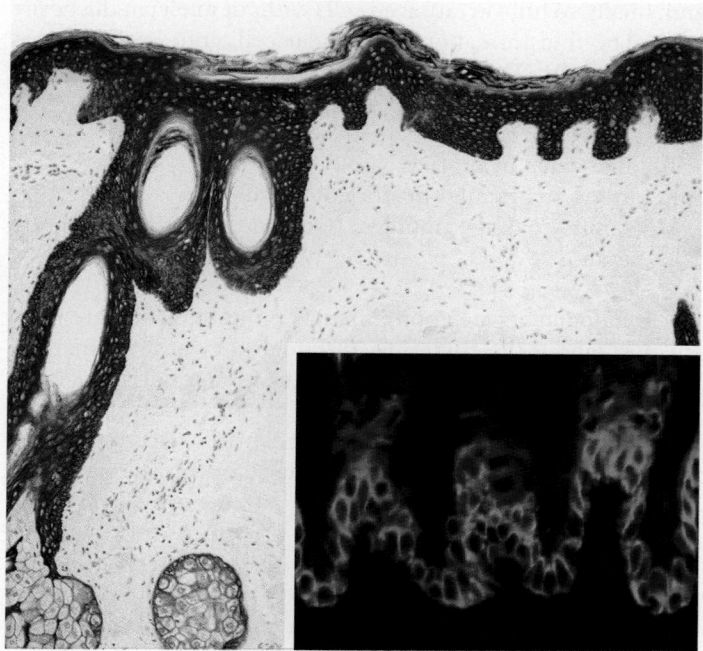

Figure 3-12 Immunohistochemistry for a pan-keratin (including low- and high-molecular-weight keratins) showing diffuse expression in the epidermis and adnexal structures. Inset: Preferential expression of keratin 14 by the basal and parabasal layers (immunofluorescence).

Stratum Basalis

The basal cells form a single layer, are ovoid in contour, and lie with their long axes perpendicular to the underlying basement membrane. They have a more basophilic cytoplasm than cells of the stratum spinosum, often contain melanin pigment, particularly in supranuclear regions transferred from adjacent melanocytes, and contain dark-staining round to oval nuclei (Fig. 3-5). They are connected with each other and with the overlying squamous cells by intercellular bridges united by desmosomes (discussed in detail later). At their base, the basal cells are attached to the subepidermal basement membrane zone by modified desmosomes, termed hemidesmosomes. Basal cells and overlying squamous cells contain keratin intermediate filaments termed tonofilaments, which form the developing cytoskeleton; these cells and related cytoskeletal proteins ultimately give rise to the normally anucleate stratum corneum at the epidermal surface (Figs. 3-6 and 3-8).

Most of the mitotic activity in normal human epidermis occurs in the basal cell layer (8). By tritiated thymidine labeling of cells in the S phase of DNA synthesis, which is approximately seven times longer than the mitotic or M phase, many more tritiated-thymidine-labeled basal cells can be visualized than mitotically active basal cells. Ki-67 labeling is a useful way of determining cycling cells in paraffin sections, and, as with tritiated thymidine, the vast majority of labeled cells in normal skin are within the basal cell layer of the epidermis (Fig. 3-9).

Stratum Spinosum

The polyhedral cells of the stratum spinosum overlying the basal cell layer form a mosaic usually 5 to 10 layers thick. They become progressively flattened toward the skin surface as they mature (Fig. 3-6). The cells are separated by spaces that are traversed by intercellular bridges united by desmosomes. These intercellular

spaces contain neutral mucopolysaccharides and acid mucopolysaccharides (glycosaminoglycans). Hyaluronic acid, an important component of the glycosaminoglycans, is quite abundant in the matrix between keratinocytes, occurring predominantly in the spinous layers but also in the basal layer and the stratum corneum (9). The intercellular cement substance between two adjacent keratinocytes, also referred to as glycocalyx, has a gel-like consistency. On the one hand, it provides cohesion between the epidermal cells, and, on the other hand, it allows the rapid passage of water-soluble substances through the intercellular spaces; furthermore, it allows the opening up of desmosomes and individual cell movement (10–12).

The tonofilaments within the cytoplasm of the keratinocytes of the stratum spinosum are loose bundles of electron-dense filaments, each filament measuring 7 to 8 nm in diameter. These structures correlate with keratin proteins, as may be demonstrated by immunohistochemistry (see later discussion on Immunohistochemistry) (Fig. 3-12).

The tonofilaments at one end are attached to the attachment plaque of a desmosome, and the tonofilaments at the other end form the cytoskeleton within the cytoplasm. Electron microscopy shows that the intercellular junctions (desmosomes) consist of two dense plaques 10 to 15 nm thick on adjacent cell membranes. A 30-nm-wide multilayered zone is present between them (Fig. 3-11). The binding of adjacent keratinocytes via interaction of these ultrastructurally complex adjacent desmosomal plaques (10,11) has recently been understood at a molecular level (Fig. 3-11; see also Fig. 3-23). A key family of molecules is the cadherins, derived from multiple genes and representing Ca^{2+}-dependent cell adhesion molecules with a characteristic single-spanning transmembrane structure (13). Desmosomal cadherins are desmogleins and desmocollins (14) that localize to desmosomes and are linked to intracytoplasmic intermediate filaments by plakoglobin and desmoplakin. Within the desmosome complex, desmogleins within the cell membrane bind to plakoglobin through their cytoplasmic domain. Intermediate keratin filaments anchor at the desmosomal plaque, possibly by way of the carboxy-terminal domain of plakoglobin. Functionally, we now know that disengaging desmosomes from intermediate filaments results in the expression of differentiation markers via activation of ErbB2 by Src family kinase-mediated phosphorylation, suggesting that the desmosome-intermediate filament complex is critical to supporting the differentiation and molecular polarization implicit to the normal epidermis (15). The structural importance of these molecules in uniting keratinocyte cytoskeletons within the epidermis is indicated by the disorders pemphigus vulgaris and pemphigus foliaceus, in which autoantibodies to desmoglein 3 and desmoglein 1, respectively, result in clinical blisters owing to loss of cell–cell adherence (Fig. 3-23) (see Chapter 9) (16,17). Desmoglein 3 is normally concentrated between immediately suprabasal keratinocytes, whereas desmoglein 1 is distributed preferentially among keratinocytes directly beneath the stratum corneum. Indeed, a remarkable correlation has been established between desmoglein expression in normal skin and pathologic lesions in which specific desmogleins are disrupted with regard to the plane of blister formation owing to loss of cell–cell adhesion.

Stratum Granulosum

The cells of the granular cell layer are flattened, and their cytoplasm contains keratohyalin granules that are deeply basophilic and irregular in size and shape (Fig. 3-6). The thickness of the granular layer in normal skin is generally proportional to the thickness of the horny layer (stratum corneum): It is only one to three cell layers thick in areas in which the horny layer is thin but measures up to 10 layers in regions with a thick, horny layer, such as the palms and soles (Figs. 3-5 and 3-7). In the process of keratinization, the keratohyalin granules form two structures: the interfibrillary matrix, or filaggrin, which cements the keratin filaments together, and the inner lining of the horny cells, the so-called marginal band. Whereas the tonofibrils contain only small amounts of sulfur as sulfhydryl groups, the interfibrillary matrix and the marginal band contain about 10 times the amount of sulfur that is present in the tonofibrils, predominantly as disulfide bonds of cystine (18,19). Consequently, the tonofibrils are soft and flexible, whereas the matrix and marginal band provide necessary strength and stability (19). Thus, the keratin of the epidermis represents "soft" keratin, in contrast to the "hard" keratin of the hair and nails, in which keratohyalin granules are lacking and the tonofibrils themselves harden through the incorporation of disulfide bonds (20). "Soft" keratin desquamates as the result of enzymatic action, but the "hard" keratin of the hair and nails does not and thus requires periodic cutting, save for follicular cycling, whereby hair shafts are periodically jettisoned as follicles evolve from anagen to telogen phases.

The granular cell layer represents the mature keratin-forming transitional zone of the epidermis, in which the dissolution of the nucleus and other cell organelles is prepared. In contrast to the stratum basalis and stratum spinosum, in which lysosomal enzymes, such as acid phosphatase and aryl sulfatase are present as only a few granular aggregates, there is diffuse staining for lysosomal enzymes in the granular cell layer. These diffusely staining lysosomal enzymes probably play an important role in the autolytic changes occurring in the granular layer (21).

Stratum Corneum

Unlike the nucleated cells of the other epidermal layers, the cell remnants of the normal stratum corneum are anucleate. Thus, the normal horny layer is eosinophilic. The thickness of the horny layer is often difficult to ascertain in formalin-fixed specimens because the outer cell layers may become detached. The portion of the horny layer cytoplasm that contains disulfide bonds of cystine tends to shrink on formalin fixation to form a shell along the cell membrane, resulting in the characteristic basket-weave architecture of nonacral stratum corneum in routine sections (Fig. 3-6) (22). In contrast, glutaraldehyde fixation used for electron microscopy causes precipitation of the formalin-soluble substances within the horny cells and allows staining of the contents of the horny cells with reagents such as uranyl acetate and lead citrate. With a fluorescent stain, it can be shown that the cells of the horny layer are arranged in orderly vertical stacks (23).

Maturation and Terminal Differentiation

Maturation of keratinocytes from basal cells to the horny layer normally takes approximately 30 days, although this may be radically altered in certain disease states. The process involves transition from vertically oriented ovoid basal cells to polyhedral cells in the squamous cell layer, to more horizontally flattened cells associated with acquisition of keratohyalin granules,

and, finally, to fully keratinized cells without nuclei in the horny layer. The transformation of granular cells into horny cells is usually abrupt. The keratinization process during maturation involves three intracellular organelles:

- Tonofilaments in stratum basalis
- Keratohyalin granules in stratum granulosum
- Membrane-coating granules (Odland bodies) in stratum corneum

Tonofilaments are approximately 8 nm thick and are present throughout the epidermis, although they become increasingly prominent as they approach the epidermal surface. By electron microscopy, the cytoplasm of the cells in the lower portion of the horny layer shows relatively electron-lucent tonofilaments embedded in an interfilamentous substance (Fig. 3-8) (24). In the upper portions of the horny layer, however, the cells lose their filamentous structure. Together with the sudden keratinization of the horny cells, an electron-dense, homogeneous marginal band forms in their peripheral cytoplasm in close approximation to the trilaminar plasma membrane. In the lowermost horny layer, the trilaminar plasma membrane is preserved outside of the marginal band; in the midportion of the horny layer, it becomes discontinuous and then desquamates so that the marginal band serves as the real cell membrane (25).

Keratohyalin granules are biochemically complex and composed of profilaggrin, loricrin, and keratin filaments. Profilaggrin is a filaggrin precursor, which is a histidine-rich protein (26). When granular cells are converted to cornified cells, the filaggrin precursor is broken down into many units of filaggrin. Immunohistochemistry reveals that involucrin, a structural component of mature squamous epithelium, is incorporated into the marginal band as part of the formation of the protein envelope that characterizes squamous cells immediately before terminal differentiation (27). Desmosomal contacts are at first still present in the horny layer but disappear before desquamation of the horny cells. Keratohyalin granules may become abnormally shaped (rounded rather than angulated in the setting of human papillomavirus infection) and may be especially helpful as markers of the stratum granulosum, which is thickened or thinned in certain inflammatory disorders and which becomes more prominent with chronic rubbing.

Odland bodies, also called membrane-coating granules, lamellar granules, or keratinosomes are small (not visible by routine microscopy) organelles that are discharged from the granular cells into the intercellular space and that have two important functions: they establish a barrier to water loss, and they mediate stratum corneum cell cohesion. Lamellar granules appear first in the perinuclear cytoplasm in the stratum spinosum. Higher up in the epidermis, they rapidly increase in number and size (28). Both within and outside the granular cells, lamellar granules are round or oval, measure approximately 300 to 500 nm in diameter, and, by electron microscopy, are observed to possess a trilaminar membrane and a laminated interior. During maturation, the lamellar granules fuse with the plasma membrane of a granular cell, secreting its contents into the intercellular spaces, an event associated with establishing a permeability barrier near the epidermal surface (see later) (29).

Regional Variation

Skin shows considerable variation among different body sites, and appreciation of such normal differences is critical to accurate diagnostic assessment. Perhaps the most profound differences exist at *mucosal and paramucosal* sites. For example, with the exception of the dorsum of the tongue and the hard palate, the mucous membrane of the mouth possesses neither a granular nor a horny layer (Fig. 3-10). When these layers are absent, the epithelial cells may appear vacuolated, largely as a result of their glycogen content. Electron microscopic examination reveals that the number of tonofilaments diminishes in the upper layers and become dispersed. Large aggregates of glycogen are present in the cells. The epithelial cells of the oral mucosa show only few well-developed desmosomes. Instead, they show numerous microvilli at their borders. They are held together by an amorphous, moderately electron-dense intercellular cement substance, the dissolution of which causes the detachment of the uppermost cells (25).

In contrast to mucosal epithelium, *acral skin* has a thick stratum granulosum and stratum corneum. Stratum lucidum, forming the lowest portion of the horny layer, can be best recognized in acral skin, especially on the palms and soles (Fig. 3-7).

Specialized Structure and Function
Superficial Cellular Cohesion

The number of tonofilaments in the epidermis increases in the upper portion of the squamous layer. The earliest formation of keratohyalin granules consists of the aggregation of electron-dense ribonucleoprotein particles largely along tonofilaments. The keratohyalin granules increase in size through peripheral aggregation of ribonucleoprotein particles, and they surround more and more tonofilaments (30). By extending along numerous tonofilaments, the keratohyalin granules assume an irregular, often star-shaped outline and may reach a size of 1 to 2 μm. After ultimately ensheathing all tonofilaments, they form in the horny cells the electron-dense interfilamentous protein matrix of mature epidermal keratin. Profilaggrin in keratohyalin granules at the level of the stratum granulosum breaks down into many units of filaggrin in the stratum corneum, where filaggrin then aggregates with keratin filaments and acts as "glue" for keratin filaments. Recent studies indicate a filaggrin gene mutation occurring in up to 10% of the European population, an event associated with increased risk of developing atopic dermatitis with asthma (31), as well as ichthyosis vulgaris (32). Indeed, murine models where filaggrin gene expression is knocked out display skin lesions with features strikingly similar to those of atopic disease (33).

Barrier Function

Odland granules fuse and completely fill the intercellular spaces at the level of the granular layer, thus establishing a barrier to water loss. They contain neutral sugars linked to lipids and/or proteins; hydrolytic enzymes, possibly charged with degrading intercellular materials; and free sterols. The stratum granulosum interstices contain free sterols and sugars; the stratum corneum intercellular spaces stain as a pure neutral lipid mixture with abundant free sterols but no sugars (29). Sugars are cleaved at the granular-cornified layer interface by sugar-specific glycosidases. The lipids formed in these organelles act as hydrophobic material, which is important to the barrier function (34,35).

A similar permeability barrier exists in the oral mucosa. Lamellar granules may also contribute to cohesion between the cells of the lower stratum corneum as a result of the lipids that they contain. The action of enzymes, such as steroid sulfatase, removes the lipids from the upper stratum corneum and brings about desquamation of the cells there (36).

Enzyme Activity

Primary lysosomes that are membrane bound and contain a variety of hydrolytic enzymes, such as acid phosphatase, aryl sulfatase, and β-galactosidase, are seen in small numbers within keratinocytes, largely but not exclusively in the basal cell layer and lower squamous cell layer (12). A great number of lysosomal enzymes, primarily located free within the cytoplasm, are demonstrable in the granular layer and in the lowermost horny layer. Lysosomal enzymes are also found in the lamellar granules and are located within granular cells and after their discharge into the intercellular space (37). Secondary lysosomes, also called phagolysosomes, are present in the lower epidermis, especially in the basal cells, where they digest phagocytized melanosomes, usually as melanosome complexes (see later discussion). In cases of epidermal injury, such as sunburn or interface dermatitis, numerous phagosomes are observed that contain remnants of organelles from damaged cells (37).

Immune Functions of Keratinocytes

In recent years, the epidermal keratinocyte has been recognized as a potent source of immunogenic molecules. Keratinocytes are capable of producing interleukins (ILs) (IL-1α, IL-1β, IL-6, IL-8), colony-stimulating factors (CSFs) (IL-3, granulocyte-macrophage-CSF, granulocyte-CSF, macrophage-CSF), interferons (IFNs) (IFNα, IFNβ), tumor necrosis factors (TNFs), transforming growth factors (TGFs) (TGFα, TGFβ), and growth factors (platelet-derived growth factor, fibroblast growth factor, melanocyte-stimulating hormone) (38). Some of these substances are expressed constitutively, whereas others are synthesized only after signal transduction initiated by external or systemic cues (39). Accordingly, keratinocytes may play an active role in elaboration of molecular signals that facilitate lymphocyte homing and local activation, enabling certain dermal cells to mature and regulating synthesis of extracellular matrix molecules.

Immunohistochemistry

Immunohistochemical techniques have become an important part of the diagnostic arsenal of pathologists, and the expression of keratin by poorly differentiated tumor cells is considered an important marker of epithelial differentiation. Keratins consist of two families of intermediate filament proteins, with type I and type II members always occurring as pairs (40,41). In humans, keratin genes are clustered as families in two regions of the genome, the type I genes on chromosome 17q21.2, and those encoding type II keratins on chromosome 12q13.13. There are 54 functional keratin genes, 27 in each of these domains (41). Different epithelia express different keratins. In addition, different keratins are expressed by the different layers of the human epidermis, reflecting the variable degree of differentiation in keratinocytes. Keratin 5 (K5) and keratin 14 (K14) are predominantly expressed by basal cells (42) (Fig. 3-12). When these cells differentiate, they downregulate expression of mRNAs encoding these two keratins and induce expression of new sets of keratins specific for individual programs of epithelial differentiation (Fig. 3-12). Moreover, unlike other basal cells that express K14, basal cells in the general region where stem cells reside also express keratin 15, indicating that biosynthetic heterogeneity exists within the basal layer with regard to expression of cytoskeletal elements (43,44). Suprabasal keratinocytes predominantly express keratin 1 and keratin 10. Keratin 2 is expressed by terminally differentiated keratinocytes. Keratin 9 is expressed by suprabasal keratinocytes in palmar and plantar epidermis. The pattern and type of keratin expression is different in the epidermis and adnexal structures. It is important to be familiar with the expression of keratin by normal structures because specific mutations are associated with different conditions (e.g., epidermolysis bullosa simplex variants are associated with mutations in keratin 5 and 14 genes, whereas mutations for keratin 1 and 10 genes are associated with bullous ichthyosiform erythroderma; mutations in the keratin 2 gene result in bullous ichthyosis of Siemens, and mutations of keratin 9 genes are responsible for epidermolytic palmoplantar keratoderma) (Table 3-2).

A more novel epithelial immunohistochemical marker is p63, a member of the p53 gene family implicated in both the development and maintenance of stratified epithelial tissues, including the epidermis. Increasing data support p63 function in the regenerative capacity of basal keratinocytes by maintaining cell proliferation (45) as well as inducing epidermal commitment of embryonic stem cells (46,47). The critical contribution of p63 to embryonic development is underscored by the severe abnormalities seen at birth in mice null for p63, including lack of epidermis. Mutations in p63 have been linked to ectodermal dysplasia syndromes with a skin phenotype, indicating the relevance of p63 to normal epidermal development in humans (48). In normal human epidermis, in hair follicles, and in stratified epidermal cultures, p63 protein is principally restricted to cells with high proliferative potential and is absent from the cells that are undergoing terminal differentiation. Accordingly, p63 expression is seen in basal/suprabasal cells of the epidermis, outer root sheath, and hair matrix cells of the hair follicle, basal cells situated in the outermost layer of sebaceous glands, and outer layer cells of the ductal portion and myoepithelial cells of the secretory portion of the sweat glands (Fig. 3-13). p63 is overexpressed in the vast majority of squamous cell carcinomas and basal cell carcinomas and appears to be an especially helpful marker for poorly differentiated squamous cell carcinomas, including the sarcomatoid variant (49).

Melanocytes

Embryology

The appearance of melanocytes in the epidermis takes place in a craniocaudal direction, in accordance with the development of the neural crest, from which the melanocytes are derived. By enzyme histochemistry, melanocytes can be identified in the epidermis of the head region during the latter part of the third fetal month; in the more caudal body regions, the earliest formed melanin can be observed only in the latter part of the fourth month. Because melanocytes are functionally immature during their migration through the fetal dermis, they cannot be identified by histochemical methods until they have reached the epidermis (50). Electron microscopy and immunohistochemical approaches (e.g., stain for HMB-45 protein) allow for an earlier recognition of melanocytes in the epidermis than is possible by light microscopy (51,52).

The tyrosine kinase receptor KIT and its ligand stem cell factor play a critical role in melanocyte physiology, influencing migration, proliferation, differentiation, and survival (53–55). Piebaldism, a genetic disorder, results from KIT receptor defects secondary to mutations of the c-kit proto-oncogene. Patients with piebaldism present at birth with white patches of skin and hair that lack melanocytes, supporting the major role of KIT in melanocyte migration from the neural crest to the skin (56).

Microphthalmia transcription factor (MITF) is a nuclear protein involved in the embryonic development of melanocytes and the regulation of transcription of genes involved in melanin synthesis, such as tyrosinase. The microphthalmia (mi) gene is located on chromosome 3p. Since its discovery as a mutant allele producing mice devoid of viable melanocytes, mi has emerged as the gene whose mutation is responsible for the human pigmentation condition Waardenburg syndrome IIa, as well as a variety of cellular defects involving retinal pigment epithelium, osteoclasts, and mast cells (57).

Normal Microanatomy

Mature melanocytes are melanin-synthesizing dendritic cells located within the basal layer of the epidermis, hair bulb, and outer root sheath of hair follicles (Figs. 3-14 to 3-17). In sections stained with hematoxylin–eosin, the dendrites of epidermal melanocytes are usually not seen, and the cell bodies are randomly dispersed within the basal cell layer. They contain round to oval, dark-stained nuclei that are generally smaller than those of basal keratinocytes and what may appear as a clear

Table 3-2			
Diseases Associated with Keratin Defects			
	Type I	Type II	Diseases
Suprabasal keratinocyte	1	10	Epidermolytic hyperkeratosis, bullous congenital ichthyosiform erythroderma
Basal keratinocyte	5	14	Epidermolysis bullosa simplex
Palmoplantar suprabasal keratinocyte		9	Epidermolytic palmoplantar keratoderma (Vorner syndrome)
Outer root sheath	6a	16	Pachyonychia congenita type 1
Nail bed	6b	17	Pachyonychia congenita type 2
Nonkeratinizing stratified squamous epithelium/mucosa	4	13	White sponge nevus

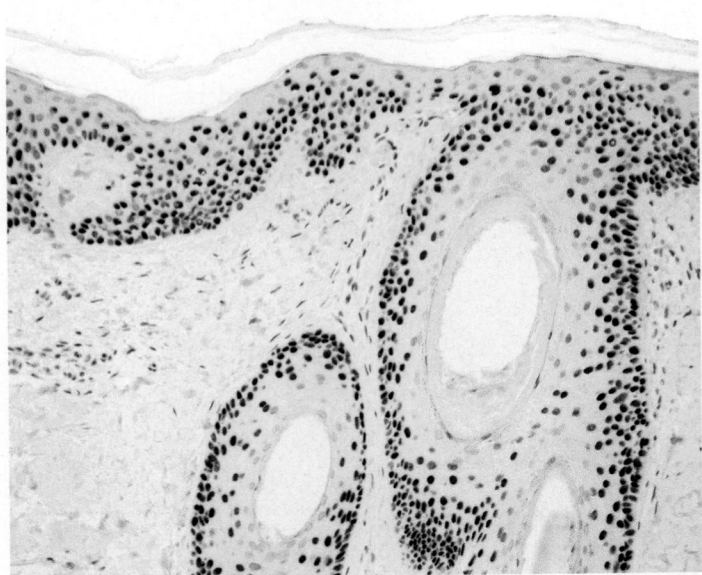

Figure 3-13 p63 immunostain shows intense nuclear positivity in all epithelial compartments, including the epidermis and adnexal structures. The staining is more intense in basal and parabasal areas.

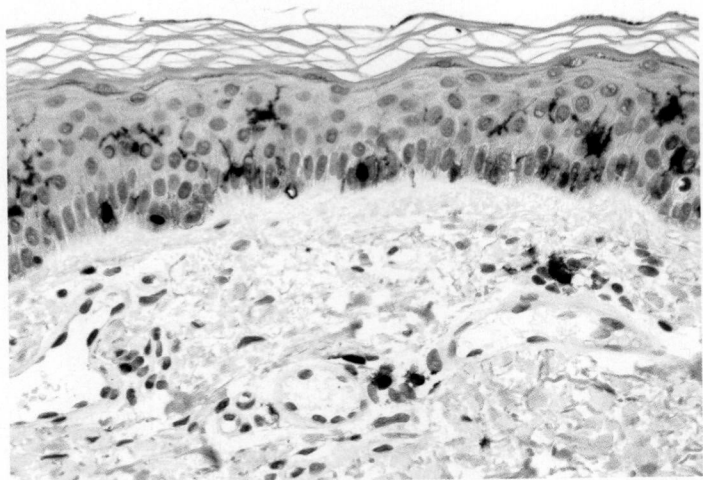

Figure 3-14 S100 immunostain is expressed by junctional melanocytes and also by Langerhans cells in the midepidermis and dermis.

halo of surrounding cytoplasm, largely as the result of shrinkage during tissue processing. Although the number of melanocytes in relation to basal cells varies with the body region and increases with repeated exposure to ultraviolet (UV) light, the average number of clear cells in hematoxylin–eosin-stained vertical sections is 1 of 10 cells in the basal layer, and a similar ratio was found with immunohistochemical studies (58,59). Melanin is transferred by means of the dendritic processes (Figs. 3-14 and 3-15A, B) from the melanocytes to the basal keratinocytes, where it is first stored and later degraded. As a rule, a greater amount of melanin is present in the basal keratinocytes than in the melanocytes, and often basal cells at the tips of rete ridges are preferentially more melanized. Because only about 10% of the cells in the basal layer are melanocytes, each melanocyte supplies several keratinocytes with melanin, forming with them an epidermal-melanin unit (60).

In persons with light skin color, staining with hematoxylin–eosin may reveal few or no melanin granules in the basal cell layer. In persons with dark skin color, especially individuals of African heritage, melanin granules are present in the basal cell layer as well as throughout the epidermis, including the horny layer, and, in some instances, in the upper dermis within macrophages, called melanophages. Accordingly, ethnic background and body site are critical in separating normal variations from true pathology.

Special Stains

Melanocytes may be difficult to appreciate on hematoxylin–eosin-stained sections, and there are several special stains that can facilitate their detection by light microscopy. Silver stains indicate the presence of melanin, which is both argyrophilic and argentaffin. Argyrophilia is based on the ability of melanin to be impregnated with silver nitrate solutions, which, on reduction with hydroquinone to silver, stain black. Because melanin is argentaffin, ammoniated silver nitrate may be reduced by phenolic groups in the melanin, forming black silver precipitate (e.g., the Fontana-Masson method). Neither of these methods is entirely specific for melanin, however. Melanin may be bleached by a strong oxidizing agent, such as hydrogen peroxide or potassium permanganate, a method that permits more specific identification (61) and that is used in heavily melanized tumors, where pigment may obscure nuclear detail.

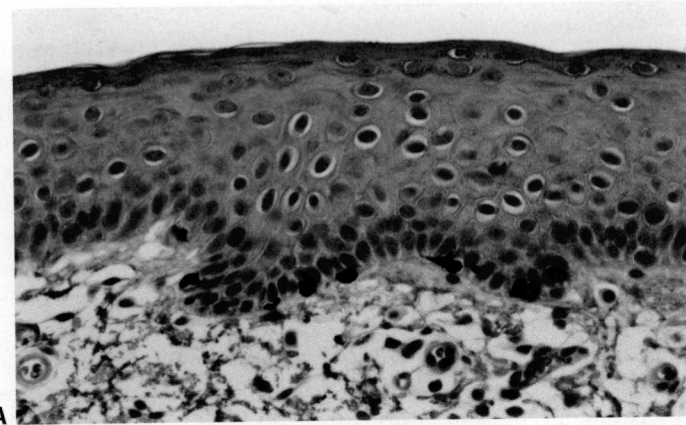

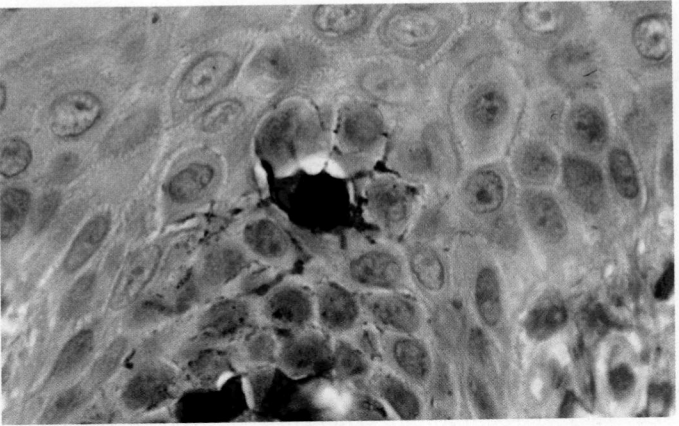

A   B

Figure 3-15 Melan-A/MART-1 immunostain demonstrates normal melanocytes within the epidermal basal layer. This is a more specific melanocytic marker compared with S100 (A). Note the dendritic extension at higher magnification (B). This melanocyte appears to be suprabasal as a result of the tangential plane of the section.

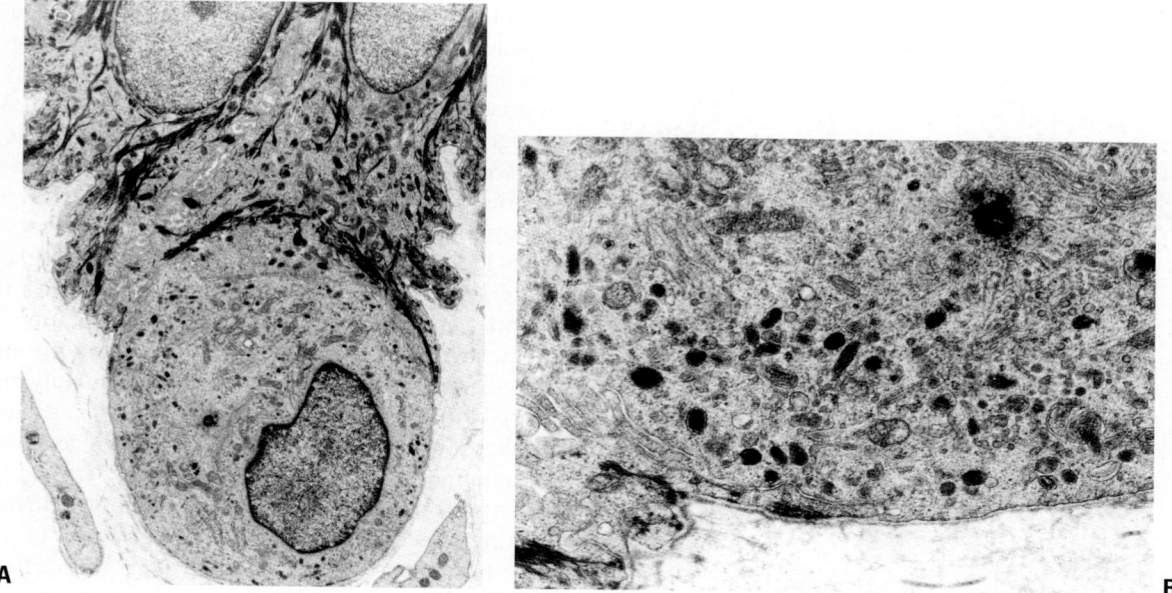

Figure 3-16 Ultrastructure of melanocytes. These cells characteristically "hang down" from the basal cell layer and are devoid of tonofilaments of desmosomes (**A**). They contain characteristic melanosomes in varying stages of melanization (**B**).

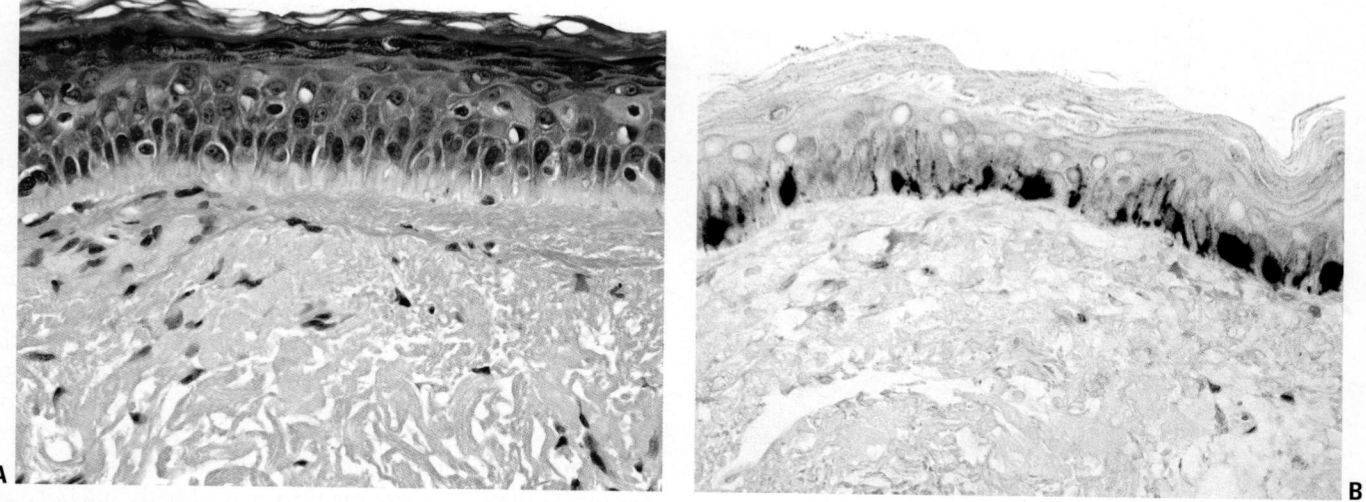

Figure 3-17 **A:** Melanocytes in sun-damaged skin may be increased in number and size, as depicted in this microphotograph. Note the marked dermal solar elastosis. **B:** MART-1 immunostain highlights an increase in melanocyte density in sun-damaged skin.

The dihydroxyphenylalanine (dopa) reaction, which stains melanocytes dark brown to black, imitates physiologic melanin formation, which begins by tyrosinase-dependent hydroxylation of tyrosine to dopa and the oxidation of dopa to dopaquinone, which is subsequently polymerized into melanin. Thus, the dopa reaction is, in essence, an assay for tyrosinase activity in melanosomes (61).

The use of immunohistochemical techniques for labeling melanocytes is now increasingly important, and several melanocytic markers that work in paraffin-embedded tissues are available (Table 3-3). Immunohistochemical detection of melanocytes has been classically accomplished by polyclonal antibodies to S100 protein. The antigen S100, a family of calcium-binding proteins (molecular weight 21,000), originally isolated from bovine brain extract (62), is present in the cytoplasm and nucleus of a variety of cells, including those of

neural melanocytic lineage (63). The function of S100 within melanocytes is unclear, although different subtypes of S100 appear to have different functions in different cell types. The member of the S100 family predominantly expressed in normal melanocytes is S100B (64), whereas S100A subtypes have been reported in various skin lesions. In the skin, in addition to melanocytes, S100 labels Langerhans cells, specialized macrophages, Schwann cells, sweat glands, and adipocytes, and therefore, although it is a sensitive marker, it lacks specificity (Fig. 3-14; see also Figs. 3-35F, 3-52C, 3-53A, and 3-54B).

The search for new targets for immunotherapy in patients with melanoma generated several reagents valuable for diagnostic pathology. By using cytotoxic T-cell assays, various antigens that are recognized by autologous cytotoxic T lymphocytes were identified (65). A group of these antigens is referred to as melanocyte differentiation antigens because their expression is restricted

Table 3-3

Immunohistochemical Expression of S100 and Most Common Melanocytic Differentiation Markers in Normal Skin

Antigen	Antibody	Positive Cells	Antigen Location
S100 protein	Anti-S100 protein	Melanocytes, Langerhans cells, macrophages, Schwann cells, adipocytes, myoepithelial cells of sweat glands	Nuclear and cytoplasmic (primarily nuclear)
gp100	HMB-45	Fetal melanocytes, activated melanocytes	Cytoplasmic
Melan-A/MART-1	A103/M2-7C10	Melanocytes	Cytoplasmic
Tyrosinase	T311	Melanocytes	Cytoplasmic
PNL2 antigen	PNL2 antibody	Melanocytes, neutrophils	Cytoplasmic
MITF	MITF antibody	Melanocytes, macrophages, Schwann cells, smooth muscle cells	Nuclear

MART, melanoma antigen recognized by T cells; MITF, microphthalmia transcription factor.

to cells of melanocytic lineage. A number of reagents to melanocyte differentiation antigens suitable for analysis of paraffin-embedded material have become available, including the classically used monoclonal antibody HMB-45 and additional reagents such as monoclonal antibodies to Melan-A/MART-1 (66,67) (Fig. 3-15), tyrosinase, and PNL2. HMB-45 antibody reacts with a cytoplasmic epitope, the premelanosome glycoprotein gp100 (75 to 100 kDa), in cells of most but not all melanomas and in a minority of nevi (68,69). HMB-45 is negative in normal epidermal melanocytes in adults; however, it is expressed by melanocytes in fetal skin and stimulated adult melanocytes and is considered a highly specific antibody for the immunocytochemical substantiation of the diagnosis of malignant melanoma.

The advantage of the newer melanocyte differentiation antigens (e.g., Melan-A/MART-1) is a stronger sensitivity when dealing with melanocytic neoplasms compared with HMB-45 and a stronger specificity when compared with S100. The gene for Melan-A/MART-1 was independently cloned by two groups of scientists, which explains the two different designations (MART stands for Melanoma Antigen Recognized by T cells) (70). This melanocytic differentiation antigen is a small cytoplasmic protein (22 kDa) with distinctive nucleotide sequences and genetic organization that is believed to be a melanosomal component. Tyrosinase is a key enzyme in melanin biosynthesis and represents a marker of melanocytic differentiation. T311, a murine monoclonal antibody to tyrosinase, is a reliable marker of melanocytes in paraffin-embedded sections (71). PNL2 is a monoclonal antibody directed against a fixative-resistant melanocyte antigen. The exact nature of the antigen recognized by PNL2 remains to be defined. The analysis of PNL2 immunostaining on a broad range of normal or malignant human tissues and on various melanocytic lesions revealed its high specificity (72). Despite the advent of these new markers, S100 and HMB-45 remain very important tools when dealing with tumors, and S100 remains the more sensitive (although not very specific marker) for neoplastic melanocytes, especially spindle cell lesions (e.g., desmoplastic melanoma), now supplemented by SOX10, which is both sensitive and quite specific (73), although staining also occurs in normal structures, including sweat glands, neural structures (including nerves and neural tumors), and nonspecific cells in lymph nodes and in granulomatous infiltrates (74).

MITF, another novel melanocyte differentiation marker, was shown to be less sensitive and not restricted to melanocytes. D5 (monoclonal antibody to MITF) was generated from the consensus region shared by various isoforms of MITF. Only one isoform, MITF-M, is melanocyte specific. Other isoforms that are recognized by D5 can be found in various nonmelanocytic cell types (Table 3-3) (75).

Ultrastructure

Melanocytes differ from keratinocytes by possessing no tonofilaments or desmosomes (Fig. 3-16A). At their base, where they lie in close apposition to the lamina densa, melanocytes show structures resembling, yet smaller than, hemidesmosomes of basal keratinocytes (76). Melanosomes are the most characteristic organelles of the melanocyte, and identification of various stages of their formation within a cell assists in its ultrastructural identification as a melanocyte (in contrast to keratinocytes that contain via transfer only fully melanized organelles) (Fig. 3-16B). Melanosomes are membrane-bound organelles that in their development from stage I to stage IV gradually move from the cytoplasm of the melanocyte into the dendritic processes. As melanosomes mature, their content of melanin increases, and their concentration of melanogenic enzyme decreases (77).

Stage I melanosomes are round, 0.3 μm in diameter, and contain no melanin (78). Stage II–IV melanosomes are ellipsoid and measure approximately 0.5 μm in length. They contain longitudinal filaments that are cross-linked with one another. Enzyme activity is present both on the enveloping membrane and on the filaments. Melanin deposition on the cross-linked filaments begins at stage II. Stage III melanosomes have only little tyrosinase activity but show continued melanin deposition, partially through nonenzymatic polymerization. Stage IV melanosomes are fully melanized and no longer possess tyrosinase activity. Melanin, which is homogeneous and electron dense, fills the entire organelle at this stage, obscuring its internal structure.

Regional and Racial Variation

The highest concentration of melanocytes is found on the face and the male genitals, about 2,000/mm^2, and the lowest on the trunk, about 800/mm^2 (79–81). No significant difference in the density of distribution of melanocytes for any given area of the skin exists between African American and Caucasoid skin. In the former, the melanocytes are uniformly highly enzymatically reactive, whereas the melanocytes of Caucasoids, when not exposed to sunlight, are highly variable in dopa reactivity (82). In addition, African American skin contains larger and more highly dendritic melanocytes than does Caucasoid skin (80,81). Finally, transferred melanosomes within keratinocytes of people of African descent tend to be individually distributed, whereas those in keratinocytes of Caucasians are packaged in membrane-enclosed aggregates (83–86). The melanocortin 1 receptor gene (MC1R) is responsible for normal pigment variation in humans and is highly polymorphic with numerous population-specific alleles. Some MC1R variants have been associated with skin cancer risk (86).

Melanocytes in Sun-Exposed Areas

Regional variation of melanocyte number and morphology may also be influenced by environmental factors, such as sun exposure. After a single exposure to UV light *in vivo*, the skin of Caucasoids, when examined with the dopa reaction, shows no increase in the density of the melanocyte population but does show an increase in the size and functional activity of the existing melanocytes (87). Repeated exposure to UV light, however, causes an increase in the concentration of dopa-positive melanocytes, as well as an increase in their size and functional activity (82,88). Thus, examination of habitually exposed and of unexposed skin from adjacent anatomic sites, such as the lateral and medial aspects of the upper arm, has shown a twofold-higher concentration of melanocytes in the former, and the melanocyte concentration is even higher in areas such as the head and neck (89).

Surgical pathologists and dermatopathologists often face the difficulty of having to distinguish melanocyte hyperplasia of sun-damaged skin from melanoma *in situ* (e.g., when evaluating surgical margins in melanoma excisions). It is known that melanocytes increase in number and size in sun-damaged skin (Fig. 3-17A, B). On immunohistochemical studies, long-standing sun-exposed skin has been reported to have an average of 15 to 20 melanocytes per high-power field (in 0.5 mm of skin) (89,90), some degree of contiguous growth (up to 9 adjacent melanocytes), and melanocytes extending to hair follicles but not reaching the level of the uppermost portion of sebaceous glands. However, there should not be significant confluence, deep follicular penetration, nesting, or pagetoid spread.

Specialized Structure and Function
Melanogenesis

Enzymatic melanogenesis involves tyrosinase as the melanogenic enzyme (81,91). Tyrosinase is a copper-containing enzyme that catalyzes the hydroxylation of tyrosine to dopa and the oxidation of dopa to dopa-quinone. However, before tyrosinase can act on tyrosine, two cupric atoms present in tyrosinase must be reduced to cuprous atoms. It is believed that, in addition to being a substrate, dopa activates this reduction, thereby acting as a cofactor in the reaction. The conversion of tyrosine to melanin by tyrosinase is characterized by a variable lag period. When tyrosinase is present in low concentrations, as in epidermal melanocytes of nonirradiated skin, this lag period is markedly prolonged, and no use of tyrosine by tyrosinase is detectable. In contrast, in skin exposed *in vivo* to UV light, as well as in epidermal sheets and in hair bulbs, tyrosinase activity is

detectable with tyrosine as substrate (60,81,92). Because there is no lag period with dopa as substrate, tyrosinase in epidermal melanocytes can be readily demonstrated even in nonirradiated skin when skin sections are incubated in dopa rather than in tyrosine. The enzyme acting on dopa is therefore thought to be tyrosinase rather than dopa-oxidase.

The melanogenic enzyme tyrosinase is synthesized in the Golgi-associated endoplasmic reticulum, in which tyrosinase condenses in membrane-limited vesicles. This process has been observed by electron microscopy in epidermal melanocytes after *in vivo* UV irradiation with either dopa or tyrosine as substrate (93). Subsequently, these tyrosinase units are transferred to dilated tubules of the smooth endoplasmic reticulum. There, tyrosinase is incorporated into a structural protein matrix containing filaments that have a distinctive periodicity. This then represents a stage I melanosome (94). Few stage I and II melanosomes have acid phosphatase activity, but the proportion of acid phosphatase–positive melanosomes increases in stage III, reaching a maximum in stage IV (95). This enzyme may play a role in the degradation or transfer of melanosomes. Detailed analysis of nonmelanosomal regulatory factors in melanogenesis has revealed coated vesicles to be richest in tyrosinase and catalase, whereas premelanosomes have the highest concentrations of peroxidase (96). Among relevant metal ions, premelanosomes contain higher amounts of copper, zinc, and iron than do coated vesicles.

Melanin Transfer

The transfer of melanosomes from melanocytes to epidermal keratinocytes and to hair cortex cells is the result of active phagocytosis of the tips of melanocytic dendrites by keratinocytes and hair cortex cells, as demonstrated in tissue cultures (97) and in epidermal reconstructs seeded with melanocytes (98). Once incorporated into keratinocytes, melanosomes aggregate to form protective parasols above the keratinocyte nuclei. As previously noted, melanin in Caucasoids is concentrated in basal keratinocytes, whereas in people of African ancestry, distribution is more diffuse within the epidermis (99,100). Both melanin formation and melanin transfer are enhanced by various stimuli, notably by skin exposure to UV light. Data suggest a central role for p53 in UV-induced skin melanization and potentially certain forms of pathologic hyperpigmentation (101). UV-induced melanization, or sun tanning, requires the induction of α-melanocyte-stimulating hormone (α-MSH) secretion by epidermal keratinocytes. This phenomenon requires α-MSH generation as a cleavage product of pro-opiomelanocortin (POMC), and the interaction of α-MSH with its highly pleomorphic receptor MC1R, which mediates melanocyte functions, including pigmentary phenotype and proliferation (86). p53 is believed to stimulate the POMC promoter in response to UV exposure, and mice genetically deficient in p53 fail to exhibit the normal tanning response. Accordingly, it is possible that p53 may function as, in addition to an inducer of apoptosis in UV-damaged cells, a sensor/effector of the tanning response, and even potentially as a trigger for certain pathologic forms of melanization.

Merkel Cells
Embryology

Although the origin of Merkel cells is unclear, it seems likely that they are differentiated from stem cells in the epidermis (102,103). The alternative hypothesis is that Merkel cells derive from the neural crest (102,104,105). The favored hypothesis, however, is that they arise between weeks 8 and 12 of gestational age from precursor stages of epithelial cells of early fetal epidermis that still express simple epithelial cytokeratins. *In situ* differentiation from epidermal ectoderm versus immigration of cells from the neural crest is supported by studies of fetal skin without Merkel cells transplanted to nude mice and subsequently found to contain mature Merkel cells within the engrafted tissue (106). Some Merkel cells detach from the epidermis and migrate temporarily into the upper dermis, where some of them associate with small nerves.

Normal Microanatomy

Merkel cells are present within the basal cell layer of the epidermis, oral mucosa, and the bulge region of hair follicles (107). They are quite scarce, irregularly distributed, and occasionally arranged in groups, often at tips of rete ridges (Fig. 3-18A), in eccrine glandular ridges of glabrous skin, in "Haarscheiben" of hairy skin, within beltlike clusters of hair follicles, and in certain mucosal tissues (108). It is assumed that the Merkel cell may represent a rudimentary touch receptor, more important in lower vertebrates (e.g., particularly in relationship to vibrissa hairs). The Merkel cell cannot be recognized in light microscopic sections; however, in silver-impregnated sections, the meniscoid neural terminal that covers the basal portion of each Merkel cell can be seen as a Merkel disk (109). A sensory nerve fiber may terminate at the disk. Immunohistochemistry for low-molecular-weight cytokeratins (CKs) such as CK8, -18, -19, and -20 more typical of simple epithelial cells than keratinocytes permits differential identification of Merkel cells in tissue sections (82). The most useful of these filamentous proteins is CK20, which has been shown to be a highly specific marker for Merkel cells because in human skin no other cell type expressing CK20 exists (107) (Fig. 3-18A). A novel immunohistochemical marker for Merkel cell is INSM1 (insulinoma associated protein 1), a zinc-finger transcriptional factor expressed in tissues undergoing terminal neuroendocrine differentiation (Fig. 3-18B) (110,111).

By electron microscopic examination, Merkel cells are usually located directly above the basement membrane (112). They possess small, electron-dense, membrane-bound neurosecretory-type granules, strands of perinuclear intermediate filaments, and occasional desmosomes on their cell membranes connecting them with neighboring keratinocytes (Fig. 3-18C). The electron-dense granules vary in size between 80 and 200 nm and tend to be located at the side of cytoplasm in contact with axon terminals. Intermediate-type junctions are noted between axon terminals and Merkel cells.

Regional Variation

Merkel cells are most heavily concentrated in skin with high hair density and in glabrous epithelium of the digits, lips,

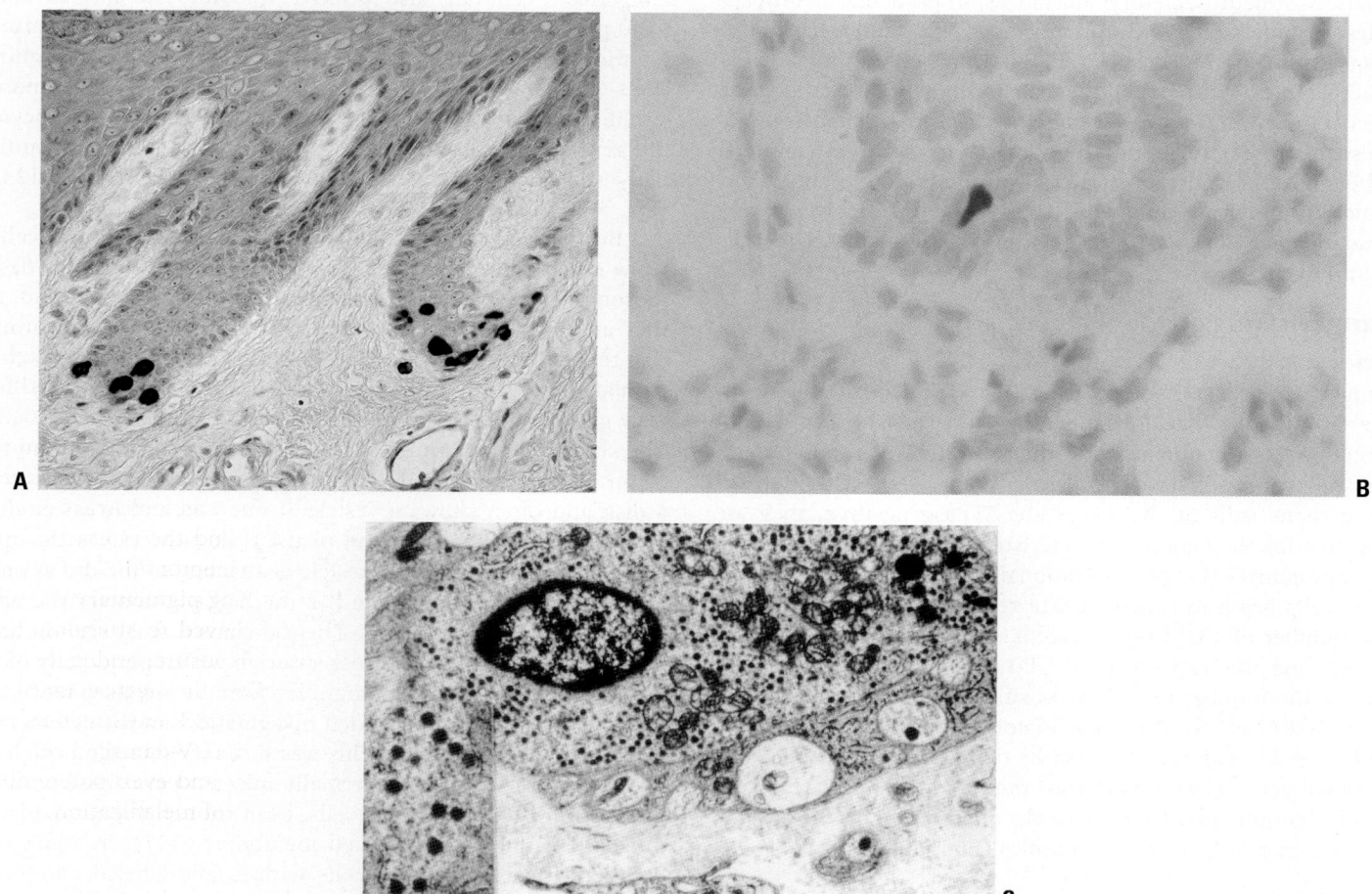

Figure 3-18 Immunohistochemistry with cytokeratin 20 (A) and INSM1 (B) highlights Merkel cells in the glabrous epithelium of the digit. They are often distributed, forming small groups at the tip of the rete ridges. C: By electron microscopy, Merkel cells contain characteristic neurosecretory granules.

regions of the oral cavity, and the outer root sheath of the hair follicle. These cells are present in mammals as so-called "touch-domes," also known as "Haarscheiben," a form of type I mechanoreceptor that surrounds tylotrich (large touch-sensitive) hairs and the rete ridge collars about external root sheaths of hair follicles.

An increase in Merkel cells is seen after chronic sun exposure and has also been described in the epidermal basal layer adjacent to prurigo nodularis, actinic keratoses, and tumors such as basal cell carcinomas (108).

Specialized Structure and Function

Merkel cells are specialized epithelial cells that react with the intermediate filament CTK and desmosomal proteins (113,114). Of note, Merkel cells also express neuroendocrine markers such as chromogranin A, the matrix substance of the dense-core granules, as well as synaptophysin, supporting the view that they are epithelial neuroendocrine cells and that they may possess a neurosecretory function (108,115). Merkel cells also contain neuron-specific enolase and neurofilaments in their cytoplasm (116,117). The characteristic presence of specific cytokeratins (CK20) and neuroendocrine markers in Merkel cells is relevant to the diagnosis of Merkel cell carcinoma (primary neuroendocrine tumor of the skin), perhaps the only practical reason for the diagnostician to know about this mysterious cell type.

In addition to the expression of neuroendocrine markers, a variety of neurosecretory substances, in particular neuropeptides, that are stored within the dense-core granules have been demonstrated in Merkel cells. These neuropeptides include vasoactive intestinal polypeptide, calcitonin gene-related peptide (CGRP), serotonin, and substance P (108). Although some of these neurosecretory substances work as neurotransmitters, others have been demonstrated to promote growth and differentiation of various cutaneous cell types (108). However, any functional significance to their presence in human Merkel cells is unproven.

Langerhans Cells

Embryology

Langerhans cells are bone marrow–derived, dendritic, antigen-presenting cells that appear in the epidermis by 7 weeks of gestation, as documented by their positive staining for adenosine triphosphatase (ATPase) (Fig. 3-19). Although all Langerhans cells at this stage are ATPase positive, they are negative for their more characteristic and specific cell surface glycoprotein CD1a. At a gestational stage of 60 days, Langerhans cells begin to express CD1a reactivity. By 80 to 90 days, the number of CD1a-positive cells increases abruptly, and after 90 days, the expression of CD1a is approximately equivalent to the number of ATPase-positive Langerhans cells (118) (Fig. 3-20A, B). S100 protein is not found in the Langerhans cells of fetal epidermis but can be demonstrated within 1 day after delivery (119). By electron microscopy, Langerhans cells can be identified by 10 to 11 weeks of gestation on the basis of the presence of Langerhans granules (Fig. 3-20C).

Normal Microanatomy

Langerhans cells may be presumptively observed in histologic sections stained with hematoxylin–eosin as clear cells in the suprabasal epidermis. However, they cannot be reliably

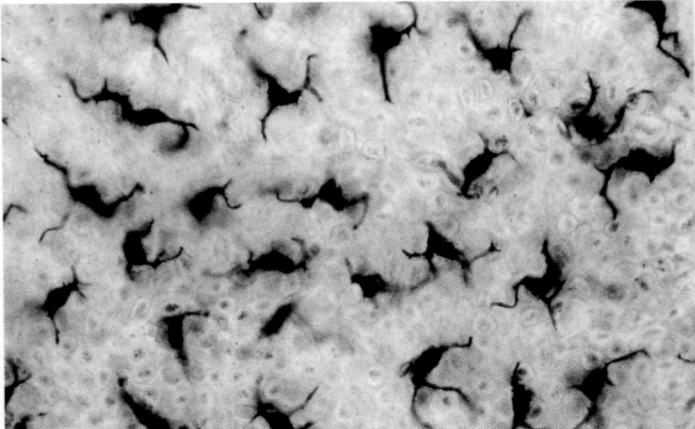

Figure 3-19 An epidermal sheet, removed and viewed en face, after adenosine triphosphatase enzyme histochemical staining. Note numerous, evenly distributed dendritic Langerhans cells.

distinguished from occasional intraepidermal T lymphocytes and macrophages, and their dendritic cytoplasmic processes cannot be resolved. Because Langerhans cell detection is difficult in conventional sections, special stains are generally required for their detection and enumeration. Several enzyme histochemical stains have historically been used to identify Langerhans cells and to differentiate them from melanocytes. These include ATPase (Fig. 3-19) and aminopeptidase (120). Langerhans cells are also positive for HLA-DR antigen and S100 protein, although the former also reacts with cells forming the acrosyringium (121), and the latter is found in melanocytes (Fig. 3-14). Langerhans cells can be demonstrated more specifically with monoclonal antibody to the prothymocyte differentiation cell surface glycoprotein CD1a when the antibody is labeled with either peroxidase or fluorescein (122–124) (Fig. 3-20A, B).

By electron microscopic examination, Langerhans cells show a markedly folded nucleus and no tonofilaments or desmosomes. Melanosomes are only rarely found in them, and, if they are, they are always located within lysosomes, indicating that they have been phagocytized (125). Of great interest is the regular presence of an organelle called the Langerhans or Birbeck granule in the cytoplasm of Langerhans cells (Fig. 3-20C). The size of these granules varies considerably, from 100 nm to 1 μm (126). The granule has the three-dimensional shape of a disk and often shows a vesicle at one end and occasionally at both ends. A cross section of the disk portion has the appearance of a rod, and, if a vesicle is attached to the rod at one end, the Langerhans granule has the highly characteristic appearance of a tennis racquet. The rod-shaped cross section has a central lamella showing cross striation with a periodicity of 6 nm (126). Langerhans cell granules form as a consequence of endocytotic, clathrin-associated invaginations of the cell membrane of Langerhans cells. This was first recognized on the basis of the presence of intradermally injected peroxidase within the granules of Langerhans cells, even though the peroxidase molecule cannot cross the cell membrane (127). In addition, on incubating Langerhans cells with a gold-labeled antibody directed against the CD1a glycoprotein of the cell membrane of the Langerhans cell, it was found that the labeled CD1a was internalized and appeared within Langerhans granules (128). The histiocytes present in the cutaneous and visceral lesions

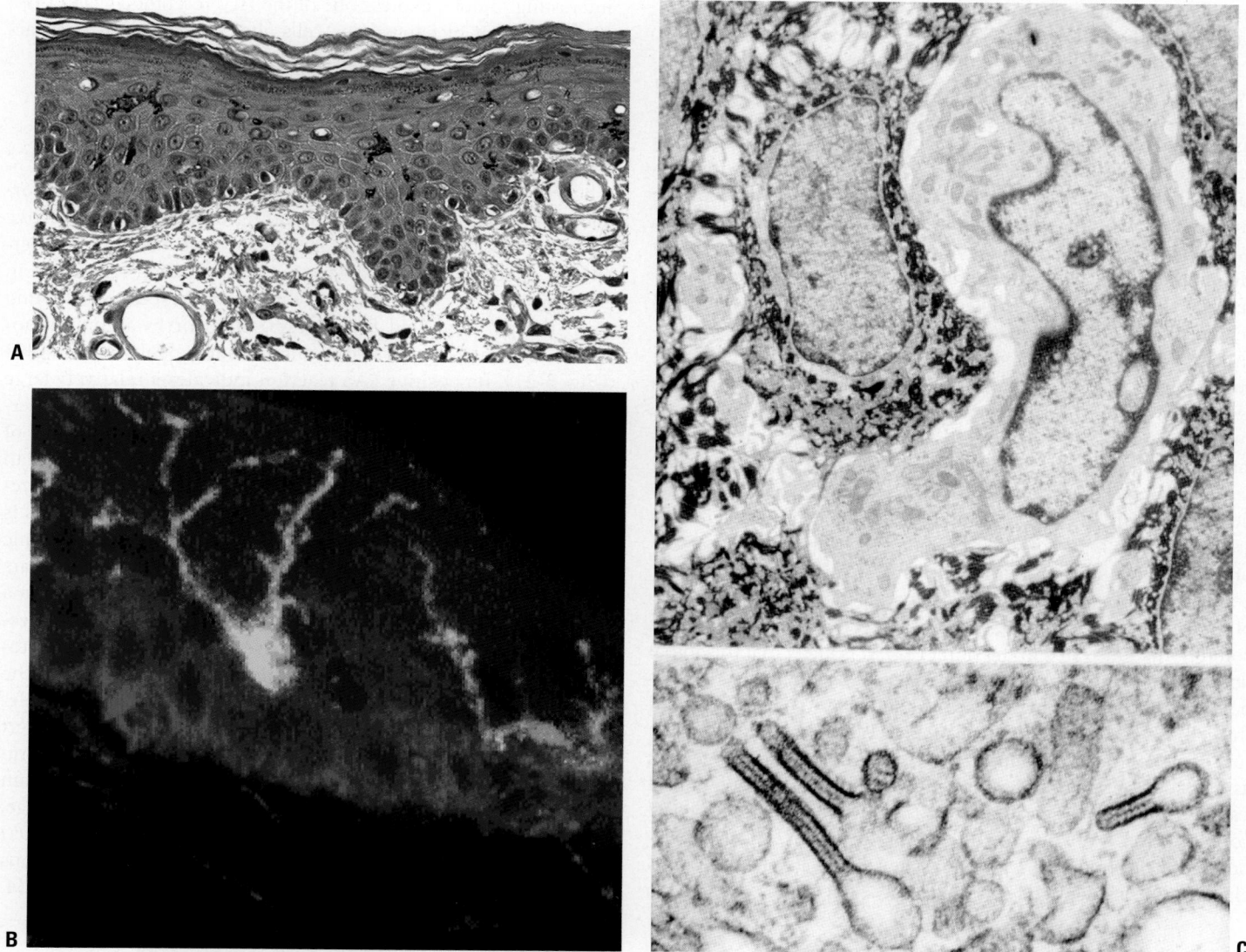

Figure 3-20 A: Anatomy of a human Langerhans cell. B: Typical dendritic morphology seen with immunohistochemical stain for CD1a and immunofluorescence detection of CD1a glycoprotein by confocal scanning laser microscopy. C: Transmission electron micrograph of Langerhans cell (**top**) and characteristic cytoplasmic granules (Birbeck granules) (**bottom**).

of histiocytosis X contain Langerhans granules. These granules are indistinguishable in their electron microscopic appearance from those seen in epidermal Langerhans cells (129,130). Cells that have the ultrastructural features of Langerhans cells but lack the Langerhans granule have been called indeterminate cells. They react specifically with the monoclonal antibody to CD1a (131,132).

Regional Variation

Langerhans cells are present in the epidermis in a concentration similar to that of melanocytes, between 460 and 1,000/mm². In contrast to melanocytes, their number does not increase but may instead decrease with repeated exposure to UV light (120). CD1a-positive Langerhans cells have been found to be less plentiful in trunk skin than extremity skin (133). However, there appears to be considerable site variation among individuals, and the best comparison for the determination of site-matched normal Langerhans cell numbers may be uninvolved skin directly adjacent to the lesion under study (133).

Langerhans cells are present not only in the skin but also in the oral mucosa, the vagina, the lymph nodes, and the thymus; occasionally, they are seen in the dermis (134). Their numbers may vary significantly in pathologic processes, partly as a result of local accumulation or their tendency to actually migrate on stimulation (135).

Specialized Structure and Function

Langerhans cells originate in the bone marrow and are functionally and immunologically related to the monocyte–macrophage–histiocyte series (136). Langerhans cells constitute 2% to 4% of the total epidermal cell population and tend to be evenly distributed such that their dendrites extend uniformly toward the epidermal surface (137). A few Langerhans cells are present in the dermis of normal skin. Langerhans cells express immune response–associated antigens class II (HLA-DR in humans, Ia in mice) (138,139), leukocyte common antigen (140) Fc and C3 receptors, CD1a antigen (123–125), CD1c (M241) antigen (141), a membrane-bound ATPase (137), S100 protein, and actin-like and vimentin filaments. These markers are compatible with an active role in cutaneous immunity.

Langerhans cells have antigen-processing and antigen-presenting capacity. The recognition of a soluble protein and haptenized antigens by T lymphocytes requires the initial uptake and processing by an HLA-DR–positive cell like the Langerhans cell, which then presents immunologically relevant signals to the T lymphocytes. This often involves active migration of the antigen-bearing Langerhans cell from the epidermis into the dermis, where transit to draining lymph nodes occurs via lymphatic channels. In the lymph node, naive T cells are plentiful for receipt of the antigenic signals communicated by the Langerhans cells in a class II (HLA-DR)–dependent manner. Such T-cell sensitization results in the formation of memory T cells with the ability to recall and respond to the specific antigenic peptide on re-exposure or challenge. This mechanism is believed to provide an important component to normal cutaneous immunosurveillance, as well as the underpinning of the contact hypersensitivity reaction. However, recent studies suggest a more complex function for Langerhans cells in normal skin homeostasis, where they are involved in maintenance of tolerance through activation and proliferation of skin-resident regulatory T cells (142).

UV radiation interferes with the antigen-presenting capacity of Langerhans cells. After UV irradiation, fewer Langerhans cells could be demonstrated in the skin (143). It is likely that this initial decrease in the number of Langerhans cells is attributable to a temporary loss of membrane markers rather than to a destruction of the cells. Chronic repeated exposure to UV light may result in actual depletion of cells, contributing to potential for carcinogenesis as a result of impaired immunosurveillance. Similar depletion of Langerhans cells may result from the application of potent topical corticosteroids (144) and in the setting of acquired immunodeficiency syndrome (145). With respect to the latter, viral particles have been identified in Langerhans cells (146), which, it is

interesting to note, express one of the HIV receptors, CD4 (147). Replenishment of Langerhans cells after depletion has been accomplished by the application of topical retinoids (148).

Basement Membrane Zone

Normal Microanatomy, Ultrastructure, and Molecular Structure

The basement membrane is an inconspicuous structure of enormous functional significance, bonding together the protective epidermal layer and adnexal structures with the adjacent dermis. A subepidermal basement membrane zone not visible in sections stained with hematoxylin–eosin is seen on staining with the periodic acid Schiff (PAS) stain or by immunofluorescence as a 0.5- to 1.0-μm-thick homogeneous band (149) (Fig. 3-21). Its positive PAS reaction indicates a relatively large number of neutral mucopolysaccharides in this zone. Furthermore, impregnation with silver nitrate reveals a meshwork of reticulum fibers in the uppermost dermis. Staining with alcian blue, which identifies the band of polysaccharides and the reticulum meshwork, reveals that the band of polysaccharides is located above the reticulum layer (150). The light microscopic PAS-positive subepidermal basement membrane zone appears heterogeneous on electron microscopy (Fig. 3-22). The plasma membrane at the undersurface of basal cells shows hemidesmosomes ("half-desmosomes") possessing only one intracytoplasmic attachment plaque, to which tonofilaments from the interior of the basal cell are attached (Fig. 3-22). The cytoskeletal intermediate filaments within basal keratinocytes that insert into hemidesmosomes are composed predominantly of keratins 14 and 5 (151,152) (Fig. 3-23). Hemidesmosomes contain plaque proteins involved in intermediate filament anchorage, including bullous pemphigoid antigen 1 (BPAG1; 230 kDa) and plectin, transmembranous proteins, including bullous pemphigoid antigen 2 (BPAG2; 180 kDa), and integrin α6β4.

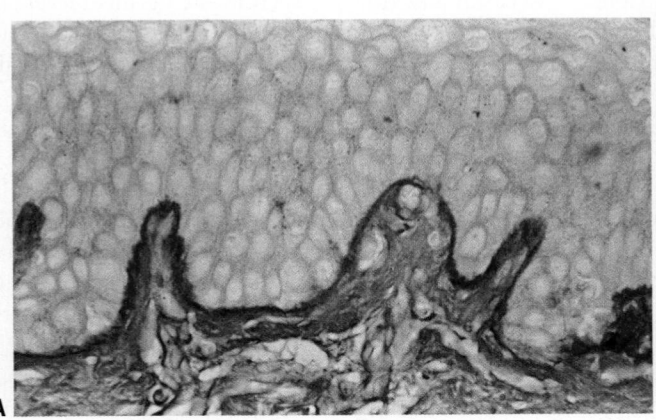
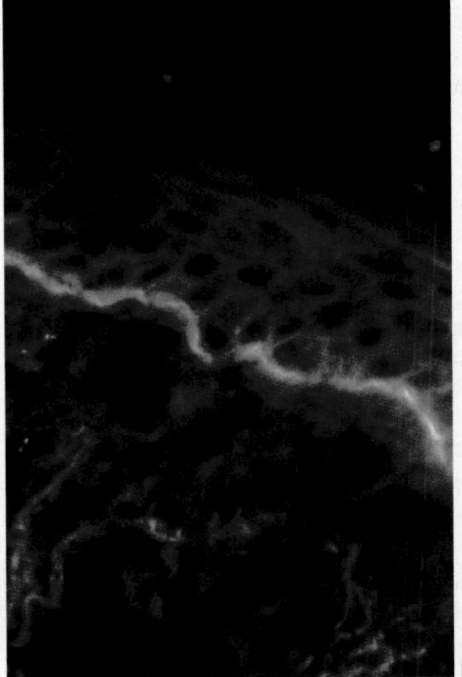

Figure 3-21 **A:** Demonstration of normal basement membrane zone separating epidermal and dermal layers by periodic acid Schiff stain. **B:** By direct immunofluorescence staining for the basement membrane–associated structural protein bullous pemphigoid antigen, a linear band is observed along the dermal–epidermal junction.

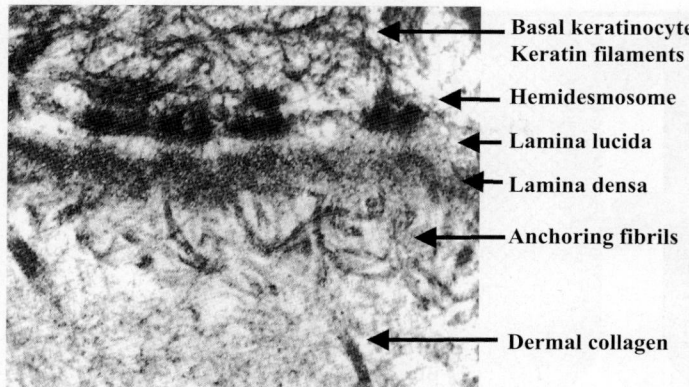

Figure 3-22 Transmission electron microscopy of the basement membrane separating the epidermis and dermis. Hemidesmosomes, lamina lucida, lamina densa, and anchoring fibrils can all be seen in this image.

Additional components of the hemidesmosomes include p200, a noncollagenous N-glycosylated acidic protein that is distinct from subunits of type VI collagen (153), and other molecules not yet fully characterized. Bullous pemphigoid antigens are easily demonstrated by immunofluorescence as a smooth linear band that separates the epidermal and dermal layers (Fig. 3-21B). Beneath the plasma membrane of the basal cells, a rather electron-lucent zone, called the lamina lucida, separates the trilaminar plasma membrane, about 8 nm wide, from the more electron-dense component of the basement membrane, or lamina densa (149). Anchoring filaments extend from the basal cell plasma membrane to the lamina densa, traversing the lamina lucida (Fig. 3-23). Anchoring filament components include BPAG2 and α6β4 integrin, which extend from the basal cell membrane into the lamina lucida. BPAG2 exhibits features of a collagen molecule, and it is also referred to as collagen XVII. The 97-/120-kDa protein ladinin, an important antigen in linear immunoglobulin A (IgA) dermatosis (lamina lucida type), is considered to represent a degradation product of the 180-kDa bullous pemphigoid antigen (BPAG2) (154). Other proteins in the lamina lucida that are associated with these anchoring filaments include laminin 5 (also called kalinin, nicein, or epiligrin), uncein (defects in uncein are known to be involved in the recessive junctional type of epidermolysis bullosa), laminin 1, and nidogen (entactin). Although the molecular binding interactions are undoubtedly complex, it is known that α6β4 integrin is a receptor for laminin 1 and 5 and that laminin 5 (epiligrin) is a ligand for α3β1 integrin, which is also expressed by basal keratinocytes. Such adhesive interactions are likely to contribute to the anchoring of basal cells to underlying lamina lucida. Nidogen within the lamina lucida is a 150-kDa protein that facilitates adhesion between specific domains of laminin and type IV collagen within the adjacent lamina densa. Anchoring fibrils are short, curved structures with an irregularly spaced cross-banding of their central portions (155). They fan out at either end, the distal part inserting into the lamina densa and the proximal part terminating in the papillary dermis or looping around and merging in the lamina densa. They insert into amorphous patches containing type IV collagen, which is the main component of the lamina densa (155). The lamina densa itself is anchored to the underlying dermis in part by anchoring fibrils. The anchoring fibrils derive, at least in part, from the dermis and contain type VII collagen (156). The anchoring fibrils connect with islet-like anchoring plaques in the subjacent dermis. These anchoring plaques have a basement membrane-like composition (152). These anchoring structures are interwoven with the dermal interstitial type I and type III collagen fibers, resulting in the adhesion of the basement membrane to the dermis.

In addition to anchoring fibrils, elastic fibers consisting of microfibril bundles and individual microfibrils approximately 10 nm in diameter are attached to the undersurface of the lamina densa. Three varieties of elastic tissue exist: oxytalan, elaunin, and elastic fibers (157). The oxytalan fibers consisting of microfibrils form a thin, superficial network perpendicular to the dermoepidermal junction. They originate from a plexus of elaunin fibers located parallel to the dermoepidermal junction in the upper dermis. The elaunin fibers are connected with the thicker elastic fibers of the middle and deep dermis. Effective anchoring of the epidermis to the dermis is a function largely of the anchoring fibrils; anchoring of the basement membrane by oxytalan fibers is quite sparse (158). Defects in basement membrane zone adhesive molecules attributable to autoantibodies or gene defects may result in disorders characterized by dermal–epidermal separation, as in bullous pemphigoid (BPAG1 and 2 = targets), cicatricial pemphigoid and Herlitz-type junctional epidermolysis bullosa (laminin 5 and uncein = target), and epidermolysis bullosa acquisita, dystrophic epidermolysis bullosa, bullous systemic lupus erythematosus, and some cases of linear IgA disease (type VII collagen = target). There are likely to be numerous other antigenic targets in the basement membrane zone that are relevant to human disease, and our understanding of these new molecules is actively evolving. For example, the 200 kDa protein p200 has recently been implicated in a disorder initially named anti-p200 pemphigoid. This autoimmune subepidermal blistering disease was originally thought to target p200 (159,160), although, recently, the C-terminus of laminin γ1 has been identified as target antigen in anti-p200 pemphigoid, and the disease was renamed anti-laminin γ1 pemphigoid (161). The immunobullous disorders with their respective targets are summarized in Fig. 3-23, and discussed further in Chapters 6 and 9.

In addition to their critical adhesive junctions, basement membrane–related proteins have recently been shown to subserve other important functions. Certain protein components of the hemidesmosomes have more than just a structural role; for example, integrin α6β4 is able to transduce signals from the extracellular matrix to the interior of the basal cells modulating the organization of their cytoskeleton and their proliferation, apoptosis, and differentiation (162). Moreover, the basement membrane may also play a key role in the maintenance of epidermal stem cells required for normal skin integrity and function. One recent study, for example, showed that photoaging is associated with a decrease in basement membrane laminin-511, resulting in a reduction of epidermal stem/progenitor cells and thus potentially relating to the skin atrophy that characterizes the photoaging process (163).

Hair Follicles

Embryology

Hair germs, or primary epithelial germs, are first observed in embryos in the eyebrow region and the scalp during the third month of gestation (164). The general development of hair begins in the fourth fetal month in the face and scalp and gradually extends in a cephalocaudal direction. Thus, during the fourth month, while some hair follicles on the head are already well matured and are

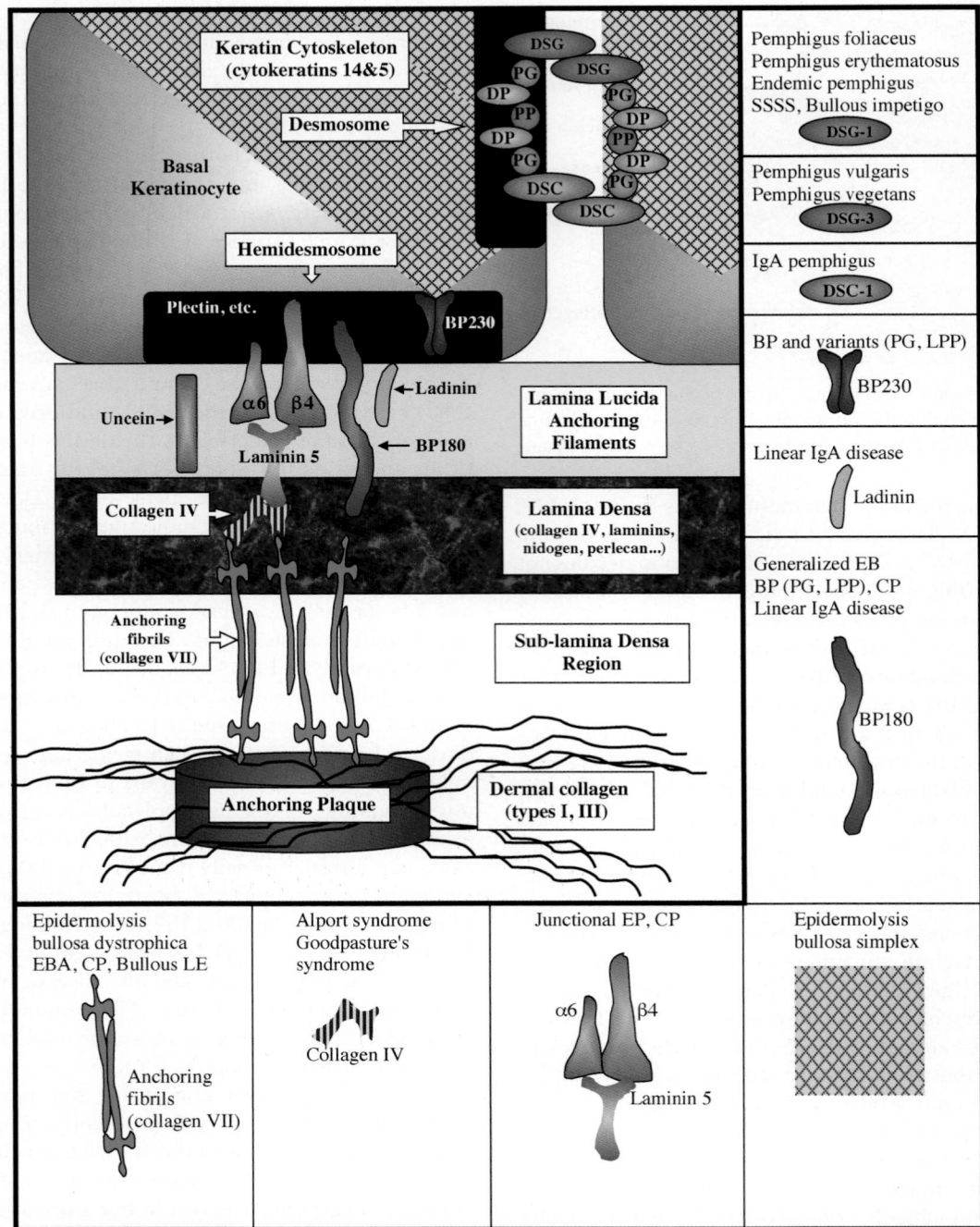

Figure 3-23 Diagram illustrating the different components of the desmosome and basement membrane zone. *BP*, bullous pemphigus; *CP*, cicatricial pemphigus; *DP*, desmoplakin; *DSC*, desmocollin; *DSC-1*, desmocollin-1; *DSG*, desmoglein; *DSG-1*, desmoglein-1; *DSG-3*, desmoglein-3; *EB*, epidermolysis bullosa; *EBA*, epidermolysis bullosa acquisita; *EBS*, epidermolysis bullosa simplex; *LPP*, lichen planus pemphigoides; *PG*, pemphigoid gestationis; *PG*, plakoglobin; *PP*, plakophilin; *SSSS*, staphylococcal scalded skin syndrome.

producing hair, most of those on the trunk are barely differentiated (165). In addition, new primary epithelial germs continue to form adjacent to more established ones so that, in any section obtained from the beginning of the fifth month up to birth, hair structures in different stages of development are found (166).

Hair germs, or primary epithelial germs, in their earliest stage of development consist of a cluster of tightly aggregated, deeply basophilic cells in the basal cell layer of the epidermis. Subsequently, these develop into buds that protrude into the dermis (Figs. 3-24 and 3-25). Beneath each bud lies a zone of plump mesenchymal cells from which the dermal hair papilla is later formed. As the primary epithelial germ grows deeper

into the dermis under the inductive influence of the underlying mesenchymal cells, it forms first the hair peg and then, as the hair matrix cells and the dermal hair papilla develop, the bulbous hair peg (167). Ultrastructural observations suggest that the "hair germ mesenchymal cells" pull down the hair germ as they move deeper in the dermal mesenchyme (164).

As the bulbous peg stage is reached, differentiation occurs in the lower and upper portions of the hair follicle and in the overlying epidermis. Differentiation in the lower portion of the follicle leads to the formation of the hair cone and subsequently to the formation of the hair, the cuticle, and the two inner root sheaths. The hair canal in the upper portion of the hair follicle,

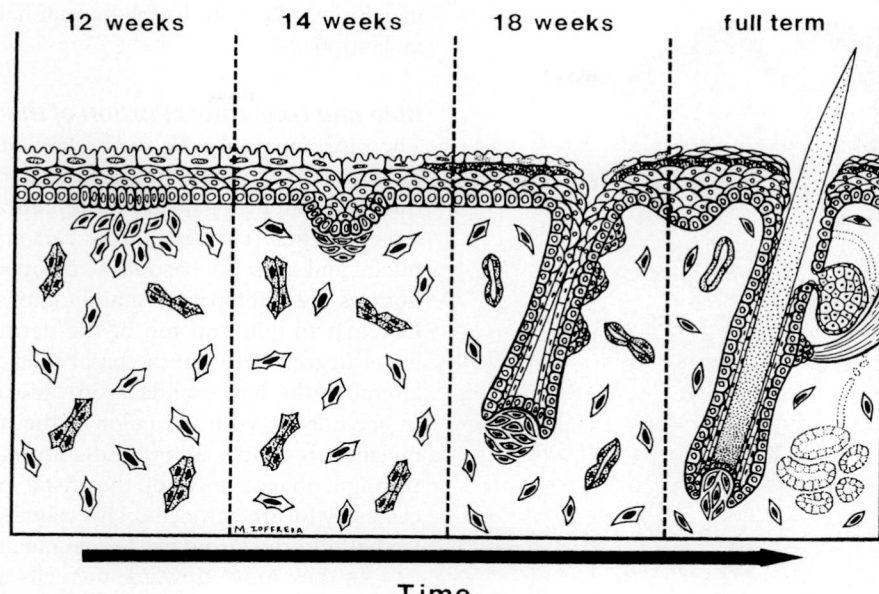

Figure 3-24 Schematic overview of embryonic trichogenesis in human skin. (Courtesy of Dr. Michael Ioffreda.)

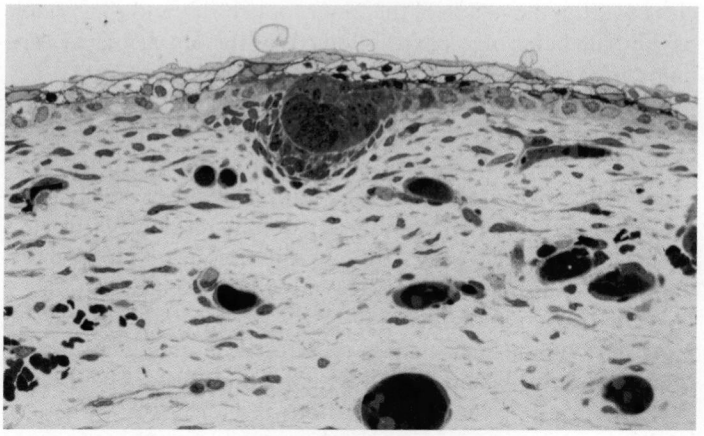

Figure 3-25 Histology of early trichogenesis, showing the formation of a primary epithelial germ with associated underlying mesenchymal condensation (1-μm-thick, plastic-embedded section).

located at the level of the upper dermis, is formed by the premature death of the central core cells before they have become keratinized. In contrast, the intraepidermal portion of the hair canal is produced by means of premature keratinization and subsequent dissolution of the matrix cells of the cordlike hair canal extending obliquely through the epidermis. By the time the hair cone has reached the upper portion of the hair follicle, the hair canal is already open within the dermis and epidermis (168).

The hair follicles grow at a slant and, in the late hair peg or early bulbous stage, develop two or three bulges on their undersurface. The lowest of the three bulges develops into the attachment for the arrector pili muscle and is associated with the follicular stem cell niche; the middle bulge differentiates into the sebaceous gland. The uppermost bulge, if present, either involutes or develops into an apocrine gland. Apocrine glands develop only in certain regions (169). The intraepidermal portion of the hair canal seems to form by lysosomal digestion of cellular cytoplasm analogous to the formation of the intraepidermal eccrine duct and of the intrafollicular apocrine duct (168).

In sections treated with the dopa reaction or stained with ammoniated silver nitrate, melanocytes are distributed at random in primary epithelial germs and in hair pegs. During the bulbous peg stage, the melanocytes concentrate in the so-called pigment matrix region (the basal cell layer lying on top of the dermal hair papilla) and, to a lesser degree, in the lower hair bulb located lateral to the dermal hair papilla (166).

Normal Microanatomy
General Anatomic Features
The hair follicle, with its hair in longitudinal sections, consists of three parts: the lower portion, extending from the base of the follicle to the insertion of the arrector pili muscle; the middle portion, or isthmus, a rather short section, extending from the insertion of the arrector pili to the entrance of the sebaceous duct; and the upper portion, or infundibulum, extending from the entrance of the sebaceous duct to the follicular orifice (Figs. 3-26 to 3-33). The lower portion of the hair follicle is composed of five major portions: the dermal hair papilla; the hair matrix; the hair, consisting inward to outward of medulla, cortex, and hair cuticle; the inner root sheath, consisting inward to outward of inner root sheath cuticle, Huxley layer, and Henle layer; and the outer root sheath (Figs. 3-27 and 3-28). This bulb region gives rise to the formation of the hair shaft that occupies the overlying follicular canal (Figs. 3-27 and 3-28). The hair shaft is composed predominantly of keratin. The large keratin multigene family comprises the epithelial keratins and the hair keratins, the latter involved in the formation of hard keratinized structures such as hair and nail. The human hair keratin family consists of nine type I and six type II members, whose genes are organized as distinct clusters within the type I and type II epithelial keratin gene domains (170,171).

Cycles of Hair Growth
The size of the hair follicles varies from long and thick terminal hairs with their bulbs in the fat to thin, short, and often hypopigmented vellus hairs with bulbs located in the upper dermis (Fig. 3-31). Regardless of size, every follicle goes through

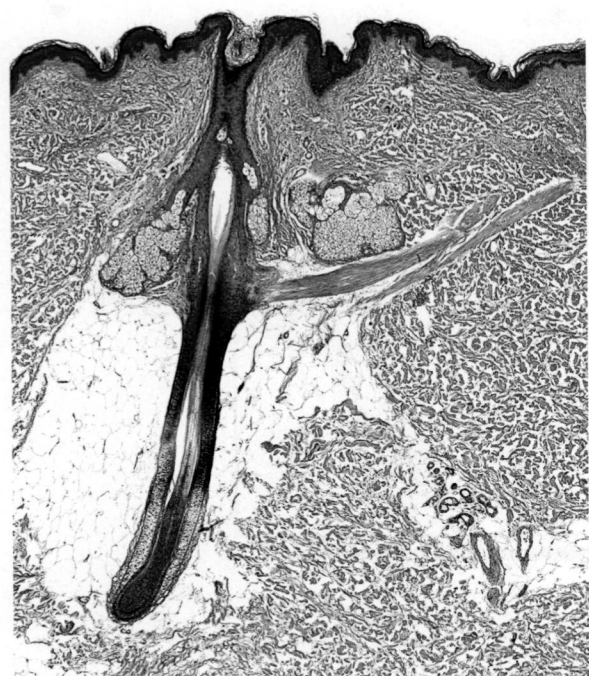

Figure 3-26 Low-power view of a hair follicle to illustrate its four zones. From **bottom** to **top**: the hair bulb, the suprabulbar zone (at which point the various layers of the follicle start to differentiate), the isthmus (located between the arrector pili muscle and entrance of the sebaceous duct), and the infundibulum (the uppermost zone of the follicle, whose inferior boundary is represented by the entrance of the sebaceous duct).

the three phases of the "hair cycle." The histologic appearance of the hair follicle changes considerably during the hair cycle, which causes the hair to turn from an anagen hair into a catagen hair, then into a telogen hair, and, finally, into a new anagen hair (Chapter 18). In the adult scalp, the anagen stage—the phase of active growth—lasts at least 3 years; catagen—the phase of regression—lasts about 3 weeks; and telogen—the resting period—lasts about 3 months. At any one time, approximately 84% of scalp hairs are in anagen stage, 2% in catagen, and 14% in telogen (172). These ratios are important in evaluating abnormalities in the hair cycle in biopsies of partially alopecic scalp. The daily hair growth rate averages about 0.4 mm on the scalp.

During its active growth, or anagen, stage the hair follicle shows at its lower pole a knoblike expansion, the hair bulb, composed of matrix cells and melanocytes. A small, egg-shaped dermal structure, the dermal hair papilla, protrudes into the hair bulb (Fig. 3-27). The papilla induces and maintains the growth of the hair follicle (173). Because of the presence of large amounts of acid mucopolysaccharides in its ground substance, the dermal hair papilla stains positively with alcian blue and metachromatically with toluidine blue. Because positive staining with alcian blue takes place at pH 2.5 and 0.5, it can be concluded that the ground substance of the hair papilla contains nonsulfated acid mucopolysaccharides, such as hyaluronic acid, and sulfated acid mucopolysaccharides, such as chondroitin sulfate (174,175). In addition, there is considerable alkaline phosphatase activity in the hair papilla during the anagen stage as a result of the presence of large numbers of capillary loops (175,176). In persons with dark hair, large amounts of

melanin can be seen in the dermal hair papilla situated within melanophages.

Bulb and Lowermost Portion of the Hair Follicle

The pluripotential cells of the hair matrix present in the hair bulb give rise to the hair and to the inner root sheath. In contrast, the outer root sheath represents a downward extension of the epidermis. The cells of the hair matrix have large vesicular nuclei and a deeply basophilic cytoplasm. Dopa-positive melanocytes are interspersed mainly between the basal cells of the hair matrix lying on top of the dermal hair papilla and, to a lesser degree, between the basal cells of the hair matrix located lateral to the hair papilla (166). Melanin, varying in quantity in accordance with the color of the hair, is produced in these melanocytes and is incorporated into the future cells of the hair through phagocytosis of the distal portion of dendritic processes by future hair cells. This transfer of melanin is analogous to that observed from epidermal melanocytes to keratinocytes.

As they move upward, the cells arising from the hair matrix differentiate into six different types of cells, each of which keratinizes at a different level. The outermost layer of the inner root sheath, the Henle layer, keratinizes first, thus establishing a firm coat around the soft central parts. The two apposed cuticles covering the inside of the inner root sheath and the outside of the hair keratinize next, followed by the Huxley layer. The hair cortex then follows, and the medulla is last (177).

The hair medulla of human hair is often difficult to find by routine light microscopy because it may be discontinuous or even absent. It is more readily recognizable by polariscopic examination because, unlike the cortex, the only partially keratinized medulla contains hardly any doubly refractile structures (178). If the medulla is seen by light microscopy in human hairs, it appears amorphous because of only partial keratinization.

The hair cortex consists of cells that, during their upward growth from the hair matrix, keratinize gradually by losing their nuclei and become filled with keratin fibrils. The process of keratinization takes place without the formation of keratohyalin granules, as seen in the keratinizing epidermis, or of trichohyalin granules, as seen in the inner root sheath. Thus, the keratin of the hair cortex represents hard keratin, in contrast to the keratin of the inner root sheath, which, like that of the epidermis, represents soft keratin (179).

The hair cuticle (Fig. 3-28), located peripheral to the hair cortex, consists of overlapping cells arranged like shingles and pointing upward with their peripheral portion. The cells of the hair cuticle are tightly interlocked with the cells of the inner root sheath cuticle, resulting in the firm attachment of the hair to its inner root sheath. The hair and the inner root sheath move upward in unison (180).

The inner root sheath is composed of three concentric layers; from the inside to the outside, these are the inner root sheath cuticle, the Huxley layer, and the Henle layer (Fig. 3-28). None of these three layers contain melanin. All three layers keratinize, unlike the cells of the hair cortex and of the hair cuticle, by means of trichohyalin granules. These granules resemble the keratohyalin granules of the epidermis, although they stain eosinophilic, in contrast to the basophilic-staining keratohyalin granules of the epidermis. Similar granules may be noted in the pathologic process of epidermolytic hyperkeratosis. Closest to the hair is the single-layered inner root sheath cuticle, consisting of flattened overlapping cells that point downward

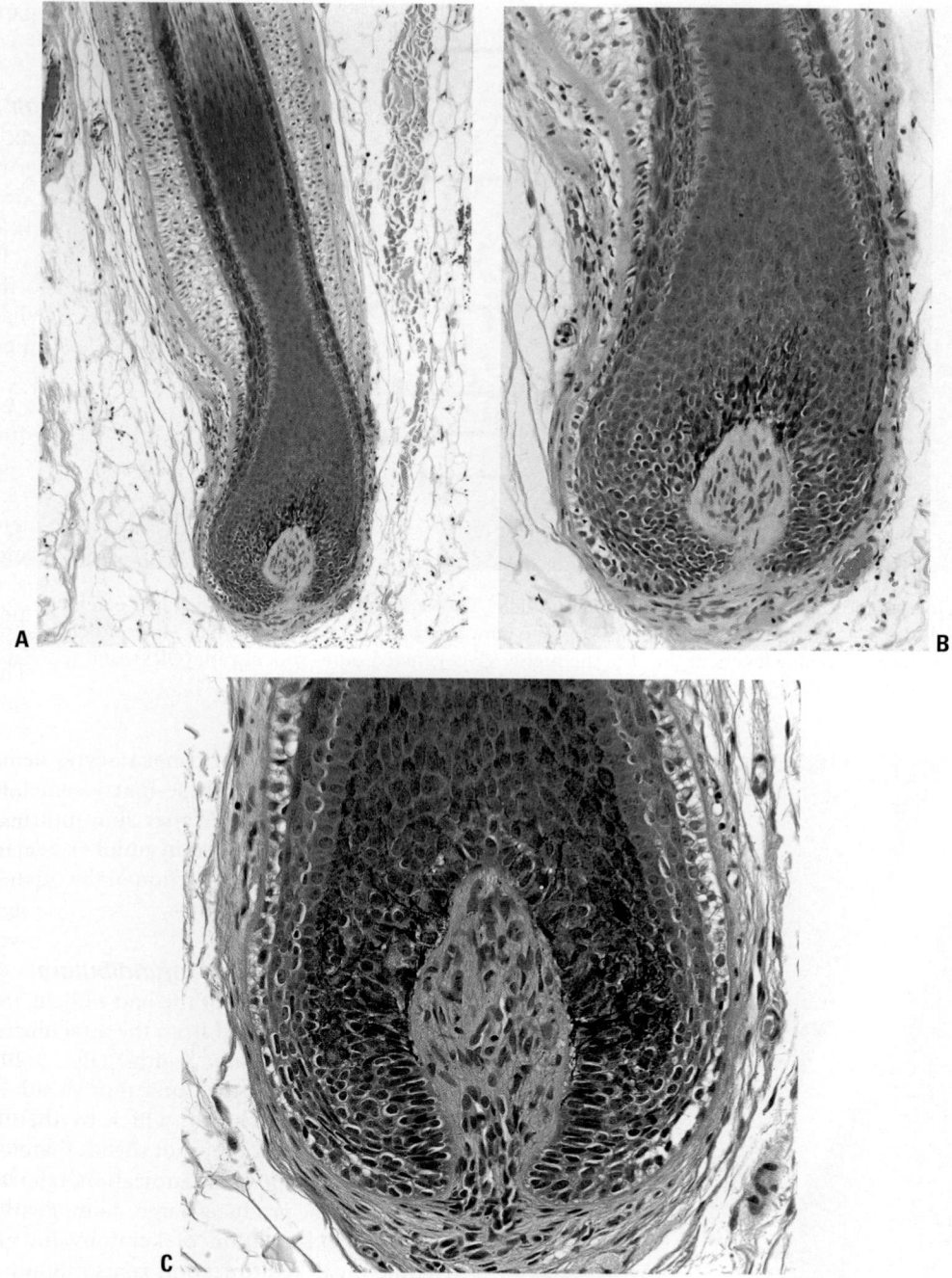

Figure 3-27 Histology of the lower portion of the human hair follicle. **A:** The terminal anagen hair bulb is usually located in the deep dermis or superficial subcutaneous tissue. **B:** The basophilic hair matrix surrounds the dermal papillae. **C:** Note the pigmented and dendritic melanocytes in the suprapapillary matrix. The typically mucinous inferior portion of the follicular papilla (stalk) is continuous with the fibrous root sheath.

in the direction of the hair bulb. Because the cells of the hair cuticle point upward, these two types of cells interlock tightly. There are only a few trichohyalin granules in the inner root sheath cuticle cells. The Huxley layer, which usually consists of two rows of cells, develops numerous trichohyalin granules at the level of the keratogenous zone of the hair. The Henle layer, which is only one cell layer thick and the first layer to undergo keratinization, already has many trichohyalin granules at its emergence from the hair matrix (181) (Fig. 3-27). After having become fully keratinized, the cells of all three layers composing the inner root sheath disintegrate when they reach the isthmus

of the hair follicle, which extends from the area of attachment of the arrector pili muscle to the entrance of the sebaceous duct. The cells of the inner root sheath thus do not contribute to the emerging hair (182).

The outer root sheath extends upward from the matrix cells at the lower end of the hair bulb to the entrance of the sebaceous duct, where it changes into surface epidermis, which lines the upper portion, or infundibulum, of the hair follicle. The outer root sheath is thinnest at the level of the hair bulb, gradually increases in thickness, and is thickest in the middle portion of the hair follicle, the isthmus. In its lower portion,

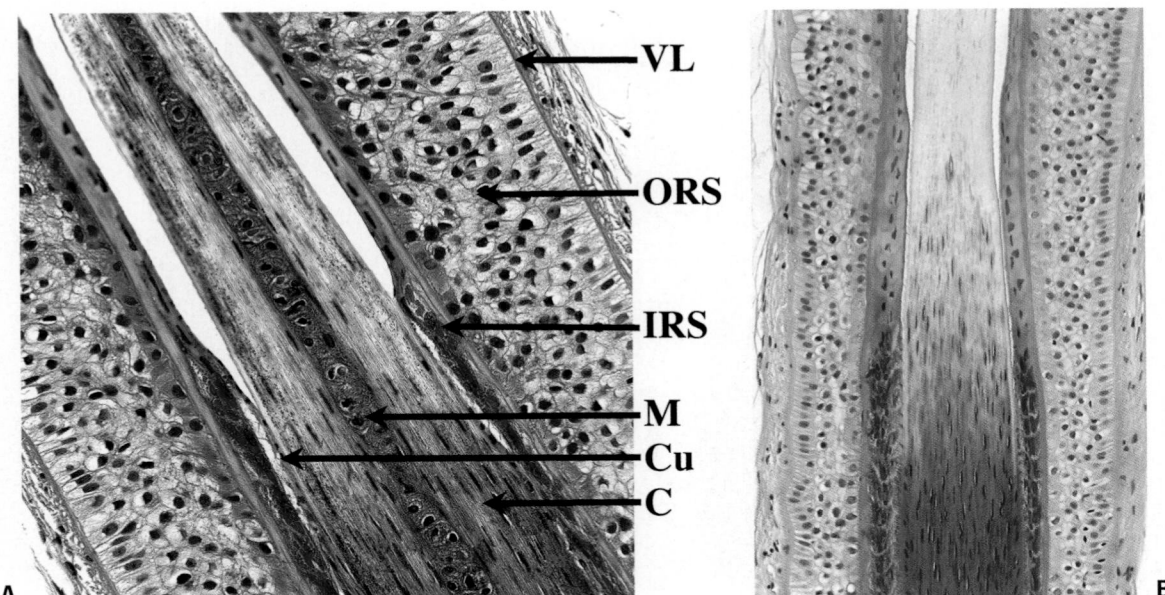

Figure 3-28 A: Suprabulbar portion (lower segment) of the hair follicle. The various layers of the anagen hair can be recognized. From the inside to the periphery: the medulla (*M*) when present, the cortex (*C*), the cuticle (*Cu*) that includes the hair shaft cuticle and the cuticle of the inner root sheath (*IRS*), the Huxley and Henley layers of the IRS, the highly glycogenated outer root sheath (*ORS*), and the glassy vitreous layer (*VL*). B: Note the loss of nuclei in the hair shaft and inner root sheath.

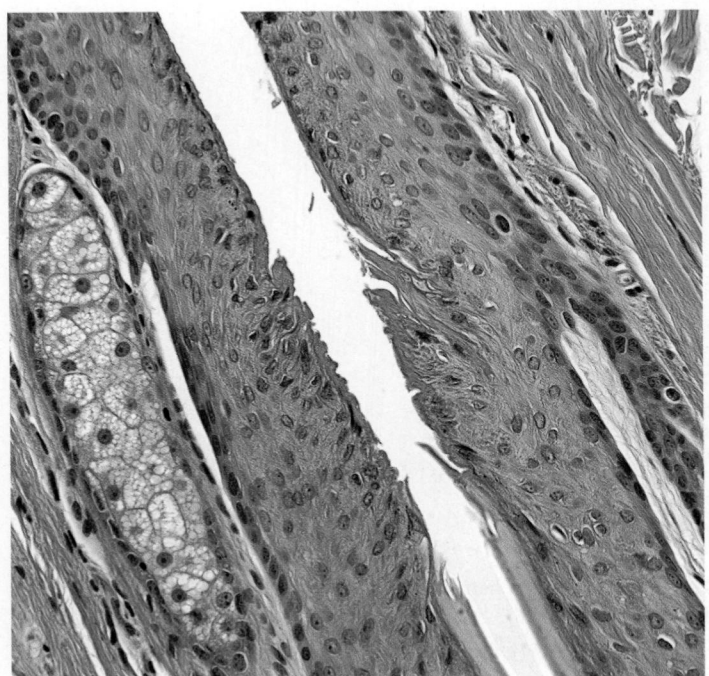

Figure 3-29 Isthmus of a hair follicle. Its upper limit is marked by the sebaceous gland opening. In the midportion of the isthmus, the abrupt desquamation of the inner root sheath (*gray blue*) takes place. Above it, the outer root sheath cornifies (*dark pink*) without formation of a granular layer (trichilemmal keratinization).

below the isthmus, the outer root sheath is covered by the inner root sheath and does not undergo keratinization. The outer root sheath cells have a clear, vacuolated cytoplasm because of the presence of considerable amounts of glycogen (Fig. 3-28). In contrast to the surface epidermis lining the infundibulum, which contains active, melanin-producing melanocytes in its basal layer, the basal layer of the outer root sheath contains

only inactive, amelanotic melanocytes demonstrable with toluidine blue. However, these inactive melanocytes can become melanin-producing cells after skin injuries, such as dermabrasion, when they increase in number and migrate upward into the regenerating upper portion of the outer root sheath and into the regenerating epidermis.

Follicular Isthmus and Infundibulum

In the middle portion of the hair follicle, the so-called isthmus, which extends upward from the attachment of the arrector pili muscle (so-called bulge region) (Fig. 3-29) to the entrance of the sebaceous duct, the outer root sheath is no longer covered by the inner root sheath, which by then has keratinized and disintegrated. The outer root sheath therefore undergoes keratinization. This type of keratinization, referred to as trichilemmal keratinization, produces large, homogeneous keratinized cells without the formation of keratohyalin granules (Fig. 3-29). Trichilemmal keratinization is also found in catagen and telogen hairs and in trichilemmal cysts and trichilemmal tumors. The bulge region at the site of the arrector pili muscle insertion is poorly defined in human follicles and difficult to detect in routine sections. When it is visualized, it consists of several knobby protuberances and ridges composed of relatively undifferentiated follicular keratinocytes with putative stem cell capability. Stem cells in the bulge region participate in the regeneration of the hair follicle during cycling. The cells reside in a niche that includes the dermal papilla and dermal sheath. Interactions between hair follicle epithelial and dermal cells are necessary for hair follicle morphogenesis during development and in the hair cycle (183).

The upper portion of the hair follicle above the entrance of the sebaceous duct, the infundibulum, is lined by surface epidermis, which, like the sebaceous duct, undergoes keratinization with the formation of keratohyalin granules. The infundibulum contains a number of dendritic nonkeratinocytes on ultrastructural examination, and immunohistochemistry

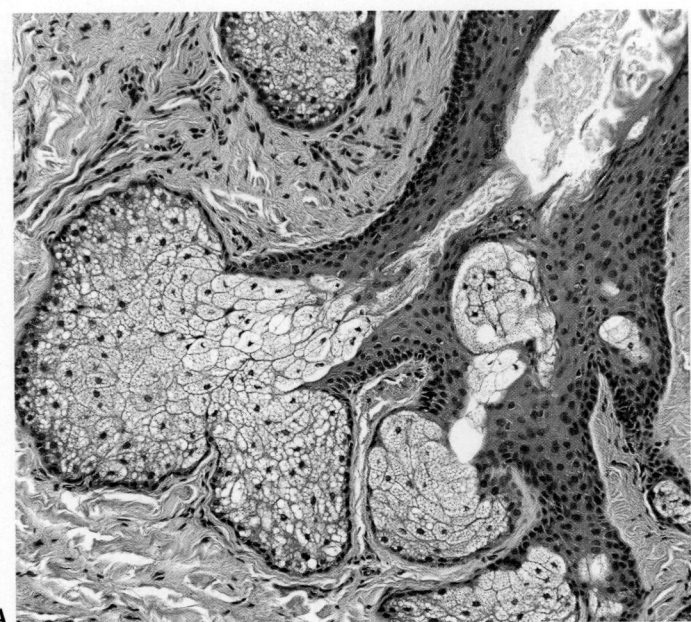
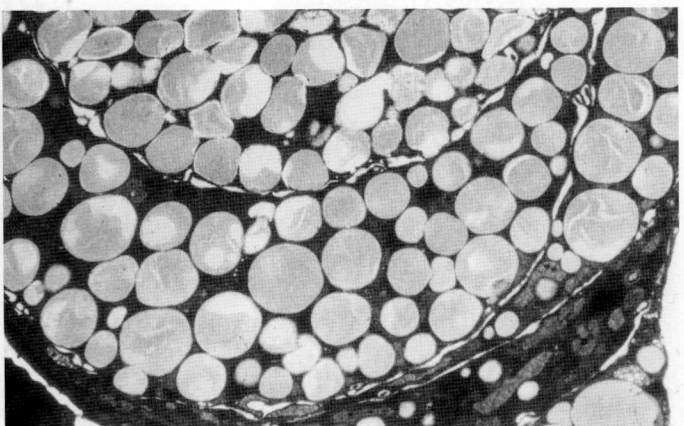

Figure 3-30 **A:** Sebaceous gland and sebaceous duct opening into a hair follicle. **B:** Transmission electron microscopy of a sebaceous lobule. Lipid is visible as rounded, homogeneous bodies filling the cytoplasm of mature sebocytes.

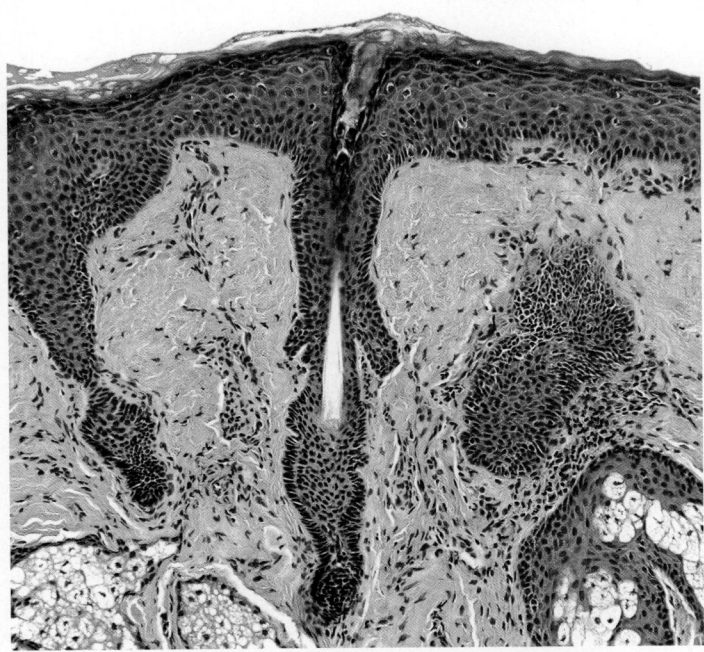

Figure 3-31 Vellus hair. The bulb of these small hair follicles is located in the upper dermis. As terminal hairs, vellus hairs go through the entire hair cycle.

reveals numerous CD1a-positive Langerhans cells within the infundibula of normal adult anagen hairs.

The glassy or vitreous layer forms a homogeneous, eosinophilic zone peripheral to the outer root sheath (Fig. 3-28). Like the subepidermal basement membrane zone, it is PAS positive and diastase resistant, but it differs from the subepidermal basement membrane zone by being thicker and visible with routine stains. It is thickest around the lower one-third of the hair follicle. Peripheral to the vitreous layer lies the fibrous root sheath, which is composed of thick collagen bundles.

Sebaceous Glands

The sebaceous glands are well developed at the time of birth, most likely because of maternal hormones. After a few months, they undergo considerable involution. At puberty, as a result of increased androgen output, the sebaceous glands become greatly enlarged (184). This normal cycle may also occur in certain pathologic conditions, such as nevus sebaceus.

A sebaceous gland may consist of only one lobule but often has several lobules leading into a common excretory duct composed of stratified squamous epithelium (Fig. 3-30A). Sebaceous glands, being holocrine glands, form their secretion by decomposition of their cells. In sebaceous glands of the skin, the pilosebaceous follicle into which the sebaceous duct leads may possess a large hair or a vellus hair that may be too small to reach the skin surface. There is no relationship between the size of the sebaceous gland and the size of the associated hair. For example, in the center of the face and on the forehead, where the sebaceous glands are very large, the associated hairs are of the vellus type. Each sebaceous lobule possesses a peripheral layer of cuboidal, deeply basophilic cells that usually contain no lipid droplets (Fig. 3-30B). The more centrally located cells contain lipid droplets, which can be detected if lipid stains are used on formalin-fixed frozen sections, but in routinely processed sections in which the lipid has been extracted, the cytoplasm of these cells appears as a delicate network of fine cytoplasmic vacuoles. The nucleus is centrally located. In the portion of the lobule located closest to the duct, the cells disintegrate.

The composition of lipids in the sebaceous glands is not uniform. Thus, under polarized light, doubly refractile lipids may be present in small-to-moderate amounts or may be absent (185). Histochemical examination reveals the presence of triglycerides and small amounts of phospholipids. Esterified cholesterol is present, but there is no free cholesterol. Waxes are also present, but they are not identifiable by histochemical means (185). Evidence of active lipid synthesis and storage may be observed by electron microscopy (186,187).

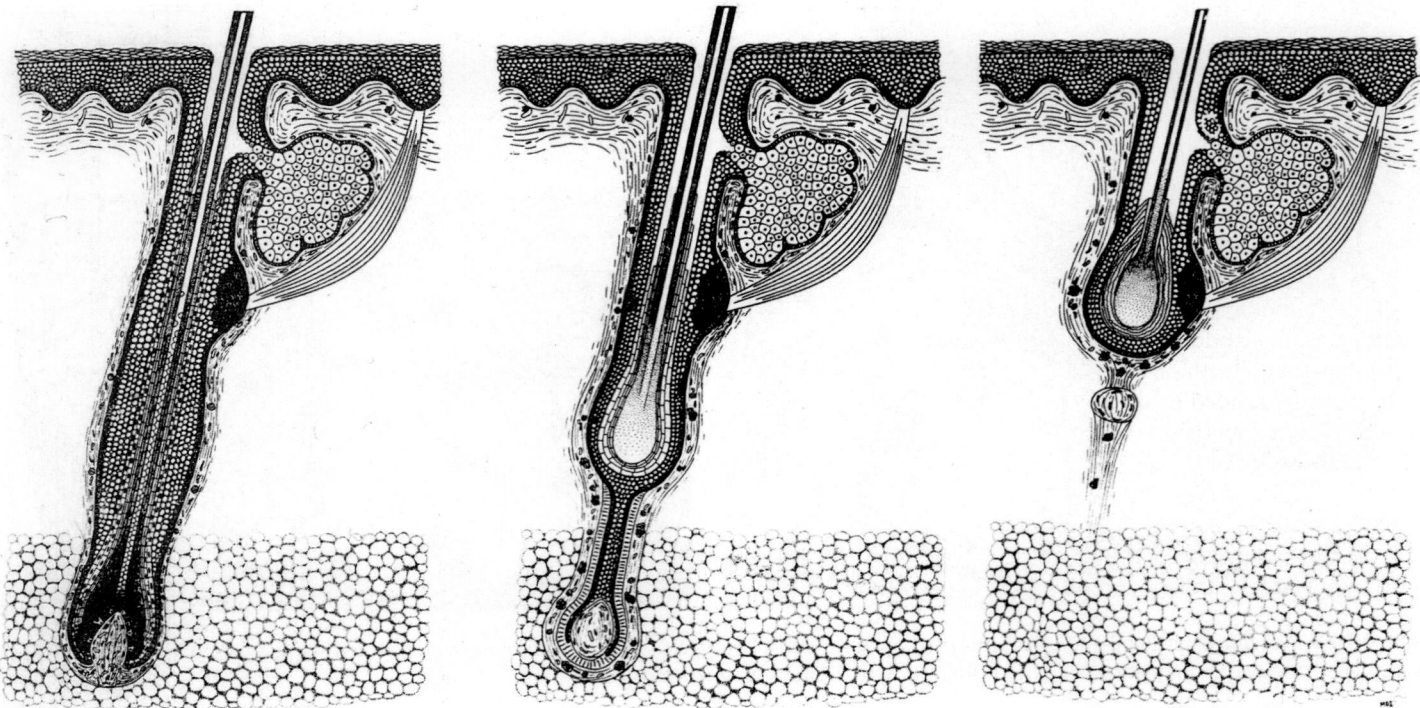

Figure 3-32 Diagram of the hair cycle. From **left** to **right**: anagen hair, catagen hair, and telogen hair.

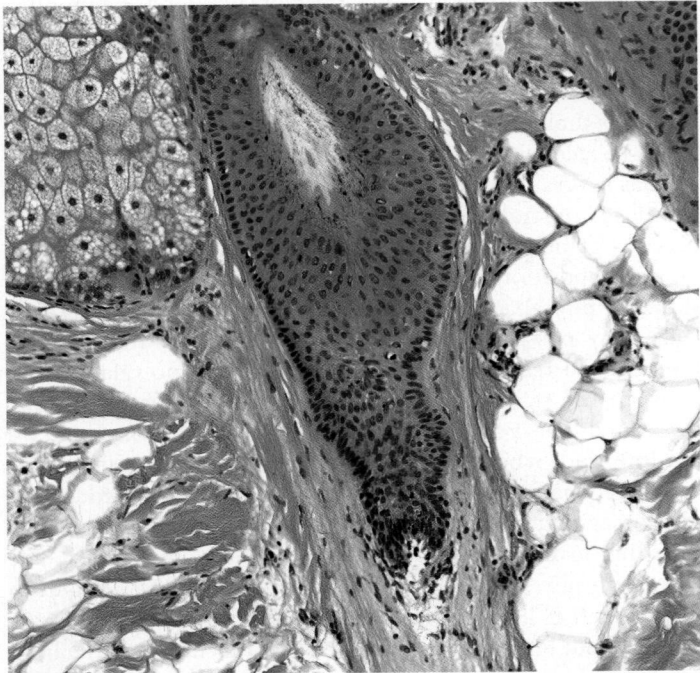

Figure 3-33 Section of a catagen/telogen hair. Note the club-shaped cornifying hair shaft with serrated borders. There are numerous apoptotic nuclei in the hair epithelium.

Lysosomal enzymes bring about the physiologic autolysis that occurs in the holocrine secretion. Histochemical staining of electron microscopic sections for lysosomal enzymes, such as acid phosphatase and aryl sulfatase, reveals an increasing number of lysosomes as the sebaceous cells become more lipidized. In the disintegrating cells located in the preductal region, the acid phosphatase and aryl sulfatase activity is most pronounced, but this activity is largely outside of lysosomes because the lysosomes

have released their contents in their function as "suicide bags" (188). Prior to the sudden disintegration of the sebaceous cells, an abrupt conversion of –SH to S–S linkages of proteins occurs in sebaceous glands just as in the epidermis and hair (189).

Regional Variation

Hair follicles vary considerably in different anatomic regions and according to age and sex. In adults, deep anagen hairs (extending into subcutaneous fat) are typically found on the scalp (see Fig. 3-59) and male beard area, whereas vellus hairs typify the female face and nonbeard-area facial regions of men. Hair of extremities and trunk can generally be differentiated from the scalp by the more superficial location of the bulbs and diminished density. Sebaceous glands are present everywhere on the skin except on the palms and soles. On the skin, they are found in association with hair structures. In addition, free sebaceous glands that are not associated with hair structures occur in some areas of modified skin, such as the nipple and areola of both the male and female breasts. There, they occur over the entire surface of the nipple and in Montgomery areolar tubercles, each of which contains several sebaceous lobules in association with a lactiferous duct. Free sebaceous glands may also be found on the labia minora and the inner aspect of the prepuce. Modified sebaceous glands called Tyson glands have been reported to occur on the coronal sulcus of the penis (190). The not infrequent presence of free sebaceous glands on the vermilion border of the lips and on the buccal mucosa is known as Fordyce condition. The meibomian glands of the eyelids are modified sebaceous glands (see Fig. 3-62A).

Specialized Structure and Function
Hair Cycle

The hair cycle ensures that entirely new hair shafts are produced periodically and also serves as an intrinsic regulator of maximum hair length The hair cycle consists of the involutionary stage (catagen) and the end stage (telogen) of the old hair and its replacement by a young, new hair (early anagen) (Fig. 3-32). At the onset of the catagen stage, mitotic activity and melanin production in the hair bulb cease. Next, the bulb shrinks and becomes separate from the dermal hair papilla (181). As the hair moves upward, the lower portion of the follicle involutes (Fig. 3-33). The reduction in follicle size results from cell deletion by apoptosis, or programmed cell death (191). The lower follicle thus becomes a thin cord of epithelial cells surrounded by the fibrous root sheath, which is wrinkled in thick folds. In addition, as the hair moves upward, growth of the inner root sheath ceases, so the lower end of the hair shaft becomes surrounded by dense keratin, referred to as trichilemmal keratin, which is formed by the outer root sheath without the interposition of keratohyalin granules. This then represents the club hair of the catagen stage.

Next, the thin cord of epithelial cells retracts upward, faithfully followed by the underlying dermal hair papilla, which also moves upward. The cord of epithelial cells shortens until it forms only a small, nipple-like downward protrusion from the club hair, called the secondary hair germ. Under it lies the dermal hair papilla. With the hair follicle decreased to about one-third of its former length, the lowest portion of the hair follicle lies at the level of the attachment of the arrector pili. The lower portion of the hair is encased in trichilemmal keratin and completely surrounded by the outer root sheath. Folds of the fibrous root sheath extend downward from the hair follicle. At this point, the hair has reached the telogen stage (192).

When regrowth of the hair begins, the secondary hair germ where the stem cell cluster is preserved begins to elongate by cell division and grows down as an epithelial column together with the dermal hair papilla inside of the old, collapsed fibrous root sheath of the previous hair (so-called "bulge activation" stage) (183). As it is growing down, the lower end of the epithelial column becomes invaginated by the dermal hair papilla. A new hair bulb is formed, representing the early anagen stage. By subsequent differentiation, a new hair arises. Thus, the formation of an active hair follicle from the secondary germ recapitulates the embryonic pattern of development of the hair from the primary hair germ (192). Experimental and observational data suggest that the primary site that gives rise to new hair germ during follicular regrowth is the bulge region of the follicle, where a population of normally slow-cycling, relatively undifferentiated cells with features of stem cells resides (183). Stimulation of the bulge region, which persists throughout telogen, then gives rise to new hair germ and the developing anagen follicle (bulge activation hypothesis). Although the precise pathways involved in bulge activation are incompletely understood, this event appears to be associated with epigenetic changes in DNA hydroxymethylation (193). Moreover, the production of stem cell progeny (transit amplifying cells) during follicular cycling may have implications beyond hair shaft production, because it has also been shown that these cells regulate proliferation of underlying adipocyte proliferation via the sonic hedgehog pathway (194).

Hair Color

Three types of melanosomes are present in hair. Erythromelanin granules, seen in red hair, are polymorphous and have an irregular internal structure. The other two types of granules, homogeneous eumelanin granules and lamellated pheomelanin granules—are found in varying proportions in blond and dark hair and are round to oval. Dark hair contains more melanosomes than light hair, and the melanosomes are largely of the homogeneous eumelanin type; in light hair, lamellated pheomelanin melanosomes predominate (195).

In gray and white hair, the melanocytes in the basal layer of the hair matrix are greatly reduced in number or are absent. The melanocytes that are present show degenerative changes, especially of their melanosomes (196). Such changes appear to affect melanocyte stem cells, resulting in permanent hair graying (197). The hair shafts contain only detritus of melanin or none at all (195). The regulation of melanogenesis is complex, however, and deficiencies may also potentially produce hair graying and whitening independent of melanocyte depletion. Recently, it has been shown in animal models that activation of sympathetic nerves responsible for activation of the melanocyte stem cell niche in the bulge region of the hair follicle results in local release of neuroadrenaline, which ultimately depletes melanocyte stem cells from the niche, thus establishing a link between emotional stress and some instances of hair depigmentation (198).

Follicular Immunity

The number of CD1a-positive Langerhans cells in normal follicular infundibula raises questions concerning their role in follicular immunity. Such populations could be appropriately sequestered from harmful environmental agents, such as UV light, and thus serve as a reservoir of antigen-presenting cells, as well as an evolutionary rationale for the preservation of hair follicles in Homo sapiens no longer in need of the thermal or protective benefits of hair shafts. Such follicle-associated immune tissue has been evidenced in clinical settings of primarily follicular pathology in contact dermatitis, as well as in sequential studies of human, experimentally induced contact allergy, where the first sentinel lymphocytes selectively home to follicular infundibula (199). Chronic UV exposure may deplete epidermal Langerhans cells, whereas follicular Langerhans cells remain intact, resulting in a protected niche that may be stimulated to replenish sun-damaged skin (148).

Eccrine and Apocrine Glands

The apocrine glands differ from eccrine glands in origin, distribution, size, and mode of secretion. The eccrine glands serve primarily in the regulation of heat, and the apocrine glands represent scent glands. A third type of sweat gland, called the apoeccrine gland, has been described in the axillae (200).

Embryology

Eccrine glands are present in mammals, with the exception of anthropoid apes, only on the soles. Their presence in other parts of the skin in humans is a late development from the phylogenetic point of view. Accordingly, the eccrine glands develop in humans earlier on the palms and soles than elsewhere. On the palms and soles, eccrine gland germs are first seen early in the fourth gestational month (201). In the early part of the fifth fetal month, they develop in the axillae, and near the end of the fifth month, they begin to appear over the remainder of the body (165). The eccrine gland germs begin as areas of crowding of deeply basophilic cells in the basal layer of the epidermis. They differ from primary epithelial germs only slightly by being narrower and by showing fewer mesenchymal cells at their base. Like hair follicles, eccrine glands may be seen at one time in different stages of development. In 16-week-old embryos, some eccrine glands are already beginning to form coils on the palms and soles, whereas new eccrine gland germs are still forming in the epidermis (202).

At the time of lumen formation, the intradermal duct and the secretory segment show a wall composed of two layers of cells—an inner layer of luminal cells and an outer layer of basal cells. Although the dermal duct continues to consist of these two layers of cells throughout life, the two layers in the secretory segment undergo differentiation: The luminal cells differentiate into tall, columnar secretory cells extending from the basement membrane to the luminal border, and the basal cells differentiate into secretory cells or into myoepithelial cells, which appear as pyramidal, relatively small cells wedged at the base between secretory cells (201). The differentiation into secretory and myoepithelial cells in the secretory segment is well advanced on the palms and soles of embryos 22 weeks old. At the time of birth, the appearance of the eccrine glands resembles that of adult eccrine glands.

In contrast to eccrine glands, apocrine glands develop only in certain areas. Wherever they form, they develop from the upper bulge of hair follicles that are in the early bulbous peg stage and show a hair cone. The formation of apocrine glands begins late in the fourth month and continues until late in embryonic life, as long as new hair follicles develop. In the earliest stage, a solid epithelial cord projects into the perifollicular mesenchyme at a right angle to the long axis of the hair follicle and then grows downward past the developing sebaceous gland and arrector pili bulge. By the time the tip of the epithelial cord has reached the level of the sebaceous gland, the intradermal ductal lumen begins to form, as does the intrafollicular lumen (169). At the time of birth, there is no recognizable myoepithelial layer of cells around the secretory portion of the apocrine glands (165).

Eccrine glands apparently give rise to apoeccrine axillary glands during puberty (200).

Normal Microanatomy

Eccrine glands are composed of three segments: the intraepidermal duct, the intradermal duct, and the secretory portion (Fig. 3-34). The secretory portion makes up about one-half of the basal coil, the other half being composed of duct. The basal coil lies either at the border between the dermis and the subcutaneous fat or in the lower one-third of the dermis. When located in the lower dermis, it is surrounded by fatty tissue that connects with the subcutaneous fat. Eccrine glands are highlighted by immunohistochemical stains for S100 protein and carcinoembryonic antigen (Fig. 3-35).

The intraepidermal eccrine duct extends from the base of a rete ridge to the surface and follows a spiral course (Fig. 3-34A). The cells composing the duct are different from the cells of the surrounding epidermis in that they are derived from dermal duct cells through mitosis and upward migration (203). For this reason, the intraepidermal eccrine duct has been referred to as acrosyringium or the epidermal sweat duct unit. The intraepidermal eccrine duct consists of a single layer of inner or luminal cells and two or three rows of outer cells. The ductal cells begin to keratinize, as evidenced by the presence of keratohyalin granules, at a lower level than the cells of the

surrounding epidermis, in the middle squamous layer, and are fully keratinized at the level of the stratum granulosum of the surrounding epidermis (204). Before keratinization, the intraepidermal lumen is lined by an eosinophilic cuticle.

The intradermal eccrine duct is composed of two layers of small, cuboidal, deeply basophilic epithelial cells (Fig. 3-34B). Unlike the secretory portion of the eccrine gland, the eccrine duct has no peripheral hyaline basement membrane zone, but the lumen of the duct is lined with a deeply eosinophilic, homogeneous cuticle that is PAS positive and diastase resistant.

The secretory portion of the eccrine gland shows only one distinct layer composed of secretory cells (Fig. 3-34C). The presence of only one distinct layer is attributable to the fact that the cells of the outer layer have become differentiated into either secretory or myoepithelial cells during the sixth to eighth months of embryonic life. The secretory cells lining the lumen consist equally of two types—clear cells and dark cells. The clear cells are generally broader at the base than near the lumen, appear somewhat larger than the dark cells, and contain very faint, small granules. The dark cells are broadest near the lumen and contain numerous basophilic granules (205). The clear cells contain PAS-positive, diastase-labile glycogen, and the dark cells contain PAS-positive, diastase-resistant mucopolysaccharides. The clear cells secrete abundant amounts of aqueous material together with glycogen; the dark cells secrete sialomucin. This substance contains both neutral and nonsulfated acid mucopolysaccharides, is positive for PAS and for alcian blue at pH 2.4, and is resistant to diastase and hyaluronidase. Prolonged sweating leads to a depletion of glycogen in the clear cells (206). The myoepithelial cells possess a small spindle-shaped nucleus and long contractile fibrils. The fibrils run in a spiral, their long axes aligned obliquely to the direction of the secretory tubule. Delivery of sweat to the skin surface is greatly aided by myoepithelial contraction (207). Peripheral to the myoepithelial cells lies a hyaline basement membrane zone containing collagen fibers. The transition from the secretory to the ductal epithelium is abrupt (Fig. 3-34B). The lumen of the secretory portion of the eccrine gland, measuring approximately 20 μm in diameter, is small in comparison with that of the apocrine gland (compare Figs. 3-34C and 3-36). The lumen of the eccrine duct measures about 15 μm across.

Apocrine glands are tubular glands, the secretory cells of which pass through various stages. Schiefferdecker (208), who in 1917 first described these glands, observed that during secretion part of the cell was pinched off and released into the lumen. He referred to this process as decapitation secretion. He chose the name *apocrine* for these glands to indicate that part of the cytoplasm of the secretory cells was pinched off ("apo" means "off").

Apocrine glands, like eccrine glands, are composed of three segments: the intraepidermal duct, the intradermal duct, and the secretory portion. Because apocrine glands originate from the hair germ, or primary epithelial germ, the duct of an apocrine gland usually leads to a pilosebaceous follicle, entering it in the infundibulum, above the entrance of the sebaceous duct. An occasional apocrine duct, however, opens directly on the skin surface close to a pilosebaceous follicle. In contrast to eccrine glands, the basal coil of apocrine glands, which is located in the subcutaneous fat, is composed entirely of secretory cells and contains no ductal cells.

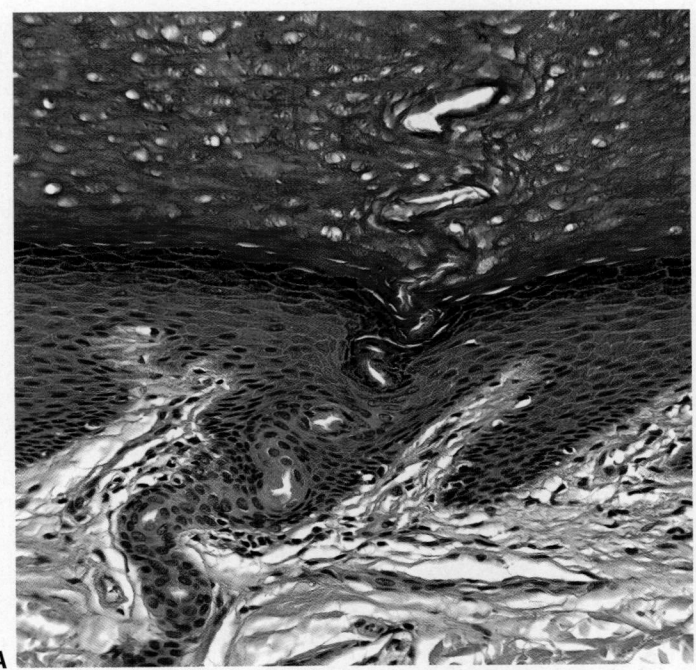

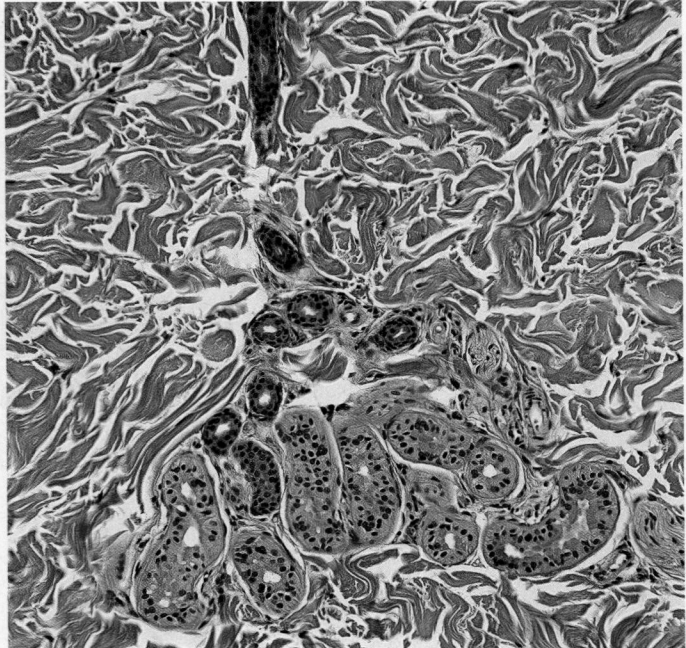

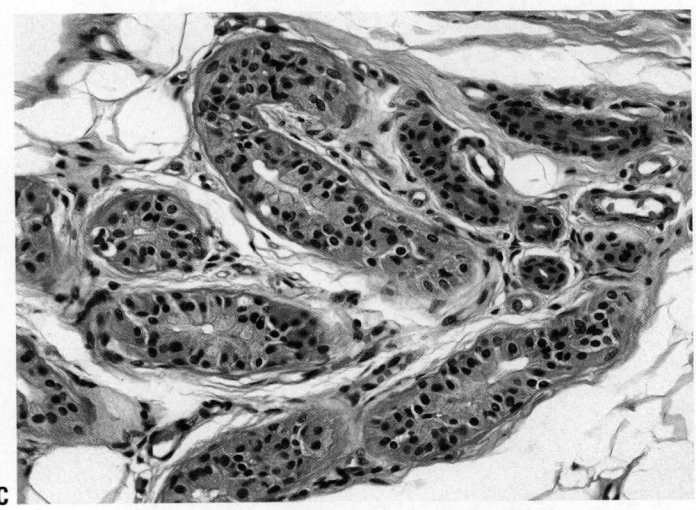

Figure 3-34 A: Acrosyringium with characteristic spiraling course within the epidermis and acellular lining cuticle. **B:** Junction between the straight dermal eccrine duct (**top half**) and the coiled secretory segment (**lower half**). **C:** The secretory portion of the gland comprises a mixture of dark and pale secretory cells.

The ductal portion of the apocrine glands has the same histologic appearance as the eccrine duct, showing a double layer of basophilic cells and a periluminal eosinophilic cuticle (Fig. 3-36). The intrafollicular or intraepidermal portion of the apocrine duct is straight and not spiral in appearance, as is the intraepidermal eccrine duct.

The secretory portion of the apocrine gland shows a single layer of secretory cells because the outer layer of cells consists of myoepithelial cells, just as in the eccrine gland. The secretory cells vary greatly in height, depending on the stage of secretion. Variation in height may be seen even in the cross section of the same secretory tubule (209). The secretory cells possess an eosinophilic cytoplasm. Except in the apical portion, they contain in their cytoplasm fairly large, PAS-positive, diastase-resistant granules, which appear much larger than similar granules seen in the dark secretory cells of eccrine glands. In addition, the apocrine granules frequently contain iron. Maturation of the secretory cells is indicated by the formation of a dome-shaped apical cap (Fig. 3-36). The type of secretion occurring in apocrine glands consists of the release of portions of cytoplasm into the lumen. Because of the cytoplasm in the secretion, apocrine secretion, in contrast to eccrine secretion, is visible in histologic sections stained with hematoxylin–eosin. The apocrine secretion contains amorphous, PAS-positive, diastase-resistant material originating from the granules that have dissolved in the apical portion of the secretory cells (210). This PAS-positive material, like the secretion of the dark cells in eccrine glands, consists of sialomucin.

The third type of sweat gland, designated as the apoeccrine sweat gland, shows a segmental or diffuse, apocrine-like dilation of its secretory tubule but has a long and thin duct that does not open into a hair follicle. The electron microscopy of its dilated segment is often indistinguishable from that of the classical apocrine gland. The less remarkably dilated segment of the apoeccrine gland tends to retain intercellular canaliculi and/or dark cells (200).

Regional Variation

Eccrine glands are present everywhere in the human skin; however, they are absent in areas of modified skin that lack all

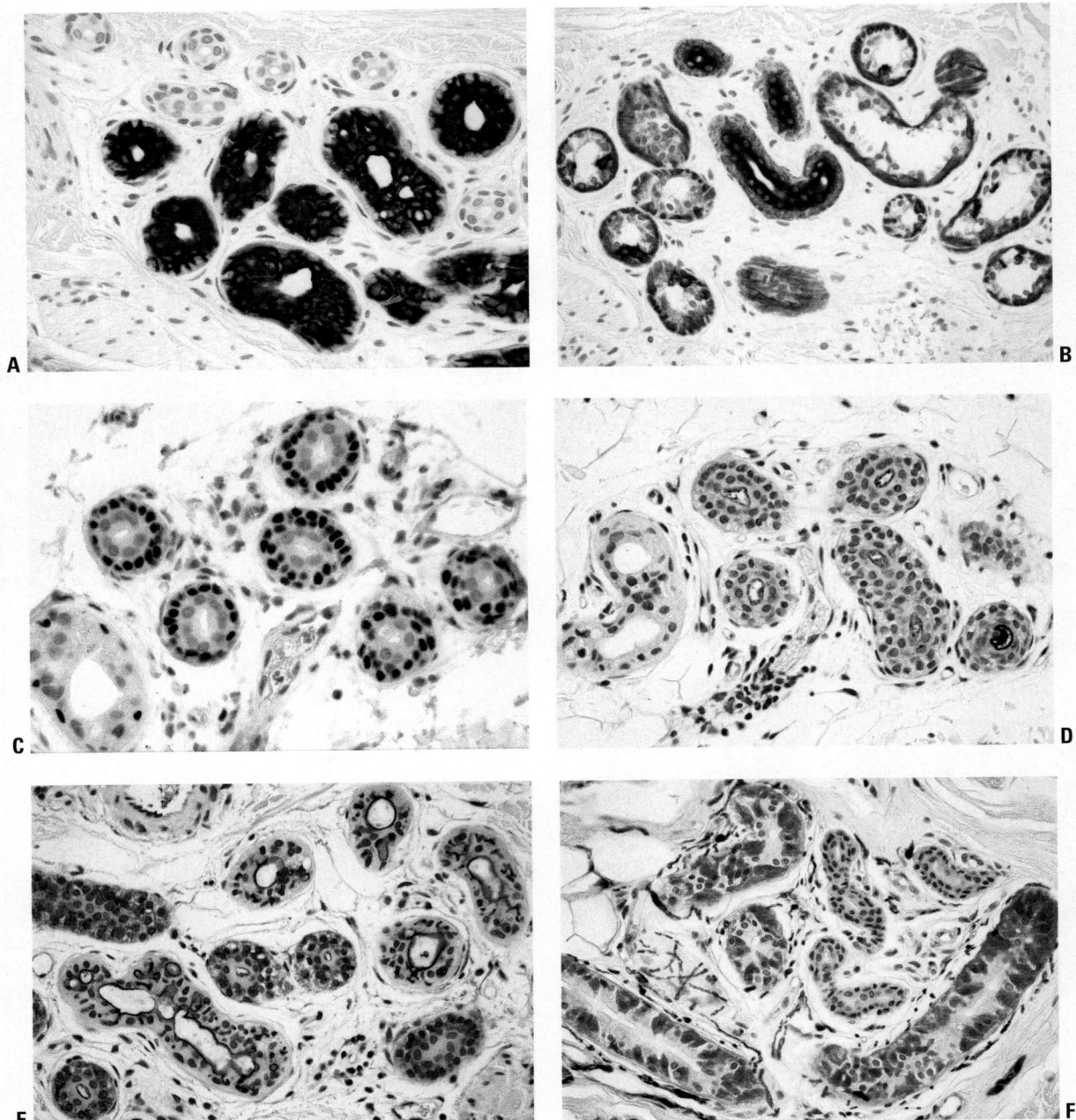

Figure 3-35 Immunohistochemistry of eccrine glands. **A:** Cytokeratin 7 shows strong immunopositivity of the secretory portion, whereas the ductal portion is negative. **B:** With cytokeratin 34 β E12, there is a preferential staining of the most basally located cells in the secretory portion. The ductal cells are strongly positive. **C:** p63 immunostain shows strong expression by the most basally located cells in the ductal portion, scattered positive nuclei in the secretory portion of the eccrine glands. **D:** Carcinoembryonic antigen immunostain shows a classical luminal expression pattern. **E:** Epithelial membrane antigen immunohistochemistry. Characteristic canalicular pattern. **F:** S100 protein is expressed by some of the secretory cells. The surrounding stroma contains delicate S100-positive nerves.

cutaneous appendages, that is, the vermilion border of the lips, the nail beds, the labia minora, the glans penis, and the inner aspect of the prepuce. They are found in greatest abundance on the palms and soles and in the axillae.

Apocrine glands are encountered in only a few areas: in the axillae, in the anogenital region, and as modified glands in the external ear canal (ceruminous glands) (Fig. 3-37), in the eyelid (Moll glands) (see Fig. 3-62D), and in the breast (mammary glands). Occasionally, a few apocrine glands are found on the face, in the scalp, and on the abdomen; they are usually small and nonfunctional (211). Apocrine glands develop their

secretory portion and become functional only at puberty. Each of the multiple protuberances present in the areola of the female breast and referred to as Montgomery areolar tubercles contains a lactiferous duct and several superficially located sebaceous lobules whose ducts lead into the lactiferous duct (212,213).

Specialized Structure and Function

The eccrine sweat gland is engineered for temperature regulation (208). With approximately 3 million glands in the human integument, weighing 35 μg/gland, the average human boasts about 100 g of eccrine glands capable of producing a

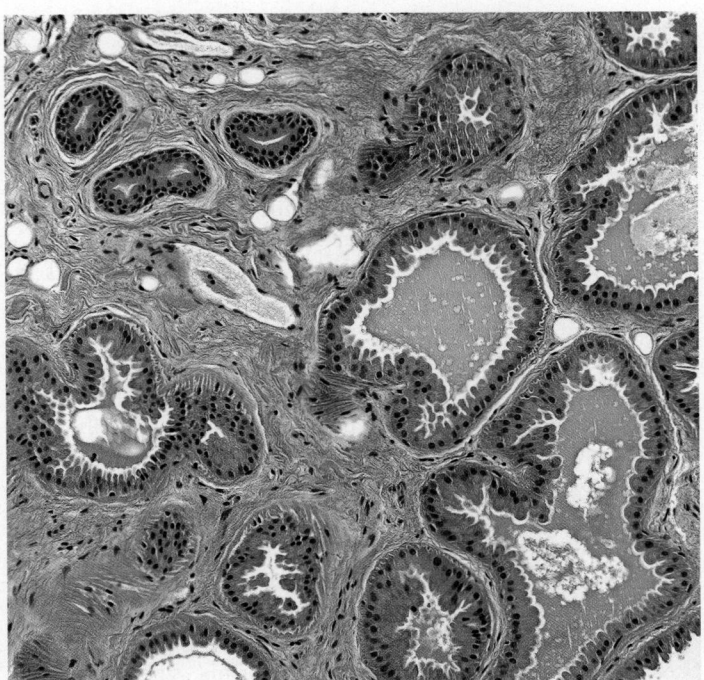

Figure 3-36 Apocrine glands. The secretory portion shows typical decapitation-type secretion. The ductal portion is indistinguishable from the ductal portion of the eccrine glands.

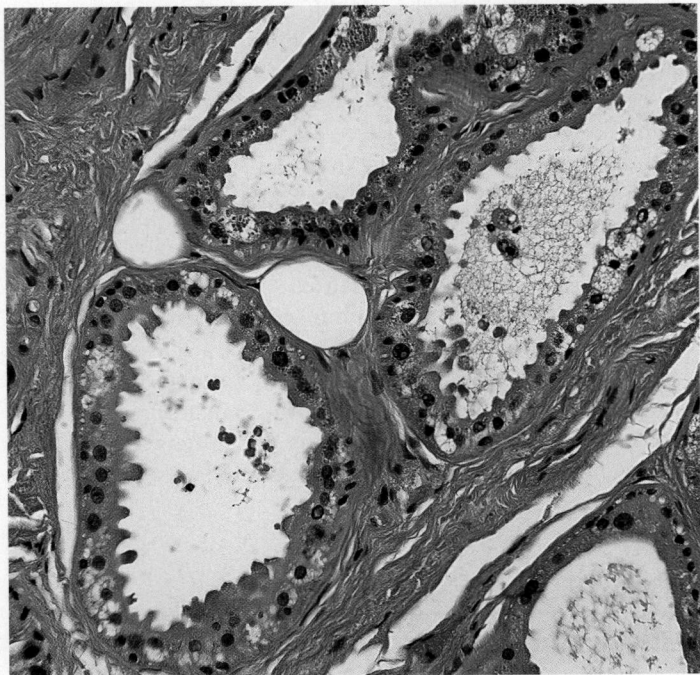

Figure 3-37 Ceruminous glands are modified apocrine glands found in the external ear canal. Note the lipofuscin pigment in the cytoplasm of apocrine cells.

maximum of approximately 1.8 L of sweat/hour! The eccrine secretory coil is richly invested with a stroma rich in unmyelinated nerve fibers, which are believed to play an important role in the regulation of sweat production. Cholinergic stimulation of eccrine clear cells has been shown to increase cytosolic Ca^{2+} in a biphasic manner. This results in stimulation of both K^+ and Cl^- membrane channels, resulting in a net efflux of KCl along with Na^+ from the cell. Such electrolyte shifts, associated with water loss, underscore major metabolic implications of

excessive eccrine sweating. Aside from potentially critical temperature regulation, the eccrine gland may contribute to general cutaneous homeostasis. For example, patients with congenital anhidrotic ectodermal dysplasia suffer from heat intolerance that cannot be alleviated by simply adding moisture to the skin surface, suggesting that vasodilation associated with sweating may in some way be linked to eccrine function (214). There is abundant biologically active IL-1 in sweat (215), as well as numerous proteolytic enzymes, raising the possibility that eccrine sweat may possess proinflammatory or protective functions.

The mechanisms and rationale for apocrine-type secretion remain elusive. Schaumburg-Lever and Lever found three types of secretion (209): merocrine, apocrine, and holocrine. In the apocrine type of secretion, three stages were observed: formation of an apical cap, formation of a dividing membrane at the base of the apical cap, and formation of tubules above and parallel to the dividing membrane, supplying a new plasma membrane for both the undersurface of the apical cap and the top of the residual cell, bringing about detachment of the apical cap. Convincing proof of the detachment of entire apical caps in apocrine glands was provided through scanning microscopy by Inoue (216), who observed on each secretory cell a cytoplasmic luminal protuberance about 2 μm in diameter. In the early stage of secretion, the protuberance was hemispheric, but it later increased in height to form a linguiform process.

Why apocrine glands undergo the cellular complexities of decapitation secretion and the functional raison d'être for apocrine secretion in humans remain an enigma, although they may simply be an evolutionary vestige (musk glands of the deer and scent glands of the skunk are modified apocrine-type structures). The characteristic odor in human axillary sweat has recently been shown to reside in volatile C_6–C_{11} acids, with the most abundant being 3-methyl-2-hexenoic acid (217). This initially odorless apocrine secretion is formed at the skin surface from protein precursors via saponification or bacteriolysis. Such chemical interactions are similar to those in lower mammals, in which secreted proteins act as carriers of one or more pheromone signals.

Special Stains

Eccrine and apocrine glands and their products can be identified using special histochemical, enzymatic, and immunohistochemical stains (218,219). With the PAS stain the clear secretory cells show a dense, globular PAS-positive material when glycogen is present (there is a depletion of glycogen after sweating). The dark cells show a finely granular, PAS-positive and diastase-resistant cytoplasm that is also seen with acid-fast stains. The ductal cells of eccrine and apocrine glands show a more variable staining with PAS (220). PAS stains the basement membrane of both eccrine and apocrine ducts. PAS stains of the secretory apocrine component vary from negative to focally positive; they can show a markedly positive granularity with iron and acid-fast stains. The mucicarmine stain is usually noncontributory. Enzymatic stains in fresh tissue such as amylophosphorylase and succinic dehydrogenase are very rarely used in routine surgical pathology (220).

Immunohistochemical stains (Fig. 3-35A–F) show that carcinoembryonic antigen is expressed in the luminal border of eccrine and apocrine ducts; it is also expressed in the intercellular canaliculi and cytoplasm of some eccrine secretory cells but is usually negative in secretory apocrine cells (Fig. 3-35D).

A characteristic canalicular pattern is observed with epithelial membrane antigen (Fig. 3-35E). CTK of low molecular weight such as CK7 and CAM 5.2 are expressed only by the secretory portion of both eccrine and apocrine glands (Fig. 3-35A) but not by their excretory ducts. Keratin AE1 stains the secretory and ductal cells of both eccrine and apocrine glands. Keratin 34 β E12 is expressed by ductal cells and basal cells of the secretory portion (Fig. 3-35B). p63 is expressed by basal cells (but not luminal cells) of the ductal portion and only scattered cells of the secretory portion (Fig. 3-35C). The expression of S100 protein is seen in some of the secretory cells of the eccrine glands (Fig. 3-35F) but not in apocrine glands. However, in sections of the axilla, some larger glands do show S100 staining; these may represent apoeccrine glands (220). The myoepithelial cells express smooth muscle actins. Eccrine glands strongly express SOX10, and this must be considered when using this biomarker for the detection of cells of melanocytic lineage in biopsy specimens (221).

Specialized Keratinization: Nails

The nail unit is a region of specialized keratinization of practical importance because dermatosis, infections, and neoplasms may affect this region, prompting histologic sampling (222). The nail unit has six main components (Figs. 3-38 and 3-39): (a) the nail matrix, which gives rise to the nail plate; (b) the nail plate; (c) the cuticular system, consisting of the dorsal component, or cuticle, and the distal component, or hyponychium; (d) the nail bed, which includes the dermis and underlying bone and soft tissue beneath the nail plate; (e) an anchoring system of ligaments between bone and matrix proximally and between distal grooves distally; and (f) the nail folds proximally, laterally, and distally.

The proximal nail fold is a wedge-shaped fold of the skin on the dorsum of the distal digit underneath where the nail plate arises. It consists of two layers of epidermis, both of which show a granular layer. The dorsal surface proximal nail fold contains eccrine but not pilosebaceous units and undergoes epidermal-type keratinization with an intervening granular cell layer, resulting in the production of soft keratin. Its ventral surface or eponychium is devoid of rete ridges and appendages. Keratohyalin granules are present in the epidermis of the ventral proximal nail fold, which produces the semihard keratin of the cuticle. The ventral surface of the proximal nail fold forms the roof of the proximal nail groove. The floor of the proximal nail groove is formed by the nail matrix, and the nail plate lies between the two (Figs. 3-38 and 3-39B).

The nail matrix is responsible for the production of the "hard keratin" of the nail plate. This occurs via a process termed onychokeratinization, and, as in trichilemmal keratinization, it occurs by accretion of tonofilaments without the formation of intervening keratohyalin granules (223,224). This process involves thickening of the cellular envelope of the keratinizing cells to form a marginal band, analogous to similar changes in the surface epidermis (225). The nail matrix may be divided into two regions—one distal, responsible for the formation of the ventral portion of the nail plate, and clinically visible (the lunula) and the other proximal and responsible for the formation of the dorsal surface of the nail plate. The nail thickness is determined predominantly by the matrix, although one study suggested that the nail bed may contribute up to 20% as the nail grows (226). The matrix epithelium contains an upper, broad keratogenous zone containing flattened eosinophilic keratinocytes and a basal compartment with active germinative cells (Fig. 3-39C). Compared with the epidermis, this basal compartment is multilayered (227). Melanocytes are present in the distal portion of the nail matrix (228), and Langerhans cells and Merkel cells have also been identified in this region (223).

The nail bed begins at the distal lunula and ends distally at the hyponychium. It also exhibits onycholemmal-type keratinization. The nail bed epidermis is usually thinner than the matrix epidermis, with less prominent basal layer and no melanocytes (Fig. 3-39D). The surface of the bed typically shows parallel longitudinal grooves that correlate with interdigitation of underlying rete ridges and dermal papillae. Clinically, the onychodermal band signifies the separation of the nail plate from the hyponychium, where the normal volar epidermis and epidermal-type keratinization resumes.

The nail plate consists of closely packed, adherent, interdigitating corneocytes lacking nuclei or organelles. Desmosomal junctions are identified.

Immunohistochemical studies have revealed two types of tissue compartments in the nail unit—compartments that exclusively express epidermal keratins and others exhibiting a varying, mixed expression of epidermal and hair keratins (227).

DERMIS

Cellular Components

The cellular components (resident cells) of the dermis comprise the following:

- Fibroblasts
- Dermal dendritic cells
- Macrophages
- Mast cells

The dermis is a dynamic, supportive connective tissue composed of an extracellular matrix that includes collagen, elastic fibers, and ground substance intimately associated with a cellular component that is mainly composed of fibroblasts, myofibroblasts, macrophages, dermal dendritic cells, and mast cells (Figs. 3-40 to 3-55). Within the dermis, there are also

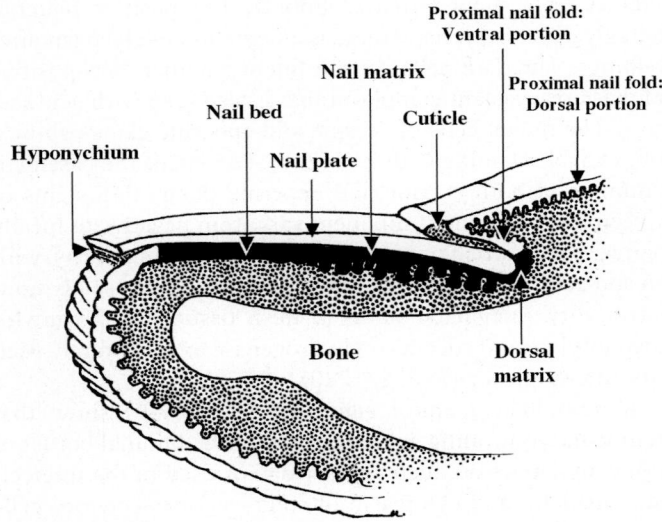

Figure 3-38 Diagram of the nail unit.

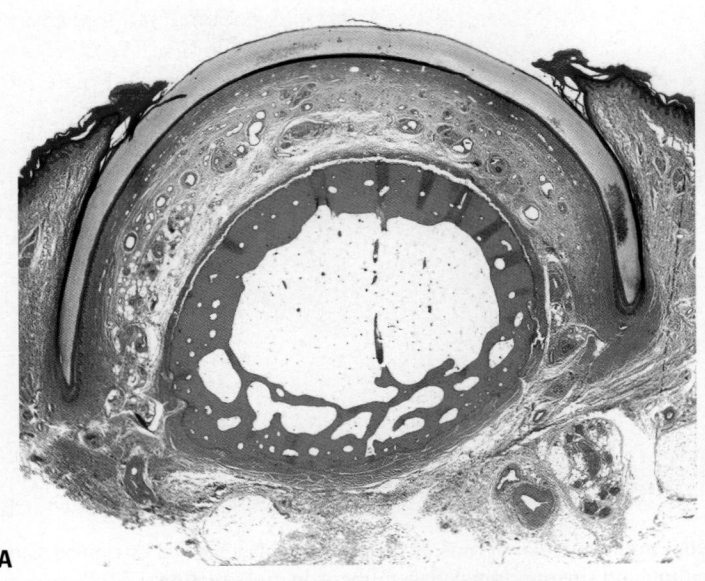

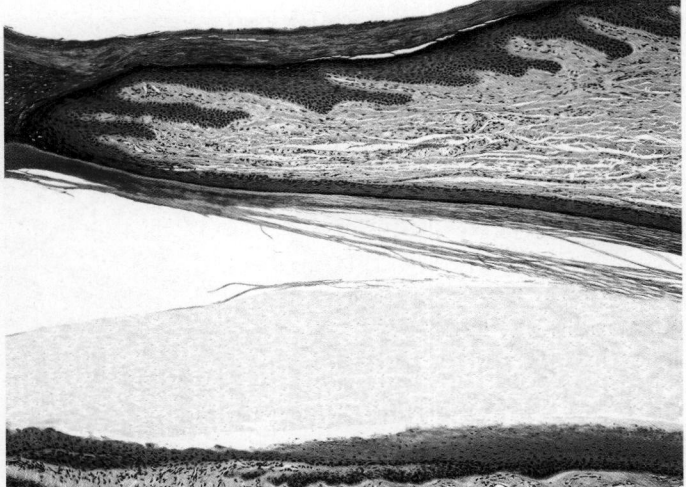

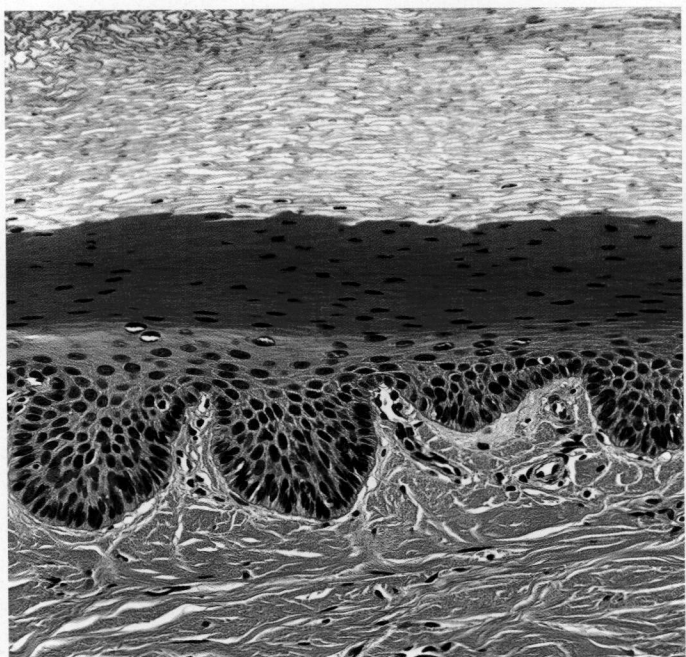

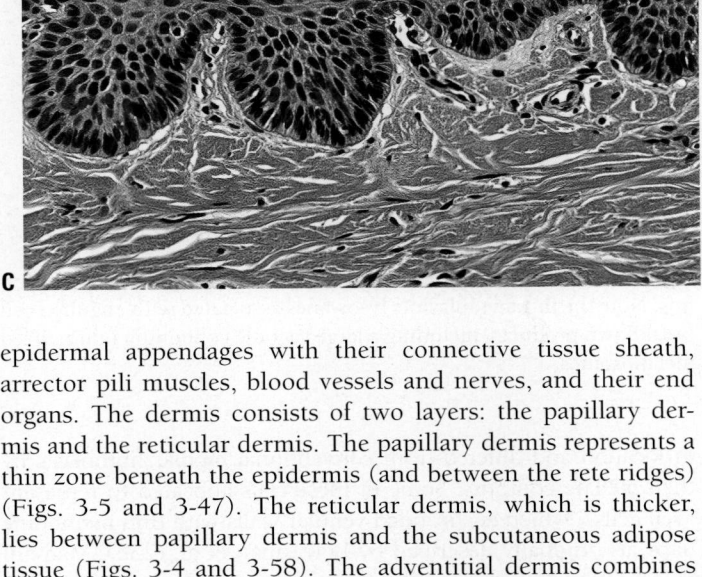

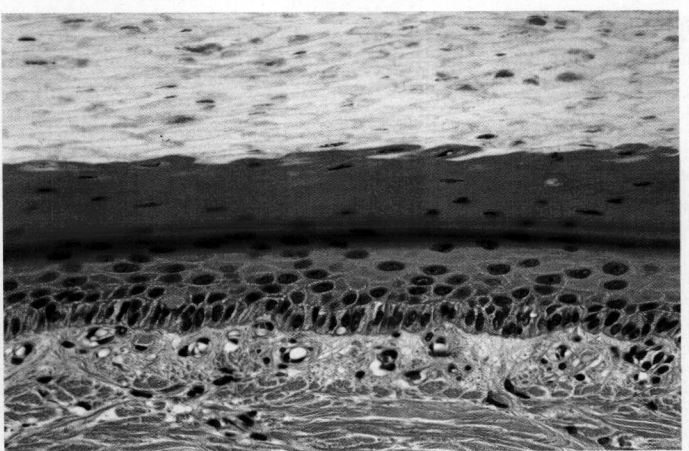

Figure 3-39 **A:** Low-power view of a transverse section of the distal portion of a finger, including the nail unit. Overlying the nail bed is a thick, acellular nail plate. The lateral folds can be appreciated on both sides. **B:** Proximal nail fold forming the roof of the nail groove. Note the presence of granular layer on the dorsal and ventral surfaces. The floor of the nail groove corresponds to the nail matrix. Between the two structures lies the nail plate. **C:** Nail matrix. Note the lack of granular layer and presence of multilayered germinative basal cells. **D:** Nail bed. Note the lack of granular layer. The epithelium shows a paucity of germinative basal cells.

epidermal appendages with their connective tissue sheath, arrector pili muscles, blood vessels and nerves, and their end organs. The dermis consists of two layers: the papillary dermis and the reticular dermis. The papillary dermis represents a thin zone beneath the epidermis (and between the rete ridges) (Figs. 3-5 and 3-47). The reticular dermis, which is thicker, lies between papillary dermis and the subcutaneous adipose tissue (Figs. 3-4 and 3-58). The adventitial dermis combines the papillary and periadnexal dermis. The papillary dermis and the epidermis together form a morphologic and functional unit whose interrelatedness is reflected in their alteration jointly in various inflammatory processes, for example, interface dermatitides such as lichen planus and erythema multiforme (Chapters 7 and 9). An analogous relationship exists between adnexal epithelium and periadnexal connective tissue (the "adventitial dermis") (229).

Dermal Fibroblasts

The dermis of a 2-month-old embryo consists of loosely arranged mesenchymal cells that are embedded in ground substance.

During the third month, argyrophilic reticulum fibers appear. As these fibers increase in number and in thickness, they arrange themselves in bundles that can no longer be impregnated with silver and, instead, stain with the methods for collagen. Simultaneously, the mesenchymal cells develop into fibroblasts. Electron microscopic examination of the fetal dermis from week 6 to 14 reveals, apart from Schwann cells identified by their association with neuraxons, three main types of cells: (a) stellate mesenchymal cells with long processes, (b) phagocytic macrophages of probable yolk-sac origin, and (c) cells containing granules, which could be either melanoblasts or mast precursors. From week 14 on, fibroblasts become numerous. In the normal adult dermis, fibroblasts appear as inconspicuous bipolar spindle cells with elongated ovoid nuclei. They cannot be reliably distinguished from other dermal spindle-shaped and dendritic cells. By electron microscopy, fibroblasts that actively synthesize collagen have a prominent rough endoplasmic reticulum composed of many membrane-lined cisternae with large numbers of attached ribosomes (Fig. 3-40B). The dilated cisternae are filled with an amorphous material produced by

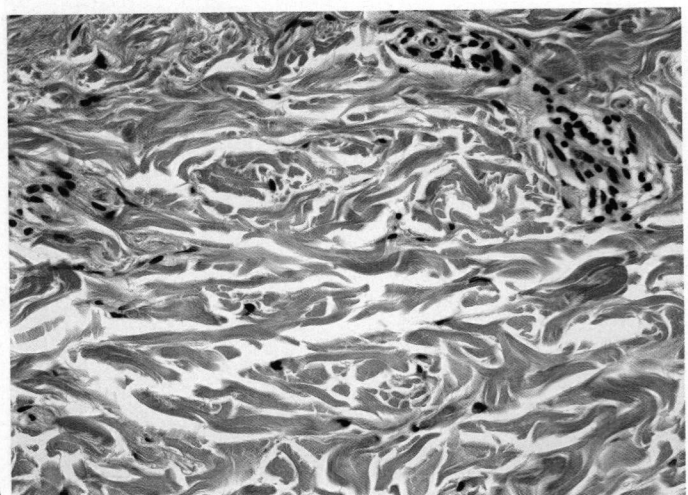
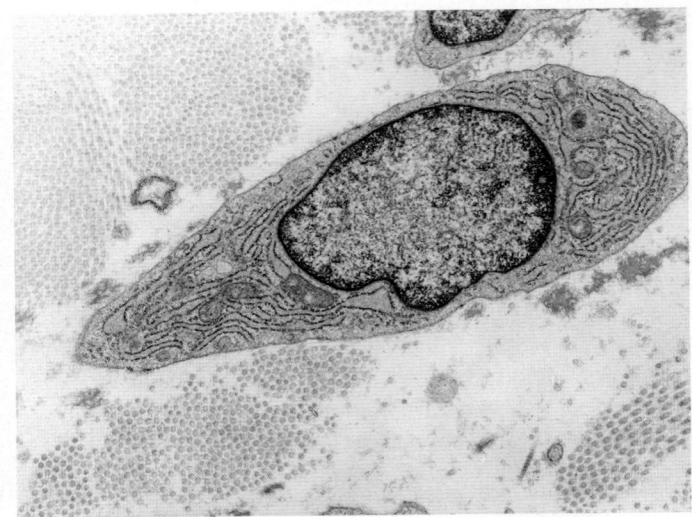

Figure 3-40 A: Scattered fibroblasts are present among thick collagen bundles in the reticular dermis. B: Dermal fibroblast viewed by transmission electron microscopy, showing dilated cisternae of rough endoplasmic reticulum and surrounding collagen fibers on cross section.

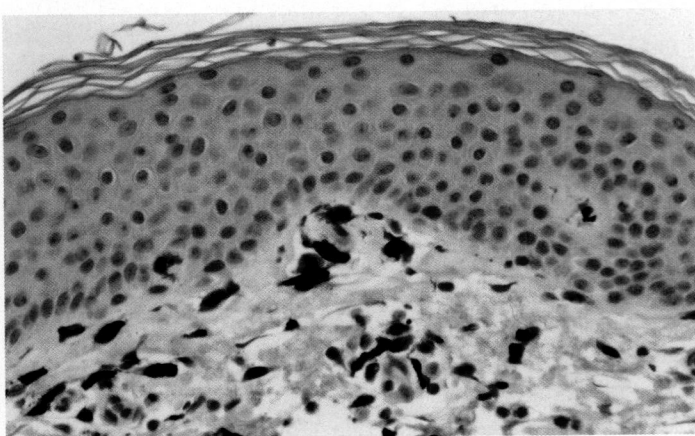

Figure 3-41 Factor XIIIa–positive "dermal dendrocytes" concentrated beneath the epidermal layer and about the dermal microvascular unit.

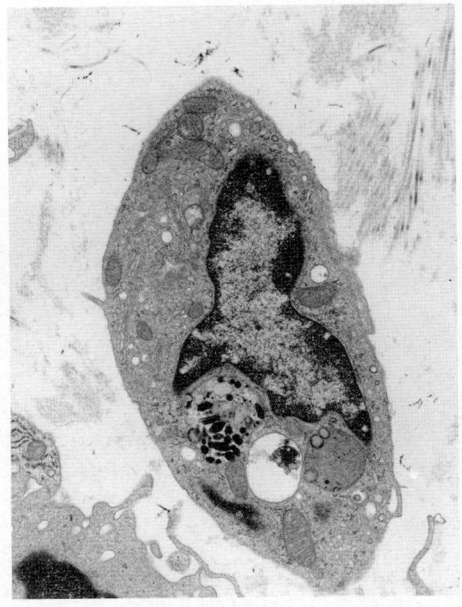

Figure 3-42 Ultrastructure of phagocytic macrophage within the dermis. Note the intracytoplasmic lysosomes associated with engulfed cell breakdown products, including a large vacuole containing internalized melanosomes.

the ribosomes lining the cisternae (230). This apparently amorphous material consists of triple-helical procollagen molecules, each molecule being composed of three pro–α-polypeptide chains. The procollagen molecules pass from the cisternae of the rough endoplasmic reticulum to the Golgi area, whence they are excreted into the extracellular space by means of secretory vesicles (231,232). Conversion of procollagen molecules into collagen molecules composed of three α chains then occurs outside the cell (233). Immunohistochemically, fibroblasts express vimentin. CD10 immunoreactivity is normally found in periadnexal fibroblasts. Active, regenerative fibroblasts (e.g., in granulation tissue) disclose ultrastructural and immunohistochemical features of myofibroblasts (234). Myofibroblasts may express, in addition to vimentin, smooth muscle actin and desmin. Whereas resting fibroblasts may be difficult to differentiate from other dermal spindle cell elements, stimulated fibroblasts may be detected at transcriptional and posttranscriptional levels by probes that identify components involved in active collagen synthesis.

Perivascular and Interstitial Dendritic Cells

In 1986, Headington (235) introduced the term "dermal dendrocyte" to denote newly recognized dendritic cells in the human dermis. These cells were primarily, but not exclusively, perivascular

in location and differed from conventional bipolar fibroblasts by their stellate contours. Some of these cells appeared to represent "veil cells," which enshrouded venular walls with thin membrane flaps, as originally described by Braverman et al. (236). Many of these cells were subsequently shown to express the membrane glycoprotein CD1c (237), HLA-DR, and certain macrophage markers as well as the cytoplasmic transglutaminase, factor XIIIa (238) (Fig. 3-41). Heterogeneity of dermal dendrocytes within different dermal strata with regard to their expression of the hematopoietic progenitor antigen, CD34, and FXIIIa has been described (239). Per conventional immunohistochemistry, factor XIIIa–positive cells are predominantly found in perivascular distribution in the papillary dermis and around sweat glands. Although their presence is not specific, factor XIIIa–positive cells have been detected in increased numbers in numerous pathologic conditions, including Kaposi sarcoma, dermatofibroma, and scar formation.

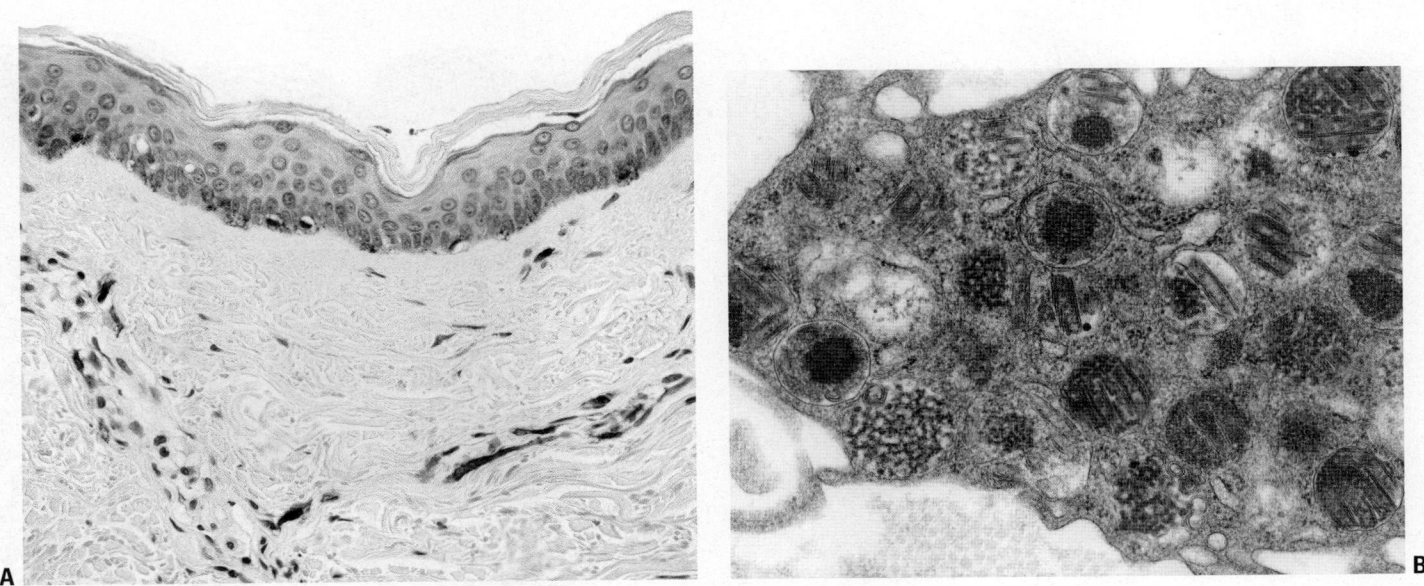

Figure 3-43 **A:** KIT (CD117) highlights dermal mast cells and junctional melanocytes. **B:** Transmission electron micrograph of a granulated mast cell.

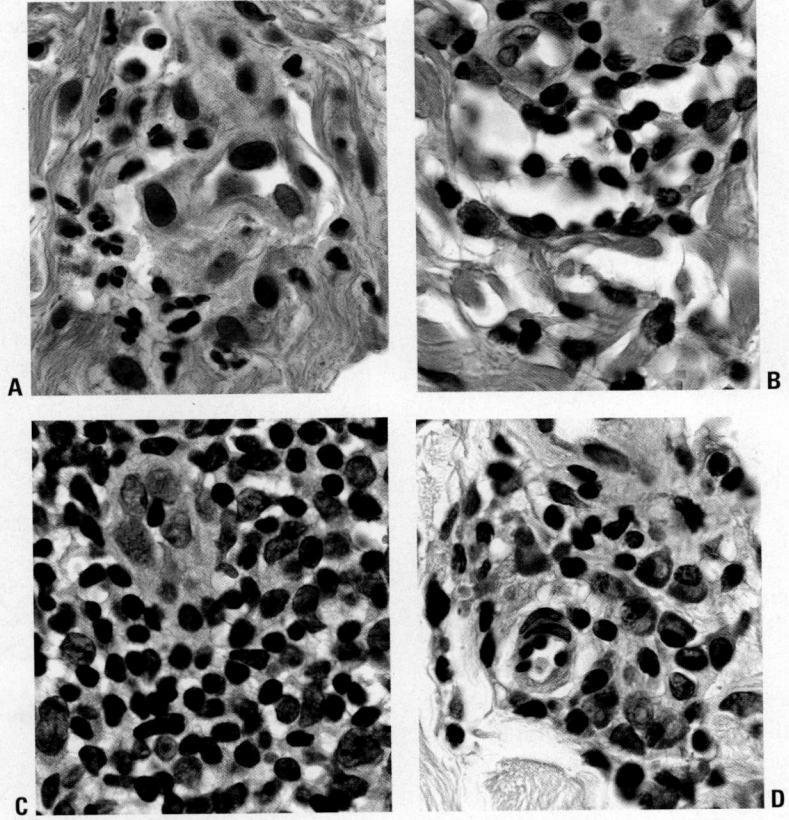

Figure 3-44 Emigrant inflammatory cells found in different common dermatitides include neutrophils (**A**), eosinophils (**B**), lymphocytes and histiocytes (**C**), and plasma cells (**D**).

CD34-positive cells are more numerous in the mid- and deep dermis and around adnexa (240).

Whereas dermal dendrocytes are dendritic only in cross section, with three-dimensional reconstructions showing elaborate membranous flaps (239), truly dendritic cells also exist in the perivascular space. These cells are Langerhans cell-like, although they generally do not contain Birbeck granules, strongly express

HLA-DR, and are believed to be involved in dermal antigen presentation (241). Considerable plasticity among the various subpopulations of dermal perivascular dendritic cells may exist, and alterations in local microenvironment may induce phenotypic transformation from one subtype to another (242).

In general, perivascular dendritic cells are not identifiable as such in routinely prepared and stained sections, although

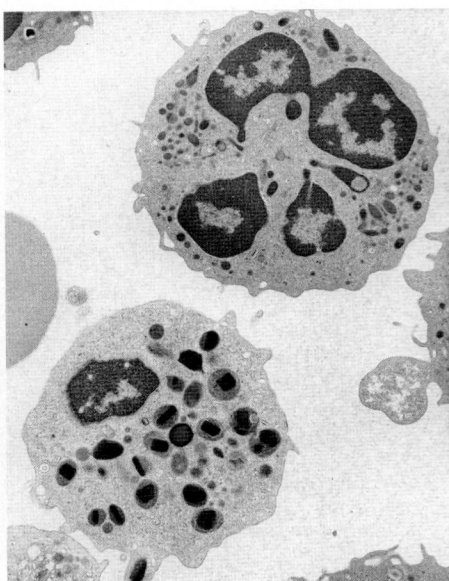

Figure 3-45 Ultrastructural comparison between neutrophilic (**uppermost cell**) and eosinophilic (**lowermost cell**) granulocytes.

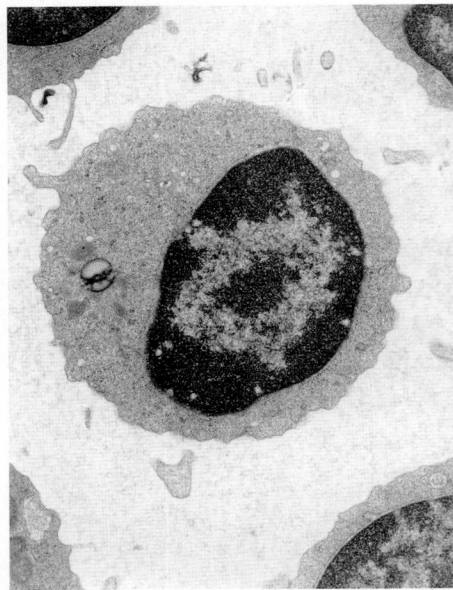

Figure 3-46 Transmission electron micrograph of a mature lymphocyte; note the chromatin-rich nucleus and organelle-poor cytoplasm.

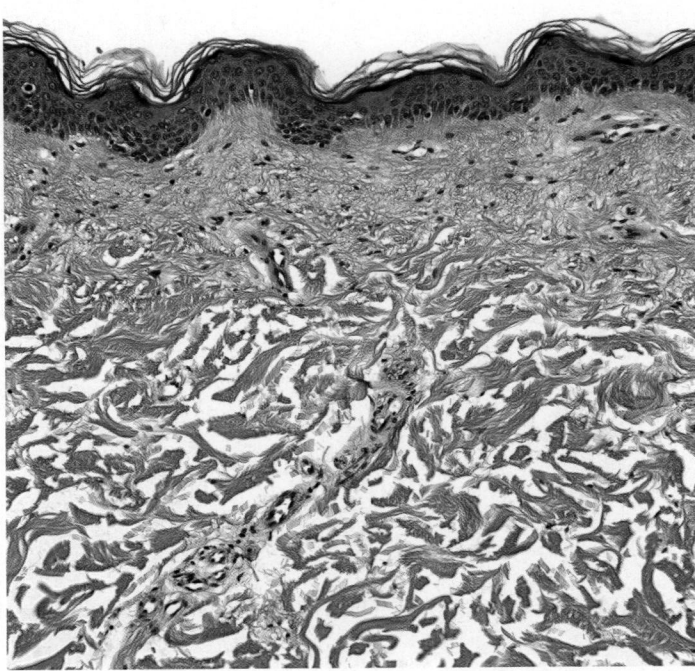

Figure 3-47 Conventional histology of the transition between papillary (**top**) and reticular (**bottom**) dermis. The dermal collagen in the papillary dermis is more delicate and thin than the thicker collagen bundles in the papillary dermis.

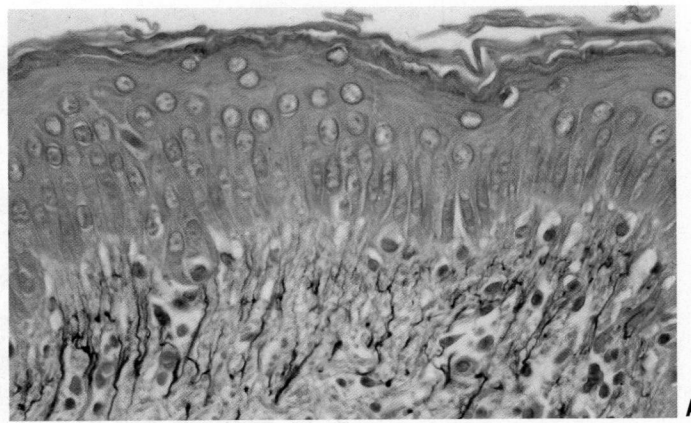

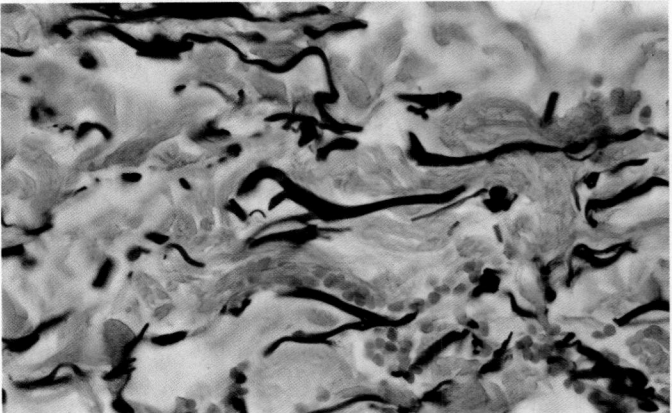

Figure 3-48 Histochemical demonstration of elastin fibers within papillary dermis (**A**) and reticular dermis (**B**). Silver stain.

immunohistochemistry for the relevant markers permits the ready identification and classification of these cell types. Dermal dendrocytes may be observed in certain situations in which they acquire avid phagocytic potential, taking up hemosiderin, for example. Such phagocytic perivascular dendritic cells have been termed "dendrophages" (243).

Phagocytic Macrophages

Macrophages, also called histiocytes, are of bone marrow origin, circulate in the blood as precursors, and enter the tissue as monocytes (244). On proper stimulation, monocytes can develop into macrophages in the skin, which involves a considerable increase in cell size and changes in cellular composition and architecture, including increases in lysosomal enzymes, such as β-glucuronidase, acid phosphatase, lysozyme, and aryl sulfatase (245). Macrophages may develop further into

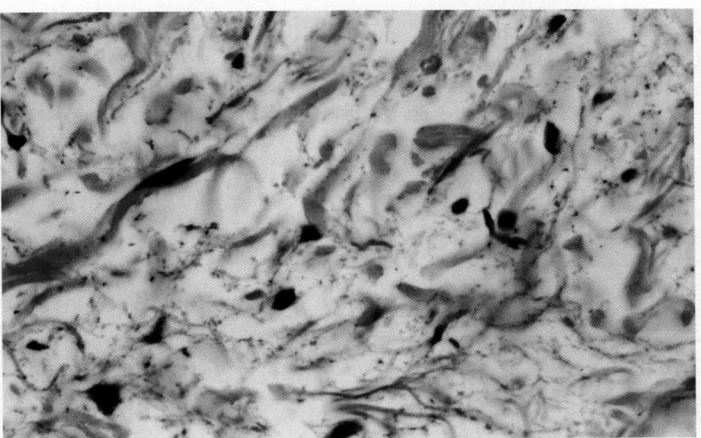

Figure 3-49 Ground substance. Although these mucopolysaccharides are normally inconspicuous by conventional light microscopy, in this case, they are pathologically increased and thus visible as thin, pale blue-gray strands within widened spaces separating reticular dermal collagen.

epithelioid histiocytes and foreign body giant cells. Aggregates of activated macrophages are referred to as granulomas. Macrophages are most often concentrated in the perivascular space of normal skin, although, depending on the nature and location of

the stimulus for their activation, they may be found anywhere in the dermis (or epidermis).

Macrophages constitute the "mononuclear phagocytic system," a concept that has replaced that of the reticuloendothelial system. The macrophages of the mononuclear phagocytic system, including the alveolar phagocytes in the lungs and the Kupffer cells in the liver, are the "professional" phagocytes, whereas the reticuloendothelial cells, including the dendritic reticulum cells in lymph nodes and the endothelial cells of blood vessels, are merely "facultative" phagocytes and are comparatively inadequate (245). As "professional" phagocytes, macrophages are capable of ingesting large particles and developing a high concentration of lysosomal enzymes, which combine with the particles to form phagolysosomes. In contrast, the facultative phagocytosis carried out by endothelial cells consists merely of pinocytosis of small particles without immune stimulation (245). Macrophages can also be stimulated by immunologic factors having surface receptors for the Fc portion of IgG, for C3, and for immune-associated HLA-DR antigen (human leukocyte antigen-D subregion of the major histocompatibility complex) (246).

Monocytes are indistinguishable from lymphocytes by routine histology because both cells have a small, dark, rounded nucleus and very scanty cytoplasm that cannot be recognized in routine sections. Only slightly larger than lymphocytes,

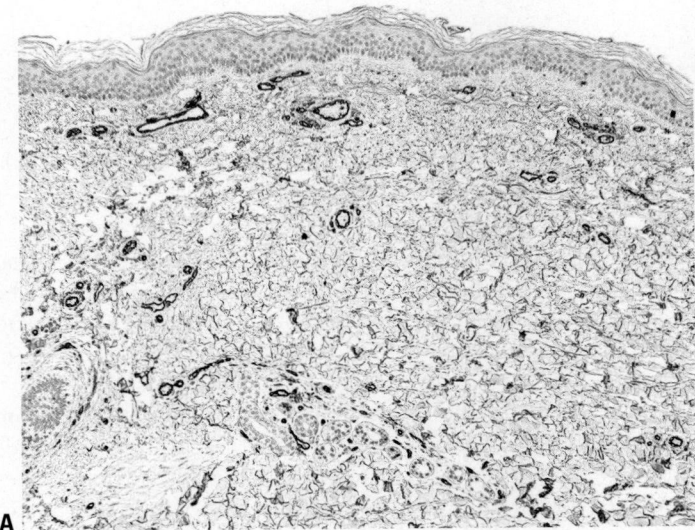

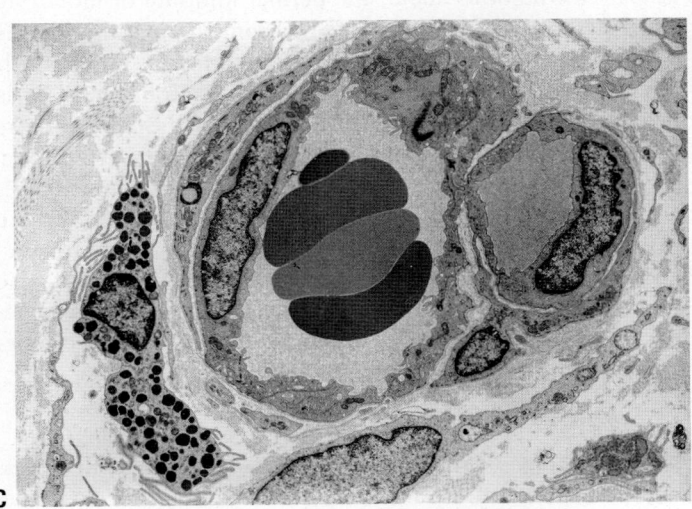

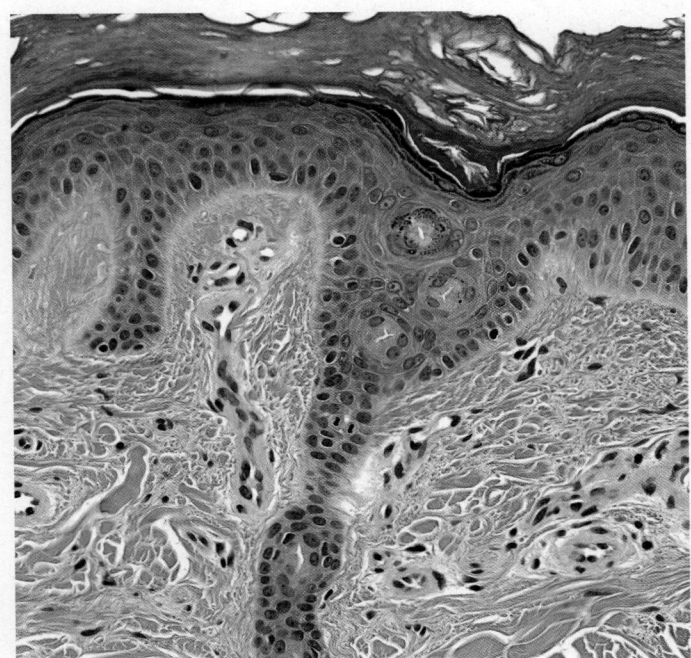

Figure 3-50 A: Immunohistochemical stain with CD31 highlights the vascular pattern in the dermis. B: Histology of a capillary loop originating from underlying superficial vascular plexus and extending into the dermal papilla. C: Transmission electron micrograph of dermal microvascular unit consisting of a plexus of central vessels and surrounding cells that form the junction between the papillary and reticular dermis. Note the endothelial cells lining the central postcapillary venule surrounded by pericytes and dermal immune cells, including granulated mast cells.

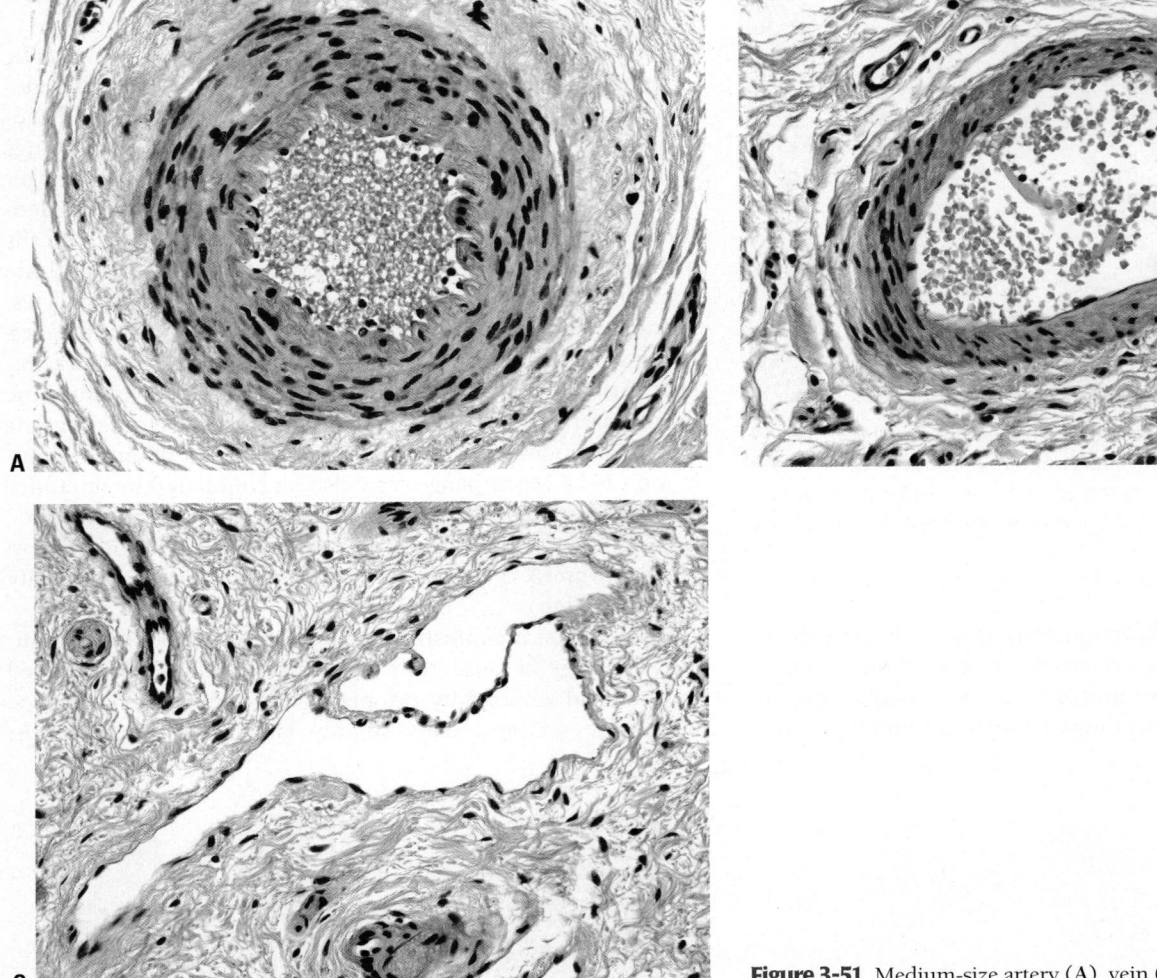

Figure 3-51 Medium-size artery (A), vein (B), and lymphatic vessel (C).

monocytes measure 12 to 15 μm in diameter (246). They can be differentiated from lymphocytes in histologic sections through staining for lysosomal enzymes, such as acid phosphatase, which are present in monocytes and absent in lymphocytes. In addition, monocytes, but not lymphocytes, express intracytoplasmic molecules, such as CD68 and KP1, probably associated with lysosomes. Such molecules, however, are generally regarded as organelle rather than cell lineage specific and are not considered exclusive markers of cells of monocyte/macrophage derivation (247). A more recently described monocytic/macrophagic marker is CD163, which is a glycoprotein belonging to the scavenger receptor cysteine-rich superfamily. CD163 is of particular interest because its expression has been shown by *in situ* hybridization, immunofluorescent, and immunohistochemical techniques to be largely restricted to monocytes and tissue macrophages (247). CD68, KP1, and CD163 may be detected immunohistochemically in paraffin sections (248).

Macrophages, because they are activated monocytes, are larger cells than monocytes and measure from 20 to 80 μm in diameter (246). They possess a vesicular, lightly staining, elongated nucleus with a clearly visible nuclear membrane. It is often impossible in routinely stained sections to distinguish macrophages from fibroblasts or from endothelial cells except through their respective locations or phagocytic activities. Macrophages that have ingested melanin are referred to as melanophages and may be observed normally within the papillary

dermis of darkly pigmented individuals. Macrophages that have ingested hemosiderin are termed *siderophages* and may be suspected because of the characteristic yellow-green color and refractile nature of particulate hemosiderin. Iron stains (e.g., Prussian blue) are confirmatory.

The origin of the tissue monocytes in human skin from blood monocytes has been established in healthy probands through transfusion of tritiated-thymidine-labeled monocytes and their observation 3 hours later in skin window exudates (249). On the other hand, the dermal infiltrate of monocytes and macrophages in patients with chronic dermatitis is largely self-renewing because the monocyte recruitment rate from the blood is low in these patients after the autotransfusion of labeled monocytes (249). Electron microscopic examination reveals in monocytes many primary lysosomes scattered through their cytoplasm as small dense bodies (250). Macrophages, which represent stimulated monocytes, differ from monocytes in that they are larger, show longer processes, and contain a greater number of lysosomes (251) (Fig. 3-42). Many macrophages contain phagocytized material within phagosomes, which, through the influx of the contents of primary lysosomes, have become phagolysosomes.

Mast Cells

Mast cells (Fig. 3-43) are bone marrow–derived cells that occur in the normal dermis in small numbers as oval to spindle-shaped

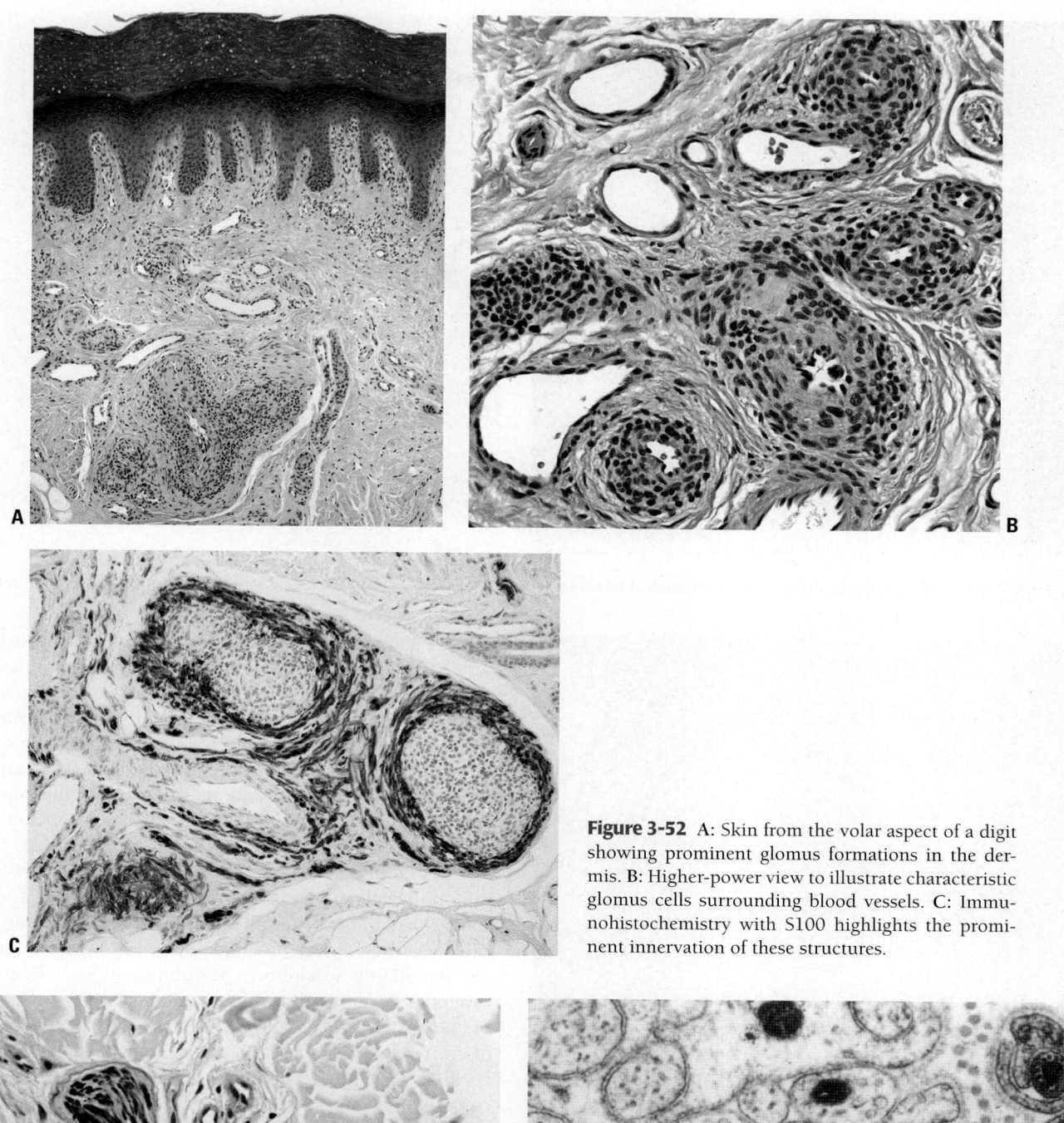

Figure 3-52 A: Skin from the volar aspect of a digit showing prominent glomus formations in the dermis. B: Higher-power view to illustrate characteristic glomus cells surrounding blood vessels. C: Immunohistochemistry with S100 highlights the prominent innervation of these structures.

Figure 3-53 Dermal nerve fibers demonstrated by S100 immunohistochemical staining (A) and by transmission electron microscopy as individual axons enveloped by Schwann cells (B).

cells with a centrally located round to oval nucleus. They are generally concentrated about blood vessels, specifically postcapillary venules (one to three cells per cross-sectional vessel profile). They contain in their cytoplasm numerous granules that do not stain with routine stains like hematoxylin–eosin. Therefore, mast

cells in normal skin are not reliably distinguishable from other perivascular cells, although one can occasionally recognize in mast cells a small amount of cytoplasm and the cell membrane. The granules stain with methylene blue, which is present in the Giemsa stain, with toluidine blue, and with alcian blue. They also

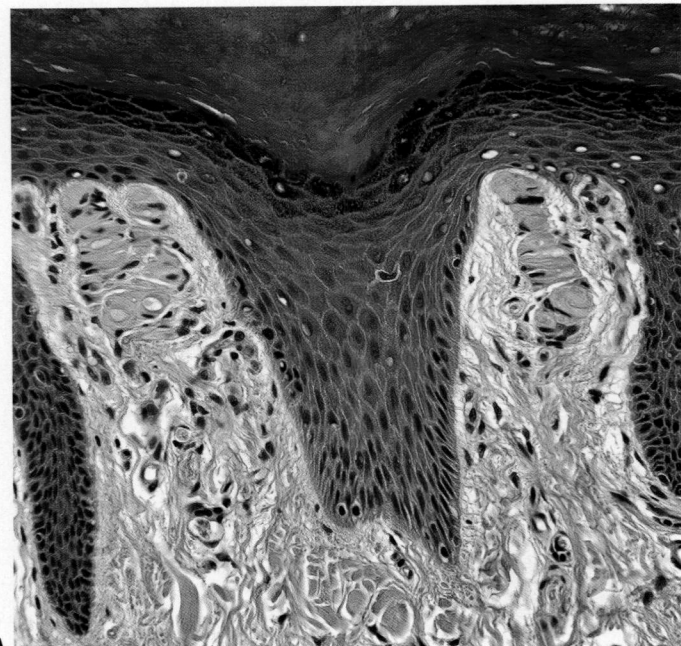
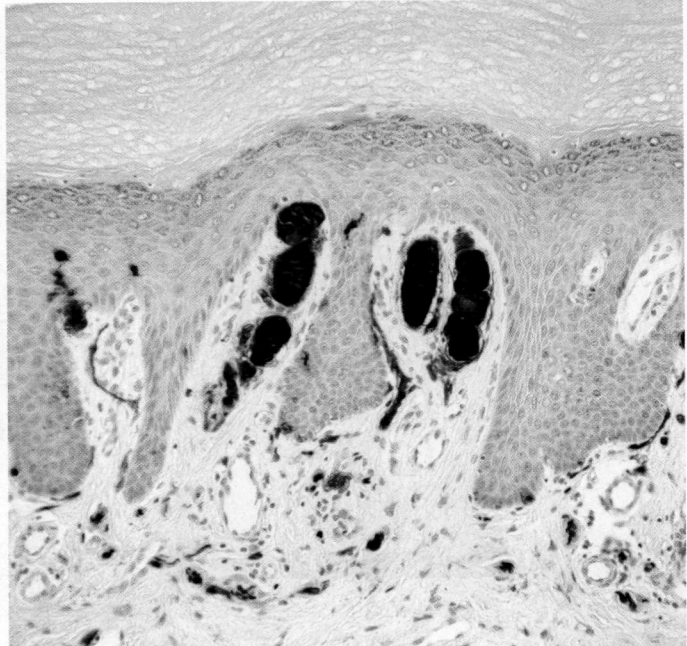

Figure 3-54 **A:** Meissner corpuscle within dermal papillae of human palm skin. **B:** Meissner corpuscles are strongly positive with S100 immunostain.

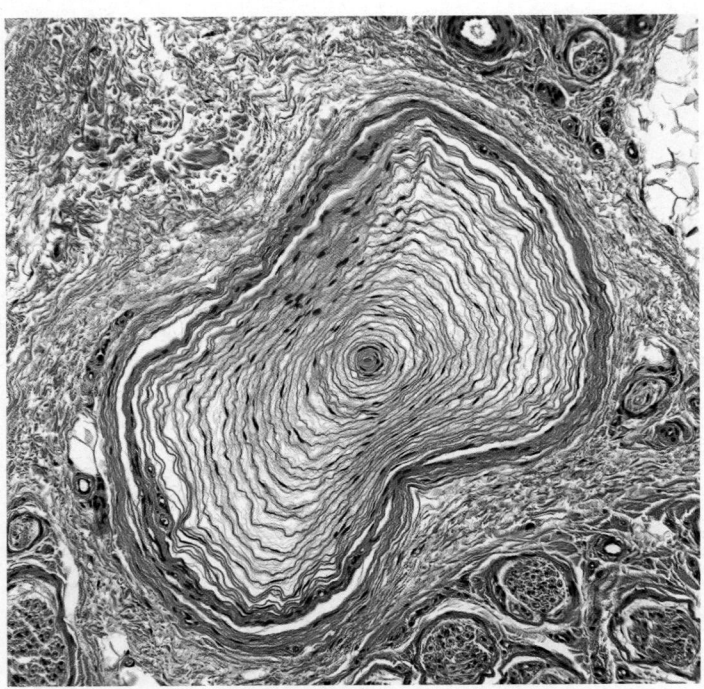

Figure 3-55 Vater–Pacini structure with characteristic concentric pattern.

stain metachromatically with methylene blue and toluidine blue, that is, they stain in a color different from that possessed by the dye and appear purplish red rather than blue.

Electron microscopic examination of mast cells reveals numerous large and long villi at their periphery. The mast cell granules appear as round, oval, or angular-shaped, membrane-bound structures. Mature granules measure up to 0.8 μm in diameter (252) (Fig. 3-43B). They contain two components: lamellae and electron-dense, finely granular material (253). Tangential sectioning of the lamellae reveals paracrystalline lattices as a result of transverse banding. Immunoultrastructural observations indicate that the

various granule subcompartments correlate with distribution of serine proteinases tryptase and chymase within granules (254). In addition, mast cells that populate connective tissue environments like dermis tend to contain granules with poorly formed scrolls and express both chymase and tryptase, whereas mast cells found primarily in mucosae and associated lamina propria have granules with well-formed scrolls and express tryptase but not chymase (255,256). Of interest, one of these two granule types may be preferentially expressed in some cases of mastocytosis (257).

Degranulation of mast cells occurs after cross-linking of IgE on the cell surface, exposure to neuropeptides such as substance P, after nonspecific mechanical or thermal stimuli, or after exposure to a variety of exogenous secretagogues (compound 48/80, calcium ionophore, morphine sulfate). Degranulation generally occurs within minutes of exposure of the cell membrane to the secretagogue and usually consists in the extrusion of entire granules, but some granules may undergo intracellular disintegration (252,258,259). Initial stages of degranulation consist in granule swelling with loss of internal substructure and electron density. Extrusion of granules takes place through extensive membrane fusion between the plasma membrane and perigranular membranes and is associated with the formation of conduits resulting from fusion of the membranes of multiple granules. This results in extensive labyrinthine channels in the cell through which swollen, less electron-dense granules, all of which have lost their individual surrounding membranes, are released into the extracellular space (253,260). Concomitant with their release into the extracellular space, the granules release their preformed and stored mediators histamine, heparin, serine proteinases, and certain cytokines.

Immediate hypersensitivity reactions can be triggered by mast cells and basophils in "anaphylactically" sensitized persons through the presence on their cell surfaces of specific antibodies of the IgE type. When the specific antigen combines with these antibodies, an anaphylactic reaction is elicited through the degranulation of mast cells and the release of histamine from the granules (261). Histamine increases the permeability of postcapillary venules and, if released in sufficient amounts, may produce an anaphylactic shock. In delayed hypersensitivity reactions and in experimental allogeneic cytotoxic reactions, mast cells degranulate early, often preceding the initial influx of pioneer lymphocytes (262,263). Part of the reason for this lies in the fact that human mast cells contain TNFα (264) and local release of TNFα as a consequence of mast cell degranulation induces expression of adhesion molecules such as E-selectin in adjacent postcapillary venules (265), with resultant leukocyte binding to the endothelial luminal membrane (266). Cooperation between the mast cell and the endothelial cell is also underscored by the observations that mast cells appear to situate in the laminin-rich perivascular space in association with expression of specific laminin receptors on their membranes (267) and that endothelial cells express mast cell growth factor (also known as c-kit ligand or stem cell factor) (268). CD117 (KIT) is a type III receptor tyrosine kinase operating in cell signal transduction in several cell types. Normally, KIT is activated (phosphorylated) by binding of its ligand, the stem cell factor. This leads to a phosphorylation cascade, ultimately activating various transcription factors in different cell types. Such activation regulates apoptosis, cell differentiation, proliferation, chemotaxis, and cell adhesion. KIT-dependent cell types in the skin include mast cells, some hematopoietic stem cells, melanocytes, scattered basal keratinocytes, and epithelial cells of skin adnexa (269) (Fig. 3-43A).

Emigrant Inflammatory Cells

Various types of cells, largely derived from the bone marrow, infiltrate the dermis and occasionally also the epidermis in the inflammatory dermatoses. Infiltration is initiated at the level of the dermal microvascular unit, accounting for the observation that on detection, such cells are often partially or exclusively perivascular in location (Fig. 3-44A–D). Such cells may also be present in normal skin in low numbers as part of the skin immune system. It is important for diagnostic purposes to identify the cell types because many diagnostic algorithms for dermatitis classification and identification depend on initial categorization by architecture followed by recognition of inflammatory cell type(s) (see Chapter 5) (270). Three groups of cells are derived from the bone marrow: the granulocytic group (Table 3-4);

the lymphocytic group, including plasma cells; and the monocytic or macrophagic group (discussed earlier).

Neutrophilic Granulocytes

The neutrophilic granulocyte, also called a neutrophil or polymorphonuclear leukocyte, has a lobated nucleus consisting of several segments that are connected only by narrow bridges of nucleoplasm (Fig. 3-44A). The cytoplasm contains numerous neutrophilic to slightly eosinophilic granules. Two types of membrane-bound cytoplasmic granules or lysosomes are found to be present in neutrophils on electron microscopic examination: azurophilic and specific granules (271) (Fig. 3-45 and Table 3-4). These granules contain lysosomal enzymes and thus represent primary lysosomes that have bacteriostatic properties and play important roles in degradation and lysis of dead bacteria or other necrotic materials. In tissue sections, neutrophils are often recognized by virtue of their "popcorn"-shaped nuclei within pale pink, faintly granular cytoplasm. Nuclear breakdown caused by local necrosis or autodigestion results in fragmentation of the multiple nuclear lobes, resulting in the characteristic "nuclear dust" of vasculitis. Neutrophils are unusual in normal skin but occur typically in a relatively small subset of dermatitides, including various cutaneous infections, urticaria, immune complex–mediated necrotizing vasculitis, and the spectrum of neutrophilic dermatosis (e.g., *Sweet syndrome, pyoderma gangrenosum*). Neutrophils may participate, along with other cell types, in other inflammatory processes, such as *psoriasis, seborrheic dermatitis*, and *pityriasis lichenoides et varioliformis acuta (PLEVA)*.

Functionally, neutrophilic granulocytes play an important role in (a) certain inflammatory responses, (b) the phagocytosis and killing of microorganisms, and (c) the immobilization and phagocytosis of antigen–antibody complexes in the presence of complement (272). Neutrophils fail to kill bacteria in chronic granulomatous disease, where they are congenitally incapable of oxygen uptake from the surrounding media (273). Phagocytosis of organisms and antigen–antibody complexes by neutrophils is accompanied by their partial or complete degranulation, with associated discharge of lysosomal enzymes (274). Endocytotic uptake of microorganisms by neutrophils results in

Table 3-4

Inflammatory Cells of Granulocytic Group

Cell Type	Diameter (μm)	Granules	Major Components of Granules	Stains to Highlight Granules
Neutrophilic granulocytes	10–15	Azurophilic (20%)	Myeloperoxidase, acid hydrolases, neutral proteases, cationic proteins, lysozyme	Leder (CAE—chloroacetate esterase)
		Specific (80%)	Lysozyme, collagenase, alkaline phosphatase, and lactoferrin, an iron-binding protein	
		Metachromatic	Inorganic phosphate polymer, heparin	
Eosinophilic granulocytes	12–17	Eosinophilic	Hydrolytic enzymes, particularly eosinophil peroxidase and arylsulfatase, ribonuclease, plasminogen, deoxyribonucleases, lipase	H&E
Basophilic granulocytes	10–14	Metachromatic	Inorganic phosphate polymer	H&E, Giemsa
Mast cells	8–10	Metachromatic	Inorganic phosphate polymer, heparin, histamines	Toluidine blue, Giemsa, methylene blue, c-kit, tryptase

H&E, hematoxylin–eosin.

the formation of intracytoplasmic phagolysosomes, where high enzyme concentrations facilitate microbial degradation. Immune complexes, after activation of complement, may induce the local accumulation of neutrophils via chemotaxis. Phagocytosis of immune complexes by neutrophils and/or neutrophil degranulation may then occur (275). Exocytosis of neutrophil granules containing collagenase and elastase may cause local tissue damage, including necrosis of vessels containing immune complexes in their basement membranes (276).

Eosinophilic Granulocytes

The eosinophil is characterized by strongly eosinophilic granules in the cytoplasm and a characteristically bilobed nucleus (277). Eosinophil granules are larger than the granules of neutrophils (Table 3-4). Although visible with routine H&E sections (Fig. 3-44B), these granules stand out more clearly in brilliant red when a Giemsa stain is used. They consist of two components—a central, angular-shaped core, often referred to as the crystalloid, and a surrounding matrix. In electron microscopic sections stained with lead compounds, the crystalloid is more darkly stained than the matrix (278) (Fig. 3-45). Diseases in which deposition of antigen–antibody complexes is the cause of eosinophilia include *pemphigus vulgaris, particularly pemphigus vegetans, pemphigus foliaceus, bullous pemphigoid* (see Chapter 9), and *granuloma faciale* (see Chapter 8). The reasons for the occasional presence of tissue eosinophilia in *histiocytosis X* (see Chapter 6) and in *Hodgkin disease* (see Chapter 31) are not fully apparent. Parasitic infestations are often associated with eosinophilia both in the peripheral blood and in the tissue (see Chapter 24). It is likely that eosinophils function as effector cells in parasite destruction (279).

Functionally, the phagocytic potential of eosinophils seems to be limited to immune complexes and mast cell granules. During phagocytosis, which is analogous to that seen in neutrophils, the content of the eosinophilic granules is discharged into phagosomes (279). Because eosinophils can phagocytize mast cell granules and certain antigen–antibody complexes, tissue eosinophilia in the skin can occur (a) as a result of anaphylactic or atopic hypersensitivity, (b) subsequent to the degranulation of mast cells, and (c) in certain diseases associated with deposits of antigen–antibody complexes in the skin. The tissue eosinophilia appearing in anaphylactic reactions and other forms of "immediate" allergy such as atopy is based on antibodies of the IgE type on the surface of mast cells. The anaphylactic reaction, classified as type I hypersensitivity reaction (280), occurs after the binding of a specific antigen to a specific antibody on the surface of the mast cells. This leads to degranulation of mast cells and to the release of vasoactive substances, especially histamine. Wherever degranulation of mast cells occurs, eosinophils may appear and phagocytize the released mast cell granules (274). Eosinophils may thus modify an anaphylactic reaction (281). Eosinophils are attracted in an anaphylactic reaction by sensitized mast cells, which release an eosinophil chemotactic factor of anaphylaxis. Eosinophils thus attracted to the site of an anaphylactic reaction accumulate around degranulating mast cells and phagocytize the free mast cell granules (282).

Basophilic Granulocytes and Mast Cells

Although basophils and mast cells have similar or identical functions and supplement each other, they are different cells both in origin and in anatomy (Table 3-4) (283). Both cells have their origin in the bone marrow, although basophils circulate in the peripheral blood, and mature mast cells are confined to connective tissue and mucosal tissue compartments. Basophils are relatively rare in human dermatitis, although they are active participants in certain forms of dermatitis in rodents (283). The demonstration of basophils in light microscopic sections requires the use of electron microscopic fixation and processing techniques; biopsy specimens must be embedded in plastic resin and sectioned at 1 μm. The sections are then stained with the Giemsa stain. Basophils possess a multilobed nucleus and large, diffusely arranged metachromatic granules, whereas mast cells have a unilobed nucleus and smaller, peripherally located metachromatic granules (284).

Lymphocytes

There are two main types of peripheral lymphocytes—T and B lymphocytes—both of which arise in the bone marrow. One type migrates to the thymus, where it differentiates into a mature lymphocyte and then proceeds to the peripheral lymphoid tissues as a thymus-derived or T lymphocyte. In lymph nodes, T lymphocytes are located predominantly in the interfollicular cortex, also called the paracortical areas. The other type of lymphocyte—the B lymphocyte—matures in the bone marrow (285). The term B lymphocyte, meaning bursa-derived lymphocyte, was originally used because in birds the bursa of Fabricius is held responsible for B-cell maturation (285). In humans, the term B lymphocyte is used to indicate a bone marrow–derived lymphocyte. In lymph nodes, B lymphocytes largely occupy the lymphoid follicles, including their germinal centers. Whereas the T lymphocyte is the effector cell for cellular immunity, the B lymphocyte mediates humoral immunity. T cells can exert important regulating functions on both T cells and B cells in the form of specific functional subsets termed helper T cells and cytotoxic/suppressor T cells (286). The lymph nodes and other lymphoid organs share three principal functions to (a) concentrate within them antigens from all parts of the body, (b) expose these antigens to naive and antigen-specific lymphocytes that circulate within them, and (c) deliver products of the immune response, namely, the antibodies and cells mediating humoral and cellular immunity, respectively, to the blood and peripheral nonlymphoid tissues (285). Tissues that represent significant host–environmental interfaces, like skin and gut, are regular targets for physiologic T-cell trafficking mediated by tissue-specific homing receptors that interact with endothelial adhesion molecules (e.g., T-cell cutaneous lymphocyte–associated antigen and endothelial E-selectin in skin). This intimate homing relationship between central lymphoid organs and tissues like skin, in addition to resident populations of dendritic antigen-presenting cells (Langerhans cells) and effector cells (mast cells, see later discussion) is responsible for the concept of skin-associated lymphoid tissue.

Resting lymphocytes measure on average 8 to 10 μm in diameter and possess a relatively small, round nucleus that appears deeply basophilic because of the presence of numerous chromatin particles (Fig. 3-46). They have only a very narrow rim of cytoplasm that is difficult to delineate by conventional light microscopy. It is also usually not possible by light microscopy to distinguish lymphocytes from monocytes in routinely stained histologic sections. It is therefore preferable to refer to cells with a histologic appearance of lymphocytes as lymphoid cells, and infiltrates likely to contain significant admixtures of both lymphocytes and monocytes are sometimes referred to as involving mononuclear cells or described as "lymphohistiocytic infiltrates." Ultrastructurally, resting lymphocytes contain relatively few organelles within a thin cytoplasmic rim that surrounds a nucleus with coarsely aggregated heterochromatin (Figs. 3-44C and 3-46). Activated lymphocytes, on the other hand, may show enlarged, vesicular nuclei, visible nucleoli, and/or elaborately infolded nuclear contours that may bear some resemblance to Lutzner–Sézary cells.

The patterns of T- and B-cell infiltration in the skin are also of interest. In most inflammatory conditions, T cells are present primarily around blood vessels within the dermis and periadnexal adventitia. Migration into the epidermis (exocytosis) is generally accompanied by related pathologic changes affecting adjacent keratinocytes (e.g., spongiosis, apoptosis). In cutaneous T-cell lymphoma, migration of neoplastic lymphocytes into the epidermis is commonly termed "epidermotropism," and spongiosis is usually absent. Although interstitial infiltrates of T cells may occur, this pattern is less commonly encountered. B cells, on the other hand, tend not to migrate into the epidermis. When significant dermal B-cell infiltration exists, nodular aggregates replete with actual lymphoid follicles may develop.

Although T and B cells are indistinguishable by light microscopy, they can be differentiated by *in vitro* tests and immunohistochemical studies. Human T lymphocytes have receptors for sheep erythrocytes (E), so, in the historically important E rosette assay, sheep erythrocytes form rosettes around T lymphocytes (287,288). Antibodies are available for the identification of T cells and B cells in routine paraffin sections (e.g., CD3 for T cells and L26 [CD20] and CD79a for B cells). Immunohistochemically specific detection of cell surface glycoproteins that correlate with T-cell functional subsets (CD4 for helper/inducer, CD8 for cytotoxic/suppressor) is also possible on paraffin-embedded tissues. The T-cell receptor (TCR) consists of either $\alpha\beta$ or $\gamma\delta$ heterodimer expressed on the cell surface in association with CD3. The majority of the peripheral T lymphocytes express the $\alpha\beta$ TCR and are CD4$^+$ or CD8$^+$. In 1970, Gershon and Kondo (289) and, in 2007, Sakaguchi et al. (290) observed that T cells not only augmented but also dampened immune responses and that this downregulation was mediated by T cells that were different from helper T cells. The phenotype of suppressor T cells corresponded for the most part to CD8$^+$, whereas some of them, in particular those suppressing delayed-type hypersensitivity, were CD4$^+$ cells.

There are an estimated 2×10^{10} T cells in the entire integument, almost twice the number of T cells in the circulation (291). These T cells provide protection by patrolling for pathogens and other noxious antigens (292,293). In recent years, interest has been rekindled in the biology of T cells resident in the skin (294). In 2003, the replicative potential of resident T cells in healthy-appearing "normal" human skin exposed to a diverse array of immunologic stimuli was established (295). More recently, it has been shown that noncirculating pools of resident CD8$^+$ T cells are abundant in human skin and are capable of cytotoxic responses against certain microbes, such as vaccinia (292). Such local cutaneous T-cell responses can initiate and perpetuate immune reactions in the absence of T-cell recruitment from the blood (291). Resident memory T cells in the skin also have been shown to respond to Herpes simplex virus (HSV) infection, where the CD8$^+$ phenotype mediates epidermal involvement, and the CD4$^+$ subset is involved in deeper dermal interactions. Moreover, skin immunity regulated by resident memory T cells may be suppressed by the influx of recipient circulating FoxP3+ regulatory T cells (T$_{reg}$) that express skin-homing receptors (296). T$_{reg}$ are a subset of T lymphocytes that express CD25 (IL-2 receptor), as well as the FoxP3 marker, in addition to CD4. Such "regulatory" T cells serve to limit/suppress the immune response and may be detected in tissue by conventional immunohistochemical markers (290).

An additional lymphocytic lineage closely related to T cells is composed of the natural killer (NK) cells. These cells represent approximately 10% of the circulating lymphocytes and are reactive to glycolipids presented in the context of the major histocompatibility complex (MHC) class I-like molecule CD1d. NK cells are characterized by the expression of CD56, CD57, and CD16. They lack B-cell markers and surface CD3 but express cytoplasmic CD3ε. They are usually CD4$^-$/CD8$^-$ but can rarely express CD8. NK cells do not demonstrate rearrangement of immunoglobulin heavy-chain genes or TCR genes (297).

T cells play an important role in normal cutaneous immunosurveillance and in delayed hypersensitivity reactions. Initial antigen uptake by Langerhans cells occurs during sensitization. After their migration to draining lymph nodes via dermal lymphatics (see later discussion), Langerhans cells present antigen to naive T cells, which undergo initial clonal expansion to become memory cells. In the challenge reaction, the dermal microvascular unit is activated (possibly in part owing to mast cell degranulation stimulated by antigen-specific IgE-like molecules generated during sensitization) (298), resulting in display of leukocyte adhesion molecules on the endothelial luminal surface that facilitate the recruitment of antigen-specific, skin-homing memory T cells. On local antigen presentation at the challenge site, these pioneer memory cells, now capable of antigen recognition, respond by elaboration of a cascade of cytokines that result in recruitment of secondary inflammatory cells.

The B lymphocyte is the effector cell of humoral immunity. On antigenic stimulation, the primary follicles in lymph nodes, composed of small B lymphocytes, develop into secondary follicles, consisting of a germinal center surrounded by a rim of small B lymphocytes (285). In the germinal centers, small B lymphocytes enlarge through an intermediate stage of centrocytes with cleaved nuclei into centroblasts, which are large cells with noncleaved nuclei (299). The centroblasts become immunoblasts as a result of antigenic stimulation and produce a clone of daughter cells that mature into immunoglobulin-secreting plasma cells (300,301). The differentiation of B lymphocytes into plasma cells is facilitated by helper T cells and is suppressed by suppressor T cells (302). The plasma cells collect in the medullary cords of lymph nodes without entering the bloodstream but secrete immunoglobulins that circulate as "humoral" antibodies. Although these events occur most commonly in lymph nodes, identical alterations may take place in the dermis in response to locally introduced antigen, as is the case in cutaneous lymphoid hyperplasia with prominent germinal center formation (303,304). In clonal neoplasms of B cells, there may be an arrest at any of these differentiation stages, producing a monotonous infiltrate typical of the various categories of lymphoma cutis (see Chapter 31).

Plasma Cells

Plasma cells have an abundant cytoplasm that is deeply basophilic, homogeneous, and sharply defined. The round nucleus is eccentrically placed, and along its membrane, it shows coarse, deeply basophilic, regularly distributed chromatin particles, which give the nucleus a cartwheel appearance (Fig. 3-44D). The fact that patients with agammaglobulinemia lack plasma cells was responsible for early recognition of the fact that the plasma cell is the site of formation of all immunoglobulins that circulate as humoral antibodies. The synthesis of immunoglobulins takes place in plasma cells located mainly in the lymph nodes, the spleen, and the bone marrow. Because plasma cells are tissue cells and are not seen in the peripheral circulation, it can be assumed that, if they are present in the dermis, they have developed there from B lymphocytes. Intracytoplasmic immunoglobulins may be demonstrated immunohistochemically in paraffin-embedded tissue. Subclassification of cells according to κ (approximately two-thirds of reactive plasma cells) and γ (approximately one-third of reactive plasma cells) is also possible and may, in some instances, facilitate detection of a neoplastic clone where only one of the light chains is produced exclusively. On electron microscopy, plasma cells are characterized by the presence in their cytoplasm of an extensive system of cisternae lined by a ribosome-associated rough endoplasmic reticulum.

Plasma cells are apt to be present in conspicuous numbers in several infectious diseases, such as early syphilis, rhinoscleroma, and granuloma inguinale (see Chapters 21 and 22). In the presence of many plasma cells, but especially in rhinoscleroma, round, hyaline, eosinophilic bodies, called Russell bodies, may be found inside and outside of plasma cells. They form within plasma cells as the result of a very active synthesis of immunoglobulins and may ultimately completely replace the plasma cells in which they have formed (305). They may possess a size twice that of normal plasma cells, measuring up to 20 μm in diameter. They contain varying amounts of glycoproteins and are as a rule gram positive as well as PAS positive and diastase resistant (306). Russell bodies are initiated by intracisternal secretion, analogous to the secretion of immunoglobulins. When the plasma cell is overloaded with this material, first, the nucleus and, ultimately, the entire cell lyses (305). Immunofluorescence and immunohistochemical stains show the presence of immunoglobulins within the Russell bodies, especially on their surface (307,308).

Dermal Muscle Cells
Smooth Muscle
Smooth or involuntary muscle of the skin occurs as arrectores pilorum, tunica dartos of the external genitals, and in the areola of the nipples. The muscle fibers of the arrectores pilorum arise in the connective tissue of the upper dermis and are attached to the hair follicle below the sebaceous glands (Fig. 3-26). They are situated in the obtuse angle of the hair follicle. Thus, when contracted, they pull the hair follicle into a vertical position and produce the perifollicular elevations of "gooseflesh."

Smooth muscle is characterized by the absence of striation and by the location of the nucleus in the center of the muscle cell. Typically, the nuclei are cigar shaped with rounded ends, a feature that may be diagnostically helpful in assessing dermal spindle cell proliferations and neoplasms. Argyrophilic reticulum fibers surround each muscle cell. Electron microscopic examination reveals that smooth muscle cells possess a basement membrane peripheral to the plasma membrane. The cytoplasm of the cells is filled with myofilaments 5 nm in diameter that form cytoplasmic and peripheral dense bodies as a result

of condensations, just as the myofilaments do in myoepithelial cells, vascular smooth muscle cells, and glomus cells. The rather narrow spaces between the muscle cells are occupied by collagen fibrils and by Schwann cells with associated nonmyelinated axons.

Smooth muscle cells contain vimentin and desmin as intermediate filaments and smooth muscle actin (240).

Striated Muscle
Striated or voluntary muscle is found in the skin of the neck as platysma and in the skin of the face as muscles of expression. The striated muscle bundles take their origin either from a fascia or from the periosteum, or they form a closed ring, as in the musculus sphincter oris. They extend through the subcutaneous tissue into the lower dermis (see Fig. 3-62C). The muscle fibers, like skeletal muscle, show characteristic cytoplasmic cross-striations. Their nuclei are located at the periphery of the fibers immediately beneath the sarcolemma, the limiting membrane of the fibers.

Extracellular Matrix
The extracellular matrix of the dermis consists of three components:

- Collagen fibers
- Elastic fibers
- Ground substance

All the three components are formed by fibroblasts. Collagenous and elastic fibers are embedded within the ground substance.

Collagen Fibers
Collagen represents by far the most abundant constituent of the connective tissue of the dermis. On light microscopy, collagen consists of fibers (Figs. 3-47 to 3-50). The diameter of collagen fibers is quite variable, ranging from 2 to 15 μm. The collagen fibers are present either as a finely woven network or as thick bundles. Collagen as a finely woven meshwork of collagen fibers is found in the papillary layer of the dermis, which includes not only the subepidermal papillae situated between the rete ridges, but also the subpapillary layer forming a narrow ribbon between the rete ridges and the subpapillary blood vessels (Figs. 3-5, 3-47, and 3-50B). This is referred to as the papillary dermis. In addition, the pilosebaceous units and the eccrine and apocrine glands are encircled by a thin meshwork of collagen fibers similar to that present in the papillary dermis. Therefore, the papillary and the periadnexal dermis is regarded as an anatomic unit, the adventitial dermis. The blood vessels of the dermis are also surrounded by a thin layer of fine collagen fibers. Biochemically, the papillary dermis is composed primarily of type III collagen.

The rest of the dermis, constituting by far the largest portion of the dermis and referred to as the reticular dermis, shows the collagen fibers united into thick bundles (Figs. 3-40A and 3-47). These collagen bundles extend horizontally in various directions, and thus some are cut lengthwise and others across in histologic sections. As a rule, collagen bundles that are cut lengthwise appear slightly wavy. Biochemically, reticular dermal collagen is composed primarily of type I collagen.

Reticulum fibers are not recognizable with routine stains, but, being argyrophilic, they can be impregnated with silver nitrate, which, by being subsequently reduced to silver, stains black. Reticulum fibers represent a special type of thin collagen fiber that measures from 0.2 to 1 μm in diameter. The argyrophilia shown by reticulum fibers, in contrast to collagen fibers, is probably related to the fact that reticulum fibers correspond to the distribution of type III collagen rather than type I collagen.

Argyrophilic reticulum fibers are the first-formed fibers during embryonic life and in various pathologic conditions associated with increased fibroblastic activity. In normal skin, even though collagen is being continuously replaced, the formation of new collagen is not preceded by an argyrophilic phase. Instead, all newly formed collagen consists of large fibers. However, there are a few areas in which normally small collagen fibers are present as reticulum fibers without transforming into larger, nonargyrophilic collagen fibers. This occurs above all in the basement membrane zone, the region of the adventitial dermis that lies closest to the epidermis and its appendages. In addition, reticulum fibers are present normally around blood vessels and as a basket-like capsule around each fat cell.

The biosynthesis of collagen begins within the fibroblast by the assembly of three pro–α-polypeptide chains into a triple-helical procollagen molecule (233). After excretion into the extracellular space, the three pro-α chains of each procollagen molecule are shortened by 30% to 40% through the removal of the carboxy-terminal and amino-terminal peptide extensions brought about by the action of two enzymes produced by the fibroblast: carboxy-terminal peptidase and amino-terminal peptidase (232). This results in conversion of the procollagen molecule into the collagen molecule. Although the additional peptides present in procollagen keep it soluble and prevent its intracellular polymerization, collagen molecules polymerize readily. The collagen molecule is a rigid rod in which each of the three coiled α chains consists of about 1,000 amino acids (233). The collagen molecule is about 300 nm long and 1.5 nm wide (309–311). Collagen fibrils form by both lateral and longitudinal association of collagen molecules. However, the collagen fibrils vary in diameter as a result of varying degrees of polymerization of collagen molecules, with younger collagen fibrils being thinner than older fibrils. In the normal dermis, the thickness of collagen fibrils ranges from 70 to 140 nm; most of the fibrils are approximately 100 nm thick (312).

Collagen fibrils possess characteristic cross-striations with a periodicity of 68 nm. The periodicity of the cross-striations in the collagen fibrils can be explained as follows. Each collagen molecule possesses along its length of 300 nm five charged regions 68 nm apart, and although neighboring collagen molecules overlap each other, they always have their charged regions lying side by side. This parallel alignment of the charged regions produces the cross-striations (310). Reticulum fibrils possess the same 68-nm periodicity of their cross-striations as collagen fibrils but have a smaller diameter than collagen fibrils, varying between 40 and 65 nm rather than between 70 and 140 nm (313). Furthermore, reticulum and collagen differ in the number of fibrils present in the cross section of each fiber and in the amount of ground substance present within and around each fiber. The amount of ground substance around the fibrils and on the surface of the fiber may explain the presence of argyrophilia in reticulum fibers and its absence in collagen fibers (313).

Seven types of collagen have been recognized that differ in composition and antigenicity. Type I collagen, the predominant collagen in postfetal skin, is found in the large fiber bundles of the reticular dermis. Reticulum fibers are composed of type III collagen. Although type III collagen is the prevalent type of collagen in early fetal life, in postfetal life it is limited to the subepidermal and periappendageal regions, that is, the basement membrane zones and the perivascular region or the "papillary" and "adventitial" dermis (314). Basement membrane collagen (basal lamina collagen) is type IV, and the collagen of cartilage is type II. Type V collagen has been recognized in fetal membranes and vascular tissue (315). Type VI collagen is a major component of microfibrils and is important in muscle function. Type VII collagen occurs in different basement membranes, including those of the skin, and forms a major structural component of anchoring fibrils (316). The skin of the human fetus contains a large percentage of type III collagen, in contrast to the skin of the adult, which contains a large proportion of type I collagen (317).

Among the differences in composition relevant to collagen in skin are the following. In type I collagen, the three α chains in the collagen molecule consist of two different kinds: two identical α chains designated as α-1(I) and a third chain called α-2. In type II collagen, the collagen molecules are composed of three identical, genetically distinct α chains, α-1(II). Type III collagen is also composed of three identical, distinct α chains (232). Type IV collagen consists of procollagen composed of three identical pro-α chains that have retained their nonhelical extensions. Type VII collagen consists of three α chains, with the terminal regions being noncollagenous (316).

Elastic Fibers

Elastic fibers appear in the dermis at 22 weeks, much later than the collagen fibers. At this time, acid orcein stains show elastic tissue in the reticular dermis either as granular material interspersed with occasional short fibers or as a delicate network of branching fibers. As gestation progresses, elastic fibers increase in quantity. At 32 weeks, a well-developed network of elastic fibers indistinguishable from that seen in term infants is present in both the papillary and the reticular dermis (318). Young elastic fibers, as seen in a 22-week-old fetal dermis, show masses of peripheral microfibrils surrounding a small, amorphous, electron-lucent core representing elastin, with only a few internal microfibrils. As the embryo matures, the amount of elastin and the number of microfibrils within the elastin increase, whereas the number of peripheral microfibrils decreases (319).

In light microscopic sections that are routinely stained, elastic fibers are inconspicuous. With special elastic tissue stains, such as orcein or resorcin-fuchsin, or in plastic-embedded sections they are found entwined among the collagen bundles (Fig. 3-48). Because elastic fibers are thin in comparison with collagen bundles, measuring from 1 to 3 μm in diameter, and are wavy, only a small portion of any fiber is seen in histologic sections, giving even normal elastic fibers a fragmented appearance. The elastic fibers are thickest in the lower portion of the dermis, where they are arranged, like collagen bundles, chiefly parallel to the surface of the skin. Elastic fibers become thinner as they approach the epidermis. In the papillary dermis, they form an intermediate plexus of thinner elaunin fibers running parallel to the dermal–epidermal junction (Fig. 3-48). From this plexus, thin fibers termed oxytalan fibers run upward in the papillary dermis perpendicular to the dermal–epidermal junction and terminate at the PAS-positive basement membrane zone.

The elastic fibers of the dermis consist of two components: the microfibrils and the matrix elastin. The microfibrils are electron dense and measure 10 to 12 nm in diameter. They are aggregated at the periphery of the elastic fiber, giving the fiber its characteristic frayed appearance by ultrastructure. In addition, microfibrils are present within the elastin as strands 15 to 80 nm in diameter extending in a longitudinal direction (311). The microfibril component amounts to only 15% of the elastic fiber, whereas the amorphous, electron-lucid elastin makes up 85% of the fiber (319). It is the elastin that stains with elastic tissue stains, is removable by elastase, and is markedly extensible, whereas the microfibrils are the elastic resilient component of the elastic fiber (320).

Elastic fibers undergo significant changes during life. One change, representing aging, is best studied in nonexposed skin. The other change, elastotic degeneration, is the result of chronic sun exposure and is described in Chapter 15. In young children up to the age of 10 years, the elastic fibers may not be fully matured, so that microfibrils predominate (321). Physiologic aging is a gradual process and usually becomes quite apparent by age 30 to 50 years. There is a gradual decrease in the number of peripheral microfibrils so that ultimately there may be none; instead, the surface of the elastic fiber appears irregular and granular (312). The microfibrils within the elastin matrix become thicker and show electron-lucent holes of varying sizes (322). In very old persons, fragmentation and disintegration of some of the elastic fibers may be observed. Oxytalan fibers that consist of microfibrils diminish and ultimately disappear in aging skin.

Ground Substance

The ground substance, an amorphous substance that fills the spaces between collagen fibers and collagen bundles, contains glycosaminoglycans, or acid mucopolysaccharides (Fig. 3-49). These glycosaminoglycans are covalently linked to peptide chains to form high-molecular-weight complexes called proteoglycans (323). Glycosaminoglycans are present in normal skin in such small amounts that they cannot be demonstrated with either routine or special histologic staining methods except in the hair papilla of anagen hair, which contains both nonsulfated and sulfated acid mucopolysaccharides. However, through the study of tissues with an active growth of fibroblasts, as seen in the papillary dermis in dermatofibroma and in the connective tissue around the tumor islands of basal cell epithelioma, it is known that the dermal ground substance consists largely of nonsulfated acid mucopolysaccharides such as hyaluronic acid (174). In healing wounds, however, in which new collagen is laid down, the ground substance contains sulfated and nonsulfated acid mucopolysaccharides (324).

The nonsulfated acid mucopolysaccharides consist largely of hyaluronic acid, are stainable with alcian blue at pH 3.0 but not at pH 0.5, and show metachromasia with toluidine blue at pH 3.0 but not at pH 1.5. The sulfated acid mucopolysaccharides consist largely of chondroitin sulfate, are stainable with alcian blue at pH 0.5 and at pH 3.0, and show metachromasia with toluidine blue at pH 1.5 and at pH 3.0. Both nonsulfated and sulfated acid mucopolysaccharides stain with colloidal iron. Testicular hyaluronidase hydrolyzes hyaluronic acid but not the sulfated acid mucopolysaccharides (174).

Dermal Microvascular Unit

Not long ago, the dermis was considered to be a leathery cutaneous layer primarily responsible for housing and protecting vessels that served to nourish the keratinizing epidermis. Today, we realize that the dermis is a dynamic microenvironment containing a repertoire of cells and matrix molecules arguably more complex and sophisticated than the epidermis and its appendages. The dermal microvascular unit is the heart of this new concept of the dermis, for it represents an intricate assemblage of cells responsible not only for cutaneous nutrition but also for immune cell trafficking, regulation of vessel tone, and local hemostasis.

Endothelial Cells
General Microanatomy

The dermal microvasculature is divided into two important strata. The first, the superficial vascular plexus, defines the boundary between the papillary and the reticular dermis and extends within an adventitial mantle to envelop adnexal structures (Figs. 3-5 and 3-50A). This plexus forms a layer of anastomosing arterioles and venules in close approximation to the overlying epidermis and is normally surrounded by other cellular components of the dermal microvascular unit (see later discussion). Small capillary loops emanate from the superficial vascular plexus and extend into each dermal papilla (Fig. 3-50B, C). The second plexus—the deep vascular plexus—is connected to the first by vertically oriented reticular dermal vessels and separates the reticular dermis from the subcutaneous fat. Many of these vessels are of larger caliber and communicate with branches that extend within fibrous septae that separate lobules of underlying subcutaneous fat.

The small arteries of the deep vascular plexus and the arterioles of the dermis possess three layers: an intima, composed of endothelial cells, and an internal elastic lamina that stains for elastic tissue; a media, which contains two or more layers of muscle cells in the small arteries but only a single layer of muscle cells in the arterioles of the lower dermis and a discontinuous layer of muscle cells in the arterioles of the upper dermis; and an adventitia of connective tissue (325) (Fig. 3-51A). The capillaries that are present throughout the dermis, but especially in the papillary dermis, are composed of a layer of endothelial cells surrounded by an incomplete layer of pericytes. A basement membrane, which stains positive with PAS, is present peripheral to the endothelial cells and surrounds the pericytes. There is alkaline phosphatase activity in the endothelial cells of all capillaries (326). Staining for alkaline phosphatase thus clearly demonstrates the capillary loop in each subepidermal dermal papilla, with the ascending, arterial limb of the loop staining more heavily than the descending, venous limb. The abundant capillaries present in the hair papillae of anagen hairs also stain heavily (175,326).

The walls of veins are generally thinner than those of arteries and less clearly divided into the three classic layers (Fig. 3-51B). The postcapillary venules resemble capillaries because they consist of endothelial cells, pericytes, and a basement membrane (Fig. 3-50C). The arteriolar and venous segments can be distinguished from each other on the basis of the basement membrane, which has a homogeneous appearance in the former and is multilaminated in the latter. Furthermore, terminal arterioles have elastin and smooth muscle cells in their walls, whereas postcapillary venules have only pericytes in their walls (327). The capillary loops leading from the subpapillary plexus to the dermal papillae and back can be divided into an intrapapillary portion and an extrapapillary portion. The extrapapillary ascending limb and the intrapapillary portion have the characteristics of an arterial capillary, that is, a homogeneous basement membrane, whereas the extrapapillary descending limb has venous characteristics, that is, a multilayered basement membrane (328). Although some investigators have observed areas of fenestration at the tips of the capillary loops between the endothelial cells (329), others have failed to find them (328). Endothelial cells characteristically show a well-developed endoplasmic reticulum, bundles of fairly thick cytoplasmic filaments with a diameter of 5 to 10 nm, and many pinocytotic vesicles at their luminal surface. Frequently, one can observe in endothelial cells a unique structure, the Weibel–Palade body. It is an electron-dense, rod-shaped cytoplasmic organelle measuring approximately 0.1 μm in diameter and up to 3 μm in length. It is composed of a number of small tubules, approximately 15 nm thick, arranged in the long axis of the rod (329). Peripheral to the endothelium lies a basement membrane. The peripheral row of cells—the pericytes—have long cytoplasmic processes and form a discontinuous layer. They are completely surrounded by the capillary basement membrane. In larger capillaries, more than one layer of pericytes may be present, and transitional forms between pericytes and smooth muscle cells may be seen (330).

Endothelial cells of blood capillaries contain α-L-fucose, which can be demonstrated with *Ulex europaeus* (331), and they contain factor VIII–related antigen. *U. europaeus* and an antibody against factor VIII–related antigen have been used as endothelial markers for the identification of neoplastic endothelial cells. Endothelial cells also express CD31 (332,333), a marker that may be the most sensitive for normal and neoplastic endothelial cells. In addition, endothelial cells of blood capillaries contain class I antigens (HLA-A, B, C) and class II antigen (HLA-DR) (334). HLA-DR is considered to play a role in antigen presentation and elicitation of an immune response (335), and endothelial cells and perivascular dermal dendritic cells are capable of dermal antigen presentation (see later discussion). Laminin and type IV collagen are present within the vascular basement membranes. Blood capillaries contain vimentin intermediate filaments.

Specialized Structure and Function

Recent evidence indicates that endothelial cells are active participants in transmural shuttling of macromolecules, as well as facilitators of normal and pathologic trafficking of immune cells. The luminal surface of the endothelial cell that lines the superficial postcapillary venule is the primary site of adhesive interactions that initiate subsequent diapedesis of leukocytes. The outer membrane of the Weibel–Palade body contains a glycoprotein termed CD62, which is rapidly transported to the luminal endothelial membrane on exposure to histamine or thrombin (336,337). This molecule mediates the initial loose rolling adhesion between circulating leukocytes and the endothelial surface. Subsequently, other cytokine-inducible glycoproteins are expressed in a cascade (E-selectin, vascular cell adhesion molecule-1, intercellular adhesion molecule-1) on the endothelial surface, resulting in orchestrated and progressively stable leukocyte-endothelial adhesion (338–342). Some luminal molecules that are constitutively and diffusely expressed (e.g., CD31) redistribute to cell–cell junctions on endothelial stimulation, thus creating a situation potentially conducive to concentrating adherent leukocytes at sites where transmural diapedesis may occur (342). Provocative signals for such events may come from

inflammatory cells themselves or from native cells in the perivascular space (see Mast Cells, earlier discussion).

Glomus Cells

A special vascular structure, the glomus, is located within the reticular dermis in certain areas. Glomus formations occur most abundantly in the pads and nail beds of the fingers and toes but also elsewhere on the volar aspect of the hands and feet, in the skin of the ears, and in the center of the face (Fig. 3-52A). The glomus is concerned with temperature regulation and represents a special arteriovenous shunt that, without the interposition of capillaries, connects an arteriole with a venule. When open, these shunts cause a great increase in blood flow in the area. Each glomus consists of an arterial and a venous segment. The arterial segment, called the Sucquet–Hoyer canal, branches from an arteriole and has a narrow lumen and a thick wall measuring 20 to 40 μm in diameter. The wall shows a single layer of endothelium, surrounded by a PAS-positive, diastase-resistant basement membrane zone, and a media that is densely packed with four to six layers of glomus cells (Fig. 3-52B). These are large cells with a clear cytoplasm resembling epithelioid cells. Although myofibrils cannot be recognized within glomus cells with light microscopic staining methods, these cells have generally been regarded as smooth muscle cells (343). Peripheral to the glomus cells is a zone of loose connective tissue. Staining with silver salts or antineurofilament antibody shows many nerve fibers extending to the glomus cells within this zone. The venous segment of the glomus is thin walled and has a wide lumen. This wide collecting venule functions as a reservoir and drains into a dermal venule. As many as four Sucquet–Hoyer canals may be found in a single glomus body, which is encapsulated (344).

Electron microscopic study of the Sucquet–Hoyer canal reveals the glomus cells to be vascular smooth muscle cells. As such, each glomus cell is surrounded by a basement membrane. The cytoplasm of the glomus cells is filled with filaments with a diameter of about 5 nm. Cytoplasmic and peripheral dense bodies, 300 to 400 nm in diameter, are present in the glomus cells as a result of condensations of the myofilaments. Numerous nonmyelinated nerves ensheathed by Schwann cells are present peripheral to the glomus cells (345) (Fig. 3-52C).

Dermal Lymphatics

Dermal lymphatics are often inconspicuous in normal skin because they do not have a well-developed wall, as is the case with blood vessels. They are easily detected, however, when they become slightly ectatic as a result of increased lymphatic drainage, as in urticaria. Lymph vessels are typically not rounded in contour, but instead show angulations dictated by the fact that their lining lymphatics are buttressed by adjacent collagen bundles (Fig. 3-51C). In normal skin, the perilymphatic space is relatively devoid of other cells, and the lumen is lined by relatively flattened endothelial cells. Occasional valves may be observed emanating from the endothelial lining. By electron microscopy, the thin layer of endothelium does not contain Weibel–Palade bodies and is devoid of a basement membrane or surrounding pericytes. Lymphatic vessels show a negative or weakly positive reaction when incubated with *U. europaeus* and no reaction with an antibody against factor VIII–related antigen in most instances. They do not contain class I (HLA-A, B, C) or class II

(HLA-DR) antigens (325). Endothelial cells of lymphatic vessels contain cytoplasmic filaments (346), which probably represent vimentin filaments. Like vascular endothelial cells, they stain positively with CD312. Lymphatic vessels contain podoplanin and can be specifically labeled using an antibody such as D2-40 or LYVE-1 (346).

Neural Network

In sections stained with routine methods, one can recognize only the larger myelinated nerve bundles and the Meissner and Vater–Pacini end organs. The finer nerves require special staining, and, accordingly, the critical importance of these structures to cutaneous homeostasis and pathology has been overlooked. Among the staining methods used are impregnation with silver salts (347), vital staining with methylene blue (348), and *in vitro* staining of thick sections with methylene blue (349). More recently, nerves have been identified by the S100 technique (Fig. 3-53A) and by using antibodies to specific neurofilaments, neuropeptides, and adhesion molecules (neural cell adhesion molecule 1). Nerves are composed of neuraxons, a cytoplasmic process that conducts neural impulses from cell bodies in the central nervous system, and Schwann cells (sheath cells or neurilemmal cells) enveloping the neuraxons (Fig. 3-53A,B). This primary functioning unit may or may not be myelinated and is surrounded by an endoneurium—a mucinous or fibrous matrix containing fibroblasts—which supports the primary functioning unit. A perineurium composed of elongated, flattened cells surrounds several primary functioning units and their endoneurial matrix (350).

The skin is supplied with sensory nerves and autonomic nerves, which permeate the entire dermis with nerve fibers and show frequent branching. Sensory and autonomic nerves differ in that sensory nerves possess a myelin sheath up to their terminal ramifications, but autonomic nerves do not. The autonomic nerves, derived from the sympathetic nervous system, supply the blood vessels, the arrectores pilorum, and the eccrine and apocrine glands. The sebaceous glands possess no autonomic innervation, and their functioning depends on endocrine stimuli. All autonomic nerves end in fine arborizations. So do the sensory nerves, except in a few areas in which there are, in addition to fine arborizations, special nerve end organs. Hair follicles, especially large hair follicles, are also surrounded below the entry of the sebaceous duct by a network of sensory nerves that lose their myelin sheaths a short distance from the outer root sheath and end in numerous arborizations of fine nonmyelinated fibers.

The papillary dermis is richly invested in unmyelinated nerve fibers, particularly about the dermal microvascular unit, where axons often terminate in proximity to mast cells (351). This relationship is of interest inasmuch as small neurosecretory granules within axons contain a variety of mediators, including neuropeptides that may serve as mast cell secretagogues, such as substance P. The development of confocal scanning laser microscopy has permitted the assessment of complicated spatial relationships between axons and skin cells. Recently, superficial dermal axons containing another neuropeptide, CGRP, were documented to enter the epidermis and to associate selectively with the cell bodies of Langerhans cells (352). Substance P–induced mast cell degranulation may elicit expression of endothelial-leukocyte adhesion molecules and thus be proinflammatory (353), and CGRP has been shown to diminish antigen presentation by Langerhans cells (354). Thus, the superficial dermal plexus of unmyelinated axons may represent

a heretofore unappreciated influence of normal and perturbed cutaneous immunity.

Special Nerve End Organs

In the areas of hairless skin on the palms and the soles and in the areas of modified hairless skin at the mucocutaneous junctions, some of the sensory nerves end in special nerve end organs. They are of three types: mucocutaneous end organs, Meissner corpuscles (Fig. 3-54A,B), and Vater–Pacini corpuscles (Fig. 3-55). Although it is customary to speak of them as end organs, they actually represent starting organs in a functional sense because nerve impulses start there and are transmitted to the sensory cells of the spinal cord (355).

The mucocutaneous end organs, which are on average 50 µm in diameter, are found in the modified hairless skin at the mucocutaneous junctions, namely, the glans, the prepuce, the clitoris, the labia minora, the perianal region, and the vermilion border of the lip. They are in the papillary dermis. They cannot be recognized in routinely stained sections, in contrast to the Meissner corpuscles in the dermal papillae. Impregnation with silver nitrate reveals that from two to six myelinated nerve fibers enter each mucocutaneous end organ and, after losing their myelin sheaths, form many loops of nerve fibers, resembling an irregularly wound ball of yarn. The electron microscopic features of mucocutaneous end organs are similar to those of Meissner corpuscles (356), despite minor differences in their light microscopic appearance. They show a subdivision into lobules, each containing a complex arrangement of axon terminals. These axon terminals are surrounded by concentric lamellar processes derived from so-called laminar cells, the nuclei of which are situated toward the periphery of the lobules. It is assumed that the laminar cells represent modified Schwann cells. The mucocutaneous end organs are always separated from the basal layer of the epidermis by a band of papillary dermal collagen.

Meissner corpuscles are located in dermal papillae (Fig. 3-54A, B) and mediate a sense of touch. They occur exclusively on the ventral aspects of the hands and feet, their number increasing distally. There are more Meissner corpuscles on the hands than on the feet. At the site of their greatest concentration, the fingertips, approximately every fourth papilla contains a Meissner corpuscle. The size of the Meissner corpuscles averages 30 by 80 µm in diameter. Owing to their size and their elongated shape, resembling that of a pine cone, they occupy the greater part of the papilla in which they are located. They possess a capsule composed of several layers of flattened Schwann cells that are arranged transverse to the long axis of the corpuscle. Impregnation with silver salts reveals that several myelinated nerves, as they approach the base or the side of the corpuscle, lose their myelin sheaths and then enter it. Within the corpuscle, the nerves take a meandering course upward. Electron microscopic studies reveal that the principal part of the Meissner corpuscle is made up of irregular layers of flattened, greatly elongated laminar cells. The nuclei of the laminar cells are located largely at the periphery of the corpuscle. The axons terminating within the Meissner corpuscle are surrounded by slender processes of the laminar cells. This enveloping of axons by laminar cells or their lamellar processes is analogous to the enveloping of axons by infolding of the plasma membrane of Schwann cells and indicates that the laminar cells are modified Schwann cells (357). The axon terminals and laminar cells are in direct contact with the epidermal basal cells at the upper end of the Meissner corpuscle without interposition of a basement membrane (358).

Vater–Pacini corpuscles are large nerve end organs that are located in the subcutis and mediate a sense of pressure. They measure up to 1 mm in diameter and are thus detected easily by light microscopy (Fig. 3-55). They are found most commonly below the skin of the volar aspects of the palms and soles, showing their greatest concentration at the tips of the fingers and toes. In addition, a few Vater–Pacini corpuscles occur in the subcutis of the nipple and of the anogenital region (356). Vater–Pacini corpuscles vary in shape. Some are ovoid, others have the appearance of a flattened sphere, and still others have an irregular shape. They consist of a stalk and of the body proper, the latter having a small core and a thick capsule. In the stalk, the single thick nerve supplying the Vater–Pacini corpuscle makes several turns and, just after entering the stalk, loses its myelin sheath. The core shows a granular substance surrounding the ascending meandering nerve. The thick capsule consists of 30 or more concentric, loosely arranged lamellae. On electron microscopic examination, the single nerve fiber present in the inner portion of the core retains its Schwann cell cytoplasmic covering for a short distance. The outer portion of the core shows closely packed, greatly elongated laminar cells. The thick capsule consists of at least 30 layers of flattened laminar cells separated from one another by fluid-filled spaces (359). The laminar cells of the Vater–Pacini corpuscle, analogous to those of the Meissner corpuscle, are modified Schwann cells.

SUBCUTANEOUS FAT

Fat cells begin to develop in the subcutaneous tissue toward the end of the fifth month. Histologic examination at that time shows (a) spindle-shaped, lipid-free mesenchymal cells as precursor cells, (b) young-type fat cells containing two or more small lipid droplets, and (c) mature fat cells possessing one large central lipid droplet and a peripherally located nucleus, so-called signet-ring cells. Although some of the cells containing multiple small lipid droplets resemble the multivacuolated mulberry cells present in brown fat and in hibernoma, only few such cells occur in embryonic white fat. Brown and white fat are two separate entities incapable of interconversion (360).

Mature subcutaneous fat consists of lobules composed of adipocytes with cytoplasm markedly expanded by nonvacuolated or membrane-bound lipid that displaces the cell nucleus eccentrically to produce a thin, fusiform contour compressed along the inner plasma membrane. The lipid dissolves in routinely processed specimens, although it is visible in glutaraldehyde-fixed, plastic-embedded specimens. It may be stained histochemically in frozen section obtained from fresh or "wet" tissue retrieved while still in formalin. The lobules that form the subcutis are separated by thin fibrous septae through which small vessels course (Fig. 3-56). The septae provide structural stability to the subcutaneous layer by compartmentalizing it and by connecting the lowermost reticular dermis to the fascial planes that underlie the subcutis.

CUTANEOUS STEM CELLS

Epidermal Stem Cells

Only the subset of cells termed "stem cells" retain the capability of self-renewal and differentiation required to potentially reconstitute the epidermis and cutaneous appendages after injury or

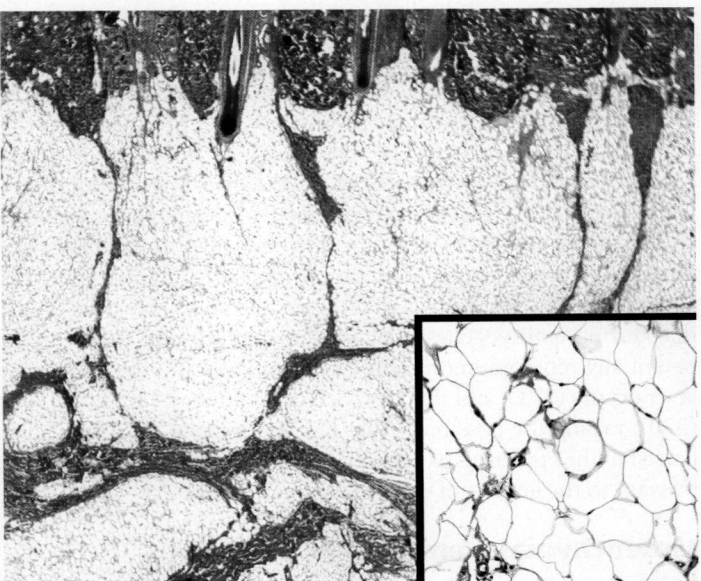

Figure 3-56 Low-power view of the subcutaneous tissue. Lobules of adipose tissue are separated by fibrous septa. Inset: A higher-power view of a subcutaneous lobule.

depletion (361,362). They participate in tissue repair and, more recently, have been of great interest with regard to tissue regeneration and neoplasia. Thus, in the skin they have relevance to a wide variety of disorders where skin is lost or damaged or when it undergoes neoplastic transformation. The epidermal stem cells are located in at least two distinct locations, the basal cell layer of the epidermis and the hair follicle bulge region near the insertion site of the arrector pili muscle. A specialized adjacent compartment, the so-called niche, is composed of a variety of differentiated cell types (363); these provide a microenvironment that allows the stem cells to maintain their unique characteristics, which include (364) the following:

- Normally slow-cycling kinetics
- Ability to self-renew as well as produce progeny that differentiate
- Pluripotency, the ability to form epidermal, dermal, and adnexal structures
- Potential for activation on demand
- Innate protective strategies to prevent apoptosis, toxin influx, and immune-mediated injury

Within the epithelial layers, the bulge stem cell is thought to be of the higher hierarchy in terms of the "stemness" than the epidermal stem cells, because the bulge stem cells can give rise to both the skin and hair epithelia, while the epidermal stem cells differentiate only into the epidermis under physiologic conditions (361,362,364). The bulge stem cells in early development express four key transcription factors: Sox9, Tcf3, Lhx2, and NFATc1 (365). Within several weeks of postnatal life, bulge cells acquire expression of two markers widely: CD34 and cytokeratin 15. In addition, K15, Sox 9, Lgr5, and Lgr6 mark both bulge stem cells and hair germ cells, and these are thus often considered to represent the hair follicle stem cell markers (361,366). However, despite tremendous efforts in identifying epidermal stem cell markers, none can be considered to be specific stem cell markers at this juncture (364). Recent studies, however, have shown a few promising candidates as putative epidermal stem cell markers, including integrins α6 and β1 and Lrig1, Rac1, and p63 in epidermal growth factor receptor (EGFR) pathways (367,368).

Melanocytic Stem Cells

It has been proposed that normal melanocytic stem cells reside in the bulge region of the hair follicle, where they exist as a reservoir for replenishing the epidermis on demand (197,369). Dermal cells with potential for melanocytic differentiation, however, also exist (370). Although rigorous proof that these cells represent primary physiologic stem cells is accruing, whether melanomas arise from altered physiologic stem cells or transform to a more stemlike phenotype as a consequence of mutations affecting a more differentiated melanocyte (or both) remain open questions. We have found that during embryogenesis, significant migration of dermal cells potentially representing melanocyte stem cells into the epidermal layer occurs (371), and this has been substantiated experimentally (370), raising the possibility that rare melanocyte stem cells may persist in the epidermis as potential targets for oncogenic mutation relevant to the genesis of early melanoma (372).

Mesenchymal Stem Cells

Mesenchymal stem cells (MSCs) are multipotent stromal cells that can differentiate into a variety of cell types, including osteoblasts, adipocytes, and chondrocytes *in vitro* (373,374). Recent evidence has suggested that MSCs can transdifferentiate to epidermal cells, keratinocytes, and microvascular endothelial cells under defined conditions *in vitro* (375–377) and that they resemble resident dermal fibroblasts in the wound environment (378). In addition, when under conditions that permit interactions with native epidermal cells, MSCs have been purported to also transdifferentiate into keratinocytes (379). These studies suggest that MSCs could participate directly in the structural regeneration of dermal and epidermal tissues, thus representing an additional mechanism by which the MSCs may promote cutaneous wound healing (380). However, radical transitions of mesenchymal to nonmesenchymal phenotypes must be established with experimental rigor, and confirmatory studies are needed to fully understand the extent of plasticity of MSCs. Finally, recent studies also demonstrate that MSCs are involved in immunosuppressive biochemical signaling in response to inflammatory cytokines by modulating the expression levels of Toll-like receptors (381). MSCs may function similarly to T cells and macrophages by polarizing their phenotype in the context of inflammatory environments (382).

More recent data have demonstrated more precisely that a subpopulation of dermal mesenchymal stem cells (DMSCs) are nondescript by routine staining and are thus likely to be confused with fibroblasts or dendritic macrophages. These recently recognized cells express the multidrug resistance marker, ABCB5, are immunosuppressive, and possess potential differentiation plasticity that appear to promote effective wound healing in experimental models (383).

AGE- AND ENVIRONMENTAL-RELATED VARIATIONS

Structural and functional alterations caused by intrinsic aging and independent of environmental insults are now recognized in the skin of elderly individuals and must be considered a fundamental component of "normal" histology (384). Changes associated with skin aging include a thinner epidermis with flattened dermal–epidermal junction (384–386). The keratinocytes become less adherent to one another and tend to be arranged haphazardly because of the aberrant proliferation of basal cells. Because DMSCs are depleted in older skin, their significance in terms of skin alterations that accompany chronologic aging, as well as their potential for therapeutic manipulation to promote regenerative healing and rejuvenative responses are only now beginning to be explored (387).

The melanocyte density also declines slowly with aging, and a reduction in the number of melanosomes leads to reduced pigmentation (386). Although it is conceptually important to distinguish between the effects of true biologic aging and environmental factors such as sun exposure, the observed changes are, in general, a practical consequence of the combined effect of both. Despite the decreased melanocyte density, photoaged skin has irregular or heterogeneous pigmentation. Heterogeneity in skin color in exposed areas of skin is attributable to uneven distribution of pigment cells. Associated with a local loss of melanocytes are noncontiguous areas where melanocytes are increased in number and size (Fig. 3-17A, B) (388,389). Langerhans cells decrease in number and function with age and chronic sun damage, which partially contributes to age-associated deterioration of the immune system. In general, the dermis becomes atrophic, and it is relatively acellular and avascular. Dermal changes involve alteration and reduction of collagen, elastin, and ground substance. There is attenuation in the number and diameter of elastic fibers in the papillary dermis, an increase in number and thickness of the same fibers in the reticular dermis, and a coarsening of collagen fibers, which become thicker and stiffer (385). Fibroblasts, dendritic cells, and mast cells are reduced in number. In chronically sun-damaged skin, however, the dermis may be rich in cells showing some enlarged, angulated fibroblast/myofibroblast (386). The hallmark of sun-damaged skin is the presence of solar elastosis characterized by a fibrillary basophilic material present in the upper dermis (Fig. 3-57). The elastotic material is composed of elastin, fibronectin, fibrillin (microfibrillary proteins), and

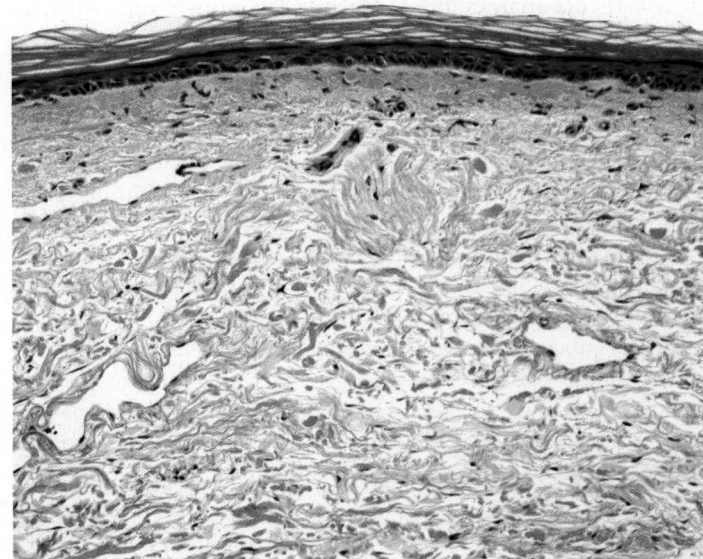

Figure 3-57 Changes associated with skin aging include a thinner epidermis with flattened dermal–epidermal junction and telangiectatic dermal vessels associated with marked solar elastosis in the form of bluish-gray fibers, the latter related to chronic sun damage.

Table 3-5		
Regional Variation of Skin and Potential Diagnostic Pitfalls		
Site	Histologic Features	Diagnostic Pitfalls
Back and trunk	Thick reticular dermis	Morphea, scleroderma
Acral skin (palm and sole)	Compact and thick stratum corneum	Lichen simplex chronicus
Mucosa	Diminished stratum corneum and granulosum; pale, glycogenated cytoplasm; highly vascularized	Ichthyosis, psoriasis, nutritional deficiency, clear cell acanthoma, white sponge nevus; hemangioma
Eyelid	Thin epidermis, basaloid follicular buds, and small rudimentary hairs	Atrophy, basal cell carcinoma
Nose	Prominent sebaceous glands	Sebaceous hyperplasia
Axilla	Apocrine glands, verrucoid epidermis	Nevus sebaceus, keratosis, acanthosis nigricans
Nipple/areola	Numerous smooth muscle fibers, lactiferous ducts	Leiomyoma, eccrine hamartoma
Foreskin/scrotum	Numerous smooth muscle fibers; numerous thin-walled vessels	Leiomyoma
Leg	Relatively thick basement membranes in superficial dermal microvessels	Diabetes, porphyria

glycosaminoglycans. The pathogenesis of solar elastosis is complex and not fully understood, but it appears to include both *de novo* synthesis of elastotic material and degradation of previously synthesized dermal matrix proteins (390).

A consistent finding in aged skin everywhere is the dilation of lymphatic channels, which is especially evident in areas where elastosis has taken place (354) (Fig. 3-57). Eccrine and apocrine glands are reduced in number and function. Sebaceous glands may remain unchanged or may increase in size; they are, however, less active (384). There is a progressive reduction in the density of hair follicles per unit area on the face and scalp and a decline in the rate of growth. The hair shaft diameter is generally reduced, but in some areas, especially the ears, nose, and eyebrows of men and the upper lip and chin in women, it is increased as vellus hairs convert to cosmetically compromising terminal hairs (384).

The subcutaneous tissue is diminished in some areas, especially the face, shins, hands, and feet, whereas in others, particularly the abdomen in men and the thighs in women, it is increased (384).

The nail plate is generally thinned, the surface ridged and lusterless, and the lunula decreased in size; these structural changes are associated with a slowing of the rate of nail growth (384).

REGIONAL VARIATION OF THE SKIN

As a final consideration in the context of the many different components of the skin discussed to this point, it is important to emphasize that although the skin has basically the same components at different anatomic sites, the distribution of these components is variable, so that recognition of different background morphologies at different sites is important to avoid diagnostic pitfalls (Table 3-5). The skin of the trunk and especially the back has a significantly thicker reticular dermis compared with that of other regions (Fig. 3-58), and the skin

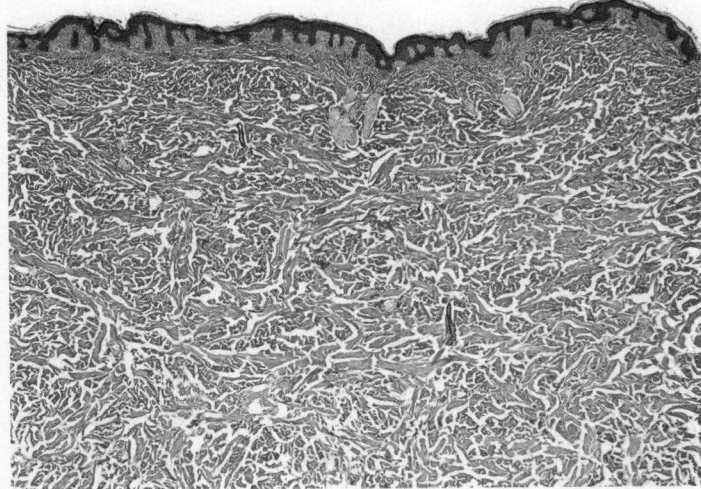

Figure 3-58 Skin from the back, showing a significantly thicker reticular dermis compared with most other regions.

of the umbilical area also shows a thick and fibrotic dermis. Acral skin from palms and soles has a typical thickened and compact stratum corneum containing a stratum lucidum, numerous eccrine glands, and no pilosebaceous units (Figs. 3-7 and 3-52A). Glomus structures and nerve end organs are seen in the dermis (Figs. 3-52B and 3-54A, B). The scalp is characterized by numerous terminal hair follicles, with most of their bulbs in the subcutaneous tissue (Fig. 3-59). The skin from the face has prominent sebaceous glands in vellus hairs and especially on the nose (Fig. 3-60). Anywhere in hairy skin, but especially in the beard area, it is possible to find pili multigemini characterized by more than one hair shaft emerging from a single infundibulum. Although classically considered a rare developmental defect of hair, recent studies suggest that they are commonly present in variable numbers in otherwise normal skin (391) (Fig. 3-61). Skeletal muscle is more superficial on the face, including lips and periorbital areas; skeletal

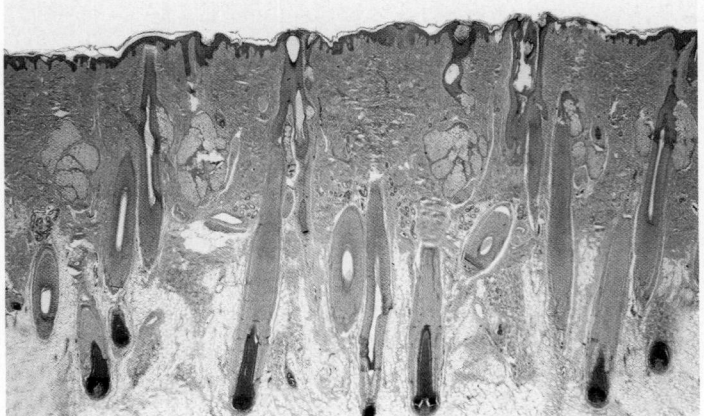

Figure 3-59 The scalp is characterized by numerous terminal hair follicles with most of their bulbs in the subcutaneous tissue, as also illustrated in Figure 3-27.

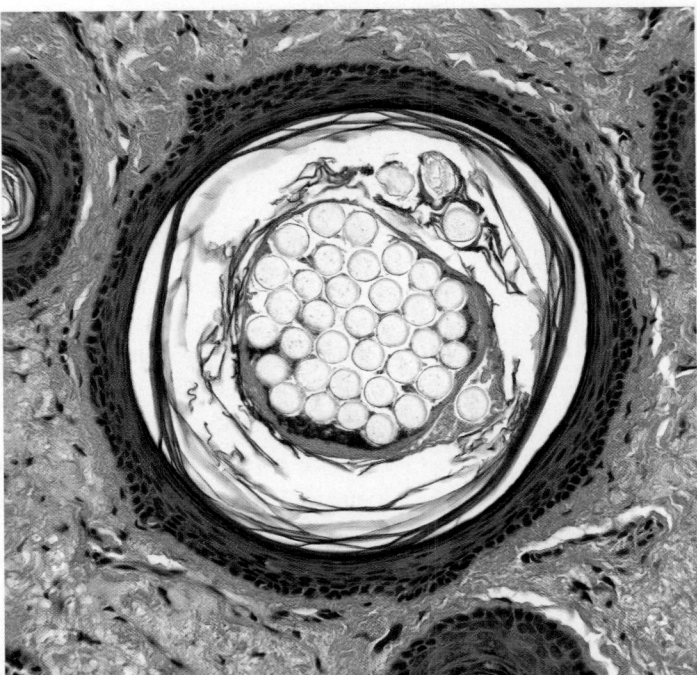

Figure 3-61 Pili multigemini, showing clusters of shafts emerging from a single follicular canal. They are typically found in the beard area of males.

dartos layer (underneath the dermis) in foreskin and scrotum (Fig. 3-63). Skin biopsies from the legs, especially in adults, may show prominent thick-walled blood vessels because of gravity and stasis (Fig. 3-64).

INCIDENTAL FINDINGS IN SKIN SPECIMENS

"Normal" skin is seldom perfect and pristine, and it can be argued that the only time skin is truly normal is at birth. As discussed earlier, it must be viewed in the context of alterations implicit to normal aging, unavoidable environmental agents, and anatomic site. In this section, some of the "incidental findings" in normal skin that may at times be confused with pathologic and clinically significant changes are briefly discussed.

Focal Epidermolytic Hyperkeratosis

Incidental (focal) epidermolytic hyperkeratosis is a common, nonspecific finding that may be seen in normal and especially sun-damaged skin (392). It has also been described adjacent or within different unrelated lesions such as seborrheic keratosis, scars, fibrous histiocytomas, actinic keratosis, carcinomas, and melanocytic lesions. Incidental epidermolytic hyperkeratosis is characterized by a focal area showing hyperkeratosis, acanthosis, thickened and abnormal granular layer containing irregular, enlarged, and deeply eosinophilic intracytoplasmic inclusions resembling trichohyalin granules, and suprabasal keratinocytes showing marked intracellular edema (cytolysis). There is no clinical correlate, and the pathogenesis is unclear. Incidental epidermolytic hyperkeratosis should be distinguished from *congenital bullous ichthyosiform*

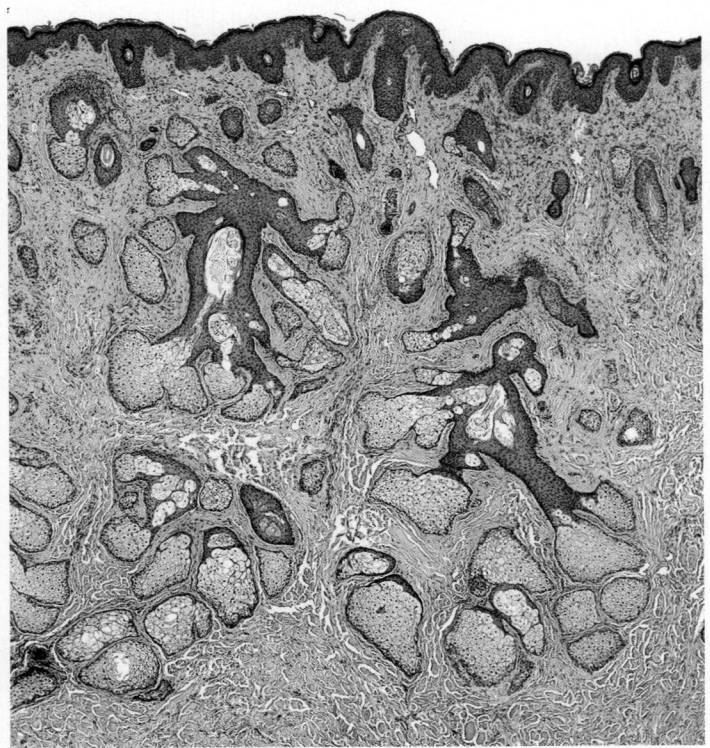

Figure 3-60 Skin from the nose, showing villous hairs and prominent sebaceous glands.

muscle fibers may be seen in the dermis in these areas (Fig. 3-62D). Numerous vellus hairs are seen in the ear. The eyelid epidermis is thin (two to three layers thick) with basaloid buds (Fig. 3-62A, B). The basal layer tends to show increased pigmentation and more melanocytes compared with specimens from other anatomic locations from the same person. Modified apocrine glands (Moll glands) and vellus hairs are seen in the dermis (Fig. 3-62D). The mucosal portion of the eyelid is lined by a nonkeratinizing stratified epithelium with scattered goblet cells (Fig. 3-62C). Smooth muscle fibers are numerous in the dermis of the areola and nipple and are also seen in the

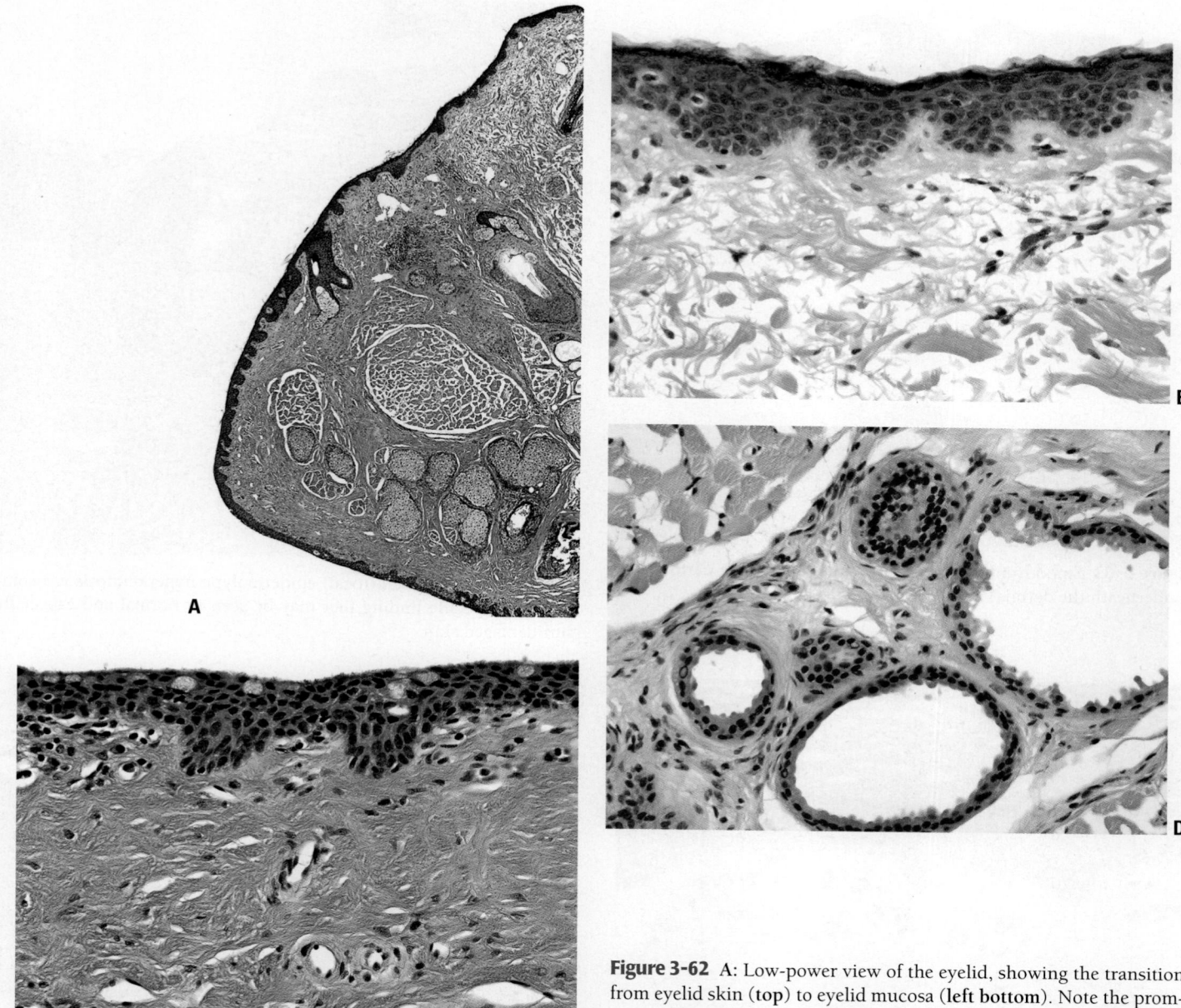

Figure 3-62 A: Low-power view of the eyelid, showing the transition from eyelid skin (**top**) to eyelid mucosa (**left bottom**). Note the prominent Meibomian sebaceous glands. **B:** The eyelid epidermis is thin (2–3 layers thick) with basaloid buds. The basal layer tends to show increased pigmentation and more melanocytes compared with specimens from other regions. **C:** The mucosal (conjunctiva) epithelium shows scattered goblet cells. **D:** Note the modified apocrine glands (glands of Moll) and the presence of superficial skeletal muscle fibers in the dermis.

erythroderma, linear verrucous epidermal nevus, epidermolytic keratoderma, and *epidermolytic acanthoma* (see Chapter 6). The changes in the incidental form are less extensive and limited to the epidermis (Fig. 3-65).

Focal Acantholytic Dyskeratosis

Another incidental finding that can be seen in normal skin is focal acantholytic dyskeratosis. Like incidental epidermolytic hyperkeratosis, focal acantholytic dyskeratosis is a subclinical condition of unknown pathogenesis frequently identified in normal skin or adjacent to unrelated pathologic conditions, including dermatitis, benign tumors, carcinomas, and melanomas (393,394). Histologically, there is a focal area of hyperkeratosis, parakeratosis, and suprabasal cleft formation with dyskeratosis and acantholysis (393) (Fig. 3-66). The differential diagnosis includes *Darier disease, Grover disease, warty dyskeratoma, acantholytic acanthoma, epidermal nevus,* and others.

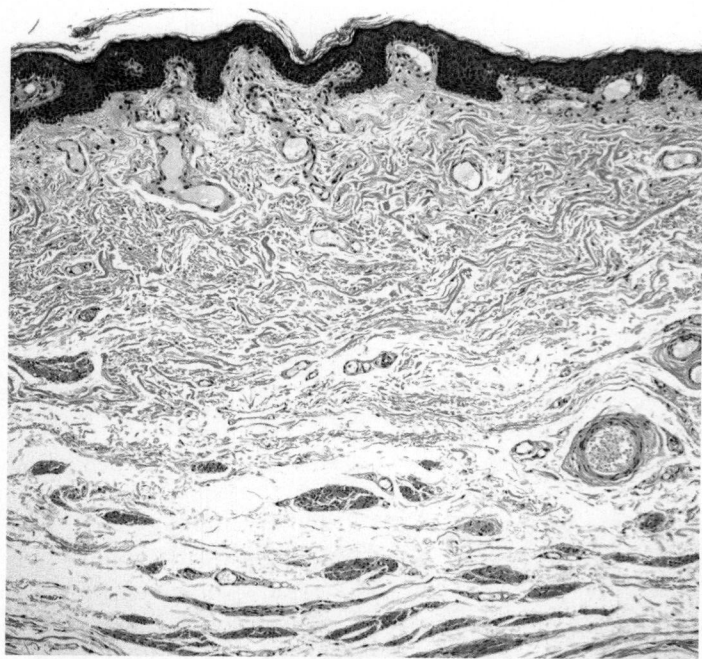

Figure 3-63 Smooth muscle fibers are numerous in the dartos layer (underneath the dermis) in foreskin.

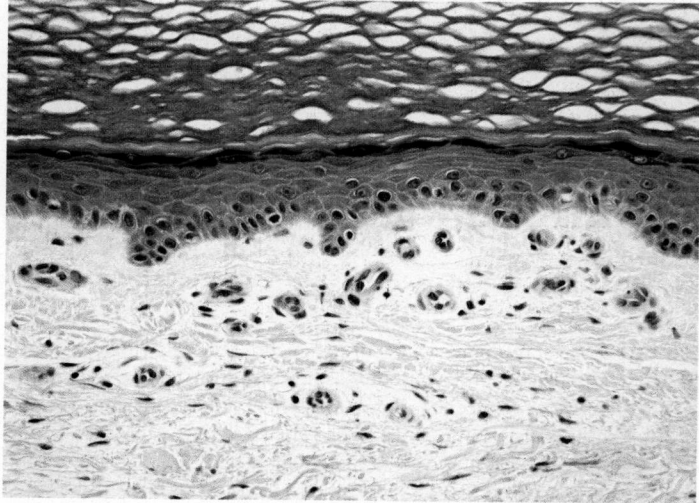

Figure 3-64 Skin biopsies from the legs, especially in adults, may show prominent thick-walled blood vessels owing to gravity and stasis.

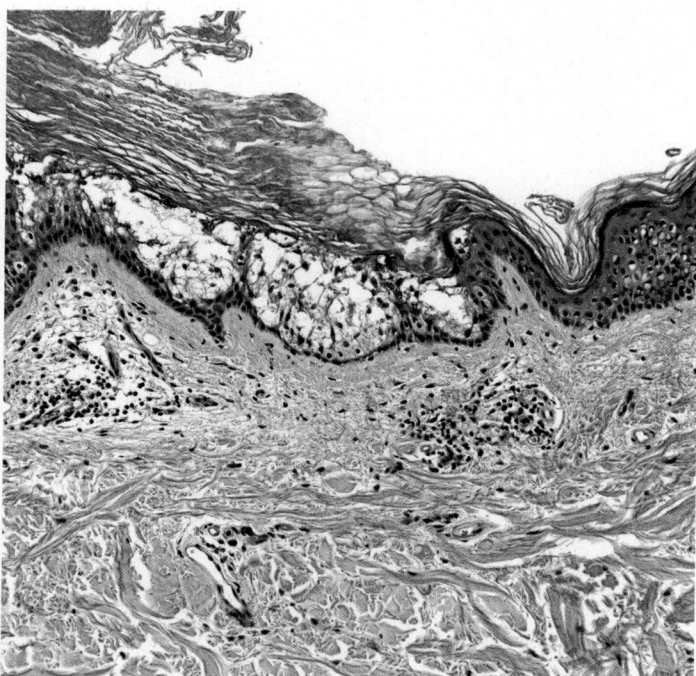

Figure 3-65 Incidental (focal) epidermolytic hyperkeratosis is a common, nonspecific finding that may be seen in normal and especially sun-damaged skin.

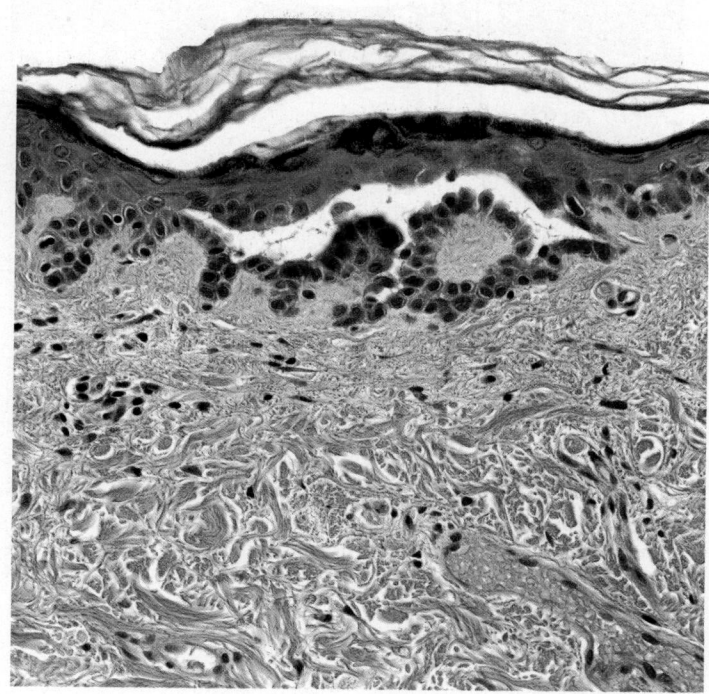

Figure 3-66 Focal acantholytic dyskeratosis represents another incidental finding that can be seen in normal skin.

MICROORGANISMS PRESENT IN NORMAL SKIN

Microorganisms such as *Staphylococcus epidermidis*, yeast forms of *Malassezia furfur* (*Pityrosporum ovale*) (395), and *Demodex folliculorum* mites can normally be found in the follicular infundibulum, and the colonization is usually asymptomatic (Fig. 3-67A–C). The role of *D. folliculorum* in rosacea and other skin disorders is controversial. *Malassezia* yeasts are residents of normal human skin with a fine balance between commensalism and pathogenicity. They may play a role in seborrheic dermatitis and atopic eczema, and a form of *Pityrosporum* folliculitis has been described. They are the cause of tinea versicolor (in this last condition, however, hyphae are found admixed with yeasts in the cornified layer).

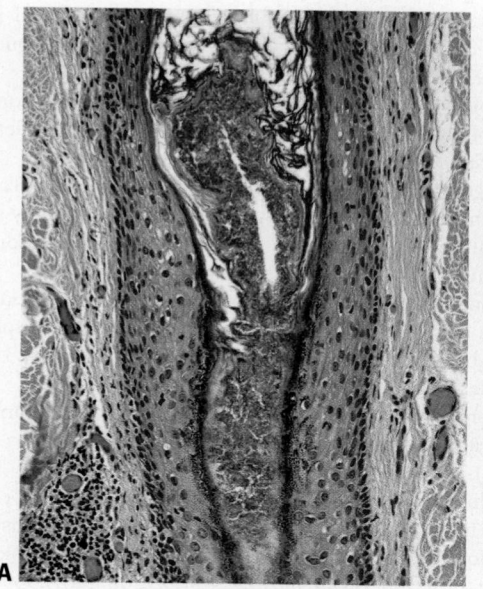
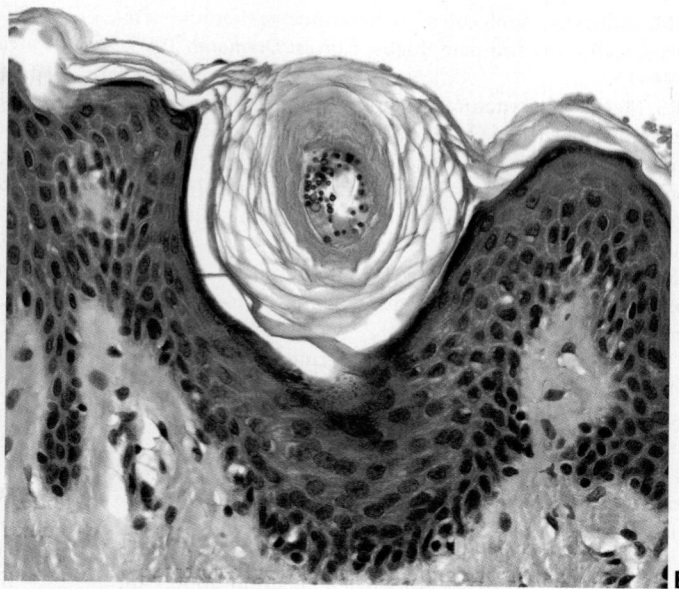
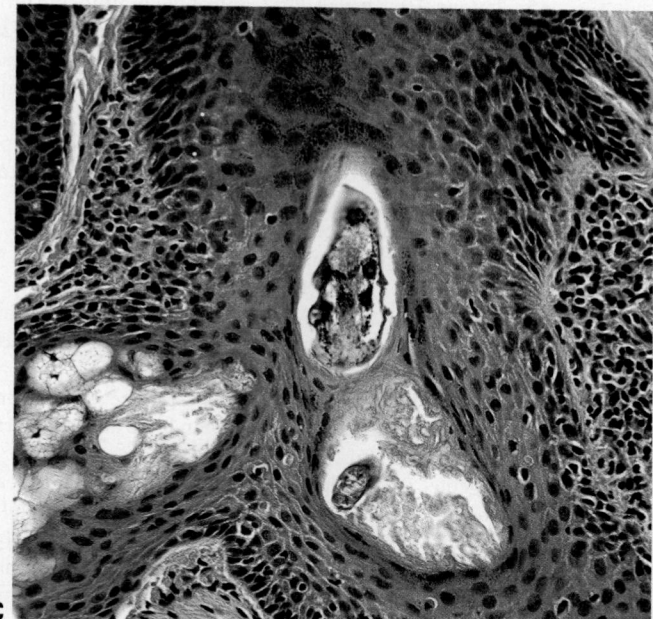

Figure 3-67 Bacteria (A), fungi (yeast forms of *Pityrosporum ovale*) (B), and parasites (*Demodex folliculorum* mites) (C) can be normally found in the follicular infundibulum, and the colonization is usually asymptomatic.

REFERENCES

1. Morrison P. *Powers of Ten*. Scientific American Library; 1994.
2. Toker C. Clear cells of the nipple epidermis. *Cancer*. 1970;25(3):601–610.
3. Lundquist K, Kohler S, Rouse RV. Intraepidermal cytokeratin 7 expression is not restricted to Paget cells but is also seen in Toker cells and Merkel cells. *Am J Surg Pathol*. 1999;23(2):212–219.
4. Breathnach AS. The Herman Beerman lecture: embryology of human skin, a review of ultrastructural studies. *J Invest Dermatol*. 1971;57(3):133–143.
5. Holbrook KA, Odland GF. The fine structure of developing human epidermis: light, scanning, and transmission electron microscopy of the periderm. *J Invest Dermatol*. 1975;65(1):16–38.
6. Hashimoto K, Gross BG, DiBella RJ, et al. The ultrastructure of the skin of human embryos, IV: the epidermis. *J Invest Dermatol*. 1966;47(4):317–335.
7. Matsunaka M, Mishima Y. Electron microscopy of embryonic human epidermis at seven and ten weeks. *Acta Derm Venereol*. 1969;49(3):241–250.
8. Penneys NS, Fulton JE Jr, Weinstein GD, et al. Location of proliferating cells in human epidermis. *Arch Dermatol*. 1970; 101(3):323–327.
9. Maytin EV, Chung HH, Seetharaman VM. Hyaluronan participates in the epidermal response to disruption of the permeability barrier in vivo. *Am J Pathol*. 2004;165(4):1331–1341.
10. Hashimoto K, Lever WF. The cell surface coat of normal keratinocytes and of acantholytic keratinocytes in pemphigus: an electron microscopic study. *Br J Dermatol*. 1970;83(2):282–290.
11. Odland GF. The fine structure of the interrelationship of cells in the human epidermis. *J Biophys Biochem Cytol*. 1958;4(5):529–538.
12. Wolff K, Wolff-Schreiner EC. Trends in electron microscopy of skin. *J Invest Dermatol*. 1976;67(1):39–57.

13. Amagai M. Adhesion molecules. I: keratinocyte–keratinocyte interactions; cadherins and pemphigus. *J Invest Dermatol.* 1995; 104(1):146–152.

14. Buxton RS, Magee AI. Structure and interactions of desmosomal and other cadherins. *Semin Cell Biol.* 1992;3(3):157–167.

15. Broussard JA, Koetsier JL, Hegazy M, Green KJ. Desmosomes polarize and integrate chemical and mechanical signaling to govern epidermal tissue form and function. *Curr Biol.* 2021;31(15):3275–3291.e5.

16. Amagai M, Klaus-Kovtun V, Stanley JR. Autoantibodies against a novel epithelial cadherin in pemphigus vulgaris, a disease of cell adhesion. *Cell.* 1991;67(5):869–877.

17. Shimizu H, Masunaga T, Ishiko A, et al. Demonstration of desmosomal antigens by electron microscopy using cryofixed and cryosubstituted skin with silver-enhanced gold probe. *J Histochem Cytochem.* 1994;42(5):687–692.

18. Matoltsy AG. Desmosomes, filaments, and keratohyaline granules: their role in the stabilization and keratinization of the epidermis. *J Invest Dermatol.* 1975;65(1):127–142.

19. Matoltsy AG. Keratinization. *J Invest Dermatol.* 1976;67(1):20–25.

20. Schwarz E. Biochemie der epidermalen keratinisation. In: Marchionini A, ed. *Handbuch der Haut-und Geschlechtskrankheiten.* Vol 1, Part 4A. Springer-Verlag; 1979.

21. Lazarus GS, Hatcher VB, Levine N. Lysosomes and the skin. *J Invest Dermatol.* 1975;65(3):259–271.

22. Spearman RI. Some light microscopical observations on the stratum corneum of the guinea-pig, man and common seal. *Br J Dermatol.* 1970;83(5):582–590.

23. Christophers E. Cellular architecture of the stratum corneum. *J Invest Dermatol.* 1971;56(3):165–169.

24. Brody I. An electron microscopic study of the fibrillar density in the normal human stratum corneum. *J Ultrastruct Res.* 1970;30(1):209–217.

25. Hashimoto K. Cellular envelopes of keratinized cells of the human epidermis. *Arch Klin Exp Dermatol.* 1969;235:374–385.

26. Dale BA. Filaggrin, the matrix protein of keratin. *Am J Dermatopathol.* 1985;7(1):65–68.

27. Murphy GF, Flynn TC, Rice RH, et al. Involucrin expression in normal and neoplastic human skin: a marker for keratinocyte differentiation. *J Invest Dermatol.* 1984;82(5):453–457.

28. Wolff-Schreiner EC. Ultrastructural cytochemistry of the epidermis. *Int J Dermatol.* 1977;16(2):77–102.

29. Elias PM. Epidermal lipids, barrier function, and desquamation. *J Invest Dermatol.* 1983;80(suppl):44–49.

30. Bell RF, Kellum RE. Early formation of keratohyalin granules in rat epidermis. *Acta Derm Venereol.* 1967;47(5):350–353.

31. van den Oord RA, Sheikh A. Filaggrin gene defects and risk of developing allergic sensitisation and allergic disorders: systematic review and meta-analysis. *BMJ.* 2009;339:b2433.

32. Thyssen JP, Godoy-Gijon E, Elias PM. Ichthyosis vulgaris: the filaggrin mutation disease. *Br J Dermatol.* 2013;168(6):1155–1166.

33. Oyoshi MK, Murphy GF, Geha RS. Filaggrin-deficient mice exhibit TH17-dominated skin inflammation and permissiveness to epicutaneous sensitization with protein antigen. *J Allergy Clin Immunol.* 2009;124:485–493.

34. Elias PM, Goerke J, Friend DS. Mammalian epidermal barrier layer lipids: composition and influence on structure. *J Invest Dermatol.* 1977;69(6):535–546.

35. Feingold KR. The outer frontier: the importance of lipid metabolism in the skin. *J Lipid Res.* 2009;50(suppl):S417–S422.

36. Epstein EH Jr, Williams ML, Elias PM. Steroid sulfatase, X-linked ichthyosis, and stratum corneum cell cohesion. *Arch Dermatol.* 1981;117(12):761–763.

37. Wolff K, Schreiner E. Epidermal lysosomes: electron microscopic-cytochemical studies. *Arch Dermatol.* 1970;101(3):276–286.

38. Bos JD, Kapsenberg ML. The skin immune system: progress in cutaneous biology. *Immunol Today.* 1993;14(2):75–78.

39. Katz SI. Dohi Memorial lecture. The skin as an immunological organ: allergic contact dermatitis as a paradigm. *J Dermatol.* 1993;20(10):593–603.

40. Moll R. Cytokeratins as markers of differentiation: expression profiles in epithelia and epithelial tumors [in German]. *Veroff Pathol.* 1993;142:1–197.

41. Rogers MA, Edler L, Winter H, et al. Characterization of new members of the human type II keratin gene family and a general evaluation of the keratin gene domain on chromosome 12q13.13. *J Invest Dermatol.* 2005;124(3):536–544.

42. Coulombe PA, Kopan R, Fuchs E. Expression of keratin K14 in the epidermis and hair follicle: insights into complex programs of differentiation. *J Cell Biol.* 1989;109(5):2295–2312.

43. Lyle S, Christofidou-Solomidou M, Liu Y, et al. The C8/144B monoclonal antibody recognizes cytokeratin 15 and defines the location of human hair follicle stem cells. *J Cell Sci.* 1998;111(pt 21):3179–3188.

44. Whitaker-Menezes D, Jones SC, Friedman TM, et al. An epithelial target site in experimental graft-versus-host disease and cytokine-mediated cytotoxicity is defined by cytokeratin 15 expression. *Biol Blood Marrow Transpl.* 2003;9(9):559–570.

45. Truong AB, Khavari PA. Control of keratinocyte proliferation and differentiation by p63. *Cell Cycle.* 2007;6(3):295–299.

46. Senoo M, Pinto F, Crum CP, et al. p63 is essential for the proliferative potential of stem cells in stratified epithelia. *Cell.* 2007;129(3):523–536.

47. Aberdam E, Barak E, Rouleau M, et al. A pure population of ectodermal cells derived from human embryonic stem cells. *Stem Cells.* 2008;26(2):440–444.

48. King KE, Weinberg WC. p63: defining roles in morphogenesis, homeostasis, and neoplasia of the epidermis. *Mol Carcinog.* 2007;46(8):716–724.

49. Di Como CJ, Urist MJ, Babayan I, et al. p63 expression profiles in human normal and tumor tissues. *Clin Cancer Res.* 2002; 8(2):494–501.

50. Becker SW Jr, Zimmermann AA. Further studies on melanocytes and melanogenesis in the human fetus and newborn. *J Invest Dermatol.* 1955;25(2):103–112.

51. Sagebiel RW, Odland GF. Ultrastructural identification of melanocytes in early human embryos. *J Invest Dermatol.* 1970;54:96.

52. Holbrook KA, Underwood RA, Vogel AM, et al. The appearance, density and distribution of melanocytes in human embryonic and fetal skin revealed by the anti-melanoma monoclonal antibody, HMB-45. *Anat Embryol (Berl).* 1989;180(5):443–455.

53. Grabbe J, Welker P, Dippel E, et al. Stem cell factor, a novel cutaneous growth factor for mast cells and melanocytes. *Arch Dermatol Res.* 1994;287(1):78–84.

54. Wehrle-Haller B, Weston JA. Soluble and cell-bound forms of steel factor activity play distinct roles in melanocyte precursor dispersal and survival on the lateral neural crest migration pathway. *Development.* 1995;121(3):731–742.

55. Grichnik JM. Kit and melanocyte migration. *J Invest Dermatol.* 2006;126(5):945–947.

56. Spritz RA. Molecular basis of human piebaldism. *J Invest Dermatol.* 1994;103(suppl 5):137S–140S.

57. Fisher DE. Microphthalmia: a signal responsive transcriptional regulator in development. *Pigment Cell Res.* 2000;13(suppl 8): 145–149.

58. Cochran AJ. The incidence of melanocytes in normal human skin. *J Invest Dermatol.* 1970;55(1):65–70.

59. Dean NR, Brennan J, Haynes J, et al. Immunohistochemical labeling of normal melanocytes. *Appl Immunohistochem Mol Morphol.* 2002;10(3):199–204.

60. Fitzpatrick TB. Human melanogensis. *Arch Dermatol Syph.* 1952;65:379–391.

61. Pearse AGE. *Histochemistry: Theoretical and Applied.* 3rd ed. Churchill Livingstone; 1972.

62. Moore BW. A soluble protein characteristic of the nervous system. *Biochem Biophys Res Commun.* 1965;19(6):739–744.

63. Nakajima T, Watanabe S, Sato Y, et al. An immunoperoxidase study of S-100 protein distribution in normal and neoplastic tissues. *Am J Surg Pathol.* 1982;6(8):715–727.

64. Donato R. Functional roles of S100 proteins, calcium-binding proteins of the EF-hand type. *Biochim Biophys Acta.* 1999;1450(3): 191–231.

65. Boon T, Old LJ. Cancer tumor antigens. *Curr Opin Immunol.* 1997;9(5):681–683.

66. Marincola FM, Hijazi YM, Fetsch P, et al. Analysis of expression of the melanoma-associated antigens MART-1 and gp100 in metastatic melanoma cell lines and in in situ lesions. *J Immunother Emphasis Tumor Immunol.* 1996;19(3):192–205.

67. Jungbluth AA, Busam KJ, Gerald WL, et al. A103: an anti-melan-a monoclonal antibody for the detection of malignant melanoma in paraffin-embedded tissues. *Am J Surg Pathol.* 1998;22(5):595–602.

68. Gown AM, Vogel AM, Hoak D, et al. Monoclonal antibodies specific for melanocytic tumors distinguish subpopulations of melanocytes. *Am J Pathol.* 1986;123(2):195–203.

69. Adema GJ, de Boer AJ, van't Hullenaar R, et al. Melanocyte lineage-specific antigens recognized by monoclonal antibodies NKI-beteb, HMB-50, and HMB-45 are encoded by a single cDNA. *Am J Pathol.* 1993;143(6):1579–1585.

70. Chen YT, Stockert E, Jungbluth A, et al. Serological analysis of Melan-A(MART-1), a melanocyte-specific protein homogeneously expressed in human melanomas. *Proc Natl Acad Sci U S A.* 1996;93(12):5915–5919.

71. Jungbluth AA, Iversen K, Coplan K, et al. T311-an anti-tyrosinase monoclonal antibody for the detection of melanocytic lesions in paraffin embedded tissues. *Pathol Res Pract.* 2000;196:235–242.

72. Rochaix P, Lacroix-Triki M, Lamant L, et al. PNL2, a new monoclonal antibody directed against a fixative-resistant melanocyte antigen. *Mod Pathol.* 2003;16(5):481–490.

73. Szumera-Ciećkiewicz A, Bosisio F, et al. EORTC Melanoma Group. SOX10 is as specific as S100 protein in detecting metastases of melanoma in lymph nodes and is recommended for sentinel lymph node assessment. *Eur J Cancer.* 2020;137:175–182.

74. Merelo Alcocer V, Flamm A, Chen G, Helm K. SOX10 Immunostaining in granulomatous dermatoses and benign reactive lymph nodes. *J Cutan Pathol.* 2019;46(8):586–590.

75. Busam KJ, Iversen K, Coplan KC, et al. Analysis of microphthalmia transcription factor expression in normal tissues and tumors, and comparison of its expression with S-100 protein, gp100, and tyrosinase in desmoplastic malignant melanoma. *Am J Surg Pathol.* 2001;25(2):197–204.

76. Tarnowski WM. Ultrastructure of the epidermal melanocyte dense plate. *J Invest Dermatol.* 1970;55(4):265–268.

77. Fitzpatrick TB, Miyamoto M, Ishikawa K. The evolution of concepts of melanin biology. *Arch Dermatol.* 1967;96(3):305–323.

78. Toshima S, Moore GE, Sandberg AA. Ultrastructure of human melanoma in cell culture: electron microscopy studies. *Cancer.* 1968;21(2):202–216.

79. Gilchrest BA, Blog FB, Szabo G. Effects of aging and chronic sun exposure on melanocytes in human skin. *J Invest Dermatol.* 1979;73(2):141–143.

80. Staricco RJ, Pinkus H. Quantitative and qualitative data on the pigment cells of adult human epidermis. *J Invest Dermatol.* 1957;28(1):33–45.

81. Fitzpatrick TB, Szabo G. The melanocyte: cytology and cytochemistry. *J Invest Dermatol.* 1959;32(2, Pt 2):197–209.

82. Quevedo WC Jr, Szabó G, Virks J, et al. Melanocyte populations in UV-irradiated human skin. *J Invest Dermatol.* 1965;45(4):295–298.

83. Szabo G, Gerald AB, Pathak MA, et al. The ultrastructure of racial color differences in man. *J Invest Dermatol.* 1970;54:98.

84. Flaxman BA, Sosis AC, Van Scott EJ. Changes in melanosome distribution in Caucasoid skin following topical application of nitrogen mustard. *J Invest Dermatol.* 1973;60(5):321–326.

85. Toda K, Pathak MA, Parrish JA, et al. Alteration of racial differences in melanosome distribution in human epidermis after exposure to ultraviolet light. *Nat New Biol.* 1972;236(66):143–145.

86. Savage SA, Gerstenblith MR, Goldstein AM, et al. Nucleotide diversity and population differentiation of the melanocortin 1 receptor gene, MC1R. *BMC Genet.* 2008;9:31.

87. Pathak MA, Sinesi SJ, Szabo G. The effect of a single dose of ultraviolet radiation on epidermal melanocytes. *J Invest Dermatol.* 1965;45(6):520–528.

88. Mishima Y, Tanay A. The effect of alpha-methyldopa and ultraviolet irradiation on melanogenesis. *Dermatologica.* 1968; 136(2):105–114.

89. Hendi A, Brodland DG, Zitelli JA. Melanocytes in long-standing sun-exposed skin: quantitative analysis using the MART-1 immunostain. *Arch Dermatol.* 2006;142(7):871–876.

90. Weyers W, Bonczkowitz M, Weyers I, et al. Melanoma in situ versus melanocytic hyperplasia in sun-damaged skin: assessment of the significance of histopathologic criteria for differential diagnosis. *Am J Dermatopathol.* 1996;18(6):560–566.

91. Lerner AB, Fitzpatrick TB. Biochemistry of melanin formation. *Physiol Rev.* 1950;30(1):91–126.

92. Szabo G. Tyrosinase in epidermal melanocytes of white human skin. *Arch Dermatol.* 1967;76:324–329.

93. Hunter JA, Mottaz JH, Zelickson AS. Melanogeneisis: ultrastructural histochemical observations on ultraviolet irradiated human melanocytes. *J Invest Dermatol.* 1970;54:213–221.

94. Jimbow K, Quevedo WC Jr, Fitzpatrick TB, et al. Some aspects of melanin biology: 1950–1975. *J Invest Dermatol.* 1976;67(1):72–89.

95. Nakagawa H, Rhodes AR, Fitzpatrick TB, et al. Acid phosphatase in melanosome formation: a cytochemical study in normal human melanocytes. *J Invest Dermatol.* 1984;83(2):140–144.

96. Shibata T, Prota G, Mishima Y. Non-melanosomal regulatory factors in melanogenesis. *J Invest Dermatol.* 1993;100:274S–280S.

97. Cruickshank CN, Harcourt SA. Pigment donation in vitro. *J Invest Dermatol.* 1964;42:183–184.

98. Valyi-Nagy IT, Murphy GF, Mancianti ML, et al. Phenotypes and interactions of human melanocytes and keratinocytes in an epidermal reconstruction model. *Lab Invest.* 1990;62(3):314–324.

99. Mottaz JH, Zelickson AS. Melanin transfer: a possible phagocytic process. *J Invest Dermatol.* 1967;49(6):605–610.

100. Olson RL, Nordquist J, Everett MA. The role of epidermal lysosomes in melanin physiology. *Br J Dermatol.* 1970;83(1):189–199.

101. Cui R, Widlund HR, Feige E, et al. Central role of p53 in the suntan response and pathologic hyperpigmentation. *Cell.* 2007;128(5):853–864.

102. Tachibana T, Nawa T. Recent progress in studies on Merkel cell biology. *Anat Sci Int.* 2002;77(1):26–33.

103. Moll I, Zieger W, Schmelz M. Proliferative Merkel cells were not detected in human skin. *Arch Dermatol Res.* 1996;288(4):184–187.

104. Halata Z, Grim M, Bauman KI. Friedrich Sigmund Merkel and his "Merkel cell," morphology, development, and physiology: review and new results. *Anat Rec A Discov Mol Cell Evol Biol.* 2003;271(1):225–239.

105. Szeder V, Grim M, Halata Z, et al. Neural crest origin of mammalian Merkel cells. *Dev Biol.* 2003;253(2):258–263.

106. Moll I, Lane AT, Franke WW, et al. Intraepidermal formation of Merkel cells in xenografts of human fetal skin. *J Invest Dermatol.* 1990;94(3):359–364.

107. Moll I. Merkel cell distribution in human hair follicles of the fetal and adult scalp. *Cell Tissue Res.* 1994;277(1):131–138.

108. Moll I, Roessler M, Brandner JM, et al. Human Merkel cells—aspects of cell biology, distribution and functions. *Eur J Cell Biol.* 2005;84(2–3):259–271.

109. Smith KR Jr. The ultrastructure of the human Haarscheibe and Merkel cell. *J Invest Dermatol.* 1970;54(2):150–159.

110. Rosenbaum JN, Guo Z, Baus RM, et al. INSM1: a novel immunohistochemical and molecular marker for neuroendocrine and neuroepithelial neoplasms. *Am J Clin Pathol.* 2015;144(4):579–591.

111. Leblebici C, Yeni, B, Savli TC, et al. A new immunohistochemical marker, insulinoma-associated protein 1 (INSM1), for Merkel cell carcinoma: evaluation of 24 cases. *Ann Diagn Pathol.* 2019;40:53–58.

112. Hashimoto K. Fine structure of Merkel cell in human oral mucosa. *J Invest Dermatol.* 1972;58(6):381–387.

113. Moll R, Moll I, Franke WW. Identification of Merkel cells in human skin by specific cytokeratin antibodies: changes of cell density and distribution in fetal and adult plantar epidermis. *Differentiation.* 1984;28(2):136–154.

114. Ortonne JP, Darmon M. Merkel cells express desmosomal proteins and cytokeratins. *Acta Derm Venereol.* 1985;65(2):161–164.

115. Ortonne JP, Petchot-Bacque JP, Verrando P, et al. Normal Merkel cells express a synaptophysin-like immunoreactivity. *Dermatologica.* 1988;177:110.

116. Masuda T, Ikeda S, Tajima K, et al. Neuron-specific enolase (NSE): a specific marker for Merkel cells in human epidermis. *J Dermatol.* 1986;13(1):67–69.

117. Narisawa Y, Hashimoto K, Kohda H. Immunohistochemical demonstration of the expression of neurofilament proteins in Merkel cells. *Acta Derm Venereol.* 1994;74(6):441–443.

118. Foster CA, Holbrook KA, Farr AG. Ontogeny of Langerhans cells in human embryonic and fetal skin: expression of HLA-DR and OKT-6 determinants. *J Invest Dermatol.* 1986;86(3):240–243.

119. Penneys NS, Stoer C, Buck B, et al. Langerhans' cells in fetal and newborn skin and newborn thymus. *Arch Dermatol.* 1984;120:1082.

120. Wolff K, Winkelmann RK. The influence of ultraviolet light on the Langerhans cell population and its hydrolytic enzymes in guinea pigs. *J Invest Dermatol.* 1967;48(6):531–539.

121. Murphy GF, Shepard RS, Harrist TJ, et al. Ultrastructural documentation of HLA-DR antigen reactivity in normal human acrosyringial epithelium. *J Invest Dermatol.* 1983;81(2):181–183.

122. Murphy GF, Bhan AK, Sato S, et al. A new immunologic marker for human Langerhans cells. *N Engl J Med.* 1981;304(13):791–792.

123. Fithian E, Kung P, Goldstein G, et al. Reactivity of Langerhans cells with hybridoma antibody. *Proc Natl Acad Sci U S A.* 1981;78(4):2541–2544.

124. Murphy GF, Bhan AK, Sato S, et al. Characterization of Langerhans cells by the use of monoclonal antibodies. *Lab Invest.* 1981;45(5):465–468.

125. Breathnach AS, Wyllie LM. Melanin in Langerhans cells. *J Invest Dermatol.* 1965;45(5):401–403.

126. Niebauer G, Krawczyk W, Wilgram GF. The Langerhans cell organelle in Letterer Siwe's disease [in German]. *Arch Klin Exp Dermatol.* 1970;239(2):125–137.

127. Hashimoto K. Langerhans' cell granule: an endocytotic organelle. *Arch Dermatol.* 1971;104(2):148–160.

128. Hanau D, Fabre M, Schmitt DA, et al. Human epidermal Langerhans cells internalize by receptor-mediated endocytosis T6 (CD1 "NA1/34") surface antigen: Birbeck granules are involved in the intracellular traffic of the T6 antigen. *J Invest Dermatol.* 1987;89(2):172–177.

129. Wolff K. The Langerhans cell. *Curr Probl Dermatol.* 1972;4:79–145.

130. Nezelof C, Basset F, Rousseau MF. Histiocytosis X histogenetic arguments for a Langerhans cell origin. *Biomedicine.* 1973; 18(5):365–371.

131. Murphy GF, Bhan AK, Harrist TJ, et al. In situ identification of T6-positive cells in normal human dermis by immunoelectron microscopy. *Br J Dermatol.* 1983;108(4):423–431.

132. Chu A, Eisinger M, Lee JS, et al. Immunoelectron microscopic identification of Langerhans cells using a new antigenic marker. *J Invest Dermatol.* 1982;78(2):177–180.

133. Horton JJ, Allen MH, MacDonald DM. An assessment of Langerhans cell quantification in tissue sections. *J Am Acad Dermatol.* 1984;11(4, pt 1):591–593.

134. Kiistala U, Mustakallio KK. The presence of Langerhans cells in human dermis with special reference to their potential mesenchymal origin. *Acta Derm Venereol.* 1968;48(2):115–122.

135. Mackie RM, Turbitt ML. The use of a double-label immunoperoxidase monoclonal antibody technique in the investigation of patients with mycosis fungoides. *Br J Dermatol.* 1982;106(4):379–384.

136. Tamaki K, Stingl G, Katz SI. The origin of Langerhans cells. *J Invest Dermatol.* 1980;74(5):309–311.

137. Wolff K, Stingl G. The Langerhans cell. *J Invest Dermatol.* 1983;80(1 suppl):17S–21S.

138. Shimada S, Katz SI. The skin as an immunologic organ. *Arch Pathol Lab Med.* 1988;112(3):231–234.

139. Breathnach SM, Katz SI. Cell-mediated immunity in cutaneous disease. *Hum Pathol.* 1986;17(2):161–167.

140. Flotte TJ, Murphy GF, Bhan AK. Demonstration of T200 on human Langerhans cell surface membranes. *J Invest Dermatol.* 1984;82(5):535–537.

141. Murphy GF, Bronstein BR, Knowles RW, et al. Ultrastructural documentation of M241 glycoprotein on dendritic and endothelial cells in normal human skin. *Lab Invest.* 1985;52(3):264–269.

142. Seneschal J, Clark RA, Gehad A, et al. Human epidermal Langerhans cells maintain immune homeostasis in skin by activating skin resident regulatory T cells. *Immunity.* 2012;36(5):873–884.

143. Krueger GG, Emam M. Biology of Langerhans cells: analysis by experiments to deplete Langerhans cells from human skin. *J Invest Dermatol.* 1984;82(6):613–617.

144. Belsito DV, Flotte TJ, Lim HW, et al. Effect of glucocorticosteroids on epidermal Langerhans cells. *J Exp Med.* 1982;155(1):291–302.

145. Belsito DV, Sanchez MR, Baer RL, et al. Reduced Langerhans' cell Ia antigen and ATPase activity in patients with the acquired immunodeficiency syndrome. *N Engl J Med.* 1984;310(20):1279–1282.

146. Tschachler E, Groh V, Popovic M, et al. Epidermal Langerhans cells—a target for HTLV-III/LAV infection. *J Invest Dermatol.* 1987;88(2):233–237.

147. Wood GS, Warner NL, Warnke RA. Anti-Leu-3/T4 antibodies react with cells of monocyte/macrophage and Langerhans lineage. *J Immunol.* 1983;131(1):212–216.

148. Murphy GF, Katz S, Kligman AM. Topical tretinoin replenishes CD1a-positive epidermal Langerhans cells in chronically photodamaged human skin. *J Cutan Pathol.* 1998;25(1):30–34.

149. Bourlond A, Vandooren-Deflorenne R. The sub-epidermal basal membrane: its structure and ultrastructure [in French]. *Arch Belg Dermatol Syphiligr.* 1968;24:119–135.

150. Cooper JH. Microanatomical and histochemical observations on the dermal-epidermal junction. *AMA Arch Derm.* 1958;77(1):18–22.

151. Yancy K. Adhesion molecules, II: interactions of keratinocytes with epidermal basement membrane. *Prog Dermatol.* 1995; 104:1008–1014.

152. Moll R, Moll I. Epidermal adhesion molecules and basement membrane components as target structures of autoimmunity. *Virchows Arch.* 1998;432(6):487–504.

153. Shimanovich I, Hirako Y, Sitaru C, et al. The autoantigen of anti-p200 pemphigoid is an acidic noncollagenous N-linked glycoprotein of the cutaneous basement membrane. *J Invest Dermatol.* 2003;121(6):1402–1408.

154. Nie Z, Nagata Y, Joubeh S, et al. IgA antibodies of linear IgA bullous dermatosis recognize the 15th collagenous domain of BP180. *J Invest Dermatol.* 2000;115(6):1164–1166.

155. Eady RA. The basement membrane. Interface between the epithelium and the dermis: structural features. *Arch Dermatol.* 1988;124(5):709–712.

156. Bruckner-Tuderman L, Rüegger S, Odermatt B, et al. Lack of type VII collagen in unaffected skin of patients with severe

recessive dystrophic epidermolysis bullosa. *Dermatologica*. 1988; 176(2):57–64.

157. Frances C, Robert L. Elastin and elastic fibers in normal and pathologic skin. *Int J Dermatol*. 1984;23(3):166–179.

158. Kobayasi T. Dermo-epidermal junction of normal skin. *J Dermatol*. 1978;5(4):157–165.

159. Zillikens D, Kawahara Y, Ishiko A, et al. A novel subepidermal blistering disease with autoantibodies to a 200-kDa antigen of the basement membrane zone. *J Invest Dermatol*. 1996; 106(6):1333–1338.

160. Chen KR, Shimizu S, Miyakawa S, et al. Coexistence of psoriasis and an unusual IgG-mediated subepidermal bullous dermatosis: identification of a novel 200-kDa lower lamina lucida target antigen. *Br J Dermatol*. 1996;134(2):340–346.

161. Vafia K, Groth S, Beckmann T, et al. Pathogenicity of autoantibodies in anti-p200 pemphigoid. *PLoS One*. 2012;7(7):e41769.

162. Fassihi H, Wong T, Wessagowit V, et al. Target proteins in inherited and acquired blistering skin disorders. *Clin Exp Dermatol*. 2006;31(2):252–259.

163. Iriyama S, Yasuda M, Nishikawa S, Takai E, Hosoi J, Amano S. Decrease of laminin-511 in the basement membrane due to photoaging reduces epidermal stem/progenitor cells. *Sci Rep*. 2020;10:12592.

164. Hashimoto K. The ultrastructuref the skin of human embryos. V: The hair germ and perifollicular mesenchymal cells. Hair germ-mesenchyme interaction. *Br J Dermatol*. 1970;83(1): 167–176.

165. Serri F, Montagna W, Mescon H. Studies of the skin of the fetus and the child. II: Glycogen and amylophos-phorylase in the skin of the fetus. *J Invest Dermatol*. 1962;39:199–217.

166. Mishima Y, Widlan S. Embryonic development of melanocytes in human hair and epidermis: their cellular differentiation and melanogenic activity. *J Invest Dermatol*. 1966;46(3):263–277.

167. Pinkus H. Embryology of hair. In: Montagna W, Ellis R, eds. *The Biology of Hair Growth*. Academic Press; 1958.

168. Hashimoto K. The ultrastructure of the skin of human embryos. IX: Formation of the hair cone and intraepidermal hair canal. *Arch Klin Exp Dermatol*. 1970;238(4):333–345.

169. Hashimoto K. The ultrastructure of the skin of human embryos. VII: Formation of the apocrine gland. *Acta Derm Venereol*. 1970;50(4):241–251.

170. Rogers MA, Winter H, Wolf C, et al. Characterization of a 190-kilobase pair domain of human type I hair keratin genes. *J Biol Chem*. 1998;273(41):26683–26691.

171. Rogers MA, Winter H, Langbein L, et al. Characterization of a 300 kbp region of human DNA containing the type II hair keratin gene domain. *J Invest Dermatol*. 2000;114(3):464–472.

172. Thiers BH, Galbraith GMP. Alopecia areata. In: Thiers BH, Dobson RL, eds. *Pathogenesis of Skin Disease*. Churchill Livingstone; 1986:57–64.

173. Kollar EJ. The induction of hair follicles by embryonic dermal papillae. *J Invest Dermatol*. 1970;55(6):374–378.

174. Johnson WC, Helwig EB. Histochemistry of the acid mucopolysaccharides of skin in normal and in certain pathologic conditions. *Am J Clin Pathol*. 1963;40:123–131.

175. Kopf AW, Orentreich N. Alkaline phosphatase in alopecia areata. *AMA Arch Derm*. 1957;76(3):288–295.

176. Cormia FE. Vasculature of the normal scalp. *Arch Dermatol*. 1963;88:692–701.

177. Pinkus H. Anatomy and histology of skin. In: Graham JH, Johnson WC, Helwig EB, eds. *Dermal Pathology*. Harper & Row; 1972.

178. Garn SM. The examination of hair under the polarizing microscope. *Ann N Y Acad Sci*. 1951;53(3):649–652.

179. Leppard BJ, Sanderson KV, Wells RS. Hereditary trichilemmal cysts. *Clin Exp Dermatol*. 1976;2:23–32.

180. Bandmann HJ, Bosse K. Histology and anatomy of the hair follicle in the course of the hair cycle [in German]. *Arch Klin Exp Dermatol*. 1966;227(1):390–409.

181. Montagna W. *The Structure and Function of Skin*. 2nd ed. Academic Press; 1962.

182. Parakkal PF, Matoltsy AG. A study of the differentiation products of the hair follicle cells with the electron microscope. *J Invest Dermatol*. 1964;42:23–34.

183. Yang CC, Cotsarelis G. Review of hair follicle dermal cells. *J Dermatol Sci*. 2010;57(1):2–11.

184. Strauss JS, Pochi PE. Histology, histochemistry, and electron microscopy of sebaceous glands in man. In: Marchionini A, ed. *Handbuch der Haut-und Geschlechtskrankheiten, Erganzungswerk*. Vol 1, Part 1. Springer-Verlag; 1968.

185. Suskind RR. The chemistry of the human sebaceous gland. I: Histochemical observations. *J Invest Dermatol*. 1951;17(1):37–54.

186. Cashion PD, Skobe Z, Nalbandian J. Ultrastructural observations on sebaceous glands of the human oral mucosa (Fordyce's "disease"). *J Invest Dermatol*. 1969;53(3):208–216.

187. Niizuma K. Lipid droplets of the sebaceous gland: some new observations from tannic acid fixation. *Acta Derm Venereol*. 1979;59(5):401–405.

188. Rupec M, Braun-Falco O. On the problem of lysosomal activity in normal human sebaceous glands [in German]. *Arch Klin Exp Dermatol*. 1968;232(3):312–324.

189. Ito M, Suzuki M, Motoyoshi K, et al. New findings on the proteins of sebaceous glands. *J Invest Dermatol*. 1984;82(4):381–385.

190. Hyman AB, Brownstein MH. Tyson's "glands": ectopic sebaceous glands and papillomatosis penis. *Arch Dermatol*. 1969;99(1):31–36.

191. Weedon D, Strutton G. Apoptosis as the mechanism of the involution of hair follicles in catagen transformation. *Acta Derm Venereol*. 1981;61(4):335–339.

192. Kligman AM. The human hair cycle. *J Invest Dermatol*. 1959;33:307–316.

193. Leavitt D, Wells P, Abarzua P, Murphy GF, Lian CG. Differential distribution of the epigenetic marker 5-hydroxymethylcytosine occurs in hair follicle stem cells during bulge activation. *J Cutan Pathol*. 2019;46:327–334.

194. Zhang B, Tsai P-C, Gonzalez-Celero M, et al. Hair follicles' transit-amplifying cells govern concurrent dermal adipocyte production through sonic hedgehog. *Genes Dev*. 2016;30:2325–2338.

195. Mahrle G, Orfanos CE. Hair colour and hair pigment: electron-microscopic investigations on natural and bleached hair [author's transl]. *Arch Dermatol Forsch*. 1973;248(2):109–122.

196. Herzberg J, Gusek W. The greying of hair: histochemical and electronmicroscopical investigations. *Arch Klin Exp Dermatol*. 1970;236(4):368–384.

197. Nishimura EK, Granter SR, Fisher DE. Mechanisms of hair graying: incomplete melanocyte stem cell maintenance in the niche. *Science*. 2005;307(5710):720–724.

198. Zhang B, Rachmin, He M, et al. Hyperactivation of sympathetic nerves drives depletion of melanocyte stem cells. *Nature*. 2020;577:676–681.

199. Waldorf HA, Walsh LJ, Schechter NM, et al. Early cellular events in evolving cutaneous delayed hypersensitivity in humans. *Am J Pathol*. 1991;138(2):477–486.

200. Sato K, Leidal R, Sato F. Morphology and development of an apoeccrine sweat gland in human axillae. *Am J Physiol*. 1987;252(1, pt 2):R166–R180.

201. Hashimoto K, Gross BG, Lever WF. The ultrastructure of the skin of human embryos. I: The intraepidermal eccrine sweat duct. *J Invest Dermatol*. 1965;45(3):139–151.

202. Hashimoto K, Gross B, Lever W. The ultrastructure of human embryo skin. II: The formation of intradermal portion of the eccrine sweat duct and of the secretory segment during the first half of embryonic life. *J Invest Dermatol*. 1966;46:513–529.

203. Christophers E, Plewig G. Formation of the acrosyringium. *Arch Dermatol*. 1973;107(3):378–382.

204. Hashimoto K, Gross BG, Lever WF. Electron microscopic study of the human adult eccrine gland, I: the duct. *J Invest Dermatol*. 1966;46(2):172–185.

205. Montagna W, Chase HB, Lotiz WE Jr. Histology and cytochemistry of human skin, IV: the eccrine sweat glands. *J Invest Dermatol.* 1963;20:415–423.

206. Dobson RL, Sato K. The secretion of salt and water by the eccrine sweat gland. *Arch Dermatol.* 1972;105(3):366–370.

207. Hurley HJ, Witkowski JA. The dynamics of eccrine sweating in man. I: Sweat delivery through myoepithelial contraction. *J Invest Dermatol.* 1962;39:329–338.

208. Schiefferdecker P. Die Hautdrusen des Menschen und der Saugetier, ihre biologische und rassenanatomische Bedeuturng, sowie die Muscularis sexualis. *Biol Ztrbl.* 1917;37:534–562.

209. Schaumberg-Lever G, Lever WF. Secretion from human apocrine glands. *J Invest Dermatol.* 1975;64:38–41.

210. Montes LF, Baker BL, Curtis AC. The cytology of the large axillary sweat glands in man. *J Invest Dermatol.* 1960;35:273–291.

211. Hurley HJ, Shelley WB. *The Human Apocrine Sweat Gland in Health and Disease.* Charles C Thomas; 1960.

212. Montagna W, Yun JS. The glands of Montgomery. *Br J Dermatol.* 1972;86(2):126–133.

213. Smith DM Jr, Peters TG, Donegan WL. Montgomery's areolar tubercle: a light microscopic study. *Arch Pathol Lab Med.* 1982;106(2):60–63.

214. Sato K, Kane N, Soos G, et al. The eccrine sweat gland: basic science and disorder of eccrine sweating. In: Moshell AN, ed. *Progress in Dermatology.* Vol 29. Dermatology Foundation; 1995:1–11.

215. Sato K, Sato F. Interleukin-1 alpha in human sweat is functionally active and derived from the eccrine sweat gland. *Am J Physiol.* 1994;266:950–959.

216. Inoue T. Scanning electron microscopic study of the human axillary apocrine glands. *J Dermatol.* 1979;6(5):299–308.

217. Spielman AI, Zeng XN, Leyden JJ, et al. Proteinaceous precursors of human axillary odor: isolation of two novel odor-binding proteins. *Experientia.* 1995;51(1):40–47.

218. Wollina U, Schaarschmidt H, Knopf B. Immunolocalization of cytokeratins in human eccrine sweat glands. *Acta Histochem.* 1990;88(2):125–129.

219. Watanabe S, Ichikawa E, Takanashi S, et al. Immunohistochemical localization of cytokeratins in normal eccrine glands, with monoclonal antibodies in routinely processed, formalin-fixed, paraffin-embedded sections. *J Am Acad Dermatol.* 1993;28(2, pt 1):203–212.

220. Urmacher C. Histology of normal skin. *Am J Surg Pathol.* 1990;14(7):671–686.

221. Cassarino DS, Su A, Robbins BA, Altree-Tacha D, Ra S. SOX10 immunohistochemistry in sweat ductal/glandular neoplasms. *J Cutan Pathol.* 2017;44(6):544–547.

222. Scher RK, Daniel CR III. *Nails: Therapy, Diagnosis, Surgery.* WB Saunders; 1990.

223. Hashimoto K. Ultrastructure of the human toenail. I: Proximal nail matrix. *J Invest Dermatol.* 1971;56(3):235–246.

224. Hashimoto K. Ultrastructure of the human toenail. II: Keratinization and formation of the marginal band. *J Ultrastruct Res.* 1971;36(3):391–410.

225. Hashimoto K. The marginal band: a demonstration of the thickened cellular envelope of the human nail cell with the aid of lanthanum staining. *Arch Dermatol.* 1971;103(4):387–393.

226. Johnson M, Shuster S. Continuous formation of nail along the bed. *Br J Dermatol.* 1993;128(3):277–280.

227. Perrin C, Langbein L, Schweizer J. Expression of hair keratins in the adult nail unit: an immunohistochemical analysis of the onychogenesis in the proximal nail fold, matrix and nail bed. *Br J Dermatol.* 2004;151(2):362–371.

228. Higashi N. Melanocytes of nail matrix and nail pigmentation. *Arch Dermatol.* 1968;97(5):570–574.

229. Ackerman AB, Chongchitnant N, Sanchez J, et al. *Histologic Diagnosis of Inflammatory Skin Disease.* 2nd ed. Lippincott Williams & Wilkins; 1997.

230. Scarpelli DG, Goodman RM. Observations on the fine structure of the fibroblast from a case of Ehlers-Danlos syndrome with the Marfan syndrome. *J Invest Dermatol.* 1968;50(3):214–219.

231. Ross R, Benditt EP. Wound healing and collagen formation. V: Quantitative electron microscope radioautographic observations of proline-H3 utilization by fibroblasts. *J Cell Biol.* 1965;27(1):83–106.

232. Uitto J, Lichtenstein JR. Defects in the biochemistry of collagen in diseases of connective tissue. *J Invest Dermatol.* 1976;66(02):59–79.

233. Nigra TP, Friedland M, Martin GR. Controls of connective tissue synthesis: collagen metabolism. *J Invest Dermatol.* 1972;59(1):44–49.

234. Eyden B. The myofibroblast: an assessment of controversial issues and a definition useful in diagnosis and research. *Ultrastruct Pathol.* 2001;25(1):39–50.

235. Headington JT. The dermal dendrocyte. *Adv Dermatol.* 1986;1:159–171.

236. Braverman IM, Sibley J, Keh-Yen A. A study of the veil cells around normal, diabetic, and aged cutaneous microvessels. *J Invest Dermatol.* 1986;86(1):57–62.

237. Nestle FO, Zheng XG, Thompson CB, et al. Characterization of dermal dendritic cells obtained from normal human skin reveals phenotypic and functionally distinctive subsets. *J Immunol.* 1993;151(11):6535–6545.

238. Cerio R, Griffiths CE, Cooper KD, et al. Characterization of factor XIIIa positive dermal dendritic cells in normal and inflamed skin. *Br J Dermatol.* 1989;121(4):421–431.

239. Sueki H, Whitaker D, Buchsbaum M, et al. Novel interactions between dermal dendrocytes and mast cells in human skin: implications for hemostasis and matrix repair. *Lab Invest.* 1993;69(2):160–172.

240. Kanitakis J. Anatomy, histology and immunohistochemistry of normal human skin. *Eur J Dermatol.* 2002;12(4):390–399; quiz 400–401.

241. Meunier L, Gonzalez-Ramos A, Cooper KD. Heterogeneous populations of class II MHC+ cells in human dermal cell suspensions: identification of a small subset responsible for potent dermal antigen-presenting cell activity with features analogous to Langerhans cells. *J Immunol.* 1993;151(8):4067–4080.

242. Murphy GF, Messadi D, Fonferko E, et al. Phenotypic transformation of macrophages to Langerhans cells in the skin. *Am J Pathol.* 1986;123(3):401–406.

243. Nickoloff BJ, Griffiths CE. Not all spindled-shaped cells embedded in a collagenous stroma are fibroblasts: recognition of the "collagen-associated dendrophage." *J Cutan Pathol.* 1990;17(4):252–254.

244. Hirsh BC, Johnson WC. Concepts of granulomatous inflammation. *Int J Dermatol.* 1984;23(2):90–100.

245. Wells GC. The pathology of adult type Letterer-Siwe disease. *Clin Exp Dermatol.* 1979;4(4):407–412.

246. Lasser A. The mononuclear phagocytic system: a review. *Hum Pathol.* 1983;14(2):108–126.

247. Lau SK, Chu PG, Weiss LM. CD163: a specific marker of macrophages in paraffin-embedded tissue samples. *Am J Clin Pathol.* 2004;122(5):794–801.

248. Pulford KA, Rigney EM, Micklem KJ, et al. KP1: a new monoclonal antibody that detects a monocyte/macrophage associated antigen in routinely processed tissue sections. *J Clin Pathol.* 1989;42(4):414–421.

249. Meuret G, Marwendel A, Brand ET. Macrophage-recruitment from blood monocytes in inflammatory skin reactions [in German]. *Arch Dermatol Forsch.* 1972;245(3):254–266.

250. Papadimitriou JM, Spector WG. The origin, properties and fate of epithelioid cells. *J Pathol.* 1971;105(3):187–203.

251. Spector WG. Immunologic components of granuloma formation: epithelioid cells, giant cells, and sarcoidosis. *Ann N Y Acad Sci.* 1976;278:3–6.

252. Hashimoto K, Tarnowski WM, Lever WF. Maturation and degranulation of mast cells in the human skin: electron microscopic studies [in German]. *Hautarzt.* 1967;18(7):318–324.

253. Lagunoff D. Contributions of electron microscopy to the study of mast cells. *J Invest Dermatol.* 1972;58(5):296–311.

254. Whitaker-Menezes D, Schechter NM, Murphy GF. Serine proteinases are regionally segregated within mast cell granules. *Lab Invest.* 1995;72(1):34–41.

255. Irani AM, Bradford TR, Kepley CL, et al. Detection of MCT and MCTC types of human mast cells by immunohistochemistry using new monoclonal anti-tryptase and anti-chymase antibodies. *J Histochem Cytochem.* 1989;37(10):1509–1515.

256. Craig SS, Schechter NM, Schwartz LB. Ultrastructural analysis of human T and TC mast cells identified by immunoelectron microscopy. *Lab Invest.* 1988;58(6):682–691.

257. Mirowski G, Austen KF, Chiang L, et al. Characterization of cellular dermal infiltrates in human cutaneous mastocytosis. *Lab Invest.* 1990;63(1):52–62.

258. Kobayasi T, Asboe-Hansen G. Degranulation and regranulation of human mast cells: an electron microscopic study of the whealing reaction in urticaria pigmentosa. *Acta Derm Venereol.* 1969;49(4):369–381.

259. Kaminer MS, Lavker RM, Walsh LJ, et al. Extracellular localization of human connective tissue mast cell granule contents. *J Invest Dermatol.* 1991;96(6):857–863.

260. Uvnas B. Chemistry and storage function of mast cell granules. *J Invest Dermatol.* 1978;71(1):76–80.

261. Kaliner MA. The mast cell–a fascinating riddle. *N Engl J Med.* 1979;301(9):498–499.

262. Lewis RE, Buchsbaum M, Whitaker D, et al. Intercellular adhesion molecule expression in the evolving human cutaneous delayed hypersensitivity reaction. *J Invest Dermatol.* 1989;93(5):672–677.

263. Murphy GF, Sueki H, Teuscher C, et al. Role of mast cells in early epithelial target cell injury in experimental acute graft-versus-host disease. *J Invest Dermatol.* 1994;102(4):451–461.

264. Walsh LJ, Trinchieri G, Waldorf HA, et al. Human dermal mast cells contain and release tumor necrosis factor alpha, which induces endothelial leukocyte adhesion molecule 1. *Proc Natl Acad Sci U S A.* 1991;88(10):4220–4224.

265. Klein LM, Lavker RM, Matis WL, et al. Degranulation of human mast cells induces an endothelial antigen central to leukocyte adhesion. *Proc Natl Acad Sci U S A.* 1989;86(22):8972–8976.

266. Christofidou-Solomidou M, Murphy GF, Albelda SM. Induction of E-selectin-dependent leukocyte recruitment by mast cell degranulation in human skin grafts transplanted on SCID mice. *Am J Pathol.* 1996;148(1):177–188.

267. Walsh LJ, Kaminer MS, Lazarus GS, et al. Role of laminin in localization of human dermal mast cells. *Lab Invest.* 1991;65(4):433–440.

268. Weiss RR, Whitaker-Menezes D, Longley J, et al. Human dermal endothelial cells express membrane-associated mast cell growth factor. *J Invest Dermatol.* 1995;104(1):101–106.

269. Miettinen M, Lasota J. KIT (CD117): a review on expression in normal and neoplastic tissues, and mutations and their clinicopathologic correlation. *Appl Immunohistochem Mol Morphol.* 2005;13(3):205–220.

270. Murphy GF. *Dermatopathology.* WB Saunders; 1995.

271. Weissmann G, Smolen JE, Hoffstein S. Polymorphonuclear leukocytes as secretory organs of inflammation. *J Invest Dermatol.* 1978;71(1):95–99.

272. Wilkinson DS. Pustular dermatoses. *Br J Dermatol.* 1969;81(suppl 3):38–45.

273. Wade BH, Mandell GL. Polymorphonuclear leukocytes: dedicated professional phagocytes. *Am J Med.* 1983;74(4):686–693.

274. Parish WE. Investigations on eosinophilia: the influence of histamine, antigen-antibody complexes containing gamma-1 or gamma-2 globulins, foreign bodies (phagocytosis) and disrupted mast cells. *Br J Dermatol.* 1970;82(1):42–64.

275. Henson PM. Pathologic mechanisms in neutrophil-mediated injury. *Am J Pathol.* 1972;68(3):593–612.

276. Lazarus GS, Daniels JR, Lian J, et al. Role of granulocyte collagenase in collagen degradation. *Am J Pathol.* 1972;68(3):565–578.

277. Berretty PJ, Cormane RH. The eosinophilic granulocyte. *Int J Dermatol.* 1978;17(10):776–784.

278. Poole JC. Electron microscopy of polymorphonuclear leucocytes. *Br J Dermatol.* 1969;81(suppl 3):11–18.

279. Zucker-Franklin D. Eosinophil function related to cutaneous disorders. *J Invest Dermatol.* 1978;71(1):100–105.

280. Gell PGH, Coombs RRA. Classification of hypersensitivity reactions. In: Gell PGH, Coombs RRA, eds. *Clinical Aspects of Immunology.* 2nd ed. Blackwell Scientific; 1968.

281. Berretty PJ, Cormane RH. Eosinophilic granulocytes and skin disorders. *Int J Dermatol.* 1981;20(8):531–540.

282. Goetzl EJ, Wasserman SI, Austen F. Eosinophil polymorphonuclear leukocyte function in immediate hypersensitivity. *Arch Pathol.* 1975;99(1):1–4.

283. Dvorak HF, Dvorak AM. Basophils, mast cells, and cellular immunity in animals and man. *Hum Pathol.* 1972;3(4):454–456.

284. Katz SI. Recruitment of basophils in delayed hypersensitivity reactions. *J Invest Dermatol.* 1978;71(1):70–75.

285. Weissman IL, Warnke R, Butcher EC, et al. The lymphoid system: its normal architecture and the potential for understanding the system through the study of lymphoproliferative diseases. *Hum Pathol.* 1978;9(1):25–45.

286. Stingl G, Knapp W. Immunological markers for characterization of subpopulations of mononuclear cells. *Am J Dermatopathol.* 1981;3(2):215–223.

287. Claudy AL. The immunological identification of the Sezary cell. *Br J Dermatol.* 1974;91(5):597–600.

288. Luckasen JR, Sabad A, Goltz RW, et al. T and B lymphocytes in atopic eczema. *Arch Dermatol.* 1974;110(3):375–377.

289. Gershon RK, Kondo K. Cell interactions in the induction of tolerance: the role of thymic lymphocytes. *Immunology.* 1970;18(5):723–737.

290. Sakaguchi S, Wing K, Miyara M. Regulatory T cells—a brief history and perspective. *Eur J Immunol.* 2007;37(suppl 1):S116–S123.

291. Clark RA, Chong B, Mirchandani N, et al. The vast majority of CLA+ T cells are resident in normal skin. *J Immunol.* 2006;176(7):4431–4439.

292. Jiang X, Clark RA, Liu L, et al. Skin infection generates non-migratory memory CD8+ T(RM) cells providing global skin immunity. *Nature.* 2012;483(7388):227–231.

293. Zhu J, Peng T, Johnston C, et al. Immune surveillance by CD8αα+ skin-resident T cells in human herpes virus infection. *Nature.* 2013;497(7450):494–497.

294. Hayday A, Theodoridis E, Ramsburg E, et al. Intraepithelial lymphocytes: exploring the Third Way in immunology. *Nat Immunol.* 2001;2(11):997–1003.

295. Curry JL, Qin JZ, Bonish B, et al. Innate immune-related receptors in normal and psoriatic skin. *Arch Pathol Lab Med.* 2003;127(2):178–186.

296. Hirahara K, Liu L, Clark RA, et al. The majority of human peripheral blood CD4+CD25^{high}Foxp3+ regulatory T cells bear functional skin-homing receptors. *J Immunol.* 2006;177(7):4488–4494.

297. Spits H, Lanier LL, Phillips JH. Development of human T and natural killer cells. *Blood.* 1995;85(10):2654–2670.

298. Askenase PW. Delayed-type hypersensitivity (DTH) recruitment of T cell subsets via antigen-specific non-IgE factors, and IgE antibodies: relevance to asthma, autoimmunity and immune resistance to tumors and parasites. In: Coffman R, ed. *The Regulation and Functional Significance of T Cell Subsets: Progress in Chemical Immunology.* Karger Publishers; 1993.

299. Gerard-Marchant R, Hamilin I, Lenner K, et al. Classification of non-Hodgkin's lymphoma. *Lancet.* 1974;2:406–408.

300. Wilson JE. Prospectives in mycosis fungicides in relation to other lymphomas. *Trans St John's Hosp Dermatol Soc.* 1975;61:16–30.

301. Rywlin AM. Non-Hodgkin's malignant lymphomas: brief historical review and simple unifying classification. *Am J Dermatopathol.* 1980;2(1):17–25.

302. Aisenberg AC. Cell lineage in lymphoproliferative disease. *Am J Med.* 1983;74(4):679–685.

303. Murphy GF, Mihm MC Jr. Benign, dysplastic, and malignant lymphoid infiltrates of the skin: an approach based on pattern analysis. In: Murphy GF, Mihm MC Jr, eds. *Lymphoproliferative Disorders of the Skin.* Butterworths; 1986:123–141.

304. Murphy GF, Elder D. *Non-Melanocytic Tumors of the Skin (Atlas of Tumor Pathology).* Vol 1. Armed Forces Institute of Pathology; 1990.

305. Erlach E, Gebhart W, Niebauer G. Ultrastructural investigations on the morphogenesis of Russell bodies. *J Cutan Pathol.* 1976;3:145.

306. Tappeiner J, Pfleger L, Wolff K. The presence and histochemical behavior of Russell's bodies in plasma cell skin infiltrates [in German]. *Arch Klin Exp Dermatol.* 1965;222:71–90.

307. Blom J, Wiik A. Russell bodies: immunoglobulins? *Am J Clin Pathol.* 1983;79:262–263.

308. Matthews JB. The immunoglobulin nature of Russell bodies. *Br J Exp Pathol.* 1983;64(3):331–335.

309. Lazarus GS. Collagen, collagenase and clinicians. *Br J Dermatol.* 1972;86(2):193–199.

310. Grant ME, Prockop DJ. The biosynthesis of collagen, 1. *N Engl J Med.* 1972;286(4):194–199.

311. Grant ME. From collagen chemistry towards cell therapy—a personal journey. *Int J Exp Pathol.* 2007;88(4):203–214.

312. Hayes RL, Rodnan GP. The ultrastructure of skin in progressive systemic sclerosis (scleroderma). I: Dermal collagen fibers. *Am J Pathol.* 1971;63(3):433–442.

313. Schmidt W. Die normale Histologic von Corium und Subcutis. In: Marchionini A, ed. *Hanbuch der Haut-und Geschlechskrankheiten, Erganzungswerk.* Vol 1, Part 1. Springer-Verlag; 1968.

314. Meigel WN, Gay S, Weber L. Dermal architecture and collagen type distribution. *Arch Dermatol Res.* 1977;259(1):1–10.

315. Byers PH, Barsh GS, Holbrook KA. Molecular pathology in inherited disorders of collagen metabolism. *Hum Pathol.* 1982; 13(2):89–95.

316. Leigh IM, Eady RA, Heagerty AH, et al. Type VII collagen is a normal component of epidermal basement membrane, which shows altered expression in recessive dystrophic epidermolysis bullosa. *J Invest Dermatol.* 1988;90(5):639–642.

317. Stenn K. Collagen heterogeneity of skin. *Am J Dermatopathol.* 1979;1(1):87–88.

318. Deutsch TA, Esterly NB. Elastic fibers in fetal dermis. *J Invest Dermatol.* 1975;65(3):320–323.

319. Varadi DP. Studies on the chemistry and fine structure of elastic fibers from normal adult skin. *J Invest Dermatol.* 1972;59(3):238–246.

320. Hashimoto K, DiBella RJ. Electron microscopic studies of normal and abnormal elastic fibers of the skin. *J Invest Dermatol.* 1967;48(5):405–423.

321. Stadler R, Orfanos CE. Maturation and aging of elastic fibers [authors transl, in German]. *Arch Dermatol Res.* 1978;262(1):97–111.

322. Marsch WC, Schober E, Nurnberger F. Ultrastructure and morphogenesis of the elastic fibers and actinic elastosis [in German]. *Z Hautkr.* 1979;54(2):43–46.

323. Winand R. Biosynthesis, organization and degradation of mucopolysaccharides. *Arch Belg Dermatol Syphiligr.* 1972;28(1):35–40.

324. Jacques J, Cameron HC. Changes in the ground-substance of healing wounds. *J Pathol.* 1969;99(4):337–340.

325. Moretti G. The blood vessels of the skin. In: Marchionini A, ed. *Handbuch der Haut-und Geschlechtskrankheiten, Erganzungswerk.* Vol 1, Part 1. Springer-Verlag; 1968.

326. Kopf AW. The distribution of alkaline phosphatase in normal and pathologic human skin. *AMA Arch Derm.* 1957;75(1):1–37.

327. Yen A, Braverman IM. Ultrastructure of the human dermal microcirculation: the horizontal plexus of the papillary dermis. *J Invest Dermatol.* 1976;66(3):131–142.

328. Braverman IM, Yen A. Ultrastructure of the human dermal microcirculation. II: The capillary loops of the dermal papillae. *J Invest Dermatol.* 1977;68(1):44–52.

329. Seifert HW, Klingmuller G. Electron microscopic structure of normal skin-capillaries and the alkaline phosphatase pattern [in German]. *Arch Dermatol Forsch.* 1972;242(2):97–110.

330. Weber K, Braun-Falco O. Ultrastructure of blood vessels in human granulation tissue. *Arch Dermatol Forsch.* 1973;248(1):29–44.

331. Holthofer H, Virtanen I, Kariniemi AL, et al. *Ulex europaeus* I lectin as a marker for vascular endothelium in human tissues. *Lab Invest.* 1982;47(1):60–66.

332. Albelda SM, Oliver PD, Romer LH, et al. EndoCAM: a novel endothelial cell-cell adhesion molecule. *J Cell Biol.* 1990; 110(4):1227–1237.

333. Berger R, Albelda SM, Berd D, et al. Expression of platelet-endothelial cell adhesion molecule-1 (PECAM-1) during melanoma-induced angiogenesis in vivo. *J Cutan Pathol.* 1993; 20(5):399–408.

334. Suzuki Y, Hashimoto K, Crissman J, et al. The value of blood group-specific lectin and endothelial associated antibodies in the diagnosis of vascular proliferations. *J Cutan Pathol.* 1986;13(6):408–419.

335. Smolle J. HLA-DR antigen-bearing keratinocytes in various dermatologic diseases. *Acta Derm Venereol (Stockholm).* 1985; 65:9–13.

336. Jones DA, Abbassi O, McIntire LV, et al. P-selectin mediates neutrophil rolling on histamine-stimulated endothelial cells. *Biophys J.* 1993;65:1560–1569.

337. Thorlacius H, Raud J, Rosengren-Beezley S, et al. Mast cell activation induces P-selectin-dependent leukocyte rolling and adhesion in postcapillary venules in vivo. *Biochem Biophys Res Commun.* 1994;203(2):1043–1049.

338. Albelda SM, Smith CW, Ward PA. Adhesion molecules and inflammatory injury. *FASEB J.* 1994;8(8):504–512.

339. Butcher EC. Leukocyte-endothelial cell recognition: three (or more) steps to specificity and diversity. *Cell.* 1991;67(6):1033–1036.

340. Walsh LJ, Murphy GF. Role of adhesion molecules in cutaneous inflammation and neoplasia. *J Cutan Pathol.* 1992;19(3):161–171.

341. McEever RP. Selectins: novel receptors that mediate leukocyte adhesion during inflammation. *Thromb Haemost.* 1991;65:225–228.

342. Ioffreda MD, Elder DE, Albelda SM, et al. TNFα induces E-selectin expression and PECAM-1 (CD31) redistribution in extracutaneous tissues. *Endothelium.* 1993;1:47–54.

343. Hurley HJ Jr, Mescon H, Moretti G. The anatomy and histochemistry of the arteriovenous anastomosis in human digital skin. *J Invest Dermatol.* 1956;27(3):133–145.

344. Pepper MC, Laubenheimer R, Cripps DJ. Multiple glomus tumors. *J Cutan Pathol.* 1977;4(5):244–257.

345. Goodman TF. Fine structure of the cells of the Suquet-Hoyer canal. *J Invest Dermatol.* 1972;59(5):363–369.

346. Ji RC. Lymphatic endothelial cells, lymphangiogenesis, and extracellular matrix. *Lymphat Res Biol.* 2006;4(2):83–100.

347. Winkelmann RK. A silver impregnation method for peripheral nerve endings. *J Invest Dermatol.* 1955;24(1):57–64.

348. Woollard HH, Weddell G, Harpman JA. Observations on the neurohistological basis of cutaneous pain. *J Anat.* 1940;74(Pt 4):413–440.7.

349. Arthur RP, Shelley WB. The innervation of human epidermis. *J Invest Dermatol.* 1959;32(3):397–411.

350. Reed RJ. Cutaneous manifestations of neural crest disorders (neurocristopathies). *Int J Dermatol.* 1977;16(10):807–826.

351. Wiesner-Menzel L, Schulz B, Vakilzadeh F, et al. Electron microscopical evidence for a direct contact between nerve fibres and mast cells. *Acta Derm Venereol.* 1981;61(6):465–469.

352. Hosoi J, Murphy GF, Egan CL, et al. Regulation of Langerhans cell function by nerves containing calcitonin gene-related peptide. *Nature*. 1993;363(6425):159–163.

353. Matis WL, Lavker RM, Murphy GM. Substance P induces the expression of an endothelial-leukocyte adhesion molecule by microvascular endothelium. *J Invest Dermatol*. 1990;94(4):492–495.

354. Ashina A, Hosoi I, Bruyers S, et al. Regulation of Langerhans cell protein antigen presentation by calcitonin gene-related peptide, granulocyte-macrophage colony stimulating factor, and tumor necrosis factor α. *J Invest Dermatol*. 1993;100:489.

355. Orfanos CE, Mahrle G. Ultrastructure and cytochemistry of human cutaneous nerves: with special reference to the ultrastructural localization of the specific and nonspecific cholinesterases in human skin. *J Invest Dermatol*. 1973;61(2):108–120.

356. MacDonald DM, Schmitt D. Ultrastructure of the human mucocutaneous end organ. *J Invest Dermatol*. 1979;72(4):181–186.

357. Cauna N, Ross LL. The fine structure of Meissner's touch corpuscles of human fingers. *J Biophys Biochem Cytol*. 1960;8:467–482.

358. Hashimoto K. Fine structure of the Meissner corpuscle of human palmar skin. *J Invest Dermatol*. 1973;60:20–28.

359. Pease DC, Quilliam TA. Electron microscopy of the Pacinian corpuscle. *J Biophys Biochem Cytol*. 1957;3(3):331–342.

360. Seemayer TA, Knaack J, Wang NS, et al. On the ultrastructure of hibernoma. *Cancer*. 1975;36(5):1785–1793.

361. Fuchs E. The tortoise and the hair: slow-cycling cells in the stem cell race. *Cell*. 2009;137(5):811–819.

362. Cotsarelis G, Kaur P, Dhouailly D, et al. Epithelial stem cells in the skin: definition, markers, localization and functions. *Exp Dermatol*. 1999;8(1):80–88.

363. Fuchs E, Tumbar T, Guasch G. Socializing with the neighbors: stem cells and their niche. *Cell*. 2004;116(6):769–778.

364. Barthel R, Aberdam D. Epidermal stem cells. *J Eur Acad Dermatol Venereol*. 2005;19(4):405–413.

365. Nowak JA, Polak L, Pasolli HA, et al. Hair follicle stem cells are specified and function in early skin morphogenesis. *Cell Stem Cell*. 2008;3(1):33–43.

366. Snippert HJ, Haegebarth A, Kasper M, et al. Lgr6 marks stem cells in the hair follicle that generate all cell lineages of the skin. *Science*. 2010;327(5971):1385–1389.

367. Nanba D, Toki F, Barrandon Y, et al. Recent advances in the epidermal growth factor receptor/ligand system biology on skin homeostasis and keratinocyte stem cell regulation. *J Dermatol Sci*. 2013;72(2):81–86.

368. Page ME, Lombard P, Ng F, et al. The epidermis comprises autonomous compartments maintained by distinct stem cell populations. *Cell Stem Cell*. 2013;13(4):471–482.

369. Nishimura EK. Melanocyte stem cells: a melanocyte reservoir in hair follicles for hair and skin pigmentation. *Pigment Cell Melanoma Res*. 2011;24(3):401–410.

370. Li L, Fukunaga-Kalabis M, Herlyn M. Isolation and cultivation of dermal stem cells that differentiate into functional epidermal melanocytes. *Methods Mol Biol*. 2012;806:15–29.

371. Gleason BC, Crum CP, Murphy GF. Expression patterns of MITF during human cutaneous embryogenesis: evidence for bulge epithelial expression and persistence of dermal melanoblasts. *J Cutan Pathol*. 2008;35(7):615–622.

372. Girouard SD, Murphy GF. Melanoma stem cells: not rare, but well done. *Lab Invest*. 2011;91(5):647–664.

373. Beyer Nardi N, da Silva Meirelles L. *Mesenchymal Stem Cells: Isolation, In Vitro Expansion and Characterization*. Springer; 2006.

374. Wobus AM, Boheler KR, eds. *Stem Cells: Handbook of Experimental Pharmacology*. Vol 174. Springer; 2006.

375. Sasaki M, Abe R, Fujita Y, et al. Mesenchymal stem cells are recruited into wounded skin and contribute to wound repair by transdifferentiation into multiple skin cell type. *J Immunol*. 2008;180(4):2581–2587.

376. Fu X, Fang L, Li X, et al. Enhanced wound-healing quality with bone marrow mesenchymal stem cells autografting after skin injury. *Wound Repair Regen*. 2006;14(3):325–335.

377. Lozito TP, Kuo CK, Taboas JM, et al. Human mesenchymal stem cells express vascular cell phenotypes upon interaction with endothelial cell matrix. *J Cell Biochem*. 2009;107(4):714–722.

378. Yamaguchi Y, Kubo T, Murakami T, et al. Bone marrow cells differentiate into wound myofibroblasts and accelerate the healing of wounds with exposed bones when combined with an occlusive dressing. *Br J Dermatol*. 2005;152(4):616–622.

379. Wu Y, Chen L, Scott PG, et al. Mesenchymal stem cells enhance wound healing through differentiation and angiogenesis. *Stem Cells*. 2007;25(10):2648–2659.

380. Jackson WM, Nesti LJ, Tuan RS. Mesenchymal stem cell therapy for attenuation of scar formation during wound healing. *Stem Cell Res Ther*. 2012;3(3):20.

381. Raicevic G, Rouas R, Najar M, et al. Inflammation modifies the pattern and the function of Toll-like receptors expressed by human mesenchymal stromal cells. *Hum Immunol*. 2010;71(3):235–244.

382. Bunnell BA, Betancourt AM, Sullivan DE. New concepts on the immune modulation mediated by mesenchymal stem cells. *Stem Cell Res Ther*. 2010;1(5):34.

383. VanderBeken S, De Vries JC, Meier-Schiesser B, et al. Newly defined ABCB5+ dermal mesenchymal stem cells promote healing of chronic iron overload wounds via secretion of interleukin-1 receptor antagonist. *Stem Cells*. 2019;37:1057–1074.

384. Fenske NA, Lober CW. Structural and functional changes of normal aging skin. *J Am Acad Dermatol*. 1986;15(4, pt 1):571–585.

385. Kurban RS, Bhawan J. Histologic changes in skin associated with aging. *J Dermatol Surg Oncol*. 1990;16(10):908–914.

386. Montagna W, Carlisle K. Structural changes in ageing skin. *Br J Dermatol*. 1990;122(suppl 35):61–70.

387. Murphy GF, Russell-Goldman E. The pathobiology of skin aging: new insights into an old dilemma. *Am J Pathol*. 2020;190;1356–1369.

388. Ortonne JP. Pigmentary changes of the ageing skin. *Br J Dermatol*. 1990;122(*suppl 35*):21–28.

389. Bhawan J, Andersen W, Lee J, et al. Photoaging versus intrinsic aging: a morphologic assessment of facial skin. *J Cutan Pathol*. 1995;22(2):154–159.

390. Sellheyer K. Pathogenesis of solar elastosis: synthesis or degradation? *J Cutan Pathol*. 2003;30(2):123–127.

391. Lester L, Venditti C. The prevalence of pili multigemini. *Br J Dermatol*. 2007;156(6):1362–1363.

392. Mahaisavariya P, Cohen PR, Rapini RP. Incidental epidermolytic hyperkeratosis. *Am J Dermatopathol*. 1995;17(1):23–28.

393. Waldo ED, Ackerman AB. Epidermolytic hyperkeratosis and focal acantholytic dyskeratosis: a unified concept. *Pathol Annu*. 1978;13(pt 1):149–175.

394. Hutcheson AC, Nietert PJ, Maize JC. Incidental epidermolytic hyperkeratosis and focal acantholytic dyskeratosis in common acquired melanocytic nevi and atypical melanocytic lesions. *J Am Acad Dermatol*. 2004;50(3):388–390.

395. Ashbee HR. Update on the genus *Malassezia*. *Med Mycol*. 2007;45(4):287–303.

Chapter 4

Laboratory Methods

ROSALIE ELENITSAS AND JOHN T. SEYKORA

INTRODUCTION

There are a number of important steps in accessioning and preparing histologic sections prior to their interpretation by the dermatopathologist. Failure to handle the tissue properly may make it difficult to provide an accurate diagnosis or appropriate margins. Attention to each step is critical to the final step in providing a pathology report (Table 4-1).

PREPARATION OF SPECIMENS

Specimen Accessioning

Skin biopsies received by the histopathology laboratory are typically logged into an electronic medical record system that will link the patient's demographic data with the specimen and a unique "barcode" that will label the specimen bottle, tissue block, and all slides associated with the case. Careful identification of specimens using multiple factors is important at all stages of the diagnostic process, including sign-out.

Fixation

It is important to properly fix a skin biopsy to stabilize cellular macromolecules, including proteins, and prevent tissue decay. The specimen should be placed in a fixative immediately after it is removed from the patient, as artifacts may result if it is allowed to dry. The fixative of choice is a 10% neutral-buffered formalin solution. The volume of formalin should be 10 to 20 times the volume of the specimen. During winter, if the specimen might be exposed to subfreezing temperatures, either 95% ethyl alcohol, 10% by volume, should be added to the formalin solution, or the specimen should be allowed to stand in the formalin solution at room temperature for at least 6 hours before mailing.

Adequate time should be allowed for fixation. Fixation time is 1 to 2 hours/mL thickness. Large specimens, such as excised tumors, should be cut in the laboratory into slices 4 to 5 mm to promote fixation, which typically takes overnight and requires greater volumes of formalin.

Grossing

After fixation, ink should be applied to the deep and lateral margins of an excisional specimen requiring examination of tissue margins. The specimen should be appropriately cut for the examination of margins. Some examples are provided in Figure 4-1. It is important to remember that these cuts are only representative of the margins because it is almost impossible to evaluate every marginal cell. If a localizing suture has been placed by the surgeon, ink of a different color should be applied to that margin, or some other method of labeling should be used to identify the margins. Both 4- and 6-mm punch biopsies are generally bisected, and specimens 3 mm in size or smaller should be submitted in toto. If a laboratory does not handle many skin specimens, discussion with the embedding technician may be appropriate to facilitate optimal orientation of the blocks.

Table 4-1
Source of Error in the Laboratory

Labeling specimen at accessioning

Grossing, specimen switch

Tissue processor malfunction affecting tissue quality

Embedding, malorientation

Sectioning, cut away tissue

Staining quality

Failure to do quality assurance before sending slides to pathologist

Pathologist identification of correct slides for patient

Pathologist diagnosis

Transcription

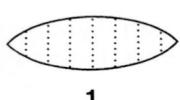 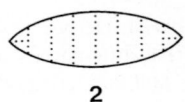 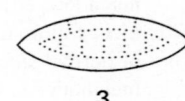

1 2 3

Figure 4-1 Preparation of blocks from a skin ellipse. After the margins have been painted with ink, the specimen is sectioned for processing and later embedding. In example 1, the tissue is cut as if one is slicing a loaf of bread; this is one of the most common methods used in dermatopathology laboratories. Example 2 allows for better evaluation of the "tips" of the ellipse; however, embedding of these small pieces is more difficult. Often, only the center section of the "tips" is embedded, or the tips may be cut in half and embedded flat, especially for smaller specimens. In example 3, the entire margin is theoretically visualized; however, this method requires the technician to meticulously embed and orient small pieces of tissue and is not recommended for most specimens in most routine laboratories. (Reprinted from Rapini RP. Comparison of methods for checking surgical margins. *J Am Acad Dermatol*. 1990;23(2 Pt 1):288–294. Copyright © 1990 Elsevier. With permission.)

Demonstration of Enzyme Activities

With few exceptions, specimens should not be placed in formalin for the demonstration of enzyme activities. Instead, they should be delivered to the laboratory wrapped in water-moistened gauze and placed in a clean container because frozen sections cut on a cryostat are usually used to detect enzyme activity. Because detecting enzyme activities is not routinely done, it is best to first check with the laboratory prior to submitting a sample.

Although immunohistochemistry has largely replaced histochemistry for routine diagnostic use, certain enzymes, such as succinic dehydrogenase and phosphorylase (eccrine), and acid phosphatase and β-glucuronidase (apocrine), can be detected in glandular tumors. However, these differentials are not usually significant clinically.

Enzyme reactions can be carried out on formalin-fixed, paraffin-embedded tissue, an example being demonstration of naphthol AS-D chloroacetate esterase activity, with naphthol AS-D chloroacetate as substrate (present in mature and immature granulocytes, except in myeloblasts and mast cells).

In two diseases—scleredema of Buschke and amyloidosis—unfixed frozen sections may show a stronger reaction to specific staining methods than is obtainable with formalin-fixed material. It is recommended that in these two diseases only part of the tissue be fixed in formalin and the remainder be used for frozen sections. In scleredema, demonstration of hyaluronic acid with toluidine blue at pH 7.0 may be more intense in unfixed, frozen sections than in formalin-fixed sections; in amyloidosis, the reactions of the amyloid with crystal violet or Congo red may be stronger in unfixed, frozen sections (see Chapter 17).

Processing

The purpose of processing is to extract water and lipids from the skin samples and to provide a supporting matrix (paraffin) so that thin tissue sections can be cut with minimal distortion. After fixation, routine specimens are processed in machines programmed to serially change the alcohol and xylene exchanges. Alternative methods are required for specimens that are to be stained for lipids. Because lipids are extracted by xylene during processing, frozen sections are cut and postfixed in 10% neutral-buffered formalin to preserve tissue lipids.

In the automated histology processor, the specimens pass through a series of increasing concentrations of ethanol for dehydration, then through xylene for lipid extraction and clearing of alcohol. Finally, the tissues are infiltrated with several changes of hot, liquid paraffin (or Paraplast) to provide a matrix so that the tissue can be stabilized and cut easily. This processing takes between 3 and 12 hours; in most laboratories, processing is run overnight. Other methodology includes microwave-assisted tissue processing, application of microwave irradiation accelerates tissue fixation and processing, allowing processing times of 1 to 2 hours (1). This rapid tissue processing, when optimized, can yield histologic sections and immunohistochemical staining comparable in quality to conventional tissue processing (2). In the authors' experience, rapid tissue processing yields comparable results in most tissues except for very small specimens or larger specimens with substantial fatty tissue.

Following processing, the specimens are embedded with the cutting surface face down into the cassette base mold, in the liquid paraffin, which is allowed to harden. To prevent tangentially oriented sections, it is important that the cutting surface be firmly embedded in the base of this mold. The specimens are then cut on a rotary microtome into sections ~5 μm thick.

Staining

Routine sections are usually stained with hematoxylin and eosin, the most widely used routine stain. With this staining method, nuclei stain blue or "basophilic," and keratins, collagen, muscles, and nerves stain red or "eosinophilic." Special stains are employed when particular structures need to be demonstrated (for details, see later discussion and Ref. (3)).

HISTOCHEMICAL STAINING

Histochemistry, especially immunohistochemistry, at both the light microscopic and electron microscopic levels has gained increasing importance in recent years and has been largely responsible for the expansion of histopathology from a purely descriptive science to one that is more analytic. Many enzyme histochemical methods are used only for research and typically perform better on fresh tissue compared with formalin-fixed tissue.

However, most histochemical "special" stains can be carried out on formalin-fixed, paraffin-embedded material. Their primary uses in dermatopathology are listed in Table 4-2.

The *periodic acid–Schiff* (*PAS*) *stain* demonstrates the presence of certain polysaccharides, particularly glycogen and mucoproteins containing neutral mucopolysaccharides, by staining them magenta. The PAS reaction consists in the oxidation of adjacent hydroxyl groups in 1,2-glycols to aldehydes and the staining of the aldehydes with fuchsin-sulfuric acid. The PAS reaction is also of value in the study of basement membrane thickening, such as in lupus erythematosus (Fig. 4-2) or porphyria cutanea tarda. Furthermore, because the cell walls of fungi are composed of a mixture of cellulose and chitin and thus contain polysaccharides, fungi stain magenta with the PAS reaction.

For the distinction of neutral mucopolysaccharides and fungi from glycogen deposits, it is necessary to compare two serial sections, one exposed to diastase before staining and the other not. Because glycogen is digested by the diastase and is thus no longer detected by the PAS reaction, it can be easily distinguished from neutral mucopolysaccharides and fungi that are diastase resistant. Because glycogen is present in outer root sheath cells and eccrine gland cells, demonstration of glycogen may be of diagnostic value in adnexal tumors with outer root sheath or eccrine differentiation. Demonstration of neutral mucopolysaccharides is of value in Paget disease of the breast and in extramammary Paget disease.

The *alcian blue reaction* demonstrates the presence of acid mucopolysaccharides by staining them blue. Acid mucopolysaccharides are present in the dermal ground substance but in amounts too small to be demonstrable in normal skin. However, in the dermal mucinoses, there is a considerable increase in nonsulfated acid mucopolysaccharides, mainly

Table 4-2

Histochemical Stains Used in Dermatopathology

Stain	Purpose of Stain	Results
Hematoxylin–eosin	Routine	Nuclei: blue Collagen, muscles, nerves: red
Masson trichrome	Collagen	Collagen: blue or green Nuclei, muscles, nerves: dark red
Verhoeff-van Gieson	Elastic fibers	Elastic fibers: black Collagen: red Nuclei, muscles, nerves: yellow
Pinkus acid orcein	Elastic fibers	Elastic fibers: dark brown
Silver nitrate	Melanin, reticulum fibers (argyrophilic)	Melanin, reticulum fibers: black
Fontana-Masson	Melanin (argentaffin)	Melanin: black
Methenamine silver	Fungi, Donovan bodies, Frisch bacilli (rhinoscleroma), basement membranes	Black
Grocott	Fungi	Fungus cell walls: black
PAS	Glycogen, neutral MPS, fungi	Glycogen: red; diastase labile Neutral MPS, fungi: red; diastase resistant
Alcian blue, pH 2.5	Acid MPS	Blue
Alcian blue, pH 0.5	Sulfated MPS	Blue
Toluidine blue	Acid MPS	Blue
Colloidal iron	Acid MPS	Blue
Mucicarmine	"Epithelial" mucin	Red
Giemsa	Mast cell granules, acid MPS, myeloid granules, Leishmania	MCG, acid MPS: metachromatically purple Myeloid granules, Leishmania: red
Fite	Acid-fast bacilli	Red
Perls potassium ferrocyanide	Hemosiderin (iron)	Blue
Congo red	Amyloid	Pink-red, green birefringence in polarized light
Von Kossa	Calcium	Black
Scarlet red	Lipids	Red
Oil red O	Lipids	Red
Naphthol-AS-D-chloroacetate esterase	Mast cells, neutrophils, myelocytes	Granules stain red
Warthin–Starry	Spirochetes	Black
Dieterle and Steiner	Spirochetes, bacillary angiomatosis	Black
Ziehl–Neelson	Acid-fast bacilli	Red

Note: All stains, except those for lipids, can be carried out on formalin-fixed, paraffin-embedded specimens. The stains for lipids require formalin-fixed frozen sections.
MCG, mast cell granules; MPS, mucopolysaccharides; PAS, periodic acid–Schiff.

hyaluronic acid, so that the mucin stains with alcian blue (see Chapter 17). In extramammary Paget disease of the anus with rectal carcinoma (see Chapter 29) and in cutaneous metastases of carcinoma of the gastrointestinal tract containing goblet cells (see Chapter 38), tumor cells in the skin, like their parent cells, secrete sialomucin. Sialomucin contains nonsulfated acid mucopolysaccharides staining with alcian blue, as well as PAS-positive neutral mucopolysaccharides. Whereas non-sulfated acid mucopolysaccharides stain with alcian blue at pH 2.5 but not at pH 0.5, strongly acidic sulfated acid mucopolysaccharides, such as heparin in mast cell granules and chondroitin sulfate in cartilage, stain with alcian blue both at pH 2.5 and at pH 0.5.

Several special stains for elastic tissue are available. The most commonly used stains are the Verhoeff-van Gieson stain (Fig. 4-3) or Weigert resorcin-fuchsin. Additional techniques, such as the Luna stain and the Miller stain, may allow better visualization of elastic fibers than traditional methods (4). These

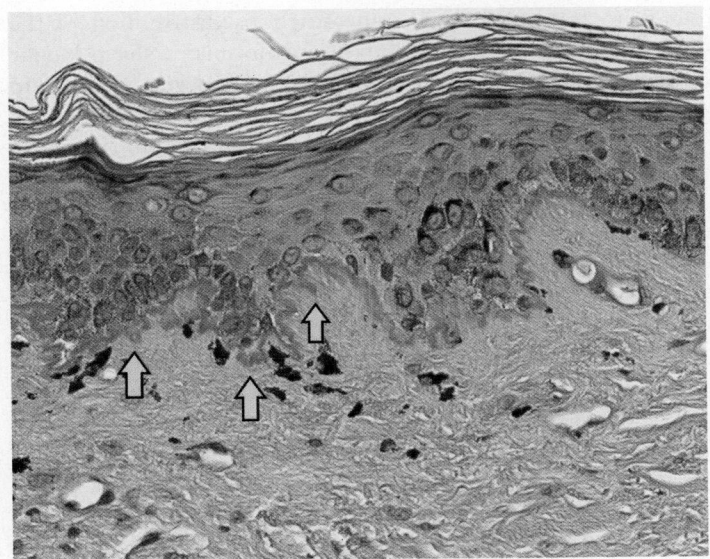

Figure 4-2 PAS stain. In this case of discoid lupus erythematosus, PAS staining highlights a thickened basement membrane (*arrows*).

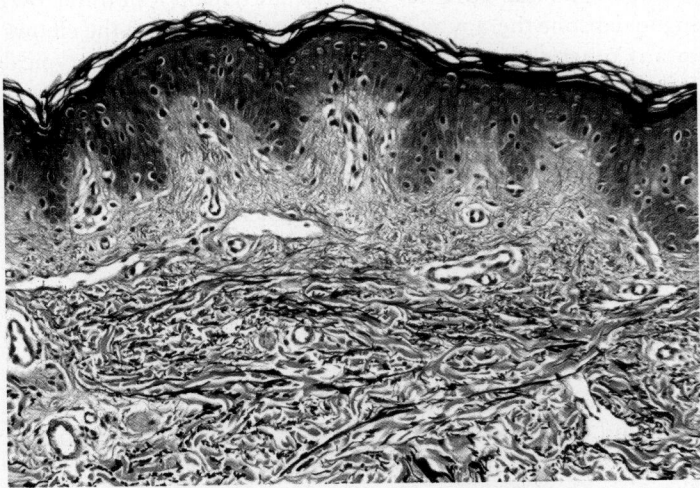

Figure 4-3 Elastic fibers. This Verhoeff-van Gieson stain demonstrates the darkly staining normal elastic fibers of the skin.

stains are beneficial in the diagnosis of anetoderma, connective tissue nevi, middermal elastolysis, and other alterations of elastic tissue.

The Giemsa stain is frequently used to highlight mast cells. Giemsa contains methylene blue, a metachromatic stain. The granules of a mast cell stain metachromatically purple.

POLARISCOPIC EXAMINATION

Polariscopic examination is the examination of histologic sections under the microscope with polarized light, that is, light from which all waves except those vibrating in one plane are excluded.

For polariscopic examination, two filter disks made of polarizing plastics or glass are placed on the microscope. One disk is placed below the condenser of the microscope and acts as the polarizer. The other disk is placed in the eyepiece of the microscope or on top of the glass slide and acts as the analyzer. When one of the two disks is rotated so that the path of the light through the two disks is broken at a right angle, the field is dark. However, when doubly refractile substances are introduced between the two disks, they break the polarization and are visible as bright white bodies in the dark field.

Polariscopic examination is useful in evaluating lipid deposits, certain foreign bodies, gout, and amyloid.

With regard to lipids, it is not fully known why certain lipids are doubly refractile and others are not. In general, cholesterol esters are doubly refractile, but free cholesterol, phospholipids, and neutral fat are not. Only formalin-fixed, frozen sections can be used for a polariscopic examination for lipids.

Doubly refractile lipids are regularly present in the tuberous and plane xanthomas and xanthelasmata (but not always in the eruptive xanthomas) of hyperlipoproteinemia, in the cutaneous lesions of diffuse normolipemic plane xanthoma, and in the vascular walls of angiokeratoma corporis diffusum (Fabry disease) (see Chapter 33). Doubly refractile lipids are present, as long as the cutaneous lesions contain a sufficient amount of lipids, in histiocytosis X (Hand–Schüller–Christian type) (see Chapter 26), in juvenile xanthogranuloma (see Chapter 26), in erythema elevatum diutinum (extracellular cholesterosis) (see Chapter 8), and in dermatofibroma (lipidized "histiocytoma") (see Chapter 32).

Among foreign bodies, silica causes granulomas showing doubly refractile spicules. These granulomas are caused either by particles of soil or glass (silicon dioxide) or by talcum powder (magnesium silicate) (see Chapter 14). Wooden splinters, suture material, and starch granules are also doubly refractile. An example of polariscopic examination is seen in Figure 4-4.

Gouty tophi show double refraction of the urate crystals if the crystals are sufficiently preserved. They are preserved by the use of alcohol rather than formalin for fixation (see Chapter 17).

Amyloid shows a characteristic green birefringence in polarized light after staining with alkaline Congo red (see Chapter 17).

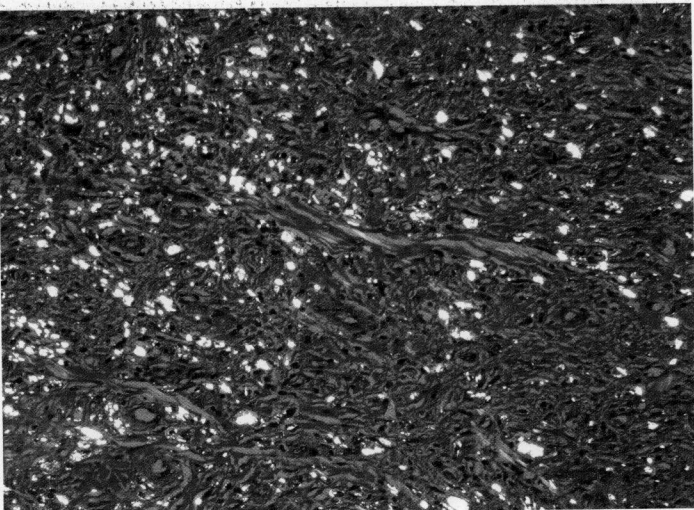

Figure 4-4 Polariscopic examination. In this talc granuloma, polariscopy reveals hundreds of refractile foreign bodies within the dermis.

IMMUNOFLUORESCENCE TESTING

Immunofluorescence testing is a specialized technique that is beneficial in the diagnosis of certain skin disorders. Two immunofluorescence methods are commonly used in dermatology: direct immunofluorescence testing (DIF), which probes for immunoreactants localized in patients' skin or mucous membranes, and indirect immunofluorescence testing, which is used to identify and titer circulating autoantibodies in the patient's serum. A modified indirect immunofluorescence technique using the patient's skin as a substrate, known as immunomapping, is used to determine the site of cleavage or abnormalities in the distribution of mutated proteins in forms of hereditary epidermolysis bullosa.

Direct Immunofluorescence

DIF has a valuable diagnostic role in several autoimmune and inflammatory mucocutaneous diseases, including autoimmune-mediated blistering diseases, dermatitis herpetiformis, Henoch–Schönlein purpura (immunoglobulin [Ig] A vasculitis), and cutaneous lupus erythematosus. The role of DIF as a diagnostic procedure is important but not critical in other dermatoses, such as dermatomyositis, cutaneous porphyrias, pseudoporphyria, lichen planus, and vasculitides other than Henoch–Schönlein purpura. Table 4-3 illustrates a stepwise schematic for the evaluation of immunofluorescence sections prior to making an immunopathologic diagnosis.

Biopsy Techniques

A 3- to 4-mm punch biopsy is generally adequate. In the group of autoimmune blistering diseases, an inflamed but unblistered perilesional area is the ideal specimen. Blistered-lesional sampling is the most common cause of false-negative results. On the other hand, sampling too distant from the blistering can also cause false-negative results. In some cases of pemphigus, pemphigoid, and epidermolysis bullosa acquisita, false-positive results can occur if blistered lesions are analyzed. Of note,

owing to the often focal, noncontiguous distribution of the immunoreactants in dermatitis herpetiformis, a shave biopsy provides a broader surface containing more dermal papillae to assess than a punch biopsy.

The performance of an adequate perilesional biopsy in mucosal lesions is often not feasible, and thus a high incidence of false negatives and even false positives may occur in these specimens. In patients with desquamative gingivitis secondary to mucous membrane pemphigoid, an easy way to obtain sampling is by the so-called peeling technique, in which rubbing the perilesional affected gingivae with a cotton swab induces a "fresh peeling of the mucosa." In most cases of mucous membrane pemphigoid, the 180- and 230-kDa hemidesmosomal antigens are the autoantigens; therefore, the hemidesmosomes will be available for interpretation in the peeled gingivae specimens, and a linear immunostaining with "capping" phenomenon is observed (5).

It has been reported that there is a theoretical higher incidence of false-negative results in bullous pemphigoid lesions from lower extremities; however, this finding has not been confirmed by others.

In asymptomatic dermatitis herpetiformis patients who have strictly adhered to a gluten-free diet for <6 months, or even patients that have not done so but remain lesion free owing to dapsone therapy, wide-shaved specimens from the elbows or any other classically affected area will still show the typical IgA deposits at the tips of dermal papillae (6).

In autoimmune and inflammatory disorders other than autoimmune blistering diseases in which DIF plays an important role, the specimens should be taken from lesional areas, including cutaneous lupus erythematosus, dermatomyositis, vasculitides, lichen planus, cutaneous porphyria, and pseudoporphyria.

Transport and Laboratory Handling of Biopsy Specimens

Tissue for immunofluorescence studies should be obtained fresh and kept moist until it is quickly frozen. Skin specimens can be kept on saline-moistened gauze and transported immediately to the laboratory if it is nearby. If it cannot be transported in <24 hours, the specimen should be put into Michel transport medium. This medium is composed of 5% ammonium sulfate, the potassium inhibitor N-ethylmaleimide, and magnesium sulfate in citrate buffer (pH 7.25). This solution is stable at room temperature but must be kept in a tightly capped container to prevent absorption of CO_2 and acidification. Specimens stored in Michel medium are stable for at least 4 weeks, and potentially up to 6 months, at room temperature. Specimens for immunofluorescence that were inadvertently put into formalin may produce nonspecific staining as well as false-negative results. The use of Michel medium has made the DIF technique much more readily applicable. When the specimen is received in a laboratory, the ammonium sulfate is washed out, and the specimen is oriented and embedded in OCT (optimal cutting temperature) compound, and then the specimen is snap frozen. The tissue is then sectioned at 6 μm. The frozen sections are incubated with antihuman antibodies to IgG, IgA, IgM, C3, and fibrinogen. Some laboratories also utilize C5b-9. These antibodies are linked to a fluorescent label such as fluorescein isothiocyanate (FITC) to allow visualization using a fluorescence microscope. Slides should be stored in darkness

Table 4-3
Multistep Scheme for the Interpretation of Cutaneous Direct Immunofluorescence

Real vs. artifact

Specific vs. nonspecific

↓

Location of immunofluorescence
(Epithelial, basement membrane zone, vascular)

↓

Dominant immunoreactant(s)
IgG, IgA, IgM, C3, Fibrinogen

↓

Characteristics
(Granular, linear, continuous, or patchy)

↓

Diagnostic algorithm based on IF patterns

IF, immunofluorescence; Ig, immunoglobulin.

because light exposure can cause fading of the stain. The use of permanent mounting medium with antifade ingredients has allowed for longer storage times, although continued storage in darkness is recommended (7).

Direct Immunofluorescence Interpretation
Autoimmune Blistering Diseases

Cell Surface Membrane (intercellular) Pattern. Sensitivity of DIF with active autoimmune blistering disease is high, over 90%. If it is not, it may be attributable to technical factors. In pemphigus vulgaris (PV) and pemphigus foliaceus (PF), the IgG immunostaining on the epithelial cell surfaces can be granular and/or linear, giving a characteristic "chicken wire" pattern. C3 staining may also be detected and, rarely, IgA. Nonspecific patchy granular staining along the basement membrane is not uncommon, especially in mucosal lesions. In paraneoplastic pemphigus the IgG "chicken wire" immunostaining tends to be linear, thick, and homogeneous throughout the epidermis and mucosal specimens, including those from bronchi with or without a concomitant linear basement membrane staining. Lichenoid mucosal and even cutaneous lesions in paraneoplastic pemphigus tend to show focal granular IgG and other immunoreactants along the basement membrane without the typical "chicken wire" pattern.

Linear Basement Membrane Pattern. A variety of blistering disorders produce linear basement membrane staining: pemphigoid, epidermolysis bullosa acquisita, linear IgA disease, pemphigoid gestationis, and bullous lupus erythematosus. These disorders can be differentiated by determining which antibodies are present and correlating with routine histopathology and clinical presentation. Some cases of subepidermal blistering disorders with deposition of immune reactants may be difficult to differentiate from one another. The typical example is pemphigoid and epidermolysis bullosa acquisita, both subepidermal blistering diseases with C3 and/or IgG deposition on DIF (Fig. 4-5). In these cases, a technique called salt-split direct immunofluorescence often circumvents this problem. Direct immunofluorescence salt-split skin analysis can be performed only if the specimen sent for DIF is not already blistered. This technique consists of thawing the frozen specimen formerly used for routine DIF and incubating it in 1 M NaCl for 48 to 72 hours, allowing for separation of the epidermis from the dermis. Following the incubation in NaCl, new sections of frozen skin are cut and incubated with antibodies linked to FITC, similar to the

standard DIF testing. This salt cleaves the basement membrane zone through the lamina lucida, leaving the hemidesmosomes on the epidermal side and deeper-seated proteins such as type VII collagen and epiligrin on the dermal side of an artificially induced blister. Therefore, in virtually all cases of bullous pemphigoid, the linear IgG immunostaining will be localized on the epidermal side (occasionally epidermal and dermal) and in epidermolysis bullosa acquisita on the dermal side. Exceptions include p200 pemphigoid and anti–laminin-332 mucosal pemphigoid, which show staining on the dermal side (8). Some authors have recommended evaluation of the serration pattern of DIF (9). The pemphigoid group of diseases will produce an n-serrated pattern (Fig. 4-6); epidermolysis bullosa acquisita and bullous lupus erythematosus will produce a u-serrated pattern.

Cutaneous Lupus Erythematosus

DIF has a significant value in the evaluation of patients with active cutaneous connective tissue disease. The intensity of the deposits of immunoreactants along the basement membrane in these patients correlates with the degree of interface/lichenoid dermatitis/mucositis.

In discoid lupus erythematosus, granular immune reactants (IgG, IgA, IgM, and C3) are present along the dermal–epidermal junction. The most common immunoreactant visualized with DIF is IgM; in systemic lupus erythematosus and in subacute cutaneous lupus erythematosus, it is IgG (Fig. 4-7). Of note, most patients with anti–Ro-positive subacute cutaneous lupus erythematosus may have a characteristic granular IgG-speckling pattern along the basement membrane and throughout the epidermis. The lupus band test, originally described as positive when granular IgG is present along the basement membrane zone in specimens from sun-protected nonlesional areas, is rapidly being abandoned owing to its unreliability and the availability of more reliable methods for the early diagnosis and prediction of systemic disease in lupus erythematosus (Chapter 10).

In cutaneous lesions of dermatomyositis, dense, granular C5b-9 (membrane attack complex) deposition at the basement membrane zone and upper dermal vessels along with that of

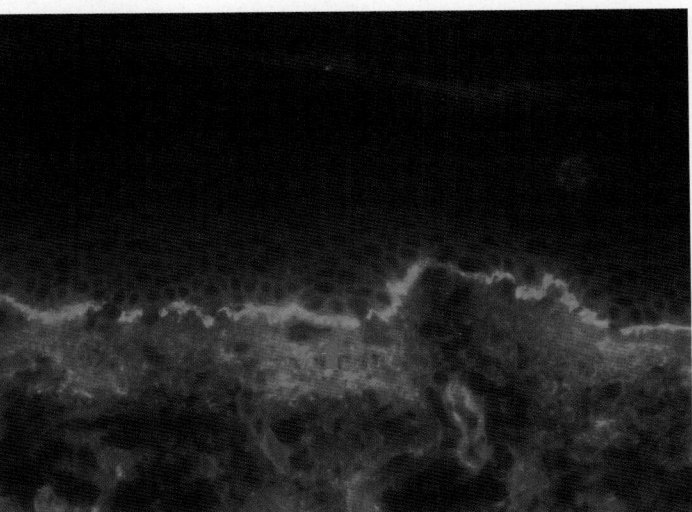

Figure 4-6 Direct immunofluorescence: n-serrated pattern of pemphigoid. Anti-C3 shows linear basement membrane staining with areas resembling a lower case "n" (*arrow*).

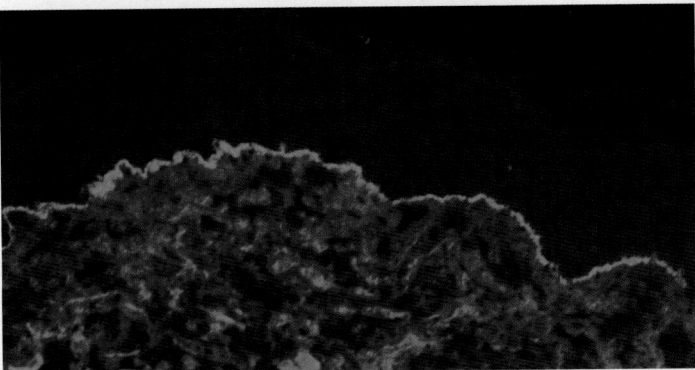

Figure 4-5 Direct immunofluorescence. Bullous pemphigoid. Continuous linear C3 staining along the basement membrane zone.

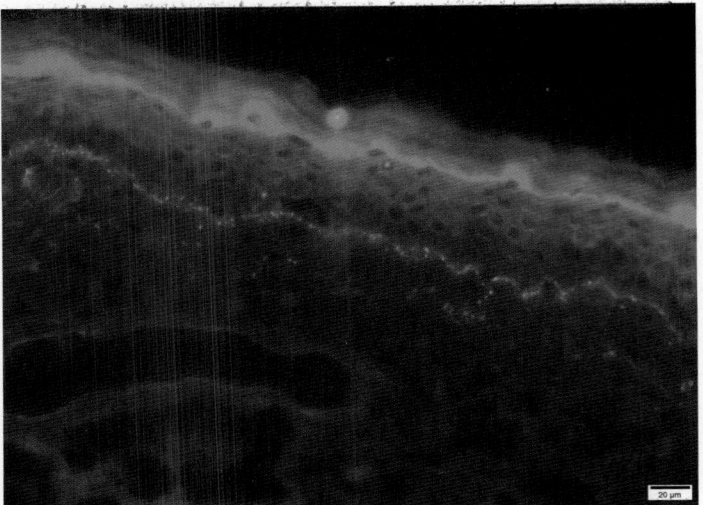

Figure 4-7 Lupus erythematosus. Direct immunofluorescence shows granular IgG along the dermal–epidermal junction.

weaker C3, IgG, and IgM deposits is an immunofluorescence pattern that may help to distinguish dermatomyositis from lupus erythematosus spectrum (10).

Cutaneous Vasculitides

DIF evaluation is an important diagnostic tool in the workup of cutaneous small-vessel vasculitis, especially Henoch–Schönlein purpura. The best immunofluorescence diagnostic yield in Henoch–Schönlein purpura is obtained from 1- to 2-day-old lesions. As lesions get older, the IgA deposits get degraded and cleared. Because most patients have older lesions at the time of the evaluation, a high index of suspicion is required and an exhaustive search for scant granular IgA deposits in very superficial papillary dermis is mandatory before ruling out Henoch–Schönlein purpura.

Hypocomplementemic urticarial vasculitis is another small-vessel vasculitis in which DIF plays a diagnostic role. In this type of cutaneous vasculitis, granular IgG and C3 deposits are seen in and around small dermal vessels and along the basement membrane zone.

Other Autoimmune and Inflammatory Skin Diseases

Lichen planus lesions, mainly the mucosal variant, are characterized by typical yet not pathognomonic, linear and shaggy fibrinogen deposits and patchy granular IgM and C3 along the basement membrane. Colloid bodies, often present in lichenoid tissue reactions, are often positive on DIF. They are most frequently positive with antibodies to IgM but may stain with other antibodies as well. In lichen planus pemphigoides, one will see immunofluorescent staining that is indistinguishable from pemphigoid.

The DIF findings in cutaneous porphyrias are indistinguishable from those seen in pseudoporphyria. These findings are characterized by thick and glassy linear IgG and IgA deposits in superficial dermal vessels in a "doughnut pattern" and along the basement membrane. It is believed that immunoglobulins become trapped and bound to glycoproteins in a thickened basement membrane zone and degenerated blood vessels in this disorder.

Indirect Immunofluorescence

Indirect immunofluorescence is a semiquantitative procedure in which immunolabeling is carried out to evaluate the presence and titer of circulating antibodies or specifically to localize antigen in the skin.

Indirect Immunofluorescence in the Evaluation of Circulating Antiepithelial Antibodies

Blood is drawn into a tube without anticoagulant, and the serum is serially diluted. Substrates most commonly used are 6-μm frozen sections of monkey esophagus, human salt-split skin, and murine bladder. The substrate is incubated with serum dilutions for 30 minutes at room temperature and then washed; antibodies bound to the substrates are detected by incubation with FITC-labeled goat antihuman IgG and/or IgA.

Monkey esophagus is probably the best substrate for the evaluation of antiepithelial surface antibodies specifically for PV. PF may show false-negative results with this substrate, and normal human skin can be used as a substrate if PF is suspected and there is a negative result using monkey esophagus. Low titers of antiepithelial surface antibodies up to 1:80 or even higher can also be seen in control sera (11). In PV and PF, antidesmoglein antibodies give a "chicken wire" staining pattern (Fig. 4-8). It may be more prominent on superficial epithelial cells, whereas in paraneoplastic pemphigus the antiplakin antibodies give a pattern that is consistently homogeneous throughout the epithelium and sometimes even associated with immunostaining along the basement membrane zone.

Transitional epithelium is a plakin-rich substrate, and thus murine bladder is a common substrate for the screening of circulating antiplakin antibodies in paraneoplastic pemphigus. Exceptional cases of PV and PF and pemphigoid can have concomitant low-titer antidesmoplakin antibodies.

Monkey esophagus is also a useful substrate in the indirect immunofluorescence screening for subepidermal autoimmune blistering disease. Basement membrane staining on monkey esophagus can be seen in both pemphigoid and epidermolysis bullosa acquisita. However, human salt-split skin renders better definition of the subtypes of subepidermal blistering disorders. In this technique, normal human skin is incubated in NaCl, separating the epidermis from the dermis. Patient serum is

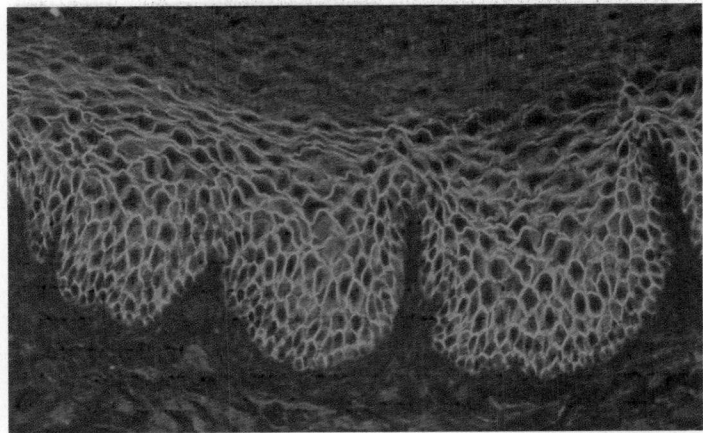

Figure 4-8 Pemphigus vulgaris. Indirect immunofluorescence with monkey esophagus substrate. Anti-IgG staining of epithelium showing a "chicken wire" pattern.

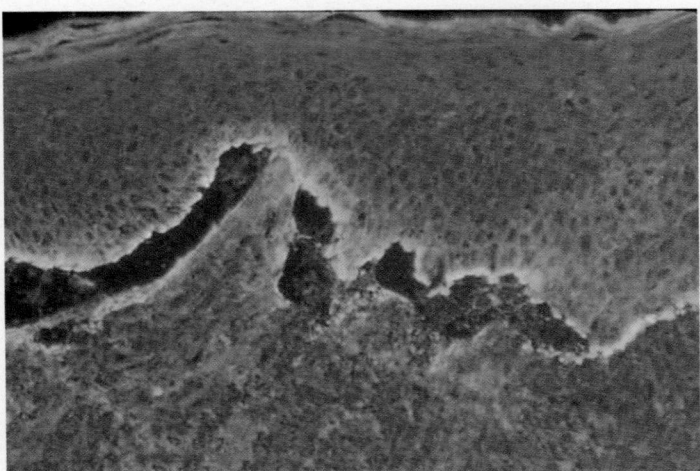

Figure 4-9 Bullous pemphigoid: thin wavy linear IgG deposition along the epidermal (roof) side of salt-split basement membrane zone.

incubated with tissue sections of the human split skin and subsequently incubated with a fluorescent label. Disorders characterized by antibodies to hemidesmosomal proteins BP180 and BP230, including those seen in bullous and gestational pemphigoid, some cases of mucous membrane pemphigoid, and linear IgA bullous disease, are associated with a linear immunostaining on the epidermal side (roof) of the salt-split human skin (Fig. 4-9).

On the other hand, patients with circulating antibodies reacting against type VII collagen and antiepiligrin (laminin 5), as is seen in epidermolysis bullosa acquisita (Fig. 4-10) and antiepiligrin mucous membrane pemphigoid respectively, have circulating IgG autoantibodies that bind the dermal side of the salt-split human skin. In bullous systemic lupus erythematosus, staining is also seen on the floor of the salt-split skin, and nuclear staining of keratinocytes may be present (Fig. 4-11).

More sensitive and specific assays for the evaluation of circulating autoantibodies, including enzyme-linked immunosorbent assay (ELISA) for antidesmoglein and anti-BP180 antibodies, immunoblotting and immunoprecipitation for pemphigoid, epidermolysis bullosa acquisita, and antiepiligrin, and

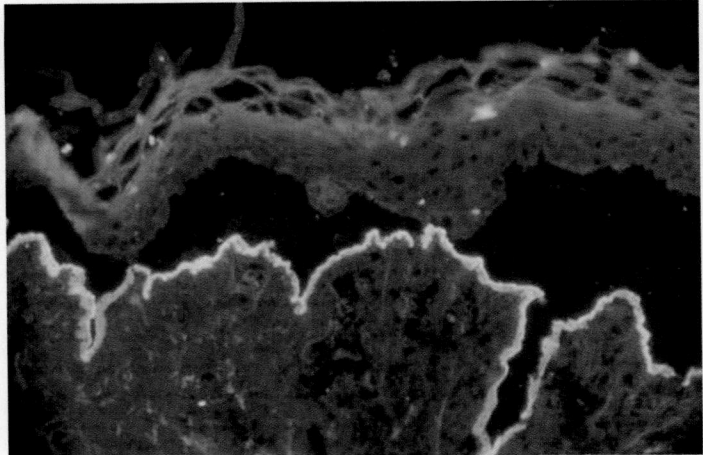

Figure 4-10 Epidermolysis bullosa acquisita: thick "ribbon type" linear IgG deposition along the dermal (floor) side of salt-split basement membrane zone.

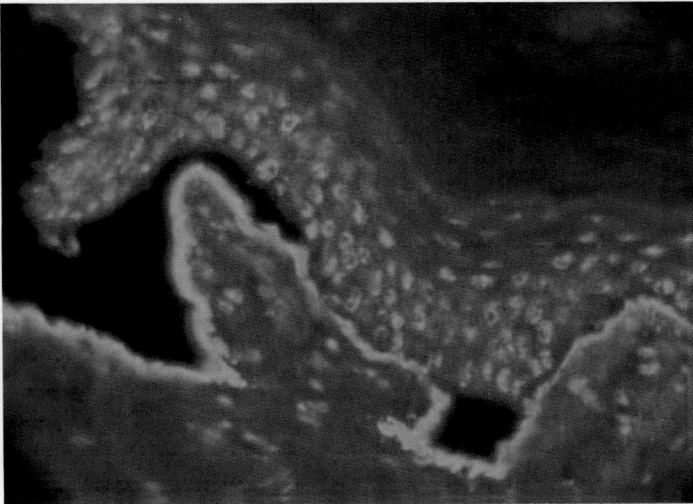

Figure 4-11 Bullous systemic lupus erythematosus: thick "ribbon type" linear IgG deposition along the dermal (floor) side of salt-split basement membrane zone in combination with strong *in vivo* antinuclear antibody pattern in keratinocytes and dermal cells.

immunoprecipitation for paraneoplastic pemphigus, have been recently incorporated into the diagnostic armamentarium of autoimmune blistering diseases.

ELISA Testing for Immunobullous Disorders

Most pemphigus patients' sera have autoantibodies to Dsg1 and/or Dsg3. In pemphigoid, most patients have antibodies to hemidesmosome proteins BP180 and/or BP230. The ELISA test applied to immunobullous disorders uses the autoantigen as the target and screens the patient's sera for these autoantibodies. When evaluating for pemphigus, ELISA for anti-Dsg1 and anti-Dsg3 has a sensitivity of 85% to 100% and specificity of 96% to 100%. This testing may also assist in distinguishing PV from PF. ELISA for anti-BP180 has a sensitivity of 54% to 100% and a specificity of 90% to 100% (12). Overall, ELISA has greater sensitivity and specificity for BP or PV than IF. It is recommended that diagnostic ELISA testing be utilized in conjunction with routine pathology, as well as direct and indirect immunofluorescence. Antibody titers to Dsg1, Dsg3, and BP180 have shown correlation with disease activity, and, therefore, monitoring of titers may be used as an adjunct to clinical assessment (12).

Immunofluorescence for the Evaluation of Site of Cleavage in Hereditary Epidermolysis Bullosa

This technique offers a practical, yet useful, diagnostic tool in hereditary epidermolysis bullosa by revealing the site of the defect in these mechanobullous disorders. Thus, this technique classifies these disorders into epidermolytic, functional, and dermolytic categories (Table 4-4).

In brief, this technique is performed as follows: A freshly induced blister is obtained by twisting a rubber-ended pencil, and then incubating this artificially induced blister skin specimen with anti-type IV collagen and anti-BP180 antigen. Then, according to localization of the immunolabeling of these antibodies, the site of cleavage can be deduced.

In some cases of generalized atrophic benign epidermolysis bullosa where the mutated protein is the BP180 antigen,

Table 4-4

Indirect Immunofluorescence for the Evaluation of Site of Cleavage in HEB

Type of HEB	Anti-BP180 Immunostaining	Anti-type IV Collagen Immunostaining
Epidermolytic (simplex)	Floor	Floor
Junctional	Roof	Floor
Dermolytic	Roof	Roof

HEB, hereditary epidermolysis bullosa.

the immunostaining in the floor of the induced blister given by the anti-BP180 may be focal or absent. Specific antibodies to the mutated protein are also used for complementary diagnostic purposes. These antibodies include antiplectin antibodies for epidermolysis bullosa simplex with muscular dystrophy, anti-$\alpha 6\beta 4$ for junctional epidermolysis bullosa with pyloric atresia, antilaminin 5 antibodies for most cases of junctional epidermolysis bullosa, and anti-type VII collagen for most cases of the dystrophic form of hereditary epidermolysis bullosa. These specific antibodies are intended to identify a disrupted linear staining owing to an even distribution of the probed mutated protein (13). The definite diagnosis of hereditary epidermolysis bullosa is made with electron microcopy and genetic analysis.

IMMUNOHISTOCHEMISTRY

Introduction, Techniques

Immunohistochemistry techniques (IHC) have been available since the early 1970s, but they have been used widely for diagnostic pathology since the early 1980s. IHC are mainly used to diagnose poorly differentiated malignant tumors and lymphoma but can be beneficial in the diagnosis of bullous diseases. With continued refinement of techniques, IHC have achieved the same sensitivity for many antigens in paraffin-embedded tissues as DIF on frozen sections. The paraffin-embedded tissues offer the advantage over frozen sections of better preservation of cellular details and permanency of the reaction so that the specimens can be preserved and stored. Most monoclonal antibodies, especially those necessary for the diagnosis of lymphoma, required frozen section studies when first introduced, but monoclonal and polyclonal antibodies are now available that can be applied to formalin-fixed, paraffin-embedded tissue (e.g., antibodies for the identification of B cells, T cells, macrophages, and many other cell types).

Sections that will be incubated with polyclonal or monoclonal antibodies should be mounted on glass slides specially coated or charged to ensure better adherence (14).

Certain antibodies, including antibodies against keratins, lysozyme, or chymotrypsin, require protease digestion if formalin-fixed, paraffin-embedded sections are used. Other "antigen retrieval" methods include the use of heat, either by microwaving or steaming the sections, and pretreatment of the sections with acid (HCl).

Immunohistologic Techniques

In most laboratories, immunopathology techniques are well established. Historically, several techniques have been used; the peroxidase–antiperoxidase technique has been replaced by more sensitive techniques, namely, techniques using avidin–biotin–peroxidase complex, alkaline phosphatase/anti-alkaline phosphatase, and streptavidin peroxidase or alkaline phosphatase. In all of these methods, the antibody is used to localize an enzyme (peroxidase or phosphatase) to sites of the antigen in the tissue section. An appropriate "chromogen" is then added—a reagent that has the property of developing a color that can be visualized at sites of localization of the enzyme–antibody–antigen complex.

The Alkaline Phosphatase/Anti-alkaline Phosphatase Technique

This is an unlabeled antibody bridge technique that uses three antibodies; the first and third antibodies are from the same species and are monoclonal. The second antibody is polyclonal, from the rabbit, and forms a bridge between the first and the third antibodies (15). The third antibody is linked to the enzyme alkaline phosphatase. After applying these antibodies with the linked enzyme, an alkaline phosphatase substrate is added containing a compatible indole chromogen such as 2-(4-iodophenyl)-3-(4-nitrophenyl)-5-phenyltetrazolium chloride (INT)/5-bromo-4-chloro-3′-indolyl phosphate p-toluidine salt (BCIP) (which yields a red color after the phosphatase-catalyzed reaction), naphthol fast red (red color), or nitro-blue tetrazolium chloride (NBT)/BCIP (blue). These chromogens may be useful for pigmented tumors because the blue or red reagents can be distinguished easily from melanin (14).

The Avidin–Biotin–Peroxidase Complex and Streptavidin Peroxidase or Alkaline Phosphatase Techniques

The avidin–biotin technique takes advantage of the strong binding of avidin to biotin (16,17). Avidin is a glycoprotein found in egg white that has a strong affinity to biotin, a vitamin of low molecular weight. The streptavidin technique is exactly analogous but achieves sensitivity one to two orders of magnitude greater by using streptavidin in place of avidin. In these techniques, the primary antibody (which may be monoclonal or polyclonal) binds directly with the specific antigen, in or on the cells, to form a stable antigen–antibody complex on the tissue section. A secondary antibody that has been labeled with biotin (biotinylated) and is directed against the same species and immunoglobulin type binds to the primary antibody, leaving the biotinylated end accessible for a chromogenic reagent. For the next step, either a peroxidase or an alkaline phosphatase detection system can be used. For a peroxidase method, the biotinylated complex is detected by avidin or streptavidin conjugated to the peroxidase enzyme. A peroxidase-compatible chromogen is then added, such as diaminobenzidine (yielding a brown color) or aminoethylcarbazole (red color and therefore useful for pigmented lesions). The alkaline phosphatase–streptavidin method is analogous to the streptavidin peroxidase method, but in this case the biotinylated complex is detected with an alkaline phosphatase–linked streptavidin and requires indole reagents such as INT/BCIP (red color), naphthol fast red (red), or NBT/BCIP (blue). This technique in the authors' experience achieves the greatest sensitivity of the described immunohistochemical methods.

The biologic origin of an undifferentiated cell can usually be determined with the application of monoclonal or polyclonal antibodies. A "panel approach" using multiple markers is the best method for evaluating problem neoplasms. Positive and negative controls should be used. If tumor cells unexpectedly do not show a positive reaction with a certain antibody, several possibilities exist, including technical difficulties with the assay. One may encounter nonspecific staining as well as aberrant immunoreactivity (observed staining with a particular antibody where it is theoretically unexpected). Caution should be taken not to make a diagnosis based on IHC alone. Unfortunately, there is no antibody that reliably distinguishes between benign and malignant cells.

APPLICATIONS OF IMMUNOHISTOPATHOLOGY

Diagnosis of Tumors (Excluding Lymphomas)

Commonly used antibodies for routine dermatopathology and their occurrence in certain cells and tissues are listed in Table 4-5. Some of the most frequently used antibodies in dermatopathology are discussed later. The list of available antibodies is extensive; detailed information is available in the literature and text reviews (18–22).

Antibodies Against Cytoskeletal Antigens

The cytoskeleton of a cell consists of intermediate filaments (IFs) measuring 7 to 11 nm in diameter, actin-containing microfilaments, and tubulin-containing microtubules (23–25). IFs are smaller than microtubules (25 nm) but larger than microfilaments (6 nm), and hence the designation intermediate.

Antibodies against IFs help to identify the biologic origin of an anaplastic cell. Malignant tumors often retain the IF-type characteristic of the tissue of origin, and metastases generally continue to express these IFs (26). There are six groups of IFs. Type 1 and 2 IFs include cytokeratins, which are present in epithelia. Type 3 IFs include vimentin, found in mesenchymal cells and melanocytes; desmin, found in most muscle cells; and glial fibrillary acidic protein, found in glial cells and astrocytes. Type 4 IFs include neurofilaments, which are components of neurons. Nuclear lamins constitute type 5 IFs, and nestin comprises type 6 and is found in some stem cells.

Keratins

In dermatopathology, keratin antibodies are used to differentiate epithelial from nonepithelial (melanocytic, hematopoietic, and mesenchymal) tumors. A mixture of antibodies against low and intermediate keratins such as AE1 and AE3 (AE1/3) is commonly used (27). An additional antibody to low-molecular-weight keratins such as CAM 5.2 may be beneficial in poorly differentiated carcinomas (28). CK7 staining may support a diagnosis of adenocarcinoma, including mammary ductal carcinoma and pigmented extramammary Paget disease, which can mimic melanoma (29). The keratin marker CK20 has useful specificity for Merkel cell carcinoma (30).

Atypical spindle cell tumors, for example, are often difficult to diagnose with routine stains. The differential diagnosis for such lesions includes spindle cell squamous cell carcinoma, atypical fibroxanthoma, leiomyosarcoma, and spindle cell malignant melanoma. Table 4-6 lists the most important antibodies to use (31).

Vimentin

Vimentin is an IF originally isolated from chick embryo fibroblasts. It is found in fibroblasts, endothelial cells, macrophages, melanocytes, lymphocytes, and smooth muscle cells. Detection of vimentin is found in both benign and malignant counterparts of these cells (32). There have been reports of vimentin positivity in epithelial tumors, typically higher-grade lesions (33); however, unremarkable epidermis is negative with this antibody. Because of the widespread expression of vimentin in many cell types, it is used as a component of a panel to support mesenchymal or melanocytic differentiation.

Carcinoembryonic Antigen and Epithelial Membrane Antigen

Carcinoembryonic antigen (CEA) is detected in eccrine and apocrine cells, in benign sweat gland tumors, and in mammary carcinoma and extramammary Paget disease of the skin. Incubation with anti-CEA can be helpful in distinguishing Paget cells from atypical melanocytes in melanoma in situ. However, reactivity of melanomas with CEA has been reported (34). CEA typically stains adenocarcinomas from most organ systems. Most epithelial tumors react with antibodies against epithelial membrane antigen (EMA), including squamous cell carcinoma, breast carcinoma, and large cell lung carcinoma. EMA will also stain sweat and sebaceous glands, although epidermis is nonreactive with this antibody. Epithelioid sarcoma is also stained by EMA (see Chapter 32).

Neuron-Specific Enolase

Neuron-specific enolase (NSE) is an acidic enzyme found in neuroendocrine cells, neurons, and tumors derived from them. Merkel cell carcinoma contains NSE; however, NSE can be detected in a variety of other tumors, including malignant melanoma, and therefore has low specificity. The keratin marker CK20 has better specificity for Merkel cell tumor than for melanoma and other neuroendocrine tumors (35).

Chromogranin and Synaptophysin

The soluble proteins of chromaffin granules are called chromogranin (36). Chromogranins are normally found in most endocrine cells (e.g., thyroid, parathyroid, anterior pituitary). Synaptophysin is a 38-kDa glycoprotein that participates in calcium-dependent release of neurotransmitters (37). It is a neuroendocrine antigen with a distribution similar to chromogranin. Positive staining with antibodies to chromogranin and synaptophysin is useful in the diagnosis of neuroendocrine tumors such as Merkel cell carcinoma (38). Of interest, normal Merkel cells are negative with synaptophysin, and melanocytic tumors do not stain with chromogranin or synaptophysin.

S100 Protein

S100 proteins are acidic proteins that bind Ca^{2+} and Zn^{2+}. They are called S100 because of their solubility in 100% ammonium sulfate at neutral pH. S100 proteins are found in the cytoplasm and in the nucleus. S100 proteins can be detected in many cell types, including melanocytes, Langerhans cells, eccrine and apocrine

Table 4-5

Common Antigens That Can Be Detected in Formalin-Fixed, Paraffin-Embedded Sections

Antigen	Location
Cytokeratins, including AE1, AE3, CAM 5.2	Epidermis and its appendages and their tumors
CK20	Merkel cells and Merkel cell carcinoma, metastatic gastrointestinal adenocarcinoma
CK7	Cells of Paget disease, metastatic breast carcinoma
Vimentin	Mesenchymal cells, melanocytes, lymphomas, sarcomas, melanomas
Desmin	Smooth and skeletal muscle, muscle tumors
Leukocyte common antigen (LCA)	Benign leukocytes, lymphoma, leukemia
CD3 and CD45-RO (UCHL-1)	T lymphocytes
CD20 (L-26) and PAX5	B lymphocytes
Epithelial membrane antigen (EMA)	Sweat and sebaceous glands, carcinoma, epithelioid sarcoma
Carcinoembryonic antigen (CEA)	Eccrine and apocrine glands and their tumors, Paget cells
S100 protein	Melanocytes, Langerhans cells, eccrine and apocrine glands and their tumors, Schwann cells, nerves, interdigitating reticulum cells, chondrocytes, melanomas, adipose tissue, liposarcomas, Langerhans cell histiocytosis
Sox10	Melanocytes, melanomas, Schwann cells in nerves and tumors, sweat gland and mammary tumors
HMB-45	Melanoma cells, some nevus cells
Chromogranin	Neuroendocrine cells, Merkel cell carcinoma, eccrine gland cells
Synaptophysin	Neuroendocrine cells, Merkel cell carcinoma
Lysozyme	Macrophages, granulocytes, myeloid cells
Factor VIII–related antigen	Endothelial cells, angiosarcomas, Kaposi sarcoma
HHV-8	Kaposi sarcoma
CD31	Endothelial cells
CD34	Endothelial cells, bone marrow progenitor cells, cells of dermatofibrosarcoma protuberans
Smooth muscle actin	Smooth muscle cells and tumors, myofibroblastic cells
MART-1/Melan-A/MITF/SOX-10	Melanocytes, nevi, melanoma
Factor XIIIa	Dermatofibromas, certain fibrohistiocytic cells (see text)
CD1a	Langerhans cells
CD163 and CD68	Histiocytic tumors, dermal macrophages, and dendrocytes
MIB-1/Ki-67	All stages of mitosis except G0
Phospho-Histone H3 (pHH3)	Mitotic figures
D2-40	Lymphatic endothelium
GLUT-1	Juvenile hemangiomas, erythrocytes
Fli-1	Ewing sarcoma, lymphocytes, endothelial cells
Gross cystic disease fluid protein-15	Tumors with apocrine differentiation, breast carcinoma
Ber-EP4	Basal cell carcinoma and sebaceous tumors
Thyroid transcription factor-1	Metastatic thyroid and lung tumors

Note: Few, if any, of these reagents are perfectly specific for their target antigens. Every test must be interpreted in the context of all of the available histologic and clinical information.

HHV, human herpesvirus; MITF, microphthalmia transcription factor.

gland cells, nerves, muscles, Schwann cells, myoepithelial cells, chondrocytes, adipocytes, and their malignant counterparts. The polyclonal antibody against S100 works well on paraffin sections. Its high sensitivity contrasts with a low specificity, a feature that supports a "panel" approach to immunohistochemistry.

Useful applications of the antibody against S100 protein include (a) diagnosing spindle cell melanoma and desmoplastic melanoma, (b) distinguishing between melanocytes and lymphocytes in halo nevi, and (c) diagnosing poorly differentiated cutaneous metastases.

Table 4-6
Differential Diagnosis of Malignant Spindle Cell Tumors

Diagnosis	Keratin	Vimentin	Desmin	S100/Sox10	HMB-45	ERG/CD31	P63
Squamous cell carcinoma	+	−	−	−	−	−	+
Atypical fibroxanthoma	−	+	−	−	−	−	±
Melanoma	−	+	−	+	+	−	−
Leiomyosarcoma	−	+	+	−	−	−	−
Angiosarcoma	±	±	−	−	−	+	−

Note: Few, if any, of these reagents are perfectly specific for their target antigens. Every test must be interpreted in the context of all of the available histologic and clinical information.

Sox10

Sox10 is a nuclear antigen that has specificity for melanocytes and also for Schwann cells, and their tumors, including nevi and melanomas, neurofibromas and related lesions, and malignant peripheral nerve sheath tumors. In skin, there is also reactivity in sweat gland epithelial cells and in sweat gland tumors as well as in metastatic mammary carcinoma. This marker has been especially useful in the delineation of the extension of invasion in desmoplastic melanomas (39).

HMB-45

HMB-45 is a monoclonal antibody that was initially generated from an extract of metastatic melanoma (40). Both primary and metastatic melanomas demonstrate cytoplasmic staining with HMB-45; spindle cell melanomas and desmoplastic melanomas are frequently negative. This antibody reacts with a melanosomal protein, GP-100, which tends to be expressed in immature or proliferating cells (41). Unfortunately, HMB-45 may react with melanocytes in some nevi, including dysplastic nevi and Spitz nevi (42). Therefore, it should not be used in isolation for the differential diagnosis between a malignant melanoma and a benign nevus. Most desmoplastic melanomas, as well as some metastatic melanomas, may show negative staining with HMB-45 (42). Cutaneous PEComas, rare tumors exhibiting myomelanocytic differentiation, usually stain positively with HMB-45 (43).

MART-1/Melan-A

Melanoma antigen recognized by T cells (MART-1) is a well-established melanocytic differentiation marker. The antigen is expressed in melanocytes, common nevi, Spitz nevi, and malignant melanoma (Fig. 4-12). Monoclonal antibodies to MART-1/Melan-A are commercially available and are suitable for both frozen tissue and formalin-fixed, paraffin-embedded tissue. Negative staining is frequently seen in neurotized nevi and desmoplastic melanomas (44). In the skin, Melan-A mRNA has been found only in melanocytic lesions and angiomyolipomas (45). Immunoreactivity can also be seen in the adrenal cortex, Leydig cells of the testes, granulosa cells of the ovary, and tumors derived from these cells. This antibody is a useful addition when evaluating intraepidermal melanocytes (vitiligo, early melanoma *in situ*), as well as amelanotic melanomas.

PRAME

Gene expression profiling experiments have identified PRAME (PReferentially expressed Antigen in MElanoma) as being highly overexpressed in melanomas and other tumors compared

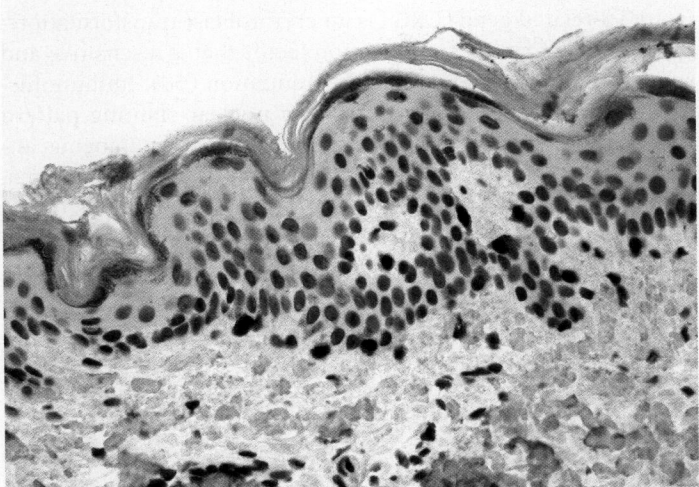

Figure 4-12 MART-1/Melan-A immunoperoxidase staining highlights normal melanocytes in the basal layer of the epidermis.

with benign tissue counterparts (46). Such data suggest that PRAME immunostaining may be helpful in distinguishing nevi from melanoma. Recent studies have indicated that PRAME immunostaining is helpful in distinguishing metastatic melanoma from nodal nevi (47).

CD34

CD34 is a heavily glycosylated molecule that is expressed on most human hematopoietic progenitor cells. Expression is typically not found on more mature hematopoietic cells in the skin. Both benign and malignant vascular tumors express this antigen. In dermatopathology, CD34 positivity in dermatofibrosarcoma protuberans is useful in differentiating these lesions from dermatofibromas, which are CD34 negative and factor XIIIa positive (48). Other cutaneous neoplasms that express CD34 include dermal dendrocytic lesions (49,50), solitary fibrous tumor (51), giant cell fibroblastoma (52), neurofibroma, epithelioid sarcoma, spindle cell lipoma (53), sclerotic fibroma, cellular digital fibromas (54), and fibrous papule of the nose.

Factor VIII–Related Antigen Factor VIII–Related Antigen (von Willebrand Factor)

This is a large glycoprotein produced by endothelial cells and therefore useful in benign and malignant vascular neoplasms. However, some studies have demonstrated factor VIII positivity in only 50% of hemangiomas and 5% to 25% of malignant endothelial tumors (55,56).

CD31, D2-40, and ERG

CD31 is a marker of endothelial differentiation that is typically expressed in endothelial cells and selected hematopoietic elements (Fig. 4-13) (57). This 130-kDa glycoprotein, whose major function is to mediate platelet adhesion in vascular endothelial cells, is also known as platelet endothelial cell adhesion molecule (PECAM). CD31 is a sensitive marker for vascular tumors, except Kaposi sarcoma (58). It is a more sensitive marker for cutaneous angiosarcoma than factor VIII–related antigen. D2-40 has similar sensitivity for lymphatic endothelium and stains a subset of angiosarcomas, implying that lymphatic or mixed lymphatic and blood vascular differentiation is common in these tumors (59).

ETS-related gene (ERG) is an erythroblast transformation–specific (ETS) family transcription factor that is a sensitive and specific marker of endothelial differentiation (60). Immunohistochemistry for ERG demonstrates a nuclear staining pattern that has shown strong utility in the diagnosis of cutaneous angiosarcoma, in particular, poorly differentiated angiosarcoma. In some studies, ERG has outperformed FLI1 in diagnostic studies of angiosarcoma.

Human Herpesvirus 8

Human herpesvirus 8 (HHV-8), also known as Kaposi sarcoma–associated herpesvirus (KSHV), was first discovered in Kaposi sarcoma tissue from patients with acquired immune deficiency syndrome. In addition to Kaposi sarcoma, HHV-8 has been detected in certain lymphomas, in some cases of multicentric Castleman disease (MCD), and in a condition known as KSHV inflammatory cytokine syndrome. Immunostaining for HHV-8 has proven to be extremely helpful in the diagnosis of Kaposi sarcoma, including early and equivocal cases (61).

Factor XIIIa

Factor XIIIa, a blood coagulation factor, is responsible for stabilizing newly formed clots by cross-linking fibrin. It is present in fibroblast-like mesenchymal cells, dermal dendrocytes, platelets, megakaryocytes, peritoneal and alveolar macrophages, normal adipose tissue, monocytes, and placenta, uterine, and prostate tissue. As noted earlier, using factor XIIIa in combination with

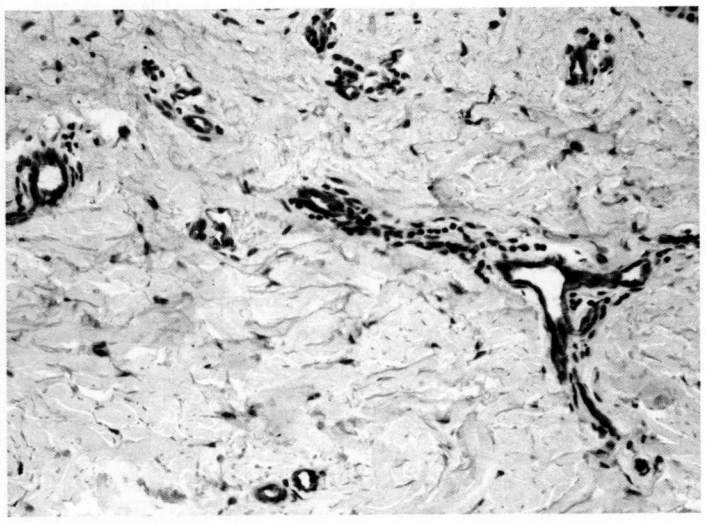

Figure 4-13 CD31 staining of vascular endothelium.

CD34 can be helpful in differentiating dermatofibroma from dermatofibrosarcoma protuberans. Factor XIIIa has also been reported to be positive in a multitude of other lesions, including fibrous papule, atypical fibroxanthoma, xanthogranuloma, multinucleate cell angiohistiocytoma, epithelioid cell histiocytoma, and atypical cells in radiation dermatitis (62,63).

Antibodies Against Lysozyme, α_1-Antitrypsin, and α_1-Antichymotrypsin

These antibodies have been regarded as markers of mononuclear phagocytic cells. Although once felt to be markers for "fibrohistiocytic" neoplasms, they have also been identified in carcinomas and melanomas, making them less specific.

CD163

The CD163 antigen is also known as M130. It is a hemoglobin scavenger receptor expressed in monocytes and tissue macrophages (64). In the skin, the CD163 monoclonal antibody is expressed in dermal dendritic cells and neoplasms with histiocytic differentiation, including dermatofibroma/fibrous histiocytoma, atypical fibroxanthoma, Rosai–Dorfman disease, and acute myeloid leukemia. This antigen can be expressed in nonhistiocytic tumors, so it should be utilized in a panel approach.

c-kit (CD117)

The human proto-oncogene c-kit is a member of the type III receptor tyrosine kinase family that includes macrophage growth factor, platelet-derived growth factor, and flt-3/flk-2 receptors. It is present on a number of cell types, including mast cells, melanocytes, hematopoietic stem cells, immature myeloid cells, and myeloid and lymphoid progenitors, and in germ cell lineages, and it plays a crucial role in their activation and growth. Constitutively active c-kit has been implicated in the pathogenesis of several disorders, including systemic mastocytosis and gastrointestinal stromal tumors, whereas impairment of kinase activity has been implicated in a number of developmental disorders (65,66). Increased c-kit expression has been seen on malignant cells from many acute myeloid leukemia subtypes and chronic myelogenous leukemia; in addition, several solid tumor cells have been shown to express high-affinity c-kit receptors, including breast, lung, and gastric carcinoma, as well as some melanomas, especially of the acral, lentigo maligna, mucosal, and ocular subtypes.

CD1a

CD1a is a transmembrane glycoprotein, structurally related to major histocompatibility class I, and it is found as a heterodimer associated with β_2-microglobin (67). CD1a is localized to the plasma membrane, with a small fraction of internalized CD1a restricted to the perinuclear recycling vesicles of endosomal sorting machinery. Like other members of the CD1 family, CD1a functions to mediate the presentation of lipid and glycolipid antigens to T cells. In pathology, CD1a has become a marker of Langerhans cells (Fig. 4-14) and blood monocyte–derived dendritic cells. CD1a is also expressed on double-positive (CD4$^+$CD8$^+$) cortical thymocytes and with less-intense expression on CD4 or CD8 single-positive thymocytes. As a diagnostic tool, it has been used together with S100 to define dendritic cell populations in tumors and other tissues, as well as for the diagnosis of Langerhans cell histiocytosis (histiocytosis X) (68).

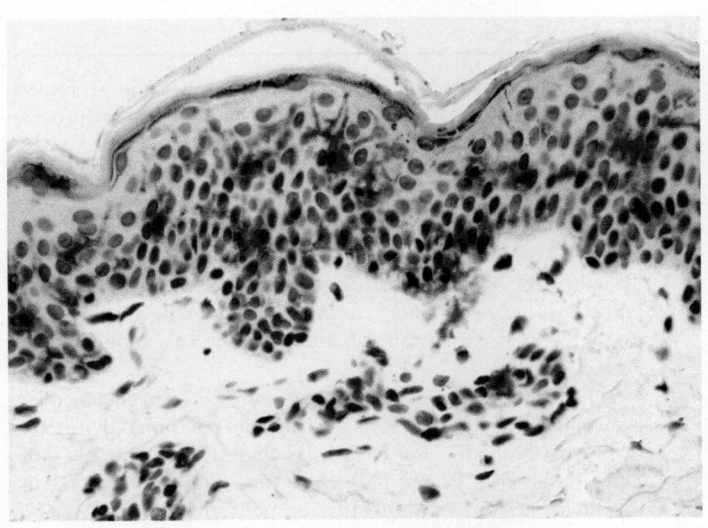

Figure 4-14 CD1a immunoperoxidase stain highlights Langerhans cells in the epidermis.

Antibodies Against Leukocyte Common Antigen (CD45)

This antibody helps to distinguish between undifferentiated lymphomas and poorly differentiated carcinomas. CD45 is found on all leukocytes, including granulocytes, lymphocytes, monocytes, macrophages, mast cells, and Langerhans cells. The lymphomas and leukemias react with the antibody against CD45; carcinomas and melanomas are negative. In addition to CD45, lysozyme and chloroacetate esterase aid in the diagnosis of leukemia cutis (69). CD45 is particularly useful in the evaluation of tumors composed of small atypical basophilic cells in the dermis (Table 4-7). Other antigens useful in the analysis of suspected lymphomas include the B- and T-cell markers L-26 (CD20, B cells) or CD79a (B cells) and UCHL-1 (CD45-RO, T cells) (see Chapter 31).

Diagnosis of Lymphomas

Immunohistochemistry. The application of monoclonal antibodies for the diagnosis of lymphomas is expanding. However, there is no antibody that distinguishes between benign and malignant lymphocytes. Hence, the difficult distinction between lymphoma and pseudolymphoma remains.

Although many antibodies were originally developed using frozen sections, a large number of commonly available antibodies work very well on formalin-fixed, paraffin-embedded tissue. The quality of certain markers, such as κ and λ light chains, may be variable in paraffin sections, and their cognate mRNAs are more reliably detected utilizing *in situ* hybridization. Monoclonal antibodies can determine the cell types in a lymphoma or pseudolymphoma: helper or suppressor T cells, B cells, plasma cells, or macrophages. One potentially confusing issue is that B-cell lymphomas may contain reactive T-cell infiltrates, which can outnumber the B cells. The predominance of a T-helper lymphocytic infiltrate with epidermotropism of the T-helper subtype is suggestive of cutaneous T-cell lymphoma. In contrast, a mixture of T-helper and T-suppressor phenotypes is most consistent with a reactive profile (e.g., spongiotic dermatitis). In dense nodular infiltrates, the presence of germinal center formation with B-lymphocyte aggregates surrounded by a mantle of T cells favors lymphocytoma cutis over lymphoma. A detailed discussion of antibodies helpful in the diagnosis of cutaneous hematopoietic processes has been reviewed (70) and can also be found in Chapter 31.

Molecular studies can provide additional information in the evaluation of atypical lymphoid infiltrates. Detection of a characteristic gene rearrangement coding for B- and T-cell antigen receptors can identify the presence or absence of a clonal population of lymphocytes (71). These applications are an important supplement to routinely available technology; however, they need to be interpreted in the context of the clinical presentation and findings on routine histology. Although clonality studies can assist in early detection of cutaneous T-cell lymphoma, nonneoplastic processes such as pityriasis lichenoides, pseudolymphoma, and lichen planus occasionally show T-cell clonality (72–74).

Diagnosis of Infectious Agents in the Skin

The diagnosis of infections in dermatopathology is often challenging with current routine histology and histochemical stains. There are an increasing number of immunoperoxidase stains, *in situ* hybridization (ISH), and polymerase chain reactions for identification of cutaneous infections (75). The antibodies for immunoperoxidase staining are commercially available and are used in many laboratories. Commonly used immunoperoxidase stains include antibodies against herpes simplex virus (HSV), varicella-zoster virus (VZV), Epstein–Barr virus (EBV), cytomegalovirus, human herpesvirus 8, and *Treponema pallidum* (Fig. 4-15). Because HSV and VZV infection can show identical changes on routine histology, these stains add specificity to the diagnosis.

Table 4-7				
Immunohistochemistry of Basophilic Small Cells in the Dermis				
Diagnosis	S100	Synaptophysin	Leukocyte Common Antigen	Keratin
Lymphoma	−	−	+	−
Merkel cell carcinoma	−	+	−	+*
Carcinoma	±	−	−	+
Melanoma	+	−	−	−

Note: Few, if any, of these reagents are perfectly specific for their target antigens. Every test must be interpreted in the context of all of the available histologic and clinical information. Poorly differentiated carcinoma may be keratin negative or only positive with low-molecular-weight keratin antibodies.
*Perinuclear staining.

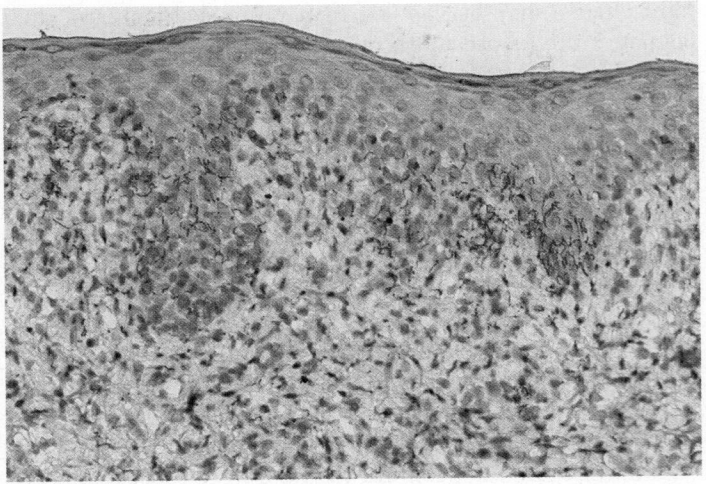

Figure 4-15 Secondary syphilis. Immunoperoxidase stain (red chromogen) for *T. pallidum* highlights spirochetes in the epidermis.

Sensitivities for HSV and VZV via immunohistochemistry have been shown to be higher than routine hematoxylin–eosin staining (76).

Some of these infectious agents can also be detected using *in situ* hybridization. This technique can be performed using a fluorochrome (FISH) or chromogen (CISH), with the latter resulting in a slide that resembles immunoperoxidase staining. Some of the agents that can be detected via ISH include human papillomavirus, EBV, pox virus, Hepatitis C virus, HIV, Nocardia, Candida, Cryptococcus, Aspergillus, Fusarium, and Leishmania.

Polymerase chain reaction (PCR) is a highly sensitive technique that can detect DNA or RNA in skin biopsies or other tissues. PCR for infectious agents can be performed using fresh/frozen tissue or formalin-fixed, paraffin-embedded tissue. PCR has been utilized to detect bacteria (Rickettsia, mycobacteria, borrelia, *T. pallidum*), viruses (human papillomavirus, HHV-8, herpes simplex, varicella zoster, Epstein–Barr), fungi (candida, blastomyces, sporothrix, dermatophytes), and parasites (leishmania).

ELECTRON MICROSCOPY

Transmission electron microscopy, although rarely used today because of the availability of additional markers, especially immunohistochemistry, may be beneficial in the diagnosis of poorly differentiated skin neoplasms for which immunohistochemistry is negative (77). Using electron microscopy, the identification of intercellular junctions (epithelial tumors), melanosomes (melanocytic tumors), or Weibel–Palade bodies (endothelial cells) can provide important diagnostic information. Other uses of diagnostic electron microscopy include the subtype determination of epidermolysis bullosa and the diagnosis of metabolic storage diseases (e.g., Fabry disease) or amyloidosis. For optimum results, fresh tissue should be fixed in Karnovsky medium (paraformaldehyde–glutaraldehyde) and stored in the refrigerator until processing; although electron microscopy can rarely be performed from paraffin-embedded tissue, there may be extensive distortion precluding interpretation.

REFERENCES

1. Morales AR, Nassiri M, Kanhoush R, Vincek V, Nadji M. Experience with an automated microwave-assisted rapid tissue processing method. *Am J Clin Pathol.* 2004;121:528–536.
2. Emerson LL, Tripp SR, Baird BC, Layfield LJ, Rohr LR. A comparison of immunohistochemical stain quality in conventional and rapid microwave processed tissues. *Am J Clin Pathol.* 2006;125(2):176–183.
3. Luna LG, ed. *Manual of Histologic Staining Methods of the Armed Forces Institute of Pathology.* 3rd ed. McGraw-Hill; 1968.
4. Roten SV, Bhat S, Bhawan J. Elastic fibers in scar tissue. *J Cutan Pathol.* 1996;23:37.
5. Siegel MA, Anhalt GJ. Direct immunofluorescence of detached gingival epithelium for diagnosis of cicatricial pemphigoid: report of five cases. *Oral Surg Oral Med Oral Pathol.* 1993;75(3):296–302.
6. Zone JJ, Meyer LJ, Petersen MJ. Deposition of granular IgA relative to clinical lesions in dermatitis herpetiformis. *Arch Dermatol.* 1996;132(8):912–918.
7. Elbendary A, Zhou C, Truong T, Elston DM. Durability of direct immunofluorescence (DIF) slides stored at room temperature. *J Am Acad Dermatol.* 2015;73:1021–1024.
8. Goletz S, Hashimoto T, Zellikens D, Schmidt S. Anti-p200 pemphigoid. *J Am Acad.* 2014;71:185–191.
9. Meijer JM, Atefi I, Diercks GFH et al. Serration pattern analysis for differentiating epidermolysis bullosa acquisita from other pemphigoid diseases *J Am Acad Dermatol.* 2018:78:754–759.
10. Magro CM, Crowson AN. The immunofluorescent profile of dermatomyositis: a comparative study with lupus erythematosus. *J Cutan Pathol.* 1997;24(9):543–552.
11. Collins BA, Colvin RB, Nousari HC, Anhalt GJ. Immunofluorescence methods for diagnosis of renal and skin diseases. In: Rose NR, RG, Detrick B, eds. *Manual of Clinical Laboratory Immunology.* ASM Press; 2002:393–401.
12. Saschenbreckers S, Ingolf K, Komorowski L, et al. Serological diagnosis of autoimmune bullous skin disease. *Front Immunol.* 2019;10:1–18.
13. Pardo RJ, Penneys NS. Location of basement membrane type IV collagen beneath subepidermal bullous diseases. *J Cutan Pathol.* 1990;17:336.
14. Schaumburg-Lever G. The alkaline phosphatase anti-alkaline phosphatase technique in dermatopathology. *J Cutan Pathol.* 1987;14:6.
15. Cordell JL, Falini B, Erber WN, et al. Immunoenzymatic labeling of monoclonal antibodies using immune complexes of alkaline phosphatase and monoclonal anti-alkaline phosphatase (APAAP complexes). *J Histochem Cytochem.* 1984;32:219.
16. Hsu SM, Raine L. Protein A, avidin and biotin in immunohistochemistry. *J Histochem Cytochem.* 1981;29:1349.
17. Elias JM. Immunohistochemical methods. In: Elias JM, ed. *Immunohistology: A Practical Approach to Diagnosis.* ASCP Press; 1990:1.
18. Hoang MP, Mahalingam M, Selim MA. Immunohistochemistry in the diagnosis of cutaneous neoplasms. *Future Oncol.* 2010;6(1):93–109.
19. Ferringer T. Update on immunohistochemistry in melanocytic lesions. *Dermatol Clin.* 2012;30(4):567–579.
20. Hoang MP. Role of immunohistochemistry in diagnosing tumors of cutaneous appendages. *Am J Dermatopathol.* 2011;33(8):765–771.
21. Robson A. Immunocytochemistry and the diagnosis of cutaneous lymphoma. *Histopathology.* 2010;56(1):71–90.
22. Alcaraz I, Cerroni L, Rutten A, Kutzner H, Requena L. Cutaneous metastases from internal malignancies: a clinicopathologic and immunohistochemical review. *Am J Dermatopathol.* 2012;34(4):347–393.
23. Murphy GF. Cytokeratin typing of cutaneous tumors: a new immunochemical probe for cellular differentiation and malignant transformation. *J Invest Dermatol.* 1985;84:1.

24. Ho CL, Liem RK. Intermediate filaments in the nervous system: implications in cancer. *Cancer Metastasis Rev.* 1996;15(4):483–497.

25. Fuchs E. The cytoskeleton and disease: genetic disorders of intermediate filaments. *Annu Rev Genet.* 1996;30:197–231.

26. Osborn M. Component of the cellular cytoskeleton: a new generation of markers of histogenetic origin. *J Invest Dermatol.* 1984; 82:443.

27. Nelson WG, Sun TT. The 50 and 58-kdalton keratin classes as molecular markers for stratified squamous epithelia: cell culture studies. *J Cell Biol.* 1983;97(1):244–251.

28. Inaloz HS, Ayyalaraju RS, Holt PJ, et al. A case of sarcomatoid carcinoma of the skin. *J Eur Acad Dermatol Venereol.* 2003; 17(1):59–61.

29. DeLa Garza Bravo MM, Curry JL, Torres-Cabala CA, et al. Pigmented extramammary Paget disease of the thigh mimicking a melanocytic tumor: report of a case and review of the literature. *J Cutan Pathol.* 2014;41(6):529–535.

30. Chan JK, Suster S, Wenig BM, Tsang WY, Chan JB, Lau AL. Cytokeratin 20 immunoreactivity distinguishes Merkel cell (primary cutaneous neuroendocrine) carcinomas and salivary gland small cell carcinomas from small cell carcinomas of various sites. *Am J Surg Pathol.* 1997;21(2):226–234.

31. Argenyi ZB. Spindle cell neoplasms of the skin: a comprehensive diagnostic approach. *Semin Dermatol.* 1989;8:283.

32. Leader M, Collins M, Patel J, Henry K. Vimentin: an evaluation of its role as a tumour marker. *Histopathology.* 1987;11:63.

33. Iver PV, Leong AS. Poorly differentiated squamous cell carcinomas of the skin can express vimentin. *J Cutan Pathol.* 1992; 19(1):34–39.

34. Sanders DSA, Evans AT, Allen CA, et al. Classification of CEA-related positivity in primary and metastatic malignant melanoma. *J Pathol.* 1994;172:343.

35. Moll R, Lowe A, Laufer J, Franke WW. Cytokeratin 20 in human carcinomas. A new histodiagnostic marker detected by monoclonal antibodies. *Am J Pathol.* 1992;140:427.

36. Schober M, Fischer-Colbrie R, Schmid KW, Bussolati G, O'Connor DT, Winkler H. Comparison of chromogranin A, B, and secretogranin II in human adrenal medulla and phaeochromocytoma. *Lab Invest.* 1987;57:385.

37. Weidenmann B, Franke WW. Identification and localization of synaptophysin: an integral membrane glycoprotein of MW 38,000 characteristic of presynaptic vesicles. *Cell.* 1985;45:1017.

38. Lloyd RV, Cano M, Rosa P, Hille A, Huttner WB. Distribution of chromogranin A and chromogranin I (chromogranin B) in neuroendocrine cells and tumors. *Am J Pathol.* 1988;130:296.

39. Ordóñez NG. Value of melanocytic-associated immunohistochemical markers in the diagnosis of malignant melanoma: a review and update. *Hum Pathol.* 2014;45(2):191–205.

40. Gown AM, Vogel AM, Hoak D, Gough F, McNutt MA. Monoclonal antibodies specific for melanocytic tumors distinguish subpopulations of melanocytes. *Am J Pathol.* 1986;123(2):195–203.

41. Adema GJ, de Boer AJ, Vogel AM, Loenen WA, Figdor CG. Molecular characterization of the melanocyte lineage-specific antigen gp100. *J Biol Chem.* 1994;269(31):20126–20133.

42. Wick MR, Swanson PE, Rocamora A. Recognition of malignant melanoma by monoclonal antibody HMB-45: an immunohistochemical study of 200 paraffin-embedded cutaneous tumors. *J Cutan Pathol.* 1988;15:201.

43. Mentzel T, Reisshauer S, Rütten A, Hantschke M, Soares de Almeida LM, Kutzner H. Cutaneous clear cell myomelanocytic tumour: a new member of the growing family of perivascular epithelioid cell tumours (PEComas). Clinicopathological and immunohistochemical analysis of seven cases. *Histopathology.* 2005;46(5):498–504.

44. Busam KJ, Chen YT, Old LJ, et al. Expression of melan-A (MART-1) in benign melanocytic nevi and primary cutaneous malignant melanoma. *Am J Surg Pathol.* 1998;22:976–982.

45. Jungbluth AA, Busam KJ, Gerald WL, et al. A103, an anti melan-A monoclonal antibody for the detection of malignant melanoma in paraffin-embedded tissues. *Am J Surg Pathol.* 1998;22:595–602.

46. Beard RE, Abate-Daga D, Rosati SF, et al. Gene expression profiling using nanostring digital RNA counting to identify potential target antigens for melanoma immunotherapy. *Clin Cancer Res.* 2013;19(18):4941–4950.

47. Lezcano C, Pulitzer M, Moy AP, Hollmann TJ, Jungbluth AA, Busam KJ. Immunohistochemistry for PRAME in the distinction of nodal nevi from metastatic melanoma. *Am J Surg Pathol.* 2020;44(4):503–508.

48. Goldblum JR, Tuthill RJ. CD34 and factor XIIIa immunoreactivity in dermatofibrosarcoma protuberans and dermatofibroma. *Am J Dermatopathol.* 1997;19:147–153.

49. Sueki H, Whitaker D, Buchsbaum M, Murphy GF. Novel interactions between dermal dendrocytes and mast cells in human skin. Implications for hemostasis and matrix repair. *Lab Invest.* 1993;69:160–172.

50. Cowper SE, Kilpatrick T, Proper S, Morgan MB. Solitary fibrous tumor of the skin. *Am J Dermatopathol.* 1999;21(3):213–219.

51. Okamura JM, Barr RJ, Battifora H. Solitary fibrous tumor of the skin. *Am J Dermatopathol.* 1997;19(5):515–518.

52. Cohen PR, Rapini RP, Farhood AI. Expression of the human hematopoietic progenitor cell antigen CD34 in dermatofibrosarcoma protuberans, other spindle cell tumors, and vascular lesions. *J Am Acad Dermatol.* 1994;30(1):147–148.

53. Silverman JS, Tamsen A. Fibrohistiocytic differentiation in subcutaneous fatty tumors. Study of spindle cell, pleomorphic, myxoid, and atypical lipoma and dedifferentiated liposarcoma cases composed in part of CD34+ fibroblasts and FXIIIa+ histiocytes. *J Cutan Pathol.* 1997;24(8):484–493.

54. McNiff JM, Subtil A, Cowper SE, Lazova R, Glusac EJ. Cellular digital fibromas: distinctive CD34-positive lesions that may mimic dermatofibrosarcoma protuberans. *J Cutan Pathol.* 2005;32(6):413–418.

55. Swanson PE, Wick MR. Immunohistochemical evaluation of vascular neoplasms. *Clin Dermatol.* 1991;9:243.

56. Wick MR, Manivel JC. Vascular neoplasms of the skin: a current perspective. *Adv Dermatol.* 1989;4:185.

57. Albelda SM, Muller WA, Buck CA, Newman PJ. Molecular and cellular properties of PECAM-1 (ends CAM/CD31): a novel vascular cell–cell adhesion molecule. *J Cell Biol.* 1991;115:1059.

58. DeYoung BR, Swanson PE, Argenyi ZB, et al. CD31 immunoreactivity in mesenchymal neoplasms of the skin. *J Cutan Pathol.* 1995;22:215–222.

59. Mankey CC, McHugh JB, Thomas DG, Lucas DR. Can lymphangiosarcoma be resurrected? A clinicopathological and immunohistochemical study of lymphatic differentiation in 49 angiosarcomas. *Histopathology.* 2010;56(3):364–371.

60. McKay KM, Doyle LA, Lazar AJ, Hornick JL. Expression of ERG, an Ets family transcription factor, distinguishes cutaneous angiosarcoma from histological mimics. *Histopathology.* 2012;61(5):989–991.

61. Katano H. Pathological features of Kaposi's sarcoma-associated herpesvirus infection. *Adv Exp Med Biol.* 2018;1045:357–376.

62. Nemeth AJ, Penneys NS. Factor XIIIa is expressed by fibroblasts in fibrovascular tumors. *J Cutan Pathol.* 1989;16:266–271.

63. Moretto JC, Soslow RA, Smoller BR. Atypical cells in radiation dermatitis express factor XIIIa. *Am J Dermatopathol.* 1998;20:370–372.

64. Nguyen TT, Schwartz EJ, West RB, Warnke RA, Arber DA, Natkunam Y. Expression of CD163 (hemoglobin scavenger receptor) in normal tissues, lymphomas, carcinomas, and sarcomas is largely restricted to the monocyte/macrophage lineage. *Am J Surg Pathol.* 2005;29:617.

65. Miettinen M, Lastoa J. KIT (CD117): a review on expression in normal and neoplastic tissues, and mutations and their

clinicopathologic correlation. *Appl Immunohistochem Mol Morphol.* 2005;13(3):205–220.

66. Hornick JL, Fletcher CD. The significance of KIT (CD117) in gastrointestinal stromal tumors [review]. *Int J Surg Pathol.* 2004; 12(2):93–97.

67. Coventry B, Heinzel S. CD1a in human cancers: a new role for an old molecule. *Trends Immunol.* 2004;25:242–248.

68. Querings K, Starz H, Balda BR. Clinical spectrum of cutaneous Langerhans' cell histiocytosis mimicking various diseases [case report]. *Acta Derm Venereol.* 2006;86(1):39–43.

69. Ratnam KV, Su WPD, Ziesmer SC, Li CY. Value of immunohistochemistry in the diagnosis of leukemia cutis: study of 54 cases using paraffin-section markers. *J Cutan Pathol.* 1992;19:193.

70. Willemze R, Cerroni L, Kempf W, et al. The 2018 update of the WHO-EORTC classification for primary cutaneous lymphomas. *Blood.* 2019;133(16):1703–1714.

71. Weinberg JM, Rook AH, Lessin SR. Molecular diagnosis of lymphocytic infiltrates of the skin. *Arch Dermatol.* 1993;129:1491.

72. Weiss LM, Wood GS, Ellisen LW, Reynolds TC, Sklar J. Clonal T-cell populations in pityriasis lichenoides et varioliformis acuta (Mucha-Haberman disease). *Am J Pathol.* 1987;126:417–421.

73. Schiller PI, Flaig MJ, Puchta U, et al. Detection of clonal T-cells in lichen planus. *Arch Dermatol Res.* 2000;292:568–569.

74. Ponti R, Quaglino P, Novelli M, et al. T-cell receptor gamma gene rearrangement by multiplex polymerase chain reaction/heteroduplex analysis in patients with cutaneous T-cell lymphoma (mycosis fungoides/Sezary syndrome) and benign inflammatory disease: correlation with clinical, histological and immunophenotypical findings. *Br J Dermatol.* 2005;153:565–573.

75. Abbas O, Bhawan J. Infections in dermatopathology: emerging frontiers. *Am J Dermatopathol.* 2012;34:789–799.

76. Nikkels AF, Debrus S, Sadzot-Delvaux C, Piette J, Rentier B, Piérard GE. Immunohistochemical identification of varicella-zoster virus gene 63-encoded protein (IE63) and late (gE) protein on smears and cutaneous biopsies: implications for diagnostic use. *Mod Virol.* 1995;47:342–347.

77. Murphy GF, Dickersin GR, Harrist TJ, Mihm MC Jr. The role of diagnostic electron microscopy in dermatology. In: Moschella S, ed. *Dermatology Update.* Elsevier Press; 1981:355.

Outline of Cutaneous Pathology

DAVID E. ELDER, ROSALIE ELENITSAS, MISHA ROSENBACH, GEORGE F. MURPHY, ADAM I. RUBIN, AND XIAOWEI XU

Chapter

5

INTRODUCTION

The diagnosis of disease concerns the ability to classify disorders into categories that predict clinically important attributes such as prognosis or response to therapy. This permits appropriate interventions to be employed for particular patients. Understanding this process involves mastery of the stages of disease; the mechanisms of changes in morphology over time; and the molecular, cellular, clinical, and epidemiologic reasons for the differences among diseases.

The process of cutaneous diagnosis at its simplest level might involve the matching of a large number of attributes contained in classical descriptions of skin diseases with the presence or absence of the same attributes in a particular case under consideration. As there are hundreds of potential diagnostic categories, each having potentially scores of attributes, it is evident that an efficient strategy must be employed to enable diagnoses to be considered, dismissed, or retained for further consideration. Observation of an experienced dermatopathologist reveals a rapidity of accurate diagnosis that precludes the simultaneous consideration of more than a few variables. Indeed, the process of diagnosis by an experienced observer is quite different from that employed by the novice and is based on the rapid recognition of combinations or patterns of criteria (1,2). Just as the recognition of an old friend occurs by a process that does not require the serial enumeration of particular facial features, this process of pattern recognition occurs almost instantly and is based on broad parameters that do not at least initially require detailed evaluation.

In clinical medicine, patterns may present as combinations of symptoms and signs, or even of laboratory values, but in dermatopathology, the most predictive diagnostic patterns are recognized through the scanning lens of the microscope, or even before microscopy, as the microscopist holds the slide up to the light, to evaluate the tissue profile(s) and distribution of colors. Occasionally, a specific diagnosis can be made during this initial stage of pattern recognition, by a process of "gestalt" or instant recognition, but this should be tempered with a subsequent moment of healthy analytical scrutiny. More often, the scanning magnification pattern suggests a small list of possible diagnoses, a "differential diagnosis." Then, features that are more readily recognized at higher magnification may be employed to differentiate among the possibilities. Put in the language of science, the scanning magnification pattern suggests a series of hypotheses, which are then tested by additional observations (1). The tests may be observations made at higher magnification, the results of special studies such as immunohistochemistry, external findings such as the clinical appearance of the patient, or the results of laboratory investigations. For example, a broad plaque-like configuration of small blue dots near the dermal–epidermal junction could represent lichenoid dermatitis or lichenoid actinic keratosis. At higher magnification, the blue dots are confirmed to be lymphocytes, and one might seek evidence of parakeratosis, atypical keratinocytes, and plasma cells in the lesion, a combination that would rule out lichen planus and establish a diagnosis of actinic keratosis.

Most diagnoses in dermatopathology are established either by the "gestalt" method or by the process of hypothesis generation and testing (differential diagnosis and investigation) just described, but in either case, the basis of the methods is the identification of simple patterns recognizable with the scanning lens that suggest a manageably short list of differential diagnostic considerations. This pattern recognition method was first developed for dermatopathology in a series of lectures given in Boston by Wallace Clark (3) and has been refined since for inflammatory skin disease by Ackerman (4), for inflammatory and neoplastic skin disease by Mihm (5), and more recently by Murphy (6), Barnhill (7,8), Maize and colleagues (9), Weedon (10,11), and McKee (12,13). In addition, our *Atlas of Dermatopathology: Synopsis* and *Atlas of Lever's Histopathology of the Skin*, now in its fourth edition, is organized strictly along pattern recognition lines (14,15).

Some of these published texts, including the Atlas, are based more or less extensively on pattern classification. The present work, however, has been organized upon more traditional "pathophysiologic" lines, in which diseases are discussed on the basis of pathogenesis (mechanisms) or etiology as well as upon reaction patterns. Such a classification has the advantage of placing disorders such as infections in a common relationship to one another, facilitating the description of their many common attributes. From a histopathologic point of view, however, the novice must learn that some infections, such as syphilis, can resemble disorders as disparate as psoriasis, as lichen planus, as a cutaneous lymphoma, or as a granulomatous dermatitis.

Because there is a limited number of reaction patterns in the skin, morphologic simulants of disparate disease processes are common in the skin, as elsewhere. For this reason, classification methods based on patterns and those based on pathogenesis are incompatible with each other. To partially circumvent this problem, the present section of this book presents a pattern-based classification of cutaneous pathology based on location in the skin, on reaction patterns, and where applicable on cell type, indexed to the more detailed descriptions of the disease entities discussed in other sections of the text. The section was originally based (with permission) on the original lecture notes prepared by Wallace H. Clark Jr., M.D., in 1965, and on the published works cited above, especially that of Hood, Kwan, Mihm, and Horn (5).

The classification is presented here in tabular form and is redundant, in that a particular disease entity may appear in several positions in the table. This is because of the morphologic heterogeneity of disease processes, which are often based on evolutionary or involutional morphologic changes as a disease waxes and wanes. The order of presentation of particular entities in any given position in the table reflects the authors' general opinion of the relative frequency of the entities in the list, as encountered in a typical dermatopathology practice. For example, lichenoid drug eruption may be more common than lichen planus in most hospital-based practices. However, lichen planus is the "prototypic" lichenoid dermatitis, whereas drug eruptions may adopt any of a number of morphologies as reflected by their appearance in the psoriasiform, lichenoid, perivascular, and bullous categories as well as elsewhere. The "prototypic" member of each category is underlined for easy reference to the detailed descriptions because such entities constitute the descriptive standard in a given category, and they are also the standard against which other entities are evaluated. For example, a "naked" epithelioid cell granuloma may suggest sarcoidosis, whereas the presence of lymphocytes and necrosis in addition to granulomas might suggest tuberculosis, plasma cells might suggest syphilis, and neuritis might suggest leprosy.

The classification tables may be used as the basis of an algorithmic approach to differential diagnosis and as a guide to the descriptions in the other sections of this book. For example, psoriasiform dermatitis with plasma cells may represent syphilis or mycosis fungoides, whose descriptions are to be found in Chapters 21 and 31, respectively. Terms such as "psoriasiform" and "lichenoid" are defined briefly, and appropriate page references are provided in this section so that the reader may review more specific criteria for the distinctions among morphologic simulants. This system of hypothesis generation and testing should lead not only to more efficient use of this book in the evaluation and diagnosis of an unknown case but also should facilitate the development of pattern recognition skills as increasingly subtle diagnostic clues are absorbed into the diagnostic repertoire to allow for "tempered gestalt" diagnosis in an increasing percentage of cases.

The schema presented here is also the basis of the classification presented in our *Atlas of Dermatopathology: Synopsis* and *Atlas of Lever's Histopathology of the Skin*, which is organized strictly along pattern recognition lines and is intended to be a more richly illustrated companion to this present volume, with a more synoptic text relating to the disease entities that are illustrated (14,15).

Although this chapter is intended as a guide to differential diagnosis, it should not be construed as an infallible diagnostic tool. Diagnosis should be based not only on the diagnostic considerations presented here but also on those discussed elsewhere in this book and in the literature, all considered in a clinical and epidemiologic context appropriate to the individual patient.

HOW TO USE THIS CLASSIFICATION SYSTEM

In this System, diseases are classified not by the usual pathophysiologic classification but also according to the pattern classification, more fully discussed above. The diseases are grouped first as to their location in the skin, then according to morphologic patterns that may present in those particular locations, and finally according to the cell types involved. Generally speaking, these classifiers can be thought of as low-power, medium-power, and high-power microscopic features, or as Site, Pattern, and Cytology classifiers.

There are eight specified locations, which are assigned Roman Numerals I through VIII, as follows:

   I. Disorders Mostly Limited to the Epidermis and Stratum Corneum
  II. Localized Superficial Epidermal or Melanocytic Proliferations
 III. Disorders of the Superficial Cutaneous Reactive Unit
  IV. Epidermal Acantholytic, Vesicular, and Pustular Disorders
   V. Perivascular, Diffuse, and Granulomatous Infiltrates of the Reticular Dermis
  VI. Tumors and Cysts of the Dermis and Subcutis
 VII. Inflammatory and Other Benign Disorders of Skin Appendages
VIII. Disorders of the Subcutis

Some of these "locations" also combine patterns where these have particularly broad significance. For example, "II. Localized Superficial Epidermal or Melanocytic Proliferations," "IV. Epidermal Acantholytic, Vesicular, and Pustular Disorders," and "V. Perivascular, Diffuse, and Granulomatous Infiltrates of the Reticular Dermis" are all terms that combine a location and one or more patterns, namely, proliferations of cells to form plaques or superficial nodules (II); separation of epidermal cells either from each other or from the underlying dermis to form spaces termed vesicles, bullae, or pustules (IV); granulomas which are collections of epithelioid histiocytes (V); or tumors which are mass lesions formed by neoplastic cells (VI), and so on. In this book, it is generally assumed that basic pathologic processes like cell identification, suppuration, granulomatous inflammation, and neoplasia can be recognized by the reader.

The major subheadings and their first-level subdivisions are presented beginning on Part 1 of this chapter, with photomicrographs selected to illustrate a few of the important patterns of skin diseases. Subsequently, in Part 2, the full listings of Site, Pattern, and Cytology are presented, with itemization of the major diseases that fall into each category. The same classification, with expanded discussion and illustration of the disease entities, is presented in the fourth edition of the volume *Atlas of Dermatopathology: Synopsis* and *Atlas of Lever's Histopathology of the Skin* (15, which is designed to be a companion to this present more comprehensive text).

In these roman numeral–designated sections, the various patterns that may occur in the various locations are designated by capital letters, A, B, C, etc. These patterns differ from one location to another. For example, within the very important group of inflammatory disorders of the superficial cutaneous reactive unit, the patterns include reactions involving the epidermis such as spongiosis which is a basic pattern of the common eczematous disorders; reactions involving these highly reactive superficial vessels such as perivascular lymphocytic inflammation, which is frequent in many diseases; reactions at the dermal–epidermal interface such as vacuolar or lichenoid patterns, and changes in the interstitium such as sclerosis, to name a few. All of these patterns have their own associations that are redundant and not specific. For example, a lichenoid pattern, discussed in section IIIF, can be shared by lichen planus (its prototypic disorder), a lichenoid drug reaction, a lichenoid actinic keratosis, and other conditions. As is often the case in dermatopathology, the term "lichenoid" is not intuitive histologically but is derived from the clinical appearance of the lesion and from clinical terminology.

The third level of classification is by cell type, designated by Arabic numerals 1, 2, 3, etc. The cell types in question in the same superficial inflammatory disorders discussed above include among others lymphocytes only (e.g., lichen planus, which is section IIIF1), lymphocytes with eosinophils (e.g., lichenoid drug eruption IIIF2a), lymphocytes with plasma cells (e.g., syphilis IIIF2b), or in other patterns the cytologic choices might include neutrophils predominating (e.g., Sweet syndrome, VC2), eosinophils predominating (e.g., Wells syndrome, VC6), and so on. Neoplasms also often have quite specific cytology. The addition of the cytologic classifier to the location and pattern classifiers can often lead to a very narrow differential diagnosis or even a specific diagnosis.

For each of the subsets of disease at this level, a condition considered to be prototypic is emphasized by underlining in the detailed listings, as these conditions (such as for example lichen planus) form the basis for description of a group of conditions that resemble them, in this case, lichenoid disorders.

Even if a specific diagnosis cannot be made histopathologically, it is always useful to generate a differential diagnosis that can be correlated with the clinical impressions, often leading to a unified diagnosis based on clinicopathologic correlation. In this book, conditions that may be considered in the differential diagnosis are listed at the end of each section, and these lists may serve as the basis for crafting a pathology report that considers, as completely as possible, the range of possibilities for any given case. In addition, page references are given to discussions of the various entities elsewhere in this volume.

The companion Atlas can be used as a visual indexing system. When looking at a microscopic slide of an unknown disorder using this classification, the first approach is to determine what part of the skin is primarily involved in that process. Next, the relevant sections of the Atlas can be scanned in an effort to identify the predominant pattern of the abnormality. This can be done by scanning the table of contents or by checking the images to find ones that look similar to the microscopic image. This process may seem difficult at first; however, this pattern recognition method has the potential to lead quite rapidly to the section that contains the disease in question.

We have found in practice that trainees who use this system can develop more comprehensive differential diagnoses as they preview cases for signout with their teachers. Similarly, experienced dermatopathologists can use this method to ensure that their differential diagnostic considerations are complete and also to illustrate to their trainees the range of lesions that can have a morphology similar to that which is visualized under the microscope. We hope and expect that using these principles will increase the value of the signout process as a learning experience and ultimately may make itself superfluous as the patterns become ingrained into the experience of the learner, who may then begin to perceive diseases like lichen planus, lupus profundus, bullous pemphigoid, superficial spreading melanoma, and so on, in a flash of recognition or "gestalt," similar to how old friends can be rapidly picked out of a crowd of otherwise generally similar human beings. When this stage is reached, our work can be considered to be done and a lifetime of continued learning, useful productivity, and fun, will follow.

Diagnosis as always should be based not only on the diagnostic considerations presented here but also on those discussed elsewhere in this book and in the literature, all considered in a clinical and epidemiologic context appropriate to the individual patient. It is essential to remember that dermatopathologists work as part of a patient care team and that clear and accurate communication with clinicians and incorporation of clinical information into the diagnostic process will allow diagnostic precision. Although the dermatopathologist may be separated physically from clinical colleagues, it is this interaction and collaboration that allows for the best service to the patient, who is the reason for our efforts. In our hospital-based practice, an interactive clinicopathologic correlation conference occurs weekly for selected cases, with great benefits for the quality of patient care and also for the continuing education of dermatopathologists and dermatologists alike.

REFERENCES

1. Sackett DL, Haynes RB, Guyatt GH, Tugwell P. *Clinical Epidemiology. A Basic Science for Clinical Medicine.* 2nd ed. Little Brown; 1991.
2. Foucar E. Diagnostic decision-making in surgical pathology. In: Weidner N, ed. *Difficult Diagnosis in Surgical Pathology.* W.B. Saunders; 1996.
3. Reed RJ, Clark WH Jr. Pathophysiologic reactions of the skin. In: Fitzpatrick TB, ed. *Dermatology in General Medicine.* McGraw-Hill; 1971:192–216.
4. Ackerman AB. *Histologic Diagnosis of Inflammatory Skin Diseases. A Method by Pattern Analysis.* Lea & Febiger; 1978.
5. Hood AF, Kwan TH, Mihm MC, Horn TD. *Primer of Dermatopathology.* Little, Brown & Company; 1993.
6. Murphy GF. *Dermatopathology.* Saunders; 1995.
7. Barnhill RL, ed. *Textbook of Dermatopathology.* McGraw-Hill; 1998.
8. Barnhill RL, Crowson AN, Magro CM, Piepkorn MW, Kutzner H, Desman GT. eds. *Barnhill's Dermatopathology.* 4th ed. McGraw-Hill; 2020.
9. Maize JC, ed. *Cutaneous Pathology.* Churchill Livingstone; 1998.
10. Weedon D. *Skin Pathology.* Churchill Livingstone; 2002.
11. Paterson JW. *Weedon's Skin Pathology.* 5th ed. Elsevier; 2021.
12. McKee P. *Pathology of the Skin, with Clinical Correlations.* JB Lippincott Co.; 1989.
13. Calonje E, Brenn T, Lazar AJ, Billings S. *McKee's Pathology of the Skin, with Clinical Correlations.* 5th ed. Elsevier; 2020.
14. Elder DE, Elenitsas R, Johnson BL, Ioffreda MD, Miller J, Miller OF. *Synopsis and Atlas of Lever's Histopathology of the Skin.* Lippincott Williams and Wilkins; 2007.
15. Elder DE, Elenitsas R, Rubin AI, et al. *Atlas of Dermatopathology. Synopsis and Atlas of Lever's Histopathology of the Skin.* 4th ed. Wolters Kluwer; 2021.

PART 1. SITE CATEGORIES OF CUTANEOUS PATHOLOGY

In this part, the major categories of cutaneous disease based on their location in the skin and subcutis are briefly discussed.

I. DISORDERS MOSTLY LIMITED TO THE STRATUM CORNEUM

The stratum corneum is usually arranged in a delicate mesh-like or "basket-weave" pattern. It may be shed (exfoliated) or thickened (hyperkeratosis) with or without retention of nuclei (parakeratosis or orthokeratosis, respectively). Usually, alterations in the stratum corneum result from inflammatory or neoplastic changes that affect the whole epidermis and, more often than not, the superficial dermis. Only a few conditions, mentioned in this section, show pathology mostly or entirely limited to the stratum corneum.

II. NEOPLASTIC LOCALIZED EPITHELIAL OR MELANOCYTIC PROLIFERATIONS

Localized proliferations may be reactive but are often neoplastic. The epidermis (keratinocytes) may proliferate without extension into the dermis or extend into the dermis where it may be squamous or basaloid. Melanocytes within the epidermis may proliferate with or without cytologic atypia (nevi, dysplastic nevi, melanoma *in situ*), in a proliferative epidermis (superficial spreading melanoma *in situ*, Spitz nevi), or an atrophic epidermis (lentigo maligna); they can also extend into the dermis as proliferative infiltrates (invasive melanoma with or without vertical growth phase). There may be an associated variably cellular often mixed inflammatory infiltrate, or inflammation may be essentially absent.

III. INFLAMMATION OF THE SUPERFICIAL CUTANEOUS REACTIVE UNIT

The epidermis, papillary dermis, and superficial capillary–venular plexus at the interface of the papillary and superficial reticular dermis react together in many dermatologic conditions and have been termed the "superficial cutaneous reactive unit" by Clark. Many dermatoses are associated with infiltrates of lymphocytes with or without other cell types, around the superficial vessels. The epidermis in pathologic conditions can be thinned (atrophic), thickened (acanthosis), edematous (spongiosis), dyshesive (acantholysis), and/or infiltrated by inflammatory cells (exocytosis). The epidermis may proliferate in response to chronic irritation and infection (bacterial, yeast, deep fungal, or viral). The epidermis also may proliferate in response to dermatologic conditions (psoriasis, atopic dermatitis, prurigo). The papillary dermis and superficial vascular plexus may have a variety of inflammatory cells, can be edematous, may have increased ground substance (hyaluronic acid), or may be sclerotic or homogenized.

IV. ACANTHOLYTIC, VESICULAR, AND PUSTULAR DISORDERS

Keratinocytes may separate from each other, resulting in dyshesion and rounding-up of their cell bodies (acantholysis). This may occur on the basis of immunologic antigen–antibody-mediated damage, on the basis of edema and inflammation (spongiosis), infections (impetigo or herpes viral infection), or on the basis of structural deficiencies of cell adhesion (Darier disease). These processes produce spaces within the epidermis (vesicles, bullae, pustules).

V. INFLAMMATION OF THE RETICULAR DERMIS

The dermis serves as a reaction site for a variety of inflammatory, infiltrative, and desmoplastic (fibrogenic) processes. These include infiltrations of a variety of cells (lymphocytes, histiocytes, eosinophils, plasma cells, melanocytes, etc.); perivascular and vascular reactions; infiltration with organisms and foreign bodies; and proliferations of dermal fibers and precursors of dermal fibers as reactions to a variety of stimuli. The infiltrates may be characterized as perivascular, diffuse, or granulomatous.

VI. NEOPLASTIC NODULES AND CYSTS OF THE RETICULAR DERMIS

Neoplasms of the reticular dermis may arise from any of the tissues included in the dermis—lymphoreticular tissue, connective tissue, and epithelial tissue of the skin appendages. In addition, metastases commonly present in the dermis.

VII. INFLAMMATORY DISORDERS OF SKIN APPENDAGES

The hair, sebaceous glands, eccrine glands, apocrine glands, and nails may be involved in inflammatory processes (hidradenitis, folliculitis). Some neoplasms may masquerade as inflammatory processes.

VIII. DISORDERS OF THE SUBCUTIS

The reactions in the subcutis are mostly inflammatory, although neoplastic proliferations of the subcutis do occur (lipoma). Pathologic conditions centered in the dermis may infiltrate the subcutis.

PART 2. **SITE, PATTERN, AND CYTOLOGIC CATEGORIES OF CUTANEOUS PATHOLOGY**

In the following listings, the categories of cutaneous disease based on location in the skin (categories I, II, III, etc.), architectural pattern (categories A, B, C, etc.), and cytology (categories 1, 2, 3, etc.) are presented. A single prototypic example of each disease category is listed, and a prototypic example of each major pattern category is illustrated.

I. DISORDERS MOSTLY LIMITED TO THE EPIDERMIS AND STRATUM CORNEUM

A. Hyperkeratosis with Hypogranulosis

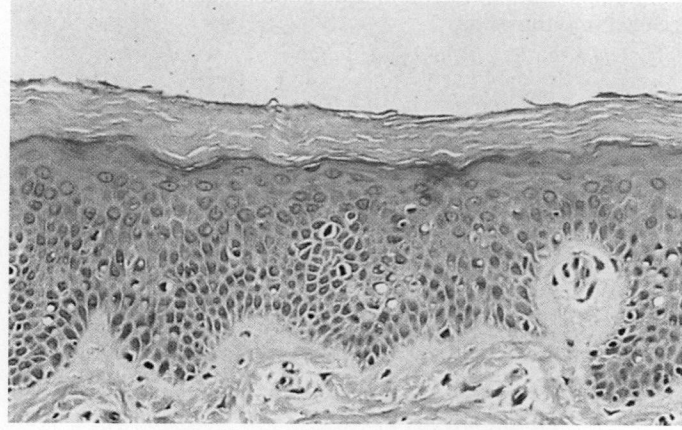

1. No Inflammation
ichthyosis vulgaris

B. Hyperkeratosis with Normal or Hypergranulosis

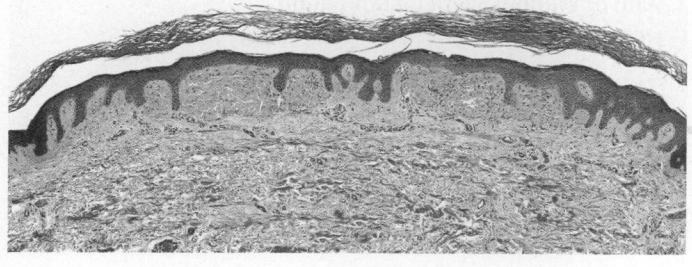

1. No Inflammation
lamellar ichthyosis

2. Scant Inflammation
lichen amyloidosis

C. Hyperkeratosis with Parakeratosis

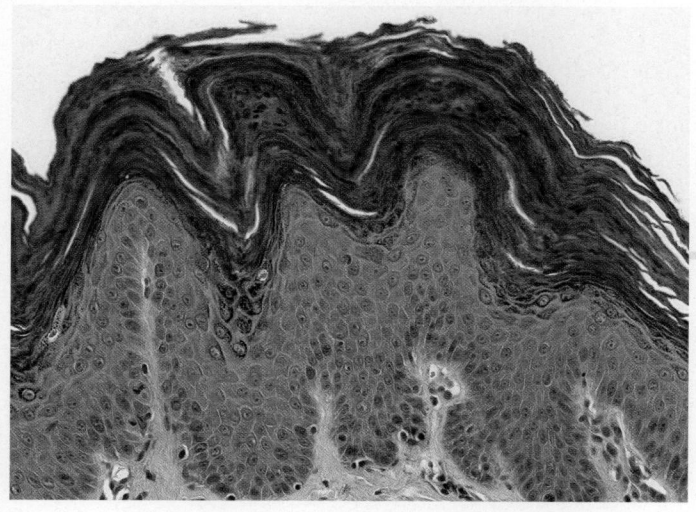

1. No Inflammation
granular parakeratosis

2. Scant Inflammation
scurvy

3. With Epidermal Pallor or Necrosis ("Nutritional Dermatosis")
pellagra

D. Localized or Diffuse Hyperpigmentations

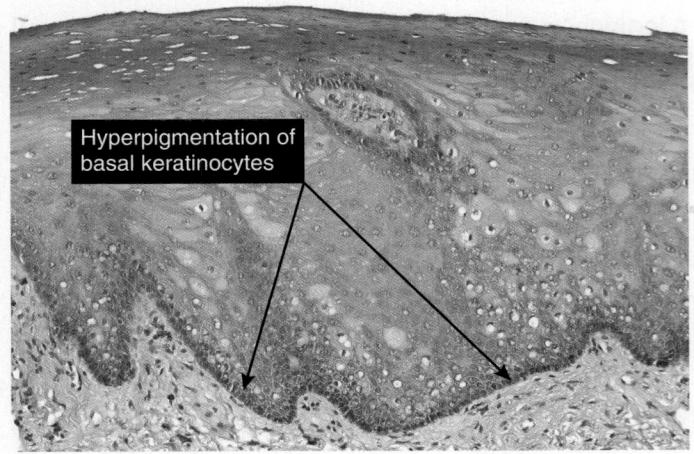

Hyperpigmentation of basal keratinocytes

1. No Inflammation
mucosal melanotic macule

2. Scant Inflammation
postinflammatory hyperpigmentation

E. Localized or Diffuse Hypopigmentation/Depigmentation

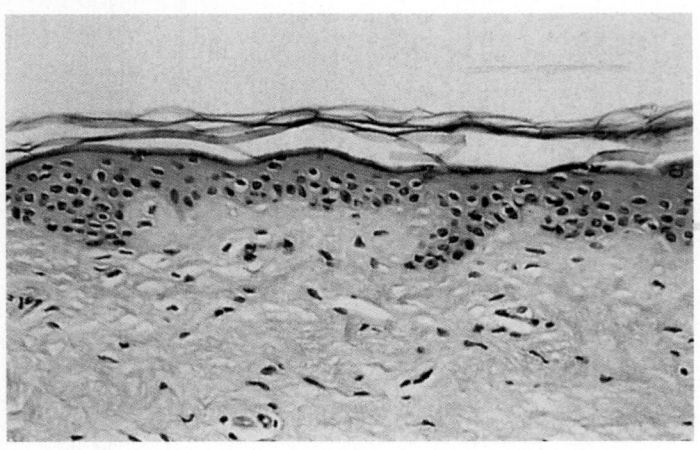

1. With or Without Slight Inflammation
vitiligo

II. LOCALIZED SUPERFICIAL EPIDERMAL OR MELANOCYTIC PROLIFERATIONS

A. Localized Irregular Thickening of the Epidermis

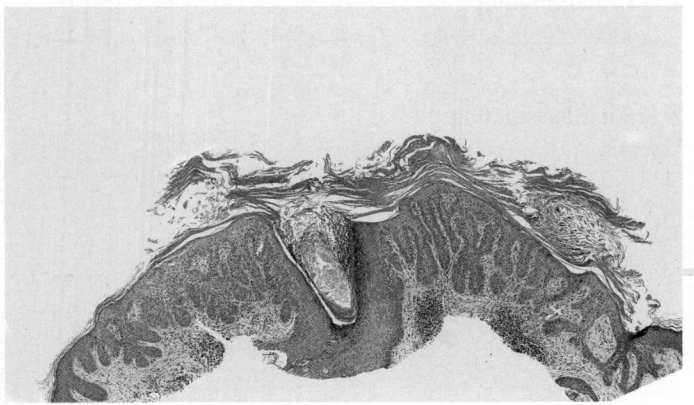

1. Localized Epidermal Proliferations
actinic keratosis

2. Superficial Melanocytic Proliferations
melanoma in situ *(superficial spreading type)*

B. Localized Lesions with Thinning of the Epidermis

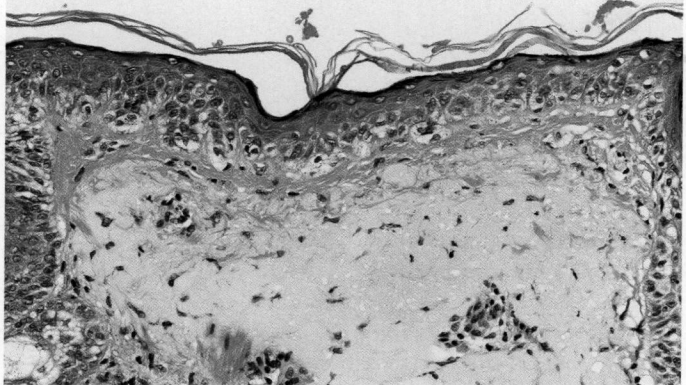

1. With Melanocytic Proliferation
melanoma in situ *(lentigo maligna type)*

2. Without Melanocytic Proliferation
solar keratosis

C. Localized Lesions with Elongated Rete Ridges

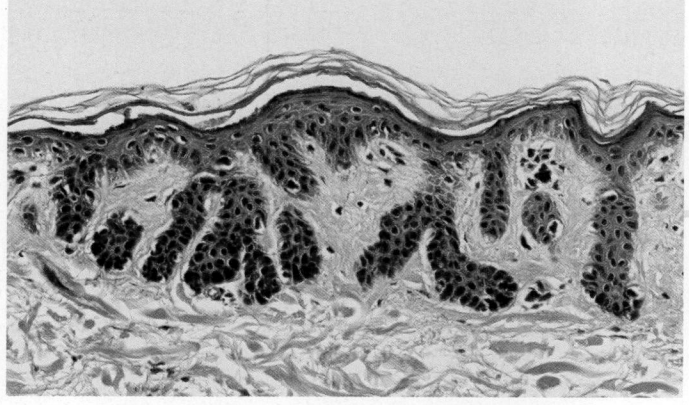

1. With Melanocytic Proliferation
solar lentigo

2. Without Melanocytic Proliferation
epidermal nevi

D. Localized Lesions with Pagetoid Epithelial Proliferation

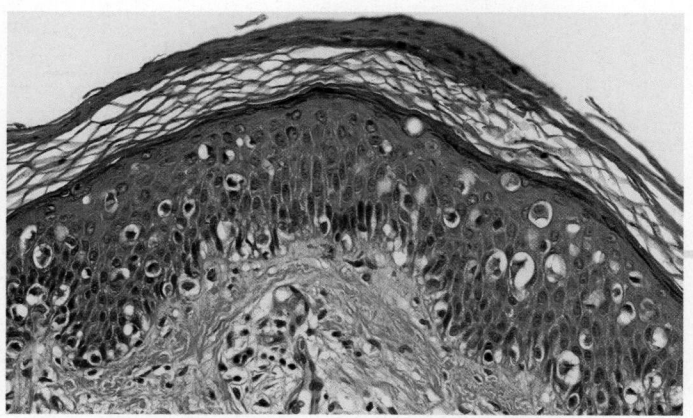

1. Keratinocytic Proliferations
pagetoid squamous cell carcinoma in situ

2. Melanocytic Proliferation
melanoma in situ *(superficial spreading type, pagetoid)*

3. Glandular Epithelial Proliferations
Paget disease (mammary or extramammary)

4. Lymphoid Proliferations
Pagetoid reticulosis, localized (Woringer–Kolopp)

E. Localized Papillomatous Epithelial Lesions

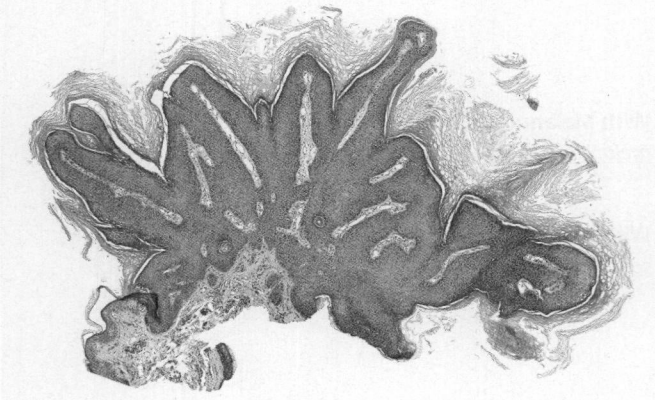

1. With Viral Cytopathic Effects
verruca vulgaris

2. No Viral Cytopathic Effect
seborrheic keratosis

F. Irregular Proliferations Extending into the Dermis

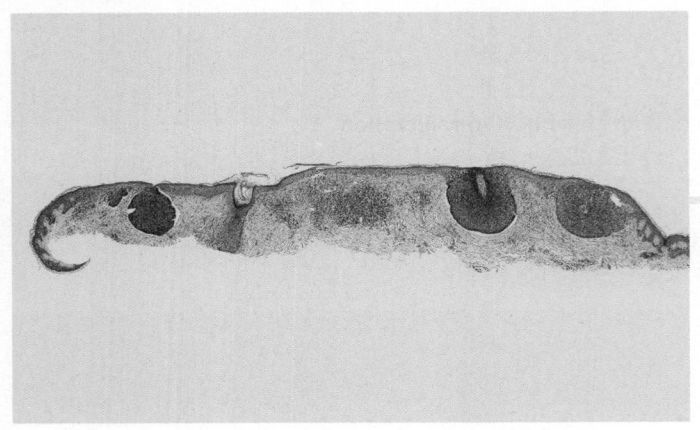

1. Squamous Differentiation
squamous cell carcinoma, superficial

2. Basaloid Differentiation
basal cell carcinoma, superficial type

G. Superficial Polypoid Lesions

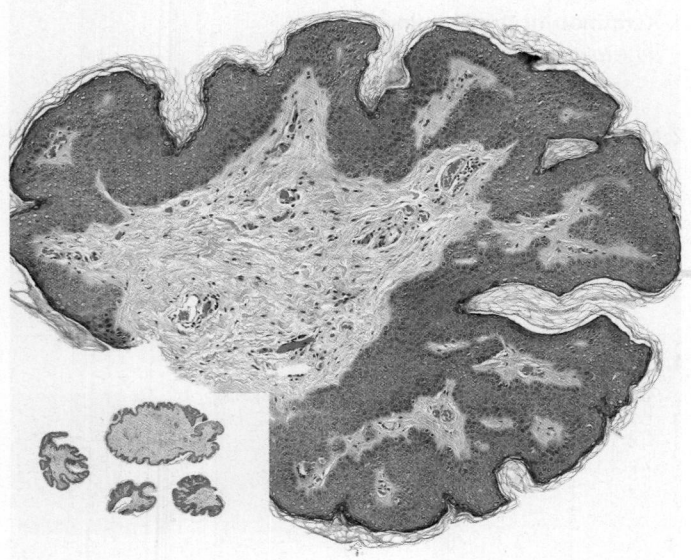

1. Melanocytic Lesions
polypoid dermal and compound nevi

2. Stromal Lesions
fibroepithelial polyp

III. DISORDERS OF THE SUPERFICIAL CUTANEOUS REACTIVE UNIT

A. Superficial Perivascular Dermatitis

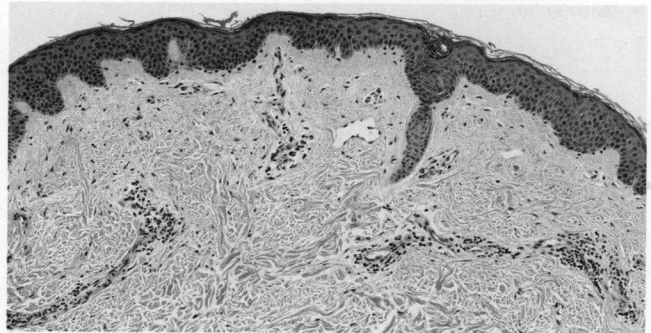

1. Lymphocytes Predominant
morbilliform viral exanthem
1a. With Eosinophils
  morbilliform drug eruption
1b. With Neutrophils
  erysipelas
1c. With Plasma Cells
  secondary syphilis
1d. With Extravasated Red Cells
  pigmented purpuric dermatosis
1e. Melanophages Prominent
  postinflammatory pigmentation

2. Mast Cells Predominant
telangiectasia macularis eruptiva perstans

B. Superficial Perivascular Dermatitis with Spongiosis (Spongiotic Dermatitis)

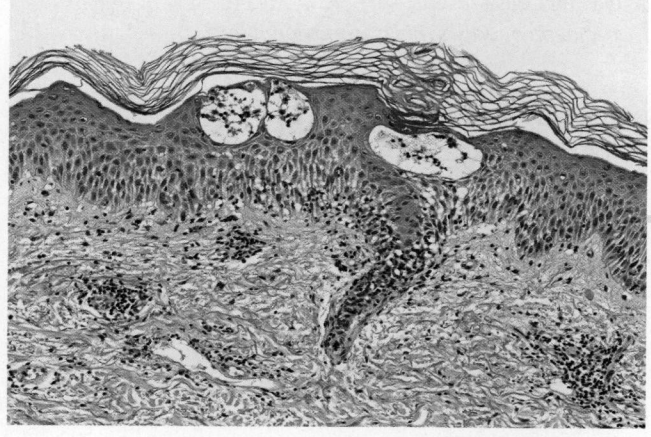

1. Lymphocytes Predominant
nummular dermatitis (eczema)
1a. With Eosinophils
  allergic contact dermatitis
1b. With Plasma Cells
  syphilis, primary or secondary lesions
1c. With Neutrophils
  seborrheic dermatitis

C. Superficial Perivascular Dermatitis with Epidermal Atrophy (Atrophic Dermatitis)

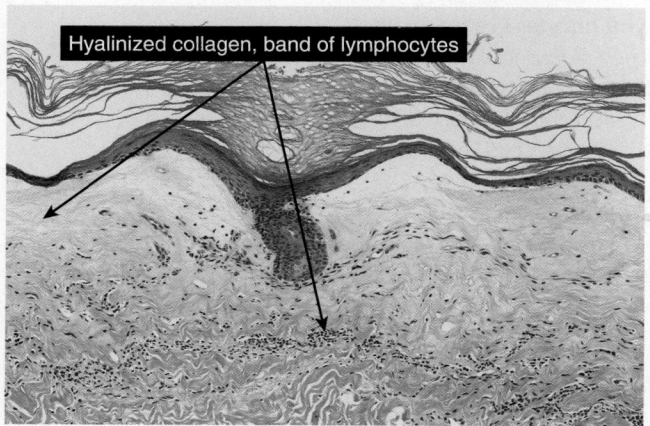

Hyalinized collagen, band of lymphocytes

1. Scant Inflammatory Infiltrates
radiation dermatitis

2. Lymphocytes Predominant
parapsoriasis/early mycosis fungoides
2a. With Papillary Dermal Sclerosis
  lichen sclerosus et atrophicus

D. Superficial Perivascular Dermatitis with Psoriasiform Proliferation (Psoriasiform Dermatitis)

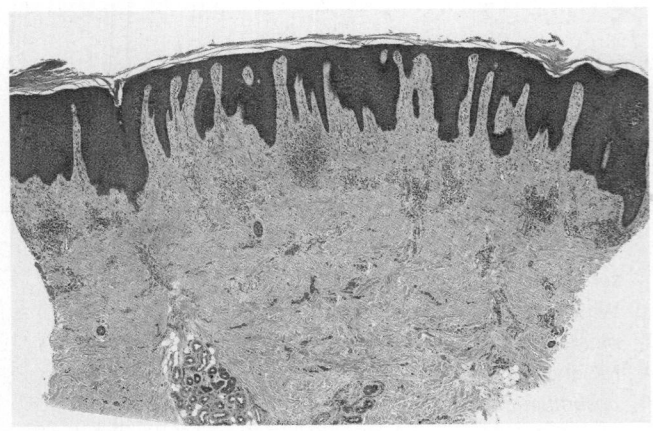

1. Lymphocytes Predominant
chronic atopic dermatitis
  1a. With Plasma Cells
     secondary syphilis
  1b. With Eosinophils
     chronic allergic dermatitis

2. Neutrophils Prominent
psoriasis vulgaris

3. Psoriasiform Epidermal Proliferation, with Epidermal Pallor or Necrosis ("Nutritional Dermatosis")
pellagra

E. Superficial Perivascular Dermatitis with Irregular Epidermal Proliferation (Hypertrophic Dermatitis)

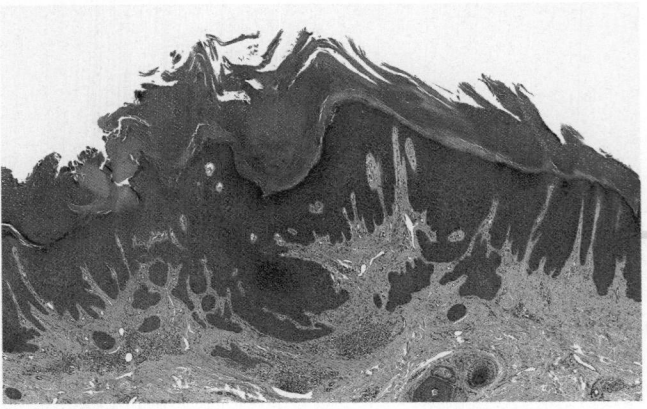

1. Lymphocytes Predominant
prurigo nodularis
  1a. Plasma Cells Present
     rupial secondary syphilis, condyloma lata

2. Neutrophils Prominent
impetigo contagiosa

3. Neoplastic
malignant melanoma ("verrucous" pattern)

F. Superficial Dermatitis with Lichenoid Infiltrates (Lichenoid Dermatitis)

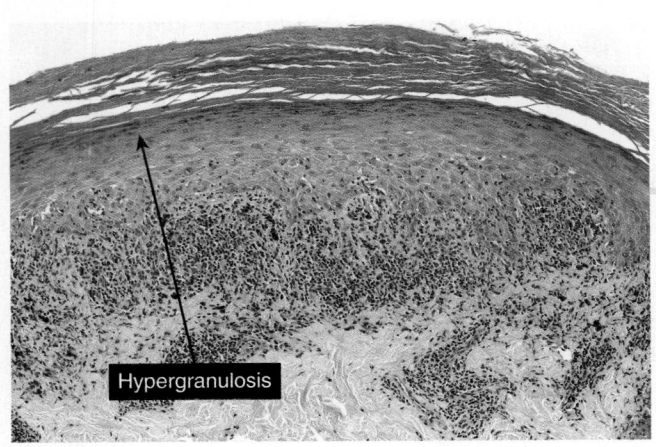

Hypergranulosis

1. Lymphocytes Exclusively
lichen planus

2. Lymphocytes Predominant
lichen planus–like keratosis (benign lichenoid keratosis)
  2a. Eosinophils Present
     lichenoid drug eruptions
  2b. Plasma Cells Present
     secondary syphilis
  2c. With Melanophages
     postinflammatory hyperpigmentation
  2d. With Lymphocytic Atypia
     mycosis fungoides

3. Histiocytes Predominant
lichen nitidus

G. Superficial Vasculitis and Vasculopathies

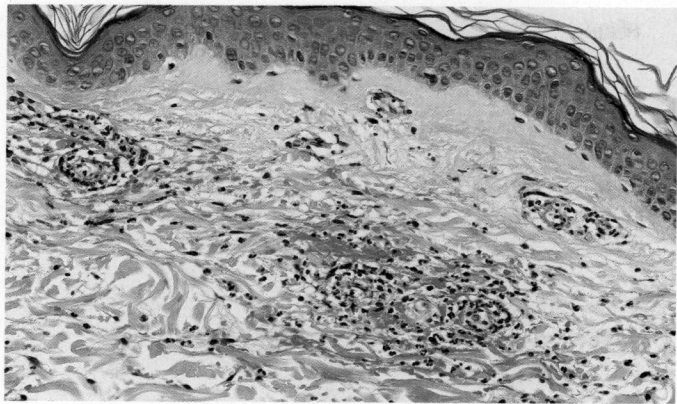

1. Neutrophilic Vasculitis
cutaneous necrotizing (leukocytoclastic) vasculitis

2. Mixed Cell and Granulomatous Vasculitis
Churg–Strauss vasculitis

3. Vasculopathies with Scant Inflammation
malignant atrophic papulosis (Degos)

4. Thrombotic, Embolic, and Other Microangiopathies
disseminated intravascular coagulation

H. Superficial Perivascular Dermatitis with Interface Vacuoles (Interface Dermatitis)

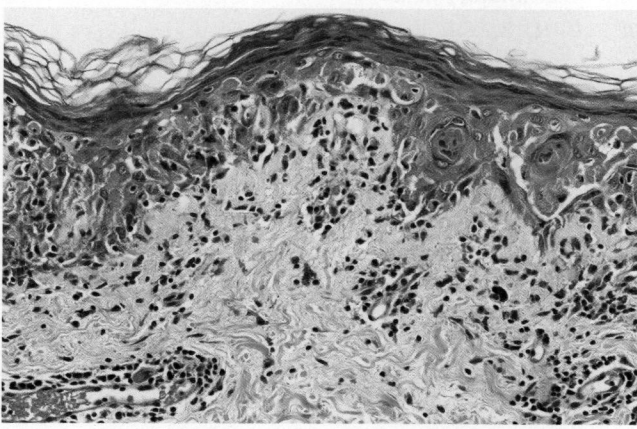

1. Apoptotic Cells Prominent (Cytotoxic Dermatitis)
erythema multiforme

2. Apoptotic Cells Usually Absent
dermatomyositis

3. Variable Apoptosis
cytotoxic drug eruptions

4. Basement Membranes Thickened
lupus erythematosus

IV. ACANTHOLYTIC, VESICULAR, AND PUSTULAR DISORDERS

A. Subcorneal or Intracorneal Separation

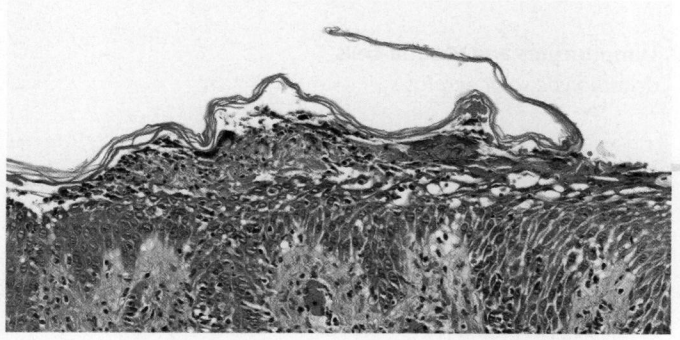

1. Scant Inflammatory Cells
staphylococcal scalded skin

2. Neutrophils Prominent
impetigo contagiosa

3. Eosinophils Predominant
erythema toxicum neonatorum

B. Intraspinous Keratinocyte Separation, Spongiotic

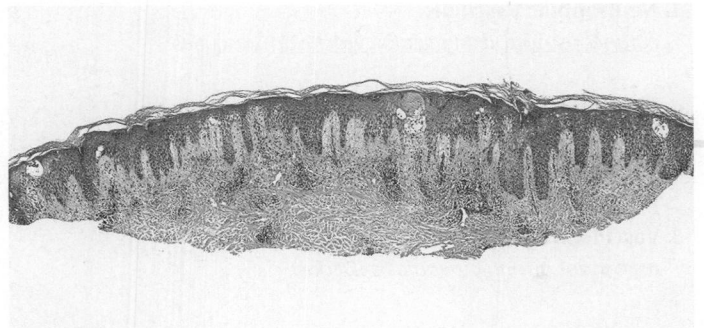

1. Scant Inflammatory Cells
focal acantholytic dyskeratosis

2. Lymphocytes Predominant
nummular eczema
2a. Eosinophils Present
    allergic contact dermatitis

3. Neutrophils Predominant
pustular psoriasis

C. Intraspinous Keratinocyte Separation, Acantholytic

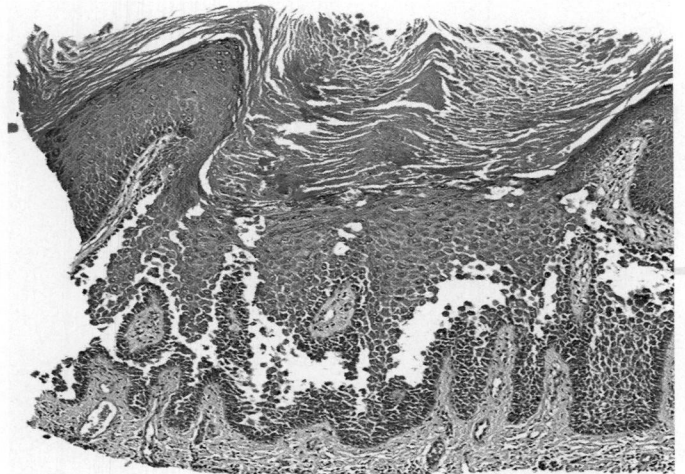

1. Scant Inflammatory Cells
Hailey–Hailey disease

2. Predominant Lymphocytes
herpes simplex, varicella-zoster
2a. Eosinophils Present
    pemphigus vegetans

3. Mixed Cell Types
acantholytic solar keratosis

D. Suprabasal Keratinocyte Separation

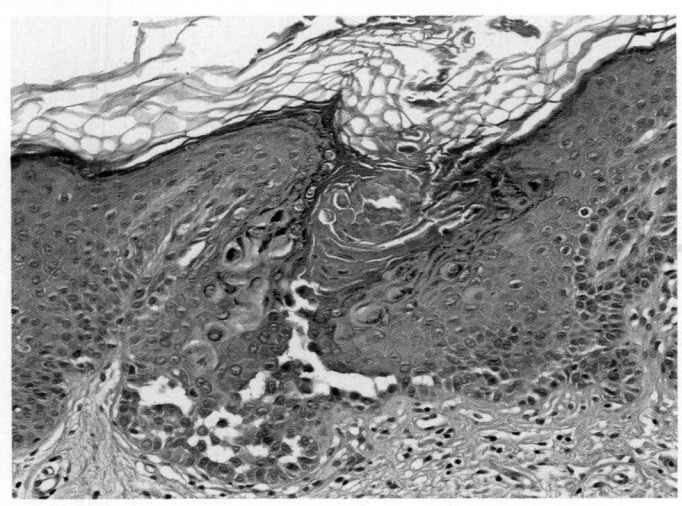

1. Scant Inflammatory Cells
focal acantholytic keratosis (Darier-like)

2. Lymphocytes and Plasma Cells
acantholytic solar keratosis

3. Lymphocytes and Eosinophils
pemphigus vulgaris

E. Subepidermal Vesicular Dermatitis

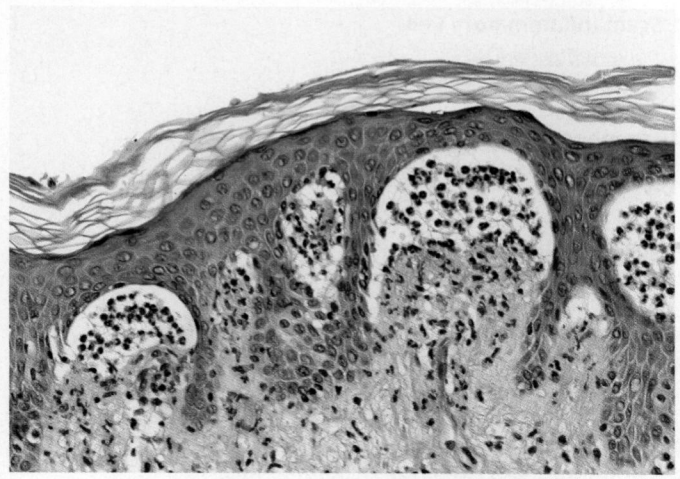

1. Scant/No Inflammation
porphyria cutanea tarda

2. Lymphocytes Predominant
bullous lichen planus

3. Eosinophils Prominent
bullous pemphigoid

4. Neutrophils Prominent
dermatitis herpetiformis

5. Mast Cells Prominent
bullous mastocytosis

V. PERIVASCULAR, DIFFUSE, AND GRANULOMATOUS INFILTRATES OF THE RETICULAR DERMIS

A. Superficial and Deep Perivascular Infiltrates without Vascular Damage or Vasculitis

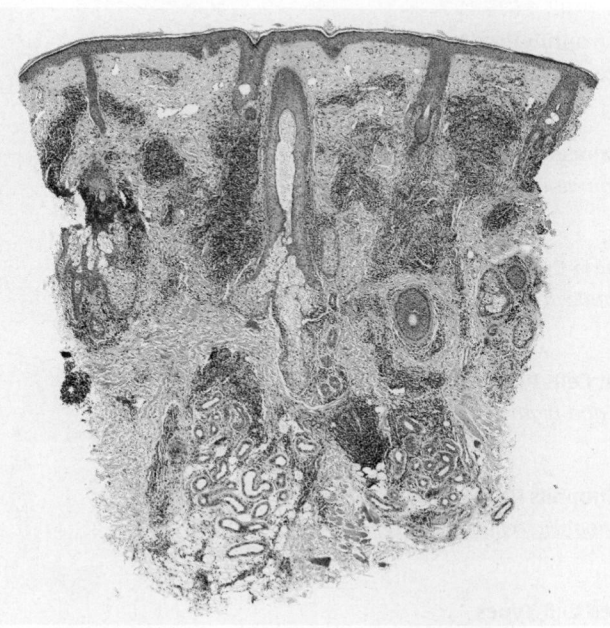

1. Lymphocytes Predominant
tumid lupus erythematosus

2. Neutrophils Predominant
acute febrile neutrophilic dermatosis (Sweet)

3. Lymphocytes and Eosinophils
papular urticaria

4. With Plasma Cells
scleroderma/morphea

5. Mixed Cell Types
erythema chronicum migrans

B. Vasculitis and Vasculopathies

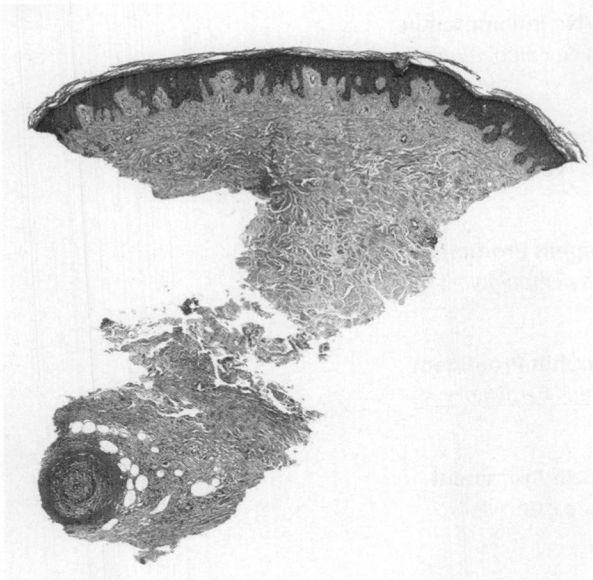

1. Scant Inflammatory Cells
polyarteritis nodosa

2. Lymphocytes Predominant
"lymphocytic vasculitis"

3. Neutrophils Prominent
leukocytoclastic vasculitis

4. Mixed Cell Types and/or Granulomas
allergic granulomatosis (Churg–Strauss)

5. Thrombotic and Other Microangiopathies
disseminated intravascular coagulation

C. Diffuse Infiltrates of the Reticular Dermis

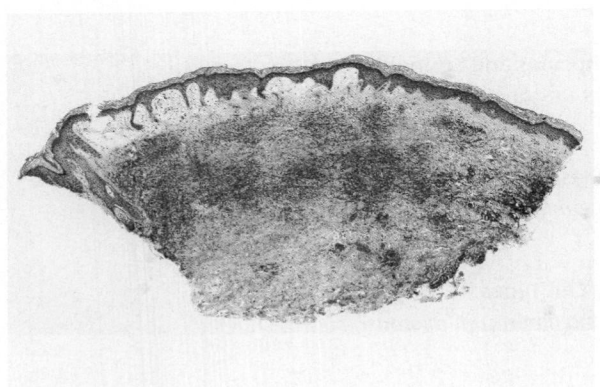

1. Lymphocytes Predominant
cutaneous lymphoid hyperplasia/lymphocytoma cutis

2. Neutrophils Predominant
acute neutrophilic dermatosis (Sweet)

3. "Histiocytoid" Cells Predominant
lepromatous leprosy

4. Plasma Cells Prominent
plasmacytoma, myeloma

5. Mast Cells Predominant
urticaria pigmentosa

6. Eosinophils Predominant
eosinophilic cellulitis (Wells syndrome)

7. Mixed Cell Types
syphilis, primary, secondary, or tertiary

8. Pigment Cells
nevus of Ota, nevus of Ito

9. Extensive Necrosis
calciphylaxis

D. Diffuse or Nodular Infiltrates of the Reticular Dermis with Epidermal Proliferation

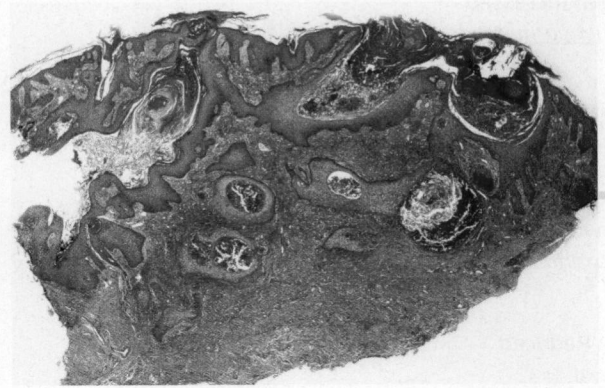

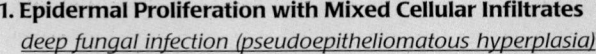

1. Epidermal Proliferation with Mixed Cellular Infiltrates
deep fungal infection (pseudoepitheliomatous hyperplasia)

E. Nodular Inflammatory Infiltrates of the Reticular Dermis—Granulomas, Abscesses, and Ulcers

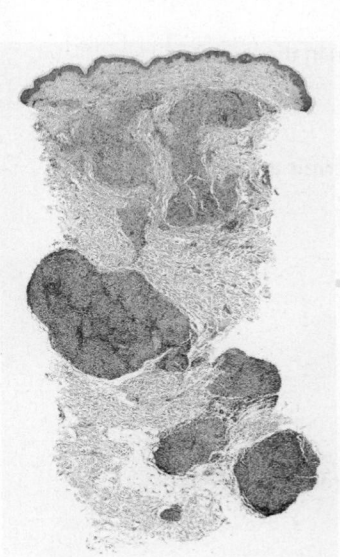

1. Epithelioid Cell Granulomas without Necrosis
sarcoidosis (lupus pernio and other types)

2. Epithelioid Cell Granulomas with Necrosis
tuberculosis (lupus vulgaris and other types)

3. Palisading Granulomas
granuloma annulare

4. Mixed Cell Granulomas
keratin granuloma (ruptured cyst)

5. Inflammatory Nodules with Prominent Eosinophils
angiolymphoid hyperplasia with eosinophils

6. Inflammatory Nodules with Mixed Cell Types
sporotrichosis

7. Abscesses
acute or chronic bacterial abscesses

8. Inflammatory Nodules with Prominent Necrosis
aspergillosis

9. Chronic Ulcers and Sinuses
pyoderma gangrenosum

F. Dermal Matrix Fiber Disorders

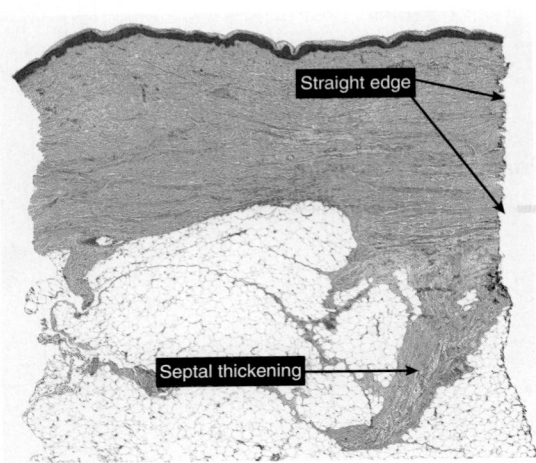

1. Collagen Increased
scleroderma/morphea

2. Collagen Reduced
scleroderma/morphea

3. Elastin Increased or Prominent
pseudoxanthoma elasticum

4. Elastin Reduced
cutis laxa

5. Perforating
elastosis perforans serpiginosa

G. Deposition of Material in the Dermis

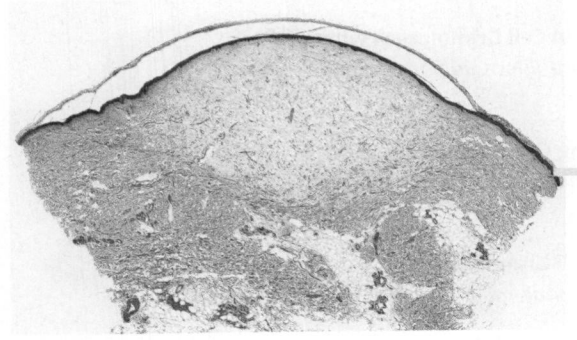

1. Increased Normal Matrix Constituents
focal dermal mucinosis

2. Material Not Normally Present in the Dermis
gout

3. Parasitic Infestations of the Dermis and/or Subcutis
myiasis

VI. TUMORS AND CYSTS OF THE DERMIS AND SUBCUTIS

A. Small Cell Tumors

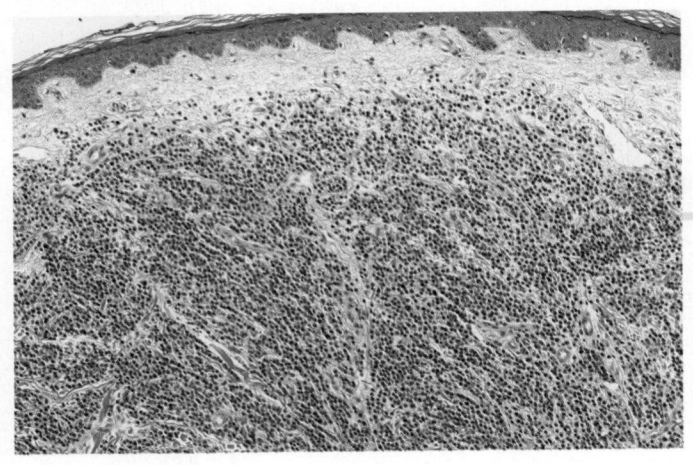

1. Tumors of Lymphocytes or Hemopoietic Cells
tumor-stage mycosis fungoides

2. Tumors of Lymphocytes and Mixed Cell Types
cutaneous lymphoid hyperplasia/lymphocytoma cutis

3. Tumors of Plasma Cells
cutaneous plasmacytoma

4. Small Round Cell Tumors
eccrine spiradenoma

B. Large Polygonal and Round Cell Tumors

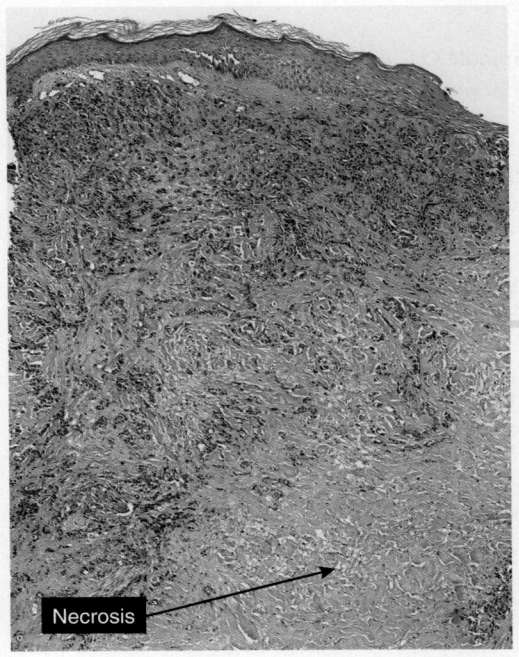

Necrosis

1. Squamous Cell Carcinomas
primary squamous cell carcinoma

2. Adenocarcinomas
metastatic mammary adenocarcinoma (as in the previous edition)

3. Melanocytic Tumors
metastatic melanoma

4. Eccrine Tumors
nodular hidradenoma (eccrine acrospiroma)

5. Apocrine Tumors
hidradenoma papilliferum

6. Pilar Tumors
trichoepithelioma

7. Sebaceous Tumors
sebaceous adenoma and epithelioma

8. "Histiocytoid" Tumors
xanthomas—eruptive, plane, tuberous, tendon

9. Tumors of Large Lymphoid Cells
cutaneous anaplastic large cell lymphoma

10. Mast Cell Tumors
mastocytosis

11. Tumors with Prominent Necrosis
epithelioid sarcoma

12. Miscellaneous and Undifferentiated Epithelial Tumors
undifferentiated carcinoma (large cell, small cell)

C. Spindle Cell, Pleomorphic, and Connective Tissue Tumors

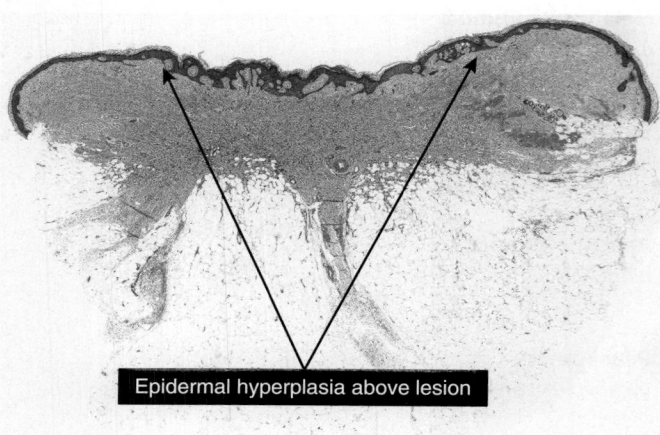

Epidermal hyperplasia above lesion

1. Fibrohistiocytic Spindle Cell Tumors
benign fibrous histiocytoma (dermatofibroma)

2. Schwannian/Neural Spindle Cell Tumors
neurofibromas

3. Spindle Cell Tumors of Muscle
leiomyoma

4. Melanocytic Spindle Cell Tumors
desmoplastic melanoma, including amelanotic

5. Tumors and Proliferations of Angiogenic Cells
pyogenic granuloma

6. Tumors of Adipose Tissue
nevus lipomatosus superficialis

7. Tumors of Cartilaginous Tissue
soft tissue chondroma

8. Tumors of Osseous Tissue
osteoma cutis

D. Cysts of the Dermis and Subcutis

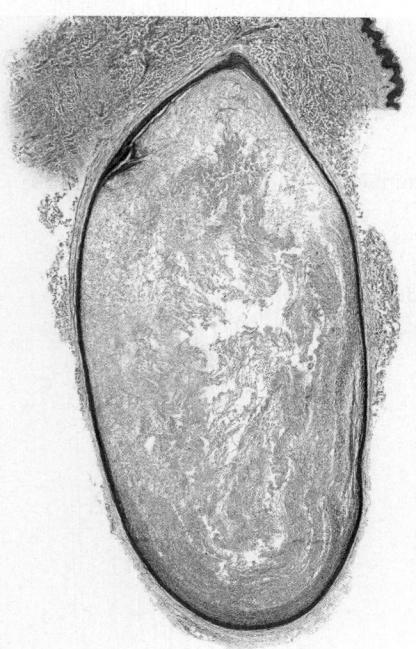

1. Pilar Differentiation
epidermal cyst

2. Eccrine and Similar Differentiation
eccrine hidrocystoma

3. Apocrine Differentiation
apocrine hidrocystoma

VII. INFLAMMATORY DISORDERS OF SKIN APPENDAGES

A. Pathology Involving Hair Follicles

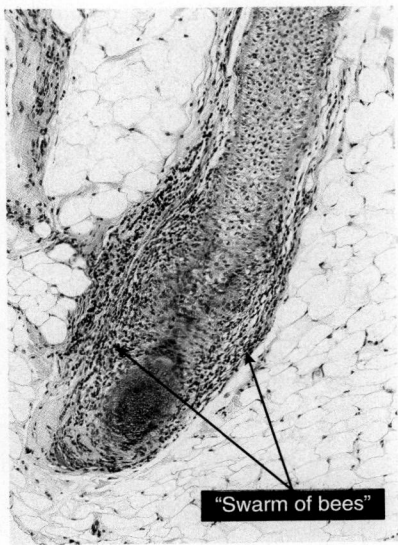

"Swarm of bees"

1. Scant Inflammation
androgenic alopecia

2. Lymphocytes Predominant
<u>*alopecia areata*</u>
2a. With Eosinophils Present
eosinophilic pustular folliculitis

3. Neutrophils Prominent
acute bacterial folliculitis

4. Plasma Cells Prominent
acne keloidalis

5. Fibrosing and Suppurative Follicular Disorders
hidradenitis suppurativa

B. Pathology Involving Sweat Glands

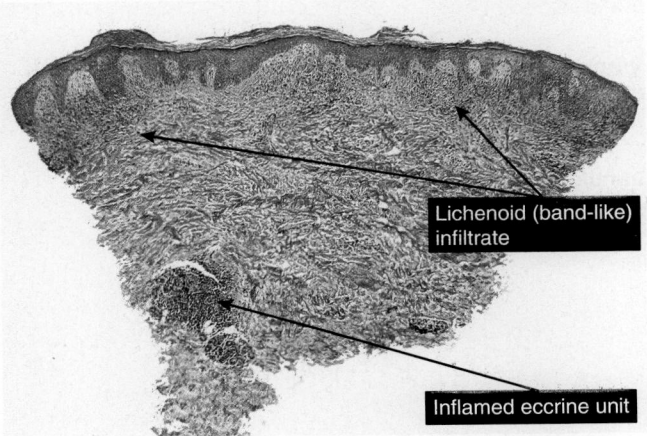

Lichenoid (band-like) infiltrate

Inflamed eccrine unit

1. Scant Inflammation
eccrine nevus

2. Lymphocytes Predominant
<u>*lichen striatus*</u>
2a. With Plasma Cells
cheilitis glandularis
2b. With Eosinophils
insect bite reactions
2c. With Neutrophils
neutrophilic eccrine hidradenitis

C. Pathology Involving Nerves

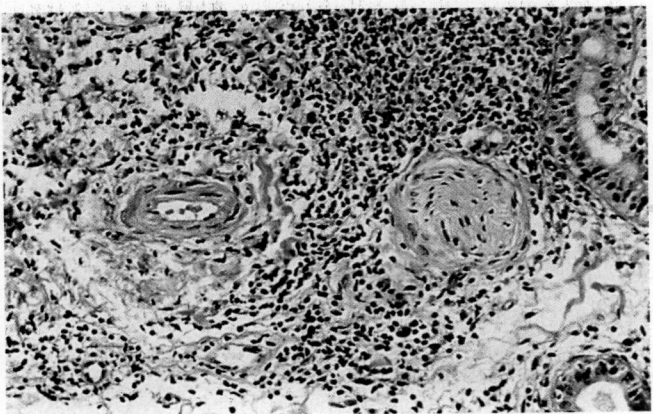

1. Lymphocytic Infiltrates
neurotropic melanoma

2. Mixed Inflammatory Infiltrates
<u>*leprosy*</u>

3. Neoplastic Infiltrates
neurotropic melanoma

D. Pathology of the Nails

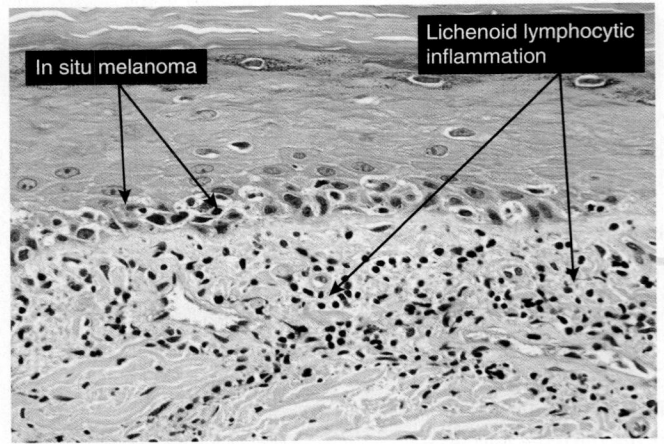

In situ melanoma

Lichenoid lymphocytic inflammation

1. Lymphocytic Infiltrates
melanoma in situ, acral-lentiginous type

2. Lymphocytes with Neutrophils
tinea unguium, onychomycosis

3. Bullous Diseases
Darier disease

4. Parasitic Infestations
scabies

VIII. DISORDERS OF THE SUBCUTIS

A. Subcutaneous Vasculitis and Vasculopathy (Septal or Lobular)

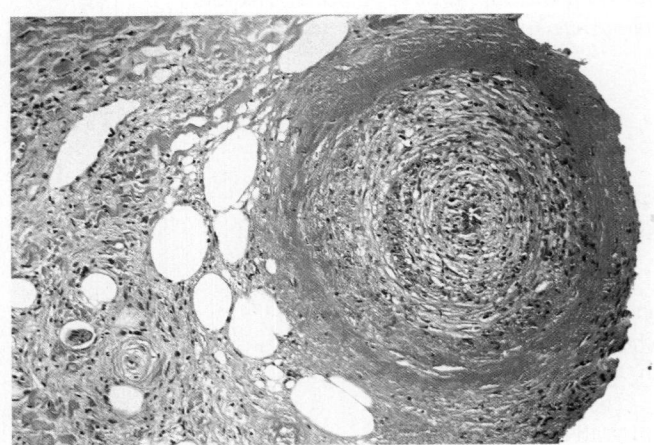

1. Neutrophilic
subcutaneous polyarteritis nodosa

2. Lymphocytic
nodular vasculitis

3. Granulomatous
eosinophilic granulomatosis with polyangiitis

B. Septal Panniculitis without Vasculitis

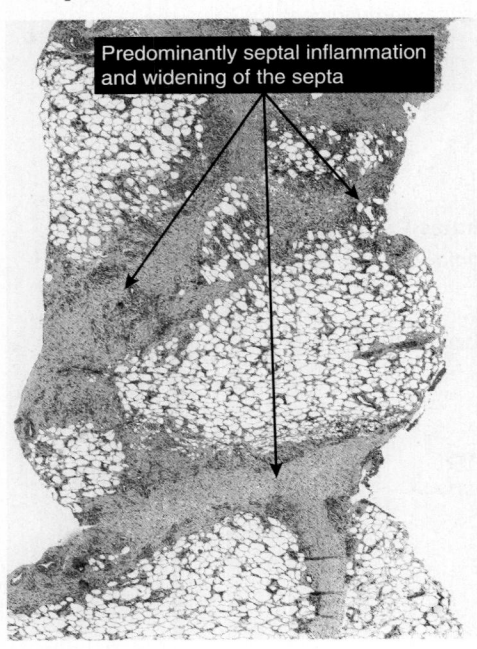

Predominantly septal inflammation and widening of the septa

1. Lymphocytes and Mixed Infiltrates
erythema nodosum and variants

2. Granulomatous
subcutaneous granuloma annulare

3. Sclerotic
scleroderma, morphea

C. Lobular Panniculitis without Vasculitis

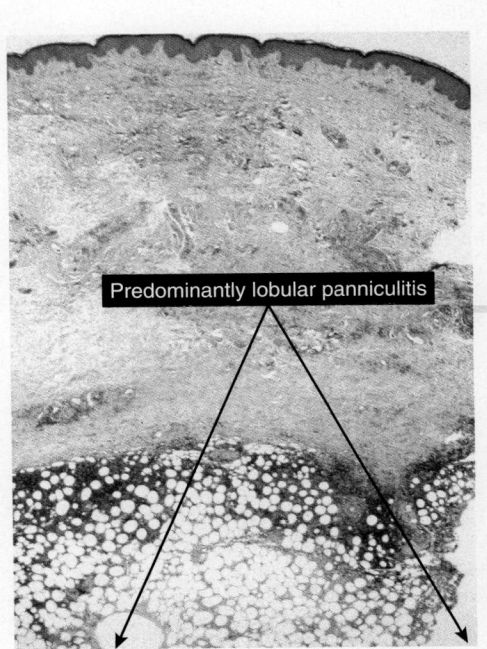

Predominantly lobular panniculitis

1. Lymphocytes Predominant
lupus panniculitis

2. Lymphocytes and Plasma Cells
scleroderma

3. Neutrophilic
infection (cellulitis)

4. Eosinophils Prominent
eosinophilic fasciitis

5. Histiocytes Prominent
cytophagic histiocytic panniculitis

6. Mixed with Foam Cells
Weber–Christian disease

7. Granulomatous
subcutaneous sarcoidosis

8. Crystal Deposits, Calcifications
sclerema neonatorum

9. Necrosis Prominent
pancreatic panniculitis

10. Embryonic Fat Pattern
lipoatrophy

11. Miscellaneous
lipomembranous panniculitis

D. Mixed Lobular and Septal Panniculitis

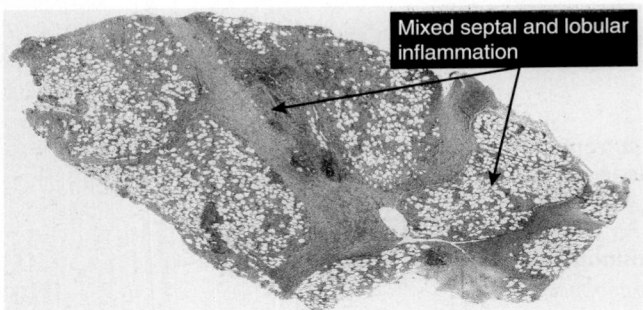

Mixed septal and lobular inflammation

1. With Hemorrhage or Sclerosis
traumatic panniculitis

2. With Many Neutrophils
necrotizing fasciitis (bacterial infection)

3. With Many Lymphocytes
nonspecific panniculitis

4. With Cytophagic Histiocytes
histiocytic cytophagic panniculitis (late lesion)

5. With Granulomas
mycobacterial panniculitis

E. Subcutaneous Abscesses

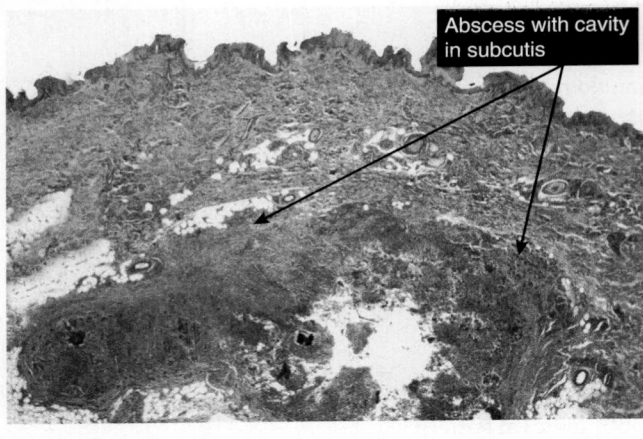

Abscess with cavity in subcutis

1. With Neutrophils
<u>*deep fungal infection*</u>
(Image Courtesy Waine Johnson, MD)

PART 3. DISEASE LISTINGS CATEGORIZED BY SITE, PATTERN, AND CYTOLOGY

In this section, the cutaneous diseases are listed in categories based on their location in the skin, their architectural patterns, and their cytology. One or more prototypic conditions are underlined in each category. The listings may be used as a basis for differential diagnosis generation and for review of material covered elsewhere in this text.

I. DISORDERS MOSTLY LIMITED TO THE EPIDERMIS AND STRATUM CORNEUM†

The stratum corneum is usually arranged in a delicate mesh-like or "basket-weave" pattern. It may be shed (exfoliated) or thickened (hyperkeratosis) with or without retention of nuclei (parakeratosis or orthokeratosis, respectively). The granular layer may be normal, increased (hypergranulosis), or reduced (hypogranulosis). Usually, alterations in the stratum corneum result from inflammatory or neoplastic changes that affect the entire epidermis and, more often than not, the superficial dermis. Only a few conditions, mentioned in this section, show pathology mostly or entirely limited to the stratum corneum.

A. Hyperkeratosis with Hypogranulosis..............91

1. No Inflammation 91

B. Hyperkeratosis with Normal or Hypergranulosis...................................91

The stratum corneum is thickened, the granular cell layer is normal or thickened, and the dermis shows only sparse perivascular lymphocytes. There is no epidermal spongiosis or exocytosis.

1. No Inflammation 91
The upper dermis contains only sparse perivascular lymphocytes.

†In the lists that follow, the term "predominant" is used to describe an infiltrate in which the majority of the cells are of a certain type, usually lymphocytes or neutrophils. Many dermatoses are composed of infiltrates that are predominantly lymphocytic, with only an occasional other cell type; these are listed as, for example, "1. lymphocytes predominant." Many other dermatoses contain a diagnostically significant admixture of other cell type(s) as a minority population; these are listed in subsequent sections as "1a. with eosinophils," "1b. with plasma cells," etc., it being understood that lymphocytes predominate in these dermatoses also. Infiltrates in which there is an approximately equal admixture of multiple cell types are listed as "mixed" infiltrates.

2. Scant Inflammation 91
Lymphocytes are minimally increased about the superficial plexus. There may be a few neutrophils in the stratum corneum.

C. Hyperkeratosis with Parakeratosis 91

The stratum corneum is thickened, the granular cell layer is reduced, and there is parakeratosis. The dermis may show only sparse perivascular lymphocytes, although some of these conditions in other instances may show more substantial inflammation. There is no epidermal spongiosis or exocytosis.

1. Scant or No Inflammation 91
The upper dermis contains only sparse perivascular lymphocytes.

2. Scant Inflammation 91
Lymphocytes are minimally increased about the superficial plexus. There may be a few lymphocytes and/or neutrophils in the stratum corneum.

3. With Epidermal Pallor or Necrosis ("Nutritional Dermatosis") 91
There may be psoriasiform epidermal hyperplasia, and there is hyperkeratosis with parakeratosis and with pallor, swelling, or necrosis of superficial keratinocytes.

D. Localized or Diffuse Hyperpigmentations 92

Increased melanin pigment is present in keratinocytes or in the superficial dermis, without melanocytic proliferation.

1. No Inflammation 92

The upper dermis contains only sparse perivascular lymphocytes.

2. Scant Inflammation. 92

Lymphocytes are minimally increased about the superficial plexus. There may be a few lymphocytes and/or neutrophils in the stratum corneum. Melanophages may be present in the papillary dermis.

E. Localized or Diffuse Hypopigmentations 92

Melanin pigment is reduced in basal keratinocytes with (vitiligo) or without (early stages of chemical depigmentation) a reduction in the number of melanocytes.

1. With or without Slight Inflammation 92

Lymphocytes may be minimally increased about the dermal–epidermal junction, as in the active phase of vitiligo, or may be absent, as in albinism.

II. LOCALIZED SUPERFICIAL EPIDERMAL OR MELANOCYTIC PROLIFERATIONS

Localized proliferations may be reactive but are often neoplastic. The epidermis (keratinocytes) may proliferate without extension into the dermis, extend into the dermis, and may be squamous or basaloid. Melanocytes within the epidermis may proliferate with or without cytologic atypia (nevi, dysplastic nevi, melanoma *in situ*) in a proliferative epidermis (superficial spreading melanoma *in situ*, Spitz nevi) or an atrophic epidermis (lentigo maligna); they can also extend into the dermis as proliferative infiltrates (invasive melanoma with or without vertical growth phase). There may be an associated variably cellular often mixed inflammatory infiltrate, or inflammation may be essentially absent.

A. Localized Irregular Thickening of The Epidermis 92

Localized irregular epidermal proliferations are usually neoplastic.

1. Localized Epidermal Proliferations 92

The epidermis is thickened secondary to a localized proliferation of keratinocytes (acanthosis). The proliferation can be cytologically atypical, as in squamous cell carcinoma *in situ*, or bland, as in eccrine poroma.

1a. No Cytologic Atypia 90

1b. With Cytologic Atypia 90

1c. Pseudoepitheliomatous Hyperplasia. 29-988

2. Superficial Melanocytic Proliferations. 92

The epidermis may be thickened (acanthosis) and is associated with a proliferation of single or nested melanocytic cells. The proliferation can be malignant as in superficial spreading melanoma or benign as in nevi.

B. Localized Lesions with Thinning of the Epidermis. 93

A thinned epidermis is characteristic of aged or chronically sun-damaged skin. The epidermis is thinned secondary to diminished number and to decreased size of keratinocytes.

1. With Melanocytic Proliferation. 93

The epidermis is thinned (atrophic), and there is proliferation of single or small groups of atypical melanocytes, resulting in the localization of melanocytes in contiguity with one another, in the basal layer of the epidermis.

2. Without Melanocytic Proliferation **93**

The epidermis is thinned without proliferation of keratinocytes or melanocytes. Each melanocyte is separated from the next by several keratinocytes.

C. Localized Lesions with Elongated Rete Ridges **93**

Elongation of the rete ridges without melanocytic proliferation is termed "psoriasiform hyperplasia" because this pattern is seen in psoriasis. Elongated rete may accompany a proliferation of melanocytes within the basal layer as single cells over nests, termed a "lentiginous" pattern. The prototype of this pattern, also seen in a more exaggerated form in dysplastic nevi and in the "lentiginous" melanomas, is the lentigo simplex.

1. With Melanocytic Proliferation...........................**93**

The epidermal rete ridges are elongated and within these there is melanocytic proliferation.

2. Without Melanocytic Proliferation **93**

The epidermis is thickened (acanthotic). Melanocytes are normal as are keratinocytes. The only change is acanthosis.

D. Localized Lesions with Pagetoid Epithelial Proliferation...**93**

A neoplastic proliferation of one cell type distributed as single cells or nests within a benign epithelium is termed "Pagetoid" after Paget disease of the breast (mammary carcinoma cells proliferating in skin of the nipple).

1. Keratinocytic Proliferation **93**

The epidermis has atypical keratinocytes scattered within mature epithelium at all or multiple levels; there is loss of normal maturation. Mitoses are increased, and there may be individual cell necrosis.

2. Melanocytic Proliferation...**93**

Atypical melanocytes are seen at all levels within the otherwise mature but often hyperplastic epidermis.

3. Glandular Epithelial Proliferations **93**

Atypical large clear cells with glandular differentiation (mucin production, occasionally lumen formation) proliferate in a normally maturing epidermis.

4. Lymphoid Proliferations.......................................**93**

Atypical large clear lymphoid cells proliferate in a normally maturing epidermis.

E. Localized Papillomatous Epithelial Lesions......... **94**

A "papilla" may be likened to a "finger" of stroma with a few blood vessels, collagen fibers, and fibroblasts, covered by a "glove" of epithelium, which may be reactive or neoplastic, benign or malignant.

1. With Viral Cytopathic Effects **94**

The epidermis is acanthotic with vacuolated cells often having enlarged and somewhat irregular nuclei (koilocytes), the granular cell layer is usually thickened with enlarged, often rounded keratohyalin granules, and there is parakeratosis in tall columns overlying the thickened epidermis at the tops of the papillae. Large cytoplasmic inclusions are seen in molluscum contagiosum.

2. No Viral Cytopathic Effect.....................................**94**

The epidermis proliferates. The cells may be basophilic or "basaloid" in type (seborrheic keratoses). There may be increased stratum corneum and elongation of the dermal papillae (squamous papilloma), or there may be basilar keratinocyte atypia (actinic keratosis).

F. Irregular Proliferations Extending into the Dermis...................................... **94**

Irregular or asymmetrical proliferations of keratinocytes extending into the dermis are usually neoplastic. The differential diagnosis includes reactive pseudoepitheliomatous hyperplasia, which may be seen around chronic ulcers or in association with other inflammatory conditions.

The epidermis is irregularly thickened, the maturation is abnormal, and there may be keratinocyte atypia (squamous cell carcinoma). The proliferation is often associated with a thick parakeratotic scale.

The proliferation is of basal cells from the epidermis, extending into the dermis. The epidermis can be thickened, normal, or atrophic.

A polyp is any lesion that protrudes from a surface. Although a papilloma consists of elongated papillae representing a "finger" of stroma covered by a "glove" of epithelium, a polyp is more like a hand within which the papillae ("fingers") may be elongated or, more usually, normal or attenuated. Thus, polypoid lesions may or may not also be papillomatous. Many of the neoplasms listed in Section VI may also present as polypoid neoplasms.

III. DISORDERS OF THE SUPERFICIAL CUTANEOUS REACTIVE UNIT

The epidermis, papillary dermis, and superficial capillary–venular plexus react together in many dermatologic conditions and have been termed the *superficial cutaneous reactive unit* by Clark. Many dermatoses are associated with infiltrates of lymphocytes with or without other cell types, around the superficial vessels.

The epidermis in pathologic conditions can be thinned (atrophic), thickened (acanthosis), edematous (spongiosis), and/or infiltrated (exocytosis). The epidermis may proliferate in response to chronic irritation and infection (bacterial, yeast, deep fungal, or viral). The epidermis may proliferate in response to dermatologic conditions (psoriasis, atopic dermatitis, prurigo). The papillary dermis and superficial vascular plexus may have a variety of inflammatory cells, can be edematous, may have increased ground substance (hyaluronic acid), and may be sclerotic or homogenized.

Many dermatoses are associated with infiltrates of lymphocytes with or without other cell types, around the vessels of the superficial capillary–venular plexus. The vessel walls may be quite unremarkable, or there may be slight-to-moderate endothelial prominence. Eosinophilic change ("fibrinoid necrosis"), a hallmark of true vasculitis, is not seen. The term "lymphocytic vasculitis" may encompass some of the conditions mentioned here, but is of doubtful validity in the absence of vessel wall damage. The epidermis is variable in its thickness, amount and type of exocytotic cells, and in the integrity of the basal cell zone (liquefaction degeneration). In some of the entities listed here, the perivascular infiltrate may in some examples also involve vessels of the mid and deep dermis. These conditions are also listed in Section V: Perivascular, Diffuse and Granulomatous Infiltrates of the Reticular Dermis.

Lymphocytes are seen about the superficial vascular plexus. Other cell types are rare or absent.

In addition to lymphocytes, eosinophils are present in varying numbers, with both a perivascular and interstitial distribution.

1b. Superficial Perivascular Dermatitis with Neutrophils 95

In addition to lymphocytes, neutrophils are present in varying numbers, with both a perivascular and interstitial distribution.

1c. Superficial Perivascular Dermatitis with Plasma Cells 95

Plasma cells are seen about the dermal vessels as well as in the interstitium. They are most often admixed with lymphocytes.

1d. Superficial Perivascular Dermatitis, with Extravasated Red Cells 95

A perivascular lymphocytic infiltrate is associated with extravasation of erythrocytes, without fibrinoid necrosis of vessels.

1e. Superficial Perivascular Dermatitis, Pigmented Histiocytes Prominent 95

There is a perivascular infiltrate of lymphocytes, with an admixture of pigment-laden melanophages, indicative of prior damage to the basal layer and "pigmentary incontinence." Some degree of residual interface damage may also be evident.

2. Superficial Perivascular Dermatitis, Mast Cells Predominant 95

Mast cells are the main infiltrating cells seen in the dermis. Lymphocytes are also present, and there may be a few eosinophils.

B. Superficial Dermatitis with Spongiosis (Spongiotic Dermatitis) 95

Spongiotic dermatitis is characterized by intercellular edema in the epidermis. In mild or early lesions, the intercellular space is increased with stretching of desmosomes, but the integrity of the epithelium is intact. In more severe spongiotic conditions, there is separation of keratinocytes to form spaces (vesicles). For this reason, the spongiotic dermatoses are also discussed later in Section IV: Acantholytic, Vesicular, and Pustular Disorders.

1. Spongiotic Dermatitis, Lymphocytes Predominant 95

There is marked intercellular edema (spongiosis) within the epidermis. In the dermis, perivascular lymphocytes are predominant.

1a. Spongiotic Dermatitis, with Eosinophils 95

There is marked intercellular edema (spongiosis) within the epidermis. In the dermis, lymphocytes are predominant. Eosinophils can be found in most examples of atopy and allergic contact dermatitis and are numerous in incontinentia pigmenti.

1b. Spongiotic Dermatitis with Plasma Cells 95

There is marked intercellular edema (spongiosis) within the epidermis. In the dermis, perivascular lymphocytes are predominant, and plasma cells are present.

1c. Spongiotic Dermatitis with Neutrophils 95

There is marked intercellular edema (spongiosis) within the epidermis. Lymphocytes are present in the dermis. There is focal and shoulder parakeratosis, with a few neutrophils in the stratum corneum.

C. Superficial Dermatitis with Epidermal Atrophy (Atrophic Dermatitis) 95

Most inflammatory dermatoses are associated with epithelial hyperplasia. Only a few chronic conditions exhibit epidermal atrophy.

1. Epidermal Atrophy, Scant Inflammatory Infiltrates........... 95

The epidermis is thinned, only a few cell layers thick. There is a scanty lymphocytic infiltrate about the superficial capillary–venular plexus.

2. Epidermal Atrophy, Lymphocytes Predominant.............. 95

The epidermis is thinned, but not as marked as in aged or irradiated skin. In the dermis, there are many lymphocytes about the superficial capillary–venular plexus.

2a. Epidermal Atrophy with Papillary Dermal Sclerosis/Matrix Changes 95

The epidermis is thinned, and there can be hyperkeratosis. The dermis is homogenized and edematous; inflammation is minimal.

D. Superficial Dermatitis with Psoriasiform Proliferation (Psoriasiform Dermatitis) 96

Psoriasiform proliferation is a form of epithelial hyperplasia characterized by uniform elongation of rete ridges. Although the surface may be slightly raised to form a plaque, the epidermal proliferation tends to extend downward into the dermis, in contrast to a papillomatous pattern in which the dermal papillae and overlying epidermis are elongated upward above the plane of the epidermal surface and a papilloma (such as a wart) is formed. The prototype of psoriasiform proliferation is psoriasis, in which the suprapapillary plates are thinned. In most other psoriasiform conditions, the suprapapillary plates are thickened, but not as much as the elongated rete. Because of the increased epithelial turnover, there is often associated hypogranulosis and parakeratosis.

1. Psoriasiform Epidermal Proliferation, Lymphocytes Predominant... 96

The epidermis is evenly and regularly thickened in a psoriasiform pattern, and spongiosis is variable (rare to absent in psoriasis, common in seborrheic and inflammatory dermatoses). There is an infiltrate of lymphocytes about dermal vessels.

1b. Psoriasiform Epidermal Proliferation, with Plasma Cells....... 96

The epidermis is evenly thickened and may be spongiotic. There may be exocytosis of lymphocytes. The stratum corneum is variable, often parakeratotic. Plasma cells are found about the superficial vessels in varying numbers, admixed with lymphocytes.

1c. Psoriasiform Epidermal Proliferation, with Eosinophils....... 96

The epidermis is evenly thickened and may be spongiotic, and there may be exocytosis of inflammatory cells, including eosinophils. Eosinophils are easily identified in the dermis and may be numerous in some conditions (e.g., incontinentia pigmenti).

2. Psoriasiform Epidermal Proliferation, Neutrophils Prominent (Neutrophilic/Pustular Psoriasiform Dermatitis) 96

The epidermis is evenly thickened, and there is exocytosis (migration of inflammatory cells through the epidermis) of neutrophils. These may collect into abscesses in the epidermis at the level of the stratum corneum (Munro microabscess). The stratum corneum is thickened, parakeratotic, and contains neutrophils.

3. Psoriasiform Epidermal Proliferation, with Epidermal Pallor or Necrosis ("Nutritional Dermatosis") 96

There may be psoriasiform epidermal hyperplasia, and there is hyperkeratosis with parakeratosis and with pallor, swelling, or necrosis of superficial keratinocytes.

E. Superficial Dermatitis with Irregular Epidermal Proliferation (Hypertrophic Dermatitis) 96

Irregular thickening and thinning of the epidermis is seen in some reactive conditions, but the possibility of squamous cell carcinoma should also be considered. As in other conditions associated with increased epithelial turnover, there may be hypogranulosis and parakeratosis.

1. Irregular Epidermal Proliferation, Lymphocytes Predominant 96

The epidermis is irregularly thickened, with areas of normal thickness, acanthosis, and thinning. Lymphocytes are the predominant inflammatory cell in the dermal vessels.

1a. Irregular Epidermal Proliferation, Plasma Cells Present 96

The epidermis is irregularly acanthotic. Plasma cells are found about the dermal vessels admixed with lymphocytes.

2. Irregular Epidermal Proliferation, Neutrophils Prominent 96

The epidermis has focal areas of acanthosis, neutrophils can be seen as exocytotic cells, and are found in the dermis in abscesses and about dermal vessels without there being a primary vasculitis.

3. Irregular Epidermal Proliferation, above a Neoplasm 96

The epidermis is irregularly acanthotic. There is an associated neoplastic infiltrate, in the epidermis or dermis, or in both.

F. Superficial Dermatitis with Lichenoid Infiltrates (Lichenoid Dermatitis) 96

Lichenoid inflammation is a dense "bandlike" infiltrate of small lymphocytes clustered about the dermal–epidermal junction and obscuring the interface. The epidermis is variable in its thickness, amount of exocytotic lymphocytes, and the integrity of the basal cell zone (liquefaction degeneration). Hypergranulosis owing to delayed epidermal maturation is a commonly associated feature. For the same reason, there may be orthokeratotic hyperkeratosis. Apoptotic or necrotic keratinocytes are often present. In lichen planus, these are called Civatte bodies. Pigmentary incontinence (melanin-laden macrophages in the papillary dermis) is common, as in any condition in which there is destruction of basal keratinocytes.

1. Lichenoid Dermatitis, Lymphocytes Exclusively 96

The bandlike infiltrate is composed almost exclusively of lymphocytes. Eosinophils and plasma cells are essentially absent.

2. Lichenoid Dermatitis, Lymphocytes Predominant 96

The bandlike lichenoid infiltrate is composed almost exclusively of lymphocytes. A few plasma cells and eosinophils may also be present.

2a. Lichenoid Dermatitis, Eosinophils Present 96

Eosinophils are found in the lichenoid dermal infiltrate, about the dermal vessels and in some instances around the adnexal structures.

2b. Lichenoid Dermatitis, Plasma Cells Present **96**

Plasma cells are found in the lichenoid infiltrate; their number is variable, but they do not as a rule comprise the major portion of the dermal infiltrate.

2c. Lichenoid Dermatitis, with Melanophages **96**

Most of the conditions listed as lichenoid dermatoses may be associated with the release of pigment from damaged basal keratinocytes into the papillary dermis "pigmentary incontinence." If a specific dermatosis cannot be identified, the appearances may be classified as postinflammatory hyperpigmentation.

3. Lichenoid Dermatitis, Histiocytes Prominent **96**

Histiocytes are the predominant or a prominent cell type in the dermal infiltrate.

4. Lichenoid Dermatitis, Mast Cells Predominant **96**

5. Lichenoid Dermatitis with Dermal Fibroplasia **96**

G. Superficial Vasculitis and Vasculopathies

Endothelial swelling, eosinophilic degeneration of the vessel walls ("fibrinoid necrosis"), and infiltration of the vessel wall by neutrophils, with nuclear fragmentation or leukocytoclasia resulting in "nuclear dust," define true vasculitis. There are extravasated red cells in the vessel walls and adjacent dermis. If the vasculitis is severe, secondary luminal thrombi and/or ulceration or subepidermal separation ("bullous vasculitis") can occur. "Lymphocytic vasculitis" in which there is no vessel wall damage is a controversial term and is discussed under lymphocytic infiltrates. A "vasculopathy" includes any abnormality of the vessel wall that does not meet the criteria above for vasculitis, such as fibrosis or hyalinization of the vessel wall without inflammation or necrosis.

1. Neutrophilic Vasculitis **97**

In the dermis, vessels are necrotic, fibrinoid is present, and there are perivascular and intravascular neutrophils with leukocytoclasia and nuclear dust.

2. Mixed Cell and Granulomatous Vasculitis **97**

There is vessel wall damage, and a mixed infiltrate in the dermis that includes eosinophils, plasma cells, histiocytes, and giant cells.

3. Vasculopathies with Lymphocytic Inflammation **97**

4. Vasculopathies with Scant Inflammation **97**

There is fibrosis or hyalinization of the vessel walls, with few inflammatory cells.

5. Thrombotic, Embolic, and Other Microangiopathies **97**

There are thrombi or emboli within the lumens of small vessels. In other microangiopathies, the vessel walls may be thickened with compromise of the lumen (amyloidosis, calciphylaxis).

H. Superficial Dermatitis with Interface Vacuoles (Interface Dermatitis) 97

1. Vacuolar Dermatitis, Apoptotic/Necrotic Cells Prominent. 97

Lymphocytes approximate the dermal–epidermal junction. Vacuolar degeneration is present in the basal cell zone. Apoptotic keratinocytes are found in the epidermis in variable numbers, visualized as round eosinophilic anuclear structures. The dermis usually has perivascular lymphocytes and may show pigment incontinence.

2. Vacuolar Dermatitis, Apoptotic Cells Usually Absent. 97

There is basilar keratinocyte vacuolar destruction; apoptotic cells are rare or absent. The dermis has perivascular lymphocytes and may show pigment incontinence.

3. Vacuolar Dermatitis, Variable Apoptosis 97

Vacuolar degeneration is associated with variable numbers of apoptotic cells in the epidermis. The dermis may have increased ground substance, and there may be pigmentary incontinence.

4. Vacuolar Dermatitis, Basement Membranes Thickened 97

Vacuolar degeneration is associated with variable numbers of apoptotic cells in the epidermis. The basement membrane zone is thickened by deposition of eosinophilic hyaline material.

IV. ACANTHOLYTIC, VESICULAR, AND PUSTULAR DISORDERS

Keratinocytes may separate from each other on the basis of immunologic antigen–antibody mediated damage resulting in separation and rounding-up of keratinocyte cell bodies (acantholysis), on the basis of edema and inflammation (spongiosis), or perhaps on the basis of structural deficiencies of cell adhesion (Darier disease). These processes produce intraepidermal spaces (vesicles, bullae, pustules).

A. Subcorneal or Intracorneal Separation

There is separation within or just below the stratum corneum. Inflammatory cells may be sparse or may consist predominantly of neutrophils.

1. Sub/Intracorneal Separation, Scant Inflammatory Cells 97

There is separation within or just below the stratum corneum, associated with scant inflammation, usually lymphocytic.

2. Sub/Intracorneal Separation, Neutrophils Prominent 97

There is separation in or just below the stratum corneum. Neutrophils are prominent in the stratum corneum and in the superficial epidermis and can often be found in the dermis.

3. Sub/Intracorneal Separation, Eosinophils Predominant 97

There is separation in or just below the stratum corneum, with (pemphigus) or without acantholytic keratinocytes. Eosinophils are present in the epidermis, and occasionally there is eosinophilic spongiosis. The separation is associated with a dermal infiltrate that contains eosinophils.

B. Intraspinous Keratinocyte Separation, Spongiotic. 98

There are spaces within the epidermis (vesicles, bullae). There may be dyskeratosis or acantholysis, and a few eosinophils may be present in the epidermis.

1. Intraspinous Spongiosis, Scant Inflammatory Cells 98

The infiltrate in the dermis is scant, lymphocytic, or eosinophilic.

2. Intraspinous Spongiosis, Lymphocytes Predominant 98

In the dermis, lymphocytes predominate. Eosinophils can be found in most examples of atopy and allergic contact dermatitis.

2a. Intraspinous Spongiosis, Eosinophils Present 98

The number of eosinophils seen is variable from many in incontinentia pigmenti and pemphigus vegetans to few in atopic dermatitis.

3. Intraspinous Spongiosis, Neutrophils Predominant. 98

Neutrophils are seen in the epidermis, stratum corneum, and dermis. Aggregations of neutrophils in the superficial spinous layer constitute the spongiform pustules of Kogoj characteristic of psoriasis.

C. Intraspinous Keratinocyte Separation, Acantholytic

There are spaces within the epidermis (vesicles, bullae). The process of separation is acantholysis. Keratinocytes within the spinous layer detach or separate from each other or from basal keratinocytes. There may be dyskeratosis, and a few eosinophils may be present in the epidermis. The infiltrate in the dermis is variable, composed of lymphocytes with or without eosinophils.

1. Intraspinous Acantholysis, Scant Inflammatory Cells 98

The infiltrate in the dermis is scant, lymphocytic, or eosinophilic.

2. Intraspinous Acantholysis, Predominant Lymphocytes 98

In the dermis, lymphocytes are predominant. In erythema multiforme and related lesions, there is necrosis of individual cells (apoptosis) that may become confluent.

2a. Intraspinous Acantholysis, Eosinophils Present 98

The number of eosinophils seen is variable from many in incontinentia pigmenti and pemphigus vegetans to few in atopic dermatitis.

3. Intraspinous Separation, Neutrophils or Mixed Cell Types 98

Inflammatory cells in the dermis include lymphocytes and plasma cells, with or without eosinophils, neutrophils, mast cells, and histiocytes.

D. Suprabasal Keratinocyte Separation

There is separation between the keratinocytes of the basal layer and those of the spinous layer.

1. Suprabasal Vesicles, Scant Inflammatory Cells. 98

The suprabasal separation may be associated with scant inflammation and frequently with dyskeratotic or atypical keratinocytes.

2. Suprabasal Separation, with Keratinocytes Atypia, Lymphocytes, and Often Plasma Cells **98**

Suprabasal separation is associated with keratinocyte atypia.

3. Suprabasal Vesicles/Bullae, Lymphocytes, and Eosinophils **98**

There is suprabasal separation with eosinophils in the epidermis (eosinophilic spongiosis) and in the dermis.

E. Subepidermal Vesicular Dermatitis **99**

A subepidermal blister refers to the separation of the epidermis from the dermis. The roof of the blister is composed of an intact or (partially) necrotic epithelium.

1. Subepidermal Vesicles, Scant/No Inflammation **99**

The infiltrate in the dermis in most of these conditions is scant (few lymphocytes, eosinophils, neutrophils).

2. Subepidermal Vesicles, Lymphocytes Predominant **99**

The epidermis is separated from the dermis, predominantly owing to liquefaction of the basal cell layer. In PMLE, massive papillary dermal edema is the cause of this separation. The infiltrate in the dermis is primarily lymphocytic.

3. Subepidermal Vesicles, Eosinophils Prominent **99**

The subepidermal blister is associated with a dermal infiltrate rich in eosinophils. Eosinophils may extend into the overlying epidermis.

4. Subepidermal Vesicles, Neutrophils Prominent **99**

A neutrophilic infiltrate is seen often in dermal papillae at the dermal–epidermal junction adjacent to the subepidermal blister or in the blister.

5. Subepidermal Vesicles, Mast Cells Prominent **99**

The epidermis is separated from the dermis. There is an infiltrate in the superficial dermis composed almost entirely of mast cells, with or without a few eosinophils. This may be associated with separation of the epidermis from the dermis.

V. PERIVASCULAR, DIFFUSE, AND GRANULOMATOUS INFILTRATES OF THE RETICULAR DERMIS

The dermis serves as a reaction site for numerous inflammatory, infiltrative, and desmoplastic processes. These include infiltrations of a variety of cells (lymphocytes, histiocytes, eosinophils, plasma cells, melanocytes, etc.); perivascular and vascular reactions; infiltration with organisms and foreign bodies; and proliferations of dermal fibers and precursors of dermal fibers as reactions to a variety of stimuli.

A. Superficial and Deep Perivascular Infiltrates without Vascular Damage or Vasculitis **99**

In some of the diseases considered here, the infiltrates are predominantly in the upper reticular dermis (urticarial eruptions), whereas others are both superficial and deep (gyrate erythemas). Most of these also involve the superficial plexus. A few diseases are mainly deep (some examples of lupus erythematosus, scleroderma).

1. Perivascular Infiltrates, Lymphocytes Predominant **99**

In the dermis, there is no vasculitis, only a perivascular surround of lymphocytes as the predominant cell.

2. Perivascular Infiltrates, Neutrophils Predominant **99**

Neutrophils are seen in perivascular or perivascular and diffuse patterns in the dermis. Edema is prominent in some instances (Sweet).

neutrophil-rich urticaria 7-222
solar urticaria 12-416
rheumatoid neutrophilic dermatosis
neutrophilic dermatosis of the dorsal hands
Behcet disease
Bowel bypass syndrome (Bowel-associated dermatosis–arthritis syndrome)
Erythema elevatum diutinum
VEXAS syndrome UBA1 mutation systemic inflammation
if vasculitis is present, refer to V.B.

3. Perivascular Infiltrates, Lymphocytes and Eosinophils 99
Lymphocytes and eosinophils are mixed in the infiltrate. Lymphocytes are always seen; eosinophil numbers may vary, being greatest in bite reactions and often (though variable and sometimes very few) in eosinophilic fasciitis.

4. Perivascular Infiltrates, with Plasma Cells 99
In addition to lymphocytes, plasma cells are found in the dermal infiltrate.

5. Perivascular Infiltrates, Mixed Cell Types 99
In addition to lymphocytes, plasma cells and eosinophils are found in the dermal infiltrate.

B. Vasculitis and Vasculopathies 100
True vasculitis is defined by eosinophilic degeneration of the vessel wall ("fibrinoid necrosis"), infiltration of the vessel wall by neutrophils, with neutrophils, nuclear dust, and extravasated red cells in the vessel walls and adjacent dermis. Some of the conditions mentioned here lack these prototypic findings and may be termed "vasculopathies" (e.g., Degos disease).

1. Vascular Damage, Scant Inflammatory Cells 100
Although there is significant vascular damage, there is little early inflammatory response.

2. Vasculitis, Lymphocytes Predominant 100
The term "lymphocytic vasculitis" is controversial, but there are some conditions in which perivascular and intramural lymphocytes may be associated with some degree of vasculopathy, not usually including frank fibrinoid necrosis. Most of these conditions are discussed elsewhere as "perivascular lymphocytic infiltrates." In angiocentric lymphomas, the cells infiltrating the vessel walls are neoplastic, but the process may be mistaken for an inflammatory reaction.

3. Vasculitis, Neutrophils Prominent 100
Neutrophils are prominent in the infiltrate, with fibrinoid necrosis and nuclear dust; eosinophils and lymphocytes are also found.

4. Vasculitis, Mixed Cell Types and/or Granulomas 100
Histiocytes and giant cells are a part of the infiltrate. Lymphocytes and eosinophils can also be found depending on the diagnosis. Giant cell arteritis is a true inflammation of the artery wall (true arteritis), although there is no fibrinoid necrosis.

5. Thrombotic and Other Microangiopathies 100
The dermal vessels contain fibrin, red cells and platelet thrombi, and/or eosinophilic protein precipitates.

C. Diffuse Infiltrates of the Reticular Dermis. 100

Diffuse infiltrates of the reticular dermis may show some relation to vessels or to skin appendages or may be randomly distributed in the reticular dermis.

1. Diffuse Infiltrates, Lymphocytes Predominant. 100

Lymphocytes are seen almost to the exclusion of other cell types.

2. Diffuse Infiltrates, Neutrophils Predominant 100

Neutrophils are the main infiltrating cell, although lymphocytes can be found.

3. Diffuse Infiltrates, "Histiocytoid" Cells Predominant 100

Histiocytes or histiocytoid cells are found in great numbers in the dermal infiltrate. Some may be foamy; others may contain organisms. The leukemic cells of myeloid leukemia may be easily mistaken for histiocytes and may have histiocytic differentiation (myelomonocytic leukemia).

4. Diffuse Infiltrates, Plasma Cells Prominent 100

Plasma cells are found in the diffuse dermal infiltrate, though they may not be the predominant cell.

5. Diffuse Infiltrates, Mast Cells Predominant 100

Mast cells compose almost the entire dermal infiltrate. There may be an admixture of eosinophils.

6. Diffuse Infiltrates, Eosinophils Predominant. 100

Eosinophils are prominent, although not the only infiltrating cell. Lymphocytes are also found, and plasma cells may also be present.

7. Diffuse Infiltrates, Mixed Cell Types 100

The diffuse infiltrate contains plasma cells, lymphocytes, histiocytes, and a variety of acute inflammatory cells.

8. Diffuse Infiltrates, Pigment Cells 100

The diffuse infiltrate contains bipolar, cuboidal, or dendritic cells with brown cytoplasmic pigment.

9. Diffuse Infiltrates, Extensive Necrosis 100

Vascular and dermal necrosis are found secondary to vascular occlusion or to destruction by organisms.

D. Diffuse or Nodular Infiltrates of the Reticular Dermis with Epidermal Proliferation..................101

Ill-defined nodules or diffuse infiltrates of inflammatory cells, usually including lymphocytes, plasma cells, and neutrophils, are present in the dermis, and the epidermis is irregularly thickened.

1. Epidermal Proliferation with Mixed Cellular Infiltrates 101

E. Nodular Inflammatory Infiltrates of the Reticular Dermis—Granulomas, Abscesses, and Ulcers 101

A granuloma is defined as a collection of histiocytes that may have abundant cytoplasm and confluent borders ("epithelioid histiocytes"), often with Langhans-type giant cells. Granulomas may be associated with necrosis or may palisade around areas of necrobiosis, may be mixed with other inflammatory cells, may include foreign-body giant cells, or may contain ingested foreign material or pathogens (acid-fast bacilli, fungi). An abscess is a localized area of suppurative necrosis, containing abundant neutrophils mixed with necrotic debris, and usually surrounded by a reaction of granulation tissue and fibrosis.

1. Epithelioid Cell Granulomas without Necrosis 101

Large epithelioid histiocytes are common in the infiltrate as well as giant cells. The infiltrate may also contain a few plasma cells as well as lymphocytes.

2. Epithelioid Cell Granulomas with Necrosis 101

The presence of necrosis in an epithelioid cell granuloma of the skin strongly suggests tuberculosis except in lesions of the face. Epithelioid sarcoma may simulate a necrotizing granuloma.

3. Palisading Granulomas 101

There are foci of altered collagen ("necrobiosis") surrounded by histiocytes and lymphocytes. Histiocytic giant cells may also be seen in the infiltrate. The lesions of epithelioid sarcoma are associated with true tumor necrosis, but may superficially resemble rheumatoid nodules.

4. Mixed Cell Granulomas 101

Lymphocytes and plasma cells are present in addition to epithelioid histiocytes, which may form loose clusters, and giant cells, which may be quite inconspicuous. In many of these granulomatous infiltrates, organisms are found. Keratin granuloma is the most common mixed granuloma. Flakes of keratin may be appreciated as fibers, often gray rather than pink, in the cytoplasm of giant cells.

5. Inflammatory Nodules with Prominent Eosinophils 101

The nodular dermal infiltrates contain many eosinophils often admixed with lymphocytes.

6. Inflammatory Nodules with Mixed Cell Types 101

A variety of cells are seen in the infiltrate, including neutrophils, histiocytes, plasma cells, giant cells, and lymphocytes.

7. Inflammatory Nodules with Necrosis and Neutrophils (Abscesses) 101

Inflammatory nodules characterized by central suppurative necrosis, with neutrophils adjacent to the necrosis, and often with granulation tissue, mixed inflammatory cells including epithelioid histiocytes and giant cells, and fibrosis at the periphery.

8. Inflammatory Nodules with Prominent Necrosis 101

Necrosis is a striking feature along with variable but sometimes sparse infiltrates of inflammatory cells, which may include plasma cells, epithelioid histiocytes, neutrophils, lymphocytes, and hemorrhage. Organisms may be demonstrable. Epithelioid sarcoma may simulate an inflammatory lesion.

9. Chronic Ulcers and Sinuses Involving the Reticular Dermis . . 101

A chronic ulcer is characterized by central suppurative necrosis, with neutrophils adjacent to the necrosis, and often with granulation tissue, fibrosis, and reactive epithelium at the periphery. A sinus extends deeper into the dermis than most ulcers in a serpentine fashion. A fistula is an abnormal communication between two epithelial-lined surfaces. The histologic architecture of fistulas and sinuses is similar to that of chronic ulcers.

F. Dermal Matrix Fiber Disorders 102

The dermis serves as a reaction site for a variety of inflammatory, infiltrative, and desmoplastic processes. These may include accumulations or deficiencies of dermal fibrous and nonfibrous matrix constituents as reactions to a variety of stimuli.

1. Fiber Disorders, Collagen Increased 102

Dermal collagen is increased with production at the dermal subcutaneous interface. Inflammation is seen at this site. The inflammatory cells are lymphocytes, plasma cells, and eosinophils. Fibroblasts in some instances are increased.

Collagen may be reduced focally or diffusely as part of an inborn error of collagen fiber metabolism or as an acquired phenomenon.

Abnormal elastic fibers are increased focally in the dermis and may become calcified (PXE), or there is diffuse elastosis in the superficial reticular dermis of sun-exposed skin.

Elastin may be reduced focally or diffusely as part of an inborn error of its metabolism or as an acquired phenomenon.

Abnormal elastin or collagen fibers may be extruded through the epidermis, which may form channels that extend down into the dermis.

G. Deposition of Material in the Dermis 102

The dermis serves as a reaction site for a variety of inflammatory, infiltrative, and desmoplastic processes, which may include accumulations of matrix molecules that may be either indigenous to the normal dermis or foreign to it.

1. Increased Normal Nonfibrous Matrix Constituents 102

Ground substance (hyaluronic acid) is increased, associated with a varying inflammatory infiltrate that can include lymphocytes, plasma cells, and eosinophils.

Materials not present in substantial amounts in the normal dermis are deposited, as crystals (gout), amorphous deposits (calcinosis), hyaline material (colloid milium, amyloidosis, porphyria), or as pigments.

Macroscopically visible parasitic agents may infest the dermis and subcutis.

VI. TUMORS AND CYSTS OF THE DERMIS AND SUBCUTIS

Neoplasms in the reticular dermis may arise from any of the tissues included in the dermis—lymphoreticular tissue, connective tissue, and epithelial tissue of the skin appendages. In addition, metastases commonly present in the dermis and subcutis.

A. Small Cell Tumors................................. 102

A neoplastic nodule is a circumscribed collection of neoplastic cells in the dermis. Abscesses, granulomas, and cysts may also present as nodules. Cysts are considered separately. In general, neoplastic nodules can be differentiated from reactive and inflammatory nodules by the presence of a monotonous population of cells consistent with a clonal proliferation, whereas inflammatory nodules are composed of inflammatory cell types (lymphocytes, neutrophils, histiocytes, etc.), generally in a heterogeneous mixture.

1. Tumors of Lymphocytes or Hemopoietic Cells.............. 102

Nodular infiltrates or extensive diffuse infiltrates of normal and/or atypical lymphocytes are found in the dermis.

2. Tumors of Lymphocytes and Mixed Cell Types.............. 102

Nodular infiltrates or extensive diffuse infiltrates of normal lymphocytes are found in the dermis. Other reactive cell types (plasma cells, histiocytes) are admixed.

3. Tumors of Plasma Cells................................... 102

Nodular plasma cell infiltrates, with scattered lymphocytes.

4. Small Round Cell Tumors 102

Tumors of small cells with scant cytoplasm, and with small dark nuclei, constitute a group of tumors that can usually be distinguished from one another with appropriate immunohistochemical investigations, in conjunction with light microscopic and clinical information. Some of these tumors arise in the deep soft tissue, but they may rarely present in a deep skin biopsy.

B. Large Polygonal and Round Cell Tumors 103

1. Squamous Cell Carcinomas 103

Proliferations of atypical cells with more or less abundant cytoplasm, contiguous cell borders, evidence of keratinization, and/or desmosomes occupy the dermis as nodular masses. Most primary squamous cell carcinomas show evidence of epidermal origin, often with associated squamous cell carcinoma *in situ*.

2. Adenocarcinomas 103

Proliferations of atypical cells with more or less abundant cytoplasm and with evidence of gland formation and/or mucin production occupy the dermis as nodular masses. Possibility of metastatic adenocarcinoma must be considered and differentiated from the possibility of a primary cutaneous adenocarcinoma of skin appendages (refer to eccrine, apocrine, pilar, sebaceous tumor sections below)

3. Melanocytic Tumors 103

The proliferations in the dermis are melanocyte derived, pigmented or amelanotic, benign, atypical, or malignant. Superficial lesions may involve the epidermis (junctional component). There may be a fibrous and inflammatory host response. S100 and HMB45 stains may be of value in recognizing melanocytic differentiation in amelanotic tumors.

Superficial Melanocytic Nevi

4. Eccrine Tumors **103**

Proliferations of eccrine ductal (small dark cells usually forming tubules at least focally) or glandular tissue or both in a hyalinized or sclerotic dermis. The inflammatory infiltrate is mainly lymphocytic.

5. Apocrine Tumors **103**

Tumors in the dermis are composed of proliferation of apocrine ductal and glandular epithelium (large pink cells with decapitation secretion). The stroma is sclerotic and well vascularized, and the inflammatory cells are mainly lymphocytes.

6. Pilar Tumors. **103**

The dermal infiltrating tumor is composed of epithelium that differentiates toward hair follicle or is a proliferation of portions of the follicular structure and its stroma. The inflammatory cell infiltrate is mainly lymphocytic, and the dermis is fibrocellular.

7. Sebaceous Tumors **103**

The dermal masses are proliferations of the germinative epithelium and of mature sebocytes. The admixture of these cells varies from one tumor to the other. The dermis is fibrocellular.

8. "Histiocytoid" Tumors. **103**

"Histiocytes" may have foamy cytoplasm reflecting the accumulation of lipids or may have eosinophilic or amphophilic cytoplasm surrounding an ovoid nucleus with open chromatin. Some nonhistiocytic lesions whose cells may simulate histiocytes are also included here.

9. Tumors of Large Hemato-Lymphoid Cells **103**

Large lymphoid cells may be mistaken for carcinoma or melanoma cells but may be distinguished morphologically by their tendency to less cohesive growth in large sheets, by the absence of epithelial or melanocytic differentiation, and by immunopathology.

10. Mast Cell Tumors **103**

Mast cells predominate in a nodular dermal infiltrate, with scattered eosinophils.

11. Tumors with Prominent Necrosis **103**

Necrosis is a striking feature in epithelioid sarcoma, which may be in consequence be mistaken for a granulomatous process. In addition, many advanced malignancies, often metastatic, have prominent necrosis.

12. Miscellaneous and Undifferentiated Epithelial Tumors **103**

Proliferations of atypical cells with more or less abundant cytoplasm and contiguous cell borders occupy the dermis as nodular masses.

C. Spindle Cell, Pleomorphic, and Connective Tissue Proliferations **104**

In the dermis is a proliferation of elongated tapered "spindle cells"; these may be of fibrohistiocytic, muscle, neural (Schwannian), melanocytic, or unknown origin. Immunohistochemistry may be essential in making these distinctions.

1. Fibrohistiocytic Spindle Cell Proliferations..................104
There is a proliferation of spindle to pleomorphic cells that may synthesize collagen or be essentially undifferentiated. In the absence of specific markers for fibroblasts, immunohistochemistry is of little diagnostic utility except to rule out non-fibrous spindle cell tumors. Morphology is critical for accurate diagnosis.

2. Schwannian/Neural Spindle Cell Tumors...................104
These tumors are composed of elongated, narrow spindle cells that tend to have serpentine S-shaped nuclei and to be arranged in "wavy" fiber bundles. Immunohistochemistry for S100 is useful, but not specific.

3. Spindle Cell Tumors of Muscle 104
Smooth muscle cells have more abundant cytoplasm than fibroblasts or Schwann cells. The cytoplasm is trichrome positive and reacts with muscle markers—desmin, muscle-specific actin. The nuclei tend to have blunt ends. In neoplasms, the cells tend to be arranged in whorled bundles.

4. Melanocytic Spindle Cell Tumors...........................104
Melanocytic spindle cell tumors may have many attributes of schwannian tumors described above. S100 is positive, and HMB45 is often negative in the spindle cell melanomas. Diagnosis of melanoma then depends on recognizing melanocytic

differentiation—pigment synthesis or a characteristic intraepidermal *in situ* or microinvasive component.

5. Tumors and Proliferations of Angiogenic Cells 104

There is a dermal proliferation of vascular endothelium. Factor VIII staining may be helpful in demonstrating endothelial differentiation. The many variants of benign hemangiomas should be carefully considered in the differential diagnosis of Kaposi sarcoma and angiosarcoma.

Hyperplasias

Angiomas

Lymphangiomas

Telangiectases

Vascular Malformations

Glomus Tumors

Vascular Lipomas

Angiosarcomas

Kaposi Sarcoma

6. Tumors of Adipose Tissue 104

Lipomas

Liposarcomas

Miscellaneous

7. Tumors of Cartilaginous Tissue 104

8. Tumors of Osseous Tissue 104

D. Cysts of the Dermis and Subcutis 104

A cyst is a space lined by epithelium; its contents are usually a product of its lining. Some cysts are inclusion or retention cysts of normal structures (hair follicle–related cysts). Others are benign neoplasms. Some malignant neoplasms may be cystic. These tend to be larger and asymmetric, with a poorly circumscribed and infiltrative border. Their epithelial lining is proliferative, with cytologic atypia. A sinus is an invagination of a surface epithelium, which in some cases may be a precursor of a cyst.

1. Pilar Differentiation..........................104

Cystic proliferations are present in the dermis; these show spaces surrounded by the epithelium of follicular origin and differentiation. Keratin is usually seen in the cystic cavity. Associated cells may be sparse or may include lymphocytes and plasma cells.

2. Eccrine and Similar Differentiation.........................104

Cystic proliferations are present in the dermis; these show spaces surrounded by eccrine epithelium (small dark epithelial cells). The epithelium of ciliated and bronchogenic cysts is not eccrine but may resemble that of an eccrine cyst.

3. Apocrine Differentiation....................................104

Cystic proliferations are present in the dermis; these show spaces surrounded by apocrine epithelium (large pink cells with decapitation secretion). There may be lymphocytes and plasma cells (syringocystadenoma).

VII. INFLAMMATORY AND OTHER BENIGN DISORDERS OF SKIN APPENDAGES

The hair, sebaceous glands, eccrine glands, apocrine glands, and nails may be involved in inflammatory processes (hidradenitis, folliculitis). Some neoplasms may masquerade as inflammatory processes.

A. Pathology Involving Hair Follicles 105

Inflammatory processes may present as alopecia or as follicular localization of inflammatory rashes. Acne and related conditions present as dilatation of follicles which are filled with keratin.

1. Scant Inflammation 105

There is follicular alteration with a sparse infiltrate of cells, mainly lymphocytes.

Follicular Maturation Disorders

Follicular Keratinization Disorders

2. Lymphocytes Predominant..................................105

There is follicular alteration with an inflammatory infiltrate mainly of lymphocytes.

2a. With Eosinophils Present 105

Eosinophils are prominent in the infiltrate and may infiltrate the follicular structures.

3. Neutrophils Prominent 105

There is a follicular alteration with an inflammatory infiltrate containing neutrophils, which may result in disruption of the follicle.

Superficial Folliculitis

Deep Folliculitis

Follicular Occlusion Disorders

Fungal Folliculitis

4. Plasma Cells Prominent **105**
Plasma cells are seen in abundance in the infiltrate. In most instances, they are admixed with lymphocytes.

5. Fibrosing and Suppurative Follicular Disorders **105**
In follicular occlusion disorders and acne keloidalis, there is extensive fibrosis of the dermis, often with keratin tunnels of follicular origin, and with embedded hairs with associated foreign-body inflammation. Neutrophils and plasma cells are seen in abundance in the infiltrate in addition to lymphocytes. In scarring alopecias, the follicles become replaced by a delicate fibrous track.

Follicular Occlusion Disorders

Deep Folliculitis

Scarring Alopecias

B. Pathology Involving Sweat Glands **105**
The sebaceous glands, eccrine glands, and apocrine glands may be involved in inflammatory processes (hidradenitis).

1. Scant Inflammation. **105**
Sweat glands are abnormal in color or size and number, but there is little or no inflammation.

2. Lymphocytes Predominant **105**
There is a predominantly lymphocytic infiltrate in and around the sweat glands.

2a. With Plasma Cells. **105**
There is a predominantly lymphocytic infiltrate in and around the sweat glands. Plasma cells are also present as a minority population.

2b. With Eosinophils **105**
There is an inflammatory infiltrate with eosinophils in and around the sweat glands.

3. Neutrophils Predominant. **105**
There is an inflammatory infiltrate with neutrophils in and around the sweat glands.

C. Pathology Involving Nerves **105**
Specific inflammatory involvement of nerves is uncommon in dermatopathology.

1. Lymphocytic Infiltrates **105**
Neurotropic spread of neoplasms, especially neurotropic melanoma, may be associated with a dense lymphocytic infiltrate that may tend to obscure a subtle infiltrate of neoplastic spindle cells. Certain infections may also be associated with inflammation of nerves.

2. Mixed Inflammatory Infiltrates **105**
There is a mixed inflammatory infiltrate involving nerves.

3. Neoplastic Infiltrates. **105**
Many neoplasms may occasionally involve nerves. The involvement by carcinomas (basal cell, squamous cell, metastatic) is common in the perineural space, while involvement by neurotropic melanoma tends to occupy the endoneurium and to be associated with a dense lymphocytic infiltrate that may tend to obscure a subtle infiltrate of neoplastic spindle cells.

D. Pathology of the Nail Unit. **106**
Several inflammatory dermatoses more often seen elsewhere in the skin may present incidentally or exclusively in the nails. The reaction patterns may vary from those seen elsewhere because of the unique responses of the nail unit to injury.

1. Lymphocytic Infiltrates **106**

2. Lymphocytes with Neutrophils. **106**

VIII. DISORDERS OF THE SUBCUTIS

The reactions in the subcutis are mostly inflammatory, although tumors (proliferations) of the subcutis do occur (lipoma). Pathologic conditions arising in the dermis may infiltrate the subcutis.

A. Subcutaneous Vasculitis and Vasculopathy (Septal or Lobular) 106

True vasculitis is defined by the presence of necrosis and inflammation in vessel walls. Other forms of vasculopathy include thrombosis and thrombophlebitis, fibrointimal hyperplasia, and neoplastic infiltration of vessel walls.

1. Neutrophilic 106

Neutrophils and disrupted nuclei are present in the wall of the vessel, with associated eosinophilic "fibrinoid" necrosis.

2. Lymphocytic. 106

The concept of "lymphocytic vasculitis" is a controversial one. Many disorders characterized by lymphocytes within the walls of vessels are best classified as lymphocytic infiltrates. The term "vasculitis" may be appropriate when there is vessel wall damage, as in nodular vasculitis, even in the absence of neutrophils and "fibrinoid."

3. Granulomatous. 106

The inflammatory infiltrate in the vessel walls is composed of mixed cells including more or less epithelioid histiocytes and giant cells. Other cell types including lymphocytes and plasma cells, and sometimes neutrophils and eosinophils, are commonly present also.

B. Septal Panniculitis without Vasculitis 106

1. Septal Panniculitis, Lymphocytes, and Mixed Infiltrates. 106

The inflammation predominantly involves the subcutaneous septa, although there may be "spillover" into the fat lobules.

The infiltrate is mainly lymphocytic, although other cells can be found including plasma cells and acute inflammatory cells.

2. Septal Panniculitis, Granulomatous 106

Subcutaneous granulomas may present as ill-defined collections of epithelioid histiocytes, as well-formed epithelioid cell granulomas, and as palisading granulomas in which histiocytes are radially arranges around areas of necrosis or necrobiosis.

3. Septal Panniculitis, Sclerotic. 106

Sclerosis of the panniculitis may begin as a septal process and extend into the lobules

C. Lobular Panniculitis without Vasculitis. 107

The inflammation is mainly confined to the lobules, although there may be some septal involvement.

1. Lobular Panniculitis, Lymphocytes Predominant 107

Lymphocytes are the primary infiltrating cells.

2. Lobular Panniculitis, Lymphocytes, and Plasma Cells 107

Lymphocytes and plasma cells are the primary infiltrating cells.

3. Lobular Panniculitis, Neutrophilic 107

Lymphocytes and neutrophils are the primary infiltrating cells.

4. Lobular Panniculitis, Eosinophils Prominent. 107

Lymphocytes and eosinophils are the primary infiltrating cells.

5. Lobular Panniculitis, Histiocytes Prominent **107**

Lymphocytes and histiocytes are the primary infiltrating cells.

6. Lobular Panniculitis, Mixed with Foam Cells. **107**

Lymphocytes, plasma cells, and a variety of infiltrating cells can be seen, including giant cells and foamy histiocytes.

7. Lobular Panniculitis, Granulomatous **107**

Lymphocytes and histiocytes are the primary infiltrating cells.

8. Lobular Panniculitis, Crystal Deposits, Calcifications **107**

Crystalline deposits derived from free fatty acids or other precipitated salts are present in the fat lobules.

9. Lobular Panniculitis, Necrosis Prominent. **107**

There is fat necrosis with a resulting infiltrate that is mixed.

10. Lobular Panniculitis, Embryonic Fat Pattern. **107**

Owing to atrophy or failure of normal morphogenesis, immature small fat cells are present in the lobules.

11. Lobular Panniculitis, Miscellaneous **107**

Lymphocytes, plasma cells, and a variety of infiltrating cells can be seen including giant cells and histiocytes.

D. Mixed Lobular and Septal Panniculitis. **108**

Neoplastic infiltrates and inflammation owing to trauma or infection do not respect anatomic compartments of the subcutis.

1. With Hemorrhage or Sclerosis **108**

Inflammation owing to trauma is likely to be associated with hemorrhage, neutrophilic inflammation, and sclerosis in late lesions.

2. With Many Neutrophils **108**

Neutrophilic inflammation diffusely involves the subcutis.

3. With Many Eosinophils **108**

Few to many eosinophils are present in subcutaneous lobules and septa.

4. With Many Lymphocytes **108**

Lymphocytic infiltrates diffusely involve the subcutis.

Histiocytes with phagocytized erythrocytes diffusely infiltrate the subcutis.

There is granulomatous inflammation diffusely involving the subcutis.

A collection of neutrophils in the subcutis, usually surrounded by granulation tissue and fibrosis.

The center of the abscess contains pus, which is viscous because of the presence of DNA fragments derived from neutrophils and dead organisms.

Congenital diseases, Genodermatoses, and Selected Pediatric Conditions

Chapter 6

ALEJANDRO A. GRU AND ADNAN MIR

HEREDITARY DISORDERS OF CORNIFICATION

Ichthyoses are disorders of the epidermis characterized by hyperkeratosis and scaling, which are distinguished by their clinical phenotype, histopathology, and underlying genetic defect. Normal desquamation requires orderly keratinocyte differentiation and functional enzymes to degrade corneocytes. Both are required for adequate epidermal turnover and a functional skin barrier. Recently, genetic mutations in epidermal proteins or abnormalities in lipid metabolism have been identified to cause many of these disorders, resulting in poor barrier function, predisposition to influx of pathogens and antigens, and increased transepidermal water loss.

The most recent classification of the ichthyoses is derived on the basis of clinical phenotype, histopathology, and biochemical and genetic features. They are divided into syndromic and nonsyndromic ichthyoses, depending on whether the disorder is associated with significant extracutaneous manifestations (syndromic) or not (nonsyndromic). (Note that it is possible for a disorder to fall into both categories because individual patients with a particular disorder vary in their degree of extracutaneous involvement.) There are four typically nonsyndromic ichthyoses, which will be addressed first: (a) *ichthyosis vulgaris*; (b) *X-linked recessive ichthyosis* (XLRI); (c) *epidermolytic ichthyosis*; and (d) *autosomal recessive congenital ichthyosis* (*ARCI*, including lamellar ichthyosis, congenital ichthyosiform erythroderma, and Harlequin ichthyosis) (1).

Nonsyndromic Ichthyoses

Ichthyosis Vulgaris
Clinical Summary. Ichthyosis vulgaris (IV) is the most common form of ichthyosis. Typically, it develops within the first few months of life, although some patients may not manifest features of the disease until adolescence or even early adulthood. The disorder is caused by mutations in the profilaggrin gene, and IV is inherited in an autosomal semidominant fashion. Milder manifestations can be seen with a single mutation, but the severity increases with two affected alleles (2). Clinically, patients develop large, plate-like adherent scales on the extensor surfaces of the extremities. The flexural surfaces are typically spared. Keratosis pilaris and atopic dermatitis are often an accompanying feature, and the palms and soles may show hyperlinearity. Most children improve in the summer and with age.

Histopathology. The characteristic finding is a reduced or absent granular layer in association with a mild-to-moderate degree of hyperkeratosis, which helps to distinguish IV from other forms of ichthyosis (Fig. 6-1). The hyperkeratosis often extends into the hair follicles, resulting in large keratotic follicular plugs. The dermis is unremarkable.

Pathogenesis. A defect in the synthesis of filaggrin, which is the major component of the granular layer, is responsible for the characteristic reduction of this layer on histopathology. Ultrastructurally, keratohyalin granules appear small and crumbly or spongy, which is evidence of defective synthesis. Defective profilaggrin expression in IV may be a result of selectively impaired posttranscriptional control (3). In addition, filaggrin links proteins of the corneocyte envelope. Dysfunctional filaggrin leads to an impaired skin barrier with increased penetration of allergens, which may predispose to epicutaneous sensitization and the development of atopic disorders, including atopic dermatitis and asthma. Studies suggest that approximately 25% to 50% of patients with atopic dermatitis and secondary asthma harbor

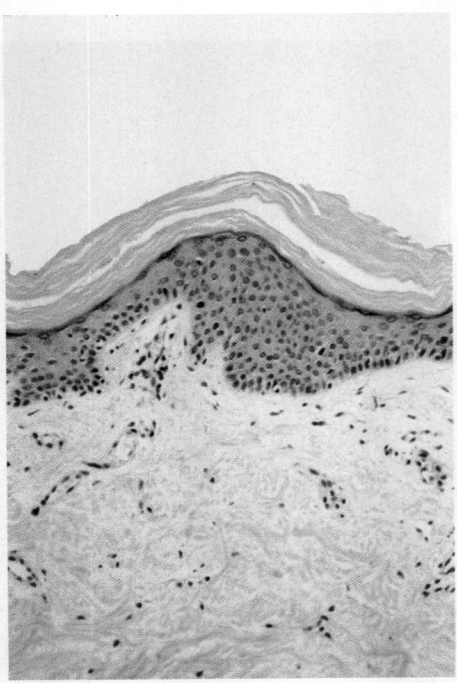

Figure 6-1 Ichthyosis vulgaris. Hyperkeratosis with a diminished and focally absent granular cell layer (original magnification ×100).

filaggrin mutations, approximately 40 of which have been identified as pathogenic (4).

Differential Diagnosis. Although the noninflamed but dry skin of patients with atopic dermatitis clinically resembles IV, on histologic examination, atopic dermatitis more commonly demonstrates epidermal hyperplasia, spongiosis, patchy parakeratosis, and slight hypergranulosis.

X-Linked Recessive Ichthyosis

Clinical Summary. X-linked recessive ichthyosis (XLRI) is caused by a mutation in the *ARSC1* gene encoding steroid sulfatase, which in nearly 90% of cases results from gene deletion. It rarely presents at birth and most frequently develops in the first few months of life. Males are invariably affected. Female carriers do not tend to manifest the clinical cutaneous phenotype because the gene is located at the distal tip of the X chromosome, which typically escapes random X-inactivation. As a result, both genes are expressed in each cell, providing sufficient enzyme despite the mutated allele that the skin remains largely unaffected. However, female carriers who are pregnant often have prolonged labor and may fail to progress secondary to insufficient placental steroid sulfatase. Affected females with Turner syndrome or those with homozygous mutations in the *ARSC1* gene have been described, and those so affected have more typical features of the disorder (5). Patients tend to develop diffuse plate-like brown scale on the trunk and extremities, with accentuation on the neck and sparing of the flexural areas (as in ichthyosis vulgaris), palms, soles, and central face (Fig. 6-2). Asymptomatic corneal opacities have been described in 25% to 50% of patients, and they can be seen in unaffected carrier females as well (6). Boys may also be affected with isolated cryptorchidism or hypogonadism (7). A contiguous gene syndrome has been observed in patients with clinical findings of XLRI and Kallmann syndrome (hypogonadotropic hypogonadism associated with mental retardation and anosmia) (8).

In the uncommon instances where extracutaneous features are identified, they are considered examples of syndromic ichthyosis. Prolonged labor with affected fetuses is common. An association with chondrodysplasia punctate is also noted (9).

Histopathology. Hyperkeratosis, with or without parakeratosis, is present along with a granular layer that is normal or slightly thickened, in contrast to IV (Fig. 6-2B). The epidermis may be slightly acanthotic as well (10). Hyperkeratosis of the follicular and sweat duct orifices can be seen. Electron microscopy shows increased size and number of keratohyalin granules (11).

Pathogenesis. Steroid sulfatase is concentrated in lamellar bodies and degrades cholesterol sulfate, which provides the cholesterol "mortar" between "brick" corneocytes in the cornified envelope. Cholesterol sulfate also functions as a serine protease inhibitor in the epidermis and is required for orderly corneocyte degradation and normal desquamation. Increased cholesterol sulfate leads to persistent cell cohesion with delayed dissolution of desmosomes in the stratum spinosum, leading to retention hyperkeratosis (12,13). This was first recognized in skin fibroblasts but was also found subsequently in the entire epidermis and in leukocytes (12,14).

Keratinopathic Ichthyosis

Keratinopathic ichthyosis is the updated terminology for ichthyoses resulting from mutations in keratin genes, which include epidermolytic ichthyosis (the most common subtype and previously referred to as *bullous congenital ichthyosiform erythroderma [BCIE], ichthyosis en confetti, and superficial epidermolytic ichthyosis [previously called ichthyosis bullosa of Siemens]*).

Epidermolytic Ichthyosis

Clinical Summary. Epidermolytic ichthyosis (EI) is caused by mutations in the keratin 1 (*KRT1*) or keratin 10 (*KRT10*) genes and is typically inherited in an autosomal dominant fashion,

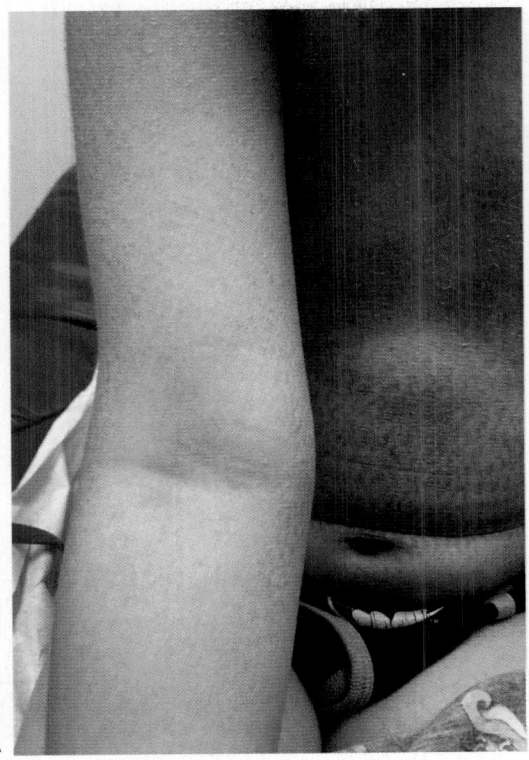

A

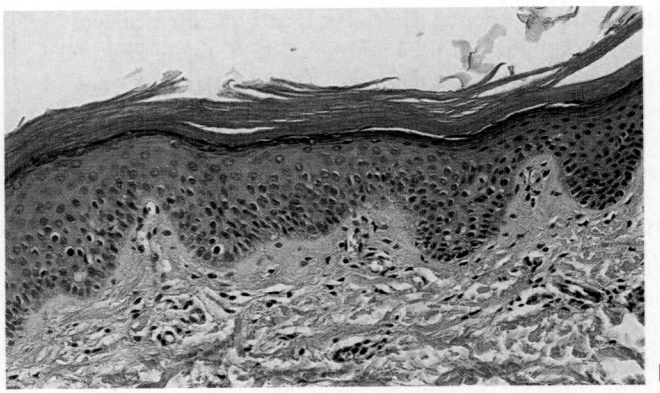

B

Figure 6-2 **A:** X-linked recessive ichthyosis sparing the flexural area. (Reprinted with permission from Gru AA. *Pediatric Dermatopathology and Dermatology.* Wolters Kluwer; 2019.) **B:** X-linked recessive ichthyosis. Hyperkeratosis with preservation of the granular cell layer and hyperorthokeratosis (original magnification ×200). (Digital slides courtesy of Path Presenter.com.)

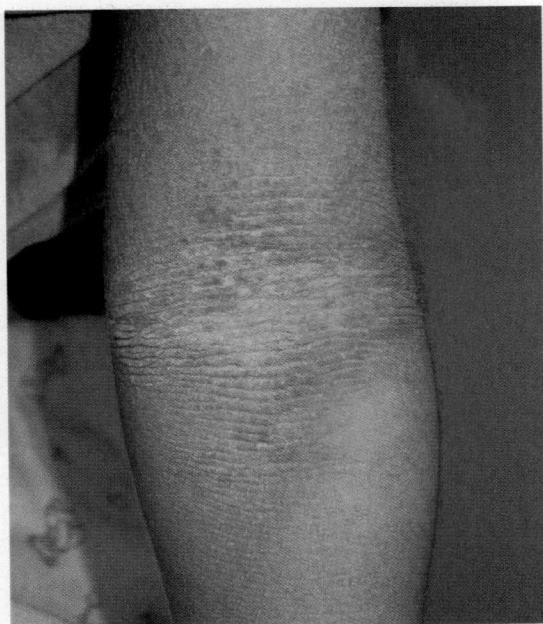

Figure 6-3 Epidermolytic ichthyosis. Linear scaling reminiscent of "corrugated cardboard." (Courtesy of Albert Yan, CHOP Dermatology.)

although recessive forms have also been reported (1). Infants show generalized tender erythema from the time of birth, with the development of superficial bullae and erosions that can be confused with staphylococcal scalded skin syndrome. Vesicles, bullae, and erosions typically resolve within the first few years, to be replaced by thick brown, verrucous scaling that predominates over time (Fig. 6-3). The flexural surfaces show marked involvement with furrowed hyperkeratosis, particularly in flexural areas, leading to the appearance of "corrugated cardboard." Patients with severe disease are commonly colonized with bacteria and may exhibit a characteristic odor.

Histopathology. Epidermolytic hyperkeratosis (EHK) is a characteristic histologic finding in the epidermis (Fig. 6-4). There are variously sized clear spaces around the nuclei in the upper stratum spinosum and in the stratum granulosum. Peripheral to the clear spaces, the cells show indistinct boundaries formed by lightly staining material or by keratohyalin granules. A markedly thickened granular layer containing an increased number

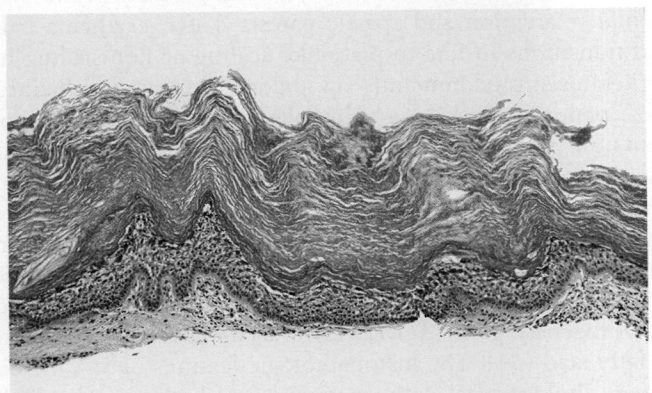

Figure 6-4 Epidermolytic hyperkeratosis. There is vacuolization of the upper spinus and mid-spinus layer, with hyperkeratosis and large keratohyalin granules in the vacuolated expanded granular cell layer (original magnification ×100).

of irregularly shaped keratohyalin granules and compact hyperkeratosis is observed (15). When bullae form, they arise intraepidermally through separation of edematous cells from one another. The upper dermis shows a moderately severe, chronic inflammatory infiltrate (16).

Pathogenesis. Mutations are predominantly point mutations that occur in the carboxy terminal of the rod domain of keratin 1 and the amino terminal of the rod domain of keratin 10, producing an abnormal keratin network that leads to blistering and skin fragility (17). The essential electron microscopic features are excessive production of tonofilaments and premature formation of keratohyalin granules. At the periphery of the cells, numerous keratohyalin granules are embedded in thick shells of irregularly clumped tonofilaments. The desmosomes appear normal, but the tonofilament–desmosomal interaction is disturbed, so many desmosomes are attached to only one keratinocyte instead of connecting two neighboring keratinocytes, with resultant clinically observed blister formation and sometimes histologic features of acantholysis.

Differential Diagnosis. Although EHK is found in all cases of EI, it can also be seen as an isolated histologic finding in other benign dermatoses and neoplasms, including *epidermolytic palmoplantar keratoderma* (detailed below); solitary epidermolytic acanthoma, disseminated epidermolytic acanthoma; and an epidermal nevus, usually of the systematized type. In the latter case, it represents a mosaic finding where only affected skin (but not normal surrounding skin) contains a mutation in the keratin 1 or 10 genes (18). Patients with extensive epidermal nevi exhibiting EHK may possess germline mutations, which may place them at risk for transmitting germline mutations to their offspring, resulting in generalized *EI* (19).

Ichthyosis En (With) Confetti

Clinical Summary. Ichthyosis with confetti is an autosomal dominant disorder also caused by mutations in *KRT1* or *KRT10*. Affected patients are born with exfoliative erythroderma and palmoplantar keratoderma, which—over many years—become peppered with numerous pale "confetti-like" islands of normal skin during childhood (20).

Histopathology. Histology of the erythrodermic skin shows epidermal acanthosis with disordered differentiation above the basal layer, perinuclear vacuolization, hypogranulosis, and hyperkeratosis with retained nuclei in the stratum corneum (21).

Pathogenesis. Ichthyosis with confetti has been shown to result from revertant mosaicism, where islands of normal intervening skin appear secondary to loss of heterozygosity in the *KRT10* gene via mitotic recombination (21). This form of "natural gene therapy" results from genetic events in a single somatic cell, causing loss of the disease-causing phenotype, followed by expansion of the reverted cell. Revertant mosaicism has been reported in other skin diseases, including epidermolysis bullosa as well as in primary immunodeficiencies and muscular dystrophy (22).

Superficial Ichthyosis

Clinical Summary. Superficial ichthyosis, previously called *ichthyosis bullosa of Siemens*, is caused by mutations in the *KRT2e* gene and is marked by more superficial blistering than *EI*, which is consistent with localization of KRT2 in the upper spinous and granular layers. Intact bullae can occur, but denuded peeling skin more commonly predominates. Hyperkeratosis of the palms and soles is rare.

Histopathology. Skin biopsies are similar to EI with EHK in the upper spinous and granular layers. The diagnosis is often a clinical one, with genetic confirmation of mutations in *KRT2* (23).

Autosomal Recessive Congenital Ichthyosis

Clinical Summary. ARCI is a collection of various disorders that includes a range of phenotypes including *harlequin ichthyosis (HI)*, *lamellar ichthyosis (LI)*, and *nonbullous congenital ichthyosiform erythroderma (CIE)*, but some patients may have overlapping features. The diagnosis is exclusively a clinical one, although biopsy can be helpful to exclude other diagnoses. *HI* is the most severe ARCI phenotype, and patients are born with thick, yellow/brown plates of scale interspersed with large, deep, bright red fissures, ectropion, eclabium, ear abnormalities, and common prematurity. Such features mimic the costume of a harlequin (Fig. 6-5). The mortality in the neonatal period is very high, typically secondary to sepsis or respiratory failure. Patients with the *CIE* phenotype demonstrate fine white scales with fairly pronounced erythroderma that may improve with age. The *LI* phenotype is characterized by large, plate-like "fish" scales, although there is a spectrum of severity ranging from mild disease to more severe involvement with ectropion (eversion of the eyelid resulting in exposure of the conjunctiva), eclabium (eversion of the lips), and scarring alopecia (Fig. 6-6). In all forms, the flexural surfaces and the palms and soles are involved. Both CIE and LI manifest with collodion membrane at birth. This is a taut, shiny membrane covering the infant's entire body, derived from thickened stratum corneum (Fig. 6-7A, B).

Pathogenesis. Six genes have been implicated in ARCI. Most patients with the lamellar phenotype have mutations in the gene encoding transglutaminase 1 (*TGM1*), which cross-links proteins in the cornified envelope (24). HI results from truncating mutations or deletions in the *ABCA12* transporter gene, leading to deficiency of proteases in the stratum corneum, dysregulated lipid transport with abnormal lamellar bodies, and premature differentiation of keratinocytes. Massive orthokeratosis results (25). Missense mutations in *ABCA12* produce milder LI or CIE phenotypes secondary to the presence of some functioning protein (26). Mutations in *ALOX12B* (12(R)-lipoxygenase), *TGM1*,

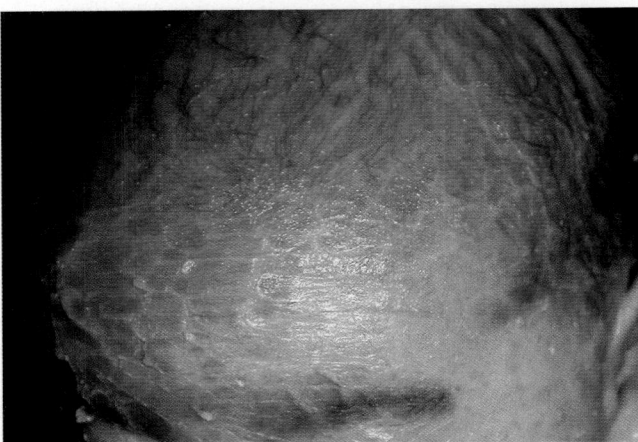

Figure 6-6 Lamellar ichthyosis phenotype of autosomal recessive congenital ichthyosis. Plate-like scaling on the forehead of a patient with confirmed TGM-1 mutation. (Courtesy of Albert Yan, CHOP Dermatology.)

ALOXE3 (lipoxygenase-3), *CYP4F22* (cytochrome p450 subunit), *ABCA12, PNPLA1, LIPM, CerS3,* and *NIPAL4* (ichthyin) also lead to ARCI through disruption of lipid synthesis and/or processing of filaggrin (27–30).

Histopathology. The histologic findings are nonspecific and include massive hyperorthokeratosis with follicular plugging. Typically, histopathology of *CIE* shows mild thickening of the stratum corneum with foci of parakeratosis, whereas *LI* demonstrates a markedly thickened stratum corneum without areas of parakeratosis (Fig. 6-8). On electron microscopy, *HI* demonstrates absent lamellar granules in the stratum granulosum (31). *LI* shows elongated cholesterol clefts, variable translucent lipid droplets in the corneal layer, and a thin-to-absent cornified envelope (such features are also shared by *CIE*) (32).

Syndromic Ichthyoses

Clinical Summary. There is an expanding list of syndromes that combine ichthyosis with neuroectodermal and mesodermal defects. Most of these syndromes demonstrate nonspecific orthokeratosis with the exception of Refsum disease, for which the histopathologic skin findings are specific and diagnostic, and CHILD syndrome (see below).

Sjögren–Larsson syndrome (SLS) is an autosomal recessive disorder characterized by erythroderma early in life, with mental retardation and spastic paresis. Later, erythema fades and transitions to fine to plate-like scaling or non-scaling hyperkeratosis, predominantly on abdomen, neck, and flexures. Most patients also have a palmoplantar keratoderma. *SLS* patients are photophobic, but "retinal glistening dots" are not always present in childhood. Collodion presentation is rare. With age, these patients develop generalized lamellar thickening, which is most pronounced on the neck and trunk, sparing the face. Pruritus is invariably present and can be severe (33). The disorder is secondary to mutations in the fatty aldehyde dehydrogenase gene (*ALDH3A2*), which converts fatty alcohol to fatty acid (34). The histopathologic features of *SLS* include hyperorthokeratosis with scattered parakeratosis, a mildly papillated surface, and variable changes in the granular layer, features that are different from most ichthyoses in the skin. Ultrastructural analysis reveals lamellar inclusions in the upper layers of the epidermis.

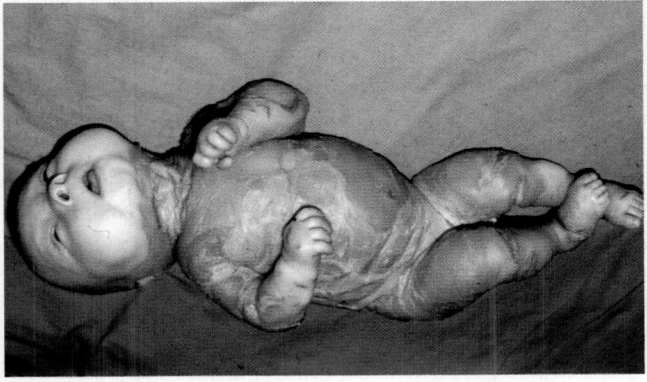

Figure 6-5 Harlequin ichthyosis phenotype. (Courtesy of Dr Kenneth Greer, Department of Dermatology, University of Virginia.)

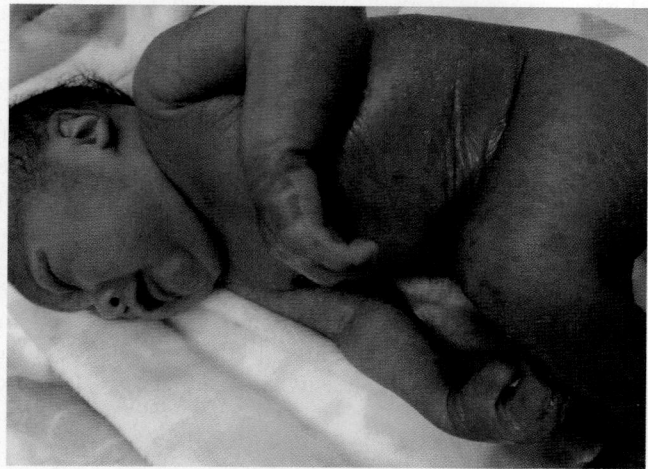 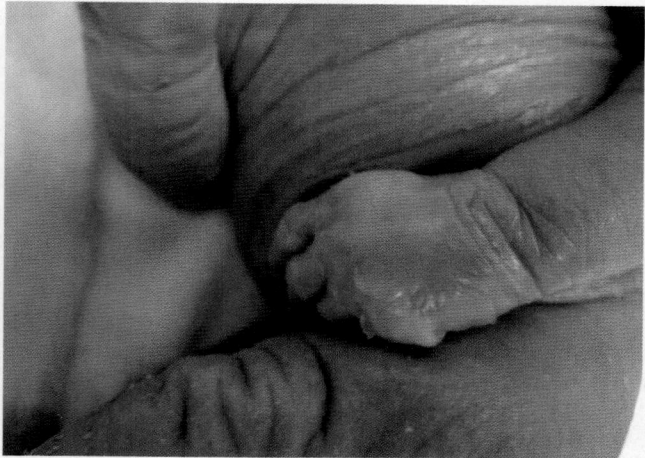

A   B

Figure 6-7 A, B: Separate examples of collodion membranes. (Reprinted with permission from Gru AA. *Pediatric Dermatopathology and Dermatology*. Wolters Kluwer; 2019.)

Conradi–Hünermann–Happle syndrome (*CHHS, chondrodysplasia punctata type 2*) is an X-linked dominant form of chondrodysplasia punctata, which is characterized by punctate epiphyseal calcifications, asymmetric skeletal abnormalities, ichthyosiform areas in a Blaschkoid distribution (termed ptychotropism), and cataracts. This ichthyosiform erythroderma resolves over time, and older children develop linear plaques of follicular atrophoderma in the same distribution (Fig. 6-9). Additional cutaneous findings include linear dyspigmentation, patchy scarring alopecia, course hair, and onychoschizia. X-chromosomal inactivation in girls produces the Blaschkoid skin findings and asymmetric bone involvement, and the underlying defect occurs in the pathway of cholesterol synthesis and metabolism. Mutations have been found in the emopamil-binding protein (*EBP*) gene, which encodes 3β-hydroxysteroid delta 8, delta 7 sterol isomerase (35). Mutations cause accumulation of abnormal sterols in tissue and plasma. Some forms are associated with peroxisome abnormalities (35). Biopsy specimens from ichthyotic plaques in patients with CHHS display dilated follicular ostia, hyperorthokeratosis, and occasional hypergranulosis. Early lesions show calcification within corneocytes, which can be demonstrated with von Kossa staining.

Netherton syndrome (*NS*) is an autosomal recessive condition marked by the combination of CIE, severe atopic diathesis, immune dysregulation, and hair shaft deformities, most commonly trichorrhexis invaginata. Most patients present in the newborn period with an exfoliative erythroderma and failure to thrive, and they are at high risk for sepsis and electrolyte

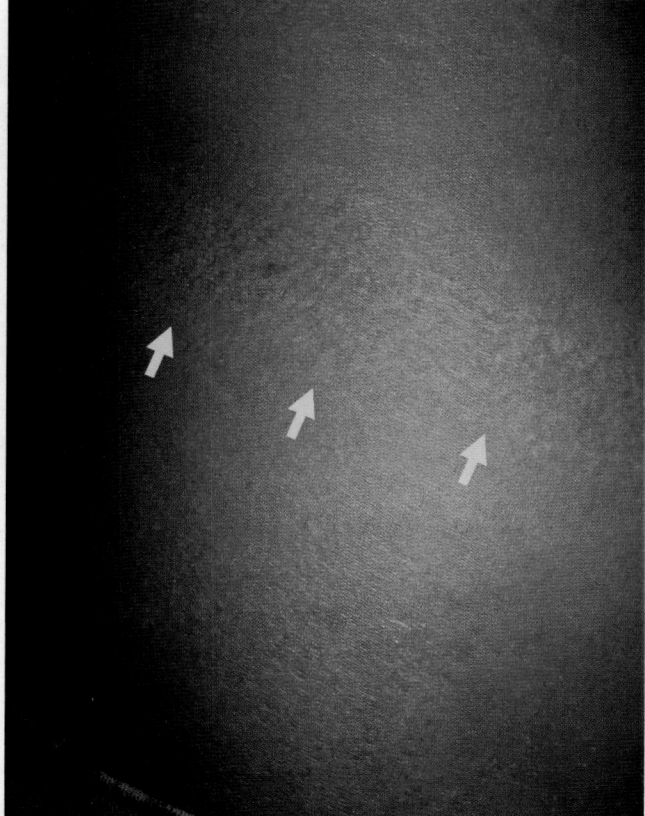

Figure 6-8 Lamellar ichthyosis. Epidermal acanthosis and massive hyperkeratosis (original magnification ×200). (Reprinted with permission from Gru AA. *Pediatric Dermatopathology and Dermatology*. Wolters Kluwer; 2019.)

Figure 6-9 Conradi–Hünermann–Happle syndrome. Linear plaques of follicular atrophoderma in the same distribution (*arrow heads*). (Courtesy of Dr. Nnenna Agim, Department of Dermatology, University of Texas Southwestern Medical Center.)

abnormalities secondary to dehydration. The classic skin finding in *NS* is ichthyosis linearis circumflexa, which is not typically seen until early childhood and manifests as extensive migratory polycyclic lesions of erythema and scaling (Fig. 6-10A). At their periphery, some of the areas show a distinctive "double-edged" scale (36). Trichorrhexis invaginata (so-called bamboo-hair, Fig. 6-10B) is the classic hair shaft deformity, giving the hair the appearance of bamboo. This finding is thought to represent a defect involving the inner root sheath (37). Patients typically have elevated eosinophils and IgE with severe atopy including eczema, asthma, food allergies, and anaphylaxis (38). The skin barrier dysfunction in these patients results in a high risk for percutaneous absorption of topically applied medicaments.

Histopathology. The areas of erythema and scaling show non-specific changes with some resemblance to psoriasis, such as elongation of the rete ridges, exocytosis of neutrophils, and hyperkeratosis, as well as parakeratosis (Fig. 6-10C). The double-edged scale frequently manifests as spongiosis in the upper stratum spinosum, resulting in multilocular vesicles or vesiculopustules (39). Erythroderma cases can show confluent parakeratosis.

Pathogenesis. NS is caused by mutations in the gene *SPINK5*, which encodes LEKTI (Lymphoepithelial Kazal-Type Inhibitor), a serine protease inhibitor. Deficiency of LEKTI causes epidermal protease hyperactivity, leading to desmosomal

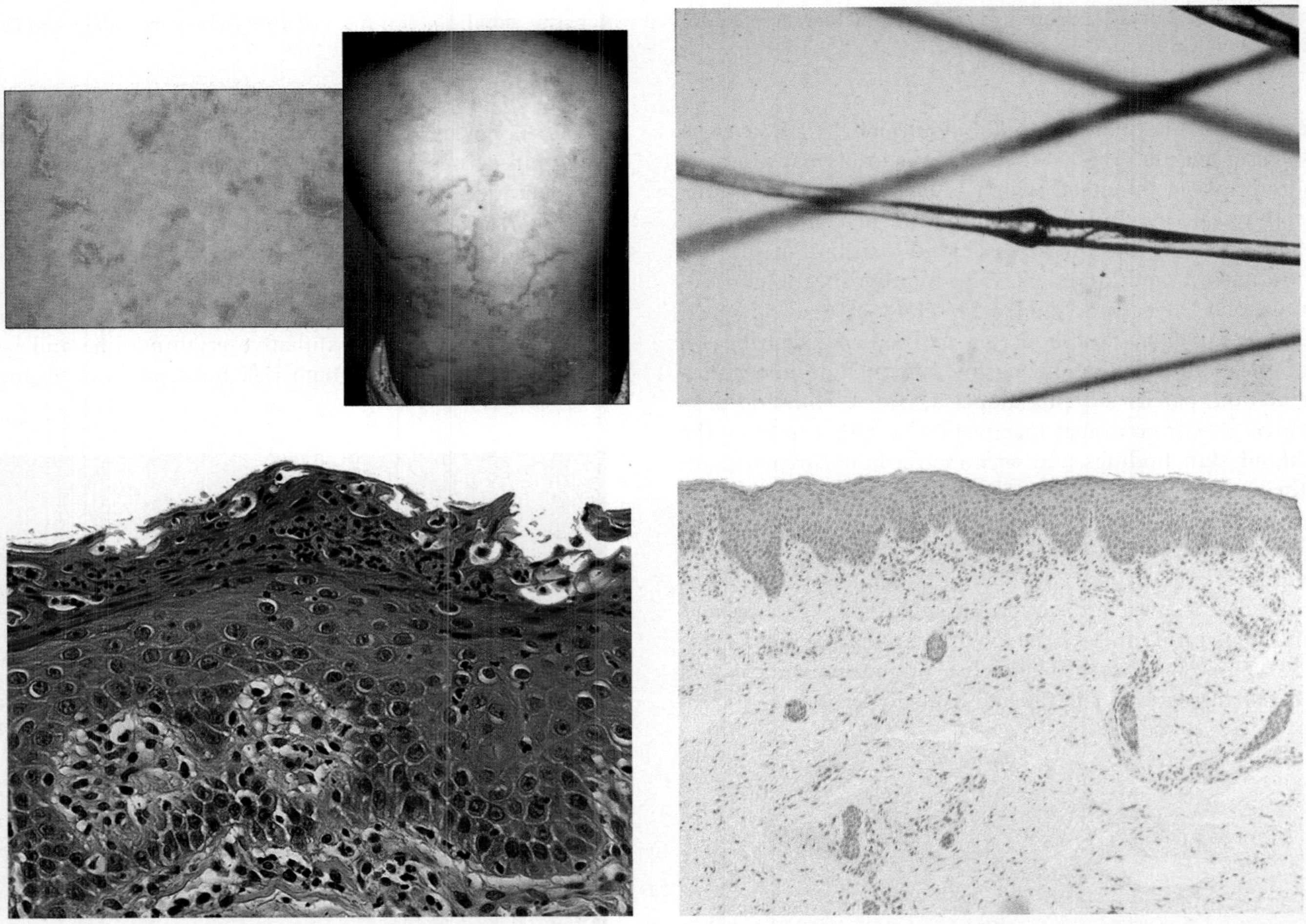

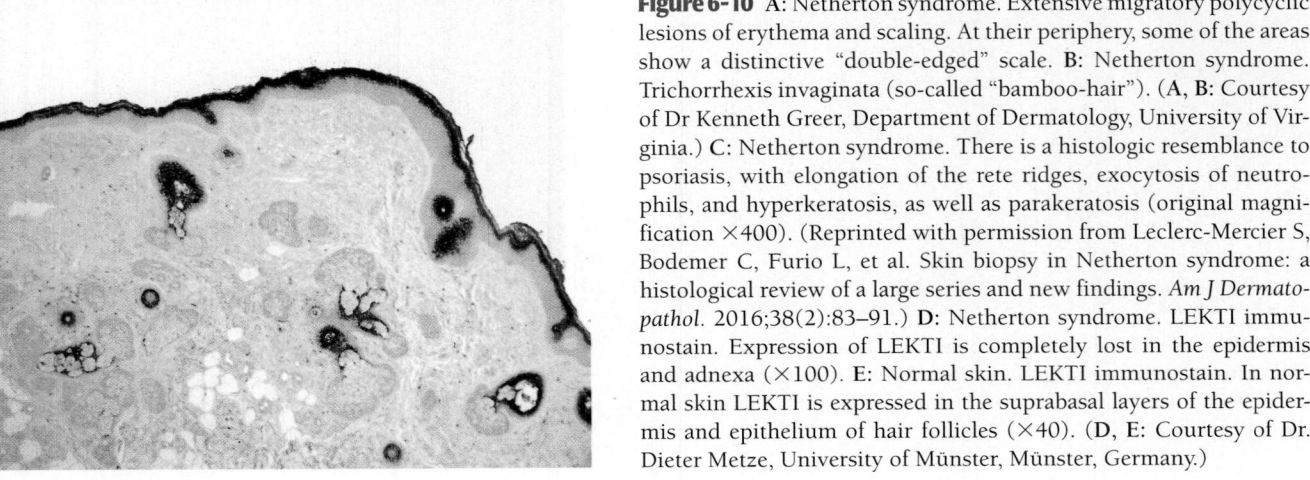

Figure 6-10 **A:** Netherton syndrome. Extensive migratory polycyclic lesions of erythema and scaling. At their periphery, some of the areas show a distinctive "double-edged" scale. **B:** Netherton syndrome. Trichorrhexis invaginata (so-called "bamboo-hair"). (**A, B:** Courtesy of Dr Kenneth Greer, Department of Dermatology, University of Virginia.) **C:** Netherton syndrome. There is a histologic resemblance to psoriasis, with elongation of the rete ridges, exocytosis of neutrophils, and hyperkeratosis, as well as parakeratosis (original magnification ×400). (Reprinted with permission from Leclerc-Mercier S, Bodemer C, Furio L, et al. Skin biopsy in Netherton syndrome: a histological review of a large series and new findings. *Am J Dermatopathol.* 2016;38(2):83–91.) **D:** Netherton syndrome. LEKTI immunostain. Expression of LEKTI is completely lost in the epidermis and adnexa (×100). **E:** Normal skin. LEKTI immunostain. In normal skin LEKTI is expressed in the suprabasal layers of the epidermis and epithelium of hair follicles (×40). (**D, E:** Courtesy of Dr. Dieter Metze, University of Münster, Münster, Germany.)

degradation, detachment of the stratum corneum, and activation of TH$_2$ cytokines, in turn leading to atopy (36,40). More recently, immunohistochemical stains have been introduced to help in the diagnosis of NS. In NS, expression of LEKTI is completely lost in the epidermis and adnexa. In normal skin, LEKTI is expressed in the suprabasal layers of the epidermis and epithelia of hair follicles (Fig. 6-10D).

Trichothiodystrophy is otherwise known as **IBIDS syndrome** secondary to characteristic features of Ichthyosis, Brittle hair, Impaired intelligence, Decreased fertility, and Short stature. Some patients also demonstrate photosensitivity (which is referred to as **PIBIDS syndrome**). Patients with these syndromes have sulfur-deficient, sparse hair, which demonstrates a characteristic "tiger tail" appearance under polarized microscopy (41).

Refsum disease is an autosomal recessive disorder characterized by generalized ichthyosis, cerebellar ataxia, progressive paresis of the extremities, and retinitis pigmentosa, which typically manifests in late childhood or adolescence. Patients typically present with neurologic manifestations, and a delay in diagnosis can lead to irreversible damage. Cutaneous findings include fine, white scaling on the trunk and extremities and hyperlinear palmoplantar markings, similar to that seen in ichthyosis vulgaris. This generally begins concurrently or after neurologic symptoms.

Histopathology. Skin biopsy specimens from patients with Refsum disease may show mild hyperorthokeratosis and a diminished granular layer, similar to the changes seen in ichthyosis vulgaris. Accumulation of lipid droplets can be appreciated in specimens fixed in alcohol with lipid stains such as Sudan black or ultrastructural analysis with electron microscopy (42–44).

Pathogenesis. Refsum disease is caused by mutations in two genes: the *PAHX* gene, which encodes the peroxisomal enzyme phytanoyl-CoA hydroxylase, and the *PEX7* gene, which encodes the PTS2 (peroxisomal targeting signal 2) receptor, both of which lead to the accumulation of phytanic acid (45,46). Treatment includes avoidance of phytanic acid-containing foods.

CHILD syndrome is an X-linked dominant disease characterized by Congenital Hemidysplasia with Ichthyosiform erythroderma and Limb Defects (CHILD). Affected patients present at, or soon, after birth with striking unilateral musculoskeletal, cutaneous, and visceral abnormalities. Cutaneous manifestations include thick, scaly, erythematous plaques that are Blaschkoid to nearly confluent in nature and are unilateral with a sharp midline demarcation (Fig. 6-11). Patients may also have unilateral alopecia and onychorrhexis of the affected side. Internal abnormalities are also frequent, including unilateral brain, lung, renal, and endocrine gland hypoplasia as well as cardiovascular defects. Sensorineural hearing loss and mild intellectual impairment are also seen. Nearly all published cases have been female, and it is presumed to be lethal in the hemizygote male fetus. The disorder is secondary to mutations in the *NSHDL* gene, which encodes the enzyme 3β-hydroxysteroid dehydrogenase that converts lanosterol to cholesterol (47). Ultrastructural analysis of affected skin has demonstrated *both* cholesterol depletion and accumulation of toxic metabolites. Application of topical lovastatin/cholesterol compound (but not cholesterol alone) has resulted in virtual clearance of affected skin, with normalization of histologic and ultrastructural skin, presumably secondary to therapy that not only replenished the deficient end product but also prevented generation of toxic metabolites (48).

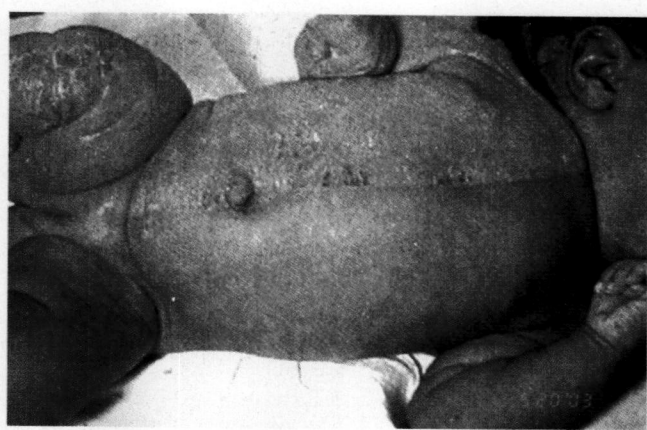

Figure 6-11 CHILD syndrome. Note unilateral erythema, scaling, and ipsilateral limb hypoplasia.

Histopathology. The epidermis is acanthotic with alternating layers of orthokeratosis and parakeratosis in the stratum corneum. Neutrophils are often present within the zones of parakeratosis. Numerous lipid-laden vesicles can be noted in the lower stratum corneum, with elongation of the rete ridges and an inflammatory infiltrate (49). Histologic features of verruciform xanthoma (VX) can be seen in the areas of ichthyosiform erythroderma, and isolated VX can also be seen in CHILD syndrome. Histologically, VX is characterized by infiltration of papillary dermal tips with foamy macrophages (50).

Principles of Management: The current standard for treating all forms of ichthyosis includes keratolytics and emollients containing urea, lactic or glycolic acid, or propylene glycol to restore the epidermal barrier (51,52). Salicylic acid–based products can also be effective, but they should be used with great caution in these disorders where percutaneous absorption can be significant and can lead to potential toxicity. There is emerging evidence for use of topical N-acetyl cysteine, a glutathione precursor, which serves various functions as a potent antioxidant and may also have effects on improving keratinocyte differentiation (52). Topical steroids are often ineffective because there is minimal epidermal hyperproliferation or inflammation. CHILD syndrome has responded to topical application of 2% lovastatin/2% cholesterol compound to affected skin to bypass the defective cholesterol synthesis pathway and reduce toxic metabolites associated with NSDHL deficiency (53).

MEDNIK syndrome is an autosomal recessive disorder with a constellation of symptoms including Mental retardation, Enteropathy, Deafness, Neuropathy, Ichthyosis, and Keratoderma. It is caused by mutation in adapter protein complex subunit a1 (*AP1S1*) (54–56). Infants present at birth or within the first few weeks of life. Cutaneous manifestations include erythematous patches and hyperkeratotic plaques of variable size (Fig. 6-12). Mucosal and nail involvement are common. Other findings include sensorineural deafness, delayed psychomotor development, growth retardation, and peripheral neuropathy. Severe life-threatening diarrhea is a major complication. Cutaneous histopathologic findings include hyperkeratosis, gentle papillomatosis, and focal parakeratosis.

Arthrogryposis-renal dysfunction-cholestasis (ARC) syndrome is a multisystem, life-threatening, autosomal recessive disorder arising from mutations in *VPS33B* or *VIPAR* (57–59). Cutaneous findings are seen in about 50% of affected patients and are evident within the first few days or weeks of life. Infants

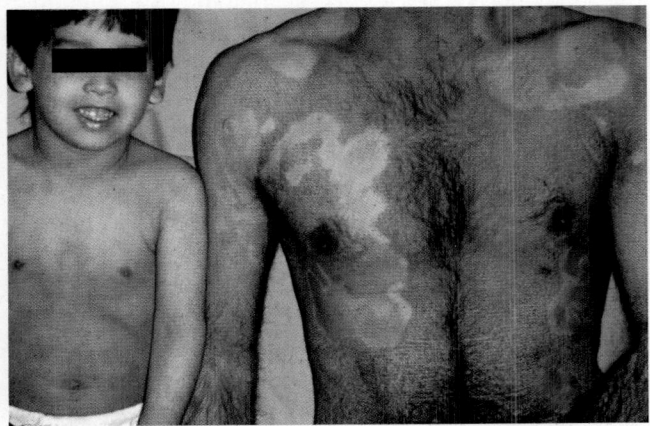

Figure 6-12 MEDNIK syndrome. Father and son with erythrokeratoderma variabilis. Circinated patches and plaques with erythema and hyperkeratosis. (Courtesy of Dr Kenneth Greer, Department of Dermatology, University of Virginia.)

develop generalized scaling on trunk and extremities. There is relative sparing of skin folds (Fig. 6-13). Affected infants present with arthrogryposis (congenital joint contracture) and develop renal tubular acidosis, as well as cholestasis, secondary to intrahepatic bile duct hypoplasia. Aminoaciduria can be seen. The hallmark neuromuscular finding is arthrogryposis or severe congenital contractures. Other findings include failure to thrive, sensorineural hearing loss, central nervous system anomalies, congenital heart defects, and platelet abnormalities leading to hemorrhage. The histopathologic findings of ARC syndrome are not well characterized.

Pathogenesis: Vacuolar protein sorting 33 homolog B (VPS33B) regulates SNARE protein-mediated fusion of membrane vesicles. VPS33B-interacting protein, apical-basolateral polarity regulatory (VIPAR) is a protein that complexes with VPS33B and is involved in orienting cells to apical-basolateral polarity. The pathogenic role in ichthyosis is related to altered lamellar body secretion.

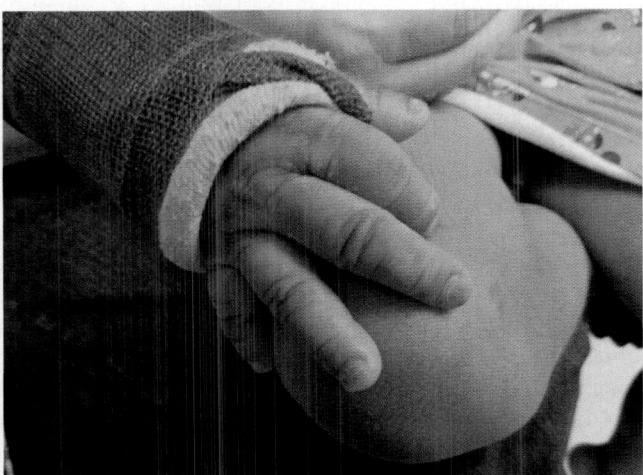

Figure 6-13 Arthrogryposis-renal dysfunction-cholestasis (ARC) syndrome. Generalized scaling on extremities with relative sparing of skin folds. (Courtesy of Dr. Nnenna Agim, Department of Dermatology, University of Texas Southwestern Medical Center.)

OTHER DISORDERS OF KERATINOCYTE DIFFERENTIATION

Erythrokeratoderma Variabilis and Progressive Symmetric Erythrokeratoderma

Clinical Summary. A rare, autosomal dominant, inherited disorder, *erythrokeratoderma variabilis (EKV)*, typically starts in infancy and is characterized by two striking morphologies. First, areas of erythema expand centrifugally and coalesce into circinate figures. These lesions fluctuate over days to weeks in their configuration and extent and thus are "variable." Second, persistent yellow-to-brown hyperkeratotic plaques develop both within the areas of erythema and in areas of apparently normal skin. The trunk, buttocks, and limbs are typically affected with relative sparing of the face (60). *Progressive symmetric erythrokeratoderma (PSEK)* is a variant of EKV characterized by *fixed,* symmetric hyperkeratotic plaques involving the extensor surfaces, the face, and buttocks. The disorder is inherited with variable penetrance and is best distinguished from EKV by the facial involvement and absence of migratory erythema, although overlap phenotypes have been reported (61,62).

Histopathology. The changes are nonspecific in both EKV and PSEK. The hyperkeratotic plaques consist of hyperkeratosis with moderate papillomatosis and acanthosis. The granular layer appears normal, being two to three cell layers thick (60).

Pathogenesis. EKV is caused by mutations I *GJB3* encoding connexin 31 (63) and *GJB4* encoding connexin 30.3 (64,65). Labeling with tritiated thymidine shows a normal rate of proliferation, and it is likely that the hyperkeratosis is secondary to retention of corneocytes because of decreased shedding of horny cells. The genetics of PSEK are still poorly understood, although missense mutations in connexin 30.3 and the loricrin gene have previously been reported in some patients (66–68).

Principles of Management: Patients tend to improve with age and during warmer months, and many are asymptomatic. Liberal use of emollients is a mainstay of treatment. Systemic retinoids have been used in some cases with improvement.

Palmoplantar Keratodermas

Clinical Summary. The palmoplantar keratodermas (PPKs) (Table 6-1) represent a heterogeneous group of diseases that share the clinical characteristic of prominent thickening of palmoplantar skin. The molecular pathogenesis of the inherited forms is linked to abnormalities in intracellular structural proteins (keratins); cornified envelope proteins (loricrin, transglutaminase); cell–cell connections (desmoglein, desmoplakin, plakophilin, connexins); and enzymatic signaling transduction (cathepsins) (69–73). They are typically classified as diffuse or focal. They may be isolated to the palmoplantar surfaces (non-transgradient) or may extend to the dorsal surfaces of the hands and feet (transgradient). The most frequent form of diffuse PPK is epidermolytic PPK, caused by mutations in the keratin-1 and keratin-9 genes. Defects in these cytoskeletal elements lead to intraepidermal blistering and subsequent hyperkeratosis. Affected patients present during infancy with thick, yellow hyperkeratosis of the palms and soles that are sharply demarcated at the borders with peripheral erythema and do not

Table 6-1

Palmoplantar Keratodermas

Type	Clinical Pattern	Inheritance	Histologic Pattern	Genetics
Unna-Thost	Diffuse	AD	Nonepidermolytic	Keratin 1
Vorner	Diffuse	AD	Epidermolytic	Keratin 9
Vohwinkel	Diffuse	AD	Nonepidermolytic	Connexin 26; Loricrin
Mal de Meleda	Diffuse	AR	Nonepidermolytic	SLURP1
Papillon-Lefevre	Diffuse	AR	Nonepidermolytic	Cathepsin C
Haim Munk	Diffuse	AR	Nonepidermolytic	Cathepsin C
Olmsted	Diffuse	AD	Nonepidermolytic	TRPV3
Carvajal	Diffuse	AR	Epidermolytic	Desmoplakin
Naxos	Diffuse	AR	Nonepidermolytic	Plakoglobin
Norrbotten	Diffuse	AR	Nonepidermolytic	Unknown
Clouston	Diffuse	AD	Nonepidermolytic	Connexin 30; Connexin 26
Richner-Hanhart	Diffuse	AR	Nonepidermolytic	TAT
Keratosis punctate palmaris et plantaris	Focal or punctate	AD	Nonepidermolytic	AAGAB
Pachyonychia congenita	Focal	AD	Non-epidermolytic	Keratins: 6a, 6b, 6c, 16, 17

AD, autosomal dominant; AR, autosomal recessive.

extend onto the dorsa of the hands and feet (non-transgradient). The major forms of diffuse PPK include the following:

1. **Diffuse epidermolytic palmoplantar keratoderma**, otherwise known as **Unna-Thost type**, is an autosomal dominant disorder characterized by diffuse hyperkeratosis of the palms and soles (Fig. 6-14). It is caused by mutations in the gene encoding keratin-1 and keratin-9 (74).

2. **Diffuse epidermolytic palmoplantar keratoderma**, otherwise known as the **Vorner type**, is clinically indistinguishable from the Unna-Thost type but histologically demonstrates epidermolytic hyperkeratosis. This disorder is inherited in an autosomal dominant fashion and is often associated with hyperhidrosis and secondary bacterial infection. This variant has been associated with mutations in keratin type 9 localized within the keratin gene cluster on chromosome 17q 12-q21 (69,75).

3. **Vohwinkel syndrome** is an autosomal dominant disorder associated with sensorineural deafness, severe mutilating PPK with a characteristic *honeycomb* pattern, and constrictions called pseudoainhum that may lead to auto-amputation. Hyperkeratotic starfish-like plaques are commonly observed on the knees, elbows, and dorsal hands. It is caused by mutations in the *GJB2* gene, which encodes connexin 26 (76,77). Mutations in the gene encoding loricrin result in a variant of *Vohwinkel syndrome* with prominent PPK and ichthyosis but normal hearing (78).

4. **Mal de Meleda** is an autosomal recessive PPK with diffuse inflammatory keratoderma of the palms and soles that extends to involve the dorsal hands (transgradient spread), feet, ankles, and wrists. Flexion contractures may occur when keratoderma overlies joints, and auto-amputation is a rare complication. The disorder is caused by mutations in *SLURP1*, a secreted epidermal neuromodulator that regulates epidermal homeostasis and inhibits macrophage-induced tumor necrosis factor (TNF)-α release, accounting for its inflammatory and hyperproliferative phenotype (79).

5. Like Mal de Meleda, **Papillon–Lefèvre syndrome** is a transgradient PPK with hyperkeratosis of the palms and soles that extends to the dorsal hands and feet. Patients often have psoriasiform plaques on the elbows and knees. Its distinguishing feature is early-onset, severe periodontitis, resulting in loss of both deciduous and permanent teeth with secondary changes in alveolar bone (80). **Haim Munk syndrome** (reported in individuals from a single religious isolate in Cochin, India) is a variant characterized by periodontitis, with additional findings of acroosteolysis, onychogryphosis, and arachnodactyly. Both disorders have been localized to abnormalities in cathepsin C localized to chromosome 11q14.1 and result from activation of serine proteases, leading to premature desquamation (75).

6. **Olmsted syndrome** (mutilating palmoplantar keratoderma with periorificial plaques) is an autosomal dominant PPK characterized by mutilating keratoderma of the palms and soles, periorificial and often intertriginous inflammatory

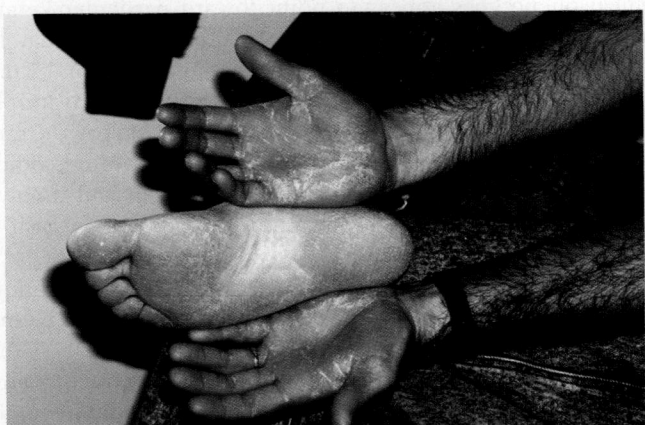

Figure 6-14 Keratosis palmaris et plantaris of Unna-Thost. Thickened palms and soles of the father, whose child has similar findings.

plaques, and alopecia that begins in infancy. The disorder can be complicated by severe contractures with auto-amputation from progressive constriction. Recently, mutations have been found in the *TRPV3* gene, which encodes a transient receptor potential vanilloid-3 cation channel, leading to apoptosis of keratinocytes with reactive hyperplasia of the epidermis (81).

Histopathology. The histopathology for all the diffuse PPKs except for *diffuse epidermolytic palmoplantar keratoderma* is nonspecific, consisting of considerable hyperkeratosis, hypergranulosis, acanthosis, and a sparse inflammatory infiltrate of lymphocytes in the upper dermis (82). *Diffuse epidermolytic palmoplantar keratoderma* demonstrates an identical histology to that seen in epidermolytic hyperkeratosis. Many cells in the middle and upper stratum spinosum appear vacuolated, and scattered cavities are present as a result of ruptured cell walls, with numerous large keratohyalin granules (83,84).

The focal (or punctate) PPKs include:

Keratosis Punctata Palmaris et Plantaris

Clinical Summary. This is an autosomal dominant disorder characterized by multiple discrete keratotic plugs on the palms and soles, which typically manifests in adolescence.

Histopathology. There is massive hyperkeratosis over a sharply limited area, with depression of the underlying malpighian layer below the general level of the epidermis. There is an increase in the thickness of the granular layer. The dermis is free of inflammation (85).

Pathogenesis. At least three forms of the disorder have been described, some of which have been mapped to the *AAGAB* gene, which encodes an alpha-and-gamma-adaptin-binding protein p34 that serves as a chaperone for membrane trafficking (86,87).

Pachyonychia Congenita

Clinical Summary. Pachyonychia congenita (PC) refers to a collection of autosomal dominant disorders characterized by early-onset nail dystrophy followed by the development of focal painful palmoplantar keratoderma sometimes with secondary bullae formation. Other notable findings include mucosal leukokeratosis (Fig. 6-15), occasionally cysts, follicular keratoses on the elbows and knees, and natal teeth. Unlike other

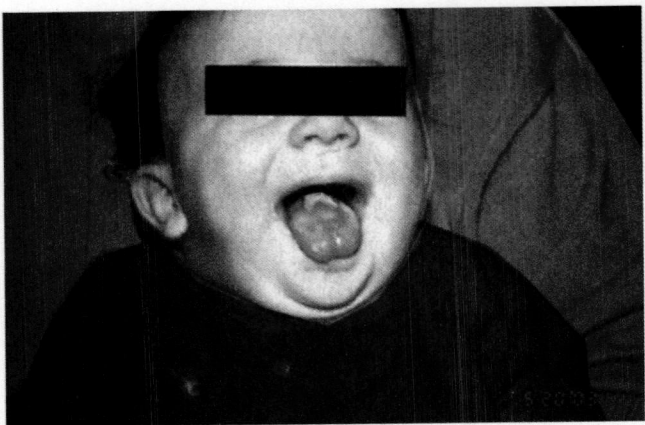

Figure 6-16 Pachyonychia congenita. Note whitened mucosa at back of tongue.

conditions associated with oral leukokeratoses, the mucosal changes in PC are benign and do not predispose to malignant degeneration (Fig. 6-16).

Histopathology. The nail bed shows marked hyperkeratosis. As in the normal nail bed, there is no granular layer. The blisters that may be seen beneath and around the plantar callosities arise in the upper layers of the stratum spinosum through increasing intracellular edema and vacuolization. Unlike friction blisters, they show no areas of necrosis (88). The oral lesions show thickening of the oral epithelium with extensive intracellular vacuolization, exactly as seen in white sponge nevus and without evidence of dyskeratosis (89).

Pathogenesis. Genetic mutations have been described in the paired keratin genes 6a, 6b, 6c, 16, and 17, which are variably expressed in the nail bed, mucosa, and palmoplantar epithelium, and lead to epidermolysis with compensatory reactive hyperkeratosis. The historical terms Jadassohn–Lewandowsky syndrome (PC-1) and Jackson–Lawler syndrome (PC-2) have been abandoned secondary to considerable overlap between subtypes in favor of a new classification scheme that categorizes disease phenotype based on specific keratin mutations. The presence of cysts, previously thought to be pathognomonic of PC-2, associated with keratin 17 mutations has now been documented in patients with keratin 6a mutations. Genotype–phenotype investigation is still ongoing through the International Pachyonychia Congenita Research Registry, but certain clinical phenotypes appear to point toward particular keratin mutations. For example, congenital nail dystrophy that involves all nails is most likely to indicate keratin 6a or 17 mutations. The concurrent presence of congenital nail dystrophy and natal teeth strongly suggests keratin 17 mutations. Childhood PPK with later development of associated features points toward keratin 16 mutations, and isolated focal nail involvement is rare but most likely to indicate underlying keratin 6c mutations (90).

PPK can also be seen in association with other unique identifying features, for example, Norrbotten recessive palmoplantar keratoderma (associated with knuckle pads). Those inherited disorders featuring PPK along with extracutaneous signs include Carvajal syndrome (dilated cardiomyopathy with epidermolytic keratoderma), Naxos disease (woolly hair, diffuse nonepidermolytic palmoplantar keratoderma, with arrhythmogenic cardiomyopathy), hidrotic ectodermal dysplasia

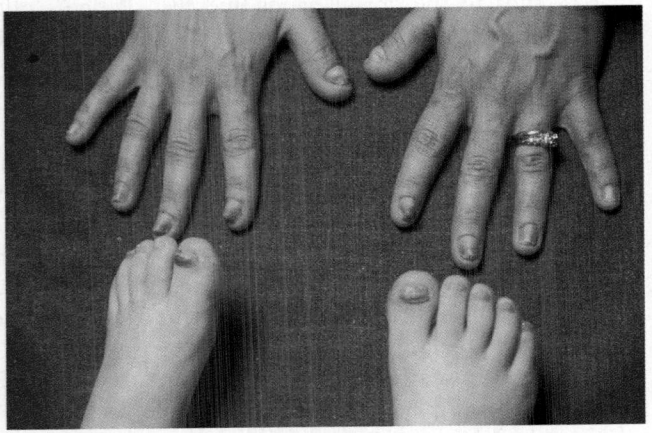

Figure 6-15 Pachyonychia congenita. Thickened nails in infant with this syndrome.

(Clouston syndrome), and Richner-Hanhart syndrome (tyrosinemia type II).

Principles of Management: Treatment of all forms of PPK includes keratolytics, soaks, and debridement as necessary, particularly for the mutilating disorders. Systemic retinoids can be helpful but should be reserved for those with severe disease and disability, given their long-term side effects.

Acrokeratoelastoidosis

Clinical Summary. Acrokeratoelastoidosis is a rare condition characterized by shiny, firm, yellow-to-translucent, sometimes umbilicated papules, which develop at the periphery of the palms and soles with extension to the dorsa of the fingers and the sides of the feet (Fig. 6-17) (91). Autosomal dominant inheritance is most common, although some cases appear to be sporadic. Most patients develop the disorder in childhood or adolescence, but presentation in adulthood has also been reported. Associated findings may include diffuse palmoplantar keratoderma and hyperhidrosis (92).

Histopathology. Elastorrhexis is the essential histologic feature of acrokeratoelastoidosis, with diminution and fragmentation of the elastic fibers, especially in the deeper portions of the papillary dermis sparing the reticular dermis (91). Some of the fragmented elastic fibers may appear thickened and tortuous (93). Additional histopathologic findings include focal hyperkeratosis, acanthosis, and hypergranulosis (94).

Pathogenesis. The pathogenesis remains speculative. There are some data to suggest that acrokeratoelastoidosis results from failed secretion of elastin from fibroblasts, rather than from degeneration of elastic fibers (95). Formation of the discrete papules may result from filaggrin aggregation (96).

Differential Diagnosis. Focal acral hyperkeratosis looks identical clinically but lacks elastorrhexis on histopathology (94). *Degenerative collagenous plaques of the hands* are typically concentrated on the index finger and opposing thumb in white men with chronic sun exposure and repetitive trauma from manual labor. There is no familial predisposition. Histologic changes consist of basophilic degeneration of the elastic tissue (91).

Principles of Management: Most patients are asymptomatic and require no treatment. Topical keratolytics such as urea 40% cream have been reported to be helpful to some patients.

The Porokeratoses

The term "porokeratosis" refers to a group of disorders characterized by a distinct "thread-like" peripheral hyperkeratotic ridge that histologically corresponds to the cornoid lamella, a column of parakeratosis arising from an invagination of the epidermis (Fig. 6-12). It was originally coined by Mibelli in 1893, who erroneously believed that the cornoid lamella arose from sweat pores (97).

Clinical Summary. The porokeratoses are speculated to arise from a local clonal proliferation of abnormal keratinocytes, although the genetics are still incompletely understood. Five different forms have been described (98).

One or more annular, hyperkeratotic plaques that develop in childhood and subsequently enlarge from the periphery over years characterize classic **porokeratosis of Mibelli**. Lesions initiate as hyperkeratotic papules that can enlarge to several centimeters in diameter. The characteristic keratotic border has been likened to the "Great Wall of China" and correlates to the cornoid lamella on histopathology. Rarely, numerous lesions may develop, and these are typically unilateral. Boys are more commonly affected. Transmission may be autosomal dominant with incomplete penetrance, or through a sporadic event (99). Porokeratosis can be caused by several different somatic mutations that result in clonal proliferation of keratinocytes with abnormal maturation. Among the genes implicated are *PMVK* (phosphomevalonate kinase), *MVD* (mevalonate phosphate decarboxylase), *MVK* (mevalonate kinase), and *SLC17A9* (100–103).

Disseminated superficial actinic porokeratosis (DSAP), the most common of the porokeratoses, is an autosomal dominant disorder with incomplete penetrance that typically manifests in the third or fourth decade of life (104). Multiple (>50) atrophic circinate plaques with a thread-like border occur most commonly on sun-exposed surfaces, typically the lower legs and arms, and may be exacerbated by exposure to sun (Fig. 6-18). However, the

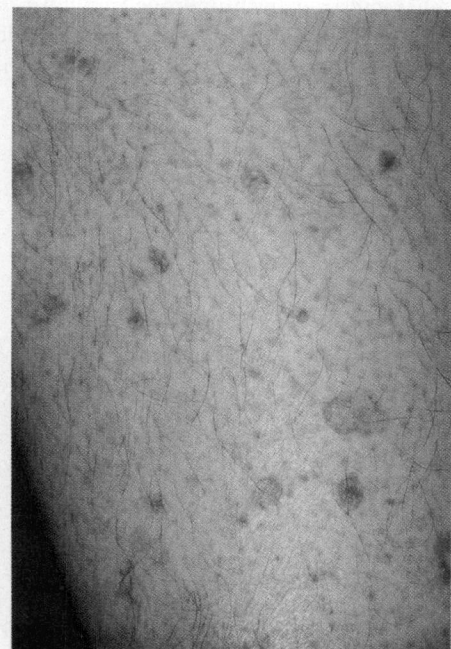

Figure 6-18 Disseminated actinic porokeratosis. Numerous pink-brown plaques on the leg, with a characteristic raised peripheral rim. (Photograph by William K. Witmer.)

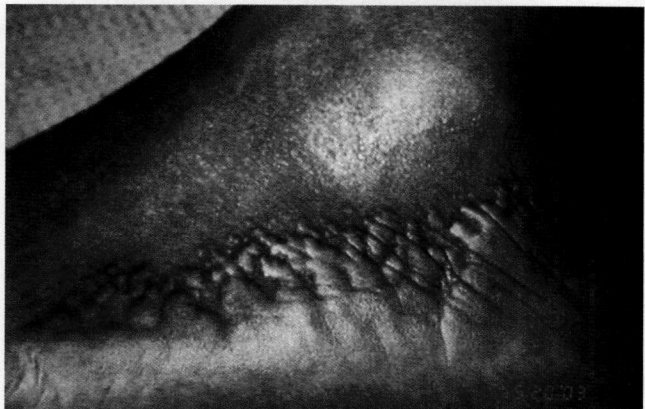

Figure 6-17 Acrokeratoelastoidosis. Firm papules on the lateral foot.

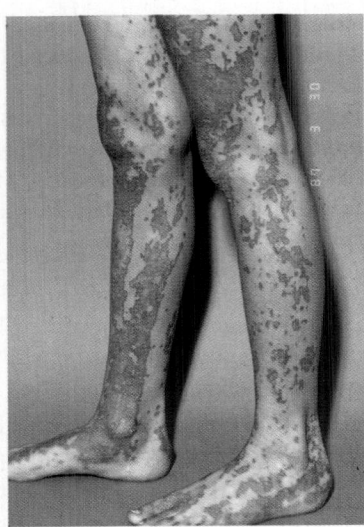

Figure 6-19 Linear porokeratosis. Linear hyperkeratosis along the feet and legs.

term *actic* cannot be applied to all cases. The main risk factors for DSAP include sun exposure, genetic susceptibility, and immunosuppression, presumably because of reduced immune surveillance (98). Interestingly, immunosuppressed patients with DSAP do not appear at greater risk for malignant transformation than other patients, in spite of a higher risk of *de novo* skin cancers (105). Mutations in the mevalonate kinase (*MVK*) gene have been found in some patients, although the function of this enzyme in DSAP pathogenesis is unclear (106).

Linear porokeratosis may involve only a segment of the body or may be generalized, but it typically follows Blaschko lines (Fig. 6-19). Presentation in infancy or childhood is most common. It likely represents a form of type II mosaicism, reflecting loss of heterozygosity in early development with proliferation of a single-cell clone (107).

Punctate porokeratosis, with onset in childhood or adolescence, is characterized by numerous punctate 1- to 2-mm seed-like keratotic plugs limited to the palms and soles, without tendency to centrifugal enlargement. They may be moderately tender to pressure (108).

Porokeratosis plantaris, palmaris, et disseminata is an autosomal dominant variant of punctate porokeratosis characterized by keratotic papules on the palms and soles in childhood or early adolescence with subsequent generalization to other areas of the body. Both sun-exposed and sun-protected skin may be involved. Males are more commonly affected, but the genetic cause remains unknown (109,110).

The development of nonmelanoma skin cancers (predominantly squamous cell carcinoma or Bowen disease) within lesions of porokeratosis is well documented, with increased p53 expression found in some cases (111,112). A review of 281 individuals with porokeratosis from 1964 to 1994 found the highest incidence of skin carcinoma development in patients with linear porokeratosis (19%), followed by porokeratosis palmaris and plantaris (9.5%), porokeratosis of Mibelli (7.6%), DSAP (3.4%), and punctate porokeratosis (0%) (105). None of the patients who developed cutaneous malignancies were iatrogenically immunosuppressed, although two patients had congenital genodermatoses (Werner and Bloom syndromes).

Histopathology. It is important that the biopsy specimen include the peripheral, raised, hyperkeratotic ridge. On histologic examination, the ridge correlates to a keratin-filled invagination of the epidermis. In classic porokeratosis of Mibelli, the invagination extends deeply downward at an angle, the apex of which points away from the central portion of the lesion. In the center of this keratin-filled invagination rises a parakeratotic column, the cornoid lamella, representing the most characteristic feature of porokeratosis (Fig. 6-20A, B) (97). Within the parakeratotic column, the cells appear homogeneous and possess pyknotic nuclei. In the epidermis beneath the parakeratotic column, the keratinocytes are irregularly arranged and have pyknotic nuclei with perinuclear edema. Dyskeratotic keratinocytes can be seen in the epithelium at the base of the cornoid lamella. In the upper stratum spinosum, some cells possess an eosinophilic cytoplasm as a result of premature keratinization (113). Typically, the site at which the parakeratotic column arises lacks a granular layer, but elsewhere the granular layer is preserved. The histologic changes in the other forms of porokeratosis are similar but less pronounced than those seen in classic porokeratosis of Mibelli (Fig. 6-19).

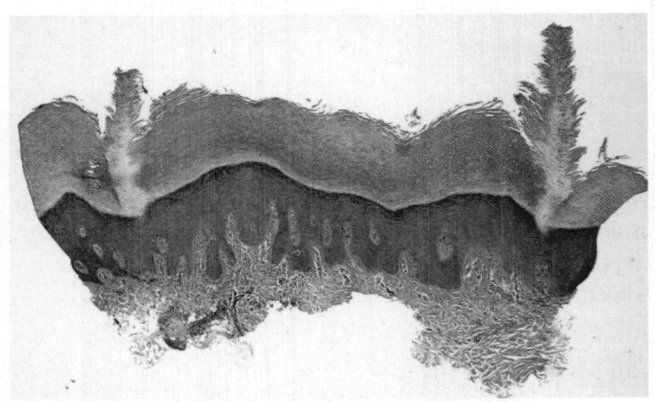

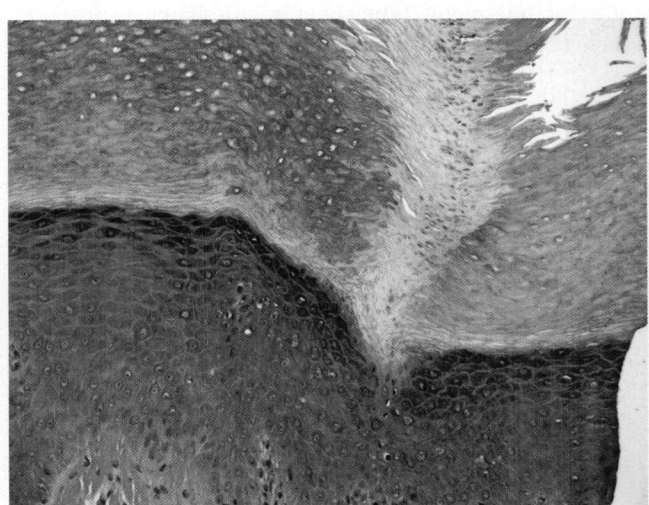

Figure 6-20 **A:** Porokeratosis. Prominent cornoid lamellae at the edges of the biopsy (original magnification ×40). **B:** Porokeratosis. A cornoid lamella consists of a column of parakeratosis and hypogranulosis underneath (original magnification ×100). (Reprinted with permission from Gru AA. *Pediatric Dermatopathology and Dermatology*. Wolters Kluwer; 2019.)

Because the peripheral raised ridge in porokeratosis slowly moves centrifugally, it stands to reason that the invagination is not bound to a definite structure, such as the sweat pore, as originally assumed by Mibelli. Although the invagination may be seen occasionally within a sweat pore or a pilosebaceous follicle, it is found most commonly in the epidermis independent of these cutaneous appendages (114). The epidermis overlying the central portion of a lesion of porokeratosis may be atrophic, normal in thickness, or rarely, acanthotic. A nonspecific perivascular infiltrate of chronic inflammatory cells is present in the dermis.

Transmission electron microscopic examination reveals signs of degeneration in keratinocytes beneath the parakeratotic column, with pyknotic nuclei, large perinuclear vacuoles that are separated from one another by cytoplasmic strands, and condensation of tonofilaments at their periphery (115). At the base of the parakeratotic column, dyskeratotic cells composed of nuclear remnants and aggregated tonofilaments are seen. The parakeratotic column is composed chiefly of cells with a pyknotic nucleus and a cytoplasm possessing high electron density because of the presence of many partially degraded organelles (116).

Differential Diagnosis. Although the presence of cornoid lamella is essential for the diagnosis of porokeratosis, it is not a specific finding, and it can be seen in other conditions including verruca vulgaris and actinic keratosis (117). The histologic differential diagnosis of punctate porokeratosis may include plantar or palmar verrucae. Clinical information, including age of onset, inheritance, and number and size of lesions, may be helpful in establishing a specific diagnosis.

Principles of Management: A variety of destructive therapies can be tried for cosmesis, including topical retinoids, topical 5-fluorouracil, cryotherapy, photodynamic therapy, or electrodesiccation. All patients with persistent porokeratosis should be monitored for the development of secondary skin cancers, particularly as they reach adulthood.

CONGENITAL BULLOUS DISORDERS

Epidermolysis Bullosa

Clinical Summary. Epidermolysis bullosa (EB) refers to a group of heritable skin fragility disorders caused by mutations in at least 18 genes (118). This group of disorders is further divided based on the clinical, histologic, and electron microscopic findings. Four subcategories of EB are recognized: epidermal, junctional, dermal, and Kindler syndrome (Table 6-2) (119). In general, patients with EB develop blistering at site of minor

Table 6-2

Epidermolysis Bullosa

Location of Cleavage	EB Type	EB Subtypes	Gene Product
Intraepidermal	Suprabasal EBS	Lethal acantholytic EB	Desmoplakin
		Plakophilin deficiency	Plakophilin1
	Basal EBS	Localized EBS	Keratin 5 and 14
		Dowling-Meara EBS	Keratin 14
		Other generalized EBS	Keratin 5 and 14
		EBS with mottled pigmentation	Keratin 5
		EBS with muscular dystrophy	Keratin 5 and 14
		EBS with pyloric atresia	Plectin
		Autosomal recessive EBS	$\alpha6\beta4$ integrin
		Migratory circinate EBS	Keratin 5
		EBS Ogna	Keratin 5, tail
			Plectin
Lamina lucida	Junctional EB	Herlitz JEB	Laminin 332
		Non-Herlitz JEB	Laminin 332
			Type 17 Collagen
		JEB with pyloric atresia	$\alpha6\beta4$ integrin
		JEB inversa	Laminin 332
		LOC syndrome	Laminin 332, $\alpha3$ chain
Sublamina densa	Dystrophic EB	Dominant DEB	Type VII Collagen
		Recessive DEB	
Mixed	Kindler		Kindlin-1

AD, autosomal dominant; AR, autosomal recessive; DEB, dystrophic epidermolysis bullosa; EB, epidermolysis bullosa; EBS, epidermolysis bullosa simplex; JEB, junctional EB.

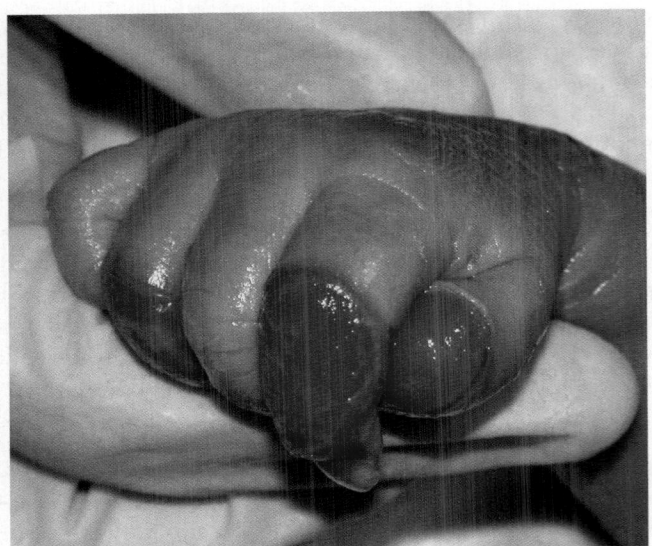

Figure 6-21 Epidermal bullosa simplex. Superficial blistering on the hand in a child with epidermolysis bullosa simplex confirmed with genetic testing. (Courtesy of Albert Yan, CHOP Dermatology.)

friction or trauma. Identification of the subtype of EB is important to guide medical management for patients and provides valuable information for prognosis, surveillance, and genetic counseling in affected families.

Epidermolysis bullosa acquisita (EBA) is an immunobullous disorder that may present in childhood but occurs more commonly in adults; it is fully discussed in Chapter 9.

Epidermolysis bullosa simplex (EBS) refers to the EB subtypes demonstrating intraepidermal bulla formation. Most patients present symptoms at birth, but a small subset may not develop clinically appreciable skin fragility until adolescence. The cleavage plane is within the epidermis and healing occurs spontaneously without scarring (Fig. 6-21). EB simplex is further classified by the extent of involvement and other associations (120,121). The most prevalent subtypes are in the basal category and include localized EBS (66% of cases), generalized severe EBS (7%), generalized intermediate EBS (6%), EBS with mottled pigmentation (0.4%), and EBS with muscular dystrophy. The Dowling-Meara variant may show generalized blistering, including involvement of the mucous membranes that at times is associated with mortality during early infancy (122,123). High mortality is also seen in lethal acantholytic EB (LAEB). There is generalized epidermolysis of the skin and respiratory and gastrointestinal tracts (124).

Junctional EB (JEB) presents with cleavage through the lamina lucida and therefore heals with scarring (Fig. 6-22A, B). Classic signs in the neonatal period include blistering in the diaper area or along the back. The blisters may have a "herpetiform" or raised appearance resulting from the granulation tissue. Fingernails and hair abnormalities are also present. Widespread ulceration is often seen in the most severe variant Herlitz JEB, and respiratory and gastrointestinal tract involvement leads to high mortality (123). Less severe presentations have a higher survival rate. Periorificial blistering is particularly prominent in JEB with excessive granulation tissue noted in variants associated with laminin 332 mutation (125). Perioral granulation tissue associated with respiratory granulation

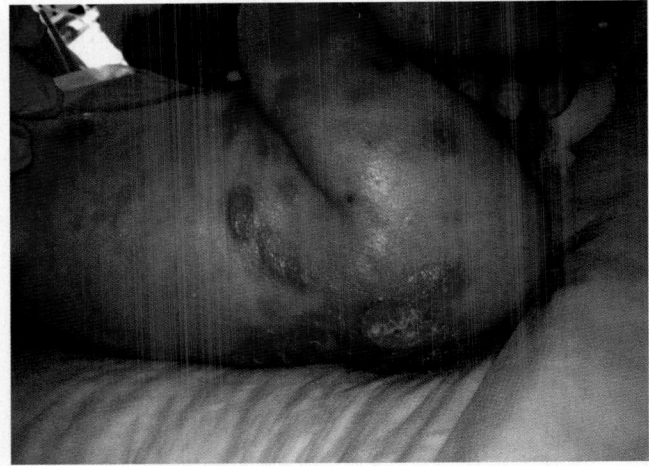

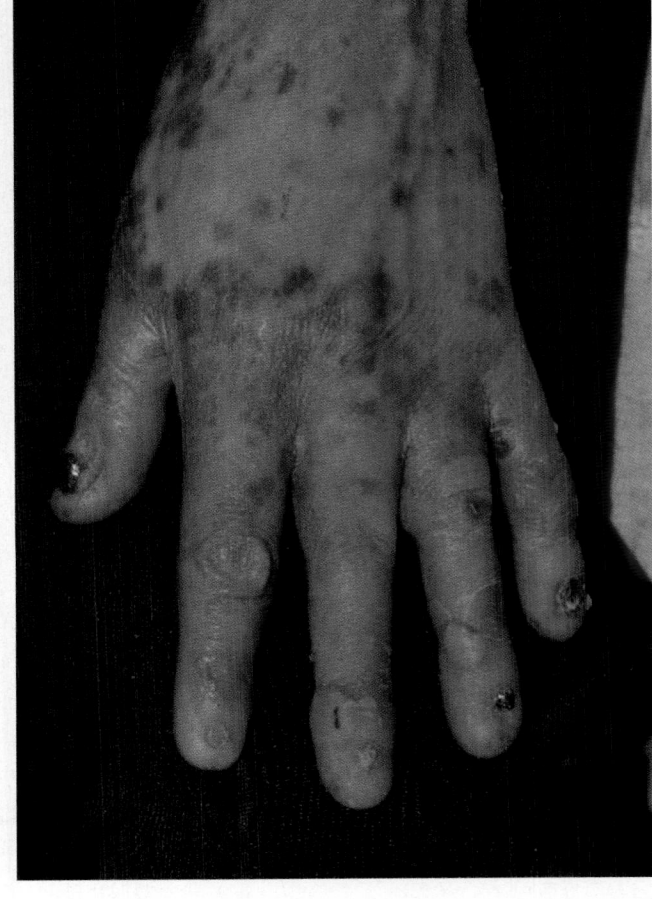

Figure 6-22 A: Junctional epidermolysis bullosa. Granulation tissue present in the wounds. **B:** Junctional epidermolysis bullosa. Finger nail involvement and dyspigmentation. (Courtesy of Kristen Hook, MD.)

tissue formation is characteristic of laryngo–onycho–cutaneous syndrome, also secondary to mutations in laminin 332. Patients with JEB have an especially high risk of highly aggressive squamous cell carcinomas (126,127).

Subepidermal blistering and ulceration is seen in dystrophic EB, including recessive and dominant variants. Dominant dystrophic EB has an acral predilection and often heals with milia and scarring. Recessive dystrophic EB is the most severe of the congenital bullous disorders. Blistering is generalized and patients may have severe involvement of the mucosal surfaces as well. Severe scarring leads to fusion of the fingers in toes, resulting in pseudosyndactyly (Fig. 6-23). Patients are at risk of recurrent skin infections and nutritional deficiency, which may necessitate placement of a feeding tube. In early adulthood, the ulcers, milia formation, and scars of the skin, mouth, and esophagus may give rise to aggressive squamous cell carcinomas (126). Rarely, EB may be transient and heal within a few months and has been termed bullous dermolysis in newborns (128). It is likely that most cases published as Bart syndrome, which was originally described as congenital absence of the skin (129), belong in this group.

Like other forms of EB, neonates with Kindler syndrome present with trauma-induced blistering most predominately in acral locations (130). The blistering dramatically improves or resolves with age. Photosensitivity with the development of poikiloderma is progressive. These cutaneous features are associated with mucosal involvement of the gingiva and anogenital mucosa. Severe colitis may result (131). Pseudosyndactyly and squamous cell carcinoma can be seen in areas of scarring but is less severe than in recessive dystrophic EB (132,133).

Histopathology. A biopsy is best taken from an induced blister because it will show a blister free of secondary changes. In an existing blister, the location of the blister may have changed as a result of regeneration of keratinocytes at the base of the blister or degeneration of the keratinocytes over the blister. The mode of artificially producing a blister depends on the degree of vulnerability of the skin. However, in most instances, gentle friction with a pencil eraser is used, or in older children, an activity that is known to induce blisters (134). Transmission electron microscopic examination has traditionally been the standard criterion for diagnosis of EB subtypes, but increased availability of immunofluorescence mapping techniques has added to the histologic diagnosis of EB and is able to guide more targeted genetic testing (135). Light microscopic features seen in the various forms of EB can be of additional diagnostic value. If possible, specimens of artificially induced blisters should be subjected to electron microscopic examination or immunofluorescence mapping to help guide diagnosis and therapy (134,136).

In EB simplex, the primary separation in induced blisters occurs within the basal cell layer. Spontaneously arising blisters may be found subepidermally as the result of complete disintegration of the basal cell layer. In bullae of more than a day's duration, the cleavage may be found intraepidermally or subcorneally because of epidermal regeneration, thereby confusing the interpretation. Faint remnants of basal keratinocyte cytoplasm may remain attached to the dermis. Blisters are also often multiloculated, particularly in early lesions. Very early lesions may show only prominent vacuolization (sometimes referred to as "cytolysis") of the basal layer keratinocyte cytoplasm just below the nucleus.

In JEB, the trauma of having a specimen taken for biopsy generally is sufficient to induce separation. This separation is located between the epidermis and the dermis (Fig. 6-24).

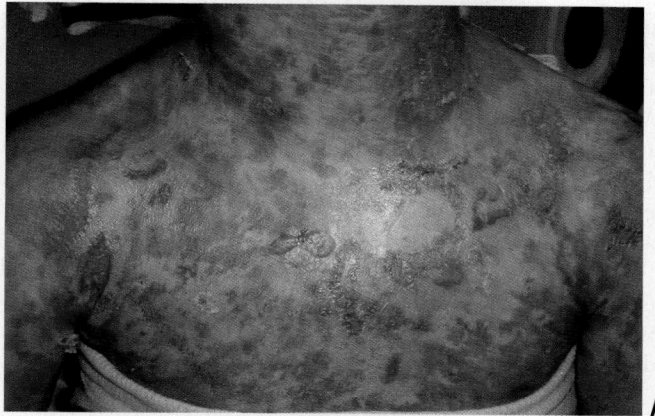

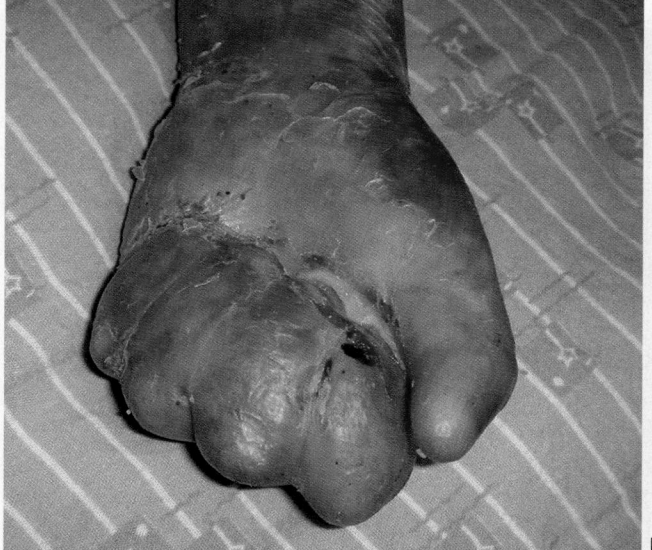

A

B

Figure 6-23 Recessive dystrophic epidermolysis bullosa. Child with generalized blisters and scarring (**A**) as well as mitten deformity of hands (**B**). (Courtesy of Albert Yan, CHOP Dermatology.)

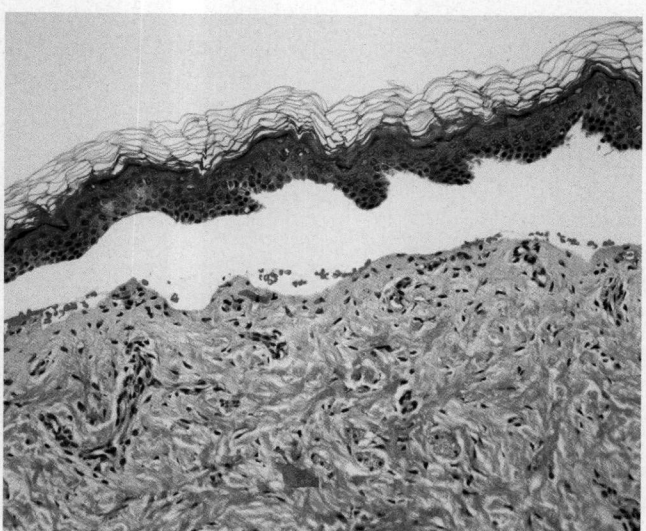

Figure 6-24 Junctional epidermolysis bullosa. A pauci-cellular subepidermal blister is present (original magnification ×200).

In Herlitz JEB, autopsy experience has revealed extensive sub-epithelial separation in the gastrointestinal, respiratory, and urinary tracts also. There are no morphologic or enzymatic abnormalities that can help distinguish the atrophic benign form of JEB from Herlitz JEB. In contrast to EBS, JEB lesions lack cells or debris within the blister cavity. There is typically no significant associated inflammatory infiltrate. Absence of hypoplastic hemidesmosomes can be noted with ultrastructural examination. IHC or DIF mapping identifies BP antigen-180 on the roof of the blister, whereas laminin or collagen IV is identified along the floor of the blister (137,138).

In dominant dystrophic EB and recessive dystrophic EB, light microscopy shows dermal–epidermal separation. The split occurs below the lamina densa, and there is a subepidermal vesicle that lacks significant inflammation. Scar tissue is a frequent finding in these biopsies. Many times biopsies are taken to exclude the possibility of squamous cell carcinoma. Despite the relative low-grade appearance of these tumors, most patients will develop metastatic squamous cell carcinoma within 5 years after the diagnosis.

The histology of Kindler syndrome depends on the characteristics of the lesion that is biopsied. A skin biopsy from an area of poikiloderma will show epidermal atrophy and loss of the rete ridges. Hyperkeratosis is variable (130,139). Pigmentary incontinence, blood vessel dilation, and elastosis may be found in the dermis. Abnormal distribution of melanosomes may be seen (139). A biopsy of a bullous area shows the cleavage plane on different levels.

The immunomapping procedure for diagnosis of EB consists of exposing cryostat sections to EB-relevant antibodies (119,140). The panel of antibodies used can define a more precise level of cleavage. Additional information is gained by looking at relative staining intensity of the targeted antibodies that can reveal the underlying molecular defects causing skin fragility in patients with EB (Fig. 6-25). Using an expanded panel of antibodies, higher sensitivity and specificity were demonstrated with immunofluorescence mapping over electron microscopy, in at least one center's experience (140).

Pathogenesis. In the epidermal types of EB, microscopic examination most frequently shows cleavage resulting from degenerative cytolytic changes occurring in the lower portion of the basal cells between the dermal–epidermal junction and the nucleus. Immunofluorescence mapping shows that all three antigens (type IV collagen, laminin, bullous pemphigoid antigen) are located beneath the cleavage. Mutations of keratin genes for *KRT5* and *KRT14* on chromosomes 12 and 17, respectively, have been demonstrated in EBS and these proteins can be demonstrated to be reduced or absent. The perturbation of keratin filament assembly results in the clumping of tonofilaments in basal keratinocytes. Rarer subtypes of EBS (Table 6-2) have identified mutations in α6β4 integrin, transglutaminase 5, desmoplakin, plakoglobin, plakophilin 1, exophilin, bullous pemphigoid antigen-1, and plectin, resulting in poor integration of keratin filaments into hemidesmosomes (121,141). Intraepidermal cleavage is seen in subtypes caused by plakophilin and desmoplakin deficiency. EM examination demonstrates perinuclear retraction of keratin filaments (140).

In the junctional types of EB, electron microscopic examination often shows abnormal hemidesmosomes, especially in Herlitz JEB. They may be reduced in size or number and may lack their subbasal cell-dense plaque (141). Immunofluorescence mapping shows type IV collagen and laminin on the floor of the blister. Bullous pemphigoid antigen is present mainly on the blister roof with a patchy and far lesser distribution on the blister floor. Mutations have been found in any of three polypeptides of laminin 332 (formerly laminin 5): α-3 (LAMA3), BETA-3 (LAMB3), and GAMMA-2 (LAMC2). This mutation reduces adhesion between the epidermis and dermis (142). In Herlitz JEB, laminin 332 is absent or more severely affected, leading to the more severe clinical phenotype. Non-Herlitz JEB may be caused by missense laminin 332, collagen 17, or α6β4 integrin mutations. Here, the relevant gene products are reduced on immunofluorescence (140). Electron microscopy shows more variability in the hemidesmosomal size and number (141).

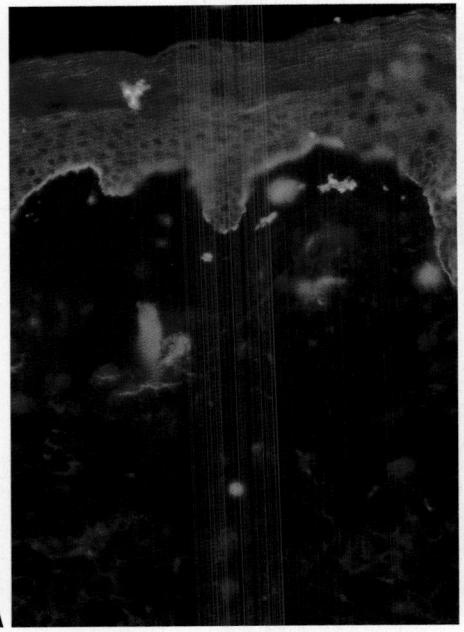
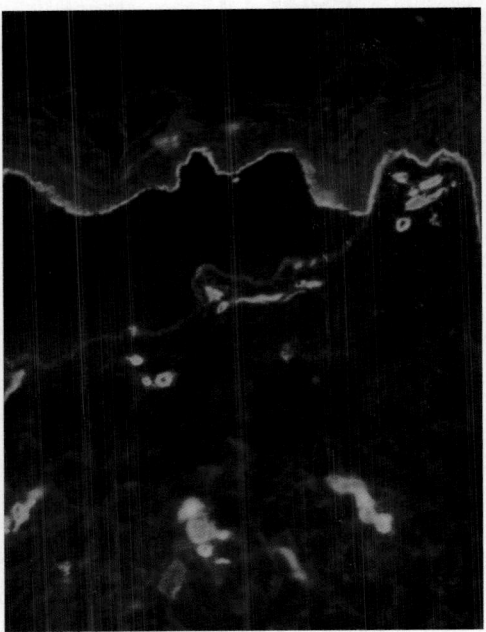

Figure 6-25 Immunofluorescence mapping for epidermolysis bullosa. In this case of dystrophic epidermolysis bullosa, BP180 (**A**) and laminin (**B**) can be seen on the roof of the blister (original magnification ×200). (These images are courtesy of Lori Prok, MD, University of Colorado and Children's Hospital Colorado.)

On electron microscopy, the dermal types of EB show abnormalities in anchoring fibrils. Generalized recessive dystrophic EB demonstrates absence of the anchoring fibrils even in nonlesional skin, which is established through the lack of a reaction with monoclonal antibodies to the anchoring fibrils. Mutations in the gene encoding type VII collagen (*COL 7A1*) located at chromosome band 3p21 have been reported to cause these abnormal findings in the dystrophic forms of EB (143,144). Because type VII collagen is a major structural component of the anchoring fibrils, immunofluorescence staining with polyclonal antibodies to type VII collagen reveals complete absence of staining, even in the unaffected skin of patients with severe dystrophic recessive EB (140). Similarly, there is no reaction with periodic acid–thiosemicarbazide–silver proteinate, which stains anchoring fibrils selectively (145). In both dominant dystrophic EB and in localized recessive dystrophic EB, structurally normal anchoring fibrils are present but are reduced in number and function (146). Immunofluorescence mapping shows all three basement membrane zone constituents—bullous pemphigoid antigen, laminin, and type IV collagen—on top of the cleavage (140).

Kindler syndrome is unique among EB subtypes in that the layer of separation is variable. The *FERMT1* gene, which is mutated, plays important roles in keratinocyte migration, adhesion, and proliferation. This effect is at least in part through the activation of integrin function. Loss of FERMT1 activity leads to loss of cell adhesion as seen by electron microscopy as clefting within the basal keratinocytes, lamina lucida, or below the lamina densa. Hemidesmosomes and anchoring fibrils remain intact. There is disorganization of the basement membrane zone with characteristic reduplication of the lamina densa (147). Diminished integrin function may also account for epidermal atrophy through decreased epidermal proliferation.

Differential Diagnosis. Clinically, the distinction among the subtypes of EB can sometimes be challenging at birth. Diagnostic biopsies and genetic testing can aid in securing the diagnosis that is critical for management and prognostic significance. When presenting in a neonate, infectious etiologies of bulla must be considered excluded, including, but not limited to, congenital varicella, herpes simplex viral infection, and *Staphylococcus aureus* infection, leading to bullous impetigo or staph scalded skin syndrome. Autoimmune bullous disorders should also be considered. Infants born to mothers with pemphigus foliaceus, pemphigus vulgaris, and bullous pemphigoid may have transplacental passage of antigens and transient disease. Infants with epidermolytic hyperkeratosis may present with flaccid bullae or erosions that may mimic EB. Histologically, when confronted with a paucicellular vesicular process, one could consider entities such as cell poor bullous pemphigoid, porphyria, EBA, and friction blisters. However, clinical correlation and additional targeted testing as described above will assist in establishing a final diagnosis.

Principles of Management: The mainstay of EB management continues to be meticulous wound care and infection control. Nutritional support is important for the more severe forms. For scarring forms of EB, monitoring the development of cutaneous malignancy and conservative management when they do arise is of utmost importance. Allogeneic bone marrow transplant has been reported to improve fragility in some patients with recessive dystrophic EB (126). Experimental methods of gene correction and protein replacement for severe, scarring EB are emerging (148).

Familial Benign Pemphigus (Hailey–Hailey Disease)

Clinical Summary. Familial benign pemphigus is an autosomal dominant genodermatosis, with a family history obtainable in about two-thirds of patients. It presents in teenagers and young adults, usually at or after puberty, although presentation in infants has been infrequently described (149). It is characterized by a localized, recurrent eruption of small vesicles, erosions, and crusted plaques in the intertriginous areas, typically the lateral neck, in the axillae, groin, and perianal areas (Fig. 6-26). The scalp, chest, antecubital fossae, and popliteal fossae are less commonly involved. Mucosal involvement is rare. By peripheral extension, the lesions may assume a circinate configuration. The predilection of Hailey–Hailey disease for intertriginous areas, especially the axillae and the groin, likely has to do with the contribution of heat, moisture, and friction to the development of the erosions. Bacterial and candida superinfection is common. Rare instances of mucosal involvement have been reported, including the mouth, the labia majora, and the esophagus. The disease follows a chronic relapsing and remitting course, and it can be triggered by factors such as trauma, sweating, infection, pregnancy, and UV exposure.

Histopathology. Whereas early lesions may show small suprabasal separations, so-called lacunae, fully developed lesions show large separations in a predominantly suprabasal position

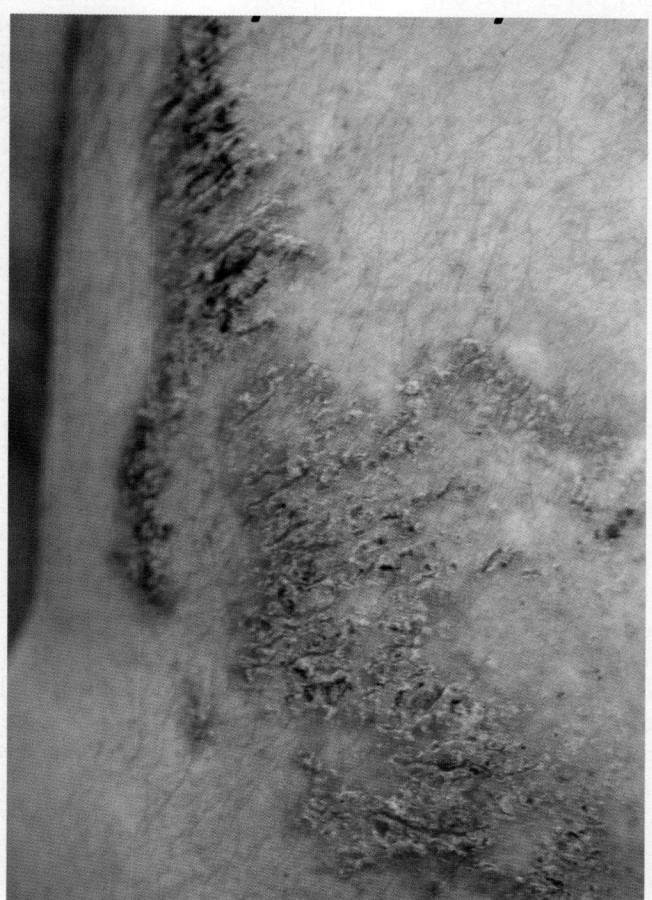

Figure 6-26 Familial benign pemphigus (Hailey–Hailey). Recurrent eruption of small vesicles, erosions, and crusted plaques in the intertriginous areas, typically the lateral neck, in the axillae, groin, and perianal areas. (Reprinted with permission from Gru AA. *Pediatric Dermatopathology and Dermatology.* Wolters Kluwer; 2019.)

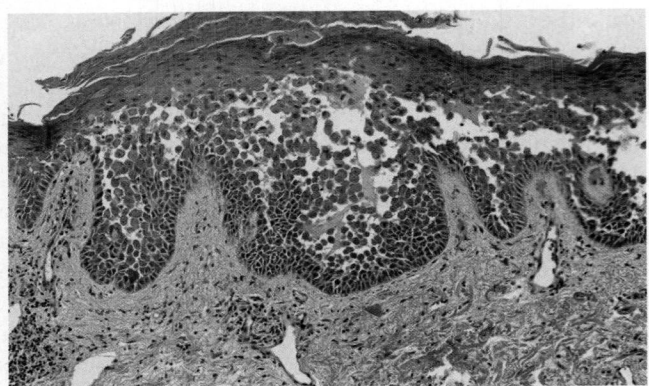

Figure 6-27 Familial benign pemphigus (Hailey–Hailey). The bulla is largely in a suprabasal position. The extensive loss of intercellular bridges with partial coherence of cells gives the detached epidermis the appearance of a dilapidated brick wall (original magnification ×40).

(Fig. 6-27). Villi, which are elongated papillae lined by a single layer of basal cells, protrude upward into the bulla, and in some cases, narrow strands of epidermal cells proliferate downward into the dermis. Many cells of the detached stratum malpighii show loss of their intercellular bridges with acantholysis affecting large portions of the epidermis. Despite the extensive loss of intercellular bridges, the cells of the detached epidermis in many places show only slight separation from one another because a few intact intercellular bridges still hold them loosely together, leading to the so-called "dilapidated brick wall" appearance of the disease. Large numbers of individual and groups of cells are often seen in the bulla cavity. Unlike Darier disease, adnexal involvement is not common. The coexistence of HHD and infection from herpes simplex viruses have been subject to case reports (150,151).

Many of the cells of the stratum malpighii that have lost their intercellular bridges show a relatively normal cytoplasm and a normal nucleus in which mitotic activity is preserved. Some of the acantholytic cells, however, have a homogenized cytoplasm, suggesting premature partial keratinization. Such acantholytic cells with premature keratinization resemble the grains of Darier disease. Occasionally, a few corps ronds are present in the granular layer.

Pathogenesis. Genetic studies have localized the key mutations to the *ATP2C1* gene on chromosome 3q, specifically 3q21-q24 (152). Clinical variability is attributed to haploinsufficiency (153). This locus encodes the SPCA pumps that are responsible for ATP-dependent calcium transport along with the SERCA proteins that are mutated in Darier disease (154,155). The defective pump protein leads to decreased calcium content in the usually calcium-rich basal keratinocytes (156). It is hypothesized that the calcium defect disrupts protein processing, leading to a failure to process desmosomal proteins and, therefore, to a loss of cell–cell adhesion (154). Keratin expression and keratinocyte differentiation may also be affected (156). Exacerbation by physical stress such as heat and friction may lead to an additive decrease in SPCA expression.

Differential Diagnosis. Histologically, familial benign pemphigus shares certain features with Darier disease and pemphigus vulgaris, vegetans, and foliaceous. In all the diseases, one finds predominantly suprabasal separation of the epidermis caused by acantholysis and resulting in lacunae or bullae and villi

formation. Infections such as erythrasma and intertrigo with candidiasis, in addition to extramammary Paget disease, may also show overlapping features.

Several features can distinguish familial benign pemphigus from Darier disease because in Darier disease, the suprabasal separations are usually smaller, thus appearing as lacunae rather than as bullae; acantholysis is less pronounced, being limited to the lower epidermis, especially the suprabasal region; and dyskeratosis consisting of the formation of corps ronds and grains is much more evident.

Pemphigus vulgaris often resembles familial benign pemphigus, and the histologic differentiation of these two diseases may be impossible. There is generally less extensive acantholysis in pemphigus vulgaris, and it is limited largely to the suprabasal region. Therefore, the detached epidermis appears normal and lacks the appearance of a dilapidated brick wall. There is more severe degeneration of the acantholytic cells within and near the bulla cavity. The presence of eosinophils in the bulla points toward a diagnosis of pemphigus vulgaris, but their absence does not rule it out. Correlation of the findings on the routinely prepared sections with immunofluorescence and/or ELISA testing can establish a specific diagnosis.

Principles of Management: Reduction of triggering factors such as heat, friction, and moisture is the mainstay of treatment. Topical steroids and other anti-inflammatory preparations can be useful in reducing symptoms. Bacterial and fungal infections may exacerbate symptoms and require topical or systemic antimicrobial therapy.

Keratosis Follicularis (Darier Disease)

Clinical Summary. Darier disease is an autosomal dominant genodermatosis characterized by progressive hyperkeratotic or crusted papules in a seborrheic distribution (Fig. 6-28A, B). The peak age of onset is near the time of puberty, although congenital cases have also been described (157). The disease presents typically in the second decade of life, with pruritic, red-brown to yellowish papules on the scalp, forehead, alar creases, ears, and upper trunk. Mild axillary involvement is common, although there is a small subset of patients in which flexural disease predominates. The oral mucosa may be involved (158). Flexural involvement often results in vegetative lesions with maceration and superinfection that can lead to distressing malodor. In some cases of Darier disease, keratotic papules that resemble those seen in acrokeratosis verruciformis of Hopf may be found on the dorsal hands and feet. Nails show longitudinal erythronychia, longitudinal leukonychia, and distal V-shaped nicks in the nail plate secondary to nail fragility. These nail findings are sometimes referred to as "candy cane nails."

Keratosis follicularis may occur as a number of clinical variants including hypertrophic, vesiculobullous, and segmental Darier disease. In the hypertrophic type, widespread, markedly thickened, and hyperkeratotic lesions are seen, especially in the intertriginous areas. In the vesiculobullous type, vesicles and small bullae are seen in addition to papules. Segmental Darier disease is usually limited to one side in a blaschkolinear distribution and may be present at birth or acquired. The designation acantholytic dyskeratotic epidermal nevus has been suggested; however, mutations in *ATP2A2* found in these specimens suggest that this is a form of mosaic Darier disease (159).

Histopathology. The characteristic changes in Darier disease include the following: a specific pattern of dyskeratosis resulting

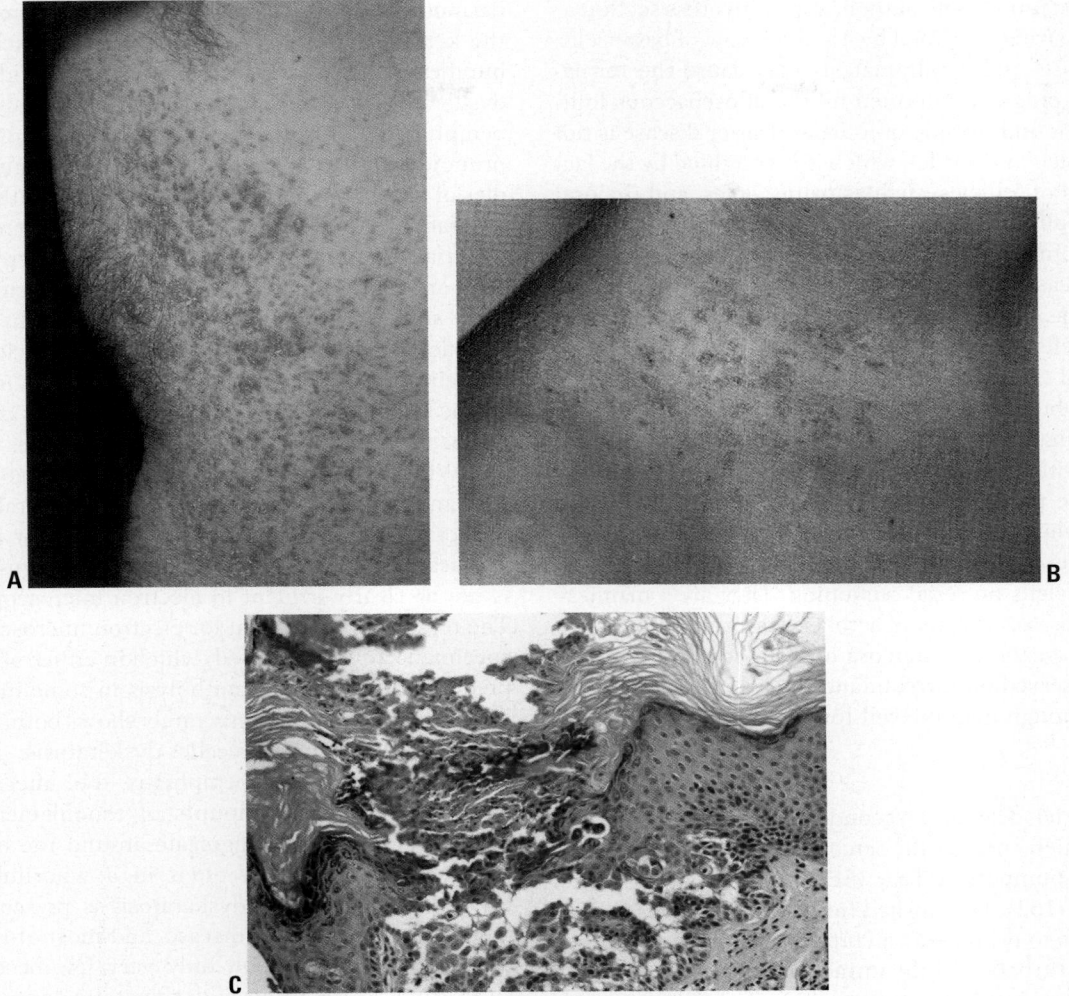

Figure 6-28 A: Darier disease. Multiple tiny hyperkeratotic papules that coalesce into plaques present on the trunk. B: Crusted papules in a follicular distribution at the base of the neck and upper chest. C: Darier disease, low magnification. Hyperkeratosis and papillomatosis are evident. Numerous lacunae are present. On the left are elongated papillae lined by a single layer of cells, so-called villi. Corps ronds are present in the granular layer and grains are seen in the horny layer. The lacunae contain desquamated cells (original magnification ×100).

in the formation of corps ronds and grains; suprabasal acantholysis resulting in suprabasal clefts or lacunae; and irregular upward proliferation into the lacunae of papillae lined with a single layer of basal cells, so-called villi (Fig. 6-28C). There are also papillomatosis, acanthosis, and hyperkeratosis. The dermis shows a chronic inflammatory infiltrate. In some cases, there is a downward proliferation of epidermal cells into the dermis.

The corps ronds occur in the upper stratum malpighii, particularly in the granular and horny layers. Grains are found in the horny layer and as acantholytic cells within the lacunae. Corps ronds possess a central homogeneous, basophilic, pyknotic nucleus that is surrounded by a clear halo. By virtue of their size and the conspicuous halo, corps ronds stand out clearly (Fig. 6-29). Peripheral to the halo lies a basophilic dyskeratotic material as a shell. The nonstaining halo in some instances is partially replaced by homogeneous, eosinophilic dyskeratotic material. Compared with the corps ronds, the grains are much less conspicuous. They resemble parakeratotic cells but are somewhat larger. The nuclei of grains are elongated and are surrounded by homogeneous dyskeratotic material that usually stains basophilic but may also stain eosinophilic. The lacunae represent small, slit-like intraepidermal vesicles most

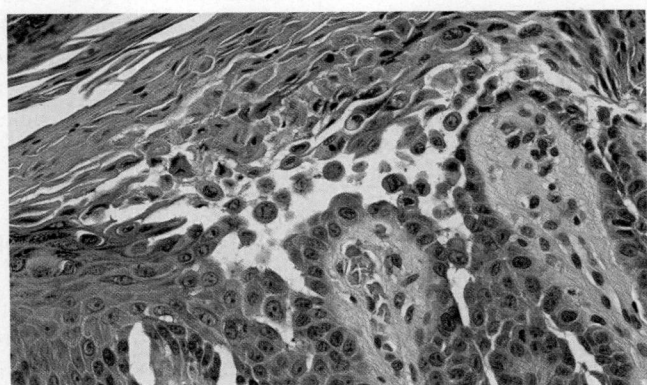

Figure 6-29 Darier disease. Hyperkeratosis is present with corps ronds in the thickened stratum corneum and epidermis. Suprabasal acantholysis is present (original magnification ×400).

commonly located directly above the basal layer. They contain acantholytic cells and show premature partial keratinization. Because of shrinkage, some of them are elongated, and these then appear identical with the grains in the horny layer. The villi projecting into the lacunae may be quite tortuous; so on histologic examination, some of them appear in cross section as rounded dermal structures lined by a solitary row of basal cells.

Hyperkeratosis and papillomatosis may cause the formation of keratotic plugs, which often fill the pilosebaceous follicles but are also found outside of follicles. Darier disease is not exclusively a follicular disorder, which is highlighted by the fact that areas devoid of follicles, such as palms, soles, and the oral mucosa, may be affected.

In hypertrophic lesions of Darier disease, considerable acanthosis may occasionally be observed, either as proliferations of basal cells or as pseudocarcinomatous hyperplasia. Proliferations of basal cells consist of long, narrow cords composed of two rows of basal cells separated by a narrow lacunar space.

The vesiculobullous lesions, which occur in rare instances, differ from lacunae merely in size; they contain numerous shrunken cells with the appearance of grains.

The keratotic papules that may occur on the dorsa of the hands and feet, which clinically resemble those seen in acrokeratosis verruciformis of Hopf, show mild dyskeratotic changes and often suprabasal clefts on serial sectioning. They are a manifestation of Darier disease and not of acrokeratosis verruciformis.

The lesions on the oral mucosa are analogous in appearance to those observed on the skin and thus show lacunae and dyskeratosis, although definite well-formed corps ronds generally are absent.

Pathogenesis. Darier disease is secondary to mutations in the *ATP2A2* gene, which encodes the sarcoplasmic/endoplasmic reticulum calcium pumping ATPase (SERCA2) on chromosome 12q23-24.1 (160–162). Diminished functioning of this ubiquitous protein leads to decreased calcium content in the stratum basalis (156). Perturbation of the intracellular calcium disrupts calcium-dependent signaling, resulting in loss of adhesion and dyskeratosis. In addition, transduction of SERCA2 mutant protein into human keratinocytes caused cells to detach and be resistant to apoptosis in the face of a second endoplasmic reticulum stress, explaining a possible gain-of-function mechanism for the acantholysis and dyskeratosis in Darier disease (163).

Acantholysis has been thought by some authors to be secondary to the loss of the intercellular contact layer within desmosomes, both in Darier disease and in familial benign pemphigus. The two halves of the desmosomes then pull apart, after which the tonofilaments become detached from them. Another group of authors believes that there is some basic defect in the tonofilament–desmosome complex in Darier disease and in familial benign pemphigus, resulting in the separation of tonofilaments from the attachment plaques of desmosomes. It is likely that both processes take place simultaneously in both Darier disease and familial benign pemphigus.

The cause for the acantholysis in Darier disease and familial benign pemphigus is not definitely known yet. Faulty synthesis of the intercellular substance has long been suspected. Further studies have suggested that intercellular communication is crucial for epidermal differentiation. This was corroborated when mutations in *ATP2A2* were found to cause Darier disease and disclosed a role for the SERCA2 pump in the calcium signaling pathway that regulates cell-to-cell adhesion and differentiation of the epidermis (164).

Loss of calcium homostasis via inhibition of SERCA2 is sufficient to disrupt desmosome assembly and leads to loss of intracellular adhesion (165). In association with the loss of

desmosomes, excessive amounts of tonofilaments form within the keratinocytes around the nucleus as thick, electron-dense bundles. A defect of the tonofilaments would best explain the dyskeratotic features of both Darier disease and familial benign pemphigus. In Darier disease, the dyskeratosis is much more pronounced than in familial benign pemphigus, and thick bundles of tonofilaments, often in association with large keratohyalin granules, form large aggregates of homogenized dyskeratotic material. The corps ronds, on electron microscopic examination, are characterized by extensive cytoplasmic vacuolization. They show, in their center, an irregularly shaped nucleus surrounded by a halo of autolyzed electron-lucid cytoplasm and, at their periphery, a shell of tonofilaments. On electron microscopic examination, the grains are seen to consist of nuclear remnants surrounded by dyskeratotic bundles of tonofilaments.

Whereas histologically a distinction between Darier disease and familial benign pemphigus is generally possible, with dyskeratosis being the predominating factor in Darier disease and acantholysis in familial benign pemphigus, this distinction is not as clearly evident in electron microscopic examination. The reason for this is that for electron microscopy, only a small specimen can be processed, which in either of the two diseases predominantly shows acantholysis in some instances and dyskeratosis in others and only rarely shows both. In both diseases, however, acantholysis precedes dyskeratosis.

In familial benign pemphigus, too, after loss of the desmosomes, excessive amounts of tonofilaments form within the keratinocytes and aggregate around the nucleus as thick, electron-dense bundles, often in a whorling configuration. However, even though dyskeratosis is present, it is less pronounced than in Darier disease, and most of the keratinocytes keratinize normally, with only very few becoming grains or corps ronds as the result of dyskeratotic degeneration.

Differential Diagnosis. Although acantholytic dyskeratosis in association with corps ronds is highly characteristic of Darier disease, it also occurs in several other conditions: in warty dyskeratoma, a solitary lesion with a deep central invagination; in transient or persistent acantholytic dermatosis (Grover disease), in which the lesions consist of discrete papules; in focal acantholytic dyskeratoma, manifesting itself as a solitary papule; and as an incidental small focus in a variety of unrelated lesions. Occasionally, a few corps ronds are also seen in familial benign pemphigus.

Principles of Management: Topical or systemic retinoids can effectively control Darier disease. Topical corticosteroids can also be helpful. Bacterial or fungal overgrowth may be treated with topical antimicrobial preparations.

MISCELLANEOUS CONDITIONS

Acrokeratosis Verruciformis of Hopf

Clinical Summary. In acrokeratosis verruciformis (AKV), an autosomal dominant disorder, numerous flat, hyperkeratotic, occasionally verrucous papules are present on the distal part of the extremities, predominantly on the dorsa of the hands and feet (Fig. 6-30A). It is considered to be a form fruste of Darier disease. They may also be found on the knees and hands. Nail changes of longitudinal striations and thinning may be seen. Punctate keratosis of the palms is an additional feature that may be seen in affected individuals.

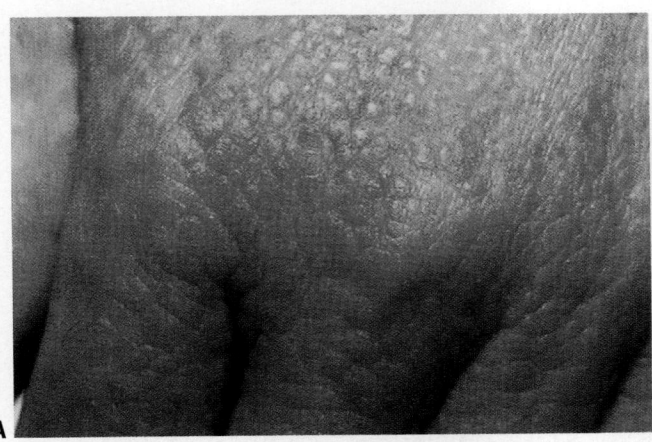
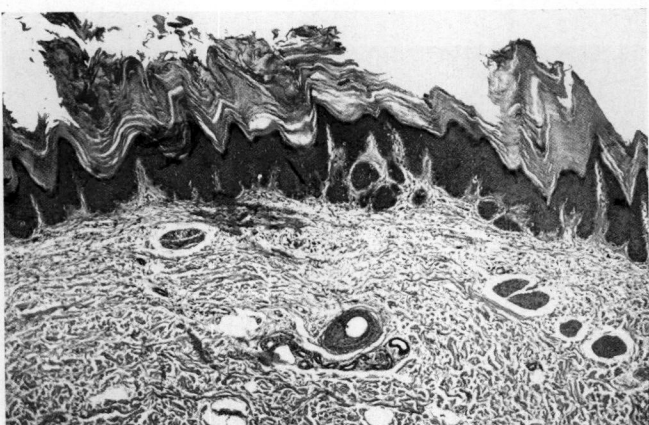

Figure 6-30 **A:** Acrokeratosis verruciformis of Hopf. **B:** A well-circumscribed lesion shows hyperkeratosis and papillomatosis. The latter is associated with elevations of the epidermis resembling church spires (original magnification ×100).

Histopathology. The papules show considerable hyperkeratosis, an increase in thickness of the granular layer, and acanthosis. In addition, there is slight papillomatosis, which is frequently but not always associated with circumscribed elevations of the epidermis resembling church spires (Fig. 6-30B). The rete ridges are slightly elongated and extend to a uniform level. In some sections, focal areas of mild acantholysis and dyskeratosis were found in patients with AKV and mutations in *ATP2A2* (166). It is not known if these histologic features can be found in AKV in the absence of *ATP2A2* mutations. A central cup-like epidermal depression with compact hyperkeratosis may be an additional feature.

Pathogenesis. A possible relationship between AKV and Darier disease has long been debated. There is no question that AKV usually occurs as an independent entity with both autosomal dominant and sporadic cases reported. Identification of mutations in *ATP2A2* in both familial and sporadic cases of AKV suggests that it may be allelic with Darier disease, explaining the clinical association (167,168). However, the mutations appear to be distinct from those seen in Darier disease, further separating these as distinct but related clinical entities (168). Additional genes responsible for AKV are yet to be identified.

Differential Diagnosis. Although elevations of the epidermis with the configuration of church spires are quite typical of AKV, they may be absent and are not specific for that disease. Particularly, they are present in the hyperkeratotic type of seborrheic keratosis. Even though seborrheic keratoses usually are larger than the lesions of AKV, clinical data may be necessary for the differentiation of these two conditions. Also, AKV may resemble verrucae clinically, but it differs from verruca plana by the absence of vacuolization in the cells of the upper epidermis and from verruca vulgaris by the absence of parakeratosis.

Principles of Management: Therapeutic options are poor and recurrence is common. Destructive methods such as cryosurgery, shave excision, and CO_2 laser ablation may have some palliative effects. Acitretin has been used successfully (169).

Incontinentia Pigmenti

Incontinentia pigmenti (IP) is an X-linked dominantly inherited disorder. It is secondary to a mutation in the *IKBKG* gene as part of the NEMO complex localized to the Xq28 region. Heterozygous females are variably affected, likely given X-inactivation. Hemizygous males typically die *in utero*. However, male patients with IP have been reported (170). Male patients may survive through hypomorphic mutations, postzygotic mosaicism, or the presence of a compensatory X chromosome, as in cases of 47, XXY, or Klinefelter syndrome (171,172).

Clinical Summary. The disorder has four stages. The first stage, consisting of erythema and bullae arranged in lines of Blaschko, either is present at birth or starts shortly thereafter (Fig. 6-31A). The extremities are predominantly affected. There is typically a marked blood eosinophilia. In the second stage, which begins after about 2 months, linear, verrucous lesions that persist for several months gradually supersede the vesicular lesions. As the verrucous lesions wane, widely disseminated areas of irregular, splattered, or whorled pigmentation develop. This pigmentation, representing the third stage, is most pronounced on the trunk. It diminishes gradually after several years and may even clear completely. The fourth stage is seen in adult females. Subtle, faint, hypochromic, or atrophic lesions in an irregular, streaky, linear pattern are most apparent on the lower extremities. There is often significant overlap among the clinical stages.

Although the characteristic skin findings are the major criteria for IP diagnosis, numerous other systems may also be affected, compromising the proposed minor diagnostic criteria (173). In about 80% of the cases, IP is associated with congenital abnormalities, including those of the central nervous system, eyes, and teeth. The associated cutaneous findings tend to be less severe than in classic ectodermal dysplasias (EDs), but alopecia, dental anomalies, nail, and breast changes are common. Seizures and motor and cognitive impairments may be present. Peripheral eosinophilia is supportive of the diagnosis.

Histopathology. The vesicles seen during the first stage arise within the epidermis and are associated with eosinophilic spongiosis (Fig. 6-31B). The epidermis between the vesicles often shows single dyskeratotic cells and whorls of squamous cells with central keratinization. Like the epidermis, the dermis shows an infiltrate containing many eosinophils and some mononuclear cells.

The alterations in the second stage consist of acanthosis, irregular papillomatosis, and hyperkeratosis (Fig. 6-31C, D). Intraepidermal keratinization, consisting of whorls of keratinocytes and of scattered dyskeratotic cells, is often more

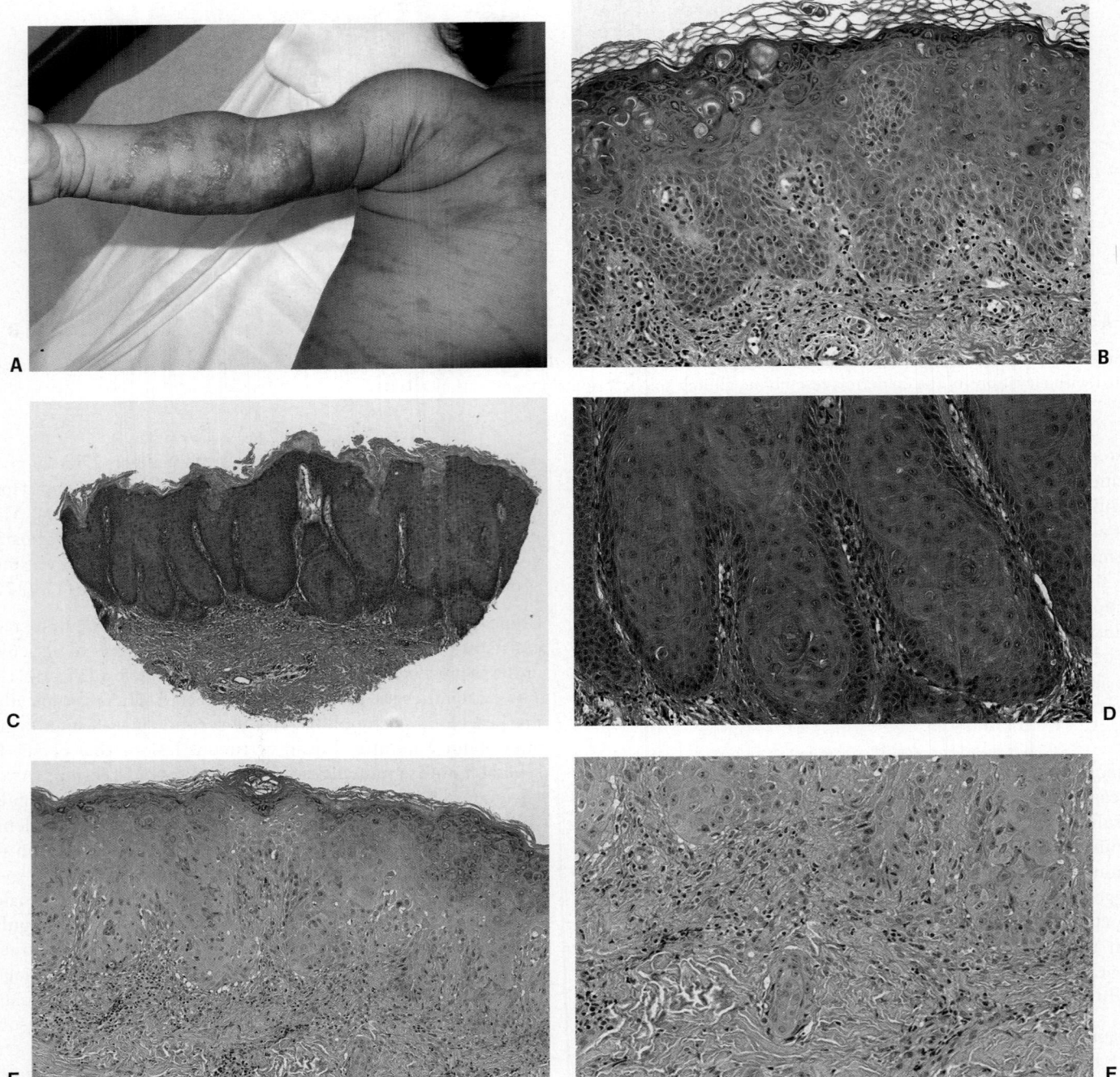

Figure 6-31 Incontinentia pigmenti. **A:** Characteristic vesicles with underlying erythema along lines of Blaschko. (Courtesy of Albert Yan, CHOP Dermatology.). **B:** The epidermis shows eosinophilic spongiosis, dyskeratotic individual keratinocytes, and whorls of dyskeratotic keratinocytes in the epidermis. Prominent eosinophils are also seen in the dermis (original magnification ×200). **C:** Incontinentia pigmenti, second stage. Acanthosis, irregular papillomatosis, and hyperkeratosis (original magnification ×40). **D:** Incontinentia pigmenti, second stage. Numerous dyskeratotic cells are present at all levels of the epidermis (original magnification ×400). **E, F:** Incontinentia pigmenti, third stage. Prominent interface changes are still present with abundant pigmented melanophages. (**C–F:** Digital slides courtesy of Path Presenter.com.)

pronounced than in the first stage. The basal cells show vacuolization and a decrease in melanin content. The dermis shows a mild, chronic inflammatory infiltrate intermingled with melanophages. This infiltrate extends into the epidermis in many places.

The areas of pigmentation seen in the third stage show extensive deposits of melanin within melanophages located in the upper dermis. Usually, this dermal hyperpigmentation is found in association with a diminution of pigment in the basal

layer, the cells of which show vacuolization and degeneration (Fig. 6-31E, F). In some cases, however, the cells of the basal layer contain abundant amounts of melanin. Apoptotic cells may be found in the epidermis but are reduced in number.

The final stage with hypopigmentation and alopecia shows a marked reduction in basal layer melanin and an atrophic epidermis. Appendageal structures are variably reduced. Apoptotic cells may be located but continue to be in reduced number. Dermal fibrosis may be present (174).

Pathogenesis. The fact that the first two stages of IP are seen predominantly on the extremities and the third stage mainly on the trunk has led to the assumption by some authors that the pigmentary changes of the third stage occur independently of the bullous and verrucous lesions of the first two stages and represent some sort of nevoid anomaly. However, electron microscopic studies have revealed common features, albeit to varying extents, in all three stages of IP and thus suggest that the three stages are related to each other (174–176). Even in the first stage, many keratinocytes and melanocytes show degenerative changes, resulting in the migration of macrophages to the epidermis, where they phagocytize dyskeratotic keratinocytes and melanosomes. Subsequently, the macrophages return to the dermis. The macrophages seen in the dermis in the second and third stages contain many melanosome complexes and thus are easily recognizable as melanophages even by light microscopy, whereas the macrophages in the first stage contain only few melanosome complexes and therefore can be identified as melanophages only with an electron microscope. The phagocytosis of melanin by dermal macrophages in the first stage of the disease and the presence of dyskeratotic keratinocytes in the epidermis during all stages of the disease has been confirmed.

The presence of eosinophils in epidermal and dermal infiltrates can be explained by the presence of basophils in the early vesicular stage, which release eosinophil chemotactic factor of anaphylaxis (177). Eosinophil chemotactic activity has been demonstrated in patients with IP in the blister fluid and in eluates of crusted scales overlying the lesions.

Differential Diagnosis. From a clinical perspective, the vesicular stage must be differentiated from mechanobullous disease such as EB and infectious causes such as herpes simplex, varicella virus, and bacterial infections need to be considered. In general, the broadest histopathologic differential diagnosis should be entertained with the vesicular stage, which is characterized by spongiotic dermatitis with eosinophils. The presence of dyskeratotic keratinocytes will help favor IP. However, other causes of spongiotic dermatitis with eosinophils should also be considered, including contact dermatitis, arthropod bites, and autoimmune bullous disorders such as bullous pemphigoid and pemphigus vulgaris. The second stage should be differentiated from verrucous epidermal nevi by the presence of dyskeratosis and the presence of eosinophils. The hyperpigmented stage may resemble findings in the blaschkolinear pigmentary disorders such as hypomelanosis of Ito and pigmentary mosaicism. The final stage may resemble other forms of ED, and often the clinical context is necessary to secure the diagnosis.

Principles of Management: Use of topical steroids or topical calcineurin inhibitors may lessen the vesicular phase, although no treatment is necessary because the cutaneous findings spontaneously resolve.

DNA REPAIR DISORDERS

Xeroderma Pigmentosum

Clinical Summary. Xeroderma pigmentosum, a rare autosomal recessive disorder, is characterized by extreme photosensitivity, leading to early actinic damage and risk of cutaneous neoplasms. Eight complementation groups are identified (XPA through XPG and XP variant). Three clinical stages are recognized.

Photosensitivity typically first manifests during the period from infancy to 3 years of age, and it is characterized by slight diffuse erythema, associated scaling, followed by small areas of hyperpigmentation resembling freckles. Not all groups show severe photosensitivity (178). Photophobia and chronic conjunctivitis may be early presenting signs (179). In early childhood, the second stage presents with skin atrophy, mottled pigmentation, and telangiectasia, giving the skin an appearance similar to chronic severe actinic damage. Actinic keratoses arise in areas of scaling. The final stage is characterized by multiple malignant tumors of the skin appearing in late childhood. The tumors include squamous cell carcinoma; basal cell carcinoma; melanoma; and, rarely, fibrosarcoma and atypical fibroxanthoma. In some patients, neoplasms progress rapidly and represent the major cause of early mortality (180). The eyes are also progressively affected, showing conjunctivitis, keratitis with corneal opacities and palpebral scarring (179). Ocular neoplasms may also occur. Oral and visceral neoplasms occur with a higher incidence in patients with XP. Progressive neurologic degeneration in up to 30% of patients is seen in the rare type of XP, DeSanctis–Cacchione syndrome, and in Cockayne–XP overlap syndrome (180). The median age for the initial diagnosis of non-melanoma skin cancer (NMSC) in XP patients is 9 years, with patients under the age of 20 years having a 10,000-fold increased risk of NMSC (basal cell and squamous cell carcinomas). The median age for a melanoma diagnosis is 22 years, with a risk 2,000 times the typical population (181–183).

Histopathology. In the first stage, the histopathologic appearance is not specific, but the diagnosis is suggested by a combination of changes that are normally not seen in the skin of young persons. These include hyperkeratosis, thinning of the stratum malpighii, with atrophy of some of the rete ridges and elongation of others; a chronic inflammatory infiltrate in the upper dermis; and irregular accumulations of melanin in the basal cell layer, with or without an increase in the number of melanocytes.

In the second stage, the hyperkeratosis and irregular hyperpigmentation already present in the first stage become more pronounced. The epidermis shows atrophy in some areas and acanthosis in others. There may be disorder in the arrangement of the epidermal nuclei, and in some areas, the epidermis may show atypical downward growth, so the histologic picture in such areas is identical with that of an actinic keratosis. The upper dermis shows basophilic degeneration of the collagen and solar elastosis, as is also seen in solar degeneration.

In the third, or tumor, stage, histologic evidence of the various malignant tumors mentioned earlier is found (Fig. 6-32 and Fig. 6-33).

In pigmented areas, electron microscopic examination of the epidermis reveals marked pleomorphism and increased number of melanosomes. In some cases, very large melanosomes, referred to as giant melanosomes, are present in both melanocytes and keratinocytes. Even epidermis that is protected from light and shows no clinical abnormalities exhibits significant cellular alterations.

Pathogenesis. In patients with xeroderma pigmentosum (with the exception of those who have the so-called XP variant; see below), cells of the skin in tissue culture show a decrease in their ability to repair the DNA damage induced by sunlight secondary to a genetic defect in one of the components of the

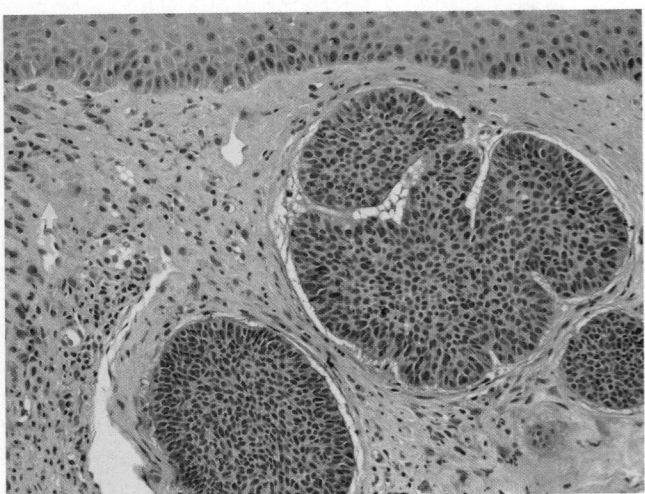

Figure 6-32 Basal cell carcinoma in the setting of xeroderma pigmentosum. Typical basaloid neoplasm, in the context of prominent solar elastosis in a child (original magnification ×200). (Reprinted with permission from Gru AA. *Pediatric Dermatopathology and Dermatology.* Wolters Kluwer; 2019.)

nucleotide excision repair complex (181,183–187). In unaffected individuals, repair of damaged DNA is brought about by a system whereby damaged single-strand regions of DNA are excised and replaced with new sequences of bases. Specifically, DNA damage is recognized by the *XPC* and *XPE* (DDB2; DNA-damage binding protein 2) gene products. Following recognition of the damage, the surrounding DNA is unwound by helicases, ERCC3 (excision repair cross-complementing) and ERCC2, which are products of the *XPB* and *XPD* genes, respectively. The *XPA* gene product, DDB1, assembles the repair complex at the site of the damage. The *XPF* and *XPG* gene products, ERCC4 and ERCC5 nucleases, incise the damaged DNA. *In vitro* testing of skin fibroblasts from different patients with xeroderma pigmentosum shows considerable variation in the excision defect. Affected siblings are usually similar to each other in the degree of repair replication. However, no correlation

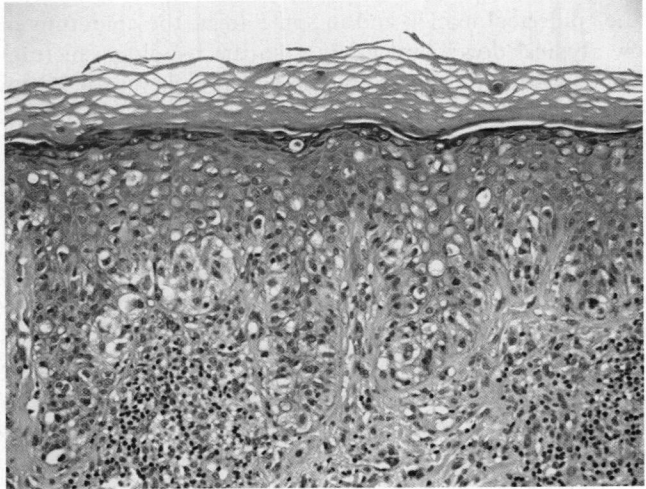

Figure 6-33 Melanoma *in situ* in a patient with xeroderma pigmentosum. Prominent pagetoid spreading and malignant cytologic features of individual melanocytes (original magnification ×200). (Reprinted with permission from Gru AA. *Pediatric Dermatopathology and Dermatology.* Wolters Kluwer; 2019.)

exists between the level of repair replication and the severity of clinical symptoms.

Some patients present with features clinically consistent with XP but normal excision repair and have defective DNA repair referred to as post-replication repair. Regular DNA polymerases are unable to replicate through areas with UV-induced DNA damage. DNA polymerase eta (encoded by the *POLH* gene) replicates through unrepaired UV-induced thymine dimers, correcting the UV-induced damage (188). *POLH* is mutated in the XP variant form.

Differential Diagnosis. Patients with trichothiodystrophy and Cockayne syndrome show photosensitivity and early actinic damage; however, the risk of malignancy is not present. Histopathology is not distinct to distinguish the actinic damage from that seen in XP. Other disorders of early-onset photosensitivity may be considered as well, such as Rothmund–Thomson, Bloom syndrome, dyskeratosis congenita, and poikiloderma with neutropenia. Severe drug-induced photosensitivity, such as that seen in patients receiving voriconazole, may also have similar clinical and histologic features. However, characteristic dysmorphisms and associated clinical characteristics can differentiate these disorders. Patients with porphyria present with photosensitivity and can be differentiated based on biochemical analysis and histologic examination of the skin.

Principles of Management: Strict photoprotection is the mainstay of XP treatment. Surveillance and treatment of premalignant and malignant skin tumors can increase patient survival. Systemic retinoids can be used to decrease cutaneous cancer development.

Dyskeratosis Congenita

Clinical Summary. Dyskeratosis congenita (DKC) usually is inherited as an X-linked recessive disorder; but in some instances, it is transmitted in an autosomal dominant fashion. Female carriers may have a mild phenotype. The following triad characterizes DKC: nail dystrophy, mucosal leukoplakia, and reticulate pigmentation. The reticulate hyperpigmentation, primarily of the neck, chest, and arms, occurs within the first decade and progresses to intermixed hypopigmentation, mild atrophy, and telangiectasia characteristic of poikiloderma. Nail dystrophy is also progressive, resulting in pterygium formation. In the X-linked form, testicular atrophy is common. Carcinoma may develop in areas of mucosal leukoplakia, and it most commonly affects the oral mucosa. However, the gynecologic and gastrointestinal mucosae are also at risk. Greater than 50% to 90% of patients with DKC develop progressive bone marrow failure, with fewer at risk for myelodysplasia, leukemia, and Hodgkin disease (189).

Histopathology. In dyskeratosis congenita, the areas of net-like pigmentation show melanophages in the upper dermis as the only constant feature. In contrast to poikiloderma atrophicans vasculare, atrophy of the epidermis, dilated capillaries, vacuolization of basal cells, and inflammatory infiltration of the upper dermis are either absent or are mild and thus not diagnostic. Mucosal biopsies show abnormalities of keratins 10, 13, and 16 (190). More advanced lesions may show squamous cell carcinoma *in situ* or invasive squamous cell carcinoma. Telomere length can be assayed by *in situ* hybridization on leukocytes from DKC patients (191,192).

Pathogenesis. Cell division causes shortening of the telomeres that, if progressive, would lead to loss of vital DNA. Telomerase adds noncoding repeats to the telomere regions of DNA, which is then protected from further degradation by protein complexes involving shelterin. Seven gene defects have been identified in dyskeratosis congenita, all of which encode proteins that are involved in telomere maintenance (193). These defects lead to variable degrees of telomere shortening with the most severe phenotypes correlating with greater degree of telomere truncation (192,194). Because telomere shortening is most pronounced during cell division, rapidly dividing tissues are at greatest risk, explaining the phenotypic spectrum of DKC.

The gene responsible for the most common type, X-linked DKC, encodes a protein called dyskerin, which is essential for telomerase RNP assembly and stability and is located on Xq28. Autosomal dominant DKC may be caused by defects in genes encoding telomerase components TERT and TERC. Shelterin protects telomere ends, and mutations in one of its components, TINF2, have also been implicated in autosomal dominant DKC. Autosomal recessive inheritance has been seen secondary to mutations in *NOP10* and *NHP2*, which encode proteins that associate with the telomerase complex. About 50% of patients have an identified mutation, and novel mutations are likely to be found but will undoubtedly encode proteins involved in telomere maintenance also (191).

Differential Diagnosis. Other causes of poikiloderma must be distinguished on clinical grounds, and histopathology is not distinct. Bloom syndrome, Rothmund–Thomson, and poikiloderma with neutropenia show poikilodermatous changes; but they are more commonly located on the face and extremities. Laboratory values and associated findings such as the nail dystrophy and leukoplakia in DKC may help distinguish among this group. Pathology of advanced poikilodermatous lesions can overlap. The dermal melanophages of earlier changes in DKC may be more pronounced. Fanconi anemia may present with hyperpigmentation and hematologic abnormalities that are similar to DKC, but limb defects are also evident.

Principles of Management: Treatment is mainly aimed at detection and management of the complications of DKC. Biannual blood counts and yearly bone marrow aspiration are advised by the consensus guidelines (189). Sun protection and skin cancer screening are critical as is surveillance for SCC formation of the mouth and anogenital mucosa. Yearly liver ultrasound and pulmonary function tests monitor for development and allow early management of fibrosis that may complicate the disease. Bone marrow transplant has been used to manage bone marrow failure.

Rothmund–Thomson Syndrome (Poikiloderma Congenitale)

Clinical Summary. Rothmund–Thomson syndrome is an autosomal recessive genodermatosis secondary to mutations in the DNA helicase gene *RECQL4* on chromosome 8q24.3. It begins a few months after birth with erythema on the face (Fig. 6-34) and subsequently extends to the dorsa of the hands and feet and occasionally also to the arms, legs, and buttocks. Slight atrophy develops with telangiectasia and mottled pigmentation, giving the appearance of poikiloderma often within the first year of life, which leads to an aged appearance of skin with scarring (Fig. 6-35). Keratotic skin lesions can also arise that

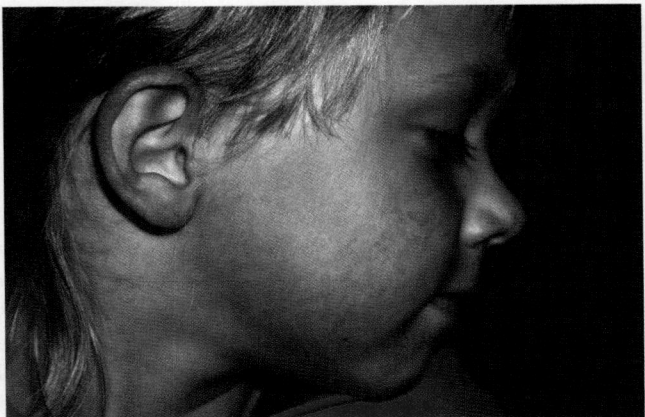

Figure 6-34 Rothmund–Thompson syndrome. Poikilodermatous changes of the cheek and ear.

may represent either benign keratoses or premalignant keratoses. Skeletal defects are seen, including radial defects and proportional short stature. Hypogonadism is common. Sparse hair and nail hypoplasia is progressive. Risk of malignancy presents most commonly as osteosarcoma and squamous cell carcinoma of the skin, although other cutaneous neoplasms are also reported (195–198).

Histopathology. During the early phase occurring in infancy and early childhood, there is hydropic degeneration of the basal layer, leading to "pigment incontinence" with presence of melanophages in the upper dermis. A mild chronic inflammatory infiltrate is intermingled with the melanophages and may show a bandlike arrangement close to the flattened epidermis. The histologic changes thus may be identical with those seen in the early stage of poikiloderma atrophicans vasculare. In later childhood and adult life, the epidermis is flattened, and dilated capillaries as well as melanophages are present in the upper dermis, but there is no longer any inflammatory infiltrate. Keratoses may show varying degrees of epidermal dysplasia, including frank SCC formation.

Pathogenesis. RECQL4 is a member of the DNA helicases, which initiate unwinding of double-stranded DNA and is responsible for the majority of cases of Rothmund–Thomson (199,200).

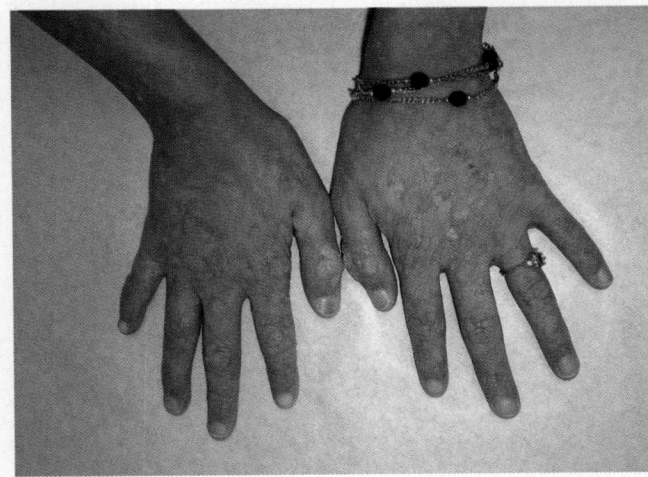

Figure 6-35 Poikiloderma and scarring on the hands of a child with Rothman-Thompson syndrome. (Courtesy of Albert Yan, CHOP Dermatology.)

The loss of RECQL4 helicase activity leads to chromosome instability and decreased ability for DNA repair that may be important for the malignancy risk. RECQL4 associates with the shelterin complex and reduction of function leads to telomere fragility (201).

Differential Diagnosis. Rothmund–Thomson may be confused with the allelic disorders RAPADILINO and Baller–Gerold syndromes, although poikiloderma and hair and nail changes are not common. The poikiloderma may be similar in presentation to that in Werner syndrome, Bloom syndrome, poikiloderma with neutropenia, and DKC. The histopathology cannot differentiate these entities. However, timing and progression of the skin changes, associated findings, and genetics will elucidate the diagnosis. Radial ray defects may be seen in Fanconi anemia, but poikiloderma is not characteristic.

Principles of Management: As with similar poikilodermatous conditions, sun protection is important. Surveillance and treatment of malignancy are the most important therapeutic interventions.

Poikiloderma With Neutropenia, Clericuzio-Type

Clinical Summary. Clericuzio-type poikiloderma with neutropenia is a rare autosomal recessive disorder characterized by progressive cutaneous findings of poikiloderma, nail dystrophy, and chronic neutropenia manifesting as recurrent infections (202). First described among the Native American Navajo population, it is now recognized in other ethnic groups (203). Patients have characteristic facial features, including a high, bossed forehead; saddle nose; and midface hypoplasia. Poikiloderma is progressive even with sun protection. Prior to the onset of poikiloderma, eczematous erythema is seen on the extremities with progressive centripetal spread. Mild keratoderma of the palms and soles is also seen (Fig. 6-36). Neutropenia secondary to maturation arrest and decreased oxidative burst activity leads to recurrent pyogenic infections (204). Growth and developmental delay and bone marrow failure may be seen in a subset of patients (205). Squamous cell carcinoma has been reported at a young age (206).

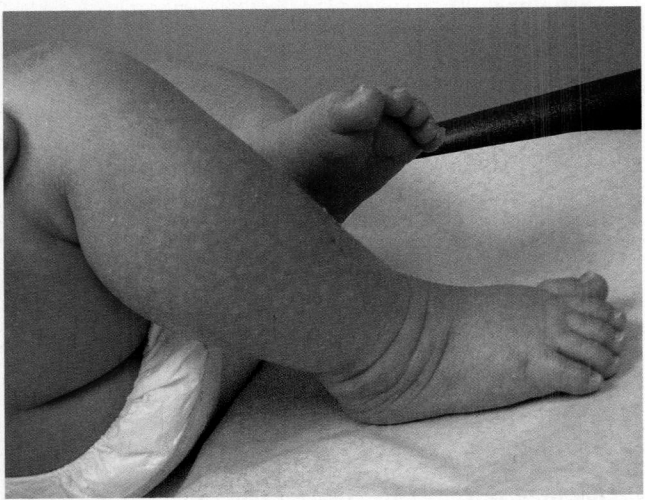

Figure 6-36 Poikiloderma with neutropenia. Early eczematous erythema with poikilodermatous change on the legs. (Courtesy of Albert Yan, CHOP Dermatology.)

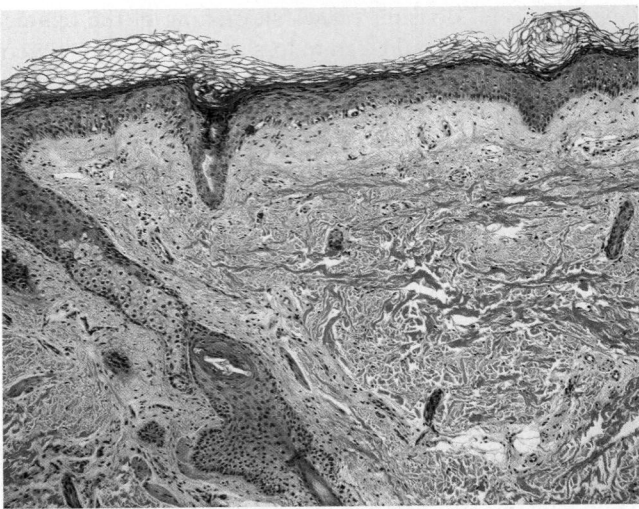

Figure 6-37 Poikiloderma with neutropenia. There is epidermal atrophy associated with vacuolar degeneration of basilar keratinocytes and rare dyskeratotic keratinocytes. Telangiectasias are present in the papillary and upper dermis.

Histopathology. Few biopsies of this condition have been documented in the literature. A biopsy of poikilodermatous change may show an interface dermatitis with lymphohistiocytic infiltration and other characteristic features of poikiloderma, including telangiectasia and epidermal atrophy (Fig. 6-37). Pigment incontinence can also be noted.

Pathogenesis. Mutations in the *C16orf57* gene are responsible for poikiloderma with neutropenia (207). The *C16orf57* gene encodes the USB1 (U6 biogenesis 1) protein, a phosphodiesterase responsible for posttranscriptional 3' end modification of the U6 small nuclear ribonucleoproteins (snRNPs) (208). The modifications protect U6 snRNPs from destruction by nuclear exosomes (209). The exact mechanism by which gene disruption leads to the clinical phenotype of poikiloderma with neutropenia is unknown.

Differential Diagnosis. The histologic features are nonspecific in differentiating poikiloderma with neutropenia. The finding of persistent neutropenia differentiates poikiloderma with neutropenia from other genodermatosis presenting with poikiloderma that are discussed in this chapter.

Principles of Management: Sun protection may decrease development of poikiloderma and cutaneous malignancy risk. Neutropenia is responsive to granulocyte-stimulating factors.

Bloom Syndrome (Congenital Telangiectatic Erythema)

Clinical Summary. Bloom syndrome is a rare autosomal recessive disorder caused by mutations in the gene *BLM*. It is characterized by photosensitivity and telangiectatic erythema of sun-exposed surfaces starting early in infancy, similar to Rothmund–Thomson (Fig. 6-38). However, patients with Bloom syndrome have more severe intrauterine and postnatal growth restriction. Patients are developmentally appropriate. Café-au-lait macules may be present adjacent to areas of hypopigmentation. Typical facial dysmorphisms include dolichocephaly and malar hypoplasia, leading to an elongated face and a prominent nose. Hypogonadism results

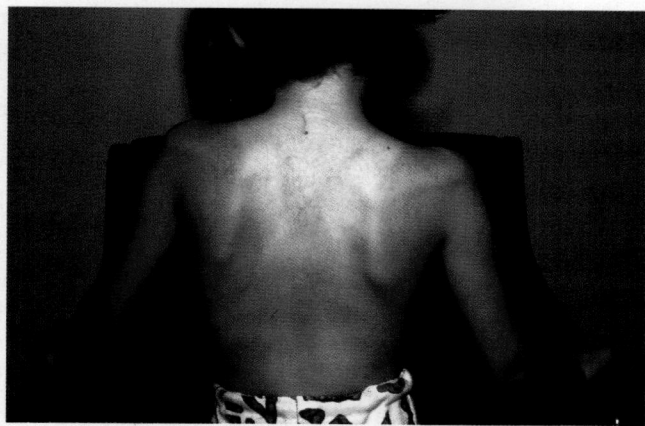

Figure 6-38 Bloom syndrome. Photo-distributed erythema of the shoulders and upper back.

in decreased fertility in male and female patients; sterility in male patients may arise secondary to sperm defects. Bloom syndrome shows impairment of both cellular and humoral immunity, although this is not as pronounced as in ataxia–telangiectasia.

Immunoglobulin deficiencies, especially of IgA and IgM, may lead to an increased risk of infection. Although many cancer types have been reported, malignancy risk is best characterized by an increased risk of leukemia, lymphoma, carcinoma of the alimentary tract, and cutaneous malignancy (210).

Histopathology. The epidermis is flattened and may show hydropic degeneration of the basal cell layer. There is dilatation of the capillaries in the upper dermis, which may be associated with a perivascular mononuclear infiltrate; however, there may be absence of any infiltrate. Quadriradial configuration of the chromosomes, resulting from aberrant sister chromatid exchange, is diagnostic, although rarely used in clinical practice since the advent of molecular testing.

Pathogenesis. The Bloom syndrome gene, *BLM*, encodes a DNA helicase RecQ protein-like 2 on gene map locus 15q26.1. *BLM* is expressed in actively replicating cells and the gene product is known to collect at sites of DNA damage. It is part of a complex that repairs DNA structures and intermediates arising from recombination (211). *BLM* often co-localizes with *WRN*, the gene responsible for Werner syndrome. Loss of the BLM helicase function leads to somatic mutations and chromosome instability, specifically with a high incidence of nonspecific chromosomal breakage and an increase in sister chromatid exchanges. Increased malignancy risk arises from this failure of proper DNA surveillance and repair.

Differential Diagnosis. Pigmentary incontinence is not as pronounced in Bloom syndrome as in Rothmund–Thompson syndrome. The presence of hydropic degeneration of the basal cell layer and of a perivascular infiltrate may cause difficulties in differentiation from lupus erythematous. However, no linear deposits of immunoglobulin are seen at the dermal–epidermal junction in Bloom syndrome.

Principles of Management: Sun protection may prevent progression of cutaneous findings. Exposures leading to risk of chromosomal instability, such as radiation, should be avoided. Screening and treatment of malignancy are paramount.

Ataxia–Telangiectasia

Clinical Summary. Ataxia–telangiectasia is an autosomal recessive disorder of immunodeficiency, ocular and cutaneous telangiectasia, and hematologic malignancy predisposition. Patients first present with progressive cerebellar ataxia within the first 5 years of life (212). With progression of ataxia, patients tend to lose the ability to walk by the teenage years. Ocular telangiectasia is a universal feature and is reported to occur by age of 4 to 6 years (213). Telangiectasias usually appear first on the bulbar conjunctiva. Cutaneous telangiectasias also develop in a subset of patients and may be found on the cheeks, ears, and neck and, less commonly, on the buttocks and extremities. Other cutaneous manifestations include café-au-lait macules, pigmented nevi, and hypopigmentation (213). Noninfectious cutaneous granulomas are a variable, but can be a presenting, feature of ataxia–telangiectasia (214). Features of immunodeficiencies are found in patients with ataxia–telangiectasia, including lymphopenia, impaired cell-mediated and humoral immunity with decreased or absent immunoglobulin (215). An increased susceptibility to infections, particularly sinopulmonary infections, exists. Death from chronic respiratory infection or hematologic malignancy is common in the second or third decade of life (216). Heterozygous carriers of the disease show an increased risk of visceral malignancy (217).

Histopathology. The upper dermis shows numerous markedly dilated vessels that belong to the subpapillary venous plexus consistent with telangiectasia. Biopsy of infiltrated plaques shows lymphohistiocytic granulomatous inflammation palisading around areas of necrobiosis. Mucin is not present (214,218,219). Infectious organisms should be ruled out with tissue culture but have yet to be identified in patients with granulomas associated with ataxia–telangiectasia.

Pathogenesis. Mutations in the *ATM* gene have been mapped to gene locus 11q22.3 and lead to inactivation of the ATM kinase. ATM protein kinase is activated in response to double-stranded DNA breaks and is part of a cascade that leads to cell cycle arrest, repair, and/or apoptosis (220). In addition, many of the substrates of the ATM kinase are tumor-suppressor genes such as *BRCA1*. The loss of ATM kinase makes cells particularly susceptible to ionizing radiation. It is hypothesized that accumulated DNA damage leads to apoptosis of cerebellar neurons, which in turn leads to the cardinal feature of ataxia–telangiectasia (221). Immunodeficiency and malignancy risk are further attributed to the defect in DNA repair. It is less clear how *ATM* mutation leads to telangiectasia, although upregulation of vascular endothelial growth factor (VEGF) and hypoxia inducible factor 1 (HIF1) suggest that oxidative stress may play a role (222,223).

Differential Diagnosis. Findings and histopathology of telangiectasia are not specific for ataxia–telangiectasia and may be differentiated from other DNA repair disorders such as Rothmund–Thomson, Bloom syndrome, and DKC by the lack of other poikilodermatous features. Ataxia–telangiectasia is distinct from benign disorders of telangiectasia such as generalized essential telangiectasia by the associated features of ataxia and immunodeficiency. Histopathologically, the cutaneous granulomas that may be present can resemble granuloma annulare or sarcoidosis. However, unlike granuloma annulare, mucin is not a prominent feature of granulomas in ataxia–telangiectasia. Predominance of CD8+ cells differentiated specimens from sarcoidal granulomas in one small series (218). Moreover, granulomas of ataxia–telangiectasia are sometimes tender, and often violaceous, ulcerated plaques, making them clinically distinct from granuloma annulare. However, they may be histopathologically and clinically indistinguishable from granulomas associated with other immunodeficiency syndromes.

Principles of Management: Treatment is largely symptom directed. Appropriate antimicrobial therapy and prevention are needed. Immune replacement therapy with intravenous immune globulin may be warranted. Cutaneous granulomas are generally resistant to treatment. Topical, intralesional, and systemic glucocorticoids may have some benefit. Efficacy of TNF inhibitors has been reported (224). Periodic routine malignancy screening and avoidance of ionizing radiation are of central importance.

Hutchinson–Gilford Progeria

Clinical Summary. Hutchinson–Gilford progeria is a rare autosomal dominant condition of premature senility. Although the phenotype is not evident at birth, cutaneous findings manifest often within the first few months of life (225). Sclerodermoid changes of the skin with soft cutaneous outpouchings give a pseudocellulite appearance most prominent on the abdomen and lower extremities. There is a severe loss of subcutaneous fat leading to prominent veins on the scalp and other body areas. Alopecia and mottled dyspigmentation are progressively found. Growth failure is profound. Bony abnormalities, including joint contractures, dental changes, and laboratory abnormalities are also features of the disease (226). Characteristic facies of a proportionally large cranium, beaked nose, frontal bossing, and prominent eyes are typically seen by the age of 3 years but may be absent in younger children. Hutchinson–Gilford progeria is fatal within the second decade of life secondary to cardiovascular and cerebrovascular complications from premature atherosclerosis.

Histopathology. Histopathology may vary depending on the site and age of the patient. In areas of sclerodermoid change, the biopsy shows epidermal atrophy and thickened collagen throughout the dermis. Epidermal appendages are decreased in number or absent with more advanced disease. Histopathology is often not diagnostic, and molecular verification of the gene defect must be undertaken.

Pathogenesis. Hutchinson–Gilford progeria results from a specific point mutation (1824C->T) in *LMNA,* which encodes lamin A, leading to abnormal splicing of this component of the nuclear lamina. Mature lamin A protein is formed following farnesylation and subsequent cleavage that removes the farnesylation. The mutated gene product lacks the cleavage site, resulting in the mutant protein, also known as progerin, which is permanently farnesylated (227). Farnesylation of progerin results in permanent insertion within the nuclear envelope, preventing interaction with the nuclear lamina, which is believed to account for dominant negative expression of the progeria phenotype. There is progressive irregularity of the nuclei in Hutchinson–Gilford progeria, which is diagnostic of the disease (228).

Differential Diagnosis. Hutchinson–Gilford progeria may be differentiated from other progeroid syndromes secondary to mutations in *LMNA* by the clinical features, and histopathology is rarely helpful among this group. Sclerodermoid changes in an infant may also be seen in restrictive dermopathy, which, unlike Hutchinson–Gilford progeria, is present at birth. Histopathologic

overlap of features is seen; however, collagen is compact and there are sparse elastic fibers in restrictive dermopathy. Skin appendages are rudimentary. Sclerema neonatorum, occurring in ill, premature infants may have sclerotic skin changes but biopsy shows sparse inflammation of the subcutaneous fat and needle-shaped clefts. Stiff skin syndrome can rarely present in the neonatal period, but biopsy will show hyalinization of the fascia with overlying dermal collagen thickening.

Principles of Management: Management of the comorbidities of Hutchinson–Gilford progeria is the mainstay of treatment. A clinical trial of a farnesyltransferase inhibitor improved growth, vascular compliance, hearing, and bony changes in children with progeria (229).

Progeria of the Adult (Werner Syndrome)

Clinical Summary. Werner syndrome, an autosomal recessive condition, does not manifest itself until the second or third decade of life (230,231). Patients first exhibit a lack of the pubertal growth spurt and therefore reach a decreased adult height. The subcutaneous fat and musculature of the extremities undergo atrophy. Sclerodermoid changes of the skin on the extremities and cutaneous ulcerations are progressive. Signs of premature aging appear with patients showing alopecia, graying of the hair, and atherosclerosis in early adult life. Cataracts, a hoarse or high-pitched voice, soft-tissue calcification and a bird-like facies are other cardinal features (231). Metabolic syndrome, including diabetes, and hypogonadism secondary to interstitial fibrosis of the testes are common. Death usually occurs in the fifth decade of life because of atherosclerosis or an increased incidence of malignancy (232).

Histopathology. On the arms and legs, where the skin is taut, the epidermis is thin and devoid of rete ridges, and the dermis shows fibrosis with or without hyalinization of the collagen. The pilosebaceous structures degenerate. The subcutaneous fatty tissue is largely replaced by newly synthesized, hyalinized collagen that merges with the collagen of the overlying dermis. Vessels may show advanced angiopathy.

Pathogenesis. Causative mutations in the *WRN* or *RECQL2* gene on chromosome 8p12-11.2 are identified in the majority of cases. WRN protein is a homolog of the *Escherichia coli* RecQ DNA helicase and displays both helicase and exonucleus activity (233). It plays an important role in DNA replication and recombination repair with loss, resulting in chromosome instability (234). Telomere maintenance is also affected by loss of WRN activity (235). The accumulation of genomic instability is thought to lead to premature senescence of cells and malignancy predisposition in patients. A subset of patients with atypical Werner syndrome, characterized by earlier age of onset, have heterozygous mutations in *LMNA* (236).

Differential Diagnosis. The major differential includes other syndromes of premature aging. However, the clinical features are usually diagnostic and histopathology does not often aid in the distinction. Differentiation from a late lesion of scleroderma may be difficult because fibrosis and hyalinization of the collagen are also seen in scleroderma. In its late stage, scleroderma may also show no inflammatory infiltrate so that differentiation has to be made on the basis of the patient's history and clinical manifestations.

Principles of Management: Treatment is largely aimed at managing the complications of Werner syndrome. Appropriate malignancy and health maintenance surveillance should be undertaken. Vitamin C supplementation was found to increase the life span and rescue both the clinical and molecular phenotypes in a mouse model of Werner syndrome (237).

DISORDERS OF CONNECTIVE TISSUE

Ectodermal Dysplasias

Clinical Summary. EDs are a large heterogeneous group of diseases that share common abnormalities of the hair, nails, teeth, and sweat glands (238,239). Over 200 different clinical conditions have been reported as EDs, many of which have clinical overlap. To date, greater than 60 gene defects have been identified as causative in the EDs. To qualify as an ED, at least two of the four major ectodermal derivatives must be affected—hair, teeth, nails, and eccrine glands. Disorders are classified based on which of these are affected and the presence or absence of associated immune dysregulation. In general, EDs are grouped into two large categories (240). Group I EDs are secondary to defects in epithelial mesenchymal interactions. Mutations have been identified in several important pathways. The prototypical group I ED is hypohidrotic ED. Group II EDs are secondary to functional defects in structural proteins, affecting cell adhesion or communication. The prototypical group II ED is hidrotic ED. EDs are caused by mutations in genes encoding signaling pathway components, adhesion molecules, and transcription factors important during embryologic development

The X-linked hypohidrotic ED is the most common ED, and it is characterized by the tetrad of hypohidrosis, hypotrichosis, dental hypoplasia, and a characteristic facies (Fig. 6-39). Patients have distinct facial features, including frontal bossing, a depressed nasal bridge, periorbital hyperpigmentation, and low-set ears (Fig. 6-40). Skin fragility (Fig. 6-41)

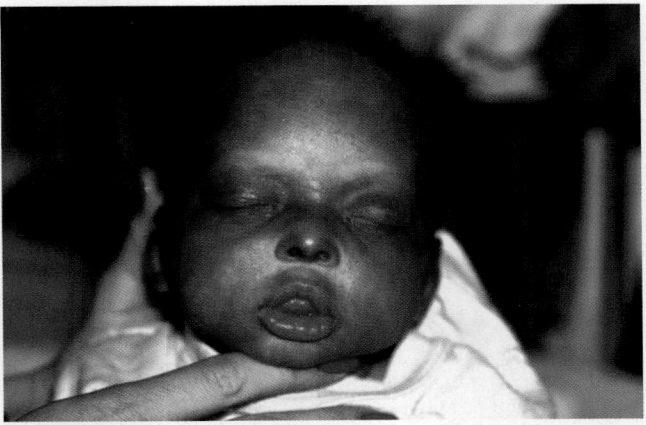

Figure 6-40 X-linked hypohidrotic ectodermal dysplasia. In addition to frontal bossing and a flat nasal bridge, this infant demonstrates hyperpigmentation of the eyelids and surrounding skin as well as patulous lips.

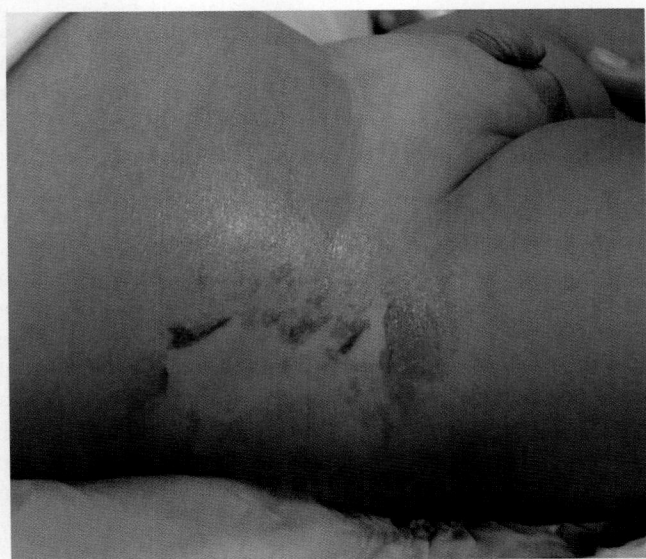

Figure 6-41 X-linked hypohidrotic ectodermal dysplasia. Prominent skin fragility is present. (Reprinted with permission from Gru AA. *Pediatric Dermatopathology and Dermatology*. Wolters Kluwer; 2019.)

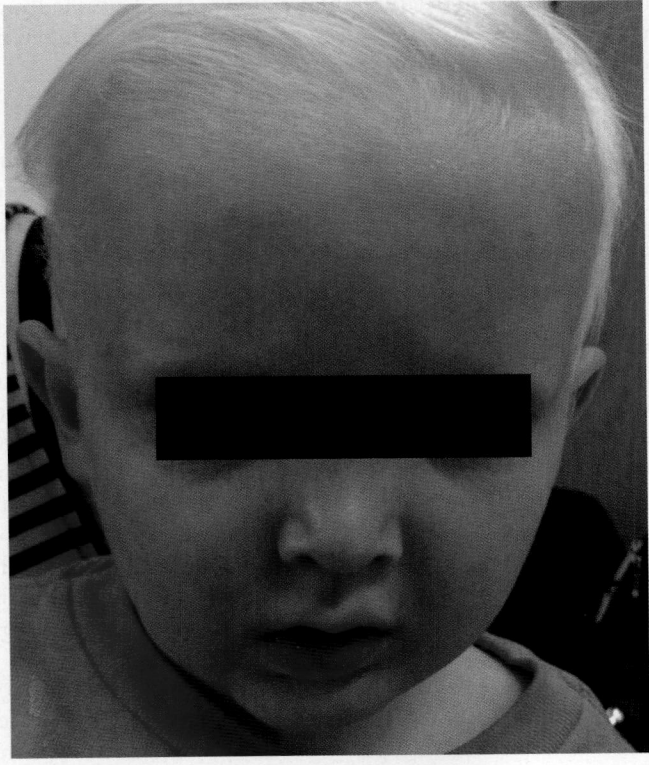

Figure 6-39 X-linked hypohidrotic ectodermal dysplasia. Characteristic facies. (Reprinted with permission from Gru AA. *Pediatric Dermatopathology and Dermatology*. Wolters Kluwer; 2019.)

and sebaceous gland hyperplasia are present (Fig. 6-42). Hair is sparse to absent, and often light in color. Teeth, when they do develop, are small and peg-shaped. The decreased ability to sweat leads to unexplained fevers in infants and severe hyperthermia. Inheritance is most commonly X-linked recessive. However, autosomal recessive and autosomal dominant forms have been described. In X-linked recessive variants of ED, female heterozygotes may be mildly affected, with reduced sweating and faulty dentition. In addition, the mucous glands of the mouth and respiratory tract may be absent, leading to respiratory tract infections (241). Developmental abnormality of mammary glands and nipples has been noted (242). A subset of patients with clinical manifestations of hypohidrotic ED present with recurrent and serious infections, so-called hypohidrotic ED with immunodeficiency. These patients are susceptible to bacterial and mycobacterial infections. Hypogammaglobulinemia is often present.

The final major grouping of type I ED presents with ectodermal, orofacial, and limb defects (243). The most severe limb defects are split hand/foot malformations or ectrodactyly.

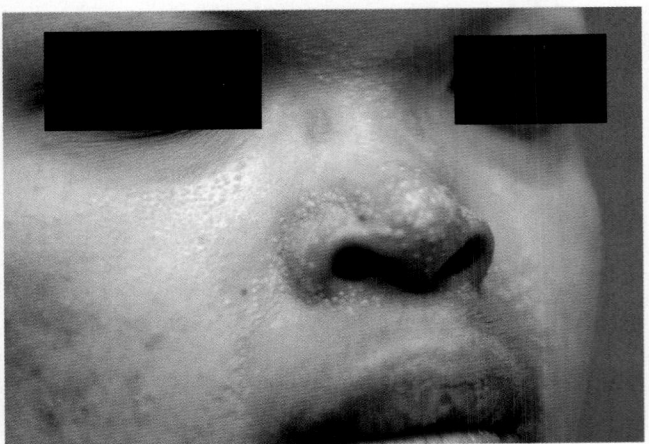

Figure 6-42 X-linked hypohidrotic ectodermal dysplasia. Prominent sebaceous gland hyperplasia is present. (Reprinted with permission from Gru AA. *Pediatric Dermatopathology and Dermatology.* Wolters Kluwer; 2019.)

Cleft lip and/or palate are also common associations. Although sparse hair and misshapen teeth do characterize these disorders, the defects are often less severe (244). These disorders occur on a spectrum with much phenotypic overlap. Examples of this group include AEC (ankyloblepharon–ectodermal dysplasia–clefting) and EEC (ectrodactyly–ectodermal dysplasia–clefting) syndromes. In AEC syndrome, extensive erosions of the scalp place patients at risk of infection (Fig. 6-43) (245).

The hidrotic form, which has an autosomal dominant inheritance, is primarily a disorder of keratinization that is characterized by hypotrichosis, dystrophic nails, and palmoplantar hyperkeratosis (240). The degree of alopecia varies from slight to total. It is sometimes associated with dental hypoplasia. Palmoplantar keratoderma is progressive. Nail dystrophy is the most common clinical manifestation and may be the presenting complaint in patients. The nails may show lateral convexity, hypoplasia, and subungual hyperkeratosis.

Histopathology. Both the hidrotic and the anhidrotic forms show hypoplasia of the hair and the sebaceous glands. There is

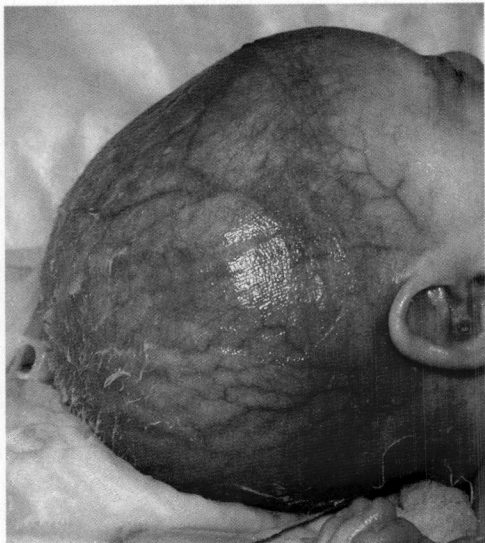

Figure 6-43 Ankyloblepharon–ectodermal dysplasia–clefting syndrome (AEC). Extensive scalp erosions are commonly observed. (Courtesy of Albert Yan, CHOP Dermatology.)

a variable degree of reduction in their number, size, and degree of maturation. In the hypohidrotic form, there is either a total absence or severe hypoplasia of the eccrine glands. In the case of hypoplasia, eccrine glands are present in only a few areas, especially the axillae and palms; but even in these areas, they are sparse and poorly developed. The secretory cells may be small and flat so that they resemble endothelial rather than epithelial cells, and the excretory ducts may be composed of a single instead of a double layer of epithelial cells. The apocrine glands of the axillae are present in some patients with the hypohidrotic form. In others, these glands are hypoplastic and cannot be distinguished from hypoplastic eccrine glands. In still others, both eccrine and apocrine glands are absent.

Histopathology of the scalp dermatitis in AEC is nonspecific. Mild epidermal atrophy, a superficial perivascular lymphocytic infiltrate, focal hyperkeratosis, and pigment incontinence have been reported (246). The erosions on the scalp and at other sites highlight the skin fragility seen in these patients, and they may be associated with decreased basal and suprabasal keratins.

Pathogenesis. The pathogenic mutations present in ED can be best divided according to (1) genes encoding cell signaling and communication molecules; (2) adhesion-related molecules; (3) developmental signal molecules; and (4) others. The most common form of hypohidrotic ED is an X-linked recessive disorder caused by mutations in the genes for ectodysplasin (EDA) localized to Xq12-q13.1. Autosomal dominant and autosomal recessive forms are caused by mutations in the ectodysplasin receptor (EDAR), or mediating proteins (EDARADD), localized to 2q13 and 1q42.2-q43, respectively (240). These genes are expressed early in embryonic ectoderm with continued expression in ectodermal derivatives. The EDA pathway has early importance in the proper formation of the epithelial placodes, which give rise to skin appendages (247). Expression in postnatal appendageal structures likely affects the continued morphogenesis of the skin appendages, with defects resulting in the tooth and hair hypoplasia seen in hypohidrotic ED (248).

Activation of the NF-κB signaling pathway is essential for EDA signal transduction, thus explaining the phenotypic overlap of mutations in EDA pathway and NF-κB pathway mutations. It has been demonstrated that patients with hypohidrotic ED with immunodeficiency have hypomorphic mutations in the NF-κB essential modulator (NEMO) located on Xq28 and more rarely in IκBA on 14q13 (249).

Mutations in *TP63* have been identified in the spectrum of disorders with abnormalities of the ectoderm, limb, and orofacial development such as AEC and EEC (250). These autosomal dominant disorders are secondary to well-characterized mutations in p63 on chromosome 3q27. P63 is important for early epidermal differentiation and appendage formation, including a role in expression of keratin proteins (251). Postnatal expression of p63 in basal keratinocytes is believed to be critical for basement membrane formation and cell adhesion. The phenotypic variation of mutations in p63 is hypothesized to be secondary to differential effects on p63 downstream mediators (243,251).

A mutated gene gap junction protein beta-6 (GJB6) on chromosome 13q12, which encodes connexin 30, is implicated in hidrotic ectodermal dysplasia (252). Connexin 30 is a member of the gap junction protein family that is important for intracellular communication. It is expressed in the hair follicle, nail unit, and palmoplantar epidermis and thereby accounts for the spectrum of clinical findings in hidrotic ED (253).

Differential Diagnosis. Differentiating among the numerous types of ED can be challenging as clinical and histopathologic features are shared. Known genetic mutations aid in diagnosis, although great clinical overlap and incomplete penetrance complicate definitive diagnosis.

Principles of Management: In hypohidrotic ED, heat regulation with avoidance and cooling strategies is an important therapeutic challenge. Dental prosthetics are often necessary. For erosive dermatitis, local wound care and infection control are needed.

Aplasia Cutis Congenita

Clinical Summary. Aplasia cutis congenita (ACC) consists of a localized absence of skin with or without underlying bone and meningeal defects (Fig. 6-44). ACC is a finding associated with a number of pathologic conditions. ACC is most commonly characterized by a single lesion 1 to 3 cm in diameter that is located on the vertex scalp. Multiple areas may also be seen. The initial clinical appearance varies and includes ulcerated; eroded; bullous; nodular; or, if intrauterine healing has occurred, scarred areas. When ACC presents with a thin, moist-appearing surface, it is referred to as membranous ACC. ACC surrounded by thick, terminal hairs has been termed the "hair collar sign" and may represent a sign of heterotopic brain tissue or an occult neural tube defect. The hair collar sign is a marker for cranial dysraphism. Rarely, large defects of the skin are present, which increases the likelihood of underlying soft-tissue or bony defects. Exposure and injury of the sagittal sinus have been reported for exceptionally deep lesions that involve the dura. Bullous ACC is a variant presenting with a serous fluid-filled vesicle with surface telangiectasias (254). If the skin alone is affected, healing takes place over several days to several months, depending on the size of the defect. Large areas of ACC may also present on the trunk and extremities. The condition includes a diverse group of disorders in which localized absence of skin occurs alone or in association with a wide variety of abnormalities (255). *In utero* fetal demise of one

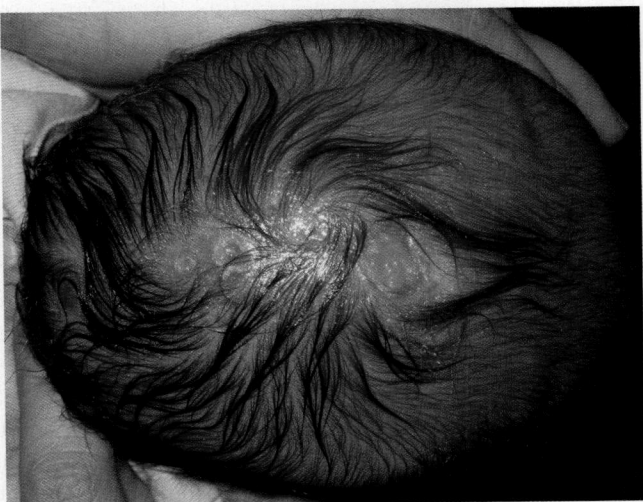

Figure 6-44 Aplasia cutis congenita. Multiple areas of congenitally absent skin with overlying membranous change (membranous aplasia cutis). (Courtesy of Albert Yan, CHOP Dermatology.)

fetus in a multiparous pregnancy may result in the surviving infant experiencing large areas of stellate truncal aplasia cutis termed fetus papyraceus (256).

Histopathology. Ulcers may extend through the entire thickness of the dermis, exposing the subcutaneous fat. Healed areas show, besides a flattened epidermis, fibrosis in the dermis and complete absence of adnexal structures with scar formation.

Pathogenesis. The cause of ACC is unknown and likely multifactorial. Most cases are believed to be sporadic and likely represent a developmental anomaly. Syndromic cases of ACC can be associated with known genetic defects such as seen with trisomy 13 and Adams-Oliver syndrome. ACC has also been associated with medications, most notably intrauterine exposure to methimazole for the treatment of hyperthyroidism.

Differential Diagnosis. Aplasia cutis should not be confused with congenital absence of the skin, where only epidermis is absent. The scarring features of ACC are missing in the latter. This is a variant of EB (Bart syndrome) (257). Differentiation from acute infectious etiologies is also of critical importance.

Principles of Management: Generally, local wound care is the only treatment indicated. In cases with a hair collar present, neuroimaging should be completed to evaluate for an associated neurologic defect.

Focal Dermal Hypoplasia Syndrome

Clinical Summary. The focal dermal hypoplasia (FDH) syndrome, or Goltz syndrome, is a rare X-linked dominant disorder characterized by cutaneous, skeletal, ocular, and dental abnormalities. It is caused by mutations in the gene *PORCN*, which encodes a protein necessary for the secretion of Wnt and is critical for ectodermal–mesodermal communication in early development (258–260). The cutaneous hallmarks of this disorder are widely distributed telangiectatic patches of dermal hypoplasia (resembling striae distensae); soft, yellow outpouchings in a linear arrangement (consistent with subcutaneous fat herniation through a thinned dermis); spotty or streaky hyperpigmentation or hypopigmentation; fleshy papillomas in the oral, anal, and genital regions; and cutaneous ulcerations that heal with atrophy (Fig. 6-45A–C). The cutaneous findings follow Blaschko lines, which are thought to represent the clonal expansion and migration of ectodermal cells during embryologic development. Additional developmental defects include hypodontia with enamel hypoplasia, alopecia, dystrophic nails, colobomas or microopthalmia, and skeletal defects including syndactyly and ectrodactyly (261). Radiographs typically reveal fine linear striations in the metaphyses of long bones, termed *osteopathic striata*, which is consistent with thinning of the bone and supportive of the diagnosis (262,263). Females are almost exclusively affected, and the disease is presumed to be lethal in hemizygous males. Postzygotic somatic mutation reflecting type II mosaicism is causative in affected males, and the timing of this mutation likely determines the severity of disease manifestations, with earlier defects causing more extensive findings (260,264). Additional cases have been seen in males with XXY or Klinefelter syndrome (265).

Histopathology. The linear areas of hypoplasia of the skin show a marked diminution in the thickness of the dermis, with the collagen being present as thin fibers not united into bundles. The soft, yellow nodules represent accumulations of fat that largely

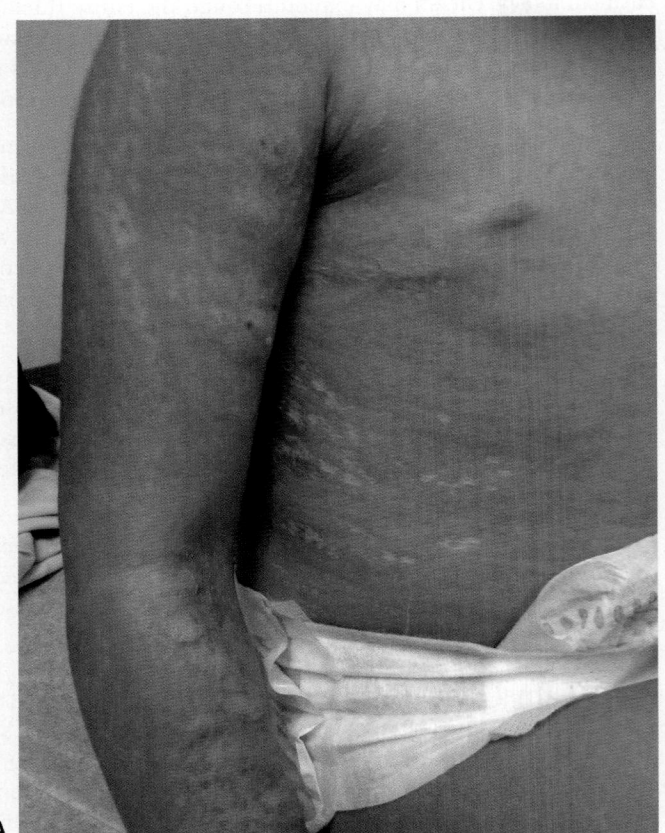

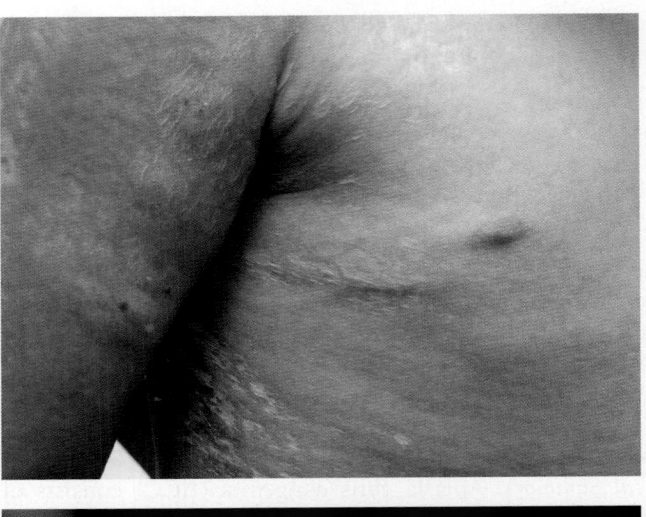

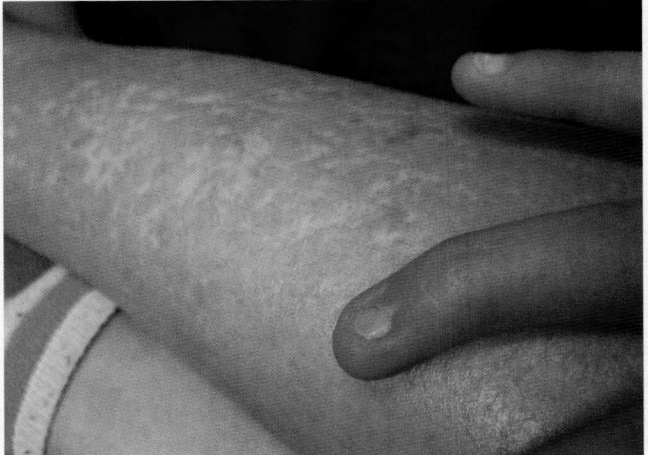

Figure 6-45 A–C: Goltz syndrome. Numerous atrophic patches with scarring in a Blaschkoid distribution. Panel C also shows micronichia. (Courtesy of Dr. Nnenna Agim, Department of Dermatology, University of Texas Southwestern Medical Center.)

replace the dermis; thus, the subcutaneous fat extends upward to the epidermis in some areas (Fig. 6-46) (266). Thin fibers of collagen and even some bundles of collagen resembling those of normal dermis may be located between the subepidermal adipose tissue and the subcutaneous fat.

Pathogenesis. Mutations in *PORCN*, which are involved in the Wnt signaling pathway, have been identified as causal

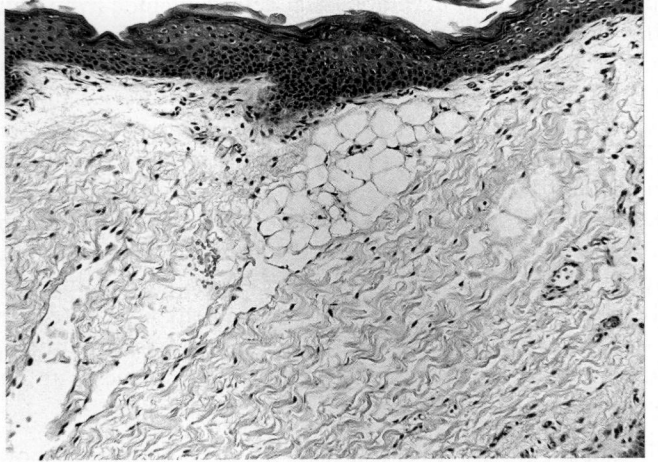

Figure 6-46 Focal dermal hypoplasia. Adipose tissue is present very near the epidermis, separated from it by only a few collagen fibers (original magnification ×100). (Courtesy of Albert Yan, CHOP Dermatology.)

in Goltz syndrome (258,259,267,268). *PORCN* encodes an O-acyltransferase that is critical in Wnt protein secretion. Wnt proteins are critical mediators of cutaneous development, particularly ectodermal–mesenchymal interactions. Electron microscopic examination shows, in addition to collagen fibrils 70 nm or more in diameter, many fine filamentous structures measuring 5 to 70 nm in diameter. There are two types of fat cells, one unilocular and the other multilocular, the latter representing young lipocytes.

Differential Diagnosis. Fat cells in the dermis may also be seen in nevus lipomatosus superficialis, but the extreme attenuation of the collagen is only seen in the skin of patients with FDH.

Principles of Management: Surgical intervention can ameliorate symptomatic areas.

PSEUDOXANTHOMA ELASTICUM

Clinical Summary. Pseudoxanthoma elasticum (PXE) is an autosomal recessive disorder featuring calcification and fragmentation of elastic fibers with cutaneous, ocular, and cardiovascular manifestations (269). Initial skin findings include soft, yellowish coalescent papules, which often appear in childhood on the lateral neck but may be missed until the second or third decade of life, when they generalize to involve the axillae, below the clavicle, antecubital fossa, and perineum. The

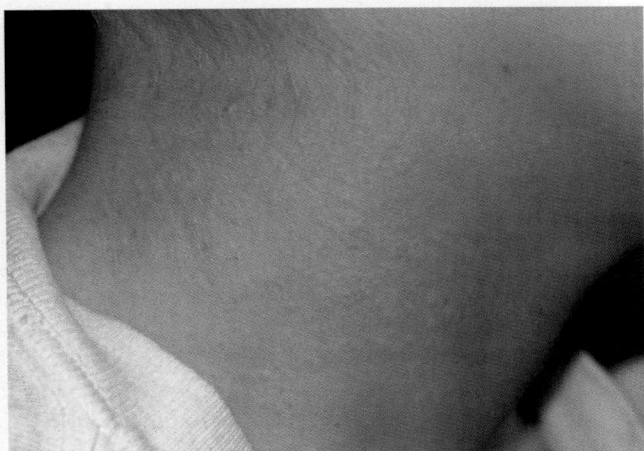

Figure 6-47 Pseudoxanthoma elasticum. Yellow coalescing papules on the lateral neck. (Courtesy of Albert Yan, CHOP Dermatology.)

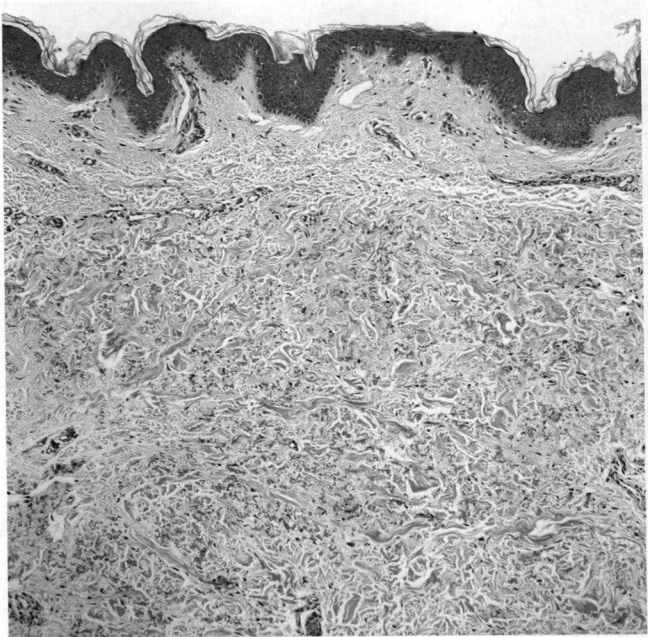

Figure 6-48 Pseudoxanthoma elasticum, medium magnification, hematoxylin–eosin (H&E) stained tissue showing calcified altered elastic fibers in the mid-reticular dermis (original magnification ×100).

affected skin appears loose and wrinkled and has been likened to "plucked chicken skin" (Fig. 6-47) (270,271). Mucosal involvement appears as yellow papules on the lower lip and the genitals. Patients with *GGCX* mutations have more extensive PXE-like lesions over the trunk with more severe cutis laxa (272). Ocular findings include angioid streaks in the fundus, which typically develop in the second and third decades of life and are caused by pathologic breaks in Bruch membrane, an elastin-rich layer. Retinal epithelial mottling (*peau d'orange* change) often precedes the development of angioid streaks and is secondary to degenerated elastic tissue. Other reported ocular manifestations include choroidal neovascularizations, chorioretinal atrophy, and reticular drusen (273). Cardiovascular involvement results from accelerated atherosclerosis secondary to degenerated elastic lamina and may manifest as claudication, stroke, or myocardial infarction (271). Arterial rupture also occurs with resultant hemorrhage, presumably secondary to abnormal stiffening of the vasculature, resulting in defective contraction. Gastrointestinal hemorrhage has been reported in 8% to 19% of patients (274).

Pathogenesis. Pseudoxanthoma elasticum is primarily a disease of anti-mineralization factor deficiency. Mutations in the gene *ABCC6*, which encodes an ATP-binding cassette transporter protein, cause PXE in 80% of cases (275–277). To date, there are over 300 loss-of-function mutations in *ABCC6*, which encodes multidrug resistance-associated protein 6 (MRP6). MRP6 is expressed in the liver and kidney and results in the down-regulation of systemic anti-mineralization factors inorganic pyrophosphate (PPi) and fetuin-A. Dysregulation of PPi can also be caused by homozygous inactivating mutations in the gene product of *ENPP1*, leading to a subset of PXE or generalized arterial calcification of infancy (278,279). Initially, PXE was speculated to result from a primary connective tissue defect. However, LeSaux et al. found that in the presence of normal human serum, PXE fibroblasts produced increased elastic fibers that were structurally normal. In contrast, incubation of *either* PXE fibroblasts or normal fibroblasts with *serum* from PXE patients produced abnormal aggregates of degenerated, calcified elastin, suggesting the presence of a circulating metabolite that was required for PXE mineralization. As a result of this and other work, PXE is now presumed to be a primary metabolic disorder with secondary connective tissue manifestations (278,280). Finally, compound mutations in γ-glutamyl carboxylase (GGCX)

and ABCC6 can also cause PXE. GGCX is responsible for the γ-glutamyl carboxylation of the anti-mineralization factor matrix gla protein and vitamin K–dependent coagulation factors. Double mutations in GGCX cause PXE skin lesions with primary coagulopathy (279).

Histopathology. The histopathologic hallmark of PXE in the skin is accumulation of fragmented, "elastotic" material in the middle and lower thirds of the dermis, with calcification of the elastic structures (Figs. 6-48 and 6-49). The abnormal elastic fibers stain deeply black with orcein or Verhoeff stain. Although normally elastic fibers do not stain with hematoxylin and eosin, the altered elastic fibers in PXE stain faintly basophilic because of their calcium imbibition. Staining for calcium with the von Kossa method also shows these fibers well (Fig. 6-50). Near the altered elastic fibers, there may be accumulations of a slightly basophilic mucoid material, which stains strongly positive with colloidal iron or with Alcian blue stains (281). The number of

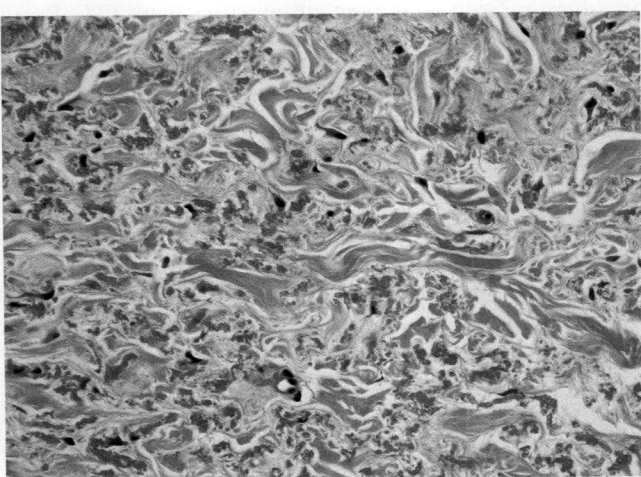

Figure 6-49 Pseudoxanthoma elasticum, high magnification. High-power view of the calcified elastic fibers (original magnification ×200).

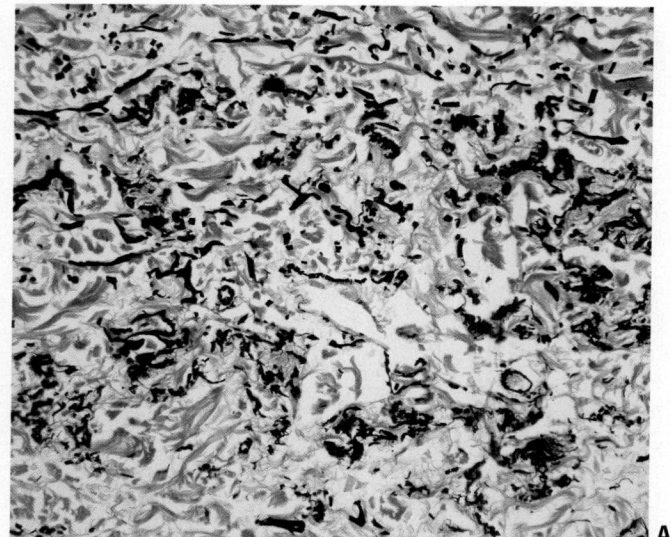

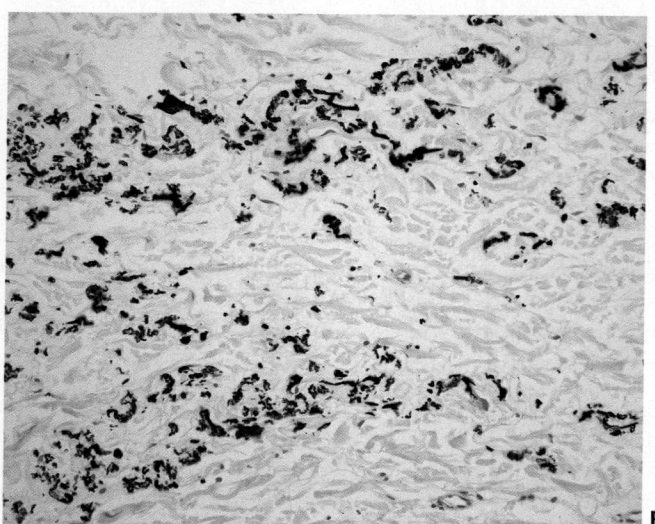

Figure 6-50 A: Pseudoxanthoma elasticum, elastic tissue stain. The elastic fibers show marked degeneration (original magnification ×200). B: Von Kossa. Von Kossa-stained sections demonstrate the calcium deposition on the fragmented elastic fibers (original magnification ×200).

collagen bundles is reduced in such areas, and numerous reticulum fibers are seen on impregnation with silver (282). In some cases with pronounced elastic tissue calcification, a macrophage and giant-cell reaction may be present (283). PXE-like changes can also occur in association with calciphylaxis (284,285), papillary dermal elastolysis (286,287), nephrogenic systemic fibrosis (288), and others.

The angioid streaks occur in Bruch membrane, which is located between the retina and the choroid and contains numerous elastic fibers in its outer portion, the lamina elastica. Calcification of these fibers causes fissure formation, resulting in hemorrhages and exudates, which in turn cause degenerative changes in the retina (283,289).

Gastric bleeding is the result of calcification of elastic fibers in the thin-walled arteries located immediately beneath the gastric mucosa. The internal elastic lamina is particularly affected. In muscular arteries, such as the coronary arteries and the large peripheral arteries, calcification begins in the internal and external elastic laminae, leading to their fragmentation,

and subsequently extends to the media and intima (290). Calcification of the elastic fibers in the endocardium is a common occurrence but is clinically silent (291).

Histogenesis. Electron microscopic examination shows that calcification occurs in normal-appearing elastic fibers (282,291,292). In young patients, only some of the elastic fibers in the lower dermis are calcified, and the calcification may be variable in degree. However, in adult patients, most elastic fibers show considerable calcification and, as a result, degeneration. Early calcification of elastic fibers consists either of diffuse granular deposits throughout the elastic fiber or of dense aggregates that may be in the center or near the margin of the fiber. Elastic fibers ultimately become fully calcified, showing marked swelling and bizarre distortions. In addition, heavy calcium deposits may be seen in the ground substance adjacent to elastic fibers and free in the ground substance. The presence of calcified material outside of elastic fibers can be explained by the disintegration of completely calcified elastic fibers (292).

Differential Diagnosis. Fundoscopic signs, vascular disease, and ectopic calcification of lesional skin are keys to diagnosing pseudoxanthoma elasticum. Cutis laxa secondary to other disorders may be considered if PXE-like papules are not present. Fibroelastolytic papulosis is a spectrum of noninflammatory fibroelastolytic disorders (PXE-like papillary dermal elastolysis and white fibrous papulosis of the neck) and can present with similar papules and plaques. The latter can be differentiated by loss of elastic fibers in the papillary dermis and lack of calcification of the elastic fibers. Late-onset focal dermal elastosis and elastosis perforans serpinginosa also lack dermal calcium deposits. Perforating calcific elastosis occurs in multiparous women around the periumbilical region and has identical histologic findings to PXE, with the lack of systemic involvement being the only reliable distinction.

Principles of Management: Presently, there is no cure for PXE and treatment is supportive. Patients should avoid contact sports and intense exercise secondary to the risk of traumatizing already-calcified vessels. Close follow-up with ophthalmology and cardiology is imperative to screen for progressive vascular disease.

Elastosis Perforans Serpiginosa

Clinical Summary. Elastosis perforans serpiginosa (EPS) is a rare cutaneous disorder characterized by transepidermal elimination of elastin. It represents one of the primary perforating dermatoses, which also includes reactive perforating collagenosis (collagen), Kyrle disease (mixed connective tissue), and acquired perforating dermatosis. EPS typically presents during childhood or young adulthood. Groups of erythematous or hyperpigmented papules are arranged in annular or serpiginous patterns usually found on the neck, face, and flexural surfaces of the arm (Fig. 6-51, EPS). A central keratotic plug in each papule represents the hyperkeratotic epidermis and the transepidermal eruption of elastic fibers. Lesions can be pruritic or asymptomatic (293–295).

Histopathology. An acanthotic epidermis with hyperparakeratosis houses a keratin plug within a central depression. Transepidermal channels connecting to the plug are filled by eosinophilic aggregates of elastin with basophilic debris of inflammatory cells and keratinocytes. Channels may be contained within hair follicles. On the papillary dermis side of the channel, elastosis

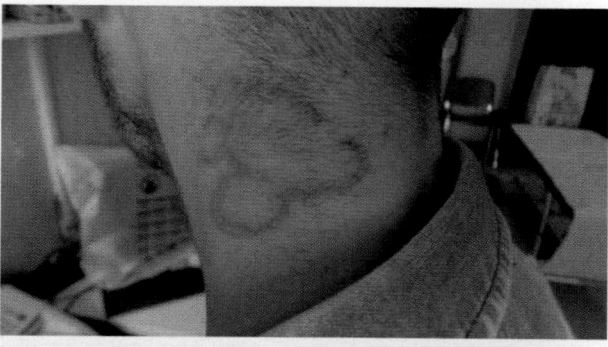
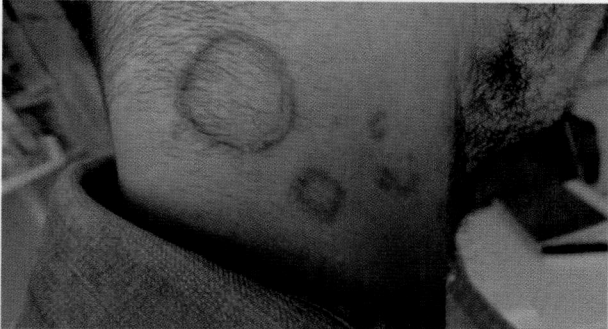
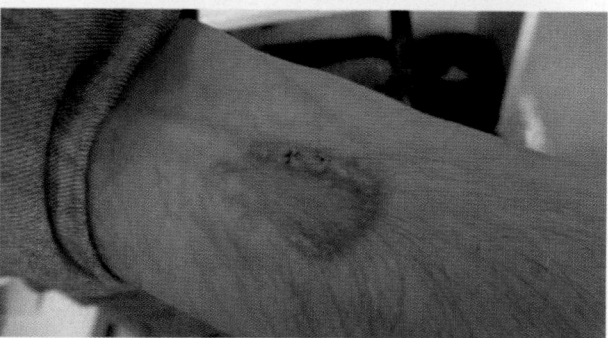

Figure 6-51 Elastosis perforans serpinginosa (EPS). Groups of erythematous or hyperpigmented papules are arranged in annular or serpiginous patterns usually found on the neck, face, and flexural surfaces of the arm. (Reprinted with permission from Ranucci G, Di Dato F, Leone F, et al. Penicillamine-induced elastosis perforans serpiginosa in Wilson disease: is useful switching to zinc? *J Pediatr Gastroenterol Nutr.* 2017;64(3):e72–e73.)

is prominent with twisted and thickened elastic fibers. At the dermal opening of the channel, individual elastic fibers are positioned vertically toward the route of elimination. A mixed dermal infiltrate of lymphocytes, histiocytes, and multinucleated giant cells are present. "Bramble bush"-appearing elastic fibers can be seen in both lesional and nonlesional dermis of penicillamine-induced EPS (Fig. 6-52A, B).

Pathogenesis. EPS is often associated with genetic diseases such as Ehlers-Danlos syndrome, osteogenesis imperfecta, Marfan syndrome, pseudoxanthoma elasticum, and acrogeria. Long-term use of penicillamine and chronic kidney disease are thought to be causes of acquired EPS. Isolated reports show a potential autosomal dominant pattern of inheritance (92).

Connective Tissue Nevi

Clinical Summary. Connective tissue nevi are dermal hamartomas composed of extracellular dermal matrix proteins, including collagen, elastin, or both. The lesions consist of slightly elevated, dermal papules or plaques, whose surface may appear cerebriform or cobblestoned (Fig. 6-53). They can be solitary or multiple and occur as sporadic finding or as part of various syndromes (296). The plantar cerebriform connective tissue nevus is one of the most characteristic findings of Proteus syndrome, a postnatal overgrowth disorder affecting multiple tissues including skin, bone, and soft tissue, caused by mutations in *AKT1* (297). The fibrous forehead plaque and shagreen patch seen in tuberous sclerosis also represent connective tissue nevi. Buschke–Ollendorff syndrome (BOS) is an autosomal dominant disorder characterized by areas of focal bone opacification (osteopoikilosis) in association with multiple connective tissue nevi (elastomas, collagenomas, of mixed connective tissue nevi) composed primarily of elastin (dermatofibrosis lenticularis disseminata), caused by mutations in the gene *LEMD3*, which encodes an inner nuclear membrane protein (298–300). The skin lesions in this syndrome consist of firm, pale papules and plaques, which are often grouped on the trunk but may be seen on the extremities. Individual members of affected families may have skin lesions without bone lesions and vice versa. The bone lesions of osteopoikilosis are asymptomatic but are seen radiographically as round or oval densities 2 to 10 mm in

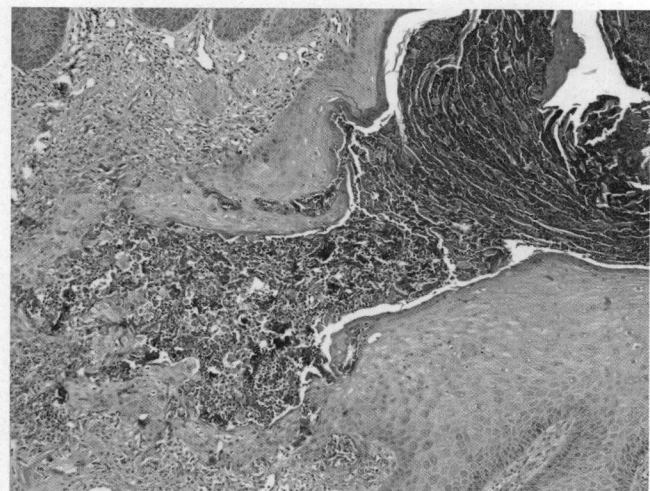
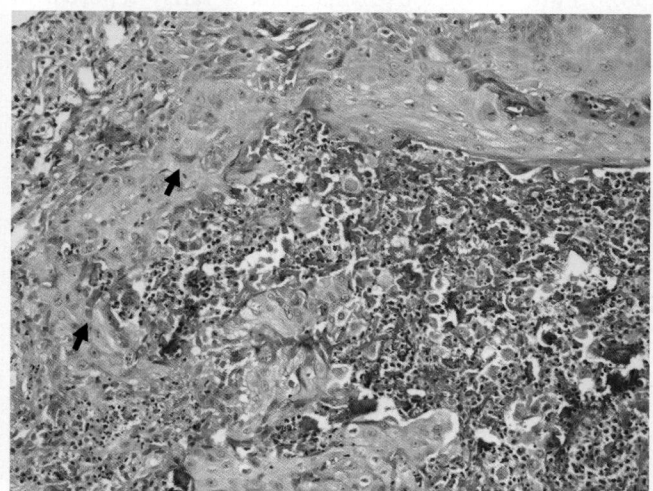

Figure 6-52 A, B: Elastosis perforans serpinginosa (EPS). Transepidermal channels connecting to the plug are filled by eosinophilic aggregates of elastin with basophilic debris of inflammatory cells and keratinocytes. Channels may be contained within hair follicles (original magnification ×400). (Digital slides courtesy of Path Presenter.com.)

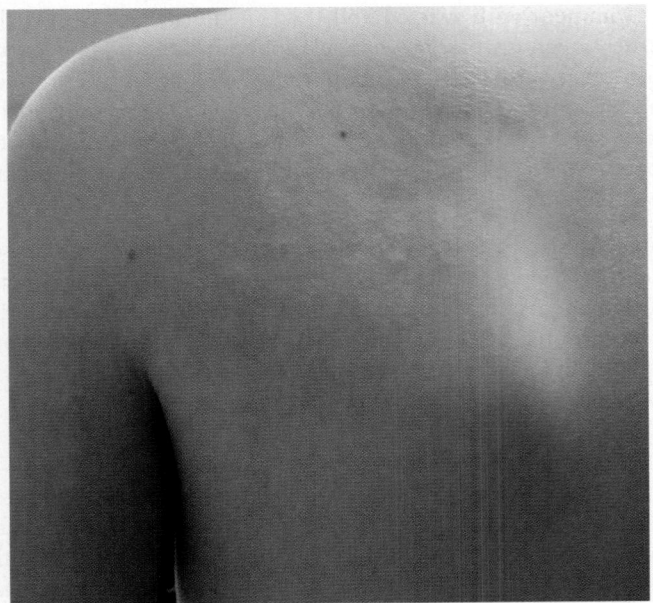

Figure 6-53 Connective tissue nevi. Grouped flesh-colored papules producing an irregular contour on the left upper back. (Courtesy of Albert Yan, CHOP Dermatology.)

diameter in the long bones and in the bones of the hands, feet, and pelvis (300). Melorheostosis, hyperostotic cortical bone that takes on a dripping wax appearance is also sometimes seen on imaging. Other rare reported findings include short stature, diabetes, craniosynostosis, and otosclerosis.

Histopathology. A clear separation of collagenoma and elastoma is not always possible because, in many instances, both collagenous and elastic fibers are increased, as indicated by the fact that most lesions of connective tissue nevus feel firm to the touch (Figs. 6-54 and 6-55). Elastomas are characterized by clumped fragments or a thickened, interlaced meshwork of elastic fibers in the mid-to-deep dermis. Collagenomas feature dermal accumulation of hypertrophic collagen bundles with a relative dilution of normal elastic fibers. Most cases of the Buschke–Ollendorff syndrome clearly show a marked increase in the amount of elastic fibers, which are present as broad, interfacing bands, without showing signs of degeneration (Fig. 6-56) (301,302). Pure collagenous hamartoma is rarely reported in

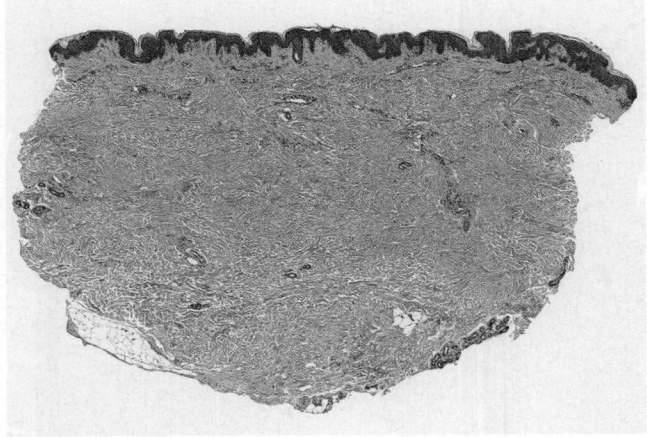

Figure 6-54 Low-power image: connective tissue nevus. This low-power image shows mildly thickened collagen bundles in the dermis and a sparse inflammatory infiltrate (original magnification ×40).

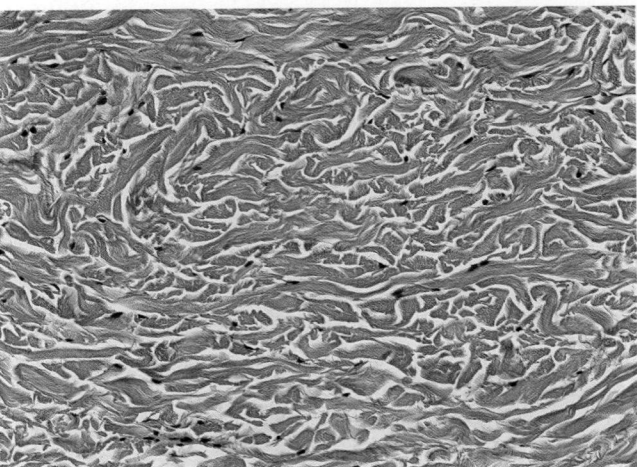

Figure 6-55 High-power image: connective tissue nevus. This high-power view shows an increased density of thickened collagen bundles and a mildly increased population of fibroblasts (original magnification ×200).

BOS. Multiple collagenomas with mucin deposition have been reported recently (303).

Pathogenesis. On electron microscopic examination, connective tissue nevi may be variable. In some cases, the elastic fibers appear thick and are surrounded by a thready material (304). In the Buschke–Ollendorff syndrome, the elastic fibers lack their microfibrillar component, so only electron-lucent elastin is present (302).

Differential Diagnosis. Histologically, the changes of a connective tissue nevus can be subtle. Because of this, the histologic differential diagnosis would include entities with mild changes in the "normal skin" differential diagnosis list.

Principles of Management: Connective tissue nevi are benign and require no treatment.

Stiff Skin Syndrome
Clinical Summary. Stiff skin syndrome (SSS) is a rare autosomal dominant disorder characterized by noninflammatory fibrosis

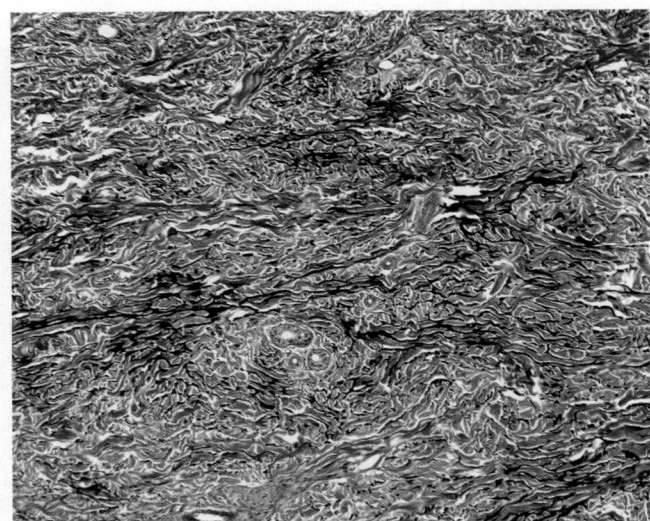

Figure 6-56 Connective tissue nevus. With a Verhoeff van Gieson stain, areas of increased density of thickened elastic fibers are seen in the dermis (original magnification ×100).

of the skin. Often presenting in late infancy and early childhood, typical skin plaques and nodules are woody to palpation with frequent involvement of deep subcutaneous tissue. The overlying skin could appear normal or with mild hypertrichosis and hyperpigmentation. Joint immobility favoring the limb girdles and contractures sometimes become significant secondary to the thickened, constricting skin. Both segmental and generalized forms have been described (305–307).

Histopathology. Horizontally oriented to the normal epidermis, thickened dermal collagen bundles extend down to a sclerotic fascia with an associated increase in fibroblast cellularity (Fig. 6-57A, B). There are no inflammatory changes in the dermis, but accumulation of mucin may be prominent within the collagen clefts, and it can be detected by acid Alcian blue or colloidal iron staining. Elastic fibers have normal morphology. In the dermis and subcutis, entrapment of adipocytes by collagen bundles is a distinctive feature (306,307).

Pathogenesis. It is caused by mutations in the TGF-β-binding protein-like domain 4 (TB4) of fibrillin-1 (*FBN1*). Marfan syndrome (MFS) is also associated with nonoverlapping *FBN1* mutations. Key functional differences exist between the mutated fibrillin-1 found in MFS and SSS. MFS mutations result in loss of fibrillin-1 expression. In contrast, SSS skin demonstrates large deposits of abnormal fibrillin-1 at the dermal–epidermal junction and increased expression throughout the dermis, leading to the sequestration of inactive TGF-β at these sites. In these mutations, fibrillin is prevented from binding to integrin, resulting in TGF-β activation and profibrotic signaling (308–310).

Winchester Syndrome and Multicentric Osteolysis, Nodulosis, and Arthropathy

Clinical Summary. Winchester syndrome is a heritable disease of connective tissue that has significant clinical overlap with multicentric osteolysis, nodulosis, and arthropathy (MONA). Both Winchester syndrome and MONA feature generalized osteoporosis and symmetric osteolysis of the carpal and tarsal bones that lead to joint contractures beginning during the first 6 years of life. Coarse facial features, corneal opacity, EKG changes, and gum hypertrophy are variable findings. Winchester syndrome features more severe, progressive bone disfigurement. Patches of thick, hyperpigmented skin with hypertrichosis can develop over the trunk and limbs, which become softer and paler over time. The presence of subcutaneous nodules favors the diagnosis of MONA (311,312).

Histopathology. Histopathologic findings in both conditions include deep dermal proliferation of fibroblasts with thickened collagen bundles. The dermis of older lesions evolves to become hypocellular and with homogenized collagen bundles.

Pathogenesis. The genetic basis of Winchester syndrome is not firmly established, but it is likely caused by mutation in membrane type-1 metalloproteinase (*MT1-MMP*). The mutation results in decreased expression of both the zymogen and active MT1-MMP, which leads to reduced activation *of* matrix metalloproteinase-2 (MMP2). Homozygous mutations in the *MMP2* gene are associated with MONA. MMPs proteolyze and remodel the extracellular matrix, which broadly regulates the function of epithelial and mesenchymal tissue. Ultrastructural studies have demonstrated abnormal fibroblasts with vacuolation of the mitochondria (313).

Primary Idiopathic Osteoarthropathy

Clinical Summary. Primary hypertrophic osteoarthropathy (PHO), or pachydermoperiostosis, is a rare disease caused by disruptions in prostaglandin metabolism (314). PHO can be inherited in an autosomal dominant or recessive fashion. Disease onset typically occurs in infancy (PHOAR1) or adolescence (PHOAR2) with common findings of digital clubbing, pachydermia, and periostitis. Cutaneous manifestations include cutis verticis gyrata (CVG), thickened facial skin with the appearance of premature deep furrowing, seborrhea, blepharoptosis, acne,

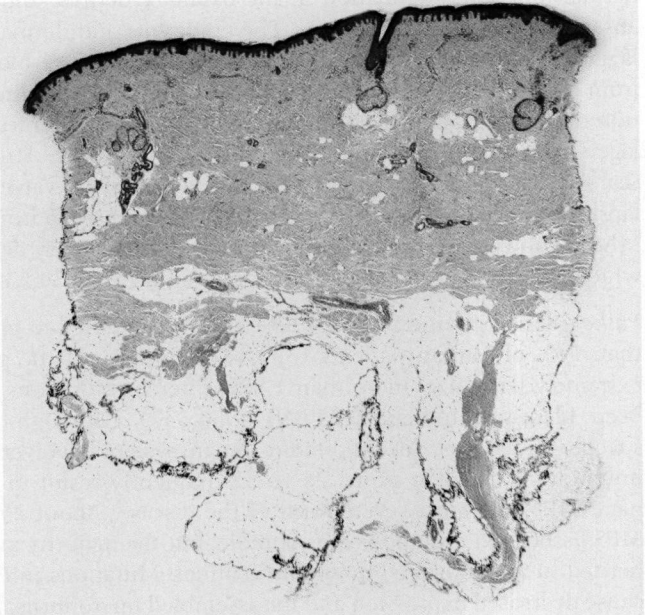

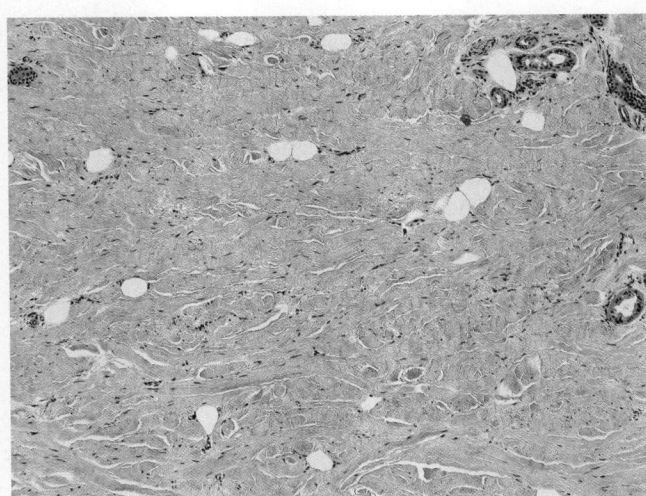

A   **B**

Figure 6-57 A, B Stiff skin syndrome. Horizontally oriented to the normal epidermis, thickened dermal collagen bundles extend down to a sclerotic fascia with an associated increase in fibroblast cellularity (original magnifications ×20 and ×100). (Reprinted with permission from Gru AA. *Pediatric Dermatopathology and Dermatology*. Wolters Kluwer; 2019.)

atopic dermatitis, and hyperhidrosis. Severe CVG occurs only with PHOAR2 (315). Skeletal involvement results in noninflammatory arthralgia, acroosteolysis, tendon ossification, and radiographic evidence of endosteal and periosteal hyperostosis. Gastrointestinal disease, patent ductus arteriosus (PHOAR1), and myelofibrosis (PHOAR2) have also been documented.

Histopathology. Histologic examination of normal-appearing skin may show acanthosis with underlying dermal edema and increased connective tissue mucin. Biopsy samples from the thickened skin show a normal epidermis overlying an edematous dermis, within which there is increased connective tissue mucin. Sebaceous gland hyperplasia, elastin degeneration, and dermal fibrosis are variable, and they tend to be more marked with increasing clinical severity of pachydermia (316,317).

Pathogenesis. Mutations in the *HPGD* (PHO autosomal recessive, type 1, PHOAR1) and *SLCO2A1* (PHO autosomal recessive, type 2, PHOAR2) genes have been identified as the cause of the recessive primary hypertrophic osteoarthropathy (318,319). Based on the clinical severity, PHO is delineated into a complete form (the classical phenotype), an incomplete form (isolated bone involvement with limited skin involvement), and a form fruste (pachydermia and minimal bone disease).

Restrictive Dermopathy

Clinical Summary. Restrictive dermopathy (RD), a rare and lethal progeroid laminopathy, is characterized by pathologically tight skin leading to fetal akinesia and neonatal demise from pulmonary failure. Patients are born prematurely with taut, translucent skin with prominent vasculature. Generalized alopecia sparing the head is seen. Characteristic facial features are microstomia fixed in the "O" position, micrognathia, pinched nose, and wide cranial sutures (320–322).

Histopathology. Biopsy specimens show flattened rete overlying a thinned dermis. There is scar-like dermal fibrosis, in which collagen bundles are arranged in parallel to the epidermis with sparse elastic fibers. Adnexal structures are uniformly poorly differentiated. The subcutis appears normal.

Pathogenesis. RD is the most severe form of the lamin-associated disorder that also includes mandibuloacral dysplasia, Hutchinson–Gilford progeria syndrome, and others. RD results from heterozygous or homozygous mutations of the *LMNA* gene or, more commonly, null mutations of the *ZMPSTE24* gene (encoding zinc metalloprotease STE24) (323,324). Lamin A is a structural constituent of the inner nuclear envelope. STE24 is responsible for processing and maturation of lamin A. There are isolated cases of RD for which causative mutations have not been identified. Mutations in *LMNA* and *ZMPSTE24* result in abnormal nuclear morphology and an accumulation of unprocessed prelamin A. Ultrastructural studies confirm the proliferation of small-caliber collagen fibrils, the presence of degenerated fibroblasts, and the near absence of elastic fibers.

Marfan Syndrome

Clinical Summary. The classic signs of Marfan syndrome are reduced upper segment-to-lower segment ratio, severe pectum excavatum, scoliosis, ectopia lentis, dilatation and dissection of the ascending aorta, and lumbosacral dural ectasia (325,326). Patients present with a typical habitus characterized by tall, thin stature with long arms, legs, fingers, and toes (Fig. 6-58)

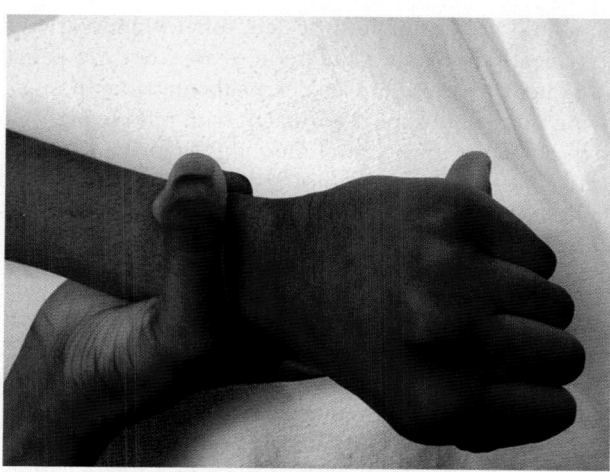

Figure 6-58 Marfan syndrome. Long fingers result in the thumb sign, in which the thumb protrudes from a closed fist, and the wrist sign, in which the thumb and the fifth fingers overlap when encircling the opposite wrist. (Reprinted with permission from Bitterman AD, Sponseller PD. Marfan syndrome: a clinical update. *J Am Acad Orthop Surg.* 2017;25(9):603–609. Copyright 2017 by the American Academy of Orthopaedic Surgeons.)

(325,327,328). The prevalence of striae increases with age and is present in the vast majority of adult Marfan patients, appearing as atrophic, linear plaques ranging from erythematous to white in color (329,330). Presence in locations other than the thighs, buttocks, and hips occurs significantly more frequently in affected patients than in the general population. Infantile striae have been reported in the neonatal form of MFS (331). Abnormal wound healing is a common finding, with wide or atrophic scarring, dyspigmentation, and recurrent incisional hernias (325,326,329).

Histopathology. Clinically normal-appearing skin of patients with Marfan syndrome may have characteristic histologic dermal findings. Elastic fibers appear fragmented with some scattering in orientation (332,333). Immunohistochemical evaluation for fibrillin protein shows discontinuous staining of the dermoepidermal junction, attenuation in the papillary dermis, and near absence in the reticular dermis. The epidermis and dermal collagen appear normal. As in striae from normal patients, biopsies from MFS patients show thinning of the epidermis with attenuation of the rete. The dermis is also thin, with hypertrophied collagen and elastic fibers run in parallel with the surface. Atrophic scars in a patient with incomplete MFS (i.e., *mitral valve prolapse, aortic enlargement, skin and skeletal findings syndrome* or MASS) show short, broken elastic fibers in the papillary dermis, which formed large aggregates in older lesions (332,334,335).

Pathogenesis. Mutation in the *FBN1* gene is identified in greater than 90% of Marfan patients (336,337). Because of the gene's extremely large size, more than 1,800 different mutations have been identified to date in *FBN1* (336,337). Although most specific mutations do not predict organ system involvement, mutations located in exons 24 to 32 frequently result in neonatal MFS, the most severe form of the disease. About 25% of MFS-associated mutations are sporadic, but the majority are inherited in an autosomal dominant manner. Mutations in *FBN1* cause decreased expression and misassembled microfibrils, leading to errors in elastic fiber formation and compromise of the mechanical integrity of connective tissues (338). FBN1 has also been strongly implicated in the regulation of TGF-β signaling.

Ehlers-Danlos Syndrome

Clinical Summary. Ehlers-Danlos syndrome (EDS) is a heterogeneous group of inherited disorders of collagen characterized by joint hypermobility, increased cutaneous elasticity, and skin fragility associated with poor wound healing and formation of wide atrophic scar (Table 6-3). Other clinical features include the presence of wrinkled subcutaneous nodules (pseudotumors) secondary to resolution of traumatic hematomas with accompanying fibrosis (Fig. 6-59) (339). Particularly on the shins and forearms, these may calcify or undergo traumatic fat

---

Table 6-3

Categorization and Features of Ehlers-Danlos Syndrome

Type (Historic Category)	Genetic Mutations	Major Features	Inheritance Pattern	Salient Histologic/Ultra-structural Features
Classic˙(I, II)	COL5A1, COL5A2. COL1A1	Skin hyperextensibility with atrophic scarring, GJH	AD	Flower like collagen fibrils
Classic-like	TNXB	Skin hyperextensibility without atrophic scarring, easy bruising, GJH	AR	
Cardiac valvular	COL1A2	Cardiac valvular disease, classic skin involvement, joint hypermobility	AR	
Hypermobile (III)	Mostly unknown, partially secondary to TNXB heterozygous	Joint hypermobility, less skin involvement, abdominal hernia, pelvic organ prolapse, aortic root dilatation	AD	Calcified deposits within amorphous matrix of elastic fibers and clusters of hyaluronic acid
Vascular (IV)	COL3A1	Early arterial rupture, sigmoid colon perforation, gestational uterine rupture, peripartum perineum laceration, carotid-cavernous sinus fistula, family history of vEDS	AD	Thin dermis, irregular thickness of dermal–epidermal junction, fibroblasts with lysosome
Kyphoscoliotic (VIA)	PLOD1. FKBP14	Congenital hypotonia, congenital or early-onset kyphoscoliosis, GJH	AR	Subtle irregularities in collagen fibril contour and spacing
Musculocontractural (VIB)	CHST14. DSE	Characteristic congenital contractures, characteristic facies, classic skin involvement with palmar wrinkling	AR	Dispersal of collagen fibrils
Arthrochalasia (VIIA, VIIB)	COL1A1, COL1A2	Congenital bilateral hip dislocation, severe GJH, skin hyperextensibility	AD	Collagen fibrils with variable diameter and highly irregular contour
Dermatosparaxis (VIIC)	ADAMTS2	Extreme congenital skin fragility, characteristic facies, lax skin with palmar wrinkling, severe bruisability, umbilical hernia, growth retardation, short appendages, perinatal complications	AR	Hieroglyphic collagen fibrils
Periodontal (VIII)	C1R, C1S	Severe periodontitis, detached gingiva, pretibial plaques, family history of pEDS	AD	
Spondylodysplastic	B4GALT7. B3GALT6. SLC39A13	Short stature, congenital hypotonia, limb bowing	AR	
Brittle cornea syndrome	ZNF469. PRDM5	Thin cornea, keratoconus, keratoglobus, blue sclera	AR	
Myopathic	COL12A1	Congenital hypotonia with/without atrophy, joint contractures, hypermobility of distal joints	AD or AR	

Abbreviations: AD, autosomal dominant; AR, autosomal recessive; GJH, generalized joint hypermobility.

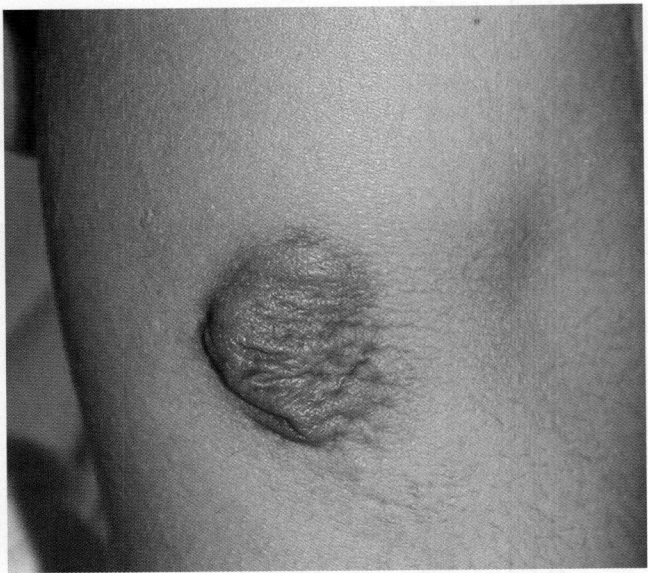

Figure 6-59 Ehlers-Danlos syndrome. Pseudo-molluscoid scarring.

necrosis and are called spheroids. In 1998, the classification scheme was revised to include six main subgroups on the basis of clinical, molecular, and biochemical findings (340). The clinical spectrum of disease severity ranges from mild, asymptomatic skin and joint laxity to severe physical disability with life-threatening arterial complications.

Classical type EDS is the most common form and is characterized by velvety skin that is hyperextensible, easy bruising, impaired wound healing with "cigarette paper scars," and small and large joint laxity, which may be complicated by recurrent joint dislocations. Gorlin sign, characterized by the ability to touch the tip of the nose with the tongue, may be present (Fig. 6-60). The disorder is inherited in an autosomal dominant fashion and is caused by mutations in the COL5A1 and COL5A2 genes (341).

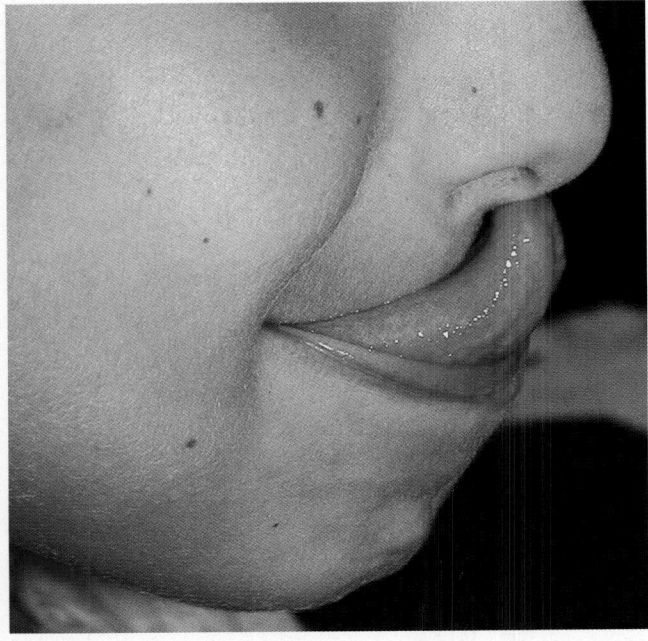

Figure 6-60 Ehlers-Danlos syndrome. Gorlin sign consistent with increased elasticity in Ehlers-Danlos syndrome.

Patients with **hypermobility type EDS** demonstrate generalized joint hypermobility, joint instability complications, and musculoskeletal pain. The skin manifestations are a minor feature and include velvety soft skin, although cutaneous hyperextensibility and impaired wound healing are less common features (342). The molecular basis of the disorder remains unknown, although approximately 5% of patients have been found to have homozygous or compound heterozygous mutations in the enzyme tenascin X (TNXB) (343).

Vascular type EDS is an autosomal dominant disorder caused by mutations in the COL3A1 gene. The earliest manifestations are cutaneous and include thin, translucent skin with easy bruising despite normal coagulation and hemostasis studies. Many patients have a characteristic facial appearance that includes a pinched nose, sunken eyes, thin lips, fine telangiectasias of the eyelids, and decreased facial fat (344). Spontaneous arterial rupture is the most common cause of death and can rarely occur in childhood. Arterial or gastrointestinal rupture may present with severe flank pain mimicking an acute surgical abdomen, and rupture of intracranial aneurysms may lead to hemorrhagic stroke (345).

Kyphoscoliosis type EDS is an autosomal recessive disorder characterized by hypotonia and scoliosis at birth, generalized joint laxity and skin fragility with atrophic scarring (340). Decreased muscle tone leads to delay in gross motor skills, and scoliosis is typically progressive and disabling. Osteopenia, blue sclerae, and a marfanoid habitus are associated features. Rupture of the globe is a rare finding. The disease is caused by mutations in the gene PLOD1, which encodes collagen lysyl hydroxylase 1. Deficiency of this enzyme leads to impaired collagen cross-linking and mechanical weakness of affected tissues (340,346).

Arthrochalasia type EDS is characterized by generalized joint hypermobility, joint instability, (particularly congenital bilateral hip dislocations), hypotonia, and facial dysmorphisms (347). The disease is inherited as an autosomal dominant trait secondary to mutations in the COL1A1 or COL1A2 gene (348). The skin and tendons of patients with this form of EDS contain collagen polypeptides with a length intermediate between procollagen chains and fully formed collagen chains secondary to a structural mutation that prevents normal enzymatic removal of an amino-propeptide (349).

Patients with **dermatosparaxis type EDS** demonstrate extreme skin fragility with easy bruising and joint hypermobility, which becomes more pronounced with age. In contrast to other types of EDS, the skin of affected patients is lax and sagging but not hyperextensible (i.e., it does not snap back into place). Patients are at risk for life-threatening visceral organ rupture. Characteristic features include blue sclerae, micrognathia, gingival hyperkeratosis, umbilical and inguinal hernias, delayed fontanelle closure, and postnatal growth failure (350). The disease is inherited as an autosomal recessive trait caused by mutations in the gene ADAMTS-2, which encodes the enzyme procollagen 1 N-proteinase, and functions to excise the N-terminal propeptide in procollagen types I, II, and III (351,352). As a consequence, there is an accumulation of abnormal collagen fibrils, which on electron microscopy appear thin, branched, irregular, and have been likened to "hieroglyphics" (353,354).

Histopathology. Vascular EDS demonstrates dermal thinning, usually to half or three-quarters of normal thickness. There is a relative abundance of elastic fibers that appear shortened and fragmented, likely secondary to changes in collagen fiber morphology. Most other subtypes of EDS demonstrate normal skin thickness and appearance of collagen and elastic fibers. Occasionally, biopsies will demonstrate thin collagen fibers that are not united into bundles. In these cases, the skin may also be reduced in thickness and show a relative increase in the amount of elastic fibers. They are often seen best in the collagen bundles of the connective tissue septae of the subcutaneous fat (355).

The raisin-like pseudotumors that arise at the site of hematomas often show fibrosis and numerous capillaries and occasionally show foreign-body giant cells. The spheroid subcutaneous nodules consist of partially necrotic fat that may contain areas of dystrophic calcification (356).

Principles of Management: Management is generally supportive and varies by severity of disease and subtype. A multidisciplinary approach, including dermatology, rheumatology, and sometimes cardiology, neurology, and orthopedic surgery, is ideal for integrative patient care. Genetic counseling should be offered to patients and families. Those with skin fragility issues should be protected as much as possible from laceration or bruising.

Cutis Laxa (Elastolysis)

Clinical Summary. Cutis laxa, also called *generalized elastolysis,* is characterized by redundant, inelastic pendulous skin, resulting in a prematurely aged appearance. The disease may be congenital or acquired, with variable systemic manifestations. The congenital types may be autosomal dominant or recessive and result from mutations that affect elastic fibers, including mutations in elastin, fibulin-4, fibulin-5, latent transforming growth factor-β binding protein-4, among others (357–359). Recessive disease is caused by mutations in elastin support proteins (*FBLN4* and *FBLN5*), the TGF-β pathway (*LTBP4*), vesicular ATPase (*ATP6V0A2, ATP6V1E1, ATP6V1A*), vesicular trafficking proteins (*GORAB, RIN2*), and mitochondrial components (*PYCR1, ALDH18A1*) (360–362). Patients with fibulin gene mutations are more likely to have associated arterial tortuosity, stenosis, and aneurysms (363). Acquired forms typically present in adulthood are associated with exposure to certain drugs or underlying malignancy, and they are typically preceded by an inflammatory dermatosis (357,364,365).

In both the congenital and acquired types, visceral involvement may occur, including pulmonary emphysema, diverticula in the gastrointestinal tract or bladder, rectal prolapse, and inguinal, umbilical and hiatal hernias (357,366). Radiographically, the congenital forms may reveal Wormian bones of the lambdoidal suture and osteoporosis.

The occipital horn syndrome (X-linked cutis laxa) shows moderate skin extensibility, joint hypermobility, bladder diverticula, herniae, and rhizomelic limb shortening. The defect is inherited as an X-linked recessive trait and has a mutation in the *ATP7A* gene, which results in deficiency of lysyl oxidase and abnormal copper metabolism. This disorder may be allelic with Menkes syndrome and was previously classified as EDS type IX (367,368).

Histopathology. In cases without an inflammatory infiltrate, the changes are limited to the elastic fibers and depend on the stage and the severity of the disease. Microscopic findings include loss of elaunin fibers and sparse fragmented elastic fibers, which are best visualized with an elastic fiber stain

such as Verhoeff van Gieson. In the early stage, the elastic fibers are diminished either throughout the dermis or largely in the papillary or reticular dermis (369). Elastic fibers may be considerably thickened in their midportion and may taper to a point at either end. Their borders may be indistinct, and they may stain unevenly, showing a granular appearance. Ultimately, no intact elastic fibers may be identifiable, with only fine, dust-like orceinophilic granules remaining in the dermis. In patients with involvement of internal organs, the lungs and gastrointestinal tract show the same granular changes in the elastic fibers as seen in the skin.

Pathogenesis. Electron microscopic examination shows degenerative changes in the elastic fibers that vary somewhat from case to case. In some instances, the elastic fibers show normal microfibrils but a deficiency of the amorphous, electron-lucent elastin; in other instances, the elastin is preserved and the microfibrils are absent (369,370). In most electron microscopic examinations, the most significant finding is the presence of electron-dense amorphous or granular aggregates in the vicinity of the elastic fibers (371). The presence of this electron-dense material outside of elastic fibers suggests that instead of a primary elastolysis, as generally assumed, a defect in the synthesis of elastic fibers causes the disease (370).

Principles of Management: Plastic surgery may improve patients' cosmetic appearance and there is no contraindication as these patients have normal wound healing. Surgical intervention may be necessary for a variety of complications, including the presence of diverticula, uterine or rectal prolapse, and hernias. Treatment is supportive.

Pachydermoperiostosis

Clinical Summary. Both genetic and acquired forms of pachydermoperiostosis exist, the latter being secondary to carcinoma of the lung. The idiopathic form is transmitted as an autosomal dominant or autosomal recessive trait, with males being more severely affected than females (372). Manifestations include clubbing of the digits, with periosteal proliferation of the bones of the hands and feet; hyperplasia of the soft parts of the forearms and legs, with periosteal proliferation of the corresponding bones; and thickening and furrowing of the skin of the face and scalp (CVG). In abortive forms, the only manifestations may include clubbing of the fingers with periosteal proliferation of the bones in the hands and forearms. The recessive form is secondary to homozygous or compound heterozygous mutations in the *SLCO2A1* gene, which encodes a prostaglandin transporter (373).

Histopathology. The skin of the face shows thickening of the dermis, with thick fibrous bands extending into the subcutaneous tissue. In addition to an increase in the amount and size of the collagen bundles in the dermis, there is an increase in the number of fibroblasts and in the amount of ground substance (11). The latter stains with colloidal iron, and because it is composed largely of hyaluronic acid, it stains with Alcian blue at pH 2.5 but not at pH 0.45.

Principles of Management: The polyarthritis associated with pachydermoperiostosis may be treated with a variety of agents, including nonsteroidal anti-inflammatories and/or corticosteroids. Cosmetic treatment of cutis vertices gyrate may include dermal fillers or fractional laser.

DISORDERS OF ABNORMAL PIGMENTATION

Oculocutaneous Albinism

This is a group of autosomal dominant, inherited disorders of melanin synthesis (374–376). Patients typically present at birth with variable hypopigmentation of the skin, hair, and eyes. Several gene-encoding proteins crucial for melanin synthesis have been identified as etiologic factors for oculocutaneous albinism (OCA). Absence or deficiency of tyrosinase (TYR) activity, as seen in OCA1a and OCA1b, results in diffuse depigmentation (377). Patients typically present with variable degrees of congenital pigmentary dilution of the skin, eyes, and hair. Ocular involvement includes translucent blue irides, hypopigmented retina, and nystagmus. Accelerated photoaging occurs, which include the development of skin cancers. Melanomas are also common and are typically amelanotic (378). The histopathologic changes include a normal number and density of melanocytes, but there is reduced-to-absent melanin pigmentation of the basal layer (379).

Hermansky-Pudlak Syndrome

This is a group of autosomal recessive hereditary disorders characterized by pigmentary changes, platelet abnormalities, and accumulation of ceroid-lipofuscin within internal organs (380–382). This condition is more common in Puerto Ricans (383). The genes involved in Hermansky-Pudlak syndrome (HPS) encode proteins involved in the regulation of vesicular trafficking within lysosome-related organelles, including platelet granules and melanosomes. The involved genes are typically organized into functional structures of interacting proteins known as BLOC (biogenesis of lysosome-related organelles complex). These patients exhibit variable pigmentary dilution of the skin and eyes, nystagmus, photophobia, and visual loss. Life-threatening pulmonary fibrosis can occur. The dysfunction of the platelets leads to bleeding diathesis with ecchymosis, epistaxis, and heavy menstrual periods. Uncommon complications include granulomatous colitis, cardiomyopathy, and renal failure. There are no distinctive histopathologic findings typical of HPS.

Chediak–Higashi Syndrome

This is an autosomal recessive, genetic disorder characterized by silvery hair, grayish skin pigmentation, and immunodeficiency secondary to mutations in the LYST gene (384–386). The gene product is a lysosomal transport protein. LYST regulates the fusion of primary lysozyme-like structures within cells, and its dysfunction results in an inability to properly target and transfer lysosomal vesicles. Giant granules accumulate within cells, and they typically include giant melanosomes in melanocytes, dense granules in platelets, and abnormal ones within neutrophils.

The clinical findings include pigmentary dilution and silvery hair (387,388). Dark-skinned patients can have acral hyperpigmentation. Photophobia, strabismus, and nystagmus are present. The primary morbidity from Chediak–Higashi syndrome (CHS) results from hematologic and immunodeficiency states. Recurrent skin, upper respiratory, and pulmonary infections occur. Most patients succumb to a life-threatening accelerated phase in the first decade of life, involving diffuse visceral infiltration by lymphoid and histiocytic cells, representing an inherited form of hemophagocytic lymphohistiocytosis (HLH).

Microscopic evaluation of the affected hairs shows clumping of melanin in the shaft (382,388,389). The clumping is evenly spaced, as opposed to Griscelli syndrome (GS).

Griscelli Syndrome

This is a group of rare, autosomal recessive genetic disorders with cutaneous findings of silvery hair and pigmentary dilution (382,390). Type 1 GS, including the variant Elejalde syndrome, presents with neurologic deficits; type 2 GS with immunodeficiency and risk for HLH; and type 3 GS with pigmentary changes only. Type 1 GS is caused by a mutation in myosin Va (MYO5A), expressed in melanocytes and the CNS, and it binds melanosomes to actin filaments for transportation. Type 2 GS results from a mutation in RAB27A (melanosome transfer). Type 3 GS is associated with mutations in melanophilin, only present in the skin, and interacts with MYO5A and RAB27A to facilitate melanosome transport in the cells (391).

Cutaneous manifestations include the presence of grayish pigment dilution, blue irides, and silvery hair (all three subtypes of GS). Granulomatous skin disorders are seen in types 1 and 2 GS. The characteristic finding on hair examination includes clumped melanin within the hair shafts (392). Absence of melanin is seen in individual keratinocytes, but it is present in melanocytes.

Piebaldism

This is an autosomal dominant disorder that presents with congenital depigmented patches on the skin and focal patches of white hair caused by an absence of melanosomes. The causative mutations have been shown to occur in the KIT gene as well as Snail homolog 2 (SNAI2/SLUG) (393–395). KIT is essential for neural crest migration during embryogenesis. Failure of the cells to complete migration to the anterior midline results in the characteristic clinical findings. The most typical clinical finding is a white forelock, leukoderma in the face midline, on the anterior trunk, and ventral extremities (Fig. 6-61A, B). Histopathologic changes reveal an absence of melanocytes in the skin and hair follicles of the affected skin (396,397).

Waardenburg Syndrome

This syndrome includes a group of autosomal dominant genodermatoses characterized by irides with heterochromia, piebald depigmentation, and often congenital deafness (398,399). The most common form is WS1. Four major types are described in the literature. Waardenburg syndrome (WS) is caused by abnormalities in the development of neural crest derivatives. Biopsies of patients with WS show a lack of melanocytes (400,401); differential diagnosis of WS includes vitiligo and piebaldism.

Alkaptonuria

Alkaptonuria is caused by a mutation in the homogentisic acid oxidase (402,403). The resultant buildup of homogentisic acid in tissue leads to oxidation of benzoquinone acetic acid. Such product binds to collagen in the skin, sclerae, and cartilage irreversibly to produce the brown-black pigment that is typical of the disease. The cutaneous findings are typically more pronounced in photoexposed areas (404–406). The pigmentary changes in alkaptonuria are seen in the sclerae in the fifth decade of life and subsequently on the face, ears, buccal mucosa, nail beds, and intertriginous areas (Fig. 6-62A–C). The pigmentary changes include blue-black deep macules and patches.

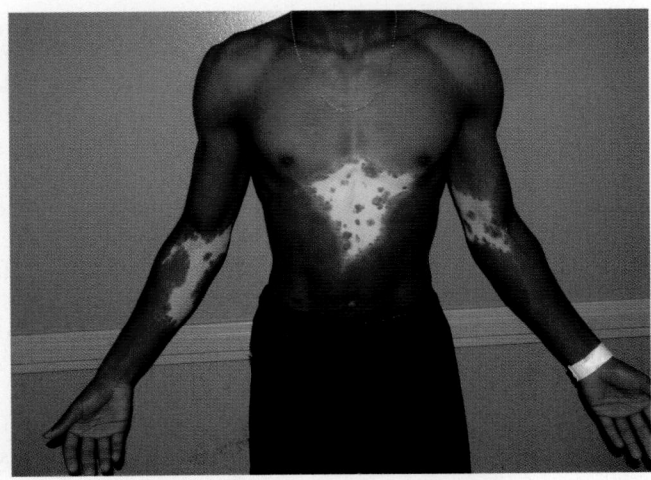

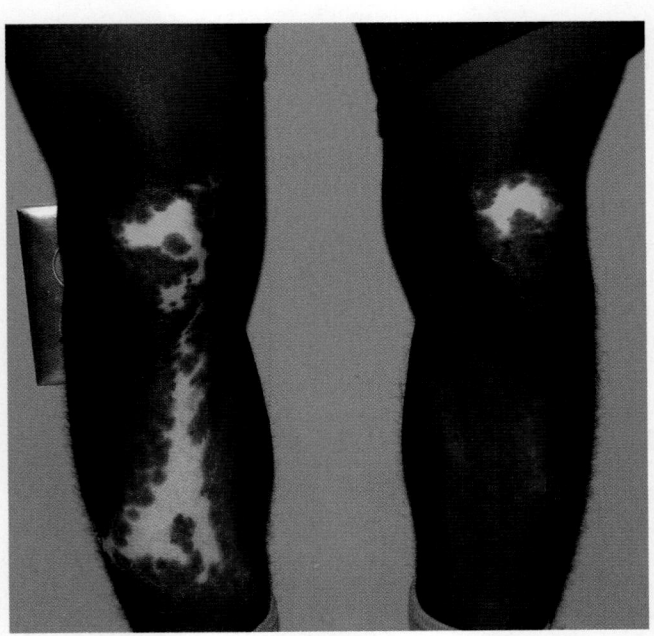

Figure 6-61 A, B: Piebaldism. Leukoderma of anterior trunk and extremities. Poliosis of the lower extremities is present. (Reprinted with permission from Gru AA. *Pediatric Dermatopathology and Dermatology*. Wolters Kluwer; 2019.)

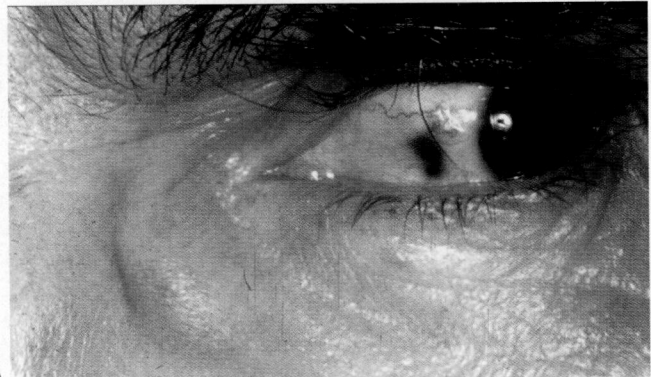

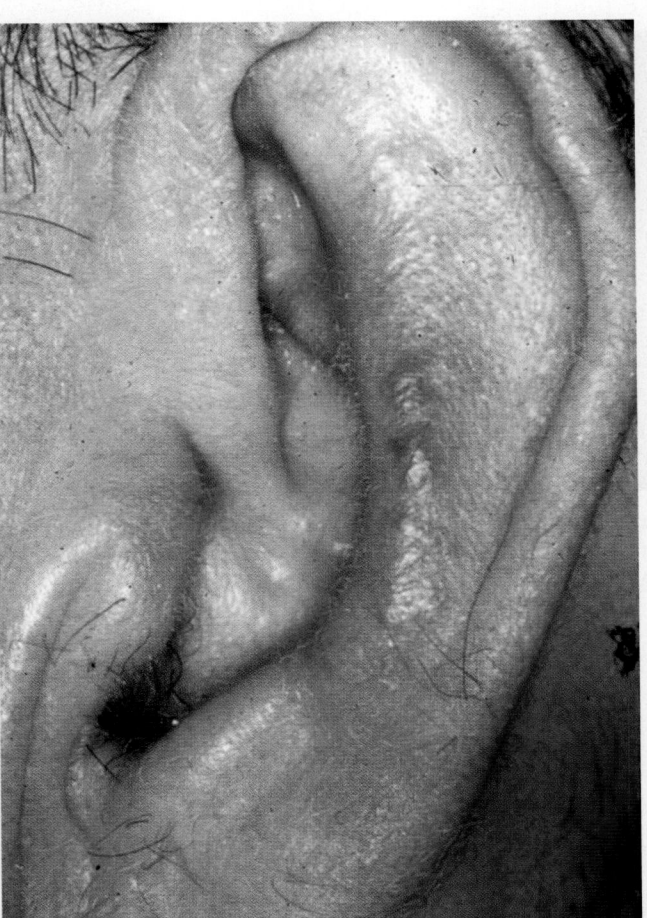

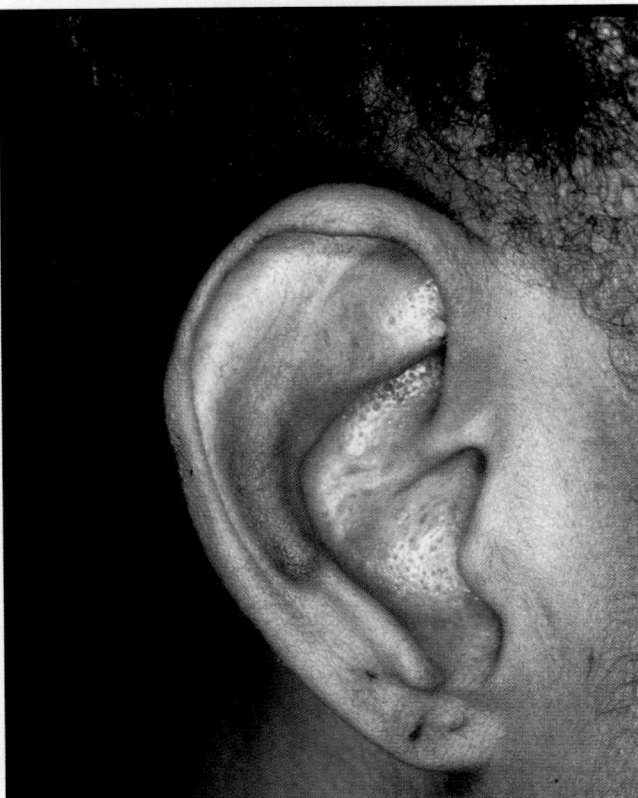

Figure 6-62 A–C: Alkaptonuria. The pigmentary changes in alkaptonuria are seen in the sclerae in the fifth decade of life, and subsequently on the face, ears, buccal mucosa, nail beds, and intertriginous areas. (Courtesy of Dr Kenneth Greer, Department of Dermatology, University of Virginia.)

Dark coloration of the urine occurs after prolonged exposure of wet diapers to air, and it represents the first sign of the disease. The tympanic membrane, tendons, and cartilage are also involved. The latter leads to arthritis and degenerative disk disease. Hearing impairment and pain are also common. Cardiac dysfunction from valvular alterations can also be present. Biopsies of patients with alkaptonuria show the typical findings of ochronosis: There are distinctive yellow-brown, or ochre, deposits within the dermis, often referred to as "banana bodies." Pigment may be also seen in the basement membrane at the dermoepidermal junction, and surrounding adnexa.

DEPOSITION DISORDERS

Lipoid Proteinosis

Clinical Summary. Lipoid proteinosis (*hyalinosis cutis et mucosae*) is a rare autosomal recessive condition characterized by thickening of the skin and mucosae (407–409). The majority of the patients are of European ancestry (410). Males and females are equally affected, and the disease usually presents during early childhood (411). A hoarse or weak cry is common, usually at birth or within the first few years of life. The cutaneous findings vary with the patient's age. Infants and young children show vesicles or bullae with hemorrhagic crusting on the face and upper extremities. The lesions heal with varioliform scarring. Later in childhood, the patients develop yellow papules and plaques on the face, eyelids, neck, and hands. The scalp is also affected, leading to alopecia. Waxy plaques are more frequent in the flexural surfaces, whereas verrucous plaques favor the extensor surface (Fig. 6-63). Fifty percent of patients show a string of bead-like papules on the free eyelid margins, often leading to loss of hair. Corneal ulcers can also develop. A cobblestone appearance of the oral mucosa can also be seen. The systemic complications of the hyaline material deposition can lead to dysphagia, respiratory obstruction, premature loss of teeth, and neurologic complications. A characteristic finding on radiologic examination is the presence of bilateral, intracranial, single or bean-shaped calcification of the temporal lobes (412).

Histopathology. Pathologically, there is prominent deposition of pale, eosinophilic, amorphous material surrounding small capillaries and eccrine ducts in the superficial dermis (413,414). More developed lesions show prominent thickening of the walls with an "onion-skinning" appearance (Fig. 6-64A, B). Hyperkeratosis and papillomatosis are present in verrucous lesions. Such deposits are positive with periodic acid-schiff (PAS) and are diastase resistant. They are negative for Congo Red.

Pathogenesis. Lipoid proteinosis is caused by a mutation in the ECM1 protein (415,416). This is normally found within the basement membrane zone and acts as a scaffolding molecule that binds to numerous structural proteins, including collagen IV and laminin 332. LP patients show loss of functional ECM1, resulting in hyalinized deposition of protein material at the dermoepidermal junction and within the papillary dermis. Interestingly, dysfunction of such protein has also been implicated in the pathogenesis of lichen sclerosus.

Gaucher Disease

Gaucher disease (GD) is an autosomal recessive lysosomal storage disorder caused by mutations in β-glucosidase (417). Such mutations result in the accumulation of the glycolipid

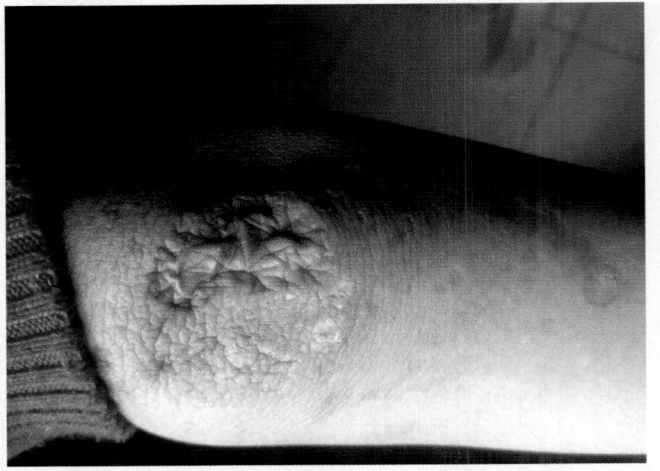

Figure 6-63 Lipoid proteinosis. Waxy plaques present in flexural areas. (Reprinted with permission from Gru AA. *Pediatric Dermatopathology and Dermatology.* Wolters Kluwer; 2019.)

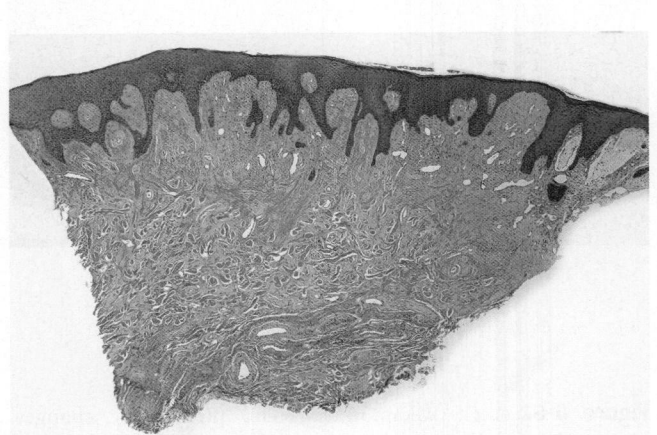

A

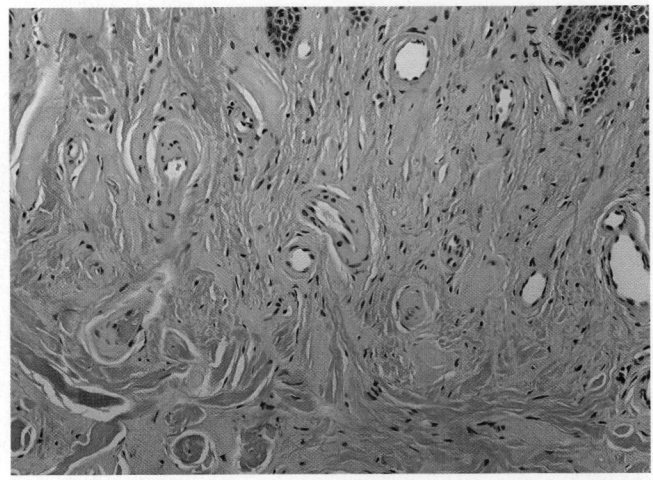

B

Figure 6-64 A, B: Lipoid proteinosis. There is prominent deposition of pale, eosinophilic, amorphous material surrounding small capillaries and eccrine ducts in the dermis. More developed lesions show prominent thickening of the walls with an "onion-skinning" appearance (original magnifications ×40 and ×200). (Courtesy of Dr. Travis Vandergriff, Department of Dermatology, UT Southwestern Medical Center.)

glucocerebrosidase, which leads to a variety of complications involving the skin, bones, and liver (418,419). GD is relatively common and is classically divided into three clinical subtypes. Type 1 GD is the most frequent, affecting 1/800 births in the Ashkenazi Jewish population. Types 2 and 3 are rare. The accumulation of the protein leads to the formation of Gaucher cells, which generate bone destruction. Type 1 is non-neuronopathic, and the skin findings include hyperpigmentation and purpura. Infiltration by macrophages in the bone marrow produces pancytopenia and associated thrombocytopenia, which leads to the petechial rash. These patients also have an increased risk of multiple myeloma. Type 2 is the acute neuronopathic type, which is rapidly progressive and lethal by the age of 2 years (420,421). It is characterized by a triad of opisthotonos, severe dysphagia, and oculomotor palsy. A rare subtype of type 2 is fetal GD, which presents with a collodion membrane and arthrogryposis. There are no specific histopathologic findings of GD in the skin, but the classic Gaucher cells, which show a "crumpled tissue paper" appearance, can be seen in the bone, liver, and bone marrow but not in the skin.

Hyaline Fibromatosis Syndrome

Clinical Summary. This entity includes infantile systemic hyalinosis (ISH) and juvenile hyaline fibromatosis (JHF). It is a rare autosomal recessive disorder of connective tissue that leads to deposition of hyaline material in the dermis and other organs (422–423). The early-onset form (ISH) has a more severe course, where patients present at birth with diffuse thickening of the skin, and hyperpigmentation over the joints of the dorsal hands and ankles (424,426). ISH patients have malabsorption, protein-losing enteropathy, diarrhea, and recurrent infections, which can be lethal. JHF manifests during early childhood with progressive development of disfiguring nodules and papules on the face, scalp, ears, and hands (Fig. 6-65) (427,428). The lesions can be hard and fixed, or mobile. Oral mucosal involvement can also occur. Visceral symptoms of chronic diarrhea and malabsorption are not seen, in contrast to ISH. Patients also develop contractures, lytic bone lesions, osteopenia, and osteoporosis.

Histopathology. HFS is characterized by ill-defined dermal deposits of brightly eosinophilic hyaline material, which is variably sized, and contains interspersed plump spindle cells, which can be arranged in pseudovascular cords (Fig. 6-66). The hyaline material is PAS+ and diastase resistant (429,430).

Pathogenesis. Both conditions are associated with mutations of the anthrax toxin receptor-2 (*ANTXR2*), which encodes a transmembrane receptor that likely plays a role in vasculogenesis and basement membrane integrity (431–433). The loss or reduction of functional ANTXR2 leads to deposition of hyaline material within the dermis and viscera.

AUTOINFLAMMATORY DISORDERS

Cryopyrin-Associated Periodic Syndrome

Clinical Summary. Cryopyrin-associated periodic syndrome (CAPS) is a rare disorder of childhood onset, characterized by systemic and tissue-specific inflammation of the integumentary, nervous, and musculoskeletal systems (434–436). Three related, but distinct, phenotypes encompass the clinical spectrum

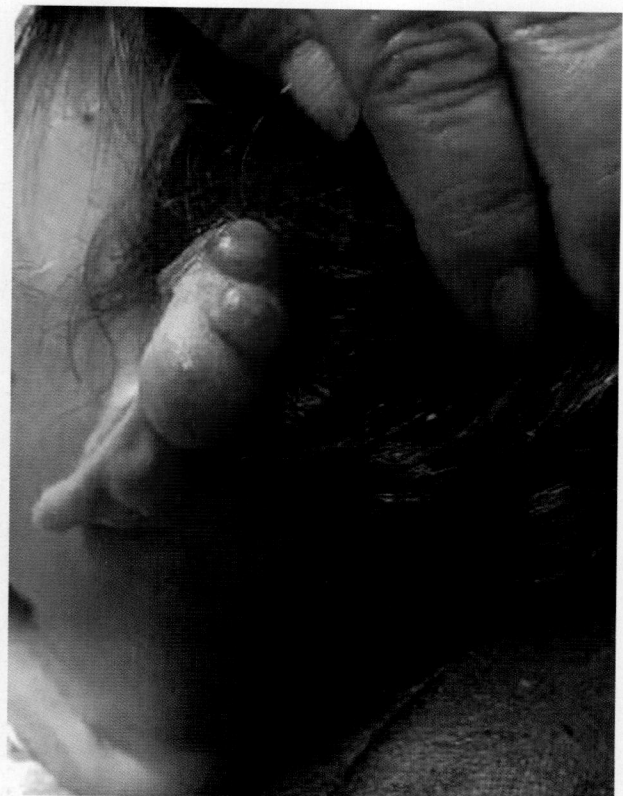

Figure 6-65 Juvenile hyaline fibromatosis. A 20-year-old woman with waxy nodules on the helix. (Reprinted with permission from Rahvar M, Teng J, Kim J. Systemic hyalinosis with heterozygous CMG2 mutations: a case report and review of literature. *Am J Dermatopathol.* 2016;38(5):e60–e63.)

of CAPS and are referred to as cryopyrinopathies (437–439) because they have all been linked to mutations in the gene encoding cryopyrin (*CIAS1* [cold-induced autoinflammatory syndrome 1], also known as *NLRP3* [NACHT domain, leucine-rich repeat, and pyrin-containing protein 3]). The mildest phenotype is familial cold autoinflammatory syndrome (FCAS) followed by Muckle–Wells syndrome (MWS), which is associated with more systemic inflammation (Fig. 6-67). The most severe phenotype is neonatal-onset multisystem inflammatory disease (NOMID), which is sometimes referred to in Europe as chronic infantile neurological cutaneous and articular (CINCA) syndrome (Fig. 6-68) (440,441). A defining feature of NOMID is central nervous system inflammation, resulting in chronic aseptic meningitis, seizures, cognitive impairment, and hearing and vision loss. CAPS presents with urticaria-like papules and plaques, conjunctivitis, fevers, arthralgia, and constitutional symptoms. Symptoms are triggered within hours of exposure to cold temperatures, resulting in an effervescent urticarial rash followed by scleral injection, fever, and arthralgia, which typically lasts less than 24 hours.

Histopathology. Skin biopsy of the erythematous and edematous papules and plaques in patients with CAPS shows superficial perivascular and perieccrine infiltrate predominately composed of mature neutrophils and dilated superficial dermal lymphatics (Fig. 6-69, B) (442–444). This contrasts with the typical superficial perivascular lymphocytic inflammatory infiltrate of classic allergic urticaria. In addition, a helpful identifying feature is characteristic perieccrine neutrophilic infiltration like neutrophilic eccrine hidradenitis. There is an absence of karyorrhexis

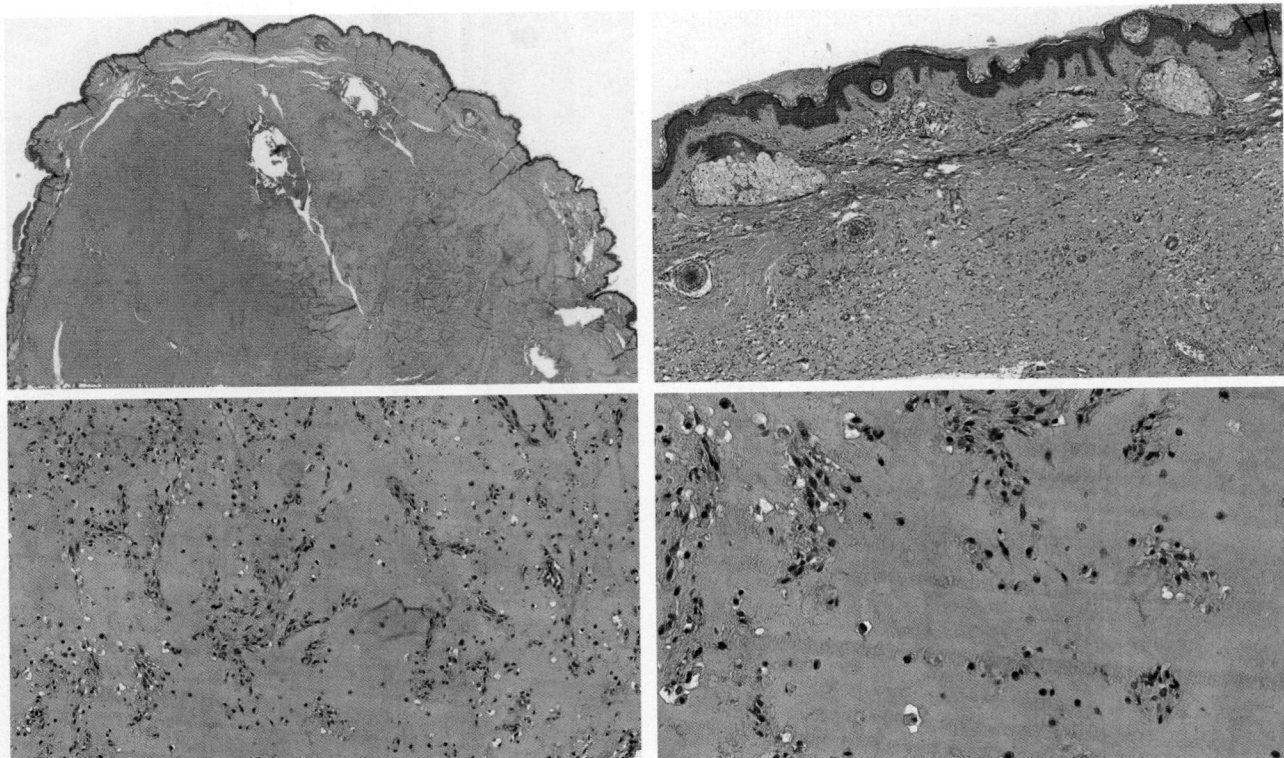

Figure 6-66 Juvenile hyaline fibromatosis. Hyaline fibromatosis syndrome is characterized by ill-defined dermal deposits of brightly eosinophilic hyaline material, which is variably sized, and contains interspersed plump spindle cells, which can be arranged in pseudovascular cords. (Digital slides courtesy of Path Presenter.com.)

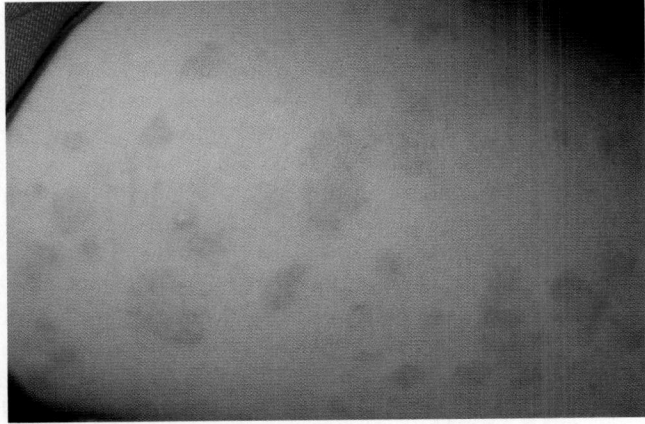

Figure 6-67 Muckle–Wells syndrome. Urticarial papules and plaques. (Reprinted with permission from Gru AA. *Pediatric Dermatopathology and Dermatology*. Wolters Kluwer; 2019.)

or leukocytoclasis and vasculitis. There are no epidermal changes and no eosinophils.

Pathogenesis. The cryopyrinopathies are associated with autosomal dominant or *de novo* mutations of *NLRP3/CIAS1*, which encodes the protein cryopyrin (440,445–448). The hallmark of the innate immune dysregulation of CAPS is excessive production of interleukin-1β (IL-1β). Cryopyrin is a critical component of the inflammasome, a multi-protein complex responsible for generation of IL-1β in response to pathogens or "danger signals" from dead or dying host cells. *NLRP3* mutations in patients with CAPS appear to activate the inflammasome in the absence of pathogenic insults. Nearly all patients with FCAS

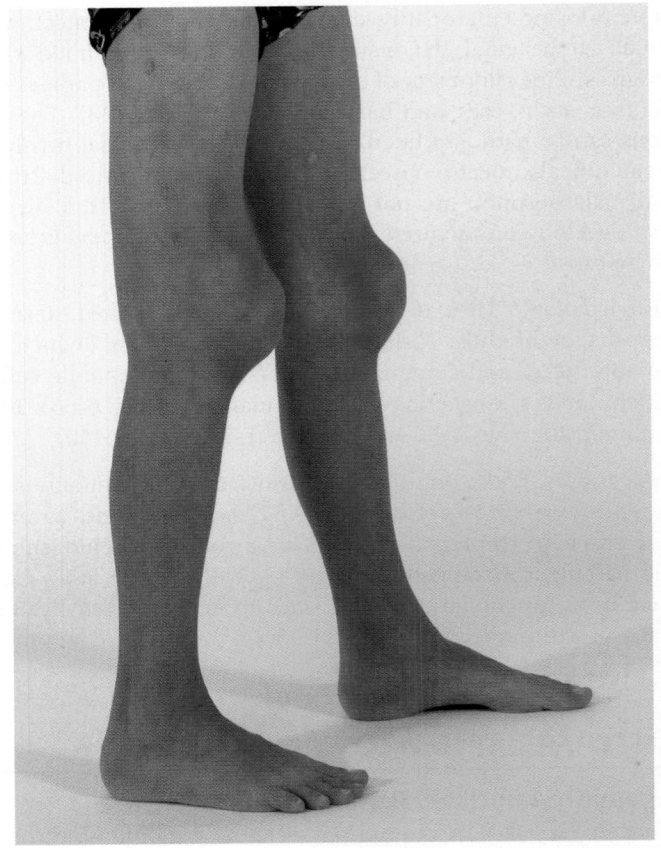

Figure 6-68 Neonatal-onset multisystem inflammatory disease (NOMID). Extensive joint and bone involvement resulting in bone deformities. (Reprinted with permission from Gru AA. *Pediatric Dermatopathology and Dermatology*. Wolters Kluwer; 2019.)

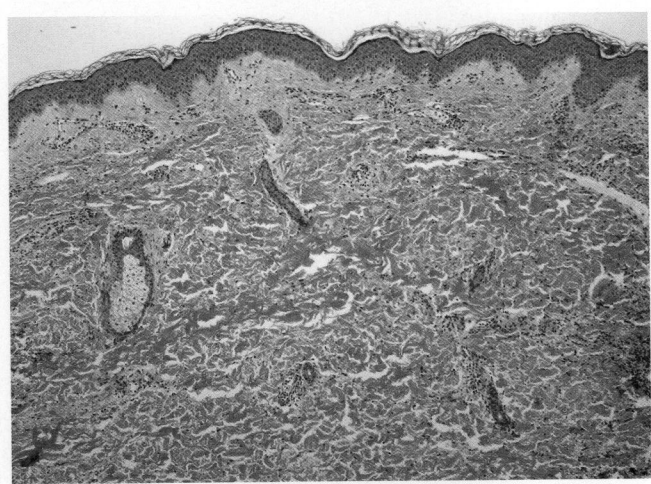
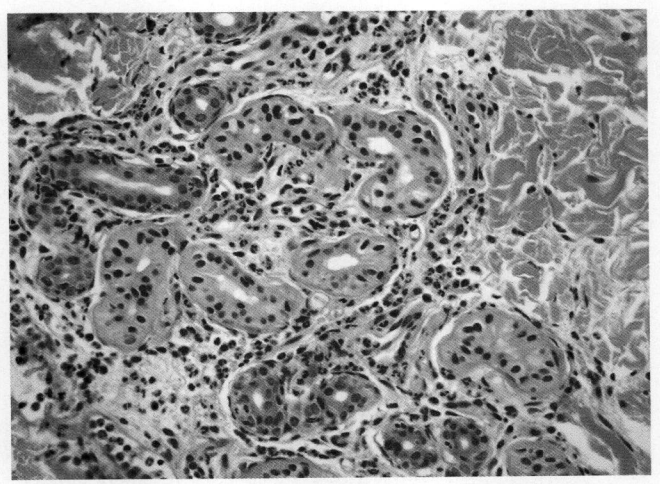

Figure 6-69 A, B: Cryopyrin-associated periodic syndrome (CAPS). Mild papillary dermal edema and unremarkable epidermis. There is a superficial and deep, perivascular, interstitial, and perieccrine infiltrate. Characteristic perieccrine neutrophilic inflammation is present (original magnification ×40 and ×200). (Reprinted with permission from Gru AA. *Pediatric Dermatopathology and Dermatology*. Wolters Kluwer; 2019.)

and MWS have inherited mutations in *NLRP3*, whereas *NLRP3* mutations found in NOMID patients tend to occur *de novo*. Furthermore, about half of the patients with NOMID do not have detectable germline *NLRP3* mutations; however, many somatic mutations have been found in these patients.

Deficiency of the Interleukin-1 Receptor Antagonist

Clinical Summary. Deficiency of the interleukin-1 receptor antagonist (DIRA) is a rare autoinflammatory disorder characterized by sterile multifocal osteomyelitis and periostitis with skin lesions resembling pustular psoriasis in the neonatal period (449,450). Autosomal recessive mutations in interleukin-1 receptor antagonist (*IL1RN*) result in uncontrolled IL-1α/β signaling (451). Reports of DIRA to date are predominately described in patients of Puerto Rican, Newfoundland, Lebanese, Dutch, and Brazilian descent. The condition is associated with an estimated 30% mortality during infancy if untreated. It is estimated that 0.2% of the population in Newfoundland are carriers of the mutation with likely similar rates in Lebanon, Brazil, and the Netherlands (449,450,452,453).

At birth or within a few weeks of age, neonates with DIRA develop a pustular rash, swollen joints, pain with movement, and oral mucosal ulcers (Fig. 6-70). Of note, fever is characteristically absent despite elevation of inflammatory markers and acute phase reactants. The rash may consist of discrete erythematous plaques studded with follicular pustules or evolve to generalized pustulosis. Less commonly, ichthyosiform skin changes and nail changes including pitting and onychomadesis are present. The early onset of disease together with neonatal distress and markers of systemic inflammation, including periostitis, multifocal sterile osteomyelitis, and hepatosplenomegaly are characteristic of DIRA. The most common radiographic findings include balloon widening of the anterior rib ends, multifocal osteolytic lesions, and periosteal elevation (454,455). Treatment with IL-1 blockers is life-saving.

Histopathology. Cutaneous biopsies of the pustular rash show dense infiltrate of mature neutrophils throughout the dermis with acanthosis, intraepidermal neutrophils, prominent

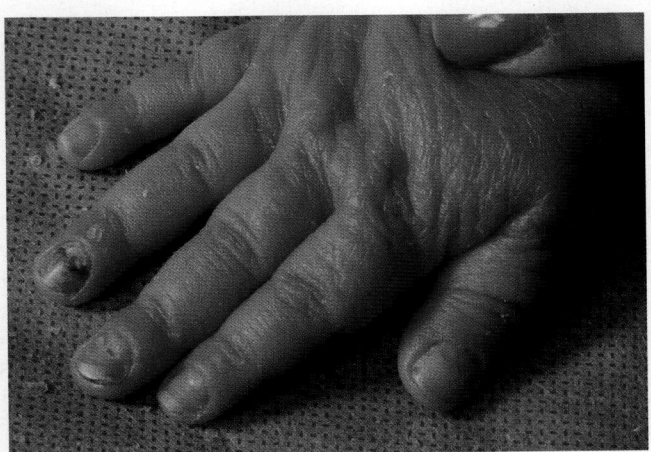

Figure 6-70 Deficiency of the interleukin-1 receptor antagonist (DIRA). Nail dystrophic changes. (Reprinted with permission from Gru AA. *Pediatric Dermatopathology and Dermatology*. Wolters Kluwer; 2019.)

papillary dermal edema, and pustule formation along the hair follicular infundibulum (Fig. 6-71A, B). Notably, there is a combination of subcorneal pustules as well as dense neutrophilic infiltrate with destruction of hair follicular infundibula (449,450).

Pathogenesis. DIRA is caused by autosomal recessive mutations in the IL-1 receptor antagonist (*IL1RN*). The lack of a functional IL-1 receptor antagonist in DIRA patients results in unopposed stimulation of the IL-1 receptor by IL-1α and IL-1β. IL-1β is processed by myeloid cells of the innate immune system by the inflammasome whereas IL-1α is preformed and can be released by nonimmune cells such as keratinocytes and endothelial cells. Downstream effects of IL-1α/β result in the production of additional proinflammatory cytokines including TNF and IL-17. DIRA is the result of an inability to terminate signaling from both IL-1β and IL-1α. In addition, the IL-1 receptor is highly expressed within the epidermis and unopposed signaling by IL-1α may be responsible for the epidermal changes including hyperkeratosis and subcorneal pustulosis seen in DIRA (451).

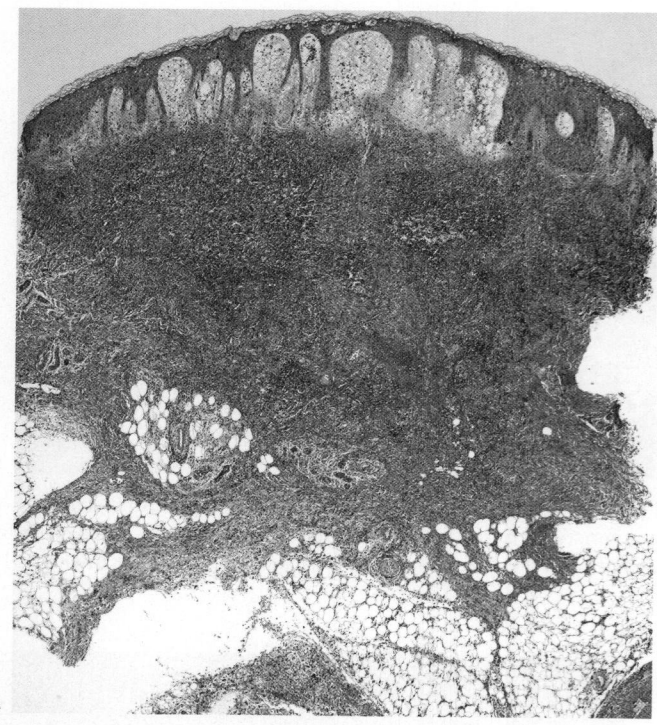

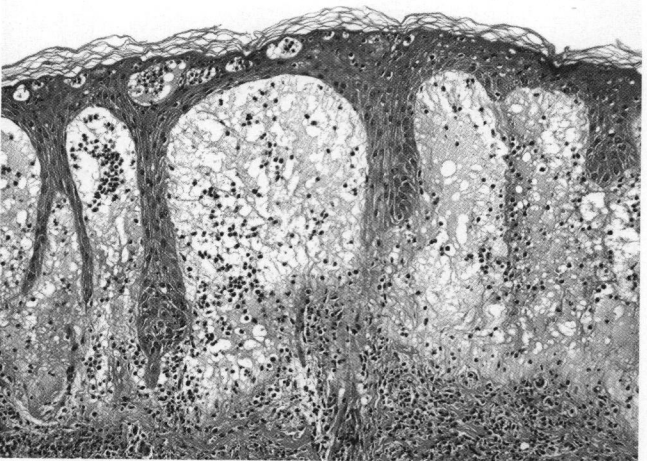

Figure 6-71 A, B: Deficiency of the interleukin-1 receptor antagonist (DIRA). Dense infiltrate of mature neutrophils throughout the dermis with acanthosis, intraepidermal neutrophils, prominent papillary dermal edema, and pustule formation along the hair follicular infundibulum (original magnification ×40 and ×200). (Reprinted with permission from Gru AA. *Pediatric Dermatopathology and Dermatology.* Wolters Kluwer; 2019.)

Deficiency of Adenosine Deaminase-2

Clinical Summary. Deficiency of adenosine deaminase 2 (DADA2) is a recently identified autoinflammatory syndrome characterized by intermittent fevers, livedo racemosa, and systemic vasculopathy/vasculitis (456,457). Since the initial description of DADA2 in 2014, more than 50 cases have been reported (458). A significant number of cases of DADA2 have been reported in individuals of Georgian Jewish ancestry (456). Livedo racemosa, polyarteritis nodosa, and early-onset stroke are the distinguishing early features of DADA2 (Fig. 6-72). In addition, intermittent fevers, splenomegaly with consumptive thrombocytopenia, portal hypertension with esophageal varices, hypocellular bone marrow with anemia, and mild immunodeficiency with hypogammaglobulinemia are also commonly present. Livedo racemosa, which is most prominent on the trunk and extremities, is composed of broad, interrupted pink to violaceous patches in a branching or net-like configuration. Discrete, firm, painful pink nodules on the extremities resembling PAN occur in some patients in early childhood. Recurrent early-onset hemorrhagic and ischemic strokes are a potentially devastating clinical feature and may lead to neurologic deficits in childhood. Another particular association of these patients is with multicentric dermatofibrosarcoma protuberans (459).

Histopathology. Histopathologic examination of the painful, pink subcutaneous nodules demonstrates medium-sized vessel vasculitis at the dermal subcutaneous junction consistent with polyarteritis nodosa (Fig. 6-73A, B) (456,460,461). A dense, transmural neutrophilic and lymphohistiocytic infiltrate with fibrinoid necrosis of the vessel wall is present. Cutaneous biopsies of the livedo racemosa rash may show a mild interstitial neutrophilic and mononuclear infiltration with perivascular lymphocytes without vasculitis. However, many biopsies of the livedoid pattern only show dilated superficial small blood vessels with thickening of the vascular wall.

Pathogenesis. Loss-of-function, autosomal recessive mutations in *CERC1* (cat eye syndrome chromosome region, candidate

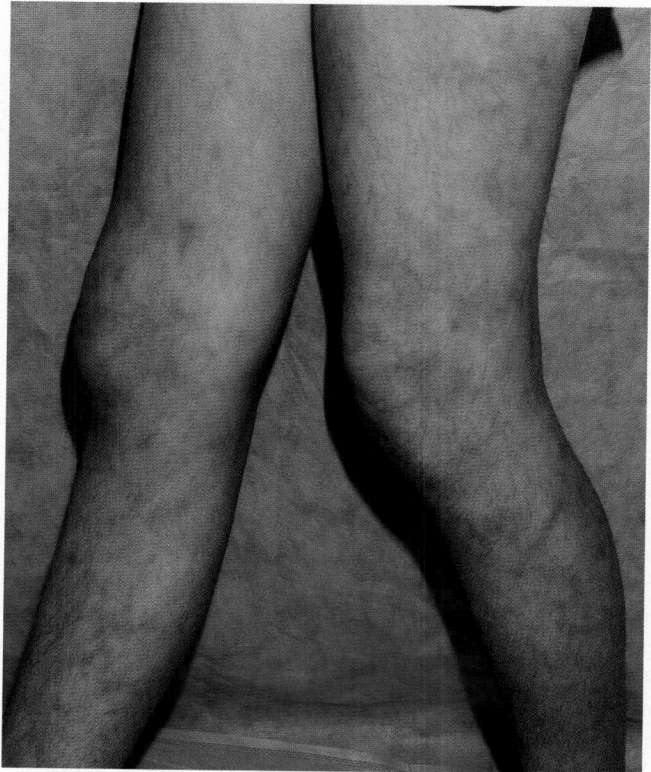

Figure 6-72 Deficiency of adenosine deaminase-2 (DADA2). Livedo racemosa on the extremities. (Reprinted with permission from Gru AA. *Pediatric Dermatopathology and Dermatology.* Wolters Kluwer; 2019.)

1), which encodes ADA2, have been identified in patients with DADA2. In one study, all 19 Georgian Jewish DADA2 patients shared the same homozygous p.Gly47Arg mutation. ADA2 is a secreted protein of the myeloid cell lineage that helps differentiate monocytes into macrophages and dendritic cells. In addition, ADA2 may also play a role in the development

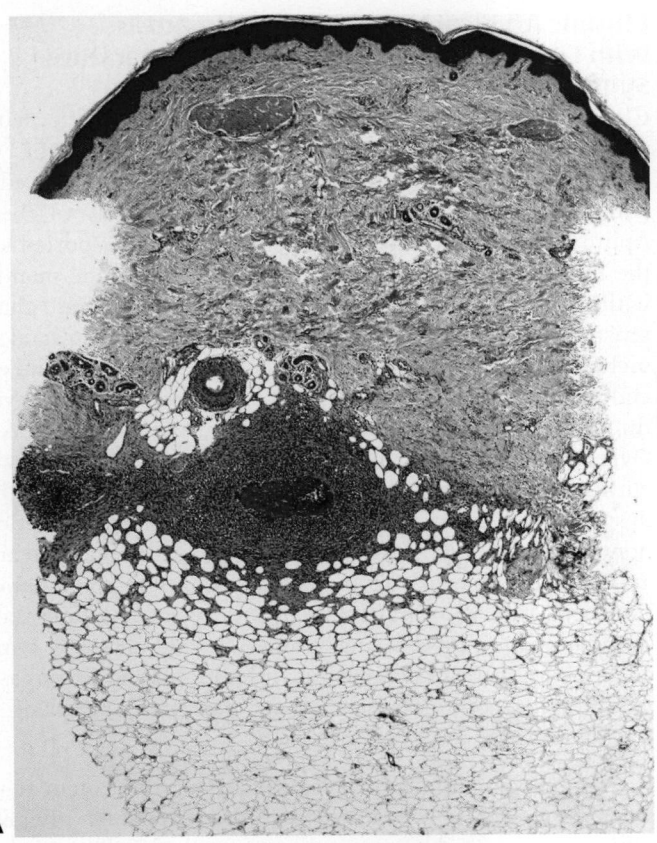

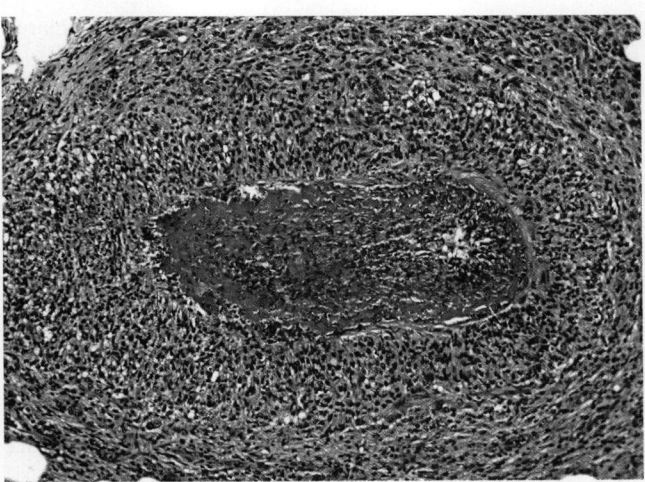

Figure 6-73 A, B: Deficiency of adenosine deaminase-2 (DADA2). Histopathologic examination of the painful, pink subcutaneous nodules demonstrates medium-sized vessel vasculitis at the dermal subcutaneous junction consistent with polyarteritis nodosa (original magnification ×40 and ×200). (Reprinted with permission from Gru AA. *Pediatric Dermatopathology and Dermatology*. Wolters Kluwer; 2019.)

and differentiation of endothelial cells. However, very little is known regarding how the loss of ADA2 function results in vasculopathy and vasculitis. Analysis of blood from DADA2 patients reveals an elevated neutrophil and interferon signature, suggesting that there is excessive neutrophil activation in the absence of ADA2 (456,462,463).

STING-Associated Vasculopathy With Onset in Infancy

Clinical Summary. stimulator of interferon genes (STING)-associated vasculopathy with onset in infancy (SAVI) is characterized by severe cutaneous vasculopathy, small vessel vasculitis, interstitial lung disease, and systemic inflammation (464).

Approximately 30 cases of SAVI have been reported since its initial description in 2014 (465–467). The earliest clinical manifestations of SAVI occur within the first 6 months of life and include telangiectatic-purpuric patches and plaques on cold-sensitive areas such as cheeks, nose, ears, hands, and feet (Fig. 6-74A, B). Pustular and blistering rashes on acral sites that worsen with cold exposure have also been described. Over time, these lesions progress to painful ulcerations with eschar formation. Cartilage resorption of the ear and nasal septum are common sequelae. In addition, distal digit gangrene may require surgical amputation. Chronic disease is marked by atrophic scars with telangiectasia. Most patients develop interstitial lung disease and hilar or paratracheal lymphadenopathy, which

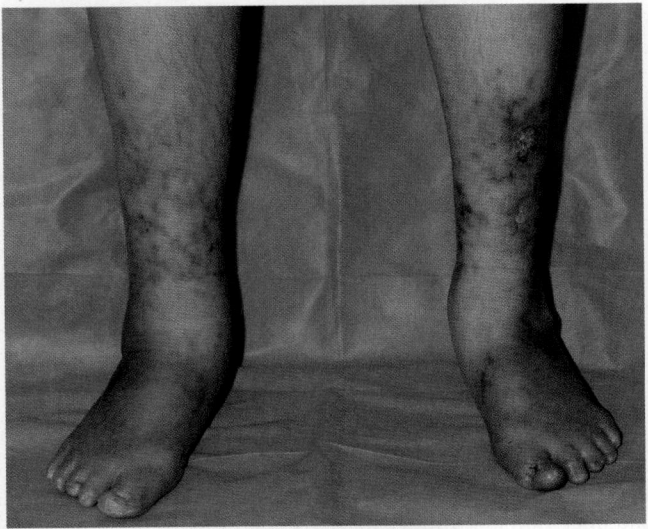

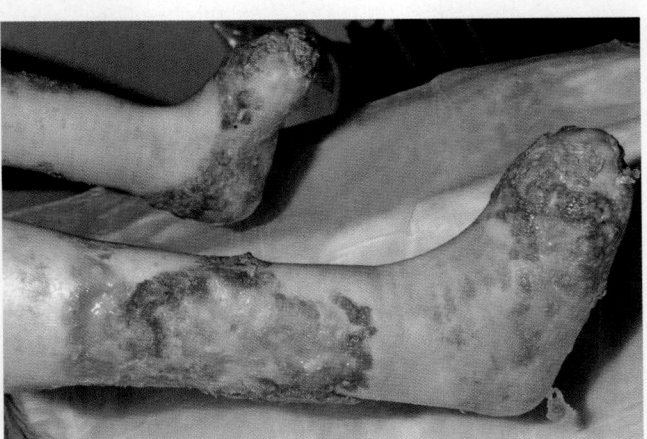

Figure 6-74 A, B: STING-associated vasculopathy with onset in infancy (SAVI). Painful ulcerations with eschar formation. Pernio-like lesions on the toes are present. Distal necrosis leads to digit loss. (Reprinted with permission from Gru AA. *Pediatric Dermatopathology and Dermatology*. Wolters Kluwer; 2019.)

often presents as tachypnea. Systemic inflammation associated with intermittent fevers, anemia of chronic disease, and failure to thrive is present in all patients. Some patients succumb to severe pulmonary complications from chronic inflammation and subsequent fibrosis and die in their teenage years (464).

Histopathology. Biopsy of early skin lesions shows intense inflammation of cutaneous small vessels including a dense neutrophilic and mononuclear inflammatory infiltrate with karyorrhexis and fibrin deposits within the vessel lumen (Fig. 6-75A, B) (464,467). Chronic cutaneous lesions show variable amounts of intraluminal thrombi within cutaneous small vessels, fibrinoid necrosis of the vessel wall, and a mild dermal neutrophilic infiltrate with sparse leukocytoclasis. In addition, there is a perivascular lymphocytic infiltrate and rare epidermal necrotic keratinocytes. Vasculopathy appears to primarily involve small-caliber vessels of the skin, but occasional involvement of medium-sized vessels has been observed.

Pathogenesis. SAVI is caused by gain-of-function mutations (autosomal dominant) in TMEM173 (transmembrane protein 173), which encodes STING, resulting in excessive interferon-β (IFN-β) production and stimulation (464,465,468,469). Unlike DADA2, there does not appear to be a population with enriched mutation frequency for SAVI, suggesting that most cases of SAVI are likely secondary to *de novo* mutations. The interferon pathway is critical for host protection against pathogens, especially viruses. STING is downstream of the type 1 IFN receptor, and when activated, STING induces transcription of type I IFNs and IFN-response genes. Thus, gain-of-function mutations in STING, which cause SAVI, result in uncontrolled IFN production, particularly IFN-$\beta\beta$. In addition, STING is expressed in endothelial cells and in skin biopsies from lesional skin, endothelial cells show increased expression of certain inflammatory markers, suggesting a possible etiology for the vasculitis and vasculopathy in patients with SAVI. Furthermore, STING is expressed by type II pneumocytes and alveolar macrophages, which likely contributes to the pulmonary disease by an unknown mechanism(s).

Chronic Atypical Neutrophilic Dermatosis With Lipodystrophy and Elevated Temperature Syndrome

Clinical Summary. Chronic Atypical Neutrophilic Dermatosis with Lipodystrophy and Elevated Temperature (CANDLE) syndrome is characterized by recurrent fevers, periorbital edema with violaceous plaques, and facial lipodystrophy (470,471). Approximately 60 cases of CANDLE have been reported since the initial description in 2010. CANDLE syndrome manifests within the first 6 months of life with recurrent fever and characteristic intense, red-violaceous edematous plaques on acral sites including nose, ears, fingers, and toes. Later in infancy and early childhood, annular, purpuric, and edematous plaques develop throughout the body and resolve with purpura (Fig. 6-76A, B). Over time, persistent violaceous, periorbital edema develops with occasional perioral involvement. Progressive facial lipodystrophy begins in early childhood with subsequent development of more generalized lipodystrophy, disabling arthritis, and delayed physical development with systemic inflammation occurring in nearly every organ. Systemic manifestation of inflammation includes hepatomegaly, splenomegaly, lymphadenopathy, arthritis, chondritis, aseptic meningitis, myositis, pneumonitis, conjunctivitis, nodular episcleritis, nephritis, and epididymitis (472).

Histopathology. Pathologic examination of the cutaneous lesions of CANDLE shows a dense, predominantly interstitial infiltrate composed of atypical mononuclear cells with karyorrhexis throughout the papillary and reticular dermis with extension into the subcutaneous fat with perivascular lymphocytes. Characteristically, this mononuclear cell infiltrate is composed of atypical (immature) myeloid cells with large, vesicular, elongated or kidney-shaped nuclei, conspicuous nucleoli, mixed with rare mature neutrophils, eosinophils, and scattered mature lymphocytes (Fig. 6-77A–C). There is leukocytoclasis in the dermis but an absence of vasculitis. The epidermis is spared, and if subcutaneous tissue is present, then a lobular pattern panniculitis with lipodystrophy is sometimes

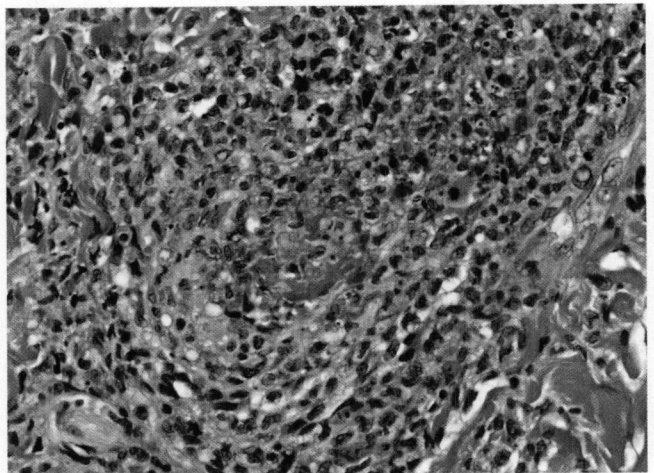
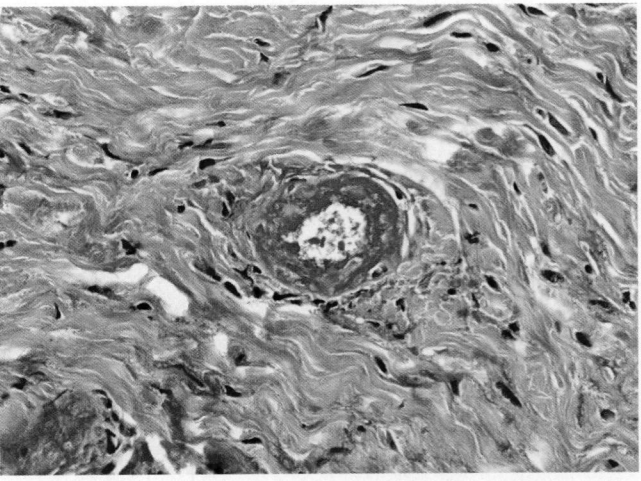

Figure 6-75 A, B: STING-associated vasculopathy with onset in infancy (SAVI). Biopsy of early skin lesions shows intense inflammation of cutaneous small vessels including a dense neutrophilic and mononuclear inflammatory infiltrate with karyorrhexis and fibrin deposits within the vessel lumen (**A**). Chronic cutaneous lesions show variable amounts of intraluminal thrombi within cutaneous small vessels, fibrinoid necrosis of the vessel wall, and a mild dermal neutrophilic infiltrate with sparse leukocytoclasis (**B**) (original magnification ×400). (Reprinted with permission from Gru AA. *Pediatric Dermatopathology and Dermatology.* Wolters Kluwer; 2019.)

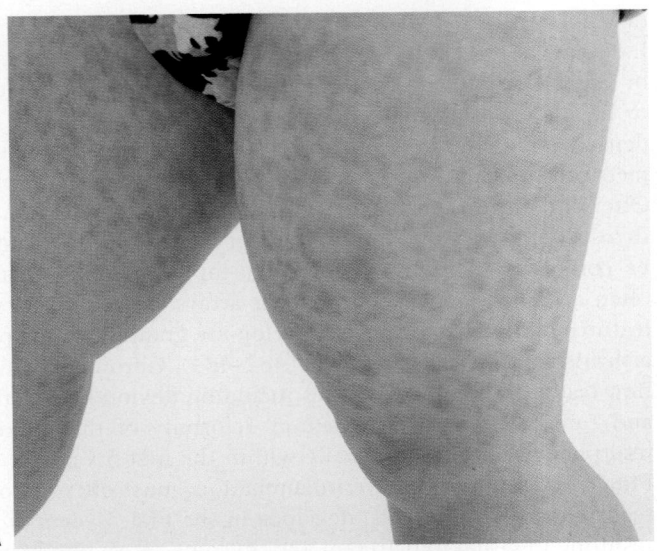
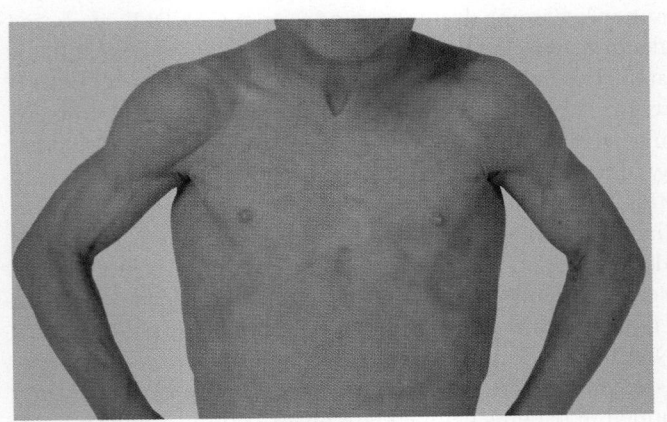

Figure 6-76 A, B: Chronic atypical neutrophilic dermatosis with lipodystrophy and elevated temperature (CANDLE) syndrome. Annular, purpuric, and edematous plaques that resolve with purpura (A). Progressive facial and generalized lipodystrophy (B). (Reprinted with permission from Gru AA. *Pediatric Dermatopathology and Dermatology*. Wolters Kluwer; 2019.)

observed. Histopathologic studies have confirmed the presence of myeloid lineage cells (positive for Leder stain) and further immunophenotypic analysis has confirmed an infiltrate comprised of CD68⁺ and CD163⁺ macrophages as well as clusters of CD123-positive plasmacytoid dendritic cells, which are the major producers of type I IFN (470,473).

Pathogenesis. CANDLE is caused by homozygous or compound heterozygous mutations in the proteasome or immunoproteasome subunits *PSMB8*, *PSMB3*, *PSMB4*, *PSMB9*, and *PROM* (proteasome maturation protein) (474–477). Under steady-state conditions, multiple subunits come together within cells to form the proteasome, which degrades and recycles intracellular

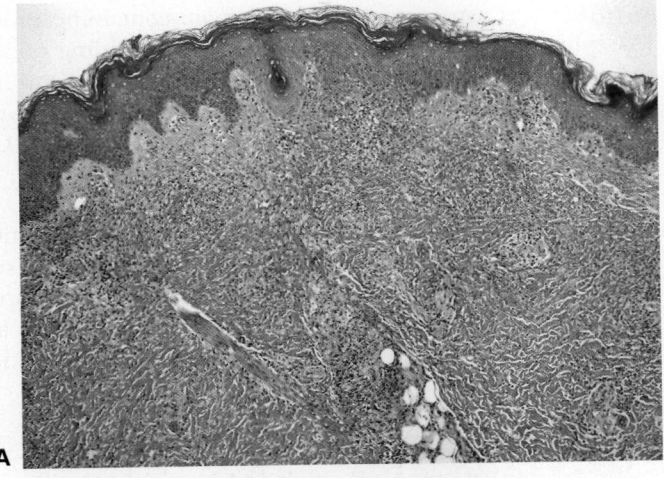
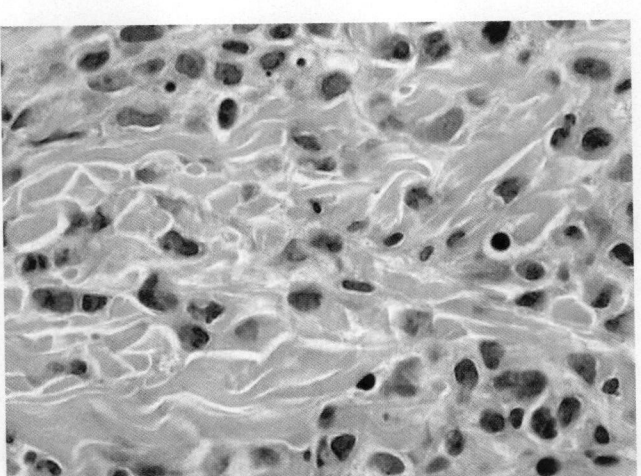
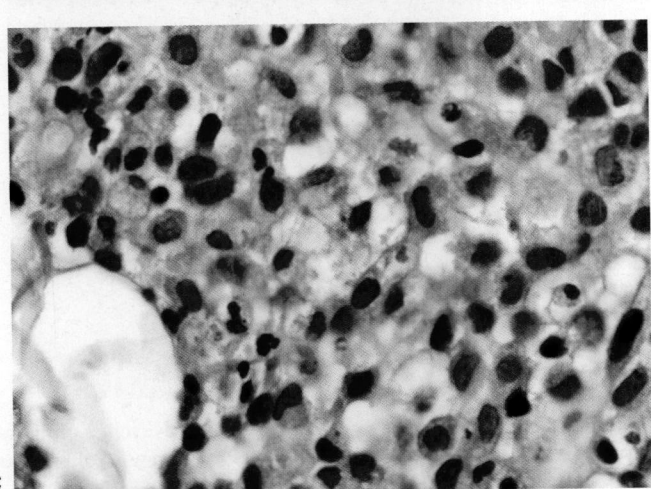

Figure 6-77 A–C: Chronic neutrophilic dermatosis with lipodystrophy and elevated temperature (CANDLE) syndrome. Dense, predominantly interstitial infiltrate composed of atypical mononuclear cells with karyorrhexis throughout the papillary and reticular dermis (A). The mononuclear cell infiltrate is composed of atypical (immature) myeloid cells with large, vesicular, elongated or kidney-shaped nuclei, conspicuous nucleoli, mixed with rare mature neutrophils, eosinophils, and scattered mature lymphocytes (B, C) (original magnifications ×100 and ×600). (Reprinted with permission from Gru AA. *Pediatric Dermatopathology and Dermatology*. Wolters Kluwer; 2019.)

waste proteins. Under inflammatory conditions, such as a viral infection within a cell, a variant of the proteasome called the immunoproteasome is formed to degrade foreign (i.e., viral) proteins for antigen processing and presentation. Proteasome-immunoproteasome dysfunction as seen in CANDLE syndrome results in accumulation of protein waste; cellular stress; and, ultimately, hypersecretion of type I interferons. Thus, CANDLE represents in inherited interferonopathy that acutely worsens during periods of cellular stress such as viral infections. The majority of patients with CANDLE have heterozygous mutations in *PSMB8* (proteasome subunit beta type-8 precursor). This protein is a key component of the proteasome, an organelle responsible for degrading and recycling of intracellular protein products. A subset of patients has now been described with mutations in other proteasome components. The majority of patients with CANDLE have homozygous or compound heterozygous mutations in proteasome subunits that arise *de novo* and have been identified in patients belonging to diverse ethnic groups including mixed European, Hispanic, and Japanese (478,479).

Blau Syndrome

Clinical Summary. Blau syndrome is an autosomal dominantly inherited autoinflammatory disorder characterized by granulomatous dermatitis, uveitis, and polyarthritis as independently

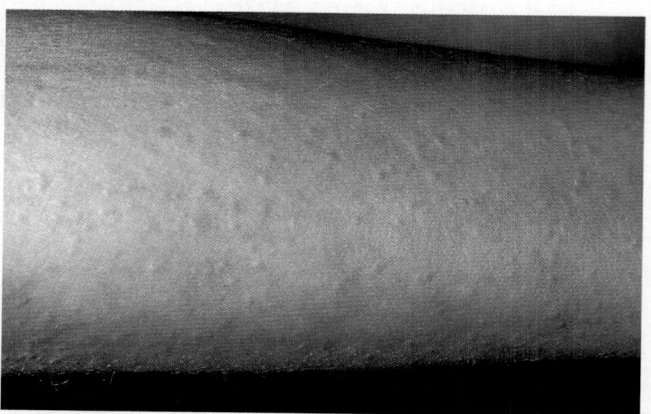

Figure 6-78 Blau syndrome. Discrete, small, flat-topped papules that are often arranged in clusters or linear arrays. (Reprinted with permission from Gru AA. *Pediatric Dermatopathology and Dermatology.* Wolters Kluwer; 2019.)

described in 1985 by Dr. Jabs and Dr. Blau (480,481). The earliest clinical presentation of Blau syndrome is the development of slightly scaly, red-brown to dark-red papular, eczematous, or lichenoid rash within the first year of life (Fig. 6-78). This densely populated, erythematous papular eruption occurs symmetrically on trunk and extremities and spontaneously resolves. Often, infants are misdiagnosed with atopic dermatitis or ichthyosis vulgaris. However, the rash of Blau syndrome tends to be composed of discrete, small, flat-topped papules that are often arranged in clusters or linear arrays. The next classical features of Blau syndrome to develop are granulomatous polyarthritis and intermittent fevers (482–484). Chronic inflammation results in joint deformities including flexion contractures and camptodactyly (fixed flexion deformity of the proximal interphalangeal joints), usually within the first 5 years of age. Finally, granulomatous eye inflammation, most often chronic, recurrent bilateral uveitis, develops in the first 5 years of life, resulting in visual impairment and, in some cases, blindness.

Histopathology. Skin biopsy of rash during infancy shows noncaseating, sarcoid-type granulomas in a polycyclic configuration (Fig. 6-79A, B) (482,485). Granulomas are a universal feature in all skin biopsies despite an eczematous or lichenoid clinical appearance. Janssen and colleagues characterized the polycyclic granulomas of Blau syndrome with large lymphocytic coronas, extensive emperipolesis of lymphocytes within multinucleated giant cells, multinucleated giant-cell death, fibrinoid necrosis, and fibrosis. Some reports demonstrate the epithelioid granulomas of Blau syndrome in a periadnexal or perifollicular pattern.

Pathogenesis. Blau syndrome is caused by activating mutations in *CARD15* (Caspase recruitment domain-containing protein 15), which is also called NOD2 (nucleotide-binding oligomerization domain protein 2) (486–488). Blau syndrome is a monogenic autoinflammatory disorder characterized by predominantly granulomatous inflammation (489–491). Currently, it is thought that Blau syndrome affects all races, but the exact incidence remains unknown, and it is considered very rare. CARD15/NOD2 is an intracellular protein that functions as a pathogen recognition receptor within immune cells such as macrophages, monocytes, and dendritic cells. The normal function of CARD15/NOD2 is to recognize pathogens such as viruses and bacteria and activate proinflammatory cytokines

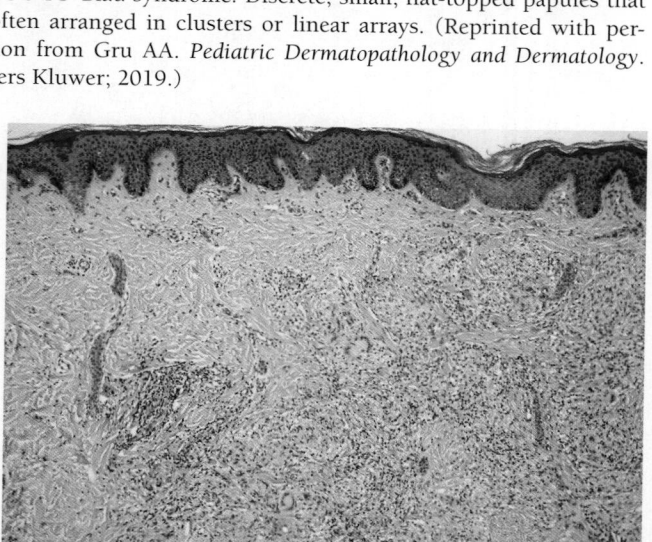

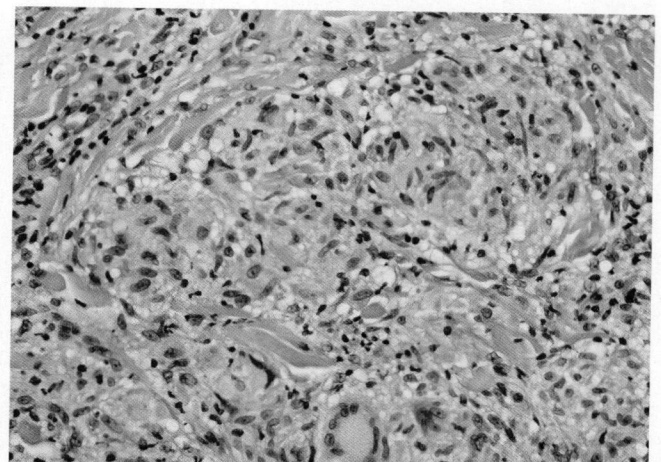

A   **B**

Figure 6-79 A, B: Blau syndrome. Skin biopsy of rash during infancy shows noncaseating, sarcoid-type granulomas in a polycyclic configuration (original magnification ×100 and ×400). (Reprinted with permission from Gru AA. *Pediatric Dermatopathology and Dermatology.* Wolters Kluwer; 2019.)

(e.g., IL-1, IL-6, TNF) through nuclear factor κB (NF-κB). Patients with Blau syndrome have an activating, gain-of-function mutation in *CARD15/NOD2* that results in constitutive activation of NF-κB, resulting in overproduction of proinflammatory cytokines.

MASTOCYTOSIS

Clinical Summary. Mastocytosis can be divided into cutaneous mastocytosis and systemic mastocytosis (492). For the purposes here, we will focus on cutaneous mastocytosis. The main subtypes of cutaneous mastocytosis, per WHO criteria (2018), include solitary *mastocytoma, maculopapular cutaneous mastocytosis* (urticaria pigmentosa, monomorphic and polymorphic subtypes), *diffuse cutaneous mastocytosis,* and *mast cell sarcoma* (492–494). It is strongly recommended that pathologists recognizing cutaneous involvement by mastocytosis should use the preliminary and descriptive term *mastocytosis in the skin* (MIS). This term is particularly of preferred use, until a complete workup that excludes systemic disease is achieved. Urticaria pigmentosa is most commonly a sporadic childhood disorder, but autosomal dominant inheritance with incomplete penetrance has also been reported (495). Sporadic and familial cases have been associated with *c-kit* mutations. Many dermatologists recognize a form of cutaneous mastocytosis called *telangiectasia eruptiva macularis perstans* (TMEP).

In classic childhood urticaria pigmentosa, the cutaneous lesions often improve or even clear at puberty (496). Systemic involvement is typically absent. Progression into systemic mast cell disease is very rare (497). In urticaria pigmentosa arising later, in adolescence or adult life, systemic disease is more likely to be present, but a minority show progression to systemic mast cell disease, which is characterized by extensive and progressive involvement of internal organs (498).

Patients with extensive mast cell infiltration of the skin and/or the internal organs commonly have attacks of flushing, palpitation, or diarrhea because of degranulation of mast cells and the release of histamine.

The lesions of *urticaria pigmentosa* (UP) are usually red or brown and oval-shaped and typically vary in size. Most of the lesions are larger than 0.5 mm and may be macules, papules, nodules, or plaques. The lesions can be sharply demarcated or have indistinct borders. The lesions are typically symmetrically distributed on the head, neck, and extremities. The lesions usually urticate on stroking (Darier sign) (Fig. 6-80A). The individual lesions often have a so-called *peau d'orange* texture. Sometimes multiple brown nodules or plaques that, on stroking, urticate and occasionally form blisters (Fig. 6-80B) occur. Patients with isolated cutaneous mastocytosis generally have lower serum tryptase levels than those with systemic mastocytosis. Most children with UP have normal tryptase levels, as children usually have skin-limited disease (499,500). Some congenital UP cases can present with alopecia (501). The prognosis in children is good. In most patients, the rash regresses by the time the patient reaches puberty. On the other hand, adults with UP are more likely to have persistent disease and systemic involvement (493). When bullae are a predominant clinical feature, the term bullous mastocytosis has been applied. Hartmann et al. have suggested that UP can be subdivided into two clinically distinct variants based on the morphology of the lesions (493): Most children with UP have a *polymorphic* variant, which is characterized by large lesions (usually nodules and plaques) of varying shapes and sizes; these lesions show a benign behavior and spontaneously resolve by puberty. A smaller percentage of pediatric patients with UP show lesions that are monomorphic and small (monomorphic variant). Children with the monomorphic variant often have increased tryptase levels and systemic involvement. The childhood monomorphic variant of UP also frequently persists into adulthood.

Solitary mastocytomas are typically brown or yellow-brown macules, plaques, or nodules. The lesions are most commonly distributed on the trunk, but they also occur frequently on the face and limbs. Typically, solitary mastocytomas are 1 cm in diameter or less. The Darier sign can also occur in these lesions. Patients with solitary mastocytomas have an excellent prognosis. Strictly speaking, cutaneous mastocytomas are a form of isolated cutaneous mastocytosis (499,502,503). Thus, by

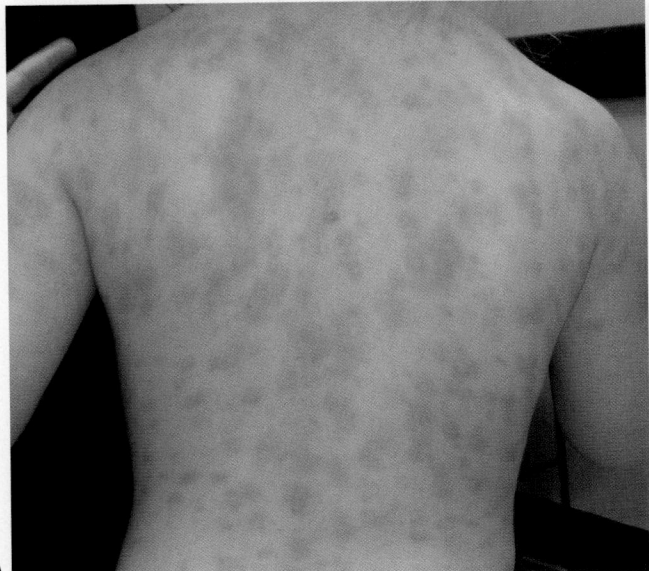
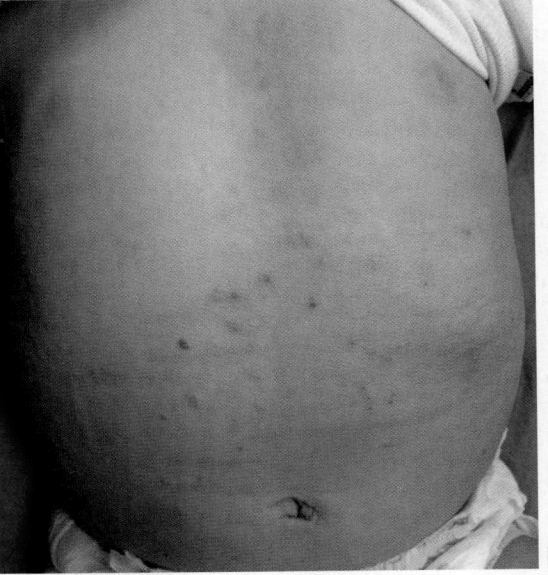

Figure 6-80 **A:** Urticaria pigmentosa. Multiple red-brown papules of urticaria pigmentosa. **B:** Bullous mastocytosis. Scattered edematous papules and flaccid bullae, which urticate with stroking.

definition, patients do not have systemic disease. The majority of mastocytomas will resolve spontaneously—in most cases within 4 to 10 years, and often by the time the patient reaches puberty. In contrast, mastocytomas in adults are less likely to regress (503,504). Cases without regression are often treated with surgical management.

Diffuse cutaneous mastocytosis (DCM) is the rarest form of cutaneous mastocytosis. The disease is often present at birth and most frequently occurs in the first 6 months of life. It is the most severe clinical presentation of cutaneous mastocytosis and is characterized by mast cell infiltration of the entire skin (505). Patients typically present with widespread erythema, erosions, or thickened skin. Generalized blistering can be present and should not be confused with primary blistering disease. Most patients have systemic symptoms, and its prognosis is worse.

Telangiectasia eruptiva macularis perstans (TMEP) typically occurs in adults and consists of an extensive eruption of brownish-red macules showing fine telangiectasias, with little or no urtication on stroking. TMEP is very rare, and less than 1% of all patients with mastocytosis have this specific variant (506,507). Rare familial forms of mastocytosis can present with TMEP. The lesions are typically distributed symmetrically over the proximal extremities and trunk. The palms, soles, and face are generally not involved. As opposed to other forms of cutaneous mastocytosis, Darier sign is usually not seen.

Systemic mastocytosis (SM) is defined as the involvement of one or more extracutaneous sites by an abnormal proliferation of mast cells. It is a group of diseases that includes indolent *systemic mastocytosis* (ISM), *aggressive systemic mastocytosis* (ASM), *systemic mastocytosis with associated clonal hematologic non–mast cell lineage disease* (SM-AHNMD), and *mast cell leukemia* (MCL). The clinical presentation of SM depends on the subtype (496,508–511). The skin is often involved, especially in ISM. UP is the most common pattern of cutaneous involvement in SM. UP is seen in 90% of patients with SM. TMEP is also associated with SM. SM can involve multiple organs, and the disease manifestations differ depending on which organs are involved. Fatigue is the most commonly reported symptom in patients with SM. Most adult patients have bone marrow involvement. Most adult patients have bone marrow involvement, with progression of disease leading to lymph node involvement. Involvement of the gastrointestinal tract is frequent, and symptoms such as abdominal pain, diarrhea, nausea, and vomiting may occur. Hepatomegaly and abnormal liver function tests have also been documented. Fifty to 60% of patients with SM will also develop splenomegaly. In SM, massive infiltration of the bones may cause collapse of several vertebrae or fracture of long bones. Myelofibrosis may occur, resulting in anemia, leukopenia, and thrombocytopenia. Pancytopenia may cause death. On rare occasions, MCL (with circulating mast cells) can occur.

Very rare, isolated case reports of *mast cell sarcoma* (MCS) have been reported in the literature. Less than 10 cases have been reported in the literature and the usual locations included colon, larynx, brain, retroperitoneal area, atrium, and bone (512).

Histopathology. In all types of lesions, the histologic picture shows an infiltrate composed chiefly of mast cells, which are characterized by the presence of metachromatic granules in their cytoplasm. These granules are not visible with routine stains but can be seen well after staining with a Giemsa stain or with toluidine blue. Also, the method using naphthol AS-D chloroacetate esterase, often called Leder's method, makes mast cell granules appear red and thus quite conspicuous.

Biopsies of *UP* lesions show an increase in dermal mast cells that is "4 to 8 times higher than that seen in normal skin and 2 to 3 times higher than that seen in inflamed skin." In the maculopapular type and in TMEP, the mast cells are more limited to the upper third of the dermis and are generally located around capillaries (493). The presence of more than 5 to 10 mast cells per high-power field is considered abnormal and can help confirm the diagnosis of TMEP. At times, the infiltrate can be more localized to the dermal–epidermal junction. In some mast cells, the nuclei may be round or oval, but in most mast cells, they are spindle-shaped (Fig. 6-81). Because the mast cells may be present only in small numbers, and because in sections stained with hematoxylin–eosin, their nuclei resemble those of fibroblasts or pericytes, the diagnosis may be missed unless special staining is employed.

In cases with multiple nodules or plaques or with a solitary large nodule, the mast cells lie closely packed in tumor-like aggregates (Figs. 6-82 and 6-83). The infiltrate may extend through the entire dermis and even into the subcutaneous fat (493). Whenever the mast cells lie in dense aggregates, their nuclei are cuboidal rather than spindle-shaped, and they show ample eosinophilic cytoplasm and a well-defined cell border. Because of the shape of their nuclei and ample cytoplasm, they have a rather distinctive appearance; so, the diagnosis can usually be made even before special staining has been carried out. Cutaneous *mastocytomas* tend to have a denser, nodular aggregate of mast cells in the dermis, which can extend into the subcutaneous tissue. Histologic sections of DCM show a diffuse infiltrate of loosely arranged mast cells throughout the dermis (513). Mast cells in *DCM* tend to aggregate close to vessels within the superficial dermis and within the dermal papillae (514). Biopsies of SM show similar histologic changes to cases of TMEP, UP, mastocytomas, and DCM. *Mast cell sarcomas* have

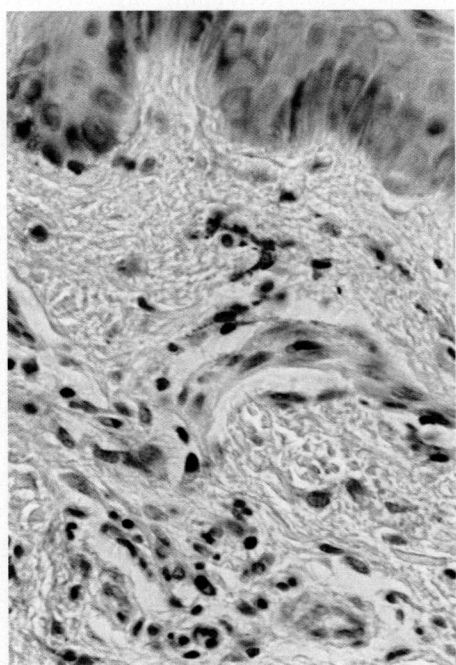

Figure 6-81 Urticaria pigmentosa. Scattered mast cells are seen, some cuboidal in shape. The greatest numbers are about dermal vessels. The epidermis is hyperpigmented (original magnification ×100).

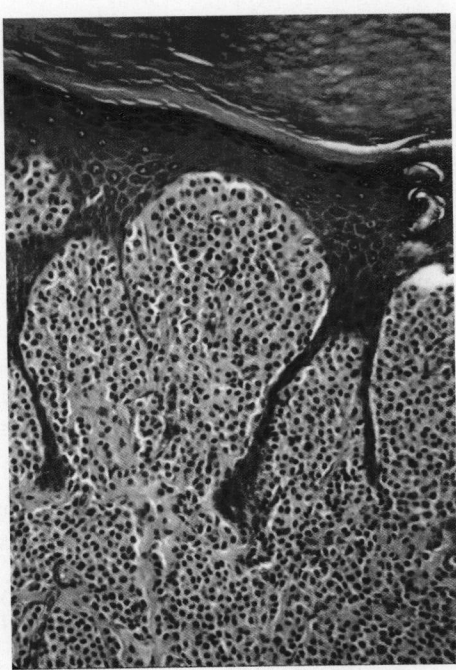

Figure 6-82 Urticaria pigmentosa. Mast cells fill the expanded papillary dermis (original magnification ×100).

a highly pleomorphic morphology. Frequent mitoses and areas of necrosis can be present (515).

Eosinophils may be present in small numbers in all types of UP with the exception of TMEP, in which eosinophils are generally absent because of the small numbers of mast cells within the lesions. If a biopsy is taken shortly after the lesion has been stroked, an increased number of eosinophils and extracellular mast cell granules is observed, which is an indication that granules have been released by the cells.

The bullae that may occur in infants with multiple or solitary nodules or with the diffuse type arise subepidermally. Because of regeneration of the epidermis at the base of the bulla, older bullae may be located intraepidermally. The bullous cavity often contains mast cells as well as eosinophils. The pigmentation of lesions of UP is caused by the presence of increased amounts of melanin in the basal cell layer and, occasionally, also by the presence of melanophages in the upper dermis.

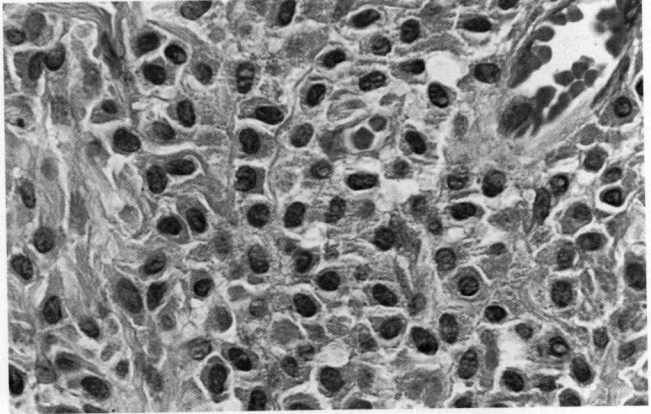

Figure 6-83 Urticaria pigmentosa. Cuboidal mast cells that fill and expand the papillary dermis. These cells closely resemble nevus cells. Special stains will differentiate (original magnification ×400).

The immunophenotype of mastocytomas includes the expression of normal mast cell markers such as CD33, CD5, CD68, CD117, tryptase, and chymase (516,517). Mast cells also express CD45 (common leukocyte antigen). Histochemical stains such as toluidine blue, Giemsa, and chloroacetate esterase (the Leder stain) may also be used to highlight mast cells (492,493). CD117 is the most sensitive marker for mast cells but is not entirely specific. Conversely, chymase is highly specific for mast cells, but less sensitive. Childhood mastocytoses very rarely express aberrant immunohistochemical markers such as CD25 or CD2 (518,519). However, those cases are frequently expressed in cases of SM and in adult patients with UP. Recently, an increased expression of CD30 in mast cells of the aggressive subtypes of SM has been reported. CD30 positivity may indicate more aggressive disease in patients with SM (520).

Pathogenesis. As seen by both light microscopy and electron microscopy, the mast cells of UP do not differ from normal mast cells either in structure or in their mode of degranulation. Because mast cells contain histamine and release it during degranulation, chemical analysis of cutaneous lesions of UP reveals a considerably higher level of histamine than is found in normal skin.

The increased melanin pigmentation in lesions of UP is a result of stimulation of epidermal melanocytes by mast cells and is not caused by any substance present within the mast cells. In one case of nodular UP, however, some mast cells showed dual granulation containing both mast cell granules and melanosomes, as well as granules representing intergrades between mast cell granules and melanosomes.

Activating mutations of the *KIT* gene are particularly common across all subtypes of mastocytosis (493,521,522). KIT is a receptor tyrosine kinase and proto-oncogene that is normally expressed by mast cells. *KIT* activating mutations are key molecular carcinogenic events in gastrointestinal stromal tumors (GISTs) as well as in some melanomas and acute myeloid leukemias. Both sporadic and germline activating mutations in the *KIT* proto-oncogene have been demonstrated in UP (522,523). Over 80% of adults with mastocytosis show a specific *KIT* mutation: D816V on exon 17 (493). In contrast, only 35% of childhood mastocytosis cases (most of which are UP) have D816V *KIT* mutations. The majority of familial cases of UP follow an autosomal dominant pattern of inheritance. Solitary mastocytomas show mutations in the *KIT* gene in approximately 67% of cases (524). Similar to UP and isolated mastocytomas, many cases of DCM also have *KIT* mutations. Familial forms of DCM have been identified and show germline mutations in *KIT* (525,526). It has been reported that up to 50% of cases of TMEP also show mutations in the *KIT* gene (506). The vast majority of patients with SM have activating mutations in the *c-KIT* proto-oncogene, the most common of which is the point mutation D816V (527,528). In patients with advanced forms of SM, especially AHNMD, the activation mutation in c-*KIT* occurs late in the disease after other mutations causing the clonal myeloid neoplasm have occurred (508). Other mutations have been identified in advanced SM, including *CBLB*, *RUNX1*, *TET2*, *ASXL1*, and *SRSF2* (such mutations are common to myeloid neoplasms). The additional mutations are associated with a more aggressive disease course and worse outcome. The pathogenesis of MCS is poorly understood.

Differential Diagnosis. Even if numerous mast cells are present, a reliable diagnosis of UP requires the demonstration of mast cell granules with the Giemsa stain, Leder's method, or toluidine blue stain. On routine staining, the mast cells in macular lesions may resemble fibroblasts or pericytes, but those in nodular or erythrodermic lesions may resemble the histiocytes that are seen in Langerhans cell histiocytosis. Differentiation of UP from Langerhans cell histiocytosis on routine staining can be particularly difficult because in all three diseases, the infiltrate may contain eosinophils. In contrast with Langerhans cell histiocytosis, the cells of UP have no tendency to invade the epidermis. Occasionally, the cuboidal mast cells in nodular UP resemble nevus cells, but they show no tendency to lie in nests and show no junction activity. LCH is positive for Langerhans cell markers (CD1a, langerin, S100), which are negative in mastocytosis.

The macular type of UP, especially TMEP, occasionally may be difficult to diagnose even with the Giemsa stain because the number of mast cells may be so small that it does not differ significantly from the number normally present. Some inflammatory dermatoses, such as atopic dermatitis, lichen simplex chronicus, and lichen planus, may contain a high percentage of mast cells in their inflammatory cell infiltrates. However, in UP, the infiltrate consists exclusively of mast cells, except for a slight admixture of eosinophils as a result of the degranulation of some of the mast cells.

Principles of Management: Patients with mastocytosis should be advised to avoid mast cell degranulators and environmental triggers. Symptoms of mastocytosis can be controlled with the use of antihistamines, often in combination, with long-acting H1 antagonists being most effective. Addition of H2 blockers may be helpful for refractory symptoms. For local relief of cutaneous symptoms, topical steroids may be used. Oral cromolyn may have additional benefits for patients with gastrointestinal symptoms. More severe attacks with systemic manifestations may require injected epinephrine if life-threatening symptoms are present. Phototherapy, either narrow-band ultraviolet B or Psoralens with ultraviolet A (PUVA), may be warranted for difficult-to-control cutaneous disease (529,530). Patients with a high mast cell burden may benefit from cytoreductive therapies, including the use of the tyrosine kinase inhibitor, imatinib (531). However, imatinib does not act against the most common D816 c-kit mutation, but these may be dasatinib-responsive (532,533). The more aggressive forms of SM (SM-AHNMD, ASM, and MCL) often require treatment with cytotoxic chemotherapy and hematopoietic stem cell transplant. Clinical trials with the use of anti-CD30 therapy are currently underway.

REFERENCES

1. Oji V, Tadini G, Akiyama M, et al. Revised nomenclature and classification of inherited ichthyoses: results of the First Ichthyosis Consensus Conference in Soreze 2009. *J Am Acad Dermatol.* 2010;63:607–641.
2. McGrath JA, Uitto J. The filaggrin story: novel insights into skin-barrier function and disease. *Trends Mol Med.* 2008;14:20–27.
3. Nirunsuksiri W, Presland RB, Brumbaugh SG, Dale BA, Fleckman P. Decreased profilaggrin expression in ichthyosis vulgaris is a result of selectively impaired posttranscriptional control. *J Biol Chem.* 1995;270:871–876.
4. Osawa R, Akiyama M, Shimizu H. Filaggrin gene defects and the risk of developing allergic disorders. *Allergol Int.* 2011;60:1–9.
5. Mevorah B, Frenk E, Muller CR, Ropers HH. X-linked recessive ichthyosis in three sisters: evidence for homozygosity. *Br J Dermatol.* 1981;105:711–717.
6. Costagliola C, Fabbrocini G, Illiano GM, Scibelli G, Delfino M. Ocular findings in X-linked ichthyosis: a survey on 38 cases. *Ophthalmologica.* 1991;202:152–155.
7. Traupe H, Happle R. Clinical spectrum of steroid sulfatase deficiency: X-linked recessive ichthyosis, birth complications and cryptorchidism. *Eur J Pediatr.* 1983;140:19–21.
8. Maya-Nunez G, Cuevas-Covarrubias S, Zenteno JC, Ulloa-Aguirre A, Kofman-Alfaro S, Méndez JP. Contiguous gene syndrome due to deletion of the first three exons of the Kallmann gene and complete deletion of the steroid sulphatase gene. *Clin Endocrinol (Oxf).* 1998;48:713–718.
9. Jeong HS, Funari T, Gordon K, Richard G, Agim NG. Concurrent chondrodysplasia punctata type 2 (Conradi-Hunermann-Happle Syndrome) and ichthyosis vulgaris in teenaged twin girls. *Pediatr Dermatol.* 2017;34(5):e245–e248.
10. Feinstein A, Ackerman AB, Ziprkowski L. Histology of autosomal dominant ichthyosis vulgaris and X-linked ichthyosis. *Arch Dermatol.* 1970;101:524–527.
11. Chan A, Godoy-Gijon E, Nuno-Gonzalez A, et al. Cellular basis of secondary infections and impaired desquamation in certain inherited ichthyoses. *JAMA Dermatol.* 2015;151(3):285–292. doi:10.1001/jamadermatol.2014.3369
12. Webster D, France JT, Shapiro LJ, Weiss R. X-linked ichthyosis due to steroid-sulphatase deficiency. *Lancet.* 1978;1:70–72.
13. Williams ML. Ichthyosis: mechanisms of disease. *Pediatr Dermatol.* 1992;9:365–368.
14. Elias PM, Williams ML, Maloney ME, et al. Stratum corneum lipids in disorders of cornification. Steroid sulfatase and cholesterol sulfate in normal desquamation and the pathogenesis of recessive X-linked ichthyosis. *J Clin Invest.* 1984;74:1414–1421.
15. Ackerman AB. Histopathologic concept of epidermolytic hyperkeratosis. *Arch Dermatol.* 1970;102:253–259.
16. McCurdy J. Congenital bullous ichthyosiform erythroderma. *Br J Dermatol.* 1967;79:294–297.
17. Rothnagel JA, Dominey AM, Dempsey LD, et al. Mutations in the rod domains of keratins 1 and 10 in epidermolytic hyperkeratosis. *Science.* 1992;257:1128–1130.
18. Paller AS. Expanding our concepts of mosaic disorders of skin. *Arch Dermatol.* 2001;137:1236–1238.
19. Paller AS, Syder AJ, Chan YM, et al. Genetic and clinical mosaicism in a type of epidermal nevus. *N Engl J Med.* 1994;331:1408–1415.
20. Burger B, Spoerri I, Schubert M, Has C, Itin PH. Description of the natural course and clinical manifestations of ichthyosis with confetti caused by a novel KRT10 mutation. *Br J Dermatol.* 2012;166:434–439.
21. Choate KA, Lu Y, Zhou J, et al. Mitotic recombination in patients with ichthyosis causes reversion of dominant mutations in KRT10. *Science.* 2010;330:94–97.
22. Jonkman MF, Pasmooij AM. Revertant mosaicism—patchwork in the skin. *N Engl J Med.* 2009;360:1680–1682.
23. Ross R, DiGiovanna JJ, Capaldi L, Argenyi Z, Fleckman P, Robinson-Bostom L. Histopathologic characterization of epidermolytic hyperkeratosis: a systematic review of histology from the National Registry for Ichthyosis and Related Skin Disorders. *J Am Acad Dermatol.* 2008;59:86–90.
24. Laiho E, Niemi KM, Ignatius J, Kere J, Palotie A, Saarialho-Kere U. Clinical and morphological correlations for transglutaminase 1 gene mutations in autosomal recessive congenital ichthyosis. *Eur J Hum Genet.* 1999;7:625–632.
25. Thomas AC, Cullup T, Norgett EE, et al. ABCA12 is the major harlequin ichthyosis gene. *J Invest Dermatol.* 2006;126:2408–2413.

26. Akiyama M. ABCA12 mutations and autosomal recessive congenital ichthyosis: a review of genotype/phenotype correlations and of pathogenetic concepts. *Hum Mutat.* 2010;31:1090–1096.

27. Epp N, Furstenberger G, Muller K, et al. 12R-lipoxygenase deficiency disrupts epidermal barrier function. *J Cell Biol.* 2007;177:173–182.

28. Eckl KM, de Juanes S, Kurtenbach J, et al. Molecular analysis of 250 patients with autosomal recessive congenital ichthyosis: evidence for mutation hotspots in ALOXE3 and allelic heterogeneity in ALOX12B. *J Invest Dermatol.* 2009;129:1421–1428.

29. Lefevre C, Bouadjar B, Ferrand V, et al. Mutations in a new cytochrome P450 gene in lamellar ichthyosis type 3. *Hum Mol Genet.* 2006;15:767–776.

30. Dahlqvist J, Klar J, Hausser I, et al. Congenital ichthyosis: mutations in ichthyin are associated with specific structural abnormalities in the granular layer of epidermis. *J Med Genet.* 2007;44:615–620.

31. Williams ML, Elias PM. Heterogeneity in autosomal recessive ichthyosis. Clinical and biochemical differentiation of lamellar ichthyosis and nonbullous congenital ichthyosiform erythroderma. *Arch Dermatol.* 1985;121:477–488.

32. Gruber R, Rainer G, Weiss A, et al. Morphological alterations in two siblings with autosomal recessive congenital ichthyosis associated with CYP4F22 mutations. *Br J Dermatol.* 2017;176(4):1068–1073. doi:10.1111/bjd.14860

33. Jagell S, Liden S. Ichthyosis in the Sjogren-Larsson syndrome. *Clin Genet.* 1982;21:243–252.

34. Rizzo WB, Dammann AL, Craft DA, et al. Sjogren-Larsson syndrome: inherited defect in the fatty alcohol cycle. *J Pediatr.* 1989;115:228–234.

35. Derry JM, Gormally E, Means GD, et al. Mutations in a delta 8-delta 7 sterol isomerase in the tattered mouse and X-linked dominant chondrodysplasia punctata. *Nat Genet.* 1999;22:286–290.

36. Fartasch M, Williams ML, Elias PM. Altered lamellar body secretion and stratum corneum membrane structure in Netherton syndrome: differentiation from other infantile erythrodermas and pathogenic implications. *Arch Dermatol.* 1999;135:823–832.

37. Mevorah B, Frenk E. Ichthyosis linearis circumflexa comel with trichorrhexis invaginata (Netherton's syndrome): a light microscopical study of the skin changes. *Dermatologica.* 1974;149:193–200.

38. Hovnanian A. Netherton syndrome: skin inflammation and allergy by loss of protease inhibition. *Cell Tissue Res.* 2013;351:289–300.

39. Zina AM, Bundino S. Ichthyosis linearis circumflexa Comel and Netherton's syndrome; an ultrastructural study. *Dermatologica.* 1979;158:404–412.

40. Briot A, Lacroix M, Robin A, Steinhoff M, Deraison C, Hovnanian A. Par2 inactivation inhibits early production of TSLP, but not cutaneous inflammation, in Netherton syndrome adult mouse model. *J Invest Dermatol.* 2010;130:2736–2742.

41. Faghri S, Tamura D, Kraemer KH, Digiovanna JJ. Trichothiodystrophy: a systematic review of 112 published cases characterises a wide spectrum of clinical manifestations. *J Med Genet.* 2008;45:609–621.

42. Davies MG, Marks R, Dykes PJ, Reynolds D. Epidermal abnormalities in Refsum's disease. *Br J Dermatol.* 1977;97:401–406.

43. Warren M, Shimura M, Wartchow EP, Yano S. Use of electron microscopy when screening liver biopsies from neonates and infants: experience from a single tertiary children's hospital (1991-2017). *Ultrastruct Pathol.* 2020;44 (1):32–41. doi:10.1080/01913123.2019.1709934

44. Warren M, Mierau G, Wartchow EP, Shimada H, Yano S. Histologic and ultrastructural features in early and advanced phases of Zellweger spectrum disorder (infantile Refsum disease). *Ultrastruct Pathol.* 2018;42(3):220–227. doi:10.1080/01913123.2018.1440272

45. Mihalik SJ, Morrell JC, Kim D, Sacksteder KA, Watkins PA, Gould SJ. Identification of PAHX, a Refsum disease gene. *Nat Genet.* 1997;17:185–189.

46. Jansen GA, Waterham HR, Wanders RJ. Molecular basis of Refsum disease: sequence variations in phytanoyl-CoA hydroxylase (PHYH) and the PTS2 receptor (PEX7). *Hum Mutat* .2004;23:209–218.

47. Konig A, Happle R, Bornholdt D, Engel H, Grzeschik KH. Mutations in the NSDHL gene, encoding a 3beta-hydroxysteroid dehydrogenase, cause CHILD syndrome. *Am J Med Genet.* 2000;90:339–346.

48. Paller AS, van Steensel MA, Rodriguez-Martin M, et al. Pathogenesis-based therapy reverses cutaneous abnormalities in an inherited disorder of distal cholesterol metabolism. *J Invest Dermatol.* 2011;131:2242–2248.

49. Hashimoto K, Topper S, Sharata H, Edwards M. CHILD syndrome: analysis of abnormal keratinization and ultrastructure. *Pediatr Dermatol.* 1995;12:116–129.

50. Hashimoto K, Prada S, Lopez AP, Hoyos JG, Escobar M. CHILD syndrome with linear eruptions, hypopigmented bands, and verruciform xanthoma. *Pediatr Dermatol.* 1998;15:360–366.

51. Rubeiz N, Kibbi AG. Management of ichthyosis in infants and children. *Clin Dermatol.* 2003;21:325–328.

52. Deffenbacher B. Successful experimental treatment of congenital ichthyosis in an infant. *BMJ Case Rep.* 2013;2013:bcr2013008688.

53. Seeger MA, Paller AS. The role of abnormalities in the distal pathway of cholesterol synthesis in the Congenital Hemidysplasia with Ichthyosiform erythroderma and Limb Defects (CHILD) syndrome. *Biochim Biophys Acta.* 2014;1841(3):345–352.

54. Alsaif HS, Al-Owain M, Barrios-Llerena ME, et al. Homozygous loss-of-function mutations in AP1B1, Encoding beta-1 subunit of adaptor-related protein complex 1, cause MEDNIK-like syndrome. *Am J Hum Genet.* 2019;105(5):1016–1022. doi:10.1016/j. ajhg.2019.09.020

55. Incecik F, Bisgin A, Yılmaz M. MEDNIK syndrome with a frame shift causing mutation in AP1S1 gene and literature review of the clinical features. *Metab Brain Dis.* 2018;33(6):2065–2068. doi:10.1007/s11011-018-0313-4

56. Martinelli D, Dionisi-Vici C. AP1S1 defect causing MEDNIK syndrome: a new adaptinopathy associated with defective copper metabolism. *Ann N Y Acad Sci.* 2014;1314:55–63. doi:10.1111/ nyas.12426

57. Agakidou E, Agakidis C, Kambouris M, et al. A novel mutation of VPS33B gene associated with incomplete arthrogryposis-renal dysfunction-cholestasis phenotype. *Case Rep Genet.* 2020;2020: 8872294. doi:10.1155/2020/8872294.eCollection

58. Lee MJ, Suh CR, Shin JH, et al. A novel VPS33B variant identified by exome sequencing in a patient with arthrogryposis-renal dysfunction-cholestasis syndrome. *Pediatr Gastroenterol Hepatol Nutr.* 2019;22(6):581–587. doi:10.5223/pghn.2019.22.6.581

59. Chai M, Su L, Hao X, et al. Identification of genes and signaling pathways associated with arthrogryposis–renal dysfunction–cholestasis syndrome using weighted correlation network analysis. *Int J Mol Med.* 2018;42(4):2238–2246. doi:10.3892/ijmm.2018.3768

60. Vandersteen PR, Muller SA. Erythrokeratodermia variabilis: an enzyme histochemical and ultrastructural study. *Arch Dermatol.* 1971;103:362–370.

61. Hirano SA, Harvey VM. From progressive symmetric erythrokeratoderma to erythrokeratoderma variabilis progressiva. *J Am Acad Dermatol.* 2011;64:e81–e82.

62. Common JE, O'Toole EA, Leigh IM, et al. Clinical and genetic heterogeneity of erythrokeratoderma variabilis. *J Invest Dermatol.* 2005;125:920–927.

63. Richard G, Smith LE, Bailey RA, et al. Mutations in the human connexin gene GJB3 cause erythrokeratodermia variabilis. *Nat Genet.* 1998;20:366–369.

64. Macari F, Landau M, Cousin P, et al. Mutation in the gene for connexin 30.3 in a family with erythrokeratodermia variabilis. *Am J Hum Genet.* 2000;67:1296–1301.

65. Richard G, Brown N, Rouan F, et al. Genetic heterogeneity in erythrokeratodermia variabilis: novel mutations in the connexin gene GJB4 (Cx30.3) and genotype-phenotype correlations. *J Invest Dermatol.* 2003;120:601–609.

66. Ishida-Yamamoto A, McGrath JA, Lam H, Iizuka H, Friedman RA, Christiano AM. The molecular pathology of progressive symmetric erythrokeratoderma: a frameshift mutation in the loricrin gene and perturbations in the cornified cell envelope. *Am J Hum Genet.* 1997;61:581–589.

67. Wei S, Zhou Y, Zhang TD, et al. Evidence for the absence of mutations at GJB3, GJB4 and LOR in progressive symmetrical erythrokeratodermia. *Clin Exp Dermatol.* 2011;36:399–405.

68. van Steensel MA, Oranje AP, van der Schroeff JG, Wagner A, van Geel M. The missense mutation G12D in connexin30.3 can cause both erythrokeratodermia variabilis of Mendes da Costa and progressive symmetric erythrokeratodermia of Gottron. *Am J Med Genet A.* 2009;149A:657–661.

69. Kimyai-Asadi A, Kotcher LB, Jih MH. The molecular basis of hereditary palmoplantar keratodermas. *J Am Acad Dermatol.* 2002;47:327–343; quiz 344–326.

70. Itin PH, Fistarol SK. Palmoplantar keratodermas. *Clin Dermatol.* 2005;23:15–22.

71. Sperelakis-Beedham B, Lopez M, Girodon E, Hickman G, Bourrat E, Bienvenu T. Genetics of complex and syndromic palmoplantar keratoderma [in French]. *Ann Biol Clin (Paris).* 2021;79(6):551–565. doi:10.1684/abc.2021.1688

72. Knop M, Alelq N, Kubieniec ME, Giehl K. Palmoplantar dermatoses in children [in German]. *Hautarzt.* 2021;72(3):215–224. doi:10.1007/s00105-021-04765-w

73. Bodemer C, Steijlen P, Mazereeuw-Hautier J, O'Toole EA. Treatment of hereditary palmoplantar keratoderma: a review by analysis of the literature. *Br J Dermatol.* 2021;184(3):393–400. doi:10.1111/bjd.19144

74. Kimonis V, DiGiovanna JJ, Yang JM, Doyle SZ, Bale SJ, Compton JG. A mutation in the V1 end domain of keratin 1 in non-epidermolytic palmar-plantar keratoderma. *J Invest Dermatol.* 1994;103:764–769.

75. Hart TC, Hart PS, Michalec MD, et al. Haim-Munk syndrome and Papillon-Lefevre syndrome are allelic mutations in cathepsin C. *J Med Genet.* 2000;37:88–94.

76. Iossa S, Chinetti V, Auletta G, et al. New evidence for the correlation of the p.G130V mutation in the GJB2 gene and syndromic hearing loss with palmoplantar keratoderma. *Am J Med Genet A.* 2009;149A:685–688.

77. Lee JR, White TW. Connexin-26 mutations in deafness and skin disease. *Expert Rev Mol Med.* 2009;11:e35.

78. O'Driscoll J, Muston GC, McGrath JA, Lam HM, Ashworth J, Christiano AM. A recurrent mutation in the loricrin gene underlies the ichthyotic variant of Vohwinkel syndrome. *Clin Exp Dermatol.* 2002;27:243–246.

79. Chimienti F, Hogg RC, Plantard L, et al. Identification of SLURP-1 as an epidermal neuromodulator explains the clinical phenotype of Mal de Meleda. *Hum Mol Genet.* 2003;12:3017–3024.

80. Ochiai T, Nakano H, Rokunohe D, et al. Novel p.M1T and recurrent p.G301S mutations in cathepsin C in a Japanese patient with Papillon-Lefevre syndrome: implications for understanding the genotype/phenotype relationship. *J Dermatol Sci.* 2009;53:73–75.

81. Lin Z, Chen Q, Lee M, et al. Exome sequencing reveals mutations in TRPV3 as a cause of Olmsted syndrome. *Am J Hum Genet.* 2012;90:558–564.

82. Bach JN, Levan NE. Papillon-Lefevre syndrome. *Arch Dermatol.* 1968;97:154–158.

83. Klaus S, Weinstein GD, Frost P. Localized epidermolytic hyperkeratosis: a form of keratoderma of the palms and soles. *Arch Dermatol.* 1970;101:272–275.

84. Fritsch P, Honigsmann H, Jaschke E. Epidermolytic hereditary palmoplantar keratoderma: report of a family and treatment with an oral aromatic retinoid. *Br J Dermatol.* 1978;99:561–568.

85. Buchanan RN Jr. Keratosis punctata palmaris et plantaris. *Arch Dermatol.* 1963;88:644–650.

86. Eytan O, Sarig O, Israeli S, Mevorah B, Basel-Vanagaite L, Sprecher E. A novel splice-site mutation in the AAGAB gene segregates with hereditary punctate palmoplantar keratoderma and congenital dysplasia of the hip in a large family. *Clin Exp Dermatol.* 2014;39(2):182–186.

87. Giehl KA, Eckstein GN, Pasternack SM, et al. Nonsense mutations in AAGAB cause punctate palmoplantar keratoderma type Buschke-Fischer-Brauer. *Am J Hum Genet.* 2012;91:754–759.

88. Schonfeld PH. The pachyonychia congenita syndrome. *Acta Derm Venereol.* 1980;60:45–49.

89. Witkop CJ Jr, Gorlin RJ. Four hereditary mucosal syndromes: comparative histology and exfoliative cytology of Darier-White's disease, hereditary benign intraepithelial dyskeratosis, white sponge nevus, and pachyonychia congenita. *Arch Dermatol.* 1961;84:762–771.

90. Shah S, Boen M, Kenner-Bell B, Schwartz M, Rademaker A, Paller AS. Pachyonychia congenita in pediatric patients: natural history, features, and impact. *JAMA Dermatol.* 2014;150(2):146–153.

91. Lewis KG, Bercovitch L, Dill SW, Robinson-Bostom L. Acquired disorders of elastic tissue, part II: decreased elastic tissue. *J Am Acad Dermatol.* 2004;51:165–185; quiz 186–168.

92. Nelson-Adesokan P, Mallory SB, Leonardi CL, Lund R. Acrokeratoelastoidosis of Costa. *Int J Dermatol.* 1995;34:431–433. doi:10.1111/j.1365-4362.1995.tb04448.x

93. Bogle MA, Hwang LY, Tschen JA. Acrokeratoelastoidosis. *J Am Acad Dermatol.* 2002;47:448–451.

94. Erkek E, Kocak M, Bozdogan O, Atasoy P, Birol A. Focal acral hyperkeratosis: a rare cutaneous disorder within the spectrum of Costa acrokeratoelastoidosis. *Pediatr Dermatol.* 2004;21:128–130.

95. Masse R, Quillard A, Hery B, Toudic L, Le Her G. Costa's acrokerato-elastoidosis: ultrastructural study (author's transl) [in French]. *Ann Dermatol Venereol.* 1977;104:441–445.

96. Abulafia J, Vignale RA. Degenerative collagenous plaques of the hands and acrokeratoelastoidosis: pathogenesis and relationship with knuckle pads. *Int J Dermatol.* 2000;39:424–432.

97. V. M. Contributo allo studio della ipercheratosi dei canali sudoriferi (porokeratosi). *G It Mal Vener Pelle.* 1893;28:313–355.

98. Murase J, Gilliam AC. Disseminated superficial actinic porokeratosis co-existing with linear and verrucous porokeratosis in an elderly woman: update on the genetics and clinical expression of porokeratosis. *J Am Acad Dermatol.* 2010;63:886–891.

99. Ferreira FR, Santos LD, Tagliarini FA, Lira ML. Porokeratosis of Mibelli—literature review and a case report. *An Bras Dermatol.* 2013;88:179–182.

100. Vargas-Mora P, Morgado-Carrasco D, Fustà-Novell X. Porokeratosis: a review of its pathophysiology, clinical manifestations, diagnosis, and treatment [in English, Spanish]. *Actas Dermosifiliogr (Engl Ed).* 2020;111(7):545–560. doi:10.1016/j.ad.2020.03.005

101. Li L, Zuo N, Yang D, Zhang D, Feng Y, Li X. Novel missense mutations of MVK and FDPS gene in Chinese patients with disseminated superficial actinic porokeratosis. *Clin Chim Acta.* 2021;523:441–445. doi:10.1016/j.cca.2021.10.026

102. Arisawa Y, Ito Y, Tanahashi K, et al. Two cases of porokeratosis with MVD mutations, in association with bullous pemphigoid. *Acta Derm Venereol.* 2021;101(3):adv00423. doi:10.2340/00015555-3764

103. Leng Y, Yan L, Feng H, et al. Mutations in mevalonate pathway genes in patients with familial or sporadic porokeratosis. *J Dermatol.* 2018;45(7):862–866. doi:10.1111/1346-8138.14343

104. Kanitakis J, Euvrard S, Faure M, Claudy A. Porokeratosis and immunosuppression. *Eur J Dermatol.* 1998;8:459–465.

105. Sasson M, Krain AD. Porokeratosis and cutaneous malignancy: a review. *Dermatol Surg.* 1996;22:339–342.

106. Zhang SQ, Jiang T, Li M, et al. Exome sequencing identifies MVK mutations in disseminated superficial actinic porokeratosis. *Nat Genet.* 2012;44:1156–1160.

107. Happle R. Mibelli revisited: a case of type 2 segmental porokeratosis from 1893. *J Am Acad Dermatol.* 2010;62:136–138.

108. Himmelstein R, Lynfield YL. Punctate porokeratosis. *Arch Dermatol.* 1984;120:263–264.

109. Guss SB, Osbourn RA, Lutzner MA. Porokeratosis plantaris, palmaris, et disseminata. A third type of porokeratosis. *Arch Dermatol.* 1971;104:366–373.

110. Neumann RA, Knobler RM, Gebhart W. Unusual presentation of porokeratosis palmaris, plantaris et disseminata. *J Am Acad Dermatol.* 1989;21:1131–1133.

111. Vivas AC, Maderal AD, Kirsner RS. Giant ulcerating squamous cell carcinoma arising from linear porokeratosis: a case study. *Ostomy Wound Manage.* 2012;58:18–20.

112. Arranz-Salas I, Sanz-Trelles A, Ojeda DB. p53 alterations in porokeratosis. *J Cutan Pathol.* 2003;30:455–458.

113. Braun-Falco O, Balsa RE. Histochemistry of cornoid lamella. Pathogenesis of porokeratosis Mibelli [in German]. *Hautarzt.* 1969;20:543–550.

114. Reed RJ, Leone P. Porokeratosis: a mutant clonal keratosis of the epidermis. I. Histogenesis. *Arch Dermatol.* 1970;101:340–347.

115. Mann PR, Cort DF, Fairburn EA, Abdel-Aziz A. Ultrastructural studies on two cases of porokeratosis of Mibelli. *Br J Dermatol.* 1974;90:607–617.

116. Sato A, Anton-Lamprecht I, Schnyder UW. Ultrastructure of inborn errors of keratinization, VII: porokeratosis Mibelli and disseminated superficial actinic porokeratosis. *Arch Dermatol Res.* 1976;255:271–284.

117. Wade TR, Ackerman AB. Cornoid lamellation. A histologic reaction pattern. *Am J Dermatopathol.* 1980;2:5–15.

118. Bruckner-Tuderman L, Has C. Molecular heterogeneity of blistering disorders: the paradigm of epidermolysis bullosa. *J Invest Dermatol.* 2012;132:E2–E5.

119. Fine JD, Eady RAJ, Bauer EA, et al. The classification of inherited epidermolysis bullosa (EB): report of the Third International Consensus Meeting on Diagnosis and Classification of EB. *J Am Acad Dermatol.* 2008;58(6):931–950.

120. Sprecher E. Epidermolysis bullosa simplex. *Dermatol Clin.* 2010;28:23–32.

121. Bardhan A, Bruckner-Tuderman L, Chapple ILC, et al. Epidermolysis bullosa. *Nat Rev Dis Primers.* 2020;6(1):78. doi:10.1038/s41572-020-0210-0

122. Fine J-D, Johnson LB, Weiner M, Suchindran C. Cause-specific risks of childhood death in inherited epidermolysis bullosa. *J Pediatr.* 2008;152:276–280.

123. Shemanko CS, Horn HM, Keohane SG, et al. Laryngeal involvement in the Dowling-Meara variant of epidermolysis bullosa simplex with keratin mutations of severely disruptive potential. *Br J Dermatol.* 2000;142:315–320.

124. McGrath JA, Bolling MC, Jonkman MF. Lethal acantholytic epidermolysis bullosa. *Dermatol Clin.* 2010;28:131–135.

125. Schneider H, Mühle C, Pacho F. Biological function of laminin-5 and pathogenic impact of its deficiency. *Eur J Cell Biol.* 2007;86:701–717.

126. Fine JD, Johnson LB, Weiner M, Li KP, Suchindran C. Epidermolysis bullosa and the risk of life-threatening cancers: the National EB Registry experience, 1986–2006. *J Am Acad Dermatol.* 2009;60:203–211.

127. Yuen WY, Jonkman MF. Risk of squamous cell carcinoma in junctional epidermolysis bullosa, non-Herlitz type: report of 7 cases and a review of the literature. *J Am Acad Dermatol.* 2011;65:780–789.

128. Radkevich-Brown O, Shwayder T. Bullous dermolysis of the newborn: four new cases and clinical review. *Pediatr Dermatol.* 2013;30(6):736–740.

129. Bart BJ, Gorlin RJ, Anderson VE, Lynch FW. Congenital localized absence of skin and associated abnormalities resembling epidermolysis bullosa: a new syndrome. *Arch Dermatol.* 1966;93:296–304.

130. Lai-Cheong JE, Tanaka A, Hawche G, et al. Kindler syndrome: a focal adhesion genodermatosis. *Br J Dermatol.* 2009;160:233–242.

131. Sadler E, Klausegger A, Muss W, et al. Novel KIND1 gene mutation in Kindler syndrome with severe gastrointestinal tract involvement. *Arch Dermatol.* 2006;142:1619–1624.

132. Mizutani H, Masuda K, Nakamura N, Takenaka H, Tsuruta D, Katoh N. Cutaneous and laryngeal squamous cell carcinoma in mixed epidermolysis bullosa, kindler syndrome. *Case Rep Dermatol.* 2012;4:133–138.

133. Has C, Castiglia D, del Rio M, et al. Kindler syndrome: extension of FERMT1 mutational spectrum and natural history. *Hum Mut.* 2011;32:1204–1212.

134. Intong LRA, Murrell DF. How to take skin biopsies for epidermolysis bullosa. *Dermatol Clin.* 2010;28:197–200, vii.

135. Pohla-Gubo G, Cepeda-Valdes R, Hintner H. Immunofluorescence mapping for the diagnosis of epidermolysis bullosa. *Dermatol Clin.* 2010;28:201–210, vii.

136. Murrell DF. The pitfalls of skin biopsies to diagnose epidermolysis bullosa. *Pediatr Dermatol.* 2013;30:273–275.

137. Rao R, Shetty VM. Utility of immunofluorescence antigen mapping in hereditary epidermolysis bullosa. *Indian J Dermatol.* 2021;66(4):360–365. doi:10.4103/ijd.IJD_131_20

138. Phillips GS, Huang A, Augsburger BD, et al. A retrospective analysis of diagnostic testing in a large North American cohort of patients with epidermolysis bullosa. *J Am Acad Dermatol.* 2022;86(5):1063–1071. doi:10.1016/j.jaad.2021.09.065

139. Lai-Cheong JE, Parsons M, Tanaka A, et al. Loss-of-function FERMT1 mutations in kindler syndrome implicate a role for fermitin family homolog-1 in integrin activation. *Am J Pathol.* 2009;175:1431–1441.

140. Berk DR, Jazayeri L, Marinkovich MP, Sundram UN, Bruckner AL. Diagnosing epidermolysis bullosa type and subtype in infancy using immunofluorescence microscopy: the Stanford experience. *Pediatr Dermatol.* 2013;30:226–233.

141. Shinkuma S, McMillan JR, Shimizu H. Ultrastructure and molecular pathogenesis of epidermolysis bullosa. *Clin Dermatol.* 2011;29:412–419.

142. McGrath JA, Pulkkinen L, Christiano AM, Leigh IM, Eady RA, Uitto J. Altered laminin 5 expression due to mutations in the gene encoding the beta 3 chain (LAMB3) in generalized atrophic benign epidermolysis bullosa. *J Invest Dermatol.* 1995;104:467–474.

143. Ryynänen M, Knowlton RG, Parente MG, Chung LC, Chu ML, Uitto J. Human type VII collagen: genetic linkage of the gene (COL7A1) on chromosome 3 to dominant dystrophic epidermolysis bullosa. *Am J Hum Genet.* 1991;49:797–803.

144. Dunnill MG, Richards AJ, Milana G, et al. Genetic linkage to the type VII collagen gene (COL7A1) in 26 families with generalised recessive dystrophic epidermolysis bullosa and anchoring fibril abnormalities. *J Med Genet.* 1994;31:745–748.

145. Nanchahal J, Tidman MJ. A study of the dermo-epidermal junction in dystrophic epidermolysis bullosa using the periodic acid-thiosemicarbazide-silver proteate technique. *Br J Dermatol.* 1985;113:397–404.

146. Tidman MJ, Eady RA. Evaluation of anchoring fibrils and other components of the dermal-epidermal junction in dystrophic epidermolysis bullosa by a quantitative ultrastructural technique. *J Invest Dermatol.* 1985;84:374–377.

147. Forman AB, Prendiville JS, Esterly NB, et al. Kindler syndrome: report of two cases and review of the literature. *Pediatr Dermatol.* 1989;6:91–101.

148. Bruckner-Tuderman L, McGrath JA, Robinson EC, Uitto J. Progress in epidermolysis bullosa research: summary of DEBRA International Research Conference 2012. *J Invest Dermatol.* 2013;133:2121–2126.

149. Xu Z, Zhang L, Xiao Y, et al. A case of Hailey-Hailey disease in an infant with a new ATP2C1 gene mutation. *Pediatr Dermatol.* 2011;28:165–168.

150. Nikkels AF, Delvenne P, Herfs M, Pierard GE. Occult herpes simplex virus colonization of bullous dermatitides. *Am J Clin Dermatol.* 2008;9(3):163–168. doi:10.2165/00128071-200809030-00004

151. Chin AGM, Asif M, Hultman C, Caffrey J. Hailey-Hailey disease with superimposed eczema herpeticum caused by herpes simplex virus type 2 infection in a burn unit: a case report and literature review. *Cureus.* 2019;11(10):e5907. doi:10.7759/cureus.5907

152. Yang L, Zhang Q, Zhang S, Liu Y, Liu Y, Wang T. Generalized Hailey-Hailey disease: novel splice-site mutations of ATP2C1 gene in Chinese population and a literature review. *Mol Genet Genomic Med.* 2021;9(2):e1580. doi:10.1002/mgg3.1580

153. Ben Lagha I, Ashack K, Khachemoune A. Hailey-Hailey disease: an update review with a focus on treatment data. *Am J Clin Dermatol.* 2020;21(1):49–68. doi:10.1007/s40257-019-00477-z

154. Szigeti R, Kellermayer R. Autosomal-dominant calcium ATPase disorders. *J Invest Dermatol.* 2006;126:2370–2376.

155. Hu Z, Bonifas JM, Beech J, et al. Mutations in ATP2C1, encoding a calcium pump, cause Hailey-Hailey disease. *Nat Genet.* 2000;24:61–65.

156. Leinonen PT, Hägg PM, Peltonen S, et al. Reevaluation of the normal epidermal calcium gradient, and analysis of calcium levels and ATP receptors in Hailey-Hailey and Darier epidermis. *J Invest Dermatol.* 2009;129:1379–1387.

157. Fong G, Capaldi L, Sweeney SM, Wiss K, Mahalingam M. Congenital Darier disease. *J Am Acad Dermatol.* 2008;59:S50–S51.

158. Ferris T, Lamey PJ, Rennie JS. Darier's disease: oral features and genetic aspects. *Br Dent J.* 1990;168:71–73.

159. Sakuntabhai A, Dhitavat J, Burge S, Hovnanian A. Mosaicism for ATP2A2 mutations causes segmental Darier's disease. *J Invest Dermatol.* 2000;115:1144–1147.

160. Bachar-Wikström E, Wikström JD. Darier disease—a multi-organ condition? *Acta Derm Venereol.* 2021;101(4):adv00430. doi:10.2340/00015555-3770

161. Nellen RG, Steijlen PM, van Steensel MA, et al. Mendelian disorders of cornification caused by defects in intracellular calcium pumps: mutation update and database for variants in ATP2A2 and ATP2C1 associated with Darier disease and Hailey-Hailey disease. *Hum Mutat.* 2017;38(4):343–356. doi:10.1002/humu.23164

162. Takagi A, Kamijo M, Ikeda S. Darier disease. *J Dermatol.* 2016;43(3):275–279. doi:10.1111/1346-8138.13230

163. Wang Y, Bruce AT, Tu C, et al. Protein aggregation of SERCA2 mutants associated with Darier disease elicits ER stress and apoptosis in keratinocytes. *J Cell Sci.* 2011;124:3568–3580.

164. Sakuntabhai A, Ruiz-Perez V, Carter S, et al. Mutations in ATP2A2, encoding a Ca2+ pump, cause Darier disease. *Nat Genet.* 1999;21:271–277.

165. Hobbs RP, Amargo EV, Somasundaram A, et al. The calcium ATPase SERCA2 regulates desmoplakin dynamics and intercellular adhesive strength through modulation of PKC signaling. *FASEB J.* 2011;25:990–1001.

166. Bergman R, Sezin T, Indelman M, Helou WA, Avitan-Hersh E. Acrokeratosis verruciformis of Hopf showing P602L mutation in ATP2A2 and overlapping histopathological features with Darier disease. *Am J Dermatopathol.* 2012;34:597–601.

167. Berk DR, Taube JM, Bruckner AL, Lane AT. A sporadic patient with acrokeratosis verruciformis of Hopf and a novel ATP2A2 mutation. *Br J Dermatol.* 2010;163:653–654.

168. Wang PG, Gao M, Lin GS, et al. Genetic heterogeneity in acrokeratosis verruciformis of Hopf. *Clin Exp Dermatol.* 2006;31:558–563.

169. Serarslan G, Balci DD, Homan S. Acitretin treatment in acrokeratosis verruciformis of Hopf. *J Dermatolog Treat.* 2007;18:123–125.

170. Fusco F, Fimiani G, Tadini G, Michele D, Ursini MV. Clinical diagnosis of incontinentia pigmenti in a cohort of male patients. *J Am Acad Dermatol.* 2007;56:264–267.

171. Pacheco TR, Levy M, Collyer JC, et al. Incontinentia pigmenti in male patients. *J Am Acad Dermatol.* 2006;55:251–255.

172. Minic S, Trpinac D, Obradovic M. Incontinentia pigmenti diagnostic criteria update. *Clin Genet.* 2014;85(6):536–542.

173. Nazzaro V, Brusasco A, Gelmetti C, Ermacora E, Caputo R. Hypochromic reticulated streaks in incontinentia pigmenti: an immunohistochemical and ultrastructural study. *Pediatr Dermatol.* 1990;7:174–178.

174. Caputo R, Gianotti F, Innocenti M. Ultrastructural findings in incontinentia pigmenti. *Int J Dermatol.* 1975;14:46–55.

175. Guerrier CJ, Wong CK. Ultrastructural evolution of the skin in incontinentia pigmenti (Bloch-Sulzberger): study of six cases. *Dermatologica.* 1974;149:10–22.

176. Schmalstieg FC, Jorizzo JL, Tschen J, Subrt P. Basophils in incontinentia pigmenti. *J Am Acad Dermatol.* 1984;10:362–364.

177. Frieden IJ. Aplasia cutis congenita: a clinical review and proposal for classification. *J Am Acad Dermatol.* 1986;14:646–660.

178. Brooks BP, Thompson AH, Bishop RJ, et al. Ocular manifestations of xeroderma pigmentosum: long-term follow-up highlights the role of DNA repair in protection from sun damage. *Ophthalmology.* 2013;120:1324–1336.

179. Bradford PT, Goldstein AM, Tamura D, et al. Cancer and neurologic degeneration in xeroderma pigmentosum: long term follow-up characterises the role of DNA repair. *J Med Genet.* 2011;48:168–176.

180. Cleaver JE, Lam ET, Revet I. Disorders of nucleotide excision repair: the genetic and molecular basis of heterogeneity. *Nat Rev Genet.* 2009;10:756–768.

181. Rizza ERH, DiGiovanna JJ, Khan SG, Tamura D, Jeskey JD, Kraemer KH. Xeroderma pigmentosum: a model for human premature aging. *J Invest Dermatol.* 2021;141(4S):976–984. doi:10.1016/j.jid.2020.11.012

182. Masaki T, Wang Y, DiGiovanna JJ, et al. High frequency of PTEN mutations in nevi and melanomas from xeroderma pigmentosum patients. *Pigment Cell Melanoma Res.* 2014;27(3):454–464. doi:10.1111/pcmr.12226

183. Digiovanna JJ, Kraemer KH. Shining a light on xeroderma pigmentosum. *J Invest Dermatol.* 2012;132:785–796.

184. Hentosh P, Benjamin T, Hall L, et al. Xeroderma pigmentosum variant: complementary molecular approaches to detect a 13 base pair deletion in the DNA polymerase eta gene. *Exp Mol Pathol.* 2011;91:528–533.

185. Martens MC, Emmert S, Boeckmann L. Xeroderma pigmentosum: gene variants and splice variants. *Genes (Basel).* 2021;12(8):1173. doi:10.3390/genes12081173

186. Sharma R, Lewis S, Wlodarski MW. DNA repair syndromes and cancer: insights into genetics and phenotype patterns. *Front Pediatr.* 2020;8:570084. doi:10.3389/fped.2020.570084

187. Lehmann AR, Fassihi H. Molecular analysis directs the prognosis, management and treatment of patients with xeroderma pigmentosum. *DNA Repair (Amst).* 2020;93:102907. doi:10.1016/j.dnarep.2020.102907

188. Savage SA, Alter BP. Dyskeratosis congenita. *Hematol Oncol Clin North Am.* 2009;23:215–231.

189. Ogden GR, Chisholm DM, Leigh IM, Lane EB. Cytokeratin profiles in dyskeratosis congenita: an immunocytochemical investigation of lingual hyperkeratosis. *J Oral Pathol Med.* 1992;21:353–357.

190. Alter BP, Baerlocher GM, Savage SA, et al. Very short telomere length by flow fluorescence in situ hybridization identifies patients with dyskeratosis congenita. *Blood.* 2007;110:1439–1447.

191. Alter BP, Rosenberg PS, Giri N, et al. Telomere length is associated with disease severity and declines with age in dyskeratosis congenita. *Haematologica.* 2012;97:353–359.

192. Mason PJ, Bessler M. The genetics of dyskeratosis congenita. *Cancer Genet.* 2011;204:635–645.

193. Vulliamy TJ, Marrone A, Knight SW, Walne A, Mason PJ, Dokal I. Mutations in dyskeratosis congenita: their impact on

telomere length and the diversity of clinical presentation. *Blood.* 2006;107:2680–2685.

194. Stinco G, Governatori G, Mattighello P, Patrone P. Multiple cutaneous neoplasms in a patient with Rothmund-Thomson syndrome: case report and published work review. *J Dermatol.* 2008;35:154–161.

195. Hicks MJ, Roth JR, Kozinetz CA, Wang LL. Clinicopathologic features of osteosarcoma in patients with Rothmund-Thomson syndrome. *J Clin Oncol.* 2007;25:370–375.

196. Piquero-Casals J, Okubo AY, Nico MMS. Rothmund-Thomson syndrome in three siblings and development of cutaneous squamous cell carcinoma. *Pediatr Dermatol.* 2002;19:312–316.

197. Siitonen HA, Sotkasiira J, Biervliet M, et al. The mutation spectrum in RECQL4 diseases. *Eur J Hum Genet.* 2009;17:151–158.

198. Kitao S, Shimamoto A, Goto M, et al. Mutations in RECQL4 cause a subset of cases of Rothmund-Thomson syndrome. *Nat Genet.* 1999;22:82–84.

199. Larizza L, Magnani I, Roversi G. Rothmund-Thomson syndrome and RECQL4 defect: splitting and lumping. *Cancer Lett.* 2006;232:107–120.

200. Ghosh AK, Rossi ML, Singh DK, et al. RECQL4, the protein mutated in Rothmund-Thomson syndrome, functions in telomere maintenance. *J Biol Chem.* 2012;287:196–209.

201. Clericuzio C, Hoyme HE, Aase JM. Immune deficient poikiloderma: a new genodermatosis. *Am J Hum Genet.* 1991;49:A661.

202. Chantorn R, Shwayder T. Poikiloderma with neutropenia: report of three cases including one with calcinosis cutis. *Pediatr Dermatol.* 2012;29:463–472.

203. Van Hove JLK, Jaeken J, Proesmans M, et al. Clericuzio type poikiloderma with neutropenia is distinct from Rothmund-Thomson syndrome. *Am J Med Genet A.* 2005;132A:152–158.

204. Arnold AW, Itin PH, Pigors M, Kohlhase J, Bruckner-Tuderman L, Has C. Poikiloderma with neutropenia: a novel C16orf57 mutation and clinical diagnostic criteria. *Br J Dermatol.* 2010;163:866–869.

205. Rodgers W, Ancliff P, Ponting CP, et al. Squamous cell carcinoma in a child with Clericuzio-type poikiloderma with neutropenia. *Br J Dermatol.* 2013;168:665–667.

206. Volpi L, Roversi G, Colombo EA, et al. Targeted next-generation sequencing appoints c16orf57 as clericuzio-type poikiloderma with neutropenia gene. *Am J Hum Genet.* 2010;86:72–76.

207. Mroczek S, Krwawicz J, Kutner J, et al. C16orf57, a gene mutated in poikiloderma with neutropenia, encodes a putative phosphodiesterase responsible for the U6 snRNA 3' end modification. *Genes Dev.* 2012;26:1911–1925.

208. Hilcenko C, Simpson PJ, Finch AJ, et al. Aberrant 3' oligoadenylation of spliceosomal U6 small nuclear RNA in poikiloderma with neutropenia. *Blood.* 2013;121:1028–1038.

209. German J. Bloom's syndrome. XX. The first 100 cancers. *Cancer Genet Cytogenet.* 1997;93:100–106.

210. Cheok CF, Bachrati CZ, Chan KL, Ralf C, Wu L, Hickson ID. Roles of the Bloom's syndrome helicase in the maintenance of genome stability. *Biochem Soc Transac.* 2005;33:1456–1459.

211. Nissenkorn A, Levi YB, Vilozni D, et al. Neurologic presentation in children with ataxia-telangiectasia: is small head circumference a hallmark of the disease? *J Pediatr.* 2011;159:466–471.e1.

212. Greenberger S, Berkun Y, Ben-Zeev B, Levi YB, Barziliai A, Nissenkorn A. Dermatologic manifestations of ataxia-telangiectasia syndrome. *J Am Acad Dermatol.* 2013;68:932–936.

213. Paller AS, Massey RB, Curtis MA, et al. Cutaneous granulomatous lesions in patients with ataxia-telangiectasia. *J Pediatr.* 1991;119:917–922.

214. Nowak-Wegrzyn A, Crawford TO, Winkelstein JA, Carson KA, Lederman HM. Immunodeficiency and infections in ataxia-telangiectasia. *J Pediatr.* 2004;144:505–511.

215. Micol R, Ben Slama L, Suarez F, et al. Morbidity and mortality from ataxia-telangiectasia are associated with ATM genotype. *J Allergy Clin Immunol.* 2011;128:382–389.e1.

216. Thompson D, Duedal S, Kirner J, et al. Cancer risks and mortality in heterozygous ATM mutation carriers. *J Allergy Clin Immunol.* 2005;97:813–822.

217. de Jager M, Blokx W, Warris A, et al. Immunohistochemical features of cutaneous granulomas in primary immunodeficiency disorders: a comparison with cutaneous sarcoidosis. *J Cutan Pathol.* 2008;35:467–472.

218. Mitra A, Pollock B, Gooi J, Darling JC, Boon A, Newton-Bishop JA. Cutaneous granulomas associated with primary immunodeficiency disorders. *Br J Dermatol.* 2005;153:194–199.

219. McKinnon PJ. ATM and the molecular pathogenesis of ataxia telangiectasia. *Ann Rev Pathol.* 2012;7:303–321.

220. Hoche F, Seidel K, Theis M, et al. Neurodegeneration in ataxia telangiectasia: what is new? What is evident? *Neuropediatrics.* 2012;43:119–129.

221. Raz-Prag D, Galron R, Segev-Amzaleg N, et al. A role for vascular deficiency in retinal pathology in a mouse model of ataxia-telangiectasia. *Am J Pathol.* 2011;179:1533–1541.

222. Ousset M, Bouquet F, Fallone F, et al. Loss of ATM positively regulates the expression of hypoxia inducible factor 1 (HIF-1) through oxidative stress: role in the physiopathology of the disease. *Cell Cycle.* 2010;9:2814–2822.

223. Mitra A, Gooi J, Darling J, Newton-Bishop JA. Infliximab in the treatment of a child with cutaneous granulomas associated with ataxia telangiectasia. *J Am Acad Dermatol.* 2011;65:676–677.

224. Rork JF, Huang JT, Gordon LB, Kleinman M, Kieran MW, Liang MG. Initial cutaneous manifestations of Hutchinson-Gilford progeria syndrome. *Pediatr Dermatol.* 2014;31(2):196–202.

225. Merideth MA, Gordon LB, Clauss S, et al. Phenotype and course of Hutchinson-Gilford progeria syndrome. *N Engl J Med.* 2008;358:592–604.

226. Capell BC, Tlougan BE, Orlow SJ. From the rarest to the most common: insights from progeroid syndromes into skin cancer and aging. *J Invest Dermatol.* 2009;129:2340–2350.

227. Kudlow BA, Kennedy BK, Monnat RJ. Werner and Hutchinson-Gilford progeria syndromes: mechanistic basis of human progeroid diseases. *Nat Rev Mol Cell Biol.* 2007;8:394–404.

228. Gordon LB, Kleinman ME, Miller DT, et al. Clinical trial of a farnesyltransferase inhibitor in children with Hutchinson-Gilford progeria syndrome. *Proc Natl Acad Sci U S A.* 2012;109:16666–16671.

229. Muftuoglu M, Oshima J, von Kobbe C, Cheng WH, Leistritz DF, Bohr VA. The clinical characteristics of Werner syndrome: molecular and biochemical diagnosis. *Hum Genet.* 2008;124:369–377.

230. Takemoto M, Mori S, Kuzuya M, et al. Diagnostic criteria for Werner syndrome based on Japanese nationwide epidemiological survey. *Geriatr Gerontol Int.* 2013;13:475–481.

231. Lauper JM, Krause A, Vaughan TL, Monnat RJ Jr. Spectrum and risk of neoplasia in Werner syndrome: a systematic review. *PloS One.* 2013;8:e59709.

232. Friedrich K, Lee L, Leistritz DF, et al. WRN mutations in Werner syndrome patients: genomic rearrangements, unusual intronic mutations and ethnic-specific alterations. *Hum Genet.* 2010;128:103–111.

233. Kamenisch Y, Berneburg M. Progeroid syndromes and UV-induced oxidative DNA damage. *J Investig Dermatol Symp Proc.* 2009;14:8–14.

234. Rossi ML, Ghosh AK, Bohr VA. Roles of Werner syndrome protein in protection of genome integrity. *DNA Repair.* 2010;9:331–344.

235. Chen L, Lee L, Kudlow BA, et al. LMNA mutations in atypical Werner's syndrome. *Lancet.* 2003;362:440–445.

236. Massip L, Garand C, Paquet ER, et al. Vitamin C restores healthy aging in a mouse model for Werner syndrome. *FASEB J.* 2010;24:158–172.

237. Wang X, Reid Sutton V, Omar Peraza-Llanes J, et al. Mutations in X-linked PORCN, a putative regulator of Wnt signaling, cause focal dermal hypoplasia. *Nat Genet.* 2007;39:836–838.

238. Ruggieri M, Gentile AE, Ferrara V, et al. Neurocutaneous syndromes in art and antiquities. *Am J Med Genet C Semin Med Genet.* 2021;187(2):224–234. doi:10.1002/ajmg.c.31917

239. Steele L, Shipman AR. Neuroimaging in infants and children in select neurocutaneous disorders. *Clin Exp Dermatol.* 2021;46(3):438–443. doi:10.1111/ced.14471

240. Callea M, Teggi R, Yavuz I, et al. Ear nose throat manifestations in hypoidrotic ectodermal dysplasia. *Int J Pediatr Otorhinolaryngol.* 2013;77:1801–1804.

241. Mégarbané H, Cluzeau C, Bodemer C, et al. Unusual presentation of a severe autosomal recessive anhydrotic ectodermal dysplasia with a novel mutation in the EDAR gene. *Am J Med Genet A.* 2008;146A:2657–2662.

242. Rinne T, Brunner HG, van Bokhoven H. p63-associated disorders. *Cell Cycle.* 2007;6:262–268.

243. Rinne T, Hamel B, van Bokhoven H, Brunner HG. Pattern of p63 mutations and their phenotypes—update. *Am J Med Genet A.* 2006;140:1396–1406.

244. Knaudt B, Volz T, Krug M, Burgdorf W, Röcken M, Berneburg M. Skin symptoms in four ectodermal dysplasia syndromes including two case reports of Rapp-Hodgkin-Syndrome. *Eur J Dermatol.* 2012;22:605–613.

245. Dishop MK, Bree AF, Hicks MJ. Pathologic changes of skin and hair in ankyloblepharon-ectodermal defects-cleft lip/palate (AEC) syndrome. *Am J Med Genet A.* 2009;149A:1935–1941.

246. Millar SE. Molecular mechanisms regulating hair follicle development. *J Invest Dermatol.* 2002;118:216–225.

247. Mikkola ML. Molecular aspects of hypohidrotic ectodermal dysplasia. *Am J Med Genet A.* 2009;149A:2031–2036.

248. Zonana J, Elder ME, Schneider LC, et al. A novel X-linked disorder of immune deficiency and hypohidrotic ectodermal dysplasia is allelic to incontinentia pigmenti and due to mutations in IKK-gamma (NEMO). *Am J Hum Genet.* 2000;67:1555–1562.

249. Koster MI. p63 in skin development and ectodermal dysplasias. *J Invest Dermatol.* 2010;130:2352–2358.

250. Sutton VR, van Bokhoven H. TP63-related disorders. In: Adam MP, Ardinger HH, Pagon RA, et al, eds. *GeneReviews®.* University of Washington, Seattle; 2010.

251. Lamartine J, Munhoz Essenfelder G, Kibar Z, et al. Mutations in GJB6 cause hidrotic ectodermal dysplasia. *Nat Genet.* 2000;26:142–144.

252. Fujimoto A, Kurban M, Nakamura M, et al. GJB6, of which mutations underlie Clouston syndrome, is a potential direct target gene of p63. *J Dermatol Sci.* 2013;69:159–166.

253. Ardelean D, Pope E. Incontinentia pigmenti in boys: a series and review of the literature. *Pediatr Dermatol.* 2006;23:523–527.

254. Steele L, Shipman AR. Neuroimaging in infants and children in select neurocutaneous disorders. *Dermatol Pract Concept.* 2021;11(2):e2021012. doi:10.5826/dpc.1102a12

255. Mazza JM, Klein JF, Christopher K, Silverberg NB. Aplasia cutis congenita in a setting of fetus papyraceus associated with small fetal abdominal circumference and high alpha-fetoprotein and amniotic acetylcholinesterase. *Pediatr Dermatol.* 2015;32(1):138–140. doi:10.1111/pde.12228

256. Bart BJ. Epidermolysis bullosa and congenital localized absence of skin. *Arch Dermatol.* 1970;101:78–81.

257. Sethi M, Lehmann AR, Fawcett H, et al. Patients with xeroderma pigmentosum complementation groups C, E and V do not have abnormal sunburn reactions. *Br J Dermatol.* 2013;169:1279–1287.

258. Grzeschik KH, Bornholdt D, Oeffner F, et al. Deficiency of PORCN, a regulator of Wnt signaling, is associated with focal dermal hypoplasia. *Nat Genet.* 2007;39:833–835.

259. Paller AS. Wnt signaling in focal dermal hypoplasia. *Nat Genet.* 2007;39:820–821.

260. Clements SE, Mellerio JE, Holden ST, McCauley J, McGrath JA. PORCN gene mutations and the protean nature of focal dermal hypoplasia. *Br J Dermatol.* 2009;160:1103–1109.

261. Knockaert D, Dequeker J. Osteopathia striata and focal dermal hypoplasia. *Skeletal Radiol.* 1979;4:223–227.

262. Howell JB, Reynolds J. Osteopathia striata. A diagnostic osseous marker of focal dermal hypoplasia. *Trans St Johns Hosp Dermatol Soc.* 1974;60:178–182.

263. Yoshihashi H, Ohki H, Torii C, Ishiko A, Kosaki K. Survival of a male mosaic for PORCN mutation with mild focal dermal hypoplasia phenotype. *Pediatr Dermatol.* 2011;28:550–554.

264. Alkindi S, Battin M, Aftimos S, Purvis D. Focal dermal hypoplasia due to a novel mutation in a boy with Klinefelter syndrome. *Pediatr Dermatol.* 2013;30:476–479.

265. Goltz RW, Henderson RR, Hitch JM, Ott JE. Focal dermal hypoplasia syndrome: a review of the literature and report of two cases. *Arch Dermatol.* 1970;101:1–11.

266. Naouri M, Boisseau C, Bonicel P, et al. Manifestations of pseudoxanthoma elasticum in childhood. *Br J Dermatol.* 2009;161:635–639.

267. Yu J, Liao PJ, Xu W, et al. Structural model of human PORCN illuminates disease-associated variants and drug-binding sites. *J Cell Sci.* 2021;134(24):jcs259383. doi:10.1242/jcs.259383

268. Happle R. The PORCN non-Goltz spectrum (PONGOS): a new group of genetic disorders. *Am J Med Genet A.* 2021;185(1):13–14. doi:10.1002/ajmg.a.61984

269. McCuaig CC, Vera C, Kokta V, et al. Connective tissue nevi in children: institutional experience and review. *J Am Acad Dermatol.* 2012;67:890–897.

270. Neldner KH. Pseudoxanthoma elasticum. *Clin Dermatol.* 1988;6:1–159.

271. Gliem M, Zaeytijd JD, Finger RP, Holz FG, Leroy BP, Charbel Issa P. An update on the ocular phenotype in patients with pseudoxanthoma elasticum. *Front Genet.* 2013;4:14.

272. Li D, Ryu E, Saeidian AH, et al. GGCX mutations in a patient with overlapping pseudoxanthoma elasticum/cutis laxa-like phenotype. *Br J Dermatol.* 2021;184(6):1170–1174. doi:10.1111/bjd.19576

273. Plomp AS, Toonstra J, Bergen AA, van Dijk MR, de Jong PT. Proposal for updating the pseudoxanthoma elasticum classification system and a review of the clinical findings. *Am J Med Genet A.* 2010;152A:1049–1058.

274. Bergen AA, Plomp AS, Schuurman EJ, et al. Mutations in ABCC6 cause pseudoxanthoma elasticum. *Nat Genet.* 2000;25:228–231.

275. Ringpfeil F, Lebwohl MG, Christiano AM, Uitto J. Pseudoxanthoma elasticum: mutations in the MRP6 gene encoding a transmembrane ATP-binding cassette (ABC) transporter. *Proc Natl Acad Sci USA.* 2000;97:6001–6006.

276. Li Q, Jiang Q, Pfendner E, Váradi A, Uitto J. Pseudoxanthoma elasticum: clinical phenotypes, molecular genetics and putative pathomechanisms. *Exp Dermatol.* 2009;18:1–11.

277. Jiang Q, Uitto J. Pseudoxanthoma elasticum: a metabolic disease? *J Invest Dermatol.* 2006;126:1440–1441.

278. Saux OL, Urban Z, Tschuc C, et al. Mutations in a gene encoding an ABC transporter cause pseudoxanthoma elasticum. 2000;25:223–227.

279. Omarjee L, Nitschke Y, Verschuere S, et al. Severe early-onset manifestations of pseudoxanthoma elasticum resulting from the cumulative effects of several deleterious mutations in ENPP1, ABCC6 and HBB: transient improvement in ectopic calcification with sodium thiosulfate. *Br J Dermatol.* 2020;183(2):367–372. doi:10.1111/bjd.18632

280. Huang SN, Steele HD, Kumar G, Parker JO. Ultrastructural changes of elastic fibers in pseudoxanthoma elasticum: a study of histogenesis. *Arch Pathol.* 1967;83:108–113.

281. Danielsen L, Kobayasi T, Larsen HW, Midtgaard K, Christensen HE. Pseudoxanthoma elasticum: a clinico-pathological study. *Acta Derm Venereol.* 1970;50:355–373.

282. Goodman RM, Smith EW, Paton D, et al. Pseudoxanthoma elasticum: a clinical and histopathological study. *Medicine (Baltimore).* 1963;42:297–334.

283. Kreysel HW, Lerche W, Janner M. Observations on the Gronblad-Strandberg syndrome (angioid streaks—pseudoxanthoma elasticum) [in German]. *Hautarzt.* 1967;18:24–28.

284. Chen EL, Altman I, Braniecki M. A helpful clue to calciphylaxis: subcutaneous pseudoxanthoma elasticum-like changes. *Am J Dermatopathol.* 2020;42(7):521–523. doi:10.1097/DAD.0000000000001577

285. Penn LA, Brinster N. Calciphylaxis with pseudoxanthoma elasticum-like changes: a case series. *J Cutan Pathol.* 2018;45(2):118–121. doi:10.1111/cup.13075

286. Atzori L, Ferreli C, Pilloni L, Rongioletti F. Pseudoxanthoma elasticum-like papillary dermal elastolysis: a mimicker of genetic pseudoxanthoma elasticum. *Clin Dermatol.* 2021;39(2):206–210. doi:10.1016/j.clindermatol.2020.10.018

287. Oiso N, Kato M, Kawada A. Fibroelastolytic papulosis in an elderly woman with a 30-year history: overlapping between pseudoxanthoma elasticum-like papillary dermal elastolysis and white fibrous papulosis of the neck. *Eur J Dermatol.* 2014;24(6):688–689. doi:10.1684/ejd.2014.2470

288. Ishikawa M, Motegi SI, Toki S, Endo Y, Yasuda M, Ishikawa O. Calciphylaxis and nephrogenic fibrosing dermopathy with pseudoxanthoma elasticum-like changes: successful treatment with sodium thiosulfate. *J Dermatol.* 2019;46(7):e240–e242. doi:10.1111/1346-8138.14780

289. Mendelsohn G, Bulkley BH, Hutchins GM. Cardiovascular manifestations of pseudoxanthoma elasticum. *Arch Pathol Lab Med.* 1978;102:298–302.

290. Akhtar M, Brody H. Elastic tissue in pseudoxanthoma elasticum: ultrastructural study of endocardial lesions. *Arch Pathol.* 1975;99:667–671.

291. McKee PH, Cameron CH, Archer DB, Logan WC. A study of four cases of pseudoxanthoma elasticum. *J Cutan Pathol.* 1977;4:146–153.

292. Lebwohl M, Neldner K, Pope FM, et al. Classification of pseudoxanthoma elasticum: report of a consensus conference. *J Am Acad Dermatol.* 1994;30:103–107.

293. Montesu MA, Onnis G, Gunnella S, Lissia A, Satta R. Elastosis perforans serpiginosa: causes and associated disorders. *Eur J Dermatol.* 2018;28(4):476–481. doi:10.1684/ejd.2018.3355

294. Ramírez-Bellver JL, Bernárdez C, Macías E, et al. Dermoscopy and direct immunofluorescence findings of elastosis perforans serpiginosa. *Clin Exp Dermatol.* 2016;41(6):667– 670. doi:10.1111/ced.12882

295. Navarrete-Dechent C, Puerto Cd, Bajaj S, Marghoob AA, González S, Jaque A. Dermoscopy of elastosis perforans serpiginosa: a useful tool to distinguish it from granuloma annulare. *J Am Acad Dermatol.* 2015;73(1):e7–e9. doi:10.1016/j.jaad.2015.02.1132

296. Beachkofsky TM, Sapp JC, Biesecker LG, Darling TN. Progressive overgrowth of the cerebriform connective tissue nevus in patients with Proteus syndrome. *J Am Acad Dermatol.* 2010;63:799–804.

297. Uitto J, Santa Cruz DJ, Starcher BC, Whyte MP, Murphy WA. Biochemical and ultrastructural demonstration of elastin accumulation in the skin lesions of the Buschke-Ollendorff syndrome. *J Invest Dermatol.* 1981;76:284–287.

298. Hellemans J, Preobrazhenska O, Willaert A, et al. Loss-of-function mutations in LEMD3 result in osteopoikilosis, Buschke-Ollendorff syndrome and melorheostosis. *Nat Genet.* 2004;36:1213–1218.

299. Morrison JG, Jones EW, MacDonald DM. Juvenile elastoma and osteopoikilosis (the Buschke—Ollendorff syndrome). *Br J Dermatol.* 1977;97:417–422.

300. Cole GW, Barr RJ. An elastic tissue defect in dermatofibrosis lenticularis disseminata. Buschke-Ollendorff syndrome. *Arch Dermatol.* 1982;118:44–46.

301. Verbov J, Graham R. Buschke-Ollendorff syndrome—disseminated dermatofibrosis with osteopoikilosis. *Clin Exp Dermatol.* 1986;11:17–26.

302. Danielsen L, Kobayasi T, Jacobsen GK. Ultrastructural changes in disseminated connective tissue nevi. *Acta Derm Venereol.* 1977;57:93–101.

303. Xu Z, Yang C, Xue R. Buschke-Ollendorff syndrome with LEMD3 germline stopgain mutation p.R678* presenting as multiple subcutaneous nodules with mucin deposition. *J Cutan Pathol.* 2021;48(1):77–80. doi:10.1111/cup.13771

304. Fogel S. Surgical failures: is it the surgeon or the patient? The all too often missed diagnosis of Ehlers-Danlos syndrome. *Am Surg.* 2013;79:608–613.

305. Quintana Castanedo L, Rodríguez Bandera AI, Feito Rodríguez M, González García MC, Stewart N, de Lucas Laguna R. Clinical presentation, sonographic features and treatment options of segmental stiff skin syndrome. *Clin Exp Dermatol.* 2021;46(1):135–141. doi:10.1111/ced.14394

306. Ko CJ, Atzmony L, Lim Y, et al. Review of genodermatoses with characteristic histopathology and potential diagnostic delay. *J Cutan Pathol.* 2019;46(10):756–765. doi:10.1111/cup.13520

307. Myers KL, Mir A, Schaffer JV, Meehan SA, Orlow SJ, Brinster NK. Segmental stiff skin syndrome (SSS): a distinct clinical entity. *J Am Acad Dermatol.* 2016;75(1):163–168. doi:10.1016/j.jaad.2016.01.038

308. Fusco C, Nardella G, Augello B, et al. Pro-fibrotic phenotype in a patient with segmental stiff skin syndrome via tgf-β signaling overactivation. *Int J Mol Sci.* 2020;21(14):5141. doi:10.3390/ijms21145141

309. Jensen SA, Iqbal S, Bulsiewicz A, Handford PA. A microfibril assembly assay identifies different mechanisms of dominance underlying Marfan syndrome, stiff skin syndrome and acromelic dysplasias. *Hum Mol Genet.* 2015;24(15):4454–4463. doi:10.1093/hmg/ddv181

310. Loeys BL, Gerber EE, Riegert-Johnson D, et al. Mutations in fibrillin-1 cause congenital scleroderma: stiff skin syndrome. *Sci Transl Med.* 2010;2(23):23ra20. doi:10.1126/scitranslmed.3000488

311. de Vos IJHM, Wong ASW, Welting TJM, Coull BJ, van Steensel MAM. Multicentric osteolytic syndromes represent a phenotypic spectrum defined by defective collagen remodeling. *Am J Med Genet A.* 2019;179(8):1652–1664. doi:10.1002/ajmg.a.61264

312. Bhavani GS, Shah H, Shukla A, et al. Clinical and mutation profile of multicentric osteolysis nodulosis and arthropathy. *Am J Med Genet A.* 2016;170A(2):410–417. doi:10.1002/ajmg.a.37447

313. Evans BR, Mosig RA, Lobl M, et al. Mutation of membrane type-1 metalloproteinase, MT1-MMP, causes the multicentric osteolysis and arthritis disease Winchester syndrome. *Am J Hum Genet.* 2012;91(3):572–576.

314. Manuel Martínez-Lavín. Hypertrophic osteoarthropathy. *Best Pract Res Clin Rheumatol.* 2020;34(3):101507. doi:10.1016/j.berh.2020.101507

315. Oikarinen A, Palatsi R, Kylmäniemi M, Keski-Oja J, Risteli J, Kallioinen M. Pachydermoperiostosis: analysis of the connective tissue abnormality in one family. *J Am Acad Dermatol.* 1994;31(6):947–953. doi:10.1016/s0190-9622(94)70262-4

316. Tanese K, Niizeki H, Seki A, et al. Pathological characterization of pachydermia in pachydermoperiostosis. *J Dermatol.* 2015;42(7):710–714. doi:10.1111/1346-8138.12869

317. Diggle CP, Parry DA, Logan CV, et al. Prostaglandin transporter mutations cause pachydermoperiostosis with myelofibrosis. *Hum Mutat.* 2012;33(8):1175–1181. doi:10.1002/humu.22111

318. Uppal S, Diggle CP, Carr IM, et al. Mutations in 15-hydroxyprostaglandin dehydrogenase cause primary hypertrophic osteoarthropathy. *Nat Genet.* 2008;40(6):789–793. doi:10.1038/ng.153

319. Alessandrella A, Della Casa R, Alessio M, Puente Prieto J, Strisciuglio P, Melis D. A novel homozygous mutation in the SLCO2A1 gene causing pachydermoperiostosis:

efficacy of hydroxychloroquine treatment. *Am J Med Genet A.* 2018;176(5):1253–1257. doi:10.1002/ajmg.a.38677

320. Wesche WA, Cutlan RT, Khare V, Chesney T, Shanklin D. Restrictive dermopathy: report of a case and review of the literature. *J Cutan Pathol.* 2001;28(4):211–218. doi:10.1034/j .1600-0560.2001.028004211.x

321. Morais P, Magina S, Ribeiro Mdo C, et al. Restrictive dermopathy—a lethal congenital laminopathy. Case report and review of the literature. *Eur J Pediatr.* 2009;168(8):1007–1012. doi:10.1007/s00431-008-0868-x

322. Schreiber KH, Kennedy BK. When lamins go bad: nuclear structure and disease. *Cell.* 2013;152(6):1365–1375. doi:10.1016/j .cell.2013.02.015

323. Navarro CL, Cadiñanos J, De Sandre-Giovannoli A, et al. Loss of ZMPSTE24 (FACE-1) causes autosomal recessive restrictive dermopathy and accumulation of Lamin A precursors. *Hum Mol Genet.* 2005;14(11):1503–1513. doi:10.1093/hmg/ddi159

324. Navarro CL, De Sandre-Giovannoli A, Bernard R, et al. Lamin A and ZMPSTE24 (FACE-1) defects cause nuclear disorganization and identify restrictive dermopathy as a lethal neonatal laminopathy. *Hum Mol Genet.* 2004;13(20):2493–2503. doi:10.1093/hmg/ddh265

325. Judge DP, Dietz HC. Therapy of Marfan syndrome. *Annu Rev Med.* 2008;59:43–59. doi:10.1146/annurev.med.59.103106 .103801.

326. Loeys BL, Dietz HC, Braverman AC, et al. The revised Ghent nosology for the Marfan syndrome. *J Med Genet.* 2010;47(7): 476–485. doi:10.1136/jmg.2009.072785.

327. Faivre L, Masurel-Paulet A, Collod-Béroud G, et al. Clinical and molecular study of 320 children with Marfan syndrome and related type I fibrillinopathies in a series of 1009 probands with pathogenic FBN1 mutations. *Pediatrics.* 2009;123(1):391–398. doi:10.1542/peds.2008-0703.

328. Faivre L, Collod-Beroud G, Adès L, et al. The new Ghent criteria for Marfan syndrome: what do they change? *Clin Genet.* 2012;81(5):433–442. doi:10.1111/j.1399-0004.2011.01703.x

329. Grahame R, Pyeritz RE. The Marfan syndrome: joint and skin manifestations are prevalent and correlated. *Br J Rheumatol.* 1995;34(2):126–131.

330. Ledoux M, Beauchet A, Fermanian C, Boileau C, Jondeau G, Saiag P. A case-control study of cutaneous signs in adult patients with Marfan disease: diagnostic value of striae. *J Am Acad Dermatol.* 2011;64(2):290–295.

331. Ghandi Y, Zanjani KS, Mazhari-Mousavi SE, Parvaneh N. Neonatal Marfan syndrome: report of two cases. *Iran J Pediatr.* 2013;23(1):113–117.

332. Tsuji T. Marfan syndrome: demonstration of abnormal elastic fibers in skin. *J Cutan Pathol.* 1986;13(2):144–153.

333. Hollister DW, Godfrey M, Sakai LY, Pyeritz RE. Immunohistologic abnormalities of the microfibrillar-fiber system in the Marfan syndrome. *N Engl J Med.* 1990;323(3):152–159.

334. Pinkus H, Keech MK, Mehregan AH. Histopathology of striae distensae, with special reference to striae and wound healing in the Marfan syndrome. *J Invest Dermatol.* 1966;46(3):283–292.

335. Bergman R, Nevet MJ, Gescheidt-Shoshany H, Pimienta AL, Reinstein E. Atrophic skin patches with abnormal elastic fibers as a presenting sign of the MASS phenotype associated with mutation in the fibrillin 1 gene. *JAMA Dermatol.* 2014;150(8):885–889.

336. Tiecke F, Katzke S, Booms P, et al. Classic, atypically severe and neonatal Marfan syndrome: twelve mutations and genotype-phenotype correlations in FBN1 exons 24-40. *Eur J Hum Genet.* 2001;9(1):13–21.

337. Martinez-Quintana E, Caballero-Sanchez N, Rodriguez-Gonzalez F, Garay-Sanchez P, Tugores A. Novel Marfan syndrome-associated mutation in the FBN1 gene caused by parental mosaicism and leading to abnormal limb patterning. *Mol Syndromol.* 2017;8(3):148–154.

338. Faivre L, Collod-Beroud G, Child A, et al. Contribution of molecular analyses in diagnosing Marfan syndrome and type I fibrillinopathies: an international study of 1009 probands. *J Med Genet.* 2008;45(6):384–390.

339. Beighton P, De Paepe A, Steinmann B, Tsipouras P, Wenstrup RJ. Ehlers-Danlos syndromes: revised nosology, Villefranche, 1997. Ehlers-Danlos National Foundation (USA) and Ehlers-Danlos Support Group (UK). *Am J Med Genet.* 1998;77:31–37.

340. Schwarze U, Atkinson M, Hoffman GG, Greenspan DS, Byers PH. Null alleles of the COL5A1 gene of type V collagen are a cause of the classical forms of Ehlers-Danlos syndrome (types I and II). *Am J Hum Genet.* 2000;66:1757–1765.

341. Castori M. Ehlers-Danlos syndrome, hypermobility type: an underdiagnosed hereditary connective tissue disorder with mucocutaneous, articular, and systemic manifestations. *ISRN Dermatol.* 2012;2012:751768.

342. Schalkwijk J, Zweers MC, Steijlen PM, et al. A recessive form of the Ehlers-Danlos syndrome caused by tenascin-X deficiency. *N Engl J Med.* 2001;345:1167–1175.

343. Germain DP, Herrera-Guzman Y. Vascular Ehlers-Danlos syndrome. *Ann Genet.* 2004;47:1–9.

344. Germain DP. Clinical and genetic features of vascular Ehlers-Danlos syndrome. *Ann Vasc Surg.* 2002;16:391–397.

345. Rohrbach M, Vandersteen A, Yis U, et al. Phenotypic variability of the kyphoscoliotic type of Ehlers-Danlos syndrome (EDS VIA): clinical, molecular and biochemical delineation. *Orphanet J Rare Dis.* 2011;6:46.

346. Klaassens M, Reinstein E, Hilhorst-Hofstee Y, et al. Ehlers-Danlos arthrochalasia type (VIIA-B)—expanding the phenotype: from prenatal life through adulthood. *Clin Genet.* 2012;82:121–130.

347. Byers PH, Duvic M, Atkinson M, et al. Ehlers-Danlos syndrome type VIIA and VIIB result from splice-junction mutations or genomic deletions that involve exon 6 in the COL1A1 and COL1A2 genes of type I collagen. *Am J Med Genet.* 1997;72:94–105.

348. Prockop DJ, Kivirikko KI, Tuderman L, Guzman NA. The biosynthesis of collagen and its disorders (first of two parts). *N Engl J Med.* 1979;301:13–23.

349. Malfait F, De Coster P, Hausser I, et al. The natural history, including orofacial features of three patients with Ehlers-Danlos syndrome, dermatosparaxis type (EDS type VIIC). *Am J Med Genet A.* 2004;131:18–28.

350. Wang WM, Lee S, Steiglitz BM, et al. Transforming growth factor-beta induces secretion of activated ADAMTS-2. A procollagen III N-proteinase. *J Biol Chem.* 2003;278:19549–19557.

351. Colige A, Sieron AL, Li SW, et al. Human Ehlers-Danlos syndrome type VII C and bovine dermatosparaxis are caused by mutations in the procollagen I N-proteinase gene. *Am J Hum Genet.* 1999;65:308–317.

352. Nusgens BV, Verellen-Dumoulin C, Hermanns-Le T, et al. Evidence for a relationship between Ehlers-Danlos type VII C in humans and bovine dermatosparaxis. *Nat Genet.* 1992;1:214–217.

353. Pierard GE, Lapiere M. Skin in dermatosparaxis. Dermal microarchitecture and biomechanical properties. *J Invest Dermatol.* 1976;66:2–7.

354. Pierard GE, Pierard-Franchimont C, Lapiere CM. Histopathological aid at the diagnosis of the Ehlers-Danlos syndrome, gravis and mitis types. *Int J Dermatol.* 1983;22:300–304.

355. Cullen SI. Localized Ehlers-Danlos syndrome. *Arch Dermatol.* 1979;115:332–333.

356. Berk DR, Bentley DD, Bayliss SJ, Lind A, Urban Z. Cutis laxa: a review. *J Am Acad Dermatol.* 2012;66:842 e841–e817.

357. Van Maldergem L, Loeys B. FBLN5-related cutis laxa. In: Pagon RA, Adam MP, Bird TD, et al, eds. *Gene Reviews.* University of Washington, Seattle; 1993.

358. Urban Z, Davis EC. Cutis laxa: intersection of elastic fiber biogenesis, TGFbeta signaling, the secretory pathway and metabolism. *Matrix Biol.* 2014;33:16–22.

359. Renard M, Holm T, Veith R, et al. Altered TGFbeta signaling and cardiovascular manifestations in patients with autosomal recessive cutis laxa type I caused by fibulin-4 deficiency. *Eur J Hum Genet.* 2010;18:895–901.

360. Morlino S, Nardella G, Castellana S, et al. Review of clinical and molecular variability in autosomal recessive cutis laxa 2A. *Am J Med Genet A.* 2021;185(3):955–965. doi:10.1002/ajmg.a.62047

361. Zhang Q, Qin Z, Yi S, Wei H, Zhou XZ, Su J. Two novel compound heterozygous variants of LTBP4 in a Chinese infant with cutis laxa type IC and a review of the related literature. *BMC Med Genomics.* 2020;13(1):183. doi:10.1186/s12920-020-00842-6

362. Mohamed M, Voet M, Gardeitchik T, Morava E. Cutis laxa. *Adv Exp Med Biol.* 2014;802:161–184. doi:10.1007/978-94-007-7893-1_11

363. New HD, Callen JP. Generalized acquired cutis laxa associated with multiple myeloma with biphenotypic IgG-lambda and IgA-kappa gammopathy following treatment of a nodal plasmacytoma. *Arch Dermatol.* 2011;147:323–328.

364. Tan JK, Lipworth AD, Nelson AA, Zembowicz A, Moschella SL. Part III: cutaneous hypersensitivity during selective serotonin reuptake inhibitor therapy resulting in acquired cutis laxa. *J Drugs Dermatol.* 2011;10:215–216.

365. Goltz RW, Hult AM, Goldfarb M, Gorlin RJ. Cutis laxa: a manifestation of generalized elastolysis. *Arch Dermatol.* 1965;92:373–387.

366. Yasmeen S, Lund K, De Paepe A, et al. Occipital horn syndrome and classical Menkes syndrome caused by deep intronic mutations, leading to the activation of ATP7A pseudo-exon. *Eur J Hum Genet.* 2014;22(4):517–521.

367. Tumer Z. An overview and update of ATP7A mutations leading to Menkes disease and occipital horn syndrome. *Hum Mutat.* 2013;34:417–429.

368. Ledoux-Corbusier M. Cutis laxa, congenital form with pulmonary emphysema: an ultrastructural study. *J Cutan Pathol.* 1983;10:340–349.

369. Hashimoto K, Kanzaki T. Cutis laxa. Ultrastructural and biochemical studies. *Arch Dermatol.* 1975;111:861–873.

370. Sayers CP, Goltz RW, Mottiaz J. Pulmonary elastic tissue in generalized elastolysis (cutis laxa) and Marfan's syndrome: a light and electron microscopic study. *J Invest Dermatol.* 1975;65:451–457.

371. Rimoin DL. Pachydermoperiostosis (idiopathic clubbing and periostosis): genetic and physiologic considerations. *N Engl J Med.* 1965;272:923–931.

372. Zhang Z, He JW, Fu WZ, Zhang CQ, Zhang ZL. Mutations in the SLCO2A1 gene and primary hypertrophic osteoarthropathy: a clinical and biochemical characterization. *J Clin Endocrinol Metab.* 2013;98:E923–E933.

373. Hambrick GW Jr, Carter DM. Pachydermoperiostosis: Touraine-Solente-Gole syndrome. *Arch Dermatol.* 1966;94:594–607.

374. Fernández A, Hayashi M, Garrido G, et al. Genetics of non-syndromic and syndromic oculocutaneous albinism in human and mouse. *Pigment Cell Melanoma Res.* 2021;34(4):786–799. doi:10.1111/pcmr.12982

375. Marçon CR, Maia M. Albinism: epidemiology, genetics, cutaneous characterization, psychosocial factors. *An Bras Dermatol.* 2019;94(5):503–520. doi:10.1016/j.abd.2019.09.023

376. Kubasch AS, Meurer M. Oculocutaneous and ocular albinism [in German]. *Hautarzt.* 2017;68(11):867–875. doi:10.1007/s00105-017-4061-x

377. Teramae A, Kobayashi Y, Kunimoto H, et al. The molecular basis of chemical chaperone therapy for oculocutaneous albinism type 1A. *J Invest Dermatol.* 2019;139(5):1143–1149. doi:10.1016/j.jid.2018.10.033

378. Ruiz-Sanchez D, Garabito Solovera EL, Valtueña J, et al. Amelanotic melanoma in a patient with oculocutaneous albinism. *Dermatol Online J.* 2020;26(5):13030/qt2gv5w93x.

379. Grønskov K, Ek J, Brondum-Nielsen K. Oculocutaneous albinism. *J Eur Acad Dermatol Venereol.* 2003;17(3):251–256. doi:10.1046/j.1468-3083.2003.00767.x

380. Nurden P, Stritt S, Favier R, Nurden AT. Inherited platelet diseases with normal platelet count: phenotypes, genotypes and diagnostic strategy. *Haematologica.* 2021;106(2):337–350. doi:10.3324/haematol.2020.248153

381. El-Chemaly S, Young LR. Hermansky-Pudlak syndrome. *Semin Respir Crit Care Med.* 2020;41(2):238–246. doi:10.1055/s-0040-1708088

382. Fukuda M. Rab GTPases: key players in melanosome biogenesis, transport, and transfer. *Pigment Cell Melanoma Res.* 2021;34(2):222–235. doi:10.1111/pcmr.12931

383. Santiago Borrero PJ, Rodríguez-Pérez Y, Renta JY, et al. Genetic testing for oculocutaneous albinism type 1 and 2 and Hermansky-Pudlak syndrome type 1 and 3 mutations in Puerto Rico. *J Invest Dermatol.* 2006;126(1):85–90. doi:10.1038/sj.jid.5700034

384. Sharma P, Nicoli ER, Serra-Vinardell J, et al. Chediak-Higashi syndrome: a review of the past, present, and future. *Drug Discov Today Dis Models.* 2020;31:31–36. doi:10.1016/j.ddmod.2019.10.008

385. Fukuchi K, Tatsuno K, Sakaguchi K, et al. Novel gene mutations in Chédiak-Higashi syndrome with hyperpigmentation. *J Dermatol.* 2019;46(11):e416–e418. doi:10.1111/1346-8138.14987

386. Gomaa NS, Lee JYW, El Sharkawy A, et al. Genetic analysis in Egyptian patients with Chediak-Higashi syndrome reveals new LYST mutations. *Clin Exp Dermatol.* 2019;44(7):814–817. doi:10.1111/ced.13937

387. Gironi LC, Zottarelli F, Savoldi G, et al. Congenital hypopigmentary disorders with multiorgan impairment: a case report and an overview on gray hair syndromes. *Medicina (Kaunas).* 2019;55(3):78. doi:10.3390/medicina55030078

388. Ridaura-Sanz C, Durán-McKinster C, Ruiz-Maldonado R. Usefulness of the skin biopsy as a tool in the diagnosis of silvery hair syndrome. *Pediatr Dermatol.* 2018;35(6):780–783. doi:10.1111/pde.13624

389. Wang Z, Liang Y, Xu Z. Silvery Gray Hair: a clue to diagnosing Chédiak-Higashi syndrome. *J Pediatr.* 2019;209:255–255.e1.

390. Castaño-Jaramillo LM, Lugo-Reyes SO, Cruz Muñoz ME, et al. Diagnostic and therapeutic caveats in Griscelli syndrome. *Scand J Immunol.* 2021;93(6):e13034

391. Nouriel A, Zisquit J, Helfand AM, Anikster Y, Greenberger S. Griscelli syndrome type 3: two new cases and review of the literature. *Pediatr Dermatol.* 2015;32(6):e245–e248. doi:10.1111/pde.12663

392. Bhattarai D, Banday AZ, Sadanand R, et al. Hair microscopy: an easy adjunct to diagnosis of systemic diseases in children. *Appl Microsc.* 2021;51(1):18. doi:10.1186/s42649-021-00067-6

393. Oiso N, Fukai K, Kawada A, Suzuki T. Piebaldism. *J Dermatol.* 2013;40(5):330–335. doi:10.1111/j.1346-8138.2012.01583.x

394. Spritz RA. Molecular basis of human piebaldism. *J Invest Dermatol.* 1994;103(5 suppl):137S–140S. doi:10.1111/1523-1747.ep12399455

395. Tomita Y. The molecular genetics of albinism and piebaldism. *Arch Dermatol.* 1994;130(3):355–338.

396. Hattori M, Shimizu A, Ishida-Yamamoto A, Wakamatsu K, Ishikawa O. Melanocyte lineage cells in piebald skin. *J Dermatol.* 2019;46(9):816–818. doi:10.1111/1346-8138.14999

397. Spritz RA. Piebaldism, Waardenburg syndrome, and related disorders of melanocyte development. *Semin Cutan Med Surg.* 1997;16(1):15–23. doi:10.1016/s1085-5629(97)80031-4

398. Huang S, Song J, He C, Cai X, Yuan K, Mei L, Feng Y. Genetic insights, disease mechanisms, and biological therapeutics for Waardenburg syndrome. *Gene Ther.* 2021. doi:10.1038/s41434-021-00240-2. Online ahead of print.

399. Lee TL, Lin PH, Chen PL, Hong JB, Wu CC. Hereditary hearing impairment with cutaneous abnormalities. *Genes (Basel).* 2020;12(1):43. doi:10.3390/genes12010043

400. Sleiman R, Kurban M, Succaria F, Abbas O. Poliosis circumscripta: overview and underlying causes. *J Am Acad Dermatol.* 2013;69(4):625–633. doi:10.1016/j.jaad.2013.05.022

401. Read AP, Newton VE. Waardenburg syndrome. *J Med Genet.* 1997;34(8):656–665. doi:10.1136/jmg.34.8.656

402. Aquaron R. Alkaptonuria: a very rare metabolic disorder. *Indian J Biochem Biophys.* 2013;50(5):339–344.

403. Ranganath LR, Jarvis JC, Gallagher JA. Recent advances in management of alkaptonuria (invited review; best practice article). *J Clin Pathol.* 2013;66(5):367–373. doi:10.1136/jclinpath-2012-200877

404. Grosicka A, Kucharz EJ. Alkaptonuria. *Wiad Lek.* 2009;62(3):197–203.

405. Lubics A, Schneider I, Sebök B, Havass Z. Extensive bluish gray skin pigmentation and severe arthropathy. Endogenous ochronosis (alkaptonuria). *Arch Dermatol.* 2000;136(4):548–549, 551–552. doi:10.1001/archderm.136.4.547-b

406. Touart DM, Sau P. Cutaneous deposition diseases. Part II. *J Am Acad Dermatol.* 1998;39(4 Pt 1):527–44; quiz 545-6. doi:10.1016/s0190-9622(98)70001-5

407. Wei Z, Labbe A, Liang Q. Lipoid proteinosis presenting as beaded papules of the eyelid: report of three cases. *BMC Ophthalmol.* 2021;21(1):35. doi:10.1186/s12886-021-01802-z

408. Aksoy M, An I. Evaluation of inflammatory parameters in lipoid proteinosis patients. *Dermatol Ther.* 2020;33(6):e14495. doi:10.1111/dth.14495

409. Frenkel B, Vered M, Taicher S, Yarom N. Lipoid proteinosis unveiled by oral mucosal lesions: a comprehensive analysis of 137 cases. *Clin Oral Investig.* 2017;21(7):2245–2251. doi:10.1007/s00784-016-2017-7

410. Konstantinov K, Kabakchiev P, Karchev T, Kobayasi T, Ullman S. Lipoid proteinosis. *J Am Acad Dermatol.* 1992;27(2, pt 2):293–297. doi:10.1016/0190-9622(92)70183-g

411. Touart DM, Sau P. Cutaneous deposition diseases. Part I. *J Am Acad Dermatol.* 1998;39(2, pt 1):149–171; quiz 172–174. doi:10.1016/s0190-9622(98)70069-6

412. Oguz Akarsu E, Dinçsoy Bir F, Baykal C, et al. The characteristics and long-term course of epilepsy in lipoid proteinosis: a spectrum from mild to severe seizures in relation to ECM1 mutations. *Clin EEG Neurosci.* 2018;49(3):192–196. doi:10.1177/1550059417705280

413. Brar BK, Jain S, Brar SK. Lipoid proteinosis: a case with distinct histopathological and radiological findings. *J Cutan Pathol.* 2017;44(10):887–891. doi:10.1111/cup.13002

414. Ranjan R, Goel K, Sarkar R, Garg VK. Lipoid proteinosis: a case report in two siblings. *Dermatol Online J.* 2014;21(3):13030/qt72c3461z.

415. Patel N, Nabil A, Alshammari M, Alkuraya FS. Hoarse voice in children as the presenting feature of ECM1-related lipoid proteinosis. *Am J Med Genet A.* 2021;185(12):3924–3925. doi:10.1002/ajmg.a.62406

416. Dertlioğlu SB, Edgünlü TG, Şen DE, Süzek TÖ. Extracellular matrix protein 1 gene mutation in Turkish patients with lipoid proteinosis. *Indian J Dermatol.* 2019;64(6):436–440. doi:10.4103/ijd.IJD_365_18

417. Grabowski GA. Phenotype, diagnosis, and treatment of Gaucher's disease. *Lancet.* 2008;372(9645):1263–1271. doi:10.1016/S0140-6736(08)61522-6

418. Stirnemann J, Vigan M, Hamroun D, et al. The French Gaucher's disease registry: clinical characteristics, complications and treatment of 562 patients. *Orphanet J Rare Dis.* 2012;7:77. doi:10.1186/1750-1172-7-77

419. Sidransky E, Fartasch M, Lee RE, et al. Epidermal abnormalities may distinguish type 2 from type 1 and type 3 of Gaucher disease. *Pediatr Res.* 1996;39(1):134–141. doi:10.1203/00006450-199601000-00020

420. Chan A, Holleran WM, Ferguson T, et al. Skin ultrastructural findings in type 2 Gaucher disease: diagnostic implications. *Mol Genet Metab.* 2011;104(4):631–636. doi:10.1016/j.ymgme.2011.09.008

421. Holleran WM, Ziegler SG, Goker-Alpan O, et al. Skin abnormalities as an early predictor of neurologic outcome in Gaucher disease. *Clin Genet.* 2006;69(4):355–357. doi:10.1111/j.1399-0004.2006.00589.x

422. Raeeskarami SR, Aghighi Y, Afshin A, et al. Infantile systemic hyalinosis: report of 17-year experience. *Iran J Pediatr.* 2014;24(6):775–778.

423. Al-Mayouf SM, AlMehaidib A, Bahabri S, Shabib S, Sakati N, Teebi AS. Infantile systemic hyalinosis: a fatal disorder commonly diagnosed among Arabs. *Clin Exp Rheumatol.* 2005;23(5):717–720.

424. Hanks S, Adams S, Douglas J, et al. Mutations in the gene encoding capillary morphogenesis protein 2 cause juvenile hyaline fibromatosis and infantile systemic hyalinosis. *Am J Hum Genet.* 2003;73(4):791–800. doi:10.1086/378418

425. Al Kaissi A, Hilmi M, Betadolova Z, et al. Infantile systemic hyalinosis: variable grades of severity. *Afr J Paediatr Surg.* 2021;18(4):224–230. doi:10.4103/ajps.AJPS_162_20

426. Folpe AL, Schoen M, Kang S. Juvenile hyaline fibromatosis. *Mayo Clin Proc.* 2020;95(2):328–329. doi:10.1016/j.mayocp.2019.11.021

427. Ribeiro SL, Guedes EL, Botan V, Barbosa A, Freitas EJ. Juvenile hyaline fibromatosis: a case report and review of literature. *Acta Reumatol Port.* 2009;34(1):128–133.

428. Muniz ML, Lobo AZ, Machado MC. Exuberant juvenile hyaline fibromatosis in two patients. *Pediatr Dermatol.* 2006;23(5):458–464. doi:10.1111/j.1525-1470.2006.00283.x

429. Lyra ALCO, Razo LM, Estrella RR, Pantaleão L. Juvenile hyaline fibromatosis: an unusual clinical presentation. *Dermatol Online J.* 2019;25(7):13030/qt75082292.

430. Marques SA, Stolf HO, Polizel JO. Hyaline fibromatosis syndrome: cutaneous manifestations. *An Bras Dermatol.* 2016;91(2):226–229. doi:10.1590/abd1806-4841.20163799

431. Liu Y, Zeng X, Ding Y, Xu Y, Duan D. Hyaline fibromatosis syndrome: a case presenting with gingival enlargement as the only clinical manifestation and a report of two new mutations in the ANTXR2 gene. *BMC Oral Health.* 2021;21(1):508. doi:10.1186/s12903-021-01840-5

432. Härter B, Benedicenti F, Karall D, et al. Clinical aspects of hyaline fibromatosis syndrome and identification of a novel mutation. *Mol Genet Genomic Med.* 2020;8(6):e1203. doi:10.1002/mgg3.1203

433. Cozma C, Hovakimyan M, Iuraşcu MI, et al. Genetic, clinical and biochemical characterization of a large cohort of patients with hyaline fibromatosis syndrome. *Orphanet J Rare Dis.* 2019;14(1):209. doi:10.1186/s13023-019-1183-5

434. Borst C, Symmank D, Drach M, Weninger W. Cutaneous signs and mechanisms of inflammasomopathies. *Ann Rheum Dis.* 2022;81(4):454-465. doi:10.1136/annrheumdis-2021-220977

435. Welzel T, Kuemmerle-Deschner JB. Diagnosis and management of the cryopyrin-associated periodic syndromes (CAPS): what do we know today? *J Clin Med.* 2021;10(1):128. doi:10.3390/jcm10010128

436. Oldham J, Lachmann HJ. The systemic autoinflammatory disorders for dermatologists. Part 1: overview. *Clin Exp Dermatol.* 2020;45(8):962–966. doi:10.1111/ced.14250

437. Gupta A, Tripathy SK, Phulware RH, Arava S, Bagri NK. Cryopyrin-associated periodic fever syndrome in children: a case-based review. *Int J Rheum Dis.* 2020;23(2):262–270. doi:10.1111/1756-185X.13772

438. Tartey S, Kanneganti TD. Inflammasomes in the pathophysiology of autoinflammatory syndromes. *J Leukoc Biol.* 2020;107(3):379–391. doi:10.1002/JLB.3MIR0919-191R

439. Nishikomori R, Izawa K, Kambe N, Ohara O, Yasumi T. Low-frequency mosaicism in cryopyrin-associated periodic fever syndrome: mosaicism in systemic autoinflammatory diseases. *Int Immunol.* 2019;31(10):649–655. doi:10.1093/intimm/dxz047

440. Aksentijevich I, Nowak M, Mallah M, et al. De novo CIAS1 mutations, cytokine activation, and evidence for genetic heterogeneity in patients with neonatal-onset multisystem inflammatory disease (NOMID): a new member of the expanding family of pyrin-associated autoinflammatory diseases. *Arthritis Rheum.* 2002;46(12):3340–3348.

441. Farasat S, Aksentijevich I, Toro JR. Autoinflammatory diseases: clinical and genetic advances. *Arch Dermatol.* 2008;144(3):392–402.

442. Aubert P, Suarez-Farinas M, Mitsui H, et al. Homeostatic tissue responses in skin biopsies from NOMID patients with constitutive overproduction of IL-1beta. *PLoS One.* 2012;7(11):e49408.

443. Jacob SE, Cowen EW, Goldbach-Mansky R, Kastner D, Turner ML. A recurrent rash with fever and arthropathy. *J Am Acad Dermatol.* 2006;54(2):318–321.

444. Huttenlocher A, Frieden IJ, Emery H. Neonatal onset multisystem inflammatory disease. *J Rheumatol.* 1995;22(6):1171–1173.

445. Cuisset L, Drenth JP, Berthelot JM, et al. Genetic linkage of the Muckle-Wells syndrome to chromosome 1q44. *Am J Hum Genet.* 1999;65(4):1054–1059.

446. Hoffman HM, Mueller JL, Broide DH, Wanderer AA, Kolodner RD. Mutation of a new gene encoding a putative pyrin-like protein causes familial cold autoinflammatory syndrome and Muckle-Wells syndrome. *Nat Genet.* 2001;29(3):301–305.

447. Hoffman HM, Wanderer AA, Broide DH. Familial cold autoinflammatory syndrome: phenotype and genotype of an autosomal dominant periodic fever. *J Allergy Clin Immunol.* 2001;108(4):615–620.

448. Feldmann J, Prieur AM, Quartier P, et al. Chronic infantile neurological cutaneous and articular syndrome is caused by mutations in CIAS1, a gene highly expressed in polymorphonuclear cells and chondrocytes. *Am J Hum Genet.* 2002;71(1):198–203.

449. Aksentijevich I, Masters SL, Ferguson PJ, et al. An autoinflammatory disease with deficiency of the interleukin-1-receptor antagonist. *N Engl J Med.* 2009;360(23):2426–2437.

450. Reddy S, Jia S, Geoffrey R, et al. An autoinflammatory disease due to homozygous deletion of the IL1RN locus. *N Engl J Med.* 2009;360(23):2438–2444.

451. Jesus AA, Goldbach-Mansky R. IL-1 blockade in autoinflammatory syndromes. *Annu Rev Med.* 2014;65:223–244.

452. Minkis K, Aksentijevich I, Goldbach-Mansky R, et al. Interleukin 1 receptor antagonist deficiency presenting as infantile pustulosis mimicking infantile pustular psoriasis. *Arch Dermatol.* 2012;148(6):747–752.

453. Jesus AA, Osman M, Silva CA, et al. A novel mutation of IL1RN in the deficiency of interleukin-1 receptor antagonist syndrome: description of two unrelated cases from Brazil. *Arthritis Rheum.* 2011;63(12):4007–4017.

454. Naik HB, Cowen EW. Autoinflammatory pustular neutrophilic diseases. *Dermatol Clin.* 2013;31(3):405–425.

455. Altiok E, Aksoy F, Perk Y, et al. A novel mutation in the interleukin-1 receptor antagonist associated with intrauterine disease onset. *Clin Immunol.* 2012;145(1):77–81.

456. Navon Elkan P, Pierce SB, Segel R, et al. Mutant adenosine deaminase 2 in a polyarteritis nodosa vasculopathy. *N Engl J Med.* 2014;370(10):921–931.

457. Zhou Q, Yang D, Ombrello AK, et al. Early-onset stroke and vasculopathy associated with mutations in ADA2. *N Engl J Med.* 2014;370(10):911–920.

458. Pichard DC, Ombrello AK, Hoffmann P, Stone DL, Cowen EW. Early-onset stroke, polyarteritis nodosa (PAN), and livedo racemosa. *J Am Acad Dermatol.* 2016;75(2):449–453.

459. Kesserwan C, Sokolic R, Cowen EW, et al. Multicentric dermatofibrosarcoma protuberans in patients with adenosine deaminase-deficient severe combined immune deficiency. *J Allergy Clin Immunol.* 2012;129(3):762–769.e1. doi:10.1016/j.jaci.2011.10.028

460. Zhou Q, Yang D, Ombrello AK, et al. Early-onset stroke and vasculopathy associated with mutations in ADA2. *N Engl J Med.* 2014;370(10):911–920.

461. Pichard DC, Ombrello AK, Hoffmann P, Stone DL, Cowen EW. Early-onset stroke, polyarteritis nodosa (PAN), and livedo racemosa. *J Am Acad Dermatol.* 2016;75(2):449–453.

462. Zhou Q, Yang D, Ombrello AK, et al. Early-onset stroke and vasculopathy associated with mutations in ADA2. *N Engl J Med.* 2014;370(10):911–920.

463. Pichard DC, Ombrello AK, Hoffmann P, Stone DL, Cowen EW. Early-onset stroke, polyarteritis nodosa (PAN), and livedo racemosa. *J Am Acad Dermatol.* 2016;75(2):449–453.

464. Liu Y, Jesus AA, Marrero B, et al. Activated STING in a vascular and pulmonary syndrome. *N Engl J Med.* 2014;371(6):507–518.

465. Jeremiah N, Neven B, Gentili M, et al. Inherited STING-activating mutation underlies a familial inflammatory syndrome with lupus-like manifestations. *J Clin Invest.* 2014;124(12):5516–5520.

466. Melki I, Rose Y, Uggenti C, et al. Disease-associated mutations identify a novel region in human STING necessary for the control of type I interferon signaling. *J Allergy Clin Immunol.* 2017;140(2):543–552 e545.

467. Chia J, Eroglu FK, Ozen S, et al. Failure to thrive, interstitial lung disease, and progressive digital necrosis with onset in infancy. *J Am Acad Dermatol.* 2016;74(1):186–189.

468. Seo J, Kang JA, Suh DI, et al. Tofacitinib relieves symptoms of stimulator of interferon genes (STING)-associated vasculopathy with onset in infancy caused by 2 de novo variants in TMEM173. *J Allergy Clin Immunol.* 2017;139(4):1396–1399 e1312.

469. Jain A, Misra DP, Sharma A, Wakhlu A, Agarwal V, Negi VS. Vasculitis and vasculitis-like manifestations in monogenic autoinflammatory syndromes. *Rheumatol Int.* 2017.

470. Torrelo A, Patel S, Colmenero I, et al. Chronic atypical neutrophilic dermatosis with lipodystrophy and elevated temperature (CANDLE) syndrome. *J Am Acad Dermatol.* 2010;62(3):489–495.

471. Garg A, Hernandez MD, Sousa AB, et al. An autosomal recessive syndrome of joint contractures, muscular atrophy, microcytic anemia, and panniculitis-associated lipodystrophy. *J Clin Endocrinol Metab.* 2010;95(9):E58–E63.

472. Torrelo A. CANDLE syndrome as a paradigm of proteasome-related autoinflammation. *Front Immunol.* 2017;8:927.

473. Torrelo A, Colmenero I, Requena L, et al. Histologic and immunohistochemical features of the skin lesions in CANDLE syndrome. *Am J Dermatopathol.* 2015;37(7):517–522.

474. Kanazawa N. Nakajo-Nishimura syndrome: an autoinflammatory disorder showing pernio-like rashes and progressive partial lipodystrophy. *Allergol Int.* 2012;61(2):197–206.

475. McDermott A, Jacks J, Kessler M, Emanuel PD, Gao L. Proteasome-associated autoinflammatory syndromes: advances in pathogeneses, clinical presentations, diagnosis, and management. *Int J Dermatol.* 2015;54(2):121–129.

476. Touitou I, Galeotti C, Rossi-Semerano L, et al. The expanding spectrum of rare monogenic autoinflammatory diseases. *Orphanet J Rare Dis.* 2013;8:162.

477. Brehm A, Liu Y, Sheikh A, et al. Additive loss-of-function proteasome subunit mutations in CANDLE/PRAAS patients promote type I IFN production. *J Clin Invest.* 2015;125(11):4196–4211.

478. Patel PN, Hunt R, Pettigrew ZJ, Shirley JB, Vogel TP, de Guzman MM. Successful treatment of chronic atypical neutrophilic dermatosis with lipodystrophy and elevated temperature (CANDLE) syndrome with tofacitinib. *Pediatr Dermatol.* 2021;38(2):528–529. doi:10.1111/pde.14517

479. de Jesus AA, Hou Y, Brooks S, et al. Distinct interferon signatures and cytokine patterns define additional systemic autoinflammatory diseases. *J Clin Invest.* 2020;130(4):1669–1682. doi:10.1172/JCI129301

480. Blau EB. Familial granulomatous arthritis, iritis, and rash. *J Pediatr.* 1985;107(5):689–693.

481. Jabs DA, Houk JL, Bias WB, Arnett FC. Familial granulomatous synovitis, uveitis, and cranial neuropathies. *Am J Med.* 1985;78(5):801–804.

482. Schaffer JV, Chandra P, Keegan BR, Heller P, Shin HT. Widespread granulomatous dermatitis of infancy: an early sign of Blau syndrome. *Arch Dermatol.* 2007;143(3):386–391.

483. Rose CD, Pans S, Casteels I, et al. Blau syndrome: cross-sectional data from a multicentre study of clinical, radiological and functional outcomes. *Rheumatology (Oxford).* 2015;54(6):1008–1016.

484. Sarens IL, Casteels I, Anton J, et al. Blau syndrome-associated uveitis: preliminary results from an international prospective interventional case series. *Am J Ophthalmol.* 2018;187:158–166.

485. Janssen CE, Rose CD, De Hertogh G, et al. Morphologic and immunohistochemical characterization of granulomas in the nucleotide oligomerization domain 2-related disorders Blau syndrome and Crohn disease. *J Allergy Clin Immunol.* 2012; 129(4):1076–1084.

486. Miceli-Richard C, Lesage S, Rybojad M, et al. CARD15 mutations in Blau syndrome. *Nat Genet.* 2001;29(1):19–20.

487. Kanazawa N, Matsushima S, Kambe N, Tachibana T, Nagai S, Miyachi Y. Presence of a sporadic case of systemic granulomatosis syndrome with a CARD15 mutation. *J Invest Dermatol.* 2004;122(3):851–852.

488. Rose CD, Doyle TM, McIlvain-Simpson G, et al. Blau syndrome mutation of CARD15/NOD2 in sporadic early onset granulomatous arthritis. *J Rheumatol.* 2005;32(2):373–375.

489. Manouvrier-Hanu S, Puech B, Piette F, et al. Blau syndrome of granulomatous arthritis, iritis, and skin rash: a new family and review of the literature. *Am J Med Genet.* 1998;76(3):217–221.

490. Saini SK, Rose CD. Liver involvement in familial granulomatous arthritis (Blau syndrome). *J Rheumatol.* 1996;23(2):396–399.

491. Kanazawa N, Okafuji I, Kambe N, et al. Early-onset sarcoidosis and CARD15 mutations with constitutive nuclear factor-kappaB activation: common genetic etiology with Blau syndrome. *Blood.* 2005;105(3):1195–1197.

492. Valent P, Horny HP, Escribano L, et al. Diagnostic criteria and classification of mastocytosis: a consensus proposal. *Leuk Res.* 2001:603–625.

493. Hartmann K, Escribano L, Grattan C, et al. Cutaneous manifestations in patients with mastocytosis: consensus report of the European Competence Network on mastocytosis; the American Academy of Allergy, Asthma & Immunology; and the European Academy of Allergology and Clinical Immunology. *J Allergy Clin Immunol.* 2016;137(1):35–45. doi:10.1016/j.jaci.2015.08.034

494. Horny HP, Valent P. Diagnosis of mastocytosis: general histopathological aspects, morphological criteria, and immunohistochemical findings. *Leuk Res.* 2001;25(7):543–551.

495. Fett NM, Teng J, Longley BJ. Familial urticaria pigmentosa: report of a family and review of the role of KIT mutations. *Am J Dermatopathol.* 2013;35:113–116.

496. Uzzaman A, Maric I, Noel P, Kettelhut BV, Metcalfe DD, Carter MC. Pediatric-onset mastocytosis: a long term clinical follow-up and correlation with bone marrow histopathology. *Pediatr Blood Cancer.* 2009;53:629–634.

497. Kiszewski AE, Durán-Mckinster C, Orozco-Covarrubias L, Gutiérrez-Castrellón P, Ruiz-Maldonado R. Cutaneous mastocytosis in children: a clinical analysis of 71 cases. *J Eur Acad Dermatol Venereol.* 2004;18:285–290.

498. Noack F, Escribano L, Sotlar K, et al. Evolution of urticaria pigmentosa into indolent systemic mastocytosis: abnormal immunophenotype of mast cells without evidence of c-kit mutation ASP-816-VAL. *Leuk Lymphoma.* 2003;44:313–319.

499. Longley BJ, Henz BM. Mastocytosis. In: LeBoit PE, Burg G, Weedon D, Sarasin A, eds. *World Health Organization Classification of Tumors: Pathology and Genetics of Skin Tumors.* IARC Press; 2006:226–228.

500. Wiechers T, Rabenhorst A, Schick T, et al. Large maculopapular cutaneous lesions are associated with favorable outcome in childhood-onset mastocytosis. *J Allergy Clin Immunol.* 2015;136(6):1581–1590.e3. doi:10.1016/j.jaci.2015.05.034

501. Kim CR, Kim HJ, Jung MY, et al. Cutaneous mastocytosis associated with congenital alopecia. *Am J Dermatopathol.* 2012;34(5):529–532.

502. Hartmann K, Bruns SB, Henz BM. Mastocytosis: review of clinical and experimental aspects. *J Investig Dermatol Symp Proc.* 2001;6(2):143–147.

503. Schena D, Galvan A, Tessari G, Girolomoni G. Clinical features and course of cutaneous mastocytosis in 133 children. *Br J Dermatol.* 2016;174(2):411–413. doi:10.1111/bjd.14004

504. Pandhi D, Singal A, Aggarwal S. Adult onset, hypopigmented solitary mastocytoma: report of two cases. *Indian J Dermatol Venereol Leprol.* 2008;74(1):41–43.

505. Lange M, Niedoszytko M, Nedoszytko B, et al. Diffuse cutaneous mastocytosis: analysis of 10 cases and a brief review of the literature. *J Eur Acad Dermatol Venereol.* 2012;26(12):1565–1571.

506. Watkins CE, Bokor WB, Leicht S, et al. Telangiectasia macularis eruptiva perstans: more than skin deep. *Dermatol Rep.* 2011;3(1):e12. doi:10.4081/dr.2011.e12.

507. Costa DL, Moura HH, Rodrigues R, et al. Telangiectasia macularis eruptiva perstans: a rare form of adult mastocytosis. *J Clin Aesthet Dermatol.* 2011;4(10):52–54.

508. Tremblay D, Carreau N, Kremyanskaya M, et al. Systemic mastocytosis: clinical update and future directions. *Clin Lymphoma Myeloma Leuk.* 2015;15(12):728–738.

509. Valent P, Akin C, Escribano L, et al. Standards and standardization in mastocytosis: consensus statements on diagnostics, treatment recommendations and response criteria. *Eur J Clin Invest.* 2007;37(6):435–453.

510. Lim KH, Tefferi A, Lasho TL, et al. Systemic mastocytosis in 342 consecutive adults: survival studies and prognostic factors. *Blood.* 2009;113(23):5727–5736.

511. Andersen CL, Kristensen TK, Severinsen MT, et al. Systemic mastocytosis—a systematic review. *Dan Med J.* 2012;59(3):A4397.

512. Swerdlow SH, Campo E, Harris NL, et al., eds. *WHO Classification of Tumours of Haematopoietic and Lymphoid Tissues.* 4th ed. IARC; 2008

513. Mihm MC, Clark WH, Reed RJ, et al. Mast cell infiltrates of the skin and the mastocytosis syndrome. *Hum Pathol.* 1973;4(2):231–239.

514. Willemze R, Ruiter DJ, Scheffer E, et al. Diffuse cutaneous mastocytosis with multiple cutaneous mastocytomas. Report of a case with clinical, histopathological and ultrastructural aspects. *Br J Dermatol.* 1980;102(5):601–607.

515. Wardle CLW, Oldhoff JM, Diepstra A, et al. Case report of a clinically indolent but morphologically high-grade cutaneous mast cell tumor in an adult: atypical cutaneous mastocytoma or mast cell sarcoma? *J Cutan Pathol.* 2021;48(11):1404–1409. doi:10.1111/cup.14088

516. Horny HP, Valent P. Diagnosis of mastocytosis: general histopathological aspects, morphological criteria, and immunohistochemical findings. *Leuk Res.* 2001;25(7):543–551.

517. Li WV, Kapadia SB, Sonmez-Alpan E, et al. Immunohistochemical characterization of mast cell disease in paraffin sections using tryptase, CD68, myeloperoxidase, lysozyme, and CD20 antibodies. *Mod Pathol.* 1996;9(10):982–988.

518. Hu S, Kuo TT, Hong HS. Mast cells with bilobed or multilobed nuclei in a nodular lesion of a patient with urticaria pigmentosa. *Am J Dermatopathol.* 2002;24(6):490–492.

519. Tran DT, Jokinen CH, Argenyi ZB. Histiocyte-rich pleomorphic mastocytoma: an uncommon variant mimicking juvenile xanthogranuloma and Langerhans cell histiocytosis. *J Cutan Pathol.* 2009;36(11):1215–1220.

520. Sotlar K, Cerny-Reiterer S, Petat-Dutter K, et al. Aberrant expression of CD30 in neoplastic mast cells in high-grade mastocytosis. *Mod Pathol.* 2011;24(4):585–595.

521. Meni C, Bruneau J, Georgin-Lavialle S, et al. Paediatric mastocytosis: a systematic review of 1747 cases. *Br J Dermatol.* 2015;172(3):642–651.

522. Pollard WL, Beachkofsky TM, Kobayashi TT. Novel R634W c-kit mutation identified in familial mastocytosis. *Pediatr Dermatol.* 2015;32(2):267–270.

523. Beghini A, Tibiletti MG, Roversi G, et al. Germline mutation in the juxtamembrane domain of the kit gene in a family with gastrointestinal stromal tumors and urticaria pigmentosa. *Cancer.* 2001;92(3):657–662.

524. Ma D, Stence AA, Bossler AB, et al. Identification of KIT activating mutations in paediatric solitary mastocytoma. *Histopathology.* 2014;64(2):218–225.

525. Wang HJ, Lin ZM, Zhang J, et al. A new germline mutation in KIT associated with diffuse cutaneous mastocytosis in a Chinese family. *Clin Exp Dermatol.* 2014;39(2):146–149.

526. Tang X, Boxer M, Drummond A, et al. A germline mutation in KIT in familial diffuse cutaneous mastocytosis. *J Med Genet.* 2004;41(6):e88.

527. Cruse G, Metcalfe DD, Olivera A. Functional deregulation of KIT: link to mast cell proliferative diseases and other neoplasms. *Immunol Allergy Clin North Am.* 2014;34(2):219–237.

528. Furitsu T, Tsujimura T, Tono T, et al. Identification of mutations in the coding sequence of the proto-oncogene c-kit in a human mast cell leukemia cell line causing ligand-independent activation of c-kit product. *J Clin Invest.* 1993;92(4):1736–1744.

529. Prignano F, Troiano M, Lotti T. Cutaneous mastocytosis: successful treatment with narrowband ultraviolet B phototherapy. *Clin Exp Dermatol.* 2010;35:914–915.

530. Morren MA, Hoppé A, Renard M, et al. Imatinib mesylate in the treatment of diffuse cutaneous mastocytosis. *J Pediatr.* 2013;162:205–207.

531. Vega-Ruiz A, Cortes JE, Sever M, et al. Phase II study of imatinib mesylate as therapy for patients with systemic mastocytosis. *Leuk Res.* 2009;33:1481–1484.

532. Purtill D, Cooney J, Sinniah R, et al. Dasatinib therapy for systemic mastocytosis: four cases. *Eur J Haematol.* 2008;80: 456–458.

533. Priolo M. Ectodermal dysplasias: an overview and update of clinical and molecular-functional mechanisms. *Am J Med Genet A.* 2009;149A:2003–2013.

Noninfectious Erythematous, Papular, and Squamous Diseases

AMRITA GOYAL, RUTH K. FOREMAN, AND LYN M. DUNCAN

INTRODUCTION

This group of "papulosquamous" disorders is defined clinically and is rather heterogeneous in terms of pathogenesis. Histopathologically, these disorders are characterized by superficial predominantly lymphocytic inflammation, with variable effects on the structures of the superficial integument—the epidermis, the vessels of the superficial capillary–venular plexus, and the papillary dermis. Perivascular inflammation is usually manifested clinically by erythema or blanchable redness of the skin. For dermal edema and more significant inflammatory infiltrates, clinical correlates include raised lesions, either papules or plaques. Abnormalities of keratinocytic maturation may lead to epidermal hyperplasia or atrophy. Hyperkeratosis of the stratum corneum clinically appears as scaling and may be referred to as a "squamous" disorder. When the epidermal alteration involves damage to basal keratinocytes, one sees hyperkeratosis without parakeratosis, owing to delayed epidermal maturation.

Lichen planus is the prototypic disorder in this category, and the pattern of bandlike inflammation obscuring the dermal–epidermal junction in this disorder is termed "lichenoid." In other epidermal proliferative disorders, there may be hyperkeratosis with retention of the epidermal nuclei in the thickened keratin layer, called parakeratosis. The prototype of these conditions is psoriasis vulgaris, which, is characterized by loss of the granular cell layer and a characteristic pattern of epidermal hyperplasia with regularly elongated rete ridges termed "psoriasiform." Erythematous papular and squamous disorders are characterized by variations in these patterns of perivascular, lichenoid, and psoriasiform dermatitis.

PSORIASIS

Psoriasis may be divided primarily into psoriasis vulgaris, generalized pustular psoriasis, and localized pustular psoriasis, though other variants (guttate, erythrodermic, inverse) exist.

Clinical summary

Psoriasis Vulgaris

Psoriasis vulgaris is a common chronic inflammatory skin disorder that affects approximately 1.5% to 2% of the population in the Western countries. It is characterized by pink to red scaly papules and plaques (Fig. 7-1). The lesions are of variable size, sharply demarcated, and usually with fine, silvery scale. Gentle scraping to remove the surface scale reveals fine

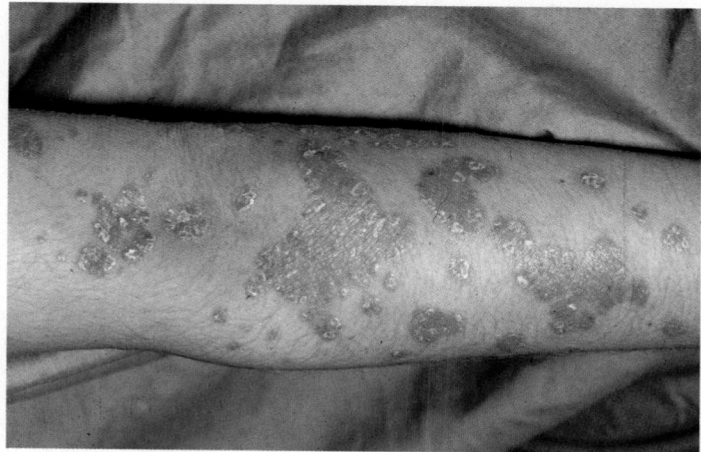

Figure 7-1 Psoriasis vulgaris. Sharply demarcated erythematous scaly papules and plaques on the upper extremity. (Courtesy of Department of Dermatology, University of Pennsylvania School of Medicine, Philadelphia, Pennsylvania.)

bleeding points—the so-called Auspitz sign. The scalp, sacral region, and extensor surfaces of the extremities are commonly involved, although in some patients the flexural and intertriginous areas are primarily affected (inverse psoriasis). An acute variant—guttate or eruptive psoriasis—is often seen in younger patients, and may be characterized by an abrupt eruption of small lesions associated with acute group A β-hemolytic streptococcal infections (1). Involvement of the nails is common; the most frequent alteration of the nail plate surface is the presence of pits, although onycholysis and oil spots are also common (2). In severe cases, the disease may present as generalized erythroderma. Pustules are generally absent in psoriasis vulgaris, although pustules on palms and soles occasionally occur. Rarely, one or a few areas show pustules, and this is referred to as "psoriasis with pustules." Severe psoriasis vulgaris may very rarely develop into generalized pustular psoriasis. Oral lesions such as stomatitis areata migrans (geographic stomatitis) and benign migratory glossitis (geographic tongue) may be seen in psoriasis vulgaris and in generalized pustular psoriasis (3,4).

Generalized Pustular Psoriasis

Generalized pustular psoriasis includes (a) acute generalized pustular psoriasis (von Zumbusch type and acute exanthematous type), (b) generalized pustular psoriasis of pregnancy (impetigo herpetiformis), (c) infantile and juvenile pustular psoriasis, and (d) subacute annular or circinate pustular psoriasis (5).

Generalized pustular psoriasis is characterized by the presence of variable numbers of sterile pustules appearing in erythematous and scaly lesions associated with moderate-to-severe constitutional symptoms (6). Recurrent exacerbations may occur, and lesions of ordinary psoriasis may be seen in the intervals between them.

The four variants of generalized pustular psoriasis show considerable resemblance and overlapping in their clinical picture and also have a similar histopathologic appearance. They differ mainly in the mode of onset and the distribution of the lesions. Frequently, all four diseases show oral pustules, particularly on the tongue (7).

Acute generalized pustular psoriasis of von Zumbusch is generally diagnosed when the pustular eruption occurs in patients with preexisting psoriasis, either of the plaque (8) or erythrodermic type (9). Frequently, the eruption occurs after systemic steroid therapy withdrawal (5,10). The differential diagnosis may include acute generalized exanthematous pustulosis (AGEP), a severe acute cutaneous eruption commonly associated with medications, including aminopenicillins, pristinamycin, sulfonamides, quinolones, hydroxychloroquine, terbinafine, and diltiazem. It has also been associated with infections including parvovirus B19, mycoplasma, cytomegalovirus, coxsackie B4, *Chlamydia pneumoniae*, and *E. coli* (11). The *exanthematous type of generalized pustular psoriasis* refers to a group of patients with later onset of psoriasis, atypical distribution of the lesions, and a rapid and apparently spontaneous pustular eruption (12).

Generalized pustular psoriasis of pregnancy is a rare pustular eruption that appears during the last trimester of pregnancy. It starts with flexural lesions of psoriasis followed by a generalized pustular eruption. It may recur during subsequent pregnancies (13). Some authors have considered it to be the same disease as *impetigo herpetiformis* (5), but others claim that they stand as separate entities (14,15). This condition is notable because it is the only form of psoriasis which is treated with systemic steroids. Unlike the pruritic and urticarial papules and plaques of pregnancy (PUPPP), impetigo herpetiformis is associated with increased risk of stillbirth, perinatal mortality owing to placental insufficiency, preterm labor, and intrauterine growth restriction (16).

In some instances of *subacute annular pustular psoriasis*, the annular or gyrate lesions show a clinical resemblance to subcorneal pustular dermatosis (17,18). Figurate lesions are more frequently seen in subacute or chronic forms of generalized pustular psoriasis (5). Annular pustular psoriasis, although usually generalized, in some instances may be localized (19).

Very rarely, children develop generalized pustular psoriasis, also known as *infantile and juvenile pustular psoriasis*. In these patients, the disease has a benign course with frequent spontaneous remissions (20).

Localized Pustular Psoriasis

There are three types of localized pustular psoriasis: (a) "psoriasis with pustules" (10,12), in which only one or a few areas of psoriasis show pustules and the tendency to change into generalized pustular psoriasis is low; (b) localized acrodermatitis continua of Hallopeau, which occasionally evolves into generalized acrodermatitis continua; and (c) pustular psoriasis of the palms and soles, with two variants: the chronic palmoplantar pustulosis, also called pustulosis palmaris et plantaris, and the

acute palmoplantar pustulosis, or "pustular bacterid." Both are occasionally seen in association with psoriasis vulgaris (5).

Acrodermatitis continua of Hallopeau is the term used when the pustular eruption involves the distal portions of the hands and feet. In this manifestation of psoriasis, the pustular eruption begins in the tips of the fingers and toes, most commonly in the thumb. The chronic eruption of sterile pustules is associated with hyperkeratosis and skin atrophy. Nail involvement is central to this pathology: There is pustulation of the nail bed, and this can result in onychodystrophy, onycholysis, onychomadesis, and ultimately, anonychia, with "lakes of pus" or the evocative "fingernail floating away in a sea of pus." Local inflammation may result in sclerosis of soft tissue, muscular atrophy, arthropathy, and osteolysis, resulting in disability and pain. In the localized type of acrodermatitis continua, these are the only areas affected, whereas in the generalized type of acrodermatitis continua, extensive areas of the skin in addition to the acral portions of extremities are involved (12). Atrophy of the skin and permanent nail loss may occur.

Pustulosis palmaris et plantaris is a chronic, relapsing disorder that involves the palms and or soles (Fig. 7-2). Crops of small, deep-seated sterile pustules are seen within areas of erythema and scaling. In the earliest stage, the lesions appear as vesicles or vesiculopustules. During the subsiding stage, the pustules appear as brown macules. The sites of predilection are the mid-palms and thenar eminences of the hands and the heels and insteps of the feet (21). In pustulosis palmaris et plantaris, in contrast to acrodermatitis continua of Hallopeau, the acral portions of the fingers and toes are spared. An acute variant called "pustular bacterid" (22) describes a rare eruption of large and sterile pustules on hands and feet. Although tumor necrosis factor (TNF)-α inhibitors can induce multiple subtypes of psoriasis, palmoplantar pustular eruptions are not uncommon.

Extracutaneous Manifestations of Psoriasis

Patients with psoriasis often suffer from other medical comorbidities. Approximately 20% to 35% of patients have psoriatic arthritis (PsA), a seronegative inflammatory arthritis characteristically involving the terminal interphalangeal joints and frequently the large joints (23). The clinical differential for PsA includes rheumatoid arthritis; presence of rheumatoid

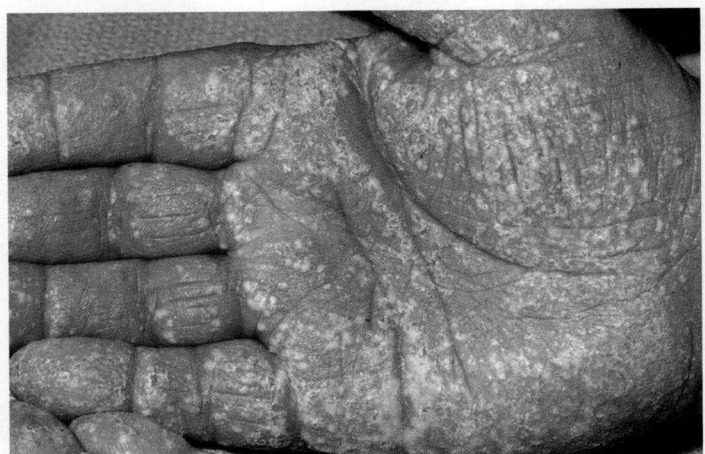

Figure 7-2 Pustular psoriasis (palmar pustulosis). Confluent pustules on erythematous scaly skin of the palm. (Courtesy of Department of Dermatology, University of Pennsylvania School of Medicine, Philadelphia, Pennsylvania.)

factor (positive in RA and absent in PsA) and a history of psoriasis (typically present in PsA) are helpful in differentiating these disorders. Psoriasis is a chronic inflammatory condition and can lead to premature atherogenic inflammation and advanced vascular aging and markedly increased cardiovascular risks. Patients with psoriasis have been found to have higher rates of the metabolic syndrome and obesity, type 2 diabetes, cardiovascular disease, depression, lymphoma, and inflammatory bowel disease than the general population (24). These comorbid conditions may all be driven by increased expression of inflammatory cytokine mediators at the root of their pathogenesis.

Histopathology

Psoriasis Vulgaris

The histopathologic picture of psoriasis vulgaris varies considerably with the stage of the lesion and usually is diagnostic only in early, scaling papules and near the margin of advancing plaques.

The earliest pinhead-sized macules or smooth-surfaced papules show subtle histopathologic changes (25,26). Initially, there is papillary dermal capillary dilation and edema, with a superficial dermal perivascular lymphocytic infiltrate. The lymphocytes extend to the lower portion of the epidermis, which may display slight spongiosis. Changes then occur in the upper epidermis, with loss of the granular cells and formation of mounds of parakeratosis. Neutrophils may be seen at the surface of the parakeratotic mounds and scattered through the orthokeratotic cornified layer (Fig. 7-3). Mounds of parakeratosis with neutrophils are an early manifestation of psoriasis known as Munro microabscesses (26). In some cases, neutrophils may aggregate in the upper epidermis and form small spongiform pustules of Kogoj (Fig. 7-4). Lymphocytes remain confined to the lower epidermis, which, as more and more mitoses occur, becomes increasingly hyperplastic. The epidermal changes are at first focal, but later become confluent, leading clinically to plaques.

In the fully developed lesions of psoriasis, as best seen at the margin of enlarging plaques, the histopathologic picture is

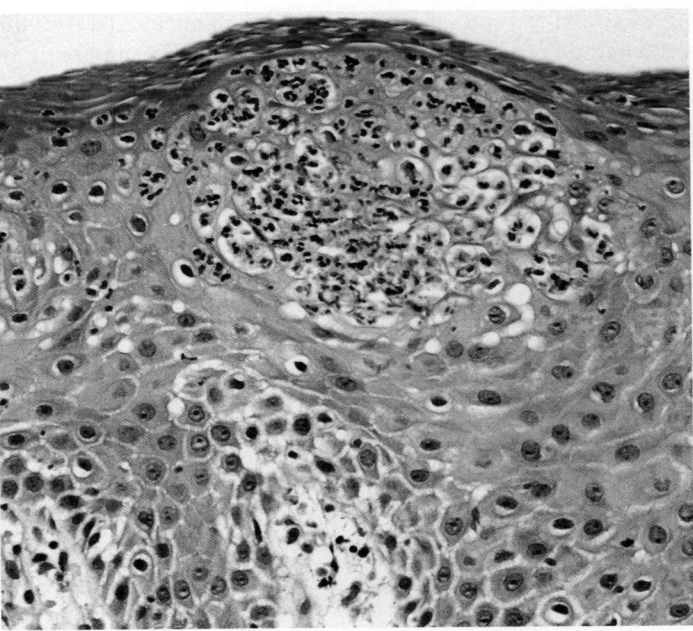

Figure 7-4 Psoriasis. Higher power view of a spongiform pustule of Kogoj formed by collections of neutrophils in the spinous and granular layers.

characterized by (a) acanthosis with regular elongation of the rete ridges with thickening in their lower portion; (b) thinning of the suprapapillary epidermis with the occasional presence of small spongiform pustules of Kogoj; (c) pallor of the upper layers of the epidermis; (d) diminished to absent granular layer; (e) confluent parakeratosis; (f) the presence of Munro microabscesses (Fig. 7-6); (g) elongation and edema of the dermal papillae; and (h) dilated and tortuous papillary dermal capillaries (Fig. 7-5).

Of the listed features, only the spongiform pustules of Kogoj and Munro microabscesses are truly diagnostic of psoriasis, and, in their absence, the diagnosis can rarely be made with certainty on a histopathologic basis.

The rete ridges show considerable elongation and extend downward to a uniform level, resulting in regular acanthosis. They are often slender in their upper portion but show thickening termed "clubbing" in their lower portion. Not infrequently, adjacent rete ridges seem to coalesce at their bases. Usually, there is minimal spongiosis, and keratinocytes located well above the basal layer show deep basophilia. In addition, mitoses are not limited to the basal layer as in normal skin but are also seen above the basal layer. This, together with a considerable lengthening of the basal cell layer owing to elongation of the rete ridges, results in a marked increase in the number of mitoses, more than 25 times the number of mitoses in uninvolved skin (27).

The suprapapillary epidermis appears relatively thin in comparison with the markedly elongated rete ridges, whereas keratinocytes in the upper layers of the epidermis may appear enlarged and pale as a result of intracellular edema and hypogranulosis. Keratinocytes beneath the parakeratotic cornified layer may be intermingled with neutrophils (28). The histopathologic picture is then that of a small spongiform pustule of Kogoj. Such a spongiform pustule, highly diagnostic for psoriasis and its variants, shows aggregates of neutrophils within the interstices of a sponge-like network formed by degenerated and thinned epidermal cells (29).

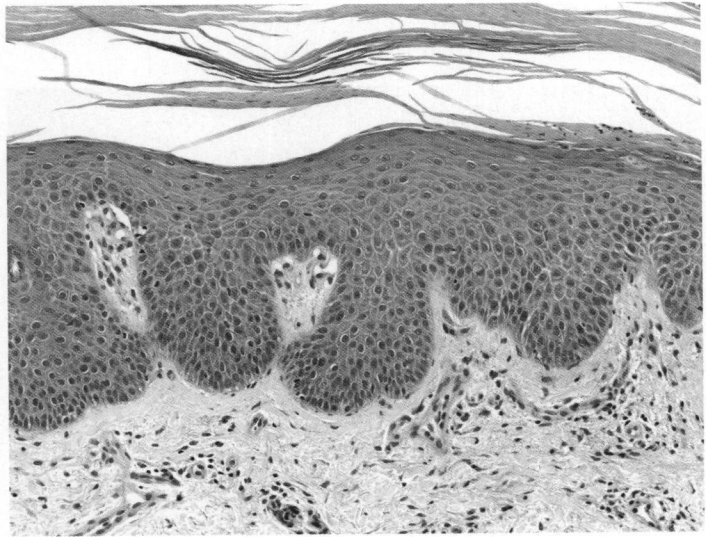

Figure 7-3 Early psoriasis. Parakeratosis with neutrophils, thinned granular layer, mild acanthosis, focal spongiosis, dilated blood vessels at the tip of the dermal papillae, and perivascular infiltrate of lymphocytes with rare neutrophils.

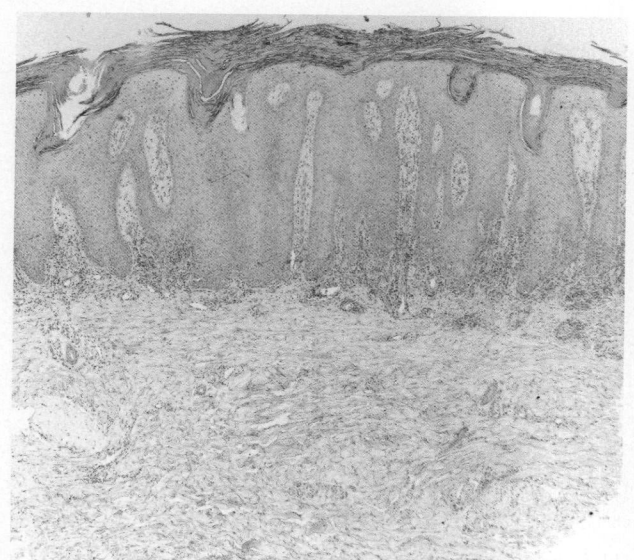
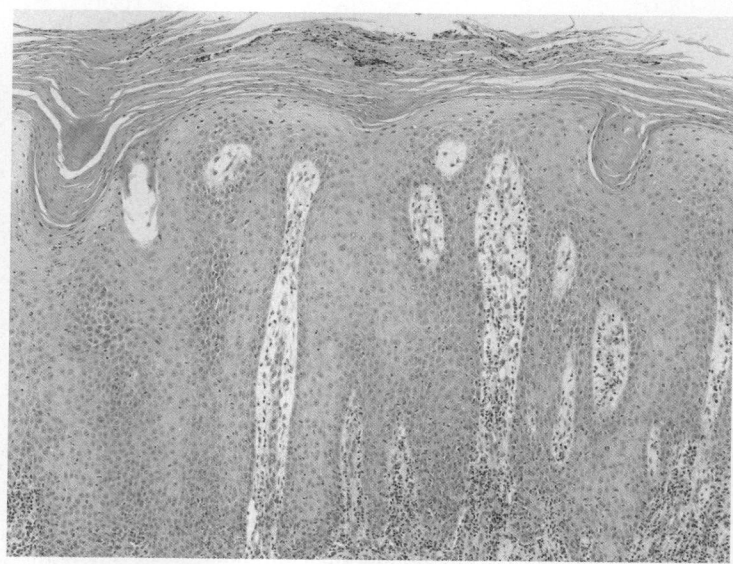

Figure 7-5 Psoriasis, well-developed plaque. (**A**, **B**) Classic features, including neutrophilic scale, hypogranulosis, suprapapillary plate thinning, and regular acanthosis.

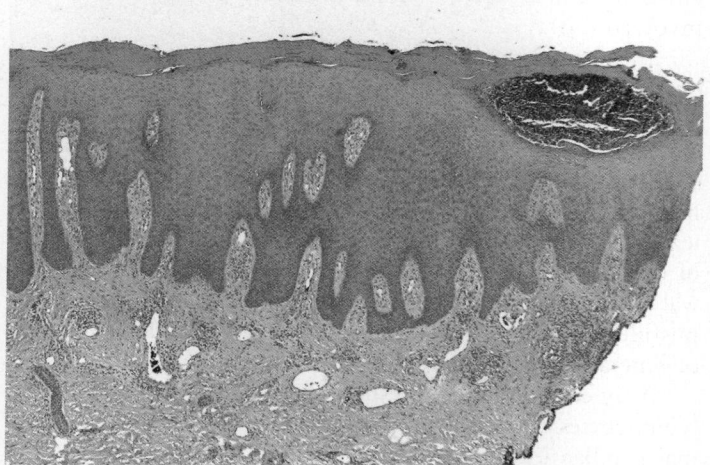

Figure 7-6 Psoriasis. Prominent Munro microabscess and regular acanthosis.

In some instances, the cornified layer consists entirely of confluent parakeratosis forming a plate-like scale with an underlying reduced or absent granular layer. However, occasional focal orthokeratosis with preservation of the underlying granular cells is present, particularly in treated psoriasis.

Munro microabscesses are located within the parakeratotic areas of the cornified layer (Fig. 7-6). They consist of accumulations of neutrophils and pyknotic nuclei of neutrophils that have migrated there capillaries in the papillae through the suprapapillary epidermis. As a rule, Munro microabscesses are easily found in early lesions but are few in number or absent in long-standing lesions (30).

The dermal papillae complement the elongation and basal thickening of the rete ridges; as such, they are also elongated and club shaped. There is papillary edema with dilated and tortuous capillaries. A relatively mild lymphocytic infiltrate is present in the upper dermis and the papillae. In early lesions, neutrophils are also present in the upper portion of the papillae (31).

An entirely typical histopathologic picture as described earlier is not always found, even if the biopsy specimens are

taken from clinically typical lesions of psoriasis (32). Orthokeratosis often appears intermingled with parakeratosis. In such cases, one may see vertically adjoining areas of orthokeratosis and parakeratosis, focal parakeratosis, or, occasionally, alternating layers of orthokeratosis and parakeratosis. The last-named pattern indicates a fluctuation in the activity of psoriasis.

The bleeding points that may be produced by gentle scraping of the skin (Auspitz sign) correspond to the tips of dermal papillae and exposure of the thin suprapapillary epidermal plate and underlying dilated capillaries.

Guttate or eruptive psoriasis shows the histopathologic features of an early or active lesion of psoriasis, where there is more pronounced inflammatory infiltrate and less acanthosis as compared with a well-developed chronic plaque of psoriasis. Because of its acute onset, one may observe the remaining normal basket-weave orthokeratotic cornified layer overlying the mounds of parakeratosis with neutrophils, which, in turn, may appear loosely arranged (Fig. 7-7).

The histopathologic picture of *erythrodermic psoriasis* in some instances shows enough of the characteristics of psoriasis to allow this diagnosis. Frequently, however, the histopathologic appearance is indistinguishable from that of chronic eczematous dermatitis (33).

Generalized Pustular Psoriasis

Whereas in ordinary psoriasis the spongiform pustule of Kogoj is a micropustule seen only in early, active lesions, it occurs as a macropustule in all variants of generalized pustular psoriasis and represents their characteristic histopathologic lesion. The spongiform pustule forms through the migration of neutrophils from the papillary dermal capillaries to the upper layer of epidermis, where they aggregate within the interstices of a sponge-like network formed by degenerated and thinned epidermal cells (29). As the size of the pustule increases, the epidermal cells in the center of the pustule undergo complete cytolysis so that a large single cavity forms (Fig. 7-8). As the neutrophils of the spongiform pustule move up into the cornified layer, they become pyknotic and assume the appearance of a larger Munro microabscess (8,34).

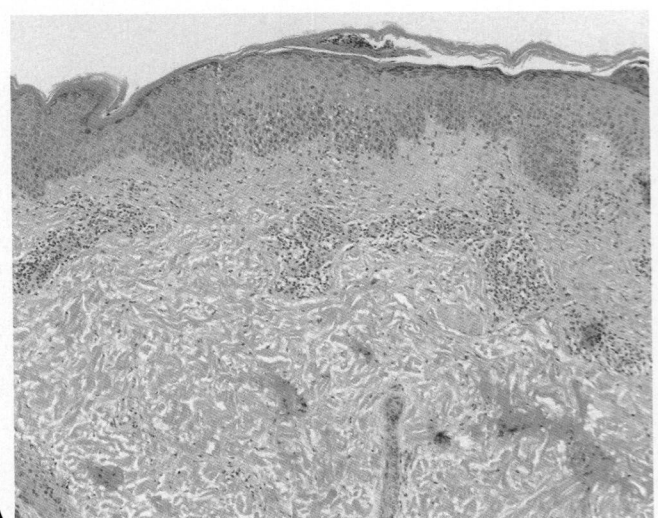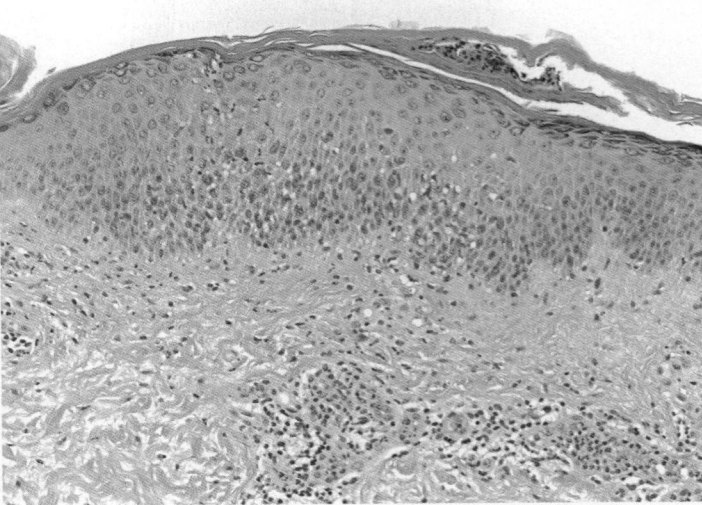

Figure 7-7 Guttate psoriasis. **A:** Mounds of neutrophilic parakeratotic scale, mild acanthosis. **B:** Neutrophilic exocytosis and spongiosis.

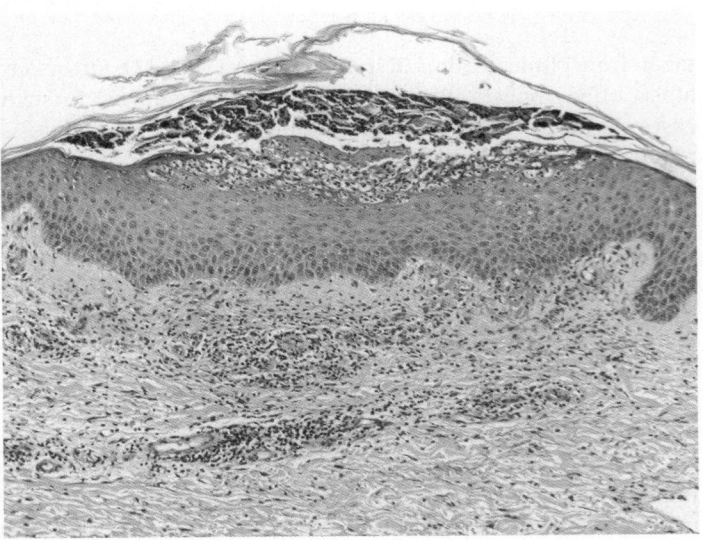

Figure 7-8 Pustular psoriasis. Subcorneal neutrophilic pustule, and lacking other classic features of psoriasis.

In addition to the large spongiform pustules, the epidermal changes in generalized pustular psoriasis are very much like those seen in psoriasis vulgaris, consisting of parakeratosis and elongation of the rete ridges. The upper dermis contains an infiltrate of lymphocytes, and neutrophils can often be seen migrating from the capillaries in the papillae into the epidermis (35). The oral lesions show the same spongiform pustule formation as those seen on the skin (7).

In the healing stage, the lesions of all types of generalized pustular psoriasis may present the same histopathologic appearance as ordinary psoriasis (8).

Localized Pustular Psoriasis

In the variants of localized pustular psoriasis "psoriasis with pustules" (10,12) and localized annular pustular psoriasis, the histopathologic picture is the same as that described for generalized pustular psoriasis.

In localized acrodermatitis continua of Hallopeau, the nail bed is mainly affected, showing marked epithelial hyperplasia with variable numbers of spongiform pustules, hypogranulosis, and hyperkeratosis with mounds of parakeratosis with neutrophils. The nail matrix is only occasionally involved (36).

In pustulosis palmaris et plantaris, there is a fully developed large intraepidermal unilocular neutrophilic pustule. It is elevated only slightly above the surface but impinges on the underlying dermis. The epidermis surrounding the pustule shows slight acanthosis, and an inflammatory infiltrate can be seen beneath the pustule (37). In many instances, one can observe typical, although small, spongiform pustules in the epidermal wall of the pustule, most commonly at the junction of the lateral walls and the overlying epidermis (37–41). These spongiform pustules are identical to those seen in the walls of the pustules of generalized pustular psoriasis.

Very early lesions may show spongiosis and exocytosis of lymphocytes in the lower epidermis overlying the tips of dermal papillae (40). This may be followed by the formation of a small intraepidermal vesicle containing mostly lymphocytes (37,40). Subsequently, there is a massive exocytosis of neutrophils, which penetrate the intercellular spaces of the vesicle wall, where the histopathologic picture of spongiform pustules is then seen (37). In the acute form, pustular bacterid, leukocytoclastic vasculitis has been described (42).

Pathogenesis

Psoriasis Vulgaris

Although the cause of psoriasis is unknown, there is increasing evidence of a complex interaction among altered keratinocytic proliferation and differentiation, inflammation, and immune dysregulation.

Epidermal Cell Cycle Kinetics

The rate of epidermal cell replication is markedly accelerated in active lesions of psoriasis, as shown by increased numbers of intraepidermal mitotic figures (43). The mitotic activity within different lesions of psoriasis and even within the same lesion can vary considerably and seems to be correlated with the degree of parakeratosis. The frequent finding in psoriasis of alternating layers of orthokeratosis and parakeratosis suggests that epidermal growth activity fluctuates in the lesions (32). Step sections of early "punctate" papules show a mitotically very active parakeratotic center surrounded by a zone of a thickened granular layer with a relatively low mitotic rate (44).

Psoriatic lesions demonstrate a great acceleration of the transit time of cells from the basal cell layer to the uppermost row of the squamous cell layer, from approximately 53 days in normal epidermis to only 7 days in the epidermis of active psoriatic lesions (43).

Psoriatic epidermis shows aberrant expression of apoptosis-related molecules representing a suppressed apoptotic process, which may contribute to the proliferative nature of the epidermis in this disease (45).

Immunopathology

Psoriasis is an immune-mediated chronic inflammatory skin condition characterized by sustained chronic inflammation resulting in keratinocyte proliferation and dysfunctional cellular differentiation. For many years, psoriasis was characterized as a TH1-driven disease. Although disturbances in both innate and adaptive immunity contribute to the pathogenesis of psoriasis, this condition is now largely regarded as a T-cell-mediated disorder driven by pathogenic T cells that produce high levels of IL-17 in response to IL-23. This central role of the IL-17/23 axis has led to major advances in our understanding of disease pathogenesis and treatment (46).

Pre-psoriatic skin demonstrates upregulation of IL-17, which drives a keratinocyte inflammatory response that is self-amplifying and ultimately results in epidermal hyperplasia, epidermal cell proliferation, and the recruitment of lymphocytes and neutrophils into the skin (47). It is believed that dermal dendritic cells produce IL-23, which drives the production of IL-17, TNF, IL-26, and IL-29 by CD4+ T cells (Th17), CD8+ T cells (Tc17), and γ/δ cells (47). This generates a feed-forward mechanism that results in upregulation of keratinocyte-derived inflammatory products and ultimately generates the phenotype of the psoriatic plaque. IL-17 and TNF potentiate IL-17-induced synthesis of proinflammatory peptides including TNF, IL-1β, IL-6, and IL-8, which in turn activate dendritic cells and promote further differentiation of T cells along the Th17 axis in the skin and lymph nodes (48). A large number of novel biologic medications targeting the IL-17/23 axis have been released in recent years and are mainstays of current psoriasis treatment.

The role of TNF in the pathogenesis of psoriasis is underscored by the tremendous success of TNF blockers in the treatment of both psoriasis and PsA. In psoriatic skin, in response to trauma, plasmacytoid dendritic cells may release TNF, which causes the release of IL-23 from monocytoid dendritic cells—this serves as a major source of IL-23 in psoriatic skin and feeds into the IL-17/23 axis described earlier (49).

Autoreactivity and autoimmunity play a key role in the pathogenesis of psoriasis: A recent study demonstrated that 75% of patients with moderate-to-severe psoriasis possessed autoreactive CD4+ or CD8+ T cells against LL-37/cathelicidin, a protein produced by keratinocytes and neutrophils in response to infections and trauma; LL-37/cathelicidin has been demonstrated to be upregulated in psoriatic plaques. These T cells demonstrate a strong IFN-γ and IL-17 phenotype (50). ADAMTSL5 (ADAMTS-like protein 5) is another key potential psoriasis autoantigen. This zinc metalloprotease-related protein may play a role in regulating components of the extracellular matrix. Presentation of this antigen may lead to activation of IL-17 producing T cell in psoriatic skin (51). PLA2G4D (phospholipase A1 group IVD) has also recently been implicated as possible psoriasis autoantigen and has been found to be upregulated in psoriatic skin (52).

The critical role of the skin microbiome in health and disease has experienced significant recognition in the last several years. The organisms in the microbiome play an active role in immune regulation and pathogen defense via stimulation of the production of antibacterial peptides and through the generation of biofilms. Aberrant immune activation triggered by skin microbes may be involved in the pathogenesis of a number of autoimmune diseases, including psoriasis, which is characterized by an autoimmune diathesis. The role of bacterial infection or colonization in the initiation and propagation of psoriasis is under significant investigation. Bacterial superantigens, such as those of group A β-hemolytic streptococci, may activate T lymphocytes. The streptococcal M-protein has been found to share sequences with keratin 17, suggesting that an epitope on keratin 17 or keratin 6 may be a target for autoreactive lymphocytes in psoriasis (53,54). There is an overall increase in microbial diversity in psoriatic plaques compared with normal skin, although the specific composition of that flora varies by study.

Differential Diagnosis

Two histopathologic features are of great value in the diagnosis of psoriasis vulgaris: (a) mounds of parakeratosis with neutrophils (Munro microabscesses) and (b) spongiform micropustules of Kogoj in the uppermost layers of the spinous layer. Dilation and tortuosity of capillaries in the dermal papillae may also help in the diagnosis. All other features, such as acanthosis with elongation of the rete ridges and parakeratosis, can be found also in chronic eczematous dermatitis, such as *atopic dermatitis*, *nummular dermatitis*, or *allergic contact dermatitis*, which then may appear to be "psoriasiform." However, in those conditions, the elongation of rete ridges is often uneven, as compared to the regular acanthosis of psoriasis. Although mild spongiosis may be seen in psoriasis, the presence of marked spongiosis and especially of coagulated serum as evidence of crusting in the cornified layer are features speaking against psoriasis, except in psoriasis on volar skin, in which spongiosis may be prominent. In addition, eosinophils, which are commonly found in allergic contact dermatitis and often in HIV-positive patients, are rarely seen in the psoriatic infiltrate. Difficulties may arise in treated lesions of psoriasis and in those with superimposed allergic contact dermatitis secondary to topical treatments.

Lichen simplex chronicus is considered in the differential diagnosis of fully developed psoriatic plaques. In contrast to psoriasis, it shows a prominent granular layer, more irregular acanthosis, and fibrosis of the papillary dermis with collagen bundles aligned perpendicular to the skin surface.

Seborrheic dermatitis may be very difficult to distinguish from psoriasis vulgaris, especially if the overlap occurs on the scalp as sebopsoriasis. Accentuated spongiosis, mounds of parakeratosis with neutrophils predominantly at the follicular ostia, and more irregular acanthosis are histopathologic features that support a diagnosis of seborrheic dermatitis.

Pityriasis rubra pilaris shares some histopathologic features with psoriasis—namely, acanthosis and parakeratosis. However, it can be differentiated from well-developed lesions of psoriasis by the presence of thick suprapapillary plates, broader and shorter rete ridges, and a preserved granular layer and alternating ortho- and parakeratosis. Munro microabscesses and neutrophilic infiltrates are usually absent in pityriasis rubra pilaris (55).

Although the Kogoj spongiform pustule is highly diagnostic of the psoriasis group of diseases, including reactive arthritis, histopathologically typical spongiform pustules may occur also in *pustular dermatophytosis*, *bacterial impetigo*, *pustular drug eruptions*, and *candidiasis*, particularly if pustules are clinically present (56). Periodic acid–Schiff (PAS) and Gram stains are useful for identifying infectious microorganisms. Aggregates of neutrophils with pyknotic nuclei within areas of parakeratosis may occur in conditions other than psoriasis, but they generally differ from Munro microabscesses by being larger and less well circumscribed.

Because of the clinical and the histopathologic resemblance of the tongue lesions in pustular psoriasis to those seen in geographic tongue, it has been suggested that geographic tongue represents an abortive form of pustular psoriasis (57).

Principles of Management

The treatment of psoriasis is based on the type of psoriasis, the extent of cutaneous involvement, presence of joint and other systemic symptoms, and patient comorbidities. Additional factors include patient age, gender, complexity of the treatment regimen, practicality, tolerability, safety, and patient preference. Psoriasis is a chronic illness, and the selected treatments should be sustainable in terms of patient lifestyle.

Topical agents are the mainstay of treatment for psoriasis for limited disease severity (usually <10% of the body surface area) and for patients with mild-to-moderate psoriasis, which account for approximately 80% of patients (58). Commonly used topical agents include topical corticosteroids, vitamin D analogs, retinoids, calcineurin inhibitors, coal tar, anthralin, and keratolytics. Small, resistant plaques may respond to intralesional steroid injections.

Phototherapy using narrow-band (NB)-UVB plays an integral role in psoriasis treatment and can be used for both extensive disease and for limited disease with debilitating symptoms (58). In the management of localized plaque-type lesions, 308-nm excimer laser phototherapy can be used to deliver targeted high UVB doses while sparing adjacent healthy skin. Ultraviolet light is locally immunosuppressive but typically lacks the cutaneous adverse effects of long-term corticosteroid use and the immunosuppression encountered with systemic agents and biologics. Anti-inflammatory agents and immunosuppressive agents such as retinoids and methotrexate still are helpful for subsets of patients, sometimes in combination with phototherapy. Apremilast is a newer oral agent that has been helpful for select populations of patients with psoriasis.

However, psoriasis management has been transformed with the advent of targeted biologic therapies. The TNF-inhibitor class of agents remains highly effective, but in recent years the development of IL12/23, IL23, and IL17 inhibitors has added a number of highly effective, well-tolerated treatments to the therapeutic toolbox.

Psoriasis is a condition of chronic systemic inflammation. Patients with psoriasis are subject to increased risk of severe vascular disease including myocardial infarctions and stroke. Patients also have an increased prevalence of hypertension, diabetes mellitus, dyslipidemia, obesity, and metabolic syndrome, all further contributors to cardiovascular disease. The theoretical mechanisms of this association include chronic inflammatory pathways, adipokine secretion, insulin resistance, angiogenesis, oxidative stress, and hypercoagulability. Studies have demonstrated that systemic treatment for psoriasis, including methotrexate and TNF-α inhibitors, may significantly decrease the risk of cardiovascular events in patients with psoriasis. Amelioration of cardiovascular risk is becoming a key factor in the selection of treatment options, as more aggressive systemic treatment may be utilized in patients with moderate skin disease but significant cardiovascular risk (59).

PITYRIASIS RUBRA PILARIS

Clinical Summary

Pityriasis rubra pilaris (PRP) is an erythematous papulosquamous disorder characterized by follicular keratotic papules and perifollicular erythema that coalesce to form orange-red scaly plaques with islands of normal-appearing skin (Fig. 7-9). As the erythema extends, the follicular component is often lost, but it persists longest on the dorsal aspect of the proximal phalanges. The lesions spread caudally and may progress to a generalized erythroderma (60). Other clinical findings are palmoplantar keratoderma and scaling of the face and scalp. There are six types of PRP:

- Type I: Classical adult onset. This type of PRP accounts for 50% of all cases and has an excellent prognosis; 80% of patients go into spontaneous remission with rare relapses. Pruritic follicular keratotic papules and plaques may coalesce to form erythematous or salmon-colored plaques with scaling, which may expand to cover the entire body. Erythroderma may occur. Islands of sparing and red-orange palmoplantar keratoderma are characteristic clinical findings. Pityriasiform scaling of the face and scalp may occur (61). In the setting of prolonged facial erythroderma, ectropion has been reported. Other ocular complications include peripheral ulcerative keratitis, corneal perforation, and xeropthalmia (62). Because type I PRP may be associated with underlying malignancy, age-appropriate cancer screenings should be performed.
- Type II: Atypical adult onset. Accounting for only 5% of cases, this rare form of PRP may persist for 20 or more years. This type often has an eczematous component and with ichthyosiform scales, patches of alopecia, and palmoplantar keratoderma with lamellated scales (61).

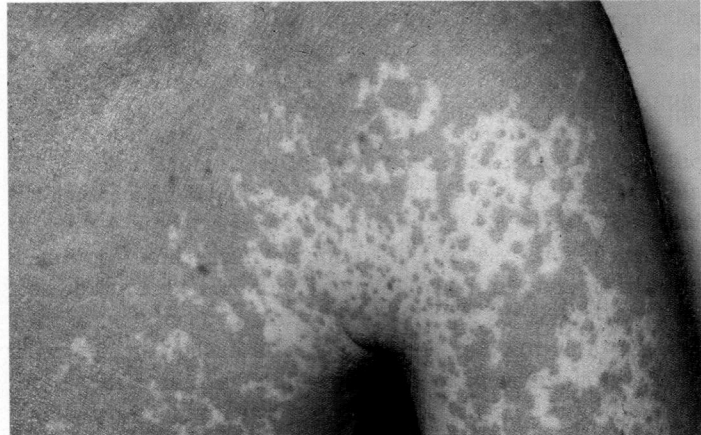

Figure 7-9 Pityriasis rubra pilaris. Confluent orange-red scaly plaques with islands of normal-appearing skin. (Courtesy of Department of Dermatology, University of Pennsylvania School of Medicine, Philadelphia, Pennsylvania.)

- Type III: Classical juvenile onset. This form of PRP accounts for 10% of all cases and occurs in children 5 to 10 years old. It often follows an acute infection and typically remits spontaneously within a year. The clinical presentation is similar to that of type I PRP, with the exception that in adults PRP typically starts on the face and scalp and spreads in a caudal direction, whereas in children it typically begins on the lower body. As with type I PRP, islands of sparing and red-orange palmoplantar keratoderma are characteristic clinical findings (61).
- Type IV: Circumscribed juvenile. This variant of PRP accounts for 25% of all cases, occurs in prepubertal children, and is characterized by sharply demarcated areas of follicular hyperkeratosis and erythema of the knees and elbows. As the name suggests, lesions are typically confined to palms, soles, knees, and elbows. The long-term outcome of this type of PRP is varied, but patients may experience improvement with age (61).
- Type V: Atypical juvenile onset. This rare form of PRP accounts for only 5% of cases and is mostly characterized by follicular hyperkeratosis. It typically occurs at birth or in early childhood and is generally very persistent (61). It may be inherited and shows some overlap with hereditary ichthyoses. Familial cases have been reported in association with mutations in the *CARD14* gene (63).
- Type VI: HIV associated. This very rare form of PRP has been presented in case reports and responds poorly to treatment (64). Presentation is similar to that of type I PRP but with prominent follicular plugging and the formation of spicules. Other disease associations include acne conglobata, hidradenitis suppurativa, and lichen spinulosus. The prognosis of this type of PRP is variable. Given the existence of this form of PRP, HIV testing is recommended in all patients with new-onset PRP (61).

Histopathology

Fully developed erythematous lesions of PRP show acanthosis with broad and short rete ridges, slight spongiosis, thick suprapapillary plates, focal or confluent hypergranulosis, and alternating orthokeratosis and parakeratosis oriented in both vertical and horizontal directions (Fig. 7-10). In the dermis, there is a mild superficial perivascular lymphocytic infiltrate and moderately dilated blood vessels (65).

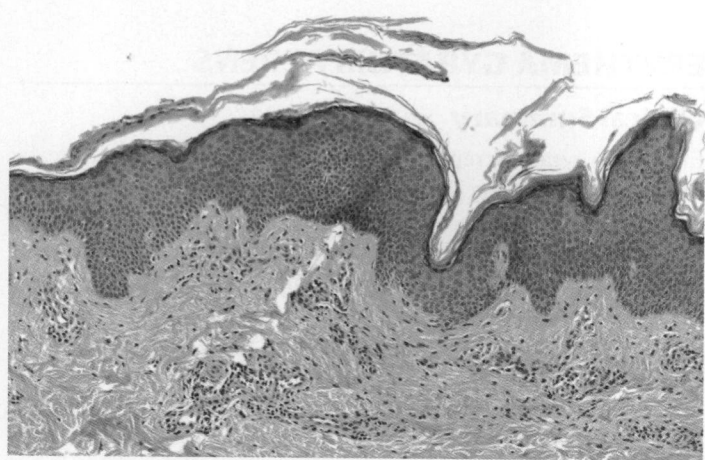

Figure 7-10 Pityriasis rubra pilaris. Alternating orthokeratosis and parakeratosis with mild acanthosis and superficial perivascular lymphocytic infiltrate.

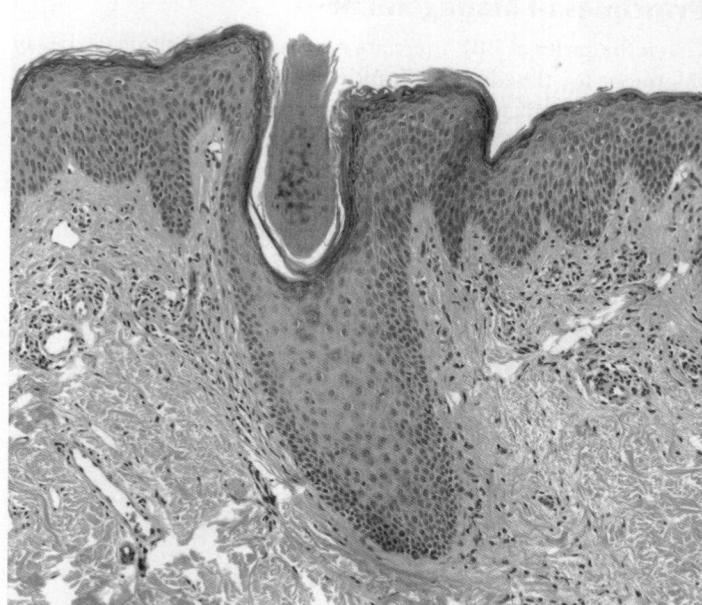

Figure 7-11 Pityriasis rubra pilaris. Dilated follicular infundibulum with hyperkeratotic plug.

Areas corresponding to follicular papules show dilated infundibula filled with an orthokeratotic plug and often display perifollicular shoulders of parakeratosis and a sparse perifollicular lymphocytic infiltrate (Fig. 7-11). Erythrodermic lesions have a thinned or absent cornified layer with serum exudate and a diminished granular zone. Acantholysis may also be seen, focally or extensively, in a suprabasal or subcorneal location.

Differential Diagnosis

Although PRP and psoriasis may be difficult to distinguish clinically, they may demonstrate significant histopathologic differences. Psoriasis is characterized by the presence of neutrophils and Munro microabscesses, more pronounced mounds of parakeratosis, thin suprapapillary plates, elongated rete ridges, and rete papillae with tortuous blood vessels (65). PRP has a prominent granular layer with less epidermal spongiosis and inflammatory infiltrate. The hyperkeratotic scale of PRP may display alternating orthokeratosis and parakeratosis with more widely spaced retained keratinocytic nuclei creating an intracorneal pattern resembling notes on a musical scale or a checkerboard. Additionally, the follicular hyperkeratosis seen clinically is associated with parakeratosis at the shoulders of follicular ostia in PRP.

Pathogenesis

The cause of PRP is unknown. There is evidence that suggests an abnormal epidermal differentiation based on the presence of suprabasal staining with monoclonal antibody against keratin AE1 and the detection of cytokeratins K6 and K16, which are not expressed in normal skin. In familial PRP, there are mutations in the *CARD14* gene, which encodes an activator of nuclear factor kappa B (NFκB) signaling. *CARD14* levels are increased (mostly in basal and suprabasal locations) and p65 is activated, resulting in the recruitment of inflammatory cells by keratinocytes (66).

Principles of Management

Given the rarity of PRP, there are no randomized clinical trials of treatment for this disease. Topical therapy is primarily targeted at ameliorating pruritus, including emollients and topical corticosteroids. Narrowband and UVB therapy may result in disease exacerbation and should be used cautiously. Oral retinoids are the mainstay of treatment for type I and III PRP. Methotrexate, TNF-α inhibitors, ustekinumab, secukinumab, and apremilast have been used with some success (67–69). More targeted biologics have been reported with increasing frequency as effective therapeutic options for patients with PRP. It is important to carefully exclude cutaneous T-cell lymphoma (CTCL) in patients with PRP, as initiation of select immune-modulating agents in the setting of CTCL can lead to disease progression. Data on treatment are generally anecdotal and limited to case reports and case series.

POLYMORPHIC ERUPTION OF PREGNANCY/PRURITIC URTICARIAL PAPULES AND PLAQUES OF PREGNANCY

Clinical Summary

Polymorphic eruption of pregnancy (PEP), previously known as pruritic urticarial papules and plaques of pregnancy (PUPPP), is a fairly common benign entity, first described by Lawley et al. in 1979 (70). The condition has a predilection for primigravidas in the third trimester of pregnancy, particularly in twin/triplet pregnancies. The rash usually starts on the abdomen, sparing the umbilicus (as compared to pemphigoid gestationis, which classically involves the umbilicus), and then spreads to proximal parts of the extremities and buttocks. The eruption may involve any body area. It is composed of intensely pruritic erythematous urticarial papules and vesicles. There is no increased incidence of the rash in subsequent pregnancies (71), and it usually resolves spontaneously after delivery. Fetal outcome appears to be unaffected, without evidence of increased risk of premature delivery, intrauterine growth restriction, or fetal demise. Unusual clinical presentations have been reported, including involvement of palmoplantar surfaces and initial manifestation of the disease in the postpartum period (72,73).

Histopathology

Microscopic findings most commonly show a superficial and mid-dermal perivascular lymphocytic and histiocytic infiltrate with variable numbers of eosinophils and neutrophils with superficial dermal edema. Epidermal involvement is variable and may consist of focal spongiosis, parakeratosis, and mild acanthosis (70,71,74).

Pathogenesis

An association between PEP and increased maternal weight and twin/triplet pregnancies has been identified (75,76), suggesting a relationship between skin distention and the development of PEP (77). In cultures of human keratinocytes, lesional epidermis of PEP has shown progesterone receptor (PR) expression detected by immunohistochemistry and reverse transcriptase-polymerase chain reaction (RT-PCR), whereas PR is not detected in nonlesional epidermis (78). A paternal factor hypothetically generated or expressed by the fetal portion of the placenta has been invoked as the cause of PEP in two families with unusual conjugal patterns (79). Direct immunofluorescence studies may be negative or show nonspecific immunoreactants around the superficial dermal blood vessels or at the dermoepidermal junction (80).

Differential Diagnosis

Specific dermatoses associated with pregnancy should be considered in the differential diagnoses and include pemphigoid gestationis, atopic eruption of pregnancy (AEP), and intrahepatic cholestasis of pregnancy (81). Other items on the differential include skin lesions that may occur in nonpregnant patients, including drug reactions, viral exanthemas, contact dermatitis, and scabies. Pemphigoid gestationis (PG) is a blistering dermatosis with a preliminary urticarial phase. Unlike PEP, it may develop in subsequent pregnancies, and the rash often involves the umbilicus. Histopathologically, more eosinophils are present along the dermoepidermal junction in PG than in PUPPP. Direct immunofluorescence studies usually show linear deposition of C3 and IgG along the basement membrane zone in perilesional skin (82). Whereas PEP has an indolent course, PG is associated with a greater prevalence of decreased gestational age at delivery and low birth weight (83).

Patients with AEP usually have personal or familial history of atopic dermatitis. As opposed to PEP, skin lesions in AEP commonly start during early pregnancy. In intrahepatic cholestasis of pregnancy, patients present with intense pruritus, skin excoriations, and lichenification. Histopathologically, in both entities, epidermal changes such as acanthosis, hypergranulosis, and hyperkeratosis are much more pronounced because of chronic scratching (81).

Principles of Management

Because PEP tends to resolve spontaneously shortly after delivery, treatment is mainly focused on relieving the associated pruritus, including emollients and soothing baths. Topical corticosteroids or even systemic steroids may be needed to ameliorate the symptoms (84). Use of high-potency topical steroids over large surface areas in pregnancy is controversial; systemic absorption may increase the risk of low birth weight, and treatment should be conducted in close collaboration with the obstetrician. Antihistamines with sedative effects can be effective against pruritus and serve as a sleep aid (85).

ERYTHEMA GYRATUM REPENS

Clinical Summary

Erythema gyratum repens (EGR) is a very rare but clinically highly characteristic figurate erythema that was originally reported in 1952 by Gammel (86). It most often occurs as a paraneoplastic syndrome associated with internal malignancy in 82% of patients, including lung/bronchial, esophageal, and breast carcinomas (87). Occurrence of EGR as a nonparaneoplastic phenomenon has also been described in the setting of tuberculosis, hypereosinophilic syndrome, bullous pemphigoid, pemphigus vulgaris, systemic lupus erythematosus, and ulcerative colitis (88–90). The eruption typically is very pruritic and is composed of concentric and parallel bands of erythema and scale, producing a pattern resembling wood grain. The trunk and extremities are preferentially involved; however, the skin eruption may be generalized. The rash of EGR constantly migrates rapidly (up to 1 cm/day). Concomitant ichthyosis and palmar/plantar hyperkeratosis have been observed in 16% and 10% of patients, respectively (91). Paraneoplastic EGR may precede the diagnosis of cancer by several months (92). The average age of onset is in the seventh decade of life, and it is twice as common in males than in females.

Histopathology

The histopathologic picture of EGR usually shows mild acanthosis, spongiosis, focal parakeratosis, and a superficial perivascular lymphohistiocytic infiltrate that may also include eosinophils, neutrophils, and melanophages (91,93).

Pathogenesis

Several authors have described granular deposition of C3, C4, or IgG at the basement membrane zone on direct immunofluorescence, suggesting that EGR may have an immunologic basis (94,95). In particular, Caux et al. (95), using immunoelectron microscopy, noted that the deposits are located in the sublamina densa region. Given nonspecific immunofluorescence findings in EGR, immunofluorescence is most useful in excluding other blistering conditions.

Differential Diagnosis

Clinical differential diagnosis of these peculiar polycyclic lesions includes unusual forms of tinea corporis (specifically tinea imbricata secondary to *Trichophyton concentricum*), urticaria, necrolytic migratory erythema, subacute cutaneous lupus erythematosus, and atypical cases of bullous pemphigoid or linear immunoglobulin A (IgA) (96). Other gyrate erythemas including erythema annular centrifugum, erythema marginatum rheumaticum (associated with rheumatic fever), and erythema chronicum migrans (associated with Lyme disease) may also be considered. In parsing this clinical and histopathologic differential diagnosis, EGR lacks PAS-positive hyphae in the cornified layer and does not have marked dermal edema, necrotic keratinocytes, interface dermatitis, or subepidermal blistering. Patients presenting with lesions suspicious for EGR should be evaluated for the presence of an underlying malignancy, including assessment for systemic symptoms and imaging. Underlying malignant lesions may be small, and identification of an occult malignancy may be challenging, requiring a combination of imaging and bloodwork as well as more invasive techniques such as endoscopy or cystoscopy. It is important to communicate openly with the care team and patient about the suspicion of malignancy.

Principles of Management

The condition is known to remit with the treatment of the associated malignancy (91). Antihistamines and topical or systemic corticosteroids have been reported to be beneficial in some cases (97,98).

ERYTHEMA DYSCHROMICUM PERSTANS

Clinical Summary

Erythema dyschromicum perstans (EDP), also called ashy dermatosis, was first described by Oswaldo Ramirez in 1957 (99). It is an asymptomatic form of acquired dermal macular

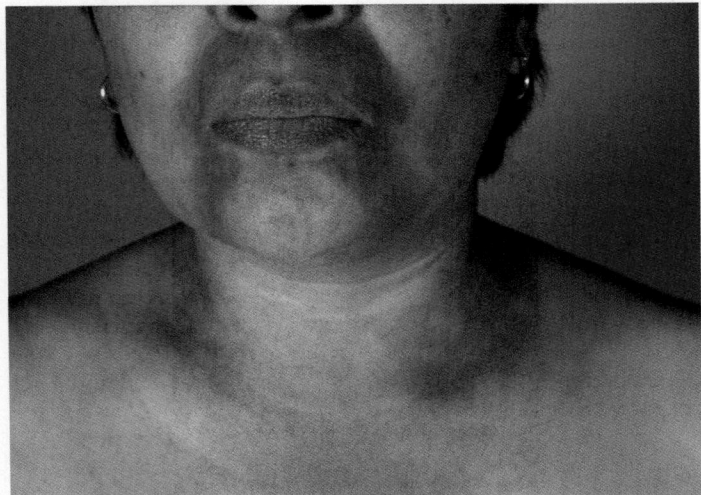

Figure 7-12 Erythema dyschromicum perstans. Disseminated blue-gray macules on face, neck, and chest. (Courtesy of Ronald O. Perelman Department of Dermatology, New York University School of Medicine, New York, New York.)

hyperpigmentation characterized by well-circumscribed, round-to-oval, grayish patches on the trunk and proximal extremities, with variable erythema and papule formation. Lesions begin as disseminated macules with an elevated red active border, which may coalescence and form large patches with a polycyclic outline (Fig. 7-12). Although the macules may at first be erythematous before assuming their characteristic bluish gray color, they may appear blue-gray from the very beginning. The disease progresses slowly, and discoloration may be persistent. Most patients with this disorder have darker skin tones, often hailing from Latin America (100) and Asia (101,102). A genetic susceptibility to develop the disease in Mexican mestizo patients has been associated with the HLA-DR4 DRB1(*)0407 allele (103).

Histopathology

Biopsies taken during early active stage or at the erythematous active border demonstrate basal layer epidermal vacuolization with a sparse-to-moderate superficial perivascular infiltrate of lymphocytes and histiocytes with papillary dermal melanophages (104). Lymphocytic exocytosis into the basal layers of the epidermis with occasional necrotic keratinocytes and colloid bodies resembling those of lichen planus may be present. Late lesions are characterized by less inflammation and more prominent collections of papillary dermal melanophages (104) (Fig. 7-13).

Pathogenesis

Direct immunofluorescence studies have shown IgG deposition on necrotic keratinocytes at the dermal–epidermal junction, suggesting an immune-mediated disease mechanism. Immunohistochemical studies have revealed that in early lesions, the dermal inflammatory infiltrate is composed primarily of T lymphocytes, both CD4+ (helper-inducer) and CD8+ (cytotoxic-suppressor) subtypes (105). Some authors have found predominance of CD8+ lymphocytes in the inflammatory dermal infiltrate (106).

Basal layer keratinocytes in EDP demonstrate increased expression of ICAM-1 and HLA-DR (106,107). The

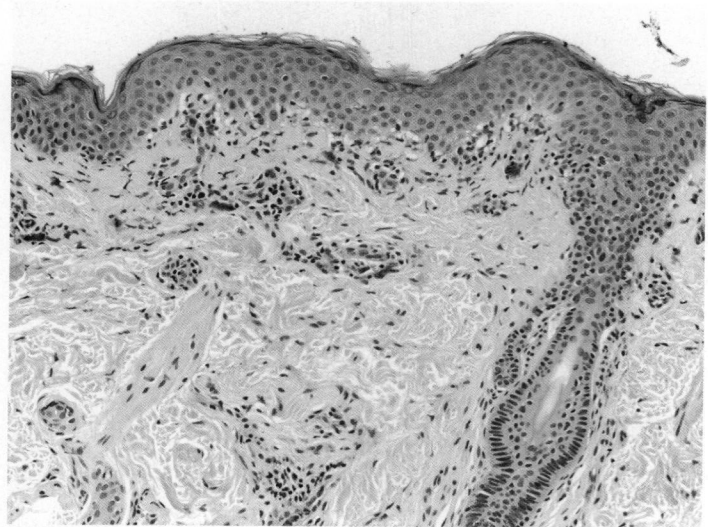

Figure 7-13 Erythema dyschromicum perstans. Vacuolar interface change and prominent dermal melanophages.

activation molecule AIM/CD69 and the cytotoxic cell marker CD94 have been seen to be expressed in the inflammatory cell infiltrate (107).

Differential Diagnosis

Disorders of pigmentation included in the differential diagnosis are postinflammatory hyperpigmentation, lichen planus pigmentosus, occupational dermatosis with hyperpigmentation, fixed-drug reactions, and drug-induced hyperpigmentation (e.g., owing to minocycline or antimalarials) (102). It is important to distinguish EDP from the late stage of pinta; serologic testing for treponemes may be necessary.

EDP may show histopathologic overlap with interface drug reactions, particularly the late stage of fixed-drug eruption; clinical correlation is usually necessary. Damage to and necrosis of the basal keratinocytes resulting in the formation of colloid bodies and pigmentary incontinence suggests a possible relationship of EDP to lichen planus pigmentosus (also called lichen planus actinicus or subtropicus) (108). However, lichen planus pigmentosus characteristically has a different clinical presentation with pruritic dark brown macules located predominantly on exposed areas and flexural folds. Histopathologically, lichen planus pigmentosus shows a more pronounced lichenoid distribution of the infiltrate and some effacement of rete ridges resulting in epidermal atrophy (104,109). Although EDP and lichen planus pigmentosus may be difficult to distinguish clinically and histopathologically, a recent consensus statement concluded that EDP and lichen planus pigmentosus are distinct forms of acquired macular hyperpigmentation based largely on differences in clinical appearance and distribution (110).

Principles of Management

Therapeutic options for EDP are limited and primarily rely on camouflage creams. Reported therapeutic options are predominantly based on anecdotal evidence and may include topical corticosteroids, antihistamines, topical tacrolimus, isotretinoin, dapsone, oral steroids, or clofazimine. However, none produce satisfactory results (111,112). As with other forms of skin darkening, patients may benefit from photoprotection, although this too may be ineffective.

CHRONIC PRURIGO (PRURIGO NODULARIS)

Clinical Summary

Prurigo nodularis is a chronic dermatitis characterized by raised, firm hyperkeratotic or excoriated papulonodules, usually from 5 to 12 mm in diameter but occasionally larger. They occur chiefly on the extensor surfaces of the extremities and are intensely pruritic (113). The disease usually begins in middle age, and women are more frequently affected than men (114). Prurigo nodularis may coexist with lesions of lichen simplex chronicus (113).

The exact cause is typically unknown, but local trauma, insect bites, atopic background, and infectious, metabolic, or systemic diseases may be predisposing factors and may be implicated in the pathogenesis and persistence of the disease (113,115–119). Predisposing factors contributing to disease can be identified in up to 87% of the patients with prurigo nodularis (120). A recent psychometric study has shown that psychological factors such as anxiety and depression were more severe in patients with prurigo nodularis than in the control group (121).

Histopathology

Prurigo nodularis is characterized histopathologically by hyperkeratosis, epidermal hyperplasia, and reactive fibrosis and inflammation in the dermis. There is often pronounced hyperorthokeratosis with focal parakeratosis, hypergranulosis, and irregular acanthosis (122). In addition, there may be papillomatosis and irregular downward proliferation of the epidermis and adnexal epithelium (123) approaching pseudoepitheliomatous hyperplasia (124) (Fig. 7-14). The papillary dermis shows vertically oriented collagen bundles with increased numbers of fibroblasts and capillaries and a perivascular inflammatory infiltrate of lymphocytes and to a lesser extent eosinophils and neutrophils (122). Occasionally, prominent neural hyperplasia may be observed (124); however, this uncommon finding is not an essential feature for the diagnosis (122,125). Eosinophils and marked eosinophil degranulation may be seen more frequently in patients with an atopic background (115). Dermal Langerhans cells are shown to be increased in prurigo nodularis compared to normal controls (126). The identification of enlarged dendritic mast cells containing fewer cytoplasmic granules within the lesional dermis has also been described (127).

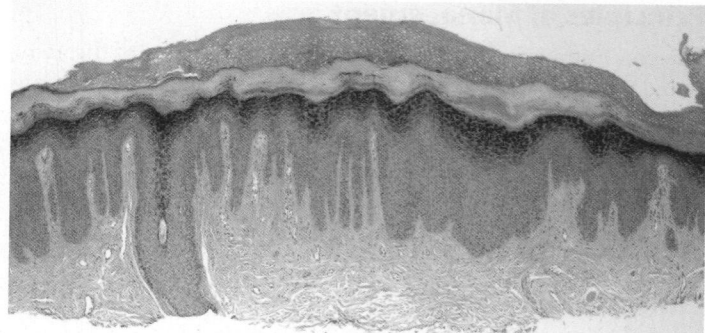

Figure 7-14 Prurigo nodularis. Dome-shaped papule with hyperkeratosis, hypergranulosis, epidermal acanthosis, and dermal fibrosis.

Pathogenesis

Immune and neural dysregulation have been implicated in the pathogenesis of prurigo nodularis, and immune cells and neuropeptides may play a critical role in the cutaneous inflammation and altered neural pathways that drive the pruritus that contributes to and results from prurigo nodularis. The itch–scratch cycle is a critical component of the pathogenesis of prurigo nodularis, and breaking this cycle is of utmost importance in treatment (128). Prurigo nodularis is histopathologically characterized by dense dermal, interstitial, and perivascular infiltrates of T cells, mast cells, and eosinophils, which together generate an inflammatory response by releasing a variety of mediators, including IL-31, tryptase, eosinophil cationic protein, histamine, prostaglandins, and neuropeptides (129). Eosinophils play a key role in releasing a number of these mediators (11). Th2 cytokines such as IL-4 have also been demonstrated to be elevated in the skin lesions of prurigo nodularis (130).

Alterations to neural architecture in the skin lesions of prurigo nodularis have also been implicated in disease pathogenesis. Neuronal hyperplasia in prurigo nodularis was first described by Pautrier in 1934 (Pautrier neuroma) (131). The epidermis of patients with prurigo nodularis has a lower density of nerve growth factor receptor immunoreactive nerve fibers and fewer PGP9.5+ nerve fibers (132). However, functional small fiber neuropathy has not been identified in patients with prurigo nodularis, which argues against an intrinsic neuropathy as a cause of prurigo nodularis; these findings rather may be secondary to scratching. Other contributors to pruritus include neuropeptide dysregulation (particularly calcitonin gene-related peptide and substance P) as has dysregulation of μ and κ opioid receptors.

Differential Diagnosis

Lichen simplex chronicus may have a similar histopathologic picture, although in most cases lichen simplex chronicus is less exuberant and less circumscribed (122,125). Multiple keratoacanthomas, which often show less of a central crater than solitary keratoacanthomas, may be difficult to distinguish from prurigo nodularis because both show marked epidermal and epithelial hyperplasia. Other causes of pseudoepitheliomatous epidermal hyperplasia including fungal infection, leishmaniasis, halogenodermas, and pemphigus vegetans may also enter the histopathologic differential diagnosis. Intraepithelial neutrophilic microabscesses are usually present in fungal infection and halogenodermas, and the presence of large yeast forms or parasites will confirm a diagnosis of infection. Suprabasal acantholysis will allow the differentiation of pemphigus vegetans from prurigo nodularis.

Principles of Management

Prurigo nodularis may have a great impact on patients' quality of life.

Chronic prurigo must be managed in a holistic manner with a focus on amelioration of symptoms, treatment of any underlying causes, and breaking of the itch–scratch cycle. Unfortunately, available treatments have shown only mild-to-moderate efficacy (133). Bland emollients and topical steroids are mainstays of treatment, as are oral antihistamines; sedating antihistamines may be particularly helpful at night. The use of occlusive dressings with topical medications may be particularly helpful in breaking the itch–scratch cycle. Oral antipruritic agents may include gabapentin, pregabalin, amitriptyline, and naltrexone.

There have been some case reports on the use of topical immunomodulators, tacrolimus and pimecrolimus, for steroid-unresponsive patients (134). NB-UVB phototherapy is an efficacious and safe treatment option, especially for widespread disease (135,136). Thalidomide has been used with good results in patients with prurigo nodularis refractory to other treatments. However, treatment may be limited by side effects, such as peripheral neuropathy and sedation, and limitations on the ability to obtain the medication (137). Antihistamines, anxiolytics, gabapentin (138), pregabalin (139), opiate receptor antagonists (140), lenalidomide (141), and the neurokinin receptor 1 antagonist, aprepitant (142) have been reported to be useful in the treatment of prurigo nodularis. Recently, dupixent has been evaluated in small case reports and case series and may be a therapeutic alternative for some patients. Multiple targeted anti-itch biologic agents are in the pipeline, and management of pruritic conditions is rapidly evolving.

REACTIVE ARTHRITIS (FORMERLY REITER SYNDROME)

Clinical Summary

Reactive arthritis, formerly called Reiter syndrome (143,144), is a seronegative spondyloarthropathy. In most cases, it occurs 2 to 4 weeks after an enteric or urogenital infection. The most commonly associated pathogens include *Yersinia, Salmonella, Shigella, Campylobacter,* and *Clostridium difficile.* The most common urogenital pathogens include *Chlamydia trachomatis, Neisseria gonorrhea,* and *Ureaplasma urealyticum.* There is no sex predilection for cases of reactive arthritis caused by enteric pathogens, but males have a higher incidence after genital *Chlamydia trachomatis* infection (145–147). The HLA-B27 allele has been associated with this condition, but it is not a diagnostic criterion.

Reactive arthritis is characterized by the triad of urethritis, oligoarthritis, and conjunctivitis. However, only one-third of the patients show the complete classic triad; diagnosis largely depends on patient history (148). There is great variation in the severity, number, and timing of clinical manifestations, and clinical findings may include ulcerative vulvitis, enthesitis, tendinitis, bursitis, anterior uveitis, and ocular keratitis. Erythema nodosum is more common in the setting of *Yersinia enterocolitica* infection (149,150).

Lesions have a predilection for glans penis (balanitis circinata), palms and soles (keratoderma blennorrhagicum), and the subungual regions (Fig. 7-15). Mucocutaneous lesions occur in about half of affected patients, including the glans, vulva, and oral mucosa.

Circinate balanitis consists of small, shallow, painless ulcers of the urethral meatus or glans penis, accompanied by characteristic circinate or gyrate white plaques. These grow centrifugally and can cover the entire surface of the glans. On an uncircumcised penis, the lesions generally remain moist, but in the setting of circumcision, they may harden and crust resulting in pain and scarring in up to half of patients. The lesions of keratoderma blenorrhagicum on the palms and soles are erythematous, thick plaques with central keratotic excrescences. Pustular lesions may also develop. Nail involvement occurs in 20% to 30% of patients and may resemble the findings of nail psoriasis including nail pitting, subungual hyperkeratosis,

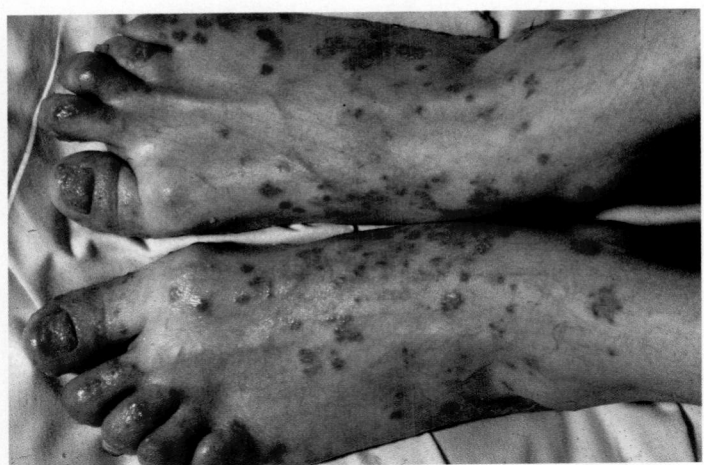

Figure 7-15 Reactive arthritis. Confluent erythematous scaly papules and plaques on the dorsum of feet and toes, with nail dystrophy. (Courtesy of Department of Dermatology, University of Pennsylvania School of Medicine, Philadelphia, Pennsylvania.)

periungual pustules, paronychia; less common are ridging, splitting, elkonyxis (loss of nail plate substance above the lunula only), and red-brown discoloration. The prevalence of reactive arthritis in HIV-infected individuals is less than 1%; however, the disease appears to be more severe in immunocompromised patients (151).

Histopathology

Early pustular lesions on the palms or soles show a spongiform macropustule in the upper epidermis with parakeratosis and elongation of the rete ridges (152,153).

As the lesions age, the parakeratotic cornified layer thickens considerably, which correlates with the keratotic excrescences seen clinically. The parakeratotic cornified layer is intermingled with the pyknotic nuclei of neutrophils. In old lesions, spongiform pustules are no longer seen, and the histopathologic picture shows acanthosis and orthokeratosis with only a few areas of parakeratosis. Occasionally, the histopathologic picture resembles that of psoriasis (152).

Pathogenesis

The pathophysiology of reactive arthritis is thought to have both infectious and immune components. It can be caused by microorganisms that infect the urogenital or gastrointestinal systems, such as *Chlamydia trachomatis*, *Ureaplasma urealyticum*, *Shigella flexneri*, *Clostridium difficile*, *Salmonella*, *Campylobacter*, *Cyclospora*, and *Yersinia* species (149).

Chlamydia trachomatis has been cultured from urethral samples in nearly half of the patients and is believed to be capable of triggering reactive arthritis in susceptible men (154). Although fluid cultured from joint aspirations are negative for bacteria in reactive arthritis, hybridization studies have detected chlamydial RNA in synovial specimens (155). The occurrence of reactive arthritis after Bacille Calmette–Guérin (BCG) immunotherapy for bladder cancer has been reported (156). Eighty percent of patients with reactive arthritis are HLA-B27 positive (151); however, the precise role of this major histocompatibility class I antigen in the development of this disease is not known. There is no proof that microbial antigens can cross-react with HLA-B27 (157). One study found decreased

IL-2 production in HLA-B27-positive and B7-positive patients who developed reactive arthritis after *Salmonella* infection. These findings suggest that impaired cellular immunity against the infectious agent may be associated with the development of the disease (158). First line of host defense involves Toll-like receptors (TLRs), which may act as pathogen sensors. Certain TLR-2 genetic variants have been associated with reactive arthritis (159).

A close relationship to psoriasis has been assumed for the cutaneous lesions because of their clinical resemblance to psoriasis and the presence of spongiform pustules (160,161). The arthritis of reactive arthritis resembles that of psoriasis both clinically and in the absence of rheumatoid factor positivity (149).

Differential Diagnosis

The early spongiform pustule seen in skin lesions of reactive arthritis is indistinguishable from the spongiform pustule seen in pustular psoriasis. Other conditions that enter the clinical differential include atopic dermatitis, Behcet disease, and contact dermatitis. Clinicopathologic correlation is often necessary to arrive at the correct diagnosis.

Principles of Management

The mucocutaneous lesions of reactive arthritis are self-limited and typically resolve within several months. HIV has been associated with severe, extensive, and chronic cutaneous manifestations, and treatment mirrors that of pustular psoriasis. Topical therapies include topical steroids, calcipotriene, tacrolimus, and tazarotene. Second-line therapies include NB-UVB and systemic steroids. Psoralen and ultraviolet A (PUVA) and immunosuppressives like methotrexate and cyclosporine may be considered in severe recalcitrant cases. TNF-α inhibitors have recently been shown to be effective and safe in this condition, although treatment may be prolonged (162). Given the self-limited nature of the cutaneous disease, treatment is typically driven by the joint symptoms. Therapies include nonsteroidal anti-inflammatories (NSAIDs) and corticosteroid injections. In severe cases, oral steroids, methotrexate, or sulfasalazine may be considered (152). TNF-α inhibitors may also be effective for joint symptoms (162).

The role of short- and long-term antibiotic therapy for reactive arthritis is controversial. Even though there is some evidence that antibiotics during the infectious phase, before the arthritis has developed, may be helpful, there is not sufficient evidence to demonstrate modification of the disease course after the development of arthritis (163). When treating a patient with reactive arthritis owing to a urogenital infection, it is also important to ensure that the patient's sexual partners are tested and treated as necessary.

DIGITATE DERMATOSIS (SMALL-PLAQUE PARAPSORIASIS)

Clinical Summary

There are three entities described as parapsoriasis: small-plaque parapsoriasis, large-plaque parapsoriasis, and parapsoriasis variegata. Many specialists in the field of cutaneous lymphoma no longer consider parapsoriasis a specific diagnosis.

Large-plaque parapsoriasis and *parapsoriasis variegata* are best considered as early stages of CTCL/mycosis fungoides and are distinct from the entity referred to as "small-plaque parapsoriasis" (164). Large-plaque parapsoriasis is discussed further in Chapter 31.

The *small-plaque parapsoriasis* is also known as digitate dermatosis (165), chronic superficial dermatitis, superficial scaly dermatitis, and less commonly as xanthoerythrodermia perstans of Crocker (166). This condition is best thought of as related to eczematous dermatitis. This condition is more common in middle-aged and elderly males, with a peak in the 40- to 50-year-old range (167). Pink-to-yellow, slightly scaly, oval or elongated, often fingerprint-like, digitate patches 1 to 5 cm in diameter are symmetrically distributed over the trunk and the proximal portions of the extremities following the tension lines of the skin (168). The eruption is usually asymptomatic without pruritus, has a chronic course, and tends to be persistent.

Histopathology

Digitate dermatosis shows histopathologic findings similar to, and often indistinguishable from, those of an eczematous dermatitis, including scant spongiosis, sparse exocytosis of lymphocytes, slight acanthosis, and parakeratosis (166,169). Elongated mounds of parakeratosis with intracorneal serum above a basket-weaved cornified layer is a characteristic finding (Fig. 7-16). In the papillary dermis, there is a sparse superficial perivascular lymphocytic infiltrate without lymphoid enlargement or significant atypia.

Pathogenesis

The inflammatory infiltrate in small-plaque parapsoriasis is dominated by CD4$^+$ (helper-inducer) T lymphocytes with a small proportion of the CD8$^+$ (cytotoxic-suppressor) T lymphocytes subset, as opposed to the hypopigmented variant where CD8$^+$ lymphocytes predominate (170). Langerhans cells are increased in the epidermis and dermis (171).

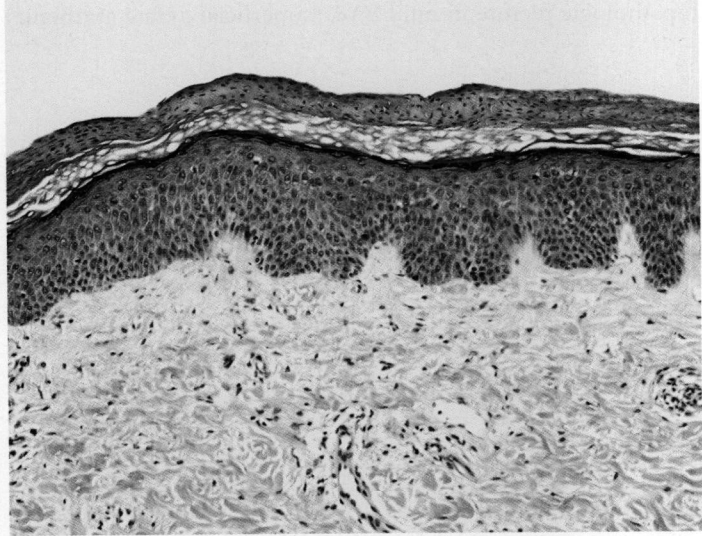

Figure 7-16 Digitate dermatosis (small-plaque parapsoriasis). Characteristic elongated mound of parakeratosis with collections of plasma above a basket-weave cornified layer, preserved granular layer, and minimal acanthosis. There is a sparse superficial perivascular lymphocytic infiltrate.

Small-plaque parapsoriasis, or digitate dermatosis, is a benign reactive dermatitis without the potential for transformation into mycosis fungoides (164,166,171–173). Although oligoclonal and monoclonal T-cell receptor gene rearrangements have been identified in small-plaque parapsoriasis, there is no convincing evidence of disease progression to lymphoma (174,175).

Differential Diagnosis

The main differential diagnosis of digitate dermatosis is with early mycosis fungoides. Patches in small-plaque parapsoriasis are generally more uniform in size, shape, and color, whereas mycosis fungoides exhibit more variability in the morphology of the lesions. Haloed atypical lymphocytes within the epidermis, formation of Pautrier microabscesses, single lymphoid cells arranged linearly along the dermoepidermal junction, and dermal fibrosis are histopathologic features considered to define early mycosis fungoides. Loss of pan-T-cell antigens such as CD2 and CD5 on immunohistochemistry is particularly helpful in arriving at a diagnosis of mycosis fungoides (176). Clinicopathologic correlation with a descriptive histopathologic diagnosis is critical to making an accurate diagnosis; molecular studies are not helpful in this setting as clonal T-cell receptor gene rearrangements may be present in a variety of reactive conditions including small-plaque parapsoriasis and mycosis fungoides.

Principles of Management

Topical treatment with emollients or mid-potency topical steroids may help to relieve scaly patches and inflammation. Phototherapy is an excellent treatment for parapsoriasis. Ultraviolet A (UVA) or UVB narrow bands are both effective and can lead to remission of the lesions (177,178). Topical nitrogen mustard may also be used as second-line therapy (179).

PITYRIASIS ROSEA

Clinical Summary

Pityriasis rosea is a self-limited papulosquamous disorder usually lasting from 4 to 7 weeks. It frequently starts with a herald patch, followed by a disseminated eruption. The lesions, found chiefly on the trunk, neck, and proximal extremities, consist of round to oval salmon-colored patches following the lines of cleavage and showing peripherally attached thin, cigarette paper—like scales (often termed trailing), a delicate annular rim of scale that trails behind the advancing edge of erythema (Fig. 7-17). Several typical and atypical clinical variants have been described, including papular, vesicular, urticarial, purpuric, and recurrent forms (180,181). Pityriasis rosea occurring during pregnancy may be associated with premature delivery, neonatal hypotonia, and miscarriage, particularly in women who developed the disease within the first 15 weeks of gestation (182).

Histopathology

The patches of the disseminated eruption of pityriasis rosea show a superficial perivascular lymphocytic dermal infiltrate with occasional eosinophils and histiocytes. Lymphocytic exocytosis is associated with spongiosis, intracellular edema, mild-to-moderate acanthosis, areas of decreased to absent granular

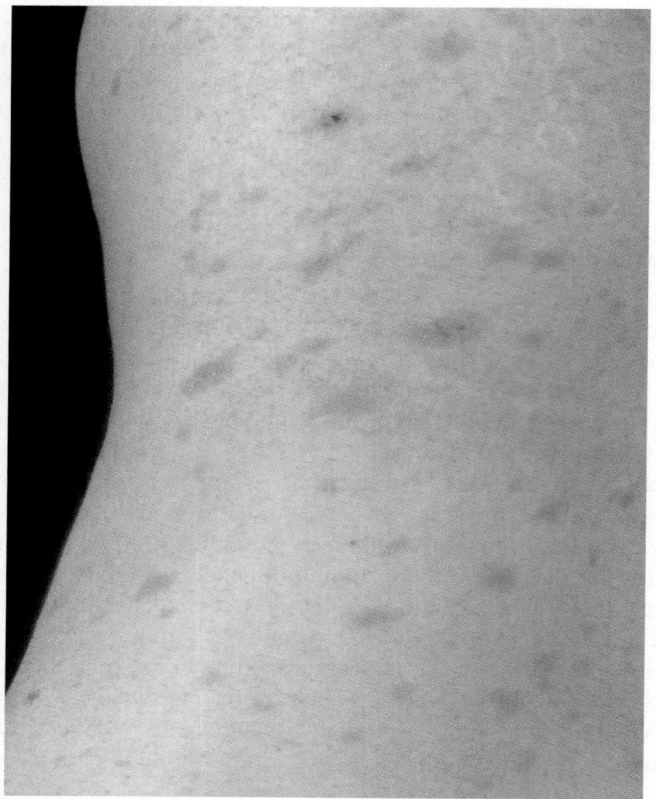

Figure 7-17 Pityriasis rosea. Round-to-oval salmon-colored patches following the lines of cleavage on the trunk. (Courtesy of Ronald O. Perelman Department of Dermatology, New York University School of Medicine, New York, New York.)

layer, and focal serum-imbued parakeratotic scale (183–185). The parakeratotic scale may appear to separate from the epidermis at one side, so-called lifting scale, correlating with the paper-thin scale observed clinically. Intraepidermal spongiotic vesicles (183,184) and a few necrotic keratinocytes (186) are found in some cases. Extravasated erythrocytes in the papillary dermis are a common feature and may extend into the overlying epidermis (186,187) (Fig. 7-18). Occasionally, multinucleated

keratinocytes in the affected epidermis can be seen (187). Late lesions from the disseminated eruption are more likely to have a psoriasiform pattern (183) and a slightly increased number of eosinophils in the inflammatory infiltrate (185). The herald patch may additionally have more pronounced acanthosis, deeper and denser perivascular inflammatory infiltrate, and papillary dermal edema (187). Immunohistochemical studies have shown, in both herald patch and secondary lesions, a predominant T-cell dermal infiltrate, with an increased CD4/CD8 ratio. There was also enhanced staining for Langerhans cells within the dermis of lesional skin (188).

Pathogenesis

The cause of pityriasis rosea is unknown, although a viral etiology such as human herpesvirus (HHV) 6 and/or 7 is highly suspected (189). Polymerase chain reaction (PCR) reveals higher frequency of HHV-6 and HHV-7 DNA in tissue and blood samples from patients with pityriasis rosea compared with healthy controls (190). However, there is controversy whether skin lesions are the result of direct infection or rather a reactive response to systemic HHV-6 and HHV-7 (191).

Enterovirus and influenza H1N1 have also been proposed as a possible cause of the disease (192,193). Several drugs including anti-TNF-α agents may produce pityriasis rosea–like reactions (194–196). PR has incidentally been reported in the setting of vaccination for SARS-CoV-2.

Cell-mediated immunity may be involved in the pathogenesis of pityriasis rosea. The infiltrate is predominantly composed of activated CD4$^+$/HLA-DR+ helper-inducer T lymphocytes (197), in association with increased numbers of CD1a+ Langerhans cells (198) and surface HLA-DR expression on keratinocytes located around the area of lymphocytic exocytosis (199). In addition, absence of natural killer (NK) and B-cell activity in pityriasis rosea lesions has been reported (188).

Differential Diagnosis

The differential diagnosis for pityriasis rosea includes erythema annulare centrifugum (EAC), digitate dermatosis (small-plaque parapsoriasis), drug eruptions, and secondary syphilis. The histopathologic picture in mild EAC (superficial gyrate erythema)

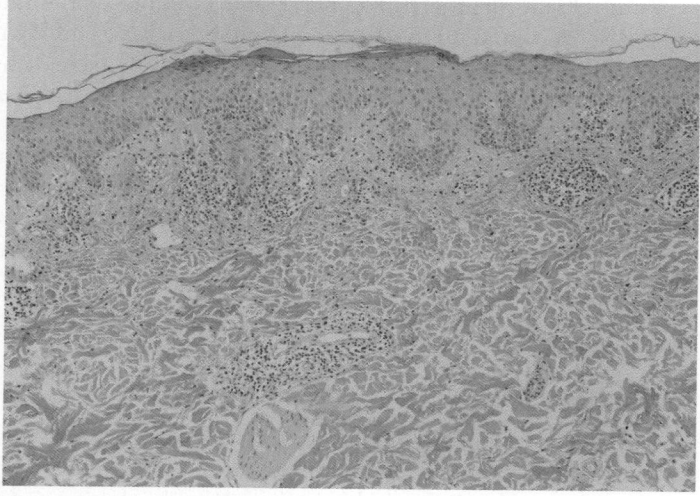
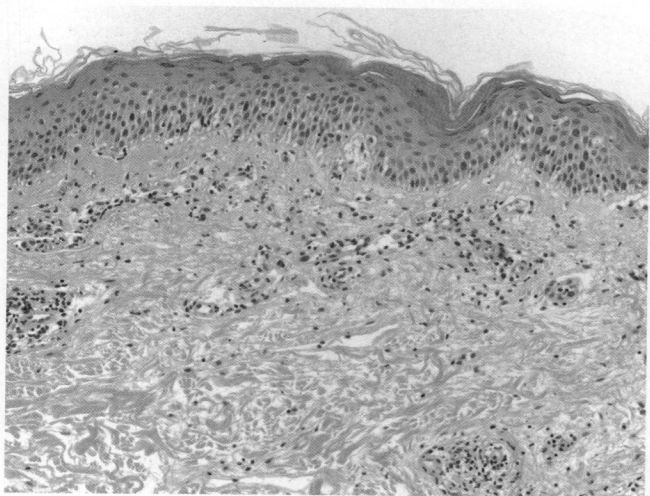

Figure 7-18 Pityriasis rosea. A: Mound-like scale, spongiosis, and superficial perivascular lymphocytic infiltrate. B: Prominent erythrocyte extravasation.

could be identical to that seen in pityriasis rosea. Elongated mounds of parakeratosis with serum, sparse superficial perivascular lymphocytic infiltrate, minimal exocytosis, and spongiosis are features of digitate dermatosis (small-plaque parapsoriasis) that distinguish it from pityriasis rosea (169). A detailed history of the patient's prescription medications, over-the-counter medications, and supplements will help in the evaluation of suspected drug eruption. Given the increasing incidence of syphilis around the world, a high index of suspicion for secondary syphilis should be maintained; although secondary syphilis is typically associated with an infiltrate of plasma cells, a spirochete stain and/or peripheral blood serologies should be performed in any case in which concern is raised.

Principles of Management

Pityriasis rosea is a self-limited disease and typically resolves within 6 weeks; reassurance is typically all that is needed (191). There is no need for isolation or restricted activities. Excessive sweating and use of soap may cause further irritation and should be avoided. Pruritus is usually mild; topical lotions with zinc oxide and calamine can help to alleviate it. In more severe and inflammatory cases, topical or oral corticosteroids can be used. Antibiotics and antivirals have not been shown to be effective in speeding recovery (200,201). Recalcitrant cases have been treated with phototherapy. As clinically pityriasis rosea can closely resemble secondary syphilis, some advocate for routine testing in patients with a diagnosis of pityriasis rosea.

GIANOTTI–CROSTI SYNDROME (PAPULAR ACRODERMATITIS OF CHILDHOOD AND PAPULOVESICULAR ACROLOCATED SYNDROME)

Clinical Summary

Papular acrodermatitis of childhood was first described by Gianotti in 1955 (202). It is clinically characterized by an exanthematous, symmetric papular rash of nonpruritic, monomorphic erythematous papules or papulovesicles on the face, extremities, and buttocks. It may be associated with mild constitutional symptoms and has a benign, albeit protracted course (lasting about 3 weeks). The eruption occurs usually in children 3 months to 15 years of age; however, rare adult cases have been reported especially in women (203–205). Synonyms for this entity include papular acrodermatitis of childhood, infantile papular acrodermatitis, and papulovesicular acrolocated syndrome. The diagnosis of Gianotti–Crosti syndrome is clinical, although biopsies may occasionally be performed.

Papular acrodermatitis was originally described in association with lymphadenopathy and hepatitis B viral infection (206). However, in recent years, it has become apparent that similar acral papular eruptions may occur with several other viruses, such as Epstein–Barr virus, coxsackie virus, parainfluenza virus, vaccine-related virus, cytomegalovirus, among others (207–210). In such cases, there is often no hepatitis or lymphadenopathy. These eruptions were classified by Gianotti (206) in a separate category as "papular or papulovesicular acrolocated syndrome." However, further studies (210,211) failed to identify repeatable clinical differences between popular acrodermatitis of childhood and papulovesicular acrolocated

syndrome. The term *Gianotti–Crosti syndrome* now applies to all self-limited, acrolocated, papular eruptions that occur in association with an underlying viral or other infectious agent, such as *Mycoplasma pneumoniae, Mycobacterium avium-intracellulare, Neisseria meningitidis,* coxsackievirus, enterovirus, HHV6, reovirus, varicella, roseola, rotavirus, respiratory syncytial virus, and Lyme borreliosis (205,212,213). Gianotti–Crosti syndrome has also been reported to occur following immunizations (214,215). Atopic background has been shown to have a significant association with this syndrome (216).

The eruption of Gianotti–Crosti is that of monomorphic, lentil-size lesions symmetrically located on the face, extremities, and buttocks. They are papular or papulovesicular and may occasionally be edematous and rarely purpuric. A transient truncal rash may occur in early stages. There is no mucous membrane involvement. Lesions may koebnerize. Skin lesions typically begin on the thighs and buttocks, then extend to the extensor aspect of the arms, and finally the face. Pruritus is mild, and excoriation is rare. Lesions fade with mild desquamation, and relapse is unusual. Inguinal and axillary lymphadenopathy are common, self-limited findings. In cases associated with hepatitis B virus (HBV), the hepatitis typically coincides with the skin lesions, with an enlarged and nontender liver, with elevated liver enzymes but absent jaundice.

Histopathology

Characteristically, epidermal changes are mild with focal spongiosis and parakeratosis. There is a superficial and mid-dermal perivascular infiltrate of lymphocytes and histiocytes with some exocytosis of lymphocytes in the overlying epidermis. In some cases, there is associated papillary dermal edema and extravasation of erythrocytes. Occasionally, lymphocytic vasculitis has been described with lymphocytes in the vessel walls and extravasated erythrocytes into the upper dermis (207). Gianotti–Crosti syndrome associated with Epstein–Barr virus is reported to have marked papillary dermal edema with minimal spongiosis and rare eosinophils in the dermal infiltrate (217). The inflammatory pattern may also present as a lichenoid interface dermatitis (218).

Pathogenesis

Immunohistochemical stains have shown that the inflammatory infiltrate is composed predominantly of $CD4^+$ (helper-inducer) T lymphocytes with a minor component of $CD8^+$ (suppressor-cytotoxic) T lymphocytes. There is also an increased number of Langerhans cells in the epidermis. A virus-induced type IV hypersensitivity reaction has been proposed (219).

Differential Diagnosis

The histopathologic differential diagnosis of Gianotti–Crosti syndrome includes other dermatitides with spongiosis, such as pityriasis rosea, EAC, allergic contact dermatitis, and nummular dermatitis. Papular lesions of Gianotti–Crosti exhibit more spongiosis and dermal edema than pityriasis rosea or EAC. Allergic contact dermatitis and nummular dermatitis tend to have more prominent eosinophils in the infiltrate (220).

Principles of Management

Reassurance for the child's parents is usually sufficient for this self-limited process. Therapeutic interventions for pruritus include soothing topical preparations and oral antihistamines (221).

Administration of oral ribavirin has been reported to be effective in one case of long-lasting and disabling Gianotti–Crosti syndrome, although this has not been recommended as a regular therapy (222). In cases associated with hepatitis B, the underlying hepatitis can be treated with antivirals; family members should also be screened for infection and vaccinated as needed.

MUCOCUTANEOUS LYMPH NODE SYNDROME (KAWASAKI DISEASE)

Clinical Summary

The mucocutaneous lymph node syndrome, first reported by Kawasaki in 1967 (223), is an acute, febrile, multiorgan vasculitic process of childhood best known for its mucocutaneous and nodal involvement. It is often associated with vasculitis that affects medium-sized arteries, particularly the coronary arteries (224). It is most common in Japanese or Korean children younger than 5 years of age, although it can occur in all races (225) either sporadically or epidemically. A definitive diagnosis is established by the presence of unexplained fever lasting 5 or more days and of at least four of five clinical criteria: (a) bilateral conjunctivitis; (b) erythematous oral mucosa, injected or dry fissured lips, and "strawberry tongue"; (c) erythema and indurated edema of hands and feet, often followed by periungual desquamation; (d) polymorphous skin rash; and (e) cervical nonsuppurative lymphadenopathy (226). Measles and group A β-hemolytic streptococcal infections may closely resemble Kawasaki disease and must be excluded (227). Recently, there have been limited reports of Kawasaki disease identified in HIV-infected individuals.

The course of the disease is divided into three clinical phases: acute, subacute, and convalescent. The acute phase lasts from the onset of fever to resolution (average 11 days). The subacute phase lasts until all clinical features of Kawasaki disease are resolved (average 2 weeks), and the convalescent phase is complete when erythrocyte sedimentation rate (ESR) and platelet count are normalized (4 to 8 weeks after fever onset). During the acute phase, 80% to 90% of patients experience a high-grade fever that does not respond to antipyretic medications; this may last 10 to 14 days or longer without treatment (228). Thrombocytosis develops during the second week of illness and typically resolves in 4 to 8 weeks; patients with thrombocytopenia at presentation are at significantly increased risk of coronary aneurysms. Eosinophils are elevated early in the disease course and continue to rise. ESR and C-reactive protein (CRP) levels are elevated at presentation and return to normal in 6 to 10 weeks. Up to 90% of patients will develop a cutaneous eruption, which usually appears around days 3 to 5. A wide array of dermatologic findings has been described in Kawasaki disease, ranging from a polymorphous erythematous diffuse eruption that may be macular, scarlatiniform, or erythema multiforme-like, to a papulosquamous presentation with scaling plaques. Urticarial exanthem, erythroderma, and micropustular eruptions are rare; vesicles and bullae are never present (229). Up to two-thirds of patients with Kawasaki disease develop a perineal rash which is typically scarlatiniform, may be tender, and desquamates during the acute phase of disease (230). Psoriasiform skin lesions may develop during any portion of the disease, potentially owing to the proinflammatory cytokine milieu (231,232). Erythema and edema of the hands and feet seen at presentation in 80% to 90% of patients and may be painful; erythema is typically well demarcated with a sharp division between the involved acral skin and the wrist or ankle. Periungual desquamation is one of the most common findings and occurs during the subacute phase, 2 to 3 weeks after fever onset, following erythema and edema of the hands and feet. Conjunctival injection, predominantly involving the bulbar conjunctiva rather than the palpebral conjunctiva and with sparing of the limbus, is common. Lymphadenopathy occurs in 50% to 60% of patients and is almost always unilateral and cervical; tenderness and overlying edema may be present. Oral mucosal findings are present in 80% to 90% of patients and may include lip fissuring, erythema of the oropharynx, nonexudative inflammation of the throat, and strawberry tongue. Nail findings may include red-brown chromonychia, leukonychia striata, Beau lines, onychomadesis, detachment of the hyponychium, and pincer-nail deformity. All of these nail manifestations resolve over time and nails regrow normally (233).

There are other associated systemic manifestations, with many of them being severe. Nearly 2% of children with Kawasaki disease die of cardiovascular complications (223). Twenty percent of untreated patients may develop coronary artery aneurysms (234); myocardial infarction secondary to aneurysmal thrombosis is the principal cause of death (235). The development of peripheral ischemia and gangrene are rare and serious complications (236).

Histopathology

The cutaneous histopathologic changes in Kawasaki disease consist of a sparse perivascular infiltrate of lymphocytes and histiocytes (223), marked papillary dermal edema, and dilation of blood vessels (237). Mild exocytosis of lymphocytes can be seen (230). An uncommon pustular variant of Kawasaki disease shows sterile intraepidermal spongiform pustules with neutrophils (238). Occasionally, cutaneous leukocytoclastic vasculitis can be seen in patients with peripheral gangrene (239).

Pathogenesis

Electron microscopic studies have revealed swelling and focal degenerative changes of endothelial cells in the superficial and deep vascular plexuses of the skin (237). Immunohistochemical stains have shown that the inflammatory infiltrate has predominantly CD4[+] (helper-inducer) T lymphocytes and CD13[+] macrophages, with only a few CD8[+] (suppressor-cytotoxic) T lymphocytes and no CD20[+] B lymphocytes. There is also expression of HLA-DR by keratinocytes and endothelial cells (240). In the acute stage of the disease, IL-1α and TNF-α can be detected in the epidermis. TNF-α is also found on blood vessel walls (240). All of these findings support the hypothesis of a cell-mediated immune reaction in the pathogenesis of the disease, possibly triggered by a virus (241), conventional antigen (242), or superantigen (243) in a genetically susceptible host (244). Recently, viral-like cytoplasmic inclusion bodies were found in tissues of patients with Kawasaki disease. These particles appear to contain proteins and RNA that may derive from an etiologic agent (245).

It has been suggested that vascular endothelial growth factor and hepatocyte growth factor might play important roles in the pathophysiology of Kawasaki disease (246). Autoantibodies against a 70-kDa protein from vascular smooth muscle cells may also contribute to the coronary and systemic vasculitis in Kawasaki disease (247).

Differential Diagnosis

The primary clinical differential diagnosis for Kawasaki disease includes viral exanthems, acute streptococcal and staphylococcal infections (particularly scarlet fever and staphylococcal scalded skin syndrome), and drug hypersensitivity reactions. Histopathologic features of cutaneous lesions in Kawasaki disease are not pathognomonic and can be similar to those of viral exanthems, drug eruptions, EAC, and polymorphous light eruption, particularly in cases with marked dermal edema.

Principles of Management

The primary goal of treatment in Kawasaki disease is to prevent cardiac complications, including coronary artery disease, aneurysm formation, myocardial infarction, and sudden death. Salicylates and intravenous immunoglobulin (IVIg) are used to manage the acute inflammatory aspects of the condition and prevent cardiovascular sequelae. Treatment should be started within the first 10 days of illness and ideally within the first 7 days to reduce the likelihood of the development of coronary abnormalities (248,249). IVIg is the predominant first-line therapy and can lead to rapid defervescence (250). It neutralizes circulating anti-myelin antibodies and downregulates proinflammatory cytokines including interferon gamma (IFN-γ). Failure of IVIg therapy has been associated with a gene polymorphism in plasma platelet-activating factor acetylhydrolase (251).

Approximately 10% to 15% of patients are refractory to conventional treatment and may require additional therapy such as intravenous pulse methylprednisolone (252) or infliximab (253). Patients with coronary abnormalities should receive antiplatelet agents or anticoagulants (249).

ADULT-ONSET STILL DISEASE

Clinical Summary

Adult-onset Still disease (AOSD) is a rare, idiopathic, systemic inflammatory disorder characterized by spiking fevers, a pink or salmon-colored rash, arthralgias, myalgias, striking neutrophilic leukocytosis, hyperferritinemia with low glycosylated ferritin (<20%), abnormal liver function tests, sore throat, abdominal pain, nausea, anorexia, hepatosplenomegaly, lymphadenopathy, and other stigmata of systemic inflammatory disease. The fever of AOSD is typically greater than 102.2°F (39°C). The rash typically develops during a fever episode and is classically pink or salmon in color; it may be pruritic and is generally evanescent. Inflammatory arthritis of the knees, wrists, ankles, and hips may occur, and if untreated, can result in destruction and long-term severe, disabling complications. Patients may rarely develop pericarditis or myocarditis. Rare but dangerous sequelae of AOSD include macrophage activation syndrome (MAS) or hemophagocytic lymphohistiocytosis (HLH) (254). Triggers of AOSD may include infection and malignancy.

The symptoms, frequency of episodes, and progression of the disorder are variable between patients and difficult to predict. AOSD may be considered the adult form of systemic juvenile idiopathic arthritis. Although AOSD was first reported in 1971, cases fitting the description of the disease date back to the late 1800s. There are three patterns of presentation of patients with AOSD (254):

- Monophasic: Patients have a single episode of symptoms lasting weeks to months but typically less than a year.
- Polyphasic (intermittent): recurrent episodes of symptoms. Patients are often symptom-free for weeks to years. Subsequent episodes tend to be more mild and shorter in duration compared to the initial episode.
- Chronic: patients have persistent episodes over time.

Histopathology

The histopathology of AOSD is varied and includes neutrophil-rich, lymphocyte-rich, and mixed neutrophilic and lymphocytic patterns. More specific histopathologic features may include intraepidermal neutrophils, epidermal acanthosis with dyskeratotic keratinocytes, vacuolar interface dermatitis, neutrophilic eccrine hidradenitis, and dermal mucin (255).

Pathogenesis

The pathogenesis of AOSD is multifactorial and poorly understood. Patients are believed to have a genetic predisposition to the development of autoinflammatory reactions to environmental triggers. Macrophage and neutrophil activation are hallmarks of the disease. Pathogen-associated or damage-associated molecular patterns trigger the dysregulated NLRP3 inflammasome, which triggers activation and secretion of proinflammatory cytokines including IL-1β and IL-18. This results in Th1 polarization of CD4+ lymphocytes. Activation of TLR-7 results in induction of the Th17 response in dendritic cells and neutrophil recruitment. The increased IL-1β results in increased production of TNF-α, IL-8, and IL-6. In turn, IL-6 is responsible for hepatic synthesis and release of ferritin. IL-18 triggers a NK cell–mediated interferon γ production, which increases macrophage activation. In some cases, macrophage activation can lead to MAS or hemophagocytic lymphohistiocytosis (HLH).

Differential Diagnosis

Given the variability of presentations, the differential diagnosis of AOSD is broad and includes viral infections, autoinflammatory disorders, lymphoma, Castleman disease, drug reaction with eosinophilia and systemic symptoms (DRESS), systemic lupus erythematosus, idiopathic inflammatory myositis, rheumatoid arthritis, systemic vasculitis, reactive arthritis, sarcoidosis, neutrophilic dermatosis, and Kikuchi–Fujimoto disease.

Principles of Management

In AOSD, it is believed that early treatment may mitigate some of the long-term or chronic sequelae of disease.

SYMMETRICAL DRUG-RELATED INTERTRIGINOUS AND FLEXURAL EXANTHEMA

Clinical Summary

Symmetrical drug-related intertriginous and flexural exanthema (SDRIFE) is a symmetrical erythematous eruption that occurs on the gluteal and intertriginous areas after exposure to one of many systemic medications. SDRIFE was initially described in

1984 as "baboon syndrome," a reference to the characteristic marked gluteal and thigh erythema (256). The term SDRIFE was proposed by Hausermann et al. in 2004 (258). SDRIFE is a clinical diagnosis based on a characteristic physical examination and a history of a systemically administered drug in the absence of contact allergens. Patients present with well-demarcated erythema in the gluteal, perianal, inguinal, or perigenital region, with involvement of at least one intertriginous area. Symmetry is required, as is an absence of systemic symptoms (257). Lesions are typically erythematous or maculopapular in nature, although reports of atypical presentations with pustules, papules, blisters, and purpuric lesions exist. Mucosal involvement is typically absent, as are facial and palmoplantar involvement.

The most commonly implicated medications include β-lactam antibiotics (particularly amoxicillin), non-β-lactam antibiotics (including pristinamycin, clindamycin, erythromycin, cotrimoxazole), anti-infectives (nystatin, terbinafine, fluconazole, metronidazole, valacyclovir), and assorted other medications including codeine, pseudoephedrine, cimetidine, allopurinol, heparin, hydroxyurea, oxycodone, naproxen, risperidone, antihypertensives, chemotherapeutic agents, and infliximab (258).

Histopathology

The histopathologic features of SDRIFE are nonspecific and highly variable; as such, SDRIFE is a clinical diagnosis, and biopsy is typically performed to rule out other causes of intertriginous exanthematous eruptions. There is typically a superficial perivascular mononuclear cell infiltrate containing scattered neutrophils and eosinophils (259). However, subcorneal pustules, epidermal keratinocytic necrosis, vacuolar interface dermatitis, and subepidermal bullae have been reported (260).

Pathogenesis

The pathogenic mechanisms underlying the development of SDRIFE are currently unclear, but it is thought to develop as a result of a type IV delayed hypersensitivity response. There is immunohistochemical evidence for CD4+ T-cell infiltration as well as increased endothelial and keratinocyte expression of CD26P-selectin, a protein that helps recruit helper T cells to sites of inflammation (259). Some data suggest that the pathogenesis of SDRIFE involves both a type IVa reaction involving CD4+ Th1 cells and macrophages and type IVc involving cytotoxic CD8+ T cells (261).

Differential Diagnosis

The differential diagnosis for SDRIFE includes other drug hypersensitivity reactions, seborrheic dermatitis, intertrigo, allergic contact dermatitis, inverse psoriasis, granular parakeratosis, Darier disease, and Hailey–Hailey. Other considerations include AGEP, DRESS, and fixed-drug eruption (FDE). Notably, AGEP and DRESS are characteristically widespread and accompanied by systemic symptoms.

Principles of Management

As with other drug hypersensitivity reactions, the main principle of treatment of SDRIFE is identification and removal of the offending agent. Topical corticosteroids, emollients, and antipruritic agents like pramoxine may be helpful in ameliorating symptoms. Skin patch testing after the resolution of the rash may be helpful in identifying the causative agent for future reference.

URTICARIA

Clinical Summary

Urticaria is characterized by the presence of abrupt-onset transient and recurrent wheals, which are raised erythematous and edematous areas of skin that are often pruritic. When large wheals occur and the edema extends to the subcutaneous or submucosal tissues, the process is referred to as angioedema (262). A large survey of nearly 1,000 patients revealed that angioedema can occur without urticarial flares (263).

Acute urticaria is a condition characterized by the transient appearance of smooth, erythematous, intensely pruritic elevated plaques or papules known as wheals. Lesions resolve without scarring over the course of hours. Acute urticaria lasts less than 6 weeks, although any individual lesion lasts only several hours.

When episodes of urticaria recur over more than 6 to 8 weeks, the condition is considered *chronic urticaria.*

When urticaria and angioedema occur simultaneously, the condition tends to have a chronic course. In approximately 15% to 25% of patients with chronic urticaria, an eliciting stimulus or underlying predisposing condition can be identified (264). The various causes of urticaria include soluble antigens in foods, drugs, and insect venom; contact allergens; physical stimuli such as pressure, vibration, solar radiation, or cold temperature; occult infections and malignancies; and some hereditary syndromes such as familial cold urticaria and Muckle–Wells syndrome (amyloidosis, nerve deafness, and urticaria), which are both inherited as an autosomal dominant trait and linked to chromosome 1q44. Schnitzler syndrome is characterized by a chronic urticaria and an IgM monoclonal gammopathy with evolution in 15% of patients to lymphoplasmacytic neoplasms (265,266). Recent evidence suggests that more than a third of chronic idiopathic urticarias may have an autoimmune basis for their condition (267) (see Pathogenesis discussion).

In *hereditary angioedema*, a rare form of dominantly inherited angioedema, recurrent attacks of edema involve not only the skin but also the oral, upper respiratory, and gastrointestinal tracts. Itching is absent, and there is no associated urticaria. Although not pruritic, lesions may be painful. Attacks are commonly precipitated by trauma such as dental extraction or emotional stress. Hereditary angioedema manifesting in late middle age after angiotensin-converting enzyme inhibitor therapy has been reported (268). Patients may later manifest autoimmune disorders such as systemic or discoid lupus erythematosus (269).

Urticarial vasculitis is a syndrome consisting of recurrent episodes of urticarial lesions often associated with arthralgia and abdominal pain and rarely with glomerulonephritis and obstructive pulmonary disease (270). The individual skin lesions tend to persist for 1 to 3 days and may resolve with purpura or hyperpigmentation (271). Lesions in urticarial vasculitis are not necessarily acral in distribution. Urticarial vasculitis should be suspected when individual lesions persist for more than 24 hours and produce burning or stinging sensations (272).

Urticarial vasculitis may be normo- or hypocomplementemic. Organ involvement is more common in hypocomplementemic urticarial vasculitis than in the normocomplementemic form (271). Hypocomplementemic vasculitis accounts for approximately 30% of cases of urticarial vasculitis (273). Hypocomplementemic urticarial vasculitis is characterized by low C1q and C4 levels, with variably decreased C3 (274).

C1q autoantibodies are commonly identified but are not specific and are found in 30% of cases of systemic lupus erythematosus (SLE) and 80% of SLE patients with glomerulonephritis (275).

Urticarial vasculitis is usually idiopathic but may be associated with SLE, infectious mononucleosis, infectious hepatitis, serum sickness, Sjögren syndrome, mixed cryoglobulinemia, polycythemia rubra vera (276), and B-cell lymphoma (277).

Urticarial vasculitis may antedate other manifestations of collagen vascular disease by months or years (278). Accordingly, the appropriate serologic studies should be performed and periodically monitored. Other associations with urticarial vasculitis include drugs, especially selective serotonin reuptake inhibitors (279).

Histopathology

In *acute urticaria*, there may be interstitial dermal edema, dilated venules with endothelial swelling, and a paucity of inflammatory cells. The histopathologic features of urticaria maybe subtle in some cases; urticaria is in the differential diagnosis of histopathologically normal skin. When there are significant histopathologic changes, one of two patterns is usually seen; a predominantly lymphoid infiltrate or more prominently neutrophilic. Lymphocyte-predominant urticaria is typically characterized by a perivascular infiltrate, whereas neutrophil-predominant is most often interstitial (280). The age of the lesion may impact the intensity of inflammatory changes. Changes are typically most prominent in the upper dermis, but deep dermal involvement may be present and the cellular infiltrate is generally mild. The presence of neutrophils in the lumen of small vessels may be a useful clue to the diagnosis of acute urticaria. Leukocytoclastic vasculitis is not present in acute urticaria.

In *chronic urticaria*, interstitial dermal edema and a perivascular and interstitial mixed-cell infiltrate with variable numbers of lymphocytes and a mixture of eosinophils and neutrophils are present (281) (Fig. 7-19).

In *angioedema*, the edema and infiltrate extend into the subcutaneous tissue. In *hereditary angioedema*, there is subcutaneous and submucosal edema without significant inflammatory infiltrate (282).

In *urticarial vasculitis*, the dermis shows leukocytoclastic vasculitis characterized by a superficial perivascular neutrophilic infiltrate with nuclear fragmentation (leukocytoclasis),

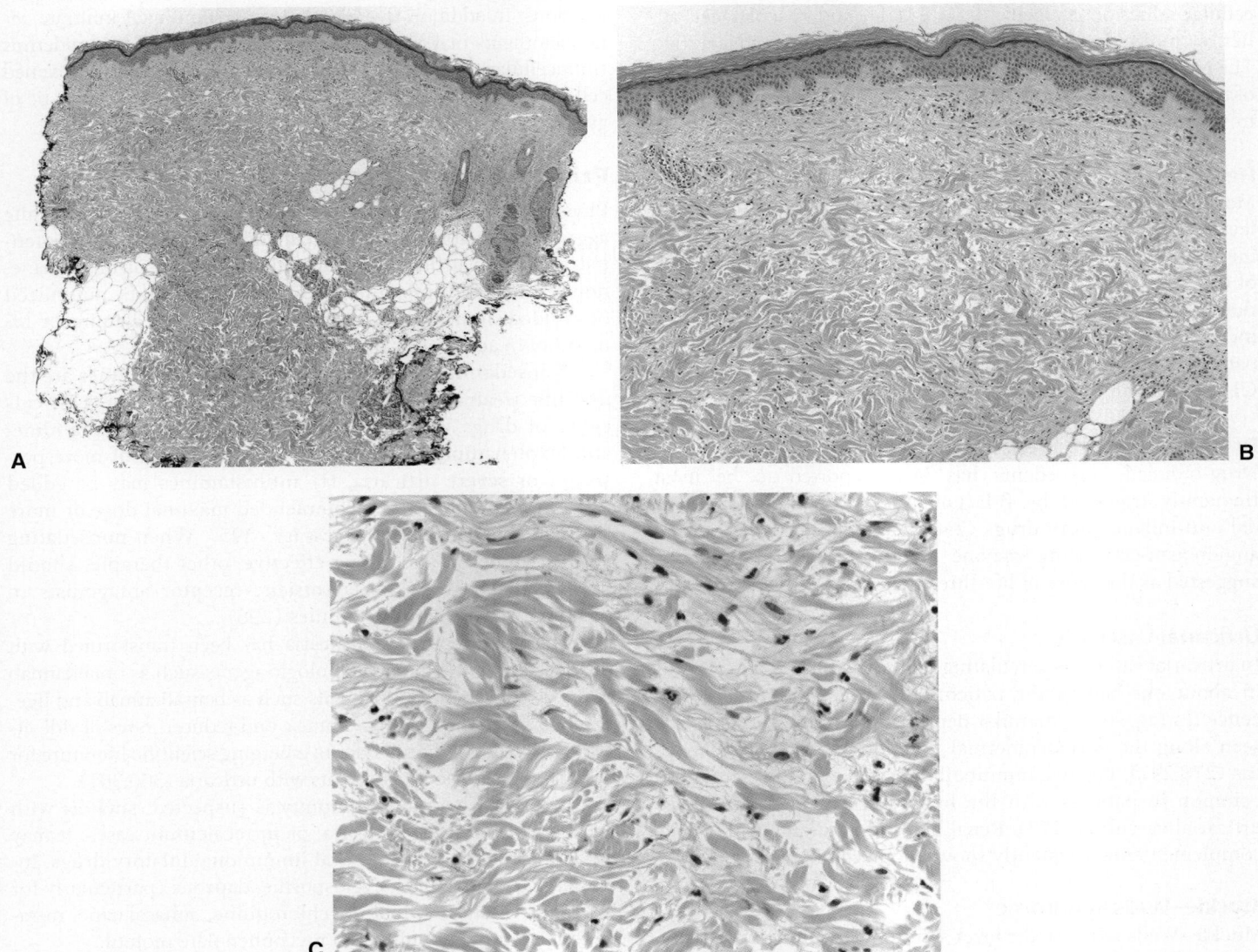

Figure 7-19. Urticaria. **A:** Sparse superficial perivascular and interstitial inflammatory infiltrate with dermal edema. **B:** Medium power image showing an interstitial infiltrate. **C:** Composed predominantly of neutrophils.

focal fibrinoid degeneration of vascular endothelia, and erythrocyte extravasation (283).

The urticarial lesions of *Muckle–Wells syndrome* are characterized by vasodilation and marked infiltration of neutrophils and monocytes/macrophages. There is increased expression of $\beta2$ integrins (284).

This histopathology of the urticarial lesions of *Schnitzler syndrome* is that of a neutrophilic urticaria.

Pathogenesis

Classic Urticaria

Electron microscopic examination reveals mast cell and eosinophil degranulation in common urticaria. Tryptase and FXIIIa have been identified within the granules of mast cells (285). In chronic urticaria, IgG autoantibodies cross-link the α chain of the high-affinity receptor for IgE on mast cells (FcϵRI), which results in histamine release. It appears that complement, especially C5a, augments histamine release (286,287). In addition, studies have shown that CD203c is a basophil activation marker that is upregulated by cross-linking of the FcϵRI α-receptor and may serve as a useful marker to identify patients with chronic urticaria (288). Chemotactic mediators are released from mast cells that induce a sequential upregulation of endothelial adhesion molecules (P-selectin, E-selectin, intercellular adhesion molecule 1 [ICAM-1], and vascular cell adhesion molecule 1) and of β_2-integrins on leukocytes (289). The presence of these autoantibodies against the FcϵRI α-subunit of the IgE receptor or IgE itself is detected in approximately 30% to 40% of patients with chronic urticaria (288).

Hereditary Angioedema

Most patients with hereditary angioedema have a low serum level of the esterase inhibitor of the first component of complement (C1-INH). Exhaustion of this inhibitor allows activation of C1. This leads to activation of C4 and C2, with the generation of a C2 fragment possessing kinin-like activity and causing increased vascular permeability (264). A smaller proportion of patients with hereditary angioedema have a deficit in functional C1-esterase inhibitor.

Drug-Induced Angioedema

Drug-induced angioedema has been reported to be most frequently triggered by β-lactam antibiotics and nonsteroidal anti-inflammatory drugs (290), and the increasing role of angiotensin-converting enzyme inhibitors (ACEIs) has been suggested as the cause of life-threatening angioedema (291).

Urticarial Vasculitis

In urticarial vasculitis, circulating immune complexes are found in about one-half of the patients. By direct immunofluorescence testing, strong granular deposits of immunoreactants are seen along the dermoepidermal junction and perivascular areas (278,292). Positive immunofluorescence findings are more common in patients with the hypocomplementemic form of urticarial vasculitis (273). Renal biopsy in patients with hypocomplementemia frequently shows glomerulonephritis (270).

Muckle–Wells Syndrome

Muckle–Wells is a periodic fever syndrome resulting from autosomal dominant mutation in *CIAS1*, which encodes the protein cryopyrin.

Schnitzler Syndrome

Schnitzler syndrome is an autoinflammatory disease, the etiology of which is just beginning to be understood. This condition is mediated by a number of mechanisms, including inappropriate inflammasome-mediated production of IL-1β and abnormalities in NFkB signaling, ubiquitination, cytokine signaling, and protein folding (293).

Differential Diagnosis

Clinical appearance and evolution of urticarial wheals are often very characteristic and diagnostic of the disease. Differential diagnosis of urticaria may include dermal hypersensitivity reactions to drugs or insect bites, contact dermatitis, gyrate erythema, viral exanthema, and the urticarial phase of bullous pemphigoid. Biopsy with direct immunofluorescence testing (DIF) is critical to differentiating the urticarial phase of bullous pemphigoid from chronic urticaria or urticarial vasculitis.

The absence of epidermal changes with the presence of dermal edema and a mixed infiltrate of neutrophils and eosinophils favor the diagnosis of urticaria. The infiltrate is more interstitial in urticaria than in drug reactions. A predominance of eosinophils within the inflammatory infiltrate is more common in drug and insect bite reactions (294). Epidermal changes, including focal necrosis and spongiosis, are characteristically seen in insect bite reactions. In addition to a lymphocyte-predominant infiltrate, viral exanthems may show reticular degeneration of the epidermis (intracellular edema leading to a fenestrated pattern of retained cell membranes). A tight perivascular infiltrate is characteristic of gyrate erythemas.

Principles of Management

Physical triggers (e.g., cold, overheating, pressure), nonspecific aggravating factors (e.g., stress, alcohol), and drugs with potential to worsen urticaria or angioedema (e.g., aspirin, codeine, nonsteroidal anti-inflammatories, ACEIs) should be minimized or avoided. Topical antipruritic lotions, such as calamine or 1% menthol in aqueous cream, can be soothing (295).

Nonsedating second generation H_1 antihistamines are the first-line treatment in most cases of acute urticaria. This category of drugs includes loratidine, cetirizine, desloratidine, and fexofenadine among others (296). In cases of more persistent or severe urticaria, H_2 antihistamines may be added (297). Doses above the recommended maximal dose or more frequent dosing may be necessary (295). When nonsedating antihistamines are no longer effective, other therapies should be considered, such as leukotriene receptor antagonists in combination with antihistamines (298).

The management of urticaria has been transformed with the development of targeted biologic agents such as omalizumab (299). Second-generation agents such as benralizumab and ligelizumab show tremendous promise and reduced rates of side effects, and readers should refer to emerging scientific literature for optimal management of patients with urticaria (300,301).

In cases where autoimmunity is suspected, such as with an abnormal chronic urticaria, or in recalcitrant cases, it may be appropriate to consider oral immunomodulatory drugs, including corticosteroids, cyclosporine, dapsone (particularly for urticarial vasculitis), hydroxychloroquine, sulfasalazine, intravenous immunoglobulin, and mycophenolate mofetil.

Intramuscular epinephrine can be lifesaving in anaphylaxis and in severe laryngeal angioedema (295), and patients with a suggestive history should be counseled to carry epi-pens for self-administration.

Given the autoinflammatory etiology of Schnitzler syndrome, treatment with IL-1 receptor antagonist anakinra offers complete control of symptoms in 80% of patients. Other options include canakinumab, an anti-IL1β antibody and rilonacept, a fusion protein that neutralizes IL-1 (302). Rilonacept and canakinumab have also been approved for the treatment of Muckle–Wells syndrome.

ERYTHEMA ANNULARE CENTRIFUGUM

Clinical Summary

EAC is considered a chronic reactive form of gyrate erythema and represents a hypersensitivity reaction manifesting as arcuate and polycyclic areas of erythema, typically in response to an underlying trigger. Triggers may include cutaneous fungal infections; internal malignancy; adverse medication reactions; pregnancy; and a variety of hematologic, endocrine, and

rheumatic disorders. Resolution of the underlying condition typically results in resolution of the EAC, although in the majority of cases the trigger remains unknown.

The condition has been categorized into superficial and deep variants. The superficial variant is more common, comprising up to 80% of cases, and is characterized by the presence of trailing scale—a delicate annular rim of scale that trails behind the advancing edge of erythema (303) (Fig. 7-20). Small vesicles may occur. The deep form was originally described by Darier and is characterized by annular areas of palpable erythema with central clearing and absence of surface changes (304).

The lesions may attain considerable size (up to 10 cm in diameter) over a period of several weeks, expanding up to 2 to 3 mm/day. They may be mildly pruritic and have a predilection for the trunk and proximal extremities. Most cases resolve spontaneously within 6 weeks; however, the condition may persist or recur for years. In a study of 66 patients with EAC, the lower extremities were the most frequently involved area and the superficial variant was more common than the deep form, 78% versus 22%, respectively (305).

Histopathology

In the superficial variant of EAC, there is a superficial perivascular tightly cuffed lymphohistiocytic infiltrate with endothelial cell swelling and focal extravasation of erythrocytes in the papillary dermis (Fig. 7-21). In addition, there is focal epidermal spongiosis and parakeratosis (303).

In the classic deep form, or indurated type, of EAC, a superficial and deep perivascular lymphocytic infiltrate characterized by a tightly cuffed "coat-sleeve–like" pattern is present in the mid- and deep dermis (Fig. 7-22). Occasionally, focal vacuolar alteration of the basal layer keratinocytes may be noted in the deep variant (306).

Pathogenesis

The exact pathogenesis of EAC is not clear. It has been associated with occult infections, dermatophytosis, candidiasis, medications, hormonal changes and, rarely, an underlying malignancy (307–309). Because a patient responded with complete clearance with etanercept, it has been suggested that it may be a TNF-dependent process (310).

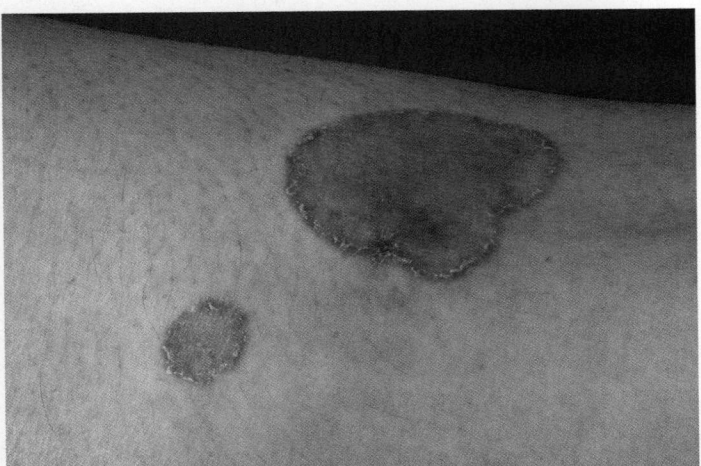

Figure 7-20 Erythema annulare centrifugum. Characteristic delicate annular rim of scale trailing behind the edge of erythema. (Courtesy of Ronald O. Perelman Department of Dermatology, New York University School of Medicine, New York, New York.)

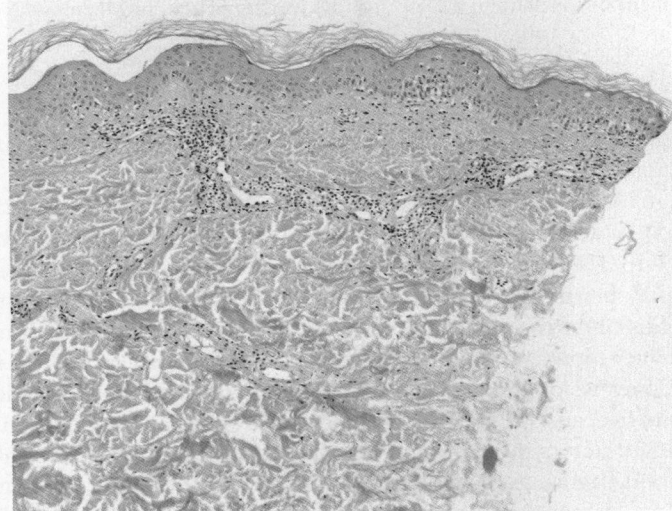 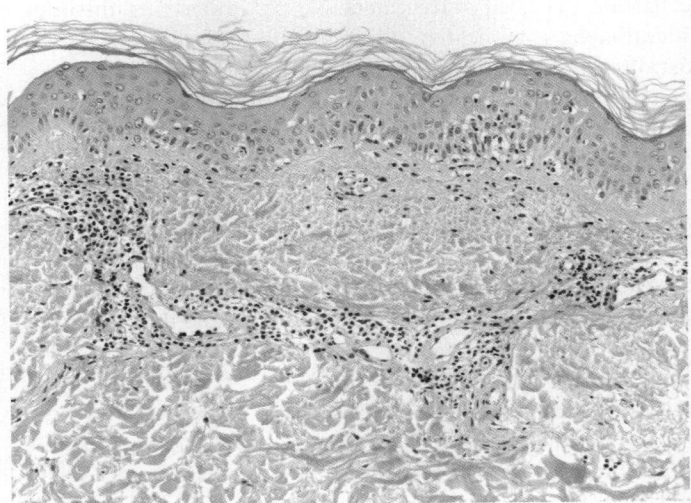

A   B

Figure 7-21 Erythema annulare centrifugum, superficial form. Medium power (A) and higher power (B) images showing spongiosis with "tightly cuffed" perivascular lymphocytic infiltrate.

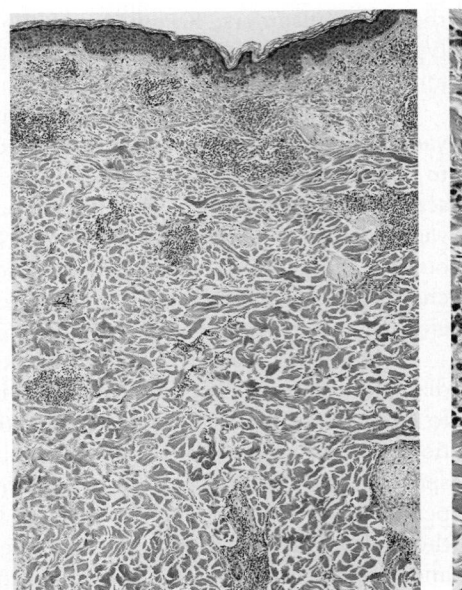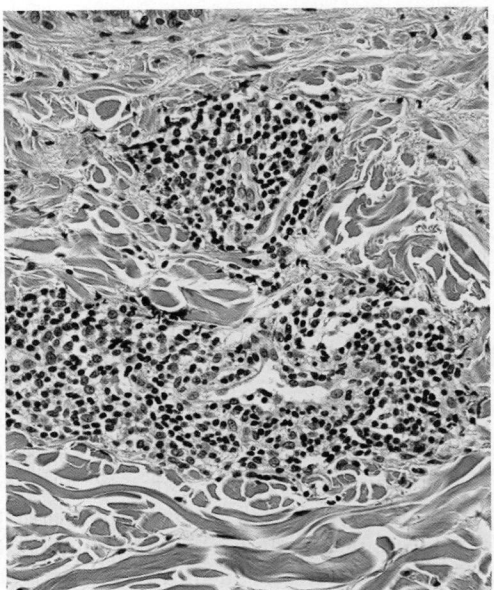

Figure 7-22 Erythema annulare centrifugum, deep form. **A:** Superficial and deep, dense perivascular lymphocytic infiltrate. **B:** Dense "tightly cuffed" perivascular lymphocytic infiltrate.

Differential Diagnosis

The rather striking coat-sleeve–like tightly perivascular arrangement of the infiltrate seen in the deep form of gyrate erythema is encountered also in secondary syphilis. However, in secondary syphilis, plasma cells and histiocytes, with endothelial cell edema, are usually present. The presence of increased deposits of connective tissue mucin and periadnexal lymphoid infiltrates may help to distinguish tumid lupus erythematosus from EAC.

Principles of Management

EAC is usually a self-limited process and may not require any treatment. In the case of EAC associated with fungal infection, treatment of the underlying infection may result in clearance of the gyrate erythema. Topical and systemic steroids and calcipotriol may ameliorate pruritus, and there have been reports of efficacy of metronidazole and etanercept in the resolution of the lesions (310,311). Treatment of any underlying disorder, if identifiable, is indicated, although the underlying trigger is most often not identified. Given the low incidence of EAC associated with malignancy, most do not consider EAC alone a reason to embark on a paraneoplastic workup.

LICHEN PLANUS

Lichen planus is a common subacute or chronic dermatosis that may involve skin, mucous membranes, hair follicles, and nails (312).

Clinical Summary

The eruption is characterized by small, flat-topped, shiny, polygonal, violaceous papules that may coalesce into plaques. The papules often show a network of white lines known as Wickham striae (Fig. 7-23). Pruritus is usually pronounced. The disease has a predilection for the flexor surfaces of the forearms, legs, and glans penis; palmoplantar involvement is rare. Lichen

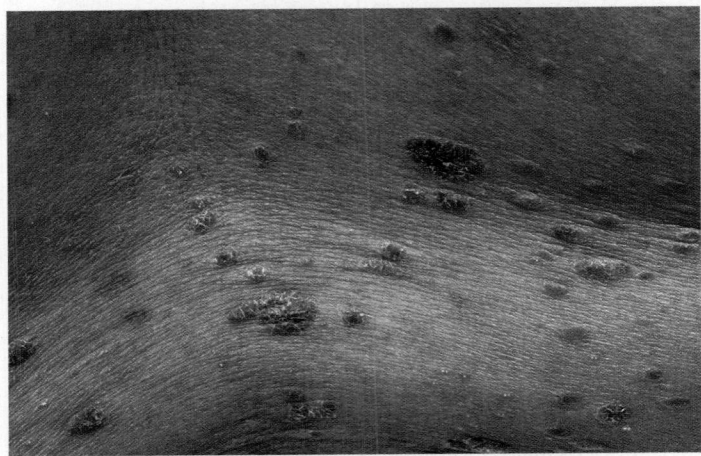

Figure 7-23 Lichen planus. Flat-topped, shiny, violaceous papules with white Wickham striae. (Courtesy of Ronald O. Perelman Department of Dermatology, New York University School of Medicine, New York, New York.)

planus may be localized or extensive, and Koebner phenomenon is commonly seen.

Mucosal involvement in lichen planus can be seen in the oral cavity, esophagus, or genitals including the glans and labia (313,314). Oral lesions of lichen planus are frequently seen and may be the sole manifestation of the disease. The buccal and glossal mucosa are commonly involved with lesions displaying a lacy reticular network of white coalescent papules (Fig. 7-24). Other lesional patterns include plaque-like, atrophic, papular, erosive, and bullous (315). Among the aggravating and/or etiologic factors in oral lesions are stress, contact allergy to metals, food flavorings, spicy foods, and poor oral hygiene (315,316). Involvement of esophagus may occur, affecting more females and frequently presenting as the initial manifestation of mucocutaneous lichen planus (314,317).

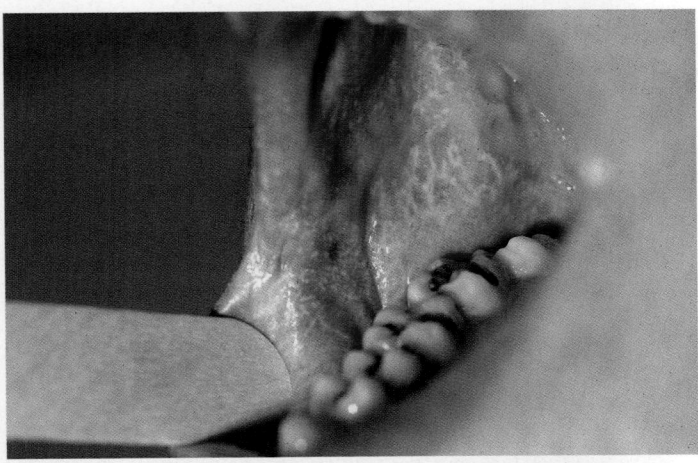

Figure 7-24 Oral lichen planus. Lacy reticular network of white coalescent papules involving the buccal and labial mucosa. (Courtesy of Department of Dermatology, University of Pennsylvania School of Medicine, Philadelphia, Pennsylvania.)

The nails are involved in about 10% of cases and show roughening, longitudinal ridging, and rarely, thinning with destruction. Dorsal pterygium formation is a frequent finding. Fingernails are more frequently involved than toenails (318).

Clinical cutaneous subtypes include hypertrophic, atrophic, annular, vesicular, eruptive, linear, erosive/ulcerative, lichen planus actinicus, lichen planus pigmentosus, lichen planopilaris, lichen planus pemphigoides, and overlap syndrome with lupus erythematosus. A rare variant, eruptive or exanthematous lichen planus has also been described, with generalized erythematous polygonal or umbilicated papules and macules (319).

Hypertrophic lichen planus is a common variant that is usually found on the shins and consists of thickened, often verrucous plaques. Although often characteristic clinically, these lesions may be challenging to differentiate from squamous cell carcinoma histopathologically, with histopathologic overlap, especially in superficial shave biopsies. The *atrophic* variant is usually the result of resolution of hypertrophic or annular lesions. In the *annular* subtype, male genitalia and intertriginous areas such as axilla and groins are usually involved. Less commonly, the trunk or eyelids are affected (320).

Vesicular/bullous lichen planus is rare and shows vesicles situated only on some of the preexisting lesions. It is different from *lichen planus pemphigoides*, in which the eruption is more disseminated and the bullae are more extensive, arising from both the papules of lichen planus or from normal-appearing skin (321,322). Although lichen planus pemphigoides manifesting exclusively in the oral mucosa has been reported (322), the bullous lesions are more acrally distributed, and involvement of palms and soles are reported more frequently in children (323). There are also several reports of this variant being induced by various drugs (323,324). Although lichen planus pemphigoides and bullous pemphigoid manifest in different ways clinically, the same antigen may be involved in the immunopathogenesis of these two diseases (see the Direct Immunofluorescence Studies in Lichen Planus section below for details).

Lichen planopilaris (see also discussion in Chapter 18) designates the folliculotropic variant of lichen planus, which predominantly involves the scalp. Initially, there may only be

follicular papules or perifollicular erythema; however, with progressive hair loss, irregularly shaped atrophic patches of scarring alopecia develop on the scalp. The axillae and the pubic region may also be affected, and the alopecia in these areas may be cicatricial (325). Hyperkeratotic follicular papules may also be seen, particularly on the face. The association of scarring alopecia and hyperkeratotic follicular papules is known as Graham-Little syndrome. Lichen planopilaris may coexist with typical lesions of lichen planus on skin, mucous membranes, or nails, but these findings are not always present, which can make differentiating lichen planopilaris from other scarring alopecias challenging. Linear lichen planopilaris of the face resolving with scarring has also been described.

Ulcerative/erosive lichen planus, a rare but quite characteristic variant of lichen planus, manifests as bullae, erosions, and painful ulcerations on the feet and toes, resulting in atrophic scarring and permanent loss of the toenails. It is highly resistant to therapy and usually associated with patches of atrophic alopecia of the scalp and with cutaneous and oral lesions of lichen planus (326,327).

Lichen planus actinicus or *subtropicus*, also known as *lichen planus pigmentosus*, occurs mainly in Middle Eastern countries, where between 20% and 30% of the cases of lichen planus are of this type (328). This condition may be closely related to EDP or ashy dermatosis, discussed later. Lichen planus pigmentosus tends to be more common in children or young adults. The lesions develop in spring and summer on sun-exposed areas, especially the face. Three different forms have been described: annular (the most common type), pigmented (resembling melasma), and dyschromic (329,330). The lesions are typically annular plaques with central slate blue to light brown pigmentation and well-defined, slightly raised hypopigmented borders. Pruritus is minimal or absent.

The *overlap syndrome* or *lichen planus/lupus erythematosus* refers to a heterogeneous group of patients bearing simultaneous lesions with clinical, histopathologic, and/or immunologic features typical of both diseases (331). The cutaneous findings include erythematous to purplish scaly patches and plaques, some of which show central atrophy, with a predilection for photodistributed areas or acral portions of extremities (331).

Twenty-nail dystrophy may be encountered in adults as well as children. The nails have longitudinal ridging and distal notching and splitting. With time, they become thin and roughened. Clinically, the nail changes resemble those seen in lichen planus (332). Other manifestations of lichen planus are usually absent. In children, the nail changes tend to resolve spontaneously after a few years. In familial cases, it tends to have an unremitting course. Congenital cases have been described (333). The clinical finding of diffuse trachyonychia is not specific to lichen planus and may be associated with other conditions, such as atopic dermatitis, psoriasis, alopecia areata, and more rare genetic syndromes.

Lichen Planus in Childhood. Lichen planus is more common in adults; however, the disease occurring in children has also been reported. The largest series from India, consisting of 316 children, reported the mean age of 10, with the classic type as the commonest manifestation, followed by eruptive, hypertrophic, linear, and lichen planopilaris variants. Cutaneous lesions were seen in the majority, followed by oral mucosa, nails, and genitalia (334).

Malignant transformation of cutaneous lichen planus occurs in less than 1% of cases (335). In hypertrophic lichen planus of the leg, development of squamous cell carcinoma, verrucous carcinoma, or keratoacanthoma is a rare occurrence (336,337). There have been reports of squamous cell carcinoma arising occasionally on long-standing lesions of lichen planus on mucous membranes or the vermillion border of the lips (338,339). The incidence of carcinoma evolving in oral lichen planus is about 0.5% (340), with a range of 0.3% to 3%. Development of squamous cell carcinoma in association with esophageal lichen planus has been recently reported, highlighting the importance of timely diagnosis of lichen planus in esophagus and its follow-up (317). It seems that expression of desmocollin 1 in the atrophic variant of oral lichen planus may be a predictor of the dysplasia, and expression of E-cadherin is a predictor of squamous cell carcinoma (341). Development of carcinoma in ulcers of the feet in ulcerative lichen planus has been reported in lesions that had not been previously grafted (342).

Lichen planus has been reported to be associated with several entities including but not limited to chronic hepatitis C infection, hepatitis B vaccination, vitiligo, and radiation therapy (343–348). An erosive lichen planus–like dermatitis has been reported in association with long-term hydroxyurea treatment (349). Drug-induced lichenoid eruptions that can resemble lichen planus are not uncommon, with a long and growing list of offending agents (see discussion in Chapter 11). The coexistence of lichen nitidus with lichen planus is frequent enough, suggesting that both entities are variants of the same disease.

Histopathology

Typical papules of lichen planus show (a) compact orthokeratosis, (b) wedge-shaped hypergranulosis, (c) irregular acanthosis, (d) vacuolar alteration of the basal layer, and (e) a bandlike dermal lymphocytic infiltrate in close approximation to the epidermis (Fig. 7-25). This constellation of findings is sufficiently diagnostic that a histopathologic diagnosis can be rendered in more than 90% of the cases.

The cornified layer shows compact orthokeratosis and contains very few, if any, parakeratotic cells, a fact that is important for the diagnosis. The thickening of the granular layer is uneven and wedge shaped. The granular cells appear increased in size and contain coarse and more abundant keratohyalin granules. On step sectioning, the areas of wedge-shaped hypergranulosis are found to be contiguous to intraepidermal adnexal structures—namely, acrosyringia and acrotrichia. Wickham striae are believed to be caused by focal increase in the thickness of the granular layer and the stratum spinosum.

The acanthosis in lichen planus is irregular and affects the stratum spinosum and the suprapapillary plates. Keratinocytes of the stratum spinosum often appear larger with more eosinophilic cytoplasm, consistent with increased cytoplasmic keratin. The rete ridges are irregularly hyperplastic, some with jagged or pointed interface with the underlying dermis, giving them a saw-toothed appearance. The dermal papillae between elongated rete ridges are often dome shaped.

The basal layer keratinocytes are not clearly visible in early lesions because the dense dermal infiltrate obscures the dermal–epidermal junction with vacuolar alteration and necrosis of these cells. In fully developed lesions, basal layer keratinocytes resemble the keratinocytes of the upper epidermis, so-called squamatized.

The lymphoid and histiocytic infiltrate in the upper dermis is bandlike and sharply demarcated at its lower border. A few

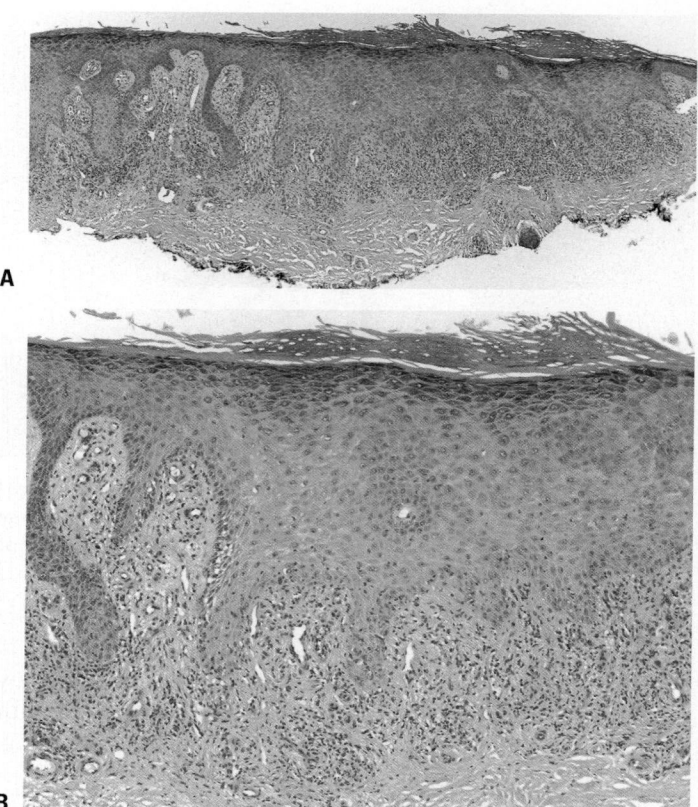

Figure 7-25 Lichen planus. Dense, bandlike infiltrate predominantly of lymphocytes in the papillary dermis (**A**), with wedge-shaped hypergranulosis, compact orthokeratosis, and irregular acanthosis, and vacuolar alteration of the basal layer (**B**).

rare eosinophils and/or plasma cells may be seen. Papillary dermal melanophages are present, often in considerable number, as a result of damage to the basal cells and pigment incontinence. In some instances, the dermal lymphocytic infiltrate is seen in juxtaposition to the acrosyringium, and vacuolar alteration of the acrosyringeal basal cell layer is a prominent finding (*acrosyringeal lichen planus*) (350).

In old lesions, the cellular infiltrate decreases in density, but the number of melanophages increases. In areas in which a basal cell layer has regenerated, the dermal infiltrate no longer lies in close approximation to the epidermis.

Hypertrophic lichen planus shows considerable acanthosis, papillomatosis, hypergranulosis, and hyperkeratosis and may mimic well-differentiated invasive squamous cell carcinoma. The interface vacuolar changes are discrete and often limited to the base of the rete ridges.

Necrotic keratinocytes are present in most of the cases in the lower epidermis and especially in the papillary dermis. Homogeneous eosinophilic deposits, referred to as apoptotic, dyskeratotic, colloid, hyaline, cytoid, or Civatte bodies, may have a diameter of up to 20 μm. These PAS-positive and diastase-resistant aggregates of keratin and immunoglobulin are most commonly seen in lichen planus. However, colloid bodies are characteristically seen in any interface dermatitis in which damage to the basal cells occurs, including graft-versus-host disease, lichen nitidus, lupus erythematosus, and drug reactions, as well as in inflamed keratoses such as lichenoid actinic keratosis and lichen planus–like keratosis. They may even be seen in normal skin. In lichen planus, the colloid bodies may be numerous and form clusters in the uppermost dermis. Their aggregation may result in the perforation of the epidermis with subsequent transepidermal elimination (351).

When there is extensive damage to the basal layer keratinocytes, clefting between the epidermis and the dermis, known as Max Joseph spaces, may occur. When extensive, this may form subepidermal blisters as is seen in *vesicular lichen planus*.

Oral Lichen Planus

The oral lesions of lichen planus differ in their histopathologic appearance from those of the skin because the granular cell layer is normally absent in the oral mucosa. Indeed, the presence of a granular cell layer in mucosa is one of the histopathologic hallmarks of oral lichen planus. Additionally, lichen planus in the oral mucosa may show parakeratosis rather than orthokeratosis without a granular layer, although alternating areas of both types of keratinization with the presence of a granular layer may also be observed (Fig. 7-26). Epidermal atrophy and ulceration are more common in oral lichen planus than in cutaneous lesions.

Lichen Planopilaris

Most early lesions of lichen planopilaris show a perifollicular lymphocytic infiltrate at the level of the infundibulum and the isthmus where the hair "bulge" is located (Fig. 7-27). Initially, the inferior segment of the hair follicle is spared. Vacuolar changes of the basal layer of the outer root sheath and necrotic keratinocytes are often seen. In addition, orthokeratosis, follicular plugging, and wedge-shaped hypergranulosis of the infundibulum may be seen. The interfollicular epidermis is often spared, but it can occasionally be involved (352). In more developed lesions, perifollicular fibrosis and epithelial atrophy at the level of the infundibulum and isthmus are characteristic findings (Fig. 7-28) and give rise to an hourglass configuration. It is hypothesized that damage to the hair bulge, where the stem cells of the hair follicle supposedly reside, results in permanent scarring alopecia (353). Advanced cases show alopecia with vertically oriented fibrotic tracts containing clumps of degenerated elastic fibers that had replaced the destroyed hair follicles. This end-stage scarring alopecia in which no visible hair

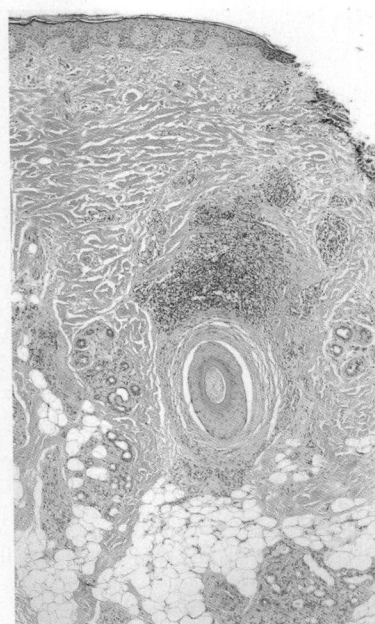

Figure 7-27 Lichen planopilaris, vertical section. Dense perifollicular lymphocytic infiltrate and fibrosis at the level of the isthmus.

follicles remain is called pseudopelade of Brocq and may occur after any form of scarring alopecia (354).

The hyperkeratotic follicular papules that are occasionally seen in association with lichen planopilaris of the scalp exhibit similar changes; however, perifollicular fibrosis is usually slight, and the process does not eventuate in scarring (355).

Ulcerative/Erosive Lichen Planus

In ulcerative lichen planus, samples taken from the tissue adjacent to the ulcer generally show histopathologic changes diagnostic of lichen planus; biopsy of the ulcer will yield nonspecific findings.

Lichen Planus Actinicus

In some instances, the histopathologic picture of lichen planus actinicus is similar to that of the typical lichen planus but with epidermal atrophy at the center of the lesion and more papillary dermal melanophages (348). Because of the histopathologic resemblance in some cases, a relationship between lichen planus actinicus and EDP has been postulated (356); however, they have significant clinical differences, mostly the more widespread and non–sun-exposed distribution of the lesions in the latter.

Overlap Syndrome–Lichen Planus/Lupus Erythematosus

In some cases of the overlap syndrome, the histopathologic features and direct immunofluorescence findings are more consistent with lichen planus. In others, the immunofluorescence testing favors lupus erythematosus, and still in another subset of patients, there are lesions of lichen planus that coexist rather than overlap with those of lupus erythematosus (357).

Twenty-Nail Dystrophy

Histopathologic data on twenty-nail dystrophy are sparse, and vary based on the underlying cause (333). Biopsies may show typical lichen planus involving the nail matrix (332); however, spongiosis may be prominent as in cases associated with atopic dermatitis.

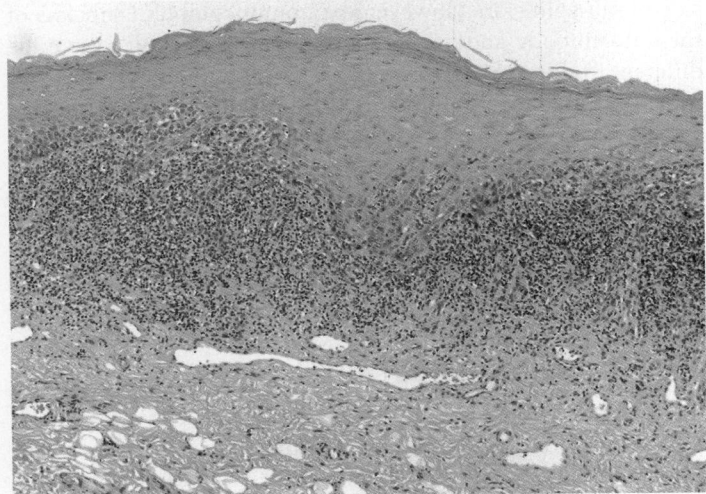

Figure 7-26 Oral lichen planus. Similar lichenoid inflammatory pattern, but with less hypergranulosis than the skin. Also note the focal granular cell layer that is normally absent in oral mucosa.

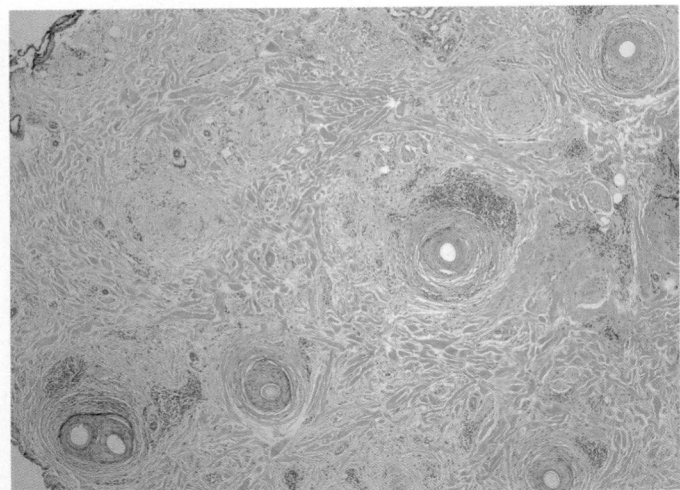 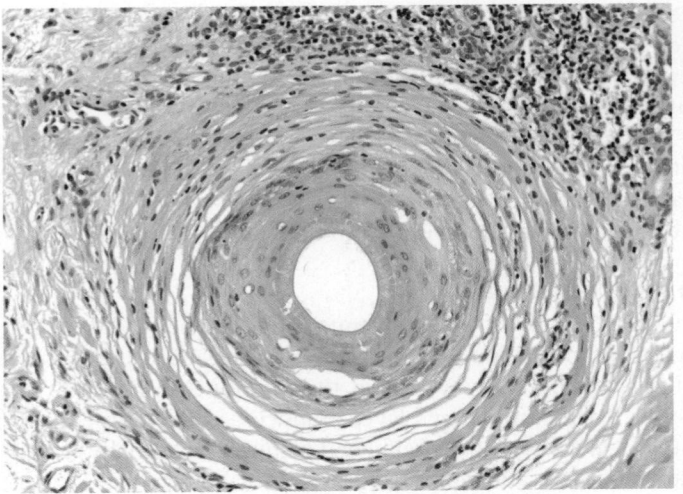

Figure 7-28 Lichen planopilaris, horizontal section. (A) Circumferential perifollicular fibrosis with associated lymphocytic infiltrate, fibrous stellae, and absence of sebaceous glands, and fusion of follicles. (B) Perifollicular fibrosis and interface changes, including dyskeratosis.

Lichen Planus Pemphigoides

In lichen planus pemphigoides, biopsies taken from blisters arising from uninvolved skin show subepidermal bullae with an infiltrate that contains eosinophils (358).

Electron Microscopy of Lichen Planus

Basal keratinocytes in lichen planus, together with their desmosomes and hemidesmosomes, show degenerative changes (359). Whereas the tonofilaments in the basal cells are decreased in early lesions, they are increased in later lesions (360). Because of the presence of degenerated and necrotic keratinocytes in the basal layer, it is assumed that the basal cells in later lesions are largely regenerated cells. The dermal infiltrate, extending to the epidermis, causes damage to the lamina densa such as fragmentation. This may be followed by duplication and irregular folding of the lamina densa. The dermal infiltrate contains mainly lymphocytes, but it also contains macrophages. Some of the lymphocytes have hyperconvoluted nuclei and may be indistinguishable from Sézary cells.

Colloid bodies are located largely in the papillary dermis but also in the lowermost epidermis. These aggregates of filament bundles, with each filament measuring approximately 10 nm in diameter, stain positively for keratins (361). Colloid bodies often still contain cell organelles, such as melanosomes and mitochondria, but only rarely contain nuclear material. Fibrin deposits in the upper dermis are a common finding in electron microscopy studies. In the vesicular lesions of lichen planus, electron microscopic examination shows cytolysis of basal keratinocytes with the blister cavity situated below the spinous layer.

Direct Immunofluorescence Studies in Lichen Planus

Classically, the direct immunofluorescence findings of lichen planus are characterized by fibrinogen deposition as shaggy deposits at the dermal–epidermal junction and numerous colloid bodies (362). Only occasionally are there granular deposits of IgM or linear deposits of C3, or both IgG and C3 in the basement membrane zone (363). Nearly 90% of cases will show colloid bodies staining predominantly for IgM but often also for IgG, IgA, C3, and fibrin. Although colloid bodies are found occasionally in many other conditions with damage

to the basal cell layer, such as lupus erythematosus, they are highly suggestive of lichen planus if present in large numbers or arranged in clusters.

In lichen planopilaris, direct immunofluorescence in many specimens shows deposition of IgM and/or IgA, IgG, and, rarely, C3 at the level of the infundibulum and isthmus (364). There is often deposition of fibrinogen in a shaggy pattern surrounding the affected follicles. The dermal–epidermal junction is virtually always negative for deposition of immunoreactants (352).

In lichen planus pemphigoides, direct immunofluorescence of perilesional skin shows the presence of IgG and C3 in a linear arrangement along the basement membrane zone (365). On immunoelectron microscopy, C3 is localized within the lamina lucida, analogous to its location in bullous pemphigoid. It has been shown that circulating IgG autoantibodies are directed against the bullous pemphigoid antigen 180 (BP180, type XVII collagen), a transmembrane hemidesmosomal glycoprotein of the basal keratinocytes that spans the lamina lucida (366,367). Immunoelectron microscopic studies have also confirmed that the location of the antigen is at the same site as the bullous pemphigoid antigen, the basal cell hemidesmosomes on the epidermal side of salt-split skin. However, the immunoglobulin subclass of the autoantibody and/or the epitope that is recognized may be different in these two diseases (366). One study in lichen planus has shown that in addition to BP180 antigen, the autoantibodies were directed against a 200-kDa antigen (368).

In the overlap syndrome–lichen planus/lupus erythematosus, some patients show immunofluorescence testing consistent with lichen planus; yet another group demonstrates deposition of immunoglobulins and C3 at the dermal–epidermal junction in a linear granular pattern as in cutaneous lupus erythematosus.

Differential Diagnosis

It should be emphasized that parakeratosis is not a feature of lichen planus of the skin and that if more than focal parakeratosis is present, a diagnosis of lichen planus should not be made on histopathologic grounds.

Focal parakeratosis and adjacent solar elastosis in an otherwise typical histopathologic picture of lichen planus may be regarded as lichen planus–like keratosis, even more so if there is a solitary and nonpruritic lesion (369). Lichenoid drug eruptions may be differentiated from lichen planus by the presence of focal parakeratosis with concomitant absence of the granular layer, intraepidermal colloid bodies, exocytosis of lymphocytes to the upper layers of the epidermis, and a deeper inflammatory infiltrate with eosinophils (370).

Differentiation from lichenoid lupus erythematosus is based on (a) atrophy of the epidermis in addition to acanthosis, (b) minimal squamotization of basal layer keratinocytes, (c) a superficial bandlike infiltrate with a superficial and deep perivascular and periadnexal infiltrate, (d) the presence of a thickened, PAS-positive basement membrane, and (e) increased dermal connective tissue mucin. Direct immunofluorescence findings may also be helpful; in lupus erythematosus linear or granular deposits of immunoglobulins and C3 predominate in lesional skin, whereas in lichen planus clusters of necrotic keratinocytes with absorbed immunoglobulins and complement are found. Langerhans cells are decreased in number in discoid and SLE; in contrast, they are increased in early lichen planus (371).

The epidermal changes in chronic graft-versus-host disease may be similar to those in lichen planus; however, the inflammatory infiltrate tends to be perivascular instead of bandlike. In addition, the number of Langerhans cells in graft-versus-host disease is decreased, and nearly all intraepidermal lymphocytes are cytotoxic-suppressor T cells.

In long-standing hypertrophic lichen planus, the basal layer may minimal residual damage, and the infiltrate may no longer be bandlike, rendering differentiation from lichen simplex chronicus and well-differentiated invasive squamous cell carcinoma at times difficult. However, in hypertrophic lichen planus, damage to the basal layer at the base of the rete ridges is often seen; colloid bodies and pigment incontinence are additional clues. Absence of perforating elastic fibers has been suggested as a method to distinguish hypertrophic lichen planus from invasive squamous cell carcinoma, but significant histopathologic overlap can remain between these entities, necessitating clinicopathologic correlation to reach a diagnosis (372,373).

On the lips and in the mouth, the differentiation of lichen planus from early squamous cell carcinoma in situ ("dysplastic leukoplakia") may be clinically and histopathologically challenging. Both diseases may show hyperkeratosis and an inflammatory infiltrate close to the epidermis/epithelium. However, thorough microscopic study reveals more atypical keratinocytes in squamous cell carcinoma in situ. Furthermore, squamous cell carcinoma in situ is more likely than lichen planus to show irregular downward proliferation of the rete ridges and numerous plasma cells. A broad range of inflammatory disorders that can mimic oral lichen planus, including chronic graft-versus-host disease, orofacial granulomatosis, lupus erythematosus, mucous membrane pemphigoid, chronic ulcerative stomatitis, lichen planus pemphigoides, and lichen sclerosus (374).

Lichen planopilaris of the scalp must be differentiated in its early phase from discoid lupus erythematosus, which affects the hair follicles as well as the interfollicular epidermis. Lupus erythematosus shows vacuolar alteration of the basal cells both in the epidermis and in the hair follicles with less squamotization of basal layer keratinocytes. The presence of basement membrane zone thickening, an interfollicular patchy superficial and deep perivascular infiltrate, and increased connective tissue mucin are also characteristic of lupus. In their late stages, both lichen planopilaris and lupus erythematosus may show permanent scarring alopecia, or pseudopelade of Brocq (354).

Principles of Management

First-line therapies for cutaneous and oral lichen planus include topical corticosteroids, intralesional corticosteroids, and antihistamines for symptomatic treatment of associated pruritus. For more generalized disease, additional treatment considerations include oral metronidazole, sulfasalazine, isotretinoin, acitretin, and methotrexate. Narrowband UVB phototherapy is an excellent nonpharmacotherapeutic option for more generalized disease. Oral lichen planus is typically treated with a combination of topical steroids and topical analgesics. Lichen planopilaris remains a therapeutic challenge, and antimalarials are felt to be the most effective treatment. Alternate immunosuppressive (e.g., mycophenolate mofetil) agents have been reported for patients with recalcitrant lichen planus. The identification of IFNγ as a key inflammatory signal in some patients with lichen planus has led to use of JAK inhibitors, with promising results in isolated early case reports (375,376).

LICHEN PLANUS–LIKE KERATOSIS

Lichen planus–like keratosis (LPLK), also known as "benign lichenoid keratosis," was originally described in 1966 as "solitary lichen planus" (377) and as "solitary lichen planus–like keratosis" (378).

Clinical Summary

This is a common lesion that occurs predominantly on the trunk and upper extremities of adults between the fifth and seventh decades. Occurrence on the face and lower extremities has also been reported (379,380). LPLK consists of a nonpruritic papule or slightly indurated plaque that is nearly always solitary, although cases with more than one skin lesion have been reported (381). It usually measures 5 to 20 mm in diameter, and its color varies from bright red to violaceous and brown. Its surface may be smooth or slightly verrucous. Lichen planus–like keratosis may represent the inflammatory stage of involuting solar lentigines (382). Because clinically it can be confused with basal cell carcinoma, this lesion is frequently biopsied.

Histopathology

Histopathologic examination shows a lichenoid inflammatory pattern indistinguishable from lichen planus with vacuolar alteration of the basal cell layer epidermal keratinocytes, a bandlike lymphocytic infiltrate that obscures the dermal–epidermal junction, and numerous colloid bodies (369,378). As in lichen planus, the epidermis often shows increased eosinophilic cytoplasm of keratinocytes (termed squamatization), hypergranulosis, and hyperkeratosis in LPLK (Fig. 7-29). In contrast to lichen planus, parakeratosis is fairly common and ranges from focal to prominent. In addition, eosinophils and plasma cells in the infiltrate are more frequently found in LPLK than in lichen planus, in which they are rarely seen (369). A residual solar lentigo at the edge of the lesion may support the diagnosis of LPLK (383).

Direct immunofluorescence studies may reveal a linear deposition of IgM at the basement membrane zone (384). Even though some keratinocytes may show pyknotic hyperchromatic nuclei, no definite nuclear atypia is seen. If marked keratinocytic atypia is present in the setting of solar elastosis, a lichenoid actinic keratosis should be considered in the differential diagnosis.

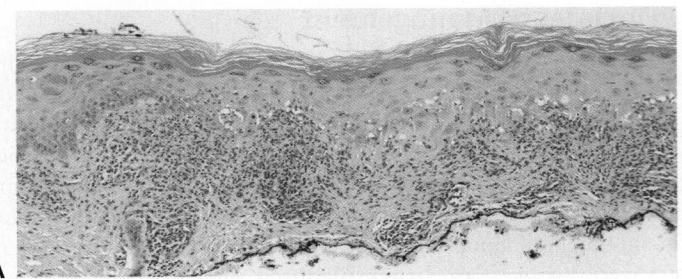

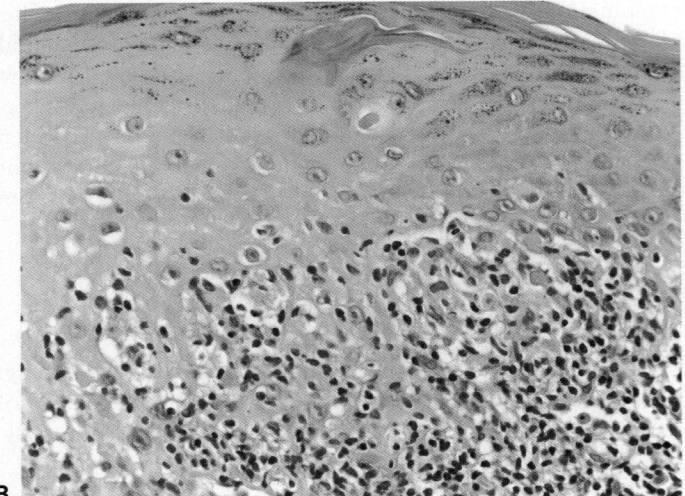

Figure 7-29 Lichen planus–like keratosis. Lichenoid inflammatory pattern with vacuolar change, orthokeratosis (**A**) and numerous necrotic keratinocytes and colloid bodies, and irregular pigmentation (**B**).

Pathogenesis

LPLK may represent the inflammatory stage of regressing solar lentigines and macular seborrheic keratoses (383). These precursor lesions could be the targets of an immune cell–mediated reaction (369).

Principles of Management

LPLK usually involutes spontaneously without need for specific clinical intervention.

KERATOSIS LICHENOIDES CHRONICA

A rare asymptomatic dermatosis, keratosis lichenoides chronica, was first described by Kaposi in 1895 as "lichen ruber acuminatus verrucosus et reticularis" (385) and received its present name in 1972 (386–388).

Clinical Summary

The disease usually starts in adulthood between 20 to 50 years of age and is extremely rare in children. Pediatric-onset keratosis lichenoides chronica may represent a different disease or a subset of the adult type, with special genetic and clinical features. Adult-onset disease is clinically characterized by an extensive, symmetrically distributed eruption of red to violaceous papulonodules with thick, adherent scale, predominantly on the dorsal aspects of extremities and the trunk. Lesions are often arranged in a linear and occasionally reticular pattern. The lesions may coalesce to form erythematous scaly or hyperkeratotic plaques (389,390). Very frequently, there is associated seborrheic dermatitis–like eruption of the face and palmoplantar hyperkeratosis. Nail changes may occur and are characterized by warty hypertrophy of the periungual tissues, which has been described as a distinctive feature of the disease (391). Mucosal membrane involvement is common and includes oral ulcers, nodular infiltration of the epiglottis and larynx, blepharitis, and keratoconjunctivitis, among others. Palmoplantar keratoderma, mucosal involvement, ocular symptoms, and nail dystrophy are reported in approximately 20% to 30% of patients (392). In pediatric patients, familial occurrence with a probable autosomal recessive inheritance, early-onset facial erythematous and purpuric macules on the forehead, eyelash alopecia, and pruritus have been reported (393). The disease has been reported in association with lymphoma (394), following trauma (395), and after a drug-induced erythroderma (396), although these associations are not well validated.

Histopathology

In most cases, a lichenoid inflammatory infiltrate composed of lymphocytes, histiocytes, and numerous plasma cells obscures the dermal–epidermal junction with vacuolar alteration of the basal cell layer epidermal keratinocytes and papillary dermal colloid bodies (389). The epidermis shows areas of acanthosis and atrophy with overlying hyperkeratosis, focal parakeratosis, and follicular plugging. Prominent dilated dermal capillaries are seen in cases with associated telangiectasias.

Differential Diagnosis

Although the histopathologic picture may closely resemble that of lichen planus, the presence of parakeratosis, alternating areas of atrophy and acanthosis, numerous plasma cells, and a denser lymphocytic infiltrate than is usually seen in lichen planus may help in the differentiation. In addition, the clinical appearance of keratosis lichenoides chronica is different from that of lichen planus; hence, clinicopathologic correlation is of utmost importance.

Principles of Management

The disease is characterized by a chronic and progressive course and, is notoriously difficult to treat. Evidence is limited to case reports and small case series. The most effective treatment options include phototherapy and systemic retinoids, alone or in combination. One literature review reported that up to half of patients are able to achieve complete remission with these methods. Notably, systemic corticosteroids, antibiotics, and antimalarials are not effective (392). Occasionally, spontaneous resolution may occur.

LICHEN NITIDUS

Lichen nitidus is a chronic and usually asymptomatic dermatitis that commonly begins in childhood or early adulthood.

Clinical Summary

The lesions are characterized by round, flat-topped, flesh-colored papules 1 to 3 mm in diameter that may occur in groups but do not coalesce (Fig. 7-30). They appear frequently as a localized eruption affecting predominantly the arms, trunk, or penis. A rare facial variant has been reported (397). The eruption may become generalized, and Koebner phenomenon may be observed (398,399). Purpuric generalized variant has also been reported (400). In addition, lesions occurring on the palms, soles, nails, and mucous membranes have been described (401). Palmar lesions may be more likely to be hemorrhagic.

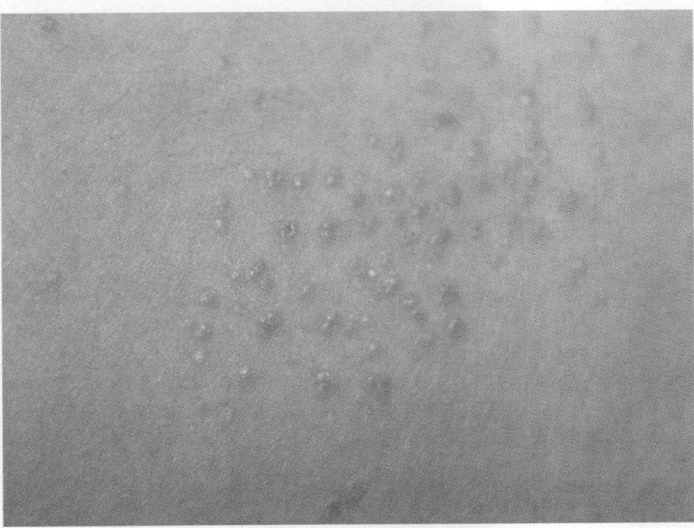

Figure 7-30 Lichen nitidus. Cluster of round, flat-topped, flesh-colored papules of a few millimeters in diameter. (Courtesy of Ronald O. Perelman Department of Dermatology, New York University School of Medicine, New York, New York.)

Histopathology

Each papule of lichen nitidus consists of a well-circumscribed, mixed-cell granulomatous infiltrate that abuts lower surface of the epidermis and is confined to widened dermal papillae. The infiltrate is composed of lymphocytes and a few multinucleated epithelioid histiocytes. The dermal infiltrate often extends slightly into the overlying epidermis, which is flattened and shows vacuolar alteration of the basal cell layer, focal subepidermal clefting, diminished granular layer, and focal parakeratosis. Transepidermal perforation of the infiltrate through the thinned epidermis may occur (402). At each lateral margin of the infiltrate, the epidermal rete ridges extend downward and surround the infiltrate resembling a claw clutching a ball (Fig. 7-31). The palmar lesions have the infiltrate mostly disposed around the bases of the rete ridges, similar to that found in hypertrophic lichen planus. Follicular involvement in lichen nitidus has also been described (403).

Principles of Management

The clinical course is unpredictable. Given that the rash is typically asymptomatic, treatment is generally not required. First-line therapies include topical corticosteroids and narrowband UVB phototherapy, although evidence is limited to case series and case reports. Second-line therapies vary and include topical tacrolimus, topical pimecrolimus, antihistamines, PUVA, oral retinoids, and cyclosporine (404–406). Spontaneous resolution of individual lesions may occur.

LICHEN STRIATUS

Lichen striatus is a fairly uncommon dermatitis that typically occurs in children from 5 to 15 years of age but may be seen in adults.

Clinical Summary

Lichen striatus usually manifests as a unilateral Blaschkoid eruption on the extremities, trunk, or neck, as a continuous or an interrupted band composed of minute, slightly raised erythematous papules, which may have a scaly surface (407,408) (Fig. 7-32). The lesions appear abruptly and usually involute within a year. They are occasionally pruritic. Hypopigmented lesions may be seen in dark-skinned patients. Uncommon presentations include associated onychodystrophy, multifocal or bilateral presentation, and simultaneous occurrence of lichen striatus in siblings (409–412). Facial lichen striatus in children has been reported. Some of these cases were associated with atopy (413).

Histopathology

Although the histology of lichen striatus is variable, there is usually a vacuolar interface dermatitis with a superficial perivascular predominantly lymphocytic infiltrate (Fig. 7-33) (414). Plasma cells and eosinophils are rare (Fig. 7-33). A lichenoid pattern, colloid bodies and papillary dermal melanophages may be seen. There may be epidermal spongiosis, lymphocytic exocytosis, and focal parakeratosis. Less frequently, there are scattered necrotic keratinocytes in the spinous layer as well as subcorneal spongiotic vesicles

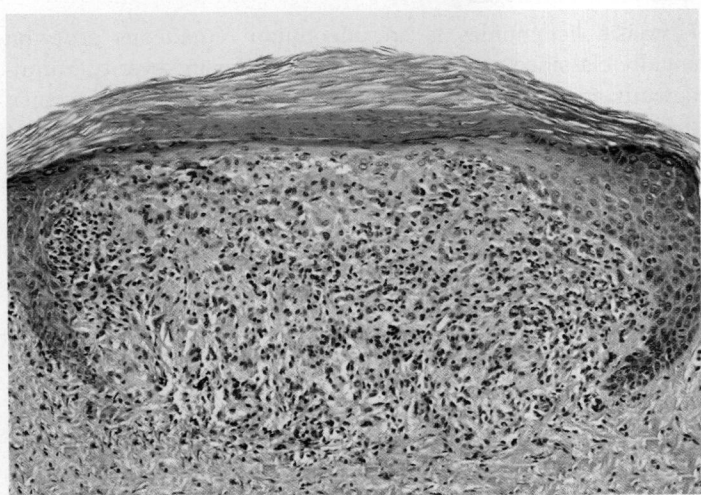

Figure 7-31 Lichen nitidus. Dense infiltrate of lymphocytes and histiocytes in an expanded dermal papilla, thin suprapapillary epidermis with vacuolar alteration of the basal layer, and focal parakeratosis.

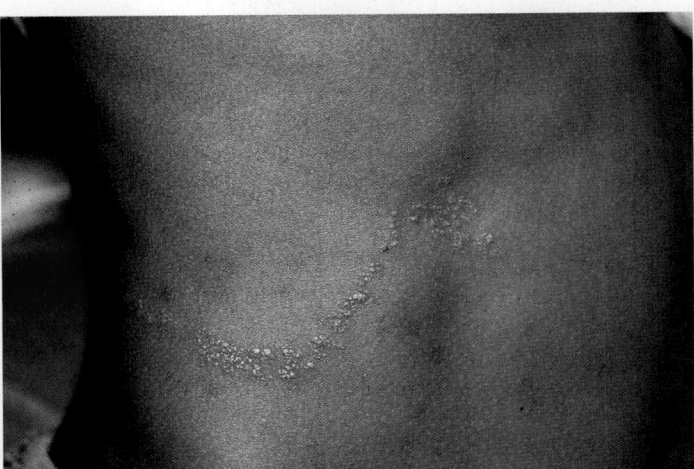

Figure 7-32 Lichen striatus. Linear band of confluent small papules following a Blaschko line. (Courtesy of Department of Dermatology, University of Pennsylvania School of Medicine, Philadelphia, Pennsylvania.)

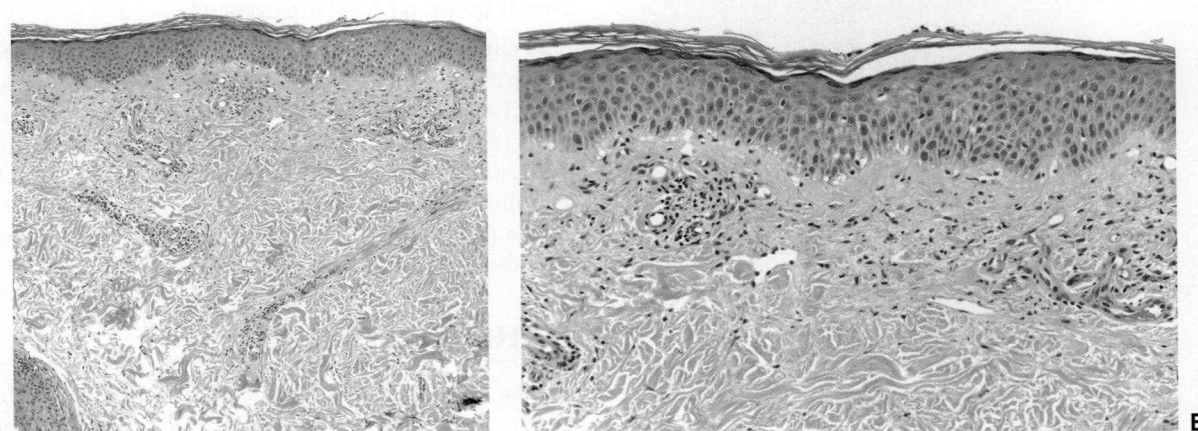

Figure 7-33 Lichen striatus. (A, B) Vacuolar interface change, spongiosis, and perivascular lymphocytic infiltrate.

filled with Langerhans cells. The most distinctive feature of lichen striatus is the presence of inflammatory infiltrate in the reticular dermis around hair follicles and eccrine glands (Fig. 7-34) (414). An unusual perforating variant of lichen striatus has been described, which shows transepidermal elimination of clusters of necrotic keratinocytes (415).

Pathogenesis

The inflammatory infiltrate of lichen striatus is composed of CD8+ lymphocytes and variable numbers of Langerhans cells (416). These findings suggest a cell-mediated immunologic mechanism in which cytotoxic events against keratinocytes occur.

Differential Diagnosis

Lichen striatus may show histopathologic features similar to those of other interface dermatitides including lichen planus, lichen nitidus, and graft-versus-host disease. The presence of

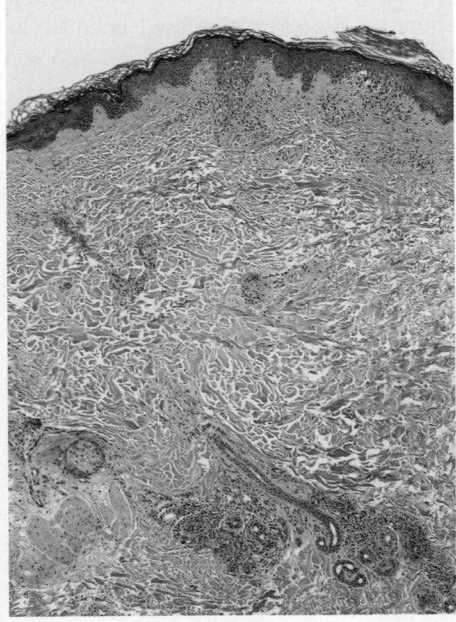

Figure 7-34 Lichen striatus. Superficial and deep perivascular, perieccrine, and perifollicular infiltrate of lymphocytes and histiocytes, with overlying spongiosis.

epidermal spongiosis, parakeratosis, and a deeper dermal inflammatory infiltrate around adnexal structures are features rarely seen in lichen planus. In secondary syphilis, the infiltrate usually contains plasma cells. In contrast to lichen striatus, the inflammatory infiltrate of lichen nitidus is typically present in a widened dermal papilla and contains more histiocytes and the characteristic claw and ball relationship of hyperplastic epidermis to dermal inflammatory infiltrate. "Periappendageal lichen nitidus" has been reported in patients with clinical lesions of lichen nitidus, that histopathologically displayed perifollicular and perieccrine inflammation, in addition to typical interface changes of lichen nitidus. This may support an overlap or a morphologic spectrum between lichen nitidus and lichen striatus (417).

Principles of Management

Lichen striatus is typically self-limited, and treatment is not required. A short course of low-dose systemic corticosteroids and photodynamic therapy have been reported in case reports and small case series (418,419).

PITYRIASIS LICHENOIDES CHRONICA

Clinical Summary

Pityriasis lichenoides is an uncommon cutaneous eruption usually classified into two forms that differ in severity. Simultaneous appearance of the two types and transitions between them often occur, suggesting that they are variants of the same disease (420). Both are rarely pruritic or painful, with crops of self-healing lesions affecting mainly young adults and occasionally children (420,421).

The milder form, called *pityriasis lichenoides chronica* (PLC), is characterized by recurrent crops of brown-red papules 4 to 10 mm in size, mainly on the trunk and extremities, that are covered with a scale and generally involute within 3 to 6 weeks with postinflammatory pigmentary changes.

Histopathology

PLC presents with a superficial perivascular and occasionally lichenoid infiltrate composed of lymphocytes that extends into the epidermis, where there is vacuolar alteration of the basal layer, mild spongiosis, a few necrotic keratinocytes, and confluent parakeratosis. Melanophages and small numbers of extravasated erythrocytes are commonly seen in the papillary dermis.

Differential Diagnosis

The clinical differential diagnosis for PLC is broad and includes guttate psoriasis, lichen planus, pityriasis rosea, varicella, lymphomatoid papulosis, erythema multiforme, leukocytoclastic vasculitis, secondary syphilis, and neurotic excoriation. Histopathologically, differentiating PLC from lymphomatoid papulosis may be particularly challenging.

Pathogenesis

Most of the cells in the inflammatory infiltrate are activated T lymphocytes (HLA-DR$^+$/CD3$^+$) that express CD7 and do not have loss of other pan-T-cell antigens (CD2, CD5) (422,423). In PLC, CD4$^+$ lymphocytes and FOXP3-positive regulatory T cells predominate (424). Some cases of PLC exhibit a clonal T-cell receptor gene rearrangement (425,426). PLC is considered by most to be a T-cell dyscrasia not associated with an increased risk of lymphoma.

Principles of Management

Give the rarity of this condition, evidence for treatment of PLC is limited to case reports and case series. Although topical corticosteroids are often prescribed, there is little evidence of efficacy. PUVA is strongly recommended. Antibiotics may be helpful in some cases, particularly in pediatric patients. Methotrexate and etanercept have been reported as effective in severe, refractory cases (427–429).

PITYRIASIS LICHENOIDES ET VARIOLIFORMIS ACUTA

Clinical Summary

The more severe form of *pityriasis lichenoides et varioliformis acuta* (PLEVA), also referred to as Mucha–Habermann disease, consists of a fairly extensive eruption present mainly on the trunk and proximal extremities. It is characterized by erythematous papules that develop into papulonecrotic, occasionally hemorrhagic, or vesiculopustular lesions that resolve within a few weeks, usually with little or no scarring. Occasionally, some lesions increase in size to necrotic ulcers 1 to 2 cm in diameter, which heal with an atrophic or varioliform scar. Although the individual lesions follow an acute course, the disorder is chronic, extending over several months or even years with development of new lesions and variable periods of remission. Cases of PLEVA occurring during pregnancy and affecting the vagina/cervical mucosa with resultant premature rupture of the membranes and/or premature labor have been reported (430). Very rarely, patients with PLEVA have a sudden, severe flare of their disease, characterized by innumerable coalescent necrotic ulcerations associated with high fever and systemic manifestations (431,432). Pityriasis lichenoides occurring concurrently with idiopathic thrombocytopenic purpura in childhood has been reported (433). Associations of pityriasis lichenoides with measles, mumps, and rubella vaccination, and statin use (434,435).

Histopathology

In PLEVA, there is a perivascular and dense, bandlike, predominantly lymphocytic infiltrate in the papillary dermis that extends into the reticular dermis in a wedge-shaped pattern

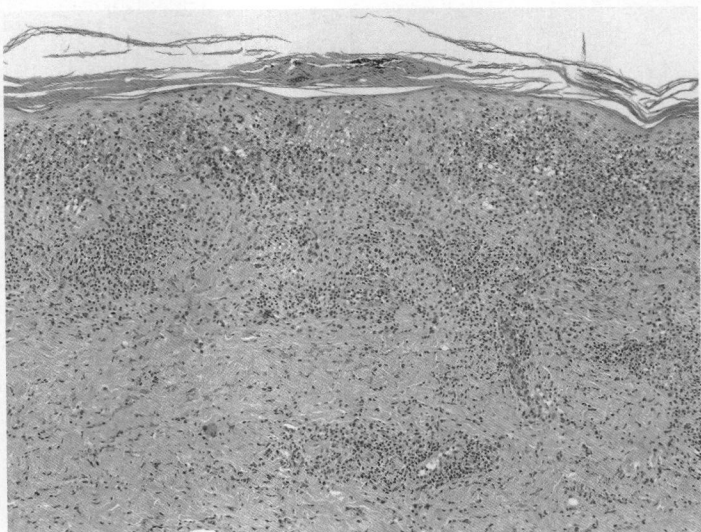

Figure 7-35 Pityriasis lichenoides et varioliformis acuta (PLEVA). Wedge-shaped, lichenoid inflammatory infiltrate with parakeratosis and prominent erythrocyte extravasation.

(Figs. 7-35 and 7-36). The infiltrate obscures the dermal–epidermal junction with pronounced vacuolar alteration of the basal layer, marked exocytosis of lymphocytes and erythrocytes, and intercellular and intracellular edema leading to variable degree of epidermal necrosis (Fig. 7-37). Ultimately, erosion or even ulceration may occur. The overlying cornified layer shows parakeratosis and a scaly crust with neutrophils in the more severe cases (422).

Variable degrees of papillary dermal edema, endothelial swelling, and extravasated erythrocytes are seen in the majority of cases (Fig. 7-38). Although occasionally small deposits of fibrin are present within the vessel walls, severe vascular damage is rarely found, except in the severe febrile ulceronecrotic variant of PLEVA, in which lymphocytic vasculitis with leukocytoclasia is a fairly common feature (431).

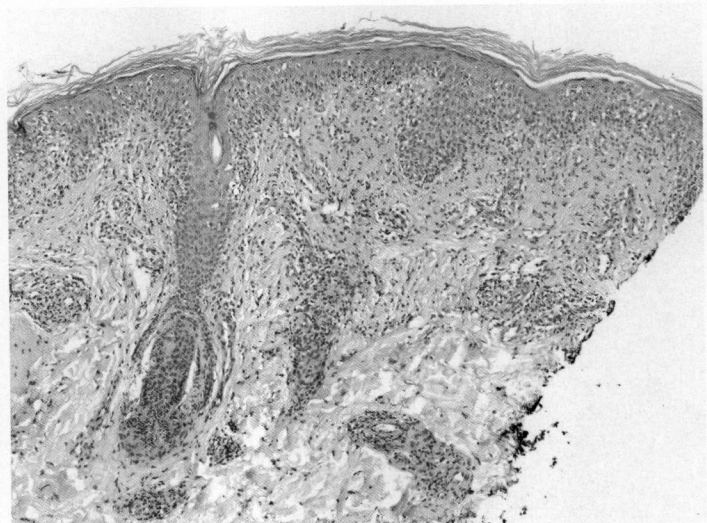

Figure 7-36 Pityriasis lichenoides et varioliformis acuta (PLEVA). Lichenoid and wedge-shaped lymphocytic infiltrate without prominent erythrocytes.

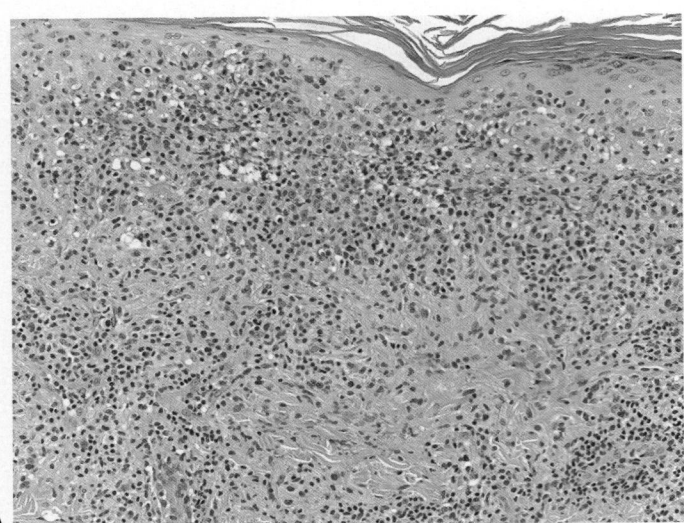 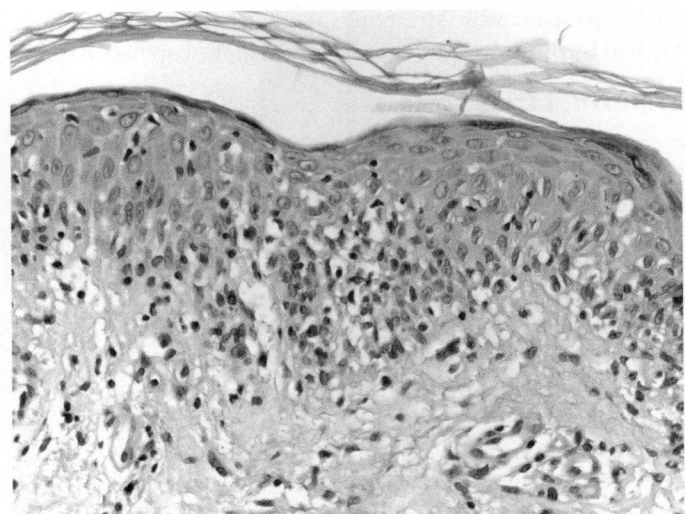

Figure 7-37 Pityriasis lichenoides et varioliformis acuta (PLEVA). Vacuolar change of the basal layer with erythrocyte extravasation (**A**) and prominent lymphocytic exocytosis (**B**).

Differential Diagnosis

Occasionally, the histopathologic picture of PLEVA can be mimicked by other diseases such as pityriasis rosea, vesicular insect bites, and subacute eczematous dermatitis. The presence of a deeper inflammatory infiltrate, extensive epidermal necrosis, and the absence of intraepidermal spongiotic microvesicles may help to distinguish PLEVA from pityriasis rosea and subacute eczematous dermatitis. Numerous eosinophils in a vertically oriented dermal infiltrate are more commonly seen in insect bites (436).

Pathogenesis

Recent studies have suggested that PLEVA is a clonal T-cell disorder (425,437). Malignant transformation in pityriasis lichenoides is controversial. It does not appear that cases of clonal PLEVA have a higher risk of developing malignant lymphoma (438). However, there are a few reports of cases with pityriasis lichenoides that have been associated with cutaneous lymphoma (439–441). It is proposed that pityriasis lichenoides represents an indolent T-cell dyscrasia (442). Monoclonal expansion of T cells results most likely from a cellular host immune response to an as-yet-unidentified antigen; proposed triggers include parvovirus B19 or HHV8 (424,425,443).

Principles of Management

As with PLC, treatment data are mostly limited to case reports and case series (444). In infants, observation is typically sufficient. However, children are recommended to receive a 6-week course of high-dose erythromycin (429). As with PLC, efficacy of topical corticosteroids is questionable. Although antihistamines may improve symptomatic pruritus, they do not change the disease course. PUVA is strongly recommended in both adult and pediatric patients (446). In extensive or systematic disease, there are reports of success with methotrexate (444), cyclosporine (446), systemic corticosteroids, and intravenous immunoglobulin (447).

Two constant findings in PLEVA are the predominance of CD8$^+$ (cytotoxic-suppressor) T cells over CD4$^+$ (helper-inducer) T lymphocytes in the infiltrate and the expression of HLA-DR on the surrounding keratinocytes (422–424), suggesting a direct cytotoxic immune reaction in the pathogenesis of epidermal necrosis.

INFLAMMATORY LINEAR VERRUCOUS EPIDERMAL NEVUS

Clinical Summary

Inflammatory linear verrucous epidermal nevus (ILVEN) presents as a persistent, linear, intensely pruritic lesion composed of erythematous, slightly verrucous, scaly papules arranged in one or several linear arrays, most commonly on the lower extremity. Although lesions typically arise during childhood, adult-onset ILVEN has been reported (448,449). Vulvar and perianal involvement by ILVEN has also been reported, and rarely the lesions are bilateral (450,451).

ILVEN in association with arthritis (452) and lichen amyloidosus (453) has been reported. ILVEN is considered to be a variant of epidermal nevus; however, it is described and

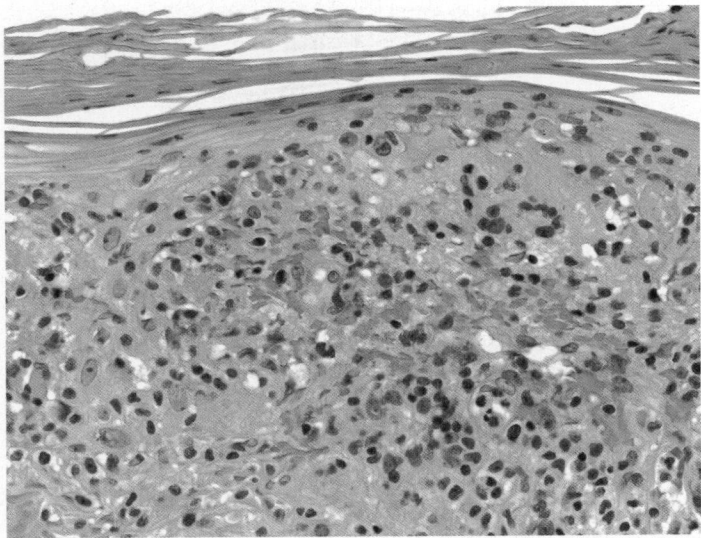

Figure 7-38 Pityriasis lichenoides et varioliformis acuta (PLEVA). Prominent erythrocyte extravasation and necrotic keratinocytes.

included in this chapter on papulosquamous disorders because of its clinical and histopathologic similarities to psoriasis and lichen striatus.

Histopathology

ILVEN is characterized by a papillated epidermal hyperplasia with a regular or psoriasiform elongation and thickening of the rete ridges, slight spongiosis, overlying foci of parakeratosis, and lymphocytic exocytosis (Fig. 7-39). There is a superficial perivascular lymphocytic and histiocytic infiltrate of variable density (454).

Sharply demarcated alternation of orthokeratosis and parakeratosis in the cornified layer is a characteristic histopathologic feature of ILVEN (Fig. 7-40). The parakeratotic areas are slightly raised, lack a granular layer, and show a compact eosinophilic cornified layer with nuclear preservation. The orthokeratotic areas are slightly depressed with underlying hypergranulosis (451,455).

Pathogenesis

Electron microscopy and immunohistochemical studies have shown altered keratinocyte differentiation in the

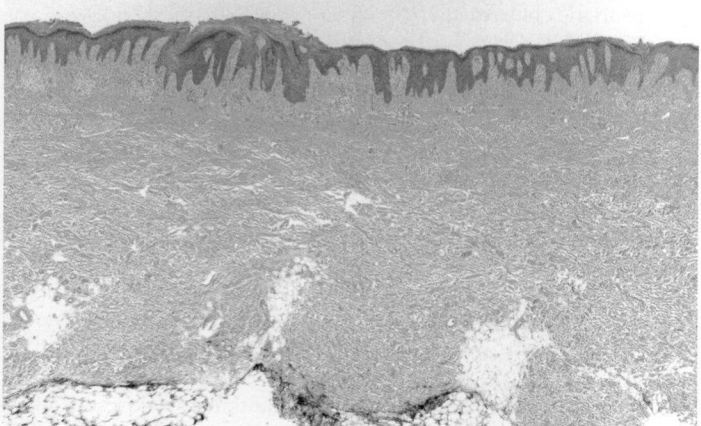

Figure 7-39 Inflammatory linear verrucous epidermal nevus (ILVEN). Epidermal acanthosis, orthokeratosis, and parakeratosis.

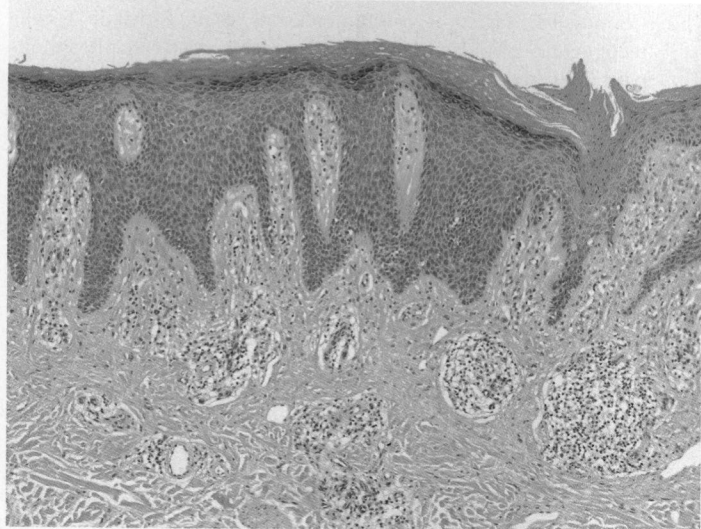

Figure 7-40 Inflammatory linear verrucous epidermal nevus (ILVEN). Sharply demarcated parakeratosis with acanthosis and superficial perivascular lymphohistiocytic inflammatory infiltrate.

parakeratotic areas. Ultrastructurally, keratinocytes have prominent Golgi apparatus and vesicles in their cytoplasm. The intercellular spaces in upper layers of the epidermis are widened by deposits of an electron-dense homogeneous substance. The cytoplasm of parakeratotic corneocytes contains remnants of nucleus and membrane structures and a few lipid droplets. The marginal band formation inside the plasma membrane is incomplete, suggesting a deficient keratinization process (455).

Involucrin expression has a very characteristic pattern in ILVEN: The orthokeratotic epidermis shows increased involucrin expression, whereas the parakeratotic areas are almost negative for involucrin staining. This pattern differs from that of psoriasis, in which involucrin is expressed prematurely in most of the suprabasal keratinocytes.

More than 90% of the mononuclear cells in the dermal infiltrate are CD4$^+$ T lymphocytes; in contrast, the majority of the epidermal infiltrating T lymphocytes are CD4 negative (456).

Differential Diagnosis

The clinical appearance of lichen striatus and that of ILVEN may be indistinguishable. However, ILVEN, in contrast to lichen striatus, is pruritic and persistent. Histopathologically, lichen striatus tends to have a lichenoid pattern and ILVEN a psoriasiform pattern. Furthermore, ILVEN is characterized by alternating areas of orthokeratosis/hypergranulosis and parakeratosis/hypogranulosis.

Given that alternating orthokeratosis and parakeratosis may be seen in psoriasis and occasionally Munro microabscesses are observed in ILVEN, the differential diagnosis of these two entities could be sometimes difficult, and clinicopathologic correlation is usually necessary.

Principles of Management

ILVEN is relatively resistant to therapy and several treatment options have been used, not only to relieve the discomfort but also to help with the cosmetic appearance of the lesions. These include topical steroids, tacrolimus, calcipotriol, retinoids, surgical excisions and laser therapies with different success rates (457–459).

ACKNOWLEDGMENT

The Editors and Authors wish to acknowledge the contributions of previous authors of this chapter: Narciss Mobini, Sonia Toussaint Caire, Stephanie Hu, and Hideko Kamino.

REFERENCES

1. Telfer NR, Chalmers RJG, Whale K, Colman G. The role of streptococcal infection in the initiation of guttate psoriasis. *Arch Dermatol.* 1992;128:39–42.
2. Faber EM, Nall ML. Natural history of psoriasis in 5,600 patients. *Dermatologica.* 1974;148:1–18.
3. Morris LF, Phillips CM, Binnie WH, Sander HM, Silverman AK, Menter MA. Oral lesions in patients with psoriasis: a controlled study. *Cutis.* 1992;49:339–344.
4. Pogrel MA, Cram D. Intraoral findings in patients with psoriasis with a special reference to ectopic geographic tongue (erythema circinata). *Oral Surg Oral Med Oral Pathol.* 1988;66:184–189.
5. Baker H. Pustular psoriasis. *Dermatol Clin.* 1984;2:455–470.

6. Zelickson BD, Muller SA. Generalized pustular psoriasis. *Arch Dermatol.* 1991;127:1339–1345.

7. Wagner G, Luckasen JR, Goltz RW. Mucous membrane involvement in generalized pustular psoriasis. *Arch Dermatol.* 1976;112:1010–1014.

8. Shelley WB, Kirschbaum JO. Generalized pustular psoriasis. *Arch Dermatol.* 1961;84:73–78.

9. Braverman IM, Cohen I, O'Keefe EO. Metabolic and ultrastructural studies in a patient with pustular psoriasis (Von Zumbusch). *Arch Dermatol.* 1972;105:189–196.

10. Schuppener JH. Ausdrucksformen pustulöser psoriasis. *Dermatol Wochenschr.* 1958;138:841–854.

11. Feldmeyer L, Heidemeyer K, Yawalkar N. Acute generalized exanthematous pustulosis: pathogenesis, genetic background, clinical variants and therapy. *Int J Mol Sci.* 2016;17(8):1214. doi:10.3390/ijms17081214

12. Baker H, Ryan TJ. Generalized pustular psoriasis. *Br J Dermatol.* 1968;80:771–793.

13. Katzenellenbogen I, Feuerman EI. Psoriasis pustulosa and impetigo herpetiformis: single or dual entity? *Acta Dermatol Venereol (Stockholm).* 1966;46:86.

14. Pierard GE, Pierard-Franchimont C, de la Brassine M. Impetigo herpetiformis and pustular psoriasis during pregnancy. *Am J Dermatopathol.* 1983;5:215–220.

15. Lotem M, Katzenelson V, Rotem A, Hod M, Sandbank M. Impetigo herpetiformis: a variant of pustular psoriasis or a separate entity? *J Am Acad Dermatol.* 1989;20:338–341.

16. Namazi N, Dadkhahfar S. Impetigo herpetiformis: review of pathogenesis, complication, and treatment. *Dermatol Res Pract.* 2018;2018:1–4. doi:10.1155/2018/5801280

17. Resneck JS, Cram DL. Erythema annulare-like pustular psoriasis. *Arch Dermatol.* 1973;108:687–688.

18. Adler DJ, Rower JM, Hashimoto K. Annular pustular psoriasis. *Arch Dermatol.* 1981;117:313–314.

19. Zala L, Hunziker T. Lokalisierte form der psoriasis von typ des erythema annulare centrifugum mit pustulation. *Hautarzt.* 1984;35:53–55.

20. Zelickson BD, Muller SA. Generalized pustular psoriasis in childhood: report of thirteen cases. *J Am Acad Dermatol.* 1991; 24:186–194.

21. Ashhurst PJC. Relapsing pustular eruptions of the hands and feet. *Br J Dermatol.* 1964;776:169–180.

22. Andrews GC, Machacek GF. Pustular bacterids of the hands and feet. *Arch Dermatol Syphilol.* 1935;32:837–847.

23. Patel RV, Lebwohl M. In the clinic: psoriasis. *Ann Intern Med.* 2011;155(3):ITC2-1–ICT2-15.

24. Levine D, Gottlieb A. Evaluation and management of psoriasis: an internist's guide. *Med Clin North Am.* 2009;93:1291–1303.

25. Braun-Falco O, Christophers E. Structural aspects of initial psoriatic lesions. *Arch Dermatol Forsch.* 1974;251:95–110.

26. Ragaz A, Ackerman AB. Evolution, maturation, and regression of lesions of psoriasis. *Am J Dermatopathol.* 1979;1:199–214.

27. Van Scott EJ, Ekel TW. Kinetics of hyperplasia in psoriasis. *Arch Dermatol.* 1963;88:373–381.

28. Gordon M, Johnson WC. Histopathology and histochemistry of psoriasis. *Arch Dermatol.* 1967;95:402–407.

29. Rupec M. Zur ultrastruktur der spongiformen pustel. *Arch Klin Exp Dermatol.* 1970;239:30–49.

30. Burks JW, Montgomery H. Histopathologic study of psoriasis. *Arch Dermatol Syphilol.* 1943;48:479–493.

31. Pinkus H, Mehregan AH. The primary histologic lesion of seborrheic dermatitis and psoriasis. *J Invest Dermatol.* 1966;46:109–116.

32. Cox AH, Watson W. Histological variations in lesions of psoriasis. *Arch Dermatol.* 1972;106:503–506.

33. Abrahams J, McCarthy JT, Sanders ST. 101 cases of exfoliative dermatitis. *Arch Dermatol.* 1963;87:96–101.

34. Muller SA, Kitzmiller KW. Generalized pustular psoriasis. *Acta Dermatol Venereol (Stockholm).* 1962;42:504.

35. Kingery FAJ, Chinn HD, Saunders TS. Generalized pustular psoriasis. *Arch Dermatol.* 1961;84:912–919.

36. Piraccini BM, Fanti PA, Morelli R, Tosti A. Hallopeau's acrodermatitis continua of the nail apparatus: a clinical and pathological study of 20 patients. *Acta Dermatol Venereol (Stockholm).* 1994;74:65–67.

37. Pierard J, Kint A. La pustulose palmo-plantaire chronique et recidivante. *Ann Dermatol Venereol.* 1978;105:681–688.

38. Pierard J, Kint A. Les "bacterides pustuleuses" d'Andrews. *Arch Belg Dermatol Syphiligr.* 1966;22:83.

39. Lever WF. In discussion with pay D: pustular psoriasis. *Arch Dermatol.* 1969;99:641–642.

40. Uehara M, Ofuji S. The morphogenesis of pustulosis palmaris et plantaris. *Arch Dermatol.* 1974;109:518–520.

41. Thorman J, Heilesen B. Recalcitrant pustular eruptions of the extremities. *J Cutan Pathol.* 1975;2:19–24.

42. Tan RS. Acute generalized pustular bacterid. *Br J Dermatol.* 1974;91:209–215.

43. Weinstein GD, Van Scott EJ. Autoradiographic analysis of turnover times of normal and psoriatic epidermis. *J Invest Dermatol.* 1965;45:257–262.

44. Soltani K, Van Scott EJ. Patterns and sequence of tissue changes in incipient and evolving lesions of psoriasis. *Arch Dermatol.* 1972;106:484–490.

45. Takahashi H, Manabe A, Ishida-Yamamoto A, Hashimoto Y, Iizuka H. Aberrant expression of apoptosis-related molecules in psoriatic epidermis. *J Dermatol Sci.* 2002;28:187–197.

46. Hawkes JE, Chan TC, Krueger JG. Psoriasis pathogenesis and the development of novel targeted immune therapies. *J Allergy Clin Immunol.* 2017;140(3):645–653. doi:10.1016/j.jaci.2017.07.004

47. Kim J, Krueger JG. Highly effective new treatments for psoriasis target the IL-23/Type 17 T cell autoimmune axis. *Annu Rev Med.* 2017;68(1):255–269. doi:10.1146/annurev-med-042915-103905

48. Chiricozzi A, Guttman-Yassky E, Suárez-Fariñas M, et al. Integrative responses to IL-17 and TNF-α in human keratinocytes account for key inflammatory pathogenic circuits in psoriasis. *J Invest Dermatol.* 2011;131(3):677–687. doi:10.1038/jid.2010.340

49. Zaba LC, Krueger JG, Lowes MA. Resident and "inflammatory" dendritic cells in human skin. *J Invest Dermatol.* 2009;129(2): 302–308. doi:10.1038/jid.2008.225

50. Lande R, Botti E, Jandus C, et al. The antimicrobial peptide LL37 is a T-cell autoantigen in psoriasis. *Nat Commun.* 2014;5(1):5621. doi:10.1038/ncomms6621

51. Arakawa A, Siewert K, Stöhr J, et al. Melanocyte antigen triggers autoimmunity in human psoriasis. *J Exp Med.* 2015; 212(13):2203–2212. doi:10.1084/jem.20151093

52. Cheung KL, Jarrett R, Subramaniam S, et al. Psoriatic T cells recognize neolipid antigens generated by mast cell phospholipase delivered by exosomes and presented by CD1a. *J Exp Med.* 2016;213(11):2399–2412. doi:10.1084/jem.20160258

53. Gudmundsdottir AS, Sigundsdottir H, Sigurgeirsson B, Good MF, Valdimarsson H, Jonsdottir I. Is an epitope on keratin 17 a major target for autoreactive T lymphocytes in psoriasis? *Clin Exp Immunol.* 1999;117:580–586.

54. Valdimarsson H, Sigmundsdottir H, Jonsdottir I. Is psoriasis induced by streptococcal superantigens and maintained by M-protein–specific T cells that cross-react with keratin? *Clin Exp Immunol.* 1997;107(suppl 1):21–24.

55. Soeprono FF. Histologic criteria for the diagnosis of pityriasis rubra pilaris. *Am J Dermatopathol.* 1986;8:277–283.

56. Degos R, Garnier G, Civatte J. Pustulose par *Candida albicans* avec lésions psoriasiformes rappelant le psoriasis pustuleux. *Bull Soc Fr Dermatol Syphiligr.* 1962;69:231–233.

57. Dawson TAJ. Tongue lesions in generalized pustular psoriasis. *Br J Dermatol.* 1974;91:419–424.

58. Ladizinski B, Lee KC, Wilmer E, Alavi A, Mistry N, Sibbald RG. A review of the clinical variants and the management of psoriasis. *Adv Skin Wound Care.* 2013;26:271–284.

59. Hu S, Lan C-CE. Psoriasis and cardiovascular comorbidities: focusing on severe vascular events, cardiovascular risk factors and implications for treatment. *Int J Mol Sci.* 2017;18(10):2211. doi:10.3390/ijms18102211

60. Griffiths WAD. Pityriasis rubra pilaris. *Clin Exp Dermatol.* 1980; 5:105.

61. Wang D, Chong VC-L, Chong W-S, Oon HH. A review on pityriasis rubra pilaris. *Am J Clin Dermatol.* 2018;19(3):377–390. doi:10.1007/s40257-017-0338-1

62. Haridas AS, Sullivan TJ. Surgical management of cicatricial ectropion in pityriasis rubra pilaris. *Ophthalmic Plast Reconstr Surg.* 2016;32(1):e12–e15. doi:10.1097/IOP.0000000000000385

63. Craiglow BG, Boyden LM, Hu R, et al. CARD14-associated papulosquamous eruption: a spectrum including features of psoriasis and pityriasis rubra pilaris. *J Am Acad Dermatol.* 2018;79(3): 487–494. doi:10.1016/j.jaad.2018.02.034

64. De D, Dogra S, Narang T, Radotra BD, Kanwar AJ. Pityriasis rubra pilaris in a HIV-positive patient (Type 6 PRP). *Skinmed.* 2008;7(1):47–50. doi:10.1111/j.1540-9740.2007.07167.x

65. Braun-Falco O, Ryckmanns F, Schmoeckel C, Landthaler M. Pityriasis rubra pilaris: a clinico-pathological and therapeutic study with special reference to histochemistry, autoradiography, and electron microscopy. *Arch Dermatol Res.* 1983;275:287.

66. Fuchs-Telem D, Sarig O, van Steensel MA, et al. Familial pityriasis rubra pilaris is caused by mutations in CARD14. *Am J Hum Genet.* 2012;91:163–170.

67. Klein A, Landthaler M, Karrer S. Pityriasis rubra pilaris: a review of diagnosis and treatment. *Am J Clin Dermatol.* 2010;11:157–170.

68. Adnot-Desanlis L, Antonicelli F, Tabary T, Bernard P, Reguiaï Z. Effectiveness of infliximab in pityriasis rubra pilaris is associated with pro-inflammatory cytokine inhibition. *Dermatology.* 2013;226:41–46.

69. Di Stefani A, Galluzzo M, Talamonti M, Chiricozzi A, Costanzo A, Chimenti S. Long-term Ustekinumab treatment for refractory type I pityriasis rubra pilaris. *J Dermatol Case Rep.* 2013;7:5–9.

70. Lawley TJ, Hertz HC, Wade TR, Ackerman AB, Katz SI. Pruritic urticarial papules and plaques of pregnancy. *JAMA.* 1979; 241:1696–1699.

71. Callen JP, Hanno R. Pruritic urticarial papules and plaques of pregnancy (PUPPP). *J Am Acad Dermatol.* 1981;5:401–405.

72. High WA, Hoang MP, Miller MD. Pruritic urticarial papules and plaques of pregnancy with unusual and extensive palmoplantar involvement. *Obstet Gynecol.* 2005;105:1261–1264.

73. Buccolo LS, Viera AJ. Pruritic urticarial papules and plaques of pregnancy presenting in the postpartum period: a case report. *J Reprod Med.* 2005;50:61–63.

74. Yancey KB, Russel RP, Lawley TJ. Pruritic urticarial papules and plaques of pregnancy. *J Am Acad Dermatol.* 1984;10:473–480.

75. Cohen LM, Capeless EL, Krusinski PA, Maloney ME. Pruritic urticarial papules and plaques of pregnancy and its relationship to maternal–fetal weight gain and twin pregnancy. *Arch Dermatol.* 1989;125:1534–1536.

76. Elling SV, McKenna P, Powell FC. Pruritic urticarial papules and plaques of pregnancy in twin and triplet pregnancies. *J Eur Dermatol Venereol.* 2000;14:378–381.

77. Rudolph CM, Al-Fares S, Vaughan-Jones SA, Müllegger RR, Kerl H, Black MM. Polymorphic eruption of pregnancy: clinicopathology and potential trigger factors in 181 patients. *Br J Dermatol.* 2006;154:54–60.

78. Im S, Lee ES, Kim W, et al. Expression of progesterone receptor in human keratinocytes. *J Korean Med Sci.* 2000;15:647–654.

79. Weiss R, Hull P. Familial occurrence of pruritic urticarial papules and plaques of pregnancy. *J Am Acad Dermatol.* 1992;26: 715–717.

80. Aronson IK, Bond S, Fiedler VC, Vomvouras S, Gruber D, Ruiz C. Pruritic urticarial papules and plaques of pregnancy: clinical and immunopathologic observations in 57 patients. *J Am Acad Dermatol.* 1998;39:933–939. Erratum in: *J Am Acad Dermatol.* 1999;40:611.

81. Ambros-Rudolph CM, Müllegger RR, Vaughan-Jones SA, Kerl H, Black MM. The specific dermatoses of pregnancy revisited and reclassified: results of a retrospective two-center study on 505 pregnant patients. *J Am Acad Dermatol.* 2006;54:395–404.

82. Semkova K, Black M. Pemphigoid gestationis: current insights into pathogenesis and treatment. *Eur J Obstet Gynecol Reprod Biol.* 2009;145:138–144.

83. Chi CC, Wang SH, Charles-Holmes R, et al. Pemphigoid gestationis: early onset and blister formation are associated with adverse pregnancy outcomes. *Br J Dermatol.* 2009;160:1222–1228.

84. Scheinfeld N. Pruritic urticarial papules and plaques of pregnancy wholly abated with one week twice daily application of fluticasone propionate lotion: a case report and review of the literature. *Dermatol Online J.* 2008;14:4.

85. Ahmadi S, Powell FC. Pruritic urticarial papules and plaques of pregnancy: current status. *Australas J Dermatol.* 2005;46:53–58.

86. Gammel JA. Erythema gyratum repens. *Arch Dermatol.* 1952; 66:494–505.

87. Eubanks LE, McBurney E, Reed R. Erythema gyratum repens. *Am J Med Sci.* 2001;321:302–305.

88. Bryan ME, Lienhart K, Smoller BR, Johnson SM. Erythema gyratum repens in a case of resolving psoriasis. *J Drugs Dermatol.* 2003;2:315–317.

89. Rongioletti F, Fausti V, Parodi A. Erythema gyratum repens is not an obligate paraneoplastic disease: a systematic review of the literature and personal experience. *J Eur Acad Dermatol Venereol.* 2014;28(1):112–115. doi:10.1111/j.1468-3083.2012.04663.x

90. Gore M, Winters M. Erythema gyratum repens: a rare paraneoplastic rash. McPheeters R, ed. *West J Emerg Med.* 2011;12(4): 556–558. doi:10.5811/westjem.2010.11.2090

91. Boyd AS, Neldner KH, Menter A. Erythema gyratum repens: a paraneoplastic eruption. *J Am Acad Dermatol.* 1992;26:757–762.

92. Kleyn CE, Lai-Cheong JE, Bell HK. Cutaneous manifestations of internal malignancy. *Am J Clin Dermatol.* 2006;7(2):71–84. doi:10.2165/00128071-200607020-00001

93. Leavell UW, Winternitz WW, Black JH. Erythema gyratum repens and undifferentiated carcinoma. *Arch Dermatol.* 1967;95(1):69–72.

94. Albers SE, Fenske NA, Glass LF. Erythema gyratum repens: direct immunofluorescence microscopic findings. *J Am Acad Dermatol.* 1993;29:493–494.

95. Caux F, Lebbe C, Thomine E, et al. Erythema gyratum repens. A case studied with immunofluorescence, immunoelectron microscopy and immunohistochemistry. *Br J Dermatol.* 1994;131:102–107.

96. Sharma A, Lambert PJ, Maghari A, Lambert WC. Arcuate, annular, and polycyclic inflammatory and infectious lesions. *Clin Dermatol.* 2011;29:140–150.

97. Miyagawa F, Danno K, Uehara M. Erythema gyratum repens responding to cetirizine hydrochloride. *J Dermatol.* 2002; 29:731–734.

98. Naveen KN, Kalinga B, Pai VV, et al. Erythema gyratum repens like figurate erythema responding to topical steroid in an healthy individual. *Indian J Dermatol.* 2013;58:329.

99. Ramirez CO. *Los cenicientos: problema clínico. Presented at: Proceedings of the First Central American Congress of Dermatology;* December 5–8, 1957; 122–130.

100. Dominguez-Soto L, Hojyo-Tomoka T, Vega-Memije E, Arenas R, Cores-Franco R. Pigmentary problems in the tropics. *Dermatol Clin.* 1994;12(4):777–784.

101. Oiso N, Tsuruta D, Imanishi H, Kobayashi H, Kawada A. Erythema dyschromicum perstans in a Japanese child. *Pediatr Dermatol.* 2012;29:637–640.

102. Chakrabarti N, Chattopadhyay C. Ashy dermatosis: a controversial entity. *Indian J Dermatol.* 2012;57:61–62.

103. Correa MC, Vega-Memije E, Vargas-Alarcon G, et al. HLA-DR association with the genetic susceptibility to develop ashy dermatosis in Mexican Mestizo patients. *J Am Acad Dermatol.* 2007;56:617–620.

104. Vega-Memije E, Waxtein L, Arenas R, Hojyo T, Dominguez-Soto L. Ashy dermatosis and lichen planus pigmentosus: a clinicopathologic study of 31 cases. *Int J Dermatol.* 1992;31:90–94.

105. Miyagawa S, Komatsu M, Okuchi T, Shirai T, Sakamoto K. Erythema dyschromicum perstans: immunopathologic studies. *J Am Acad Dermatol.* 1989;20:882–886.

106. Vásquez-Ochoa LA, Isaza-Guzmán DM, Orozco-Mora B, Restrepo-Molina R, Trujillo-Perez J, Tapia FJ. Immunopathologic study of erythema dyschromicum perstans (ashy dermatosis). *Int J Dermatol.* 2006;45:937–941.

107. Baranda L, Torres-Alvarez B, Cortes-Franco R, Moncada B, Portales-Perez DP, Gonzalez-Amaro R. Involvement of cell adhesion and activation molecules in the pathogenesis of erythema dyschromicum perstans (ashy dermatitis). The effect of clofazimine therapy. *Arch Dermatol.* 1997;133:325–329.

108. Bhutani LK, Bedi TR, Pandhi RK, Nayak NC. Lichen planus pigmentosus. *Dermatologica.* 1974;149(1):43–50.

109. Sanchez NP, Pathak MA, Sato SS, Sánchez JL, Mihm MC, Fitzpatrick TB. Circumscribed dermal melaninoses: classification, light, histochemical, and electron microscopic studies on three patients with the erythema dyschromicum perstans type. *Int J Dermatol.* 1982;21:25–31.

110. Kumarasinghe SPW, Pandya A, Chandran V, et al. A global consensus statement on ashy dermatosis, erythema dyschromicum perstans, lichen planus pigmentosus, idiopathic eruptive macular pigmentation, and Riehl's melanosis. *Int J Dermatol.* 2019;58(3):263–272. doi:10.1111/ijd.14189

111. Keisham C, Sarkar R, Garg VK, Chugh S. Ashy dermatosis in an 8-year-old Indian child. *Indian Dermatol Online J.* 2013;4:30–32.

112. Bahadir S, Cobanoglu U, Cimsit G, Yayli S, Alpay K. Erythema dyschromicum perstans: response to dapsone therapy. *Int J Dermatol.* 2004;43:220–222.

113. Rowland Payne CME, Wilkinson JD, McKee PH, Jurecka W, Black MM. Nodular prurigo: a clinicopathological study of 46 patients. *Br J Dermatol.* 1985;113:431–439.

114. Ständer S, Stumpf A, Osada N, Wilp S, Chatzigeorgakidis E, Pfleiderer B. Gender differences in chronic pruritus: women present different morbidity, more scratch lesions and higher burden. *Br J Dermatol.* 2013;168:1273–1280.

115. Tanaka M, Aiba S, Matsumura N, Aoyama H, Tagami H. Prurigo nodularis consists of two distinct forms: early-onset atopic and late-onset non-atopic. *Dermatology.* 1995;190:269–276.

116. Rien BE, Lemont H, Cohen RS. Prurigo nodularis in association with uremia. *J Am Podiatry Assoc.* 1982;72:321–323.

117. Fina L, Grimalt R, Berti E, Caputo R. Nodular prurigo associated with Hodgkin's disease. *Dermatologica.* 1991;182:243–246.

118. Katotomichelakis M, Balatsouras DG, Bassioukas K, Kontogiannis N, Simopoulos K, Danielides V. Recurrent prurigo nodularis related to infected tonsils: a case report. *J Med Case Rep.* 2008;2:243.

119. Saporito L, Florena AM, Colomba C, Pampinella D, Di Carlo P. Prurigo nodularis due to *Mycobacterium tuberculosis. J Med Microbiol.* 2009;58:1649–1651.

120. Iking A, Grundmann S, Chatzigeorgakidis E, Phan NQ, Klein D, Ständer S. Prurigo as a symptom of atopic and non-atopic diseases: aetiological survey in a consecutive cohort of 108 patients. *J Eur Acad Dermatol Venereol.* 2013;27:550–557.

121. Dazzi C, Erma D, Piccinno R, Veraldi S, Caccialanza M. Psychological factors involved in prurigo nodularis: a pilot study. *J Dermatolog Treat.* 2011;22:211–214.

122. Weigelt N, Metze D, Ständer S. Prurigo nodularis: systematic analysis of 58 histological criteria in 136 patients. *J Cutan Pathol.* 2010;37:578–586.

123. Miyauchi H, Uehara M. Follicular occurrence of prurigo nodularis. *J Cutan Pathol.* 1988;15:208–211.

124. Runne U, Orfanos CE. Cutaneous neural proliferation in highly pruritic lesions of chronic prurigo. *Arch Dermatol.* 1977;113:787–791.

125. Lindley RP, Rowland P. Neural hyperplasia is not a diagnostic prerequisite in nodular prurigo. *J Cutan Pathol.* 1989;16:14–18.

126. Johansson O, Liang Y, Heilborn JD, Marcusson JA. Langerhans cells in prurigo nodularis investigated by HLA-DR and S-100 immunofluorescence double staining. *J Dermatol Sci.* 1998;17:24–32.

127. Liang Y, Jacobi HH, Marcusson JA, Haak-Frendscho M, Johansson O. Dendritic mast cells in prurigo nodularis skin. *Eur J Dermatol.* 1999;9:297–299.

128. Kwatra SG. Breaking the itch–scratch cycle in prurigo nodularis. *N Engl J Med.* 2020;382(8):757–758. doi:10.1056/NEJMe1916733

129. Siiskonen H, Harvima I. Mast cells and sensory nerves contribute to neurogenic inflammation and pruritus in chronic skin inflammation. *Front Cell Neurosci.* 2019;13:422. doi:10.3389/fncel.2019.00422

130. Williams KA, Huang AH, Belzberg M, Kwatra SG. Prurigo nodularis. *J Am Acad Dermatol.* 2020;83(6):1567–1575. doi:10.1016/j.jaad.2020.04.182

131. Hirschel-Scholz S, Salomon D, Merot Y, Saurat J-H. Anetodermic prurigo nodularis (with Pautrier's neuroma) responsive to arotinoid acid. *J Am Acad Dermatol.* 1991;25(2):437–442. doi:10.1016/0190-9622(91)70224-P

132. Schuhknecht B, Marziniak M, Wissel A, et al. Reduced intraepidermal nerve fibre density in lesional and nonlesional prurigo nodularis skin as a potential sign of subclinical cutaneous neuropathy. *Br J Dermatol.* 2011;165(1):85–91. doi:10.1111/j.1365-2133.2011.10306.x

133. Fostini AC, Girolomoni G, Tessari G. Prurigo nodularis: an update on etiopathogenesis and therapy. *J Dermatolog Treat.* 2013;24(6):458–462.

134. Edmonds EV, Riaz SN, Francis N, Bunker CB. Nodular prurigo responding to topical tacrolimus. *Br J Dermatol.* 2004;150:1216–1217.

135. Gambichler T, Hyun J, Sommer A, Stücker M, Altmeyer P, Kreuter A. A randomised controlled trial on photo(chemo)therapy of subacute prurigo. *Clin Exp Dermatol.* 2006;31:348–353.

136. Bruni E, Caccialanza M, Piccinno R. Phototherapy of generalized prurigo nodularis. *Clin Exp Dermatol.* 2010;35:549–550.

137. Andersen TP, Fogh K. Thalidomide in 42 patients with prurigo nodularis Hyde. *Dermatology.* 2011;223:107–112.

138. Gencoglan G, Inanir I, Gunduz K. Therapeutic hotline: treatment of prurigo nodularis and lichen simplex chronicus with gabapentin. *Dermatol Ther.* 2010;23:194–198.

139. Mazza M, Guerriero G, Marano G, Janiri L, Bria P, Mazza S. Treatment of prurigo nodularis with pregabalin. *Clin Pharm Ther.* 2013;38:16–18.

140. Phan NQ, Lotts T, Antal A, Bernhard JD, Ständer S. Systemic kappa opioid receptor agonists in the treatment of chronic pruritus: a literature review. *Acta Derm Venereol.* 2012;92:555–560.

141. Liu H, Gaspari AA, Schleichert R. Use of lenalidomide in treating refractory prurigo nodularis. *J Drugs Dermatol.* 2013;12:360–361.

142. Ständer S, Siepmann D, Herrgott I, Sunderkötter C, Luger TA. Targeting the neurokinin receptor 1 with aprepitant: a novel antipruritic strategy. *PLoS One.* 2010;5:e10968.

143. Lu DW, Katz KA. Declining use of the eponym "Reiter's syndrome" in the medical literature, 1998–2003. *J Am Acad Dermatol.* 2005;53:720–723.

144. Wallace DJ, Weismann M. Should a war criminal be rewarded with eponymous distinction? *J Clin Rheumatol.* 2000;6:49–54.

145. Keat A. Reiter's syndrome and reactive arthritis in perspective. *N Engl J Med.* 1983;309:1606–1615.

146. Arora S, Arora G. Reiter's disease in a six-year-old girl. *Indian J Dermatol Venereol Leprol.* 2005;71:285–286.

147. Cuttica RJ, Scheines EJ, Garay SM, Romanelli MC, Maldonado Cocco JA. Juvenile onset Reiter's syndrome: a retrospective study of 26 patients. *Clin Exp Rheumatol.* 1992;10:285–288.

148. Rothe MJ, Kerdel FA. Reiter syndrome. *Int J Dermatol.* 1991;30:173–180.

149. Wu IB, Schwartz RA. Reiter's syndrome: the classic triad and more. *J Am Acad Dermatol.* 2008;59:113–121.

150. Luqmani RA, Dawes PT. Yersinia arthritis with erythema nodosum. *Postgrad Med J.* 1986;62(727):405. doi:10.1136/pgmj.62.727.405

151. Altman EM, Centeno LV, Mahal M, Bielory L. AIDS-associated Reiter's syndrome. *Ann Allergy.* 1994;72:307–316.

152. Perry HO, Mayne JG. Psoriasis and Reiter's syndrome. *Arch Dermatol.* 1965;92:129–136.

153. Weinberger HW, Ropes MW, Kulka JP, Bauer W. Reiter's syndrome, clinical and pathologic observations (review). *Medicine (Baltimore).* 1962;41:35–91.

154. Martin DH, Pollock S, Kuo CC, Wang SP, Brunham RC, Holmes KK. *Chlamydia trachomatis* infections in men with Reiter's syndrome. *Ann Intern Med.* 1984;100:207–213.

155. Rahman MU, Cheema MA, Schumacher HR, Hudson AP. Molecular evidence for the presence of chlamydia in the synovium of patients with Reiter's syndrome. *Arthritis Rheum.* 1992;35:521–529.

156. Hogarth MB, Thomas S, Seifert MH, Tariq SM. Reiter's syndrome following intravesical BCG immunotherapy. *Postgrad Med J.* 2000;76:791–793.

157. Ringrose JH. HLA-B27 associated spondyloarthropathy, an autoimmune disease based on crossreactivity between bacteria and HLA-B27? *Ann Rheum Dis.* 1999;58:598–610.

158. Inman RD, Chiu B, Johnston ME, Vas S, Falk J. HLA class I-related impairment in IL-2 production and lymphocyte response to microbial antigens in reactive arthritis. *J Immunol.* 1989;142:4256–4260.

159. Tsui FW, Xi N, Rohekar S, et al. Toll-like receptor 2 variants are associated with acute reactive arthritis. *Arthritis Rheum.* 2008;58:3436–3438.

160. Ackerman AB. Reiter syndrome and Hans Reiter: neither legitimate! *J Am Acad Dermatol.* 2009;60:517–518.

161. Ingram GJ, Scher RK. Reiter's syndrome with nail involvement: is it psoriasis? *Cutis.* 1985;36:37–40.

162. Thorsteinsson B, Geirsson AJ, Krogh NS, Gudbjornsson B. Outcomes and safety of tumor necrosis factor inhibitors in reactive arthritis: a nationwide experience from Iceland. *J Rheumatol.* 2020;47(10):1575–1581. doi:10.3899/jrheum.191307

163. Barber CE, Kim J, Inman RD, Esdaile JM, James MT. Antibiotics for treatment of reactive arthritis: a systematic review and metaanalysis. *J Rheumatol.* 2013;40(6):916–928. doi:10.3899/jrheum.121192

164. Burg B, Dummer R, Nestle FO, Doebbeling U, Haeffner A. Cutaneous lymphomas consist of a spectrum of nosologically different entities including mycosis fungoides and small plaque parapsoriasis. *Arch Dermatol.* 1996;132:567–572.

165. Hu CH, Winkelmann RK. Digitate dermatosis: a new look at symmetrical small plaque parapsoriasis. *Arch Dermatol.* 1973;107:65–69.

166. Radcliffe-Crocker H. Xanthoerythrodermia perstans. *Br J Dermatol.* 1905;17:119–134.

167. Lewin J, Latkowski JA. Digitate dermatosis (small-plaque parapsoriasis). *Dermatol Online J.* 2012;18:3.

168. Yeager JK, Posnak EJ, Cobb MW. Digitate dermatosis. *Cutis.* 1991;48:457–458.

169. Benmaman O, Sanchez JL. Comparative clinicopathological study on pityriasis lichenoides chronica and small plaque parapsoriasis. *Am J Dermatopathol.* 1988;10:189–196.

170. El-Darouti MA, Fawzy MM, Hegazy RA, Abdel Hay RM. Hypopigmented parapsoriasis en plaque, a new, overlooked member of the parapsoriasis family: a report of 34 patients and a 7-year experience. *J Am Acad Dermatol.* 2012;67:1182–1188.

171. Bonvalet D, Colau-Gohm K, Belaich S, et al. Les differentes formes du para-psoriasis en plaques. *Ann Dermatol Venereol.* 1977;104:18–25.

172. Samman PD. The natural history of parapsoriasis en plaques (chronic superficial dermatitis) and prereticulotic poikiloderma. *Br J Dermatol.* 1972;87:405–411.

173. Heid E, Desvaux J, Brändle J, Grosshans E. Der verlauf der parapsoriasis en plaques (Brocq'sche Krankheit). *Z Hautkr.* 1977;52:658.

174. Belousova IE, Vanecek T, Samtsov AV, Michal M, Kazakov DV. A patient with clinicopathologic features of small plaque parapsoriasis presenting later with plaque-stage mycosis fungoides: report of a case and comparative retrospective study of 27 cases of 'nonprogressive' small plaque parapsoriasis. *J Am Acad Dermatol.* 2008;59:474–482.

175. Liu V, McKee PH. Cutaneous T-cell lymphoproliferative disorders: recent advances and clarification of confusing issues. *Adv Anat Pathol.* 2002;9:79–100.

176. Pimpinelli N, Olsen EA, Santucci M, et al. Defining early mycosis fungoides. *J Am Acad Dermatol.* 2005;53:1053–1063.

177. Duarte IA, Korkes KL, Amorim VA, Kobata C, Buense R, Lazzarini R. An evaluation of the treatment of parapsoriasis with phototherapy. *An Bras Dermatol.* 2013;88:306–308.

178. Takahashi H, Takahashi I, Tsuji H, Ishida-yamamoto A, Iizuka H. Digitate dermatosis successfully treated by narrowband ultraviolet B irradiation. *J Dermatol.* 2011;38:923–924.

179. Lindahl LM, Fenger-Gron M, Iversen L. Topical nitrogen mustard therapy in patients with mycosis fungoides or parapsoriasis. *J Eur Acad Dermatology Venereol.* 2013;27(2):163–168. doi:10.1111/j.1468-3083.2011.04433.x

180. Parsons JM. Pityriasis rosea update. *J Am Acad Dermatol.* 1986;15:159–167.

181. Chuh A, Zawar V, Lee A. Atypical presentations of pityriasis rosea: case presentations. *J Eur Acad Dermatol Venereol.* 2005;19:120–126.

182. Drago F, Broccolo F, Zaccaria E, et al. Pregnancy outcome in patients with pityriasis rosea. *J Am Acad Dermatol.* 2008;58:S78–S83.

183. Bunch LW, Tilley JC. Pityriasis rosea. *Arch Dermatol.* 1961;84:79–86.

184. Aiba S, Tagami H. Immunohistologic studies in pityriasis rosea. *Arch Dermatol.* 1985;121:761–765.

185. Panizzon R, Bloch PH. Histopathology of pityriasis rosea Gibert: qualitative and quantitative light-microscopic study of 62 biopsies of 40 patients. *Dermatologica.* 1982;165:551–558.

186. Okamoto H, Imamura S, Aoshima T, Komura J, Ofuji S. Dyskeratotic degeneration of epidermal cells in pityriasis rosea: light and electron microscopic studies. *Br J Dermatol.* 1982;107:189–194.

187. Bonafe JL, Icart J, Perpere M, Oksman F, Divoux D. Etude histopathologique, ultrastructurale, immunologique et virologique du pityriasis rose de Gibert. *Ann Dermatol Venereol.* 1982;109:855–861.

188. Neoh CY, Tan AW, Mohamed K, Sun YJ, Tan SH. Characterization of the inflammatory cell infiltrate in herald patches and fully developed eruptions of pityriasis rosea. *Clin Exp Dermatol.* 2010;35:300–304.

189. Blauvett A. Skin diseases associated with human herpesvirus 6, 7, and 8 infection. *J Invest Dermatol Symp Proc.* 2001;6:197–202.

190. Canpolat Kirac B, Adisen E, Bozdayi G, et al. The role of human herpesvirus 6, human herpesvirus 7, Epstein-Barr virus and cytomegalovirus in the aetiology of pityriasis rosea. *J Eur Acad Dermatol Venereol.* 2009;23:16–21.

191. Drago F, Broccolo F, Rebora A. Pityriasis rosea: an update with a critical appraisal of its possible herpesviral etiology. *J Am Acad Dermatol.* 2009;61:303–318.

192. Chia JK, Shitabata P, Wu J, Chia AY. Enterovirus infection as a possible cause of pityriasis rosea: demonstration by immunochemical staining. *Arch Dermatol.* 2006;142:942–943.

193. Kwon NH, Kim JE, Cho BK, Park HJ. A novel influenza a (H1N1) virus as a possible cause of pityriasis rosea? *J Eur Acad Dermatol Venereol.* 2011;25:368–369.

194. Atzori L, Pinna AL, Ferreli C, Aste N. Pityriasis rosea–like adverse reaction: review of the literature and experience of an Italian drug-surveillance center. *Dermatol Online J.* 2006;12:1.

195. Rajpara SN, Ormerod AD, Gallaway L. Adalimumab-induced pityriasis rosea. *J Eur Acad Dermatol Venereol.* 2007;21:1294–1296.

196. Guarneri C, Polimeni G, Nunnari G. Pityriasis rosea during etanercept therapy. *Eur Rev Med Pharmacol Sci.* 2009;13: 383–387.

197. Yoshiike T, Aikawa Y, Wongwaisayawan H, Ogawa H. HLA-DR antigen expression on peripheral T cell subsets in pityriasis rosea and herpes zoster. *Dermatologica.* 1991;82:160–163.

198. Bos JD, Huisman PM, Kreg SR, Faber WR. Pityriasis rosea (Gibert): abnormal distribution pattern of antigen presenting cells in situ. *Acta Dermatol Venereol (Stockholm).* 1985;65:132–137.

199. Aiba S, Tabami H. HLA-DR antigen expression on the keratinocyte surface in dermatoses characterized by lymphocytic exocytosis (e.g., pityriasis rosea). *Br J Dermatol.* 1984;3:285–294.

200. Rasi A, Tajziehchi L, Savabi-Nasab S. Oral erythromycin is ineffective in the treatment of pityriasis rosea. *J Drugs Dermatol.* 2008;7:35–38.

201. Chuh AA, Dofitas BL, Comisel GG, et al. Interventions for pityriasis rosea. *Cochrane Database Syst Rev.* 2007;(2):CD005068.

202. Gianotti F. Rilievi di una particolare casistica tossinfettiva caratterizzata de eruzione eritemato-infiltrativa desquamativa a focolai lenticolari, a sede elettiva acroesposata. *G Ital Dermatol.* 1955;96:678–697.

203. Turhan V, Ardic N, Besirbellioglu B, Dogru T. Gianotti-Crosti syndrome associated with HBV infection in an adult. *Ir J Med Sci.* 2005;174:92–94.

204. Ting PT, Barankin B, Dytoc MT. Gianotti-Crosti syndrome in two adult patients. *J Cutan Med Surg.* 2008;12:121–125.

205. Manoharan S, Muir J, Williamson R. Gianotti-Crosti syndrome in an adult following recent *Mycoplasma pneumoniae* infection. *Australas J Dermatol.* 2005;46:106–109.

206. Gianotti F. Papular acrodermatitis of childhood and other papulo-vesicular acro-located syndromes. *Br J Dermatol.* 1979;100:49–59.

207. Spear KL, Winkelmann RK. Gianotti-Crosti syndrome: a review of ten cases not associated with hepatitis B. *Arch Dermatol.* 1984;120:891–896.

208. Taieb A, Plantin P, Du Pasquier P, Guillet G, Maleville J. Gianotti-Crosti syndrome: a study of 26 cases. *Br J Dermatol.* 1986;115: 49–59.

209. Baldari U, Monti A, Righini MG. An epidemic of infantile papular acrodermatitis (Gianotti-Crosti syndrome) due to Epstein-Barr virus. *Dermatology.* 1994;188:203–204.

210. Draelos ZK, Hansen RC, James WD. Gianotti-Crosti syndrome associated with infections other than hepatitis B. *JAMA.* 1986;256:2386–2388.

211. Caputo R, Gelmetti C, Ermacora E, Gianni E, Silvestri A. Gianotti-Crosti syndrome: a retrospective analysis of 308 cases. *J Am Acad Dermatol.* 1992;26:207–210.

212. Blauvelt A, Turner ML. Gianotti-Crosti syndrome and human immunodeficiency virus infection. *Arch Dermatol.* 1994;130: 481–483.

213. Khan I, Gleeson J, McKenna D. Gianotti-Crosti syndrome following meningococcal septicaemia. *Ir Med J.* 2007;100:373.

214. Atanasovski M, Dele-Michael A, Dasgeb B, Ganger L, Mehregan D. A case report of Gianotti-Crosti post vaccination with MMR and dTaP. *Int J Dermatol.* 2011;50:609–610.

215. Tay YK. Gianotti-Crosti syndrome following immunization. *Pediatr Dermatol.* 2001;18:262.

216. Ricci G, Patrizi A, Neri I, Specchia F, Tosti G, Masi M. Gianotti-Crosti syndrome and allergic background. *Acta Dermatol Venereol.* 2003;83:202–205.

217. Smith KJ, Skelton H. Histopathologic features seen in Gianotti-Crosti syndrome secondary to Epstein-Barr virus. *J Am Acad Dermatol.* 2000;43:1076–1079.

218. Stefanato CM, Goldberg LJ, Andersen WK, Bhawan J. Gianotti-Crosti syndrome presenting as lichenoid dermatitis. *Am J Dermatopathol.* 2000;22:162–165.

219. Margyarlaki M, Drobnitsch I, Schneider I. Papular acrodermatitis of childhood: Gianotti-Crosti disease. *Pediatr Dermatol.* 1991;8:224–227.

220. Ackermann AB, Chongchitnant N, Sanchez J, et al. Gianotti-Crosti's disease syndrome. In: *Histologic Diagnosis of Inflammatory Skin Diseases.* 2nd ed. Williams and Wilkins; 1997:403.

221. Boeck K, Mempel M, Schmidt T, Abeck D. Gianotti-Crosti syndrome: clinical, serologic, and therapeutic data from nine children. *Cutis.* 1998;62:271–274.

222. Zawar V, Chuh A. Efficacy of ribavirin in a case of long lasting and disabling Gianotti-Crosti syndrome. *J Dermatol Case Rep.* 2008;2:63–66.

223. Kawasaki T, Kosaki F, Owaka S, Shigematsu I, Yanagawa H. A new infantile acute febrile mucocutaneous lymph node syndrome (MLNS) prevailing in Japan. *Pediatrics.* 1974;54:271–276.

224. Genizi J, Miron D, Spiegel R, Fink D, Horowitz Y. Kawasaki disease in very young infants: high prevalence of atypical presentation and coronary arteritis. *Clin Pediatr.* 2003;42:263–267.

225. Melish ME, Hicks RV. Kawasaki syndrome: clinical features, pathophysiology, etiology and therapy. *J Rheumatol.* 1990;17:2–10.

226. Dajani AS, Bisno AL, Chung KJ, et al. Diagnostic guidelines for Kawasaki disease. American Heart Association Committee on Rheumatic fever, endocarditis, and Kawasaki disease. *Am J Dis Child.* 1990;144:1218–1219.

227. Burns JC, Mason WH, Glode MP, et al. Clinical and epidemiologic characteristics of patients referred for evaluation of possible Kawasaki disease. *J Pediatr.* 1991;118:680–686.

228. Wortmann DW. Kawasaki syndrome. *Semin Dermatol.* 1992;11:37–47.

229. Ducos MH, Taieb A, Sarlangue J, et al. Manifestations cutanees de la maladie de Kawasaki: a propos de 30 observations. *Ann Dermatol Venereol.* 1993;120:589–597.

230. Friter BS, Lucky AW. The perineal eruption of Kawasaki syndrome. *Arch Dermatol.* 1988;124:1805–1810.

231. Eberhard BA, Sundel RP, Newuger JW, et al. Psoriatic eruption in Kawasaki disease. *J Pediatr.* 2000;137:578–580.

232. Zvulunov A, Greenberg D, Cagnano E, Einhorn M. Development of psoriatic lesions during acute and convalescent phases of Kawasaki disease. *J Pediatr Child Health.* 2003;39:229–231.

233. Bayers S, Shulman ST, Paller AS. Kawasaki disease. *J Am Acad Dermatol.* 2013;69(4):501.e1–501.e11. doi:10.1016/j.jaad.2013.07.002

234. Suzuki A, Kamiya T, Kuwahara N, et al. Coronary arterial lesions of Kawasaki disease: cardiac catheterization findings of 1100 cases. *Pediatr Cardiol.* 1986;7:3–9.

235. Kato H, Ichinose E, Kawasaki T. Myocardial infarction in Kawasaki disease: clinical analyses in 195 cases. *J Pediatr.* 1986; 108:923–927.

236. Tomita S, Chung K, Mas M, Gidding S, Shulman ST. Peripheral gangrene associated with Kawasaki disease. *Clin Infect Dis.* 1992;14:121–126.

237. Hirose S, Hamashima Y. Morphological observations on the vasculitis in the mucocutaneous lymph node syndrome: a skin biopsy study of 27 patients. *Eur J Pediatr.* 1978;129:17–27.

238. Kimura T, Miyazawa H, Watanabe K, Moriya T. Small pustules in Kawasaki disease: a clinicopathological study of four patients. *Am J Dermatopathol.* 1988;10:218–223.

239. Gomez-Moyano E, Vera Casaño A, Camacho J, Sanz Trelles A, Crespo-Erchiga V. Kawasaki disease complicated by cutaneous vasculitis and peripheral gangrene. *J Am Acad Dermatol.* 2011;64(5): e74–e75.

240. Sato N, Sagawa K, Sasaguri Y, Inoue O, Kato H. Immunopathology and cytokine detection in the skin lesions of patients with Kawasaki disease. *J Pediatr.* 1993;122:198–203.

241. Shingadia D, Bose A, Booy R. Could a herpes virus be the cause of Kawasaki disease? *Lancet Infect Dis.* 2002;2:310–313.

242. Shulman ST, De Inocencio J, Hirsch R. Kawasaki disease. *Pediatr Clin North Am.* 1995;42:1205–1222.

243. Leung DY, Meissner HC, Fulton DR, et al. Superantigens in Kawasaki syndrome. *Clin Immunol Immunopathol.* 1995;77:119–126.

244. Burgner D, Davila S, Breunis WB, et al. A genome-wide association study identifies novel and functionally related susceptibility Loci for Kawasaki disease. *PLoS Genet.* 2009;5(1):e1000319.

245. Rowley AH, Baker SC, Orenstein JM, Shulman ST. Searching for the cause of Kawasaki disease—cytoplasmic inclusion bodies provide new insight. *Nat Rev Microbiol.* 2008;6(5):394–401.

246. Ohno T, Yuge T, Kariyazono H, et al. Serum hepatocyte growth factor combined with vascular endothelial growth factor as a predictive indicator for the occurrence of coronary artery lesions in Kawasaki disease. *Eur J Pediatr.* 2002;161:105–111.

247. Suzuki H, Muragaki Y, Uemura S, et al. Detection of autoantibodies against a 70 kDa protein derived from vascular smooth muscle cells in patients with Kawasaki disease. *Eur J Pediatr.* 2002;161:324.

248. Rowley AH, Shulman ST. Pathogenesis and management of Kawasaki disease. *Expert Rev Anti Infect Ther.* 2010;8:197.

249. Newburger JW, Takahashi M, Gerber MA, et al. Diagnosis, treatment, and long-term management of Kawasaki disease. *Circulation.* 2004;110:2747.

250. Newburger JW, Takahashi M, Beiser AS, et al. A single intravenous infusion of globulin as compared with four infusions in the treatment of acute Kawasaki syndrome. *N Engl J Med.* 1991;324:1633.

251. Minami T, Suzuki H, Takeuchi T, Uemura S, Sugatani J, Yoshikawa N. A polymorphism in plasma platelet-activating factor acetylhydrolase is involved in resistance to immunoglobulin treatment in Kawasaki disease. *J Pediatr.* 2005;147(1):78–83. doi:10.1016/j.jpeds.2005.03.037

252. Newburger JW, Sleeper LA, McCrindle BW, et al. Randomized trial of pulsed corticosteroid therapy for primary treatment of Kawasaki disease. *N Engl J Med.* 2007;356:663–675.

253. Burns JC, Best BM, Mejias A, et al. Infliximab treatment of intravenous immunoglobulin-resistant Kawasaki disease. *J Pediatr.* 2008;153:833–838.

254. Gerfaud-Valentin M, Jamilloux Y, Iwaz J, Sève P. Adult-onset Still's disease. *Autoimmun Rev.* 2014;13(7):708–722. doi:10.1016/j.autrev.2014.01.058

255. Larson AR, Laga AC, Granter SR. The spectrum of histopathologic findings in cutaneous lesions in patients with still disease. *Am J Clin Pathol.* 2015;144(6):945–951. doi:10.1309/AJCPZE77UAPSMDCD

256. Andersen KE, Hjorth N, Menné T. The baboon syndrome: systemically-induced allergic contact dermatitis. *Contact Dermatitis.* 1984;10(2):97–100. doi:10.1111/j.1600-0536.1984.tb00343.x

257. Hausermann P, Harr T, Bircher AJ. Baboon syndrome resulting from systemic drugs: is there strife between SDRIFE and allergic contact dermatitis syndrome? *Contact Dermatitis.* 2004;51(5–6): 297–310. doi:10.1111/j.0105-1873.2004.00445.x

258. Magnolo N, Metze D, Ständer S. Pustulobullous variant of SDRIFE (symmetrical drug-related intertriginous and flexural exanthema). *JDDG J der Dtsch Dermatologischen Gesellschaft.* 2017;15(6):657–659. doi:10.1111/ddg.13031

259. Nespoulous L, Matei I, Charissoux A, Bédane C, Assikar S. Symmetrical drug-related intertriginous and flexural exanthema (SDRIFE) associated with pristinamycin, secnidazole, and nefopam, with a review of the literature. *Contact Dermatitis.* 2018;79(6):378–380. doi:10.1111/cod.13084

260. Bulur I, Keseroglu HO, Saracoglu ZN, Gönül M. Symmetrical drug-related intertriginous and flexural exanthema (Baboon syndrome) associated with infliximab. *J Dermatol Case Rep.* 2015;9(1):12–14. doi:10.3315/jdcr.2015.1190

261. Huynh T, Hughey LC, McKay K, Carney C, Sami N. Systemic drug-related intertriginous and flexural exanthema from radio contrast media: a series of 3 cases. *JAAD Case Reports.* 2015;1(3):147–149. doi:10.1016/j.jdcr.2015.03.007

262. Zuberbier T, Asero R, Bindslev-Jensen C, et al. EAACI/GA(2) LEN/EDF/WAO guideline: definition, classification and diagnosis of urticaria. *Allergy.* 2009;64(10):1417–1426.

263. Zingale LC, Beltrami L, Zanichelli A, et al. Angioedema without urticaria: a large clinical survey. *CMAJ.* 2006;175:1065–1070.

264. Cooper KD. Urticaria and angioedema: diagnosis and evaluation. *J Am Acad Dermatol.* 1991;25:166–174.

265. Lipsker D, Veran Y, Grunenberger F, Cribier B, Heid E, Grosshans E. The Schnitzler syndrome. Four new cases and review of the literature. *Medicine (Baltimore).* 2001;80:37–44.

266. Kacar M, Pathak S, Savic S. Hereditary systemic autoinflammatory diseases and Schnitzler's syndrome. *Rheumatology.* 2019;58(suppl 6):vi31–vi43. doi:10.1093/rheumatology/kez448

267. Marsland AM. Autoimmunity and complement in the pathogenesis of chronic urticaria. *Curr Allergy Asthma Rep.* 2006;6:265–269.

268. Ricketti AS, Cleri DJ, Ramos-Bonner LS, Vernaleo JR. Hereditary angioedema presenting in late middle age after angiotensin-converting enzyme inhibitor treatment. *Ann Allergy Asthma Immunol.* 2007;98:397–401.

269. Gallais Sérézal I, Bouillet L, Dhôte R, et al. Hereditary angioedema and lupus: a French retrospective study and literature review. *Autoimmun Rev.* 2015;14(6):564–568. doi:10.1016/j.autrev.2015.02.001

270. Soter NA. Chronic urticaria as a manifestation of necrotizing venulitis. *N Engl J Med.* 1977;296:1440–1442.

271. Sanchez NP, Winkelmann RK, Schroeter AL, Dicken CH. The clinical and histopathologic spectrums of urticarial vasculitis: study of forty cases. *J Am Acad Dermatol.* 1982;7:599–605.

272. Venzor J, Lee WL, Huston DP. Urticarial vasculitis. *Clin Rev Allergy Immunol.* 2002;23:201–216.

273. Mehregan DR, Hall MJ, Gibson LE. Urticarial vasculitis: a histopathologic and clinical review of 72 cases. *J Am Acad Dermatol.* 1992;26:441–448.

274. Wisnieski JJ, Naff GB. Serum IgG antibodies to C1q in hypocomplementemic urticarial vasculitis syndrome. *Arthritis Rheum.* 1989;32(9):1119–1127. doi:10.1002/anr.1780320910

275. Siegert C, Kazatchkine MD, Sjöholm A, Würzner R, Loos M, Daha MR. Autoantibodies against C1q: view on clinical relevance and pathogenic roles. *Clin Exp Immunol.* 1999;116(1):4–8. doi:10.1046/j.1365-2249.1999.00867.x

276. Farell AM, Sabroe RA, Bunker CB. Urticarial vasculitis associated with polycythemia rubra vera. *Clin Exp Dermatol.* 1996;21:302–304.

277. Wilson D, McCluggage WG, Wright GD. Urticarial vasculitis: a paraneoplastic presentation of B-cell non Hodgkin's lymphoma. *Rheumatology (Oxford).* 2002;41(4):476–477.

278. Bisaccia E, Adamo V, Rozan SW. Urticarial vasculitis progressing to systemic lupus erythematosus. *Arch Dermatol.* 1988;124:1088–1090.

279. Welsh JP, Cusack KA, Ko C. Urticarial vasculitis secondary to paroxetine. *J Drugs Dermatol.* 2006;5:1012–1014.

280. Barzilai A, Sagi L, Baum S, et al. The histopathology of urticaria revisited—clinical pathological study. *Am J Dermatopathol.* 2017;39(10):753–759. doi:10.1097/DAD.0000000000000786

281. Huston DP, Bressler RB. Urticaria and angioedema. *Med Clin North Am.* 1992;76:805–840.

282. Soter NA, Wasserman SI. Urticaria, angioedema (review). *Int J Dermatol.* 1979;18:517–532.

283. Soter NA, Austen KF, Gigli I. Urticaria and arthralgias as manifestations of necrotizing angiitis (vasculitis). *J Invest Dermatol.* 1974;63:485–490.

284. Haas N, Kuster W, Zuberbier T, Henz BM. Muckle-Wells syndrome: clinical and histological skin findings compatible with cold air urticaria in a large kindred. *Br J Dermatol.* 2004;151(1): 99–104. doi:10.1111/j.1365-2133.2004.06001.x

285. Criado PR, Criado RF, Takakura CF, et al. Ultrastructure of vascular permeability in urticaria. *Isr Med Assoc J.* 2013;15: 173–177.

286. Monroe EW, Schulz CI, Maize JC, Jordon RE. Vasculitis in chronic urticaria: an immunopathologic study. *J Invest Dermatol.* 1981;76:103–107.

287. Kikuchi Y, Kaplan AP. A role for C5a in augmenting IgG-dependent histamine release from basophils in chronic urticaria. *J Allergy Clin Immunol.* 2002;109:114–118.

288. Yasnowsky KM, Dreskin SC, Efaw B, et al. Chronic urticaria sera increase basophil CD203c expression. *J Allergy Clin Immunol.* 2006;117:1430–1434.

289. Haas N, Hermes B, Henz BM. Adhesion molecules and cellular infiltrate: histology of urticaria. *J Invest Dermatol Symp Proc.* 2001;6:137–138.

290. Lerch M. Drug-induced angioedema. *Chem Immunol Allergy.* 2012;97:98–105.

291. Sánchez-Borges M, González-Aveledo LA. Angiotensin-converting enzyme inhibitors and angioedema. *Allergy Asthma Immunol Res.* 2010;2:195–198.

292. Davis MD, Daoud MS, Kirby B, Gibson LE, Rogers RS 3rd.. Clinicopathologic correlation of hypocomplementemic and normocomplementemic urticarial vasculitis. *J Am Acad Dermatol.* 1998;38:899–905.

293. Manthiram K, Zhou Q, Aksentijevich I, Kastner DL. The monogenic autoinflammatory diseases define new pathways in human innate immunity and inflammation. *Nat Immunol.* 2017;18(8):832–842. doi:10.1038/ni.3777

294. Miteva M, Elsner P, Zieme M. A histopathologic study of arthropod bite reactions in 20 patients highlights relevant adnexal involvement. *J Cutan Pathol.* 2009;36:26–33.

295. Grattan CE, Humphreys F. Guidelines for evaluation and management of urticaria in adults and children. *Br J Dermatol.* 2007;157:1116–1123.

296. Simons FE. H1-Antihistamines: more relevant than ever in the treatment of allergic disorders. *J Allergy Clin Immunol.* 2003;112:S42–S52.

297. Lin RY, Curry A, Pesola GR, et al. Improved outcomes in patients with acute allergic syndromes who are treated with combined H$_1$ and H$_2$ antagonists. *Ann Emerg Med.* 2000;36:462–468.

298. Wan KS. Efficacy of leukotriene receptor antagonist with an anti-H1 receptor antagonist for treatment of chronic idiopathic urticaria. *J Dermatolog Treat.* 2009;20:194–197.

299. Nam YH, Kim JH, Jin HJ, et al. Effects of omalizumab treatment in patients with refractory chronic urticaria. *Allergy Asthma Immunol Res.* 2012;4:357–361.

300. Bernstein JA, Singh U, Rao MB, Berendts K, Zhang X, Mutasim D. Benralizumab for chronic spontaneous urticaria. *N Engl J Med.* 2020;383(14):1389–1391.

301. Cohen JM. Ligelizumab for chronic spontaneous urticaria. *N Engl J Med.* 2020;382(6):579.

302. Palladini G, Merlini G. The elusive pathogenesis of Schnitzler syndrome. *Blood.* 2018;131(9):944–946. doi:10.1182/blood-2018-01-824862

303. Bressler GS, Jones RE Jr. Erythema annulare centrifugum. *J Am Acad Dermatol.* 1981;4:597–602.

304. Darier J. De l'erythema annulaire centrifuge. *Ann Dermatol Syphilol.* 1916;6:57–76.

305. Kim KJ, Chang SE, Choi JH, Sung KJ, Moon KC, Koh JK. Clinicopathologic analysis of 66 cases of erythema annulare centrifugum. *J Dermatol.* 2002;29:61–67.

306. Weyers W, Diaz-Cascajo C, Weyers I. Erythema annulare centrifugum: results of a clinicopathologic study of 73 patients. *Am J Dermatopathol.* 2003;25:451–462.

307. High WA, Cohen JB, Wetherington W, Cockerell CJ. Superficial gyrate erythema as a cutaneous reaction to alendronate for osteoporosis. *J Am Acad Dermatol.* 2003;48:945–946.

308. Ural AU, Ozcan A, Avcu F, et al. Erythema annulare centrifugum as the presenting sign of CD 30 positive anaplastic large cell lymphoma: association with disease activity. *Hematologica (Budapest).* 2001;31:81–84.

309. Ravic-Nikolic A, Milicic V, Jovovic-Dagovic B, Ristić G. Gyrate erythema associated with metastatic tumor of gastrointestinal tract. *Dermatol Online J.* 2006;12:11.

310. Minni J, Sarro R. A novel therapeutic approach to erythema annulare centrifugum. *J Am Acad Dermatol.* 2006;54:S134–S135.

311. De Aloe G, Rubegni P, Risulo M, Sbano P, Poggiali S, Fimiani M. Erythema annulare centrifugum successfully treated with metronidazole. *Clin Exp Dermatol.* 2005;30:583–584.

312. Boyd AS, Neldner KH. Lichen planus. *J Am Acad Dermatol.* 1991;25:93.

313. Bricker SL. Oral lichen planus: a review. *Semin Dermatol.* 1994;13:87.

314. Fox LP, Lightdale CJ, Grossman ME. Lichen planus of the esophagus: what dermatologists need to know. *J Am Acad Dermatol.* 2011;65:175–183.

315. Bajaj DR, Khoso NA, Devrajani BR, Matlani BL, Lohana P. Oral lichen planus: a clinical study. *J Coll Physicians Surg Pak.* 2010;20(3):154–157.

316. Eisen D. The clinical features, malignant potential, and systemic associations of oral lichen planus: a study of 723 patients. *J Am Acad Dermatol.* 2002;46:207–214.

317. Nielsen JA, Law RM, Fiman KH, Roberts CA. Esophageal lichen planus: a case report and review of the literature. *World J Gastroenterol.* 2013;19:2278–2281.

318. Goettmann S, Zaraa I, Moulonguet I. Nail lichen planus: epidemiological, clinical, pathological, therapeutic and prognosis study of 67 cases. *J Eur Acad Dermatol Venereol.* 2012;26: 1304–1309.

319. Liu KC, Lee JY, Hsu MM, Hsu CK. The evolution of clinicopathologic features in eruptive lichen planus: a case report and review of literature. *Dermatol Online J.* 2013;19:8.

320. Reich HL, Nguyen JT, James WD. Annular lichen planus: a case series of 20 patients. *J Am Acad Dermatol.* 2004;50:595–599.

321. Mora RG, Nesbitt LT Jr, Brantley JB. Lichen planus pemphigoides: clinical and immunofluorescence findings in four cases. *J Am Acad Dermatol.* 1983;8:331.

322. Solomon LW, Helm TN, Stevens C, Neiders ME, Kumar V. Clinical and immunopathologic findings in oral lichen planus pemphigoides. *Oral Surg Oral Med Oral Pathol Oral Radiol Endod.* 2007;103:808.

323. Zaraa I, Mahfoudh A, Sellami MK, et al. Lichen planus pemphigoides: four new cases and a review of the literature. *Int J Dermatol.* 2013;52:406–412.

324. Ben SC, Chenguel L, Ghariani N, Denguezli M, Hmouda H, Bouraoui K. Captopril-induced lichen planus pemphigoides. *Pharmacoepidemiol Drug Saf.* 2008;17:722–724.

325. Silvers DN, Katz BE, Young AW. Pseudopelade of Brocq is lichen planopilaris: report of four cases that support this nosology. *Cutis.* 1993;51:99.

326. Chopra A, Jain C, Mamta I, Bahl RK. Ulcerative lichen planus of the foot. *Indian J Dermatol Venereol Leprol.* 1996;62:60–61.

327. Renner R, Treudler R, Gebhardt C, Simon JC. Ulcerated plantar lichen planus. Successful treatment with cyclosporine. *Hautarzt.* 2009;60:647–650.

328. Dilaimy M. Lichen planus subtropicus. *Arch Dermatol.* 1976; 112:125.

329. Salman SM, Kibbi AG, Zaynoun S. Actinic lichen planus: a clinicopathologic study of 16 patients. *J Am Acad Dermatol.* 1989;20:226.

330. Bouassida S, Boudaya S, Turki H, Gueriani H, Zahaf A. Actinic lichen planus: 32 cases. *Am J Dermatol Venereol.* 1998;125:408.

331. Camisa C, Neff JC, Olsen RG. Use of indirect immunofluorescence in the lupus erythematosus/lichen planus overlap syndrome: an additional diagnostic clue. *J Am Acad Dermatol.* 1984;11:1050.

332. Scher RK, Fischbein R, Ackerman AB. Twenty-nail dystrophy: a variant of lichen planus. *Arch Dermatol.* 1978;114:612.

333. Kechijian P. Twenty nail dystrophy of childhood. *Cutis.* 1985;35:38.

334. Pandhi D, Singal A, Bhattacharya SN. Lichen planus in childhood: a series of 316 patients. *Pediatr Dermatol.* 2014;31(1): 59–67. doi:10.1111/pde.12155

335. Sigurgeirsson B, Lindelof B. Lichen planus and malignancy: an epidemiologic study of 2071 patients and a review of the literature. *Arch Dermatol.* 1991;127:1684.

336. Allen JV, Callen JP. Keratoacanthomas arising in hypertrophic lichen planus. *Arch Dermatol.* 1981;117:519.

337. Castano E, Lopez-Rios F, Alvarez-Fernandez JG, Rodríguez-Peralto JL, Iglesias L. Verrucous carcinoma in association with hypertrophic lichen planus. *Clin Exp Dermatol.* 1997;22:23.

338. Fowler CB, Rees TD, Smith BR. Squamous cell carcinoma on the dorsum of the tongue arising in a long-standing lesion of erosive lichen planus. *J Am Dent Assoc.* 1987;115:707.

339. Katz RW, Brahim JS, Travis WD. Oral squamous cell carcinoma arising in a patient with long-standing lichen planus: a case report. *Oral Surg Oral Med Oral Pathol.* 1990;70:282.

340. Murti PR, Daftary DK, Bhonsle RB, Gupta PC, Mehta FS, Pindborg JJ. Malignant potential of oral lichen planus: observation in 722 patients from India. *J Oral Pathol.* 1986;15:71.

341. Mattila R, Alanen K, Syrjanen S. Desmocollin expression in oral atrophic lichen planus correlates with clinical behavior and DNA content. *J Cut Pathol.* 2008;35:832–838.

342. Crotty CP, Su WP, Winkelmann RK. Ulcerative lichen planus: follow-up of surgical excision and grafting. *Arch Dermatol.* 1980;116:1252.

343. Carrozzo M, Pellicano R. Lichen planus and hepatitis C virus infection: an updated critical review. *Minerva Gastroenterol Dietol.* 2008;54:65–74.

344. Lodi G, Pellicano R, Carrozzo M. Hepatitis C virus infection and lichen planus: a systematic review with meta-analysis. *Oral Dis.* 2010;16:601–612.

345. Shengyuan L, Songpo Y, Wen W, Wenjing T, Haitao Z, Binyou W. Hepatitis C and lichen planus: a reciprocal association determined by meta-analysis. *Arch Dermatol.* 2009;145:1040–1047.

346. Calista D, Morri M. Lichen planus induced by hepatitis B vaccination: a new case and review of the literature. *Int J Dermatol.* 2004;43:562–564.

347. Baghestani S, Moosavi A, Eftekhari T. Familial colocalization of lichen planus and vitiligo on sun exposed areas. *Ann Dermatol.* 2013;25:223–235.

348. Morar N, Francis ND. Generalized lichen planus induced by radiotherapy: shared molecular mechanisms? *Clin Exp Dermatol.* 2009;34:434–435.

349. Renfro L, Kamino H, Raphael B, Moy J, Sanchez M. Ulcerative lichen planus-like dermatitis associated with hydroxyurea. *J Am Acad Dermatol.* 1991;24:143–145.

350. Enhamre A, Lagerholm B. Acrosyringeal lichen planus. *Acta Dermatol Venereol (Stockholm).* 1987;67:346.

351. Hanau D, Sengel D. Perforating lichen planus. *J Cutan Pathol.* 1984;11:176.

352. Mehregan DA, Van Hale HM, Muller SA. Lichen planopilaris: clinical and pathologic study of forty-five patients. *J Am Acad Dermatol.* 1992;27:935.

353. Mobini N, Tam S, Kamino H. Possible role of the bulge region in the pathogenesis of inflammatory scarring alopecia: lichen planopilaris as the prototype. *J Cutan Pathol.* 2005;32:675.

354. Dawber PRP. What is pseudopelade? *Clin Exp Dermatol.* 1992;17:305.

355. Matta M, Kibbi AG, Khattar J, Salman SM, Zaynoun ST. Lichen planopilaris: a clinicopathologic study. *J Am Acad Dermatol.* 1990;22:594.

356. Tschen JA, Tschen EA, McGavran MH. Erythema dyschromicum perstans. *J Am Acad Dermatol.* 1980;2:295.

357. Van der Horst JC, Cirkel PKS, Nieboer C. Mixed lichen planus–lupus erythematosus disease: a distinct entity? *Clin Exp Dermatol.* 1983;8:631.

358. Saurat JH, Guinepain MT, Didierjean L, Sohier J, Puissant A. Coexistence d'un lichen plan et d'un pemphigoide bulleuse. *Ann Dermatol Venereol.* 1977;104:368.

359. Medenica M, Lorincz A. Lichen planus: an ultrastructural study. *Acta Dermatol Venereol (Stockholm).* 1977;57:55.

360. Clausen J, Kjaergaard J, Bierring F. The ultrastructure of the dermo-epidermal junction in lichen planus. *Acta Dermatol Venereol (Stockholm).* 1981;61:101.

361. Gomes MA, Staquet MJ, Thivolet J. Staining of colloid bodies by keratin antisera in lichen planus. *Am J Dermatopathol.* 1981;3:341.

362. Abell E, Presbury DG, Marks R, Ramnarain D. The diagnostic significance of immunoglobulin and fibrin deposition in lichen planus. *Br J Dermatol.* 1975;93:17.

363. Morel P, Perron J, Crickx B, Barrandon Y, Civatte J. Lichen plan avec depots lineaires d'IgG et de C3 a la junction dermo-epidermique. *Dermatologica.* 1981;163:117.

364. Ioannades D, Bystryn JC. Immunofluorescence abnormalities in lichen planopilaris. *Arch Dermatol.* 1992;128:214.

365. Sobel S, Miller R, Shatin H. Lichen planus pemphigoides. *Arch Dermatol.* 1976;112:1280.

366. Zillikens D. BP 180 as the common autoantigen in blistering diseases with different clinical phenotypes. *Keio J Med.* 2002; 51:21.

367. Hsu S, Ghohestani RF, Uitto J. Lichen planus pemphigoides with IgG autoantibodies to the 180 kD bullous pemphigoid antigen (type XVII collagen). *J Am Acad Dermatol.* 2000;42:136.

368. Yoon KH, Kim SC, Kang DS, Lee IJ. Lichen planus pemphigoides with circulating autoantibodies against 200 and 180 kDa epidermal antigens. *Eur J Dermatol.* 2000;10:212.

369. Prieto VG, Casal M, McNutt NS. Lichen planus–like keratosis: a clinical and histological reexamination. *Am J Surg Pathol.* 1993;17:259.

370. Van den Haute V, Antoine JL, Lachapelle JM. Histopathological discriminant criteria between lichenoid drug eruption and idiopathic lichen planus: retrospective study on selected samples. *Dermatologica.* 1989;179:10.

371. Shiohara T, Moriya N, Tanaka K, et al. Immunopathologic study of lichenoid skin diseases: correlation between HLA-DR positive keratinocytes or Langerhans' cells and epidermotropic T cells. *J Am Acad Dermatol.* 1988;18:67.

372. Bowen AR, Burt L, Boucher K, Tristani-Firouzi P, Florell SR. Use of proliferation rate, p53 staining and perforating elastic fibers in distinguishing keratoacanthoma from hypertrophic lichen planus: a pilot study. *J Cutan Pathol.* 2012;39(2):243–250. doi:10.1111/j.1600-0560.2011.01834.x

373. Astudillo MG, Hoang MP, Nazarian RM, Foreman RK. Distinction between hypertrophic lichen planus and squamous cell carcinoma requires clinicopathologic correlation in difficult cases. *Am J Dermatopathol.* 2021;43(5):349–355. doi:10.1097/DAD.0000000000001776

374. Woo S-B. *Oral Pathology.* 2nd ed. Elsevier; 2017.

375. Shao S, Tsoi LC, Sarkar MK, et al. IFN-γ enhances cell-mediated cytotoxicity against keratinocytes via JAK2/STAT1 in lichen planus. *Sci Transl Med.* 2019;11(511):eaav7561.

376. Damsky W, Wang A, Olamiju B, Peterson D, Galan A, King B. Treatment of severe lichen planus with the JAK inhibitor tofacitinib. *J Allergy Clin Immunol.* 2020;145(6):1708–1710.e2.

377. Lumpkin LR, Helwig EB. Solitary lichen planus. *Arch Dermatol.* 1966;93:54.

378. Shapiro L, Ackerman AB. Solitary lichen planus-like keratosis. *Dermatologica.* 1966;132:386.

379. Le Coz CJ. Lichen planus-like keratosis or (solitary) benign lichenoid keratosis. *Ann Dermatol Venereol.* 2000;127:219.

380. Jang KA, Kim SH, Choi JH. Lichenoid keratosis: a clinicopathologic study of 17 patients. *J Am Acad Dermatol.* 2000;43:511.

381. Morgan MB, Stevens GL, Switlyk S. Benign lichenoid keratosis. *Am J Dermatopathol.* 2005;27:387.

382. Goldenhersh MA, Barnhill RL, Rosenbaum HM, Stenn KS. Documented evolution of a solar lentigo into a solitary lichen planus-like keratosis. *J Cutan Pathol.* 1986;13:308.

383. Mehregan AH. Lentigo senilis and its evolution. *J Invest Dermatol.* 1975;65:429.

384. Inui S, Itami S, Kobayashi T, Yoshikawa K. A case of lichen planus–like keratosis: deposition of IgM in the basement membrane zone. *J Dermatol.* 2000;27:615.

385. Kaposi M. Lichen ruber acuminatus and lichen ruber planus. *Arch Dermatol Syphilol.* 1895;31:1.

386. Torrelo A, Mediero IG, Zambrano A. Keratosis lichenoides chronica in a child. *Pediatr Dermatol.* 1994;11:46.

387. van der Kerkhof PCM. Spontaneous resolution of keratosis lichenoides chronica. *Dermatology.* 1993;187:200.

388. Margolis MG, Cooper GA, Johnson SAM. Keratosis lichenoides chronica. *Arch Dermatol.* 1972;105:739.

389. Masouye I, Saurat JH. Keratosis lichenoides chronica: the century of another Kaposi's disease. *Dermatology.* 1995;191:188.

390. Braun-Falco O, Bieber T, Heider L. Chronic lichenoid keratosis: disease variant or disease entity? *Hautarzt.* 1989;40:614.

391. Baran R, Panizzon R, Goldberg L. The nails in keratosis lichenoides chronica: characteristics and response to treatment. *Arch Dermatol.* 1984;120:1471.

392. Pistoni F, Peroni A, Colato C, Schena D, Girolomoni G. Keratosis lichenoides chronica: case-based review of treatment options. *J Dermatolog Treat.* 2016;27(4):383–388. doi:10.3109/09546634.2015.1115818

393. Ruiz-Maldonado R, Duran-McKinster C, Orozco-Covarrubias L, Saez-de-Ocariz M, Palacios-Lopez C. Keratosis lichenoides chronica in pediatric patients: a different disease? *J Am Acad Dermatol.* 2007;56:S1–S5.

394. Lombardo GA, Annessi G, Baliva G, Monopoli A, Girolomoni G. Keratosis lichenoides chronica. Report of a case associated with B-cell lymphoma and leg panniculitis. *Dermatology.* 2000;201:261.

395. Haas N, Czaika V, Sterry W. Keratosis lichenoides chronica following trauma. A case report and update of the last literature review. *Hautarzt.* 2001;52:629.

396. Criado PR, Valente NY, Sittart JA, Juang JM, Vasconcellos C. Keratosis lichenoides chronica: report of a case developing after erythroderma. *Australas J Dermatol.* 2000;41:247.

397. Dar NR, Rao SU. Facial lichen nitidus. *Australas J Dermatol.* 2012;53:e16–17.

398. Al-Mutiri N, Hassanein A, Nour-Eldin O, et al. Generalized lichen nitidus. *Pediatr Dermatol.* 2005;22:158.

399. Maeda M. A case of generalized lichen nitidus with Koebner's phenomenon. *J Dermatol.* 1994;21:273.

400. Rallis E, Verros C, Moussatou V, Sambaziotis D, Papadakis P. Generalized purpuric lichen nitidus. Report of a case and review of the literature. *Dermatol Online J.* 2007;13:5.

401. Munro CS, Cox NH, Marks JM, Natarajan S. Lichen nitidus presenting as palmoplantar hyperkeratosis and nail dystrophy. *Clin Exp Dermatol.* 1993;18:381.

402. Itami A, Ando I, Kukita A. Perforating lichen nitidus. *Int J Dermatol.* 1994;33:382.

403. Madhok R, Winkelmann RK. Spinous, follicular lichen nitidus associated with perifollicular granulomas. *J Cutan Pathol.* 1988;15:248.

404. Bilgili SG, Karadag AS, Calka O, Ozdemir S, Kosem M. A case of generalized lichen nitidus successfully treated with narrow-band ultraviolet B treatment. *Photodermatol Photoimmunol Photomed.* 2013;29:215–217.

405. Topal IO, Gokdemir G, Sahin IM. Generalized lichen nitidus: successful treatment with systemic isotretinoin. *Indian J Dermatol Venereol Leprol.* 2013;79:554.

406. Farshi S, Mansouri P. Generalized lichen nitidus successfully treated with pimecrolimus 1 percent cream. *Dermatol Online J.* 2011;17:11.

407. Momin SB, Hawkes S, Mobini N. Large linear papular eruption on the forearm. Diagnosis: lichen striatus. *Int J Dermatol.* 2012;51:369–371.

408. Taieb A, el Youbi A, Grosshans E, Maleville J. Lichen striatus: a Blaschko linear acquired inflammatory skin eruption. *J Am Acad Dermatol.* 1991;25:637.

409. Karp DL, Cohen BA. Onychodystrophy in lichen striatus. *Pediatr Dermatol.* 1993;10:359.

410. Tosti A, Peluso AM, Misciali C, Cameli N. Nail lichen striatus: clinical features and long-term follow-up of five patients. *J Am Acad Dermatol.* 1997;36:908.

411. Aloi F, Solaroli C, Pippione M. Diffuse and bilateral lichen striatus. *Pediatr Dermatol.* 1997;14:36.

412. Racette AJ, Adams AD, Kessler SE. Simultaneous lichen striatus in siblings along the same Blaschko lines. *Pediatr Dermatol.* 2009;26:50–54.

413. Mu EW, Abuav R, Cohen BA. Facial lichen striatus in children: retracing the line of Blaschko. *Pediatr Dermatol.* 2013;30:364–366.

414. Gianotti R, Restano L, Grimalt R, Berti E, Alessi E, Caputo R. Lichen striatus-a chameleon: a histopathological and immunohistological study of forty-one cases. *J Cutan Pathol.* 1995;22:18.

415. Pujol RM, Toneu A, Moreno A, de Moragas JM. Perforating lichen striatus. *Acta Dermatol Venereol (Stockholm).* 1988;68:171.

416. Zhang Y, McNutt NS. Lichen striatus. Histological, immunohistochemical and ultrastructural study of 37 cases. *J Cutan Pathol.* 2001;28:65.

417. Sanders S, Collier DA, Scott R, Wu H, MeNutt NS. Periappendageal lichen nitidus: report of a case. *J Cutan Pathol.* 2002;29:125–128.

418. Lee DY, Kim S, Kim CR, Kim HJ, Byun JY, Yang JM. Lichen striatus in an adult treated by a short course of low dose systemic corticosteroids. *J Dermatol.* 2011;38:298–299.

419. Park JY, Kim YC. Lichen striatus successfully treated with photodynamic therapy. *Clin Exp Dermatol.* 2012;37:570–572.

420. Gelmetti C, Rigoni C, Alessi E, Ermacora E, Berti E, Caputo R. Pityriasis lichenoides in children: a long-term follow-up of eighty-nine cases. *J Am Acad Dermatol.* 1990;23:473.

421. Ersoy-Evans S, Greco MF, Mancini AJ, Subaşi N, Paller AS. Pityriasis lichenoides in childhood: a retrospective review of 124 patients. *J Am Acad Dermatol.* 2007;56:205.

422. Muhlbauer JE, Bhan AK, Harrist TJ, et al. Immunopathology of pityriasis lichenoides acuta. *J Am Acad Dermatol.* 1984;10:783.

423. Giannetti A, Girolomoni G, Pincelli C, Benassi L. Immunopathologic studies in pityriasis lichenoides. *Arch Dermatol Res.* 1988;280:S61.

424. Kim JE, Yun WJ, Mun SK, et al. Pityriasis lichenoides et varioliformis acuta and pityriasis lichenoides chronica: comparison of lesional T-cell subsets and investigation of viral associations. *J Cutan Pathol.* 2011;38:649–656.

425. Weinberg JM, Kristal L, Chooback L, Honig PJ, Kramer EM, Lessin SR. The clonal nature of pityriasis lichenoides. *Arch Dermatol.* 2002;138:1063.

426. Shieh S, Mikkola DL, Wood GS. Differentiation and clonality of lesional lymphocytes in pityriasis lichenoides chronica. *Arch Dermatol.* 2001;137:305.

427. Hapa A, Ersoy-Evans S, Karaduman A. Childhood pityriasis lichenoides and oral erythromycin. *Pediatr Dermatol.* 2012;29:719–724.

428. Park JM, Jwa SW, Song M, et al. Is narrowband ultraviolet B monotherapy effective in the treatment of pityriasis lichenoides? *Int J Dermatol.* 2013;52:1013–1018.

429. Meziane L, Caudron A, Dhaille F, et al. Febrile ulceronecrotic Mucha-Habermann disease: treatment with infliximab and intravenous immunoglobulins and review of the literature. *Dermatology.* 2012;225:344–348.

430. Brazzini B, Gheresetich I, Urso C, Cianferoni L, Lotti T. Pityriasis lichenoides et varioliformis acuta during pregnancy. *J Eur Acad Dermatol Venereol.* 2001;15:458.

431. Maekawa Y, Nakamura T, Nogami R. Febrile ulceronecrotic Mucha-Habermann's disease. *J Dermatol.* 1994;21:46.

432. De Cuyper C, Hindryckx P, Deroo N. Febrile ulceronecrotic pityriasis lichenoides et varioliformis acuta. *Dermatology.* 1994; 189:50.

433. Garcia B, Connelly EA, Newbury R, Friedlander SF. Pityriasis lichenoides and idiopathic thrombocytopenia in a young girl. *Pediatr Dermatol.* 2006;23:21.

434. Gunatheesan S, Ferguson J, Moosa Y. Pityriasis lichenoides et varioliformis acuta: a rare association with measles, mumps and rubella vaccine. *Australas J Dermatol.* 2012;53:76–78.

435. Massay RJ, Maynard AA. Pityriasis lichenoides chronica associated with use of HMG-CoA reductase inhibitors. *West Indian Med J.* 2012;61:743–745.

436. Hood AF, Mark EJ. Histopathologic diagnosis of pityriasis lichenoides et varioliformis acuta and its clinical correlation. *Arch Dermatol.* 1982;118:478.

437. Dereure O, Levi E, Kadin ME. T cell clonality in pityriasis lichenoides et varioliformis acuta: a heteroduplex analysis of 20 cases. *Arch Dermatol.* 2000;136:1483.

438. Kadin ME. T-cell clonality in pityriasis lichenoides: evidence for a premalignant or reactive immune disorder? *Arch Dermatol.* 2002;138:1089.

439. Panizzon RC, Speich R, Dassi H. Atypical manifestations of pityriasis lichenoides chronica: development into paraneoplasia and non-Hodgkin lymphomas of the skin. *Dermatology.* 1992;184:65.

440. Tomasini D, Zampatti C, Palmedo G, Bonfacini V, Sangalli G, Kutzner H. Cytotoxic mycosis fungoides evolving from pityriasis lichenoides in a 17-year-old girl. *Dermatology.* 2002;205:176.

441. Cozzio A, Hafner J, Kempf W, et al. Febrile ulcernecrotic Mucha-Habermann disease with clonality: a cutaneous T-cell lymphoma entity? *J Am Acad Dermatol.* 2004;51:1014.

442. Magro CM, Crowson AN, Morrison C, Li J. Pityriasis lichenoides chronica: stratification by molecular and phenotypic profile. *Hum Pathol.* 2007;38:479.

443. Tomasini D, Tomasini CF, Cerri A, et al. Pityriasis lichenoides: a cytotoxic T-cell–mediated skin disorder. Evidence of human parvovirus B19 DNA in nine cases. *J Cutan Pathol.* 2004;31:531.

444. Bellinato F, Maurelli M, Gisondi P, Girolomoni G. A systematic review of treatments for pityriasis lichenoides. *J Eur Acad Dermatology Venereol.* 2019;33(11):2039–2049. doi:10.1111/jdv.15813

445. Maranda EL, Smith M, Nguyen AH, Patel VN, Schachner LA, Joaquin JJ. Phototherapy for pityriasis lichenoides in the pediatric population: a review of the published literature. *Am J Clin Dermatol.* 2016;17(6):583–591. doi:10.1007/s40257-016-0216-2

446. Lis-Święty A, Michalska-Bańkowska A, Zielonka-Kucharzewska A, Pypłacz-Gumprecht A. Successful therapy of cyclosporin A in pityriasis lichenoides et varioliformis acuta preceded by hand, foot and mouth disease. *Antivir Ther.* 2015;20(3):273–275. doi:10.3851/IMP3012

447. Xing C, Shen H, Xu J, Liu Z, Zhu J, Xu A. A fatal case of febrile ulceronecrotic Mucha-Habermann disease which presenting as toxic epidermal necrolysis. *Indian J Dermatol.* 2017;62(6):675. doi:10.4103/ijd.IJD_631_16

448. Goldman K, Don PC. Adult onset of inflammatory linear verrucous epidermal nevus in a mother and her daughter. *Dermatology.* 1994;189:170.

449. Kawaguchi H, Takeuchi M, Ono H, Nakajima H. Adult onset of inflammatory linear verrucous epidermal nevus. *J Dermatol.* 1999;26:599–602.

450. Le K, Wong LC, Fischer G. Vulval and perianal inflammatory linear verrucous epidermal nevus. *Australas J Dermatol.* 2009;50:115–117.

451. Landwehr AJ, Starink TM. Inflammatory linear verrucous epidermal naevus. *Dermatologica.* 1983;166:107.

452. Al-Enezi S, Huber AM, Krafchick BR, Laxer RM. Inflammatory linear verrucous epidermal nevus and arthritis: a new association. *J Pediatr.* 2001;138:602.

453. Zhuang L, Zhu W. Inflammatory linear verrucous epidermal nevus coexisting with lichen amyloidosus. *J Dermatol.* 1996;23:415.

454. Altman J, Mehregan AH. Inflammatory linear verrucous epidermal nevus. *Arch Dermatol.* 1971;104:385.

455. Ito M, Shimizu N, Fujiwara H, Maruyama T, Tezuka M. Histopathogenesis of inflammatory linear verrucose epidermal naevus: histochemistry, immunohistochemistry and ultrastructure. *Arch Dermatol Res.* 1991;283:491.

456. Welch ML, Smith KJ, Skelton HG, et al. Immunohistochemical features in inflammatory linear verrucous epidermal nevi suggest a distinctive pattern of clonal dysregulation of growth. *J Am Acad Dermatol.* 1993;29:242.

457. Mutasim DF. Successful treatment of inflammatory linear verrucous epidermal nevus with tacrolimus and fluocinonide. *J Cutan Med Surg.* 2006;10:45–47.

458. Lee BJ, Mancini AJ, Renucci J, Paller AS, Bauer BS. Full-thickness surgical excision for the treatment of inflammatory linear verrucous epidermal nevus. *Ann Plast Surg.* 2001;47:285–292.

459. Conti R, Bruscino N, Campolmi P, Bonan P, Cannarozzo G, Moretti S. Inflammatory linear verrucous epidermal nevus: why a combined laser therapy. *J Cosmet Laser Ther.* 2013;15:242–245.

Chapter

8

Vascular Diseases

GARRETT T. DESMAN, XIAOWEI XU, AND RAYMOND L. BARNHILL

INTRODUCTION

Cutaneous vascular injury can be divided into two basic categories: vasculitis and vasculopathy. Vasculitis is characterized by blood vessels that are both damaged and inflamed, naturally with much of the damage being related to the inflammation. In vasculopathy, blood vessel damage without inflammation is observed, often with much of the damage related to vascular occlusion. Histopathologic findings that assist in the subclassification of the vasculitides include the caliber of blood vessel involved (small, medium, or large), the type of blood vessel involved (arterial or venous), and the anatomic location of the vessel injury (dermal or subcutaneous). A biopsy indicating vascular injury must be interpreted in light of the clinical scenario and laboratory findings. Two clinical considerations are key: What is the distribution of the disease (systemic or localized), and could the vascular process be secondary to an underlying disease state, such as external trauma or ulceration? (1–13).

In general, any vascular disease (occlusive or nonocclusive) associated with damage to the structural integrity of the vessel wall may lead to leakage of blood into the interstitial space, resulting in hemorrhage and edema. Cutaneous hemorrhage is clinically seen as purpura. Areas of hemorrhage less than 3 mm in diameter are called petechiae, whereas lesions 3 to 10 mm in diameter are called purpura. Larger hemorrhages, 10 mm in diameter, are called ecchymoses. If an inflammatory infiltrate is present, the purpura may become palpable. Severe vascular damage leading to vascular occlusion often causes ischemic damage and may result in necrosis, blister formation, and ulceration, often confounding the distinction between primary and secondary processes.

CRITERIA FOR VASCULITIS

The dynamic nature of vascular injury may cause difficulties in diagnosis because the appearance of the injured vessel and the nature of the associated inflammatory cells change as the lesions evolve. Furthermore, the degree of vascular injury varies depending on the severity of the insult. The spectrum of vascular reaction to injury ranges from endothelial cell swelling and increased permeability to frank fibrinoid necrosis and fibrin deposition.

In general, vasculitis must have two components: (a) an inflammatory cell infiltrate and (b) evidence of vascular injury (Table 8-1). As vasculitis is an inflammatory process, the

---

Table 8-1

Definitions of Vascular Injury

Primary vascular injury
Vasculopathy

  Fibrinoid deposition, thrombosis with limited to no inflammation

  Infiltration of vessel wall by inflammatory cells with otherwise minimal alteration

  Leukocytoclasis of tissue infiltrate with minimal alteration of vessel, that is, swelling only, absence of fibrinoid necrosis

Vasculitis

  Perivascular inflammatory cell infiltrate (neutrophilic, eosinophilic, lymphocytic, histiocytic, or mixed)

  Fibrinoid necrosis: necrosis of vessel wall with deposition of fibrinoid material

  Other changes often present but not essential: edema, extravasation of erythrocytes, leukocytoclasis, infiltration of vessel wall by inflammatory cells, swelling of endothelial cells, luminal thrombosis

---

absence of inflammation precludes the diagnosis even though vascular alterations may be present; however, in the late healing state, the inflammatory cell infiltrate may be minimal. Neutrophils, eosinophils, lymphocytes, or monocytes/macrophages may be present, and the type of infiltrating cell may correlate to some extent with the chronology of the process.

Evidence of vascular injury is the second major component of vasculitis. Criteria for vascular injury include (a) evidence of vessel leakiness such as edema and extravasation of erythrocytes, (b) evidence of vessel destruction such as necrosis of endothelium and deposition of fibrinoid material within the vascular lumina or vessel walls, and (c) evidence of inflammatory compromise of the vascular walls, including infiltration by inflammatory cells and leukocytoclasis of the surrounding inflammatory cell infiltrate (Fig. 8-1). As mentioned, there is a continuum of injury. However, for several years, pathologists have required a certain degree of injury, as manifested by deposition of fibrinoid material and/or necrosis of the vessel itself, as a primary indicator of a true vasculitis. Certain changes, including edema, extravasation of erythrocytes, infiltration of vessel walls, leukocytoclasis, and thrombosis, may occur with minimal evidence of vascular injury. Pathologists should strive not to overinterpret such changes as vasculitis when definitive

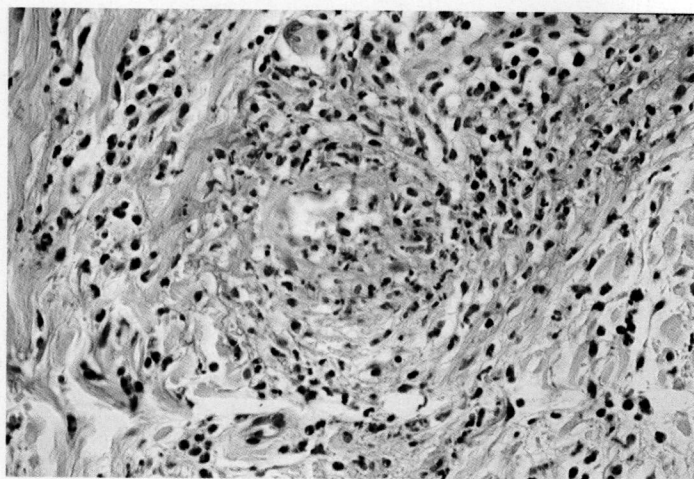

Figure 8-1 Vascular injury. Hypersensitivity vasculitis showing an upper dermal small blood vessel with full-blown features of neutrophil-rich vasculitis: neutrophilic permeation of vessel walls, leukocytoclasis, fibrinoid necrosis of vessel wall, fibrin thrombus formation, and red blood cell extravasation. The specimen was obtained from a 2-day-old purpuric papule.

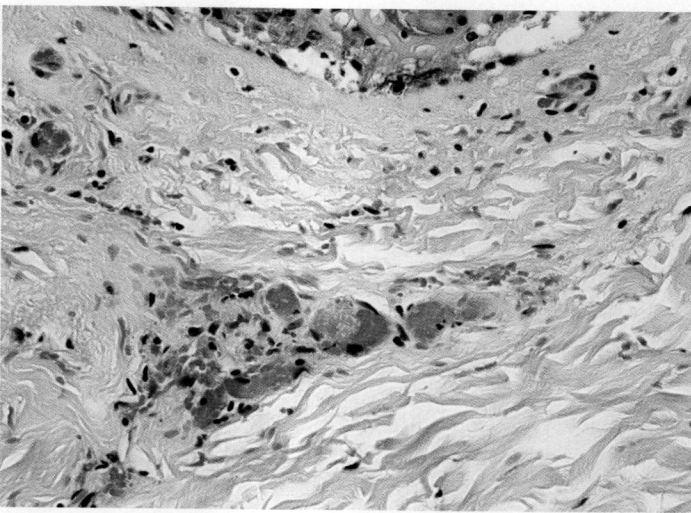

Figure 8-2 Vasculopathic reaction, disseminated intravascular coagulation. Pink fibrin thrombi are present within vessels that do not show evidence of damage or inflammation in their walls.

evidence of vessel injury is lacking. For instance, leukocytoclasis may result from degranulation of a neutrophilic infiltrate by itself without accompanying fibrinoid necrosis of surrounding vessels. Similarly, fibrin thrombi may be present in noninflamed vessels in the setting of hypercoagulable states.

Secondary Vasculitis, Incidental Vasculitis, Vasculopathy, Pseudovasculitis

Terminology has been developed to describe whether vascular injury or vasculitis is primary or secondary (incidental), the degree of injury present, and conditions or disorders mimicking vasculitis (2–13). Primary vascular injury implies that the vascular insult is the predominant disease process. Secondary or incidental vascular injury indicates that an underlying non-vascular disease process is the primary pathologic process. The context of the histologic findings is important. For example, an ulcer, folliculitis, herpes virus infection, or trauma may cause secondary vasculitic changes in nearby blood vessels. Sometimes, the primary lesion may be hidden deeper in the tissue, and additional sections may be revelatory. In many instances, distinguishing clearly between a primary and a secondary vascular insult is not possible. However, secondary vascular injury is often variable, with sparing of some vessels within the zone of tissue injury. Other indications of secondary vascular injury include deposition of fibrinoid material at the periphery of the vessel wall and focal thrombosis without significant infiltration by inflammatory cells.

The term *vasculopathy* or *pseudovasculitis* may be used to describe certain degrees of vascular alteration and injury that fail to satisfy the criteria for vasculitis (Table 8-1). Such histopathologic alterations might include hemorrhage, vascular thrombosis (hypercoagulable states), embolic phenomena with little additional evidence of vascular injury (Fig. 8-2), deposition of fibrinoid material with little or no inflammation, minimal infiltration of vessel walls with little or no leukocytoclasis, pathologic alterations of the vessel wall, vasospasm, and repetitive vascular trauma (2,8–10).

EVALUATION OF VASCULITIS

In an attempt to provide a structure for more consistency in the diagnosis of vasculitides, a consensus nomenclature and categorization has been developed. The consensus document "The International Chapel Hill Consensus Conference Nomenclature of Vasculitis" was updated in 2012 and later addended in 2018, in an effort to adopt widely accepted names and definitions(4,12). The new naming system uses the size of the involved blood vessel (small, medium, large) as an important organizing principle (Table 8-2). Thus, the standardized nomenclature for vasculitis is based on vessel size (3,14,15). Large vessels are considered to include the aorta and large named arteries and veins. Medium-sized vessels include medium-sized and small arteries and veins located in the subcutis or near the dermal–subcutis junction in the skin. Small vessels include arterioles, venules, and capillaries of the dermis. Classification based on vessel size is helpful because there is some correlation with the clinical presentation. Macular purpura, palpable purpura, urticaria, vesicles and bullae, and splinter hemorrhages typically reflect small-vessel injury. Cutaneous nodules, ulcers, livedo reticularis, and digital gangrene suggest the involvement of medium-sized arteries. However, classification based on vessel size alone is of limited value in dermatopathology because most cutaneous vasculitides affect primarily small dermal vessels. Small-vessel vasculitides are subclassified according to the composition of the inflammatory infiltrate (neutrophilic/leukocytoclastic, lymphocytic, or granulomatous) in combination with data from clinical and laboratory findings. In addition, terminology has been proposed and widely accepted to replace nomenclature for two important conditions, formerly known as Wegener granulomatosis and Churg–Strauss syndrome (see later and Table). A practical approach (Table 8-3) for the histopathologist in evaluating vascular inflammatory reactions is to decide whether clear-cut vascular damage is present and sufficient for a designation as vasculitis, assess the cellular composition of the inflammatory infiltrate, and define the anatomic

Table 8-2

Skin Involvement Status by Vasculitis Category and Disease

CHCC2012 (4) Vasculitis category, name	Skin Involvement Status	
	Cutaneous component of systemic vasculitis	Skin-limited or skin-dominant variant
Large-vessel vasculitis		
Takayasu arteritis	No	No
Giant cell arteritis	Rare	No
Medium vessel vasculitis		
Polyarteritis nodosa	Yes	Yes
Kawasaki disease	No	No
Small-vessel vasculitis		
Microscopic polyangiitis	Yes	Yes
Granulomatosis with polyangiitis (Wegener granulomatosis)	Yes	Yes
Eosinophilic granulomatosis with polyangiitis (Churg–Strauss syndrome)	Yes	Yes
Antiglomerular basement membrane disease (Goodpasture syndrome)	No	No
Cryoglobulinemic vasculitis	Yes	Yes
IgA vasculitis (Henoch–Schönlein purpura)	Yes	Yes
Hypocomplementemic urticarial vasculitis (anti-C1q vasculitis)	Yes	Yes
Variable vessel vasculitis		
Behçet disease	Yes	Yes
Cogan syndrome	Rare	No
Vasculitis associated with systemic disease		
SLE, rheumatoid arthritis, sarcoidosis, etc.	Yes	Yes
Vasculitis associated with probable etiology		
Drugs, infections, sepsis, autoimmune disease, etc.	Yes	Yes
Cutaneous SOV (12)		
IgM/IgG vasculitis	No (NYO)	Yes (as SOV)
Nodular vasculitis (erythema induratum)	No	Yes (as SOV)
Erythema elevatum diutinum	No	Yes (as SOV)
Hypergammaglobulinemic macular vasculitis	No	Yes (as SOV)
Normocomplementemic urticarial vasculitis	No	Yes (as SOV)

CHCC2012, 2012 revised International Chapel Hill Consensus Nomenclature of Vasculitides; NYO, not yet observed; SLE, systemic lupus erythematosus; SOV, single-organ involvement.

distribution of the infiltrate within the skin. Associated findings, such as microorganisms, may narrow the differential diagnosis. During evaluation, the evanescent quality of vascular damage should be kept in mind as lesions also have life spans; a neutrophilic vasculitis with leukocytoclasia may evolve into a predominantly lymphocytic or even granulomatous process.

Histopathology alone is inadequate to classify a vasculitic disease process. Integration of data from clinical history and physical examination, other laboratory tests, and even arteriography may be critical to arrive at a final diagnosis. In particular, clinical and radiographic findings are needed to assess the degree of systemic involvement and range in size of arteries involved. Infection must be excluded via special stains, cultures, and other laboratory studies. Evidence for specific systemic conditions, such as collagen vascular diseases, hepatitis, and

ingestion of certain medications or illicit drugs that may be associated with vasculitis must be evaluated.

Antineutrophil cytoplasmic antibodies (ANCAs) are serologic markers that have allowed classification of a subset of vasculitides. These markers may reflect biologic relationships between disease processes (14–18). ANCAs are best demonstrated by a combination of indirect immunofluorescence of normal peripheral blood neutrophils followed by enzyme-linked immunosorbent assay (ELISA) to detect specific autoantibodies. Indirect immunofluorescence assays reveal two staining patterns: cytoplasmic (c-ANCA) and perinuclear (p-ANCA). ELISAs show that most c-ANCAs are autoantibodies to proteinase 3 and that most p-ANCAs are specific for myeloperoxidase (MPO). These antibodies are especially helpful, in combination with clinical features, in the differential diagnosis of three

Table 8-3
Approach to Vasculitis

1. Determine whether vasculitis or vasculopathy is present or absent
2. Primary or secondary
3. Size of vessel and type
   a. Large
   b. Medium
   c. Small
4. Composition of infiltrate
   a. Neutrophilic/leukocytoclastic
   b. Eosinophilic
   c. Lymphocytic
   d. Histiocytic/granulomatous
5. Evaluation for infection
6. Serologic and immunopathologic evaluation
   a. Evaluation for ANCA, antinuclear antibodies, rheumatoid factor, cryoglobulins
   b. Immunofluorescence and other studies for the detection of immune complexes, for example, immunoglobulin A-fibronectin aggregates
7. Clinical context
   a. Cutaneous involvement only
   b. Extent of systemic involvement

small-vessel vasculitides: granulomatosis with polyangiitis (formerly Wegener granulomatosis) (GPA), eosinophilic granulomatosis with polyangiitis (formerly Churg–Strauss syndrome) (EGPA), and microscopic polyangiitis (MPA). GPA is usually associated with c-ANCA, MPA with either p- or c-ANCA, and EGPA with p-ANCA (see following discussion and Table 8-4). These three syndromes are termed "pauci-immune vasculitides" because vascular injury is not associated with immunoglobulin deposition in vessel walls, in contrast to the immune complex–mediated small-vessel injury seen in entities such as Henoch–Schönlein purpura. The role of ANCAs in these disease processes is unclear; however, a combination of predisposing genetic factors and exposure to environmental factors is likely involved. ANCAs may induce vasculitis by excessively activating circulating neutrophils and monocytes, allowing adherence to vessels, degranulation, and release of toxic metabolites. Additionally, activation of neutrophils by ANCAs has been shown to result in the formation of neutrophil extracellular traps (NETs), which are fused phagolysosomal products released into the microenvironment following phagocytosis (19). These

NETs are a potent form of innate immunity where they bind various microbes and virulence factors. Excessive NET formation has been shown to be injurious to small vessels as well as being responsible for the production of ANCAs, creating a positive feedback loop (20). Other complex genetic and epigenetic mechanisms, including barrier dysfunction, auto-amplification of cellular death and inflammation, altered autoantigen presentation, and alternative complement pathway activation, have also been implicated (15).

The following sections discuss the histologic features and clinical differential diagnoses of inflammatory vascular reactions affecting the skin.

VASCULITIS OF LARGE AND MEDIUM-SIZED VESSELS

Large-vessel vasculitides with cutaneous or subcutaneous findings include temporal (giant cell) arteritis and Takayasu arteritis (TA) (21,22). Vasculitis affecting medium-sized and small arteries and, in particular, small-vessel vasculitides are discussed in more detail (23–25).

Temporal (Giant Cell) Arteritis

Clinical Summary. The clinical presentation may include pain and tenderness of the forehead and sudden visual impairment. Erythema and edema of the skin overlying the involved arteries are commonly seen, and occasionally the scalp may ulcerate (21,26). The involved artery may be palpable. Clinical laboratory data include a significantly elevated erythrocyte sedimentation rate. Although the clinical presentation is strongly suggestive of the diagnosis, a biopsy is considered the gold standard for diagnostic confirmation and must be performed as early as possible. However, false-negative biopsy results have been reported to range from 5% to 13% (27). An emerging role of state-of-the-art time-of-flight positron emission tomography/computed tomography (PET/CT) as an adjunct diagnostic test has shown promising results (28). In 2016, the American College of Rheumatology revised early diagnostic criteria for giant-cell (temporal) arteritis (Table 8-5) (29). In a study in which the diagnosis of giant-cell arteritis was confirmed by temporal artery biopsy, the presence of three or more criteria yielded a sensitivity of 97.5% and a specificity of 78.9% (30).

Pathogenesis. Giant-cell arteritis primarily affects large or medium-sized arteries in the temporal region of elderly individuals. Although the etiology of temporal arteritis is not clearly understood, multiple factors such as genetic and environmental

Table 8-4
Antineutrophil Cytoplasmic Antibody (ANCA)–Positive Vasculitides

Disease Process	Antimyeloperoxidase (p-ANCA)	Antiserine Proteinase (c-ANCA)
Granulomatosis with polyangiitis (GPA)	Rare (5%)	Common (80%)
Microscopic polyangiitis (polyarteritis)	Common (50%–60%)	Common (45%)
Eosinophilic granulomatosis with polyangiitis (EGPA)	Common (70%)	Rare (7%)

c-ANCA, cytoplasmic ANCA; p-ANCA, perinuclear ANCA.

Table 8-5

The 2016 ACR Revised Classification Criteria for Giant-Cell (Temporal) Arteritis (29)

Early Criteria:
- Age at onset ≥50 years old
- Absence of exclusion criteria[b]

Domain I criteria[a]:
- New onset localized headache[c] = 1.p
- Sudden onset of visual disturbances[c] = 1.p
- Polymyalgia Rheumatica (PMR) = 2.p
- Jaw Claudication[c] = 1.p
- Abnormal temporal artery[d] = Up to 2.p

Domain II criteria:
- Unexplained fever and/or anemia = 1.p
- ESR ≥ 50 mm/hour[e] = 1.p
- Compatible pathology[f] = Up to 2.p

[a]In the presence of 3 points or more out of 11 with at least one point derived from domain I along with all entry criteria, the diagnosis of giant-cell arteritis can be established.

[b]Exclusion criteria include ENT and eye inflammation, kidney, skin and peripheral nervous system involvement, lung infiltration, lymphadenopathies, stiff neck and digital gangrene or ulceration.

[c]No other etiology can better explain any one of the criteria.

[d]Enlarged and/or pulseless temporal artery: 1.p. / tender temporal artery: 1.p.

[e]It must be ignored in the presence of PMR.

[f]Vascular and/or perivascular fibrinoid necrosis along with leukocyte infiltration: 1.p. /and granuloma: 1.p.

From Salehi-Abari I. 2016 ACR revised criteria for early diagnosis of giant cell (temporal) arteritis. *Autoimmune Dis Ther Approach.* 2016;3(1):119–122. https://creativecommons.org/licenses/by/3.0/

influences affect susceptibility and severity of disease (26). The arteritis may be unilateral or bilateral and associated with involvement of other cranial arteries, notably the retinal arteries.

Histopathology. Involved arteries show an inflammatory process of mainly lymphocytes and macrophages that may extend throughout the entire arterial wall (Fig. 8-3). Classically, fragmentation of the lamina elastica and elastophagocytosis by multinucleated giant cells are seen. However, depending on the stage of the disease process, giant cells may not be present, and the inflammatory infiltrate is often unevenly distributed. Step sections may be needed to reveal diagnostic features. In some instances, neutrophils may be present; thus, some neutrophils in a background of findings otherwise typical for giant-cell arthritis should not exclude the diagnosis. An elastica van Gieson stain greatly facilitates the evaluation of elastic fibers. Disruption of the internal elastic lamina is not sufficient for diagnosis because this is nonspecific. In late stages, thickening of the intima by deposits of fibrin-like material and myofibroblastic proliferation with subsequent luminal narrowing may be the only findings. Classic histologic findings may become difficult to recognize following steroid treatment. Three reliable histopathologic parameters of corticosteroid-treated temporal arteritis have been identified, including (a) complete or incomplete mantle of lymphocytes and epithelioid histiocytes located between the outer muscular layer and the adventitia; (b) large circumferential defects in the elastic lamina (best seen with the Movat pentachrome); and (c) absent or few small multinucleated giant cells (31). The CD68 immunostain may aid in the identification of rare histiocytes.

Differential Diagnosis. Not all cases of arteritis involving the temporal artery represent examples of temporal arteritis. Infection-related vasculitis, connective tissue disease, and polyarteritis nodosa (PAN) might enter into the differential diagnosis. The latter processes often show necrotizing neutrophilic vasculitides (depending on the stage), and diagnosis depends on serologic studies, the absence of infection, and clinical findings.

Principles of Management: Urgent treatment with high-dose systemic steroids is necessary to decrease the risk of blindness secondary to retinal artery occlusion. Tocilizumab (interleukin-6 receptor α inhibitor) has recently been shown to increase the rate of sustained remission and reduce the cumulative exposure to glucocorticoid therapy (32).

Takayasu Arteritis

Clinical Summary. The principal clinical manifestations of TA, usually in women younger than 40 years, include erythematous nodules often of the lower extremities (easily misdiagnosed as erythema nodosum or erythema induratum) and pyoderma

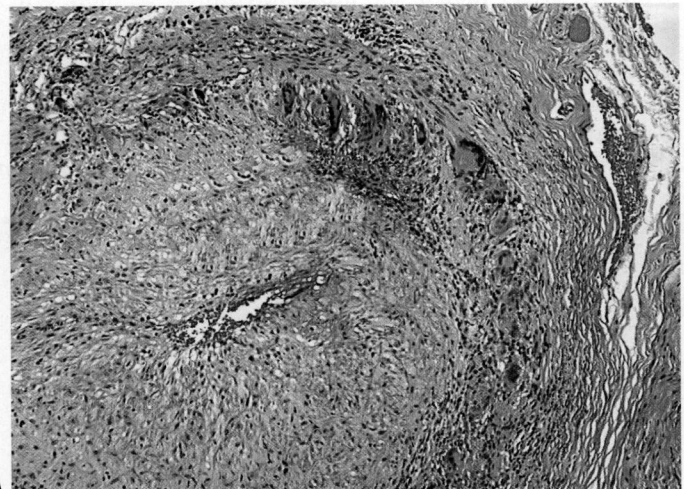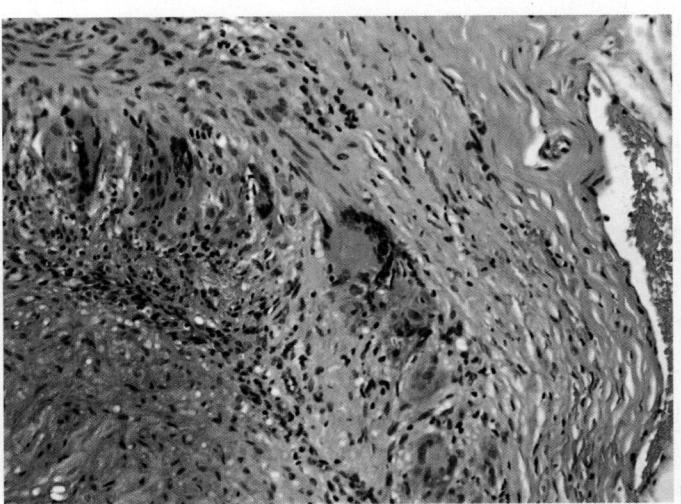

Figure 8-3 Giant-cell arteritis. **A and B:** Biopsy of the temporal artery shows a predominantly mononuclear cell infiltrate with a few giant cells in the region of the internal elastic lamina.

gangrenosum (PG)–like ulcers (33). Because this form of vasculitis is associated with visceral involvement and leads to stenosis, occlusion, and/or aneurysmal degeneration of large arteries, the gold standard for diagnosis and for topographical classification is angiography, which correlates with symptoms and prognosis (34).

Pathogenesis. A chronic, fibrosing large-vessel vasculitis primarily involving the aorta. TA may rarely have cutaneous involvement (33,35).

Histopathology. Small and medium arteries of the subcutaneous fat usually show a necrotizing panarteritis with fibrinoid necrosis and sparse inflammatory infiltrates containing lymphocytes and neutrophils. Additional findings may include granulomatous vasculitis, fibrin thrombi without vasculitis, neutrophilic abscesses, and septal and lobular panniculitis.

Differential Diagnosis. PAN, PG, and erythema nodosum may be histologically indistinguishable. Additional clinical findings and angiography should facilitate differentiation of TA from other entities.

Principles of Management: First-line treatment is with oral corticosteroids, although other immunosuppressants such as methotrexate and biologics are acceptable. For severely narrowed or acutely blocked arteries, surgery may be required. Biologic agents may be used in refractory or relapsing patients. Antiplatelet and anticoagulant therapies are no longer recommended for routine treatment (36).

VASCULITIS AFFECTING MEDIUM-SIZED AND SMALL VESSELS

Vasculitides affecting medium-sized vessels include Kawasaki syndrome, TA, infections, Buerger disease, PAN, MPA, GPA (WG), EGPA (Churg–Strauss Syndrome [CSS]), rheumatoid vasculitis, lupus vasculitis, and giant-cell (temporal) arteritis. A variety of data are used to subclassify this group, including laboratory findings such as ANCA, the composition of the inflammatory infiltrate, and the type of blood vessel (artery or vein) involved. The presence of an internal elastic lamina, visualized as a wavy layer of elastic fibers, between the intima and the media characterize an artery. Another feature of an artery is a prominent concentric muscular layer. In many circumstances,

the distinction between vein and artery is straightforward; however, persistent hydrostatic pressure in the lower extremities may result in hypertrophy of the medial musculature of subcutaneous veins. In this location, the muscular layer of the vein may be thicker than its arterial counterpart. Knowledge of this pitfall and an appropriately interpreted elastic stain can prevent misidentification of entities in this category (37,38).

Kawasaki Disease (Mucocutaneous Lymph Node Syndrome)

Clinical Summary. Kawasaki disease is a necrotizing arteritis that usually affects young children, with a peak incidence at 1 year of age (25). Mucocutaneous findings are common and include a polymorphous exanthematous macular rash, conjunctival congestion, dry reddened lips, "strawberry tongue," oropharyngeal reddening, and swelling of the hands and feet—especially the palms and soles. Typically, a nonpurulent cervical lymphadenopathy is associated. Desquamation of the skin of the fingers typically occurs after 1 to 2 weeks, often followed by thrombocytosis. The most serious clinical complications are related to arteritis and thrombosis of the coronary arteries with frequent aneurysm formation (Table 8-6). Patients not fulfilling the complete diagnostic criteria are referred to as having Kawasaki-like disease or atypical Kawasaki disease. Recently, cases have been reported in association with viral infections, such as SARS-CoV-2 ("pediatric inflammatory multisystem syndrome") in children and adolescents and human immunodeficiency virus (HIV) infection in adults (23,39–41). The former coronavirus disease 2019 (COVID-19)–related condition has also been associated with systemic circulatory collapse (Kawasaki shock syndrome) and macrophage activation syndrome (MAS) (39,42).

Pathogenesis. The cause of Kawasaki disease is currently unknown, although most believe it is caused by both genetic predisposition and environmental factors, such as viral infection.

Histopathology. Cutaneous vasculitis is rare. The macular rash is usually accompanied by nonspecific histologic changes. Characteristic arteritis is typically found in visceral sites such as the coronary arteries (see also Chapter 7).

Principles of Management: Administration of corticosteroids, intravenous immunoglobulin (IVIG), tocilizumab, anakinra, enoxaparin, and aspirin are currently the treatment guidelines,

Table 8-6
Diagnostic Criteria for Kawasaki Disease (43)

Criteria	Clinical Features
1. Mucosal Changes	Erythema and cracking of lips; "strawberry tongue" with erythema and prominent fungiform papillae and/or erythema of the oral and pharyngeal mucosa.
2. Conjunctivitis	Bilateral bulbar nonexudative conjunctival injection, often sparing the limbus
3. Polymorphous rash	Diffuse maculopapular erythroderma or erythema multiforme–like presentation. Less commonly, urticarial or micropustular eruptions
4. Extremity changes	Acute phase: erythema and edema of the hands and feet Subacute phase: periungual desquamation
5. Lymphadenopathy	Acute, nonsuppurative, cervical lymphadenopathy (≥1.5 cm diameter), typically unilateral

Note: To be diagnosed with classic KD, the patient must have ≥5 days of fever as well as ≥4 of the 5 principal clinical features.
Reprinted by permission from Springer: Rife E, Gedalia A. Kawasaki disease: an update. *Curr Rheumatol Rep.* 2020;22(10):75. Copyright © 2020 Springer Nature.

although aspirin must be cautiously used given its association with Reye syndrome in children with viral infection (44).

Superficial Thrombophlebitis

Clinical Summary. Superficial thrombophlebitis (STP) of small to medium-sized veins is a common condition usually involving the lower extremities and presents as a painful or tender erythematous cordlike structure or nodule (45). Ultrasonography usually provides the diagnosis.

Pathogenesis. STP is associated with increased risk of clotting. Affected individuals often have predisposing factors such as varicose veins, a hypercoagulable state, ingestion of oral contraceptives, or an underlying malignancy. Variants of STP include Mondor disease and superficial septic thrombophlebitis (usually secondary to peripheral venous infusion).

Histopathology. Small and medium-sized veins of the lower dermis and subcutaneous fat are involved by an acute vasculitis and thrombosis that occludes the vessel lumina. Early lesions demonstrate dense inflammatory infiltrates composed primarily of neutrophils within the vessel wall. The venous wall is significantly thickened by this influx of leukocytes and edema fluid. In later stages, one may observe other inflammatory cells, including lymphocytes, histiocytes, and multinucleate giant cells within the walls of veins. Recanalization of the affected veins ultimately occurs with resolution of the process. A Gram stain is indicated for the assessment of septic STP.

Differential Diagnosis. PAN, the principal entity to be distinguished, involves medium-sized arteries rather than veins. PAN is more inflammatory and less thrombogenic than STP to the extent that thrombi are usually absent in PAN. PAN shows conspicuous fibrinoid necrosis, whereas STP usually does not. An elastic tissue stain, especially if the lower extremity is biopsied, to fully characterize the involved vessels may facilitate the differentiation of PAN and STP.

Principles of Management: Local care with warm compresses and gentle compression stockings and nonsteroidal anti-inflammatory drugs (NSAIDs) for tenderness associated with clots are reasonable initial approaches. Patients at high risk of clotting may warrant anticoagulation therapy. Superficial thrombophlebitis can be an initial manifestation of a deep vein thrombosis, and consideration should be given to Doppler ultrasonography when clinically indicated.

Mondor Disease

Clinical Summary. This condition is often manifested clinically by a cordlike induration on the body surface. Mondor disease (MD) can be roughly categorized into three different groups based on lesion site: anterolateral thoracoabdominal wall, dorsum and dorsolateral aspects of the penis, and axillary web syndrome with mid–upper arm involvement after axillary surgery (46). Generalized symptoms are usually not a feature, and resolution within weeks is the norm. Ultrasonography usually provides the diagnosis.

Pathogenesis. MD is a thrombophlebitis of the subcutaneous veins of the chest region or dorsal vein of the penis (formerly termed sclerosing lymphangitis). In most cases, the etiology is unknown; however, local interference with venous flow may be a factor. Trauma, connective tissue disease, breast carcinoma

(in rare cases), and a variety of other conditions have been associated.

Histopathology. In early lesions, a polymorphonuclear infiltrate may be present. Later, a sparse inflammatory infiltrate composed of lymphocytes, histiocytes, and plasma cells can be observed. Most biopsied lesions show prominent subcutaneous vessels with plump endothelial cells. Characteristic organizing thrombi and thickened fibrous walls give these vessels a cordlike appearance at scanning magnification (47).

Principles of Management: Management is with warm compresses and NSAIDs.

Thromboangiitis Obliterans (Buerger Disease)

Clinical Summary. Buerger disease is a distinctive condition characterized by a segmental, thrombosing inflammatory process affecting intermediate and small arteries and sometimes veins. It may be closely related to STP (45). The vessels of the upper and lower extremities are most commonly involved. Distal extremity disease is characteristic. The condition almost exclusively affects smokers of tobacco and cannabis under 50, with the cannabis smokers tending to be younger. Cutaneous findings are manifestations of ischemic injury.

Pathogenesis. The specific cause is unknown; however, the arteritis is attributed to immunoglobulins (IgG, IgA, IgM) and complement deposition along the internal elastic lamina of arterial walls (48). It is believed that tobacco or related products may trigger an immune response in susceptible individuals, leading to vasculopathic changes and occlusion in fingers and toes.

Histopathology. Active lesions are characterized by luminal thrombotic occlusion and a mixed inflammatory cell infiltrate of the vessel wall, characteristically with microabscesses. Later, the thrombus is organized, and its lumen may be recanalized (Fig. 8-4). A granulomatous reaction may be present as well.

Differential Diagnosis. The histologic findings in Buerger disease are nonspecific, and knowledge of the clinical scenario would most likely be required to trigger consideration of a diagnosis of Buerger disease. As smoking cessation may dramatically reverse symptoms, Buerger disease represents another example of the importance of adequate clinical information being provided to the dermatopathologist. If extensive neutrophilia is present, infection should be excluded.

Principles of Management: Smoking cessation is essential but may not lead to resolution of the symptoms. Notably, there is some concern that nicotine replacement therapy can continue the vascular process. Drugs and procedures to help with vasodilation may be effective. Anticoagulation has not been found to be effective.

Polyarteritis Nodosa

Clinical Summary. In 1866, Kussmaul and Maier reported the case of a 27-year-old man with fever, abdominal pain, muscle weakness, peripheral neuropathy, and renal disease. They termed the fatal illness *periarteritis nodosa*, referring to nodular protuberances along the course of medium-sized muscular arteries, which were histologically characterized by inflammation predominantly at the periphery of the vessel walls with vessel-wall destruction (49). Ferrari noted in 1903 the more characteristic presence of inflammatory cells within all levels of

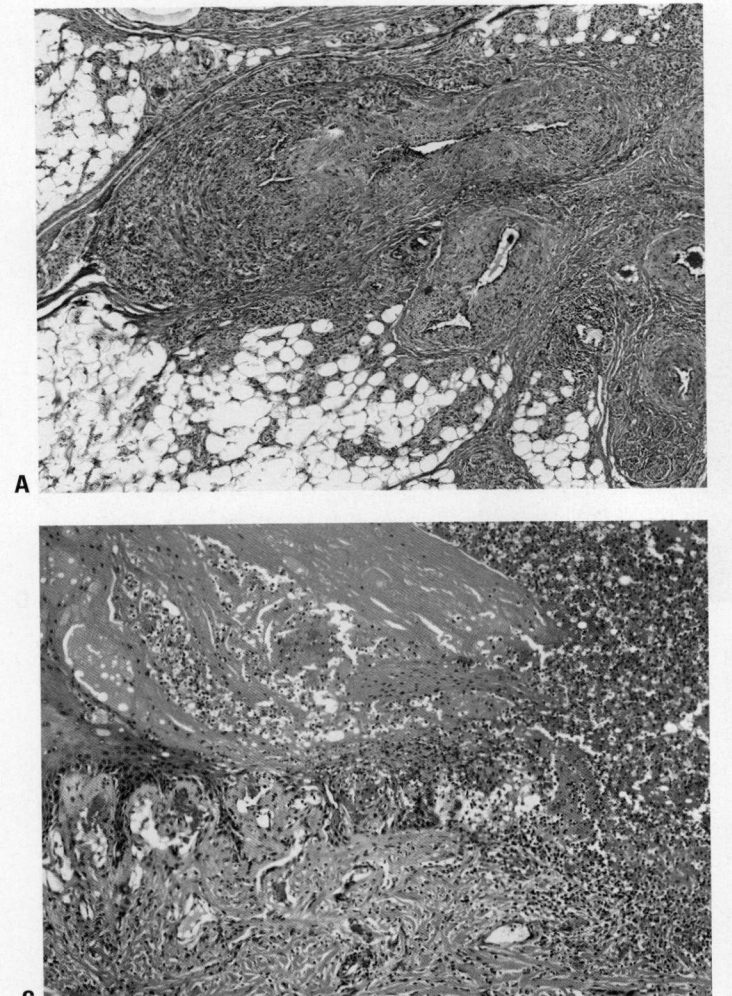

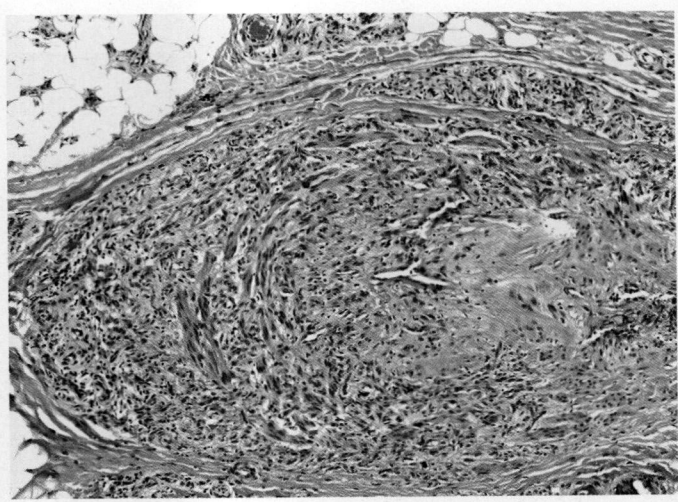

Figure 8-4 Thromboangiitis obliterans (Buerger disease). A mixed inflammatory infiltrate is present in the wall of a large vein, and its lumen is recanalized in a 35-year-old man (**A, B**) with associated ischemic ulceration in the distal extremity (**C**).

the affected vessels and suggested the term *polyarteritis* instead of *periarteritis*. The term PAN is believed to subsume three entities: (a) classic systemic PAN, (b) cutaneous PAN, and (c) MPA (50,51). Classic PAN is a multisystem disorder characterized by inflammatory vasculitis involving arterioles and small and medium-sized arteries. According to some authors, cutaneous PAN is the only variety of PAN consistently involving the deep dermis and subcutaneous fat with diagnostic features of arteritis. Some authors maintain that if there is no evidence of systemic involvement by (skin-limited) PAN at the time of initial diagnosis, then the condition will remain confined to the skin despite a potentially prolonged clinical course with multiple recurrences (52).

Clinical Features. PAN is more common in men than women and usually occurs between the ages of 20 and 60 years. Clinical manifestations may be dramatic and protean. Fever, malaise, weight loss, weakness, myalgias, arthralgias, and anorexia are common symptoms, reflecting the systemic nature of the disease. Other findings may reflect infarction of specific organs. Renal involvement, present in about 75% of patients, is the most common cause of death. Hematuria, proteinuria, hypertension, and azotemia may result from both infarction owing to disease of renal arteries and sometimes focal, segmental necrotizing glomerular lesions suggesting involvement of small vessels. Acute abdominal crises, strokes, myocardial infarction, and mononeuritis multiplex result from involvement of the relevant

arteries. Arteriography of visceral arteries often shows multiple aneurysms that are highly suggestive of PAN. ANCAs are generally absent in patients with predominately medium-sized vessel involvement. Symptoms such as asthma, Löffler syndrome, and rashes may be related to the hypereosinophilia sometimes seen in these patients. Cutaneous manifestations include nondescript subcutaneous nodules (Fig. 8-5A) that may rarely pulsate or ulcerate, ecchymoses, livedo reticularis, bullae, papules, scarlatiniform lesions, atrophie blanche-like lesions, and urticaria (53). End-stage lesions include gangrene of toes and fingers (Fig. 8-5B). A limited form of PAN without visceral involvement, referred to as benign cutaneous PAN, presents with subcutaneous nodules and livedo reticularis most frequently on the lower extremities (52,54). The so-called cutaneous polyarteritis nodosum may not be limited to the skin but may also affect muscle, peripheral nerve, and joints. The course of disease is described as benign but protracted with steroid dependence.

Pathogenesis. The pathogenesis of classic PAN is poorly understood. Direct immunofluorescence testing of skin lesions of PAN shows some immune deposits in dermal vessels. However, they may reflect a secondary event after vascular injury from another cause. ANCAs are generally absent in patients with predominantly medium-sized vessel involvement and are thus not involved in the pathogenesis of all cases of PAN. Drug-induced cases have been reported, such as from minocycline and other agents, and infection-associated cases (hepatitis B virus [HBV], TB) exist as well.

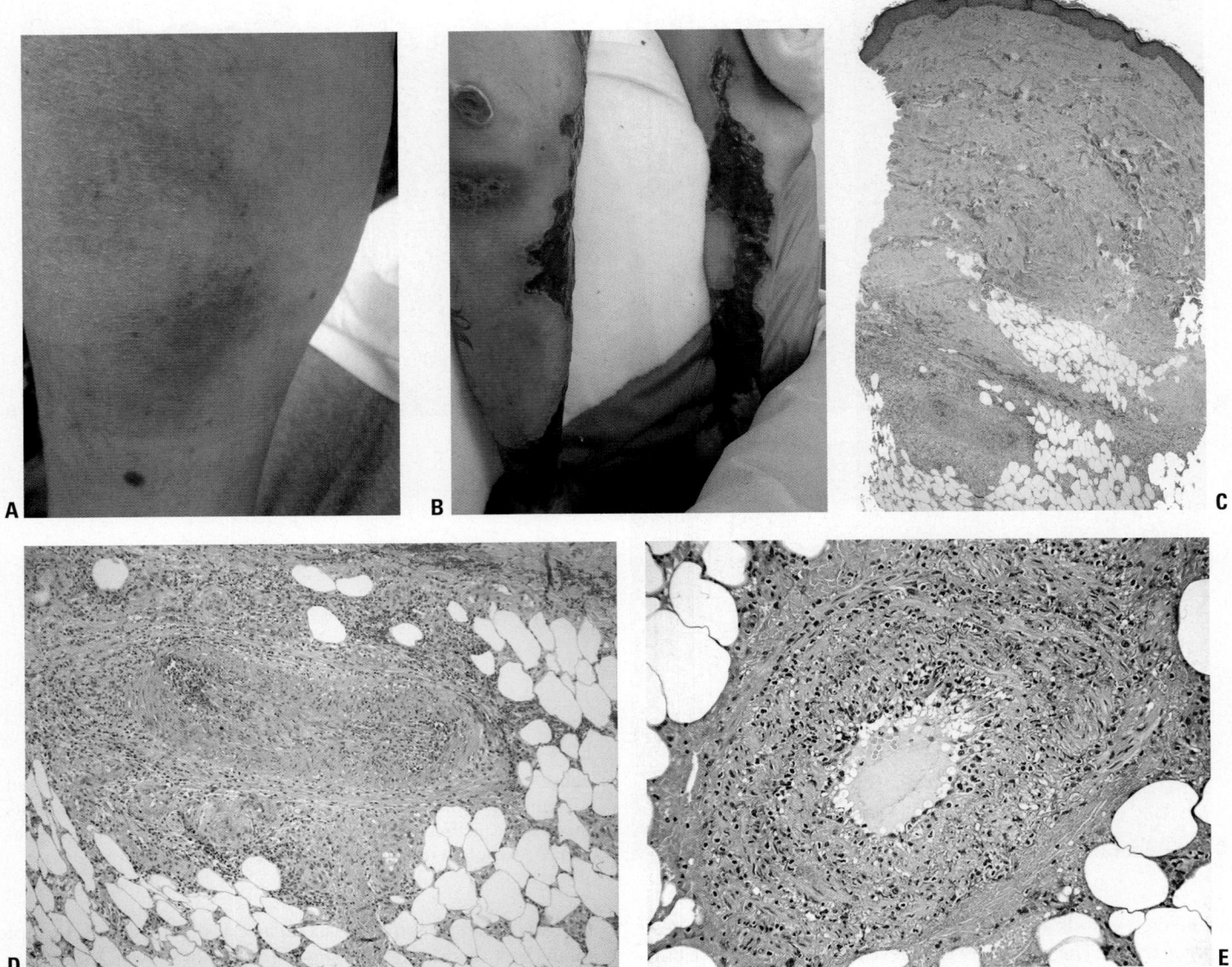

Figure 8-5 Polyarteritis nodosa. **A:** Early-stage lesion showing subcutaneous nodules with overlying color change probably related to telangiectasias and/or hemorrhage. **B:** Late-stage lesion showing epidermal necrosis and eschar formation. **C:** A small artery in the subcutis is surrounded and partially obliterated by a cellular inflammatory infiltrate. **D:** Necrotizing leukocytoclastic vasculitis, with eosinophilic change of the vessel wall, neutrophilic infiltration, and leukocytoclasia. **E:** Another example of neutrophil-rich, medium-sized vasculitis with focal necrotizing features in a subcutaneous vessel in a patient with polyarteritis nodosa.

Histopathology. The characteristic lesion of classic PAN is a panarteritis involving medium-sized and small arteries, and arterioles (33) (Fig. 8-5B,C). Even though in classic PAN the arteries show the characteristic changes in many visceral sites, affected skin often shows only small-vessel disease, and arterial involvement is typically focal. The changes affecting cutaneous small vessels are usually those of a necrotizing leukocytoclastic vasculitis (LCV). If there is a clinical presentation of cutaneous nodules, panarteritis similar to visceral lesions is usually detected. In classic PAN, the lesions typically are in different stages of development (i.e., fresh and old). Early lesions show degeneration of the arterial wall with deposition of fibrinoid material. There is partial to complete destruction of the external and internal elastic laminae. An infiltrate present within and around the arterial wall is composed largely of neutrophils, showing evidence of leukocytoclasis, although it often contains eosinophils. At a later stage, intimal proliferation and thrombosis lead to complete occlusion of the lumen with subsequent

ischemia and possibly ulceration. The infiltrate may also contain a significant number of lymphocytes, histiocytes, and some plasma cells, which may extend far into the surrounding perivascular tissue and may be predominant at a certain stage. In the healing stage, there is fibroblastic proliferation extending into the perivascular area. The small vessels of the middle and upper dermis often exhibit a nonspecific lymphocytic perivascular infiltrate.

Differential Diagnosis. Vasculitis indistinguishable from PAN may be observed in infections (bacterial, e.g., pseudomonas; viral, e.g., hepatitis B or HIV), connective tissue diseases (lupus erythematosus, rheumatoid arthritis), TA, GPA, EGPA, and other settings—for example, acute myelogenous leukemia. MPA can overlap considerably with PAN, as discussed later.

Principles of Management: As with all potentially systemic vasculitides, the first step is to determine which organs are involved and make treatment decisions based on the severity of internal organ involvement. First-line treatments include oral corticosteroids as well as cyclophosphamide, although other immunosuppressants have been shown to be effective. The treatment of HBV-associated PAN is centered on the use of an antiviral agent to control the infection (54). Cutaneous PAN may be managed less aggressively, as with NSAIDs.

Microscopic Polyangiitis

Clinical Summary. Davson et al. distinguished *classic PAN* from MPA (55). *Classic PAN* is to a greater degree a disease of medium-sized vessels so that ischemic glomerular lesions are common but glomerulonephritis is rare. *MPA* refers to a systemic small-vessel vasculitis primarily affecting arterioles and capillaries that is typically associated with focal crescentic necrotizing glomerulonephritis and presence of serum p-ANCA autoantibodies. Involvement of the small vessels of the kidneys, lungs, and skin gives MPA a particular clinical picture and separates MPA from classic polyarteritis nodosum (56–58).

Clinical Features. Most patients with MPA are men older than 50 years of age. Prodromal symptoms include fever, myalgias, arthralgias, and sore throat. The most common clinical feature is renal disease, manifesting as micro-hematuria, proteinuria, or acute oliguric renal failure. Although cutaneous involvement is rare in classic PAN, at least 30% to 40% of patients with MPA have skin changes. These include erythematous macules (100% in one study), livedo reticularis, palpable purpura, splinter hemorrhages, and ulcerations. Tender erythematous nodules are exceedingly rare in MPA. Pulmonary involvement without granulomatous tissue reaction occurs in approximately one-third of patients. Other organ systems (e.g., gastrointestinal tract, central nervous system, serosal and articular surfaces) may also be affected, but this is less common. Serious clinical complications usually arise from renal and pulmonary disease.

Pathogenesis. The exact mechanism for initial ANCA formation has not been elucidated. However, it is believed that primed neutrophils (i.e., potentially primed by infection, drug, proinflammatory cytokines) express MPO and PR3 on their cell surfaces and once bound to corresponding ANCAs (p-ANCA/anti-MPO) degranulate and cause vascular injury through lytic enzymes and free radicals. This collection of damaged tissue mixed with degenerated neutrophil debris creates NETs that concentrate MPO and PR3 and stimulate humoral production of additional ANCAs, creating a positive feedback loop of neutrophil-mediated vascular injury (59).

Histopathology. An LCV primarily affecting arterioles, venules, and capillaries is observed. Necrotizing vasculitis of medium-sized arteries typical of classic PAN is present on occasion. Cutaneous palisading granulomatous inflammation may be seen rarely.

Differential Diagnosis. MPA and classic PAN may not be distinguishable in every case, practically speaking. Glomerulonephritis, typical skin signs, ANCA positivity, and lack of arteriography findings (aneurysms and stenoses reflecting medium-sized vessel involvement) favor MPA over classic PAN (56). MPA also tends not to be associated with viral hepatitis, in contrast to some cases of classic PAN. Biopsy findings are less useful in distinguishing between these two syndromes because the size of diseased vessels detected is highly dependent on biopsy site, size of specimens, and number of tissue samples. Thus, lack

of medium-size vessel involvement in a biopsy by no means excludes classic PAN. Conversely, detection of small-vessel involvement also does not exclude classic PAN, which may show small-vessel disease. A number of cases of vasculitis show overlapping features, leading to the introduction of the term "overlapping syndrome of vasculitis" to encompass vasculitides affecting both small and medium-sized arteries (56). The differential diagnosis also includes GPA and other small-vessel vasculitides that are occasionally ANCA-positive, such as certain drug reactions. The granulomatous inflammation of GPA should be lacking in MPA; however, these two entities share many features, and some researchers believe that the distinction of MPA from GPA is largely artificial (60).

Principles of Management: Oral corticosteroids, cyclophosphamide, and rituximab have proven useful in the treatment of this condition. The 2011 revised five-factor scoring system for prognosticating systemic necrotizing vasculitides is covered under eosinophilic granulomatosis with polyangiitis (EGPA) (see Table 8-8).

GRANULOMATOUS VASCULITIS AND GRANULOMATOUS VASCULAR REACTIONS

Granulomatous inflammation may be a part of many inflammatory cutaneous infiltrates, and some of the granulomas may occur around blood vessels (Fig. 8-6) (1,4). When fibrinoid degeneration of the vessel wall is also observed, the process is termed granulomatous vasculitis. The main disease entities that need to be considered in the differential diagnosis of a granulomatous vascular reaction are listed in Table 8-7.

The two main disease processes in which granulomatous vasculitis has been described as prominent and fairly characteristic are GPA and EGPA, which are discussed in more detail here. However, the most common cutaneous histologic finding in both diseases is LCV. The granulomatous inflammation seen in the skin in these conditions is usually not angio-destructive.

Eosinophilic Granulomatosis with Polyangiitis

Clinical Summary. The classic clinicopathologic syndrome of eosinophilic granulomatosis with polyangiitis (formerly Churg–Strauss syndrome), or EGPA, is characterized by asthma, fever, hypereosinophilia, eosinophilic tissue infiltrates, necrotizing vasculitis, and extravascular granuloma formation (61). Short of an autopsy, the classic pathologic triad of necrotizing vasculitis, eosinophilic tissue infiltration, and extravascular granulomas is extremely difficult to demonstrate because of the focality of the process (62). A broader definition of EGPA, requiring asthma, hypereosinophilia greater than 1.5×10^9/L, and systemic vasculitis involving two or more extrapulmonary organs, has been suggested (63). Considerable overlap with other systemic vasculitides and with other inflammatory disorders associated with eosinophils, such as eosinophilic pneumonitis, has brought the legitimacy of the concept of EGPA into question.

Clinical Features. Despite multiple reports, EGPA appears to be rare. Between 1950 and 1995, only 120 cases were identified at the Mayo clinic (64). The incidence of EGPA is similar in males and females. It typically presents in the third or fourth

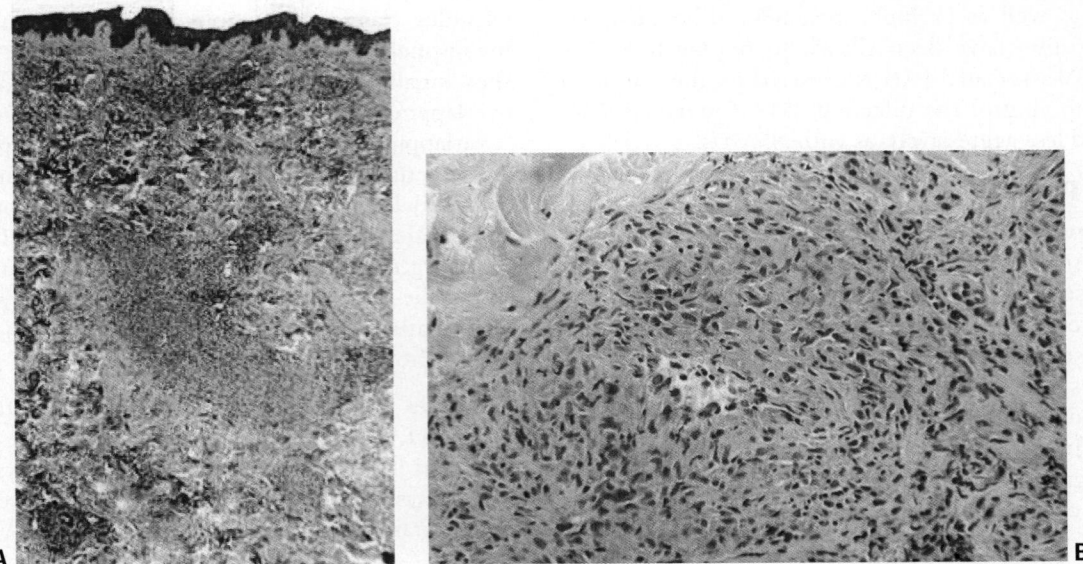

Figure 8-6 Granulomatous vasculitis. Note perivascular histiocytic/granulomatous infiltrate (A) and focal vascular damage (B).

Table 8-7

Differential Diagnosis of Granulomatous Vascular Reactions

Infection

Granulomatosis with polyangiitis (Wegener syndrome)

Eosinophilic granulomatosis with polyangiitis (Churg–Strauss syndrome)

Polyarteritis nodosa

Cutaneous Crohn disease

Drug reaction

Connective tissue disease

Granuloma annulare

Necrobiosis lipoidica

Paraneoplastic phenomena

Angiocentric T-cell lymphoma (lymphomatoid granulomatosis)

Erythema nodosum and erythema nodosum–like reactions

---

decade of life. Patients tend to display several phases of disease development, from nonspecific symptoms of asthma and allergic rhinitis (prodromal phase) to a phase of hypereosinophilia with eosinophilic pneumonitis or gastroenteritis (second phase) and, finally, to systemic vasculitis (third phase). The internal organs most commonly involved are the lungs, the gastrointestinal tract, and, less commonly, the peripheral nerves and heart. In contrast to PAN, renal failure is rare. The three disease phases do not always occur sequentially but may on occasion present simultaneously. There is also a limited form of allergic granulomatosis in which, in addition to preexisting asthma, the lesions are confined to the conjunctiva, the skin, and subcutaneous tissue. Certain medications have been associated with EGPA, including leukotriene modifying agents, inhaled corticosteroids, and omalizumab (65).

Two types of cutaneous lesions occur in about two-thirds of all patients: (a) hemorrhagic lesions varying from petechiae or extensive ecchymoses to palpable purpura and necrotic ulcers with associated areas of erythema (similar to Henoch–Schönlein purpura), and (b) cutaneous–subcutaneous nodules. The most common sites of skin lesions are the extremities, but the trunk may also show involvement. In some instances, the petechiae and ecchymoses are generalized. Other skin manifestations include urticaria, erythematous macules, and livedo reticularis.

Diagnostically helpful laboratory findings include an elevated peripheral eosinophil count. EPGA is also associated with ANCA positivity. Serum samples from patients with EGPA obtained during an active phase of the disease contain anti-MPO (p-ANCA) in most cases (~70%). The levels of anti-MPO have been found to correlate with disease activity. Anti-MPO is found less often in patients with limited forms of the disease. Anti-serine proteinase antibodies (c-ANCA) may infrequently be found in patients with CSS (~7%) (14).

Pathogenesis. The pathogenesis is currently unknown. The vascular damage is secondary to deposition of antibodies in the vessel walls with subsequent migration of neutrophils, which then degranulate and damage the endothelium (see Pathogenesis of Microscopic Polyarteritis for additional proposed mechanisms of ANCA-associated vasculitis).

Histopathology. The areas of cutaneous hemorrhage typically show LCV. However, eosinophils may be conspicuous. In some instances, the dermis contains palisading necrotizing granulomas composed predominantly of radially arranged histiocytes and, frequently, multinucleated giant cells centered around degenerated collagen fibers (Fig. 8-7). The central portions of the granulomas contain degenerated collagen fibers and disintegrated cells, particularly eosinophils, in great numbers—the so-called "red" palisading granulomas. These palisading granulomas can be embedded in a diffuse inflammatory exudate rich in eosinophils. In the subcutaneous tissue, the granulomas may attain considerable size through expansion and confluence, giving rise to the clinically apparent cutaneous–subcutaneous nodules. Initially believed to be characteristic histologic features, these granulomas were referred to as Churg–Strauss granulomas. However, they are not always present and are not a prerequisite for the diagnosis. Moreover, more recent studies have shown that similar findings can also be observed in other disease processes, such as connective tissue diseases (rheumatoid arthritis and lupus erythematosus), GPA (Wegener), PAN, lymphoproliferative disorders, subacute bacterial endocarditis, chronic active hepatitis, and inflammatory bowel disease (Crohn disease and ulcerative colitis) (66). Despite the common occurrence of LCV and Churg-Strauss (CS) granulomas in EGPA, granulomatous arteritis may also be observed (67).

Differential Diagnosis. EGPA is a clinicopathologic entity. As such, a diagnosis of EGPA depends on the clinical picture of respiratory disease, particularly a history of asthma, p-ANCA positivity, and histology compatible and supportive of this diagnosis, especially granulomatous inflammation, necrotizing angiitis, and eosinophilia. The principal differential diagnosis is with PAN, MPA, GPA, and the conditions mentioned previously that sometimes demonstrate extravascular necrotizing granulomas. There appears to be significant overlap with GPA and PAN. Particular patients may shift from one disease category to another over time.

Principles of Management: As with all potentially systemic vasculitides, the first step is to determine which organs are involved and make treatment decisions based on the severity of internal organ involvement. Like many vasculitides, high-dose corticosteroid is first-line treatment. In more severe cases, pulsed cyclophosphamide should be initiated. The management of systemic vasculitides is an area of active investigation, and consultation with rheumatology and an up-to-date review of the literature is recommended when treating patients with these potentially life-threatening systemic inflammatory syndromes. In 2011, the French Vasculitis Group revised their five-factor scoring system to improve the prognostication of systemic necrotizing vasculitides (Table 8-8). This scoring system may be applied to polyarteritis nodosa (PAN), microscopic polyangiitis (MPA), eosinophilic granulomatosis with polyangiitis (EGPA), and granulomatosis with polyangiitis (GPA). They found that the 5-year mortality rates for scores of 0, 1, and ≥2 were 9%, 21%, and 40%, respectively (68).

Granulomatosis with Polyangiitis

Granulomatosis with polyangiitis (formerly Wegener granulomatosis) (GPA) was first recognized as a distinct clinicopathologic disease process in 1936, when Wegener reported three patients with a "peculiar rhinogenic granulomatosis." Goodman and Churg summarized postmortem studies in 1954, from which evolved the classic triad of this clinicopathologic complex characterized by (a) necrotizing and granulomatous inflammation of the upper and lower respiratory tracts,

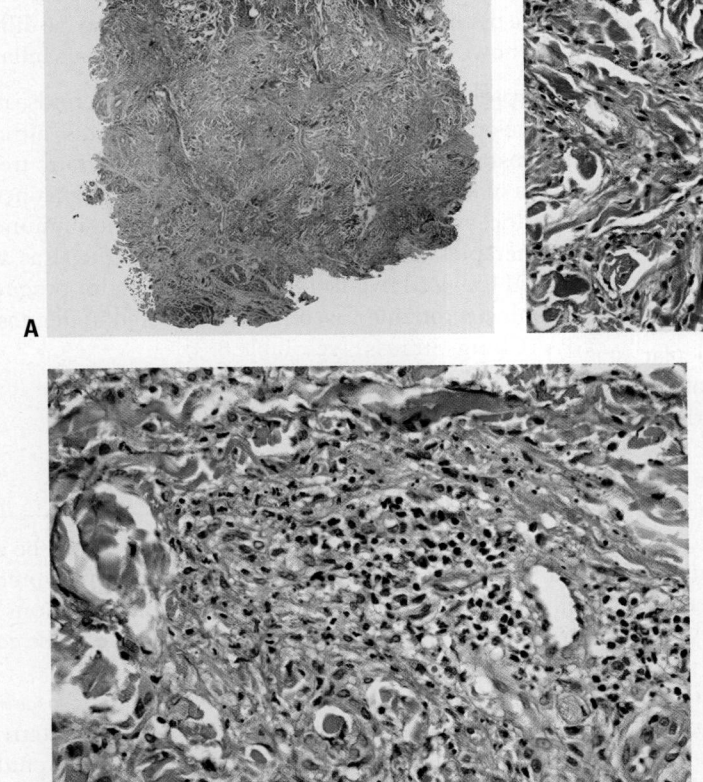

Figure 8-7 Palisading necrotizing granuloma. **A:** Scanning magnification shows a moderately dense cellular infiltrate with an ill-defined palisading pattern around areas of collagen degeneration. **B:** The infiltrate comprises mainly histiocytes, and collagen degeneration is prominent. **C:** Degenerating cells, including eosinophils, are present in some foci. This lesion, formerly called Churg–Strauss granuloma, is not diagnostic of any particular entity and, in addition to granulomatosis with polyangiitis (Wegener), may also be seen in connective tissue diseases, polyarteritis nodosa, lymphoproliferative disorders, subacute bacterial endocarditis, chronic active hepatitis, and inflammatory bowel disease (see text).

Table 8-8

Revised Five-Factor Scoring in Systemic Necrotizing Vasculitides (68)

Age >65 years = 1

Cardiac insufficiency = 1

Renal insufficiency (stabilized peak creatinine 1.7 mg/dL [150 μmol/L]) = 1

Gastrointestinal involvement = 1

Absence of ENT manifestations (presence is associated with a better prognosis) = 1

Score ranges from 0 to 2;

0 when no factors are present

1 when 1 factor is present

2 when ≥2 factors are present.

(b) glomerulonephritis, and (c) systemic vasculitis (69). Liebow and Carrington (62) and later Deremee et al. (70) described limited variants of the disease involving the respiratory tract only.

With the recognition of an association between ANCAs and GPA, the concept of GPA has been modified and the necessity of demonstrating granulomatous inflammation as a prerequisite for the diagnosis of GPA has been challenged. A less restrictive definition was proposed in the Third International Workshop on ANCA in 1991 (3) as *Wegener vasculitis.* Subsumed under this less restrictive category are ANCA-positive patients with clinical presentations of GPA, such as sinusitis, pulmonary infiltrates, and nephritis, and documented necrotizing vasculitis, but without biopsy-proven granulomatous inflammation. Both classic WG and Wegener vasculitis are considered different manifestations of *Wegener syndrome,* a more generic term, which was more recently renamed "granulomatosis with polyangiitis," or GPA (71).

Two-thirds of patients with GPA are male, and the mean age of diagnosis is 35 to 54 years. Most patients are white. The clinical presentation is extremely variable, ranging from an insidious course with a prolonged period of nonspecific constitutional symptoms and upper respiratory tract findings to an abrupt onset of severe pulmonary and renal disease. The most commonly involved anatomic sites include the upper respiratory tract, lower respiratory tract, and kidneys. Other organ systems that are commonly affected include joints and skin. Migratory, polyarticular arthralgia of large and small joints is found in up to 85% of patients with GPA. Cutaneous involvement is extremely variable in different series, ranging from about 10% to more than 50% of patients. Skin involvement presents most commonly as palpable purpura. Other cutaneous manifestations include macular erythematous eruptions, papules, papulonecrotic lesions, subcutaneous nodules with and without ulceration, and PG-like ulcerations. Occasionally, cutaneous lesions are the first manifestation of GPA, but, because of their nonspecific appearance, they are infrequently recognized as presentations of GPA.

The development of assays for ANCA has greatly facilitated the diagnosis of GPA and the monitoring of disease activity. In a study of 502 patients with biopsy-proven

ANCA-associated vasculitis, ANCA specificity was predictive of relapse. The relapse rate in c-ANCA–positive (anti-PR3)

patients was almost twice that of those with p-ANCA (anti-MPO) (72).

Pathogenesis. ANCAs are believed to be the primary mediators of inflammation and result in neutrophil-mediated vessel damage. The cause of elevated ANCAs, however, remains unclear (see pathogenesis of microscopic polyarteritis for further proposed mechanisms of ANCA-associated vasculitis).

Histopathology. Most skin biopsies in patients with GPA show nonspecific histopathology, and not all of them are directly related to the pathophysiology of GPA (73–75). Such nonspecific reaction patterns include perivascular lymphocytic infiltrates. However, in about 25% to 50% of patients, cutaneous lesions have fairly characteristic histopathologic findings. The more frequent distinct reaction patterns include necrotizing/leukocytoclastic small-vessel vasculitis and granulomatous inflammation. Minute foci of tissue necrosis are surrounded by histiocytes and are similar to lesions described in open lung biopsies from GPA patients. The palisading granulomas resembling those of EGPA (CSS) may occur, except that the center of the GPA granuloma contains necrobiotic collagen and basophilic fibrillar necrotic debris admixed with neutrophils (the "blue" palisading granulomas) (Fig. 8-7). True granulomatous vasculitis appears to be rare.

Differential Diagnosis. Other conditions causing LCV and granulomatous reactions include EGPA, metastatic Crohn disease, rheumatoid arthritis, and sarcoidosis. Granulomatous vascular reactions may also be a manifestation of T-cell lymphomas such as angiocentric T-cell lymphoma or panniculitic T-cell lymphoma. The distinction between EGPA and GPA relies primarily on the clinical findings. In contrast to GPA, EGPA is associated with asthma, lacks lesions in the upper respiratory tract, rarely shows severe renal involvement, and is typically accompanied by eosinophilia or eosinophilic infiltrates and p-ANCA positivity. The distinction between MPA and GPA may be difficult clinically; however, MPA should lack granulomatous inflammation.

Principles of Management: Oral corticosteroids, rituximab, and cyclophosphamide are standard treatments, although specific dosing regimens and mono- or dual-therapy treatment is an area of rapid evolution in the literature. Plasmapheresis, azathioprine, and other immunomodulatory and immunosuppressive therapies have been found to be beneficial as well (76). The 2011 revised five-factor scoring system for prognosticating systemic necrotizing vasculitides is covered under eosinophilic GPA (Churg–Strauss) (see Table 8-8).

SMALL-VESSEL NEUTROPHILIC/LEUKOCYTOCLASTIC VASCULITIS

A large number of different disease processes can be accompanied by small-vessel vasculitis with a neutrophil-predominant infiltrate. The clinical and histologic manifestations are thus fairly nonspecific (Fig. 8-8). The main diseases to be considered are listed in Table 8-9 (4,77).

Histopathology of Neutrophilic Small-Vessel Vasculitis. Neutrophilic small-vessel vasculitis is a reaction pattern of small dermal vessels, almost exclusively postcapillary venules, characterized by a combination of vascular damage and an infiltrate composed largely of neutrophils (Fig. 8-8). Because there is

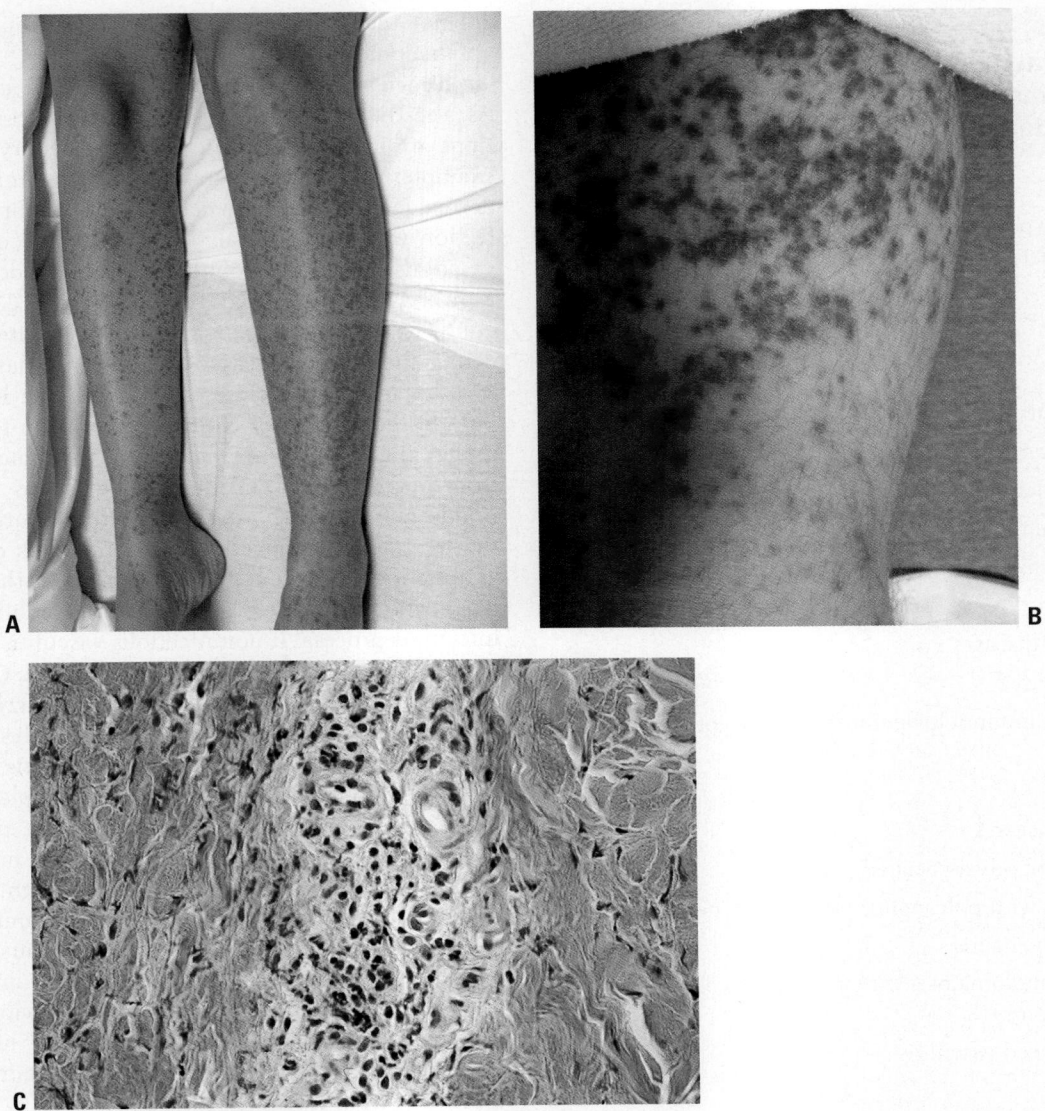

Figure 8-8 **A:** Extensive palpable purpura associated with leukocytoclastic vasculitis. (Courtesy of Melvin Chiu, MD.) **B:** Close-up view of lesions of leukocytoclastic vasculitis. **C:** Hypersensitivity vasculitis showing an upper dermal small blood vessel with neutrophil-rich vasculitis and other adjacent postcapillary venules with a perivascular mononuclear cell infiltrate without features of vasculitis. The specimen was obtained from a 6-day-old purpuric macule.

often fragmentation of neutrophil nuclei (karyorrhexis or leukocytoclasis), the term *leukocytoclastic vasculitis* is frequently used. Depending on its severity, this process may be subtle and limited to the superficial dermis or severe, manifesting as a fulminant pandermal reaction leading to necrosis and ulceration. If edema is prominent, a subepidermal blister may form. If the neutrophilic infiltrate is dense and there is pustule formation, the term *pustular vasculitis* may be applied (Fig. 8-9). In a typical case of LCV, the dermal vessels show swelling of the endothelial cells and presence of strongly eosinophilic strands of fibrin within the vessels and around their walls. The deposits of fibrin and the marked edema together give the vessel walls a "smudgy" appearance referred to as *fibrinoid degeneration*. Actual necrosis of the perivascular collagen, however, is seen only rarely in conjunction with ulcerative lesions. If the vascular changes are severe, luminal occlusion of vessels may be observed. The cellular infiltrate is present predominantly around the dermal blood vessels or within the vascular walls so that the outline of the blood vessels may appear indistinct. The infiltrate

consists mainly of neutrophils and varying numbers of eosinophils and mononuclear cells. The infiltrate can also be scattered throughout the upper dermis in association with fibrin deposits between and within collagen bundles. Extravasation of erythrocytes is commonly present.

As with any inflammatory process, the appearance of the reaction pattern depends on the stage at which the biopsy is taken. In older lesions, the number of neutrophils may be decreased, and the number of mononuclear cells increased to such an extent that mononuclear cells predominate, leading to a designation of a lymphocytic or even granulomatous vasculitis.

Pathogenesis. Many disease processes may exhibit LCV. The major causes of vasculitis are infection and immune-mediated inflammation. Table 8-6 categorizes vasculitides on the basis of suggested pathogenetic mechanisms. Although T-cell–mediated inflammation has been implicated in large-vessel vasculitides, antibody-mediated inflammation seems to play a prominent role in small-vessel vasculitis. Its final common pathway typically

Table 8-9

Differential Diagnosis of Cutaneous Neutrophilic Small-Vessel Vasculitis, Categorized on the Basis of Proposed Pathogenic Mechanisms

Infection

   Bacterial (gram-positive/gram-negative organisms, mycobacteria, spirochetes)

   Rickettsial

   Fungal

   Viral

Immunologic injury

Immune complex mediated

   Henoch–Schönlein purpura

   Urticarial vasculitis

   Cryoglobulinemia

   Serum sickness

Connective tissue diseases

Autoimmune diseases

Infection-induced immunologic injury (e.g., hepatitis B or C, streptococcal)

Drug induced

Paraneoplastic processes

Antineutrophil antibody associated

   Granulomatosis with polyangiitis (Wegener syndrome)

   Microscopic polyangiitis

   Eosinophilic granulomatosis with polyangiitis (Churg–Strauss syndrome)

   Some drug-induced vasculitis

Unknown

   Behçet disease

   Erythema elevatum diutinum

   Polyarteritis nodosa

involves neutrophil and monocyte activation with adherence to endothelial cells, infiltration of the vessel wall, and release of lytic enzymes and toxic-free radical metabolites. This final pathway of vascular injury may be initiated by (a) the deposition of immune complexes, (b) direct binding of antibodies to antigens in vessel walls, and (c) activation of leukocytes by antibodies with specificity for leukocyte antigens (ANCAs).

For example, hepatitis C virus (HCV) is directly linked to a subset of mixed cryoglobulinemia, which is an immune complex–mediated vasculitis (53). HCV particles and nonenveloped nucleocapsid protein participate in the formation of immune complexes. Clonal expansion of rheumatoid factor–synthesizing B lymphocytes is fundamental to the development of mixed cryoglobulinemia. Such B-cell clonal expansion takes place primarily in the liver and correlates directly with intrahepatic HCV viral load, indicating the critical role of HCV in the pathogenesis of such B-cell clonality.

However, it must be stressed that an immune complex etiology has too often been invoked for vasculitis, particularly small-vessel vasculitis. In many instances, immune complexes are not the primary event in vascular injury but are simply epiphenomena.

Diagnostic Approach to Neutrophilic Small-Vessel Vasculitis. As already mentioned, the clinical and histologic manifestations are fairly nonspecific for this category of vasculitis. For example, palpable purpura may be the clinical appearance of dermal leukocytoclastic small-vessel vasculitis secondary to infection (e.g., gonococcal sepsis), immune complex–mediated vasculitis (e.g., cryoglobulinemia or Henoch–Schönlein purpura), ANCA-associated vasculitis (e.g., GPA), allergic vasculitis (e.g., reaction to a drug), vasculitis associated with connective tissue disease, or a paraneoplastic phenomenon. It is important, therefore, to interpret the histologic findings only in the context of clinical information to reach an appropriate diagnosis. Often, additional laboratory data, such as from microbiologic cultures, special stains for organisms, or immunofluorescence or serologic studies, are needed. Because the treatment for infectious vasculitides is different from the treatment for immune-mediated diseases, the most important diagnostic step in the evaluation of a vasculitis is to rule out an infectious process. If noninfectious vasculitis is suspected, evidence for systemic vasculitis must be sought. Clinical findings—such as hematuria, arthritis, myalgia, enzymatic assays for muscle or liver enzymes, and serologic analysis for ANCAs, antinuclear antibodies, cryoglobulins, hepatitis B and C antibodies, IgA-fibronectin aggregates, and complement levels—are important to further delineate the disease process. Exposure to potential allergens, such as a drug, that might have elicited a hypersensitivity reaction should be sought, including illicit drugs such as cocaine with or without levamisole. Evidence of an allergic pathogenesis is reassuring because it suggests that the vasculitic process may be self-limited and not associated with systemic vasculitis. As mentioned previously, it is also important to address the possibility that the histologic findings of vasculitis may be a secondary phenomenon, for example, in ulceration from localized trauma.

The following subsections discuss the main clinical settings in which LCV occurs.

Infectious Vasculitis

An infectious process must be ruled out early in the evaluation of an LCV (1,7).

Clinical Summary. The spectrum of changes ranges from small macules and papules to purpura and necrosis. Biopsies show vascular damage, including LCV.

Histopathology. In most cases of infectious vasculitis, there are neutrophils and fibrin in vessel lumens, and there is usually also some degree of damage to the vessel wall, which may be indistinguishable from LCV, also usually being of lesser degree. Ischemia and necrosis of the epidermis, dermis, and adnexal structures occur often, and ulcerations are seen. Some researchers have suggested that the massive endothelial mycobacterial burden in the Lucio phenomenon may directly lead to vascular damage (78,79).

Pathogenesis. Microorganisms may invade vessels directly or damage them by an immune-mediated mechanism (80). *Neisseria meningitides* is a common cause of infectious cutaneous LCV. Meningococci may be found within endothelial cells and neutrophils at sites of vascular inflammation. However, other

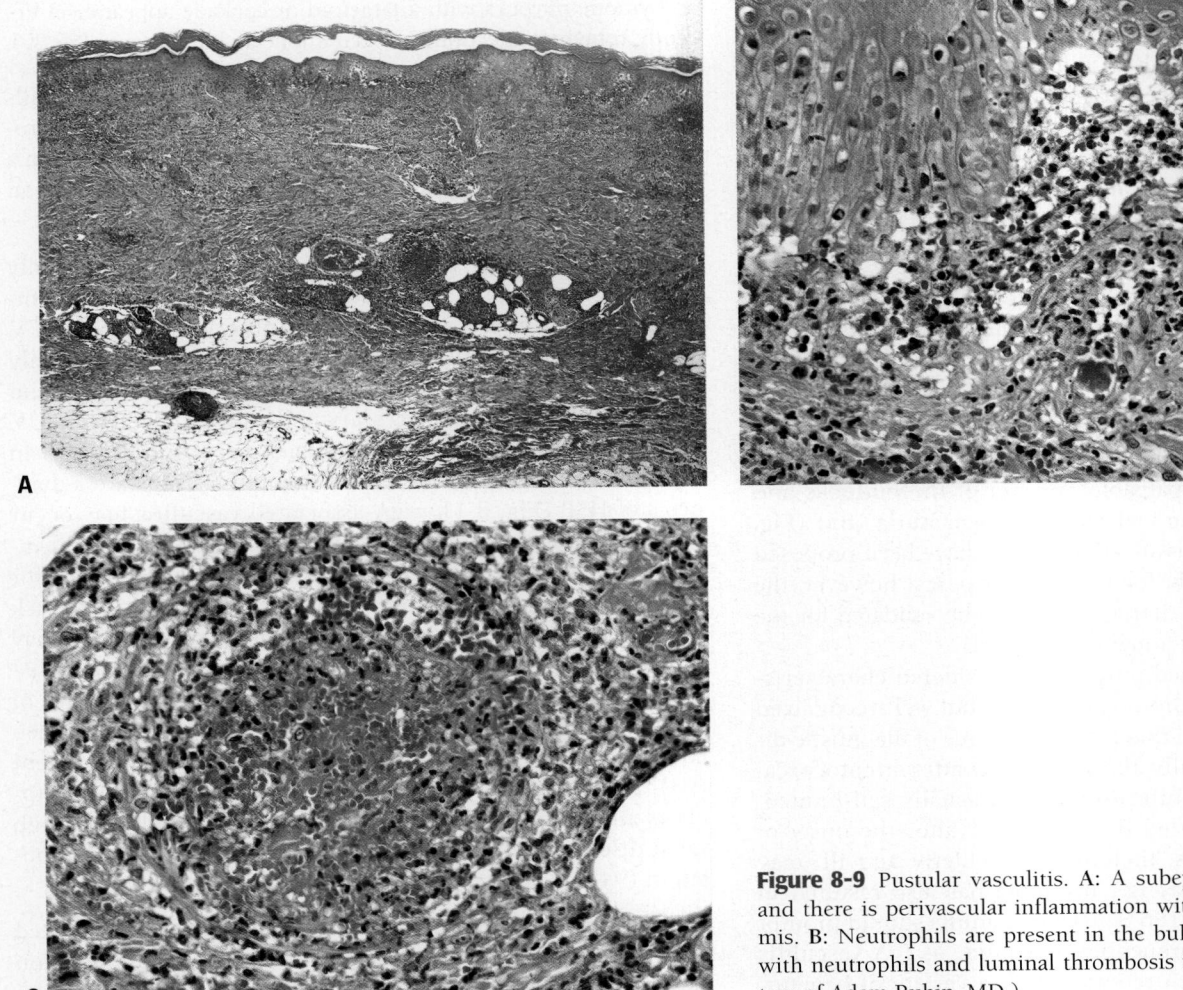

Figure 8-9 Pustular vasculitis. **A:** A subepidermal bulla is present, and there is perivascular inflammation with hemorrhage in the dermis. **B:** Neutrophils are present in the bulla. **C:** Vessel wall damage with neutrophils and luminal thrombosis in a dermal vessel. (Courtesy of Adam Rubin, MD.)

gram-positive or gram-negative bacteria and fungi may also cause cutaneous small-vessel vasculitis (Fig. 8-10). Staphylococcal sepsis with or without endocarditis can lead to neutrophilic vasculitis with purpura or nodular lesions, which may contain microabscesses. Rickettsial infections, such as Rocky Mountain spotted fever (RMSF), are characterized by invasion of endothelial cells by organisms causing vascular damage. Inflammation, however, is often minimal in RMSF. Direct immunofluorescence microscopy may demonstrate the organism. Lucio phenomenon (erythema necroticans) and erythema

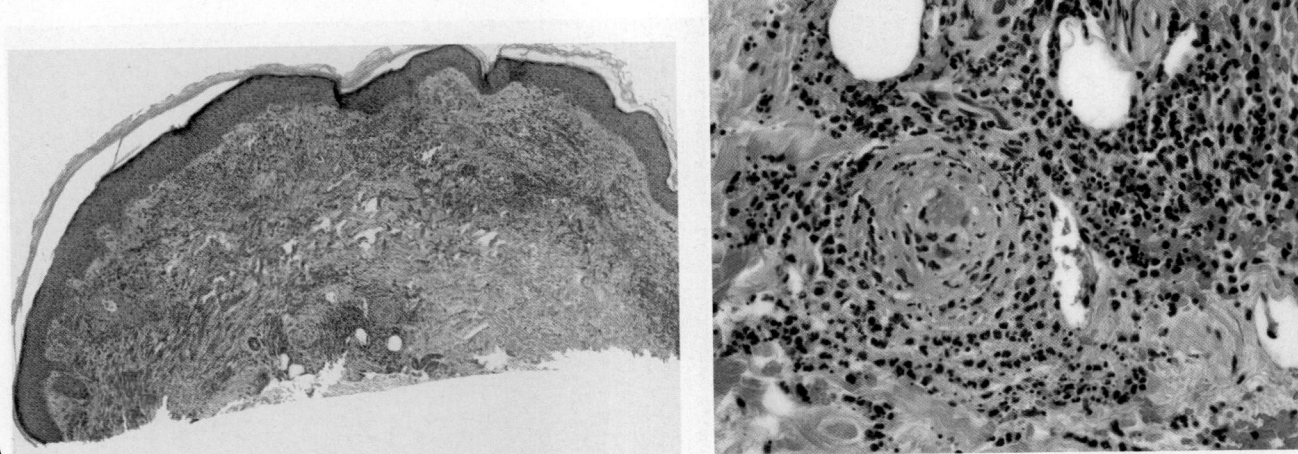

Figure 8-10 Septic vasculitis. **A:** Multiple vessels are surrounded by a dense inflammatory infiltrate and/or contain eosinophilic thrombotic material. It is associated with marked purpuric hemorrhage. **B:** A small vessel contains fibrin in its lumen and shows fibrinoid change of its wall, with a prominent neutrophilic infiltrate in the wall and in the adjacent tissue. Culture was positive for *Pseudomonas*. Organisms are difficult to appreciate in the figure.

nodosum leprosum are syndromes that may arise during the course of lepromatous leprosy. Lucio phenomenon shows necrotizing small-vessel vasculitis, and Fite-Faraco staining reveals large aggregates of acid-fast bacilli within the vascular walls, endothelium, and throughout the dermis.

Many viral organisms, such as HIV, hepatitis B, Epstein–Barr virus (EBV), HCV, cytomegalovirus (CMV), herpesvirus, parvovirus B19, and SARS-CoV-2 (81,82), may result in LCV on occasion.

Principles of Management: Treatment of the underlying infection with the appropriate antimicrobial agent will resolve the associated vasculitis.

Henoch–Schönlein Purpura (IgA Vasculitis)

Clinical Summary. Henoch–Schönlein purpura (HSP) is clinically characterized by palpable purpura of the buttocks and lower extremities, abdominal pain, and hematuria (83) (Fig. 8-11A). A number of classification criteria have been proposed for IgA vasculitis, mostly for research purposes; however, the clinical utility of these criteria have yet to be validated for the clinical diagnosis in individual patients (84).

Retiform or patterned purpura is considered characteristic of HSP. Bullous evolution is an unusual but well-recognized cutaneous manifestation that may be a source of diagnostic dilemma (85). HSP typically affects children after streptococcal upper respiratory tract infections and is usually self-limited, with a resolution expected 6 to 16 weeks after the onset of symptomatology. Adults, including the elderly and ill, may also develop this disease. IgA myeloma has also resulted in HSP-like manifestations (86,87). HSP in adults should prompt a consideration for a paraneoplastic source, as IgA vasculitis resembling HSP has been reported with a variety of hematologic and solid-organ malignancies. Complications generally arise from renal involvement that may even necessitate kidney transplantation.

Acute infantile hemorrhagic edema (AHE) is an uncommon benign form of cutaneous vasculitis occurring in children younger than 2 years of age and is considered by some to be a variant of HSP. AHE often presents with striking inflammatory edema and ecchymotic purpura with a targetoid or cockade appearance. Recently, rotavirus infection has been implicated in one case (88,89).

Pathogenesis. Complexes of IgA and C3 deposit in vessel walls in multiple organs, including the skin, connective tissue, scrotum, joints, gastrointestinal tract, and kidneys. This results in a type III hypersensitivity reaction, vascular injury, and end-organ damage.

Histopathology. HSP cannot be distinguished histologically from other forms of LCV, although the degree of vascular damage is often not as great as that usually observed in typical LCV. Such a limited extent of vascular damage is also commonly observed in urticarial vasculitis (UV) (see text following), and clinical findings may be necessary to distinguish HSP from UV. Immunofluorescence demonstrating the deposition of IgA in capillaries and the clinical scenario would lead toward a diagnosis of HSP (Fig. 8-11). IgA-associated vasculitis may occur outside of the symptom complex of HSP (90,91). Several investigations have attempted to identify prognostic markers for HSP to permit stratification of affected individuals into risk groups. Serologic detection of IgA-fibronectin aggregates may be associated with greater likelihood of renal or systemic disease in patients with cutaneous LCV (92), and a paucity of eosinophils in skin biopsies from adults with HSP has been correlated with a higher likelihood of renal involvement (93). Relapse may be predicted by the severity of leukocytoclasis and absence of IgM deposits on vessel walls, although renal disease does not seem to be associated with IgM deposition (94,95).

Principles of Management: Patients should be evaluated for a streptococcal infection, and, if present, such an infection should be treated appropriately with antibiotics. Patients require evaluation for renal disease in all cases, which in some patients, particularly those with extensive cutaneous vasculitis (lesions above the buttocks/extending to the abdomen or upper extremities), may occur weeks to months after the initial episode of HSP vasculitis. Because of the high recovery rate, treatment is not necessary in most cases except for symptomatic control of abdominal and joint pains with NSAIDs. However,

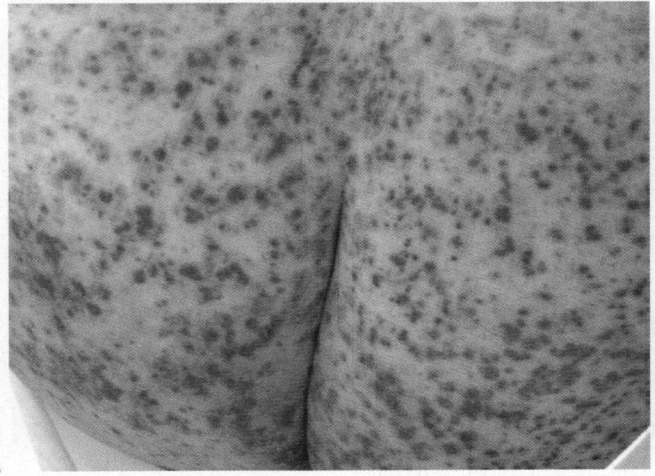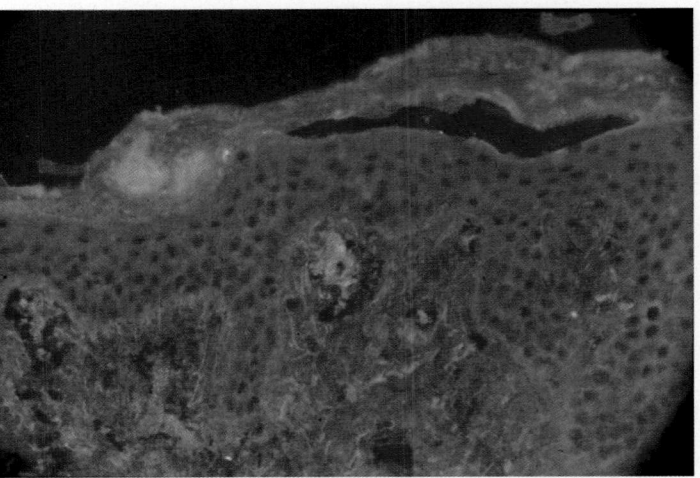

A **B**

Figure 8-11 **A:** Palpable purpura of sudden onset affecting the buttocks and lower extremities. (Courtesy of Rahat S. Azfur, MD.) **B:** Direct immunofluorescence showing granular immunoglobulin A (IgA) deposits in very superficial dermal vessels. This immunofluorescence finding is diagnostic of IgA vasculitis (Henoch–Schönlein purpura). Other immunoreactants were negative or significantly weaker.

in severe cases, or in those with renal injury or other systemic vasculitis, corticosteroids, cyclophosphamide, and IVIG can be used. Controversy exists over the use of corticosteroids to prevent renal involvement.

Urticarial Vasculitis

Clinical Summary. Persistent wheals (lasting more than 24 hours by convention) that burn rather than itch are a typical clinical finding of UV (96,97). Residual purpura is often seen after resolution of the urticarial lesions. The course of UV is generally benign and episodic, lasting several months. However, UV sometimes occurs in lupus erythematosus and may be the initial clinical manifestation of that disease. Approximately one-third of all patients with vasculitic urticaria have decreased complement levels (hypocomplementemic vasculitis) (Fig. 8-12). They may have systemic findings, such as arthralgias and adenopathy and may be more likely to have underlying systemic lupus erythematosus (98). Low complement levels and positive anti-C1q antibodies may indicate greater likelihood of more severe systemic disease.

Pathogenesis. UV is not a specific disease but rather a manifestation of a vasculitis that is associated with increased vascular permeability. The exact cause is unknown, although autoimmune diseases, cancers, and medications are associated.

Histopathology. The histology of UV is characterized by scant perivascular and interstitial neutrophilic infiltrates ranging from mild to fully developed LCV (Fig. 8-13). The minimal essential criteria for UV include neutrophilic infiltration of vessel walls with extravasation of erythrocytes. Nuclear debris and/or fibrinoid alteration of microvessels may be seen in fully developed lesions.

Principles of Management: All patients with UV warrant evaluation for underlying systemic lupus erythematosus. In isolated UV, in nonsevere cases, NSAIDs and/or antihistamines may be effective. Many cases will prove recalcitrant, and refractory and severe cases may require dapsone, oral corticosteroids, or cytotoxic agents.

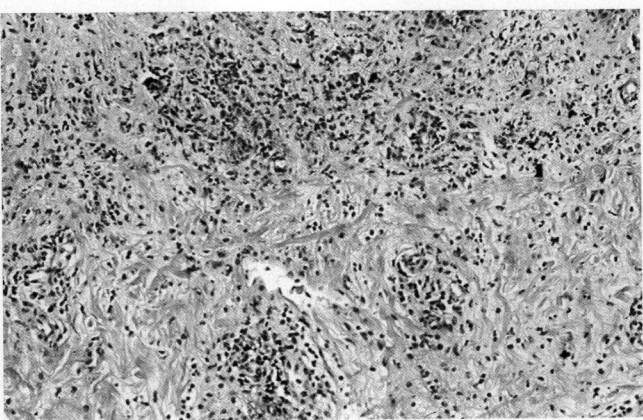

Figure 8-13 Neutrophil-rich small-vessel vasculitis of upper- and middermal vessels associated with interstitial spillage of neutrophils from a patient with hypocomplementemic urticarial vasculitis.

Cryoglobulinemias and Other Small-Vessel Vasculitides Associated with Paraproteins

Small-vessel vasculitis may be associated with paraproteins—that is, abnormal serum proteins (1,99,100). Such paraproteins include cryoglobulins, cryofibrinogens, macroglobulins, and gamma heavy chains. Cryoglobulins are serum immunoglobulins that precipitate when the serum is cooled and redissolve on rewarming. There are three major types of cryoglobulinemia: In type I cryoglobulinemia, monoclonal IgG or IgM cryoglobulins are found, often associated with lymphoma, leukemia, Waldenström macroglobulinemia, multiple myeloma, or without known underlying disease. In type II cryoglobulinemia, the cryoprecipitate consists of both monoclonal and polyclonal cryoglobulins, with one cryoglobulin acting as an antibody against the other. These cryoglobulins are circulating immune complexes. The most common combination is IgG–IgM (Fig. 8-14). In type III cryoglobulinemia, the immunoglobulins are polyclonal. Type II and III or mixed cryoglobulinemias are frequently seen in connective tissue disorders, such as lupus

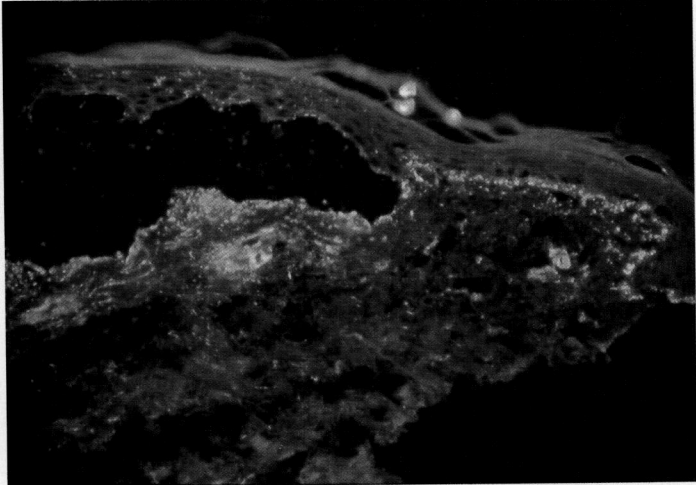

Figure 8-12 Direct immunofluorescence showing granular immunoglobulin G deposits in superficial dermal vessels and along the basement membrane zone. This combined vasculitic and lupus type of immunofluorescence finding is characteristic of hypocomplementemic urticarial vasculitis.

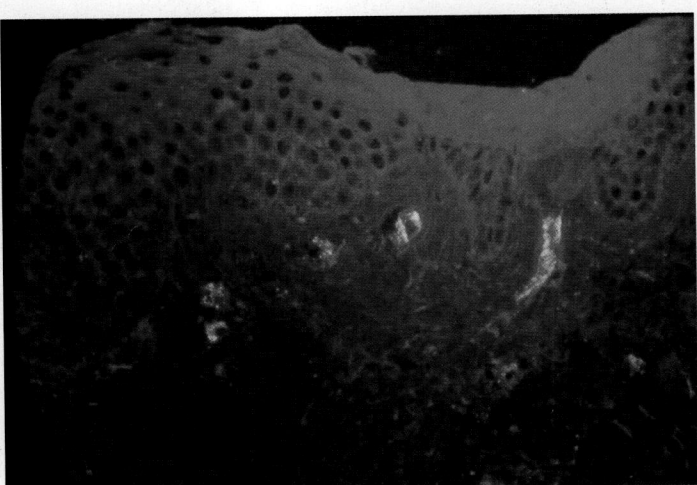

Figure 8-14 Direct immunofluorescence showing dense granular immunoglobulin M deposits in superficial small vessels in a patient with cryoglobulinemia type 2. This specimen also showed concomitant dense granular C3 in the same blood vessels.

erythematosus, rheumatoid arthritis, and Sjögren syndrome, or may be related to infection—in particular, hepatitis C infection. Idiopathic forms of type II and III cryoglobulinemias are also termed essential mixed cryoglobulinemia (101,102).

Clinically, cutaneous lesions in patients with cryoglobulinemia may manifest as chronic palpable purpura, urticaria-like lesions, livedo reticularis, PAN-like lesions, leg ulcers, splinter hemorrhages, palmar erythema, acrocyanosis, and digital gangrene. Raynaud phenomenon is common. Systemic manifestations may include arthralgia, hepatosplenomegaly, lymphadenopathy, and glomerulonephritis.

Histopathology. In type I cryoglobulinemia, amorphous material (precipitated cryoglobulins) is deposited subjacent to endothelium and throughout the vessel wall as well as within the vessel lumen, resulting in a thrombus-like appearance (Fig. 8-15). These precipitates stain pink with hematoxylin and eosin and bright red with periodic acid–Schiff (PAS) stain, as opposed to less intense staining of fibrinoid material. Some capillaries are filled with red blood cells, and extensive extravasation of erythrocytes may be present. An inflammatory infiltrate is usually lacking, in contrast to mixed cryoglobulinemia, which typically shows an LCV (Fig. 8-16). PAS-positive intramural and intravascular cryoprecipitates may also be found in mixed cryoglobulinemia, although less frequently than in type I cryoglobulinemia.

Other small-vessel vasculitides with the histologic pattern of an LCV may be found in association with Waldenström hyperglobulinemia (hyperglobulinemic purpura) and in Schnitzler syndrome, which manifests as chronic urticaria with macroglobulinemia (usually monoclonal IgM) and other paraproteinemias.

Serum Sickness

This syndrome of a morbilliform urticarial eruption, fever, and lymphadenopathy occurs 7 to 10 days after a primary antigen exposure or 2 to 4 days after a repeat exposure. The antigen may be a drug, from an arthropod sting or a previous infection, or therapeutic serum globulins (103). Serum sickness is usually a self-limited condition. The LCV of serum sickness has no distinctive histologic features.

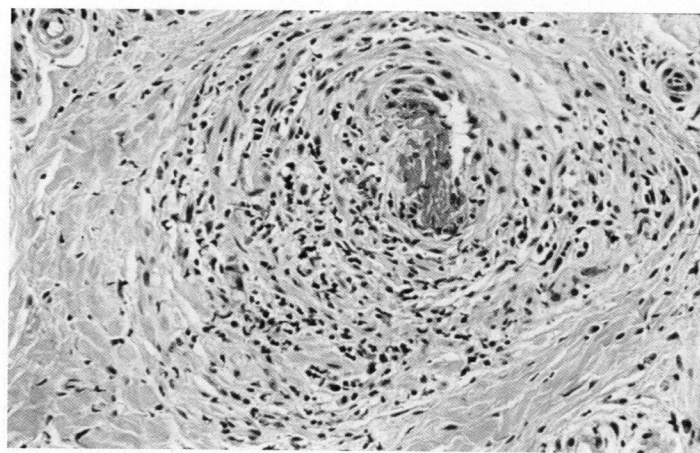

Figure 8-16 Cryoglobulinemia. A small middermal artery showing neutrophil-rich vasculitis secondary to hepatitis C–associated cryoglobulinemia type 2.

Connective Tissue Disease

Rheumatoid arthritis, lupus erythematosus, and other diseases in the spectrum of connective tissue disease may develop LCV (104-107). Patients with systemic lupus erythematosus may develop a lupus-nonspecific skin eruption with a vasculitis that may be neutrophil or lymphocyte predominant. Leukocytoclastic vasculitis may also occur in patients with antiphospholipid antibody syndrome (108). Clinical and serologic information is critical to the correct interpretation of the cutaneous findings in these clinical settings.

Autoimmune Diseases

Primary Sjögren syndrome is not associated with connective tissue disease but may present with purpura in addition to ocular and glandular involvement (1). The histologic reaction pattern is often an LCV or lymphocytic vasculitis.

Antineutrophil Cytoplasmic Antibodies–Associated Vasculitis

The pauci-immune vasculitides associated with ANCA were discussed in more detail earlier. MPA, GPA, and EGPA syndrome may all be associated with cutaneous LCV.

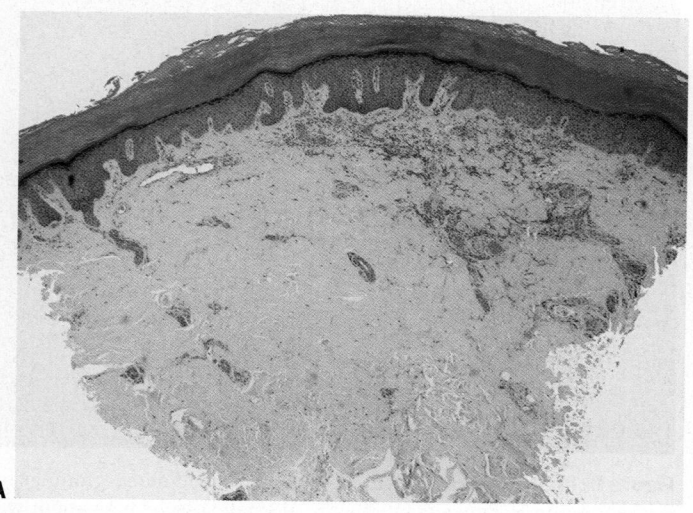

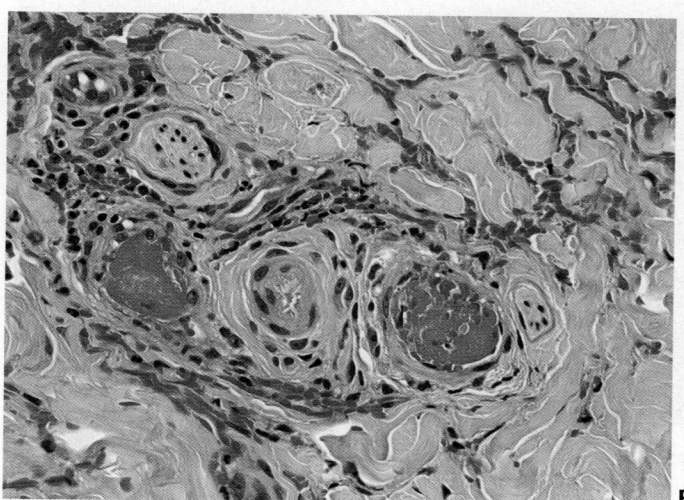

Figure 8-15 A: Cryoglobulinemia. Vessels in the reticular dermis contain brightly eosinophilic material. B: The deposition is associated with little or no damage to the vessel walls in this case.

Drug-Induced Vasculitis

A hypersensitivity reaction to a drug may result in an LCV (1,109). Penicillin, thiazides, and sulfonamides are the most common drugs used to induce LCV. Other medications include propylthiouracil, rifampin, pyrazinamide, and, more recently, checkpoint inhibitors and epidermal growth factor receptor inhibitors (110–112). The list of medications that can induce a vasculitis is long and growing. Drugs may also induce the pattern of pustular vasculitis. Increased tissue eosinophil counts (5.2 vs. 1.05 per 10 high-power fields) have recently been suggested to correlate with drug-induced versus non–drug-induced LCV (113).

Paraneoplastic Vasculitis

A wide spectrum of vasculitic processes has been associated with neoplastic disorders (114,115). Sixty patients with cancer-related vasculitis demonstrated the following vasculitic patterns: 45% LCV, 36.7% PAN, 6.7% GPA, 5% MPA, and 5% HSP (115). The distribution of malignancies among these patients was as follows: 63.1% with hematologic (including 32.3% with myelodysplastic syndromes and with 29.2% lymphoid neoplasms) and 36.9% with solid malignancies. Common associations include PAN with hairy cell leukemia and cutaneous small-vessel vasculitis with lymphoproliferative disorders and some carcinomas.

Localized Fibrosing Small-Vessel Vasculitis

Erythema elevatum diutinum (EED), granuloma faciale (GF), and some examples of cutaneous inflammatory pseudotumor are very similar chronic fibrosing conditions that show evidence of vascular damage (116). Sometimes, they may be classified with the neutrophilic dermatoses. These entities are hypothesized to be reactions to localized persistent immune complex deposition or hypersensitivities to a persistent antigen. EED- and GF-like reactions may occasionally be seen in clinical settings atypical for either entity.

Erythema Elevatum Diutinum

Clinical Summary. This rare condition is characterized by persistent, initially red to violaceous and later brown to yellow papules, nodules, and plaques (117,118). The lesions, typically distributed symmetrically on the extensor surfaces of the extremities, are initially soft and then evolve into fibrous nodules. Extracutaneous associations include arthralgias, scleritis, panuveitis, peripheral ulcerative keratitis, oral and genital ulcers, and neuropathy. Additionally, associations with various systemic diseases, including HIV, IgA paraproteinemia, myeloma, neutrophilic dermatoses, systemic lupus erythematosus, and inflammatory bowel diseases have been reported (119).

Histopathology. In the early stage of EED, nonspecific LCV is observed. In later stages, granulation tissue and fibrosis form with a diffuse mixed-cell infiltrate showing a predominance of neutrophils. Granuloma formation is occasionally present (117). The capillaries may still show deposits of fibrinoid material or merely fibrous thickening. Fully developed lesions of EED may be indistinguishable from neutrophilic dermatoses, Behçet disease, or neutrophilic drug reaction. GF may also resemble EED but is distinguished by clinical localization to the face, sparing of the superficial papillary dermis (a grenz zone), and prominence of eosinophils and plasma cells in addition to neutrophils.

Occasional cases show neutrophilic microabscesses in the tips of dermal papillae that might suggest dermatitis herpetiformis (118). In old, fibrotic lesions of EED, there is an orderly array of spindle cells and collagen bundles often parallel to the skin surface with vertically arranged capillaries similar to a scar. Lipid material may also be present as cholesterol clefts. Serial sections may be required to demonstrate vascular damage in late lesions. These older lesions of EED must be differentiated from Kaposi sarcoma, dermatofibroma, or granuloma annulare. Neutrophils, nuclear dust, and fibrin owing to persistent vascular damage may be present, helping to distinguish these lesions from dermatofibromas or scars. The irregularly arranged, jagged vascular spaces of Kaposi sarcoma are absent, and many of the spindle cells have the immunohistochemical and electron microscopic features of macrophages. Focal areas of basophilic collagen caused by nuclear dust in EED can resemble the mucin seen in granuloma annulare but do not stain with Alcian blue. Direct immunofluorescence studies reveal perivascular deposition of IgM, IgA, IgG, C3, and fibrin (120).

Pathogenesis. EED probably is not a distinct disease entity but rather a clinicopathologic reaction pattern of chronic immune complex–mediated vasculitis with scarring, most often developing in the setting of either a monoclonal or polyclonal gammopathy, in particular IgA hyperglobulinemia. Inflammatory bowel disease, rheumatoid arthritis, and systemic lupus erythematosus may also be associated with EED. HIV-infected patients also develop EED, which can clinically mimic Kaposi sarcoma (121).

Principles of Management: Dapsone has been shown to be effective for this condition.

Granuloma Faciale

Clinical Summary. GF presents as one or several asymptomatic, soft, brown-red, slowly enlarging papules or plaques with dilated follicular ostia and telangiectasias, almost always on the face of older individuals (122). Less commonly, multiple facial and even extrafacial lesions may occur (123). Rare forms affecting the upper respiratory tract have been described. Multiple case reports have demonstrated an association with eosinophilic angiocentric fibrosis of mucosal surfaces, resulting in sinonasal tumors, epistaxis, dyspnea, and proptosis (124).

Pathogenesis. Vascular damage may be important to the pathogenesis of this lesion because direct immunofluorescence data suggest an immune complex–mediated event with deposition of mainly IgG in and around vessels. A significant number of GF cases have been shown to be associated with an increase in IgG4 plasma cells, especially in male patients and cases with multiple or recurrent lesions. Obliterative vascular inflammation and storiform sclerosis are also features of IgG4-associated sclerosing diseases, suggesting that some cases of GF might represent a localized form of IgG4-related disease (125).

Histopathology. A dense polymorphous infiltrate is present mainly in the upper half of the dermis but may extend into the lower dermis and, occasionally, even into the subcutaneous tissue. Quite characteristically, the infiltrate does not invade the epidermis or the pilosebaceous appendages but is separated from them by a narrow grenz zone of normal collagen (Fig. 8-17). The pilosebaceous structures tend to remain intact. The polymorphous infiltrate consists primarily of neutrophils

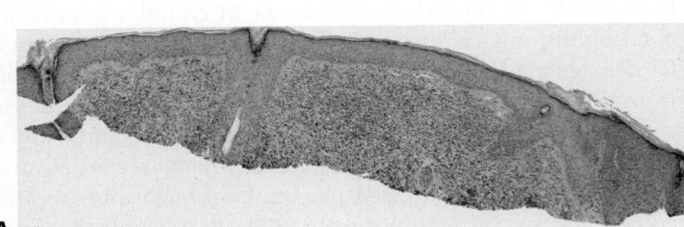
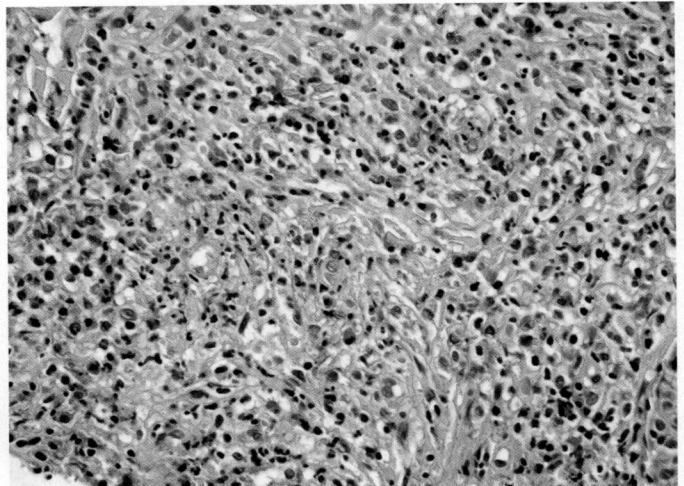

Figure 8-17 Granuloma faciale. **A:** There is a cellular infiltrate in the dermis, separated from the epidermis by an uninvolved or grenz zone. **B:** The infiltrate contains numerous neutrophils and eosinophils. Vascular damage is minimal.

and eosinophils, but mononuclear cells, plasma cells, and mast cells are also present. Vascular damage in GF is seen but often limited, and thus perhaps GF is best termed a neutrophilic vascular reaction (126). Frequently, the nuclei of some of the neutrophils are fragmented, especially in the vicinity of the capillaries, thus forming nuclear dust. Often, there is some evidence of vasculitis with deposition of fibrinoid material within and around vessel walls. Occasionally, some hemorrhage is noted. Foam cells and fibrosis are frequently observed in older lesions.

Differential Diagnosis. Histologic overlap between GF and EED is substantial. Formerly, a grenz zone, the prevalence of eosinophils and plasma cells and the degree of fibrosis were believed to distinguish GF and EED; however, a recent review suggests that none of these features are helpful. Only granulomatous nodules are limited to EED, and those are not an especially frequent finding (126). The characteristic clinical presentations do help separate these entities; however, clinical overlap from atypical cases has been described. Other neutrophilic dermatoses can be distinguished from GF by the lack of a grenz zone and clinical features. Frank LCV should not be seen in GF. In acneiform lesions and folliculitides, pilosebaceous units are invaded by inflammatory cells and may be destroyed or disrupted.

Principles of Management: Multiple modalities can be used to remove or lessen the appearance of this lesion, including intralesional corticosteroids, lasers, dermabrasion, cryotherapy, and surgical excision. Some patients have responded to dapsone, colchicine, or antimalarial medications in limited reports.

NEUTROPHILIC DERMATOSES

These are lesions that consist of a neutrophilic infiltrate, sometimes even with leukocytoclasis, and some degree of vascular damage in up to one-third of cases (127). Microvascular injury is most likely secondary to the dense neutrophilic infiltrates; the extent of vascular damage is insufficient for necrotizing vasculitis—that is, fibrinoid necrosis is lacking. Occasionally, such a histologic picture may be seen in an early lesion of vasculitis. However, several clinical conditions characterized by neutrophilic infiltrates rarely develop necrotizing vasculitis

and need to be distinguished from vasculitis. These entities are categorized as neutrophilic dermatoses and are characterized by (a) a neutrophilic infiltrate histologically, (b) a lack of microorganisms on special stains and cultures, and (c) clinical improvement on systemic steroid treatment (128,129). Vascular damage has been observed in these conditions, but it remains unclear whether the vascular injury plays an etiologic role or is merely an epiphenomenon. A relationship between these entities may be indicated by their occasional co-occurrence in patients with predisposing conditions. Relatively recent insights suggest some of these entities may be classified as autoinflammatory disorders related to dysfunction of the innate immune system (130).

Acute Febrile Neutrophilic Dermatosis (Classic Sweet Syndrome and Sweet-Like Neutrophilic Dermatosis)

Clinical Summary. Dr. R.D. Sweet described, in 1964, a disease process, which he termed "acute febrile neutrophilic dermatosis," that was characterized by abrupt onset of fever, leukocytosis, and erythematous plaques infiltrated by neutrophils (129). This condition typically occurs in middle-aged women after nonspecific infections of the respiratory or gastrointestinal tract. The lesions tend to be found on the face or extremities and only rarely involve the trunk and respond to steroid treatment. Despite the numerous neutrophils, the lesions are sterile. Vesicles and pustules may also arise. Involvement of noncutaneous sites, such as eyes, joints, oral mucosa, and visceral sites (lungs, liver, kidneys), has been reported. A variety of disorders have been associated with neutrophilic dermatoses similar to those seen in Sweet syndrome (Sweet-like neutrophilic dermatosis). About 20% of cases are associated with malignancy. Cutaneous eruptions with inflammatory vascular reactions, which on occasion simulate the lesions of Sweet syndrome, may also occur in association with hereditary periodic fever, which comprises several syndromes, including familial Mediterranean fever, the hyper-IgD syndrome, and the tumor necrosis factor receptor-associated periodic syndrome (131).

Pathogenesis. Sweet syndrome's etiology is unknown, but theories have included immune complex vasculitis, altered T-cell activation, and altered function of neutrophils. All, however, lack sufficient experimental support. The vascular alterations seen in Sweet syndrome may be secondary to the massive extravasation of activated neutrophils. Direct immunofluorescence studies are generally negative in Sweet syndrome (131). New emerging autoinflammatory mechanisms involve polymorphisms of the innate immune system that react to infectious, drug, tumor, and other antigens and the stimulation and overproduction of cytokines (e.g., granulocyte colony-stimulating factor [G-CSF], IL-1, IL-3, IL-6, and IL-8) that promote neutrophil activation and infiltration (132,133).

Histopathology. Typically, a dense perivascular infiltrate composed largely of neutrophils is seen assuming a bandlike distribution throughout the papillary dermis (Fig. 8-18). Some of the neutrophils may show nuclear fragmentation (leukocytoclasis). In addition, the infiltrate may contain scattered lymphocytes and histiocytes and occasional eosinophils. The density of the infiltrate varies and may be limited in a small proportion of cases. Vasodilation and swelling of endothelium with moderate erythrocyte extravasation and prominent edema of the upper dermis are characteristic. In some instances, subepidermal blister formation may result. Extensive vascular damage is not a feature of Sweet syndrome. The histologic appearance varies depending on the stage of the process. In later stages, lymphocytes and histiocytes may predominate. Sweet's-like neutrophilic dermatoses often show a similar histologic picture. However, the reaction pattern may, on occasion, be quite different, manifesting, for instance, as deep subcutaneous localized suppurative panniculitis. The infiltrate of Sweet syndrome is not characteristic enough to exclude infection on histologic findings alone. As always, to arrive at the correct interpretation of a neutrophilic infiltrate, cultures need to be obtained and special stains need to be performed to exclude an infectious etiology (although it should be recognized that these stains in isolation are not sensitive for this purpose). Rarely, subcutaneous neutrophilic infiltrates with a lobular or, less frequently, septal pattern with minimal dermal involvement occur in a clinical setting identical to Sweet syndrome. These infiltrates have been termed "subcutaneous Sweet syndrome" or neutrophilic panniculitis (134). Some cutaneous lesions of Sweet syndrome are histopathologically characterized by an infiltrate mostly composed of histiocytoid cells that are actually immature myeloid cells. This variant is termed histiocytoid Sweet syndrome and may be mistaken for leukemia cutis or other inflammatory dermatoses that are histopathologically characterized by histiocytes interstitially arranged between collagen bundles of the dermis (135).

Principles of Management: Oral corticosteroids are the "gold standard" treatments, although other options such as potassium iodide, colchicine, doxycycline, clofazimine, cyclosporine, and dapsone can also be efficacious. A response to steroid treatment is part of the diagnostic criteria and is usually rapid.

Bowel-Associated Dermatosis–Arthritis Syndrome

This syndrome was initially described in patients after jejuno-ileal bypass surgery. Subsequently, however, the spectrum of the syndrome has expanded to include other disease processes with typical cutaneous findings and associated bowel disease (1). Patients may have inflammatory bowel disease or a blind loop after peptic ulcer surgery.

Clinical Summary. The cutaneous lesions are characterized by initial small macules that develop through a papular phase into pustules on a purpuric base. The evolution usually occurs within a 2-day period. The lesions typically reach a size of 0.5 to 1.5 cm. They are typically distributed on the upper part of the body, especially the arms, rather than on the dependent sites of the legs. Cutaneous lesions often occur in crops and are episodic (1 to 2 weeks), with a tendency to recur within months. Fever, myalgias, and arthralgias may accompany the disease process.

Pathogenesis. One suggested etiology involves antigens derived from an overgrowth of intestinal bacteria triggering an immune complex–mediated reaction with vascular insults. The peptidoglycan antigens of bacteria, specifically group A streptococci, are thought to be responsible (136).

Histopathology. The histopathologic changes are usually those of neutrophilic vascular reactions with little or none of the vascular damage observed in Sweet syndrome and other neutrophilic dermatoses. However, frank necrotizing small-vessel vasculitis may occasionally be noted. In fully developed lesions,

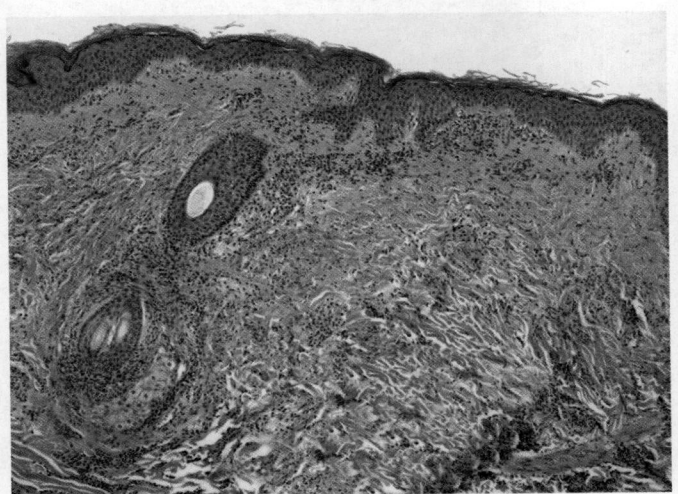
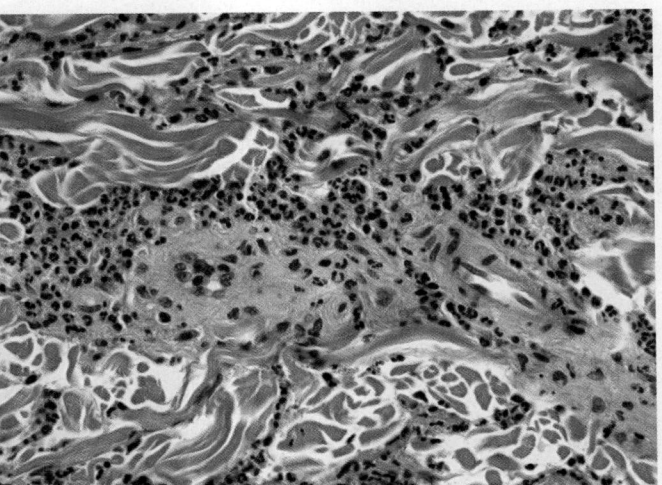

Figure 8-18 Sweet syndrome. **A:** There is a dense infiltrate in the upper dermis, consisting mainly of neutrophils, without leukocytoclasia. Derma edema is not prominent in this example. **B:** Vascular damage is slight.

the neutrophilic infiltrate and papillary dermal edema may be florid, and subepidermal pustule formation is seen. If vascular damage is observed in such a context, the term "pustular vasculitis" is applied.

Principles of Management: Oral antibiotics and corticosteroids have been helpful, as has surgical repair to improve bowel function.

Pyoderma Gangrenosum

PG is included in this chapter as well as in Chapter 16 because in these and other authors' opinions it represents a clinicopathologic manifestation that falls within the spectrum of neutrophilic dermatoses (1). As with other neutrophilic dermatoses, infection must be excluded to arrive at the correct diagnosis.

Clinical Summary. Several clinical types have been described: ulcerative PG with an undermined border; pustular PG with discrete, painful pustules; painful bullae with progression to a superficial ulceration; and vegetative PG with a painless ulcer

and a nonundermined exophytic border (Fig. 8-19A) (137). Classically, lesions begin as tender papulopustules or folliculitis that eventually may ulcerate. In the fully developed stage, the lesions have a distinctive raised, undermined border with a dusky purple hue. The process of tissue breakdown, perhaps as a response to minor trauma, is known as pathergy, which is considered to be primarily a clinical term. As pathergy is clinically demonstrable only in 20% to 30% of patients with PG, its absence should not be used to exclude this diagnosis, and its presence should not deter clinicians from performing diagnostic biopsies to exclude PG-mimics.

Pathogenesis. The exact pathogenesis is unknown, but an autoinflammatory process is favored (see pathogenesis of Sweet syndrome). Again, as with neutrophilic dermatoses, in general, PG may occur as an isolated cutaneous phenomenon or may be a cutaneous manifestation associated with various systemic disease processes, such as inflammatory bowel disease and inflammatory arthritis, lymphoproliferative lesions

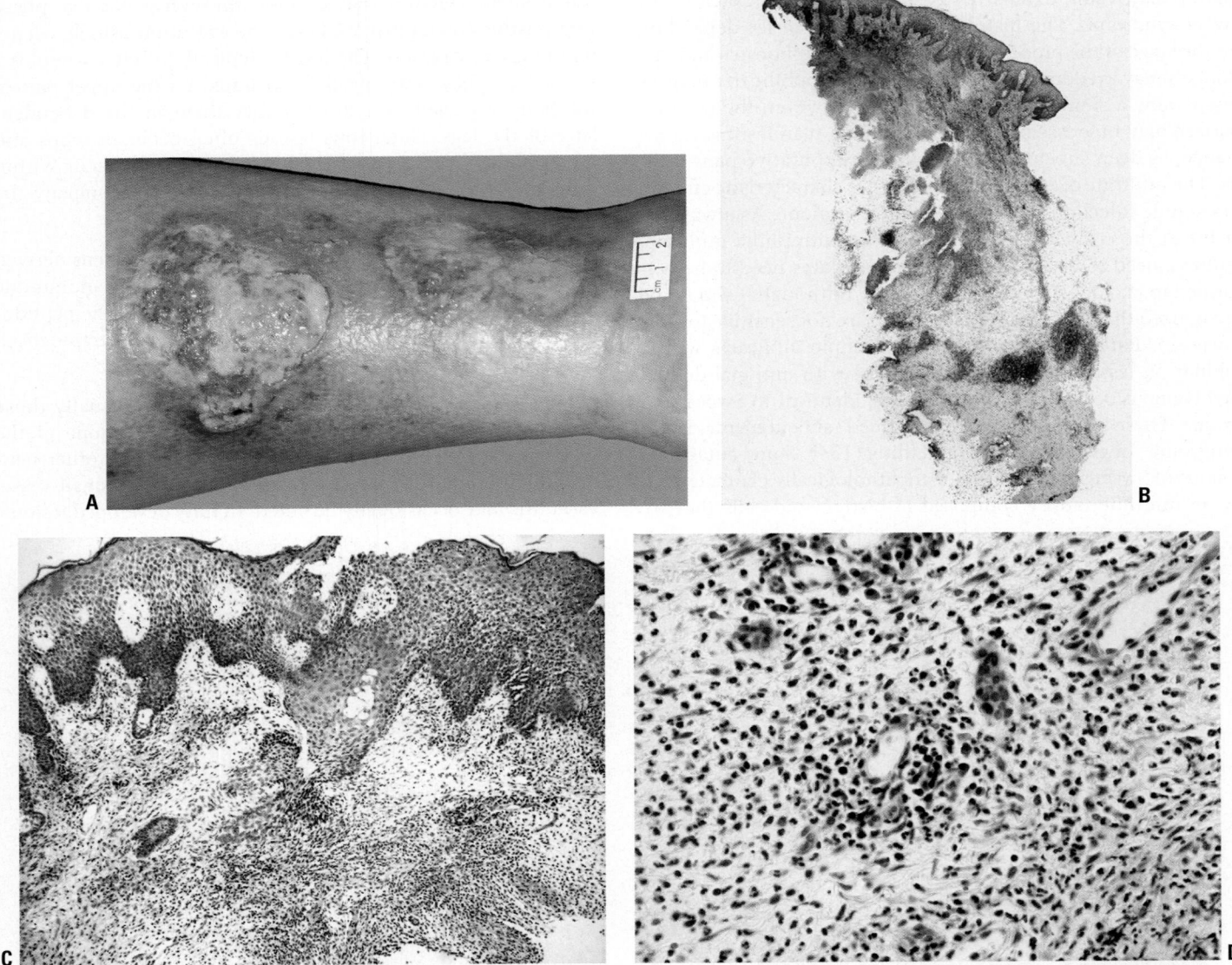

Figure 8-19 Pyoderma gangrenosum. **A:** Superficial ulcers with central suppurative exudate and a peripheral raised and slightly undermined border. (Courtesy of Adam Rubin, MD.) **B:** Punch biopsy from the edge of an ulcer shows a mixed inflammatory infiltrate spanning the dermis and the panniculus. The infiltrate is deeper and more extensive than that in classic Sweet syndrome. **C:** A mixed inflammatory infiltrate in the dermis with spongiosis of the epidermis at the edge of the ulcer. **D:** Neutrophils and lymphocytes surround a vessel, but there is no frank vasculitis.

(particularly in older patients), and less commonly in association with connective tissue disease (129). Drug-induced cases are rare but have been reported, including with levamisole-tainted cocaine.

Histopathology. The histologic findings are nonspecific, and the diagnosis is primarily clinical. Most authors studying early lesions have reported a primarily neutrophilic infiltrate, which frequently involves follicular structures (138). Others, however, have stated that the lesions begin with a lymphocytic reaction (139). The degree of vessel involvement ranges from none to fibrinoid necrosis. In the majority of biopsied lesions, a neutrophilic infiltrate is present with some, but limited, vascular damage. Outright vasculitis has been reported and has led to speculations about its possible role in the etiology of PG. Focal vasculitis is often observed in fully developed lesions but appears secondary to the inflammatory process. The infiltrate tends to be deeper and more extensive than that in classic Sweet syndrome. The pattern of pustular vasculitis may be present. Fully developed lesions exhibit ulceration, necrosis, and a mixed inflammatory cell infiltrate (Fig. 8-19). Involvement of the deep reticular dermis and subcutis may exhibit primarily mononuclear cell and granulomatous inflammatory reactions.

Principles of Management: Treatment is centered on: (1) stopping the inflammation, (2) healing the wound. Treatment of PG with systemic corticosteroids, cyclosporine, or infliximab is considered first-line. Multiple additional therapeutic agents have been reported to be beneficial, ranging from anti-inflammatory antibiotics to alternative immunosuppressive agents. Local treatment with intralesional corticosteroids, potent topical corticosteroids, topical dapsone, or topical tacrolimus can be used for localized lesions. Appropriate wound care is an essential component of therapy for all PG, including, in particular, removing any microbial superinfection or biofilm/colonization. Surgical debridement or trauma can worsen the condition ("pathergy") and is not recommended. An appropriate response to treatment may be regarded as part of the diagnostic criteria.

Behçet Disease

Clinical Summary. Behçet disease is a multisystem autoinflammatory disease characterized by oral aphthous lesions and at least two of the following criteria: genital aphthae, synovitis, posterior uveitis, cutaneous pustular vasculitis, and meningoencephalitis (127,140). This HLA-B51–associated disease is common in the Middle East and Japan but rare in northern Europe and the United States. This entity is positioned at the intersection of vasculitis and neutrophilic dermatoses. Behçet disease may be heterogeneous as separate phenotypic expressions have been shown to cluster in familial cases (141). These findings correlate with an extremely variable clinical presentation and a varying degree of vascular involvement, ranging from active inflammatory lesions to aneurysms, arterial or venous occlusions, or varices.

Pathogenesis. The etiology of Behçet disease is unknown, but an autoinflammatory pathogenesis is favored (128). The vascular injury is presumably immune-mediated because immune complex deposition has been demonstrated in vessel walls. Disorders of neutrophils and dysregulation of innate immunity are also discussed with regard to the etiology of this disease.

However, the occurrence of cutaneous vasculitis together with the vascular injury seen in other organ systems suggests that Behçet disease is best classified as a systemic vasculitis (142). The process of tissue breakdown in Behçet disease and also in PG (discussed previously) is known as pathergy and often appears to be a response to minor trauma. Induction of a pathergy reaction with a needle prick may be used as a diagnostic test for Behçet disease.

Histopathology. The histopathologic spectrum of mucocutaneous inflammatory vascular lesions includes, depending on the stage and activity of the lesion, neutrophilic, lymphocytic, and granulomatous vascular reactions. Biopsy specimens of early lesions typically show a neutrophilic vascular reaction. However, fully developed necrotizing LCV may develop. If the neutrophilic infiltrate is very dense, the pattern of pustular vasculitis may be found (see Fig. 8-9).

Principles of Management: Dapsone may be a particularly effective drug in some patients with Behçet disease. Many patients may require treatment with immunosuppressive agents such as corticosteroid therapy, azathioprine, and anti-TNF therapy. Additional therapies include colchicine, thalidomide, and other anti-inflammatory and immunosuppressive agents.

LYMPHOCYTIC SMALL-VESSEL VASCULITIS

A histologic diagnosis of a lymphocytic vasculitis may be made if there is sufficient evidence of vascular damage and the inflammatory infiltrate is predominantly lymphocytic (Fig. 8-20). Often, the vascular damage is subtle, and in many cases there may be disagreement among dermatopathologists on whether the term "vasculitis" is warranted (143). Clear-cut evidence of vasculitis is indisputable if dermal hemorrhage and an inflammatory infiltrate are present together with fibrinoid necrosis of the vascular wall or fibrin thrombi. However, these findings are rarely or only focally present in most conditions that have been said to manifest lymphocytic vasculitis.

The disease processes in which lymphocytic vasculitis is commonly observed are listed in Table 8-10. Lymphocytic vasculitis may also be seen in a stage of an otherwise leukocytoclastic or granulomatous vasculitis or in a process that at other times may even be noninflammatory and manifested perhaps as a vasculopathy (e.g., atrophie blanche).

COVID-19-Related Chilblains (Pernio)

The emergence of the SARS-Cov-2 and the COVID-19 pandemic has resulted in the appearance of many different cutaneous and systemic clinical–pathologic phenomena, most relating to various forms of vascular injury.

Clinical Summary. At the time of this writing, the American Academy of Dermatology's COVID-19 Registry contained 171 patients with laboratory-confirmed SARS-Cov-2 infection and cutaneous manifestations. Within this group, the second most common cutaneous manifestation (after morbilliform rash) was erythematous-violaceous purpuric macules on the fingers, toes, elbows, and lateral aspects of the feet without accompanying edema or pruritus (Fig. 8-21A) (144). These pernio-like lesions have been reported in a wide age range of patients and without

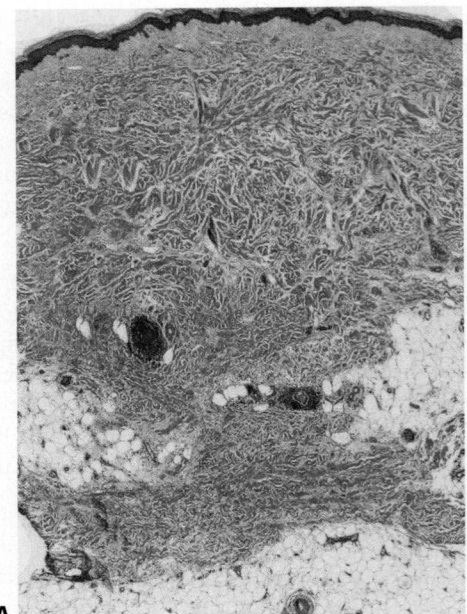
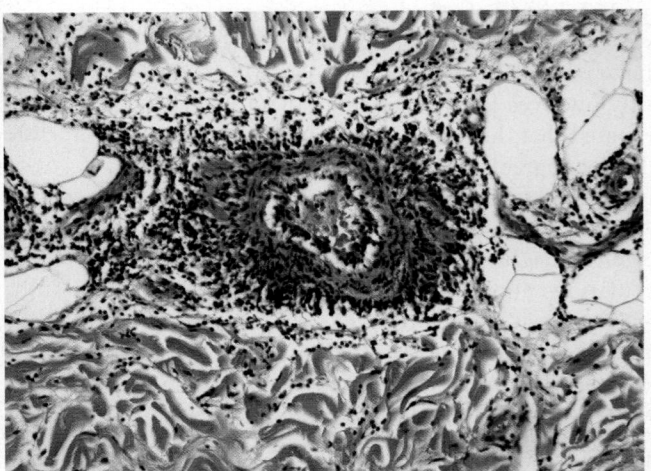

Figure 8-20 Lymphocytic vasculitis. **A:** A small vessel in the reticular dermis is surrounded by an inflammatory infiltrate. **B:** The infiltrate is composed of lymphocytes. There is damage to the vessel

Table 8-10
Differential Diagnosis of Lymphocytic Vasculitis and Lymphocytic Vascular Reactions

Arthropod bites

Drug-induced and other hypersensitivity reactions

Infection-associated reactions (e.g., viral)

Connective tissue diseases

Behçet disease

Purpuric dermatitides

PLEVA/PLC/LYP

Cutaneous lymphoma

Autoimmune diseases

Pernio

Polymorphous light eruption

Atrophie blanche

Infestations (e.g., scabies)

LYP, lymphomatoid papulosis; PLC, pityriasis lichenoides chronica; PLEVA, pityriasis lichenoides et varioliformis acuta.

cold or other systemic associations of conventional chilblains. Preliminary data indicate that a pernio-like cutaneous presentation may be associated with a mild course of disease, because 55% of patients in this group were otherwise asymptomatic (145). Controversy exists over whether the initial observation of pernio-like lesions at the start of the pandemic represented instead an epiphenomenon, with patients staying home, walking barefoot, and having expanded access to teledermatology. Pernio-like lesions have been reported following vaccination against SARS-CoV-2 as well.

Pathogenesis. The precise pathogenesis of these COVID-19 related lesions is unclear, although preliminary reports indicate shared histopathologic and direct immunofluorescence findings with idiopathic and secondary chilblains (146). A recent French study revealed a viral-induced type I interferonopathy, suggesting an innate immune response in these patients that may lead to rapid control of the virus, and a potential explanation for the mild course of infection frequently seen in these patients (147).

Histopathology. Most cases have demonstrated robust perivascular and perieccrine lymphocytic infiltrates accompanied by superficial dermal edema and increased dermal mucin. Vacuolar interface dermatitis with scattered dyskeratotic basilar keratinocytes is commonly present. Vascular changes include endothelialitis, microthromboses, and fibrin deposition (Fig. 8-21B,C) (146).

Principles of Management: No treatment recommendations have been established for COVID-19–related pernio; however, high potency topical corticosteroids may be helpful in symptomatic patients.

Lymphomatoid Vasculitis and Vascular Reactions

The terms "lymphomatoid vasculitis" and "lymphomatoid vascular reaction" may be used if there is a lymphocytic vasculitis or lymphocytic vascular reaction with significant cytologic atypia of the lymphoid cells (Table 8-11). Although lymphoid nuclear irregularities of some degree may be present in many lymphocytic vascular reactions, probably as a reflection of an activated state of the lymphocytes, lymphoid atypia tends to be particularly well developed in lymphomatoid papulosis and some viral processes. The differential diagnosis includes vascular damage in the context of cutaneous lymphoma, such as angiocentric T-cell lymphoma and other lymphomas (148).

Pigmented Purpuric Dermatitis

Historically, four variants of purpura pigmentosa chronica have been described: purpura annularis telangiectoides of Majocchi, progressive pigmentary dermatosis of Schamberg, pigmented purpuric dermatitis (PPD) of Gougerot and Blum, and eczematoid-like purpura of Doucas and Kapetanakis. These entities are all closely related and often cannot be reliably distinguished on clinical and

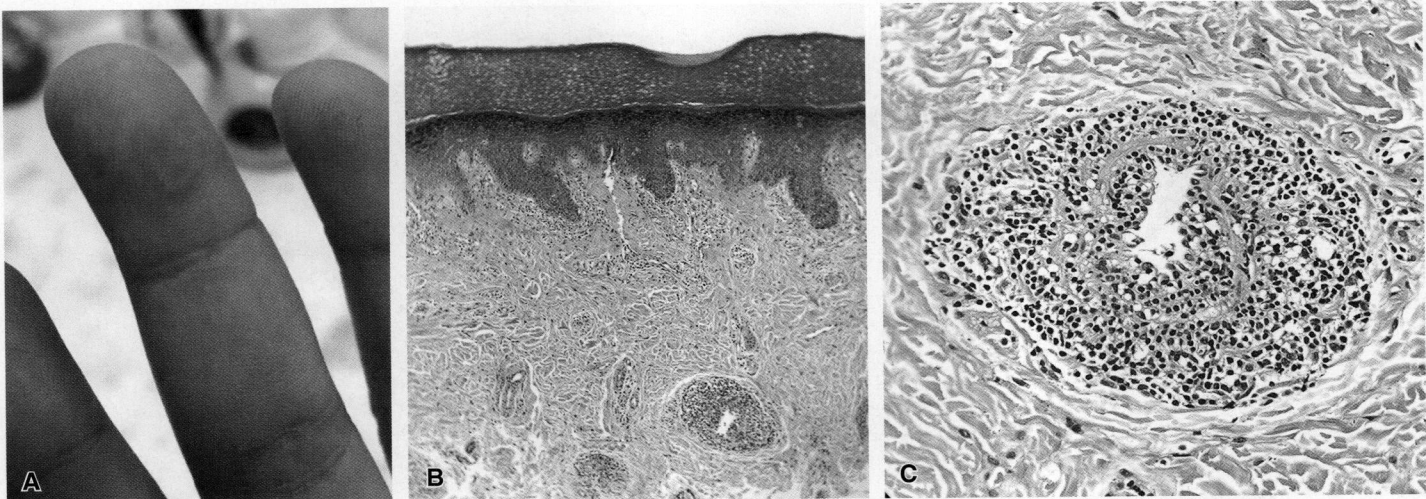

Figure 8-21 COVID-19–Related Chilblains. **A:** Painful erythematous to violaceous purpuric macules on the fingers. **B:** Vacuolar interface dermatitis involving volar skin with a superficial and deep perivascular and periadnexal lymphocytic infiltrate. **C:** The vessels are surrounded and permeated by lymphocytes (endothelialitis). (Courtesy of Patrick Emanuel, MD, Clinica Ricardo Palma, Lima, Peru; Adjunct Assistant Professor of Dermatology and Pathology, Icahn School of Medicine at Mount Sinai, New York, NY.)

Table 8-11

Differential Diagnosis of Lymphomatoid Vasculitis and Vascular Reaction

T-cell lymphoproliferative disorders

Peripheral T-cell lymphoma

Angiocentric T-cell lymphoma

Lymphomatoid papulosis

Lymphomatoid granulomatosis

Angioimmunoblastic lymphadenopathy

PPD-like eruptions

Lymphomatoid drug eruptions

Lymphomatoid contact dermatitis

Connective tissue disease

Viral processes

Florid hypersensitivity reactions

Arthropod bites

Scabies infestations

histologic grounds (149). In practice, subclassification may not be necessary. Lichen aureus is a closely related localized variant. The general terms "pigmented purpuric dermatitis," "chronic purpuric dermatitis," and "purpura pigmentosa chronica" appear suitable for this disease spectrum.

Clinical Summary. The primary lesion consists of discrete puncta. Gradually, telangiectatic puncta may appear as a result of capillary dilation, with pigmentation as a result of hemosiderin deposits. In some cases, telangiectasia (Majocchi disease) predominates; in others, pigmentation (Schamberg disease) predominates. In Majocchi disease, the lesions are usually irregular in shape and occur predominantly on the lower legs. In some cases, the findings may mimic those of stasis. Not infrequently, clinical signs of inflammation are present, such as erythema, papules, and scaling (Gougerot–Blum disease) or papules, scaling, and lichenification (eczematoid-like purpura). The disorder is often limited to the

lower extremities, but it may be extensive. Mild pruritus may be present. There are no systemic symptoms related to this disease process. A localized variant of PPD is lichen aureus, in which one or a few patches are present, most commonly on the legs (150). The patches are composed of closely set, flat papules of a rust, copper, or orange color. In some cases, petechiae are present within the patches. Lichen aureus shows a male predilection and a peak incidence in the fourth decade. The lesions of lichen aureus tend to persist. They typically occur on the lower legs but may affect many other sites (151).

Pathogenesis. The etiology of PPD is essentially unknown, and there are probably several factors involved. Some cases of chronic purpuric dermatitis may be related to a hypersensitivity reaction to drugs. However, in most cases, the etiology of this process is unclear. Stasis changes are seen in some individuals with PPD, suggesting that venous insufficiency may be a contributing factor (139). Eruptions with the clinical and histologic appearance of a PPD have also been associated with subsequent development of a T-cell lymphoproliferative disorder in some patients. Thus, it is possible that some PPD may be the initial manifestation of T-cell lymphoproliferative disease (152,153).

Histopathology. The basic process is a lymphocytic perivascular infiltrate limited to the papillary dermis (Fig. 8-22). Epidermal alterations may include slight acanthosis and basal layer vacuolopathy. There is also some variability in the pattern of the dermal infiltrate. In some instances, the infiltrate may assume a band-like or lichenoid pattern, particularly in the lichenoid variant of Gougerot–Blum disease and may involve the reticular dermis in a perivascular distribution. Evidence of vascular damage may be present, and the reaction pattern may then be termed lymphocytic vasculopathy, vasculitis, or capillaritis. However, the extent of vascular injury is usually mild and often insufficient to justify the term "vasculitis." Vascular damage commonly consists only of endothelial cell swelling and dermal hemorrhage. Extravasated red blood cells and subtle deposits of hemosiderin are usually found in the vicinity of the capillaries. Less commonly, however, fibrinoid material is deposited in vessel walls. In some instances, the infiltrate involves the epidermis and may be associated with mild spongiosis and patchy parakeratosis, particularly in some

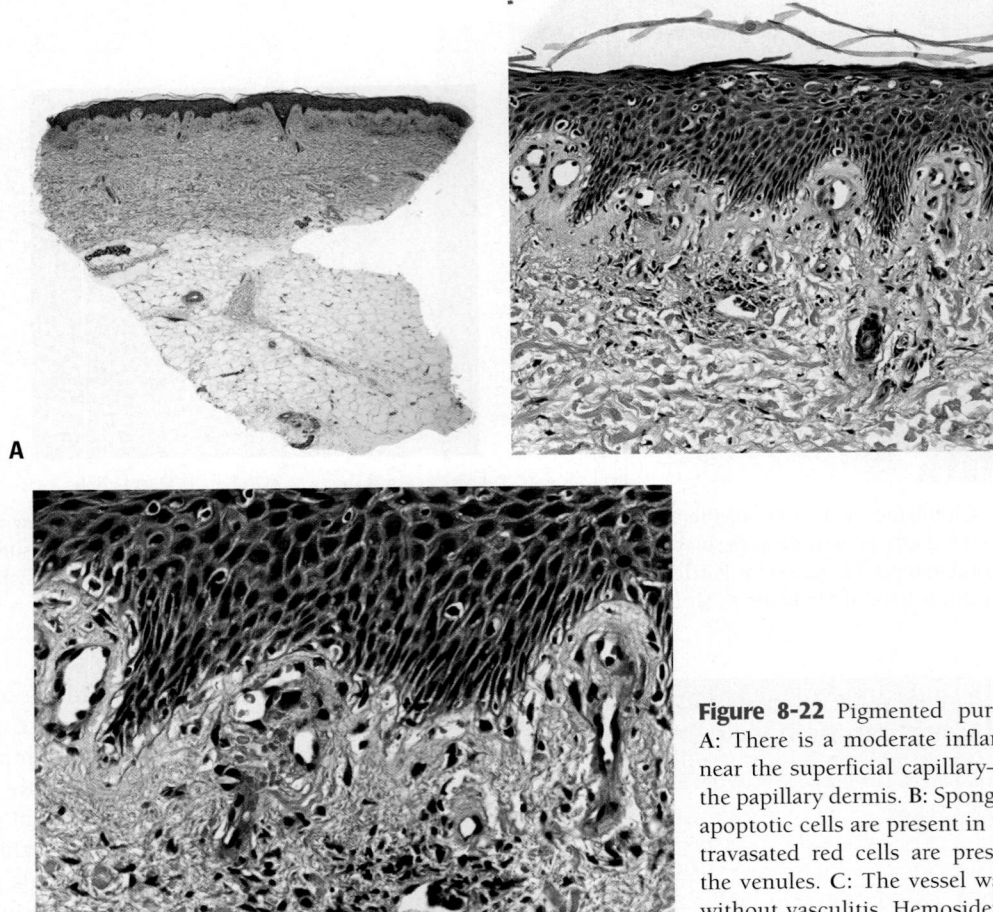

Figure 8-22 Pigmented purpuric dermatosis. **A:** There is a moderate inflammatory infiltrate near the superficial capillary–venular plexus in the papillary dermis. **B:** Spongiosis and scattered apoptotic cells are present in the epidermis. Extravasated red cells are present near some of the venules. **C:** The vessel walls are thickened, without vasculitis. Hemosiderin pigment is not prominent in this example.

cases of pigmented purpuric lichenoid dermatitis of Gougerot and Blum and eczematoid-like purpura of Doucas and Kapetanakis. The pattern of the infiltrate is often both perivascular and interstitial, infiltrating the papillary dermis between vessels. Rare, atypical histologic variants, such as granulomatous PPD, have also been reported.

In old lesions, the capillaries often show dilation of their lumen and proliferation of their endothelium. Extravasated red blood cells may no longer be present, but one frequently finds hemosiderin, albeit in varying amounts. The inflammatory infiltrate is less pronounced than in the early stage.

In lichen aureus, a dense lymphohistiocytic infiltrate is present in the superficial dermis, typically distributed in a bandlike fashion and often associated with an increase in dermal capillaries. Exocytosis of mononuclear cells into the epidermis may be seen. Scattered within the infiltrate are hemosiderin-laden macrophages (Fig. 8-23). The absence or near absence of Civatte bodies or basal layer vasculopathy facilitates the differential

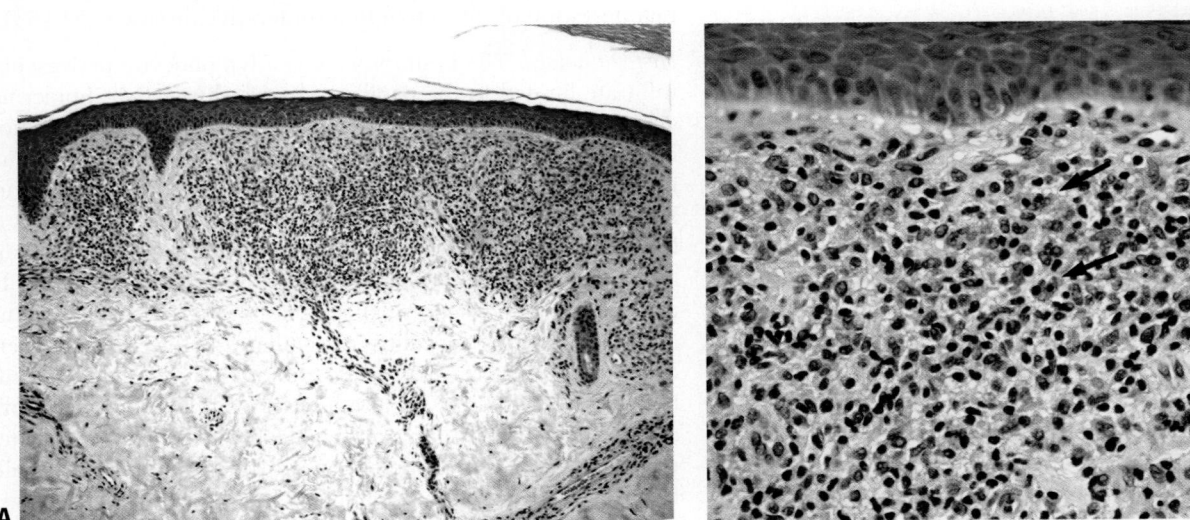

Figure 8-23 Lichen aureus. A dense lichenoid infiltrate in the papillary dermis (A), with hemosiderin-laden macrophages (B).

diagnosis from lichenoid dermatitides, such as lichen planus or lichen striatus.

Very rarely, pigmented purpura demonstrates a granulomatous dermatitis with extravasated erythrocytes, melanophages, and vascular proliferation (152).

Differential Diagnosis. PPD may resemble stasis dermatitis because inflammation, dilation of capillaries, extravasation of erythrocytes, and deposits of hemosiderin occur in both. However, in stasis dermatitis, the process extends much deeper into the dermis, and more pronounced epidermal changes and fibrosis of the dermis are usually present. Changes of intravascular red blood cell sludge and some fibrin deposits may also be seen in stasis, indicating a low flow state. As mentioned earlier, the histologic pattern of PPD may resemble or possibly be an abnormal T-cell process. Evidence of T-cell clonality may even be demonstrated in some examples of PPD that otherwise lack sufficient criteria for T-cell lymphoma. Careful evaluation of the lesion for epidermotropism and lymphoid atypia and (of particular importance) good clinicopathologic correlation are needed to arrive at the correct diagnosis. However, suspicious or equivocal lesions require monitoring and possibly further evaluation for possible progression to cutaneous T-cell lymphoma.

Principles of Management: Treatment is symptomatic, with topical steroids and antihistamines for pruritus. Avoidance of lower extremity edema, through use of compression, as well as light therapy may be beneficial in some circumstances. Vitamin C and rutoside have been described in isolated case reports as helpful to some patients.

VASCULOPATHIC REACTIONS AND PSEUDOVASCULITIS

Vasculopathic processes, as defined in Table 8-12, refer to the histologic finding of vascular damage in the absence of vasculitis. As already mentioned, the term pseudovasculitis has been used to describe a closely related group of conditions that mimic or exhibit some attributes of vasculitis. Vasculopathic reactions (and pseudovasculitis) may be associated with (a) coagulopathies, (b) pathologic alterations of the vessel wall, (c) embolic phenomena, (d) structural deficiencies of the perivascular connective tissue, or (e) miscellaneous other disease processes, including drug-induced vasospasm and repetitive vascular injury.

Coagulopathies and Vascular Thrombosis

Any coagulopathy may be accompanied by vasculopathic changes. The extent of vascular damage is variable. Vascular damage may occur in the setting of altered platelet counts, such as in idiopathic thrombocytopenic purpura, in coagulation factor deficiencies (e.g., inherited or acquired protein C and S deficiencies), in coagulopathies associated with connective tissue disease (e.g., lupus anticoagulant, antiphospholipid antibody syndrome; Fig. 8-24), and platelet thrombosis in heparin-induced skin necrosis. Extensive vascular damage with luminal occlusion by thrombotic material may develop in coumarin/warfarin-induced skin necrosis, in thrombotic thrombocytopenic purpura, and in disseminated intravascular coagulation—specifically in the setting of purpura fulminans (154).

Table 8-12

Vasculopathic Reactions and Pseudovasculitis

Mechanism	Condition
Coagulopathies	Idiopathic thrombocytopenic purpura
	Coagulation factor deficiencies (e.g., proteins C and S deficiencies)
	Antiphospholipid antibody syndrome
	Thrombotic thrombocytopenic purpura
	Coumadin/warfarin-induced skin necrosis
	Heparin-induced skin necrosis
	Calciphylaxis
	Purpura fulminans
	Disseminated intravascular coagulation
	Monoclonal gammopathy
	Sickle cell disease
	Livedo vasculopathy
Pathologic alterations of the vessel wall	Calciphylaxis
	Primary hyperoxaluria
	Diabetes mellitus
	Amyloidosis
	Porphyria
	Radiation vasculopathy
Embolic phenomena	Cholesterol embolism
	Atrial myxoma
Structural deficiencies of the perivascular connective tissue	Solar/senile purpura
	Scurvy
Vasospasm	Ergot derivatives
	Cocaine
	Methamphetamines
Repetitive vascular trauma	Hypothenar hammer syndrome

Clinical Summary. In mild forms, the clinical manifestations may be subtle and limited to petechiae. In severe forms of coagulopathies, large areas of ecchymosis may be present, typically located on the extremities. Large hemorrhagic bullae may overlie the ecchymoses, and some of the ecchymotic areas may undergo necrosis. Retiform purpura (a livedoid pattern of cutaneous hemorrhage) in palpable plaques is characteristic of antiphospholipid antibody syndrome, heparin-induced skin necrosis, Coumadin/warfarin-induced skin necrosis, and calciphylaxis (155).

Histopathology. The histologic features are nonspecific for any particular disorder. In mild forms of coagulopathies, the only histologic manifestation may be dermal hemorrhage, that is,

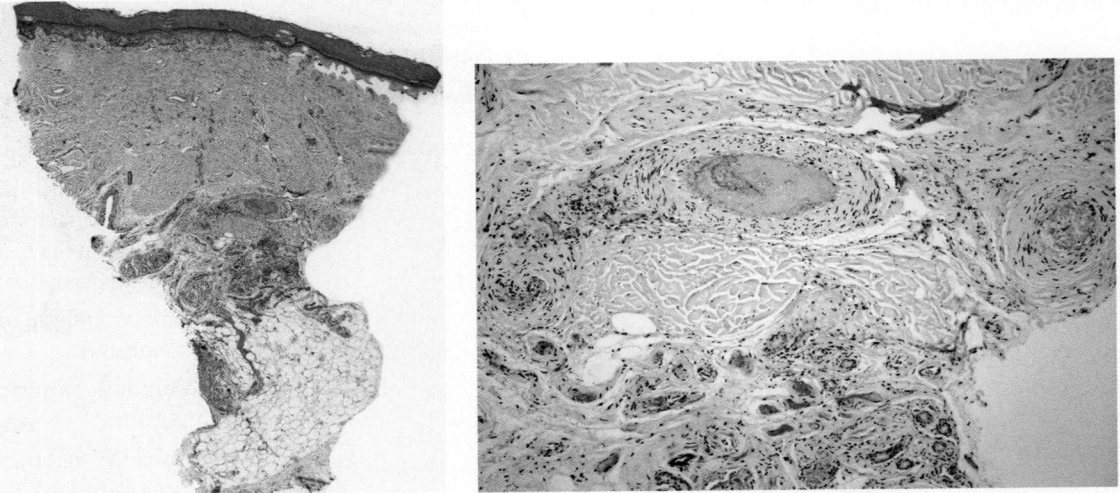

Figure 8-24 Antiphospholipid syndrome. **A:** A vessel in the deep dermis contains an eosinophilic fibrin thrombus. The affected vessels are commonly more superficial in this condition. **B:** The thrombus is not associated with inflammation of the vessel wall. Other small vessels in the vicinity are also affected. (*arrows*), accounting for the golden clinical color of these lesions.

extravasation of red blood cells into perivascular connective tissue. With increasing severity of the disease process, intravascular fibrin thrombi may be found (Fig. 8-2). In severe forms (e.g., thrombotic thrombocytopenic purpura, coumarin necrosis, and purpura fulminans), thrombotic vascular occlusion may lead to hemorrhagic infarcts, epidermal and dermal necrosis, or subepidermal bulla formation. In severe systemic intravascular coagulation, internal organs may also show widespread thrombosis of small vessels and hemorrhagic necrosis.

Calciphylaxis

Calciphylaxis or calcific uremic arteriolopathy is a multifactorial cutaneous vascular disease characterized by chronic nonhealing painful ulcers, most commonly associated with chronic renal failure, dialysis, and usually in combination with secondary or tertiary hyperparathyroidism. Obesity, female gender, and poor nutritional status are putative risk factors (156). Nonuremic calciphylaxis has been reported as well, with risk factors including some of the foregoing, but notably also use of corticosteroids or warfarin as potential triggers (157).

Clinical Summary. Painful violaceous lesions that may be indurated often develop in areas of livedo reticularis on the trunk and extremities and can rapidly progress to form bullae, ulcers, eschars, and gangrene. The prognosis is extremely poor, especially for proximal disease, even with aggressive treatment by parathyroidectomy (156). Fulminant sepsis may develop from infection of necrotic or gangrenous tissue.

Pathogenesis. The relationships among the calcification, thrombosis, and ischemic necrosis in calciphylaxis are poorly understood. Although vascular calcification is common in uremic patients, calciphylaxis is rare. Elevation of the calcium and phosphorous product along with a poorly defined precipitating or challenging event or agent is hypothesized to be necessary for calcium deposition in cutaneous tissues. The combination of uremia and decreased local vascular calcification inhibitory proteins initiate the differentiation of vascular smooth muscle cells into osteoblast-like and chondroblast-like phenotypes (156). Chronic inflammatory states, such as chronic renal failure, are associated with increased

activity of NF-kB (nuclear factor-kappa B), RANK (receptor activator of nuclear factor-kappa B)) and RANKL (receptor activator of nuclear factor-kappa B ligand), resulting in increased activity of transcription factors, such as bone morphogenic protein-4 (BMP-4), and osteogenic differentiation. The list of putative sensitizing agents is long, and the calcium and phosphorus product may be within normal limits. The development of a hypercoagulable state may be an additional important element in the pathogenesis of this entity but is not present in all cases (158,159). Finally, calciphylaxis may mimic vasculitis clinically (160).

Histopathology. The principal histologic findings include (a) calcification of soft tissue and small vessels (von Kossa and Alizarin red stains might increase the detection of calcium deposits), (b) nonspecific fibrous intimal proliferation of small vessels, often resulting in luminal narrowing, (c) variable fibrin thrombi, and (d) frequent ischemic necrosis of skin and subcutis (Fig. 8-25). Small-vessel microthrombi are

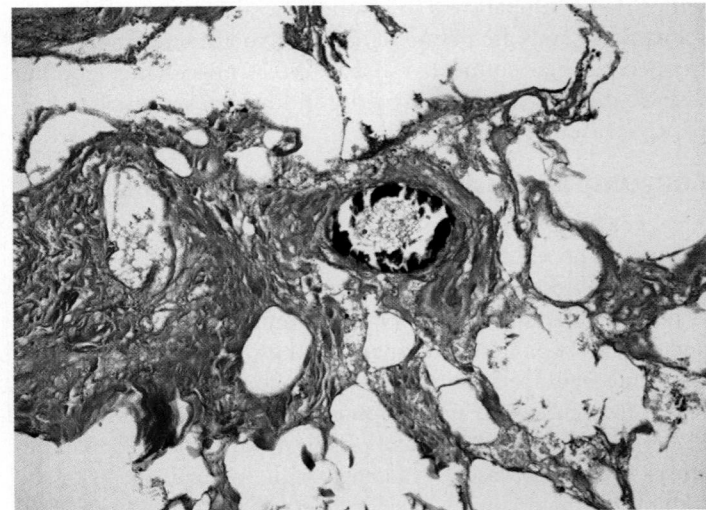

Figure 8-25 Calciphylaxis. There is calcification of the media of a small vessel in the panniculus, with delicate fibroplasia of the intima. There may be interstitial deposition of calcium as well.

commonly present, and also changes of small-vessel vasculitis. Occasionally, perieccrine calcium deposition, highly specific to calciphylaxis, is the only form of calcium deposition in the specimen (161). The small vessels involved by this process cannot be identified as either arterial or venous. Foreign-body giant-cell reaction to calcium and mixed inflammatory cell infiltrates that are neutrophil rich may be seen.

Cutaneous calcium deposits may be seen in many other conditions, especially cutaneous calcinosis and metastatic calcifications. Calcinosis usually lacks prominent vascular involvement. Other crystal-induced inflammatory diseases such as gout, pseudogout, or oxalosis that are associated with a giant-cell reaction to crystal deposits and surrounding fibrosis may resemble calciphylaxis. Histopathologically, pancreatic panniculitis may suggest calciphylaxis. However, the polymorphous infiltrate and ghostlike cells seen in panniculitis are absent in calciphylaxis (161). If a biopsy of calciphylaxis lacks significant calcium deposits owing to sampling error, the findings may be considered limited to ischemic damage or mimic a coagulopathy.

Principles of Management: Once calcium is deposited, lesions of calciphylaxis may persist. It is important to prevent further deposition of calcium by adequately controlling serum calcium and phosphate balance with phosphate binding agents, dialysis, or possible chemical parathyroid hormone control or parathyroidectomy. Sodium thiosulfate may liberate vascular and tissue calcium and may be beneficial. Some authors have described the use of thrombolytic agents, which carry a significant risk of bleeding. Hyperbaric oxygen, surgical debridement, and adjustments to systemic medications that can contribute to disease pathogenesis should be considered. More recently, some have focused on vitamin K as a potential factor in calciphylaxis, and many experts advocate for avoidance of warfarin in patients. Pentoxifylline has been used in some cases, along with bisphosphonates, although their use should be carefully monitored in renal disease. Appropriate wound care is essential, and patients should be monitored for signs of infection. Avoidance of additional trauma to the skin is also important (162).

Pathologic Alterations of the Vessel Wall, Including Metabolic Vasculopathies

Vasculopathies may also arise from metabolic disorders. Deposition of endogenously produced material, as in diabetes mellitus, amyloidosis, or porphyria, may lead to vessel fragility. Hemorrhage and ischemic damage to the area of skin supplied by the affected vessels is seen. The basic histologic vascular alteration in the aforementioned disorders is the deposition of amorphous material in the walls of dermal capillaries. The details of the histopathology of these disorders are discussed in more detail elsewhere.

Atherosclerosis is by far the most common form of vasculopathy. However, atherosclerosis is primarily a disease of large vessels supplying visceral organs and is thus not discussed here in detail. Cutaneous changes are usually secondary manifestations of peripheral ischemia. Luminal occlusion may result from intimal thickening and lipid deposition, superimposed thrombosis, or, less frequently, cholesterol emboli. Because cholesterol microemboli can cause cutaneous findings mimicking

vasculitis, this phenomenon is discussed in more detail in the next subsection.

Embolic Phenomena

Microemboli may be involved in the pathogenesis of septic vasculitis and related findings associated with endocarditis, as discussed previously. Embolization of cholesterol fragments from severely atherosclerotic large vessels to the distal extremity is another important example.

Cutaneous Cholesterol Embolism

Clinical Summary. Cutaneous manifestations are common, often affect the lower extremities, and include livedo reticularis, "blue toe syndrome," purple discoloration, gangrene of toes, and small, painful ulcerations on the legs. Occasionally, a few nodules or indurated plaques may occur. A typical clinical sign is adequate distal pulsation, indicating that the ischemia is arteriolar rather than arterial.

Pathogenesis. Cholesterol crystal embolization is usually a disease of the elderly with significant atherosclerosis (163,164). Atheromatous plaque material may erupt or detach spontaneously. However, more commonly, plaque material is dislodged by an invasive procedure, such as arterial catheterization. Microemboli or cholesterol crystals typically lead to ischemic changes.

Histopathology. Cholesterol emboli may be found as needle-shaped clefts within the lumina of small vessels. The intravascular clefts, which are in effect dissolved cholesterol crystals, may be single or multiple and are commonly associated with amorphous eosinophilic material, macrophages, or foreign-body giant-cell reactions. Vascular walls exhibit intimal fibrosis and often obliteration of lumina in older lesions. In many instances, only fibrin thrombi are observed. Often, a deep biopsy and multiple sections of biopsy material are needed to reveal such emboli, which are distributed focally and are therefore difficult to find. Viewing the cholesterol deposits themselves is nearly impossible with standard specimen processing; some have described delivering frozen tissue to preserve the cholesterol crystals, which, if present, are birefringent on polarized microscopy.

Principles of Management: The phenomenon cannot be reversed. Treatment should focus on addressing the symptoms and complications. Supportive care is essential. Although medical therapy is limited with no controlled trials, statins may improve the condition and have been reported to decrease the need for dialysis in those with kidney failure secondary to cholesterol emboli.

Vasculopathy Resulting from Deficiencies in Connective Tissue

Structural deficiencies in the perivascular connective tissue may cause vascular fragility and lead to dermal hemorrhage. Such alterations underlie the hemorrhages that accompany senile purpura and scurvy.

Histopathology. In senile purpura, extravasation of red blood cells is encountered in atrophic skin with solar elastosis and normal-appearing capillaries. In scurvy, dermal hemorrhage is found predominantly in the vicinity of hair follicles without evidence of capillary changes. Hemosiderin-laden macrophages are usually noted (165). Other findings associated with scurvy include intrafollicular keratotic plugs and coiled hair.

Other Clinical Presentations Associated with Vasculopathic Reactions

Livedo Reticularis

Clinical Summary. Livedo reticularis is persistent red-blue mottling of the skin in a netlike pattern and differs from cutis marmorata, which does not subside with warming of the skin.

Pathogenesis. This condition is a nonspecific sign of sluggish blood flow from any cause. Associations include vasculitis or vasculopathy in the context of several different systemic or localized disease processes, such as infection, atrophie blanche, cholesterol emboli, and connective tissue disease (166). Underlying coagulopathy might be a consideration, and cases of livedo reticularis associated with factor V Leiden heterozygous mutation, antithrombin III mutation, and other inherited forms of hypercoagulability have been reported (166). Frequently, however, the condition is idiopathic and limited to the lower extremities. Generalized livedo reticularis has also been described as part of a potentially severe arterio-occlusive syndrome (Sneddon syndrome) that is often complicated by cerebrovascular disease and seizures (167). Antiphospholipid antibody syndrome may present initially with isolated livedo reticularis.

Histopathology. A biopsy specimen taken from an erythematous area may be normal, whereas a biopsy specimen from a white area may show a vessel with a thickened wall and the lumen occluded by a thrombus. In other cases, deeply situated dermal arterioles have shown obliterative changes. Intravascular aggregates of red blood cells, suggesting a low flow state, may be seen.

Principles of Management: Treating the underlying condition in secondary livedo may help resolve the condition. Otherwise, keeping the affected area warm should diminish the appearance of the livedo.

Atrophie Blanche

Atrophie blanche is a common condition that usually affects middle-aged or elderly women (168). Synonymous terms are *livedoid vasculitis, livedo reticularis with seasonal ulceration*, and *segmental hyalinizing vasculitis.*

Clinical Summary. Typically located on the lower portions of the legs, particularly on the ankles and the dorsa of the feet, this condition begins as purpuric macules and papules, which develop into small, painful ulcers with a tendency to recur. Healing of the ulcers results in the white atrophic areas that have given the disease its name. A fully developed case of atrophie blanche shows irregularly outlined, whitish atrophic areas with peripheral hyperpigmentation and telangiectasia. Many of the patients have associated livedo reticularis. The condition may also be seasonal, the disease activity being greatest in the summer and winter months.

Pathogenesis. The etiology of atrophie blanche is unknown. Immune complex deposits that have been observed in late lesions are likely secondary changes (169). A primary disturbance of fibrinolysis in the endothelium of affected microvessels has been postulated (170).

Histopathology. The histologic findings are nonspecific and vary with the stage of the lesion. However, in all stages, vascular changes are present. In early lesions, fibrinoid material may be noted in the vessel wall or vessel lumen (Fig. 8-26). Infarction with hemorrhage and an inflammatory infiltrate may be present as well. In late atrophic lesions, the epithelium is thinned, and the dermis is sclerotic, with little, if any, cellular infiltrate. The walls of the dermal vessels may show thickening and hyalinization of the intima. Luminal occlusion by intimal proliferation and/or fibrinoid material is seen. Recanalized thrombotic vessels may be a feature. In some cases, the vessels in the superficial dermis are predominantly affected; in others, the vessels in the middle and even deep dermis are mostly affected. Among 29 consecutive patients with atrophie blanche, 6 manifested a necrotizing medium-sized arteritis consistent with PAN (53).

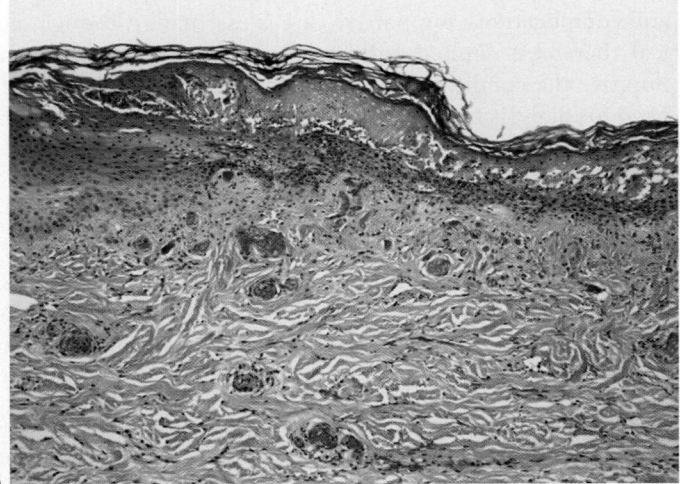
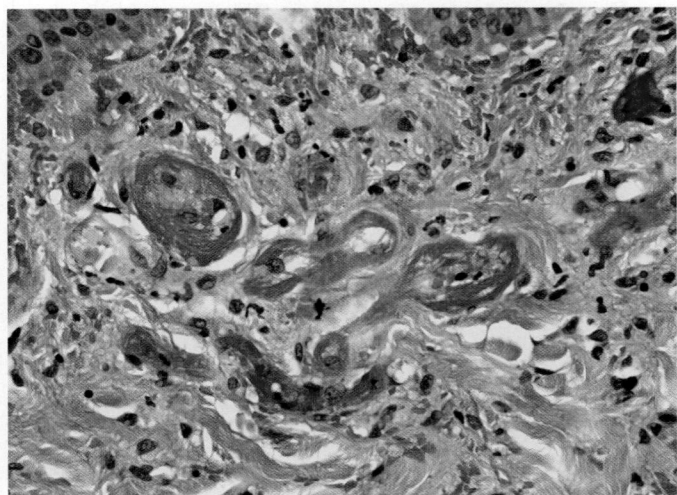

Figure 8-26 Atrophie blanche. **A:** An early lesion characterized by an area of epidermal necrosis with underlying vasculopathy. **B:** The superficial portion of the epidermis is necrotic. Vessel walls are thickened and contain fibrinoid/thrombotic material.

Principles of Management: There has not been any consistent treatment for this condition, although corticosteroids and anticoagulation medications have been tried.

Degos Syndrome

Degos had initially described a cutaneointestinal syndrome in which distinct skin findings ("drops of porcelain") were associated with recurrent attacks of abdominal pain that often ended in death from intestinal perforations (171).

Clinical Summary. The skin lesions of this syndrome arise in crops of asymptomatic, slightly raised, yellowish red papules that gradually develop an atrophic porcelain-white center. These papules tend to affect the trunk and proximal extremities. Degos chose the name *malignant atrophic papulosis* (MAP) for these lesions to emphasize the serious clinical course of the cutaneointestinal disease he was describing. At that time, the cutaneous lesions were then thought to be specific and pathognomonic for this unique disease entity (Degos disease). However, skin-limited forms of Degos disease have been described (172,173), and currently such skin lesions are considered to be a clinicopathologic reaction pattern that can be associated with a number of conditions (174). Lesions similar, if not identical, to MAP have been noted in connective tissue diseases such as lupus erythematosus, dermatomyositis, and progressive systemic sclerosis, in atrophie blanche, and in Creutzfeldt–Jakob disease (175,176).

Pathogenesis. The etiology of Degos syndrome is unclear. The findings have been ascribed to a coagulopathy, vasculitis, or mucinosis (174). Emerging evidence of a type I interferon signature (endothelial and inflammatory cells expression of myxovirus resistance protein A (MXA) and endothelial tubuloreticular inclusions on electron microscopy) combined with C5b-9 deposition in microvessels has been reported (177).

Histopathology. The classic lesion shows a wedge-shaped area of altered dermis covered by atrophic epidermis with slight hyperkeratosis. Dermal alterations may include frank necrosis. More common, however, are edema, extensive mucin deposition, and slight sclerosis (Fig. 8-27). A sparse perivascular lymphocytic infiltrate may be seen, although the dermis is largely acellular. Typically, vascular damage is noted in the vessels at the base of the "cone of necrobiosis." Vascular alterations may be subtle and manifest as endothelial swelling or demonstrate lymphocytic vasculitis. However, more characteristically, intravascular fibrin thrombi may be noted, suggesting that the dermal and epidermal changes result from ischemia. Altered vessels may lack an inflammatory infiltrate (177). The histopathology observed may vary with the evolution of the lesions. Early lesions may be more mucinous and mimic tumid lupus. Significant clinical overlap with lupus has also been reported (178) and may lead to diagnostic confusion. More evolved lesions are sclerotic and could suggest lichen sclerosus et atrophicus (172).

Principles of Management: Options are limited and consist of anticoagulants, antiplatelet drugs, and immunosuppressants (179). The use of eculizumab in preventing C5b-9 activation in a small series of patients was shown to be useful as salvage therapy for critically ill patients with thrombotic microangiopathy (180).

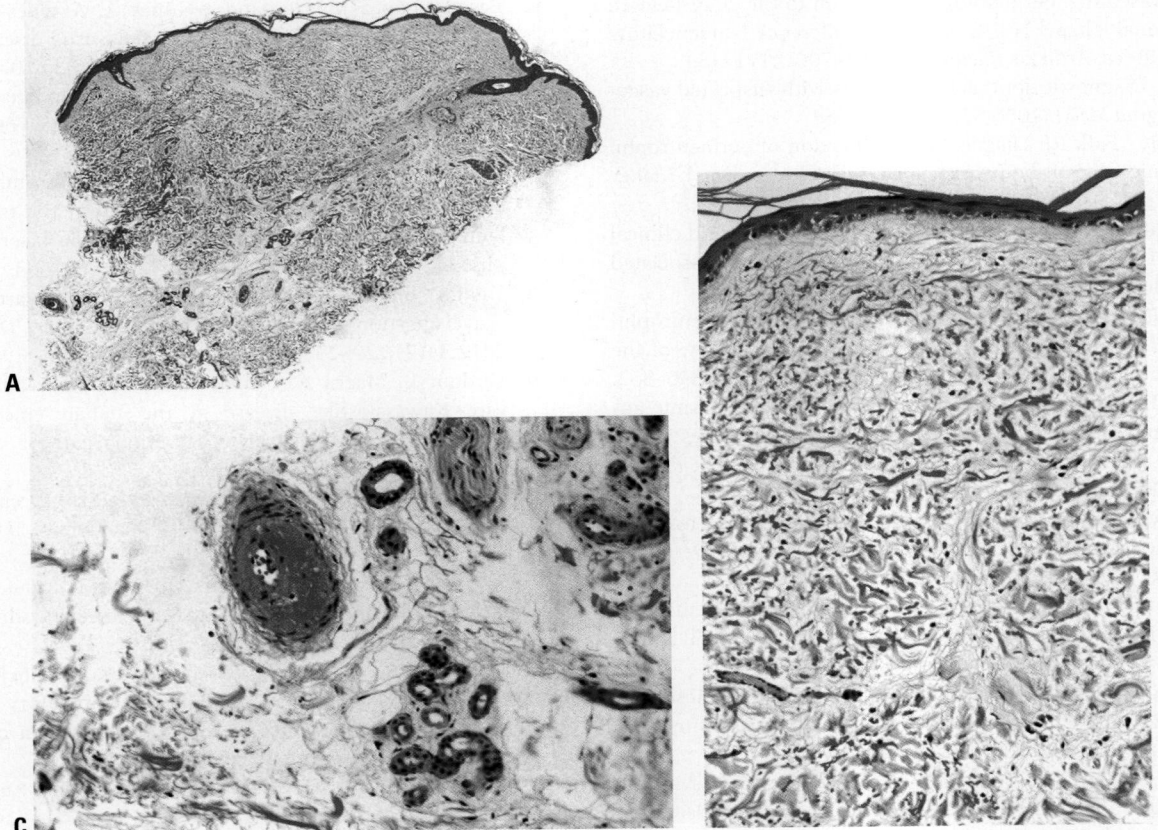

Figure 8-27 Degos lesion. Atrophic epidermis overlies a wedge-shaped area of dermis (A) with mucin deposition (B) and a thrombosed vessel at the base (C). This Degos lesion was observed in a patient with dermatomyositis.

REFERENCES

1. Callen JP. Cutaneous vasculitis and its relationship to systemic disease. *Dis Mon.* 1981;28(1):1–48.
2. Fauci AS, Haynes B, Katz P. The spectrum of vasculitis: clinical, pathologic, immunologic and therapeutic considerations. *Ann Intern Med.* 1978;89(5, pt 1):660–676.
3. Jennette JC, Falk RJ, Andrassy K, et al. Nomenclature of systemic vasculitides. Proposal of an international consensus conference. *Arthritis Rheum.* 1994;37(2):187–192.
4. Jennette JC, Falk RJ, Bacon PA, et al. 2012 revised International Chapel Hill Consensus Conference Nomenclature of Vasculitides. *Arthritis Rheum.* 2013;65(1):1–11.
5. Carlson JA, Chen KR. Cutaneous vasculitis update: small vessel neutrophilic vasculitis syndromes. *Am J Dermatopathol.* 2006;28(6):486–506.
6. Carlson JA, Chen KR. Cutaneous vasculitis update: neutrophilic muscular vessel and eosinophilic, granulomatous, and lymphocytic vasculitis syndromes. *Am J Dermatopathol.* 2007;29(1):32–43.
7. Carlson JA, Ng BT, Chen KR. Cutaneous vasculitis update: diagnostic criteria, classification, epidemiology, etiology, pathogenesis, evaluation and prognosis. *Am J Dermatopathol.* 2005;27(6):504–528.
8. Gonzalez-Gay MA, Garcia-Porrua C, Pujol RM. Clinical approach to cutaneous vasculitis. *Curr Opin Rheumatol.* 2005;17(1):56–61.
9. Hayat S, Berney SM. Cutaneous vasculitis. *Curr Rheumatol Rep.* 2005;7(4):276–280.
10. Russell JP, Gibson LE. Primary cutaneous small vessel vasculitis: approach to diagnosis and treatment. *Int J Dermatol.* 2006;45(1):3–13.
11. Sunderkötter C, Sindrilaru A. Clinical classification of vasculitis. *Eur J Dermatol.* 2006;16(2):114–124.
12. Sunderkötter CH, Zelger B, Chen KR, et al. Nomenclature of cutaneous vasculitis: dermatologic addendum to the 2012 Revised International Chapel Hill Consensus Conference Nomenclature of Vasculitides. *Arthritis Rheumatol.* 2018;70(2):171–184.
13. Suresh E. Diagnostic approach to patients with suspected vasculitis. *Postgrad Med J.* 2006;82(970):483–488.
14. Jennette JC, Falk RJ. Diagnostic classification of antineutrophil cytoplasmic autoantibody-associated vasculitides. *Am J Kidney Dis.* 1991;18(2):184–187.
15. Lamprecht P, Kerstein A, Klapa S, et al. Pathogenetic and clinical aspects of anti-neutrophil cytoplasmic autoantibody-associated vasculitides. *Front Immunol.* 2018;9:680.
16. Savige J, Davies D, Falk RJ, Jennette JC, Wiik A. Antineutrophil cytoplasmic antibodies and associated diseases: a review of the clinical and laboratory features. *Kidney Int.* 2000;57(3):846–862.
17. Sinclair D, Stevens JM. Role of antineutrophil cytoplasmic antibodies and glomerular basement membrane antibodies in the diagnosis and monitoring of systemic vasculitides. *Ann Clin Biochem.* 2007;44(pt 5):432–442.
18. Sais G, Vidaller A. Role of direct immunofluorescence test in cutaneous leukocytoclastic vasculitis. *Int J Dermatol.* 2005;44(11):970–971; author reply 971.
19. Brinkmann V, Reichard U, Goosmann C, et al. Neutrophil extracellular traps kill bacteria. *Science.* 2004;303(5663):1532–1535.
20. Nakazawa D, Masuda S, Tomaru U, Ishizu A. Pathogenesis and therapeutic interventions for ANCA-associated vasculitis. *Nat Rev Rheumatol.* 2019;15(2):91–101.
21. Baum EW, Sams WM Jr, Payne RR. Giant cell arteritis: a systemic disease with rare cutaneous manifestations. *J Am Acad Dermatol.* 1982;6(6):1081–1088.
22. de Souza AW, de Carvalho JF. Diagnostic and classification criteria of Takayasu arteritis. *J Autoimmun.* 2014;48-49:79–83.
23. Whittaker E, Bamford A, Kenny J, et al. Clinical characteristics of 58 children with a pediatric inflammatory multisystem syndrome temporally associated with SARS-CoV-2. *JAMA.* 2020;324(3):259–269.
24. Berardicurti O, Conforti A, Ruscitti P, Cipriani P, Giacomelli R. The wide spectrum of Kawasaki-like disease associated with SARS-CoV-2 infection. *Expert Rev Clin Immunol.* 2020;16(12):1205–1215.
25. Landing BH, Larson EJ. Pathological features of Kawasaki disease (mucocutaneous lymph node syndrome). *Am J Cardiovasc Pathol.* 1987;1(2):218–229.
26. Ciofalo A, Gulotta G, Iannella G, et al. Giant cell arteritis (GCA): pathogenesis, clinical aspects and treatment approaches. *Curr Rheumatol Rev.* 2019;15(4):259–268.
27. Wang X, Hu ZP, Lu W, et al. Giant cell arteritis. *Rheumatol Int.* 2008;29(1):1–7.
28. Serling-Boyd N, Stone JH. Recent advances in the diagnosis and management of giant cell arteritis. *Curr Opin Rheumatol.* 2020;32(3):201–207.
29. Salehi Abari I. 2016 ACR revised criteria for early diagnosis of giant cell (temporal) arteritis. *Autoimmune Dis Ther Approaches Open Access.* 2016;3:119–122.
30. Strady C, Arav E, Strady A, et al. Diagnostic value of clinical signs in giant cell arteritis: analysis of 415 temporal artery biopsy findings [in French]. *Ann Med Interne (Paris).* 2002;153(1):3–12.
31. Font RL, Prabhakaran VC. Histological parameters helpful in recognising steroid-treated temporal arteritis: an analysis of 35 cases. *Br J Ophthalmol.* 2007;91(2):204–209.
32. Stone JH, Tuckwell K, Dimonaco S, et al., Trial of tocilizumab in giant-cell arteritis. *N Engl J Med.* 2017;377(4):317–328.
33. Dourmishev AL, Serafimova DK, Vassileva SG, Dourmishev LA, Schwartz RA. Segmental ulcerative vasculitis: a cutaneous manifestation of Takayasu's arteritis. *Int Wound J.* 2005;2(4):340–345.
34. Maffei S, Di Renzo M, Bova G, Auteri A, Pasqui AL. Takayasu's arteritis: a review of the literature. *Intern Emerg Med.* 2006;1(2):105–112.
35. Pascual-López M, Hernández-Núñez A, Aragüés-Montañés M, Daudén E, Fraga J, García-Díez A. Takayasu's disease with cutaneous involvement. *Dermatology.* 2004;208(1):10–15.
36. Hellmich B, Agueda A, Monti S, et al. 2018 Update of the EULAR recommendations for the management of large vessel vasculitis. *Ann Rheum Dis.* 2020;79(1):19–30.
37. Chen KR. The misdiagnosis of superficial thrombophlebitis as cutaneous polyarteritis nodosa: features of the internal elastic lamina and the compact concentric muscular layer as diagnostic pitfalls. *Am J Dermatopathol.* 2010;32(7):688–693.
38. Yus ES, Simón RS, Requena L. Vein, artery, or arteriole? A decisive question in hypodermal pathology. *Am J Dermatopathol.* 2012;34(2):229–232.
39. Verdoni L, Mazza A, Gervasoni A, et al. An outbreak of severe Kawasaki-like disease at the Italian epicentre of the SARS-CoV-2 epidemic: an observational cohort study. *Lancet.* 2020;395(10239):1771–1778.
40. Viner RM, Whittaker E. Kawasaki-like disease: emerging complication during the COVID-19 pandemic. *Lancet.* 2020;395(10239):1741–1743.
41. Stankovic K, Miailhes P, Bessis D, Ferry T, Broussolle C, Sève P. Kawasaki-like syndromes in HIV-infected adults. *J Infect.* 2007;55(6):488–494.
42. Koné-Paut I, Cimaz R. Is it Kawasaki shock syndrome, Kawasaki-like disease or pediatric inflammatory multisystem disease? The importance of semantic in the era of COVID-19 pandemic. *RMD Open.* 2020;6(2):e001333.
43. Rife E, Gedalia A. Kawasaki disease: an update. *Curr Rheumatol Rep.* 2020;22(10):75.
44. Akca UK, Kesici S, Ozsurekci Y, et al. Kawasaki-like disease in children with COVID-19. *Rheumatol Int.* 2020;40(12):2105–2115.
45. Luis Rodríguez-Peralto J, Carrillo R, Rosales B, Rodríguez-Gil Y. Superficial thrombophlebitis. *Semin Cutan Med Surg.* 2007;26(2):71–76.

46. Amano M, Shimizu T. Mondor's disease: a review of the literature. *Intern Med.* 2018;57(18):2607–2612.

47. Kumar B, Narang T, Radotra BD, Gupta S. Mondor's disease of penis: a forgotten disease. *Sex Transm Infect.* 2005;81(6):480–482.

48. Kobayashi M, Ito M, Nakagawa A, Nishikimi N, Nimura Y. Immunohistochemical analysis of arterial wall cellular infiltration in Buerger's disease (endarteritis obliterans). *J Vasc Surg.* 1999;29(3):451–8.

49. Matteson EL. A history of early investigation in polyarteritis nodosa. *Arthritis Care Res.* 1999;12(4):294–302.

50. Diaz-Perez JL, Winkelmann RK. Cutaneous periarteritis nodosa. *Arch Dermatol.* 1974;110(3):407–414.

51. Díaz-Pérez JL, De Lagrán ZM, Díaz-Ramón JL, Winkelmann RK. Cutaneous polyarteritis nodosa. *Semin Cutan Med Surg.* 2007;26(2):77–86.

52. Rogalski C, Sticherling M. Panarteritis cutanea benigna—an entity limited to the skin or cutaneous presentation of a systemic necrotizing vasculitis? Report of seven cases and review of the literature. *Int J Dermatol.* 2007;46(8):817–821.

53. Mimouni D, Ng PP, Rencic A, Nikolskaia OV, Bernstein BD, Nousari HC. Cutaneous polyarteritis nodosa in patients presenting with atrophie blanche. *Br J Dermatol.* 2003;148(4):789–94.

54. De Virgilio A, Greco A, Magliulo G, et al. Polyarteritis nodosa: a contemporary overview. *Autoimmun Rev.* 2016;15(6):564–570.

55. Davson J, Ball J, Platt R. The kidney in periarteritis nodosa. *Q J Med.* 1948;17(67):175–202.

56. Morgan AJ, Schwartz RA. Cutaneous polyarteritis nodosa: a comprehensive review. *Int J Dermatol.* 2010;49(7):750–756.

57. Watts R, Lane S, Hanslik T, et al. Development and validation of a consensus methodology for the classification of the ANCA-associated vasculitides and polyarteritis nodosa for epidemiological studies. *Ann Rheum Dis.* 2007;66(2):222–227.

58. Niiyama S, Amoh Y, Tomita M, Katsuoka K. Dermatological manifestations associated with microscopic polyangiitis. *Rheumatol Int.* 2008;28(6):593–595.

59. Kronbichler A, Lee KH, Denicolò S, et al. Immunopathogenesis of ANCA-Associated Vasculitis. *Int J Mol Sci.* 2020;21(19):7319.

60. Guillevin L, Lhote F, Amouroux J, Gherardi R, Callard P, Casassus P. Antineutrophil cytoplasmic antibodies, abnormal angiograms and pathological findings in polyarteritis nodosa and Churg-Strauss syndrome: indications for the classification of vasculitides of the polyarteritis Nodosa Group. *Br J Rheumatol.* 1996;35(10):958–964.

61. Churg J, Strauss L. Allergic granulomatosis, allergic angiitis, and periarteritis nodosa. *Am J Pathol.* 1951;27(2):277–301.

62. Liebow AA, Carrington CB. Hypersensitivity reactions involving the lung. *Trans Stud Coll Physicians Phila.* 1966;34(2):47–70.

63. Masi AT, Hunder GG, Lie JT, et al. The American College of Rheumatology 1990 criteria for the classification of Churg-Strauss syndrome (allergic granulomatosis and angiitis). *Arthritis Rheum.* 1990;33(8):1094–1100.

64. Kallenberg CG, Stegeman CA, Abdulahad WH, Heeringa P. Pathogenesis of ANCA-associated vasculitis: new possibilities for intervention. *Am J Kidney Dis.* 2013;62(6):1176–1187.

65. Keogh KA. Leukotriene receptor antagonists and Churg-Strauss syndrome: cause, trigger or merely an association? *Drug Saf.* 2007;30(10):837–843.

66. Davis MD, Daoud MS, McEvoy MT, Su WP. Cutaneous manifestations of Churg-Strauss syndrome: a clinicopathologic correlation. *J Am Acad Dermatol.* 1997;37(2 pt 1):199–203.

67. Chen KR, Sakamoto M, Ikemoto K, Abe R, Shimizu H. Granulomatous arteritis in cutaneous lesions of Churg-Strauss syndrome. *J Cutan Pathol.* 2007;34(4):330–337.

68. Guillevin L, Pagnoux C, Seror R, et al. The Five-Factor Score revisited: assessment of prognoses of systemic necrotizing vasculitides based on the French Vasculitis Study Group (FVSG) cohort. *Medicine (Baltimore).* 2011;90(1):19–27.

69. Godman GC, Churg J. Wegener's granulomatosis: pathology and review of the literature. *AMA Arch Pathol.* 1954;58(6):533–553.

70. DeRemee RA, McDonald TJ, Harrison EG Jr, Coles DT. Wegener's granulomatosis. Anatomic correlates, a proposed classification. *Mayo Clin Proc.* 1976;51(12):777–781.

71. Falk RJ, Gross WL, Guillevin L, et al. Granulomatosis with polyangiitis (Wegener's): an alternative name for Wegener's granulomatosis. *Arthritis Rheum.* 2011;63(4):863–864.

72. Lionaki S, Blyth ER, Hogan SL, et al. Classification of antineutrophil cytoplasmic autoantibody vasculitides: the role of antineutrophil cytoplasmic autoantibody specificity for myeloperoxidase or proteinase 3 in disease recognition and prognosis. *Arthritis Rheum.* 2012;64(10):3452–3462.

73. Barksdale SK, Hallahan CW, Kerr GS, Fauci AS, Stern JB, Travis WD. Cutaneous pathology in Wegener's granulomatosis. A clinicopathologic study of 75 biopsies in 46 patients. *Am J Surg Pathol.* 1995;19(2):161–172.

74. Montero-Vilchez T, Martinez-Lopez A, Salvador-Rodriguez L, et al. Cutaneous manifestations of granulomatosis with polyangiitis: a case series Study. *Acta Derm Venereol.* 2020;100(10):adv00150.

75. Comfere NI, Macaron NC, Gibson LE. Cutaneous manifestations of Wegener's granulomatosis: a clinicopathologic study of 17 patients and correlation to antineutrophil cytoplasmic antibody status. *J Cutan Pathol.* 2007;34(10):739–747.

76. Guillevin L, Pagnoux C, Karras A, et al. Rituximab versus azathioprine for maintenance in ANCA-associated vasculitis. *N Engl J Med.* 2014;371(19):1771–1780.

77. Tai YJ, Chong AH, Williams RA, Cumming S, Kelly RI. Retrospective analysis of adult patients with cutaneous leukocytoclastic vasculitis. *Australas J Dermatol.* 2006;47(2):92–96.

78. Pursley TV, Jacobson RR, Apisarnthanarax P. Lucio's Phenomenon. *Archives of Dermatology.* 1980;116(2):201–204.

79. Al-Mayouf SM, Bahabri S, Majeed M. Cutaneous leukocytoclastic vasculitis associated with mycobacterial and salmonella infection. *Clin Rheumatol.* 2007;26(9):1563–1564.

80. Sansonno D, Dammacco F. Hepatitis C virus, cryoglobulinaemia, and vasculitis: immune complex relations. *Lancet Infect Dis.* 2005;5(4):227–236.

81. Sanz-Sánchez T, Daudén E, Moreno de Vega MJ, García-Díez A. Parvovirus B19 primary infection with vasculitis: DNA identification in cutaneous lesions and sera. *J Eur Acad Dermatol Venereol.* 2006;20(5):618–620.

82. Becker RC. COVID-19-associated vasculitis and vasculopathy. *J Thromb Thrombolysis.* 2020;50(3):499–511.

83. Yang YH, Yu HH, Chiang BL. The diagnosis and classification of Henoch-Schönlein purpura: an updated review. *Autoimmun Rev.* 2014;13(4-5):355–358.

84. Mills JA, Michel BA, Bloch DA, et al. The American College of Rheumatology 1990 criteria for the classification of Henoch-Schönlein purpura. *Arthritis Rheum.* 1990;33(8):1114–1121.

85. Trapani S, Mariotti P, Resti M, Nappini L, de Martino M, Falcini F. Severe hemorrhagic bullous lesions in Henoch Schonlein purpura: three pediatric cases and review of the literature. *Rheumatol Int.* 2010;30(10):1355–1359.

86. Audemard-Verger A, Pillebout E, Guillevin L, Thervet E, Terrier B. IgA vasculitis (Henoch-Shönlein purpura) in adults: diagnostic and therapeutic aspects. *Autoimmun Rev.* 2015;14(7):579–585.

87. Magro CM, Crowson AN. A clinical and histologic study of 37 cases of immunoglobulin A-associated vasculitis. *Am J Dermatopathol.* 1999;21(3):234–240.

88. Saraçlar Y, Tinaztepe K. Infantile acute hemorrhagic edema of the skin. *J Am Acad Dermatol.* 1992;26(2 pt 1):275–276.

89. Di Lernia V, Lombardi M, Lo Scocco G. Infantile acute hemorrhagic edema and rotavirus infection. *Pediatr Dermatol.* 2004;21(5):548–550.

90. Podjasek JO, Wetter DA, Pittelkow MR, Wada DA. Henoch-Schönlein purpura associated with solid-organ malignancies: three case reports and a literature review. *Acta Derm Venereol.* 2012;92(4):388–392.

91. Birchmore D, Sweeney C, Choudhury D, Konwinski MF, Carnevale K, D'Agati V. IgA multiple myeloma presenting as Henoch-Schönlein purpura/polyarteritis nodosa overlap syndrome. *Arthritis Rheum.* 1996;39(4):698–703.

92. Jennette JC, Wieslander J, Tuttle R, Falk RJ. Serum IgA-fibronectin aggregates in patients with IgA nephropathy and Henoch-Schönlein purpura: diagnostic value and pathogenic implications. The Glomerular Disease Collaborative Network. *Am J Kidney Dis.* 1991;18(4):466–471.

93. Poterucha TJ, Wetter DA, Gibson LE, Camilleri MJ, Lohse CM. Histopathology and correlates of systemic disease in adult Henoch-Schönlein purpura: a retrospective study of microscopic and clinical findings in 68 patients at Mayo Clinic. *J Am Acad Dermatol.* 2013;68(3):420–424.e3.

94. Byun JW, Song HJ, Kim L, Shin JH, Choi GS. Predictive factors of relapse in adult with Henoch-Schönlein purpura. *Am J Dermatopathol.* 2012;34(2):139–144.

95. Poterucha TJ, Wetter DA, Gibson LE, Camilleri MJ, Lohse CM. Correlates of systemic disease in adult Henoch-Schönlein purpura: a retrospective study of direct immunofluorescence and skin lesion distribution in 87 patients at Mayo Clinic. *J Am Acad Dermatol.* 2012;67(4):612–616.

96. Mehregan DR, Hall MJ, Gibson LE. Urticarial vasculitis: a histopathologic and clinical review of 72 cases. *J Am Acad Dermatol.* 1992;26(3 pt 2):441–448.

97. Davis MD, Daoud MS, Kirby B, Gibson LE, Rogers RS 3rd. Clinicopathologic correlation of hypocomplementemic and normocomplementemic urticarial vasculitis. *J Am Acad Dermatol.* 1998;38(6 pt 1):899–905.

98. Davis MDP, van der Hilst JCH. Mimickers of urticaria: urticarial vasculitis and autoinflammatory diseases. *J Allergy Clin Immunol Pract.* 2018;6(4):1162–1170.

99. Cohen SJ, Pittelkow MR, Su, WP. Cutaneous manifestations of cryoglobulinemia: clinical and histopathologic study of seventy-two patients. *J Am Acad Dermatol.* 1991;25(1 pt 1):21–27.

100. De Vita S, Soldano F, Isola M, et al. Preliminary classification criteria for the cryoglobulinaemic vasculitis. *Ann Rheum Dis.* 2011;70(7):1183–1190.

101. Damoiseaux J. The diagnosis and classification of the cryoglobulinemic syndrome. *Autoimmun Rev.* 2014;13(4-5):359–362.

102. Braun GS, Horster S, Wagner KS, Ihrler S, Schmid H. Cryoglobulinaemic vasculitis: classification and clinical and therapeutic aspects. *Postgrad Med J.* 2007;83(976):87–94.

103. Patel A, Prussick R, Buchanan WW, Sauder DN. Serum sickness-like illness and leukocytoclastic vasculitis after intravenous streptokinase. *J Am Acad Dermatol.* 1991;24(4):652–653.

104. Sharma A, Dhooria A, Aggarwal A, Rathi M, Chandran V. Connective tissue disorder-associated vasculitis. *Curr Rheumatol Rep.* 2016;18(6):31.

105. Lakhanpal S, Conn DL, Lie JT. Clinical and prognostic significance of vasculitis as an early manifestation of connective tissue disease syndromes. *Ann Intern Med.* 1984;101(6):743–74.

106. Chen KR, Toyohara A, Suzuki A, Miyakawa S. Clinical and histopathological spectrum of cutaneous vasculitis in rheumatoid arthritis. *Br J Dermatol.* 2002;147(5):905–913.

107. Ramos-Casals M, Nardi N, Lagrutta M, et al. Vasculitis in systemic lupus erythematosus: prevalence and clinical characteristics in 670 patients. *Medicine (Baltimore).* 2006;85(2):95–104.

108. Kawakami T, Soma Y, Mizoguchi, M. Initial cutaneous manifestations associated with histopathological leukocytoclastic vasculitis in two patients with antiphospholipid antibody syndrome. *J Dermatol.* 2005;32(12):1032–1037.

109. Grau RG. Drug-induced vasculitis: new insights and a changing lineup of suspects. *Curr Rheumatol Rep.* 2015;17(12):71.

110. Ayturk S, Demir MV, Yaylacı S, Tamer A. Propylthiouracil induced leukocytoclastic vasculitis: a rare manifestation. *Indian J Endocrinol Metab.* 2013;17(2):339–340.

111. Kim JH, Moon JI, Kim JE, et al. Cutaneous leukocytoclastic vasculitis due to anti-tuberculosis medications, rifampin and pyrazinamide. *Allergy Asthma Immunol Res.* 2010;2(1):55–58.

112. Uchimiya H, Higashi Y, Kawai K, Kanekura T. Purpuric drug eruption with leukocytoclastic vasculitis due to gefitinib. *J Dermatol.* 2010;37(6):562–564.

113. Bahrami S, Malone JC, Webb KG, Callen JP. Tissue eosinophilia as an indicator of drug-induced cutaneous small-vessel vasculitis. *Arch Dermatol.* 2006;142(2):155–561.

114. Solans-Laqué R, Bosch-Gil JA, Pérez-Bocanegra C, Selva-O'Callaghan A, Simeón-Aznar CP, Vilardell-Tarres M. Paraneoplastic vasculitis in patients with solid tumors: report of 15 cases. *J Rheumatol.* 2008;35(2):294–304.

115. Fain O, Hamidou M, Cacoub P, et al. Vasculitides associated with malignancies: analysis of sixty patients. *Arthritis Rheum.* 2007;57(8):1473–1480.

116. Carlson JA, LeBoit PE. Localized chronic fibrosing vasculitis of the skin: an inflammatory reaction that occurs in settings other than erythema elevatum diutinum and granuloma faciale. *Am J Surg Pathol.* 1997;21(6):698–705.

117. LeBoit PE, Yen TS, Wintroub B. The evolution of lesions in erythema elevatum diutinum. *Am J Dermatopathol.* 1986;8(5):392–402.

118. Sangüeza OP, Pilcher B, Martin Sangüeza J. Erythema elevatum diutinum: a clinicopathological study of eight cases. *Am J Dermatopathol.* 1997;19(3):214–222.

119. Sandhu JK, Albrecht J, Agnihotri G, Tsoukas MM. Erythema elevatum et diutinum as a systemic disease. *Clin Dermatol.* 2019;37(6):679–683.

120. Shimizu S, Nakamura Y, Togawa Y, Kamada N, Kambe N, Matsue H. Erythema elevatum diutinum with primary Sjögren syndrome associated with IgA antineutrophil cytoplasmic antibody. *Br J Dermatol.* 2008;159(3):733–73.

121. Requena L, Sánchez Yus E, Martín L, Barat A, Arias D. Erythema elevatum diutinum in a patient with acquired immunodeficiency syndrome. Another clinical simulator of Kaposi's sarcoma. *Arch Dermatol.* 1991;127(12):1819–1822.

122. Marcoval J, Moreno A, Peyr J. Granuloma faciale: a clinicopathological study of 11 cases. *J Am Acad Dermatol.* 2004;51(2):269–73.

123. Pratap DV, Putta S, Manmohan G, Aruna S, Geethika M. Granuloma faciale with extra-facial involvement. *Indian J Dermatol Venereol Leprol.* 2010;76(4):424–426.

124. Stelini RF, Moysés MD, Cintra ML, et al. Granuloma faciale and eosinophilic angiocentric fibrosis: similar entities in different anatomic sites. *Appl Immunohistochem Mol Morphol.* 2017;25(3):213–220.

125. Cesinaro AM, Lonardi S, Facchetti F. Granuloma faciale: a cutaneous lesion sharing features with IgG4-associated sclerosing diseases. *Am J Surg Pathol.* 2013;37(1):66–73.

126. Ziemer M, Koehler MJ, Weyers W. Erythema elevatum diutinum—a chronic leukocytoclastic vasculitis microscopically indistinguishable from granuloma faciale? *J Cutan Pathol.* 2011;38(11):876–883.

127. Jorizzo JL, Solomon AR, Zanolli MD, Leshin B. Neutrophilic vascular reactions. *J Am Acad Dermatol.* 1988;19(6):983–1005.

128. Nelson CA, Stephen S, Ashchyan HJ, James WD, Micheletti RG, Rosenbach M. Neutrophilic dermatoses: pathogenesis, sweet syndrome, neutrophilic eccrine hidradenitis, and Behçet disease. *J Am Acad Dermatol.* 2018;79(6):987–1006.

129. von den Driesch P. Sweet's syndrome (acute febrile neutrophilic dermatosis). *J Am Acad Dermatol.* 1994;31(4):535–556; quiz 557–560.

130. Marzano AV, Ishak RS, Saibeni S, Crosti C, Meroni PL, Cugno M. Autoinflammatory skin disorders in inflammatory bowel diseases, pyoderma gangrenosum and Sweet's syndrome: a comprehensive review and disease classification criteria. *Clin Rev Allergy Immunol.* 2013;45(2):202–210.

131. Naik HB, Cowen EW. Autoinflammatory pustular neutrophilic diseases. *Dermatol Clin.* 2013;31(3):405–425.

132. Voelter-Mahlknecht S, Bauer J, Metzler G, Fierlbeck G, Rassner G. Bullous variant of Sweet's syndrome. *Int J Dermatol.* 2005;44(11):946–947.

133. Kawakami T, Ohashi S, Kawa Y, et al. Elevated serum granulocyte colony-stimulating factor levels in patients with active phase of sweet syndrome and patients with active Behcet disease:

implication in neutrophil apoptosis dysfunction. *Arch Dermatol.* 2004;140(5):570–574.

134. Chan MP, Duncan LM, Nazarian RM. Subcutaneous Sweet syndrome in the setting of myeloid disorders: a case series and review of the literature. *J Am Acad Dermatol.* 2013;68(6):1006–1015.

135. Requena L, Kutzner H, Palmedo G, et al. Histiocytoid Sweet syndrome: a dermal infiltration of immature neutrophilic granulocytes. *Arch Dermatol.* 2005;141(7):834–842.

136. Ely PH. The bowel bypass syndrome: a response to bacterial peptidoglycans. *J Am Acad Dermatol.* 1980;2(6):473–487.

137. Powell FC, Su WP, Perry HO. Pyoderma gangrenosum: classification and management. *J Am Acad Dermatol.* 1996;34(3):395–409; quiz 410–412.

138. Ashchyan HJ, Nelson CA, Stephen S, James WD, Micheletti RG, Rosenbach M. Neutrophilic dermatoses: pyoderma gangrenosum and other bowel-and arthritis-associated neutrophilic dermatoses. *J Am Acad Dermatol.* 2018;79(6):1009–1022.

139. Su WP, Schroeter AL, Perry HO, Powell FC. Histopathologic and immunopathologic study of pyoderma gangrenosum. *J Cutan Pathol.* 1986;13(5):323–330.

140. Bulur I, Onder M. Behçet disease: new aspects. *Clin Dermatol.* 2017;35(5):421–434.

141. Karaca M, Hatemi G, Sut N, Yazici H. The papulopustular lesion/arthritis cluster of Behçet's syndrome also clusters in families. *Rheumatology (Oxford).* 2012;51(6):1053–1060.

142. Chen KR, Kawahara Y, Miyakawa S, Nishikawa T. Cutaneous vasculitis in Behçet's disease: a clinical and histopathologic study of 20 patients. *J Am Acad Dermatol.* 1997;36(5, pt 1):689–696.

143. Massa MC, Su WP. Lymphocytic vasculitis: is it a specific clinicopathologic entity? *J Cutan Pathol.* 1984;11(2):132–139.

144. Freeman EE, McMahon DE, Fitzgerald ME, et al. The American Academy of Dermatology COVID-19 registry: crowdsourcing dermatology in the age of COVID-19. *J Am Acad Dermatol.* 2020;83(2):509–510.

145. Freeman EE, McMahon DE, Lipoff JB, et al. Pernio-like skin lesions associated with COVID-19: a case series of 318 patients from 8 countries. *J Am Acad Dermatol.* 2020;83(2):486–492.

146. Kanitakis J, Lesort C, Danset M, Jullien D. Chilblain-like acral lesions during the COVID-19 pandemic ("COVID toes"): histologic, immunofluorescence, and immunohistochemical study of 17 cases. *J Am Acad Dermatol.* 2020;83(3):870–875.

147. Hubiche T, Cardot-Leccia N, Le Duff F, et al. Clinical, laboratory, and interferon-alpha response characteristics of patients with chilblain-like lesions during the COVID-19 pandemic. *JAMA Dermatol.* 2021;157(2):202–206.

148. Thomas R, Vuitch F, Lakhanpal S. Angiocentric T cell lymphoma masquerading as cutaneous vasculitis. *J Rheumatol.* 1994;21(4):760–762.

149. Randall SJ, Kierland RR, Montgomery H. Pigmented purpuric eruptions. *AMA Arch Derm Syphilol.* 1951;64(2):177–191.

150. Waisman M, Waisman M. Lichen aureus. *Arch Dermatol.* 1976;112(5):696–697.

151. Huang YK, Lin CK, Wu YH. The pathological spectrum and clinical correlation of pigmented purpuric dermatosis—a retrospective review of 107 cases. *J Cutan Pathol.* 2018;45(5):325–332.

152. Kaplan J, Burgin S, Sepehr A. Granulomatous pigmented purpura: report of a case and review of the literature. *J Cutan Pathol.* 2011;38(12):984–989.

153. Barnhill RL, Braverman IM. Progression of pigmented purpura-like eruptions to mycosis fungoides: report of three cases. *J Am Acad Dermatol.* 1988;19(1, pt 1):25–31.

154. Martinez-Mera C, Fraga J, Capusan TM, et al. Vasculopathies, cutaneous necrosis and emergency in dermatology. *G Ital Dermatol Venereol.* 2017;152(6):615–637.

155. Jones A, Walling H. Retiform purpura in plaques: a morphological approach to diagnosis. *Clin Exp Dermatol.* 2007;32(5):596–602.

156. García-Lozano JA, Ocampo-Candiani J, Martínez-Cabriales SA, Garza-Rodríguez V. An update on calciphylaxis. *Am J Clin Dermatol.* 2018;19(4):599–608.

157. Yu WY, Bhutani T, Kornik R, et al. Warfarin-associated nonuremic calciphylaxis. *JAMA Dermatol* 2017;153(3):309–313.

158. Harris RJ, Cropley TG. Possible role of hypercoagulability in calciphylaxis: review of the literature. *J Am Acad Dermatol.* 2011;64(2):405–412.

159. Lugo-Somolinos A, Sánchez JL, Méndez-Coll J, Joglar F. Calcifying panniculitis associated with polycystic kidney disease and chronic renal failure. *J Am Acad Dermatol.* 1990;22(5, pt 1):743–747.

160. Jacobs-Kosmin D, Dehoratius RJ. Calciphylaxis: an important imitator of cutaneous vasculitis. *Arthritis Rheum.* 2007;57(3):533–537.

161. Mochel MC, Arakaki RY, Wang G, Kroshinsky D, Hoang MP. Cutaneous calciphylaxis: a retrospective histopathologic evaluation. *Am J Dermatopathol.* 2013;35(5):582–586.

162. Seethapathy H, Noureddine L. Calciphylaxis: approach to diagnosis and management. *Adv Chronic Kidney Dis.* 2019;26(6):484–490.

163. Falanga V, Fine MJ, Kapoor WN. The cutaneous manifestations of cholesterol crystal embolization. *Arch Dermatol.* 1986;122(10):1194–1198.

164. Yücel AE, Kart-Köseoglu H, Demirhan B, Ozdemir FN. Cholesterol crystal embolization mimicking vasculitis: success with corticosteroid and cyclophosphamide therapy in two cases. *Rheumatol Int.* 2006;26(5):454–460.

165. Walker A. Chronic scurvy. *Br J Dermatol.* 1968;80(10):625–630.

166. Gan EY, Tang MB, Tan SH, Chua SH, Tan AW. A ten-year retrospective study on livedo vasculopathy in Asian patients. *Ann Acad Med Singap.* 2012;41(9):400–406.

167. Sneddon IB. Cerebro-vascular lesions and livedo reticularis. *Br J Dermatol.* 1965;77:180–185.

168. Stiefler RE, Bergfeld WF. Atrophie blanche. *Int J Dermatol.* 1982;21(1):1–7.

169. Amato L, Chiarini C, Berti S, Massi D, Fabbri P. Idiopathic atrophie blanche. *Skinmed.* 2006;5(3):151–154.

170. McCalmont CS, McCalmont TH, Jorizzo JL, White WL, Leshin B, Rothberger H. Livedo vasculitis: vasculitis or thrombotic vasculopathy? *Clin Exp Dermatol.* 1992;17(1):4–8.

171. Black MM. Malignant atrophic papulosis (Degos'disease). *Int J Dermatol.* 1976;15(6):405–411.

172. Harvell JD, Williford PL, White WL. Benign cutaneous Degos' disease: a case report with emphasis on histopathology as papules chronologically evolve. *Am J Dermatopathol.* 2001;23(2):116–123.

173. Loewe R, Palatin M, Petzelbauer P. Degos disease with an inconspicuous clinical course. *J Eur Acad Dermatol Venereol.* 2005;19(4):477–480.

174. Ball E, Newburger A, Ackerman AB. Degos' disease: a distinctive pattern of disease, chiefly of lupus erythematosus, and not a specific disease per se. *Am J Dermatopathol.* 2003;25(4):308–320.

175. Wallace MP, Thomas JM, Meligonis G, Ha T. Systemic lupus erythematosus, following prodromal idiopathic thrombocytopenic purpura, presenting with skin lesions resembling malignant atrophic papulosis. *Clin Exp Dermatol.* 2017;42(7):774–776.

176. Magrinat G, Kerwin KS, Gabriel DA. The clinical manifestations of Degos' syndrome. *Arch Pathol Lab Med.* 1989;113(4):354–362.

177. Magro CM, Poe JC, Kim C, et al. Degos disease: a C5b-9/interferon-α-mediated endotheliopathy syndrome. *Am J Clin Pathol.* 2011;135(4):599–610.

178. Ortiz A, Ceccato F, Albertengo A, Roverano S, Iribas J, Paira S. Degos cutaneous disease with features of connective tissue disease. *J Clin Rheumatol.* 2010;16(3):132–134.

179. Scheinfeld N. Commentary on 'Degos disease: a C5b-9/interferon-α-mediated endotheliopathy syndrome' by Magro et al: a reconsideration of Degos disease as hematologic or endothelial genetic disease. *Dermatol Online J.* 2011;17(8):6.

180. Magro CM, Wang X, Garrett-Bakelman F, Laurence J, Shapiro LS, DeSancho MT. The effects of Eculizumab on the pathology of malignant atrophic papulosis. *Orphanet J Rare Dis.* 2013;8:185.

Chapter 9

Noninfectious Vesiculobullous and Vesiculopustular Diseases

BEVERLY E. FAULKNER-JONES, EMILY M. ALTMAN, CHARLES H. PALMER, AND TERENCE J. HARRIST

CLASSIFICATION OF BLISTERS

Definition

A blister is a fluid-filled cavity formed within or beneath the epidermis. The fluid consists of tissue fluid and plasma. A variable component of inflammatory cells may also be present. Blisters may occur in many dermatoses. At first glance, this observation seems to imply that blistering is too general or nonspecific for use in clinical gross evaluation. However, the character of blisters in a given disorder tends to be uniform and to have reproducible characteristics. One useful distinction is the categorization of blisters into *vesicles* (blisters < 0.5 cm in diameter) and *bullae* (blisters > 0.5 cm in diameter). For example, vesicles characteristically occur in dermatitis herpetiformis (DH) as opposed to pemphigoid, in which bullae are most commonly observed.

Mechanisms of Blister Formation

The mechanisms observable in routine sections for some diseases are shown in Table 9-1.

Spongiosis is the accumulation of extracellular fluid within the epidermis with resultant separation of the keratinocytes (Fig. 9-1A). Pronounced spongiosis gives the keratinocytes a stellate appearance and subsequently leads to disruption of desmosomes and blister formation. Thus, the epidermis has a "spongy" appearance microscopically, and the increasing accumulation of fluid leads to a vesicle and, in some instances, to a bulla. Marked spongiosis may terminate in reticular degeneration (see later). Spongiosis is almost always associated with an infiltrate of lymphocytes within the epidermis and around superficial vessels. Diagnostically important are the types of inflammatory cells in the spongiosis—lymphocytes, neutrophils, and eosinophils (Tables 9-2 and 9-3). In addition, the pityriasiform spongiosis and parakeratosis (regularly separated foci) as in pityriasis rosea, pityriasis rosea–like drug eruption, miliaria, and erythema annulare centrifugum are important. Spongiosis is a passive event associated with increased permeability of the superficial vascular plexus, particularly the postcapillary venules. Spongiotic keratinocytes are viable cells.

Acantholysis results from the loss of appropriate keratinocyte cell–cell contact (Fig. 9-1B, C). Histologic evidence of acantholysis includes the presence of rounded keratinocytes with condensed cytoplasm and large nuclei with peripheral condensation of chromatin and prominent nucleoli. Acantholytic keratinocytes are, at least initially, viable and may mimic cytopathic changes of herpesvirus infection. The rounded keratinocytes of acantholysis differ strikingly from the stellate keratinocytes of spongiotic dermatitis.

Table 9-1		
Diseases and Their Mechanisms of Blister Formation		
Spongiosis	"Eczematous" dermatitis	
	Miliaria	
	Pemphigus (early)	
	Transient acantholytic dermatosis (one pattern)	
Acantholysis	Pemphigus	
	Transient acantholytic dermatosis (some patterns)	
	Hailey–Hailey disease	
	Darier disease	
	Irritant dermatitis (some) such as Cantharidin and other contactants	
Reticular degeneration	Viral infections	
	Eczematous dermatitis (late stage)	
Cytolysis	Epidermolysis bullosa simplex	
	Epidermolytic hyperkeratosis	
	Friction blister	
	Erythema multiforme (in part)	
	Irritant dermatitis (some)	
Basement membrane zone destruction	Bullous pemphigoid	
	Mucous membrane (cutaneous cicatricial) pemphigoid	
	Linear IgA dermatosis (probably IgA EBA)	
	Dermatitis herpetiformis (later lesions)	
	Epidermolysis bullosa acquisita	
	Epidermolysis bullosa letalis	
	Epidermolysis bullosa dystrophica	

Cytolysis is the disruption of keratinocytes. It occurs in the normal epidermis when the structural (keratin) matrix and desmosomal plaques of the keratinocyte are overwhelmed by high levels of physical agents such as friction and heat. Friction (mechanical energy applied parallel to the epidermis) leads to the shearing of keratinocytes one from another and

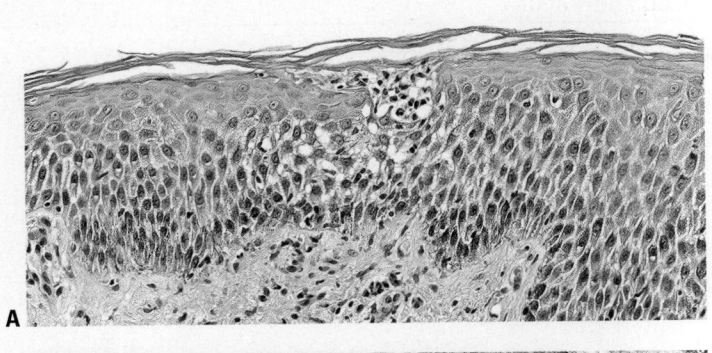
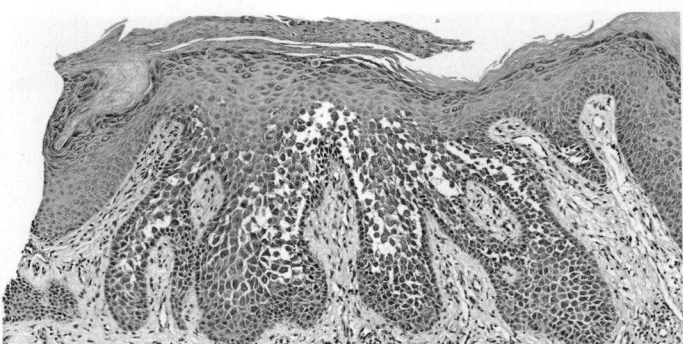
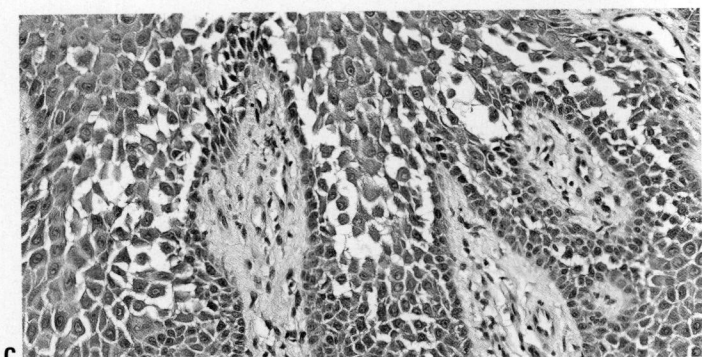

Figure 9-1 Mechanisms of blister formation. **A:** Spongiosis. As extracellular fluid accumulates between keratinocytes, it causes their separation and stellate appearance and may lead to vesicle or even bulla formation. In this example, there are also intraepidermal lymphocytes, a surface collection of Langerhans cells and eosinophils in the epidermis and dermis. **B, C:** Acantholysis. Keratinocyte cell–cell adhesion is lost. The cells have a rounded outline, in contrast to the keratinocytes in spongiosis. Acantholysis in familial benign chronic pemphigus (Hailey–Hailey disease). **B:** Low-power architecture. **C:** Medium power highlights acantholytic cells.

of the keratinocytes themselves, giving the characteristic clear fluid-filled blisters unless extending into the dermis, leading to hemorrhagic blisters. In mechanobullous diseases, minimal friction may lead to cytolysis because the keratinocytes do not have normal structural matrix and desmosomes, such as in epidermolysis bullosa (EB) simplex and EB of the Cockayne–Weber type.

Reticular degeneration, a subset of cytolysis, results from ballooning degeneration (intracellular edema) with secondary rupture and death of the keratinocytes. The remaining desmosomal attachments often connect strands of ruptured keratinocytic membranes and cytoplasm to intact keratinocytes, giving the epidermis an irregular meshwork (reticulated) appearance.

Basement membrane zone disruption or destruction results from primary structural deficiencies as well as from both humoral and cellular immunologically mediated damage. When blisters arise at the epidermal basement membrane zone, any of the specific subanatomic compartments can be affected: (a) the basal keratinocytes, in particular their lower portions; (b) the lamina lucida, an electron-lucid area immediately subjacent to the plasma membrane; (c) the lamina densa, composed principally of type IV collagen; and (d) the sublamina densa zone, largely Type VII collagen, with other components.

Pathologic Evaluation

When blisters are encountered microscopically, systematic analysis can lead to the correct diagnosis in most cases. The critical interpretive assessments to be approached in sequence are as follows: (a) the blister separation plane (Table 9-4); (b) the mechanism(s) of blister formation (Table 9-1); and (c) the character of the inflammatory infiltrate, including its presence or absence, its pattern, and the specific cell types involved (Tables 9-1 to 9-3 and 9-5).

Table 9-2
Spongiosis Associated with Neutrophils
Psoriasis
Seborrheic dermatitis
Reiter disease
Pemphigus (IgG and IgA mediated)
Superficial fungal infection (dermatophytes/*Candida* sp.)
Acute generalized exanthematous pustulosis
Phototoxic dermatitis
Contact reactions, especially irritant type
Acrodermatitis enteropathica/glucagonoma
Toxic shock syndrome
Impetigo/bullous impetigo
Infantile acropustulosis
Transient neonatal pustular melanosis
Idiopathic pustular dermatitis of the intertriginous zones
Connective tissue disease (uncommon)
Prurigo pigmentosa
Bacterial infections
Pustular secondary lues
Pustular drug eruption
Subcorneal pustular dermatosis
Id reaction
Kawasaki disease

Table 9-3
Spongiosis Associated with Eosinophils

Pemphigus (early lesions)

Pemphigoid (bullous, mucous membrane, gestationis)

Itchy red/pink bump disease

Pruritic and urticarial papules and plaques of pregnancy/
   polymorphous eruption of pregnancy

Eczematous dermatitis (contact, +/−atopy, id)

Incontinentia pigmentosa (first stage)

Drug eruptions

Photoallergic dermatitis

Arthropod assaults

Grover disease

Well syndrome

Scabies

Erythema toxicum neonatorum

Table 9-4
Some Diseases with Their Specific Separation Planes
Intraepidermal

Subcorneal/Granular

Miliaria crystallina

Staphylococcal scalded skin syndrome

Pemphigus foliaceus and variants

Bullous impetigo

IgA pemphigus (some variants)

Subcorneal pustular dermatosis

Erythema toxicum neonatorum

Transient neonatal pustular melanosis

Acropustulosis of infancy

Spinous

Spongiotic dermatitis

Grover disease

Friction blister (may extend into dermis)

Miliaria rubra

Incontinentia pigmenti

IgA pemphigus (some variants)

Epidermolytic hyperkeratosis

Hailey–Hailey disease

Suprabasal

Pemphigus vulgaris

Pemphigus vegetans

Grover disease

Hailey–Hailey disease

Paraneoplastic autoimmune multiorgan syndrome/
   Paraneoplastic pemphigus (PNP/PAMS)

Darier disease

Subepidermal

Basal Keratinocyte Necrosis, Cytolysis, or Damage

Epidermolysis bullosa simplex

Thermal injury (some)

Erythema multiforme

Epidermal Basement Membrane Zone Destruction or Disruption

Lamina Lucida

Bullous pemphigoid

Mucous membrane pemphigoid

Cutaneous cicatricial pemphigoid

Pemphigoid gestationis

Dermatitis herpetiformis, early

Linear IgA dermatosis

Epidermolysis bullosa letalis (junctional)

Suction blister

Thermal injury (some)

Sublamina Densa

Bullous systemic lupus erythematosus

Epidermolysis bullosa acquisita (EBA)

Linear IgA dermatosis (IgA-mediated epidermolysis bullosa
   acquisita)

Epidermolysis bullosa dystrophica

Porphyria cutanea tarda/pseudoporphyria

Dermatitis herpetiformis, late

Mucous membrane pemphigoid

Cutaneous cicatricial pemphigoid

Dermal

Penicillamine-induced blisters (iatrogenic)

Bullous amyloidosis (primary systemic)

Six principal problems are encountered using this algorithm. The first is that the separation plane may change as blisters age (Fig. 9-2A). Spongiotic microvesicles may move into the stratum corneum as crust. The epidermal blister roofs may become necrotic, not allowing assessment of the original blister plane. However, the basal keratinocytes may retain their columnar appearance in the blister roof (or base), allowing for separation into either suprabasal or subbasal blister formation. Also, basal keratinocytes (stratum basalis) are the most melanized cells in the epidermis. Search for the melanized basal keratinocytes (i.e., the basal unit), even if they are necrotic, may allow assessment of the original blister plane. Immunohistochemical study for type IV collagen is sometimes useful in subepidermal blistering disorders because type IV collagen may be detectable on the base of subepidermal blister roofs even when the blister roof is necrotic and blister bases where the split is in the lamina lucida. Some blister roofs may be viable for a week or so; in this case, the viable keratinocytes may become elongated and line the base of the blister roof. Similarly, the reepithelialized subepidermal or suprabasal blister bases are initially lined by flat squamous keratinocytes rather

Table 9-5
Principal Infiltrating Inflammatory Cells in Some Vesiculobullous Dermatoses*

Dermatosis	Characteristic Cell Type	Infiltrate
Porphyria		Absent
Variegate		
Cutanea tarda		
Epidermolysis bullosa acquisita (classic)		Absent
Bullous pemphigoid (cell-poor)	Eosinophils	Minimal
Spongiotic dermatitis	Lymphocytes	Present
Erythema multiforme	Lymphocytes	Present
Bullous pemphigoid (cell-rich)	Eosinophils	Present
Pemphigoid gestationis	Eosinophils	Present
Linear IgA dermatosis	Neutrophils	Present
Epidermolysis bullosa acquisita (inflammatory)	Neutrophils or Mixed neutrophils and eosinophils	Present
Anti-p200 pemphigoid	Neutrophils or Mixed neutrophils and eosinophils	Present
Bullous SLE	Neutrophils Interface dermatitis	Present
Mucous membrane pemphigoid/cutaneous cicatricial pemphigoid	Mixed neutrophils and eosinophils Lymphocytic, bandlike (mucosa only) Eosinophils	Present
Paraneoplastic autoimmune multiorgan syndrome/paraneoplastic pemphigus (PNP/PAMS)	Lymphocytes—interface dermatitis (lichen planus or erythema multiforme–like)	Present

SLE, systemic lupus erythematosus.

*These descriptions are accurate in most of the cases in each dermatosis; however, the cell types may occasionally differ, rendering IF testing mandatory. Other inflammatory cells may be present as a minor component but on occasion are of significant number. The inflammatory cells in old/healing lesions are often not cells characteristic of the specific primary disease but represent the inflammatory cells present during healing or responding to secondary effects (ulceration, etc.) of the vesiculobullous disorder.

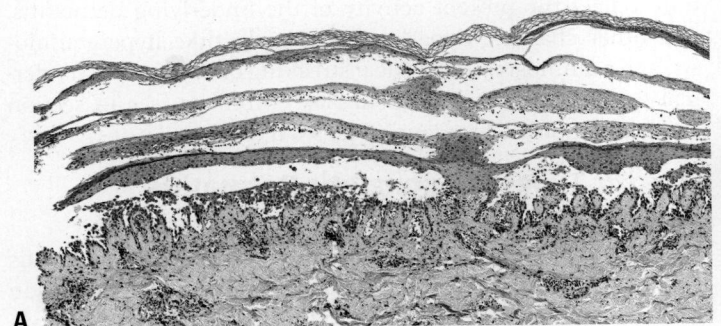

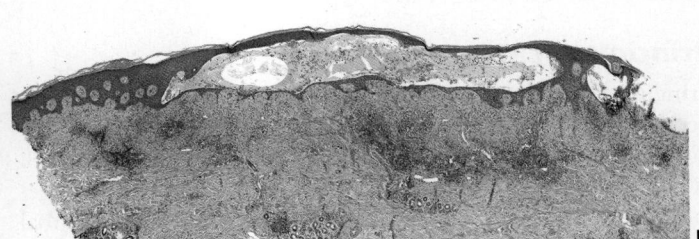

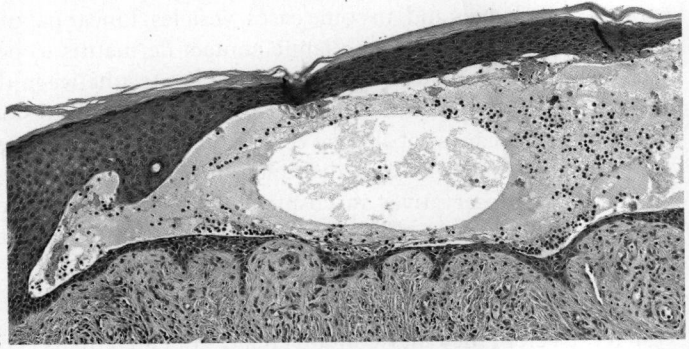

Figure 9-2 Pathologic evaluation. Secondary epithelial regeneration, trauma, or infection can obscure the original separation plane. **A:** Pemphigus vulgaris with typical intraepidermal suprabasal acantholysis exhibiting four repeated bouts of blister formation but with four overlying levels of epidermal regeneration (low power). **B, C:** Subepidermal vesicle with reepithelialized bulla floor. The vesicle contains fibrin and eosinophils. **B:** Low-power architecture. **C:** Medium power.

than columnar or cuboidal keratinocytes. When reepithelialization occurs first, there are no normal rete ridges, and the flat squamous keratinocytes migrate on a matrix of fibrinogen, not normal papillary dermis (Fig. 9-2B, C). Second, microscopic slit-like spaces occur within the epidermis in the group of clefting diseases—Darier disease, Hailey–Hailey disease, and Grover disease (GD)—mimicking true blisters. However, these clefts are small and most of them do not contain fibrin and tissue fluid. Furthermore, this group of disorders only rarely presents clinically with blisters. Third, evaluation of routine histologic preparations may not allow one to accurately assess the specific mechanism of blister formation. This is particularly true in subepidermal vesiculobullous disorders. Fourth, the cell types infiltrating the lesions in the vesiculobullous diseases change as the lesions age. Fifth, the histologic descriptions of many of the subepidermal blistering disorders are not accompanied by the rigorous immunologic evaluation required. For example, many cases originally reported as bullous pemphigoid and mucous membrane pemphigoid (cicatricial pemphigoid) (MMP/CP) are now known to be better classified as EB acquisita or linear IgA bullous dermatosis (LABD). Many of the subepidermal blistering disorders may strikingly mimic each other clinically, leading to inappropriate diagnosis and making the histologic descriptions in the literature suspect. Finally, in order to rapidly improve the rash and symptomology of the patient, clinicians often embark on therapeutic regimens for the presumed clinical diagnosis. The therapy often consists of topical or systemic steroids and inhibitors of inflammation. Histopathologic examination of a biopsy is pursued only when the therapeutic response is nil or partial, calling into question the clinical diagnosis. Many submit biopsies without notifying the dermatopathologist of the therapy. Such therapy often suppresses the inflammatory infiltrate and the epidermal response and produces other histopathologic changes. The evolution and temporal relationship of histologic changes of dermatitides under various therapies are *not* sufficiently documented to allow optimal or, perhaps, even accurate diagnostic study. Biopsies should be taken of nontreated (locally or systemically) disease that has not been therapeutically altered, if possible. If therapy has been instituted, it should, ideally, be stopped at least a week, and optimally several weeks, before repeat biopsy.

Principles of Management

Principles of management for bullous disorders are diverse, reflecting their differing pathophysiologies. In the following sections, the management principles are briefly discussed for each of the major disease entities. In the final section, the management of immunobullous disorders is discussed in a more global manner.

SPONGIOTIC DERMATITIS

Definition and Evaluation

Spongiotic dermatitis may be acute, subacute, or chronic from a histologic perspective. The process is dynamic, and each specific type of dermatitis may or may not progress from the histologic acute to the chronic phase. Although the term *spongiotic dermatitis* is occasionally used interchangeably with *eczema*, the word *eczema* lacks specific meaning. *Spongiosis* refers to the accumulation of edema fluid between keratinocytes, in some

cases progressing to vesicle or even bulla formation. In most spongiotic dermatitis, lymphocytes are the primary infiltrating cell; however, neutrophilic spongiosis and eosinophilic spongiosis may be prominent in some cases (Tables 9-2 and 9-3). The categories of neutrophilic spongiosis and eosinophilic spongiosis are important because of the relatively small subset of diseases that produce these findings.

In *acute spongiotic dermatitis*, the stratum corneum is normal, and the epidermis is of normal thickness. The degree of spongiosis is variable, extending from slight to marked, with intraepidermal vesiculation in the latter instance. The surrounding keratinocytes may be stellate, surrounded by clear spaces representing the site of fluid collection (Fig. 9-1A and 9-3C). Papillary dermal edema is present, correlating with the degree of spongiosis. A lymphohistiocytic infiltrate is present around the superficial plexus, with exocytosis of lymphocytes into spongiotic foci. When biopsies are performed for diagnostic purposes, the acute stage is often over.

In *subacute spongiotic dermatitis*, there is usually mild-to-moderate spongiosis, occasionally with microvesiculation. The epidermis is moderately acanthotic. The parakeratotic stratum corneum may contain aggregates of plasma that is sometimes coagulated, as well as scattered lymphocytes and neutrophils, forming a crust (Fig. 9-4B, C). There is a superficial perivascular lymphohistiocytic infiltrate, which may be less prominent than in the acute phase. Impetiginization by gram-positive cocci (Staphylococci and Streptococci) may lead to neutrophilic crust. Excoriation and lichen simplex chronicus may develop in all forms of spongiotic dermatitis. Postinflammatory pigmentation may develop with melanophages with either hypermelanosis or hypomelanosis present clinically.

In *chronic dermatitis*, there is hyperkeratosis with areas of parakeratosis, often wedge-shaped hypergranulosis, and moderate to marked acanthosis. Spongiosis may be present focally, often minimal in degree clinically. The inflammatory infiltrate is often sparse, and papillary dermal fibrosis may be a prominent feature. The degree of spongiosis and quantity of the infiltrate reflect the present activity of the underlying dermatitis. The other changes, hyperkeratosis, wedge-like hypergranulosis, and acanthosis with vertical streaking of thick papillary dermal collagen, reflect lichen simplex chronicus (see in section "Lichen Simplex Chronicus"; Fig. 9-7B, C).

Specific Types of Spongiotic Dermatitis
Allergic Contact Dermatitis

Clinical Summary. The prototype of acute spongiotic dermatitis is allergic contact dermatitis, secondary to exposure to poison ivy. Usually between 24 and 72 hours after exposure to the antigen, the patient develops pruritic, edematous, erythematous papules and plaques and, in some cases, vesicles. Linear papules and vesicles are common in allergic contact dermatitis to poison ivy (urushiol), reflecting the points of contact between the plants or antigen-contaminated hands and the uninvolved skin. Other common causes of allergic contact dermatitis (Fig. 9-3A) include nickel, paraphenylenediamine, rubber compounds, fragrances, and preservatives in cosmetics. The histologic alterations to these antigens are often less striking in degree than those secondary to poison ivy.

Histopathology. Early lesions are acute spongiotic dermatitis. If vesicles develop, they may contain clusters of Langerhans cells,

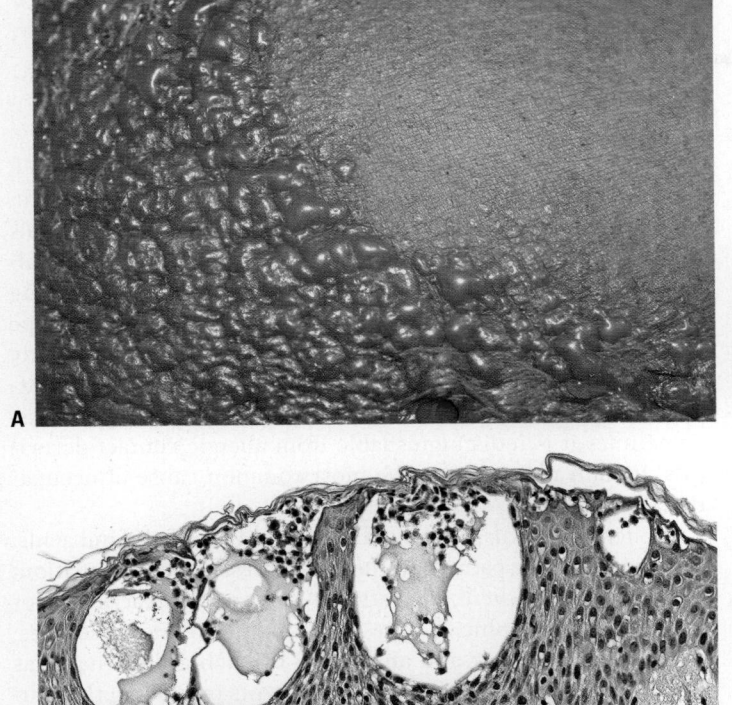

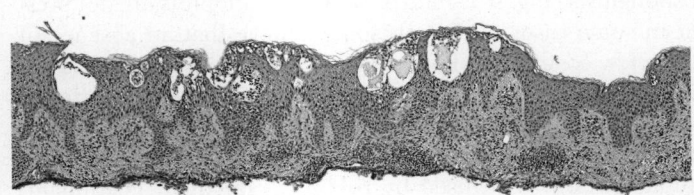

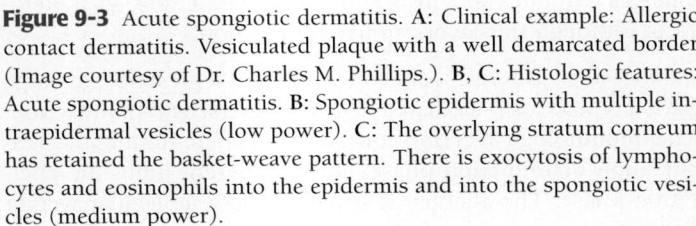

Figure 9-3 Acute spongiotic dermatitis. **A:** Clinical example: Allergic contact dermatitis. Vesiculated plaque with a well demarcated border (Image courtesy of Dr. Charles M. Phillips.). **B, C:** Histologic features: Acute spongiotic dermatitis. **B:** Spongiotic epidermis with multiple intraepidermal vesicles (low power). **C:** The overlying stratum corneum has retained the basket-weave pattern. There is exocytosis of lymphocytes and eosinophils into the epidermis and into the spongiotic vesicles (medium power).

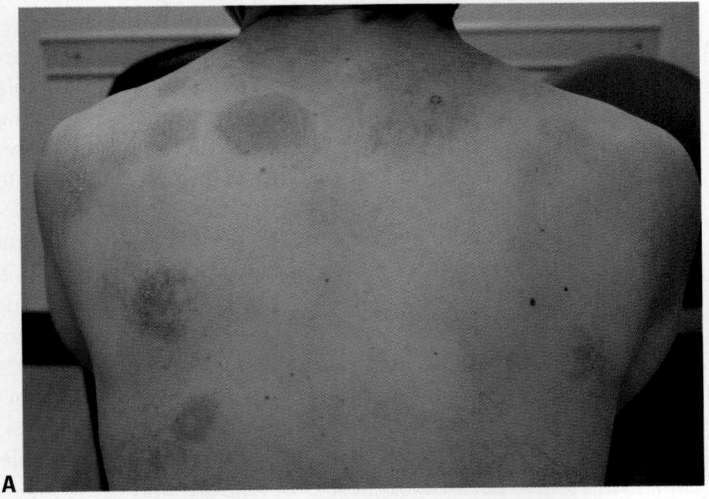

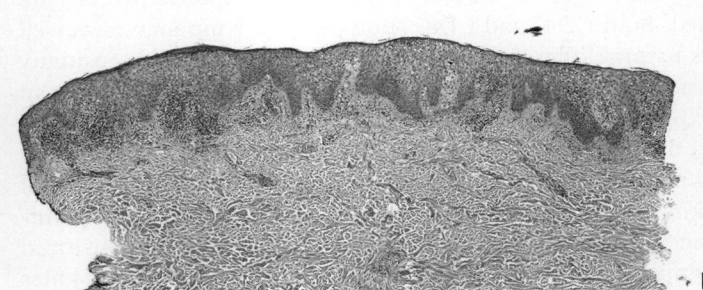

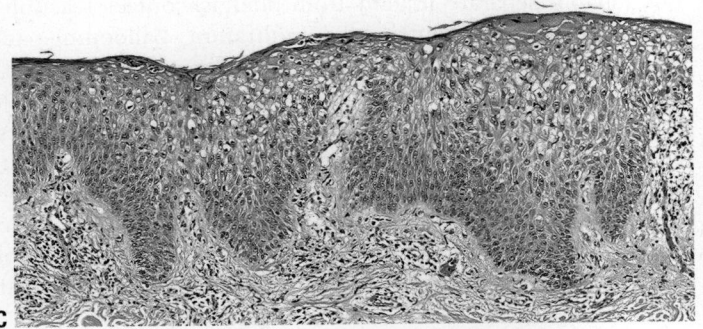

Figure 9-4 Subacute spongiotic dermatitis. **A:** Clinical example: Nummular dermatitis. Multiple round "coin-shaped" plaques on the back. **B, C:** Histologic features: Subacute spongiotic dermatitis. **B:** There is irregular acanthosis, spongiosis, and a superficial perivascular inflammatory infiltrate (low power). **C:** The spongiosis is accompanied by exocytosis of mostly lymphocytes. Parakeratosis containing serum crust is also present (medium power).

some of which are flask shaped. Some have stated that these Langerhans cell clusters, or "granulomas," are specific to acute allergic contact dermatitis; however, other spongiotic dermatitis variants may have these clusters. There is a superficial dermal infiltrate of lymphocytes, macrophages, and Langerhans cells with accentuation around the small vessels. Eosinophils may be present in the dermal infiltrate as well as within areas of spongiosis (Fig. 9-1A and 9-3B, C). Eosinophils are not present in some cases. Although some believe that an absence or only a few eosinophils favor nummular dermatitis, this has not been the author's experience (TJH). In patients with continued exposure to the antigen, the biopsy may show subacute dermatitis or, later, a chronic spongiotic dermatitis, often with lichen simplex chronicus caused by rubbing/scratching. Postinflammatory pigment alterations may develop.

The histopathologic features, as outlined, are idealized and, in any instance, reflect the character of the hapten, its resultant hapten–protein complex, and the particular immune response to that antigen. Some antigens may produce but minimal changes without spongiosis and only hyperkeratosis/parakeratosis, although this favors an irritant reaction.

Pathogenesis. Allergic contact dermatitis represents, in large part, a type IV cell–mediated delayed hypersensitivity reaction. The immunologic reaction consists of an afferent limb, the sensitization or induction phase, and an efferent limb, the elicitation phase. The allergen is usually of low molecular weight (a hapten) and lipid soluble. After penetrating the skin, the hapten binds covalently to a carrier protein to form a complete antigen, which is processed by antigen-presenting cells, principally the epidermal Langerhans cells, and other cutaneous dendritic cells. Keratinocytes are the second most important antigen-presenting cell in the epidermis. Langerhans cells/dendritic cells then migrate to the draining lymph nodes, where they present the antigen to T lymphocytes. The process triggers antigen-specific commitment and production of memory and effector T cells. Following subsequent exposure of the sensitized subject to the same allergen, an accelerated and more aggressive secondary immune response will be elicited. Both CD4+ and CD8+ subtypes of T lymphocytes as well as natural killer T cells participate in contact hypersensitivity reactions (1). The homing of lymphocytes to the antigen in exposed skin requires various cell adhesion molecules, such as lymphocyte function–associated antigen-1 (LFA-1) (2). Lymphocytes liberate various cytokines in the affected area of skin, including several interleukins, TNF-α, leading to a further influx of inflammatory cells, particularly nonsensitized lymphocytes and eosinophils (3,4). Furthermore, chemokines (CCL20 and CXCL) appear to be crucial regulators of both induction and expression of allergic contact dermatitis (5). In contrast to lipid-soluble haptens, metal ions activate inflammatory response through different mechanisms. Nickel, for example, directly activates Toll-like receptor 4 (TLR4) and generates a signal that promotes inflammation (6).

Principles of Management: Contact dermatitis is best managed through avoidance. Patch testing to environmentally relevant allergens can help identify causative agents. Registries of safe-to-use products, such as Contact Allergen Management Program (CAMP) are available through contact dermatitis societies (https://www.contactderm.org/resources/acds-camp).

Active lesions often require treatment with topical corticosteroids and/or topical calcineurin inhibitors; widespread or severe eruptions may warrant systemic corticosteroid therapy.

Irritant Contact Dermatitis

Clinical Summary. Ten clinical subsets have been described (7). This inflammatory reaction occurs after exposure to an irritant, a toxic compound that causes a reaction in most individuals who come into contact with it. Common irritants include alkalis, such as soaps, detergents, lye, and ammonia-containing compounds. The irritant response is determined by the type of chemical, its concentration, the mode of exposure, the body site, the barrier function locally, and the age of the patient. Atopy is a predisposing factor. The clinical morphology varies. Sometimes it is indistinguishable from allergic contact dermatitis. Irritant reactions are the most common cause of occupational dermatitis.

Chemical burns, usually caused by strong alkalis and acids, lead to immediate painful erythema progressing to vesiculation, necrosis, and, if severe, ulceration. Acute irritant reactions produce a monomorphic picture with scaling, redness, vesicles, pustules, or erosions, and are caused by such mild irritants as detergents and water with additives. Agents producing this pattern include tretinoin, benzalkonium chloride, dithranol, adhesive tapes, and cosmetics. Dryness, chapping, and absence of vesicles characterize chronic irritant contact dermatitis. This reaction pattern is often produced by repetitive contact with water, detergent, and solvents.

Histopathology. The histologic picture varies from extensive ulceration, to simply diffuse hyperkeratosis or parakeratosis with congestion and ectasia, to a spongiotic pattern essentially identical to that of allergic contact dermatitis. Langerhans cell clusters, eosinophils, and follicular spongiosis favor an allergic contact dermatitis over an irritant etiology. The variable features reflect the protean factors discussed previously. Some correlations are worthy of note. In some instances, there is significant necrosis with nuclear karyorrhexis and cytoplasmic pallor, apoptosis, and reticular degeneration. In severe reactions, the necrosis may extend into the dermis. Some irritants such as cantharidin and trichloroethylene produce acantholysis and neutrophilic infiltration in the epidermis (8). Other contactants may specifically target vascular endothelium. If ulcers are present, the exudate may produce an irritant effect in adjacent skin (eczematoid reaction). Some reactions may be entirely spongiotic, such as those attributable to weak irritants, strong irritants in low concentration, and those in the "irritable skin syndrome." Because of these observations and those made in positive patch test sites, routine histopathologic changes do not reliably separate irritant from allergic contact reactions, although necrosis, neutrophilic infiltration, ballooning, and acantholysis are more frequent in the former (Fig. 9-5A, B). In the recovery and chronic phase of irritant dermatitis, mild epidermal hyperplasia, sometimes psoriasiform, is often present. In other words, most common irritants lead to subacute and chronic spongiotic dermatitis histologic features essentially identical to those of allergic contact reactions. Some contact reactions may be lymphomatoid, granulomatous (chewing gum, etc.), pigmentary purpuric dermatosis–like, pustular, and urticarial in type.

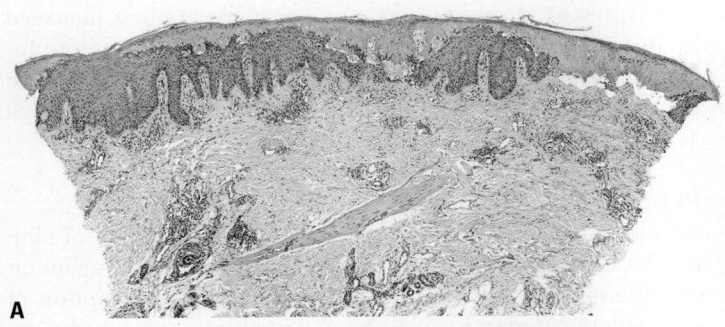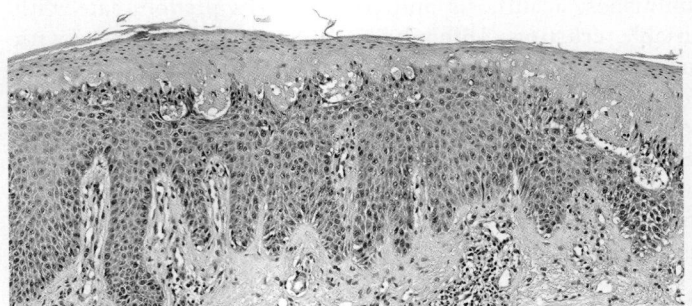

Figure 9-5 Irritant contact dermatitis. **A:** Surface necrosis with underlying epidermal spongiosis secondary to application of rubbing alcohol and vinegar (low power). **B:** Confluent surface necrosis (medium power).

Pathogenesis. The pathogenesis at the cellular and molecular levels of irritant contact dermatitis is not completely understood. Some individuals have increased stratum corneum permeability owing to loss of the filaggrin gene, giving rise to an increase in irritant reactions (9). Mechanisms of damage are variable with different irritants; these include keratin denaturation, damage of the permeability barrier through removal of surface lipid and water-holding substances, disruption of cell membranes and direct cytotoxic effects. Indeed, some contactants may cause both an allergic contact dermatitis and irritant contact dermatitis simultaneously. Recent studies indicate that very complex reaction patterns involving immunologic components occur in the irritant response. There are surprisingly more similarities than differences between irritant contact dermatitis and allergic contact dermatitis in morphology (10), clinical manifestation, chemokine expression, especially interleukins, and involvement of T cells (11–13), facilitated by chemokines secreted by lymphatic epithelium that promotes T-cell exodus.

Principles of Management: Avoidance of exposure to irritants is essential. Often, irritant dermatitis can be managed through use of appropriate protective equipment (such as a combination of cotton and rubber gloves) and aggressive emollient use. Dimethicone is a silicone-based polymer that is often used as a skin protectant in skincare products.

Pompholyx (Acral Vesicular Dermatitis, Dyshidrotic Dermatitis)

Clinical Summary. This entity is characterized by recurrent, severely pruritic, tense vesicles that classically involve the volar and lateral aspects of the fingers, palms, and, in some cases, the plantar surface and toes. Hands are much more frequently involved (70% vs. 20%) (14). Episodes may be precipitated/caused by drugs, foods, infections, "id" reactions, contact reactions, and emotional stress, oftentimes associated with atopic dermatitis (15). Many have precipitating conditions such as contactants (some systemic) at other cutaneous sites. In chronic cases, there may be more extensive involvement of the palms and soles. Although the eruption develops acutely, it may become chronic with erythema, lichenification, and fissuring. Secondary impetiginization is common. Exclusion of the precipitating factors, including the above considerations, is important therapeutically.

Histopathology. Spongiosis and intraepidermal vesiculation occur in acute lesions (Fig. 9-6A, B). There is a superficial perivascular lymphohistiocytic infiltrate with exocytosis of lymphocytes into spongiotic zones. Eosinophils are few or absent. The infiltration is usually mild, often less than expected given the degree of spongiosis. In acute lesions, the compact, thickened stratum corneum of acral skin remains intact, and the epidermal thickness is normal. With chronicity, spongiosis

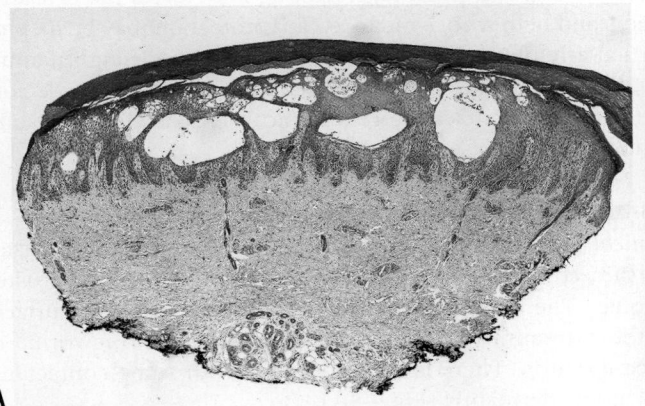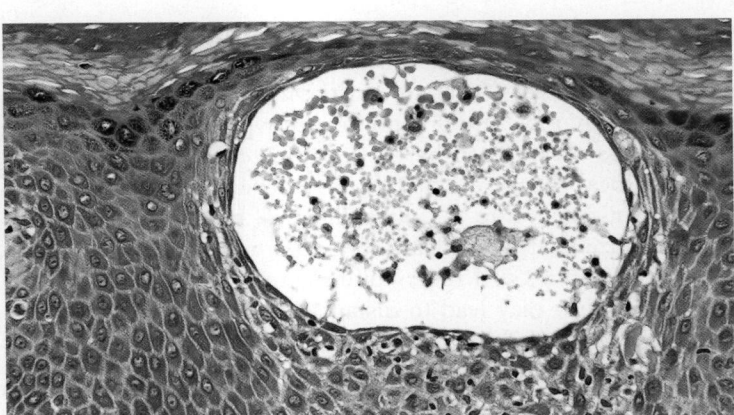

Figure 9-6 Pompholyx. Histologic features: Spongiosis with intraepidermal vesiculation, lymphocyte exocytosis, and a scant superficial perivascular lymphocytic infiltrate. In acral skin, the large intraepidermal vesicles are held intact by the thick stratum corneum **A:** Scanning power. **B:** High power. Intraepidermal vesicle containing fibrin, serum, and lymphocytes.

diminishes; acanthosis and parakeratosis predominate with variable crusting. Difficulty in differential diagnosis with pustular psoriasis may occur because of the formation of vesiculopustules in older lesions. A periodic acid–Schiff (PAS) stain (with or without diastase digestion) should always be performed on spongiotic vesicular lesions of the palms and soles, as tinea manuum and tinea pedis may mimic dyshidrotic dermatitis and other hand/foot spongiotic dermatitis histologically.

Principles of Management: Maintaining the skin barrier function through avoidance of irritants and consistent use of moisturizers is important. Mid- to high-potency topical steroids are the first line of treatment of dyshidrotic dermatitis. Topical calcineurin inhibitors, such as tacrolimus or pimecrolimus, may be helpful alone or, more often, in combination with topical steroids. Ultraviolet light in the form of UVA or narrow band UVB may help control chronic dyshidrosis. For severe disease, systemic agents such as prednisone and other immunosuppressive agents (mycophenolate mofetil (MMF), cyclosporine, methotrexate, azathioprine) may be required. Case reports and case series of successful use of dupilumab in dyshidrotic dermatitis have been published recently (16).

Autoeczematization or "Id" Reaction

Clinical Summary. A sudden generalized or localized vesicular dermatitis developing in association with a defined local dermatitis or infection is known as an "id" reaction. The lesions are pinhead-sized, acuminate, or flat-topped papules. The patient often has bullous tinea pedis or kerion; hence the name "*dermatophytid.*" In some cases, patients have a severe localized dermatitis, such as stasis dermatitis, with subsequent development of widespread papulovesicular lesions (17). Other forms of id reaction exist, such as that attributable to ionizing radiation therapy, bacterial infections, infestations, and contact dermatitis.

Histopathology. The features are those of acute spongiotic dermatitis, often with micro- or macrovesiculation. Eosinophils may be present. There is often some edema of the superficial papillary dermis with some large lymphocytes (presumably activated) in the upper dermis (18). The infiltrating cells are T cells: Those within the epidermis are principally CD8$^+$, and those within the dermis are principally CD4$^+$.

Pathogenesis. Id reactions have been postulated to represent hypersensitivity dermatitis to an autoantigen; however, this has never been proven. Several other possibilities exist. First, the reaction may represent a conditioned hyperirritability or responsiveness precipitated by the local infection or dermatitis. Acute local chemical irritation may lower the threshold for an irritant reaction to the same chemical at remote sites. Second, localized dermatitis leads to local production of cytokines by keratinocytes. If the cytokines are hematogenously disseminated, they may lead to distant skin hyperirritability. Circulating activated T lymphocytes may play a role in "id" reaction associated with allergic contact dermatitis. Lastly, dissemination of antigen (but not of whole infectious agents) from the local site may occur with a secondary response developing at a site of distant deposition. Microbial antigens have been identified in an id reaction in a patient with tuberculoid leprosy (19).

Principles of Management: "Id" reactions are best managed by treating the inciting localized eruption and treating the inflamed skin with topical steroids and emollients. Depending on the extent and severity of the id reaction, systemic agents such as prednisone may be required.

Photoallergic Dermatitis

Clinical Summary. Photoallergy is increased reactivity of skin to UVA and visible light, brought about by a chemical agent on an immunologic basis (Type 1 and IV) (20). The eruption of photoallergic dermatitis may be attributable to topical application of, or oral ingestion of, a photosensitizing agent, resulting in a photocontact dermatitis or photodrug eruption, respectively. Agents that may elicit photocontact dermatitis include soaps and cleansers (containing halogenated salicylanilides), perfumes (such as Musk ambrette), topical sulfonamides, sunscreens, benzocaine, and diphenhydramine. Common causes of photodrug eruption include thiazide diuretics, oral hypoglycemics, nonsteroidal anti-inflammatory drugs (NSAIDs), oral sulfonamides, and phenothiazines. The eruption is pruritic and composed of erythematous papules and confluent plaques on sun-exposed skin, usually the face, dorsal aspect of the arms, and the "V" of the neck.

Histopathology. The features are similar to those of an acute allergic contact dermatitis, showing variable spongiosis, in some cases with vesiculation, and a superficial perivascular lymphohistiocytic infiltrate with exocytosis. A deeper perivascular infiltrate and eosinophils are more common in photoallergic dermatitis induced by systemic ingestion of medications. With chronic exposure to the antigen, there is progression to subacute spongiotic chronic dermatitis, with diminished spongiosis, less intense inflammation, and more acanthosis.

Pathogenesis. In contrast, phototoxic reactions are "sunburn" reactions with epidermal apoptosis and necrosis with intraepidermal to subepidermal blisters, with the changes parallel to the degree of damage. Neutrophils may be prominent. The changes are similar to those of an irritant, in this case, light. Topical or systemic agents "sensitize" the skin to UVA/UVB (phytophotodermatitis, thiazides, NSAIDs).

Principles of Management: A thorough history of exposures, patch testing, and photopatch testing may reveal the causative agents and help with avoidance. Sun protection may be helpful, particularly physical blockers, such as zinc oxide and titanium dioxide. Some sunscreen ingredients may actually cause contact and photocontact allergies. Topical steroids may offer some benefit in select cases (21).

Nummular Dermatitis

Clinical Summary. The eruption is characterized by intensely pruritic, coin-shaped (nummular), erythematous, scaly, crusted plaques. The lesions tend to develop on the extensor surfaces of the extremities and are often mistaken for "ringworm" or tinea corporis. There is an association with some contactants and atopic dermatitis (Fig 9-4A).

Histopathology. Nummular dermatitis is the prototype of subacute spongiotic dermatitis; but it may proceed from acute to chronic stages. There is mild-to-moderate spongiosis, usually without vesiculation. Irregular acanthosis with some exocytosis of inflammatory cells is usually present. The parakeratotic stratum corneum contains aggregates of coagulated plasma, forming a crust. Mild papillary dermal edema and vascular dilatation may be present. There is a superficial perivascular infiltrate of lymphocytes, some eosinophils, and occasional neutrophils, with only uncommon progression to a lichenoid pattern.

Pathogenesis. The etiology of this entity is unknown. The routine and ultrastructural changes in nummular dermatitis resemble those of contact dermatitis. Intercellular edema is the most conspicuous finding. There is shearing and loss of desmosomes as spongiosis becomes marked.

Principles of Management: A search for associated conditions (atopy, contact reaction, drug, etc.) is required with the treatment of the underlying etiology. Nummular dermatitis often requires high-potency topical steroids to achieve relief.

Atopic Dermatitis

Clinical Summary. The eruption is characterized by areas of severe pruritus, erythema, scaling, excoriation, and with chronicity, lichenification. Acute lesions of atopic dermatitis begin as erythematous papules with serous exudates. Secondary lesions include excoriations and crusted erosions attributable to scratching. Subacute lesions appear as erythematous scaling papules and plaques. If the itch and rash progress uncontrolled, chronic lichenified atopic dermatitis develops, featuring accentuated skin markings and hyperpigmentation. Most patients are diagnosed in childhood; approximately one-third of cases are diagnosed before 1 year of age (22). There is a female predominance, and many patients have other atopic disorders such as allergic rhinitis or asthma. Increased incidence of contact dermatitis and susceptibility to cutaneous infection is also noted among patients with atopic dermatitis. In infants, the lesions predominate on the face and extensor surfaces of the extremities but later affect the flexural surfaces. The classically involved sites in older children and adults are the popliteal and antecubital fossae as well as the sides of the neck. Secondary bacterial infection with pustules is common. Approximately 50% resolve by the early teenage years.

Histopathology. In early phases, there is mild spongiosis, exocytosis of lymphocytes, and parakeratosis. Lymphocytes and scattered histiocytes are present around the superficial vascular plexus. In long-standing lesions, the rete ridges are regularly elongated, with less prominent spongiosis and cellular infiltrate. Hyperkeratosis and wedge-shaped hypergranulosis with areas of parakeratosis develop (lichen simplex chronicus). There appear to be an increased number of small vessels with thickened walls. Eosinophils may be present, although they are said to be fewer than in most cases of allergic contact dermatitis.

Pathogenesis. The current understanding remains incomplete. Atopic dermatitis develops as a result of complex interactions of genetic, environmental, and immunologic factors. Both abnormalities of immune regulation and barrier functions of the epidermis are involved. The immune factors include the differentiation of helper T cells, increased life span of eosinophils, multiple roles of IgE, the pattern of local cytokine expression, infectious agents, and superantigens (23). The initiation of atopic dermatitis appears to be driven by allergen-induced activation of type 2 T helper cells (T_H2 cells), leading to increased levels of interleukin-4, -10, and

-13. Elevated IgE ensues. IgE contributes to the inflammatory cell infiltrate by several mechanisms, including immediate/late phase reaction, allergen presentation by IgE-bearing Langerhans cells, and allergen-induced activation of IgE-bearing macrophages.

The mononuclear cell infiltrate in the lesions probably reflects a combination of both IgE-dependent mast cell/basophil degranulation, and T_H2 cell–mediated responses elicited during acute exposure to allergens, which include ingestants, inhalants, or contact aeroallergens such as human dander, grass pollens, and house dust mites (24).

The pattern of local cytokine expression plays an important role in modulating tissue inflammation and depends on the activity and/or duration of the lesion. Acute skin inflammation is associated with a predominance of interleukin IL-4 and IL-13 expression, and little INF-γ. But in chronic lesions, there are increased INF-γ-producing cells (25,26).

Abnormal epidermal barrier function is a well-recognized clinical association of atopic dermatitis. Filaggrin gene mutations (inherited or acquired), which result in impairment in barrier function and increased ease of allergen presentation to epidermal dendritic cells, may potentiate contact reactions (27).

No specific single gene is a unique marker for atopic dermatitis. Genomic screens of families with atopic dermatitis have implicated chromosomal regions that overlap with other skin diseases, including inflammatory and autoimmune skin diseases (28). The abnormal skin barrier genes, which lead to loss of functional filaggrin, reside on chromosome 1q21 (29). Increased protease activity and a lack of protease inhibitors predispose patients to the harmful effects of environmental agents (30). Chromosome 5q31 contains the IL-4 gene cluster family. Because IL-4 is central to the induction of IgE synthesis by B cells, it has been suggested that polymorphisms in the chromosome 5q31 region may be linked to the gene controlling total serum IgE in atopic individuals. Another possible candidate gene found on chromosome 11q13 is the high-affinity IgE receptor (31,32).

Principles of Management: Successful therapy of atopic dermatitis requires multiple modalities. Patients should use good bathing practices to improve epidermal barrier function. Lukewarm baths, moisturizing nonsoap cleansers (used without sponges or washcloths), avoidance of harsh abrasive scrubs, and extensive moisturization with thick, bland emollients are essential. Avoidance of fragrances and dyes in all products that contact the skin, including laundry products, is helpful. Humidification of room air during winter months will also help prevent excessive skin xerosis. First-line treatment for inflammation and pruritus is topical corticosteroids. Topical calcineurin inhibitors may be used in addition to, or instead of, topical steroids. Topical calcineurin inhibitors have the advantage of not causing skin atrophy and may be used for long-term control of chronic atopic dermatitis. Patients should be evaluated for superinfection, including both bacterial and, sometimes, viral infections. Dilute bleach baths may help control superinfections. Phototherapy with narrow band UVB may be helpful with widespread disease. Severe atopic dermatitis may require systemic agents. Systemic steroids should be used only in "crisis" situations because they will rapidly improve the disease; however, atopic dermatitis tends to flare quickly on discontinuation of steroid therapy. Other systemic therapies include cyclosporine, methotrexate, azathioprine, MMF, and systemic biologic therapies, such as dupilumab, which blocks IL-4 and IL-13. Other directed therapies for atopic dermatitis are in clinical trials.

Lichen Simplex Chronicus

Clinical Summary. Most patients with pruritus who chronically rub the skin may develop lichen simplex chronicus. It often develops in the setting of atopic dermatitis or allergic contact dermatitis. The lesions are pruritic, thick plaques, often with excoriation. The normal skin markings are accentuated; this finding is known as lichenification (Fig. 9-7A). Uncommonly, some patients develop macular or lichen amyloidosis.

Histopathology. Lichen simplex chronicus is the prototype or end stage of chronic dermatitis (Fig. 9-7B, C). There is hyperkeratosis interspersed with areas of parakeratosis, acanthosis with irregular elongation of the rete ridges, wedge-shaped hypergranulosis, and broadening of the dermal papillae. Slight spongiosis may be observed, but vesiculation is absent. Minimal papillomatosis is sometimes present. There may be a sparse superficial perivascular infiltrate without exocytosis. In the papillary dermis, there are an increased number of fibroblasts and vertically oriented collagen bundles. As rubbing increases in intensity and chronicity, epidermal hyperplasia becomes more florid and the fibrosis more marked.

Excoriations, which are punctate ulcerations lined by necrotic superficial papillary dermis, fibrin, and neutrophils, are often present; however, they may be present in many pruritic dermatoses, such as stasis dermatitis.

Pathogenesis. Features associated with a specific dermatitis may allow identification of the underlying cause.

Principles of Management: Management of lichen simplex chronicus requires mid- to high-potency topical steroids, often in an ointment form, and aggressive skin moisturization. Longer-term treatment with topical calcineurin inhibitors may be needed.

Seborrheic Dermatitis

Clinical Summary. Clinically, patients develop erythema and greasy scale symmetrically on the scalp, ears, eyebrows, nasolabial areas, and central chest (Fig. 9-8A). Rarely, patients with seborrheic dermatitis develop generalized lesions. In infants, the scalp ("cradle cap"), face, and diaper areas are often involved. It is said to be a rare cause of erythroderma. Seborrheic dermatitis is seen with increased frequency in patients with Parkinson disease, epilepsy, congestive heart failure, chronic alcoholism, zinc deficiency, and HIV infection. Patients with HIV infection often have severe refractory disease and atypical distribution of lesions (33).

Histopathology. The histopathologic features are a combination of those observed in psoriasis and spongiotic dermatitis. Mild cases may exhibit only slight subacute spongiotic dermatitis. The stratum corneum contains focal parakeratosis, with a predilection for the follicular ostia, a finding known as "shoulder parakeratosis" (Fig 9-8B). Occasional pyknotic neutrophils are present within parakeratotic foci (neutrophilic parakeratosis), sometimes with fluid (neutrophilic crust). There is moderate acanthosis with regular elongation of the rete ridges, mild spongiosis, and focal exocytosis of lymphocytes. The dermis contains a sparse mononuclear cell infiltrate and may be edematous (Fig. 9-8C). In HIV-infected patients, the epidermis contains apoptotic keratinocytes and expresses heat shock proteins, and the dermal infiltrate usually contains plasma cells.

Pathogenesis. The pathogenesis is unknown; the role of *Malassezia* sp. (*Pityrosporum*) in the etiology is controversial even though many patients have a good response to oral or topical ketoconazole (34,35).

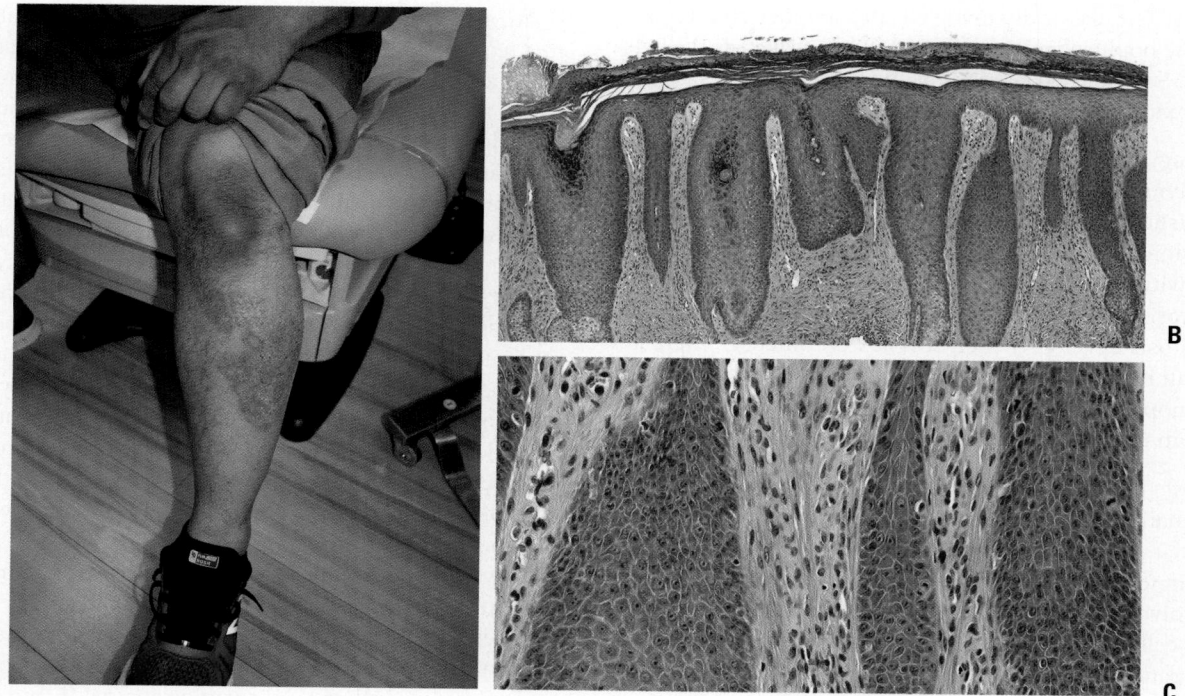

Figure 9-7 Lichen simplex chronicus. **A:** Clinical example: Sharply defined, lichenified plaques over the anterior leg. **B, C:** Histologic features. **B:** Psoriasiform epidermal hyperplasia with hyperkeratosis, parakeratosis, hypergranulosis, and dermal fibrosis (low power). **C:** Characteristic vertical collagen streaking in the papillary dermis (medium power).

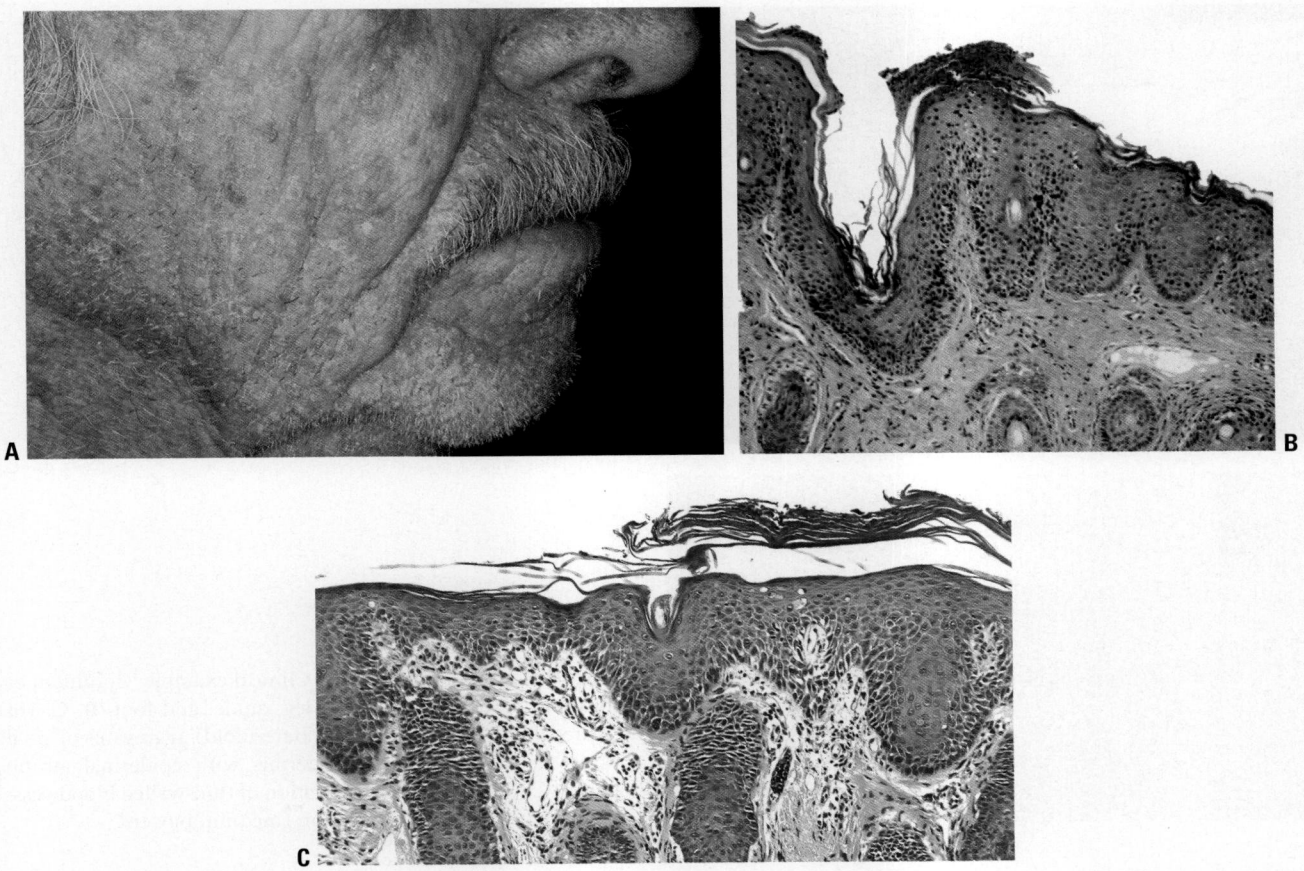

Figure 9-8 Seborrheic dermatitis. A: Clinical example. Erythematous scaly pink thin papules and plaques of the cheeks and nasolabial folds. (Courtesy of Dr. Charles M. Phillips.) B, C: Histologic features. B: There is follicular neutrophilic parakeratosis and hyperplastic epidermis with minimal spongiosis. C: Focally, there is more spongiosis and papillary dermal edema (both B and C: low-medium power).

Principles of Management: Seborrheic dermatitis may improve with zinc pyrithione, selenium sulfide, ketoconazole, corticosteroid, or tar shampoos. Topical antifungal creams, low-potency topical corticosteroids, and/or topical calcineurin inhibitors are also helpful. Seborrheic dermatitis of the scalp may require mid- to high-potency steroid solutions or lotions to achieve control. Extensive or recalcitrant seborrheic dermatitis should prompt a search for associated conditions, such as HIV, or neurologic diseases such as Parkinson disease and strokes.

Stasis Dermatitis

Clinical Summary. Patients with long-standing venous insufficiency and lower extremity edema may develop pruritic, erythematous, scaly papules and plaques on the lower legs, often in association with brown pigmentation and hair loss (Fig 9-9A). Ulceration is a frequent complication of long-standing stasis dermatitis.

Histopathology. The variable epidermis may be hyperkeratotic with focal parakeratosis and acanthotic to atrophic with focal spongiosis. There is proliferation of small thick-walled blood vessels in the papillary dermis, forming lobular aggregates (glomeruloid proliferation, Fig. 9-9B). The proliferation may be florid, mimicking Kaposi sarcoma, both clinically and pathologically (acroangiodermatitis) (36). Dermatoliposclerosis may develop with subcutaneous fibrosis with lipomembranous change (pseudocysts lined by thick walls of PAS-positive material, i.e., fibrinogen). There is a superficial perivascular lymphocytic

infiltrate that surrounds thickened capillaries and venules. The reticular dermis is often fibrotic. Extravasated erythrocytes and hemosiderin are usually present superficially, but they may be identified about the deep vascular plexus as well (Fig. 9-9C). Fibrin thrombi may be observed in the small vessels, likely reflecting flow disruption (loss of laminar flow) and anoxia. They do not indicate a concurrent systemic coagulopathy. Endothelial necrosis and neutrophils may be present as well, reflecting similar changes, and do not indicate leukocytoclastic vasculitis.

Principles of Management: Compression therapy is the mainstay of stasis dermatitis management. Compression stockings should be put on as soon as the patient wakes up to avoid the accumulation of fluid in the legs. Acute weeping stasis dermatitis benefits from astringent soaks, such as Burow's solution and short-term application of mid- to high-potency topical steroids. Topical calcineurin inhibitors may be helpful in longer-term therapy. The patient may also benefit from treatment of varicose veins. It is essential to check what products patients are applying to the inflamed area. Over-the-counter topical antibiotics are frequent causes of allergic contact dermatitis.

Spongiotic Drug Eruption

Spongiosis, although often a minor component, may occur in response to ingestants, drug administration, or internal parasites as type IV hypersensitivity reactions. Spongiotic dermatitis may occur in association with other reaction patterns (interface, lichenoid, superficial perivascular dermatitis, superficial and

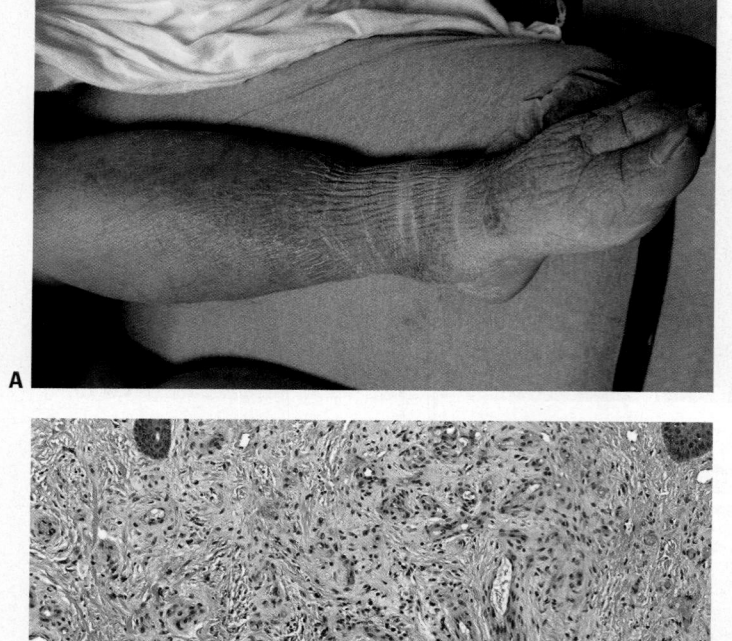

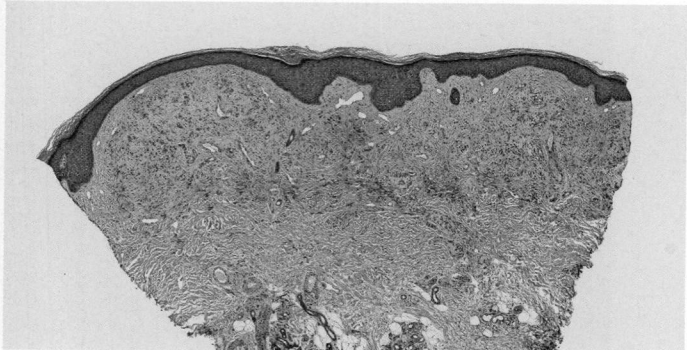

Figure 9-9 Stasis dermatitis. **A:** Clinical example. Confluent erythematous and scaly plaques of the leg, ankle, and foot. **B, C:** Histologic features. **B:** There are lobular (glomeruloid) aggregates of small blood vessels in the fibrotic upper dermis with epidermal atrophy (low power). **C:** Glomeruloid proliferation of thin-walled blood vessels with extensive hemosiderin deposition (medium power).

deep perivascular dermatitis, and pityriasis lichenoides-like). When multiple patterns are present, a drug etiology may be favored. The presence of eosinophils is often stressed, but they may be few or absent. The expanded use of immunomodulatory inhibitors targeting PD-1 and PDL-1 has led to the recognition of a wide range of secondary dermatologic manifestations, including psoriasis, acneiform reactions, bullous pemphigoid, autoimmune processes such as alopecia areata and dermatomyositis, sarcoidal reactions, and spongiotic and lichenoid hypersensitivity patterns in the drug-associated rashes (see also discussion in Chapter 11) (37).

Differential Diagnosis of Spongiotic Dermatitis

Acute spongiotic dermatitis may be seen histologically in pityriasis rosea, guttate parapsoriasis, digitate dermatitis, spongiotic drug eruptions, arthropod bite reactions, and dermatophyte infections initially. Later lesions show a subacute spongiotic dermatitis. Lesions of pityriasis rosea contain periodic discontiguous suprapapillary spongiosis (pityriasiform spongiosis), exocytosis of lymphocytes, and regularly disposed overlying mounds of (lenticular) parakeratosis. The spongiosis varies from micro- to macrovesicular. In addition, extravasated erythrocytes may be present in the involved papillae and overlying epidermis. Guttate parapsoriasis is similar to pityriasis rosea, but it lacks the intraepidermal erythrocytes and often has less spongiosis and less lymphohistiocytic infiltrate. Spongiotic drug eruptions tend to have a deeper infiltrate with eosinophils than other forms of acute spongiotic dermatitis. They usually do not vesiculate. In arthropod assaults, the epidermal changes are focal, corresponding to the site of attack (punctum), and

the infiltrate is often wedge-shaped. Bite or sting parts are often not found.

Pityriasis lichenoides, dermatophyte infection, or an arthropod bite reaction may show histopathologic features similar to those of *subacute spongiotic dermatitis*. In pityriasis lichenoides et varioliformis acuta, the lesions are sharply circumscribed. Apoptotic keratinocytes, dry neutrophil-rich scale, bandlike interface dermatitis, areas of epidermal necrosis, and a deeper perivascular infiltrate are present. Dermatophyte infections may have neutrophils within the stratum corneum, along with fungal hyphae (Gottlieb sign). However, PAS stain is often necessary to identify the fungal hyphae. PAS stain with diastase digestion removes glycogen and background "noise," allowing easier recognition of fungi. In addition, the reaction to superficial fungal infection has great variability with spongiotic, interface, and lichenoid reactions as well.

Conditions that have features of a *chronic dermatitis* include pellagra and other nutritional deficiencies, mycosis fungoides, and psoriasis, particularly if altered by therapy. In the nutritional deficiencies, upper epidermal pallor, necrosis, and neutrophilic infiltrate are characteristic. In mycosis fungoides, psoriasiform epidermal hyperplasia may be present, but the lymphocytes may have nuclear atypia and cerebriform morphology with epidermotropism, often "tagging along" in the basal unit most frequently in the absence of spongiosis. Owing to chronicity, there is "ropy" fibrosis of the papillary dermis. Lesions of psoriasis may resemble lichen simplex chronicus, but thinning of the suprapapillary plates, confluent parakeratosis, neutrophils layered between flat parakeratotic keratinocytes within the stratum corneum and neutrophilic exocytosis into the upper epidermis (spongiform pustules) with dilated tortuous capillaries juxtaposed to the suprapapillary epidermis are distinctive.

Other Disorders with Spongiotic Dermatitis
Erythroderma and Generalized Exfoliative Dermatitis
Clinical Summary. Erythroderma is characterized by generalized erythema over more than 70% to 80% of the body surface area, accompanied by scale, often in association with fever. The eruption is nonspecific and may be caused by various underlying conditions. In one study, 74.4% were associated with a preexisting dermatosis, 14.6% were idiopathic, 5.5% were related to drugs and malignancy (38). Psoriasis is the most common preexisting dermatosis; others include spongiotic "eczematous" dermatitis, pityriasis rubra pilaris, photosensitivity syndromes, and, rarely, scabies infestation, dermatophytosis, dermatomyositis, acute graft-versus-host (AGVH), pemphigus foliaceus, and even bullous pemphigoid. Many drugs have been incriminated, such as phenytoin, thiazides, NSAIDs, and recombinant cytokines; erythrodermatous drug eruptions should be considered severe, and patients should be evaluated for signs of systemic inflammation. A small percentage of erythroderma is associated with lymphoma, either paraneoplastic or more frequently cutaneous T-cell lymphoma, in the form of Sézary syndrome or erythrodermic mycosis fungoides.

Histopathology. A careful search for histologic features of any of the previously listed etiologies must be undertaken; however, the nature of the underlying dermatosis is not always discernible in the erythrodermic phase, and the changes are often those of nonspecific subacute spongiotic dermatitis. Erythrodermic lesions associated with underlying psoriasis (39) resemble early lesions of psoriasis with only mild epidermal hyperplasia, mild spongiosis, mounds of parakeratosis with a few neutrophils, and red cell extravasation in the papillary dermis (Auspitz sign). Blood vessels in the upper dermis are usually dilated. In cases of erythroderma related to mycosis fungoides, atypical lymphocytes with cerebriform nuclei are present in the infiltrate and epidermis. Eosinophils may be present. Drug-related cases might simulate mycosis fungoides with exocytosis, lymphocytic atypia (lymphomatoid), and presence of eosinophils. The presence of rare apoptotic keratinocytes may be a clue to the drug etiology.

The histopathologic findings are helpful in establishing the etiologic diagnosis in only about 40% of cases (40). Repeat biopsies and hematologic studies at regular intervals are recommended in patients without definitive diagnosis.

Principles of Management: The underlying cause of the erythroderma must be identified and treatment tailored toward that condition. The initial management of erythroderma regardless of etiology is the replacement of fluid, electrolyte, and nutritional losses the patient is experiencing owing to the exfoliative process and increased blood flow to the skin caused by dilatation of superficial blood vessels (41). Erythrodermic patients are at risk for secondary infection and bacteremia, high output heart failure, and significant metabolic disturbances. Aggressive topical care, often with wet wraps or baths, thick layers of low- to mid-potency topical steroid ointments, and a protective wrap such as a "sauna suit," may lead to rapid clinical improvement while the underlying cause is being evaluated.

Miliaria
Miliaria develops when sweating is associated with obstruction of the intraepidermal sweat duct. There are three types: miliaria crystallina, miliaria rubra, and miliaria profunda.

Clinical Summary. Miliaria crystallina develops when the sweat duct is obstructed within the stratum corneum. Asymptomatic, small, superficial, noninflammatory vesicles resembling dewdrops develop, mainly on the trunk, after severe sunburn or with profuse sweating during a febrile illness (Fig. 9-10A). The vesicles rapidly subside when sweating ceases or the horny layer overlying the vesicles exfoliates. In some cases, the eruption may be present at birth (42).

Miliaria rubra (prickly heat) ensues when the sweat duct is obstructed within the deeper layers of the epidermis. It generally develops during and after excessive sweating in skin covered by clothing. It may also occur after prolonged covering of the skin by occlusive polyethylene wraps. Anhidrosis and heat intolerance result, particularly when the trunk is occluded. The lesions consist of pruritic small papulovesicles surrounded by erythema. Pustules may develop.

Miliaria profunda usually develops after recurrent episodes of miliaria rubra, particularly in tropical climates. The sweat duct is occluded at the dermal–epidermal junction. Lesions are nonpruritic, flesh-colored papules and can result in widespread anhidrosis.

Histopathology. In *miliaria crystallina*, one observes intracorneal or subcorneal vesicles that are in continuity with the underlying sweat duct. A sparse to moderate infiltrate of neutrophils is seen at the periphery of the vesicle. The surrounding epidermis is spongiotic, and there is papillary dermal edema and sparse superficial perivascular inflammation.

In *miliaria rubra*, spongiotic vesicles are found in the stratum malpighii. Serial sectioning shows these vesicles to be in continuity with a sweat duct. Periductal lymphocyte infiltration and spongiosis are seen, as is an infiltrate in the underlying dermis (Fig. 9-10B). In many instances, the distal intraepidermal sweat duct is filled with amorphous "casts" that are PAS positive and diastase resistant. Miliaria pustulosa is a variant of miliaria rubra, with pustule formation in the superficial aspect of the eccrine duct (Fig. 9-10C).

In *miliaria profunda,* the features are similar to those of miliaria rubra, but the inflammatory changes involve the lower epidermis and superficial dermis.

Pathogenesis. In *miliaria crystallina,* the obstruction of the sweat duct within the stratum corneum is caused either by mild damage to the epidermis from a preceding sunburn or by excessive hydration of the stratum corneum. In neonates, excess hydration of the stratum corneum *in utero* in combination with immature eccrine ducts may cause swelling of the ductal epithelial cells and occlusion of the duct (43). In *miliaria rubra*, increased environmental temperature plays an important role (43). Aerobic bacteria are thought to contribute to the obstruction of the acrosyringium. In favor of this view are the frequent presence of *Staphylococcus aureus* within the sweat ducts and the fact that the development of miliaria rubra under an occlusive polyethylene film can be prevented by the application of antibacterial solutions.

The PAS-positive, diastase-resistant, amorphous plug within the acrosyringium may occur as a result of injury to the luminal cells. The inflammation, casts, and spongiosis occur

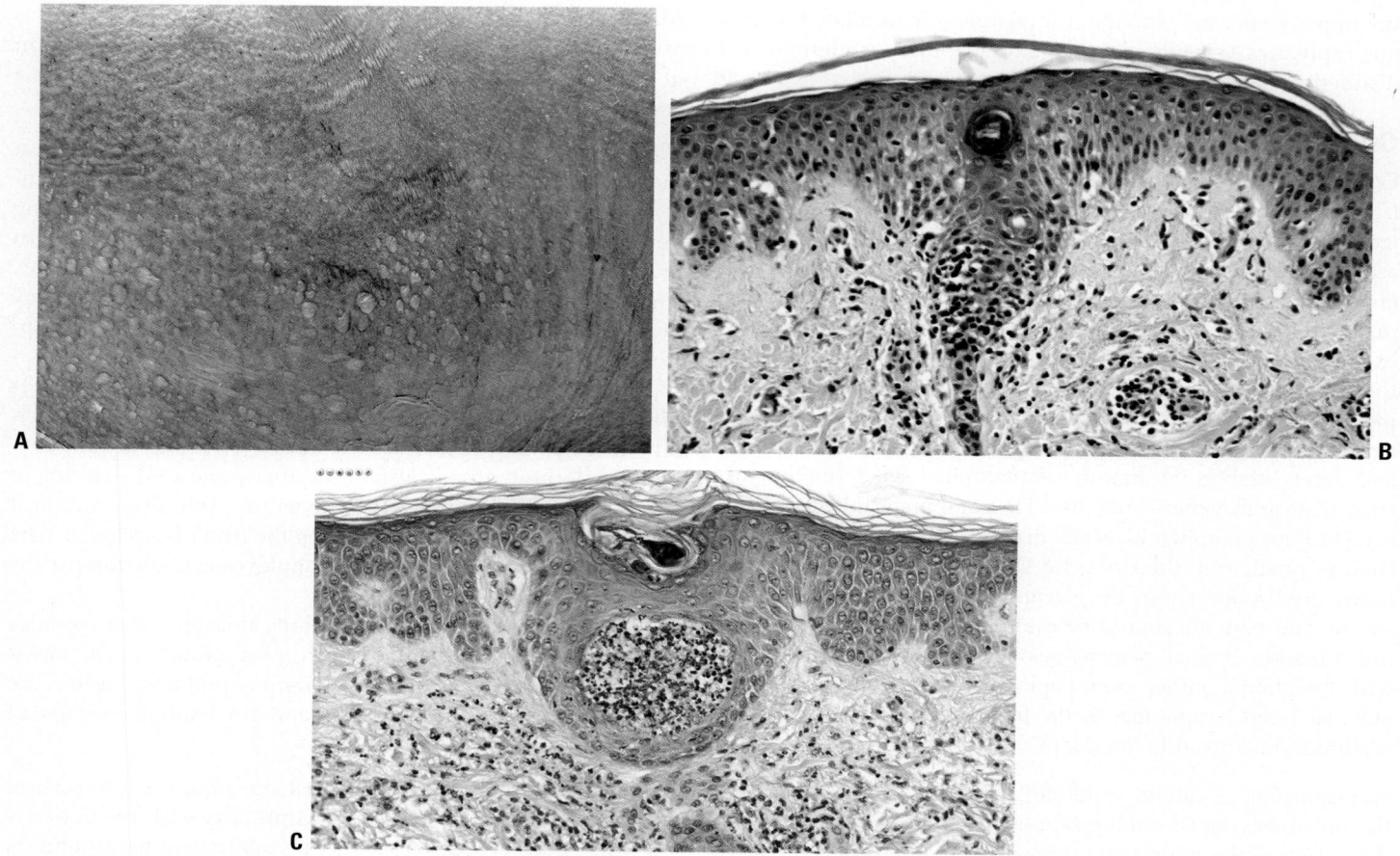

Figure 9-10 Miliaria crystallina, rubra, and pustulosa. A: Crystallina. Clinical example. Multiple, superficial pinpoint vesicles. B, C: Histologic features. B: Rubra. There is spongiosis adjacent to and within the acrosyringium and upper eccrine duct containing lymphocytes. C: Pustulosa. Neutrophilic pustule in the lower acrosyringium and superficial portion of the eccrine duct (both B and C: medium power).

after 48 hours of occlusion and resolve after 14 days. When old, the damaged stratum corneum is desquamated. Tape stripping can restore sweating, supporting a reversible, high-level poral blockage.

Principles of Management: Miliaria can often be prevented with a cooler environment, showering, frequent positional changes, and antipyretics (if needed). Most miliaria will improve when patients are more mobile and their environments and skin are cooled off. Some patients benefit from either low- or mid-potency topical steroids.

Immunologic Deficiency Diseases Associated with Spongiotic Dermatitis

Familial Leiner Disease
In this syndrome, infants develop generalized seborrheic dermatitis, severe diarrhea, recurrent local and systemic infections, and marked wasting. Death is usually caused by septicemia. Biotin deficiency–associated dysfunction of the components of complement (C3, C4, C5) exists, in addition to other cellular and humoral immune defects.

Hyperimmunoglobulin E Syndrome (Job Syndrome)
In this autosomal dominant (STAT3) or recessive (DOCS, PGM3, SPINKS, TRK) disease, patients have recurrent pyogenic infections, atopic dermatitis, extreme elevation of serum IgE, and defective neutrophil chemotaxis attributable to decreased production of interferon-*gamma* (IFN-γ) (44). The infectious

complications include recurrent cold staphylococcal abscesses, furunculosis, otitis, sinusitis, and staphylococcal pneumonia in the various subtypes. It is associated with abnormal neutrophil chemotaxis secondary to decreased interferon-γ secreted by T lymphocytes.

Wiscott–Aldrich Syndrome
This X-linked recessive disorder affects males and is characterized by recurrent, systemic bacterial and viral infections, purpura caused by thrombocytopenia, and an atopic dermatitis-like eruption because of progressive depletion of nodal and circulating T cells; death due to infection or lymphoma often ensues in the first decade of life. There is association with spindle cell hemangioma.

Chronic Granulomatous Disease
This X-linked recessive disorder affects males, beginning in infancy with perioral dermatitis. The dermatitis often progresses to granulomatous lesions accompanied by cervical adenitis. Suppurative and granulomatous infections develop in the skin, lungs, bone, and liver, most commonly owing to *S. aureus*. Death occurs in most cases in childhood or adolescence. The defect lies in decreased capacity of neutrophils to generate hydrogen peroxide and kill catalase-positive bacteria and fungi. *In vitro*, neutrophils are unable to reduce nitroblue tetrazolium dye after phagocytosis, a useful screening test for the disease. The X-linked disease arises because of mutations and deletions

for the gene that codes gp91 protein (p91-PHOX). Other autosomal recessive gene defects affecting PHOX proteins play a role in some patients.

Rare disorders may give rise to spongiotic blisters, including acrodermatitis enteropathica/glucagonoma syndrome, and acrokeratosis paraneoplastica (Bazex syndrome). Graft-versus-host disease (GVHD) has been reported to have a spongiotic dermatitis, as may the eruption of lymphocyte recovery.

PEMPHIGUS GROUP

As first demonstrated in 1943, acantholysis is the characteristic feature of the bullae of pemphigus, of which the vulgaris variant is by far the most common (80%). Pemphigus has been associated with several autoimmune diseases, malignancies (not limited to paraneoplastic autoimmune multiorgan syndrome [PAMS], also known as paraneoplastic pemphigus [PNP] variant), and other immunobullous diseases (bullous pemphigoid, etc.). The acantholysis appears to result from *in vivo* bound antibodies first discovered in 1964 (45); however, the exact mechanism is disputed. Pemphigus is characterized as an autoimmune blistering disease presenting clinically with flaccid intraepithelial blisters, erosions, and ulcerations of the skin and mucous membranes—histologically with acantholysis and immunologically with *in vivo* bound and circulating autoantibodies against the cell membrane components of

keratinocytes important in cell–cell adhesion. Circulating autoantibodies are present in almost 100% of patients with active disease, and their titer usually correlates with disease activity. These antibodies are demonstrable by direct immunofluorescence (DIF) testing of skin and indirect immunofluorescence (IIF) testing of serum or enzyme-linked immunosorbent (ELISA) assay. The use of these techniques is now the accepted practice in the diagnosis of all antibody-mediated primary vesiculobullous disorders (see Table 9-6). Pemphigus can be divided into, at least, six types: (a) pemphigus vulgaris, with its reactive state, pemphigus vegetans; (b) pemphigus foliaceus, with its lupus-like variant, pemphigus erythematosus, and its endemic variant, fogo selvagem (several varieties—Brazil, Tunisia, and Columbia); (c) drug-induced pemphigus, (d) IgA pemphigus; (e) PNP; and (f) herpetiform pemphigus (HP), which has grouped small vesicles that simulate DH, thus giving its name, but is a variant of pemphigus vulgaris or foliaceus.

Pathophysiology of Pemphigus

The following pathogenetic mechanism is the one that is currently generally accepted, but newer data indicate it is incomplete and that other mechanisms may be more integral or, at least, complementary to this standard model elaborated in what follows.

The most important target antigens originally described for pemphigus (Table 9-7) are located in the desmosomes, the

Table 9-6

Direct Immunofluorescence in Vesiculobullous Dermatoses*

Dermatosis	Principal Immunoreactant(s)	Site	Pattern
Pemphigus, all variants except:	IgG	ICS	Lacelike, dot-like
IgA pemphigus	IgA	ICS	Lacelike, dot-like
	IgG	ICS	Lacelike, dot-like
PNP/PAMS	IgG	ICS	Lacelike, dot-like
	C3, IgG	BMZ	Linear
	C3, IgG	BMZ	Granular
Bullous pemphigoid	C3, IgG	BMZ	Linear
Mucous membrane pemphigoid	C3, IgG	BMZ	Linear
Cutaneous cicatricial pemphigoid			
Anti-p200 pemphigoid	C3, IgG	BMZ	Linear
Pemphigoid gestationis	C3	BMZ	Linear
Epidermolysis bullosa acquisita	C3, IgG	BMZ	Linear
Bullous LE	C3, IgG	BMZ	Linear
	C3, IgG	BMZ	Granular
Dermatitis herpetiformis	IgA	BMZ	Granular/Thready"
Linear IgA dermatosis	IgA	BMZ	Linear
Erythema multiforme	C3, IgM	BMZ	Granular
	C3, IgM, fibrinogen	Vessels	Granular
Porphyria/pseudoporphyria/bullous dermatosis of hemodialysis	IgG, C3	BMZ	Glassy, broad
		Vessels	Glassy, broad

*Other immunoglobulins may be present, but they are less intense when present and less frequently observed.

ICS, squamous intercellular substance; LE, lupus erythematosus; PNP/PAMS, paraneoplastic pemphigus/paraneoplastic autoimmune multiorgan syndrome; BMZ, epidermal basement membrane zone.

Table 9-7

Principal Target Antigens in Pemphigus

Disease	Autoantibodies	Antigens	Location of Antigens
Pemphigus vulgaris:			
Mucosal mainly	IgG	Desmoglein 3 (130 kDa)	Desmosomes
Mucocutaneous	IgG	Desmoglein 3 (130 kDa)	
		Desmoglein 1 (160 kDa)	
Pemphigus foliaceus	IgG	Desmoglein 1 (160 kDa)	Desmosomes
Herpetiform pemphigus	IgG	Desmoglein 1 (160 kDa, most common)	Desmosomes
		Desmoglein 3 (130 kDa)	
Paraneoplastic pemphigus (PNP/PAMS)	IgG	Desmoglein 1 (160 kDa)	Desmosomes or hemidesmosomes
		Desmoglein 2 (122 kDa)	
		Desmoglein 3 (130 kDa)	
		Desmoplakin 1 (250 kDa)	
		Desmoplakin 2* (170 kDa)	
		Desmocollin 1 (100 kDa)	
		Desmocollin 2 (100 kDa)	
		Desmocollin 3 (130 kDa)	
		Envoplakin (210 kDa)	
		Periplakin (190 kDa)	
		Plectin (450 kDa)	
		BPAG1 (230 kDa)**	
		Plakoglobin (184 kDa, 115 kDa).	
		γ-Catenin (plakoglobin, 82 kDa)	
Drug-induced pemphigus (autoimmune variants)	IgG	Desmoglein 3 (130 kDa)	Desmosomes
		Desmoglein 1 (160 kDa)	
Drug-induced pemphigus (toxic variant)	–	–	–
IgA Pemphigus:			
SPD type**	IgA	Desmocollin 1 (110/100 kDa)	Desmosomes
IEN type**	IgA	Desmoglein 1 (160 kDa)	
		Desmoglein 3 (130 kDa)	
IgG/IgA pemphigus	IgG/IgA	Desmoglein 1 (160 kDa)	Desmosomes
		Desmoglein 3 (130 kDa)	
		Desmocollins (rare)	

*a-macroglobulin-like.

**BPAG1, bullous pemphigoid antigen; SPD, subcorneal pustular dermatosis; IEN, intraepithelial neutrophilic.

most prominent adhesion junctions in stratified squamous epithelium. The desmosome complex contains desmogleins and desmocollins as transmembrane constituents and plakoglobin, plakophilin, and desmoplakins as cytoplasmic constituents (Fig. 9-11). Desmogleins and desmocollins are members of the cadherin supergene family (46,47), a group of calcium-dependent proteins that play an important role in the formation and maintenance of tissue integrity. The cadherin molecules form dimers as their functional unit, with the extracellular domain from one cell binding to an opposing cell. The cytoplasmic domain of the cadherin associates with plakoglobin, which links intermediate filaments (i.e., keratins) to the desmosome through desmoplakin. The extracellular epitopes of the desmogleins and desmocollins are the most frequent targets of the antibodies. Of these, desmoglein 1 and desmoglein 3 are the best characterized and most important diagnostically. Desmoglein 1 is a 160-kDa molecule that is expressed in greater intensity in the upper layers of the epidermis but in only small quantities in squamous mucosa. It is the primary target antigen in pemphigus foliaceus. Desmoglein 3 is a 130-kDa molecule that localizes primarily in the deeper layer of epidermis and throughout the thickness of squamous mucosa.

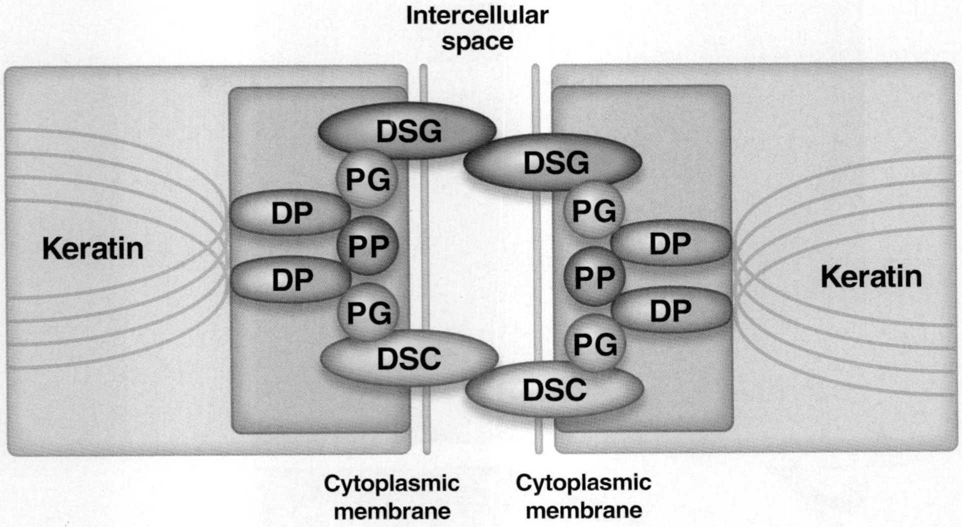

Figure 9-11 Schematic model of the desmosome. The desmosome complex includes desmogleins and desmocollins as transmembrane components and plakoglobin, plakophilin, and desmoplakin as cytoplasmic components. The cytoplasmic domains of desmoglein and desmocollin associate with plakoglobin, which links intermediate filaments (keratin) to the desmosome through desmoplakin. DSC, desmocollin; DSG, desmoglein; DP, desmoplakin; PG, plakoglobin; PP, plakophilin. (Courtesy of Dr. H. Wu.)

It is the principal target antigen in pemphigus vulgaris (48). Because mucosal epithelium expresses mainly desmoglein 3 but skin expresses both desmoglein 1 and 3, damage by antibodies to desmoglein 3 alone results in oral lesions with or without skin lesions. If both desmoglein 3 and desmoglein 1 antibodies are present, cutaneous lesions, as well as mucosal lesions, appear, and the disease tends to be more severe (49). Some patients have had antibodies to the desmocollins as well. IgE antibodies have been detected (50,51).

In summary, the localization and the degree of expression of desmogleins 1 and 3 along with the presence of anti-desmoglein 1 antibodies alone, anti-desmoglein 3 antibodies alone, or both antibodies together reliably predict the mucosal and/or cutaneous involvement and the severity of pemphigus in each patient. Less is known about the desmocollins (52). IgA pemphigus has had autoantibodies to desmocollins. Lastly, we have observed conversion of the vulgaris to foliaceus variant with change in antibody profile and hybrid cases. Pemphigus vulgaris and pemphigus foliaceus, in general, cannot be separated on DIF study because full-thickness squamous intercellular substance deposition of IgG is present in most cases owing to the ubiquity of desmogleins 1 and 3 in the epidermis, albeit in apparently different concentrations. On occasion, pemphigus foliaceus will exhibit only superficial epidermal IgG intercellular substance deposition, allowing a definitive diagnosis.

Lastly, a panoply of antibodies directed against other desmosomal and cytoplasmic constituents has been described whose role in producing lesions may be contributory, in particular to acetylcholine receptors (53). Furthermore, compensating cellular processes play a role in adhesion such that acantholysis develops only after they are overwhelmed and includes keratin production and/or keratin retraction triggered by the desmosomal binding of IgG (54). A role for T cells has been confirmed as well (55,56). Apoptosis may be a contributing factor even though it is not prominent in routine study (except basal apoptosis in PAMS/PNP). There is upregulation of apoptotic genes by pemphigus antibodies with clustering of FasR, FasL, and caspase-8 on the cell surface before the lesions develop. Caspase 3 may directly cleave Dsq3 and other desmosomal proteins (57–59). The exact immune mechanism of the loss of tolerance for Dsq3 or Dsq1 is unclear. In addition, the

intracellular signaling pathways that alter other events/proteins necessary for adhesion may be important. The different views on the exact pathogenesis of pemphigus have been covered in detail (60).

Pemphigus Vulgaris

Clinical Summary. Pemphigus vulgaris develops primarily in older individuals, presenting with large and flaccid bullae. They break easily and leave denuded areas that tend to increase in size by progressive peripheral detachment of the epidermis, leading, in some cases, to widespread cutaneous involvement. Any age may be affected, and rarely familial cases have occurred, for which a genetic marker has been described (HLA-E*0103X) (61), and there is association with human leukocyte antigens (HLA) haplotypes (62). The lesions characteristically involve the oral mucosa (Fig. 9-12A), scalp, midface, sternum, groin, and pressure points (Fig. 9-12B). Oral lesions are almost always present and may be the first manifestation of the disease (10% of cases) (63). Before corticosteroids became available, the mortality of this disease was high because of fluid loss and superinfection. Even today, death from these latter issues is not uncommon (up to 20%) (63–65). Some (not just the PNP variant, to be discussed later) cases of classic pemphigus vulgaris and pemphigus foliaceus have been associated with malignancies that will be discussed later.

Histopathology. It is important that early blisters, preferably small ones, are selected for biopsy. Care should be given to keeping the epidermis attached to the dermis, because the torque applied in punch biopsies may separate the blister roof from the blister base. Therefore, one may use a refrigerant spray before excising the blister with a punch biopsy. A shave biopsy is a good method of obtaining an appropriate sample if delicately performed and the specimen is handled with care. If no recent blister is available, an old one may be moved into the neighboring skin by gentle vertical pressure with a finger (positive Asboe–Hansen sign). The newly created cleavage will reveal early and specific histologic changes.

The earliest recognized change may be either eosinophilic spongiosis or, more commonly, "spongiosis" in the lower epidermis (Fig. 9-12C). This "spongiosis" may actually represent

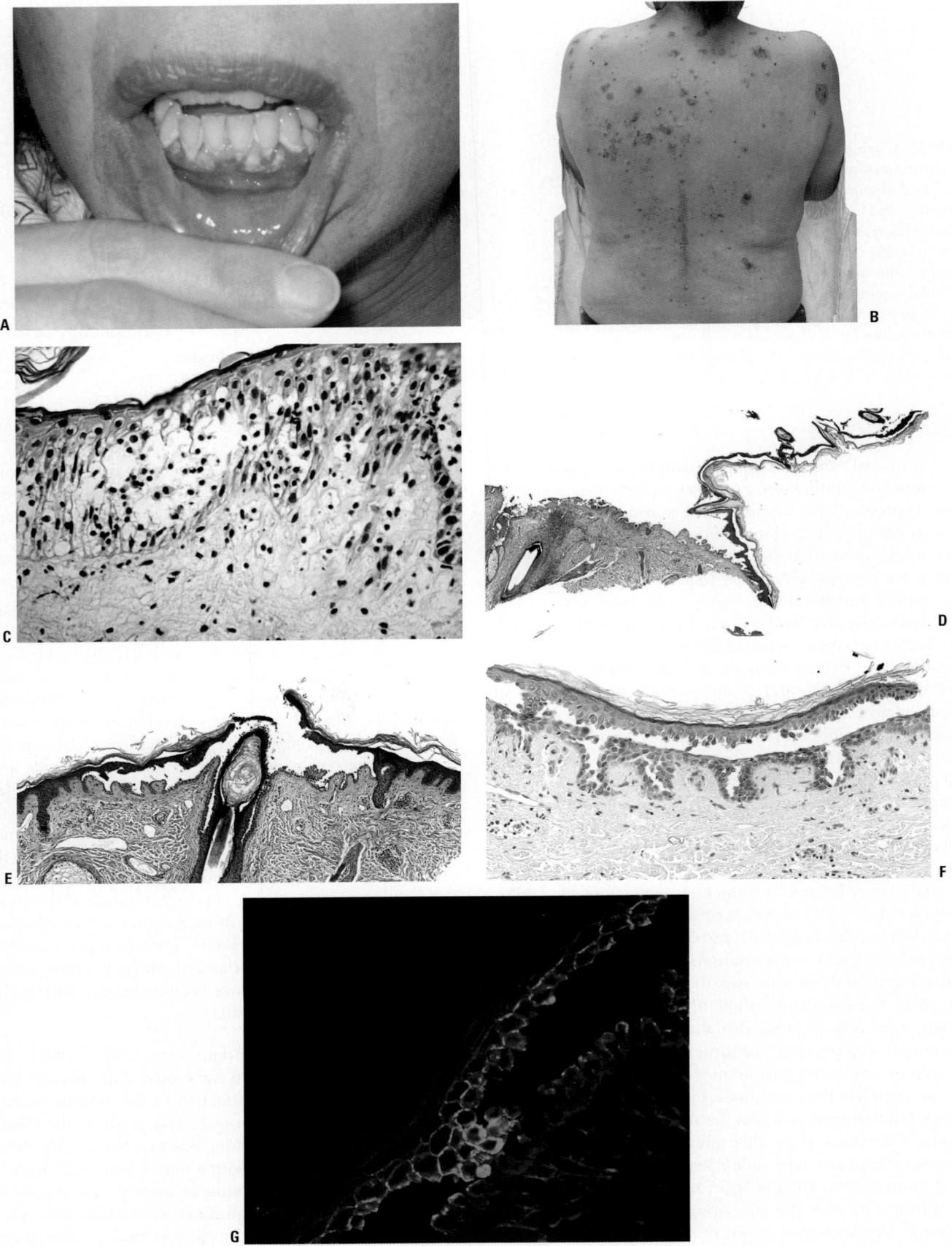

Figure 9-12 Pemphigus vulgaris. **A, B:** Clinical examples. **A:** Multiple gingival erosions with white fibrinous bases. (Courtesy of Kenneth Tsai, MD, PhD.) **B:** Eroded plaques, some confluent, on the back. **C–F:** Histologic Features. **C:** Skin. The earliest changes consist of intercellular edema with eosinophilic spongiosis and loss of the integrity of intercellular bridges in the lower epidermis (high power). **D:** The "roof" of the bulla, "peeled off" to the right, contains the upper portion of hair follicles in this image (scanning power). **E:** A suprabasal intraepidermal acantholytic vesicle extends into the upper hair follicle. Elongate dermal papillae lined by a single layer of basal keratinocyte, so-called villi, are seen in the bulla floor (low power). **F:** The suprabasal blister contains acantholytic cells (medium power). **G:** There is lacelike squamous intercellular space deposition of IgG.

the earliest manifestation of acantholysis rather than true spongiosis as defined earlier. Acantholysis leads first to the formation of clefts and then to blisters in a predominantly suprabasal location (Fig. 9-12D–F). The intraepithelial acantholysis extends into adnexal structures, and occasionally into the stratum spinosum. The basal keratinocytes, although separated from one another through the loss of attachment, remain firmly attached to the dermis like a "row of tombstones." Within the blister cavity, the acantholytic keratinocytes, singularly or in clusters, have rounded condensed cytoplasm about an enlarged nucleus with peripherally palisaded chromatin and enlarged nucleoli. In some patients, there are varying quantities of anti-desmoglein 1 and anti-desmoglein 3 antibodies, leading to variable planes of acantholysis. There is little inflammation in the early phase of blister formation. If present, it is usually a sparse, lymphocytic perivascular infiltrate accompanied by dermal edema. If, however, eosinophilic spongiosis is apparent, few to numerous eosinophils may infiltrate the dermis. Neutrophilic spongiosis may be the initial lesion rarely (and characteristically present in IgA pemphigus).

The phenomenon of eosinophilic spongiosis occurs occasionally in other blistering diseases, particularly in their early phases, including contact dermatitis, pemphigus foliaceus, bullous pemphigoid, pemphigoid (herpes) gestationis, drug eruptions, spongiotic arthropod bite reactions, and transient acantholytic dermatosis (TAD) (Table 9-3). Several important changes ensue as the lesions age. First, a mixed inflammatory cell reaction consisting of neutrophils, lymphocytes, macrophages, and eosinophils may develop. Because of the instability of the blister roof, erosion and ulceration may occur. Older blisters may also have several layers of keratinocytes at the blister base because of keratinocyte migration and proliferation. Lastly, there may be considerable downward growth of epidermal retia, giving rise to so-called "villi" (Fig. 9-12F). Follicular acantholysis is an important diagnostic feature.

The evaluation of patients with only oral lesions is difficult because intact blisters are rarely encountered owing to the trauma of mastication, and biopsies may show only erosion and ulceration. Indeed, it is best to sample the edge of a denuded area with intact mucosa in an attempt to demonstrate the typical pathologic changes. Clinicians frequently cannot distinguish between an ulcer and the intact inflamed mucosa, because both are often white and shaggy. In patients with only oral lesions, biopsies of intact oral mucosa for DIF testing are more sensitive than biopsies of lesions for routine light microscopic evaluation. Therefore, biopsy for DIF study from the upper buccal cheek mucosa is necessary when there is extensive ulceration. Serum contents may insudate into the squamous intercellular substance, particularly into the lower portion of the mandibular mucosa yielding false positive DIF tests.

Cytologic examination using a Tzanck preparation is useful for the rapid demonstration of acantholytic epidermal keratinocytes in the blisters of pemphigus vulgaris. For this purpose, a smear is taken from the underside of the roof and from the base of an early freshly opened bulla. Giemsa stain is applied with subsequent rinsing and air-drying. Because acantholytic keratinocytes are occasionally seen in various nonacantholytic vesiculobullous or pustular diseases as a result of secondary acantholysis, cytologic examination represents merely a preliminary test and should not supplant histologic examination. The acantholytic keratinocytes often mimic herpetically infected cells and may result in misdiagnosis.

Immunofluorescence (IF) Testing. The edge of a blister with intact surrounding normal skin, uninvolved skin adjacent to a blister, or adjacent erythematous skin should be supplied for study. The tissue may be snap-frozen or transported in Michel medium. DIF testing is a very reliable and sensitive diagnostic test for pemphigus vulgaris in that it demonstrates lacelike IgG in the squamous intercellular/cell surface areas in up to 95% of cases, including early cases and those with very few lesions, and in up to 100% of cases with active disease (Fig. 9-12G) C3 may be identified in up to 50% of cases. When routine DIF study is negative, immunofluorescence trichoscopy may demonstrate IgG intercellular substance deposition (66). Routine DIF study may remain positive after clinical disease has subsided. In late lesions, when acantholysis is well developed, the lacelike intercellular/cell surface pattern of IgG may become dot-like, paralleling electron microscopic findings and correlating with aggregation of desmosomes on the cell surface. Negative DIF findings when the patient is in remission may be a good prognostic indicator (67). False positives on DIF study may occur. On occasion, it may be difficult to distinguish intercellular staining of pemphigus from nonspecific staining; for example, epidermis in spongiotic dermatitis, psoriasis, bullous impetigo, and adjacent to ulcers secondary to a number of disorders may have insudation of serum into the intercellular substance. Often IgM, IgA, fibrinogen, and albumin are present as well, indicating nonspecific trapping in the false-positive tests. Immunoperoxidase methods have achieved roughly the same sensitivity as the IF method, but they have not replaced IF testing as the prime diagnostic tool.

For IIF testing of serum, unfixed frozen sections of monkey esophagus or normal human skin have been used as substrate because they yield the most sensitive substrates for indirect IF tests. Polyclonal circulating IgG autoantibody (mostly IgG4) is demonstrated in the squamous intercellular substance in 80% to 90% of cases (68), and the titer correlates with disease activity. Some data indicate that antiDsg1 antibody level may be the best predictor of recurrent disease (69), and ELISA study results have shown to correlate best with disease activity (66). False-positive IIF tests occur. In a series of 1,500 patients with circulating pemphigus antibodies, approximately 1% had no evidence of clinical disease. False-negative tests may occur in 5% of cases. Antibodies that mimic or that may give *in vitro* deposition in stratified squamous epithelium in the absence of pemphigus have been reported in burns, penicillin allergy, toxic epidermal necrolysis (TEN), systemic lupus erythematosus (SLE), myasthenia gravis, bullous pemphigoid, CP, lichen planus (LP), and in patients with antibodies directed against blood groups A and B. Such antibodies are present in low titer and are thought to be nonpathogenic. Anti-desmoglein autoantibodies are sometimes found in patients with no bullous disease. For example, they have been found in patients with silicosis (70) and in relatives of patients with pemphigus vulgaris (71). Pemphigus may evolve in some of these patients, and so follow-up evaluations are key in this latter setting.

Pathogenesis. The originally described and most important target antigens in pemphigus (Table 9-7) are located in the desmosome. Now there are over 40 pemphigus antigens described (72). It is clear that pemphigus antibodies are integral to the pathogenesis of pemphigus.

Several antibody binding mechanisms, with some experimental support, have been suggested:

1. Desmoglein compensation. This is the standard model in which the distribution of Dsg1 and Dsg3 in the epidermis and mucosa and the antibodies directed against these targets determine the planes of cleavage and initiate acantholysis.
2. Multiple hit hypothesis. Acantholysis develops only after the mechanisms of adhesion and repair are overcome by multiple antibodies binding to structures that incapacitate normal adhesion.
3. Antibody-induced apoptosis. Markers of apoptosis appear before acantholysis in some systems studied.
4. Steric hindrance. Antibody binding does not allow normal structure and function of desmosomes leading to acantholysis.
5. Basal cell shrinkage. Collapse of cytoskeletal structures caused by the retraction of tonofilaments from desmosomes precedes desmosomal loss of integrity and function, resulting in basal cell shrinkage (53,73–75).

Compelling evidence has accumulated that IgG autoantibodies against desmoglein 3 and desmoglein 1 are pathogenic and play a primary role in inducing the blister formation in pemphigus. Affinity-purified IgG from pemphigus vulgaris sera recognizes the extracellular domain of desmoglein 3 and causes suprabasal acantholysis when injected into neonatal mice (60,76). Furthermore, when anti-desmoglein 3 IgG from pemphigus vulgaris is immunoabsorbed with the extracellular domains of desmoglein 3, those sera no longer have the ability to cause blisters in neonatal mice (60). Although the pathogenic role of anti-desmoglein autoantibodies in blister formation is assured, the exact sequence of events that occur after antibody binding is not totally understood. Conformational epitope mapping of desmoglein 3 in pemphigus vulgaris suggests that the aminoterminal residue 1–161 is the target of autoantibodies (77). This segment is in the extracellular domain that is essential for cell–cell adhesion. One possibility is that these antibodies interfere directly with the adhesive interaction of desmogleins between cells by steric hindrance. Another possibility is that the disruption of cell–cell adhesion is mediated by signal transduction. Proteinases, likely induced by pemphigus antigen–antibody union, may play an important role in acantholysis. However, some evidence speaks against this possibility (78). Although complement fixation (79) and cytokine production play a part in the final pathway of acantholysis by pemphigus antibodies and may promote acantholysis, acantholysis occurs in experimental systems in the absence of complement. Of course, cytokine production in such keratinocyte culture systems occurs. The stimulus for the formation of autoantibodies is unknown, although drugs, viral infection, trauma, ionizing radiation, and PUVA therapy have been implicated because they have preceded the onset of pemphigus. Pemphigus vulgaris is rarely associated with internal cancer. Castleman disease, multiple myeloma, thymoma, myasthenia gravis, localized scleroderma, Graves disease, SLE, and interstitial lung disease are known associations (63,80–84). The involvement of the oral mucosa in pemphigus vulgaris is attributable to the high expression of desmoglein 3 and the much lower expression of desmoglein 1 in the squamous mucosa. A serologic biochip assay (not only in pemphigus) has shown great promise in the diagnosis of multiple specific antibodies in primary immunobullous diseases (85).

Ultrastructural Study. The intercellular cement substance, or glycocalyx, is partially or entirely lysed in lesions with early acantholysis. There is widening of the intercellular spaces with intact desmosomes. As the intercellular space is widened, there is separation of the two opposing attachment plaques of the desmosomes, so single attachment plaques, with adherent tonofilaments, are seen at the periphery of keratinocytes. As acantholysis progresses, the desmosomes are gradually endocytosed, and their production cannot keep up with their destruction. The keratinocytes develop numerous cytoplasmic processes that often interdigitate with one another. All of the early ultrastructural changes in pemphigus vulgaris are extracellular. Only after the dissolution of the desmosomes does retraction of the tonofilaments to the perinuclear area develop with ultimate degeneration of the acantholytic cells in most studies. The cohesion of the basal keratinocytes with the basement membrane zone is not affected in pemphigus vulgaris because of the preservation of structures connecting the basal keratinocytes with the dermis. Immunoelectron microscopy shows that the immunoglobulins are deposited on the surface of the keratinocytes in a discontinuous globular pattern in the extracellular domains of desmosomes (85).

Differential Diagnosis. In early blisters that are free of secondary changes, such as the degeneration or regeneration of epidermal cells, the histopathology of pemphigus vulgaris is characteristic. Important differential diagnoses include Hailey–Hailey disease and TAD. Hailey–Hailey disease has full-thickness ("dilapidated brick wall") acantholysis, epidermal hyperplasia, and an impetiginized scale crust. The acantholysis in Hailey–Hailey does *not* extend down follicles as it does in pemphigus. TAD may exhibit small foci of intraepidermal acantholysis, but these are only a few rete wide in contrast to the uniform widespread acantholysis observed in biopsies of pemphigus vulgaris. Disorders that are characterized by focal acantholytic dyskeratosis are readily separated from pemphigus vulgaris by the presence of abnormal granular keratinocytes and parakeratotic cells, "corps ronds" and "corps grains," respectively. Although light microscopic examination of pemphigus lesions is important, positive DIF study is the gold standard in diagnosis at this time and must be pursued in all cases in which pemphigus vulgaris is considered.

Principles of Management: Prior to initiating treatment for pemphigus vulgaris, patients must be assessed for secondary infections and any potentially causative medications. The first line of treatment of extensive pemphigus vulgaris is systemic steroids and a steroid-sparing agent. In a network meta-analysis–based comparison of first-line steroid-sparing adjuvants for the treatment of pemphigus vulgaris and pemphigus foliaceus, the authors evaluated conventional immunosuppressive agents versus rituximab as the best first-line steroid-sparing agent. Steroid-sparing agents included azathioprine, cyclophosphamide, dexamethasone–cyclophosphamide pulse, and MMF. Rituximab was determined to be the best choice for first-line pemphigus treatment in terms of efficacy and safety (86). In a letter to the editor of the *New England Journal of Medicine (NEJM)*, Ahmed et al. reported long-term remissions in patients with recalcitrant pemphigus vulgaris after treatment with a combination of rituximab and IVIG (87).

Pemphigus Vegetans

Clinical Summary. This is an uncommon variant of pemphigus vulgaris, comprising only 1% to 2% of cases (70). Historically, pemphigus vegetans has been divided into the Neumann type and Hallopeau type. In the more severe Neumann type, the disease begins and ends as pemphigus vulgaris, but many of the denuded areas heal with verrucous vegetations that may contain small pustules in early stages. The Hallopeau type is relatively benign, having pustules as the primary lesions instead of bullae. Their development is followed by the formation of gradually enlarging verrucous vegetations, especially in intertriginous areas. Oral involvement is almost always present (88).

Histopathology. In the Neumann type, the early lesions consist of bullae and denuded areas that have the same histologic picture as that of pemphigus vulgaris. As the lesions age, however, there is formation of "villi" and verrucous epidermal hyperplasia (Fig. 9-13A). Numerous eosinophils are present within the epidermis and dermis, producing both eosinophilic spongiosis and eosinophilic pustules accompanied by neutrophilic abscesses on occasion (Fig. 9-13B, C). Acantholysis may not be present in older lesions. In the Hallopeau type, the early lesions consist of pustules arising on normal skin with acantholysis in small clefts, many in a suprabasal location. The clefts are filled with numerous eosinophils and degenerated acantholytic epidermal cells. Early lesions may reveal more eosinophilic abscesses than in the Neumann type. The subsequent verrucous lesions are histologically identical to the Neumann type.

Pathogenesis. Pemphigus vegetans is a variant of pemphigus vulgaris in which verrucous vegetations develop. It is unclear why such vegetations develop in some cases of pemphigus vulgaris and not in others. However, they tend to develop in areas of relative occlusion and maceration with subsequent bacterial infection, suggesting a response to superinfection.

Differential Diagnosis. The principal differential diagnosis is pyoderma (or pyostomatitis) vegetans, a condition often associated with inflammatory bowel disease, particularly ulcerative colitis. It can mimic pemphigus vegetans clinically and histologically (89). In pyoderma vegetans, neutrophils are more commonly found, and intraepidermal eosinophilic abscesses and acantholysis are rare. DIF study is negative in pyoderma vegetans (90). Halogenoderma and blastomycosis-like pyoderma must be excluded as well.

Principles of Management: Treatment is similar to that of pemphigus vulgaris, although local care with appropriate topical antimicrobials and in some cases anti-inflammatory therapies may be beneficial. Systemic retinoids and dapsone may also be helpful (91). Surgical modalities, such as excision, intralesional triamcinolone, or chemical cautery of vegetative lesions, should be considered in addition to systemic therapies (92).

Pemphigus Foliaceus

Clinical Summary. Usually developing in middle-aged individuals, pemphigus foliaceus may have a chronic localized, chronic generalized course or may rarely present as an exfoliative dermatitis/erythroderma. Patients may present with flaccid bullae that usually arise on an erythematous base or as scaly, crusted erosions without evident blisters (Fig. 9-14A). Because of their superficial location, the blisters break easily, leaving shallow erosions more commonly rather than the ulcerations seen in pemphigus vulgaris. Oral lesions are uncommon to rare. The Asboe–Hansen sign is positive, and Tzanck preparation reveals acantholytic granular keratinocytes. Fogo selvagem (endemic pemphigus foliaceus) is clinically, histologically, and

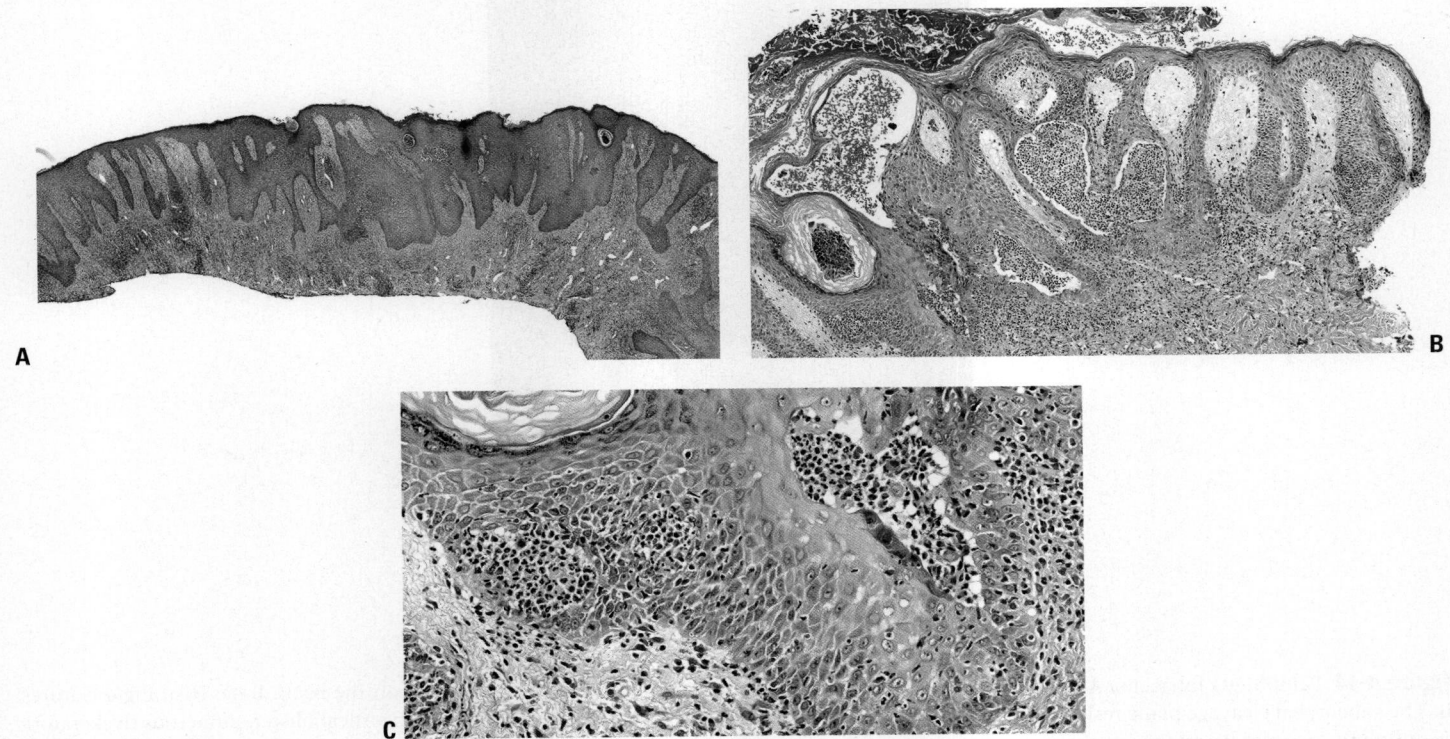

Figure 9-13 Pemphigus vegetans. **A:** There is marked vegetative epidermal hyperplasia with intraepidermal eosinophilic abscesses and dermal fibrosis (scanning power). **B:** Epidermal hyperplasia with several intraepidermal abscesses and dermal edema in this example (low power). **C:** The intraepidermal abscesses are composed of eosinophils and a few acantholytic keratinocytes (medium power).

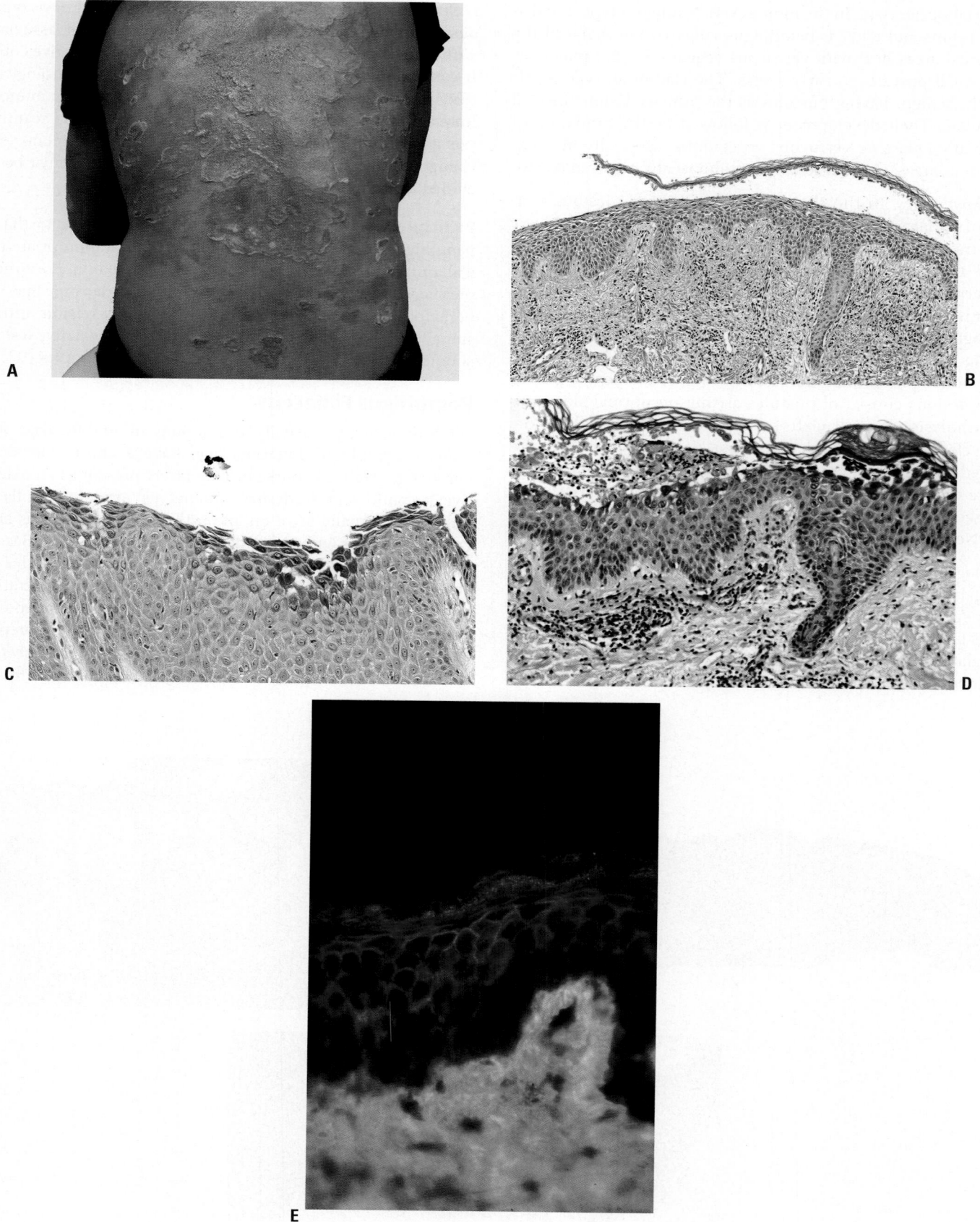

Figure 9-14 Pemphigus foliaceus. **A:** Clinical example. Confluent scaly eroded thin plaques are present on the back. **B–D:** Histologic features. **B:** The subcorneal cleavage plane resides beneath the thin blister roof (low power). **C:** In the setting of a subcorneal blister, numerous dyskeratotic acantholytic granular keratinocytes are diagnostic of pemphigus foliaceus. The blister roof is not present. Acantholytic dyskeratotic keratinocytes on the surface of the epidermis (high power). **D:** A subcorneal blister contains acantholytic cells and neutrophils (high power). **E:** Direct immunofluorescence. The IgG is deposited in the intercellular spaces throughout the epidermis. Rarely, as in this case, the IgG is present in greater quantity in the superficial layers. In this biopsy, the roof of the blister is absent, a frequent event secondary to trauma, leaving an artifactual loss during tissue processing.

on routine immunologic studies indistinguishable from pemphigus foliaceus and rarely pemphigus vulgaris as well (90). It develops in those who live or visit areas close to rivers and streams in Brazil, Columbia, other South American countries, and Tunisia, the peak incidence being at the end of the rainy season. The cause of endemic pemphigus foliaceus is unknown, but substantial epidemiologic evidence suggests that it is precipitated by an environmental factor. A case control study found that farmers exposed to black fly (*Simulium* sp.) bites were much more likely to develop fogo selvagem than farmers who were not bitten (93). Sunlight may exacerbate the condition (94). A protein from the saliva of one sandfly species reacts with anti-desmoglein antibodies, suggesting this as a pathogenetic factor (95). There appears to be epitopic spreading because some cases have had antibodies to desmocollins. There are clinical and immunologic differences between the Columbian fogo selvagem, Brazilian fogo selvagem, and nonendemic pemphigus foliaceus. Whereas the principal autoantibodies are reactive with Dsg1, the pemphigus foliaceus antigen, the Columbian variant much more frequently had antibodies to desmoplakin I and envoplakin (96). The Brazilian variant had antibodies to Dsg3 much more frequently; 51% had IgM antiDsg1 in contrast to other forms of pemphigus foliaceus and the Columbian variant (97). Both variants are associated with interaction with hematophagous insects.

Histopathology. The earliest change consists of acantholysis in the upper epidermis, within or adjacent to the granular layer, leading to a subcorneal bulla in some instances (Fig. 9-14B–D). More commonly, enlargement of the cleft leads to detachment of the stratum corneum without bullae observed clinically. The acantholytic granular cells may be spindled and not round because their cell shape is fixed at the time of IgG binding to the desmoglein or that the binding to the desmoglein permits differentiation to a granular keratinocyte architecture. The number of acantholytic keratinocytes is usually small, often requiring a careful search to identify them. Secondary clefts may develop, leading to detachment of the epidermis in its midlevel. These clefts may extend to above the basal layer, rarely giving rise to limited areas of suprabasal separation. In the setting of a subcorneal acantholytic blister, dyskeratotic granular keratinocytes are diagnostic for this disorder. Eosinophilic spongiosis may be prominent with intraepidermal eosinophilic pustules. Thus, the histologic features of pemphigus foliaceus may have three patterns: (a) eosinophilic spongiosis; (b) a subcorneal blister, often with few acantholytic keratinocytes; and (c) a subcorneal blister with dyskeratotic granular keratinocytes (Fig. 9-12C). The character of the inflammatory infiltrate is variable and depends on the age of the lesion, whether a blister is present, whether the superficial portion of the epidermis has been detached, and whether there is impetiginization or necrosis of the blister roof.

IF Testing. DIF testing of perilesional or lesional skin is positive in most of the cases. Two patterns of pemphigus antibody deposition have been described. In most cases, there is full-thickness squamous intercellular substance deposition of IgG (Fig. 9-14E). Rarely, IgG may be localized only to the superficial portion of the epidermis. IIF testing of serum reveals squamous intercellular substance deposition of IgG in 80% to 90% of cases. Diaz and others have found IgM-antiDsq1 antibodies are present in Brazilian fogo selvagem in much greater incidence than in other forms of pemphigus vulgaris and pemphigus foliaceus (97).

Pathogenesis. As in pemphigus vulgaris, the autoantibodies of pemphigus foliaceus appear to be pathogenic (IgG4). During the course of the disease, the antibody levels fluctuate and have some correlation with disease activity. The aminoterminal end of the pemphigus foliaceus antigen, desmoglein 1, is expressed more intensely in the upper layers of the epidermis (47,48), which explains the superficial cleavage plane of pemphigus foliaceus. Interestingly, in staphylococcal scalded skin syndrome (SSSS), and its localized form, bullous impetigo, the exfoliative exotoxin produced by *S. aureus* specifically binds and cleaves desmoglein 1, resulting in blister formation at identical levels of the epidermis as pemphigus foliaceus (98,99). In addition, desmoglein 1 is concentrated in the upper torso and is less prominent in the buccal mucosa, scalp, and lower torso, correlating with lesion distribution (100).

Ultrastructural Study. There is early loss of intercellular cement substance within the lower epidermis, associated with a decrease in the number of desmosomes and the formation of tortuous microvilli from the keratinocyte surface. However, acantholysis is most pronounced in the upper layers of the epidermis. In the midepidermis, many keratinocytes have perinuclear arrangement of the tonofilaments and homogenization of the perinuclear tonofilament bundles as evidence of dysmaturation.

Differential Diagnosis. The differential diagnosis includes SSSS, impetigo, subcorneal pustular dermatosis (SPD; Sneddon–Wilkinson), and IgA pemphigus (see differential diagnosis of IgA pemphigus). IF testing may be required to separate SSSS from pemphigus foliaceus, because a few acantholytic cells may be observed in SSSS. The lesions of pemphigus foliaceus may become impetiginized and secondarily altered, producing pustules as in impetigo, SPD, and IgA pemphigus. Pemphigus foliaceus contains more acantholytic keratinocytes than do the other two disorders, and pustules are the primary lesions in SPD. Because the lesions of pemphigus foliaceus may become superinfected, the finding of bacteria does not confirm a diagnosis of bullous impetigo; therefore, IF testing is critical. SPD usually produces large dome-shaped subcorneal pustules rather than the flaccid flat blisters and pustules of pemphigus foliaceus.

Principles of Management: Treatment of pemphigus foliaceus is similar to that of pemphigus vulgaris (86). Patients are also at risk for viral or bacterial superinfection of open areas, particularly when immunosuppressed.

Pemphigus Erythematosus

Clinical Summary. Also known as Senear–Usher syndrome, pemphigus erythematosus is a variant of pemphigus foliaceus that gets its name from its lupus erythematosus–like clinical appearance, in which the erythematous plaques and patches are in a butterfly distribution. It commonly arises in middle age and has a female predominance, further complicating the differential diagnosis of lupus erythematosus. There appears to be a predilection for black individuals (101). Pemphigus erythematosus, infrequently drug-associated, may occur in association with subacute cutaneous lupus erythematosus with these drugs: oral antifungals, especially terbinafine, biologics, including TNF-α inhibitors, antiepileptics, proton pump inhibitors (e.g., omeprazole), thrombocyte inhibitors, penicillamine, atorvastatin, captopril, NSAIDs, and thiol-containing drugs (102). There is an association with hyperimmune HLA haplotypes (103).

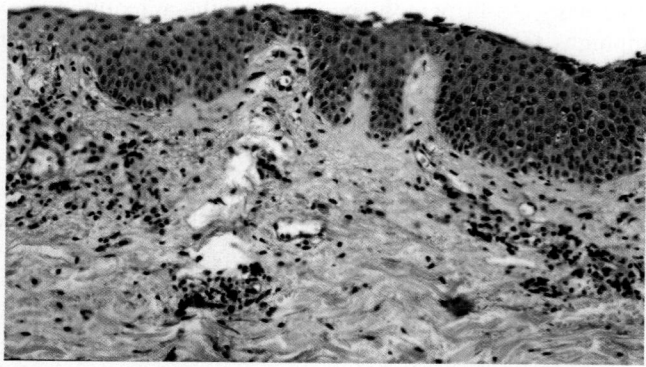

Figure 9-15 Pemphigus erythematosus. The histologic appearance is identical to those of pemphigus foliaceus. In this biopsy, the roof of the vesicle is not present (possibly secondary to processing), which is a frequent event, leaving a diminished but acantholytic granular layer (low-medium power).

They most commonly remain localized to the face, but it may become generalized. No oral lesions are observed.

Histopathology. The light microscopic features are identical to those of pemphigus foliaceus in most cases (Fig. 9-15). Interface dermatitis has been apparent in rare cases, making it difficult to distinguish it from lupus erythematosus.

IF Testing. DIF testing of perilesional or lesional skin reveals squamous intercellular substance deposition of IgG in greater than 75% of cases and granular deposition of IgM and IgG (i.e., a positive lupus band test) at the dermoepidermal junction. IIF study using monkey esophagus or normal human skin as substrate reveals squamous intercellular substance deposition of IgG in 80% of cases. Serologically, antinuclear antibodies are observed in 30% to 80% of cases, as may anti-DNA and anti–extractable nuclear antigen (ENA) antibodies rarely.

Ultrastructural Study. Pemphigus erythematosus is identical to pemphigus foliaceus in its epidermal ultrastructural alterations. An intriguing study with UVA in pemphigus foliaceus found that fragmented desmoglein bound anti-desmoglein-1 IgG at the dermoepidermal junction, a mechanism similar to that observed in lupus erythematosus, where DNA binds with IgG anti-DNA at the dermoepidermal junction.

Differential Diagnosis. The differential diagnosis is the same as in pemphigus foliaceus. The presence of interface dermatitis in some cases leads to confusion with lupus erythematosus and PNP/PAMS. Subcorneal acantholysis is not a feature of lupus erythematosus. PNP/PAMS has linear C3 and IgG at the dermoepidermal junction, in contrast to pemphigus erythematosus, in which deposition is granular in pattern. PNP has erythema multiforme (EM)/LP-like features at the dermoepidermal junction and within the papillary dermis.

Principles of Management: Immunosuppressive therapy with systemic steroids and a steroid-sparing agent is the mainstay. In some patients, topical steroids have been used (104).

Pemphigus Herpetiformis

Clinical Summary. Pemphigus herpetiformis combines the clinical features of DH with the immunologic and histologic features of pemphigus, usually the foliaceus type (105). This variant deserves recognition only because of its clinical presentation. Patients often present with very pruritic, erythematous, vesicular, or papular lesions, often in herpetiform pattern. Mucous membranes are uncommonly involved. Associations with SLE, malignancies, and psoriasis have been reported as well as one case of an infant whose mother had B-cell lymphoma (106–109).

Histopathology. There is eosinophilic spongiosis with or without acantholysis. Variable numbers of neutrophils may be present, leading to neutrophilic spongiosis or subcorneal pustules, with both eosinophils and neutrophils. Both suprabasal and subcorneal splits have been reported.

IF Testing. Because the clinical presentation and histologic findings are often atypical, the most reliable basis for diagnosis of pemphigus herpetiformis is IF study. DIF of perilesional or lesional skin shows deposition of IgG on the surface of keratinocytes primarily in the upper epidermis in most cases (110). IIF has demonstrated circulating IgG antisquamous cell surface autoantibodies, most directed against desmoglein 1, the pemphigus foliaceus antigen. A few cases with antibodies to the pemphigus vulgaris antigen, desmoglein 3, have been reported (110,111). Rare cases have had antibodies to the desmocollins and BP180 (112). Hybrid cases of pemphigus herpetiformis and other vesiculobullous diseases have been reported (112,113).

Principles of Management: Treatment of pemphigus herpetiformis often includes dapsone alone or in combination with systemic steroids (105).

Drug-Induced Pemphigus

Although immunologic features identical to those of idiopathic pemphigus are reported in most cases of drug-induced pemphigus (114), evidence indicates that some drugs may induce acantholysis without the production of antibodies (115). The offending drugs, most frequently penicillamine, captopril, and penicillin derivatives, contain sulfhydryl groups (116). Indeed, chronic penicillamine therapy leads to pemphigus foliaceus in 10%. Some foods containing sulfhydryl groups may produce pemphigus as well. The earliest clinical manifestation is a nonspecific morbilliform or urticarial eruption. In penicillamine-induced pemphigus, the eruption is characteristic and has been labeled "toxic pre-pemphigus rash" (116). Subsequently, the characteristic lesions of pemphigus develop. On cessation of drug therapy, the rash regresses in those patients who do *not* have pemphigus antibodies, in contrast to those patients with pemphigus antibodies, in whom the rash frequently persists. This latter subset has the clinical waxing and waning course of pemphigus.

Rarely, locally applied drugs such as imiquimod, 5-FU, and some contactants such as pesticides (117,118) have been associated with subsequent pemphigus in which lesions are localized to the site of application with subsequent generalization. The mechanism is unclear. Several mechanisms may be at play, including precipitating subclinical pemphigus or autoantigen induction secondary to agents applied.

Histopathology. The findings in the early eruption are nonspecific, consisting of spongiosis, parakeratosis, and a variable dermal infiltrate. Well-developed lesions are essentially identical to those of pemphigus foliaceus or pemphigus vulgaris. Eosinophilic spongiosis may be prominent.

IF Testing. DIF testing is positive in approximately 90% of patients with drug-induced pemphigus (116). IIF study of serum reveals circulating squamous intercellular substance IgG antibodies in 70% of cases. The antibody titers are usually of low titer and do not appear to correlate with the severity of the disease. Both anti-desmoglein 1 and 3 antibodies have been demonstrated by the ELISA technique, which is more sensitive than routine IF studies.

Pathogenesis. In those cases in which there is antibody production and *in vivo* deposition with subsequent acantholysis, the pathogenesis appears to be identical to that of idiopathic pemphigus. Because the pemphigus antigens have disulfide bonds, sulfhydryl-containing drugs may bind to them. These drugs have been shown to localize in high concentration in the epidermis. Therefore, the drug appears to directly affect the keratinocyte adhesion molecules, interferes with their function, and causes subsequent acantholysis, explaining those cases of drug-induced pemphigus that do not have pemphigus antibodies.

Principles of Management: Cessation of the causative agent is essential, although many patients may have drug-"unmasked" disease and require treatment as with *de novo* autoimmune pemphigus.

IgA Pemphigus

Clinical Summary. IgA pemphigus is a pruritic vesiculopustular eruption characterized by squamous intercellular IgA deposits and intraepidermal neutrophils. It occurs in primarily middle-aged and elderly individuals, but several cases have been described in children (119,120). The clinical findings are similar to those in pemphigus foliaceus or SPD most frequently. There are flaccid pustules that arise on an erythematous base. They often appear in an annular arrangement. The most common sites of involvement are the axilla and groin, but trunk, proximal extremities, and lower abdomen can also be involved. Mucous membrane involvement overall is rare. Mild leukocytosis, eosinophilia, IgA paraproteinemia, IgA multiple myeloma, and B-cell lymphoma may be present (121,122). Rare cases have been associated with ulcerative colitis, particularly the pemphigus vegetans variant. Drug association has been reported (123). Rarely, the rash may have extensive mucosal involvement.

Table 9-8	
IgA Pemphigus Subtypes and Autoantigens	
Superficial pustular dermatosis (SPD) type	Dsc1
Intraepidermal neutrophilic IgA dermatosis (IEN)	Dsc1,3
IgA pemphigus vegetans (P. Vegetans–like)	Dsc2
IgA pemphigus foliaceus (P. Foliaceus–like)	Dsg1
IgA pemphigus vulgaris (P. Vulgaris–like)	Dsg3
Unclassified (U/C) IgA dermatosis	Dsg1, Dsg3, desmocollins

Dsc1, desmocollin 1; Dsc-3, desmocollin 3; Dsc2, desmocollin-2; Dsg1, desmoglein-1; Dsg3, desmoglein-3.

IgA pemphigus is clinically heterogeneous, reflecting differences in the autoantigens involved (124). Hashimoto et al. (125) have reported on clinical grounds, histologic appearance, and the autoantigens (ELISA) into six types (Table 9-8). However, most patients develop one of the two histologic types that were initially described: an SPD type or an intraepidermal neutrophilic dermatosis (IEN) type (120,121,126). The presence of cases with overlapping features supports the notion that this is one disease with variable expression. Some associations differ between the proposed variants. In general, the clinical findings parallel the distribution and character of the other pemphigus variants to which they are similar (SPD, pemphigus vulgaris (PV), pemphigus vegetans (PVe), pemphigus foliaceus (PF)). Much more work is needed to validate this assessment.

Histopathology. In the SPD type, there are subcorneal vesicopustules or pustules with minimal acantholysis (Fig. 9-16A). In the IEN type, there are intraepidermal vesicopustules or pustules containing variable numbers of neutrophils (Fig. 9-16B, C).

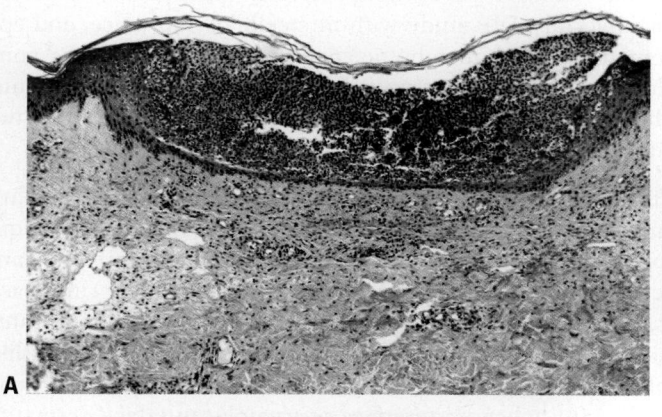

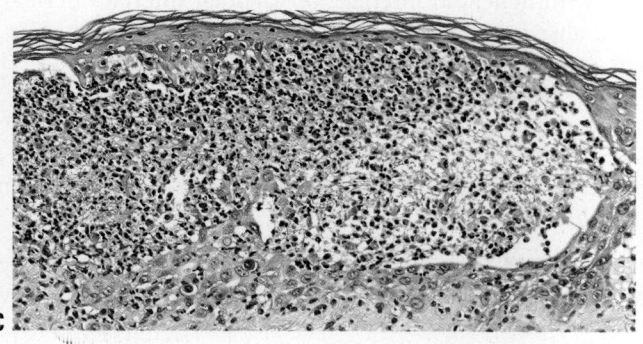

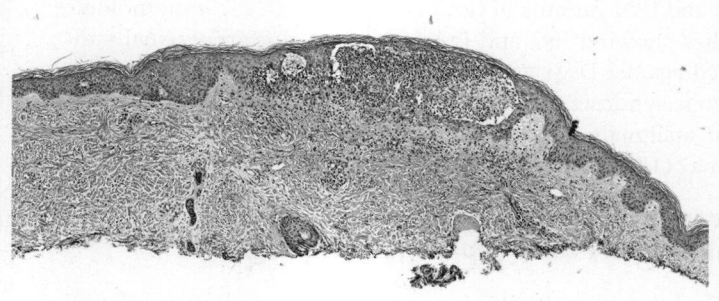

Figure 9-16 IgA pemphigus. **A:** In the subcorneal pustular dermatosis (SPD) type, a subcorneal intraepidermal pustule with numerous neutrophils is seen (medium power). **B and C:** In the intraepidermal neutrophilic (IEN) type, the neutrophils are suprabasal and below the stratum corneum (B—low power, C—high power). (Whole Slide Image Courtesy of Dr. H. Wu.)

The other cases have features of the pemphigus variant to which they are similar. One case of IgA pemphigus, which resembled pemphigus foliaceus without neutrophil infiltration, has been described (127). Early lesions may consist of neutrophilic spongiosis. The differential diagnosis of other variants are the IgG-mediated pemphigus variants (PF, PV, PVe, etc.).

IF Testing. DIF testing reveals IgA deposition in the squamous intercellular substance throughout the epidermis with increased intensity in the upper layers in some cases of the subcorneal pustular type. Complement and other immunoglobulins are usually not present (121). However, some cases may have both IgG and IgA present and may thus make a specific diagnosis difficult (i.e., IgG/IgA pemphigus) unless evaluation for antigen specificity is available (128). IIF results are positive in fewer than 50% of reported cases. In the SPD type, IgA autoantibodies were shown to recognize desmocollin 1 (129). In the IEN type, the antibodies have been variously characterized as reacting to desmoglein 1 or desmoglein 3; however, further study is needed (124,126,130).

Differential Diagnosis. The SPD variant is identical to Sneddon–Wilkinson disease. Indeed, many cases reported as Sneddon–Wilkinson disease, in which IF testing was not performed, likely represent the SPD variant of IgA pemphigus. Pustular psoriasis, bullous impetigo, and PV are the principal differential diagnoses. Pustular psoriasis may not be distinguishable on routine light microscopic study, and IF testing is therefore required. Lastly, as previously mentioned, exclusion by IF testing (and ELISA study if available) is required to exclude IgG pemphigus variants.

Principles of Management: In a systematic review of IgA pemphigus, Kridin et al. compiled data from 119 eligible studies, where oral dapsone was the most frequent treatment, followed by systemic steroids used concurrently or as primary treatment (131).

IgA/IgG Pemphigus

IgG/IgA pemphigus clinically appears similar to classic pemphigus in most cases rather than IgA pemphigus. Histologically, it is often similar to classic pemphigus foliaceus and PV, but there may be more neutrophilic infiltrate, some mimicking the SPD and IEN variants of IgA pemphigus with the immunologic studies showing IgG and IgA in intercellular array usually directed against Dsg1 and Dsg3 (132). There is association with Sjogren syndrome and ulcerative colitis (133,134) as well as solid malignancies (lung, uterine, gallbladder, ovary, and thymoma) (132,135).

Paraneoplastic Autoimmune Multiorgan Syndrome: Paraneoplastic Pemphigus

Clinical Summary. PAMS, first described as, and often referred to as, paraneoplastic pemphigus (PNP), is a complex autoimmune vesiculobullous and erosive mucocutaneous disease associated with an underlying malignancy (Fig. 9-17A). The most commonly associated neoplasms included non-Hodgkin lymphoma (42%), chronic lymphocytic leukemia (29%), Castleman disease (10%), thymoma (6%), sarcoma (6%), Waldenström macroglobulinemia (6%) as well as malignant melanoma, and other carcinomas (lung, breast, etc.). Several other carcinomas and sarcomas have been associated as well. Approximately 10% (136,137) may not have overt malignancy at presentation.

However, follow-up evaluations for occult malignancy over time are necessary (137–139). The age of onset is variable, although most patients are between the ages of 45 and 70 years. Cutaneous lesions are polymorphic. The most consistent clinical feature of PNP/PAMS is the presence of intractable stomatitis, which presents as erosions and ulcerations, often hemorrhagic, that affect all surfaces of the oropharynx and characteristically extend onto the lips mimicking Stevens–Johnson syndrome (SJS). Multiple organ systems (conjunctiva, bronchi, vaginal, anal) may be involved, and the high rate of mortality often stems from constrictive bronchiolitis obliterans (140). If the associated malignancy is in remission, PNP/PAMS may relent. Autoantibodies are deposited in the kidneys, bladder, muscle, heart, lung, mucous membrane, and skin. The extent and diversity of the clinical presentations and immunopathologic mechanisms led to the suggestion that PNP/PAMS, a disease of epithelial adhesion, represents one manifestation of a heterogeneous autoimmune syndrome, PAMS, a term that the author (TJH) prefers (141). At least seven different clinical variants of PNP/PAMS are recognized: bullous pemphigoid-like, MMP-like, pemphigus-like, EM-like, graft-versus-host disease–like, CP-like, and LP-like (142–146).

A recent review by Svoboda et al. has published a revised panel of diagnostic criteria to include approximately 90% of PAMS/PNP cases (147). They propose three major criteria, including mucous membrane involvement with or without cutaneous involvement, concomitant internal neoplasia, and serologic antiplakin antibodies (ELISA and immunoblot techniques). Minor criteria include acantholysis and/or lichenoid interface dermatitis as well as DIF study with intercellular substance or epidermal basement membrane zone antibody/complement deposition. Having three major criteria or two major criteria and both minor criteria confirms a diagnosis of PAMS/PNP.

The previous report generally used paradigms by Camisa and Helm (147) proposing three major criteria, namely, polymorphous mucocutaneous eruptions, concomitant internal neoplasia, and serum antibodies with specific immunoprecipitation findings. Three minor criteria included acantholysis histologically, DIF study with intercellular substance, and epidermal basement membrane zone deposition of IgG and complement and IIF deposition of IgG on rat bladder epithelium. They required three major criteria or two major criteria and two minor criteria for a diagnosis of PAMS/PNP.

Histopathology. The histologic features are variable, depending on the various clinical presentations. The lesions show a unique combination of EM-like, LP-like, pemphigus vulgaris-like, and pemphigoid-like features. The principal findings are suprabasal acantholysis with basal apoptosis, in association with an interface dermatitis (EM-like) with or without an LP-like bandlike infiltrate (Fig. 9-17B, C) (148). PNP/PAMS may present exclusively with lichenoid interface or vacuolar interface dermatitis in the absence of acantholysis (149). In pemphigoid-like lesions, subepidermal blisters are present.

The TEN-like and EM-like variants may be associated with a much worse prognosis (150). Rare cases of GVH-like PNP/PAMS and LP-like PNP/PAMS have been described without antibodies. However, these may represent drug-associated dermatitis, which must be excluded.

IF Testing. DIF testing of perilesional skin and mucosa reveals IgG in the squamous intercellular substance in concert with

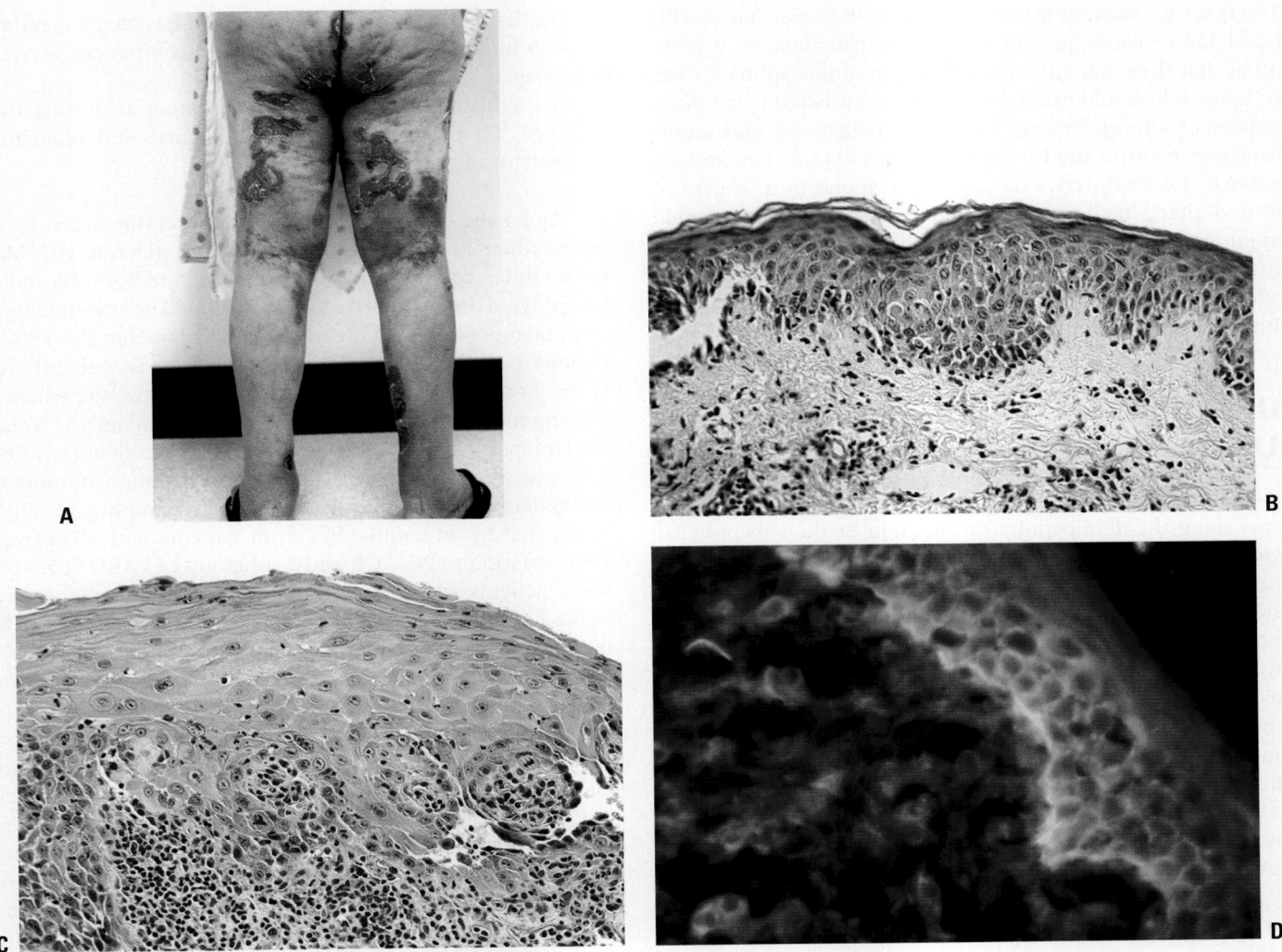

Figure 9-17 Paraneoplastic autoimmune multiorgan syndrome/paraneoplastic pemphigus. **A:** Clinical example. Crusted large plaques are present on the lower extremities. **B, C:** Histologic features. **B:** Erythema multiforme–like pattern. There is a cell-poor interface dermatitis with apoptosis of keratinocytes. There are also pemphigus vulgaris–like changes with a suprabasal blister (low-medium power). **C:** Lichen planus–like pattern. There is a cell-rich lichenoid dermatitis associated with a suprabasal blister (medium power). **D:** Direct Immunofluorescence. There are both intercellular lacelike and epidermal linear basement membrane deposition of IgG.

immune reactant deposition at the dermoepidermal junction (Fig. 9-17D). At the dermoepidermal junction, granular deposition of complement is noted most frequently (144). Linear deposition of complement, IgG, and IgM and granular deposition of complement and IgG have also been identified (138). When present, basement membrane zone immunoglobulin and complement deposition helps to distinguish PNP/PAMS from other forms of pemphigus in which basement membrane zone antibodies and complement are generally not present (151). In most cases, circulating PNP/PAMS antibodies bind to squamous keratinocytes in routine substrates, whereas the antibodies bind to rat bladder epithelium. However, false-positive (patients with other variants of pemphigus) and false-negative (up to ~25%) results do occur using this substrate.

Pathogenesis. Patients with PNP/PAMS develop IgG autoantibodies against multiple antigens (Table 9-7). It appears that all the members of the plakin family, as well as desmogleins, desmocollins, plakoglobin, and others have been reported to be targeted by IgG autoantibodies in PNP. Although anti-desmoglein antibodies play a role in inducing the loss of cellular adhesion of keratinocytes and blister formation, the pathophysiologic relevance of the antiperiplakin autoantibodies is unclear. PNP often has antibodies directed against several of these antigens. In addition to the humoral autoimmunity, mounting evidence suggests that cytotoxic T cells play a prominent role (CD8 positive cells). In cases with TEN-like features, there have been IgG antibodies directed against a periplakin and plectin (152). Proteases may play a role as in the classic pemphigus disease. Cases with clinical features of PNP in the absence of detectable autoantibodies have been reported (153). In those patients, the affected areas had high levels of CD8+ cytotoxic T cells, which mediated damage, including interface dermatitis with dyskeratosis/apoptosis (152). IL-6, which activates CD8+ T cells and CD56+ natural killer (NK) cells, has been reported to be significantly increased in the blood of PNP/PAMS patients (154). The association of PNP with bronchiolitis obliterans provides additional evidence that cytotoxic T cells may play a critical role in PNP/PAMS.

Principles of Management: Because PNP is associated with underlying hematologic and solid organ malignancies, it is essential that these patients receive rapid multidisciplinary care. The approach should be focused on the identification and management of any underlying triggering malignancy and monitoring and treating any lung disease. There is no standardized treatment for PNP. Active disease may respond to treatment of the underlying malignancy or may require local or systemic immunomodulatory or suppressive therapy as well. Systemic corticosteroids, azathioprine, MMF, cyclosporine, rituximab, cyclophosphamide, plasmapheresis, and IVIG have been tried with variable results (155).

SUBEPIDERMAL/SUBEPITHELIAL BULLOUS DISEASE

Subepidermal bullous diseases are disorders in which a blister forms along the dermoepidermal junction or the subepithelial zone in mucosa. This group of diseases includes conditions with different clinical presentations, histologic findings, and pathogenesis. Both inherited and acquired alterations in key adhesion proteins at or in the dermoepidermal junction result in blister formation. In the subgroup of autoimmune subepidermal bullous diseases, major target antigens bound by autoantibodies from patients have been characterized (Table 9-9). Importantly, some of the genes encoding these autoantigens harbor mutations responsible for the various mechanobullous diseases, that is, the EB variants. To understand subepidermal bullous disease, it is essential to have some knowledge of the epidermal basement membrane zone and its various target proteins (Fig. 9-18).

Proceeding from the epidermis to the dermis, there are four distinct structural components of the epidermal basement membrane:

1. The intermediate filament, hemidesmosomal plaques, and plasma membranes of the basal keratinocytes.
2. The lamina lucida that contains delicate anchoring filaments connecting hemidesmosomes (HD) in basal keratinocytes to the underlying lamina densa.

3. The lamina densa that provides the basement membrane with much of its strength. The main component is type IV collagen.
4. The sublaminar densa region containing anchoring fibrils (type VII collagen), anchoring plaques, and filamentous proteins of the papillary dermis.

Along the deep surface of the basal keratinocytes, keratin intermediate filaments (keratin 5 and 14) attach to HD. Major intracellular components of HD include the 230-kDa bullous pemphigoid antigen (BPAg1) and plectin. The transmembrane components of the HD include $\alpha_6\beta_4$ integrin and the 180-kDa bullous pemphigoid antigen (BPAg2), that is, collagen XVII (156). Both extend into the lamina lucida at the site where anchoring filaments are located. The anchoring filaments straddle the lamina lucida between HD and the lamina densa. Antibodies to the BPAg1 are present in the most common autoimmune subepidermal bullous disease, bullous pemphigoid. BPAg2 is targeted by autoantibodies from patients with BP, pemphigoid gestationis (PG), CP, and a subgroup of LABD (157–159). Some patients with generalized atrophic benign epidermolysis bullosa (GABEB) have a congenital deficiency of BPAg2. Mutation of the β_4 subunit of $\alpha_6\beta_4$ integrin leads to junctional EB associated with pyloric atresia (160). Patients with one form of ocular CP have autoantibodies directed against the β_4 subunit and B6 integrin (161).

The lamina lucida is the weakest link in the dermoepidermal junction, and it is the cleavage plane in the salt-split skin test. Multiple antigens are associated with the lamina lucida, particularly the anchoring filaments. The antigens include laminin 5, laminin 6, uncein, nidogen, epiligrin, and P200 (162,163). Autoantibodies to epiligrin, the α_3 subunit of laminin 5, result in one form of CP. Nonsense mutation of the laminin 5 gene is associated with the Herlitz subtype of junctional EB (164).

The lamina densa is an electron-dense layer that lies deep and parallel to and contiguous to the lamina lucida. The main component is type IV collagen, which is thought to provide the basement membrane with much of its strength. Other antigenic components are laminin 1, nidogen, and heparan sulfate proteoglycans.

Table 9-9
Targets Common to Autoimmune and Inherited Blistering Diseases*

Protein Target/Deficiency	Structural Target	Autoimmune Disease	Genetic Disease
BPAG1 (BP230)	HD	BP	None identified
BPAG2 (BP180, type XVII collagen)	HD-anchoring filament complexes	BP, PG, MP, LABD	GABEB
A6β4 integrin, subunit β4	HD-anchoring filament complexes	Ocular MP	Junctional EB with pyloric atresia
Laminin 5, 6	Lamina lucida–lamina densa interface	Antiepiligrin MP, PNP	Junctional EB-Herlitz
P200	Lower lamina lucida	Anti-p200 pemphigoid	None identified
Type VII collagen	Anchoring fibrils	EB acquisita	Dystrophic EB, multiple types, Bart Syndrome
		Bullous SLE	

*The targets are bound by antibody in autoimmune disease, but in genetic disease the target components are absent or aberrantly synthesized.
BP, bullous pemphigoid; EB, epidermolysis bullosa; GABEB, generalized atrophic benign EB; HD, hemidesmosome; LABD, linear IgA bullous dermatosis; MP, mucous membrane (cicatricial) pemphigoid; PG, pemphigoid gestationis.

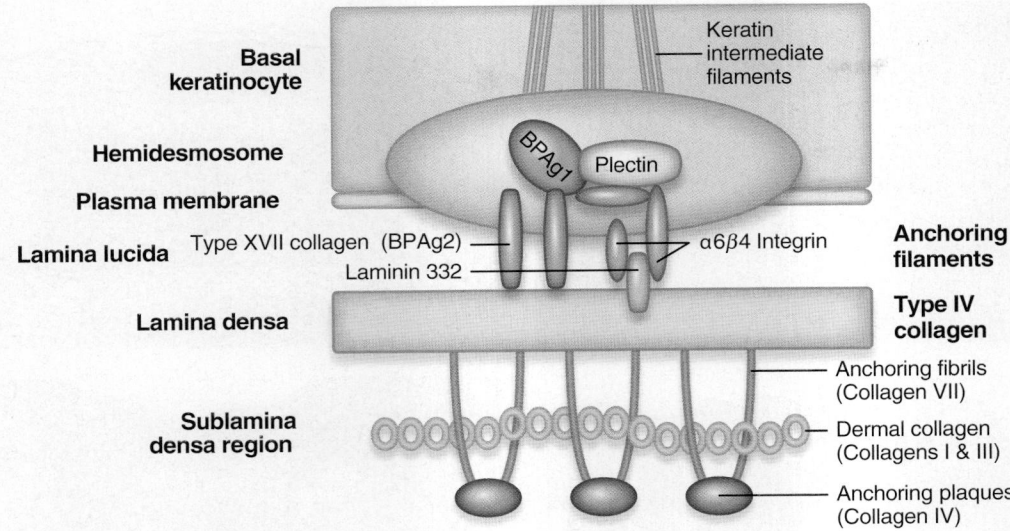

Figure 9-18 Schematic model of dermoepidermal junction. Along the basal surface of the keratinocytes, keratin intermediate filaments attach to HD on the basal plasma membrane. Major intracellular components of HD include the bullous pemphigoid antigen (BPAg1) and plectin. The transmembrane components of the HD include $\alpha_6\beta_4$ integrin and the bullous pemphigoid antigen (BPAg2). Both extend to the lamina lucida at the site where anchoring filaments are located. The anchoring filaments straddle the lamina lucida between HD and the lamina densa. Multiple antigens are associated with the lamina lucida, including laminin 5 and epiligrin. The lamina densa is an electron-dense layer that lies parallel to and contiguous to the lamina lucida. The main component is type IV collagen. In the sublamina densa region, the lamina densa and the overlying epidermis are tethered to the papillary dermis by anchoring fibrils. Type VII collagen is the major component of anchoring fibrils. HD, hemidesmosome. (Courtesy of Dr. H. Wu.)

In the sublamina densa region, the lamina densa is tethered to the papillary dermis by anchoring fibrils, a series of looping elements along the underside of the lamina densa that serve as attachment sites for collagens in the papillary dermis. Type VII collagen is the major component of anchoring fibrils. Autoantibodies against type VII collagen have been identified in epidermolysis bullosa acquisita (EBA), bullous systemic lupus erythematosus (BSLE), and some variants of Linear IgA disease (IgA-mediated EBA) (165). Nonsense mutation of type VII collagen gene (COL7A1) is associated with dystrophic EB.

Bullous Pemphigoid

Clinical Features. First described in 1953, bullous pemphigoid, by far the most common primary immunobullous disease, affects primarily elderly patients with large tense bullae arising on urticarial erythematous bases or on nonerythematous skin (Fig. 9-19A) (166). In contrast to pemphigus, the Asboe–Hansen/Nikolsky sign is negative. It may rarely be present in younger adults and children. The lesions involve the trunk, the extremities, and the intertriginous areas, with the oral mucosa involved in about one-third of the cases. Bullous pemphigoid may start as a nonspecific eruption suggestive of urticaria or dermatitis, which can persist for weeks or months. Rarely, bullous pemphigoid may present as erythroderma. Drug-induced forms of bullous pemphigoid do occur, and a thorough medication history is essential. There are reports of elderly patients with pruritus who undergo biopsy for DIF and are found to have antibodies to the BP antigens in the absence of classic skin lesions. Just as pemphigus is associated with malignancy, so are bullous pemphigoid and other pemphigoid variants, although this is debated and some recent studies indicate the association may be spurious (167,168). The malignancies most commonly

include hematopoietic proliferations as well as carcinomas and sarcomas. Because most patients are elderly, they often have other diseases, and any association may be coincidental. Interestingly, multiple sclerosis (and other neurodegenerative diseases) is statistically associated with bullous pemphigoid. This may be explained by exposure of neuronal BPAg2 to the immune system, leading to bullous pemphigoid as a secondary event (169). Some elderly patients have circulating anti-BPAg1/anti-BPAg2 antibodies associated with pruritus but with negative DIF findings.

Histopathology. In early lesions, papillary dermal edema, in combination with a cell-poor or cell-rich perivascular lymphocytic and eosinophilic infiltrate, is present (Fig. 9-19B). The blister arises at the dermoepidermal junction (170). In the cell-rich pattern, which correlates clinically with blisters arising on erythematous skin (Fig. 9-19C–E), eosinophilic papillary abscesses may develop with numerous perivascular and interstitial eosinophils intermingled with lymphocytes and a few neutrophils in the superficial and deep dermis. Early lesions may have the histologic features of eosinophilic cellulitis (Wells Syndrome). Eosinophilic spongiosis may occur. When blisters develop on relatively normal skin, a cell-poor pattern is observed in which there is usually a scant perivascular lymphocytic infiltrate with few eosinophils, some scattered throughout the dermis and others near the epidermis. The blister lumen contains few inflammatory cells. Epithelial migration and regeneration may result in an intraepidermal blister in older blisters, and other secondary lesions such as erosions and ulcerations are common. Similar to pemphigus vegetans, a pseudocarcinomatous hyperplasia of the epidermis, subepidermal bullae, and accumulations of eosinophils and lymphocytes may be seen (pemphigoid vegetans).

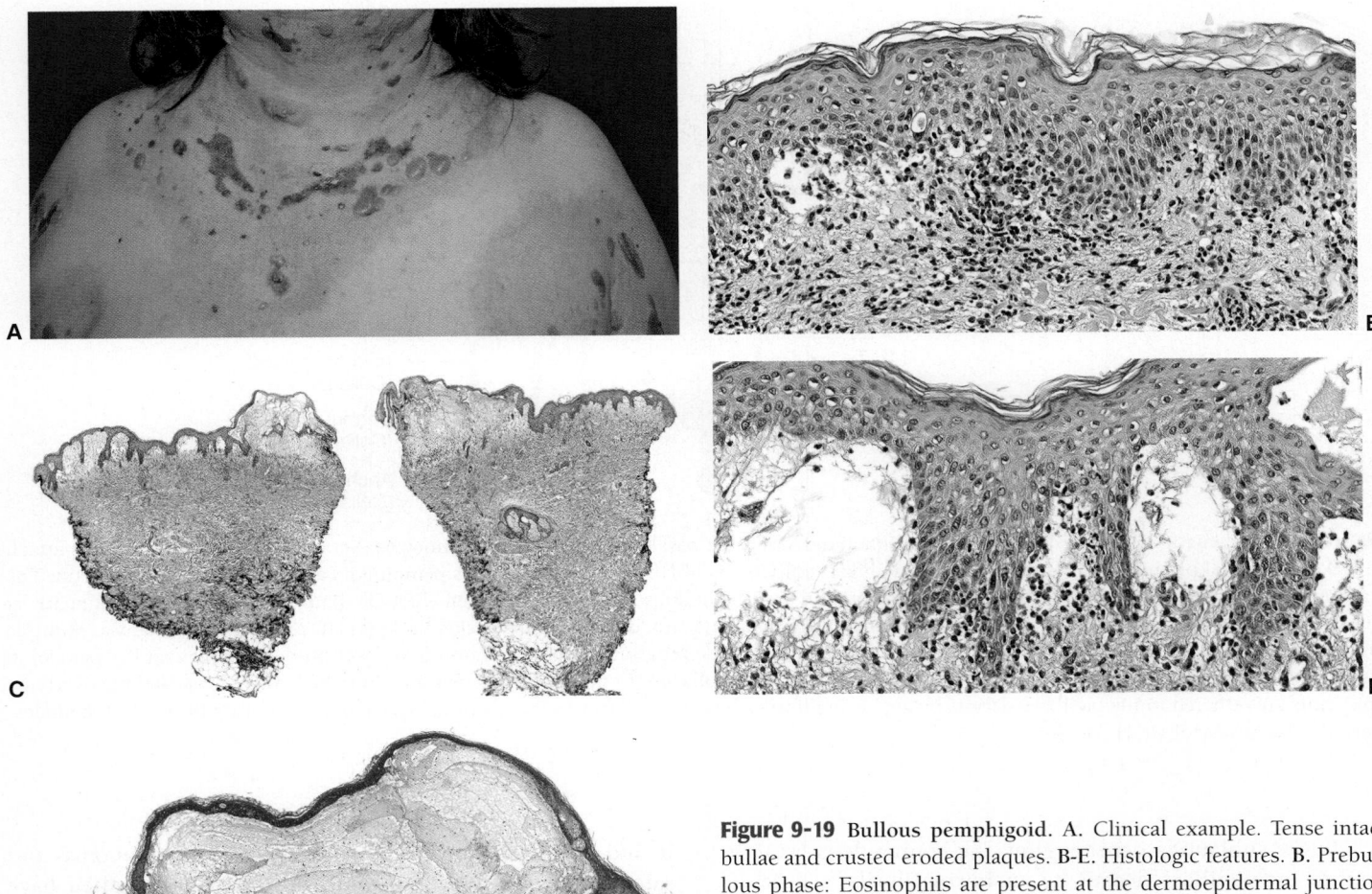

Figure 9-19 Bullous pemphigoid. **A.** Clinical example. Tense intact bullae and crusted eroded plaques. **B-E.** Histologic features. **B.** Prebullous phase: Eosinophils are present at the dermoepidermal junction and in the dermis. There is early subepithelial separation in this image (low-medium power). **C-E.** Bullous phase. **C.** Skin with inflammation, papillary dermal edema, and more developed bullae than in B (scanning power). **D.** In the same biopsy at higher power numerous eosinophils can be seen in the dermis, bulla cavity, and epidermis. **E.** Scanning power of a unilocular subepithelial bulla.

IF Testing. DIF testing of perilesional skin (peribullous erythematous skin as well) in active disease has shown linear C3 deposition (Table 9-9) at the dermoepidermal junction in virtually 100% of cases and IgG in up to 95% (Fig. 9-20A, B). Linear C3 at the dermoepidermal junction without IgG (or IgM or IgA) is sufficient for a diagnosis of bullous pemphigoid in the appropriate clinical setting. Similarly deposited IgA and IgM are observed in about 25% of cases. Use of fluoresceinated anti-IgG type 4 antibodies in DIF testing may be more sensitive than routine fluoresceinated anti-IgG in identifying deposition and diminishes the background fluorescence commonly present in routine IgG preparations. Importantly, recent studies have shown that C4b persists longer than C3b and that its presence is likely a more sensitive indicator of bullous pemphigoid (171). IIF studies reveal circulating anti–basement membrane zone IgG antibodies in 70% to 80%. No correlation exists between the overall antibody titer (Anti-BPAg1, Anti-BPAg2) and the clinical severity of the disease. However, titers of anti-BPAg2 alone may overall correlate with disease activity. The IgG is located within the lamina lucida, where it binds specifically to the HD. It is in the "n-serrated" pattern. Rare cases of IgM-mediated bullous pemphigoid have been reported (172).

Salt-split skin IF studies are an important diagnostic tool. The technique was first developed in 1984 in which normal human skin was used as a substrate and patient serum as test (indirect salt-split skin technique) (170). Incubation of normal or patient skin in 1 mol/L NaCl results in a split in the lamina lucida. Bullous pemphigoid antibodies bind solely to the lower aspect of the basal keratinocytes (the blister roof) in 80% of cases; in about 20% of cases, the antibodies bind to both the lower basal keratinocytes (the roof) and the superior aspect of the dermis (the blister floor) (Table 9-10). It must be made clear that the antigenic specificity of IgG binding to the base or roof is unknown. The IgG cannot be said to be directly against BPAg 1, 2, or other antigens. As time goes on to as research proceeds, it is likely that it will be found that the IgG, in some cases, may have different antigenic specificities (as in anti-p200 pemphigoid and Chan disease) and should be labeled different diseases defining additional autoimmune subepidermal blistering diseases (see comments on vesicular pemphigoid). On IIF study, salt-split skin is more sensitive as a substrate, in contrast to nonsplit normal human skin, monkey and guinea pig esophagus and showed deposition in all cases of suspected pemphigoid (Table 9-10).

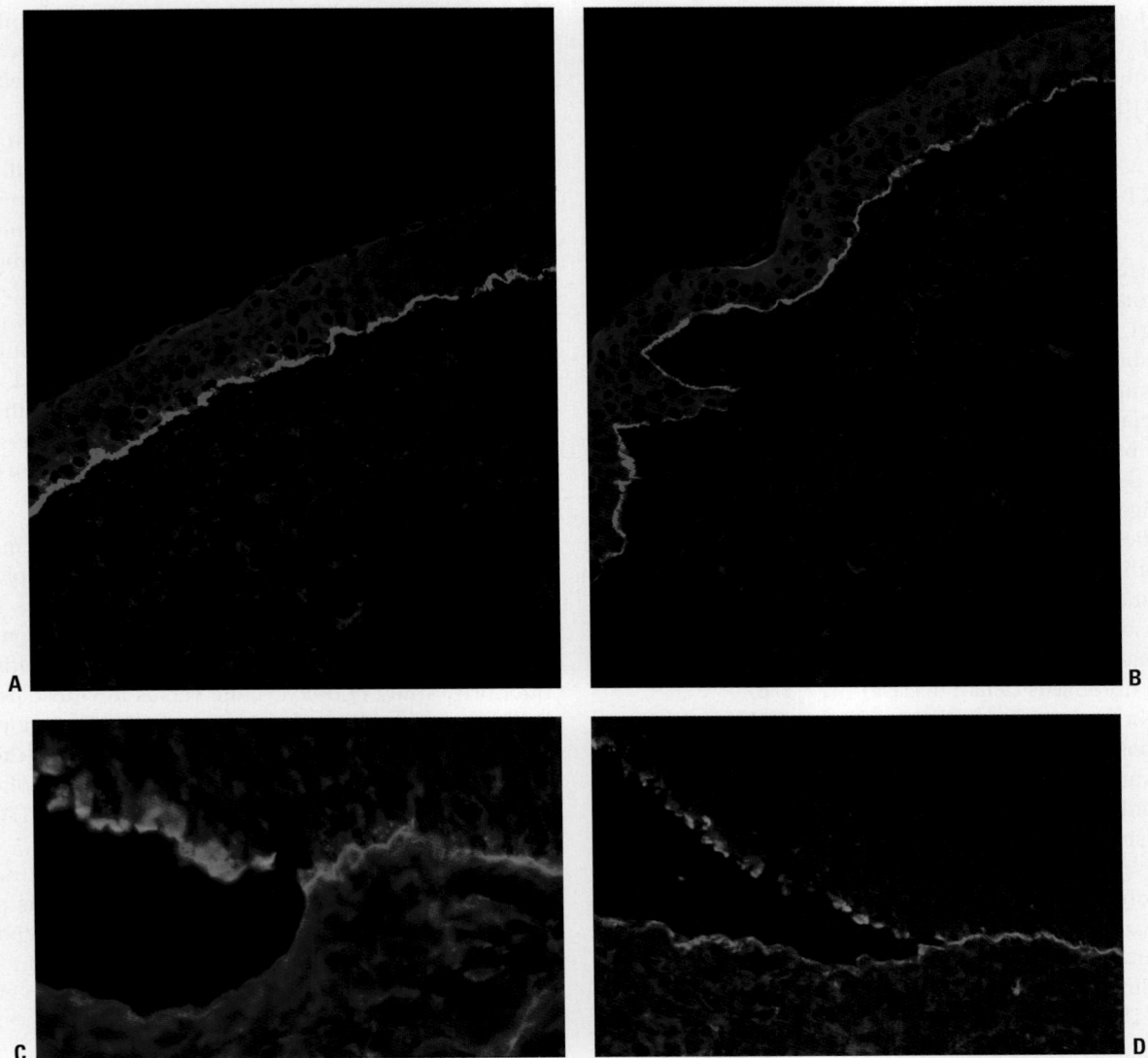

Figure 9-20 Bullous pemphigoid Direct Immunofluorescence. There is linear deposition of IgG (A) and C3 (B) along the basement membrane zone. C, D: Salt-split skin, direct immunofluorescence. C: IgG deposition on the epidermal side of the blister. D: IgG deposition on the epidermal and dermal sides of the blister. When present on the roof, note the semilunar pattern, corresponding to the curvature of the basal keratinocytes.

Table 9-10

Split-Skin Immunofluorescence Results (Indirect Method)

Roof Only	Roof and Base	Base Only	IR
Bullous pemphigoid (80%)	Bullous pemphigoid (~15%)	Anti-p200 pemphigoid	IgG
Pemphigoid gestationis	Pemphigoid gestationis		
MMP/CCP	MMP/CCP	Antiepiligrin cicatricial pemphigoid	C3
		Epidermolysis bullosa acquisita	IgG
		Bullous systemic lupus erythematosus	
		Porphyria cutanea tarda	
Linear IgA dermatosis	Linear IgA dermatosis	IgA epidermolysis bullosa acquisita	IgA

IR, immune reactants; MMP/CCP, mucous membrane pemphigoid/cutaneous cicatricial pemphigoid.

Perilesional skin submitted for DIF examination may also be salt-split (direct salt-split skin technique) (173,174). When this technique is used in pemphigoid, IgG is present on the roof or on the roof and the floor (Fig. 9-20C, D). Localization to only the dermal base is characteristic of MMP, EBA (see Fig. 9-23D) anti-P200 pemphigoid, and some variants of MMP and CP.

Pathogenesis. Pemphigoid antibodies bind predominantly to two antigens, a 230-kDa protein (BPAg1) and a second, 180-kDa protein (BPAg2) (175,176). The initially reported antigen, BPAg1, is associated with the cytoplasmic attachment site of HD and is largely within the basal keratinocyte. BPAg2, the most important antigen pathogenetically, is transmembrane collagen XVII, which extends through the lamina lucida. Anti-BPAg2 produces disease in experimental models, whereas anti-BPAg1 does not. The distribution/apparent concentration of these antigens within the skin correlates with lesion location. IgE antibodies directed against the bullous pemphigoid antigens are pathogenic as well, correlating with disease activity, and are bound to mast cells and eosinophils via a receptor. A blistering disorder clinically similar to pemphigoid has antibodies that recognize a 105-kDa protein synthesized by both keratinocytes and fibroblasts (Chan disease) (177,178).

Given the known data, a sequence of pathogenetic events may be proposed. Pemphigoid antibodies bind with BPAg1 and BPAg2, activating the complement cascade leading to mast cell activation and eosinophilic infiltration or IgE binding to mast cells and eosinophils. Eosinophil infiltration ensues with subsequent degranulation and release of major basic protein and other proteolytic enzymes. The vessels are hyperpermeable, probably because of the release of vascular permeability factor (VPF) by keratinocytes (179). Lamina lucida separation develops from injury of basal keratinocytes, disruption of HD, and proteolysis (180). The role of infiltrating lymphocytes, that are predominantly CD4+, is unclear. IL-1 and IL-2, as well as IFN-γ, have been identified in blister fluids (181).

Ultrastructural Study. Pemphigoid antibodies bind within the lamina lucida, in particular, to the HD. The blister arises within the lamina lucida in both the cell-poor and cell-rich lesions. In cell-poor lesions, there is disruption of the anchoring filaments without lamina densa fragmentation. In contrast, inflammatory lesions of bullous pemphigoid with numerous eosinophils and mononuclear cells in the dermis result in greater local destruction or blister formation in the lamina lucida with the fragmentation of the lamina densa.

Differential Diagnosis of Bullous Pemphigoid. Histologic differentiation of bullous pemphigoid from PV is not difficult because of the difference in cleavage planes and the mechanism of blister formation in well-established lesions. Initially, however, bullous pemphigoid may be heralded by eosinophilic spongiosis, engendering its differential diagnosis. Bullous pemphigoid is frequently indistinguishable from PG; however, PG may have greater quantities of infiltrating neutrophils and more basal keratinocyte damage. EBA (inflammatory variant) may have greater numbers of infiltrating neutrophils, but differentiation may be impossible on routine histopathologic study. DH is characterized by a subepidermal infiltrate of neutrophils with papillary microabscesses. Similarly, linear IgA dermatosis (LAD) is characterized, in most cases, by a neutrophil-rich infiltrate. EM is an interface dermatitis characterized by basal vasculopathy,

basal apoptosis, and a tagging lymphohistiocytic infiltrate along the dermoepidermal junction. Diabetic blisters are noninflammatory, subepithelial in location, and often associated with fibrosis and microangiopathy.

Some patients with pemphigoid may present only with a superficial perivascular lymphoeosinophilic infiltrate without migration of eosinophils to the dermoepidermal junction. This histologic reaction pattern is most commonly associated with morbilliform drug eruptions. Rarely, the changes of eosinophilic cellulitis (Wells syndrome) may also herald the presence of pemphigoid. Bullous drug eruptions may present with subepidermal vesicles and eosinophils and cannot be separated from bullous pemphigoid, and later lesions of DH may contain eosinophils. IF study is necessary to make a specific diagnosis.

Some patients will present only with pruritus and no clinical lesions. Lastly, drug-induced pemphigoid must always be excluded as in pemphigus.

Principles of Management: The initial management of mild/localized bullous pemphigoid is with potent topical steroids, such as clobetasol. Several published guidelines recommend concomitant use of oral dapsone, low-dose systemic steroids, or anti-inflammatory antibiotics (182). In a multicenter non-inferiority study of doxycycline versus low-dose prednisolone, Williams et al. showed that doxycycline was not inferior to low-dose prednisolone and significantly safer in the long term (183). Second-line therapies for BP include dapsone, MMF, cyclophosphamide, intravenous immunoglobulin (IVIG), rituximab, and plasmapheresis (182).

Omalizumab (anti-IgE) appears to have a significant disease-modifying effect in patients with bullous pemphigoid (184). In a five-center case series, Abdat et al. reported a 92% disease clearance or satisfactory response rate in 13 patients with bullous pemphigoid treated with dupilumab (185).

Clinical Variants
Drug-Associated Bullous Pemphigoid
Statins, protein pump inhibitors, vitamin supplements, β-blockers, angiotensin-converting enzyme (ACE) inhibitors, furosemide, phenacetin, psoralen-boosted phototherapy, some antibiotics, and various penicillins have been associated with bullous pemphigoid (186,187). It is possible that drug hypersensitivity may not be a cause of pemphigoid but that the patients had subclinical pemphigoid with a superimposed drug eruption, which also produces damage to the dermoepidermal junction similar to pemphigoid. The combination hits the threshold of basal damage necessary to produce subepidermal blister formation, or the damage to the dermoepidermal junction leads to exposure of the BP-antigen to the immune system (similar to LP pemphigoides). BP has developed after rechallenge, with some drugs showing a clear-cut association.

Pemphigoid Localized to the Lower Extremities
Some patients, usually women, present with tense bullae localized to the lower extremities. Histologically, these reveal a cell-poor pattern and have positive IF findings less frequently (50%) than routine bullous pemphigoid. At least in one instance, it has been shown that the IgG is directed against BPAg1 (188). The exact nosology of the DIF-negative cases is unclear. In our estimation, they likely represent subepidermal blisters in ischemic lower extremities secondary to bullous edema or chronic ischemic dermatitis such as diabetic microangiopathy,

owing to the high metabolic activity of basal keratinocytes and inhibition of HD formation and maintenance. The HD turnover rate in normal skin is quite rapid, 4 to 6 hours.

Vesicular Pemphigoid

This variant is worthy of designation because of its clinical similarity to DH with small, grouped blisters, which may lead to clinical misdiagnosis. Most has autoantibodies against BPA1/BPA2. While labeled "vesicular pemphigoid," some cases have had antibodies directed against a number of epidermal basement membrane zone components (189,190) and should perhaps be considered a different disease rather than pemphigoid.

Prurigo Pemphigoides/Pemphigoid Nodularis

This is a rare pemphigoid variant in which clinical lesions of prurigo nodularis develop without blisters, at least initially. Often, both blisters and prurigo nodularis are present. Histologically, there are findings of lichen simplex chronicus/prurigo nodularis superimposed on an infiltrate of lymphocytes and eosinophils and subsequent subepidermal blister development.

Lichen Planus Pemphigoides

This rare disorder may be a variant of pemphigoid, LP, or a separate disease sui generis. It develops in a younger age group with a median age of 35 to 46 years of age; but it has occurred in children and elderly adults as well. The patient usually presents with typical lichenoid papules in which blisters develop. The blisters may occur simultaneously with the papules or develop later and even develop in clinically normal skin. When the latter occurs, it is a clinical marker for LP pemphigoides, in contrast to bullous LP. There is a slight female predilection and with the trunk, extremities, and oral mucosa as common sites.

Histologically, the lichenoid papules and plaques are identical to classic LP, sometimes with eosinophils. The blister roof has the characteristics of the altered epidermis in LP while those arising in clinically normal skin have a perivascular and interstitial infiltrate of lymphocytes and eosinophils often minimal in intensity similar to bullous pemphigoid. There is linear C3 and IgG in all cases characteristically directed against BP180 antigen (BPAg2), but some cases have demonstrated antibodies against BPAg1, desmoglein 1, a 200 kDa protein, and a 130 kDa protein. There is linear IgG and C3 at the dermoepidermal junction with the IgG directed against BPAg2 and BPAg1, in contrast to bullous LP, in which there are colloid bodies, granular C3, and possibly trace to moderately dense granular IgM and linear/shaggy fibrinogen. IIF of serum studies on normal skin (split and nonsplit) is less sensitive, being positive in approximately 60% to 65% of cases (191).

T-cell response to BPAg2 has been demonstrated and linked to antibody production. The blister separation is in the lamina lucida, and IgG splits to the blister roof. ELISA and Western blot studies confirm the target antigen is BPAg2, a 180 kDa protein (192). Evidence of a drug association is best with ACE inhibitors. Many drugs have been implicated, but evidence of rechallenge with the production of new lesions is largely lacking.

Anti-p200 Pemphigoid

Patients with anti-p200 pemphigoid, a disorder less frequent than BP, usually present with a generalized eruption composed of urticarial papules and plaques in combination with tense blisters, closely mimicking BP. In Asian patients, an association with coexisting psoriasis has been reported (163). Mucosal involvement is not uncommon (164). It is important to recognize the entity because it shares similar histologic features and an immunofluorescence pattern with EBA. In contrast to EBA, anti-p200 pemphigoid was initially reported to have had a self-limiting course and rapid resolution without scarring. Later studies reveal mortality in more than 30% (193). Until further immunoblot or ELISA studies are performed, anti-p200 pemphigoid is indistinguishable from EBA and CP (194).

p200 is a glycoprotein localized to the lower lamina lucida of the basement membrane zone. It has been shown to be the laminin γ-1 chain (195). However, it is unclear if these are pathogenic, because one study implicates antibodies to the α-3 chain of laminin 5 (196).

Histopathology. The lesions are characterized by subepidermal blistering and a superficial inflammatory infiltrate, usually of neutrophils, but occasionally containing significant numbers of eosinophils. Microabscesses form in the papillary dermis adjacent to the blister cavity, and, in addition, eosinophilic or neutrophilic spongiosis may be observed. A moderate-to-dense inflammatory infiltrate in the upper dermis is usually present (197).

Immunofluorescence Testing. DIF study shows linear IgG and C3 deposition at the basement membrane zone, whereas IIF study of patient sera demonstrates IgG labeling exclusively the dermal side (floor) of salt-split human skin. By indirect immunogold electron microscopy, immunoreactants are localized to the lower lamina lucida.

Principles of Management: Therapies for anti-p200 pemphigoid are similar to those for bullous pemphigoid (198).

Mucous Membrane Pemphigoid/Cicatricial Pemphigoid

Clinical Features. The MMP variant of CP is a bullous disorder characterized by a chronic course, scarring, and predilection for mucosal surfaces. Most patients are elderly, and there is a male predilection. Oral blisters are present in virtually all cases, and ocular involvement is observed in 75%, with cutaneous involvement in 33% or less. The oral lesions are usually small blisters that subsequently often erode and ulcerate rapidly (Fig. 9-21A). Other mucosal surfaces, including the larynx, esophagus, nose, vulva, and anus, may also be involved. Scarring is less evident in these locations than in the conjunctiva, where erythema, without blisters and ulceration, and subsequent scarring are the rule. Unilateral blindness occurs in up to 20% of cases. In cutaneous CP, the cutaneous lesions are of two types: (a) an extensive eruption of bullae that heals without scarring initially and (b) areas of erythema mainly on the face and scalp in which bullae erupt intermittently followed by atrophy and scarring. Both types of lesions may be present in the same patient. In the Brunsting–Perry variant of CP, there are no mucosal lesions but rather one to several circumscribed erythematous patches on which recurrent crops of blisters appear with atrophic scarring. The patches are usually confined to the head and neck area but may generalize. Other clinical variants include a widespread generally nonscarring bullous eruption in which scarring lesions develop only on the head and widespread bullae that

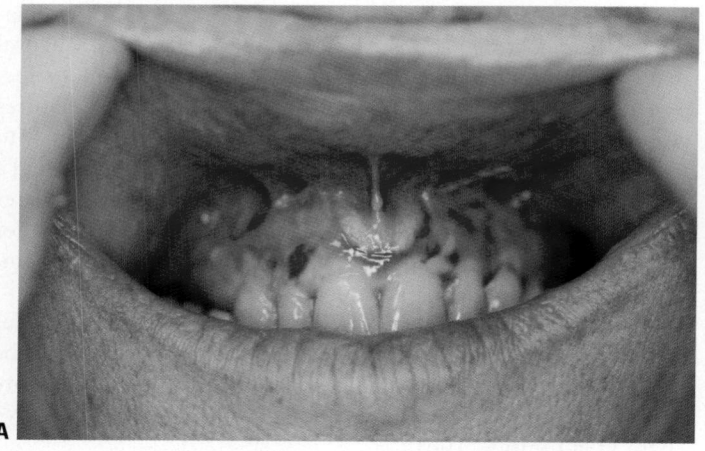

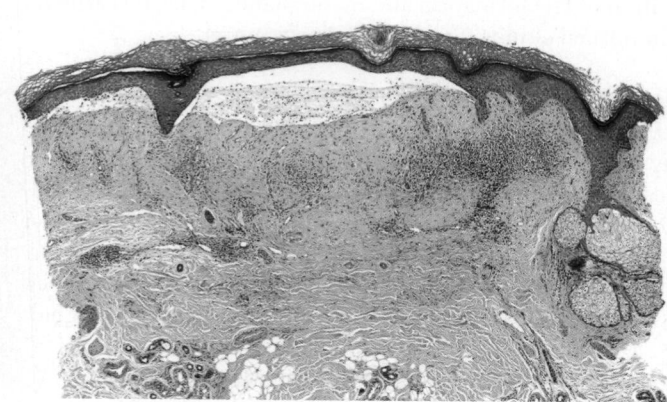

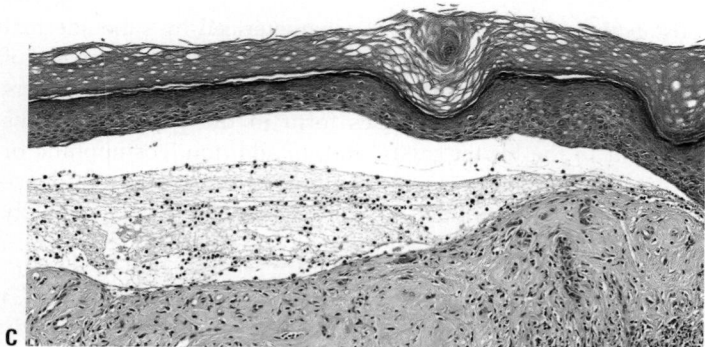

Figure 9-21 Mucous membrane pemphigoid. **A:** Clinical example. Gingival eroded and ulcerated plaque along the gum margin. (Courtesy of Dr. Charles M. Phillips.) **B and C:** Histologic features, cutaneous lesion (scalp), from a patient with coexistent ocular involvement. **B:** There is a subepidermal blister with underlying fibrosis and inflammation (low power). **C:** The bulla cavity contains fibrin and inflammatory cells, including eosinophils (medium power).

heal with atrophic scars. Paraneoplastic CP, in particular the antiepiligrin variant, has been reported. All patients with CP/MMP should undergo age-appropriate and symptom-based malignancy screening.

Histopathology. In cutaneous lesions, a subepidermal blister develops that may extend down adnexa. Neutrophils and lymphocytes predominate in the inflammatory infiltrate. Eosinophils may or may not be numerous. Lamellar fibrosis beneath the epidermis is a hallmark but may not be present in the initial lesions (Fig. 9-21B, C). MMP lesions generally have a lichenoid lymphocytic infiltrate in which neutrophils or eosinophils or both may be present. The changes are often nonspecific, mimicking LP or lichenoid hypersensitivity mucositis in both mucosal and cutaneous lesions, but the above features should lead to consideration of CP/MMP.

IF Testing. In MMP, a variety of antigenic targets have been reported—β4 integrin, laminin 5, type VII collagen (MMP-like EBA), BP180, and BP230. Both IgG (most common) and IgA mediation may occur such that the latter should be labeled MMP-like IgA bullous disease (199). Other antigen targets have been described. In other words, MMP is a clinicopathologic syndrome in which several different antibody specificities to different antigens are present.

In MMP/CP, DIF studies reveal linear IgG and C3 at the squamous basement membrane zone in lesional and perilesional skin in approximately 80% of cases. In three series, a total of 35 of 46 patients had linear deposits. In most, both IgG and C3 were present, occasionally in association with IgA or

IgM. Uncommonly, only C3 was present. With respect to the Brunsting–Perry type, 9 of 10 patients had linear IgG at the dermoepidermal junction, 3 of whom had concomitant linear C3.

DIF studies are required in order to make a definitive diagnosis. As mentioned previously, in other cases labeled CP, only linear IgA was found; therefore, these cases are best considered linear IgA bullous dermatosis/mucositis (200,201). Patients with cicatricial conjunctivitis that display only linear IgA deposits are best considered a scarring variant of LAD/mucositis. IIF testing of serum yields variable results depending on the substrate used (monkey esophagus, guinea pig esophagus, normal human skin, salt-split skin). It appears that circulating antibodies in this disorder may be more readily demonstrated when normal salt-split human skin is used as substrate, in which IgG may be localized only to the roof or, as in the antiepiligrin subgroup (see later), to the base of the induced separation (see Table 9-10).

The difference in clinical presentation, as well as the localization of the immunoreactants, may be explained by differing antigenic specificity of the antibodies. The known autoantigens include the following: (a) epiligrin (202), also known as laminin 5 and 6 (the antigen is associated with the disease previously termed antiepiligrin CP laminin 6 (α 3 chain)); (b) β4 subunit of the α6β4 integrin (this antigen is predominantly associated with ocular CP) (203); (c) BPAg2 (204) and BPAg1 (177). The 6β4 integrin is closely associated with oral BP. It is noteworthy that autoantibodies from patients with CP tend to target the C-terminus of BPAg2, whereas those from patients with BP, PG, and lamina lucida type LABD typically target the NC16A domain of BPAg2. All these antigens occur within the lamina lucida, with epiligrin present in the lower lamina lucida. This likely explains the localization of the antibody to the artifactually created blister base in salt-split skin preparations (see Table 9-10). At this point in time, CP is best considered not one disease but several diseases with a similar clinical phenotype of scarring, predilection for mucosal and conjunctival surfaces, and subepidermal/subepithelial bullae. Many cases in the literature labeled CP without adequate immunologic study may be better classified as linear IgA disease or EBA involving principally mucosal surfaces. In other words, MMP/CP is a disease phenotype produced by autoimmunity directed against several different antigens and by different immunoglobulin sets.

Pathogenesis. ELISA studies are more sensitive in demonstrating the antibodies. Western blot analysis reveals bands associated with all the antigens according to the subset of CP present (130, 180, 230, 145, or 205 kDa). The immune mechanisms are similar to those of BP. At this time, BP is thought to scar only if secondarily infected. The etiology of the fibrosis in CP is unknown, but myofibroblasts and chemokines (interleukins) likely play a role.

Ultrastructural Study. Electron microscopic examination revealed in two studies that the oral and cutaneous lesions possess an intact basement membrane zone at the base of the blister (possibly early lesions). In another study of both the oral and cutaneous lesions, the basement membrane zone was destroyed.

Principles of Management: Patients with MMP require multispecialty care. The aggressiveness of management depends on the affected mucous membranes and the severity of the disease. Patients with ocular, genital, nasopharyngeal, or laryngeal involvement are considered high-risk and require early aggressive treatment (182).

Patients with mild oral disease or severe oral disease without conjunctival, laryngeal, or esophageal involvement may be treated with topical or systemic steroids, topical tacrolimus, tetracycline-class antibiotics with niacinamide, oral dapsone individually or in combination (205). The high-risk group requires treatment with a combination of rituximab and systemic steroids and dapsone. IVIG may be added if there is evidence of progression of disease or active scarring.

Pemphigoid (Herpes) Gestationis

Clinical Features. This is a blistering disorder that usually develops during the second to third trimester in pregnant women. It is estimated to occur in 1 in 50,000 pregnancies. Intensely pruritic, urticarial lesions usually develop on the abdomen with subsequent involvement of the extremities, hands, and feet (Fig. 9-22A). They usually progress to tense vesicles and bullae, some herpetiform. The disorder may recur with subsequent pregnancies, menstrual periods, or the use of birth control pills. The course for the mother is benign. There was a debate concerning the possibility of an increased incidence and risk of fetal morbidity and mortality. However, data indicate that no such risk can be confirmed (206) except for an association with prematurity and small-for-gestational-age weights (207). The infant may be born with a mild, transient, vesiculobullous eruption secondary to transplacental transfer of the mediating antibodies.

Histopathology. In zones of erythema and edema, there is a perivascular infiltrate composed of lymphocytes and eosinophils. There is marked papillary dermal edema. There may be spongiosis, which may be eosinophilic in type. Focal necrosis of the basal keratinocytes, which has been emphasized by some authors, leads to a subepidermal blister (Fig. 9-22B, C). However, in the author's (TJH) experience, it is only uncommonly documented on routine light microscopy.

IF Testing. DIF testing reveals linear deposition of C3 at the dermoepidermal junction in perilesional or erythematous skin in virtually all patients. IgG is similarly deposited in 30% to 40% (Fig. 9-22D, E). Immunoelectron microscopic study has revealed IgG and C3 to reside within the lamina lucida. Using routine IIF studies of serum, it is uncommon to demonstrate circulating anti–squamous basement membrane zone antibodies. Using *in vitro* complement fixation, a circulating anti–basement membrane zone IgG is demonstrable in most cases. At this point in time, the use of the label *HG factor* for these IgG antibodies is of historical interest only. The antibody is directed against a placental antigen that contains epitopes of BP180 (208). The BPAg2 is the principal antigen, but BPAg1 and type VII collagen are recognized in some patients as well (209,210).

Ultrastructural Study. The epidermis at the periphery of bullae shows significant damage, most pronounced in basal keratinocytes, with resultant complete or partial necrosis of epidermal cells. Even though basal keratinocytes show severe damage, the basal cell plasma membrane and the lamina densa are well preserved and are present at the floor of the blister. The HDs may be intact in some areas.

Principles of Management: PG treatment may involve mid- to high-potency topical steroids, systemic steroids, and/or oral antihistamines. Previously published studies reported systemic absorption of potent topical steroids during pregnancy, with some association with low birth weight. However, Andersson et al. (211) found no association between use of topical steroids during pregnancy and low birth weight even when large amounts of potent to very potent topical steroids were used. Treatment of the blistering disease should balance maternal and fetal concerns and should be handled with close discourse between dermatologists and obstetricians.

Differential Diagnosis. The prime differential diagnosis clinicopathologically is PUPPP syndrome (pruritic urticarial papules and plaques of pregnancy syndrome) now labeled "polymorphous eruption of pregnancy." It usually develops in late first pregnancy or even in the postpartum period associated with increased maternal weight, multiple gestational pregnancies (twins, triplets, etc.) beginning in the abdominal striae sparing the umbilicus. Later on, the rash is more polymorphic. It has a perivascular lymphohistiocytic infiltrate with dermal edema (rarely with subepidermal blisters) and spongiosis. Histologically, the changes may be identical to PG. DIF study reveals nonspecific findings, and IIF study reveals no antibodies directed against either epidermal or basement membrane zone

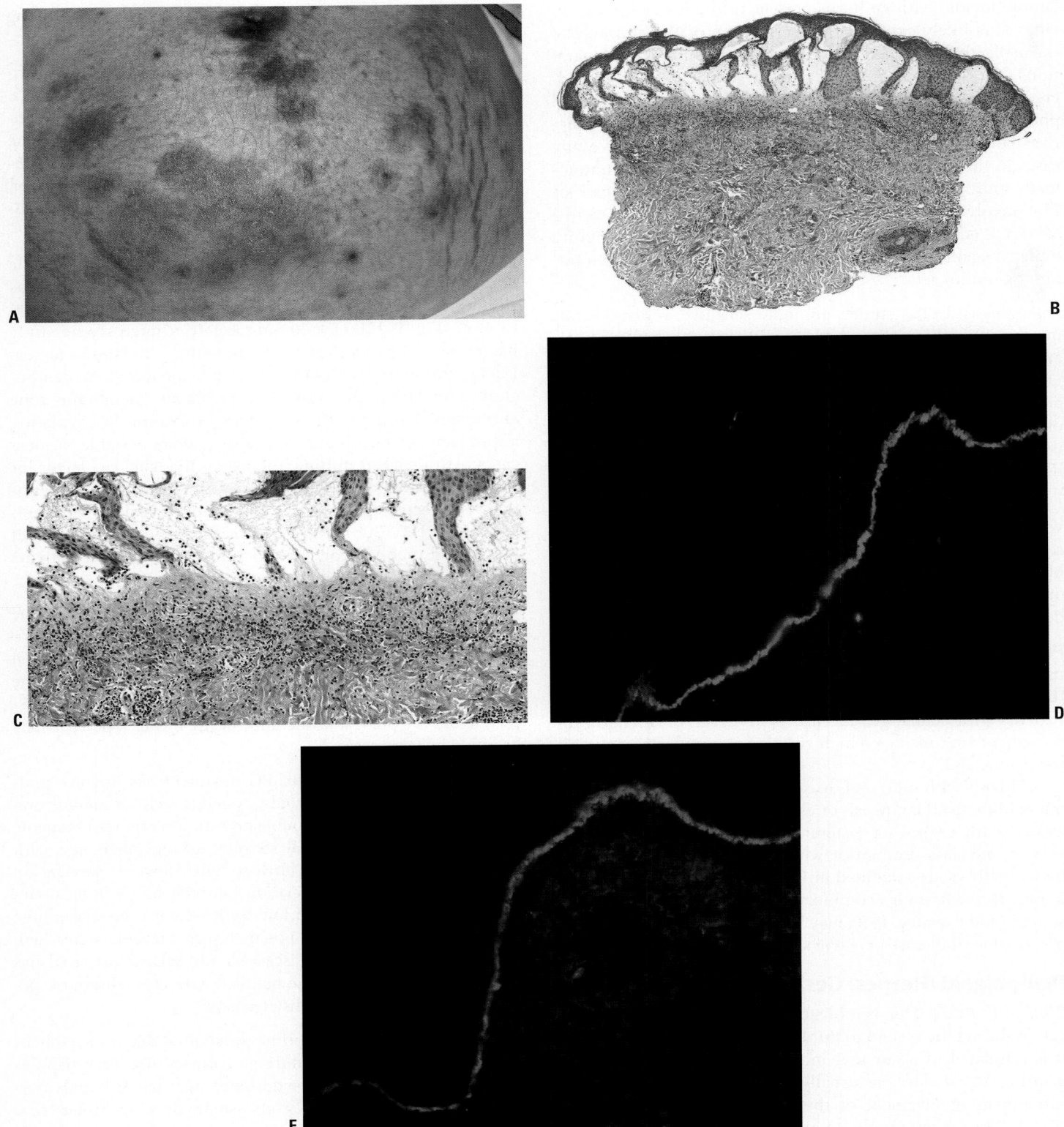

Figure 9-22 Pemphigoid gestationis. **A:** Clinical example. Erythematous and urticarial papules and plaques on the abdomen. (Courtesy of Dr. Charles M. Phillips.) **B, C:** Histologic features. **B:** Papillary dermal edema with subepidermal blister (scanning power). **C:** The bulla cavity contains fibrin and eosinophils. Eosinophils are present in and below the bulla floor (medium power). **D, E:** Direct Immunofluorescence study. There is linear deposition of IgG (D) and C3 (E) along the epidermal basement membrane zone. Oftentimes, only C3 is present using routine DIF studies.

antigens. Drug eruptions, arthropod bite reactions, atopic dermatitis (atopic eruption of pregnancy), and intrahepatic cholestasis of pregnancy (ICP) must be considered as well. Pruritus is the hallmark of ICP with secondary lesions of excoriation, nonspecific histologic changes, elevated serum bilirubin, and IF studies that are negative (i.e., nonspecific findings).

VESICULOBULLOUS DERMATOSES WITH AUTOIMMUNITY TO TYPE VII COLLAGEN AND LOWER LAMINA LUCIDA COMPONENTS

Epidermolysis Bullosa Acquisita

Clinical Features. Classically, EBA is a noninherited noninflammatory disorder of acquired skin fragility in which blisters develop on noninflammatory bases secondary to trauma with a predilection for acral areas. Scarring and milia formation ensue. A characteristic nail dystrophy and alopecia are noted. This presentation is associated with malignant lymphoma, amyloidosis, colitis or enteritis, and connective tissue disease (212–214). However, some patients with EBA may have significant involvement of oral and conjunctival mucosa and may therefore be MMP-like or CP-like (see Mucous Membrane Pemphigoid/ Cicatricial Pemphigoid, p. 317). However, acral lesions are prominent, and nail dystrophy is noted. In this type, biopsy from mucosal lesions reveals inflammatory, subepidermal bullae with scarring and milia similar to CP and MMP.

In 1984, five EBA patients with clinical and histologic features of bullous pemphigoid were described (BP-like EBA) (215). They had generalized pruritic, erythematous macules and papules on which bullae arose. There was a lesser tendency for the lesions to develop acrally or at sites of trauma and greater involvement of flexural surfaces than in the previously described forms of EBA. At presentation, neither scarring nor milia were discerned; however, delicate scars developed later at the sites of blister formation.

Histopathology. The *bullous pemphigoid-like* presentation described previously is the most common form of EBA. The subepidermal blisters are inflammatory, the differential diagnosis being BP, bullous drug eruption, linear IgA disease, and DH. The predominant infiltrating cells are lymphocytes and neutrophils in perivascular and focal interstitial array (Fig. 9-23A, B). Eosinophils are present in variable numbers such that the lesions may be indistinguishable from BP. In the *classic form* initially described, the subepidermal blisters are noninflammatory (Fig. 9-23C) with subsequent fibrosis and milia formation giving the differential diagnosis of porphyria and pseudoporphyria. In CP-like and MMP-like presentations, histologic differentiation is not possible.

IF Testing. Examination of perilesional or erythematous skin using DIF reveals linear deposition of complement at the basement membrane zone in most cases. IgG is by far the most common immunoglobulin found in the u-serrated pattern (216), but IgM and IgA may be present as well. Increasing numbers of immunoglobulin subclasses noted at the dermoepidermal

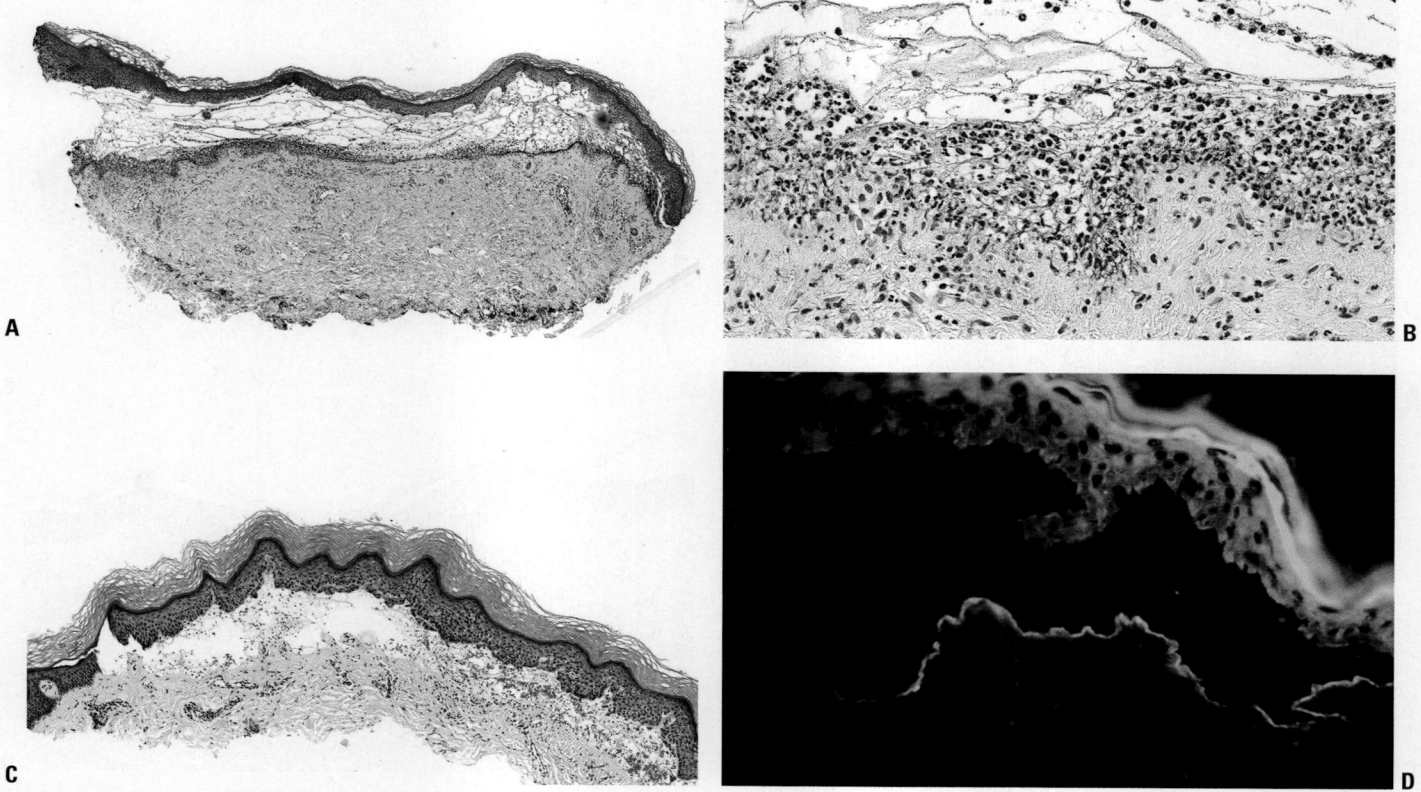

Figure 9-23 Epidermolysis bullosa acquisita. **A–C:** Histologic features. **A, B:** Inflammatory-type with some neutrophils and eosinophils in the blister cavity. **A**—Scanning power with reepithelialization of the blister base, and **B**—high power from an early blister. **C:** Noninflammatory type with a subepidermal cleft (scanning power). **D:** Salt-split direct immunofluorescence reveals linear deposition of IgG along the blister base (as it is in naturally developed blisters that arise in epidermolysis bullosa acquisita).

junction favor a diagnosis of EBA over bullous pemphigoid. The presence of linear C3 at the dermoepidermal junction alone favors bullous pemphigoid over EBA. However, use of routine DIF cannot reliably distinguish between bullous pemphigoid and EBA. IIF reveals circulating anti–basement membrane zone antibodies in up to 50%, with salt-split normal skin the most sensitive substrate.

The use of the salt-split skin technique leads to the appropriate diagnosis in most cases (217). The antibodies in EBA have specificity for the globular carboxyl terminus of type VII collagen (290 kDa protein) and are deposited beneath the lamina densa. Later studies have shown the antibodies bind with the N-terminal region, which joins the lower lamina densa (218). Therefore, in salt-split skin studies, IgG is on the floor and not on the roof of the split (Fig. 9-23D). The plane of separation is sublamina densa.

Principles of Management: EBA, particularly the noninflammatory mechanobullous subset, is often challenging to treat because it is resistant to most conventional medical therapies. It should be considered in the differential of cases of other autoimmune blistering diseases when they fail to respond to therapy because the recalcitrant nature of EBA is one of its defining features. There are no randomized controlled trials as the disease is rare. Systemic corticosteroids are the first choice

in the treatment of EBA (219). Steroid-sparing agents such as dapsone, MMF, and others are often used. Iwata et al. (220) reviewed all cases of EBA published between 1971 and 2016 and found IVIG and rituximab to be associated with complete remission.

Bullous Systemic Lupus Erythematosus

Clinical Features. Vesicles and bullae may develop in patients with SLE. In contrast to DH, the lesions are not symmetric, nor do they have a predilection for extensor surfaces of arms, elbows, or scalp (Fig. 9-24A). They may be photodistributed and widespread and are not pruritic. These patients rarely have classic lesions of discoid, systemic, or subacute cutaneous lupus erythematosus when they develop blisters. In cases from the literature, most had a previous history of lupus erythematosus, and most authors have required definitive American Rheumatologic Association (ARA) criteria before making the diagnosis of BSLE in those patients. Uncommonly, patients (who later developed other stigmata of lupus) have presented with a blistering eruption but without previous signs or symptoms of connective tissue disease. Some patients with EBA will progress to SLE, although it is possible that some of these patients had SLE all along. BSLE is most common in women, particularly black women. Most of these cases were exquisitely sensitive to dapsone therapy, with

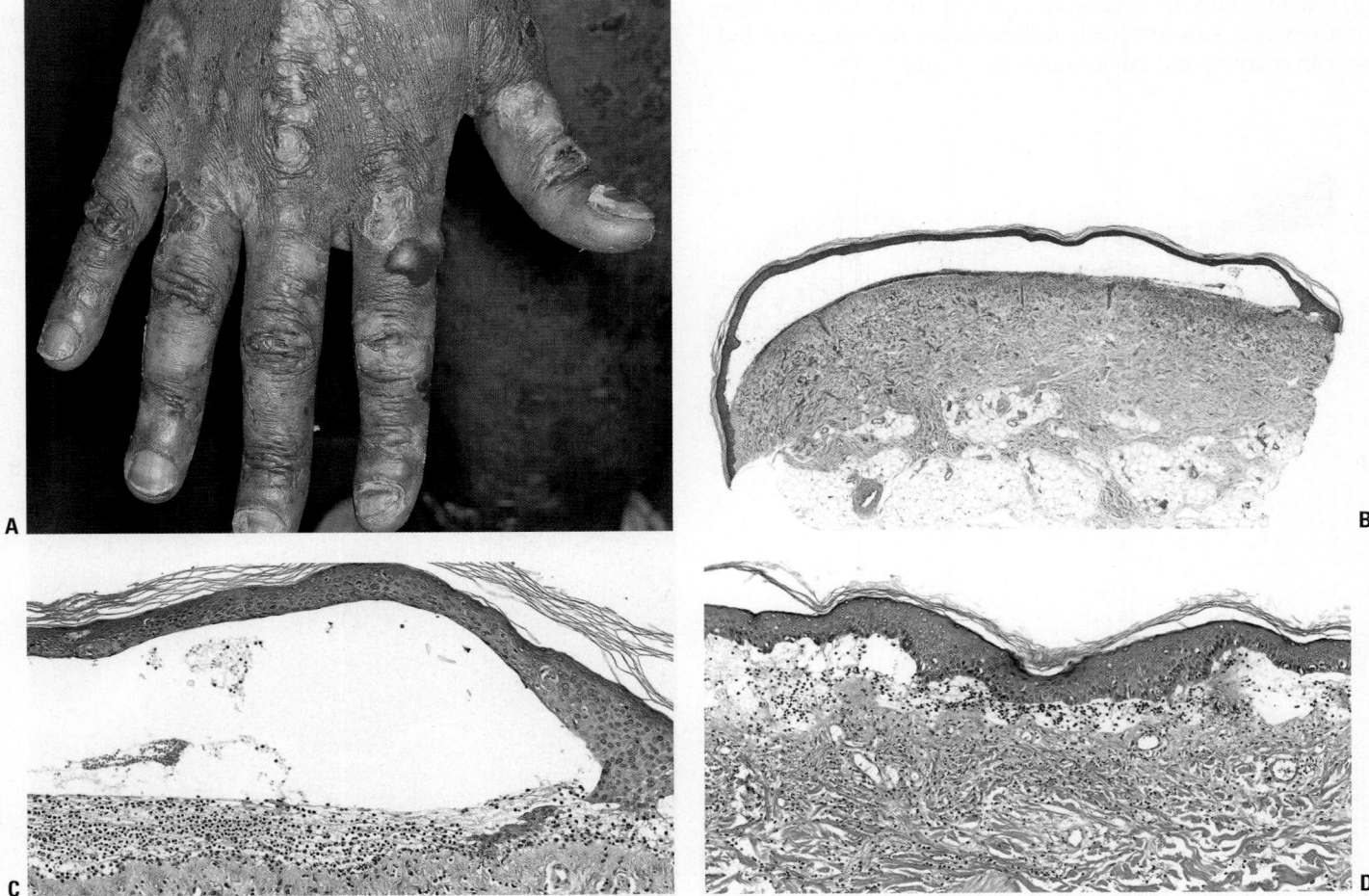

Figure 9-24 Bullous systemic lupus erythematosus. **A:** Clinical example. Tense bullae on the hands with postinflammatory pigment alteration. **B–D:** Histologic features. **B and C:** A subepidermal blister with neutrophils in the floor of the bulla. The pattern is epidermolysis bullosa acquisita–like. **B**—Scanning power, and **C**—medium power. **D:** Another case with a subepidermal split and neutrophils in the bulla and bulla floor simulating dermatitis herpetiformis (low power).

rapid involution of the lesions. No correlation with the clinical activity of lupus erythematosus was apparent.

Histopathology. Three histologic patterns have been identified in LE with blisters. The first two are not BSLE as discussed here, in which blisters are the primary lesion. The first is striking basal layer vacuolization with subsequent blister formation (classic LE lesion with a secondary blister). The second is vasculitis with subepidermal blister and pustule formation. The third is a DH-like histologic pattern true BSLE as described here, in which neutrophils predominate but do not tend to preferentially accumulate in dermal papillae (Fig. 9-24B–D). Approximately 25% of cases are said to have a small-vessel, neutrophil-rich leukocytoclastic vasculitis beneath the blister, but this may be an overinterpretation of the superficial perivascular neutrophilic infiltrate. Histologic features more routinely identified with lupus erythematosus are not present. Another histologic finding that is not emphasized in most case reports is the presence of dermal mucin/hyaluronic acid as defined by Alcian blue stain at pH 2.5 (221). The frequency of mucin deposition is unknown. Lastly, there are some patients with BSLE clinically and histologically in which no antibodies to type VII collagen are detected by routine studies (DIF, IIF).

IF Testing. In virtually all reported cases, IgG and C3 are deposited at the epidermal basement membrane zone. The pattern was linear in more than 50% and was referred to as "granular bandlike" in approximately 25%. IgM and IgA were present in approximately 50% and 60% of cases, respectively. The conflicting pattern of immune reactant deposition is difficult to explain. In these reports, the pattern varies from a "thick band" to a "fine ribbonlike" or "tubular" pattern. The ribbonlike or linear pattern represents antibodies that are bound to rigid, anatomically compartmentalized antigens such as those in BP and EBA. In general, granular patterns represent deposition of circulating immune complexes *in situ* or *in situ* binding of antigen and antibody in noncompartmentalized zones. Therefore, perhaps, some of the cases represent tubular or linear deposition obscured by confluent granular bands (positive lupus band test). IIF study of serum rarely reveals circulating anti–squamous basement membrane zone antibodies that are detected against type VII collagen. It is likely that if salt-split skin preparations were employed, the observation of IgG at the dermoepidermal junction may likely be greater. Antinuclear IgG may be observed in keratinocytic, endothelial, and other cells.

A salt-split skin preparation using patient serum reveals localization to the split floor as in EBA (Table 9-10). Lastly, Western immunoblot reveals binding to 290- or 145-kDa dermal proteins, components of type VII collagen. However, circulating antibodies to type VII collagen may not be detected.

Ultrastructural Study. Immunoelectron microscopic examination reveals electron-dense deposits of IgG at the lower edge of the basal lamina and immediately subjacent dermis in an identical location to the antibody in EBA.

Principles of Management: BSLE occurs in less than 1% of SLE patients. Patients with bullous lupus will often require treatment with neutrophil-targeting agents such as dapsone to achieve control of their skin disease. Bullous SLE is usually unresponsive to systemic corticosteroids alone or hydroxychloroquine. Responses to rituximab (222) and other agents, such as methotrexate and MMF (223), have been reported.

SUBEPIDERMAL IGA-MEDIATED VESICULOBULLOUS DERMATOSES

Dermatitis Herpetiformis

This is an intensely pruritic, chronic recurrent dermatitis that has a slight male predilection. The lesions usually develop in young to middle-aged adults as symmetric grouped erythematous papulovesicles, vesicles, or crusts (Fig. 9-25A). Oral lesions are absent. The elbows, knees, buttocks, scapula, and scalp are commonly involved. There is a high incidence (about 90%) of gluten-sensitive enteropathy, subclinical in the vast majority, and an increased, but low risk of lymphoma (224). There is usually a long course, but approximately 10% may enter remission (225).

Histopathology. The typical histologic features are best observed in erythematous skin adjacent to early blisters. In these zones, neutrophils accumulate at the tips of dermal papillae. With an increase in size to microabscesses, a significant admixture of eosinophils may be noted. As microabscesses form, a separation develops between the tips of the dermal papillae and the overlying epidermis so that early blisters are multiloculated (Fig. 9-25B–D). The presence of fibrin in the papillae may give them a blue hue. Within 1 to 2 days, the rete ridges lose their attachment to the dermis, and the blisters then become unilocular and clinically apparent. At this time, the characteristic papillary microabscesses may be observed at the blister periphery. For this reason, the inclusion of perivesicular skin in the biopsy specimen is of utmost value. The papillary dermis beneath the papillae may have a relatively intense inflammatory infiltrate of neutrophils and some eosinophils. Many neutrophils may exhibit leukocytoclasis such that neutrophil-rich "vasculitis" is present. Subjacent to this, a perivascular infiltrate composed of lymphocytes, neutrophils, and eosinophils may be apparent. In one study, the diagnostic finding of papillary microabscesses was present in all patients. In another study of 105 biopsy specimens, they were present in only 52%. Apoptotic keratinocytes may be noted above the papillary microabscesses. In our estimation, studies purporting nonspecific changes likely represent inappropriate biopsy selection or biopsy of early urticarial lesions before the development of characteristic changes or biopsy of patients with DH and other coincidental disorders (226).

IF Testing. In 1967, Cormane described the presence of granular fibrillary IgA1 in dermal papillae in dermatitis herpetiformis. It is primarily IgA in lesional and non-lesional skin (227) although IgA2 deposits have recently been described (228). IgA is found alone or in combination with other immune reactants in over 95% of cases when uninvolved skin of the forearm or buttock is tested (Fig. 9-25E). Fibrillary IgA deposits may also be present. Some recommend that biopsies be taken from clinically normal skin immediately adjacent to erythema, because false-negative results may occur when blistered or inflamed skin is evaluated. The presence of IgA within the skin is not altered by dapsone therapy. After as long as 2 years, a gluten-free diet results in the disappearance of IgA from the skin. Negative results of DIF testing of two appropriately selected biopsy sites are essentially conclusive that an untreated patient does not have DH. However, there have been DIF-negative cases in which antitransglutaminase antibodies were present serologically and the patients responded to gluten-free diet (229,230). Lastly, there is confusion

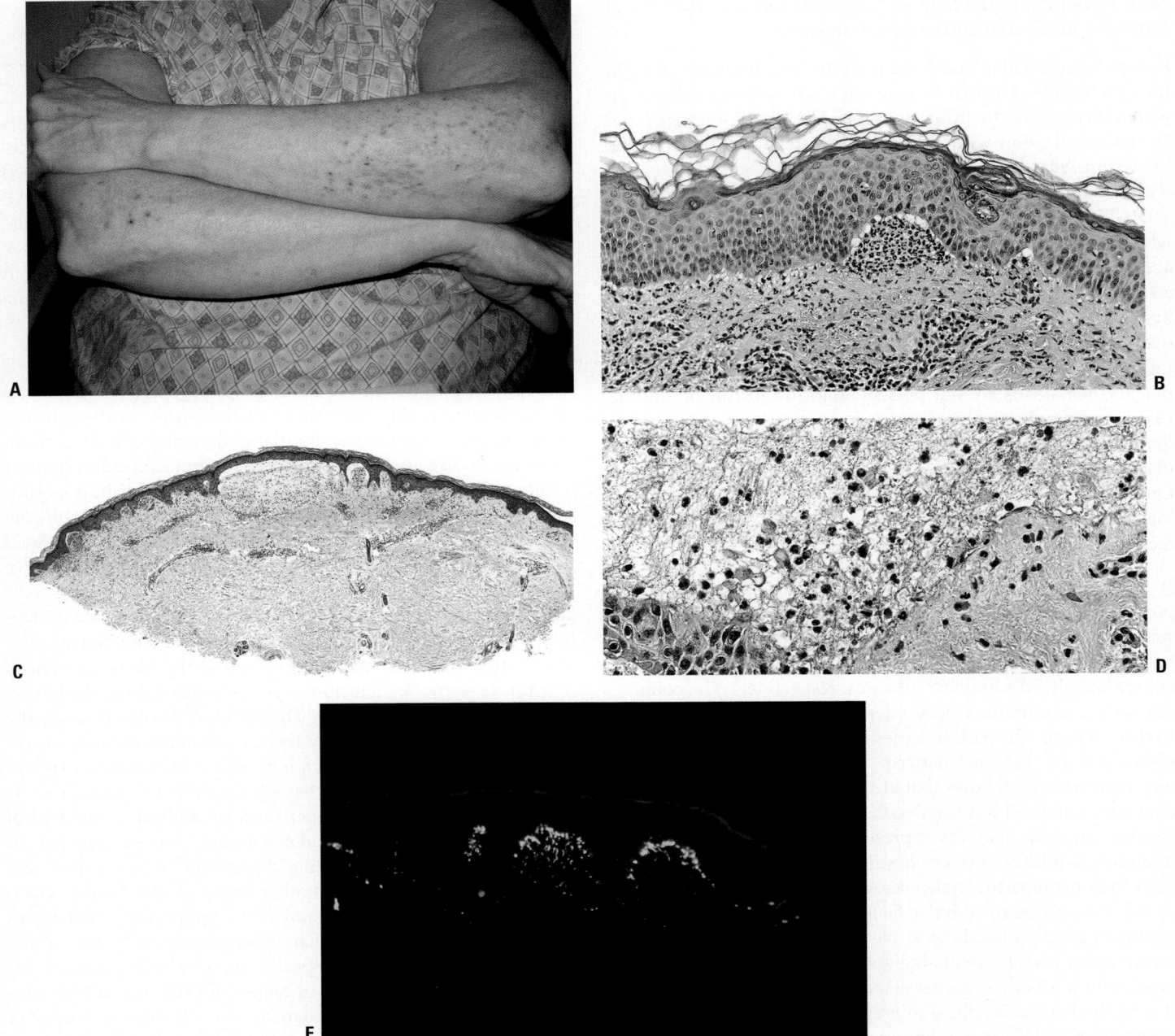

Figure 9-25 Dermatitis herpetiformis. **A.** Clinical example. Erythematous and excoriated grouped symmetrical papulovesicles on the extensor forearms. (Courtesy of KennethTsai, MD, PhD.) **B-D.** Histologic features. **B.** Papillary dermal neutrophilic microabscesses are characteristic (low-medium power). **C.** In this example of a scanning power image, there are multiple papillary dermal neutrophilic microabscesses present at the periphery of the central subepidermal vesicle. **D.** Fibrin, neutrophils, and rare eosinophils are seen in this fully developed unilocular subepidermal bulla (high power). **E.** Direct immunofluorescence. There is granular and thready IgA predominantly at the tips of dermal papillae (direct immunofluorescence).

over the status of granular IgA deposition and fibrillary IgA deposition. In the estimation of one of the authors (TJH), both represent DH, possibly with epitope spreading.

Circulating IgA antibodies that react against reticulin, smooth muscle endomysium, the dietary antigen gluten (in specific gliadin, a component of gluten), bovine serum albumin, β-lactoglobulin, and other antigens may be present. Only the presence of IgA endomysial antibodies is of diagnostic importance, but their presence is not specific or very sensitive. They are present in 70% of overall DH patients but in 100% of those with atrophy on jejunal biopsy (231). Using monkey or pig gut as substrate, IIF has been used to detect antiendomysial antibodies, which are present in 52% to 100% of patients.

Pathogenesis. Three important findings must be considered in the pathogenesis of DH. First, the disease is associated with a gluten-sensitive enteropathy; second, granular, fibrillary pattern IgA is deposited in the skin; and, third, patients have a high frequency of certain HLA alleles, DQA*0501, DQ8, DR3, and B*02. Most DH patients have focal celiac sprue-like changes on jejunal biopsy. IgA autoantibodies to tissue transglutaminase (TG2/TG3) develop, which deaminates (glutamine) gliadin. TG2 becomes bound to gliadin peptides. TG2-gliadin is recognized by B cells as foreign with subsequent differentiation into plasma cells that produce anti-TG2-gliadin protein IgA. There is also anti-TG3 IgA production. The IgA anti-TG3 circulates and binds with epidermal TG3 in the dermal papillae. Complement is fixed, and neutrophil chemotaxis ensues. Antitissue transglutaminase (TG2, TG3) antibodies and antiendomysial antibodies are detected in patients with DH (232). Papillary dermal bound IgA immune precipitates in DH have been shown to contain epidermal transglutaminase (TG3) (233). Cytokine production (CD4+ lymphocytes) appears to play a role.

The IgA deposition in those immune complexes results in activation of the complement system, followed by chemotaxis of neutrophils into the papillary dermis (234). Enzymes released from these neutrophils degrade laminin and type IV collagen, contributing to blister formation.

Ultrastructural Study. The changes in DH resemble those observed in the inflammatory bullae of bullous pemphigoid. Neutrophils are the major inflammatory cell in the former, whereas eosinophils predominate in the latter. Fibrin appears earlier and in greater amount in DH, particularly in dermal papillae. Although it has been shown immunohistochemically that the early blister forms above the apparently intact lamina densa (235), in more advanced lesions the lamina densa has been destroyed, as is noted in the "inflammatory bullae" of bullous pemphigoid.

Principles of Management: The mainstay of treatment of DH is a lifelong gluten-free diet with or without treatment with dapsone (223). Additional options include sulfasalazine, potent topical steroids, and antihistamines.

Linear IgA Dermatosis

Clinical Features
A group of bullous disorders mediated by IgA antibodies with differing specificities for epidermal basement membrane zone antigens has been labeled LAD. There are four relatively definitive clinical phenotypes that are based on patient age and clinical features—two of them are adult LAD and childhood LAD (chronic benign bullous dermatosis of childhood). They differ slightly in their clinical presentations but have identical immunopathologic features. Thirdly, a clinical phenotype similar to MMP/CP has been described. Fourthly, a subset of patients has been described with drug-induced LAD. On the basis of immunoelectron microscopic localization of the IgA deposition, there are at least two distinct types of LAD: a lamina lucida type and a sublamina densa type. Some of the sublamina densa types of LAD are best classified as IgA EBA.

Adult-Type Linear IgA Dermatosis
Clinical Features. Vesicles and bullae develop in patients usually over 40 years of age, with a slight female predilection. The lesions are less symmetric and less pruritic than those in DH but may be distributed in similar locations (Fig. 9-26A, B). Most cases resolve, but 35% are persistent. In contrast to DH, ocular and oral lesions may be present in up to 50% of cases. Plantar and palmar bullae may develop. The cutaneous lesions are heterogeneous and may mimic other bullous diseases, including EM and BP. LAD has been associated with an increased risk of lymphoma (236). Ulcerative colitis has been correlated with LAD in various studies, one of which found ulcerative colitis in 7.1% of LAD patients (237). A rare association with SLE has been reported (238).

Histopathology. The features are similar, if not identical, to DH (Fig. 9-26C, D). According to some, there is a lesser tendency for papillary microabscess formation and a greater tendency for uniform neutrophil infiltration along the entire dermoepidermal junction and rete in inflamed skin. One may uncommonly

observe a principally lymphocytic infiltrate, sometimes with numerous neutrophils (239). Neutrophilic and eosinophilic spongiosis has been reported.

IF Testing. Because, at this time, the result of this test defines the disease, DIF reveals linear IgA along the epidermal basement membrane zone in perilesional skin in 100% of cases (Fig. 9-26E). In the lamina lucida type of LAD, IgA antibodies bind to the epidermal side of salt-split skin, whereas in the sublamina densa type (and IgA-mediated EBA), IgA antibodies bind to the dermal side of salt-split skin (Table 9-7). In most cases, IgA1, but rarely IgA2, is present. When IgG and IgA are present, some detailed immunologic study may be needed to allow differential diagnosis with BP (240). It has been suggested that if the IgA deposits are more intense than the IgG deposits and C3 deposition is strong, then LAD is the best diagnosis. However, it is best considered a distinct disorder labeled *linear IgA/IgG dermatosis* until more data are available, and it may have characteristics fitting best with linear IgA disease. One patient initially presented with linearly deposited IgG and only subsequently developed linear IgA deposits. Low titers of circulating anti–squamous basement membrane zone IgA have been identified in only 20% to 30% of cases (239). Another study, however, has noted such antibodies in up to 75% of patients.

Pathogenesis. In the lamina lucida type LAD, the antigen to which the IgA is directed is a 97-kDa protein that may be found in epidermal and dermal extracts (241). It is within the cleaved ectodomain of the 180-kDa bullous pemphigoid antigen (BPAg2) (LABD97) near the carboxy-terminus or, more commonly, the adjacent portion of collagen XVII (BPAg2) (157,242,243). Some IgA antibodies bind to the lamina densa.

In the sublamina densa type, the antigen is in many instances unknown. In some cases, the antigen is type VII collagen, specifically the NC-1 domain, the immunodominant epitope for EBA (244) or LAD285 (245). However, further work is needed because some studies have not demonstrated anti–Type VII collagen antibodies. Other antigenic targets, although not characteristic, include BPAg1, BPAg2, a 255 kDa protein, a 285 kDa protein, and 95 kDa ladinin. The events of the inflammatory cascade in IgA-mediated diseases are not well understood.

Ultrastructural Study. The antibodies are deposited principally within the lamina lucida and less commonly beneath the lamina densa (IgA-mediated EBA).

Drug-Associated Linear IgA Dermatosis
It is important to note that it is not infrequent for adult-type LAD to be associated with drug therapy. Vancomycin (most commonly reported), trimethoprim/sulfamethoxazole, penicillins, lithium, diclofenac, captopril, NSAIDs, furosemide, verapamil, gemfibrozil, HPV vaccination, and cephalosporins have been associated with such presentations (246). Histologically, the changes are identical to idiopathic LAD in most cases. In some cases, there is an associated lymphoeosinophilic infiltrate in combination with the interface neutrophilic infiltration. Vancomycin has been associated with a TEN-like presentation with great morbidity and mortality. The IgA is directed against a number of antigens (247).

Childhood Type Linear IgA Dermatosis
Clinical Features. Originally known as chronic bullous dermatosis of childhood, this disorder presents in prepubertal, often preschool children, and rarely in infancy. Vesicles or bullae

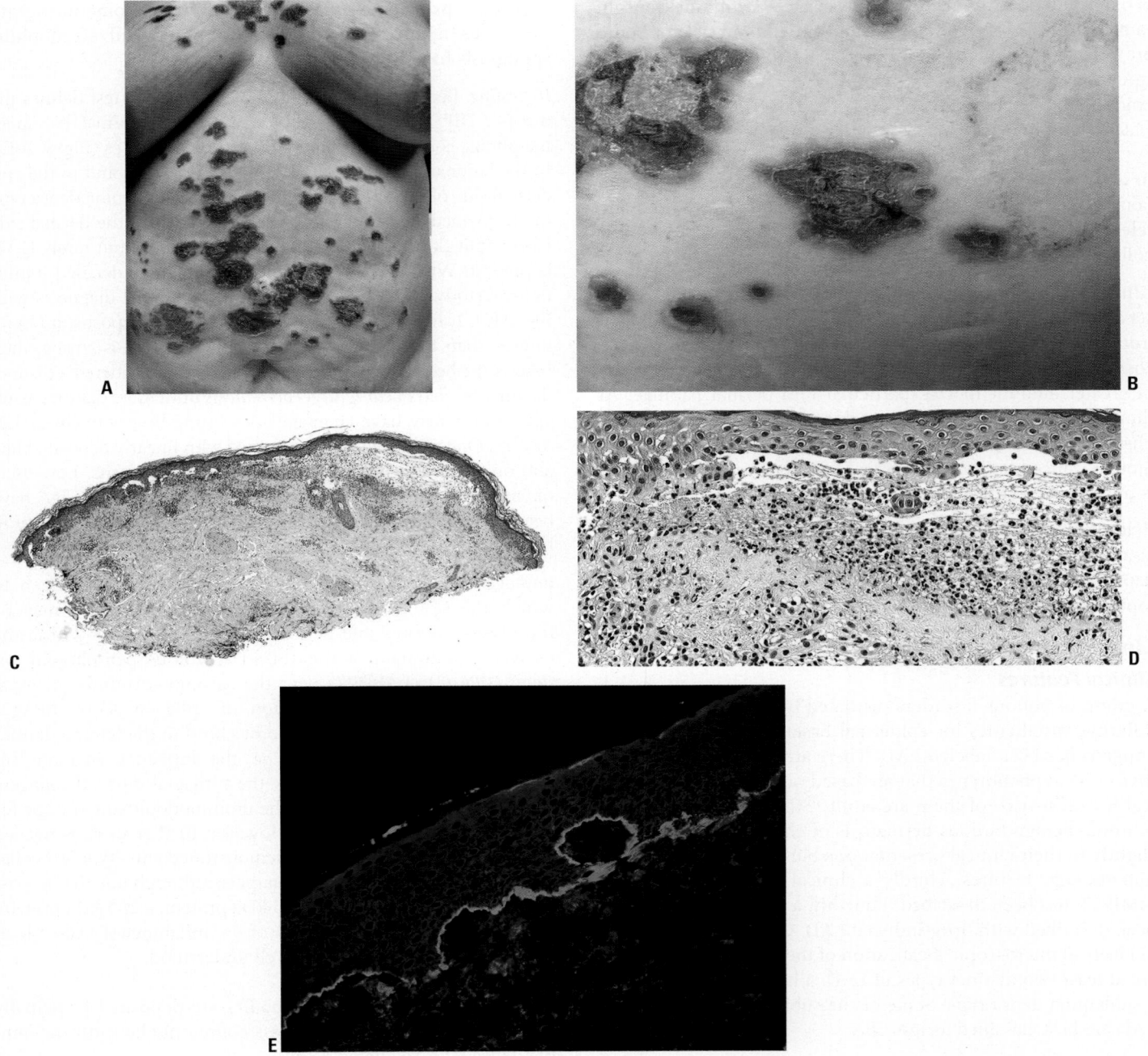

Figure 9-26 Linear IgA bullous dermatosis. A, B: Clinical example. Semiconfluent arcuate and annular plaques with peripheral bullae and crusted erosions on the abdomen, the "string of pearls" appearance. B: A closer view of A. C, D: Histologic features. C: There is a subepidermal bullae containing numerous neutrophils with papillary dermal neutrophilic microabscesses at its periphery (scanning power). D: Neutrophils, fibrin, and fluid are present in the subepidermal blister (medium power). E: Direct immunofluorescence. There is linear IgA deposition along the epidermal basement membrane zone.

develop on an erythematous or normal base, occasionally giving rise to a so-called "string of pearls," a characteristic lesion in which peripheral vesicles develop on a polycyclic plaque (Fig. 9.27). They involve the buttocks, lower abdomen, and genitalia, and characteristically have a perioral distribution on the face. Oral lesions may occur. The disorder usually remits by age 6 to 8 years; but in one series, 12% experienced persistent disease.

Histopathology. The features are similar to those of adult LAD. Some cases, however, resemble BP because of the presence of eosinophils..

IF Testing. DIF testing reveals linearly deposited IgA in virtually 100% of cases. The targeted antigens are identical to those noted in the adult-type disease. The sublamina densa type is uncommon in children [248].

Principles of Management: Multiple drugs can potentially cause linear IgA disease. Etiologic agents should be sought and discontinued. For mild cases, a potent topical steroid may be helpful. For classic cases of linear IgA disease, the treatment of choice is dapsone. Sulfapyridine may also be used [249]. For severe cases, systemic corticosteroids and other immunosuppressants may be needed.

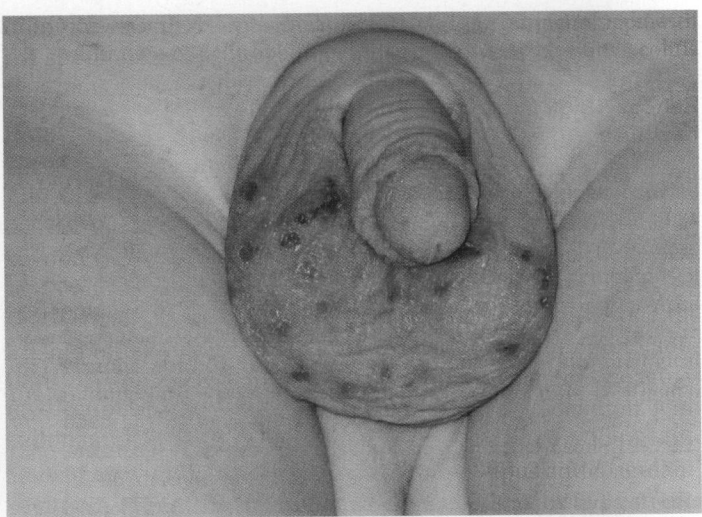

Figure 9-27 Childhood linear IgA dermatitis. Crusted erosions on the scrotum. (Courtesy of Kenneth Tsai, MD, PhD.)

TREATMENT OF IMMUNOBULLOUS DISORDERS

Autoimmune blistering disorders consist of a group of uncommon disorders characterized by the formation of antibodies to structural components of the skin and mucous membranes (250). The approach to management of immunobullous disorders starts with the establishment of the correct diagnosis based on clinical presentation, histopathology, and DIF and IIF findings described previously. Prior to initiating a disease-specific treatment strategy, disease severity, risk of permanent sequelae, and the patient's comorbidities must be taken into account. Concurrently with initiating disease-specific therapy, monitoring and prophylactic therapy for possible treatment-associated adverse effects should be instituted.

The goal of treatment in immunobullous diseases is to decrease the amount of offending autoantibodies, which then attenuates the disease and improves the patient's quality of life, while minimizing the potential adverse effects of the treatment. Preservation of function in high-risk diseases, such as MMP, involving the eyes, esophagus, and genitourinary organs, is of the highest priority and requires more aggressive treatment. There are numerous available therapeutic modalities, ranging from topical and systemic corticosteroids to antibiotics, antimetabolites, plasmapheresis, and immunomodulation with intravenous immunoglobulin (IVIg) and anti-CD20 monoclonal antibody therapy. Newer modalities for immunobullous diseases are in clinical or preclinical trials (185,251,252). First-, second-, and third-line agents are now recognized for each condition and chosen based on the individual patient's age, any underlying medical conditions, and the extent and severity of the specific disease (253,254). The first-line therapy of immunobullous diseases is systemic corticosteroids, usually combined with a steroid-sparing agent. Prior to the advent of corticosteroid therapy in the 1950s, PV was invariably fatal, 75% succumbing within one year of the diagnosis (255,256). Extensive cutaneous and mucosal erosions result in loss of fluid and electrolytes, poor nutrition, difficulties with thermoregulation, and loss of barrier function, increasing the risk of infection, including sepsis. Although the introduction of corticosteroid therapy has greatly reduced the mortality from immunobullous diseases, the adverse effects of this treatment may lead to morbidity and, infrequently, mortality.

Corticosteroids are employed in the treatment algorithms for all immunobullous disorders. Glucocorticoids have both immunosuppressive and anti-inflammatory effects, including decreased production of and response to multiple cytokines (IL-1, IL-8, TNF-α), prostaglandins, increase in apoptosis of eosinophils and autoreactive and neoplastic T cells, reduction of immunoglobulin production, and depression of neutrophil function and chemotaxis (257). Although effective in these disorders, complications from prolonged use include long-term hypothalamic–pituitary–adrenal axis suppression, fluid and electrolyte imbalance (hypokalemia, edema, hypertension, congestive heart failure), hyperglycemia, proximal myopathy, mood changes, osteoporosis, subcapsular cataracts, poor wound healing, and change in body habitus, among others. The therapeutic immunosuppressive effects increase the risk of infection, particularly staphylococcal.

In the initial management of PV, prednisone 1 to 1.5 mg/kg/day in divided dosages is given. Generally, response is seen within 4 to 6 weeks. Even those patients presenting initially with only oral lesions are started on systemic steroids in order to maintain adequate oral intake, obtain better control of the disease, and prevent epitope spreading. In a comparison of six reviewed guidelines in the treatment of PV (258), all but Brazilian Society of Dermatology also recommended rituximab as first-line treatment for moderate-to-severe PV.

The monoclonal chimeric antibody to CD20 expressed on the surface of pre-B cells and mature B cells (rituximab) has been used in the management of refractory and severe cases of several immunobullous disorders (259). The antibody causes a rapid reduction in the numbers of B cells and autoantibody production, producing an effect that can last for 6 to 10 months.

Although there is a higher risk of *Pneumocystis* pneumonia in patients on rituximab and systemic corticosteroids for hematologic malignancies, the risk was found to be 0.1% in 801 patients on rituximab/corticosteroid therapy for autoimmune blistering diseases (260). PJP prophylaxis is thus not recommended.

Other steroid-sparing agents such as antimetabolites (azathioprine, MMF, or an alkylating agent [cyclophosphamide]) may be started at the same time as the high-dose steroid therapy if rituximab is not advised or unavailable. These are slow to take effect, but once new lesions cease developing and existing lesions heal, the steroid may be slowly tapered to low-dose therapy over a period of many months. The duration of remission is unpredictable, so close clinical follow-up of these patients is needed over years. Risks of azathioprine use include bone marrow suppression, liver toxicity, and drug hypersensitivity. Cyclophosphamide is associated with myelosuppression, hemorrhagic cystitis, and urothelial carcinoma. Both drugs are associated with an increased risk of lymphoproliferative disorders.

First used for psoriasis in 1997, another agent in the therapeutic armamentarium for PV is MMF. This modified weak organic acid acts by inhibiting *de novo* purine synthesis. Because T and B cells lack the purine salvage pathway, the proliferative responses of these cells are preferentially blocked. MMF is used successfully either as an adjuvant or as monotherapy in patients with PV, EBA, CP, BP, and PNP. In fact, several case reports have documented remission in PV with this drug alone (261).

MMF is generally better tolerated than the other steroid-sparing agents, its most common side effects being GI disturbances and dose-dependent hematologic effects. Rarely, multifocal leukoencephalopathy has been reported in patients treated with this medication and other immunosuppressive agents (262).

Although most cases of PV and BP respond to the modalities described previously, in those patients with refractory or severe acute disease, removal of the offending autoantibodies with plasmapheresis, immunoadsorption, or extracorporeal photopheresis may be effective means of obtaining immediate control. These modalities are not without complications and are usually performed in an infusion center with specialized staff. In addition, because autoantibody production rebounds once this therapy is stopped, immunosuppressive agents are also generally given (263).

Another form of immunomodulation found to be effective in the management of refractory and severe PV/BP is intravenous immunoglobulin (IVIg). This modality was first used for BP in 1985 (264). Pooled IVIg from the plasma of thousands of healthy donors contains IgG classes in the same distribution as normal serum. The preparation contains antibodies to non-self and self-antigens and to other antibodies (idiotypic antibodies). The half-life is 3 weeks for IgG 1, 2, and 4 and 1 week for IgG3. Proposed mechanisms of action include blockade of neonatal Fc receptors, interference with activated components of the complement cascade, modification of cytokines, and suppression of Langerhans cell, T-cell, and B-cell function, including neutralizing and decreasing autoantibody production (265,266). Because this therapy has been associated with long-term remission in PV, the therapy is also thought to restore regulation of the patient's immune system autoreactivity. Patient's serum IgA levels should be checked because anaphylaxis can occur with IVIg treatment in IgA-deficient patients. With typically multiple cycles of therapy over many months, this treatment is expensive.

For those immunobullous disorders associated with a neutrophilic infiltrate in the skin (DH, LABD, and some cases of EBA), the first line of medication is dapsone. Dapsone inhibits the migration and binding of neutrophils to the deposits of IgA in skin and inhibits both neutrophil and eosinophil myeloperoxidase. All patients on this medication experience a mild hemolytic anemia and methemoglobinemia. A reversible peripheral neuropathy can also occur. Other idiosyncratic side effects include severe drug hypersensitivity syndrome and agranulocytosis.

In those patients with DH, strict adherence to a gluten-free diet can control the cutaneous disease without the need for dapsone, alleviate the GI symptoms, and reduce the risk of bowel lymphoma.

Treatment options for women with PG are dependent on the onset of the eruption. Before delivery, systemic corticosteroids are given. For those with refractory symptoms, plasmapheresis and IVIg may be used. After delivery, immunosuppressive agents may be employed.

Other anti-inflammatory medications used in the treatment of these diseases include antibiotics such as erythromycin and tetracycline with and without nicotinamide. These agents decrease chemotaxis of inflammatory cells and modify cytokine response (267). Given their safety profile, these adjuvants can be very useful in the appropriate clinical setting.

Cicatricial/mucosal pemphigoid requires close consultation with numerous specialists, including ophthalmologists, otolaryngologists, and gastroenterologists. High-potency topical steroids with systemic agents are used, depending on the severity and extent of the mucosal involvement. The condition is long lasting and can be debilitating.

In conclusion, since Dr. W.F. Lever published his seminal work on pemphigus over 60 years ago, considerable progress has been made in understanding the pathogenesis and treatment of these disorders (166). The therapeutic options have been broadened, and their mechanisms of action are being investigated and understood. Although many current therapies are not without significant adverse side effects, the ability to reduce the long-term exposure to systemic steroids, better monitoring of side effects, and the development of more specific methods of immunomodulation have been of great benefit to those suffering with these disorders.

OTHER NONINFECTIOUS VESICULOPUSTULAR DERMATOSES

Erythema Toxicum Neonatorum

Clinical Features. A benign, asymptomatic eruption affecting about 40% of term infants usually develops within 12 to 48 hours after birth. Erythema toxicum neonatorum lasts 2 to 3 days and consists of blotchy macular erythema, papules, and pustules that tend to develop at sites of pressure. The eruption is occasionally associated with blood eosinophilia.

Histopathology. The macular erythema is characterized by sparse eosinophils in the upper dermis, largely in a perivascular location, and mild papillary dermal edema. The papules show an accumulation of numerous eosinophils and some neutrophils in the area of the follicle and overlying epidermis. Papillary dermal edema is more intense and eosinophils more numerous. Mature pustules are subcorneal and are filled with eosinophils and occasional neutrophils. The pustules form as a result of the upward migration of eosinophils to the surface epidermis from within and around the hair follicles.

Pathogenesis. The etiology is unknown. However, two hypotheses have been offered. The first is high-viscosity ground substance in the newborn, which, because of osmotic changes at birth, causes tissue dilution and inflammation with minor trauma (268). Second, the eruption has been suggested to be a minor AGVH reaction caused by maternal–fetal transfer of lymphocytes during delivery (269).

Differential Diagnosis. Eosinophilic pustular folliculitis is similar to erythema toxicum neonatorum histologically but has completely different clinical features and has a predilection for the scalp. The subcorneal pustules of impetigo and transient neonatal pustular melanosis are not follicular in origin and contain primarily neutrophils rather than eosinophils. A smear of a pustule is helpful to characterize the predominant inflammatory cell. Although many eosinophils are present in the vesicles of incontinentia pigmenti, the vesicle is in the stratum spinosum rather than subcorneal in location, and spongiosis is present. In addition, necrotic keratinocytes may be prominent in incontinentia pigmenti but are absent in erythema toxicum neonatorum.

Principles of Management: Recognition and reassurance are advised.

Transient Neonatal Pustular Melanosis

Clinical Features. Affecting 4.4% of black newborns and 0.6% of white newborns, flaccid vesicopustules with a predilection for the face, trunk, and diaper area develop at birth. These easily rupture, leaving hyperpigmented macules with collarettes of scale. The development of typical lesions of erythema toxicum neonatorum has been observed days later (270). Perhaps the two eruptions represent the same disease in different phases, or their coexistence may be on the basis of the frequent occurrence of erythema toxicum neonatorum.

Histopathology. The vesicopustules consist of intracorneal or subcorneal aggregates of neutrophils with an admixture of eosinophils. Fragmented hair shafts may reside within the blister cavity (271). Within the dermis is an inflammatory infiltrate with some neutrophils and eosinophils. The macules show focal basal hypermelanosis. There is no melanin in the dermis.

Principles of Management: Recognition and reassurance are advised.

Acropustulosis of Infancy

Clinical Features. Intensely pruritic vesicles or pustules, 1 to 3 mm in diameter, occur most commonly on the palms and soles in recurrent crops (Fig. 9-28). The condition more commonly affects those with darker skin types, and onset is at birth or during the first year of life. The lesions heal with hyperpigmentation and resolve, in most cases, by age 2 to 3. Rare cases have

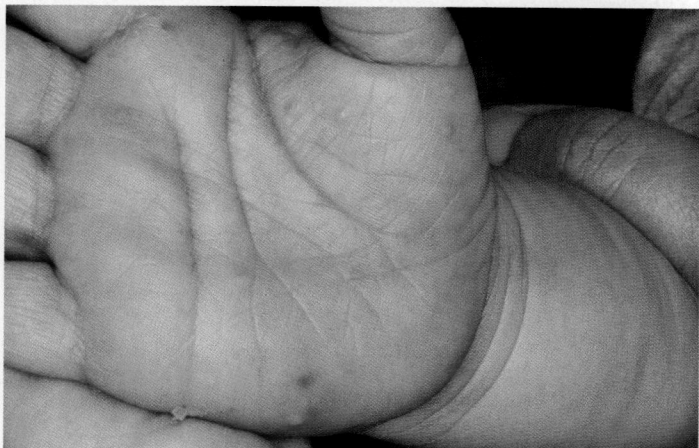

Figure 9-28 Acropustulosis. Multiple small pustules on the palm. (Courtesy of Dr. Charles M. Phillips.)

been reported in older children (272). Scabietic infestation must be considered in the differential diagnosis, and acropustulosis may be a postscabietic phenomenon.

Histopathology. The intraepidermal or subcorneal vesicopustules contain neutrophils and sparse eosinophils. There is mild papillary dermal edema and a sparse, mixed, superficial perivascular infiltrate.

Pathogenesis. The etiology of infantile acropustulosis is unknown. The disease may be associated with atopic dermatitis and elevated serum IgE levels. DIF and IIF studies have been negative. A number of reports describe a scabies infection prior to the onset of the rash; however, the relationship between the two is not clear (273,274).

Differential Diagnosis. Impetigo, SPD, candidiasis, and transient neonatal pustular melanosis may be histologically identical to acropustulosis of infancy, necessitating clinical data for differentiation. Special stains are necessary to rule out an infectious etiology.

Principles of Management: Infantile acropustulosis responds to potent topical steroids.

Subcorneal Pustular Dermatosis

Clinical Features. SPD (Sneddon–Wilkinson disease) is a chronic disorder first described in 1956 and is characterized by superficial sterile pustules that have a predilection for flexural surfaces and the axillary and inguinal folds (271,275). The pustules develop in an annular or polycyclic arrangement. Many cases have been shown to be a variant of IgA pemphigus (271,275). Several drugs have been implicated such as sorafenib, amoxicillin, cephalosporins, dapsone, and isoniazid.

SPD may be associated with a monoclonal gammopathy, most commonly an IgA paraproteinemia. Some of these cases eventuate in an IgA myeloma (276) and may have IgA squamous intercellular substance deposits (IgA pemphigus). It has been associated with pustular dermatosis, connective tissue disease, and infections ("pustular id reaction") (277–279).

Histopathology. The pustules are subcorneal and contain neutrophils, with only an occasional eosinophil (Fig. 9-29A, B). The underlying slightly edematous stratum malpighii contains a few neutrophils. Only a few spongiform pustules are formed. In some instances, a few acantholytic cells are found in the base of the pustule, most likely because of proteolytic enzymes present in the pustular contents. The dermal papillae contain dilated

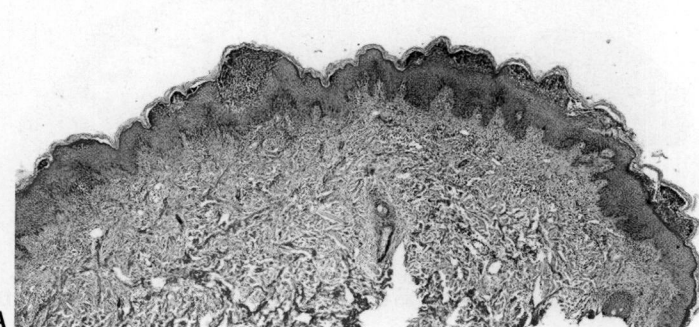
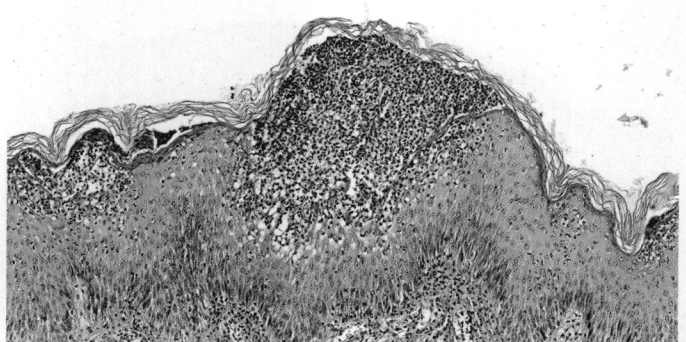

Figure 9-29 Subcorneal pustular dermatosis. There is a subcorneal vesicle filled with neutrophils. A few acanthotic keratinocytes are mixed with numerous neutrophils. Only a few spongiform pustules are formed. **A:** Low power—pustules sit "up" on the epidermal surface. **B:** Neutrophilic pustules on medium power.

capillaries and a perivascular infiltrate composed of neutrophils and a few eosinophils and mononuclear cells.

IF Testing. Although most original DIF studies were reported as negative, as more cases accumulate, many cases have squamous intercellular IgA, indicating they are best considered IgA pemphigus (intraepidermal IgA pemphigus) (276).

Pathogenesis. The squamous intercellular substance IgA leads to neutrophilic infiltration. Elevated levels of tumor necrosis factor-α in the serum and pustules may be responsible for neutrophil activation (280).

Ultrastructural Study. The edge of the pustules shows cytolytic changes in the upper epidermis, especially in the granular layer. Dissolution of the plasma membrane and of the cytoplasm of granular cells causes the formation of a subcorneal split. The transepidermal migration of neutrophils and their subcorneal accumulation are regarded as events secondary to the cellular destruction in the stratum granulosum seen in one study.

Differential Diagnosis. The differential diagnosis includes other diseases with subcorneal pustules. Histologic differentiation from impetigo may be impossible. Bacteria can be demonstrated with a Gram stain, but superinfection may occur, and the bacteria in bullous impetigo may be few. Cultures may be necessary for diagnosis. Histologic differentiation from pemphigus foliaceus or pemphigus erythematosus may also be difficult, because both diseases show subcorneal blisters with acantholysis, although the acantholysis tends to be more pronounced in pemphigus than in SPD. Clinical information, immunofluorescence testing, and a therapeutic trial of sulfones may be necessary for

definitive diagnosis. Although subcorneal pustules occur in both pustular psoriasis and SPD, spongiform pustules are much more frequent in pustular psoriasis. Some authors regard SPD as a variant of pustular psoriasis; but with the association with IgA gammopathies and squamous intercellular substance deposits of IgA, this view is discredited.

Principles of Management: Dapsone is the treatment of choice for SPD, and lesions resolve at approximately 4 weeks of treatment (281). Other agents such as prednisone and acitretin have been used but are less effective than dapsone.

Erythema Multiforme/Stevens–Johnson Syndrome/Toxic Epidermal Necrolysis

Clinical Features. There has been controversy in the literature regarding the clinical definitions of EM, SJS, and TEN and whether they are distinct entities or represent a spectrum of one disease process. EM minor is felt by many to represent classic erythema multiforme with fixed, generally acral, symmetric lesions and simple mucosal involvement. EM major is felt by many to be synonymous with SJS, although this interpretation is not universal (282). A prospective study of 500 patients with "EM major" disputes this assessment and finds that it is less severe, has multiple recurrences, and is often herpesvirus associated (283,284). SJS and TEN are widely regarded as a continuum.

EM, as classically described by von Hebra, is a benign, self-limited condition with symmetric, fixed lesions, some of which evolve into typical "target" lesions composed of three concentric rings. The lesions are located primarily on the extremities (Fig. 9-30A). Bullous EM is a more severe form,

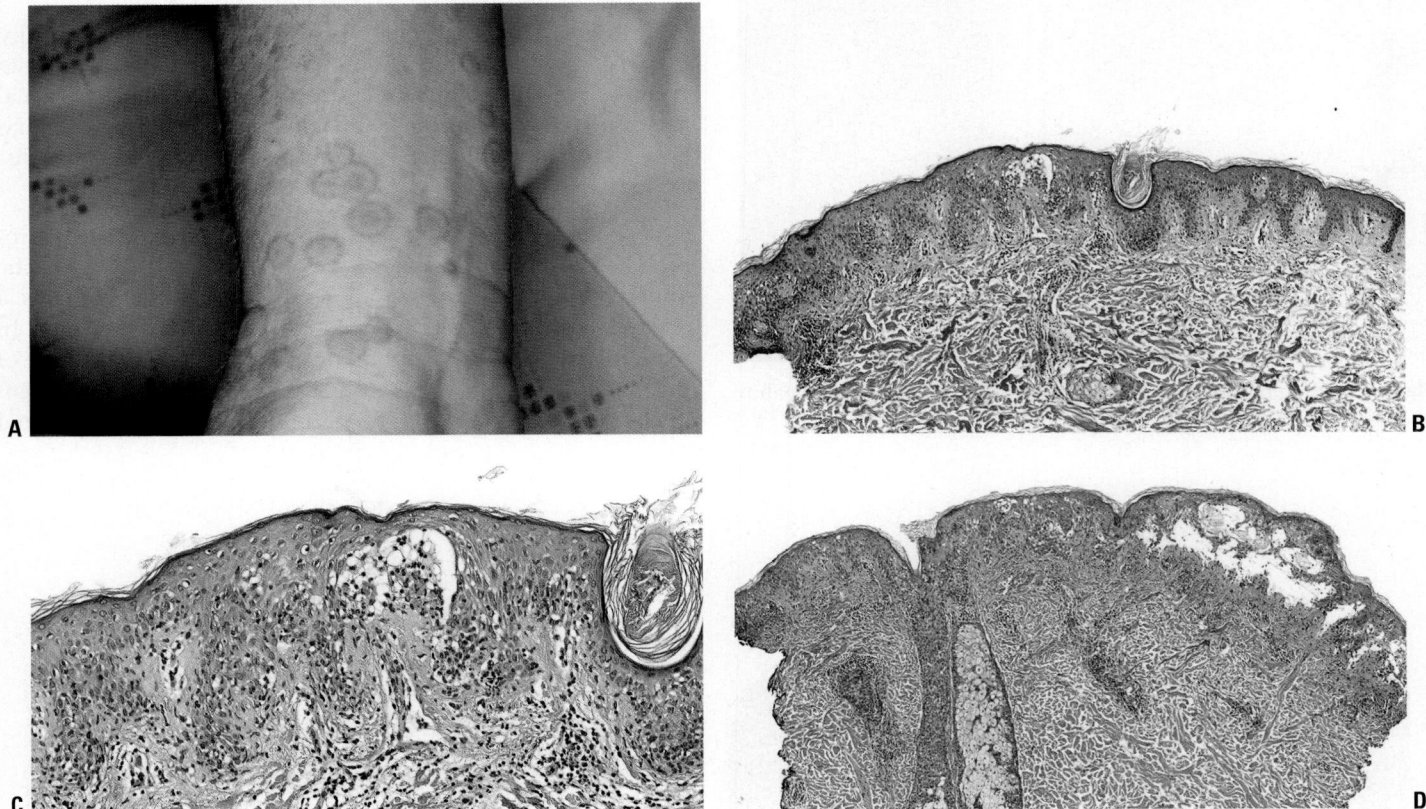

Figure 9-30 Erythema multiforme. **A:** Clinical example. Well-defined, circular target lesions on the forearm. (Courtesy of Dr. Charles M. Phillips.) **B, C:** Histologic features. **B:** Low-power image. **C:** A higher power view of the same biopsy shows numerous apoptotic keratinocytes, which have eosinophilic cytoplasm and pyknotic nuclei. Lymphocytes "tag" along the dermoepidermal junction. **D:** Perivascular and interface dermatitis with a subepidermal vesicle and a normal stratum corneum (low power).

which was defined by an international consensus group in 1993 (Bastuji-Garin classification) as having typical targets or raised atypical targets with <10% of body surface area detachment (285). Most authors ignore the pathologic findings in the individual cases, a fatal flaw to these attempts at classification in our estimation.

Patients with SJS often present with fever and malaise and develop a cutaneous eruption consisting of "flat atypical targets," or erythematous or purpuric macules, many with central epidermal necrosis or blister formation, with marked inflammation of the mucosa. The lesions usually start on the trunk and spread centrifugally (Fig. 9-31A, B). Again, epidermal detachment is <10% of the body surface area (286). TEN, also referred to as Lyell syndrome, is characterized by widespread, full-thickness epidermal necrosis involving >30% of the body surface area; mucosal inflammation is common but is not required. These patients also have systemic symptoms and may initially present with diffuse erythema and skin tenderness, followed by the development of large, flaccid bullae and detachment of the epidermis in sheets (Fig. 9-32A, B) (286). SJS/TEN overlap is used to refer to patients with epidermal detachment between 10% and 30% of the body surface area (286). TEN has a high mortality rate because of fluid loss and sepsis.

Mucosal involvement (oral, ocular, and/or genital) is common in all these severe acute bullous diseases and is a serious cause of morbidity. *Mycoplasma pneumoniae* infection has been associated with severe mucositis without skin lesions, which has been referred to by some as "atypical SJS" (287–289).

EM, which may be recurrent, is most commonly associated with herpes simplex infection (290,291). Other infections, including Epstein–Barr virus (292), cytomegalovirus (293), Lyme disease (294), and drugs have been implicated in EM. SJS is almost always drug induced (286), except in children, where most cases have been associated with infection, notably *M. pneumonia*, highlighting the confusion inherent in defining *M. pneumonia*-related disease (295,296). The most commonly implicated drugs include NSAIDs, sulfonamides, anticonvulsants, antibiotics, and allopurinol (297,298).

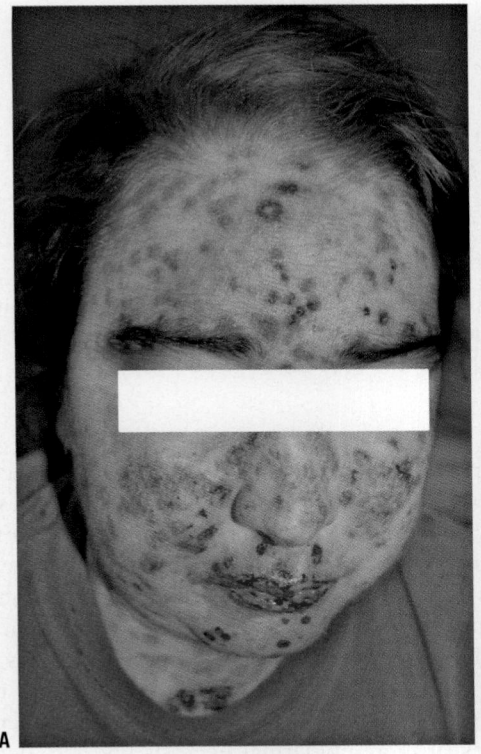

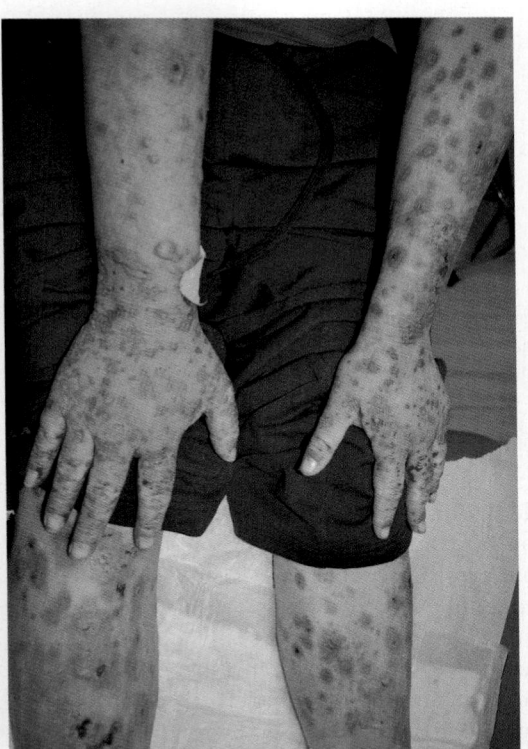

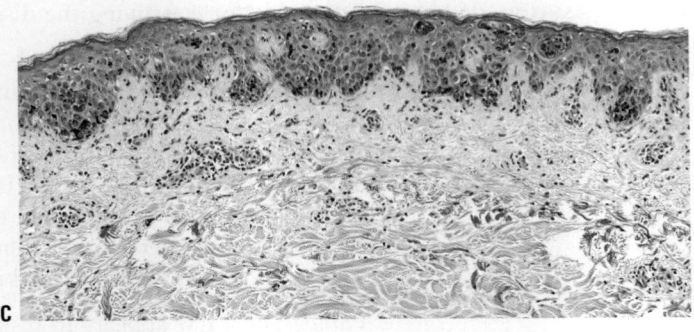

Figure 9-31 Stevens–Johnson syndrome. **A, B:** Clinical example: Face and extremities with widespread macules, plaques, and patches, some targetoid, with erosion and crusting. Intact bullae are also seen. **C:** Histologic features. In another example secondary to a drug, there is sparse lymphocytic interface dermatitis and prominent keratinocyte apoptosis (low-medium power).

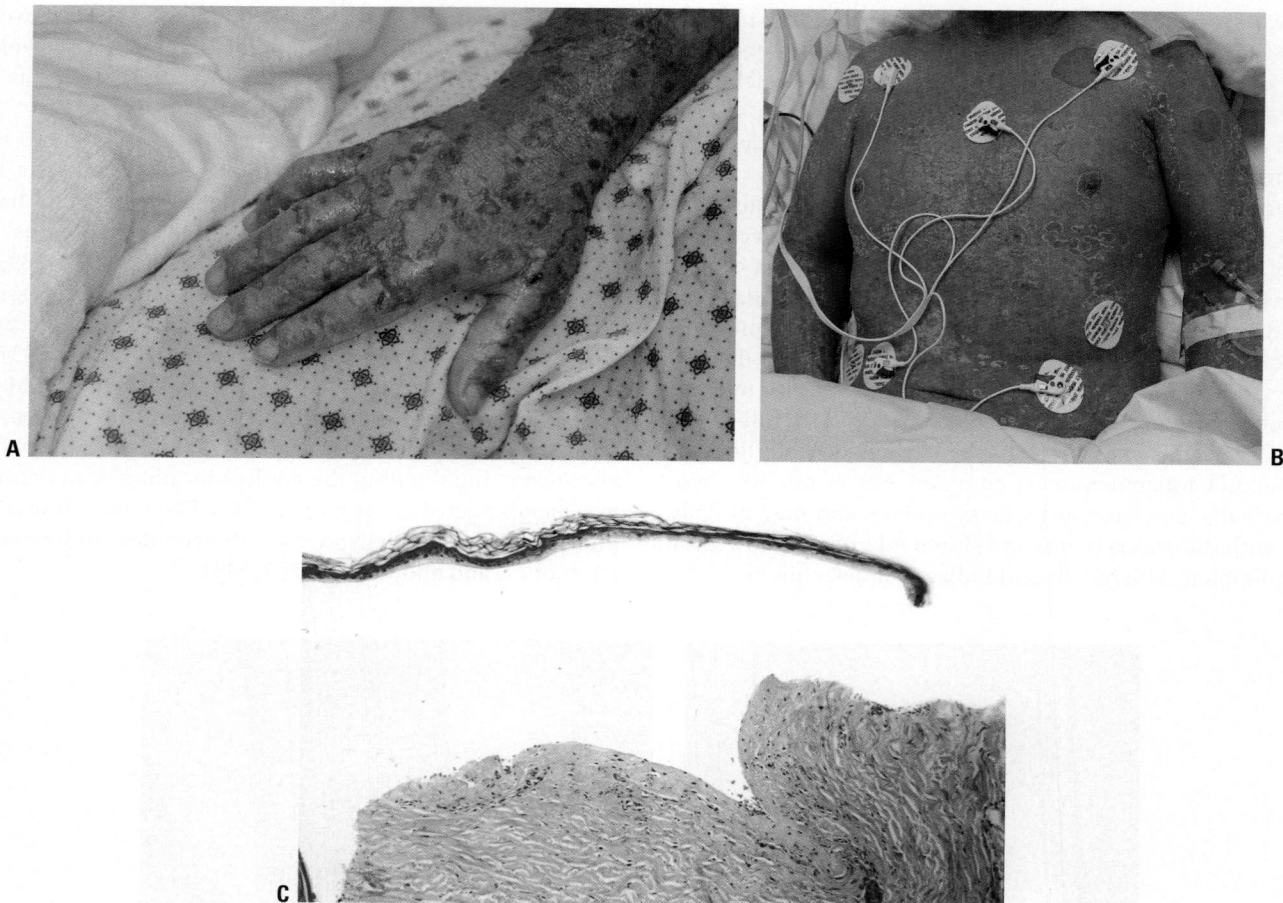

Figure 9-32 Toxic epidermal necrolysis. **A, B:** Clinical examples. **A:** Diffuse erythema of the trunk and arms with erosion and epidermal peeling. **B:** Extensive epidermal loss over the hand. **C:** Histologic features. There is a cell-poor subepidermal blister and epidermal necrosis. The dermal inflammatory infiltrate is sparse.

Histopathology. EM is considered the prototype of the vacuolar form of interface dermatitis (299). The early changes include vacuolization of the basal cell layer; tagging of lymphocytes along the dermoepidermal junction; and a sparse, superficial perivascular lymphoid infiltrate (Fig. 9-30B–D). Necrosis of individual keratinocytes in the basal unit occurs, the hallmark of EM. Because of its acute nature, there is an orthokeratotic stratum corneum. Mild spongiosis, papillary dermal edema, and red blood cell extravasation are present. As the lesion becomes more developed, there is a lichenoid infiltrate of lymphocytes and histiocytes at the dermoepidermal junction with exocytosis. More apoptotic keratinocytes within and above the basal epidermal layer are present. The intensity of epidermal necrosis varies from vacuolated individual keratinocytes surrounded by lymphocytes (satellite cell necrosis) in the basal unit to confluent necrosis in association with intraepidermal and subepidermal vesicles. The dermal infiltrate comprises lymphocytes and histiocytes. Eosinophils may also be present, usually in small numbers. Although one study has noted a significant number of eosinophils in drug-induced EM, this has not been noted by others. In our estimation, a generous number of eosinophils speaks against EM. One study has found that an acrosyringium concentration of apoptotic keratinocytes in EM is a clue to a drug etiology (300).

In early lesions of SJS/TEN, apoptotic keratinocytes are observed scattered in the basal layer of the epidermis (Fig. 9-31C).

In established lesions, there are numerous necrotic keratinocytes, even full-thickness epidermal necrosis, and a subepidermal bulla. The dermal inflammatory infiltrate is sparser in TEN than in EM (Fig. 9-32C). Extravasated erythrocytes are commonly found within the blister cavity. Melanophages within the papillary dermis occur in late lesions. Eccrine epithelium shows a variety of changes, from basal cell apoptosis to necrosis of the duct.

In general, EM shows less epidermal necrosis and more dermal inflammation and exocytosis, whereas SJS and TEN reveal more epidermal necrosis and less dermal inflammation and exocytosis. However, because of the overlapping histologic features among EM, SJS, and TEN, histologic examination, although important for recognizing the spectrum of disorders, is unreliable for classifying the disease. Correlation with clinical presentation is essential.

IF Testing. In many patients with EM, deposits of IgM and C3 are found in the walls of the superficial dermal vessels. Granular deposits of C3, IgM, and fibrinogen may also be present along the dermoepidermal junction. Nonspecific deposition of immune reactants in apoptotic or necrotic keratinocytes may be observed in other disorders that have apoptosis, lymphocyte satellite necrosis, and epidermal necrosis.

Pathogenesis. EM appears to result from a Th-1 cell–mediated immune reaction. In the case of herpes simplex, polymerase chain reaction and *in situ* hybridization have detected herpes simplex virus (HSV) DNA within lesions of EM (301). The lymphocytes attack cells with herpetic DNA polymerase gene. The virus remains in the skin for up to 3 months after the lesions have healed (302). Some authors hypothesize that disease development begins with deposition and expression of HSV genes, leading to recruitment of HSV-specific CD4+ T cells with production of IFN-γ. This step initiates an inflammatory cascade that includes increased infiltration of leukocytes, monocytes, NK cells, and T cells (303). The infiltrate consists largely of CD4+ (helper) lymphocytes in the dermis and CD8+ (cytotoxic) cells in the epidermis. The necrotic keratinocytes are surrounded by CD8 positive cytotoxic lymphocytes (so called "satellite necrosis") as in GVHD. The greater the intensity of the lymphocytic infiltrate correlates with decreasing prognosis. The pathogenesis of drug-associated TEN is uncertain, but many patients have an impaired metabolism of the offending drug that leads to increased production of toxic metabolites (304–306). Epidermal necrosis is probably mediated by cytotoxic drug–specific CD8-positive T cells and lymphokines, such as tumor necrosis factor (307).

Ultrastructural Study. The basal lamina is located on the floor or on the roof of the blister. The basal cells show marked intracytoplasmic damage with a loss of organelles. Neutrophils and macrophages, rich in lysosomes, are present in the lower epidermis, phagocytizing the damaged keratinocytes. In the midepidermis, large, electron-dense, dyskeratotic bodies correspond to the cells with eosinophilic necrosis seen by light microscopy. The damaged epidermal cells often contain few or no organelles. Large granular lymphocytes have been identified within the epidermis in close contact with keratinocytes, a finding that supports cell-mediated cytotoxic injury to keratinocytes in EM/SJS (308).

Differential Diagnosis. Necrotic keratinocytes are also a characteristic feature in drug eruption, especially fixed drug eruptions, pityriasis lichenoides, connective tissue disease, subacute radiation dermatitis and sunburn, phototoxic dermatitis, acute GVHD, and viral exanthems. Clinicopathologic correlation will help their distinction. In patients with widespread desquamation or detachment, the clinical differential diagnosis includes TEN and SSSS. Although the former splits subepidermally, the latter splits subcorneally or within the granular layer (Fig. 9-33A, B). Frozen section evaluation of the blister roof ("jelly roll") is a rapid diagnostic tool to determine the level of the split.

Principles of Management: Acute EM is most often preceded by HSV infection. Other associations, such as mycoplasma pneumoniae or medications, have also been identified. Discontinuation/treatment of etiologic factors is an important first step in the management of EM. Mild EM can be treated with oral antihistamines and/or topical steroids. For recurrent EM, chronic suppressive antiviral therapy with valacyclovir has been shown to be helpful. Resistant disease may require the addition of other immunosuppressive or immunomodulatory agents, such as MMF, dapsone, or hydroxychloroquine.

SJS/TEN management is controversial, and the detailed care of these critically ill patients is beyond the scope of this text. The core principles include cessation and avoidance of offending agents, supportive care in a skilled center (usually a burn unit), including intensive-care level therapy, consultation with ophthalmology and other appropriate services to manage the mucosal disease. Supportive care includes special attention to fluid and electrolyte balance, temperature control, skin care, and close monitoring for infection and complications.

No controlled prospective treatment studies or accepted guidelines exist for SJS/TEN. Systemic anti-inflammatory therapy with cyclosporine or TNF α inhibitors has shown decreased mortality (309,310). Treatment with systemic corticosteroids and IVIG is controversial.

Graft-Versus-Host Disease

Clinical Features. GVHD occurs in situations in which donor immunocompetent T cells are transferred into allogeneic hosts incapable of rejecting them. The sources of the T cells include primarily peripheral blood stem cell and bone marrow transplants and, infrequently, unirradiated blood products (311), solid organ transplants (312), and maternal–fetal lymphocyte engraftment. Graft-versus-host–like reaction has been reported in patients with thymoma and lymphoma (313,314).

The disease can be divided into an acute and a chronic phase. Acute GVHD (AGVHD) typically occurs between 7 and 21 days after transplantation but may be seen as late as 3 months; chronic GVHD generally arises after a mean of 4 months but may occur as soon as 40 days post transplantation. The two phases were originally defined on the basis of time of presentation (315,316). However, the use of donor lymphocytes and the withdrawal of immunosuppression in relapsed patients have obscured these time-based divisions. In addition, many patients have both phases, either merging with one another or

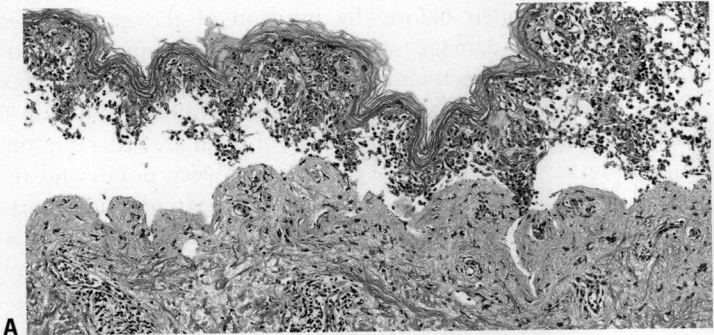 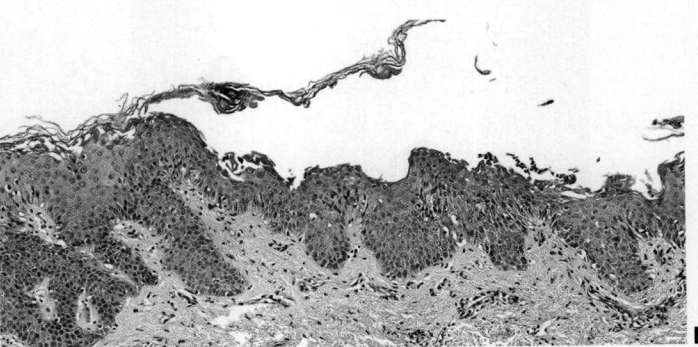

Figure 9-33 Differentiation of Stevens–Johnson syndrome (SJS)/toxic epidermal necrolysis (TEN) and staphylococcal scalded skin. **A:** Formalin-fixed, paraffin-embedded punch biopsy from a patient clinically suspected of SJS/TEN. The necrotic epidermis has separated from the underlying dermis to produce a subepidermal split. **B:** By comparison, staphylococcal scalded skin splits subcorneally or within the granular layer (both A and B are low-medium power).

separated by an asymptomatic period. The diagnosis of acute versus chronic GVHD now depends on the clinical phenotype and organs affected. The frequency of acute GVHD depends on the disparity of HLA antigens (317). The risk of chronic GVHD is much greater if the patients had prior acute GVHD.

In the *acute phase*, the classic triad includes skin lesions, hepatic dysfunction, and diarrhea. The clinical severity is judged on the basis of the extent of the cutaneous eruption, total bilirubin, and stool volume. The eruption is characterized by extensive macular erythema, a morbilliform eruption, purpuric lesions, violaceous scaly papules and plaques, bullae, or, in rare cases, a TEN-like epidermal detachment. There is a predilection for the cheeks, ears, neck, upper chest, and palms and soles. Occasionally, follicular papules are seen simulating a folliculitis. Oral lesions may be present. About 30% of patients die from complications of acute GVHD. The overall clinical stage, during the first 40 days after transplantation, is useful in identifying patients with progressive and fatal disease (317). Cutaneous GVHD may be attributable to a synergistic effect from local irradiation (318).

In the *chronic phase,* an early lichenoid stage and a late sclerodermoid stage can be distinguished (Fig. 9-34). Each stage can occur without the other. Although usually generalized, the involvement is, in rare instances, localized to a few areas. In the lichenoid stage, both the cutaneous and the oral lesions may be clinically similar to those in LP. In addition, the skin may show extensive erythema and irregular hyperpigmentation. A poikiloderma may precede the eventual sclerodermoid stage. Other late manifestations include a lupus erythematosus–like eruption, cicatricial alopecia, chronic ulcerations, pyogenic granulomas, and angiomatous lesions (319).

Histopathology. The early changes in the acute phase consist of focal basal vacuolation and sparse superficial perivascular lymphocytic infiltrate with exocytosis of individual cells into the epidermis and follicular epithelium. The number of lymphocytes correlates positively with the probability of developing

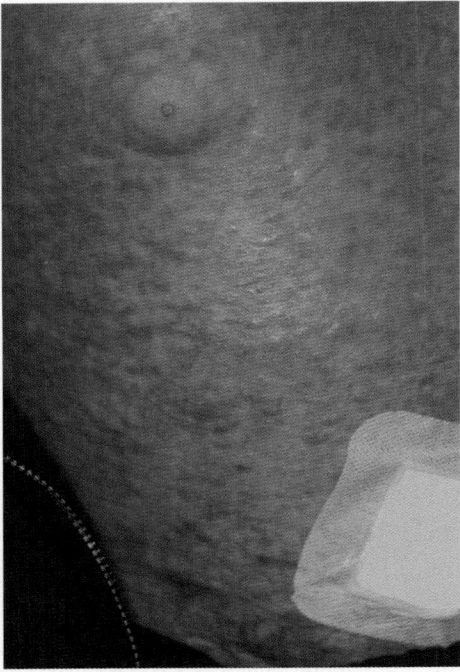

Figure 9-34 Chronic graft-versus-host disease. Clinical example. Coalescing lichenoid papules and plaques.

more severe acute GVHD (320). In association with the perivascular infiltrate, there is marked endothelial cell swelling and narrowing of the vascular lumen. Established lesions show more pronounced vacuolation, focal spongiosis, lymphocytic infiltration, and dyskeratosis at all levels of epidermis (Fig. 9-35A–C). The *acute phase* has been divided into four histopathologic grades (321). In Grade 1 disease, there is focal or diffuse vacuolization of the basal cell layer. In Grade 2 lesions, spongiosis and dyskeratotic keratinocytes are identified, some accompanied by two or more epidermal lymphocytes, a phenomenon known as "satellite cell necrosis." The necrotic keratinocytes contain a pyknotic nucleus and eosinophilic cytoplasm. Grade 3 lesions are characterized by subepidermal cleft formation, and in Grade 4 there is complete loss of the epidermis. In cases with follicular papules, the involved follicles show degenerate changes in the cells of the follicular epithelium similar to those in the epidermis. In rare cases, basal vacuolization and dyskeratosis of the follicular epithelium may be the only changes (322).

In the *chronic phase,* the early lichenoid stage may still show satellite cell necrosis within the epidermis (Fig. 9-35D). The overall histologic picture greatly resembles that of LP with hyperkeratosis, hypergranulosis, acanthosis, apoptotic keratinocytes, and a mononuclear cell infiltrate immediately below the epidermis with pigmentary incontinence. As in LP, apoptotic keratinocytes may "drop" into the upper dermis. There may be areas of separation of the basal cell layer from the dermal papillae resembling the clefts seen in severe LP. A rare manifestation is "columnar epidermal necrosis," characterized by small foci of total epidermal necrosis accompanied by a lichenoid tissue reaction (323).

In the late *sclerodermoid phase,* the epidermis is atrophic, with the keratinocytes being small, flattened, and hyperpigmented. Basal layer vacuolization, inflammation, and colloid body formation are rare or absent. The dermis is thickened, with sclerosis extending into the subcutaneous tissue, resulting in septal hyalinization. The adnexal structures are destroyed (Fig. 9-35E) (324). Subepidermal bullae were present in one reported case.

IF Testing. Epithelial basement membrane zone granular IgM and complement deposition is present in 39% of patients with the acute form and in 86% of patients with the chronic form of GVHD. In addition, IgM and C3 have been found in the walls of dermal vessels.

Pathogenesis. Acute and chronic forms of the disease have a different pathogenesis. In acute GVHD, it is believed that the preparative regimen before the infusion of the graft causes extensive tissue damage, which releases inflammatory cytokines and exposes recipient major histocompatibility complex (MHC) antigens. Recognition of the host antigen by donor T cells, and activation and proliferation of them are crucial in the initial phase. The greater the disparity between donor and recipient MHC, the greater the T-cell response. In identical pairs, the donor T cells recognize minor antigen differences. Infiltration of both CD4$^+$ and CD8$^+$ T cells or with either one of them predominating has been reported (328,325–327). T cells represent a minority of infiltrates in this setting (328,329). B cells are not found.

The inflammatory cytokines (ILs, GM-CSF, TNF-α,2 IFN-γ) produced by activated T cells and by tissue damage during the preparative regimen also activate mononuclear phagocytes and

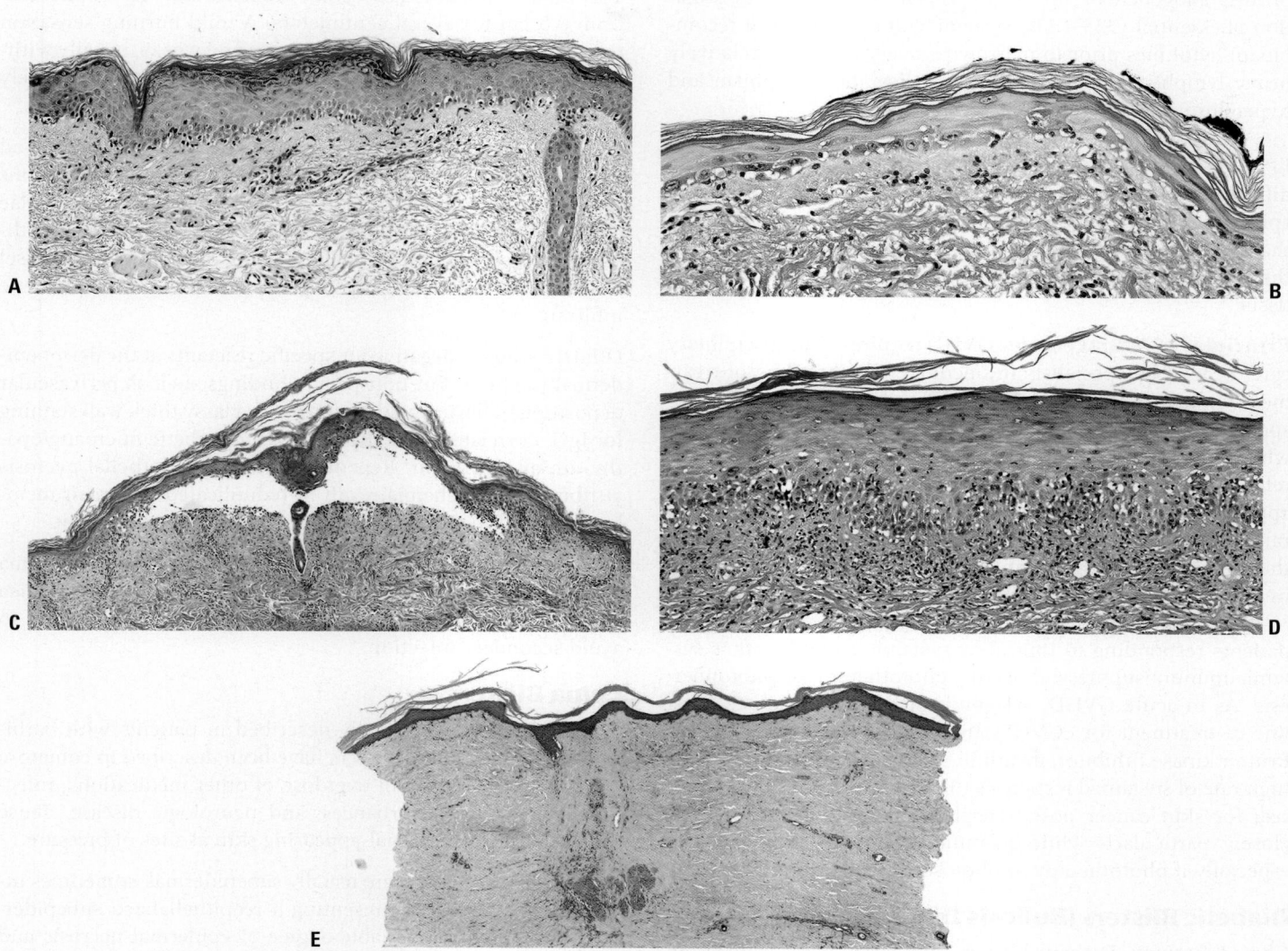

Figure 9-35 Graft-versus-host disease (GVHD)—histologic features. **A:** Paucicellular lymphocytic interface dermatitis with sparse dyskeratosis (low-medium power). **B:** GVHD with prominent basal vacuolar change (medium power). **C:** GVHD with subepidermal vesiculation (low power). **D:** Lichenoid GVHD with satellite cell necrosis (medium power). **E:** Sclerodermoid GVDH (scanning power).

NK cells (330). Both Fas/FasL-dependent apoptosis and perforin/granzyme-dependent killing are important in GVHD-induced damage (331). In skin, young rete ridge keratinocytes, follicular stem cells (332), and Langerhans cells are preferred targets. However, the exact mechanisms by which the skin, liver, and gastrointestinal (GI) tract are targeted are not clear.

Less is understood about the pathophysiology of chronic GVHD. The role of donor T cells against the recipient's tissue has been demonstrated. In addition, autoreactivity has also been suggested. Most immunohistochemical studies have shown that CD8$^+$ T cells predominate. Tumor necrosis factor-α and IL-1α are produced by keratinocytes in skin lesions (333).

Ultrastructural Study. The necrotic keratinocytic cytoplasm is filled with numerous aggregated tonofilaments. Granule-producing cytotoxic lymphocytes, NK-like cells, have been identified in direct cytolytic attack on epithelial cells undergoing apoptosis.

Differential Diagnosis. The AGVHD is similar to EM, with scattered necrotic keratinocytes and the formation of subepidermal clefts through hydropic degeneration of basal cells.

In severe cases, the fulminant lesions are identical to TEN. These patients are also at increased risk for drug eruptions, chemotherapy-induced eruptions, and radiation dermatitis, all of which may be indistinguishable from acute GVHD. If there is follicular dyskeratosis, the diagnosis is said to be more likely to be AGVHD. The presence of eosinophils is not necessarily in favor of drug reaction, because eosinophils are occasionally observed in GVHD. Subtle epidermal changes identical to acute/early GVHD may be seen in bone marrow transplant patients without cutaneous lesions.

The *eruption of lymphocyte recovery* occurs predominantly in patients after receiving cytoreductive therapy (without bone marrow transplant) for acute myelogenous leukemia. The eruption is typically morbilliform and develops between 6 and 21 days of chemotherapy, correlating with the earliest recovery of lymphocytes to the circulation. In contrast to patients with GVHD, these patients do not develop diarrhea or liver abnormalities. Resolution occurs over several days. Histopathologically, a superficial perivascular mononuclear cell infiltrate, basal vacuolization, spongiosis, and rare dyskeratotic keratinocytes are present. The changes may be indistinguishable from those of early allogeneic or autologous GVHD, and clinical information is essential (334). The systemic administration of recombinant cytokines prior to marrow recovery leads to a relatively heavy lymphocytic infiltrate with nuclear pleomorphism and hyperchromasia (335).

Distinguishing between the lichenoid lesions of GVHD and LP is often impossible. However, late sclerotic lesions can be differentiated from scleroderma by the marked atrophy of the epidermis. Active synthesis of collagen takes place largely in the upper third of the dermis; in scleroderma, collagen is synthesized mainly in the lower dermis and in the subcutaneous tissue.

Principles of Management: GVHD requires multidisciplinary care, headed by specialists in oncology. The first line of treatment for acute GVHD is high-dose systemic corticosteroids. Response to steroids should be seen within 3 to 5 days. Patients who do not respond in that time frame are considered steroid refractory. In 2019, a Janus kinase 1/2 inhibitor, ruxolitinib, was approved as second-line treatment of acute GVHD. In 2020, a randomized study that compared ruxolitinib with best available therapy showed a clear advantage to the use of ruxolitinib, both in overall response and in durability of the response (336).

Chronic GVHD may require multimodality care, with some patients responding to topical or systemic steroids, other systemic immunosuppressive agents, phototherapy, or photopheresis. As in acute GVHD, systemic corticosteroids are the first line of treatment for cGVHD. In steroid-refractory patients, a Bruton kinase inhibitor, ibrutinib, has been shown to induce a high rate of sustained responses (337). Patients are at increased risk for skin cancer post transplant and should be screened closely, particularly while on immunosuppressive agents and especially if phototherapy or photosensitizing drugs are used.

Diabetic Blisters (Bullosis Diabeticorum)

Clinical Features. Diabetic blisters (bullosis diabeticorum) is an uncommon condition associated with chronic diabetes mellitus. It usually presents as spontaneous blisters on the distal extremities (Fig. 9-36). The most frequent locations are the feet, lower legs, hands, forearms, and, rarely, the trunk. The lesions

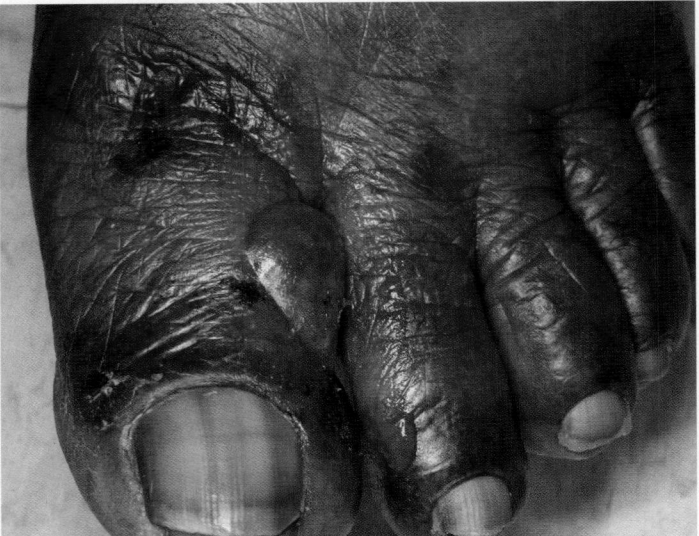

Figure 9-36 Bullosis diabeticorum. Tense, noninflammatory bulla on the great toe.

arise on a noninflamed base; they are tense and vary in diameter from 0.5 cm to several centimeters. A mild burning sensation may be present. The blisters heal in several weeks, usually without scarring. The cause of diabetic bullae is unclear but is likely to be chronic ischemia.

Histopathology. The level of cleavage is subepidermal, and earlier reported intraepidermal blisters represent old lesions undergoing reepithelialization of the blister base. The bullae contain fibrin and a few inflammatory cells. There may be diabetic microangiopathy with thickening of small dermal vessel walls. There is usually only a sparse perivascular lymphocytic infiltrate.

DIF. DIF study is negative for specific reactants at the dermoepidermal junction. But nonspecific findings such as perivascular deposition of fibrin and C3, along with glassy thick wall staining for IgG, correlated with the underlying diabetic microangiopathy, are often present. Repetitive bouts of endothelial necrosis attributable to ischemia result in reduplicated basement membrane zone/Type IV collagen trapping Ig and complement.

Principles of Management: Patients should avoid trauma and maintain good glycemic control. Presence of bullous tinea should be excluded. Local supportive care should be used to avoid secondary infection.

Coma Blisters

Clinical Features. Classically described in patients with barbiturate overdose, these blisters have been described in comatose patients in the setting of overdose of other medications, infections, metabolic disturbances, and neurologic disease. Tense bullae develop on normal-appearing skin at sites of pressure.

Histopathology. Blisters are usually subepidermal, sometimes intraepidermal (likely representing a reepithelialized subepidermal blister), with a variable degree of epidermal necrosis and a sparse inflammatory cell infiltrate (338,339). Eccrine gland necrosis is a characteristic finding (340), but other appendages may be necrotic as well.

Pathogenesis. The exact pathogenesis of these blisters is unknown. Pressure, friction, and local hypoxia have all been implicated as causative factors. The pressure may decrease blood flow, with secondary endothelial damage and microthrombus formation. In cases involving drug overdose, a direct toxic effect has been postulated to explain the eccrine gland necrosis and blister formation. Many drugs are excreted by the eccrine glands.

Principles of Management: Patients should receive supportive care, local wound care, and prevention with frequent turning and pressure-offloading techniques.

Edema Blisters

Clinical Features. Tense bullae can occur in the setting of acute edema, most commonly on the lower extremities of elderly patients, with acute exacerbation of chronic edema. Bullae can range in size up to several centimeters and are usually filled with clear serous fluid. They resolve with treatment of the underlying cause of the edema (341).

Histopathology. There is marked epidermal spongiosis. The dermis is edematous with dilated blood vessels and a mild lymphohistiocytic infiltrate. In some cases, subepidermal blisters can be found. DIF and IIF studies reveal no specific findings.

Principles of Management: The management is generally focused on the source of the edema, with patients benefiting from diuresis, improved nutrition, improved mobility, and locally from supportive garments or compression therapy.

Grover Disease (Transient Acantholytic Dermatosis)

Clinical Features. First described in 1970, TAD is characterized by pruritic, discrete papules and scaly macules on the chest, back, and thighs. In rare instances, vesicles and even bullae are seen (Fig. 9-37A). Most patients are middle-aged or elderly men. Although the disorder may be transient in most patients, lasting from 2 weeks to 3 months, it can persist for several years. The condition has been reported to coexist with other dermatoses, such as asteatotic eczema, allergic contact dermatitis, atopic eczema, psoriasis, and pemphigus foliaceus. There have been reports of patients with TAD and malignancy, most commonly lymphoproliferative and genitourinary neoplasms, stem cell therapy, chemotherapy, and radiation therapy (342–344).

Histopathology. Focal acantholysis and dyskeratosis ("focal acantholytic dyskeratosis—FAD") are present. Because these foci are small (often 0.5 mm in diameter or less), they are sometimes found only when serial sections are obtained. The acantholysis may occur in four histologic patterns, resembling Darier disease (Fig. 9-37B, C), Hailey–Hailey disease, PV, or spongiotic

dermatitis. Two or more of these patterns may be found in the same specimen. There is usually a superficial dermal infiltrate of lymphocytes and often eosinophils.

IF Testing. In general, IF results are often said to be negative. However, C3 deposition may occur in the epidermis. Granular C3 and IgM may be observed at the dermoepidermal junction. A few "colloid bodies" and superficial focal perivascular C3 and IgM may be present.

Pathogenesis. Despite the histologic similarity to Darier disease, GD does not share an abnormality in the ATP2A2 gene (345), which encodes a keratinocyte Ca^{2+} pump. Although GD pathogenesis remains unknown, there appears to be a relationship to excessive sweating, fever, and bed confinement. Some authors have hypothesized that urea in sweat leaks from the intraepidermal portion of the sweat duct into the surrounding epidermis, causing acantholysis. Others dispute this theory and have found the sweat duct to be intact. Finally, IL-4 may be responsible for acantholysis, either by induction of plasminogen activator or by stimulation of antibody production (346). The expression of Syndecan-1, a proteoglycan important for keratinocytes intercellular adhesion, is markedly decreased in GD. The same phenomenon also occurs in other acantholytic conditions such as pemphigus and herpes simplex infection, suggestive of decreased intercellular adhesion, characteristic of this disease (347).

Ultrastructural Study. In the pemphigus-like zones, there is intradesmosomal separation, fewer desmosomes, and perinuclear aggregation of tonofilament bundles. In the Darier type, features similar to those of Darier disease are present.

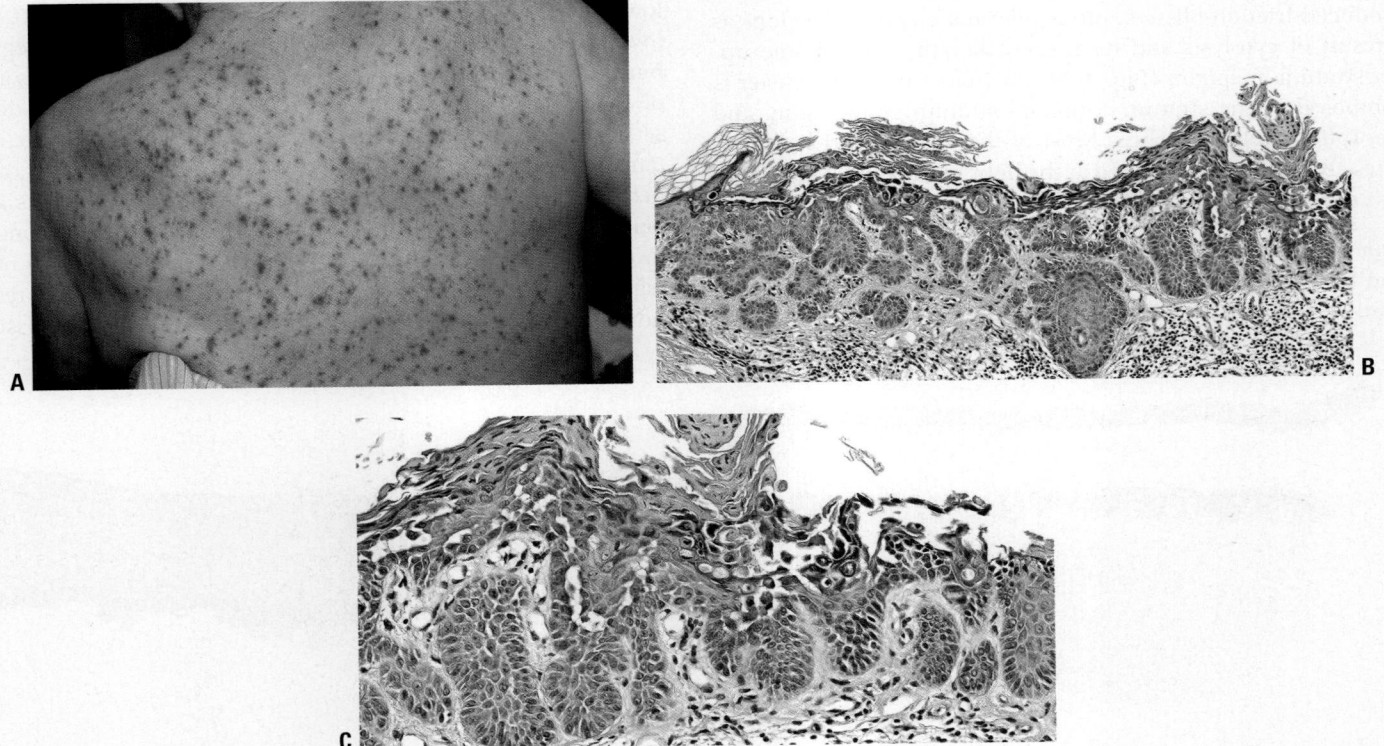

Figure 9-37 Transient acantholytic dyskeratosis. **A:** Clinical example: Widespread papules and papulovesicles on the back. (Courtesy of Dr. Charles M. Phillips.) **B, C:** Histologic features. There is hyperkeratosis with hypergranulosis, acantholysis, and dyskeratosis. The intraepidermal clefts extend to the suprabasilar zone. **B:** Low power. **C:** Medium power.

Differential Diagnosis. The features that help differentiate TAD from the four diseases that it resembles are the focal nature of the histologic changes (often 0.5 mm or less) and the mixture of the four patterns. The presence of eosinophils in the superficial dermal infiltrate of GD serves as a distinguishing feature from Darier disease, in which they are usually absent. It is important to have clinical information for a definitive diagnosis. IF studies are rarely necessary to exclude pemphigus. If only one biopsy of a rash is taken, it should be remembered that foci of TAD-like change may be incidental and occur as small foci in "normal" skin (often in melanoma reexcisions, perhaps because of the large area of skin sampled).

Principles of Management: The evidence base for treatment of GD is anecdotal. There should be strict avoidance of heat and sweating. Topical corticosteroids, topical calcipotriene, and oral retinoids have been reported as successful therapy. Oral antihistamines may help with the intense pruritus. Oral corticosteroids help reduce the discomfort; however, relapses are common after discontinuation. May patients are unaware of their lesions, or only slightly annoyed by them.

DERMATOPATHIES PRODUCED BY EXTERNAL ENERGY

Friction Blisters

Clinical Features. These blisters develop mainly on the soles as a result of prolonged walking and on the palms and the palmar surfaces of the fingers as a result of repetitive actions required in certain occupations or sports. They may also occur as self-inflicted artifacts.

Histopathology. In both naturally occurring and experimentally produced friction blisters, intraepidermal cleavage develops as a result of cytolysis and necrosis of keratinocytes in the upper stratum malpighii (Fig. 9-38A, B). The roof of the blister is composed of the stratum corneum, stratum granulosum, and amorphous cellular debris. Most of the degenerated keratinocytes are pale and are located at the floor of the cleft. The deeper part of the epidermis consists of undamaged cells.

Pathogenesis. Shearing forces within the epidermis cause friction blisters. They form only where the epidermis is thick and firmly attached to the underlying tissue.

Ultrastructural Study. Electron microscopy reveals clumped tonofilaments, intracellular edema, small vacuoles at the cell periphery, and areas devoid of organelles.

Principles of Management: In general, the management is avoidance. Improved footwear, sometimes supplemented by podiatric inserts or areas of pressure-offloading, may reduce future episodes of friction blisters on the feet.

Electric Burns

It is important that dermatopathologists be familiar with the cutaneous effects of electric current because of the electrodesiccation and electrocautery used in therapy.

Histopathology. Electrodesiccation and electrocautery cause a separation of the epidermis from the dermis. A diagnostic histologic feature is the fringe of elongated, degenerated cytoplasmic processes that protrudes from the lower end of the detached basal cells into the subepidermal space (Fig. 9-39A–C). The nuclei of the basal cells appear stretched vertically. In addition, the upper dermis is homogenized because of coagulation necrosis.

Thermal Burns

In the evaluation of thermal burns, the depth of penetration is of great importance because first- and second-degree burns heal readily, whereas third-degree burns require grafting.

Histopathology. First-degree burns are those in which the lower epidermis, particularly the basal cell layer, remains viable, and only the upper epidermis is affected by heat coagulation. In the affected areas, coagulative necrosis with nuclear pyknosis and cytoplasmic eosinophilia is present.

Second-degree burns often show subepidermal blisters and are characterized by partial-thickness dermal necrosis. The lower portion of the cutaneous appendages remains intact, allowing reepithelialization to occur. Superficial second-degree burns are associated with necrosis of the surface epidermis and of only a small amount of superficial dermal collagen; in deep second-degree burns, much of the dermal collagen and the cutaneous appendages are injured. In partial-thickness dermal necrosis, the depth of epithelial damage in the cutaneous appendages is a good indicator of the depth of irreversible damage to the collagen. The border between heat-coagulated and normal epithelium is sharp. At a later stage, an inflammatory reaction develops at the junction of the viable and nonviable tissue.

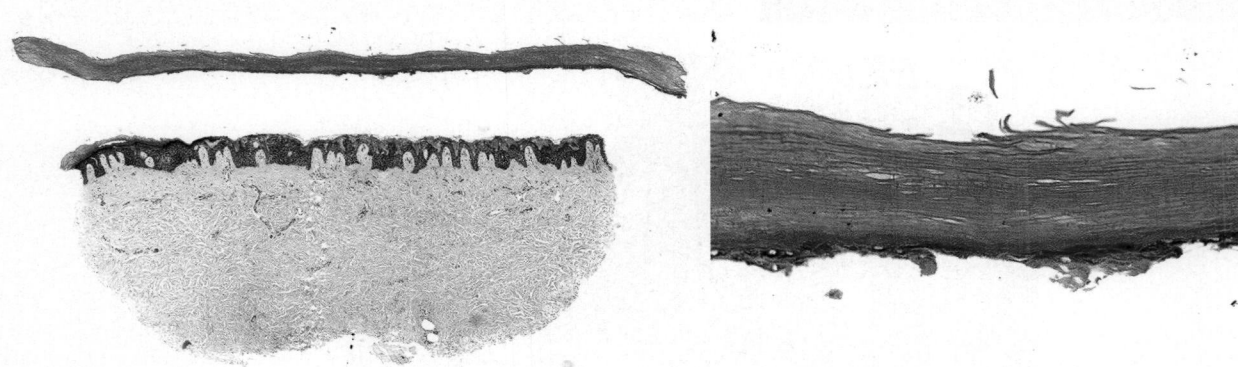

A   **B**

Figure 9-38 Friction blister. **A:** In this case, the level of split for the intraepidermal blister is just beneath the stratum granulosum. In this scanning power image, the blister roof is completely detached from the underlying stratum malpighii and dermis. **B:** The stratum corneum and, focally, the underlying stratum granulosum form the blister roof. These blisters may extend into the papillary dermis, giving hemorrhagic blisters often noted clinically (medium power).

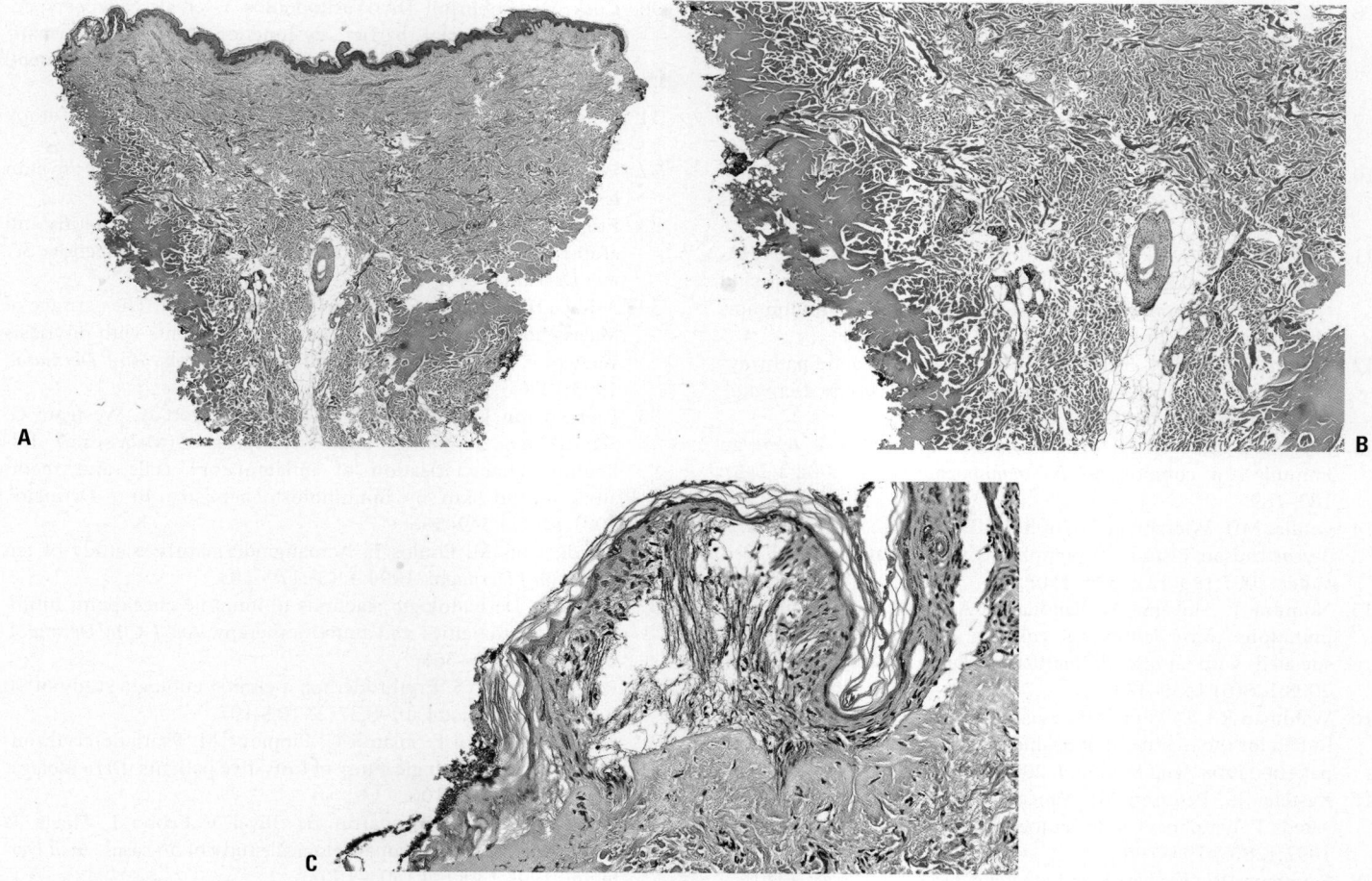

Figure 9-39 Electrodessication. **A:** Cautery artifact along the edge of a skin excision—scanning power. **B:** The dermis on the left-hand side is densely eosinophilic and coagulated with loss of the normal fiber pattern (low power). **C:** The surface epidermis has an artifactual subepidermal cleft. There is also keratinocyte elongation with nuclear pyknosis and cytoplasmic eosinophilia (medium power). (Whole slide image courtesy of Dr. H. Wu.)

Third-degree burns show full-thickness dermal necrosis with destruction of all cutaneous appendages. The coagulation necrosis may extend to the subcutaneous tissue and to the underlying muscle.

Suction Blisters and Purpura

Negative pressure applied over a circumscribed area may form a subepidermal blister that arises in the lamina lucida. Noninflammatory purpura may also result (348).

ACKNOWLEDGMENTS (INCLUDING SUPPORTING RESEARCH GRANTS)

ACKNOWLEDGMENT: We thank Mrs. Phyllis Gilardi for her expert help during the preparation of this book chapter.

DEDICATION: We dedicate this work to Dr. Lisa Harbury Lerner, our skilled colleague from whom we learned so much, being in receipt of her encyclopedic knowledge of dermatology and dermatopathology, and her generosity of spirit.

REFERENCES

1. Kimber I, Dearman RJ. Allergic contact dermatitis: the cellular effectors. *Contact Dermatitis.* 2002;46(1):1–5.
2. Kondo S, Kono T, Brown WR, Pastore S, McKenzie RC, Sauder DN. Lymphocyte function-associated antigen-1 is required for maximum elicitation of allergic contact dermatitis. *Br J Dermatol.* 1994;131(3):354–359.
3. Sar-Pomian M, Kurzeja M, Rudnicka L, Olszewska M. The value of trichoscopy in the differential diagnosis of scalp lesions in pemphigus vulgaris and pemphigus foliaceus. *An Bras Dermatol.* 2014;89(6):1007–1012.
4. Kurzeja M, Rakowska A, Rudnicka L, Olszewska M. Criteria for diagnosing pemphigus vulgaris and pemphigus foliaceus by reflectance confocal microscopy. *Skin Res Technol.* 2012;18(3):339–346.
5. Shklar G, Cataldo E. Histopathology and cytology of oral lesions of pemphigus. *Arch Dermatol.* 1970;101(6):635–641.
6. Schmidt M., Raghavan B, Muller V, et al. Crucial role for human Toll-like receptor 4 in the development of contact allergy to nickel. *Nat Immunol.* 2010;11(9):814–819.
7. Akiyama M, Hashimoto T, Sugiura M, Nishikawa T. Ultrastructural localization of Brazilian pemphigus foliaceus (fogo selvagem) antigens in cultured human squamous cell carcinoma cells. *Br J Dermatol.* 1993;128(4):378–383.

8. Willis CM, Stephens CJ, Wilkinson JD. Differential patterns of epidermal leukocyte infiltration in patch test reactions to structurally unrelated chemical irritants. *J Invest Dermatol.* 1993;101(3):364–370.

9. Matsuo K, Komai A, Ishii K, et al. Pemphigus foliaceus with prominent neutrophilic pustules. *Br J Dermatol.* 2001;145(1):132–136.

10. Timóteo RP, Silva MV, da Silva DAA, et al. Cytokine and chemokines alterations in the endemic form of pemphigus foliaceus (fogo selvagem). *Frontiers in Immunology.* 2017;8:978.

11. Brand CU, Hunziker T, Schaffner T, Limat A, Gerber HA, Braathen LR. Activated immunocompetent cells in human skin lymph derived from irritant contact dermatitis: an immunomorphological study. *Br J Dermatol.* 1995;132(1):39–45.

12. Brasch J, Burgard J, Sterry W. Common pathogenetic pathways in allergic and irritant contact dermatitis. *J Invest Dermatol.* 1992;98(2):166–170.

13. Levin CY, Maibach HI. Irritant contact dermatitis: is there an immunologic component? *Int Immunopharmacol.* 2002;2(2–3): 183–189.

14. Guillet MH, Wierzbicka E, Guillet S, Dagregorio G, Guillet G. A 3-year causative study of pompholyx in 120 patients. *Arch Dermatol.* 2007;143(12):1504–1508.

15. Nomura T, Akiyama M, Sandilands A, et al. Specific filaggrin mutations cause ichthyosis vulgaris and are significantly associated with atopic dermatitis in Japan. *J Invest Dermatol.* 2008;128(6):1436–1441.

16. Waldman RA, DeWane ME, Sloan B, Grant-Kels JM, Lu J. Dupilumab for the treatment of dyshidrotic eczema in 15 consecutive patients. *J Am Acad Dermatol.* 2020;82(5):1251–1252.

17. Kasteler JS, Petersen MJ, Vance JE, Zone JJ. Circulating activated T lymphocytes in autoeczematization. *Arch Dermatol.* 1992;128(6):795–798.

18. Patterson JW. *Weedon's Skin Pathology.* 6th ed. Elsevier; 2020.

19. Choudhri SH, Magro CM, Crowson AN, Nicolle LE. An Id reaction to *Mycobacterium leprae*: first documented case. *Cutis.* 1994;54(4):282–286.

20. Epstein JH. Phototoxicity and photoallergy. *Semin Cutan Med Surg.* 1999;18(4):274–284.

21. Heurung AR, Raju SI, Warshaw EM. Adverse reactions to sunscreen agents: epidemiology, responsible irritants and allergens, clinical characteristics, and management. *Dermatitis.* 2014;25(6):289–326.

22. Diepgen TL, Fartasch M. Recent epidemiological and genetic studies in atopic dermatitis. *Acta Derm Venereol Suppl (Stockh).* 1992;176:13–18.

23. Leung DY, Soter NA. Cellular and immunologic mechanisms in atopic dermatitis. *J Am Acad Dermatol.* 2001;44(1, suppl):S1–S12.

24. Ring J, Darsow U, Behrendt H. Role of aeroallergens in atopic eczema: proof of concept with the atopy patch test. *J Am Acad Dermatol.* 2001;45(1, suppl):S49–S52.

25. Teraki Y, Hotta T, Shiohara T. Increased circulating skin-homing cutaneous lymphocyte-associated antigen (CLA)+ type 2 cytokine-producing cells, and decreased CLA+ type 1 cytokine-producing cells in atopic dermatitis. *Br J Dermatol.* 2000;143(2):373–378.

26. Cooper KD, Stevens SR. T cells in atopic dermatitis. *J Am Acad Dermatol.* 2001;45(1, suppl):S10–S12.

27. Irvine AD, McLean WH, Leung DY. Filaggrin mutations associated with skin and allergic diseases. *N Engl J Med.* 2011; 365(14):1315–1327.

28. Morar N, Willis-Owen SA, Moffatt MF, Cookson WO. The genetics of atopic dermatitis. *J Allergy Clin Immunol.* 2006;118(1): 24–34; quiz 35–36.

29. Weidinger S, Illig T, Baurecht H, et al. Loss-of-function variations within the filaggrin gene predispose for atopic dermatitis with allergic sensitizations. *J Allergy Clin Immunol.* 2006;118(1):214–219.

30. Cork MJ, Robinson DA, Vasilopoulos Y, et al. New perspectives on epidermal barrier dysfunction in atopic dermatitis: gene-environment interactions. *J Allergy Clin Immunol.* 2006;118(1):3–21; quiz 22–23.

31. Coleman R, Trembath RC, Harper JI. Genetic studies of atopy and atopic dermatitis. *Br J Dermatol.* 1997;136(1):1–5.

32. Wollenberg A, Bieber T. Atopic dermatitis: from the genes to skin lesions. *Allergy.* 2000;55(3):205–213.

33. Froschl M, Land HG, Landthaler M. Seborrheic dermatitis and atopic eczema in human immunodeficiency virus infection. *Semin Dermatol.* 1990;9(3):230–232.

34. Ashbee HR, Ingham E, Holland KT, Cunliffe WJ. The carriage of Malassezia furfur serovars A, B and C in patients with pityriasis versicolor, seborrhoeic dermatitis and controls. *Br J Dermatol.* 1993;129(5):533–540.

35. Faergemann J, Bergbrant IM, Dohse M, Scott A, Westgate G. Seborrhoeic dermatitis and *Pityrosporum* (Malassezia) folliculitis: characterization of inflammatory cells and mediators in the skin by immunohistochemistry. *Br J Dermatol.* 2001;144(3):549–556.

36. Rao B, Unis M, Poulos E. Acroangiodermatitis: a study of ten cases. *Int J Dermatol.* 1994;33(3):179–183.

37. Sibaud V. Dermatologic reactions to immune checkpoint inhibitors: skin toxicities and immunotherapy. *Am J Clin Dermatol.* 2018;19(3):345–361.

38. Pal S, Haroon TS. Erythroderma: a clinico-etiologic study of 90 cases. *Int J Dermatol.* 1998;37(2):104–107.

39. Tomasini C, Aloi F, Solaroli C, Pippione M. Psoriatic erythroderma: a histopathologic study of forty-five patients. *Dermatology.* 1997;194(2):102–106.

40. Botella-Estrada R, Sanmartin O, Oliver V, Febrer I, Aliaga A. Erythroderma. A clinicopathological study of 56 cases. *Arch Dermatol.* 1994;130(12):1503–1507.

41. Okoduwa C, Lambert WC, Schwartz RA, et al. Erythroderma: review of a potentially life-threatening dermatosis. *Indian J Dermatol.* 2009;54(1):1–6.

42. Straka BF, Cooper PH, Greer KE. Congenital miliaria crystallina. *Cutis.* 1991;47(2):103–106.

43. Lillywhite LP. Investigation into the environmental factors associated with the incidence of skin disease following an outbreak of Miliaria rubra at a coal mine. *Occup Med (Lond).* 1992; 42(4): 183–187.

44. Borges WG, Augustine NH, Hill HR. Defective interleukin-12/interferon-gamma pathway in patients with hyperimmunoglobulinemia E syndrome. *J Pediatr.* 2000;136(2):176–180.

45. Beutner EH, Jordon RE. Demonstration of skin antibodies in sera of pemphigus vulgaris patients by indirect immunofluorescent staining. *Proc Soc Exp Biol Med.* 1964;117:505–510.

46. Amagai M, Klaus-Kovtun V, Stanley JR. Autoantibodies against a novel epithelial cadherin in pemphigus vulgaris, a disease of cell adhesion. *Cell.* 1991;67(5):869–877.

47. Koch PJ, Walsh MJ, Schmelz M, Goldschmidt MD, Zimbelmann R, Franke WW. Identification of desmoglein, a constitutive desmosomal glycoprotein, as a member of the cadherin family of cell adhesion molecules. *Eur J Cell Biol.* 1990;53(1):1–12.

48. Kowalczyk AP, Anderson JE, Borgwardt JE, Hashimoto T, Stanley JR, Green KJ. Pemphigus sera recognize conformationally sensitive epitopes in the amino-terminal region of desmoglein-1. *J Invest Dermatol.* 1995;105(2):147–152.

49. Harman KE, Gratian MJ, Bhogal BS, Challacombe SJ, Black MM. A study of desmoglein 1 autoantibodies in pemphigus vulgaris: racial differences in frequency and the association with a more severe phenotype. *Br J Dermatol.* 2000;143(2):343–348.

50. Spaeth S, Riechers R, Borradori L, Zillikens D, Büdinger L, Hertl M. IgG, IgA and IgE autoantibodies against the ectodomain of desmoglein 3 in active pemphigus vulgaris. *Br J Dermatol.* 2001;144(6):1183–1188.

51. Mentink LF, de Jong MC, Kloosterhuis GJ, Zuiderveen J, Jonkman MF, Pas HH. Coexistence of IgA antibodies to desmogleins 1 and 3 in pemphigus vulgaris, pemphigus foliaceus and paraneoplastic pemphigus. *Br J Dermatol.* 2007;156(4):635–641.

52. Makino T, Hara H, Mizawa M, et al. Detection of IgG antibodies to desmoglein 3 and desmocollins 2 and 3 in mucosal dominant-type pemphigus vulgaris with severe pharyngalgia and hyperemia of the bulbar conjunctiva. *Eur J Dermatol.* 2015;25(6):619–620.

53. Grando SA. Autoimmunity to keratinocyte acetylcholine receptors in pemphigus. *Dermatology.* 2000;201(4):290–295.

54. Bystryn JC, Grando SA. A novel explanation for acantholysis in pemphigus vulgaris: the basal cell shrinkage hypothesis. *J Am Acad Dermatol.* 2006;54(3):513–516.

55. Hertl M, Amagai M, Sundaram H, Stanley J, Ishii K, Katz SI. Recognition of desmoglein 3 by autoreactive T cells in pemphigus vulgaris patients and normals. *J Invest Dermatol.* 1998;110(1):62–66.

56. Eming R, Budinger L, Riechers R, et al. Frequency analysis of autoreactive T-helper 1 and 2 cells in bullous pemphigoid and pemphigus vulgaris by enzyme-linked immunospot assay. *Br J Dermatol.* 2000;143(6):1279–1282.

57. Wang X, Bregegere F, Frusic-Zlotkin M, Feinmesser M, Michel B, Milner Y. Possible apoptotic mechanism in epidermal cell acantholysis induced by pemphigus vulgaris autoimmunoglobulins. *Apoptosis.* 2004;9(2):131–143.

58. Puviani M, Marconi A, Cozzani E, Pincelli C. Fas ligand in pemphigus sera induces keratinocyte apoptosis through the activation of caspase-8. *J Invest Dermatol.* 2003;120(1):164–167.

59. Weiske J, Schoneberg T, Schroder W, Hatzfeld M, Tauber R, Huber O. The fate of desmosomal proteins in apoptotic cells. *J Biol Chem.* 2001;276(44):41175–41181.

60. Amagai M, Ahmed AR, Kitajima Y, et al. Are desmoglein autoantibodies essential for the immunopathogenesis of pemphigus vulgaris, or just "witnesses of disease"? *Exp Dermatol.* 2006;15(10):815–831.

61. Bhanusali DG, Sachdev A, Rahmanian A, et al. HLA-E*0103X is associated with susceptibility to Pemphigus vulgaris. *Exp Dermatol.* 2013;22(2):108–112.

62. Capon F, Bharkhada J, Cochrane NE, et al. Evidence of an association between desmoglein 3 haplotypes and pemphigus vulgaris. *Br J Dermatol.* 2006;154(1):67–71.

63. Younus J, Ahmed AR. The relationship of pemphigus to neoplasia. *J Am Acad Dermatol.* 1990;23(3, pt 1):498–502.

64. Seidenbaum M, David M, Sandbank M. The course and prognosis of pemphigus. A review of 115 patients. *Int J Dermatol.* 1988;27(8):580–584.

65. Martin FJ, Perez-Bernal AM, Camacho F. Pemphigus vulgaris and disseminated nocardiosis. *J Eur Acad Dermatol Venereol.* 2000;14(5):416–418.

66. Daneshpazhooh M, Chams-Davatchi C, Khamesipour A, et al. Desmoglein 1 and 3 enzyme-linked immunosorbent assay in Iranian patients with pemphigus vulgaris: correlation with phenotype, severity, and disease activity. *J Eur Acad Dermatol Venereol.* 2007;21(10):1319–1324.

67. Ratnam KV, Pang BK. Pemphigus in remission: value of negative direct immunofluorescence in management. *J Am Acad Dermatol.* 1994;30(4):547–550.

68. Korman NJ. Pemphigus. *Dermatol Clin.* 1990;8(4):689–700.

69. Abidi NY, Lainiotis I, Malikowski G, Seiffert-Sinha K, Sinha AA. Longitudinal tracking of autoantibody levels in a pemphigus vulgaris patient: support for a role of anti-desmoglein 1 autoantibodies as predictors of disease progression. *J Drugs Dermatol.* 2017;16(2):135–139.

70. Ueki H, Kohda M, Nobutoh T, et al. Antidesmoglein autoantibodies in silicosis patients with no bullous diseases. *Dermatology.* 2001;202(1):16–21.

71. Brandsen R, Frusic-Zlotkin M, Lyubimov H, et al. Circulating pemphigus IgG in families of patients with pemphigus: comparison of indirect immunofluorescence, direct immunofluorescence, and immunoblotting. *J Am Acad Dermatol.* 1997;36(1):44–52.

72. Grando SA. Pemphigus autoimmunity: hypotheses and realities. *Autoimmunity.* 2012;45(1):7–35.

73. Mahoney MG, Wang Z, Rothenberger K, Koch PJ, Amagai M, Stanley JR. Explanations for the clinical and microscopic localization of lesions in pemphigus foliaceus and vulgaris. *J Clin Invest.* 1999;103(4):461–468.

74. Amagai M. Autoimmunity against desmosomal cadherins in pemphigus. *J Dermatol Sci.* 1999;20(2):92–102.

75. Udey MC, Stanley JR. Pemphigus—diseases of antidesmosomal autoimmunity. *JAMA.* 1999;282(6):572–576.

76. Amagai M, Karpati S, Prussick R, Klaus-Kovtun V, Stanley JR. Autoantibodies against the amino-terminal cadherin-like binding domain of pemphigus vulgaris antigen are pathogenic. *J Clin Invest.* 1992;90(3):919–926.

77. Futei Y, Amagai M, Sekiguchi M, Nishifuji K, Fujii Y, Nishikawa T. Use of domain-swapped molecules for conformational epitope mapping of desmoglein 3 in pemphigus vulgaris. *J Invest Dermatol.* 2000;115(5):829–834.

78. Mahoney MG, Wang ZH, Stanley JR. Pemphigus vulgaris and pemphigus foliaceus antibodies are pathogenic in plasminogen activator knockout mice. *J Invest Dermatol.* 1999;113(1):22–25.

79. Amagai M, Hashimoto T, Green KJ, Shimizu N, Nishikawa T. Antigen-specific immunoadsorption of pathogenic autoantibodies in pemphigus foliaceus. *J Invest Dermatol.* 1995;104(6):895–901.

80. Patten SF, Dijkstra JW. Associations of pemphigus and autoimmune disease with malignancy or thymoma. *Int J Dermatol.* 1994;33(12):836–842.

81. Kurokawa M, Koketsu H, Oda Y, et al. A case of pemphigus vulgaris accompanied by multiple myeloma. *Int J Dermatol.* 2005;44(10):873–875.

82. Gili A, Ngan BY, Lester R. Castleman's disease associated with pemphigus vulgaris. *J Am Acad Dermatol.* 1991;25(5, pt 2):955–959.

83. Vetters JM, Saikia NK, Wood J, Simpson JA. Pemphigus vulgaris and myasthenia gravis. *Br J Dermatol.* 1973;88(5):437–441.

84. Chan LS, Cooper KD. Coexistence of pemphigus vulgaris and progressive localized scleroderma. *Arch Dermatol.* 1989;125(11):1555–1557.

85. Adaszewska A, Kalinska-Bienias A, Jagielski P, Wozniak K, Kowalewski C. The use of BIOCHIP technique in diagnosis of different types of pemphigus: vulgaris and foliaceus. *J Immunol Methods.* 2019;468:35–39.

86. Lee MS, Yeh YC, Tu YK, Chan TC. Network meta-analysis-based comparison of first-line steroid-sparing adjuvants in the treatment of pemphigus vulgaris and pemphigus foliaceus. *J Am Acad Dermatol.* 2021;85(1):176–186.

87. Ahmed AR, Kaveri S, Spigelman, Z. Long-term remissions in recalcitrant pemphigus vulgaris. *N Engl J Med.* 2015;373(27):2693–2694.

88. Woo TY, Solomon AR, Fairley JA. Pemphigus vegetans limited to the lips and oral mucosa. *Arch Dermatol.* 1985;121(2):271–272.

89. Bianchi L, Carrozzo AM, Orlandi A, Campione E, Hagman JH, Chimenti S. Pyoderma vegetans and ulcerative colitis. *Br J Dermatol.* 2001;144(6):1224–1227.

90. Crosby DL, Diaz LA. Endemic pemphigus foliaceus. Fogo selvagem. *Dermatol Clin.* 1993;11(3):453–462.

91. Ichimiya M, Yamamoto K, Muto M. Successful treatment of pemphigus vegetans by addition of etretinate to systemic steroids. *Clin Exp Dermatol.* 1998;23(4):178–180.

92. Ruocco V, Ruocco E, Caccavale S, Gambardella A, Lo Schiavo A. Pemphigus vegetans of the folds (intertriginous areas). *Clin Dermatol.* 2015;33(4):471–476.
93. Lombardi C, Borges PC, Chaul A, et al. Environmental risk factors in endemic pemphigus foliaceus (Fogo selvagem). "The Cooperative Group on Fogo Selvagem Research." *J Invest Dermatol.* 1992;98(6):847–850.
94. Reis VM, Toledo RP, Lopez A, Diaz LA, Martins JE. UVB-induced acantholysis in endemic Pemphigus foliaceus (Fogo selvagem) and Pemphigus vulgaris. *J Am Acad Dermatol.* 2000;42(4):571–576.
95. Aoki V, Rivitti EA, Diaz LA; Cooperative Group on Fogo Selvagem Research. Update on fogo selvagem, an endemic form of pemphigus foliaceus. *J Dermatol.* 2015;42(1):18–26.
96. Abreu-Velez AM, Beutner EH, Montoya F, Bollag WB, Hashimoto T. Analyses of autoantigens in a new form of endemic pemphigus foliaceus in Colombia. *J Am Acad Dermatol.* 2003;49(4):609–614.
97. Diaz LA, Prisayanh PS, Dasher DA, et al. The IgM anti-desmoglein 1 response distinguishes Brazilian pemphigus foliaceus (fogo selvagem) from other forms of pemphigus. *J Invest Dermatol.* 2008;128(3):667–675.
98. Amagai M. Desmoglein as a target in autoimmunity and infection. *J Am Acad Dermatol.* 2003;48(2):244–252.
99. Stanley JR, Amagai M. Pemphigus, bullous impetigo, and the staphylococcal scalded-skin syndrome. *N Engl J Med.* 2006;355(17):1800–1810.
100. Ioannides D, Hytiroglou P, Phelps RG, Bystryn JC. Regional variation in the expression of pemphigus foliaceus, pemphigus erythematosus, and pemphigus vulgaris antigens in human skin. *J Invest Dermatol.* 1991;96(2):159–161.
101. Hobbs LK, Noland MB, Raghavan SS, Gru AA. Pemphigus erythematosus: a case series from a tertiary academic center and literature review. *J Cutan Pathol.* 2021;48(8):1038–1050.
102. Lo Schiavo A, Puca RV, Romano F, Cozzi R. Pemphigus erythematosus relapse associated with atorvastatin intake. *Drug Des Devel Ther.* 2014;8:1463–1465.
103. Pritchett EN, Hejazi E, Cusack CA. Pruritic, pink scaling plaques on the face and trunk. Pemphigus erythematosus. *JAMA Dermatol.* 2015;151(10):1123–1124.
104. Forsti AK, Vuorre O, Laurila E, Jokelainen J, Huilaja L, Tasanen K. Pemphigus foliaceus and pemphigus erythematosus are the most common subtypes of pemphigus in Northern Finland. *Acta Derm Venereol.* 2019;99(12):1127–1130.
105. Robinson ND, Hashimoto T, Amagai M, Chan LS. The new pemphigus variants. *J Am Acad Dermatol.* 1999;40(5, pt 1):649–671; quiz 672–673.
106. Morita E, Amagai M, Tanaka T, Horiuchi K, Yamamoto S. A case of herpetiform pemphigus coexisting with psoriasis vulgaris. *Br J Dermatol.* 1999;141(4):754–755.
107. Palleschi GM, Giomi B. Herpetiformis pemphigus and lung carcinoma: a case of paraneoplastic pemphigus. *Acta Derm Venereol.* 2002;82(4):304–305.
108. Marzano AV, Tourlaki A, Cozzani E, Gianotti R, Caputo R. Pemphigus herpetiformis associated with prostate cancer. *J Eur Acad Dermatol Venereol.* 2007;21(5):696–698.
109. Schoch JJ, Boull CL, Camilleri MJ, Tollefson MM, Hook KP, Polcari IC. Transplacental transmission of pemphigus herpetiformis in the setting of maternal lymphoma. *Pediatr Dermatol.* 2015;32(6):e234–e237.
110. Ishii K, Amagai M, Komai A, et al. Desmoglein 1 and desmoglein 3 are the target autoantigens in herpetiform pemphigus. *Arch Dermatol.* 1999;135(8):943–947.
111. Yamamoto A, Harada S, Nakada T, Iijima M. Contact dermatitis to phenylephrine hydrochloride eyedrops. *Clin Exp Dermatol.* 2004;29(2):200–201.
112. Kurashige Y, Mitsuhashi Y, Saito M, Fukuda S, Hashimoto T, Tsuboi R. Herpetiform pemphigus with anti-Dsg 1 and full-length BP180 autoantibodies. *Eur J Dermatol.* 2012;22(2):269–270.
113. Ohata C, Koga H, Teye K, et al. Concurrence of bullous pemphigoid and herpetiform pemphigus with IgG antibodies to desmogleins 1/3 and desmocollins 1–3. *Br J Dermatol.* 2013;168(4):879–881.
114. Korman NJ, Eyre RW, Zone J, Stanley JR. Drug-induced pemphigus: autoantibodies directed against the pemphigus antigen complexes are present in penicillamine and captopril-induced pemphigus. *J Invest Dermatol.* 1991;96(2):273–276.
115. Pisani M, Ruocco V. Drug-induced pemphigus. *Clin Dermatol.* 1986;4(1):118–132.
116. Ruocco V, Sacerdoti G. Pemphigus and bullous pemphigoid due to drugs. *Int J Dermatol.* 1991;30(5):307–312.
117. Vozza A, Ruocco V, Brenner S, Wolf R. Contact pemphigus. *Int J Dermatol.* 1996;35(3):199–201.
118. Michailidou EZ, Belazi MA, Markopoulos AK, Tsatsos MI, Mourellou ON, Antoniades DZ. Epidemiologic survey of pemphigus vulgaris with oral manifestations in northern Greece: retrospective study of 129 patients. *Int J Dermatol.* 2007;46(4):356–361.
119. Hodak E, David M, Ingber A, et al. The clinical and histopathological spectrum of IgA-pemphigus—report of two cases. *Clin Exp Dermatol.* 1990;15(6):433–437.
120. Ebihara T, Hashimoto T, Iwatsuki K, et al. Autoantigens for IgA anti-intercellular antibodies of intercellular IgA vesiculopustular dermatosis. *J Invest Dermatol.* 1991;97(4):742–745.
121. Miyagawa S, Hashimoto T, Ohno H, et al. Atypical pemphigus associated with monoclonal IgA gammopathy. *J Am Acad Dermatol.* 1995;32(2, pt 2):352–357.
122. Espana A, Gimenez-Azcarate A, Ishii N, Idoate MA, Panizo C, Hashimoto T. Antidesmocollin 1 autoantibody negative subcorneal pustular dermatosis-type IgA pemphigus associated with multiple myeloma. *Br J Dermatol.* 2015;172(1):296–298.
123. Belloni Fortina A, Romano I, Peserico A. Contact sensitization to compositae mix in children. *J Am Acad Dermatol.* 2005;53(5):877–880.
124. Harman KE, Holmes G, Bhogal BS, McFadden J, Black MM. Intercellular IgA dermatosis (IgA pemphigus)—two cases illustrating the clinical heterogeneity of this disorder. *Clin Exp Dermatol.* 1999;24(6):464–466.
125. Hashimoto T, Teye K, Ishii N. Clinical and immunological studies of 49 cases of various types of intercellular IgA dermatosis and 13 cases of classical subcorneal pustular dermatosis examined at Kurume University. *Br J Dermatol.* 2017;176(1):168–175.
126. Teraki Y, Amagai N, Hashimoto T, Kusunoki T, Nishikawa T. Intercellular IgA dermatosis of childhood. Selective deposition of monomer IgA1 in the intercellular space of the epidermis. *Arch Dermatol.* 1991;127(2):221–224.
127. Neumann E, Dmochowski M, Bowszyc J, Bowszyc-Dmochowska M, Raptis M. The occurrence of IgA pemphigus foliaceus without neutrophilic infiltration. *Clin Exp Dermatol.* 1994;19(1):56–58.
128. Ohno H, Miyagawa S, Hashimoto T, et al. Atypical pemphigus with concomitant IgG and IgA anti-intercellular autoantibodies associated with monoclonal IgA gammopathy. *Dermatology.* 1994;189(suppl 1):115–116.
129. Hashimoto T, Kiyokawa C, Mori O, et al. Human desmocollin 1 (Dsc1) is an autoantigen for the subcorneal pustular dermatosis type of IgA pemphigus. *J Invest Dermatol.* 1997;109(2):127–131.
130. Hashimoto T, Komai A, Futei Y, Nishikawa T, Amagai. Detection of IgA autoantibodies to desmogleins by an enzyme-linked immunosorbent assay: the presence of new minor subtypes of IgA pemphigus. *Arch Dermatol.* 2001;137(6):735–738.
131. Kridin K, Patel PM, Jones VA, Cordova A, Amber KT. IgA pemphigus: a systematic review. *J Am Acad Dermatol.* 2020;82(6):1386–1392.
132. Lane N, Parekh P. IgG/IgA pemphigus. *Am J Dermatopathol.* 2014;36(12):1002–1004.

133. Uchiyama R, Ishii N, Arakura F, et al. IgA/IgG pemphigus with infiltration of neutrophils and eosinophils in an ulcerative colitis patient. *Acta Derm Venereol.* 2014;94(6):737–738.

134. Furuya A, Takahashi E, Ishii N, Hashimoto T, Satoh T. IgG/IgA pemphigus recognizing desmogleins 1 and 3 in a patient with Sjogren's syndrome. *Eur J Dermatol.* 2014;24(4):512–513.

135. Toosi S, Collins JW, Lohse CM, et al. Clinicopathologic features of IgG/IgA pemphigus in comparison with classic (IgG) and IgA pemphigus. *Int J Dermatol.* 2016;55(4):e184–e190.

136. Camisa C, Helm TN, Liu YC, et al. Paraneoplastic pemphigus: a report of three cases including one long-term survivor. *J Am Acad Dermatol.* 1992;27(4):547–553.

137. Ohzono A, Sogame R, Li X, et al. Clinical and immunological findings in 104 cases of paraneoplastic pemphigus. *Br J Dermatol.* 2015;173(6):1447–1452.

138. Anhalt GJ. Paraneoplastic pemphigus. *Adv Dermatol.* 1997;12: 77–96; discussion 97.

139. Kitagawa C, Nakajima K, Aoyama Y, et al. A typical case of paraneoplastic pemphigus without detection of malignancy: effectiveness of plasma exchange. *Acta Derm Venereol.* 2014;94(3):359–361.

140. Kartan S, Shi VY, Clark AK, Chan LS. Paraneoplastic pemphigus and autoimmune blistering diseases associated with neoplasm: characteristics, diagnosis, associated neoplasms, proposed pathogenesis, treatment. *Am J Clin Dermatol.* 2017;18(1): 105–126.

141. Nguyen VT, Ndoye A, Bassler KD, et al. Classification, clinical manifestations, and immunopathological mechanisms of the epithelial variant of paraneoplastic autoimmune multiorgan syndrome: a reappraisal of paraneoplastic pemphigus. *Arch Dermatol.* 2001;137(2):193–206.

142. Mutasim DF, Pelc NJ, Anhalt GJ. Paraneoplastic pemphigus. *Dermatol Clin.* 1993;11(3):473–481.

143. Anhalt GJ, Kim SC, Stanley JR, et al. Paraneoplastic pemphigus. An autoimmune mucocutaneous disease associated with neoplasia. *N Engl J Med.* 1990;323(25):1729–1735.

144. Bystryn JC, Hodak E, Gao SQ, Chuba JV, Amorosi EL. A paraneoplastic mixed bullous skin disease associated with anti-skin antibodies and a B-cell lymphoma. *Arch Dermatol.* 1993;129(7):870–875.

145. Musette P, Joly P, Gilbert D, et al. A paraneoplastic mixed bullous skin disease: breakdown in tolerance to multiple epidermal antigens. *Br J Dermatol.* 2000;143(1):149–153.

146. Setterfield J, Shirlaw PJ, Lazarova Z, et al. Paraneoplastic cicatricial pemphigoid. *Br J Dermatol.* 1999;141(1):127–131.

147. Svoboda SA, Huang S, Liu X, Hsu S, Motaparthi K. Paraneoplastic pemphigus: revised diagnostic criteria based on literature analysis. *J Cutan Pathol.* 2021;48(9):1133–1138.

148. Horn TD, Anhalt GJ. Histologic features of paraneoplastic pemphigus. *Arch Dermatol.* 1992;128(8):1091–1095.

149. Stevens SR, Griffiths CE, Anhalt GJ, Cooper KD. Paraneoplastic pemphigus presenting as a lichen planus pemphigoides-like eruption. *Arch Dermatol.* 1993;129(7):866–869.

150. Leger S, Picard D, Ingen-Housz-Oro S, et al. Prognostic factors of paraneoplastic pemphigus. *Arch Dermatol.* 2012;148(10): 1165–1172.

151. Mehregan DR, Oursler JR, Leiferman KM, Muller SA, Anhalt GJ, Peters MS. Paraneoplastic pemphigus: a subset of patients with pemphigus and neoplasia. *J Cutan Pathol.* 1993;20(3): 203–210.

152. Reich K, Brinck U, Letschert M, et al. Graft-versus-host disease-like immunophenotype and apoptotic keratinocyte death in paraneoplastic pemphigus. *Br J Dermatol.* 1999;141(4):739–746.

153. Cummins DL, Mimouni D, Tzu J, Owens N, Anhalt GJ, Meyerle JH. Lichenoid paraneoplastic pemphigus in the absence of detectable antibodies. *J Am Acad Dermatol.* 2007;56(1): 153–159.

154. Nousari HC, Kimyai-Asadi A, Anhalt GJ. Elevated serum levels of interleukin-6 in paraneoplastic pemphigus. *J Invest Dermatol.* 1999;112(3):396–398.

155. Maruta CW, Miyamoto D, Aoki V, Carvalho RGR, Cunha BM, Santi CG. Paraneoplastic pemphigus: a clinical, laboratorial, and therapeutic overview. *An Bras Dermatol.* 2019;94(4):388–398.

156. Li K, Tamai K, Tan EM, Uitto J. Cloning of type XVII collagen. Complementary and genomic DNA sequences of mouse 180-kilodalton bullous pemphigoid antigen (BPAG2) predict an interrupted collagenous domain, a transmembrane segment, and unusual features in the 5'-end of the gene and the 3'-untranslated region of the mRNA. *J Biol Chem.* 1993;268(12):8825–8834.

157. Marinkovich MP, Taylor TB, Keene DR, Burgeson RE, Zone JJ. LAD-1, the linear IgA bullous dermatosis autoantigen, is a novel 120-kDa anchoring filament protein synthesized by epidermal cells. *J Invest Dermatol.* 1996;106(4):734–738.

158. Zillikens D, Giudice GJ. BP180/type XVII collagen: its role in acquired and inherited disorders or the dermal-epidermal junction. *Arch Dermatol Res.* 1999;291(4):187–194.

159. Schmidt E, Zillikens D. Autoimmune and inherited subepidermal blistering diseases: advances in the clinic and the laboratory. *Adv Dermatol.* 2000;16:113–157; discussion 158.

160. Vidal F, Aberdam D, Miquel C, et al. Integrin beta 4 mutations associated with junctional epidermolysis bullosa with pyloric atresia. *Nat Genet.* 1995;10(2):229–234.

161. Tyagi S, Bhol K, Natarajan K, Livir-Rallatos C, Foster CS, Ahmed AR. Ocular cicatricial pemphigoid antigen: partial sequence and biochemical characterization. *Proc Natl Acad Sci U S A.* 1996;93(25):14714–14719.

162. Chen KR, Shimizu S, Miyakawa S, Ishiko A, Shimizu H, Hashimoto T. Coexistence of psoriasis and an unusual IgG-mediated subepidermal bullous dermatosis: identification of a novel 200-kDa lower lamina lucida target antigen. *Br J Dermatol.* 1996;134(2):340–346.

163. Zillikens D, Kawahara Y, Ishiko A, et al. A novel subepidermal blistering disease with autoantibodies to a 200-kDa antigen of the basement membrane zone. *J Invest Dermatol.* 1996;106(3):465–470.

164. Pulkkinen L, Christiano AM, Gerecke D, et al. A homozygous nonsense mutation in the beta 3 chain gene of laminin 5 (LAMB3) in Herlitz junctional epidermolysis bullosa. *Genomics.* 1994;24(2):357–360.

165. Chorzelski TP, Jablonska S, Maciejowska E. Linear IgA bullous dermatosis of adults. *Clin Dermatol.* 1991;9(3):383–392.

166. Lever WF. Pemphigus. *Medicine (Baltimore).* 1953;32(1):1–123.

167. Lindelof B, Islam N, Eklund G, Arfors L. Pemphigoid and cancer. *Arch Dermatol.* 1990;126(1):66–68.

168. Taylor G, Venning V, Wojnarowska F. Bullous pemphigoid and associated autoimmune thrombocytopenia: two case reports. *J Am Acad Dermatol.* 1993;29(5, pt 2):900–902.

169. Kibsgaard L, Rasmussen M, Lamberg A, Deleuran M, Olesen AB, Vestergaard C. Increased frequency of multiple sclerosis among patients with bullous pemphigoid: a population-based cohort study on comorbidities anchored around the diagnosis of bullous pemphigoid. *Br J Dermatol.* 2017;176(6):1486–1491.

170. Gammon WR, Briggaman RA, Inman AO 3rd, Queen LL, Wheeler CE. Differentiating anti-lamina lucida and anti-sublamina densa anti-BMZ antibodies by indirect immunofluorescence on 1.0 M sodium chloride-separated skin. *J Invest Dermatol.* 1984;82(2):139–144.

171. Good LM, Good TJ, High WA. Infantile acropustulosis in internationally adopted children. *J Am Acad Dermatol.* 2011; 65(4):763–771.

172. Baardman R, Horvath B, Bolling MC, Pas HH, Diercks GFH. Immunoglobulin M bullous pemphigoid: an enigma. *JAAD Case Rep.* 2020;6(6):518–520.

173. Wuepper KD. Repeat direct immunofluorescence to discriminate pemphigoid from epidermolysis bullosa acquisita. *Arch Dermatol.* 1990;126(10):1365.

174. Gammon WR, Kowalewski C, Chorzelski TP, Kumar V, Briggaman RA, Beutner EH. Direct immunofluorescence studies of sodium chloride-separated skin in the differential diagnosis of bullous pemphigoid and epidermolysis bullosa acquisita. *J Am Acad Dermatol.* 1990;22(4):664–670.

175. Mueller S, Klaus-Kovtun V, Stanley JR. A 230-kD basic protein is the major bullous pemphigoid antigen. *J Invest Dermatol.* 1989;92(1):33–38.

176. Labib RS, Anhalt GJ, Patel HP, Mutasim DF, Diaz LA. Molecular heterogeneity of the bullous pemphigoid antigens as detected by immunoblotting. *J Immunol.* 1986;136(4):1231–1235.

177. Cotell SL, Lapiere JC, Chen JD, et al. A novel 105-kDa lamina lucida autoantigen: association with bullous pemphigoid. *J Invest Dermatol.* 1994;103(1):78–83.

178. Chan LS, Cooper KD. A novel immune-mediated subepidermal bullous dermatosis characterized by IgG autoantibodies to a lower lamina lucida component. *Arch Dermatol.* 1994;130(3):343–347.

179. Brown LF, Harrist TJ, Yeo KT, et al. Increased expression of vascular permeability factor (vascular endothelial growth factor) in bullous pemphigoid, dermatitis herpetiformis, and erythema multiforme. *J Invest Dermatol.* 1995;104(5):744–749.

180. Stahle-Backdahl M, Inoue M, Guidice GJ, Parks WC. 92-kD gelatinase is produced by eosinophils at the site of blister formation in bullous pemphigoid and cleaves the extracellular domain of recombinant 180-kD bullous pemphigoid autoantigen. *J Clin Invest.* 1994;93(5):2022–2030.

181. Kaneko F, Minagawa T, Takiguchi Y, Suzuki M, Itoh N. Role of cell-mediated immune reaction in blister formation of bullous pemphigoid. *Dermatology.* 1992;184(1):34–39.

182. Patel PM, Jones VA, Murray TN, Amber KT. A review comparing international guidelines for the management of bullous pemphigoid, pemphigoid gestationis, mucous membrane pemphigoid, and epidermolysis bullosa acquisita. *Am J Clin Dermatol.* 2020;21(4):557–565.

183. Williams HC, Wojnarowska F, Kirtschig G, et al. Doxycycline versus prednisolone as an initial treatment strategy for bullous pemphigoid: a pragmatic, non-inferiority, randomised controlled trial. *Lancet.* 2017;389(10079):1630–1638.

184. Lonowski S, Sachsman S, Patel N, Truong A, Holland V. Increasing evidence for omalizumab in the treatment of bullous pemphigoid. *JAAD Case Rep.* 2020;6(3):228–233.

185. Abdat R, Waldman RA, de Bedout V, et al. Dupilumab as a novel therapy for bullous pemphigoid: a multicenter case series. *J Am Acad Dermatol.* 2020;83(1):46–52.

186. Tan CW, Pang Y, Sim B, Thirumoorthy T, Pang SM, Lee HY. The association between drugs and bullous pemphigoid. *Br J Dermatol.* 2017;176(2):549–551.

187. Hodak E, Ben-Shetrit A, Ingber A, Sandbank M. Bullous pemphigoid—an adverse effect of ampicillin. *Clin Exp Dermatol.* 1990;15(1):50–52.

188. Soh H, Hosokawa H, Miyauchi H, Izumi H, Asada Y. Localized pemphigoid shares the same target antigen as bullous pemphigoid. *Br J Dermatol.* 1991;125(1):73–75.

189. Ohnishi Y, Tajima S, Ishibashi A, Fujiwara S. A vesicular bullous pemphigoid with an autoantibody against plectin. *Br J Dermatol.* 2000;142(4):813–815.

190. Okura M, Tatsuno Y, Sato M, et al. Vesicular pemphigoid with antidesmoplakin autoantibodies. *Br J Dermatol.* 1997;136(5):794–796.

191. Hsu S, Ghohestania RF, Uitto J. Lichen planus pemphigoides with IgG antibodies to the 180 kd bullous pemphigoid antigen (type XII collagen). *J Am Acad Dermatol.* 2000;42(1Pt 1): 136–141.

192. Zillikens D, Mascaro JM, Rose PM, et al. A highly sensitive enzyme-linked immunosorbent assay for the detection of circulating anti-BP180 autoantibodies in patients with bullous pemphigoid. *J Invest Dermatol.* 1997;109:679–683.

193. Velthuis PJ, Hendrikse JC, Nefkens JJ. Combined features of pemphigus and pemphigoid induced by penicillamine. *Br J Dermatol.* 1985;112(5):615–619.

194. Groth S, Recke A, Vafia K, et al. Development of a simple enzyme-linked immunosorbent assay for the detection of autoantibodies in anti-p200 pemphigoid. *Br J Dermatol.* 2011;164(1):76–82.

195. Goletz S, Hashimoto T, Zillikens D, Schmidt E. Anti-p200 pemphigoid. *J Am Acad Dermatol.* 2014;71(1):185–191.

196. Shimanovich I, Petersen EE, Weyers W, Sitaru C, Zillikens D. Subepidermal blistering disease with autoantibodies to both the p200 autoantigen and the alpha3 chain of laminin 5. *J Am Acad Dermatol.* 2005;52(5, suppl 1):S90–S92.

197. Rose C, Weyers W, Denisjuk N, Hillen U, Zillikens D, Shimanovich I. Histopathology of anti-p200 pemphigoid. *Am J Dermatopathol.* 2007;29(2):119–124.

198. Meijer JM, Diercks GF, Schmidt E, Pas HH, Jonkman MF. Laboratory diagnosis and clinical profile of anti-p200 pemphigoid. *JAMA Dermatol.* 2016;152(8):897–904.

199. Mostafa MI, Hassib NF, Nemat AH. Oral mucous membrane pemphigoid in a 6-year-old boy: diagnosis, treatment and 4 years follow-up. *Int J Paediatr Dent.* 2010;20(1):76–79.

200. Leonard JN, Hobday CM, Haffenden GP, et al. Immunofluorescent studies in ocular cicatricial pemphigoid. *Br J Dermatol.* 1988;118(2):209–217.

201. Smith EP, Taylor TB, Meyer LJ, Zone JJ. Identification of a basement membrane zone antigen reactive with circulating IgA antibody in ocular cicatricial pemphigoid. *J Invest Dermatol.* 1993;101(4):619–623.

202. Domloge-Hultsch N, Anhalt GJ, Gammon WR, et al. Antiepiligrin cicatricial pemphigoid. A subepithelial bullous disorder. *Arch Dermatol.* 1994;130(12):1521–1529.

203. Bhol KC, Dans MJ, Simmons RK, Foster CS, Giancotti FG, Ahmed AR. The autoantibodies to alpha 6 beta 4 integrin of patients affected by ocular cicatricial pemphigoid recognize predominantly epitopes within the large cytoplasmic domain of human beta 4. *J Immunol.* 2000;165(5):2824–2829.

204. Bernard P, Prost C, Lecerf V, et al. Studies of cicatricial pemphigoid autoantibodies using direct immunoelectron microscopy and immunoblot analysis. *J Invest Dermatol.* 1990;94(5): 630–635.

205. Montagnon CM, Tolkachjov SN, Murrell DF, Camilleri MJ, Lehman JS. Subepithelial autoimmune blistering dermatoses: clinical features and diagnosis. *J Am Acad Dermatol.* 2021;85(1):1–14.

206. Shornick JK. Herpes gestationis. *Dermatol Clin.* 1993;11(3):527–533.

207. Shornick JK, Black MM. Fetal risks in herpes gestationis. *J Am Acad Dermatol.* 1992;26(1):63–68.

208. Kelly SE, Black MM. Pemphigoid gestationis: placental interactions. *Semin Dermatol.* 1989;8(1):12–17.

209. Kelly SE, Bhogal BS, Wojnarowska F, Whitehead P, Leigh IM, Black MM. Western blot analysis of the antigen in pemphigoid gestationis. *Br J Dermatol.* 1990;122(4):445–449.

210. Yang B, Wang C, Wu M, et al. A case of pemphigoid gestationis with concurrent IgG antibodies to BP180, BP230 and type VII collagen. *Australas J Dermatol.* 2014;55(1):e15–e18.

211. Andersson NW, Skov L, Andersen JT. Evaluation of topical corticosteroid use in pregnancy and risk of newborns being small for gestational age and having low birth weight. *JAMA Dermatol.* 2021;157(7):788–795.

212. Dotson AD, Raimer SS, Pursley TV, Tschen J. Systemic lupus erythematosus occurring in a patient with epidermolysis bullosa acquisita. *Arch Dermatol.* 1981;117(7):422–426.

213. Boh E, Roberts LJ, Lieu TS, Gammon WR, Sontheimer RD. Epidermolysis bullosa acquisita preceding the development of systemic lupus erythematosus. *J Am Acad Dermatol.* 1990;22(4):587–593.

214. Rencic A, Goyal S, Mofid M, Wigley F, Nousari HC. Bullous lesions in scleroderma. *Int J Dermatol.* 2002;41(6):335–339.

215. Gammon WR, Briggaman RA, Woodley DT, Heald PW, Wheeler CE Jr. Epidermolysis bullosa acquisita—a pemphigoid-like disease. *J Am Acad Dermatol.* 1984;11(5, pt 1):820–832.

216. Vodegel RM, Jonkman MF, Pas HH, de Jong MC. U-serrated immunodeposition pattern differentiates type VII collagen targeting bullous diseases from other subepidermal bullous autoimmune diseases. *Br J Dermatol.* 2004;151(1):112–118.

217. Gammon WR, Fine JD, Briggaman RA. Autoimmunity to type VII collagen: features and roles in basement membrane zone injury. In: Fine JD, ed. *Bullous Diseases.* Igaka Shoin; 1993:75.

218. Ishii N, Yoshida M, Hisamatsu Y, et al. Epidermolysis bullosa acquisita sera react with distinct epitopes on the NC1 and NC2 domains of type VII collagen: study using immunoblotting of domain-specific recombinant proteins and postembedding immunoelectron microscopy. *Br J Dermatol.* 2004;150(5):843–851.

219. Koga H, Prost-Squarcioni C, Iwata H, Jonkman MF, Ludwig RJ, Bieber K. Epidermolysis bullosa acquisita: the 2019 update. *Front Med (Lausanne).* 2018;5:362.

220. Iwata H, Vorobyev A, Koga H, et al. Meta-analysis of the clinical and immunopathological characteristics and treatment outcomes in epidermolysis bullosa acquisita patients. *Orphanet J Rare Dis.* 2018;13(1):153.

221. Tsuchida T, Furue M, Kashiwado T, Ishibashi Y. Bullous systemic lupus erythematosus with cutaneous mucinosis and leukocytoclastic vasculitis. *J Am Acad Dermatol.* 1994;31(2, pt 2):387–390.

222. Lowe CD, Brahe CA, Green B, Lam TK, Meyerle JH. Bullous systemic lupus erythematosus successfully treated with rituximab. *Cutis.* 2019;103(6):E5–E7.

223. Duan L, Chen L, Zhong S, et al. Treatment of bullous systemic lupus erythematosus. *J Immunol Res.* 2015;2015:167064.

224. Bose SK, Lacour JP, Bodokh I, Ortonne JP. Malignant lymphoma and dermatitis herpetiformis. *Dermatology.* 1994;188(3):177–181.

225. Paek SY, Steinberg SM, Katz SI. Remission in dermatitis herpetiformis: a cohort study. *Arch Dermatol.* 2011;147(3):301–305.

226. Ceri M, Unverdi S. IgA nephropathy coexisting with linear IgA bullous disease. *Ren Fail.* 2011;33(1):101.

227. Olbricht SM, Flotte TJ, Collins AB, Chapman CM, Harrist TJ. Dermatitis herpetiformis. Cutaneous deposition of polyclonal IgA1. *Arch Dermatol.* 1986;122(4):418–421.

228. Wojnarowska F, Delacroix D, Gengoux P. Cutaneous IgA subclasses in dermatitis herpetiformis and linear IgA disease. *J Cutan Pathol.* 1988;15(5):272–275.

229. Huber C, Trueb RM, French LE, Hafner J. Negative direct immunofluorescence and nonspecific histology do not exclude the diagnosis of dermatitis herpetiformis Duhring. *Int J Dermatol.* 2013;52(2):248–249.

230. Beutner EH, Baughman RD, Austin BM, Plunkett RW, Binder WL. A case of dermatitis herpetiformis with IgA endomysial antibodies but negative direct immunofluorescent findings. *J Am Acad Dermatol.* 2000;43(2, pt 2):329–332.

231. Reunala T, Chorzelski TP, Viander M, et al. IgA anti-endomysial antibodies in dermatitis herpetiformis: correlation with jejunal morphology, gluten-free diet and anti-gliadin antibodies. *Br J Dermatol.* 1987;117(2):185–191.

232. Kumar V, Jarzabek-Chorzelska M, Sulej J, Rajadhyaksha M, Jablonska S. Tissue transglutaminase and endomysial antibodies-diagnostic markers of gluten-sensitive enteropathy in dermatitis herpetiformis. *Clin Immunol.* 2001;98(3):378–382.

233. Sardy M, Karpati S, Merkl B, Paulsson M, Smyth N. Epidermal transglutaminase (TGase 3) is the autoantigen of dermatitis herpetiformis. *J Exp Med.* 2002;195(6):747–757.

234. Graeber M, Baker BS, Garioch JJ, Valdimarsson H, Leonard JN, Fry L. The role of cytokines in the generation of skin lesions in dermatitis herpetiformis. *Br J Dermatol.* 1993;129(5):530–532.

235. Pardo RJ, Penneys NS. Location of basement membrane type IV collagen beneath subepidermal bullous diseases. *J Cutan Pathol.* 1990;17(6):336–341.

236. Godfrey K, Wojnarowska F, Leonard J. Linear IgA disease of adults: association with lymphoproliferative malignancy and possible role of other triggering factors. *Br J Dermatol.* 1990;123(4):447–452.

237. Paige DG, Leonard JN, Wojnarowska F, Fry L. Linear IgA disease and ulcerative colitis. *Br J Dermatol.* 1997;136(5):779–782.

238. Lau M, Kaufmann-Grunzinger I, Raghunath M. A case report of a patient with features of systemic lupus erythematosus and linear IgA disease. *Br J Dermatol.* 1991;124(5):498–502.

239. Wojnarowska F, Whitehead P, Leigh IM, Bhogal BS, Black MM. Identification of the target antigen in chronic bullous disease of childhood and linear IgA disease of adults. *Br J Dermatol.* 1991;124(2):157–162.

240. Adachi A, Tani M, Matsubayashi S, et al. Immunoelectronmicroscopic differentiation of linear IgA bullous dermatosis of adults with coexistence of IgA and IgG deposition from bullous pemphigoid. *J Am Acad Dermatol.* 1992;27(3):394–399.

241. Zone JJ, Taylor TB, Kadunce DP, Meyer LJ. Identification of the cutaneous basement membrane zone antigen and isolation of antibody in linear immunoglobulin A bullous dermatosis. *J Clin Invest.* 1990;85(3):812–820.

242. Zone JJ, Taylor TB, Meyer LJ, Petersen MJ. The 97 kDa linear IgA bullous disease antigen is identical to a portion of the extracellular domain of the 180 kDa bullous pemphigoid antigen, BPAg2. *J Invest Dermatol.* 1998;110(3):207–210.

243. Ishii N, Ohyama B, Yamaguchi Z, Hashimoto T. IgA autoantibodies against the NC16a domain of BP180 but not 120-kDa LAD-1 detected in a patient with linear IgA disease. *Br J Dermatol.* 2008;158(5):1151–1153.

244. Zambruno G, Kanitakis J. Linear IgA dermatosis with IgA antibodies to type VII collagen. *Br J Dermatol.* 1996;135(6):1004–1005.

245. Allen J, Zhou S, Wakelin SH, Collier PM, Wojnarowska F. Linear IgA disease: a report of two dermal binding sera which recognize a pepsin-sensitive epitope (NC-1 domain) of collagen type VII. *Br J Dermatol.* 1997;137(4):526–533.

246. Carpenter S, Berg D, Sidhu-Malik N, Hall RP 3rd, Rico MJ. Vancomycin-associated linear IgA dermatosis. A report of three cases. *J Am Acad Dermatol.* 1992;26(1):45–48.

247. Paul C, Wolkenstein P, Prost C, et al. Drug-induced linear IgA disease: target antigens are heterogeneous. *Br J Dermatol.* 1997;136(3):406–411.

248. Lally A, Chamberlain A, Allen J, Dean D, Wojnarowska F. Dermal-binding linear IgA disease: an uncommon subset of a rare immunobullous disease. *Clin Exp Dermatol.* 2007;32(5):493–498.

249. Vale E, Dimatos OC, Porro AM, Santi CG. Consensus on the treatment of autoimmune bullous dermatoses: dermatitis herpetiformis and linear IgA bullous dermatosis—Brazilian Society of Dermatology. *An Bras Dermatol.* 2019;94(2, suppl 1):48–55.

250. Zhao C, Murrel D. Approach and management of autoimmune blistering diseases. *Current Dermatol Rep Vol.* 2016;5:105–114.

251. Garrido PM, Queiro SC, Travassos AR, Borges-Costa J, Filipe P. Emerging treatments for bullous pemphigoid. *J Dermatolog Treat.* 2021:1–13.

252. Altman EM. Novel therapies for pemphigus vulgaris. *Am J Clin Dermatol.* 2020;21(6):765–782.

253. Mutasim DF. Management of autoimmune bullous diseases: pharmacology and therapeutics. *J Am Acad Dermatol.* 2004;51(6):859–877; quiz 878–880.

254. Lebwohl MG, Heymann WR, Berth-Jones J, Coulson I. *Treatment of Skin Disease: Comprehensive Therapeutic Strategies.* 3rd ed. Saunders; 2010.

255. Bystryn JC, Steinman NM. The adjuvant therapy of pemphigus. An update. *Arch Dermatol.* 1996;132(2):203–212.

256. Lever WF, White H. Treatment of pemphigus with corticosteroids. Results obtained in 46 patients over a period of 11 years. *Arch Dermatol.* 1963;87:12–26.

257. Wolverton S. *Comprehensive Dermatologic Drug Therapy.* 4th ed. Elsevier; 2020.

258. Zhao W, Wang J, Zhu H, Pan M. Comparison of guidelines for management of pemphigus: a review of systemic corticosteroids, rituximab, and other immunosuppressive therapies. *Clin Rev Allergy Immunol.* 2021;61(3):351–362.

259. Lunardon L, Payne AS. Rituximab for autoimmune blistering diseases: recent studies, new insights. *G Ital Dermatol Venereol.* 2012;147(3):269–276.

260. Amber KT, Lamberts A, Solimani F, et al. Determining the incidence of pneumocystis pneumonia in patients with autoimmune blistering diseases not receiving routine prophylaxis. *JAMA Dermatol.* 2017;153(11):1137–1141.

261. Grundmann-Kollmann M, Korting HC, Behrens S, et al. Mycophenolate mofetil: a new therapeutic option in the treatment of blistering autoimmune diseases. *J Am Acad Dermatol.* 1999;40(6, pt 1):957–960.

262. Schmelt N, Anderson JE, Garbe E. Signals of progressive multifocal leukoencephalopathy for immunosuppresants: a disproportionality analysis of spontaneous reports with the US Adverse Event Reporting system (AERS). *Pharmacoepidemiol Drug Saf.* 2012;21:1216–1220.

263. Euler HH, Loffler H, Christophers E. Synchronization of plasmapheresis and pulse cyclophosphamide therapy in pemphigus vulgaris. *Arch Dermatol.* 1987;123(9):1205–1210.

264. Godard W, Roujeau JC, Guillot B, Andre C, Rifle G. Bullous pemphigoid and intravenous gammaglobulin. *Ann Intern Med.* 1985;103(6, pt 1)):964–965.

265. Mouthon L, Kaveri SV, Spalter SH, et al. Mechanisms of action of intravenous immune globulin in immune-mediated diseases. *Clin Exp Immunol.* 1996;104(suppl 1):3–9.

266. Durandy A, Kaveri SV, Kuijpers TW, et al. Intravenous immunoglobulins—understanding properties and mechanisms. *Clin Exp Immunol.* 2009;158(suppl 1):2–13.

267. Sapadin AN, Fleischmajer R. Tetracyclines: nonantibiotic properties and their clinical implications. *J Am Acad Dermatol.* 2006;54(2):258–265.

268. Stone OJ. High viscosity of newborn extracellular matrix is the etiology of erythema toxicum neonatorum: neonatal jaundice?: hyaline membrane disease? *Med Hypotheses.* 1990;33(1):15–17.

269. Bassukas ID. Is erythema toxicum neonatorum a mild self-limited acute cutaneous graft-versus-host-reaction from maternal-to-fetal lymphocyte transfer? *Med Hypotheses.* 1992;38(4):334–338.

270. Ferrandiz C, Coroleu W, Ribera M, Lorenzo JC, Natal A. Sterile transient neonatal pustulosis is a precocious form of erythema toxicum neonatorum. *Dermatology.* 1992;185(1):18–22.

271. Wallach D. Intraepidermal IgA pustulosis. *J Am Acad Dermatol.* 1992;27(6, pt 1):993–1000.

272. Dromy R, Raz A, Metzker A. Infantile acropustulosis. *Pediatr Dermatol.* 1991;8(4):284–287.

273. Prendiville JS. Infantile acropustulosis—how often is it a sequela of scabies? *Pediatr Dermatol.* 1995;12(3):275–276.

274. Mancini AJ, Frieden IJ, Paller AS. Infantile acropustulosis revisited: history of scabies and response to topical corticosteroids. *Pediatr Dermatol.* 1998;15(5):337–341.

275. Gniadecki R, Bygum A, Clemmensen O, Svejgaard E, Ullman S. IgA pemphigus: the first two Scandinavian cases. *Acta Derm Venereol.* 2002;82(6):441–445.

276. Atukorala DN, Joshi RK, Abanmi A, Jeha MT. Subcorneal pustular dermatosis and IgA myeloma. *Dermatology.* 1993;187(2):124–126.

277. Lombart F, Dhaille F, Lok C, Dadban A. Subcorneal pustular dermatosis associated with Mycoplasma pneumoniae infection. *J Am Acad Dermatol.* 2014;71(3):e85–e86.

278. Bohelay G, Duong TA, Ortonne N, Chosidow O, Valeyrie-Allanore L. Subcorneal pustular dermatosis triggered by *Mycoplasma pneumoniae* infection: a rare clinical association. *J Eur Acad Dermatol Venereol.* 2015;29(5):1022–1025.

279. Iyengar S, Chambers CJ, Chang S, Fung MA, Sharon VR. Subcorneal pustular dermatosis associated with Coccidioides immitis. *Dermatol Online J.* 2015;21(8):13030/qt35r6z6bx.

280. Grob JJ, Mege JL, Capo C, et al. Role of tumor necrosis factor-alpha in Sneddon-Wilkinson subcorneal pustular dermatosis. A model of neutrophil priming in vivo. *J Am Acad Dermatol.* 1991;25(5, pt 2):944–947.

281. Cohen PR. Neutrophilic dermatoses: a review of current treatment options. *Am J Clin Dermatol.* 2009;10(5):301–312.

282. Assier H, Bastuji-Garin S, Revuz J, Roujeau JC. Erythema multiforme with mucous membrane involvement and Stevens-Johnson syndrome are clinically different disorders with distinct causes. *Arch Dermatol.* 1995;131(5):539–543.

283. Mabuchi E, Umegaki N, Murota H, Nakamura T, Tamai K, Katayama I. Oral steroid improves bullous pemphigoid-like clinical manifestations in non-Herlitz junctional epidermolysis bullosa with COL17A1 mutation. *Br J Dermatol.* 2007;157(3):596–598.

284. Laimer M, Bauer JW, Klausegger A, et al. Skin grafting as a therapeutic approach in pretibially restricted junctional epidermolysis bullosa. *Br J Dermatol.* 2006;154(1):185–187.

285. Bastuji-Garin S, Rzany B, Stern RS, Shear NH, Naldi L, Roujeau JC. Clinical classification of cases of toxic epidermal necrolysis, Stevens-Johnson syndrome, and erythema multiforme. *Arch Dermatol.* 1993;129(1):92–96.

286. Lyell A. Toxic epidermal necrolysis: an eruption resembling scalding of the skin. *Br J Dermatol.* 1956;68(11):355–361.

287. Ravin KA, Rappaport LD, Zuckerbraun NS, Wadowsky RM, Wald ER, Michaels MM. *Mycoplasma pneumoniae* and atypical Stevens-Johnson syndrome: a case series. *Pediatrics.* 2007;119(4):e1002–e1005.

288. Tay YK, Huff JC, Weston WL. *Mycoplasma pneumoniae* infection is associated with Stevens-Johnson syndrome, not erythema multiforme (von Hebra). *J Am Acad Dermatol.* 1996;35(5, pt 1):757–760.

289. Schalock PC, Dinulos JG, Pace N, Schwarzenberger K, Wenger JK. Erythema multiforme due to *Mycoplasma pneumoniae* infection in two children. *Pediatr Dermatol.* 2006;23(6):546–555.

290. Schofield JK, Tatnall FM, Leigh IM. Recurrent erythema multiforme: clinical features and treatment in a large series of patients. *Br J Dermatol.* 1993;128(5):542–545.

291. Weston WL, Brice SL, Jester JD, Lane AT, Stockert S, Huff JC. Herpes simplex virus in childhood erythema multiforme. *Pediatrics.* 1992;89(1):32–34.

292. Hughes J, Burrows NP. Infectious mononucleosis presenting as erythema multiforme. *Clin Exp Dermatol.* 1993;18(4):373–374.

293. Koga T, Kubota Y, Nakayama J. Erythema multiforme-like eruptions induced by cytomegalovirus infection in an immunocompetent adult. *Acta Derm Venereol.* 1999;79(2):166.

294. Schuttelaar ML, Laeijendecker R, Heinhuis RJ, Van Joost T. Erythema multiforme and persistent erythema as early cutaneous manifestations of Lyme disease. *J Am Acad Dermatol.* 1997;37(5, pt 2):873–875.

295. Leaute-Labreze C, Lamireau T, Chawki D, Maleville J, Taïeb A. Diagnosis, classification, and management of erythema multiforme and Stevens-Johnson syndrome. *Arch Dis Child.* 2000;83(4):347–352.

296. Schopf E, Stuhmer A, Rzany B, Victor N, Zentgraf R, Kapp JF. Toxic epidermal necrolysis and Stevens-Johnson syndrome. An epidemiologic study from West Germany. *Arch Dermatol.* 1991;127(6):839–842.

297. Chan HL, Stern RS, Arndt KA, et al. The incidence of erythema multiforme, Stevens-Johnson syndrome, and toxic epidermal necrolysis. A population-based study with particular reference to reactions caused by drugs among outpatients. *Arch Dermatol.* 1990;126(1):43–47.

298. Rzany B, Correia O, Kelly JP, Naldi L, Auquier A, Stern R. Risk of Stevens-Johnson syndrome and toxic epidermal necrolysis during first weeks of antiepileptic therapy: a case-control study. Study Group of the International Case Control Study on Severe Cutaneous Adverse Reactions. *Lancet.* 1999;353(9171):2190–2194.

299. LeBoit PE. Interface dermatitis. How specific are its histopathologic features? *Arch Dermatol.* 1993;129(10):1324–1328.

300. Zohdi-Mofid M, Horn TD. Acrosyringeal concentration of necrotic keratinocytes in erythema multiforme: a clue to drug etiology. Clinicopathologic review of 29 cases. *J Cutan Pathol.* 1997;24(4):235–240.

301. Aslanzadeh J, Helm KF, Espy MJ, Muller SA, Smith TF. Detection of HSV-specific DNA in biopsy tissue of patients with erythema multiforme by polymerase chain reaction. *Br J Dermatol.* 1992;126(1):19–23.

302. Brice SL, Leahy MA, Ong L, et al. Examination of non-involved skin, previously involved skin, and peripheral blood for herpes simplex virus DNA in patients with recurrent herpes-associated erythema multiforme. *J Cutan Pathol.* 1994;21(5):408–412.

303. Aurelian L, Ono F, Burnett J. Herpes simplex virus (HSV)-associated erythema multiforme (HAEM): a viral disease with an autoimmune component. *Dermatol Online J.* 2003;9(1):1.

304. Wolkenstein P, Charue D, Laurent P, Revuz J, Roujeau JC, Bagot M. Metabolic predisposition to cutaneous adverse drug reactions. Role in toxic epidermal necrolysis caused by sulfonamides and anticonvulsants. *Arch Dermatol.* 1995;131(5):544–551.

305. Shaw DW, Fine JD, Piacquadio DJ, Greenberg MJ, Wang-Rodriguez J, Eichenfield LF. Gastric outlet obstruction and epidermolysis bullosa. *J Am Acad Dermatol.* 1997;36(2, pt 2):304–310.

306. Hammami-Hauasli N, Raghunath M, Kuster W, Bruckner-Tuderman L. Transient bullous dermolysis of the newborn associated with compound heterozygosity for recessive and dominant COL7A1 mutations. *J Invest Dermatol.* 1998;111(6):1214–1219.

307. Paquet P, Paquet F, Al Saleh W, Reper P, Vanderkelen A, Piérard GE. Immunoregulatory effector cells in drug-induced toxic epidermal necrolysis. *Am J Dermatopathol.* 2000;22(5):413–417.

308. Ford MJ, Smith KL, Croker BP, Hacker SM, Flowers FP. Large granular lymphocytes within the epidermis of erythema multiforme lesions. *J Am Acad Dermatol.* 1992;27(3):460–462.

309. Kirchhof MG, Miliszewski MA, Sikora S, Papp A, Dutz JP. Retrospective review of Stevens-Johnson syndrome/toxic epidermal necrolysis treatment comparing intravenous immunoglobulin with cyclosporine. *J Am Acad Dermatol.* 2014;71(5):941–947.

310. Zhang S, Tang S, Li S, Pan Y, Ding Y. Biologic TNF-alpha inhibitors in the treatment of Stevens-Johnson syndrome and toxic epidermal necrolysis: a systemic review. *J Dermatolog Treat.* 2020;31(1):66–73.

311. Anderson KC, Weinstein HJ. Transfusion-associated graft-versus-host disease. *N Engl J Med.* 1990;323(5):315–321.

312. Schmuth M, Vogel W, Weinlich G, Margreiter R, Fritsch P, Sepp N. Cutaneous lesions as the presenting sign of acute graft-versus-host disease following liver transplantation. *Br J Dermatol.* 1999;141(5):901–904.

313. Holder J, North J, Bourke J, et al. Thymoma-associated cutaneous graft-versus-host-like reaction. *Clin Exp Dermatol.* 1997;22(6):287–290.

314. Scarisbrick JJ, Wakelin SH, Russell-Jones R. Cutaneous graft-versus-host-like reaction in systemic T-cell lymphoma. *Clin Exp Dermatol.* 1999;24(5):382–384.

315. Darmstadt GL, Donnenberg AD, Vogelsang GB, Farmer ER, Horn TD. Clinical, laboratory, and histopathologic indicators of the development of progressive acute graft-versus-host disease. *J Invest Dermatol.* 1992;99(4):397–402.

316. Fujii H, Hiketa T, Matsumoto Y, et al. Clinical characteristics of chronic cutaneous graft-versus-host disease in Japanese leukemia patients after bone marrow transplantation: low incidence and mild manifestations of skin lesions. *Bone Marrow Transplant.* 1992;10(4):331–335.

317. Johnson ML, Farmer ER. Graft-versus-host reactions in dermatology. *J Am Acad Dermatol.* 1998;38(3):369–392; quiz 393–396.

318. Desbarats J, Seemayer TA, Lapp WS. Irradiation of the skin and systemic graft-versus-host disease synergize to produce cutaneous lesions. *Am J Pathol.* 1994;144(5):883–888.

319. Barnadas MA, Brunet S, Sureda A, et al. Exuberant granulation tissue associated with chronic graft-versus-host disease after transplantation of peripheral blood progenitor cells. *J Am Acad Dermatol.* 1999;41(5, pt 2):876–879.

320. Horn TD, Bauer DJ, Vogelsang GB, Hess AD. Reappraisal of histologic features of the acute cutaneous graft-versus-host reaction based on an allogeneic rodent model. *J Invest Dermatol.* 1994;103(2):206–210.

321. Horn TD. Acute cutaneous eruptions after marrow ablation: roses by other names? *J Cutan Pathol.* 1994;21(5):385–392.

322. Chaudhuri SP, Smoller BR. Acute cutaneous graft versus host disease: a clinicopathologic and immunophenotypic study. *Int J Dermatol.* 1992;31(4):270–272.

323. Saijo S, Honda M, Sasahara Y, Konno T, Tagami H. Columnar epidermal necrosis: a unique manifestation of transfusion-associated cutaneous graft-vs-host disease. *Arch Dermatol.* 2000;136(6):743–746.

324. Tanaka K, Sullivan KM, Shulman HM, Sale GE, Tanaka A. A clinical review: cutaneous manifestations of acute and chronic graft-versus-host disease following bone marrow transplantation. *J Dermatol.* 1991;18(1):11–17.

325. Murphy GF, Whitaker D, Sprent J, Korngold R. Characterization of target injury of murine acute graft-versus-host disease directed to multiple minor histocompatibility antigens elicited by either CD4+ or CD8+ effector cells. *Am J Pathol.* 1991;138(4):983–990.

326. Kawai K, Matsumoto Y, Watanabe H, Ito M, Fujiwara M. Induction of cutaneous graft-versus-host disease by local injection of unprimed T cells. *Clin Exp Immunol.* 1991;84(2):359–366.

327. Sakamoto H, Michaelson J, Jones WK, et al. Lymphocytes with a CD4+ CD8-CD3-phenotype are effectors of experimental cutaneous graft-versus-host disease. *Proc Natl Acad Sci U S A.* 1991;88(23):10890–10894.

328. Horn TD, Farmer ER. Distribution of lymphocytes bearing TCR gamma/delta in cutaneous lymphocytic infiltrates. *J Cutan Pathol.* 1990;17(3):165–170.

329. Norton J, al-Saffar N, Sloane JP. An immunohistological study of gamma/delta lymphocytes in human cutaneous graft-versus-host disease. *Bone Marrow Transplant.* 1991;7(3):205–208.

330. Acevedo A, Aramburu J, Lopez J, Fernández-Herrera J, Fernández-Rañada JM, López-Botet M. Identification of natural killer (NK) cells in lesions of human cutaneous graft-versus-host disease: expression of a novel NK-associated surface antigen (Kp43) in mononuclear infiltrates. *J Invest Dermatol.* 1991;97(4):659–666.

331. Vogelsang GB, Lee L, Bensen-Kennedy DM. Pathogenesis and treatment of graft-versus-host disease after bone marrow transplant. *Annu Rev Med.* 2003;54:29–52.

332. Murphy GF, Lavker RM, Whitaker D, Korngold R. Cytotoxic folliculitis in GvHD. Evidence of follicular stem cell injury and recovery. *J Cutan Pathol.* 1991;18(5):309–314.

333. Aractingi S, Chosidow O. Cutaneous graft-versus-host disease. *Arch Dermatol.* 1998;134(5):602–612.

334. Bauer DJ, Hood AF, Horn TD. Histologic comparison of autologous graft-vs-host reaction and cutaneous eruption of lymphocyte recovery. *Arch Dermatol.* 1993;129(7):855–858.

335. Horn T, Lehmkuhle MA, Gore S, Hood A, Burke P. Systemic cytokine administration alters the histology of the eruption of lymphocyte recovery. *J Cutan Pathol.* 1996;23(3):242–246.

336. Zeiser R, von Bubnoff N, Butler J, et al. Ruxolitinib for glucocorticoid-refractory acute graft-versus-host disease. *N Engl J Med.* 2020;382(19):1800–1810.

337. Miklos D, Cutler CS, Arora M, et al. Ibrutinib for chronic graft-versus-host disease after failure of prior therapy. *Blood.* 2017;130(21):2243–2250.

338. Kato N, Ueno H, Mimura M. Histopathology of cutaneous changes in non-drug-induced coma. *Am J Dermatopathol.* 1996;18(4):344–350.

339. Sanchez YE, Requena L, Simon P. Histopathology of cutaneous changes in drug-induced coma. *Am J Dermatopathol.* 1993;15(3):208–216.

340. Wenzel FG, Horn TD. Nonneoplastic disorders of the eccrine glands. *J Am Acad Dermatol.* 1998;38(1):1–17; quiz 18–20.

341. Bhushan M, Chalmers RJ, Cox NH. Acute oedema blisters: a report of 13 cases. *Br J Dermatol.* 2001;144(3):580–582.

342. Roger M, Valence C, Bressieux JM, Bernard P, Fur A. Grover's disease associated with Waldenstrom's macroglobulinemia and neutrophilic dermatosis. *Acta Derm Venereol.* 2000;80(2):145–146.

343. Guana AL, Cohen PR. Transient acantholytic dermatosis in oncology patients. *J Clin Oncol.* 1994;12(8):1703–1709.

344. Manteaux AM, Rapini RP. Transient acantholytic dermatosis in patients with cancer. *Cutis.* 1990;46(6):488–490.

345. Powell J, Sakuntabhai A, James M, Burge S, Hovnanian A. Grover's disease, despite histological similarity to Darier's disease, does not share an abnormality in the ATP2A2 gene. *Br J Dermatol.* 2000;143(3):658.

346. Mahler SJ, De Villez RL, Pulitzer DR. Transient acantholytic dermatosis induced by recombinant human interleukin 4. *J Am Acad Dermatol.* 1993;29(2, pt 1):206–209.

347. Bayer-Garner I, Dilday B, Sanderson R, Smoller B. Acantholysis and spongiosis are associated with loss of syndecan-1 expression. *J Cutan Pathol.* 2001;28(3):135–139.

348. Metzker A, Merlob P. Suction purpura. *Arch Dermatol.* 1992;128(6):822–824.

Connective Tissue Diseases (Syn. Collagen Vascular Disease)

ROSALYNN M. NAZARIAN AND LYN M. DUNCAN

Chapter

10

INTRODUCTION

The skin is not infrequently the presenting site of signs of connective tissue diseases (CTDs). These disorders, which target the connective tissues of the body, usually have an underlying autoimmune pathogenesis. Although many of these diseases have systemic manifestations, initial clinical findings may occur in the skin, heightening the importance of histopathologic diagnosis. Nevertheless, given the varied clinical signs and overlapping features, precise diagnosis always requires careful clinical pathologic correlation. Additionally, serologic testing may be necessary for diagnosis. Although the pathogenesis of some CTDs remains unclear, genetic factors and environmental exposures may contribute to the development of pathogenic autoantibodies. Immune complex deposition and cell-mediated immunity contribute to the pathogenesis of these diseases. In addition to CTDs driven by autoimmunity, there are genetic disorders that lead to connective tissue abnormalities that usually present early in life and are congenital. These conditions are discussed elsewhere, especially in Chapter 6. The related term "collagen vascular disease" refers to disorders that are typically associated with collagen and blood vessel abnormalities and that are usually autoimmune in nature. They may or may not be associated with vasculitides.

LUPUS ERYTHEMATOSUS

Lupus erythematosus (LE) may occur as a skin-localized disease or develop systemic signs with the involvement of multiple organ systems. Thus, the clinical manifestations range from an erythematous cutaneous rash to fatal systemic illness. Fortunately, skin-limited cutaneous LE is more common than systemic lupus. Regardless of the organ systems involved, the underlying mechanism and pathogenesis of LE are similar. For those patients who develop systemic LE, the disease presents in the skin in 23% to 28% of cases, and 72% to 82% of patients with systemic lupus manifest at least one cutaneous symptom through the course of their illness (1).

Clinical Summary

In 1972, the American Rheumatism Association (ARA) developed clinical and laboratory criteria for the classification of systemic LE. In 1982 and 1997, modifications reflected changes in diagnostic technology (2–4). Two more recent classification schemes form the backbone of current clinical care, the Systemic Lupus International Collaborating Clinics classification criteria

set (SLICC 2012) and the European League Against Rheumatism (EULAR) and the ACR in 2019 (5,6). The initial 1972 ARA criteria were developed primarily for the distinction of patients with systemic lupus erythematosus (SLE) from those with other autoimmune diseases. This initial classification was based on 11 criteria, not restrictive or exclusive to the diagnosis of SLE:

1. Malar rash
2. Discoid rash
3. Photosensitivity
4. Oral ulcers, usually painless
5. Arthritis, not erosive, involving two or more peripheral joints, with tenderness, swelling, or effusion
6. Serositis (pleurisy or pericarditis)
7. Renal disorder (persistent proteinuria exceeding 0.5 g/day or cellular casts)
8. Neurologic disorders (seizures or psychosis)
9. Hematologic disorders (hemolytic anemia, leukopenia of $<4,000/mm^3$, lymphopenia of $<1,500/mm^3$, or thrombocytopenia of $<100,000/mm^3$)
10. Immunologic disorder (positive LE cell preparation, anti-DNA in abnormal titer, antibody to Sm nuclear antigen, or false-positive serologic test for syphilis)
11. Antinuclear antibody

The diagnosis of systemic LE was applied if four or more of the 11 criteria were present serially or simultaneously. A diagnosis of SLE was also possible if a patient had at least three of the following four symptoms: (a) a cutaneous eruption consistent with LE, (b) renal involvement, (c) serositis, or (d) joint involvement (5). There was also the recognition that the diagnosis of SLE requires serologic abnormality.

The 2019 EULAR/ACR classification criteria for systemic LE include positive ANA (>1:80); without the ANA, a diagnosis of systemic LE is not made. In patients with positive ANA, additional weighted criteria (2 to 10) in seven clinical (constitutional, hematologic, neuropsychiatric, mucocutaneous, serosal, musculoskeletal, and renal) and three immunologic (antiphospholipid antibodies, complement proteins, and SLE-specific antibodies) categories are scored and patients with greater than 10 points are classified with SLE. These criteria had a sensitivity of 96% and specificity of 93%, compared to 83% sensitivity and 93% specificity of the ACR 1997 and 97% sensitivity and 84% specificity of the SLICC 2012 criteria (6) (Table 10-1). A comparison of these criteria with the original 11 criteria reveals that the clinical manifestations of systemic LE

Table 10-1			
Criteria for Systemic Lupus Erythematosus			

Entry Criterion

Antinuclear antibodies (ANA) at a titer of >1:80

If absent, not SLE

Additive Criteria

Do not count a criterion if there is a more likely explanation than SLE

SLE requires at least one clinical criterion and >10 points

Within each domain, only the highest weighted criterion is counted toward the total score.

Clinical Domains and Criteria	Weight	Immunology Domains and Criteria	Weight
Constitutional		*Antiphospholipid antibodies*	
Fever	2	Anti cardiolipin antibodies *or*	2
Hematologic		Anti-b2GP1 antibodies *or*	
Leukopenia	3	Lupus anticoagulant	
Thrombocytopenia	4		
Autoimmune hemolysis	4		
Neuropsychiatric		*Complement proteins*	
Delirium	2	Low C3 OR low C4	3
Psychosis	3	Low C3 AND C4	4
Seizure	5		
Mucocutaneous		*SLE-specific antibodies*	
Nonscarring alopecia	2	Anti-dsDNA antibody *or*	6
Oral ulcers	2	Anti-Smith antibody	
Subacute cutaneous *or* discoid lupus	4		
Acute cutaneous lupus	6		
Serosal			
Pleural or pericardial effusion	5		
Acute pericarditis	6		
Musculoskeletal			
Joint involvement	6		
Renal			
Proteinuria >0.5 g/24 h	4		
Renal Biopsy Class II or V lupus nephritis	8		
Renal Biopsy Class III or IV lupus nephritis	10		
Total Score:			

Classify as systemic lupus erythematosus with a total score of >10

Adapted from Aringer M, Costenbader K, Daikh D, et al. 2019 European League Against Rheumatism/American College of Rheumatology classification criteria for systemic lupus erythematosus. *Arthritis Rheumatol.* 2019;71(9):1400–1412. Copyright © 2019 American College of Rheumatology. Reprinted by permission of John Wiley & Sons, Inc.

have been well known for half a century; this algorithmic and weighted analysis may lead to a higher sensitivity and specificity in the diagnosis of systemic LE.

Even though the prognosis of systemic LE has been improved by early diagnosis and new treatments, the mortality rate of the disease is between 15% and 25% (5). Death usually results from infection or severe nephritis (7). A meta-analysis of lupus patients showed that patients with systemic LE are at increased risk of lymphomas, specifically non-Hodgkin lymphoma, independent of the risk associated with chronic immunosuppressive therapy (8).

Cutaneous changes of LE may be subdivided according to the morphology of the clinical lesion and/or its duration (acute, subacute, or chronic). Differentiation between LE subtypes is based on the constellation of clinical, histologic, and immunofluorescence findings (9). Histologic findings alone may not be sufficient to correctly classify the subtype of the eruption (10); additionally, intermediate forms and transitions from one type to another occur. Although some cases defy subtyping, clinically distinct subtypes are addressed in the following section.

Discoid Lupus Erythematosus

Clinical Summary. Characteristically, lesions of discoid lupus erythematosus (DLE) consist of well-demarcated, erythematous, slightly infiltrated, disk-like plaques with prominent adherent thick scale and follicular plugging. Early and active lesions are erythematous, corresponding to cutaneous inflammation (Fig. 10-1A). Old lesions often appear atrophic and have hypo- or hyperpigmentation and may have scarring. Occasionally, lesions may show verrucous epidermal hyperplasia, especially at their periphery (11). Uncommonly, malignant neoplasms have been reported in lesions of DLE, including basal cell carcinoma, squamous cell carcinoma, and atypical fibroxanthoma (12).

In many instances, the discoid cutaneous lesions are limited to the face, most commonly the malar areas and the nose. In some cases, the scalp, ears, oral mucosa, and vermilion border of the lips may be involved. In patients with discoid lupus limited to the head and neck, conversion to SLE is rare (5% to 10%) (13).

In patients with *disseminated DLE*, discoid lesions are seen on the upper trunk and upper limbs, usually, but not always, in association with lesions on the head (14). Systemic LE may eventually

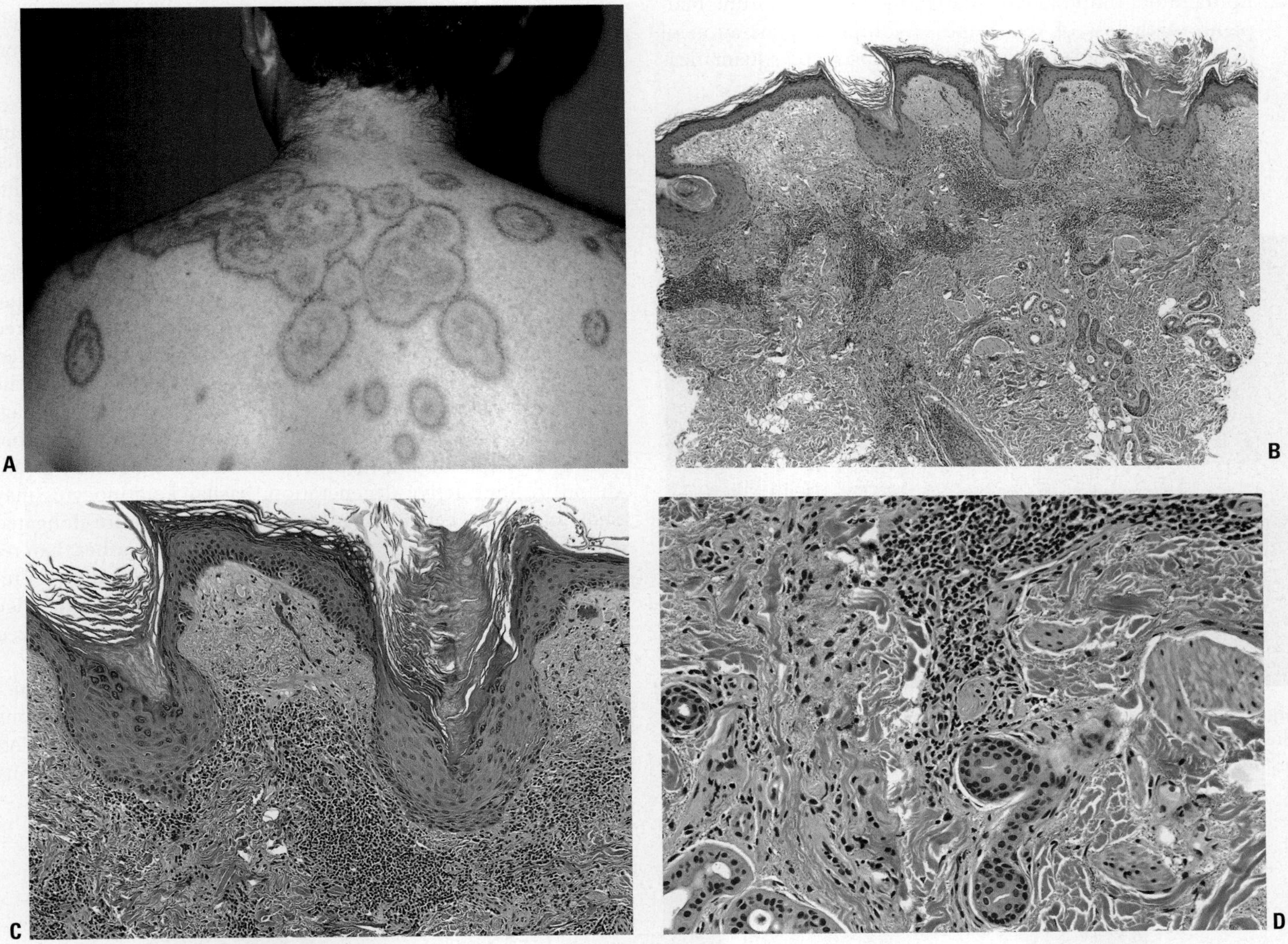

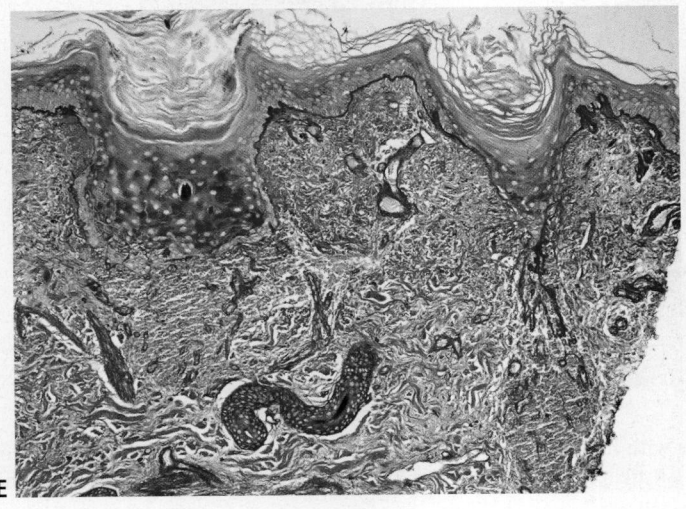

Figure 10-1 Discoid lupus erythematosus. **A:** An adult with discoid plaques of lupus erythematosus on the upper back: Areas of erythema show stromal inflammation, and paler zones demonstrate scarring. **B:** The epidermis has lost its rete ridge pattern and shows follicular plugging. There is a brisk mononuclear inflammatory infiltrate near the dermal–epidermal junction and around appendages. The faint bluish background is mucin among collagen bundles. **C:** Focal subepidermal vacuolization and lymphoplasmacytic infiltrates approximating squamatized basilar keratinocytes. Thickening of the basement membrane is noticeable around follicular ostia. **D:** Lymphoplasmacytic infiltrates surround eccrine coils in the deep dermis. Interstitial mucin deposits are present in the adjacent stroma. **E:** Combination Alcian blue–periodic acid–Schiff stain demonstrating a thickened and tortuous basement membrane zone and abundant interstitial mucin deposits among collagen bundles.

develop in up to 20% of these patients (15). Although discoid cutaneous lesions are typical of patients with chronic cutaneous LE, they are also seen in 14% of patients with systemic LE (16).

Histopathology. In most instances of *discoid lesions*, a combination of histopathologic findings allows for a diagnosis of LE (Fig. 10-1B–E). The following changes may be apparent at all levels of the skin, but all need not be present in every case:

1. Stratum corneum: hyperkeratosis with follicular hyperkeratosis (plugging)
2. Epithelium: thinning and flattening of the stratum malpighii, with loss of rete ridges, hydropic degeneration of basal cells (vacuolar change), dyskeratosis, and squamatization of basilar keratinocytes
3. Basement membrane: thickening and tortuosity, correlating with deposition of immune reactants (immunoglobulins and complement) (Fig. 10-2)

4. Dermal changes: predominantly lymphocytic and plasmacellular infiltrate arranged along the dermal–epidermal junction, around hair follicles and eccrine units, and in an interstitial pattern; interstitial mucin deposition; edema, vasodilation, slight extravasation of erythrocytes
5. Subcutaneous: possible sparse extension of the inflammatory infiltrate

The stratum corneum is usually hyperkeratotic. Parakeratosis is not conspicuous, and it may be absent. Keratotic plugs are found mainly in dilated follicular openings (Fig. 10-1B, C), but they may occur in the openings of eccrine ducts as well. Follicular channels in the dermis may contain concentric layers of keratin instead of hairs.

The epidermal changes vary with the clinical character of lesions. A clinically verrucous lesion shows a hyperplastic epidermis with hyperkeratotic scale that, given the maturation disarray and dyskeratosis seen in LE, may simulate a hypertrophic actinic keratosis or even a superficially invasive squamous cell carcinoma (Fig. 10-3A, B) (17).

The most significant histopathologic change in LE is hydropic degeneration of the basal layer, also referred to as liquefactive or vacuolar degeneration. This change is characterized by vacuolar spaces beneath and between basilar keratinocytes. This vacuolar degeneration is particularly evident on periodic acid–Schiff (PAS) stains. In its absence, a histopathologic diagnosis of LE should be made with caution and only when other histopathologic findings greatly favor such a diagnosis. In addition to liquefactive degeneration, basilar keratinocytes may show individual cell necrosis (apoptosis) and acquire elongated contours similar to their superficial counterparts rather than retain their normal columnar appearance (squamatization). Frequently, there is epidermal atrophy; the undulating rete ridge pattern is lost and is replaced by a linear array of squamatized keratinocytes (Fig. 10-1C) (10).

The basement membrane, normally delicate and inconspicuous, appears thickened and tortuous in long-standing lesions (Fig. 10-1E). This change becomes more apparent with the PAS stain and may be found along the follicular–dermal junctions

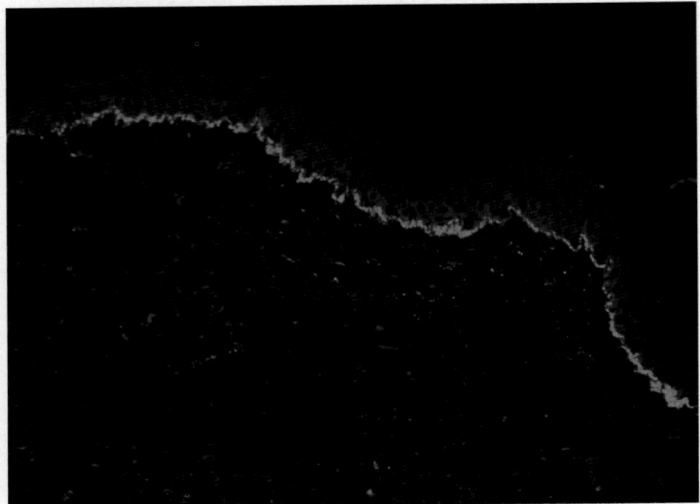

Figure 10-2 Positive lupus band test. Granular deposits of C3 in the basement membrane zone on direct immunofluorescence of lesional skin.

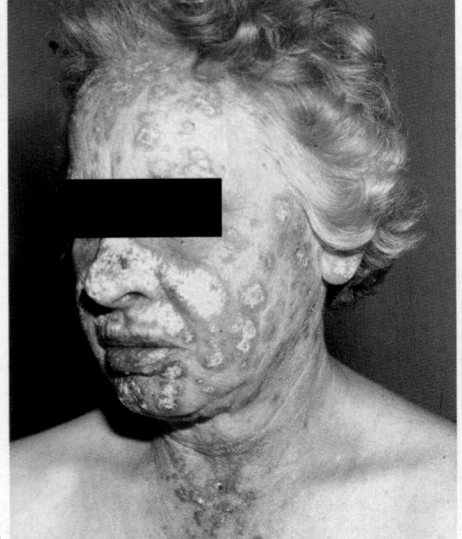

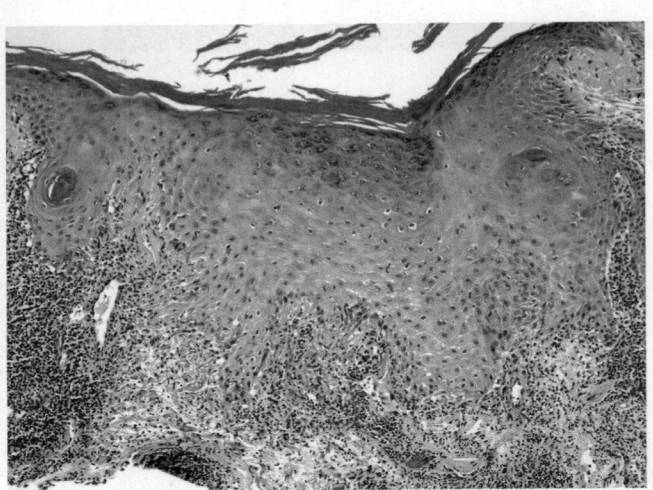

Figure 10-3 Hypertrophic or verrucous lupus erythematosus. **A:** A woman with hyperkeratotic scaly plaques on an erythematous base in a photo distribution. **B:** A hyperplastic epidermis with hypergranulosis and a brisk lichenoid mononuclear infiltrate, histologically mimicking lichen planus.

as well. These findings correlate with locations of immunoreactant deposits found on direct immunofluorescence testing of
the affected skin (Fig. 10-2). By contrast, in areas of pronounced
hydropic degeneration of the basal cells, the PAS-positive
subepidermal basement zone may be fragmented and even absent (18). Capillary walls may also show thickening, homogenization, and an increase in the intensity of the PAS reaction.

The inflammatory infiltrate in the dermis is predominantly composed of lymphocytes admixed with plasma cells
(Fig. 10-1C, D). Vacuolar interface dermatitis with a periadnexal
lymphoid infiltrate is a clue to the diagnosis of LE. In active
lesions, the infiltrate can be found approximating the dermal–
epidermal junction associated with hydropic degeneration (vacuolar interface dermatitis). In hair-bearing areas, the infiltrate
is located around folliculosebaceous units and eccrine glands
(Fig. 10-1C, D). Frequently, hydropic changes in the basal layer
of the hair follicles may be seen. This may be of diagnostic value
in the absence of dermal–epidermal changes. Ongoing inflammation results in atrophy and eventual dropout of the pilosebaceous
units. A patchy inflammatory infiltrate may also be present in the
upper dermis in an interstitial pattern and around eccrine coils.
Occasionally, the infiltrate extends into the subcutaneous fat.

The dermis may show edema, ectatic vessels, and foci of
erythrocyte extravasation. In dark-skinned persons, papillary
dermal melanophages are commonly seen. Increased connective tissue mucin (hyaluronic acid) is common in the middle
and lower dermis and is best demonstrated with colloidal iron
or Alcian blue stains (Fig. 10-1E) (19). Fibrinoid deposits in
the dermis are encountered only rarely in discoid lesions.

Colloid bodies, referred to in lichen planus as Civatte bodies,
are apoptotic keratinocytes that present as round-to-ovoid, homogeneous, eosinophilic structures. They may be seen in lesions of
DLE and in other inflammatory processes where there is damage
to basilar keratinocytes (poikiloderma, lichen planus, fixed drug
eruption, and lichenoid keratoses). Colloid bodies range in size,
but usually measure approximately 10 μm in diameter and are
present in the lower epidermis or in the papillary dermis. When
located in the dermis, colloid bodies are PAS positive and diastase
resistant and, on direct immunofluorescence staining, are often
found to contain immunoglobulins (Igs) (IgG, IgM, IgA), complement, and fibrin. This staining does not represent an immunologic
phenomenon but is the result of passive adsorption of Ig.

Pathogenesis. Refer to the end of the discussion of systemic LE.

Differential Diagnosis. The epidermal changes seen in DLE must
be differentiated from lichen planus because both diseases may
show hydropic degeneration of the basal cell layer. In lichen
planus, there is wedge-shaped hypergranulosis and triangular
elongation of rete ridges described as "saw-toothing," which are
not characteristic of DLE; in DLE, the rete ridge pattern frequently appears flat. In addition, lichen planus shows a superficial infiltrate (not superficial and deep) and lacks plasma cells
and stromal mucin. (For a discussion of the overlap of lichen
planus with LE, see Chapter 7.)

Patchy predominantly dermal lymphocytic infiltrates may
be seen in five disorders that begin with the letter *L* (called the
five *L*s). They are LE, lymphocytic lymphoma, lymphocytoma
cutis, polymorphous light eruption of the plaque type, and lymphocytic infiltrate of Jessner. Some may also add lues (syphilis)
and Lyme disease.

In cases of LE without significant vacuolar interface
changes, other factors may assist in the differential diagnosis:

- In *lymphocytic lymphoma*, atypical lymphocytes are present,
are tightly packed, have an interstitial distribution ("single fil-
ing"), and usually do not have the characteristic periadnexal
infiltrates of LE. Immunohistochemical stains are necessary
to allow for a definitive diagnosis of cutaneous lymphoma.
- In *lymphocytoma cutis* (cutaneous lymphocytic hyperplasia) (see
Chapter 31), the infiltrate usually is heavier than in LE, may
have an interstitial component, is rarely arranged around pilosebaceous structures, and may contain reactive lymphoid follicles.
- In the plaque type of *polymorphous light eruption*, there is
often a prominent band of papillary dermal edema and endothelial cell prominence of the superficial vascular plexus.
The infiltrate is more intense in the superficial dermis than in
deep dermis and is occasionally admixed with neutrophils. It
rarely has a folliculocentric arrangement or increased stromal
mucin deposition, in contrast to LE where these are characteristic findings (see Chapter 12).
- In *Jessner lymphocytic infiltration of the skin*, the dermal infiltrate may be indistinguishable from that seen in early, nonscarring, or purely dermal lesions of LE; however, plasma
cells and mucin are generally absent. The presence of increased numbers of B lymphocytes in the infiltrate may also
help distinguish this from LE (see later text) (20).
- In *lues*, lichenoid lymphoplasmacytic infiltrates are not associated with mucin deposits. Confirmatory antitreponemal
antibody immunohistochemical stains or silver stains, such
as a Steiner stain, when positive are helpful in distinguishing
lues from LE.
- In *Lyme disease*, there are lymphoplasmacytic infiltrates
around dermal vessels. Silver, Dieterle, or Steiner stains may
reveal spirochetal organisms, although they are sparse and
difficult to detect. Serologic studies and clinical history are
usually necessary to arrive at a diagnosis of Lyme disease.

As will be discussed in "Systemic Lupus Erythematosus"
sections, particular forms of LE may be associated with certain
drug exposures. 5-Fluorouracil (5-FU) and capecitabine (a pro-
drug of 5-FU) have been associated with the induction of DLE-
like lesions. Other reported causes of drug-induced discoid
lupus include uracil-tegafur (UTF) and infliximab.

Principles of Management: Refer to the end of discussion of systemic LE.

Verrucous Lupus Erythematosus

Clinical Summary. An exaggerated proliferative epithelial response may occur in approximately 2% of patients with chronic
cutaneous LE. These are manifest as verrucous-appearing lesions (Fig. 10-3A). Clinically, two types of lesions have been
reported in this subset of LE. Lesions may simulate hypertrophic lichen planus or keratoacanthomas. They occur on the
face (nose, chin, and lips), arms, dorsal aspects of the hands,
and occasionally the back. The presence of typical DLE lesions
elsewhere is a helpful clue to the diagnosis.

Histopathology. Histopathologically, the epidermis is papillomatous and hyperplastic with overlying hyperkeratotic scale.
Large numbers of dyskeratotic keratinocytes are seen in the
lower portion of the epithelium, associated with a bandlike
mononuclear infiltrate (Fig. 10-3B). Older lesions show a thickened basement membrane zone. A second pattern consists of a
cup-shaped, keratin-filled crater surrounded by an acanthotic

epidermis with elongated rete ridges and a sparse mononuclear infiltrate. These changes, in the presence of a deep dermal perivascular, periappendageal, and interstitial infiltrate and mucin deposition, suggest a diagnosis of verrucous LE. CD123, a marker for plasmacytoid dendritic cells, typically marks large numbers of mononuclear cells in LE. The marker has been reported to be of utility in distinguishing hypertrophic LE from squamous cell carcinomas (21).

Pathogenesis. Refer to the end of discussion of systemic LE.

Differential Diagnosis. Histopathologically, lesions may simulate hypertrophic lichen planus, keratoacanthomas, and squamous cell carcinomas. Careful examination of the basement membrane zone for thickening and tortuosity and for stromal mucin deposition helps distinguish these entities.

Principles of Management: Refer to the end of discussion of systemic LE.

Tumid Lupus Erythematosus

Clinical Summary. The dermal form of LE without epithelial changes is known as tumid LE or lupus erythematosus tumidus. Clinically, affected patients display indurated urticarial papules, plaques, and nodules without erythema, atrophy, or ulceration (Fig. 10-4A).

Histopathology. Histopathologically, superficial and deep dermal perivascular, interstitial, and periappendageal lymphocytic infiltrates associated with stromal mucin deposits are observed (Fig. 10-4B, C) (22). Unlike discoid lupus, in which

discoid lesions may coexist with systemic LE, the diagnosis of tumid LE typically excludes the presence of systemic LE (23). Changes at the dermal–epidermal junction, such as liquefaction degeneration or basement membrane thickening, are not seen.

Pathogenesis. Refer to the end of discussion of systemic LE.

Differential Diagnosis. As described later, there is a significant overlap of tumid LE with other entities such as lymphocytic infiltrate of Jessner (24).

Principles of Management: Refer to the end of discussion of systemic LE.

Lupus Erythematosus Profundus (Lupus Panniculitis)

Clinical Summary. LE may show changes in adipose tissue associated with the chronic cutaneous or systemic forms in 1% to 3% of patients. Two-thirds of the affected patients have DLE lesions, which may be present either directly overlying the area affected by deeper inflammation or remote from it. A minority of patients have only panniculitis without other cutaneous involvement. Women are affected three to four times more often than men. Typically, multiple discrete, firm, deep nodules arise on the face, arms (particularly the deltoid area), chest, and/or buttocks. The legs and back may be affected as well. The overlying skin may be normal, erythematous, or atrophic. The panniculitis resolves, leaving depressed atrophic scars owing to loss of fat with minimal epidermal change.

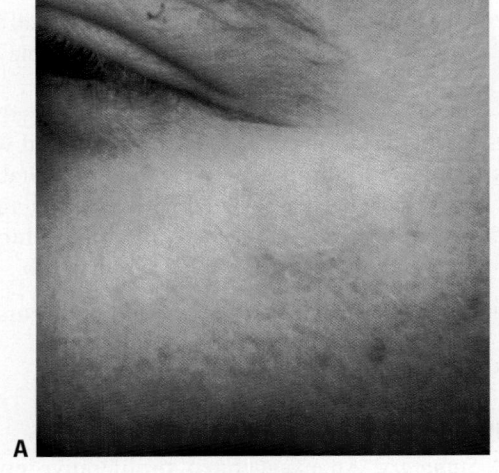

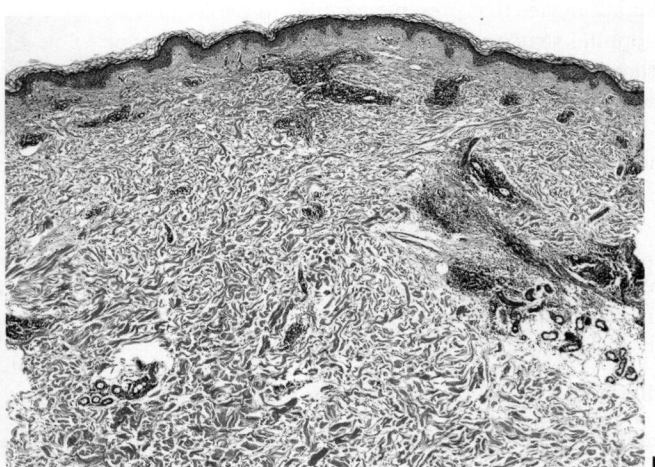

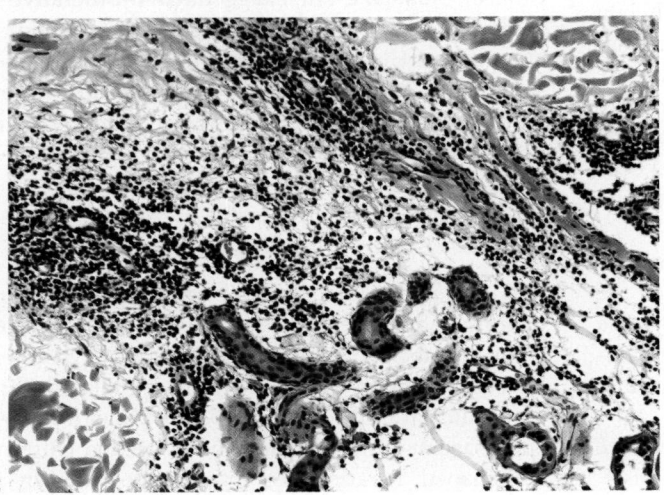

Figure 10-4 Tumid lupus erythematosus. **A:** A barely raised, slightly hyperpigmented plaque on the cheek, without significant scaling, erythema, or atrophy. **B:** An angiocentric and periappendageal dermal inflammatory infiltrate. The dermal–epidermal junction of this specimen fails to show interface alterations. **C:** A lymphocytic infiltrate admixed with plasma cells surrounds and separates eccrine glands and adjacent collagen bundles. The faint bluish hue of the matrix is indicative of mucin deposition.

Histopathology. Subcutaneous adipose tissue may be involved with or without inflammation in the dermis or dermal–epidermal junction. Salient histopathologic findings include a predominantly lobular panniculitis with lymphocytic infiltrates and plasma cells, occasionally forming germinal centers. Although typically described as a lobular panniculitis, septal involvement is reported in 82% of patients in one study (25). Vascular changes include endothelial prominence, thrombosis, calcification, or perivascular fibrosis ("onion-skin" appearance). Fat necrosis occurs with fibrin deposition and lymphocytic nuclear dust, which eventuates into hyalinization of adipose lobules (Fig. 10-5A, B). Stromal mucin deposition is conspicuous in well-established lesions. The intensity of the infiltrate lessens over time as the hyalinization progresses.

Pathogenesis. Refer to the end of discussion of systemic LE.

Differential Diagnosis. Some observers believe that LE profundus may represent a subcuticular T-cell dyscrasia related to CTD, which has an indolent biologic behavior (26). Others feel that lupus panniculitis may be differentiated from subcutaneous panniculitis-like T-cell lymphoma (SPTCL) by histopathologic features: The absence of other features of LE and the presence of a predominantly α/β CD8 cytotoxic T-cell lobular panniculitis with rimming of adipocyte spaces by atypical lymphocytes favors SPTCL (25). CD123 immunohistochemistry has been reported to be a helpful adjunct for differentiating LE from SPTCL, with higher percentages of CD123-positive plasmacytoid dendritic cells, often comprising more than 20% of the inflammatory infiltrate and forming clusters, identified in LE, but rarely seen in SPTCL (27). Generally, the presence of reactive lymphoid follicles, stromal mucin, and eosinophilic hyaline change of the subcutis also favors the diagnosis of lupus profundus over SPTCL.

Principles of Management: Refer to the end of discussion of systemic LE.

Subacute Cutaneous Lupus Erythematosus

Clinical Summary. Subacute cutaneous lupus erythematosus (SCLE), described in 1979, represents about 9% of all cases of LE. It is characterized by extensive, erythematous, symmetric nonscarring, and nonatrophic lesions that arise abruptly on the upper trunk, extensor surfaces of the arms, and dorsa of the hands and fingers. This eruption has two clinical variants:

(a) papulosquamous lesions and (b) annular to polycyclic lesions (Fig. 10-6A). Frequently, both types of lesions are seen. In some instances, vesicular and discoid lesions with scarring may coexist.

Patients with SCLE may have mild systemic involvement, particularly arthralgias. Approximately 50% fulfill at least four of the criteria for systemic LE. Conversely, 10% to 15% of systemic LE patients exhibit cutaneous lesions of SCLE (28). Severe systemic LE, with renal or cerebrovascular disease, develops in only 10% of SCLE cases (29,30). Serologic studies show 70% of affected patients to have the anti-Ro (SSA) antibody. Patients with SCLE often bear the HLA-DR2 and HLA-DR3 phenotypes. SCLE may occur asynchronously with other CTDs such as Sjögren syndrome and morphea.

Histopathology. See the Histopathology section of Neonatal LE and Fig. 10-6B.

Pathogenesis. Refer to the end of discussion of systemic LE.

Differential Diagnosis. Subacute LE is a commonly reported phenotype in drug-induced LE. About 25% to 30% of cases of SCLE may be attributable to medications, and numerous medications have been reported to cause drug-induced LE with a subacute morphology (31). Distinguishing a medication-induced reaction can be difficult, though systemic symptoms are typically absent in drug-induced LE as opposed to SCLE. The most common medications implicated include hydrochlorothiazide, ACE inhibitors, calcium channel blockers, tumor necrosis factor (TNF) inhibitors, terbinafine, and chemotherapeutic agents (32), though the list is long and ever-expanding (31).

Principles of Management: If the onset of the eruption coincides with the administration of a new medication, particularly one on the above list, discontinuation may permit the resolution of the eruption. Notably, some patients may have "drug-unmasked" lupus rather than pure "drug-induced" lupus. If the eruption persists, sunscreens and therapeutic agents as discussed at the end of the section on systemic lupus are used.

Neonatal Lupus Erythematosus

Clinical Summary. Neonatal LE has clinical and histopathologic skin changes and serologic findings similar to those of SCLE. Children of mothers with active systemic LE or Sjögren syndrome may develop LE-like symptoms in the neonatal period. Anti-Ro/

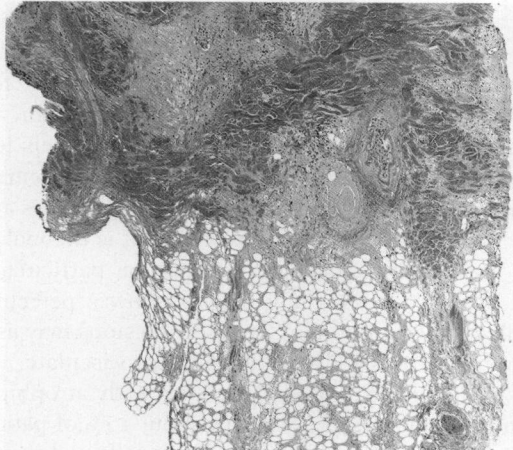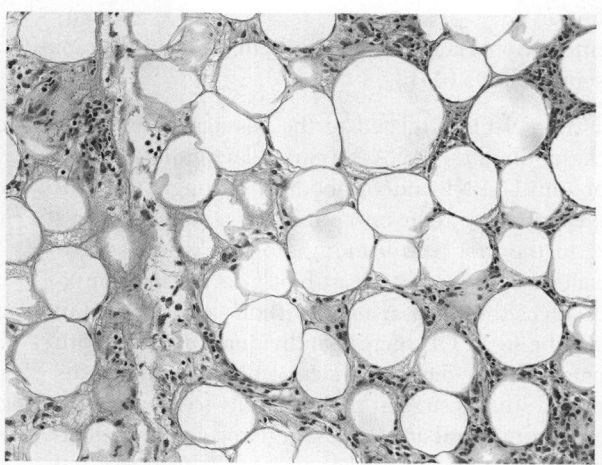

Figure 10-5 Lupus panniculitis. **A:** A perivascular and perifollicular inflammatory infiltrate is present in the deep dermis and extends into adipose tissue in an interstitial pattern. **B:** Adipocytes vary in size and are embedded in a hyalinized matrix. Long-standing lesions show minimal inflammation and prominent hyalinization.

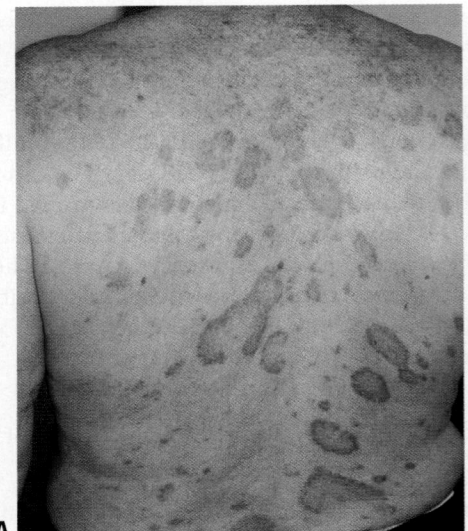
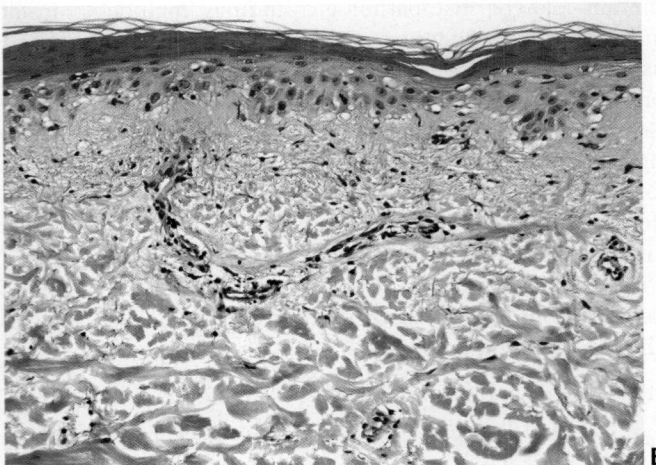

Figure 10-6 Subacute lupus erythematosus. **A:** Variably sized annular scaly patches on the upper back. Scarring and atrophy, as commonly seen in discoid/chronic cutaneous lupus, are uncommon. **B:** A sparse mononuclear inflammatory infiltrate in the upper dermis associated with pronounced dermal edema. There is continuous subepidermal vacuolization, focal hemorrhage, and slight mucin deposition.

SSA is the predominant autoantibody and is found in approximately 95% of cases. This may result in a transient syndrome characterized by widespread erythematous desquamative polycyclic, annular, usually nonscarring lesions. Atrophy may be present in some cases. There is typically central facial involvement. Less common cutaneous manifestations include urticarial lesions (33). There is associated photosensitivity, transient thrombocytopenia, mild hemolytic anemia, leukopenia, and congenital heart block.

Histopathology of SCLE and Neonatal LE. Histopathologic changes differ in degree from those in the discoid lesions and are most intense at the dermal–epidermal interface (Fig 10-6B). They consist of the following:

1. Hydropic degeneration of the basilar epithelial layer, sometimes severe enough to form clefts and subepidermal vesicles
2. Colloid bodies in the lower epidermis and papillary dermis (common)
3. Edema of the dermis, which is more pronounced than in discoid lesions
4. Focal extravasation of erythrocytes and dermal fibrinoid deposits (common)
5. Less prominent hyperkeratosis and inflammatory infiltrate than in discoid lesions (34)

Pathogenesis. Neonatal LE is related to the passage of maternal IgG antinuclear antibodies (ANAs) (particularly anti-Ro/SSA, anti-La/SSB, or anti-U1RNP autoantibodies) through the placenta. These changes have their onset at birth to 2 months and usually resolve in the first 6 to 9 months of life with decreasing levels of maternal antibodies. Heart block occurs in approximately 50% of affected infants, usually without associated skin lesions, and may be fatal. Of interest, individuals affected with transient neonatal LE may develop systemic LE as young adults (22). Animal model studies suggest that reactivity to the p200 region of the Ro52 protein and antibodies targeting calcium channel blockers may have a role in cardiac involvement in affected children (35). Of interest, multigenerational genetic studies suggest that mothers of neonates with lupus accumulate genetic risk preferentially from neonatal lupus children's grandparents (35).

Differential Diagnosis. The eruption in the clinical setting of a neonate born to a mother with LE and interface changes on biopsy is characteristic.

Principles of Management: Treatment includes management of the cutaneous eruption as well as cardiomyopathy. All children with suspected neonatal lupus require immediate evaluation of the cardiac conduction system. Parents of children with neonatal lupus should be evaluated, as this may be the presenting sign of previously subclinical disease. Fluorinated steroids, intravenous immunoglobulin, and hydroxychloroquine are used in the prevention and treatment of the disease.

Systemic Lupus Erythematosus

Clinical Summary. In systemic LE, the cutaneous manifestations usually appear less suddenly than in SCLE and are less pronounced, such that the signs and symptoms of systemic disease usually overshadow the often subtle form of skin involvement. Usually, systemic manifestations, especially arthritis, precede the cutaneous lesions. Only 20% of systemic LE patients demonstrate prominent cutaneous features at the onset of their disease, but approximately 80% will exhibit cutaneous lesions in the course of their disease (36,37).

The cutaneous manifestations consist of malar erythema, photosensitivity, palmar erythema, periungual telangiectasia, diffuse hair loss as a result of telogen effluvium, and urticarial vasculitis or bullous lesions. The erythematous lesions of systemic LE consist of erythematous, slightly edematous patches without scaling or atrophy. As a rule, the patches are ill-defined. The most common site of involvement is the malar region, but any area of the skin may be involved, particularly the palms and fingers. Occasionally, lesions show a petechial, vesicular, or ulcerative component. Senescent lesions may assume the appearance of poikiloderma atrophicans vasculare.

Well-defined "discoid" lesions with atrophic scarring, as seen typically in DLE, occur in about 15% of patients with systemic LE. They may precede all other clinical manifestations of systemic LE. A relatively benign course characterizes systemic LE in most patients with preceding DLE (38); however, many patients have had persistent multiple abnormal laboratory findings from the beginning. This is in contrast to cases of simple DLE, in which most abnormal laboratory findings are transient.

Two variants of systemic LE—*systemic LE with genetic deficiency of complement components* and *bullous systemic LE*—bear mention. In the former, the onset of systemic LE occurs in early childhood, is transmitted in an autosomal recessive fashion, and often affects several siblings (39). Deficiencies of C2 and C4 result in extensive lesions similar to DLE, with scaling, atrophy, and scarring associated with sensitivity to sunlight. There can be associated central nervous system involvement and glomerulonephritis, which may be fatal (40).

In *bullous systemic LE*, subepidermal blisters may arise in previously involved or uninvolved areas. They may form large hemorrhagic bullae or herpetiform vesicles, which arise suddenly, and are clinically similar to lesions of bullous pemphigoid or dermatitis herpetiformis.

Rowell syndrome is a distinct clinical presentation of lupus with erythema multiforme-like lesions. Patients have speckled antinuclear and anti-La antibodies and test positive for rheumatoid factor (41).

The coexistence of systemic LE and diffuse systemic sclerosis (scleroderma) or dermatomyositis has often been described. It is known as overlap syndrome and refers to the coexistence of two related but separate diseases. Similarly, there are reports of systemic lupus and coexistent eosinophilic fasciitis (42,43). Such instances of overlap are in contrast to *mixed connective tissue disease* (MCTD), which is recognized as a separate disease entity.

Many drugs are associated with the induction of LE, the majority of which induce predominantly systemic symptoms such as arthritis, serositis, lymphadenopathy, and fever. A few are associated with specific cutaneous manifestations. Select drugs are listed in Table 10-2 and are discussed further in the section on drug-induced LE in Chapter 11.

Histopathology. Early lesions of systemic LE of the erythematous, edematous type may show only mild, nonspecific changes. In well-developed lesions, the histopathologic changes correspond to those described for SCLE (Fig. 10-6B): Hydropic degeneration of the basal cell layer occurs in association with edema of the upper dermis and extravasation of erythrocytes. Fibrin deposits in the connective tissue of the skin are often seen in erythematous lesions. They appear as granular, strongly eosinophilic, PAS-positive, diastase-resistant deposits between collagen bundles, in the walls

Table 10-2
Drugs Related to Induction of Lupus Erythematosus

Antiarrhythmics	Procainamide	Anticholesterol	Statins
	Quinidine		Gemfibrozil
	Tocainide	Biologic agents	Interleukin 2
Antihypertensive	Hydralazine		Etanercept
	Methyldopa		Infliximab†
	β-Blockers		Interferon α
	Hydrochlorothiazide*		Efalizumab*
	Calcium channel blockers	Hormones	Estrogen
			Leflunomide*
	Angiotensin-converting	Other	Sulfasalazine
	enzyme inhibitors		Penicillamine
	Clonidine		Fluorouracil agents†
Antibiotics	Isoniazid		Gold salts
	Minocycline		Sertraline†
	Penicillin		Ticlopidine*
	Streptomycin		Bupropion*
	Tetracycline		Lansoprazole*
	Griseofulvin		Docetaxel*
	Terbinafine		Reserpine
	Ciprofloxacin		Lithium
	Rifampicin		Clonidine
Antithyroid	Propylthiouracil	Hydroxyurea	
	Methimazole	Clozapine	
	Thiamazole	Zafirlukast	
Anticonvulsants	Carbamazepine		
	Ethosuximide		
	Phenytoin*		
	Valproate		

*Associated with subacute cutaneous lupus-like syndrome.
†Associated with chronic cutaneous lupus-like syndrome

of dermal vessels, in the papillary dermis, or beneath the epidermis in the basement membrane zone. Fibrinoid deposits are not specific for LE. They are seen in association with vascular injury, particularly in leukocytoclastic vasculitis.

Subcutaneous fat is often involved in systemic LE. Changes similar to those in lupus profundus may be seen but are usually milder: There may be focal mucin deposition associated with a predominantly lymphocytic infiltrate. Adipocytes may be separated by edema and fibrinoid deposits. These histopathologic changes in subcutaneous fat produce no clinically apparent lesions.

Occasionally, palpable purpuric lesions in systemic LE patients show a leukocytoclastic vasculitis histopathologically indistinguishable from leukocytoclastic vasculitis of other causes. There is endothelial cell swelling, a neutrophilic inflammatory infiltrate, nuclear dust, perivenular fibrin deposition, and stromal hemorrhage. Urticaria-like lesions may occur and show either a leukocytoclastic vasculitis or a perivascular mononuclear infiltrate not diagnostic of LE (44). In addition, white atrophic lesions may

occur in systemic LE that both clinically and histopathologically resemble those of malignant atrophic papulosis of Degos (45).

Bullous systemic LE shows two histopathologic inflammatory patterns: one neutrophilic and one mononuclear. The neutrophilic type simulates dermatitis herpetiformis or linear IgA disease with the formation of papillary microabscesses (Fig. 10-7A, B) (46). Nuclear dust is seen in the papillary microabscesses and in the upper dermis around and within the walls of blood vessels. Direct immunoelectron studies have localized immunoreactant deposits beneath the lamina densa and consist of IgG with or without IgM—and often IgA in a linear or granular pattern. Some patients may also have circulating anti-basement zone antibodies and antibodies directed against type VII collagen. The latter antibodies are similar but not identical to those in epidermolysis bullosa acquisita (47).

The subepidermal blister associated with a mononuclear inflammatory infiltrate arises in long-standing lesions of cutaneous LE (Fig. 10-8A, B). It likely corresponds to an altered dermal–epidermal interface resulting from inflammation and

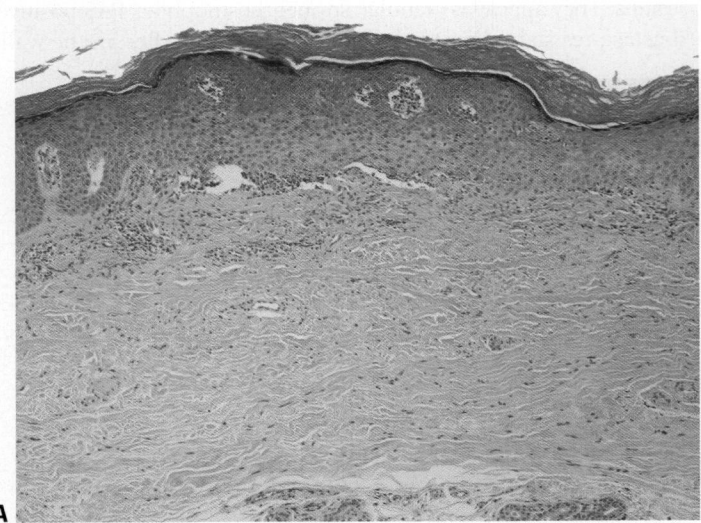
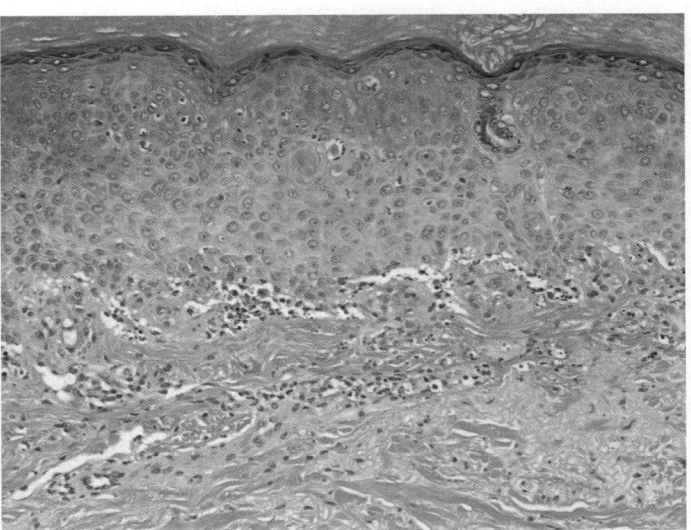

A   **B**

Figure 10-7 Bullous lupus erythematosus, neutrophilic. **A:** There are broad-based subepidermal blisters associated with mild papillary dermal edema and prominent neutrophils. Neutrophils are also present around vessels and among collagen bundles throughout the superficial dermis. Erythrocyte extravasation is seen. Faint interstitial mucin deposits and nuclear dust are present. **B:** The papillary dermal neutrophil aggregates simulate findings of dermatitis herpetiformis. The dermal changes as noted in **A**, however, would not be seen in dermatitis herpetiformis.

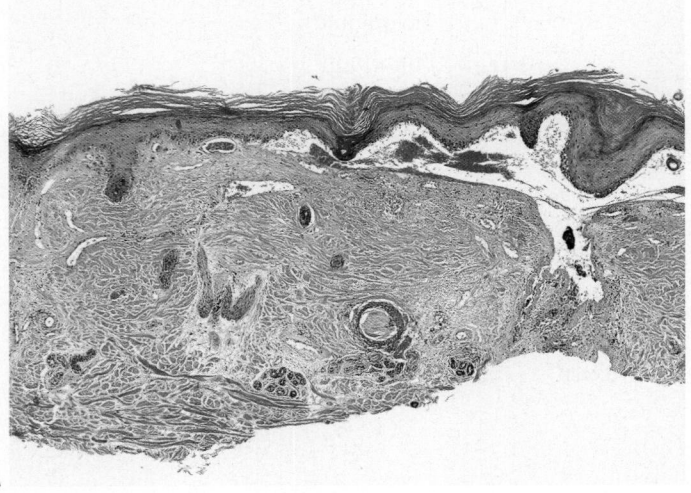
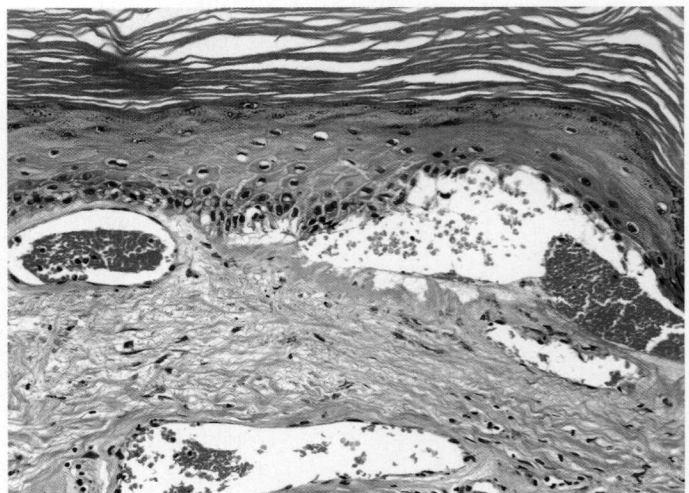

A   **B**

Figure 10-8 Bullous lupus erythematosus, mononuclear. **A:** A broad subepidermal cleft is present beneath an epidermis that has lost its rete ridge pattern and is surmounted by hyperkeratotic scale. The stroma contains perivascular and periappendageal inflammatory infiltrates. **B:** Adjacent to the zone of dermal–epidermal separation is a thickened eosinophilic basement membrane zone. Melanophages are scattered in the superficial dermis.

immune complex deposition. This type of change is a part of the spectrum of LE rather than a distinct entity.

Systemic Lesions. Much of the tissue damage in systemic LE results from deposition of antibody–antigen complexes in affected organ systems.

A detailed presentation of the arthritic, serosal, and cardiac manifestations and classifications of glomerulonephritides is beyond the scope of this section but can be found in the review by Dooley et al. (47).

Antiphospholipid syndrome occurs in patients with systemic LE and other autoimmune diseases that develop immunoglobulins capable of prolonging phospholipid-dependent coagulation tests. These immunoglobulins occur in association with systemic LE and other autoimmune diseases but are found unassociated with them as well. One of these, lupus anticoagulant, occurs in about 10% of systemic LE patients. Affected patients are at greater risk for thromboembolic disease, including deep venous thrombosis, pulmonary emboli, and other large-vessel thrombosis (48). Other findings include recurrent fetal wastage, renal vascular thrombosis, thrombosis of dermal vessels (Fig. 10-9A, B), and thrombocytopenia. Anticardiolipin antibody, a second type of antiphospholipid antibody, occurs five times more often than lupus anticoagulant antibody. It is associated with recurrent arterial and venous thrombosis, valvular abnormalities, cerebrovascular thromboses, and essential hypertension (Sneddon syndrome) (49). Other cutaneous findings include livedo reticularis, necrotizing purpura, disseminated intravascular coagulation, and stasis ulcers of the ankles (50).

Pathogenesis. The etiology of LE is considered to be multifactorial (Table 10-3). Studies have demonstrated numerous defects in the innate and adaptive immune system resulting in a widespread loss of self-tolerance. These abnormalities include but are not limited to abnormal responses to ultraviolet radiation, abnormal antigen-presenting cell function, plasmacytoid dendritic cell function, numerous HLA associations, polymorphisms in TNF-α promoters, abnormal keratinocyte apoptosis, and polymorphisms in the genes coding for interleukin 1 (IL-1) receptor antagonist and IL-10 promoter sequence (51). Aberrant stimulation of intracellular Toll-like receptors (TLRs), specifically TLR7 and TLR9, by endogenous antigens may play

a crucial role in the autoimmune feedback loop between T cells and B cells (52). The common final pathway involves the production of autoantibodies that mediate tissue damage (53).

The initial screening test for ANAs is indirect immunofluorescence, which provides limited but clinically useful information. Many other assays are available for more specific characterization of ANAs and include immunodiffusion, enzyme-linked immunosorbent assays, immunoprecipitation, and immunoblots.

Indirect immunofluorescence detects nuclear, homogeneous, rim, speckled, and nucleolar patterns. The fluorescence ANA test can be regarded as a specific marker for systemic LE in a rim pattern with a titer of 1:160 or higher and is indicative of the presence of anti-native or double-stranded (ds) DNA antibodies. Although anti-dsDNA has generally been regarded as the most specific marker of systemic LE, the lack of sensitivity makes a negative test unhelpful. Other markers that have been examined include antinucleosome antibodies, which may be more prevalent in systemic LE patients and may develop earlier than anti-dsDNA antibodies. This assay, however, is not widely available and has not been rigorously evaluated (54). At a titer of 1:20, about 20% of patients with DLE, most patients with systemic scleroderma, and as many as 5% of normal persons may have a positive reaction. The presence of anti-Sm is indicative of associated lupus nephritis. Anti-nRNP antibodies are of diagnostic significance only at high titers where they indicate MCTD. ANA-negative sera should be examined for the presence of anti-Ro/SSA and La/SSB antibodies, characteristic of subacute and neonatal LE and systemic LE with genetic deficiency of complement components.

Direct immunofluorescence studies detect immunoreactant deposits in affected tissues, particularly the skin and kidneys. A skin biopsy (3- to 4-mm punch) is submitted in saline-impregnated gauze, Zeus, Michel's or phosphate-buffered saline, snap frozen, sectioned, and incubated with fluorescein-conjugated antisera to IgA, IgM, IgG, and the third component of complement (C3). In a positive test, there is a continuous granular deposition of usually two or more immunoreactants in a band along the dermal–epidermal junction (Fig. 10-2). Variables that affect test results are the site of the biopsy (sun exposed vs. sun protected), duration of the lesion (acute,

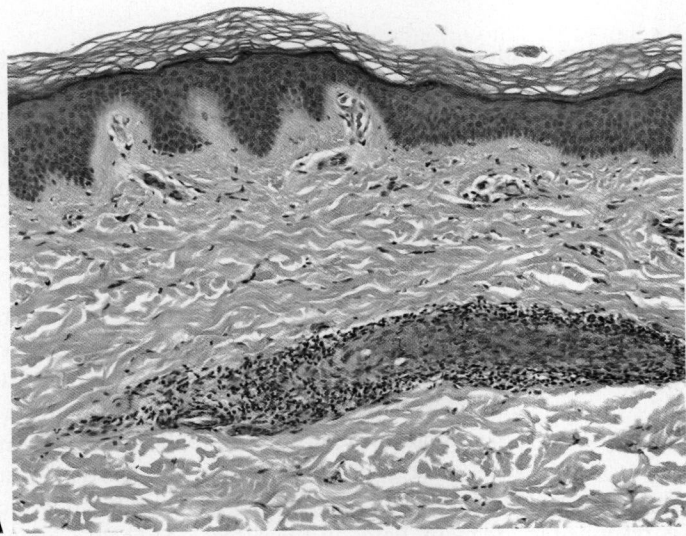

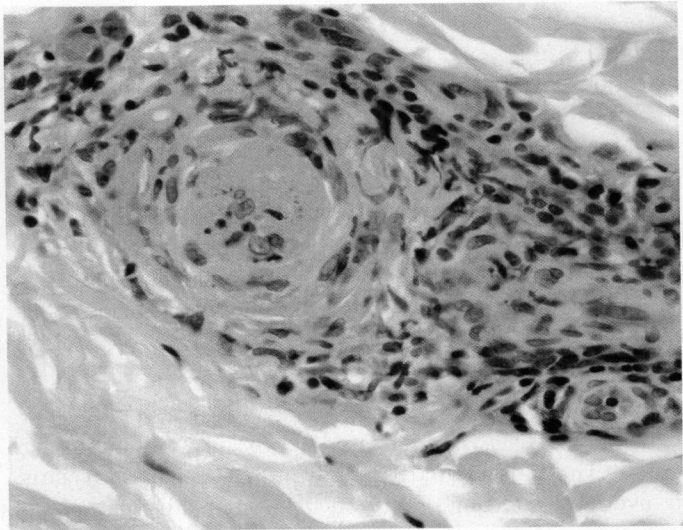

A   B

Figure 10-9 Lupus anticoagulant syndrome. **A:** A superficial dermal vessel is surrounded by lymphocytes. **B:** High magnification of pale eosinophilic intravascular thrombus.

Table 10-3

Lupus Erythematosus: Etiologic Factors

Genetic	HLA-DR2	Mothers with newborns with neonatal LE
		Patients positive for anti-Ro/SSA
		Older patients with SLE
	HLA-DR3	Younger SLE patients with anti-native DNA antibodies
	HLA-B8	Increased frequency in:
	HLA-DR3	Mothers with newborns with neonatal LE
	HLA-DQ23	Female patients with primary Sjögren syndrome
	HLA-DRw52	Female patients with Sjögren syndrome/LE
Environmental precipitants	Drugs	See Table 10-2
	Ultraviolet light	
	Possibly diet	
Hormonal influences	Predisposition of women in childbearing years	
Autoimmunity	Every aspect of immune system affected:	
	B cells	Abnormal B-lymphocyte maturation and activation
		Hypergammaglobulinemia
	T cells	Decreased peripheral T lymphocytes
		T-cell hyperactivity
		Increased percentage of CD29$^+$ (memory helper) T cells
		Preferential loss of CD4, CD45R$^+$ (suppressor inducer) cells in active LE
	Other	Defective T-suppressor function CD123$^+$ plasmacytoid dendritic cells
	Natural killer (NK) cell	Normal number of NK cells but decreased NK-cell activity (deficient in active cytotoxicity)
	Antilymphocyte antibody	Lymphocytotoxic antibodies in sera of 80% of SLE patient
	Antinuclear antibodies	Nuclear membrane targets
		Chromatin targets
		Ribonucleoprotein targets
	Abnormal feedback loop	Abnormal stimulation of TLR7 and TLR9 by endogenous antigens

LE, lupus erythematosus; SLE, systemic lupus erythematosus.

subacute, chronic), and preceding therapy. The frequency and implications of positive results in DLE and systemic LE are summarized in Table 10-4 (55–57).

Cautious sampling and interpretation of findings are necessary to avoid false-positive and false-negative results. The presence of only one type of immunoreactant, particularly in an intermittent distribution, may be seen in chronically sun-exposed skin or with underlying disorders such as rosacea. False-negative results are often found in acute or subacute lesions and treated lesions. Optimally, an established lesion—present for 3 months or longer—that has not been treated is submitted for study (58).

Differential Diagnosis. Lichenoid eruptions, including lichenoid eruptions related to medications, dermatomyositis, and overlap syndromes may show similar histopathologic features. Correlation with clinical presentation and serologic studies is necessary.

Principles of Management: The treatment modalities for LE cover a wide range of immunosuppressant topical and systemic agents. Typically, the extent of disease dictates the course of therapy. All patients benefit from sun protection with broad-spectrum UV-blocking chemical and physical agents. Limited cutaneous disease of discoid lupus can be treated with topical mid- to high-potency steroids. This is often insufficient, however, and systemic therapy with hydroxychloroquine or other antimalarials is necessary; some feel that the administration of hydroxychloroquine may decrease progression to overt systemic LE. Patients who fail to respond or with extensive, disfiguring, or symptomatic disease may require more aggressive therapy. These may include methotrexate, thalidomide, prednisone, azathioprine, or mycophenolate mofetil. Of particular importance in discoid lupus is meticulous sun avoidance, which is responsible for many flares in the disease. Subacute cutaneous lupus is similarly treated, though in this instance the strong

Table 10-4

Direct Immunofluorescence in Lupus Erythematosus

Site		Result	
		Discoid LE	Systemic LE
Sun exposed (e.g., dorsal forearm)	Involved	Positive in >90% of untreated	Positive in 80%–90% of untreated lesions
Sun exposed (e.g., volar forearm)	Uninvolved	Almost always negative	Positive in >80% of untreated SLE
Non-sun exposed (e.g., buttock)	Uninvolved	Negative	With active LE: positive in >91%
			With inactive SLE: positive in 33%
			Positive result may indicate renal involvement.

LE, lupus erythematosus; SLE, systemic lupus erythematosus.

association with medication-induced disease warrants a thorough review of the patients' medication list to identify potential triggers. Lupus profundus, owing to the subcuticular location of the disease process, is not amenable to topical steroids, and patients typically are treated with antimalarials. Systemic lupus is typically treated with systemic immunosuppressants including prednisone, cyclophosphamide, mycophenolate mofetil, methotrexate, azathioprine, and/or belimumab (59). Case reports and small studies have examined the efficacy of thalidomide and lenalidomide, high-dose intravenous immunoglobulins, and rituximab or TNF inhibitors, with varying response rates (60). Bullous lupus is often particularly responsive to dapsone and other anti-neutrophilic agents but may require rituximab.

Jessner Lymphocytic Infiltration of the Skin

Clinical Summary. Jessner lymphocytic infiltration of the skin, first described in 1953 (61), is not a well-understood entity. It is characterized by asymptomatic papules or well-demarcated, slightly infiltrated red plaques, which may develop central clearing. In contrast to lesions of chronic LE, the surface shows no follicular plugging or atrophy. Lesions arise most often on the face but may also involve the neck and upper trunk (62). Although this disorder has been reported to occur in childhood (63), affected patients are usually middle-aged men and women. Some authors consider this entity to exist on the spectrum of LE, and some consider it to be identical to tumid lupus (64,65).

Variable numbers of lesions persist for several months or several years. They may disappear without sequelae or recur at previously involved sites. The eruption may be precipitated or aggravated by sunlight.

Histopathology. The epidermis may be normal or slightly flattened. In the dermis, there are dense perivascular and interstitial infiltrates composed of small, mature lymphocytes admixed with occasional histiocytes and plasma cells (Fig. 10-10A, B). The infiltrate may extend around folliculosebaceous units and into subcutaneous adipose tissue.

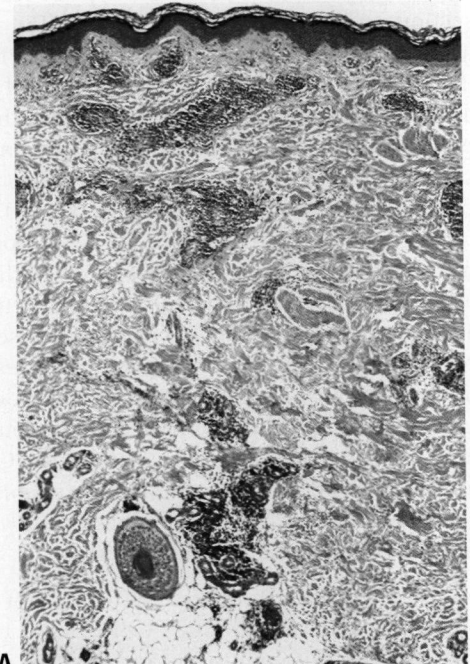
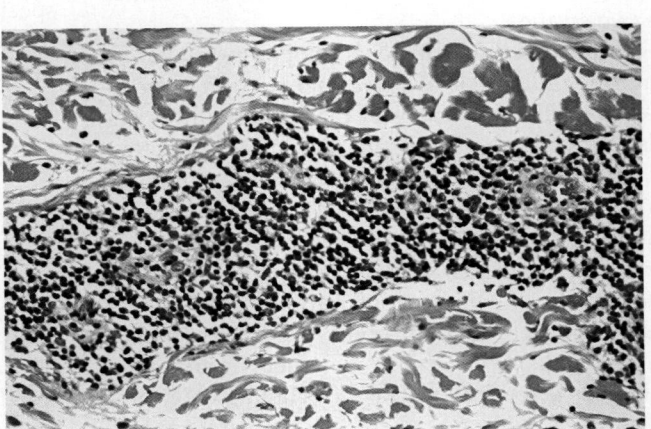

Figure 10-10 Jessner lymphocytic infiltrate. **A:** The epidermis is normal. The dermis contains tightly cuffed lymphocytic infiltrates following blood vessels and focally surrounding appendages. **B:** Higher magnification shows a purely lymphocytic infiltrate around vascular channels.

Pathogenesis. Opinion varies as to whether Jessner lymphocytic infiltrate of the skin is a distinct entity. The following four views have been expressed: (a) Clinical, histopathologic, and immunohistochemical findings warrant its distinction as a separate entity (66). (b) Although some cases represent a distinct entity, others are LE. (c) All cases are LE. (d) It represents an abortive or initial phase of LE, plaque type of polymorphous light eruption, lymphocytoma cutis, or lymphocytic lymphoma. In support of the notion that Jessner lymphocytic infiltrate is a form of LE, studies of CD123, a plasmacytoid dendritic cell marker, known to have an effector role in lupus, have shown similar patterns of staining in the inflammatory cells (64). Isolated reports of Jessner lymphocytic infiltrate have been reported in association with angiotensin-converting enzyme inhibitor, enalapril, and a synthetic polypeptide, glatiramer acetate, used to treat multiple sclerosis (67,68). Isolated familial cases have also been reported (69).

Immunohistochemical studies indicate that the predominant cells of lymphocytic infiltrate of the skin are mature T lymphocytes. Phenotyping studies predominantly show CD4[+] T-helper cells (70). Other studies have suggested a CD8[+] cytotoxic phenotype (69). Rearrangement of the T-cell receptor gene has not been detected in the limited number of cases studied. The relative paucity of B lymphocytes may assist in the separation of this entity from cutaneous lymphoid hyperplasia, which usually displays larger B-cell components, with or without associated germinal center formation. Immunophenotypic analysis will assist in distinction from cutaneous lymphoma.

Differential Diagnosis. The histopathologic differential diagnosis of Jessner lymphocytic infiltration of the skin includes the other six of the seven *L*s: LE, polymorphous light eruption, lymphocytoma cutis, lues, Lyme disease, and lymphoma. Jessner lymphocytic infiltrate is limited to sun-exposed skin and lacks the hyperkeratosis, atrophy, interface changes, and direct immunofluorescence findings noted in lupus. Therefore, lupus should be excluded with serologic and direct immunofluorescence studies. Serologic studies and the clinical distribution of lesions allow the separation of lues and Lyme disease from Jessner lymphocytic infiltrates.

Approximately 10% of cases of lupus lack interface alterations and show negative direct immunofluorescence studies. Polymorphous light eruptions usually show prominent papillary dermal edema; however, plaque-type polymorphous light eruption may histopathologically overlap with Jessner lymphocytic infiltration of the skin. Clinical features may sometimes separate these two entities.

A poorly understood entity histopathologically similar to Jessner lymphocytic infiltrate is *palpable migratory arciform erythema*. This entity differs clinically in that it is slightly pruritic and tends to involve the trunk and proximal extremities. It waxes and wanes over days to weeks rather than months. Differences in histology have been reported but have not been validated by multiple studies (71).

The differential diagnosis includes primary cutaneous CD4[+] small/medium T-cell lymphoproliferative disorder, which usually occurs on the face, neck, or upper trunk. Histopathologically, there is overlap with Jessner lymphocytic infiltrate; however, T follicular helper cell markers (including PD1) predominate in this CD4[+] infiltrate, whereas periadnexal inflammation is less commonly seen.

The absence of epidermotropism and significant lymphocytic atypia allows differentiation from cutaneous T-cell lymphoma. Additionally, immunophenotypic analysis of Jessner lymphocytic infiltrate reveals a mixed lymphocytic infiltrate without loss of CD2 or CD5 expression by T cells.

Principles of Management: Mid-potency topical steroids are typically utilized for symptomatic management. Sun avoidance is encouraged. In recalcitrant cases, antimalarial drugs and/or corticosteroids are useful in controlling this disorder. Other therapies have included methotrexate, gold, thalidomide, and photodynamic therapy.

MIXED CONNECTIVE TISSUE DISEASE

Clinical Summary. Overlapping findings of systemic LE, scleroderma (systemic sclerosis), and polymyositis associated with the presence of high titers of anti-U1 ribonucleoprotein (RNP) antibodies have been recognized since 1972 as MCTD (72). The first clue to the diagnosis is usually a positive, high-titer speckled ANA. The clinical presentation includes, but is not limited to, edema of the hands, acrosclerosis, Raynaud phenomenon, synovitis of one or more joints, and myositis that is documented with biopsy or serum elevations of muscle enzymes. Esophageal hypomotility and pulmonary disease may be seen as well. The diagnosis of MCTD may not be made at the outset because symptoms may present in an asynchronous fashion.

Cutaneous LE lesions are found in approximately half of the patients. They cover the entire spectrum of cutaneous LE. Most commonly, there are diffuse, nonscarring, poorly demarcated subacute lesions, but some patients show malar eruptions as seen in systemic LE or persistent scarring lesions of DLE.

Patients with high-titer anti-U1 RNP antibodies have a low prevalence of renal disease and life-threatening neurologic complications. Although the prognosis of MCTD is comparable to that of systemic LE, death may occur from progressive pulmonary hypertension and cardiac complications (73).

Histopathology. If cutaneous lesions of LE are present, the histopathologic findings correspond to the type of lesion described in the section on DLE and Systemic LE. MCTD, in contrast to most cases of systemic LE, has no antibodies to DNA. The absence of such antibodies accounts for the rarity of renal disease.

Indirect immunofluorescence studies show the presence of very high titers of serum antibodies directed against extractable ribonuclease-sensitive antigens known as small nuclear ribonucleoproteins (snRNPs). They characterize MCTD but are not specific for it, and produce a fine speckled ANA pattern at high dilutions. This speckled pattern corresponds to the widespread distribution of snRNP in the nucleus at sites of active gene transcription, where messenger RNA is being processed.

Direct immunofluorescence staining of normal skin shows deposition of IgG in a speckled pattern in epidermal nuclei. Although this finding is typical of MCTD, it is found occasionally also in patients with systemic LE and other CTDs (74). In addition, patients with MCTD may show a subepidermal lupus band in normal skin. Such a band has been observed in normal sun-exposed skin in about 20% of the cases.

Pathogenesis. The pathogenesis of MCTD is not fully understood but shows some similarities to LE. Like LE, MCTD is a manifestation of autoimmunity and loss of self-tolerance, driven by aberrations in both innate and adaptive arms of the immune system. Triggering of this process, similar to LE, occurs through interactions of the innate immune system, through TLR with apoptotic cells that have undergone antigen structural modification.

Differential Diagnosis. The differential diagnosis includes many stand-alone diseases that make up the constellation of MCTD. These include polymyositis, systemic LE, and systemic sclerosis. Although there are distinct serologic patterns that distinguish systemic LE from MCTD, the underlying immunologic aberration is believed to be similar.

Principles of Management: Similar to other CTDs, the extent of disease dictates the treatment course, and sun protection is essential. For mild disease with arthritic symptoms and cutaneous lesions, nonsteroidal anti-inflammatory agents and topical steroids may be all that is required. Hydroxychloroquine may be used as an adjuvant. For more aggressive disease, systemic steroids and alternate immunosuppressive agents may be required. Pulmonary involvement, in the form of pulmonary hypertension, is treated with phosphodiesterase inhibitors and the endothelin receptor antagonist ambrisentan and the synthetic prostaglandin epoprostenol. Phosphodiesterase inhibitors and calcium channel blockers may be used for the treatment of Raynaud phenomenon. Intravenous immunoglobulin has been used in recalcitrant cases with success (75).

DERMATOMYOSITIS

Clinical Summary. Dermatomyositis manifests as an inflammatory myopathy with characteristic cutaneous findings. In the absence of cutaneous findings, the diagnosis of polymyositis is applied. Cutaneous findings alone, without muscular involvement, have been termed *amyopathic dermatomyositis* or *dermatomyositis sine myositis* (76).

Both dermatomyositis and polymyositis are uncommon diseases that have a similar incidence. Both have two peaks of occurrence: one in childhood and one between the ages of 45 and 65 years (77). The cutaneous eruption and inflammatory myositis may occur asynchronously. Their appearance may be separated by months to years.

The four systemic and single cutaneous diagnostic criteria for dermatomyositis are symmetric proximal muscle weakness, elevated muscle enzymes, an abnormal electromyogram in the absence of neuropathy, consistent muscle biopsy changes, and cutaneous findings (77). Involvement of the skeletal muscles causes progressive weakness, pain, and eventual muscle atrophy. The proximal muscles of the extremities and the anterior neck muscles often are the first to be involved. Involvement of the pharynx may result in dysphagia and aspiration. Involvement of the diaphragm and the intercostal muscles may lead to respiratory failure. Arthritis and arthralgias occur in up to 25% of cases. Interstitial lung disease is becoming increasingly recognized as a frequent occurrence in patients with dermatomyositis, particularly among those with anti-MDA5 antibodies (78,79). Less common systemic manifestations include dysphagia, dysphonia, and cardiac conduction abnormalities, which portend a worse prognosis. Both traditional dermatomyositis and amyopathic dermatomyositis are strongly associated with internal malignancies, as discussed below.

Two distinctive cutaneous lesions are found in dermatomyositis. The heliotrope rash appears as violaceous, slightly edematous periorbital patches involving the eyelids. The other manifestation Gottron papules manifested as discrete red-purple papules over the knuckles, knees, and elbows. These may evolve into atrophic plaques with pigmentary alterations and telangiectasia and are then known as Gottron sign. Patients also frequently display a diffuse, purple-tinted violaceous erythema over their scalp, face, anterior neck and upper chest ("V sign"), upper back and deltoids ("shawl sign"), or lateral hips ("holster sign") (80).

Other cutaneous findings include periungual telangiectasia, hypertrophy of cuticular tissues associated with splinter hemorrhages, photosensitivity, and poikiloderma. Often, lesions resembling the erythematous–edematous lesions seen in SCLE or systemic LE may be found. Subcutaneous and periarticular calcification may occur, particularly in children, or rarely in adults, particularly with NXP2 autoantibodies. Calcinosis is usually seen in the proximal muscles of the shoulders and pelvic girdle. Childhood onset may also be associated with lipodystrophy and insulin resistance (81). Uncommon cutaneous findings include gingival telangiectasia, angiokeratomas, panniculitis, flagellate erythema on the back, follicular hyperkeratosis ("Wong-type dermatomyositis"), hyperkeratosis and fissuring involving the palms and lateral aspects of the fingers (mechanic's hands) seen in Jo-1/antisynthetase antibody disease, scleromyxedematous lesions, and pityriasis rubra pilaris-like lesions (82–86). Specific subtypes of dermatomyositis may show unique clinical findings, such as the "inverse Gottron" involvement of volar skin folds and presence of ulcerations in MDA-5 dermatomyositis associated with rapidly progressive interstitial lung disease (79).

Retrospective analyses indicate an increased risk of development of neoplasms during the first and—to a lesser degree—in the second year after a diagnosis of dermatomyositis is rendered (87). Incidences range from 6% to 50% in various reports, likely owing to the asynchronous development of malignancy in relation to the dermatomyositis. Some series fail to show a significant difference between affected patients and the control population. If malignancy arises with dermatomyositis, it usually occurs in adults. Paraneoplastic dermatomyositis may be more common in patients with certain autoantibody profiles, such as anti-TIF1-γ. Various tumors have been reported. Cancers of the lung, ovary, and lymphatic and hematopoietic systems are most frequently reported (88). Larger population-based studies have suggested an incidence of carcinoma at between 20% and 25% (89). The association with ovarian malignancy may be particularly strong and should not be overlooked, because screening for ovarian neoplasms is not often included in standard age-appropriate malignancy screening. Other tumors reported include lung, prostatic, pancreatic, and gastrointestinal carcinomas. In younger males, testicular carcinoma is more prevalent. In Asians, there is an increased association with nasopharyngeal carcinoma (90).

Histopathology. Dermatomyositis may show only nonspecific inflammation, but frequently the histopathologic changes are indistinguishable from those seen in systemic LE. There is epidermal atrophy, basement membrane degeneration, vacuolar alteration of basilar keratinocytes, a sparse lymphocytic inflammatory infiltrate around blood vessels, and interstitial mucin deposition (Fig. 10-11A, B) (91). With severe inflammatory changes, they may be associated subepidermal fibrin deposition. Although immune complexes are not detected at the dermal–epidermal junction in dermatomyositis, the absence of these immunoreactants does not exclude a diagnosis of LE. Up to 50% of subacute cutaneous lupus biopsies can also have a negative direct immunofluorescence. Serologic studies may

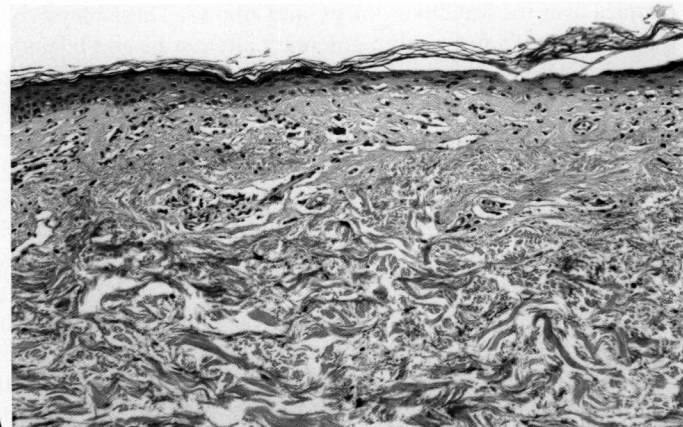 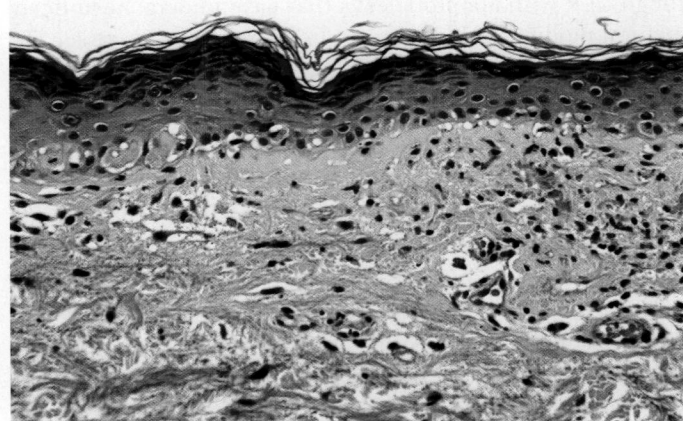

Figure 10-11 Dermatomyositis. **A:** An atrophic epidermis shows marked vacuolar alteration of basilar keratinocytes associated with a sparse lymphocytic inflammatory infiltrate around superficial dermal vessels. **B:** Marked vacuolar alteration of basilar keratinocytes associated with sparse lymphocytic infiltrates and papillary dermal melanophages.

help in this differential diagnosis. Patients with anti-MDA5-dermatomyositis have higher rates of vasculopathy (vessel wall thickening) (79).

Old cutaneous lesions with the clinical appearance of poikiloderma atrophicans vasculare usually show a bandlike infiltrate under an atrophic epidermis with hydropic degeneration of the basal cell layer (see also the section on Poikiloderma Atrophicans Vasculare). Gottron papules overlying the knuckles also show vacuolization of the basal cell layer with acanthosis rather than epidermal atrophy (92). Subcutaneous tissue may show focal areas of panniculitis associated with degeneration of adipocytes in early lesions. Extensive areas of calcification may be present in the subcutis at a later stage (see Calcinosis Cutis, Chapter 17).

Magnetic resonance imaging permits noninvasive assessment of muscle inflammation and may serve as a guide in locating a site for muscle biopsy. Tender proximal muscles of an extremity yield more useful information than atrophic, weak muscles, which show end-stage changes. Three types of changes may be observed in active diseases: (a) interstitial inflammatory infiltrates composed of lymphocytes and macrophages; (b) segmental muscle fiber necrosis (loss of skeletal muscle transverse striation, hyalinization of the sarcoplasm, fragmentation and/or phagocytosis of degenerated muscle fragments); and (c) vasculopathy (93). The latter entity may be seen in the childhood form and shows immune complex deposition in vessel walls (94). Old lesions usually show a rather nonspecific picture of atrophy of the muscle fibers and diffuse interstitial fibrosis with relatively little inflammation.

Systemic Lesions. Changes in organs other than the skin and the striated muscles occur only rarely in dermatomyositis, in contrast to systemic LE and systemic scleroderma. The myocardium may show changes identical to those in the skeletal muscle but less severe. Ulcerative lesions in the gastrointestinal tract, caused by vascular occlusions, have also been described (95).

Pathogenesis. As with LE, the pathogenesis of the disease is uncertain. Associated antibodies include PM1, Jo1 (correlates with pulmonary fibrosis), Ku (associated with sclerodermatomyositis), and Mi2 (associated with a more favorable prognosis and therapeutic responsiveness) (80). Other reported markers include autoantibodies to SAE (reported to be associated with

amyopathic dermatomyositis) and antibodies to TIF-1γ (anti-p155, anti-p155/140) and NXP-2 (anti-MJ or anti-p140) (associated with severe disease and higher malignancy risk) (80,96). Recent studies have shown that titers of anti-CADM140/MDA5 autoantibodies predict worse outcomes in patients with dermatomyositis and interstitial lung disease (80,97).

The landscape of antibody-specific associations is rapidly changing, and readers are encouraged to consult the primary literature. A single case of a cutaneous eruption mimicking dermatomyositis after treatment with imatinib mesylate has been reported (98). Medications, including hydroxyurea, quinidine, nonsteroidal anti-inflammatory agents, D-penicillamine, isoniazid, TNF-α inhibitors, and 3-hydroxy-3-methylglutaryl coenzyme A reductase inhibitors, have been reported to induce or exacerbate dermatomyositis.

Differential Diagnosis. Differentiation of the cutaneous lesions of dermatomyositis from those of SCLE or systemic LE may be impossible on a histopathologic basis. One study indicates possible differences in lymphocyte populations present in skin biopsies. CD4/CXCR-3+ lymphocytes predominate, as compared with lupus, where CD8 and CD20 lymphocytes predominate (99). It may also be impossible to distinguish between dermatomyositis and lupus on clinical grounds in cases where muscular weakness is mild or absent, as may be seen in the early stage of dermatomyositis. The most important laboratory test in such cases is the lupus band test, which is always negative in lesions of dermatomyositis (100), whereas in lesions of LE it is positive in 90% of the cases. Other tests that are usually negative in dermatomyositis and often positive in LE include urinalysis and renal function tests, as well as tests for ANA, anti-native DNA antibodies, and antibodies to RNP. Rarely, patients with dermatomyositis demonstrate a positive Ro antibody titer. Patients with active myositis show an elevation of serum creatine kinase and aldolase.

Principles of Management: On the whole, the prognosis of dermatomyositis is favorable, especially when treatment with corticosteroids is used. Sun protection is essential. Antimalarial agents can be tried, though notably about 25% of patients with dermatomyositis will develop a morbilliform exanthema in response. Other therapeutic agents include mycophenolate mofetil, methotrexate, azathioprine, dapsone, intravenous immunoglobulins, cyclophosphamide, rituximab (generally for muscle disease), tacrolimus, and cyclosporine. Novel treatments, including targeted therapeutics, are on the horizon. The mortality has been reported to be approximately 14% in some series, with metastatic malignancy a frequent cause of death (101). Different manifestations of dermatomyositis may require different treatments, and it is essential to evaluate patients thoroughly for internal disease and direct treatment accordingly.

POIKILODERMA ATROPHICANS VASCULARE

Clinical Summary. Clinically, the term poikiloderma atrophicans vasculare is applied to lesions that, in the early stage, show erythema with slight, superficial scaling, a mottled pigmentation, and telangiectases. In the late stage, the skin appears atrophic and the erythema is less pronounced, and the mottled pigmentation and the telangiectases are more pronounced. The late-stage clinical picture resembles that of chronic radiation dermatitis. Poikiloderma atrophicans vasculare may be seen in three different settings: (a) in association with genodermatoses, (b) as an early stage of mycosis fungoides, and (c) in association with dermatomyositis and, less commonly, LE.

Histopathology. In early-stage poikiloderma atrophicans vasculare, there is moderate thinning of the stratum malpighii, effacement of the rete ridges, and hydropic degeneration of the basal layer keratinocytes. In the upper dermis, there is a band-like infiltrate, which in places extends into the epidermis. The infiltrate consists mainly of lymphoid cells, but it also contains a few histiocytes. Melanophages, a result of pigmentary incontinence, are found in varying numbers within the infiltrate. In addition, there is papillary dermal edema and ectasia of the superficial venules. In the late stage, the epidermis is markedly atrophic with hydropic degeneration of basal layer keratinocytes. Melanophages and edema of the upper dermis are still present, and telangiectasia may be pronounced.

The amount and type of dermal infiltrate vary with the underlying cause. In poikiloderma atrophicans vasculare associated with one of the genodermatoses, the mononuclear infiltrate is mild and may be absent in the late stage (102). Similarly, in the late stage of poikiloderma seen in association with dermatomyositis or systemic LE, there is only slight dermal inflammation (91). In contrast, the amount of inflammatory infiltrate seen in poikiloderma associated with early mycosis fungoides increases rather than decreases with time (Fig. 10-12A, B). In addition, enlarged lymphocytes with densely chromatic nuclei and irregular nuclear contours are likely to be present. Epidermotropism of the infiltrate may result in the formation of Pautrier microabscesses, and atypical lymphocytes may line up along the dermal–epidermal junction, so-called tagging. Cell-marker analysis of such cases has shown most cells to be T-helper/inducer (CD4⁺) lymphocytes that lack expression of pan-T-cell antigen CD2, CD5, or CD7 (103). Loss of CD2 or CD5 expression by T cells is consistent with cutaneous T-cell lymphoma, whereas loss of CD7 is not a diagnostic finding and may be observed in reactive lymphoid infiltrates (see also Chapter 31).

Pathogenesis. The pathogenesis of poikiloderma atrophicans vasculare is dependent upon the underlying disease process. The genodermatoses in which the cutaneous lesions have the appearance of poikiloderma atrophicans vasculare are (a) poikiloderma congenitale of Rothmund–Thomson (see Chapter 6), with the lesions of poikiloderma present largely on the face, hands, and feet, and occasionally also on the arms, legs, and buttocks; (b) Bloom syndrome (see Chapter 6), with poikiloderma-like lesions on the face, hands, and forearms; and (c) dyskeratosis congenita (see Chapter 6), in which there may be extensive netlike pigmentation of the skin suggestive of poikiloderma atrophicans vasculare.

Poikiloderma-like lesions as features of early mycosis fungoides may be seen in one of two clinical forms: either as the large plaque type of parapsoriasis en plaques—also known as poikilodermatous parapsoriasis (see Chapter 7)—or as parapsoriasis variegata, which shows papules arranged in a netlike pattern (see Chapter 7). Although these two types of parapsoriasis may represent an early stage of mycosis fungoides, not all cases progress clinically into fully developed mycosis fungoides (104). Cases in which no progression toward mycosis fungoides

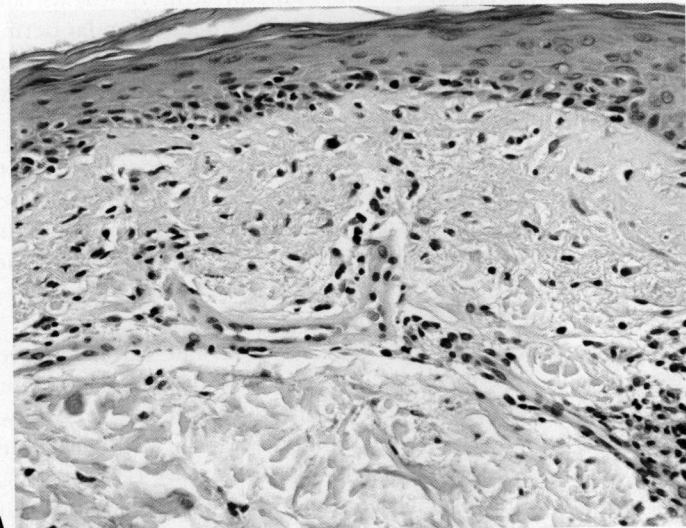
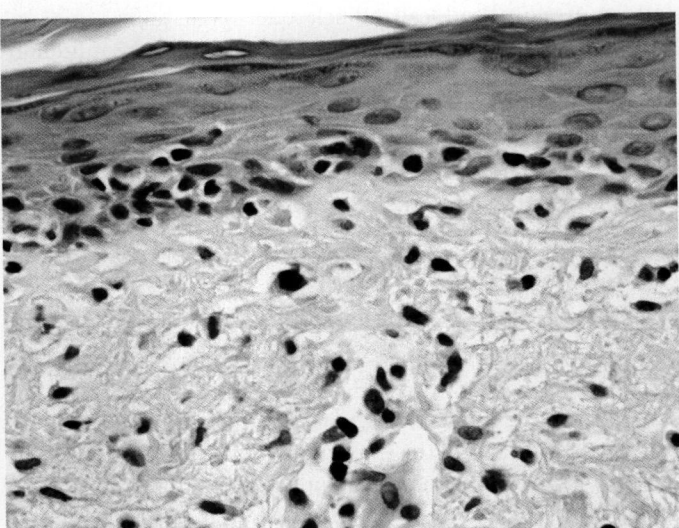

Figure 10-12 Poikiloderma. **A:** The epidermis appears flattened and shows hydropic degeneration of basal cells. **B:** The upper superficial contains a bandlike infiltrate, which in places extends into the epidermis.

is observed have been described also as *idiopathic poikiloderma atrophicans vasculare* (105).

The third group of diseases in which poikiloderma atrophicans vasculare occurs is dermatomyositis and systemic LE. Dermatomyositis is much more commonly seen as the primary disease than LE, and the association with dermatomyositis often is referred to as poikilodermatomyositis. In contrast to mycosis fungoides, in which poikilodermatous lesions are seen in the early stage, the lesions found in dermatomyositis and systemic LE generally represent a late stage.

Differential Diagnosis. As discussed earlier, changes of poikiloderma atrophicans vasculare may be seen in genodermatoses, parapsoriasis, early stages of cutaneous T-cell lymphoma, in association with dermatomyositis and, less commonly, LE.

Principles of Management: Therapy is driven by the underlying cause and extent of disease. With predominantly cutaneous disease, sun avoidance, topical steroids, and disease-modifying agents such as methotrexate, mycophenolate mofetil, or antimalarials are commonly employed. For significant muscle involvement, systemic steroids are the treatment of choice. Other agents used to treat myositis include intravenous immunoglobulin or biologics, including rituximab and TNF antagonists.

SYSTEMIC AND LOCALIZED SCLEROSIS (SCLERODERMA/MORPHEA)

Clinical Summary. Scleroderma (from the Greek *skleros*, hard, and *derma*, skin) is the principal clinical finding in a group of disorders characterized by thickening and fibrosis of the skin. This group of disorders is divided into the systemic form (systemic sclerosis, emphasizing coexistent visceral involvement) and the localized form (linear, including en coup de sabre and localized/generalized morphea). Because there is significant histopathologic overlap between systemic sclerosis (scleroderma) and morphea (localized scleroderma), they will be discussed together in this section. They are somewhat analogous to the purely cutaneous form of LE (DLE) and the cutaneous plus visceral involvement in systemic LE. Localized and systemic scleroderma may coexist. In such instances, the manifestations of morphea/localized scleroderma arise first and are extensive, whereas those of systemic scleroderma are mild and nonprogressive (106). Rarely, the manifestations of systemic scleroderma precede those of morphea (107).

Variants of morphea include circumscribed morphea, linear morphea (includes coup de sabre), pansclerotic morphea, atrophoderma of Pasini and Pierini, and eosinophilic fasciitis of Shulman. The latter disease differs sufficiently from morphea and will be discussed separately.

Morphea/Localized Scleroderma

Clinical Summary. In morphea, or localized scleroderma, the lesions usually are limited to the skin and to the subcutaneous tissue beneath the cutaneous lesions. Occasionally, the underlying muscles and rarely the underlying bones are also affected.

Morphea may be clinically divided according to morphology and number, or extent, of lesions. Variable classifications exist. According to morphology, lesions have been described as guttate, plaque, linear, segmental, subcutaneous, and generalized. More recently, lesions have been categorized as circumscribed, generalized, linear, mixed, and pansclerotic. Eosinophilic fasciitis (EF) is discussed separately because of its different clinical and histopathologic appearance.

Guttate, or drop-like, lesions typically occur in association with lesions of the plaque type. Guttate lesions are small and superficial; they resemble the lesions of lichen sclerosus et atrophicus but do not show hyperkeratosis or follicular plugging. Lesions of the plaque type, the most common manifestation of morphea, are round or oval but may assume an irregular configuration through coalescence. They are indurated, have a smooth surface, and are ivory colored. As long as they are enlarging, they may show a violaceous border, the so-called lilac ring. Both types of lesions may be seen in circumscribed and generalized morphea (108).

Lesions of the linear type occur predominantly on the extremities and on the anterior scalp. When one or several extremities are involved, there is often, in addition to induration of the skin, marked atrophy of the subcutaneous fat and of the muscles, resulting in contractures of muscles and tendons and ankyloses of joints. In children, it may result in impaired growth of the affected limb (109). On the anterior scalp and forehead, linear morphea may have the configuration of the stroke of a saber (*coup de sabre*).

Segmental morphea occurs on one side of the face, resulting in hemiatrophy. Occasionally, morphea en coup de sabre and facial hemiatrophy occur together (110). This manifestation of morphea typically occurs in children and can be associated with neurologic deficits (111). Because of a high incidence of overlap between the two conditions and the similar histopathology, some authors feel that they represent slightly different manifestations of the same process. Retrospective studies have estimated the coincidence of the conditions at between 36% and 42% (112,113).

In subcutaneous morphea (morphea profunda), the involved skin feels thickened and bound to the underlying fascia and muscle. The involved plaques are ill-defined, and the skin of these plaques is smooth and shiny. Occasionally, the lesions may become bullous (114).

Generalized morphea comprises very extensive cases showing a combination of several types described above. It is seen mainly in children, in whom it has been described as disabling pansclerotic morphea, but may also occur in adults. Rarely, bullous lesions are seen in patients with generalized morphea (115).

There are several reported cases of morphea that involve the superficial reticular dermis (superficial morphea) as contrasted with its usual involvement of the deep reticular dermis (116). The clinical impact of the depth of involvement is unclear. The coexistence of lesions of morphea and lichen sclerosus et atrophicus is worthy of note.

Histopathology. The different types of morphea/localized scleroderma cannot be differentiated histopathologically. Rather, they differ in regard to severity and depth of involvement of the skin. It is of great importance that the biopsy specimen includes adequate subcutaneous tissue because most of the diagnostic alterations are seen in the lower dermis and in the subcutis.

Early inflammatory, intermediate, and late sclerotic stages exist. In the early inflammatory stage, found particularly at the violaceous border of enlarging lesions, the reticular dermis shows interstitial lymphoplasmacytic infiltrates with or without eosinophils among slightly thickened collagen bundles (Fig. 10-13A). As lesions become established, the inflammatory infiltrates surround eccrine coils and are associated with hypocellular collagen bundles and reduced numbers of surrounding adipocytes (Fig. 10-13B). A much more pronounced inflammatory infiltrate

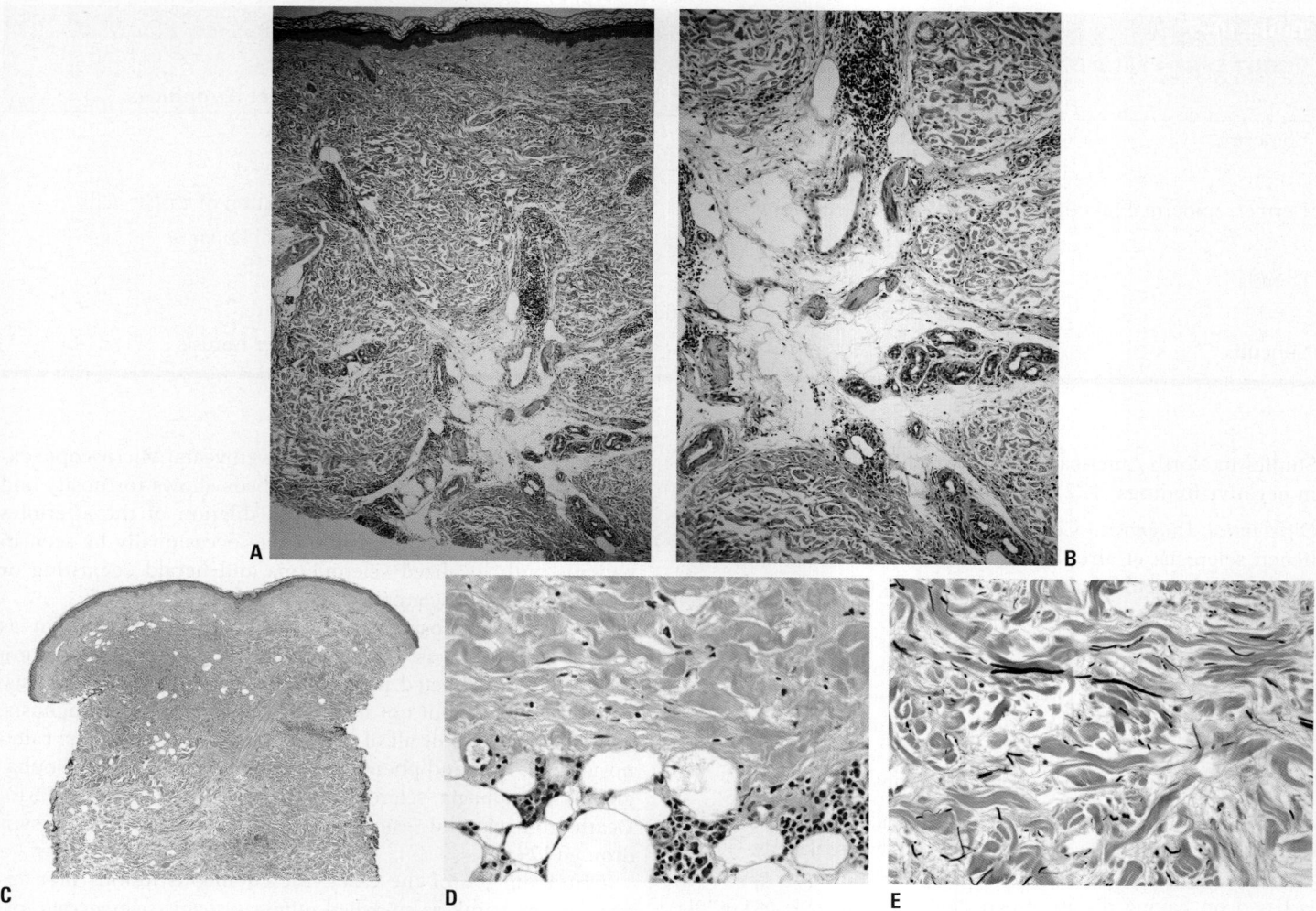

Figure 10-13 Morphea. **A:** The early inflammatory phase of morphea, where there is an interstitial lymphoplasmacytic infiltrate distributed among deep dermal collagen bundles. Collagen bundles are minimally swollen. **B:** Over time, collagen bundles become thickened, hypocellular, and swollen. Lymphoplasmacytic inflammatory infiltrates separate such collagen strands, surround eccrine coils in the deep dermis, and are associated with loss of adipocytes around eccrine apparatus. **C:** An established lesion of morphea: a "square" appearance in a punch biopsy. Note that appendages such as pilar apparatus are absent. **D:** There is a patchy lymphoplasmacytic infiltrate at the dermal–subcutaneous interface. Pale, thickened collagen bundles appear arranged parallel to each other. **E:** Elastic stains demonstrate straightened and elongated elastic fibers separated by collagen. They have a somewhat parallel array.

than that seen in the dermis often involves the subcutaneous fat and extends upward toward the eccrine glands. Trabeculae subdividing the subcutaneous fat are thickened because of the presence of an inflammatory infiltrate and deposition of new collagen. Large areas of subcutaneous fat are replaced by newly formed collagen, which is composed of fine, wavy fibers rather than bundles and stains only faintly with hematoxylin–eosin (117). Vascular changes in the early inflammatory stage generally are mild both in the dermis and in the subcutaneous tissue. They may consist of endothelial swelling and edema of the walls of the vessels (118).

In the late sclerotic stage, as seen in the center of old lesions, the inflammatory infiltrate has disappeared almost completely, except in some areas of the subcutis. The epidermis is normal. The collagen bundles in the reticular dermis often appear thickened, closely packed, and hypocellular. They stain more deeply eosinophilic than in normal skin (Fig. 10-13C, D). In the papillary dermis, where the collagen normally consists of loosely arranged fibers, the collagen may appear homogeneous.

Eccrine glands appear markedly atrophic, have few or no adipocytes surrounding them, and appear to be surrounded by newly formed collagen (Fig. 10-13B). Instead of lying near the dermal–subcutaneous junction as in normal skin,

eccrine glands appear higher in the dermis as a result of the replacement of most of the subcutaneous fat by newly formed collagen. This collagen consists of thick, pale, sclerotic, homogeneous, or hyalinized bundles with only few fibroblasts (hypocellular). Few blood vessels are seen within the sclerotic collagen; they often have a fibrotic wall and a narrowed lumen. Elastic stains show thick elastic fibers arranged parallel to hypocellular collagen strands and parallel to the epidermal surface (Fig. 10-13E) (119).

The fascia and striated muscles underlying lesions of morphea may be affected in the linear, segmental, subcutaneous, and generalized types. The fascia shows fibrosis and sclerosis similar to that seen in subcutaneous tissue. The muscle fibers appear vacuolated and separated from one another by edema and focal collections of inflammatory cells (120).

Bullae, seen only on rare occasions in generalized and in subcutaneous morphea, arise subepidermally, probably as a result of lymphatic obstruction, causing subepidermal edema.

Pathogenesis. There are conflicting data regarding *Borrelia burgdorferi* infection in cases of morphea. Studies indicating that such a relationship exists are primarily from Europe (121).

Table 10-5

Contrasting Features of Morphea and Lichen Sclerosus et Atrophicus

	Morphea	Lichen Sclerosus et Atrophicus
Epidermis	Relatively normal	Thinning of rete
	No follicular plugging	Follicular plugging
Dermal–epidermal junction	No hydropic degeneration	Hydropic degeneration of basilar cells
	Subepidermal separation infrequent	Often subepidermal bullae
Dermis	Appears homogenized	Marked edema
	Papillary dermal collagen and elastic fibers present	Elastic fibers absent
Subcutis	Inflammation	No inflammation or fibrosis

Studies in North America and some from Europe have resulted in negative findings (122).

Differential Diagnosis. Contrasting features of morphea and lichen sclerosus et atrophicus are summarized in Table 10-5. They include relatively little epidermal change in morphea, as compared with thinning of the rete ridges, follicular plugging, and interface alterations of lichen sclerosus (LS). The reticular dermal changes of fibrosis and inflammation in morphea contrast with the edema and loss of elastic tissue in LS. Histopathologic differentiation of the late stage of morphea from lichen sclerosus et atrophicus may cause difficulties, particularly in view of the fact that the two conditions may coexist.

Principles of Management: Treatment depends on the depth of inflammation, extent of disease, location, and disease activity. Generally, inactive disease leaves permanent fibrosis; therefore, treatment is based on halting disease progression. Involvement over joints should prompt consideration for more rapid or aggressive treatment and inclusion of physical therapy to preserve the range of motion. Topical agents, intralesional agents, and phototherapy (narrow-band ultraviolet B [NB-UVB] for some, though psoralen and ultraviolet A [PUVA] and especially UVA1 may be more effective) may be options for patients with limited disease, whereas systemic immunosuppressive agents may be required for patients with more widespread involvement. This may include methotrexate with or without corticosteroids, mycophenolate, or other suppressive drugs (122).

Systemic Scleroderma

Clinical Summary. In systemic scleroderma, in addition to the involvement of the skin and the subcutaneous tissue, visceral lesions are present, leading to death in some patients. The indurated lesions of the skin are not sharply demarcated or "circumscribed," as in morphea, although a few well-demarcated morphea-like patches may occasionally be seen.

Cutaneous involvement usually starts peripherally on the face and hands, gradually extending to the forearms. Facial changes include a mask-like, expressionless face; inability to wrinkle the forehead; a beak-like nose; and tightening of the skin around the mouth associated with radial folds. The upper extremities show nonpitting edema involving the dorsa of the fingers, hands, and forearms; this may be one of the first signs of the systemic inflammation of this disease, and physicians should be alert to this possibility. Gradually, the fingers become tapered, the skin becomes hard, and flexion contractures form. These changes are referred to as acrosclerosis and are associated with Raynaud phenomenon, which may precede other manifestations by months or even years. Microscopic examination of the nail fold capillary beds shows tortuosity and redundancy of capillary loops with dilation of the arterioles and venules. Such abnormalities may occasionally be seen in patients with localized scleroderma and herald coexisting or evolving systemic sclerosis (123).

Systemic sclerosis with limited scleroderma, known as CREST syndrome, is associated with Raynaud phenomenon in virtually all affected patients. This variant of acrosclerosis, which frequently but not invariably has a favorable prognosis, consists of several or all of the following manifestations: calcinosis cutis, Raynaud phenomenon, involvement of the esophagus with dysphagia, sclerodactyly, and telangiectases (CREST). Death from visceral lesions is infrequent in the CREST syndrome (124).

In about 5% of the cases, the cutaneous lesions first appear on the trunk as so-called *diffuse systemic scleroderma*, often sparing the peripheral portions of the extremities. Raynaud phenomenon is absent in such patients. There are, however, transitional forms starting out as acrosclerosis with Raynaud phenomenon but then extending to the proximal portions of the arms and to the trunk. In both forms of systemic scleroderma, the skin in the involved areas is diffusely indurated and, as a result of diffuse fibrosis of the subcutaneous fat, becomes firmly bound to underlying structures. The skeletal musculature is affected, resulting in weakness and atrophy. Contractures of the muscles and tendons and ankyloses of the joints may develop.

Occasional manifestations pertaining to the skin include diffuse hyperpigmentation, which is seen mainly in diffuse systemic scleroderma. Macular telangiectases on the face and hands, calcinosis cutis located on the extremities, and ulcerations, especially on the tips of the fingers and over the knuckles, occur predominantly in acrosclerosis. In addition, vascular ulcers on the lower extremities resembling those seen in atrophie blanche may occur in patients with acrosclerosis.

Histopathology. The histopathologic appearance of skin lesions in systemic scleroderma is similar to that of morphea, so that histopathologic differentiation of the two types is not possible. One small study stated that the two conditions may be differentiated based upon the pattern of the inflammatory infiltrate and presence or absence of papillary dermal involvement (125). In early lesions of systemic scleroderma, the inflammatory reaction is less pronounced than in morphea, so that only a mild inflammatory infiltrate is present around the dermal vessels, around the eccrine coils, and in the subcutaneous tissue. The vascular changes in early lesions are slight, as in morphea (126). By contrast, in the late stage, systemic scleroderma shows more pronounced vascular changes than morphea, particularly in the subcutis. These changes consist of a paucity of blood vessels, thickening and hyalinization of their walls, and narrowing of the lumen. Even in the late stage of systemic scleroderma, the epidermis appears normal, only occasionally showing disappearance of the rete ridges. Aggregates of calcium may also be seen in the late stage within areas of sclerotic, homogeneous collagen of the subcutaneous tissue (see also Calcinosis Cutis, Chapter 17).

Systemic Lesions. Internal organs are often affected in scleroderma, but their involvement varies greatly in extent and degree. Involvement does not necessarily imply functional compromise, and in many affected patients systemic scleroderma ultimately comes to a standstill. The clinical symptoms produced by reduced pliability, vascular compromise, and subsequent loss of function can be found in the gastrointestinal tract, lungs, heart, and kidneys, as well as the skin. In the gastrointestinal tract, submucosal fibrosis and replacement of the muscularis by fibrosis with intimal thickening of blood vessels give rise to difficulties in swallowing, regurgitation, and malabsorption and eventually ileus. In the lungs, interstitial fibrosis, degeneration of alveolar spaces, and intimal thickening of arteries result in dyspnea and cor pulmonale. Cases of pulmonary carcinoma (predominantly bronchioloalveolar) have been observed and are associated with the presence of pulmonary fibrosis (127). The most serious consequences arise in the kidneys. Adventitial fibrosis may affect interlobar, arcuate, and interlobular arteries, and mucoid degeneration affects arcuate and interlobular arteries. Uremia occurs more frequently than rapidly evolving renal failure and hypertension. The latter entity, termed scleroderma renal crisis, is associated with "onion-skin" hyperplasia of arterial walls and may be fatal (128).

Pathogenesis. The pathogenesis of systemic scleroderma/morphea, as with LE, is uncertain and may be multifactorial.

The triad of vascular compromise, collagen matrix aberrations, and presence of serologic autoimmune mediators contributes in variable degrees to symptoms and clinical findings in scleroderma and morphea (Table 10-6). Although a relationship to retroviral disease has been suggested, it is speculative and may reflect molecular mimicry of viral antigens (129). Genetic markers of scleroderma have been studied with DNA microarrays and indicate differential expression of genes in endothelial cells, B lymphocytes, and fibroblasts between scleroderma and normal biopsies (130).

Microvascular Changes. The involved vessels are primarily precapillary arterioles. Changes in the microvasculature have been noted in clinically normal skin. Perivascular edema and functional changes in endothelial cells can be detected early (131). Precapillary arterioles then show endothelial proliferation and mononuclear inflammatory infiltrates, followed by intimal proliferation and luminal narrowing (132). The corresponding electron microscopic findings include vacuolization and destruction of endothelial cells, reduplication of the basement membrane, enlargement of the rough endoplasmic reticulum in pericytes and fibroblasts, and perivascular fibrosis. Some data suggest that hyperplasia of the pericytic cells at the peripheral superficial aspect of the advancing border of the sclerosis may

Table 10-6
Pathogenic Factors in Scleroderma

Vascular aberrations	Raynaud phenomenon
	Intimal hyperplasia of blood vessels
	Adventitial fibrosis
	Vascular abnormalities in other visceral organs
	Enlargement and tortuosity of capillary loops
	Capillary loop dropout
	Thickened and reduplicated basement membrane
	Loss of endothelium
Immunologic factors	T-helper cell (CD4$^+$) infiltrates
	Reduction in T-suppressor (CD8$^+$) cells
	Increased soluble interleukin 2 receptors correlate with disease progression and mortality
	Decreased interleukin 1 production by peripheral mononuclear cells
Serologic markers	ANA$^+$ in more than 90% of patients
	Low/absent anti-native (double-stranded) DNA, anti-Sm, rare anti-nRNP
	Speckled ANA pattern correlates with anticentromere antibody on HEp-2 cells and CREST and a relatively favorable prognosis
	Anti–DNA topoisomerase 1 (Sci-70)

ANA, antinuclear antibody; CREST, calcinosis cutis, Raynaud phenomenon, involvement of the esophagus with dysphagia, sclerodactyly, and telangiectases.

play a role in the fibrosing process through synthesis of collagenous matrix material and recruitment of fibroblasts through release of cytokines (133). Although widespread arteriolitis may be present in early stages, only rarely does it progress to a necrotizing arteriolitis and eventuate in periarteritis nodosa (134).

A role for adhesion molecules in the evolution of lesions of scleroderma has been suggested: They are believed to bind mononuclear cells to endothelial cells and facilitate diapedesis of inflammatory cells into the connective tissue. Interactions with connective tissue components may lead to the release of cytokines and growth factors, resulting in upregulation of matrix production by fibroblasts and changes in fibroblast phenotype, resulting in fibrosis (135).

Collagen Matrix Aberrations. Analysis of collagen in affected skin has shown excess production of connective tissue components normally present in the dermis, including types I, III, V, VI, and VII collagen, fibronectin, and proteoglycans (136,137). Other studies suggest that fibroblasts in localized and systemic scleroderma express markers of smooth muscle differentiation (myofibroblasts), which may account for their different biologic behavior (138). Some observers have found loss of CD34$^+$ dendritic cells in affected areas, a finding of uncertain significance (139).

Serologic/Immunologic Markers. Most patients with systemic sclerosis (>90%) and approximately 50% of those with localized scleroderma (morphea) have a positive ANA. The pattern may be homogeneous, speckled, or nucleolar. When using the human laryngeal carcinoma cell line HEp-2, more than 90% of patients with morphea or acrosclerosis have a detectable anticentromere antibody. In patients with systemic sclerosis, this antibody is not usually detected. Instead, 20% to 40% of them have antibodies to Scl-70. This antigen has been identified as DNA topoisomerase I, an intracellular enzyme involved in the uncoiling of DNA before it is transcribed. Antibodies to this enzyme hinder its function. The presence of antibodies to Scl-70 correlates with systemic sclerosis, whereas the presence of anticentromere antibodies correlates with morphea or CREST and suggests a more favorable prognosis (140). Antihistone antibodies have been shown to be positive in cases of morphea, particularly in generalized morphea and linear scleroderma. Although not particularly sensitive, anti–single-stranded DNA is considered very specific for linear scleroderma (141).

In some cases of systemic scleroderma, epidermal nucleolar IgG deposition is seen by immunofluorescence even in clinically normal skin as a result of high serum concentrations of antibody to nucleolar antigen (142). Although subepidermal and vascular deposits are regularly absent in the skin in scleroderma, kidney biopsies in patients with renal involvement show diffuse vascular deposits of immunoglobulins, predominantly IgM, or of complement in the intima of the interlobular and arcuate arteries, which by light microscopy often exhibit fibromucinous alterations (143).

Differential Diagnosis. Sclerodermoid changes in the skin may be seen unassociated with scleroderma or morphea in numerous other settings. These include changes in association with genetic, metabolic, neurologic, and immunologic disorders, with occupational or chemical exposures, in association with malignancy, or as sequelae of infection (76). Genetic disorders that may show sclerodermatous cutaneous changes include phenylketonuria, progeria, Rothmund–Thomson syndrome, and Werner syndrome. Individuals at risk of occupational scleroderma include jackhammer and chain saw operators and those exposed to polyvinyl chloride, silica, and epoxy resins. Patients with metabolic disorders such as porphyria cutanea tarda, primary systemic amyloidosis, Hashimoto disease, carcinoid syndrome, and childhood diabetes mellitus may show similar cutaneous changes. Chronic graft-versus-host disease frequently shows scleroderma-like changes, and scattered reports in the literature indicate such changes may arise subsequent to silicone and paraffin injections in cosmetic procedures (144). Chemical agents have been known to induce thickening and hardening of the skin. Specific compounds include polyvinyl chloride, bleomycin, pentazocine, L-5 hydroxytryptophan and carbidopa (145), Spanish rapeseed oil (146), and L-tryptophan (eosinophilia–myalgia syndrome) (147).

Chemotherapy-associated sclerodermoid changes in the skin have been reported with balicatib, taxane, mitomycin C, paclitaxel, and carboplatin. Of note, sclerodermoid changes may arise in association with plasma cell dyscrasias. Although there are increased numbers of IgG₄ plasma cells in immunoglobulin G₄-related disease that affects visceral organs with lymphoplasmacytic infiltrates and fibrosis, IgG₄ plasma cells are not seen in greater numbers in scleroderma (148,149).

Principles of Management: Optimal management of Raynaud phenomenon involves a multidisciplinary approach including lifestyle modifications to prevent triggering factors (e.g., cold or wet environmental conditions) and prompt initiation of pharmacologic therapy (e.g., calcium channel blockers such as nifedipine and phosphodiesterase-5 inhibitors). Intravenous prostanoids such as iloprost have a role in the treatment of Raynaud phenomenon after failed calcium channel blockers or phosphodiesterase-5 inhibitors and in the treatment of digital ulcerations. Hematopoietic stem cell transplantation and methotrexate among other systemic therapies including mycophenolate mofetil have shown benefit in patients with cutaneous sclerosis and systemic scleroderma. Note the potential for methotrexate-associated pneumonitis in patients with underlying interstitial lung disease (ILD). Phototherapy with PUVA or UVA1 has also shown benefit in patients with systemic scleroderma (150). Studies examining anti-TNF agents, including infliximab and etanercept, have shown variable improvement (151). In cases where morphea or scleroderma compromise joint mobility with contractures, physical therapy and/or surgical intervention are used. Physical therapy should be initiated early as a preventive measure when joints are involved.

Postirradiation Morphea

Clinical Summary. Postirradiation morphea (PIM) is an underrecognized late complication of radiotherapy with the vast majority of cases occurring in women on the breast (152). Neither age nor radiation dose has been shown to correlate with the incidence of PIM (152). PIM arises abruptly with an initial erythema and induration progressing to violaceous plaques with peau d'orange skin changes and contractures resulting in pain and disfigurement (152). PIM has an estimated incidence of 1 in 500 patients in contrast to morphea of any etiology, which is far less common (153). The onset of PIM can occur at an interval of 1 month to as many as 32 years following radiotherapy (153). Systemic sclerosis is believed to be a risk factor for subsequent development of PIM. PIM predominantly involves the radiation portal, although extension beyond the radiation portal to other sites has also been reported (153).

Histopathology. Skin biopsy of PIM reveals a superficial and deep perivascular and periadnexal inflammatory infiltrate composed of lymphocytes and plasma cells in the early stage that gradually disappears. The late sclerosing phase that follows is characterized by dermal expansion with presence of thickened collagen bundles. Skin biopsy typically captures PIM in a mixed inflammatory and sclerosing phase (Fig. 10-14A–C) (153). Epidermal changes are not characteristic although overlapping features and co-occurrence with lichen sclerosus (which can also be radiation induced) may be seen (discussed below) (153).

Pathogenesis. The pathophysiology of PIM remains unclear. However, it has been posited that radiation may induce the creation of neoantigens that subsequently stimulate the secretion of TGF-β, a growth factor that plays a role in collagen synthesis and fibrosis via fibroblast activation (152).

Differential Diagnosis. Skin biopsy is critical for diagnosing PIM and excluding other similar appearing dermatologic findings including cellulitis, radiation dermatitis, and cancer recurrence (154). Certain characteristics can help distinguish PIM from the more commonly described phenomenon of radiation-induced fibrosis (RIF). Whereas RIF shows no significant inflammatory

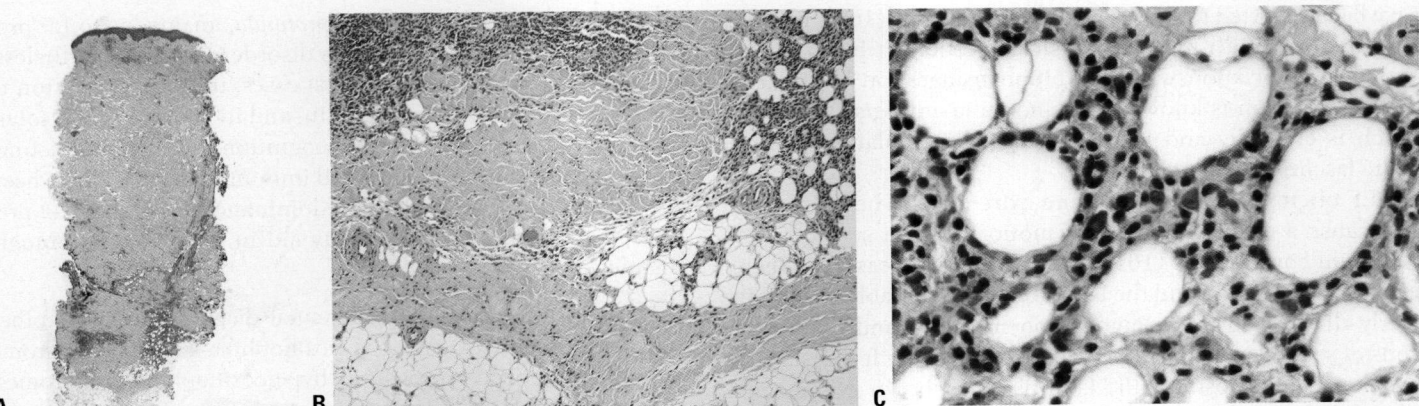

Figure 10-14 Postirradiation morphea. A: Skin biopsy reveals dermal expansion with superficial and deep perivascular and periadnexal inflammation. B: A mixed phase of dermal sclerosis and inflammation at the dermal–subcutaneous junction is seen. Subcutaneous septae are thickened. C: The inflammatory infiltrate is composed of lymphocytes and plasma cells.

infiltrate, involves a deeper subcutaneous or fascial fibrosis, and generally appears within the first 3 months after radiotherapy, PIM demonstrates a strong inflammatory component, involves a predominantly dermal fibrosis, and usually occurs at a later interval following radiotherapy (155). The cutaneous findings of RIF are generally limited to the area of skin exposed to radiation, whereas those of PIM can extend beyond the irradiated area (152).

Principles of Management: There are no clear treatment guidelines for PIM. Lesions are treated similar to those of idiopathic morphea with variable efficacy, including topical, intralesional, and systemic steroids; topical hyaluronidase; calcineurin inhibitors; systemic immunosuppressants such as methotrexate and tacrolimus; phototherapy (UVA, UVA1, UVB, PUVA); systemic antibiotics; and plasmapheresis (154,155). To date, clinical outcomes following therapy have been reported to be unsatisfactory (155).

ATROPHODERMA OF PASINI AND PIERINI

Clinical Summary. In atrophoderma of Pasini and Pierini, there are areas on the trunk, particularly the back, in which the skin appears slightly depressed with a slate-gray color but without surface changes. The lesions are asymptomatic, bilateral, symmetric, and sharply and irregularly demarcated, measuring from 1 to 10 cm in diameter. In late lesions, the center of the depressed area may feel slightly indurated.

Histopathology. The histopathologic changes in early lesions usually are slight and nonspecific, consisting of some thickening of the collagen bundles and a mild, scattered, chronic inflammatory infiltrate (156). With time, lesions show less inflammatory infiltrate and deep dermal changes including collagen bundles that appear thickened and tightly packed. In addition, indurated areas may show homogeneous, hyalinized collagen bundles.

Because the collagen bundles in the skin of the back normally are rather thick, it may be difficult to determine whether the collagen shows any changes. It is therefore desirable to take a biopsy specimen not only from the lesion but also from normal skin, either from an area nearby or from the opposite side with subcutaneous fat for comparison.

Pathogenesis. Some authors believe that atrophoderma of Pasini and Pierini is a disease entity, sui generis, as suggested by the original describers. This is supported by the fact that in atrophoderma, the atrophy comes first and the sclerosis possibly appears later, whereas in morphea, the sclerosis comes first and the atrophy appears later (157).

Differential Diagnosis. Most observers view the clinical presentation of atrophoderma to be distinct from that of morphea: Atrophoderma has an earlier onset (second to third decade) and protracted course of 10 to 20 years, and lesions lack a violaceous ring, which characteristically surrounds lesions of morphea. Microscopic findings show similarities to morphea, suggesting that atrophoderma of Pasini and Pierini may be a distinct, abortive variant of morphea (158). To support this view, there are instances of coexistent morphea and atrophoderma, as well as reports of transformation of lesions of morphea into atrophoderma. A relationship of this disorder to *B. burgdorferi* infection has been reported but needs more studies to be confirmed (159).

Principles of Management: There are presently no randomized placebo-controlled studies showing efficacy of any one agent. Variable success has been reported using topical steroids, penicillin, tetracycline, and antimalarials. In instances where serologic studies are positive for *B. burgdorferi*, treatment with oral doxycycline for several weeks led to clinical improvement (160).

EOSINOPHILIC FASCIITIS (SHULMAN SYNDROME)

Clinical Summary. First described in 1974 (161), eosinophilic fasciitis is a scleroderma-like disorder characterized by inflammation and thickening of the deep fascia. It has a rapid onset associated with pain, swelling, and progressive induration of the skin leading to exaggerated deep grooving of the skin around superficial veins. This disorder is often accompanied by a peripheral eosinophilia, hypergammaglobulinemia, and elevated erythrocyte sedimentation rate and has been associated with aplastic anemia. Other rare associations include polycythemia rubra vera, cutaneous T-cell lymphoma, borreliosis, and autoimmune thyroid disease (162). Simvastatin and phenytoin have been reported to cause eosinophilic fasciitis (163). EF may have its onset with unusual physical exertion. It has been reported in association with L-tryptophan ingestion (164). The latter association is known as eosinophilia–myalgia syndrome, which is clinically and histopathologically similar to eosinophilic fasciitis.

EF often involves one or more extremities. The induration may cause a decreased range of motion and, in severe cases, even joint contractures (165,166). In only a few cases are there lesions on the trunk, and the face is almost invariably spared. In nearly all reported cases, Raynaud phenomenon and visceral lesions of scleroderma have been absent. Only very few instances of incontestable eosinophilic fasciitis have shown evidence of Raynaud phenomenon (167) or mild pulmonary fibrosis (168), and in general experts feel the absence of Raynaud is a helpful diagnostic clue for EF. The disorder has a varied course: Some patients improve spontaneously, others improve with corticosteroids, and still others may have relapses and remissions.

Histopathology. A deep wedge biopsy to skeletal muscle including fascia is essential for the diagnosis of eosinophilic fasciitis. The fascia is markedly thickened, appears homogeneous, and is permeated by a mononuclear inflammatory infiltrate (Fig. 10-15A–C). The infiltrate in the fascia may contain an admixture of eosinophils (169). The underlying skeletal muscle in some cases shows myofiber degeneration, severe inflammation with a component of eosinophils, and focal scarring; in other cases, skeletal muscle is not involved.

In most cases, the adipose tissue shows no significant changes, except that the fibrous septa separating deeply located fat lobules are thicker, paler staining, and more homogeneous and hyalinized than normal dermal connective tissue. In other cases, however, the collagen in the lower reticular dermis appears pale and homogeneous, and the entire subcutaneous fat is replaced by horizontally oriented, thick, homogeneous collagen containing only few fibroblasts and merging with the fascia (170).

Pathogenesis. Although it was initially thought that eosinophilic fasciitis was a distinct syndrome, it soon became apparent that the disorder may lie on a spectrum with morphea. EF may show overlapping clinical and morphologic features with generalized morphea, including inflammation and fibrosis of the fascia, peripheral eosinophilia, and hypergammaglobulinemia (171,172). ANAs are present in a significant number of

cases (173). The term *morphea profunda*, analogous to LE profundus, has been applied to this disorder (174). Nevertheless, because of its acute onset in most cases, its usual limitation to the structures underlying the skin, and its tendency to resolve, eosinophilic fasciitis deserves recognition as a disorder distinct from morphea (175). Polar T-cell immune infiltrates have been reported with Th1 and Th17 predominance in EF and Th2 predominance in morphea and may aid in their histopathologic distinction (172).

Differential Diagnosis. The differential diagnosis includes other sclerosing disorders, such as eosinophilia–myalgia syndrome after L-tryptophan ingestion, hypereosinophilic syndromes, systemic sclerosis, Churg–Strauss syndrome, and/or peripheral T-cell lymphomas with cutaneous involvement (166).

Principles of Management: The first-line therapy for eosinophilic fasciitis is systemic corticosteroids, though often combination therapy with methotrexate or mycophenolate is used. Remission of symptoms can be achieved in 3 to 6 months. Numerous alternative therapies have been examined in steroid-refractory cases; however, none have shown reliable and durable responses.

NEPHROGENIC SYSTEMIC FIBROSIS

Clinical Summary. Nephrogenic systemic fibrosis, previously referred to as nephrogenic fibrosing dermopathy, is a systemic disorder characterized by symmetric thickening of the skin of the trunk and extremities. It was first recognized in a group of renal transplant patients in 1997 (176). The nomenclature changed when respiratory symptoms and related cardiac changes were recognized. All patients have some degree of renal impairment (177). Initially, dialysis was suspected as a predisposing factor; however, up to 10% of patients had never received dialysis (178). There are equal sex and age distributions, and children have been affected. The cause is believed to be exposure to low-stability gadolinium-based contrast agents in association with impaired renal function. Genetic predisposition may be a factor as well (179,180).

Clinically, nephrogenic systemic fibrosis presents as limited or widespread areas of symmetric thickening and hardening of the skin that may resemble scleroderma. The borders of involved

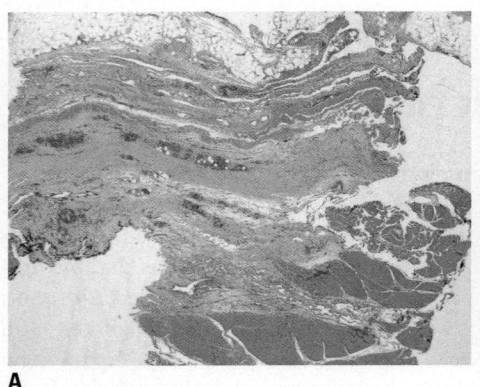 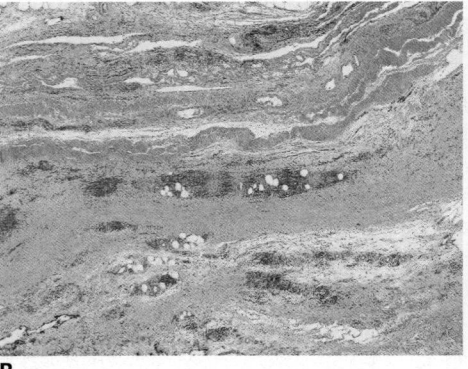 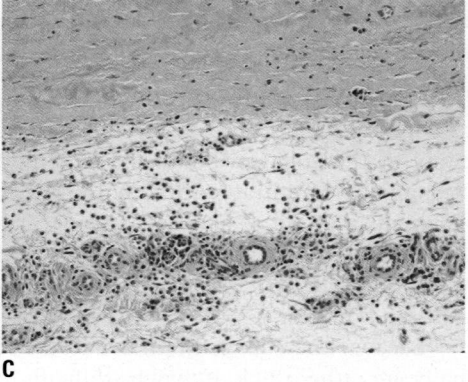

A   **B**   **C**

Figure 10-15 Eosinophilic fasciitis. **A:** A deep biopsy including fascia. The subcutaneous septum and the fascia appear thickened and contain an inflammatory infiltrate. **B:** A widened fascia contains an interstitial inflammatory infiltrate and alternating sclerosis that extends to involve the adipose tissue. **C:** Among sclerotic and edematous bands of collagen is an infiltrate composed of lymphocytes, plasma cells, and conspicuous eosinophils.

areas may be sharply demarcated, serpentine, or ameboid. The skin becomes smooth and shiny or may acquire a peau d'orange appearance. Involvement over joints may lead to contractures. Although typically asymptomatic, patients may complain of muscular weakness, pruritus, and pain (178,180–182). In contrast to scleromyxedema, the face is typically spared. Pulmonary involvement may give rise to respiratory symptoms. Muscle weakness occurs with the involvement of skeletal muscles and fascia. Patients with muscle weakness may have sensory motor polyneuropathy by electromyography and nerve conduction

studies. Although cardiac fibrosis has been reported, impaired cardiac function has not been documented (182–185).

Histopathology. Histopathologic findings of nephrogenic systemic fibrosis may be subtle and require incisional biopsies to include fascia (Fig. 10-16A–C). Sections show spindled fibroblasts that extend into subcutaneous septa and subjacent fascia (Fig 10-16B). Collagen bundles are thickened. Cytoplasmic processes of fibrocytes surround collagen bundles. Such areas may demonstrate factor XIIIa-positive stellate fibroblastic cells and CD68-positive multinucleated giant cells (Fig. 10-16C–E).

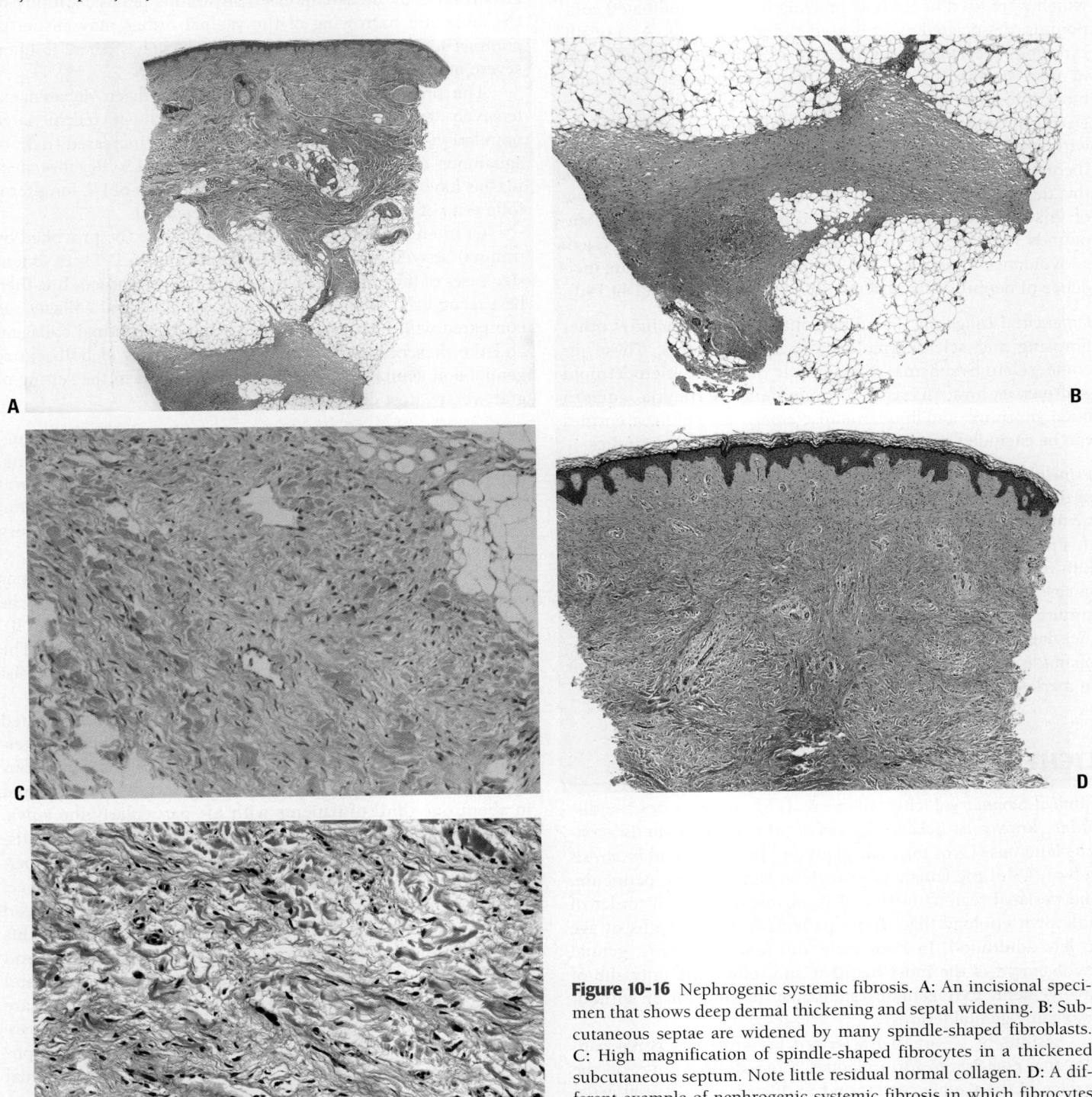

Figure 10-16 Nephrogenic systemic fibrosis. **A:** An incisional specimen that shows deep dermal thickening and septal widening. **B:** Subcutaneous septae are widened by many spindle-shaped fibroblasts. **C:** High magnification of spindle-shaped fibrocytes in a thickened subcutaneous septum. Note little residual normal collagen. **D:** A different example of nephrogenic systemic fibrosis in which fibrocytes are distributed diffusely throughout the dermis. **E:** High magnification shows multinucleated fibroblastic cells. Note the spindle-shaped fibrocyte proliferation and thickened collagen bundles with adjacent clefting.

Immunohistochemical stains show fibrocyte reactivity with CD34 in a membranous pattern and procollagen I in a cytoplasmic pattern (178,179). Such cells may represent a class of circulating fibrocytes that are home to areas of cutaneous injury and play a crucial role in wound healing. One study showed the presence of myofibroblastic cells in early lesions of nephrogenic systemic fibrosis (186).

Pathogenesis. In vitro and *in vivo* studies have been undertaken to explain the etiopathogenesis of nephrogenic systemic fibrosis. It appears that low-stability gadolinium–chelate complexes, which were used in contrast imaging instead of iodinated compounds, dissociated and released gadolinium ions. As a result, cytokines are released by the free or complexed gadolinium, in turn stimulating peripheral blood monocytes. Stimulated monocytes activate fibroblasts, resulting in fibrosis of the skin. Detection and quantification of gadolinium in skin biopsies with synchrotron x-ray fluorescence spectroscopy support the theory that tissue deposits of gadolinium are associated with the development of tissue fibrosis (187,188). As awareness of this disorder has increased and alternate gadolinium compounds have been administered under strict guidelines (such as avoidance in patients undergoing chronic dialysis), the incidence of nephrogenic systemic fibrosis has declined (189,190).

Differential Diagnosis. The differential diagnosis includes other fibrosing and sclerodermoid cutaneous disorders. These include scleromyxedema, eosinophilic fasciitis, sclerodermoid graft-versus-host disease, sclerodermoid porphyria cutanea tarda, morphea, and lipodermatosclerosis. Most of these entities can be excluded based on the history and laboratory studies.

Principles of Management: Owing to the elucidation of the cause of the disease and its rarity, there are numerous case studies of treatments but no controlled trials. The primary treatment at this point is prevention, through careful avoidance of gadolinium in patients with renal failure, and adequate IV hydration in cases where its use cannot be avoided. Treatments in the literature have included extracorporeal photopheresis, imatinib mesylate, UVA1, systemic steroids, plasmapheresis, cyclophosphamide, and topical steroids. Renal transplantation may result in marked improvements in appropriate patients.

LICHEN SCLEROSUS ET ATROPHICUS

Clinical Summary. Lichen sclerosus (LS) encompasses the disorders known as *lichen sclerosus et atrophicus, balanitis xerotica obliterans* (LS of the male glans and prepuce), and *kraurosis vulvae* (LS of the female labia majora, labia minora, perineum, and perianal region) (191). LS is an inflammatory disorder of unknown etiology that affects patients from 6 months of age to late adulthood. In both male and female patients, genital involvement is the most frequent and, often, the only site of involvement. Extragenital lesions may occur with or without coexisting genital lesions.

Lesions of LS are characterized by white polygonal papules that coalesce to form plaques. Comedo-like plugs on the surface of the plaque correspond to dilated appendageal ostia. The plugs may disappear as the lesion ages, leaving a smooth, porcelain-white plaque. Solitary or generalized lesions may become bullous and hemorrhagic.

In male patients, involvement of the glans and prepuce often results in phimosis. Although the literature is dominated by reports of LS in incompletely or uncircumcised men (192), occurrences in circumcised men are reported as well (193). Neoplasms have been infrequently documented in association with LS; however, a cause-and-effect relationship has not been established.

In female patients, contiguous involvement of the labial, perineal, and anal areas has been described clinically as "figure 8" or "keyhole" lesions (194). Many cases of childhood LS in girls resolve by menarche (195). If lesions persist, atrophy of the labia and narrowing of the vaginal orifice may ensue. In contrast to LS of the skin, which rarely itches, there is often severe pruritus in the vulvar region.

The premalignant potential in LS has been debated extensively and remains ill-defined. The most recent large population-based study detected a small increased risk of squamous cell carcinoma in patients with LS. Because neoplasms have arisen in areas adjacent to lesions of LS, long-term follow-up of patients with LS is recommended.

Of interest, lesions of LS may koebnerize (be provoked by trauma) as well as coexist with morphea (196,197). In extensive cases of morphea, LS may become superimposed. It is then best recognized by finding pale superficial dermal collagen, as compared with hypocellular compacted deep dermal collagen, and the presence of follicular plugging. Cases of both extragenital and genital LS have also been reported in the setting of graft-versus-host disease (198).

Histopathology. The salient histopathologic findings in cutaneous lesions of LS are (a) hyperkeratosis with follicular plugging, (b) atrophy of the stratum malpighii with hydropic degeneration of basal cells, (c) pronounced edema and homogenization of the collagen in the upper dermis, and (d) an inflammatory infiltrate in the mid-dermis.

The hyperkeratosis is so marked that the stratum corneum is often thicker than the atrophic stratum malpighii, which may be reduced to a few layers of flattened keratinocytes (Fig. 10-17A, B). The basal layer keratinocytes show hydropic degeneration. The rete ridges often are completely absent, although they may persist in a few areas and show irregular downward proliferation.

Keratotic plugging of appendageal ostia is often associated with atrophy and disappearance of appendageal structures. Keratotic plugging is not apparent in mucosal lesions. Squamous hyperplasia adjacent to the atrophic epidermis can be found in about one-third of patients with LS, particularly the vulva. There may be varying degrees of maturation disarray with disorderly arrangement of the keratinocytes and enlarged, hyperchromatic nuclei giving the epithelium a dysplastic appearance.

Beneath the epidermis, there is characteristically a broad zone of pronounced lymphedema (Fig. 10-17A, B). Within this zone, the collagenous fibers are swollen and homogeneous and contain only a few nuclei. They stain poorly with eosin and other connective tissue stains. The blood and lymph vessels are dilated, and there may be areas of hemorrhage. Elastic fibers are sparse and, in old lesions, are absent within the area of lymphedema (199). In areas of severe lymphedema, subepidermal blistering may lead to clinically visible bullae (200). Shrinkage within the area of lymphedema may occur during the process of dehydration of the specimen, resulting in the formation of pseudobullae, which often are located intradermally.

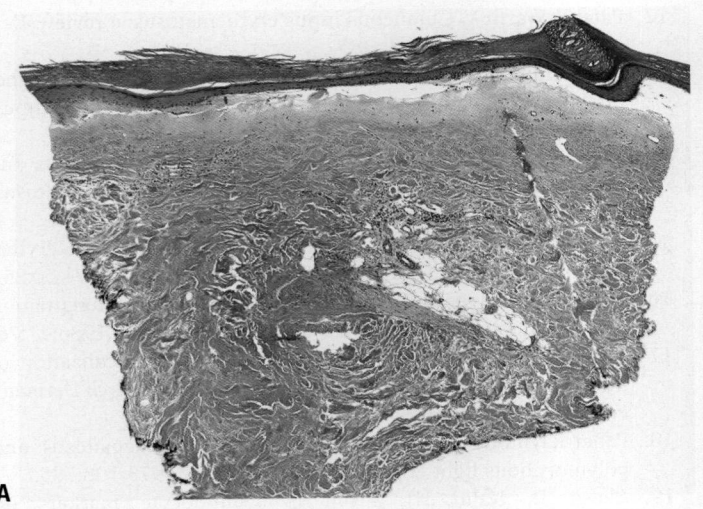
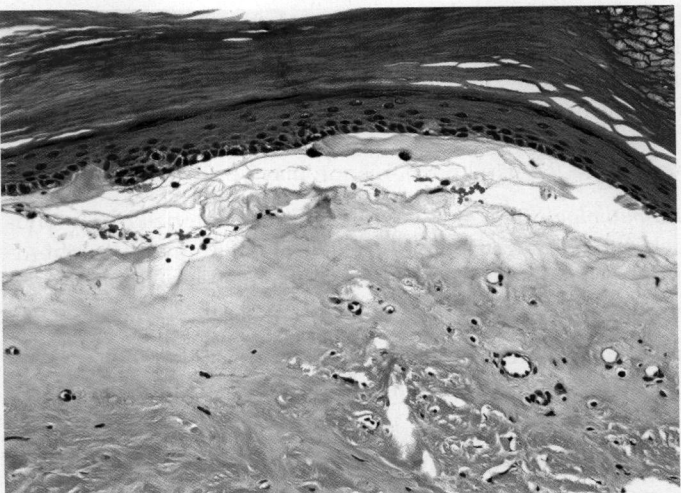

Figure 10-17 Lichen sclerosus. **A:** Lichen sclerosus showing a subepidermal zone of pallor. A "tri-layered" or "striped" appearance: compact hyperorthokeratotic scale and atrophic epidermis (dark pink/red), a pale dermis (white), and subjacent, variably dense interstitial lymphocytic inflammatory infiltrate (blue) delineating the depth of this process. **B:** An established lesion, showing a thick hyperkeratotic scale, an atrophic epidermis, and pale superficial dermal stroma with rare lymphocytes and plasma cells. A cleft-like space separates an atrophic epidermis from a pale dermis.

Except in lesions of long duration, an inflammatory infiltrate is present in the dermis. The earlier the lesion, the more superficial is the location of the infiltrate. In very early lesions and at the periphery of somewhat older lesions, a lichenoid inflammatory infiltrate may be found in the uppermost dermis, in direct apposition to the basal layer. Shortly thereafter, a narrow zone of edema and homogenization of the collagen displaces the inflammatory infiltrate further down, so that, in well-developed lesions, the infiltrate is found in the mid-dermis. The infiltrate can be patchy, but it is often bandlike or lichenoid and composed of lymphoid cells admixed with plasma cells and histiocytes. In well-developed lesions in which the infiltrate is slight or absent, the collagen bundles in the midportion and lower dermis may appear swollen, homogeneous, and eosinophilic, thus appearing sclerotic (hence lichen *sclerosus*). Cases of overlap of morphea and LS may be seen and demonstrate the histopathologic changes of both disorders in their respective locations of the dermis.

Pathogenesis. Studies suggest an increased rate of matrix turnover or a dysregulated remodeling response in LS. There are reports of increased dermal matrix proteins tenascin and fibrinogen, which serve as scaffold proteins on which new collagen is deposited. Although, similar increases in tenascin and fibrinogen have been demonstrated in scleroderma and morphea, suggesting that this is may be a nonspecific change (201).

Investigations into the presence of papillomavirus in vulvar and penile LS have shown no relationship between the two. One study showed 26.5% of cases of vulvar LS to contain Epstein–Barr virus with polymerase chain reaction. A causal relationship has not been established (202,203).

In the epidermis, intercellular edema separates epidermal cells that show degenerative changes. There is nearly a complete absence of melanosomes within the keratinocytes. Immunoperoxidase and Fontana–Masson stains of melanocytes have shown that there is both a loss of melanocytes and decreased transfer of melanosomes to keratinocytes (204). In contrast to morphea, where the basement membrane zone is continuous,

in LS numerous invaginations and holes have been noted at the level of the lamina lucida and lamina densa (204,205).

Differential Diagnosis. Very early lesions may resemble lichen planus because of the apposition of the inflammatory infiltrate to the basal layer. However, the basal cells are not replaced by flattened squamous cells as in lichen planus but appear hydropic, and a subepidermal zone of edema usually has already begun to form in some areas in LS.

Old lesions of LS may resemble morphea, with thickening and eosinophilia of the collagen bundles in the midportion and lower dermis and only a slight inflammatory infiltrate. Nevertheless, the epidermis in morphea, although it may be thin, shows neither hydropic degeneration of the basal cells nor follicular plugging, and the upper dermis in morphea has intact elastic fibers and shows no edema. In lesions in which LS develops either secondarily to morphea or simultaneously with it, there are, in addition to the epidermal and subepidermal changes of LS, changes indicative of morphea in the lower dermis and in the subcutaneous fat. A definite diagnosis of both LS and morphea in the same lesion can be made only if both superficial and deep dermal collagen abnormalities are detected (206).

Principles of Management: Topical corticosteroids are the mainstay of therapy in LS. Use of high-potency topical steroids for long periods of time is the primary treatment. Calcineurin inhibitors tacrolimus and pimecrolimus have been used in steroid-resistant disease or as steroid-sparing agents. Calcineurin inhibitors should be used with caution, however, because of concerns regarding malignant potential with the use of these agents and the potential of development of squamous cell carcinoma in lesions of LS (207).

FIBROBLASTIC RHEUMATISM

Clinical Summary. This rare condition is characterized by a combination of progressive inflammatory arthritis and fibrotic nodules typically involving the skin of the hands. It may occur in children as well as adults. Patients typically present with the sudden onset of polyarthralgia and develop a progressive inflammatory polyarthritis, with cutaneous nodules typically in the form of periungual papules that may mimic multicentric reticulohistiocytosis. Patches or plaques of erythema, sclerodactyly, and Raynaud phenomenon may be associated findings.

Histopathology. The skin nodules are characterized by mononuclear cell infiltrates, fibroblastic proliferation with myofibroblastic differentiation (208,209), dermal fibrosis with thickened collagen fibers, and decreased or absent elastic fibers.

Pathogenesis. The pathogenesis of fibroblastic rheumatism is unknown. There are no significant laboratory findings.

Differential Diagnosis. The differential diagnosis includes rheumatoid nodules and rheumatoid arthritis, which show different histopathologic and serologic findings.

Principles of Management: This condition is variably but often inexorably progressive, but it may be responsive to immunosuppressive therapy, especially in its early stages (210). Corticosteroids and methotrexate are the mainstays of therapy. Earlier therapeutic intervention correlates with a better response.

ACKNOWLEDGMENT

The Authors and Editors gratefully acknowledge the contributions of Christine Jaworsky and Harry Winfield to previous editions of this Chapter.

REFERENCES

1. Albrecht J, Berlin JA, Braverman IM, et al. Dermatology position paper on the revision of the 1982 ACR criteria for systemic lupus erythematosus. *Lupus.* 2004;13:839–849.
2. Tan EM, Cohen AS, Fries JF, et al. The 1982 revised criteria for the classification of systemic lupus erythematosus. *Arthritis Rheum.* 1982;25:1271.
3. Hochberg MC. Updating the American College of Rheumatology revised criteria for the classification of systemic lupus erythematosus [letter]. *Arthritis Rheum.* 1997;40:1725.
4. Petri M, Orbai AM, Alarcon GS, Gordon C, et al. Derivation and validation of the Systemic Lupus International Collaborating Clinics classification criteria for systemic lupus erythematosus. *Arthritis Rheum.* 2012;64:2677–86.
5. Aringer M, Costenbader K, Daikh D, et al. 2019. European League Against Rheumatism/American College of Rheumatology classification criteria for systemic lupus erythematosus. *Arthritis Rheumatol.* 2019;71(9):1400–1412.
6. Ginzler EM, Schorn K. Outcome and prognosis in systemic lupus erythematosus. *Rheum Dis Clin North Am.* 1988;14:67.
7. Zintzaras E, Voulgarelis M, Moutsopoulos HM. The risk of lymphoma development in autoimmune diseases: a meta-analysis. *Arch Intern Med.* 2005;165:2337–2344.
8. David-Bajar KM, Bennion SD, DeSpain JD, Golitz LE, Lee LA. Clinical, histologic, and immunofluorescent distinctions between subacute cutaneous lupus erythematosus and discoid lupus erythematosus. *J Invest Dermatol.* 1992;99:251.
9. Jerdan MS, Hood AF, Moore GW, Callen JP. Histopathologic comparison of the subsets of lupus erythematosus. *Arch Dermatol.* 1990;126:52.
10. Uitto J, Santa-Cruz DJ, Eisen AZ, Leone P. Verrucous lesions in patients with discoid lupus erythematosus. *Br J Dermatol.* 1978;98:507.
11. de Berker D, Dissaneyeka M, Burge S. The sequelae of chronic cutaneous lupus erythematosus. *Lupus.* 1992;1:181.
12. Patel P, Werth V. Cutaneous lupus erythematosus: a review. *Dermatol Clin.* 2002;20:373–385.
13. O'Loughlin S, Schroeter AL, Jordon RE. A study of lupus erythematosus with particular reference to generalized discoid lupus. *Br J Dermatol.* 1978;99:1.
14. Millard LG, Rowell NR. Abnormal laboratory test results and their relationship to prognosis in discoid lupus erythematosus. *Arch Dermatol.* 1979;115:1055.
15. Estes D, Christian CL. The natural history of systemic lupus erythematosus by prospective analysis. *Medicine (Baltimore).* 1971;50:85.
16. Vinciullo C. Hypertrophic lupus erythematosus: differentiation from squamous cell carcinoma. *Australas J Dermatol.* 1986;27:76.
17. Ueki H, Wolff HH, Braun-Falco O. Cutaneous localization of human gamma globulins in lupus erythematosus. *Arch Dermatol Forsch.* 1974;248:297.
18. Panet-Raymond G, Johnson WC. Lupus erythematosus and polymorphous light eruption. *Arch Dermatol.* 1973;108:785.
19. Akasu R, Kahn HJ, From L. Lymphocyte markers on formalin-fixed tissue in Jessner's lymphocytic infiltrate and lupus erythematosus. *J Cutan Pathol.* 1992;19:59.
20. Ko CJ, Srivastava B, Braverman I, Antaya RJ, McNiff JM. Hypertrophic lupus erythematosus: the diagnostic utility of CD123 staining. *J Cutan Pathol.* 2011;38(11):889–892.
21. Ruiz H, Sanchez JL. Tumid lupus erythematosus. *Am J Dermatopathol.* 1999;12:356.
22. Alexiades-Armenakas MR, Baldassano M, Bince BH, et al. Tumid lupus erythematosus: criteria for classification with immunohistochemical analysis. *Arthritis Rheum.* 2003;49:494–500.
23. Kuhn A, Sonntag M, Ruzicka T, Lehmann P, Megahed M. Histopathologic findings in lupus erythematosus tumidus: review of 80 patients. *J Am Acad Dermatol.* 2003;48(6):901–908.
24. Park HS, Choi JW, Kim BK, Cho KH. Lupus erythematosus panniculitis: clinicopathological, immunophenotypic, and molecular studies. *Am J Dermatopathol.* 2010;32(1):24–30.
25. Magro CM, Crowson AN, Kovatich AJ, Burns F. Lupus profundus, indeterminate lymphocytic lobular panniculitis and subcutaneous T-cell lymphoma: a spectrum of subcuticular T-cell lymphoid dyscrasia. *J Cutan Pathol.* 2001;28:235.
26. Gilliam JN, Sontheimer RD. Distinctive cutaneous subsets in the spectrum of lupus erythematosus. *J Am Acad Dermatol.* 1981;4:471–475.
27. Chen SJT, Tse JY, Harms PW, Hristov AC, Chan MP. Utility of CD123 immunohistochemistry in differentiating lupus erythematosus from cutaneous T cell lymphoma. *Histopathology.* 2019;74:908.
28. Sontheimer RD. Subacute cutaneous lupus erythematosus: a decade's perspective. *Med Clin North Am.* 1989;73:1073.
29. Font J, Cervera R. 1982 revised criteria for classification of systemic lupus erythematosus—ten years later. *Lupus.* 1993;2:339–341.
30. Grönhagen CM, Fored CM, Linder M, Granath F, Nyberg F. Subacute cutaneous lupus erythematosus and its association with drugs: a population-based matched case-control study of 234 patients in Sweden. *Br J Dermatol.* 2012;167(2):296–305.
31. Funke AA, Kulp-Shorten CL, Callen JP. Subacute cutaneous lupus erythematosus exacerbated or induced by chemotherapy. *Arch Dermatol.* 2010;146(10):1113–1116.
32. Peñate Y, Guillermo N, Rodríguez J, et al. Histopathologic characteristics of neonatal cutaneous lupus erythematosus: description of five cases and literature review. *J Cutan Pathol.* 2009;36(6):660–667.
33. Lee LA. Neonatal lupus erythematosus. *J Invest Dermatol.* 1993;100:9S.
34. Izmirly PM, Buyon JP, Saxena A. Neonatal lupus: advances in understanding pathogenesis and identifying treatments of cardiac disease. *Curr Opin Rheumatol.* 2012;24(5):466–472.
35. Provost TT. Subsets in systemic lupus erythematosus. *J Invest Dermatol.* 1979;72:110.
36. Gilliam JN. Systemic Lupus Erythematosus and the Skin. In: Lahita RG, ed. *Systemic Lupus Erythematosus.* Wiley; 1987:615.
37. Callen JP. Chronic cutaneous lupus erythematosus. *Arch Dermatol.* 1982;118:412.

38. Mascart-Lemone F, Hauptmann G, Goetz J, et al. Genetic deficiency of C4 presenting with recurrent infections and a systemic lupus erythematosus-like disease. *Am J Med.* 1983;75:295.

39. Tappeiner G, Hintner H, Scholz S, Albert E, Linert J, Wolff K. Systemic lupus erythematosus in hereditary deficiency of the fourth component of complement. *J Am Acad Dermatol.* 1982;7:66.

40. Zeitouni NC, Funaro D, Cloutier RA, Gagné E, Claveau J. Redefining Rowell's syndrome. *Br J Dermatol.* 2000;142(2):343–346.

41. Kitamura Y, Hatamochi A, Hamasaki Y, Ikeda H, Yamazaki S. Association between eosinophilic fasciitis and systemic lupus erythematosus. *J Dermatol.* 2007;34(2):150–152.

42. Baffoni L, Frisoni M, Maccaferri M, Ferri S. Systemic lupus erythematosus and eosinophilic fasciitis: an unusual association. *Clin Rheumatol.* 1995;14(5):591–592.

43. Provost TT, Zone JJ, Synkowski D, Maddison PJ, Reichlin M. Unusual cutaneous manifestations of systemic lupus erythematosus, I: urticaria-like lesions—correlation with clinical and serologic abnormalities. *J Invest Dermatol.* 1980;75:495.

44. Callen JP. Mucocutaneous changes in patients with lupus erythematosus: the relationship of these lesions to systemic disease. *Rheum Dis Clin North Am.* 1988;14:79.

45. Camisa C. Vesiculobullous systemic lupus erythematosus: a report of four cases. *J Am Acad Dermatol.* 1988;18:93.

46. Gammon WR, Briggaman RA. Bullous SLE: a phenotypically distinctive but immunologically heterogeneous bullous disorder. *J Invest Dermatol.* 1993;100:28S.

47. Dooley MA, Aranow C, Ginzler EM. Review of ACR renal criteria in systemic lupus erythematosus. *Lupus.* 2004;13:857–860.

48. Asherson RA, Baguley E, Pal C, Hughes GR. Antiphospholipid syndrome: five year follow up. *Ann Rheum Dis.* 1991;50:805.

49. Bick RL, Baker WF Jr. The antiphospholipid and thrombosis syndromes. *Med Clin North Am.* 1994;78:667.

50. Angotti C. Immunology of cutaneous lupus erythematosus. *Clin Dermatol.* 2004;22:105–112.

51. Christensen SR, Shlomchik MJ. Regulation of lupus-related autoantibody production and clinical disease by Toll-like receptors. *Semin Immunol.* 2007;19:11–23.

52. Craft J, Choi J, Kim ST. The pathogenesis of systemic lupus erythematosus, an update. *Curr Opin Immunol.* 2012;24:651–657.

53. Gutierrez-Andrianzen OA, Koutouzov S, Mota RMS, das Chagas Medeiros MM, Bach JF, de Holanda Campos H. Diagnostic value of antinucleosome antibodies in the assessment of disease activity of systemic lupus erythematosus: a prospective study comparing antinucleosome with anti-dsDNA antibodies. *J Rheumatol.* 2006;33:8.

54. Tuffanelli DL. Cutaneous immunopathology: recent observations. *J Invest Dermatol.* 1975;65:143.

55. Provost TT, Andres G, Maddison PJ, Reichlin M. Lupus band test in untreated SLE patients. *J Invest Dermatol.* 1980;74:407.

56. Gately LE, Nesbitt LT. Update on immunofluorescent testing in bullous diseases and lupus erythematosus. *Dermatol Clin.* 1994;1:133.

57. Jaworsky C, Murphy GF. Special techniques in dermatology. *Arch Dermatol.* 1989;125:963.

58. Hahn BH. Belimumab for systemic lupus erythematosus. *N Engl J Med.* 2013;368(16):1528–1535.

59. De Souza A, Ali-Shaw T, Strober BE, Franks AG Jr. Successful treatment of subacute lupus erythematosus with ustekinumab. *Arch Dermatol.* 2011;147(8):896–898.

60. Jessner M, Kanof NB. Lymphocytic infiltration of the skin. *Arch Dermatol Syphiligr.* 1953;68:447.

61. Toonstra J, Wildschut A, Boer J, et al. Jessner's lymphocytic infiltration of the skin. *Arch Dermatol.* 1989;125:1525.

62. Higgins CR, Wakeel RA, Cerio R. Childhood Jessner's lymphocytic infiltrate of the skin. *Br J Dermatol.* 1994;131:99.

63. Tomasini D, Mentzel T, Hantschke M, et al. Plasmacytoid dendritic cells: an overview of their presence and distribution in different inflammatory skin diseases, with special emphasis on Jessner's lymphocytic infiltrate of the skin and cutaneous lupus erythematosus. *J Cutan Pathol.* 2010;37(11):1132–1139.

64. Rémy-Leroux V, Léonard F, Lambert D, et al. Comparison of histopathologic-clinical characteristics of Jessner's lymphocytic infiltration of the skin and lupus erythematosus tumidus: multicenter study of 46 cases. *J Am Acad Dermatol.* 2008;58(2):217–223.

65. Konttinen YT, Bergroth V, Johansson E, Nordström D, Malmström M. A long-term clinicopathologic survey of patients with Jessner's lymphocytic infiltration of the skin. *J Invest Dermatol.* 1987;89:205.

66. Schepis C, Lentini M, Siragusa M, Batolo D. ACE-inhibitor-induced drug eruption resembling lymphocytic infiltration of Jessner-Kanof and lupus erythematosus tumidus. *Dermatology.* 2004;208:354–355.

67. Nolden S, Casper C, Kuhn A, Petereit HF. Jessner-Kanof lymphocytic infiltration of the skin associated with glatiramer acetate. *Mult Scler.* 2005;11(2):245–248.

68. Dippel E, Poenitz N, Klemke CD, Orfanos CE, Goerdt S. Familial lymphocytic infiltration of the skin: histochemical and molecular analysis in three brothers. *Dermatology.* 2002;204:12–16.

69. Willemze R, Dijkstra A, Meijer CJ. Lymphocytic infiltrate of the skin (Jessner): a T cell lymphoproliferative disease. *Br J Dermatol.* 1984;110:523–529.

70. Dietrich A, Ollert MW, Eckert F, et al. Palpable migratory arciform erythema. *Arch Dermatol.* 1997;133:763–766.

71. Sharp GC, Irvin WS, Tan EM, Gould RG, Holman HR. Mixed connective tissue disease: an apparently distinct rheumatic disease syndrome associated with a specific antibody to an extractable nuclear antigen (ENA). *Am J Med.* 1972;52:148.

72. Ueda N, Mimura K, Meada H, et al. Mixed connective tissue disease with fatal pulmonary hypertension and a review of the literature. *Virchows Arch A Pathol Anat Histopathol.* 1984;404:335.

73. Burrows NP, Bhogal BS, Russel Jones R, Black MM. Clinicopathological significance of cutaneous epidermal nuclear staining by direct immunofluorescence. *J Cutan Pathol.* 1993;20:159.

74. Ulmer A, Kötter I, Pfaff A, Fierlbeck G. Efficacy of pulsed intravenous immunoglobulin therapy in mixed connective tissue disease. *J Am Acad Dermatol.* 2002;46(1):123–127.

75. Callen JP, Tuffanelli DL, Provost TT. Collagen vascular disease: an update. *J Am Acad Dermatol.* 1994;28:477.

76. Bohan A, Peter JB. Polymyositis and dermatomyositis. *N Engl J Med.* 1975;292:344–347, 403–407.

77. Morganroth PA, Kreider ME, Okawa J, Taylor L, Werth VP. Interstitial lung disease in classic and skin-predominant dermatomyositis: a retrospective study with screening recommendations. *Arch Dermatol.* 2010;146(7):729–738.

78. Shakshouk H, Deschaine MA, Wetter DA, Drage LA, Ernste FC, Lehman JS. Clinical and histopathological features of adult patients with dermatomyositis and MDA5 autoantibody seropositivity status, as determined by commercial-based testing: a retrospective, single-institution comparative cohort study. *Clin Exp Dermatol.* 2022;47(2):282–288. doi:10.1111/ced.14870

79. Cobos GA, Femia A, Vleugels RA. Dermatomyositis: an update on diagnosis and treatment. *Am J Clin Dermatol.* 2020;21:339.

80. Huemer C, Kitson H, Malleson PN, et al. Lipodystrophy in patients with juvenile dermatomyositis—evaluation of clinical and metabolic abnormalities. *J Rheumatol.* 2001;28:610–615.

81. Requena L, Grilli R, Soriano L, Escalonilla P, Fariña C, Martín L. Dermatomyositis with a pityriasis rubra pilaris–like eruption: a little-known distinctive cutaneous manifestation of dermatomyositis. *Br J Dermatol.* 1997;136:768–771.

82. Kaufmann R, Greiner D, Schmidt P, Wolter M. Dermatomyositis presenting as plaque-like mucinosis. *Br J Dermatol.* 1998;138:889–892.

83. Launay D, Hatron PY, Delaporte E, Hachulla E, Devulder B, Piette F. Scleromyxedema (lichen myxedematosus) associated with dermatomyositis. *Br J Dermatol.* 2001;144:359–362.

84. Kimyai-Asadi A, Tausk FA, Nousari HC. A patient with dermatomyositis and linear streaks on the back: centripetal flagellate erythema (CFE) associated with dermatomyositis. *Arch Dermatol.* 2000;136(5):667–670.

85. Bonnetblanc JM, Bernard P, Fayol J. Dermatomyositis and malignancy. *Dermatologica.* 1990;180:212–216.

86. DeWane ME, Waldman R, Lu J. Dermatomyositis: clinical features and pathogenesis. *J Am Acad Dermatol.* 2020;82:267.

87. Chow WH, Gridley G, Mellemkjaer L, McLaughlin JK, Olsen JH, Fraumeni JF Jr. Cancer risk following polymyositis and dermatomyositis: a nationwide cohort study in Denmark. *Cancer Causes Control.* 1995;6:9–13.

88. Hill CL, Zhang Y, Sigurgeirsson B, et al. Frequency of specific cancer types in dermatomyositis and polymyositis: a population-based study. *Lancet.* 2001;357:96–100.

89. Peng J-C, Sheem T-S, Hsu M-M. Nasopharyngeal carcinoma with dermatomyositis: analysis of 12 cases. *Arch Otolaryngol Head Neck Surg.* 1995;121:1298–1301.

90. Janis JF, Winkelmann RK. Histopathology of the skin in dermatomyositis. *Arch Dermatol.* 1968;97:640.

91. Hanno R, Callen JP. Histopathology of Gottron's papules. *J Cutan Pathol.* 1985;12:389.

92. DeGirolami UU, Smith TW. Teaching monograph: pathology of skeletal muscle diseases. *Am J Pathol.* 1982;107:231.

93. Kissel JT, Mendell JR, Rammohan KW. Microvascular deposition of complement membrane attack complex in dermatomyositis. *N Engl J Med.* 1986;314:329.

94. Wainger CK, Lever WF. Dermatomyositis: a report of three cases with postmortem observations. *Arch Dermatol Syph.* 1949;59:196.

95. Targoff IN, Trieu EP, Sontheimer RD. Autoantibodies to 155 kd and Se antigens in patients with clinically-amyopathic dermatomyositis. *Arthritis Rheum.* 2000;43:S194A.

96. Sato S, Kuwana M, Fujita T, Suzuki Y. Anti-CADM-140/MDA5 autoantibody titer correlates with disease activity and predicts disease outcome in patients with dermatomyositis and rapidly progressive interstitial lung disease. *Mod Rheumatol.* 2013;23(3):496–502.

97. Kuwano Y, Asahina A, Watanabe R, Fujimoto M, Ihn H, Tamaki K. Heliotrope-like eruption mimicking dermatomyositis in a patient treated with imatinib mesylate for chronic myeloid leukemia. *Int J Dermatol.* 2006;45(10):1249–1251.

98. Magro CM, Segal JP, Crowson AN, Chadwick P. The phenotypic profile of dermatomyositis and lupus erythematosus: a comparative analysis. *J Cutan Pathol.* 2010;37:659–671.

99. Harrist TJ, Mihm MC Jr. Cutaneous immunopathology: the diagnostic use of direct and indirect immunofluorescence techniques in dermatologic diseases [review]. *Hum Pathol.* 1979;10:625.

100. Bohan A, Peter JB, Bowman RL, Pearson CM. A computer-assisted analysis of 153 patients with polymyositis and dermatomyositis. *Medicine (Baltimore).* 1977;56:255.

101. Braun-Falco O, Marghescu S. Kongenitales teleangiektatisches erythem (Bloom-syndrom) mit diabetes insipidus. *Hautarzt.* 1966;17:155.

102. Lindae ML, Abel EA, Hoppe RT, Wood GS. Poikilodermatous mycosis fungoides and large-plaque parapsoriasis exhibit similar abnormalities of T-cell antigen expression. *Arch Dermatol.* 1988;124:366.

103. Samman PD. The natural history of parapsoriasis en plaques (chronic superficial dermatitis) and prereticulotic poikiloderma. *Br J Dermatol.* 1972;87:405.

104. Steigleder GK. Die poikilodermien-genodermien und genodermatosen? *Arch Dermatol Syph (Berlin).* 1952;194:461.

105. Lindae JL, Connolly SM, Winkelmann RK. Disabling pansclerotic morphea of children. *Arch Dermatol.* 1980;116:169.

106. Ikai K, Tagami H, Imamura S, Hayakawa M. Morphea-like cutaneous changes in a patient with systemic scleroderma. *Dermatologica.* 1979;158:438.

107. Fett N. Scleroderma: nomenclature, etiology, pathogenesis, prognosis, and treatments: facts and controversies. *Clin Dermatol.* 2013;31(4):432–437.

108. Falanga V, Medsger TA Jr, Reichlin M, Rodnan GP. Linear scleroderma: clinical spectrum, prognosis, and laboratory abnormalities. *Ann Intern Med.* 1986;104:849.

109. Dilley JJ, Perry HO. Bilateral linear scleroderma en coup de sabre. *Arch Dermatol.* 1968;97:688.

110. Zulian F, Athreya BH, Laxer R, et al. Juvenile localized scleroderma: clinical and epidemiological features in 750 children—an international study. *Rheumatology (Oxford).* 2005;45:614–620.

111. Tollefson MM, Witman PM. En coup de saber morphea and Parry-Romberg syndrome: a retrospective review of 54 patients. *J Am Acad Dermatol.* 2007;56:257–263.

112. Sommer A, Gambichler T, Bacharach-Buhles M, von Rothenburg T, Altmeyer P, Kreuter A. Clinical and serological characteristics of progressive facial hemiatrophy: a case series of 12 patients. *J Am Acad Dermatol.* 2006;54:227–233.

113. Su WPD, Greene SL. Bullous morphea profunda. *Am J Dermatopathol.* 1986;8:144.

114. Synkowski DR, Lobitz WC Jr, Provost TT. Bullous scleroderma. *Arch Dermatol.* 1981;117:135–137.

115. McNiff JM, Glusac EJ, Lazova RZ, Carroll CB. Morphea limited to the superficial reticular dermis: an under recognized histologic phenomenon. *Am J Dermatopathol.* 1999;21:315.

116. Taylor RM. Sclerosing disorders. In: Farmer ER, Hood AF, eds. *Pathology of the Skin.* Appleton and Lange; 1990:275.

117. O'Leary PA, Montgomery H, Ragsdale WE. Dermatohistopathology of various types of scleroderma [review]. *Arch Dermatol.* 1957;75:78.

118. Walters R, Pulitzer M, Kamino H. Elastic fiber patterns in scleroderma/morphea. *J Cutan Pathol.* 2009;36(9):952–957.

119. Hickman JW, Sheils WS. Progressive facial hemiatrophy. *Arch Intern Med.* 1964;113:716.

120. Buechner SA, Winkelmann RK, Lautenschlager S, Gilli L, Rufli T. Localized scleroderma associated with Borrelia burgdorferi infection: clinical, histologic, and immunohistochemical observations. *J Am Acad Dermatol.* 1993;29:190.

121. Zollinger T, Mertz KD, Schmid M, Schmitt A, Pfaltz M, Kempf W. *Borellia* in granuloma annulare, morphea and lichen sclerosus: aPCR-based study and review of the literature. *J Cutan Pathol.* 2010;37:571–577.

122. Florez-Pollack S, Kunzler E, Jacobe HT. Morphea: current concepts. *Clin Dermatol.* 2018;36:475–486.

123. Maricq HR. Capillary abnormalities, Raynaud's phenomenon, and systemic sclerosis in patients with localized scleroderma. *Arch Dermatol.* 1992;128:630.

124. Medsger TA, Masi AT, Rodnan GP, Benedek TG, Robinson H. Survival with systemic sclerosis (scleroderma). *Ann Intern Med.* 1971;75:369.

125. Torres JE, Sanchez JL. Histopathologic differentiation between localized and systemic scleroderma. *Am J Dermatopathol.* 1998;20(3):242–245.

126. Fleischmajer R, Nedwich A. Generalized morphea. I: Histology of the dermis and subcutaneous tissue. *Arch Dermatol.* 1972; 106:509.

127. Abu-Shakra M, Guillemin F, Lee P. Cancer in systemic sclerosis. *Arthritis Rheum.* 1993;36:460.

128. Tuffanelli DL. Systemic scleroderma. *Med Clin North Am.* 1989;73:1167.

129. Jablonska S, Blaszczyk M, Chorzelski TP, Jarzabek-Chorzelska M, Kumar V, Beutner EH. Clinical relevance of immunologic findings in scleroderma. *Clin Dermatol.* 1993;10:407.

130. Whitfield ML, Finlay DR, Murray JI, et al. Systemic and cell type-specific gene expression patterns in scleroderma skin. *Proc Natl Acad Sci U S A.* 2003;100(21):12319–12324.

131. Prescott RJ, Freemont AJ, Jones CJ, Hoyland J, Fielding P. Sequential dermal microvascular and perivascular changes in the development of scleroderma. *J Pathol.* 1992;166:255.

132. Haustein UF, Herrmann K, Böhme HJ. Pathogenesis of progressive systemic sclerosis [review]. *Int J Dermatol*. 1986;25:286.

133. Helmbold P, Fiedler E, Fischer M, Marsch WCh. Hyperplasia of dermal microvascular pericytes in scleroderma. *J Cutan Pathol*. 2004;31(6):431–440.

134. Toth A, Alpert LI. Progressive systemic sclerosis terminating as periarteritis nodosa. *Arch Pathol*. 1971;92:31.

135. Postlewaithe AE. Connective tissue metabolism including cytokines in scleroderma. *Curr Opin Rheumatol*. 1993;5:766.

136. Rudnicka L, Varga J, Christiano AM, Iozzo RV, Jimenez SA, Uitto J. Elevated expression of type VII collagen in the skin of patients with systemic sclerosis: regulation by transforming growth factor-beta. *J Clin Invest*. 1994;93:1709.

137. Varga J, Rudnicka L, Uitto J. Connective tissue alterations in systemic sclerosis [review]. *Clin Dermatol*. 1994;12:387.

138. Sappino AP, Masouyé I, Saurat JH, Gabbiani G. Smooth muscle differentiation in scleroderma fibroblastic cells. *Am J Pathol*. 1990;137:585.

139. Aiba S, Tabata N, Ohtani H, Tagami H. CD34+ spindle-shaped cells selectively disappear from the skin lesion of scleroderma. *Arch Dermatol*. 1994;130:593.

140. Aeschlimann A, Meyer O, Bourgeois P, et al. Anti-Scl-70 antibodies detected by immunoblotting in progressive systemic sclerosis: specificity and clinical correlations. *Ann Rheum Dis*. 1989;48:992–997.

141. El-Azhary RA, Aponte CC, Nelson AM, Weaver AL, Homburger HA. Antihistone antibodies in linear scleroderma variants. *Int J Dermatol*. 2006;45:1296–1299.

142. Prystowsky SD, Gilliam JN, Tuffanelli D. Epidermal nucleolar IgG deposition in clinically normal skin. *Arch Dermatol*. 1971;114:536.

143. Lapenas D, Rodnan GP, Cavallo T. Immunopathology of the renal vascular lesion of progressive systemic sclerosis (scleroderma). *Am J Pathol*. 1978;91:243.

144. Sahn EE, Garen PD, Silver RM, Maize JC. Scleroderma following augmentation mammoplasty. *Arch Dermatol*. 1990;126:1198.

145. Joly P, Lampert A, Thomine E, Lauret P. Development of pseudobullous morphea and scleroderma-like illness during therapy with L-5 hydroxytryptophan and carbidopa. *J Am Acad Dermatol*. 1991;25:332.

146. Toxic Epidemic Syndrome Study Group. Toxic epidemic syndrome: Spain, 1981. *Lancet*. 1982;2:697.

147. Oursler JR, Farmer ER, Roubenoff R, Mogavero HS, Watson RM. Cutaneous manifestations of the eosinophilia-myalgia syndrome. *Br J Dermatol*. 1992;127:138.

148. Magro CM, Iwenofu H, Nuovo GJ. Paraneoplastic scleroderma-like tissue reactions in the setting of underlying plasma cell dyscrasia: a report of 10 cases. *Am J Dermatopathol*. 2013;35:561–568.

149. Pearson DR, Werth VP, Pappas-Taffer L. Systemic sclerosis: current concepts of skin and systemic manifestations. *Clin Dermatol*. 2018;36:459–474.

150. Reddi DM, Cardona DM, Burchette JL, Puri PK. Scleroderma and IgG$_4$ related disease. *Am J Dermatopathol*. 2013;35:458–462.

151. Kreuter A. Localized scleroderma. *Dermatol Ther*. 2012;25(2):135–147.

152. Alhathlool A, Hein R, Andres C, Ring J, Eberlein B. Post-irradiation morphea: case report and review of the literature. *J Dermatol Case Rep*. 2012;3:73.

153. Walsh N, Rheaume D, Barnes P, Tremaine R, Reardon M. Post-irradiation morphea: an underrecognized complication of treatment for breast cancer. *Hum Pathol*. 2008;39:1680.

154. Spalek M, Jonska-Gmyrek J, Galecki J. Radiation-induced morphea—a literature review. *J Eur Acad Dermatol Venereol*. 2015;29:197.

155. Gonzalez-Ericsson PI, Estrada MV, Al-Rohil R, Sanders ME. Post-irradiation morphoea of the breast: a case report and review of the literature. *Histopathology*. 2018;72:342.

156. Quiroga ML, Woscoff A. L'atrophodermie idiopathique progressive (Pasini-Pierini) et la sclérodermie atypique lilacée non indurée (Gougerot). *Ann Dermatol Syphiligr*. 1961;88:507.

157. Murphy PK, Mymes SR, Fenske NA. Concomitant unilateral idiopathic atrophoderma of Pasini and Pierini (IAPP) and morphea: observations supporting IAPP as a variant of morphea. *Int J Dermatol*. 1990;29:281–283.

158. Kencka D, Blaszczyk M, Jablonska S. Atrophoderma Pasini-Pierini is a primary atrophic abortive morphea. *Dermatology*. 1995;190:203.

159. Buechner SA, Rufli T. Atrophoderma of Pasini and Pierini: clinical and histopathologic findings and antibodies to Borrelia burgdorferi in thirty-four patients. *J Am Acad Dermatol*. 1994;30:441.

160. Lee Y, Oh Y, Ahn SY, Park HY, Choi EH. A case of atrophoderma of Pasini and Pierini associated with Borrelia burgdorferi infection successfully treated with oral doxycycline. *Ann Dermatol*. 2011;23(3):352–356.

161. Shulman L. Diffuse fasciitis with hypergammaglobulinemia and eosinophilia: a new syndrome? [abstract]. *J Rheumatol*. 1974;1:46.

162. Jacob SE, Lodha R, Cohen JJ, Romanelli P, Kirsner RS. Paraneoplastic eosinophilic fasciitis: a case report. *Rheumatol Int*. 2003;23:262–264.

163. Antic M, Lautenschlager S, Itin PH. Eosinophiic fasciitis 30 years after—what do we really know? *Dermatology*. 2006;213:93–101.

164. Freundlich B, Werth VP, Rook AH, et al. L-Tryptophan ingestion associated with eosinophilic fasciitis but not progressive systemic sclerosis. *Ann Int Med*. 1990;112:758.

165. Moulin C, Cavailhes A, Balme B, Skowron F. Eosinophilic fasciitis (Shulman disease): morphoea-like plaques revealing an eosinophilic (Shulman) fasciitis. *Clin Exp Dermatol*. 2009;34(8):e851–e853.

166. Lebeaux D, Sene D. Eosinophilic fasciitis (Shulman disease). *Best Pract Res Clin Rheumatol*. 2012;26(4):449–458.

167. Barriere H, Stalder JF, Berger M, Chupin M, Rodat O. Syndrome de Shulman. *Ann Dermatol Venereol (Stockholm)*. 1980;107:643.

168. Tamura T, Saito Y, Ishikawa H. Diffuse fasciitis with eosinophilia. *Acta Dermato Venereol (Stockholm)*. 1979;59:325.

169. Weinstein D, Schwartz RA. Eosinophilic fasciitis. *Arch Dermatol*. 1978;114:1047.

170. Lupton GP, Goette DK. Localized eosinophilic fasciitis. *Arch Dermatol*. 1979;115:85.

171. Valentini F, Rossiello R, Gualdieri L, Tirri G, Gerster JC, Frenck E. Morphea developing in patients previously affected with eosinophilic fasciitis: report of two cases. *Rheumatol Int*. 1988;8:235–237.

172. Moy AP, Maryamchik E, Nikolskaia OV, et al. Th1-and Th17-polarized immune infiltrates in eosinophilic fasciitis—a potential marker for histopathologic distinction from morphea. *J Cutan Pathol* 2017;44:548.

173. Jablonska S, Hamm G, Kencka D, Sieminska S. Fasciitis eosinophilica, Übergang in eine eigenartige sklerodermie (sklerodermie-fasciitis). *Z Hautkr*. 1984;59:711.

174. Su WPD, Person JR. Morphea profunda. *Am J Dermatopathol*. 1981;3:251.

175. Helfman T, Falanga V. Eosinophilic fasciitis. *Clin Dermatol*. 1994;12:449.

176. LeBoit PE. What nephrogenic fibrosing dermopathy might be. *Arch Dermatol*. 2003;139:928–930.

177. Cowper SE. Nephrogenic systemic fibrosis: the nosological and conceptual evolution of nephrogenic fibrosing dermopathy. *Am J Kidney Dis*. 2005;46:763–765.

178. Cowper SE, Su L, Bhawan J, Robin HS, LeBoit PE. Nephrogenic fibrosing dermopathy. *Am J Dermatopathol*. 2001;23:383–393.

179. Cowper SE, Bucala R. Nephrogenic fibrosing dermopathy: suspect identified, motive unclear. *Am J Dermatopathol*. 2003;25:358.

180. DeHoratius DM, Cowper SE. Nephrogenic systemic fibrosis: an emerging threat among renal patients. *Semin Dial.* 2006;19: 191–194.

181. Mackay-Wiggan JM, Cohen DJ, Hardy MA, Knobler EH, Grossman ME. Nephrogenic fibrosing dermopathy (scleromyxedema-like illness of renal disease). *J Am Acad Dermatol.* 2003;48:55–60.

182. Cowper SE. Nephrogenic fibrosing dermopathy: the first six years. *Curr Opin Rheumatol.* 2003;15:785–790.

183. Cowper SE, Boyer PJ. Nephrogenic systemic fibrosis: an update. *Curr Rheumatol Rep.* 2006;8:151–157.

184. Ortonne N, Lipsker D, Chantrel F, Boehm N, Grosshans E, Cribier B. Presence of CD45RO+ CD34+ cells with collagen synthesis activity in nephrogenic fibrosing dermopathy: a new pathogenic hypothesis. *Br J Dermatol.* 2004;150:1050–1052.

185. Gibson SE, Farver CF, Prayson RA. Multiorgan involvement in nephrogenic fibrosing dermopathy: an autopsy case and review of the literature. *Arch Pathol Lab Med.* 2006;130:209–212.

186. Swartz RD, Crofford LJ, Phan SH, Ike RW, Su LD. Nephrogenic fibrosing dermopathy: a novel cutaneous fibrosing disorder in patients with renal failure. *Am J Med.* 2003;114:563–572.

187. Chopra T, Kandukurti K, Shah S, Ahmed R, Panesar M. Understanding nephrogenic systemic fibrosis. *Int J Nephrol.* 2012;2012: 912189.

188. High WA, Ranville JF, Brown M, Punshon T, Lanzirotti A, Jackson BP. Gadolinium deposition in nephrogenic systemic fibrosis: an examination of tissue using synchrotron x-ray fluorescence spectroscopy. *J Am Acad Dermatol.* 2010;62(1):38–44.

189. Igreja AC, Mesquita KC, Cowper SE, Costa IM. Nephrogenic systemic fibrosis: concepts and perspectives. *An Bras Dermatol.* 2012;87(4):597–607.

190. Wang Y, Alkasab TK, Narin O, et al. Incidence of nephrogenic systemic fibrosis after adoption of restrictive gadolinium-based contrast agent guidelines. *Radiology* 2011;260:105.

191. Meffert JJ, Davis BM, Grimwood RE. Lichen sclerosus. *J Am Acad Dermatol.* 1995;32:393.

192. Ledwig PA, Weigand DA. Late circumcision and lichen sclerosus et atrophicus of the penis. *J Am Acad Dermatol.* 1989;20:211.

193. Loening-Baucke V. Lichen sclerosus et atrophicus in children. *Am J Dis Child.* 1991;145:1058.

194. Clark JA, Muller SA. Lichen sclerosus et atrophicus in children. *Arch Dermatol.* 1967;95:476.

195. Helm KF, Gibson LE, Muller SA. Lichen sclerosus et atrophicus in children and young adults. *Pediatr Dermatol.* 1991;8:97.

196. Pock L. Koebner phenomenon in lichen sclerosus et atrophicus [letter]. *Dermatologica.* 1990;181:76.

197. Shono S, Imura M, Ota M, Osaku A, Shinomiya S, Toda K. Lichen sclerosus et atrophicus, morphea and coexistence of both diseases: histologic studies using lectins. *Arch Dermatol.* 1991;127:1352.

198. Schaffer JV, McNiff JM, Seropian S, Cooper DL, Bolognia JL. Lichen sclerosus and eosinophilic fasciitis as manifestations of chronic graft-versus-host disease: expanding the sclerodermoid spectrum. *J Am Acad Dermatol.* 2005;53:591–601.

199. Steigleder GK, Raab WP. Lichen sclerosus et atrophicus. *Arch Dermatol.* 1961;84:219.

200. Gottschalk HR, Cooper ZK. Lichen sclerosus et atrophicus with bullous lesions and extensive involvement. *Arch Dermatol.* 1947;55:433.

201. Farrell AM, Dean D, Charnock FM, Wojnarowska F. Alterations in distribution of tenascin, fibronectin and fibrinogen in vulval lichen sclerosus. *Clin Lab Invest.* 2000;201:223–229.

202. Aide S, Lattario FR, Almeida G, do Val IC, da Costa Carvalho M. Epstein-Barr virus and human papilloma virus infection in vulvar lichen sclerosus. *J Low Genit Tract Dis.* 2010;14(4):319–322.

203. D'Hauwers KW, Depuydt CE, Bogers JJ, et al. Human papillomavirus, lichen sclerosus and penile cancer: a study in Belgium. *Vaccine.* 2012;30(46):6573–6577.

204. Carlson JA, Grabowski R, Mu XC, Del Rosario A, Malfetano J, Slominski A. Possible mechanisms of hypopigmentation in lichen sclerosus. *Am J Dermatopathol.* 2002;24:97–107.

205. Kowalewski C, Kozlowska A, Gorska M, et al. Alterations of basement membrane zone and cutaneous microvasculature in morphea and extragenital lichen sclerosus. *Am J Dermatopathol.* 2005;27:489–496.

206. Uitto J, Santa Cruz DJ, Bauer EA, Eisen AZ. Morphea and lichen sclerosus et atrophicus: clinical and histopathologic studies in patients with combined features. *J Am Acad Dermatol.* 1980;3:271.

207. Yesudian PD. The role of calcineurin inhibitors in the management of lichen sclerosus. *Am J Clin Dermatol.* 2009;10(5):313–318.

208. Lee JM, Sundel RP, Liang MG. Fibroblastic rheumatism: case report and review of the literature. *Pediatr Dermatol.* 2002;19:532–535.

209. du Toit R, Schneider JW, Whitelaw DA. Fibroblastic rheumatism. *J Clin Rheumatol.* 2006;12:201–203.

210. Jurado SA, Alvin GK, Selim MA, et al. Fibroblastic rheumatism: a report of 4 cases with potential therapeutic implications. *J Am Acad Dermatol.* 2012;66(6):959–965.

Cutaneous Toxicities of Drugs

CUONG V. NGUYEN, JONATHAN L. CURRY, AND EMILY Y. CHU

Chapter

11

INTRODUCTION

The skin is the most common site of drug reactions (1). Cutaneous eruptions attributed to drugs occur at a rate of 0.1% to 2% of all hospitalized patients, with a higher rate of 12% reported in the intensive care setting (2,3). Morbilliform and urticarial eruptions are the most common patterns of cutaneous adverse drug eruptions. Skin eruptions are most often seen in response to antibiotics and antiepileptics, although they can occur in the setting of almost any drug or treatment regimen (4). Fortunately, the incidence of severe cutaneous adverse reactions (SCAR) (Stevens–Johnson syndrome [SJS], toxic epidermal necrolysis [TEN], exfoliative dermatitis, and drug reaction with eosinophilia and systemic symptoms [DRESS]) is lower. These severe reactions are attributed most commonly to the same class of drugs, although the incidence ranges from 1 in 1,000–10,000 for DRESS to nearly 1–2 in 1,000,000 for TEN (5). The risk of developing an adverse drug reaction is higher in women and patients with altered immune systems, in particular in patients with systemic lupus erythematosus (SLE) and acquired immunodeficiency syndrome (5,6).

Drug-related eruptions are attributed to immunologic as well as nonimmunologic mechanisms. Nonimmunologic mechanisms encompass the pharmacokinetics of drugs, such as absorption, plasma protein binding, distribution, metabolism, elimination, and oxidative stress (7). Genetic factors influence metabolic pathways, specifically oxidation, hydrolysis, and acetylation, and are suggested to be the mechanisms of toxicity reactions, such as those that occur in sulfonamide and anticonvulsant toxicities (8). Theories regarding immunologic mechanisms of drug-induced disease include (a) cell-mediated reactions to altered cell-surface proteins, affecting lymphocytic response; (b) a complex interaction of drug-induced immunoalteration, leading to viral replication and robust host-and-virus response; and (c) direct toxic effects of lymphocytes themselves. Drug–protein interactions may lead to immunoglobulin E (IgE)-mediated anaphylactic-type reactions, IgG-mediated direct tissue or complement-activated injury, or T-cell–induced injury. Immune complex mechanisms rely on persistence of drug antigen in the serum long enough to elicit an antibody response. Depending on the type of T-effector cell elicited, different cutaneous reactions may range from a morbilliform exanthem to SJS/TEN (9). New drug formulations, in particular liposomal and transdermal delivery systems, and the introduction of numerous chemotherapeutic and immune response modulators, are accountable for increasing numbers of cutaneous reactions primarily by the nature of their preferential accumulation in target tissues, such as skin (10–12). Several medication-related cutaneous eruptions are considered in depth elsewhere in this text but are mentioned briefly in this context.

Principles of Management for Drug Eruptions. For most of the entities, the treatment of choice is drug withdrawal. As the drug is metabolized and cleared, the eruption resolves. For more severe eruptions, such as SJS or DRESS, intensive supportive care may be necessary. Immunomodulating therapies, including systemic corticosteroids, intravenous immunoglobulins (IVIG), cyclosporine, etanercept, and plasmapheresis, have been used, although evidence from randomized trials is sparse. Anaphylactic reactions may require acute intervention with supportive care, epinephrine, and corticosteroids. Specific disorders induced by drugs, such as SLE, bullous pemphigoid (BP), or linear IgA dermatosis, are generally managed in ways similar to those for the "spontaneous" forms of these diseases, with the obvious addition of withdrawal of the triggering agent. Pigment alteration, in the form of melanophages or drug deposition, takes significantly longer to clear, and fibrosing lesions may never clear, although progression can be halted with discontinuation of the offending drug.

Drug eruptions in this section are covered based on histologic patterns, followed by those eruptions that have classic clinical presentations.

HISTOLOGIC PATTERNS OF DRUG-INDUCED SKIN DISORDERS

Some drug eruptions present with specific histopathologic patterns that can support the diagnosis and perhaps help in identifying the responsible agent(s).

Lymphocytic Drug Eruptions

The histologic response in these conditions is mediated primarily by lymphocytes.

Interface Dermatitis

The histologic features comprising interface dermatitis (see Chapter 7) include vacuolar alteration of the basilar epidermis, flattening of basilar keratinocytes, necrotic keratinocytes, variable infiltration of the upper dermis by lymphocytes and histiocytes, variable exocytosis, and melanophages.

Erythema Multiforme

Clinical Summary. Erythema multiforme (EM) is characterized by an abrupt onset of self-limited and occasionally recurring edematous papulovesicles and erythematous macules with concentric zones of color change described as targetoid lesions or a "bull's eye" (Fig. 11-1). The distribution varies but shows a predilection for the palms and soles and usually occurs symmetrically. Mucosal involvement and systemic symptoms, such as fever, myalgia, and arthralgia, may develop. As in the other drug-related cutaneous eruptions, the list of offending agents continues to expand, but it is most commonly attributed to nonsteroidal anti-inflammatory drugs (NSAIDs), antiepileptics, sulfonamides, and other antibiotics (13) and includes diverse agents such as selective serotonin reuptake inhibitors, chemotherapeutics, and radiographic contrast (14–16). EM is most frequently triggered by herpes simplex virus, mycoplasma, or other infections, and a thorough investigation for triggers is warranted.

Histopathology. In EM, there is a mild lichenoid infiltrate with dyskeratotic keratinocytes, characteristically found at all epidermal levels in the fully evolved lesion. Dyskeratosis may become confluent to form a thoroughly necrotic blister roof (Fig. 11-2) (see Chapter 9). Exocytosis of lymphocytes is also present. The dermis shows a mild perivascular inflammatory infiltrate. Although the etiology of the process often cannot be determined by the histology, the presence of eosinophils and acrosyringeal keratinocyte necrosis would suggest a drug-mediated process (17).

Principles of Management: EM is often managed with topical corticosteroids or topical analgesics, such as viscous lidocaine for oral ulcers. A concurrent infection warrants targeted treatment.

Toxic Epidermal Necrolysis and Stevens–Johnson Syndrome

Clinical Summary. At the other end of the interface dermatitis spectrum, SJS and TEN are both severe cutaneous eruptions that display diffuse, tender erythema, which may take the form of bright red "spots," or targetoid lesions, which may partially blanch; mucosal inflammation is common and may be the first and most severe finding. Blisters may develop in both disorders, as well as mucosal and conjunctival involvement (Fig. 11-3). Fortunately, their incidence is low: 1.2 to 6 cases per million persons per year for SJS and 0.4 to 1.2 cases per million persons per year for TEN (18). TEN is associated with therapeutic drugs in 95% of cases and with immunizations and infections in the other instances. SJS, on the other hand, is reported to be associated with drugs in only 50% of cases, though this may be an underestimation owing to SJS historically being classified with EM. Viruses and other infections can also trigger the syndrome, particularly in children (18). An overwhelming number of drugs have been associated with SJS and TEN, most commonly antibiotics, NSAIDs, and anticonvulsants. In a multi-institutional study of 338 cases of SJS and TEN, trimethoprim–sulfamethoxazole was the most common culprit (19).

Pathogenesis. The mechanism of epithelial destruction is not clearly defined. However, drug-specific, CD8+ lymphocytes

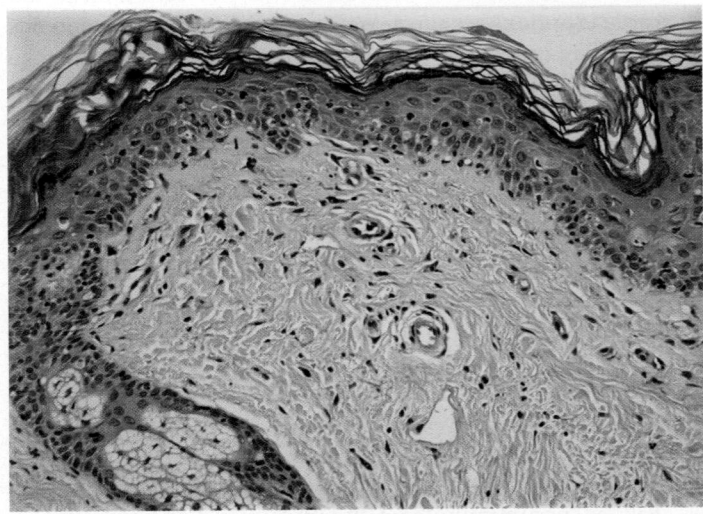

Figure 11-2 Drug-induced erythema multiforme. The epidermis has necrotic keratinocytes at all levels of the epidermis and a minimal dermal inflammatory infiltrate. The eosinophils suggest the drug-induced etiology.

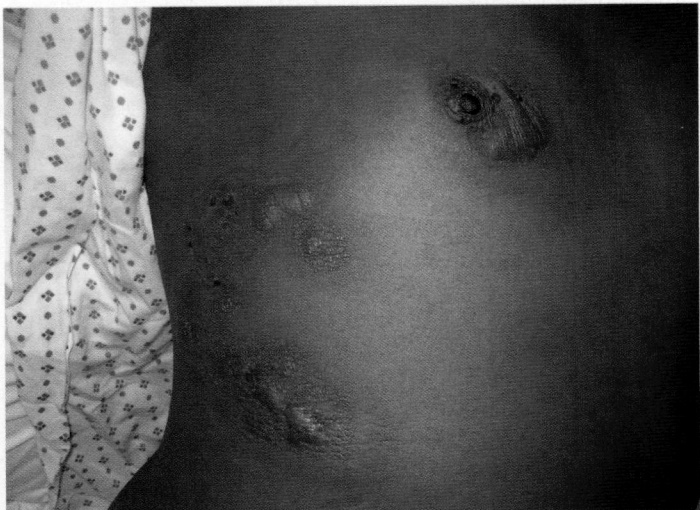

Figure 11-1 Drug-induced erythema multiforme shows targetoid lesions with edematous, violaceous centers, and erythematous halos. In this lesion, caused by carbamazepine, the extent of interface degeneration also resulted in blister formation.

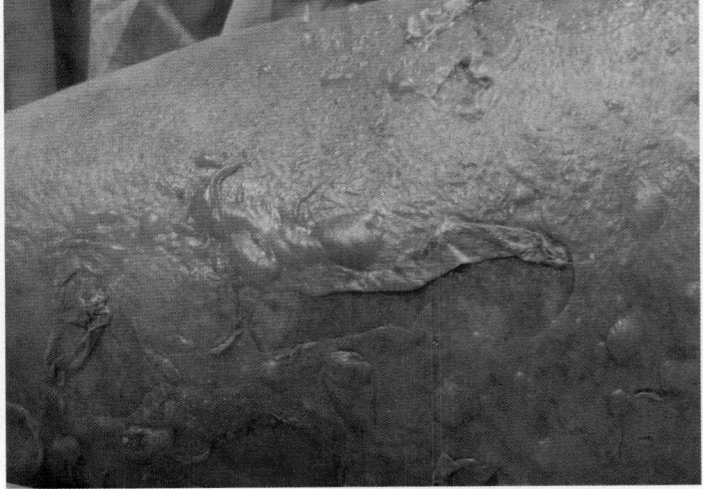

Figure 11-3 Toxic epidermal necrolysis. Diffuse blisters with sloughing skin secondary to allopurinol.

with granzyme-mediated cytotoxicity are suggested to have a role in the pathogenesis of SJS and TEN (20).

Histopathology. In the spectrum of interface dermatitides, SJS and TEN display greater keratinocyte necrosis and less inflammation than other disorders. Necrotic keratinocytes are found at all epidermal levels and, as in EM, may become confluent to form a thoroughly necrotic blister roof (Fig. 11-4). Eventual subepidermal bullae may form (see Chapter 9). The etiology of the process often cannot be determined by histology. As there is considerable overlap with the histology of EM, the diagnosis cannot be reliably made without detailed clinicopathologic correlation.

Principles of Management: There exists controversy over the optimal management for patients with SJS and TEN. All patients should be cared for in an intensive care setting by a multidisciplinary team. All suspect drugs should be stopped, and supportive care is essential. Systemic treatment options include IVIG, cyclosporine, etanercept, or corticosteroids, although there is no high-quality comparative evidence suggesting one agent over the others or that any of these options is conclusively effective.

Lichenoid Drug Eruption

Clinical Summary. Similar to lichen planus, erythematous to violaceous papules and plaques develop on the trunk and extremities, in association with drug ingestion. Implicated agents most commonly include quinacrine, quinidine, and gold but also NSAIDs, antihypertensive medications (especially captopril), penicillamine, chloroquine, etanercept, imatinib, sildenafil, terazosin, infliximab, and hepatitis B vaccine (21–27).

Histopathology. Lichenoid drug eruption is similar to lichen planus histologically (Fig. 11-5). In comparison with EM and TEN, lichenoid drug eruptions are more heavily inflamed, with a more prominent interstitial pattern. Differentiation from lichen planus may not be possible. Numerous eosinophils, parakeratosis, and perivascular inflammation around the mid- and deep dermal plexuses may be seen in lichenoid drug eruptions and are generally absent in lichen planus.

Principles of Management: Cessation of likely causative agents is essential. Topical corticosteroids may offer some relief; widespread, severe cases may warrant systemic or phototherapy.

Fixed Drug Eruption

Clinical Summary. Fixed drug eruptions (FDEs) show circumscribed erythematous patches that recur persistently at the same site with each administration of the implicated drug. Increasing numbers of lesions may occur with each successive administration. The most common type of FDE consists of one or several slightly edematous, erythematous patches that may develop dusky centers, become bullous, and, on healing, leave pigmented macules. FDEs occur most commonly after the ingestion of trimethoprim–sulfamethoxazole, tetracyclines, NSAIDs, acetylsalicylic acid, phenolphthalein, barbiturates, and phenylbutazone, but they also occur after ingestion of various other drugs (28).

Histopathology. The histologic changes observed in FDE resemble those of EM and TEN. The frequent presence of hydropic degeneration of the basal cell layer leads to "pigmentary incontinence," which is characterized by the presence of melanin within macrophages in the upper dermis; this may be more prominent in FDE as the eruption is, by definition, recurrent in the same site (Fig. 11-6). Scattered necrotic keratinocytes with eosinophilic cytoplasm and pyknotic nuclei (often referred to as civatte bodies, colloid bodies, or dyskeratotic or apoptotic cells) are frequently seen in the epidermis and represent apoptosis. Bullae form by the detachment of the epidermis from the underlying dermis. Not infrequently, the epidermis shows extensive confluent necrosis, even in areas in which it has not yet become detached. Confident distinction among FDE, EM, and TEN based on examination of a skin biopsy specimen alone is not possible. The inflammatory infiltrate may be composed purely of mononuclear cells or may be polymorphous.

Pathogenesis. On electron microscopic examination, the necrotic keratinocytes are filled with thick, homogenized keratin tonofilaments and show only sparse remnants of organelles and nuclei. Keratinocytes located in the basal cell layer are often

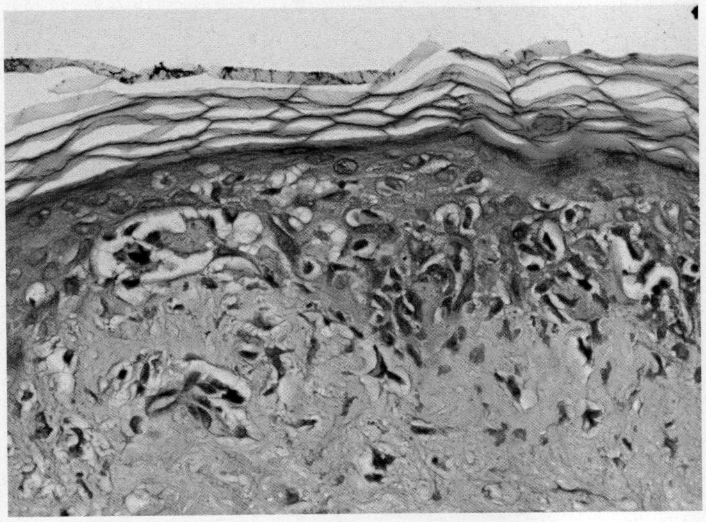

Figure 11-4 Toxic epidermal necrolysis. There is extensive dyskeratosis of the epidermis with early blister formation. A mild perivascular lymphocytic infiltrate is seen in the superficial dermis.

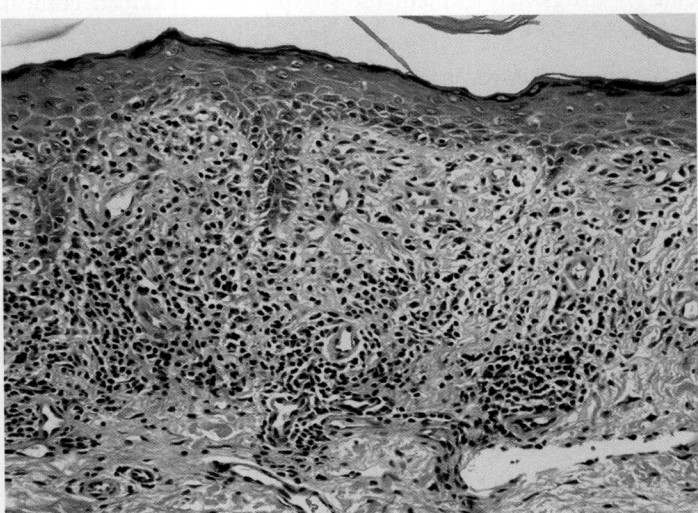

Figure 11-5 ■ Lichenoid drug reaction. There is a vacuolar change of the basilar layer and scattered apoptotic keratinocytes. Eosinophils in the dermal infiltrate and melanin incontinence are not characteristically seen in the clinically and histologically similar lichen planus.

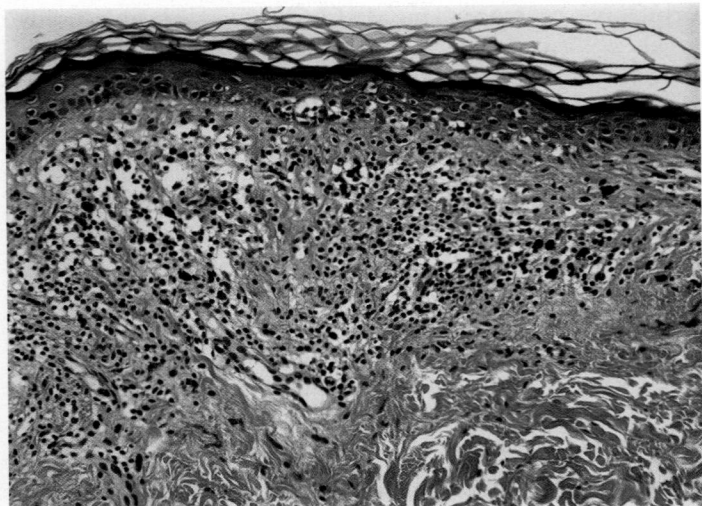

Figure 11-6 Fixed drug eruption. This section shows the characteristic lichenoid lymphocytic infiltrate and abundant pigment incontinence with scattered melanophages. In addition, basal vacuolar alteration and dyskeratotic cells occur in the epidermis.

the most severely affected cells. The pigmentary incontinence develops when (a) lymphocytes migrate into the epidermis and cause damage to keratinocytes, which become necrotic; (b) macrophages invade the epidermis and phagocytize the necrotic keratinocytes together with their melanosomes; and (c) the macrophages return to the dermis, where they are able to digest all cellular remnants, except for the melanosomes, which are resistant to digestion. The intraepidermal lymphocytes are largely represented by CD8+ T cells, whereas the dermal perivascular and interstitial lymphocytes are predominantly CD4+, phenotypically resembling effector memory cells (29). In addition, these CD8+ intraepidermal lymphocytes demonstrate keratinocyte cytolytic activity, indicating their role in the pathogenesis of FDE lesions (30). The process of pigmentary incontinence in FDE is similar to that occurring in incontinentia pigmenti (see Chapter 6). Expression of keratinocyte intercellular adhesion molecule-1 (CD54) is sharply limited to lesional epidermis in FDE. Localized induction of this adhesion molecule by drugs may explain the sharply circumscribed clinical lesions (30–33).

Principles of Management: Cessation of likely causative agents is essential. If multiple culprits are considered, targeted patch testing within the affected area may help elucidate the true causative agent (34). Patch testing for the culprit drug may be most useful when either an antiepileptic or contrast media are suspected (35). Topical corticosteroids may offer some relief; widespread, severe cases may warrant systemic therapy.

Drug-Induced Lupus

Clinical Summary. There are two major forms of drug-induced lupus: drug-induced systemic lupus erythematosus (DI-SLE) and drug-induced subacute cutaneous lupus erythematosus (DI-SCLE). DI-SLE is characterized by arthralgia, arthritis, myalgia, serositis, fever, hepatomegaly, splenomegaly, weight loss, pericarditis, and skin manifestations. The cutaneous lesions of DI-SLE are less likely to present with malar rash and oral ulcers, but instead present with erythema nodosum, purpura, and photodistributed erythema, which may erupt days to years after the onset of treatment (36–38). Central nervous system and renal

involvement are rare. The drugs most commonly implicated include procainamide, hydralazine, quinidine, chlorpromazine, isoniazid, methyldopa, minocycline, quinine, penicillamine, propylthiouracil, and antitumor necrosis factor-α (TNF-α) agents (39–41). The presence of antihistone antibodies may be a clue to diagnosing DI-SLE but is also found in up to 75% of patients with idiopathic SLE (42). It is possible that the development of an SLE-like syndrome in a patient treated with these drugs represents the uncovering of latent SLE. Cutaneous eruptions in DI-SLE are far less common than they are in DI-SCLE.

DI-SCLE is characterized by erythematous annular or psoriasiform plaques usually located on the upper trunk and extensor surfaces in conjunction with anti-Ro, SSA, and anti-La, SSB, antibodies (Fig. 11-7). Antihistone antibodies are uncommon. Antihypertensives are the most likely agents known to induce SCLE. Although hydrochlorothiazide is the most common offending drug, other hypertension medications, including calcium channel blockers, diuretics, β-blockers, and angiotensin-converting enzyme (ACE) inhibitors, are reported triggers. Antifungals (e.g., terbinafine, griseofulvin), chemotherapeutics (e.g., docetaxel), immunomodulators (e.g., interferon [IFN]), antiepileptics, statins, biologics, proton-pump inhibitors, H2 blockers (e.g., ranitidine), NSAIDs, hormone-altering drugs, TNF-α inhibitors, and ultraviolet (UV) therapy (e.g., PUVA) have also been described.

Histopathology. The histologic picture of the cutaneous lesions is the same as in lupus erythematosus (see Chapter 10; Fig. 11-8).

Pathogenesis. As in other autoimmune-related disorders, genetic predisposition, in particular HLA-DR4, has a role in DI-SLE. Antinuclear antibodies are usually present and directed against single-stranded DNA or histones (43). Different drugs appear to be associated with different antihistone profiles (39). Anti–double-stranded DNA antibodies are usually absent. Hypocomplementemia is rare. The occurrence of a lupus band on direct immunofluorescence testing of normal-appearing skin is uncommon (44). The rate of drug acetylation has also been associated with disease onset. Rapid acetylators have a much lower incidence of hydralazine-induced lupus, whereas slow

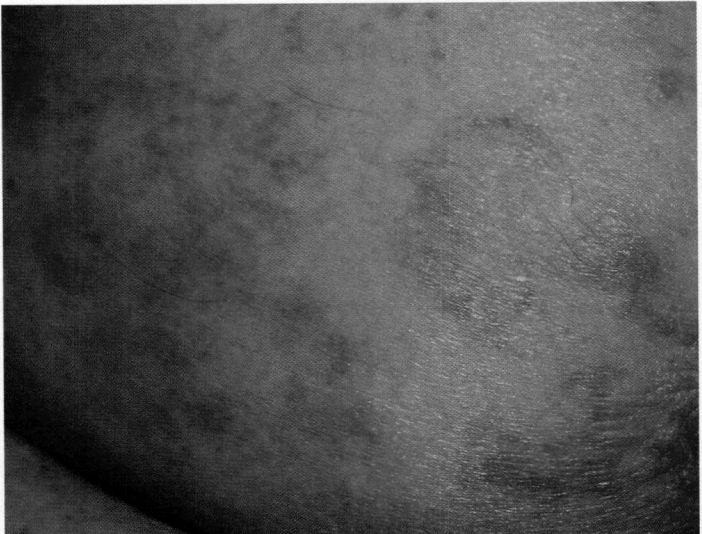

Figure 11-7 Drug-induced subacute cutaneous lupus erythematosus. Annular erythematous plaques with mild peripheral scale are seen in this patient on an angiotensin-converting enzyme inhibitor.

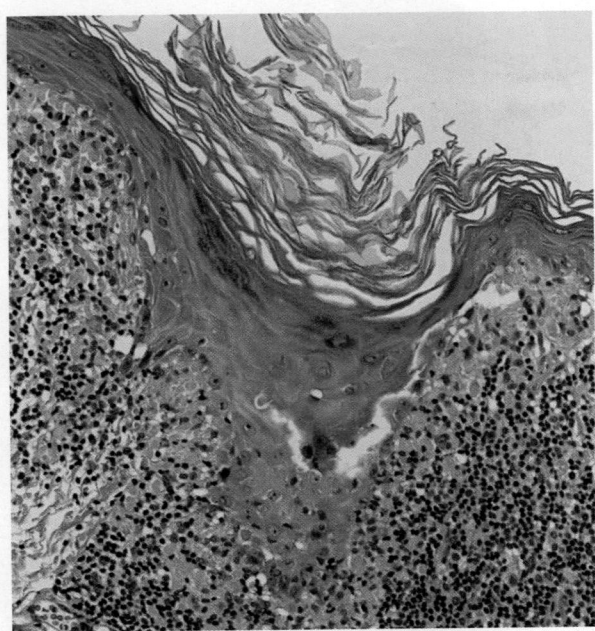

Figure 11-8 Drug-induced subacute cutaneous lupus erythematosus. Vacuolar change of the follicular basilar layer with scattered apoptotic keratinocytes, colloid bodies, and mild hyperkeratosis of the infundibulum.

acetylators are at higher risk. In addition, there is evidence that certain drugs can activate neutrophils to form neutrophil extracellular traps (NETs) to release autoantigen-rich proteins and nuclear DNA that induce autoimmunity (45). The pathogenesis of DI-SCLE has not been well elucidated.

Principles of Management: Discontinuation of likely causative agents is essential. All patients should be evaluated for signs and symptoms of systemic lupus—some patients may have true drug-induced lupus, whereas others may have drug "unmasked" lupus and should be treated as though they have lupus. Smoking cessation, sun avoidance, topical steroids, antimalarials, and systemic immunomodulatory or immunosuppressive agents may be indicated.

Noninterface Lymphocytic Drug Eruptions

A dense lymphocytic infiltrate with atypia may be termed "pseudolymphoma" if a true lymphoma can be ruled out.

Drug-Induced Pseudolymphoma

Clinical Summary. Anticonvulsants (e.g., phenobarbital, phenytoin, ethosuximide, lamotrigine, carbamazepine, valproate sodium), antipsychotics (chlorpromazine, promethazine), gemcitabine, imatinib, gold, allopurinol, amiloride, diltiazem, clomipramine, cyclosporine, and vaccinations are among the agents that have been associated with a pseudolymphoma syndrome, characterized by generalized lymphadenopathy, hepatosplenomegaly, fever, arthralgia, and eosinophilia (46–49). Cutaneous findings range from a few erythematous plaques or nodules to a generalized macular and papular eruption and generalized exfoliative dermatitis (48). In all cases, there is improvement and ultimate clearing when the offending agent is discontinued.

Histopathology. In plaque-like lesions, the infiltrate is often indistinguishable from that of mycosis fungoides (this syndrome is also known as "pseudomycosis fungoides"), in that there

are cerebriform nuclei in the dermal infiltrate and Pautrier microabscesses in the epidermis (Fig. 11-9). In nodular lesions (cutaneous lymphoid hyperplasia), the infiltrate may suggest a cutaneous lymphoma of the non-Hodgkin type because large masses of atypical lymphocytes are present in the dermis and subcutaneous tissue. T- and B-cell receptor monoclonality has been demonstrated in some cases (50,51).

Principles of Management: Cessation of likely causative agents is essential. Therapy should be directed at the remaining inflammation and may require either topical or intralesional steroids, or, in severe cases, systemic treatment.

Neutrophilic Drug Eruptions

Drugs have been implicated in cutaneous eruptions with a neutrophilic infiltrate; these conditions include acneiform eruptions, neutrophilic FDE, neutrophilic eccrine hidradenitis, acute generalized exanthematous pustulosis (AGEP), Sweet syndrome, serum sickness–like reaction, and dermatitis herpetiformis–like eruption. The neutrophilic dermatitis seen as a result of granulocyte repopulation owing to exogenous granulocyte colony-stimulating factor (G-CSF) is described in the section of this chapter pertaining to eruptions resulting from human recombinant proteins.

Acute Generalized Exanthematous Pustulosis

Clinical Summary. In AGEP, widespread nonfollicular, sterile pustules develop on the face (Fig. 11-10) or in intertriginous areas and disseminate over a few hours. This is often associated with high fever and leukocytosis and can be mistaken for an infection. The pinpoint pustules may run together and form "lakes of pus," which can be mistaken for bullae or even for sheets of epidermal necrosis. As the inflammation in AGEP is more superficial than that in SJS/TEN, any resultant epidermal loss is at a superficial layer, with intact epidermis below the area of superficial desquamation. Although enteroviral infection and mercury exposure are cited as causes, β-lactam and macrolide antibiotics (penicillin, aminopenicillins, cephalosporins) are most often implicated, with a broad range of other medications, including acetaminophen, quinolones, hydroxychloroquine,

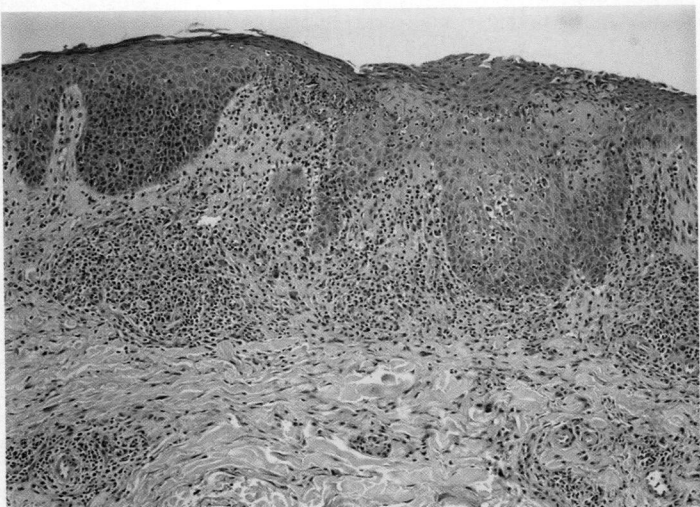

Figure 11-9 Cutaneous pseudolymphoma. There is a dense inflammatory infiltrate with exocytosis of atypical-appearing lymphocytes and absence of spongiosis in this Dilantin-induced pseudolymphoma.

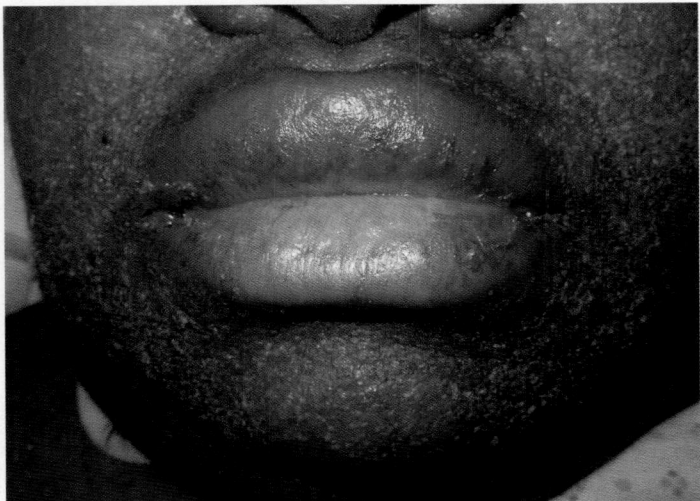

Figure 11-10 Acute generalized exanthematous pustulosis. Small, sterile pustules developed on the face in this patient on allopurinol.

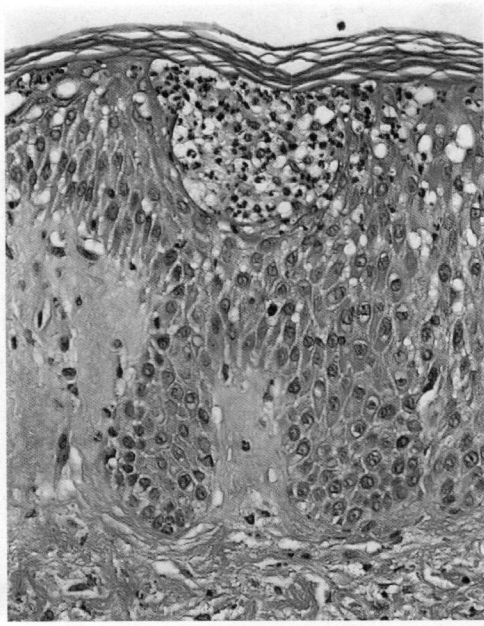

Figure 11-12 Acute generalized exanthematous pustulosis. Diffuse spongiosis and a mild upper dermal perivascular inflammatory infiltrate are seen in this case caused by amoxicillin.

sulfonamides, terbinafine, diltiazem, antimalarials, carbamazepine, nystatin, metronidazole, vancomycin, and doxycycline. AGEP has been reported after spider bites and in the setting of certain contrast dyes and dialysates as well (52). Acute localized exanthematous pustulosis (ALEP) is a variant of AGEP with sterile pustules localized most commonly to just the face, neck, or chest (57).

Histopathology. Biopsies of AGEP or ALEP have subcorneal pustules, papillary dermal edema, and a lymphohistiocytic perivascular infiltrate with sparse-to-moderate infiltrate of eosinophils and neutrophils (Figs. 11-11 and 11-12). Vasculitis and/or single-cell keratinocyte necrosis may rarely be present. Histologic features of AGEP may be indistinguishable from pustular psoriasis, though the presence of eosinophilic spongiosis or dermal eosinophilia may favor the former.

Pathogenesis. In vitro studies have shown this to be a drug-specific process affected by CD4+ T-cell–mediated release of the neutrophil chemoattractant interleukin-8 (IL-8) (53). T cells from

patients with AGEP secrete high levels of IL-8/CXCL8, a potent neutrophil attractant. In addition, these T cells produce large quantities of granulocyte–macrophage colony-stimulating factor (GM-CSF) (53). Unlike drug-induced macular and papular eruptions, there is no upregulation of major histocompatibility complex (MHC) class II expression on keratinocytes in AGEP.

Principles of Management: Patients generally improve when the causative agent is stopped. Topical steroids may offer some relief. Most patients experience extensive superficial desquamation and may require aggressive emollient use. Pustular psoriasis, which has higher morbidity and a more prolonged course, must be considered if there is no improvement following drug withdrawal.

Sweet Syndrome

Clinical Summary. Drug-induced acute febrile neutrophilic dermatosis, or Sweet syndrome, is clinically identical to the non–drug-induced variant of Sweet syndrome (see Chapter 8). It presents with fever, peripheral blood neutrophilia, and tender erythematous plaques that favor the face and upper extremities. Drug-induced Sweet syndrome is most commonly associated with all-*trans*-retinoic acid, G-CSF, and GM-CSF. Other implicated drugs include furosemide, oral contraceptives, nitrofurantoin, trimethoprim–sulfamethoxazole, clindamycin, celecoxib, and tetracyclines (54,55,58). Neutrophilic dermatosis of the dorsal hands (NDDH) is a localized variant of Sweet syndrome, which presents as pustules and ulcerative plaques on the dorsal hands. Some patients have lesions distributed at sites other than just the dorsal hands (Fig. 11-13) (59).

Histopathology. Histologic sections show papillary dermal edema and a dense dermal neutrophilic infiltrate, identical to non–drug-induced Sweet syndrome (see Chapter 8). Leukocytoclasia and plump, reactive endothelial cells may be seen. Leukocytoclastic vasculitis may be present in Sweet syndrome or NDDH (59,60).

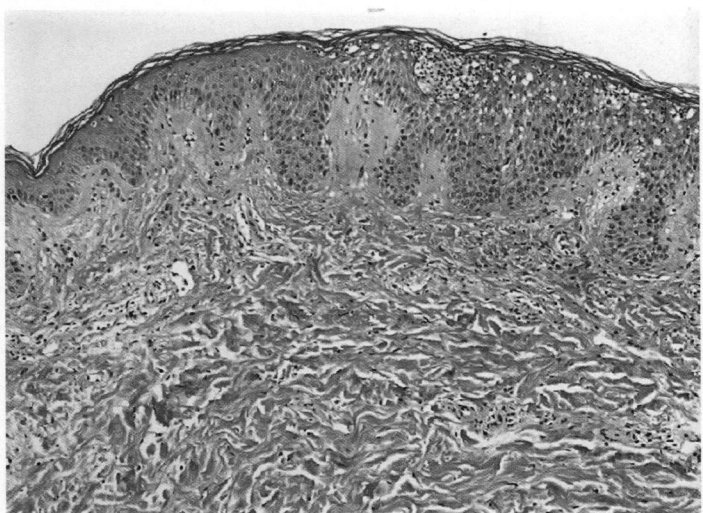

Figure 11-11 Acute generalized exanthematous pustulosis. A subcorneal and intraspinous collection of neutrophils is present in the background of mild epidermal spongiosis.

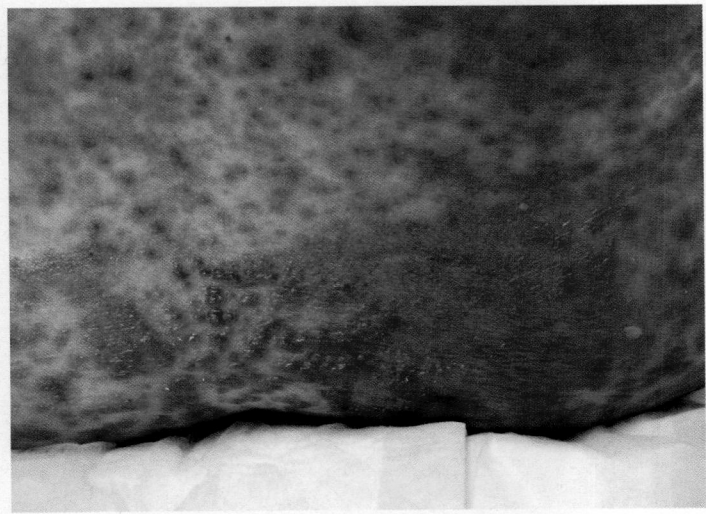

Figure 11-13 In Sweet syndrome, patients have tender, erythematous plaques that favor the face and upper extremities, but spread to other sites.

Principles of Management: Cessation of likely causative agents is essential. Topical corticosteroids may offer some relief, with many patients requiring systemic therapy. Corticosteroids are the mainstay of treatment; other options include dapsone, colchicine, saturated solution of potassium iodide (SSKI), or thalidomide.

Halogenodermas

Clinical Summary. Halogenodermas are rare dermatoses that develop following exposure to bromide, fluorides, and iodides. Common sources of exposure are radiation protectants, SSKI, contrast media, povidone-iodine, amiodarone, and potassium bromide used for seizure control (61,62). Bromoderma is characterized by a pustular eruption or vegetating, papillomatous plaques on the lower extremities that can have pustules at their periphery. Iododerma is usually seen in areas of dense sebaceous glands, such as the face, and consists of pustules, pustulonodules, and vegetative plaques. Like bromoderma, the plaques of iododerma typically show pustules at their peripheries, but they usually show less papillomatous proliferation and a softer consistency than bromoderma, and they often ulcerate. Iododerma is frequently associated with severe systemic signs and symptoms and may be fatal in rare instances (63). Other variants include vesicles, urticaria, and hemorrhagic and ulcerative plaques. Fluoroderma presents with exudative plaques, fungating nodules, necrotic ulcers, and acneiform eruptions.

Histopathology. The histologic picture in the halogen eruptions is suggestive rather than diagnostic. The epidermal changes in bromoderma are typically more exuberant than in iododerma; dermal changes are essentially the same and vary with the age of the lesion.

In early lesions, the dermis in both bromoderma and iododerma shows a dense infiltrate of neutrophils, which, in areas of dermal necrosis, show nuclear dust. There may be intradermal abscesses. Eosinophils are present in most cases and may be numerous. Extensive extravasation of erythrocytes may also be seen. At a later stage, the proportion of mononuclear cells increases, and histiocytes may show abundant cytoplasm or large nuclei. The blood vessels are increased in number and dilated and may show proliferation of endothelium.

The epidermal changes in bromoderma are often pronounced. In addition to papillomatosis, there is considerable downward epidermal proliferation, occasionally to such a degree as to produce the picture of pseudocarcinomatous hyperplasia. The acanthosis may center on the follicular epithelium. Frequently, intraepidermal abscesses are present (Fig. 11-14). The intraepidermal abscesses are filled with neutrophils, eosinophils, and some desquamated keratinocytes, most of which appear necrotic, although some resemble acantholytic cells. Some epithelial islands in the upper dermis, instead of enclosing an abscess, are filled with keratin.

In iododerma, the epidermis may be eroded or ulcerated. At the margin of the ulcers, one may find intraepidermal abscesses. In old lesions, pseudoepitheliomatous hyperplasia may be encountered, although usually less than in bromoderma. Fluoroderma has been described only as a mild eruption in a few cases, but it shares with iododerma and bromoderma the presence of eosinophils, neutrophils, and erythrocytes in the dermis and of microabscesses in the epidermis (64,65).

Pathogenesis. It has been suggested that halogenodermas represent delayed hypersensitivity reactions or inflammatory reactions caused by the elimination of the drug through eccrine and sebaceous glands (66). Accumulation of the halogen seems to be important with renal disease, potentially increasing the risk. Lesions normally appear after long-term exposure, although they can occur as rapidly as in a few days. Even though there is often a very long interval between the first ingestion of iodides or bromides and the appearance of the cutaneous lesion, halogen eruptions appear to be an allergic phenomenon; once a person has become sensitized, the eruption recurs within a few days on the readministration of iodides or bromides. Fluoroderma has been described after the frequent application of a fluoride gel to the teeth for the purpose of preventing caries during ionizing radiation to the face (64).

Drug-Induced Fibrosing Disorders

Scleroderma and nephrogenic system fibrosis are examples of drug-induced fibrosing disorders that affect the skin and may be seen in skin biopsies.

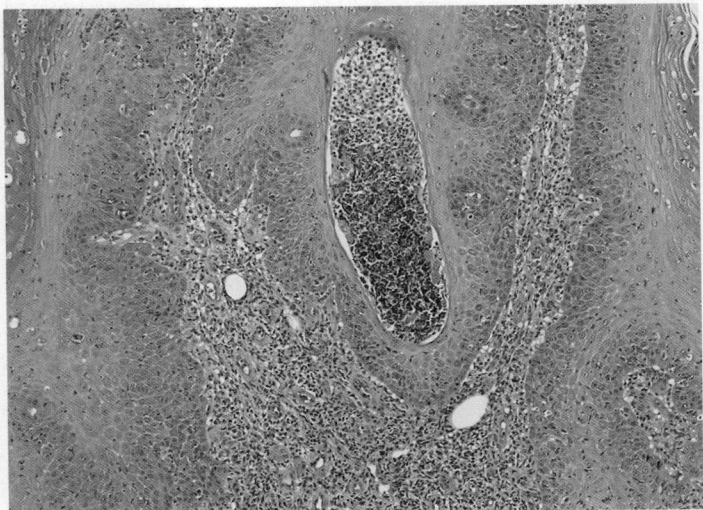

Figure 11-14 Bromoderma. There is downward proliferation of the epidermis with a large intraepidermal abscess. A dense inflammatory infiltrate is present in the dermis.

Scleroderma-Like Conditions

Clinical Summary. Scleroderma-like conditions have been attributed to numerous exogenous agents. Although the pathophysiology is unclear, disturbances in the vasculature and immune system leading to fibroblastic dysregulation and subsequent deposition of intercellular matrix proteins have been proposed, and telomerase activity appears to serve a protective role (67). Bleomycin, an antitumor agent, is known to cause similar changes in a reversible, dose-dependent manner in both the skin and the lung because of drug accumulation in these organs deficient in specific metabolic enzymes (67). Scleroderma-like changes have also been associated with other agents, including phytonadione (vitamin K1), L-tryptophan, pentazocine, taxanes (docetaxel, paclitaxel), penicillamine, ergot, bromocriptine, ketobemidone, morphine, cocaine, toxic oil/Spanish oil, and appetite suppressants (68–70).

Histopathology. The features are those of idiopathic scleroderma (see Chapter 10), including fibrosis of the dermis and subcutis, adnexal structure entrapment, and atrophy and mild vascular dilation with variable lymphoplasmacytic inflammatory infiltrate, which may extend into the subcutis and surround vessels, adnexal structures, and nerves.

Principles of Management: Treatment of fibrosing disorders may be challenging and requires a combination of topical therapy, phototherapy, and physical therapy and often mandates systemic immunomodulatory and/or immunosuppressive therapy.

Nephrogenic Systemic Fibrosis

Clinical Summary. Nephrogenic systemic fibrosis (NSF), previously referred to as *nephrogenic fibrosing dermopathy*, is a progressive multiorgan fibrosing disorder. Although the precise cause and pathogenesis remain elusive, it has been closely linked to patients with compromised renal function and gadolinium exposure. The incidence of this condition has been greatly reduced because of changes in radiologic practice. High morbidity and mortality are associated with NSF. The fibrosis most commonly affects the lower extremities and manifests as dense induration, papules, or plaques. A role for gadolinium in routing the collagen-producing circulating fibrocyte has been proposed (71). A gadolinium-associated systemic inflammatory process that results in mobilization of iron and subsequent tissue injury has also been proposed (71). NSF is also discussed elsewhere in the book (Chapters 10, 17, and 20).

Histopathology. The biopsy specimen shows mild-to-moderate increased cellularity in the mid- to deep reticular dermis. The cellularity is composed of fibroblasts with activated morphology, large nuclei, occasional multinucleation, and abundant angulated cytoplasm (Fig. 11-15). Increased collagen and dermal mucin are also characteristically seen. The cellularity and collagen deposition may extend along the subcutaneous septa and fascia. The fibrocytes may stain positive for CD34.

Principles of Management: Avoidance of gadolinium in the setting of renal insufficiency is the most important step in preventing the development of this devastating disease. Although multiple treatments have been described, renal transplant and restoration of normal function is the only modality with compelling results (72).

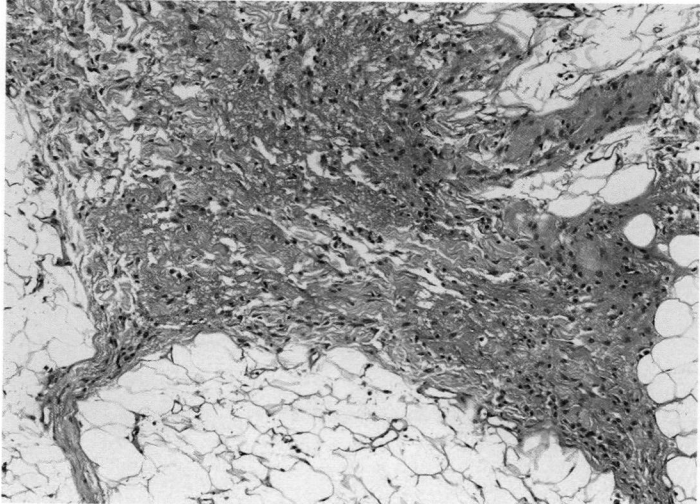

Figure 11-15 Nephrogenic systemic fibrosis. The deep dermis shows increased cellularity composed of activated fibroblasts with stellate morphology and increased collagen. Occasional multinucleation and dermal mucin may also be present.

Drug-Induced Bullous Disorders

Drugs can be involved in bulla formation through various mechanisms (see also Chapter 9).

Coma Blister

Clinical Summary. A patient who is in a coma as a result of an accident, illness, carbon monoxide poisoning, or a large dose of a narcotic drug may show, within a few hours, areas of erythema at sites of pressure (73). Usually within 24 hours, vesicles and bullae develop in the erythematous patches. The incidence of bullae depends on the severity of the coma and is highest in patients who subsequently die. The bullae are located at sites subjected to pressure, such as the hands, wrists, scapulae, sacrum, knees, legs, ankles, and heels.

Histopathology. The epidermis shows varying degrees of necrosis and can be full thickness. Intraepidermal or subepidermal bullae or vesicles develop and may contain some acantholytic cells (Fig. 11-16).

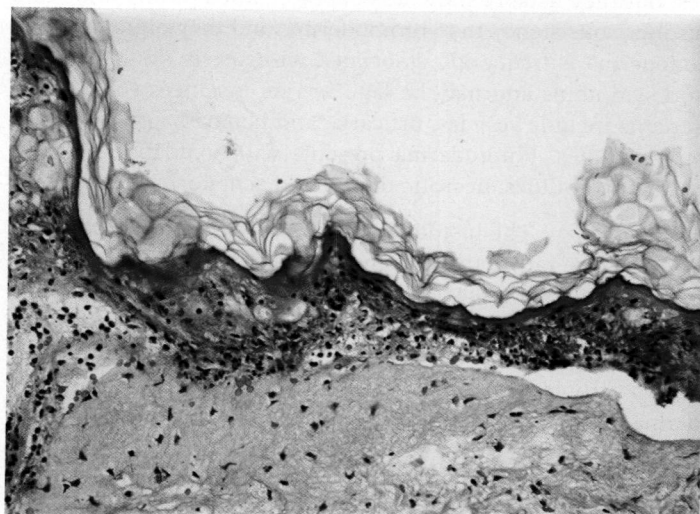

Figure 11-16 Drug-induced coma bulla. There is extensive necrosis of the epidermis with subepidermal blister formation. Inflammation in the blister cavity is secondary to adjacent ulceration. The dermis shows only a mild inflammatory infiltrate.

The secretory cells of the sweat coil are the most suscepti-ble to necrosis, which is characterized by eosinophilic homoge-nization of their cytoplasm and pyknosis or the absence of their nuclei. The sweat ducts usually appear less severely damaged but may also show pale staining or necrosis similar to that of the secretory cells (Fig. 11-17) (73). Sweat gland necrosis is limited to areas in which there are skin lesions. Necrosis may also be seen in the hair follicle, sebaceous gland, and, as men-tioned, the epidermis. In patients who survive, the necrotic sweat gland epithelium is replaced by normal-appearing epi-thelial cells within about 2 weeks.

The dermis beneath the bullae, and occasionally also the dermis around the sweat glands, contains a sparse polymor-phous infiltrate composed of neutrophils, eosinophils, lym-phocytes, and histiocytes. In addition, some extravasated erythrocytes are often present.

Vascular changes consist of vessel wall damage associated with a neutrophilic infiltrate. Lesions caused by a non–drug-induced coma characteristically show fibrinoid thrombi in the vascular lumina (73).

Pathogenesis. The necrosis of the epidermis and sweat glands is a result of both generalized and local hypoxia. The bullae, in turn, are the result of epidermal damage. Coma, whether the result of an accident, an illness, or a drug, causes generalized hypoxia by depressing blood circulation and respiration. In the case of poisoning with carbon monoxide, its binding to hemo-globin acts as an additional factor. Pressure causes further local hypoxia by decreasing blood flow.

Pseudoporphyria

Clinical Summary. NSAIDs (e.g., naproxen, nabumetone, keto-profen, celecoxib), diuretics (e.g., furosemide, chlorthalidone, bumetanide, hydrochlorothiazide/triamterene), antimicrobials (e.g., nalidixic acid, tetracycline, dapsone, ampicillin/sulbac-tam, voriconazole), retinoids (e.g., isotretinoin, etretinate), and oral contraceptive pills are among the medications reported to cause cutaneous lesions, resembling the skin fragility and scarring of porphyria cutanea tarda (74–79). Unlike porphyria cutanea tarda, no biochemical abnormalities in porphyrin me-tabolism exist.

Histopathology. The blisters resemble the pauci-inflammatory or non-inflammatory subepidermal bullae of non–drug-induced porphyria cutanea tarda (see Chapter 17). Direct immunoflu-orescence demonstrates similar deposition to porphyria (80).

Histogenesis. The mechanism by which this reaction occurs is unknown. Pseudoporphyria is usually seen in patients with chronic renal insufficiency, undergoing hemodialysis, and with excessive sun or tanning bed exposure.

Principles of Management: Treatment consists of sun avoidance and discontinuing the causative medication. How-ever, cutaneous lesions may continue for months after drug discontinuation.

Drug-Induced Pemphigus

Clinical Summary. Pemphigus is an autoimmune blistering dis-order that has been linked to several medications (Table 11-1). Among these, penicillamine is perhaps the most common; however, the growing list of implicated agents includes other thiol-, sulfur-, and amide-containing drugs (81). The majority of cases of penicillamine, and other thiol-induced pemphigus eruptions, present as pemphigus foliaceus and have fewer im-munofluorescence findings and a more favorable prognosis on drug withdrawal. Those cases attributed to nonthiol drugs, in particular, those with an active amide group, may provoke dis-ease indistinguishable from spontaneously occurring pemphi-gus vulgaris (82). Oropharyngeal pemphigus secondary to IFN alfa-2a has also been reported (Fig. 11-18) (83).

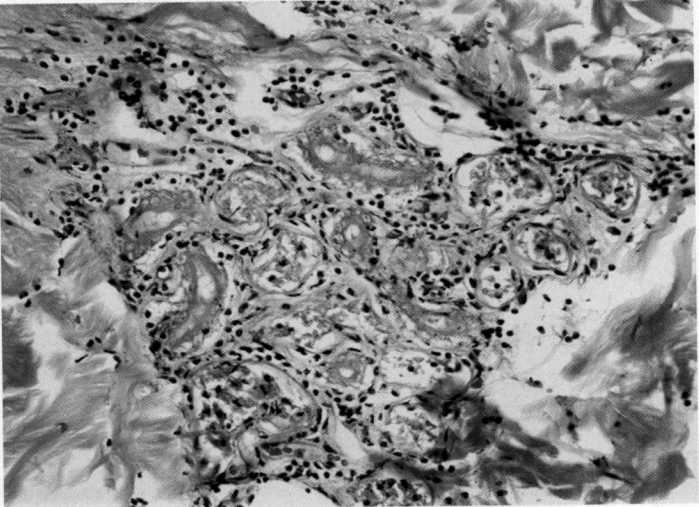

Figure 11-17 Coma bulla and sweat gland necrosis. This image shows necrosis of the eccrine coil with cytoplasmic eosinophilia along with absent and pyknotic nuclei.

Table 11-1
Drugs Causing Pemphigus
Penicillamine
Pyritinol
Gold sodium thiomalate
Captopril
Piroxicam
Bucillamine
Penicillin
Ampicillin
Rifampin
Cefadroxil
Cephalexin
Ceftazidime
Pyrazolone derivatives
Interleukin-2
Interferon-α
Propranolol
Phenobarbital
Levodopa
Nifedipine
Glibenclamide
Cilazapril
Lisinopril

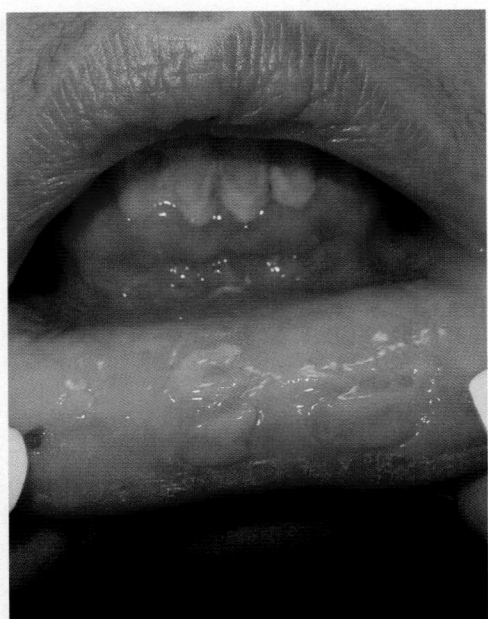

Figure 11-18 Drug-induced pemphigus vulgaris presents with cutaneous and mucosal shallow blisters.

Histopathology. Histologic examination reveals a picture identical to that seen in pemphigus vulgaris and/or pemphigus foliaceus not associated with drugs (see Chapter 9). The autoantibody response to desmoglein 1 and desmoglein 3 is similar in both spontaneous and drug-induced disease (84).

Pathogenesis. Both biochemical and immunologic mechanisms, not mutually exclusive, have been proposed. In the subset of patients in which tissue-bound antibodies cannot be found, a biochemical mechanism has been suggested. These drugs directly bind to keratinocyte membranes, forming bonds that interfere with cell–cell adhesion and resulting in acantholysis (81). Biochemical events can also trigger immunologic acantholysis, leading to the formation of a neoantigen, with consequent autoantibody production (84). In most thiol drug–related cases, intercellular antibodies can be demonstrated, indicating that this class of drugs acts primarily through immunologically mediated acantholysis. In addition, pemphigus vulgaris development is linked to MHC II, specifically human leukocyte antigen (HLA) DRB1 and DQB1 (85), though it is unclear whether drug-induced pemphigus also carries this genetic risk factor. It has been postulated that polymorphisms of the DR4 β-chain impart T-cell recognition of exogenous peptides that stimulate autoantibody production by B lymphocytes.

Drug-Induced Bullous Pemphigoid

Clinical Summary. BP is an autoimmune, subepidermal blistering disease that typically affects the elderly, but may rarely present in adolescents or children. Drug-induced BP resembles the "classic" form of the disease, with tense blisters on erythematous or normal-looking skin of the trunk and limbs. Bullae and/or erosions may rarely present in the oral and genital mucosa. Pruritus or urticarial plaques may also be seen and can precede the formation of bullae.

The most commonly implicated medications in drug-induced BP are gliptins, programmed cell death protein-1/programmed death-ligand 1 (PD-1/PD-L1) inhibitors, loop diuretics, penicillin and its derivatives, psoralen with ultraviolet A (UVA),

sulfasalazine, enalapril, NSAIDs, penicillamine, cephalexin, fluoxetine, spironolactone, and gabapentin (86).

Histopathology. Histologic examination reveals a picture identical to that seen in BP not associated with drugs (see Chapter 9).

Pathogenesis. The majority of implicated drugs contain free sulfhydryl groups. It has been proposed that the thiol group may allow the molecule to combine with proteins in the lamina lucida, act as a hapten, and result in autoantibody formation to BMZ proteins (86).

Linear IgA Bullous Dermatosis

Clinical Summary. Linear IgA bullous dermatosis (LABD) is an autoantibody-mediated subepidermal blistering disease characterized by linear deposits of IgA along the dermoepidermal junction. The typical clinical presentation is a polycyclic grouping of bullae with central crusting termed a "crown of jewels." Clinical, histologic, and immunofluorescence features of drug-induced LABD are often indistinguishable from the idiopathic subtype. However, in contrast to the persistent, difficult-to-treat idiopathic form of LABD, the drug-induced LABD generally occurs within 24 hours to 15 days following administration of the offending drug and resolves within 2 weeks of its discontinuation. Drug-induced LABD has been reported to be more atypical, severe, with cases mimicking TEN, to have larger erosions and Nikolsky sign–positive bullae (87). The most commonly implicated drug is vancomycin, followed by β-lactam antibiotics, captopril, NSAIDs, phenytoin, rifampin, sulfonamides, amiodarone, furosemide, lithium, and G-CSF.

Histopathology. Histologic examination reveals a picture identical to that seen in LABD not associated with drugs (see Chapter 9). Interestingly, vancomycin has been reported to cause a drug-induced morbilliform eruption, which has the same immunofluorescence findings of LABD (88).

Pathogenesis. The etiology of LABD is not fully understood. Antigenic targets are localized to the basement membrane zone. Antibodies in drug-induced LABD are targeted most commonly to type VII collagen, the 230-kDa antigen, the 97-kDa antigen with less frequent involvement against the BP 180- and 285-kDa antigen (89,90).

Principles of Management: For all drug-induced bullous diseases, cessation of likely causative agents is essential. Similar to drug-induced lupus, it may be challenging to distinguish between cases of drug-induced disease from drug "unmasked" disease, and many patients with drug-induced blistering disorders require treatment similar to patients with frank autoimmune blistering diseases, including systemic immunosuppressive agents. Patients with LABD typically respond best to dapsone or sulfapyridine.

CLINICAL PATTERNS OF DRUG-INDUCED SKIN DISORDERS

Clinicopathologic correlation is of vital importance in establishing the diagnosis of most if not all biopsies of potential drug eruptions, and histopathologic examination alone is rarely if ever pathognomonic. Hence, it is important for the histopathologist to have a good understanding of the clinical patterns of these conditions and good communication with the clinicians.

Exanthematous Drug Eruptions

Clinical Summary. Eruptive and efflorescent cutaneous drug reactions are the most common adverse effects of medications (4,6,91–93). Virtually, any drug may be associated with a morbilliform rash, which consists of brightly erythematous macules and/or papules that appear suddenly, are symmetric, and become confluent with time. The rash often starts on the trunk and spreads centrifugally (Fig. 11-19). The mucous membranes are characteristically not involved, and generally, most common morbilliform drug eruptions spare the face, palms, and soles. The nonspecific clinical and histologic changes make definitive implication of a specific agent difficult. The most common medications causing morbilliform eruptions are antibacterial sulfonamides, aminopenicillins, antiepileptic agents, cephalosporins, and allopurinol (4,92). The presence of facial edema, fever, systemic hypereosinophilia, and signs of organ inflammation (such as a transaminitis) in conjunction with the morbilliform eruption is a signal to consider a more serious drug eruption: DRESS, which occurs most commonly with antiepileptics, sulfonamides, allopurinol, and minocycline, although it may occur with a number of other agents as well (1,94–97).

Histopathology. The typical morbilliform drug eruption displays a variable, often sparse, mainly perivascular infiltrate of lymphocytes and eosinophils. Eosinophils may be absent. Some vacuolization of the dermal–epidermal junction with few apoptotic epidermal cells may be observed, but not to the degree typical of EM or TEN.

In a study of 32 cases of DRESS, compared to 17 cases of maculopapular exanthem, DRESS most commonly demonstrated perivascular lymphocytic infiltration (97%), dyskeratosis (97%), interface vacuolization (91%), epidermal spongiosis (78%), and eosinophilic infiltration (72%). Many pathologic features were common between the two conditions. However, severe dyskeratosis, epidermal spongiosis, and severe interface vacuolization were more prominent in DRESS. The interface reaction in DRESS syndrome can resemble a lichenoid process or resemble EM or SJS/TEN (98). The presence of severe dyskeratosis is associated with the clinical severity of hepatic disease, renal impairment, and high risk for intensive care unit admission or death (97,99,100).

Differential Diagnosis. The distinction of morbilliform drug eruption from viral exanthem in the absence of eosinophils is generally not possible. More than occasional dyskeratotic epidermal cells should prompt consideration of EM, SJS/TEN, DRESS, or FDE.

Principles of Management: For mild morbilliform exanthems, many patients can potentially continue on their treatment regimen without modification, while being monitored for signs or symptoms indicative of a more severe reaction. In widespread morbilliform exanthems, cessation of causative agents and supportive care with systemic antihistamines and topical steroids may offer relief. In DRESS, systemic corticosteroids or other immunosuppressives are needed.

Photoallergic Drug Eruption

Clinical Summary. Photoallergic reactions occur as a result of T-cell–mediated hypersensitivity to an antigen that is either activated or produced by the effect of UV light on a drug or its metabolite (101). Photoallergic drug eruptions are caused by sulfonamide antibiotics, thiazide diuretics, sulfonylureas, and phenothiazines, which all contain sulfur moieties. Other implicated medications are NSAIDs, antimalarials, antidepressants, griseofulvin, chlorpromazine, and sunscreens (101,102). Clinically, the eruption occurs gradually, and lesions are pruritic and resemble dermatitis or lichen planus in sun-exposed areas. Over time, lesions may become lichenified and may spread to non–sun-exposed areas.

Histopathology. The histologic appearance of a photoallergic dermatitis is that of an allergic contact dermatitis and includes spongiosis, mild acanthosis, and a superficial perivascular lymphocytic infiltrate with eosinophils (Fig. 11-20).

Principles of Management: For photo-associated reactions, aggressive sun protection and adjusting the causative agent are the mainstays of treatment. Photo-testing, photopatch testing, or rechallenge can help determine the culprit drug.

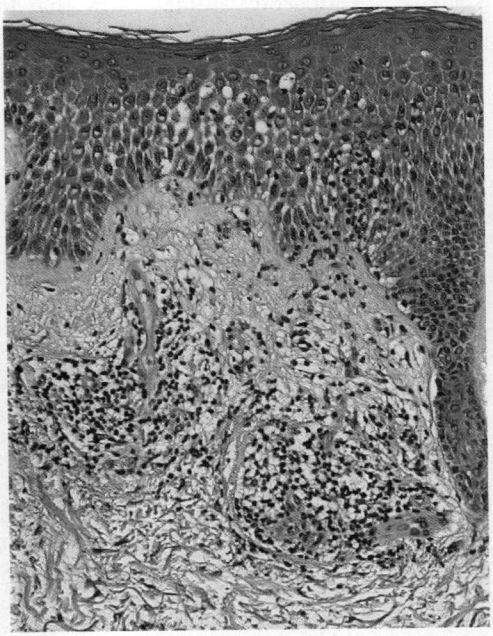

Figure 11-20 Photoallergic dermatitis. There is spongiosis with microvesicle formation, exocytosis of lymphocytes, and a perivascular lymphocytic infiltrate admixed with scattered eosinophils.

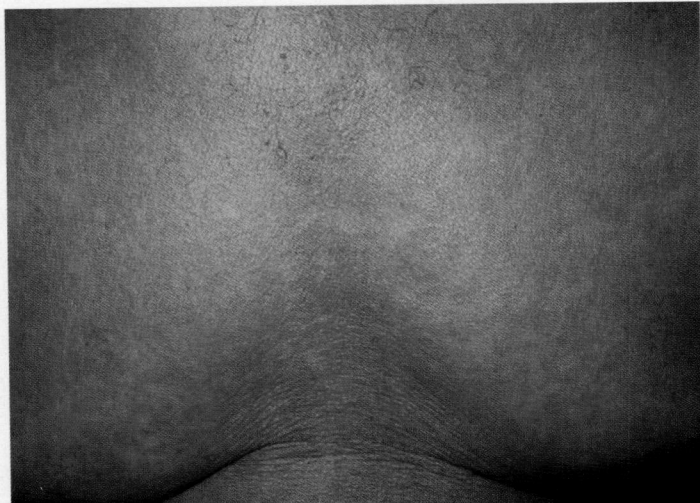

Figure 11-19 Morbilliform drug eruption. This eruption occurred in a patient with systemic symptoms (drug rash with eosinophilia and systemic symptoms). (Courtesy of Frances Ramos-Ceballos, MD.)

Phototoxic Drug Eruption

Clinical Summary. Phototoxic reactions occur when a person receives a sufficient amount of a phototoxic drug together with a sufficient amount of UV light. The drug absorbs radiation energy and results in free radicals or oxygen radical formation, resulting in cellular injury. The eruption clinically resembles a sunburn, which often resolves, leaving hyperpigmentation. All the drugs capable of producing a photoallergic reaction can also cause a phototoxic eruption when given in a sufficiently high concentration. Drugs commonly associated with phototoxic reactions are tetracyclines, particularly demeclocycline and doxycycline, fluoroquinolones, amiodarone, and psoralens (102). Multiple chemotherapeutic agents may induce a radiation or UV-recall phenomenon, an erythematous cutaneous eruption that appears in an area of previous exposure to radiation or UV light, including sunburn. This can be indistinguishable from phototoxic eruptions (103,104).

Histopathology. A phototoxic drug eruption, like a sunburn reaction, shows both vacuolated keratinocytes (sunburn cells) characterized by abundant, pale cytoplasm and apoptotic keratinocytes characterized by reduced, eosinophilic cytoplasm. The dermis shows edema and enlargement of endothelial cells (Fig. 11-21).

Principles of Management: Aggressive sun protection and adjusting the causative agent are the mainstays of treatment.

Photodistributed Hyperpigmentation

Clinical Summary. Certain drugs, in particular tetracycline, chlorpromazine, diltiazem, amiodarone, imipramine, and desipramine, are known to produce cutaneous discoloration on sun-exposed areas of the skin (105–107). This pigment change results from overproduction of melanin in melanocytes, specifically stimulated by the offending drug, lack of melanin clearance owing to stable complex formation with the drug, or dermal deposition of the drug, which undergoes a UV-related change that inhibits clearance (106). In imipramine hyperpigmentation, dispersive spectroscopy studies show that the dermal granules have copper and sulfur, elements normally found in tyrosinase and pheomelanin as well as melanin (108,109). This pigment alteration results in blue, blue-gray, or brown hues. Exposed parts of the bulbar conjunctivae may show brownish pigmentation. Similarly, photodistributed slate-gray, reticulated pigmentation has been described in patients on long-acting diltiazem hydrochloride (106).

Histopathology. In chlorpromazine, amiodarone, imipramine, and desipramine reactions, there is a variable amount of melanin in the basal layer of the epidermis. Throughout the dermis, there is a considerable accumulation of pigment-laden macrophages, predominantly in a perivascular pattern (Fig. 11-22). The pigment has the staining properties of melanin, in that it stains black with the Fontana–Masson silver stain and is decolorized by hydrogen peroxide. Hyperpigmentation from imipramine results from melanin complexed with drug metabolite, which causes refractile golden yellow granules that deposit in the superficial and papillary dermis and are visible on light microscopy (Fig. 11-23) (110). In addition, on electron microscopy,

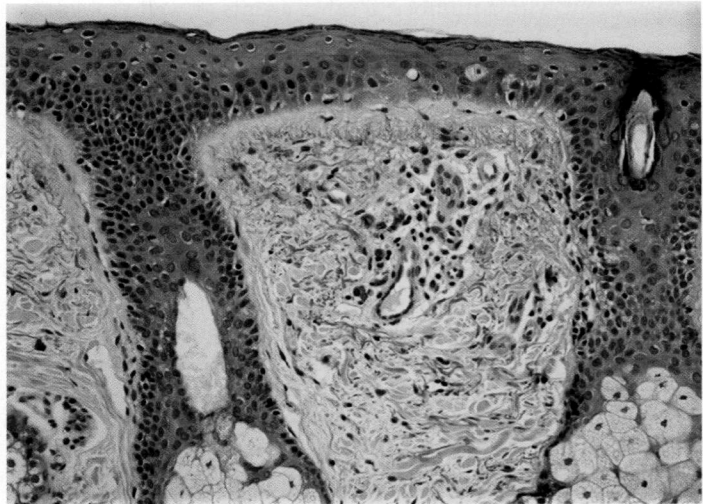

Figure 11-22 Chlorpromazine pigmentation. Perivascular pigment-laden macrophages are seen in this case of chlorpromazine pigmentation.

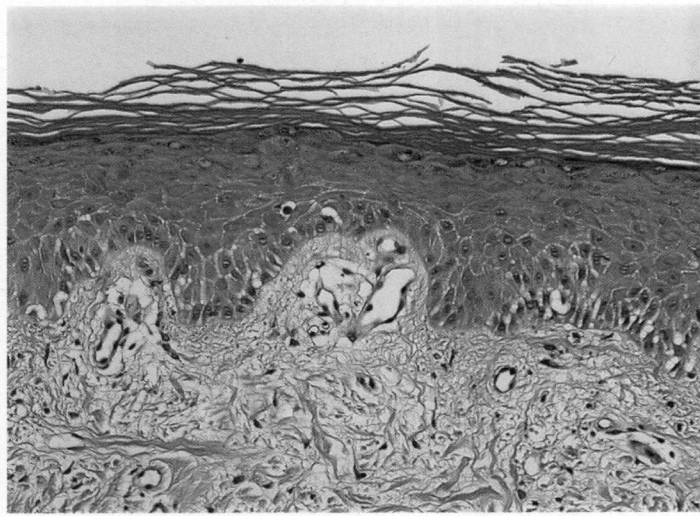

Figure 11-21 Phototoxic dermatitis. There are vacuolated basilar keratinocytes and apoptotic keratinocytes in the epidermis. Dermal edema and enlarged endothelial cells are also characteristic.

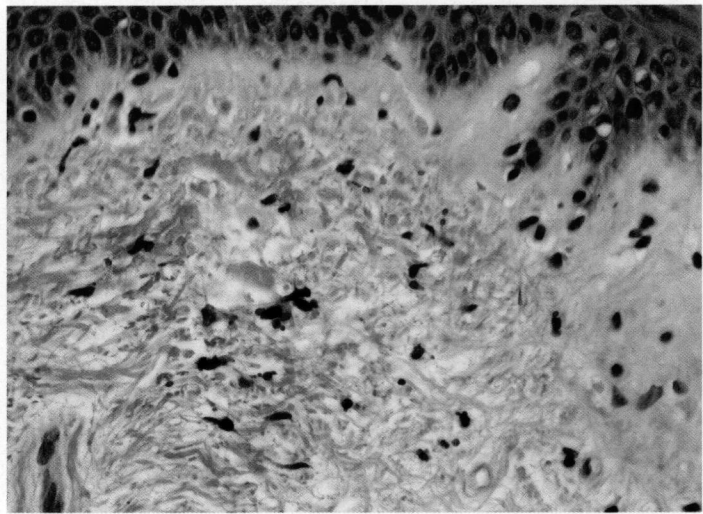

Figure 11-23 Imipramine pigmentation. Photodistributed slate-gray pigmentation is caused by round, yellow-brown globules in the dermis.

electron-dense granules are present within macrophages (108). In patients on long-term chlorpromazine, this melanin-like material is found in many internal organs, throughout the entire mononuclear-phagocyte system and, to a lesser degree, in the parenchymal cells of the liver, kidneys, and endocrine glands; myocardial fibers; and cerebral neurons (111).

In contrast, the diltiazem reactions reveal lichenoid dermatitis with atrophic epidermis and basal vacuolar change. The papillary dermis is expanded with prominent and dilated thin-walled vessels and a sparse perivascular and periadnexal lymphocytic infiltrate (107).

Pathogenesis. Electron microscopic examination has confirmed the presence of many melanosome complexes within the lysosomes of dermal macrophages. In addition, 0.2- to 3-μm-diameter, round or bizarrely-shaped electron-dense bodies may be seen in macrophages, endothelial cells, pericytes, Schwann cells, and fibroblasts, usually within lysosomes (112,113). Both electron-dense bodies and melanosome complexes may be found within the same lysosome. Although the dense bodies histochemically react like melanin, the striking sulfur peak on microprobe analysis strongly suggests the drug or its metabolite (113) is also present. Because some drugs do bind to melanin (113), it seems likely that the electron-dense bodies represent complexes of melanin with drug. These complexes are subsequently carried from the dermis by way of the circulating blood leukocytes to the various internal organs. In diltiazem-related hyperpigmentation, only melanosomes, without drug or drug metabolite, are seen (114).

Principles of Management: For photo-associated reactions, aggressive sun protection and adjusting the causative agent are the mainstays of treatment.

Pigmentary Disorders

Hyperpigmentation is a side effect of various therapeutic agents (in addition to photo-associated reactions discussed earlier), detailed in the next few sections.

Principles of Management: Pigmentary changes may resolve over time if the causative agent is stopped. Some may improve with aggressive sun protection, whereas others may be amenable to select laser treatments in the appropriate setting.

Minocycline Pigmentation

Clinical Summary. The prolonged administration of minocycline, a semisynthetic tetracycline, may result in three distinct types of cutaneous pigmentation: I—blue-black pigmentation occurring within areas of inflammation or scarring, usually on the face, especially in active or healed acne lesions; II—a blue-gray pigmentation of previously normal skin, most commonly seen on the legs but also occurring on the forearms; and III—a diffuse, muddy brown discoloration, sometimes accentuated in sun-exposed areas (115). In addition to that of the skin, nail and scleral pigmentation also occur (116). Pigmentation may extend into the subcutaneous tissue or be limited to the subcutaneous tissue. A systemic minocycline-induced hypersensitivity syndrome can present 2 to 4 weeks after the start of therapy. Symptoms include fever, rash, peripheral eosinophilia, and internal organ involvement (117). Internal organ involvement includes hepatitis or abnormal liver function test results, pneumonitis, and renal abnormalities (117,118).

Histopathology. The histologic picture shows differences among the three types of pigmentation. The focal blue-black pigmentation of the face in type I is associated with hemosiderin-laden macrophages (Fig. 11-24). In contrast, the blue-gray pigmentation in type II, most commonly observed on the legs, shows staining for iron and also reacts with the Fontana–Masson stain. The muddy brown pigmentation in type III reveals increased melanization of the basal cell layer and melanin within macrophages in the upper dermis. Pigmentation limited to the subcutaneous tissue is green-brown granules in macrophages, around vessels, between lipocytes, and in the septa. The subcutaneous pigment may be negative for both iron and melanin stains (119) or may be accentuated with Fontana–Masson stain (120).

Pathogenesis. The iron-containing pigment in types I and II pigmentation represents a drug metabolite–protein complex (121). The pigment in type II also reacts with the Fontana–Masson stain and does not bleach with hydrogen peroxide as melanin would, indicating that this stain is not melanin. The pigment in type III reacts like melanin and may represent a phototoxic phenomenon. Mass spectroscopy analysis of cutaneous minocycline pigmentation indicates the presence of iron and calcium. Radiographic techniques have confirmed that the clinical coloration is a result of a minocycline derivative chelated with iron that is stored within lysosomes of macrophages (119). The pathogenesis of minocycline-induced hypersensitivity reaction has not been elucidated.

Clofazimine-Induced Pigmentation

Clinical Summary. Clofazimine is administered to patients with leprosy and drug-resistant tuberculosis. It causes a pink to red-brown coloration of the skin, eyes, and gastrointestinal (GI) tract and dark pigmentation of the hair (122). The pigmentation resolves slowly after discontinuation of clofazimine. The most notably involved areas are the obvious leprosy lesions (123,124).

Histopathology. The upper dermis contains numerous foamy macrophages with cytoplasmic brown granular pigment. This pigment stains for lipofuscin, but not for melanin or iron.

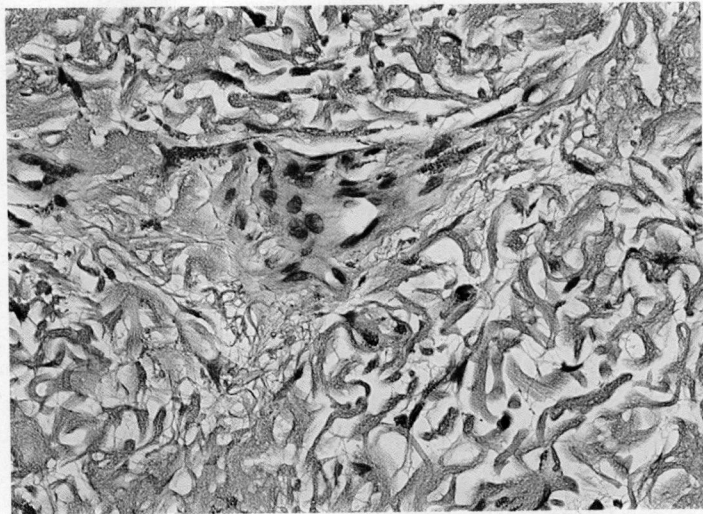

Figure 11-24 Minocycline hyperpigmentation. Pigment is present in dermal melanophages and dendritic cells, with a perivascular predominance.

Pathogenesis. On electron microscopy, the macrophages have phagolysosomes with either lipid or electron-dense granules with a lamellar substructure consistent with lipofuscin or ceroid pigment (124). The mechanism by which clofazimine causes these changes is unclear.

Amiodarone Pigmentation

Clinical Summary. Amiodarone is a class III anti-arrhythmic and coronary vasodilator that is well known to cause a photosensitivity and a blue-gray or purple discoloration in sun-exposed areas, especially the face with prominent involvement of the nose and ears (125). Corneal pigmentation is often associated with skin changes. The risk factors for developing the pigmentary changes include a daily dosage of more than 200 mg, long duration of treatment, fair skin, and excessive sun exposure (126).

Histopathology. Light microscopy of discolored skin shows aggregates of granular yellow-brown pigment in the cytoplasm of dermal histiocytes at the junction of the papillary and reticular dermis. Electron microscopy of affected skin reveals lysosomal membrane–bound dense bodies within the cytoplasm of histiocytes (127). The mechanism involved in amiodarone-induced pigmentation is unknown but may involve the deposition of lipofuscin in dermal histiocytes. Pigmentation is usually slowly reversible after discontinuation of the medication.

Bleomycin and Hydroxyurea Pigmentation

Clinical Summary. Hyperpigmentation is a common cutaneous side effect of cancer chemotherapeutic agents. Skin, hair, nails, and mucous membranes may all be affected. Grouped linear streaks, or "flagellate" hyperpigmentation, on the trunk and extremities are characteristic of bleomycin hyperpigmentation (128,129) (Fig. 11-25). Hyperpigmentation after long-term hydroxyurea therapy is well documented (130,131). The pigmentation may be diffuse or localized to a specific pattern that correlates with an anatomic feature or with external materials, such as occlusive dressings.

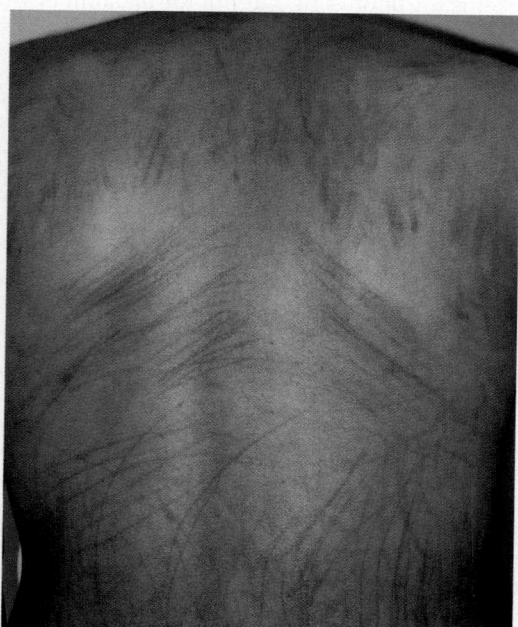

Figure 11-25 Bleomycin pigmentation. The characteristic linear "flagellate" streaks on the trunk of this patient on bleomycin.

Histopathology. Increased melanin pigmentation in basilar melanocytes, without an increase in melanocyte number, along with upper dermal melanophages is seen histologically. Ultrastructural studies show damage to subcellular organelles in the same distribution (132). Lymphocytic vasculitis along with the dermal melanophages has also been described (133).

Diltiazem Pigmentation

Clinical Summary. Diltiazem is a benzothiazepine calcium channel blocker widely used to treat hypertension and angina. Adverse effects of the drug include morbilliform eruptions, urticaria, pruritus, subacute lupus erythematosus, SJS/TEN, and vasculitis. Diltiazem has also been reported to induce a gray-brown, reticulated hyperpigmentation in sun-exposed areas (114). It is seen more frequently in older female patients with darker skin types who have taken the drug for at least 6 months.

Histopathology. Histologic examination shows a lichenoid eruption with necrotic keratinocytes, pigmentary incontinence, and lymphocytic infiltration. The pathogenesis is unknown, but it has been proposed that the drug or a metabolite may be a photosensitizer (107). However, electron microscopy of affected skin showed fully melanized melanosomes compatible with pigmentary incontinence without deposits of the drug or its metabolites (114).

Antimalarial Pigmentation

Clinical Summary. Antimalarials are a class of drugs that includes chloroquine, hydroxychloroquine, quinacrine, and mefloquine. Antimalarials have been reported to cause hyperpigmentation in up to 25% of patients (134). The pigmentation ranges from blue gray to purple to black and can appear on the anterior side of the legs, nose, cheeks, forehead, ears, and oral mucosa, especially the hard palate and nail bed, causing transverse bands or diffuse pigmentation. Antimalarials are also known to cause hypopigmentation, xerosis, pruritus, exacerbation of preexisting psoriasis, urticaria, lichenoid skin rashes, SJS, and hair loss or discoloration (135). Quinacrine pigmentation has a unique presentation, causing a lemon-yellow discoloration, which may involve the whole body and appear similar to jaundice.

Histopathology. Histopathology of affected skin consists of yellow to dark brown granules within macrophages and extracellularly in the dermis. Melanin can be present in the deeper dermis and in a perivascular distribution (136). The pathogenesis of antimalarial-induced pigmentation is not fully understood. Four basic mechanisms have been described: first, the accumulation of melanin usually results from either hyperproduction by epidermal melanocytes or in response to a nonspecific cutaneous inflammation. Second, hyperpigmentation results from the accumulation of the triggering drug itself. Third, some of the drugs synthesize special pigments, such as lipofuscin. Fourth, iron deposits occur in the dermis, usually as a result of drug-induced damage of dermal vessels with leakage of red blood cells (106).

Argyria

Clinical Summary. Argyria is skin discoloration related to the absorption of silver. When ingested, or after mucosal application, there is a slate-blue discoloration on the skin, especially in the sun-exposed areas. The oral mucosa, conjunctivae, fingernail beds (but not toenail), intestines, liver, spleen, and peritoneum may also be involved (137–139). The most common risk factor for argyria is now occupational exposure, including, but not limited to, dietary supplements, mining, welding, silversmithing, antique restoration, jewelry manufacturing, and photographic development. It has also been reported after acupuncture and in a silversmith following multiple cutaneous punctures by a silver filament (140–144). Pseudo-ochronosis has also been reported to occur in association with localized argyria (145).

Histopathology. In the dermis, there are extracellular fine, small, round, uniformly sized brown-black silver granules, both singly and clustered. The deposition is predominantly extracellular and found in both sun-exposed and sun-unexposed skin. They are present in the greatest numbers not only in the basement membrane zone surrounding the sweat glands (Fig. 11-26) but also in the connective tissue sheaths around the hair follicles and sebaceous glands, the walls of capillaries, arrectores pilorum, and nerves (146). Silver granules are also found in the dermal papillae and scattered diffusely throughout the dermis. Elastic tissue stains reveal a predilection of the granules for elastic fibers, which explains the presence of finger-like chains of granules projecting into the dermal papillae (146). In contrast, silver is not seen in the epidermis or its appendages. Although visible in routine stains, dark-field microscopy reveals brilliantly refractile, white particles against a dark background. In addition to silver, there is an increase in the amount of epidermal melanin, particularly in sun-exposed skin. Melanophages may also be scattered throughout the upper dermis. Deposits of silver are also found in internal organs. Incubation of sections in a solution consisting of 1% potassium ferricyanide in 20% sodium thiosulfate results in decolorization of silver.

Pathogenesis. The slate-blue discoloration is believed to stem from absorption of silver that complexes with proteins, DNA, and RNA. UV light causes these complexes to form metallic silver, which can then be oxidized to black silver sulfide deposits. Silver sulfide can stimulate melanocyte activity, leading to an increase in melanin deposition (138). Electron microscopy reveals extracellular aggregates of irregularly shaped granules varying in size from 200 to 400 nm in diameter but ranging up to 1,000 nm (147).

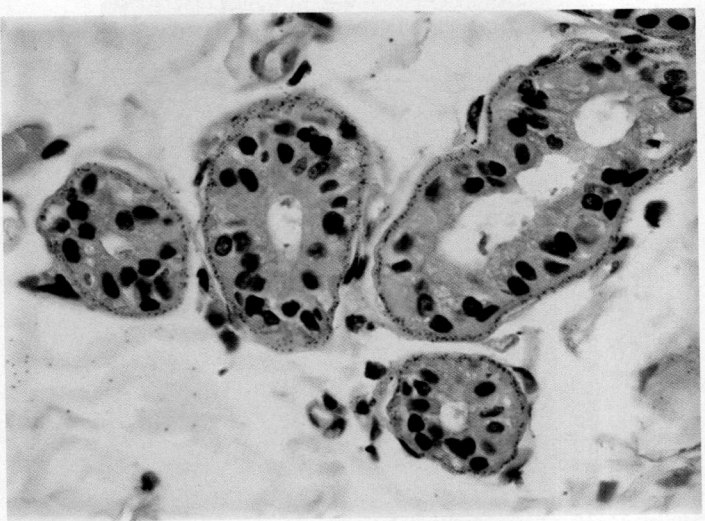

Figure 11-26 Argyria. Silver granules are present in the basement membrane surrounding the sweat glands.

Chrysiasis

Clinical Summary. Chrysiasis is slate-blue discoloration on sun-exposed skin caused by the prolonged parenteral administration of gold salts, generally for the treatment of rheumatoid arthritis and secondary to Q-switched ruby laser treatment (148,149).

Histopathology. Gold granules are found predominantly within cells, particularly within endothelial cells and macrophages (150). Extracellular granules may also be observed. Gold granules are larger and more irregularly shaped than silver granules. They are light refractile with dark-field examination, orange-red birefringent on fluorescence microscopy (151).

Pathogenesis. The exact cause of pigmentation is not known. Patients have a higher concentration of melanin in the epidermis and dermis. Gold deposits in the dermis may enhance melanogenesis by indirectly increasing tyrosinase activity. UV light may stimulate preferential uptake of gold by the skin.

Electron microscopic examination shows the presence of electron-dense, angulated particles within phagolysosomes of endothelial cells and macrophages. X-ray spectroscopic analysis demonstrates a spectrum consistent with the presence of gold (151).

Mercury Pigmentation

Clinical Summary. Regular application of a mercury-containing cream to the face and neck over many years may produce a slate-gray pigmentation of the skin in the areas to which the cream has been applied. Generally, the pigmentation is most pronounced on the eyelids, in the nasolabial folds, and in the folds of the neck (152). A systemic contact dermatitis can also occur (153). Most mercury-containing creams have been banned from therapeutic use in Western countries (154). However, mercury can be found both deliberately and as a contaminant in traditional medicines. Exposure to mercury can also occur through topical antiseptics, inhalation, traumatic implantation, and in over-the-counter skin lightening products used worldwide (156).

Histopathology. Irregular, brown-black granules are found in the upper dermis, both extracellularly and within macrophages. In rare instances, granules are seen also in the basal cell layer of the epidermis. As in argyria and chrysiasis, dark-field microscopy reveals brilliantly refractile granules. Silver staining reveals normal or increased basilar melanin (155). Traumatic implantation of mercury results in variably sized, often large amorphous deposits of mercury in the dermis and subcutis. Chronic changes include dermal fibrosis and granulomatous inflammation (Fig. 11-27).

Pathogenesis. Electron microscopic examination shows the mercury particles, which are approximately 14 nm in diameter, to be aggregated into irregular granules with diameters of up to 340 nm. The granules are associated with elastic fibers as well as along the collagen fibers. In macrophages, they are present within lysosomes or free in the cytoplasm. When seen in the epidermis, the mercury granules lie in the intercellular spaces of the basal cell layer (155).

Because the pigmentation is most pronounced in skin folds that are protected from the sun and there may be no increase in the amount of melanin, it can be concluded that most of the pigmentation is caused by mercury rather than melanin.

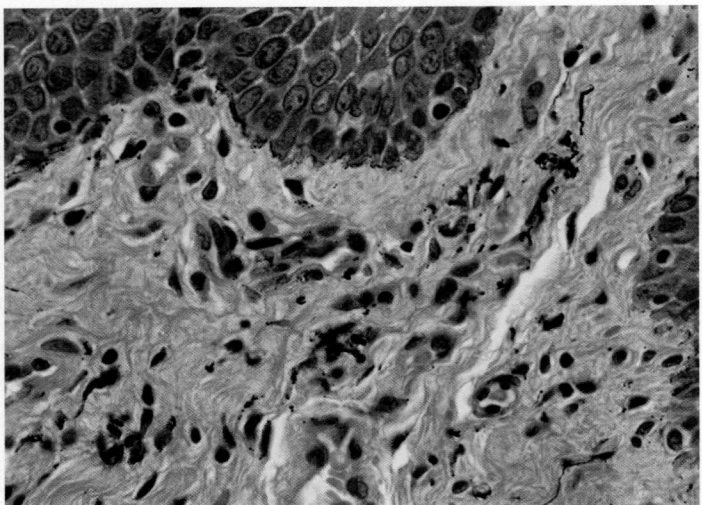

Figure 11-27 Mercury deposition. Large, black-brown mercury deposits along with multinucleate foreign-body giant cells are seen in the papillary dermis and along the basement membrane in this case of traumatic mercury implantation in the buccal mucosa.

REACTIONS TO CHEMOTHERAPEUTIC AGENTS

In general, the cutaneous changes brought about by antineoplastic chemotherapeutic agents are the result of their antiproliferative effects disrupting cutaneous cellular metabolism. Clinical manifestations vary. Anagen effluvium is a well-established effect of the antiproliferative nature of many chemotherapeutic agents. Neutrophilic eccrine hidradenitis presents with erythematous, often acral, plaques several days after cytoreductive chemotherapy. Acral erythema unassociated with primary eccrine changes also occurs after chemotherapy (see previous discussion). Some authors group the common reactions caused by chemotherapeutic agents under the unifying term "toxic erythema of chemotherapy," in an attempt to encompass hand–foot syndrome, eccrine syringosquamous metaplasia, and other alternative terms for chemotherapy reactions into a common umbrella syntax (156). Hyperpigmentation caused by these agents is discussed earlier.

Principles of Management: The changes generally resolve over time after the causative agent is stopped. Symptomatic therapy may be necessary in the acute phase.

Dysmaturation

Clinical Summary. Cytoreductive chemotherapy may cause a disruption of the normal pattern of keratinocyte maturation. These changes, referred to as *epidermal dysmaturation*, may be observed in the epidermis after any significant cytoreductive therapy and are not necessarily associated with clinical lesions.

Histopathology. There is a loss of the normal keratinocyte maturation from small cuboidal cells in the basilar epidermis to flattened squamous cells in the stratum corneum. Keratinocytes are separated by widened intercellular spaces, lose polarity, and display irregular large nuclei, mid-epidermal mitotic figures, and apoptosis (Figs. 11-28 and 11-29). These changes, when severe, may be mistaken for squamous cell carcinoma (SCC), *in situ*. "Starburst" mitotic figures are described after systemic etoposide administration (157). Etoposide is a vinca alkaloid

derivative that disrupts mitotic spindle formation by attaching to microtubule proteins. Papillary dermal melanophages are also often present.

Neutrophilic Eccrine Hidradenitis

Clinical Summary. Neutrophilic eccrine hidradenitis often manifests as slightly violaceous, erythematous papules, plaques, and nodules, more common on the head and upper trunk, particularly on the face and axilla, approximately 2 to 3 weeks after initiation of chemotherapy. The eruption occurs classically with cytarabine but can occur in the setting of numerous chemotherapeutic regimens.

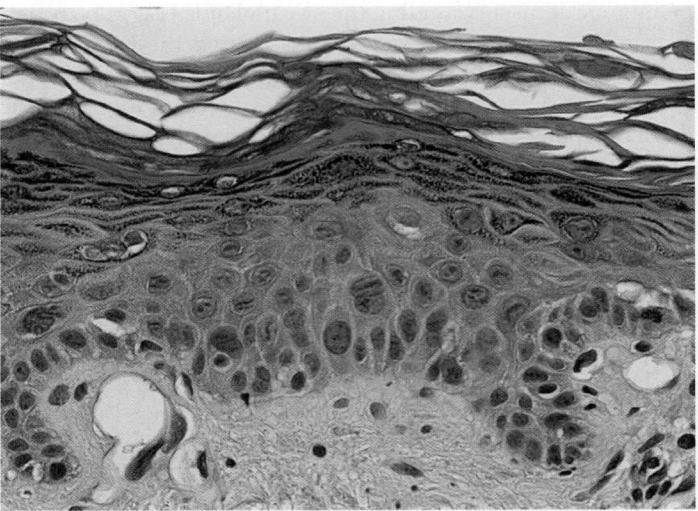

Figure 11-28 Mild epidermal dysmaturation owing to antineoplastic chemotherapy. Loss of polarity and disorganization of keratinocytes is minimal and confined to the lower and mid-epidermal layers in this specimen.

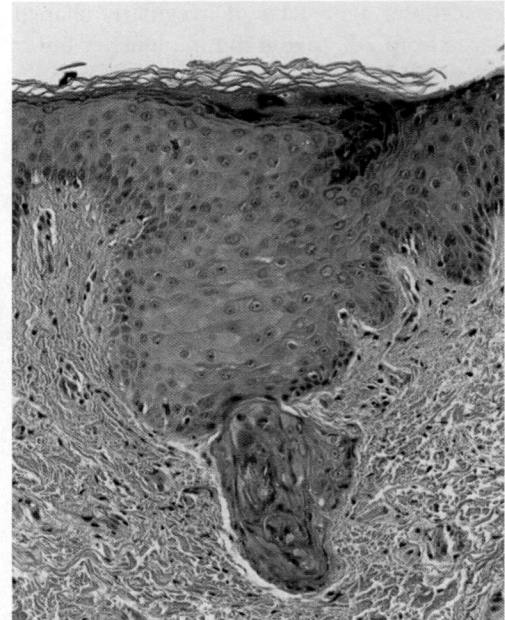

Figure 11-29 Severe epidermal dysmaturation owing to antineoplastic chemotherapy. Loss of polarity and disorganization of keratinocytes are advanced in this specimen.

Histopathology. Several entities in this section are unified by the theory of drug concentration in eccrine sweat. Specimens from patterned *postchemotherapy hyperpigmentation* show vacuolization of basilar epidermis, melanin incontinence, and apoptosis in occluded skin after administration of alkylating agents (158). Inflammation is sparse or absent. Squamous metaplasia of the upper eccrine ducts, *syringosquamous metaplasia,* is described after cytoreductive therapies. The normally cuboidal cells lining the duct display irregularly increased amounts of eosinophilic cytoplasm with associated polymorphous inflammation, fibrosis, and necrosis (Fig. 11-30). *Neutrophilic eccrine hidradenitis* consists of variable infiltration of the eccrine coil by neutrophils and lymphocytes with necrosis of secretory epithelium. Individual cells or whole coils show increased cytoplasmic eosinophilia, degeneration of nuclei, and loss of integrity of cell walls (Fig. 11-31). Edema and mucinous change may be seen in the perieccrine adipose tissue.

Pathogenesis. The notion of concentration of antineoplastic chemotherapeutic agents in sweat serves to unify the clinical observation of patterned hyperpigmentation (beneath bandages and electrocardiogram pads in the case of thiotepa) and the histologic observations of neutrophilic eccrine hidradenitis

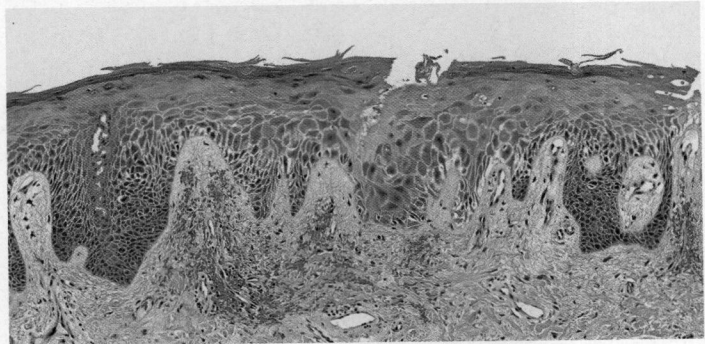

Figure 11-30 Syringosquamous metaplasia. This eccrine duct is lined by squamoid cells with ample eosinophilic cytoplasm and large nuclei rather than the normal cuboidal cells.

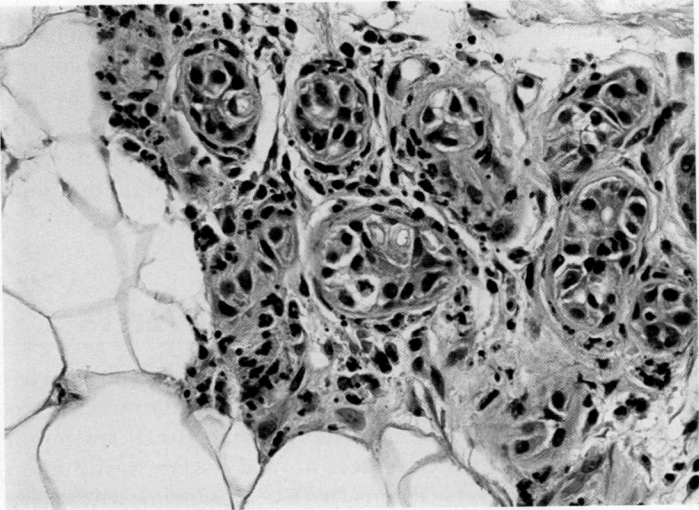

Figure 11-31 Neutrophilic eccrine hidradenitis. Neutrophils and lymphocytes are present in the perieccrine adventitia and eccrine coil. Increased cytoplasmic eosinophilia and pyknotic nuclei characterize eccrine necrosis.

and syringosquamous metaplasia. Changes after antineoplastic chemotherapy likely represent a mix of direct toxic effect on the various constituent cells of the skin with secondary inflammation incited by cell damage. Other chemotherapy-related cutaneous changes may also involve similar mechanisms—namely, intertriginous erosion/ulceration after isophosphamide (159) and flagellate hyperpigmentation after bleomycin. Why specific agents affect specific cell populations in the skin in a repeatable manner is unclear. It is important to note that identification of epidermal dysmaturation assumes considerable importance in establishing the diagnosis of acute graft-versus-host reaction (160). When possible, the inflammation and apoptosis of a graft-versus-host reaction should be sought in areas unaffected or less affected by dysmaturation.

Toxic Acral Erythema

Clinical Summary. Hand–foot syndrome, palmar–plantar erythrodysesthesia syndrome, or toxic acral erythema refers to a transient painful erythema of the palms and soles that becomes edematous and ultimately desquamates. Blisters may form, leaving ulcerated epithelium. Numerous chemotherapeutic agents, including cytarabine, docetaxel, and 5-fluorouracil, have been implicated. The cutaneous lesions attributable to docetaxel—an antineoplastic agent that interferes with normal microtubule function—are not limited to acral sites (161).

Histopathology. The skin displays vacuolar degeneration of basilar keratinocytes with eventual cleft formation. Mild epidermal dysmaturation may be seen. Keratinocyte necrosis is also present in the lower third of the epidermis. In the dermis, there is a mild perivascular infiltrate of lymphocytes with few eosinophils.

REACTIONS TO TARGETED AGENTS

Clinical Summary. There is an ever-expanding list of novel chemotherapeutic agents, particularly small molecule inhibitors and targeted therapeutics, many of which are associated with an array of cutaneous findings. Although an exhaustive discussion of these findings is outside the scope of a dermatopathology text, readers should be aware of the cutaneous and pathologic findings that may occur in the setting of these therapies.

Epidermal Growth Factor Receptor Inhibitors

Clinical Summary. Inhibitors of the epidermal growth factor receptor (EGFR) have increasing importance in the treatment of solid tumors. These receptors are integral to epidermal development and maintenance and are commonly expressed in basal layer keratinocytes, sebaceous gland epithelium, and the outer root sheath of hair follicles. Accordingly, cutaneous reactions owing to the inhibition of the receptors are common. Most of these reactions (85%) occur as an acneiform eruption (162–164). Patients present with a seborrheic distribution of pruritic folliculocentric papulopustules without comedones. Lesions may become secondarily infected, most commonly with *Staphylococcus aureus.* Other cutaneous reactions may include xerosis, photosensitivity, hair changes, mucositis, paronychia, onycholysis, and pyogenic granuloma–like lesions.

Histopathology. In the acneiform eruption, there is follicular ectasia with a neutrophil-predominant inflammatory infiltrate. Follicular rupture may result in a granulomatous reaction.

Multikinase Inhibitors

Clinical Summary. The tyrosine kinase inhibitors are small molecules, which affect multiple target receptors. Sorafenib inhibits RAF, vascular endothelial growth factor receptor (VEGFR), and platelet derived growth factor receptor (PDGFR), among others (165). Similarly, sunitinib and regorafenib also affect multiple kinase receptors. Patients on sorafenib and sunitinib develop hand–foot–skin reaction (HFSR) in 36% to 48% of cases. They present with hyperkeratotic, often yellow, tender papules and plaques on the knuckles and pressure sites of the hands and feet. Bullae formation may also occur. Patients may also develop xerosis, eruptive pigmented lesions, keratoacanthoma-like SCC, seborrheic dermatitis–like eruption, acneiform dermatitis, yellow discoloration of the skin, and hair and nails changes.

Histopathology. An interface dermatitis presenting with a band-like layer of necrosis is noted in HFSR. The degree and level of epidermal necrosis is dependent on the duration and dosage of therapy, with higher levels of epidermal involvement noted with continued length of therapy. Epidermal vesiculation, dermal telangiectasias, and cystic degeneration of eccrine glands may also be identified (165,166).

Kit and BCR-ABL inhibitors

Clinical Summary. Medications such as imatinib, dasatinib, and nilotinib have been utilized to treat malignancies with *bcr-abl* fusion gene caused by chromosome 9:22 translocation, such as chronic myeloid leukemia, or c-Kit mutation, such as GI stromal tumor. Dose-dependent facial and generalized edema may develop (167). As c-Kit is integral in melanocyte physiology and melanogenesis, dyspigmentation or vitiligo of the skin and hair can be seen. Patients may also develop a morbilliform exanthem, lichenoid drug reaction, or, more rarely, SCAR like SJS/TEN or DRESS (168–170).

Histopathology. The histopathologic features of c-Kit or *bcr-abl* inhibitors are similar to the *de novo* reactions.

BRAF and MEK Inhibitors

Clinical Summary. Mutations in BRAF are common in malignancies, such as hairy cell leukemia and melanoma, but may also be seen in common and dysplastic nevi. BRAF is involved in the RAS-RAF-MEK-ERK-MAP kinase signaling pathway, which is integral in regulating proliferation and growth. MEK inhibitors (MEKi) block downstream of BRAF inhibitors (BRAFi) in this pathway. Vemurafenib, a selective BRAFi, can induce a host of skin changes, such as curling of the hair, keratosis pilaris, thickening of the palms and soles, darkening or eruption of nevi with rare instances of atypia, involution of nevi, development of verrucous keratoses, and, most notably, development of SCC in nearly a quarter of patients, often of the keratoacanthoma type (171,172) (Figs. 11-32 and 11-33). The majority, 61%, of SCC develop within 3 months of therapy. The development of these keratinocytic tumors may be related to paradoxical activation of the MAP kinase pathway. As such, the addition of MEKi with BRAFi may reduce the incidence of SCC development, while improving progression-free survival in melanoma (173). MEKi may result in similar cutaneous reactions as the EGFRi with an acneiform eruption, xerosis, hair and nail changes, as well as a dose-dependent morbilliform exanthem (174).

Histopathology. Verrucous lesions in the setting of BRAFi demonstrate acanthosis, papillomatosis, hypergranulosis, and

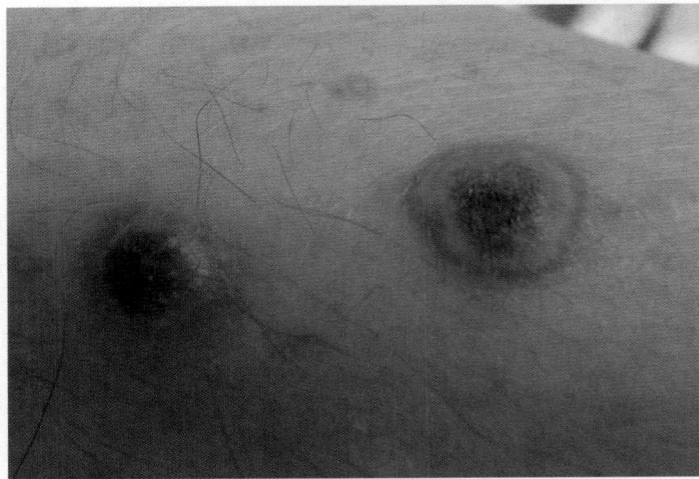

Figure 11-32 Keratoacanthoma-type squamous cell carcinomas arising in a patient treated with vemurafenib.

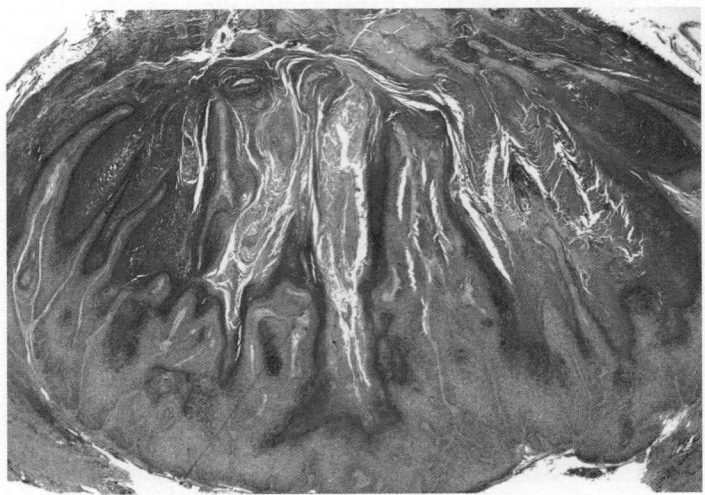

Figure 11-33 Keratoacanthoma-type squamous cell carcinoma showing central hyperkeratosis and surrounding lobules of glassy keratinocytes.

hyperkeratosis. The lesions are often negative for human papillomavirus (HPV) immunostaining but have demonstrated positivity for p16 (175). Nevi that develop with BRAFi may lack BRAFV600E mutation and demonstrate hypermelanosis of the epidermis, including the stratum corneum, increased melanophages, and an atypical pattern of HMB-45 immunostaining with deep dermal positivity (176).

IMMUNE-RELATED ADVERSE EVENTS

Clinical Summary. By targeting cytotoxic T-lymphocyte–associated antigen-4 (CTLA-4) or PD-1/PDL1, immune checkpoint inhibitors (ICIs) upregulate cytotoxic T-cell antitumor activity. However, this can affect normal tissues, resulting in immune-related adverse events (irAEs). Cutaneous irAEs have been estimated to occur in one-third to nearly half of patients on anti–CTLA-4 or anti–PD-1/PD-L1 therapy, with the former being more likely to develop reactions (177,178). Common irAEs are a morbilliform exanthem and pruritus. In one study, lichen planus–like or lichenoid dermatitis associated with PD-1/PD-L1 inhibitors are the most commonly biopsied adverse reaction (Coleman et al., 2019) (Figs. 11-34 and 11-35). Other reactions that have been documented include, but are not limited to, eczematous, psoriasiform, sarcoidosis, and other granulomatous, autoimmune blistering dermatoses such as BP (Fig. 11-36), vitiligo, alopecia areata, vasculitis, panniculitis, sclerodermoid reactions, vasculitis, Grover disease, Sweet syndrome, pyoderma gangrenosum, graft-versus-host disease, or severe drug reactions like SJS/TEN or DRESS (179). The development of lichenoid and spongiotic reactions may indicate a positive prognosis and survival (180). Patients with irAEs in more than two organs demonstrated improved overall survival (181).

Histopathology. The histopathologic features of the irAEs are similar to their non–drug-associated versions. Multiple biopsies from different anatomic sites may be helpful in better identifying cutaneous irAEs. Variability among biopsies in the degree of eosinophilic infiltrate and/or spongiosis can help differentiate a lichenoid irAE from lichen planus or a psoriasiform eruption from psoriasis (182).

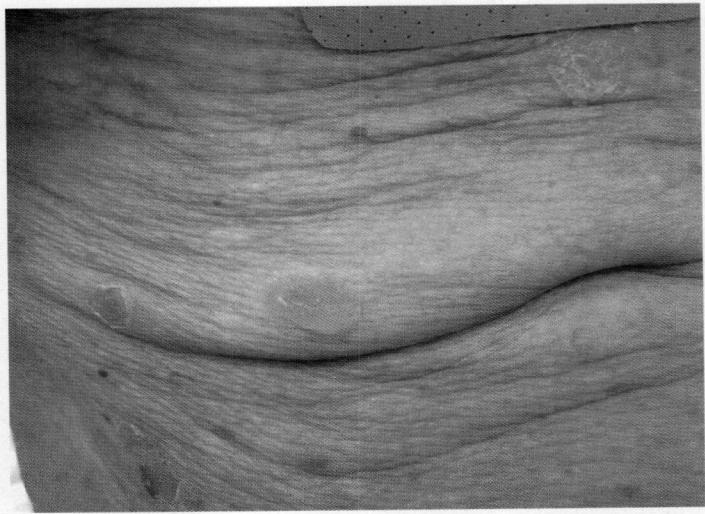

Figure 11-36 PD-1 inhibitor–associated bullous pemphigoid.

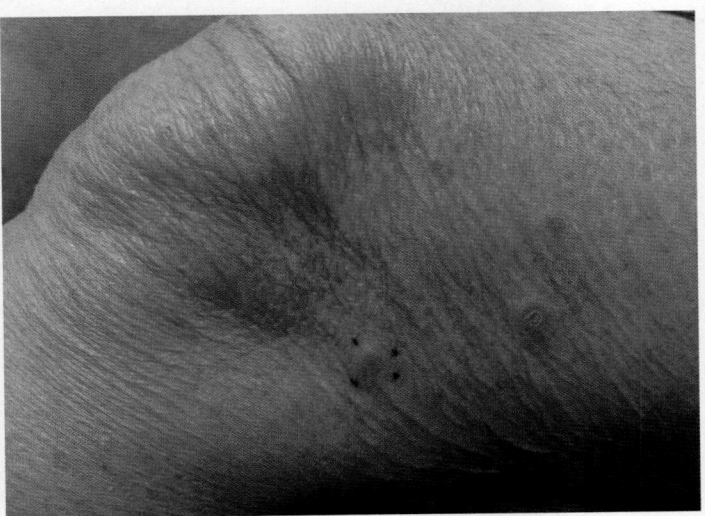

Figure 11-34 Lichenoid dermatitis secondary to PD-1 inhibitor use.

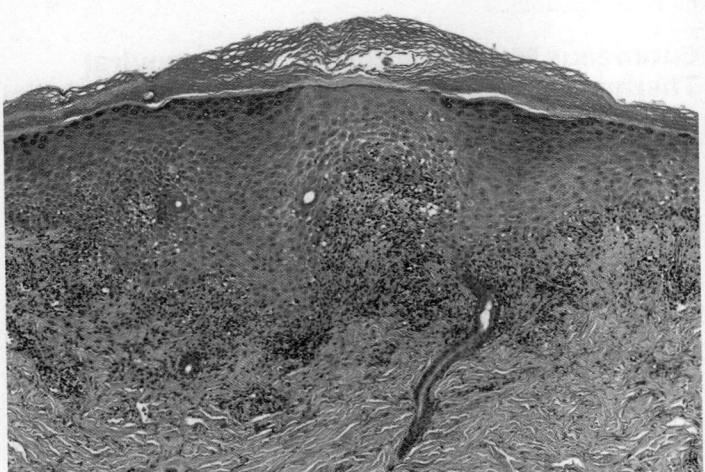

Figure 11-35 Lichenoid dermatitis secondary to PD-1 inhibitor use showing a band-like lymphocytic inflammatory infiltrate in the superficial dermatitis.

Readers evaluating patients on novel chemotherapeutic and immunotherapy regimens are encouraged to examine the emerging primary literature for an up-to-date discussion on this rapidly changing field.

REACTION TO BIOLOGIC AGENTS

Technological advances in recombinant DNA research have resulted in the availability of biologic agents: proteins, cytokines, antibodies, and fusion protein or soluble receptors. These agents are administered to patients to provide immunologic manipulation for therapeutic benefit.

Mucocutaneous effects of systemic administration of cytokines and monoclonal antibodies have been described. The findings generally occur (a) at injection sites, (b) as variably distributed eruptions, or (c) as exacerbation or induction of other dermatologic disorders, such as psoriasis.

Etanercept, a recombinant TNF-α receptor fused to the Fc fragment of IgG2, and recombinant IFN β-1a and IFN β-1b, has been associated with injection-site reactions, lichenoid dermatitis, urticaria, leukocytoclastic vasculitis, EM, SJS and TEN, and granulomatous reactions, which can resemble sarcoidosis (21,183). Both etanercept and other TNF inhibitors have been reported to induce psoriasiform eruptions, which may be limited to palmoplantar pustular eruptions or more widespread eruptions of psoriasiform dermatitis.

Recombinant human/mouse monoclonal anti-EGFR causes a variety of cutaneous eruptions, as might be anticipated based on the role of EGFR in cutaneous homeostasis; 85% of these eruptions are acneiform (163). This eruption of erythematous follicular papules and plaques may occur on the face, trunk, or extremities and is associated with intense pruritis and fever. Other less common mucocutaneous reactions are erythema, xerosis, mucositis, pruritus, paronychia, hair changes, and anaphylactoid reactions (184,185).

G-CSF is used to accelerate repopulation of the granulocytic lineage of hematopoietic cells after bone marrow depletion, either from chemotherapy or from bone marrow transplantation. Large dermal histiocytes intercalating collagen bundles are characteristically seen as a result of the neutrophil recovery process. In addition, injection-site reaction, pyoderma gangrenosum, Sweet syndrome–like eruption, leukocytoclastic vasculitis, and folliculitis have been attributed to hematopoietic growth factors (186).

Correlating the temporal relation between drug administration, peripheral leukocyte count, and onset of the eruption is helpful. The eruption begins soon after initiation of drug, and the histopathology of the eruption will relate to recognized effects of the drug.

Histopathology. The morbilliform eruption induced by pharmacologic doses of human recombinant GM-CSF is characterized by a perivascular and interstitial infiltrate of neutrophils, eosinophils, and lymphocytes in the upper dermis (Fig. 11-37). The relative proportion of cell types varies. Macrophages are increased in number and size and may contain melanin when situated in the upper dermis. The epidermis may display intercellular edema with exocytosis of inflammatory cells. Vasculitis is absent.

The erythematous plaques associated with G-CSF contain numerous neutrophils and upper dermal edema, thus resembling the skin lesions of Sweet syndrome (187) (Fig. 11-38).

Findings at the site of etanercept injection include a superficial perivascular inflammatory infiltrate composed primarily of lymphocytes, with eosinophils admixed with small numbers of neutrophils and macrophages. Mild dermal edema and vasodilation are also noted (188). IFN injection sites have shown a mild perivascular lymphocytic infiltrate and thrombosis of deep vessels without fibrinoid necrosis (189).

The acneiform eruptions associated with anti-EGFR show florid suppurative superficial folliculitis with disruption of the epithelial lining (190).

TNF-α inhibitor–induced palmoplantar pustulosis and psoriasiform dermatitis often display classic histologic findings of psoriasis.

Pathogenesis. In the case of eruptions associated with GM-CSF and G-CSF, the histologic findings relate to the administration and known actions of the cytokine. In a period of peripheral neutropenia, the lesional tissue will have numerous granulocytes. In addition, the effects of GM-CSF on macrophages are demonstrable in the skin by observing their expanded number

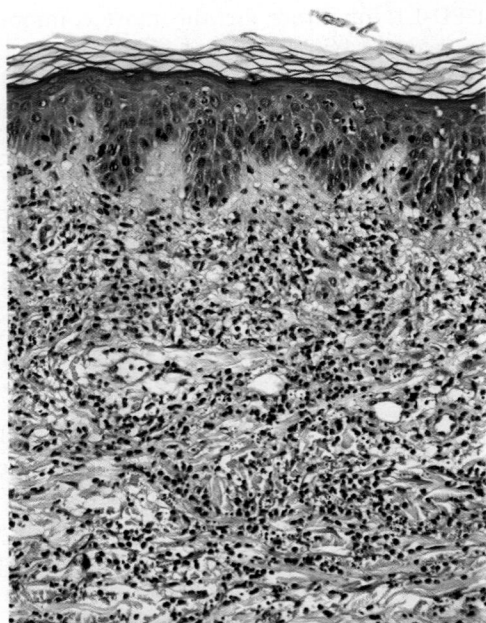

Figure 11-38 Granulocyte-macrophage colony-stimulating factor. The density of the neutrophilic infiltrate may be florid, resembling Sweet syndrome, as in this case.

and size. Immunohistochemical stains to macrophage/monocyte markers may be useful to highlight this finding. Injection-site reactions with etanercept are suggestive of a delayed-type hypersensitivity reaction, whereas those of IFN β suggest enhancement of preexisting disease-related platelet activation (191). TNF-induced psoriasis develops through unclear mechanisms, as the TNF inhibitors are often used to treat psoriasis; some have hypothesized that there may be alterations in IFN levels that contribute to TNF inhibitor–induced psoriasis.

Principles of Management: The changes generally resolve over time after the causative agent is stopped. Symptomatic therapy may be necessary in the acute phase.

CUTANEOUS MANIFESTATIONS OF ANTIRETROVIRAL THERAPY

Antiretroviral therapy is not uncommonly associated with cutaneous reactions.

Cutaneous Manifestations of Antiretroviral Therapy for Hepatitis C Virus

Clinical Summary. A variety of cutaneous eruptions have been associated with treatment for hepatitis C virus (HCV) using pegylated IFN alfa-2a or IFN alfa-2b plus ribavirin. These account for more than 10% of all IFN-associated side effects. Common cutaneous events include injection-site reactions, psoriasis, alopecia, sarcoidosis, and, most commonly, generalized pruritus and xerosis, with eczematous lesions accentuated by erythematous papules and microvesicles that are often excoriated, predominately located on the trunk and extremities (Fig. 11-39) (192). The new HCV protease inhibitors, such as boceprevir, telaprevir, and sofosbuvir, when used in combination with IFN and ribavirin, have higher rates of dermatologic adverse events. In recent clinical trials, 55% of patients treated with telaprevir developed a rash. More than 90% of events were grade 1 or 2

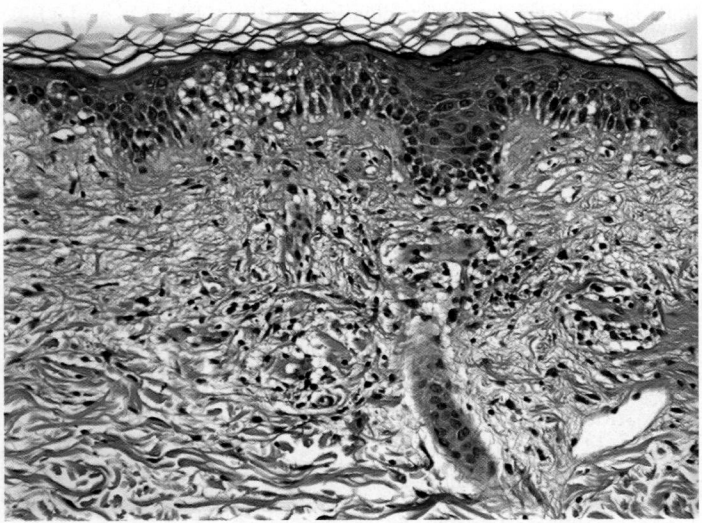

Figure 11-37 Granulocyte-macrophage colony-stimulating factor. A mild, diffuse perivascular and interstitial neutrophilic infiltrate is present with associated vascular dilation and spongiosis.

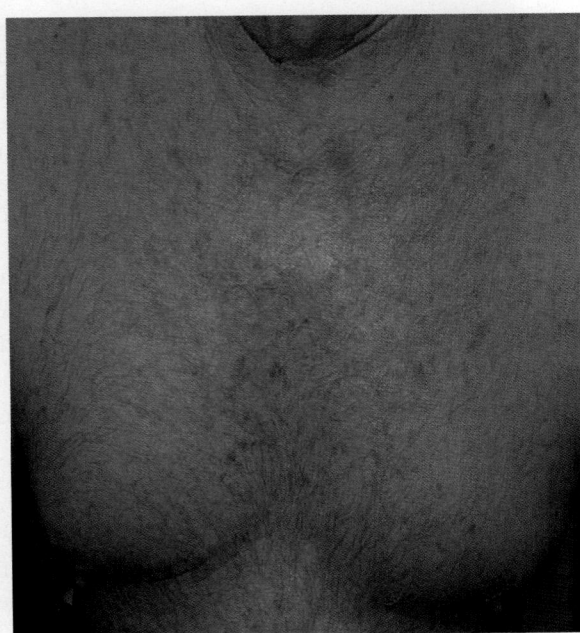

Figure 11-39 Hepatitis C treatment. This patient developed erythematous papules and microvesicles on the trunk during treatment with pegylated interferon alfa and boceprevir.

reactions and consisted of a pruritic, erythematous dermatitis, affecting less than 50% of body surface area. However, cases of leukocytoclastic vasculitis, DRESS, and SJS were also seen (193,194).

Histopathology. There are no uniquely identifying features of the eruptions caused by antiviral therapy. Histologic features are identical to the nonantiviral therapy–associated eruption.

Pathogenesis. The mechanism of adverse dermatologic events remains unknown, and no predictors have been identified.

Principles of Management: Milder reactions may be treated symptomatically during the course of therapy, whereas severe reactions necessitate drug withdrawal.

Cutaneous Manifestations of Antiretroviral Therapy for HIV

Clinical Summary. Antiretroviral therapy options include protease inhibitors, non-nucleoside reverse transcriptase inhibitors, and nucleoside reverse transcriptase inhibitors. Although exanthematous eruptions and urticaria have been most commonly described with the use of these agents, they have also been associated with several unique findings. The lipodystrophy syndrome, identified originally with the use of protease inhibitors and subsequently with the use of reverse transcriptase inhibitors, is characterized by peripheral lipoatrophy, central adiposity, and metabolic abnormalities. Protease inhibitors and reverse transcriptase inhibitors are associated with paronychia with pyogenic granulomas of the lateral nail fold (195). Unique patterns of hyperpigmentation involving the nails, palms, soles, and mucous membranes are seen secondary to melanocyte stimulation by zidovudine and emtricitabine (196). Hypersensitivity reactions such as leukocytoclastic vasculitis and DRESS are also associated with nucleoside reverse transcriptase inhibitors, especially nevirapine and abacavir (197). Non-nucleoside reverse transcriptase inhibitors are the most frequent class of

antiretrovirals to cause morbilliform exanthems (198). Nevirapine is associated with systemic hypersensitivity reactions and is one of the most common causes of SJS in the developing world (199). The fusion inhibitor, enfuvirtide, requires subcutaneous administration and has a very high incidence of injection-site reactions. The immune reconstitution syndrome, an inflammatory response to infectious agents such as viruses, mycobacteria, and fungi, occurs during initiation of antiretroviral therapy and can mimic a drug reaction (198,200).

Histopathology. Histologic features of the lipodystrophy syndrome and other conditions mentioned previously as secondary to protease inhibitors are the same as those from other causes (see Chapter 20).

Principles of Management: The changes generally resolve over time after the causative agent is stopped. Symptomatic therapy may be necessary in the acute phase.

MISCELLANEOUS DRUGS

Among a large potential variety of disease-causing reagents, the following are especially likely to be associated with changes that may present in skin biopsies.

Penicillamine-Induced Dermatoses

Penicillamine, a degradation product of penicillin that is used in the treatment of rheumatoid arthritis, and as a chelating agent, has many documented cutaneous side effects, including dermatoses resulting from interference with collagen and elastin, such as anetoderma, elastosis perforans serpiginosa (EPS), excessive wrinkling, cutis laxa, and pseudoxanthoma elasticum; acute sensitivity reactions, such as urticaria; autoimmune diseases, such as pemphigus, BP, SLE, and dermatomyositis; lichen planus; psoriasiform dermatitis; seborrheic dermatitis–like eruption; alopecia; hypertrichosis; and nail changes (201).

Penicillamine-Induced Atrophy of the Skin
Clinical Summary. Patients on prolonged penicillamine therapy may show atrophy of the skin of the face and neck; light blue, atrophic macules resembling anetoderma; easy bruising; and small, white papules at sites of venipuncture in the antecubital fossae (202).

Histopathology. Histologic features are similar to their non–penicillamine-associated lesions. Accordingly, anetoderma shows diminution or absence of elastic tissue, areas of bruising and the papules at sites of venipuncture show diminution or degeneration and homogenization of collagen.

Penicillamine-Induced Elastosis Perforans Serpiginosa
Clinical Summary. EPS is a rare condition affecting the cutaneous elastic tissue. It is associated with systemic diseases such as Down syndrome, Ehlers-Danlos syndrome, Rothman-Thomson syndrome, acrogeria, scleroderma, osteogenesis imperfecta, pseudoxanthoma elasticum, and Marfan syndrome. The acquired form is secondary to prolonged treatment with penicillamine. The clinical picture does not differ from that of idiopathic EPS (see Chapter 15).

Histopathology. In comparison with the idiopathic type of EPS, the penicillamine-induced type, on staining for elastic tissue, shows less hyperplasia of elastic fibers in the papillary dermis, except in areas of active transepidermal elimination (Fig. 11-40). However, in the middle and deep layers of the dermis, a greater number of hyperplastic elastic fibers are present than in idiopathic EPS. These fibers have an appearance that is specific for penicillamine-induced EPS. Lateral budding is noted, with the buds arranged perpendicular to the principal fibers. The coarse elastic fibers thus show a serrated, sawtooth-like border and have been aptly compared to the twigs of a bramble bush or have been referred to as "lumpy-bumpy" (202) (Fig. 11-41). Similar changes in individual elastic fibers are observed in nonlesional skin and have been seen in a skeletal artery (203).

Pathogenesis. Penicillamine affects the middle and deep dermal elastic fibers. Two mechanisms have been proposed: first, copper deficiency secondary to penicillamine treatment impairs lysyl oxidase function on elastic fiber cross-linking, a crucial process to stabilize and compact the fibers. Second, direct penicillamine post-translational inhibition of type I collagen synthesis results in abnormal fiber deposition (204). On electron microscopic examination, the affected elastic fibers show an inner core that closely resembles a normal elastic fiber with dark microfibrils embedded in electron-lucent elastin. Peripheral to this, a wide, homogeneous, electron-lucent coat is seen that has the appearance of elastin and shows numerous sac-like projections.

Principles of Management: The changes tend to be persistent once established.

Levamisole

Levamisole is an antiparasitic medication used in livestock. It is now a common adulterant added to cocaine. The U.S. Drug Enforcement Agency reported that 70% of the cocaine seized in 2009 contained levamisole (205).

Clinical Summary. Adverse reactions to levamisole-tainted cocaine may be associated with fever, agranulocytosis, antineutrophil cytoplasmic antibodies (ANCAs) (usually dual-positive cANCA and pANCA), and a distinct mixed vasculitis and vasculopathy characterized by retiform purpuric lesions, most often involving the ears, face, and extremities (Fig. 11-42). The purpuric lesions are nonblanching centrally and erythematous at the periphery. The purpura can develop overlying bulla and is often followed by necrosis and ulceration.

Histopathology. Biopsy specimens show leukocytoclastic vasculitis, thrombotic vasculitis, vascular occlusion, and/or a combination of these (Fig. 11-43) (206).

Pathogenesis. The exact mechanism is not fully understood. The drug is thought to promote the normal activities of macrophages and T lymphocytes, enhancing immune system

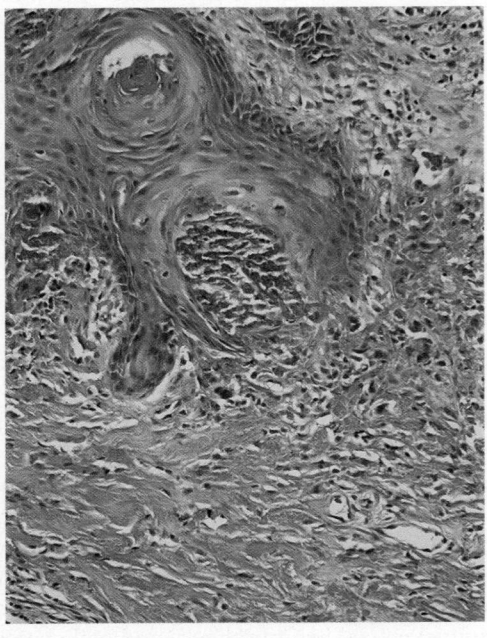

Figure 11-40 Penicillamine-induced elastosis perforans serpiginosa. This image shows thickened elastic fibers in the process of transepidermal elimination. The papillary dermal elastic fibers otherwise appear normal on routine-stained sections.

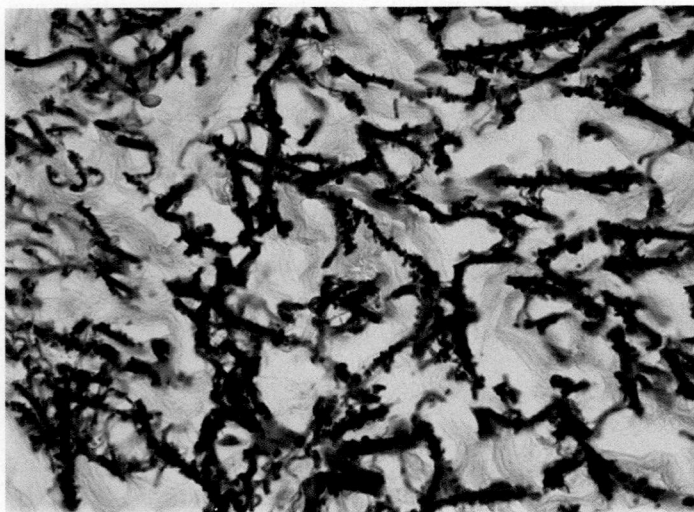

Figure 11-41 Elastosis perforans serpiginosa. The classic fibers in the mid dermis show lateral budding characteristic of penicillamine effect. Verhoeff-van Gieson elastic stain.

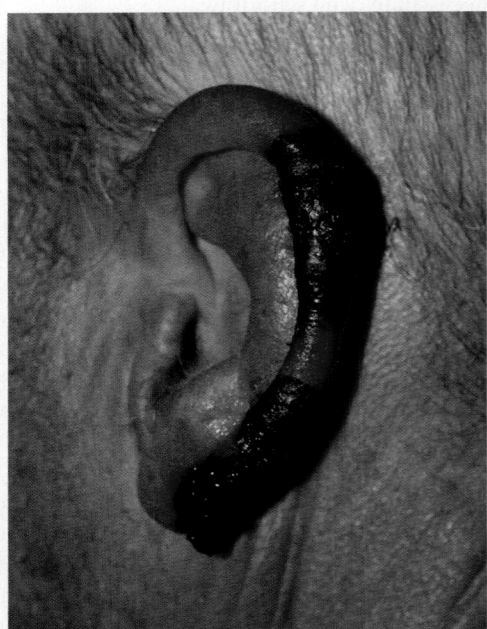

Figure 11-42 Levamisole-induced vasculitis. Levamisole eruption presents with purpuric lesions, classically on the ears.

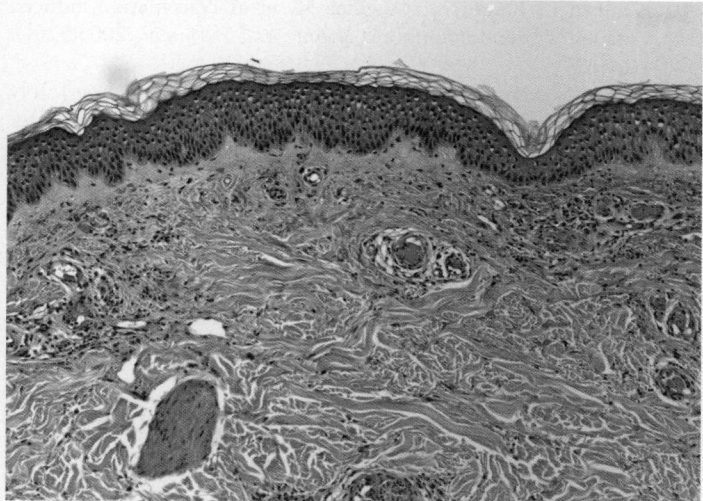

Figure 11-43 Levamisole eruption. A biopsy of the purpuric lesion shows occlusive thrombi in many small vessels throughout the dermis.

response by affecting the activation and maturation of human monocyte-derived dendritic cells and inhibiting the production of endogenous immunosuppressive factors (207).

Principles of Management: Withdrawal of the agent and management of complications.

Krokodil

Krokodil is a drug composed of a mixture of several chemicals, including paint thinner, gasoline, and other toxic ingredients, with the principal active agent being desomorphine, a synthetic derivative of morphine. Desomorphine has an 8 to 10 times higher analgesic potency, faster onset of action, and shorter half-life compared with morphine, which accounts for its increased addictive potential. The use of this drug was first reported in Russia and then across Europe, but has recently been reported in the United States (208).

Clinical Summary. Regular use results in damage to vasculature, muscles, and bones and can lead to multiorgan failure. It can cause abscesses, thrombophlebitis, and turn a user's skin dark, scaly, and necrotic, hence its colloquial name that corresponds to the crocodile-like skin lesions (209).

Principles of Management: Withdrawal of the agent and management of complications.

REFERENCES

1. Roujeau J-C. Clinical heterogeneity of drug hypersensitivity. *Toxicology.* 2005;209(2):123–129.
2. Naldi L, Crotti S. Epidemiology of cutaneous drug-induced reactions. *G Ital Dermatol Venereol.* 2014;149(2):207–218. http://www.ncbi.nlm.nih.gov/pubmed/24819642.
3. Campos-Fernández M del M, Ponce-De-León-Rosales S, Archer-Dubon C, Orozco-Topete R. Incidence and risk factors for cutaneous adverse drug reactions in an intensive care unit. *Rev Invest Clin.* 2014;57(6):770–774. http://www.ncbi.nlm.nih.gov/pubmed/16708902.
4. Breathnach SM. Adverse cutaneous reactions to drugs. *Clin Med (Northfield Il).* 2002;2(1):15–19.
5. Duong TA, Valeyrie-Allanore L, Wolkenstein P, Chosidow O. Severe cutaneous adverse reactions to drugs. *Lancet.* 2017;390(10106):1996–2011.
6. Hernandez-Salazar A, de Leon-Rosales SP, Rangel-Frausto S, Criollo E, Archer-Dubon C, Orozco-Topete R. Epidemiology of adverse cutaneous drug reactions. A prospective study in hospitalized patients. *Arch Med Res.* 2006;37(7):899–902.
7. Verma P, Bhattacharya SN, Banerjee BD, Khanna N. Oxidative stress and leukocyte migration inhibition response in cutaneous adverse drug reactions. *Indian J Dermatol Venereol Leprol.* 2012;78(5):664.
8. Pavlos R, Mallal S, Phillips E. HLA and pharmacogenetics of drug hypersensitivity. *Pharmacogenomics.* 2012;13(11):1285–1306.
9. Meth MJ, Sperber KE. Phenotypic diversity in delayed drug hypersensitivity: an immunologic explanation. *Mt Sinai J Med.* 2006;73(5):769–776. http://www.ncbi.nlm.nih.gov/pubmed/17008937.
10. Lotem M, Hubert A, Lyass O, et al. Skin toxic effects of polyethylene glycol-coated liposomal doxorubicin. *Arch Dermatol.* 2000;136(12):1475–1480.
11. Hashimoto Y, Kanto H, Itoh M. Adverse skin reactions due to pegylated interferon alpha 2b plus ribavirin combination therapy in a patient with chronic hepatitis C virus. *J Dermatol.* 2007;34(8):577–582.
12. Kawada K, Maeda N, Kobayashi S, Sowa J, Tsuruta D, Kawada N. Injection site with generalized rash caused by pegylated interferon alpha 2a injection. *Dermatology.* 2005;212(1):82–83.
13. Ernst EJ, Egge JA. Celecoxib-induced erythema multiforme with glyburide cross-reactivity. *Pharmacotherapy.* 2002;22(5):637–640.
14. Krasowska D, Szymanek M, Schwartz RA, Myśliński W. Cutaneous effects of the most commonly used antidepressant medication, the selective serotonin reuptake inhibitors. *J Am Acad Dermatol.* 2007;56(5):848–853.
15. Thomson LEJ, Allman KC. Erythema multiforme reaction to sestamibi. *J Nucl Med.* 2001;42(3):534.
16. Han JH, Yun SJ, Nam T-K, Choi Y-D, Lee J-B, Kim S-J. Erythema multiforme after radiotherapy with 5-fluorouracil chemotherapy in a rectal cancer patient. *Ann Dermatol.* 2012;24(2):230–232.
17. Zohdi-Mofid M, Horn TD. Acrosyringeal concentration of necrotic keratinocytes in erythema multiforme: a clue to drug etiology. Clinicopathologic review of 29 cases. *J Cutan Pathol.* 1997;24(4):235–240.
18. French LE. Toxic epidermal necrolysis and Stevens Johnson syndrome: our current understanding. *Allergol Int.* 2006;55(1):9–16.
19. Micheletti RG, Chiesa-Fuxench Z, Noe MH, et al. Stevens-Johnson syndrome/toxic epidermal necrolysis: a multicenter retrospective study of 377 adult patients from the United States. *J Invest Dermatol.* 2018;138(11):2315–2321.
20. Nassif A, Bensussan A, Boumsell L, et al. Toxic epidermal necrolysis: effector cells are drug-specific cytotoxic T cells. *J Allergy Clin Immunol.* 2004;114(5):1209–1215.
21. Bovenschen JH, Kop EN, Van De Kerkhof PCM, Seyger MMB. Etanercept-induced lichenoid reaction pattern in psoriasis. *J Dermatolog Treat.* 2006;17(6):381–383.
22. Bodmer M, Egger SS, Hohenstein E, Beltraminelli H, Krähenbühl S. Lichenoid eruption associated with the use of nebivolol. *Ann Pharmacother.* 2006;40(9):1688–1691.
23. Dalmau J, Peramiquel L, Puig L, Fernández-Figueras MT, Alomar ERA. Imatinib-associated lichenoid eruption: acitretin treatment allows maintained antineoplastic effect. *Br J Dermatol.* 2006;154(6):1213–1216.
24. Goldman BD. Lichenoid drug reaction due to sildenafil. *Cutis.* 2000;65(5):282–283.
25. Koh MJA, Seah PP, Tay YK, Mancer K. Lichenoid drug eruption to terazosin. *Br J Dermatol.* 2008;158(2):426–427.

26. Devos SA, Van Den Bossche N, De Vos M, Naeyaert JM. Adverse skin reactions to anti-TNF-alpha monoclonal antibody therapy. *Dermatology*. 2003;206(4):388–390.

27. Jenerowicz D, Czarnecka-Operacz M, Górecka A, Stawny M. Drug-related hospital admissions—an overview of frequency and clinical presentation. *Acta Pol Pharm*. 2006;63(5):395–399.

28. Sehgal VN, Srivastava G. Fixed drug eruption (FDE): changing scenario of incriminating drugs. *Int J Dermatol*. 2006;45(8): 897–908.

29. Shiohara T, Mizukawa Y, Teraki Y. Pathophysiology of fixed drug eruption: the role of skin-resident T cells. *Curr Opin Allergy Clin Immunol*. 2002;2(4):317–323.

30. Shiohara T, Mizukawa Y. Fixed drug eruption: a disease mediated by self-inflicted responses of intraepidermal T cells. *Eur J Dermatology*. 2007;17(3):201–208.

31. Shiohara T. Fixed drug eruption: pathogenesis and diagnostic tests. *Curr Opin Allergy Clin Immunol*. 2009;9(4):316–321.

32. Mizukawa Y, Shiohara T. Fixed drug eruption: a prototypic disorder mediated by effector memory T cells. *Curr Allergy Asthma Rep*. 2009;9(1):71–77.

33. Teraki Y, Kokaji T, Shiohara T. Expansion of IL-10-producing CD4+ and CD8+ T cells in fixed drug eruption. *Dermatology*. 2006;213(2):83–87.

34. Andrade P, Brinca A, Gonçalo M. Patch testing in fixed drug eruptions-a 20-year review. *Contact Dermatitis*. 2011;65(4): 195–201.

35. Ohtoshi S, Kitami Y, Sueki H, Nakada T. Utility of patch testing for patients with drug eruption. *Clin Exp Dermatol*. 2014;39(3): 279–283.

36. Pelizza L, De Luca P, La Pesa ML, Minervino A. Drug-induced systemic lupus erythematosus after 7 years of treatment with carbamazepine. *Acta Biomed l'Ateneo Parm*. 2006;77(1):17–19.

37. Amerio P, Innocente C, Feliciani C, Angelucci D, Gambi D, Tulli A. Drug-induced cutaneous lupus erythematosus after 5 years of treatment with carbamazepine. *Eur J Dermatology*. 2006;16(3):281–283.

38. Katz U, Zandman-Goddard G. Drug-induced lupus: an update. *Autoimmun Rev*. 2010;10(1):46–50.

39. Sarzi-Puttini P, Atzeni F, Capsoni F, Lubrano E, Doria A. Drug-induced lupus erythematosus. *Autoimmunity*. 2005;38(7): 507–518.

40. Costa MF, Said NR, Zimmermann B. Drug-induced lupus due to anti-tumor necrosis factor α agents. *Semin Arthritis Rheum*. 2008; 37(6):381–387.

41. Spillane AP, Xia Y, Sniezek PJ. Drug-induced lupus erythematosus in a patient treated with adalumimab. *J Am Acad Dermatol*. 2007;56(5, suppl):S114–S116.

42. Almoallim H, Al-Ghamdi Y, Almaghrabi H, Alyasi O. Anti-tumor necrosis factor-α induced systemic lupus erythematosus. *Open Rheumatol J*. 2012;6:315–319.

43. Vaglio A, Grayson PC, Fenaroli P, et al. Drug-induced lupus: traditional and new concepts. *Autoimmun Rev*. 2018;17(9): 912–918.

44. Grossman J, Callerame ML, Condemi JJ. Skin immunofluorescence studies on lupus erythematosus and other antinuclear antibody positive diseases. *Ann Intern Med*. 1974;80(4):496–500.

45. He Y, Sawalha AH. Drug-induced lupus erythematosus: an update on drugs and mechanisms. *Curr Opin Rheumatol*. 2018;30(5): 490–497.

46. Masruha MR, Marques CM, Vilanova LCP, De Seixas Alves MT, Peres MFP, Rodrigues MG. Drug induced pseudolymphoma secondary to ethosuximide. *J Neurol Neurosurg Psychiatry*. 2005;76(11):1610.

47. Scheinfeld N. Impact of phenytoin therapy on the skin and skin disease. *Expert Opin Drug Saf*. 2004;3(6):655–665.

48. Albrecht J, Fine LA, Piette W. Drug-associated lymphoma and pseudolymphoma: recognition and management. *Dermatol Clin*. 2007;25(2):233–244.

49. Maubec E, Pinquier L, Viguier M, et al. Vaccination-induced cutaneous pseudolymphoma. *J Am Acad Dermatol*. 2005;52(4): 623–629.

50. Cordel N, Lenormand B, Courville P, Helot MF, Benichou J, Joly P. Usefulness of cutaneous T-cell clonality analysis for the diagnosis of cutaneous T-cell lymphoma in patients with erythroderma. *Arch Pathol Lab Med*. 2005;129(3):372–376.

51. Böer A, Tirumalae R, Bresch M, Falk TM. Pseudoclonality in cutaneous pseudolymphomas: a pitfall in interpretation of rearrangement studies. *Br J Dermatol*. 2008;159(2):394–402.

52. Sidoroff A, Dunant A, Viboud C, et al. Risk factors for acute generalized exanthematous pustulosis (AGEP)—results of a multinational case-control study (EuroSCAR). *Br J Dermatol*. 2007;157(5):989–996.

53. Britschgi M, Pichler WJ. Acute generalized exanthematous pustulosis, a clue to neutrophil-mediated inflammatory processes orchestrated by T cells. *Curr Opin Allergy Clin Immunol*. 2002;2(4):325–331.

54. Clark BM, Homeyer DC, Glass KR, D'Avignon LC. Clindamycin-induced Sweet's syndrome. *Pharmacotherapy*. 2007;27(9, pt 1): 1343–1346.

55. Thompson DF, Montarella KE. Drug-induced Sweet's syndrome. *Ann Pharmacother*. 2007;41(5):802–811.

56. Nguyen CV, Miller DD. Serum sickness-like drug reaction: two cases with a neutrophilic urticarial pattern. *J Cutan Pathol*. 2017;44(2):177–182.

57. Villani A, Baldo A, De Fata Salvatores G, Desiato V, Ayala F, Donadio C. Acute localized exanthematous pustulosis (ALEP): review of literature with report of case caused by amoxicillin-clavulanic acid. *Dermatol Ther (Heidelb)*. 2017;7(4):563–570.

58. Govindarajan G, Bashir Q, Kuppuswamy S, Brooks C. Sweet syndrome associated with furosemide. *South Med J*. 2005;98(5): 570–572.

59. Larsen HK, Danielsen AG, Krustrup D, Weismann K. Neutrophil dermatosis of the dorsal hands. *J Eur Acad Dermatology Venereol*. 2005;19(5):634–637.

60. Malone JC, Slone SP, Wills-Frank LA, et al. Vascular inflammation (vasculitis) in Sweet syndrome: a clinicopathologic study of 28 biopsy specimens from 21 patients. *Arch Dermatol*. 2002;138(3): 345–349.

61. Massé M, Falanga V, Zhou LH. Use of topical povidone-iodine resulting in an iododerma-like eruption. *J Dermatol*. 2008;35(11): 744–747.

62. Paloni G, Mattei I, Ravagnan E, Cutrone M. Infantile bromoderma. *J Pediatr*. 2013;163(3):920–920.e1.

63. Runge M, Williams K, Scharnitz T, et al. Iodine toxicity after iodinated contrast: new observations in iododerma. *JAAD Case Rep*. 2020;6(4):319–322.

64. Blasik LG, Spencer SK. Fluoroderma. *Arch Dermatol*. 1979;115(11):1334–1335.

65. Perbet S, Salavert M, Amarger S, Constantin J-M, D'Incan M, Bazin J-E. Fluoroderma after exposure to sevoflurane. *Br J Anaesth*. 2011;107(1):106–107.

66. Maffeis L, Musolino MC, Cambiaghi S. Single-plaque vegetating bromoderma. *J Am Acad Dermatol*. 2008;58(4):682–684.

67. Fridlender ZG, Cohen PY, Golan O, Arish N, Wallach-Dayan S, Breuer R. Telomerase activity in bleomycin-induced epithelial cell apoptosis and lung fibrosis. *Eur Respir J*. 2007;30(2):205–213.

68. Kupfer I, Balguerie X, Courville P, Chinet P, Joly P. Scleroderma-like cutaneous lesions induced by paclitaxel: a case study. *J Am Acad Dermatol*. 2003;48(2, suppl):279–281.

69. Yang J-Q, Dou T-T, Chen X-B, et al. Docetaxel-induced scleroderma: a case report and its role in the production of extracellular matrix. *Int J Rheum Dis*. 2017;20(11):1835–1837.

70. Ferreli C, Gasparini G, Parodi A, Cozzani E, Rongioletti F, Atzori L. Cutaneous manifestations of scleroderma and scleroderma-like

disorders: a comprehensive review. *Clin Rev Allergy Immunol.* 2017;53(3):306–336.

71. Bucala R. Circulating fibrocytes: cellular basis for NSF. *J Am Coll Radiol.* 2008;5(1):36–39.

72. Cuffy MC, Singh M, Formica R, et al. Renal transplantation for nephrogenic systemic fibrosis: a case report and review of the literature. *Nephrol Dial Transplant.* 2011;26(3):1099–1101.

73. Dinis-Oliveira RJ. Drug overdose-induced coma blisters: pathophysiology and clinical and forensic diagnosis. *Curr Drug Res Rev.* 2019;11(1):21–25.

74. Bryant P, Lachman P. Pseudoporphyria secondary to non-steroidal anti-inflammatory drugs. *Arch Dis Child.* 2003;88(11):961.

75. DeGiovanni CV, Darley CR. Pseudoporphyria occurring during a course of ciprofloxacin. *Clin Exp Dermatol.* 2008;33(1):109–110.

76. Kwong WT, Hsu S. Pseudoporphyria associated with voriconazole. *J Drugs Dermatol.* 2007;6(10):1042–1044. http://www.ncbi.nlm.nih.gov/pubmed/17966183.

77. Silver EA, Silver AH, Silver DS, McCalmont TH. Pseudoporphyria induced by oral contraceptive pills. *Arch Dermatol.* 2003;139(2):227–228.

78. Werth VP. Dermatology vignette. *J Clin Rheumatol.* 2001;7(2):123.

79. Kalivas J. Pseudoporphyria. *Int J Dermatol.* 2006;45(12):1455.

80. de Groot HJ, Jonkman MF, Pas HH, Diercks GFH. Direct immunofluorescence of mechanobullous epidermolysis bullosa acquisita, porphyria cutanea tarda and pseudoporphyria. *Acta Derm Venereol.* 2019;99(1):26–32.

81. Brenner S, Goldberg I. Drug-induced pemphigus. *Clin Dermatol.* 2011;29(4):455–457.

82. Saito Y, Hayashi S, Yamauchi A, et al. Tracing the origins of active amide group-positive drug-induced pemphigus vulgaris along the Silk Road: a case report of candesartan-induced pemphigus vulgaris and review of nonthiol drug-induced pemphigus. *Int J Dermatol.* 2018;57(11):e131–e134.

83. Marinho RT, Johnson NW, Fatela NM, et al. Oropharyngeal pemphigus in a patient with chronic hepatitis C during interferon alpha-2a therapy. *Eur J Gastroenterol Hepatol.* 2001;13(7):869–872.

84. Ghaedi F, Etesami I, Aryanian Z, et al. Drug-induced pemphigus: a systematic review of 170 patients. *Int Immunopharmacol.* 2021;92:107299.

85. Lee E, Lendas KA, Chow S, et al. Disease relevant HLA class II alleles isolated by genotypic, haplotypic, and sequence analysis in North American Caucasians with pemphigus vulgaris. *Hum Immunol.* 2006;67(1–2):125–139.

86. Verheyden MJ, Bilgic A, Murrell DF. A systematic review of drug-induced pemphigoid. *Acta Derm Venereol.* 2020;100(15):adv00224.

87. Chanal J, Ingen-Housz-Oro S, Ortonne N, et al. Linear IgA bullous dermatosis: comparison between the drug-induced and spontaneous forms. *Br J Dermatol.* 2013;169(5):1041–1048.

88. Billet SE, Kortuem KR, Gibson LE, El-Azhary R. A morbilliform variant of vancomycin-induced linear IgA bullous dermatosis. *Arch Dermatol.* 2008;144(6):774–778.

89. Yamagami J, Nakamura Y, Nagao K, et al. Vancomycin mediates IgA autoreactivity in drug-induced linear IgA bullous dermatosis. *J Invest Dermatol.* 2018;138(7):1473–1480.

90. Palmer RA, Ogg G, Allen J, et al. Vancomycin-induced linear IgA disease with autoantibodies to BP180 and LAD285. *Br J Dermatol.* 2001;145(5):816–820.

91. Sushma M, Noel M V, Ritika MC, James J, Guido S. Cutaneous adverse drug reactions: a 9-year study from a South Indian Hospital. *Pharmacoepidemiol Drug Saf.* 2005;14(8):567–570.

92. Borch JE, Andersen KE, Bindslev-Jensen C. The prevalence of suspected and challenge-verified penicillin allergy in a university hospital population. *Basic Clin Pharmacol Toxicol.* 2006;98(4):357–362.

93. Puavilai S, Noppakun N, Sitakalin C, et al. Drug eruptions at five institutes in Bangkok. *J Med Assoc Thail.* 2005;88(11):1642–1650.

94. Markel A. Allopurinol-induced DRESS syndrome. *Isr Med Assoc J.* 2005;7(10):656–660.

95. Michel F, Navellou J-C, Ferraud D, Toussirot E, Wendling D. DRESS syndrome in a patient on sulfasalazine for rheumatoid arthritis. *Joint Bone Spine.* 2005;72(1):82–85.

96. Syn W-K, Naisbitt DJ, Holt AP, Pirmohamed M, Mutimer DJ. Carbamazepine-induced acute liver failure as part of the DRESS syndrome. *Int J Clin Pract.* 2005;59(8):988–991.

97. Chi M-H, Hui RC-Y, Yang C-H, et al. Histopathological analysis and clinical correlation of drug reaction with eosinophilia and systemic symptoms (DRESS). *Br J Dermatol.* 2014;170(4):866–873.

98. Cho YT, Yang CW, Chu CY. Drug reaction with eosinophilia and systemic symptoms (DRESS): an interplay among drugs, viruses, and immune system. *Int J Mol Sci.* 2017;18(6).

99. Skowron F, Bensaid B, Balme B, et al. Drug reaction with eosinophilia and systemic symptoms (DRESS): clinicopathological study of 45 cases. *J Eur Acad Dermatol Venereol.* 2015;29(11):2199–2205.

100. Walsh S, Diaz-Cano S, Higgins E, et al. Drug reaction with eosinophilia and systemic symptoms: is cutaneous phenotype a prognostic marker for outcome? A review of clinicopathological features of 27 cases. *Br J Dermatol.* 2013;168(2):391–401.

101. Lozzi F, Di Raimondo C, Lanna C, et al. Latest evidence regarding the effects of photosensitive drugs on the skin: pathogenetic mechanisms and clinical manifestations. *Pharmaceutics.* 2020;12(11):1104.

102. Hofmann GA, Weber B. Drug-induced photosensitivity: culprit drugs, potential mechanisms and clinical consequences. *J Dtsch Dermatol Ges.* 2021;19(1):19–29.

103. Goldfeder KL, Levin JM, Katz KA, Clarke LE, Loren AW, James WD. Ultraviolet recall reaction after total body irradiation, etoposide, and methotrexate therapy. *J Am Acad Dermatol.* 2007;56(3):494–499.

104. Hird AE, Wilson J, Symons S, Sinclair E, Davis M, Chow E. Radiation recall dermatitis: case report and review of the literature. *Curr Oncol.* 2008;15(1):53–62.

105. Boyer M, Katta R, Markus R. Diltiazem-induced photodistributed hyperpigmentation. *Dermatol Online J.* 2003;9(5):89–95.

106. Dereure O. Drug-induced skin pigmentation epidemiology, diagnosis and treatment. *Am J Clin Dermatol.* 2001;2(4):253–262.

107. Saladi RN, Cohen SR, Phelps RG, Persaud AN, Rudikoff D. Diltiazem induces severe photodistributed hyperpigmentation: case series, histoimmunopathology, management, and review of the literature. *Arch Dermatol.* 2006;142(2):206–210.

108. Angel TA, Stalkup JR, Hsu S. Photodistributed blue-gray pigmentation of the skin associated with long-term imipramine use. *Int J Dermatol.* 2002;41(6):327–329.

109. Sicari MC, Lebwohl M, Baral J, Wexler P, Gordon RE, Phelps RG. Photoinduced dermal pigmentation in patients taking tricyclic antidepressants: histology, electron microscopy, and energy dispersive spectroscopy. *J Am Acad Dermatol.* 1999;40(2, pt 2):290–293.

110. Ming ME, Bhawan J, Stefanato CM, McCalmont TH, Cohen LM. Imipramine-induced hyperpigmentation: four cases and a review of the literature. *J Am Acad Dermatol.* 1999;40(2, pt 1):159–166.

111. Greiner AC, Nicolson GA. Pigment deposition in viscera associated with prolonged chlorpromazine therapy. *Can Med Assoc J.* 1964;91:627–635.

112. Waitzer S, Butany J, From L, Hanna W, Ramsay C, Downar E. Cutaneous ultrastructural changes and photosensitivity associated with amiodarone therapy. *J Am Acad Dermatol.* 1987;16(4):779–787.

113. Benning TL, Mccormack KM, Ingram P, Kaplan DL, Shelburne JD. Microprobe analysis of chlorpromazine pigmentation. *Arch Dermatol.* 1988;124(10):1541–1544.

114. Scherschun L, Lee MW, Lim HW. Diltiazem-associated photodistributed hyperpigmentation: a review of 4 cases. *Arch Dermatol.* 2001;137(2):179–182.

115. Mehrany K, Kist JM, Ahmed DDF, Gibson LE. Minocycline-induced cutaneous pigmentation. *Int J Dermatol.* 2003;42(7):551–552.

116. Angeloni VL, Salasche SJ, Ortiz R. Nail, skin, and scleral pigmentation induced by minocycline. *Cutis.* 1987;40(3):229–233.

117. de Paz S, Pérez A, Gómez M, Trampal A, Domínguez Lázaro A. Severe hypersensitivity reaction to minocycline. *J Investig Allergol Clin Immunol.* 1999;9(6):403–404.

118. Lefebvre N, Forestier E, Farhi D, et al. Minocycline-induced hypersensitivity syndrome presenting with meningitis and brain edema: a case report. *J Med Case Rep.* 2007;1:22.

119. Bowen AR, McCalmont TH. The histopathology of subcutaneous minocycline pigmentation. *J Am Acad Dermatol.* 2007;57(5): 836–839.

120. Rahman Z, Lazova R, Antaya RJ. Minocycline hyperpigmentation isolated to the subcutaneous fat. *J Cutan Pathol.* 2005;32(7): 516–519.

121. Argenyi ZB, Finelli L, Bergfeld WF, et al. Minocycline-related cutaneous hyperpigmentation as demonstrated by light microscopy, electron microscopy and X-ray energy spectroscopy. *J Cutan Pathol.* 1987;14(3):176–180.

122. Philip M, Samson JF, Simi PS. Clofazimine-induced hair pigmentation. *Int J Trichology.* 2012;4(3):174–175.

123. Cholo MC, Steel HC, Fourie PB, Germishuizen WA, Anderson R. Clofazimine: current status and future prospects. *J Antimicrob Chemother.* 2012;67(2):290–298.

124. Job CK, Yoder L, Jacobson RR, Hastings RC. Skin pigmentation from clofazimine therapy in leprosy patients: a reappraisal. *J Am Acad Dermatol.* 1990;23(2):236–241.

125. Rappersberger K, Hönigsmann H, Ortel B, Tanew A, Konrad K, Wolff K. Photosensitivity and hyperpigmentation in amiodarone-treated patients: incidence, time course, and recovery. *J Invest Dermatol.* 1989;93(2):201–209.

126. Kounis NG, Frangides C, Papadaki PJ, Zavras GM, Goudevenos J. Dose-dependent appearance and disappearance of amiodarone-induced skin pigmentation. *Clin Cardiol.* 1996;19(7):592–594.

127. Granstein RD, Sober AJ. Drug-and heavy metal-induced hyperpigmentation. *J Am Acad Dermatol.* 1981;5(1):1–18.

128. Kumar R, Pai V. Bleomycin induced flagellate pigmentation. *Indian Pediatr.* 2006;43(1):74–75.

129. Pavithran K, Doval DC, Talwar V, Vaid AK. Flagellate hyperpigmentation from bleomycin. *Indian J Dermatol Venereol Leprol.* 2004;70(1):46–47.

130. Koley S, Choudhary S, Salodkar A. Melanonychia and skin hyperpigmentation with hydroxyurea therapy. *Indian J Pharmacol.* 2010;42(1):60–61.

131. Zargari O, Kimyai-Asadi A, Jafroodi M. Cutaneous adverse reactions to hydroxyurea in patients with intermediate thalassemia. *Pediatr Dermatol.* 2004;21(6):633–635.

132. Wright AL, Bleehen SS, Champion AE. Reticulate pigmentation due to bleomycin: light-and electron-microscopic studies. *Dermatologica.* 1990;180(4):255–257.

133. Duhra P, Ilchyshyn A, Das RN. Bleomycin-induced flagellate erythema. *Clin Exp Dermatol.* 1991;16(3):216–217.

134. Hendrix JR JD, Greer K. Cutaneous hyperpigmentation caused by systemic drugs. *Int J Dermatol.* 1992;31(7):458–466.

135. Sharma AN, Mesinkovska NA, Paravar T. Characterizing the adverse dermatologic effects of hydroxychloroquine: a systematic review. *J Am Acad Dermatol.* 2020;83(2):563–578.

136. Puri PK, Lountzis NI, Tyler W, Ferringer T. Hydroxychloroquine-induced hyperpigmentation: the staining pattern. *J Cutan Pathol.* 2008;35(12):1134–1137.

137. Park S-W, Shin H-T, Lee K-T, Lee D-Y. Medical concern for colloidal silver supplementation: argyria of the nail and face. *Ann Dermatol.* 2013;25(1):111–112.

138. McClain CM, Kantrow SM, Abraham JL, Price J, Parker ER, Robbins JB. Localized cutaneous argyria: two case reports and clinicopathologic review. *Am J Dermatopathol.* 2013;35(7):e115-e118.

139. Massi D, Santucci M. Human generalized argyria: a submicroscopic and X-ray spectroscopic study. *Ultrastruct Pathol.* 1998;22(1): 47–53.

140. Kamiya K, Yamasaki O, Tachikawa S, Iwatsuki K. Localized cutaneous argyria in a silversmith. *Eur J Dermatol.* 2013;23(1): 112–113.

141. Bowden LP, Royer MC, Hallman JR, Lewin-Smith M, Lupton GP. Rapid onset of argyria induced by a silver-containing dietary supplement. *J Cutan Pathol.* 2011;38(10):832–835.

142. Thompson R, Elliott V, Mondry A. Argyria: permanent skin discoloration following protracted colloid silver ingestion. *BMJ Case Rep.* 2009;2009:bcr0820080606.

143. Cho EA, Lee WS, Kim KM, Kim S-Y. Occupational generalized argyria after exposure to aerosolized silver. *J Dermatol.* 2008; 35(11):759–760.

144. Rackoff EM, Benbenisty KM, Maize JC, Maize Jr. Localized cutaneous argyria from an acupuncture needle clinically concerning for metastatic melanoma. *Cutis.* 2007;80(5):423–426.

145. Lee J, Korgavkar K, DiMarco C, Robinson-Bostom L. Localized argyria with pseudo-ochronosis. *J Cutan Pathol.* 2020;47(8): 671–674.

146. White JML, Powell AM, Brady K, Russell-Jones R. Severe generalized argyria secondary to ingestion of colloidal silver protein. *Clin Exp Dermatol.* 2003;28(3):254–256.

147. Pezzarossa E, Alinovi A, Ferrari C. Generalized argyria. *J Cutan Pathol.* 1983;10(5):361–363.

148. Geist DE, Phillips TJ. Development of chrysiasis after Q-switched ruby laser treatment of solar lentigines. *J Am Acad Dermatol.* 2006;55(2, suppl):S59–S60.

149. Almoallim H, Klinkhoff AV, Arthur AB, Rivers JK, Chalmers A. Laser induced chrysiasis: disfiguring hyperpigmentation following Q-switched laser therapy in a woman previously treated with gold. *J Rheumatol.* 2006;33(3):620–621.

150. Smith RW, Cawley MID. Chrysiasis. *Br J Rheumatol.* 1997;36(1):3–5.

151. Pelachyk JM, Bergfeld WF, McMahon JT. Chrysiasis following gold therapy for rheumatoid arthritis: ultrastructural analysis with x-ray energy spectroscopy. *J Cutan Pathol.* 1984;11(6):491–494.

152. Lamar LM, Bliss BO. Localized pigmentation of the skin due to topical mercury. *Arch Dermatol.* 1966;93(4):450–453.

153. Winnicki M, Shear NH. A systematic approach to systemic contact dermatitis and symmetric drug-related intertriginous and flexural exanthema (SDRIFE): a closer look at these conditions and an approach to intertriginous eruptions. *Am J Clin Dermatol.* 2011;12(3):171–180.

154. Wu M-L, Deng J-F, Lin K-P, Tsai W-J. Lead, mercury, and arsenic poisoning due to topical use of traditional Chinese medicines. *Am J Med.* 2013;126(5):451–454.

155. Burge KM, Winkelmann RK. Mercury pigmentation: an electron microscopic study. *Arch Dermatol.* 1970;102(1):51–61.

156. Bolognia JL, Cooper DL, Glusac EJ. Toxic erythema of chemotherapy: a useful clinical term. *J Am Acad Dermatol.* 2008;59(3): 524–529.

157. Yokel BK, Friedman KJ, Farmer ER, Hood AF. Cutaneous pathology following etoposide therapy. *J Cutan Pathol.* 1987;14(6): 326–330.

158. Horn TD, Beveridge RA, Egorin MJ, Abeloff MD, Hood AF. Observations and proposed mechanism of N,N′,N″-triethylenethiophosphoramide (thiotepa)-induced hyperpigmentation. *Arch Dermatol.* 1989;125(4):524–527.

159. Linassier C, Colombat P, Reisenleiter M, et al. Cutaneous toxicity of autologous bone marrow transplantation in nonseminomatous germ cell tumors. *Cancer.* 1990;65(5):1143–1145.

160. Hymes SR, Simonton SC, Farmer ER, Beschorner WB, Tutschka PJ, Santos GW. Cutaneous busulfan effect in patients

eruption normally allow distinction. Just histologically, PMLE must be differentiated from lupus erythematosus, the porphyrias, AP, Jessner lymphocytic infiltrate, cutaneous T-cell lymphoma, chilblains, rosacea, and dermatophyte infections with prominent papillary dermal edema (7,9,14). In cutaneous lupus erythematosus, the interface change is more prominent not only in the epidermis but also in adnexal structures, apoptotic keratinocytes are often seen, and papillary dermal edema is not usually a feature. In addition, dermal mucin deposition may be seen in lupus and is absent in PMLE. A further finding that may aid in the differential diagnosis is that in lupus erythematosus there are numerous CD123 positive plasmacytoid dendritic cells, whereas in PMLE they tend to be absent (15). AP usually displays changes secondary to excoriation, variable epidermal hyperplasia, and more prominent lymphocyte spongiosis and exocytosis; however, early lesions in both conditions may show very similar microscopic findings, except that dermal edema is usually absent in AP. In Jessner lymphocytic infiltrate, epidermal changes are absent, there is no papillary dermal edema, and the dermal mononuclear cell infiltrate tends to be more prominent. Cutaneous T-cell lymphoma is only rarely included in the differential diagnosis of PMLE, mainly when the dermal infiltrate is prominent and the eruption very prolonged; however, the exocytosis of lymphocytes with irregular nuclear outlines is not a feature of the latter, which usually also shows variable spongiosis. The histology of chilblains is almost identical to that of PMLE, particularly when there is prominent papillary dermal edema, but, fortunately, the clinical setting of each disease usually allows distinction. Rosacea shows no epidermal change, dermal edema is absent, the dermal infiltrate is mild and surrounds superficial small blood vessels and adnexal structures, and focal lymphocytic exocytosis into hair follicles is often seen. In dermatophyte infections with prominent papillary dermal edema, a periodic acid–Schiff (PAS) stain allows identification of the fungal organisms in the stratum corneum.

Principles of Management: Treatment, either prophylactic or remedial, is for the most part effective. Often, the restriction of UVR exposure, use of appropriate clothing, and regular application of high-protection, broad-spectrum sunscreens during exposure are satisfactory preventive therapies for mild disease. In more severe instances, prior to the end of winter, before periods of increased sun exposure, four to six weekly courses of broadband or, more commonly, low-dose narrowband (311 to 312 nm) UVB phototherapy, or slightly more reliably, low-dose psoralen photochemotherapy (PUVA), are usually effective in inducing skin immunologic tolerance and preventing the eruption of PMLE (16). If the eruption should develop despite these measures, a short course of systemic steroid therapy (20 to 30 mg prednis(ol)one daily) usually abolishes it quickly (17). Azathioprine and cyclosporine have rarely been used with effect for very severe disease but if needed does suggest the possibility of severe light-exacerbated eczema or even CAD instead. The value of other previously advocated medications, such as antimalarials and beta-carotene, has not been supported in controlled trials.

ACTINIC PRURIGO

Clinical Summary. AP is an itchy, papular or nodular, excoriated, symmetric, chronic eruption, which is usually much worse in summer. It affects the light-exposed and, to a lesser extent, covered skin of children, usually girls, occurring relatively rarely worldwide, although it is comparatively common among native and mixed-race Americans (1,2). It may often, but by no means always, resolve by early adulthood, and most often affects the face and distal limbs, whereas the proximal limbs and forehead beneath the hair fringe, which are less often exposed, are mostly spared. However, the buttocks are sometimes involved through apparent internal, sympathetic spread of the immunologic effect. Superficial, pitted, or linear scars may affect the face at sites of previous lesions, whereas chronic cheilitis and conjunctivitis, sometimes severe, are also possible, particularly in native and mixed-race Americans. In addition, some patients describe acute attacks of rash development following specific sunlight exposure similar to the eruption that occurs in PMLE (18).

Histology. The histology varies according to the clinical evolution (19). Thus, early intact lesions show variable, often mild, epidermal spongiosis and a superficial and deep dermal, perivascular, mononuclear cell infiltration similar to that of PMLE albeit in the absence of substantial papillary dermal edema (Fig. 12-5). However, this latter finding may be seen in occasional biopsies, and histologic distinction from PMLE may then be impossible, requiring close clinicopathologic correlation (19). Occasional eosinophils are often seen. The lesions of AP are frequently excoriated, such that careful attention should be paid when biopsy is performed to avoid lesions with such prominent secondary changes (Fig. 12-6). Evolving lesions may also occasionally display focal interface change with hydropic degeneration of basal cells, such that distinction from cutaneous lupus may then be difficult (Fig. 12-7). In rare cases, there may be a heavy, superficial and deep dermal, mononuclear cell infiltrate with difficulty in distinction from lymphoma, especially if associated interface changes are present. In older lesions, there is usually variable lichenification (Fig. 12-8), focal papillary dermal fibrosis, a moderately heavy mononuclear cell infiltrate, and irregular epithelial hyperplasia similar to the features of chronic eczema, or even prurigo nodularis. The AP inflammatory cell infiltrate has a T-helper phenotype (CD3/CD4 positive). AP must thus

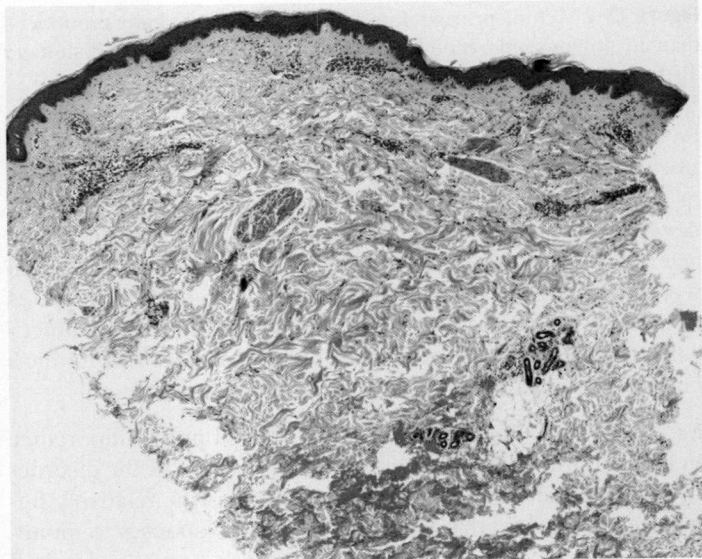

Figure 12-5 Actinic prurigo. Early lesion with absence of epidermal change, and mild to moderate, superficial and deep, perivascular and periadnexal, mononuclear inflammatory cell infiltrate.

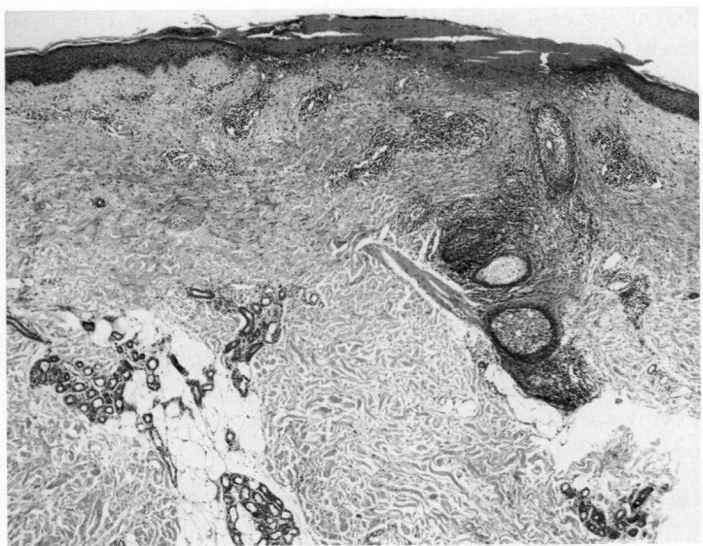

Figure 12-6 Actinic prurigo. Prominent superficial necrosis secondary to excoriation and fairly heavy perivascular and periadnexal inflammatory cell infiltrate.

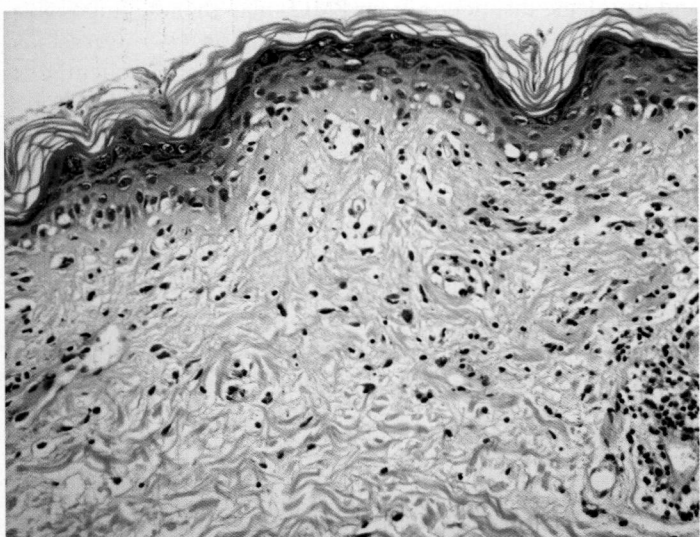

Figure 12-7 Actinic prurigo. Interface change may be more prominent than in polymorphic (polymorphous) light eruption and histologic distinction from lupus more difficult.

be differentiated from the same disorders as PMLE in its more uncommon acute form and from other causes of chronic eczema or prurigo in its chronic forms. Finally, although AP histology may often be fairly nonspecific, the lesions of AP cheilitis characteristically show a dense lymphocytic infiltrate with frequent well-formed lymphoid follicles (20,21), a finding regarded as potentially very helpful in cases of diagnostic doubt. Conjunctival and lip lesions may very rarely display changes that mimic a cutaneous low-grade B-cell marginal zone lymphoma.

Pathogenesis. UVR exposure appears to be of prime importance in the causation of AP, given the greater severity of the disorder in summer and after sun exposure as well as the relatively frequent abnormal erythemal or papular skin responses to monochromatic irradiation (1,2). Such reactions occur in one-half to two-thirds of patients, often to UVB wavelengths alone but sometimes also to UVA, while responses to broad-spectrum irradiation have not yet been reported. Further, the clinical

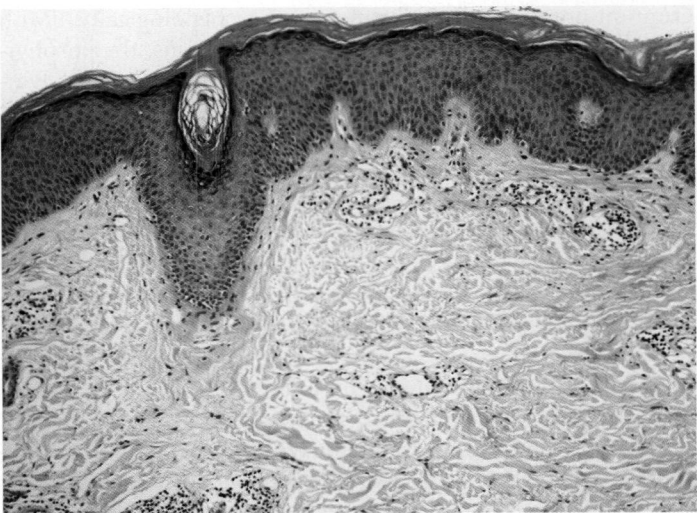

Figure 12-8 Actinic prurigo. Older lesion showing lichenification.

behavior of acute attacks of AP, its histologic appearances, its marked familial association with PMLE, and its differentiation from PMLE in large part by the HLA (human leukocyte antigen) subtypes DRB1*04 (DR4) and, more specifically, DRB1*0407 (18), all strongly suggest that it is very likely a genetically prolonged form of PMLE. It is therefore most probably also a DTH reaction against UVR-induced, cutaneous autoantigen, but without the isolation so far of any proven causative antigen, this statement must remain ultimately speculative, although the abnormal keratinocyte apoptotic findings noted previously for PMLE (3) very likely apply in AP as well.

Differential Diagnosis. AP must be differentiated from PMLE, lupus erythematosus, insect bites, scabies, lymphoma, nodular prurigo, and eczema. However, its seasonal variation, affected sites, usual characteristic HLA abnormalities, and sometimes positive light tests normally assist in this differentiation, and so may its histology, particularly if a lesion is fresh. Close clinicopathologic correlation is essential for reliable diagnosis. In biopsies with interface change, distinction from lupus erythematosus may be difficult, but in AP, such change is usually very patchy, focal, and limited to the epidermis, whereas apoptotic keratinocytes are usually absent. If a prominent dermal infiltrate is seen, the diagnosis of T-cell lymphoma may well come into consideration, but cytologic atypia and epidermotropism are lacking in AP. Finally, in its usual chronic forms, the distinction of AP from chronic eczema is impossible on histologic grounds alone.

Principles of Management: Therapy is often helpful, consisting in mild cases of restricted sun exposure, the use of protective clothing, the application of high-protection, broad-spectrum sunscreens, and the use of emollients and topical steroids on affected sites. However, in some cases, prophylactic, low-dose narrowband UVB phototherapy or PUVA, as for PMLE, may be useful, particularly in spring, for patients who have been cleared of their eruption in winter (22). Topical calcineurin inhibitors may also help in such rash-free patients, although not confirmed by formal studies, whereas oral thalidomide clears most affected subjects, albeit with a marked risk of teratogenicity and a moderate possibility of peripheral neuropathy, which necessitates great care in its use (23). Oral immunosuppressive therapy, such as with cyclosporine, has also been reported to help in some cases and may be considered if clinically appropriate, although not formally shown in controlled studies.

HYDROA VACCINIFORME

Clinical Summary. HV is a very rare, intermittent, UVR-induced, blistering, scarring eruption of only some exposed skin, usually in white children and only rarely in adults (1,2,24,25). The condition generally has onset by 10 years of age, with resolution often by early adulthood. It has recently been shown that EBV infection of T and/or natural killer (NK) cells plays a causative role in HV development, viral particles in the skin perhaps having a permissive, conceivably immunologic, effect after sun exposure (5,26–29). This is of particular interest, because it has been proposed that HV is at the benign end of the spectrum of what is now known as HV EBV-lymphoproliferative disorder. Severe forms of the disease that may be associated with systemic involvement (fever, lymphadenopathy, and hepatosplenomegaly) or even full-blown T- or NK-cell lymphoma/leukemia, affect mainly Asian and native Central and South Americans (5,28,29) (see Chapter 31, p. 1150). The latter patients usually have much higher levels EBV DNA in blood compared to white patients with the more benign form of the disease. In both groups a T-cell clone can be demonstrated, and this finding does not correlate with behavior. Usually sparse, occasionally coalescent, symmetrically scattered, sometimes hemorrhagic vesicles and bullae occurring within hours of sun exposure are characteristic, particularly of the face, ears, and limbs. These then umbilicate and crust over days, healing thereafter in weeks to leave persistent, disfiguring pock scars (Fig. 12-9).

Histology. The main, very characteristic, histologic abnormality is that of progressive intra- and intercellular epidermal edema, leading to prominent reticular degeneration, vesiculation, and, finally, confluent epidermal necrosis (Figs. 12-10 and 12-11). The vesicles contain fibrin and acute inflammatory cells and overlie a dermal cellular infiltrate of predominantly perivascular lymphocytes, histiocytes, and neutrophils (2,24). A vasculitis is not seen. In some cases, there is focal necrosis of the superficial dermis. Prominent secondary changes in late lesions may obscure the characteristic findings. EBV can be detected by in-situ hybridization in the nuclei of the lymphocytes in the

infiltrate. The virus has also been identified at an ultrastructural level in keratinocytes of involved skin (5).

Pathogenesis. The eruption of HV is clearly inducible by sunlight exposure, whereas artificial induction is more difficult, requiring repeated broad-spectrum or, less reliably, monochromatic skin exposure, short wavelength UVA abnormalities in particular being present on occasion, although exact action spectra have not been determined (24,25). Blood, urine, and stool porphyrin concentrations and extractable nuclear antibody titers are normal. Further, the very PMLE-like clinical features of HV apart from its scarring and PMLE-like dermal perivascular mononuclear cell infiltration together strongly suggest similar pathogeneses for the two disorders. HV may therefore also be a DTH-type immunologic response to UVR-induced, endogenous, cutaneous auto-antigen, mediated by the presence of Epstein–Barr viral particles

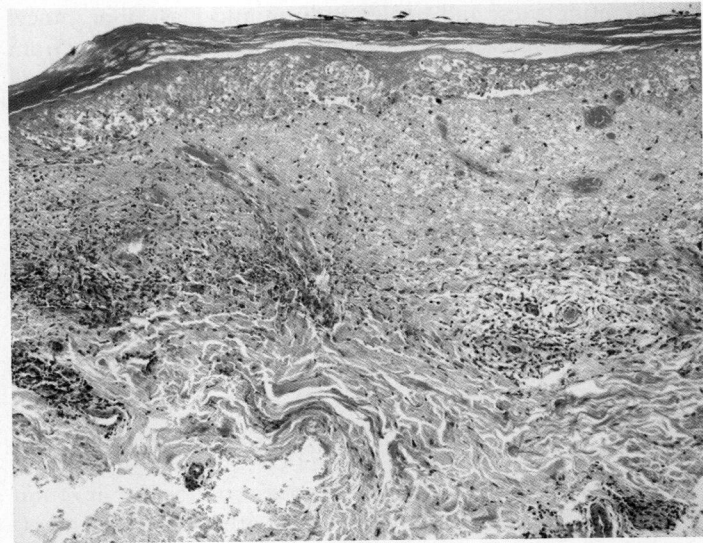

Figure 12-10 Hydroa vacciniforme. Prominent confluent epidermal necrosis associated with dermal perivascular inflammatory cell infiltrate.

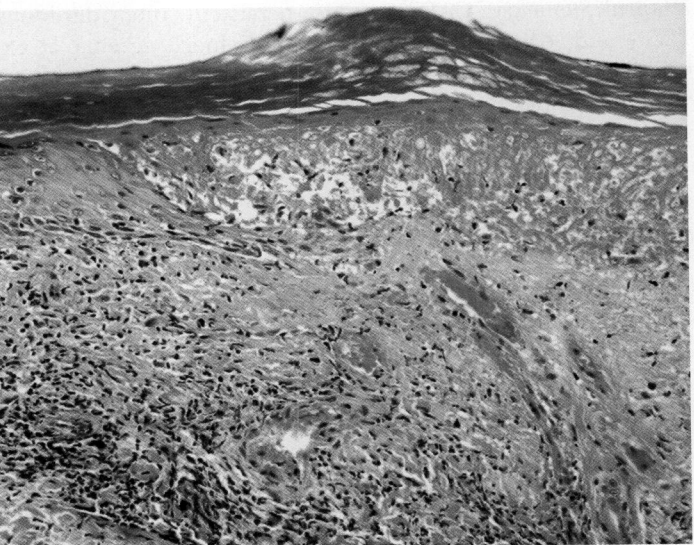

Figure 12-11 Hydroa vacciniforme. Marked reticular degeneration of the epidermis at the edge of the lesion and very superficial dermal necrosis with fibrin deposition.

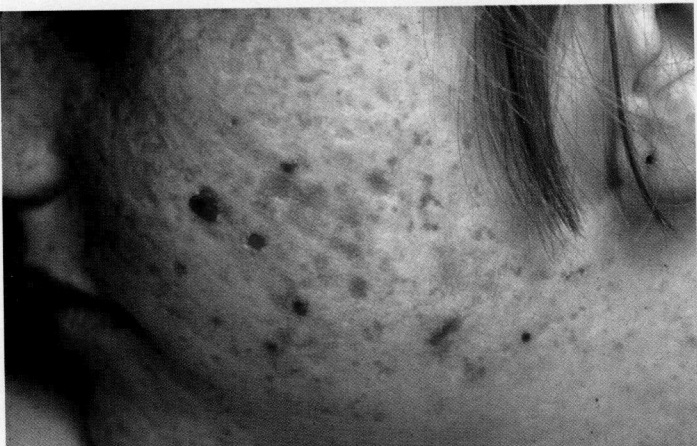

Figure 12-9 Hydroa vacciniforme. Scarring is seen in late stages.

in the exposed skin (5,26–29). In HV, however, the location of the putative antigen, the presence of a toxic photoproduct, or the intensity of the reaction may conceivably contribute to the characteristic scarring. In a single patient, lesional skin demonstrated increased expression of interferon gamma and chemokines that attract T cells and NK cells (28).

Differential Diagnosis. HV must be differentiated from cutaneous viral disorders, the porphyrias, lupus erythematosus, and the other immunologically based photodermatoses by its clinical features and largely diagnostic histopathology, provided that appropriate viral studies, blood, urine, and stool porphyrin concentrations as well as circulating antinuclear factor and extractable nuclear antibody titers are also normal. The pattern of necrosis is remarkably similar to that seen in viral (including herpetic) infections and hand, foot, and mouth disease. Nevertheless, distinction from herpetic infection is easy, as HV lesional biopsies lack obvious viral inclusions, multinucleated keratinocytes, and nuclei with ground glass appearance; also, hair follicle necrosis is lacking. However, distinction from hand, foot, and mouth disease is more difficult, but the clinical settings of the two diseases are totally different. Lesions in the severe form of the disease presenting in Asian and native Central American children, and rarely in adults, may show a more prominent, superficial, and deep dermal lymphoid infiltrate associated with marked necrosis and ulceration and cytologic atypia.

Principles of Management: Treatment is usually difficult. The restriction of UVR exposure and use of clothing cover are helpful, whereas the careful, regular application of high-protection, broad-spectrum but particularly UVA-efficient sunscreens also frequently has efficacy. In resistant cases, courses of prophylactic low-dose UVB phototherapy or PUVA are also helpful on occasion, but care must be taken not to induce the eruption with too high irradiation doses (30). All other suggested therapies have, in practice, seemed unhelpful.

CHRONIC ACTINIC DERMATITIS

Clinical Summary. CAD is a rare, persistent, often disabling, UVR- and, occasionally, visible light–induced eczema of exposed, and sometimes also covered, sites (1,2,31). It is most common in older men at temperate latitudes and most severe in summer. It may affect previously normal subjects or patients with prior endogenous eczema, photoallergic or allergic contact dermatitis, perhaps oral drug photosensitivity, or maybe rarely PMLE. Allergic contact sensitivity to ubiquitous, often airborne, perhaps occasionally photoactive agents often coexist. There is itchy, scattered or confluent, subacute or chronic eczema of the exposed skin, which may be lichenified (Fig. 12-12), excoriated, or more severely, erythematous, shiny, infiltrated, discrete or coalescent papules or plaques on a background of erythema, eczema, or just normal skin. Erythroderma is also rarely possible. Malignant transformation has been claimed on occasion but never convincingly substantiated, although a CAD-like photoresponse as part of cutaneous T-cell lymphoma itself may perhaps rarely occur (32). UVB-, UVA-, and occasionally also visible light–induced pseudolymphomatous CAD has previously been described as actinic reticuloid and as persistent light reaction (reactivity).

Histology. In early CAD, the histology (33,34) may resemble that of any other spongiotic process, including eczema and contact dermatitis, with epidermal spongiosis, lymphocytic exocytosis, and a superficial and deep, perivascular, lymphohistiocytic, inflammatory cell infiltrate. In older lesions, however, there is variable, often marked, acanthosis of the epidermis and infundibular portions of hair follicles (Fig. 12-13), while spongiosis and lymphocytic exocytosis may be focally prominent (Fig. 12-14). Secondary changes from excoriation are also frequent in both early and late disease and consist of focal epidermal necrosis, scale-crust formation, dermal–epidermal junction fibrin deposition, and neutrophils with nuclear dust. In addition, there may be occasional aggregates of cells mimicking Pautrier microabscess, and these usually represent collections cells of Langerhans type. In the papillary dermis, vertically streaked collagen, stellate fibroblasts, and small multinucleated cells, often described as Montgomery giant cells (Fig. 12-15), are frequently present; these latter, however, may commonly

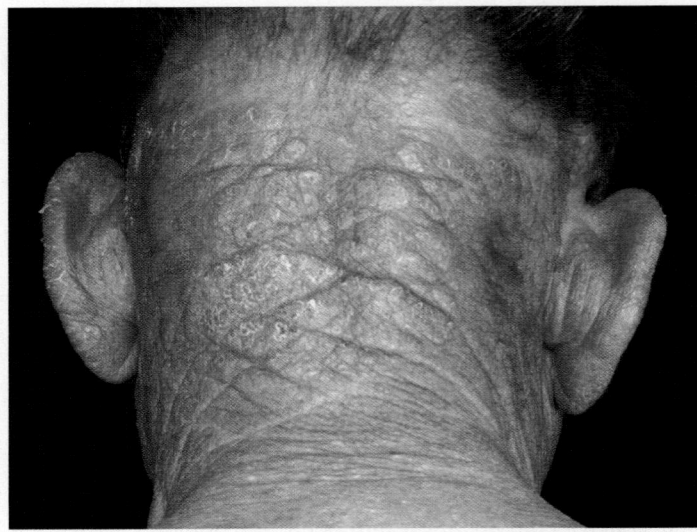

Figure 12-12 Chronic actinic dermatitis. Extensive lichenification and excoriation.

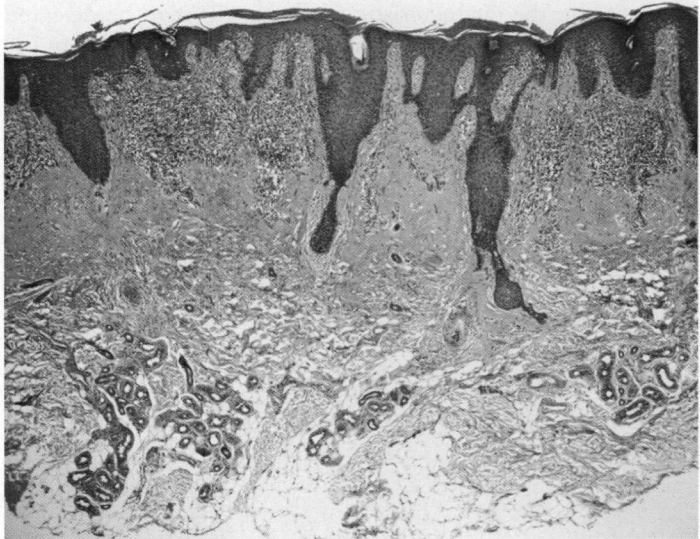

Figure 12-13 Chronic actinic dermatitis. Older lesion with prominent hyperplasia of epidermis and infundibular portion of hair follicles.

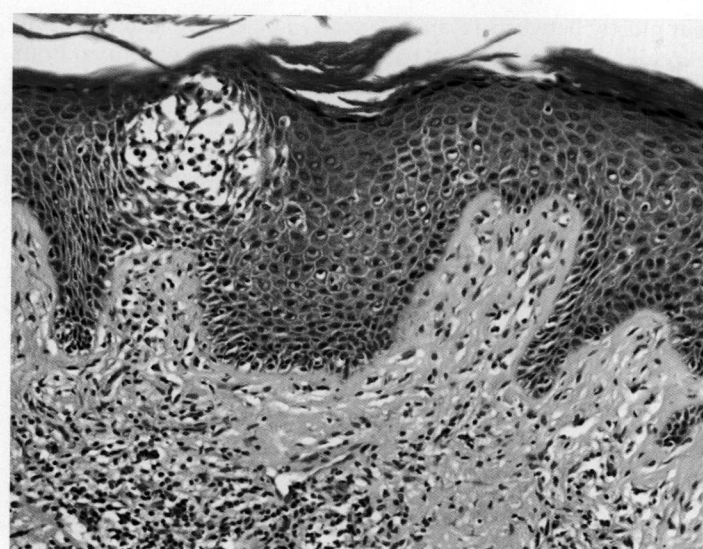

Figure 12-14 Chronic actinic dermatitis. Lichenification in association with prominent spongiotic changes and exocytosis of lymphocytes.

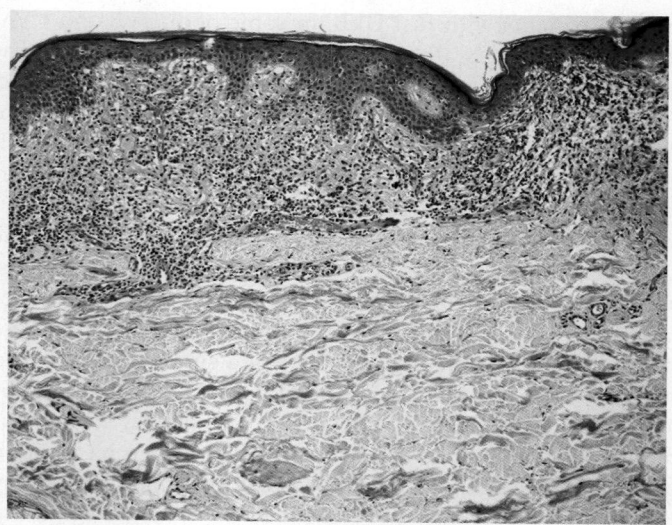

Figure 12-16 Chronic actinic dermatitis (actinic reticuloid variant). Prominent superficial dermal mononuclear cell infiltrate focally obscuring the dermal–epidermal junction.

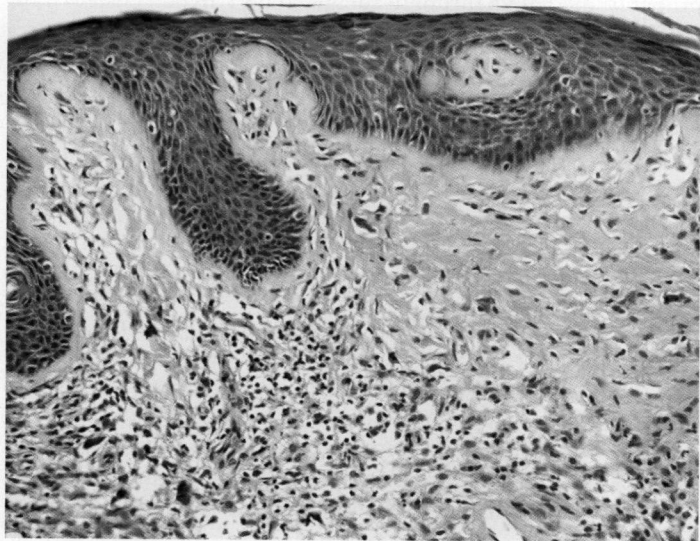

Figure 12-15 Chronic actinic dermatitis. Fibrosis of papillary dermis with mononuclear inflammatory cells and scattered small giant cells.

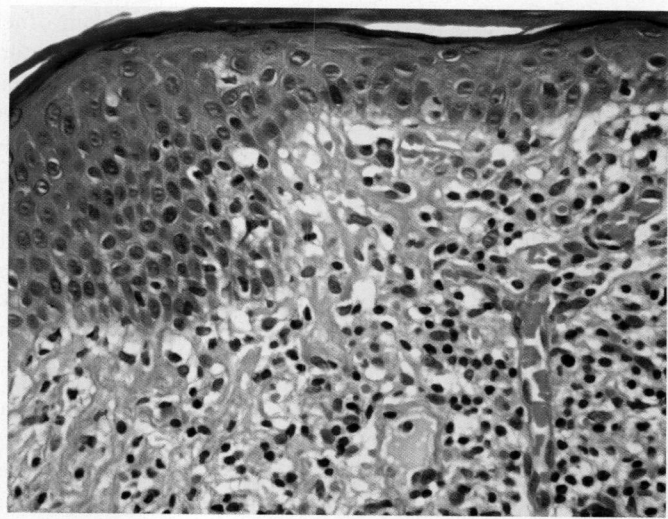

Figure 12-17 Chronic actinic dermatitis (actinic reticuloid variant). Focal epidermal exocytosis of lymphocytes, with some displaying irregular nuclear outlines.

occur in any chronic inflammatory process. Deep in the dermis, there is often a predominantly perivascular, usually dense, mononuclear cell infiltrate of mainly T lymphocytes, histiocytes, eosinophils, and plasma cells; in severe CAD, this may be even more prominent, along with marked focal epidermal lymphocyte exocytosis (Fig. 12-16), and a degree of irregularity of nuclear outline (Figs. 12-17 and 12-18). In such cases, formerly included within the term actinic reticuloid, distinction from cutaneous T-cell lymphoma may often be difficult. It has been suggested that the T lymphocytes in such cases have a diagnostically helpful (predominantly CD8 [cytotoxic] positive) phenotype and that most other reactive infiltrates and cutaneous T-cell lymphomas are instead mostly CD4 (helper) positive (34). However, personal experience suggests that this is not always so and that infiltrating helper T lymphocytes are often prominent in CAD as well.

Pathogenesis. CAD is clinically and histologically reproducible at all skin sites in the absence of exogenous photosensitizer,

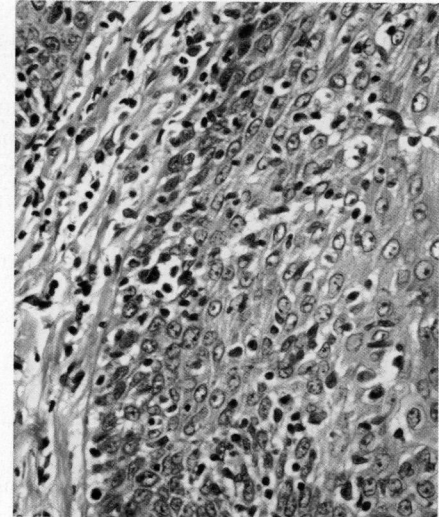

Figure 12-18 Chronic actinic dermatitis (actinic reticuloid variant). A Pautrier-like microabscess within the infundibulum of a hair follicle.

in some patients with just UVB; in some both UVB and UVA; and rarely in others all of UVB, UVA, and short visible radiation; or even more rarely, just visible light. However, otherwise, the clinical features and pattern of dermal cellular infiltration, cytokine production, and adhesion molecule activation are all essentially indistinguishable from those of allergic contact dermatitis (2). Since the latter is a known DTH response, it therefore seems highly likely that the same situation applies in the CAD reaction, presumably against photoactivated endogenous, cutaneous autoantigen. Furthermore, action spectrum studies have suggested that the UVR absorber initiating the process may conceivably sometimes be DNA or a similar or associated molecule (35). In addition, it is possible that the airborne allergic contact dermatitis common in CAD may increase cutaneous immune responsiveness and thus putative antigen recognition or else that the frequently photoaged skin in the disease may lead to diminished normal UVR-induced cutaneous immunosuppression, as occurs genetically in PMLE as described earlier, and again greater antigen recognition. Finally, slower clearance of antigen may also occur in the aged skin of CAD, arguably again potentiating disease development.

Differential Diagnosis. CAD must be distinguished from other eczemas, in particular the seborrheic and atopic forms, from airborne and topical medicament contact dermatitis, and from cutaneous T-cell lymphoma. However, as the histologic appearances are indistinguishable from those of other subacute or chronic spongiotic processes, or in its severe forms from cutaneous T-cell lymphoma, a careful clinical history, patch and photopatch testing and monochromatic or broad-spectrum irradiation phototesting are essential for firm diagnosis as well. Nevertheless, severe CAD is generally separable from lymphoma by its superficial dermal fibrosis, paucity of cytologically atypical lymphocytes, and at least focal prominent spongiosis.

Principles of Management: CAD treatment requires great care, with the restriction of UVR exposure, wearing of appropriately protective clothing, application of high-protection broad-spectrum sunscreens, and avoidance of exacerbating contact or photocontact allergens all being necessary but often of only partial help. Topical moisturizers and intermittent potent topical steroid use on affected sites also help, whereas topical calcineurin inhibitors may be useful in some cases, even those that are severe (36), and intermittent oral steroid therapy, low-dose narrowband UVB phototherapy, or probably more reliably PUVA, initially under high-dose oral steroid cover, may also be very effective (37). Failing this, oral immunosuppressive therapy with azathioprine, cyclosporine, or occasionally mycophenolate generally clears or nearly clears the condition fully, if tolerated (38). In addition, dupilumab, helpful in atopic eczema, has recently been shown to improve, if not necessarily fully abate, CAD (39). Finally, CAD may often eventually remit spontaneously (40).

SOLAR URTICARIA

Clinical Summary. SU is a rare UVR- or visible radiation–induced whealing of exposed skin. The more common primary SU occurs spontaneously, and the very rare secondary form follows photosensitization to drugs or chemicals (41). Primary SU is slightly more common in women, with onset at any age but mostly between 10 and 50 years. The eruption develops on exposed skin within 5 to 10 minutes and fades within an hour or 2. Regularly uncovered sites such as the face and backs of hands are occasionally spared. A tingling sensation and patchy erythema generally precede separate or confluent whealing, the latter sometimes generalized and in severe instances occasionally associated with headache, nausea, bronchospasm, faintness, or systemic collapse. Secondary SU generally follows exposure to substances such as tar, pitch, dyes, drugs such as the long-discontinued benoxaprofen, or, very rarely, endogenous porphyrin in the porphyrias.

Histopathology. The epidermis appears unremarkable. In the dermis, there is edema as evidenced by mild collagen bundle separation, along with slight, rarely moderate, perivascular and interstitial inflammatory cell infiltration with eosinophils and occasionally also neutrophils and lymphocytes (41,42) (Fig. 12-19).

Pathogenesis. Any UVR- or visible radiation waveband, specific for a given patient, though occasionally broadening or contracting over time (43), may induce primary SU (41). Whealing is probably mediated through allergic type I hypersensitivity to cutaneous or circulating, irradiation-induced allergen. Presumed circulating antibodies have also been identified, very likely of the immunoglobulin E type. In secondary SU, the eruption apparently follows direct nonimmunologic injury after UVR absorption by the responsible chemical or drug and its secondary transfer to adjacent mast cells to stimulate histamine release, such histamine being the major chemical mediator in both forms (44).

Differential Diagnosis. Clinically, SU must be differentiated from other light-induced eruptions by its much shorter time course and characteristic whealing and from other forms of urticaria, particularly the rare localized heat urticaria. Histologic distinction, however, is not possible. The porphyrias (particularly, very rarely, erythropoietic protoporphyria) (45), drug and chemical photosensitivity, and lupus erythematosus, must also be excluded, usually easily, for final diagnosis.

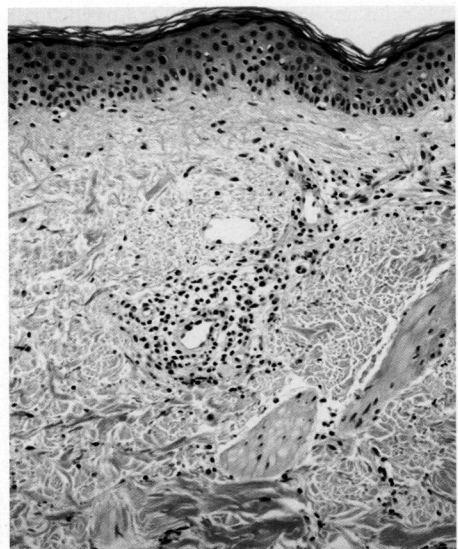

Figure 12-19 Solar urticaria. Dermal edema and a mild interstitial and perivascular inflammatory cell infiltrate of lymphocytes and eosinophils.

Principles of Management: Avoidance of the inducing radiation, the use of appropriate sunscreens, or in particular adequate, usually high, doses of nonsedating antihistamines, help approximately half of patients. Resistant cases sometimes respond to low-dose narrowband UVB phototherapy, low-dose PUVA (46) or, more often, plasmapheresis (47), whereas up to several linked short courses of intravenous immunoglobulin (48) are also reasonably often helpful. Cyclosporine may very rarely be effective. However, a proportion of SU patients do poorly with all therapy, whereas a moderate number resolve spontaneously. Relatively recently, however, omalizumab, very useful in other forms of resistant urticaria, has been shown to be helpful in up to three-quarters of SU patients and may quite possibly become the next treatment choice if initial sunscreen and high-dose nonsedating antihistamine use are insufficient (49).

REFERENCES

1. Lim HW, Hawk JLM. Evaluation of the photosensitive patient. In: Lim HW, Hönigsmann H, Hawk JLM, eds. *Photodermatology*. Informa Healthcare; 2007:139.
2. Gambichler T, Al-Muhammadi R, Boms S. Immunologically mediated photodermatoses. *Am J Clin Dermatol*. 2012;10:169.
3. Lembo S, Hawk JLM, Murphy GM, et al. Aberrant gene expression with deficient apoptotic keratinocyte clearance may dispose to polymorphic light eruption. *Br J Dermatol*. 2017;177:1450.
4. Hirai Y, Yamamoto T, Kimura H, et al. Hydroa vacciniforme is associated with increased numbers of Epstein–Barr virus-infected γδT cells. *J Invest Dermatol*. 2012;22:380.
5. Verneuil L, Gouarin S, Comoz F, et al. Epstein–Barr virus involvement in the pathogenesis of hydroa vacciniforme: an assessment of seven adult patients with long-term follow-up. *Br J Dermatol*. 2010;163:174–182.
6. Dover JS, Hawk JLM. Polymorphic light eruption sine eruptione. *Br J Dermatol*. 1988;118:73.
7. Epstein JH. Polymorphous light eruption. *J Am Acad Dermatol*. 1980;3:329.
8. Hölzle E, Plewig G, Hofmann C, Roser-Maass E. Polymorphous light eruption-experimental induction of lesions. *J Am Acad Dermatol*. 1982;7:111.
9. Norris PG, Morris J, McGibbon DM, Chu AC, Hawk JL. Polymorphic light eruption: an immunopathological study of evolving lesions. *Br J Dermatol*. 1989;120:173.
10. Su W, Hall BJ IV, Cockerell CJ. Photodermatitis with minimal inflammatory infiltrate: clinical inflammatory conditions with discordant histologic findings. *Am J Dermatopathol*. 2006;28:482.
11. van de Pas CB, Kelly DA, Seed PT, Young AR, Hawk JL, Walker SL. Patients with polymorphic light eruption are resistant to UVR-induced suppression of the contact hypersensitivity response. *J Invest Dermatol*. 2004;122:295.
12. Palmer RA, Hawk JL, Young AR, Walker SL. The effect of solar-simulated on the elicitation phase of contact hypersensitivity does not differ between controls and patients with polymorphic light eruption. *J Invest Dermatol*. 2005;124:1308.
13. Palmer RA, Hawk, JL. Light-induced seborrhoeic eczema: severe provocation from subclinical disease. *Photodermatol Photoimmunol Photomed*. 2004;20:62.
14. Hoss D, Berke A, Kerr P, Grant-Kels J, Murphy M. Prominent papillary dermal edema in dermatophytosis (tinea corporis). *J Cutan Pathol*. 2010;37:237.
15. Wackernagel A, Massone C, Hoefler G, Steinbauer E, Kerl H, Wolf P. Plasmacytoid dendritic cells are absent in skin lesions of polymorphic light eruption. *Photodermatol Photoimmunol Photomed*. 2007;23:24.
16. Murphy GM, Logan RA, Lovell CR, Morris RW, Hawk JL, Magnus IA. Prophylactic PUVA and UVB therapy in polymorphic light eruption—a controlled trial. *Br J Dermatol*. 1987;116:531.
17. Patel DC, Bellaney GJ, Seed PT, McGregor JM, Hawk JL. Efficacy of short-course oral prednisolone in polymorphic light eruption: a randomized controlled trial. *Br J Dermatol*. 2000;143:828.
18. Grabczynska SA, McGregor JM, Kondeatis E, Vaughan RW, Hawk JL. Actinic prurigo and polymorphic light eruption: common pathogenesis and the importance of HLA-DR4/DRB1*0407. *Br J Dermatol*. 1999;140:232.
19. Lane PR, Murphy F, Hogan DJ, Hull PR, Burgdorf WH. Histopathology of actinic prurigo. *Am J Dermatopathol*. 1993;15:326.
20. Herrera-Geopfert R, Magaña M. Follicular cheilitis: a distinctive histopathologic finding in actinic prurigo. *Am J Dermatopathol*. 1995;17:357.
21. Vega-Memije ME, Mosqueda-Taylor A, Irigoyen-Camacho ME, Hojyo-Tomoka MT, Domínguez-Soto L. Actinic prurigo cheilitis: clinicopathologic analysis and therapeutic results in 116 cases. *Oral Surg Oral Med Oral Pathol Oral Radiol Endod*. 2002;94:83.
22. Farr PM, Diffey BL. Treatment of actinic prurigo with PUVA: mechanism of action. *Br J Dermatol*. 1989;120:411.
23. Lovell, CR, Hawk JL, Calnan CD, Magnus IA. Thalidomide in actinic prurigo. *Br J Dermatol*. 1983;108:467.
24. Sonnex TS, Hawk JLM. Hydroa vacciniforme: a review of ten cases. *Br J Dermatol*. 1988;118:101.
25. Gupta G, Man I, Kemmett D. Hydroa vacciniforme: a clinical and follow-up study of 17 cases. *J Am Acad Dermatol*. 2000;42:208.
26. Sangueza M, Plaza JA. Hydroa vacciniforme-like cutaneous T-cell lymphoma: clinicopathologic and immunohistochemical study of 12 cases. *J Am Acad Dermatol*. 2013;69:112.
27. Quintanilla-Martinez L, Ridaura C, Nagl F, et al. Hydroa vacciniforme-like lymphoma: a chronic EBV+ lymphoproliferative disorder with risk to develop a systemic lymphoma. *Blood*. 2013;122:3101.
28. Cohen JI, Manoli I, Dowdell K, et al. Hydroa vacciniforme-like lymphoproliferative disorder: an EBV disease with a low risk to systemic illness in Caucasians. *Blood*. 2019;133:2753.
29. Quitanilla-Martinez L, Fend F. Deciphering hydroa vacciniforme. *Blood*. 2019;133:2735.
30. Jaschke E, Hönigsmann H. Hydroa vacciniforme-action spectrum. UV-tolerance following photochemotherapy. *Hautarzt*. 1981;32:350.
31. Hawk JL. Chronic actinic dermatitis. *Photoderm Photoimmunol Photomed*. 2004;20:312.
32. Morris SD, Hawk JLM, Russell-Jones R, Whittaker SJ. Severe photosensitivity in four patients with erythrodermic cutaneous T-cell lymphoma. *Br J Dermatol*. 2002;147:36.
33. Toonstra J. Actinic reticuloid. *Semin Diagn Pathol*. 1991;8:109.
34. Chu AC, Robinson D, Hawk JLM, Meacham R, Spittle MF, Smith NP. Immunologic differentiation of the Sézary syndrome due to cutaneous T-cell lymphoma and chronic actinic dermatitis. *J Invest Dermatol*. 1986;86:134.
35. Menagé HduP, Harrison GI, Potten CS, Young AR, Hawk JL. The action spectrum for induction of chronic actinic dermatitis is similar to that for sunburn inflammation. *Photochem Photobiol*. 1995;62:976.
36. Evans AV, Palmer RA, Hawk JL. Erythrodermic chronic actinic dermatitis responding only to tacrolimus. *Photodermatol Photoimmunol Photomed*. 2004;20:59.
37. Hindson C, Spiro J, Downey A. PUVA therapy of chronic actinic dermatitis, *Br J Dermatol*. 1985;113:157.
38. Murphy GM, Maurice PD, Norris PG, Morris RW, Hawk JL. Azathioprine treatment in chronic actinic dermatitis: a double-blind controlled trial with monitoring of exposure to ultraviolet radiation. *Br J Dermatol*. 1989;121:639.
39. Patel N, Konda S, Lim HW. Dupilumab for the treatment of chronic actinic dermatitis. *Photodermatol Photoimmunol Photomed*. 2020;36:398.

40. Dawe RS, Crombie IK, Ferguson J. The natural history of chronic actinic dermatitis. *Arch Dermatol.* 2000;136:1215.

41. Horio T, Hölzle E. Solar urticaria. In: Lim HW, Hönigsmann H, Hawk JLM, eds. *Photodermatology.* Informa Healthcare; 2007:183.

42. Leiferman K, Norris PG, Murphy GM, Hawk JL, Winkelmann RK. Evidence for eosinophil degranulation with deposition of granule major basic protein in solar urticaria. *J Am Acad Dermatol.* 1989;21:75–80.

43. Murphy GM, Hawk JL. Broadening of action spectrum in a patient with solar urticaria. *Clin Exp Dermatol.* 1987;12:455.

44. Hawk JL, Eady RA, Challoner AV, Kobza-Black A, Keahey TM, Greaves MW. Elevated blood histamine levels and mast cell degranulation in solar urticaria. *Br J Clin Pharmacol.* 1980;9:183.

45. Magnus IA, Jarrett A, Prankerd TA, Rimington C. Erythropoietic protoporphyria: a new porphyria syndrome due to protoporphyrinaemia. *Lancet.* 1961;26:448.

46. Calzavara-Pinton P, Zane C, Rossi M, Sala R, Venturini M. Narrow-band ultraviolet B phototherapy is a suitable treatment option for solar urticaria. *J Am Acad Dermatol.* 2012;67:e5.

47. Leenutaphong V, Hölzle E, Plewig G, Kutkuhn B, Grabensee B. Plasmapheresis in solar urticaria. *Dermatologica.* 1991;182:35.

48. Adamski H, Bedane C, Bonnevalle A, et al. Solar urticaria treated with intravenous immunoglobulins. *J Am Acad Dermatol.* 2011;65:336.

49. Morgado-Carrasco D, Fustà-Novell X, Podlipnik S, Combalia A, Aguilera P. Clinical and photobiological response in eight patients with solar urticaria under treatment with omalizumab, review of the literature. *Photoderm Photoimmunol Photomed.* 2018;34:194.

Disorders Associated with Physical Agents: Heat, Cold, Radiation, and Trauma

SUSAN PEI AND EMILY Y. CHU

Chapter
13

INTRODUCTION

Physical injury to the skin can result in a number of disorders of the epidermis, dermis, and/or subcutis, depending on the type of agent exposure. Direct injury to the skin by radiation- and temperature-associated exposure results in distinct histopathologic skin alterations, which are discussed in this chapter. Disorders due to direct physical injury and surgical-related injury are also discussed; however, cutaneous alterations associated with cosmetic-associated procedures such as reactions to injectable material (e.g., silicone) are discussed elsewhere. Conditions that have other pathogenesis but may be related to temperature or physical exposure, such as physical urticaria, Raynaud phenomenon, and cold panniculitis, are discussed in Chapters 7, 10, and 20, respectively.

HEAT-ASSOCIATED INJURIES

The effect of heat on the skin is determined by the skin thickness and degree, extent, and duration of the heat exposure. The source of the heat also influences the degree of tissue injury. For instance, dry heat results in charring and desiccation, whereas moist heat results in opaque coagulation. Immersion burns are more severe than flash and splatter burns, and electrical burns result in deep tissue necrosis (1). Exposure of the skin to extreme heat results in a first-, second-, or third-degree burn, whereas prolonged or repetitive exposure to less intense heat results in changes of erythema ab igne. Surgery-related electrodesiccation-induced injury also has distinct histopathologic features and is discussed at the end of the chapter.

Burns

Clinical Summary. Burns to the skin may be due to *thermal injury* from flames or hot substances such as scalding water, contact, or flash burns from explosions; *chemical burns*, such as wet cement (2) or mustard gas (3); and *electrical injury*. The end result is similar in all burns, and these are classified according to the depth of injury (4).

Tissue injury from direct exposure to heat is the most common and is defined by the depth (partial or full thickness) or extent (first, second, or third degree) of tissue injury. The resultant tissue injury is a sequela of the release of inflammatory and vasoactive mediators released due to denaturation and coagulation of proteins and to edema from increased capillary permeability (5). Painful erythema and edema without vesiculation is

seen in first-degree burns; vesiculation and blisters characterize superficial second-degree burns, which progress to pallor and anesthesia if both the epidermis and the dermis are injured; and third-degree burns show massive necrosis with charring, denuded superficial tissue, granulation tissue, and scar formation (1). Deep second- and third-degree burns show overlapping features. Secondary bacterial infections may cause the injury of a superficial second-degree burn to extend deeper, with changes similar to a third-degree burn.

Chemical burns may be due to acid or alkalis, the latter of which penetrate more deeply, with delayed pain. Cement burns are an example and tend to occur on the lower extremities, associated with accidental seepage of cement onto clothing or boots (2). Occasionally, there may be burns from marking lines on playing fields. There is burning, pain, erythema, and vesiculation within about 6 to 48 hours of exposure (mean, 38 hours). Erosions and necrosis similar to heat burns ensue. Mustard gas (yperite) burns in chemical warfare may be seen even with less than 1 hour of exposure, with a latent period of less than 6 hours. Patients present with pruritus, burning, pain, erosions, erythema, vesicles, bulla, ulceration, edema, and dyschromia, especially hyperpigmentation (3). Involvement of groin and axilla is more common, owing to moisture. There may be a toxic epidermal necrolysis–like picture. Chemical burns due to commercially available vinegar (acetic acid 4% to 8%) can occur with patient application of vinegar as "natural home remedies" to warts, lice, molluscum contagiosum (6), and nevi (7,8).

Secondary inflammatory events or malignant conditions may arise at burn sites (see later discussion), and rarely, neutrophilic dermatosis may be induced by thermal burn injury (9). Eccrine poroma (10), sarcoidosis, neurothekeoma, schwannoma (11), and pemphigus vulgaris (12) may also be seen. In addition, delayed postburn blistering can occur up to 1 year or more after healing of partial-thickness burn wounds and should be differentiated from autoimmune blistering dermatoses (13).

Histopathology. The histopathology depends on the degree of tissue damage. There is variable necrosis of the epidermis, dermis, and adnexal structures, with necrosis and eventual sclerotic changes of the dermis. The inflammatory infiltrate is variable and includes neutrophils, lymphocytes, and macrophages. Attempts have been made to estimate the age of the burn wound based on the degree of neutrophilic and macrophage infiltration (14). Acute inflammation tends to predominate in the first 6 hours to 2 days after injury; however, neutrophils can also be seen in later lesions. The latter may possibly be related to infection, which can often occur. Macrophages tend to be encountered from days 2 to 20, but many cases show a minimal or absent macrophage response. Lymphocytes typically appear later.

The degree of burn is defined more specifically by the following features:

First-degree burns: Vasodilation is the predominant feature. Epidermal and subepidermal edema may progress to partial-thickness superficial epidermal necrosis. Full-thickness epidermal necrosis differentiates second-degree burns from first-degree burns.

Second-degree burns: In superficial second-degree burns, partial- to full-thickness necrosis and edema of the epidermis and subepidermal stroma result in blister formation. Typically, epidermal necrosis and separation from the dermis at the dermal–epidermal junction or within necrotic basilar keratinocytes are seen (Fig. 13-1). Although initially vasoconstriction occurs, the biopsies show prominent vasodilation and edema in the dermis. Necrotic changes may extend into the lower reticular dermis in deep second-degree burns, but the appendages tend to be

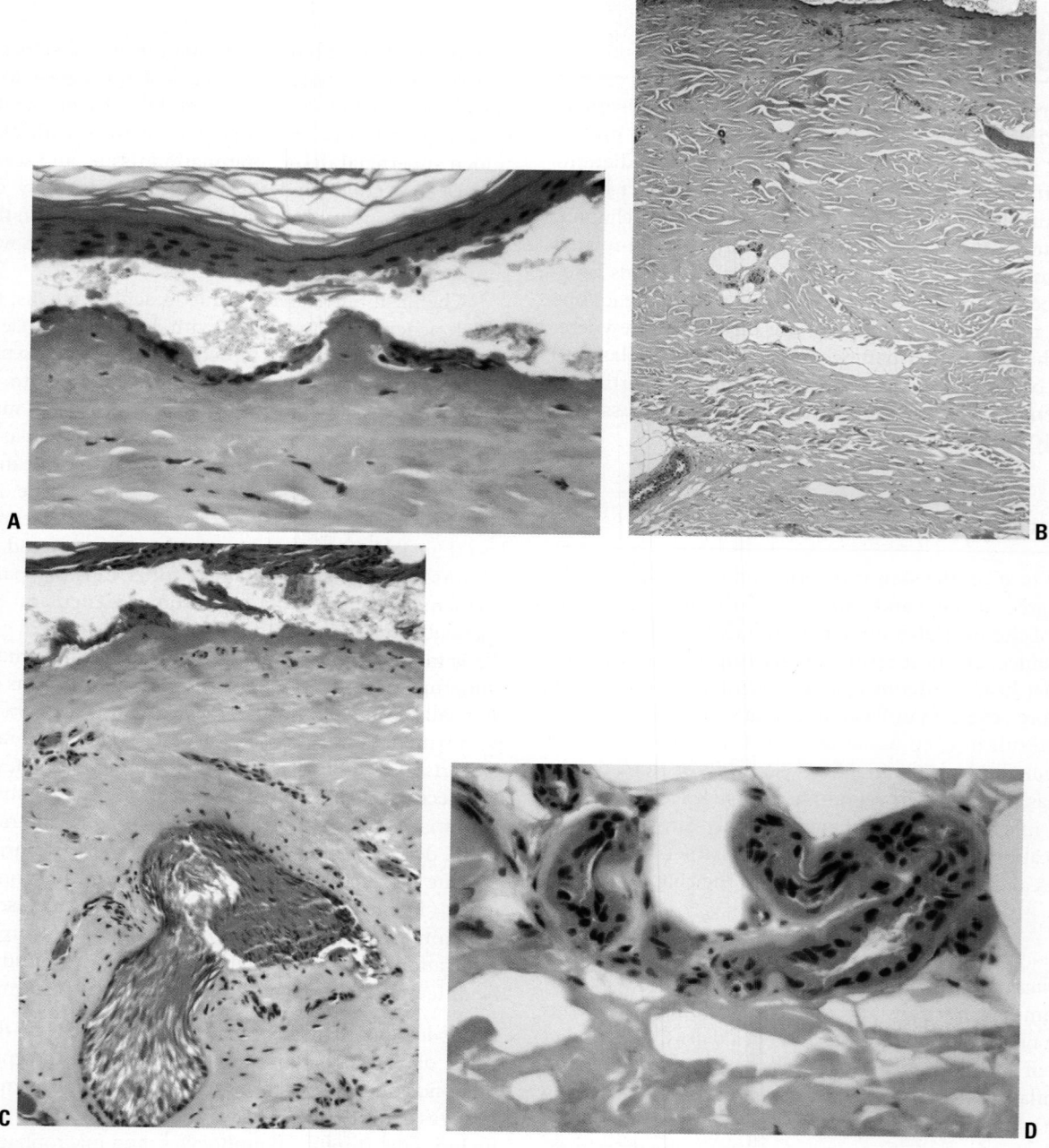

Figure 13-1 Third-degree burn. **A:** The epidermis shows full-thickness eosinophilic necrosis, resulting in bullous disassociation from the dermis and incipient demotion. This bulla formation can be seen in second- and third-degree burns. The collagen shows homogenized necrosis, with loss of distinction between collagen bundles. The fibroblasts are nonatypical, differentiating this from chronic radiation injury. **B:** There is pandermal eosinophilic homogenized alteration collagen, with necrosis of an eccrine gland. The epidermis shows bulla formation. **C:** Extension of the injury involving the pilosebaceous units, differentiating a third-degree burn from a superficial second-degree burn. Burn injury to the pilosebaceous unit results in eosinophilic necrosis of the epithelium and elongation of the nuclei. The surrounding stroma shows coagulation of the collagen and vascular thrombosis. **D:** Eosinophilic alteration of an injured eccrine gland, differentiating third-degree burn from second- and first-degree burns.

spared, differentiating a second-degree from a third-degree burn. Apoptosis can be seen in the adnexal structures and dermal fibroblasts of deep partial burns (15).

Third-degree burns: Full-thickness coagulation necrosis of the epidermis and dermis, including the appendages, is seen (Fig. 13-1). The resultant scar is characterized by hyalinized collagen and an absence of adnexal structures (Fig. 13-2).

Chemical burns: Chemical burns may vary, depending on the substance. Dermal and adnexal necrosis similar to thermal burns may be seen. Histopathology of sulfur mustard shows four patterns:

1. Interface dermatitis, with or without necrosis, similar to toxic epidermal necrolysis or erythema multiforme, with hyperpigmentation of the epidermal roof
2. Spongiotic dermatitis, similar to acute contact dermatitis. Bulla formation is often at the dermal–epidermal junction, with or without acantholytic cells. The epidermal roof shows dysmaturation with cellular atypia.
3. Hyperpigmentation of the basal layer of the epidermis with dermal melanophages
4. Dermal alteration, including coagulation necrosis, low-grade fibrosis with sclerodermoid changes, telangiectases, and perivascular inflammation, without vasculitis (3)

Histopathology of burns due to vinegar "home remedies" shows abrupt epidermal necrosis with neutrophils and fibrinoid vascular changes (6) and scar formation in the mid-dermis with distinct borders (8). When vinegar is used to treat nevi, recurrent nevus phenomenon may occur as a result (8).

Differential Diagnosis. Radiation dermatitis is differentiated from burn scars by the presence of atypical radiation fibroblasts in the former. Complete absence of the adnexal structures favors a burn scar because the eccrine glands may be spared with radiation. In morphea/scleroderma, there is preservation of eccrine coils, and a lymphoplasmacellular infiltrate may be seen.

Principles of Management: Management of burns is dependent on the extent of injury—the degree of burn (first, second, or third), the body surface area involved, and the anatomic region affected. Superficial burns are improved by application of ice, cold water, and/or cold compresses. Prevention of infection is of paramount importance, especially for patients affected by deeper burns. Topical antimicrobial agents are commonly used for this reason, including silver sulfadiazine. Excision of burn wounds that extend into the deep reticular dermis and subcutaneous fat may be performed to prevent wound infection and limit morbidity. Careful attention should be given to the cardiopulmonary status of a patient with extensive injury (>10% to 15% body surface area) and/or deep burn wounds, given the risk of insensible water losses and sepsis as a result of compromised skin-barrier function. Such patients may be best managed in the setting of a burn center.

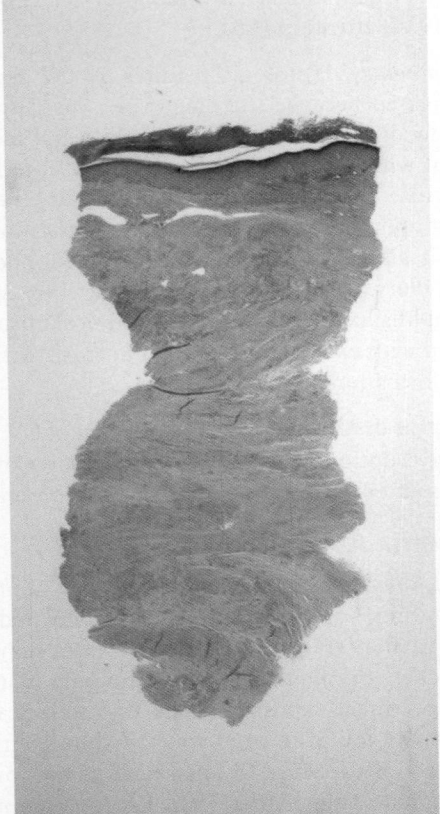
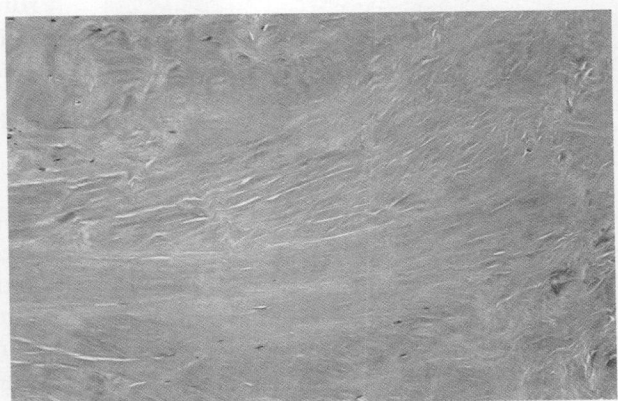

A   B

Figure 13-2 Chronic burn scar. **A:** The dermis and subcutis are diffusely sclerotic and homogenized, with complete absence of adnexal structures, including arrector pili muscles, differentiating this from radiation injury and scleroderma/morphea. The absence of vascular proliferation and presence of homogenized thickening of the collagen differentiate a chronic burn from a scar from other reparative causes. **B:** The sclerotic collagen is nearly devoid of fibroblasts, in particular atypical ones, differentiating this from chronic radiation injury.

Burn Scar–Associated Malignancy

Chronic burn scars are subject to the development of dystrophic calcinosis cutis (16), and carcinomas, especially basal cell carcinomas, may arise acutely within 2 to 3 months after the injury (1). Delayed carcinomas arise after a latency that ranges from 10 to 70 years, with an average of approximately 30 years. Of the delayed carcinomas, basal cell carcinomas have the shortest latency period (17). There may be a shorter lag time (19 years) if there is poor wound care (18). The tumors most often arise on the extremities but may also arise on the head and trunk. Burn scar–associated cancers include squamous more often than basal cell carcinomas, but malignant melanoma (19), sarcomas (including malignant fibrous histiocytoma, fibrosarcoma, liposarcoma, dermatofibrosarcoma protuberans, malignant schwannoma, leiomyosarcoma, osteosarcoma, and angiosarcoma (17,20), and primary cutaneous lymphomas (21,22) may be seen. Squamous cell carcinomas are more often seen with scalding burns, whereas basal cell carcinomas are associated with burns from flames. Welders are also at risk of getting both basal and squamous cell carcinomas because of chronic exposure to both high temperatures and nonsolar ultraviolet (UV) radiation (23,24). The occurrence of cancer developing in burn scars was noted in 1860 by Heurteux, and trauma-induced carcinomas were described by Marjolin in 1828; these cancers are more aggressive than their sun-induced counterparts. Metastases may occur in up to approximately one-third of the cases. Recurrence is also higher in cancers due to these chronic ulcers. The term "Marjolin ulcer" has been applied to cancers related to either burn or trauma-related chronic wounds. The carcinomas arise from the edges of wounds or from epithelial remnants entrapped in the scar; thus, they may not occur as frequently if there has been grafting (1).

Acute Ultraviolet Burn

Mild UV-induced burns are commonly referred to as "sunburns." The resulting erythema is characterized by the presence of scattered apoptotic keratinocytes on histopathology, termed "sunburn cells." Variable subepidermal edema is seen. Clinical blistering may result from severe burns due to full-thickness epidermal necrosis and/or dermal edema (Fig. 13-3). The preservation of appendages allows for epidermal regeneration.

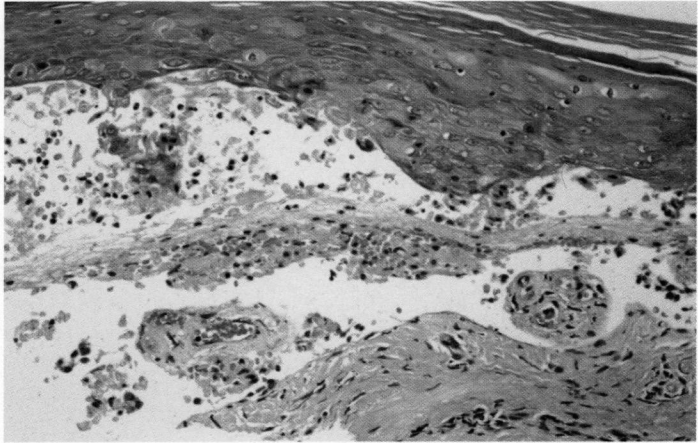

Figure 13-3 Acute ultraviolet (UV) radiation burn. This is an example of a UVA-induced burn showing full-thickness dyskeratotic keratinocytes throughout all layers of the epidermis, with subepidermal blister formation.

Ultraviolet Recall

Clinical Summary. UV recall refers to the phenomenon in which a medication induces an acute cutaneous eruption restricted to the area of previous sunburn or UV light therapy (25). Other names for this phenomenon include sunburn reactivation, sunburn recall, photo recall, and photodermatitis reactivation. UV recall is seen after methotrexate use, but it can also be associated with other chemotherapeutic agents, targeted therapy agents (including sorafenib), and antibiotics, such as ampicillin and trimethoprim–sulfamethoxazole (26). Two clinical presentations may be seen, depending on whether the UV recall reaction occurs days after UV exposure, as is seen with methotrexate, or weeks to months later, as is typically seen with antibiotics. Methotrexate-induced recall phenomenon generally occurs if methotrexate is given 1 to 5 days after sunburn occurs, but not if the burn is concomitant or much earlier. This UV recall tends to be associated with pain and burning, with an erythematous to violaceous vesiculobullous eruption (25), and in most cases, it is more severe than the initial sunburn. UV recall reactions associated with antibiotics (27,28) differ from the methotrexate reaction. These tend to occur at a later interval—weeks to months from the sunburn—with a less severe, pruritic macular, papular or morbilliform-like drug reaction (28). The UV reaction with either presentation presents within a few hours or days of the medication intake. Rechallenge may occur at a shorter interval than the initial reaction and with a more severe blistering reaction (29). It has been proposed that the methotrexate-induced reaction be considered a UV enhancement reaction and those associated with a delayed interval of UV exposure be considered UV reactivation (25).

Histopathology. Histologic features of UV recall are not well documented because the diagnosis is usually made clinically. A review of the literature described several histologic features, most of which indicate a component of interface or cytotoxic dermatitis, characterized by hydropic degeneration, dyskeratotic or apoptotic keratinocytes, dysmaturation, or acanthosis. There is also a variable perivascular lymphocytic infiltrate in the papillary dermis, sometimes with erythrocyte extravasation. Neutrophils have been described. Clinical blisters have been associated with extensive epidermal necrosis with intraepidermal bullae formation (25).

Principles of Management: Treatment of UV recall is supportive. The eruption will spontaneously resolve over time. Topical steroids and emollients may provide symptomatic relief.

Erythema Ab Igne

Clinical Summary. Erythema ab igne is a clinically distinctive skin finding, which manifests as reticulated, dusky red to brown patches (Fig. 13-4). Telangiectases may be seen within the patches. Erythema ab igne commonly manifests following repetitive, direct exposure of the skin to a heat source. It was traditionally found to occur on the shins, buttocks, and back as a result of exposure to open hearths or stoves, steam heaters, and hot water bottles (30). Laptop computers have been more recently reported to induce erythema ab igne, often on the thighs (31). Heated car seats and recliners are also newer associations (32–34). Patients with altered mental status may be at increased risk of erythema ab igne, given decreased awareness of prolonged exposure to heat sources, including heating

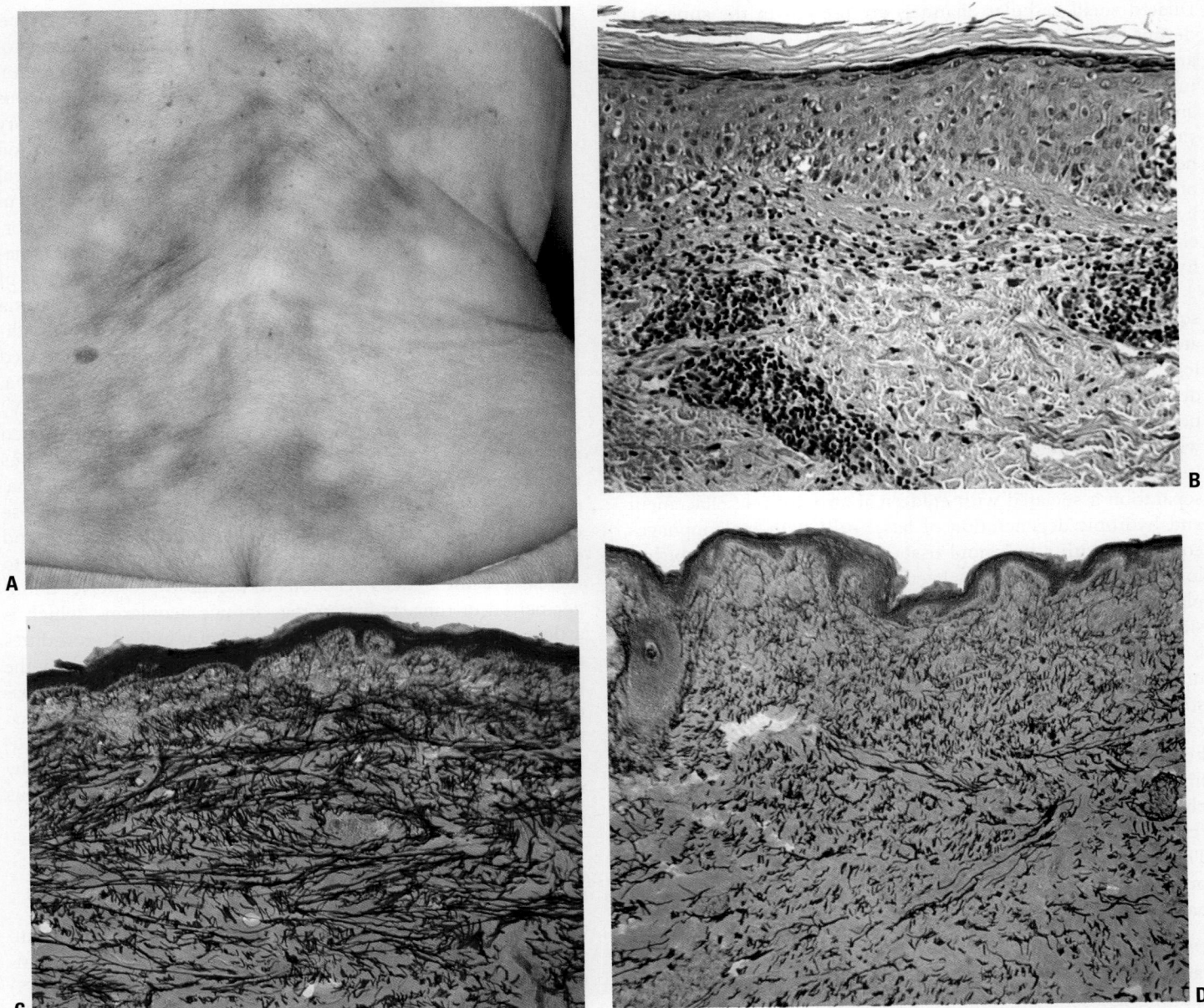

Figure 13-4 Erythema ab igne. **A:** Clinically, reticulated brown patches are seen in erythema ab igne. This may present on the lower back, where there has been frequent use of a heating pad. **B:** Erythema ab igne has variable histologic features. This hematoxylin and eosin–stained biopsy shows a perivascular lymphocytic infiltrate in the superficial dermis that focally disrupts the dermal–epidermal interface. There is no discernible elastic fiber abnormality noted on routine staining. The absence of clumped basophilic elastic tissue differentiates erythema ab igne from solar elastosis. **C:** Staining for elastic tissue highlights the increased amount of elastic tissue in comparison to uninvolved skin (see **D**), characteristic of erythema ab igne. **D:** Elastic staining of uninvolved skin, showing a normal distribution of elastic fibers, as compared with **C**. (Photographs courtesy of Waine Johnson, MD.)

blankets (35). More recently, rare reports of widespread erythema ab igne due to compulsive hot showering and use of heating pads to relieve nausea in cannabinoid hyperemesis syndrome have been reported (36,37).

In addition to pigmentary alternation, secondary clinical findings may occur in erythema ab igne. Specifically, formation of bullae has been observed (38,39). Thermal keratoses (which histologically show partial-thickness epidermal atypia, akin to actinic keratoses) and squamous cell carcinomas may arise in areas of erythema ab igne (40). Merkel cell carcinoma, poorly differentiated carcinoma, and cutaneous marginal zone lymphoma have also been described to occur in erythema ab igne (41–44).

Histopathology. The histopathologic findings of erythema ab igne are often subtle and may be nonspecific in the absence of correlative clinical information. The epidermis may be normal or atrophic, with effacement of the epidermal rete. Interface dermatitis, featuring mild basovacuolar change, dyskeratotic keratinocytes, and a squamatized basal epidermal layer, is observed. There is mild spongiosis and prominent papillary dermal edema (45,46). Pigment incontinence is frequently seen, and it consists of melanin-laden macrophages as well as extracellular melanin granules (47). Hemosiderin deposition has been described, although this may be attributed to the fact that many biopsies of erythema ab igne are taken from the lower legs and are more likely to display extravasated red blood cells (45).

Dilated small vascular channels are present in the superficial dermis, sometimes engorged with red blood cells. Enlarged, atypical endothelial cells have been observed, demonstrating hyperchromatic, irregularly shaped nuclei (46). A mixed angiocentric infiltrate of variable intensity is observed in the superficial dermis, composed of lymphocytes, macrophages, neutrophils, plasma cells, and mast cells. Increased numbers of elastic fibers are seen in biopsies of erythema ab igne, highlighted by elastic stains (30) (Fig. 13-4), and fragmentation of elastic fibers may occur (39). Alcian blue stains detect increased hyaluronic acid in the papillary and reticular dermis (30).

Thermal keratoses showing basal keratinocytic atypia and squamous cell carcinoma *in situ* have been documented to arise within erythema ab igne, often occurring on the lower leg (40,48). A case of cutaneous marginal zone lymphoma, demonstrating a dermal infiltrate consisting of a diffuse, monotonous proliferation of CD20$^+$ CD5$^-$ CD10$^-$ lymphoid cells with round to slightly irregular nuclei, has been reported (44). In bullous erythema ab igne, there is a subepidermal plane of separation associated with epidermal atrophy, rete effacement, and hydropic degeneration of basal cells with melanophages, consistent with a lichenoid tissue reaction (39). Cases of bullous erythema ab igne have been attributed to coexisting lichen planus (49), but may simply represent a manifestation of intrinsic blistering. Direct immunofluorescence on these cases either is negative or shows a pattern of immunoglobulin M staining in the papillary dermis, consistent with colloid bodies. Ultrastructural investigations of erythema ab igne have been reported (50) and show changes consistent with apoptosis of the basal keratinocytes, functional activation of melanocytes, and elastic fiber alterations indistinguishable from actinic elastosis due to chronic UV radiation. The keratinocyte change appears to represent heat-related damage and not a preneoplastic alteration. The vessels are dilated and increased in number. This may rarely present as cutaneous reactive angiomatosis, mimicking a malignant vascular neoplasm or diffuse dermal angiomatosis (51).

Differential Diagnosis. The elastic tissue alteration induced by UV radiation in solar elastosis is apparent, on hematoxylin and eosin staining, as a solid and homogenized material, as opposed to erythema ab igne, which, on routine staining, shows no perceptible elastic tissue changes. Erythema dyschromicum perstans may also show subtle interface dermatitis with pigment dropout, but is distinguished from erythema ab igne by the clinical presentation and the absence of increased elastic fibers. A hypersensitivity reaction with interface changes may show some overlapping features with erythema ab igne, but the clinical history should prompt elastic tissue staining, differentiating the two entities.

Principles of Management: Withdrawal of the offending heat source is essential to prevent worsening or recurrence of erythema ab igne. The pigmentary changes will resolve slowly over time. Treatment with Nd-YAG (neodymium-doped yttrium aluminum garnet) lasers has been reported to be beneficial for pigmentary alteration (52).

RADIATION-INDUCED SKIN ALTERATIONS

Radiation is frequently administered therapeutically for diagnostic purposes or for the treatment of primary and metastatic malignancies. In the past, it had been used to treat inflammatory

conditions of the skin, including acne and eczema, although this is no longer a common practice. Radiation-induced dermatoses are commonly seen and include acute and chronic radiation dermatitis, radiation recall dermatitis, and secondary cutaneous neoplasms. Radiation dermatitis is a common inflammatory skin finding that is the direct result of exposure to radiation and is dose dependent. The injury is the result of biochemical changes in x-ray–penetrated cells without a concomitant rise in temperature. Changes of radiation dermatitis appear at the portal of radiation entry or exit. In addition to the dose of irradiation, additional host factors play a role in the development of radiation dermatitis. Patients with the inherited condition ataxia telangiectasia (A-T) syndrome display greater-than-normal radiation sensitivity (53); other DNA repair disorders characterized by exaggerated responses to radiation include Fanconi anemia, Nijmegen breakage syndrome, and DNA ligase intravenous (IV) deficiency (54). Acute and chronic radiation toxicity has been reported in individuals with rheumatoid arthritis, systemic lupus erythematosus, mixed connective tissue disease, scleroderma, diabetes mellitus, and hyperthyroidism (55). Concomitant use of radiation-sensitizing medications, such as doxorubicin and taxane antineoplastic agents, may predispose an individual to increased acute toxicity reactions to radiation (56). Over a longer period of time, radiation may induce neoplasms, which is a dose-independent effect. Fluoroscopically guided procedures may cause radiation dermatitis in areas of skin not directly in the radiation port, usually on the back (57). Radiation recall dermatitis refers to the induction of an inflammatory reaction limited to a site of a quiescent radiation field by administration of a medication. Certain inflammatory conditions may be exacerbated by radiation, for example, vitiligo (58), lichen planus (59), bullous pemphigoid (60), and graft-versus-host disease (61).

Acute, Subacute, and Chronic Radiation Dermatitis

Clinical Summary. Radiation dermatitis can be classified into acute, subacute, and chronic phases. Acute radiation dermatitis presents within 90 days of radiation exposure (Fig. 13-5) (62). A transient erythema may appear within 24 hours of the

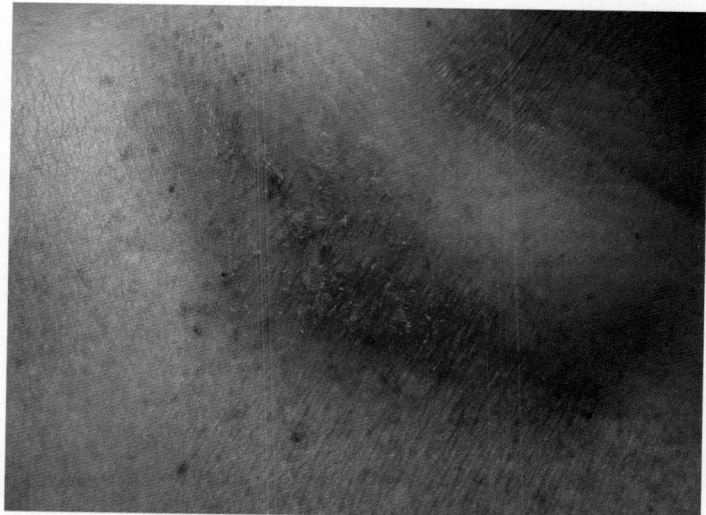

Figure 13-5 Acute radiation dermatitis. Clinically, this presents as a scaly erythematous plaque, with geographic borders defined by the radiation field.

radiation insult and resolve within several hours to days. A second, more persistent erythema is then apparent about 10 to 14 days after the initial exposure. In addition to erythema, other cutaneous changes, including desquamation, alopecia, xerosis, dyschromia, blistering, epidermal and dermal atrophy, necrosis, erosion, and ulceration, may be seen in acute radiation dermatitis. The phases of acute radiation dermatitis have been outlined in detail, and criteria have been put forth by the National Cancer Institute (62). Grade 1 radiation dermatitis includes generalized erythema with dry desquamation, which may be accompanied by pruritus and dyspigmentation. This may be concentrated in the follicles, resulting in alopecia due to injury to the pilosebaceous units. Grade 2 radiation dermatitis typically occurs in the skin folds 4 to 5 weeks after treatment of doses 40 Gy or greater. There is persistent tender edematous erythema, which may progress to bullae or focal epidermal necrosis, with fibrinous exudates, termed moist desquamation. Superinfection may occur at this stage. Grade 3 shows an increased area of moist desquamation compared to grade 2, extending beyond the skin folds. Grade 4 is characterized by ulceration, necrosis, and hemorrhage. Unresolved acute radiation results in chronic ulceration, fibrosis, and/or necrosis of the deeper structures, which is termed "consequential late" radiation dermatitis. Subacute radiation dermatitis occurs weeks to months after radiation exposure, but is otherwise not well characterized clinically (63).

Changes of chronic radiation dermatitis are noted months to years after the original insult, but often represent progression of acute and subacute radiation dermatitis and, therefore, may be evident earlier. Characteristic findings of chronic radiation dermatitis include epidermal atrophy, xerosis, hypopigmentation and hyperpigmentation, alopecia, anhidrosis, poikiloderma, hyperkeratosis, telangiectases, and fibrosis of the dermis and subcutis. Late-onset dermal necrosis and changes of chronic radiation dermatitis with or without prior acute

radiation changes may be seen years after the initial radiation. Nonhealing ulcers may be seen. Deep megavoltage radiation for noncutaneous malignancies may result in subcutaneous sclerosis that may extend into the underlying skeletal muscle (64).

Histopathology. Histopathologic changes of radiation dermatitis vary with the stage of the lesion sampled (57).

Acute radiation dermatitis shows spongiosis and scattered dyskeratotic keratinocytes in the epidermis. Depending on the dose of radiation, epidermal necrosis with blister formation and sloughing of the epidermis—which corresponds to the clinical findings of "moist desquamation"—may be seen. Hyperkeratosis is often observed. In the dermis, frequent findings include dermal edema, endothelial cell swelling, vasodilation, red blood cell extravasation, and fibrin thrombi of vessels. Variable inflammation is noted throughout the dermis, with involvement of the epidermis. Acute necrotic changes similar to those seen in the epidermis may also occur in the adnexal epithelium, eventuating in absence of pilosebaceous structures. Complete destruction of eccrine glands is infrequently observed. In severe radiation injury, necrosis of the epidermis and dermis results in persistent ulceration.

Late-stage or chronic radiation dermatitis is characterized by eosinophilic homogenized thickening of the dermal collagen, large atypical "radiation fibroblasts," lack of pilosebaceous units, and vascular changes (Fig. 13-6) (65). The superficial dermis shows thin-walled, markedly dilated vascular channels set within an edematous, homogenized stroma, whereas the deep vessels show fibrous thickening, sometimes with luminal obliteration and recanalization. The overlying epidermis may be atrophic and hyperkeratotic. Features of an interface reaction are sometimes present (Fig. 13-6). A maturation disorder with nuclear atypia and individual cell keratinization may be seen. Juxtaposed to atrophic areas may be epidermal hyperplasia that can extend downward and encase the telangiectatic vessels.

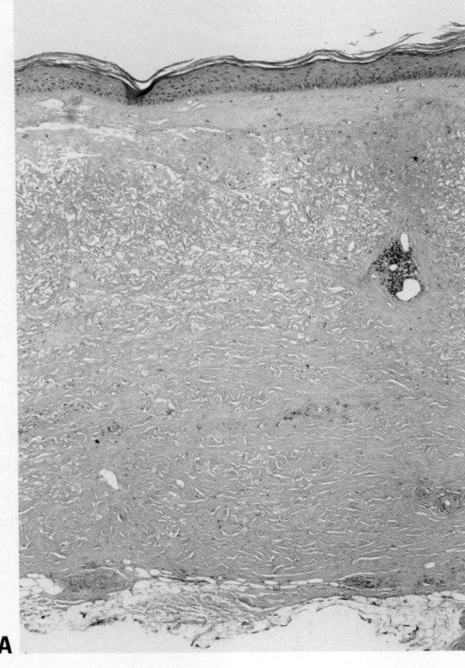
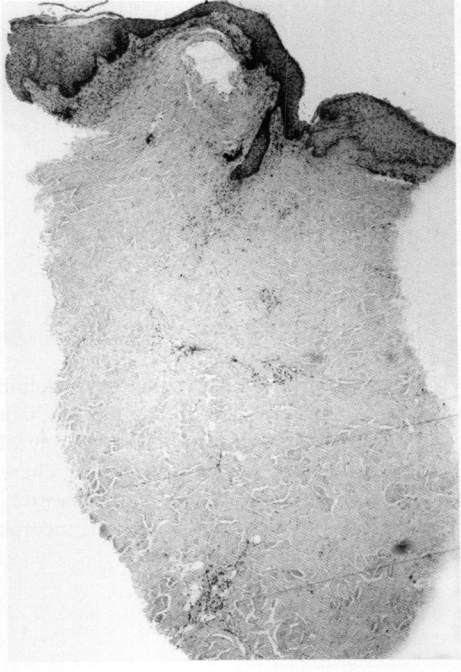

A   B

Figure 13-6 Late-stage radiation injury. **A:** This biopsy shows features of chronic radiation dermatitis, including epidermal atrophy, pandermal collagen sclerosis with mild lymphocytic inflammation, and the absence of hair follicles. **B:** A rectangular, "squared-off" silhouette due to the sclerotic collagen alteration. This biopsy also demonstrates the variation of epidermal atrophy and hyperplasia that can be seen in radiation dermatitis.

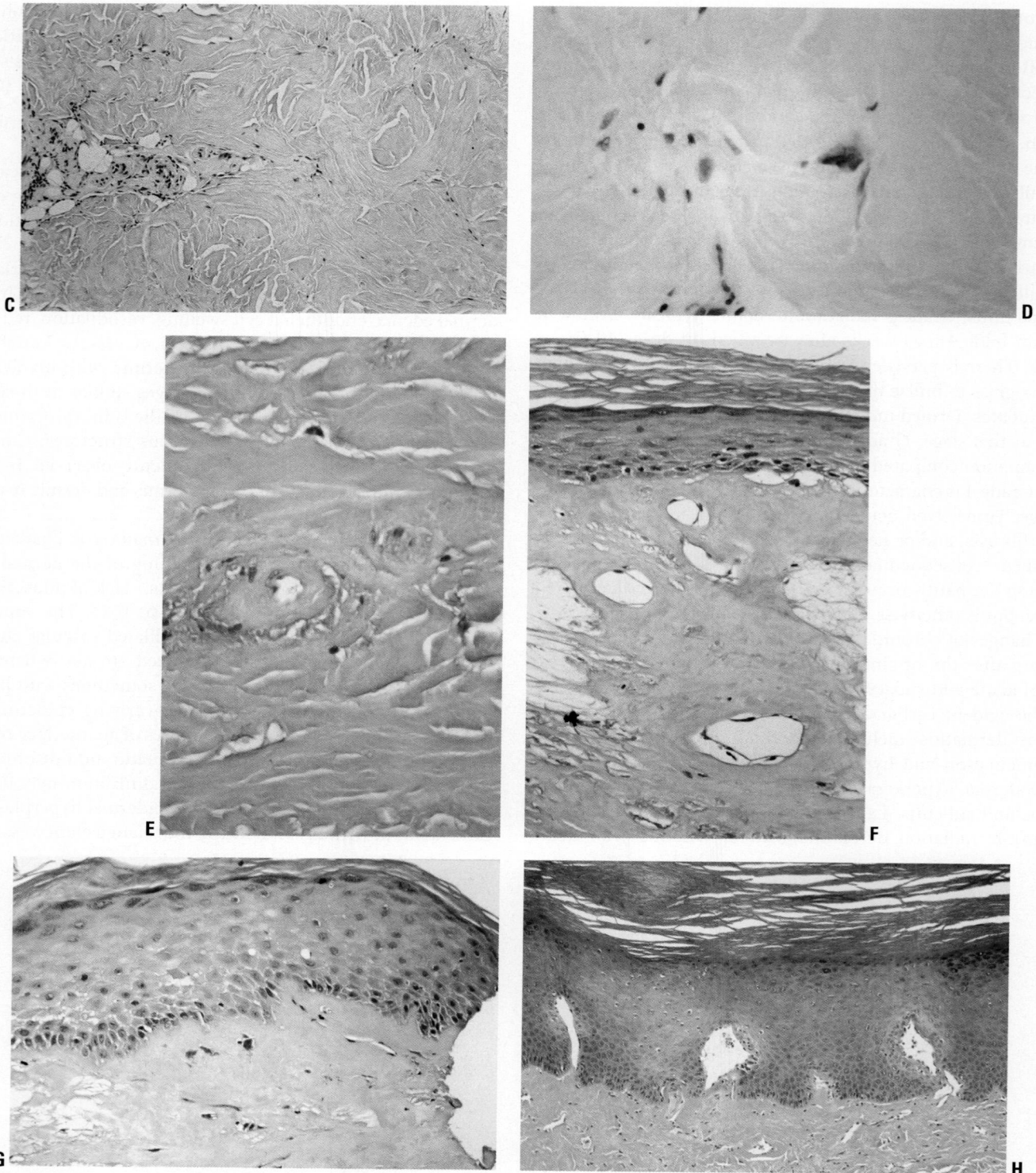

Figure 13-6 (*continued*) **C:** There is sclerotic collagen bundle thickening, with compression of eccrine glands. Preservation of eccrine glands differentiates this from a burn scar. **D:** Large, bizarre, and atypical radiation fibroblasts amid the thickened collagen bundles differentiate radiation dermatitis from morphea and third-degree burn scars. These are sparsely scattered, in contrast to atypical cells of a sarcoma. **E:** Sclerosis of endothelial cells is seen amid thickened sclerotic collagen bundles. **F:** There is telangiectasia of the upper dermal vessels, with epidermal atrophy and sclerosis of papillary dermal collagen. **G:** The epidermis shows features of interface dermatitis, with liquefaction of the basal layer, rete effacement, and pigment dropout. **H:** The epidermis may show hyperplasia, incorporating the underlying telangiectatic vessels between the rete.

The origin of the radiation fibroblast is not known. Immunohistochemical studies have shown cytoplasmic staining of radiation fibroblasts with factor XIIIa antibody and only focal CD34 positivity in some cells (66). However, factor XIIIa staining is not consistently observed in all studies. The radiation fibroblasts have been shown to be negative for HHF-35 (muscle-specific actin), Ki-67, and p53 (67).

Subacute radiodermatitis shows overlapping features of acute and chronic radiation dermatitis. There is an interface dermatitis, with basal vacuolization and keratinocyte dyskeratosis (Fig. 13-7) (68). The presence of satellite cell necrosis, characterized by close apposition of dyskeratotic keratinocytes and CD8+ TIA-1–positive T lymphocytes, suggests that cytotoxic lymphocyte–mediated apoptosis is involved in the pathogenesis of subacute radiation dermatitis (63).

Radiation-induced morphea is a rare late complication, which may occur months to years after radiation therapy (69). The majority of reported cases of radiation-induced morphea occur in conjunction with treatment for breast cancer (70). Similar to non–radiation-induced morphea, an acute phase of this process may be observed clinically with an erythematous patch or plaque, and a later phase may be observed with a hyperpigmented or hypopigmented sclerotic plaque. On histopathology, the earlier phase shows a perivascular inflammatory infiltrate composed of lymphocytes in the epidermis, whereas the later phase shows dermal collagen edema and sclerosis and loss of periecrine fat.

Radiation-induced malignancies include squamous cell carcinomas and basal cell carcinomas most commonly (71), often occurring in a background of chronic radiation dermatitis. The squamous cell carcinomas display aggressive, metastasizing behavior and include spindled variants. Radiation accelerates the development of basal cell carcinomas in patients with Gorlin syndrome, as the causative *Patched* gene mutations render their tissue radiosensitive (72). True radiation-induced sarcoma malignancies are less common and usually arise in heavily irradiated tissue, with a latent period of 3 to 24 years, including malignant fibrous histiocytoma, fibrosarcoma, osteosarcoma, liposarcoma, chondrosarcoma, and sarcomas of pluripotential mesenchymal cell derivation (73). Desmoplastic cutaneous leiomyosarcoma has also been reported (74). Mesenchymal sarcomas frequently occur on the chest wall after irradiation for breast carcinoma or Hodgkin disease (75). Angiosarcomas, including spindled cell variants, may be seen at sites of prior irradiation, usually in conjunction with lymphedematous changes (76). Adjacent changes of chronic radiation dermatitis may be seen but are not always present.

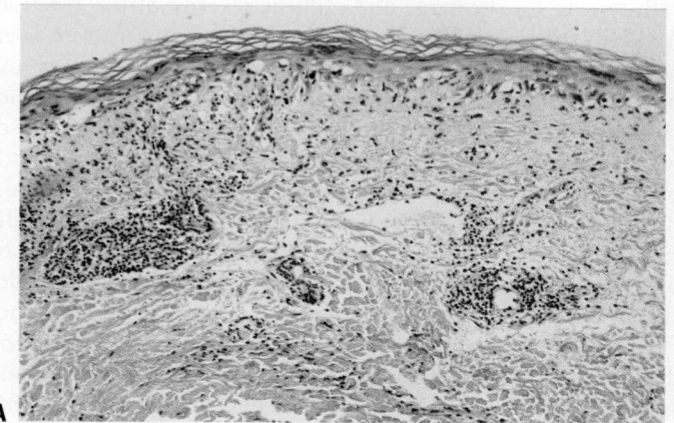
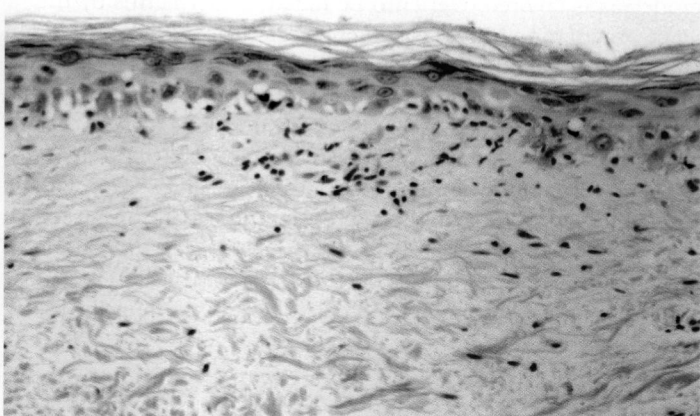
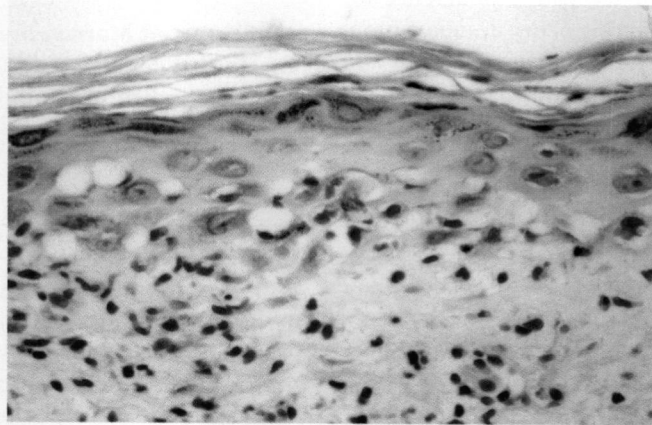

Figure 13-7 Subacute radiation dermatitis. **A:** In subacute radiation dermatitis, there is an inflammatory infiltrate involving the epidermis, papillary dermis, and vessels, without sclerotic collagen alteration. The epidermis is atrophic due to interface dermatitis. **B:** The interface dermatitis of subacute radiation dermatitis is indistinguishable from those of some other causes of interface dermatitis, such as fixed drug eruption and graft-versus-host disease, requiring clinical information to differentiate these entities. Lymphocytes disrupt the basal cell layer and are associated with vacuolization of the basal keratinocytes, dyskeratotic keratinocytes, and pigment dropout. Note that the collagen is nonsclerotic and the fibroblasts are nonatypical, in contrast to those in Figure 13-4B, C, which represent a later stage of this process. **C:** Satellite cell necrosis, or close approximation of lymphocytes with apoptotic keratinocytes, is seen in subacute radiation dermatitis, as well as in graft-versus-host disease and other cytotoxic dermatoses.

Atypical vascular lesions (AVLs) following radiation for mammary carcinoma are not uncommonly biopsied. These typically occur 3 to 4 years after radiotherapy and clinically present as solitary or multiple small, circumscribed, reddish brown papules usually less than 5 mm in diameter. In biopsies, AVLs are localized, often wedge-shaped collections of thin-walled ectatic lymphovascular channels, with irregular, angulated profiles, and focal anastomoses, generally in the superficial to mid-dermis and rarely extending more deeply. There are no mitoses, and there is no necrosis. Rare cases of angiosarcoma have developed in association with AVLs, for which complete excision and close follow-up is the treatment of choice (77).

Differential Diagnosis. Various hypersensitivity reactions may initially localize at a previous radiation port, simulating acute radiation dermatitis. This includes conditions with overlapping histology, such as erythema multiforme and toxic epidermal necrolysis, which should be differentiated by the clinical progression of the condition (78). Subacute radiation dermatitis may be indistinguishable from graft-versus-host disease and fixed drug eruption (79,80). The latter is particularly difficult to differentiate from subacute radiation dermatitis in fluoroscopy-induced cases because the changes often do not occur at the irradiation portal site and thus the clinician may be unaware of the association with radiation injury. Morphea/scleroderma is favored over chronic radiation dermatitis by the absence of radiation fibroblasts. Lichen sclerosis may show similar telangiectasia and interface alteration, and there can be similarity in the papillary dermal pallor and homogenization, but the presence of deeper, thickened eosinophilic collagen bundles with radiation fibroblasts favors radiation changes. Clinical correlation may be confirmatory. Deep burn scars show complete absence of all adnexal structures without abnormal fibroblasts, in contrast to radiation sclerosis, in which the eccrine glands are often preserved. Radiation sarcomas should be differentiated from spindled squamous cell carcinoma by immunohistochemical staining (see Chapter 32).

Principles of Management: The treatment for radiation dermatitis is primarily supportive (62). Acute radiation dermatitis is managed by using emollients, with a preference for petrolatum-based ointments in the setting of dry desquamation. Topical steroids may be beneficial for reducing erythema and for symptomatic relief (81). For radiation-induced ulcerations, appropriate wound care measures are indicated, including the use of hydrogel, hydrocolloid, alginate, and foam dressings, depending on the degree of wound exudate. Topical antiseptics and antibiotics may also be employed to prevent or treat infection.

Radiation Recall Dermatitis

Clinical Summary. Radiation recall dermatitis is a phenomenon in which an acute inflammatory reaction occurs at the site of a previously quiescent radiation field, following infusion or intake of certain medications (82,83). Commonly implicated medications include chemotherapeutic agents, including taxanes, antimetabolites (gemcitabine, capecitabine), methotrexate, and high-dose interferon-α 2b (84–86). Recently, novel kinase inhibitors used in the treatment of metastatic cancers, such as sorafenib, sunitinib, and vemurafenib, have been associated with this phenomenon (87,88). Other agents that may trigger radiation recall include several antibiotics (89–91),

statins/HMG-CoA reductase inhibitors (92,93), and lanreotide, a somatostatin analog (94). The reaction may occur days to weeks, and occasionally years, after radiation therapy, with a median time to reaction of 40 days (85). Acute toxicity need not have occurred with the initial radiation.

Clinically, early changes of radiation recall dermatitis present with a pruritic, morbilliform eruption that exhibits geographic demarcation confined to the prior field of irradiation (Fig. 13-8A). Blistering and/or desquamation are sometimes seen. A more severe reaction may occur, especially if the offending drug is administered shortly after radiation treatment, and may be associated with pain and necrosis. The dermatitis may simulate cellulitis, and fever may be rarely seen (85). Late changes of radiation recall may manifest with fibrotic, firm plaques, similar to chronic radiation dermatitis.

Extracutaneous recall reactions may involve the lung, esophagus, small intestine, musculoskeletal system, mucosa, and central nervous system (95). There may not be a cutaneous reaction in all of the previously treated radiation sites. The exact pathophysiology of the reaction is unknown. Radiation recall reactions should be differentiated from radiosensitivity and radiation enhancement, which represents a reaction induced by drugs given less than 7 to 10 days after radiotherapy (83).

Histopathology. The histopathologic features of radiation recall depend on the stage and clinical severity of the reaction. Acute to subacute radiation recall reactions demonstrate overlapping features with early stages of radiation dermatitis and may show lichenoid interface changes consisting of lymphocytes approximating the dermal–epidermal junction and basovacuolar change (Fig. 13-8B). Other features described include psoriasiform epidermal hyperplasia, follicular hyperkeratosis, pustules, and apoptotic or necrotic keratinocytes (65). Bulla formation due to prominent interface dermatitis may also be observed (96). Dermal changes include vascular dilation, endothelial cell atypia, and a perivascular and interstitial mononuclear or mixed inflammatory infiltrate. Later stages of radiation dermatitis may feature thickened, swollen collagen fibers and stellate radiation fibroblasts, findings that reflect chronic radiation damage (Fig. 13-8C, D).

Principles of Management: Reactions are managed by withdrawing offending medications. Topical steroids are beneficial for acute radiation recall dermatitis, to decrease erythema and associated pruritus.

COLD INJURY TO THE SKIN

Injury to the skin resulting from cold temperatures is categorized as either direct or indirect. Direct cold injury is a consequence solely of exposure to cold temperatures, whereas indirect cold injuries result from exacerbation of underlying diseases by low temperatures. Types of direct cold injury include frostbite and trench foot. Examples of indirect cold injury include pernio, Raynaud disease and phenomenon, cryoglobulinemia, and livedo reticularis. Cryotherapy, which is employed frequently in the practice of clinical dermatology, is a method of iatrogenically inducing cold injury, typically to treat keratoses. Direct freezing of tissue, as seen in frostbite and cryotherapy, leads to intracellular ice crystal formation and thereby tissue damage. Vascular injury is thought to play a major role

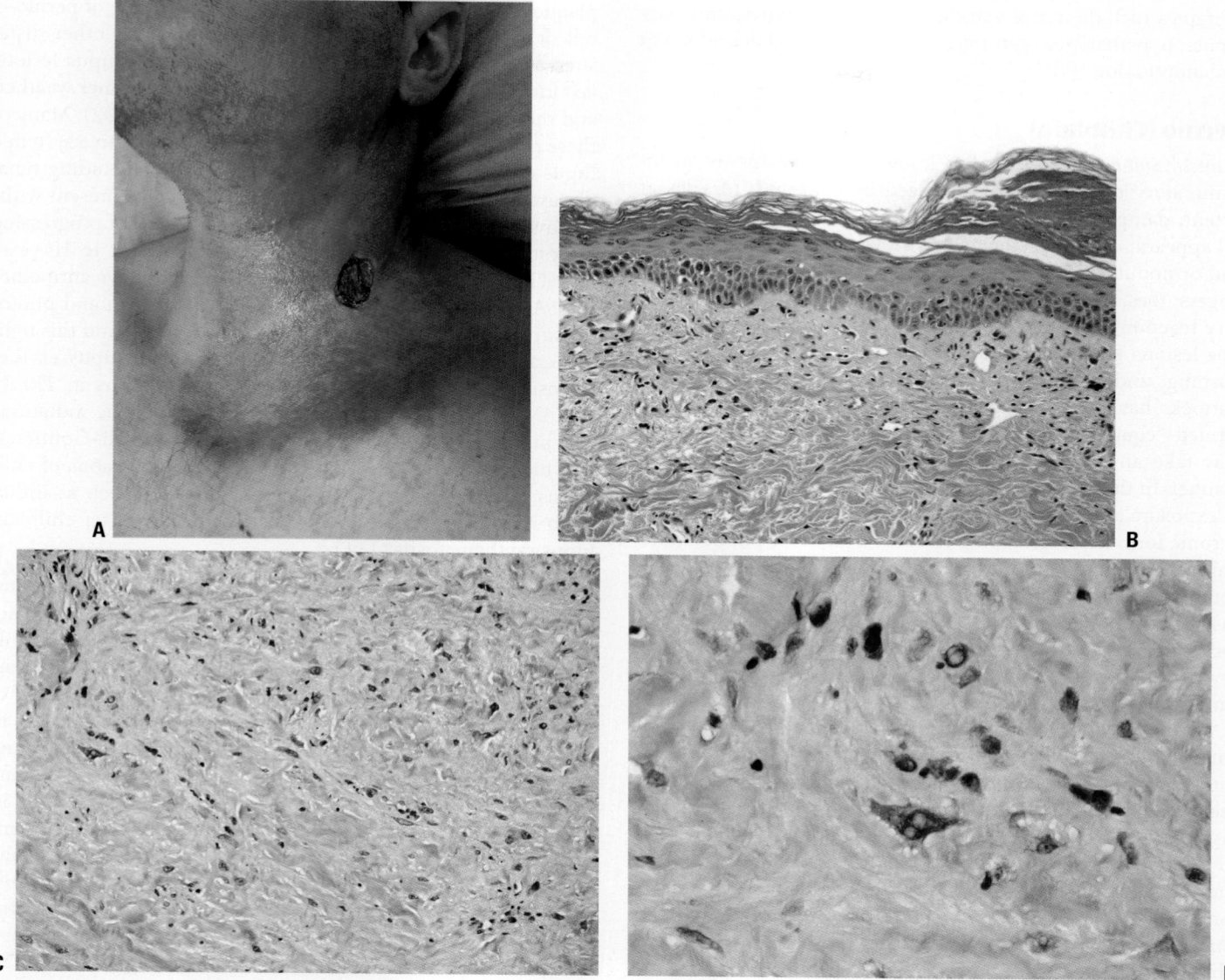

Figure 13-8 Radiation recall dermatitis. **A:** Clinical presentation of radiation recall dermatitis induced by vemurafenib, with a well-demarcated red plaque confined to the area of prior radiation therapy. **B:** Interface dermatitis is seen, featuring basovacuolar change and scattered dyskeratotic keratinocytes. **C:** In the deep reticular dermis, there are thickened collagen fibers associated with enlarged, atypical fibroblasts, features that reflect chronic radiation injury. **D:** Higher power view of stellate radiation fibroblasts.

in the pathogenesis of direct cold injury (97). Specifically, there is cyclic massive vasoconstriction and excessive vasodilation, endothelial cell leakage, erythrostasis, arteriovenous shunting, segmental vascular necrosis—possibly due to decreased clearance of toxic substances—and massive thrombosis (97).

Frostbite

Clinical Summary. Frostbite most commonly presents on the hands and feet, and the ears, nose, and chin, as a result of tissue freezing. Several risk factors for developing frostbite have been identified, including alcohol consumption, psychiatric illness, homelessness, and fatigue (98). Traditionally, military personnel were at a highest risk of developing frostbite, but civilians are increasingly affected (98). Frostbite can be categorized based on the depth of injury. First-degree frostbite, also known as frostnip, is characterized by superficial freezing of the skin. This manifests with erythema, edema, and pruritus upon rewarming and does not result in permanent skin injury.

In second-degree frostbite, freezing affects the skin and subcutaneous tissue. Blisters develop within the first day or 2 after rewarming, associated with redness and pain. The tissue becomes black and necrotic and sloughs, leaving atrophic skin behind. Hyperhidrosis and cold sensitivity are long-term sequelae. In third- and fourth-degree frostbite, deep tissue structures are affected by freezing. Hemorrhagic vesicles and bullae appear following rewarming in third-degree frostbite, which lead to eschar formation. Ulceration occurs when the eschar sloughs, revealing granulation tissue. Similar to second-degree frostbite, hyperhidrosis may appear. Fourth-degree frostbite is characterized by complete necrosis and tissue loss, and autoamputation of digits in some instances.

Principles of Management: Avoidance of frostbite is managed by addressing the risk factors discussed earlier. Once frostbite has developed, the mainstay of therapy is rapid rewarming of the affected areas, ideally at 40°C in a water bath with a mild antiseptic (98). Freeze–thaw cycles should be avoided. Adjunctive therapies include use of vasodilators, thrombolytics, anticoagulants, hyperbaric oxygen treatment, and surgical debridement and amputation (98).

Pernio (Chilblain)

Clinical Summary. Pernio, also known as chilblains, is an inflammatory disorder that is induced by cold and, to a lesser extent, damp environmental conditions (99). The usual clinical appearance is of erythema and violaceous papules, plaques, and/or nodules, affecting distal sites of the body, including the fingers, toes, heels, ears, and nose. Occasionally, the inflammatory reaction is severe enough to result in bullae and erosions. The lesions tend to be symptomatic, associated with pruritus, burning, and/or pain. Involvement of the lateral thighs and buttocks has been described in association with horse riding, termed "equestrian perniosis" (Fig 13-9A) (100,101). Pernio may take an acute, self-limited course or recur in a chronic manner. In the acute form, lesions appear within 12 to 24 hours of exposure and persist for 10 to 14 days before resolving. The chronic form has overlapping features with acute pernio and is induced by persistent and intermittent exposure to cold, wet conditions. However, older individuals who have underlying vascular disorders, including Raynaud disease and atherosclerosis, and are more likely to be affected by chronic pernio, compared to the acute form, which commonly occurs in younger patients (99). One study indicated that chronic pernio may in fact reveal an underlying connective tissue disorder (102). Rarely, chilblains-like lesions may be seen in association with leukemia cutis (103). More recently, pernio-like lesions have been reported to be associated with coronavirus infectious disease 2019 (COVID-19) (104).

The distinction between pernio (or chilblains) and chilblain lupus erythematosus often causes confusion, and in fact, some clinicians consider these conditions to be one and the same. "Chilblain lupus erythematosus" refers to instances in which pernio occurs in conjunction with histopathologic, clinical, and serologic features of lupus (102), whereas pernio or chilblains generally indicate idiopathic forms of these conditions. Patients with chilblain lupus may present with cutaneous lesions typical of lupus, including discoid and verrucous

plaques (105), in addition to lesions characteristic of pernio—red or purple plaques and nodules on acral and other distal sites. In contrast to idiopathic pernio, chilblain lupus lesions last for more than 1 month and persist during warmer weather, and there is a very strong female predominance (102). Many of these patients affected with chilblain lupus have active systemic lupus erythematosus at the time of diagnosis, including renal disease and cerebritis. Affected patients may also present without overt lupus, but these individuals are at risk of progressing to systemic lupus erythematosus approximately 1 to 10 years later (106). Many patients with chilblain lupus have antibodies to SSA/Ro, with associated Raynaud phenomenon and photosensitivity (102,106), although others have not found this tight association (107). A familial form of chilblain lupus erythematosus has been described, caused by mutations in *TREX1* or *SAMHD1* (96–110). Of note, these same genetic mutations also underlie the encephalopathy syndrome Aicardi–Goutières, in which 40% of affected patients present with lesions of chilblains (109). Tumor necrosis factor inhibitors such as infliximab have been recently associated with new-onset chilblain lupus erythematosus (111).

Histopathology. There is a superficial and deep perivascular lymphocytic infiltrate in the dermis and subcutaneous fat, with accentuation of the inflammation around the deep eccrine coils (Fig. 13-9). Interstitial inflammation may also be seen, particularly in the superficial dermis. The infiltrate tends to be of moderate intensity but may be dense. The vascular channels in the superficial dermis are often less involved by the infiltrate but may show congestion. Prominent papillary dermal edema is a characteristic finding, although its presence is variable. In some cases, only papillary dermal edema and superficial lymphocytic inflammation are seen, with little involvement of the deep reticular dermis and subcutis. Lymphocytic vasculitis, characterized by endothelial cell swelling and edema and infiltration of the vessel walls by lymphocytes, without consistent presence of fibrinoid necrosis is seen (Fig. 13-9) (112). The epidermal changes range from scattered necrotic keratinocytes to epidermal pallor or necrosis. The histopathology of pernio-like lesions associated with COVID-19 shows similar findings but with a more prominent and variable degree

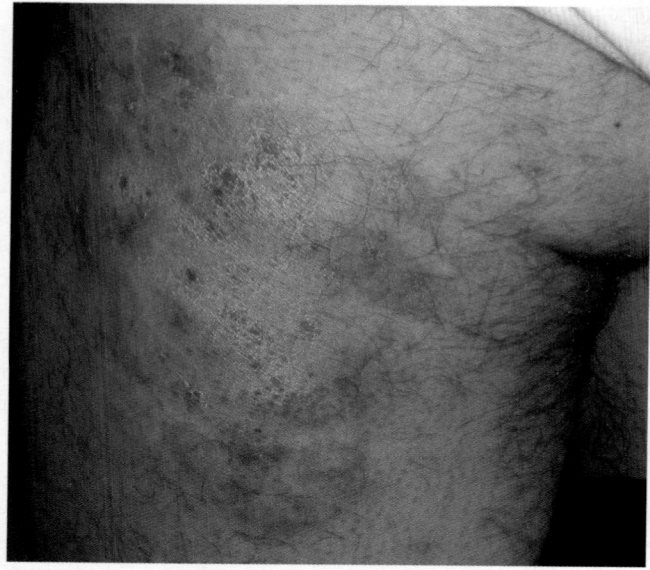

Figure 13-9 Pernio (chilblain). **A:** Indurated plaque on the lateral thigh, typical of equestrian perniosis (a nonacral presentation).

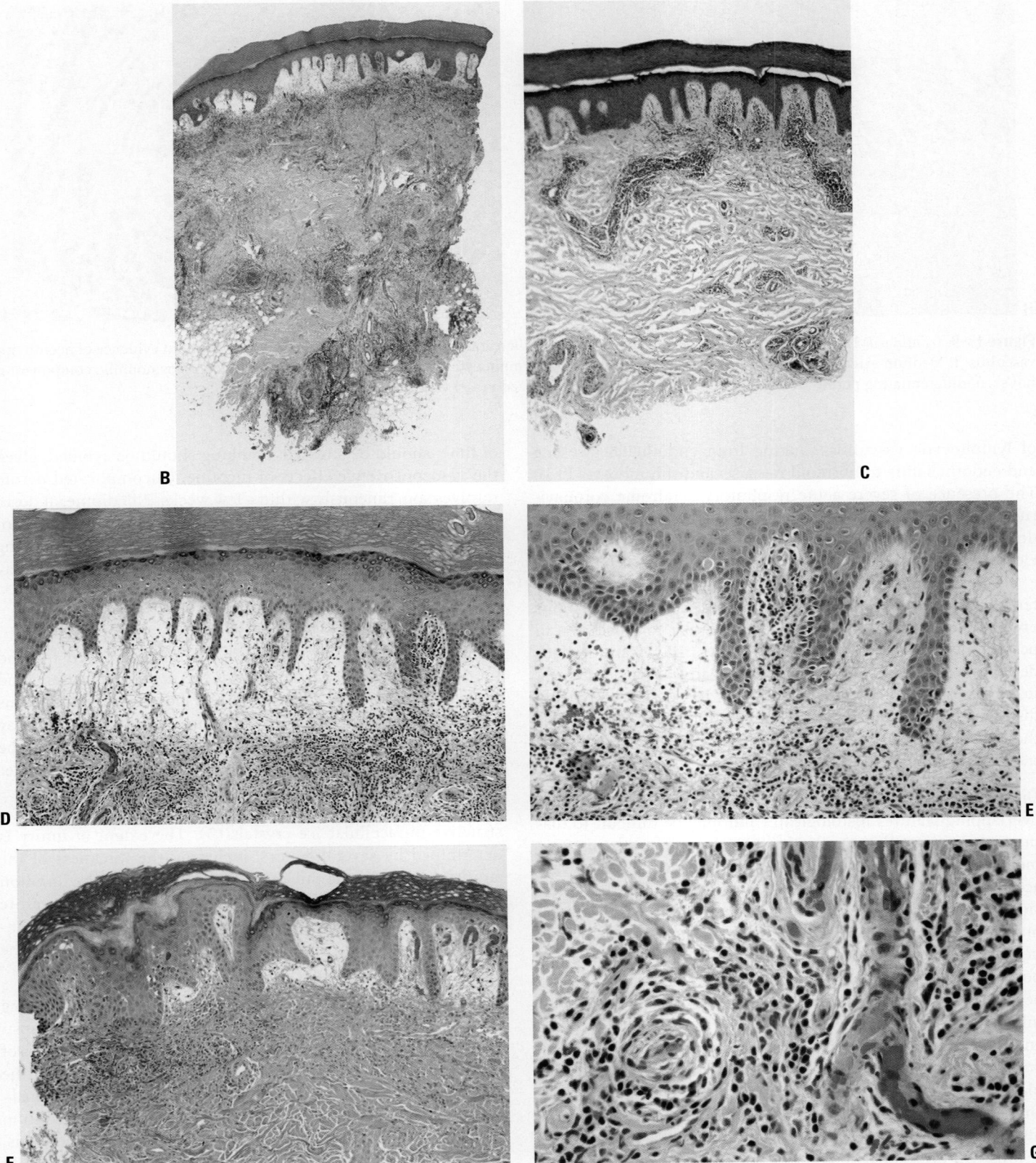

Figure 13-9 (*continued*) B: A superficial and deep perivascular and perieccrine lymphocytic infiltrate involving acral skin with striking papillary dermal edema typifies perniosis. C: Although papillary dermal edema is characteristic, some cases of pernio may lack this feature. The deep perieccrine infiltrate helps to differentiate this from conditions such as erythema multiforme, which may show some similar features. D: Striking dermal edema may result in incipient dermolytic bulla formation. E: Involvement of the dermal papillary vessels may be minimal. Dyskeratosis may be present, but a frank interface reaction is not seen. If present, lupus or chilblain lupus should be considered. F: The degree of papillary dermal edema may vary. Lymphocytes may be interstitial to band like, in addition to perivascular. Prominent vascular congestion is seen in the dermal papilla. G: Various degrees of vascular damage may be seen. Here there is congestion and vaso-occlusion with early necrosis of one small venule. In a nearby vessel, there is infiltration of the vessel wall, consistent with the lymphocytic vasculitis of pernio.

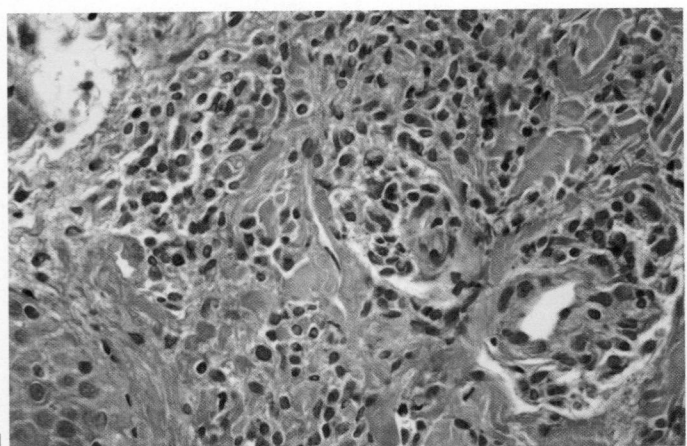
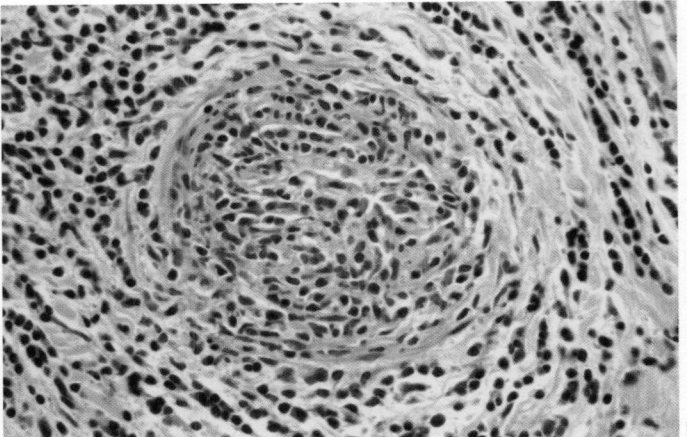

Figure 13-9 (*continued*) H: In pernio, the endothelial cells are often swollen and show infiltration by lymphocytes, without evidence of necrotizing vasculitis. I: Medium-sized vessels may occasionally be infiltrated by lymphocytes. A granulomatous, neutrophilic, or eosinophilic component is not seen, differentiating pernio from other known causes of medium-sized vessel vasculitis.

of lymphocytic vasculitis, ranging from endothelial swelling and endothelialitis to fibrinoid necrosis and thrombosis (113). The presence of severe acute respiratory syndrome coronavirus 2 (SARS-CoV-2) viral particles in the endothelium has been demonstrated with SARS-CoV-2 immunohistochemistry and on electron microscopy.

Biopsies taken from idiopathic pernio lack an effacing interface dermatitis in most cases. By contrast, chilblain lupus erythematosus reveals dermal changes similar to those seen in pernio and frequently (though not always) shows an interface dermatitis characteristic of lupus. A positive lupus band test may be seen (114). Although it may not be possible to reliably distinguish chilblains lupus from idiopathic pernio on histopathology, one study showed a more prominent perieccrine infiltrate in the latter (115).

Differential Diagnosis. Pernio and lupus erythematous show overlapping features histologically and may be difficult to distinguish. Features that suggest pernio over lupus erythematosus include the presence of prominent dermal edema, perieccrine accentuation of the infiltrate, and spongiosis (116). Papular lesions of pernio may have an appearance similar to erythema multiforme, as they both occur on acral sites (117). Biopsy helps to differentiate the two, as the deep inflammatory component of pernio is not typically seen in erythema multiforme. Several conditions that demonstrate perivascular lymphocytic inflammation, including dermal hypersensitivity, erythema annulare centrifugum, polymorphous light eruption, reticular erythematous mucinosis, and Jessner lymphocytic infiltrate, may be considered in the differential diagnosis of pernio. The latter is favored by the presence of lymphocytic vasculitis on histopathology and the clinical finding of cold-induced acral lesions. On occasion, the lymphocytic infiltrate of pernio may be intense enough to raise the possibility of cutaneous lymphoma, but the absence of atypia and presence of superficial dermal edema favor pernio. If cellular atypia is seen, immunohistochemical investigations to exclude leukemia or lymphoma should be pursued.

Principles of Management: In patients prone to developing pernio, preventive measures, including warm clothing and avoidance of cold/damp environments for prolonged periods

of time, should be stressed. Smoking should be avoided, given the vasoconstrictive effects of nicotine. Uncomplicated pernio resolves spontaneously within a few weeks. Nifedipine, at doses of 20 to 60 mg daily, has been demonstrated to speed the resolution of existing lesions and prevent new ones from occurring (118). Vasodilators, including nicotinamide and sildenafil, may be helpful.

Cryotherapy-Induced Injury

Clinical Summary. Cryotherapy is a commonly used method to destroy benign (verrucae and verrucous keratoses) and premalignant (actinic) keratoses and occasionally squamous cell carcinoma and basal cell carcinoma. This procedure may also be employed before curettage of keratoses to facilitate the procedure. As a result, the dermatopathologist may encounter freeze-related changes in this latter circumstance. Rapid freezing with liquid nitrogen results in the production of highly destructive intracellular ice crystals (5). The extent of injury is determined by several factors, including the thickness of the stratum corneum, the thickness of the epidermis, the duration of exposure to the liquid nitrogen, and the degree of pressure applied (5). Cell types differ in their susceptibility to cold injury. The hypopigmentation seen with cryotherapy reflects the susceptibility of melanocytes to this form of injury.

Histopathology. The microscopic features may vary, depending on the interval between cryotherapy and subsequent biopsy. Typically in rapid-freeze injury, the keratinocytes show a loss of cell outline, with ghostlike changes or homogenization of the epidermis (Fig. 13-10). This is associated with subepidermal–dermal bulla formation and subepidermal edema. The stratum corneum, being a devitalized structure, is not affected; thus, there is preservation of parakeratosis (5). There may be loss of melanocytes or pigment at the site of a prior cryotherapy site, with melanocytic hyperplasia or pigment dropout in the adjacent skin (119). With more intense cryotherapy, coagulation rather than edema is seen in the dermis. This may result in coagulation necrosis of hair follicles and, possibly, eccrine glands and also scar formation of the surrounding collagen. A polymorphous infiltrate, which includes eosinophils, has been described (120). Hemorrhage and thrombosis may be seen in the dermal papilla.

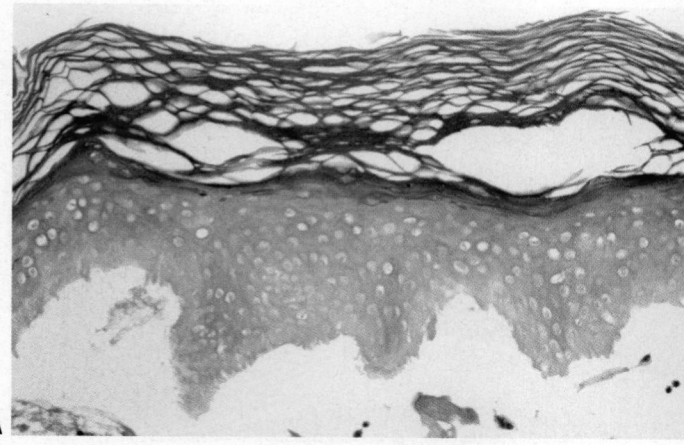
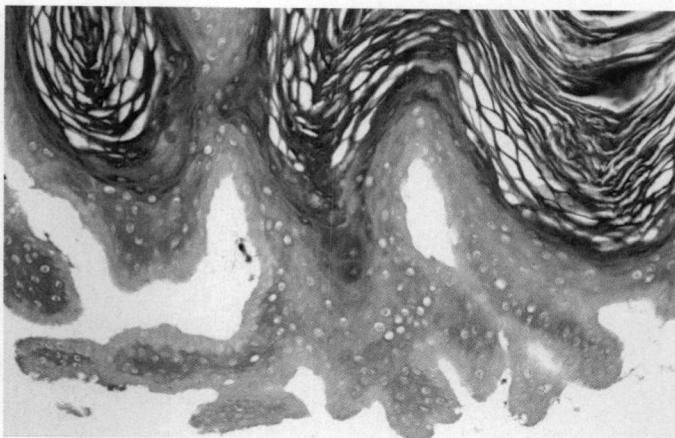

Figure 13-10 Cryotherapy-induced cold injury. **A:** There is pallor of the epidermal keratinocytes, with loss of the cellular outline. **B:** The cold injury has resulted in a subepidermal bulla. In cryotherapy of this seborrheic keratosis, there has been preservation of the stratum corneum architecture, probably due to the devitalized nature of this portion of the epidermis, whereas the remaining tissue shows homogenization of the epithelium, with disassociation of the epithelium from the dermis in a subepidermal manner.

CUTANEOUS INJURY DUE TO PHYSICAL TRAUMA

Friction-Induced Blister

Clinical Summary. Prominent or repetitive shear-induced injury, especially on acral skin, such as the hands and feet, results in bulla formation. This may or may not be accompanied by hemorrhage.

Histopathology. A friction blister has an intraepidermal plane of separation, often beneath the stratum granulosum, in the upper portions of the epidermis (Fig. 13-11). The surrounding keratinocytes show pallor and loss of the cell outline. The edge of the blister cavity shows a jagged outline. The dermis does not show significant alteration or inflammation.

Differential Diagnosis. Other causes of paucicellular blister formation should be differentiated from friction blisters. Suction blisters and porphyria cutanea tarda show subepidermal bullae histologically. Epidermolysis bullosa acquisita often appears in acral locations but shows subepidermal bullae with characteristic immunofluorescence features (see

Chapter 9). Similarly, epidermolysis bullosa simplex displays a pauci-inflammatory split through the basal layer of the epidermis, although plane of cleavage is low enough in the epidermis that this may appear to be subepidermal on paraffin sections (119); keratin tonofilament clumping is seen on electron microscopy. Although diabetic bullae are also noninflammatory blisters located on acral sites and may have a partially intraepidermal plane of separation, they tend to show a predominantly subepidermal split, without cytolytic changes in the epidermis.

Principles of Management: Friction blisters resolve spontaneously over time.

Talon Noir (Black Heel, Calcaneal Petechiae)

Clinical Summary. Talon noir typically presents as an irregular black macule or multiple black macules on thickly keratinized acral sites, such as the heels and toes. Because it may be clinically difficult to distinguish talon noir from melanoma and other atypical pigmented lesions, biopsies are frequently performed for histologic evaluation. Talon noir often occurs in association with athletic activity and results from shearing forces that lead to hemorrhage in the stratum corneum (121).

Histopathology. Frequently, only the stratum corneum is sampled and shows erythrocytes within layers of a thickened orthokeratotic stratum corneum (Fig. 13-12). Parakeratosis is often seen. There may be associated serosanguinous fluid, with superficial blister formation. When the dermis is visualized within the biopsy specimen, extravasated red blood cells may be seen in the dermal papillae and epidermis. Iron stains are typically negative, likely due to the absence of proteolytic and phagocytic activity in the stratum corneum, preventing the formation of hemosiderin (122). However, stains to detect hemoglobin, such as benzidine and patent blue V, may be positive.

Principles of Management: Treatment is unnecessary, as this process will resolve on its own.

Acanthoma Fissuratum (Granuloma Fissuratum)

Clinical Summary. Acanthoma fissuratum, sometimes called spectacle frame acanthoma (123), occurs at the site of

Figure 13-11 Friction blister. In friction blisters, one sees a noninflammatory intraepidermal blister, with pallor of the surrounding epidermis. The keratinocytes may show reticular degeneration or other sequelae of cytolysis or shearing.

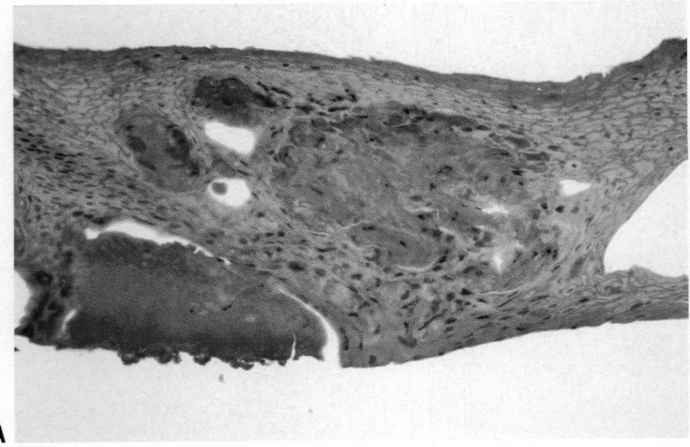
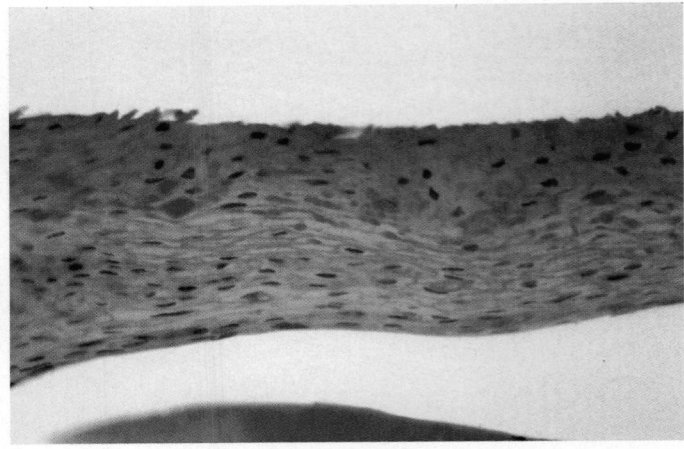
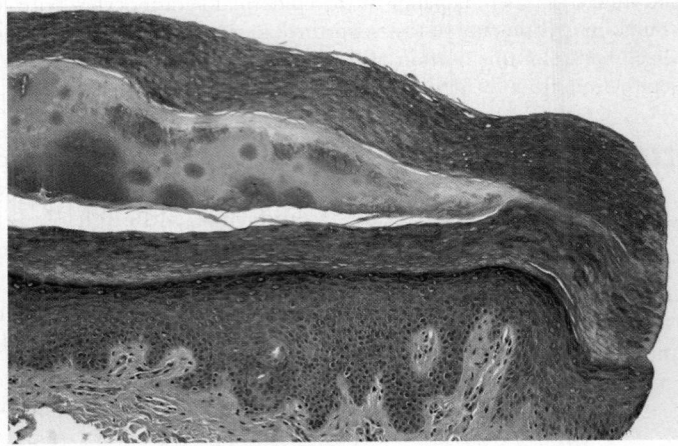

Figure 13-12 Talon noir (calcaneal petechiae). **A:** Talon noir occurs on acral skin due to shearing or rubbing trauma, and thus one sees a hyperkeratotic stratum corneum, often accompanied by parakeratosis. Often, only portions of the stratum corneum are sampled. The hemorrhage can be identified as loculated erythrocytes and serosanguinous fluid or as small collections of intracorneal erythrocytes, some of which show degeneration. **B:** The hemorrhage may present as solitary intact or degenerating erythrocytes within the corneal layers. Hemosiderin will not be apparent on hematoxylin or iron staining. **C:** There may be features of a friction blister, with intracorneal hemorrhage accompanied by serosanguinous fluid, forming an intracorneal hemorrhagic bulla.

chronic low-grade pressure or rubbing trauma at the site where eyeglasses sit on the nose or ear. Clinically, acanthoma fissuratum presents as a pink- to flesh-colored plaque or nodule with a central depression located on the lateral bridge of the nose near the medial canthus or near the cheek, or at the crease between the postauricular scalp and posterior ear, where the eyeglass stem lies. Biopsies are often performed to rule out basal cell carcinoma or squamous cell carcinoma. Lesions similar to acanthoma fissuratum may develop in the oral cavity as a result of ill-fitting dentures, referred to as epulis fissuratum (124).

Histopathology. There is prominent irregular acanthosis of the epidermis, consisting of broad and elongated rete pegs. This is associated with mild orthokeratosis and hypergranulosis. Central attenuation of the rete is observed, corresponding to the clinical depression (Fig. 13-13). Spongiosis and parakeratosis may be seen. In the underlying dermis, a proliferation of small, slightly dilated vessels with a fibrotic stroma and variable patchy chronic inflammation is seen.

Differential Diagnosis. The epidermal and dermal fibrovascular changes noted in acanthoma fissuratum are similar to those seen in chondrodermatitis nodularis helicis (see Chapter 18). The latter is distinguished by the location on the auricle and

the presence of fibrinoid dermal necrosis and cartilaginous changes. Lichen simplex chronicus has some similar features but shows more dermal fibrosis and vertical orientation of the vessels in the dermal papillae.

Principles of Management: Treatment options include surgical removal, electrodesiccation following biopsy, or CO_2 laser ablation.

Surgery-Associated Injury

Clinical Summary. Surgical curettage is often performed by dermatologists to biopsy, definitively treat, or "define" the borders of a superficial basal or squamous cell carcinoma before excision. Curettage is frequently followed by electrodesiccation to further destroy remaining tumor and/or to achieve hemostasis.

Histopathology. Electrodesiccation-induced injury results in elongation and stretch distortion of the epithelial nuclei (Fig. 13-14). Basophilic collagen necrosis can be seen beneath a recent electrodesiccation-induced surgical ulcer or scar. This may present with lacelike coagulation necrosis of the collagen and epidermis. Examination of a healing biopsy site may reveal engulfment of this injured collagen by multinucleated giant cells. The dermis beneath a recent curettage ulcer base shows edema, vascular dilation, and congestion without coagulation

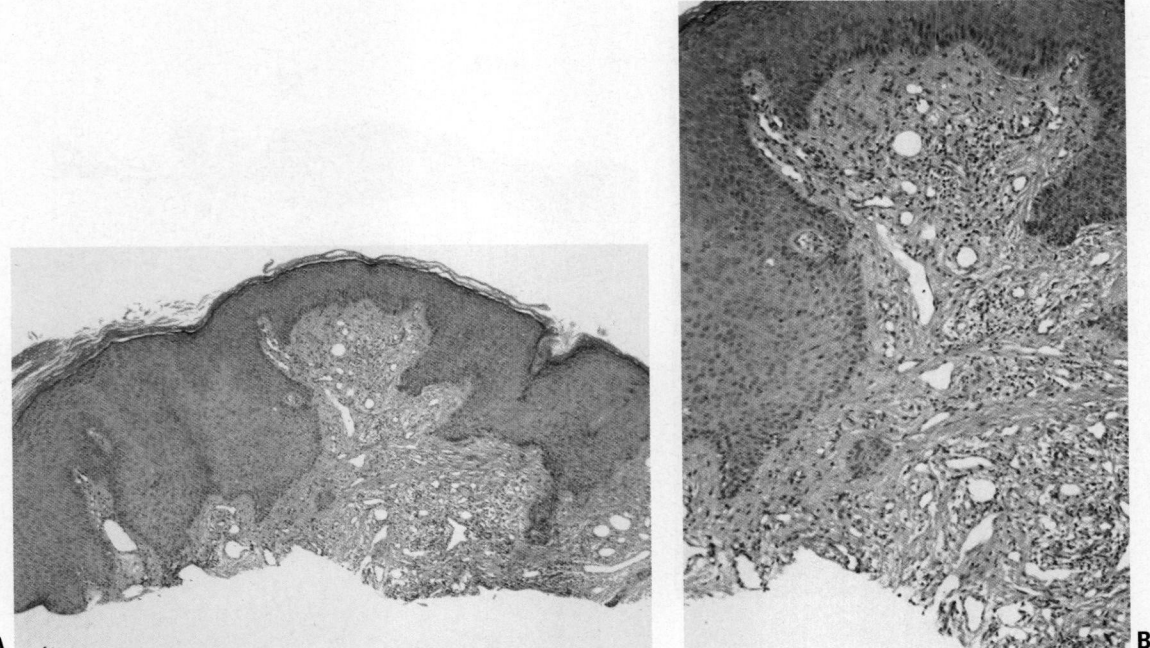

Figure 13-13 Acanthoma fissuratum (granuloma fissuratum). **A:** There is nonatypical acanthosis of the epidermis, with attenuation of the rete centrally. **B:** Within the dermis, there is a proliferation of slightly dilated small vessels, associated with fibrosis and a variable chronic inflammatory infiltrate. The term "granuloma" is a misnomer because a granulomatous infiltrate is not seen.

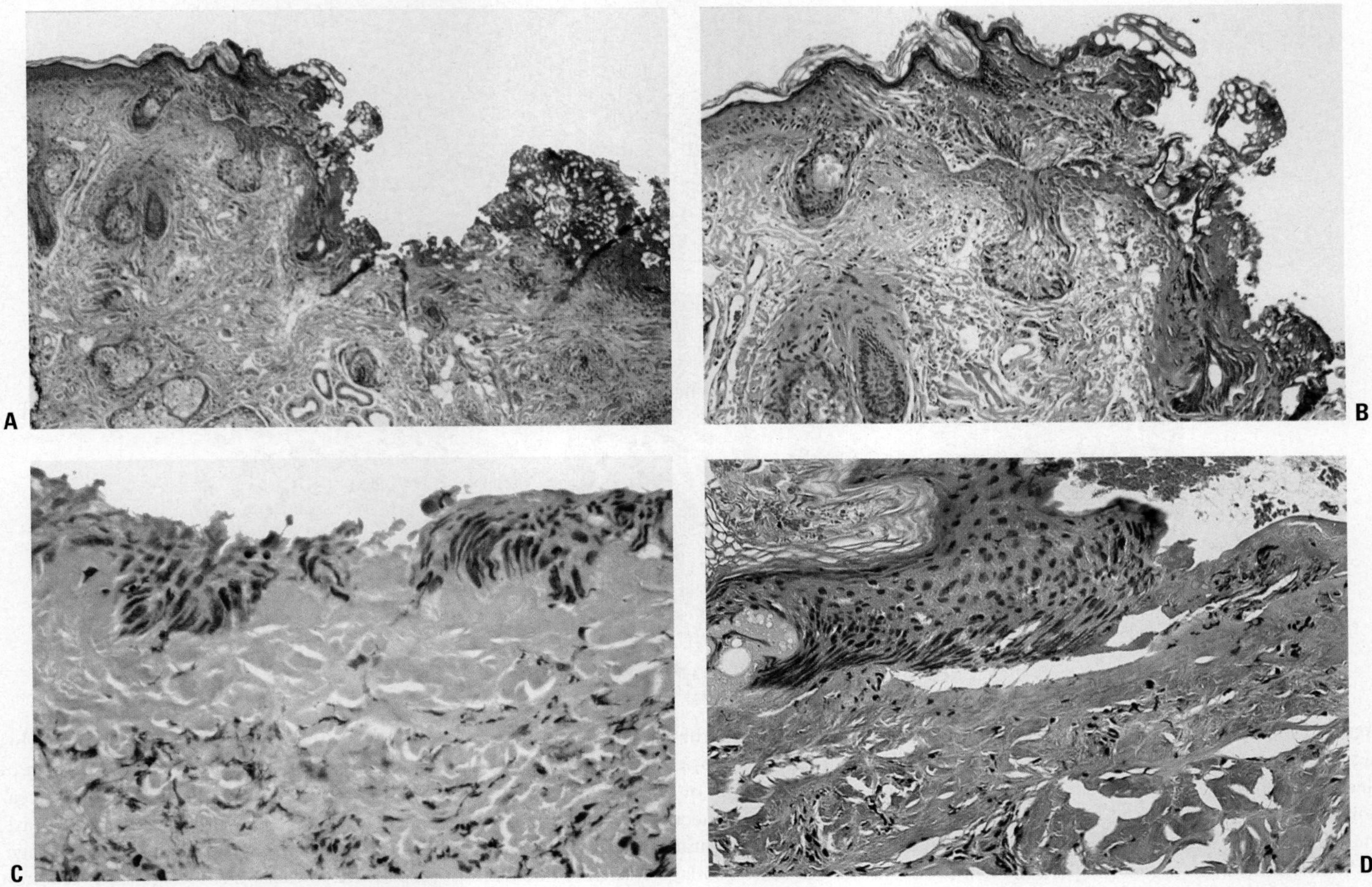

Figure 13-14 Electrodesiccation injury. **A:** There is ulceration of the epidermis and dermis with reticulated lacelike hemorrhagic and basophilic coagulation necrosis of the epidermis and superficial dermis. **B:** Near the edge of the ulcer, the epidermis and follicular epithelium show elongated alteration of the nuclei, with disassociation and blister formation. **C:** The epithelial cells typically show elongation of nuclei in electrodesiccation injury. Hyperchromasia of nuclei may be seen, simulating atypia, but the stretch artifact and absence of parakeratosis differentiate this from an actinic keratosis. **D:** Incipient blister formation can be seen in association with elongation cytolysis of keratinocytes and/or coagulation necrosis of the dermis due to electrodesiccation heat injury.

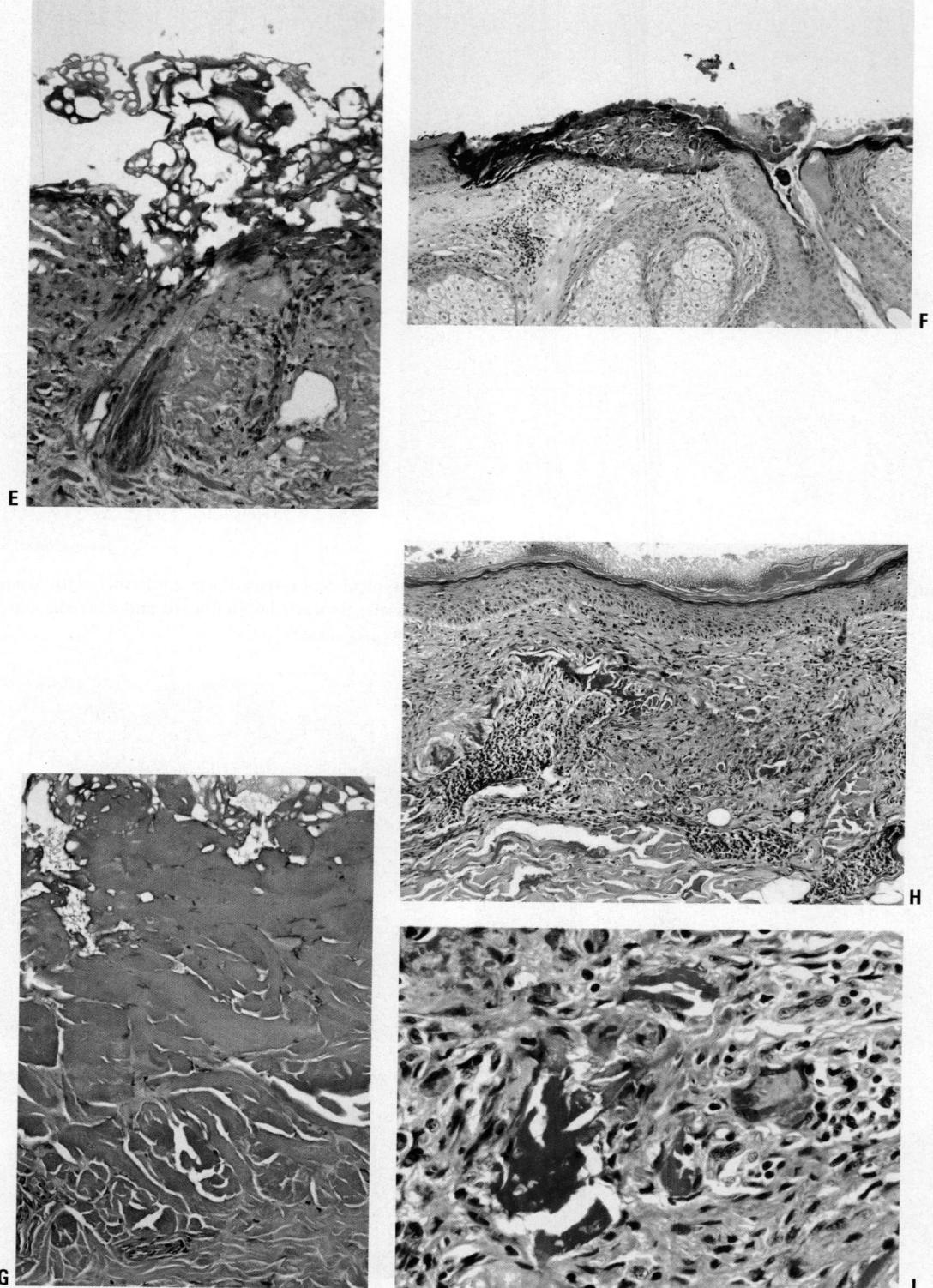

Figure 13-14 (*continued*) E: Electrodesiccation elongation effects on the follicular epithelium are similar to those seen in the epidermis. This higher power view highlights the lacelike pattern of coagulation necrosis seen in some cases of electrodesiccation injury. F: Another pattern of electrodesiccation injury, characterized by abrupt basophilic alteration of the collagen and epithelium. G: The dermal changes of electrodesiccation injury are characterized by homogenized basophilic coagulation necrosis and loss of the distinction between collagen bundles. In contrast, the deeper tissue shows minimally damaged collagen, with distinct separation of the collagen bundles. Superficially, there is mild lacelike change. H: Within a healing surgical biopsy site, foci of basophilic desiccated collagen are noted beneath the reparative fibrosis. I: A foreign-body reaction to altered collagen is noted, with engulfment of the basophilic injured collagen.

necrosis (Fig. 13-15). Dermal inflammation is typically minimal, unless there are residual biopsy site changes. Although the epidermis is typically denuded, there may be partial remnants of attached epidermis without the stretch artifact typical of electrodesiccation.

Differential Diagnosis. The nuclei elongation of electrodesiccation injury should be differentiated from atypia of an actinic keratosis. Atypical melanocytic hyperplasia may show overlap features, but this can be differentiated with immunohistochemical stains for melanocytes (see Chapter 28).

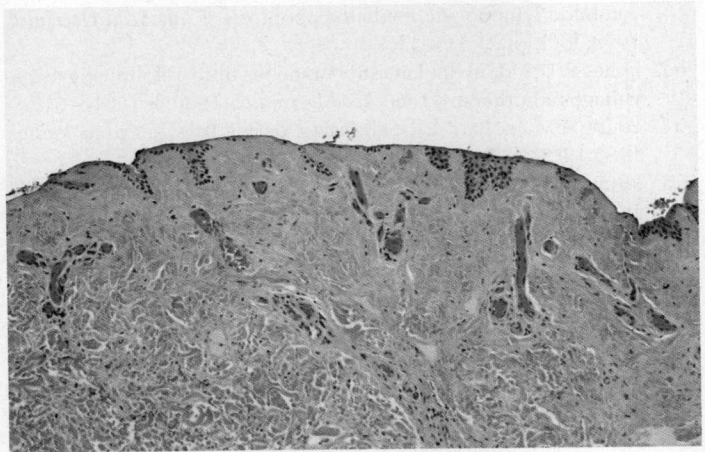

Figure 13-15 Curettage-induced ulceration. In contrast to desiccation-induced injury, there is no dermal collagen reaction. The ulcer base typically shows vascular congestion.

REFERENCES

1. Zalar GL, Harber LC. Reactions to physical agents. In: Moschella SL, Hurley HJ, eds. *Dermatology.* WB Saunders; 1985:1672–1690.
2. Spoo J, Elsner P. Cement burns: a review 1960–2000. *Contact Dermatitis.* 2001;45(2):68–71.
3. Naraghi ZS, Mansouri P, Mortazavi M. A clinicopathological study on acute cutaneous lesions induced by sulfur mustard gas (yperite). *Eur J Dermatol.* 2005;15(3):140–145.
4. Benson A, Dickson WA, Boyce DE. Burns. *BMJ.* 2006;332(7542): 649–652.
5. Page EH, Shear NH. Temperature-dependent skin disorders. *J Am Acad Dermatol.* 1988;18(5, pt 1):1003–1019.
6. Bunick CG, Lott JP, Warren CB, Galan A, Bolognia J, King BA. Chemical burn from topical apple cider vinegar. *J Am Acad Dermatol.* 2012 Oct;67(4):e143–e144.
7. Feldstein S, Afshar M, Krakowski AC. Chemical burn from vinegar following an internet-based protocol for self-removal of nevi. *J Clin Aesthet Dermatol.* 2015 Jun;8(6):50.
8. Ashchyan H, Jen M, Elenitsas R, Rubin AI. Surreptitious apple cider vinegar treatment of a melanocytic nevus: Newly described histologic features. *J Cutan Pathol.* 2018 Apr;45(4):307–309.
9. Stransky L, Broshtilova V. Neutrophilic dermatosis of the dorsal hands elicited by thermal injury. *Contact Dermatitis.* 2003; 49(1):42.
10. Wakamatsu J, Yamamoto T, Minemura T, Tsuboi R. The occurrence of eccrine poroma on a burn site. *J Eur Acad Dermatol Venereol.* 2007;21(8):1128–1129.
11. Usmani N, Akhtar S, Long E, Phipps A, Walton S. A case of sarcoidosis occurring within an extensive burns scar. *J Plast Reconstr Aesthet Surg.* 2007;60(11):1256–1259.
12. Daneshpazhooh M, Fatehnejad M, et al.. Trauma-induced pemphigus: a case series of 36 patients. *J Dtsch Dermatol Ges.* 2016;14(2):166–171.
13. Compton CC. The delayed postburn blister. A commonplace but commonly overlooked phenomenon. *Arch Dermatol.* 1992;128(2):249–252.
14. Tarran S, Langlois NE, Dziewulski P, Sztynda T. Using the inflammatory cell infiltrate to estimate the age of human burn wounds: a review and immunohistochemical study. *Med Sci Law.* 2006;46(2): 115–126.
15. Gravante G, Palmieri MB, Delogu D, Montone A. Apoptotic cells in cutaneous adnexa of burned patients. *Burns.* 2007;33(1): 129–130.
16. Lee HW, Jeong YI, Suh HS, et al. Two cases of dystrophic calcinosis cutis in burn scars. *J Dermatol.* 2005;32(4):282–285.
17. Kowal-Vern A, Criswell BK. Burn scar neoplasms: a literature review and statistical analysis. *Burns.* 2005;31(4):403–413. doi: 10.1016/j.burns.2005.02.015.
18. Copcu E, Aktas A, Sisman N, Oztan Y. Thirty-one cases of Marjolin's ulcer. *Clin Exp Dermatol.* 2003;28(2):138–141.
19. Bero SM, Busam KJ, Brady MS. Cutaneous melanoma arising in a burn scar: two recent cases and a review of the literature. *Melanoma Res.* 2006;16(1):71–76.
20. Nara T, Hayakawa A, Ikeuchi A, Katoh N, Kishimoto S. Granulocyte colony-stimulating factor-producing cutaneous angiosarcoma with leukaemoid reaction arising on a burn scar. *Br J Dermatol.* 2003;149(6):1273–1275.
21. Morihara K, Takenaka H, Morihara T, Kishimoto S. Primary cutaneous anaplastic large cell lymphoma associated with vascular endothelial growth factor arising from a burn scar. *J Am Acad Dermatol.* 2007;57(5 suppl):S103–S105.
22. Yeung CK, Ma SY, Chan HH, Trendell-Smith NJ, Au WY. Primary CD30+ve cutaneous T-cell lymphoma associated with chronic burn injury in a patient with longstanding psoriasis. *Am J Dermatopathol.* 2004;26(5):394–396.
23. Currie CL, Monk BE. Welding and non-melanoma skin cancer. *Clin Exp Dermatol.* 2000;25(1):28–29.
24. Dixon A. Arc welding and the risk of cancer. *Aust Fam Physician.* 2007;36(4):255–256.
25. Goldfeder KL, Levin JM, Katz KA, Clarke LE, Loren AW, James WD. Ultraviolet recall reaction after total body irradiation, etoposide, and methotrexate therapy. *J Am Acad Dermatol.* 2007;56(3):494–499.
26. Magne N, Chargari C, Auberdiac P, Moncharmont C, Merrouche Y, Spano JP. Ultraviolet recall dermatitis reaction with sorafenib. *Invest New Drugs.* 2011;29(5):1111–1113.
27. Garza LA, Yoo EK, Junkins-Hopkins JM, VanVoorhees AS. Photo recall effect in association with cefazolin. *Cutis.* 2004;73(1):79–80, 85.
28. Krishnan RS, Lewis AT, Kass JS, Hsu S. Ultraviolet recall-like phenomenon occurring after piperacillin, tobramycin, and ciprofloxacin therapy. *J Am Acad Dermatol.* 2001;44(6):1045–1047.
29. Shelley WB, Shelley ED, Campbell AC, Weigensberg IJ. Drug eruptions presenting at sites of prior radiation damage (sunlight and electron beam). *J Am Acad Dermatol.* 1984;11(1):53–57.
30. Johnson WC, Butterworth T. Erythema ab igne elastosis. *Arch Dermatol.* 1971;104(2):128–131.
31. Bilic M, Adams BB. Erythema ab igne induced by a laptop computer. *J Am Acad Dermatol.* 2004;50(6):973–974.
32. Adams BB. Heated car seat-induced erythema ab igne. *Arch Dermatol.* 2012;148(2):265–266.
33. Brodell D, Mostow EN. Automobile seat heater-induced erythema ab igne. *Arch Dermatol.* 2012;148(2):264–265.
34. Meffert JJ, Davis BM. Furniture-induced erythema ab igne. *J Am Acad Dermatol.* 1996;34(3):516–517.
35. Dellavalle RP, Gillum P. Erythema ab igne following heating/cooling blanket use in the intensive care unit. *Cutis.* 2000;66(2): 136–138.

36. Kraemer RR, La Hoz RM, Willig JH. Some like it hot: erythema ab igne due to cannabinoid hyperemesis. *J Gen Intern Med.* 2013;28(11):1522.

37. Sahu KK, Mishra A, Naraghi L. Erythema ab igne as a complication of cannabinoid hyperemesis syndrome. *BMJ Case Rep.* 2019;12(1):e227836.

38. Flanagan N, Watson R, Sweeney E, Barnes L. Bullous erythema ab igne. *Br J Dermatol.* 1996;134(6):1159–1160.

39. Kokturk A, Kaya TI, Baz K, Yazici AC, Apa DD, Ikizoglu G. Bullous erythema ab igne. *Dermatol Online J.* 2003;9(3):18.

40. Arrington JH III, Lockman DS. Thermal keratoses and squamous cell carcinoma in situ associated with erythema ab igne. *Arch Dermatol.* 1979;115(10):1226–1228.

41. Hewitt JB, Sherif A, Kerr KM, Stankler L. Merkel cell and squamous cell carcinomas arising in erythema ab igne. *Br J Dermatol.* 1993;128(5):591–592.

42. Jones CS, Tyring SK, Lee PC, Fine JD. Development of neuroendocrine (Merkel cell) carcinoma mixed with squamous cell carcinoma in erythema ab igne. *Arch Dermatol.* 1988;124(1):110–113.

43. Sigmon JR, Cantrell J, Teague D, Sangueza O, Sheehan DJ. Poorly differentiated carcinoma arising in the setting of erythema ab igne. *Am J Dermatopathol.* 2013;35(6):676–678.

44. Wharton J, Roffwarg D, Miller J, Sheehan DJ. Cutaneous marginal zone lymphoma arising in the setting of erythema ab igne. *J Am Acad Dermatol.* 2010;62(6):1080–1081.

45. Hurwitz RM, Tisserand ME. Erythema ab igne. *Arch Dermatol.* 1987;123(1):21–23.

46. Shahrad P, Marks R. The wages of warmth: changes in erythema ab igne. *Br J Dermatol.* 1977;97(2):179–186.

47. Finlayson GR, Sams WM Jr, Smith JG Jr. Erythema ab igne: a histopathological study. *J Invest Dermatol.* 1966;46(1):104–108.

48. Wharton JB, Sheehan DJ, Lesher JL Jr. Squamous cell carcinoma in situ arising in the setting of erythema ab igne. *J Drugs Dermatol.* 2008;7(5):488–489.

49. Horio T, Imamura S. Bullous lichen planus developed on erythema ab igne. *J Dermatol.* 1986;13(3):203–207.

50. Cavallari V, Cicciarello R, Torre V, et al. Chronic heat-induced skin lesions (erythema ab igne): ultrastructural studies. *Ultrastruct Pathol.* 2001;25(2):93–97.

51. Palmer MJ, Lee A, O'Keefe R. Cutaneous reactive angiomatosis associated with erythema ab igne. *Australas J Dermatol.* 2015;56(1):e24–e27. doi:10.1111/ajd.12118

52. Cho S, Jung JY, Lee JH. Erythema ab igne successfully treated using 1,064-nm Q-switched neodymium-doped yttrium aluminum garnet laser with low fluence. *Dermatol Surg.* 2011;37(4):551–553.

53. Busch D. Genetic susceptibility to radiation and chemotherapy injury: diagnosis and management. *Int J Radiat Oncol Biol Phys.* 1994;30(4):997–1002.

54. Pollard JM, Gatti RA. Clinical radiation sensitivity with DNA repair disorders: an overview. *Int J Radiat Oncol Biol Phys.* 2009;74(5):1323–1331.

55. Wagner LK, McNeese MD, Marx MV, Siegel EL. Severe skin reactions from interventional fluoroscopy: case report and review of the literature. *Radiology.* 1999;213(3):773–776.

56. Hanna YM, Baglan KL, Stromberg JS, Vicini FA, A Decker D. Acute and subacute toxicity associated with concurrent adjuvant radiation therapy and paclitaxel in primary breast cancer therapy. *Breast J.* 2002;8(3):149–153.

57. Koenig TR, Wolff D, Mettler FA, Wagner LK. Skin injuries from fluoroscopically guided procedures, part 1: characteristics of radiation injury. *AJR Am J Roentgenol.* 2001;177(1):3–11.

58. Pajonk F, Weissenberger C, Witucki G, Henke M. Vitiligo at the sites of irradiation in a patient with Hodgkin's disease. *Strahlenther Onkol.* 2002;178(3):159–162.

59. Shurman D, Reich HL, James WD. Lichen planus confined to a radiation field: the "isoradiotopic" response. *J Am Acad Dermatol.* 2004;50(3):482–483.

60. Parikh SK, Ravi A, Kuo DY, Nori D. Bullous pemphigoid masquerading as acute radiation dermatitis: case report. *Eur J Gynaecol Oncol.* 2001;22(5):322–324.

61. Martires KJ, Baird K, Steinberg SM, et al. Sclerotic-type chronic GVHD of the skin: clinical risk factors, laboratory markers, and burden of disease. *Blood.* 2011;118(15):4250–4257.

62. Hymes SR, Strom EA, Fife C. Radiation dermatitis: clinical presentation, pathophysiology, and treatmen. *J Am Acad Dermatol.* 2006;54(1):28–46.

63. Stone MS, Robson KJ, LeBoit PE. Subacute radiation dermatitis from fluoroscopy during coronary artery stenting: evidence for cytotoxic lymphocyte mediated apoptosis. *J Am Acad Dermatol.* 1998;38(2, pt 2):333–336.

64. James WD, Odom RB. Late subcutaneous fibrosis following megavoltage radiotherapy. *J Am Acad Dermatol.* 1980;3(6):616–618.

65. Young EM Jr, Barr RJ. Sclerosing dermatoses. *J Cutan Pathol.* 1985;12(5):426–441.

66. Moretto JC, Soslow RA, Smoller BR. Atypical cells in radiation dermatitis express factor XIIIa. *Am J Dermatopathol.* 1998;20(4):370–372.

67. Meehan SA, LeBoit PE. An immunohistochemical analysis of radiation fibroblasts. *J Cutan Pathol.* 1997;24(5):309–313.

68. LeBoit PE. Subacute radiation dermatitis: a histologic imitator of acute cutaneous graft-versus-host disease. *J Am Acad Dermatol.* 1989;20(2, pt 1):236–241.

69. Dyer BA, Hodges MG, Mayadev JS. Radiation-induced morphea: an under-recognized complication of breast irradiation. *Clin Breast Cancer.* 2016;16(4):e141–e143.

70. Spalek M, Jonska-Gmyrek J, Gałecki J. Radiation-induced morphea–a literature review. *J Eur Acad Dermatol Venereol.* 2015;29(2):197–202.

71. Totten RS, Antypas PG, Dupertuis SM, Gaisford JC, White WL. Pre-existing roentgen-ray dermatitis in patients with skin cancer. *Cancer.* 1957;10(5):1024–1030.

72. Bacanli A, Ciftcioglu MA, Savas B, Alpsoy E. Nevoid basal cell carcinoma syndrome associated with unilateral renal agenesis: acceleration of basal cell carcinomas following radiotherapy. *J Eur Acad Dermatol Venereol.* 2005;19(4):510–511.

73. Seo IS, Warner TF, Warren JS, Bennett JE. Cutaneous postirradiation sarcoma: ultrastructural evidence of pluripotential mesenchymal cell derivation. *Cancer.* 1985;56(4):761–767.

74. Diaz-Cascajo C, Borghi S, Weyers W. Desmoplastic leiomyosarcoma of the skin. *Am J Dermatopathol.* 2000;22(3):251–255.

75. Souba WW, McKenna RJ Jr, Meis J, Benjamin R, Raymond AK, Mountain CF. Radiation-induced sarcomas of the chest wall. *Cancer.* 1986;57(3):610–615.

76. Kiyohara T, Kumakiri M, Kobayashl H, et al. Spindle cell angiosarcoma following irradiation therapy for cervical carcinoma. *J Cutan Pathol.* 2002;29(2):96–100.

77. Ronen S, Ivan D, Torres-Cabala CA, et al. Post-radiation vascular lesions of the breast. *J Cutan Pathol.* 2019;46(1):52–58.

78. Chodkiewicz HM, Cohen PR. Radiation port erythema multiforme: erythema multiforme localized to the radiation port in a patient with non-small cell lung cancer. *Skinmed.* 2012;10(6):390–392.

79. Hivnor CM, Seykora JT, Junkins-Hopkins J, et al. Subacute radiation dermatitis. *Am J Dermatopathol.* 2004;26(3):210–212.

80. Schecter AK, Lewis MD, Robinson-Bostom L, Pan TD. Cardiac catheterization-induced acute radiation dermatitis presenting as a fixed drug eruption. *J Drugs Dermatol.* 2003;2(4):425–427.

81. Schmuth M, Wimmer MA, Hofer S, et al. Topical corticosteroid therapy for acute radiation dermatitis: a prospective, randomized, double-blind study. *Br J Dermatol.* 2002;146(6):983–991.

82. Azria D, Magne N, Zouhair A, et al. Radiation recall: a well recognized but neglected phenomenon. *Cancer Treat Rev.* 2005;31(7): 555–570.

83. Camidge R, Price A. Characterizing the phenomenon of radiation recall dermatitis. *Radiother Oncol.* 2001;59(3):237–245.

84. Ortmann E, Hohenberg G. Treatment side effects, case 1: radiation recall phenomenon after administration of capecitabine. *J Clin Oncol.* 2002;20(13):3029–3030.

85. Tan DH, Bunce PE, Liles WC, Gold WL. Gemcitabine-related "pseudocellulitis": report of 2 cases and review of the literature. *Clin Infect Dis.* 2007;45(5):e72–e76.

86. Thomas R, Stea B. Radiation recall dermatitis from high-dose interferon alfa-2b. *J Clin Oncol.* 2002;20(1):355–357.

87. Boussemart L, Boivin C, Claveau J, et al. Vemurafenib and radiosensitization. *JAMA Dermatol.* 2013;149(7):855–857.

88. Chung C, Dawson LA, Joshua AM, Brade AM. Radiation recall dermatitis triggered by multi-targeted tyrosine kinase inhibitors: sunitinib and sorafenib. *Anticancer Drugs.* 2010;21(2): 206–209.

89. Cho S, Breedlove JJ, Gunning ST. Radiation recall reaction induced by levofloxacin. *J Drugs Dermatol.* 2008;7(1):64–67.

90. Vujovic O. Radiation recall dermatitis with azithromycin. *Curr Oncol.* 2010;17(4):119–121.

91. Wernicke AG, Swistel AJ, Parashar B, Myskowski PL. Levofloxacin-induced radiation recall dermatitis: a case report and a review of the literature. *Clin Breast Cancer.* 2010;10(5):404–406.

92. Abadir R, Liebmann J. Radiation reaction recall following simvastatin therapy: a new observation. *Clin Oncol (R Coll Radiol).* 1995;7(5):325–326.

93. Taunk NK, Haffty BG, Goyal S. Radiation recall 5 years after whole-breast irradiation for early-stage breast cancer secondary to initiation of rosuvastatin and amlodipine. *J Clin Oncol.* 2011;29(22):e661–e663.

94. Bauza A, Del Pozo LJ, Escalas J, Mestre F. Radiation recall dermatitis in a patient affected with pheochromocytoma after treatment with lanreotide. *Br J Dermatol.* 2007;157(5):1061–1063.

95. Seidel C, Janssen S, Karstens JH, et al. Recall pneumonitis during systemic treatment with sunitinib. *Ann Oncol.* 2010;21(10): 2119–2120.

96. Castellano D, Hitt R, Cortes-Funes H, Romero A, Rodriguez-Peralto JL. Side effects of chemotherapy, case 2: radiation recall reaction induced by gemcitabine. *J Clin Oncol.* 2000;18(3):695–696.

97. Kulka JP. Cold injury of the skin: the pathogenic role of microcirculatory impairment. *Arch Environ Health.* 1965;11(4):484–497.

98. Murphy JV, Banwell PE, Roberts AH, McGrouther DA. Frostbite: pathogenesis and treatment. *J Trauma.* 2000;48(1):171–178.

99. Goette DK. Chilblains (perniosis). *J Am Acad Dermatol.* 1990; 23(2, pt 1):257–262.

100. Stewart CL, Adler DJ, Jacobson A, et al. Equestrian perniosis: a report of 2 cases and a review of the literature. *Am J Dermatopathol.* 2013;35(2):237–240.

101. Yang AY, Schwartz L, Divers AK, Sternberg L, Lee JB. Equestrian chilblain: another outdoor recreational hazard. *J Cutan Pathol.* 2013;40(5):485–490.

102. Viguier M, Pinquier L, Cavelier-Balloy B, et al. Clinical and histopathologic features and immunologic variables in patients with severe chilblains: a study of the relationship to lupus erythematosus. *Medicine (Baltimore).* 2001;80(3):180–188.

103. Affleck AG, Ravenscroft JC, Leach IH. Chilblain-like leukemia cutis. *Pediatr Dermatol.* 2007;24(1):38–41.

104. Freeman EE, McMahon DE, Lipoff JB, et al.; American Academy of Dermatology Ad Hoc Task Force on COVID-19. Pernio-like skin lesions associated with COVID-19: a case series of 318 patients from 8 countries. *J Am Acad Dermatol.* 2020;83(2):486–492.

105. Pock L, Petrovska P, Becvar R, Mandys V, Hercogová J. Verrucous form of chilblain lupus erythematosus. *J Eur Acad Dermatol Venereol.* 2001;15(5):448–451.

106. Franceschini F, Calzavara-Pinton P, Quinzanini M, et al. Chilblain lupus erythematosus is associated with antibodies to SSA/Ro. *Lupus.* 1999;8(3):215–219.

107. Bouaziz JD, Barete S, Le Pelletier F, Amoura Z, Piette JC, Francès C. Cutaneous lesions of the digits in systemic lupus erythematosus: 50 cases. *Lupus.* 2007;16(3):163–167.

108. Gunther C, Hillebrand M, Brunk J, Lee-Kirsch MA. Systemic involvement in TREX1-associated familial chilblain lupus. *J Am Acad Dermatol.* 2013;69(4):e179–e181.

109. Ravenscroft JC, Suri M, Rice GI, Szynkiewicz M, Crow YJ. Autosomal dominant inheritance of a heterozygous mutation in SAMHD1 causing familial chilblain lupus. *Am J Med Genet A.* 2011;155A(1):235–237.

110. Tungler V, Silver RM, Walkenhorst H, Günther C, Lee-Kirsch MA. Inherited or de novo mutation affecting aspartate 18 of TREX1 results in either familial chilblain lupus or Aicardi-Goutieres syndrome. *Br J Dermatol.* 2012;167(1):212–214.

111. Giraldo WAS, Lana MA, Villanueva MJG, García CG, Diaz MV. Chilblain lupus induced by TNF-alpha antagonists: a case report and literature review. *Clin Rheumatol.* 2012;31(3):563–568.

112. Herman EW, Kezis JS, Silvers DN. A distinctive variant of pernio: clinical and histopathologic study of nine cases. *Arch Dermatol.* 1981;117(1):26–28.

113. Colmenero I, Santonja C, Alonso-Riaño M, et al. SARS-CoV-2 endothelial infection causes COVID-19 chilblains: histopathological, immunohistochemical and ultrastructural study of seven paediatric cases. *Br J Dermatol.* 2020;183(4):729–737.

114. Doutre MS, Beylot C, Beylot J, Pompougnac E, Royer P. Chilblain lupus erythematosus: report of 15 cases. *Dermatology.* 1992;184(1):26–28.

115. Boada A, Bielsa I, Fernandez-Figueras MT, Ferrándiz C. Perniosis: clinical and histopathological analysis. *Am J Dermatopathol.* 2010;32(1):19–23.

116. Cribier B, Djeridi N, Peltre B, Grosshans E. A histologic and immunohistochemical study of chilblains. *J Am Acad Dermatol.* 2001;45(6):924–929.

117. Wessagowit P, Asawanonda P, Noppakun N. Papular perniosis mimicking erythema multiforme: the first case report in Thailand. *Int J Dermatol.* 2000;39(7):527–529.

118. Rustin MH, Newton JA, Smith NP, Dowd PM. The treatment of chilblains with nifedipine: the results of a pilot study, a double-blind placebo-controlled randomized study and a long-term open trial. *Br J Dermatol.* 1989;120(2):267–275.

119. Eady RA, Tidman MJ. Diagnosing epidermolysis bullosa. *Br J Dermatol.* 1983;108(5):621–626.

120. Kee CE. Liquid nitrogen cryotherapy. *Arch Dermatol.* 1967;96(2): 198–203.

121. Crissey JT, Peachey JC. Calcaneal petechiae. *Arch Dermatol.* 1961;83:501.

122. Cardoso JC, Veraitch O, Gianotti R, et al. 'Hints' in the horn: diagnostic clues in the stratum corneum. *J Cutan Pathol.* 2017; 44(3):256–278.

123. MacDonald DM, Martin SJ. Acanthoma fissuratum—spectacle frame acanthoma. *Acta Derm Venereol.* 1975;55(6):485–488.

124. Mohan RP, Verma S, Singh U, Agarwal N. Epulis fissuratum: consequence of ill-fitting prosthesis. *BMJ Case Rep.* 2013;2013. doi:10.1136/bcr-2013-200054

Chapter 14

Noninfectious Granulomas

WILLIAM DAMSKY, EARL J. GLUSAC, AND CHRISTINE J. KO

INTRODUCTION

A granuloma is a collection of epithelioid histiocytes. In some cases, these cells are abundant and closely opposed, resembling epithelium. They may form palisades around extracellular material. In other cases, the cellular aggregates are smaller and less distinct, showing histologic features that overlap with nongranulomatous histiocytic lesions. Some granulomatous infiltrates are caused by infection, and these are described in Chapters 21–24. Granulomatous conditions may also show histologic resemblance to "histiocytoses," many of which are likely neoplastic, and these are considered in Chapter 26.

GRANULOMA ANNULARE

Clinical Summary. Granuloma annulare is an idiopathic granulomatous condition. Females are affected more commonly than males. The clinical morphology of granuloma annulare can be variable, with the most common presentation consisting of asymptomatic papules and plaques that are dull pink and often annular (Fig. 14-1). The lesions are found most commonly on the arms, hands, trunk, legs, and feet. Although chronic, the lesions may subside after a number of years but may recur. Variants of granuloma annulare include (a) a generalized form, consisting of hundreds of papules that are either discrete or confluent and may not show an annular arrangement (1–4), (b) perforating granuloma annulare, with umbilicated lesions occurring usually in a localized distribution (5,6) and, rarely, in a generalized distribution (7–9), (c) erythematous or patch granuloma annulare, showing large, slightly erythematous patches, which may have a palpable border (10,11), and (d) subcutaneous/deep granuloma annulare, in which subcutaneous nodules occur, almost exclusively in children, either alone or in association with typical intradermal lesions (12–17). The subcutaneous nodules have a clinical appearance similar to that of rheumatoid nodules, although there is no history of arthritis, and there is a greater tendency to occur on the legs, feet, and, occasionally, the head (18). In adults, similar lesions may be found near the small joints of the hands (19).

Correlations between granuloma annulare and diabetes mellitus, hyperlipidemia, and thyroid disease have all been reported (2,20–24). A definitive association between granuloma annulare and internal malignancy has not been established (25). Granuloma annulare has been reported in patients with HIV or AIDS, with a greater incidence of generalized disease or GA with atypical features (including perforating) in this

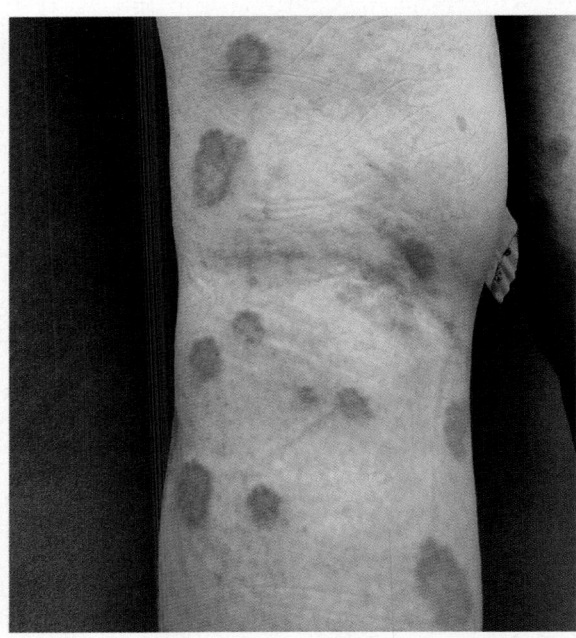

Figure 14-1 Granuloma annulare. Raised pink papules in an annular configuration in the popliteal fossa.

population (26–29). Granuloma annulare may develop in the context of both immune checkpoint inhibitors (e.g., anti-CTLA-4 and anti-PD-1) as well as paradoxically with cytokine blocking antibodies such as IL-17 inhibitors (30,31). Granuloma annulare–like lesions have also been reported to develop at sites of resolved herpes zoster (32) and, occasionally, in association with tattoos (33), necrobiosis lipoidica (34), and sarcoidosis (35).

Histopathology. Histologically, granuloma annulare shows an infiltrate of histiocytes and a perivascular infiltrate of lymphocytes that is usually sparse. The histiocytes may be present in an interstitial pattern without apparent organization or in palisades surrounding areas with prominent mucin (Figs. 14-2 to 14-5). Patterns between these two extremes occur, and a single biopsy may show interstitial, slightly palisaded, and well-palisaded histiocytes. Although altered collagen or small quantities of fibrin may be present (36), increased mucin is the hallmark of granuloma annulare. Occasionally, sections will not reveal increased mucin, particularly those lacking a palisaded arrangement of histiocytes. In biopsies with well-developed palisades, the central mucinous area is commonly accompanied by a few nuclear fragments or neutrophils. Plasma cells are rarely present.

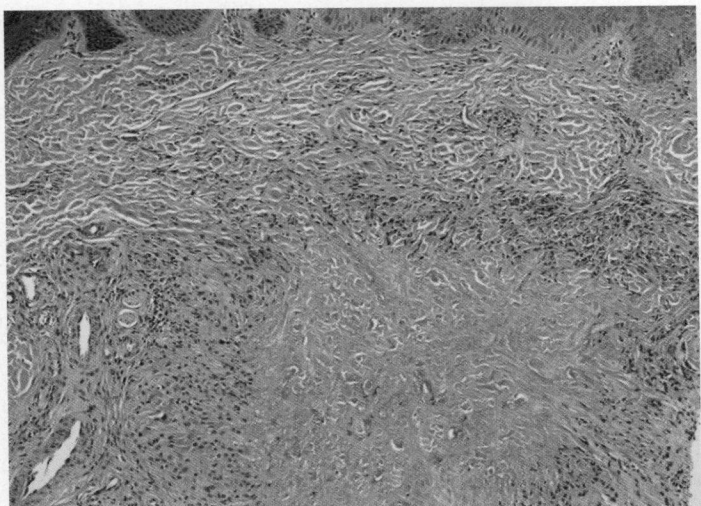

Figure 14-2 Granuloma annulare. A palisade of histiocytes surrounds mucin in the upper dermis.

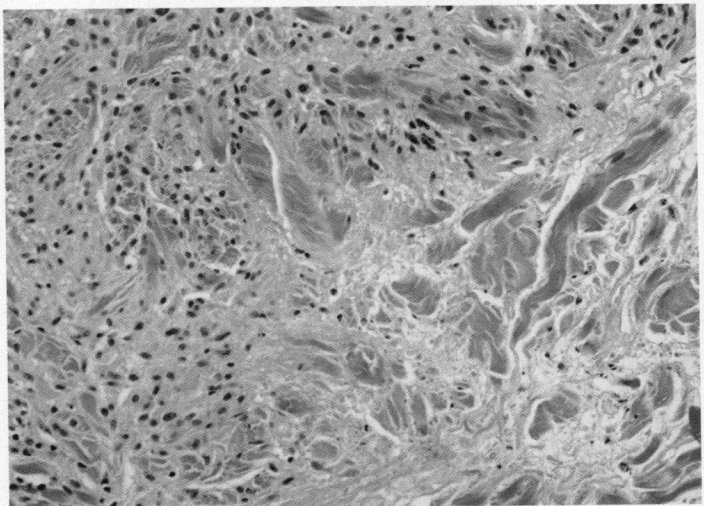

Figure 14-3 Granuloma annulare. Histiocytes surround mucin, which shows a feathery blue appearance, and a few fragments of neutrophils.

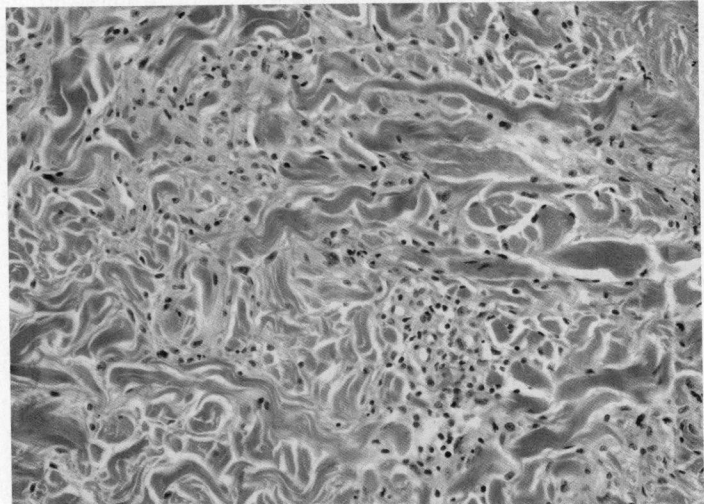

Figure 14-4 Granuloma annulare. Interstitial pattern granuloma annulare exhibits histiocytes between collagen bundles and perivascular lymphocytes.

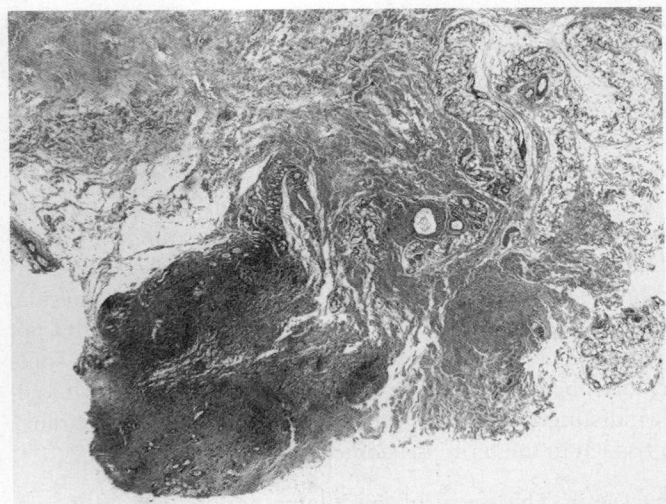

A

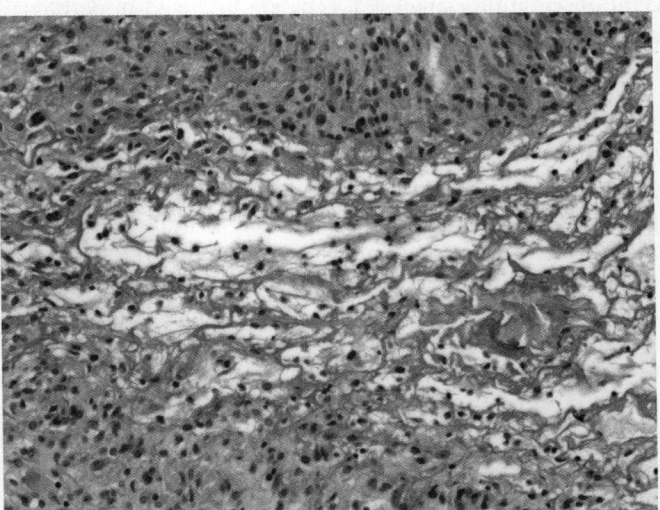

B

Figure 14-5 Deep granuloma annulare. **A:** A well-circumscribed subcutaneous nodule shows palisaded histiocytes surrounding mucin and fibrinoid material. **B:** Histiocytes in a palisade surround mucin and fibrinoid material.

A sparse infiltrate of eosinophils is seen in approximately half of cases, and occasional biopsies show abundant eosinophils (37,38). Multinucleated histiocytes are present more often than not, but they are usually few and often subtle. They can occasionally be seen to have engulfed short, thick, blue-gray elastic fibers (39). The histiocytic infiltrate is usually present throughout the full thickness of the dermis or the middle and upper dermis, but occasionally, just the superficial or the deep dermis is involved (36,40,41). Mitotic figures are usually rare (fewer than 1 per 10 high-power fields) but may be as frequent as 7 per 10 high-power fields in rare examples (42).

Rare examples of granuloma annulare show aggregates of epithelioid histiocytes, usually with some giant cells and a rim of lymphoid cells, which may resemble the granulomas of sarcoidosis (35,36,40). These usually differ from sarcoidal granulomas, however, by showing poorer circumscription and by lacking asteroid bodies. Vascular changes in granuloma annulare are variable but generally inconspicuous (43). Among the variants of granuloma annulare mentioned, the usual histologic picture of palisaded and interstitial pattern is found in the generalized form (4). Occasionally, there is a band of histiocytes and giant cells in the superficial dermis with perivascular lymphocytes (4). An interstitial pattern predominates in the erythematous and patch variants (10,11,44,45). In perforating granuloma annulare, at least part of the palisading granulomatous process is located superficially and is associated with disruption of the epidermis (5,7,8).

The subcutaneous nodules of deep granuloma annulare usually show large histiocytic palisades surrounding mucin and degenerated collagen (Fig. 14-5). These central, degenerated foci exhibit a pale appearance (46); however, examples in which mucin was not apparent or in which the central area appeared more fibrinoid have also been reported (18). Thus, some cases of subcutaneous granuloma annulare may be histologically indistinguishable from rheumatoid nodule, an appearance that has led to the term *pseudorheumatoid nodule*.

Pathogenesis. The cause of granuloma annulare is unknown. Several observations suggest T cells are involved in pathogenesis, including expansion of specific T-cell clonotypes in some granuloma annulare lesions (47), the association of granuloma annulare with particular MHC class II alleles (48), and the development of granuloma annulare in the setting of T-cell–stimulating cancer immunotherapies (30). CD4+ T cells are the predominant lymphocyte population and appear to produce factors including interferon-γ that may lead to monocyte recruitment and subsequent macrophage activation (16,47,49,50).

Electron microscopic examination reveals degeneration of both collagen and elastic fibers in granuloma annulare (36). The macrophages (histiocytes) show a high content of primary lysosomes and considerable cytoplasmic activity with the release of lysosomal enzymes into the extracellular space (51); with newer molecular studies also showing an activated phenotype in lesional macrophages (49). Histiocytic cells in granuloma annulare have generally been found to stain positively for CD68 and CD163, although in interstitial granuloma annulare they may be negative for CD68 (16,42,45). Synthesis of types I and III collagen also occurs, probably as a reparative response (52).

Blood vessel deposits of immunoglobulin M and the third component of complement (C3) have been observed by some investigators (50), but others have found them only rarely (53) or not at all (54). Thus, the existence of an immune complex vasculitis in granuloma annulare (50) appears unlikely.

Differential Diagnosis. Granuloma annulare and necrobiosis lipoidica may resemble one another histologically. Although much has been written about the difficulty of separating these disorders histologically (43), the distinction can be accomplished clinically in most circumstances (55). Furthermore, although it is true that histologic distinction may be impossible, it can usually be accomplished using the criteria in Table 14-1. Other palisading granulomas (e.g., to foreign material) can mimic granuloma annulare (see Table 14-1) (56).

The interstitial type of granuloma annulare, in which palisades of histiocytes are not well developed, is less likely to be confused with necrobiosis lipoidica. This pattern is more likely to be mistaken for a process that can also show a superficial and deep lymphocytic infiltrate, such as the inflammatory stage of morphea, but the subtle presence of histiocytes in an interstitial pattern usually allows for a diagnosis of granuloma annulare. Mycosis fungoides can have a granulomatous infiltrate with a granuloma annulare–like pattern (57,58). Such examples of this cutaneous T-cell lymphoma can usually be recognized by a dermal lymphocytic infiltrate that is denser around the superficial plexus than around the deep one, by a lichenoid component to the infiltrate, and, occasionally, by the presence of intraepidermal lymphocytes. The interstitial type of granuloma annulare may also resemble a xanthoma. Distinction is usually possible because in granuloma annulare a foamy appearance to the histiocytes is either completely lacking or very subtle; in xanthoma, at least some of the histiocytes are foamy. In addition, granuloma annulare tends to show an obvious perivascular lymphocytic infiltrate, whereas most xanthomas do not (59). Drug reactions (e.g., interstitial granulomatous drug reaction) may also mimic granuloma annulare but may show interface changes that allow for their distinction (60,61). Rarely, infection with *Mycobacterium marinum* may have relatively few neutrophils and may produce a histologic picture resembling interstitial granuloma annulare (62). *Interstitial granulomatous dermatitis* (IGD) may represent a variant of granuloma annulare or be a closely related entity. There may be associated arthritis. IGD is more strongly associated with underlying rheumatoid arthritis and inflammatory/systemic autoimmune diseases. A variety of clinical lesions have been reported in IGD and/or similar conditions. These range from linear and "ropelike" on the trunk to erythematous patches, plaques, and papules that are sometimes annular (63–67). Some authors have included IGD under the umbrella term *reactive granulomatous dermatitis* to recognize the potential clinical and histopathologic overlap of IGD with palisaded neutrophilic granulomatous dermatitis (PNGD), and interstitial granulomatous drug reaction, as discussed further on.

Differentiation of subcutaneous granuloma annulare from a rheumatoid nodule is not always possible on histologic grounds, but subcutaneous granuloma annulare is more likely than rheumatoid nodule to show prominent mucin and less likely to show foreign-body giant cells or prominent stromal fibrosis or abundant fibrin (46).

Finally, it should be remembered that granuloma annulare and other palisading granulomas may be simulated by epithelioid sarcoma, a lesion that may also contain mucin. Clues to epithelioid sarcoma include ulceration, cytologic atypia, necrotic foci that include necrotic epithelioid cells, and a history of recurrence. Although atypia tends not to be striking, the epithelioid cells in epithelioid sarcoma usually show more nuclear hyperchromasia and pleomorphism, more mitotic figures, larger size, and redder cytoplasm than do the histiocytes of granuloma annulare (68). Immunohistochemically, epithelioid sarcoma can be distinguished from granuloma annulare by positivity for epithelial membrane antigen and keratins and loss of INI1 (69–71). Whereas a variety of keratins may be present in epithelioid sarcoma, the most common is cytokeratin 8/CAM 5.2, present in 94% of cases (72).

Principles of Management: Granuloma annulare, especially if asymptomatic, does not need to be treated, particularly because lesions may resolve spontaneously. If a patient desires treatment, first-line medications include topical and intralesional corticosteroids for localized disease and a variety of treatments ranging from phototherapy to antimalarials, antibiotics, nicotinamide, systemic immunosuppressive agents, and molecularly targeted therapies, including tumor necrosis factor (TNF)-α and Janus kinase (JAK) inhibitors for more severe disease (49,73).

Table 14-1

Histopathologic Differences between Granuloma Annulare and Other Selected Palisading Entities

Entity	Pattern and Location	Material within Palisades	Inflammatory Cells	Other Distinguishing Features
Granuloma annulare	Superficial +/− deep dermis Circular palisades	Abundant mucin +/− Fragmented neutrophils	Perivascular lymphocytes Few giant cells and plasma cells	Normal collagen outside of palisades
Annular elastolytic giant-cell granuloma	Upper dermis, usually Central loss of elastic fibers, zone of giant cells with elastophagocytosis and zone of solar elastosis	Dermis lacking elastic fibers	Giant cells with engulfed elastic fibers	
Necrobiosis lipoidica	Pandermal, usually Linear arrays of histiocytes in tiers	Necrobiotic/sclerotic collagen	Prominent giant cells and plasma cells	Cholesterol clefts Dermal sclerosis Thickened blood vessel walls Lymphoid follicles
Rheumatoid nodule	Deep dermis (sometimes subcutis) Circular palisades	Fibrin	Histiocytes and giant cells	
Palisaded neutrophilic and granulomatous dermatitis	Dermal and perivascular	Fibrin and neutrophilic dust	Intact neutrophils Neutrophilic dust	Leukocytoclastic vasculitis-like changes early
Foreign-body granulomas	Variable	Foreign	Foreign-body giant cells	Often polarizable
Necrobiotic xanthogranuloma	Pandermal Palisading may be subtle	Necrotic dermis	Prominent multinucleated giant cells Foamy histiocytes Touton giant cells Plasma cells	Cholesterol clefts Lymphoid follicles
Gout	Circular to irregular palisades	Amorphous material with a feathery, crystalline outline	Histiocytes	Crystals rarely evident with polarization

ANNULAR ELASTOLYTIC GIANT-CELL GRANULOMA

Clinical Summary. Annular elastolytic giant-cell granuloma is the name that is currently favored for a condition with unclear nosologic status, and it is uncertain whether it is truly distinct from granuloma annulare (74–76). It almost always occurs on sun-exposed skin, such as the face, neck, dorsum of the hand, forearm, and upper outer arm; hence the previous name *actinic granuloma* (77,78) (Fig. 14-6); however, coincident lesions in non–sun-exposed skin may also be present in such patients. The appearance of lesions after prolonged tanning bed use has been reported (79). Overall, it remains unclear whether this entity represents a photo-induced subtype of granuloma annulare or simply granuloma annulare appearing on sun-damaged skin.

The lesions clinically resemble granuloma annulare. They are typically large, somewhat annular plaques. The border may be serpiginous and is slightly raised and pearly to pink to occasionally red-brown. The central zone may show hypopigmentation

and/or atrophy. Smaller papules may also occur, and lesions may be solitary, few, or numerous (78,80,81). Other names under which these lesions have been described include *atypical necrobiosis lipoidica of the face and scalp* (82), *Miescher granuloma of the face* (81), *granuloma multiforme* (80), and *actinic granuloma of O'Brien*.

Histopathology. The histologic features are best appreciated in a radial biopsy that contains the central zone, the elevated border, and the skin peripheral to the ring (78,80,81). The central zone shows the hallmark of the disease, that is, near or total absence of elastic fibers, best appreciated with an elastic tissue stain (e.g., Verhoeff-van Gieson) (Figs. 14-7 to 14-9). The collagen in this zone may show horizontally oriented fibers, producing a slightly scar-like appearance (Fig. 14-7). By contrast, the zone peripheral to the annulus shows an increased amount of thick elastotic material with the staining properties of elastic tissue. The transitional zone at the raised border shows a granulomatous infiltrate with either of the patterns seen in granuloma annulare, that is, histiocytes arranged interstitially between

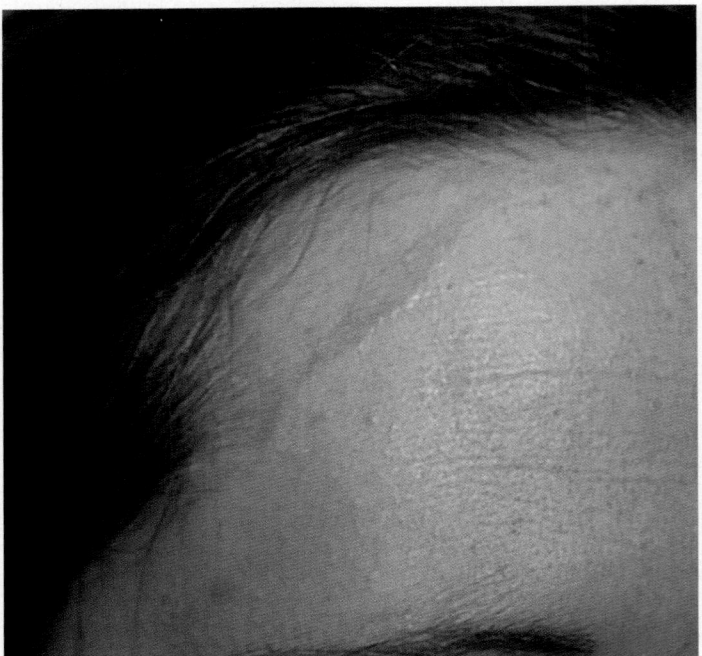

Figure 14-6 Annular elastolytic granuloma. Annular pink plaque, with somewhat serpiginous borders, on the forehead. (Courtesy of Yale Dermatology Residents' Collection.)

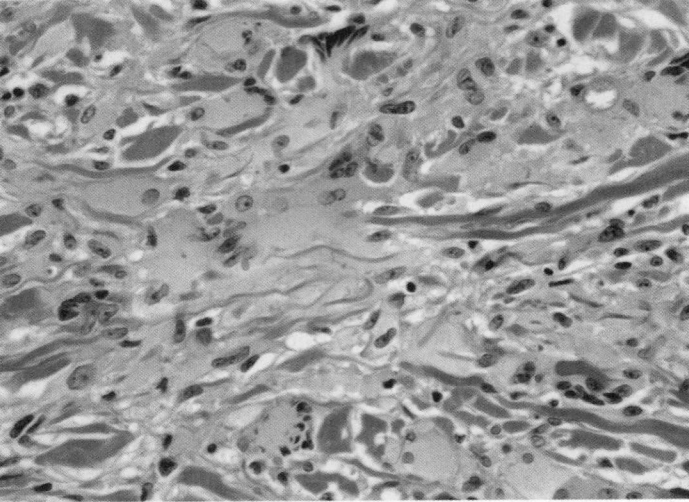

Figure 14-8 Annular elastolytic granuloma. Some multinucleated histiocytes have ingested blue-gray elastic fibers.

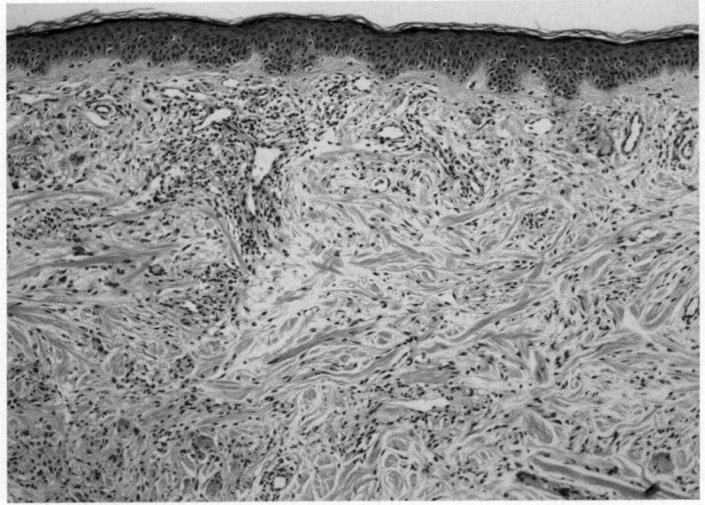

Figure 14-7 Annular elastolytic granuloma. Multinucleated histiocytes on the left abut connective tissue at the center of the lesion that is slightly fibrotic; mucin is not apparent.

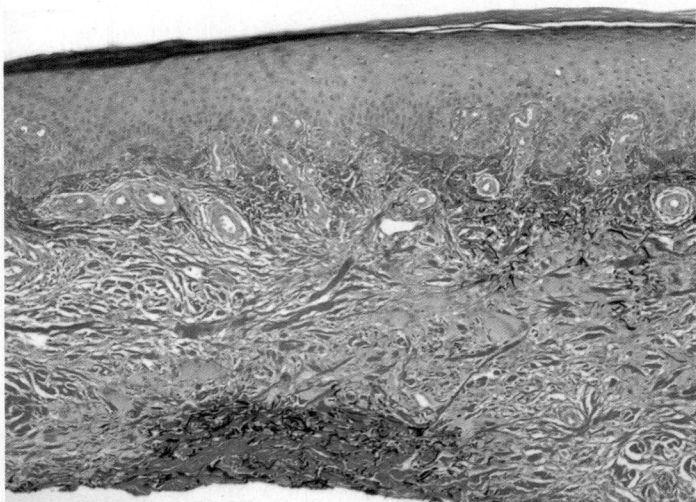

Figure 14-9 Annular elastolytic granuloma. Elastic tissue stain shows absence of elastic fibers in the center of the lesion.

collagen bundles or, less commonly, in a palisade. Occasionally, there are contiguous epithelioid histiocytes in small clusters. Multinucleated histiocytes are conspicuous, usually being large and containing as many as a dozen nuclei, mostly in haphazard arrangement but sometimes in a ringed array. Elastotic fibers are present adjacent to and within the giant cells (Fig. 14-8). Asteroid bodies that stain like elastic fibers may be found in the giant cells (81). The infiltrate also contains lymphocytes and often some plasma cells. Mucin is inapparent (74).

Differential Diagnosis. The principal differential diagnosis is granuloma annulare, which may in fact be an artificial distinction. Because engulfment of abnormal elastic fibers can also occur in granuloma annulare (39) as well as in other granulomatous processes, it has been argued that the elastophagocytosis

of annular elastolytic giant-cell granuloma does not qualify it as a distinct entity (75). Although some elastolysis has also been described in granuloma annulare (80), it is the complete loss of elastic tissue in the central zone that has been used as the primary basis for separating the diseases. Other features that have been evoked for distinguishing them are the presence of larger and more numerous giant cells, the absence of mucin in annular elastolytic giant-cell granuloma (78,83), and sparing of areas that lack elastic tissue, such as scars (84).

Necrobiosis lipoidica differs by the lack of a central zone of elastolysis and the presence of degenerated collagen, sclerosis, and, in some circumstances, lipids and vascular changes. Furthermore, annular elastolytic giant-cell granuloma involves mostly the upper and middle dermis, whereas necrobiosis lipoidica tends to affect the entire dermis and sometimes the subcutis. Foreign-body granulomas generally have more distinct collections of epithelioid histiocytes, lack zonation in the density of elastic fibers, and often have identifiable foreign material.

Principles of Management: This condition is often chronic and generally responds poorly to topical/intralesional corticosteroids.

Other treatment approaches are typically borrowed from those used in granuloma annulare and include hydroxychloroquine. Photoprotection is typically advised, whereas ultraviolet light treatment and potentially photosensitizing tetracycline antibiotics may be avoided.

NECROBIOSIS LIPOIDICA

Clinical Summary. Necrobiosis lipoidica is an idiopathic disorder typified by indurated plaques of the shins (Fig. 14-10). In 1966, Muller and Winkelman (85) reported that two-thirds of patients with necrobiosis lipoidica had overt diabetes at the time of diagnosis; however, more recent studies have suggested the number with diabetes may be significantly less (86). In a recent larger series, 56% to 58.5% of patients had diabetes; with type 2 diabetes predominating slightly over type 1 (87,88). Diabetes was more common in younger patients. However, of all patients with diabetes, fewer than 1% develop necrobiosis lipoidica (86). Some reports have suggested that necrobiosis lipoidica heralds a more rapid progression of diabetes in patients with that disorder and may suggest an increased likelihood of end-organ microvascular damage, including retinopathy and earlier renal dysfunction (89); however, this possible association needs further study. There is an approximately 5-to-1 female-to-male preponderance (85,87,88). Hyperlipidemia (52%), hypertension (44%), and thyroid disease (24.5%) are also commonly seen (87).

In well-developed necrobiosis lipoidica, one observes one or several sharply but irregularly demarcated plaques. The lower legs (especially the shins) are involved in 98% of cases (87). Usually, lesions are bilateral, but only a single lesion is present in about one-third of patients (87). Well-developed lesions appear yellow-brown in the center and more actively inflamed with pink-red, orange, or violaceous erythema at the periphery. Whereas the periphery of the lesions is raised, the center of the lesions gradually becomes atrophic, shows telangiectasia, and may ulcerate. When lesions first begin, pink-red to red-brown papules can be observed. In addition to the shins, lesions may be present elsewhere on the lower extremities, including the ankles, calves, thighs, popliteal fossae, and feet. Rarely, the head and abdomen are affected. Necrobiosis lipoidica with lesions exclusively outside the legs is extremely rare; although it is reported to occur in 1% to 2% of patients (85,87), alternate diagnoses should be considered in these instances.

Lesions located in areas other than the legs may appear raised and firm and may have a papular, nodular, or plaque-like appearance without atrophy. Clinically, they may resemble or overlap with granuloma annulare (85,90). Involvement of the scalp by large, atrophic plaques occurs occasionally and must be differentiated from sarcoidosis and necrobiotic xanthogranuloma (91–94).

In rare instances, transepidermal elimination of degenerated material takes place in necrobiosis lipoidica, producing small hyperkeratotic plugs within a plaque (95,96). Necrobiosis lipoidica is reported to occasionally coexist with sarcoidosis (97) or granuloma annulare (34). Rare examples of squamous cell carcinoma arising in lesions of necrobiosis lipoidica have been reported (98–101).

Histopathology. Usually, the entire thickness of the dermis or its lower two-thirds is affected by a process that exhibits a variable degree of granulomatous inflammation, degeneration of collagen, and sclerosis (Figs. 14-11 and 14-12). Histologic changes of necrobiosis lipoidica may be seen in subcutaneous septa (102,103). Occasionally, only the upper dermis is affected (40,43,55,85). The epidermis may be normal, atrophic, or hyperkeratotic. In some instances, the surface of the biopsy shows ulceration. The granulomatous component is usually conspicuous, and the histiocytes may or may not be arranged in a palisade. Occasionally, there are just a few scattered epithelioid histiocytes and giant cells. The latter picture is more likely to occur in sections in which sclerosis is extensive, and occasionally in such biopsies several sections must be examined before a granulomatous component becomes apparent. Giant cells are usually of the Langhans- or foreign-body type;

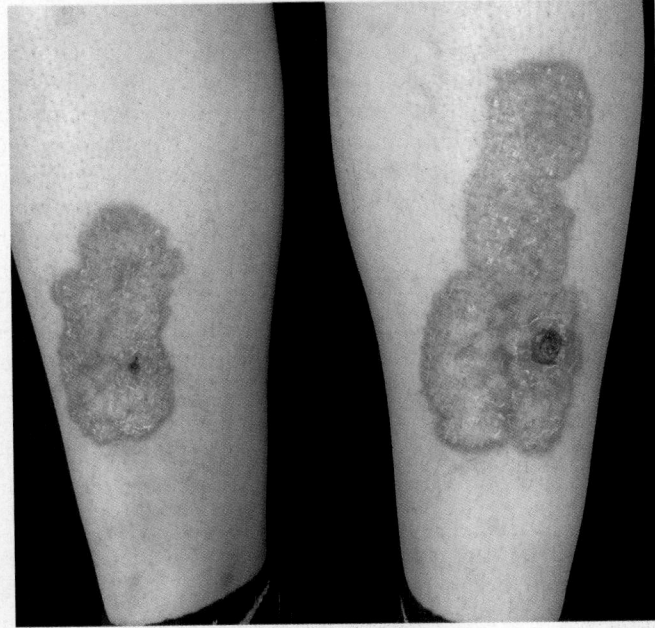

Figure 14-10 Necrobiosis lipoidica. Waxy, red-yellow plaque with raised borders, central atrophy, and fine telangiectasia on the shins. Focal ulceration is present.

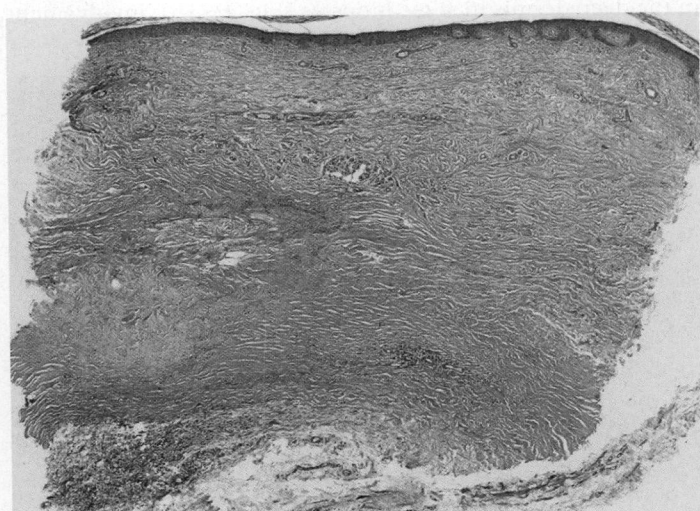

Figure 14-11 Necrobiosis lipoidica. The presence of sclerosis can be identified by the relatively straight edges of the punch biopsy. The infiltrate involves the full thickness of the dermis and is arranged in a tier-like fashion.

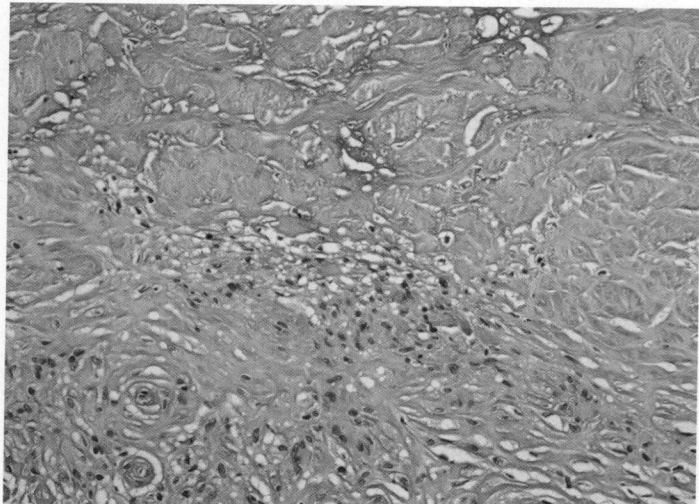

Figure 14-12 Necrobiosis lipoidica. Histiocytes, lymphocytes, and degenerated collagen are present.

occasionally, Touton cells or asteroid bodies (104) are seen. If the histiocytes are arranged in a palisade, the palisades tend to be somewhat horizontally oriented and/or vaguely tiered. Occasionally, histiocytes may be seen to completely encircle altered connective tissue, particularly degenerated collagen, but, more commonly, altered connective tissue is incompletely surrounded by histiocytes. This alteration of connective tissue has also been referred to as "necrobiosis." The altered collagen appears different from normal collagen by having a paler, grayer hue and by appearing more fragmented and haphazardly arranged; it may also appear more compact or smudged (Fig. 14-12). Areas of sclerosis with a diminished number of fibroblasts can be seen. A clue to the presence of sclerosis can be found by looking at the edges of the biopsy specimen, which tend to be straight with less of the inward retraction of the dermis ordinarily associated with punch biopsies ("squared appearance") (Fig. 14-11). Increased mucin is usually inapparent or subtle in contrast to granuloma annulare. Other findings include a sparse to moderately dense, primarily perivascular lymphocytic infiltrate, with plasma cells in the deep dermis in some biopsies (Fig. 14-13), involvement

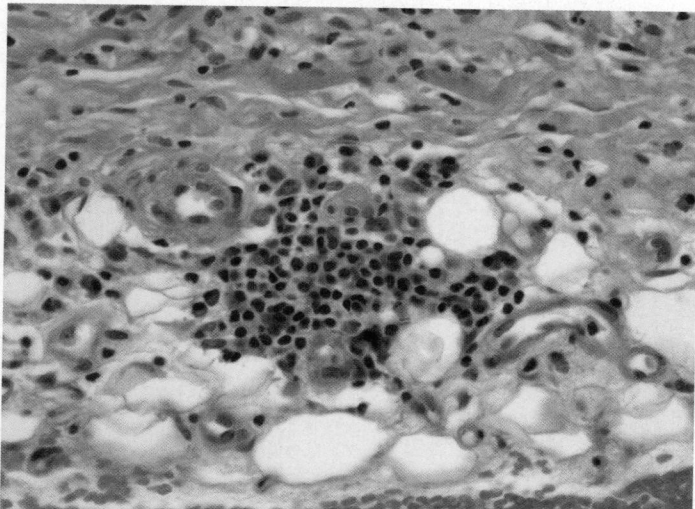

Figure 14-13 Necrobiosis lipoidica. Plasma cells at the dermal–subcutaneous junction are a typical finding.

of the upper subcutis with thickened fibrous septa, and lipid that may be present in foamy histiocytes or that may be inferred from the presence of cholesterol clefts (seen in <1% of cases) (105). Deep lymphoid follicles may be present (106). Older lesions show vascular ectasia superficially. Blood vessels, particularly in the middle and lower dermis, often exhibit thickened walls in lesions of the lower legs. The thickened walls may be infiltrated with periodic acid–Schiff (PAS)–positive, diastase-resistant material (43). Vascular changes of this type are seen particularly near foci containing thickened, hyalinized collagen bundles.

Pathogenesis. The cause of necrobiosis lipoidica is unknown. Historically, it had been postulated that degeneration of collagen could be a primary event; however, this view has largely fallen out of favor. Some authors have postulated that the degeneration of collagen is the result of vascular changes secondary to clinical or latent diabetes (107). However, evidence against a vascular cause includes (1) the absence of vascular pathology in approximately one-third of biopsies examined (85), (2) the fact that vessels that are affected are often situated in the lower dermis and are of a larger caliber than the vessels affected by diabetic microangiopathy. Further, it is now clear that many patients that develop necrobiosis lipoidica do not have diabetes (87). More recent avenues of investigation have focused on cytokine-producing lymphocyte populations in necrobiosis lipoidica lesions and frame necrobiosis as a primarily inflammatory process (108,109); there are observations showing improvement of necrobiosis lipoidica with anti-inflammatory (110,111) and cytokine inhibiting therapies (112,113).

Electron microscopic examination shows degenerative changes in collagen and elastin with loss of cross-striation in collagen fibrils. Collagen synthesis by fibroblasts is diminished (114).

Direct immunofluorescence studies have shown that necrobiotic foci contain fibrinogen. Deposits of immunoglobulin and C3 in the vessel walls have been reported (115,116) but are not a consistent finding (117).

Differential Diagnosis. See Table 14-1 for differentiation of necrobiosis lipoidica from granuloma annulare. Differentiation of necrobiosis lipoidica from annular elastolytic granuloma was discussed in the section on annular elastolytic granuloma. Occasionally, necrobiosis lipoidica shows discrete collections of epithelioid cells that may resemble those seen in sarcoidosis (93); however, significant alteration of the collagen is usually present in necrobiosis lipoidica and absent in sarcoidosis (93).

Necrobiotic xanthogranuloma with paraproteinemia can simulate necrobiosis lipoidica but differs by showing a denser, more diffuse infiltrate with many more foamy histiocytes, Touton giant cells, more extensive inflammation of the subcutis, and greater disruption of normal subcutaneous architecture. Lymphoid follicles and cholesterol clefts are more commonly seen in necrobiotic xanthogranuloma than in necrobiosis lipoidica (118).

Principles of Management: No treatment has been proven to be effective in large studies. Potent topical or intralesional corticosteroids are first-line therapy (119). In patients with diabetes, optimal glucose control is typically advised; however, the role of glucose control in the appearance and clinical course of necrobiosis lipoidica lesions remains debated (120).

RHEUMATOID NODULES

Clinical Summary. Rheumatoid nodules are deeply seated firm masses that occur in patients with rheumatoid arthritis, particularly over extensor prominences, such as the proximal ulna, the olecranon process, and the metacarpophalangeal and proximal interphalangeal joints (121). They may occur elsewhere, such as the back of the hands, over amputation stumps (122), with rare reports of extracutaneous involvement of the lung, heart, and central nervous system (123–125). The nodules vary in size from a few millimeters to several centimeters and may be solitary or numerous. Rarely, rheumatoid nodules show a central draining perforation (126). Rheumatoid factor is almost always elevated. Rarely, nodules may precede apparent joint disease (121). The rapid appearance of many small rheumatoid nodules has been reported in some patients treated with methotrexate and rarely with other disease-modifying antirheumatic drugs. This presentation has been termed accelerated rheumatoid nodulosis (127,128). The term rheumatoid nodulosis has also been proposed for the clinical presentation of multiple nodules on the hands/elbows with intermittent arthralgias/arthritis but no evidence of systemic rheumatoid arthritis (129).

Pseudorheumatoid nodule is a term that has been applied to nodules in the subcutis that mimic rheumatoid nodules histologically but that develop in the absence of joint pain, rheumatoid arthritis, or systemic lupus erythematosus (13,19). These occur in children or adults. The subsequent development of rheumatoid arthritis occurs infrequently in adults and rarely, if ever, in children. Because some of these nodules occur in patients with other lesions that are typical of dermal granuloma annulare (13), the nodules are now generally considered to represent a subcutaneous variant of granuloma annulare.

Histopathology. Rheumatoid nodules occur in the subcutis and deep dermis. They exhibit one or several areas of fibrinoid degeneration of collagen that stain homogeneously red (Fig. 14-14). Nuclear fragments and basophilic material are often present, but mucin is almost always minimal or absent (46). These foci of degenerative change are surrounded by histiocytes in a palisade. Foreign-body giant cells are present in approximately 50% of biopsies (46). In the surrounding stroma, there is a proliferation of blood vessels associated with fibrosis. A sparse infiltrate of other inflammatory cells is associated with the histiocytes and surrounding stroma. Lymphocytes and neutrophils are most common, but mast cells, plasma cells, and eosinophils may be present. Occasionally, lipid is seen (46). Vasculitis has been described (130) but is not usually encountered (46). In perforating rheumatoid nodules, the central fibrinoid material extends through the skin surface (126).

Pathogenesis. The pathogenesis of rheumatoid nodules is not well understood but appears to be the result of dysregulated inflammation, possibly related to an aberrant T-cell response (131–133) Other proposed factors include trauma and vasculitis.

Differential Diagnosis. The principal differential diagnosis is subcutaneous granuloma annulare, which was discussed in the section on granuloma annulare. A distinction should be made from epithelioid sarcoma, also covered in that section. Nonabsorbable sutures or other foreign material may produce periarticular palisaded granulomas like those of rheumatoid nodule (56,134); in such instances, there should be a history of previous surgery or trauma, and birefringent material may be visible under polarized light. Rheumatic fever may produce nodules (rheumatic nodules), especially over the elbows, knees, scalp, knuckles, ankles, and spine, which were confused with rheumatoid nodules in the early 20th century (135,136). Histologically, a rheumatic fever nodule is less likely to show central, homogeneous fibrinoid necrosis. A palisade of histiocytes is usually not as well developed, and fibrosis is minimal or absent (123,135). Rarely, an infectious process, such as cryptococcosis, can produce a deep, palisaded granuloma. It can be differentiated from rheumatoid nodule because the palisade surrounds primarily necrotic debris and organisms rather than fibrinoid material.

Principles of Management: Treatment of rheumatoid arthritis may improve rheumatoid nodules. For particularly symptomatic rheumatoid nodules, intralesional corticosteroids or surgical excision can be effective.

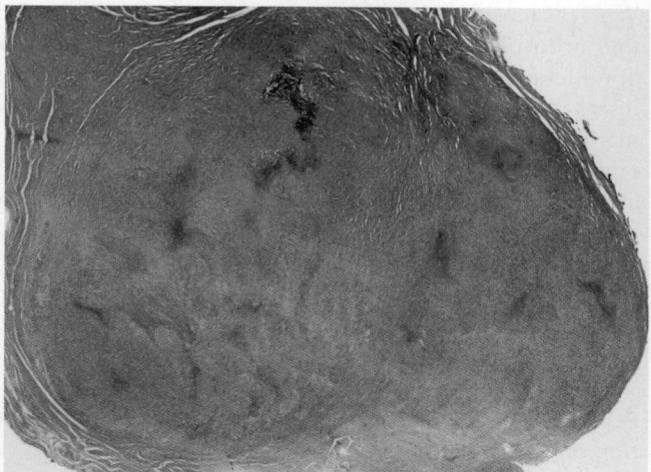
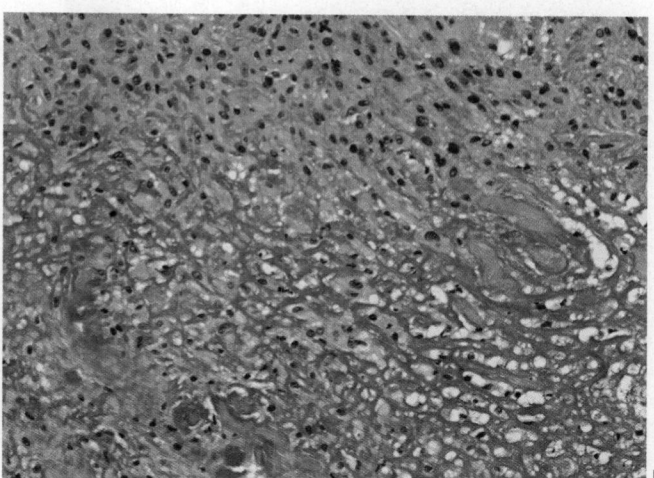

Figure 14-14 Rheumatoid nodule. **A:** A deeply seated, circumscribed nodule exhibits palisading around basophilic material. **B:** Fibrin is surrounded by histiocytes in a palisaded arrangement.

PALISADED NEUTROPHILIC & GRANULOMATOUS DERMATITIS

Clinical Summary. The classic clinical presentation is umbilicated papules on extensor surfaces, especially the elbows in a patient with an associated collagen-vascular disease (137) (Fig. 14-15). Lesions previously termed Churg–Strauss *granuloma*, Winkelmann granuloma, cutaneous extravascular necrotizing granuloma, rheumatoid papules (138,139), and superficial ulcerating rheumatoid necrobiosis (137,140,141) present in a similar fashion and may represent the same condition. Over time, small case reports and case series have expanded the clinical spectrum of PNGD from the classic lesion to additional morphologies, with PNGD diagnosed histologically. Reported clinical morphologies include erythematous nodules (142–144), pink-red plaques that may be annular (143,145–148), and even linear bands (142,149). Thus, there exists considerable overlap of this expanded concept of PNGD with IGD, and some authors have proposed the umbrella term reactive granulomatous dermatitis to address this and have also included interstitial granulomatous drug reaction within this designation (150,151).

Histopathology. There are three sometimes overlapping histologic patterns in this rare condition: (a) early lesions resembling leukocytoclastic vasculitis but with broader cuffs of fibrin around vessel walls and abundant dermal basophilic nuclear debris, (b) fully developed lesions with a granuloma annulare–like appearance but associated with prominent neutrophils and neutrophilic dust (Figs. 14-16 and 14-17), and (c) a fibrosing, necrobiosis lipoidica–like final stage, sometimes with a sparse, superficial, and deep perivascular infiltrate of lymphocytes and eosinophils (see Table 14-2) (137,142,151). These differing histologic patterns may represent a temporal evolution of the disease from early, evolving lesions to late, fully developed lesions.

Pathogenesis. Palisaded neutrophilic and granulomatous dermatitis has been associated with a wide variety of conditions and

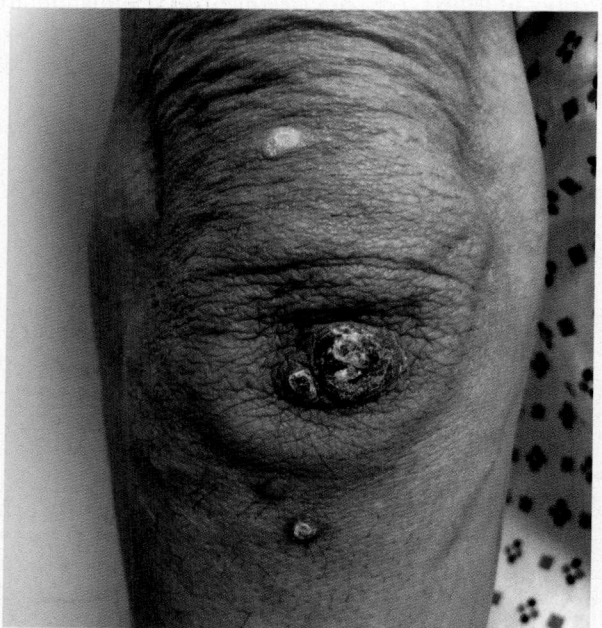

Figure 14-15 Palisaded neutrophilic and granulomatous dermatitis. Umbilicated and centrally crusted erythematous papules and plaques on the elbow. (Courtesy of Dr. Jeffrey Gehlhausen.)

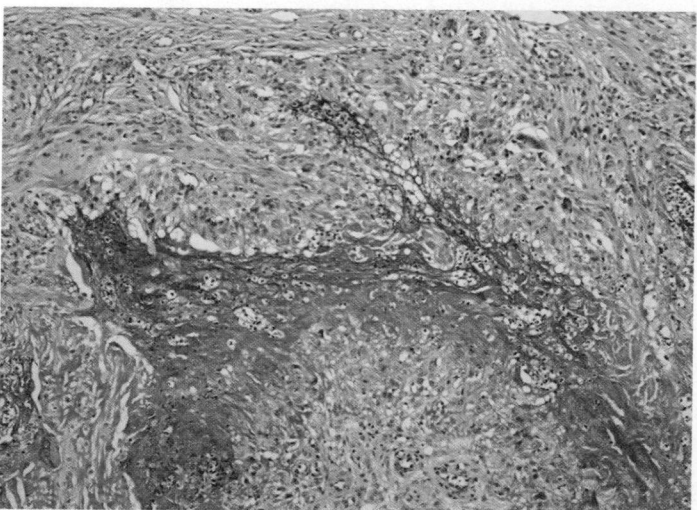

Figure 14-16 Palisaded neutrophilic and granulomatous dermatitis. This fully developed lesion exhibits palisades of histiocytes, associated with neutrophils, basophilic debris, mucin, and degenerated collagen.

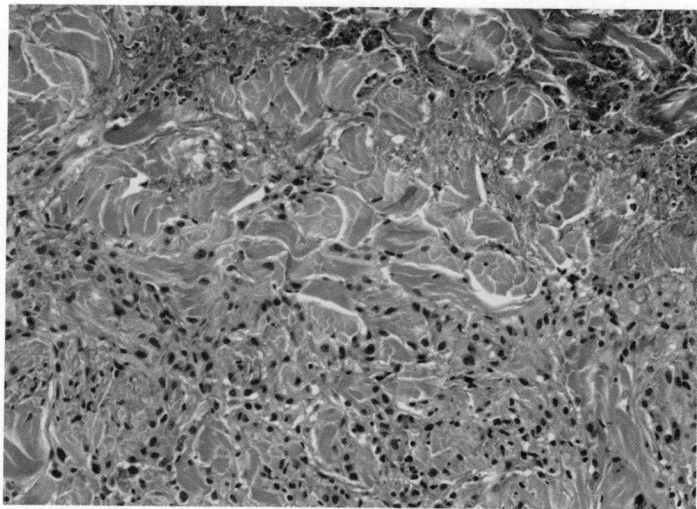

Figure 14-17 Palisaded neutrophilic and granulomatous dermatitis. Neutrophilic dust and intact neutrophils are present in the centers of the palisades, accompanied by degenerated collagen bundles, fibrin, and mucin.

is rarely reported in the absence of underlying systemic disease. Whereas most are connective tissue disorders, such as rheumatoid arthritis or lupus erythematosus, others include lymphoproliferative disorders, inflammatory bowel disease, thyroid disease, diabetes mellitus, medications, and infections, particularly bacterial endocarditis (137,152). This condition may represent an unusual immune complex–mediated vasculitis or a poorly understood primary inflammatory process. Immunoglobulin M and C3 have been identified in small-vessel walls. The changes seen in fully developed lesions are believed by some to be a response to the vasculitic changes accompanying ischemia and enzymatic degradation by neutrophils.

Differential Diagnosis. See Tables 14-1 and 14-2.

Principles of Management: PNGD usually occurs in the setting of a systemic disease, and therapy is generally targeted at the underlying disease. Treatment of localized lesions with topical or intralesional corticosteroids may be helpful. Antimalarials and dapsone have also been used successfully (153).

Table 14-2

Differential Diagnosis of Palisaded Neutrophilic and Granulomatous Dermatitis

Palisaded Neutrophilic and Granulomatous Dermatitis	Differential Diagnosis
Early lesion	Leukocytoclastic vasculitis
	Erythema elevatum diutinum
Fully developed lesion	Granuloma annulare
	Eosinophilic granulomatosis and polyangiitis (Churg–Strauss)
	Granulomatosis and polyangiitis (Wegener)
	Granulomatous drug reaction
	Infectious process
Final stage	Necrobiosis lipoidica

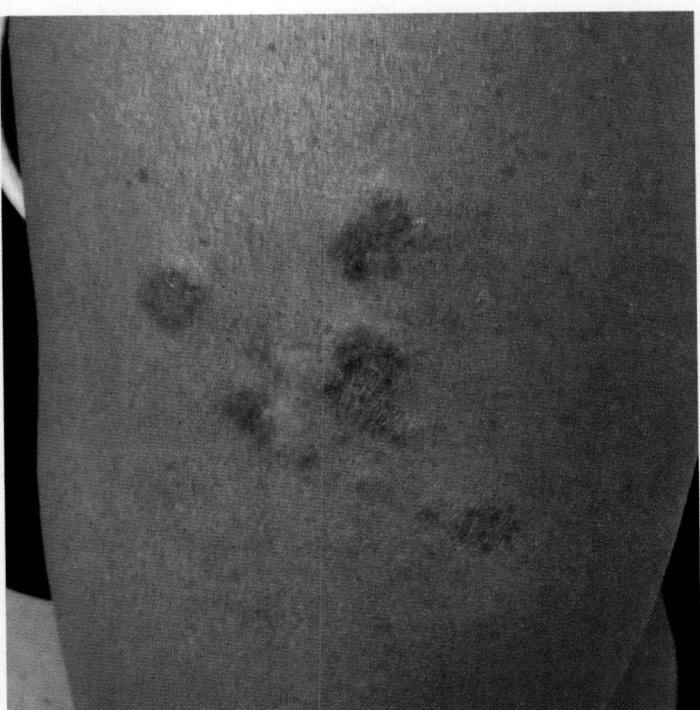

Figure 14-18 Sarcoidosis. Pink-brown papules and plaques, some with an annular configuration on the upper arm.

SARCOIDOSIS

Clinical Summary. Sarcoidosis is a granulomatous disease of undetermined cause. Although it typically affects multiple organ systems simultaneously, only individual organs, including the skin, may be involved. A distinction is made between the subacute, transient type of sarcoidosis and the chronic, persistent type.

In subacute transient sarcoidosis, erythema nodosum is associated with hilar adenopathy, fever, and, in some cases, migrating polyarthritis and acute iritis, termed Löfgren syndrome. The disease generally subsides in most patients within a few months without sequelae (154–156). Occasionally, there is an enlargement of subcutaneous lymph nodes.

In systemic sarcoidosis, cutaneous lesions are encountered in approximately 25% of patients (157–161).

The incidence of sarcoidosis is highest in Scandinavian countries and among African Americans (162–166). The average age of onset is 40 to 55 years of age; it is very rare in children (167–169). A rare genetic disorder, Blau syndrome, may present in childhood and mimic sarcoidosis. This autosomal dominant disorder, related to mutations in the *NOD2* gene (170,171), is marked by granulomatous inflammation of the skin, uveal tract, and joints, notably sparing the lungs (172,173).

The most common cutaneous lesions of sarcoidosis are pink-red to red-brown papules and plaques that are often annular (157) (Fig. 14-18). Sarcoidosis is one of the "great mimickers," and almost every cutaneous morphologic lesion type is possible. When papules or plaques of sarcoidosis are situated on the nose, cheeks, and ears, the term *lupus pernio* is applied (174). This presentation has been associated with upper respiratory involvement and greater disease severity (157,174,175).

Less common manifestations of sarcoidosis include lichenoid, ichthyosiform, psoriasiform, atrophic, ulcerative, verrucous, angiolupoid, hypopigmented, alopecic, and morpheaform variants. Sarcoidosis may also present as dactylitis and/or nail dystrophy (176). Lichenoid sarcoidosis manifests with small, flat papules that may mimic lichen planus clinically (177). In ichthyosiform sarcoidosis, ichthyotic changes favor the lower extremities (178), but at times they may also

be present elsewhere on the skin (179,180). Rarely, there are extensive atrophic lesions that may ulcerate (181–183). Multiple ulcers have also been described in plaque-like lesions (184). Angiolupoid sarcoidosis is characterized by a prominent telangiectatic component (185,186). Lesions of hypopigmented sarcoidosis appear macular with or without an associated papular or nodular component (187,188). Sarcoidosis can also present with subcutaneous nodules. Originally described by Darier and Roussy (189), they may occur in association with more typical dermally based cutaneous lesions or alone (190). Several medications have been associated with the development of sarcoidosis, including interferon-α, often in the setting of hepatitis C treatment (191), immune checkpoint inhibitor therapy (e.g., anti-CTLA-4 or anti-PD-1) (30), and, paradoxically, with cytokine blocking antibodies, including TNF-α and IL-17 inhibitors (192).

Systemic sarcoidosis has rarely been reported to coexist with granuloma annulare (35). Cutaneous lesions of sarcoidosis may localize to areas of scarring, including herpes zoster scars (193,194). Tattoos (195,196), exogenous ochronosis (197), or other exogenous materials in the skin (198) may serve as a nidus for cutaneous lesions in patients with sarcoidosis. Two studies demonstrated polarizable foreign material in approximately 20% of cutaneous sarcoidal lesions from patients with systemic sarcoidosis (199,200).

Histopathology. The lesions of erythema nodosum occurring in subacute, transient sarcoidosis have the same histologic appearance as "idiopathic" erythema nodosum (201).

Like lesions in other organs, the cutaneous lesions of chronic, persistent sarcoidosis are characterized by the presence of circumscribed collections of epithelioid histiocytes—so-called epithelioid cell tubercles—that show little or no necrosis (Figs. 14-19 and 14-20).

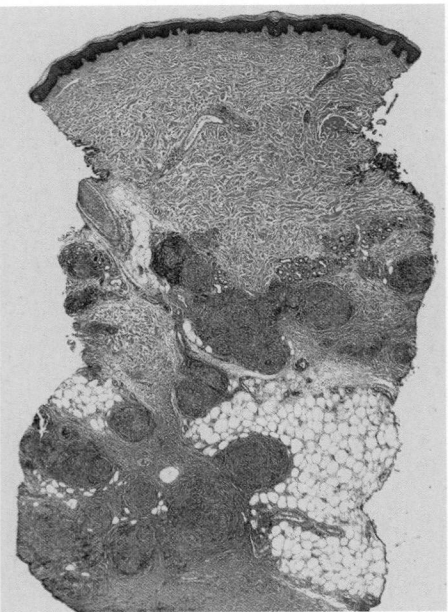

Figure 14-19 Sarcoidosis. There are well-circumscribed, nodular collections of epithelioid histiocytes in the dermis. This example also shows subcutaneous involvement, which is less common than purely dermal involvement.

The papules, plaques, and lupus pernio–type lesions show variously sized aggregates of epithelioid histiocytes scattered irregularly through the dermis with occasional extension into the subcutis (202,203). Typical sarcoidal granulomas are found in the ichthyosiform lesions (179), in ulcerated areas (184), and in atrophic lesions (204,205). Verrucous sarcoidosis exhibits prominent associated acanthosis and hyperkeratosis (206,207). Biopsies of hypopigmented sarcoidosis should reveal granulomas (188). In subcutaneous nodules, larger epithelioid cell tubercles lie in the subcutaneous fat (208).

In typical cutaneous lesions of sarcoidosis, the well-demarcated islands of epithelioid cells contain few, if any, giant cells. Those that are present are usually of the Langhans type. A moderate number of giant cells can be found in old lesions. These giant cells may be large and irregular in shape. In a minority of cases, giant cells contain asteroid bodies or

Schaumann bodies (209). Asteroid bodies (Fig. 14-21), which are more common, are star-shaped eosinophilic structures that, when stained with phosphotungstic acid–hematoxylin (PTAH), produce a center that is brown-red with radiating blue spikes (210). Schaumann bodies are round or oval, laminated, and calcified, especially at their periphery. They stain dark blue because of the presence of calcium. Neither of these two bodies is specific for sarcoidosis: They have been observed in a variety of other granulomas, including those of leprosy, tuberculosis, foreign-body reactions, and necrobiotic xanthogranuloma (210).

Classically, sarcoidosis has been associated with only a sparse lymphocytic infiltrate, particularly at the margins of the epithelioid cell granulomas (Fig. 14-20). Because of the scarcity of lymphocytes, the granulomas have been referred to as "naked" tubercles. However, lymphocytic infiltrates in sarcoidosis may occasionally be dense, as in tuberculosis (Fig. 14-22) (203). Occasionally, small foci of fibrin or necrosis showing eosinophilic staining are found in the center of some of the granulomas (Fig. 14-23) (202,211). A reticular fiber stain (reticulin, or type III collagen) of sarcoidosis revealed a network of

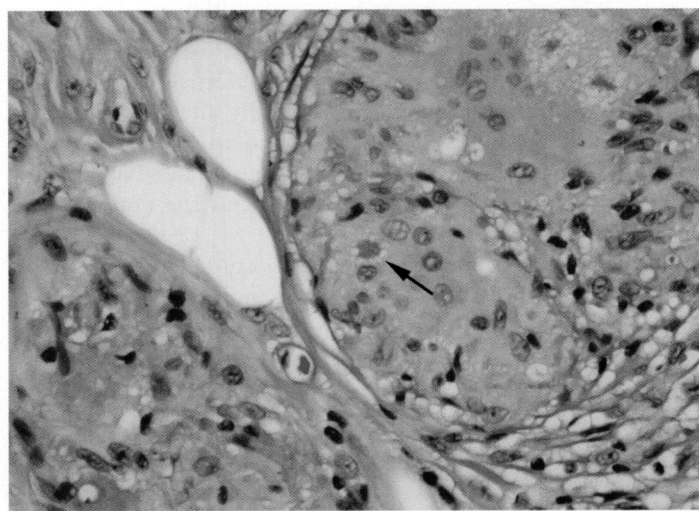

Figure 14-21 Sarcoidosis. Three star-shaped, eosinophilic asteroid bodies are present, one at the *arrow* and two in the upper right.

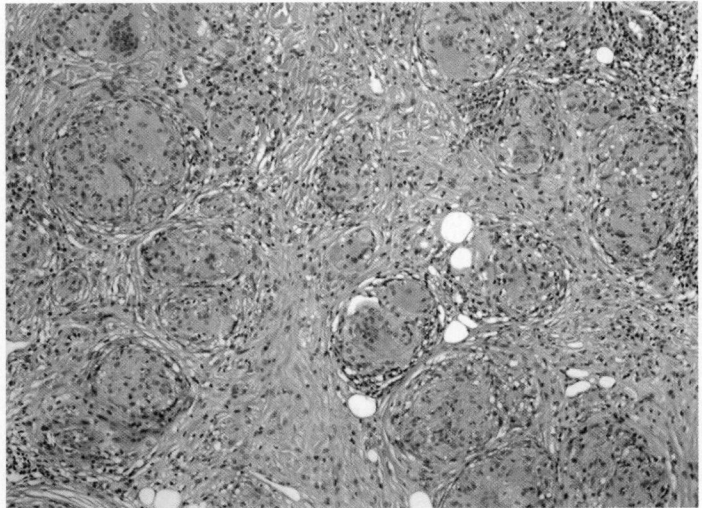

Figure 14-20 Sarcoidosis. Well-circumscribed, roundish collections of epithelioid histiocytes, some multinucleated, with few lymphocytes.

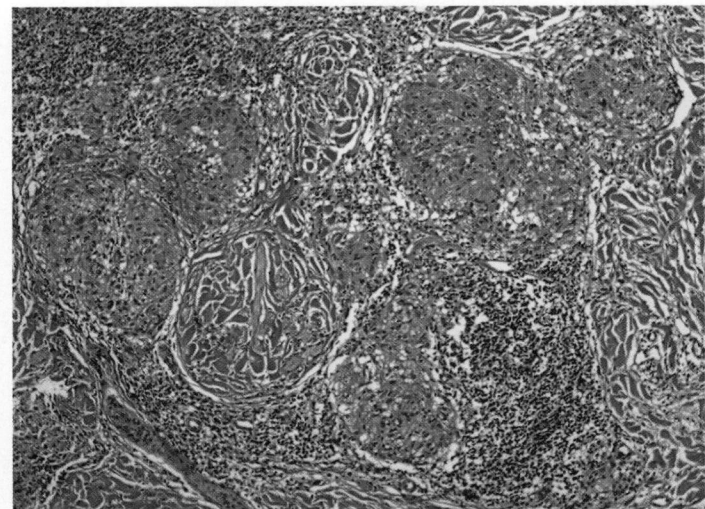

Figure 14-22 Sarcoidosis. A fairly dense lymphocytic infiltrate is associated with the epithelioid histiocytes, a less common finding than the usual "naked tubercles."

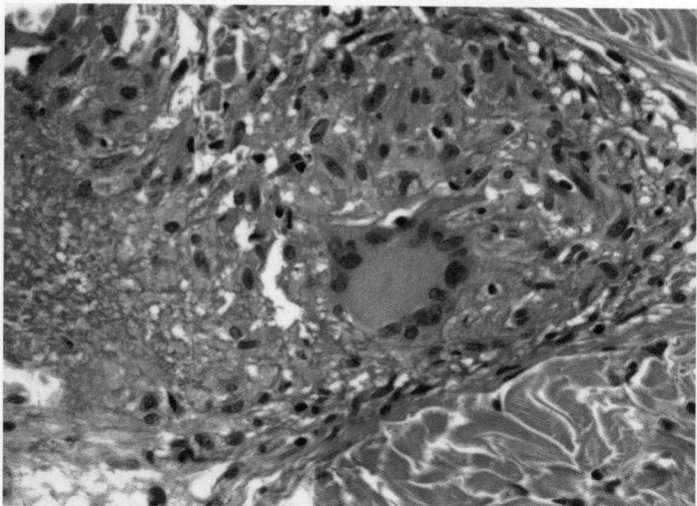

Figure 14-23 Sarcoidosis. On the left is fibrinoid material within the granulomatous component.

reticulin fibers surrounding and permeating the epithelioid cell granulomas. If the granulomas of sarcoidosis involute, fibrosis extends from the periphery toward the center, with gradual disappearance of the epithelioid cells (202). Fibrosis, however, is minimal to absent in most examples of sarcoidosis, with the exception of the uncommon morpheaform variant, where it is prominent (212). Other features that may sometimes be seen include elastophagocytosis, increased dermal mucin, and lichenoid inflammation (213).

Systemic Lesions. The lungs and mediastinal lymph nodes are involved in the vast majority of patients with the chronic, persistent type of sarcoidosis (214). The lesions may be either nodular or diffuse, and parenchymal fibrosis may be present (215,216). Ocular involvement is present in 5% to 23% of patients with sarcoidosis (161). Liver involvement can be seen in 12% to 20% of patients (161). Osseous granulomas may be present, commonly in the phalanges of the fingers and toes. Involved phalanges appear swollen and deformed, often sausage-shaped (e.g., sarcoidal dactylitis) (176). In about 3% to 9% of patients, there can be nervous system involvement, which can present with paresis of the facial nerve (161). Oral mucosal involvement occurs very rarely (199). Myocardial involvement is present in 2% to 5% of patients (161).

Sarcoidosis may be fatal, and mortality rates are significantly higher in African Americans (163). The most common causes of death in sarcoidosis are respiratory failure and cardiac arrest (163). Another serious complication is renal insufficiency resulting from hypercalcemia and hypercalciuria or from sarcoidal nephritis (217). Hypopituitarism from the involvement of either the pituitary gland or the hypothalamus is also a rare and potentially serious complication (218,219).

The diagnosis of sarcoidosis in a patient with systemic disease is based on clinical presentation, biopsy findings, and exclusion of other granulomatous processes. If skin lesions are present, they are an obvious choice for biopsy. In the absence of skin lesions, a Kveim test was frequently used in the past but is now only of historical significance. The Kveim test involved intradermal injection of a heat-sterilized suspension of sarcoidal tissue, particularly the spleen. The site was evaluated 6 weeks later, with a positive result being the formation of a sarcoidosis-like granuloma (220,221).

In the absence of cutaneous lesions, the most accepted alternative approach for confirming a presumptive diagnosis of systemic sarcoidosis is bronchoscopy with endobronchial biopsy and/or transbronchial lung parenchymal biopsy (222) and/or endobronchial ultrasound-guided transbronchial needle aspiration of lymph nodes (223). Less specific ancillary tests, such as serum angiotensin-converting enzyme levels (224) and/or soluble Interleukin 2 receptor (CD25) levels (225) can provide supportive data. Microbiology testing to rule out infectious etiologies should also be considered. Stains for organisms are also typically done; however, it should be recognized that these are not sensitive in ruling out infection.

Pathogenesis. The cause of sarcoidosis is unknown, and the disease may not have the same pathogenesis in all individuals. Seasonal and geographic variation in incidence combined with observed genetic susceptibility (214) suggest that environmental factors (which may include inorganic materials) (226) may trigger inflammation in genetically predisposed individuals. Sarcoidosis has been interpreted, at least in some cases, to be an antigen-dependent, T-cell–driven disorder based on the following observations: (1) the association of sarcoidosis with specific MHC class II alleles (227,228), (2) the presence of expanded T-cell clonotypes in lesions of some individuals, including detection of identical T-cell receptor sequences in different patients (228–231), and (3) the observation that sarcoidosis can be triggered by T-cell–stimulating cancer immunotherapy (30). The actual antigens(s) in sarcoidosis are not well understood, and both endogenous and exogenous antigens have been proposed. For example, in some patients, T-cell reactivity against vimentin has been reported and anti-vimentin autoantibodies are detected in some patients (232,233). Proposed exogenous antigens, including mycobacterial (234,235) and *Cutibacterium* (formerly *Propionibacterium*) *acnes* peptides (236,237), have been detected in lesions, but their significance is not yet resolved. Ultimately, an exaggerated T helper 1 (Th1) polarized immune response ensues and is thought to contribute to granuloma formation (214,238).

Electron microscopic examination of epithelioid cells fails to show any evidence of bacterial fragments, unlike the macrophages seen in granulomas caused by mycobacteria, although the cells contain primary lysosomes; some autophagic vacuoles; and complex, laminated residual bodies (239). The giant cells form through the coalescence of epithelioid cells with partial fusion of their plasma membranes. Schaumann bodies likely arise from laminated residual bodies of lysosomes. Asteroid bodies consist of collagen showing the typical 64 to 70 nm periodicity. It seems likely that this collagen is trapped between epithelioid cells during the stage of giant-cell formation (239).

Differential Diagnosis. The histologic differentiation of sarcoidosis from lupus vulgaris (cutaneous *Mycobacterium tuberculosis* infection) may be very difficult and occasionally impossible. There is no absolute histologic criterion by which the two diseases can be differentiated with certainty. However, as a rule, the infiltrate in sarcoidosis lies scattered throughout the dermis, whereas the infiltrate in lupus vulgaris is located close to the epidermis. Furthermore, sarcoidosis usually shows few lymphoid cells at the periphery of the granulomas, giving them the appearance of "naked" granulomas. By contrast, lupus vulgaris often shows a marked inflammatory reaction around and between the granulomas. The granulomas of sarcoidosis usually show much less central necrosis than the granulomas of lupus vulgaris (240); however, not all biopsies of tuberculosis show necrosis, and some biopsies of sarcoidosis do. The epidermis in sarcoidosis is usually normal or atrophic. In lupus vulgaris, in addition to atrophy, areas of ulceration, acanthosis, and pseudo-carcinomatous hyperplasia are not uncommon. The absence of identifiable mycobacteria with acid-fast stain cannot be used to exclude tuberculosis because the organisms in lupus vulgaris are scarce and may be difficult or impossible to find.

Foreign-body granulomas can also resemble sarcoidosis. Polariscopic examination in search of doubly refractile material, such as silica, should be performed on biopsies suspected of being sarcoidosis. The presence of foreign material does not exclude a concurrent diagnosis of sarcoidosis (209). The papular type of acne rosacea occasionally shows "naked" tubercles indistinguishable from those of sarcoidosis, but unlike sarcoidosis, they are usually perifollicular.

Tuberculoid leprosy, which may show granulomas in association with only a sparse lymphocytic infiltrate, can also be difficult to distinguish from sarcoidosis. Only 7% of cases of tuberculoid leprosy show acid-fast bacilli, and then only a few, and so may easily be overlooked (241). The most likely place to find bacilli is within degenerated dermal nerves (the granulomas of tuberculoid leprosy form around dermal nerves that are undergoing necrosis). The granulomas of tuberculoid leprosy show small areas of central necrosis more often than those of sarcoidosis. In addition, the granulomas of tuberculoid leprosy, in contrast to those of sarcoidosis, follow nerves and therefore often appear elongated (242). Clinical correlation may be required to distinguish between these two diseases. For example, in the United States, leprosy can be virtually excluded if a patient has not been in an endemic area (either in a foreign country or where it is carried in armadillos domestically, e.g., Texas and Louisiana) or has not had prolonged close contact with another individual with the disease.

Principles of Management: Limited cutaneous sarcoidosis is often treated with topical or intralesional corticosteroids. For more widespread involvement, hydroxychloroquine is the first-line choice. More severe or recalcitrant cases may require systemic corticosteroids, methotrexate, or thalidomide. Tetracycline-class antibiotics are sometimes used for skin-limited disease or where cutaneous involvement is the reason for treatment. TNF-α inhibitors (243,244) and JAK inhibitors (245,246) have been used for recalcitrant disease.

FOREIGN-BODY REACTIONS

Clinical Summary. Foreign substances, when injected or implanted accidentally into the skin, can produce a nonallergic foreign-body reaction or, in persons specifically sensitized to them, an allergic response (247). In addition, certain substances formed within the body may produce a nonallergic foreign-body reaction when deposited in the dermis or subcutis. Such endogenous foreign-body reactions are produced, for instance, by urates in gout and by keratinous material in pilomatricoma, as well as in ruptured epidermoid and trichilemmal cysts.

Histopathology. A *nonallergic* foreign-body reaction typically shows a granulomatous response marked by histiocytes and giant cells surrounding foreign material. Often, some of the giant

cells are of the foreign-body type, in which the nuclei are in haphazard array. In addition, lymphocytes are usually present, as may be plasma cells and neutrophils. Frequently, some of the foreign material is seen within macrophages and giant cells, a finding that, of course, is of great diagnostic value. The most common cause of a foreign-body granuloma is rupture of a hair follicle or follicular cyst, and sometimes only the cyst content, rather than residual cyst wall, is identifiable (Fig. 14-24). Exogenous substances producing nonallergic foreign-body reactions include silk and nylon sutures (Fig. 14-25), wood or other plant material (Fig. 14-26), paraffin and other oily substances, silicone gel, talc, surgical glove starch powder, and cactus spines. Some of these substances—nylon sutures, wood, talc, surgical glove starch powder, and sea urchin spines—are doubly refractile on polarizing examination. Double refraction is often very helpful in localizing foreign substances. Knife marks in the section may be an additional clue to the presence of particulate foreign matter (Fig. 14-27).

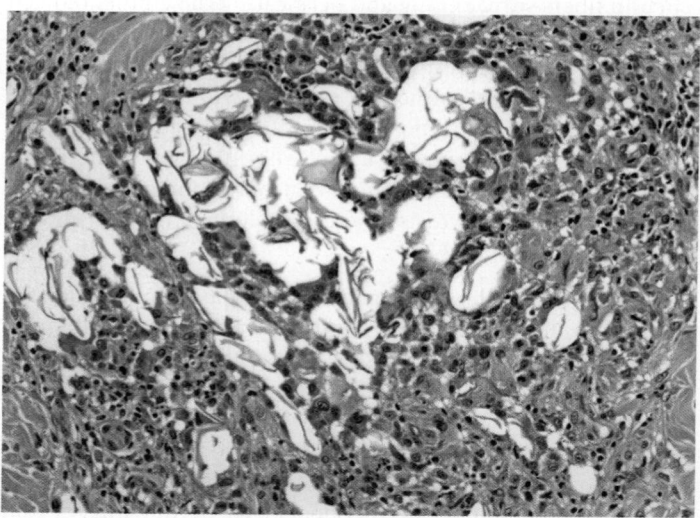

Figure 14-24 Ruptured epidermoid cyst. There are neutrophils and histiocytes surrounding cornified cells from the center of the cyst.

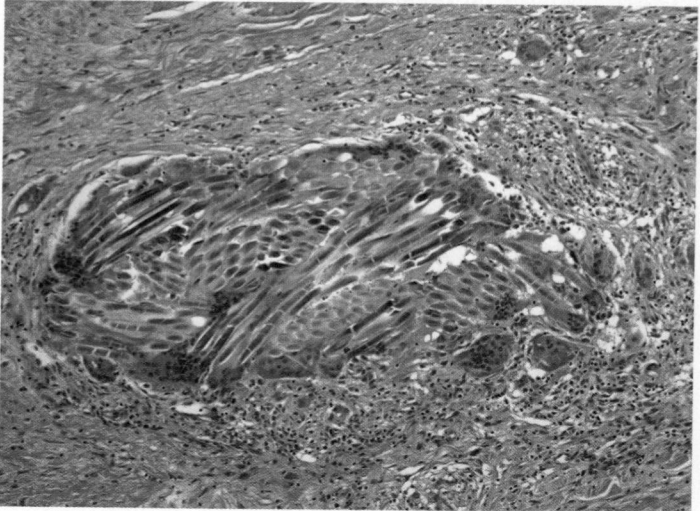

Figure 14-25 Foreign-body granuloma caused by nylon suture. The suture is composed of blue-gray, linear material and is surrounded by histiocytes, including many multinucleated foreign-body–type giant cells.

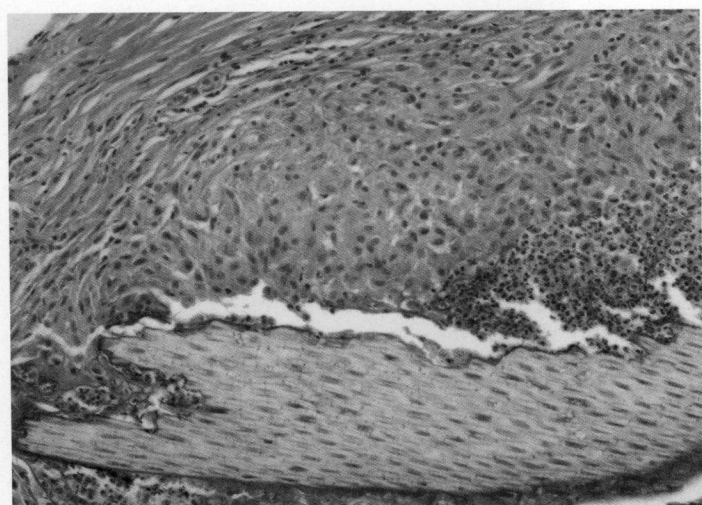

Figure 14-26 Foreign-body reaction to a wood splinter. The wood splinter shows an orderly arrangement of rectangular cells, typical of plant material, surrounded by a nodular infiltrate with histiocytes, including multinucleated histiocytes of the foreign-body type, and neutrophils.

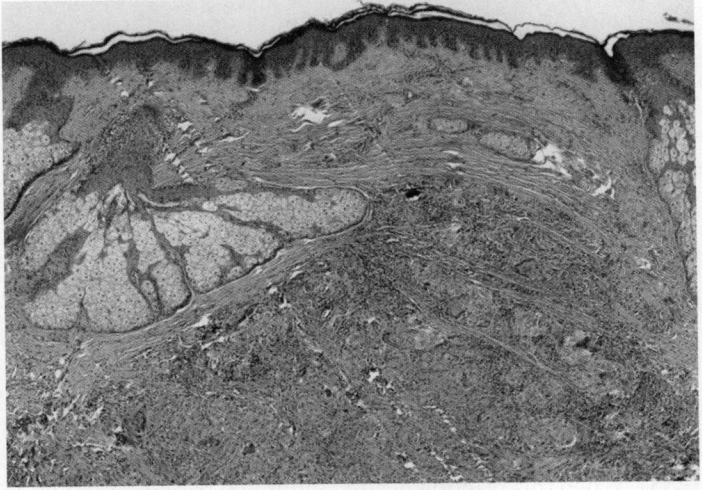

Figure 14-27 Foreign-body reaction. There are circumscribed, nodular collections of epithelioid histiocytes, similar to what may be seen in sarcoid, associated with knife marks (diagonally oriented in this photograph), which serve as a clue to the presence of the foreign material, which cannot be seen at this magnification.

An *allergic* granulomatous reaction to a foreign body typically shows a sarcoidal or tuberculoid pattern consisting of epithelioid cells with or without giant cells. Phagocytosis of the foreign substance is slight or absent. Substances that in sensitized persons produce an allergic granulomatous reaction include zirconium, beryllium, and certain dyes used in tattoos. Some substances that at first act as foreign material may later, after sensitization has occurred, act as allergens, as in the case of sea urchin spines and silica.

A histologic decision as to whether a granuloma is of the foreign-body type or of the allergic type is not always possible. A granuloma of the allergic type is more likely to show rounded, well-circumscribed collections of epithelioid histiocytes and less likely to have multinucleated histiocytes of the foreign-body type.

Principles of Management for Foreign-Body Reactions (see sections following): Foreign-body reactions may eventually improve with time. Simple excision of smaller lesions is often curative. Extensive lesions can be treated with intralesional or oral corticosteroids (247).

Paraffinoma

Clinical Summary. Foreign-body reactions may occur following injections of oily substances such as mineral oil (paraffin) typically into the breasts (248), genitalia (249), or scalp (250) for cosmetic purposes. These occur as irregular, plaque-like indurations of the skin and subcutaneous tissue (251,252). Ulcers or abscesses may develop. The interval between the time of injection and the development of induration or ulceration may be many years.

The misleading term *sclerosing lipogranuloma* was given to paraffinoma of the male genitalia because of the unproven assumption that it was a local reactive process following injury to adipose tissue (253,254).

Histopathology. Paraffinomas have a "Swiss cheese" appearance because of the presence of numerous ovoid or round cavities that show great variation in size. These cavities represent spaces occupied by the oily substance (255). The spaces between the cavities are taken up in part by fibrotic connective tissue and in part by an infiltrate of macrophages and lymphocytes. Some of the macrophages have the appearance of foam cells. Variable numbers of multinucleated foreign-body giant cells are present.

In frozen sections of paraffinoma, the foreign material stains orange with Sudan IV or oil red O, although less so than neutral fat (255).

Silicone Granuloma

Clinical Summary. Reactions to medical-grade silicone have occurred after injection of its liquid form for cosmetic purposes or from leakage or rupture of silicone gel from breast implants. Leakage from silicone breast implants can cause the development of subcutaneous nodules and plaques (256). Lesions containing silicone at sites adjacent to and, rarely, distant from areas of injection or implantation may occur (257,258). A localized reaction at injection sites by silicone-coated acupuncture or venipuncture needles has also been reported (259,260).

Histopathology. As in paraffinoma, numerous ovoid or round cavities of varying sizes are seen, resulting in a "Swiss cheese" appearance (Fig. 14-28). These spaces are what remain after the silicone has been removed during processing, although occasionally scant

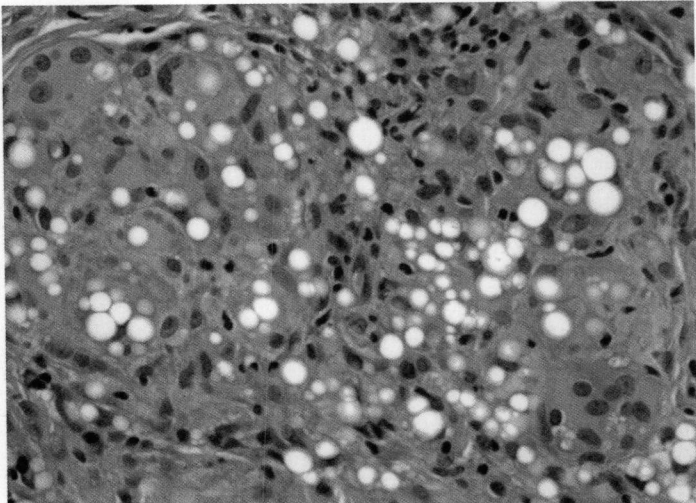

Figure 14-28 Silicone granuloma. Silicone used for cosmetic purposes may produce a granulomatous response with a "Swiss cheese" appearance. (Courtesy of John Walsh, MD.)

residual silicone is seen as colorless, irregularly shaped, refractile, nonpolarizable material within the spaces. Histiocytes may be present between the cavities; they can be foamy or multinucleated and accompanied by lymphocytes and eosinophils (256,261). In addition, varying degrees of fibrosis are present. The identification of silicone within a specimen can be facilitated via thick sectioning, dark-field microscopy, and other techniques (262).

Talc Granuloma

Clinical Summary. Talc (magnesium silicate) may produce granulomatous inflammation when introduced into open wounds. Historically, talc was used as powder on gloves, but this use has been abandoned for many years, and although starch may be used as a surgical dusting powder (263), most gloves are now powder free. Talc may also be introduced into the skin through topical application of medications (264).

Histopathology. Histologic examination reveals histiocytes and multinucleated giant cells, some of which may contain visible particles of talc. Talc crystals can be needle shaped with a yellow-brown or blue-green hue and appear as white birefringent particles with polarized light (265). Their presence can be confirmed by x-ray diffraction studies (265) or energy-dispersive x-ray analysis (265).

Starch Granuloma

Clinical Summary. Granulomas may have previously resulted from the contamination of wounds with surgical gloves powdered with corn starch; however, the use of corn starch in this setting has largely been abandoned (266).

Histopathology. A foreign-body reaction with multinucleated giant cells is present. Scattered through the infiltrate, one observes starch granules as ill-defined ovoid basophilic structures measuring 10 to 20 μm in diameter. Most of the granules are seen within foreign-body giant cells. They react with PAS and methenamine silver and, on examination in polarized light, are birefringent, showing a Maltese cross configuration (266).

Cactus Granuloma

Clinical Summary. Cactus granulomas show, within days or weeks after the injury, tender papules from which cactus spines may still protrude. They may be extruded spontaneously within a few months.

Histopathology. Early papules—a few days after the injury—show fragments of cactus spicules in the dermis that are associated with an intense, perivascular lymphohistiocytic infiltrate containing many eosinophils. After a few weeks, the infiltrate consists of lymphocytes, macrophages, and giant cells (267,268). Sharply marginated spicules are seen within giant cells and lying free in the dermis. The spicules are PAS positive (269).

Pilonidal Sinus

Clinical Summary. The pilonidal sinus is most often seen in young adult men over the sacrum (270). In barbers, the implantation of human hair in the interdigital web spaces may cause small, asymptomatic or tender sinus tracts (271,272). Similar lesions are even more common within web spaces or in other sites in dog groomers and other animal caretakers (273,274).

Histopathology. Histologic examination reveals a sinus tract lined by squamous epithelium containing one or several hairs, thus resembling a hair follicle. Either the sinus tract encases the hair completely, or, if the hair extends deeper than the sinus tract, one finds at the lower end of the hair a foreign-body giant-cell reaction intermingled with inflammatory cells (271,275).

Sea Urchin Granuloma

Clinical Summary. Injuries from the spines of sea urchins occur most commonly on the hands and feet. Even if the friable spines have been only incompletely removed, the wounds tend to heal after spontaneous extrusion of most of the foreign material (276,277). However, in some persons, violaceous nodules appear at the sites of injury after a latent period of 2 to 12 months (278).

Histopathology. The nodules are composed largely of epithelioid histiocytes and giant cells (276,279). Doubly refractile material is present in a minority of the granulomas. If remnants of a spine are still present, they are surrounded by leukocytes and many large foreign-body giant cells (277). A minority of patients show non-granulomatous findings, the most common of which is a neutrophilic infiltrate (280).

Pathogenesis. The appearance of sarcoidosis-like granulomas after a latent interval of months in only a small proportion of the injured patients suggests a delayed hypersensitivity reaction (278). The spines of sea urchins, in addition to the calcified material, contain remnants of epithelial cells (278). The double refraction that may be found in the granulomas may be attributable to the presence of a small amount of silica in the calcified spines (277).

Silica Granuloma

Clinical Summary. Silica (silicon dioxide) is present in rocks, soil, sand, and glass. It frequently contaminates accidental wounds, in which it initiates a foreign-body reaction of limited duration followed by fibrosis (281). In the vast majority of cases, silica causes no further sequelae. In exceptional cases, a granulomatous delayed hypersensitivity reaction occurs at the site of the old scar (282). The mean interval for this delayed hypersensitivity reaction is approximately 10 years, but it may be less than 1 year or more than 50 years after the original injury (283). When this reaction occurs, indurated papules or nodules develop at the site of injury.

Histopathology. In silica granuloma, there are groups of epithelioid histiocytes with a lymphocytic infiltrate that tends to be sparse (282–286). Foreign-body giant cells may be abundant or absent, and Langhans giant cells may also be present. If multinucleated histiocytes are not numerous, a picture resembling sarcoidosis is produced. However, the diagnosis of sarcoidosis may be excluded by clinical information and the presence, especially within giant cells, of crystalline particles varying in size from barely visible to 100 μm in length; they represent silica crystals. When examined with polarized light, these particles are doubly refractile (Fig. 14-29). The presence of silicon can be confirmed by x-ray spectrometric or energy-dispersive x-ray analysis (283,284,287).

Pathogenesis. Evidence suggests that the sarcoidosis-like granulomatous response to silica that occurs long after initial injury represents a delayed-type hypersensitivity reaction (282,283,285,288).

Zirconium Granuloma

Clinical Summary. Deodorant sticks containing zirconium lactate and creams containing zirconium oxide may cause a persistent eruption composed of soft, red-brown papules in the

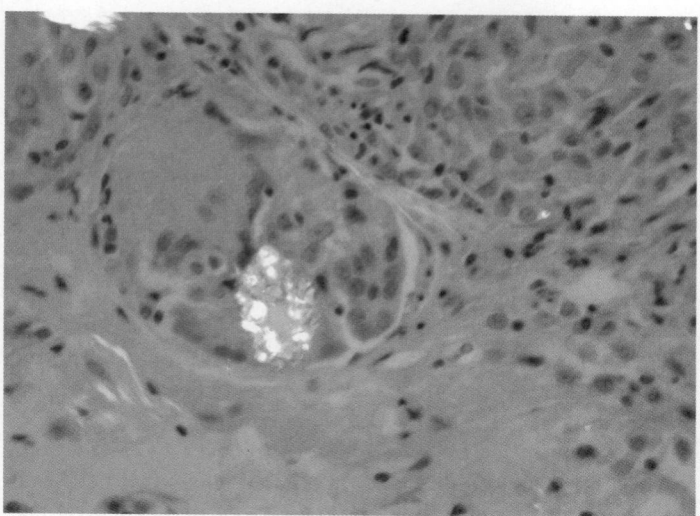

Figure 14-29 Silica. Silica, like other foreign materials with a crystalline structure, is doubly refractile when viewed under polarized light.

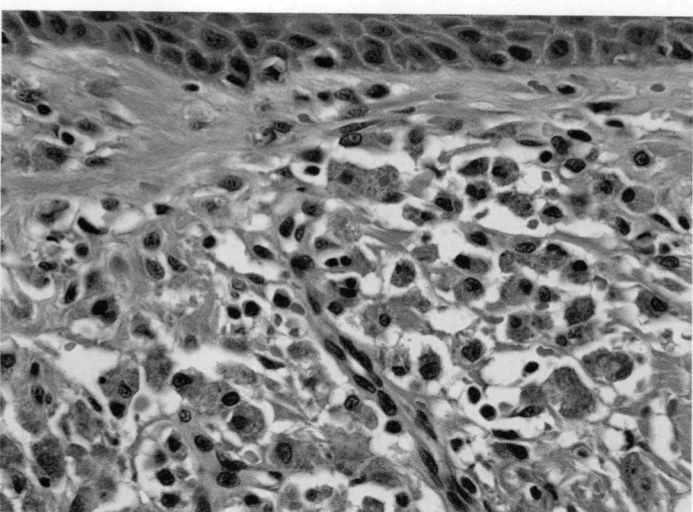

Figure 14-30 Aluminum chloride. Histiocytes with purplish granules as a consequence of aluminum chloride used for hemostasis during a previous procedure performed at this site.

areas to which they have been applied. Zirconium lactate is no longer present in antiperspirants sold in the United States; however, a granulomatous reaction has also been described in response to roll-on antiperspirant containing aluminum–zirconium complex (289,290).

Histopathology. Histologic examination shows large aggregates of epithelioid cells with a few giant cells and a sparse or moderately dense lymphocytic infiltrate, producing a picture that may be indistinguishable from sarcoidosis (291–293). Because of the small size of the zirconium particles, they cannot be detected on examination with polarized light (291). Their presence, however, can be demonstrated by spectrographic analysis (292) or energy-dispersive x-ray analysis (289).

Pathogenesis. Evidence that zirconium granulomas develop on the basis of an allergic sensitization to zirconium includes the following: (a) They occur only in persons sensitized to zirconium (294), (b) the pattern of granuloma inflammation is like that of other granulomatous dermatitides that have been attributed to delayed-type hypersensitivity reactions, and (c) autoradiographic analysis of experimentally induced lesions in sensitized individuals reveals no zirconium within histiocytes (295).

Reactions to Aluminum

Clinical Summary. Reactions to aluminum occur most often in the setting of surgical scars secondary to the use of aluminum chloride as a hemostatic agent, although these reactions are not clinically apparent. However, single or multiple persistent subcutaneous nodules may appear several months or even years after the subcutaneous injection of a variety of vaccines or allergen desensitization extracts that are aluminum adsorbed (296,297). The aluminum adjuvant is included to enhance the immunogenicity of vaccines or modify the immune response to an allergen when used in desensitization agents.

Histopathology. In surgical scars, the hemostatic agent aluminum chloride can be seen as granular violaceous-to-gray stippled deposits within macrophages (Fig. 14-30).

In subcutaneous nodules at injection sites, the most striking finding in some biopsy specimens is the presence of nodular aggregates of lymphocytes with lymphoid follicles and germinal

centers within the dermis and subcutis. There is fibrosis, which may occur in bands that separate the lymphocytic nodules. Eosinophils may be prominent, and the condition may show a pseudolymphomatous appearance (297–300). The granulomatous component consists of histiocytes with ample cytoplasm and, in some cases, a few giant cells or large areas of eosinophilic necrosis surrounded by histiocytes in a palisade (299). Early lesions tend to show a reaction that is more purely granulomatous (296). Palisading granulomatous reactions have also been reported (301). There may be prominent septal and lobular inflammation of the panniculus (302). In any of the patterns that may occur, a key to making the diagnosis is the identification of histiocytes with abundant violaceous-to-gray granular cytoplasm; these granules contain aluminum and are PAS positive and diastase resistant (298).

Pathogenesis. This condition is believed to represent a delayed hypersensitivity reaction to aluminum. Electron microscopic examination reveals irregular membrane-bound, electron-dense material within macrophages. X-ray microanalysis has shown that the electron-dense material contains aluminum (298).

Titanium Granuloma

Clinical Summary. Titanium has rarely been implicated in the formation of granulomas, internally and in the skin, the latter as a consequence of body piercing (303).

Histopathology. An infiltrate of histiocytes, lymphocytes, and plasma cells is present, and some macrophages contain minute brown-black particles (303).

Zinc-Induced Granuloma

Clinical Summary. Local reactions to subcutaneous insulin injections are not uncommon. However, the granulomatous response, which may occur with zinc-containing insulin preparations, is rare. It may begin with sterile furunculoid lesions (304,305).

Histopathology. The early furunculoid lesions show a dense neutrophilic infiltrate and many birefringent rhomboidal crystals of zinc insulin. Later, fibrosis and granulomatous inflammation develop (304).

Berylliosis

Clinical Summary. Since the 1940s (306), beryllium exposure has been known to cause berylliosis. Beryllium-containing compounds were previously widely used in the manufacture of fluorescent light tubes, and in 1949 permissible exposure limits were set in the United States. Historically, two diseases resulted from this exposure: systemic berylliosis (chronic beryllium disease) and local beryllium granulomas. Chronic beryllium disease classically developed in workers in plants manufacturing fluorescent tubes; however, occupational exposure to beryllium continues today in aerospace, construction, military, automotive, and electronics industries, where it is used as an alloy (307). Chronic beryllium disease primarily shows pulmonary involvement, and extrapulmonary manifestations are thought to be uncommon (308). Occupational permissible exposure limits were tightened in 2017 in the United States, and most workers with occupational exposure are screened for pulmonary pathology (309), yet some authors suggest this disease is still underrecognized (309). There are some reports of suspected cutaneous involvement attributable to occupational exposure (310).

Purely local beryllium granulomas occurred in persons who cut themselves on broken fluorescent tubes that were coated with a mixture containing zinc-beryllium silicate (311). The cutaneous granulomas after laceration show, as their first sign, incomplete healing of the laceration, followed by swelling, induration, tenderness, and, finally, central ulceration (312).

Histopathology. The cutaneous granulomas of chronic beryllium disease, similar to those of sarcoidosis, show very slight or no caseation (308). The cutaneous granulomas following laceration, in contrast to the cutaneous granulomas of systemic berylliosis, show central necrosis, which may be pronounced (311). A moderately dense infiltrate of lymphocytes may be present, resembling the granulomas of tuberculosis. The epidermis shows acanthosis and possibly ulceration. No particles of beryllium are seen in histologic sections, but its presence in the lesions can be demonstrated by spectrographic analysis (312).

Pathogenesis. It is now well established that beryllium directly interacts with the antigen recognition portion of the MHC class II molecule on antigen-presenting cells, resulting in a conformational change in the peptide-binding groove and facilitating responses against self-peptides. This results in the activation of a T helper 1 (Th1) polarized immune response (313,314). Chronic beryllium disease is strongly associated with HLA-DPB1 (313,314). A blood beryllium lymphocyte proliferation test can be used to support the diagnosis of chronic beryllium disease if it is suspected (315). Beryllium skin patch testing has also been reported and may result in local granuloma formation (316).

Mercury Granuloma

Clinical Summary. Mercury granuloma is generally secondary to injury (i.e., with a broken thermometer) or deliberate self-injection. Rarely, elevated serum and urine mercury can be associated with these granulomas.

Histopathology. Implanted mercury appears as dark gray to black, opaque globules and spheres of varying sizes, often surrounded by dermal necrosis. Granulomatous inflammation is present (317).

Tattoo Reactions

Clinical Summary. Clinically apparent inflammatory reactions to permanent tattoos, although uncommon, are now seen with greater frequency owing to the increased popularity of tattoos. They have been observed most commonly with red dyes containing mercuric sulfide, such as cinnabar (Chinese red). More recently, there has been a move away from using mercury-containing dyes and toward the use of dyes containing other red pigments, such as ferric hydrate (sienna or red ochre), cadmium selenide (cadmium red), and organic dyes, but such mercury-free red dyes may also produce adverse reactions (318,319). Reactions have also been reported with chrome green (320), cobalt blue (321), purple manganese salts (322), yellow cadmium sulfide (323), and iron oxide (324). In some instances, an allergic response to the pigment has been suggested by a positive patch test. Infection, particularly mycobacterial, should also be considered when seeing a tattoo reaction (325); infection may be secondary to dilution of tattoo pigment with contaminated tap water. Notably, some tattoo reactions have overlying epithelial hyperplasia that can be striking both clinically and histopathologically and mimic squamous cell carcinoma (326).

Reactions to "temporary" tattoos are rare. Usually comprised of black commercial henna, these tattoos are painted onto the skin surface. The most common reaction is allergic contact dermatitis, but a lichenoid dermatitis, a scarring reaction, and hypopigmentation have been reported (327–331).

Tattoos may also occur owing to pigmented materials accidentally implanted in the skin, such as graphite or gunpowder, or owing to solutions employed for hemostasis (332,333), particularly Monsel solution (ferric subsulfate).

Histopathology. Permanent tattoos that are not clinically inflamed show irregularly shaped granules of dye that are located within macrophages and extracellularly in the dermis (334).

Inflammatory reactions in clinically inflamed permanent tattoos may or may not be granulomatous (335). Photoexacerbation has been described with reactions to red pigments (329,330) and yellow pigments (323). Nongranulomatous reactions include a perivascular lymphocytic infiltrate with pigment-containing macrophages (319,334); a lichenoid response, which in some instances may resemble lichen planus or hypertrophic lichen planus (318,319,336,337); and a pseudolymphomatous picture with a dense, nodular, or diffuse, predominantly lymphocytic infiltrate that also contains histiocytes and coarse tattoo pigment granules (338,339). Infected tattoo reactions may not show detectable organisms (325). If present, overlying epithelial hyperplasia generally shows minimal cytologic atypia (326).

Granulomatous reactions may be either of the sarcoidal type (320,340,341) or the foreign-body type (320,324). The granulomatous responses show tattoo granules scattered throughout the infiltrate. In the sarcoidal type, the infiltrate contains nodules of epithelioid histiocytes (Figs. 14-31 and 14-32), and in the foreign-body type, there are obvious multinucleated histiocytes of the foreign-body type. A sparse or dense lymphocytic infiltrate may be present. In the sarcoidal type of reaction, regional lymph nodes may also show tattoo granules (342). Development of sarcoidal granulomas in tattoos can be associated with sarcoidosis in other organs, including lung (195,340,341,343), and it is generally recommended that patients be evaluated accordingly.

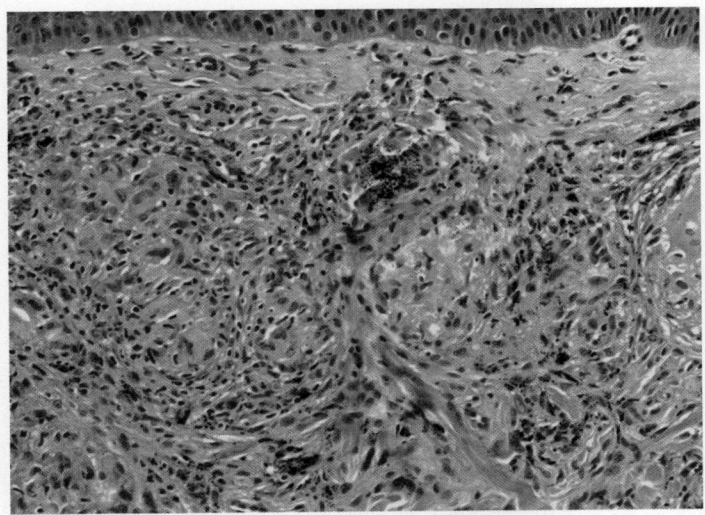

Figure 14-31 Decorative tattoo. Granulomatous inflammation in response to pigment used for a tattoo.

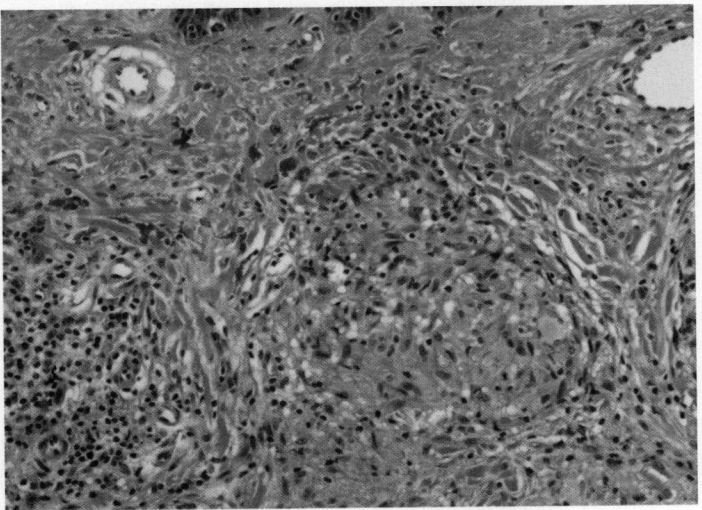

Figure 14-32 Decorative tattoo. Granulomatous response to a red tattoo.

Some authors believe this represents unmasking of true sarcoidosis when internal involvement is detected in this setting.

Traumatic graphite tattoos show black granules free in the dermis and sometimes within histiocytes (Fig. 14-33). Monsel tattoos, also typically seen in conjunction with scars, show multinucleate histiocytes containing coarse, brown, refractile pigment (Fig. 14-34), which is positive on staining for iron. Larger, brown, extracellular jagged aggregates of pigment are suggestive of Monsel tattoo (344). Ferruginization of collagen bundles is typical, and a proliferation of spindled fibrohistiocytic cells may also occur.

Electron microscopic examination of tattoos without an allergic reaction shows that most tattoo granules are located within macrophages, where they often lie within membrane-bound lysosomes. In addition, some tattoo granules are found free in the dermis (345).

Reactions to Soft Tissue Augmentation Materials

Clinical Summary. Injectable soft tissue fillers are often used to treat wrinkles and for soft tissue augmentation. Agents available for use vary in their composition and properties, and commonly used agents include hyaluronic acid, poly-L-lactic acid, calcium hydroxylapatite, and polymethylmethacrylate (346). Bovine and human-derived collagen were used in the past but are rarely used now. Hypersensitivity reactions were common with bovine collagen. With soft tissue filler use, a small minority of patients may develop a clinically apparent granulomatous response at the site of injection, and this may occur months to years later (346). Newer materials are considered less immunogenic, although reactions to these injected materials have been reported including with hyaluronic acid (347,348), poly-L-lactic acid (349–351), and calcium hydroxylapatite (352,353). Sarcoidosis-like presentations have been reported in association with hyaluronic acid (354,355). The possibility of infection must also be considered; for example, an outbreak of *Mycobacterium chelonae* infection after soft tissue filler use has been described (356).

Histopathology. Biopsies of patients with erythematous raised areas at sites of hyaluronic acid injections have revealed a granulomatous infiltrate with prominent giant cells in most patients. A mild lymphohistiocytic infiltrate without granulomas appears to be less common. The injected hyaluronic acid gel may be visible as basophilic amorphous material that stains positively for Alcian blue at pH of 2.7, but is not polarizable (357–361). Poly-L-lactic acid granuloma shows cholesterol-cleft–like spaces with translucent particles of varying sizes. There is an associated inflammatory infiltrate with histiocytes that typically contains frequent foreign-body–type giant cells, some of which may contain the translucent particles (362,363). Poly-L-lactic acid particles are birefringent with polarized light examination. Calcium hydroxylapatite particles have a bluish color histopathologically and are round to oval in shape and 25 to 40 µM in size (364,365). A granulomatous response with foreign-body–type giant cells may be apparent. Polymethylmethacrylate granuloma shows numerous sharply circumscribed, seemingly empty round spaces, uniform in size and shape, mimicking normal adipocytes (366). Epithelioid histiocytes with occasional giant cells surround these spaces. Within them, on lowering the microscope condenser, one notes vaguely visible round, sharply circumscribed, translucent, nonbirefringent foreign bodies.

Clinical and histopathologic evaluation of reactions to soft tissue fillers should include exclusion of an infectious etiology through sterile tissue culture. Stains for microorganisms may be useful for ancillary evaluation but cannot be used to exclude infection.

Corticosteroid Deposits

Clinical Summary. Corticosteroid preparations for intralesional use are suspensions of insoluble crystalline chemicals; soluble corticosteroids are not effective for intralesional use. These suspensions may be identified histologically after injection of triamcinolone or other steroids. Sites where these deposits have been described include the skin (e.g., in keloids), the nasal mucosa, and the Achilles tendon. The material may persist at the site of injection for months or years (261,367).

Histopathology. Corticosteroid deposits are recognizable by their acellular, amphophilic, granular appearance in association with clear spaces. The spaces may represent the sites of dissolved crystals. Uncommonly, birefringent crystals can be seen with polarized light. Inflammation tends to be absent or sparse, but a palisaded granuloma may develop (367–370).

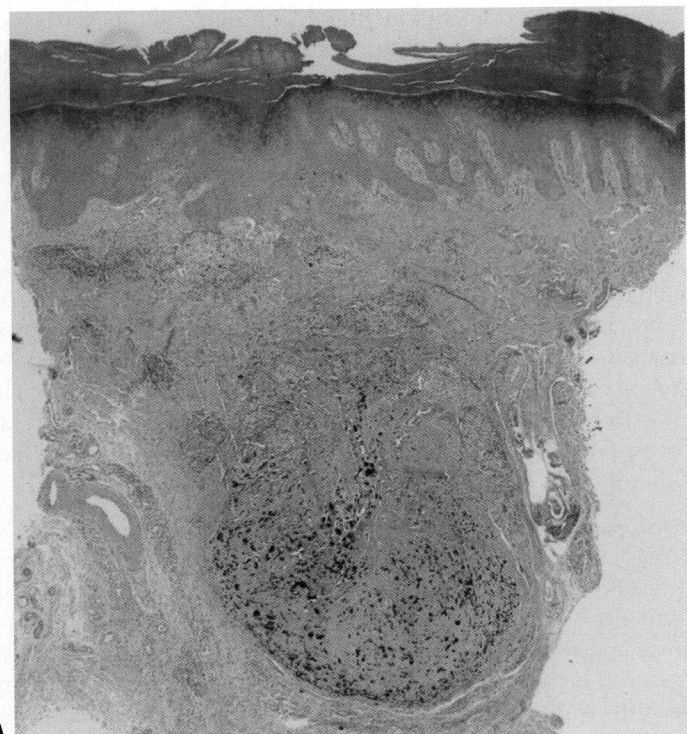

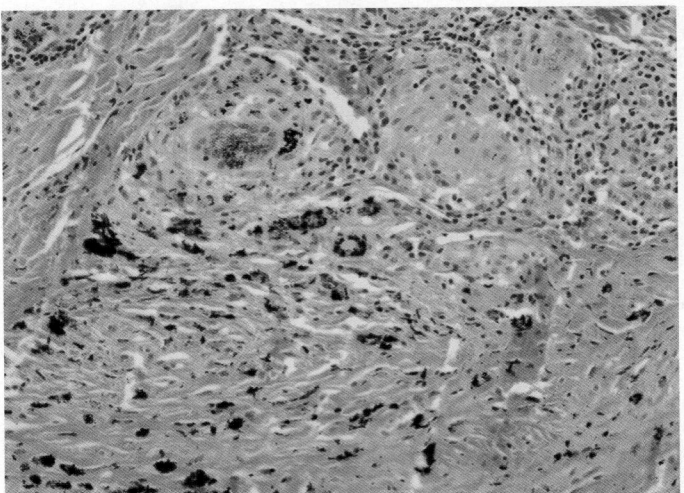

Figure 14-33 Traumatic tattoo from graphite. **A:** A circumscribed collection of black material is present in the dermis. **B:** The black material is darker than melanin, and the clumps have irregular shapes and sizes; some are intracellular and some are extracellular. There are also knife marks due to the foreign material causing the tissue to have more frictional resistance.

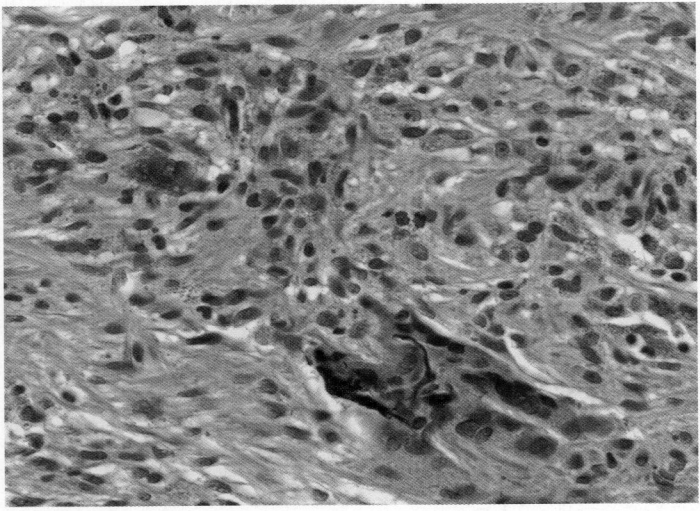

Figure 14-34 Monsel tattoo. Monsel solution may produce a granulomatous response associated with pigment that is gray-brown, with pigment sometimes in larger clumps.

CHEILITIS GRANULOMATOSA AND MIESCHER–MELKERSSON–ROSENTHAL SYNDROME

Clinical Summary. The classic triad of Miescher–Melkersson–Rosenthal syndrome consists of recurrent labial edema, relapsing facial paralysis, and fissured tongue (371). However, not all patients have the classic triad (372), and the terminology cheilitis granulomatosa (or granulomatous cheilitis) may be used when labial edema is the only sign (373). In a review of 220 patients, labial swelling was seen in 84%, facial palsy in 23%, and fissured tongue in 60% (371). Whereas monosymptomatic labial edema is recognized as part of the syndrome, lingua plicata (fissured tongue) by itself is not, because this is not uncommon in the general population. One occasionally observes, either in addition to or in place of swelling of the lips, orofacial swelling including of the forehead, chin, cheeks, eyelids, and even the tongue (371,374). Regional lymphadenopathy may be observed (375). Swelling of the buccal mucosa, gingiva, and palate can also occur (371). Given the heterogeneity in clinical presentation, the umbrella term orofacial granulomatosis has been proposed (376,377). Chronic swelling of the vulva or of the foreskin has been reported as a genital counterpart to cheilitis granulomatosa (378,379); this presentation should raise concern for underlying Crohn disease (380).

Histopathology. Granulomatous inflammation is not present in all biopsies of clinically involved lips (372). Sections may show simply edema, lymphangiectasia, and a predominately perivascular lymphoplasmacytic infiltrate. Lymphatic dilation is present in most cases (381). The infiltrate is often sparse but may be dense, producing a nodular appearance. If granulomas are present, they are noncaseating and tend to be small and scattered (Fig. 14-35). Collections of epithelioid histiocytes may be poorly circumscribed and are often associated with lymphocytes, but occasionally larger and/or "naked" tubercles are present, producing an appearance similar to that of sarcoidosis (374,381–383). Affected lymph nodes may also show granulomatous inflammation (384,385).

Pathogenesis. The cause of cheilitis granulomatosa and Miescher–Melkersson–Rosenthal is not well understood, and this terminology is typically reserved for patients with no evidence of

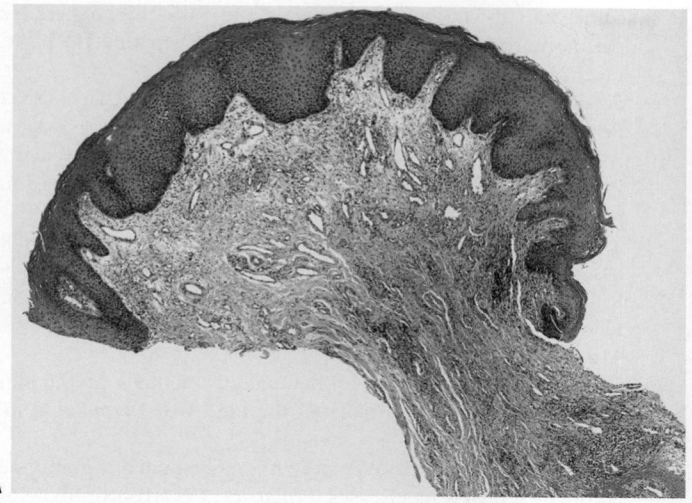
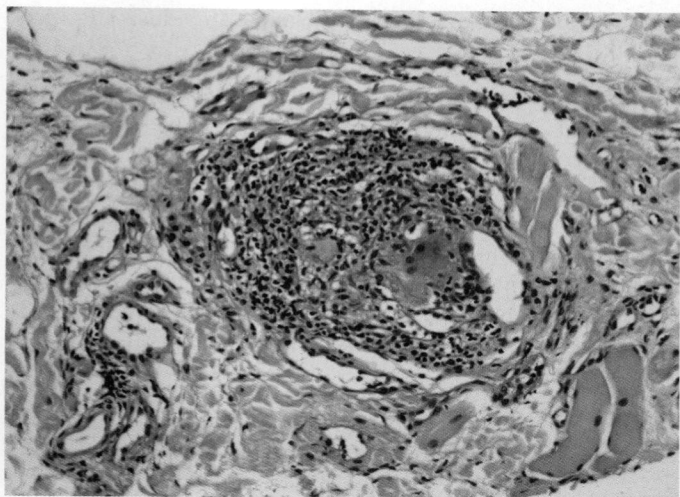

Figure 14-35 Cheilitis granulomatosa. **A:** Biopsy of lip mucosa showing slight vascular ectasia, edema, and a sparse inflammatory infiltrate including lymphocytes. **B:** A subtle granulomatous component.

underlying systemic disease. In particular, underlying sarcoidosis or Crohn disease, especially when granulomatous cheilitis is the only mucocutaneous sign, may be uncovered, and appropriate evaluation in this regard is typically recommended (373).

Principles of Management: Intralesional and oral corticosteroids as well as other oral anti-inflammatory medications have been reported as having some success in the literature, but treatment can be difficult (373,386,387).

GRANULOMA GLUTEALE INFANTUM

Clinical Summary. Granuloma gluteale infantum, first described in 1971 (388), shows asymptomatic, round to oval, smooth papules and nodules irregularly distributed over regions covered by diapers (388–391). The lesions are typically reddish blue in color, ranging from a few millimeters to a few centimeters in diameter. Although usually seen in infants, this condition has also been described in incontinent adults (391,392), and a similar process with an erosive component has been reported in adults with extensive use of benzocaine (393). Although this disorder may clinically appear similar to a granulomatous condition, histologically it is not.

Histopathology. Acanthosis is usually present. A dense, mixed infiltrate is seen throughout the dermis. Lymphocytes, histiocytes, plasma cells, neutrophils, and eosinophils may all be seen (390). In addition, there may be microabscesses composed of neutrophils and eosinophils, as well as extravasation of erythrocytes together with a proliferation of capillaries (388). Multinucleated histiocytes or well-developed granulomas are not a feature of the infiltrate. In a few instances, staining with the PAS reaction has revealed spores and pseudohyphae consistent with the presence of *Candida albicans* in the stratum corneum (394), but fungi are generally not detected.

Pathogenesis. In nearly all patients described in the literature, the development of granuloma gluteale infantum has been preceded by diaper dermatitis, which only in some instances has been associated with a *C. albicans* infection (389,394). Topical applications of fluorinated corticosteroid preparations for a prolonged period of time and prolonged wearing of plastic

diapers have been implicated, but a consistent cause has not been identified (395). It appears very likely that exogenous factors, including irritants and external trauma, contribute to this eruption (388,393).

Principles of Management: Avoidance of external irritants/trauma is important; lesions often spontaneously resolve over time (396). Candida infection, if present, should be treated appropriately.

MISCELLANEOUS GRANULOMATOUS LESIONS

Interstitial Granulomatous Drug Reaction

Clinical Summary. A limited number of patients have been described with annular to solid erythematous patches/plaques on the inner arms, proximal thighs, and intertriginous areas, often occurring symmetrically. Implicated agents include antihypertensives (particularly calcium-channel blockers), antihyperlipidemics, antihistamines, anticonvulsants, antidepressants (60,61), TNF-α inhibitors (397), and herbal medications (398).

Histopathology. An interstitial infiltrate of lymphocytes and histiocytes with slight fragmentation of collagen is reported, in conjunction with variable numbers of eosinophils and neutrophils and vacuolar interface change. Vacuolar change may not always be observed (151).

Differential Diagnosis. Clinical presentation and the presence of vacuolar interface change may be helpful in distinguishing this condition from granuloma annulare and IGD (61,137).

Principles of Management: Discontinuation of the offending medication results in the resolution of the lesions.

Zoster-Related Granulomas

Clinical Summary. Following herpes zoster, patients may present with persistent reddish papules in a zosteriform distribution.

Histopathology. A variety of reaction patterns may be found in zoster-related scars. The most common granulomatous patterns are granuloma annulare–like (399) and sarcoidosis-like patterns (400).

Principles of Management: Lesions may self-resolve; topical corticosteroids may hasten resolution (401).

Common Variable Immunodeficiency

Clinical Summary. Patients with common variable immunodeficiency often have multiple cutaneous warts and systemic signs and symptoms, which include diarrhea, chronic/recurrent bacterial infections, hepatosplenomegaly, and lymphadenopathy. Patients may also develop granulomas of the skin and other organs.

Histopathology. Biopsy of the nodules may show granuloma annulare–like (402), tuberculoid leprosy–like (403), sarcoidosis-like, and/or tuberculosis-like (404,405) granulomas.

Principles of Management: Corticosteroids, localized or systemic, are the treatment of choice, with absent to only partial responses in many cases (406).

Nonspecific Manifestation of Underlying Lymphoma

Clinical Summary. Patients with lymphoma may sometimes present with granulomatous lesions.

Histopathology. A spectrum of histologic findings has been described, including granuloma annulare–like, annular elastolytic–like, sarcoidosis-like, and tuberculoid patterns (407).

Principles of Management: Treatment of the underlying lymphoma is indicated but does not always lead to the resolution of cutaneous lesions (407).

ACKNOWLEDGMENTS

The authors would like to acknowledge and thank Dr. Philip E. Shapiro, a significant prior contributor to this chapter, for his fundamental contributions to this work. Dr. Damsky is supported by a Career Development Award from the Dermatology Foundation.

REFERENCES

1. Dicken CH, Carrington SG, Winkelmann RK. Generalized granuloma annulare. *Arch Dermatol.* 1969;99(5):556–563.
2. Yun JH, Lee JY, Kim MK, et al. Clinical and pathological features of generalized granuloma annulare with their correlation: a retrospective multicenter study in Korea. *Ann Dermatol.* 2009;21(2):113–119.
3. Haim S, Friedman-Birnbaum R, Shafrir A. Generalized granuloma annulare: relationship to diabetes mellitus as revealed in 8 cases. *Br J Dermatol.* 1970;83(2):302–305.
4. Dabski K, Winkelmann RK. Generalized granuloma annulare: histopathology and immunopathology. Systematic review of 100 cases and comparison with localized granuloma annulare. *J Am Acad Dermatol.* 1989;20(1):28–39.
5. Owens DW, Freeman RG. Perforating granuloma annulare. *Arch Dermatol.* 1971;103(1):64–67.
6. Lucky AW, Prose NS, Bove K, White WL, Jorizzo JL. Papular umbilicated granuloma annulare. A report of four pediatric cases. *Arch Dermatol.* 1992;128(10):1375–1378.
7. Duncan WC, Smith JD, Knox JM. Generalized perforating granuloma annulare. *Arch Dermatol.* 1973;108(4):570–572.
8. Samlaska CP, Sandberg GD, Maggio KL, Sakas EL. Generalized perforating granuloma annulare. *J Am Acad Dermatol.* 1992;27(2, pt 2):319–322.
9. Penas PF, Jones-Caballero M, Fraga J, Sanchez-Perez J, Garcia-Diez A. Perforating granuloma annulare. *Int J Dermatol.* 1997;36(5):340–348.
10. Aichelburg MC, Pinkowicz A, Schuster C, Volc-Platzer B, Tanew A. Patch granuloma annulare: clinicopathological characteristics and response to phototherapy. *Br J Dermatol.* 2019;181(1):198–199.
11. Khanna U, North JP. Patch-type granuloma annulare: an institution-based study of 23 cases. *J Cutan Pathol.* 2020;47(9):785–793.
12. Rubin M, Lynch FW. Subcutaneous granuloma annulare. Comment on familial granuloma annulare. *Arch Dermatol.* 1966;93(4):416–420.
13. Lowney ED, Simons HM. "Rheumatoid" nodules of the skin: their significance as an isolated finding. *Arch Dermatol.* 1963;88:853–858.
14. Felner EI, Steinberg JB, Weinberg AG. Subcutaneous granuloma annulare: a review of 47 cases. *Pediatrics.* 1997;100(6):965–967.
15. McDermott MB, Lind AC, Marley EF, Dehner LP. Deep granuloma annulare (pseudorheumatoid nodule) in children: clinicopathologic study of 35 cases. *Pediatr Dev Pathol.* 1998;1(4):300–308.
16. Stefanaki K, Tsivitanidou-Kakourou T, Stefanaki C, et al. Histological and immunohistochemical study of granuloma annulare and subcutaneous granuloma annulare in children. *J Cutan Pathol.* 2007;34(5):392–396.
17. Grogg KL, Nascimento AG. Subcutaneous granuloma annulare in childhood: clinicopathologic features in 34 cases. *Pediatrics.* 2001;107(3):E42.
18. Evans MJ, Blessing K, Gray ES. Pseudorheumatoid nodule (deep granuloma annulare) of childhood: clinicopathologic features of twenty patients. *Pediatr Dermatol.* 1994;11(1):6–9.
19. Barzilai A, Huszar M, Shpiro D, Nass D, Trau H. Pseudorheumatoid nodules in adults: a juxta-articular form of nodular granuloma annulare. *Am J Dermatopathol.* 2005;27(1):1–5.
20. Muhlemann MF, Williams DR. Localized granuloma annulare is associated with insulin-dependent diabetes mellitus. *Br J Dermatol.* 1984;111(3):325–329.
21. Veraldi S, Bencini PL, Drudi E, Caputo R. Laboratory abnormalities in granuloma annulare: a case-control study. *Br J Dermatol.* 1997;136(4):652–653.
22. Studer EM, Calza AM, Saurat JH. Precipitating factors and associated diseases in 84 patients with granuloma annulare: a retrospective study. *Dermatology.* 1996;193(4):364–368.
23. Wu W, Robinson-Bostom L, Kokkotou E, Jung HY, Kroumpouzos G. Dyslipidemia in granuloma annulare: a case-control study. *Arch Dermatol.* 2012;148(10):1131–1136.
24. Vazquez-Lopez F, Pereiro M Jr, Manjon HJA, et al. Localized granuloma annulare and autoimmune thyroiditis in adult women: a case-control study. *J Am Acad Dermatol.* 2003;48(4):517–520.
25. Hawryluk EB, Izikson L, English JC 3rd. Non-infectious granulomatous diseases of the skin and their associated systemic diseases: an evidence-based update to important clinical questions. *Am J Clin Dermatol.* 2010;11(3):171–181.
26. Toro JR, Chu P, Yen TS, LeBoit PE. Granuloma annulare and human immunodeficiency virus infection. *Arch Dermatol.* 1999;135(11):1341–1346.
27. Cohen PR. Granuloma annulare: a mucocutaneous condition in human immunodeficiency virus-infected patients. *Arch Dermatol.* 1999;135(11):1404–1407.
28. Morris SD, Cerio R, Paige DG. An unusual presentation of diffuse granuloma annulare in an HIV-positive patient—immunohistochemical evidence of predominant CD8 lymphocytes. *Clin Exp Dermatol.* 2002;27(3):205–208.
29. O'Moore EJ, Nandawni R, Uthayakumar S, Nayagam AT, Darley CR. HIV-associated granuloma annulare (HAGA): a report of six cases. *Br J Dermatol.* 2000;142(5):1054–1056.

30. Cornejo CM, Haun P, English J 3rd, Rosenbach M. Immune checkpoint inhibitors and the development of granulomatous reactions. *J Am Acad Dermatol.* 2019;81(5):1165–1175.

31. Fox JD, Aramin H, Ghiam N, Freedman JB, Romanelli P. Secukinumab-associated localized granuloma annulare (SAGA): a case report and review of the literature. *Dermatol Online J.* 2020;26(8):13030/qt1nd6p108.

32. Zanolli MD, Powell BL, McCalmont T, White WL, Jorizzo JL. Granuloma annulare and disseminated herpes zoster. *Int J Dermatol.* 1992;31(1):55–57.

33. Gradwell E, Evans S. Perforating granuloma annulare complicating tattoos. *Br J Dermatol.* 1998;138(2):360–361.

34. Crosby DL, Woodley DT, Leonard DD. Concomitant granuloma annulare and necrobiosis lipoidica. Report of a case and review of the literature. *Dermatologica.* 1991;183(3):225–229.

35. Umbert P, Winkelmann RK. Granuloma annulare and sarcoidosis. *Br J Dermatol.* 1977;97(5):481–486.

36. Umbert P, Winkelmann RK. Histologic, ultrastructural and histochemical studies of granuloma annulare. *Arch Dermatol.* 1977;113(12):1681–1686.

37. Romero LS, Kantor GR. Eosinophils are not a clue to the pathogenesis of granuloma annulare. *Am J Dermatopathol.* 1998;20(1):29–34.

38. Silverman RA, Rabinowitz AD. Eosinophils in the cellular infiltrate of granuloma annulare. *J Cutan Pathol.* 1985;12(1):13–17.

39. Burket JM, Zelickson AS. Intracellular elastin in generalized granuloma annulare. *J Am Acad Dermatol.* 1986;14(6):975–981.

40. Gray HR, Graham JH, Johnson WC. Necrobiosis lipoidica: a histopathological and histochemical study. *J Invest Dermatol.* 1965;44:369–380.

41. Gunes P, Goktay F, Mansur AT, Koker F, Erfan G. Collagen-elastic tissue changes and vascular involvement in granuloma annulare: a review of 35 cases. *J Cutan Pathol.* 2009;36(8):838–844.

42. Trotter MJ, Crawford RI, O'Connell JX, Tron VA. Mitotic granuloma annulare: a clinicopathologic study of 20 cases. *J Cutan Pathol.* 1996;23(6):537–545.

43. Wood MG, Beerman H. Necrobiosis lipoidica, granuloma annulare, and rheumatoid nodule. *J Invest Dermatol.* 1960;34:139–147.

44. Mutasim DF, Bridges AG. Patch granuloma annulare: clinicopathologic study of 6 patients. *J Am Acad Dermatol.* 2000;42(3):417–421.

45. Ronen S, Rothschild M, Suster S. The interstitial variant of granuloma annulare: clinicopathologic study of 69 cases with a comparison with conventional granuloma annulare. *J Cutan Pathol.* 2019;46(7):471–478.

46. Patterson JW. Rheumatoid nodule and subcutaneous granuloma annulare. A comparative histologic study. *Am J Dermatopathol.* 1988;10(1):1–8.

47. Mempel M, Musette P, Flageul B, et al. T-cell receptor repertoire and cytokine pattern in granuloma annulare: defining a particular type of cutaneous granulomatous inflammation. *J Invest Dermatol.* 2002;118(6):957–966.

48. Friedman-Birnbaum R, Haim S, Gideone O, Barzilai A. Histocompatibility antigens in granuloma annulare. Comparative study of the generalized and localized types. *Br J Dermatol.* 1978;98(4):425–428.

49. Wang A, Rahman NT, McGeary MK, et al. Treatment of granuloma annulare and suppression of proinflammatory cytokine activity with tofacitinib. *J Allergy Clin Immunol.* 2020.

50. Modlin RL, Vaccaro SA, Gottlieb B, et al. Granuloma annulare. Identification of cells in the cutaneous infiltrate by immunoperoxidase techniques. *Arch Pathol Lab Med.* 1984;108(5):379–382.

51. Wolff HH, Maciejewski W. The ultrastructure of granuloma annulare. *Arch Dermatol Res.* 1977;259(3):225–234.

52. Kallioinen M, Sandberg M, Kinnunen T, Oikarinen A. Collagen synthesis in granuloma annulare. *J Invest Dermatol.* 1992;98(4):463–468.

53. Thyresson HN, Doyle JA, Winkelmann RK. Granuloma annulare: histopathologic and direct immunofluorescent study. *Acta Derm Venereol.* 1980;60(3):261–263.

54. Nieboer C, Kalsbeek GL. Direct immunofluorescence studies in granuloma annulare, necrobiosis lipoidica and granulomatosis disciformis Miescher. *Dermatologica.* 1979;158(6):427–432.

55. Laymon CW, Fisher I. Necrobiosis lipoidica (diabeticorum?) A histologic study and comparison with granuloma annulare. *Arch Derm Syphilol.* 1949;59(2):150–167.

56. Shanesmith RP, Vogiatzis PI, Binder SW, Cassarino DS. Unusual palisading and necrotizing granulomas associated with a lubricating agent used in lipoplasty. *Am J Dermatopathol.* 2010;32(5):448–452.

57. Shapiro PE, Pinto FJ. The histologic spectrum of mycosis fungoides/Sezary syndrome (cutaneous T-cell lymphoma). A review of 222 biopsies, including newly described patterns and the earliest pathologic changes. *Am J Surg Pathol.* 1994;18(7):645–667.

58. Su LD, Kim YH, LeBoit PE, Swetter SM, Kohler S. Interstitial mycosis fungoides, a variant of mycosis fungoides resembling granuloma annulare and inflammatory morphea. *J Cutan Pathol.* 2002;29(3):135–141.

59. Cooper PH. Eruptive xanthoma: a microscopic simulant of granuloma annulare. *J Cutan Pathol.* 1986;13(3):207–215.

60. Magro CM, Crowson AN, Schapiro BL. The interstitial granulomatous drug reaction: a distinctive clinical and pathological entity. *J Cutan Pathol.* 1998;25(2):72–78.

61. Shah N, Shah M, Drucker AM, Shear NH, Ziv M, Dodiuk-Gad RP. Granulomatous cutaneous drug eruptions: a systematic review. *Am J Clin Dermatol.* 2021;22(1):39–53.

62. Barr KL, Lowe L, Su LD. *Mycobacterium marinum* infection simulating interstitial granuloma annulare: a report of two cases. *Am J Dermatopathol.* 2003;25(2):148–151.

63. Dykman CJ, Galens GJ, Good AE. Linear subcutaneous bands in rheumatoid arthritis. An unusual form of rheumatoid granuloma. *Ann Intern Med.* 1965;63:134–140.

64. Long D, Thiboutot DM, Majeski JT, Vasily DB, Helm KF. Interstitial granulomatous dermatitis with arthritis. *J Am Acad Dermatol.* 1996;34(6):957–961.

65. Aloi F, Tomasini C, Pippione M. Interstitial granulomatous dermatitis with plaques. *Am J Dermatopathol.* 1999;21(4):320–323.

66. Tomasini C, Pippione M. Interstitial granulomatous dermatitis with plaques. *J Am Acad Dermatol.* 2002;46(6):892–899.

67. Peroni A, Colato C, Schena D, Gisondi P, Girolomoni G. Interstitial granulomatous dermatitis: a distinct entity with characteristic histological and clinical pattern. *Br J Dermatol.* 2012;166(4):775–783.

68. Chase DR, Enzinger FM. Epithelioid sarcoma. Diagnosis, prognostic indicators, and treatment. *Am J Surg Pathol.* 1985;9(4):241–263.

69. Orrock JM, Abbott JJ, Gibson LE, Folpe AL. INI1 and GLUT-1 expression in epithelioid sarcoma and its cutaneous neoplastic and nonneoplastic mimics. *Am J Dermatopathol.* 2009;31(2):152–156.

70. Modena P, Lualdi E, Facchinetti F, et al. SMARCB1/INI1 tumor suppressor gene is frequently inactivated in epithelioid sarcomas. *Cancer Res.* 2005;65(10):4012–4019.

71. Hornick JL, Dal Cin P, Fletcher CD. Loss of INI1 expression is characteristic of both conventional and proximal-type epithelioid sarcoma. *Am J Surg Pathol.* 2009;33(4):542–550.

72. Miettinen M, Fanburg-Smith JC, Virolainen M, Shmookler BM, Fetsch JF. Epithelioid sarcoma: an immunohistochemical analysis of 112 classical and variant cases and a discussion of the differential diagnosis. *Hum Pathol.* 1999;30(8):934–942.

73. Min MS, Lebwohl M. Treatment of recalcitrant granuloma annulare (GA) with adalimumab: a single-center, observational study. *J Am Acad Dermatol.* 2016;74(1):127–133.

74. Hanke CW, Bailin PL, Roenigk HH Jr. Annular elastolytic giant cell granuloma. A clinicopathologic study of five cases and a review of similar entities. *J Am Acad Dermatol.* 1979;1(5):413–421.

75. Ragaz A, Ackerman AB. Is actinic granuloma a specific condition? *Am J Dermatopathol.* 1979;1(1):43–50.

76. Dahl MV. Is actinic granuloma really granuloma annulare? *Arch Dermatol.* 1986;122(1):39–40.

77. Meadows KP, O'Reilly MA, Harris RM, Petersen MJ. Erythematous annular plaques in a necklace distribution. Annular elastolytic giant cell granuloma. *Arch Dermatol.* 2001;137(12):1647–1652.

78. O'Brien JP. Actinic granuloma. An annular connective tissue disorder affecting sun-and heat-damaged (elastotic) skin. *Arch Dermatol.* 1975;111(4):460–466.

79. Davies MG, Newman P. Actinic granulomata in a young woman following prolonged sunbed usage. *Br J Dermatol.* 1997;136(5):797–798.

80. Steffen C. Actinic granuloma (O'Brien). *J Cutan Pathol.* 1988;15(2):66–74.

81. Mehregan AH, Altman J. Miescher's granuloma of the face. A variant of the necrobiosis lipoidica-granuloma annulare spectrum. *Arch Dermatol.* 1973;107(1):62–64.

82. Dowling GB, Jones EW. Atypical (annular) necrobiosis lipoidica of the face and scalp. A report of the clinical and histological features of 7 cases. *Dermatologica.* 1967;135(1):11–26.

83. Al-Hoqail IA, Al-Ghamdi AM, Martinka M, Crawford RI. Actinic granuloma is a unique and distinct entity: a comparative study with granuloma annulare. *Am J Dermatopathol.* 2002;24(3):209–212.

84. Ozkaya-Bayazit E, Buyukbabani N, Baykal C, Ozturk A, Okcu M, Soyer HP. Annular elastolytic giant cell granuloma: sparing of a burn scar and successful treatment with chloroquine. *Br J Dermatol.* 1999;140(3):525–530.

85. Muller SA, Winkelmann RK. Necrobiosis lipoidica diabeticorum. A clinical and pathological investigation of 171 cases. *Arch Dermatol.* 1966;93(3):272–281.

86. O'Toole EA, Kennedy U, Nolan JJ, Young MM, Rogers S, Barnes L. Necrobiosis lipoidica: only a minority of patients have diabetes mellitus. *Br J Dermatol.* 1999;140(2):283–286.

87. Hashemi DA, Brown-Joel ZO, Tkachenko E, et al. Clinical features and comorbidities of patients with necrobiosis lipoidica with or without diabetes. *JAMA Dermatol.* 2019;155(4):455–459.

88. Severson KJ, Costello CM, Brumfiel CM, et al. Clinical and morphological features of necrobiosis lipoidica. *J Am Acad Dermatol.* 2021. doi:10.1016/j.jaad.2021.04.034

89. Verrotti A, Chiarelli F, Amerio P, Morgese G. Necrobiosis lipoidica diabeticorum in children and adolescents: a clue for underlying renal and retinal disease. *Pediatr Dermatol.* 1995;12(3):220–223.

90. Rupley KA, Riahi RR, Hooper DO. Granuloma annulare and necrobiosis lipoidica with sequential occurrence in a patient: report and review of literature. *Dermatol Pract Concept.* 2015;5(1):29–34.

91. Gaethe G. Necrobiosis lipoidica diabeticorum of the scalp. *Arch Dermatol.* 1964;89:865–866.

92. Mackey JP. Necrobiosis lipoidica diabeticorum involving scalp and face. *Br J Dermatol.* 1975;93(6):729–730.

93. Mehregan AH, Pinkus H. Necrobiosis lipoidica with sarcoid reaction. A case report. *Arch Dermatol.* 1961;83:143–145.

94. Hashemi DA, Rosenbach M. Ulcerative sarcoidosis. *JAMA Dermatol.* 2019;155(2):238.

95. De la Torre C, Losada A, Cruces MJ. Necrobiosis lipoidica: a case with prominent cholesterol clefting and transepithelial elimination. *Am J Dermatopathol.* 1999;21(6):575–577.

96. Parra CA. Transepithelial elimination in necrobiosis lipoidica. *Br J Dermatol.* 1977;96(1):83–86.

97. Gudmundsen K, Smith O, Dervan P, Powell FC. Necrobiosis lipoidica and sarcoidosis. *Clin Exp Dermatol.* 1991;16(4):287–291.

98. Lim C, Tschuchnigg M, Lim J. Squamous cell carcinoma arising in an area of long-standing necrobiosis lipoidica. *J Cutan Pathol.* 2006;33(8):581–583.

99. McIntosh BC, Lahinjani S, Narayan D. Necrobiosis lipoidica resulting in squamous cell carcinoma. *Conn Med.* 2005;69(7):401–403.

100. Clement M, Guy R, Pembroke AC. Squamous cell carcinoma arising in long-standing necrobiosis lipoidica. *Arch Dermatol.* 1985;121(1):24–25.

101. Santos-Juanes J, Galache C, Curto JR, Carrasco MP, Ribas A, Sanchez del Rio J. Squamous cell carcinoma arising in long-standing necrobiosis lipoidica. *J Eur Acad Dermatol Venereol.* 2004;18(2):199–200.

102. Snow JL, Su WP. Lipomembranous (membranocystic) fat necrosis. Clinicopathologic correlation of 38 cases. *Am J Dermatopathol.* 1996;18(2):151–155.

103. Requena L, Yus ES. Panniculitis. Part I. Mostly septal panniculitis. *J Am Acad Dermatol.* 2001;45(2):163–183; quiz 84–86.

104. Smith JG Jr, Wansker BA. Asteroid bodies in necrobiosis lipoidica. *AMA Arch Derm.* 1956;74(3):276–279.

105. Gibson LE, Reizner GT, Winkelmann RK. Necrobiosis lipoidica diabeticorum with cholesterol clefts in the differential diagnosis of necrobiotic xanthogranuloma. *J Cutan Pathol.* 1988;15(1):18–21.

106. Alegre VA, Winkelmann RK. A new histopathologic feature of necrobiosis lipoidica diabeticorum: lymphoid nodules. *J Cutan Pathol.* 1988;15(2):75–77.

107. Bauer MF, Hirsch P, Bullock WK, Abul-Haj SK. Necrobiosis lipoidica diabeticorum. A cutaneous manifestation of diabetic microangiopathy. *Arch Dermatol.* 1964;90:558–566.

108. Kato M, Oiso N, Itoh T, et al. Necrobiosis lipoidica with infiltration of Th17 cells into vascular lesions. *J Dermatol.* 2014;41(5):459–461.

109. Wakusawa C, Fujimura T, Kambayashi Y, Furudate S, Hashimoto A, Aiba S. Pigmented necrobiosis lipoidica accompanied by insulin-dependent diabetes mellitus induces CD163(+) proinflammatory macrophages and interleukin-17-producing cells. *Acta Derm Venereol.* 2013;93(4):475–476.

110. Kreuter A, Knierim C, Stucker M, et al. Fumaric acid esters in necrobiosis lipoidica: results of a prospective noncontrolled study. *Br J Dermatol.* 2005;153(4):802–807.

111. Sparrow G, Abell E. Granuloma annulare and necrobiosis lipoidica treated by jet injector. *Br J Dermatol.* 1975;93(1):85–89.

112. Damsky W, Singh K, Galan A, King B. Treatment of necrobiosis lipoidica with combination Janus kinase inhibition and intralesional corticosteroid. *JAAD Case Rep.* 2020;6(2):133–135.

113. Lee JJ, English JC 3rd. Improvement in ulcerative necrobiosis lipoidica after Janus kinase-inhibitor therapy for polycythemia vera. *JAMA Dermatol.* 2018;154(6):733–734.

114. Oikarinen A, Mortenhumer M, Kallioinen M, Savolainen ER. Necrobiosis lipoidica: ultrastructural and biochemical demonstration of a collagen defect. *J Invest Dermatol.* 1987;88(2):227–232.

115. Ullman S, Dahl MV. Necrobiosis lipoidica. An immunofluorescence study. *Arch Dermatol.* 1977;113(12):1671–1673.

116. Quimby SR, Muller SA, Schroeter AL. The cutaneous immunopathology of necrobiosis lipoidica diabeticorum. *Arch Dermatol.* 1988;124(9):1364–1371.

117. Laukkanen A, Fraki JE, Vaatainen N, Korhonen T, Naukkarinen A. Necrobiosis lipoidica: clinical and immunofluorescent study. *Dermatologica.* 1986;172(2):89–92.

118. Finan MC, Winkelmann RK. Histopathology of necrobiotic xanthogranuloma with paraproteinemia. *J Cutan Pathol.* 1987;14(2):92–99.

119. Erfurt-Berge C, Seitz AT, Rehse C, Wollina U, Schwede K, Renner R. Update on clinical and laboratory features in necrobiosis lipoidica: a retrospective multicentre study of 52 patients. *Eur J Dermatol.* 2012;22(6):770–775.

120. Cohen O, Yaniv R, Karasik A, Trau H. Necrobiosis lipoidica and diabetic control revisited. *Med Hypotheses.* 1996;46(4):348–350.

121. Veys EM, De Keyser F. Rheumatoid nodules: differential diagnosis and immunohistological findings. *Ann Rheum Dis.* 1993;52(9):625–626.

122. Chalmers IM, Arneja AS. Rheumatoid nodules on amputation stumps: report of three cases. *Arch Phys Med Rehabil.* 1994;75(10):1151–1153.

123. Moore CP, Willkens RF. The subcutaneous nodule: its significance in the diagnosis of rheumatic disease. *Semin Arthritis Rheum.* 1977;7(1):63–79.

124. Suriani RJ, Lansman S, Konstadt S. Intracardiac rheumatoid nodule presenting as a left atrial mass. *Am Heart J.* 1994;127(2):463–465.

125. Jackson CG, Chess RL, Ward JR. A case of rheumatoid nodule formation within the central nervous system and review of the literature. *J Rheumatol.* 1984;11(2):237–240.

126. Horn RT Jr, Goette DK. Perforating rheumatoid nodule. *Arch Dermatol.* 1982;118(9):696–697.

127. Falcini F, Taccetti G, Ermini M, et al. Methotrexate-associated appearance and rapid progression of rheumatoid nodules in systemic-onset juvenile rheumatoid arthritis. *Arthritis Rheum.* 1997;40(1):175–178.

128. Williams FM, Cohen PR, Arnett FC. Accelerated cutaneous nodulosis during methotrexate therapy in a patient with rheumatoid arthritis. *J Am Acad Dermatol.* 1998;39(2, pt 2):359–362.

129. Gomez MT, Polo AM, Romero AM, Gutierrez JV, Garcia GM. Rheumatoid nodulosis: report of two cases. *J Eur Acad Dermatol Venereol.* 2003;17(6):695–698.

130. Sokoloff L, McCluskey RT, Bunim JJ. Vascularity of the early subcutaneous nodule of rheumatoid arthritis. *AMA Arch Pathol.* 1953;55(6):475–495.

131. Elewaut D, De Keyser F, De Wever N, et al. A comparative phenotypical analysis of rheumatoid nodules and rheumatoid synovium with special reference to adhesion molecules and activation markers. *Ann Rheum Dis.* 1998;57(8):480–486.

132. Hessian PA, Highton J, Kean A, Sun CK, Chin M. Cytokine profile of the rheumatoid nodule suggests that it is a Th1 granuloma. *Arthritis Rheum.* 2003;48(2):334–338.

133. Wikaningrum R, Highton J, Parker A, et al. Pathogenic mechanisms in the rheumatoid nodule: comparison of proinflammatory cytokine production and cell adhesion molecule expression in rheumatoid nodules and synovial membranes from the same patient. *Arthritis Rheum.* 1998;41(10):1783–1797.

134. Alguacil-Garcia A. Necrobiotic palisading suture granulomas simulating rheumatoid nodule. *Am J Surg Pathol.* 1993;17(9):920–923.

135. Dawson MH. A comparative study of subcutaneous nodules in rheumatic fever and rheumatoid arthritis. *J Exp Med.* 1933;57(5):845–858.

136. Hayes RM, Gibson S. An evaluation of rheumatic nodules in children: a clinical study of 167 cases. *JAMA.* 1942;119(7):554–555.

137. Chu P, Connolly MK, LeBoit PE. The histopathologic spectrum of palisaded neutrophilic and granulomatous dermatitis in patients with collagen vascular disease. *Arch Dermatol.* 1994;130(10):1278–1283.

138. Finan MC. Rheumatoid papule, cutaneous extravascular necrotizing granuloma, and Churg-Strauss granuloma: are they the same entity? *J Am Acad Dermatol.* 1990;22(1):142–143.

139. Higaki Y, Yamashita H, Sato K, Higaki M, Kawashima M. Rheumatoid papules: a report on four patients with histopathologic analysis. *J Am Acad Dermatol.* 1993;28(3):406–411.

140. Jorizzo JL, Olansky AJ, Stanley RJ. Superficial ulcerating necrobiosis in rheumatoid arthritis. A variant of the necrobiosis lipoidica-rheumatoid nodule spectrum? *Arch Dermatol.* 1982;118(4):255–259.

141. Patterson JW, Demos PT. Superficial ulcerating rheumatoid necrobiosis: a perforating rheumatoid nodule. *Cutis.* 1985;36(4):323–325, 328.

142. Sangueza OP, Caudell MD, Mengesha YM, et al. Palisaded neutrophilic granulomatous dermatitis in rheumatoid arthritis. *J Am Acad Dermatol.* 2002;47(2):251–257.

143. Asahina A, Fujita H, Fukunaga Y, Kenmochi Y, Ikenaka T, Mitomi H. Early lesion of palisaded neutrophilic granulomatous dermatitis in ulcerative colitis. *Eur J Dermatol.* 2007;17(3):234–237.

144. Brecher A. Palisaded neutrophilic and granulomatous dermatitis. *Dermatol Online J.* 2003;9(4):1.

145. Heidary N, Mengden S, Pomeranz MK. Palisaded neutrophilic and granulomatous dermatosis. *Dermatol Online J.* 2008;14(5):17.

146. Gordon EA, Schmidt AN, Boyd AS. Palisaded neutrophilic and granulomatous dermatitis: a presenting sign of sarcoidosis? *J Am Acad Dermatol.* 2011;65(3):664–665.

147. Mahmoodi M, Ahmad A, Bansal C, Cusack CA. Palisaded neutrophilic and granulomatous dermatitis in association with sarcoidosis. *J Cutan Pathol.* 2011;38(4):365–368.

148. Germanas JP, Mehrabi D, Carder KR. Palisaded neutrophilic granulomatous dermatitis in a 12-year-old girl with systemic lupus erythematosus. *J Am Acad Dermatol.* 2006;55(2, suppl):S60–S62.

149. Kern M, Shiver MD, Addis KM, Gardner JM. Palisaded neutrophilic and granulomatous dermatitis/interstitial granulomatous dermatitis overlap: a striking clinical and histologic presentation with "burning rope sign" and subsequent mirror image contralateral recurrence. *Am J Dermatopathol.* 2017;39(9):e141–e146.

150. Rosenbach M, English JC 3rd. Reactive granulomatous dermatitis: a review of palisaded neutrophilic and granulomatous dermatitis, interstitial granulomatous dermatitis, interstitial granulomatous drug reaction, and a proposed reclassification. *Dermatol Clin.* 2015;33(3):373–387.

151. Rodriguez-Garijo N, Bielsa I, Mascaro JM Jr, et al. Reactive granulomatous dermatitis as a histological pattern including manifestations of interstitial granulomatous dermatitis and palisaded neutrophilic and granulomatous dermatitis: a study of 52 patients. *J Eur Acad Dermatol Venereol.* 2021;35(4):988–994.

152. DiCaudo DJ, Connolly SM. Interstitial granulomatous dermatitis associated with pulmonary coccidioidomycosis. *J Am Acad Dermatol.* 2001;45(6):840–845.

153. Bremner R, Simpson E, White CR, Morrison L, Deodhar A. Palisaded neutrophilic and granulomatous dermatitis: an unusual cutaneous manifestation of immune-mediated disorders. *Semin Arthritis Rheum.* 2004;34(3):610–616.

154. James DG, Siltzbach LE, Sharma OP, Carstairs LS. A tale of two cities: a comparison of sarcoidosis in London and New York. *Arch Intern Med.* 1969;123(2):187–191.

155. Tejera Segura B, Holgado S, Mateo L, Pego-Reigosa JM, Carnicero Iglesias M, Olive A. Lofgren syndrome: a study of 80 cases [in Spanish]. *Med Clin (Barc).* 2014;143(4):166–169.

156. Mana J, Gomez-Vaquero C, Montero A, et al. Lofgren's syndrome revisited: a study of 186 patients. *Am J Med.* 1999;107(3):240–245.

157. Mana J, Marcoval J, Graells J, Salazar A, Peyri J, Pujol R. Cutaneous involvement in sarcoidosis. Relationship to systemic disease. *Arch Dermatol.* 1997;133(7):882–888.

158. Yanardag H, Pamuk ON, Karayel T. Cutaneous involvement in sarcoidosis: analysis of the features in 170 patients. *Respir Med.* 2003;97(8):978–982.

159. Baughman RP, Teirstein AS, Judson MA, et al. Clinical characteristics of patients in a case control study of sarcoidosis. *Am J Respir Crit Care Med.* 2001;164(10, pt 1):1885–1889.

160. Longcope WT, Freiman DG. A study of sarcoidosis; based on a combined investigation of 160 cases including 30 autopsies from The Johns Hopkins Hospital and Massachusetts General Hospital. *Medicine (Baltimore).* 1952;31(1):1–132.

161. Judson MA. The clinical features of sarcoidosis: a comprehensive review. *Clin Rev Allergy Immunol.* 2015;49(1):63–78.

162. Baughman RP, Field S, Costabel U, et al. Sarcoidosis in America. Analysis based on health care use. *Ann Am Thorac Soc.* 2016; 13(8):1244–1252.

163. Mirsaeidi M, Machado RF, Schraufnagel D, Sweiss NJ, Baughman RP. Racial difference in sarcoidosis mortality in the United States. *Chest.* 2015;147(2):438–449.

164. Arkema EV, Grunewald J, Kullberg S, Eklund A, Askling J. Sarcoidosis incidence and prevalence: a nationwide register-based assessment in Sweden. *Eur Respir J.* 2016;48(6):1690–1699.

165. Byg KE, Milman N, Hansen S. Sarcoidosis in Denmark 1980-1994. A registry-based incidence study comprising 5536 patients. *Sarcoidosis Vasc Diffuse Lung Dis.* 2003;20(1):46–52.

166. Milman N, Selroos O. Pulmonary sarcoidosis in the Nordic countries 1950-1982. Epidemiology and clinical picture. *Sarcoidosis.* 1990;7(1):50–57.

167. Yotsumoto S, Takahashi Y, Takei S, Shimada S, Miyata K, Kanzaki T. Early onset sarcoidosis masquerading as juvenile rheumatoid arthritis. *J Am Acad Dermatol.* 2000;43(5, pt 2):969–971.

168. Seo SK, Yeum JS, Suh JC, Na GY. Lichenoid sarcoidosis in a 3-year-old girl. *Pediatr Dermatol.* 2001;18(5):384–387.

169. O'Driscoll JB, Beck MH, Lendon M, Wraith J, Sardharwalla IB. Cutaneous presentation of sarcoidosis in an infant. *Clin Exp Dermatol.* 1990;15(1):60–62.

170. Priori R, Bombardieri M, Spinelli FR, et al. Sporadic Blau syndrome with a double CARD15 mutation. Report of a case with lifelong follow-up. *Sarcoidosis Vasc Diffuse Lung Dis.* 2004;21(3):228–231.

171. Kanazawa N, Okafuji I, Kambe N, et al. Early-onset sarcoidosis and CARD15 mutations with constitutive nuclear factor-kappaB activation: common genetic etiology with Blau syndrome. *Blood.* 2005;105(3):1195–1197.

172. Rose CD, Pans S, Casteels I, et al. Blau syndrome: cross-sectional data from a multicentre study of clinical, radiological and functional outcomes. *Rheumatology (Oxford).* 2015;54(6):1008–1016.

173. Okafuji I, Nishikomori R, Kanazawa N, et al. Role of the NOD2 genotype in the clinical phenotype of Blau syndrome and early-onset sarcoidosis. *Arthritis Rheum.* 2009;60(1):242–250.

174. Spiteri MA, Matthey F, Gordon T, Carstairs LS, James DG. Lupus pernio: a clinico-radiological study of thirty-five cases. *Br J Dermatol.* 1985;112(3):315–322.

175. Neville E, Mills RG, Jash DK, Mackinnon DM, Carstairs LS, James DG. Sarcoidosis of the upper respiratory tract and its association with lupus pernio. *Thorax.* 1976;31(6):660–664.

176. Pitt P, Hamilton EB, Innes EH, Morley KD, Monk BE, Hughes GR. Sarcoid dactylitis. *Ann Rheum Dis.* 1983;42(6):634–639.

177. Garrido-Ruiz MC, Enguita-Valls AB, de Arriba MG, Vanaclocha F, Peralto JL. Lichenoid sarcoidosis: a case with clinical and histopathological lichenoid features. *Am J Dermatopathol.* 2008; 30(3):271–273.

178. Kelly AP. Icthyosiform sarcoid. *Arch Dermatol.* 1978;114(10): 1551–1552.

179. Kauh YC, Goody HE, Luscombe HA. Ichthyosiform sarcoidosis. *Arch Dermatol.* 1978;114(1):100–101.

180. Feind-Koopmans AG, Lucker GP, van de Kerkhof PC. Acquired ichthyosiform erythroderma and sarcoidosis. *J Am Acad Dermatol.* 1996;35(5, pt 2):826–828.

181. Bazex J, Dupin P, Giordano F. Cutaneous and visceral sarcoidosis. Apropos of an exceptional form [in French]. *Ann Dermatol Venereol.* 1987;114(5):685–690.

182. Albertini JG, Tyler W, Miller OF 3rd. Ulcerative sarcoidosis. Case report and review of the literature. *Arch Dermatol.* 1997;133(2):215–219.

183. Hruza GJ, Kerdel FA. Generalized atrophic sarcoidosis with ulcerations. *Arch Dermatol.* 1986;122(3):320–322.

184. Schwartz RA, Robertson DB, Tierney LM Jr, McNutt NS. Generalized ulcerative sarcoidosis. *Arch Dermatol.* 1982;118(11):931–933.

185. Rongioletti F, Bellisomi A, Rebora A. Disseminated angiolupoid sarcoidosis. *Cutis.* 1987;40(4):341–343.

186. Wu MC, Lee JY. Cutaneous sarcoidosis in southern Taiwan: clinicopathologic study of a series with high proportions of lesions confined to the face and angiolupoid variant. *J Eur Acad Dermatol Venereol.* 2013;27(4):499–505.

187. Cornelius CE 3rd, Stein KM, Hanshaw WJ, Spott DA. Hypopigmentation and sarcoidosis. *Arch Dermatol.* 1973;108(2):249–251.

188. Clayton R, Breathnach A, Martin B, Feiwel M. Hypopigmented sarcoidosis in the negro. Report of eight cases with ultrastructural observations. *Br J Dermatol.* 1977;96(2):119–125.

189. Darier J, Roussy G. Un cas de tumeurs benignes multiples: sarcoides sous-cutanees ou tuberculides nodulaires hypodermiques. *Ann Dermatol Syph.* 1904;2:144.

190. Marcoval J, Mana J, Moreno A, Peyri J. Subcutaneous sarcoidosis—clinicopathological study of 10 cases. *Br J Dermatol.* 2005;153(4): 790–794.

191. Wendling J, Descamps V, Grossin M, et al. Sarcoidosis during combined interferon alfa and ribavirin therapy in 2 patients with chronic hepatitis C. *Arch Dermatol.* 2002;138(4):546–547.

192. Murphy MJ, Cohen JM, Vesely MD, Damsky W. Paradoxical eruptions to targeted therapies in dermatology: a systematic review and analysis. *J Am Acad Dermatol.* 2020. doi:10.1016/j .jaad.2020.12.010

193. Corazza M, Bacilieri S, Strumia R. Post-herpes zoster scar sarcoidosis. *Acta Derm Venereol.* 1999;79(1):95.

194. Bisaccia E, Scarborough DA, Carr RD. Cutaneous sarcoid granuloma formation in herpes zoster scars. *Arch Dermatol.* 1983;119(9):788–789.

195. Collins P, Evans AT, Gray W, Levison DA. Pulmonary sarcoidosis presenting as a granulomatous tattoo reaction. *Br J Dermatol.* 1994;130(5):658–662.

196. Papageorgiou PP, Hongcharu W, Chu AC. Systemic sarcoidosis presenting with multiple tattoo granulomas and an extra-tattoo cutaneous granuloma. *J Eur Acad Dermatol Venereol.* 1999;12(1):51–53.

197. Jacyk WK. Annular granulomatous lesions in exogenous ochronosis are manifestation of sarcoidosis. *Am J Dermatopathol.* 1995;17(1):18–22.

198. Walsh NM, Hanly JG, Tremaine R, Murray S. Cutaneous sarcoidosis and foreign bodies. *Am J Dermatopathol.* 1993;15(3):203–207.

199. Marcoval J, Mana J, Moreno A, Gallego I, Fortuno Y, Peyri J. Foreign bodies in granulomatous cutaneous lesions of patients with systemic sarcoidosis. *Arch Dermatol.* 2001;137(4):427–430.

200. Kim YC, Triffet MK, Gibson LE. Foreign bodies in sarcoidosis. *Am J Dermatopathol.* 2000;22(5):408–412.

201. Wood BT, Behlen CH 2nd, Weary PE. The Association of Sarcoidosis, Erythema Nodosum, and Arthritis. *Arch Dermatol.* 1966;94(4):406–408.

202. Barrie HJ, Bogoch A. The natural history of the sarcoid granuloma. *Am J Pathol.* 1953;29(3):451–469.

203. Cardoso JC, Cravo M, Reis JP, Tellechea O. Cutaneous sarcoidosis: a histopathological study. *J Eur Acad Dermatol Venereol.* 2009;23(6):678–682.

204. Okamoto H. Epidermal changes in cutaneous lesions of sarcoidosis. *Am J Dermatopathol.* 1999;21(3):229–233.

205. Chevrant-Breton J, Revillon L, Pony JC, Huguenin A. Sarcoidosis with extensive ulcerating and atrophying cutaneous manifestations (of the Pick-Herxheimer type) and with cardiac and muscular involvement. About one case (author's transl) [in French]. *Ann Dermatol Venereol.* 1977;104(12):72–811.

206. Glass LA, Apisarnthanarax P. Verrucous sarcoidosis simulating hypertrophic lichen planus. *Int J Dermatol.* 1989;28(8):539–541.

207. Smith HR, Black MM. Verrucous cutaneous sarcoidosis. *Clin Exp Dermatol.* 2000;25(1):98–99.

208. Vainsencher D, Winkelmann RK. Subcutaneous sarcoidosis. *Arch Dermatol.* 1984;120(8):1028–1031.

209. Mangas C, Fernandez-Figueras MT, Fite E, Fernandez-Chico N, Sabat M, Ferrandiz C. Clinical spectrum and histological analysis of 32 cases of specific cutaneous sarcoidosis. *J Cutan Pathol.* 2006;33(12):772–777.

210. Winkelmann RK, Dahl PR, Perniciaro C. Asteroid bodies and other cytoplasmic inclusions in necrobiotic xanthogranuloma with paraproteinemia. *J Am Acad Dermatol.* 1998;38(6, pt 1):967–970.

211. Jacyk WK. Cutaneous sarcoidosis in black South Africans. *Int J Dermatol.* 1999;38(11):841–845.

212. Burov EA, Kantor GR, Isaac M. Morpheaform sarcoidosis: report of three cases. *J Am Acad Dermatol.* 1998;39(2, pt 2):345–348.

213. Ball NJ, Kho GT, Martinka M. The histologic spectrum of cutaneous sarcoidosis: a study of twenty-eight cases. *J Cutan Pathol.* 2004;31(2):160–168.

214. Grunewald J, Grutters JC, Arkema EV, Saketkoo LA, Moller DR, Muller-Quernheim J. Sarcoidosis. *Nat Rev Dis Primers.* 2019;5(1):45.

215. Scadding JG. Sarcoidosis, with special reference to lung changes. *Br Med J.* 1950;1(4656):745–753.

216. Scadding JG. Prognosis of intrathoracic sarcoidosis in England. A review of 136 cases after five years' observation. *Br Med J.* 1961;2(5261):1165–1172.

217. Mahevas M, Lescure FX, Boffa JJ, et al. Renal sarcoidosis: clinical, laboratory, and histologic presentation and outcome in 47 patients. *Medicine (Baltimore).* 2009;88(2):98–106.

218. Langrand C, Bihan H, Raverot G, et al. Hypothalamo-pituitary sarcoidosis: a multicenter study of 24 patients. *QJM.* 2012;105(10):981–995.

219. Bihan H, Christozova V, Dumas JL, et al. Sarcoidosis: clinical, hormonal, and magnetic resonance imaging (MRI) manifestations of hypothalamic-pituitary disease in 9 patients and review of the literature. *Medicine (Baltimore).* 2007;86(5):259–268.

220. Siltzbach LE. The Kveim test in sarcoidosis. A study of 750 patients. *JAMA.* 1961;178:476–482.

221. Siltzbach LE, Ehrlich JC. The Nickerson-Kveim reaction in sarcoidosis. *Am J Med.* 1954;16(6):790–803.

222. Koonitz CH, Joyner LR, Nelson RA. Transbronchial lung biopsy via the fiberoptic bronchoscope in sarcoidosis. *Ann Intern Med.* 1976;85(1):64–66.

223. Nakajima T, Yasufuku K, Kurosu K, et al. The role of EBUS-TBNA for the diagnosis of sarcoidosis—comparisons with other bronchoscopic diagnostic modalities. *Respir Med.* 2009;103(12):1796–1800.

224. Lieberman J. Elevation of serum angiotensin-converting-enzyme (ACE) level in sarcoidosis. *Am J Med.* 1975;59(3):365–372.

225. Bargagli E, Bianchi N, Margollicci M, et al. Chitotriosidase and soluble IL-2 receptor: comparison of two markers of sarcoidosis severity. *Scand J Clin Lab Invest.* 2008;68(6):479–483.

226. Newman LS, Rose CS, Bresnitz EA, et al. A case control etiologic study of sarcoidosis: environmental and occupational risk factors. *Am J Respir Crit Care Med.* 2004;170(12):1324–1330.

227. Casanova N, Zhou T, Knox KS, Garcia JGN. Identifying novel biomarkers in sarcoidosis using genome-based approaches. *Clin Chest Med.* 2015;36(4):621–630.

228. Grunewald J, Kaiser Y, Ostadkarampour M, et al. T-cell receptor-HLA-DRB1 associations suggest specific antigens in pulmonary sarcoidosis. *Eur Respir J.* 2016;47(3):898–909.

229. Ahlgren KM, Ruckdeschel T, Eklund A, Wahlstrom J, Grunewald J. T cell receptor-Vbeta repertoires in lung and blood CD4+ and CD8+ T cells of pulmonary sarcoidosis patients. *BMC Pulm Med.* 2014;14:50.

230. Mitchell AM, Kaiser Y, Falta MT, et al. Shared alphabeta TCR usage in lungs of sarcoidosis patients with Lofgren's syndrome. *J Immunol.* 2017;199(7):2279–2290.

231. Klein JT, Horn TD, Forman JD, Silver RF, Teirstein AS, Moller DR. Selection of oligoclonal V beta-specific T cells in the intradermal response to Kveim-Siltzbach reagent in individuals with sarcoidosis. *J Immunol.* 1995;154(3):1450–1460.

232. Wahlstrom J, Dengjel J, Winqvist O, et al. Autoimmune T cell responses to antigenic peptides presented by bronchoalveolar lavage cell HLA-DR molecules in sarcoidosis. *Clin Immunol.* 2009;133(3):353–363.

233. Kinloch AJ, Kaiser Y, Wolfgeher D, et al. In situ humoral immunity to vimentin in HLA-DRB1*03(+) patients with pulmonary sarcoidosis. *Front Immunol.* 2018;9:1516.

234. Chen ES, Wahlstrom J, Song Z, et al. T cell responses to mycobacterial catalase-peroxidase profile a pathogenic antigen in systemic sarcoidosis. *J Immunol.* 2008;181(12):8784–8796.

235. Song Z, Marzilli L, Greenlee BM, et al. Mycobacterial catalase-peroxidase is a tissue antigen and target of the adaptive immune response in systemic sarcoidosis. *J Exp Med.* 2005;201(5):755–767.

236. Yamada T, Eishi Y, Ikeda S, et al. In situ localization of *Propionibacterium acnes* DNA in lymph nodes from sarcoidosis patients by signal amplification with catalysed reporter deposition. *J Pathol.* 2002;198(4):541–547.

237. Ishige I, Eishi Y, Takemura T, et al. *Propionibacterium acnes* is the most common bacterium commensal in peripheral lung tissue and mediastinal lymph nodes from subjects without sarcoidosis. *Sarcoidosis Vasc Diffuse Lung Dis.* 2005;22(1):33–42.

238. Iannuzzi MC, Rybicki BA, Teirstein AS. Sarcoidosis. *N Engl J Med.* 2007;357(21):2153–2165.

239. Azar HA, Lunardelli C. Collagen nature of asteroid bodies of giant cells in sarcoidosis. *Am J Pathol.* 1969;57(1):81–92.

240. Civatte J. Sarcoidose et infiltrats tuberculoides. *Ann Dermatol Syphiligr.* 1963;90:5.

241. Azulay RD. Histopathology of skin lesions in leprosy. *Int J Lepr Other Mycobact Dis.* 1971;39(2):244–250.

242. Wiersema JP, Binford CH. The identification of leprosy among epithelioid cell granulomas of the skin. *Int J Lepr Other Mycobact Dis.* 1972;40(1):10–32.

243. Pariser RJ, Paul J, Hirano S, Torosky C, Smith M. A double-blind, randomized, placebo-controlled trial of adalimumab in the treatment of cutaneous sarcoidosis. *J Am Acad Dermatol.* 2013;68(5):765–773.

244. Baughman RP, Drent M, Kavuru M, et al. Infliximab therapy in patients with chronic sarcoidosis and pulmonary involvement. *Am J Respir Crit Care Med.* 2006;174(7):795–802.

245. Damsky W, Thakral D, Emeagwali N, Galan A, King B. Tofacitinib treatment and molecular analysis of cutaneous sarcoidosis. *N Engl J Med.* 2018;379(26):2540–2546.

246. Kerkemeyer KL, Meah N, Sinclair RD. Tofacitinib for cutaneous and pulmonary sarcoidosis: a case series. *J Am Acad Dermatol.* 2021;84(2):581–583.

247. Epstein WL, Skahen JR, Krasnobrod H. The organized epithelioid cell granuloma: differentiation of allergic (zirconium) from colloidal (silica) types. *Am J Pathol.* 1963;43:391–405.

248. Ho WS, Chan AC, Law BK. Management of paraffinoma of the breast: 10 years' experience. *Br J Plast Surg.* 2001;54(3):232–234.

249. Cohen JL, Keoleian CM, Krull EA. Penile paraffinoma: self-injection with mineral oil. *J Am Acad Dermatol.* 2002;47(5, suppl):S251–S253.

250. Klein JA, Cole G, Barr RJ, Bartlow G, Fulwider C. Paraffinomas of the scalp. *Arch Dermatol.* 1985;121(3):382–385.

251. Behar TA, Anderson EE, Barwick WJ, Mohler JL. Sclerosing lipogranulomatosis: a case report of scrotal injection of automobile transmission fluid and literature review of subcutaneous injection of oils. *Plast Reconstr Surg.* 1993;91(2):352–361.

252. Cohen JL, Keoleian CM, Krull EA. Penile paraffinoma: self-injection with mineral oil. *J Am Acad Dermatol.* 2001;45(6, suppl):S222–S224.

253. Smetana HF, Bernhard W. Sclerosing lipogranuloma. *Arch Pathol (Chic).* 1950;50(3):296–325.

254. Newcomer VD, Graham JH, Schaffert RR, Kaplan L. Sclerosing lipogranuloma resulting from exogenous lipids. *AMA Arch Derm.* 1956;73(4):361–372.

255. Oertel YC, Johnson FB. Sclerosing lipogranuloma of male genitalia. Review of 23 cases. *Arch Pathol Lab Med.* 1977;101(6):321–326.

256. Mason J, Apisarnthanarax P. Migratory silicone granuloma. *Arch Dermatol.* 1981;117(6):366–367.

257. Brown SL, Silverman BG, Berg WA. Rupture of silicone-gel breast implants: causes, sequelae, and diagnosis. *Lancet.* 1997;350(9090):1531–1537.

258. Suzuki K, Aoki M, Kawana S, Hyakusoku H, Miyazawa S. Metastatic silicone granuloma: lupus miliaris disseminatus faciei-like facial nodules and sicca complex in a silicone breast implant recipient. *Arch Dermatol.* 2002;138(4):537–538.

259. Yanagihara M, Fujii T, Wakamatu N, Ishizaki H, Takehara T, Nawate K. Silicone granuloma on the entry points of acupuncture, venepuncture and surgical needles. *J Cutan Pathol.* 2000;27(6):301–305.

260. Tang L, Eaton JW. Inflammatory responses to biomaterials. *Am J Clin Pathol.* 1995;103(4):466–471.

261. Morgan AM. Localized reactions to injected therapeutic materials. Part 2. Surgical agents. *J Cutan Pathol.* 1995;22(4):289–303.

262. Raso DS, Greene WB, Vesely JJ, Willingham MC. Light microscopy techniques for the demonstration of silicone gel. *Arch Pathol Lab Med.* 1994;118(10):984–987.

263. Ellis H. Pathological changes produced by surgical dusting powders. *Ann R Coll Surg Engl.* 1994;76(1):5–8.

264. Lazaro C, Reichelt C, Lazaro J, Grasa MP, Carapeto FJ. Foreign body post-varicella granulomas due to talc. *J Eur Acad Dermatol Venereol.* 2006;20(1):75–78.

265. Tye MJ, Hashimoto K, Fox F. Talc granulomas of the skin. *JAMA.* 1966;198(13):1370–1372.

266. Leonard DD. Starch granulomas. *Arch Dermatol.* 1973;107(1):101–103.

267. Snyder RA, Schwartz RA. Cactus bristle implantation. Report of an unusual case initially seen with rows of yellow hairs. *Arch Dermatol.* 1983;119(2):152–154.

268. Suzuki H, Baba S. Cactus granuloma of the skin. *J Dermatol.* 1993;20(7):424–427.

269. Winer LH, Zeilenga RH. Cactus granulomas of the skin; report of a case. *AMA Arch Derm.* 1955;72(6):566–569.

270. Sondenaa K, Andersen E, Nesvik I, Soreide JA. Patient characteristics and symptoms in chronic pilonidal sinus disease. *Int J Colorectal Dis.* 1995;10(1):39–42.

271. Joseph HL, Gifford H. Barber's interdigital pilonidal sinus: the incidence, pathology, and pathogenesis. *AMA Arch Derm Syphilol.* 1954;70(5):616–624.

272. Adams CI, Petrie PW, Hooper G. Interdigital pilonidal sinus in the hand. *J Hand Surg Br.* 2001;26(1):53–55.

273. Price SM, Popkin GL. Barbers' interdigital hair sinus. *Arch Dermatol.* 1976;112(4):523–524.

274. Mohanna PN, Al-Sam SZ, Flemming AF. Subungual pilonidal sinus of the hand in a dog groomer. *Br J Plast Surg.* 2001;54(2):176–178.

275. Goebel M, Rupec M. Interdigital pilonidal sinus [in German]. *Dermatol Wochenschr.* 1967;153(13):341–345.

276. Rocha G, Fraga S. Sea urchin granuloma of the skin. *Arch Dermatol.* 1962;85:406–408.

277. Haneke E, Kolsch I. [Sea urchin granulomas]. *Hautarzt.* 1980;31(3):159–160.

278. Kinmont PD. Sea-urchin sarcoidal granuloma. *Br J Dermatol.* 1965;77:335–343.

279. Suarez-Penaranda JM, Vieites B, Del Rio E, Ortiz-Rey JA, Anton I. Histopathologic and immunohistochemical features of sea urchin granulomas. *J Cutan Pathol.* 2013;40(6):550–556.

280. De La Torre C, Toribio J. Sea-urchin granuloma: histologic profile. A pathologic study of 50 biopsies. *J Cutan Pathol.* 2001;28(5):223–228.

281. Epstein E, Gerstl B, Berk M, Belber JP. Silica pregranuloma. *AMA Arch Derm.* 1955;71(5):645–647.

282. Eskeland G, Langmark F, Husby G. Silicon granuloma of skin and subcutaneous tissue. *Acta Pathol Microbiol Scand Suppl.* 1974;248(suppl):69–73.

283. Mowry RG, Sams WM Jr, Caulfield JB. Cutaneous silica granuloma. A rare entity or rarely diagnosed? Report of two cases with review of the literature. *Arch Dermatol.* 1991;127(5):692–694.

284. Schewach-Millet M, Ziv R, Trau H, Zwas ST, Ronnen M, Rubinstein I. Sarcoidosis versus foreign-body granulomas. *Int J Dermatol.* 1987;26(9):582–585.

285. Rank BK, Hicks JD, Lovie M. Pseudotuberculoma granulosum silicoticum. *Br J Plast Surg.* 1972;25(1):42–48.

286. Arzt L. Foreign body granulomas and Boeck's sarcoid. *J Invest Dermatol.* 1955;24(3):155–166.

287. Morales-Neira D. It's elemental! Siliceous diatom frustules producing sarcoid-like granulomas in the subcutis. *J Cutan Pathol.* 2021;48(6):795–801.

288. Epstein WL. Granulomatous hypersensitivity. *Prog Allergy.* 1967;11:36–88.

289. Skelton HG 3rd, Smith KJ, Johnson FB, Cooper CR, Tyler WF, Lupton GP. Zirconium granuloma resulting from an aluminum zirconium complex: a previously unrecognized agent in the development of hypersensitivity granulomas. *J Am Acad Dermatol.* 1993;28(5, pt 2):874–876.

290. Montemarano AD, Sau P, Johnson FB, James WD. Cutaneous granulomas caused by an aluminum-zirconium complex: an ingredient of antiperspirants. *J Am Acad Dermatol.* 1997;37(3, pt 1):496–498.

291. Williams RM, Skipworth GB. Zirconium granulomas of the glabrous skin following treatment of rhus dermatitis: report of two cases. *Arch Dermatol.* 1959;80:273–276.

292. Baler GR. Granulomas from topical zirconium in poison ivy dermatitis. *Arch Dermatol.* 1965;91:145–148.

293. LoPresti PJ, Hambrick GW Jr. Zirconium granuloma following treatment of rhus dermatitis. *Arch Dermatol.* 1965;92(2):188–191.

294. Shelley WB, Hurley HJ. The allergic origin of zirconium deodorant granulomas. *Br J Dermatol.* 1958;70(3):75–101.

295. Epstein WL, Skahen JR, Krasnobrod H. Granulomatous hypersensitivity to zirconium: localization of allergen in tissue and its role in formation of epithelioid cells. *J Invest Dermatol.* 1962;38:223–232.

296. Garcia-Patos V, Pujol RM, Alomar A, et al. Persistent subcutaneous nodules in patients hyposensitized with aluminum-containing allergen extracts. *Arch Dermatol.* 1995;131(12):1421–1424.

297. Haag CK, Dacey E, Hamilton N, White KP. Aluminum granuloma in a child secondary to DTaP-IPV vaccination: a case report. *Pediatr Dermatol.* 2019;36(1):e17–e19.

298. Slater DN, Underwood JC, Durrant TE, Gray T, Hopper IP. Aluminium hydroxide granulomas: light and electron microscopic studies and X-ray microanalysis. *Br J Dermatol.* 1982;107(1):103–108.

299. Fawcett HA, Smith NP. Injection-site granuloma due to aluminum. *Arch Dermatol.* 1984;120(10):1318–1322.

300. Culora GA, Ramsay AD, Theaker JM. Aluminium and injection site reactions. *J Clin Pathol.* 1996;49(10):844–847.

301. Ajithkumar K, Anand U, Pulimood S, et al. Vaccine-induced necrobiotic granuloma. *Clin Exp Dermatol.* 1998;23(5):222–224.

302. Chong H, Brady K, Metze D, Calonje E. Persistent nodules at injection sites (aluminium granuloma)—clinicopathological study of 14 cases with a diverse range of histological reaction patterns. *Histopathology.* 2006;48(2):182–188.

303. High WA, Ayers RA, Adams JR, Chang A, Fitzpatrick JE. Granulomatous reaction to titanium alloy: an unusual reaction to ear piercing. *J Am Acad Dermatol.* 2006;55(4):716–720.

304. Jordaan HF, Sandler M. Zinc-induced granuloma—a unique complication of insulin therapy. *Clin Exp Dermatol.* 1989;14(3):227–229.

305. Morgan AM. Localized reactions to injected therapeutic materials. Part 1. Medical agents. *J Cutan Pathol.* 1995;22(3):193–214.

306. Hardy HL, Tabershaw IR. Delayed chemical pneumonitis occurring in workers exposed to beryllium compounds. *J Ind Hyg Toxicol.* 1946;28:197–211.

307. Infante PF, Newman LS. Beryllium exposure and chronic beryllium disease. *Lancet.* 2004;363(9407):415–416.

308. Stoeckle JD, Hardy HL, Weber AL. Chronic beryllium disease. Long-term follow-up of sixty cases and selective review of the literature. *Am J Med.* 1969;46(4):545–561.

309. MacMurdo MG, Mroz MM, Culver DA, Dweik RA, Maier LA. Chronic beryllium disease: update on a moving target. *Chest.* 2020;158(6):2458–2466.

310. Berlin JM, Taylor JS, Sigel JE, Bergfeld WF, Dweik RA. Beryllium dermatitis. *J Am Acad Dermatol.* 2003;49(5):939–941.

311. Neave HJ, Frank SB, Tolmach JA. Cutaneous granuloma following laceration by fluorescent light bulbs. *Arch Derm Syphilol.* 1950;61(3):401–406.

312. Dutra FR. Beryllium granulomas of the skin. *Arch Derm Syphilol.* 1949;60(6):1140–1147, illust.

313. Lombardi G, Germain C, Uren J, et al. HLA-DP allele-specific T cell responses to beryllium account for DP-associated susceptibility to chronic beryllium disease. *J Immunol.* 2001;166(5):3549–3555.

314. Fontenot AP, Torres M, Marshall WH, Newman LS, Kotzin BL. Beryllium presentation to CD4+ T cells underlies disease-susceptibility HLA-DP alleles in chronic beryllium disease. *Proc Natl Acad Sci U S A.* 2000;97(23):12717–12722.

315. Newman LS. Significance of the blood beryllium lymphocyte proliferation test. *Environ Health Perspect.* 1996;104(suppl 5):953–956.

316. Fontenot AP, Maier LA, Canavera SJ, et al. Beryllium skin patch testing to analyze T cell stimulation and granulomatous inflammation in the lung. *J Immunol.* 2002;168(7):3627–3634.

317. Lupton GP, Kao GF, Johnson FB, Graham JH, Helwig EB. Cutaneous mercury granuloma. A clinicopathologic study and review of the literature. *J Am Acad Dermatol.* 1985;12(2, pt 1):296–303.

318. Sowden JM, Byrne JP, Smith AG, et al. Red tattoo reactions: X-ray microanalysis and patch-test studies. *Br J Dermatol.* 1991;124(6):576–580.

319. Bendsoe N, Hansson C, Sterner O. Inflammatory reactions from organic pigments in red tattoos. *Acta Derm Venereol.* 1991;71(1):70–73.

320. Loewenthal LJ. Reactions in green tatoos. The significance of the valence state of chromium. *Arch Dermatol.* 1960;82:237–243.

321. Rorsman H, Brehmer-Andersson E, Dahlquist I, et al. Tattoo granuloma and uveitis. *Lancet.* 1969;2(7610):27–28.

322. Schwartz RA, Mathias CG, Miller CH, Rojas-Corona R, Lambert WC. Granulomatous reaction to purple tattoo pigment. *Contact Dermatitis.* 1987;16(4):198–202.

323. Bjornberg A. Reactions to light in yellow tattoos from cadmium sulfide. *Arch Dermatol.* 1963;88:267–271.

324. Rubianes EI, Sanchez JL. Granulomatous dermatitis to iron oxide after permanent pigmentation of the eyebrows. *J Dermatol Surg Oncol.* 1993;19(1):14–16.

325. Drage LA, Ecker PM, Orenstein R, Phillips PK, Edson RS. An outbreak of *Mycobacterium chelonae* infections in tattoos. *J Am Acad Dermatol.* 2010;62(3):501–506.

326. Fraga GR, Prossick TA. Tattoo-associated keratoacanthomas: a series of 8 patients with 11 keratoacanthomas. *J Cutan Pathol.* 2010;37(1):85–90.

327. Schultz E, Mahler V. Prolonged lichenoid reaction and cross-sensitivity to para-substituted amino-compounds due to temporary henna tattoo. *Int J Dermatol.* 2002;41(5):301–303.

328. Onder M, Atahan CC, Oztas P, Oztas MO. Temporary henna tattoo reactions in children. *Int J Dermatol.* 2001;40(9):577–579.

329. Le Coz CJ, Lefebvre C, Keller F, Grosshans E. Allergic contact dermatitis caused by skin painting (pseudotattooing) with black henna, a mixture of henna and p-phenylenediamine and its derivatives. *Arch Dermatol.* 2000;136(12):1515–1517.

330. Chung WH, Chang YC, Yang LJ, et al. Clinicopathologic features of skin reactions to temporary tattoos and analysis of possible causes. *Arch Dermatol.* 2002;138(1):88–92.

331. Lewin PK. Temporary henna tattoo with permanent scarification. *CMAJ.* 1999;160(3):310.

332. Wood C, Severin GL. Unusual histiocytic reaction to Monsel's solution. *Am J Dermatopathol.* 1980;2(3):261–264.

333. Elston DM, Bergfeld WF, McMahon JT. Aluminum tattoo: a phenomenon that can resemble parasitized histiocytes. *J Cutan Pathol.* 1993;20(4):326–329.

334. Goldstein AP. VII. Histologic reactions in tattoos. *J Dermatol Surg Oncol.* 1979;5(11):896–900.

335. Shinohara MM, Nguyen J, Gardner J, Rosenbach M, Elenitsas R. The histopathologic spectrum of decorative tattoo complications. *J Cutan Pathol.* 2012;39(12):1110–1118.

336. Clarke J, Black MM. Lichenoid tattoo reactions. *Br J Dermatol.* 1979;100(4):451–454.

337. Winkelmann RK, Harris RB. Lichenoid delayed hypersensitivity reactions in tattoos. *J Cutan Pathol.* 1979;6(1):59–65.

338. Zinberg M, Heilman E, Glickman F. Cutaneous pseudolymphoma resulting from a tattoo. *J Dermatol Surg Oncol.* 1982;8(11):955–958.

339. Blumental G, Okun MR, Ponitch JA. Pseudolymphomatous reaction to tattoos. Report of three cases. *J Am Acad Dermatol.* 1982;6(4, pt 1):485–488.

340. Sowden JM, Cartwright PH, Smith AG, Hiley C, Slater DN. Sarcoidosis presenting with a granulomatous reaction confined to red tattoos. *Clin Exp Dermatol.* 1992;17(6):446–448.

341. Weidman AI, Andrade R, Franks AG. Sarcoidosis. Report of a case of sarcoid lesions in a tattoo and subsequent discovery of pulmonary sarcoidosis. *Arch Dermatol.* 1966;94(3):320–325.

342. Hanada K, Chiyoya S, Katabira Y. Systemic sarcoidal reaction in tattoo. *Clin Exp Dermatol.* 1985;10(5):479–484.

343. Dickinson JA. Sarcoidal reactions in tattoos. *Arch Dermatol.* 1969;100(3):315–319.

344. Del Rosario RN, Barr RJ, Graham BS, Kaneshiro S. Exogenous and endogenous cutaneous anomalies and curiosities. *Am J Dermatopathol.* 2005;27(3):259–267.

345. Abel EA, Silberberg I, Queen D. Studies of chronic inflammation in a red tattoo by electron microscopy and histochemistry. *Acta Derm Venereol.* 1972;52(6):453–461.

346. Requena L, Requena C, Christensen L, Zimmermann US, Kutzner H, Cerroni L. Adverse reactions to injectable soft tissue fillers. *J Am Acad Dermatol.* 2011;64(1):1–34; quiz 5–6.

347. Tonin B, Colato C, Bruni M, Girolomoni G. Late granuloma formation secondary to hyaluronic acid injection. *Dermatol Online J.* 2020;26(7).

348. Zhang FF, Xu ZX, Chen Y. Delayed foreign body granulomas in the orofacial region after hyaluronic acid injection. *Chin J Dent Res.* 2020;23(4):289–296.

349. Lombardi T, Samson J, Plantier F, Husson C, Kuffer R. Orofacial granulomas after injection of cosmetic fillers. Histopathologic and clinical study of 11 cases. *J Oral Pathol Med.* 2004;33(2):115–120.

350. Dijkema SJ, van der Lei B, Kibbelaar RE. New-fill injections may induce late-onset foreign body granulomatous reaction. *Plast Reconstr Surg.* 2005;115(5):76e–78e.

351. Apikian M, Roberts S, Goodman GJ. Adverse reactions to poly-lactic acid injections in the periorbital area. *J Cosmet Dermatol.* 2007;6(2):95–101.

352. Moulonguet I, Arnaud E, Bui P, Plantier F. Foreign body reaction to Radiesse: 2 cases. *Am J Dermatopathol.* 2013;35(3):e37–e40.

353. Holzapfel AM, Mangat DS, Barron DS. Soft-tissue augmentation with calcium hydroxylapatite: histological analysis. *Arch Facial Plast Surg.* 2008;10(5):335–338.

354. Dal Sacco D, Cozzani E, Parodi A, Rebora A. Scar sarcoidosis after hyaluronic acid injection. *Int J Dermatol.* 2005;44(5):411–412.

355. Descamps V, Landry J, Frances C, Marinho E, Ratziu V, Chosidow O. Facial cosmetic filler injections as possible target for systemic sarcoidosis in patients treated with interferon for chronic hepatitis C: two cases. *Dermatology.* 2008;217(1):81–84.

356. Rodriguez JM, Xie YL, Winthrop KL, et al. *Mycobacterium chelonae* facial infections following injection of dermal filler. *Aesthet Surg J.* 2013;33(2):265–269.

357. Micheels P. Human anti-hyaluronic acid antibodies: is it possible? *Dermatol Surg.* 2001;27(2):185–191.

358. Zimmermann US, Clerici TJ. The histological aspects of fillers complications. *Semin Cutan Med Surg.* 2004;23(4):241–250.

359. Ghislanzoni M, Bianchi F, Barbareschi M, Alessi E. Cutaneous granulomatous reaction to injectable hyaluronic acid gel. *Br J Dermatol.* 2006;154(4):755–758.

360. Parada MB, Michalany NS, Hassun KM, Bagatin E, Talarico S. A histologic study of adverse effects of different cosmetic skin fillers. *Skinmed.* 2005;4(6):345–349.

361. Dadzie OE, Mahalingam M, Parada M, El Helou T, Philips T, Bhawan J. Adverse cutaneous reactions to soft tissue fillers—a review of the histological features. *J Cutan Pathol.* 2008;35(6):536–548.

362. Reszko AE, Sadick NS, Magro CM, Farber J. Late-onset subcutaneous nodules after poly-L-lactic acid injection. *Dermatol Surg.* 2009;35(suppl 1):380–384.

363. Wildemore JK, Jones DH. Persistent granulomatous inflammatory response induced by injectable poly-L-lactic acid for HIV lipoatrophy. *Dermatol Surg.* 2006;32(11):1407–1409; discussion 9.

364. Drobeck HP, Rothstein SS, Gumaer KI, Sherer AD, Slighter RG. Histologic observation of soft tissue responses to implanted, multifaceted particles and discs of hydroxylapatite. *J Oral Maxillofac Surg.* 1984;42(3):143–149.

365. Misiek DJ, Kent JN, Carr RF. Soft tissue responses to hydroxylapatite particles of different shapes. *J Oral Maxillofac Surg.* 1984;42(3):150–160.

366. Rudolph CM, Soyer HP, Schuller-Petrovic S, Kerl H. Foreign body granulomas due to injectable aesthetic microimplants. *Am J Surg Pathol.* 1999;23(1):113–117.

367. Balogh K. The histologic appearance of corticosteroid injection sites. *Arch Pathol Lab Med.* 1986;110(12):1168–1172.

368. Bhawan J. Steroid-induced 'granulomas' in hypertrophic scar. *Acta Derm Venereol.* 1983;63(6):560–563.

369. Santa Cruz DJ, Ulbright TM. Mucin-like changes in keloids. *Am J Clin Pathol.* 1981;75(1):18–22.

370. Weedon D, Gutteridge BH, Hockly RG, Emmett AJ. Unusual cutaneous reactions to injections of corticosteroids. *Am J Dermatopathol.* 1982;4(3):199–203.

371. Zimmer WM, Rogers RS 3rd, Reeve CM, Sheridan PJ. Orofacial manifestations of Melkersson-Rosenthal syndrome. A study of 42 patients and review of 220 cases from the literature. *Oral Surg Oral Med Oral Pathol.* 1992;74(5):610–619.

372. Greene RM, Rogers RS 3rd. Melkersson-Rosenthal syndrome: a review of 36 patients. *J Am Acad Dermatol.* 1989;21(6):1263–1270.

373. Durgin JS, Rodriguez O, Sollecito T, et al. Diagnosis, clinical features, and management of patients with granulomatous cheilitis. *JAMA Dermatol.* 2021;157(1):112–114.

374. Mahler VB, Hornstein OP, Boateng BI, Kiesewetter FF. Granulomatous glossitis as an unusual manifestation of Melkersson-Rosenthal syndrome. *Cutis.* 1995;55(4):244–246, 248.

375. Rosaria Galdiero M, Maio F, Arcoleo F, et al. Orofacial granulomatosis: clinical and therapeutic features in an Italian cohort and review of the literature. *Allergy.* 2021.

376. Wiesenfeld D, Ferguson MM, Mitchell DN, et al. Oro-facial granulomatosis—a clinical and pathological analysis. *Q J Med.* 1985;54(213):101–113.

377. Field EA, Tyldesley WR. Oral Crohn's disease revisited—a 10-year-review. *Br J Oral Maxillofac Surg.* 1989;27(2):114–123.

378. Westermark P, Henriksson TG. Granulomatous inflammation of the vulva and penis—a genital counterpart to cheilitis granulomatosa. *Dermatologica.* 1979;158(4):269–274.

379. Hoede N, Heidbuchel U, Korting GW. Chronic granulomatous vulvitis (Melkersson-Rosenthal vulvitis) [in German]. *Hautarzt.* 1982;33(4):218–220.

380. Ploysangam T, Heubi JE, Eisen D, Balistreri WF, Lucky AW. Cutaneous Crohn's disease in children. *J Am Acad Dermatol.* 1997;36(5, pt 1):697–704.

381. Ramassamy S, Van HTA, Chuang JY, Wu YH. Pathological and immunohistochemical characteristics of granuloma and lymphatics in cheilitis granulomatosa. *Am J Dermatopathol.* 2022;44(2):83–91.

382. Hornstein O. On the pathogenesis of the so-called Melkersson-Rosenthal syndrome (Miescher's cheilitis granulomatosa included) [in German]. *Arch Klin Exp Dermatol.* 1961;212:570–605.

383. Allen CM, Camisa C, Hamzeh S, Stephens L. Cheilitis granulomatosa: report of six cases and review of the literature. *J Am Acad Dermatol.* 1990;23(3, pt 1):444–450.

384. Hering H, Scheid P. [Critical remarks on the Melkersson-Rosenthal syndrome as a partial manifestation of Besnier-Boeck-Schaumann's disease]. *Arch Klin Exp Dermatol.* 1954;197(4):344–382.

385. Hernandez G, Hernandez F, Lucas M. Miescher's granulomatous cheilitis: literature review and report of a case. *J Oral Maxillofac Surg.* 1986;44(6):474–478.

386. Banks T, Gada S. A comprehensive review of current treatments for granulomatous cheilitis. *Br J Dermatol.* 2012;166(5):934–937.

387. Jaouen F, Tessier MH, Vaillant L, et al. Response to systemic therapies in granulomatous cheilitis: retrospective multicenter series of 61 patients. *J Am Acad Dermatol.* 2021.

388. Tappeiner J, Pfleger L. [Granuloma gluteale infantum]. *Hautarzt.* 1971;22(9):383–388.

389. Uyeda K, Nakayasu K, Takaishi Y, Sotomatsu S. Kaposi sarcoma-like granuloma on diaper dermatitis. A report of five cases. *Arch Dermatol.* 1973;107(4):605–607.

390. Simmons IJ. Granuloma gluteale infantum. *Australas J Dermatol.* 1977;18(1):20–24.

391. Maekawa Y, Sakazaki Y, Hayashibara T. Diaper area granuloma of the aged. *Arch Dermatol.* 1978;114(3):382–383.

392. Fujita M, Ohno S, Danno K, Miyachi Y. Two cases of diaper area granuloma of the adult. *J Dermatol.* 1991;18(11):671–675.

393. Robson KJ, Maughan JA, Purcell SD, Petersen MJ, Haefner HK, Lowe L. Erosive papulonodular dermatosis associated with topical benzocaine: a report of two cases and evidence that granuloma gluteale, pseudoverrucous papules, and Jacquet's erosive dermatitis are a disease spectrum. *J Am Acad Dermatol.* 2006;55(5, suppl):S74–S80.

394. Delacretaz J, Grigoriu D, de Crousaz H, Tapernoux B, Nicod PA, Gautier E. [Nodular candidiasis of the inguino-genital and gluteal region (granuloma glutaeale infantum)]. *Dermatologica.* 1972;144(3):143–155.

395. Sweidan NA, Salman SM, Kibbi AG, Zaynoun ST. Skin nodules over the diaper area. Granuloma gluteale infantum. *Arch Dermatol.* 1989;125(12):1703–1704, 1706–1707.

396. Bonifazi E, Garofalo L, Lospalluti M, Scardigno A, Coviello C, Meneghini CL. Granuloma gluteale infantum with atrophic scars: clinical and histological observations in eleven cases. *Clin Exp Dermatol.* 1981;6(1):23–29.

397. Deng A, Harvey V, Sina B, et al. Interstitial granulomatous dermatitis associated with the use of tumor necrosis factor alpha inhibitors. *Arch Dermatol.* 2006;142(2):198–202.

398. Lee HW, Yun WJ, Lee MW, Choi JH, Moon KC, Koh JK. Interstitial granulomatous drug reaction caused by Chinese herbal medication. *J Am Acad Dermatol.* 2005;52(4):712–713.

399. Sanli HE, Kocyigit P, Arica E, Kurtyuksel M, Heper AO, Ozcan M. Granuloma annulare on herpes zoster scars in a Hodgkin's disease patient following autologous peripheral stem cell transplantation. *J Eur Acad Dermatol Venereol.* 2006;20(3):314–317.

400. Yamauchi K, Oiso N, Iwanaga T, et al. Post-herpes zoster sarcoidosis as a recurrence. *J Dermatol.* 2018;45(6):e150–e151.

401. Kapoor R, Piris A, Saavedra AP, Duncan LM, Nazarian RM. Wolf isotopic response manifesting as postherpetic granuloma annulare: a case series. *Arch Pathol Lab Med.* 2013;137(2):255–258.

402. Abdel-Naser MB, Wollina U, El Hefnawi MA, Habib MA, El Okby M. Non-sarcoidal, non-tuberculoid granuloma in common variable immunodeficiency. *J Drugs Dermatol.* 2006;5(4):370–372.

403. Krupnick AI, Shim H, Phelps RG, Cunningham-Rundles C, Sapadin AN. Cutaneous granulomas masquerading as tuberculoid leprosy in a patient with congenital combined immunodeficiency. *Mt Sinai J Med.* 2001;68(4–5):326–330.

404. Siegfried EC, Prose NS, Friedman NJ, Paller AS. Cutaneous granulomas in children with combined immunodeficiency. *J Am Acad Dermatol.* 1991;25(5, pt 1):761–766.

405. Lun KR, Wood DJ, Muir JB, Noakes R. Granulomas in common variable immunodeficiency: a diagnostic dilemma. *Australas J Dermatol.* 2004;45(1):51–54.

406. Boursiquot JN, Gerard L, Malphettes M, et al. Granulomatous disease in CVID: retrospective analysis of clinical characteristics and treatment efficacy in a cohort of 59 patients. *J Clin Immunol.* 2013;33(1):84–95.

407. Rongioletti F, Cerroni L, Massone C, Basso M, Ciambellotti A, Rebora A. Different histologic patterns of cutaneous granulomas in systemic lymphoma. *J Am Acad Dermatol.* 2004;51(4):600–605.

Degenerative Diseases and Perforating Disorders

ADNAN MIR, MICHAEL K. MILLER, AND EDWARD R. HEILMAN

INTRODUCTION

The disorders in this chapter involve mostly the connective tissue structures and matrical elements of the skin and may rather loosely be described as "degenerative." Solar elastosis, for example, occurs as the result of chronic exposure to solar radiation and could therefore be regarded as a response to injury, rather than a degenerative condition. This process results in an increase in the amount of elastic tissue rather than in a decrease, as occurs in normal aging. Nevertheless, it seems natural to group these disorders together as they tend to present with alterations of the normal connective tissue architecture that result in loss of structure and often in functional or cosmetic abnormalities. In addition, many of them have the same overlapping differential diagnosis. Therapeutic management of these lesions also tends to overlap or to be similar among the various conditions, although in most cases, these therapeutic options have not been subjected to evidence-based scrutiny, and in many conditions therapeutic intervention is unnecessary except perhaps for cosmetic reasons or for patient reassurance.

SOLAR (ACTINIC) ELASTOSIS

Senescent changes in areas of the skin not regularly exposed to sunlight manifest themselves clinically primarily as thinning of the skin and a decrease in the amount of subcutaneous fat. In contrast, there are often pronounced changes in the appearance of the sun-exposed skin of elderly persons, especially those with fair complexions. These changes, however, are the result of chronic sun exposure (photoaging) rather than of intrinsic (chronologic) aging.

Clinical Summary. In exposed areas, especially on the face, the skin shows wrinkling, furrowing, and thinning. In addition, there may be an irregular distribution of pigment. Chronic sun exposure may also lead to more fragile skin and increased areas of purpuric ecchymoses.

Histopathology. In skin not regularly exposed to sunlight, there is a progressive loss of elastic tissue in the papillary dermis with age. Elastic fibers in the papillary dermis are composed of elaunin and oxytalan fibers. Elaunin fibers, which consist of microfibrils and a small amount of elastin, run parallel to the dermoepidermal junction. Overlying oxytalan fibers, composed solely of microfibrils, form a thin, superficial network

perpendicular to the dermal–epidermal junction that ends at the basement membrane zone (Chapter 3). In middle age, the oxytalan fibers in the papillary dermis are split and fewer than at a young age, and in old age they may be absent (1). Mature elastic fibers in the reticular dermis also undergo changes caused by intrinsic aging, becoming fragmented and porous (2). On the lower extremities, venous insufficiency may lead to stasis changes, including dermal neovascularization and fibrosis, with occasional erythrocyte extravasation and neovascularization.

In the skin of the face exposed to the sun, especially in persons with fair complexions, hyperplasia of the elastic tissue is usually evident on histologic examination, by the age of 30, even though clinically the skin may appear normal. No white person past 40 years of age has normal elastic tissue in the skin of the face (3). The elastic fibers of the reticular dermis are increased in number and are thicker, curled, and tangled.

In patients with clinically evident solar elastosis of the exposed skin, staining with hematoxylin–eosin reveals, in the upper dermis, basophilic degeneration of the collagen separated from a somewhat atrophic epidermis by a narrow band of normal collagen. In the areas of basophilic degeneration, the bundles of eosinophilic collagen have been replaced by amorphous basophilic granular material.

A grading scheme for solar elastosis (i.e., chronic solar damage [CSD]) has been developed, validated, and illustrated, and the grades are defined as follows: CSD 0, absence of elastotic fibers discernible at 200× magnification; CSD 1 (mild solar elastosis), scattered elastotic fibers lying as individual fibers, not as bunches in the reticular dermis; CSD 2 (moderate), densely scattered elastotic fibers distributed predominantly as bunches; CSD 3 (severe), amorphous deposits of blue-gray material with lost fiber texture. CSD defined in this way correlates negatively with the frequency of BRAF mutations in melanomas and with the role of the MC1R or melanocortin receptor in relation to the risk of developing melanoma (4).

The areas of basophilic degeneration stain with elastic tissue stains and are therefore referred to as elastotic material. The elastotic material usually consists of aggregates of thick, interwoven bands in the upper dermis (Fig. 15-1A) (5); but in areas of severe solar degeneration, the elastotic material may have an amorphous rather than a fibrous appearance (Fig. 15-1B) and may extend into the lower portions of the dermis rather than being confined to the upper dermis (6).

On Fontana Masson staining, the distribution of melanin in the basal cell layer may appear irregular, in that areas of hyperpigmentation alternate with areas of hypopigmentation (6).

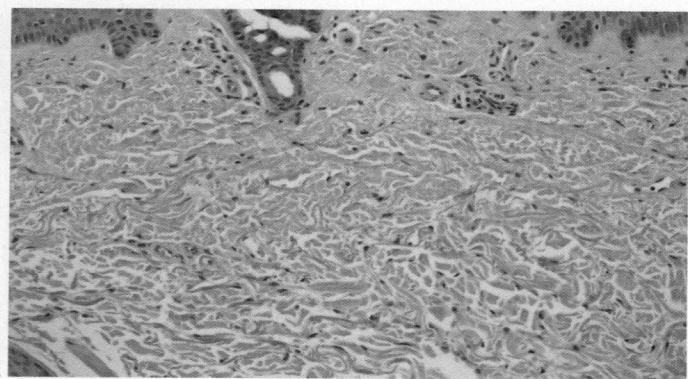
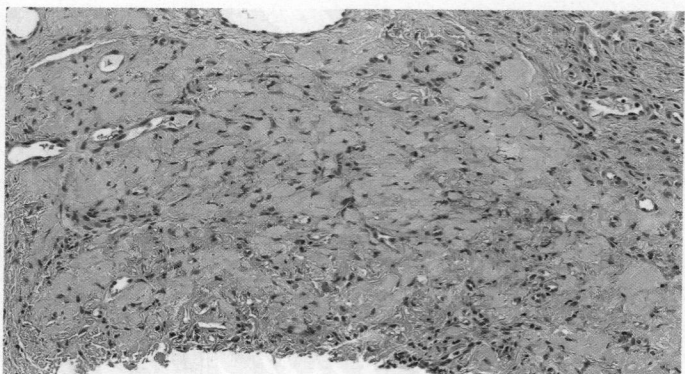

Figure 15-1 Solar (actinic) degeneration. **A:** In the upper dermis, separated from the epidermis by a narrow band of normal collagen, there are aggregates of thick, interwoven bands of the elastotic material. **B:** Extensive amorphous material can be seen around and among elastic and collagen fibers.

Pathogenesis. Electron microscopic examination of areas of solar elastosis shows elastotic material as the main component. Even though this elastotic material resembles elastic tissue in its chemical composition, it differs significantly in appearance from aged elastic fibers in unexposed, aged skin. Instead of showing amorphous electron-lucent elastin and aggregates of electron-dense microfibrils (Chapter 6), the thick fibers of elastotic material show two structural components: a fine granular matrix of medium electron density and, within this matrix, homogeneous, electron-dense, irregularly-shaped inclusions (7). Microfibrils such as those observed in normal or aged elastic fibers are absent. Immunoelectron microscopy shows that the elastotic material has retained its antigenicity for elastin but not for microfibrils (8). The number and size of elastotic fibers are greatly increased over the number and size of elastic fibers found in normal or aged skin. Extensive amorphous material can be seen around the elastotic fibers and also among the collagen fibrils. Collagen fibrils are diminished in number, with those present often showing a diminished electron density, a diminished contrast in cross striation, and a splitting up into filaments at their ends (9).

Elastotic material is not regarded as a degeneration product of preexisting elastic fibers. Most current findings indicate that elastotic material is composed primarily of elastic tissue, much of which may be newly formed as the result of an altered function of fibroblasts. Evidence of transcriptional activation of the elastin gene in biopsied tissue and fibroblast cultures from sun-damaged skin further supports this. Additional accumulation of elastotic material may be secondary to a disruption in the balance between synthesis and degradation of elastin in photodamaged skin (10).

The elastotic material that histochemically stains like elastic tissue resembles elastic tissue in its chemical composition and its physical and enzymatic reactions. Thus, the amino acid composition of the elastotic tissue resembles that of elastin and differs significantly from that of collagen. In particular, the elastotic material, like elastic tissue, has a much lower content of hydroxyproline than collagen (11). Moreover, the elastotic material in unfixed sections shows the same brilliant autofluorescence as do elastic fibers on examination with the fluorescence microscope (12), and both the elastotic material and elastic tissue are susceptible to elastase digestion (13). The elastotic material contains a large amount of acid mucopolysaccharides, as indicated by staining with alcian blue. A significant portion of

these acid mucopolysaccharides may be sulfated because prior incubation with hyaluronidase removes only 50% to 75% of the alcian blue-positive staining. The basophilia of the elastotic material, however, is not affected by incubation with hyaluronidase (14).

The irregular distribution of melanin in the epidermis observed in some patients with solar degeneration, when studied by electron microscopy, is found to be caused largely by an impairment of pigment transfer from melanocytes to keratinocytes. Although some keratinocytes contain many melanosomes, others contain few or no melanosomes. The latter are surrounded by dendrites laden with melanosomes (15).

Differential Diagnosis. For a discussion of differentiation of solar elastosis from pseudoxanthoma elasticum, see Chapter 3. Clinically, papular lesions of solar elastosis may be mistaken for basal cell carcinoma and are easily differentiated by histologic analysis.

Principles of Management: Consistent, long-term use of sunscreens and/or photoprotective clothing reduces solar elastosis significantly (16). Dermabrasion and long-term application of retinoic acid can lead to thickening of the epidermis, which may reduce the clinical appearance of photoaging (17,18). On certain sites, select lasers may ameliorate some of the accumulated photodamage as well.

LOCALIZED EXPRESSIONS OF SOLAR ELASTOSIS

Several clinically distinct forms of localized solar elastosis have been described. In the nuchal region, the skin, after many years of exposure to the sun, may appear thickened and furrowed. This is referred to as *cutis rhomboidalis nuchae. Elastotic nodules of the ears* are localized papular and nodular forms of solar elastosis usually occurring on the antihelix (19–22). Severe solar elastosis may also occur as yellowish plaques associated with small cysts and comedones. *Favre–Racouchot syndrome* (nodular elastosis with cysts and comedones) is an example occurring on facial skin lateral to the eyes (23,24). A similar condition occurring on the arms has been termed *actinic comedonal plaques* (25–27). Two other types of circumscribed solar elastosis occurring on the upper extremities are *solar elastotic bands of the forearm* (5,28) and *collagenous and elastotic marginal plaques of the hands* (29–36).

Elastotic Nodules of the Ears

Clinical Summary. Elastotic nodules are most often bilateral, small, asymptomatic, pale papules and nodules on the anterior crus of the antihelix and, occasionally, helix (21) of the ears (19,20,22).

Histopathology. Irregular elastotic fibers and clumps of elastotic material are seen in the background of marked dermal solar elastosis (Fig. 15-2A). The fibers and clumps can be highlighted with an elastic Verhoeff-van Gieson (EVG) stain (Fig. 15-2B) (21).

Differential Diagnosis. Clinically, they may mimic basal cell carcinomas, amyloidosis, gouty tophi, or chondrodermatitis nodularis helicis (19–22).

Favre–Racouchot Syndrome (Nodular Elastosis with Cysts and Comedones)

Clinical Summary. Favre–Racouchot syndrome is characterized by yellow plaques with multiple open and cystically dilated comedones. The condition typically affects the skin lateral to the eyes in elderly males (23,24,37). However, a case has also been documented on the shoulder (38). Although the condition is usually bilateral, it may be unilateral (39–41).

Histopathology. Dilated pilosebaceous openings and large, round, cystlike spaces are lined by a flattened epithelium and represent greatly distended hair follicles (23,24). Both the dilated pilosebaceous openings and the cystlike spaces are filled with layered horny material. Vellus hair shafts and bacteria have been demonstrated within the spaces as well, suggesting the cystlike spaces may represent closed comedones rather than true infundibular cysts (42). The sebaceous glands are atrophic. Solar elastosis is often pronounced (23), but it may be slight or absent (43). Because the comedones are open, they do not tend to become inflamed (44) (see the section on Acne Vulgaris, Chapter 18).

Pathogenesis. It is thought to be mainly secondary to prolonged solar exposure with the formation of comedones facilitated by an extracellular matrix of compromised structural integrity (2). Smoking may also be a contributing factor in its development (45).

Actinic Comedonal Plaques

Clinical Summary. In actinic comedonal plaques, solitary nodular plaques with a cribriform appearance and comedone-like structures occur, often unilaterally, on the arms or forearms (25–27). The plaques are composed of confluent erythematous to bluish papules and nodules. The condition has been described in fair-skinned individuals with a history of chronic sun exposure. They can be found in association with Favre–Racouchot syndrome and may, in fact, represent an ectopic expression of this entity (26).

Histopathology. Dilated corneocyte-filled follicular lumina are present within areas of elastotic, amorphous material. The overlying epidermis is usually dyskeratotic and atrophic. The histologic findings are quite similar to those seen in Favre–Racouchot syndrome (25,26).

Solar Elastotic Bands of the Forearm

Clinical Summary. Solar elastotic bands of the forearm consist of soft cordlike plaques across the flexor surface of the forearms (5,28). The bands occur in areas of actinic damage and usually with senile purpura.

Histopathology. Nodular collections of basophilic homogeneous amorphous material underlying an atrophic epidermis are conspicuous features. Thickened degenerated elastic fibers within the homogeneous material are also observed. Stellate fibroblasts and a perivascular infiltrate of lymphocytes and hemosiderin-laden macrophages are found in close apposition to the elastic fibers. The nodular collections and thickened elastic fibers stain positively with EVG stain (5).

Collagenous and Elastotic Marginal Plaques of the Hands

Collagenous and elastotic marginal plaques of the hands have been described by several names: elasto-collagenous plaques of the hands (29), degenerative collagenous plaques of the hands (30,32), and keratoelastoidosis marginalis (31).

Clinical Summary. This acquired, slowly progressive condition is usually seen in elderly males and consists of groups of linear confluent papules along the medial and lateral aspects of the hands at the juncture of the palmar and dorsal surfaces. The medial aspect of the thumb and radial aspect of the index finger are most commonly affected. The condition closely resembles the genodermatosis, acrokeratoelastoidosis (34). However, there is no familial predisposition or involvement of the plantar surfaces (31,46,47).

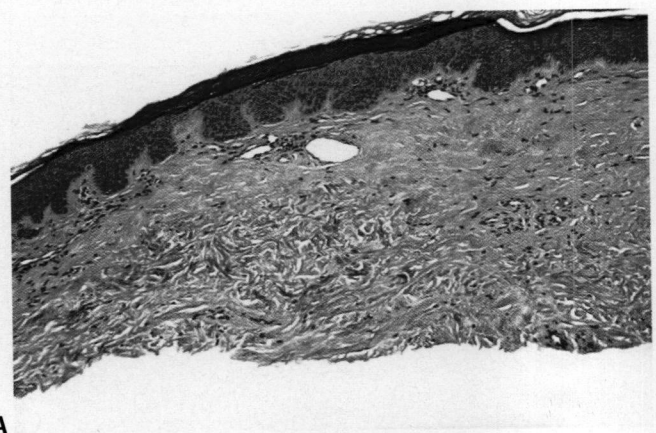

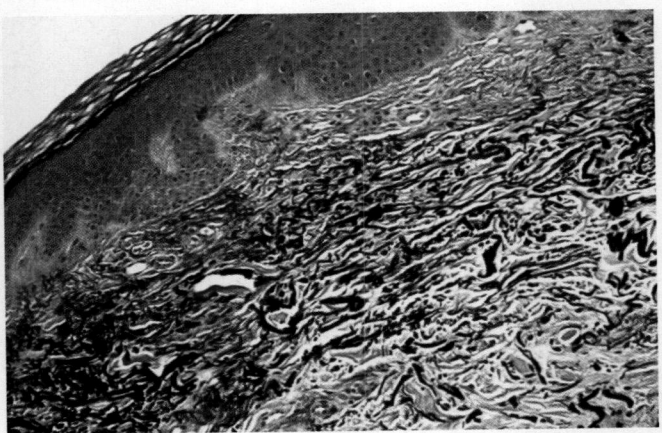

A

B

Figure 15-2 Elastotic nodule of the ear. A: A dome-shaped papule with marked solar elastosis in the dermis and clumped and irregular eosinophilic material representing degenerated elastic fibers. B: The course, clumped material is highlighted with an elastic stain.

Histopathology. The reticular dermis displays an acellular zone of haphazardly arranged collagen with some bundles running perpendicular to the epidermis (32). The bundles of collagen are admixed with fragmented elastic fibers and distinctive angulated amorphous "basophilic elastotic masses" in the upper dermis. These masses can be demonstrated to contain degenerating elastic fibers and calcium (33).

Pathogenesis. Actinic damage and chronic repetitive pressure or trauma has been implicated in its pathogenesis (31,46,47).

PERFORATING DISORDERS

The perforating disorders comprise a group of disorders sharing the common characteristic of transepidermal elimination (TEE). This phenomenon is characterized by the elimination or extrusion of altered dermal substances and, in some cases, by such material behaving as foreign material.

Traditionally, four diseases have been included in this group: *Kyrle disease* (hyperkeratosis follicularis et parafollicularis in cutem penetrans), *perforating folliculitis, elastosis perforans serpiginosa* (EPS), and *reactive perforating collagenosis* (RPC). A fifth entity, *acquired perforating dermatosis* (APD), which is usually associated with renal disease and/or diabetes mellitus, may resemble any of these four diseases clinically and histologically (48). Although TEE is a prominent feature in all of these conditions, it has also been described as a secondary phenomenon in other entities, including such inflammatory disorders as granuloma annulare, one variant of pseudoxanthoma elasticum, and chondrodermatitis nodularis helicis. Elastic fibers can be transepidermally eliminated over sites of healing wounds. Collagen may be eliminated through keratoacanthomas (49) or ulcers secondary to trauma. Needless to say, there is a long list of other conditions that can exhibit TEE as an associated reaction pattern.

Kyrle Disease

Kyrle disease is a rare disorder first described in 1916 (50). There is controversy as to whether it represents a distinct entity or an exaggerated form of perforating folliculitis (50,51) or whether it actually comprises a group of disorders with similar epidermal–dermal reaction patterns associated with chronic renal failure, diabetes, prurigo nodularis, and even keratosis pilaris. Therefore, the discussion of Kyrle disease and perforating disorders seen in chronic renal disease and/or

diabetes has a very broad overlap in terms of their clinical and pathologic features.

Clinical Features. This eruption presents with a large number of papules, some coalescing into plaques, numbering in the hundreds and often distributed on the extremities. Although some may appear to involve the follicular units, these lesions are more likely to be extrafollicular. The typical patient is young to middle-aged and often has a history of diabetes mellitus. The papules are dome shaped, 2 to 8 mm in diameter, with a central keratotic plug. Excoriations are often found in the vicinity of these lesions. Linear lesions related to possible koebnerization have been described.

Histopathology. The essential histopathologic findings include (a) a follicular or extrafollicular cornified plug with focal parakeratosis embedded in an epidermal invagination, (b) basophilic degenerated material identified in small collections throughout the plug, with absence of demonstrable collagen and elastin, (c) abnormal vacuolated and/or dyskeratotic keratinization of the epithelial cells extending to the basal cell zone, (d) irregular epithelial hyperplasia, and (e) an inflammatory component that is typically granulomatous with small foci of suppuration (Fig. 15-3). In most instances, it is important to perform elastic tissue stains and even trichrome stains to exclude perforating elastic fibers, as in EPS, or collagen fibers, as in RPC (52).

Pathogenesis. The primary event is claimed to be a disturbance of epidermal keratinization characterized by the formation of dyskeratotic foci and acceleration of the process of keratinization. This leads to the formation of keratotic plugs with areas of parakeratosis (53–55). Because the rapid rate of differentiation and keratinization exceeds the rate of cell proliferation, the parakeratotic column gradually extends deeper into the abnormal epidermis, leading in most cases to perforation of the parakeratotic column into the dermis. Perforation is not the cause of Kyrle disease, as originally thought (50), but rather represents the consequence or final event of the abnormally sped-up keratinization. This rapid production of abnormal keratin forms a plug that acts as a foreign body, penetrating the epidermis and inciting a granulomatous inflammatory reaction. A certain similarity exists between the parakeratotic column in Kyrle disease and that observed in porokeratosis of Mibelli (54). In both conditions, a parakeratotic column forms as the result of rapid and faulty keratinization of dyskeratotic cells, but, whereas in Kyrle disease the dyskeratotic cells are often used up so that disruption of the epithelium occurs, in porokeratosis of Mibelli

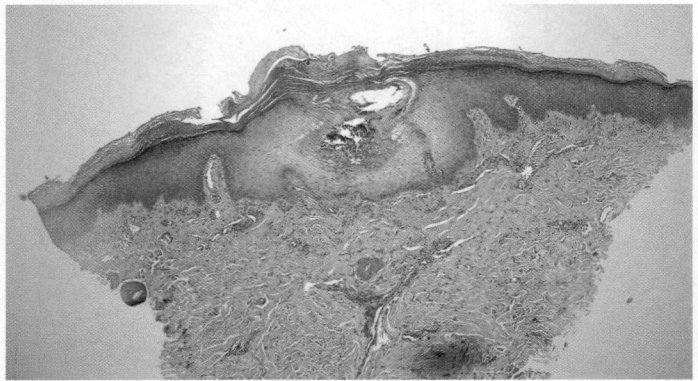
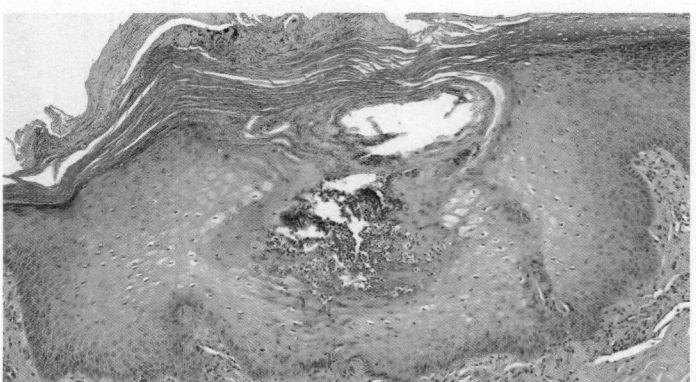

Figure 15-3 Kyrle disease. **A:** A large parakeratotic plug lies within an invagination of the epidermis. **B:** The plug contains basophilic debris. The underlying dermis displays acute and chronic inflammation.

the clone of dyskeratotic cells can maintain itself by extending peripherally.

Differential Diagnosis. See Table 15-1.

Principles of Management: Treatment is focused on the conditions underlying disease occurrence. Patients may experience reduced pruritus and decreased lesion symptomatology with regular renal-replacement therapy when the condition occurs in the setting of end-stage renal disease. Other treatment modalities are generally supported by case reports and anecdotal evidence but may include topical anti-inflammatory or antipruritic agents, including topical corticosteroids, oral and topical retinoids, systemic antibiotics, keratolytics, and systemic immunosuppressants. Limited lesions may respond to local destructive methods, including cryotherapy and laser destruction (56).

Perforating Folliculitis

Perforating folliculitis is a perforating disorder that has many features overlapping with Kyrle disease and also comprises one of the clinical and histologic patterns seen in APD.

Clinical Summary. As described by Mehregan and Coskey (57), this is a relatively uncommon disorder usually observed in the second to fourth decades and is characterized by erythematous follicular papules with central keratotic plugs. The lesions are 2 to 8 mm in diameter and tend to be localized to the extensor surfaces of the extremities and the buttocks. The key to making this diagnosis is the clinical and histologic identification of a follicular unit as the primary site for the inflammatory process. Recently, perforating folliculitis has been associated with treatment with tyrosine kinase inhibitors for cancer therapy (58,59).

Histopathology. The main pathologic abnormalities consist of (a) a dilated follicular infundibulum filled with compact ortho- and parakeratotic cornified cells (Fig. 15-4A); (b) degenerated basophilic staining material, composed of granular nuclear debris from neutrophils, other inflammatory cells, and degenerated collagen bundles (Fig. 15-4B, C); (c) one or more perforations through the follicular epithelium; and (d) an associated perifollicular inflammatory cell infiltrate composed of lymphocytes, histiocytes, and neutrophils. Additionally, altered collagen and refractile eosinophilically altered elastic fibers are found adjacent to the sites of perforation. A remnant of the hair shaft can sometimes be found.

Pathogenesis. Perforating folliculitis is the end result of abnormal follicular keratinization most likely caused by irritation, either chemical or physical, and even chronic rubbing. A portion of a curled-up hair is often seen close to or within the area of perforation or even in the dermis, surrounded by a foreign-body granuloma (55).

Differential Diagnosis. In Kyrle disease, the keratinous plug may be extrafollicular, the perforation is usually present deep in the invagination at the bottom of the keratinous plug, and no eosinophilic degeneration of elastic fibers is found. In addition, in Kyrle disease, epithelial hyperplasia is a significant feature. For a discussion of the differential diagnosis of perforating folliculitis

Table 15.1

Differential Diagnosis of Perforating Disorders

Disease	Primary Defect	Distinctive Features	Histogenesis
Kyrle disease	Focus of dyskeratotic rapidly proliferating cells in the epidermis	Follicular or extrafollicular cornified plug embedded in an epidermal invagination associated with epithelial hyperplasia and absence of demonstrable collagen and elastin	Disturbance of keratinization, forming a plug that acts as a foreign body penetrating the epidermis and inciting a granulomatous inflammatory reaction
Perforating folliculitis	Hyperkeratotic plug in follicular unit containing a retained hair	Compact ortho- and parakeratotic plug with degenerated collagen, altered elastin, and mixed inflammatory cell infiltrate, including neutrophil	A primary irritant causing follicular hyperkeratosis, resulting in a mechanical breakdown of the follicle wall by the hair shaft
Elastosis perforans serpiginosum	Formation of numerous coarse elastic fibers in the superficial dermis	Formation of narrow channel through an acanthotic epidermis with elimination of eosinophilic elastic fibers	Thickened elastic fibers act as mechanical irritants or "foreign bodies"
RPC	Subepidermal focus of altered collagen caused by trauma	Formation of cup-shaped vertically oriented channel with TEE of degenerated collagen	Histochemically altered collagen acts as "foreign body"
Acquired perforating disorder	Chronic rubbing owing to pruritis, resulting in hyperkeratosis, keratosis, and perforation, possibly in association with other factors such as accumulation of poorly dialyzable substances	A combination of features similar to any of the above disorders	Exogenously altered skin in pruritic diabetes and patients with chronic renal disease

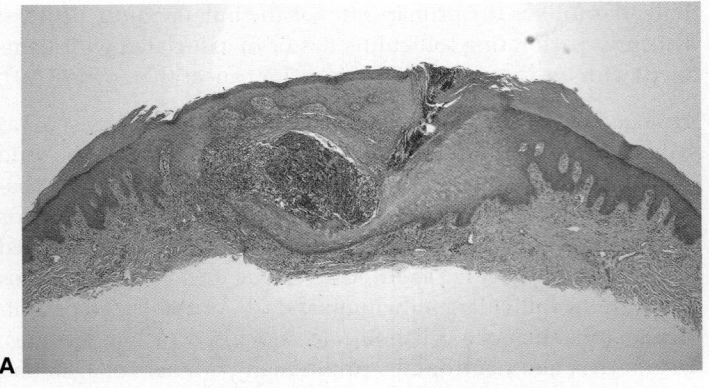

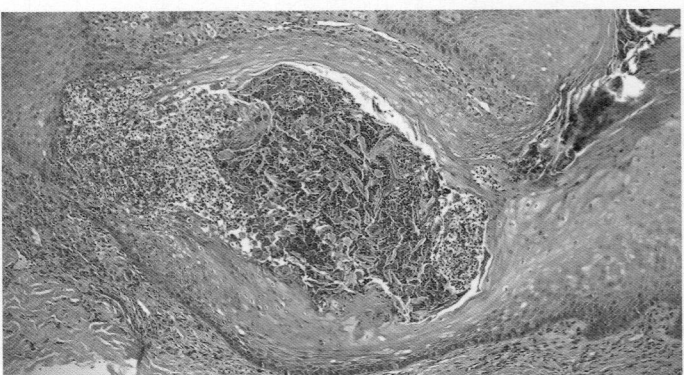

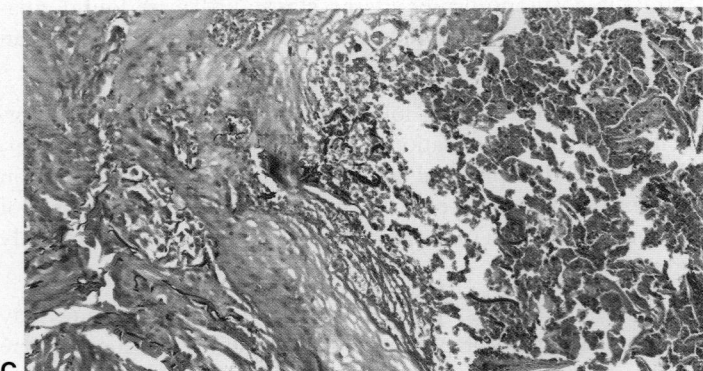

Figure 15-4 Perforating folliculitis. **A:** A widely dilated follicular unit contains a mixture of keratin, basophilic debris, inflammatory cells, and degenerated collagen fibers. **B:** An area of disrupted follicular epithelium with adjacent associated perifollicular inflammation and alteration of collagen and elastic fibers. **C:** An elastic stain highlights fibers within the debris.

from EPS, see the following section on Differential Diagnosis for Elastosis Perforans Serpiginosa. See also Table 15-1.

Principles of Management: Treatment of this condition is similar to that of Kyrle disease, discussed previously.

Elastosis Perforans Serpiginosa

EPS is the most distinctive of the perforating disorders because it demonstrates the best example of TEE. In EPS, increased numbers of thickened elastic fibers are present in the upper dermis, and altered elastic fibers are extruded through the epidermis.

Clinical Summary. EPS is a rare disorder that affects young individuals with a peak incidence in the second decade. Men are affected more often than women. It is primarily a papular eruption localized to one anatomic site and most commonly affecting the nape of the neck, the face, or the upper extremities. The papules are typically 2 to 5 mm in diameter. These papules are arranged in arcuate or serpiginous groups and may coalesce; there is often mild perilesional inflammation and erythema.

Of particular importance is the association of EPS with systemic diseases. These associations include Down syndrome, Ehlers–Danlos syndrome, osteogenesis imperfecta, pseudoxanthoma elasticum, and Marfan syndrome. In addition, on rare occasions, EPS is observed in association with Rothmund–Thompson syndrome, malignancy, or other connective tissue disorders, and as a secondary complication of penicillamine administration.

Histopathology. The essential findings include a narrow transepidermal channel that may be straight, wavy, or of corkscrew shape as well as thick, coarse elastic fibers in the channel admixed with granular basophilic staining debris (Fig. 15-5A, B). A mixed inflammatory cell infiltrate accompanies the fibers in the channel. Also observed are abnormal elastic fibers in the

upper dermis in the vicinity of the channel. In this zone, the elastic fibers are increased in size and number. As these fibers enter the lower portion of the channel, they maintain their normal staining characteristics, but as they approach the epidermal surface they may not stain as expected with elastic stains (60).

Pathogenesis. The cause of EPS is not known. Because the elastic fibers show no obvious abnormality within the dermis except hyperplasia, it is conceivable that the thickened elastic fibers act as mechanical irritants or "foreign bodies" and provoke an epidermal response in the form of hyperplasia. The epidermis then envelops the irritating material and eliminates it through transepidermal channels. The degeneration of the elastic fibers within the channels is probably caused by proteolytic enzymes set free by degenerating inflammatory cells (60). The channel is formed as a reactive phenomenon through which the "foreign bodies" are extruded. Because copper metabolism is essential to the formation of elastin (61) and because the administration of penicillamine, a copper chelating agent, has been found to induce EPS (62), it may be suggested that the primary abnormality begins with a defect in the metabolism of this essential element.

Differential Diagnosis (Table 15-1). Both Kyrle disease and perforating folliculitis have in common with EPS a central keratotic plug and a perforation through which degenerated material is eliminated. In addition, perforating folliculitis, like EPS, shows the elimination of degenerated eosinophilic elastic fibers. However, neither of the two diseases shows the great increase in elastic tissue that is observed in EPS in the uppermost dermis and particularly in the dermal papillae on staining with elastic tissue stains.

Principles of Management: Treatment modalities include local destruction with cryotherapy (63), topical medications including retinoids, corticosteroids, or salicylic acid, with rare

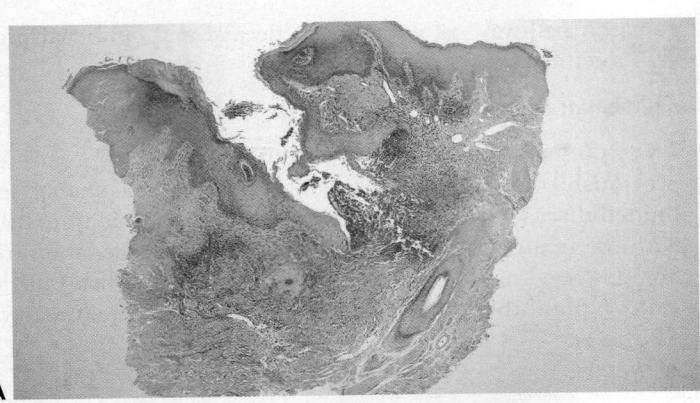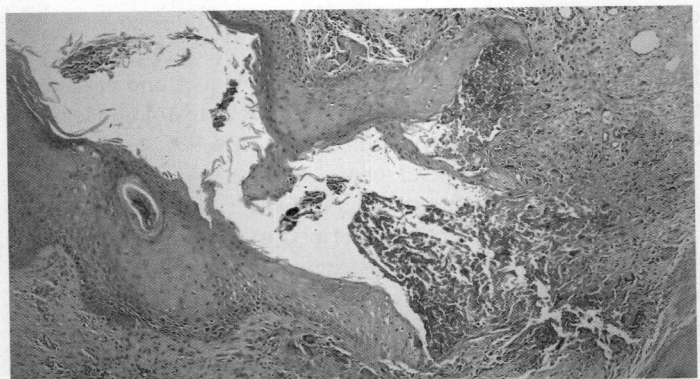

Figure 15-5 Elastosis perforans serpiginosa. A: A portion of a narrow curved channel through an acanthotic epidermis is shown. B: The lower portion of the channel contains coarse elastic fibers and basophilic debris.

reports of imiquimod (64) and photodynamic therapy (65) benefiting select patients. Systemic treatment can include retinoids (66). Other locally destructive methods such as laser therapy may be considered in select cases.

Reactive Perforating Collagenosis

RPC is a rare perforating disorder in which altered collagen is extruded by means of TEE. True, classic RPC is a genodermatosis that is inherited as an autosomal dominant or recessive trait (67,68). The lesions are precipitated by trauma, arthropod assaults, folliculitis, and even exposure to cold. RPC occurs early in life, and both genders are equally affected. An adult, acquired type of RPC has been described in association with diabetes mellitus and chronic renal failure (69–71) and may be best interpreted as an expression of APD (see text following).

Clinical Summary. The primary clinical lesion is a small papule that enlarges to a size of 5 to 10 mm with a hyperkeratotic central umbilication. Often, the lesion appears eroded. These lesions spontaneously regress, leaving superficial scars with postinflammatory pigmentary alteration. Koebnerization is common.

Histopathology. The classic lesion shows a vertically oriented, shallow, cup-shaped invagination of the epidermis, forming a short channel (Fig. 15-6A). The channel is lined by acanthotic epithelium along the sides. At the base of the invagination, there is an attenuated layer of keratinocytes that in some foci appear eroded. Within the channel, there is densely packed degenerated basophilic staining material and basophilically altered collagen bundles. Vertically oriented perforating bundles of collagen lie

interposed between the keratinocytes of the attenuated bases of the invagination (Fig. 15-6B). A Masson-trichrome stain may be performed to confirm that the fibers are collagen.

Pathogenesis. The basic process in RPC consists of the TEE of histochemically altered collagen. Nevertheless, as delineated by electron microscopy, the collagen fibrils appear intact, with regular periodicity (72).

Differential Diagnosis. See Table 15-1.

Principles of Management: Topical retinoic acid and narrow-band ultraviolet B phototherapy have been successfully used to treat familial cases (73). See also the following Principles of Management section for APD.

Acquired Perforating Dermatosis

This term was suggested by Rapini et al. (48) to describe a pathologic process encompassing the various forms of TEE seen in patients with renal disease and/or diabetes mellitus. Differences in clinical and histologic features, such as the presence of koebnerization, or histologic evidence of follicular involvement with or without collagen fibers in the epidermis have variably led to diagnoses of Kyrle disease, "acquired" RPC, or perforating folliculitis. Other terms that have been used include perforating disorder secondary to chronic renal failure and/or diabetes mellitus, perforating folliculitis of hemodialysis, Kyrle-like lesions, and uremic follicular hyperkeratosis (74–76).

Clinical Summary. Lesions are frequently pruritic and range from hyperkeratotic papules and nodules resembling Kyrle

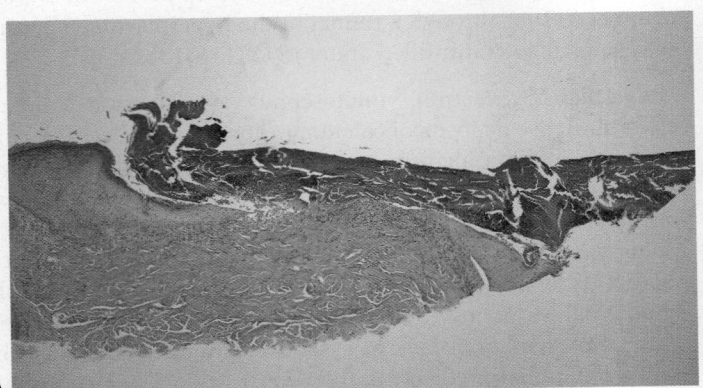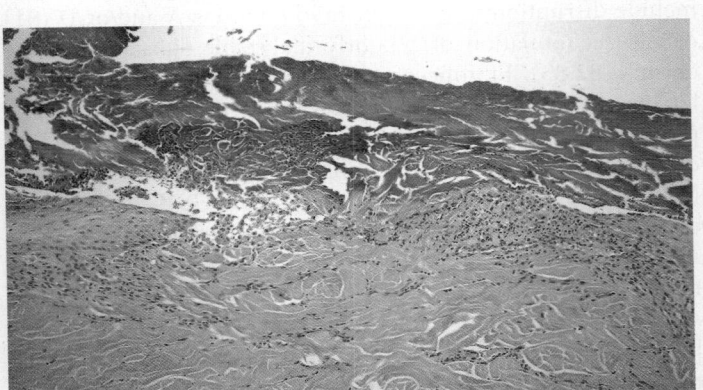

Figure 15-6 Reactive perforating collagenosis. A: A shallow cup-shaped invagination of the dermis containing a mixture of basophilic material and degenerated collagen bundles. B: Vertically oriented perforating bundles of collagen are present at the base of the invagination.

disease to RPC-like umbilicated papules, nodules, and plaques to erythematous, follicular papules and nodules mimicking perforating folliculitis (48,49,76). Annular plaques and erythematous pustules have also been described, with histologic features of RPC and perforating folliculitis, respectively (76). The most common location is the extensor surfaces of the extremities, especially lower, but the trunk and head can also be involved (48,76). APD has also been described in renal disease secondary to chronic nephritis, obstructive uropathy, anuria, and hypertension-related nephrosclerosis (49). Cases of APD have also been reported in patients with lymphoma, AIDS, hypothyroidism, hyperparathyroidism and to be associated with pruritis secondary to liver disease, neurodermatitis, atopic dermatitis, and malignant neoplasia (48,77).

Histopathology. As mentioned, the histologic features of APD are variable, even within different lesions from the same patient. When vertically oriented, Masson-trichrome positive collagen bundles are present within a perforation, the findings are suggestive of RPC. When perforation is associated with a follicle, the findings resemble perforating folliculitis. However, chronic rubbing can lead to superimposed features of prurigo nodularis, distorting the follicle and making it unrecognizable. TEE in the absence of follicular involvement, without demonstrable collagen or elastin, is reminiscent of Kyrle disease. Perforation associated with EVG-positive elastic fibers within a transepidermal canal, as seen in EPS, has also been described (76,78). Patterson et al. (79) reported a patient who had multiple lesions biopsied that variably showed histologic features of RPC, perforating folliculitis, and Kyrle disease. Combined TEE of both elastic and collagen fibers have been observed in four patients with renal disease (48), a finding that has only rarely been described in Kyrle disease or RPC (74).

Pathogenesis. RPC, EPS, and perforating folliculitis exist as distinct perforating disorders when not associated with renal disease and diabetes. At least in the setting of APD, however, the presence of various histologic patterns suggests the possibility of a common underlying mechanism (48). A nearly ubiquitous clinical feature of APD is pruritis. Certainly, lesions are often distributed in areas accessible to scratching, and reducing pruritis can lead to clearance (77). Poor blood supply secondary to diabetic microangiopathy, combined with trauma, may lead to dermal necrosis, alteration of connective tissue, and TEE (74,77,80). Others have suggested that a consequence of dialysis is the underlying cause of APD (76). Possible etiologies include disruption of metabolism of vitamins A and/or D (81) or the accumulation of a poorly dialyzable substance in the dermis (82,83). Fibronectin, a glycoprotein of the extracellular matrix, accumulates in the serum of uremic and diabetic patients. It has been suggested that transcriptional induction of fibronectin, possibly by transforming growth factor beta (TGF-β) or platelet-derived growth factor (PDGF), increases epithelial migration and proliferation and leads to TEE (81). APD has been reported in 5% to 11% of patients with chronic renal failure undergoing hemodialysis (49,82), and clearance of APD following renal transplant has been reported. However, it has also occurred following transplant, in patients with normal renal function (76). In addition, some cases have occurred prior to the start of hemodialysis or in patients who never underwent dialysis (49). Patterson suggests that TEE may represent a "final

common pathway" of a variety of dermal and epithelial processes acting alone or in concert (74).

Differential Diagnosis. See Table 15-1.

Principles of Management: A similar topical approach to previously discussed diseases may also be reasonable for limited disease or in some clinical scenarios. In conjunction with the treatment of underlying systemic disease, allopurinol, doxycycline, systemic retinoids, and narrow-band ultraviolet B phototherapy have been effective in the treatment of APD (84).

PERFORATING CALCIFIC ELASTOSIS (PERIUMBILICAL PERFORATING PSEUDOXANTHOMA ELASTICUM)

In perforating calcific elastosis, also referred to as periumbilical perforating pseudoxanthoma elasticum (PPPXE), a gradually enlarging, well-demarcated, hyperpigmented patch or plaque is usually seen in the periumbilical region in middle-aged, obese, multiparous women with hypertension (85).

Clinical Summary. Most patients described have been African American (86). The patch or plaque is in some instances atrophic with discrete keratotic papules at the periphery (87); in other instances, it has a verrucous border (88) and in still others a fissured, verrucous surface throughout (89). Lesions occurring on the breast have also been described (90–92). Perforating calcific elastosis was initially regarded as EPS coexisting with pseudoxanthoma elasticum (93–97). The disorder was later shown to be distinct from EPS (88).

Four patients with perforating calcific elastosis associated with renal failure have been described (86,91,98,99). One patient demonstrated regression of the lesions with hemodialysis (86).

Histopathology. Numerous altered elastic fibers are observed in the reticular dermis. They are short, thick, curled, and are encrusted with calcium salts, as shown by a positive von Kossa stain. They are thus indistinguishable from the elastic fibers seen in pseudoxanthoma elasticum (85). As in pseudoxanthoma elasticum, the elastic fibers are visible even in sections stained with hematoxylin–eosin, owing to their basophilia (87). The altered elastic fibers in perforating calcific elastosis are extruded to the surface either through the epidermis in a wide channel (88) or through a tunnel in the hyperplastic epidermis that ends in a keratin-filled crater (87) (Fig. 15-7A, B).

Pathogenesis. Electron microscopic examination reveals electron-dense deposits of calcium primarily in the central core of elastic fibers. Calcification of collagen bundles is also seen (90). The etiologic nature of perforating calcific elastosis has been debated. Some hypothesize it is an acquired lesion developing as a consequence of local cutaneous trauma from such factors as obesity, multiple pregnancies, ascites, or multiple abdominal surgeries (85,87,90). They cite the characteristic clinical presentation, lack of systemic manifestations, and absence of familial predisposition in most cases. The occurrence of perforating calcific elastosis in patients with renal failure may suggest that conditions resulting in an abnormal calcium

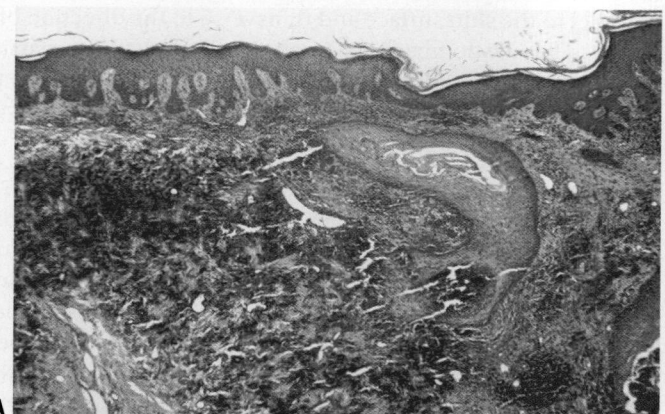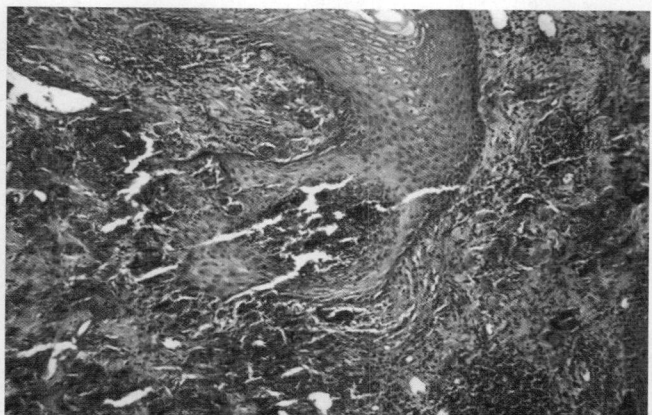

Figure 15-7 Perforating calcific elastosis. **A:** Degenerating elastic fibers encrusted with calcium salts in the reticular dermis surround a distorted transepidermal channel. **B:** The calcified fibers are in the process of being extruded through the base of the channel.

phosphate product may produce abnormal calcification of elastic fibers. The occurrence of pseudoxanthoma elasticum–like eruptions in patients exposed to saltpeter (calcium–ammonium–nitrate salts) (100), and in one patient with chronic idiopathic hyperphosphatasia (101), supports this concept. Others have argued that perforating calcific elastosis may represent a localized cutaneous expression of hereditary pseudoxanthoma elasticum (89). Arguments for the latter theory include a history of hypertension in 75% of reported patients and angioid streaks in one-third of examined patients (86). The presence of perforation is also not distinctive because the finding has also been noted to occur in lesions of classic hereditary pseudoxanthoma elasticum. The disorder may represent a spectrum ranging from a purely acquired form with no systemic manifestations to an inherited form with limited systemic expression.

Principles of Management: Topical fluocinolone acetonide therapy can be of some benefit. Spontaneous resolution without intervention has also been reported (2).

LATE-ONSET FOCAL DERMAL ELASTOSIS

Clinical Summary. Late-onset focal dermal elastosis has been described in a few elderly patients with lesions clinically resembling pseudoxanthoma elasticum (2,102–105). Patients present with slowly progressive, asymptomatic 1- to 3-mm yellow papules in healthy adults in the seventh to ninth decades. The lesions are distributed predominantly on the neck, thighs, groin, axillae, and antecubital and popliteal fossae (2,104,105). Recently, many cases in patients in the fourth to sixth decades of life have led to a proposal that the name be changed simply to focal dermal elastosis (106).

Histopathology. Focal elastosis along with an increased accumulation of normal-appearing elastic fibers in the mid- and deep dermis are seen (102). Fragmentation and calcification such as that seen in pseudoxanthoma elasticum are absent.

Pathogenesis. There is an increase in elastin and collagen contents in tested patients as compared with controls. An increase in elastin, type I and III collagen mRNAs from patients' fibroblasts has been observed. No change in excreted elastin peptides is noted in affected patients. An overexpression of elastin has been postulated (107).

HYPERKERATOSIS LENTICULARIS PERSTANS (FLEGEL DISEASE)

A rare dermatosis first described in 1958 (108), hyperkeratosis lenticularis perstans is a disorder that starts in late life and persists indefinitely. An autosomal dominant transmission has been noted in several instances (109–111).

Clinical Summary. Hyperkeratosis lenticularis perstans consists of asymptomatic, flat, hyperkeratotic papules from 1 to 5 mm in diameter, located predominantly on the dorsa of the feet and on the lower legs. Removal of the adherent, horny scale causes slight bleeding. In addition to the central horny scale, larger papules often have a peripherally attached collarette of fine scaling. In two reported instances, extensive papular lesions were present on the oral mucosa (112). Other reported sites include the thighs, upper extremities, and ears (113,114). Unilateral involvement may represent postzygotic mosaicism (115).

Histopathology. In some instances, the histologic picture is nonspecific, showing hyperkeratosis with occasional areas of parakeratosis, irregular acanthosis intermingled with areas of flattening of the stratum malpighii, and vascular dilation with a moderate amount of perivascular lymphocytic inflammation (116). It seems, however, that if the specimen is obtained from a well-developed, markedly hyperkeratotic lesion, a characteristic, although not necessarily diagnostic, histologic picture may be revealed. The lesion shows a greatly thickened, compact, strongly eosinophilic horny layer standing out in sharp contrast to the less heavily stained basket-weave keratin of the uninvolved epidermis (113). The underlying stratum malpighii appears flattened, with thinning or even absence of the granular layer (Fig. 15-8).

Acanthosis is observed at the periphery. In some instances, bordering on the central depression, the epidermis at the periphery forms a papillomatous elevation resembling a church spire (108,117,118). Vacuolar alteration and apoptotic cells in the basal layer have been seen in some cases (113,119,120). The dermal infiltrate is composed largely of lymphoid cells and is located as a narrow band fairly close to the epidermis with a rather sharp demarcation at its lower border. Immunohistochemical studies have shown the infiltrate to be predominantly T cells (121–123).

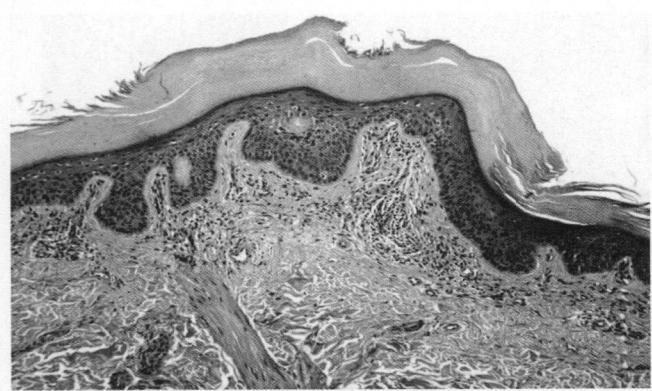

Figure 15-8 Hyperkeratosis lenticularis perstans. Dense compact orthokeratosis surmounts an epidermis, with focal flattening of the stratum malpighii. A lymphocytic infiltrate is present in the upper dermis.

Pathogenesis. Under electron microscopic examination, the absence of membrane-coating granules was noted in some cases and regarded as the primary lesion of hyperkeratosis lenticularis perstans (111,112).

A defect in the membrane-coating granules seems likely to play a role in Flegel disease, because in other cases in which membrane-coating granules were present the granules lacked a lamellar internal structure and appeared vesicular (124,125). In one case, both lamellar and vesicular bodies were observed, with lamellar bodies greatly predominating in uninvolved epidermis and vesicular bodies in lesional epidermis (126). However, one study of lesional skin from four patients found no such abnormalities in lamellar bodies (127).

Other ultrastructural findings in Flegel disease that have been described in some cases include Sézary cell–like lymphocytes (128), rodlike intracytoplasmic inclusions (129), and wormlike bodies in histiocytes (126). The significance and role of these findings in the etiology of Flegel disease are unknown.

Principles of Management: Treatment of Flegel disease is often unsuccessful. It is resistant to corticosteroids and topical keratolytic agents. Dermal abrasion and shave excision of lesions have been used. Topical 5-fluorouracil and oral retinoids have provided some benefit, but long-term results are disappointing. Topical retinoids may be of some benefit (115).

STRIAE DISTENSAE

Striae distensae, often referred to as stretch marks, are a common cutaneous disorder with no significant medical importance but can be quite disturbing to those who are afflicted (130).

Clinical Summary. Striae distensae occur most commonly on the breasts and abdomen and on the thighs, buttocks, and in the inguinal region. They are caused by stretching of the skin that occurs with pregnancy, growth spurts, obesity, and weight lifting. Use of systemic or local potent topical steroids can contribute to striae development. They consist of bands of thin, wrinkled skin that at first are red, then purple, and, finally, white, with a degree of atrophy (130).

Histopathology. The epidermis is thin and flattened. There is a decrease in the thickness of the dermis. The upper portion of the dermis shows straight, thin collagen bundles arranged

parallel to the skin surface and transverse to the direction of the striae. The elastic fibers are arranged similarly. Fine elastic fibers predominate in early lesions, whereas in older lesions they are thick (131). Within the striae, nuclei are scarce, and sweat glands and hair follicles are absent (132).

Pathogenesis. The histologic findings support the view that striae distensae are scars. They occur in conditions associated with increased production of glucocorticoids by the adrenal glands. Among these conditions are pregnancy, obesity, adolescence, and, especially, Cushing disease (133). In obesity, the increased adrenocortical activity is a consequence of the obesity, and the production of glucocorticoids returns to normal when the body weight is reduced (134). Similarly, the occurrence of striae in nonobese adolescents, as noted in 35% of the girls and 15% of the boys examined, is associated with an increase in 17-kerosteroid excretion (135). Striae may also form in response to prolonged intake of corticosteroids or following the prolonged local application of corticosteroid creams to the skin. The action of the glucocorticoids consists of an antianabolic effect suppressing both fibroblastic and epidermal activity, as tissue culture studies have shown (136).

Principles of Management: The use of topical tretinoin 0.1% cream can improve the appearance of early striae. Several types of lasers (130,137,138), platelet-rich plasma, microneedling, and dermabrasion (139) have been used to treat striae. Treatment is generally of limited benefit, but some progress has been made with combination approaches.

LINEAR FOCAL ELASTOSIS (ELASTOTIC STRIAE)

Clinical Summary. Linear focal elastosis (elastotic striae) is an uncommon, but more likely underdiagnosed or underreported, disorder presenting as palpable striae-like yellow linear bands (2). This disorder was initially described in the lumbosacral region of elderly males (140). Lesions on the thigh and legs have also been reported (141,142). Occasionally, lesions arise in association with striae distensae (143–146). Many have occurred in individuals under 30 years of age (147–149).

Histopathology. Abundant fragmented, clumped, and wavy elastic fibers are present between hypertrophic collagen bundles in the midreticular dermis (12,146). Elongated elastic fibers with split ends resembling a "paintbrush" can be seen (150). A decrease in papillary dermal elastic fibers has been demonstrated in the elastotic striae from one patient with coexistent pseudoxanthoma-like papillary dermal elastolysis (142). Unlike striae distensae, there is no decrease in thickness of the dermis or atrophy of the overlying epidermis.

Pathogenesis. Electron microscopic examination reveals fragmented elastic tissue throughout the dermis (140). Widespread elastic fiber microfibrils, some occurring in continuity with intracytoplasmic filaments of fibroblasts, along with sequential maturation of elastic fibers, have been observed, suggesting an elastogenic process (151). An increased number of elastic fibers in lesional skin have also been documented (150). It has been postulated that elastotic striae may represent a regenerative process of striae distensae (143,146). This view is supported by the presence of contiguous striae distensae and elastotic striae in several patients. Accumulations of thin elastic fibers have been observed in the late stages of striae distensae (131,132,152). Thus, linear focal elastosis may represent an excessive "keloidal" repair process occurring in striae distensae (146).

Principles of Management: There are no known efficacious treatments for this condition.

PSEUDOXANTHOMA ELASTICUM–LIKE PAPILLARY DERMAL ELASTOLYSIS

Clinical Summary. Papillary dermal elastolysis, first described in 1992 (153), is a rare, acquired condition consisting of soft coalescent yellow-white papules mainly on the lateral neck and supraclavicular regions of elderly women (142,153–161). The clinical appearance of the skin lesions closely resembles those of pseudoxanthoma elasticum (PXE). However, no other systemic features of PXE are seen. A similar and possibly related disorder, *white fibrous papulosis of the neck*, is characterized by paler, more discrete, and firm papules (162–168). The term *fibroelastolytic papulosis of the neck* has been suggested to encompass the spectrum of the two disorders (168).

Histopathology. There is a marked decrease to absence of elastic fibers in the papillary dermis (153). Focal elastotic changes in the subpapillary and mid-dermis have also been demonstrated (169). No calcification or fragmentation of elastic fibers is seen. A slight decrease in elastic fibers along with the presence of thickened collagen bundles in the papillary dermis is a differentiating feature in *white fibrous papulosis of the neck* (164,168).

Pathogenesis. Electron microscopic examination confirms the absence of elastic fibers in the papillary dermis along with the presence of immature elastic fibers in the upper reticular dermis. Fibroblasts with prominent rough endoplasmic reticulum, with numerous dilatations and elongated dendritic processes, are present (153,159). In one patient, formation of loose component fibrils of elastic fibers and elastophagocytosis were seen ultrastructurally (157). Papillary dermal elastolysis has been suggested to be a disorder of intrinsic skin aging owing to its histologic similarity (153). However, immunohistochemical studies have shown a decrease in both fibrillin-1 and elastin in affected areas, whereas aged normal-appearing skin demonstrates only a decrease in fibrillin-1. A defect in elastogenesis may contribute to the pathogenesis of the disorder (153,160). The female predominance and the report of a familial occurrence may suggest possible genetic factors (159). Immunohistochemical studies, using an antibody to serum amyloid component P, which specifically marks the peripheral mantle of microfibrils of elastic fibers in adults, underscored the absence of elastic tissue in the affected papillary dermis (170).

Principles of Management: There are no known efficacious treatments for this condition (161).

MID-DERMAL ELASTOLYSIS

Mid-dermal elastolysis is a rare disorder, first described in 1977 (171), occurring predominantly on the arms and trunk of middle-aged women.

Clinical Summary. Three patterns are seen (172). The type 1 pattern consists of widespread, large areas of fine wrinkling along skin cleavage lines. The type 2 pattern consists of small, soft, papular lesions with tiny perifollicular protrusions, leaving the hair follicle itself as an indented center (173,174). These two patterns may coexist in the same patient. Type 3 presents with persistent reticulate erythema (172,175). Urticaria (171), erythematous patches (176), granuloma annulare (177), herpes zoster, Sweet syndrome, pityriasis rosea, and many other conditions (178) may precede some of the lesions. These postinflammatory forms of mid-dermal elastolysis have some similarity to a disorder, termed *postinflammatory elastolysis and cutis laxa*, first described in young South African girls (179–181). In the latter disorder, widespread wrinkling followed an acute phase of firm, erythematous, infiltrated lesions. An overlap with another disorder described as *disseminated nevus anelasticus* is also likely (182).

Histopathology. In this condition, there is a selective absence of elastic tissue strictly limited to the mid-dermis of involved areas (171). The perifollicular protrusions around indented hair follicles result from preservation of a thin layer of elastic tissue in the immediate vicinity of the follicles. This causes the hair follicles to appear retracted while the perifollicular skin protrudes (173). A mild perivascular inflammatory infiltrate of mononuclear cells with occasional interstitial multinucleated giant cells exhibiting elastophagocytosis may be seen (183–185). Electron microscopic examination also reveals fragments of normal-appearing elastic fibers within macrophages (183,186).

Pathogenesis. The disorder likely represents a postinflammatory process, although in some cases this may be subclinical, or remote. Immunohistochemical evidence of immune activation has been observed in lesional T lymphocytes and endothelial cells (187). The cytokines and elastases produced by inflammatory cells along with elastophagocytosis by macrophages may contribute to the loss of elastic fibers (183). A possible autoimmune mechanism has been hypothesized based on its associations with rheumatoid arthritis (188), silicone mammoplasty, elevated autoantibodies, false-positive Lyme titers (189), lupus erythematosus (190), and Hashimoto thyroiditis (191). Culture studies performed with dermal fibroblasts from lesional skin showed an 80-fold increase in elastin mRNA and a 2-fold increase in elastolysis compared with normal skin (161). An idiosyncratic reaction to ultraviolet light has also been proposed as an etiologic or exacerbating factor (182,193). Recent studies suggest that UV exposure may lead to increased expression, by fibroblast-like cells, of elastin-degrading matrix metalloproteinase MMP-9 (194).

Principles of Management: There are no proven therapeutic regimens. Topical retinoids may improve wrinkling but do not alter the course of the process. A long list of treatment options such as colchicine, topical and systemic steroids, and chloroquine have not produced any benefit (172). Targeting any underlying inflammatory processes has led to a reduction in progression of the disease (178). Because sun exposure may play a role in the pathogenesis of mid-dermal elastolysis, photoprotection is strongly recommended.

MACULAR ATROPHY (ANETODERMA)

Clinical Summary. Atrophic patches located mainly on the upper trunk characterize macular atrophy or anetoderma. The skin of the patches is thin and blue-white and bulges slightly.

The lesions may give the palpating finger the same sensation as a hernial orifice.

Two types of macular atrophy are generally distinguished: the Jadassohn–Pellizzari type, in which the atrophic lesions initially appear red and, on histologic examination, show an inflammatory infiltrate; and the Schweninger–Buzzi type, which is clinically noninflammatory from the beginning. However, not every case can be clearly assigned to one or the other of these two types; many clinically noninflammatory cases show an inflammatory infiltrate when examined histologically (195). The justification for distinguishing between the inflammatory and noninflammatory types has therefore been questioned (196). In many patients, new lesions continue to appear over several years. Rare congenital and familial cases have been reported (197–201).

The so-called secondary form of macular atrophy occurs in the courses of various diseases, such as syphilis, lupus erythematosus, tuberculosis, sarcoidosis, and leprosy (202–205). The macular atrophy then represents the atrophic stage of the preceding disease (206). Other cases of secondary anetoderma have occurred in association with porphyria (207), urticaria pigmentosa (208,209), pilomatricomas (210,211), Down syndrome (212,213), acrodermatitis chronica atrophicans (196), Takayasu arteritis (214), Graves disease (215), Addison disease (215), autoimmune hemolysis (215), systemic scleroderma (215), varicella (216), anticardiolipin and antiphospholipid antibodies (217–223), HIV (224), Sjögren syndrome (225,226), α_1-antitrypsin deficiency (220), B-cell lymphoma (225,227), plasmacytoma (228,229), cutaneous lymphoid hyperplasia (228), angular cheilitis (230), juvenile xanthogranuloma (231,232), and generalized granuloma annulare (233). Macular atrophy has also been observed after iatrogenic procedures such as leech application (234), monitoring electrode placement in premature infants (235,236), hepatitis B vaccination (237), and after prolonged treatment with penicillamine (238).

Histopathology. Early, erythematous lesions usually show a moderately pronounced perivascular infiltrate of mononuclear cells (239). In a few instances, however, the early inflammatory lesions show a perivascular infiltrate in which neutrophils and eosinophils predominate and nuclear dust is present, resulting in a histologic picture of leukocytoclastic vasculitis (240,241). Microthrombosis has also been noted in patients with anetoderma and associated antiphospholipid antibodies (228–231).

The elastic tissue may still appear normal in the early stage of an erythematous lesion (232). Usually, however, it is already decreased or even absent within the lesion (242). In cases in which there is a decrease in the amount of elastic tissue, mononuclear cells may be seen adhering to elastic fibers (239). Elastophagocytosis within macrophages and giant cells may be seen (243).

Long-standing, noninflammatory lesions generally show a more or less complete loss of elastic tissue, either in the papillary and upper reticular dermis or in the upper reticular dermis only (Fig. 15-9). A perivascular and periadnexal lymphocytic infiltrate of varying intensity is invariably present, so a distinction of an inflammatory and a noninflammatory type is not justified. In some instances, the involved areas show small, normal elastic fibers, which are probably the result of resynthesis or abnormal, irregular, granular, twisted, fine fibers (195). Immunofluorescence studies of primary anetoderma have revealed immune deposits in a pattern indistinguishable from that of lupus erythematosus (244,245).

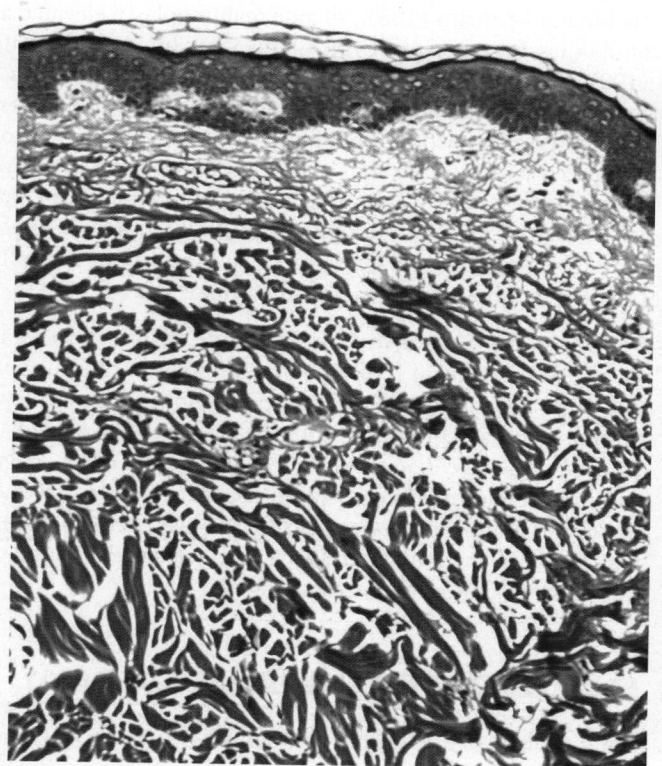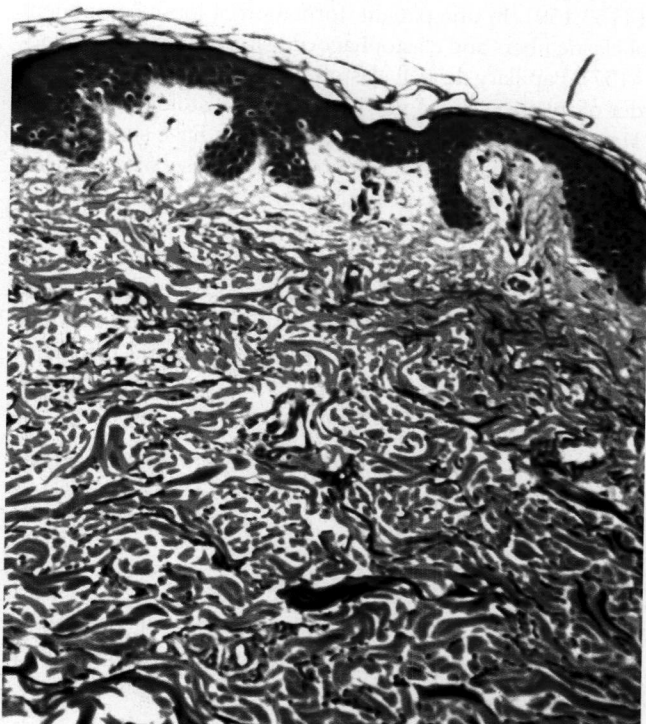

Figure 15-9 Anetoderma. Decreased to absent elastic fibers in a case of anetoderma (A) as compared with a normal control (B).

Pathogenesis. Electron microscopic examination of lesions reveals a few thin, irregular elastic fibers, with more or less complete loss of the amorphous substance elastin but with relative conservation of the microfibrils. Macrophages, lymphocytes, and some plasma cells are observed. It appears possible that partial destruction by elastases originating in the macrophages occurs because it is known that the elastases preferentially destroy the amorphous substance of the elastic fibers (245). Two elastase-type proteinases, gelatinase A (metalloproteinase 2) and B (MMP-9), have been shown to have increased expression in skin explants from patients with anetoderma (246). Morphometric analysis has demonstrated decreases in the diameter of oxytalan and dermal elastic fibers as well as the volume fractions of pre-elastic and dermal elastic fibers (247). This analysis has been used to differentiate anetoderma from other disorders of elastic tissue such as cutis laxa.

There is increasing evidence for an immunologic basis for anetoderma. In support of this hypothesis is the association of numerous autoimmune disorders and the findings of immune deposits at both the dermoepidermal junction and dermal blood vessels (215,244). In particular, the association of antiphospholipid antibodies with anetoderma is intriguing. The exact mechanism by which these antibodies may induce lesions remains to be elucidated. Some authors have postulated that microthrombosis produced by antiphospholipid antibodies with resultant ischemia of dermal tissues may induce elastic fiber degeneration (219,222). Others have hypothesized that the antibodies may alter the inhibitors of elastolytic enzymes, thus allowing the destruction of elastic fibers (248).

Principles of Management: Various modalities such as aspirin, phenytoin, dapsone, vitamin E, colchicine, and hydroxychloroquine have been tried, and may have some short-term benefits, but the long-term outcomes have been disappointing (161). Dermal fat grafting has shown some promise in localized lesions (249).

PERIFOLLICULAR ELASTOLYSIS

Clinical Summary. Perifollicular elastolysis is a relatively common condition consisting of small, hypopigmented, follicular papules on the face and upper trunk. The papules may protrude or herniate (250–253). There is a strong association with acne vulgaris, and some have suggested the term *papular acne scars* for the disorder (253).

Histopathology. There is an absence of elastic fibers localized to the regions around pilosebaceous units (250).

Pathogenesis. Perifollicular elastolysis most likely represents a form of anetoderma related to acne scarring (253). Elastase-producing strains of *Staphylococcus epidermidis* have been found in lesional hair follicles and have been proposed as the causative factor (250,252).

Principles of Management: There is no known treatment.

ACRO-OSTEOLYSIS

Clinical Summary. The term *acro-osteolysis* refers to destructive lytic changes on the distal phalanges. Three types are recognized: familial; idiopathic, nonfamilial; and occupational, which are associated with exposure to vinyl chloride gas. In addition, acro-osteolysis may be a feature of genetic syndromes such as Haim−Munk syndrome, pycnodysostosis, Hutchinson−Guilford syndrome, and Hajdu−Cheney syndrome (254−257).

The *familial type* affects mainly the phalanges of the feet and is associated with recurrent ulcers on the soles (258).

The *idiopathic type* affects the hands more severely than the feet. Involvement of the distal phalanges of the fingers causes shortening of the fingers. This variant may be associated with Raynaud phenomenon. Only one case has been described, with cutaneous lesions consisting of numerous yellow papules 2 to 4 mm in diameter and showing a linear distribution and coalescence into plaques, mainly on the arms (258).

Occupational acro-osteolysis, like the idiopathic type, causes shortening of the fingers owing to osteolysis. This variant is often associated with Raynaud phenomenon and progressive thickening of the skin of the hands and forearms simulating scleroderma. There may be erythema of the hands, and the thickening may consist of papules and plaques (259). The skin of the face may show diffuse induration (260). In addition, there may be thrombocytopenia, portal fibrosis, and impaired hepatic and pulmonary function (261). A variant of occupational acro-osteolysis has been described in guitar players and is believed to be secondary to mechanical stress (262,263).

Histopathology. The histologic changes in the papules and plaques of idiopathic and occupational acro-osteolysis consist of thickening of the dermis, with swelling and homogenization of the collagen bundles, indistinguishable from scleroderma. Staining for elastic tissue shows disorganization of the elastic fibers, which appear thin and fragmented (258−260).

Pathogenesis. Vinyl chloride disease is an immune-complex disorder associated with hyperimmunoglobulinemia, cryoglobulinemia, and evidence of *in vivo* activation of complement (261). The immunologic nature of the disease explains why it is developed by fewer than 3% of the workers exposed to vinyl chloride gas (259).

Principles of Management: Other than treatment and supportive care of the underlying cause, when one is identified, there are no specific therapeutic options.

ACKNOWLEDGMENT

The authors would like to acknowledge the work of Dr. Robert Friedman for his major contributions to this chapter in previous editions.

REFERENCES

1. Frances C, Robert L. Elastin and elastic fibers in normal and pathologic skin. *Int J Dermatol.* 1984;23:166.
2. Lewis KG, Bercovitch L, Dill SW, Robinson-Bostom L. Acquired disorders of elastic tissue, part I: increased elastic tissue and solar elastotic syndromes. *J Am Acad Dermatol.* 2004;51(1):1.
3. Kligman AM. Early destructive effect of sunlight on human skin. *JAMA.* 1969;210:2377.
4. Landi MT, Bauer J, Pfeiffer RM, et al. MC1R germline variants confer risk for BRAF-mutant melanoma. *Science.* 2006; 313(5786):521–522.
5. Raimer SS, Sanchez RL, Hubler WR, Dodson RF. Solar elastic bands of the forearm: an unusual chronic presentation of actinic elastosis. *J Am Acad Dermatol.* 1986;15:650.

6. Mitchell RE. Chronic solar dermatosis: a light and electron microscopic study of the dermis. *J Invest Dermatol.* 1967;48:203.

7. Nürnberger F, Schober E, Marsch WC, Dogliotti M. Actinic elastosis in black skin. *Arch Dermatol Res.* 1978;262:7.

8. Matsuta M, Izaki S, Ide C, et al. Light and electron microscopic immunohistochemistry of solar elastosis. *J Dermatol.* 1987;14:364.

9. Braun-Falco O. Die morphogenese der senil-aktinischen elastose. *Arch Klin Exp Dermatol.* 1969;235:138.

10. Bernstein EF, Chen YQ, Tamai K, et al. Enhanced elastin and fibrillin gene expression in chronically photodamaged skin. *J Invest Dermatol.* 1994;103(2):182.

11. Smith JG Jr, Davidson E, Sams WM Jr, Clark RD. Alterations in human dermal connective tissue with age and chronic sun damage. *J Invest Dermatol.* 1962;39:347.

12. Niebauer G, Stockinger L. Über die senile elastose. *Arch Klin Exp Dermatol.* 1965;221:122.

13. Findley GH. On elastase and the elastic dystrophies of the skin. *Br J Dermatol.* 1954;66:16.

14. Sams WM Jr, Smith JG Jr. The histochemistry of chronically sun-damaged skin. *J Invest Dermatol.* 1961;37:447.

15. Olsen RL, Nordquist J, Everett MA. The role of epidermal lysosomes in melanin physiology. *Br J Dermatol.* 1970;83:189.

16. Rabe JH, Mamelak AJ, McElugun JS, Morison WL, Sauder DN. Photoaging: mechanisms and repair. *J Am Acad Dermatol.* 2006;55:1–19.

17. Nelson BR, Majmudar G, Griffiths CEM, et al. Clinical improvement following dermabrasion of photoaged skin correlates with synthesis of collagen 1. *Arch Dermatol.* 1994;130:1136–1142.

18. Bhawan J, Gonzalez-Serva A, Nehal K, et al. Effects of tretinoin on photodamaged skin: a histologic study. *Arch Dermatol.* 1991;127:666–672.

19. Carter VH, Constantine VS, Poole WL. Elastotic nodules of the antihelix. *Arch Dermatol.* 1969;100:282.

20. Kocsard E, Ofner F, Turner B, Carter VH. Elastotic nodules of the antihelix. *Arch Dermatol.* 1970;101:370.

21. Weedon D. Elastotic nodules of the ear. *J Cutan Pathol.* 1981;8:429.

22. Requena L, Aguilar A, Sanchez Yus E. Elastotic nodules of the ears. *Cutis.* 1989;44:452–454.

23. Favre M, Racouchot J. L'élastéidose cutanée nodulaire à kystes et à comédons. *Ann Dermatol Syphiligr.* 1951;78:681.

24. Helm F. Nodular cutaneous elastosis with cysts and comedones: Favre-Racouchot syndrome. *Arch Dermatol.* 1961;84:666.

25. Eastern JS, Martin S. Actinic comedonal plaque. *J Am Acad Dermatol.* 1980;3:633.

26. John SM, Hamm H. Actinic comedonal plaque—a rare ectopic form of Favre-Racouchot syndrome. *Clin Exp Dermatol.* 1993;18:256.

27. Hauptman G, Kopf A, Rabinovitz HS, Oliviero M, Rivlin D. The actinic comedonal plaque. *Cutis.* 1997;60:145.

28. Stanford DG, Georgouroas KE, Killingsworth M. Raimer's bands: case report with a review of solar elastosis. *Acta Derm Venereol.* 1995;75:372.

29. Ackerman AB, Guo Y, Vitale PA. *Clues to Diagnosis in Dermatology.* ASCP Press; 1992:353–356.

30. Burks JW, Wise LJ, Clark WH. Degenerative collagenous plaques of the hands. *Arch Dermatol.* 1960;82:362.

31. Kocsard E. Keratoelastoidosis marginalis of the hands. *Dermatologica.* 1964;131:169.

32. Ritchle EB, Williams HM. Degenerative collagenous plaques of the hands. *Arch Dermatol.* 1966;93:202.

33. Jordaan HF, Roussouw DJ. Digital papular calcific elastosis: a histopathological, histochemical and ultrastructural study of 20 patients. *J Cutan Pathol.* 1990;17:358.

34. Rahbari H. Acrokeratoelastoidosis and keratoelastoidosis marginalis—any relation? *J Am Acad Dermatol.* 1981;5:348.

35. Rahbari H. Collagenous and elastotic marginal plaques of the hands (CEMPH). *J Cutan Pathol.* 1991;18:353.

36. Mortimore RJ, Conrad RJ. Collagenous and elastotic marginal plaques of the hands. *Australas J Dermatol.* 2001;42:211.

37. Patterson WM, Fox MD, Schwartz RA. Favre-Racouchot disease [review]. *Int J Dermatol.* 2004;43(3):167.

38. Siragusa M, Magliolo E, Batolo D, Schepis C. An unusual location of nodular elastosis with cysts and comedones (Favre-Racouchot's disease). *Acta Derm Venereol.* 2000;80:452.

39. Moulin G, Thomas L, Vigneau M, Fiere A. A case of unilateral elastosis with cysts and comedones: Favre-Racouchot syndrome. *Ann Dermatol Venereol.* 1994;121:721.

40. Stefanidou M, Ioannidou D, Tosca A. Unilateral nodular elastosis with cysts and comedones (Favre-Racouchot syndrome). *Dermatology.* 2001;202:270.

41. Mavilia L, Rossi R, Cannarozzo G, Massi D, Cappugi P, Campolmi P. Unilateral nodular elastosis with cysts and comedones (Favre-Racouchot syndrome): report of two cases treated with a new combined therapeutic approach. *Dermatology.* 2002;204:251.

42. Sanchez-Yus E, Del Rio E, Simon P, Requena L, Vázquez H. The histopathology of closed and open comedones of Favre-Racouchot disease. *Arch Dermatol.* 1997;133:1592.

43. Hassounah A, Piérard EG. Keratosis and comedos without prominent elastosis in Favre-Racouchot disease. *Am J Dermatopathol.* 1987;9:15.

44. Fanta D, Niebauer G. Aktinische (senile) komedonen. *Z Hautkr.* 1976;51:791.

45. Keough GC, Laws RA, Elston DM. Favre-Racouchot syndrome: a case for smokers' comedones. *Arch Dermatol.* 1997;133:796.

46. Sehgal VN, Singh M, Korrane RV, Nayyar M, Chandra M. Degenerative collagenous plaque of the hand (linear keratoelastoidosis of the hands): a variant of acrokeratoelastosis. *Dermatologica.* 1980;161:200.

47. Todd D, Al-Aboosi M, Hameed O, Al-Khdour M, Al-Jawamis F. The role of UV light in the pathogenesis of digital papular calcific elastosis. *Arch Dermatol.* 2001;137:379.

48. Rapini RP, Hebert AA, Drucker CR. Acquired perforating dermatosis. *Arch Dermatol.* 1989;125(8):1074.

49. Patterson JW. The perforating disorders. *J Am Acad Dermatol.* 1984;10(4):561–581.

50. Kyrle J. Hyperkeratosis follicularis et parafollicularis in cutem penetrans. *Arch Dermatol Syphilol.* 1916;123:466.

51. Ackerman AB. *Histologic Diagnosis of Inflammatory Skin Diseases.* Lea & Febieger; 1978:685–687.

52. Carter VH, Constantine VS. Kyrle's disease, I: clinical findings in five cases and review of literature. *Arch Dermatol.* 1968;97:624.

53. Constantine VS, Carter VH. Kyrle's disease, II: histopathologic findings in five cases and review of the literature. *Arch Dermatol.* 1968;97:633.

54. Tappeiner J, Wolff K, Schreiner E. Morbus kyrle. *Hautarzt.* 1969;20:296.

55. Bardach H. Dermatosen mit transepithelialer perforation. *Arch Dermatol Res.* 1976;257:213.

56. Forouzandeh M, Stratman S, Yosipovitch G. The treatment of Kyrle's disease: a systematic review. *J Eur Acad Dermatol Venereol.* 2020;34:1457.

57. Mehregan AH, Coskey RJ. Perforating folliculitis. *Arch Dermatol.* 1968;97:394.

58. Llamas-Velasco M, Steegmann JL, Carrascosa R, Fraga J, García Diez A, Requena L. Perforating folliculitis in a patient treated with nilotinib: a further evidence of C-kit involvement. *Am J Dermatopathol.* 2014;36:592.

59. Shiraishi K, Masunaga T, Tohyama M, Sayama K. A case of perforating folliculitis induced by vemurafenib. *J Dtsch Dermatol Ges.* 2018;99:230.

60. Mehregan AH. Elastosis perforans serpiginosa: a review of the literature and report of 11 cases. *Arch Dermatol.* 1968;97:381.

61. Tapiero H, Townsend DM, Tew KD. Trace elements in human physiology and pathology: copper. *Biomed Pharmacother*. 2003;57(9):386–398.

62. Iozumi K, Nakagawa H, Tamaki K. Penicillamine-induced degenerative dermatoses: report of a case and brief review of such dermatoses. *J Dermatol*. 1997;24(7):458–465.

63. Humphry S, Hemmati I, Randhawa R, Crawford RI, Hong CH. Elastosis perforans serpiginosa: treatment with liquid nitrogen cryotherapy and review of the literature. *J Cutan Med Surg*. 2010;14(1):38–42.

64. Kelly SC, Purcell SM. Imiquimod therapy for elastosis perforans serpiginosa. *Arch Dermatol*. 2006;142:829–830.

65. Alique-Garcia S, Company-Quiroga J, Horcajada-Reales C, Echeverría-García B, Tardío-Dovao JC, Borbujo J. Idiopathic elastosis perforans serpiginosa with satisfactory response after 5-ALA photodynamic therapy. *Photodiagnosis Photodyn Ther*. 2018;21:57.

66. Ratnavel RC, Norris PG. Penicillamine-induced elastosis perforans serpiginosa treated successfully with isotretinoin. *Dermatology*. 1994;189(1):81–83.

67. Weiner AL. Reactive perforating collagenosis. *Arch Dermatol*. 1970;102:540.

68. Kanan MW. Familial reactive perforating collagenosis and intolerance to cold. *Br J Dermatol*. 1974;91:405.

69. Poliak SC, Lebwohl MG, Parris A, Prioleau PG. Reactive perforating collagenosis associated with diabetes mellitus. *N Engl J Med*. 1982;306:81.

70. Cochran RJ, Tucker SB, Wilkin JK. Reactive perforating collagenosis of diabetes mellitus and renal failure. *Cutis*. 1983;31:55.

71. Beck HI, Brandrup F, Hagdrup HK, Jensen NK, Starklint H. Adult, acquired reactive perforating collagenosis. *J Cutan Pathol*. 1988;15:124.

72. Fretzin DF, Beal DW, Jao W. Light and ultrastructural study of reactive perforating collagenosis. *Arch Dermatol*. 1980;116:1054.

73. Sehgal VN, Verma P, Bhattacharya SN, Sharma S. Familial reactive perforating collagenosis in a child: response to narrow-band UVB. *Pediatr Dermatol*. 2012;30(6):762.

74. Patterson JW. Progress in the perforating dermatoses. *Arch Dermatol*. 1989;125:1121.

75. Zelger B, Hintner H, Auböck J, Fritsch PO. Acquired perforating dermatosis. *Arch Dermatol*. 1991;127:695.

76. Saray Y, Seçkin D, Bilezikçi B. Acquired perforating dermatosis: clinicopathological features in twenty-two cases. *J Eur Acad Dermatol Venereol*. 2006;20(6):679.

77. Hoque SR, Ameen M, Holden CA. Acquired reactive perforating collagenosis: four patients with a giant variant treated with allopurinol. *Br J Dermatol*. 2006;154(4):759.

78. Schamroth JM, Kellen P, Grieve TP. Elastosis perforans serpiginosa in a patient with renal disease. *Arch Dermatol*. 1986;122:82.

79. Patterson JW, Graff GE, Eubanks SW. Perforating folliculitis and psoriasis. *J Am Acad Dermatol*. 1982;7:369.

80. Kawakami T, Saito R. Acquired reactive perforating collagenosis associated with diabetes mellitus: eight cases that meet Faver's criteria. *Br J Dermatol*. 1999;140:521.

81. Morgan MB, Truitt CA, Taira J, Somach S, Pitha JV, Everett MA. Fibronectin and the extracellular matrix in the perforating disorders of the skin. *Am J Dermatopathol*. 1998;20(2):147.

82. Morton CA, Henderson IS, Jones MC, Lowe JG. Acquired perforating dermatosis in a British dialysis population. *Br J Dermatol*. 1996;135:671.

83. Haftek M, Euvrard S, Kanitakis J, Delawari E, Schmitt D. Acquired perforating dermatosis of diabetes mellitus and renal failure: further ultrastructural clues to its pathogenesis. *J Cutan Pathol*. 1993;20(4):350.

84. Karphouzis A, Giatromanolaki A, Sivridis E, Kouskoukis C. Acquired reactive perforating collagenosis: current status. *J Dermatol*. 2010;37:585–592.

85. Pruzan D, Rabbin PE, Heilman ER. Periumbilical perforating pseudo-xanthoma elasticum. *J Am Acad Dermatol*. 1992; 26:642.

86. Sapadin AN, Lebwohl MG, Teich SA, Phelps RG, DiCostanzo D, Cohen SR. Periumbilical pseudoxanthoma elasticum associated with chronic renal failure and angioid streaks—apparent regression with hemodialysis. *J Am Acad Dermatol*. 1998;39:338.

87. Hicks J, Carpenter CL Jr, Reed PJ. Periumbilical perforating pseudo-xanthoma elasticum. *Arch Dermatol*. 1979;115:300.

88. Lund HZ, Gilbert CF. Perforating pseudoxanthoma elasticum: its distinction from elastosis perforans serpiginosa. *Arch Pathol Lab Med*. 1976;100:544.

89. Schwartz RA, Richfield DF. Pseudoxanthoma elasticum with transepidermal elimination. *Arch Dermatol*. 1978;114:279.

90. Neldner KH, Martinez-Hernandez A. Localized acquired cutaneous pseudoxanthoma elasticum. *J Am Acad Dermatol*. 1979;1:523.

91. Nickoloff BJ, Noodleman R, Abel EA. Perforating pseudoxanthoma elasticum associated with chronic renal failure and hemodialysis. *Arch Dermatol*. 1985;121:1321.

92. Bressan AL, Vasconcelos BN, Silva RS, Alves Mde F, Gripp AC. Periumbilical and periareolar perforating pseudoxanthoma elasticum. *An Bras Dermatol*. 2010;85(5):705–707.

93. Smith EW, Malak JA, Goodman RM, Mckusick VA. Reactive perforating elastosis: a feature of certain genetic disorders. *Bull Johns Hopkins Hosp Med J*. 1962;111:235.

94. Schutt DA. Pseudoxanthoma elasticum and elastosis perforans serpiginosa. *Arch Dermatol*. 1965;91:151.

95. Caro I, Sher MA, Rippey JJ. Pseudoxanthoma elasticum and elastosis perforans serpiginosa. *Dermatologica*. 1975;150:36.

96. Funabashi T, Tsuyuki S. A case of elastosis perforans with pseudoxanthoma elasticum. *Jpn J Dermatol*. 1966;75:649.

97. Pai SH, Zak FG. Concurrence of pseudoxanthoma elasticum, elastosis perforans serpiginosa and systemic sclerosis. *Dermatologica*. 1970;140:54.

98. Kazakis AM, Parish WR. Periumbilical perforating pseudoxanthoma elasticum. *J Am Acad Dermatol*. 1988;19:384.

99. Toporcer MB, Kantor GR. Periumbilical hyperpigmented plaque: periumbilical perforating pseudoxanthoma elasticum (PPPXE). *Arch Dermatol*. 1990;126:1639.

100. Nielsen AO, Christensen OB, Hentzer B, Johnson E, Kobayasi T. Saltpeter-induced dermal changes electron-microscopically indistinguishable from pseudoxanthoma elasticum. *Acta Derm Venereol*. 1978;58:323.

101. Mitsudo SM. Chronic idiopathic hyperphosphatasia associated with pseudoxanthoma elasticum. *J Bone Joint Surg*. 1971;53A:303.

102. Tajima S, Shimizu K, Izumi T, Kurihara S, Harada T. Late-onset focal dermal elastosis: clinical and histological features. *Br J Dermatol*. 1995;133:303.

103. Limas C. Late onset focal dermal elastosis: a distinct clinicopathologic entity? *Am J Dermatopathol*. 1999;21:381.

104. Higgins HJ, Whitworth MW. Late-onset focal dermal elastosis: a case report and review of the literature. *Cutis*. 2010;85(4): 195–197.

105. Wang AR, Fonder MA, Telang GH, Bercovitch L, Robinson-Bostom L. Late-onset focal dermal elastosis: an uncommon mimicker of pseudoxanthoma elasticum. *J Cutan Pathol*. 2012; 39(10):957–961.

106. Knapp M, Carpenter CE, Shea K, Stowman A, Pierson JC. Focal dermal elastosis: a proposed update to the nomenclature. *Am J Dermatopathol*. 2020;42:774.

107. Tajima S, Tanaka N, Ohnishi Y, et al. Analysis of elastin metabolism in patients with late-onset focal dermal elastosis. *Acta Derm Venereol*. 1999;79:285.

108. Flegel H. Hyperkeratosis lenticularis perstans. *Hautarzt*. 1958;9:362.

109. Bean SF. The genetics of hyperkeratosis lenticularis perstans. *Arch Dermatol*. 1972;106:72.

110. Beveridge GW, Langlands AO. Familial hyperkeratosis lenticularis perstans associated with tumours of the skin. *Br J Dermatol.* 1973;88:453.

111. Frenk E, Tapernoux B. Hyperkeratosis lenticularis perstans: Flegel. *Dermatologica.* 1976;153:253.

112. Van de Staak WJBM, Bergers AMG, Bougaarts P. Hyperkeratosis lenticularis perstans: Flegel. *Dermatologica.* 1980;161:340.

113. Price ML, Wilson Jones E, MacDonald DM. A clinicopathological study of Flegel's disease: hyperkeratosis lenticularis perstans. *Br J Dermatol.* 1987;116:681.

114. Pearson LH, Smith JG, Chalker DK. Hyperkeratosis lenticularis perstans. *J Am Acad Dermatol.* 1987;16:190.

115. Miranda-Romero A, Sánchez Sambucety P, Bajo del Pozo C, Martinez Fermandez M, Esquivias Gómez JI, Garcia Muñoz M. Unilateral hyperkeratosis lenticularis perstans (Flegel's disease). *J Am Acad Dermatol.* 1998;39:655.

116. Bean SF. Hyperkeratosis lenticularis perstans. *Arch Dermatol.* 1969;99:705.

117. Raffle EJ, Rogers J. Hyperkeratosis lenticularis perstans. *Arch Dermatol.* 1969;100:423.

118. Krinitz K, Schafer I. Hyperkeratosis lenticularis perstans. *Dermatol Monatsschr.* 1971;157:438.

119. Ikada J. Hyperkeratosis lenticularis perstans. *Arch Dermatol.* 1974;110:464.

120. Hunter GA, Donald GF. Hyperkeratosis lenticularis perstans (Flegel) or dyskeratotic psoriasiform dermatosis: a single dermatosis or two? *Arch Dermatol.* 1968;98:239.

121. Jang KA, Choi JH, Sung KJ, Moon KC, Koh JK. Hyperkeratosis lenticularis perstans (Flegel's disease): histologic, immunohistochemical, and ultrastructural features in a case. *Am J Dermatopathol.* 1999;21:395.

122. Metze D, Lubke D, Luger T. Hyperkeratosis lenticularis perstans (Flegel's disease)—a complex disorder of epidermal differentiation with good response to synthetic vitamin D3 derivative. *Hautarzt.* 2000;51:31.

123. Blaheta H, Metzler G, Rassner G, Garbe C. Hyperkeratosis lenticularis perstans (Flegel's disease)—lack of response to treatment with tacalcitol and calcipotriol. *Dermatology.* 2001;202:255.

124. Squier CA, Eady RAJ, Hopps RM. The permeability of epidermis lacking normal membrane-coating granules: an ultrastructural tracer study of Kyrle-Flegel disease. *J Invest Dermatol.* 1978;70:361.

125. Tezuka T. Dyskeratotic process of hyperkeratosis lenticularis perstans: Flegel. *Dermatologica.* 1982;164:379.

126. Kanitakis J, Hermier C, Hokayem D, Schmitt D. Hyperkeratosis lenticularis: Flegel's disease: a light and electron microscopic study of involved and uninvolved epidermis. *Dermatologica.* 1987;174:96.

127. Tidman MJ, Price ML, MacDonald DM. Lamellar bodies in hyperkeratosis lenticularis perstans. *J Cutan Pathol.* 1987;14:207.

128. Langer K, Zonzits E, Konrad K. Hyperkeratosis lenticularis perstans (Flegel's disease): ultrastructural study of lesional and perilesional skin and therapeutic trial of topical tretinoin versus 5-fluorouracil. *J Am Acad Dermatol.* 1992;27:812.

129. Ikai K, Murai T, Oguchi M, Takigawa M, Komura J, Ofuji S. An ultrastructural study of the epidermis in hyperkeratosis lenticularis perstans. *Acta Derm Venereol.* 1978;58:363.

130. Kang S. Topical tretinoin therapy for management of early striae. *J Am Acad Dermatol.* 1998;39(2, pt 3):S90–S92.

131. Tsuji T, Sawabe M. Elastic fibers in striae distensae. *J Cutan Pathol.* 1988;15:215.

132. Zheng P, Lavker RM, Kligman AM. Anatomy of striae. *Br J Dermatol.* 1985;112:185.

133. Epstein NW, Epstein WL, Epstein JH. Atrophic striae in patients with inguinal intertrigo. *Arch Dermatol.* 1963;87:450.

134. Simkin B, Arce R. Steroid excretion in obese patients with colored abdominal striae. *N Engl J Med.* 1962;266:1031.

135. Sisson WR. Colored striae in adolescent children. *J Pediatr.* 1954;45:520.

136. Klehr N. Striae cutis atrophicae: morphokinetic examinations in vitro. *Acta Derm Venereol Suppl (Stockh).* 1979;85:105.

137. Jiménez GP, Flores F, Berman B, Gunja-Smith Z. Treatment of striae rubra and striae alba with the 585-nm pulsed-dye laser. *Dermatol Surg.* 2003;29(4):362–365.

138. Alexiades-Armenakas MR, Bernstein LJ, Friedman PM, Geronemus RG. The safety and efficacy of the 308-nm excimer laser for pigment correction of hypopigmented scars and striae alba. *Arch Dermatol.* 2004;140(8):955–960.

139. Seirafianpour F, Sodagar S, Mozafarpoor S, Civile VT, Lyddiatt A, Trevisani VF. Systemic review of single and combined treatments for different types of striae: a comparison of striae treatments. *J Eur Acad Dermatol Venereol.* 2021;35(11):2185–2198.

140. Burket JM, Zelickson AS, Padilla RS. Linear focal elastosis (elastotic striae). *J Am Acad Dermatol.* 1989;20:633.

141. Ramlogan D, Tan BB, Garrido M. Linear focal elastosis. *Br J Dermatol.* 2001;145:188.

142. Akagi A, Tajima S, Kawada A, Ishibashi A. Coexistence of pseudoxanthoma elasticum-like papillary dermal elastolysis and linear focal dermal elastosis. *J Am Acad Dermatol.* 2002;47:S189.

143. White GM. Linear focal elastosis: a degenerative or regenerative process of striae distensae. *J Am Acad Dermatol.* 1992;27:468.

144. Hagari Y, Norimoto M, Mihara M. Linear focal elastosis associated with striae distensae in an elderly woman. *Cutis.* 1997;60:246.

145. Chang SE, Park IJ, Moon KC, Koh JK. Two cases of linear focal elastosis (elastotic striae). *J Dermatol.* 1998;25:395.

146. Hashimoto K. Linear focal elastosis: keloidal repair of striae distensae. *J Am Acad Dermatol.* 1998;39:309.

147. Moiin A, Hashimoto K. Linear focal elastosis in a young black man: a new presentation. *J Am Acad Dermatol.* 1994;30:874.

148. Trueb RM, Fellas AS. Linear focal elastosis (elastotic striae). *Hautarzt.* 1995;46:346.

149. Tamada Y, Yokochi K, Ikeya T, Nakagomi Y, Miyake T, Hara K. Linear focal elastosis: a review of three cases in young Japanese men. *J Am Acad Dermatol.* 1997;36:301.

150. Breier F, Trautinger F, Jureck W, Hönigsmann H. Linear focal elastosis (elastotic striae): increased number of elastic fibres determined by a video measuring system. *Br J Dermatol.* 1997;137:955.

151. Hagari Y, Mihara M, Morimura T, Shimao S. Linear focal elastosis: an ultrastructural study. *Arch Dermatol.* 1991;127:1365.

152. Pinkus H, Keech MK, Mehregan AH. Histopathology of striae distensae with special reference to striae and wound healing in the Marfan syndrome. *J Invest Dermatol.* 1966;46:283.

153. Rongioletti F, Rebora A. Pseudoxanthoma elasticum-like papillary dermal elastolysis. *J Am Acad Dermatol.* 1992;26:648.

154. Patrizi A, Neri I, Trevisi P, Varotti C. Pseudoxanthoma elasticum-like papillary dermal elastolysis: another case. *Dermatology.* 1994;189:289.

155. Pirard C, Delbrouck-Poot F, Bourlond A. Pseudoxanthoma elasticum-like papillary dermal elastolysis: a new case. *Dermatology.* 1994;189:193.

156. El-Charif MA, Mousawi AM, Rubeiz NG, Kibbi AG. Pseudoxanthoma elasticum-like papillary dermal elastolysis: a report of two cases. *J Cutan Pathol.* 1994;21:252.

157. Hashimoto K, Tye MJ. Upper dermal elastolysis: a comparative study with mid-dermal elastolysis. *J Cutan Pathol.* 1994;21:533.

158. Vargaz-Diez E, Penas PF, Fraga J, Aragües M, García-Díez A. Pseudoxanthoma elasticum-like papillary dermal elastolysis: a report of two cases and review of the literature. *Acta Derm Venereol.* 1997;77:43.

159. Orlandi A, Bianchi L, Nini G, Spagnoli LG. Familial occurrence of pseudoxanthoma elasticum-like papillary dermal elastolysis. *J Eur Acad Dermatol Venereol.* 1998;10:175.

160. Ohnishi Y, Tajima S, Ishibashi A, Inazumi T, Sasaki T, Sakamoto H. Pseudoxanthoma elasticum-like papillary dermal elastolysis:

report of four Japanese cases and an immunohistochemical study of elastin and fibrillin-1. *Br J Dermatol.* 1998;139:141.

161. Lewis KG, Bercovitch L, Dill SW, Robinson-Bostom L. Acquired disorders of elastic tissue, part II: decreased elastic tissue. *J Am Acad Dermatol.* 2004;51:165.

162. Shimizu H, Kimura S, Harada T, Nishikawa T. White fibrous papulosis of the neck: a new clinicopathologic entity? *J Am Acad Dermatol.* 1989;20:1073.

163. Vermersch-Langlin A, Delaporte E, Pagniez D, et al. White fibrous papulosis of the neck. *Int J Dermatol.* 1993;32:442.

164. Joshi RK, Abanmi A, Hafeen A. White fibrous papulosis of the neck. *Br J Dermatol.* 1992;127:295.

165. Cerio R, Gold S, Wilson Jones E. White fibrous papulosis of the neck. *Clin Exp Dermatol.* 1991;16:224.

166. Zanca A, Contri MB, Carnevali C, Bertazzoni MG. White fibrous papulosis of the neck. *Int J Dermatol.* 1996;35:720.

167. Siragusa M, Batolo D, Schepis C. White fibrous papulosis of the neck in three Sicilian patients. *Australas J Dermatol.* 1996; 37:202.

168. Balus L, Amantea A, Donati P, Fazio M, Giuliano MC, Bellocci M. Fibroelastolytic papulosis of the neck: a report of 20 cases. *Br J Dermatol.* 1997;137:461.

169. Tajima S, Ohnishi Y, Akagi A, Sasaki T. Elastotic change in the subpapillary and mid-dermal layers in papillary dermal elastolysis. *Br J Dermatol.* 2000;142:586.

170. Revelles JM, Machan S, Pielasinski U, et al. Pseudoxanthoma elasticum-like papillary dermal elastolysis: immunohistochemical study using elastic fiber cross-reactivity with an antibody against amyloid P component. *Am J Dermatopathol.* 2012;34(6):637–643.

171. Shelley WB, Wood MC. Wrinkles due to idiopathic loss of mid-dermal elastic tissue. *Br J Dermatol.* 1977;97:441.

172. Gambichler T. Mid-dermal elastolysis revisited. *Arch Dermatol Res.* 2010;302(2):85–93.

173. Brenner W, Gschnait F, Konrad K, Holubar K, Tappeiner J. Non-inflammatory dermal elastolysis. *Br J Dermatol.* 1979;99:335.

174. Maghraoui S, Grossin M, Crickx B, Blanchet P, Belaich S. Mid-dermal elastolyis: report of a case with a predominant perifollicular pattern. *J Am Acad Dermatol.* 1992;26:490.

175. Bannister MJ, Rubel DM, Kossard S. Mid-dermal elastophagocytosis presenting as a persistent reticulate erythema. *Australas J Dermatol.* 2001;42:50.

176. Delacrétaz J, Perroud H, Vulliemin JF. Cutis laxa acquise. *Dermatologica.* 1977;155:233.

177. Yen A, Tschen J, Raimer SS. Mid-dermal elastolysis in an adolescent subsequent to lesions resembling granuloma annulare. *J Am Acad Dermatol.* 1997;37:870.

178. Gambichler T, Mamali K, Scheel C. A brief literature update on mid-dermal elastolysis with an emphasis on pathogenetic and therapeutic aspects. *J Clin Aesthet Dermatol.* 2020;13:E53.

179. Marshall J, Heyl T, Weber HW. Post inflammatory elastolysis and cutis laxa. *S Afr Med J.* 1966;40:1016.

180. Verhagen AR, Woederman MJ. Post-inflammatory elastolysis and cutis laxa. *Br J Dermatol.* 1975;95:183.

181. Lewis PG, Hood AF, Barnett NK, Holbrook KA. Postinflammatory elastolysis and cutis laxa. *J Am Acad Dermatol.* 1992; 26:882.

182. Crivellato E. Disseminated nevus anelasticus. *Int J Dermatol.* 1986;25:171.

183. Heudes AM, Boullie MC, Thomine E, Lauret P. Élastolyse acquise en nappe du derme moyen. *Ann Dermatol Venereol.* 1988;115:1041.

184. Larregue M, Laivre-Mathieu-Thibault M, Titi A, et al. Elastolyse en nappe superficielle acquise et inflammatoire. *J Dermatol (Paris).* 1988;13:38b.

185. Brod BA, Rabkin M, Rhodes AR, Jegasothy BV. Mid-dermal elastolysis with inflammation. *J Am Acad Dermatol.* 1992;26:882.

186. Neri I, Patrizi A, Fanti P, Passarini B, Badiali-De Giorgi L, Varotti C. Mid-dermal elastolysis: a pathological and ultrastructural study of five cases. *J Cutan Pathol.* 1996;23:165.

187. Sterling JC, Coleman N, Pye RJ. Mid-dermal elastolysis. *Br J Dermatol.* 1994;130:502.

188. Rudolph RI. Mid dermal elastolysis. *J Am Acad Dermatol.* 1990;22:203.

189. Kirsner RS, Falanga V. Features of an autoimmune process in mid-dermal elastolysis. *J Am Acad Dermatol.* 1992;27:832.

190. Boyd AS, King LE Jr. Mid dermal elastolysis in two patients with lupus erythematosus. *Am J Dermatopathol.* 2001;23:136.

191. Gambichler T, Linhart C, Wolter M. Mid-dermal elastolysis associated with Hashimoto's thyroiditis. *J Eur Acad Dermatol Venereol.* 1999;12:245.

192. Kim JM, Su WPD. Mid dermal elastolysis with wrinkling: report of two cases and review of the literature. *J Am Acad Dermatol.* 1992;26:169.

193. Snider RL, Lang PG, Maize JC. The clinical spectrum of mid-dermal elastolysis and the role of UV light in its pathogenesis. *J Am Acad Dermatol.* 1993;28:938.

194. Patroi I, Annessi G, Girolomoni G. Mid-dermal elastolysis: a clinical, histologic, and immunohistochemical study of 11 patients. *J Am Acad Dermatol.* 2003;48:846.

195. Venencie PY, Winkelmann RK. Histopathologic findings in anetoderma. *Arch Dermatol.* 1984;120:1040.

196. Venencie PY, Winkelmann RK, Moore BA. Anetoderma: clinical findings, association, and long-term follow-up evaluation. *Arch Dermatol.* 1984;120:1032.

197. Friedman SJ, Venencie PY, Bradley RR, Winkelmann RK. Familial anetoderma. *J Am Acad Dermatol.* 1987;16:341.

198. Aberer E, Weissenbacher G. Congenital anetoderma by intrauterine infection? *Arch Dermatol.* 1997;133:526.

199. Peterman A, Scheel M, Sams WM Jr, et al. Hereditary anetoderma. *J Am Acad Dermatol.* 1996;35:999.

200. Zellman GL, Levy ML. Congenital anetoderma in twins. *J Am Acad Dermatol.* 1997;36:483.

201. Gerritsen MJ, De Rooij MJ, Sybrandy-Fleuren BA, van de Kerkhof PC. Familial anetoderma. *Dermatology.* 1999;198:321.

202. Deluzenne R. Les anétodermies maculeuses. *Ann Dermatol Syphiligr (Paris).* 1956;83:618.

203. Bechelli LM, Valeri V, Pimenta WP, Tanaka AM. Schweninger-Buzzi anetoderma in women with or without lepromatous leprosy. *Dermatologica.* 1967;135:329.

204. Temime P, Baran LR, Friedmann E. Pseudotumoral anetoderma and chronic lupus erythematosus. *Ann Dermatol Syphiligr.* 1971;98:141.

205. Clement M, du Vivier A. Anetoderma secondary to syphilis. *J R Soc Med.* 1983;76:223.

206. Edelson Y, Grupper C. Anétodermie maculeuse et lupus érythémateux. *Bull Soc Fr Dermatol Syphiligr.* 1970;77:753.

207. Balina LM, Gatti JC, Cardama JE, Avila JJ, De Garrido RM. Congenital poikiloderma and anetoderma in porphyria. *Arch Argent Dermatol.* 1966;16:190.

208. Carr RD. Urticaria pigmentosa associated with anetoderma. *Acta Derm Venereol.* 1971;51:120.

209. Thivolet J, Cambazard F, Souteyrand P, Pierini AM. Mastocytosis evolving into anetoderma: review of the literature. *Ann Dermatol Venereol.* 1981;108:259.

210. Moulin G, Bouchet B, Dos Santos G. Anetodermic cutaneous changes above Malherbe's tumors. *Ann Dermatol Venereol.* 1978;105:43.

211. Shames BS, Nassif A, Bailey CS, Saltzstein SL. Secondary anetoderma involving a pilomatricoma. *Am J Dermatopathol.* 1994;16:557.

212. Kaplan H, Lacentre E, Carabelli S. Changes in the elastic tissue of patients with Down's syndrome. *Med Cutan Ibero Lat Am.* 1982;10:79.

213. Schepis C, Siragusa M. Secondary anetoderma in people with Down's syndrome. *Acta Derm Venereol.* 1999;79:245.

214. Taieb A, Dufillot D, Pellegrin-Carloz B, et al. Postgranulomatous anetoderma associated with Takayasu's arteritis in a child. *Arch Dermatol.* 1987;12:796.

215. Hodak E, Shamai-Lubovitz O, David M, et al. Immunologic abnormalities associated with primary anetoderma. *Arch Dermatol.* 1992;128:799.

216. Tousignant J, Crickx B, Grossin M, Besseige H, Lépine F, Belaïch S. Post-varicella anetoderma: 3 cases [in French]. *Ann Dermatol Venereol.* 1990;117:355.

217. Stephansson EA, Niemi KM, Jouhikainen T, Vaarala O, Palosuo T. Lupus anticoagulant and the skin: a longterm follow-up study of SLE patients with special reference to histopathologic findings. *Acta Derm Venereol.* 1991;71:416.

218. Disdier P, Harle JR, Andrac L, et al. Primary anetoderma associated with the antiphospholipid syndrome. *J Am Acad Dermatol.* 1994;30:133.

219. Gibson GE, Su WP, Pittelkow MR. Antiphospholipid syndrome and the skin. *J Am Acad Dermatol.* 1997;36:970.

220. Stephansson EA, Niemi KM. Antiphospholipid antibodies and anetoderma: are they associated? *Dermatology.* 1995;191:202.

221. Montilla C, Alarcon-Segovia D. Anetoderma in systemic lupus erythematosus: relationship to antiphospholipid antibodies. *Lupus.* 2000;9:545.

222. Romani J, Perez F, Llobet M, Planagumá M, Pujol RM. Anetoderma associated with antiphospholipid antibodies: case report and review of the literature. *J Eur Acad Dermatol Venereol.* 2000;15:175.

223. Alvarez-Cuesta CC, Raya-Aguado C, Fernandez-Rippe ML, Sánchez TS, Pérez-Oliva N. Anetoderma in a systemic lupus erythematosus patient with anti-PCNA and antiphospholipid antibodies. *Dermatology.* 2001;203:348.

224. Ruiz-Rodriguez R, Longaker M, Berger TG. Anetoderma and human immunodeficiency virus infection. *Arch Dermatol.* 1992;128:661.

225. Jubert C, Cosnes A, Clerici T, et al. Sjogren's syndrome and cutaneous B cell lymphoma revealed by anetoderma. *Arthritis Rheum.* 1993;36:133.

226. Herrero-Gonzalez JE, Herrero-Mateu C. Primary anetoderma associated with primary Sjogren's syndrome. *Lupus.* 2002;11:124.

227. Kasper RC, Wood GS, Nihal M, LeBoit PE. Anetoderma arising in cutaneous B cell lymphoproliferative disease. *Am J Dermatopathol.* 2001;23:124.

228. Jubert C, Cosnes A, Wechsler J, Andre P, Revuz J, Bagot M. Anetoderma may reveal cutaneous plasmacytoma and benign lymphoid hyperplasia. *Arch Dermatol.* 1995;131:365.

229. Child FJ, Woollons A, Price ML, Calonje E, Russell-Jones R. Multiple cutaneous immunocytoma with secondary anetoderma: a report of two cases. *Br J Dermatol.* 2000;143:165.

230. Crone AM, James MP. Acquired linear anetoderma following angular cheilitis. *Br J Dermatol.* 1998;138:923.

231. Ang P, Tay YK. Anetoderma in a patient with juvenile xanthogranuloma. *Br J Dermatol.* 1999;140:541.

232. Prigent F. Anetoderma secondary to juvenile xanthogranuloma. *Ann Dermatol Venereol.* 2001;128:291.

233. Ozkan S, Fetil E, Izler F, Pabuçcuoğlu U, Yalçin N, Güneş AT. Anetoderma secondary to generalized granuloma annulare. *J Am Acad Dermatol.* 2000;42:335.

234. Siragusa M, Batolo D, Schepis C. Anetoderma secondary to application of leeches. *Int J Dermatol.* 1996;35:226.

235. Prizant TL, Lucky AW, Frieden IJ, Burton PS, Suarez SM. Spontaneous atrophic patches in extremely premature infants: anetoderma of prematurity. *Arch Dermatol.* 1996;132:671.

236. Colditz PB, Dunster KR, Joy GJ, Robertson IM. Anetoderma of prematurity in association with electrocardiographic electrodes. *J Am Acad Dermatol.* 1999;41:479.

237. Daoud MS, Dicken CH. Anetoderma after hepatitis B immunization in two siblings. *J Am Acad Dermatol.* 1997;36:779.

238. Davis W. Wilson's disease and penicillamine-induced anetoderma. *Arch Dermatol.* 1977;113:976.

239. Kossard S, Kronman KR, Dicken CH, Schroeter AL. Inflammatory macular atrophy: immunofluorescent and ultrastructural findings. *J Am Acad Dermatol.* 1979;1:325.

240. Cramer HJ. Zur Histopathogenese der dermatitis atrophicans maculosa. *Dermatol Wochenschr.* 1963;147:230.

241. Hellwich M, Nickolay-Kiesthardt J. Kasuistischer beitrag zur anetodermia jadassohn. *Z Hautkr.* 1986;61:1638.

242. Miller WM, Ruggles CW, Rist TE. Anetoderma. *Int J Dermatol.* 1979;18:43.

243. Zaki I, Scerri L, Nelson H. Primary anetoderma: phagocytosis of elastic fibres by macrophages. *Clin Exp Dermatol.* 1994;19:388.

244. Bergman R, Friedman-Birnbaum R, Hazaz B, Cohen E, Munichor M, Lichtig C. An immunofluorescence study of primary anetoderma. *Clin Exp Dermatol.* 1990;15:124.

245. Venencie PY, Winkelmann RK. Ultrastructural findings in the skin lesions of patients with anetoderma. *Arch Dermatol.* 1984;120:1084.

246. Venencie PY, Bonnefoy A, Gogly B, et al. Increased expression of gelatinases A and B by skin explants from patients with anetoderma. *Br J Dermatol.* 1997;137:517.

247. Ghomrasseni S, Dridi M, Bonnefoix M, et al. Morphometric analysis of elastic skin fibres from patients with: cutis laxa, anetoderma, pseudoxanthoma elasticum, and Buschke-Ollendorf and Williams-Beuren syndromes. *J Eur Acad Dermatol Venereol.* 2001;15:305.

248. Lindstrom J, Smith KJ, Skelton HG, et al. Increased anticardiolipin antibodies associated with the development of anetoderma in HIV-1 disease. Military Medical Consortium for the Advancement of Retroviral research (MMCARR). *Int J Dermatol.* 1995;34:408.

249. Nomura T, Nakasone M, Okamoto T, et al. Use of dermal fat grafts for treating anetoderma with lipoatrophy following involution of hemangiomas. *Pedatr Dermatol.* 2020;37:776.

250. Varadi DP, Saqueton AC. Perifollicular elastolysis. *Br J Dermatol.* 1970;83:143.

251. Taafe A, Cunliffe WJ, Clayden AD. Perifollicular elastolysis—a common condition. *Br J Dermatol.* 1983;24S:20.

252. Lemarchand-Venencie F, Venencie PY, Foix C, Sanson MJ, Chérif F, Civatte J. Perifollicular elastolysis: discussion of the role of secretory elastase from *Staphylococcus epidermidis. Ann Dermatol Venereol.* 1985;112:735.

253. Wilson BB, Dent CH, Cooper PH. Papular acne scars: a common cutaneous finding. *Arch Dermatol.* 1990;126:797.

254. Haim S, Munk J. Periodontosis a part of an unknown familial congenital disorder. *Refuat Hapeh Vehashinayim.* 1969;18:2.

255. Lamy M, Maroteaux P. Pycnodysostosis. *Rev Esp Pediatr.* 1965;21:433.

256. Jansen T, Romiti R. Progeria infantum (Hutchinson-Gilford syndrome) associated with scleroderma-like lesions and acroosteolysis: a case report and brief review of the literature. *Pediatr Dermatol.* 2000;17:282.

257. Herrmann J, Zugibe FT, Gilbert EF, Opitz JM. Arthro-dento-osteo dysplasia (Hajdu-Cheney syndrome): review of a genetic "acro-osteolysis" syndrome. *Z Kinderheilkd.* 1973;114:93.

258. Meyerson LB, Meier GC. Cutaneous lesions in acroosteolysis. *Arch Dermatol.* 1972;106:224.

259. Markowitz SS, McDonald CJ, Fethiere W, Kerzner MS. Occupational acroosteolysis. *Arch Dermatol.* 1972;106:219.

260. Veltmann G, Lange CE, Stein G. Die Vinyl krankheit. *Hautarzt.* 1978;29:177.

261. Fine RM. Acro-osteolysis: vinyl chloride induced "scleroderma." *Int J Dermatol.* 1976;15:676.

262. Destouet JM, Murphy WA. Guitar player acro-osteolysis. *Skeletal Radiol.* 1981;6:275.

263. Baran R, Tosti A. Occupational acroosteolysis in a guitar player. *Acta Derm Venereol.* 1993;73:64.

Cutaneous Manifestations of Nutritional Deficiency States and Gastrointestinal Disease

CYNTHIA MAGRO, JASON S. STRATTON, A. NEIL CROWSON, AND MARTIN C. MIHM JR.

Chapter 16

INTRODUCTION

As a metabolically active and visible organ, the skin is often an early and prominent site of manifestation of nutritional deficiencies. These conditions and also a mixed group of conditions that are associated with other forms of gastrointestinal disease, such as hepatobiliary disease, are discussed in this chapter. The pathogenesis of these conditions may include deficiencies of essential nutrients, metabolic disturbances, derangements of the immune system, and viral infections.

Principles of Management: For all of the nutritional dermatoses in which there is a specific nutritive deficit, the key principle of management is to make a correct diagnosis and correct the specific deficit, be it of a vitamin, cofactor, protein, or lipid. These principles will not be repeated throughout this book, except where there are additional therapeutic interventions to discuss.

DEFICIENCIES OF VITAMINS, OTHER AMINO ACIDS, AND MINERALS

Scurvy

The manifestations of scurvy, which is due to vitamin C (ascorbic acid) deficiency, have been known for 3,000 years.

Clinical Summary. In 1753, Sir James Lind demonstrated the efficacy of citrus fruits in the prevention of this condition (1,2), which is characterized by follicular purpuric macules with or without follicular hyperkeratosis and corkscrew hairs; ecchymoses, particularly in the pretibial areas; and conjunctival and gingival hemorrhages, the latter associated with gingival hyperplasia (3). Subcutaneous hemorrhage with woody edema of the lower extremities and hemarthrosis may occur (4,5). Nonspecific aches and pains and impaired wound healing are frequent. Anemia, possibly related to decreased amounts of active folate and blood loss, is present in approximately 75% of individuals (4,6). For humans, the principal source of vitamin C, a substance that cannot be synthesized from glucose derivatives, is fruits and vegetables. Scurvy occurs in individuals such as patients with autism who selectively avoid these foods (7), the elderly, chronic alcoholics, patients who undergo renal dialysis, and malnourished displaced refugee populations (8,9), who also suffer other micronutrient deficiencies when dependent on food aid (10,11). Vitamin C deficiency can also be seen in cases of malabsorption secondary to diseases of the bowels, such as Crohn disease or graft-versus-host disease (12,13).

Histopathology. Follicular hyperkeratosis and perifollicular erythrocyte extravasation without an accompanying vasculopathy are characteristic. Extensive extravasations are usually associated with deposits of hemosiderin within and outside macrophages. A coiled hair may emanate from the dilated follicular orifice (14).

Differential Diagnosis. Other pauci-inflammatory hyperkeratotic dermatoses that should be considered in the differential diagnosis include keratosis pilaris, vitamin A deficiency, pityriasis rubra pilaris, ichthyosis vulgaris, and a resolving lichenoid follicular hyperkeratotic process, such as lichen planopilaris, lichen spinulosus, or lupus erythematosus. Pilotropic T-cell dyscrasia including alopecia mucinosa and frank pilotropic mycosis fungoides can demonstrate prominent follicular hyperkeratosis. Coiled or "corkscrew" hairs are not pathognomonic of scurvy and may be seen in certain ectodermal dysplasia syndromes (15).

Pathogenesis. Most manifestations of scurvy can be attributed to defective collagen synthesis. Lysine and proline hydroxylase enzymes require vitamin C to reduce Fe^{3+} during the reaction. In vitamin C deficiency, the end product, hydroxyproline, which stabilizes the collagenous domain of procollagen, is deficient (3). Individuals with the Hp 2-2 genetic polymorphism of haptoglobin, a hemoglobin-binding antioxidant, have markedly lower levels of vitamin C despite an adequate nutritional supply, establishing a basis for a potential genetic influence (16). Because of the impaired antioxidant ability of Hp 2-2 haptoglobin, there is a higher rate of vitamin C oxidation, which significantly reduces the stability of L-ascorbic acid (17) and decreases its availability to hydroxylase enzymes. Ultrastructurally, the dermal fibroblasts appear shrunken and show a decreased amount of rough endoplasmic reticulum (18). Around these fibroblasts, one observes increased amounts of extracellular filamentous or amorphous material that has failed to polymerize into normal collagen fibrils. The extravasation of red cells is caused by vacuolar degeneration and junctional separation of adjoining endothelial cells and their detachment from the basement membrane in capillaries and small venules (18).

Vitamin A Deficiency (Phrynoderma)

Seen mainly in Asia and Africa, vitamin A deficiency is rare in the United States but may occur after intestinal bypass surgery for obesity (19) or visceral myopathy (20,21).

Clinical Summary. Dryness and roughness of the skin, along with conical follicular keratotic plugs, characterize the cutaneous changes. The distribution is bilateral and symmetrical in the majority of cases and tends to be localized to the elbows, knees, extensor extremities, and/or buttocks. The elbow is the most common site of onset (22). Night blindness, xerophthalmia, and keratomalacia also occur. One reported case in France attributed the phrynoderma to severe combined endogenous deficiencies of vitamins A and C secondary to intestinal malabsorption caused by chronic intestinal parasitic infection by *Giardia intestinalis* (23). Bariatric surgery with pancreatic biliary diversion has been associated with the development of phrynoderma (21).

Histopathology. The skin shows moderate hyperkeratosis with distension of the upper part of the follicle by large, horny plugs (19). Sebaceous glands are greatly reduced in size and may exhibit epithelial atrophy (24). In severe cases, both eccrine and sebaceous glands may exhibit squamous metaplasia (25).

Differential Diagnosis. The other causes of a pauci-inflammatory interfollicular and follicular hyperkeratosis are mentioned in the prior discussion of scurvy. Striking orthohyperkeratosis with only minimal parakeratosis, hyperplasia of the epidermis, acantholysis, and a superficial dermal lymphocytic infiltrate with basilar vacuolar change are additional histologic features that distinguish pityriasis rubra pilaris from phrynoderma (26). Superficial dermal fibroplasia with melanophage accumulation is the hallmark of resolved lichen planopilaris, lupus erythematosus, and graft-versus-host disease. Sebaceous gland atrophy has been described in pellagra. Squamous metaplasia of the eccrine apparatus has been seen with methotrexate therapy and graft-versus-host disease. Lymphocyte satellitosis around eccrine ductular cells is an additional helpful clue pointing toward a diagnosis of graft-versus-host disease.

Acquired Vitamin B₃ Deficiency (Pellagra)

The word "pellagra" is derived from two Italian words *pelle*, meaning "skin," and *agra*, meaning "sharp burning" or "rough." Although primarily ascribed to niacin (vitamin B₃) deficiency, other vitamin deficiencies or protein malnutrition (27) appear integral to the development of the pellagra symptom complex.

Clinical Summary. Presenting as cutaneous lesions, gastrointestinal symptoms, and mental changes, pellagra has been ascribed the acronym of the three *D*s: dermatitis, diarrhea, and dementia; some add the fourth *D* "death," as this condition may be fatal if unrecognized. In the United States, the enrichment of whole-wheat flour with niacin has almost eliminated pellagra, but it is still prevalent in countries such as Mexico and some African nations where cornmeal is the main constituent of the diet, as well as in displaced populations (10,11). Pellagra in the United States and Europe is seen mainly in chronic alcoholics (28) and in patients with anorexia nervosa (29), malignant gastrointestinal tumors, and intestinal parasitosis (27). Its appearance in carcinoid syndrome is believed to reflect a depression of endogenous niacin production by tumor cell diversion of tryptophan toward serotonin (30). Pellagra has also been reported in patients receiving isoniazid, pyrazinamide, ethionamide, azathioprine, chloramphenicol, and anticonvulsants (31,32). Isoniazid, a structural analog of niacin, can cause suppression of endogenous niacin production.

Three basic skin eruptions occur in pellagra (33,34). The first is a photo-induced eruption that is intensely erythematous and subsequently exfoliates to yield a hyperpigmented residuum. The second eruption comprises painful erythematous erosions in genital and perineal areas, possibly induced by pressure, heat, and trauma (27). The increased skin fragility may reflect aberrations in the collagen and elastic fiber content of the skin. Patients with pellagra may develop a seborrheic dermatitis–like rash involving the face, scalp, and neck. Oral manifestations include beefy, red, cracked lips and a fissured or smooth, red, sore tongue (35). Among the neurologic symptoms are dementia, psychosis, anxiety, defective memory, burning sensations, sudden attacks of falling, dizziness, and headaches. A cause of sudden death is central pontine myelinolysis (27).

Histopathology. Psoriasiform epidermal hyperplasia with hyperkeratosis, parakeratosis, and a lymphocytic perivascular inflammatory cell infiltrate characterize initial lesions. Additional features include scattered necrotic keratinocytes, granular cell layer loss, and architectural disarray with dysmaturation of the epidermis. Depigmentation of the basal layer with accumulation of fat droplets is described, as is vacuolation of cells within the granular and spinous layers (36). The combination of confluent parakeratosis with upper epidermal pallor may be present and is a clue to a nutritional deficiency dermatosis (37). Epidermal atrophy, hypermelanosis, vascular ectasia, and sebaceous atrophy characterize end-stage lesions (36), with recent studies demonstrating a decrease in epidermal Langerhans cells (38). Seborrheic dermatitis–like lesions may show sebaceous gland hyperplasia with follicular dilation. Fragmentation, swelling, and thickening of elastic fibers; swelling of collagen fibers; and merging of elastic tissue with collagen have been described. A morphology indistinguishable from that of necrolytic migratory erythema and acrodermatitis enteropathica has been reported, comprising intracellular edema with vacuolar change of the upper stratum malpighii and keratinocyte necrosis, sometimes accompanied by neutrophilic infiltration of the upper spinous layers, subcorneal pustulation localized to or in isolation from these areas, and folliculitis (27).

Pathogenesis. A deficiency in urocanic acid caused by a reduction in histidine and histidase activity has been postulated as a possible mechanism of photosensitivity in pellagra; urocanic acid protects the skin from ultraviolet (UV) wavelengths by absorbing light in the UVB range (27,39). Kynurenic acid, a metabolic by-product of the tryptophan–kynurenine–nicotinic pathway, accumulates in pellagra as a result of a deficiency of nicotinamide, which blocks the formation of kynurenic acid. Kynurenic acid induces a phytotoxic reaction in skin subjected to long-wave UV radiation ranging from 350 to 380 nm (27). Some of the gastrointestinal symptoms may relate to degenerative changes of the dorsal vagal nuclei. The neurologic symptoms may be due to chromatolysis of various cortical and brainstem nuclei (27).

Differential Diagnosis. The histopathology is similar to that of the nutritional dermatoses acrodermatitis enteropathica and necrolytic migratory erythema. In addition, those dermatitides associated with hyperkeratosis, a maturation disarray, and/or scattered degenerating keratinocytes need to be considered, as discussed in the Differential Diagnosis section of necrolytic migratory erythema (p. 490).

Congenital Vitamin B₃ Deficiency (Hartnup Disease)

Named after the family in which it was first described in 1956, Hartnup disease is a distinctive autosomal recessive syndrome comprising pellagrinous skin (40,41), neurologic abnormalities including mental deterioration and cerebellar ataxia, and abnormal aminoaciduria (42).

Clinical Summary. The intermittent skin eruption is seen primarily in the summer at times of maximal sun exposure and at times resembles either poikiloderma vasculare atrophicans (43) or, when vesicles are prominent, hydroa vacciniforme (44). Hartnup disease, in contrast to pellagra, does not respond to treatment with niacin (44).

Histopathology. The histopathology usually resembles that of pellagra. Poikilodermatous lesions manifest flattening of the epidermis and prominent dermal melanophage accumulation (43).

Pathogenesis. An intestinal and renal tubular defect of tryptophan absorption leads to a deficiency in endogenous niacin, accounting for the pellagra-like symptomatology. The genetic abnormality involves a mutation in the gene for SCL6A19 (45,46), a transporter for monoamino-monocarboxylic acids located mainly in the kidney and intestine, which maps to chromosome 5p15 (47). Chromatographic studies of urine show persistent aminoaciduria, particularly of tryptophan and of indolic substances derived from tryptophan (41,43).

OTHER FORMS OF NUTRITIONAL DERMATOSES

Necrolytic Migratory Erythema (Glucagonoma Syndrome)

First described in 1942 in a patient with a pancreatic islet cell carcinoma (47), this distinctive dermatosis, which can precede all other symptoms of pancreatic carcinoma by several years (48), is most commonly seen in association with a glucagon-secreting α-cell tumor of the pancreas. Surgical extirpation of the neoplasm may result in resolution of the eruption, as may amino acid and fatty acid infusion (49-51). There are cases of necrolytic migratory erythema in the absence of glucagonoma. The most common association is hepatic failure and diabetes mellitus, hence resembling superficial necrolytic dermatitis of canines where the association is invariable with diabetes mellitus and hepatic failure (52). A case associated with short bowel syndrome has been described (53).

Clinical Summary. The manifestations of glucagonoma syndrome include cutaneous and mucosal lesions, weight loss, anemia, adult-onset diabetes, glucose intolerance, elevation of serum glucagon levels, and thromboembolism (54). Skin lesions are seen mainly on the face in perioral and perinasal distribution, the perineum, genitals, shins, ankles, and feet and include erythema, erosions, and flaccid vesicular–pustular lesions that rupture easily and often have a circinate appearance due to peripheral spreading (55). Rapid healing and the continuous development of new lesions result in daily fluctuations of the eruption. In some instances, the clinical lesions do not exhibit this characteristic presentation. For example, Darier-like papules may antedate the erosive necrotizing lesions, the latter of course held to be diagnostic of glucagonoma syndrome (56). Cheilitis, glossitis, brittle nails, and dyspareunia due to mucosal lesions are also reported (57).

Histopathology. The characteristic acute lesion shows abrupt necrosis of the upper layers of the stratum spinosum, which may detach from the subjacent viable epidermis. Keratinocyte degeneration varies from marked hydropic swelling to cytoplasmic eosinophilia and nuclear pyknosis. Neutrophilic chemotaxis to the necrotic epithelium may eventuate in a subcorneal pustule. Chronic lesions have psoriasiform dermatitis as their hallmark. In both acute and chronic lesions, there is architectural disarray, reflecting a maturation defect; it manifests as basal layer hyperplasia, vacuolar change, and a deficient granular layer. The epidermis is surmounted by a broad parakeratotic scale (Fig. 16-1). The combination of confluent parakeratosis with upper epidermal pallor characteristic of nutritional dermatosis may be observed in lesions that lack necrosis (37). *Candida* may be noted (58,59).

Pathogenesis. Patients with glucagonoma have sustained gluconeogenesis, resulting in a negative nitrogen balance, with protein amino acid degradation, even of epidermal proteins (60). In addition to glucagonoma, necrolytic migratory erythema has been reported with hepatic cirrhosis (61), jejunal adenocarcinoma with hepatic dysfunction, hepatitis B (62), malabsorption with villous atrophy (63), opiate dependency (64,65), and myelodysplastic syndrome (66). Glucagon levels may be normal. A comparable syndrome in dogs develops in the setting of diabetes mellitus and hepatic cirrhosis (59). In all of these conditions, malabsorption and diarrhea lead to isolated deficiencies of certain essential fatty acids, zinc, and amino acids. The pathophysiology may reflect, in part, a phospholipid fatty acid abnormality in cells due to defective Δ6-desaturase enzyme, which is known to be inhibited by zinc deficiency and excess alcohol intake. In patients with unresectable glucagonoma who manifest necrolytic migratory erythema, infusion of amino acids has resulted in rapid clearing of the cutaneous lesions (67). There is an interesting subgroup of patients with necrolytic erythema in whom the lesions are primarily confined to the dorsum of the feet. These cases are associated with hepatitis C and fall under the designation of necrolytic acral erythema (NAE) (68). The dermatitis responds to a combination of antiviral therapy and zinc.

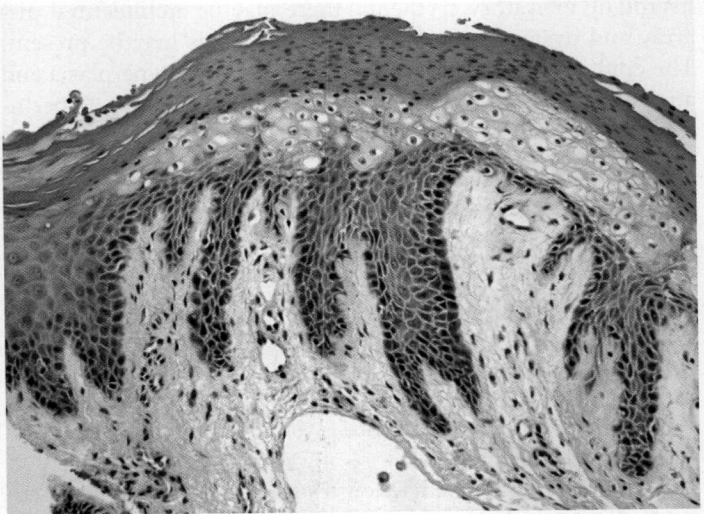

Figure 16-1 Necrolytic migratory erythema (glucagonoma syndrome). The lower portion of the stratum malpighii appears viable, whereas the upper portion shows necrolysis or "sudden death." The necrolytic portion manifests cytoplasmic eosinophilic homogenization with pyknotic nuclei.

Differential Diagnosis. The histopathology is similar to that of other nutritional dermatoses, namely, acrodermatitis enteropathica and pellagra. Other dermatoses associated with hyperkeratosis, a maturation disarray, and/or scattered degenerating keratinocytes include graft-versus-host disease, subacute cutaneous lupus erythematosus, dermatomyositis, pityriasis rubra pilaris, and toxic/irritant reactions, particularly those that are photo induced.

Principles of Management: Some patients may respond to parenteral zinc supplementation.

Acrodermatitis Enteropathica

Acrodermatitis enteropathica, first described in 1942 (69), is transmitted as an autosomal recessive trait, resulting in defective intestinal absorption of zinc (70).

Clinical Summary. The condition usually manifests in the first 4 to 10 weeks of life in bottle-fed infants as an acral and periorificial eruption with intractable diarrhea and diffuse partial alopecia. The skin exhibits areas of moist erythema, occasionally associated with vesiculobullous and/or pustular lesions (71). Untreated cases eventuate in death from malnutrition and infection because of immunologic defects reflecting zinc deficiency, the latter including decreased natural killer cell activity, impaired delayed-type hypersensitivity, and thymic atrophy (72). Paronychia, stomatitis, photophobia, blepharitis, conjunctivitis, corneal opacities, and hoarseness are additional manifestations. An acquired form occurs in patients receiving intravenous hyperalimentation with low zinc content (63), in infants who are fed breast milk low in zinc (74), in patients with Crohn disease, in patients with ornithine transcarbamylase deficiency (75), and cystic fibrosis (76) in patients with status post-pancreaticoduodenectomy (77) or sleeve gastrectomy (78) and in the setting of AIDS nephropathy when proteinuria eventuates in excessive loss of protein-bound zinc (72).

Histopathology. The upper part of the epidermis shows pallor due to intracellular edema and is surmounted by a confluent, thick, parakeratotic scale that may contain neutrophils. There is granular cell layer diminution and focal dyskeratosis. As with necrolytic migratory erythema, there may be architectural disarray and dysmaturation. Subcorneal vesicles may be present. The epidermis manifests variable psoriasiform hyperplasia and atrophy and, in a few instances, acantholysis (71,74). Superinfection with *Candida* may occur (Fig. 16-2).

Pathogenesis. Defective intestinal absorption of zinc has been demonstrated in children with acrodermatitis enteropathica (79), resulting in plasma zinc levels well below the normal range of 68 to 112 µg/dL. Oral administration of zinc sulfate results in rapid and complete resolution of the disease. Electron microscopy shows abnormal keratinization with decreased keratohyalin granules and increased number of keratinosome-derived lamellae within intercellular spaces. Keratinosomes contain several zinc-dependent enzyme systems, the metabolism of which may be affected (80).

Congenital zinc deficiency leading to acrodermatitis enteropathica shortly after birth has been linked to various mutations in the *SLC39A4* gene (81). The *SLC39A4* gene is expressed in tissues involved in zinc absorption, including the stomach, small intestine, colon, and kidney; a mutation alters the protein's function of zinc absorption, causing zinc deficiency (82).

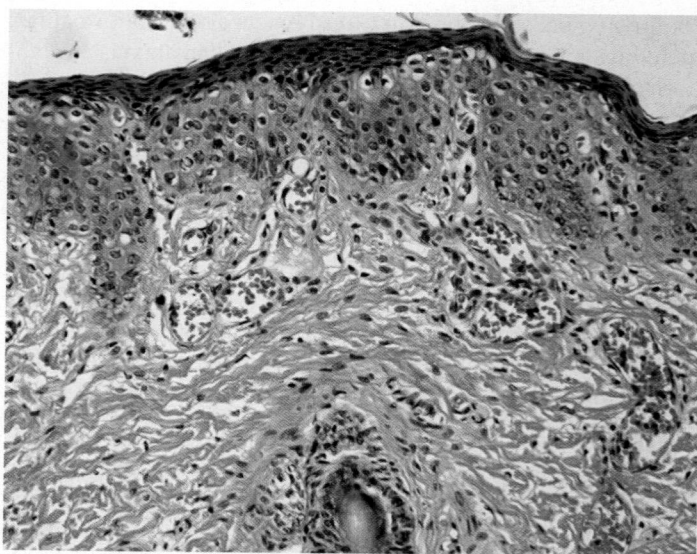

Figure 16-2 Acrodermatitis enteropathica. The epidermis demonstrates psoriasiform hyperplasia, dysmaturation, granular cell layer diminution, and vacuolar change. The epidermis is surmounted by a compact parakeratotic scale. Vascular ectasia is also present.

A case report described a 13-year-old adolescent girl with acrodermatitis enteropathica who was resistant to high-dose zinc sulfate therapy and was successfully treated with zinc gluconate and vitamin C. The authors detected a novel homozygous c.541_551dup (p.Leu186fsX38) mutation in exon 3 of her *SLC39A4* gene (83).

Differential Diagnosis. Pellagra, necrolytic migratory erythema, and acrodermatitis enteropathica share a constellation of histologic features that should suggest a diagnosis of nutritional dermatosis, namely, confluent parakeratosis, granular layer diminution, epidermal pallor and focal superficial dyskeratosis, superficial epidermal pallor, psoriasiform hyperplasia alternating with attenuation, and architectural disarray and dysmaturation of epidermal keratinocytes, the latter sometimes imparting an appearance mimicking keratinocytic dysplasia. Such cases can be misdiagnosed as eczema and psoriasis.

Principles of Management: Patients usually respond to dietary or parenteral zinc supplementation.

Kwashiorkor

Kwashiorkor is a form of protein malnutrition coupled to carbohydrate excess, resulting in the reduction of a patient's weight by 20% to 40%.

Clinical Summary. The condition is not limited to third-world countries, and risk factors include, in addition to drought and famine, conditions that interfere with protein absorption such as cystic fibrosis; dietary changes for the management of food allergies; low-protein diets, including vegan or other restricted diets; infections; parasites; lack of education; and prolonged substandard living conditions. Patients with kwashiorkor may also have other deficiencies, including zinc and vitamin deficiencies (84).

Primary manifestations include generalized hypopigmentation that begins circumorally and in the pretibial regions. With disease progression, hyperpigmented plaques with a waxy texture develop over the elbows and ankles and in the intertriginous areas. Dryness, desquamation, and decreased skin elasticity occur. "Crazy pavement" or "flaky-paint" dermatosis describes the extensive desquamation with erosions and fissuring, vesicles, and bullae that may be seen in severe cases (85). Prominent edema can mask the underlying muscle and subcutaneous tissue atrophy (86). Hair abnormalities include a diffuse alopecia, alternating bands of normal and hypopigmented hair referred to as the "flag" sign, and an unusual reddish brown discoloration called hypochromotrichia (84). Extracutaneous manifestations include cerebral atrophy secondary to loss of myelin lipid (87), diarrhea, hepatic steatosis, and mucosal abnormalities, such as a smooth tongue, angular stomatitis, and perianal and nasal erosions.

Histopathology. The histologic picture of skin lesions is not diagnostic but is said to resemble that of pellagra (36). The changes include psoriasiform hyperplasia with hyperkeratosis and increased pigmentation throughout the epidermis or atrophy with irregular shortening and flattening of the rete (87).

Pathogenesis. The etiology of the edema includes hypoalbuminemia, reduced capillary blood flow, and increased peripheral vasoconstriction (88,89).

Principles of Management: Correction of dietary protein deficiency should result in amelioration of symptoms.

CUTANEOUS MANIFESTATIONS OF GASTROINTESTINAL TRACT DISEASE

Pyoderma Gangrenosum

Pyoderma gangrenosum (PG) is a condition of poorly understood etiology and pathogenesis in which tissue necrosis results in deep ulcers, often on the legs.

Clinical Summary. First described in 1930 (90), PG was once considered pathognomonic of idiopathic ulcerative colitis but has since been described in association with a wide variety of disorders, including roughly 5% of patients with Crohn disease. Beginning as folliculocentric pustules or fluctuant nodules, the lesions ulcerate and have sharply circumscribed violaceous, raised edges in which necrotic pustules may be seen. The disease most commonly occurs on the lower extremities and trunk in adults who are 30 to 50 years old. Occasionally, it occurs in childhood, affecting the buttocks, perineal region, and head and neck area (91,92). Pathergy (development of new lesions) may occur at sites of trauma, including intravenous puncture sites, surgical wounds, and peristomal sites (93). When one examines the various etiologies for lower extremity ulcers, the vast majority are related to venous and arterial insufficiency (>75%), with PG defining the etiologic basis in only 3% of cases (94). PG is a diagnosis of exclusion, and many instances exist of incorrect diagnoses of PG being reclassified after thorough investigation. Roughly 70% of cases are associated with inflammatory bowel disease; hematologic disorders, including acute lymphoid and myeloid leukemias and myeloma (particularly immunoglobulin [Ig] A paraprotein disease); rheumatologic conditions, including rheumatoid arthritis and lupus erythematosus; and hepatopathies (95-97), including chronic active hepatitis, primary biliary cirrhosis, and sclerosing cholangitis (91,98). Both a superficial granulomatous variant (99) and a vesiculopustular variant comprising disseminated vesicles and necrotizing

pustules, some follicular based, have been observed without accompanying systemic disease. The vesiculopustular variant has also been seen in association with ulcerative colitis and/or underlying liver disease (96,100). PG has been associated with the administration of drugs, including interferon (IFN)-α in the setting of chronic granulocytic leukemia, the antipsychotic agent sulpiride (101), granulocyte colony-stimulating factor (102), the epidermal growth factor–tyrosine kinase inhibitor gefitinib (Iressa) (103), the retinoid isotretinoin (104), and the thionamide propylthiouracil (105). A recent case described the development of PG at the site of IFN-α2B injections. Tumor necrosis factor α (TNF-α) inhibitor therapy has been associated with the development of PG. Since the introduction of TNF-α inhibitors, there is a growing body of literature on the development of various autoimmune sequelae in association with their use (106). A recent study attempting to improve diagnostic criteria using Delphi consensus resulted in one major criterion of an ulcer with neutrophilic infiltrate and eight minor criteria: exclusion of infection; pathergy, history of inflammatory bowel disease or inflammatory arthritis; history of papule, pustule, or vesicle ulcerating within 4 days of appearing; peripheral erythema, undermining border, and tenderness at ulceration site; multiple ulcerations, at least one on an anterior lower leg; cribriform or "wrinkled paper" scar(s) at healed ulcer sites; and decreased ulcer size within 1 month of initiating immunosuppressive medication(s). The if one major criterion and at least four of the eight minor criteria resulted in a sensitivity and specificity of 86% and 90%, respectively (107). In addition, a clinical response to steroid therapy and a lack of response to antibiotic therapy (which has often been given empirically before consideration of the diagnosis) may be supportive.

Histopathology. PG exhibits a dichotomous tissue reaction, showing central necrotizing suppurative inflammation, usually with ulceration, and a peripheral lymphocytic vascular reaction comprising perivascular and intramural lymphocytic infiltrates, usually without fibrin deposition or mural necrosis (Figs. 16-3 and 16-4). Transitional areas show neutrophils in a loose cuff

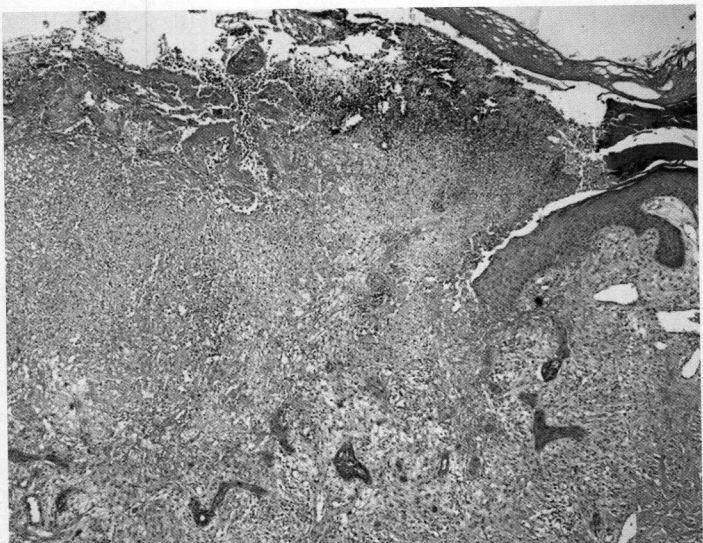

Figure 16-3 Pyoderma gangrenosum. The center of the lesion shows a neutrophilic infiltrate with leukocytoclasia and dermolysis. This biopsy is from a patient with Crohn disease, as evidenced by the presence of multinucleated histiocytes within the infiltrate.

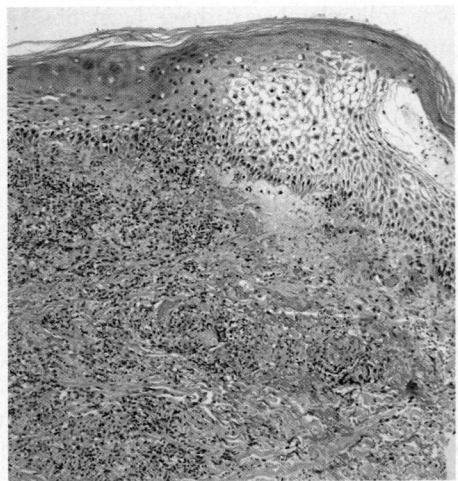

Figure 16-4 *Pyoderma gangrenosum.* The undermined epidermis often shows spongiosis or pustulation.

around the angiocentric lymphocytic infiltrates, defining a mixed lymphocytic and neutrophilic vascular reaction termed a *Sweet's-like vascular reaction* (108,109). Bullous lesions may also demonstrate a Sweet's-like vascular reaction, with perivascular disintegrating neutrophilic infiltrates and hemorrhage without mural necrosis or luminal fibrin deposition. At variance with Sweet syndrome is the destruction of the connective tissue framework with resultant tissue pathergy (110,111). Although a leukocytoclastic vasculitis may be observed in areas of maximal tissue pathology, PG does not reflect a primary vasculitis (91). In some cases, a necrotizing pustular follicular reaction may be the central nidus of the lesion, particularly in the vesicular–pustular variant associated with ulcerative colitis or hepatobiliary disease. In the superficial granulomatous variant, florid pseudoepitheliomatous hyperplasia may be observed along with the intraepithelial and superficial dermal suppurative granulomatous inflammation with admixed plasma cells and eosinophils (96). Cases of PG associated with Crohn disease may have areas of granulomatous inflammation (112).

Differential Diagnosis. Tissue neutrophilia with epithelial undermining and ulceration in the absence of leukocytoclastic vasculitis, fungal, bacterial, or mycobacterial organisms (which, if indicated, may be demonstrable with culture and special stains, e.g., periodic acid–Schiff [PAS], Gomori methenamine silver, Brown and Brenn, Gram, Ziehl–Neelsen, and auramine–rhodamine preparations) strongly implicates PG when seen in the appropriate clinical setting (91). An incipient lesion of PG, however, may be indistinguishable from Sweet syndrome, although the latter is rarely folliculocentric and does not show lysis of dermal collagen or vessel wall necrosis in areas of maximum dermal neutrophilia. In addition, clinical features usually make the distinction possible. Because of prominent follicular involvement, the differential diagnosis should also include other causes of necrotizing pustular follicular reactions with an accompanying vasculopathy, such as mixed cryoglobulinemia, Behcet disease, rheumatoid vasculitis, herpetic folliculitis, acute pustular bacterid, and pustular drug reactions (113). These other conditions frequently have a necrotizing mononuclear cell– or neutrophil-predominant vasculitis in contrast to the non-necrotizing vascular reaction of PG. Other causes of a Sweet's-like vascular reaction include the bowel arthritis

dermatosis syndrome, Behcet disease, idiopathic pustular vasculitis, rheumatoid arthritis, acute pustular bacterid, and Sweet syndrome (106,108).

Pathogenesis. Direct immunofluorescence testing supports a vasculopathy by virtue of perivascular deposition of immunoreactants, mainly IgM and C3 (114), in more than half of patients. This change occurs in nonspecific vessel injury and does not support a humoral-based pathogenesis. Defective cell-mediated immunity without humoral abnormalities has been implicated in some patients (115). Immunoelectrophoresis has revealed a monoclonal gammopathy, most commonly of the IgA type, in 10% of patients with PG (116). A polymerase chain reaction analysis demonstrated that patients with PG have clonal expansions of T cells in the peripheral blood and skin. These clonal expansions are shared between both sites, suggesting that T cells are trafficking to the skin under the influence of an antigenic stimulus (117). In further support of a potential antigenic stimulus, patients with PG have elevated levels of interleukin 8 (IL-8), a powerful neutrophilic chemoattractant, in both the serum and fibroblasts of affected skin (118).

Principles of Management: Identification and treatment of the underlying disease that is causally associated is important, particularly with respect to the potentially life-threatening malignancies and inflammatory bowel disease. Adequate treatment requires a multimodality approach: systemic anti-inflammatory drugs to stop the inflammation and localized wound therapy to aid in healing and prevent secondary infection. As regard the treatment of the skin condition, specific wound care guidelines exist (119,120). A multidisciplinary approach with close involvement of wound care and infectious disease specialists is advised. Treatment includes avoidance of trauma, local application of appropriate topical medications (which may include anti-inflammatory treatments, such as steroids and tacrolimus, or topical antibiotics when indicated [119]), and the use of systemic steroids, cyclosporine, or infliximab for disseminated or severe disease. Other options include mycophenolate mofetil, cyclosporine, dapsone, or alternate treatments (121). Surgery is generally avoided owing to the risk of pathergy, although recent literature suggests that debridement and skin graft may be useful in the appropriate clinical setting (122). PG is a challenging diagnosis and a diagnosis of exclusion; patients failing to respond to appropriate treatment warrant additional investigation and evaluation.

Bowel-Associated Dermatosis–Arthritis Syndrome (Bowel Bypass Syndrome)

Bowel-associated dermatosis–arthritis syndrome, also called bowel bypass syndrome, was first described as a complication of jejunoileal bypass surgery and is also seen in patients with diverse bowel-related disorders, including diverticulosis, peptic ulcer disease, idiopathic inflammatory bowel disease, and even cystic fibrosis (123). The syndrome includes fever and malaise, polyarthralgia, myalgia, and skin changes.

Clinical Summary. After intestinal bypass surgery for morbid obesity or after extensive small bowel resection, some patients develop an intermittent eruption, mainly on the extremities, comprising purpuric macules and papules that may evolve into necrotizing vesiculopustular lesions. Polyarthritis, malaise, and fever are often associated with, and may precede, the eruption

(124). Although originally called the bowel bypass syndrome, it now bears the more appropriate appellation *bowel arthritis dermatosis syndrome* because a similar picture may develop in patients with other bowel-related disorders (125–128).

Histopathology. Characteristically, there is a perivascular lymphocytic infiltrate with a peripheral cuff of disintegrating neutrophils, erythrocyte extravasation, and absent or minimal fibrin deposition consistent with a Sweet's-like vascular reaction; a leukocytoclastic vasculitis occurs less often (127). Papillary dermal edema may be striking and may lead to subepidermal vesiculation (118). Epidermal pustulation, variable epithelial necrosis, and massive superficial dermal neutrophilia complete the picture (Fig. 16-5) and define pustular vasculitis (118,129). In some instances, the primary pathology closely resembles bullous impetigo and/or IgA pemphigus characterized by a subcorneal pustule without the characteristic angiocentric dermal changes (130).

Pathogenesis. Circulating immune complexes, including those containing cryoproteins, are demonstrable in most patients. The antigenic trigger may be peptidoglycans from overgrowth of intestinal bacteria (124,131), which are structurally and antigenically similar to the peptidoglycan of *Streptococcus*. The latter exacerbate symptoms in patients with this condition and produce a similar syndrome in animals (124). Direct immunofluorescence testing has shown linear and granular deposits of Igs and complement along the dermal–epidermal junction and within vessels (124). One study showed *Escherichia coli* antigens in a granular array along the dermal–epidermal junction. Via an indirect methodology, a pemphigus-like pattern of intercellular staining has been reported (124), the significance of which is unclear.

Differential Diagnosis. The differential diagnosis of bowel arthritis dermatosis syndrome includes Sweet syndrome, incipient PG, and certain of the pustular vasculitides, such as acute pustular bacterid related to antecedent streptococcal infection, such as Henoch–Schönlein purpura (128), septic vasculitis due to *Meningococcus* and *Gonococcus*, Behcet syndrome, leukocytoclastic vasculitis in patients with a pustular psoriasiform

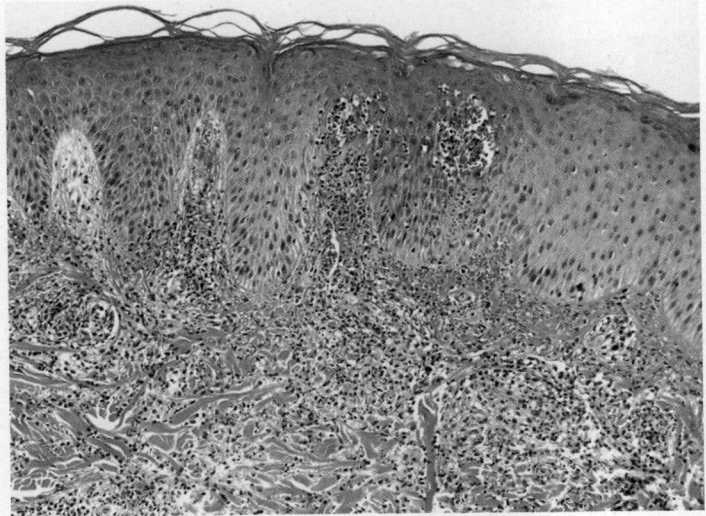

Figure 16-5 Bowel arthritis dermatosis syndrome. Pustular vasculitis characterized by dermal papillae microabscess formation along with a leukocytoclastic vasculitis.

diathesis (132), idiopathic pustular vasculitis, and acute generalized exanthematous pustulosis (108,130). The distinction may be impossible in those conditions that manifest a Sweet's-like vascular reaction (108)—namely, Behcet disease, Sweet syndrome, PG, acute pustular bacterid, idiopathic pustular vasculitis, and rheumatoid arthritis–associated neutrophilic eruptions.

Principles of Management: Once a correct diagnosis is made, a combination of steroid therapy, antibiotics, and dietary probiotics may offer empirical relief. There is no good randomized, blinded, controlled trial to generate a specific evidence-based therapeutic algorithm, however.

SPECIFIC DISEASES

Aphthosis (Behcet Disease)

Behcet disease is a symptom complex of oral and genital ulceration and iritis that has a worldwide distribution but is most common in the Pacific Rim and Eastern Mediterranean (133-136).

Clinical Summary. The presence of oral ulceration plus any two signs of genital ulceration, skin lesions (e.g., pustules or nodules), or eye lesions (e.g., uveitis or retinal vasculitis) is diagnostic. There are some patients who have complex aphthosis without the other clinical features of Behcet disease. The majority of these patients have the so-called idiopathic recurrent oral and/or genital aphthosis, whereas approximately one-quarter of these patients will have an underlying inflammatory bowel disease (137).

The cutaneous lesions include erythema nodosum–like nodules, vesicles, pustules, PG, Sweet syndrome, a pustular reaction to needle trauma, superficial migratory thrombophlebitis, ulceration, infiltrative erythema, acral purpuric papulonodular lesions, and acneiform folliculitis or pseudofolliculitis (138,139).

The extracutaneous manifestations are categorized as oral and/or genital aphthae; vasculo-, ocular-, entero-, or neuro-Behcet disease; renal disease; and arthritis. Oral aphthosis recurring at least three times over a 12-month period is essential to the diagnosis (125). In vasculo-Behcet disease, aneurysms and occlusive venous and arterial main vessel lesions occur. The ocular manifestations include uveitis, hypopyon iritis, optic neuritis, and choroiditis. Entero-Behcet disease manifests as diarrhea, constipation, abdominal pain, vomiting, and melena. Neuro-Behcet disease presents as brainstem dysfunction, meningoencephalitis, organic psychiatric symptoms, and mononeuritis multiplex (137). Asymptomatic microhematuria and/or proteinuria are among the renal manifestations. An oligoarthritis may involve the wrist, elbow, knee, or ankle joints. Morbidity and mortality in one large series of Turkish patients were greatest in young males; both the onset and the severity of ocular disease were greatest early in the course of disease, suggesting that the "disease burden" in Behcet disease is greatest early and that it tends to "burnout" over time (140). However, neurologic and major vessel disease can occur at any time and can have a late onset of 5 to 10 years into the course of illness (139). Hypercoagulability and deep vein thromboses are not uncommon.

Histopathology. The cutaneous lesions can be categorized histopathologically into two main groups: vascular and extravascular with or without vasculopathy including acneiform.

The pathologic spectrum of the cutaneous vasculopathy encompasses a mononuclear cell vasculitis with variable mural and luminal fibrin deposition; a paucicellular thrombogenic vasculopathy (Fig. 16-6); and a neutrophilic vascular reaction involving capillaries and veins of all calibers. The mononuclear cell reaction may be frankly granulomatous, or it may be lymphocyte predominant to define a lymphocytic vasculitis. The neutrophilic vascular reaction may resemble that of Sweet syndrome (Fig. 16-7) (141) or a leukocytoclastic vasculitis. Diffuse extravascular mononuclear cell– and/or neutrophil-predominant inflammation of the dermis and/or panniculus may occur with or without the aforementioned vascular changes. The histiocytes infiltrating the panniculus may manifest phagocytosis of cellular debris. Suppurative or mixed suppurative and granulomatous folliculitis with or without vasculitis characterizes the acneiform lesions. Acral purpuric papulonodular lesions show a lymphocytic interface dermatitis with lymphocytic exocytosis, dyskeratosis, and a perivascular lymphocytic infiltrate, recapitulating the mucosal histopathology (138).

Extracutaneous lesions histologically mirror the skin changes. Oral aphthous ulcers demonstrate a central diffuse neutrophilic infiltrate with necrosis of the epithelium and connective tissue pathergy of the submucosa, and peripherally a border showing dense lymphocytic infiltration with lymphocytic exocytosis and degenerative epithelial changes. Genital aphthae have the same appearance (Fig. 16-8) (137). The large-vessel arteriopathy represents an ischemic sequel of a mononuclear cell vasculitis of the vasa vasorum (142), whereas venous thrombosis may be due, in part, to an underlying hypercoagulable state. A lymphocytic vascular reaction with or without mural and intraluminal fibrin deposition is the histopathology of neuro-, entero-, ocular-, and arthritic Behcet disease, with other organ changes such as demyelination and intestinal ulceration reflecting resultant ischemia (137). The renal histopathology includes IgA nephropathy, focal and diffuse proliferative glomerulonephritis, and amyloidosis (143).

Differential Diagnosis. The lymphocytic vasculitis observed in Behcet disease may mimic that seen in association with systemic lupus erythematosus, rheumatoid arthritis (144,145), Sjögren syndrome, relapsing polychondritis, Degos disease, and paraneoplastic vasculitis in the setting of lymphoproliferative disease. Granulomatous vasculitis may also be observed in granulomatosis with polyangiitis (GPA); eosinophilic granulomatosis with polyangiitis (EGPA); Crohn disease; sarcoidosis; acquired hypogammaglobulinemia; a postherpetic eruption (146); paraneoplastic syndrome (related to underlying hematologic malignancy); rheumatoid arthritis; hypersensitivity reactions to certain infections, including syphilis and tuberculosis (147); scleroderma; and late-stage lesions of microscopic polyarteritis nodosa (108,128,144). Other causes of a Sweet's-like vasculopathy include Sweet syndrome, bowel arthritis dermatosis, PG, and idiopathic pustular vasculitis (106). Conditions that combine a vasculitis with a folliculitis include PG, mixed cryoglobulinemia, rheumatoid vasculitis, and bacterid (112).

Pathogenesis. An immunogenic basis is likely in view of the association with certain human leukocyte antigen (HLA) types, namely, HLA-B5, HLA-B12, HLA-B27, and HLA-B51 (148). A recurring association in patients of Japanese, Turkish,

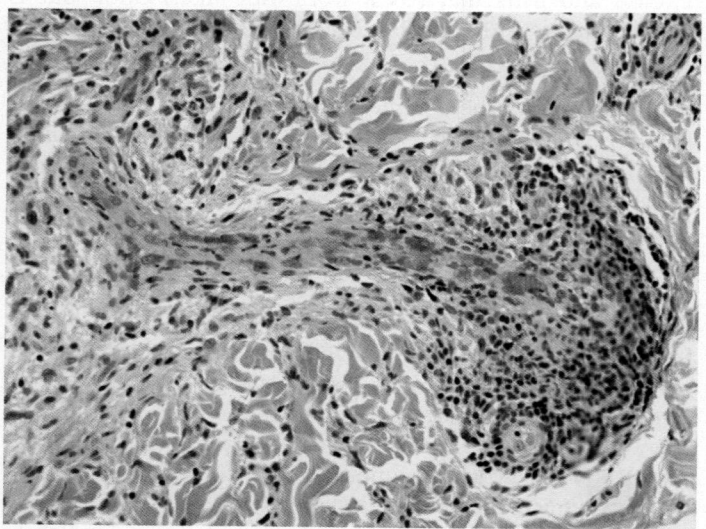

Figure 16-6 Behçet disease. A characteristic vascular reaction pattern is a lymphocytic thrombogenic vasculopathy.

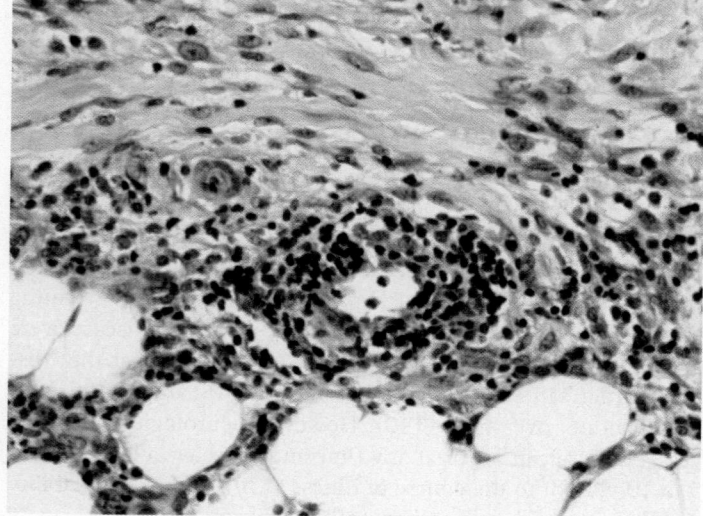

Figure 16-7 Behçet disease. There is a Sweet's-like vascular reaction manifested by angiocentric mononuclear cell and neutrophilic infiltrates with erythrocyte extravasation and leukocytoclasia but without accompanying mural and intraluminal fibrin deposition.

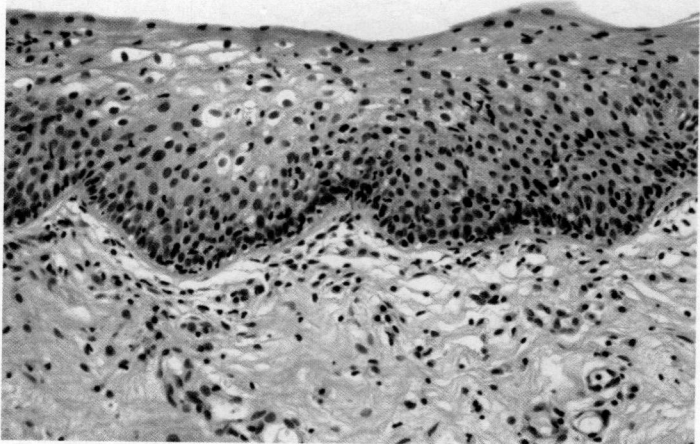

Figure 16-8 Behçet disease. Although the center of an oral or vulvar aphthous ulcer is predominated by a neutrophilic response, biopsies of the periphery typically show a lymphocyte-predominant infiltrate in both an extravascular and angiocentric disposition with variable lymphocytic exocytosis.

Korean, and Iranian ethnicities is with HLA-B51 (149,150), genetic polymorphisms in the promoter region of TNF-α (151–154), and microsatellite instabilities between these two genes (141,146,149,155). Polymorphisms of other cytokines have been identified, including IL-1 (156) and IL-18 (157). Patients with Behcet disease have elevated levels of T_H1 cytokines IL-12, IFN-γ, and TNF-α (158); increased T_H1-associated chemokine receptors CCR5 and CXCR3 (159); and a lower percentage of plasmacytoid dendritic cells in peripheral blood (160), supporting the proposed T_H1-mediated pathogenesis of the disease. Patients have shown a heightened immune response to antigenic components of certain streptococcal species (161,162), *Mycobacterium tuberculosis* (163), herpes simplex (164,165), Epstein–Barr virus, and HIV (166). The underlying abnormalities in T-lymphocyte function may be integral to an aberrant response related to the synthesis by microorganisms and mammalian tissue of a family of polypeptides termed *heat shock proteins* (HSPs) (167,168) produced by cells exposed to stresses such as increased temperature. Sensitized T cells and T-cell clones specific to the 65-kD mycobacterial HSP have been reported in rheumatoid arthritis (169). In one study, T lymphocytes from patients with Behcet disease exhibited a greater stimulation by this HSP compared to normal controls or patients with unrelated disease (170). The $\gamma\delta$ T-cell subset has been shown to be the principal populace that responds to the mycobacterial 65-kD HSP, an observation that may account for the increase in circulating $\gamma\delta$ T cells in patients with antecedent streptococcal or mycobacterial infections (171) and in those with active Behcet disease, in whom an exaggerated response to microbial products in mucosal ulcers is postulated (172). The lymphocytes themselves show resistance to Fas-mediated apoptosis, a finding that may promote lymphocyte-mediated tissue destruction in these patients (173). One study assessed the phenotypic composition in cutaneous lesions of Behcet disease. The dominant infiltrate in all lesions excluding frankly pustular ones comprised CD68-positive macrophages admixed with lymphocytes, showing a predominance of CD8$^+$ T cells over those of the CD4 subset (174).

Tissue neutrophilia may relate to the presence of HLA-B51, which has been associated with neutrophil hyperreactivity (175). Neutrophil functions are also increased in Behcet disease (176), which may be due to alteration in the expression of Toll-like receptors, regulators of innate and adaptive immunity, on both granulocytes and monocytes (177).

Vascular thrombosis has been attributed to antibody-mediated endothelial injury (178), protein C or S deficiency (179), factor XII deficiency, inhibition of plasminogen activator, and circulating lupus anticoagulant (180–182). A prothrombin gene mutation has recently been described (183). Further evidence of a genetic predisposition to thrombosis is the linkage of HLA-B51 expression and the absence of HLA-B35 as risk factors for venous thrombosis in Turkish patients (148); there is also a statistical linkage between superficial and deep venous thrombosis (184). Elevated serum levels of matrix metalloproteinases MMP-2 and MMP-9 are associated with vasculo-Behcet disease, particularly thrombotic and aneurismal involvement, respectively (185).

The role of nitric oxide (NO) is unclear. Some researchers have shown that patients with active Behcet disease have significantly higher serum levels of NO than patients with recurrent aphthous stomatitis (186), patients with inactive Behcet disease, and healthy controls (187), whereas others maintain that there is no difference in NO levels among these groups (188,189), and still others contend that the levels of NO are lower in patients with Behcet disease (190,191). Specific genetic polymorphisms have been identified in the manganese superoxide dismutase gene in Japanese patients with Behcet disease (192) and the Glu298Asp polymorphism in the endothelial nitric oxide synthase (*eNOS*) gene in Turkish (193,194), Italian (195), and Korean (196) patients with Behcet disease. One study did not identify the eNOS polymorphism in Turkish patients with Behcet disease (197). Others propose that the significantly higher levels of IL-2, IL-6, TNF-α, and NO are related to the pathogenesis of Behcet disease (198).

Principles of Management: The main aim of treatment is to prevent irreversible organ damage (199). Most of the serious manifestations respond to immunosuppressive therapy (200), namely, corticosteroids, colchicine, azathioprine, TNF-α inhibitors, and other agents. A questionnaire submitted to participants of the 2010 International Society for Behcet Disease meeting indicated that more than half would intensify immunosuppression and also anticoagulate their patients with new-onset deep vein thromboses (201). A positive pathergy test has been shown to be useful in adding specificity and sensitivity to diagnostic criteria for Behcet disease (202).

INFLAMMATORY BOWEL DISEASE

Crohn Disease (Regional Enteritis)

First described in 1932, Crohn disease is an idiopathic chronic inflammatory disorder of the gastrointestinal tract.

Clinical Summary. The diagnosis is based on a constellation of radiologic, pathologic, and endoscopic data, namely, deep mucosal fissures, fistula formation, transmural inflammation, discontinuous colonic and small bowel disease with preferential right-sided involvement, and sarcoidal granulomatous and fibrosing inflammation of the mucosa and submucosa (203). Extraintestinal manifestations include fever, anemia, lupus anticoagulant, ophthalmic disease such as uveitis and episcleritis, monoarticular large joint arthritis, polyarthritis, spondylitis, amyloidosis (204), renal lithiasis with resultant hydronephrosis (205), cerebral vascular occlusions, and a spectrum of cutaneous eruptions.

Skin manifestations, principally restricted to patients with colonic disease, occur in 14% to 44% of patients with Crohn disease, depending on whether perianal disease is considered a cutaneous manifestation (198). Ulcers, fissures, sinus tracts, abscesses, and vegetating plaques may extend in continuity from sites of intra-abdominal involvement to the perineum, buttocks, or abdominal wall, ostomy sites, or incisional scars. When sterile granulomatous skin lesions arise at sites discontinuous from the gastrointestinal tract, the appellation "metastatic Crohn disease" is applied (206). Clinically, metastatic Crohn disease presents as solitary or multiple nodules, plaques, ulcers, lichenoid lesions, or violaceous perifollicular papules involving extremities, intertriginous areas, abdominal skin folds, or genitalia (207). Erythema nodosum (208)—the most common cutaneous manifestation of Crohn disease—and PG develop in 15% and 1.5% of patients, respectively. Palmar erythema; a pustular response to trauma (207); erythema multiforme usually with mucosal involvement (207,209); epidermolysis bullosa acquisita; hidradenitis suppurative; rosacea; secondary cutaneous oxalosis; malabsorption-related acrodermatitis enteropathica (194,207); vasculitic lesions, including benign cutaneous polyarteritis nodosa; and digitate hyperkeratosis reminiscent of punctate porokeratosis are described (210). Cutaneous necrosis as a complication of circulating lupus anticoagulant may also occur. A distinct manifestation of Crohn disease is one of scrotal edema. Not surprisingly, granulomatous infiltrates are seen typically showing localization to vascular lumens of the lymphatics, in a fashion mimicking Melkersson–Rosenthal disease (211).

Oral lesions—manifesting as "cobblestone" lesions, aphthous ulcers, lip swelling, and pyostomatitis vegetans—occur in roughly 5% of patients with Crohn disease (193).

Histopathology. The perianal mucosal lesions and oral lesions of pyostomatitis vegetans show pseudoepitheliomatous hyperplasia in conjunction with suppurative granulomatous inflammation within the epithelium and subjacent corium (Fig. 16-9). The most frequent histologic patterns seen in metastatic Crohn disease are nonsuppurative granulomata, which may assume a sarcoidal or diffuse pattern, the latter often in close apposition to the epidermis in the fashion of a lichenoid and granulomatous dermatitis (212) and granulomatous vasculitis. Histologic examination of the erythema nodosum–like lesion may show one of four patterns: (a) septal panniculitis consistent with classic erythema nodosum, (b) dermal-based sarcoidal granulomata (213), (c) a dermal-based small-vessel granulomatous (214) or leukocytoclastic vasculitis, or (d) benign cutaneous polyarteritis nodosa. The latter shows mural infiltration by histiocytes and neutrophils, with variable mural fibrinoid necrosis confined to the muscular arteries of the subcutaneous fat (see Fig. 16-12); occasional vessel involvement of the peripheral nerves and skeletal muscle of the affected extremity produces mononeuritis and myositis, respectively (165). A pauci-inflammatory thrombogenic vasculopathy characterizes the cutaneous infarcts associated with lupus anticoagulant. Necrobiosis lipoidica– or granuloma annulare–like foci (215) may also be seen defined

by areas of collagen necrobiosis with concomitant mucin or fibrin deposition and a palisading histiocytic infiltrate. Unlike idiopathic granuloma annulare or necrobiosis lipoidica, there is usually an accompanying leukocytoclastic vasculitis, thrombogenic or granulomatous vasculopathy, and foci of extravascular neutrophilia (214). Dense neutrophilic infiltration of the dermis accompanied by scattered giant cells has been reported (111,216). We have also seen this pattern of suppurative granulomatous inflammation in concert with the aforementioned necrobiosis lipoidica or granuloma annulare tissue reaction. Cases of lip swelling show non-necrotizing granulomatous inflammation (194,207). The histology of PG has been discussed earlier in this chapter. A suppurative panniculitis may also be seen (217).

Differential Diagnosis. The differential diagnosis of sarcoidal granulomatous inflammation in the skin includes sarcoidosis, id reactions to antecedent streptococcal or mycobacterial infections (146), acquired hypogammaglobulinemia, rosacea, paraneoplastic histiocytopathies such as those associated with low-grade lymphoproliferative disease, rheumatoid arthritis, and granulomatous inflammatory reactions to ingested or inoculated inorganic compounds such as silica, zirconium, and beryllium. The lesions resembling benign cutaneous polyarteritis nodosa differ from systemic polyarteritis nodosa by virtue of confinement of the vasculitis to the subcutaneous fat without dermal involvement (218). The changes of pyostomatitis vegetans also should raise the possibility of GPA, mycobacterial infection, blastomycosis, and histoplasmosis. The histopathology of the lip swelling may mimic that of Melkersson–Rosenthal syndrome (207). Lichenoid and granulomatous dermatitis calls into consideration the idiopathic lichenoid disorders such as lichen nitidus, certain microbial id reaction states, and also drug reactions such as those to antibiotic, antihypertensive, lipid-lowering, and antihistaminic preparations (211).

Pathogenesis. In the development of Crohn disease, there is a complex interplay between genetic, immunologic, and environmental factors, which is not completely understood. At least 10 genes have been proposed to play a role; the best studied is *CARD15/NOD2*, a gene involved in bacterial recognition by cells involved in innate immunity (219). Three *CARD15/NOD2* mutations are associated with Crohn disease susceptibility, with approximately a two- to four fold risk in heterozygotes and 17- to 40-fold risk in homozygotes (218,220,221). This dose effect suggests a loss-of-function model and is supported by *in vitro* studies. Speculations claim that the loss of function in innate immunity allows bacterial proliferation and that a potential cytokine imbalance allows an inflammatory response from the adaptive immunity and, ultimately, causes tissue damage. *In vivo* studies have failed to confirm these speculations and have even generated other hypotheses, including a gain-of-function model (218). Even less is understood about the pathogenesis of skin lesions in Crohn disease. There is a common morphology shared by the intestinal and cutaneous disease of sarcoidal granulomatous inflammation, suggesting a pathogenetic role for cell-mediated immunity. Circulating immune complexes have been detected in some patients (207) and may play a role in the generation of necrotizing vasculitis; a subset of patients with Crohn disease has antineutrophil cytoplasmic antibodies (ANCAs). On the basis of the use of *in situ* polymerase chain reaction methods with a probe seeking bacterial 16rsRNA

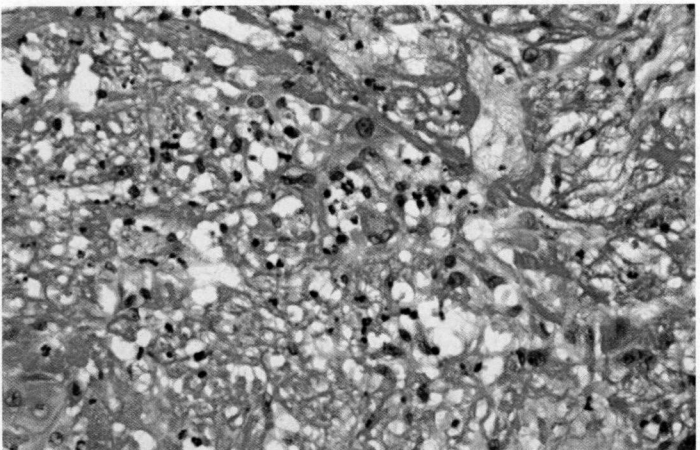

Figure 16-9 Crohn disease: pyoderma gangrenosum. Although there is suppurative granulomatous inflammation with a binucleate histiocyte in the center of the field and a mononuclear cell–predominant vasculopathic reaction pattern, biopsies of metastatic Crohn disease may show a necrotizing leukocytoclastic and granulomatous vasculitis indistinguishable from cutaneous Wegener granulomatosis and reminiscent of pyostomatitis vegetans, and a prototypic oral lesion of Crohn disease can be seen.

common to a variety of microbial pathogens implicated in Crohn disease, bacterial RNA has been shown in the vasculature of the gut in active, but not in quiescent, cases; the skin lesions are uniformly negative. It would seem, therefore, that the skin manifestations of Crohn disease are not a bacterial id reaction but rather reflect an autoimmune phenomenon, perhaps involving cross-reacting antibodies between gut- and skin-based antigens (217).

Principles of Management: Medical therapy of inflammatory bowel disease is becoming more complicated as new immunomodulatory agents come to market. First-line therapies for Crohn disease and ulcerative colitis are defined in the following categories: 5-aminosalicylates, budesonide, systemic and local steroids, azathioprine, 6-mercaptopurine, methotrexate, infliximab, adalimumab, and certolizumab pegol (222). TNF-α blockers are indicated for patients with moderately severe Crohn disease who have failed two or more courses and an 8- to 12-week course of an immunomodulator such as azathioprine or methotrexate, and those with nonresponsive perianal disease (223). Dietary modifications, including the avoidance of caffeine and alcohol and high-fiber foods during flares, are advised. Patients may do better eating smaller and more frequent meals and should empirically avoid foods that worsen their symptoms (224).

Ulcerative Colitis

Ulcerative colitis is an idiopathic chronic inflammatory bowel disease involving the large intestine, with rectal involvement being almost ubiquitous.

Clinical Summary. The disorder is characterized by glandular destruction and inflammation of variable intensity. Glandular dysplasia eventuating in carcinoma complicates the clinical course, particularly in patients with disease of pediatric onset. Extramucosal associations include chronic active hepatitis, primary sclerosing cholangitis (PSC), pulmonary vasculitis (225,226), chronic fibrosing alveolitis, limited GPA of the lung (227), pulmonary apical fibrosis, large joint monoarticular arthritis, polyarthritis, and ankylosing spondylitis. Cutaneous manifestations may occur, the spectrum of which encompasses vasculitis, erythema nodosum, PG, superficial migratory thrombophlebitis, palisaded granulomatous dermatitis (228), necrotizing neutrophilic lobular panniculitis, and cutaneous thrombosis with resultant gangrene (229); the last two named manifestations are possibly related to underlying lupus anticoagulant or cryofibrinogenemia (230,231). PG is more frequently associated with ulcerative colitis than with Crohn disease and erythema nodosum is more frequently with Crohn disease (Fig. 16-10). The lesions of PG also include an unusual disseminated vesiculopustular variant (232).

Histopathology. The histology of PG and erythema nodosum is discussed elsewhere. Cutaneous vasculitis in association with ulcerative colitis includes IgA-associated leukocytoclastic vasculitis (128,233) and benign cutaneous polyarteritis nodosa (Fig. 16-11). A pauci-inflammatory thrombogenic vasculopathy involving vessels throughout the dermis and subcutis characterizes the histomorphology of associated lupus anticoagulant and/or cryofibrinogenemia (229). The panniculitis of ulcerative colitis comprises a small-vessel vasculitis, typically in the context of a neutrophil-rich and/or granulomatous vasculitis accompanied by significant extravascular neutrophilic and granulomatous inflammation (230).

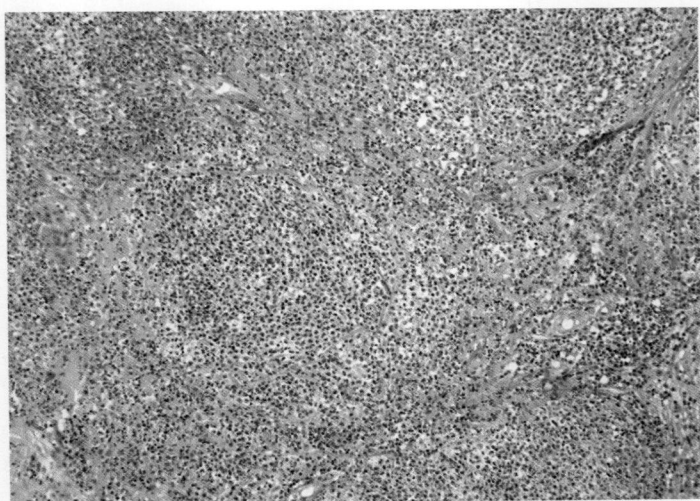

Figure 16-10 Ulcerative colitis: pyoderma gangrenosum. There is pronounced neutrophilic dermolysis.

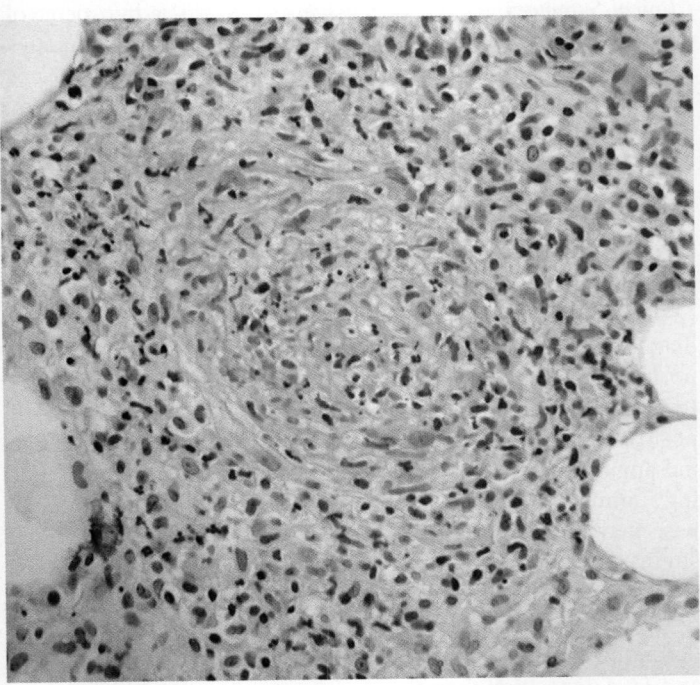

Figure 16-11 Polyarteritis nodosa in a patient with ulcerative colitis. Within the subcutaneous fat, the wall of a subcutaneous artery demonstrates striking fibrinoid necrosis and is surrounded and permeated by disintegrating neutrophilic infiltrates unaccompanied by small-vessel involvement. The findings are typical for benign cutaneous polyarteritis nodosa.

Principles of Management: There is considerable overlap as regard first-line therapies for Crohn disease and ulcerative colitis (222). In addition, one preferred option for mild left-sided ulcerative colitis is mesalazine (234). If repeated courses of systemic steroids are required for disease control, immunosuppressive therapy should be considered to minimize steroid exposure; thiopurines represent the first choice immunosuppressive agent (234). Foam preparations are effective in controlling distal left-sided disease, are more easily held within the rectum than earlier liquid preparations, and are absorbed proximally to the descending colon after endocavitary rectal installation (235). For localized ulcerative proctitis, topical therapy with 5-aminosalicylic acid may be used (236). Early escalation to anti-TNF biologics such as infliximab may be indicated for severe cases (234); other immunomodulatory agents include the calcineurin inhibitors, such as cyclosporine and tacrolimus, and immunomodulators such as azathioprine and 6-mercaptopurine (236). Many of the most severe cases may eventuate in colectomy. In that event, restorative proctocolectomy with ileal pouch–anal anastomosis is the surgical treatment of choice (237).

Celiac Disease

Celiac disease is a malabsorption syndrome, with a prevalence of up to 1% of the adult population of Western countries (238), and is associated with HLA-DQ2 (DQA1*/DQB1*2) in more than 90% of patients with celiac disease (239). It reflects small intestinal mucosal injury caused by a humoral immune response to ingested gluten and is associated with dermatitis herpetiformis in roughly 25% of cases (see Chapter 9) (233,240,241). Dietary gluten triggers the activation of CD4- and CD8-positive T cells with gut-homing CD8 $\alpha\beta$ and $\gamma\delta$ T cells in the peripheral blood (242).

Clinical Summary. A comprehensive review article by Abenavoli et al. (239) illustrates the occurrences of other skin manifestations of celiac disease, including dermatitis herpetiformis, chronic urticaria, hereditary angioneurotic edema, erythema nodosum, necrolytic migratory erythema, psoriasis, and dermatomyositis, among others. A leukocytoclastic vasculitis has also been described in patients with celiac disease (243). The presence of IgA or IgG anti-tissue transglutaminase and antiendomysial antibodies is seen in 80% to 90% of patients with active gut mucosal inflammation and has a high specificity for the diagnosis (244). A significant concern with serologic confirmation of the diagnosis is the presence of a selective IgA deficiency in a minority of patients with celiac disease; in such patients, however, IgG antitransglutaminase and antiendomysial antibodies are still positive. Underlying mixed cryoglobulinemia may occur, as may mesangial nephritis, the latter being a consequence of circulating immune complexes (240,245). Antibodies to transglutaminase may be of pathogenetic significance. Immunofluorescence studies have demonstrated IgA and epidermal transglutaminase (TG3) deposition in the papillary dermis and blood vessel walls of patients with celiac disease. Those patients with concomitant dermatitis herpetiformis showed a stronger intensity of both IgA and TG3 deposition than those without skin lesions (246).

Principles of Management: At present, the therapy of celiac disease includes a strict gluten-free diet (247), although many patients report continuing symptoms despite adherence to a gluten-free diet for 5 years or more (248). In addition to gluten-free diet for long-term disease control, the lesions of dermatitis herpetiformis can be treated with dapsone and sulfones that target the skin eruption only (249).

DERMATOPATHOLOGIC MANIFESTATIONS OF HEPATOBILIARY DISEASE

Sclerosing Cholangitis and Primary Biliary Cirrhosis

PSC is an autoimmune disease of the bile ducts causing inflammation and subsequent obstruction of bile ducts at both the intrahepatic and extrahepatic levels and can lead to primary biliary sclerosis. Many of the patients also have ulcerative colitis.

Clinical Summary. PG, particularly a disseminated superficial vesiculopustular variant (250), and dermatitis herpetiformis have been described in association with PSC (215). In addition, diffuse superficial PG has been described in patients with ulcerative colitis, an associated finding in 70% of patients with PSC. Isolated case reports of elastosis perforans serpiginosa with co-existing Down syndrome (251) and disseminated warts along with primary combined immunodeficiency and progressive multifocal leukoencephalopathy have been described in association with PSC. Lichen planus of the nail (252) and disseminated Langerhans cell histiocytosis (253) have been reported in patients with PSC. Cutaneous manifestations seen with primary biliary cirrhosis include lichen planus (254), limited cutaneous systemic sclerosis (CREST syndrome: calcinosis, Raynaud phenomenon, esophageal dysmotility, sclerodactyly, and telangiectasia), sarcoidal granulomata (255, 256), and vitiligo (254). There are reports that describe cutaneous amyloidosis (257), linear IgA bullous dermatosis (258), pustular vasculitis (259), and cutaneous fungal infections (260) in patients with primary biliary cirrhosis.

Histopathology. Vesiculopustular PG, as may be associated with PSC, is characterized by a necrolytic subepithelial blister in which massive papillary edema is accompanied by sheets of neutrophils within the blister cavity and prominent leukocytoclasia often centered around the follicles. Peripheral to the areas of neutrophilia, angiocentric mononuclear cell infiltrates with minimal accompanying vascular injury are observed (Fig. 16-12).

Pathogenesis. Although of unclear pathogenetic significance, ANCAs in a perinuclear (p) pattern have been detected in 72% of patients with PSC and ulcerative colitis (261,262). An atypical pANCA, termed xANCA, with a specificity for a 50-kD myeloid envelope protein is seen in patients with inflammatory bowel disease, autoimmune hepatitis, and PSC (263,264). ANCAs have also been described in GPA, microscopic polyarteritis nodosa, and idiopathic crescentic glomerulonephritis. Patients with PSC and concomitant ulcerative colitis (265) have circulating antibodies to colonic epithelial cells (266). An immunogenic basis has also been proposed for PSC in view of the association with HLA-B8 and/or HLA-DR3 antigens.

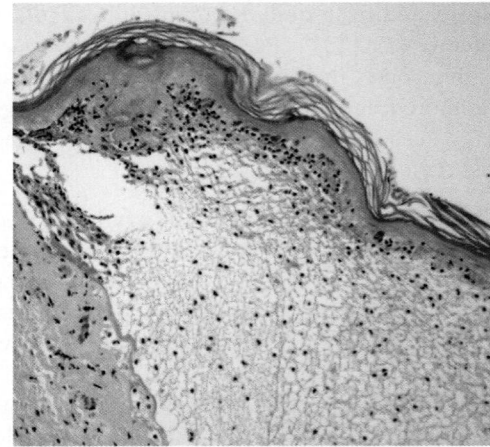

Figure 16-12 Vesicular–pustular pyoderma gangrenosum. A biopsy of the lesion demonstrated marked subepidermal edema and a subjacent intense neutrophilic and lymphocytic infiltrate with tissue pathergy confined to the superficial dermis.

Principles of Management: At present, there are no good randomized controlled trials to point toward specific medical interventions (267). That said, newer immunosuppressive agents targeting the pathogenetic mechanisms of disease can improve patient management, which, it is suggested, ought to be tailored on a case-by-case basis (268).

Cutaneous Manifestations of Hepatitis

Hepatitis can be broadly categorized into infectious and noninfectious causes. Most of the former are viral and are mediated by hepatitis A, B, and C and delta agent, cytomegalovirus, Epstein–Barr virus, and, rarely, varicella, measles, and herpes simplex virus. Chronic active hepatitis of autoimmune etiology is a necroinflammatory disorder of unknown etiology, with a predilection for young women (269). Both the clinical presentation and liver chemistry profile may resemble those of infectious hepatitis. Hepatitis C antibodies have been demonstrated in patients with classic autoimmune hepatitis, a finding reputed to represent a nonspecific response that disappears during remission. Conversely, an autoantibody profile mimicking chronic active hepatitis may be seen in hepatitis C (266). Other laboratory abnormalities include anemia, hypergammaglobulinemia, positive lupus erythematosus cell preparations, and positive antibodies to non–organ-specific antibodies, such as antinuclear antibodies, ANCAs, and antibodies to smooth muscle and liver/kidney microsomes (266).

Clinical Summary. The principal cutaneous manifestations of viral and autoimmune hepatitis are lichen planus (discussed in Chapter 7), cryoglobulinemia and leukocytoclastic vasculitis (see Chapter 8) (270), porphyria cutanea tarda (see Chapter 17) (271), erythema multiforme (see Chapter 9) (272), PG (this chapter, earlier) (273), NAE, and Gianotti–Crosti syndrome (see sections following) (274). Lichen planus has been reported in patients with hepatitis C, chronic active hepatitis of unknown etiology, and primary biliary cirrhosis (Fig. 16-13) (275). The clinical spectrum of skin lesions in patients infected with hepatitis C comprises photodistributed eruptions, palpable purpura, folliculitis, chilblains-like acral lesions, NAE, ulcers, nodules, and urticaria (276). The vasculitis may be on the basis of mixed cryoglobulinemia in the setting of hepatitis C infection. Endothelial cell swelling is common. Mixed cryoglobulinemia differs from conventional leukocytoclastic vasculitis by the presence of intraluminal eosinophilic deposits that are strongly PAS positive (269). Porphyria and erythema multiforme–like eruptions also occur in association with hepatitis C. Some patients develop a low-grade lymphoproliferative disease of B-cell lineage cognate to marginal zone lymphoma. In one study, roughly 21% of patients with hepatitis receiving pegylated IFN-α2b and ribavirin developed hyperpigmentation of oral mucous membranes in concert with acquired longitudinal melanonychia, or hyperpigmentation of the face without oral and nail involvement. Risk factors for the development of cutaneous hyperpigmentation included a darker skin type and unprotected sun exposure (277).

In our hands, the skin lesions of hepatitis C can be classified by the dominant reaction pattern, the most common being vasculopathies of neutrophilic and lymphocytic vasculitis and pauci-inflammatory subtypes; palisading granulomatous inflammation; sterile neutrophilic folliculitis; neutrophilic lobular panniculitis; benign cutaneous polyarteritis nodosa; neutrophilic dermatoses, including neutrophilic urticaria and PG; and interface dermatitis (275).

Necrolytic Acral Erythema

Clinical Summary. NAE is a papulosquamous eruption that predominantly occurs in association with hepatitis C virus infection (68,278). Many of the described cases have occurred in Egypt; however, it also occurs in the United States. The condition may appear before the discovery of the hepatitis C infection (279). Early lesions may present with erosions and flaccid blisters. Fully evolved lesions are erythematous, dusky, hyperpigmented plaques with a darker peripheral rim. Hyperkeratosis may be prominent. The characteristic distribution is the involvement of the distal extremities; however, proximal extremities and truncal lesions have also been described (Fig. 16-14).

Histopathology. Histopathologic findings of NAE include psoriasiform epidermal hyperplasia, hyperkeratosis with parakeratosis, and a diminished granular cell layer. Characteristic findings also include individual keratinocyte necrosis and pallor of the superficial epidermal layer (Fig. 16-14). Vacuolar alteration may be present. The dermis reveals a superficial perivascular mononuclear cell infiltrate. There are overlapping histologic features with psoriasis; however, the presence of spongiform pustules would favor a diagnosis of psoriasis, and individual keratinocyte necrosis favors NAE. The histologic findings of NAE may be indistinguishable from necrolytic migratory erythema, fatty acid deficiency, zinc deficiency (acrodermatitis enteropathica), pellagra, and biotin deficiency. These diagnoses must be excluded clinically.

Principles of Management: An abnormality of zinc metabolism may be involved in this condition, and zinc sulfate therapy may have some efficacy, regardless of normal or abnormal zinc levels. Clearance of lesions has also been seen in association with IFN and ribavirin-induced viral suppression (280).

Papular Acrodermatitis (Gianotti–Crosti Syndrome)

Clinical Summary. Papular acrodermatitis (273) (Gianotti–Crosti syndrome) reflects a primary infection with hepatitis B virus, acquired through the skin or mucous membranes, and comprises a

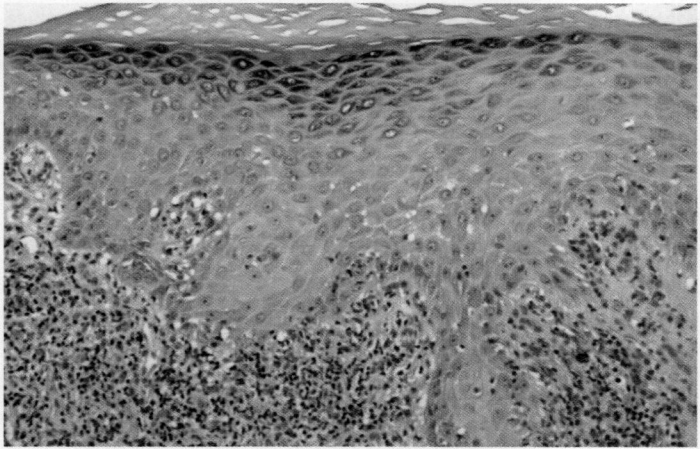

Figure 16-13 Lichenoid tissue reaction in the setting of hepatitis C infection. This patient with hepatitis C developed an eruption that was clinically compatible with lichen planus. The histomorphology confirmed the diagnosis by virtue of a dense, bandlike lymphocytic infiltrate in apposition to an epidermis showing colloid body formation.

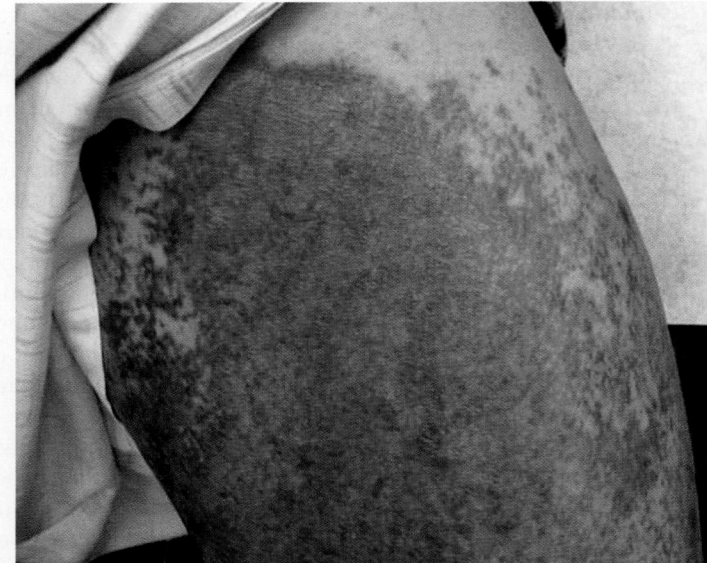

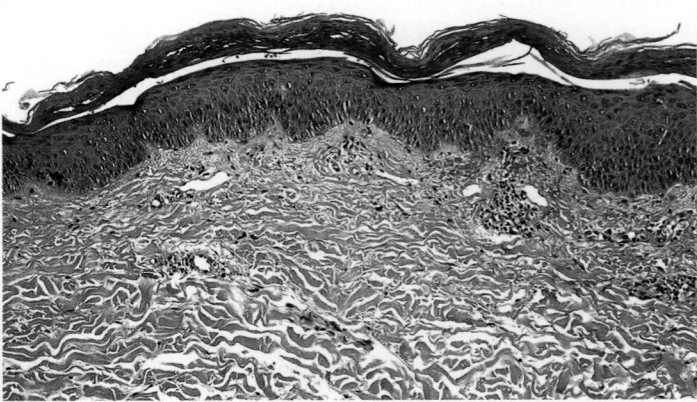

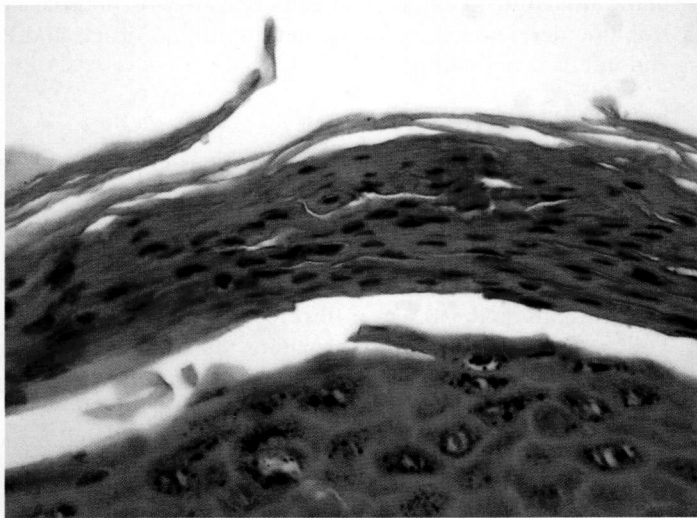

Figure 16-14 **A**: A 55-year-old man developed a progressive advancing erythematous eruption of lower extremities and was found to have a hepatitis C viral load greater than 700,000 IU/m; transaminases were elevated, and a serum Zinc level was dramatically reduced. The rash resolved following administration of parenteral zinc. **B**: Necrolytic acral erythema, medium power. A confluent parakeratotic scale crust surmounted a slightly acanthotic epidermis. **C**: Necrolytic acral erythema, high power. The parakeratotic scale contains individually necrotic keratinocytes and the epidermis shows a maturation lag.

nonpruritic, erythematous, papular eruption on the face, extremities, and buttocks. The eruption usually lasts about 3 weeks and is associated with lymphadenopathy and an acute, usually anicteric, hepatitis of at least 2 months' duration that only rarely progresses to chronic liver disease. Hepatitis B surface antigenemia is present (273). A similar eruption may be produced by several other viruses, such as Epstein–Barr virus, coxsackie B virus, and cytomegalovirus (281), in which case there is often no hepatitis or lymphadenopathy. Gianotti–Crosti syndrome has also been reported in children after immunizations with inactivated vaccines for hepatitis A (282), hepatitis B (283), Japanese encephalitis (284), diphtheria/tetanus/acellular pertussis, and *Haemophilus influenzae* B (285) and after live attenuated oral polio (286) and measles/mumps/rubella vaccines (287). It was also reported after inactivated influenza vaccine in an adult (288).

Histopathology. The histologic appearance of the papules in Gianotti–Crosti syndrome includes a moderately dense infiltrate of lymphocytes and histiocytes in the upper and mid-dermis that are found mainly around capillaries that exhibit endothelial swelling, accompanied by erythrocyte extravasation (277). Focal spongiosis, parakeratosis with mild acanthosis, and a focal interface dermatitis complete the picture, which is not specifically diagnostic in the absence of clinicopathologic correlation (277).

Pathogenesis. The sera of all patients with hepatitis B–induced papular acrodermatitis exhibit hepatitis B surface antigens by radio-immunoassay. Antibodies to hepatitis B surface antigens are not detected during the eruptive phase but only 6 to 12 months after the eruption; patients with antibodies become hepatitis B surface antigen negative, suggesting a role for humoral immunity in their recovery. As regard the skin lesions of hepatitis C infection, reverse transcriptase *in situ* polymerase chain reaction studies show expression of viral DNA in endothelia in some cases (275).

Principles of Management: Treatment of the underlying viral infection is important in management from the perspective, first, of preventing hepatic cirrhosis and, second, of controlling cutaneous manifestations, which can be treated symptomatically, if necessary.

Acrokeratosis Neoplastica (Bazex Syndrome)

Clinical Summary. First described in 1965 (289), this rare but clinically distinctive dermatosis was originally associated with either a primary malignant neoplasm of the upper aerodigestive tract—most commonly squamous cell carcinoma—or metastatic cancer to the lymph nodes of the neck. Other associated malignancies have since been described, including poorly differentiated carcinoma, adenocarcinoma, and small cell carcinoma, among others. Often, the skin changes occur before the diagnosis of the underlying malignancy and resolve if the malignancy is removed (290). More than 90% of the patients are male, and most are older than 40 years (291). Thickening of the periungual and subungual skin and of the palms and soles occurs initially when the neoplasm is silent. Subsequently, the skin of the ears, nose, face, trunk, and extremities becomes involved and shows a violaceous color, peeling, and fissuring (292,293). The palmar lesions may resemble those of Reiter disease.

Histopathology. Ill-defined perivascular lymphocytic infiltrates containing a few pyknotic neutrophils in the upper dermis along with mild acanthosis, hyperkeratosis, and scattered parakeratotic foci are described. Eosinophilic and vacuolar degeneration of the spinous layer may be noted (287).

Principles of Management: The intention is to identify and treat the underlying malignancy.

REFERENCES

1. Statters DJ, Asokan VS, Littlewood SM, Snape J. Carcinoma of the caecum in a scorbutic patient. *Br J Clin Pract.* 1990;44:738.
2. Bartholomew M. James Lind's treatise of the scurvy (1753). *Postgrad Med J.* 2002;78:695.
3. Levine M. New concepts in the biology and biochemistry of ascorbic acid. *N Engl J Med.* 1986;314:892.
4. Haslock I. Hemarthrosis and scurvy [letter]. *J Rheumatol.* 2002;29:1808.
5. Kern M, Gardner JM. Mucocutaneous manifestations of scurvy. *N Engl J Med.* 2020;382(20):e56. doi:10.1056/NEJMicm1911315
6. Stokes PL, Melikiah V, Leeming RL, Portman-Graham H, Blair JA, Cooke WT. Folate metabolism in scurvy. *Am J Clin Nutr.* 1975;28:126.
7. Monks GM, Juracek L, Weigand D, Magro C, Cornelison R, Crowson AN. A case of scurvy in an autistic boy. *J Drugs Dermatol.* 2002;1:67.
8. Ahmad K. Scurvy outbreak in Afghanistan prompts food aid concerns. *Lancet.* 2002;359:1044.
9. Colacci M, Gold WL, Shah R. Modern-day scurvy. *CMAJ.* 2020;192(4):E96. doi:10.1503/cmaj.190934
10. Mason JB. Lessons on nutrition of displaced people. *J Nutr.* 2002;132:2096s.
11. Weise Pronzo Z, de Benoist B. Meeting the challenges of micronutrient deficiencies in emergency-affected populations. *Proc Nutr Soc.* 2002;61:251.
12. Levavasseur M, Becquart C, Pape E, et al. Severe scurvy: an underestimated disease. *Eur J Clin Nutr.* 2015;69(9):1076–1077. doi:10.1038/ejcn.2015.99
13. Kletzel M, Powers K, Hayes M. Scurvy: a new problem for patients with chronic GVHD involving mucous membranes; an easy problem to resolve. *Pediatr Transplant.* 2014;18(5):524–526. doi:10.1111/petr.12285
14. Ellis CN, Vanderveen EE, Rasmussen JE. Scurvy: a case caused by peculiar dietary habits. *Arch Dermatol.* 1984;120:1212.
15. Abramovits-Ackerman W, Bustos T, Simosa-Leon V, Fernandez L, Ramella M. Cutaneous findings in a new syndrome of autosomal recessive ectodermal dysplasia with corkscrew hairs. *J Am Acad Dermatol.* 1992;27:917.
16. Langlois MR, Delanghe JR, De Buyzere ML, Bernard DR, Ouyang J. Effect of haptoglobin on the metabolism of vitamin C. *Am J Clin Nutr.* 1997;66:606–610.
17. Delanghe JR, Langlois MR, De Buyzere ML, Torck MA. Vitamin C deficiency and scurvy are not only a dietary problem but are codetermined by the haptoglobin polymorphism. *Clin Chem.* 2007;53(8):1397–1400.
18. Hashimoto K, Kitabchi AE, Duckworth WC, Robinson N. Ultrastructure of scorbutic human skin. *Acta Derm Venereol (Stockholm).* 1970;50:9.
19. Wechsler HL. Vitamin A deficiency following small-bowel bypass surgery for obesity. *Arch Dermatol.* 1979;115:73.
20. Bleasel NR, Stapleton KM, Lee MS, Sullivan J. Vitamin A deficiency phrynoderma: due to malabsorption and inadequate diet. *J Am Acad Dermatol.* 1999;41:322.
21. Ocón J, Cabrejas C, Altemir J, Moros M. Phrynoderma: a rare dermatologic complication of bariatric surgery. *JPEN J Parenter Enteral Nutr.* 2012;36(3):361–364. doi:10.1177/0148607 111422067
22. Ragunatha S, Kumar VJ, Murugesh SB. A clinical study of 125 patients with phrynoderma. *Indian J Dermatol.* 2011;56(4):389–392. doi:10.4103/0019-5154.84760
23. Girard C, Dereure O, Blatière V, Guillot B, Bessis D. Vitamin A deficiency phrynoderma associated with chronic giardiasis. *Pediatr Dermatol.* 2006;23(4):346–349.
24. Frazier CN, Hu C. Nature and distribution according to age of cutaneous manifestations of vitamin A deficiency. *Arch Dermatol Syph.* 1936;33:825.
25. Bessey OA, Wolbach SB. Vitamin A, physiology and pathology. *JAMA.* 1938;110:2072.
26. Magro CM, Crowson AN. The clinical and histomorphological features of pityriasis rubra pilaris: a comparative analysis with psoriasis. *J Cutan Pathol.* 1997;24(7):416–424.
27. Hendricks WM. Pellagra and pellagralike dermatoses: etiology, differential diagnosis, dermatopathology, and treatment. *Semin Dermatol.* 1991;10:282.
28. Wallengren J, Thelin I. Pellagra-like skin lesions associated with Wernicke's encephalopathy in a heavy wine drinker. *Acta Derm Venereol.* 2002;82:152.
29. Portale S, Sculati M, Stanford FC, Cena H. Pellagra and anorexia nervosa: a case report. *Eat Weight Disord.* 2020;25(5):1493–1496. doi:10.1007/s40519-019-00781-x
30. Castiello RJ, Lynch PJ. Pellagra and the carcinoid syndrome. *Arch Dermatol.* 1972;105:574.
31. Lyon VB, Fairley JA. Anticonvulsant-induced pellagra. *J Am Acad Dermatol.* 2002;46:597.
32. Kipsang JK, Choge JK, Marinda PA, Khayeka-Wandabwa C. Pellagra in isoniazid preventive and antiretroviral therapy. *IDCases.* 2019;17:e00550. doi:10.1016/j.idcr.2019.e00550
33. Spivak JL, Jackson DL. Pellagra: an analysis of 18 patients and a review of the literature. *Johns Hopkins Med J.* 1977;140:295.
34. Karthikeyan K, Thappa DM. Pellagra and the skin. *Int J Dermatol.* 2002;41:476.
35. Hegyi J, Schwartz RA, Hegyi V. Pellagra: dermatitis, dementia, and diarrhea. *Int J Dermatol.* 2004;43(1):1–5.
36. Montgomery H. Nutritional and vitamin deficiency. In: *Dermatopathology,* Vol 1. Harper and Row; 1967:259–266.
37. Cardoso JC, Veraitch O, Gianotti R, et al. 'Hints' in the horn: diagnostic clues in the stratum corneum. *J Cutan Pathol.* 2017;44(3):256–278.
38. Yamaguchi S, Miyagi T, Sogabe Y, et al. Depletion of epidermal Langerhans cells in the skin lesions of pellagra patients. *Am J Dermatopathol.* 2017;39(6):428–432. doi:10.1097/DAD.000000 0000000654
39. Badawy AA. Pellagra and alcoholism: a biochemical perspective. *Alcohol Alcohol.* 2014;49(3):238–250. doi:10.1093/alcalc/agu010
40. Dent CE. Hartnup disease: an inborn error of metabolism. *Arch Dis Child.* 1957;32:363.
41. Halvorsen L, Halvorsen S. Hartnup disease. *Pediatrics.* 1963;31:29.
42. Baron DN, Dent CE, Harris H, Hart EW, Jepson JB. Hereditary pellagra like skin rash with temporary cerebellar ataxia, constant renal aminoaciduria and other bizarre chemical features. *Lancet.* 1956;2:421.

43. Clodi PH, Deutsch E, Niebauer G. Krankheitsbild mit poikilo-dermieartigen hautveranderungen, aminoacidurie und Indolaceturie. *Arch Klin Exp Dermatol.* 1964;218:165.

44. Ashurst PJ. Hydroa vacciniforme occurring in association with Hartnup disease. *Br J Dermatol.* 1969;81:486.

45. Seow HF, Bröer S, Bröer A, et al. Hartnup disorder is caused by mutations in the gene encoding the neutral amino acid transporter SLC6A19. *Nat Genet.* 2004;36(9):1003–1007.

46. Kleta R, Romeo E, Ristic Z, et al. Mutations in SLC6A19, encoding B0AT1, cause Hartnup disorder. *Nat Genet.* 2004;36(9):999–1002.

47. Nozaki J, Dakeishi M, Ohura T, et al. Homozygosity mapping to chromosome 5p15 of a gene responsible for Hartnup disorder. *Biochem Biophys Res Commun.* 2001;284:255.

48. Becker SW, Kahn D, Rothman S. Cutaneous manifestations of internal malignant tumors. *Arch Dermatol Syph.* 1942;45:1069.

49. Domen RE, Shaffer MB Jr, Finke J, Sterin WK, Hurst CB. The glucagonoma syndrome. *Arch Intern Med.* 1980;140:262.

50. Alexander EK, Robinson M, Staniec M, Dluhy RG. Peripheral amino acid and fatty acid infusion for the treatment of necrolytic migratory erythema in the glucagonoma syndrome. *Clin Endocrinol (Oxf).* 2002;57:827.

51. V'lckova-Laskoska M, Balabanova-Stefanova M, Arsovska-Bezhoska I, Caca-Biljanovska N, Laskoski D. Necrolytic migratory erythema: complete healing after surgical removal of pancreatic carcinoma. *Acta Dermatovenerol Croat.* 2018;26(4):329–332

52. Brenseke BM, Belz KM, Saunders GK. Pathology in practice: superficial necrolytic dermatitis and nodular hepatopathy (lesions consistent with hepatocutaneous syndrome). *J Am Vet Med Assoc.* 2011;238(4):445–447.

53. Nakashima H, Komine M, Sasaki K, et al. Necrolytic migratory erythema without glucagonoma in a patient with short bowel syndrome. *J Dermatol.* 2006;33(8):557–562. doi:10.1111/j.1346-8138.2006.00131.x

54. Chastain MA. The glucagonoma syndrome: a review of its features and discussion of new perspectives. *Am J Med Sci.* 2001; 321:306.

55. Tolliver S, Graham J, Kaffenberger BH. A review of cutaneous manifestations within glucagonoma syndrome: necrolytic migratory erythema. *Int J Dermatol.* 2018;57(6):642–645. doi:10.1111/ijd.13947

56. Macbeth AE, James A, Rhodes M, Igali L, McGibbon D, Graham RM. Necrolytic migratory erythema with the absence of necrolysis. *Clin Exp Dermatol.* 2010;35(7):810–811.

57. Chao SC, Lee JY. Brittle nails and dyspareunia as first clues to recurrences of malignant glucagonoma. *Br J Dermatol.* 2002; 146:1071.

58. Binnick AN, Spencer SK, Dennison WL Jr, Horton ES. Glucagonoma syndrome. *Arch Dermatol.* 1977;113:749.

59. Kasper CS, McMurray K. Necrolytic migratory erythema without glucagonoma versus canine superficial necrolytic dermatitis: is hepatic impairment a clue to pathogenesis? *J Am Acad Dermatol.* 1991;25:534.

60. Kaspar CS. Necrolytic migratory erythema: unresolved problems in diagnosis and pathogenesis. A case report and literature review. *Cutis.* 1992;49:120.

61. Blackford S, Wright S, Roberts DL. Necrolytic migratory erythema without glucagonoma: the role of dietary essential fatty acids. *Br J Dermatol.* 1991;125:460.

62. Kitamura Y, Sato M, Hatamochi A, Yamazaki S. Necrolytic migratory erythema without glucagonoma associated with hepatitis B. *Eur J Dermatol.* 2005;15(1):49–51.

63. Goodenberger DM, Lawley TJ, Strober W, et al. Necrolytic migratory erythema without glucagonoma. *Arch Dermatol.* 1977; 115:1429.

64. Bencini PL, Vigo GP, Caputo R. Necrolytic migratory erythema without glucagonoma in a heroin-dependent patient. *Dermatology.* 1994;189:72–74.

65. Muller FM, Arseculeratne G, Evans A, Fleming C. Necrolytic migratory erythema in an opiate-dependent patient. *Clin Exp Dermatol.* 2008;33(1):40–42.

66. Remes-Troche JM, García-de-Acevedo B, Zuñiga-Varga J, Avila-Funes A, Orozco-Topete R. Necrolytic migratory erythema: a cutaneous clue to glucagonoma syndrome. *J Eur Acad Dermatol Venereol.* 2004;18(5):591–595.

67. Thomaidou E, Nahmias A, Gilead L, Zlotogorski A, Ramot Y. Rapid clearance of necrolytic migratory erythema following intravenous administration of amino acids. *JAMA Dermatol.* 2016;152(3):345–346. doi:10.1001/jamadermatol.2015.3538

68. el Darouti M, Abu el Ela M. Necrolytic acral erythema: a cutaneous marker of viral hepatitis C. *Int J Dermatol.* 1996;35(4):252–256.

69. Danbolt N, Closs K. Akrodermatitis enteropathica. *Acta Derm Venereol (Stockholm)* 1942;23:127.

70. Moynahan EJ. Acrodermatitis enteropathica: a lethal inherited zinc-deficiency disorder. *Lancet.* 1974;2:399.

71. Gonzalez JR, Botet MV, Sanchez JL. The histopathology of acrodermatitis enteropathica. *Am J Dermatopathol.* 1982;4:303.

72. Reichel M, Mauro TM, Ziboh VA, Huntley AC, Fletcher MP. Acrodermatitis enteropathica in a patient with the acquired immunodeficiency syndrome. *Arch Dermatol.* 1992;128:415.

73. Bernstein B, Leyden JL. Zinc deficiency and acrodermatitis enteropathica after intravenous hyperalimentation. *Arch Dermatol.* 1978;114:1070.

74. Niemi KM, Anttila PH, Kanerva L, Johansson E. Histopathological study of transient acrodermatitis enteropathica due to decreased zinc in breast milk. *J Cutan Pathol.* 1989;16:382.

75. Pascual JC, Matarredona J, Mut J. Acrodermatitis enteropathica-like dermatosis associated with ornithine transcarbamylase deficiency. *Pediatr Dermatol.* 2007;24(4):394–396.

76. Madhusudan M, Raman R, Sathyasekaran M. Acrodermatitis enteropathica as a presentation of cystic fibrosis in an infant. *Indian Pediatr.* 2020;57(6):573

77. Yu HH, Shan YS, Lin PW. Zinc deficiency with acrodermatitis enteropathica-like eruption after pancreaticoduodenectomy. *J Formos Med Assoc.* 2007;106(10):864–868.

78. Kurt BÖ, İrican CM, Ünal B, Çiftçioğlu MA, Uzun S. Acquired acrodermatitis enteropathica secondary to sleeve gastrectomy. *Indian J Dermatol Venereol Leprol.* 2019;85(2):220–223. doi:10.4103/ijdvl.IJDVL_337_18

79. Weissman K, Hoe S, Knudsen L, Sørensen SS. Zinc absorption in patients suffering from acrodermatitis enteropathica and in normal adults assessed by whole-body counting technique. *Br J Dermatol.* 1979;101:573.

80. Ortega SS, Cachaza JA, Tovar IV, Feijoo MF. Zinc deficiency dermatitis in parenteral nutrition: an electron-microscopic study. *Dermatologica.* 1985;171:163.

81. Bin BH, Bhin J, Kim NH, et al. An acrodermatitis enteropathica-associated Zn transporter, ZIP4, regulates human epidermal homeostasis. *J Invest Dermatol.* 2017;137(4):874–883. doi:10.1016/j.jid.2016.11.028

82. Küry S, Dréno B, Bézieau S, et al. Identification of SLC39A4, a gene involved in acrodermatitis enteropathica. *Nat Genet.* 2002;31:239–240.

83. Kilic M, Taskesen M, Coskun T, et al. A zinc sulphate-resistant acrodermatitis enteropathica patient with a novel mutation in SLC39A4 gene. *JIMD Rep.* 2012;2:25–28.

84. Katz KA, Mahlberg MJ, Honig PJ, Yan AC. Rice nightmare: kwashiorkor in 2 Philadelphia-area infants fed Rice Dream beverage. *J Am Acad Dermatol.* 2005;52(5, suppl 1):S69–S72.

85. Albers SE, Brozena SJ, Fenske NA. A case of kwashiorkor. *Cutis.* 1993;51:445.

86. Heath ML, Sidbury R. Cutaneous manifestations of nutritional deficiency. *Curr Opin Pediatr.* 2006;18(4):417–422.

87. Househam KC. Computed tomography of the brain in kwashiorkor: a follow up study. *Arch Dis Child.* 1991;66:623.

88. Richardson D, Iputo J. Effects of kwashiorkor malnutrition on measured capillary filtration rate in forearm. *Am J Physiol.* 1992;262:H496.

89. Coulthard MG. Oedema in kwashiorkor is caused by hypoalbuminaemia. *Paediatr Int Child Health.* 2015;35(2):83–89. doi:10.1179/2046905514Y.0000000154

90. Brunsting LA, Goeckerman WE, O'Leary PA. Pyoderma (ecthyma) gangrenosum. *Arch Dermatol.* 1930;22:655.

91. Graham JA, Hansen KK, Rabinowitz LG, Esterly NB. Pyoderma gangrenosum in infants and children. *Pediatr Dermatol.* 1994;11:10.

92. Crowson AN, Mihm MC Jr, Magro C. Pyoderma gangrenosum: a review. *J Cutan Pathol.* 2003;30(2):97–107.

93. Cairns BA, Herbst CA, Sartor BR, Briggaman RA, Koruda MJ. Peristomal pyoderma gangrenosum and inflammatory bowel disease. *Arch Surg.* 1994;129:769.

94. Körber A, Klode J, Al-Benna S, et al. Etiology of chronic leg ulcers in 31,619 patients in Germany analyzed by an expert survey. *J Dtsch Dermatol Ges.* 2011;9(2):116–121.

95. Schwaegerle SM, Bergfeld WF, Senitzer D, Tidrick RT. Pyoderma gangrenosum: a review. *J Am Acad Dermatol.* 1988;18:559.

96. Callen JP. Pyoderma gangrenosum and related disorders. *Med Clin North Am.* 1989;73:1247.

97. Montagnon CM, Fracica EA, Patel AA, et al. Pyoderma gangrenosum in hematologic malignancies: a systematic review. *J Am Acad Dermatol.* 2020;82(6):1346–1359. doi:10.1016/j.jaad.2019.09.032

98. Magro CM, Crowson AN. Vesiculopustular lesions in association with liver disease. *Int J Dermatol.* 1997;36:837.

99. Wilson-Jones E, Winkelmann RK. Superficial granulomatous pyoderma: a localized vegetative form of pyoderma gangrenosum. *J Am Acad Dermatol.* 1988;18:511.

100. Ayres S Jr, Ayres S III. Pyoderma gangrenosum with an unusual syndrome of ulcers, vesicles, and arthritis. *Arch Dermatol.* 1958;77:269–280.

101. Srebrnik A, Schachar E, Brenner S. Suspected induction of a pyoderma gangrenosum-like eruption due to sulpiride treatment. *Cutis.* 2001;67:253.

102. Ross HJ, Moy LA, Kaplan R, Figlin RA. Bullous pyoderma gangrenosum after granulocyte colony-stimulating factor treatment. *Cancer.* 1991;68:441.

103. Sagara R, Kitami A, Nakada T, Iijima M. Adverse reactions to gefitinib (Iressa): revealing sycosis-and pyoderma gangrenosum-like lesions. *Int J Dermatol.* 2006;45(8):1002–1003.

104. Freiman A, Brassard A. Pyoderma gangrenosum associated with isotretinoin therapy. *J Am Acad Dermatol.* 2006;55(5,suppl):S107–S108.

105. Gungor K, Gonen S, Kisakol G, Dikbas O, Kaya A. ANCA positive propylthiouracil induced pyoderma gangrenosum. *J Endocrinol Invest.* 2006;29(6):575–576.

106. Mir-Bonafé JM, Blanco-Barrios S, Romo-Melgar A, Santos-Briz A, Fernández-López E. Photoletter to the editor: localized pyoderma gangrenosum after interferon-alpha2b injections. *J Dermatol Case Rep.* 2012;6(3):98–99.

107. Maverakis E, Ma C, Shinkai K, et al. Diagnostic criteria of ulcerative pyoderma gangrenosum: a Delphi Consensus of International Experts. *JAMA Dermatol.* 2018;154(4):461–466. doi:10.1001/jamadermatol.2017.5980

108. Jorizzo JL, Solomon AR, Zanolli M, Leshin B. Neutrophilic vascular reactions. *J Am Acad Dermatol.* 1988;19:983.

109. Magro CM, Crowson AN. The cutaneous neutrophilic vascular injury syndromes: a review. *Semin Diagn Pathol.* 2001;18:47.

110. Pye RJ, Choudhury C. Bullous pyoderma as a presentation of acute leukemia. *Clin Exp Dermatol.* 1977;2:33.

111. Koester G, Tarnower A, Levisohn D, Burgdorf W. Bullous pyoderma gangrenosum. *J Am Acad Dermatol.* 1993;29:875.

112. Sanders S, Tahan SR, Kwan T, Magro CM. Giant cells in pyoderma gangrenosum. *J Cutan Pathol.* 2001;28:98.

113. Magro CM, Crowson AN. Sterile neutrophilic folliculitis with perifollicular vasculopathy: a distinctive cutaneous reaction pattern reflecting systemic disease. *J Cutan Pathol.* 1998;25:215.

114. Powell FC, Schroeter AL, Perry HO, Su WP. Direct immunofluorescence in pyoderma gangrenosum. *Br J Dermatol.* 1983;108:287.

115. Holt PJA, Davies MG, Saunders KC, Nuki G. Pyoderma gangrenosum: clinical and laboratory findings in 15 patients with special reference to polyarthritis. *Medicine.* 1980;59:114.

116. Powell FC, Schroeter AL, Su D, Perry HO. Pyoderma gangrenosum and monoclonal gammopathy. *Arch Dermatol.* 1983;119:468.

117. Brooklyn TN, Williams AM, Dunnill MG, Probert CS. T-cell receptor repertoire in pyoderma gangrenosum: evidence for clonal expansions and trafficking. *Br J Dermatol.* 2007;157(5):960–966.

118. Oka M. Pyoderma gangrenosum and interleukin 8. *Br J Dermatol.* 2007;157(6):1279–1281.

119. Campbell S, Cripps S, Jewell DP. Therapy insight: pyoderma gangrenosum—old disease, new management. *Nat Clin Pract Gastroenterol Hepatol.* 2005;2:587.

120. Ratnagobal S, Sinha S. Pyoderma gangrenosum: guideline for wound practitioners. *J Wound Care.* 2013;22:68.

121. Reichrath J, Bens G, Bonowitz A, Tilgen W. Treatment recommendations for pyoderma gangrenosum: an evidence-based review of the literature based on more than 350 patients. *J Am Acad Dermatol.* 2005;53:273.

122. Rosen JD, Stojadinovic O, McBride JD, Rico R, Cho-Vega JH, Nichols AJ. Bowel-associated dermatosis-arthritis syndrome (BADAS) in a patient with cystic fibrosis. *JAAD Case Rep.* 2018;5(1):37–39. doi:10.1016/j.jdcr.2018.08.029

123. Pompeo MQ. Pyoderma gangrenosum: recognition and management. *Wounds.* 2016;28(1):7–13.

124. Morrison JGL, Fourie ED. A distinctive skin eruption following small-bowel bypass surgery. *Br J Dermatol.* 1980;102:467.

125. Ely PH. The bowel bypass syndrome: a response to bacterial peptidoglycans. *J Am Acad Dermatol.* 1980;2:473.

126. Jorizzo JL, Apisarnthanarax P, Subrt P, et al. Bowel-bypass syndrome without bowel bypass: bowel-associated dermatosis-arthritis syndrome. *Arch Intern Med.* 1983;143:457.

127. Dicken CH. Bowel-associated dermatosis-arthritis syndrome: bowel bypass syndrome without bowel bypass. *J Am Acad Dermatol.* 1986;14:792.

128. Goldman JA, Casey HL, Davidson ED, Hersh T. Vasculitis associated with intestinal bypass surgery. *Arch Dermatol.* 1979;115:725.

129. Magro CM, Crowson AN. The clinical and histological spectrum of IgA-associated vasculitis. *Am J Dermatopathol.* 1999;21:234.

130. Atton T, Jukic D, Juhas E. Atypical histopathology in bowel-associated dermatosis-arthritis syndrome: a case report. *Dermatol Online J.* 2009;15(3):3.

131. Zhao H, Zhao L, Shi W, et al. Is it bowel-associated dermatosis-arthritis syndrome induced by small intestinal bacteria overgrowth? *Springerplus.* 2016;5(1):1551. doi:10.1186/s40064-016-3236-8

132. Magro CM, Crowson AN, Peeling R. Vasculitis as the pathogenetic basis of Reiter's disease. *Hum Pathol.* 1995;26:633.

133. O'Duffy JD. Behçet's syndrome. *N Engl J Med.* 1990;322:326.

134. Main DM, Chamberlain MA. Clinical differentiation of oral ulceration in Behçet's disease. *Br J Rheumatol.* 1992;31:767.

135. Scherrer MAR, Rocha VB, Garcia LC. Behçet's disease: review with emphasis on dermatological aspects. *An Bras Dermatol.* 2017;92(4):452–464. doi:10.1590/abd1806-4841.20177359

136. Alpsoy E. Behçet's disease: a comprehensive review with a focus on epidemiology, etiology and clinical features, and management of mucocutaneous lesions. *J Dermatol.* 2016;43(6):620–632. doi:10.1111/1346-8138.13381

137. Letsinger JA, McCarty MA, Jorizzo JL. Complex aphthosis: a large case series with evaluation algorithm and therapeutic ladder from topicals to thalidomide [review]. *J Am Acad Dermatol.* 2005;52(3, pt 1):500–508.

138. Magro CM, Crowson AN. Cutaneous manifestations of Behçet's disease. *Int J Dermatol.* 1995;34:159.

139. King R, Crowson AN, Murray E, Magro CM. Acral purpuric papulonodular lesions as a manifestation of Behçet's disease. *Int J Dermatol.* 1995;34:190.

140. Kural-Seyahi E, Fresko I, Seyahi N, et al. The long-term mortality and morbidity of Behçet syndrome: a 2-decade outcome survey of 387 patients followed at a dedicated center. *Medicine (Baltimore)* 2003;82:60.

141. Oguz O, Serdaroglu S, Tüzün Y, Erdoğan N, Yazici H, Savaşkan H. Acute febrile neutrophilic dermatosis (Sweet's syndrome) associated with Behçet's disease. *Int J Dermatol.* 1992;31:645.

142. Koc Y, Gullu I, Akpek G, et al. Vascular involvement in Behçet's disease. *J Rheumatol.* 1992;19:402.

143. Akutsu Y, Itami N, Tanaka M, Kusunoki Y, Tochimaru H, Takekoshi Y. IgA nephritis in Behçet's disease: case report and review of the literature. *Clin Nephrol.* 1990;34:52.

144. Sokoloff L, Bunin JJ. Vascular lesions in rheumatoid arthritis. *J Chronic Dis.* 1957;5:668.

145. Magro CM, Crowson AN. The spectrum of cutaneous lesions in rheumatoid arthritis: a clinical and pathological study of 43 cases. *J Cutan Pathol.* 2003;30:1.

146. Langenberg A, Yen TS, LeBoit PE. Granulomatous vasculitis occurring after cutaneous herpes zoster despite absence of viral genome. *J Am Acad Dermatol.* 1991;24:429.

147. Choudhri S, Magro CM, Crowson AN, Nicolle LE. A unique id reaction to Mycobacterium leprae: first documented case. *Cutis.* 1994;54:282.

148. Lehner T, Batchelor JR, Challacombe SJ, Kennedy L. An immunogenetic basis for the tissue involvement in Behçet's syndrome. *Immunology.* 1979;37:895.

149. Kaya TI, Dura H, Tursen U, Gurler A. Association of class I HLA antigens with the clinical manifestations of Turkish patients with Behçet's disease. *Clin Exp Dermatol.* 2002;27:498.

150. Mizuki N, Yabuki K, Ota M, et al. Analysis of microsatellite polymorphism around the HLA-B locus in Iranian patients with Behçet's disease. *Tissue Antigens.* 2002;60:396.

151. Duymaz-Tozkir J, Gül A, Uyar FA, Ozbek U, Saruhan-Direskeneli G. Tumour necrosis factor-alpha gene promoter region −308 and −376 G→A polymorphisms in Behçet's disease. *Clin Exp Rheumatol.* 2003;21(4, suppl 30):S15–S18.

152. Lee EB, Kim JY, Lee YJ, Park MH, Song YW. TNF and TNF receptor polymorphisms in Korean Behçet's disease patients. *Hum Immunol.* 2003;64(6):614–620.

153. Ahmad T, Wallace GR, James T, et al. Mapping the HLA association in Behçet's disease: a role for tumor necrosis factor polymorphisms? *Arthritis Rheum.* 2003;48(3):807–813.

154. Kamoun M, Chelbi H, Houman MH, Lacheb J, Hamzaoui K. Tumor necrosis factor gene polymorphisms in Tunisian patients with Behçet's disease. *Hum Immunol.* 2007;68(3):201–205.

155. Mizuki N, Inoko H, Ohno S. Molecular genetics (HLA) of Behçet's disease. *Yonsei Med J.* 1997;38(6):333–349.

156. Alayli G, Aydin F, Coban AY, et al. T helper 1 type cytokines polymorphisms: association with susceptibility to Behçet's disease. *Clin Rheumatol.* 2007;26(8):1299–1305.

157. Lee YJ, Kang SW, Park JJ, et al. Interleukin-18 promoter polymorphisms in patients with Behçet's disease. *Hum Immunol.* 2006;67(10):812–818.

158. Dalghous AM, Freysdottir J, Fortune F. Expression of cytokines, chemokines, and chemokine receptors in oral ulcers of patients with Behçet's disease (BD) and recurrent aphthous stomatitis is Th1-associated, although Th2-association is also observed in patients with BD. *Scand J Rheumatol.* 2006;35(6):472–475.

159. Suzuki N, Nara K, Suzuki T. Skewed Th1 responses caused by excessive expression of Txk, a member of the Tec family of tyrosine kinases, in patients with Behçet's disease. *Clin Med Res.* 2006;4(2):147–151.

160. Pay S, Simsek I, Erdem H, et al. Dendritic cell subsets and type I interferon system in Behçet's disease: does functional abnormality in plasmacytoid dendritic cells contribute to Th1 polarization? *Clin Exp Rheumatol.* 2007;25(4, suppl 45):S34–S40.

161. Namba K, Ueno T, Okita M. Behçet's disease and streptococcal infection. *Jpn J Ophthalmol.* 1986;30:385.

162. Yokota K, Hayashi S, Fujii N, et al. Antibody response to oral streptococci in Behçet's disease. *Microbiol Immunol.* 1992;36:815.

163. Efthimiou J, Hay PE, Spiro SG, Lane DJ. Pulmonary tuberculosis in Behçet's syndrome. *Br J Dis Chest.* 1988;82:300.

164. Studd M, McCance DJ, Lehner T. Detection of HSV-1 DNA in patients with Behçet's syndrome and in patients with recurrent oral ulcers by the polymerase chain reaction. *J Med Microbiol.* 1991;34:39.

165. Hamzaoui K, Kahan A, Ayed K, Hamsa M. Cytotoxic T cells against herpes simplex virus in Behçet's disease. *Clin Exp Immunol.* 1990;81(3):390–395.

166. Stein CM, Thomas JE. Behçet's disease associated with HIV infection. *J Rheumatol.* 1991;18:1427.

167. Lamb JR, Young DB. T cell recognition of stress proteins: a link between infectious and autoimmune disease. *Mol Biol Med.* 1990;7:311.

168. Lehner T, Lavery E, Smith R, van der Zee R, Mizushima Y, Shinnick T. Association between the 65 kilodalton heat shock protein, *Streptococcus sangui* and the corresponding antibodies in Behçet's syndrome. *Infect Immun.* 1991;59:1424.

169. Holoshitz J, Koning JE, Coligan JE, De Bruyn J, Strober S. Isolation of CD4-CD8-mycobacterial reaction T lymphocyte clones from rheumatoid arthritis synovial fluid. *Nature.* 1989;39:226.

170. Pervin K, Childerstone A, Shinnick T, et al. T cell epitope expression of mycobacterial and homologous human 65-kilodalton heat shock protein peptide in short term cell line from patient with Behçet's disease. *J Immunol.* 1993;151:2273.

171. Suzuki Y, Hoshi K, Matsuda T, Mizushima Y. Increased peripheral blood gamma delta+ T cells and natural killer cells in Behçet's disease. *J Rheumatol.* 1992;19:588.

172. Bank I, Duvdevani M, Livneh A. Expansion of gammadelta T-cells in Behçet's disease: role of disease activity and microbial flora in oral ulcers. *J Lab Clin Med.* 2003;141:33.

173. Yang P, Chen L, Zhou H, et al. Resistance of lymphocytes to Fas-mediated apopotosis in Behçet's diseases and Vogt-Koyangi-Harada syndrome. *Ocul Immunol Inflam.* 2002;10:47.

174. Cho S, Kim J, Cho SB, et al. Immunopathogenic characterization of cutaneous inflammation in Behçet's disease. *J Eur Acad Dermatol Venereol.* 2014;28(1):51–57.

175. Sensi A, Gavioli R, Spisani S, et al. HLA B51 antigen associated with neutrophil hyperactivity. *Dis Markers.* 1991;9:327.

176. Pronai L, Ichikawa Y, Nakazawa H, Arimori S. Enhanced superoxide generation and the decreased superoxide scavenging activity of peripheral blood leukocytes in Behçet's disease: effects of colchicine. *Clin Exp Rheumatol.* 1991;9:227.

177. Yavuz S, Elbir Y, Tulunay A, Eksioglu-Demiralp E, Direskeneli H. Differential expression of toll-like receptor 6 on granulocytes and monocytes implicates the role of microorganisms in Behçet's disease etiopathogenesis. *Rheumatol Int.* 2008;28(5):401–406.

178. Aydintung AO, Tokgoz G, D'Cruz DP, et al. Antibodies to endothelial cells in patients with Behçet's disease. *Clin Immunol Immunopathol.* 1993;67:157.

179. Disdier P, Harle JR, Mouly A, Aillaud MF, Weiller PJ. Case report: Behçet's syndrome and factor XII deficiency. *Clin Rheumatol.* 1992;11:422.

180. Chafa O, Fischer AM, Meriane F, et al. Behçet's syndrome associated with protein S deficiency. *Thromb Haemost.* 1992;67:1.

181. Hampton KK, Chamberlain MA, Menon DK, Davies JA. Coagulation and fibrinolytic activity in Behçet's disease. *Thromb Haemost.* 1991;66:292.

182. Al-Dalaan A, Al-Ballaa SR, Al-Janadi S, Bohlega S, Bahabri S. Association of anti-cardiolipin antibodies with vascular thrombosis

and neurological manifestation of Behçet's disease. *Clin Rheumatol.* 1993;12:28.

183. Tursen U, Irfan Kaya T, Ikizoglu G. Cardiac complications in Behcet's disease. *Clin Exp Dermatol.* 2002;27:651.

184. Tunc R, Keyman E, Melikoglu M, Fresko I, Yazici H. Target organ associations in Turkish patients with Behcet's disease: a cross sectional study by exploratory factor analysis. *J Rheumatol.* 2002;29:2393.

185. Pay S, Abbasov T, Erdem H, et al. Serum MMP-2 and MMP-9 in patients with Behçet's disease: do their higher levels correlate to vasculo-Behçet's disease associated with aneurysm formation? *Clin Exp Rheumatol.* 2007;25(4, suppl 45):S70–S75.

186. Yildirim M, Baysal V, Inaloz HS, Doguc D. The significance of serum nitric oxide levels in Behçet's disease and recurrent aphthous stomatitis. *J Dermatol.* 2004;31(12):983–988.

187. Duygulu F, Evereklioglu C, Calis M, Borlu M, Cekmen M, Ascioglu O. Synovial nitric oxide concentrations are increased and correlated with serum levels in patients with active Behçet's disease: a pilot study. *Clin Rheumatol.* 2005;24(4):324–330.

188. Gunduz K, Ozturk G, Sozmen EY. Erythrocyte superoxide dismutase, catalase activities and plasma nitrite and nitrate levels in patients with Behçet disease and recurrent aphthous stomatitis. *Clin Exp Dermatol.* 2004;29(2):176–179.

189. Aydin E, Sögüt S, Ozyurt H, Ozugurlu F, Akyol O. Comparison of serum nitric oxide, malondialdehyde levels, and antioxidant enzyme activities in Behçet's disease with and without ocular disease. *Ophthalmic Res.* 2004;36(3):177–182.

190. Ozkan Y, Yardim-Akaydin S, Sepici A, Engin B, Sepici V, Simşek B. Assessment of homocysteine, neopterin and nitric oxide levels in Behçet's disease. *Clin Chem Lab Med.* 2007;45(1):73–77.

191. Sahin M, Arslan C, Naziroglu M, et al. Asymmetric dimethylarginine and nitric oxide levels as signs of endothelial dysfunction in Behçet's disease. *Ann Clin Lab Sci.* 2006;36(4):449–454.

192. Nakao K, Isashiki Y, Sonoda S, Uchino E, Shimonagano Y, Sakamoto T. Nitric oxide synthase and superoxide dismutase gene polymorphisms in Behçet disease. *Arch Ophthalmol.* 2007;125(2):246–251.

193. Oksel F, Keser G, Ozmen M, et al. Endothelial nitric oxide synthase gene Glu298Asp polymorphism is associated with Behçet's disease [erratum in *Clin Exp Rheumatol.* 2007;25(3):507–508]. *Clin Exp Rheumatol.* 2006;24(5, suppl 42):S79–S82.

194. Karasneh JA, Hajeer AH, Silman A, Worthington J, Ollier WE, Gul A. Polymorphisms in the endothelial nitric oxide synthase gene are associated with Behçet's disease. *Rheumatology (Oxford)* 2005;44(5):614–617.

195. Salvarani C, Boiardi L, Cadsali B, et al. Endothelial nitric oxide synthase gene polymorphisms in Behçet's disease. *J Rheumatol.* 2002;29(3):535–540.

196. Kim JU, Chang HK, Lee SS, et al. Endothelial nitric oxide synthase gene polymorphisms in Behçet's disease and rheumatic diseases with vasculitis. *Ann Rheum Dis.* 2003;62(11):1083–1087.

197. Kara N, Senturk N, Gunes SO, Bagci H, Yigit S, Turanli AY. Lack of evidence for association between endothelial nitric oxide synthase gene polymorphism (glu298asp) with Behçet's disease in the Turkish population. *Arch Dermatol Res.* 2006;297(10):468–471.

198. Akdeniz N, Esrefoglu M, Keleş MS, Karakuzu A, Atasoy M. Serum interleukin-2, interleukin-6, tumour necrosis factor-alpha and nitric oxide levels in patients with Behçet's disease. *Ann Acad Med Singap.* 2004;33(5):596–599.

199. Alpsoy E, Arkman A. Behçet's disease: an algorithmic approach to its treatment. *Arch Dermatol Res.* 2009;30:693.

200. Dalvi SR, Yildirim R, Yazici Y. Behçet's disease. *Drugs.* 2012;72:2223.

201. Turkstra F, van Vugt RM, Dijkmans BA, Yazici Y, Yazici H. Results of a questionnaire on the treatment of patients with Behçet's disease: a trend for more intensive treatment. *Clin Exp Rheumatol.* 2012;30(3, suppl 72):S10–S13.

202. Davatchi F, Sadeghi Abdollahi B, Chams-Davatchi C, et al. Impact of the positive pathergy test on the performance of classification/diagnosis criteria for Behçet's disease. *Mod Rheumatol.* 2013;23(1):125–132. doi:10.1007/s10165-012-0626-9

203. Lamb CA, Kennedy NA, Raine T, et al. British Society of Gastroenterology consensus guidelines on the management of inflammatory bowel disease in adults. *Gut.* 2019;68(suppl 3):s1–s106. doi:10.1136/gutjnl-2019-318484. Erratum in: *Gut.* 2021;70(4):1.

204. Annese V. A review of extraintestinal manifestations and complications of inflammatory bowel disease. *Saudi J Med Sci.* 2019;7(2):66–73. doi:10.4103/sjmms.sjmms_81_18

205. Present DH, Rabinowitz JC, Bank PA, Janowitz HD. Obstructive hydronephropathy. *N Engl J Med.* 1969;280:523.

206. Schneider SL, Foster K, Patel D, Shwayder T. Cutaneous manifestations of metastatic Crohn's disease. *Pediatr Dermatol.* 2018;35(5):566–574. doi:10.1111/pde.13565

207. Buckley C, Bayoumi A-HM, Sarkany I. Metastatic Crohn's disease. *Clin Exp Dermatol.* 1990;15:131.

208. Greuter T, Navarini A, Vavricka SR. Skin manifestations of inflammatory bowel disease. *Clin Rev Allergy Immunol.* 2017;53(3):413–427. doi:10.1007/s12016-017-8617-4

209. Lebwohl M, Fleischmajer R, Janowitz H, Present D, Prioleau PG. Metastatic Crohn's disease. *J Am Acad Dermatol.* 1984;10:33.

210. Aloi FG, Molinero A, Pippione M. Parakeratotic horns in a patient with Crohn's disease. *Clin Exp Dermatol.* 1989;14:79.

211. Murphy MJ, Kogan B, Carlson JA. Granulomatous lymphangitis of the scrotum and penis: report of a case and review of the literature of genital swelling with sarcoidal granulomatous inflammation [review]. *J Cutan Pathol.* 2001;28(8):419–424.

212. Magro CM, Crowson AN. Lichenoid and granulomatous dermatitis: a novel cutaneous reaction pattern. *Int J Dermatol.* 2000;39:126.

213. Witkowski JA, Parish LC, Lewis JE. Crohn's disease, non-caseating granulomas on the legs. *Acta Derm Venereol (Stockholm).* 1977;57:181.

214. Burgdorf W, Orken M. Granulomatous perivasculitis in Crohn's disease. *Arch Dermatol.* 1981;117:674.

215. Magro CM, Crowson AN, Regauer S. Granuloma annulare and necrobiosis lipoidica as a manifestation of systemic disease. *Hum Pathol.* 1996;27:50.

216. Skok P, Skok K. Acute febrile neutrophilic dermatosis in a patient with Crohn's disease: case report and review of the literature. *Acta Dermatovenerol Alp Pannonica Adriat.* 2018;27(3):161–163.

217. Crowson AN, Nuovo GJ, Mihm MC Jr, Magro CM. Cutaneous manifestations of Crohn's disease, its spectrum, and its pathogenesis: intracellular consensus bacterial 16S rRNA is associated with the gastrointestinal but not the cutaneous manifestations of Crohn's disease. *Hum Pathol.* 2003;34(11):1185–1192.

218. Diaz-Perez JL, Winkelmann RK. Cutaneous polyarteritis nodosa. *Arch Dermatol.* 1974;110:407.

219. Hugot JP. CARD15/NOD2 mutations in Crohn's disease. *Ann N Y Acad Sci.* 2006;1072:9–18.

220. King K, Bagnall R, Fisher SA, et al. Identification, evolution, and association study of a novel promoter and first exon of the human NOD2 (CARD15) gene. *Genomics.* 2007;90:493–501.

221. Van Limbergen J, Russell RK, Nimmo ER, et al. Identification, evolution, and association study of a novel promoter and first exon of the human: the genetics of inflammatory bowel disease. *Am J Gastroenterol.* 2007;102(12):2820–2831.

222. Giardin M, Manz M, Manser C, et al. First-line therapies in inflammatory bowel disease. *Digestion.* 2012;86(suppl 1):6.

223. Thomson AB, Gupta M, Freeman HJ. Use of tumor necrosis factor-blockers for Crohn's disease. *World J Gastroenterol.* 2012;18:4823.

224. Brown AC, Rampertab SD, Mullin GE. Existing dietary guidelines for Crohn's disease and ulcerative colitis. *Expert Rev Gastroenterol Hepatol.* 2011;5:411.

225. Collins WJ, Bendig DW, Taylor WF. Pulmonary vasculitis complicating childhood ulcerative colitis. *Gastroenterology.* 1979; 77:1091.

226. Magro F, Gionchetti P, Eliakim R, et al.; European Crohn's and Colitis Organisation [ECCO]. Third European Evidence-based Consensus on diagnosis and management of ulcerative colitis. Part 1: Definitions, diagnosis, extra-intestinal manifestations, pregnancy, cancer surveillance, surgery, and ileo-anal pouch disorders. *J Crohns Colitis.* 2017;11(6):649–670. doi:10.1093/ecco-jcc/jjx008

227. Kedziora JA, Wolff M, Chang J. Limited forms of Wegener's granulomatosis in ulcerative colitis. *Am J Roentgenol Radium Ther Nucl Med.* 1975;125:127.

228. Stiff KM, Cohen PR. Palisaded granulomatous dermatitis associated with ulcerative colitis: a comprehensive literature review. *Cureus.* 2017;9(1):e958. doi:10.7759/cureus.958

229. Stapleton SR, Curley RK, Simpson WA. Cutaneous gangrene secondary to focal thrombosis: an important cutaneous manifestation of ulcerative colitis. *Clin Exp Dermatol.* 1989;14:387.

230. Ball GV, Goldman LN. Chronic ulcerative colitis, skin necrosis, and cryofibrinogenemia. *Ann Intern Med.* 1976;85:464.

231. Beccastrini E, Emmi G, Squatrito D, Nesi G, Almerigogna F, Emmi L. Lobular panniculitis with small vessel vasculitis associated with ulcerative colitis. *Mod Rheumatol.* 2011;21(5):528–531.

232. Barnes L, Lucky AW, Bucuvales JC, Suchy FJ. Pustular pyoderma gangrenosum associated with ulcerative colitis in childhood. *J Am Acad Dermatol.* 1986;15:608.

233. Peters AJ, van de Waal Bake AW, Daha MR, Breeveld FC. Inflammatory bowel disease and ankylosing spondylitis with cutaneous vasculitis, glomerulonephritis and circulating IgA immune complexes. *Ann Rheum Dis.* 1990;49:638.

234. Lissner D, Siegmund B. Ulcerative colitis: current and future treatment strategies. *Dig Dis.* 2013;31:91.

235. Loew BJ, Siegel CA. Foam preparations for the treatment of ulcerative colitis. *Curr Drug Deliv.* 2012;9:338–344.

236. Meier J, Sturm A. Current treatment of ulcerative colitis. *World J Gastroenterol.* 2011;17:3204.

237. Biondi A, Zoccali M, Costa S, Troci A, Contessini-Avesani E, Fichera A. Surgical treatment of ulcerative colitis in the biologic therapy era. *World J Gastroenterol.* 2012;18:1861.

238. Collin P, Reunala T. Recognition and management of the cutaneous manifestations of celiac disease: a guide for dermatologists. *Am J Clin Dermatol.* 2003;4:13.

239. Abenavoli L, Proietti I, Leggio L, et al. Cutaneous manifestations in celiac disease. *World J Gastroenterol.* 2006;12(6):843–852.

240. Reunala T, Salmi TT, Hervonen K, Kaukinen K, Collin P. Dermatitis herpetiformis: a common extraintestinal manifestation of coeliac disease. *Nutrients.* 2018;10(5):602. doi:10.3390/nu10050602

241. Moothy AV, Zimmerman SW, Maxim PE. Dermatitis herpetiformis and celiac disease: association with glomerulonephritis, hypocomplementemia and circulating immune complexes. *JAMA.* 1978;239:2019.

242. Han A, Newell EW, Glanville J, et al. Dietary gluten triggers concomitant activation of CD4+ and CD8+ αβ T cells and γδ T cells in celiac disease. *Proc Natl Acad Sci U S A.* 2013;110:13073.

243. Rodrigo L, Beteta-Gorriti V, Alvarez N, et al. Cutaneous and mucosal manifestations associated with celiac disease. *Nutrients.* 2018;10(7):800. doi:10.3390/nu10070800

244. Agardh D, Borulf S, Lernmark A, Ivarsson SA. Tissue transglutaminase immunoglobulin isotypes in children with untreated and treated celiac disease. *J Pediatr Gastroenterol Nutr.* 2003;36:77.

245. Doe WF, Evans D, Hobbs JR, Booth CC. Celiac disease, vasculitis and cryoglobulinemia. *Gut.* 1972;13:112.

246. Cannistraci C, Lesnoni La Parola I, Cardinali G, et al. Co-localization of IgA and TG3 on healthy skin of coeliac patients. *J Eur Acad Dermatol Venereol.* 2007;21(4):509–514.

247. Freeman HJ. Non-dietary forms of treatment for adult celiac disease. *World J Gastrointest Pharmacol Ther.* 2013;4:108.

248. Pulido O, Zarkadas M, Dubois S, et al. Clinical features and symptom recovery on a gluten-free diet in Canadian adults with celiac disease. *Can J Gastroenterol.* 2013;27:449.

249. Plotnikova N, Miller JL. Dermatitis herpetiformis. *Skin Therapy Lett.* 2013;18:1.

250. Laajam MA, al-Mofarreh MA, al-Zayyani NR. Primary sclerosing cholangitis in chronic ulcerative colitis: report of cases in Arabs and review. *Trop Gastroenterol.* 1992;13:106.

251. O'Donnell B, Kelly P, Dervan P, Powell FC. Generalized elastosis perforans serpiginosa in Down's syndrome. *Clin Exp Dermatol.* 1992;17:31.

252. Al-Ajroush N, Al-Khenaizan S. Isolated nail lichen planus with primary sclerosing cholangitis in a child. *Saudi Med J.* 2007;28(9):1441–1442.

253. Doganci T, Sayli T, Gulderen F, Erden E, Sencer H. Case of disseminated Langerhans' cell histiocytosis presenting with sclerosing cholangitis. *Int J Dermatol.* 2004;43(9):673–675.

254. Terziroli Beretta-Piccoli B, Guillod C, Marsteller I, et al. Primary biliary cholangitis associated with skin disorders: a case report and review of the literature. *Arch Immunol Ther Exp (Warsz).* 2017;65(4):299–309. doi:10.1007/s00005-016-0448-0

255. Harrington AC, Fitzpatrick JE. Cutaneous sarcoidal granulomas in a patient with primary biliary cirrhosis. *Cutis.* 1992;49:271.

256. Zauli D, Crespi C, Miserocchi F, et al. Primary biliary cirrhosis and vitiligo. *J Am Acad Dermatol.* 1986;15:105.

257. Tafarel JR, Lemos LB, Oliveira PM, Lanzoni VP, Ferraz ML. Cutaneous amyloidosis associated with primary biliary cirrhosis. *Eur J Gastroenterol Hepatol.* 2007;19(7):603–605.

258. Humphrey VS, Lee JJ, Supakorndej T, Malik SM, Huen AC, Jaroslaw J. Linear IgA bullous dermatosis preceding the diagnosis of primary sclerosing cholangitis and ulcerative colitis: a case report. *Am J Dermatopathol.* 2019;41(7):498–501.

259. Koulaouzidis A, Campbell S, Bharati A, Leonard N, Azurdia R. Primary biliary cirrhosis associated pustular vasculitis. *Ann Hepatol.* 2006;5(3):177–178.

260. Koulentaki M, Ioannidou D, Stefanidou M, et al. Dermatological manifestations in primary biliary cirrhosis patients: a case control study. *Am J Gastroenterol.* 2006;101(3):541–546.

261. Snook JA, Chapman RW, Fleming K, Jewell DP. Anti-neutrophil nuclear antibody in ulcerative colitis, Crohn's disease and primary sclerosing cholangitis. *Clin Exp Immunol.* 1989;76:30.

262. Hardarson S, LaBrecque DR, Mitros FA, Neil GA, Goeken JA. Antineutrophil cytoplasmic antibody in inflammatory bowel and hepatobiliary diseases: high prevalence in ulcerative colitis, primary sclerosing cholangitis, and autoimmune hepatitis. *Am J Clin Pathol.* 1993;99:277.

263. Terjung B, Spengler U, Sauerbruch T, et al. "Atypical p-ANCA" in IBD and hepatobiliary disorders react with a 50-kilodalton nuclear envelope protein of neutrophils and myeloid cell lines. *Gastroenterology.* 2000;119(2):310–322.

264. Frenzer A, Fierz W, Rundler E, Hammer B, Binek J. Atypical, cytoplasmic and perinuclear anti-neutrophil cytoplasmic antibodies in patients with inflammatory bowel disease. *J Gastroenterol Hepatol.* 1998;13:950.

265. Mohamed AK, Seow CE. Ulcerative colitis with concomitant primary sclerosing cholangitis. *Med J Malaysia.* 2020;75(6):756–758.

266. Chapman RW, Cottone M, Selby WS, Shepherd HA, Sherlock S, Jewell DP. Serum autoantibodies, ulcerative colitis and primary sclerosing cholangitis. *Gut.* 1990;27:86.

267. Trivedi PJ, Hirschfield GM. Review article: overlap syndromes and autoimmune liver disease. *Aliment Pharmacol Ther.* 2012;36:517.

268. Zachou K, Muratori P, Koukoulis GK, et al. Review article: autoimmune hepatitis—current management and challenges. *Aliment Pharmacol Ther.* 2013;38:887.

269. Gatselis NK, Zachou K, Koukoulis GK, Dalekos GN. Autoimmune hepatitis, one disease with many faces: etiopathogenetic, clinico-laboratory and histological characteristics. *World J Gastroenterol.* 2015;21(1):60–83. doi:10.3748/wjg.v21.i1.60

270. Cozzani E, Herzum A, Burlando M, Parodi A. Cutaneous manifestations of HAV, HBV, HCV. *Ital J Dermatol Venerol.* 2021;156(1): 5–12. doi:10.23736/S0392-0488.19.06488-5

271. Sastre L, To-Figueras J, Lens S, et al. Resolution of subclinical porphyria cutanea tarda after hepatitis C eradication with direct-acting anti-virals. *Aliment Pharmacol Ther.* 2020;51(10):968–973. doi:10.1111/apt.15703

272. Antinori S, Esposito R, Aliprandi C, Tadini G. Erythema multiforme and hepatitis C. *Lancet.* 1991;337:428.

273. Byrne JP, Hewitt M, Summerly R. Pyoderma gangrenosum associated with active chronic hepatitis. *Arch Dermatol.* 1976;112:1297

274. Leung AKC, Sergi CM, Lam JM, Leong KF. Gianotti-Crosti syndrome (papular acrodermatitis of childhood) in the era of a viral recrudescence and vaccine opposition. *World J Pediatr.* 2019;15(6):521–527. doi:10.1007/s12519-019-00269-9

275. Jubert C, Pawlotsky JM, Pouget F, et al. Lichen planus and hepatitis C virus–related chronic active hepatitis. *Arch Dermatol.* 1994;130:73.

276. Crowson AN, Magro CM, Nuovo GJ. The dermatopathologic manifestations of hepatitis C infection: a clinical, histological, and molecular assessment of 35 cases. *Hum Pathol.* 2003;34(6):573–579.

277. Tsilika K, Tran A, Trucchi R, et al. Secondary hyperpigmentation during interferon alfa treatment for chronic hepatitis C virus infection. *JAMA Dermatol.* 2013;149(6):675–677.

278. Abdallah MA, Ghozzi MY, Monib HA, et al. Necrolytic acral erythema: a cutaneous sign of hepatitis C virus infection. *J Am Acad Dermatol.* 2005;53:247–251.

279. Halpern AV, Peikin SR, Ferzli P, Heymann WR. Necrolytic acral erythema: an expanding spectrum. *Cutis.* 2009;84(6):301–304.

280. Grauel E, Stechschulte S, Ortega-Loayza AG, Krishna SM, Nunley JR. Necrolytic acral erythema. *J Drugs Dermatol.* 2012;11(11):1370–1371.

281. Spear RL, Winkelman RK. Gianotti-Crosti syndrome: a review of 10 cases not associated with hepatitis B infection. *Arch Dermatol.* 1984;120:891.

282. Monastirli A, Varvarigou A, Pasmatzi E, et al. Gianotti-Crosti syndrome after hepatitis A vaccination. *Acta Derm Venereol.* 2007;87:174–175.

283. Karakaş M, Durdu M, Tuncer I, Cevlik F. Gianotti-Crosti syndrome in a child following hepatitis B virus vaccination. *J Dermatol.* 2007;34(2):117–120.

284. Kang NG, Oh CW. Gianotti-Crosti syndrome following Japanese encephalitis vaccination. *J Korean Med Sci.* 2003;18(3): 459–461.

285. Murphy LA, Buckley C. Gianotti-Crosti syndrome in an infant following immunization. *Pediatr Dermatol.* 2000;17(3): 225–226.

286. Erkek E, Senturk GB, Ozkaya O, Bükülmez G. Gianotti-Crosti syndrome preceded by oral polio vaccine and followed by varicella infection. *Pediatr Dermatol.* 2001;18(6):516–518.

287. Velangi SS, Tidman MJ. Gianotti-Crosti syndrome after measles, mumps and rubella vaccination. *Br J Dermatol.* 1998;139(6): 1122–1123.

288. Cambiaghi S, Scarabelli G, Pistritto G, Gelmetti C. Gianotti-Crosti syndrome in an adult after influenza virus vaccination. *Dermatology.* 1995;191(4):340–341.

289. Bazex A, Salvador R, Dupre A, Christol B. Syndrome paranéoplastique à type d'hyperkeratose des extremitiés. *Bull Soc Fr Dermatol Syphiligr.* 1965;72:182.

290. Räßler F, Goetze S, Elsner P. Acrokeratosis paraneoplastica (Bazex syndrome)—a systematic review on risk factors, diagnosis, prognosis and management. *J Eur Acad Dermatol Venereol.* 2017;31(7):1119–1136.

291. Karabulut AA, Sahin S, Sahin M, Ekşioğlu M, Ustün H. Paraneoplastic acrokeratosis of Bazex (Bazex's syndrome): report of a female case associated with cholangiocarcinoma and review of the published work. *J Dermatol.* 2006;33(12):850–854.

292. Pecora AL, Landsman L, Imgrund SP, Lambert WC. Acrokeratosis neoplastica (Basex syndrome). *Arch Dermatol.* 1983; 119:820.

293. Bazex A, Griffith A. Acrokeratosis paraneoplastica: a new cutaneous marker of malignancy. *Br J Dermatol.* 1980;103:301.

Chapter

17

Metabolic Diseases of the Skin

JOHN C. MAIZE AND JESSICA A. FORCUCCI

AMYLOIDOSIS

Amyloid

The term *amyloid* is applied to extracellular proteinaceous deposits that are resistant to proteolytic digestion and that have distinctive physical properties. Deposits can be localized to a body site or can be "systemic," involving several organs and tissues.

By light microscopy, amyloid appears amorphous, eosinophilic, and hyaline. Characteristic staining qualities distinguish it from other glassy, pink substances. The Congo red stain results in a brick red staining reaction and apple-green birefringence and amyloid stains metachromatically with crystal violet and methyl violet stains. These staining characteristics result from the cross beta-pleated sheet conformation of the polypeptide backbones of the amyloid fibrils. These fibrils are 8 to 12 nm in width and of indeterminate length. Over 30 different proteins have been identified that amyloid deposits are derived from, and it has been recommended that classification of amyloidoses be based on the fibril protein whenever possible (1,2).

Historically, the distinction between AL amyloid (primary systemic amyloidosis resulting from a plasma cell dyscrasia) and AA amyloid (secondary systemic amyloidosis) was made utilizing the latter's sensitivity to permanganate. Immunohistochemistry, immunofluorescence microscopy, immunoelectron microscopy, Western blotting, amino acid sequencing, and mass spectrometry are techniques used in the identification of

fibril proteins, with the latter representing the current state of the art (2–6).

Cutaneous deposition of amyloid can result from any one of several systemic disease processes. However, cutaneous amyloid deposits can also result from local processes limited to the skin.

Systemic Amyloidoses That Involve the Skin
AL (Immunoglobulin Light Chains)

Clinical Summary. In its systemic form, this disease is also known as *primary systemic amyloidosis.* This uncommon disease results from a plasma cell dyscrasia with production of monoclonal light chains of kappa or lambda type (7). The heart, smooth and skeletal muscle, soft tissues, kidneys, liver, and spleen are frequently involved; however, deposits can be localized to the skin or lungs (2). When they are restricted to the skin, the terms *amyloidosis cutis nodularis atrophicans* and *nodular amyloidosis* have been applied (8,9). Heart failure, gastrointestinal bleeding, and renal failure can be fatal complications of the systemic form (10). Petechiae, purpura, and ecchymoses are the most common cutaneous lesions (11). They are the result of involvement of cutaneous blood vessels and are observed mainly on the face, especially on the eyelids and in the periorbital region (Fig. 17-1A). Minor trauma may precipitate these lesions, referred to by some as *pinch purpura* or "raccoon eyes" (12–14). In addition, there may be discrete or coalescing

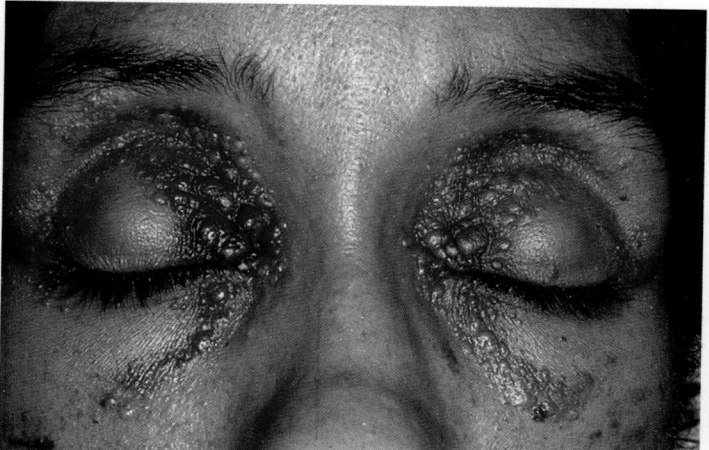
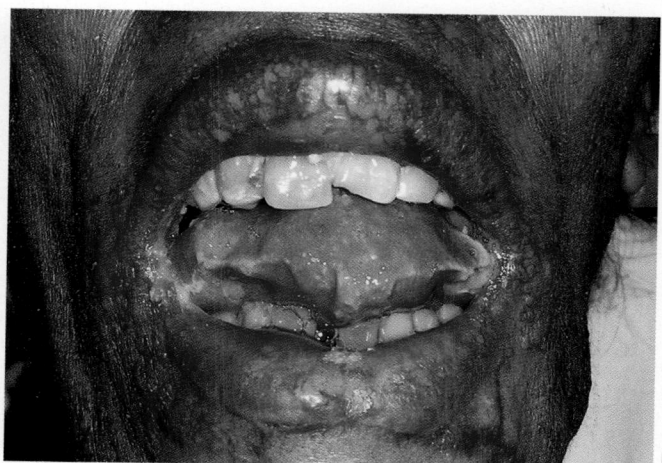

Figure 17-1 *A:* Primary systemic amyloidosis—pinch purpura. Note the papules and ecchymotic appearance in the characteristic periocular location. *B:* Primary systemic amyloidosis—macroglossia. The patient's tongue is enlarged with prominent indentations from continuous pressure against the teeth.

papules or plaques. They usually have a waxy color but may be blue-red as the result of hemorrhage into them (15). In rare instances, one observes firm cutaneous or subcutaneous nodules or plaques or areas of induration of the skin resembling morphea (16). Bullae that may be induced by minor trauma and that may be hemorrhagic occur occasionally (14). Among oral lesions, macroglossia is common, occurring in 17% of patients (10) (Fig. 17-1B).

Histopathology. Examination of cutaneous lesions in the systemic form of the disease reveals faintly eosinophilic, amorphous, often fissured masses of amyloid deposited in the dermis and subcutaneous tissue. Accumulations of amyloid are frequently deposited close to the epidermis. They may or may not be separated from the overlying epidermis by a narrow zone of collagen (Fig. 17-2).

They are rarely deposited around individual elastic fibers (17). The involvement of the walls of blood vessels is responsible for the frequent presence of extravasated erythrocytes. Inflammatory cells are lacking or scarce (14). Several mechanisms of bullous formation have been proposed: (a) the formation of clefts within large dermal amyloid deposits (18), (b) from disruption of basal keratinocytes and the basement membrane zone (14,18), or (c) secondary to inflammatory cell infiltration (18).

In the subcutaneous tissue, there may be large aggregates of amyloid with infiltration of the walls of blood vessels and so-called amyloid rings, which are formed by the deposition of amyloid around individual fat cells (19). The fat cells may then appear as if cemented together by the amyloid.

Even if there are no skin lesions, fine-needle aspirates of the abdominal fat are often of use in documenting the diagnosis, with reported sensitivities and specificities of 55% to 88% and 74% to 100%, respectively (20,21) (Fig. 17-3). Tissue biopsies of normal-appearing skin yield positive results in about 40% of all patients, showing small deposits in the walls of small blood vessels in the dermis or the subcutaneous tissue and occasionally also around eccrine glands and lipocytes. Recommended locations include the forearm (22) or abdomen (23).

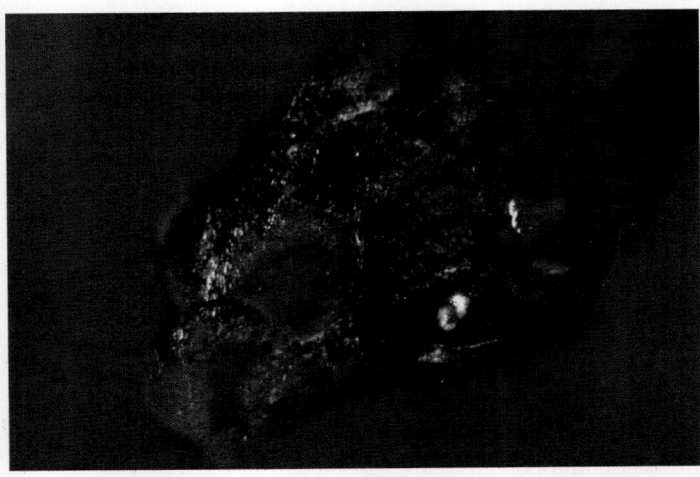

Figure 17-3 Primary systemic amyloidosis. Amyloid deposited in subcutaneous fat exhibits green birefringence under polarized light when stained with Congo red in this aspirate from the abdominal fat pad.

When localized to the skin, nodular amyloid deposits are surrounded by a dense plasmacytic infiltrate, and production of the immunoglobulin light chains is thought to occur locally.

AL amyloidosis results from the production of monoclonal immunoglobulins and/or free light chains, usually lambda light chains, by an abnormal population of plasma cells or B cells. Up to 98% of the patients have detectable monoclonal protein in urine or serum (Bence–Jones protein) (24). Appropriate clinical evaluation for an underlying plasma cell or B-cell dyscrasia is essential. Although the majority of AL amyloidosis arises in a background of monoclonal gammopathy of uncertain significance (MGUS), a subset of cases are associated with multiple myeloma, lymphoplasmacytic lymphoma (LPL), or marginal zone/mucosa-associated lymphoid tissue (MALT) lymphoma (25,26). Systemic amyloidosis is found in 5% to 15% of multiple myeloma patients (27). Additionally, patients with nodular localized cutaneous amyloidosis (see further on) may eventually develop systemic amyloidosis (28).

Pathogenesis. In the systemic form, the amyloid originates from monoclonal immunoglobulin light chains produced by plasma cells in the bone marrow. In the localized form, the amyloid is thought to be produced by the local plasma cell infiltrate, and, as in the systemic form, the amyloid protein has immunocytochemical characteristics of AL amyloid (9,11).

Ultrastructurally, amyloid deposits consist of irregularly arranged, straight, nonbranching filaments that often appear hollow because their peripheries appear electron dense in comparison with their centers. These filaments are 6 to 7 nm in diameter but are of indeterminate length (29,30).

Principles of Treatment: Treatment modalities are aimed at eradicating the pathologic plasma cells and circulating free light chains and include immunosuppressants, chemotherapy, and peripheral blood stem cell transplantation. Irreversible end organ damage may require transplantation.

AA (Serum Amyloid A) Amyloidosis

Clinical Summary. Also known as *secondary systemic amyloidosis*, AA amyloidosis can result from chronic inflammatory disease or recurring bouts of acute inflammation such as tuberculosis, complications of bronchiectasis, and chronic osteomyelitis. It is now relatively rare in industrialized countries since

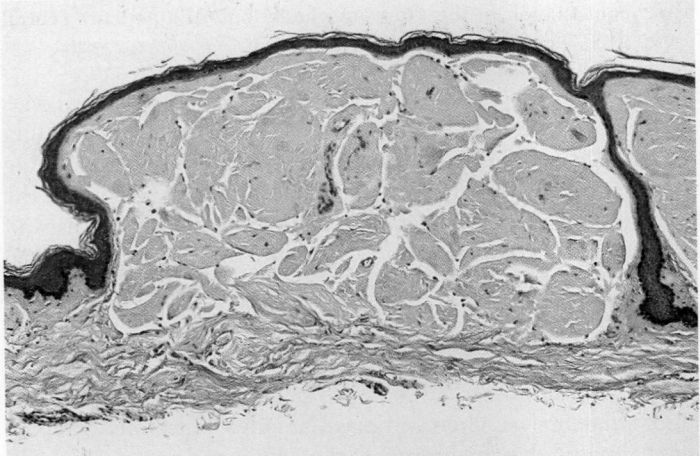

Figure 17-2 Primary systemic amyloidosis. There are amorphous, fissured masses of amyloid in the upper dermis. The amyloid material greatly resembles that observed in colloid milium (see Fig. 17-7, p. 512).

the development of modern antibiotic therapy, and most cases in the United States and Western Europe are associated with chronic rheumatoid arthritis or related disorders (31). Rare cutaneous disease processes cited as causing secondary systemic amyloidosis include vasculitis and epidermolysis bullosa (31–34). At the time of diagnosis, most patients have renal insufficiency or nephrotic syndrome (31). There are typically no cutaneous lesions, although rare reports of nodular and hemorrhagic bullous lesions of the skin containing AA amyloid have been reported (35,36).

Histopathology.   AA amyloid is deposited in parenchymatous organs such as the kidneys, liver, spleen, and adrenals. These deposits are found first in the interstitium and blood vessel walls, then gradually replacing the parenchyma. Deposits within the glomeruli and peritubular tissues result in renal failure.

Fine-needle aspiration of subcutaneous fat with Congo red staining is the most sensitive method of diagnosis (20,37). Tissue biopsy of skin with underlying subcutaneous fat demonstrates deposits of AA amyloid around lipocytes, in blood vessel walls, around eccrine glands, and sometimes free in the dermis (22).

Pathogenesis.   AA amyloid is derived from serum amyloid A (SAA), an acute phase reactant, which is produced by the liver in response to inflammation and regulated by cytokines including interleukin-1, interleukin-6, and tumor necrosis factor-alpha. AA protein is then formed when SAA undergoes carboxy terminal cleavage (38,39). This process takes place within lysosomes of macrophages that are receiving antigenic stimulation by a variety of chronic diseases. The amyloid is then deposited extracellularly using heparan sulfate as a scaffold for fibril assembly (40).

Principles of Treatment: In AA amyloidosis, treatment is generally directed at controlling the underlying infectious/inflammatory process.

Primary Localized Cutaneous Amyloidosis
Lichen Amyloidosis and Macular Amyloidosis

Clinical Summary.   Lichen amyloidosis and macular amyloidosis are best considered as different manifestations of the same disease process. Lichen amyloidosis is characterized by closely set, discrete, brown-red papules that often show some scaling and are most commonly located on the legs, especially the shins, although they may occur elsewhere (Fig. 17-4). These papules may coalesce to form plaques, often with verrucous surfaces sometimes resembling hypertrophic lichen planus or lichen simplex chronicus. Usually, the lesions of lichen amyloidosis itch severely. It is assumed by some authors that the pruritis leads to damage of keratinocytes by scratching and to subsequent production of amyloid (41,42).

Macular amyloidosis is characterized by pruritic macules showing pigmentation with a reticulated or rippled pattern (Fig. 17-5). Although macular amyloidosis may occur anywhere on the trunk or extremities, the upper back is a fairly common site (43). In Southeast Asia, where macular amyloidosis is common, prolonged friction from a rough nylon towel or a back scratcher is thought to be its cause (44). The eruption can be easily misdiagnosed as postinflammatory hyperpigmentation by physicians who are unfamiliar with the condition.

Macular amyloidosis and lichen amyloidosis sometimes occur together in the same patient (so-called biphasic

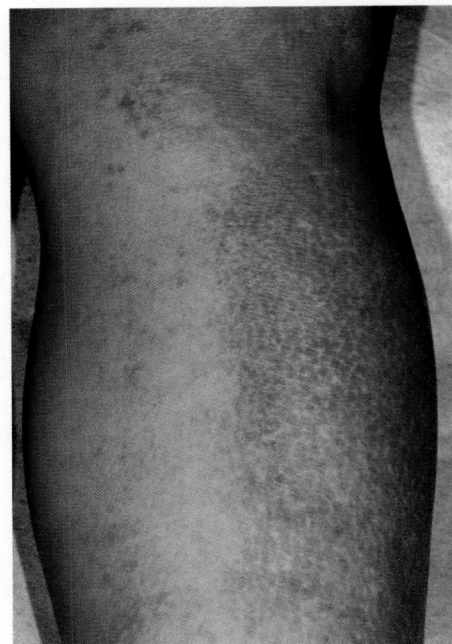

Figure 17-4 Lichen amyloidosis. There are thin, tan to brown papules coalescing into a larger plaque on the anterior lower leg.

Figure 17-5 Macular amyloidosis. Note the rippled appearance of the hyperpigmentation in this close-up photograph of a patient's central upper back, which is a characteristic location.

amyloidosis), and lichen amyloidosis can arise in a setting of macular amyloidosis, presumably because of scratching (44,45). When treated by intralesional injection of steroids, the lichenoid lesions can become macular. Up to 10% of cases of macular and lichen amyloidosis are inherited in an autosomal dominant pattern. These cases of familial primary localized cutaneous amyloidosis can be mapped to a locus on 5p13.1-q11.2 that contains the *OSMR* gene, which encodes the interleukin-6 cytokine receptor OSMRß (46).

Histopathology.   Lichen and macular amyloidosis show deposits of amyloid that are limited to the papillary dermis. Although the deposits are usually smaller in macular amyloidosis than in lichen amyloidosis, differentiation of the two based on the amount of amyloid is not possible. The two conditions differ only in the appearance of the epidermis, which is hyperplastic and hyperkeratotic in lichen amyloidosis (47). Occasionally, the amount of amyloid in macular amyloidosis is so small that it is missed, even when special stains are used. In such instances, more than one biopsy may be necessary to confirm the diagnosis (48).

In areas in which the entire dermal papilla is filled with amyloid, the amyloid appears homogeneous in both lichen and macular forms. In lesions in which the dermal papillae are only partially filled, as is seen more often in macular amyloidosis, the amyloid has a globular appearance and resembles the colloid bodies found in lichen planus (Fig. 17-6). These amyloid bodies in some areas lie in direct contact with the overlying basal cells of the epidermis. Similar colloid bodies are also found in some sections within the epidermis, but in contrast with those located at the dermal–epidermal junction, they do not stain as amyloid. In addition, there is often a striking degree of pigmentary incontinence.

Pathogenesis. The light microscopic findings in lichen and macular amyloidosis suggest that degenerating epidermal cells are discharged into the dermis, where they are converted into amyloid. This theory of primary localized cutaneous amyloid deposition, termed the fibrillar body theory, is supported by electron microscopy (49,50). Also on electron microscopy, the degenerating epidermal cells resemble the colloid bodies observed in lichen planus. They contain the following components: (a) tonofilaments; (b) degenerated, wavy tonofilaments that are thicker but less electron dense than normal tonofilaments; (c) lysosomes; and (d) typical filaments of amyloid, 6 to 10 nm thick, that are straight and nonbranching (50). It is postulated that the degenerated, wavy tonofilaments are recognized as foreign and are digested by the cell's own lysosomes, producing amyloid filaments. A conversion of tonofilaments into amyloid filaments requires that the alpha-pleated sheet configuration of the tonofilaments change into the beta configuration of amyloid (51). However, immunohistochemical studies suggest that components of the lamina densa and anchoring fibrils are also associated with amyloid deposits. Further ultrastructural examination shows disruption of the lamina densa overlying these deposits (52). As such, an alternative hypothesis of primary localized cutaneous amyloid deposition, the secretion theory, has been proposed. This theory suggests amyloid is secreted by disrupted basal cells and assembled at the dermal–epidermal junction. The amyloid then drops into the papillary dermis through a damaged lamina densa (53).

On direct immunofluorescence, all specimens of lichen or macular amyloidosis fluoresce positively for immunoglobulins or complement, particularly immunoglobulin M, complement C3, and immunoglobin A (54). Kappa and lambda light chains are negative (55,56).

The epidermal derivation of the amyloid in lichen and macular amyloidosis is supported by histochemical and immunologic findings. In contrast to the amyloid of systemic amyloidosis, the amyloid of lichenoid and macular amyloidosis shows fluorescence for disulfide bonds, as normally seen in the stratum corneum, suggesting that cross-linking of sulfhydryl groups occurs in amyloidogenesis (57). Furthermore, immunofluorescence and immunohistochemical studies have shown intense staining

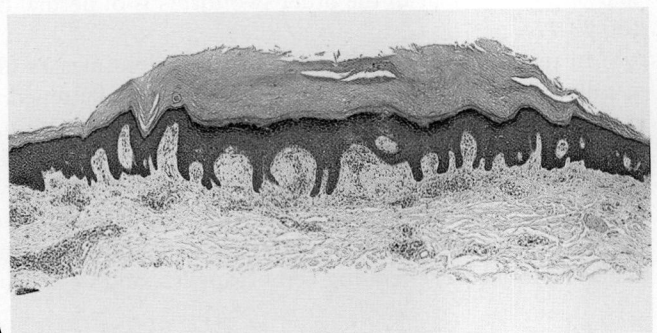

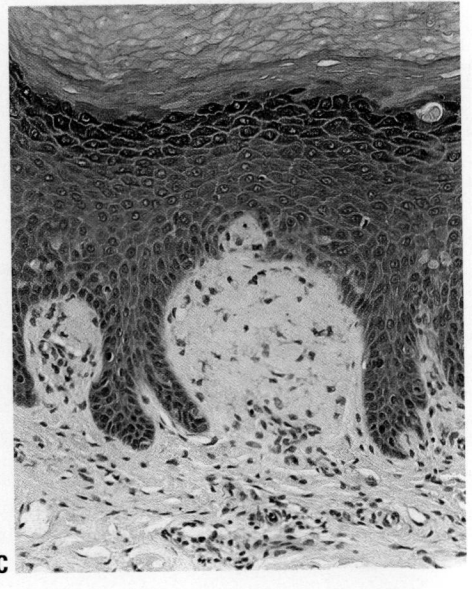

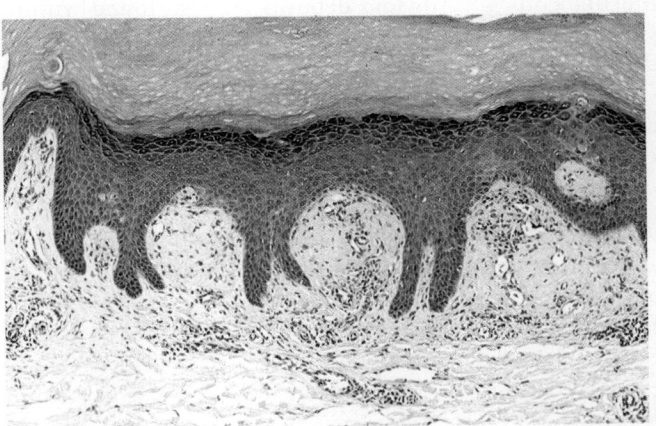

Figure 17-6 Lichen amyloidosis. There is hyperkeratosis and epidermal hyperplasia. Dermal papillae are rounded and contain globular deposits of amyloid. *A:* Hematoxylin and eosin (H&E), original magnification ×40; *B:* H&E, original magnification ×100; *C:* H&E, original magnification ×200.

of the amyloid with antikeratin antibody (58,59). Furthermore, strong cytokeratin 5 and 34ßE12 immunopositivity in lichen and macular amyloidosis suggests the amyloid is derived primarily from basal keratinocytes (59). Other investigators have found direct amyloid fibril formation at the basal surfaces of living basal cells in lichen amyloidosis (60).

The amyloid that may be found in the stroma or in the adjacent connective tissue of basal cell carcinoma and other epithelial tumors has an appearance on electron microscopy and direct immunofluorescence similar to that of lichen and macular amyloidosis, suggesting that it too is derived from tonofilaments (61). This amyloid also shows positive staining with antikeratin antiserum similar to macular and lichen amyloidosis (59).

Principles of Treatment: Treatment is directed toward the relief of pruritis.

Nodular Localized Cutaneous Amyloidosis

Clinical Summary. Nodular localized cutaneous amyloidosis is a rare condition in which nodular deposits of AL amyloid are deposited in the skin without apparent systemic involvement. One or several nodules are encountered, usually on the legs or face, but occasionally elsewhere (8,9,62,63). The nodules may measure from a few millimeters to several centimeters in diameter and typically have a waxy tumefactive appearance. In their centers, the skin may appear atrophic with a white to yellow color (9). Anetodermic and bullous lesions may be encountered, and in exceptional instances, plaques are observed (62,64).

Histopathology. Beneath an atrophic epidermis are large masses of amyloid that extend through the entire dermis into the subcutaneous fat. Amyloid deposits are also found within the walls of blood vessels, in the membrana propria of the sweat glands, and around fat cells (8,28). A lymphoplasmacytic infiltrate is scattered through the masses of amyloid and at the periphery (8,9,28). In addition to clusters of plasma cells, Russell bodies and amyloid-containing foreign-body giant cells may be seen (65).

Pathogenesis. The amyloid is AL and is thought to be derived from local plasma cells. Isolation of plasma cell clones in the cutaneous infiltrates in some cases lends support to this theory, and some have suggested these lesions be considered a form of "low grade B-cell lymphoproliferative disease" (62). Evidence that some of these lesions may be precipitated by antigenic induction in the setting of chronic inflammation is demonstrated by the close association to Sjögren syndrome in some cases (8,63).

Differential Diagnosis. On a histologic basis, differentiation of nodular amyloidosis from primary systemic amyloidosis is not possible.

Principles of Treatment: Techniques to improve the appearance of the lesion (corticosteroids, surgery, electrocautery, lasers, etc.) may be helpful, although lesions may recur.

COLLOID MILIUM AND NODULAR COLLOID DEGENERATION

Clinical Summary. There are four types of colloid degeneration of the skin: (a) juvenile colloid milium, (b) adult colloid milium, (c) nodular colloid degeneration, and (d) pigmented

colloid milium. Juvenile colloid milium and nodular colloid degeneration are very rare, and pigmented colloid milium is exceedingly rare.

Juvenile colloid milium has its onset before puberty and shows numerous round or angular, brownish, waxy papules located mainly on sun-exposed areas, particularly the face (66,67). The lesions typically begin on the face and later develop on the posterior neck and dorsal hands (67). There is a family history in nearly half of the reported cases, and the possibility of a hereditary defect has been postulated (66,68). In some cases, ligneous conjunctivitis and ligneous periodontitis are associated findings (69).

Adult colloid milium, which starts in adult life, is clinically indistinguishable from the juvenile type, except in age of onset (Fig. 17-7). Sun exposure often seems to be a precipitating factor (67). Dermoscopy has been reported to demonstrate a diffuse yellow-orange background with scattered linear and curved vessels (70,71).

Nodular colloid degeneration shows either a single large nodule on the face or multiple nodules on the face, chin, or scalp (72,73). Sun exposure does not seem to play a crucial role, because in some instances, the lesions are limited to the trunk, and a rare case involving the penis has been reported (73,74). Additionally, a case arising in herpes zoster scars has been reported (72).

Pigmented colloid milium is associated with exogenous ochronosis. This form occurs in areas subjected to application of hydroquinone, although exposure to chemical fertilizers has been rarely implicated (75,76).

Histopathology. The colloid in the juvenile form is of epidermal origin, and that in the other two forms is of dermal origin (66,73,77).

In juvenile colloid milium, fissured colloid masses fill the papillary dermis. The overlying epidermis is flattened with no grenz zone sparing, and basal cells show transformation into colloid bodies (67,69). Ultrastructurally, the colloid material is found within individual basal keratinocytes above an intact basement membrane and in extracellular aggregates in the dermis. These deposits contain remnants of nuclear membrane material, degenerating cell organelles, and desmosomes.

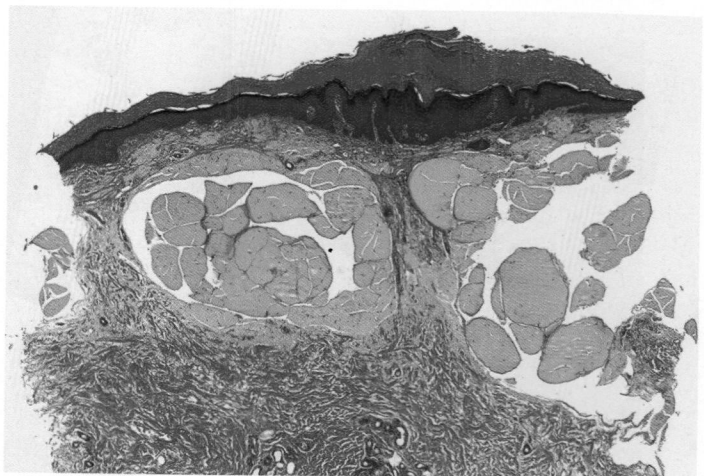

Figure 17-7 Colloid milium, adult type. Homogeneous, fissured masses of colloid are present in the uppermost dermis. The colloid material greatly resembles the amyloid material observed in primary systemic amyloidosis (see Fig. 17-2, p. 509).

The fibrillary structure is similar to that of amyloid ultrastructurally, although staining with Congo red sometimes fails to result in birefringence, and other stains for amyloid are often negative (66,69).

In adult colloid milium, a narrow zone of connective tissue usually separates the homogeneous masses of colloid located in the papillary dermis from the overlying epidermis (Fig. 17-7). Elastic tissue staining shows some elastic fibers in this narrow zone of connective tissue. In addition, solar elastotic fibers are usually seen in the background and at the base of the colloid deposits. Cleft-like spaces containing fibroblasts may be present within the deposits. The colloid deposits in adult colloid milium are usually weakly positive with Congo red and may display weak green birefringence (77).

In nodular colloid degeneration, the epidermis is flattened. The upper three-quarters of the dermis are filled with pale pink, homogeneous material; in some lesions, even the entire dermis is filled with this material (78). A grenz zone is sometimes present. Scattered nuclei of fibroblasts are present within the colloid, along with scattered clefts or fissures, and some dilated capillaries. The hair follicles and sebaceous glands appear well preserved (73).

Pigmented colloid milium is similar to adult colloid milium but contains areas of yellow-brown pigmented globules similar to ochronosis (75).

Pathogenesis. Colloid shows considerable resemblance to amyloid—not only in its histologic appearance but also in its histochemical reactions (77).

Colloid, like amyloid, is periodic acid–Schiff (PAS) positive and diastase resistant. Staining with Congo red results in green birefringence (sometimes weak), and the colloid fluoresces after staining with thioflavin T; however, it does not react with pagoda red or other cotton dyes (9,77). Serum amyloid P is not only a component of normal and abnormal dermal elastic fibers but reportedly can be stained immunocytochemically in adult colloid milium and nodular colloid degeneration (79,80). Juvenile colloid milium, however, exhibits a positive immunostaining reaction to polyclonal antikeratin antibody. This suggests that the histogenesis of this process may differ from that of the adult form in that the colloid in juvenile colloid milium is more likely derived from keratinocytes and related to amyloid K (80).

Electron microscopy in a case of juvenile colloid milium has shown that the colloid consists of tightly packed bundles of filaments, 8 to 10 nm thick, in a wavy or whorled arrangement (69,80,81). The colloid, which forms by filamentous degeneration of tonofilaments, maintains a cytoid configuration in the dermis and may contain nuclear remnants (69,81).

In adult colloid milium, the colloid masses are seen on electron microscopic examination to consist primarily of a granulofibrillar, amorphous substance. On high magnification, very fine, branching, wavy filaments, only 2 nm wide, may be seen embedded in the amorphous substance (77,79). There is rather conclusive evidence that colloid is derived from elastic fibers through sequential degenerative changes. This can be observed at the periphery of the lesion, where colloid is being produced, and within the colloid, where fibrils with a tubular structure and a diameter of 10 nm that are strikingly similar to the microfibrils of elastic fibers can be seen (82). The colloid in adult colloid milium thus represents a final product of severe solar degeneration (77,80).

The colloid in nodular colloid degeneration, similar to that in adult colloid milium, consists of an amorphous substance and short, wavy, irregularly arranged filaments (78). The diameter of these filaments is 3 to 4 nm (72). These electron microscopic findings exclude nodular amyloidosis, because in this condition the filaments have a diameter of about 6 to 7 nm and are long and straight.

Principles of Treatment: Dermabrasion, cryotherapy, photodynamic therapy, and other modalities have been used with limited success.

LIPOID PROTEINOSIS (HYALINOSIS CUTIS ET MUCOSAE; URBACH–WIETHE DISEASE)

Clinical Summary. Lipoid proteinosis is a rare autosomal recessive disorder first described by Siebenmann in 1908. It was established as a distinct clinical and histologic entity by Urbach and Wiethe in 1929. In 1932, Urbach coined the term *lipoid proteinosis* (83).

Clinically, there are papular and nodular lesions on the face. Areas of diffuse infiltration associated with hyperkeratosis are observed on the elbows, knees, hands, and occasionally elsewhere. The papules and nodules on the face cause pitted, pock-like scars, giving the skin a pigskin-leather appearance. Verrucous plaques can form in areas of friction (84). Beads of small nodules may be present along the free margins of the eyelids (moniliform blepharosis). Alopecia may be present from scalp involvement (84,85). The tongue is firm because of diffuse infiltration. Two of the hallmark findings are extension of the infiltration to the frenulum of the tongue, restricting its movement, and infiltration of the vocal cords, causing hoarseness (86). Seizures, an abnormal perception and appraisal of fear, and other neuropsychiatric symptoms are sometimes manifest (85,86).

Histopathology. There is extensive cutaneous deposition of amorphous eosinophilic material surrounding capillaries and sweat coils and in the thickened papillary dermis (Fig. 17-8). Focal deposits are found in the deeper dermis. In verrucous

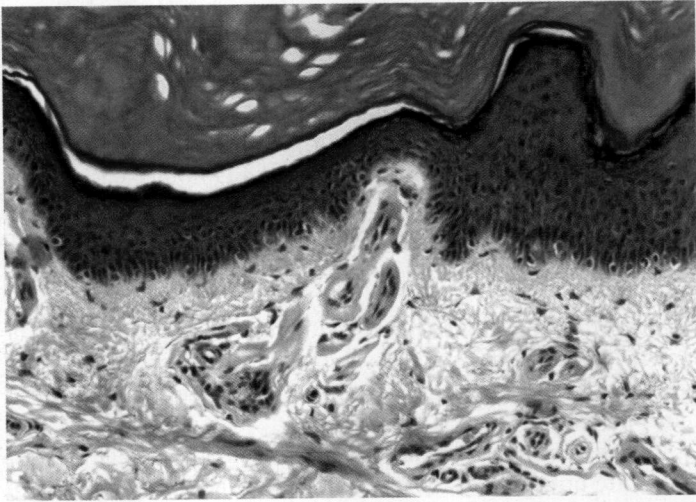

Figure 17-8 Lipoid proteinosis. The hyaline material consists of thick mantles surrounding the blood vessels.

lesions, the homogeneous bundles are often oriented perpendicular to the skin surface. This hyaline material is PAS positive and resistant to diastase digestion. Staining with Alcian blue at pH 2.5 is slightly positive and is sensitive to hyaluronidase digestion. The presence of lipids, highlighted with oil red O and Sudan black stains, is variable and likely results from the adherence of lipids to glycoproteins rather than from abnormal lipid production (87).

Systemic Lesions. Intracranial calcification, noted frequently in brain imaging of patients with lipoid proteinosis, has been held responsible for seizure activity (84,85,87). Autopsy findings have established that the calcium is deposited within the walls of capillaries located in the hippocampal gyri of the temporal lobes (88). The fact that after decalcification a mantle of PAS-positive material is observed around the endothelium of these vessels indicates that hyalinization precedes calcification of the capillary walls (89).

The widespread distribution of the pericapillary hyaline deposits has been established by biopsies and autopsies. Deposits have been found in the submucosae of the gastrointestinal and upper respiratory tracts and in the vagina; in the retina between the vitreous membrane and the pigment epithelium; and in the testes, pancreas, lungs, kidneys, and elsewhere (85,87,89).

Pathogenesis. Two different substances present in lesions of lipoid proteinosis have the light microscopic appearance of hyaline because they consist of homogeneous eosinophilic material and are PAS positive and diastase resistant; however, their different appearances and origins become evident on electron microscopy (87,90). One represents hyaline-like material consisting of multiplications of basal laminae, produced by a variety of cells. The other is true hyaline, and different studies have suggested this material is produced by fibroblasts, as denoted by distinct cytoplasmic vacuoles or by dermal eccrine glands and histiocytes (84,85,91). Abnormal lysosomes with curved tubular profiles in eccrine glands and histiocytes may reflect a defect in the degradation pathway of glycolipids and sphingolipids, similar to lysosomal storage diseases such as Farber disease (84,85). Others have suggested that defective cutaneous lymphatics or microvascular abnormalities may play a role (91).

Lipids are not an essential feature of the disease, and there is variability in the type of lipid and amount present. They can be removed with lipid solvents without damage to the protein–carbohydrate complex of the true hyaline, suggesting they are either free or loosely bound to the hyaline (87,90).

Mutations in the extracellular matrix protein 1 gene (ECM1) have been identified as the cause of lipoid proteinosis (92). The glycoprotein product of this gene is thought to play a functional role in cutaneous physiology and homeostasis. With loss of function of ECM1, there is an accumulation of lipid-like materials in various viscera as well as in the skin, as previously described (87,90). ECM1 appears to have many functions, although loss of its function in binding key components of dermal ground substance and regulation of the bioactivity of matrix components, such as matrix metalloproteinase-9, appears to have a crucial role in the development of lipoid proteinosis (84).

On electron microscopic examination, three major alterations are noted in the dermis: (a) a considerable thickening of basal laminae; (b) massive depositions of amorphous material (hyaline), predominantly in the upper dermis and around blood vessels; and (c) a marked reduction in the number and size of collagen fibrils (84,85). The thickening of the basal laminae in multiple layers is evident around small blood vessels, skin appendages, smooth muscle cells, perineuria, and Schwann cells. In contrast, there is almost no multiplication of the basal lamina of the epidermis (93). Around capillaries, basal laminae are several layers thick, arranged in a concentric "onion-skin" arrangement (85,87). Interspersed between these layers are fine collagen fibrils in an amorphous matrix. The thickened basement membranes stain intensively for laminin and collagen types IV and VII (85,90).

A unique feature of hyalinosis cutis et mucosae consists of large depositions of amorphous material in the dermis. The exact chemical nature of this hyaline material is not known, but it is a noncollagenous glycoprotein that contains neither laminin nor fibronectin (94).

The collagen within the areas of hyaline deposits appears as fine, but otherwise normal, fibrils arranged in bundles or in a random fashion. Most fibrils have a diameter of less than 50 nm, compared with the usual size of 70 to 140 nm. Involved skin shows a fivefold reduction in collagen type I, the major collagen species of normal skin, and to a lesser extent in collagen type III, as indicated by cell culture studies. As judged by the contents of glycine and hydroxyproline, normal skin contains about 80% collagen, but involved skin in lipoid proteinosis contains only 20% collagen as the result of a large accumulation of noncollagenous glycoproteins.

Cultured fibroblasts from lesions of lipoid proteinosis have shown an increased synthesis of noncollagenous proteins at the expense of newly synthesized collagens. The hyaline material in lipoid proteinosis originates from the overproduction of noncollagenous proteins, most of which are normal constituents of human skin (85,94).

Differential Diagnosis. Porphyria shows deposits of hyaline-like material around the superficial dermal capillaries that are usually less dense, but otherwise indistinguishable from the perivascular deposits of hyaline-like material seen in lipoid proteinosis. However, involvement of the membrana propria of the sweat glands is rare, and no true dermal hyaline is present. In addition, the cutaneous lesions in porphyria are limited to sun-exposed areas.

Principles of Treatment: Management depends on organ systems involved and may include dermabrasion for cutaneous lesions and surgical removal of vocal cord polyps. Variable improvement in skin lesions and hoarseness with acitretin and corticosteroids have been reported (95).

PORPHYRIA

Clinical Summary. Eight types of porphyria are recognized (Table 17-1). The light sensitivity in the six types with cutaneous lesions is caused by wavelengths that are absorbed by the porphyrin molecule. These wavelengths lie in the 400-nm range, representing long-wave ultraviolet light (UVA) and visible light (96).

In *erythropoietic porphyria* (Günther disease), a very rare disease that typically develops during infancy or childhood, recurrent vesiculobullous eruptions in sun-exposed areas of the skin gradually result in ulcerations and scarring.

Table 17-1

Classification of the Porphyrias

Porphyrias	Type; Heredity; Onset	Cutaneous Manifestations	Extracutaneous Manifestations	Urine	Feces	Erythrocytes	Enzymatic Defect
Erythropoietic porphyria	Ery; AR; Infancy	Blisters, severe scarring	Red teeth; hemolytic anemia	Uro I	Copro I	Uro I, stable fluorescence	Uroporphyrinogen cosynthase
Erythropoietic protoporphyria	Ery; AD; Childhood	Burning, edema, thickening, rarely blisters	Rarely fatal liver disease	Negative	Protoporphyrin continuously	Protoporphyrin, transient fluorescence	Ferrochelatase (Heme synthase)
Acute intermittent porphyria (AIP)	Hep; AD; Young adulthood	Negative	Abdominal pain, neuropathy, psychoses	ALA, PBG continuously	Negative	Negative	Uroporphyrinogen synthase
Porphyria variegata	Hep; AD; Young adulthood	Same as PCT	Same as AIP	ALA, PBG during attacks	Protoporphyrin continuously	Negative	Protoporphyrinogen oxidase
Porphyria cutanea tarda (PCT)	Hep; AD; Middle age	Blisters, scarring, thickening	Decreased liver function, siderosis	Uro III, continuous fluorescence	Negative	Negative	Uroporphyrinogen decarboxylase
Hepatoerythrocytic porphyria (homozygous form of PCT)	Ery and Hep; AD; Childhood	Blisters, severe scarring, thickening	Decreased liver function	Uro I, Uro III	Copro I, Copro III	Protoporphyrin	Uroporphyrinogen decarboxylase
Hereditary coproporphyria	Hep; AD; Young adulthood	Same as PCT	Same as AIP	Copro, ALA, PBG during attacks	Copro continuously	Negative	Coproporphyrinogen oxidase
Doss porphyria	Hep; AR; Childhood or adulthood	Negative	Abdominal pain, acute and chronic neuropathy	ALA, Copro III	Negative	Protoporphyrin	δ-Aminolaevulinic acid dehydratase

Ery, erythropoietic; AR, autosomal recessive; Uro, uroporphyrin; Copro, coproporphyrin; AD, autosomal dominant; Hep, hepatic; ALA, delta-aminolevulinic acid; PBG, porphobilinogen; PCT, porphyria cutanea tarda; AIP, acute intermittent porphyria.

Repeated scarring and infections in these areas can lead to disfigurement. Areas of hypo- and hyperpigmentation may also be seen. Hydrops fetalis may occur in affected embryos. Hypertrichosis, red fluorescent urine, and reddish-brown stained teeth that fluoresce are additional features (96,97).

In *erythropoietic protoporphyria*, the usual reaction to light is pruritic and burning erythema and edema followed by thickening and superficial scarring of the skin. The skin may take on a waxy or leathery appearance, particularly on the face and hands (98,99). In rare instances, vesicles are present that may resemble those seen in hydroa vacciniforme (100,101). The protoporphyrin is formed in reticulocytes in the bone marrow and is then carried in circulating erythrocytes and in the plasma. When a smear of blood from a patient is examined under a fluorescence microscope, large numbers of red-fluorescing erythrocytes are observed. The protoporphyrin is cleared from the plasma by the liver and excreted into the bile and feces (97). It is not found in the urine (101). In 1% to 4% of patients, fatal liver disease develops quite suddenly, usually in middle age (102) but occasionally only in the second decade of life (103,104).

In *porphyria variegata*, different members of the same family may have either cutaneous manifestations identical to those of porphyria cutanea tarda, systemic involvement analogous to acute intermittent porphyria, both, or the condition may remain latent. It is caused by a deficiency in the activity of protoporphyrinogen oxidase (105–107). The presence of protoporphyrin in the feces distinguishes porphyria variegata from porphyria cutanea tarda. Also, a sharp fluorescence emission peak at 626 nm is specific for the plasma of porphyria variegata (108).

Three forms of *porphyria cutanea tarda* can be distinguished: sporadic, familial, and hepatoerythropoietic (109). In the *sporadic form* (type I), which accounts for approximately 80% of cases (110), only the hepatic activity of uroporphyrinogen decarboxylase is decreased. Almost all patients are adults, and no clinical evidence of porphyria cutanea tarda is found in other members of the patient's family. Although the sporadic form can occur without any precipitating factor, in most instances, in addition to the inherited enzymatic defect, an acquired damaging factor to liver function is needed. Most commonly, this is ethanol, but iron supplements, hemochromatosis, estrogen treatment, and viral hepatitis are also frequently implicated (111–113). In some cases, porphyria cutanea tarda remission has been noted with resolution of the precipitating liver insult (114). A case of paraneoplastic exacerbation and improvement with chemoradiotherapy has also been reported (115).

The *familial form* is subdivided into types II and III and is an autosomal dominantly inherited disorder with low penetrance. In type II, in addition to the hepatic activity, the extrahepatic activity of uroporphyrinogen decarboxylase is decreased to about 50% of normal. The enzymatic activity is usually determined on the erythrocytes. Type III is very rare, and the decreased uroporphyrinogen decarboxylase activity is limited to hepatocytes. The familial form may occur at any age, including childhood, and often, but not always, there is a family history of overt porphyria cutanea tarda (111). A reliable laboratory method for the diagnosis of the porphyrias is now provided by molecular genetics (116,117).

In the very rare *hepatoerythropoietic form*, the skin lesions appear in childhood, and the activity of uroporphyrinogen

decarboxylase in all organs is decreased to 3% to 27% of normal. Family studies suggest that the inheritance pattern in these patients is autosomal recessive and they are either homozygous for the gene that causes porphyria cutanea tarda or compound heterozygous (109,118,119).

Clinically, the sporadic form of porphyria cutanea tarda, by far the most common type of porphyria, shows blisters that arise through a combination of sun exposure and minor trauma, mainly on the dorsa of the hands but sometimes also on the face (Fig. 17-9). Mild scarring may result. The skin of the face and the dorsa of the hands are often thickened and sclerotic. Hypertrichosis of the face is common. Evidence of hepatic cirrhosis with siderosis is regularly present but is generally mild (116). In rare instances, hepatocellular carcinoma or a carcinoma metastatic to the liver induces porphyria cutanea tarda (120,121). In the familial form of porphyria cutanea tarda, the clinical picture is similar to that of the sporadic form, but the changes are more pronounced. In the hepatoerythropoietic form, the manifestations are even more severe. On clinical grounds, the symptoms of most patients resemble those of erythropoietic porphyria, but when symptoms are milder, they resemble those of erythropoietic protoporphyria (122). Vesicular eruptions lead to ulceration, severe scarring, partial alopecia, and sclerosis (118,123,124). Erythrocytes and teeth may show fluorescence (118). Liver damage develops with increasing age (96,125,126). Arthritis is a rare complication (118).

In *hereditary coproporphyria*, a very rare disorder, there are episodic attacks of abdominal pain and a variety of neurologic and psychiatric disturbances analogous to those observed in acute intermittent porphyria and porphyria variegata (96,127). In some cases, there are also cutaneous manifestations indistinguishable from those of porphyria cutanea tarda and porphyria variegata (96,127).

Histopathology. The histologic changes in the skin lesions are the same in all six types of porphyria with cutaneous lesions. Differences are based on the severity rather than on the type of

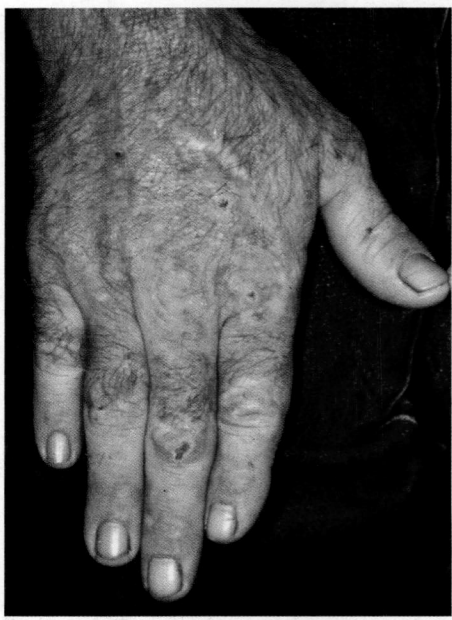

Figure 17-9 Porphyria cutanea tarda. There are crusts from healing vesicles scattered over the dorsal hand. Scars and milia are present on the middorsal hand.

porphyria. Homogeneous, eosinophilic material is regularly observed, and bullae are present in some instances (96,128,129). In addition, sclerosis of the collagen is present in old lesions (129,130).

In mild cases, homogeneous, pale, eosinophilic deposits are limited to the immediate vicinity of the blood vessels in the papillary dermis (96,128,129). These deposits are best visualized with a PAS stain, being PAS positive and diastase resistant (96,129).

In severely involved areas, which are most common in erythropoietic protoporphyria, the perivascular mantles of homogeneous material are wide enough in the papillary dermis to coalesce with those of adjoining capillaries. In addition, deeper blood vessels may show homogeneous material around them, and similar homogeneous material may be found occasionally around eccrine glands (131). PAS staining demonstrates this material particularly well. In some instances, it also contains acid mucopolysaccharides, shown with Alcian blue or colloidal iron (132), or lipids, demonstrable with Sudan IV or Sudan black B (131,133). In addition, the PAS-positive dermal–epidermal basement membrane zone may be thickened (129,132).

In areas of sclerosis, which occur especially in porphyria cutanea tarda, the collagen bundles are thickened. In contrast to scleroderma, PAS-positive, diastase-resistant material is often present in the dermis in perivascular locations (132).

The bullae, which are most common in porphyria cutanea tarda and least common in erythropoietic protoporphyria, arise subepidermally (Fig. 17-10). Some blisters are dermolytic and arise beneath the PAS-positive basement membrane zone, below the sublamina densa (129); others form in the lamina lucida and are situated above the PAS-positive basement membrane zone (129,134) (Fig. 17-11). Some demonstrate bullous pemphigoid antigen, laminin, and types IV and VII collagen on both sides of the blister and thus do not show a defined level of cleavage, whereas others show collagen IV on the roof and collagen VII on both sides, and therefore the level of cleavage is at the level of the sublamina densa. Other cases show all antigens below the plane of cleavage and are intraepidermal (129). Thus, there is no characteristic level of cleavage. It has been suggested that the blisters in porphyria cutanea tarda in mild cases arise within the junctional zone

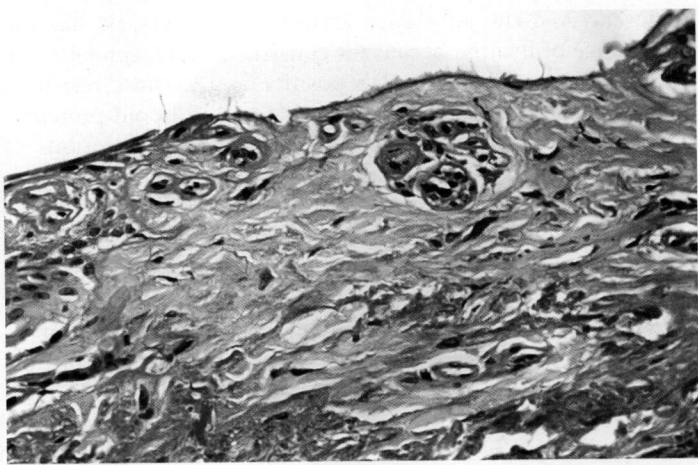

Figure 17-11 Porphyria cutanea tarda. On staining with the periodic acid–Schiff (PAS) reaction after diastase digestion, the PAS-positive basement membrane zone is observed at the floor of the blister. PAS-positive hyaline-like material is present in the walls of capillaries in the upper dermis.

but that in severe cases they form beneath the PAS-positive basement membrane zone and thus heal with scarring (135). It is quite characteristic of the bullae of porphyria cutanea tarda that the dermal papillae often extend irregularly from the floor of the bulla into the bulla cavity (129). This phenomenon, referred to as *festooning*, is explained by the rigidity of the upper dermis induced by the presence of eosinophilic material within and around the capillary walls in the papillae and the papillary dermis.

The epidermis forming the roof of the blister often contains eosinophilic bodies that are elongate and sometimes segmented (136). These "caterpillar bodies" are PAS positive and diastase resistant. Ultrastructurally, they have been found to contain three components: (a) cellular organelles, including melanosomes, desmosomes, and mitochondria; (b) colloid that may be located intracellularly or extracellularly; and (c) electron-dense material thought to be of basement membrane origin (137). Although fairly specific, these structures are not always present, and other conditions may demonstrate "caterpillar body-like" clusters (136).

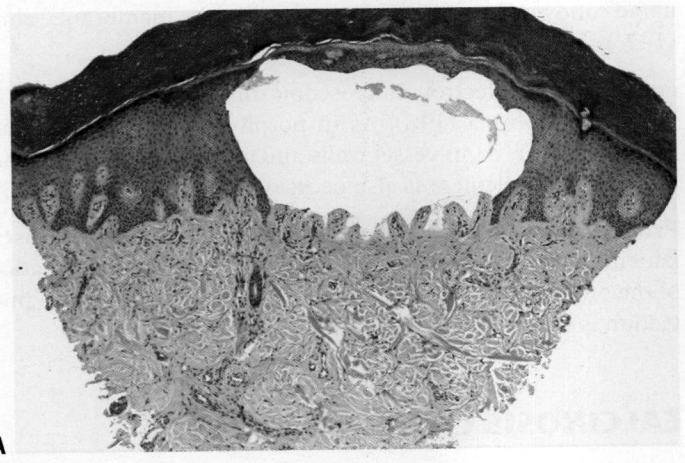

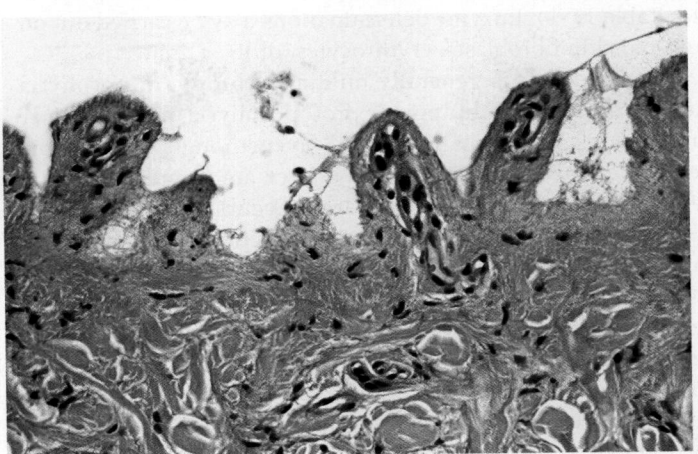

Figure 17-10 Porphyria cutanea tarda. *A:* There is a subepidermal blister. The architecture of the dermal papillae remains intact. The dermis contains no significant inflammatory infiltrate (hematoxylin and eosin [H&E]). *B:* Vessels within preserved dermal papillae at the blister base are surrounded by PAS-positive, diastase-resistant deposits.

Pathogenesis. The substance around dermal vessels has the appearance of hyaline because it consists of homogeneous, eosinophilic material and is PAS positive and diastase resistant; however, just like the perivascular material in lipoid proteinosis, it is only hyaline-like and consists of multiplications of basal laminae (128). True hyaline is absent.

On electron microscopic examination, concentric duplications of the basement membrane around the dermal blood vessels are observed. Peripheral to this multilayered basement membrane, one observes a thick mantle of unlayered material with the same filamentous and amorphous composition as that of the basement membrane (129). Often, a gradual transition from the layered to the unlayered zone can be observed (138,139). Scattered through the thick, unlayered zone are solitary collagen fibrils with an average diameter of only 35 nm, in contrast to the 100 nm of mature collagen (138,140). In cases with severe involvement, presumably from repeated injury to the vessels, intermingled filamentous and amorphous material is seen throughout the upper dermis and even in the middermis.

Because the perivascular material in porphyria represents excessively synthesized basement membrane material, it demonstrates immunofluorescence staining with anti–type IV collagen antibody (129). The presence of small collagen fibrils analogous to reticulum fibrils suggests the presence of type III collagen also (141). Tryptophan, a substance derived from blood and not present in collagen or elastic tissue, is present in the hyaline-like deposits, suggesting that the material is also derived from the vessel wall and leakiness of its contents (129).

Direct immunofluorescence studies have demonstrated deposition of immunoglobulins, particularly immunoglobulin G (IgG) and complement C3, and to a lesser extent IgA and IgM, in the vessel walls and at the dermal–epidermal junction of light-exposed skin. IgG is more persistent throughout inactive and treated phases of the disease (129). It has been deemed unlikely by some that these deposits indicate an immunologic phenomenon and that, instead, they are the result of "trapping" of immunoglobulins and complement in the filamentous material. Observations of conditions where the complement cascade has been inactivated or inhibited, however, suggest that complement activation may play a key role in the development of endothelial injury in cutaneous lesions of porphyria (129,142).

The *enzymatic defect* in each form of porphyria is known (see Table 17-1). Enzyme determinations may be carried out on cultured skin fibroblasts, erythrocytes, or liver tissue.

Liver damage is generally mild and chronic in porphyria cutanea tarda. In erythropoietic protoporphyria, however, liver function tests are usually normal, even though microscopic deposits of protoporphyrin in the liver are found frequently (98,101). Yet, in rare instances, death occurs from liver failure developing swiftly after the initial detection of hepatic dysfunction (143). Patients with liver failure have very high levels of protoporphyrin in the erythrocytes and show extensive deposits of protoporphyrin in a cirrhotic liver at the time of death. The protoporphyrin in hepatocytes and Kupffer cells appears as dark brown granules (143). This pigment exhibits birefringence on polariscopic examination, and in unstained sections viewed with ultraviolet light it shows red autofluorescence (143). In patients with normal liver function tests, biopsy of the liver may or may not show portal and periportal fibrosis (144).

Principles of Treatment: Discontinuance of risk factors (alcohol, offending drugs, iron supplements, etc.) is recommended. Administration of hemin aids in acute attacks. Avoidance of sunlight and phlebotomy are mainstays of treatment for cutaneous lesions. Low dose 4-aminoquinoline regimens (hydroxychloroquine) have been used with success, but relapse rates are higher than phlebotomy (145). Abdominal, cardiac, and nervous system manifestations are treated symptomatically.

Pseudoporphyria Cutanea Tarda

Clinical Summary. In patients with chronic renal failure who are receiving maintenance hemodialysis, an eruption indistinguishable from that of porphyria cutanea tarda may develop on the dorsa of the hands and fingers during the summer months (146). Rarely, blisters are also seen on the face, and atrophic scarring develops (147). Large case series of patients receiving hemodialysis have shown that 1% to 18% of patients showed this type of eruption (148–150). Normal porphyrin levels in urine, stool, and plasma are the rule in hemodialyzed patients developing clinical signs of porphyria cutanea tarda, although a true porphyria cutanea tarda may coexist (150,151). In such patients, if a certain degree of diuresis persists, urinalysis may not be representative of the porphyria metabolism, and the plasma and fecal porphyrins should always be measured (152).

Pseudoporphyria cutanea tarda may also occur following the ingestion of certain drugs, such as naproxen, furosemide, nalidixic acid, tetracycline hydrochloride, hydrochlorothiazide, retinoids, voriconazole, cyclosporine, oral contraceptives, finasteride, metformin, olanzapine, imatinib, sunitinib, and chlorophyll supplements (153–162). Because many patients on hemodialysis for renal failure are also receiving furosemide, withdrawal of the drug can determine whether the dialysis or the medication is the cause of the pseudoporphyria, because in drug-induced cases, withdrawal of the drug is curative (163,164).

Histopathology. In patients with pseudoporphyria, the histologic picture is indistinguishable from that seen in mild cases of porphyria. The superficial blood vessels show thickened walls, and the PAS-positive basement membrane zone is often thickened as well. Blisters are subepidermal, with festooned dermal papillae. The blisters are usually situated above the PAS-positive basement membrane zone (147,148,152,154,163).

Pathogenesis. Electron microscopic findings are identical to those of porphyria (148). As in porphyria, immunoglobulins are often observed in vessel walls and at the dermal–epidermal junction. Complement is also occasionally present (146–148).

Principles of Treatment: For hemodialysis-associated cases, patients may be treated with N-acetylcysteine. Discontinuation of the offending agents suffices in drug-induced cases. Sun protection is recommended.

CALCINOSIS CUTIS

There are four forms of calcinosis cutis: metastatic calcinosis cutis, dystrophic calcinosis cutis, idiopathic calcinosis cutis, and subepidermal calcified nodule.

Metastatic Calcinosis Cutis

Clinical Summary. Metastatic calcification develops as the result of hypercalcemia or hyperphosphatemia. Hypercalcemia may result from (a) primary hyperparathyroidism, (b) excessive intake of vitamin D, (c) excessive intake of milk and alkali (165), or (d) extensive destruction of bone by metastases (166). Other associated conditions reported include alcoholic liver disease, systemic lupus erythematosus, rheumatoid arthritis, diabetes, protein C or S deficiency, and Crohn disease (166–168). Hyperphosphatemia occurs in chronic renal failure as the result of a decrease in renal clearance of phosphorus and is associated with a compensatory drop in the serum calcium level. The low level of ionized calcium in the serum stimulates parathyroid secretion, leading to secondary hyperparathyroidism and to resorption of calcium and phosphorus from bone. The demineralization of bone causes both osteodystrophy and metastatic calcification (169).

Metastatic calcification most commonly affects the media of the arteries, periarticular regions, and the kidneys. In addition, other visceral organs, such as the myocardium, the stomach, and the lungs may be involved (170). Within the vessels, this is thought to occur primarily by osteoblastic transdifferentiation of vascular smooth muscle cells in response to uremic serum, hyperphosphatemia, and hypercalcemia (169,171).

Metastatic calcification in the subcutaneous tissue is occasionally observed in association with renal hyperparathyroidism (172), in uremia (173), in hypervitaminosis D (165), and as the result of excessive intake of milk and alkali (165) but rarely in primary hyperparathyroidism (174,175). Palpable, hard nodules, occasionally of considerable size, are located mainly in the vicinity of the large joints (165,176). With increasing size, the nodules may become fluctuant (177).

Calciphylaxis, or calcific uremic arteriolopathy, is a life-threatening condition in which there is progressive calcification of small- and medium-sized vessels of the subcutis often accompanied by necrosis. It most frequently arises in the setting of hyperparathyroidism associated with chronic renal failure, although nonuremic cases attributed to various factors, including warfarin (178), chronic corticosteroid use, and rapid weight loss (179), have been reported. Calciphylaxis is often associated with an elevated serum calcium/phosphate product, with other factors, including several glycoproteins (matrix G1a protein and glycopontin) likely playing a role in the development of vascular calcification (180).

Clinically, the lesions present as a panniculitis or vasculitis. Bullae, ulcerations, or a livedo reticularis–like eruption can be present (165,168). Potential complications of gangrene, sepsis, pancreatitis, and multisystem organ failure contribute to an overall mortality of 60% to 80% (181–184).

Instances of *cutaneous metastatic calcinosis* are rare. Most reports have concerned patients with renal hyperparathyroidism and osteodystrophy. The cutaneous lesions may consist of tender, firm, white to erythematous papules, nodules, or plaques (185,186). Papules in a linear arrangement (177) and symmetric, nodular plaques may occur (187). The lesions may ulcerate and a chalky, white substance can be expressed (185).

Mural calcification of arteries and arterioles in the deep dermis or subcutaneous tissue occurs rarely in primary hyperparathyroidism (166) but somewhat more frequently in secondary

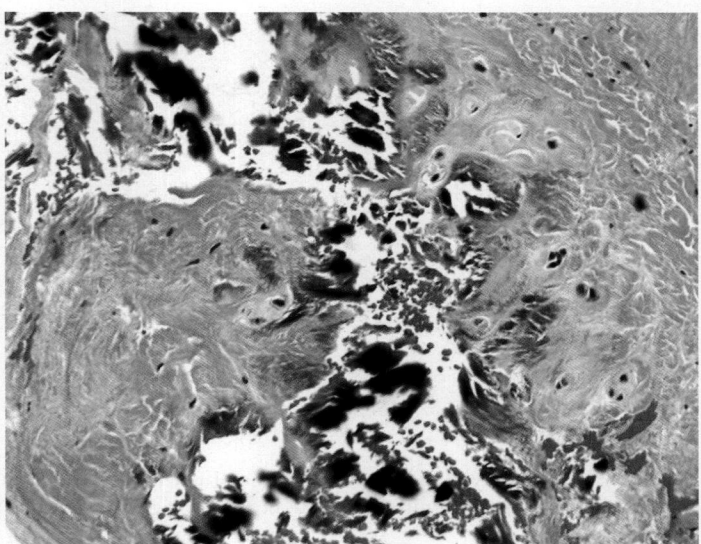

Figure 17-12 Metastatic calcinosis cutis. Amorphous deposits of basophilic material are present in the dermis.

hyperparathyroidism subsequent to renal disease, particularly if subsequent to dialysis for chronic renal disease or to renal allograft (166,188). This may lead to occlusion of these vessels and to infarctive ulcerations, especially on the legs.

Histopathology. Calcium deposits are easily recognized in histologic sections, because they stain deep blue with hematoxylin and eosin (H&E). They stain black with the von Kossa stain for calcium phosphate. As a rule, the calcium occurs as massive deposits when located in the subcutaneous fat and usually as granules and small deposits when located in the dermis (Fig. 17-12). Large deposits of calcium often evoke a foreign-body reaction; thus, giant cells, an inflammatory infiltrate, and fibrosis may be present around them (189,190).

In areas of infarctive necrosis, as a result of calcification of dermal or subcutaneous arteries or arterioles, the involved vessels show calcification of their walls and intravascular fibrosis with attempts at recanalization of the obstructed lumina (180,190). Mural calcification is often most pronounced in the internal elastic membranes of arteries or arterioles (190).

The histologic changes in calciphylaxis include calcium deposits in the subcutis, chiefly within the walls of small- and medium-sized vessels (Fig. 17-13). These deposits can be associated with endovascular fibrosis, thrombosis, or global calcific obliteration (190). The fully evolved disease process shows, in addition, areas of necrosis with a clean background or accompanied by neutrophils (189,191).

It is particularly important that these findings be recognized in order that appropriate therapy might be instituted immediately; however, the histologic changes must be considered in the context of the clinical presentation, because similar changes can be seen in asymptomatic patients with chronic kidney disease (192).

Principles of Treatment: Treatment is aimed at reducing serum calcium and phosphate levels and may include calcimimetics, bisphosphanates, and parathyroidectomy. Intravenous or intralesional sodium thiosulfate have also been used (193). Patients may also benefit from wound care, pain management, and nutrition optimization (194).

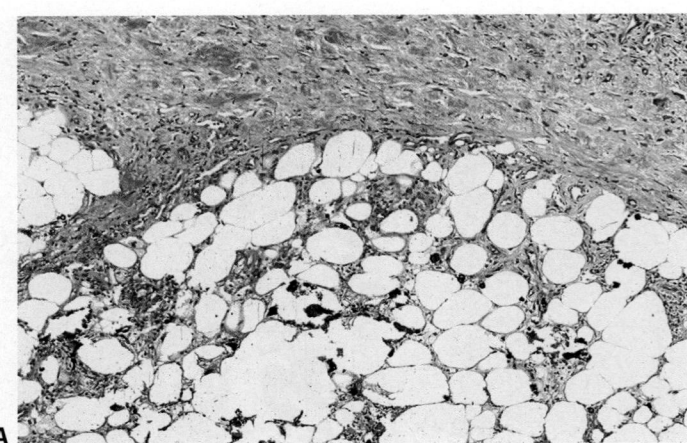
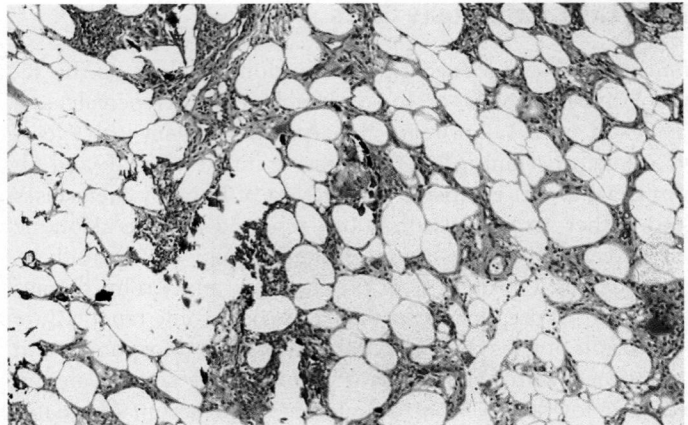

Figure 17-13 Calciphylaxis. There is a panniculitis with associated calcification of soft tissues in the walls of small vessels. *A:* Hematoxylin and eosin (H&E), original magnification ×20; *B:* H&E, original magnification ×100.

Dystrophic Calcinosis Cutis

Clinical Summary. In dystrophic calcinosis cutis, the calcium is deposited in previously damaged tissue. The values for serum calcium and phosphorus are normal, and the internal organs are spared. There may be numerous large deposits of calcium (calcinosis universalis) or only a few deposits (calcinosis circumscripta).

Calcinosis universalis occurs as a rule in patients with dermatomyositis (Fig. 17-14), but exceptionally it has also been observed in patients with systemic scleroderma, systemic lupus erythematosus, and connective tissue overlap diseases, and it may follow infections or trauma (195,196). Exceedingly rare cases may precede the onset of an underlying connective tissue disorder (197). Large deposits of calcium are found in the skin and subcutaneous tissue and often in muscles and tendons (198). In dermatomyositis, if the patient survives, the nodules of dystrophic calcinosis gradually resolve.

Calcinosis circumscripta occurs as a rule in patients with systemic scleroderma; rarely, however, it may be observed in patients with widespread morphea (199,200). Generally, in the

presence of calcinosis, systemic scleroderma manifests itself as acrosclerosis. The association of acrosclerosis and calcinosis is often referred to as the *Thibierge–Weissenbach syndrome,* or as the *CREST syndrome,* because the manifestations usually consist of calcinosis cutis, Raynaud phenomenon, esophageal dysfunction, sclerodactyly, and telangiectasia (165,201). Patients with this syndrome often have a better prognosis than those with generalized scleroderma or systemic sclerosis. Clinically, calcinosis circumscripta shows successively appearing areas of induration that often break down and extrude white, chalky material.

In addition to occurring in the connective tissue diseases, dystrophic calcinosis is often seen in subcutaneous fat necrosis of the newborn and, rarely, in inherited disorders such as Ehlers–Danlos disease, Werner syndrome, and pseudoxanthoma elasticum (202).

Histopathology. As in metastatic calcinosis cutis, the calcium in dystrophic calcinosis cutis is usually present as granules or small deposits in the dermis and as massive deposits in the subcutaneous tissue. A foreign-body giant-cell reaction with inflammation and fibrosis is often found around large deposits of calcium (165). The calcium deposits usually are located in areas in which the collagen or fatty tissue appears degenerated as a result of the disease preceding the calcinosis.

Principles of Treatment: Treatment is guided at pain relief and cosmesis. Intralesional corticosteroids have limited benefit, and other therapies such as etidronate disodium, aluminum hydroxide, calcium channel blockers, low dose anticoagulants, and bisphosphonates have shown only slightly better results. As with calciphylaxis, cases of successful intravenous or intralesional sodium thiosulfate have also been reported (203). Surgical removal may be required for severe cases and when lesions impair function, although recurrence or new lesions may result.

Idiopathic Calcinosis Cutis

Clinical Summary. Even though the underlying connective tissue disease in some instances of dystrophic calcinosis cutis may be mild and can be overlooked unless specifically searched for, there remain cases of idiopathic calcinosis cutis that resemble dystrophic calcinosis cutis but show no underlying disease (199,204,205).

Figure 17-14 Dystrophic calcinosis cutis. Granules and globules of calcium are located beneath the epidermis. This biopsy is from the buttock of a child with dermatomyositis who had extensive calcification also of muscles and tendons.

One entity is regarded as a special manifestation of idiopathic calcinosis cutis: tumoral calcinosis. It consists of solitary or numerous large, subcutaneous, calcified masses, generally along extensor surfaces of large joints, which may be associated with papular and nodular skin lesions of calcinosis (202,206,207). Dental manifestations from calcifications of the pulp may be present (206). The autosomal recessively inherited form, hyperphosphatemic familial tumoral calcinosis is caused by mutations in three genes involved in fibroblast growth factor-23 function, *FGF23*, *KL*, and *GALNT3* (202,206,208,209). Otherwise, the similarities of tumoral calcinosis to the dystrophic calcinosis universalis observed with dermatomyositis are marked.

Histopathology. Tumoral calcinosis shows large subcutaneous or intramuscular masses of calcium surrounded by a foreign-body reaction (165,202,206,210). Intradermal aggregates are present in some cases (165,206). Discharge of calcium may take place through areas of ulceration or by means of transepidermal elimination (165,207). The inactive phase of the disease typically shows dense fibrous septa without cellular elements (206,211).

Pathogenesis. Lesions of idiopathic calcinosis cutis studied by electron microscopy show that the deposits consist of pleomorphic calcium phosphate (hydroxyapatite) crystals (210). These deposits of calcium have been observed within collagen fibrils and situated in the ground substance (212,213). Many ultrastructural studies have implicated intramitochondrial calcification in histiocytes as the principal calcifying process in tumoral calcinosis (210,214).

Principles of Treatment: Surgical excision combined with phosphate deprivation and acetazolamide has proven to be effective. Successful use of topical sodium thiosulphate has also been reported (215)

Idiopathic Calcinosis of the Scrotum

Clinical Summary. Idiopathic calcinosis of the scrotum consists of multiple asymptomatic nodules of the scrotal skin. The nodules usually begin to appear in the third decade of life, although onset as early as 9 years of age or as late as 85 years has been reported. They increase in size and number, are rarely pruritic, and sometimes break down to discharge their chalky contents (216).

Histopathology. Originally, the accepted view was that some of the calcific masses in calcinosis of the scrotum were surrounded by a granulomatous foreign-body reaction and that others were not (217). However, in recent studies in which numerous scrotal nodules were examined at different times in the same patients, some of the smaller lesions were epidermal cysts, whereas other cystic lesions showed calcification of their keratin contents, and still others showed ruptures of their epithelial walls. The cyst wall seems to eventually be destroyed, leaving only dermal collections of calcium that can become larger. Thus, according to this view, calcinosis of the scrotum represents the end stage of dystrophic calcification of scrotal epidermal cysts (217). It can be assumed that many early lesions start out as cysts but, as they age and calcify, lose their cyst walls. In some cases, eccrine duct milia have been favored as the origin because of positive reactions for carcinoembryonic antigen and epithelial membrane antigen, markers of eccrine differentiation (218). Some reports have alternatively suggested dartoic muscle degeneration as a possible etiology (219). It is likely that these lesions are commonly derived from epidermal cysts, although the cause may potentially be multifactorial, and that in cases without definitive pathogenesis designation as idiopathic remains appropriate.

Principles of Treatment: Treatment is limited to surgical excision, with only rare reports of recurrence (220).

Subepidermal Calcified Nodule

Clinical Summary. In subepidermal calcified nodule, also referred to as *cutaneous calculi*, a single, small, raised, hard nodule is usually present, typically on the face. Occasionally, however, there are two or three nodules and in some instances numerous or even innumerable nodules. Most patients are children; however, in some patients, a nodule is present at birth or does not appear until adulthood (221). A male predominance with a ratio of 2:1 has been observed (222). In most instances, the surface of the nodule is verrucous, but it may be smooth, and lesions may mimic verruca vulgaris, molluscum contagiosum, or eruptive xanthoma (222–224).

Histopathology. The calcified material is located predominantly in the uppermost dermis, although in large nodules it may extend into the deep layers of the dermis. The calcium is present largely as closely aggregated globules (Fig. 17-15). In some instances, however, there is also one or several large, homogeneous masses of calcified material (222,225). Both the globules and the homogeneous masses occasionally contain well-preserved nuclei (225). A lymphohistiocytic infiltrate, macrophages, and foreign-body giant cells may be arranged around the large, homogeneous masses (222,225). The epidermis is often hypertrophic. Calcium granules may be observed within the epidermis, indicative of transepidermal elimination (222,226).

Pathogenesis. The primary event seems to be the formation of large, homogeneous masses that undergo calcification and break up into numerous calcified globules. The origin of the homogeneous masses is obscure. It is not likely that they originate from a specific preexisting structure, such as sweat ducts or nevus cells, as has been assumed. Some suggest degranulation of mast cells with subsequent calcium and phosphate deposition as the etiology (227).

Principles of Treatment: Treatment is typically surgical excision.

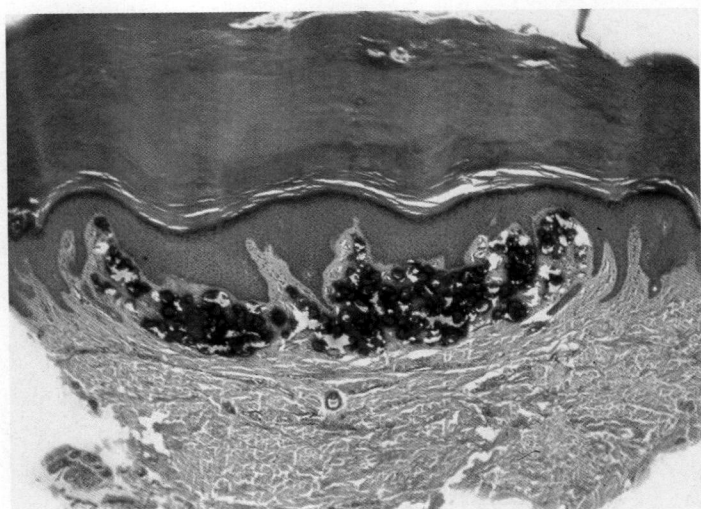

Figure 17-15 Subepidermal calcified nodule. A large deposit of calcium in the dermis distorts the overlying epidermis (hematoxylin and eosin).

GOUT

Clinical Summary. Gout was recently defined by expert consensus as "the presence of monosodium urate crystals with clinical disease" (228). In the early stage of gout, there are usually irregularly recurring attacks of acute arthritis. In the late stage, deposits of monosodium urate form within and around various joints, leading to chronic arthritis with destruction of the joints and the adjoining bone. During this late stage, urate deposits, called *tophi*, may occur in the dermis and subcutaneous tissue in 12% to 35% of patients (229). With improved treatments, the incidence of tophaceous lesions in gout significantly decreased from 14% in 1949 to 3% in 1972, even though the incidence of gout remained unchanged (230). Currently, tophi are present in less than 10% of gout patients (231). The prevalence of gout continues to increase in Western countries and Southeast Asia, along with obesity and metabolic syndrome (232). Tophaceous gout usually develops within 5 years of the initial onset of gout in 30% of untreated patients (233).

Cutaneous tophi are observed most commonly on the helix of the ears, olecranon bursae, and on the fingers and toes (233,234) (Fig. 17-16). They may attain a diameter of several centimeters. When large, tophi may discharge a chalky material (233), and may become chronic tophaceous wounds and ulcers, a sequela that can be very difficult to treat (235). In rare instances, gout may present as tophi on the fingertips or as panniculitis on the legs without the coexistence of a gouty arthritis (236,237). Exceedingly rare instances of disseminated miliarial or papulonodular lesions have been reported (238–240).

Histopathology. For the histologic examination of tophi, fixation in absolute ethanol or an ethanol-based fixative, such as Carnoy fluid, is preferable to fixation in formalin; it has been stated that aqueous fixatives such as formalin dissolve the characteristic urate crystals, leaving only amorphous material (241). However, some authors contend that formalin-fixed, paraffin-embedded tissue that is sectioned, floated in alcohol (as opposed to a water bath), and then placed onto a slide without staining will display refractile crystals when examined under polarized light (242). Unstained coverslipped thick sections of paraffin-embedded formalin-fixed tissue may preserve birefringent crystals in about 50% of cases (243). An alternate staining protocol to preserve any urate crystals remaining in formalin-fixed tissue after processing utilizes nonaqueous alcoholic eosin staining (244).

On fixation in alcohol, tophi can be seen to consist of variously sized, sharply demarcated aggregates of needle-shaped urate crystals lying closely packed in the form of bundles or sheaves (Fig. 17-17). The crystals often have a brownish color and are doubly refractile on polariscopic examination (Fig. 17-18). If a red compensator is used along with polarizing filters in tissue that has been processed to preserve crystals, the crystals will appear yellow when they are parallel to the direction of the compensator and blue when perpendicular to it (245). The aggregates of urate crystals are often surrounded by a palisaded granulomatous infiltrate containing many foreign-body giant cells (Fig. 17-17). The urate crystals appear black and the surrounding tissue yellow when the sections are stained with 20% silver nitrate solution (246).

Even when the specimen has been fixed in formalin, the diagnosis of gout can be made without difficulty because of the characteristic rim of foreign-body giant cells and macrophages surrounding the aggregates of amorphous material. As a secondary phenomenon, calcification, and occasionally ossification, may take place in the sodium urate aggregates.

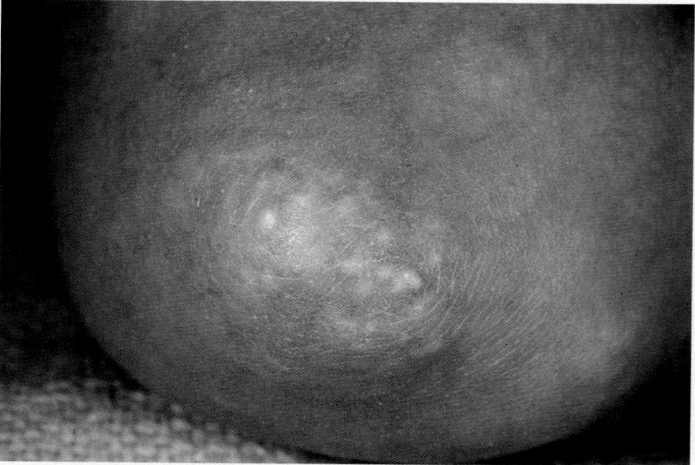

Figure 17-16 Gouty tophi. There are yellow-white urate deposits on the elbow.

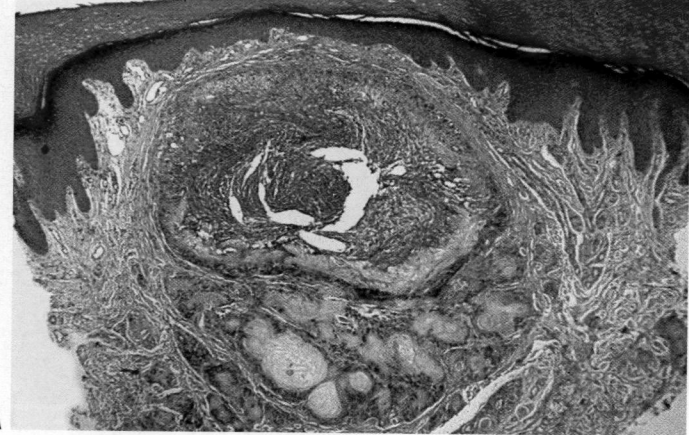
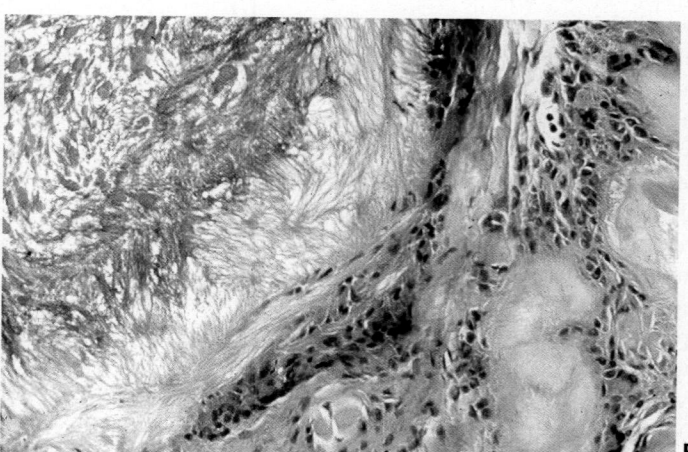

Figure 17-17 Gouty tophus. *A:* There are deposits of urate crystals in the reticular dermis that have a radial array. The lucent areas show where some urate crystals were removed during processing of the tissue (hematoxylin and eosin [H&E]). *B:* There are macrophages and multinucleated giant cells surrounding the urate deposits in the dermis (H&E).

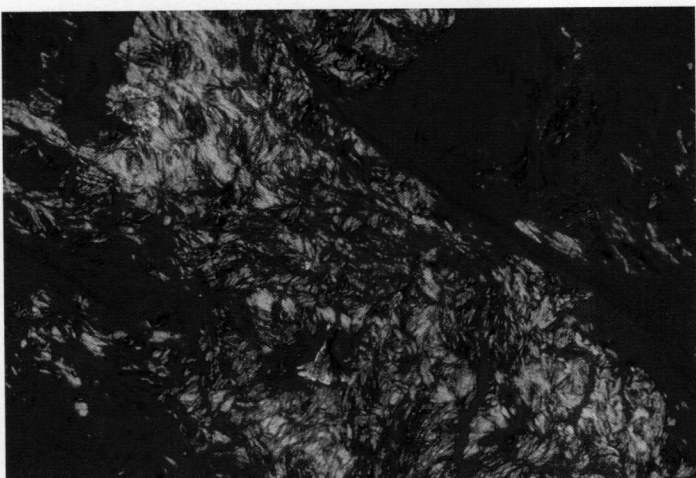

Figure 17-18 Gouty tophus. Polarization with a red filter reveals birefringent blue urate crystals in a gouty tophus.

Pathogenesis. Gout is a complex disorder characterized by hyperuricemia. An asymptomatic stage of hyperuricemia precedes the development of gouty arthritis by many years. Patients with gout are a heterogeneous group. In some patients, diminished renal excretion of uric acid accounts for the hyperuricemia; in others, an excessive production of uric acid from increased purine biosynthesis is found. In still other patients with gout, both excessive synthesis of uric acid and decreased renal excretion of uric acid are found. Gout can be secondary, as well as primary. Although there appears to be a strong heritable component that accounts for approximately 60% of the clinical variability, with multiple genes potentially involved, environmental factors also play a key role. In developed countries, obesity, diet, and medications are frequently implicated (230,233). The deposits of urate crystals stimulate cytokine production, chiefly interleukin-1β (IL-1β). IL-1β is a central mediator of the neutrophil recruitment and activation that is characteristic of joint disease (but not a feature in dermal disease) (233).

Principles of Treatment: In acute attacks, reducing pain and inflammation may be accomplished with nonsteroidal anti-inflammatory drugs, corticosteroids, and colchicine. Chronic gout is treated by reducing uric acid levels with colchicine, allopurinol, or febuxostat, in conjunction with dietary restriction, exercise, and avoidance of certain medications (247). In rare circumstances, surgical intervention can be beneficial in tophaceous gout when medical management is contraindicated or failed (229).

OCHRONOSIS

Clinical Summary. There are two types of ochronosis: endogenous ochronosis (alkaptonuria), which is inherited as an autosomal recessive trait, and localized exogenous ochronosis, which is prototypically caused by the topical application of a hydroquinone cream to exposed parts of the skin in order to lighten the color of dark skin.

As a result of the lack of homogentisate 1,2-dioxygenase (homogentisic acid oxidase) in endogenous ochronosis, homogentisic acid accumulates over the course of years in many tissues—especially in the cartilages of the joints, the ears, and

the nose; in ligaments and tendons; and in the sclerae. This results in osteoarthritis; patchy pigmentation of the sclerae; and blackening of cartilages, ligaments, and tendons. In rare cases, the presenting complaint is pigmentation of the palms and soles, sometimes with overlying hyperkeratosis and pitting (248,249). Intervertebral calcification is a characteristic x-ray finding (249–251). Cardiac valve calcifications, renal and prostate stones, and darkening of the urine following exposure to air are other common findings (251). In the course of time, homogentisic acid accumulates in the dermis in sufficient amounts to cause patchy brown pigmentation of the skin. The gene for homogentisic acid oxidase maps to chromosome 3q (251).

In localized exogenous ochronosis, there is a macular blue-black hyperpigmentation of portions of the face to which the hydroquinone cream or other responsible agent was applied (Fig. 17-19). In more severely involved areas, blue-black papules, milia, and nodules can occur (252). Cutaneous annular sarcoidosis has been reported in association with lesions of ochronosis (253). A condition termed *pseudo-ochronosis* has been described as a histopathologic finding in localized argyria occurring primarily in jewelry workers. These patients present with blue-black macules ("blue nevus-like"), typically on the upper extremities (254). A rare case of pseudo-ochronosis presumed to arise from metal-induced granule deposition other than silver, secondary to firework trauma, has been reported (255).

Dermoscopy of skin lesions in endogenous ochronosis demonstrates structureless gray-blue areas, whereas exogenous ochronosis demonstrates gray-brown globular, curvilinear, and annular structures in a brownish-black background (256).

Histopathology. Involvement of the skin is essentially identical in endogenous and exogenous ochronosis, although often more pronounced in exogenous ochronosis (257). The ochronotic pigment has a yellow-brown or ochre color when stained with H&E; hence the name *ochronosis.*

The skin shows ochronotic pigment as fine granules free in the tissue and in the endothelial cells of blood vessels, in the basement membrane and the secretory cells of sweat glands, and within scattered macrophages (258). The most striking finding, however, is the ochronotic pigment within collagen bundles, causing homogenization and swelling of the bundles. Some collagen bundles assume a bizarre shape; they appear

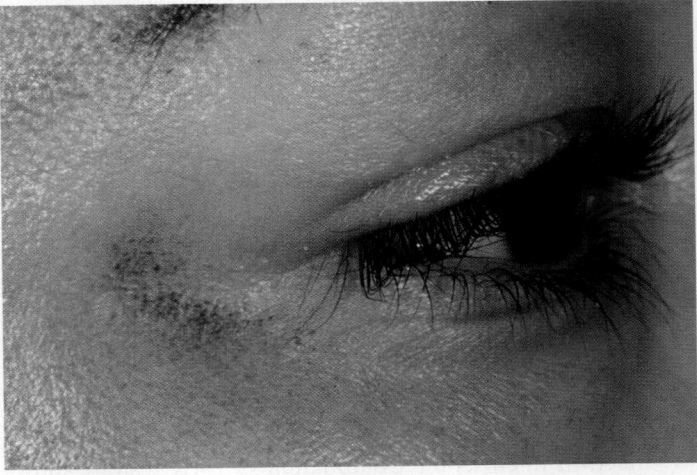

Figure 17-19 Exogenous ochronosis. There is stippled, blue-gray pigmentation following long-term use of topical hydroquinone.

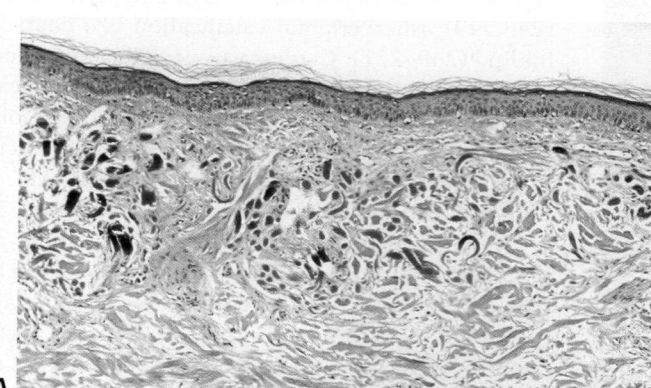
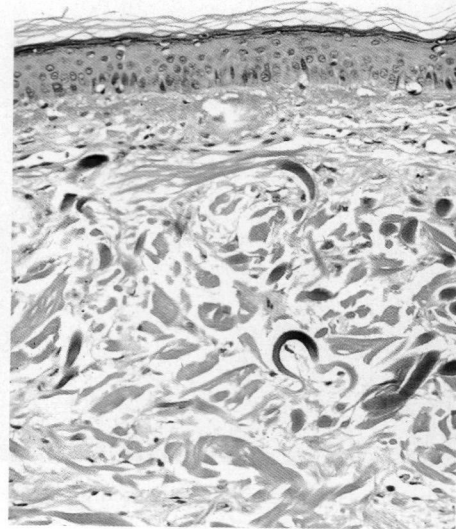

Figure 17-20 Exogenous ochronosis. Yellowish orange–colored collagen bundles are present in the superficial reticular dermis. Some are abnormally thickened. *A:* Hematoxylin and eosin (H&E), original magnification ×100; *B:* H&E, original magnification ×200.

rigid and tend to fracture transversely with jagged or pointed ends (259) (Fig. 17-20). As the result of the breaking up of degenerated collagen bundles, irregular, homogeneous, light brown clumps lie free in the tissue. The altered dermal connective tissue does not stain with silver nitrate, as melanin does, but becomes black when stained with cresyl violet or methylene blue (260). In addition, ochronotic pigment can be found within elastic fibers (258). In nodular and sarcoidal ochronosis, a granulomatous response surrounds this material (252,253). Transfollicular elimination of ochronotic fibers may occur in patients with severe disease (252).

In pseudo-ochronosis, features similar to ochronosis are present in the form of prominent collagen bundles that are yellow-brown in color. In addition, most cases have shown "ellipsoid black globules" of silver within the dermis (254).

Pathogenesis. In *endogenous ochronosis,* because of an inborn lack of homogentisic acid oxidase, the two amino acids tyrosine and phenylalanine cannot be catabolized beyond homogentisic acid. Most of the homogentisic acid is excreted in the urine. The urine, on standing or after the addition of reducing agents such as sodium hydroxide, turns black (alkaptonuria) because, through oxidation and polymerization, homogentisic acid is converted into a dark-colored insoluble product. However, some of the homogentisic acid gradually accumulates in certain tissues. It is bound irreversibly to collagen fibers as a polymer after oxidation to benzoquinone acetate (251).

In *exogenous ochronosis,* a topical agent such as hydroquinone, resorcinol, phenol, mercury, picric acid or benzene, or a systemic medication such as quinine or antimalarials inhibits the activity of homogentisic acid oxidase in the skin, resulting in the local accumulation of homogentisic acid, which polymerizes to form ochronotic pigment (261,262). In effect, this process mimics the cutaneous manifestation of endogenous ochronosis (257).

Pseudo-ochronosis appears to be attributable to deposits of traumatically implanted silver onto collagen bundles (254).

Electron microscopic examination of early lesions shows deposition of amorphous, electron-dense ochronotic pigment around individual collagen fibrils within collagen fibers (263). This causes the collagen fibrils to lose their periodicity and degenerate. Gradually, the collagen fibrils disappear as they are replaced by ochronotic pigment. Ultimately, the ochronotic pigment occupies entire collagen fibers and, by fusion, entire collagen bundles (264). Cross sections of the bundles then reveal a large, homogeneous, electron-dense aggregate that in some instances shows remnants of collagen fibrils at its periphery as well as macrophages containing particles of ochronotic pigment (252,263). Particles of ochronotic pigment can also be found in elastic fibers, and elastic fibers can show degenerative changes (252). In pseudo-ochronosis, scanning electron microscopy demonstrates silver deposited on collagen fibers (254).

Principles of Treatment: Treatment of endogenous ochronosis consists of dietary restriction of tyrosine and phenylalanine and appropriate management of arthropathy when indicated. Treatment of exogenous ochronosis begins with cessation of the offending agent. Therapies with at least mild-to-moderate reported improvement include dermabrasion with or without ablative CO_2 laser and Nd:YAG laser (265).

MUCINOSES

There are six types of cutaneous mucinosis: (a) generalized myxedema, (b) pretibial myxedema, (c) lichen myxedematosus or papular mucinosis, (d) reticular erythematous mucinosis or plaque-like mucinosis, (e) self-healing juvenile cutaneous mucinosis, and (f) scleredema.

Regular demonstration of the presence of mucin in the dermis is possible only in pretibial myxedema, self-healing juvenile cutaneous mucinosis, and lichen myxedematosus. In reticular erythematous mucinosis, it is possible in most cases. In generalized myxedema, the amount of mucin is usually too small to be demonstrable, and in scleredema, mucin may be present only in the early stage.

The mucin found in these six diseases represents an increase in the mucin that is normally present in the ground substance of the dermis. It consists of proteins bound to hyaluronic acid (hyaluronan), which is an acid mucopolysaccharide or glycosaminoglycan. As a result of the great water-binding capacity of hyaluronic acid, dermal mucin contains a considerable amount of water. This water is largely removed during the process of dehydration of the specimen; consequently, in routine sections, the mucin, because of its marked shrinkage, appears largely as threads and granules.

The mucin present in the six types of mucinosis stains a light blue in sections stained with H&E. It also stains with colloidal iron. It is Alcian blue positive at pH 2.5 but negative below pH 1.0 and shows metachromasia with toluidine blue at pH 7.0 and 4.0 but no metachromasia below pH 2.0 (266). It is PAS negative (indicating the absence of neutral mucopolysaccharides) and aldehyde fuchsin negative (indicating the absence of sulfated acid mucopolysaccharides). The mucin is completely removed on incubation of histologic sections with testicular hyaluronidase for 1 hour at 37°C (267).

Generalized Myxedema

Clinical Summary. In generalized myxedema, caused by hypothyroidism, the entire skin appears swollen, dry, pale, and waxy. It is firm to the touch. Despite its edematous appearance, the skin does not pit on pressure. There is often a characteristic facial appearance: the nose is broad, the lips are swollen, and the eyelids are puffy.

Histopathology. The epidermis may show slight orthohyperkeratosis and follicular plugging. Usually, routinely stained sections show no abnormality in the dermis, except in severe cases, in which one may observe swelling of the collagen bundles with splitting up of the bundles into individual fibers with some blue threads and granules of mucin interspersed (268,269). However, with histochemical stains, such as colloidal iron, Alcian blue, or toluidine blue, it is possible, at least in severe cases, to demonstrate small amounts of mucin, mainly in the vicinity of the blood vessels and hair follicles.

Principles of Treatment: Treatment of the underlying thyroidopathy is most important, with the addition of topical steroids in severe cases.

Pretibial Myxedema

Clinical Summary. Usually, the lesions are limited to the anterior aspects of the legs, but they may extend to the dorsa of the feet. They consist of raised, nodular, yellow, waxy plaques with prominent follicular openings that give a peau d'orange appearance (Fig. 17-21). Similar lesions rarely occur on the radial aspect of the forearms as well as the shoulders, face, and abdomen (270,271).

Pretibial myxedema usually occurs in association with Graves disease hyperthyroidism and not infrequently becomes more pronounced after treatment of the thyrotoxicosis. It nearly always occurs in association with exophthalmos, and 15% to 20% also have acropachy (272). Complete remission occurs in about 25% of cases (272). Rarely, pretibial myxedema occurs in nonthyrotoxic thyroid disease such as chronic lymphocytic thyroiditis; the patient is then either euthyroid or hypothyroid (273,274). It may also rarely occur in euthyroid or hypothyroid patients with other extrathyroidal manifestations typical of Graves disease (275,276).

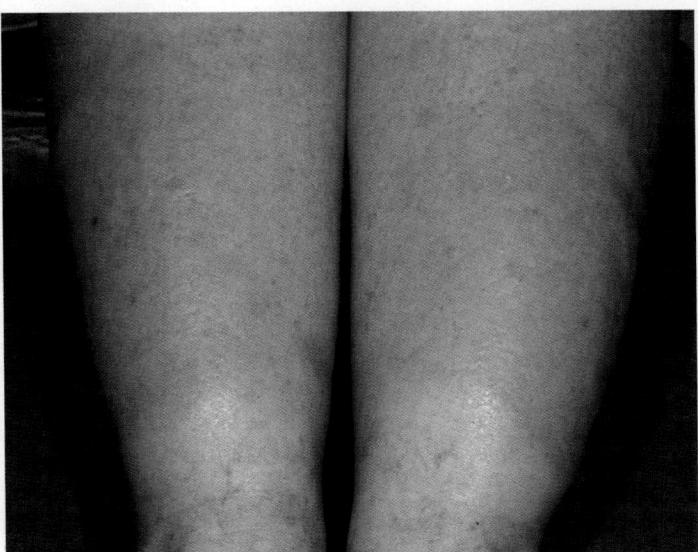

Figure 17-21 Pretibial myxedema. There are waxy infiltrated yellow-erythematous plaques on the anterior lower legs.

Histopathology. The epidermis and papillary dermis are usually normal. Mucin in large amounts is present in the dermis, particularly in the upper half (Fig. 17-22). As a result, the dermis is greatly thickened. The mucin occurs not only as individual threads and granules but also as extensive deposits, splitting up collagen bundles into widely separated fibers. As a result of shrinkage of the mucin during the process of fixation and dehydration, there are empty spaces within the mucin deposits. The number of fibroblasts is not increased, but in areas where there is much mucin, some fibroblasts have a stellate shape and are then referred to as *mucoblasts* (272,277). A perivascular infiltrate of lymphocytes may be seen, and mast cells are moderately increased in number (272,277).

Pathogenesis. On electron microscopic examination, the collagen bundles and fibers are separated by wide, electron-lucent, empty spaces. The fibroblasts that produce the mucin are stellate shaped with long, thin, cytoplasmic processes and exhibit dilated cisternae of the rough endoplasmic reticulum. An amorphous, moderately electron-dense material coats the surface of the fibroblasts. This material is also present in small, irregular clumps within the otherwise empty-appearing spaces (278). At high magnification, the amorphous material appears as a complex network of microfibrils and granules (279).

Of interest is the almost invariable presence of an immunoglobulin known as long-acting thyroid stimulator (LATS) in the serum of patients with pretibial myxedema. There is, however, a rather poor correlation between the severity of the skin lesions and serum LATS levels; furthermore, LATS is detected in about half of patients with an active exophthalmic goiter but without pretibial myxedema. Thus, LATS cannot be regarded as the cause of pretibial myxedema (280). IgG LATS likely represents an autoantibody that is produced by lymphocytes in thyroid disease, especially in thyrotoxicosis, and is a reflection rather than a cause of the underlying disease (273).

The restriction of the myxedema largely to the pretibial area may be explained by the finding that fibroblasts from the pretibial area synthesize two to three times more hyaluronic acid than fibroblasts from other areas when incubated with

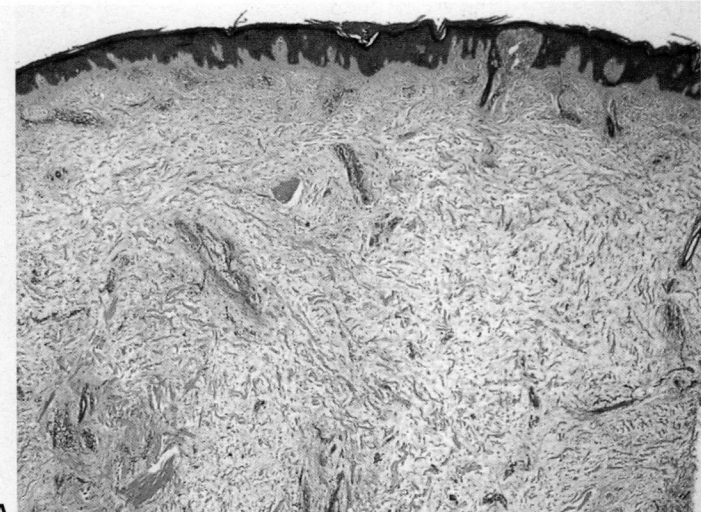
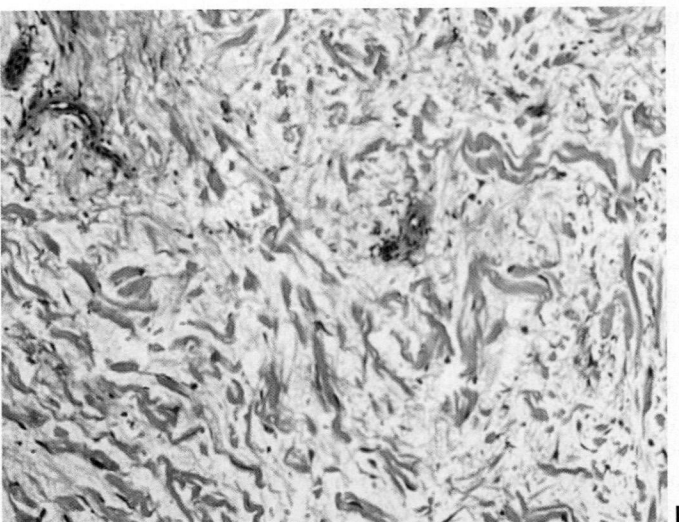

Figure 17-22 Pretibial myxedema. *A:* At scanning magnification, the epidermis and papillary dermis are normal. The collagen fibers in the reticular dermis are widely separated by deposits of mucin (hematoxylin and eosin [H&E]). *B:* At higher magnification, stellate fibroblasts are evident among the separated collagen fibers (H&E).

serum from patients with pretibial myxedema (281). The receptor for thyroid-stimulating hormone (TSH-R) appears to be the common tissue antigen in Graves disease, exophthalmos, and pretibial myxedema. TSH-R has been detected on fibroblasts in the dermis of control patients without thyroid disease, and its activation increases hyaluronic acid production in preadipocytic fibroblasts (282). Additionally, the pathophysiology may involve synergism of the TSH-R antibodies with insulin-like growth factor 1, causing fibroblast activation (283).

Differential Diagnosis. Pretibial myxedema must be differentiated from pretibial mucinosis associated with venous stasis. In pretibial mucinosis, the excess mucin is localized to the thickened papillary dermis and is accompanied by angioplasia and siderophages (284).

Principles of Treatment: Same as generalized myxedema.

Lichen Myxedematosus

Clinical Summary. Lichen myxedematosus, or papular mucinosis, is characterized by a more or less extensive eruption of asymptomatic, soft papules generally 2 to 3 mm in diameter. Although densely grouped, they usually do not coalesce. The face and arms are the most commonly affected areas (Fig. 17-23). In some instances, in addition to papules, large nodules may be present (285,286). Although the disease is very chronic, spontaneous resolution has been reported (285,286). The generalized form is almost always associated with a monoclonal gammopathy and may have systemic, even lethal, manifestations. Localized forms are not typically associated with a monoclonal gammopathy or systemic manifestations, and some of these cases have been associated with HIV and rarely hepatitis C infection. As a rule, thyroid disease is absent (285).

In the generalized variant of lichen myxedematosus, called *scleromyxedema*, a generalized eruption of papules as in lichen myxedematosus and, in addition, diffuse sclerodermoid thickening of the skin associated with erythema are found. There is marked accentuation of the skin folds,

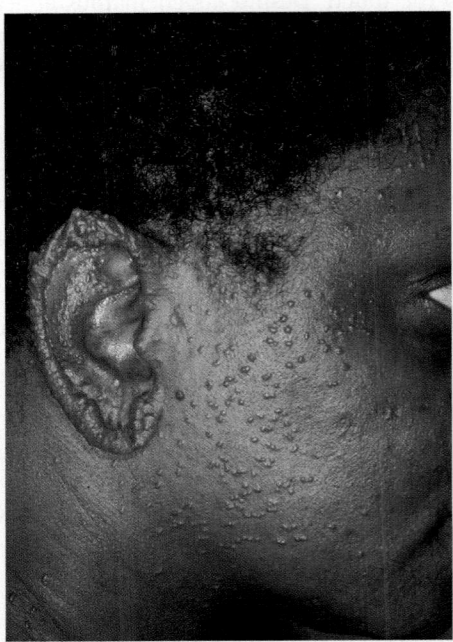

Figure 17-23 Lichen myxedematosus. There are numerous firm papules on the face and ear. Note the linear arrangement of the papules near the angle of the jaw.

particularly on the face. Sclerodactyly and decreased joint mobility may occur. Plasmacytosis that rarely progresses to multiple myeloma is sometimes seen, and other extracutaneous manifestations include muscular, neurologic, rheumatologic, pulmonary, renal, and cardiovascular complications (285). A dermato-neuro syndrome consisting of fever, convulsions, and coma, often preceded by a flu-like prodrome, portends a poor prognosis and can sometimes be fatal (287). Scleromyxedema can be differentiated from scleroderma clinically by the papular component and the absence of telangiectasias. Whether transitions of lichen myxedematosus to scleromyxedema may occur is uncertain (285).

Most cases of localized lichen myxedematosus are characterized by a discrete papular form involving the limbs and trunk in a symmetrical pattern. *Acral persistent papular mucinosis* presents as multiple small papular lesions on the extensor surfaces of the hands and forearms and demonstrates a female predominance (285). IgA monoclonal gammopathy has been reported in one case (288). *Cutaneous mucinosis of infancy* may also represent a localized form of papular mucinosis on the upper extremities unassociated with monoclonal gammopathy (285). Two reported cases have spontaneously regressed (289). *Nodular lichen myxedematosus* has been used to describe cases where nodules predominate or papules are absent (285).

Multiple dome-shaped papules with histopathologic features suggestive of papular mucinosis have been noted in Birt–Hogg–Dube syndrome (290,291).

Histopathology. In localized lichen myxedematosus, fairly large amounts of mucin are present. In contrast to pretibial myxedema, however, the mucinous infiltration is found only in circumscribed areas, is most pronounced in the upper dermis, and is associated with variably increased fibroblasts and no significant increase in dermal collagen (269,285,292) (Fig. 17-24).

The histologic picture found in the papules in scleromyxedema resembles that observed in lichen myxedematosus. In the diffusely thickened skin, there is extensive proliferation of irregularly arranged fibroblasts throughout the dermis associated with increased irregularly arranged bundles of collagen. In many areas, the collagen bundles are split into individual fibers by mucin. Elastic fibers may be fragmented and decreased in number. As a rule, the amount of mucin is greater in the upper half than in the lower half of the dermis. The overlying epidermis may be thinned, and hair follicles may be atrophic. A mild superficial perivascular lymphoplasmacytic infiltrate is often present (269,285). Two cases mimicking interstitial granuloma annulare with epithelioid histiocytes and giant cells have been reported (293,294).

Scleromyxedema may be difficult to distinguish from nephrogenic systemic fibrosis, formerly known as nephrogenic fibrosing dermopathy, without clinicopathologic correlation.

Both conditions are characterized by a dermal infiltrate of spindle cells with increased mucin and collagen. In both conditions, the spindle cells label for either factor XIIIa or CD34 and procollagen1 without demonstrating a pattern that could be utilized to discriminate between these diseases (295). However, in scleromyxedema, the infiltrate is limited to the dermis, whereas in nephrogenic systemic fibrosis the infiltrate usually also extends down the subcutaneous septa (295). Additionally, there is often iron deposition in the dermal fibroblasts in nephrogenic systemic fibrosis, which can be highlighted with iron stains and is sometimes discernible as fine dark brown pigment granules, in contrast to cases of scleromyxedema, where such deposition is not detected (296). Although it was initially thought to only involve the skin, nephrogenic systemic fibrosis has been shown to involve other tissues, including lung, liver, heart, and skeletal muscle (297), and paraproteinemia is usually absent (287).

Autopsy examination of patients with lichen myxedematosus and scleromyxedema has usually not shown mucinous deposits in any internal organs (298,299). However, in one case, mucin was detected in renal papillae, and in others it was found in the adventitia and media of blood vessels in several organs (300–303).

Pathogenesis. Electron microscopic examination of scleromyxedema reveals an increase in the number of fibroblasts. They show considerable activity, as indicated by the presence of a markedly dilated rough endoplasmic reticulum and long cytoplasmic processes (304). Phagolysosomal cytoplasmic inclusions are frequently detected in these cells (305). These fibroblasts produce both collagen and ground substance. The presence of many collagen fibrils with reduced diameter, similar to those in scleroderma, indicates that it is young collagen. In many areas, there are small bundles of young collagen fibrils, with each fibril richly coated with ground substance (304). Elastic tissue fibrils are sparse to absent (305).

The presence of a *monoclonal component* (M component) or paraprotein in the sera of patients with scleromyxedema has been noted in nearly all cases that have been adequately tested.

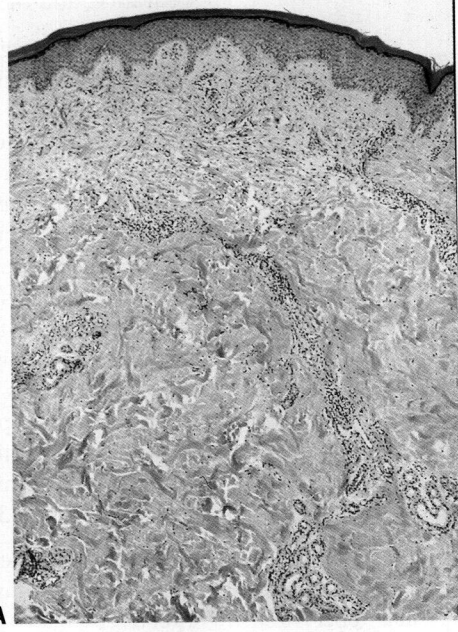
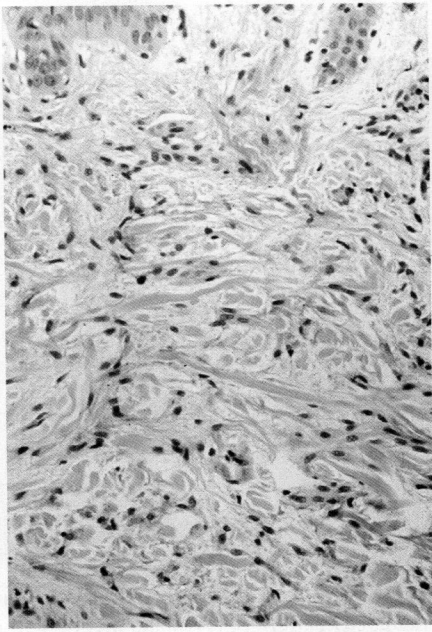

Figure 17-24 Lichen myxedematosus. *A:* At scanning power, a dome-shaped papule is evident. The papillary and superficial reticular dermis contain abundant mucin (hematoxylin and eosin [H&E]). *B:* In addition to mucin, there is an increased number of plump fibroblasts in the upper dermis (H&E).

A

B

In nearly all instances, the paraprotein is an IgG with λ light chains, although κ chains and other immunoglobulin classes occur on rare occasions (286). In addition to showing a monoclonal IgG, many cases of lichen myxedematosus show hyperplasia of plasma cells in the bone marrow (285). These plasma cells have been shown to synthesize the monoclonal IgG (306). In some cases, the plasma cells in the bone marrow have been regarded as atypical in appearance (307), and about 10% of the patients develop multiple myeloma (285).

The role of the monoclonal IgG in lichen myxedematosus is not clear. Its presence in the dermal mucin has been demonstrated by direct immunofluorescence (307). Furthermore, the serum containing the paraprotein stimulates the production of hyaluronic acid and prostaglandin E by fibroblasts *in vitro*. However, although the serum from patients with lichen myxedematosus stimulates fibroblast proliferation *in vitro*, the purified IgG paraprotein itself has no direct effect on fibroblast proliferation (286).

Recently, several reports have shown marked improvement and even complete remission of cutaneous manifestations of scleromyxedema in patients treated with agents effective against plasma cell dyscrasias, particularly combinations of bortezomib, dexamethasone, and thalidomide, sometimes in conjunction with autologous peripheral blood stem cell transplantation (308–311). Paraprotein levels did not directly correlate with response in some of these cases, suggesting that it is not the paraprotein itself but rather another factor produced by or in response to the plasma cells that could be responsible for the cutaneous manifestations (311). Circulating myeloma tumor cells have been detected by next generation flow cytometry in a scleromyxedema patient (312).

Principles of Treatment: As in the preceding case. High-dose intravenous immunoglobulins (IVIg) are the first-line treatment of choice according to European guidelines (313).

Reticular Erythematous Mucinosis

Clinical Summary. Erythematous, reticulated areas with irregular but well-defined margins are present, usually in the center of the chest and of the upper back (Fig. 17-25). This disorder was first described in 1960 as being composed of confluent papules and was called *plaque-like mucinosis*, but similar cases showing coalescent macules, rather than papules, were designated as *reticular erythematous mucinosis* in 1974 (314–317). It has since become apparent that macular and papular lesions can coexist (318). In rare instances, lesions spare the trunk and are present on the arms and face (319). The eruption is usually chronic and asymptomatic, although photoexacerbation followed by slight pruritis is sometimes present. It may be a presenting sign of systemic lupus erythematosus (320), and significant overlap with tumid lupus erythematosus has been observed (316). The lesions most frequently occur in young to middle-aged women (316). Rare cases in siblings and monozygotic twins have been reported; however, a hereditary pattern has not been proven (321,322).

Histopathology. Two histologic features are usually present: small amounts of dermal mucin and a mild or moderately pronounced mononuclear infiltrate situated predominantly around blood vessels and hair follicles (314–316,323). The infiltrate is composed of helper T cells (324).

In papular lesions, the mucin is usually fairly conspicuous. As a rule, mucin can be recognized even in routinely stained sections (Fig. 17-26). The mucin stains with Alcian blue and usually mucicarmine and is metachromatic with toluidine blue or Giemsa stains (314,315). Fibroblasts with bipolar processes are located in the mucinous deposits (325). Immunohistochemistry has revealed a significantly increased number of factor XIIIa dendritic cells in the lesional skin of a patient with reticular erythematous mucinosis but not in the patient's uninvolved skin or normal control skin samples (326). These same cells also demonstrated immunoreactivity for one isoform of hyaluronan synthase (326).

In macular lesions, the mucin may be missed in routinely stained sections and becomes apparent only on staining with Alcian blue. In some instances, no mucin is found, even on staining with Alcian blue (327). Direct immunofluorescence studies have demonstrated fine granular deposits of IgM, IgA, and C3 along the basal layer in some cases (328), which could help support the diagnosis in lesions devoid of mucin. When these findings are absent, however, the diagnosis may depend on the presence of the mononuclear infiltrate, the clinical appearance, and the response to treatment.

Differential Diagnosis. Reticular erythematous mucinosis, Jessner lymphocytic infiltrate of skin, and lupus erythematosus may share a perivascular and perifollicular lymphocytic infiltrate and increased mucin among collagen bundles. In Jessner lymphocytic infiltrate, the lymphocytic infiltrate is usually much denser than in reticular erythematous mucinosis. Lupus erythematosus usually shows vacuolar changes in the basal layer of the epidermis and follicular units, but in tumid lesions, vacuolar changes may be inconspicuous. Thus, it may not be possible to distinguish between the tumid lesions of lupus erythematosus and reticular erythematous mucinosis by conventional microscopy. Furthermore, flesh-colored papules and nodules situated on the trunk and demonstrating increased dermal mucin may precede or accompany systemic lupus erythematosus or progressive systemic sclerosis (329).

Principles of Treatment: Small doses of antimalarial drugs of the 4-aminoquinoline group, such as chloroquine, are usually effective.

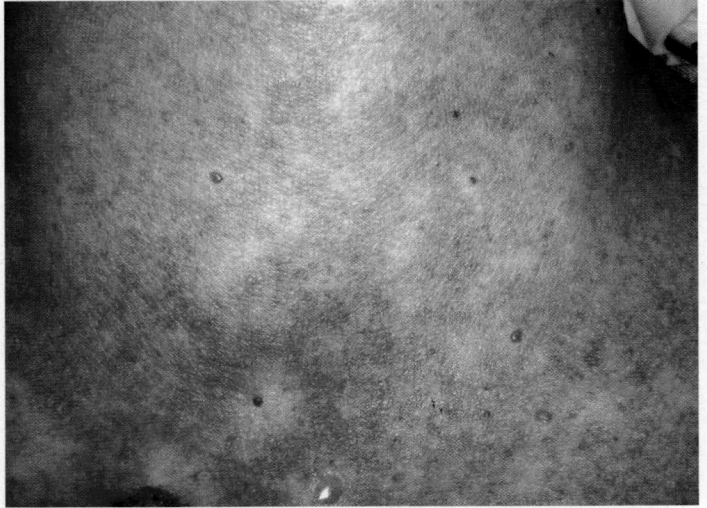

Figure 17-25 Reticular erythematous mucinosis. There is a netlike (reticulated) pattern of erythema involving the neck and upper chest.

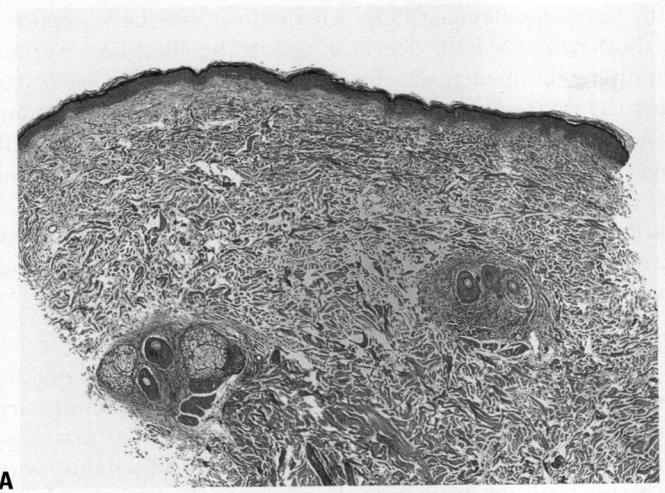
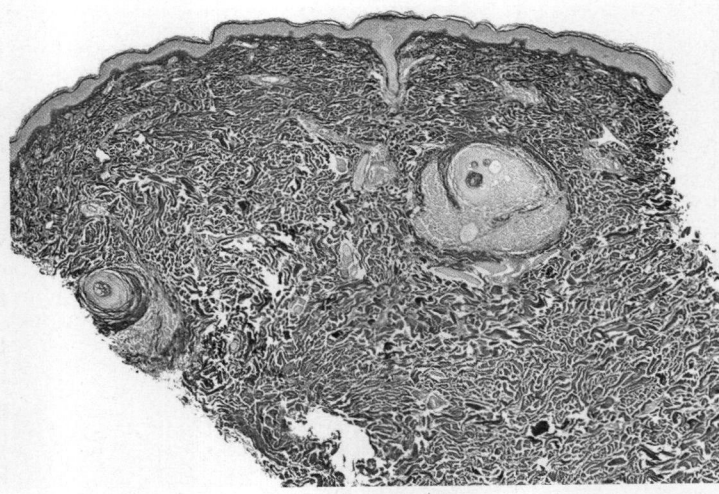

Figure 17-26 Reticular erythematous mucinosis. *A:* There is a sparse superficial perivascular and perifollicular infiltrate of lymphocytes around blood vessels in the dermis (hematoxylin and eosin). *B:* Colloidal iron staining reveals abundant mucin among collagen fibers.

Self-Healing Juvenile Cutaneous Mucinosis

Clinical Summary. Self-healing juvenile cutaneous mucinosis is a rare dermatosis with a sudden onset and spontaneous resolution within a few months. Infiltrated plaques with a corrugated surface are observed on the torso, and nodules occur on the face and in the periarticular region. Nontender ivory papules in a linear configuration may also occur. There may be associated fever, arthralgias, muscle tenderness, and weakness (330,331).

Histopathology. Abundant, Alcian blue positive, mucinous material is present mainly in the upper reticular dermis. There may be a superficial perivascular lymphocytic infiltrate and a slight increase in the number of mast cells and fibroblasts in the zone of mucin deposition. Nodular lesions may show a septolobular panniculitis-like pattern with abundant mucin in the expanded fat lobules, and epithelioid gangliocyte-like mononuclear cells may be present (332). Immunohistochemically, the spindle cells are positive for vimentin and may be variably positive for desmin and smooth muscle actin, whereas the epithelioid gangliocyte-like cells stain with CD68 and CD163 (330,333,334). The histopathologic changes can be confused with proliferative fasciitis. The presence of increased mucin in the papillary and reticular dermis favors self-healing juvenile cutaneous mucinosis.

Scleredema

Clinical Summary. Scleredema, occasionally called *scleredema adultorum,* even though it may occur in children and infants, is characterized by diffuse, nonpitting swelling and induration of the skin (335,336). Three groups are recognized (310): one with abrupt onset, one with insidious onset, and one preceded by diabetes. In the first group, the scleredema starts abruptly during or within a few weeks after a febrile illness, typically a streptococcal upper respiratory tract infection. The skin lesions may clear within a few months, or the disease may take a prolonged course. In the second group, the scleredema starts insidiously, for no apparent reason; spreads gradually; and takes a chronic course. The patients often have or subsequently develop a monoclonal gammopathy or multiple myeloma. The disease in the third group occurs mostly in men, is preceded by diabetes for years, starts insidiously, and persists indefinitely (337).

Usually, the scleredema starts on the face and extends to the neck and upper trunk. Unlike scleroderma, the hands and feet are always spared. In about 75% of patients, complete resolution takes place within a few months; in the remaining 25%, the disease may persist for as long as 40 years (338). Although visceral lesions may occur, death from scleredema is rare.

Diabetes is commonly associated with persistent scleredema and in most of these instances is quite resistant to antidiabetic therapy (339). It has been suggested that the association of persistent scleredema with maturity-onset diabetes be recognized as a special form of scleredema (340).

Histopathology. The dermis in scleredema is about three times thicker than normal (Fig. 17-27), with thickened collagen bundles separated by clear spaces, causing "fenestration" of the collagen. The secretory coils of the sweat glands, surrounded by fat tissue, are located in the upper dermis or middermis rather than, as normally, in the lower dermis or at the junction of the dermis and the subcutaneous fat. Because the distance between the epidermis and the sweat glands is unchanged, it can be concluded that much of the subcutaneous fat in scleredema has been replaced by dense collagenous bundles (341–343). No increase in the number of fibroblasts is noted in association with

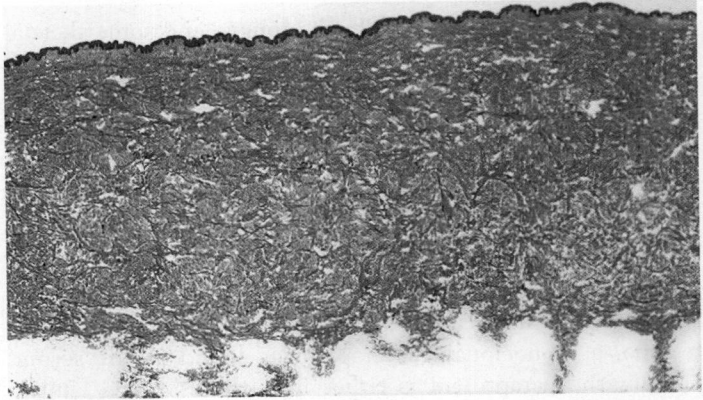

Figure 17-27 Scleredema. Panoramic view showing only a greatly thickened reticular dermis. The subcutis is not involved as in scleroderma (hematoxylin and eosin).

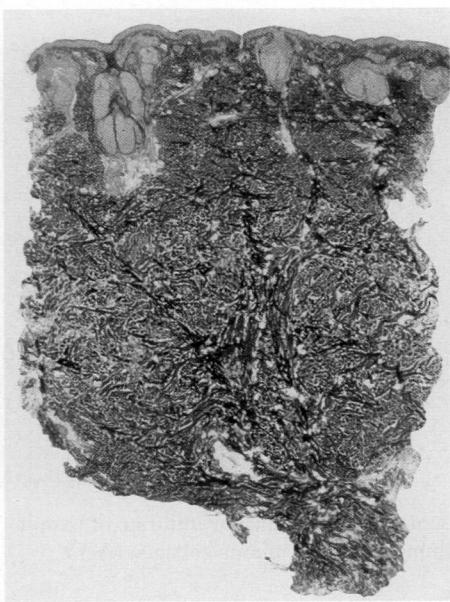

Figure 17-28 Scleredema. Colloidal iron staining of an early case reveals increased mucin in the middle and lower dermis.

the hyperplasia of the collagen; in fact, their number may be strikingly decreased (344).

In many instances, especially in early cases, histochemical staining reveals the presence of hyaluronic acid between the bundles of collagen, particularly in the areas of fenestration. Staining with toluidine blue usually reveals metachromasia, which is most evident at pH 7.0, weaker at pH 5.0, and absent at pH 1.5, indicating the presence of only nonsulfated acid mucopolysaccharides (345). Although the hyaluronic acid is usually present throughout the dermis, it may be present only in the deeper portion of the dermis (346) (Fig. 17-28).

In some cases, even frozen sections have failed to stain with Alcian blue or toluidine blue (347). It may be postulated that in long-standing cases in which the disease has reached a steady stage of collagen turnover, staining for hyaluronic acid may give negative results (341). In cases of scleredema in which formaldehyde-fixed specimens fail to show acid mucopolysaccharides, they may show them on fixation in 0.05% cetylpyridinium chloride solution and staining with Alcian blue at pH 2.5 (348). Some state that fixation with 1% cetylpyridinium chloride solution in standard formalin fixative combined with colloidal iron staining gives the best results (349).

Systemic Lesions. Occasionally, the tongue and some skeletal muscles are involved, and on histologic examination, the muscle bundles show edema and loss of striation (347,350). In a few reported cases, pleural and pericardial effusions were present (347,351). In one case, the disease terminated in death, and autopsy revealed diffuse edema of the heart, liver, and spleen in addition to pleural and pericardial effusions (352). In another case, bone marrow, nerve, liver, and salivary gland involvement was reported (342).

Pathogenesis. In many patients with long-standing scleredema, a monoclonal gammopathy is found in the serum. Usually, the paraprotein is either IgG kappa or IgG lambda (344,353). In other cases, it has been IgA kappa, IgA lambda, IgM kappa, or IgM lambda (353). There can be coexistence of scleredema with multiple myeloma in up to half of the patients

with paraproteinemia (353). Amyloidosis has been reported in three patients, with one localized to the skin; however, no immunoglobulin deposits have been found in involved skin sites (353). Complete remission of cutaneous manifestations in a patient with multiple myeloma treated with bortezomib suggests a causal relationship between scleredema and plasma cell dyscrasia in cases associated with paraproteinemia (354). A marked increase in type 1 collagen gene expression in scleroderma leads to increased collagen synthesis by dysfunctional fibroblasts (355,356).

Differential Diagnosis. It can be difficult to differentiate between end-stage scleroderma in which inflammation is no longer present and scleredema. As a rule, however, in scleroderma, the collagen in the reticular dermis and subcutaneous tissue appears homogenized and hyalinized and stains only lightly with eosin and with the Masson trichrome stain, but in scleredema, the collagen bundles are thickened without being hyalinized and stain normally with eosin and the trichrome stain (341).

Principles of Treatment: Treatment is similar to that for lichen myxedematosus/scleromyxedema and is often directed at the underlying plasma cell dyscrasia or diabetes. Spontaneous regression often occurs in infection-associated scleredema.

MUCOPOLYSACCHARIDOSIS

Clinical Summary. Mucopolysaccharidosis (MPS) comprises a group of storage diseases in which, as a result of a deficiency of specific lysosomal enzymes, there is inadequate degradation of mucopolysaccharides, or glycosaminoglycans. Consequently, this material accumulates within lysosomes of various cells in many organs, including the skin. Greatly elevated levels of mucopolysaccharides are present in the blood, serum, and urine. There are 11 different enzyme deficiencies implicated in the development of the seven major types of MPS (357). Thus, there is marked variation in the manifestations not only from type to type but also within the same type (358,359). The most common features, any or all of which may be present or absent, include dwarfism, skeletal deformities, hepatosplenomegaly, corneal clouding, and progressive mental deterioration with premature death from cardiorespiratory complications. In many instances, there is a characteristic facial appearance—thick lips, flattened nose, and hirsutism—referred to as *gargoylism*. The mode of transmission is autosomal recessive in all types of MPS except type II, the Hunter syndrome, which is X-linked recessive.

Only MPS types I to III will be discussed in this chapter. MPS I presents as three distinctive variants, even though they are all caused by a deficiency of the same enzyme. MPS I H, Hurler syndrome, causes severe mental retardation and death, usually within the first decade of life (357,360,361). In contrast, persons with MPS I S, Scheie syndrome, have normal intelligence, no dwarfism, and a normal life expectancy (360,361). MPS I H/S, the Hurler–Scheie syndrome, is intermediate between MPS I H and MPS I S. MPS II, Hunter syndrome, occurs in a severe form, with mental retardation and early death, and in a mild form, in which mental function is normal and survival to adult life is the rule (361). MPS III, Sanfilippo syndrome, has mild somatic changes but severe mental retardation (357).

The skin in all types of MPS usually appears thickened and inelastic. However, the only type in which distinctive cutaneous lesions are found frequently, although not invariably, is MPS II, Hunter syndrome. These lesions consist of ivory white papules or small nodules, usually 2 to 10 mm in diameter, which may coalesce to form ridges in a reticular pattern on the upper trunk, especially in the scapular region (362,363). This condition has been referred to as *pebbling of the skin*. Grouped papules on the extensor surfaces at the upper portions of the arms and legs have been noted in one patient with the Hurler–Scheie syndrome (MPS I H/S) (364).

Histopathology. In all types of MPS, the normal-appearing or slightly thickened skin, on staining with the Giemsa stain or toluidine blue, shows metachromatic granules within fibroblasts, so the fibroblasts resemble mast cells (365). The granules also stain with Alcian blue and with colloidal iron (366). Fixation in absolute alcohol in some instances demonstrates the metachromasia better than fixation in formalin (367). In addition, metachromatic granules are occasionally present in some epidermal cells and in the secretory and ductal cells of eccrine glands (365,368,369).

The cutaneous papules observed only in Hunter syndrome show not only metachromatic granules within dermal fibroblasts but also extracellular deposits of metachromatic material between collagen bundles and fibers (362,367,370).

In all types of MPS, metachromatic granules are also visible in the cytoplasm of circulating lymphocytes when smears of them are stained with toluidine blue after fixation in absolute methanol, a finding that aids in the rapid diagnosis of MPS (371).

Pathogenesis. Biochemical studies have shown that in MPS I, as a result of a deficiency in alpha-l-iduronidase, there is an accumulation of heparan sulfate and dermatan sulfate (chondroitin sulfate) (372). Accumulation of dermatan sulfate but not heparan sulfate is linked to impaired elastic fiber assembly, which is thought to contribute to the clinical phenotype in Hurler disease (373). In MPS II, the same two substances are excessively accumulated owing to a deficiency in iduronate sulfatase. In MPS III, there is excessive accumulation of heparan sulfate. Successful bone marrow transplantation in children with Hurler syndrome can restore the previously deficient alpha-1-iduronidase level (374). Enzyme replacement therapies have been developed for some of the mucopolysaccharidoses, including Hurler syndrome and Hunter syndrome, providing measurable and sustainable benefits (374).

By staining for acid phosphatase and by electron microscopy, the metachromatic granules in the skin and in the lymphocytes have been identified as lysosomes that contain acid mucopolysaccharides, which they are incapable of degrading (369,371).

Electron microscopic examination of the skin reveals in most fibroblasts numerous electron-lucent, greatly dilated, membrane-bound vacuoles representing lysosomes. Some of the vacuoles contain granular material or, less commonly, myelin-like structures representing residual bodies (366). Similar lysosomes are also present in macrophages (375). In addition, from 5% to 20% of the epidermal cells contain lysosomal vacuoles, with acid phosphatase activity, varying from a solitary vacuole to 20 or 30 vacuoles per cell (368).

The dermal Schwann cells also contain electron-lucent lysosomes. In addition, some Schwann cells occasionally show laminated membranous structures ("zebra bodies").

These structures resemble those found in the brains of some patients with MPS. In the brain, they contain gangliosides as a result of a deficiency in the lysosomal hydrolase beta-d-galactosidase and lead to mental deterioration through the degeneration and loss of neurons (368).

Principles of Treatment: Enzyme replacement therapy or bone marrow transplant, as stated previously, and symptomatic management of other specific conditions are currently used. Genome editing for MPSI and MPSII is under investigation as a therapeutic approach to these mucopolysaccharidoses (376).

ACANTHOSIS NIGRICANS

Clinical Summary. Acanthosis nigricans can be seen in multiple clinical settings: malignancy associated, benign, inherited, obesity associated, syndromic, drug induced, and mixed (377). The malignant type differs from the benign types by showing more extensive and more pronounced lesions, by its progressiveness, and by its onset usually after 40 years of age (377,378).

The *malignant* type is associated with a malignant tumor—usually an abdominal adenocarcinoma, particularly gastric (377,378). However, it may also occur with squamous cell carcinoma, sarcomas, Hodgkin and non-Hodgkin lymphomas, and melanoma (379–382). In some cases, the skin lesions precede the symptoms of malignancy. A possible manifestation with involvement of the palms with a velvety, white, thickened appearance with deep furrows has been termed *tripe palms*, although its occurrence in some cases without other lesions of acanthosis nigricans preferentially related to squamous cell carcinoma of the lung may warrant distinction of this entity. The sign of Leser–Trélat, which is characterized by the sudden appearance of numerous seborrheic keratoses in association with a malignant tumor, may be an early stage or incomplete form of the malignant type of acanthosis nigricans. The seborrheic keratoses observed in this sign may be accompanied or followed by lesions of acanthosis nigricans (383). Acanthosis nigricans, tripe palms, and Leser–Trélat sign may occur simultaneously, suggesting that the conditions may be related (383,384).

The *benign inherited* type usually has its onset during infancy or early childhood and is autosomal dominant (377).

Syndromic acanthosis nigricans is especially linked to syndromes associated with insulin resistance (377). In the HAIR–AN syndrome, which affects younger women, there is hyperandrogenemia (HA), insulin resistance (IR), and acanthosis nigricans (AN) (377). Another subset links autoimmune states such as lupus erythematosus with uncontrolled diabetes mellitus, acanthosis nigricans, and ovarian hyperandrogenism (377). These patients have antibodies to the insulin receptor (385). Acanthosis nigricans has also been associated with IR in obesity, hypothyroidism, and congenital generalized lipodystrophy (377).

Acanthosis nigricans–like lesions have been induced by high dosages of nicotinic acid (377). It has also occurred following the use of various drugs, including oral contraceptives, diethylstilbestrol, heroin, corticosteroids, and as a localized reaction to insulin (377).

Clinically, acanthosis nigricans presents as papillomatous hyperpigmented patches, predominantly in the intertriginous areas such as the axillae, the neck, and the genital and inframammary regions (Fig. 17-29). In extensive cases of the malignant

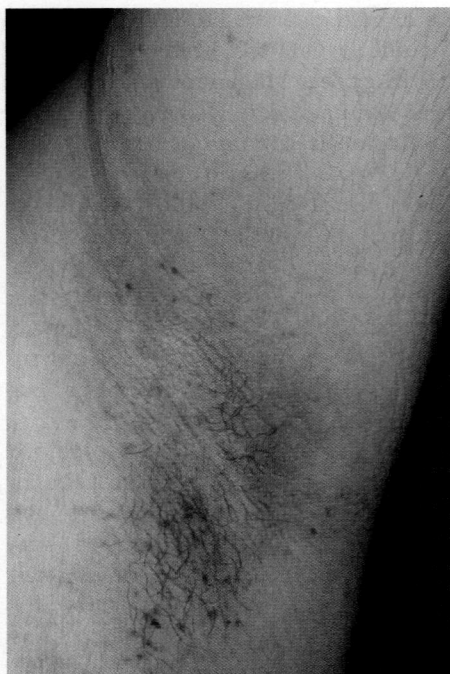

Figure 17-29 Acanthosis nigricans. There is a velvety, hyperpigmented plaque in the axillary fossa.

type, mucosal surfaces, such as the mouth, genital mucosa, and the palpebral conjunctivae, may be involved (384,386). In the acral type, there is velvety hyperpigmentation of the dorsa of the hands and feet.

Histopathology. Histologic examination is similar in all types and reveals hyperkeratosis and papillomatosis but only slight, irregular acanthosis and usually no hyperpigmentation. Thus, the term *acanthosis nigricans* has little histologic justification.

In a typical lesion, the dermal papillae project upward as finger-like projections. The valleys between the papillae show mild-to-moderate acanthosis and are filled with keratotic material (Fig. 17-30). Horn pseudocysts can occur in some cases (387). The epidermis at the tips of the papillae and often also on the sides of the protruding papillae appears thinned.

Slight hyperpigmentation of the basal layer is demonstrable with silver nitrate staining in some cases but not in others (388). The brown color of the lesions is caused more by hyperkeratosis than by melanin, although in some instances it may be the result of increased melanosomes in the stratum corneum (377,385).

Acanthosis nigricans lesions of polycystic ovary syndrome display prominent deposits of glycosaminoglycan consisting mostly of hyaluronic acid in the papillary dermis (389).

Pathogenesis. The inherited type of acanthosis nigricans can be classified as a type of epidermal nevus. In lesions associated with IR, high levels of insulin may activate insulin-like growth factor-1 receptors and thereby mediate epidermal proliferation (385). Malignant acanthosis nigricans is likely mediated by growth factors that are secreted by the associated neoplasm, such as transforming growth factor-alpha, and act on epidermal growth factor receptor (390). In some cases, the epidermal proliferation may be mediated by fibroblast growth factor receptors (385). The basal cells from one patient with syndromic acanthosis nigricans demonstrated unusually high expression of the rare keratins 18 and 19 (387).

Differential Diagnosis. Differentiation of acanthosis nigricans from other benign papillomas, particularly from linear epidermal nevi and from the hyperkeratotic type of seborrheic keratosis, may be difficult. As a rule, however, linear epidermal nevi show more marked acanthosis than acanthosis nigricans and have a more compact orthokeratotic stratum corneum. Furthermore, the pilosebaceous units in linear epidermal nevi are rudimentary. Acanthosis nigricans cannot be distinguished histologically from confluent and reticulated papillomatosis.

Principles of Treatment: Treatment is directed at correcting the underlying process.

Confluent and Reticulated Papillomatosis

Clinical Summary. Confluent and reticulated papillomatosis shows slightly hyperkeratotic and papillomatous pigmented papules that are confluent in the center and reticulated at the periphery (391). The site of predilection is the sternal

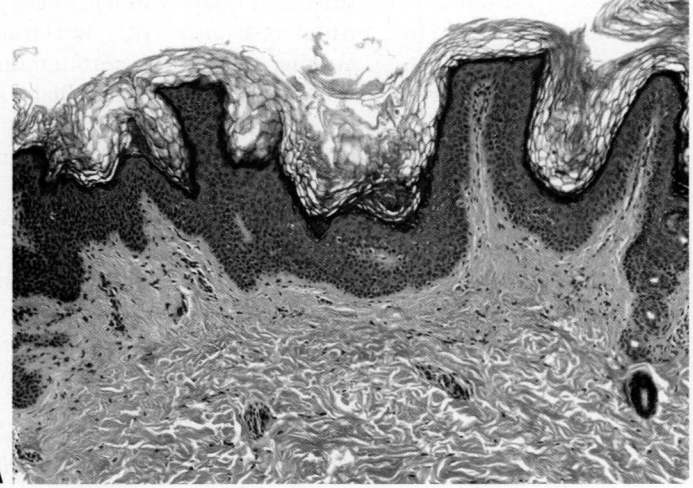
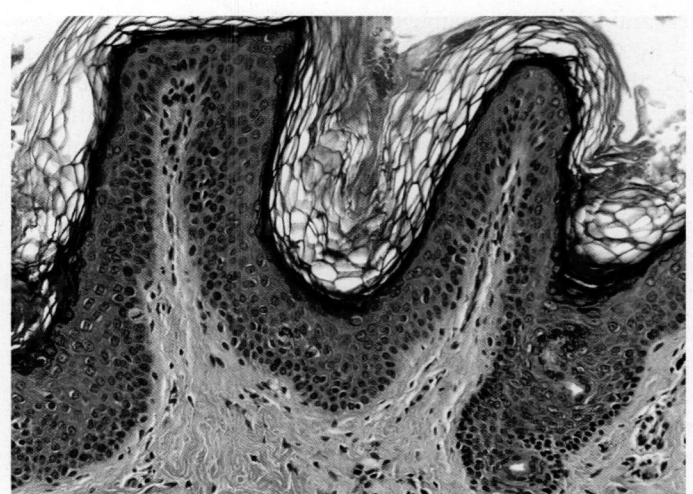

Figure 17-30 Acanthosis nigricans. *A:* There are papillomatous projections of the dermis (hematoxylin and eosin [H&E]). *B:* The epidermis is not increased in thickness above the papillomatous projections. The stratum corneum shows loose, basket-weave orthokeratosis (H&E).

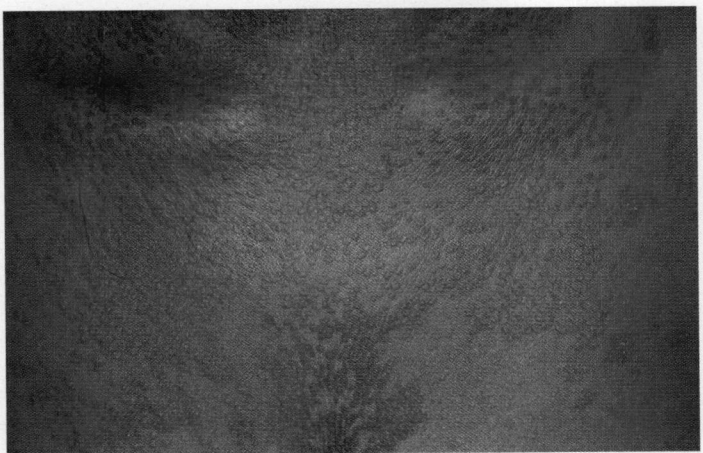

Figure 17-31 Confluent and reticulated papillomatosis. There are discrete, flat, brown papules distributed over the sternal region, a characteristic location. Note the coalescence of papules into plaques in some areas and the reticulated appearance inferiorly.

region (Fig. 17-31). Some view it as a variant of acanthosis nigricans (392). However, its location and reticulated pattern are distinctive.

Histopathology. Mild hyperkeratosis and papillomatosis are present, as is focal acanthosis, limited largely to the valleys between elongated papillae (392). Thus, the histologic changes are similar to but milder than those of acanthosis nigricans.

Pathogenesis. Heavy colonization with *Malassezia furfur* has been observed in patients with confluent and reticulated papillomatosis, leading some to regard it as potentially being a peculiar host reaction to *M. furfur* (391,393). However, in a review of the literature, it was found that even though potassium hydroxide preparations yielded positive findings for yeast in 10 cases, there were yeast and hyphae in only one case and negative results in 20 cases (394). Another report documented yeast and hyphae in two affected siblings (393). Considering the common presence of the yeast phase as a nonpathogen and the relatively ineffective treatment of these lesions with topical and oral antifungals as well as selenium sulfide, the role of *M. furfur* as the etiology can likely be discounted. Reports of a variety of antibiotics, particularly minocycline, that have been used successfully in the treatment of this condition raise the possibility that bacteria play a role in inducing the observed changes, although their utility has been regarded as more likely being due to their anti-inflammatory properties (391). A familial basis has been suggested in some studies (393,395). Increased expression of involucrin, keratin 16, and ki-67 has been demonstrated in the stratum granulosum with an increased transitional cell layer, supporting the concept of abnormal keratinocyte differentiation and maturation (395,396).

Principles of Treatment: Oral antibiotics, particularly minocycline, may eradicate the rash.

HEREDITARY HEMOCHROMATOSIS

Clinical Summary. In hereditary hemochromatosis, large amounts of iron are deposited in various organs of the body, especially in the parenchymal cells of the liver and pancreas

and in the myocardial fibers. The classic tetrad of hereditary hemochromatosis consists of hepatic cirrhosis, diabetes, hyperpigmentation of the skin, and cardiac failure.

Unless there is early recognition and adequate treatment by phlebotomy, hemochromatosis is a fatal disorder as the result of liver failure, heart disease, or hepatocellular carcinoma, which occurs in about one-third of patients with advanced hemochromatosis (397).

Pigmentation of the skin is present in 70% to 90% of patients with hereditary hemochromatosis at the time the diagnosis is made, but it is often so mild as to attract little attention (398–400). It is most pronounced in exposed areas, especially on the face. Its color is usually brown or bronze but may be blue-gray. The pigmentation is caused largely by melanin and not by iron. Ichthyosis-like changes, koilonychia, and hair loss are also common.

Histopathology. In the pigmented skin, especially from exposed areas, melanin is present in increased amounts in the basal layer of the epidermis (399,401). Hemosiderin can be demonstrated in most cases with the aid of an iron stain, such as Perls stain. It is found as blue-staining granules, mainly around blood vessels, both extracellularly and within macrophages, and in the basement membrane zone of the sweat glands and within cells of the connective tissue surrounding these glands (401). Siderosis around eccrine glands appears specific for hereditary hemochromatosis (399). In rare instances, some iron is present in the epidermis, particularly in the basal layer, and in the epithelial cells of the sweat glands (402).

It is not necessary to choose a pigmented area to biopsy, because deposits of iron are not limited to the areas of pigmentation. However, it is important not to take a specimen from the legs, where deposits of iron are frequently found in association with even minor venous stasis or as a consequence of a preceding inflammation that may no longer be evident.

A skin biopsy no longer represents an important test for establishing the diagnosis of hereditary hemochromatosis; it is merely of confirmatory value. Determinations in the serum of the level of iron, of the iron-binding capacity as measured by the degree of saturation of transferrin with iron, of the plasma ferritin concentration, and biopsy of the liver have replaced the skin biopsy in importance (403,404). Genotyping of patients who have abnormal screening exams for iron overload is now being performed before liver biopsy. If the person is homozygous for the most common mutation in the hemochromatosis gene (HFE) and has persistently elevated transaminase levels, a biopsy of the liver is considered to evaluate for fibrosis (405).

Pathogenesis. Hereditary hemochromatosis, a disease that can be caused by mutations that affect any of the proteins that limit the entry of iron into blood, is an autosomal recessive disease caused by mutation in the HFE gene in more than 80% of the cases (406). Genes that have been implicated in other cases include *TfR2* (transferrin receptor 2) and *HJV* (hemojuvelin), which are similar to HFE in that they affect the synthesis of the protein hepcidin; the gene that encodes hepcidin itself, *HAMP*; and *FPN*, which encodes ferroportin and is inherited in an autosomal dominant fashion (406). It is the most common genetically inherited disease in people of northern European ancestry (407). About 10% of the US population are carriers of the disease (404). The HFE gene is located on chromosome 6 and is most commonly altered by a point mutation that results in a cysteine to tyrosine switch at amino acid position 282 of the

HFE protein (406). Homozygosity is present in approximately 80% of affected persons of northern European descent (406).

The amino acid substitution responsible for the vast majority of cases results in the inability of HFE to bind to β-2 microglobulin, a required step in the shuttling of HFE to the cell surface, the site of interaction of HFE and transferrin. The precise role of HFE in regulating iron stores is not known, although it is likely through interaction with TfR1 and TfR2 to form a functional iron-sensing unit that regulates hepcidin synthesis (406). Although iron absorption through duodenal mucosa is excessive, it is not known if this is the primary event. The degree of saturation of transferrin with iron is very high. Consequently, not all of the iron passing from the intestinal tract can be bound to transferrin, and it is therefore deposited in a variety of organs. Iron accumulates particularly in the parenchyma of the liver and pancreas and in the myocardium, and by damaging the cells in which it accumulates, it causes hepatic cirrhosis, diabetes, and cardiac insufficiency (405,406).

Two observations indicate that the cutaneous pigmentation in hereditary hemochromatosis is caused by melanin and not by hemosiderin. The first observation concerns a patient who, in addition to having hemochromatosis, had vitiligo. The areas of vitiligo were fully depigmented despite the finding on histologic examination that they contained just as much iron as deeply pigmented areas (401). The second observation was made in a black patient with idiopathic hemochromatosis who had three epidermal cysts. Although the patient had noticed no change in his skin color, he had observed progressive darkening of the cysts, and histologic examination revealed considerable amounts of melanin both in the walls of the cysts and in their keratinous contents (408). Although pigmented epidermoid cysts have been attributed to hemochromatosis, in a series of 125 epidermal cysts in Indian patients, pigmentation was found in 79 of them, none of which was attributed to hemochromatosis or iron deposition (409).

The increase in the amount of melanin found in the skin of patients with hemochromatosis is brought about by iron in the skin. The iron stimulates melanocytic activity either by increasing oxidative processes or by reacting with epidermal sulfhydryl groups and reducing their inhibitory effect on the enzyme system governing melanin synthesis (410,411).

Principles of Treatment: Treatment generally consists of phlebotomy, iron chelation therapy, and dietary restrictions to reduce serum iron and appropriate management of end organ damage.

VITAMIN A DEFICIENCY (PHRYNODERMA)

Clinical Summary. Vitamin A deficiency is very rare in the United States, occurring mainly in Asia and Africa. It has been described, however, as occurring after small bowel bypass surgery for obesity (412). Vitamin A deficiency results in cutaneous changes to which the name *phrynoderma* (toad skin) has been given. These consist of dryness and roughness of the skin and the presence of conical, follicular keratotic lesions usually most prominent on the elbows and knees. It may clinically simulate a perforating disorder (413). Vitamin A deficiency may also cause night blindness, xerophthalmia, and keratomalacia.

Histopathology. The skin shows moderate hyperkeratosis with marked distention of the upper parts of the hair follicles by large, horny plugs (414,415). The horny plugs may perforate the follicular epithelium (416). The sebaceous gland lobules are greatly reduced in size. There may also be atrophy of the sweat glands, such as flattening of the secretory cells (417). In severe cases, the sweat glands and sebaceous glands may undergo keratinizing metaplasia (418,419). Tubular casts of keratin surrounding hair shafts were documented in one case (415).

Differential Diagnosis. Histologic differentiation of phrynoderma from ichthyosis vulgaris and keratosis pilaris is impossible, except in very severe cases of phrynoderma that show keratinizing metaplasia of the sweat glands and sebaceous glands. Pityriasis rubra pilaris differs by showing, in addition to hyperkeratosis and follicular plugging, stuttering parakeratosis, irregular epidermal hyperplasia, and an inflammatory infiltrate in the upper dermis.

Principles of Treatment: Vitamin A supplementation and ophthalmic management is standard.

PELLAGRA

Clinical Summary. Pellagra is caused by a deficiency of nicotinic acid (niacin) or its precursor, tryptophan. As a dietary deficiency disease, it may occur in chronic alcoholics and patients with anorexia nervosa (420). It may also occur in patients with the carcinoid syndrome; the tumor cells divert tryptophan toward serotonin, thus depressing endogenous niacin production (420,421). Pellagra is also a well-recognized complication of isoniazid therapy for tuberculosis. Because isoniazid is a structural analog of niacin, it can cause the suppression of endogenous niacin production (421). Because 5-fluorouracil inhibits the conversion of tryptophan to nicotinic acid, it may also precipitate pellagra (421). Multiple anticonvulsants have been reported to induce pellagra as well, although the precise mechanism for this is not known (422,423). Deficiencies of other vitamins such as B_6 and thiamine that are involved in the synthesis or utilization of niacin or excess dietary intake of substances (e.g., leucine) that directly inhibit niacin synthesis can result in clinical symptoms as well (422).

Pellagra presents with cutaneous lesions, gastrointestinal symptoms, and mental changes, resulting in the triad of the three Ds: dermatitis, diarrhea, and dementia.

Skin lesions show a symmetrical, frequently painful, photosensitive dermatitis involving mainly the dorsa of the hands, wrists, and forearms; the face; and the nape of the neck. There is erythema in the early stage that is usually sharply demarcated; in severe cases, it may be accompanied by vesicles or bullae. Later, the skin becomes thickened, scaly, and pigmented.

Histopathology. The histologic changes of the skin are nonspecific. Early lesions present a superficial perivascular lymphocytic inflammatory infiltrate in the upper dermis. Vesicles, if present, may arise either subepidermally, owing to vacuolar degeneration of the basal layer and edema in the papillary dermis, or intraepidermally, owing to excessive ballooning degeneration in the keratinocytes (421,424). Sometimes, there is a distinct pallor of the upper layers of the epidermis with or without an infiltrate of neutrophils. The differential diagnosis of this pattern includes acrodermatitis enteropathica (zinc deficiency), necrolytic migratory erythema of the glucagonoma syndrome, and occasionally psoriasis (422,425,426). There is one report of a contact dermatitis attributable to topical application of a eutectic mixture of local anesthetics (EMLA cream) that resembled pellagra microscopically (427).

In older lesions, hyperkeratosis with areas of parakeratosis and prominent but irregular epidermal hyperplasia is observed. The amount of melanin in the basal layer of the epidermis is often increased. Late lesions may show atrophy of the epidermis and sebaceous glands, and the dermis may show fibrosis in addition to chronic inflammation (421).

Principles of Treatment: Therapy consists of supplementation with niacin or nicotinamide.

Hartnup Disease

Clinical Summary. First described in 1956 and named in 1957 after the family in which it was first observed, Hartnup disease is an autosomal recessive disorder (428,429). It manifests itself in early childhood and often improves over time. A photosensitivity eruption is present that is usually indistinguishable from pellagra (421,430). In some cases, the cutaneous reaction to sun exposure resembles poikiloderma atrophicans vasculare or, because of the prominence of vesicles, hydroa vacciniforme (431,432). An acrodermatitis enteropathica-like eruption has been reported (433,434). There may also be cerebellar ataxia and mental retardation (435).

Histopathology. The cutaneous eruption in Hartnup disease usually shows the same histologic changes observed in pellagra (see previous section) (425). In patients with poikiloderma-like changes, atrophy of the epidermis and the presence of a chronic inflammatory infiltrate with melanophages in the upper dermis are observed (431).

Pathogenesis. Hartnup disease is caused by an enzymatic defect in the transport of tryptophan and a resultant decrease in the endogenous production of niacin. Specifically, the defective transporter is a transporter of monoamino-monocarboxylic acids, which is encoded by a gene that maps to chromosome 5p (436). The defect in tryptophan transport consists of both an intestinal defect in tryptophan absorption and a renal tubular defect causing inadequate reabsorption of amino acids, including tryptophan. Chromatographic study of the urine shows a constant aminoaciduria, particularly the presence of tryptophan and of indolic substances derived from tryptophan—a finding that establishes the diagnosis (431).

Principles of Treatment: Niacin or nicotinamide are used to treat Hartnup disease.

TYROSINEMIA TYPE II (OCULOCUTANEOUS TYROSINOSIS)

Clinical Summary. Tyrosinemia type II, also referred to as the *Richner–Hanhart syndrome* and *oculocutaneous tyrosinosis*, is transmitted as an autosomal recessive trait. It is characterized by very tender hyperkeratotic papules and plaques on the palms and soles arising in infancy or childhood, often associated with hyperhidrosis; bilateral keratitis, which may lead to corneal opacities; and mental retardation. Palmoplantar lesions may begin as vesicles, bullae, and erosions, and may display a linear distribution (437,438). Ocular changes are absent in about 25% of the cases (439), and skin manifestations are absent in about 20% of the cases (440).

Histopathology. In most instances, the histologic findings in the keratotic lesions are not diagnostic, showing merely orthokeratotic hyperkeratosis with hypergranulosis and acanthosis (441). In some cases, vertical parakeratotic columns are present over the openings of the acrosyringia. Multinucleated keratinocytes and dyskeratotic cells may also be noted in the spinous layer (437,441,442). A large intraepidermal bulla seen in another patient was probably also the result of irritation (443).

Pathogenesis. Tyrosinemia maps to chromosome 16q 22.1 to 16q 22.3 (440). As a result of a genetic deficiency in hepatic tyrosine aminotransferase, excessive amounts of tyrosine and its metabolites are found in the blood, urine, and tissues (440). It can be assumed that excessive amounts of intracellular tyrosine enhance cross-links between aggregated tonofilaments. On electron microscopic examination, aggregations of tonofilaments and needle-shaped tyrosine crystalline inclusions are found in keratinocytes (442).

Principles of Treatment: A diet low in tyrosine and phenylalanine improves the disease manifestations.

REFERENCES

1. Sipe JD, Benson MD, Buxbaum JN, et al. Nomenclature Committee of the International Society of Amyloidosis. *Amyloid.* 2012;19:167.
2. Picken MM. New insights into systemic amyloidosis: the importance of diagnosis of specific type. *Curr Opin Nephrol Hypertens.* 2007;16:196.
3. Linke RP. On typing amyloidosis using immunohistochemistry. Detailed illustrations, review and a note on mass spectrometry. *Prog Histochem Cytochem.* 2012;47:61.
4. Murphy C, Fulitz M, Hrncic R, et al. Chemical typing of amyloid protein contained in formalin-fixed paraffin-embedded biopsy specimens. *Am J Clin Pathol.* 2001;116:135.
5. Arbustini E, Verga L, Concardi M, Palladini G, Obici L, Merlini G. Electron and immuno-electron microscopy of abdominal fat identifies and characterizes amyloid fibrils in suspected cardiac amyloidosis. *Amyloid.* 2002;9:108.
6. Vrana JA, Gamez JD, Madden BJ, Theis JD, Bergen HR 3rd, Dogan A. Classification of amyloidosis by laser microdissection and mass spectrometry-based proteomic analysis in clinical biopsy specimens. *Blood.* 2009;114:4957.
7. Rosenzweig M, Landau H. Light chain (AL) amyloidosis: update on diagnosis and management. *J Hematol Oncol.* 2011;4:47.
8. Wey SJ, Chen YM, Lai PJ, Chen DY. Primary Sjögren syndrome manifested as localized cutaneous nodular amyloidosis. *J Clin Rheumatol.* 2011;17:368.
9. Lai KW, Lambert E, Coleman S, Scott G, Mercurio MG. Nodular amyloidosis: differentiation from colloid milium by electron microscopy. *Am J Dermatopathol.* 2009;31:472.
10. Kyle RA, Bayrd ED. Amyloidosis: review of 236 cases. *Medicine (Baltimore).* 1975;54:171.
11. Kumar S, Sengupta RS, Kakkar N, Sharma A, Singh S, Varma S. Skin involvement in primary systemic amyloidosis. *Mediterr J Hematol Infect Dis.* 2013;5:e2013005.
12. Lee HJ, Chang SE, Lee MW, Choi JH, Moon KC. Systemic amyloidosis associated with multiple myeloma presenting as periorbital purpura. *J Dermatol.* 2008;35:371.
13. Nicholson JA, Tappin J. Raccoon eyes in systemic AL amyloidosis. *Br J Haematol.* 2011;153:543.
14. Wang XD, Shen H, Liu ZH. Diffuse haemorrhagic bullous amyloidosis with multiple myeloma. *Clin Exp Dermatol.* 2008;33:94.

15. Natelson EA, Duncan EC, Macossay CR, Fred HL. Amyloidosis palpebrarum. *Arch Intern Med.* 1979;125:304.

16. Reyes CM, Rudinskaya A, Kloss R, Girardi M, Lazova R. Scleroderma-like illness as a presenting feature of multiple myeloma and amyloidosis. *J Clin Rheumatol.* 2008;14:161.

17. Bocquier B, D'Incan M, Joubert J, et al. Amyloid elastosis: a new case studied extensively by electron microscopy and immunohistochemistry. *Br J Dermatol.* 2008;158:858.

18. Asahina A, Hasegawa K, Ishiyama M, et al. Bullous amyloidosis mimicking bullous pemphigoid: usefulness of electron microscopic examination. *Acta Derm Venereol.* 2010;90:427.

19. Singh S, Kumar S, Chaudhary R. Fatigue, macroglossia, xanthomatous papules and bullae. *Indian J Dermatol Venereol Leprol.* 2010;76:216.

20. Libbey CA, Skinner M, Cohen AS. Use of abdominal fat tissue aspirate in the diagnosis of systemic amyloidosis. *Arch Intern Med.* 1983;143:1549.

21. Ansari-Lari MA, Ali SZ. Fine-needle aspiration of abdominal fat pad for amyloid detection: a clinically useful test? *Diagn Cytopathol.* 2004;30:178.

22. Rubinow A, Cohen AS. Skin involvement in generalized amyloidosis. *Ann Intern Med.* 1978;88:781.

23. Li T, Huang X, Cheng S, et al. Utility of abdominal skin plus subcutaneous fat and rectal mucosal biopsy in the diagnosis of AL amyloidosis with renal involvement [published correction appears in *PLoS One.* 2017;12(11):e0187909]. *PLoS One.* 2017;12(9):e0185078.

24. Westermark P. Localized AL amyloidosis: a suicidal neoplasm? *Ups J Med Sci.* 2012;117:244.

25. Bianchi G, Kumar S. Systemic amyloidosis due to clonal plasma cell diseases. *Hematol Oncol Clin North Am.* 2020;34(6):1009–1026.

26. Wechalekar AD, Chakraborty R, Lentzsch S. Systemic amyloidosis due to low-grade lymphoma. *Hematol Oncol Clin North Am.* 2020;34(6):1027–1039.

27. Meijer JM, Schonland SO, Palladini G, et al. Sjögren's syndrome and localized nodular cutaneous amyloidosis: coincidence or a distinct clinical entity? *Arthritis Rheum.* 2008;58:1992.

28. Katzmann JA, Kyle RA, Benson J, et al. Screening panels for detection of monoclonal gammopathies. *Clin Chem.* 2009;55:1517.

29. Mason AR, Rackoff EM, Pollack RB. Primary systemic amyloidosis associated with multiple myeloma: a case report and review of the literature. *Cutis.* 2007;80:193.

30. Lee DY, Kim YJ, Lee JY, Kim MK, Yoon TY. Primary localized cutaneous nodular amyloidosis following local trauma. *Ann Dermatol.* 2011;23:515.

31. Hashimoto K, Kumakiri M. Colloid: amyloid bodies in PUVA-treated human psoriatic patients. *J Invest Dermatol.* 1979;72:70.

32. Goldsbury C, Baxa U, Simon MN, et al. Amyloid structure and assembly: insights from scanning transmission electron microscopy. *J Struct Biol.* 2011;173:1.

33. Lachmann HJ, Goodman HJ, Gilbertson JA, et al. Natural history and outcome in systemic AA amyloidosis. *N Engl J Med.* 2007 7;356:2361.

34. Esteve V, Ribera L, Ponz E, et al. Amiloidosis secundaria asociada a vasculitis cutánea localizada. *Nefrologia.* 2007;27:634.

35. Farhi D, Ingen-Housz-Oro S, Ducret F, et al. Épidermolyse bulleuse dystrophique récessive d'Hallopeau-Siemens associée à une glomérulonéphrite à dépôts mésangiaux d'IgA: 4 cas. *Ann Dermatol Venereol.* 2004;131:963.

36. Csikós M, Orosz Z, Bottlik G, et al. Dystrophic epidermolysis bullosa complicated by cutaneous squamous cell carcinoma and pulmonary and renal amyloidosis. *Clin Exp Dermatol.* 2003;28:163.

37. Katsikas GA, Maragou M, Rontogianni D, Gouma P, Koutsouvelis I, Kappou-Rigatou I. Secondary cutaneous nodular AA amyloidosis in a patient with primary Sjögren syndrome and celiac disease. *J Clin Rheumatol.* 2008;14:27.

38. Orifila C, Giraud P, Modesto A, Suc JM. Abdominal fat tissue aspirate in human amyloidosis: light, electron, and immunofluorescence studies. *Hum Pathol.* 1986;17:366.

39. Brambilla F, Lavatelli F, Di Silvestre D, et al. Reliable typing of systemic amyloidoses through proteomic analysis of subcutaneous adipose tissue. *Blood.* 2012;119:1844.

40. Obici L, Merlini G. AA amyloidosis: basic knowledge, unmet needs and future treatments. *Swiss Med Wkly.* 2012;142:w13580.

41. Perfetto F, Moggi-Pignone A, Livi R, Tempestini A, Bergesio F, Matucci-Cerinic M. Systemic amyloidosis: a challenge for the rheumatologist. *Nat Rev Rheumatol.* 2010;6:417.

42. Obici L, Raimondi S, Lavatelli F, Bellotti V, Merlini G. Susceptibility to AA amyloidosis in rheumatic diseases: a critical overview. *Arthritis Rheum.* 2009;61:1435.

43. Jambrosic J, From L, Hanna W. Lichen amyloidosis. *Am J Dermatopathol.* 1984;6:151.

44. Leonforte JF. Sur l'origine de l'amyloidose maculeuse. *Ann Dermatol Venereol.* 1987;114:801.

45. Rasi A, Khatami A, Javaheri SM. Macular amyloidosis: an assessment of prevalence, sex, and age. *Int J Dermatol.* 2004;43:898.

46. Yoshida A, Takahashi K, Tagami H, Akasaka T. Lichen amyloidosis induced on the upper back by long-term friction with a nylon towel. *J Dermatol.* 2009;36:56.

47. Bedi TR, Datta BN. Diffuse biphasic cutaneous amyloidosis. *Dermatologica.* 1979;158:433.

48. Tanaka A, Arita K, Lai-Cheong JE, Palisson F, Hide M, McGrath JA. New insight into mechanisms of pruritus from molecular studies on familial primary localized cutaneous amyloidosis. *Br J Dermatol.* 2009;161:1217.

49. Vijaya B, Dalal BS; Sunila, Manjunath GV. Primary cutaneous amyloidosis: a clinico-pathological study with emphasis on polarized microscopy. *Indian J Pathol Microbiol.* 2012;55:170.

50. Schepis C, Siragusa M, Gagliardi ME, et al. Primary macular amyloidosis: an ultrastructural approach to diagnosis. *Ultrastruct Pathol.* 1999;23:279.

51. Kumakiri M, Hashimoto K. Histogenesis of primary localized cutaneous amyloidosis: sequential change of epidermal keratinocytes to amyloid via filamentous degeneration. *J Invest Dermatol.* 1979;73:150.

52. Hashimoto K, Kobayashi H. Histogenesis of amyloid in the skin. *Am J Dermatopathol.* 1980;2:165.

53. Glenner GG. Amyloid deposits and amyloidosis: the betafibrilloses. *N Engl J Med.* 1980;302:1283.

54. Horiguchi Y, Fine JD, Leigh IM, Yoshiki T, Ueda M, Imamura S. Lamina densa malformation involved in histogenesis of primary localized amyloidosis. *J Invest Dermatol.* 1992;99:12.

55. Bandhlish A, Aggarwal A, Koranne RV. A clinico-epidemiological study of macular amyloidosis from north India. *Indian J Dermatol.* 2012;57:269.

56. Salim T, Shenoi SD, Balachandran C, Mehta VR. Lichen amyloidosus: a study of clinical, histopathologic and immunofluorescence findings in 30 cases. *Indian J Dermatol Venereol Leprol.* 2005;71:166.

57. Looi LM. Primary localised cutaneous amyloidosis in Malaysians. *Australas J Dermatol.* 1991;32:39.

58. Ritter M, Nawab RA, Tannenbaum M, Hakky SI, Morgan MB. Localized amyloidosis of the glans penis: a case report and literature review. *J Cutan Pathol.* 2003;30:37.

59. Mukai H, Kanzaki T, Nishiyama S. Sulfhydryl and disulfide stainings in amyloids of skin-limited and systemic amyloidoses. *J Invest Dermatol.* 1984;82:4.

60. Masu S, Hosokawa M, Seiji M. Amyloid in localized cutaneous amyloidosis: immunofluorescence studies with anti-keratin antiserum. *Acta Derm Venereol (Stockh).* 1981;61:381.

61. Chang YT, Liu HN, Wang WJ, Lee DD, Tsai SF. A study of cytokeratin profiles in localized cutaneous amyloids. *Arch Dermatol Res.* 2004;296:83.

62. Westermark P, Norén P. Two different pathogenetic pathways in lichen amyloidosis and macular amyloidosis. *Arch Dermatol Res.* 1986;278:206.

63. Weedon D, Shand E. Amyloid in basal cell carcinomas. *Br J Dermatol.* 1979;101:141.

64. Criado PR, Silva CS, Vasconcellos C, Valente NY, Maito JB. Extensive nodular cutaneous amyloidosis: an unusual presentation. *J Eur Acad Dermatol Venereol.* 2005;19:481.

65. Northcutt AD, Vanover MJ. Nodular cutaneous amyloidosis involving the vulva. Case report and literature review. *Arch Dermatol.* 1985;121:518.

66. Handfield-Jones SE, Atherton DJ, Black MM, Hashimoto K, McKee PH. Juvenile colloid milium: clinical, histological and ultrastructural features. *J Cutan Pathol.* 1992;19:434.

67. Ekmekci TR, Koslu A, Sakiz D. Juvenile colloid milium: a case report. *J Eur Acad Dermatol Venereol.* 2005;19:355.

68. Martorell-Calatayud A, Balmer N, Sanmartin O, Botella-Estrada R, Requena C, Guillen-Barona C. Familial juvenile colloid milium: report of a well documented case. *J Am Acad Dermatol.* 2011;64:203.

69. Oskay T, Erdem C, Anadolu R, Peksan Y, Ozsoy N, Gül N. Juvenile colloid milium associated with conjunctival and gingival involvement. *J Am Acad Dermatol.* 2003;49:1185.

70. Figini M, De Francesco V, Finato N, Errichetti E. Dermoscopy in adult colloid milium. *J Dermatol.* 2020;47(4):e127–e128.

71. Piccolo V, Russo T, Ossola MDR, Ferrara G, Ronchi A, Argenziano G. Colloid milium: the expanding spectrum of orange color at dermoscopy. *Int J Dermatol.* 2018;57(8):e46–e48.

72. Mittal RR, Singh SP, Gupta S, Sethi PS. Nodular colloid degeneration over herpes zoster scars. *Indian J Dermatol Venereol Leprol.* 1996;62:181.

73. Choi WJ, Kim BC, Park EJ, Cho HJ, Kim KH, Kim KJ. Nodular colloid degeneration. *Am J Dermatopathol.* 2011;33:388.

74. Toossi P, Shakoei S, Hejazi S, Asadi Z, Yousefi M. Unilateral colloid milium: a rare presentation. *Dermatol Online J.* 2011;17:6.

75. Gönül M, Cakmak SK, Kiliç A, Gül U, Heper AO. Pigmented coalescing papules on the dorsa of the hands: pigmented colloid milium associated with exogenous ochronosis. *J Dermatol.* 2006;33:287.

76. Akhyani M, Hatami P, Yadegarfar Z, Ghanadan A. Pigmented colloid milium associated with exogenous ochronosis in a farmer with long-term exposure to fertilizers. *J Dermatol Case Rep.* 2015;9(2):42–45.

77. Mehregan D, Hooten J. Adult colloid milium: a case report and literature review. *Int J Dermatol.* 2011;50:1531.

78. Kawashima Y, Matsubara T, Kinbara T, et al. Colloid degeneration of the skin. *J Dermatol.* 1977;4:115.

79. Hashimoto K, Black M. Colloid milium: a final degeneration product of actinic elastoid. *J Cutan Pathol.* 1985;12:147.

80. Muscardin LM, Bellocci M, Balus L. Papuloverrucous colloid milium: an occupational variant. *Br J Dermatol.* 2000;143:884.

81. Hashimoto K, Nakayama H, Chimenti S, et al. Juvenile colloid milium: immunohistochemical and ultrastructural studies. *J Cutan Pathol.* 1989;16:164.

82. Kobayashi H, Hashimoto K. Colloid and elastic fibre: ultrastructural study on the histogenesis of colloid milium. *J Cutan Pathol.* 1983;10:111.

83. Konstantinov K, Kabakchiev P, Karchev T, Kobayasi T, Ullman S. Lipoid proteinosis. *J Am Acad Dermatol.* 1992;27:293.

84. Chan I, Liu L, Hamada T, Sethuraman G, McGrath JA. The molecular basis of lipoid proteinosis: mutations in extracellular matrix protein 1. *Exp Dermatol.* 2007;16:881.

85. Hamada T. Lipoid proteinosis. *Clin Exp Dermatol.* 2002;27:624.

86. Nasiri S, Sarrafi-Rad N, Kavand S, Saeedi M. Lipoid proteinosis: report of three siblings. *Dermatol Online J.* 2008;14:6.

87. Nanda A, Alsaleh QA, Al-Sabah H, Ali AM, Anim JT. Lipoid proteinosis: report of four siblings and brief review of the literature. *Pediatr Dermatol.* 2001;18:21.

88. Al-Natour SH. Lipoid proteinosis. A report of 2 siblings and a brief review of the literature. *Saudi Med J.* 2008;29:1188.

89. Holtz KH. Über gehirn-und augenveränderungen bei hyalinosis cutis et mucosae (lipoid-proteinose) mit autopsiebefund. *Arch Klin Exp Dermatol.* 1962;214:289.

90. Navarro C, Fachal C, Rodríguez C, Padró L, Domínguez C. Lipoid proteinosis. A biochemical and ultrastructural investigation of two new cases. *Br J Dermatol.* 1999;141:326.

91. Uchida T, Hayashi H, Inaoki M, Miyamoto T, Fujimoto W. A failure of mucocutaneous lymphangiogenesis may underlie the clinical features of lipoid proteinosis. *Br J Dermatol.* 2007;156:152.

92. Hamada T, McLean WH, Ramsay M, et al. Lipoid proteinosis maps to 1q21 and is caused by mutations in the extracellular matrix protein 1 gene (ECM1). *Hum Mol Genet.* 2002;11:833.

93. Ishibashi A. Hyalinosis cutis et mucosae. Defective digestion and storage of basal lamina glycoprotein synthesized by smooth muscle cells. *Dermatologica.* 1982;165:7.

94. Fleischmajer R, Krieg T, Dziadek M, Altchek D, Timpl R. Ultrastructure and composition of connective tissue in hyalinosis cutis et mucosae skin. *J Invest Dermatol.* 1984;82:252.

95. Loos E, Kerkhofs L, Laureyns G. Lipoid proteinosis: a rare cause of hoarseness. *J Voice.* 2019;33(2):155–158.

96. Puy H, Gouya L, Deybach JC. Porphyrias. *Lancet.* 2010;375:924.

97. Balwani M, Desnick RJ. The porphyrias: advances in diagnosis and treatment. *Blood.* 2012;120:4496.

98. Morais P, Mota A, Baudrier T, et al. Erythropoietic protoporphyria: a family study and report of a novel mutation in the FECH gene. *Eur J Dermatol.* 2011;21:479.

99. Michaels BD, Del Rosso JQ, Mobini N, Michaels JR. Erythropoietic protoporphyria: a case report and literature review. *J Clin Aesthet Dermatol.* 2010;3:44.

100. Redeker AG, Bronow RS. Erythropoietic protoporphyria presenting as hydroa aestivale. *Arch Dermatol.* 1964;89:104.

101. Lecha M, Puy H, Deybach JC. Erythropoietic protoporphyria. *Orphanet J Rare Dis.* 2009;4:19.

102. Holme SA, Anstey AV, Finlay AY, Elder GH, Badminton MN. Erythropoietic protoporphyria in the U.K.: clinical features and effect on quality of life. *Br J Dermatol.* 2006;155:574.

103. Cripps DJ, Goldfarb SS. Erythropoietic protoporphyria: hepatic cirrhosis. *Br J Dermatol.* 1978;98:349.

104. Wells MM, Golitz LE, Bender BJ. Erythropoietic protoporphyria with hepatic cirrhosis. *Arch Dermatol.* 1980;116:429.

105. Hift RJ, Peters TJ, Meissner PN. A review of the clinical presentation, natural history and inheritance of variegate porphyria: its implausibility as the source of the 'Royal Malady'. *J Clin Pathol.* 2012;65:200.

106. Hift RJ, Meissner PN. An analysis of 112 acute porphyric attacks in Cape Town, South Africa: evidence that acute intermittent porphyria and variegate porphyria differ in susceptibility and severity. *Medicine (Baltimore).* 2005;84:48.

107. Borradori L, Van Tuyll van Serooskerken AM, Abraham S, et al. Simultaneous manifestation of variegate porphyria in monozygotic twins. *Br J Dermatol.* 2008;159:503.

108. Hift RJ, Davidson BP, van der Hooft C, Meissner DM, Meissner PN. Plasma fluorescence scanning and fecal porphyrin analysis for the diagnosis of variegate porphyria: precise determination of sensitivity and specificity with detection of protoporphyrinogen oxidase mutations as a reference standard. *Clin Chem.* 2004;50:915.

109. Méndez M, Rossetti MV, Del C Batlle AM, Parera VE. The role of inherited and acquired factors in the development of porphyria

cutanea tarda in the Argentinean population. *J Am Acad Dermatol.* 2005;52:417.

110. Singal AK. Porphyria cutanea tarda: recent update. *Mol Genet Metab.* 2019;128(3):271–281.

111. Ryan Caballes F, Sendi H, Bonkovsky HL. Hepatitis C, porphyria cutanea tarda and liver iron: an update. *Liver Int.* 2012;32:880.

112. Larrondo J, Gosch M. Porphyria cutanea tarda due to primary hemochromatosis. *Am J Med.* 2020;133(11):e681–e682.

113. Jackson Cullison SR, Jedrych JJ, James AJ. Porphyria cutanea trada unmasked by supratherapeutic estrogen during gender-affirming hormone therapy. *JAAD Case Rep.* 2020;6(7):675–678.

114. Sastre L, To-Figueras J, Lens S, et al. Resolution of subclinical porphyria cutanea tarda after hepatitis C eradication with direct-acting anti-virals. *Aliment Pharmacol Ther.* 2020;51(10):968–973.

115. Hazell SZ, Fader AN, Viswanathan AN. Porphyria cutanea tarda exacerbation as a paraneoplastic syndrome in vaginal cancer resolved with chemoradiation. *Gynecol Oncol Rep.* 2020;35:100682.

116. Bygum A, Christiansen L, Petersen NE, Hørder M, Thomsen K, Brandrup F. Familial and sporadic porphyria cutanea tarda: clinical, biochemical and genetic features with emphasis on iron status. *Acta Derm Venereol.* 2003;83:115.

117. Aarsand AK, Boman H, Sandberg S. Familial and sporadic porphyria cutanea tarda: characterization and diagnostic strategies. *Clin Chem.* 2009;55:795.

118. Cantatore-Francis JL, Cohen-Pfeffer J, Balwani M, et al. Hepatoerythropoietic porphyria misdiagnosed as child abuse: cutaneous, arthritic, and hematologic manifestations in siblings with a novel UROD mutation. *Arch Dermatol.* 2010;146:529.

119. Weiss Y, Chen B, Yasuda M, Nazarenko I, Anderson KE, Desnick RJ. Porphyria cutanea tarda and hepatoerythropoietic porphyria: identification of 19 novel uroporphyrinogen III decarboxylase mutations. *Mol Gen Metab.* 2019;128(3):363–366.

120. Mosterd K, Henquet C, Frank J. Porphyria cutanea tarda as rare cutaneous manifestation of hepatic metastases treated with interferon. *Int J Dermatol.* 2007;46(suppl 3):19.

121. Sökmen M, Demirsoy H, Ersoy O, et al. Paraneoplastic porphyria cutanea tarda associated with cholangiocarcinoma: case report. *Turk J Gastroenterol.* 2007;18:200.

122. Czarnecki DB. Hepatoerythropoietic porphyria. *Arch Dermatol.* 1980;116:307.

123. Phillips JD, Whitby FG, Stadtmueller BM, Edwards CQ, Hill CP, Kushner JP. Two novel uroporphyrinogen decarboxylase (URO-D) mutations causing hepatoerythropoietic porphyria (HEP). *Transl Res.* 2007;149:85.

124. Horina JH, Wolf P. Epoetin for severe anemia in hepatoerythropoietic porphyria. *N Engl J Med.* 2000;342:1294.

125. Iglesias B, de la Torre C, Cruces MJ. Cytoplasmic birefringent needle-like inclusions in hepatocytes in a patient with hepatoerythropoietic porphyria. *Histopathology.* 2004;44:629.

126. Piñol Aguadé J, Herrero C, Almeida J, et al. Porphyrie hépato-érythrocytaire. Une nouvelle forme de porphyrie. *Ann Dermatol Syphiligr (Paris).* 1975;102:129.

127. van Tuyll van Serooskerken AM, de Rooij FW, Edixhoven A, et al. Digenic inheritance of mutations in the coproporphyrinogen oxidase and protoporphyrinogen oxidase genes in a unique type of porphyria. *J Invest Dermatol.* 2011;131:2249.

128. Kauppinen R. Porphyrias. *Lancet.* 2005;365:241.

129. Vieira FM, Aoki V, Oliveira ZN, Martins JE. Study of direct immunofluorescence, immunofluorescence mapping and light microscopy in porphyria cutanea tarda. *An Bras Dermatol.* 2010;85:827.

130. Thomas CL, Badminton MN, Rendall JR, Anstey AV. Sclerodermatous changes of face, neck and scalp associated with familial porphyria cutanea tarda. *Clin Exp Dermatol.* 2008;33:422.

131. Ozasa S, Yamamoto S, Maeda M, Inada S, Yanai S, Takagaki K. Erythropoietic protoporphyria. *J Dermatol.* 1977;4:85.

132. Epstein JH, Tuffanelli DL, Epstein WL. Cutaneous changes in the porphyrias. *Arch Dermatol.* 1973;107:689.

133. Ryan EA. Histochemistry of the skin in erythropoietic protoporphyria. *Br J Dermatol.* 1966;78:501.

134. Klein GF, Hintner H, Schuler G, Fritsch P. Junctional blisters in acquired bullous disorders of the dermal-epidermal junction zone. *Br J Dermatol.* 1983;109:499.

135. Nagato N, Nonaka S, Ohgami T, et al. Mechanism of blister formation in porphyria cutanea tarda. *J Dermatol Tokyo.* 1987;14:551.

136. Fung MA, Murphy MJ, Hoss DM, Berke A, Grant-Kels JM. The sensitivity and specificity of "caterpillar bodies" in the differential diagnosis of subepidermal blistering disorders. *Am J Dermatopathol.* 2003;25:287.

137. Raso DS, Greene WB, Maize JC, McGown ST, Metcalf JS. Caterpillar bodies of porphyria cutanea tarda ultrastructurally represent a unique arrangement of colloid and basement membrane bodies. *Am J Dermatopathol.* 1996;18:24.

138. Anton-Lamprecht I, Meyer B. Zur ultrastruktur der haut bei protoporphyrinämie. *Dermatologica.* 1970;141:76.

139. Ryan EA, Madill GT. Electron microscopy of the skin in erythropoietic protoporphyria. *Br J Dermatol.* 1968;80:561.

140. Kint A. A comparative electron microscopic study of the perivascular hyaline from porphyria cutanea tarda and from lipoid-proteinosis. *Arch Klin Exp Dermatol.* 1970;239:203.

141. Murphy GM, Hawk JLM, Magnus JA. Late-onset erythropoietic protoporphyria with unusual cutaneous features. *Arch Dermatol.* 1985;121:1309.

142. Vasil KE, Magro CM. Cutaneous vascular deposition of C5b-9 and its role as a diagnostic adjunct in the setting of diabetes mellitus and porphyria cutanea tarda. *J Am Acad Dermatol.* 2007;56:96.

143. Casanova-González MJ, Trapero-Marugán M, Jones EA, Moreno-Otero R. Liver disease and erythropoietic protoporphyria: a concise review. *World J Gastroenterol.* 2010;16:4526.

144. Wahlin S, Aschan J, Björnstedt M, Broomé U, Harper P. Curative bone marrow transplantation in erythropoietic protoporphyria after reversal of severe cholestasis. *J Hepatol.* 2007; 46:174.

145. Salameh H, Sarairah H, Rizwan M, Kuo YF, Anderson KE, Singal AK. Relapse of porphyria cutanea tarda after treatment with phlebotomy or 4-aminoquinoline antimalarial: a meta-analysis. *Br J Dermatol.* 2018;179(6):1351–1357.

146. Gilchrest B, Rowe JW, Mihm MC Jr. Bullous dermatosis in hemodialysis. *Ann Intern Med.* 1975;83:480.

147. Green JJ, Manders SM. Pseudoporphyria. *J Am Acad Dermatol.* 2001;44:100.

148. Perrot H, Germain D, Euvrard S, Thivolet J. Porphyria cutanea tardalike dermatosis by hemodialysis. *Arch Dermatol Res.* 1977;259:177.

149. Masmoudi A, Ben Hmida M, Mseddi M, et al. Manifestations cutanées chez les hémodialysés chroniques: étude prospective de 363 cas. *Presse Med.* 2006;35:399.

150. Kószó F, Földes M, Morvay M, Judák R, Vakis G, Dobozy A. Krónikus hemodialízissel kapcsolatos porphyria/pseudoporphyria. *Orv Hetil.* 1994;135:2131.

151. Huang YC, Wang CC, Sue YM. Porphyria cutanea tarda in a hemodialysis patient. *QJM.* 2013;106:591.

152. Harlan SL, Winkelmann RK. Porphyria cutanea tarda and chronic renal failure. *Mayo Clin Proc.* 1983;58:467.

153. Phung TL, Pipkin CA, Tahan SR, Chiu DS. Beta-lactam antibiotic-induced pseudoporphyria. *J Am Acad Dermatol.* 2004;51:S80.

154. Kwong WT, Hsu S. Pseudoporphyria associated with voriconazole. *J Drugs Dermatol.* 2007;6:1042.

155. Hivnor C, Nosauri C, James W, Poh-Fitzpatrick M. Cyclosporine-induced pseudoporphyria. *Arch Dermatol.* 2003;139:1373.

156. Silver EA, Silver AH, Silver DS, McCalmont TH. Pseudoporphyria induced by oral contraceptive pills. *Arch Dermatol.* 2003;139:227.

157. Santo Domingo D, Stevenson ML, Auerbach J, Lerman J. Finasteride-induced pseudoporphyria. *Arch Dermatol.* 2011; 147(6):747–748.

158. Lenfestey A, Friedmann D, Burke WA. Metformin-induced pseudoporphyria. *J Drugs Dermatol.* 2012;11(11):1272.

159. Johnson OR, Stewart MF, Bakshi A, Weston P. An unusual bullous eruption: olanzapine induced pseudoporphyria. *BMJ Case Rep.* 2019;12(11):e232263.

160. Mahon C, Purvis D, Laughton S, Bradbeer P, Teague L. Imatinib mesylate-induced pseudoporphyria in two children. *Pediatr Dermatol.* 2014;31(5):603–607.

161. Sanz-Motilva V, Martorell-Calatayud A, Llombart B, et al. Sunitinib-induced pseudoporphyria. *J Eur Acad Dermatol Venereol.* 2015;29(9):1848–1850.

162. Zhao CY, Frew JW, Muhaidat J, et al. Chlorophyll-induced pseudoporphyria with ongoing photosensitivity after cessation—a case series of four patients. *J Eur Acad Dermatol Venereol.* 2016;30(7):1239–1242.

163. Judd LE, Henderson DW, Hill DC. Naproxen-induced pseudoporphyria. *Arch Dermatol.* 1986;122:451.

164. Breier F, Feldmann R, Pelzl M, Gschnait F. Pseudoporphyria cutanea tarda induced by furosemide in a patient undergoing peritoneal dialysis. *Dermatology.* 1998;197:271.

165. Reiter N, El-Shabrawi L, Leinweber B, Berghold A, Aberer E. Calcinosis cutis: Part I. Diagnostic pathway. *J Am Acad Dermatol.* 2011;65:1.

166. Nigwekar SU, Wolf M, Sterns RH, Hix JK. Calciphylaxis from nonuremic causes: a systematic review. *Clin J Am Soc Nephrol.* 2008;3:1139.

167. Aliaga LG, Barreira JC. Calciphylaxis in a patient with systemic lupus erythematosus without renal insufficiency or hyperparathyroidism. *Lupus.* 2012;21:329.

168. Ng AT, Peng DH. Calciphylaxis. *Dermatol Ther.* 2011;24:256.

169. Hruska KA, Choi ET, Memon I, Davis TK, Mathew S. Cardiovascular risk in chronic kidney disease (CKD): the CKD-mineral bone disorder (CKD-MBD). *Pediatr Nephrol.* 2010;25:769.

170. Goel SK, Bellovich K, McCullough PA. Treatment of severe metastatic calcification and calciphylaxis in dialysis patients. *Int J Nephrol.* 2011;2011:701603.

171. Ketteler M, Rothe H, Krüger T, Biggar PH, Schlieper G. Mechanisms and treatment of extraosseous calcification in chronic kidney disease. *Nat Rev Nephrol.* 2011;7:509.

172. Howe SC, Murray JD, Reeves RT, Hemp JR, Carlisle JH. Calciphylaxis, a poorly understood clinical syndrome: three case reports and a review of the literature. *Ann Vasc Surg.* 2001;15:470.

173. Li YJ, Tian YC, Chen YC, et al. Fulminant pulmonary calciphylaxis and metastatic calcification causing acute respiratory failure in a uremic patient. *Am J Kidney Dis.* 2006;47:e47.

174. Aso Y, Sato A, Tayama K, Takanashi K, Satoh H, Takemura Y. Parathyroid carcinoma with metastatic calcification identified by technetium-99m methylene diphosphonate scintigraphy. *Intern Med.* 1996;35:392.

175. Hwang GJ, Lee JD, Park CY, Lim SK. Reversible extraskeletal uptake of bone scanning in primary hyperparathyroidism. *J Nucl Med.* 1996;37:469.

176. Katz AI, Hampers CL, Merrill JP. Secondary hyperparathyroidism and renal osteodystrophy in chronic renal failure. *Medicine (Baltimore).* 1969;48:333.

177. Putkonen T, Wangel GA. Renal hyperparathyroidism with metastatic calcification of the skin. *Dermatologica.* 1959;118:127.

178. Yu WY, Bhutani T, Kornik R, et al. Warfarin-associated nonuremic calciphylaxis. *JAMA Dermatol.* 2017;153(3):309–314.

179. Kolb L, Ellis C, Lafond A. Nonuremic calciphylaxis triggered by rapid weight loss and hypotension. *Cutis.* 2020;105(1):E11-E14.

180. Arseculeratne G, Evans AT, Morley SM. Calciphylaxis—a topical overview. *J Eur Acad Dermatol Venereol.* 2006;20:493.

181. Weenig RH, Sewell LD, Davis MD, McCarthy JT, Pittelkow MR. Calciphylaxis: natural history, risk factor analysis, and outcome. *J Am Acad Dermatol.* 2007;56:569.

182. Essary LR, Wick MR. Cutaneous calciphylaxis. An underrecognized clinicopathologic entity. *Am J Clin Pathol.* 2000;113:280.

183. McCarthy JT, El-Azhary RA, Patzelt MT, et al. Survival, risk factors, and effect of treatment in 101 patients with calciphylaxis. *Mayo Clin Proc.* 2016;91(10):1384–1394.

184. Gabel CK, Nguyen ED, Chakrala T, et al. Assessment of outcomes of calciphylaxis. *J Am Acad Dermatol.* 2021;85:770–773.

185. Tan O, Atik B, Kizilkaya A, Ozer E, Kavukcu S. Extensive skin calcifications in an infant with chronic renal failure: metastatic calcinosis cutis. *Pediatr Dermatol.* 2006;23:235.

186. Posey RE, Ritchie EB. Metastatic calcinosis cutis with renal hyperparathyroidism. *Arch Dermatol.* 1967;95:505.

187. Kolton B, Pedersen J. Calcinosis cutis and renal failure. *Arch Dermatol.* 1974;110:256.

188. Shapiro C, Coco M. Gastric calciphylaxis in a patient with a functioning renal allograft. *Clin Nephrol.* 2007;67:119.

189. Fischer AH, Morris DJ. Pathogenesis of calciphylaxis: study of three cases with literature review. *Hum Pathol.* 1995;26:1055.

190. Mwipatayi BP, Cooke C, Sinniah RH, Abbas M, Angel D, Sieunarine K. Calciphylaxis: emerging concept in vascular patients. *Eur J Dermatol.* 2007;17:73.

191. Daudén E, Oñate MJ. Calciphylaxis. *Dermatol Clin.* 2008;26:557.

192. Chaudet KM, Dutta P, Nigwekar S, Nazarian RM. Calciphylaxis-associated cutaneous vascular calcification in noncalciphylaxis patients. *Am J Dermatopathol.* 2020;42(8):557–563.

193. Strazzula L, Nigwekar SU, Steele D, et al. Intralesional sodium thiosulfate for the treatment of calciphylaxis. *JAMA Dermatol.* 2013;149(8):946–949.

194. Garcia-Lozano JA, Ocampo-Cindiani J, Martinez-Cabriales SA, Garza-Rodríguez V. An update on calciphylaxis. *Am J Clin Dermatol.* 2018;19(4):599–608.

195. Carocha AP, Torturella DM, Barreto GR, Estrella RR, Rochael MC. Calcinosis cutis universalis associated with systemic lupus erythematosus: an exuberant case. *An Bras Dermatol.* 2010;85:883.

196. Dönmez O, Durmaz O. Calcinosis cutis universalis with pediatric systemic lupus erythematosus. *Pediatr Nephrol.* 2010;25:1375.

197. Wananukul S, Pongprasit P, Wattanakrai P. Calcinosis cutis presenting years before other clinical manifestations of juvenile dermatomyositis: report of two cases. *Australas J Dermatol.* 1997;38:202.

198. Santili C, Akkari M, Waisberg G, Kessler C, Alcantara Td, Delai PL. Calcinosis universalis: a rare diagnosis. *J Pediatr Orthop B.* 2005;14:294.

199. Terranova M, Amato L, Palleschi GM, Massi D, Fabbri P. A case of idiopathic calcinosis universalis. *Acta Derm Venereol.* 2005;85:189.

200. Holmes R. Morphoea with calcinosis. *Clin Exp Dermatol.* 1979;4:125.

201. Kaiser H. Ein Dermatologe und ein Rheumatologe definieren ein Syndrom. *Z Rheumatol.* 2009;68:594.

202. Olsen KM, Chew FS. Tumoral calcinosis: pearls, polemics, and alternative possibilities. *Radiographics.* 2006;26:871.

203. Badawi AH, Patel V, Warner AE, Hall JC. Dystrophic calcinosis cutis: treatment with intravenous sodium thiosulfate. *Cutis.* 2020;106(2):E15–E17.

204. Alabaz D, Mungan N, Turgut M, Dalay C. Unusual idiopathic calcinosis cutis universalis in a child. *Case Rep Dermatol.* 2009;1:16.

205. Valdatta L, Buoro M, Thione A, et al. Idiopathic circumscripta calcinosis cutis of the knee. *Dermatol Surg.* 2003;29:1222.

206. Sprecher E. Familial tumoral calcinosis: from characterization of a rare phenotype to the pathogenesis of ectopic calcification. *J Invest Dermatol.* 2010;130:652.

207. Pursley TV, Prince MJ, Chausmer AB, Raimer SS. Cutaneous manifestations of tumoral calcinosis. *Arch Dermatol.* 1979;115:1100.

208. Esapa CT, Head RA, Jeyabalan J, et al. A mouse with an N-ethyl-N-nitrosourea (ENU) induced Trp589Arg Galnt3 mutation represents a model for hyperphosphataemic familial tumoural calcinosis. *PLoS One.* 2012;7:e43205.

209. Ramnitz MS, Gafni RI, Collins MT. Hyperphosphatemic familial tumoral calcinosis. In: Adam MP, Ardinger HH, Pagon RA, et al., eds. *GeneReviews.* University of Washington; 2018.

210. Slavin RE, Wen J, Barmada A. Tumoral calcinosis—a pathogenetic overview: a histological and ultrastructural study with a report of two new cases, one in infancy. *Int J Surg Pathol.* 2012;20:462.

211. Polykandriotis EP, Beutel FK, Horch RE, Grünert J. A case of familial tumoral calcinosis in a neonate and review of the literature. *Arch Orthop Trauma Surg.* 2004;124:563.

212. Paegle RD. Ultrastructure of mineral deposits in calcinosis cutis. *Arch Pathol.* 1966;2:474.

213. Cornelius CE III, Tenenhouse A, Weber JC. Calcinosis cutis. *Arch Dermatol.* 1968;98:219.

214. Topaz O, Bergman R, Mandel U, et al. Absence of intraepidermal glycosyltransferase ppGalNac-T3 expression in familial tumoral calcinosis. *Am J Dermatopathol.* 2005;27:211.

215. Doneray H, Ozden A, Gurbuz K. The successful treatment of deep soft-tissue calcifications with topical sodium thiosulphate and acetazolamide in a boy with hyperphosphatemic familial tumoral calcinosis due to a novel mutation in FGF23 [published online ahead of print]. *J Clin Res Pediatr Endocrinol.* 2021. doi:10.4274/jcrpe.galenos.2021.2020.0269.

216. Lei X, Liu B, Cheng Q, Wu J. Idiopathic scrotal calcinosis: report of two cases and review of literature. *Int J Dermatol.* 2012;51:199.

217. Dubey S, Sharma R, Maheshwari V. Scrotal calcinosis: idiopathic or dystrophic? *Dermatol Online J.* 2010;16(2):5.

218. Ito A, Sakamoto F, Ito M. Dystrophic scrotal calcinosis originating from benign eccrine epithelial cysts. *Br J Dermatol.* 2001;144:146.

219. Pabuççuoğlu U, Canda MS, Güray M, Kefi A, Canda E. The possible role of dartoic muscle degeneration in the pathogenesis of idiopathic scrotal calcinosis. *Br J Dermatol.* 2003;148:827.

220. Sugihara T, Tsuru N, Kume H, Homma Y, Ihara H. Relapse of scrotal calcinosis 7 years after primary excision. *Urol Int.* 2014;92(4):448–490.

221. Qader MA, Almalmi M. Diffuse cutaneous calculi (subepidermal calcified nodules): case study. *Dermatol Ther.* 2010;23:312.

222. Kim HS, Kim MJ, Lee JY, Kim HO, Park YM. Multiple subepidermal calcified nodules on the thigh mimicking molluscum contagiosum. *Pediatr Dermatol.* 2011;28:191.

223. Tharini GK, Prabavathy D, Daniel SJ, Manjula J. Congenital calcinosis cutis of the foot. *Indian J Dermatol.* 2012;57:294.

224. Ozuguz P, Balta I, Bozkurt O, Unverdi H, Dostbil A. Multiple subepidermal calcified nodule mimicking eruptive xanthoma: a case report and review of the literature. *Indian J Dermatol.* 2013;58(5):406.

225. Ahn IS, Chung BY, Lee HB, et al. A case of a subepidermal calcified nodule on the sole without trauma. *Ann Dermatol.* 2011;23(suppl 1):S116.

226. Nakamura Y, Muto M. Subepidermal calcified nodule of the knee with transepidermal elimination of calcium. *J Dermatol.* 2012;39(11):965–966.

227. Joo YH, Kwon IH, Huh CH, Park KC, Youn SW. A case of persistent subepidermal calcified nodule in an adult treated with CO2 laser. *J Dermatol.* 2004;31:480.

228. Bursill D, Taylor W, Terkeltaub R, et al. Gout, hyperuricaemia and crystal-associated disease network (G-CAN) consensus statement regarding labels and definitions of disease states of gout. *Ann Rheum Dis.* 2019;78(11)1592–1600.

229. Kasper I, Juriga M, Giurini J, Shmerling RH. Treatment of tophaceous gout: when medication is not enough. *Semin Arthritis Rheum.* 2016;45(6):669–674.

230. Bieber JD, Terkeltaub RA. Gout: on the brink of novel therapeutic options for an ancient disease. *Arthritis Rheum.* 2004;50:2400.

231. Molina-Ruiz A, Cerroni L, Kutzner H, Requena L. Cutaneous deposits. *Am J Dermatopathol.* 2014;36(1):1–48.

232. Pascart T, Liote F. Gout: state of the art after a decade of developments. *Rheumatology (Oxford).* 2019;58(1):27–44.

233. Richette P, Bardin T. Gout. *Lancet.* 2010;375:318.

234. Griffin GR, Munns J, Fullen D, Moyer JS. Auricular tophi as the initial presentation of gout. *Otolaryngol Head Neck Surg.* 2009;141:153.

235. Lam G, Ross FL, Chiu ES. Nonhealing ulcers in patients with tophaceous gout: a systematic review. *Adv Skin Wound Care.* 2017;30(5):230–237.

236. Braun-Falco M, Hofmann SC. Tophaceous gout in the finger pads. *Clin Exp Dermatol.* 2010;35:e22.

237. Ochoa CD, Valderrama V, Mejia J, et al. Panniculitis: another clinical expression of gout. *Rheumatol Int.* 2011;31:831.

238. Shukla R, Vender RB, Alhabeeb A, Salama S, Murphy F. Miliarial gout (a new entity). *J Cutan Med Surg.* 2007;11:31.

239. Lo TE, Racaza GZ, Penserga EG. 'Golden Kernels within the skin': disseminated cutaneous gout. *BMJ Case Rep.* 2013;2013.

240. Guzman R, DeClerck B, Crew A, Peng D, Adler BL. Disseminated cutaneous gout: a rare manifestation of a common disease. *Dermatol Online J.* 2020;26(1):13030/qt4m1660sp.

241. King DF, King LA. The appropriate processing of tophi for microscopy. *Am J Dermatopathol.* 1982;4:239.

242. Darby AJ, Harnes NF, Pritchard MS. Demonstration of urate crystals after formalin fixation. *Histopathology.* 1998;32:382.

243. Weaver J, Somani N, Bauer TW, Piliang M. Simple non-staining method to demonstrate urate crystals in formalin-fixed, paraffin-embedded skin biopsies. *J Cutan Pathol.* 2009;36:560.

244. Shidham V, Shidham G. Staining method to demonstrate urate crystals after formalin-fixed, paraffin-embedded tissue sections. *Arch Pathol Lab Med.* 2000;124:774.

245. Courtney P, Doherty M. Joint aspiration and injection and synovial fluid analysis. *Best Pract Res Clin Rheumatol.* 2013;27:137.

246. Orzan OA, Simion G, Tudose I, Costache. Histopathological study of cutaneous lesions in gout. *Rom J Diabetes Nutr Metab Dis.* 2013;20:11.

247. FitzGerald JD, Dalbeth N, Mikuls T, et al. 2020 American College of Rheumatology guideline for the management of gout. *Arthritis Rheumatol.* 2020;72(6):879–895.

248. Ramesh V, Avninder S. Endogenous ochronosis with a predominant acrokeratoelastoidosis-like presentation. *Int J Dermatol.* 2008;47:873.

249. Vijaikumar M, Thappa DM, Srikanth S, Sethuraman G, Nadarajan S. Alkaptonuric ochronosis presenting as palmoplantar pigmentation. *Clin Exp Dermatol.* 2000;25:305.

250. Khaled A, Kerkeni N, Hawilo A, Fazaa B, Kamoun MR. Endogenous ochronosis: case report and a systematic review of the literature. *Int J Dermatol.* 2011;50:262.

251. Keller JM, Macaulay W, Nercessian OA, Jaffe IA. New developments in ochronosis: review of the literature. *Rheumatol Int.* 2005;25:81.

252. Gil I, Segura S, Martínez-Escala E, et al. Dermoscopic and reflectance confocal microscopic features of exogenous ochronosis. *Arch Dermatol.* 2010;146:1021.

253. Moche MJ, Glassman SJ, Modi D, Grayson W. Cutaneous annular sarcoidosis developing on a background of exogenous ochronosis: a report of two cases and review of the literature. *Clin Exp Dermatol.* 2010;35:399.

254. Robinson-Bostom L, Pomerantz D, Wilkel C, et al. Localized argyria with pseudo-ochronosis. *J Am Acad Dermatol.* 2002; 46:222.

255. Shimizu I, Dill SW, McBean J, Robinson-Bostom L. Metal-induced granule deposition with pseudoochronosis. *J Am Acad Dermatol.* 2010;63:357.

256. Ankad B, Reshme A, Nikam B. Endogenous ochronosis: a dermoscopic view. *Int. J Dermatol.* 2019;58(9):e175-e178.

257. Penneys NS. Ochronosislike pigmentation from hydroquinone bleaching creams. *Arch Dermatol.* 1985;121:1239.

258. Turgay E, Canat D, Gurel MS, Yuksel T, Baran MF, Demirkesen C. Endogenous ochronosis. *Clin Exp Dermatol.* 2009;34:e865.

259. Findlay GH, Morrison JGL, Simson IW. Exogenous ochronosis and pigmented colloid milium from hydroquinone bleaching creams. *Br J Dermatol.* 1975;93:613.

260. Laymon CW. Ochronosis. *Arch Dermatol.* 1953;67:553.

261. Levin CY, Maibach H. Exogenous ochronosis. An update on clinical features, causative agents and treatment options. *Am J Clin Dermatol.* 2001;2:213.

262. Ribas J, Schettini AP, de Sousa Melo Cavalcante M. Exogenous ochronosis hydroquinone induced: a report of four cases. *An Bras Dermatol.* 2010;85:699.

263. Touart DM, Sau P. Cutaneous deposition diseases. Part II. *J Am Acad Dermatol.* 1998;39:197.

264. Attwood HD, Clifton S, Mitchell RE. A histological, histochemical and ultrastructural study of dermal ochronosis. *Pathology.* 1971;3:115.

265. Simmons B, Griffith R, Bray F, Falto-Aizpurua LA, Nouri K. Exogenous ochronosis: a comprehsive review of the diagnosis, epidemiology, causes and treatments. *Am J Clin Dermatol.* 2015;16:205–212.

266. Sawada Y, Seishima M, Funabashi M, Noda T, Maeda M, Kitajima Y. Papular mucinosis associated with scleroderma. *Eur J Dermatol.* 1998;8:497.

267. Johnson WC, Helwig EB. Cutaneous focal mucinosis. *Arch Dermatol.* 1966;93:13.

268. Cawley EP, Lupton CH Jr, Wheeler CE, McManus JF. Examination of normal and myxedematous skin. *Arch Dermatol.* 1957;76:537.

269. Rongioletti F, Rebora A. Cutaneous mucinoses: microscopic criteria for diagnosis. *Am J Dermatopathol.* 2001;23:257.

270. Ansah-Addo S, Alexis AF. Pretibial myxedema in a euthyroid patient. *J Clin Aesthet Dermatol.* 2021;14:21.

271. Verma S, Rongioletti F, Braun-Falco M, Ruzicka T. Preradial myxedema in a euthyroid male: a distinct rarity. *Dermatol Online J.* 2013;19:9.

272. Schwartz KM, Fatourechin V, Ahmed DD, Pond GR. Dermatophy of Graves' disease (pretibial myxedema): long-term outcome. *J Clin Endocrinol Metab.* 2002;87:438.

273. Lynch PJ, Maize JC, Sisson JC. Pretibial myxedema and nonthyrotoxic thyroid disease. *Arch Dermatol.* 1973;107:107.

274. Dharmalingam M, Seema G, Khaitan B, Karak A, Ammini AC. Plaque form of pretibial myxedema in hypothyroidism. *Indian J Dermatol Venereol Leprol.* 2001;67:330.

275. Senel E, Güleç AT. Euthyroid pretibial myxedema and EMO syndrome. *Acta Dermatovenerol Alp Panonica Adriat.* 2009;18:21.

276. Fatourechi V. Pretibial myxedema: pathophysiology and treatment options. *Am J Clin Dermatol.* 2005;6:295.

277. Daumerie C, Ludgate M, Costagliola S, Many MC. Evidence for thyrotropin receptor immunoreactivity in pretibial connective tissue from patients with thyroid-associated dermopathy. *Eur J Endocrinol.* 2002;146:35.

278. Konrad K, Brenner W, Pehamberger H. Ultrastructural and immunological findings in Graves' disease with pretibial myxedema. *J Cutan Pathol.* 1980;7:99.

279. Ishii M, Nakagawa M, Hamada T. An ultrastructural study of pretibial myxedema utilizing improved ruthenium red stain. *J Cutan Pathol.* 1984;11:125.

280. Schermer DR, Roenigk HH Jr, Schumacher OP, McKenzie JM. Relationship of long-acting thyroid stimulator to pretibial myxedema. *Arch Dermatol.* 1970;102:62.

281. Cheung HS, Nicoloff JT, Kamiel MB, Spolter L, Nimni ME. Stimulation of fibroblast biosynthetic activity by serum of patients with pretibial myxedema. *J Invest Dermatol.* 1978;71:12.

282. Zhang L, Bowen T, Grennan-Jones F, et al. Thyrotropin receptor activation increases hyaluronan production in preadipocyte fibroblasts: contributory role in hyaluronan accumulation in thyroid dysfunction. *J Biol Chem.* 2009;284:26447.

283. Davies TF, Andersen S, Latif R, et al. Graves' disease. *Nat Rev Dis Primers.* 2020;6:52.

284. Mir M, Jogi R, Rosen T. Pretibial mucinosis in a patient without Graves disease. *Cutis.* 2011;88:300.

285. Rongioletti F. Lichen myxedematosus (papular mucinosis): new concepts and perspectives for an old disease. *Semin Cutan Med Surg.* 2006;25:100.

286. Rongioletti F, Rebora A. Updated classification of papular mucinosis, lichen myxedematosus, and scleromyxedema. *J Am Acad Dermatol.* 2001;44:273.

287. Fleming KE, Virmani D, Sutton E, et al. Scleromyxedema and the dermato-neuro syndrome: case report and review of the literature. *J Cutan Pathol.* 2012;39:508.

288. Borradori L, Aractingi S, Blanc F, Verola O, Dubertret L. Acral persistent papular mucinosis and IgA monoclonal gammopathy. *Dermatology.* 1992;185:134.

289. Chen CW, Tsai TF, Chang SP, Chen YF, Hung CM. Congenital cutaneous mucinosis with spontaneous regression: an atypical cutaneous mucinosis of infancy? *Clin Exp Dermatol.* 2009;34:804.

290. Lindor NM, Hand J, Burch PA, Gibson LE. Birt-Hogg-Dube syndrome: an autosomal dominant disorder with predisposition to cancers of the kidney, fibrofolliculomas, and focal cutaneous mucinosis. *Int J Dermatol.* 2001;40:653.

291. Lichte V, Hanneken S, Gerber PA, van Geel M, Frank J. Faziale papeln und pneumothoraces. Birt-Hogg-Dubé syndrome. *Hautarzt.* 2012;63:762.

292. Bragg J, Soldano AC, Latkowski JA. Papular mucinosis (discrete papular lichen myxedematosus). *Dermatol Online J.* 2008;14:14.

293. Rongioletti F, Cozzani E, Parodi A. Scleromyxedema with an interstitial granulomatous-like pattern: a rare histologic variant mimicking granuloma annulare. *J Cutan Pathol.* 2010;37:1084.

294. Stetsenko GY, Vary JC Jr, Olerud JE, Argenyi ZB. Unusual granulomatous variant of scleromyxedema. *J Am Acad Dermatol.* 2008;59:346.

295. Satter EK, Metcalf JS, Maize JC. Can scleromyxedema be differentiated from nephrogenic fibrosing dermopathy by the distribution of the infiltrate? *J Cutan Pathol.* 2006;33:756.

296. Miyamoto J, Tanikawa A, Igarashi A, et al. Detection of iron deposition in dermal fibrocytes is a useful tool for histologic diagnosis of nephrogenic systemic fibrosis. *Am J Dermatopathol.* 2011;33:271.

297. Basak P, Jesmajian S. Nephrogenic systemic fibrosis: current concepts. *Indian J Dermatol.* 2011;56:59.

298. Montgomery H, Underwood LJ. Lichen myxedematosus: differentiation from cutaneous myxedemas or mucoid states. *J Invest Dermatol.* 1953;20:213.

299. Braun-Falco O, Weidner F. Skleromyxödem Arndt-Gottron mit knochenmarks-plasmocytose und myositis. *Arch Belg Dermatol Syphiligr.* 1970;26:193.

300. Perry HO, Montgomery H, Stickney JM. Further observations on lichen myxedematosus. *Ann Intern Med.* 1960;53:955.

301. McGuiston CH, Schoch EP Jr. Autopsy findings in lichen myxedematosus. *Arch Dermatol.* 1956;74:259.

302. Loggini B, Pingitore R, Avvenente A, Giuliano G, Barachini P. Lichen myxedematosus with systemic involvement: clinical and autopsy findings. *J Am Acad Dermatol.* 2001;45:606.

303. Godby A, Bergstresser PR, Chaker B, Pandya AG. Fatal scleromyxedema: report of a case and review of the literature. *J Am Acad Dermatol.* 1998;38:289.

304. Hardemeier T, Vogel A. Elektronenmikroskopische befunde beim sklerömyxodem Arndt-Gottron. *Arch Klin Exp Dermatol.* 1970;237:722.

305. Danielsen L, Kobayasi T. Ultrastructural changes in scleromyxedema. *Acta Derm Venereol.* 1975;55:451.

306. Lai A, Fat RFM, Suurmond D, Rádl J, van Furth R. Scleromyxedema (lichen myxedematosus) associated with a paraprotein, IgG1 of the type kappa. *Br J Dermatol*. 1973;88:107.

307. McCarthy JT, Osserman E, Lombardo PC, Takatsuki K. An abnormal serum globulin in lichen myxedematosus. *Arch Dermatol*. 1964;89:446.

308. Ataergin S, Arpaci F, Demiriz M, Ozet A. Transient efficacy of double high-dose chemotherapy and autologous peripheral stem cell transplantation, immunoglobulin, thalidomide, and bortezomib in the treatment of scleromyxedema. *Am J Clin Dermatol*. 2008;9:271.

309. Fett NM, Toporcer MB, Dalmau J, Shinohara MM, Vogl DT. Scleromyxedema and dermato–neuro syndrome in a patient with multiple myeloma effectively treated with dexamethasone and bortezomib. *Am J Hematol*. 2011;86:893.

310. Yeung CK, Loong F, Kwong YL. Scleromyxoedema due to a plasma cell neoplasm: rapid remission with bortezomib, thalidomide and dexamethasone. *Br J Haematol*. 2012;157:411.

311. Cañueto J, Labrador J, Román C, et al. The combination of bortezomib and dexamethasone is an efficient therapy for relapsed/refractory scleromyxedema: a rare disease with new clinical insights. *Eur J Haematol*. 2012;88:450.

312. Taha RY, Hasan S, Ibrahim F, et al. Characterization of circulating myeloma tumor cells by next generation flow cytometry in scleromyxedema patient: a case report. *Medicine*. 2020;99(27):e20726.

313. Hoffman JHO, Enk AH. Scleromyxedema. *J Dtsch Dermatol Ges*. 2020;18(12):1449–1467.

314. Perry HO, Kierland RR, Montgomery H. Plaque-like form of cutaneous mucinosis. *Arch Dermatol*. 1960;82:980.

315. Steigleder GK, Gartmann H, Linker U. REM-syndrome: reticular erythematous mucinosis (round-cell erythematosis): a new entity? *Br J Dermatol*. 1974;91:191.

316. Thareja S, Paghdal K, Lien MH, Fenske NA. Reticular erythematous mucinosis—a review. *Int J Dermatol*. 2012;51:903.

317. Wriston CC, Rubin AI, Martin LK, Kossard S, Murrell DF. Plaque-like cutaneous mucinosis: case report and literature review. *Am J Dermatopathol*. 2012;34:e50.

318. Quimby SR, Perry HO. Plaque-like cutaneous mucinosis: its relationship to reticular erythematous mucinosis. *J Am Acad Dermatol*. 1982;6:856.

319. Morison WL, Shea CR, Parrish JA. Reticular erythematous mucinosis syndrome. *Arch Dermatol*. 1979;115:1340.

320. Del Pozo J, Pena C, Almagro M, Yebra MT, Martínez W, Fonseca E. Systemic lupus erythematosus presenting with a reticular erythematous mucinosis-like condition. *Lupus*. 2000;9:144.

321. Caputo R, Marzano AV, Tourlaki A, Marchini M. Reticular erythematous mucinosis occurring in a brother and sister. *Dermatology*. 2006;212:385.

322. Fühler M, Ottmann K, Tronnier M. Reticular erythematous mucinosis—(REM syndrome) in twins. *J Dtsch Dermatol Ges*. 2009;7:968.

323. Ziemer M, Eisendle K, Müller H, Zelger B. Lymphocytic infiltration of the skin (Jessner-Kanof) but not reticular erythematous mucinosis occasionally represents clinical manifestations of Borrelia-associated pseudolymphoma. *Br J Dermatol*. 2009;161:583.

324. Braddock SW, Kay HD, Maennle D, et al. Clinical and immunologic studies in reticular erythematous mucinosis and Jessner's lymphocytic infiltrate of skin. *J Am Acad Dermatol*. 1993;28:691.

325. Herzberg J. Das REM-Syndrom. *Z Hautkr*. 1981;56:1317.

326. Tominaga A, Tajima S, Ishibashi A, Kimata K. Reticular erythematous mucinosis syndrome with an infiltration of factor XIIIa+ and hyaluronan synthase 2+ dermal dendrocytes. *Br J Dermatol*. 2001;145:141.

327. Stephens CJM, Das AK, Black MM, et al. The dermal mucinoses: a clinicopathologic and ultrastructural study. *J Cutan Pathol*. 1990;17:319.

328. Gasior-Chrzan B, Husebekk A. Reticular erythematous mucinosis syndrome: report of a case with positive immunofluorescence. *J Eur Acad Dermatol Venereol*. 2004;18:375.

329. Van Zander J, Shaw JC. Papular and nodular mucinosis as a presenting sign of progressive systemic sclerosis. *J Am Acad Dermatol*. 2002;46:304.

330. Cowen EW, Scott GA, Mercurio MG. Self-healing juvenile cutaneous mucinosis. *J Am Acad Dermatol*. 2004;50:S97.

331. Carder KR, Fitzpatrick JE, Weston WL, Morelli JG. Self-healing juvenile cutaneous mucinosis. *Pediatr Dermatol*. 2003;20(1):35.

332. Nagaraj LV, Fangeman W, White W, et al. Self-healing juvenile cutaneous mucinosis: cases highlighting subcutaneous/fascial involvement. *J Am Acad Dermatol*. 2006;55:1036.

333. Abbas O, Saleh Z, Kurban M, Al-Sadoon N, Ghosn S. Asymptomatic papules and nodules on forehead and limbs. Self-healing juvenile cutaneous mucinosis (SHJCM). *Clin Exp Dermatol*. 2010;35:e76.

334. Barreau M, Dompmartin-Blanchère A, Jamous R, et al. Nodular lesions of self-healing juvenile cutaneous mucinosis: a pitfall! *Am J Dermatopathol*. 2012;34:699.

335. Kroft EB, de Jong EM. Scleredema diabeticorum case series: successful treatment with UV-A1. *Arch Dermatol*. 2008;144:947.

336. Lewerenz V, Ruzicka T. Scleredema adultorum associated with type 2 diabetes mellitus: a report of three cases. *J Eur Acad Dermatol Venereol*. 2007;21:560.

337. Mattei P, Templet J, Cusack C. Board stiff. *Am J Med*. 2007;120:854.

338. Fleischmajer R, Raludi G, Krol S. Scleredema and diabetes mellitus. *Arch Dermatol*. 1970;101:21.

339. Martín C, Requena L, Manrique K, Manzarbeitia FD, Rovira A. Scleredema diabeticorum in a patient with type 2 diabetes mellitus. *Case Rep Endocrinol*. 2011;2011:560273.

340. Krakowski A, Covo J, Berlin C. Diabetic scleredema. *Dermatologica*. 1973;146:193.

341. Fleischmajer R, Perlish JS. Glycosaminoglycans in scleroderma and scleredema. *J Invest Dermatol*. 1972;58:129.

342. Beers WH, Ince A, Moore TL. Scleredema adultorum of Buschke: a case report and review of the literature. *Semin Arthritis Rheum*. 2006;35:355.

343. Morais P, Almeida M, Santos P, Azevedo F. Scleredema of Buschke following *Mycoplasma pneumoniae* respiratory infection. *Int J Dermatol*. 2011;50:454.

344. Kövary PM, Vakilzadeh F, Macher E, Zaun H, Merk H, Goerz G. Monoclonal gammopathy in scleredema. *Arch Dermatol*. 1981;117:536.

345. Holubar K, Mach KW. Scleredema (Buschke). *Acta Derm Venereol (Stockh)*. 1967;47:102.

346. Roupe G, Laurent TC, Malmström A, Suurküla M, Särnstrand B. Biochemical characterization and tissue distribution of the scleredema in a case of Buschke's disease. *Acta Derm Venereol (Stockh)*. 1987;67:193.

347. Curtis AC, Shulak BM. Scleredema adultorum. *Arch Dermatol*. 1965;92:526.

348. Heilbron B, Saxe N. Scleredema in an infant. *Arch Dermatol*. 1986;122:1417.

349. Matsuoka LY, Wortsman J, Dietrich JG, Kupchella CE. Glycosaminoglycans in histologic sections. *Arch Dermatol*. 1987;123:862.

350. Reichenberger M. Betrachtungen zum Skleroedema adultorum Buschke. *Hautarzt*. 1964;15:339.

351. Isaac A, Costa I, Leal I. Scleredema of Buschke in a child with cardiac involvement. *Pediatr Dermatol*. 2010;27:315.

352. Leinwand I. Generalized scleredema: report with autopsy findings. *Ann Intern Med*. 1951;34:226.

353. Dziadzio M, Anastassiades CP, Hawkins PN, et al. From scleredema to AL amyloidosis: disease progression or coincidence? Review of the literature. *Clin Rheumatol*. 2006;25:3.

354. Szturz P, Adam Z, Vašků V, et al. Complete remission of multiple myeloma associated scleredema after bortezomib-based treatment. *Leuk Lymphoma*. 2013;54:1324.

355. Varga J, Gotta S, Li L, Sollberg S, Di Leonardo M. Scleredema adultorum: case report and demonstration of abnormal expression of extracellular matrix genes in skin fibroblasts in vivo and in vitro. *Br J Dermatol.* 1995;132:992.

356. Sansom JE, Sheehan AL, Kennedy CT, Delaney TJ. A fatal case of scleredema of Buschke. *Br J Dermatol.* 1994;130:669.

357. Muenzer J. Overview of the mucopolysaccharidoses. *Rheumatology (Oxford).* 2011;50 Suppl 5:v4.

358. Maire I. Is genotype determination useful in predicting the clinical phenotype in lysosomal storage diseases? *J Inherit Metab Dis.* 2001;24(Suppl 2):57.

359. Gieselmann V. What can cell biology tell us about heterogeneity in lysosomal storage diseases? *Acta Paediatr Suppl.* 2005; 94:80.

360. Pastores GM, Meere PA. Musculoskeletal complications associated with lysosomal storage disorders: Gaucher disease and Hurler-Scheie syndrome (mucopolysaccharidosis type I). *Curr Opin Rheumatol.* 2005;17:70.

361. Giugliani R, Federhen A, Rojas MV, et al. Mucopolysaccharidosis I, II, and VI: brief review and guidelines for treatment. *Genet Mol Biol.* 2010;33:589.

362. Lonergan CL, Payne AR, Wilson WG, Patterson JW, English JC 3rd. What syndrome is this? Hunter Syndrome. *Pediatr Dermatol.* 2004;21:679.

363. Gajula P, Ramalingam K, Bhadrashetty D. A rare case of mucopolysaccharidosis: Hunter syndrome. *J Nat Sci Biol Med.* 2012;3:97.

364. Schiro JA, Mallory SB, Demmer L, Dowton SB, Luke MC. Grouped papules in Hurler-Scheie syndrome. *J Am Acad Dermatol.* 1996;35:868.

365. Hambrick GW Jr, Scheie HG. Studies of the skin in Hurler's syndrome. *Arch Dermatol.* 1962;85:455.

366. Horiuchi R, Ishikawa H, Ishii Y, Watanabe Y, Noguchi T, Suzuki S. Mucopolysaccharidosis with special reference to Scheie syndrome. *J Dermatol.* 1976;3:171.

367. Freeman RG. A pathological basis for the cutaneous papules of mucopolysaccharidosis: II. The Hunter syndrome. *J Cutan Pathol.* 1977;4:318.

368. Belcher RW. Ultrastructure of the skin in the genetic mucopolysaccharidoses. *Arch Pathol.* 1972;94:511.

369. Belcher RW. Ultrastructure and function of eccrine glands in the mucopolysaccharidoses. *Arch Pathol.* 1973;96:339.

370. Demitsu T, Kakurai M, Okubo Y, et al. Skin eruption as the presenting sign of Hunter syndrome IIB. *Clin Exp Dermatol.* 1999;24:179.

371. Belcher RW. Ultrastructure and cytochemistry of lymphocytes in the genetic mucopolysaccharidoses. *Arch Pathol.* 1972;93:1.

372. Muenzer J. The mucopolysaccharidoses: a heterogeneous group of disorders with variable pediatric presentations. *J Pediatr.* 2004;144:S27.

373. Hinek A, Wilson SE. Impaired elastogenesis in Hurler disease: dermatan sulfate accumulation linked to deficiency in elastin-binding protein and elastic fiber assembly. *Am J Pathol.* 2000;156:925.

374. Giugliani R. Mucopolysacccharidoses: from understanding to treatment, a century of discoveries. *Genet Mol Biol.* 2012;35:924.

375. Lasser A, Carter DM, Mahoney MJ. Ultrastructure of the skin in mucopolysaccharidoses. *Arch Pathol.* 1975;99:173.

376. Poleto E, Baldo G, Gomez-Ospina N. Genome editing for mucopolysaccharidoses. *Int J Mol Sci.* 2020;21(2):500.

377. Sinha S, Schwartz RA. Juvenile acanthosis nigricans. *J Am Acad Dermatol.* 2007;57:502.

378. Krawczyk M, Mykała-Cieśla J, Kołodziej-Jaskuła A. Acanthosis nigricans as a paraneoplastic syndrome. Case reports and review of literature. *Pol Arch Med Wewn.* 2009;119:180.

379. Serap D, Ozlem S, Melike Y, et al. Acanthosis nigricans in a patient with lung cancer: a case report. *Case Rep Med.* 2010; 2010.

380. McGinness J, Greer K. Malignant acanthosis nigricans and tripe palms associated with pancreatic adenocarcinoma. *Cutis.* 2006;78:37.

381. Ellis DL, Chow JC, Nanney LB, Inman WH, King LY Jr. Melanoma, growth factors, and cutaneous paraneoplastic syndromes. *Pigment Cell Res.* 1988;1:132.

382. Schulmann K, Strate K, Pox CP, Wieland U, Kreuter A. Paraneoplastic acanthosis nigricans with cutaneous and mucosal papillomatosis preceding recurrence of a gastric adenocarcinoma. *J Clin Oncol.* 2012;30:e325.

383. Ramos-E-Silva M, Carvalho JC, Carneiro SC. Cutaneous paraneoplasia. *Clin Dermatol.* 2011;29:541.

384. Pentenero M, Carrozzo M, Pagano M, Gandolfo S. Oral acanthosis nigricans, tripe palms and sign of Leser–Trélat in a patient with gastric adenocarcinoma. *Int J Dermatol.* 2004;43:530.

385. Fareau GG, Maldonado M, Oral E, Balasubramanyam A. Regression of acanthosis nigricans correlates with disappearance of anti-insulin receptor autoantibodies and achievement of euglycemia in type B insulin resistance syndrome. *Metabolism.* 2007;56:670.

386. Bottoni U, Dianzani C, Pranteda G, et al. Florid cutaneous and mucosal papillomatosis with acanthosis nigricans revealing a primary lung cancer. *J Eur Acad Dermatol Venereol.* 2000; 14:205.

387. Bonnekuh B, Wevers A, Spangenberger H, Mahrle G, Krieg T. Keratin patterns of acanthosis nigricans in syndrome-like association with polythelia, polycystic kidneys, and syndactyly. *Arch Dermatol* 1993;129:1177.

388. Brown J, Winkelmann RK. Acanthosis nigricans: a study of 90 cases. *Medicine (Baltimore).* 1968;47:33.

389. Wortsman J, Matsuoka LY, Kupchella CE, Gavin JR 3rd, Dietrich JG. Glycosaminoglycan deposition in the acanthosis nigricans lesions of the polycystic ovary syndrome. *Arch Intern Med.* 1983;143:1145.

390. Haase I, Hunzelmann N. Activation of epidermal growth factor receptor/ERK signaling correlates with suppressed differentiation in malignant acanthosis nigricans. *J Invest Dermatol.* 2002;118:891.

391. Tamraz H, Raffoul M, Kurban M, Kibbi AG, Abbas O. Confluent and reticulated papillomatosis: clinical and histopathological study of 10 cases from Lebanon. *J Eur Acad Dermatol Venereol.* 2013;27:e119.

392. Kesten BM, James HD. Pseudoatrophoderma colli, acanthosis nigricans, and confluent and reticular papillomatosis. *Arch Dermatol.* 1957;75:525.

393. Stein JA, Shin HT, Chang MW. Confluent and reticulated papillomatosis associated with tinea versicolor in three siblings. *Pediatr Dermatol.* 2005;22:331.

394. Nordby CA, Mitchell AJ. Confluent and reticulated papillomatosis responsive to selenium sulfide. *Int J Dermatol.* 1986; 25:194.

395. Inalöz HS, Patel GK, Knight AG. Familial confluent and reticulated papillomatosis. *Arch Dermatol.* 2002;138:276.

396. Kanitakis J, Zambruno G, Viac J, Thivolet J. Involucrin expression in keratinization disorders of the skin—a preliminary study. *Br J Dermatol.* 1987;117:479.

397. Harrison SA, Bacon BR. Relation of hemochromatosis with hepatocellular carcinoma: epidemiology, natural history, pathophysiology, screening, treatment, and prevention. *Med Clin North Am.* 2005;89:391.

398. Stulberg DL, Clark N, Tovey D. Common hyperpigmentation disorders in adults: Part I. Diagnostic approach, café au lait macules, diffuse hyperpigmentation, sun exposure, and phototoxic reactions. *Am Fam Phys.* 2003;68:1955.

399. Chevrant-Breton J, Simon M, Bourel M, Ferrand B. Cutaneous manifestations of idiopathic hemo-chromatosis: study of 100 cases. *Arch Dermatol.* 1977;113:161.

400. Hazin R, Abu-Rajab Tamimi TI, Abuzetun JY, Zein NN. Recognizing and treating cutaneous signs of liver disease. *Cleve Clin J Med.* 2009;76:599.

401. Perdrup A, Poulsen H. Hemochromatosis and vitiligo. *Arch Dermatol.* 1964;90:34.

402. Weintraub LR, Demis DJ, Conrad ME, Crosby WH. Iron excretion by the skin: selective localization of iron-59 in epithelial cells. *Am J Pathol.* 1965;46:121.

403. Alexander J, Kowdley KV. HFE-associated hereditary hemochromatosis. *Genet Med.* 2009;11:307.

404. Brandhagen DJ, Fairbanks VF, Baldus W. Recognition and management of hereditary hemochromatosis. *Am Fam Phys.* 2002;65:853.

405. Fletcher LM, Halliday JW. Haemochromatosis: understanding the mechanism of disease and implications for diagnosis and patient management following recent cloning of novel genes involved in iron metabolism. *J Intern Med.* 2002;251:181.

406. Pietrangelo A. Hereditary hemochromatosis: pathogenesis, diagnosis, and treatment. *Gastroenterology.* 2010;139:393.

407. Philpott CC. Molecular aspects of iron absorption: insights into the role of HFE in hemochromatosis. *Hepatology.* 2002;35:993.

408. Leyden JL, Lockshin NA, Kriebel S. The black keratinous cyst: a sign of hemochromatosis. *Arch Dermatol.* 1972;106:379.

409. Shet T, Desai S. Pigmented epidermal cysts. *Am J Dermatopathol.* 2001;23:477.

410. Robert P, Zürcher H. Pigmentstudien: I. Mitteilung: Über den einfluss von schwermetallverbindungen, hämin, vitaminen, mikrobiellen toxinen, hormonen und weiteren stoffen auf die dopamelaninbildung in vitro und die pigmentbildung in vivo. *Dermatologica.* 1950;100:217.

411. Buckley WR. Localized argyria. *Arch Dermatol.* 1963;88:531.

412. Ocón J, Cabrejas C, Altemir J, Moros M. Phrynoderma: a rare dermatologic complication of bariatric surgery. *JPEN J Parenter Enteral Nutr.* 2012;36:361.

413. Bleasel NR, Stapleton KM, Lee MS, Sullivan J. Vitamin A deficiency phrynoderma: due to malabsorption and inadequate diet. *J Am Acad Dermatol.* 1999;41:322.

414. Armstrong AW, Setyadi HG, Liu V, Strasswimmer J. Follicular eruption on arms and legs. Phrynoderma. *Arch Dermatol.* 2008;144:1509.

415. Girard C, Dereure O, Blatière V, Guillot B, Bessis D. Vitamin a deficiency phrynoderma associated with chronic giardiasis. *Pediatr Dermatol.* 2006;23:346.

416. Barr DJ, Riley RJ, Green DJ. Bypass phrynoderma: vitamin A deficiency associated with bowel-bypass surgery. *Arch Dermatol.* 1984;120:919.

417. Frazier CN, Hu C. Nature and distribution according to age of cutaneous manifestations of vitamin A deficiency. *Arch Dermatol Syph.* 1936;33:825.

418. Bessey OA, Wolbach SB. Vitamin A: physiology and pathology. *JAMA.* 1938;110:2072.

419. Maronn M, Allen DM, Esterly NB. Phrynoderma: a manifestation of vitamin A deficiency?. The rest of the story. *Pediatr Dermatol.* 2005;22:60.

420. MacDonald A, Forsyth A. Nutritional deficiencies and the skin. *Clin Exp Dermatol.* 2005;30:388.

421. Hegyi J, Schwartz RA, Hegyi V. Pellagra: dermatitis, dementia, and diarrhea. *Int J Dermatol.* 2004;43:1.

422. Lyon VB, Fairley JA. Anticonvulsant-induced pellagra. *J Am Acad Dermatol.* 2002;46:597.

423. Kaur S, Goraya JS, Thami GP, Kanwar AJ. Pellagrous dermatitis induced by phenytoin. *Pediatr Dermatol.* 2002;19:93.

424. Moore RA, Spies TD, Cooper ZK. Histopathology of the skin in pellagra. *Arch Dermatol Syph.* 1942;46:106.

425. Karthikeyan K, Thappa DM. Pellagra and skin. *Int J Dermatol.* 2002;41:476.

426. Nogueira A, Duarte AF, Magina S, Azevedo F. Pellagra associated with esophageal carcinoma and alcoholism. *Dermatol Online J.* 2009;15:8.

427. Dong H, Kerl H, Cerroni L. EMLA(r) cream-induced irritant contact dermatitis. *J Cutan Pathol.* 2002;29:190.

428. Baron DN, Dent CE, Harris H, Hart EW, Jepson JB. Hereditary pellagralike skin rash with temporary cerebellar ataxia, constant renal aminoaciduria and other bizarre chemical features. *Lancet.* 1956;2:421.

429. Patel AB, Prabhu AS. Hartnup disease. *Indian J Dermatol.* 2008;53:31.

430. Wan P, Moat S, Anstey A. Pellagra: a review with emphasis on photosensitivity. *Br J Dermatol.* 2011;164:1188.

431. Clodi PH, Deutsch E, Niebauer G. Krankheitsbild mit poikilodermieartigen hautveränderungen, aminoacidurie und indolaceturie. *Arch Klin Exp Dermatol.* 1964;218:165.

432. Ashurst PJ. Hydroa vacciniforme occurring in association with Hartnup disease. *Br J Dermatol.* 1969;81:486.

433. Seyhan ME, Selimoğlu MA, Ertekin V, Fidanoğlu O, Altinkaynak S. Acrodermatitis enteropathica-like eruptions in a child with Hartnup disease. *Pediatr Dermatol.* 2006;23:262.

434. Orbak Z, Ertekin V, Selimoglu A, Yilmaz N, Tan H, Konak M. Hartnup disease masked by kwashiorkor. *J Health Popul Nutr.* 2010;28:413.

435. Cheon CK, Lee BH, Ko JM, Kim HJ, Yoo HW. Novel mutation in SLC6A19 causing late-onset seizures in Hartnup disorder. *Pediatr Neurol.* 2010;42:369.

436. Nozaki J, Dakeishi M, Ohura T, et al. Homozygosity mapping to chromosome 5p15 of a gene responsible for Hartnup disorder. *Biochem Biophys Res Common.* 2001;284:255.

437. Tallab TM. Richner-Hanhart syndrome: importance of early diagnosis and early intervention. *J Am Acad Dermatol.* 1996;35:857.

438. Viglizzo GM, Occella C, Bleidl D, Rongioletti F. Richner-Hanhart syndrome (tyrosinemia II): early diagnosis of an incomplete presentation with unusual findings. *Pediatr Dermatol.* 2006;23:259.

439. Macsai MS, Schwartz TL, Hinkle D, Hummel MB, Mulhern MG, Rootman D. Tyrosinemia type II: nine cases of ocular signs and symptoms. *Am J Ophthalmol.* 2001;132:522.

440. Bouyacoub Y, Zribi H, Azzouz H, et al. Novel and recurrent mutations in the TAT gene in Tunisian families affected with Richner-Hanhart Syndrome. *Gene.* 2013;529:45.

441. Al-Ratrout JT, Al-Muzian M, Al-Nazer M, Ansari NA. Plantar keratoderma: a manifestation of tyrosinemia type II (Richner-Hanhart syndrome). *Ann Saudi Med.* 2005;25:422.

442. Shimizu N, Ito M, Ito K, Nakamura A, Sato Y, Maruyama T. Richner-Hanhart's syndrome: electron microscopic study of the skin lesions. *Arch Dermatol.* 1990;126:1342.

443. Zaleski WA, Hill A, Kushniruk W. Skin lesions in tyrosinosis: response to dietary treatment. *Br J Dermatol.* 1973;88:335.

Inflammatory Diseases of Hair Follicles, Sweat Glands, and Cartilage

Chapter 18

MICHAEL D. IOFFREDA

INTRODUCTION

The pilosebaceous unit, eccrine glands, apocrine glands, and superficial cartilage (ear, nose) may be involved in inflammatory processes.

INFLAMMATORY DISEASES OF HAIR FOLLICLES: FOLLICULITIS

Inflammation of hair follicles, or folliculitis, has many causes, some of which are covered in other areas of this book. Folliculitis can have an infectious etiology owing to bacteria (see Chapter 21), viruses such as herpes (see Chapter 25), and fungi, including dermatophytes (tinea capitis, tinea barbae, Majocchi granuloma), and yeast (*Pityrosporum*) (see Chapter 23). Chapter 21 discusses pseudofolliculitis barbae, folliculitis (*acne*) keloidalis nuchae (Table 21-1), and the follicular occlusion triad. Perforating folliculitis is discussed with the other perforating disorders in Chapter 15. This chapter will focus on acneiform folliculitis, alopecia, and miscellaneous follicular disorders.

Acne Vulgaris

Clinical Summary. Acne vulgaris is primarily a disease of adolescence and early adulthood that only occasionally persists into later adult life, when it is found more often in women (1). Chiefly affecting the face, upper back, and chest, it manifests as two types of lesions—comedones and inflammatory lesions, both of which are follicular based. Comedones may be closed ("whiteheads") or open ("blackheads"). In closed comedones, the follicular orifice remains more or less normal in size, but when the follicular ostium widens, an open comedone results. Inflammatory lesions evolve from ruptured comedones or microcomedones, which are not clinically apparent and originate more frequently from closed comedones. Once developed, inflammatory papules may become pustules or nodules, which are larger and develop from cystic dilatation of the follicle. Cystic acne can result in severe scarring. In acne fulminans—a rare variant occurring mainly in young male patients—lesions rapidly become tender, ulcerated, and crusted, and eventually scar (2).

Histopathology. The development of a comedone involves a complex but incompletely understood process that results in infundibular dilation and thinning of the follicular wall. A plug composed of loosely arranged keratinized cells and sebum forms (Fig. 18-1). Sebum is made up of sebaceous lipids that

empty into the follicular lumen plus microorganisms. Solvents used in histologic processing remove these lipids.

Both open and closed comedones are associated with mild mononuclear inflammation around vessels in the adjacent papillary dermis. Attenuation of the follicular wall may be so extreme as to lead to rupture. Release of follicular contents into the dermis generates an inflammatory response mediated initially by neutrophils and later by histiocytes and foreign-body giant cells. When rupture occurs superficially, it tends to lead to the development of a clinical pustule (Fig. 18-2), but when it occurs in the deeper dermis, an inflammatory nodule forms (Fig. 18-3). If the follicular damage and inflammatory response are intense, large abscesses and scarring can result. This typically occurs in severe forms of acne (cystic acne and acne fulminans).

Pathogenesis. Several reviews highlight important advances that have affected our understanding of acne (3–5). Acne vulgaris is a multifactorial condition, initially requiring sex hormone release during puberty and activation of the sebaceous glands. The major factors contributing to acne development are follicular hyperkeratinization, hormones, sebum, *Propionibacterium*

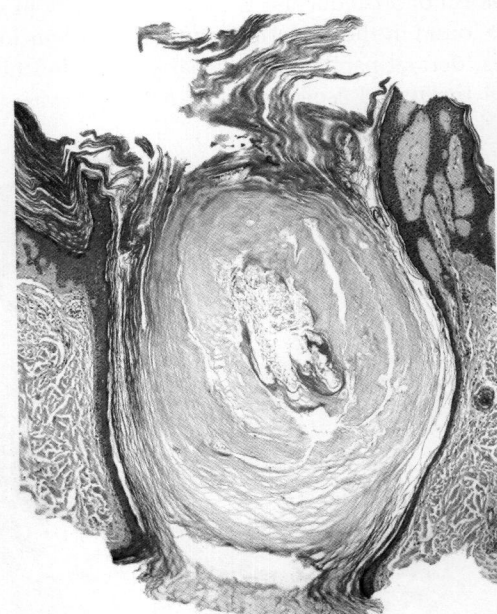

Figure 18-1 Comedone, open. A dilated follicular infundibulum with an attenuated wall is plugged with keratin and sebum. The follicular orifice is widened.

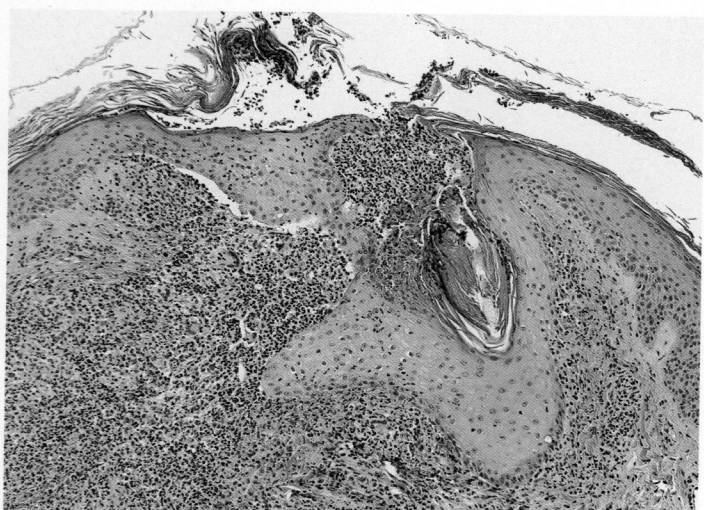

Figure 18-2 Acne vulgaris, pustule. Superficial follicular rupture incites suppurative and granulomatous inflammation, with neutrophils predominating in early lesions.

acnes, and inflammation. Generation of inflammation in acne lesions is a complex process (5,6).

Comedones exhibit hyperkeratinization, and the keratin is bound more avidly as a result of increased levels of intercellular adhesion materials (7). Ultrastructurally, follicular keratinocytes in comedones possess increased numbers of desmosomes and tonofilaments, which contribute to hypercornification (8). The black color of open comedones (blackheads) appears to be related to densely packed keratinocytes, bacteria, and bacterial products located at the surface. If dilation of the follicular orifice does not occur, continued thinning of the infundibular wall and ultimate rupture of the closed comedone becomes more probable.

There is substantial evidence linking the activation of sebum production to androgens, specifically testosterone and dihydrotestosterone (DHT). Circulating testosterone is converted in tissues to the more potent DHT by the enzyme 5α-reductase. The type 1 isoform of 5α-reductase is located primarily in sebocytes but is also found in the epidermis, infundibular hair follicle keratinocytes, dermal papilla cells, sweat glands, and fibroblasts. Activity of the type 1 isoform of 5α-reductase was greater in

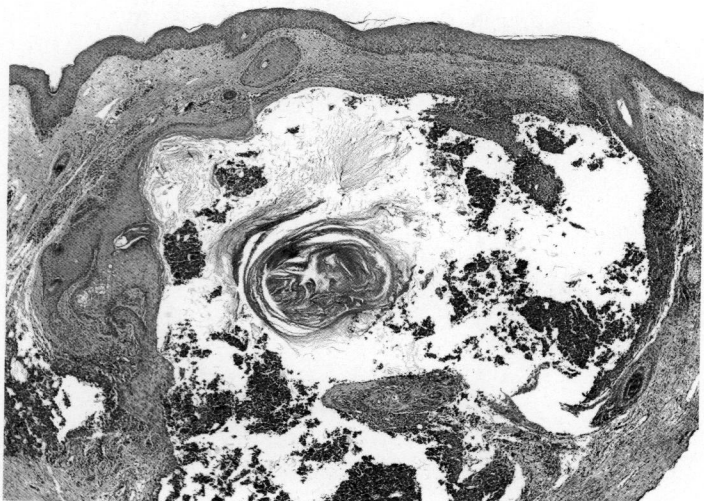

Figure 18-3 Acne vulgaris, nodule. Cystic follicular dilation with deep rupture leads to neutrophilic and granulomatous inflammation throughout the dermis.

sebaceous glands from acne-prone areas of the skin than in those from non–acne-prone areas, suggesting that regional differences in pilosebaceous production of DHT may play a role in acne (9).

Most acne patients, especially male patients, do not show abnormal serum androgen levels, although tissue androgen levels may be elevated. One study found significantly higher mean serum androgen levels in females with acne than in those without acne, although values were in the range of normal; in addition, sebaceous glands from the women with acne showed higher mean 5α-reductase type 1 activity, although the difference was not statistically significant (10). This study suggests that women with acne may have higher serum androgen levels and perhaps a greater capacity to produce DHT within sebaceous glands.

Sebum production in acne is elevated and appears to correlate with disease severity. The beneficial effect of isotretinoin (13-*cis*-retinoic acid) appears to result largely from reduction in sebum production, and after 2 months of treatment, a 70% reduction in sebum excretion is achieved (11). These changes are associated histologically with a marked reduction in sebaceous gland size.

In addition to androgens, proinflammatory hormones include insulin and insulin-like growth factor-1, which may be triggered by a high glycemic diet or dairy consumption (5). They can lead to increased sebum production, more inflammatory sebaceous lipids, *P. acnes* overgrowth, and various pathways of inflammation.

Of all the microorganisms identified in the follicular infundibulum, only *P. acnes* appears to be consistently involved in the pathogenesis of acne lesions (12). Nevertheless, levels of this organism may not be consistently greater in lesional skin than in normal skin. Immunologic reactivity to this organism may contribute to the inflammation in acne lesions.

Differential Diagnosis. When a hair follicle or follicle-derived keratin is not evident on the biopsy and the sections show only inflammation with neutrophils and histiocytes, an infectious etiology could be considered in the appropriate clinical context.

Principles of Management: Topical retinoids are a mainstay of treatment of acne vulgaris, targeting precursor microcomedones (13,14). Topical benzoyl peroxide also has comedolytic and antibacterial properties and is often used in combination with topical antibiotics. Oral antibiotics in the tetracycline class are often added for their anti-inflammatory properties when erythematous papules and pustules are present (15). In severe acne with nodulocystic lesions or scarring, oral isotretinoin may be required for adequate control (16).

Steroid Acne

Clinical Summary. Steroid acne is a folliculitis caused by the use of corticosteroids, including systemic, topical, inhaled, and intranasal (17) steroids. Despite its well-known existence, steroid acne has become more prevalent with the creation of increasingly potent topical preparations as well as various treatment regimens for cancer and organ transplantation (18). Although other medications have been implicated in acneiform eruptions, steroid acne results in a distinctive clinical picture characterized by the sudden appearance of monomorphic papulopustules predominantly on the upper trunk and arms but also on the face (19) (Fig. 18-4). Comedones are not apparent. The underlying rash for which topical steroids are used initially improves, followed by exacerbation of the rash (20).

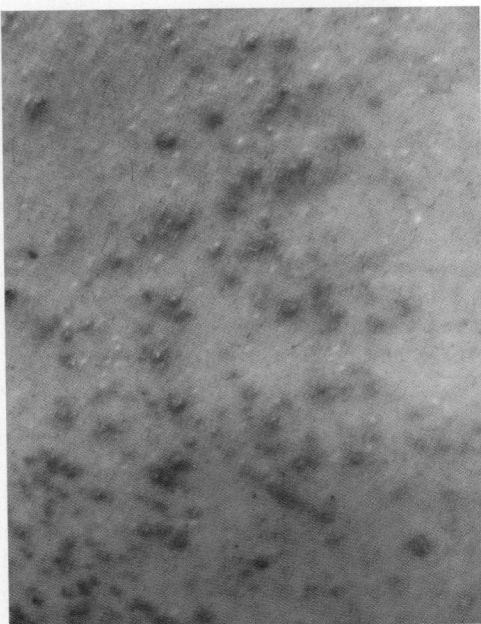

Figure 18-4 Steroid acne. Monomorphic pinpoint erythematous pustules in similar stages of development.

The exacerbation is controlled only by continued use of topical steroids (physical dependence). Resolution typically occurs without scarring. Perioral dermatitis may be caused by topical corticosteroids (see the discussion on *Perioral Dermatitis*).

Histopathology. Acne caused by both topical and systemic corticosteroids shows similar histologic features. Despite the apparent clinical absence of comedones, Hurwitz described histologic features that resembled those of acne vulgaris (Fig. 18-5), albeit with an accelerated rate of development (18). In chronologic order, biopsied flesh-colored papules that measured 1 mm showed infundibular spongiosis, hyperkeratosis, perifollicular edema, microcomedone formation, and infundibular wall thinning, sometimes with infundibular rupture. It was more common, however, to see only infundibular dilation with compact hyperkeratosis. Biopsied lesions that were 2 mm or greater and

clinically inflamed frequently showed infundibular rupture, necrotic keratinocytes, and surrounding suppurative and granulomatous inflammation that included multinucleated giant cells amid keratinous debris. Dilated blood vessels were also seen.

Pathogenesis. Although the exact pathogenesis is not known, three phases of lesion development have been described as a result of "addiction" to topical steroids (20), (a) initial improvement of the rash is attributable to the anti-inflammatory properties of topical corticosteroids, (b) local immunosuppressive effects of the steroids result in bacterial overgrowth, and (c) on withdrawal of steroids, there is rebound and flaring secondary to bacterial overgrowth. In addition to the chronologic sequence described under *Histopathology*, some authors have described a pathologic process that is the reverse of acne vulgaris, beginning with folliculitis, which proceeds to rupture and concludes with comedone formation (a so-called secondary comedone). In a study of steroid acne caused by systemic therapy, 80% of 125 patients showed significant numbers of *Pityrosporum ovale* in lesional follicles, and itraconazole, an oral antifungal agent, proved more efficacious than other medications.

Differential Diagnosis. The differential diagnosis would include acne vulgaris and other types of acute folliculitis.

Principles of Management: Withdrawal of the oral or topical corticosteroids that caused the eruption eventually results in abatement of lesions, though a rebound flare is often the norm and may require tapering of steroids. Treatment modalities used in acne vulgaris can sometimes hasten resolution.

Perioral Dermatitis

Clinical Summary. Recognition of this relatively common facial eruption is important because of its resemblance to rosacea, seborrheic dermatitis, and occasionally lupus erythematosus. Predominantly affecting women ranging in age from the midteens into middle age, it results in fine, follicular-based papules periorally and, more rarely, in a periocular distribution (*periocular dermatitis*) (21) (Fig. 18-6). The papules are single, grouped, or confluent, with minimal scaling. Pinhead-sized pustules may

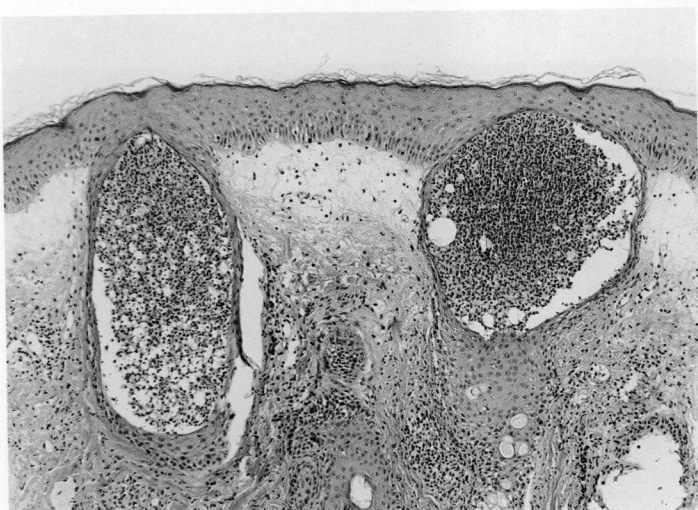

Figure 18-5 Steroid acne. Pustules in steroid acne are monomorphous and are indistinguishable from acne vulgaris.

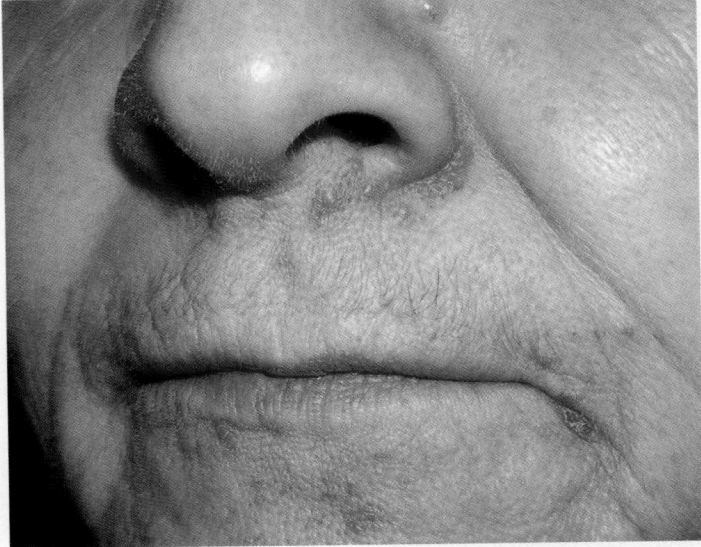

Figure 18-6 Perioral dermatitis. Erythematous papules, sometimes scaly, and small pustules are seen around the mouth and nose.

occur in more severe cases. There is sparing of a 5-mm zone around the vermilion border (19). The condition lacks significant telangiectasia. It is commonly associated with topically applied preparations, especially topical corticosteroids and cosmetics, as well as inhaled and intranasal steroids (22). Perioral dermatitis in children occurs primarily as a result of topical steroid use and is almost identical to the disease in adults (23).

Childhood granulomatous periorificial dermatitis is an acneiform facial eruption that shows some similarity to granulomatous rosacea and perioral dermatitis in children but does have some distinctive features (24). The current terminology was first coined in 1989 (24), although other terms have been proposed, such as facial Afro-Caribbean childhood eruption, reflecting its usual incidence on the face of black children (25). Other features that distinguish childhood granulomatous periorificial dermatitis from childhood perioral dermatitis and acne vulgaris include (a) exclusive incidence in healthy prepubertal children and (b) absence of pustules and lack of circumoral sparing. Clinical lesions may be flesh-colored, hypopigmented, or reddish yellow; are small (1 to 3 mm); monomorphous; and occur periorally, perinasally, and periorbitally. Lesions are asymptomatic and self-limited but may last for years, typically healing without residual except for some small, pitted scars in a few patients (26). Cases with extrafacial and generalized lesions have been reported (26).

Histopathology. Some authors consider perioral dermatitis to be a variant of rosacea, with indistinguishable histologic features (27), whereas others consider the two entities to be distinct (28,29), with some histologic overlap.

The following histologic characteristics of perioral dermatitis have been described (28). Fully developed lesions show spongiosis of the follicular infundibulum with mild mononuclear cell exocytosis (Fig. 18-7), with similar changes sometimes observed in the epidermis adjacent to the involved follicle. The epidermis may show mild acanthosis and parakeratosis, particularly about follicular ostia. The perifollicular dermis shows lymphohistiocytic inflammation around vessels, and in rare cases plasma cells may be prominent. Less developed lesions may exhibit only dermal inflammation. Lesions tend to lack the dermal edema and telangiectasias characteristic of rosacea and

show more noticeable epidermal changes. Acute folliculitis is uncommon.

Lesions of childhood granulomatous periorificial dermatitis often resemble granulomatous rosacea, with noncaseating perifollicular granulomas with some giant cells (24,26). Other features include epidermal changes consisting of mild hyperkeratosis and spongiosis, as well as dermal inflammation composed of lymphocytes and histiocytes that is mild to moderate, perivascular, and perifollicular. The granulomatous component is variable; some biopsies lacked granuloma formation or follicular involvement altogether. Some cases showed focal follicular rupture with inflammation to the released contents (24). Special stains for fungi and mycobacteria have been negative (26).

Pathogenesis. Many possible etiologies for perioral dermatitis have been proposed, including *Candida* organisms, bacteria, *Demodex* mites, a wide range of contactants, both irritant and allergic (including cosmetics and fluoride-containing toothpaste), hormones (including birth control pills), topical corticosteroids, and emotional as well as systemic conditions (30).

The etiology of childhood granulomatous periorificial dermatitis is not known, but an external contactant has been implicated in some cases, with various agents, including topical fluorinated corticosteroids, reported (26).

Differential Diagnosis. The histology may resemble rosacea, although the dermal edema and telangiectasias characteristic of rosacea are often lacking.

Principles of Management: Identification and avoidance of inciting factors, especially topical products, is foremost. Oral tetracycline antibiotics, topical antibiotics, and topical and oral retinoids can also be beneficial (31).

Rosacea

Clinical Summary. Rosacea is an acneiform inflammatory condition that primarily affects the face and is more common after the age of 30 years (32). It is characterized by background erythema within which scattered telangiectasias, papules, and occasional pustules develop (Fig. 18-8). It typically affects the nose, cheeks, glabella, and chin, and it is usually bilateral but occasionally unilateral or focal. If it is severe, lesions may

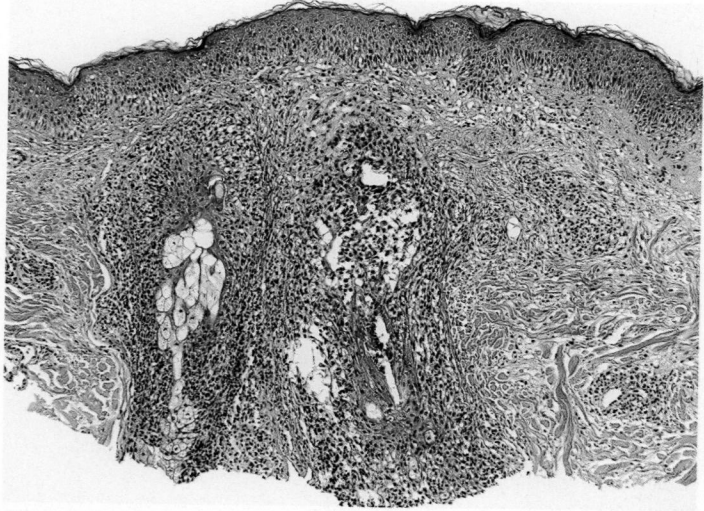

Figure 18-7 Perioral dermatitis. There is perifollicular mononuclear inflammation with infundibular spongiosis and exocytosis of lymphocytes.

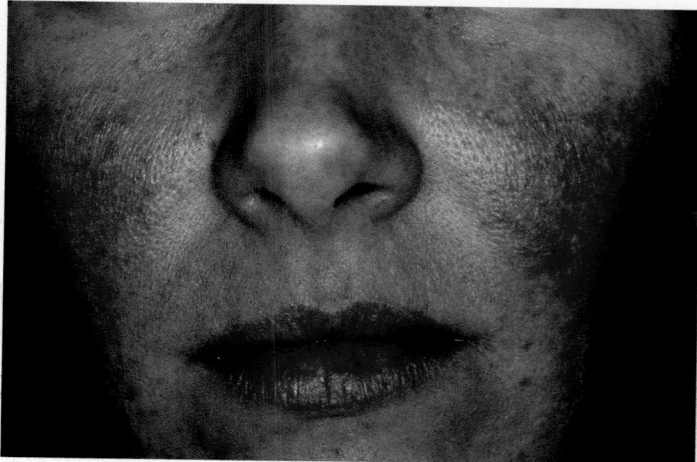

Figure 18-8 Rosacea. Scattered erythematous papules with background telangiectasias that give the face a "ruddy" appearance.

spread to the neck and, rarely, become disseminated. Rhinophyma, a bulbous swelling of the soft tissue of the nose, is a late complication that occurs almost exclusively in men. Eye changes—especially blepharitis and conjunctivitis—are quite common in rosacea, and in 5% of cases a painful keratitis can develop. Rosacea can precipitate persistent facial lymphedema.

A recently proposed clinical classification scheme for rosacea delineated four subtypes: (a) erythematotelangiectatic, (b) papulopustular, (c) phymatous, and (d) ocular (29,33).

Histopathology. Vascular dilation of upper and mid-dermal vessels with perivascular and perifollicular lymphohistiocytic inflammation (and occasional plasma cells) is generally present in all cases (Fig. 18-9). Lymphatic dilation is also common and may be prominent. With mild follicular involvement, there is infundibular spongiosis and lymphocyte exocytosis. With more extensive follicular involvement, neutrophils accumulate, resulting in a superficial pustule. Dermatoheliosis is invariably present, and *Demodex* mites are often seen within follicular infundibula. Reflecting the clinical presentation, various other pathologic changes can be seen from case to case, including organization of dermal lymphocytes into small nodular aggregates (34).

Granulomatous infiltrates are reported to occur in about 10% of all cases of rosacea (34) (Fig. 18-10), and caseation necrosis has been identified in about 10% of these patients (35). *Granulomatous rosacea* can histologically mimic mycobacterial infections, with epithelioid histiocytes forming a tuberculoid pattern (also see discussion on *Lupus Miliaris Disseminatus Faciei*). In such cases, other investigative procedures, including tissue cultures, may be necessary. Less frequently, the changes resemble cutaneous sarcoidosis. Multinucleated giant cells of the foreign-body type may aggregate around follicular contents spilled from a ruptured follicle.

In a study of rhinophyma, the classic or common type showed histologic features of fully developed rosacea, except for sebaceous gland hyperplasia, which can be prominent (36). The sebaceous ducts become dilated and filled with keratin and sebum. The same study showed that in patients with the severe form of rhinophyma, there is marked dermal thickening

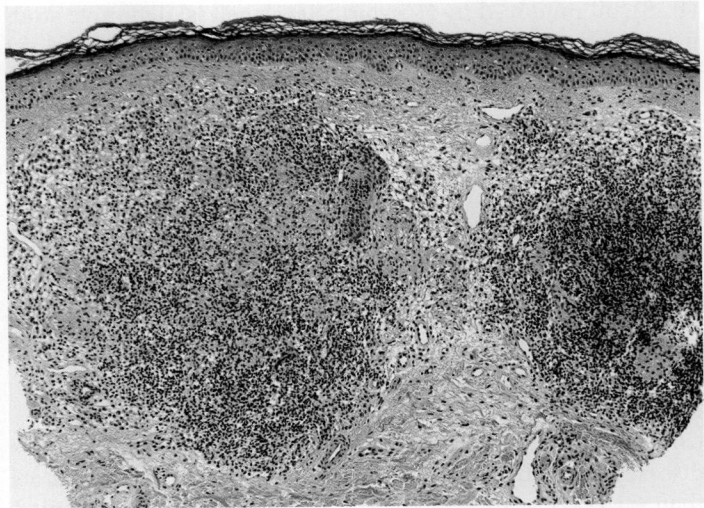

Figure 18-10 Granulomatous rosacea. The infiltrate is dense and has a prominent histiocytic component, clustered into granulomas. Telangiectatic blood vessels are present.

with sclerotic collagen bundles and large amounts of mucin, an absence of pilosebaceous structures, sparse inflammation, and telangiectasias (36). Many spindle-shaped and "bizarre" cells staining for factor XIIIa were seen in the interstitium. It was noted that the microscopic findings in the severe form of rhinophyma demonstrate many similarities to elephantiasis nostras caused by chronic lower-extremity lymphedema.

Pathogenesis. Although triggers of rosacea are well known, the pathogenesis of rosacea is multifactorial, involving genetic factors, immune and neurovascular dysregulation, microorganisms, and environmental factors, with sun damage a constant feature (37). A simplistic model by Dahl proposed that the vascular dilation leads to dermal edema, which in turn promotes the inflammation that is ultimately responsible for the sequelae of rosacea (38). In this model, warm facial skin from increased blood flow may modify the behavior of bacteria and/or *Demodex* or change the enzymatic activity of keratinocytes or other skin cells, leading to altered metabolism and inciting inflammation. Rosacea is not associated with an increase in sebum excretion.

The role of *Demodex* organisms has been debated for decades. Some reports claimed a significant association of mites in rosacea biopsies (39,40), but other studies did not support this claim (41). Although a definitive causative role for *Demodex* in rosacea is uncertain, the mites may represent an important cofactor in heightening disease severity (40).

An association with gastrointestinal *Helicobacter pylori* infection has been the subject of investigation. In one study, a number of rosacea patients had gastrointestinal symptoms related to gastritis; the prevalence of *H. pylori* in those patients with rosacea was 88%, compared to 65% in the control group without rosacea (but with nonulcer dyspepsia) (42). Furthermore, eradication of *H. pylori* with 1 week of therapy that included oral metronidazole, omeprazole, clarithromycin, and topical intraoral metronidazole resulted in marked improvement or resolution of rosacea symptoms after 2 to 4 weeks (43). Attempts to find *H. pylori* in the skin have been unsuccessful. A proposed pathogenesis is increased flushing caused by vasodilators such as nitric oxide and gastrin and inflammatory cytokines such as tissue necrosis factor-α and interleukin-8

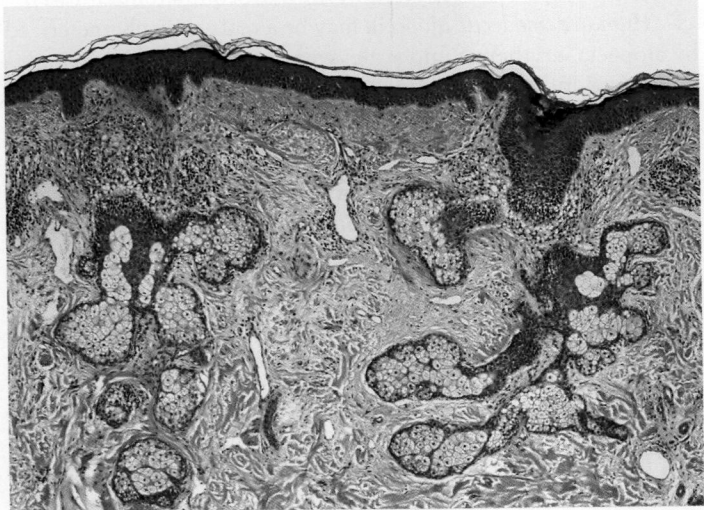

Figure 18-9 Rosacea. Patchy lymphocytic inflammation surrounds vellus hair follicles as well as some blood vessels. Telangiectasias and solar elastosis are present.

(IL-8), all produced by *H. pylori*. Nevertheless, definitive studies validating an association of *H. pylori* with rosacea have yet to be done.

Differential Diagnosis. Perioral dermatitis is histologically similar. In lesions with a prominent granulomatous component, infection can enter the differential diagnosis.

Principles of Management: (44–46). Avoidance of triggers that incite flushing, which invariably includes sunlight, is a staple of management. Topical antibiotics, sulfa products, and azelaic acid may be used. Tetracycline antibiotics are often required for papulopustular lesions.

Demodicidosis

Clinical Summary. Demodicidosis is the term for cutaneous disease caused by mites of the genus *Demodex*. Despite more than 65 years of investigation into the role of *Demodex* mites in human skin disease, questions remain. Aside from their controversial role in rosacea, *Demodex* mites have been implicated in follicular-based skin eruptions resembling rosacea, albeit with some unique features that warrant consideration as distinct entities (47). There are at least three clinical forms of demodicidosis (47). The first, *pityriasis folliculorum (aka spinulate demodicidosis)*, is characterized by facial erythema with fine follicular plugs and scale producing a "nutmeg-grater" or "sandpaper-like" appearance. It usually affects women and may be associated with itching and burning. The second, *rosacea-like demodicidosis*, resembles rosacea, in that there are papules and pustules (Fig. 18-11). In contrast to rosacea, however, there is follicular scaling, sudden onset, rapid progression, and no history of flushing. There may be eyelid involvement (demodectic blepharitis) and poor general health, such as diabetes mellitus (47). Lastly, *demodicidosis gravis* resembles severe granulomatous rosacea. An alternate classification was proposed that also included auricular demodicidosis causing external otitis (48). These forms may represent a spectrum of disease in which the clinical expression depends on the degree and duration of *Demodex* infestation and the individual's age and overall health (47). *Demodex* may also be important in the pathogenesis of nonclassic presentations involving facial pruritus and erythema and nonspecific acneiform lesions (49).

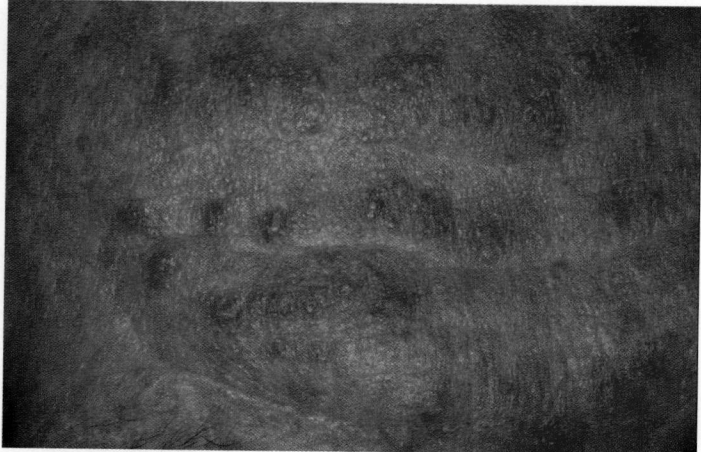

Figure 18-11 Demodicidosis, rosacea-like. Exuberant papules and minute pustules that when scraped and examined microscopically show multiple *Demodex* mites amid follicular contents.

Demodex are obligatory parasites frequently found in mammalian pilosebaceous units, and colonization is usually asymptomatic (50). The mites found in humans are of the species *Demodex folliculorum* and *D. brevis*. *D. folliculorum*, the predominant mite, has a longer body, inhabits the infundibulum of hair follicles, and is found almost exclusively on the face (51,52). *D. brevis* is smaller and lives exclusively within sebaceous glands on the face and trunk (51,52).

Demodicidosis has also been classified as *primary* or *secondary*, with the latter occurring on diseased skin (53). The primary form affects nondiseased skin, is caused by *D. folliculorum*, and causes an eruption in the T-zone of the face, involving 8% to 15% of the face. Secondary demodicidosis is characterized by a symmetric eruption of the malar region, covering 30% to 40% of the face, and is caused by *D. brevis*. There are other distinguishing features, such as onset of erythema, pruritus, and seasonality (53).

A study of consecutive biopsies submitted to one dermatopathology laboratory showed *Demodex* mites in 10% of all biopsies and 12% of all follicles (51). Their prevalence increased with age, and males were more heavily infested. In another study, there was a nonrandom association between histologic folliculitis and the presence of *Demodex* in the follicles (52); mites were found in 42% of inflamed follicles but in only 10% of noninflamed follicles, whereas 83% of follicles containing *Demodex* showed inflammation. This demonstrated a strong association but not a cause-and-effect relation because the possibility that *Demodex* could preferentially select inflamed follicles was raised. Additional support for a pathogenic role was provided by reports of sudden facial eruptions in which numerous *Demodex* mites were identified and the eruption failed to respond to therapy for rosacea but cleared quickly with treatments directed against *Demodex*, such as crotamiton or ivermectin and permethrin (54).

Some believe that *Demodex* mites are pathogenic only in large numbers (54), but an individual's overall health also appears to be important, as demonstrated by reports in immunocompromised children and multiple reports in patients with HIV and AIDS, in which the eruption may also involve the neck, upper trunk, and extremities (55). One study stated that demodicidosis is prevalent even in immunocompetent individuals (39), and it has been reported in immunocompetent children.

Human demodectic alopecia may be a real entity characterized by alopecia, erythema, and scale, with numerous *Demodex* mites in affected follicles (56). It resembles canine demodectic mange and has been successfully treated with permethrin. There are excellent reviews of human and canine demodicidosis (57,58).

Histopathology. The diagnosis can be made in the clinical setting by examining scale with 40% potassium hydroxide (KOH) or by standardized skin surface biopsy (SSSB), in which cyanoacrylate glue is used to sample the horny layer and follicular contents (59). The presence of five or more mites in a single low-power field by KOH or more than 5/cm^2 by SSSB is considered significant.

Biopsies of pityriasis folliculorum show a perivascular and diffuse dermal lymphocytic infiltrate without granuloma formation (47). Excess numbers of *Demodex* mites are present within the infundibulum of pilosebaceous units and may be associated with an infundibular pustule. Biopsies of rosacea-like demodicidosis (Fig. 18-12) show a primarily perifollicular lymphohistiocytic infiltrate, often with neutrophils or granulomatous

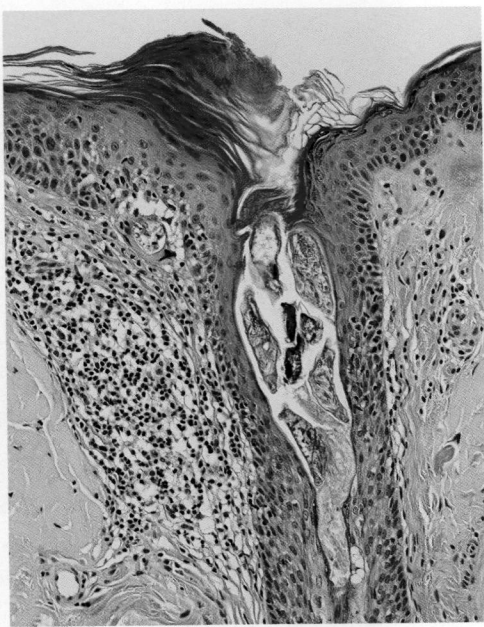

Figure 18-12 Demodicidosis. The follicular infundibulum contains multiple *Demodex* mites, and there is perifollicular lymphohistiocytic inflammation. Where the left side of the follicular epithelium meets the epidermis, an organism appears to be perforating through to the dermis.

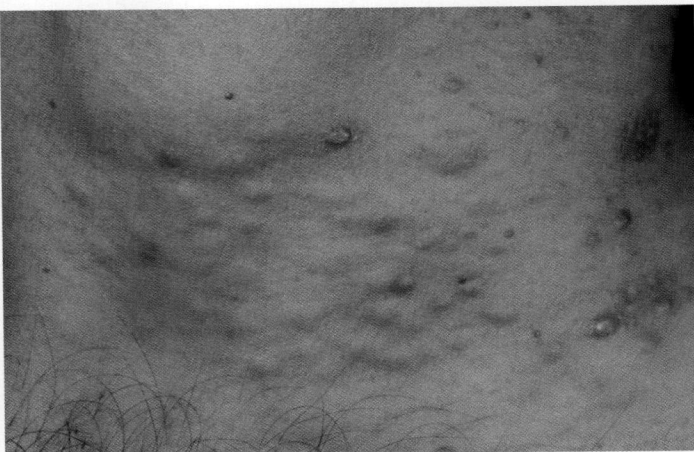

Figure 18-13 Lupus miliaris disseminatus faciei. In this atypical location, there are dermal papules that are flesh colored to red brown. Some have a yellowish hue that hints at their granulomatous histologic appearance.

inflammation containing multinucleated giant cells (47,60). Mites may be present in the dermis amid the inflammation. Demodicidosis gravis shows granulomas with central necrosis (caseation) and foreign-body–type multinucleated giant cells.

Pathogenesis. The pathogenesis of *Demodex*-related disease may be linked to one of the following: (a) blockage of hair follicles and sebaceous ducts caused by reactive epithelial hyperplasia and hyperkeratinization, (b) mites serving as vectors for bacteria, (c) a foreign-body reaction to the mite, or (d) induction of host immunity by the mites and their waste (50,58).

Differential Diagnosis. Biopsies of rosacea will commonly demonstrate organisms. The problem in *Demodex*-related skin disease is determining whether the organisms are truly pathogenic, because they are frequently seen within hair follicles, especially on the head.

Principles of Management: The mite population can be kept in check by cleansing the face regularly, by using crotamiton or permethrin cream, or oral ivermectin or metronidazole.

Lupus Miliaris Disseminatus Faciei

Clinical Summary. Some authors believe lupus miliaris disseminatus faciei to be a granulomatous variant of rosacea, but others consider it to be a separate rosacea-like syndrome (61,62). The clinical presentation is distinctive, with discrete, flesh-colored, or mildly erythematous papules—arranged singly or in small groups—typically involving facial skin, especially the eyelids and upper lip (63), although extrafacial lesions may occur in atypical presentations (Fig. 18-13). The background erythema and telangiectasias of rosacea are lacking. Papules frequently resolve spontaneously after 12 to 24 months and are resistant to treatment. One group proposed the use of equally cumbersome terminology, "facial idiopathic granulomas with regressive evolution" (F.I.GU.R.E.) (64).

Histopathology. Biopsy specimens sectioned through the central portion of a papular lesion demonstrate one of the most highly characteristic patterns of cutaneous histopathology. Surrounding a usually large area of caseous necrosis, aggregates of epithelioid histiocytes and occasional multinucleate giant cells form a "tubercle" with sparse lymphoid inflammation at the periphery (Fig. 18-14).

In one study, this characteristic histology was found only in a minority of patients in fully developed lesions, and an attempt was made to describe the histologic features of early, fully developed, and late lesions (65,66). Early, developing lesions show perivascular and perifollicular lymphocytes and some histiocytes. Fully developed lesions show a sarcoidal granuloma (first stage), sometimes accompanied by an abscess (second stage) or surrounding an area of caseation necrosis (third stage). The granuloma may be perifollicular and involve one or more hairs, and the follicle may be "ruptured" with a neutrophilic response. Granulomas may also be compact or loose and may occupy the

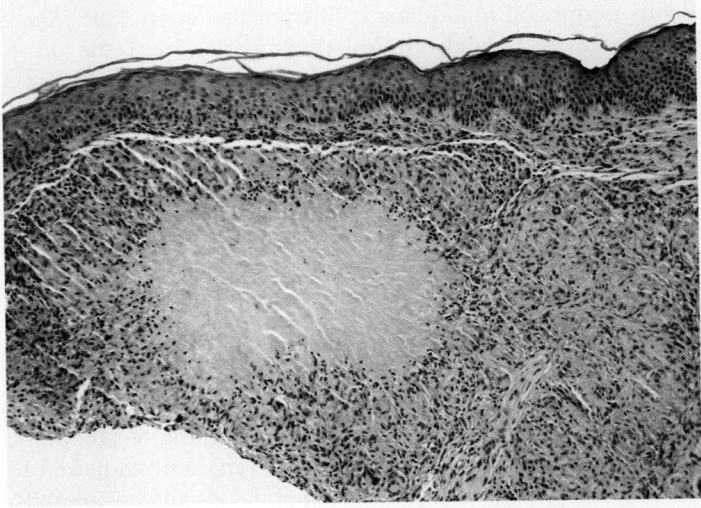

Figure 18-14 Lupus miliaris disseminatus faciei. Caseous necrosis is surrounded by epithelioid histiocytes and peripheral lymphocytes, forming a "tubercle" that mimics *Mycobacterium tuberculosis* infection.

upper or lower dermis, and some hug the epidermis. Late lesions demonstrate scattered lymphocytes, histiocytes, and neutrophils and perifollicular fibrosis. Additional findings include follicular dilation, hyperkeratosis, sometimes combined with follicular plugging and pigment incontinence (65).

Despite the histologic picture, no direct relationship with tuberculosis has been documented, including testing using polymerase chain reaction with DNA fragments specific for *Mycobacterium tuberculosis* complex (67).

Differential Diagnosis. The histology may be indistinguishable from cutaneous tuberculosis, a rare entity.

Principles of Management: Difficult to control, spontaneous resolution may occur after a couple of years. Tetracycline antibiotics are a mainstay of treatment, but there are several case reports describing other therapies in refractory cases (62,68).

Eosinophilic Pustular Folliculitis

Clinical Summary. Ofuji originally described *eosinophilic pustular folliculitis* (EPF) in immunocompetent Japanese patients as itchy follicular papules and pustules arranged in arcuate plaques with central healing and peripheral spread (69,70). Although most reported cases have been from Japan, the condition is now known to be geographically more widespread. Lesions typically involve seborrheic areas, including the face, trunk, and upper arms, with documented reports of extrafollicular lesions of the palms and soles (71). Moderate leukocytosis and eosinophilia in the peripheral blood may be present. There is usually spontaneous healing over months to years. There are reports of the eruption in children, including neonates (72), and in this subset lesions occur predominantly on the scalp. Scarring alopecia of the scalp in an adult has been reported (73). Although a cause has not been identified, rare medication-induced cases have been described (74). Cases have been associated with nevoid basal cell carcinoma syndrome (75), hepatitis C infection (76), and infestations (77).

Lesions with similar histology are well documented in patients with HIV infection (78) and other immunocompromised conditions, such as myelodysplastic syndrome, non-Hodgkin lymphoma, B-cell chronic lymphatic leukemia, polycythemia vera (79), after bone marrow transplantation, and after autologous peripheral blood stem cell transplantation (80). There appears to be enough clinical dissimilarity from the disorder described by Ofuji to consider HIV-associated disease a distinct entity, and use of the terms *eosinophilic folliculitis* or *HIV-associated eosinophilic folliculitis* was recommended to reflect this (78). Another classification scheme proposed the designations classical, infancy associated, and immunosuppression associated (mostly HIV) (69,81). In HIV patients, lesions tend to be urticarial papules with less of a tendency to become pustular (82). They are most commonly found on the face, scalp, and upper trunk and are often excoriated.

Histopathology. In Ofuji disease, there is exocytosis of eosinophils into a spongiotic follicular infundibulum and accompanying sebaceous gland, eventually forming eosinophilic micropustules (Fig. 18-15) (73,83). The epidermis adjacent to the affected follicle may contain lymphocytes and eosinophils, with the latter aggregating into small eosinophilic pustules that are subcorneal or intraepidermal; these epidermal changes reflect the histologic picture seen in palmoplantar lesions, where

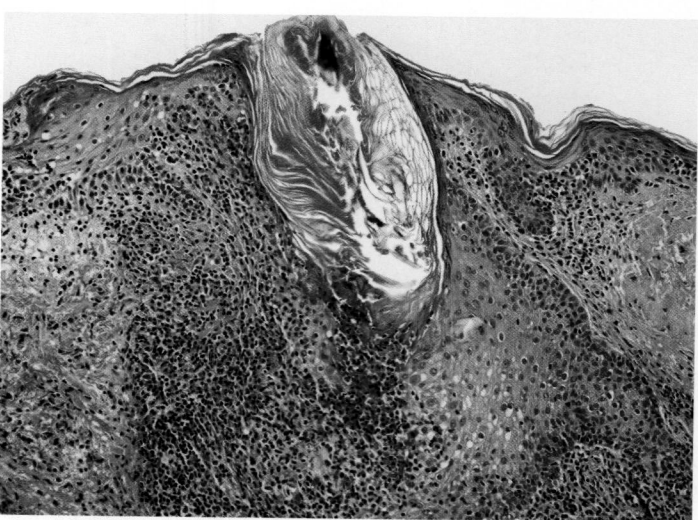

Figure 18-15 Eosinophilic pustular folliculitis. Eosinophils and lymphocytes surround and infiltrate the follicle, forming intrafollicular eosinophilic micropustules.

follicles are absent. In more inflamed lesions, neutrophils may be present. In the dermis, there are perivascular and interstitial infiltrates of lymphocytes and numerous eosinophils, which may surround the sweat glands. Associated follicular mucinosis has been reported (84).

A study of 52 biopsies in 50 HIV-positive patients best described the histology of HIV-associated eosinophilic folliculitis (82). Perifollicular and intrafollicular lymphocytes and eosinophils are concentrated about the isthmus and may involve the sebaceous duct. There is spongiosis of the follicular epithelium. Eosinophils and lymphocytes may be seen aggregating in the hair canal, but neutrophils are rare. In early lesions, lymphocytes may predominate and be distributed perifollicularly and interstitially. In more developed lesions, dermal inflammation diminishes and perifollicular/follicular inflammation increases. Less common findings include inflammation of the sebaceous gland, eosinophilic pustules, and follicular rupture (82). Dense eosinophilic infiltrates with degranulation and flame figures, resembling Wells syndrome, may sometimes be seen. A few macrophages can be present. Bacteria, yeast, or *Demodex* may be identified, albeit away from the areas of inflammation. Because the disorder is highly pruritic, excoriation is a common secondary finding.

Features that may help to distinguish suppurative folliculitis in HIV-positive patients from HIV-associated eosinophilic folliculitis have been described; suppurative folliculitis in HIV-positive patients more commonly shows an infiltrate dominated by neutrophils and macrophages, the presence of microorganisms amid the inflammation, and rupture of the involved follicle. The use of transverse histologic sections has been advocated over vertical sections for increasing diagnostic sensitivity and demonstrating the key pathologic findings in HIV-associated eosinophilic folliculitis (85).

Pathogenesis. The cause of Ofuji disease (EPF) is not known. Although the prevalence in Japan could not be explained by human leukocyte antigen (HLA) patterns (73), the occurrence in brothers in the neonatal period hints at some inherited predisposition or, possibly, an infectious etiology (86).

The perivascular infiltrating cells in EPF were found to be mostly T lymphocytes, with some CD68+ myelomonocytic cells (87). A moderate increase in the number of tryptase-positive, chymase-negative mast cells, the type predominantly found in lung and small intestine, was noted around hair follicles and sebaceous glands (83).

Ultrastructurally, in EPF lesions characterized by an infundibular pustule, acantholytic outer root sheath keratinocytes showed desmosomal cleavage with microvilli formation, and some contained sebaceous lipid droplets (88). Apposition of T lymphocytes and Langerhans cells was seen.

Differential Diagnosis. In the differential diagnosis, eosinophilic follicular pustules may be seen in erythema toxicum neonatorum, and intraepidermal eosinophilic vesicles can be seen both in acropustulosis and in the vesicular phase of incontinentia pigmenti. However, the clinical presentation of these conditions would generally be significantly different than that in EPF, although it has been suggested that EPF in infants and infantile acropustulosis may be variants of the same disorder. Identical eosinophilic pustular eruptions have been described in association with fungal infections caused by dermatophytes. A folliculocentric arthropod bite can sometimes enter into the differential diagnosis.

Principles of Management: Ofuji EPF is managed primarily with systemic steroids or dapsone. Treatments for HIV-associated eosinophilic folliculitis include topical steroids, antihistamines, phototherapy, itraconazole, topical permethrin, and isotretinoin (19).

Follicular Mucinosis and Alopecia Mucinosa

Clinical Summary. Follicular mucinosis is characterized clinically by grouped erythematous papules and/or plaques that may be markedly indurated or nodular and histologically by mucin accumulation in hair follicles (Fig. 18-16) (89). It can be classified into two types: a primary (idiopathic) type and a secondary variety. The *primary* form tends to have a shorter but benign course. The *secondary* type has been associated with numerous benign and malignant conditions, including lymphomas, most of which are mycosis fungoides. A distinct variant of mycosis fungoides—follicular mycosis fungoides—may or may not be associated with follicular mucinosis (90,91).

The primary form tends to affect children and young adults more frequently and resolves spontaneously in several months (acute benign type) or several years (chronic benign type). It is often confined to the head and neck but may be disseminated. The secondary type tends to form more widespread plaques and is almost always a disorder of adults.

The secondary type has been found in association with a number of lymphoproliferative disorders and hematologic malignancies (92), as well as inflammatory cutaneous disorders such as chronic discoid lupus erythematosus (93), angiolymphoid hyperplasia, alopecia areata (AA) (94), EPF (84), spongiotic dermatitis, lichen striatus, arthropod bites, sarcoidosis, Goodpasture syndrome (95), leprosy (96), and growths such as verrucae (95), melanocytic nevi, and squamous cell carcinoma of the tongue (97). The numerous associations with production of follicular mucin certainly suggest that this is a relatively nonspecific reaction pattern.

There has been controversy about whether the histopathology allows for distinction between the primary and secondary forms (98), and some researchers claimed that transition from the benign form to a lymphomatous type could occur (99), whereas others disputed this finding (95). In 1989, a study of 59 cases concluded that there was no clinical or pathologic pattern by which the ultimate outcome of the condition could be predicted (100).

Others have reported that adults older than 40 years with widespread follicular mucinosis are at increased risk for mycosis fungoides or Sézary syndrome (95), although Cerroni et al. (99) claimed that the criteria that purported to differentiate lymphoma-associated follicular mucinosis from the idiopathic type were not effective. A long-term follow-up study (median 10 years) of seven patients younger than 40 years with primary follicular mucinosis failed to demonstrate progression to cutaneous T-cell lymphoma, despite the presence of a T-cell clone in five of the patients (101).

In 1957, Pinkus (102) described *alopecia mucinosa,* the term used when follicular mucinosis affects terminal hair-bearing areas and is associated with hair loss (Fig. 18-17). Papules and plaques may be present or inconspicuous in this form, which may show only alopecia. Scarring is seen more commonly when alopecia mucinosa is associated with cutaneous T-cell lymphoma. Others claim that alopecia mucinosa is simply one of the many morphologic variants of mycosis fungoides (103), whereas LeBoit (104) acknowledged the

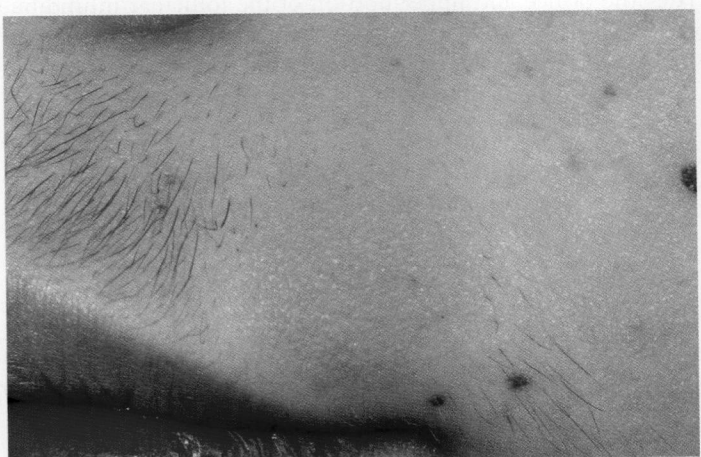

Figure 18-16 Follicular mucinosis/alopecia mucinosa. This round, slightly elevated pink plaque in an adolescent boy has resulted in clinically apparent alopecia because the hairs at this site are coarser.

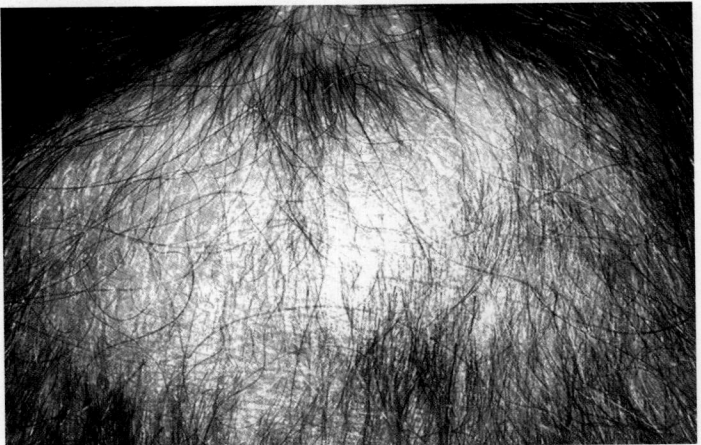

Figure 18-17 Alopecia mucinosa. Diffuse thinning of the scalp associated with slightly elevated, scaly plaques. The scalp erythema and poorly defined areas of alopecia distinguish this example from alopecia areata.

paradoxes of alopecia mucinosa that have led to the debate over classification.

Histopathology. Within the outer root sheath and sebaceous gland epithelium, there is reticular epithelial degeneration that sometimes evolves into more extensive cavitation within which mucin is deposited (Fig. 18-18). Occasionally, little mucin can be detected, perhaps because of removal of this water-soluble material in the processing procedure. The deposited mucin is an acid mucopolysaccharide that stains metachromatically with toluidine blue at pH 3.0, as well as with Alcian blue at acid pH. The fact that it can be substantially removed by digestion with hyaluronidase demonstrates that the mucin is predominantly hyaluronic acid. Colloidal iron stain may also be used for its detection.

Inflammation is perivascular and perifollicular and composed of lymphocytes and histiocytes, but there can also be eosinophils. There may be exocytosis into the outer root sheath epithelium of the infundibulum and the sebaceous gland epithelium. Although individual pathologic criteria are not absolutely diagnostic of the type of follicular mucinosis (primary or secondary), features that have been proposed as favoring a lymphoma-associated lesion include an increased density of the perifollicular infiltrate with substantial folliculotropism, a dense bandlike infiltrate containing atypical lymphocytes, epidermotropism, a predominance of CD4+ lymphocytes (vs. equal numbers of CD4 and CD8 cells), and a clonal gene rearrangement (Fig. 18-19) (105,106).

Pathogenesis. Electron microscopic studies have shown that the mucin is a product of the outer root sheath epithelial cells. The cytoplasm shows prominent, dilated, rough-surfaced endoplasmic reticulum containing fine, granular, filamentous material that is secreted into the intercellular spaces (107).

Differential Diagnosis. Determining whether follicular mucinosis is primary or an incidental, secondary finding is a diagnostic challenge. Correlation with clinical information is crucial.

Principles of Management: Although primary follicular mucinosis may spontaneously resolve, topical or systemic steroids

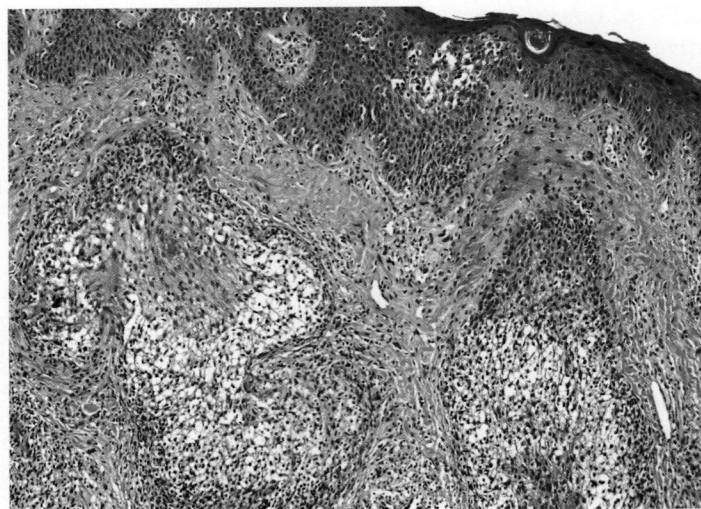

Figure 18-19 Follicular mucinosis associated with folliculotropic mycosis fungoides. In addition to changes of follicular mucinosis, there is extensive folliculotropism of lymphocytes. Epidermotropism of large lymphocytes is also present.

as a first-line treatment can help. In treating secondary follicular mucinosis, therapy is geared toward the associated condition.

Keratosis Pilaris

Clinical Summary. This common persistent condition characteristically affects the lateral aspect of the arms, thighs, and buttocks. Keratotic follicular papules, sometimes with surrounding erythema, are present. They are usually asymptomatic. Keratosis pilaris may be seen in association with ichthyosis vulgaris and appears to be more common in patients with atopic dermatitis.

Similar lesions may form as part of a variety of more extensive erythematous keratinizing disorders (108). Keratosis pilaris rubra is a variant that shows more widespread skin involvement and more prominent erythema (109). Keratosis pilaris atrophicans represents a spectrum of clinical conditions, including keratosis follicularis spinulosa decalvans (110,111), in which the involved follicle becomes atrophic and destroyed, sometimes associated with scarring alopecia of the scalp.

Histopathology. An orthokeratotic keratin plug blocks and dilates the orifice and upper portion of the follicular infundibulum (Fig. 18-20). A twisted hair shaft may be trapped within this keratin material, and a mild perivascular mononuclear cell infiltrate is usually present in the adjacent dermis.

Pathogenesis. Genetic factors may play a role in this condition. Patients with a generalized form of keratosis pilaris were found to have a chromosome 18p deletion, implicating a gene on the short arm of chromosome 18 (112).

Differential Diagnosis. A similar condition, *lichen spinulosus* (113), shows a very similar histologic picture except that the keratin plug may protrude more substantially above the skin surface and contain one or more hair shafts. Lesions similar to keratosis pilaris may also be seen in patients treated with vemurafenib (114), as well as phrynoderma (vitamin A deficiency; see Chapter 16), although the follicular keratin plug is said to be parakeratotic.

Principles of Management: Keratosis pilaris is managed primarily by topical keratolytics containing ammonium lactate, salicylic

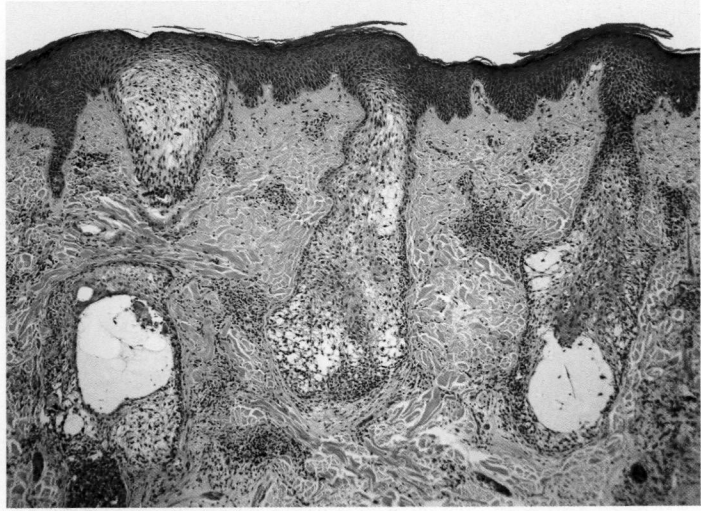

Figure 18-18 Follicular mucinosis. The outer root sheath epithelium of several follicles shows reticular degeneration with areas of cavitation. There are intercellular strands of bluish-staining mucin.

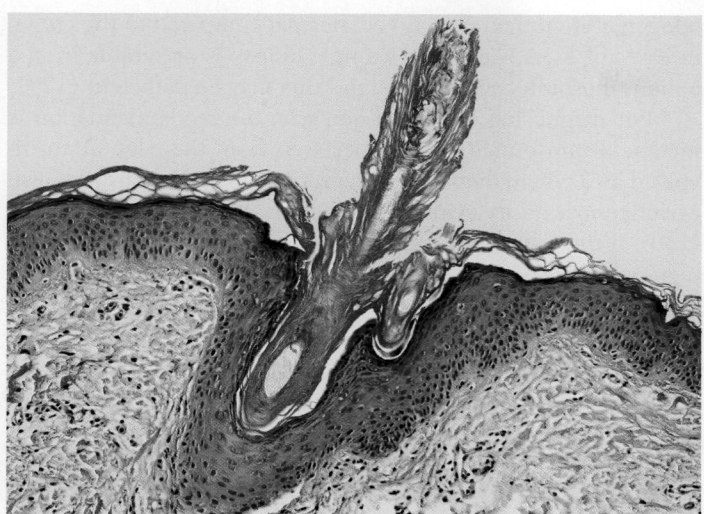

Figure 18-20 Keratosis pilaris. The follicle is plugged with compact orthokeratin that protrudes above the skin surface.

acid, or retinoids. Laser therapy is an option. Severe cases with clinical erythema may necessitate topical corticosteroids.

Trichostasis Spinulosa

Clinical Summary. Trichostasis spinulosa is a fairly common condition that may present clinically as raised follicular spicules or as open comedones or that may be inapparent (115). It occurs predominantly on the face, nose, or cheeks of middle-aged and older individuals, but it has been reported in a pediatric patient (115) and may be generalized (116,117). It can present as black dots on the scalp mimicking AA (118).

Histopathology. Affected hair follicles demonstrate retention of small hair shafts within a dilated infundibulum, sometimes enveloped in a keratinous sheath (Fig. 18-21). As many as 20 or more hair shafts may be trapped in this way, often projecting above the skin surface, reflecting the name coined by German

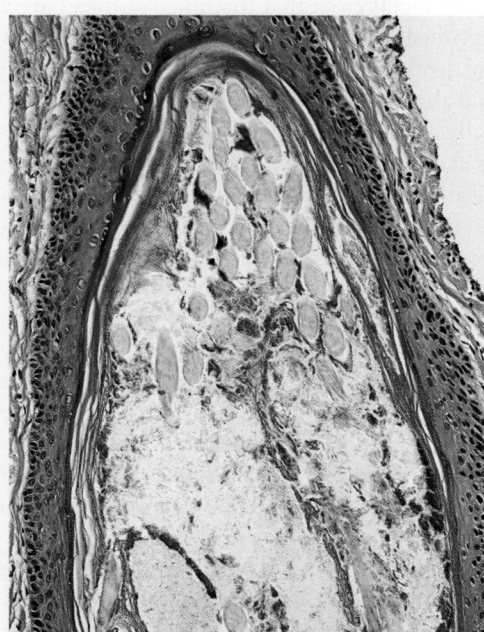

Figure 18-21 Trichostasis spinulosa. A dilated follicular infundibulum with retention of multiple vellus hair shafts. The granular blue material represents resident bacteria of the follicle.

dermatologist Felix Franke, who called it "Pinselhaar" (paintbrush hair) in 1901 (119). A perifollicular mononuclear infiltrate may be present. In the clinical setting, the follicular plugs may be easily extracted with fine forceps or a comedone extractor and examined microscopically, demonstrating a cluster of vellus hairs within a keratinous plug.

Pathogenesis. The etiology of trichostasis spinulosa is not known for certain. The retained hairs are normal telogen hairs, which suggests a normally functioning follicle. Congenital dysplasia of the hair follicles and external factors such as dust, oils, ultraviolet light, heat, and irritants have been proposed (115). One hypothesis is that hair shaft entrapment is the result of hyperkeratosis in the follicular infundibulum, thus producing an obstruction to normal hair shedding.

Differential Diagnosis. Trichostasis spinulosa may clinically resemble cutaneous spicules seen in multiple myeloma, but in the latter condition the follicles are filled with amorphous eosinophilic material, representing precipitated serum monoclonal protein, rather than hair shafts (120).

Principles of Management: Mechanical removal of entrapped hair shafts may be achieved with forceps, a comedone extractor, waxing, or adhesive strips marketed for open comedones. Topical keratolytics or retinoids may also be beneficial.

DISEASES OF HAIR FOLLICLES LEADING TO HAIR LOSS: ALOPECIA

A discussion of alopecia generally pertains to the loss of hair on the scalp, although other body sites may be affected, as can be seen in AA, trichotillomania, telogen effluvium, and lichen planopilaris (LPP), to name a few. A useful way to broadly classify the alopecias is to divide them into nonscarring and scarring types depending on their (relative) propensity to culminate in permanent hair loss. A systematic approach to alopecia can help come to the correct diagnosis (121,122). Sometimes, classification of an individual case of alopecia can be complicated by the coexistence of more than one process. For example, scarring alopecia can occur in a patient with underlying androgenetic alopecia (AGA).

Some types of alopecia are discussed elsewhere in this book, such as lupus erythematosus (Chapter 10), syphilitic alopecia (Chapter 22), perifolliculitis capitis abscedens et suffodiens (Chapter 21), folliculitis (*acne*) keloidalis nuchae (Chapter 21), and alopecia neoplastica. Although hair shaft disorders result in alopecia, a diagnosis is often made on clinical grounds and on the basis of examination of hair shafts rather than biopsy material; therefore, a discussion of hair shaft disorders is not included here but can be found in one of several review articles (123–125). Alopecia that is easily diagnosed in the clinical setting on the basis of history, physical examination, and microscopic assessment of gently pulled hairs, thereby negating the need for a scalp biopsy, is also not discussed; these include postoperative pressure-induced alopecia and loose anagen syndrome.

General Considerations in the Histologic Evaluation of Alopecia

The Scalp Biopsy

A punch biopsy or incisional biopsy extending into fat to include terminal hair bulbs is necessary for proper evaluation of alopecia. A punch biopsy is easier for the clinician to perform, and most scalp biopsies are submitted as such. It is generally accepted that at least a 4-mm punch be used to obtain a sufficient number of hairs for study. In addition, many of the published quantitative parameters for diagnosing different forms of alopecia are based on a 4-mm punch; so this is the one that is generally recommended (126).

Controversy still exists regarding the manner in which the punch biopsy should be sectioned: vertically, where the cylinder of tissue is bisected longitudinally, which is the standard way of sectioning punched specimens procured for other cutaneous disorders, or horizontally (aka transversely), in which the skin cylinder is "bread-loafed," which is the method pioneered by Headington (127). Horizontal sectioning enables visualization of all the follicles in the specimen (Fig. 18-22), whereas it has been estimated that conventional vertical sections demonstrate only 10% to 15% of the follicles in the sample (127). Dermatopathologists appear to be polarized with regard to which method of sectioning is preferable. Of dermatopathologists who favor vertical sections, some feel that they can glean as much information if serial sections are obtained, and some feel uncomfortable interpreting hair follicle anatomy and pathology in a horizontal orientation. A notable disadvantage of transverse sections is the inability to properly evaluate the epidermis (121). However, when a transversely sectioned biopsy is cut through, a portion of the epidermis can usually be seen and evaluated, albeit tangentially.

Some authors have recommended that two 4-mm punch biopsies be performed from the area of disease activity and that one biopsy be sectioned transversely and the other sectioned vertically. The latter is bisected at the time of the biopsy, with one-half sent for routine histology (embedded with the two halves of the transversely sectioned specimen) and the other half processed for direct immunofluorescence (128). In some forms of nonscarring alopecia such as telogen effluvium or early AGA, in which the histologic findings may be subtle, it may be helpful to take one specimen from the crown of the scalp and another from the occiput. On comparing the two, one should find the occipital scalp to be equally involved as the crown in

telogen effluvium and relatively normal compared to the crown in cases of AGA. Certainly, a single biopsy is preferable from a patient morbidity standpoint, and this may be sufficient (129).

For diagnosing cicatricial alopecia, the recommendation is for one 4-mm punch biopsy specimen from the edge of an involved area where there is new hair loss, a positive hair pull test, or inflammation as evidenced by clinically apparent erythema (130). If the goal of the biopsy is to assess the potential for hair regrowth (prognosis), then the optimal area to sample is an older, more central area with a "burnt-out" appearance. In 2011, the HoVert technique was introduced as a way to obtain horizontal and vertical sections from a single punch biopsy and was touted to aid in the diagnosis of scarring alopecias, particularly LPP and discoid lupus erythematosus (131). In this technique, a 4-mm punch biopsy is transected 1 mm below the epidermis to create an epidermal disk that is bisected, allowing visualization of the epidermis in vertical orientation. Transverse sections are cut from the remainder of the specimen. The "Tyler technique" also allows for horizontal and vertical sections to be prepared from a single punch biopsy; the specimen is first bisected vertically, and then one-half is sectioned horizontally (132).

In the past, serial horizontal sections would result in numerous sections and multiple slides to review, typically 12 to 20 (129). A proposed method for improving the convenience of transverse processing recommended trisecting or quadrisecting the specimen, inking one side of each resultant disk of tissue in a consistent orientation and then embedding them all in a single cassette so that several microanatomic levels can be viewed on a single slide (129). My personal experience with this technique is that, although convenient, it sometimes results in loss of tissue (often critical tissue) because laboratory personnel significantly efface some of the tissue pieces to obtain a "good" slice of *all* of the tissue disks. This can occur particularly when the pieces of tissue are embedded at slightly different depths in the paraffin block.

I have found that a safer way to process the punch specimen to avoid loss of tissue is to bisect it transversely at the dermal–subcutaneous junction, then ink the cut surfaces, and embed the two pieces together so that the inked surfaces are cut first, a method previously advocated (121,127). Deeper levels from the block reveal sections that approach the epidermis for one piece of tissue and the subcutis for the other piece of tissue. I cut six levels initially, which is often sufficient, but sometimes I cut up to 12 levels in order to visualize the infundibulum and epidermis.

The ideal way to procure a punch biopsy for transverse processing is to orient the punch tool parallel to the direction of hair growth, decreasing the frequency that hairs are transected by the biopsy procedure. The result is a cylinder of scalp skin in which the sides of the cylinder are not exactly perpendicular to the epidermal surface. With this in mind, when the specimen is bisected transversely, the cut should be angled parallel to the epidermal surface (not perpendicular to the sides of the tissue cylinder) so that each histologic section will show all of the follicles at roughly the same microanatomic level, which facilitates their interpretation. As a consequence, however, follicles and hair shafts will appear ovoid in shape under the microscope, rather than round.

My personal preference is to interpret transverse sections whenever possible, and this chapter emphasizes this method. Transversely sectioned scalp biopsies offer the following advantages (121): (a) *all* of the follicles in the biopsy specimen can be seen and studied, (b) it allows for rapid evaluation of hair density and follicular units, (c) it allows for accurate assessment of

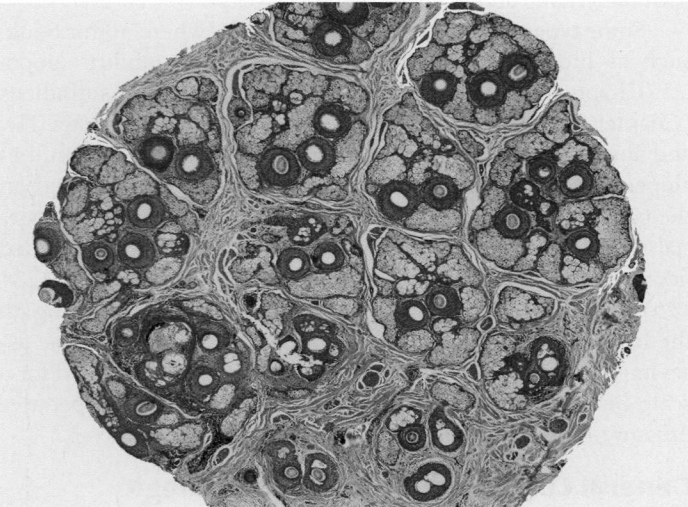

Figure 18-22 Horizontal section, scalp. This 4-mm punch biopsy was sectioned horizontally (aka transversely), enabling visualization of every follicle in the specimen. At this level, through the mid-dermis near the isthmus, arrangement of pilosebaceous structures into "follicular units" is apparent.

follicle size, (d) pathologic alterations at different levels of the follicle can easily be evaluated, and (e) it facilitates quantitative interpretation of the biopsy. In my experience, it is also a more sensitive technique for detecting tinea capitis when only scattered follicles are involved. Horizontal sections are ideal for evaluating the number of viable follicles and estimating prognosis for hair regrowth. As previously mentioned, interpretation of horizontal sections requires a thorough understanding of hair follicle microanatomy, as well as the normal hair cycle. These are superbly described in Chapter 3 and in other sources (121,127,133,134) and are not reiterated here.

Relatively new terms include *exogen*—a distinct phase of the hair cycle in which the hair shaft is actively shed, most likely by a proteolytic mechanism (135)—and *kenogen*—referring to the empty hair follicle after the telogen hair is shed (136). Kenogen is believed to represent a physiologic rest period for the follicle prior to initiation of a new growth phase.

Terminology and Definitions

Solomon and Templeton (137) noted that "working definitions" are "important in the microscopic evaluation of alopecia," although "these definitions are arbitrary and therefore debatable." Although authors differ in the definitions they use to characterize hair follicles, the following definitions are commonly employed. A terminal hair was designated by Headington (127) as having a hair shaft diameter of 0.06 mm or greater and a vellus hair as having a hair shaft diameter of 0.03 mm or less. Between terminal and vellus hairs are intermediate hairs (aka indeterminate), whose shaft diameter, i, is defined as $0.06 > i > 0.03$ mm (Fig. 18-23). A micrometer is sometimes needed to accurately assess hair shaft diameter, although without actually measuring them, hair follicles can be classified by comparing the shaft size to the width of the inner root sheath; the diameter of a vellus hair shaft should be less than or equal to the thickness of the inner root sheath (Fig. 18-23). Qualitatively, terminal hairs have their bulbs anchored in the subcutaneous fat, whereas vellus hair bulbs are in the mid- to upper dermis.

True vellus hairs lack melanin pigment and are small throughout their existence, whereas *miniaturized* vellus hairs are terminal hairs that have decreased in size. Because these are histologically identical, it is not necessary to distinguish them for the purpose of diagnosing alopecias; henceforth in this chapter, the term *vellus hairs* will encompass true vellus hairs *and* miniaturized terminal hairs. Although some authors group intermediate hairs with the terminal hair population for the purpose of quantification, I prefer to include them with the vellus group because more often they represent a transitional follicle undergoing the process of miniaturization to a vellus hair. Reversal of the process via therapy with minoxidil or finasteride, however, can confuse the picture. A cross section at the lower infundibular level is optimal for visualizing vellus hairs, allowing one to accurately count terminal and vellus hair shafts to determine the terminal-to-vellus hair ratio.

In determining the "telogen count" or "anagen-to-telogen ratio," the term *telogen* actually encompasses all phases of the nonanagen follicle, including telogen, catagen, and telogen germinal unit (Fig. 18-24), because they all represent stages in a continuum: the irreversible process of hair follicle regression and shedding. For instance, a catagen follicle, with an epithelial column in the subcutis and/or lower dermis, often shows a telogen hair near the isthmus. Although vellus hairs also cycle, only terminal-sized follicles in catagen and telogen are counted as part of the regressing/resting hair population. The telogen count derived histologically, using these definitions, reflects the count obtained in the clinical setting by forcible hair pluck (using a rubber-tipped hemostat) because this method is unsuccessful at dislodging the smaller vellus hairs (133,138).

A cross section through the isthmus is optimal for assessing the number of telogen and catagen hairs and telogen germinal units. This telogen count should be interpreted in the context of a second count at the infundibular level to assess terminal and vellus hairs because follicles in telogen or catagen according to their appearance near the isthmus show a shaft in the infundibulum that looks identical to that of a terminal anagen follicle; that is, a hair shaft with a diameter of 0.06 mm or greater situated in the infundibular hair canal. Often, the

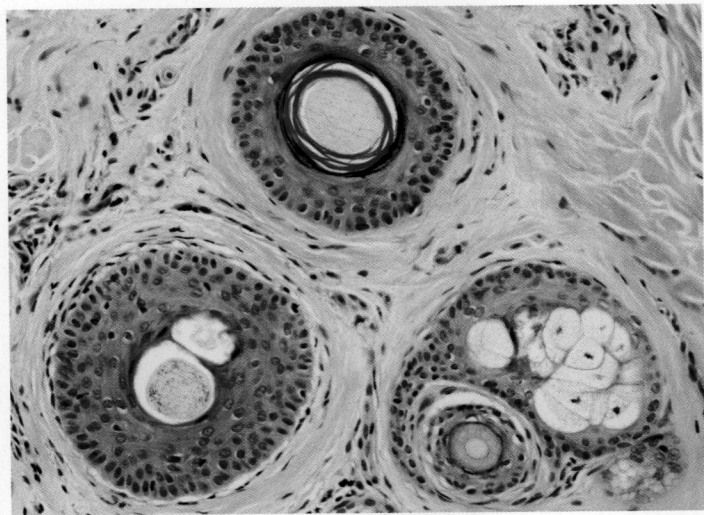

Figure 18-23 Normal variation in hair diameter (horizontal). This level is through the infundibulum of the terminal follicle, defined by a hair shaft diameter that is greater than or equal to 0.06 mm (**top**). The vellus hair (**lower right**) is readily identifiable by a shaft diameter that is equal to or less than the thickness of the inner root sheath (≤0.03 mm). An intermediate hair (**lower left**) has a shaft diameter that is between the other two.

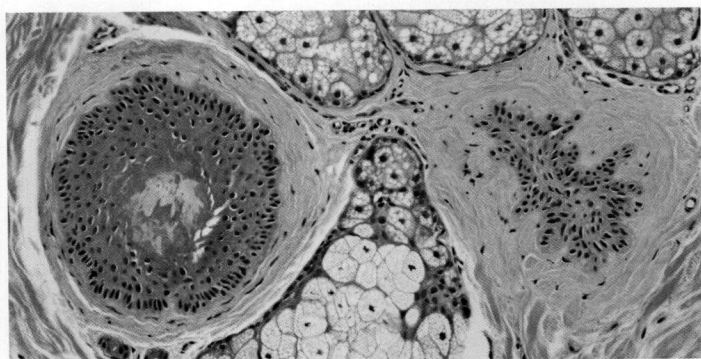

Figure 18-24 Normal resting follicles (horizontal). The follicle at left is a telogen follicle, identifiable by brightly eosinophilic trichilemmal keratinization of the proximal hair shaft. This structure is the histologic correlate of easily displaced telogen hairs viewed by microscopy in the clinical setting, so-called club hairs. To the right is a telogen germinal unit, which represents the secondary hair germ. This structure is found in the mid- to upper dermis and is characterized by follicular epithelium with radial projections. In vertical sections, it is sometimes visible just beneath the telogen hair.

infundibular portion of the hair shaft, untethered by the inner root sheath, is missing, presumably carried away by the microtome blade. In this situation, the pathologist must rely on the caliber of the follicular outer root sheath and the diameter of the empty hair canal to extrapolate the size of the hair shaft and obtain more accurate counts.

Miniaturization and conversion to catagen and telogen leave many collapsed fibrous root sheaths in the subcutis (Fig. 18-25). Also known as "stelae" and "fibrous streamers," they are found in conditions in which there is follicular miniaturization (i.e., AGA) or conditions with increased numbers of catagen and telogen hairs, such as telogen effluvium and trichotillomania.

Normal Parameters

Normal parameters as determined by examination of transversely sectioned scalp biopsies have been published in various sources and are typically based on a 4-mm punch biopsy. Most were from studies of white subjects, but ethnic differences in "normal" values have been demonstrated, and this must be taken into consideration when evaluating a scalp biopsy. Whites without alopecia should have approximately 40 total hairs in a 4-mm punch biopsy, with roughly 20 to 35 terminal hairs and 5 to 10 vellus hairs (126,127,138,139). The normal terminal-to-vellus hair ratio for adult scalp is 3:1 to 4:1 (127) but at least 2:1 (140). Another study found a normal value of 7:1 (139). A more recent study from 2013 calculated the follicular density per square centimeter along with the terminal-to-vellus ratio in scarring and nonscarring alopecias (141).

Hair density in African Americans was found to be significantly lower than in whites, with an average of 18 terminal and 3 vellus hairs in a 4-mm punch biopsy (142). However, the follicles are typically larger (143). In Koreans, the follicular density was found to be significantly lower than in whites and blacks (144).

Hair follicles on the scalp are arranged in follicular units—bundles of hairs naturally found together. They form hexagonal modules separated from one another by intervening collagen

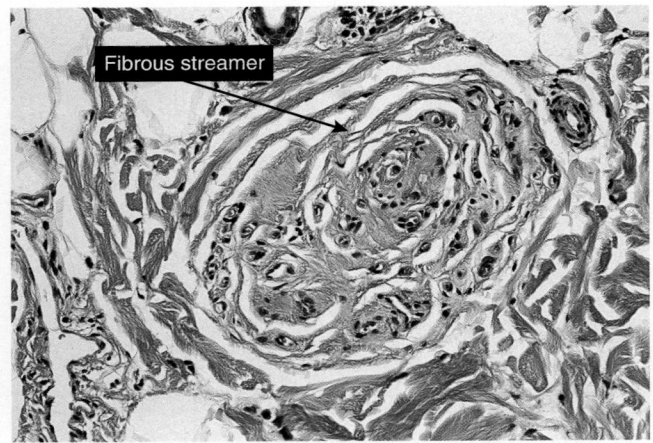

Figure 18-25 Fibrous streamer (horizontal). Also known as stelae, these collapsed fibrous sheaths are subcutaneous evidence of hairs that have moved upward through the process of miniaturization or conversion to telogen. They consist of concentrically arranged bands of collagen with numerous capillaries and an increased number of mast cells. (Reprinted with permission from Elder DE, Elenitsas R, Rubin AI, et al. *Atlas and Synopsis of Lever's Histopathology of the Skin*. 3rd ed. Wolters Kluwer Health/Lippincott Williams & Wilkins; 2013.)

and are best visualized by transverse sections through the upper dermis near the isthmus (Fig. 18-22) (145). There are typically 10 to 12 follicular units in a 4-mm punch (121). Each follicular unit normally contains two to five terminal hairs and zero to two vellus hairs, along with sebaceous glands and arrector pili muscle (126).

Nonscarring Alopecias

Alopecia that is nonscarring clinically shows intact follicular ostia and histologically shows a normal density of hair follicles (146,147). Despite being categorized as "nonscarring," conditions such as AGA, long-standing AA, and traction alopecia can lead to irreversible loss of hair follicles. Transverse sections are particularly useful in the histologic diagnosis of nonscarring alopecias because the anagen-to-telogen ratio and terminal-to-vellus hair ratio may be crucial in making an accurate diagnosis. In particular, female patients with a fairly diffuse, nonscarring alopecia can be a diagnostic dilemma based on clinical grounds alone, and a biopsy can help. The main diagnostic possibilities in this setting are (a) female-pattern hair loss, (b) acute and chronic telogen effluvium, (c) diffuse AA, and (d) loose anagen syndrome (148,149). The salient features of the most common nonscarring alopecias are listed in Table 18-1.

Alopecia Areata

Clinical Summary. AA is clinically characterized by complete or nearly complete absence of hair in one or more circumscribed areas of the scalp (Fig. 18-26) (150,151). Clinical inflammation, typically manifested by erythema, is not obvious, and the follicular openings are preserved, a clinical finding that allows the examiner to make the assessment of a nonscarring alopecia. In active areas of involvement, hair shedding is seen, as well as some short, fractured hair shafts, including the pathognomonic "exclamation point" hair. Complete scalp involvement (*alopecia totalis*) may occur suddenly or through prolonged, progressive disease. Complete or nearly complete loss of all body hair (*alopecia universalis*) can also occur. Partial scalp involvement in distinctive patterns, such as a band at the periphery of the scalp (*ophiasis*) or reverse of this pattern that spares the scalp fringe (*sisaipho*), may be seen. Losses of the eyebrows and eyelashes and regularly spaced pits on the surface of the nails are not uncommon. Most patients with localized disease undergo spontaneous resolution, but others show persistent disease, and a few patients have permanent hair loss. "The only predictable thing about the progress of AA is that it is unpredictable" (152), which means, essentially, that one cannot reliably predict which patients will have a limited disease with spontaneous resolution and which will have recurrent disease or chronic, severe disease.

Histopathology. The diagnostic pathologic feature is peribulbar lymphocytic inflammation ("swarm of bees") affecting anagen follicles (Fig. 18-27) or follicles in early catagen (Fig. 18-28). The inflammatory assault on anagen follicles induces a premature conversion to catagen. Consequently, the number of catagen and telogen follicles found may be marked, approaching 100% (Fig. 18-29) (153). Follicles may enter a persistent phase of telogen in which the hair shaft has already been shed, manifested by the *telogen germinal unit* (153). As follicles enter catagen, the lymphocytic infiltrate may persist around the epithelial remnant of the receding follicle and also within and

Table 18-1

Nonscarring Alopecia (Normal Follicular Density)

	Clinical Pattern	Degree of Miniaturization (0–111)	Telogen Count	Inflammation	Other Histologic Features
Hereditary/AGA	Males—thinning of vertex, crown, bitemporal Females—thinning of crown, retention of frontal hairline	++	16.8% avg.	Lymphocytic; superficial perivascular (37% of cases)	May have superficial perifollicular fibrosis
Alopecia areata (AA)	Round bald patches, diffuse absence of scalp hair (totalis), diffuse absence of scalp and body hair (universalis). May see exclamation point hairs	+++	27% avg.; >50% favors AA	Lymphocytic; peribulbar ("swarm of bees") around terminal hairs (acute) and miniaturized hairs (chronic, recurrent)	Nanogen hairs, pigment casts, melanin pigment deposition in fibrous tracts, intra- and intercellular edema of matrix keratinocytes
Telogen effluvium: acute	Diffuse thinning	None	>15%—suggestive >20%—presumptive >25%—definitive (usually not >50%)	Absent	May resemble normal scalp if in resolution
Telogen effluvium: chronic	Diffuse thinning	None	11% avg.	Absent	May resemble normal scalp
Trichotillomania	Patchy or diffuse. Hairs of irregular length, broken hairs	None	Elevated (>15%)	Absent	Distorted hair anatomy, empty/torn-away anagen hairs, trichomalacia, pigment casts, peribulbar hemorrhage

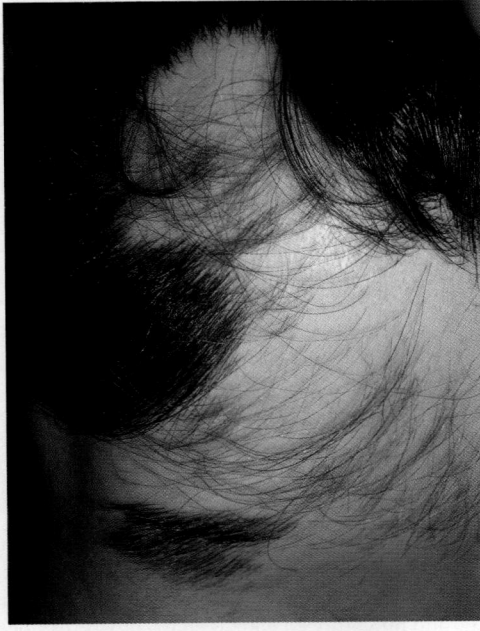

Figure 18-26 Alopecia areata. Patchy alopecia characteristic of alopecia areata, ophiasis pattern. Despite the microscopic lymphocytic infiltrate that is sometimes present, the areas lack clinical evidence of inflammation, namely erythema.

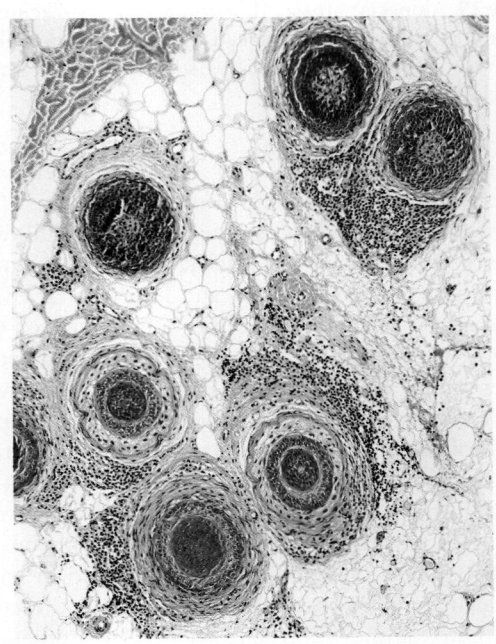

Figure 18-27 Alopecia areata (horizontal). Classic peribulbar lymphocytic inflammation likened to a "swarm of bees."

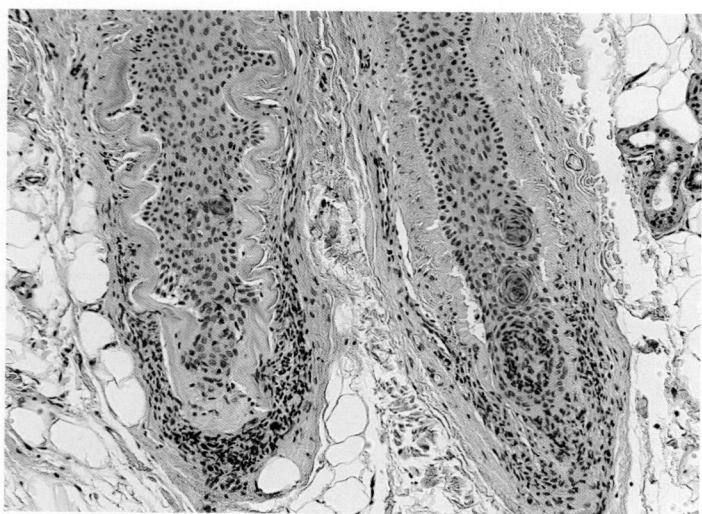

Figure 18-28 Alopecia areata (vertical). Lymphocytic inflammation surrounding catagen follicles, which are distinctive because of their eosinophilic "glassy" membrane and lack of a hair shaft.

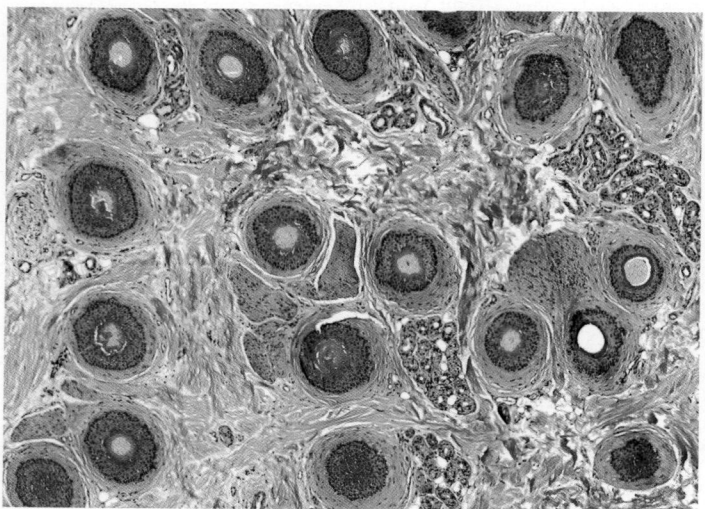

Figure 18-29 Alopecia areata (horizontal). In subacute alopecia areata, terminal anagen hairs attacked by inflammation will undergo conversion to telogen. A biopsy at this stage may show almost 100% terminal telogen hairs.

surrounding the fibrous tracts (Fig. 18-28). Telogen hairs show little to no perifollicular inflammation.

Lymphocytes may also be seen sparsely infiltrating the matrix epithelium of anagen follicles, inducing damage to the matrical cells that includes intra- and intercellular edema, cellular necrosis, and microvesicle formation. One of the earliest findings was shown to be a loss of structural integrity of bulbar keratinocytes in the central part of the supramatrical bulb and shrinkage of hair bulbs toward a club shape (154). As a result of injury to bulbar melanocytes and keratinocytes, pigment casts, which are clumps of melanin pigment, may be found within the dermal papilla, the sheath of miniaturizing or regressing follicles, the follicular epithelium, or fibrous tracts (140,155). Pigment casts are more often found in trichotillomania; one interpretation of their presence in the context of AA is that here too they represent external manipulation of the hair (27). Pigment casts have also been found in postoperative pressure-induced alopecia, leading those authors to postulate

that they resulted from the sudden conversion of follicles from anagen to catagen, as occurs in trichotillomania and AA (156).

The inflammatory assault may produce dysmorphic follicles and shafts. Anagen hairs not sufficiently damaged so as to enter prematurely into catagen may continue to manufacture a hair shaft, one that may be small, distorted, and often nonpigmented (termed *trichomalacia*). The hair shaft may taper to a point so tiny and fragile that it fractures. Small, abnormal follicles called *nanogen* hairs are a distinctive finding in long-standing cases (Fig. 18-30) (143). They are difficult to categorize as anagen, catagen, or telogen hairs, and in transverse sections they show only a minute, incompletely keratinized hair shaft or no shaft at all.

As telogen follicles reenter anagen, they again come under attack from pathogenic lymphocytes, which precipitate premature conversion to catagen once again, so that anagen duration becomes shorter and shorter and the follicles begin to miniaturize (Fig. 18-31). As the follicles decrease in size, they

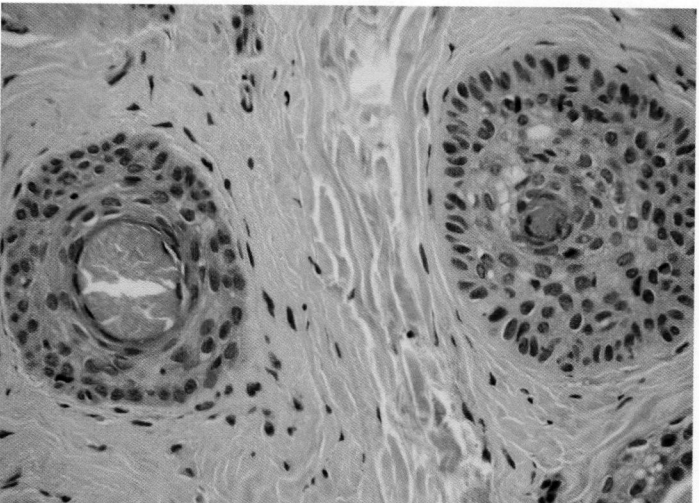

Figure 18-30 Alopecia areata (horizontal). Dystrophic hairs. The follicle at left has no shaft at all; the inner root sheath completely fills the hair canal. The follicle to the right is producing only a minute, "pencil-point" hair shaft that will break easily.

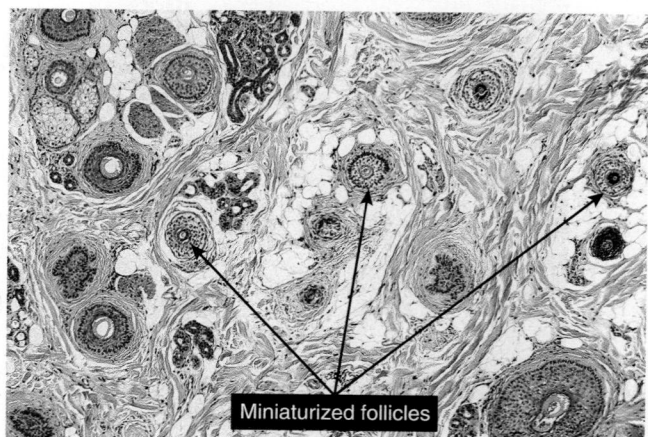

Figure 18-31 Alopecia areata (horizontal). In long-standing alopecia areata, there are an increased number of catagen and telogen follicles, and follicular miniaturization begins to occur. The combination of increased resting and miniaturized hairs is characteristic of alopecia areata, even when peribulbar inflammation is not present. (Reprinted with permission from Elder DE, Elenitsas R, Rubin AI, et al. *Atlas and Synopsis of Lever's Histopathology of the Skin.* 3rd ed. Wolters Kluwer Health/ Lippincott Williams & Wilkins; 2013.).

become situated more superficially, although often deeper than normal vellus hairs, with their bulbs situated in the mid- to lower dermis (140). With disease chronicity, most of the hairs become miniaturized. Miniaturization and conversion to catagen and telogen leave many collapsed fibrous root sheaths in the subcutis.

Whiting found that transversely sectioned scalp biopsies showed the diagnostic features of AA more often than vertically sectioned biopsies (157). He also published mean quantitative hair counts for horizontally sectioned scalp biopsies of AA. The mean terminal-to-vellus hair ratio was similar to that seen in AGA (1.1:1), reflecting extensive miniaturization. The mean anagen-to-telogen ratio was 73%:27%, and the total hair count (mean of 27 hairs) was 33% less than in the control group, with more severely affected patients (alopecia universalis) at the lower end of the spectrum. Others have also found that the follicular density can decrease in severe alopecia totalis and universalis of long duration (a decade or more), with scars replacing some of the follicular sheaths (158).

Whiting and others have emphasized the use of follicular counts to aid in the diagnosis of AA when the characteristic peribulbar inflammation is missing, with a high percentage of catagen or telogen hairs and miniaturized hairs as a strong sign of AA (Fig. 18-28) (141,155,159). In one study, the presence of eosinophils around the bulb and within fibrous tracts was found to be a helpful diagnostic feature of AA, identified in 38 of 71 patients. Eosinophils were found in fibrous tracts 44% to 50% of the time (155,160). Some plasma cells may also be present. Dilated follicular infundibula filled with orthokeratin, resembling "follicular Swiss cheese" on horizontal sections, is another histologic clue to the diagnosis of AA and correlates with yellow dots seen with dermoscopy (161,162).

Some authors claim that in long-standing AA, the inflammatory infiltrates appear to diminish, whereas others believe that the degree of inflammation found on biopsy does not depend on disease duration, citing cases of long-standing AA that showed a great deal of inflammation (140). In a reappraisal of the histopathology of AA, Whiting suggested that the key factor in the histologic picture was the duration of the attack, with lymphocytes surrounding mainly terminal hair bulbs in acute episodes and involving mainly miniaturized hair bulbs in chronic, recurrent disease (159).

Pathogenesis. The exact pathogenesis of AA is not known, but substantial evidence exists to support a role for genetic factors, nonspecific immune- and organ-specific autoimmune reactions, and environmental triggers (152,163–165). The antigenic stimulus for autoimmune attack may be the follicular keratinocyte, melanocyte, or dermal papilla. Advances in the understanding of AA in the last decade have benefited from animal models of the disease (166), including the C3H/HeJ mouse (167), the Dundee experimental bald rat (168), and the Smyth chicken (169).

Familial cases of AA are well recognized, suggesting a genetic predisposition (170). A family history of AA reportedly ranges between 10% and 42% (171), with higher incidences in patients with disease onset early in life and in identical twins (172). AA has been associated with both HLA class I and class II antigens, with different forms and severity of AA found to be associated with certain HLA types (152). The numerous genes involved in the pathogenesis of AA have recently been tabulated (173). AA has been associated with many conditions,

including Down syndrome, atopy, vitiligo, thyroid disease, pernicious anemia, diabetes, myasthenia gravis, lupus erythematosus, rheumatoid arthritis, ulcerative colitis, lichen planus, polymyalgia rheumatica, *Candida* endocrinopathy syndrome, and idiopathic thrombocytopenia purpura (152).

In a study using indirect immunofluorescence, autoantibodies to various parts of the anagen hair follicle were found in AA patients (174). Most commonly targeted were the outer root sheath, then the matrix, inner root sheath, and hair shaft. Tobin et al. (175) also found serum autoantibodies to pigmented hair follicles in 100% of AA patients but in only 44% of control patients.

Earlier experiments showed the peribulbar infiltrate to be composed predominantly of CD4$^+$ cells (helper T lymphocytes). Subsequently, CD8$^+$ cells (suppressor-cytotoxic T lymphocytes) were implicated in the pathogenesis of AA, with experiments supporting a cooperative role between CD8$^+$ and CD4$^+$ T cells (176). Expression of cell adhesion molecules in the matrix epithelium, dermal papilla, and adjacent vessels has been demonstrated, suggesting a mechanism for leukocyte binding.

The immune system of the hair follicle is unique and differs from that of the surrounding skin (177). The epithelial portion of the proximal anagen hair is immune privileged; the inner root sheath and hair matrix do not express major histocompatibility complex (MHC) class I antigens (177,178). A theory put forth by Paus, an "immune privilege collapse model," suggests that in AA, the body's immune system may begin to recognize immune-privileged hair follicle antigens as a result of upregulated MHC molecules or downregulation of local immunosuppressive factors (177,178). Also, a role for the peripheral nervous system has been postulated in AA, via neuropeptides with pro- and anti-inflammatory properties released in the vicinity of critical areas of the hair follicle (179).

Differential Diagnosis. Alopecia syphilitica may closely mimic active AA (180). Features that help to distinguish syphilitic alopecia include lymphocytes situated near the isthmus, the presence of plasma cells, an endothelial reaction, interface dermatitis, and neutrophils in the stratum corneum (160,180). AA may also look identical to the patchy, nonscarring alopecia that occurs in the setting of systemic lupus erythematosus, which shows mononuclear cell inflammation around terminal and miniaturized anagen hair bulbs, as well as an increased percentage of resting hairs, sometimes approaching 100% (143). Features favoring lupus erythematosus include increased dermal mucin, focal basal vacuolization of infundibular epithelium, and inflammation around blood vessels and eccrine glands, particularly when the infiltrate is dense. Although AGA shows diminution of follicular size, dermal infiltrates that are present in this condition are usually superficial, perivascular, and peri-infundibular. Psoriatic alopecia and TNF-inhibitor associated psoriatic alopecia may also mimic AA in terms of hair counts and pattern of inflammation, but differ with respect to psoriasiform epidermal hyperplasia and sebaceous gland atrophy (181).

Principles of Management: Alopecic patches may resolve spontaneously. For refractory patches, intralesional corticosteroids are a very effective treatment. For more widespread involvement or for patients averse to needles, topical high-potency steroids are a reasonable alternative, although penetration to the level of the hair bulbs is an issue. A topical retinoid may be added to the regimen to facilitate deeper penetration of the steroid. When larger areas are involved (i.e., alopecia totalis), topical immunotherapy with squaric acid dibutylester or *dinitrochlorobenzene (DNCB)* may be a better option. Oral and topical JAK inhibitors have recently shown promise in the treatment of AA (173).

Trichotillomania

Clinical Summary. Trichotillomania is a condition in which patients pull or manipulate hair from the scalp or other body sites (182). Persistent rubbing of an area of the scalp that may be pruritic, or compulsive avulsion of hair shafts can lead to zones of alopecia characterized by sparse, ragged, broken stubble (Fig. 18-32). Hair shaft breakage and loss may be associated with damage to the scalp, as evidenced by erosions or crusts. Trichotillomania occurs most often in children and adolescent girls. In children under the age of 6 years, the disorder may be more benign and self-limited (183). In teens and adults, it is more likely to be associated with psychopathology. Trichotillomania is part of the *Diagnostic and Statistical Manual of Mental Disorders (DSM-5)*, grouped with obsessive-compulsive disorder (184), but that association has recently been challenged (185). It is classified as a recurrent failure to resist the impulse to pull hair, with rising tension followed by relief or gratification after pulling out hair (186). In one study, a large proportion of patients with trichotillomania also had comorbid self-injurious habits (186).

Histopathology. In horizontally sectioned biopsies of trichotillomania uncomplicated by the coexistence of other types of alopecia, the density of hair follicles is normal, as is the terminal-to-vellus hair ratio. The diagnostic finding, when seen, is distorted hair follicle anatomy, without inflammation (Fig. 18-33) (140). Specifically, the pulling of hairs can leave behind empty anagen follicles and "torn-away" follicles, the result of plucked hair shafts that retain parts of the hair matrix and root sheaths (Fig. 18-34). Additional microscopic evidence of traumatic injury was published by Royer and Sperling (187) as the "hamburger sign," describing a vertically oriented split in the hair shaft containing proteinaceous material and erythrocytes, resembling a hamburger within a bun (Fig. 18-35). Distorted hair follicle anatomy may assume the appearance of

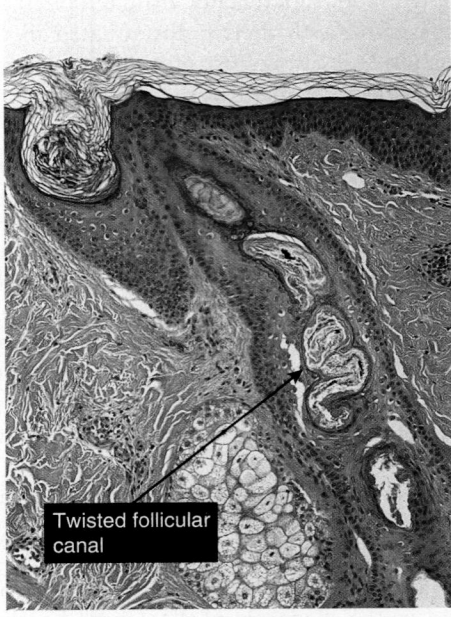

Figure 18-33 Trichotillomania (vertical). The hair canal is distorted in a spiral configuration, most likely secondary to twisting of the hair. Pigment casts, derived from bulbar or hair shaft melanin, are present. (Reprinted with permission from Elder DE, Elenitsas R, Rubin AI, et al. *Atlas and Synopsis of Lever's Histopathology of the Skin.* 3rd ed. Wolters Kluwer Health/Lippincott Williams & Wilkins; 2013.)

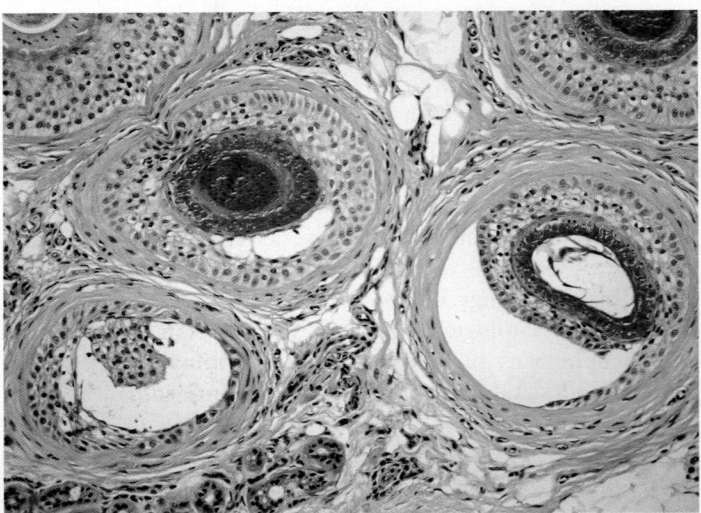

Figure 18-34 Trichotillomania (horizontal). The follicle at left shows a rim of outer root sheath epithelium that remains after the hair was forcefully pulled, taking with it the inner root sheath and part of the outer sheath. At right, the follicle is partially avulsed, and the shaft that is normally tightly anchored to the inner root sheath at this level is gone.

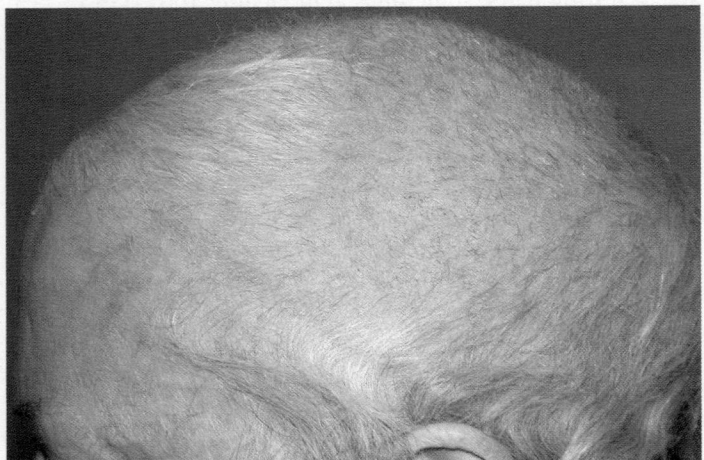

Figure 18-32 Trichotillomania. Short, broken hairs are seen diffusely over the crown and vertex, and the scalp skin is lichenified in areas, the result of compulsive rubbing of the scalp.

other food items (e.g., hot dog) (188). Damaged follicles enter the resting phase, leading to an increase in the percentage of catagen and telogen hairs, as high as 75% (Fig. 18-36) (189). Often, the hairs do not become normal catagen hairs and appear distorted and abnormal (140).

Pigment casts, which are clumps of melanin pigment, may be seen in the hair papilla and peribulbar connective tissue. They are also commonly seen in the upper portion of the hair follicle (Fig. 18-33) as a result of pigmented matrical cells being deposited distally as the hair is plucked. Pigment casts are

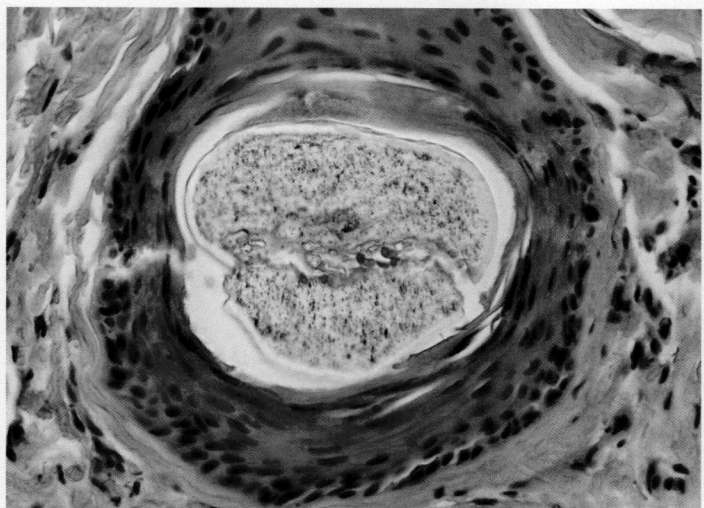

Figure 18-35 Trichotillomania (horizontal). A rare but diagnostic finding in trichotillomania is longitudinal splitting of the hair shaft. When blood and proteinaceous debris are seen in the split, it is known as the "hamburger sign."

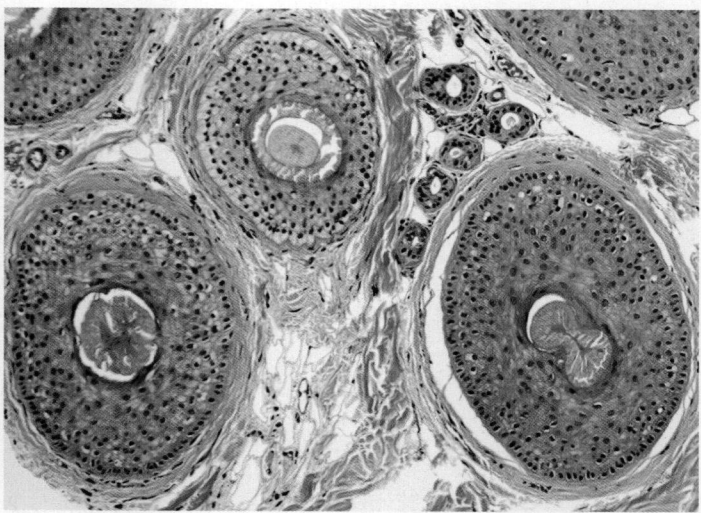

Figure 18-37 Trichotillomania (horizontal). When the hair shaft is pulled, the inner root sheath collapses and fills the empty space, forming geometric configurations, as seen in the lower two follicles.

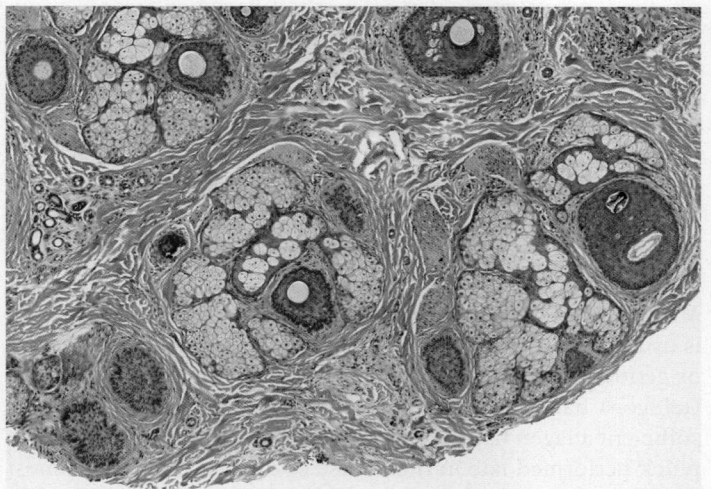

Figure 18-36 Trichotillomania (horizontal). Low-power view reveals an increased number of "resting" follicles, with catagen and telogen hairs, and telogen germinal units. A follicle to the far right contains a black pigment cast.

caused by injury to the hair matrix, although some authors have theorized that they result from the sudden conversion of anagen to catagen (156). Hair shaft changes, termed *trichomalacia*, may be seen. Characterized by diminished size, distorted and odd shape, and irregular pigmentation of the shaft, trichomalacia is additional evidence of trauma to the matrix (140,189). When the hair shaft is pulled, the inner root sheath collapses and fills the gap, often resulting in unusual geometric configurations of the inner root sheath (Fig. 18-37). Traumatized follicles can also show considerable distortion of the bulbar epithelium and conspicuous hemorrhage (189).

Because not all follicles in a given area are affected, transversely sectioned scalp biopsies may increase the yield of finding the diagnostic histologic features of trichotillomania, including increased numbers of catagen and telogen hairs (most cases) and empty or distorted follicles (>50% of cases) (140). The same study found pigment casts and trichomalacia in less than

50% of cases. When the scalp is also rubbed persistently, epidermal changes of lichen simplex chronicus may be seen.

Differential Diagnosis. The histologic differential diagnosis of increased numbers of catagen and telogen hairs, characteristic of trichotillomania, includes AA and telogen effluvium. Trichotillomania also shares with early AA the features of normal hair density and occasional trichomalacia, but trichotillomania lacks the follicular miniaturization and peribulbar infiltrates. In telogen effluvium, evidence of trauma to follicles, as discussed earlier, is not seen. The histologic findings in early traction alopecia are said to be identical with those of trichotillomania, but fewer follicles are involved, and the features are less prominent (see *Traction Alopecia*) (140).

Principles of Management: Treatment includes pharmacotherapy (*n*-acetyl cysteine or olanzapine) and behavioral therapy such as habit reversal therapy (185,190), topical adjunctive therapies, and psychotherapy (183).

Traction Alopecia

Clinical Summary. Traction alopecia is another type of mechanical alopecia, usually resulting from a variety of hair-styling practices, particularly in women of African descent (Fig. 18-38), that includes tight braids (i.e., corn rows and dreadlocks), tight buns or pony tails, hair weaves or extensions, straightening and chemical relaxers, and the use of sponge rollers (191–193). Hair follicle injury is similar to that produced in trichotillomania, but in traction alopecia there are differences that relate to the use of less force over a greater period of time (140).

Traction alopecia is often classified clinically and histologically as "early" and "late" disease. In early disease, tension on hair follicles exists over the course of months to a few years, sometimes presenting as a traction folliculitis with perifollicular erythema and pustules (192). In late disease, hair is subject to traction over many years. In early disease, discontinuation of the abnormal forces on the hair leads to regrowth, but in late disease, follicles are lost, producing a permanent alopecia. Early and late disease are commonly found together in the same patient; as permanently scarred areas develop (late disease), terminal hairs at the periphery are used in styling, becoming the

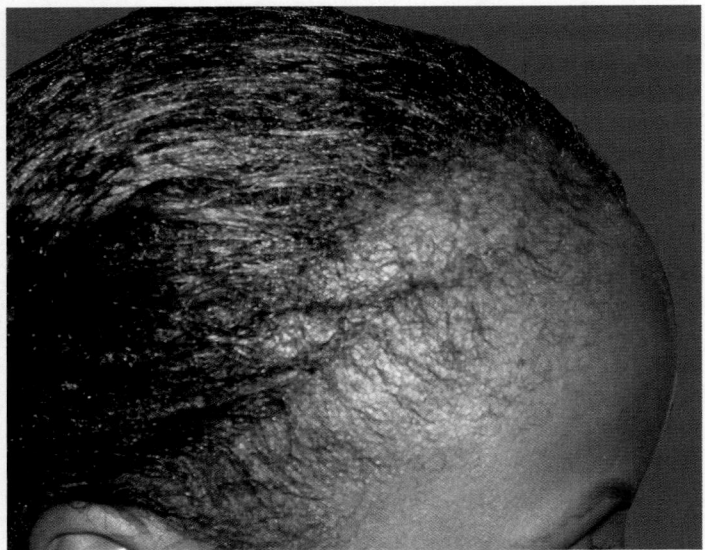

Figure 18-38 Traction alopecia. The frontotemporal hairline is mostly preserved, but there is thinning of these areas owing to chronic tension on the hair follicles as a result of hair styling.

new target of traction (early disease) (140). Occupationally related traction alopecia has been reported as a result of wearing a nurse's cap, occurring at the site of pin placement used to secure the cap (194).

Histopathology. In early traction alopecia, the histologic findings are similar to those of trichotillomania, albeit more subtle. For instance, the density of follicles is normal, with a normal number of vellus hairs. Premature conversion of anagen hairs to catagen occurs, resulting in an increased number of catagen and telogen follicles. Pigment casts and trichomalacia are sometimes found, although less often than in trichotillomania. Inflammation is absent unless traction folliculitis is sampled.

In late disease, permanent loss of terminal follicles occurs, with replacement of follicular tracts by scar tissue (Fig. 18-39). These "follicular scars" resemble columns of fibrous tissue;

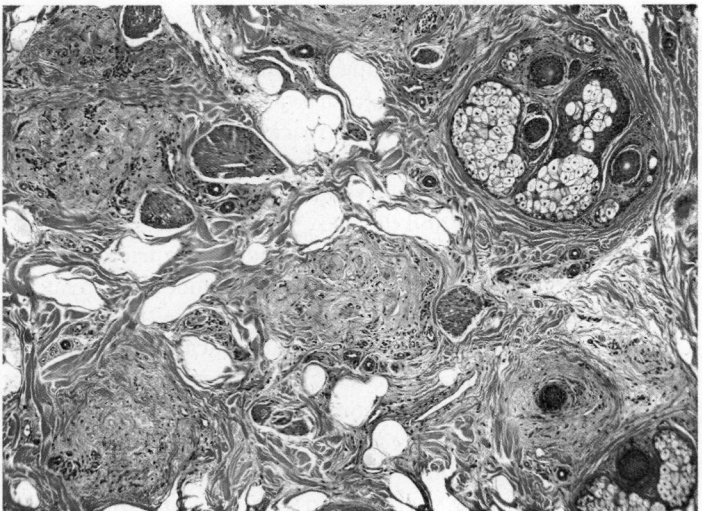

Figure 18-39 Traction alopecia, late stage (horizontal). The histologic picture is that of a burnt-out scarring alopecia. Several follicular scars are seen along with stranded arrector pili muscles and absent sebaceous glands. A few vellus follicles remain, at right. Their small size allows them to escape the mechanical forces that lead to hair follicle destruction.

interfollicular areas are uninvolved. Because vellus hairs are not sufficiently large to be included in the method of styling and be affected by tractional forces, these hairs are preserved, and this is reflected in a normal absolute number of vellus follicles, often outnumbering terminal follicles. In late disease, the pathology shows an "end-stage" scarring alopecia.

Differential Diagnosis. Late disease shows a histologic picture shared by many forms of permanent alopecia at an advanced stage. Pigment casts and trichomalacia are not seen in late traction alopecia.

Principles of Management: To avoid the permanent alopecia associated with chronic traction, early measures must be undertaken to avoid excessive tension on hair follicles by styling practices. Education at an early age is key. An excellent review of the pathogenesis and other treatment modalities that may be tried was recently published (195).

Anagen Effluvium

Clinical Summary. Acute loss of actively growing (anagen) hairs occurs as a result of a severe insult that disrupts the mitotic activity of dividing cells in the hair matrix (196), with hair shaft production suffering greatly. The shaft becomes tapered proximally, breaks at the narrowest point, and is shed. The most commonly encountered forms of anagen effluvium are from chemotherapeutic agents and radiation therapy (138), although heavy metal poisoning and other toxins should be considered (196). Rapidly progressing alopecia totalis may present as anagen effluvium. Pemphigus vulgaris may cause anagen effluvium, even from nonlesional scalp (197). Furthermore, anagen hair loss was shown to be an independent predictor of disease severity (197).

Microscopic Examination of Hairs. Diagnosis of anagen effluvium is usually made on clinical grounds with the aid of a trichogram or gentle hair pull; so scalp biopsies are seldom done. Resting (telogen) hairs are immune to the metabolic insult, so when sufficient anagen hairs are lost through shedding, a forcible hair pluck performed late in the course of disease will show almost all telogen hairs; a telogen count that approaches 100% on trichogram is a clue that a type of anagen effluvium is to blame. Early, a gentle hair pull demonstrates "pencil-point" tapered hairs with a pointed or frayed end (138).

Differential Diagnosis. In loose anagen syndrome, in contrast, the proximal portion of pulled anagen hairs shows a ruffled hair shaft cuticle because the inner and outer root sheaths are lost during extraction (138). In the setting of pemphigus vulgaris, normal-appearing anagen hairs with an intact inner root sheath and partially intact outer root sheath are lost, as the cleavage plane is in the outer root sheath (198).

Principles of Management: Treatment is geared toward the underlying cause.

Telogen Effluvium

Clinical Summary. Effluvium is a Latin term meaning "a flowing out." Telogen effluvium results from "outflowing," or shedding, of hair shafts in the telogen phase of the hair growth cycle. The concept was originally delineated by Kligman (199). This condition has many precipitating causes or associated conditions, including childbirth, serious illness, including HIV infection, high fever, life-threatening trauma, major surgery, restrictive dieting and nutritional deficiencies, hypothyroidism, iron-deficiency anemia, medications, especially hormonal drugs, allergic contact dermatitis, the onset of AGA, and psychological stress (121,199–202). The shedding tends to occur diffusely throughout the scalp and may involve hair over the rest of the body.

Telogen hairs are recognizable by the club shape of their proximal end when visualized microscopically (*club hairs*). In conjunction with the history, physical examination of the scalp, and sometimes a *trichogram* (microscopic examination of shed, pulled, or plucked hairs), a diagnosis of telogen effluvium can often be made in the clinical setting. However, in difficult cases in which the differential diagnosis includes AGA and diffuse AA, a biopsy may be done.

Chronic telogen effluvium was a concept put forth by Whiting (203,204) in 1996 after studying 355 patients with the disorder. Patients are usually middle-aged women, 30 to 60 years old, with variable shedding that persists for years. Because hairs are replaced as fast as they are shed, patients do not become bald. An obvious cause is not identified (although an initiating factor may exist), and hence the designation "idiopathic." In one long-term study, chronic telogen effluvium continued for 7 years in four of five women, and only one developed female-pattern hair loss (205). Chronic telogen effluvium has rarely been reported in men (203,206). A scalp biopsy for horizontal sections is particularly helpful in distinguishing chronic telogen effluvium from AGA (207).

Histopathology. Only a subjective assessment of the proportion of follicles in telogen can be obtained with vertical sectioning of scalp punch biopsy specimens, whereas an objective analysis can be obtained by examining horizontal sections (Fig. 18-40) (127). There is a normal number of hair follicles and an absence of follicular miniaturization, unless telogen effluvium occurs in patients with established androgenetic or another form of involutional alopecia. Inflammation is generally not seen.

Telogen follicles, characterized histologically by trichilemmal keratinization of the most proximal portion of the hair shaft, are increased (Fig. 18-40). The number of catagen follicles or telogen germinal units may also be increased (Fig. 18-41).

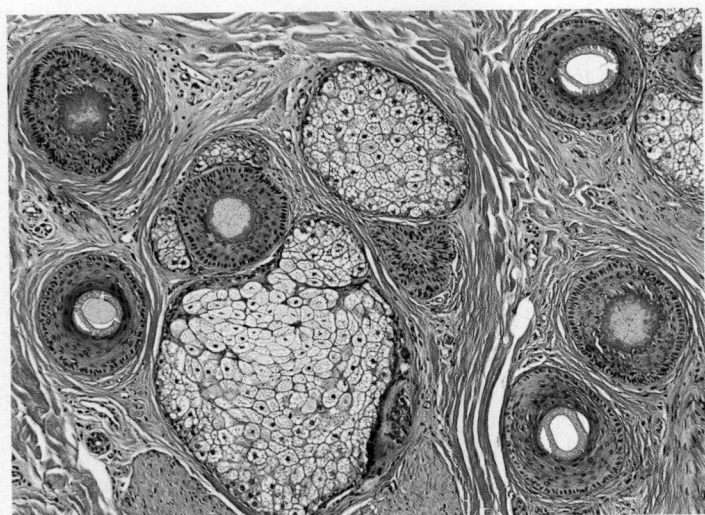

Figure 18-40 Telogen effluvium (horizontal). An increased number of telogen hairs are present. Four out of the seven follicles in this field are in a stage of telogen.

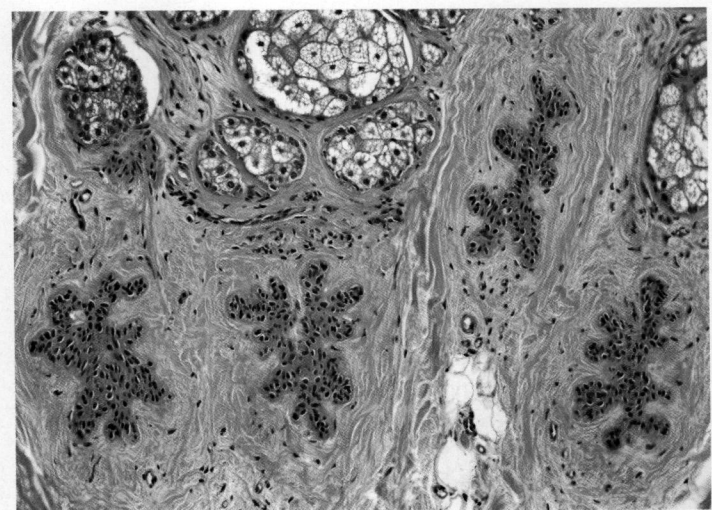

Figure 18-41 Telogen effluvium (horizontal). This field consists entirely of telogen germinal units.

According to published data, the telogen count in normal scalp may range from 0% to 25% (199), with averages of 6% (139) and 13% cited (199). Telogen follicles in excess of 15% are considered to be abnormal and suggest a diagnosis of telogen effluvium in the absence of significant inflammation and miniaturization (139,200). Others have suggested that a level of 25% is necessary for a definitive diagnosis of telogen effluvium (140,199), whereas a telogen count of 20% is "presumptive" evidence (199). Kligman also stated that telogen counts greater than 60% in telogen effluvium are rare. With a telogen count approaching 100%, one should consider anagen effluvium or AA (138,140,153).

Biopsies from the crown/vertex and occiput yield similar findings because the process is diffuse. Timing of the biopsy clearly affects the pathologic changes observed. Should a biopsy be obtained in the very early stages of recovery, follicles in early anagen will be present in addition to elevated resting follicles, but if recovery is substantial, the histopathologic assessment may be entirely normal.

In a study of chronic telogen effluvium, the average number of hairs in a 4-mm punch biopsy was normal at 39; the terminal-to-vellus hair ratio was normal; and the average telogen count was 11% (203). In comparison, the average telogen count was 16.8% in AGA and 6.5% in normal controls. Significant inflammation and fibrosis were present in only 10% to 12% of chronic telogen effluvium and control cases, as compared to 37% of AGA biopsies. Sinclair et al. (208) found that when three horizontally sectioned, 4-mm punch biopsies from the scalp were performed instead of one, diagnostic distinction between chronic telogen effluvium and female-pattern hair loss could be made with greater certainty.

Pathogenesis. In the acute form, increased shedding is noted approximately 3 months after the precipitating factor; this is the timetable for regressing anagen follicles to pass through catagen into telogen (209). Headington described five processes by which excessive telogen shedding may occur (200). Briefly, these processes depend on changes in the length of the anagen (growth) period and on the active release of hair shafts in telogen. Teloptosis is the termination of telogen with shedding of the hair, believed to be caused by loss of adhesion between the club hair and cells of the surrounding epithelium (210). These authors distinguished two kinds of telogen hairs on trichogram—those with an epithelial sheath, suggesting early telogen, and those devoid of an epithelial sheath, indicating telogen termination or teloptosis.

Differential Diagnosis. Telogen effluvium must often be differentiated from other types of diffuse nonscarring alopecia, such as AGA or diffuse AA.

Principles of Management: Identification of an underlying cause with an appropriate time frame, though not always possible, relies on a thorough history that includes medications, illnesses or hospitalizations, high fever, weight loss caused by dieting, and family history of hereditary baldness. Laboratory studies may be required to exclude thyroid abnormalities or anemia. Psychological stress may also play a role.

Androgenetic Alopecia

Clinical Summary. The hallmark of AGA is follicular miniaturization, the process by which hair follicles become progressively finer and shorter. AGA results from an androgenic influence on hair follicles in certain areas of the scalp. The pattern of involvement typically seen in the different sexes has led to the use of the terminology *male-pattern* or *female-pattern hair loss.* Some prefer this terminology over AGA because the etiologic role of androgens in women is not fully determined (211,212). AGA is the most common type of hair loss in men and women, affecting 50% of men by the age of 50 years and almost as many women, according to some reports (213), leading some to suspect that it is a physiologic process, not a pathologic one (214). AGA frequently shows a familial tendency, but inheritance does not follow simple Mendelian genetics and is most likely a polygenic trait (215).

In male patients, the process usually begins with bilateral frontotemporal thinning, often with similar changes over the vertex. In full expression of the condition, there may be almost total baldness of the entire frontal/parietal scalp. The most common pattern seen in women is one of diffuse thinning over the crown of the scalp with preservation of the frontal hairline. The process occurs with less severity in women, so significant balding is unusual.

Histopathology. Satisfactory evaluation of AGA can be achieved only from transverse sectioning of punch biopsy material (127,139,216), allowing for quantitative evaluation. Furthermore, samples smaller than 4 mm in diameter show an insufficient number of follicles for meaningful results.

Diminution of follicular size, or miniaturization, is the histologic hallmark of AGA. To fully appreciate the number of miniaturized follicles, horizontal sections at the level of the lower infundibulum of terminal hair follicles should be examined because sections below this may miss the vellus hairs whose bulbs are situated in the upper dermis. Cursory inspection at low power reveals random variation in the caliber of hair follicles, consistent with a progressive miniaturization (Fig. 18-42) (217), and absence of well-defined follicular units (216). Although vellus hairs can quickly be identified by the fact that their shaft diameter is equal to or less than the thickness of their inner root sheath, they are quantitatively defined as having a shaft diameter of 0.03 mm or less (127). In his 1984 article that laid the groundwork for horizontal interpretation of scalp biopsies, Headington also defined terminal hairs as having a shaft diameter of 0.06 mm or greater, thus recognizing an intermediate/indeterminate category in which the shaft diameter,

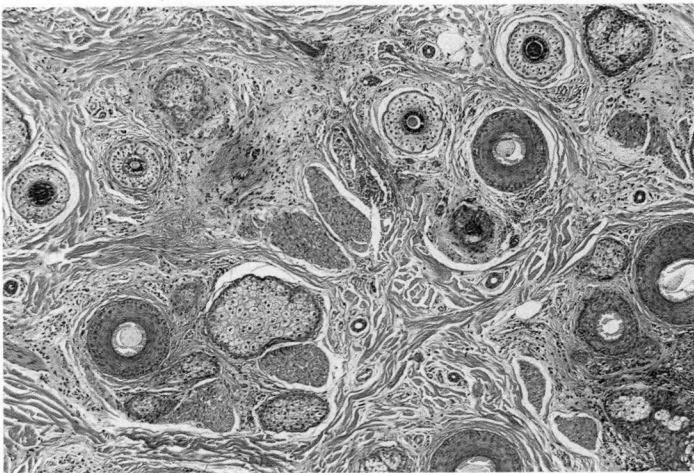

Figure 18-42 Androgenetic alopecia (horizontal). Early in the course of this disorder, the density of follicles remains normal. There is great variation in follicular size, with an increased number of intermediate and vellus follicles. An increase in the percentage of catagen and telogen follicles can sometimes be seen. (Reprinted with permission from Elder DE, Elenitsas R, Rubin AI, et al. *Atlas and Synopsis of Lever's Histopathology of the Skin.* 3rd ed. Wolters Kluwer Health/Lippincott Williams & Wilkins; 2013.)

i, measures $0.06 > i > 0.03$ mm, between terminal and vellus hairs (see Fig. 18-43) (127). An optical micrometer may be used to measure hair shaft diameter, if necessary.

However, slightly different definitions were used in subsequent articles on AGA, specifically with regard to the intermediate category. For example, Whiting (139) classified terminal hairs as having a "shaft diameter exceeding 0.03 mm ... thicker than its inner root sheath," thereby grouping intermediate hairs with the terminal hair population. He then used a 3:1 (or less) terminal-to-vellus hair ratio as being diagnostic of male-pattern AGA, although at other times he and others quoted a terminal-to-vellus hair ratio of less than or equal to 2:1 to diagnose AGA (139,140,218). Whiting (139) found the average terminal-to-vellus ratio in AGA to be 1.7:1. Using similar definitions of terminal and vellus hairs, Sperling and Winton (216) reported finding an average terminal-to-vellus ratio of 1:6.1, illustrating how, in advanced cases, miniaturized hairs outnumber terminal hairs (140). In my opinion, intermediate hairs should be grouped with the vellus hair population because more often they represent a transitional follicle undergoing miniaturization to a vellus hair (unless the patient is using agents such as minoxidil or finasteride to reverse the process). Unfortunately, ratios for normal scalp and in AGA in which vellus and intermediate hairs are lumped together are not available in the literature and necessitate further study.

It is easy to undercount the number of vellus hairs, even with horizontal sections (216). Some vellus hairs may be so small as to be mistaken for keratinous debris. The use of toluidine blue stain was reported to be superior to that of hematoxylin and eosin in identifying the tiniest of hairs because it stains the inner root sheath intensely blue (216), and the use of Ziehl–Neelsen stain has similarly been touted for counting miniaturized hair shafts, which stain intensely red (219). Modified Masson trichrome stain may be helpful in evaluating arrector pili muscle degeneration and replacement by adipose tissue, findings that have been reported in AGA (220).

The onset of AGA may be manifested by a telogen effluvium (221). Whiting found the telogen count in AGA to be

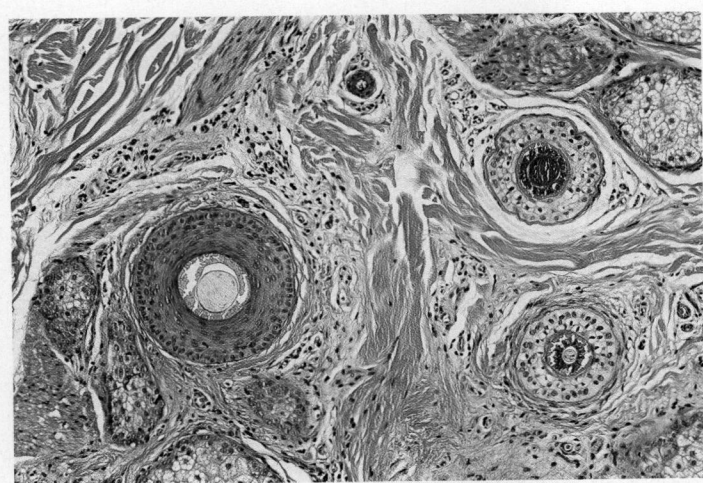

Figure 18-43 Androgenetic alopecia (horizontal). Higher magnification reveals hair follicles of varying size. This cross section is just below the level of the isthmus, as evidenced by the fact that the inner root sheath of the terminal follicle is fully keratinized but still intact. In this field, there is also an intermediate hair and a vellus hair. (Reprinted with permission from Elder DE, Elenitsas R, Rubin AI, et al. *Atlas and Synopsis of Lever's Histopathology of the Skin.* 3rd ed. Wolters Kluwer Health/Lippincott Williams & Wilkins; 2013.)

16.8%, as compared to 6.5% in controls (139), with telogen counts as high as 30% reported (216). Because the reduction in follicular size is associated with a shorter anagen phase (the smaller hairs do not grow as long), at a given point in time (for a histologic specimen this is the moment of biopsy harvest) a greater proportion of follicles will be found in telogen. There may be typical telogen hairs or, with increasing severity, telogen germinal units. A telogen germinal unit is the follicular epithelium that remains after the telogen hair shaft has been shed; it represents the secondary hair germ (Fig. 18-24) (127). Although vellus hairs continue to cycle through anagen and telogen in the papillary dermis, they are not considered to be part of the telogen count (145). Both miniaturization and increased conversion to telogen are associated with the finding of fewer terminal hair bulbs and more fibrous streamers in the deep dermis and subcutis (145). The fibrous streamers in AGA are thicker, more cellular, and, possibly, more fibrotic than those of normal follicles (222).

In advanced AGA, there may be a reduced hair density with permanent loss of follicles (139,216,223), termed cicatricial-pattern hair loss by Olsen (223). Peri-infundibular fibroplasia, ultimately leading to focal follicular scarring, may be responsible (139,224). In subtle cases of AGA, a second biopsy, taken from the occipital scalp, may be helpful for comparison because the occiput is typically uninvolved.

Lymphocytic infiltrates, defined as activated T cells in one study, are found around superficial vessels and in the vicinity of the lower infundibulum, sebaceous glands, and bulge in follicles transitioning to full miniaturization (225). The presence of inflammation has been reported in as many as 50% to 75% of cases (224) and has been linked to peripilar signs seen clinically (226). However, mild perifollicular and upper-dermal inflammation can be observed in normal scalp with a frequency similar to that of AGA (217) and is therefore of no value in diagnosing AGA. Moderate inflammation, however, was seen more often in AGA than in normal individuals (139); the infiltrate was composed primarily of lymphocytes and histiocytes,

with rare neutrophils, plasma cells, and giant cells. It has been suggested that inflammation in AGA may result from *Demodex*, seborrheic dermatitis, actinic damage, cosmetics, and grooming agents (139) and therefore should not be considered pathogenic (214). Nevertheless, its presence may have a bearing on the potential to respond to treatment; one study found that AGA patients with histologic inflammation or fibrosis showed less frequent regrowth on treatment with 2% minoxidil than AGA patients without inflammation (139), although the figures did not prove to be statistically significant. In conclusion, upper-dermal inflammation can be seen in AGA, but it does not support or discount this diagnosis.

Pathogenesis. Androgens are the primary regulators of normal human hair growth. With the arrival of puberty, they transform vellus hairs in many sites, such as the axilla, to terminal hairs but mediate the opposite effect on certain scalp follicles in predisposed individuals (227). The effects of androgens on the hair follicle are mediated via androgen receptors in the hair papilla. The primary androgen responsible for these effects is DHT, via androgen-receptor binding (228). Within the follicle, the enzyme 5α-reductase produces DHT from serum testosterone. Predisposed scalp displayed high levels of DHT and increased androgen-receptor expression in one study (228). In another study, frontal scalp follicles showed higher levels of androgen receptor and 5α-reductase than occipital scalp follicles, and men exhibited higher levels than women (229).

A group of investigators found that the predominant form of 5α-reductase in human scalp is type 1, concentrated in sebaceous glands (230). These same investigators found 5α-reductase type 2 to be present in the inner layer of the outer root sheath, the proximal inner root sheath, and the infundibulum and some in sebaceous ducts. The type 2 isozyme is responsible for AGA. It is preferentially inhibited by finasteride, which decreases scalp production of DHT and promotes hair growth in males with AGA (230).

Other serum hormones, such as adrenal-derived dehydroepiandrosterone, may also be converted to DHT by some hair follicles, and steroid sulfatase found in the dermal papilla may be the responsible enzyme (231). This may explain why males affected by X-linked recessive ichthyosis resulting from a defect in steroid sulfatase do not develop AGA or do so only mildly (232).

Whiting (145) postulated that the process of miniaturization cannot be explained simply by shortening of the anagen phase with repeated hair cycles. He suggested that miniaturization of some follicles occurred rapidly, over the course of a single hair cycle, possibly mediated by a change in the size of the dermal papilla, because vellus follicles have a smaller papilla than terminal follicles (221). In cell cultures of dermal papillae derived from balding scalp follicles, the cells were smaller and did not grow as well as those derived from nonbalding scalp follicles (233).

There is evidence that fibroplasia of the adventitial sheath surrounding the hair follicle is important to the pathogenesis of AGA (234). As previously noted, fibrous streamers in AGA may be more fibrotic than those of normal follicles (140). One study found *Demodex* to be present more frequently in patients with AGA and postulated that *Demodex*-induced inflammation could contribute to the process and possibly play a role in permanence (scarring) (235).

There exists a physiologic rest period during which the posttelogen follicle remains empty. This phase of the hair cycle is termed *kenogen* (136). It may last longer and occur with greater frequency in AGA.

Differential Diagnosis. AA, primarily the diffuse type, is the only alopecia that may clinically be confused with AGA and also demonstrate miniaturization on biopsy. In AA, peribulbar inflammation and nanogen hairs are helpful in securing the diagnosis, but in their absence a greatly elevated telogen count (especially >30%) favors AA. Owing to its prevalence, AGA may frequently coincide with other types of alopecia.

Principles of Management: Topical and oral minoxidil may be used to treat men and women with AGA. Men and postmenopausal women may respond to oral finasteride. Platelet-rich plasma (PRP) and red light laser therapy are relatively recent treatments. Hair transplantation may be an option for AGA that does not respond to medical therapies.

Scarring Alopecias

Various definitions exist for scarring (cicatricial) alopecia. A clinically relevant definition is the permanent loss of hair follicles, usually manifested on physical examination by the absence of follicular ostia, sometimes with a porcelain-white appearance (236). Histology may or may not reveal true scar formation or inflammation, although most processes resulting in permanent hair loss are inflammatory, at least initially. With this definition, we can include disorders typically classified as "nonscarring" that in late stages lead to irreversible loss of hair follicles; this biphasic pattern can be seen in AGA, long-standing AA, and traction alopecia.

Processes that specifically target the hair follicle early in the course of the disease are *primary* scarring alopecias (237,238). *Secondary* scarring alopecias result from inflammatory or neoplastic processes that secondarily involve hair follicles. Secondary scarring alopecias are not discussed here, nor is the primary scarring alopecia caused by chronic cutaneous lupus erythematosus (discussed in Chapter 10). The discussion of scarring alopecias that follows refers to *primary scarring alopecias*. Features of some common scarring alopecias are summarized in Table 18-2.

Various classification schemes have been proposed for primary scarring alopecias, including inflammatory versus noninflammatory, and neutrophil mediated versus lymphocyte mediated (239). The usefulness of these schemes is hampered by clinical and histologic overlap between the various types of scarring alopecia, as well as a lack of uniformity in the terminology used by clinicians and dermatopathologists (240). This is why clinical–pathologic correlation is so important in the interpretation of scarring alopecias. Future proposals for the definitive classification of scarring alopecias will require insight into pathogenic mechanisms or biologic markers of disease, possibly provided by molecular research (126,241). A unifying concept of *central centrifugal scarring alopecia*, discussed later, and other scarring alopecias was proposed in 2000 (242). In addition, on the basis of a workshop on cicatricial alopecia, sponsored by the North American Hair Research Society, a working classification of scarring alopecia based on clinical and pathologic features was published with hopes for an improved classification scheme pending additional, collaborative investigation (130). More importantly, however, this workshop

laid the groundwork for meaningful clinical–pathologic correlation by setting guidelines for the study of scarring alopecias to uncover etiologic factors, ultimately aiding in treatment, and facilitated collaboration between investigators. In this chapter, my goal is to present "classic" features of the more commonly encountered disorders as well as some rarer conditions.

In one published algorithm for classifying alopecia, emphasis was placed on the pattern of fibrosis (scarring), with a branch point separating follicular fibrosis from diffuse dermal fibrosis (243). The *pattern* of scarring is important in the permanent alopecias. For example, when a condition produces enough damage to completely destroy the follicle, there is replacement of the pilosebaceous structure by scar tissue (Fig. 18-44) (244). These "follicular scars" may occur without interfollicular fibrosis. Histologically, the follicular epithelium is replaced by a column of thickened collagen, sometimes surrounded by a rim of connective tissue that stains faintly blue on hematoxylin and eosin–stained sections (Fig. 18-44). Elastic tissue staining can help differentiate follicular scars from follicular streamers (245).

Clues to the histologic diagnosis of cicatricial alopecia include dilation of multiple eccrine ducts (246) and presence of naked hair shafts (247). The end stage of many forms of scarring alopecia may look similar, with the "final common pathway" characterized by decreased follicular density, absence of sebaceous glands, replacement of follicles by follicular scars that may extend into the subcutis, stranded arrector pili muscle bundles, and sometimes tufting (see later discussion of *tufted folliculitis*). Studies of elastic tissue in various forms of permanent alopecia showed distinctive staining patterns using Verhoeff-van Gieson stain (248,249). Fibrous tracts of normal follicles show an elastic tissue sheath, which may be destroyed or altered by scarring and inflammation (Fig. 18-45). Cases of end-stage LPP showed a wedge-shaped scar involving the upper one-third of the follicle where the elastic sheath was destroyed (Fig. 18-46). In addition, in well-developed lesions of lupus erythematosus, a broad pattern of scarring throughout the dermis was characteristic, with destruction of perifollicular elastic sheaths. In cases of "central progressive alopecia in black females" (*follicular degeneration syndrome*), the fibrous tracts were broad ("tree trunk") and outlined by an intact elastic sheath. Thickened elastic fibers were also found throughout the dermis, interpreted to be the result of "recoil" as the dermis became shrunken and hyalinized. "Idiopathic 'ivory white' pseudopelade" showed findings that were identical to this. In morphea, dermal elastic fibers were normal, and the fibrous tracts (with an intact elastic sheath) were narrow. Fluorescent and polarized microscopy of hematoxylin–eosin sections highlight birefringent scar tissue, and the pattern of birefringence is a clue to the type of alopecia, as with elastic tissue staining (250).

The value of transverse sections in the interpretation of nonscarring alopecias is well documented, but their value in scarring alopecias is less clear. This may be a matter of personal preference for the dermatopathologist, but one study found that when only one biopsy was available, the diagnosis made with vertical sections alone had a higher concordance rate with the original diagnosis than did transverse sections alone, although biopsies studied using vertical and transverse sections together had the highest concordance (251). A blinded, prospective study of primary cicatricial alopecia could only discriminate

Table 18-2

Scarring Alopecia (Decreased Follicular Density)

	Clinical Pattern	Inflammation Type	Site of Follicular Inflammation	Other Histologic Features	Elastic Stain (VVG)
Lichen planopilaris (LPP) (and variants)	Irregularly shaped patches of hair loss scattered over the scalp. Perifollicular scale and erythema	Lymphocytic	Isthmus and lower infundibulum; lichenoid interface with occasional colloid bodies. Sometimes interfollicular epidermis involved	Hypergranulosis of infundibula. Cleft between follicular epithelium and dermis is often found. Perivascular and perieccrine inflammation absent	Wedge-shaped scar involving upper one-third of the follicle
Discoid lupus erythematosus (DLE)*	Classic lesions show alopecic areas with erythema, atrophy, dilated and plugged infundibula. May show central hypopigmentation	Lymphoplasmacytic	Typically infundibulum but may involve entire follicle; interface—vacuolar or lichenoid; colloid bodies less common than LPP. Epidermal involvement more common than LPP	Superficial and deep perivascular and perieccrine inflammation. Dermal mucin is often increased. Epidermis may show thickened basement membrane zone.	Broad scar throughout the dermis with destruction of perifollicular elastic sheath
Central centrifugal cicatricial alopecia (CCCA)	Area of alopecia centered on the crown or vertex; progresses centrifugally	Lymphocytic	Lower infundibulum and isthmus, without interface alteration	Early finding is premature desquamation of the inner root sheath. Eccentric thinning of the outer root sheath and concentric lamellar fibrosis ensues.	Broad fibrous tracts outlined by an intact elastic sheath. Also, thickened elastic fibers throughout, due to "recoil" of the dermis
Folliculitis decalvans	Multifocal pustules, or larger alopecic patch on the crown with erythema, pustules, and crusting at the periphery	Neutrophilic and lymphocytic	Intrafollicular and perifollicular involving the infundibulum and isthmus	Resembles a bacterial folliculitis (may represent inflammatory stage of CCCA)	NA
Acne keloidalis*	Papules, pustules, and small areas of alopecia involving the posterior neck and occiput. In advanced cases, keloidal plaques form	Lymphoplasmacytic (neutrophils if a pustule is biopsied)	Lower infundibulum and isthmus	As follicles are destroyed, hair shaft fragments may serve as a stimulus for fibrosis.	NA
Dissecting scalp cellulitis*	Firm and fluctuant nodules, with areas of purulent drainage, primarily over the crown and vertex	Lymphocytic, neutrophilic, and plasmacytic	Initially, perifollicular inflammation in the lower dermis and subcutaneous fat. Later, superficial parts of follicle are affected.	Early on, alopecia is due to conversion to catagen/telogen hairs. Later, follicles are destroyed; granulation tissue, sinus tracts, and fibrosis develop. Sebaceous glands are destroyed later.	NA

*Denotes entities discussed in other chapters.

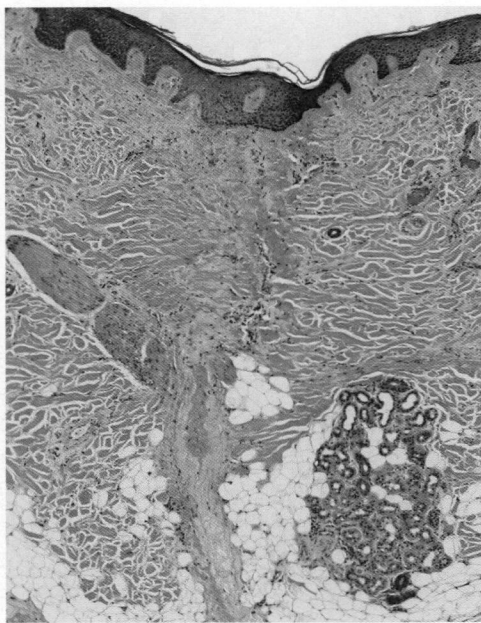

Figure 18-44 Follicular scar (vertical). A column of fibrosis replaces the hair follicle and extends into the subcutaneous fat. Note the stranded arrector pili muscle.

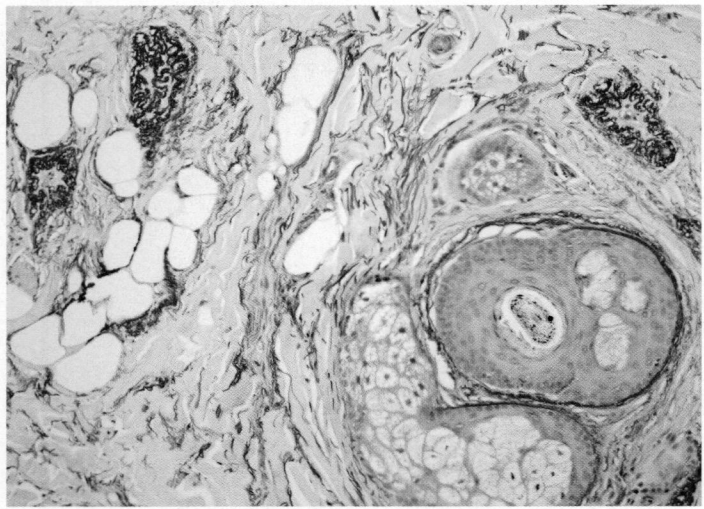

Figure 18-45 Late-stage scarring alopecia, elastic stain (horizontal). Elastic fibers that encircle normal follicles stain purple with the Luna stain. Three destroyed follicles have left behind their elastic sheath, identifiable as purple rings with a corrugated appearance.

neutrophilic types from lymphocytic types on histology but could not further differentiate clinically distinct forms of primary cicatricial alopecia (252).

Although the exact pathogenesis of each type of permanent alopecia may be different, some general pathogenic mechanisms have been proposed. For instance, Headington (253) believed that the basic pathogenesis common to cicatricial alopecias was hair follicle stem cell failure. Loss of the stem cell niche has been proposed by others, with some follicular stem cells undergoing epigenetic reprogramming to become fibroblast-like cells that may contribute to follicular fibrosis (254). In a commentary on scarring alopecias, the role of the sebaceous gland was emphasized, particularly its importance in the dissociation of the hair shaft from the inner root sheath (255); the asebia

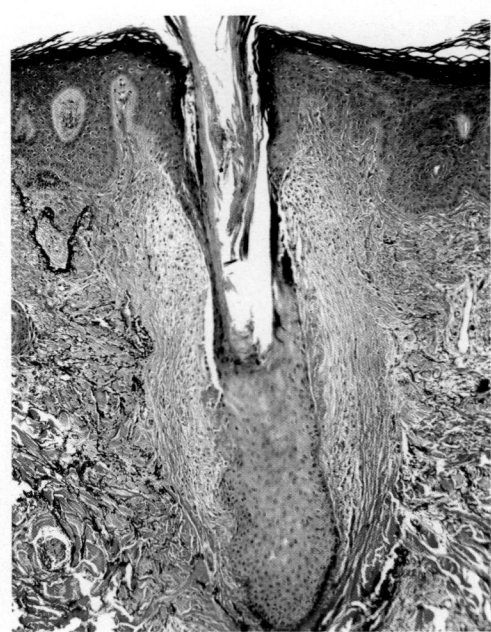

Figure 18-46 Scar in lichen planopilaris (vertical). Verhoeff-van Gieson elastic tissue stain shows a wedge-shaped perifollicular scar devoid of elastic fibers.

mouse is an animal model for scarring alopecia that is based on a sebaceous gland defect (256).

Pseudopelade of Brocq

Clinical Summary. This uncommon condition has arguably generated more controversy and confusion than any other type of alopecia (257). Many articles have been written about pseudopelade of Brocq (PPB), some classifying it as a distinct clinical–pathologic entity ("classic" or "idiopathic" PPB) (258) and others defining it as an end stage of scarring alopecia resulting from disorders such as LPP, discoid lupus erythematosus, scleroderma, folliculitis decalvans (FD), or chronic traction (259,260). Therefore, the term must be defined each time it is used anew. The salient clinical features that follow are similarly reported by both sides of the debate.

PPB in the classic definition is characterized by asymptomatic, discrete, scattered or clustered, irregularly shaped, ivory- or porcelain-white patches of alopecia predominantly over the parietal scalp and vertex (261) (Fig. 18-47) and rarely on nonscalp sites such as the beard. The patches are sometimes atrophic, producing an appearance often likened to "footprints in the snow" (253). Late-stage lesions of LPP, lupus erythematosus, or scleroderma can produce this same clinical picture. Idiopathic PPB is found mostly in whites, in women more than men, and occasionally in children. Disease progression occurs in "spurts," ultimately running its course and leaving areas of permanent alopecia. The key feature that supposedly makes idiopathic PPB distinctive is the lack of clinical inflammation throughout its course, although some theorize that an inflammatory phase exists but is fleeting (262).

In 1885, Brocq (263) first used the term *pseudopelade*, which literally means "pseudo alopecia areata" in French. Later, in 1905, Brocq et al. (264) characterized pseudopelade as a distinct entity. How the concept of PPB changed over the 20th century was chronicled in an article by Dawber (265), entitled "What is pseudopelade?".

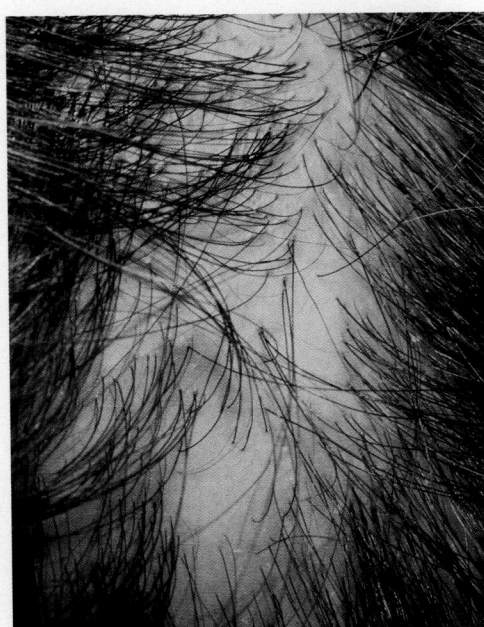

Figure 18-47 Pseudopelade of Brocq. "Ivory white," macular areas of hair loss without evidence of inflammation (erythema), likened to "footprints in the snow." This is distinguished from alopecia areata by the lack of follicular ostia.

A major publication often cited in support of PPB as a separate disorder came from Pinkus (266) in 1978, in which he noted a distinctive pattern of perifollicular and interfollicular elastic tissue in PPB and other forms of scarring alopecia, using acid orcein stain. In 180 cases that satisfied the histologic criteria for idiopathic PPB established by Brocq and others, Pinkus found that the site of destroyed hair follicles (above the level of the bulge) was marked by broad cords of collagenous and elastic fibers. He subdivided these 180 cases into classic PPB and fibrosing alopecia, the latter characterized by less perifollicular inflammation and, more importantly, the presence of prominent elastic fibers around the lower, cycling portion of the preexistent hair follicle. The major criticism of Pinkus' work is that his histologic criteria for PPB were not correlated with clinical findings (126).

Subsequently, elastic tissue staining patterns in various forms of permanent alopecia were examined using Verhoeff-van Gieson stain (248). Two cases of "idiopathic 'ivory white' pseudopelade" showed a hyalinized dermis with thickened elastic fibers and broad fibrous tracts with an intact elastic sheath, findings indistinguishable from "central progressive alopecia in black females" (*central centrifugal cicatricial alopecia* [CCCA]), and similar to the findings of Pinkus.

Braun-Falco et al. subsequently studied 26 cases believed to represent PPB (cases of scarring alopecia attributable known, identifiable causes were excluded) (259) and concluded that the clinical and histologic criteria they proposed were distinctive enough to warrant designation as a separate disease (267).

In contrast, many reports support idiopathic PPB as an end-stage scarring alopecia. In the 1950s, Degos et al. (268) noted that 70% of the time a preceding or underlying disease could be found; so he called the typically described findings a "pseudopeladic" state. One study used criteria established by Braun-Falco to diagnose PPB in 33 patients. Because two-thirds of these patients showed features of discoid lupus or LPP, the authors concluded that PPB could not be considered a distinct

entity (269). Some groups have published evidence that LPP and PPB may be variants of the same disease. One of these groups presented four alopecic patients with clinical and histologic features of PPB who also had cutaneous and mucosal findings of lichen planus (270). The authors believed that PPB represented a less inflammatory stage in the disease spectrum of LPP.

In summary, the diagnosis of idiopathic PPB is one of exclusion. The terminology has become so confusing that for cases in which an underlying disorder is not identifiable, Sperling et al. (242) proposed an alternate, more descriptive term, "patchy, scarring alopecia of unknown etiology."

Histopathology. Because the histologic findings of a typical lesion of PPB are identical to those of a burnt-out scarring alopecia (126), clinical correlation is always necessary for accurate interpretation. Classic PPB is characterized by predominantly follicular scarring, with columns of fibrosis replacing hair follicles (Figs. 18-44 and 18-48). The fibrotic columns sometimes extend into the subcutaneous fat. This is accompanied by a loss or decrease of sebaceous glands and absence of widespread (interfollicular) scarring (138,259). Normal arrector pili muscles remain, isolated in the mid-dermis or inserting on the vertically oriented fibrotic streams (Figs. 18-44 and 18-48). The epidermis may be normal or, rarely, atrophic, and sweat glands are normal. Marked inflammation is absent.

The apparent lack of inflammation in this disorder may be the result of a short, often-missed, inflammatory phase. One study targeting lesions in this short inflammatory phase found massive folliculocentric lymphocytic infiltration associated with pronounced apoptosis (271). The fact that histologic inflammation exists in some cases has led some authors to subdivide PPB into inflammatory and noninflammatory subtypes on the basis of histology (262).

In two sources, the findings of early inflammatory and more developed lesions of PPB are well described as follows (121,253). Early lesions of PPB show variable lymphocytic inflammation in the superficial dermis that is perivascular or perifollicular, centered about the infundibulum or midpoint of the follicle. The infiltrates may extend into the follicular epithelium

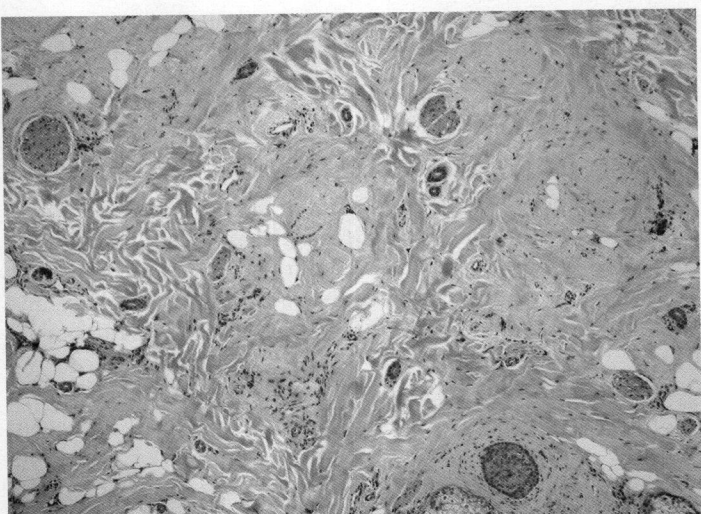

Figure 18-48 Pseudopelade of Brocq (horizontal). Viable pilosebaceous follicles are notably absent, replaced by follicular scars. Several unaffected arrector pili muscles remain.

and occasionally into sebaceous glands, but deep perifollicular inflammation or interface alteration is not detected. With disease progression there is early loss of sebaceous glands. In later, well-developed lesions, inflammation becomes patchy, mild, and perivascular and eventually disappears. There may be premature disintegration of the inner root sheath, and the infundibular epithelium may become eccentrically thinned. Concentric lamellar fibrosis may be present. Fusion of infundibular outer root sheaths ("tufting") may be seen (see *Tufted Folliculitis*). In time, follicles are destroyed, with naked hair shafts remaining and inciting a granulomatous response. Fibrous tracts mark the site of obliterated follicles. Features of this often-missed inflammatory phase of PPB are also shared by other forms of scarring alopecia (242).

Pathogenesis. As a theoretical basis for PPB, Sullivan and Kossard (260) speculated that there could occur a noninflammatory focal loss of follicles, possibly resulting from premature exhaustion or inhibition of the stem cell compartment to recycle. Headington (253) postulated that the pathogenesis of PPB is probably related to a T-cell–mediated inflammatory process involving the bulge region.

Differential Diagnosis. The histology of PPB is that of a burnt-out scarring alopecia, so the differential would include a late stage of other types of scarring alopecia.

Principles of Management: The management of all the lymphocyte-mediated scarring alopecias is similar (272). The primary objective of any treatment is to halt further loss of hair, and, second, to regrow hair if possible. Inflamed hair follicles, manifested by clinical erythema, are targeted in order to prevent their permanent destruction. Intralesional and high-potency topical corticosteroids are a first-line treatment. Reports of oral medications with anti-inflammatory properties are mostly anecdotal and include antibiotics in the tetracycline class, cyclosporine, retinoids, antimalarials, and oral steroids (short-term). A hair transplant may be considered if there are suitable donor hairs, and the hair loss is "burnt out," defined as showing no inflammation or disease progression for at least 2 years without treatment (272).

Central Centrifugal Cicatricial Alopecia

Clinical Summary. Because many forms of scarring alopecia share clinical and histologic features that make them difficult to distinguish with certainty, a unifying concept of CCCA was proposed to reflect the overlap (242); CCCA is a category that includes several types of cicatricial hair loss that have in common the following features (Fig. 18-49): (a) alopecia centered on the crown or vertex of the scalp, (b) progressive, chronic disease with eventual "burnout," the affected scalp becoming shiny and smooth, without follicular ostia, (c) fairly symmetric expansion, with the most active areas at the periphery, and (d) clinical evidence of inflammation (i.e., erythematous papules or pustules) in these active sites, corresponding to microscopic inflammation (126,242). CCCA encompasses three patterns of disease: follicular degeneration syndrome, pseudopelade pattern (a "modern" use of the term, *not* pseudopelade of Brocq), and FD. It occurs almost exclusively in females of African descent, with a reported mean age of onset of 38.2 years (273). A photographic scale was devised to assess the severity of CCCA and allow standardized assessment by investigators (274).

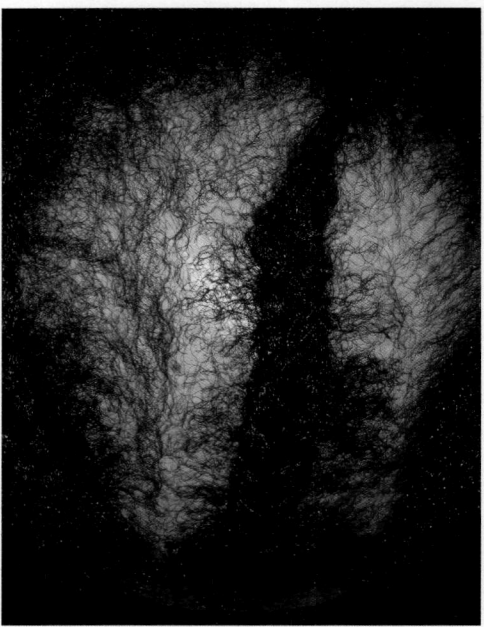

Figure 18-49 Central centrifugal cicatricial alopecia. An area of permanent alopecia on the crown of the scalp characterized by absent follicular ostia.

Histopathology. The earliest and most characteristic histologic finding of CCCA is premature desquamation of the inner root sheath (Fig. 18-50) (143), typically seen in only a few follicles. The inner root sheath normally degenerates at the isthmus, which is delimited below by the attachment point of the arrector pili muscle and above by the insertion of the sebaceous duct. "Crumbling" or absence of the inner root sheath below the isthmus, at a level through the deep dermis near the eccrine coils or in the subcutis, characterizes this finding. Some authors consider it to be a secondary phenomenon, rather than a primary event in the pathophysiology of this condition, and it has been observed in other forms of scarring alopecia (253,275). What is unique to CCCA, however, is its occurrence *early* in the disease process, particularly in noninflamed hair follicles (276,277). The inner

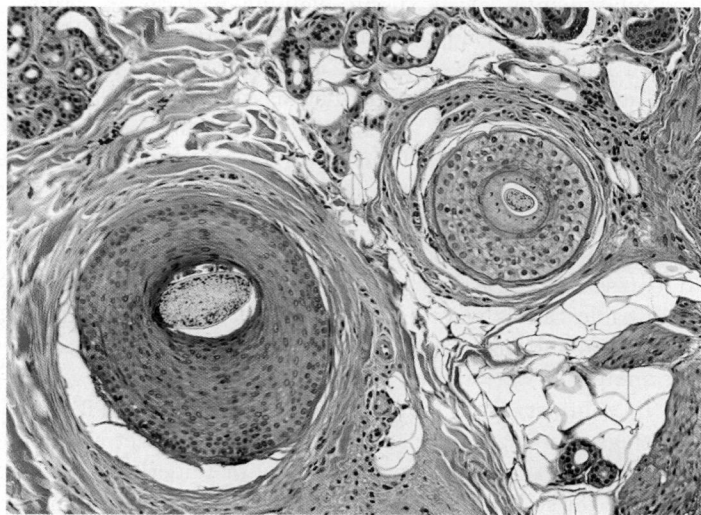

Figure 18-50 Central centrifugal cicatricial alopecia (horizontal). At a level through the superficial subcutis, the terminal follicle is missing its inner root sheath. There is mild eccentric thinning of the outer root sheath.

root sheath stains an intense blue color with Giemsa, which may be useful in assessing early desquamation (278).

Most likely as a consequence of premature loss of the inner root sheath, CCCA exhibits some or all of the following histologic features in clinically involved scalp (Fig. 18-51) (126,242): (a) eccentric thinning of the outer root sheath follicular epithelium, most prominent at the level of the isthmus and lower infundibulum, associated with (b) close apposition of the hair shaft and follicular contents to the dermis, (c) concentric lamellar fibroplasia (resembling "onion skin"), and (d) chronic inflammation composed of lymphocytes and plasma cells surrounding the zone of fibroplasia. There is (e) eventual migration of the hair shaft into the dermis, inciting granulomatous inflammation and additional epithelial damage (Fig. 18-52), and (f) replacement of the destroyed follicle by a vertical band of connective tissue, resulting in a "follicular scar." The inflammation is usually concentrated on the side opposite penetration of the shaft through the follicular epithelium. There may also be polytrichia,

whereby damaged follicles fuse their outer root sheaths at the infundibular level. Singly, these six histologic features may be found in other types of scarring alopecia. As with all scarring alopecias, sebaceous glands are eventually lost, although later in the disease course as compared with other scarring alopecias (279).

With advanced age (58–78), biopsies typically show a lower follicular density and less lymphocytic inflammation (280). It has been shown that the lymphocytic infiltrate in CCCA is primarily CD4+ and that Langerhans cells are increased in affected follicles (281). These authors also demonstrated the displacement of blood vessels away from the follicle by the lamellar fibrosis. Diseased follicles were shown to lose CK15 expression, a marker of the bulge area where stem cells reside (282).

If a clinical pustule from the expanding margin is biopsied (Fig. 18-53), there may be folliculocentric neutrophilic inflammation (Fig. 18-54), allowing for subclassification as the FD

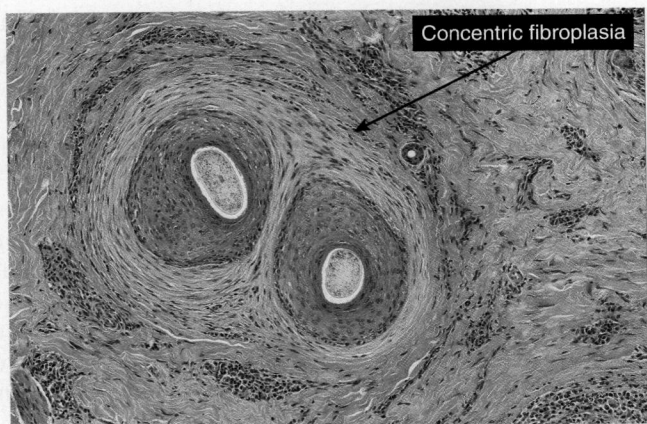

Figure 18-51 Central centrifugal cicatricial alopecia (horizontal). The affected follicles show eccentric thinning of the follicular epithelium, concentric lamellar fibroplasia, lymphoplasmacytic inflammation peripheral to the fibroplasia and perivascularly, and loss of sebaceous glands. (Reprinted with permission from Elder DE, Elenitsas R, Rubin AI, et al. *Atlas and Synopsis of Lever's Histopathology of the Skin*. 3rd ed. Wolters Kluwer Health/Lippincott Williams & Wilkins; 2013.)

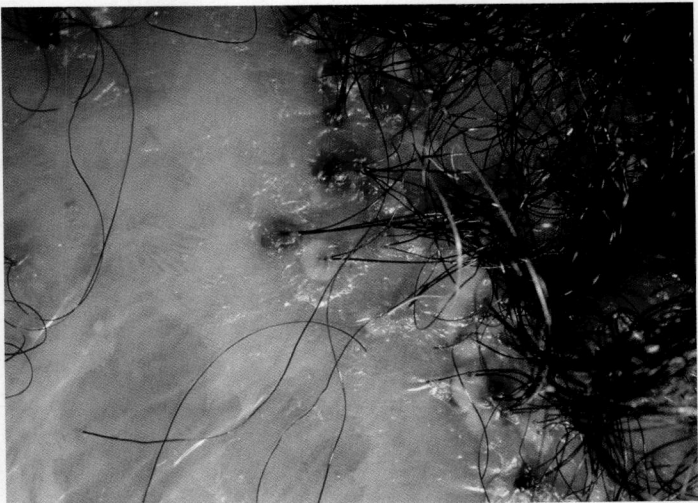

Figure 18-53 Folliculitis decalvans. The advancing edge of a scarred alopecic plaque shows the characteristic lesions of folliculitis decalvans, follicular-based pustules with crusting. (Reprinted with permission from Elder DE, Elenitsas R, Rubin AI, et al. *Atlas and Synopsis of Lever's Histopathology of the Skin*. 3rd ed. Wolters Kluwer Health/Lippincott Williams & Wilkins; 2013.)

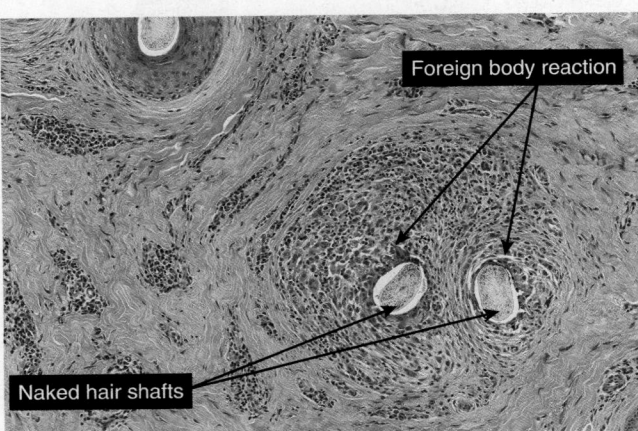

Figure 18-52 Central centrifugal cicatricial alopecia (horizontal). The follicular epithelium may be completely destroyed, resulting in dermal fibrosis and naked hair shafts that incite a granulomatous response. (Reprinted with permission from Elder DE, Elenitsas R, Rubin AI, et al. *Atlas and Synopsis of Lever's Histopathology of the Skin*. 3rd ed. Wolters Kluwer Health/Lippincott Williams & Wilkins; 2013.)

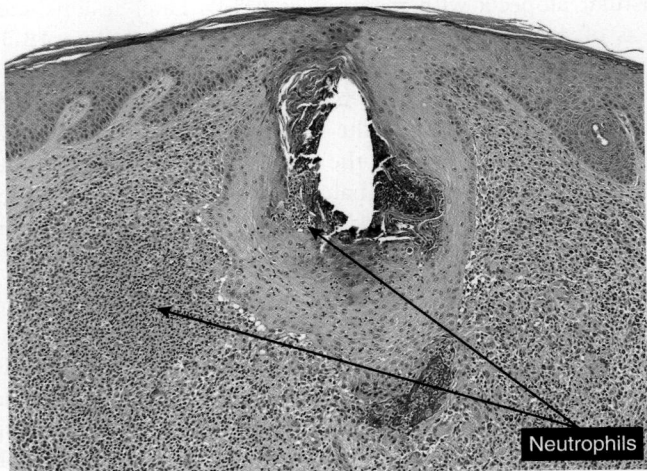

Figure 18-54 Folliculitis decalvans (vertical). Lesions start as a follicular-based pustule with perifollicular inflammation composed predominantly of neutrophils, with chronic inflammatory cells as well. (Reprinted with permission from Elder DE, Elenitsas R, Rubin AI, et al. *Atlas and Synopsis of Lever's Histopathology of the Skin*. 3rd ed. Wolters Kluwer Health/Lippincott Williams & Wilkins; 2013.)

pattern. Those cases classified as the pseudopelade pattern showed the histologic features described but were typically white patients with a clinical picture of indolent disease characterized by perifollicular scale and some papules (143).

Pathogenesis. Although the etiology is unknown, hair-care practices that include heat, bleaching, pomades, hot combs, use of relaxers, and traction (e.g., braids and weaves) have been postulated. In addition, the predominance in African Americans suggests that environmental, cultural, and genetic factors, as well as possible structural factors unique to their hair follicles, may play a role (283–286). Mutations in *PADI3*, a gene that encodes a protein involved in hair shaft formation, were shown to be associated with CCCA (287). Genes implicated in fibroproliferative disorders have been shown to be upregulated in CCCA (288), and a proposed mechanism for CCCA was influenced by studying other scarring diseases such as fibrotic kidney disease and scleroderma (289).

Special mention should be made of the follicular degeneration syndrome subtype of CCCA from a historical perspective, when it was considered a distinct clinicopathologic entity. This subtype of CCCA occurs almost exclusively in African American patients, usually women, between the second and fourth decades (283). It was originally described as "hot comb" alopecia (290), but it was subsequently shown that use of a hot comb to straighten the hair was not requisite (283).

Differential Diagnosis. CCCA shows varying degrees of histologic overlap with other forms of cicatricial alopecia, and a combination of clinical and histologic features is required to make this diagnosis (242).

Principles of Management: The treatment approach is similar to other lymphocyte-mediated scarring alopecias (291,292) and is discussed under PPB. Topical minoxidil may foster regrowth of recovering follicles (293).

Folliculitis Decalvans

Clinical Summary. FD is considered by some to represent a highly inflammatory subtype of CCCA (242). From a historical perspective, FD as a distinct entity has been described as a patchy pustular alopecia with recurrences (253). Later lesions show areas of scarring with pustules at the periphery (Fig. 18-53) (253). Cultures from the pustules usually reveal *Staphylococcus aureus*. Although some believe that the bacteria are pathogenic, others hold that they are the result of superinfection (242). When pustules are absent, the clinical picture resembles PPB (294). The finding of tufted hairs is common (295). FD has also been reported in other areas besides the scalp, including the beard, face, and nape (296).

Histopathology. Early, pustular lesions show an abscess centered about the affected follicle at the level of the lower to the upper infundibulum (Fig. 18-54) (253), which may show comedonal dilation (294). Later lesions typically show perifollicular inflammation composed predominantly of lymphocytes, with fewer plasma cells, neutrophils, eosinophils, and giant cells (297,298). There may be hyperkeratosis, follicular plugging, and evidence of tufting. Late-stage lesions show follicular destruction secondary to diffuse dermal scarring (253). In such lesions, the inflammation is less pronounced and is composed of lymphocytes, macrophages, and some giant cells in response to follicular remnants (298). Epidermal hyperplasia, which is

sometimes psoriasiform, can be a distinguishing feature of FD (299,300).

Pathogenesis. A number of authors believe that *S. aureus* is involved in the pathogenesis of FD (Fig. 18-55) (298), perhaps via bacterial superantigens that stimulate the immune system without intracellular processing (301) or an abnormal host response to *S. aureus* toxins in an otherwise straightforward infection (298). Other investigators believe the presence of pustules is attributable to secondary infection with *S. aureus* or an immune response to disrupted follicles and their contents (242). In one study, however, approximately one-third of infections were caused by gram-negative organisms (302).

Differential Diagnosis. Pustular lesions may resemble bacterial folliculitis or early lesions of dissecting cellulitis. Nonpustular lesions show histologic overlap with CCCA.

Principles of Management: Bacterial cultures with antibiotic sensitivities should be obtained from pustules, and initial treatment is aimed at eliminating bacterial infection, usually attributable to *S. aureus* (303–305). A combination of oral and topical antibiotics, along with topical treatment of colonization sites, namely the nares, is the first approach, although relapses may occur after antibiotics are stopped. Subsequent therapy is similar to other scarring alopecias and is discussed under PPB.

Tufted Hair Folliculitis

Clinical Summary. "Tufted folliculitis" refers to the clinical finding of "doll's hair deformity," resembling the clustered hairs that are characteristic of a child's doll (Fig. 18-56). Another name for this finding is "polytrichia" (290). It should be distinguished from physiologic compound hairs, where two or three hairs exit from a single infundibulum, more commonly found on the occipital scalp.

Tufted folliculitis is a finding that may be present in various forms of scarring alopecia and should not be considered a distinct entity, although some authors believe that it is, specifically characterizing it as a subset of FD (295,306). Asserting that it is a pattern that occurs in many forms of scarring alopecia

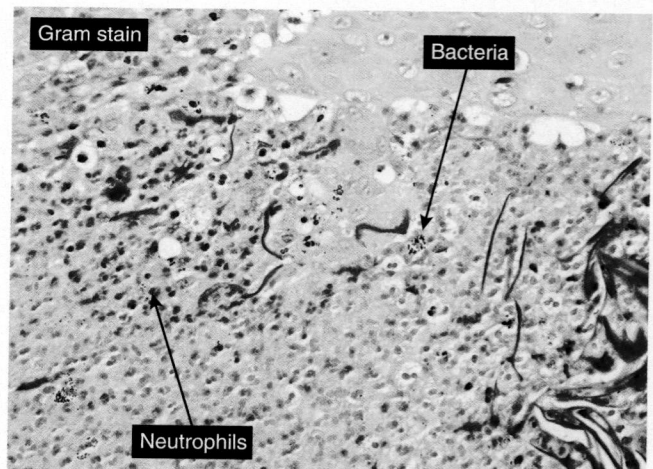

Figure 18-55 Folliculitis decalvans (Gram stain). Pustular lesions may develop as a consequence of bacterial superinfection. The Gram stain shows clusters of Gram-positive cocci amid the perifollicular neutrophils. (Reprinted with permission from Elder DE, Elenitsas R, Rubin AI, et al. *Atlas and Synopsis of Lever's Histopathology of the Skin.* 3rd ed. Wolters Kluwer Health/Lippincott Williams & Wilkins; 2013.)

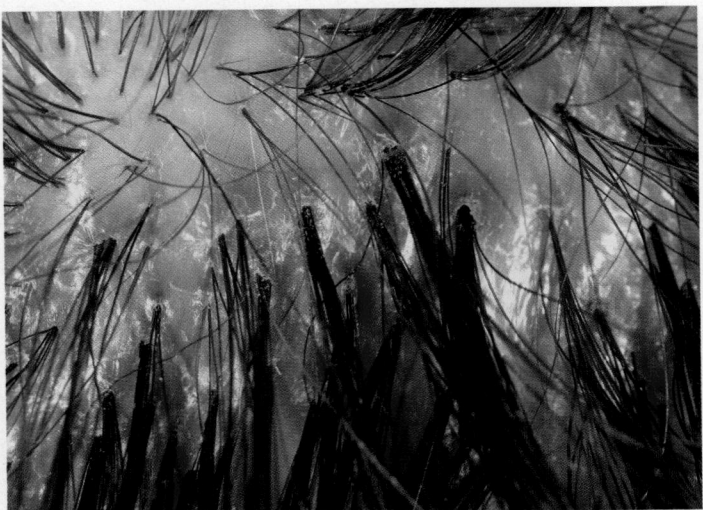

Figure 18-56 Tufted folliculitis. Groups of hairs exit the scalp through a single opening (polytrichia), producing a clinical appearance that has been likened to "doll's hair." There is interfollicular scarring and erythema.

and that it is therefore nonspecific, Sperling held that "the term tufted folliculitis should be purged from the lexicon of scarring alopecia" (126). It can be seen as a late process in several conditions, including central centrifugal scarring alopecia, FD, inflammatory tinea capitis, *S. aureus* folliculitis, LPP, dissecting cellulitis, follicular degeneration syndrome, acne keloidalis nuchae, and in lichen striatus of the scalp (307). It has also been reported after traumatic scalp laceration (308), following thermal burns (307), and after years of pemphigus vulgaris involvement of the scalp (309).

Histopathology. Histology shows a single group of three to five follicles, or several such groups of follicles, in which the infundibular epithelium of the affected hair follicles is fused together (Fig. 18-57) so that the multiple hair shafts are situated in the infundibular hair canal and exit the skin through a shared ostium, which may show hyperkeratosis and

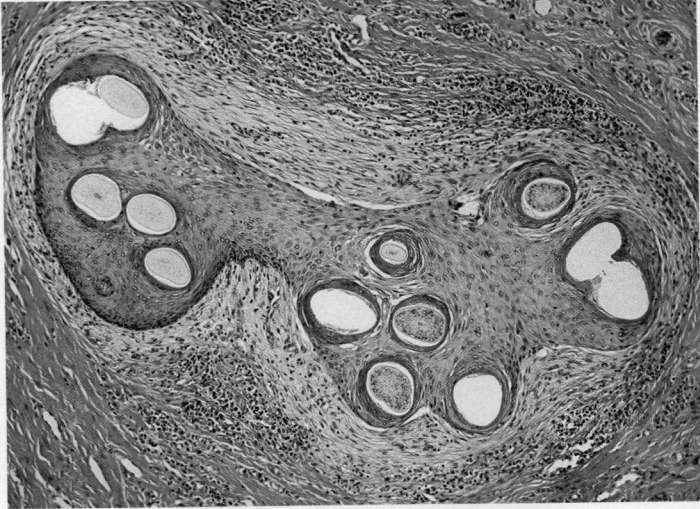

Figure 18-57 Tufted folliculitis (horizontal). In this extreme example, multiple hairs share a common outer root sheath and ultimately exit the scalp through a single opening. A "six-pack" (or more) is a clue to a later stage of a neutrophil-mediated primary scarring alopecia, according to some authors. Perifollicular fibrosis and mononuclear inflammation are present.

parakeratosis (295). A recent publication demonstrated these findings three-dimensionally (310). There is perifollicular fibroplasia superficially, as well as interfollicular fibrosis. The lower segments of the hairs are unaffected. The epidermis may be depressed from contraction of the fibrous tissue, forming a dell from which the hairs emerge. There may be variable infiltrates around the follicles and perivascularly that are composed of lymphocytes, histiocytes, and plasma cells, in addition to neutrophils when pustular lesions are biopsied. The hair tufts may eventually be destroyed by the process itself, and a foreign-body giant-cell reaction to free hair shafts may be seen. In one report, hairs were plucked from the tufts, revealing more than one-third of telogen hairs (295).

Pathogenesis. Tufting results from injury to the outer root sheath epithelium of hairs in a single follicular unit or in several adjacent follicular units, possibly from a superficial suppurative folliculitis (295). There is accompanying perifollicular and interfollicular fibroplasia, leading to contraction of the involved skin and clustering of the follicular units. In healing, the outer root sheaths of the follicles grow together at the infundibular level. Other mechanistic theories include retention of telogen hairs (311) and infection by *S. aureus* (306). Some authors suggested that when compound follicles are composed of four or more hairs melded together, it is a clue to quiescent neutrophil-mediated primary cicatricial alopecia, particularly when "six-packs" made up of at least six fused follicles are present (Fig. 18-57) (312). In contrast, tufted follicles composed of only two to three fused follicular infundibula ("two-packs" or "goggles") suggest a lymphocyte-mediated primary cicatricial alopecia.

Differential Diagnosis. Because tufting may be a secondary finding, clinical and histologic clues to an underlying condition should be sought (see discussion earlier).

Principles of Management: Treatment is geared toward the underlying condition.

Lichen Planopilaris

Clinical Summary. LPP is a primary scarring alopecia that occurs most commonly in middle-aged females, with a slight predominance in Caucasians. Several clinical subtypes exist, which are classified on the basis of the pattern of involvement on the scalp and other body sites. Common to all the subtypes is a histologic picture of lichenoid lymphocytic inflammation that targets the isthmus and infundibulum of the hair follicle (143,237,313,314). Characteristic lesions of lichen planus involve other body sites more than 50% of the time, although the alopecia usually presents first. The rare syndrome known as Graham-Little, or Graham-Little–Piccardi–Lassueur syndrome, consists of LPP that affects hair follicles on other areas of the body, particularly of the pubic area and axillae, in addition to the scalp. Lesions result in alopecia of these sites as well as keratotic follicular papules (predominantly on the trunk and extremities). Typical lichen planus of the skin or mucosa is sometimes present.

In the classic type, the vertex and parietal scalp are primarily involved, with multiple scattered alopecic patches that sometimes merge to involve the whole scalp. There may be erythematous macules and papules with accentuation around follicles, which demonstrate hyperkeratosis encircling the base of the hair (Fig. 18-58). As the affected hairs are destroyed, they leave behind irregularly shaped white patches of scarring in which follicular ostia are missing. The course of the disease

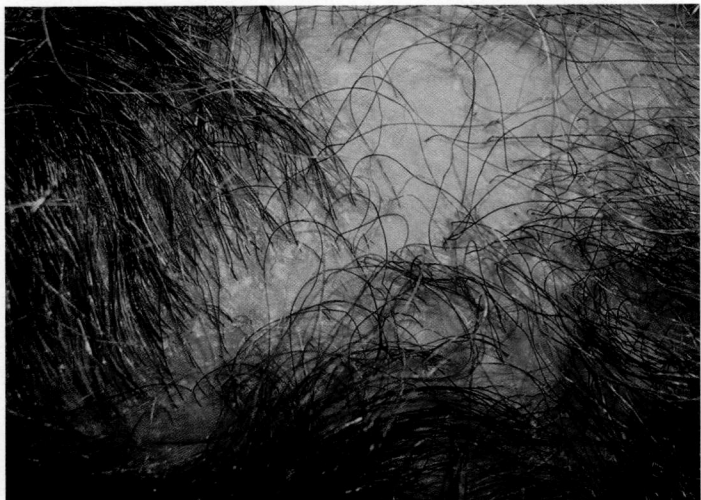

Figure 18-58 Lichen planopilaris. Areas of scarring alopecia devoid of follicular openings. At the periphery, the follicles show perifollicular erythema and scale situated at the base of the hairs.

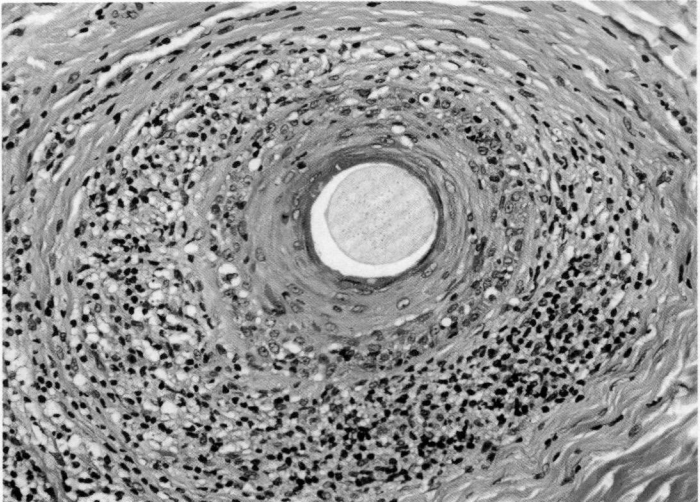

Figure 18-60 Lichen planopilaris (horizontal). At the level of the lower infundibulum, there is perifollicular lymphocytic inflammation, basal vacuolization, and eosinophilic dyskeratotic keratinocytes.

may be smoldering and slowly progressive, or fulminant. Associated symptoms may include pruritus and pain.

Histopathology. Biopsy of an inflammatory lesion of LPP shows perifollicular lymphocytic inflammation affecting the lower infundibulum and isthmus near the bulge, accompanied by hydropic degeneration of basal follicular keratinocytes and sometime necrotic keratinocytes (Civatte/colloid bodies), a key finding in making the diagnosis (Fig. 18-59) (315,316). Anti-keratin 903 antibodies have been shown to increase the sensitivity of identifying colloid bodies (317). Because only a few follicles may be involved in a single specimen, horizontal sections may demonstrate the diagnostic changes more frequently than vertical sections (Fig. 18-60). Concentric perifollicular fibrosis develops around the upper follicle, eventually creating a distance

between the infiltrate of lymphocytes and the follicular epithelium. A cleft may arise between the follicular epithelium and the surrounding dermis, the equivalent of a Max Joseph space. The infundibulum may develop hypergranulosis, and hyperkeratosis manifested by infundibular plugging by compact orthokeratin is seen. Interfollicular changes of lichen planus are seen infrequently. As lesions progress, naked hair shafts may be seen surrounded by foreign-body–type granulomatous inflammation, sebaceous glands are lost, and polytrichia can result. Late lesions resemble burnt-out scarring alopecia, with noninflammatory fibrotic tracts replacing follicles and extending into the subcutis.

Frontal fibrosing alopecia is a clinical variant of LPP that occurs predominantly in postmenopausal women (mean age, 66.8 years) and is characterized by progressive recession of the frontal hairline (Fig. 18-61) (318–320). The incidence has dramatically increased since its description in 1994 and is now the most common cause of cicatricial alopecia worldwide (321). Clinically, the involved areas are pale, without sclerosis or induration, and

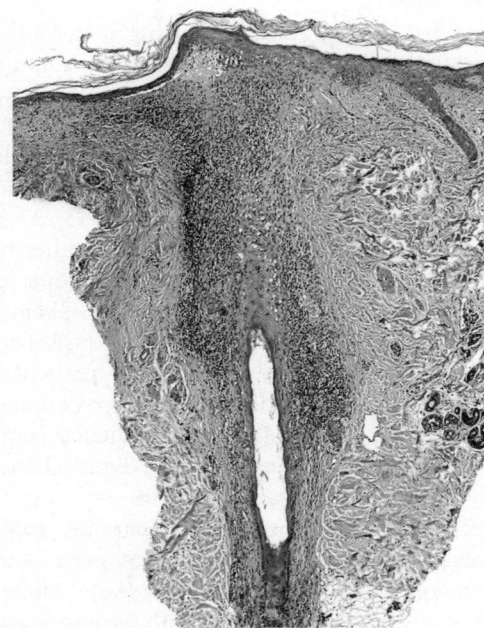

Figure 18-59 Lichen planopilaris (vertical). There is a dense perifollicular lymphocytic infiltrate that is concentrated about the lower infundibulum and isthmus and is associated with blurring of the junction between the follicular epithelium and the dermis.

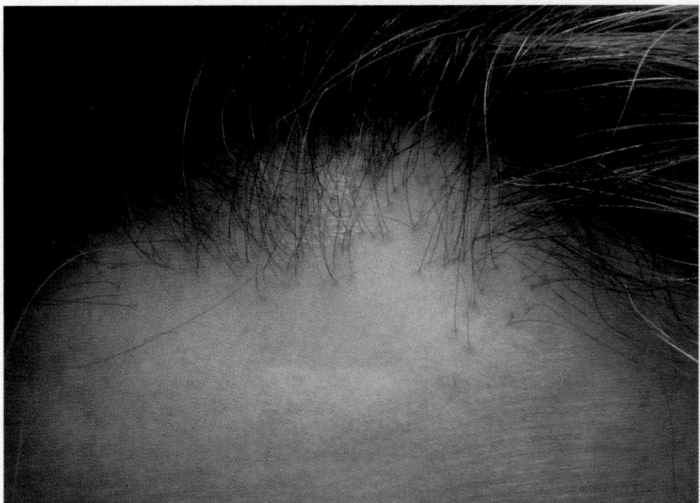

Figure 18-61 Frontal fibrosing alopecia. Hair follicles in a band along the frontal scalp are preferentially targeted, as evidenced by perifollicular erythema. The histologic changes are identical to those seen in lichen planopilaris.

show loss of follicular orifices, while follicles in the transition zone show perifollicular erythema and hyperkeratosis. A marked decrease or complete loss of the eyebrows is characteristic (322). Although signs of typical lichen planus at other body sites are lacking, there is frequent loss of body hair on the arms and facial papules on the face, representing involvement of vellus hair follicles (323,324). Biopsy of these other body sites reveals histopathologic findings of LPP (325). Frontal fibrosing alopecia is now considered a generalized variant of LPP that affects multiple body sites (322). A proposed histologic clue to the diagnosis of frontal fibrosing alopecia is the involvement of an anagen follicle, a telogen follicle, and a vellus-like follicle, the "follicular triad" (326). The greater depth of inflammation below the isthmus in frontal fibrosing alopecia (FFA) may help distinguish FFA from LPP (327), although others have argued that histologic differences between FFA and LPP are too subtle or nonspecific to reliably distinguish them (328).

Fibrosing alopecia in a pattern distribution is considered another LPP variant in which the clinically involved areas occur in androgen-dependent scalp in a pattern characteristic of AGA, and miniaturized follicles are also targeted (329,330). Patients showed progressive fibrosing alopecia of the central scalp with perifollicular erythema and follicular keratinization in the area of AGA. Multifocal lesions typical of LPP or other mucocutaneous signs of lichen planus were not seen. Women outnumbered men by roughly a 4:1 ratio, and the mean age of affected patients was 59 years. The histologic findings are identical to those of LPP in conjunction with follicular miniaturization (329). Although both terminal and vellus hairs are affected, the miniaturized follicles appear to be preferentially targeted by the inflammation.

Another variant has been described that also occurs in a female-pattern hair loss distribution and shows histologic features of LPP but *lacks* miniaturization. It has been termed *cicatricial-pattern hair loss* (CPHL) (331,332).

Pathogenesis. The inflammatory attack on the follicle in LPP targets the lower infundibulum and isthmus where follicular stem cells reside (333,334). Clues as to a potential etiology have been derived from a mouse model in which deletion of the peroxisome proliferator–activated receptor-γ in bulge stem cells causes alopecia resembling LPP in humans (326). Some cases of LPP induced by tumor necrosis factor-α inhibitors have been reported, suggesting other avenues of investigation (335), but the exact pathogenesis has yet to be elucidated.

Differential Diagnosis. In the histologic evaluation of alopecia, when a lichenoid infiltrate affecting the follicular epithelium is present, the differential diagnosis is primarily between LPP and lupus erythematosus. Max Joseph spaces and changes of lichen planus affecting the interfollicular epidermis favor LPP, while perivascular and perieccrine lymphocytic inflammation, increased reticular dermal mucin, and interfollicular changes that are more characteristic of lupus erythematosus, such as basement membrane zone thickening, favor chronic cutaneous lupus erythematosus (242). Immunohistochemistry may aid in distinguishing the two; CD123+ plasmacytoid dendritic cells are more clustered in chronic cutaneous lupus erythematosus (336), and there are differences in the number of epidermal and perifollicular CD1a+ cells (337).

Principles of Management: Therapy is similar to that for other lymphocyte-mediated scarring alopecias and is discussed under PPB (338).

Miscellaneous Alopecias

Psoriatic Alopecia

Clinical Summary. Psoriatic alopecia was first reported in 1972 (339). Three clinical patterns of scalp alopecia associated with psoriasis were described. Hair loss confined to the lesions, characterized by decreased hair density with finer hairs, is the most commonly seen pattern (Fig. 18-62). The second pattern is acute hair fallout in psoriatic plaques as well as unaffected areas, representing a telogen effluvium. The third and least common clinical presentation is a destructive alopecia. Nevertheless, that psoriasis could produce a permanent, scarring alopecia has been the subject of debate in the decades since. In a 1989 study, Headington et al. (340) found no histologic evidence to support a psoriatic cause for any form of alopecia. Nevertheless, it is now generally accepted that psoriasis on the scalp or involving other hair-bearing body sites can be associated with alopecia (341,342). Circumscribed areas of hair loss are seen 75% of the time, and 25% of cases will demonstrate diffuse hair loss (343). It can present as hair thinning or massive hair loss in tufts involving areas of psoriasis. In a study of 34 patients with psoriatic alopecia, the hair loss was considered nonscarring, defined as showing regrowth, in 70% of patients (344).

Psoriatic alopecia/AA-like reactions due to antitumor necrosis factor-α (TNF-α) therapy (345). Often used for the treatment of psoriasis, biologic therapy may paradoxically exacerbate psoriasis or cause psoriatic lesions in patients with no prior history of the condition. In the first study to report the histology of an associated alopecia, patients had no prior history of psoriasis and experienced a flare of psoriasis after newly starting TNF-α therapy (346). Some patients developed a nonscarring alopecia in which 100% of the hairs were in the resting stage (catagen/telogen), and were also miniaturized. These psoriatic alopecia/AA-like reactions secondary to TNF-α therapy demonstrated peribulbar lymphocytes around miniaturizing hairs, reminiscent of AA. The only difference from psoriatic alopecia was that this drug-induced psoriatic alopecia showed plasma cells and eosinophils (346).

Histopathology. Biopsies of psoriatic alopecia show typical psoriasiform epidermal hyperplasia (346,347). The telogen count

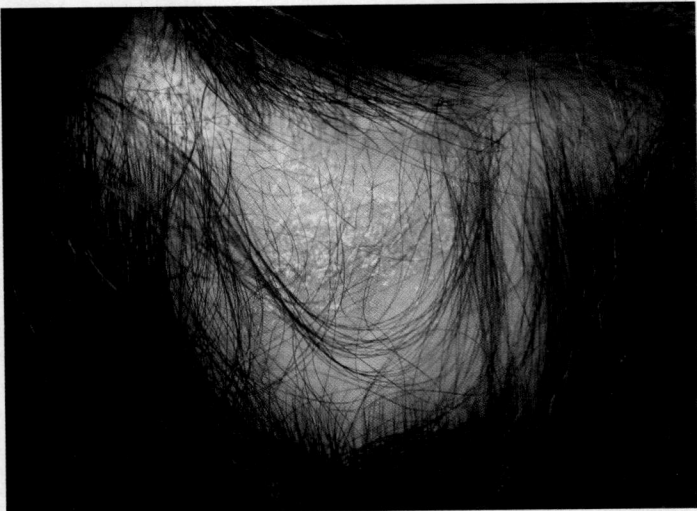

Figure 18-62 Psoriatic alopecia. An area of alopecia associated with a thin, erythematous, scaly plaque. Treatment of this area with intralesional corticosteroids resulted in regrowth.

is commonly elevated (Fig. 18-63), and an increased percentage of miniaturized follicles is seen. There is a perivascular and perifollicular lymphocytic infiltrate (Fig. 18-64), and lymphocytes may surround the bulbs of miniaturizing follicles, reminiscent of AA. Atrophic sebaceous glands are also characteristic (Fig. 18-64). Scarring psoriatic hair loss will show early signs of hair follicle damage manifested by perifollicular fibrosis and polytrichia, infundibular hyperkeratosis, and eventual follicular destruction with granuloma formation.

Pathogenesis. Although psoriasis is relatively common, associated alopecia is rare, raising the question as to whether pathogenic factors in psoriatic alopecia are the same as those for plaque-type psoriasis. One could speculate that the sebaceous gland atrophy seen histologically, unique to this form of alopecia and TNF-α inhibitor-induced variants (181), plays an important role since sebaceous gland pathology has been well documented in mouse models of alopecia (255,256).

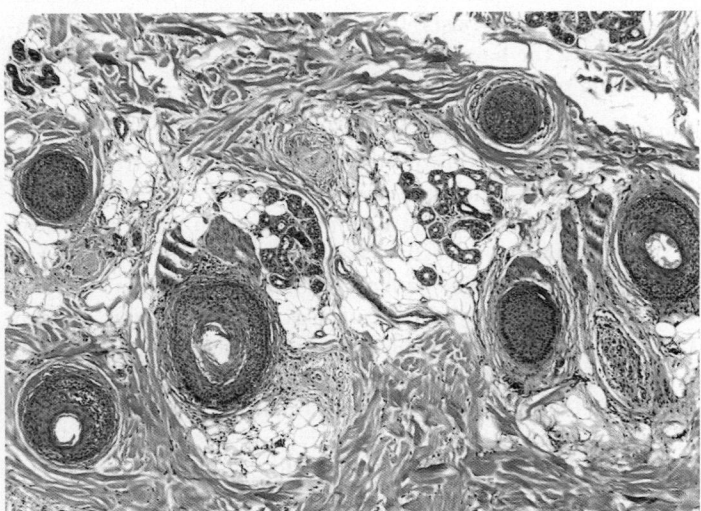

Figure 18-63 Psoriatic alopecia (horizontal). The resting hair count is elevated; this field demonstrates three of six follicles in catagen. The streamer to the right contains lymphocytes, reminiscent of alopecia areata.

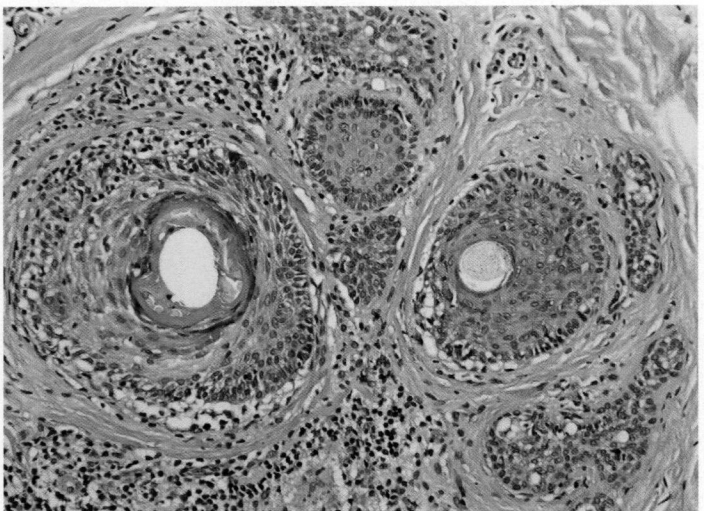

Figure 18-64 Psoriatic alopecia (horizontal). More superficially in the dermis, perifollicular lymphocytic inflammation and atrophic sebaceous glands are seen (follicle at right). The follicle at left shows spongiosis, but basal vacuolization and dyskeratosis are not present.

Differential Diagnosis. In the histologic differential diagnosis of psoriatic alopecia are AA and psoriatic alopecia/AA-like reactions secondary to anti–TNF-α therapy. AA lacks the characteristic epidermal changes of psoriasis, and anti–TNF-α alopecia reportedly shows plasma cells and eosinophils (346).

Principles of Management: High-potency topical or intralesional corticosteroids should be used in the initial treatment of psoriatic alopecia. Tar preparations may also be tried. In refractory cases, systemic therapies for psoriasis may be initiated.

Senescent Alopecia

Clinical Summary. Senescent or senile alopecia refers to the normal hair loss that occurs as a consequence of the aging process, with scalp hair becoming progressively and diffusely thinned, starting at age 50 years but more typically by the seventh or eighth decade (225,260). Both sexes are affected. All elderly individuals exhibit thinning to some degree, but in severe cases an individual may seek medical advice (138,348).

Histopathology. The most common clinical impression is that of a nonscarring alopecia, and cursory inspection of horizontal sections may appear normal. It is only through hair counts that a reduced hair density is revealed. A 4-mm punch biopsy sectioned horizontally demonstrates the following: a decrease in the total number of hairs, from a normal of 35 to 45, to 25 to 35, a normal telogen count (<20%), a terminal-to-vellus hair ratio of at least 2:1, and a lack of deep inflammation (138,140,349). The diameter of hairs may be diminished, and fibrous tracts may be seen (260). The occiput should show similar findings to those of other areas of the scalp (138).

Pathogenesis. Presumably follicles are lost forever; it is tempting to speculate that the regenerative capacity of follicular stem cells is restricted to a finite number of hair cycles.

Differential Diagnosis. Because there is follicular dropout on biopsy, the differential diagnosis may include a scarring alopecia, particularly PPB because there is little to no inflammation. However, scarring alopecias typically show sufficient histologic evidence to distinguish them as such.

Principles of Management: Active therapy is not required or available.

Chemotherapy-Induced Permanent Alopecia

Clinical Summary. Chemotherapy-induced alopecia is an anagen effluvium resulting from the toxic effects of chemotherapeutic agents that occurs in 65% of patients undergoing chemotherapy. It occurs 2 to 4 weeks after the initiation of treatment and grows back fully within 6 months of treatment cessation (350,351). Forty-seven percent of female patients consider it to be the most traumatic aspect of chemotherapy; it negatively impacts self-esteem and is a sign to others of a cancer diagnosis (350). The hair may regrow with altered color or texture. In a subset of patients, the alopecia persists beyond 6 months, and the hair fails to grow longer than 10 cm (352). Termed *chemotherapy-induced permanent alopecia (CIPAL)*, it is a rare complication that results most commonly from high-dose chemotherapy with busulphan and/or cyclophosphamide, followed by bone marrow transplantation, or from one of the taxanes (docetaxel, paclitaxel) for breast cancer, although other agents have been reported (353,354). In some patients, the alopecia is accentuated on androgen-dependent areas of the scalp (352). The persistence of the alopecia often leads to a biopsy.

Histopathology. The histologic findings in a case series of 10 patients revealed a nonscarring alopecia with a preserved number of follicular units and lack of fibrosis but a slightly decreased follicular density, with an average of 17 in a 4-mm punch biopsy (352). Hair counts demonstrated decreased terminal hairs and increased miniaturized hairs (average terminal-to-vellus ratio of ~1:1), increased telogen hairs (average anagen-to-telogen ratio of 3.6:1), and increased fibrous streamers in the reticular dermis and subcutis (352). There was a tendency of telogen hairs to group together. Only two cases showed mild perifollicular (infundibulum) and perivascular lymphocytic inflammation. Sebaceous glands were preserved in all cases. Another group found, in one case, multiple linear aggregates of basaloid epithelium resembling telogen germinal units (secondary hair germ of late-stage telogen follicles) but more slender (351). In sum, CIPAL bears striking resemblance to AGA (but with decreased density) and noninflammatory AA (Fig. 18-65).

Pathogenesis. The exact etiology of CIPAL and why some patients develop it and others do not is unknown (355). Theories include direct toxicity of high-dose chemotherapy on stem cells or hair matrix cells.

Differential Diagnosis. The clinical and histologic differential diagnosis includes **AGA** and noninflammatory AA.

Principles of Management: Some of the effects of chemotherapy may be mitigated by preventive measures such as scalp cooling during chemotherapy (356). Topical minoxidil or low-dose oral minoxidil may provide some benefit (357,358).

Temporal Triangular Alopecia

Clinical Summary. Temporal triangular alopecia (TTA) is a triangular or lancet-shaped patch of nonscarring stable alopecia that typically occurs on the frontotemporal scalp (359) (Fig. 18-66), although atypical presentations on other areas of the scalp have been reported (parietal, occipital, vertex) (360). It has also been called *congenital triangular alopecia* in the literature, but in the largest study of 53 cases only 36.5% were detected at birth, with most cases (55.8%) arising between the ages of 2 and 9, although most occur by age 6 (361). Rare cases presenting in

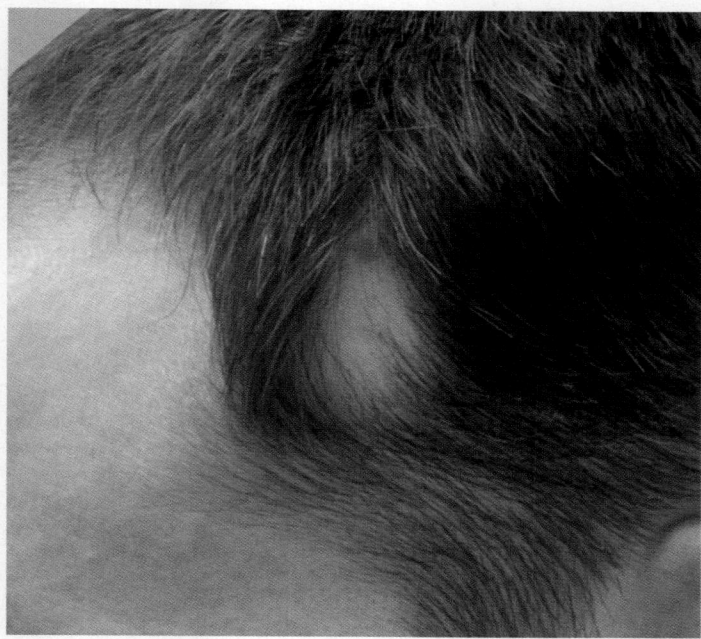

Figure 18-66 Temporal triangular alopecia. A vaguely triangular/lancet-shaped patch of nonscarring alopecia on the temple of an adult male, present for over 20 years and unchanging.

adulthood have been reported (362). Most of the time it is unilateral; of the 53 patients, 55.8% had involvement on the right side, 13.5% on the left side, and 30.8% were bilateral (361). It is most commonly mistaken for AA.

Histopathology. Horizontal sectioning of a punch biopsy is best suited for making the diagnosis histologically, revealing a normal to slightly decreased follicular density with only vellus and intermediate hairs (363,364) (Fig. 18-67). Terminal hairs are

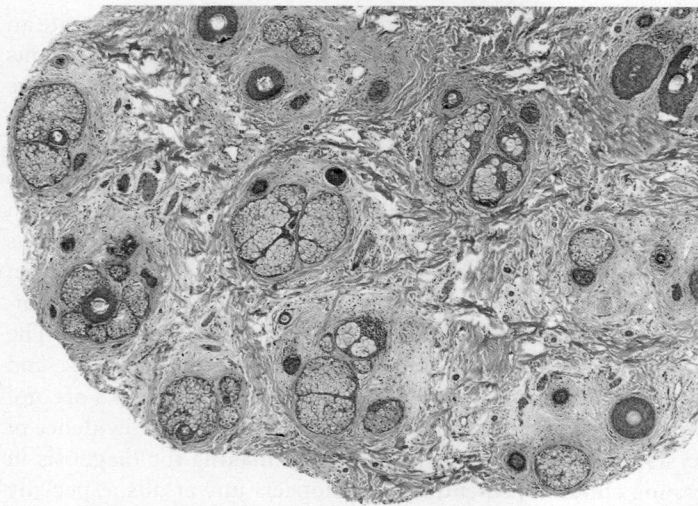

Figure 18-65 Chemotherapy-induced permanent alopecia (horizontal). These sections demonstrate a nonscarring alopecia with increased vellus-like miniaturized follicles, many of them in telogen and catagen. Sebaceous glands appear normal.

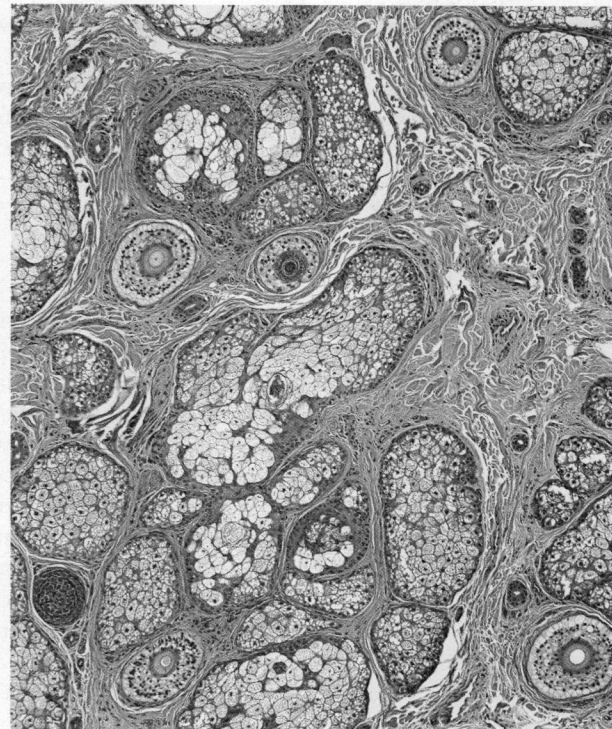

Figure 18-67 Temporal triangular alopecia (horizontal). The biopsy shows a nonscarring alopecia made up entirely of vellus and intermediate follicles. Sebaceous glands are normal.

absent except when biopsied near the edge of the patch. Inflammation is absent. The main condition in the histologic differential diagnosis is AGA. However, in contrast to AGA, the small hairs in TTA lack fibrous streamers in the deep dermis and subcutis beneath them (363).

Pathogenesis. Since most cases present in the first few years of life after a period of normal hair growth, the process represents a localized area of follicular miniaturization (363). Why this occurs, however, is unknown.

Differential Diagnosis. The differential diagnosis includes other conditions producing a clinical patch of nonscarring alopecia, namely AA, trichotillomania, traction alopecia, alopecia mucinosa, and tinea capitis (359). The clinical setting, the stable nature of the patch in TTA, and histologic findings are distinctive enough to diagnose it correctly.

Principles of Management: Treatment options include hair transplantation into the area and excision, but successful treatment with topical minoxidil has been reported (365). Camouflage with hair-styling techniques is also a viable option.

Lipedematous Alopecia

Clinical Summary. Lipedematous scalp is localized or diffuse thickening of the scalp without hair loss, a result of thickening of the subcutaneous fat layer (366,367). This finding, in association with usually diffuse or patchy alopecia, has been termed *lipedematous alopecia* (368–370). It is a rare chronic condition, with relatively few cases being reported, that occurs most often in African American females, although it has been reported in an Asian woman (371) as well as white women and men (372,373). The alopecia is characterized by short hairs that fail to grow longer than 2 cm. The scalp feels thick and boggy or spongy on palpation (370). It is smooth, without furrows, contrary to cutis verticis gyrata. Patients may complain of scalp pruritus, pain, or parasthesias. It was found in one patient with discoid lupus erythematosus (374).

Scalp thickness ranges from 10 to 15 mm, whereas normal scalp thickness averages 5.8 ± 0.12 mm, according to a study in which measurements were made at the bregma using skull x-rays (375). Scalp thickness may also be measured using computed tomography, magnetic resonance imaging (376), or ultrasound (369) or by introducing a sterile needle into the scalp (368).

Histopathology. The defining abnormality is increased thickness of the subcutaneous fat layer (377). To appreciate this on biopsy, the specimen must extend to the galea, and vertical sections are required. Superficial biopsies will not show the diagnostic finding. There is no evidence of adipose tissue hypertrophy or hyperplasia; instead, there is edema (378). The normal subcutaneous architecture of lobules separated by collagenous septae is disrupted, and septae may be absent (379). Degeneration of the adipose tissue into loosely associated collagenous strands, vessels, and aggregates of fat cells is also seen (378). Excess mucin deposition is not generally characteristic but was seen in some cases (369,372). There may be mild hyperkeratosis and acanthosis, as well as a sparse, superficial perivascular, interstitial, and perifollicular mononuclear infiltrate with occasional eosinophils (378).

When hairs appear normal, a good explanation for the associated alopecia may not be apparent, although some researchers have noted a decrease in the number of follicles and focal bulbar atrophy (378). When there is follicular dropout, vertical fibrous tracts of lamellar fibroplasia may be seen instead (379). In a study of lipedematous scalp and lipedematous alopecia, only the two cases with hair loss showed ectatic lymphatic vessels, believed to be potentially pathogenic (372). Scarring in the dermis or subcutis is generally absent, but perifollicular fibrosis has been noted (368,369). Follicular plugging and atrophic follicles have also been reported (368). Microscopic examination of hairs pulled in the clinical setting may show distal loss of the hair cuticle and changes of trichorrhexis nodosa, with hairs that break easily.

Pathogenesis. The etiology is unknown. The approximate doubling in scalp thickness is caused entirely by thickening of the adipose layer. Free-floating lipid droplets along with adipocytes in various stages of degeneration were seen using electron microscopy (378). In addition to reduced follicular density, it is postulated that alopecia from aberrant hair shaft production may occur secondary to increased tissue oncotic pressure on hair bulbs (378). Speculating that lipedematous alopecia represents an advanced stage of lipedematous scalp, some authors have proposed the unifying diagnosis of *lipedematous diseases of the scalp* (371).

Differential Diagnosis. Cutis verticis gyrata and encephalocraniocutaneous lipomatosis may enter into the clinical differential diagnosis, although the clinical setting and histologic picture of these disorders should be sufficiently characteristic to come to the correct diagnosis (379).

Principles of Management: There are no effective treatments (379).

Atrichia with Papular Lesions

Clinical Summary. Atrichia with papular lesions is a rare autosomal recessive condition characterized by total alopecia involving the scalp and body and usually the eyebrows (380), although eyelashes may be spared (381). Normal hair is present at birth but is shed within the ensuing months to years of life, never to be replaced (382). At around age 2 years, individuals start to develop generalized cystic papules. Unlike other forms of ectodermal dysplasia, defects in nails, sweat glands, or teeth are not seen (380).

Histopathology. A biopsy from affected scalp will demonstrate an absence of developed hair follicles (Fig. 18-68). Intact sebaceous glands may sometimes be seen (381). Follicular infundibula are present without the lower two-thirds of hair follicles, which are often replaced by irregular epithelial structures or cysts (383). Consequently, hair shafts are not manufactured. Cysts develop from these abnormal follicles, producing clinical papules on the scalp and elsewhere that, when biopsied, reveal keratinous cysts with differentiation toward the follicular infundibulum (epidermoid, found in the upper dermis) and isthmus (trichilemmal, found in the middle and lower dermis) (381,383). The cysts may rupture, leading to foreign-body granulomas, and eccrine glands are normal in appearance. When cysts are not apparent clinically, a biopsy may reveal microscopic evidence of cysts (384); this may be important in making the diagnosis in young children presenting with alopecia universalis, especially when genetic testing is not available.

Pathogenesis. Mutations in the human hairless (*HR*) gene on chromosome 8p12 produce the described clinical phenotype (385), although a patient with mutations in the vitamin D

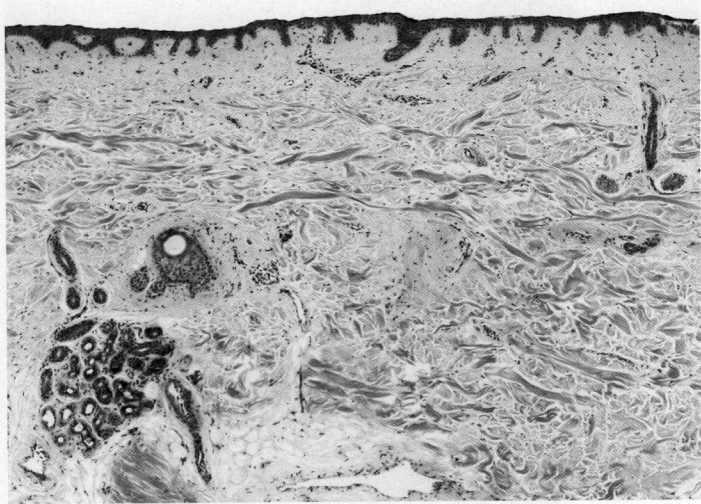

Figure 18-68 Atrichia with papular lesions (vertical). In this biopsy from the scalp, functional follicles are absent. Only a rudimentary follicle without a hair shaft is seen, near the eccrine gland, which is normal.

receptor gene has been reported (386). The hairless gene in humans is a homolog of the murine hairless gene (385). The human *HR* gene encodes an H3K9 demethylase protein that regulates epidermal homeostasis (387).

Atrichia with papular lesions is recessively inherited, requiring two defective alleles; although most of the identified mutations have been homozygous within consanguineous families, compound heterozygous mutations have also been found (382).

Differential Diagnosis. The clinical picture mimics alopecia universalis.

Principles of Management: Cysts that develop may need to be periodically removed.

INFLAMMATORY DISEASES OF SWEAT GLANDS

Neutrophilic Eccrine Hidradenitis
Clinical Summary. Neutrophilic eccrine hidradenitis (NEH) occurs in varied clinical settings (Fig. 18-69) (388,389). *Chemotherapy-associated NEH*, the most common presentation, is discussed in Chapter 11. Acute inflammation of the eccrine sweat glands

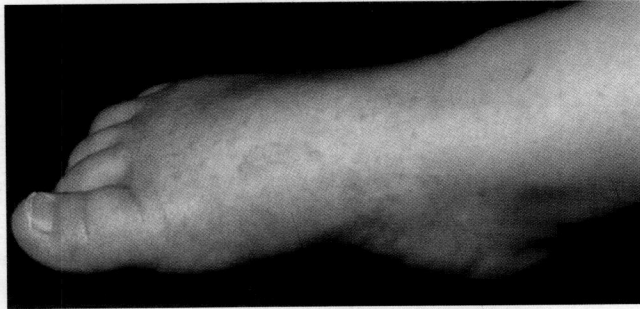

Figure 18-69 Neutrophilic eccrine hidradenitis. A young child with acute lymphocytic leukemia developed erythematous papules and plaques while on maintenance chemotherapy. (Reprinted with permission from Elder DE, Elenitsas R, Rubin AI, et al. *Atlas and Synopsis of Lever's Histopathology of the Skin*. 3rd ed. Wolters Kluwer Health/Lippincott Williams & Wilkins; 2013.)

presents as erythematous or violaceous macules, papules, nodules, or plaques occurring predominantly on the extremities and trunk. NEH has been described in conjunction with infectious agents (390,391), including *Serratia marcescens*, *Enterobacter cloacae*, *Staphylococcus aureus*, streptococcal endocarditis, *Nocardia*, *Mycobacteria chelonae*, and HIV-1 (392,393), as well as miscellaneous associations, including granulocyte colony-stimulating factor (394), BRAF inhibitors (395), and acute myelogenous leukemia in the absence of chemotherapy (396).

A subset of NEH that occurs in healthy children and young adults, *palmoplantar hidradenitis*, has been reported under many names, including "idiopathic palmoplantar eccrine hidradenitis," "juvenile neutrophilic eccrine hidradenitis," "recurrent eccrine hidradenitis," "idiopathic plantar hidradenitis," and "traumatic plantar urticaria" (79,397–400). Painful erythematous papules and nodules occur on the palms and soles. Constitutional symptoms are usually absent. In one study of 22 patients, occurrences were most frequent in the spring and fall, and almost half of the patients experienced more than one episode (401). The condition is benign and self-limited. Although the pathogenesis is unclear, temporal association with intense physical activity and exposure to cold, damp footwear have been reported (397,399).

A related condition, *Pseudomonas hot-foot syndrome*, presented as painful red to purple nodules on weight-bearing sites on the soles of 40 children within 1 to 2 days of using a community wading pool where the floor was covered with an abrasive grit (believed to be important to the pathogenesis) (402, 403). Lesions were cultured from some patients, yielding a strain of *Pseudomonas aeruginosa* identical to that found in the pool, and some of the children had associated *Pseudomonas* folliculitis (hot-tub folliculitis).

Histopathology. The histology of palmoplantar hidradenitis occurring in children is similar to that of NEH induced by certain forms of chemotherapy (see Chapter 11), except that syringosquamous metaplasia is missing. A neutrophilic infiltrate is centered on the eccrine gland coils (Figs. 18-70 and 18-71). There may be mild

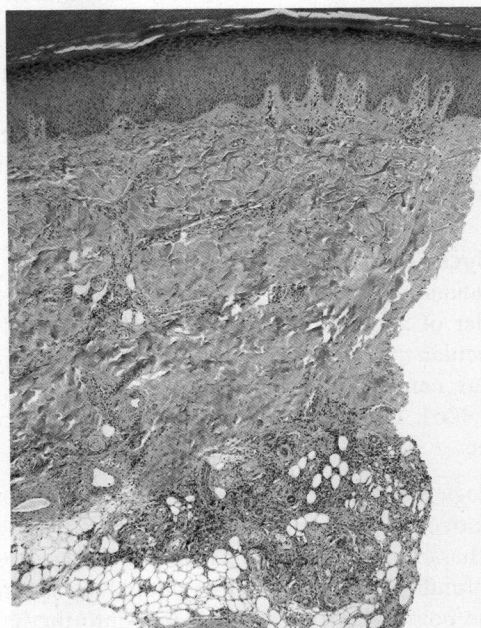

Figure 18-70 Neutrophilic eccrine hidradenitis. This biopsy from the plantar surface demonstrates an inflammatory infiltrate around eccrine glands within the subcutaneous fat.

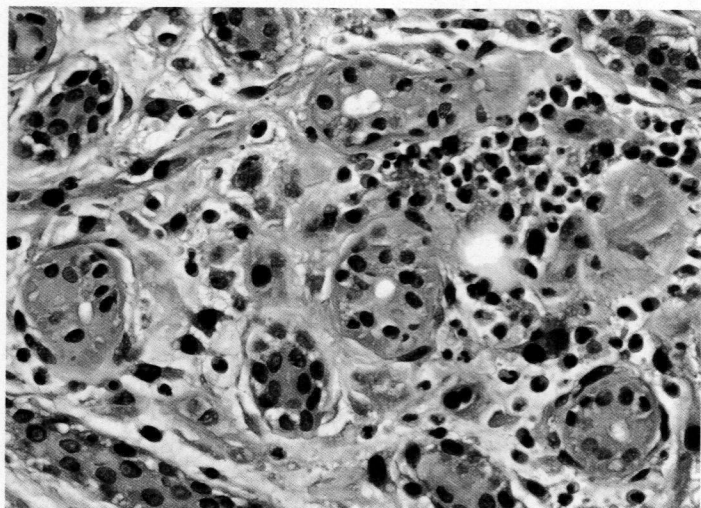

Figure 18-71 Neutrophilic eccrine hidradenitis. Neutrophils around an eccrine gland.

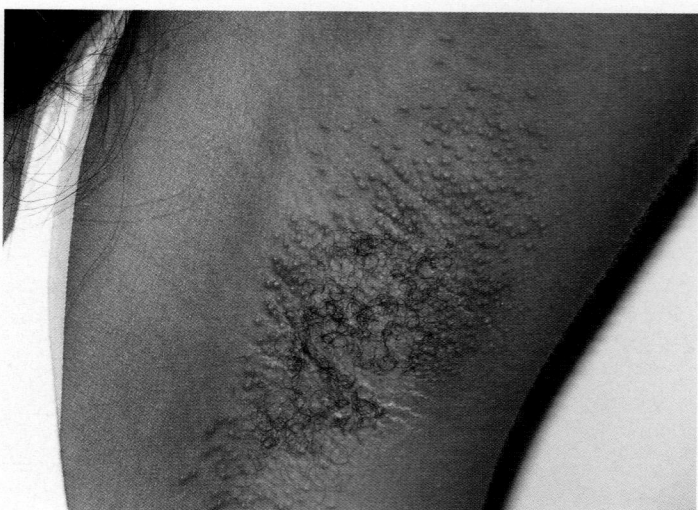

Figure 18-72 Fox–Fordyce disease. The uniform spacing of these discrete papules in the axilla is a clue to their adnexal origin.

mixed inflammation surrounding vessels in the mid- and deep dermis, without leukocytoclastic vasculitis. Neutrophilic inflammation may involve the acrosyringium or assume a nodular pattern in the reticular dermis with abscess formation (398,400). Stains for fungi and bacteria are negative, even in those cases in which cultures of lesions are positive for bacteria (388).

In the *Pseudomonas* hot-foot syndrome, biopsies from two of the patients showed superficial and deep perivascular, interstitial, and perieccrine inflammation composed of neutrophils and lymphocytes that extended into subcutaneous fat lobules. One of the cases showed a dermal microabscess with extension into the fat and focal vasculitis with an intravascular thrombus (402). The authors suggested that extension into subcutaneous fat lobules was a distinguishing feature from idiopathic NEH in children.

Differential Diagnosis. In addition to the entities discussed previously, the differential diagnosis would include infections and neutrophilic dermatoses in which deep inflammation is centered on eccrine glands.

Principles of Management: Treatment of any associated conditions is foremost. In cases that are recurrent or unavoidable with repeat courses of chemotherapy, dapsone or colchicine may be tried (404). Palmoplantar hidradenitis occurring in children is benign and self-limited.

Fox–Fordyce Disease

Clinical Summary. Fox–Fordyce disease (apocrine miliaria) is a disorder of apocrine sweat glands characterized by firm, itchy, follicular papules in anatomic sites where apocrine glands occur, namely, the axillae (Fig. 18-72), areolae, and genitalia (405,406). It occurs almost exclusively in women after adolescence.

Histopathology. Step sections of a vertically oriented biopsy specimen or horizontal sections are usually needed to adequately show the characteristic changes. There is hyperkeratosis of the follicular infundibulum and excretory duct of the apocrine sweat gland at the point where the latter inserts into the hair follicle (Fig. 18-73). The apocrine duct behind the obstructing keratin plug becomes dilated (407). A spongiotic vesicle occurs in the follicular infundibulum, possibly representing an apocrine sweat retention vesicle, with potential to rupture. Lymphocyte

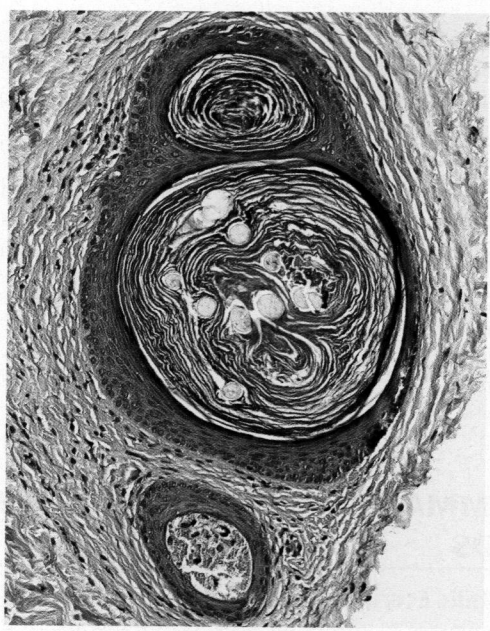

Figure 18-73 Fox–Fordyce disease (horizontal). The follicular infundibulum is dilated and hyperkeratotic and is filled with multiple vellus hair shafts. Xanthoma cells are seen within the lumen at the bottom. Mild perifollicular fibrosis is present.

exocytosis is seen in the area of spongiosis. There may also be infundibular acanthosis and mild perivascular and periadnexal lymphocytic inflammation in the adjacent upper dermis (408). A comprehensive review of the histopathology noted other possible microscopic findings, including vacuolar alteration at the dermoepithelial junction of infundibula, dyskeratotic cells in infundibula, cornoid lamella–like parakeratosis within an orthokeratotic plug filling a dilated infundibulum, and foamy macrophages surrounding follicular infundibula and apocrine ducts (perifollicular xanthomatosis) (409,410). Transverse histologic sections facilitated identification of the diagnostic histologic features in one case, and this technique was touted as the most effective way to diagnose Fox–Fordyce disease on biopsy (411).

A third type of sweat gland has been identified in the axillae; it is intermediate in size between the larger apocrine gland

and the smaller eccrine gland (412). Called the apoeccrine gland, it has a secretory coil like an apocrine gland but opens directly to the epidermal surface like an eccrine gland. A case of Fox–Fordyce disease that histologically showed blockage of the intraepidermal portion of this apoeccrine sweat duct by cells that were released from the secretory portion via a holocrine mechanism was characterized clinically by nonfollicular papules (412).

Pathogenesis. The pathogenesis appears to be related to blockage of the apocrine sweat duct. Apocrine anhidrosis results, as demonstrated by the lack of apocrine secretion following intradermal injections of an epinephrine solution into the affected area (405). There are, however, reports suggesting that mechanical obstruction alone may not explain Fox–Fordyce disease (408). Fox–Fordyce has been reported as an adverse effect of laser hair removal (413).

Differential Diagnosis. Fox–Fordyce disease may be clinically identical to axillary perifollicular xanthomatosis, which is less pruritic and confined to the axillae (414). Some consider this condition to be xanthomatous Fox–Fordyce disease, with sebum-derived lipid (415), whereas others consider it as the follicular counterpart of verruciform xanthoma (414), with keratinocyte-derived lipid.

Principles of Management: Treatment modalities may include oral contraceptives, topical antibiotics, topical and oral retinoids, topical and intralesional steroids, phototherapy, liposuction-assisted curettage, and surgery (19).

INFLAMMATORY DISEASES OF CARTILAGE

Chondrodermatitis Nodularis Helicis
Clinical Summary. Chondrodermatitis nodularis helicis (CNH) usually presents as a single, small, exquisitely tender, erythematous papule on the superior rim of the helix of the ear (Fig. 18-74) and less frequently on the antihelix or posterior ear (416). The lesion develops a crust and ulceration in the center,

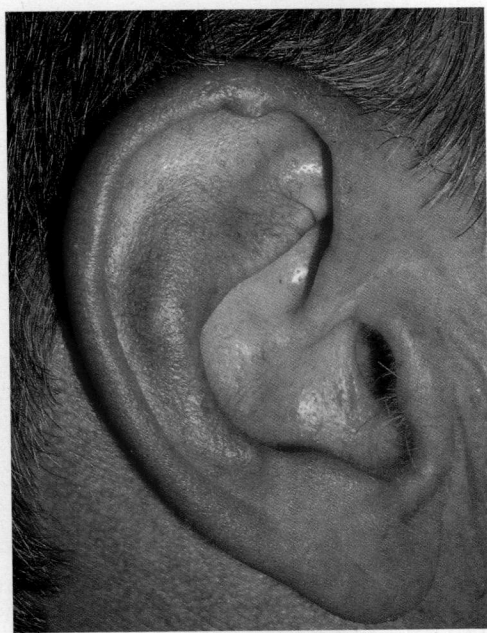

Figure 18-74 Chondrodermatitis nodularis helicis. Papule on the helical rim with a central crust.

producing elevated margins that may mimic basal cell carcinoma. CNH occurs mostly in white men older than 40 years of age. The lesion tends to persist indefinitely without treatment. *Chondrodermatitis nodularis nasi* is a rare variant affecting the skin and cartilage of the nose (417,418).

Histopathology. Epidermal ulceration or a wedge-shaped epidermal defect is usually present. The intact adjacent epidermis is hyperplastic and may contain some dyskeratotic keratinocytes. A crust of exudate, parakeratosis, and dermal debris covers the surface of the epidermal defect (419). The dermis directly below shows fibrinoid collagen degeneration that stains more deeply eosinophilic than reticular dermal collagen, is homogeneous, and is acellular; it may reach the perichondrial tissue beneath (Fig. 18-75). The stroma adjacent to the zone of degeneration shows vascular proliferation with lymphohistiocytic inflammatory cells. There may also be some fibroplasia and occasional plasma cells and neutrophils. Peripheral solar elastosis is common (419). The underlying perichondrial tissue may be thickened and appear to migrate to the base of the fibrinoid dermal necrosis. Degeneration of underlying cartilage with loss of cell nuclei can occur, although it is usually minimal. If cartilaginous degeneration is severe, there may be focal calcification and ossification. Nerve hyperplasia was found in 35 of 37 cases examined, potentially explaining the tenderness of lesions (420).

Pathogenesis. As the name implies, it was originally believed that this condition begins with cartilaginous degeneration. It is now generally considered to be an attempt at transepidermal elimination of damaged dermal collagen, a type of perforating disorder (419), although one report classified it as a necrobiotic process of collagen akin to granuloma annulare (421). The dermal collagen degeneration most likely results from vascular compromise, whether induced by trauma, pressure (during sleep or cell phone use [422]), cold, perichondrial arteriolar narrowing (423), or complications of dermatoheliosis. The limited vasculature at this anatomic site and lack of subcutaneous fat insulation may contribute to the situation.

Differential Diagnosis. Clinical lesions are often biopsied to exclude a hypertrophic actinic keratosis or carcinoma. Superficial biopsies that fail to show the characteristic fibrinoid collagen degeneration or cartilage may be mistaken for neurodermatitis when the surface is ulcerated.

Principles of Management: In addition to excluding carcinoma, a biopsy or deeper shave excision that includes cartilage may be curative (424). Offloading pressure on the ear during sleep is helpful and may be achieved by foam placed behind the ear (425), frequent repositioning, or using a doughnut-shaped pillow.

Relapsing Polychondritis
Clinical Summary. Relapsing polychondritis (RP) is a rare systemic chondromalacia that affects cartilage in multiple sites, including the ear, nose, larynx, trachea, bronchi, and joints (426,427). It also affects proteoglycan-rich tissues, such as the eyes, aorta, heart, kidneys, and skin (427). It usually starts with auricular chondritis and runs an episodic, progressively destructive course. A mortality of about 25% has been reported, most commonly from damage to the respiratory tract or heart valves, although one study estimated the survival rate to be 94% at 8 years, a result of improvements in management (427). Disorders commonly associated with RP include rheumatoid

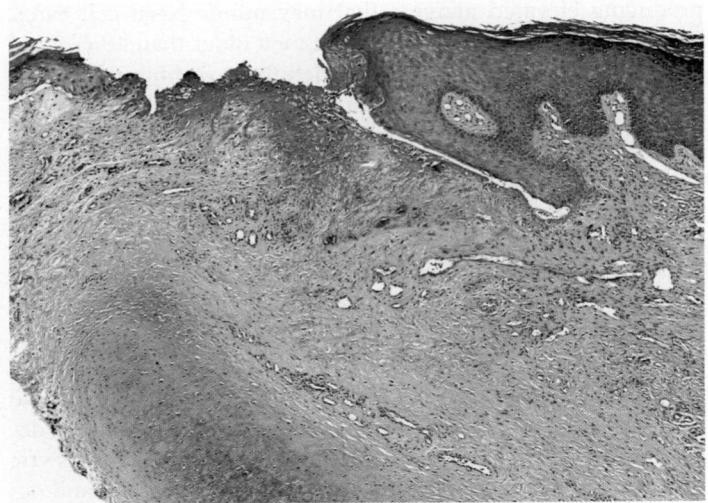

Figure 18-75 Chondrodermatitis nodularis helicis. There is a channel through the epidermis with adjacent epidermal hyperplasia. The dermis beneath shows fibrinoid degeneration of collagen that stains brightly eosinophilic and extends to the underlying perichondrium. The surrounding dermis shows a proliferation of small blood vessels and fibroplasia.

arthritis, systemic lupus erythematosus, Sjögren syndrome, and myelodysplastic syndromes (428). It may also be a paraneoplastic condition, reportedly occurring with non-Hodgkin lymphoma (429) and chronic lymphocytic leukemia (430).

Primary involvement of the ears and nose, consisting of intermittent attacks of painful erythema and swelling, may lead to a dermatology consult. Rarely, only one ear is involved. Ultimately, the ears become soft and flabby as a result of cartilage destruction, and the nose assumes a saddle nose deformity.

Nonspecific dermatologic findings associated with RP are common, varied, and found most frequently in RP patients with myelodysplasia (431). They sometimes resemble the skin findings seen in Behcet disease or inflammatory bowel disease: aphthosis, sterile pustules, limb ulcerations, or distal necrosis (431). RP has been associated with Behcet disease (432), described by the acronym MAGIC syndrome for "mouth and genital ulcers with inflamed cartilage" (433). Leukocytoclastic vasculitis is not uncommon, and, indeed, it has been suggested that the cartilaginous damage may be secondary to a primary vasculitis (434). Other associated cutaneous conditions include chronic dermatitis, superficial phlebitis, livedo reticularis (431), and panniculitides such as erythema nodosum–like lesions (435), septal and lobular panniculitis with vasculitis (436), and erythema elevatum diutinum (437).

Histopathology. In early cartilaginous lesions, only the marginal chondrocytes appear degenerate, showing vacuolization, nuclear pyknosis, and loss of basophilia, which has been shown to result from the release of chondroitin sulfate from the cartilage matrix (438). A dense inflammatory infiltrate develops in the perichondrium, which is composed primarily of neutrophils but may include lymphocytes, eosinophils, plasma cells, and macrophages. Frequently, there is edema or gelatinous cystic degeneration, and with progression, degenerated cartilage blends imperceptibly with the surrounding inflammatory cells, leading to the formation of granulation-type tissue (439). There may be fragmentation of the cartilage with necrosis and lysis of the cartilaginous plates (439). Elastic tissue stain shows

clumping and destruction of cartilaginous elastic fibers. With successive episodes, fibrosis ensues.

Pathogenesis. Circulating antibodies to type II collagen, found exclusively in cartilage, are detected in patients with RP and are generally found only in patients with active disease (440). The antibodies are directed against native and undenatured type II collagen, suggesting a primary role for these antibodies in the pathogenesis (rather than a secondary response to injured cartilage). Immunoglobulin and complement components have also been identified in the inflamed cartilage (438). RP is strongly associated with HLA-DR4 (441).

Differential Diagnosis. An infectious etiology could be considered with a neutrophil-rich infiltrate.

Principles of Management: Systemic immunosuppressants are used to manage the disease. In recent years, TNF-α blockers have been tried (442).

Pseudocyst of the Auricle
Clinical Summary. In pseudocyst of the auricle, an asymptomatic, fluctuant swelling measuring about 1 cm in diameter is observed on the upper portion of the anterior aspect of the ear, usually in young men (mean age 38.9 years) (443). It is a form of chondromalacia that arises spontaneously or sometimes after minor trauma or infection, relapses frequently, and only rarely involves both ears. Pseudocyst is caused by cavitation within the auricular cartilage, which, when punctured, releases only a few microliters of a clear, deep yellow, viscous fluid. In the differential of cystic swellings of the external ear, this feature aids in the diagnosis; so if a relatively large amount of liquid is obtained, the cavity must be located outside of the cartilage (444).

Histopathology. A small intracartilaginous cavity without an epithelial lining is found on histologic examination. The wall of the pseudocyst consists of auricular cartilage, which is partially degenerated, appearing as faintly eosinophilic amorphous material (Fig. 18-76). The overlying epidermis, reticular dermis, and perichondrium are all normal (444). Until recently,

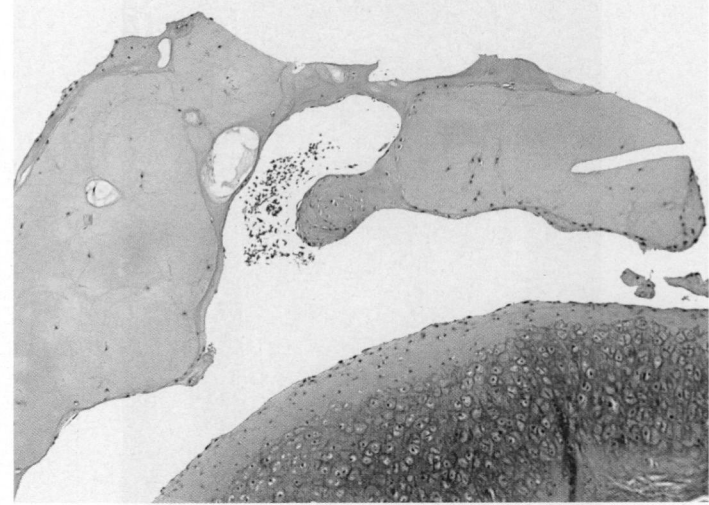

Figure 18-76 Pseudocyst of the auricle. There is an intracartilaginous cavity without an epithelial lining. The auricular cartilage is partially degenerated, appearing faintly eosinophilic and smudgy, with loss of nuclei.

inflammation was not considered a feature of this condition, but a study of 16 specimens consistently showed a perivascular lymphocytic infiltrate in the connective tissue just superficial to the cartilage (445); the authors believed that this was critical to the development of the condition.

Pathogenesis. It has been suggested that the intracartilaginous cavity forms after the release of lysosomal enzymes or overproduction of glycosaminoglycans after repeated trauma or mechanical stimulation. Compared to normal serum, aspirated fluid has been found to contain elevated levels of lactate dehydrogenase (LDH), especially the LDH-4 and LDH-5 isozymes (446), as well as the cytokines IL-6 and IL-1 (447); investigators hypothesized that these substances were released from the damaged cartilage.

Differential Diagnosis. The clinical and histopathologic features are unique.

Principles of Management: Treatment options include aspiration of fluid, followed by application of a pressure dressing, or injection of steroids, fibrin glue, or minocycline into the cystic space (442).

REFERENCES

1. Bergfeld WF. The pathophysiology of acne vulgaris in children and adolescents, part 1. *Cutis.* 2004;74(2):92–97.
2. Goldschmidt H, Leyden JJ, Stein KH. Acne fulminans. *Arch Dermatol.* 1977;113:444.
3. Harper J, Thiboutot D. Pathogenesis of acne: recent research advances. *Adv Dermatol.* 2003;19:1–10.
4. Thiboutot D. Acne: 1991–2001. *J Am Acad Dermatol.* 2002;47(1):109–117.
5. Tan JKL, Stein Gold LF, Alexis AF, Harper JC. Current concepts in acne pathogenesis: pathways to inflammation. *Semin Cutan Med Surg.* 2018;37(3S):S60–S62. doi:10.12788/j.sder.2018.024
6. Leyden JJ. New understandings of the pathogenesis of acne. *J Am Acad Dermatol.* 1995;32:15S.
7. Cunliffe WJ, Holland DB, Jeremy A. Comedone formation: etiology, clinical presentation, and treatment. *Clin Dermatol.* 2004;22(5):367–374.
8. Toyoda M, Morohashi M. Pathogenesis of acne. *Med Electron Microsc.* 2001;34(1):29–40.
9. Thiboutot D, Harris G, Iles V, Cimis G, Gilliland K, Hagari S. Activity of the type 1 5-alpha-reductase exhibits regional differences in isolated sebaceous glands and whole skin. *J Invest Dermatol.* 1995;105:209–214.
10. Thiboutot D, Gilliland K, Light J, Lookingbill D. Androgen metabolism in sebaceous glands from subjects with and without acne. *Arch Dermatol.* 1999;135:1041–1048.
11. Leyden JJ, McGinley KJ. Effect of 13-cis-retinoic acid on sebum production and *Propionibacterium acnes* in severe nodulocystic acne. *Arch Dermatol Res.* 1982;272:331.
12. Bojar RA, Holland KT. Acne and *Propionibacterium acnes. Clin Dermatol.* 2004;22(5):375–379.
13. Thiboutot DM. Overview of acne and its treatment. *Cutis.* 2008;81(1, suppl):3–7.
14. Zaenglein AL, Pathy AL, Schlosser BJ, et al. Guidelines of care for the management of acne vulgaris. *J Am Acad Dermatol.* 2016;74(5):945–973.e33. Erratum in: *J Am Acad Dermatol.* 2020;82(6):1576.
15. Zaenglein AL. Acne vulgaris. *N Engl J Med.* 2018;379(14):1343–1352.
16. Thiboutot D, Gollnick H, Bettoli V, Lookingbill D. New insights into the management of acne: an update from the Global Alliance to Improve Outcomes in Acne group. *J Am Acad Dermatol.* 2009;60(5, suppl):S1–S50.
17. Bong JL, Connell JMC, Lever R. Intranasal betamethasone induced acne and adrenal suppression. *Br J Dermatol.* 2000;142(3):579–580.
18. Hurwitz RM. Steroid acne. *J Am Acad Dermatol.* 1989;21(6):1179–1181.
19. James WD, Berger TG, Elston DM. *Andrews' Diseases of the Skin Clinical Dermatology.* 10th ed. Saunders Elsevier; 2006.
20. Brodell RT, O'Brien MJ Jr. Topical corticosteroid-induced acne: three treatment strategies to break the "addiction" cycle. *Postgrad Med.* 1999;106(6):225–226.
21. Hafeez ZH. Perioral dermatitis: an update. *Int J Dermatol.* 2003;42(7):514–517.
22. Peralta L, Morais P. Perioral dermatitis—the role of nasal steroids. *Cutan Ocul Toxicol.* 2012;31(2):160–163.
23. Nguyen V, Eichenfield LF. Periorificial dermatitis in children and adolescents. *J Am Acad Dermatol.* 2006;55(5):781–785.
24. Frieden IJ, Prose NS, Fletcher V, Turner ML. Granulomatous perioral dermatitis in children. *Arch Dermatol.* 1989;125:369–373.
25. Cribier B, Lieber-Mbomeyo A, Lipsker D. Clinical and histological study of a case of facial Afro-Caribbean childhood eruption (FACE). *Ann Dermatol Venereol.* 2008;135(10):663–667.
26. Urbatsch AJ, Frieden I, Williams ML, Elewski BE, Mancini AJ, Paller AS. Extrafacial and generalized granulomatous periorificial dermatitis. *Arch Dermatol.* 2002;138(10):1354–1358.
27. Ackerman AB. *Histologic Diagnosis of Inflammatory Skin Diseases.* 2nd ed. Williams & Wilkins; 1997.
28. Marks R, Black MM. Perioral dermatitis: a histopathological study of 26 cases. *Br J Dermatol.* 1971;84:242.
29. Wilkin J, Dahl M, Detmar M, et al. Standard classification of rosacea: report of the National Rosacea Society Expert Committee on the Classification and Staging of Rosacea. *J Am Acad Dermatol.* 2002;46(4):584–587.
30. Malik R, Quirk CJ. Topical applications and perioral dermatitis. *Australas J Dermatol.* 2000;41(1):34–38.
31. Searle T, Ali FR, Al-Niaimi F. Perioral dermatitis: diagnosis, proposed etiologies and management. *J Cosmet Dermatol.* 2021. doi:10.1111/jocd.14060
32. Baldwin HE. Diagnosis and treatment of rosacea: state of the art. *J Drugs Dermatol.* 2012;11(6):725–730.
33. Crawford GH, Pelle MT, James WD. Rosacea. I: Etiology, pathogenesis, and subtype classification. *J Am Acad Dermatol.* 2004;51(3):327–341; quiz 342–344.
34. Marks R, Harcourt-Webster JN. Histopathology of rosacea. *Arch Dermatol.* 1969;100:683.
35. Helm KF, Menz J, Gibson LE, Dicken CH. A clinical and histopathologic study of granulomatous rosacea. *J Am Acad Dermatol.* 1991;25:1038.
36. Aloi F, Tomasini C, Soro E, Pippione M. The clinicopathologic spectrum of rhinophyma. *J Am Acad Dermatol.* 2000;42(3):468–472.
37. Ahn CS, Huang WW. Rosacea pathogenesis. *Dermatol Clin.* 2018;36(2):81–86.
38. Dahl MV. Pathogenesis of rosacea. In: James WD, ed. *Advances in Dermatology.* Vol 17. Mosby; 2001:29–45.
39. Forton F, Germaux MA, Brasseur T, et al. Demodicosis and rosacea: epidemiology and significance in daily dermatologic practice. *J Am Acad Dermatol.* 2005;52(1):74–87.
40. Georgala S, Katoulis AC, Kylafis GD, Koumantaki-Mathioudaki E, Georgala C, Aroni K. Increased density of *Demodex folliculorum* and evidence of delayed hypersensitivity reaction in subjects with papulopustular rosacea. *J Eur Acad Dermatol Venereol.* 2001;15(5):441–444.
41. Ecker RI, Winkelmann RK. Demodex granuloma. *Arch Dermatol.* 1979;115:343.
42. Szlachcic A. The link between *Helicobacter pylori* infection and rosacea. *J Eur Acad Dermatol Venereol.* 2002;16(4):328–333.

43. Mayr-Kanhauser S, Kranke B, Kaddu S, Müllegger RR. Resolution of granulomatous rosacea after eradication of *Helicobacter pylori* with clarithromycin, metronidazole and pantoprazole. *Eur J Gastroenterol Hepatol.* 2001;13(11):1379–1383.

44. van Zuuren EJ, Kramer SF, Carter BR, Graber MA, Fedorowicz Z. Effective and evidence-based management strategies for rosacea: summary of a Cochrane systematic review. *Br J Dermatol.* 2011;165(4):760–781.

45. Marson JW, Baldwin HE. Rosacea: a wholistic review and update from pathogenesis to diagnosis and therapy. *Int J Dermatol.* 2020;59(6):e175–e182. doi:10.1111/ijd.14757

46. van Zuuren EJ. Rosacea. *N Engl J Med.* 2017;377(18):1754–1764. doi:10.1056/NEJMcp1506630

47. Baima B, Sticherling M. Demodicidosis revisited. *Acta Derm Venereol.* 2002;82:3–6.

48. Chen W, Plewig G. Human demodicosis: revisit and a proposed classification. *Br J Dermatol.* 2014;170(6):1219–1225. doi:10.1111/bjd.12850

49. Karincaoglu Y, Bayram N, Aycan O, Esrefoglu M. The clinical importance of *Demodex folliculorum* presenting with nonspecific facial signs and symptoms. *J Dermatol.* 2004;31(8):618–626.

50. Bonnar E, Eustace P, Powell FC. The *Demodex* mite population in rosacea. *J Am Acad Dermatol.* 1993;28(3):443–448.

51. Aylesworth R, Vance JC. *Demodex folliculorum* and *Demodex brevis* in cutaneous biopsies. *J Am Acad Dermatol.* 1982;7(6):583–589.

52. Vollmer RT. Demodex-associated folliculitis. *Am J Dermatopathol.* 1996;18(6):589–591.

53. Akilov OE, Butov YS, Mumcuoglu KY. A clinico-pathological approach to the classification of human demodicosis. *J Dtsch Dermatol Ges.* 2005;3(8):607–614.

54. Forstinger C, Kittler H, Binder M. Treatment of rosacea-like demodicidosis with oral ivermectin and topical permethrin cream. *J Am Acad Dermatol.* 1999;41(5):775–777.

55. Jansen T, Kastner U, Kreuter A, Altmeyer P. Rosacea-like demodicidosis associated with acquired immunodeficiency syndrome. *Br J Dermatol.* 2001;144(1):139–142.

56. Elston DM, Lawler KB, Iddins BO. What's eating you? *Demodex folliculorum. Cutis.* 2001;68:93–94.

57. Foley R, Kelly P, Gatault S, Powell F. Demodex: a skin resident in man and his best friend. *J Eur Acad Dermatol Venereol.* 2021;35(1):62–72. doi:10.1111/jdv.16461

58. Gazi U, Taylan-Ozkan A, Mumcuoglu KY. Immune mechanisms in human and canine demodicosis: a review. *Parasite Immunol.* 2019;41(12):e12673. doi:10.1111/pim.12673

59. Forton F, Seys B, Marchall JL, Song AM. *Demodex folliculorum* and topical treatment: acaricidal action evaluated by standardized skin surface biopsy. *Br J Dermatol.* 1998;138:461–466.

60. Hsu CK, Hsu MM, Lee JY. Demodicosis: a clinicopathological study. *J Am Acad Dermatol.* 2009;60(3):453–462.

61. van de Scheur MR, van der Waal RI, Starink TM. Lupus miliaris disseminatus faciei: a distinctive rosacea-like syndrome and not a granulomatous form of rosacea. *Dermatology.* 2003;206(2):120–123.

62. Slater N, Rapini RP. *Lupus Miliaris Disseminatus Faciei.* StatPearls Publishing; 2021.

63. Amiruddin D, Mii S, Fujimura T, Katsuoka K. Clinical evaluation of 35 cases of lupus miliaris disseminatus faciei. *J Dermatol.* 2011;38(6):618–620.

64. Skowron F, Causeret AS, Pabion C, Viallard AM, Balme B, Thomas L. F.I.GU.R.E.: facial idiopathic granulomas with regressive evolution—is "lupus miliaris disseminatus faciei" still an acceptable diagnosis in the third millenium? *Dermatology.* 2000;201(4):287–289.

65. Sehgal VN, Srivastava G, Aggarwal AK, Belum VR, Sharma S. Lupus miliaris disseminatus faciei, part I: significance of histopathologic undertones in diagnosis. *Skinmed.* 2005;4(3):151–156.

66. Sehgal VN, Srivastava G, Aggarwal AK, Belum VR, Sharma S. Lupus miliaris disseminatus faciei part II: an overview. *Skinmed.* 2005;4(4):234–238.

67. Hodak E, Trattner A, Feuerman H, et al. Lupus miliaris disseminatus faciei-the DNA of *Mycobacterium tuberculosis* is not detectable in active lesions by polymerase chain reaction. *Br J Dermatol.* 1997;137(4):614–619.

68. Al-Mutairi N. Nosology and therapeutic options for lupus miliaris disseminatus faciei. *J Dermatol.* 2011;38(9):864–873.

69. Nervi SJ, Schwartz RA, Dmochowski M. Eosinophilic pustular folliculitis: a 40 year retrospect. *J Am Acad Dermatol.* 2006;55(2):285–289.

70. Ofuji S. Eosinophilic pustular folliculitis. *Dermatologica.* 1987;174:53.

71. Tsuboi H, Niiyama S, Katsuoka K. Eosinophilic pustular folliculitis (Ofuji disease) manifested as pustules on the palms and soles. *Cutis.* 2004;74(2):107–110.

72. Buckley DA, Munn SE, Higgins EM. Neonatal eosinophilic pustular folliculitis. *Clin Exp Dermatol.* 2001;26(3):251–255.

73. Orfanos CE, Sterry W. Sterile eosinophile pustulose. *Dermatologica.* 1978;157:193.

74. Ooi CG, Walker P, Sidhu SK, Gordon LA, Marshman G. Allopurinol induced generalized eosinophilic pustular folliculitis. *Australas J Dermatol.* 2006;47(4):270–273.

75. Kishimoto S, Yamamoto M, Nomiyama T, Kawa K, Takenaka H, Tukitani K. Eosinophilic pustular folliculitis in association with nevoid basal cell carcinoma syndrome. *Acta Derm Venereol.* 2001;81(3):202–204.

76. Gul U, Kilic A, Demiriz M. Eosinophilic pustular folliculitis: the first case associated with hepatitis C virus. *J Dermatol.* 2007;34(6):397–399.

77. Opie KM, Heenan PJ, Delaney TA, Rohr JB. Two cases of eosinophilic pustular folliculitis associated with parasitic infestations. *Australas J Dermatol.* 2003;44(3):217–219.

78. Rosenthal D, LeBoit PE, Klumpp L, Berger TG. Human immunodeficiency virus associated eosinophilic folliculitis. *Arch Dermatol.* 1991;127:206.

79. Kimoto M, Ishihara S, Konohana A. Eosinophilic pustular folliculitis with polycythemia vera. *Dermatology.* 2005;210(3):239–240.

80. Keida T, Hayashi N, Kawashima M. Eosinophilic pustular folliculitis following autologous peripheral blood stem-cell transplantation. *J Dermatol.* 2004;31(1):21–26.

81. Nomura T, Katoh M, Yamamoto Y, Miyachi Y, Kabashima K. Eosinophilic pustular folliculitis: a proposal of diagnostic and therapeutic algorithms. *J Dermatol.* 2016;43(11):1301–1306. doi:10.1111/1346-8138.13359

82. McCalmont TH, Altemus O, Maurer T, Berger TG. Eosinophilic folliculitis. *Am J Dermatopathol.* 1995;17:439.

83. Ishiguro N, Shishido E, Okamoto R, Igarashi Y, Yamada M, Kawashima M. Ofuji's disease: a report on 20 patients with clinical and histopathologic analysis. *J Am Acad Dermatol.* 2002;46(6):827–833.

84. Basarab T, Jones RR. Ofuji's disease with unusual histological features. *Clin Exp Dermatol.* 1996;21:67–71.

85. Piantanida EW, Turiansky GW, Kenner JR, Mather MK, Sperling LC. HIV-associated eosinophilic folliculitis: diagnosis by transverse histologic sections. *J Am Acad Dermatol.* 1998;38(1):124–126.

86. Dupond AS, Aubin F, Bourezane Y, Faivre B, Van Landuyt H, Humbert PH. Eosinophilic pustular folliculitis in infancy: report of two affected brothers. *Br J Dermatol.* 1995;132:296–299.

87. Selvaag E, Thune P, Larsen TE, Roald B. Eosinophil cationic protein in eosinophilic pustular folliculitis: an immunohistochemical investigation. *Clin Exp Dermatol.* 1997;22:255–256.

88. Horiguchi Y, Mitani T, Ofuji S. The ultrastructural histopathology of eosinophilic pustular folliculitis. *J Dermatol.* 1992;19:201–207.

89. Anderson BE, Mackley CL, Helm KF. Alopecia mucinosa: report of a case and review. *J Cutan Med Surg.* 2003;7(2):124–128.

90. Van Doorn R, Scheffer E, Willemze R. Follicular mycosis fungoides, a distinct disease entity with or without associated follicular mucinosis: a clinicopathologic and follow-up study of 51 patients. *Arch Dermatol.* 2002;138(2):191–198.

91. Bonta MD, Tannous ZS, Demierre MF, Gonzalez E, Harris NL, Duncan LM. Rapidly progressing mycosis fungoides presenting as follicular mucinosis. *J Am Acad Dermatol.* 2000;43(4):635–640.

92. Geller S, Gomez CJ, Myskowski PL, Pulitzer M. Follicular mucinosis in patients with hematologic malignancies other than mycosis fungoides: a clinicopathologic study. *J Am Acad Dermatol.* 2019;80(6):1704–1711.

93. Cabré J, Korting GW. Zum symptomatischen charakter der "Mucinosis follicularis": Ihr Vorkommen beim Lupus erythematodes chronicus. *Dermatol Wochenschr.* 1964;149:513.

94. Fanti PA, Tosti A, Morelli R, Cameli N, Sabattini E, Pileri S. Follicular mucinosis in alopecia areata. *Am J Dermatopathol.* 1992;14:542.

95. Hempstead RW, Ackerman AB. Follicular mucinosis: a reaction pattern in follicular epithelium. *Am J Dermatopathol.* 1985;7:245.

96. Lazaro-Medina A, Tianco EA, Avila JM. Additional markers for the type I reactional states in borderline leprosy. *Am J Dermatol.* 1990;12:417.

97. Walchner M, Messer G, Rust A, Sander C, Röcken M. Follicular mucinosis in association with squamous cell carcinoma of the tongue. *J Am Acad Dermatol.* 1998;38(4):622–624.

98. Heymann WR. Predicting the nature of follicular mucinosis: still a sticky situation. *J Am Acad Dermatol.* 2019;80(6):1524–1525. doi:10.1016/j.jaad.2019.04.005

99. Cerroni L, Fink-Puches R, Back B, Kerl H. Follicular mucinosis: a critical reappraisal of clinicopathologic features and association with mycosis fungoides and Sezary syndrome. *Arch Dermatol.* 2002;138(2):182–189.

100. Gibson LE, Muller SA, Leiferman KM, Peters MS. Follicular mucinosis: clinical and histopathologic study. *J Am Acad Dermatol.* 1989;20:441.

101. Brown HA, Gibson LE, Pujol RM, Lust JA, Pittelkow MR. Primary follicular mucinosis: long-term follow-up of patients younger than 40 years with and without clonal T-cell receptor gene rearrangement. *J Am Acad Dermatol.* 2002;47(6):856–862.

102. Pinkus H. Alopecia mucinosa: inflammatory plaques with alopecia characterized by root sheath mucinosis. *Arch Dermatol.* 1957;76:419.

103. Boer A, Guo Y, Ackerman AB. Alopecia mucinosa is mycosis fungoides. *Am J Dermatopathol.* 2004;26(1):33–52.

104. LeBoit PE. Alopecia mucinosa, inflammatory disease or mycosis fungoides: must we choose? And are there other choices? *Am J Dermatopathol.* 2004;26(2):167–170.

105. Logan RA, Headington JT. Follicular mucinosis: a histologic review of 80 cases [abstract]. *J Cutan Pathol.* 1988;15:324.

106. Rongioletti F, De Lucchi S, Meyes D, Lust JA, Pittelkow MR. Follicular mucinosis: a clinicopathologic, histochemical, immunohistochemical and molecular study comparing the primary benign form and the mycosis fungoides-associated follicular mucinosis. *J Cutan Pathol.* 2010;37(1):15–19.

107. Ishibashi A. Histogenesis of mucin in follicular mucinosis: an electron microscopic study. *Acta Derm Venereol (Stockh).* 1976;56:163.

108. Wang JF, Orlow SJ. Keratosis pilaris and its subtypes: associations, new molecular and pharmacologic etiologies, and therapeutic options. *Am J Clin Dermatol.* 2018;19(5):733–757. doi:10.1007/s40257-018-0368-3

109. Marqueling AL, Gilliam AE, Prendiville J, et al. Keratosis pilaris rubra: a common but underrecognized condition. *Arch Dermatol.* 2006;142(12):1611–1616.

110. Alfadley A, Al Hawsawi K, Hainau B, Al Aboud K. Two brothers with keratosis follicularis spinulosa decalvans. *J Am Acad Dermatol.* 2002;47(5):S275–S278.

111. Romaine KA, Rothschild JG, Hansen RC. Cicatricial alopecia and keratosis pilaris: keratosis follicularis spinulosa decalvans. *Arch Dermatol.* 1997;133(3):381–384.

112. Nazarenko SA, Ostroverkhova NV, Vasiljeva EO, et al. Keratosis pilaris and ulerythema ophryogenes associated with an 18p deletion caused by a Y/18 translocation. *Am J Med Genet.* 1999;85(2):179–182.

113. Friedman SJ. Lichen spinulosus: a clinicopathologic review of thirty five cases. *J Am Acad Dermatol.* 1990;22:261.

114. Wang CM, Fleming KF, Hsu S. A case of vemurafenib-induced keratosis pilaris-like eruption. *Dermatol Online J.* 2012;18(4):7.

115. Harford RR, Cobb MW, Miller ML. Trichostasis spinulosa: a clinical simulant of acne open comedones. *Pediatr Dermatol.* 1996;13(6):490–492.

116. Kositkuljorn C, Suchonwanit P. Trichostasis spinulosa: a case report with an unusual presentation. *Case Rep Dermatol.* 2020;12(3):178–185.

117. Sidwell RU, Francis N, Bunker CB. Diffuse trichostasis spinulosa in chronic renal failure. *Clin Exp Dermatol.* 2006;31(1):86–88.

118. Chagas FS, Donati A, Soares II, Valente NS, Romiti R. Trichostasis spinulosa of the scalp mimicking alopecia areata black dots. *An Bras Dermatol.* 2014;89(4):685–687. doi:10.1590/abd1806-4841.20142407

119. Naveen KN, Shetty SR. Trichostasis spinulosa: an overlooked entity. *Indian Dermatol Online J.* 2014;5(suppl 2):S132–S133. doi:10.4103/2229-5178.146195

120. Miller JJ, Anderson BE, Ioffreda MD, Bongiovanni MB, Fogelberg AC. Hair casts and cutaneous spicules in multiple myeloma. *Arch Dermatol.* 2006;142(12):1665–1666.

121. Solomon AR. The transversely sectioned scalp biopsy specimen: the technique and an algorithm for its use in the diagnosis of alopecia. *Adv Dermatol.* 1994;9:127–157.

122. Mubki T, Rudnicka L, Olszewska M, Shapiro J. Evaluation and diagnosis of the hair loss patient. Part I: history and clinical examination. *J Am Acad Dermatol.* 2014;71(3):415.e1–415.e15. doi:10.1016/j.jaad.2014.04.070

123. Whiting DA, Dy LC. Office diagnosis of hair shaft defects. *Semin Cutan Med Surg.* 2006;25(1):24–34.

124. Whiting DA. Structural abnormalities of the hair shaft. *J Am Acad Dermatol.* 1987;16(1):1–25.

125. Dawber RPR. An update of hair shaft disorders. In: Whiting DA, ed. *Dermatologic Clinics.* Vol 14. WB Saunders; 1996:753–772.

126. Sperling LC. Scarring alopecia and the dermatopathologist. *J Cutan Pathol.* 2001;28(7):333–342.

127. Headington JT. Transverse microscopic anatomy of the human scalp. *Arch Dermatol.* 1984;120:449–456.

128. Elston DM, McCollough ML, Angeloni VL. Vertical and transverse sections of alopecia biopsy specimens: combining the two to maximize diagnostic yield. *J Am Acad Dermatol.* 1995;32(3):454–457.

129. Frishberg DP, Sperling LC, Guthrie VM. Transverse scalp sections: a proposed method for laboratory processing. *J Am Acad Dermatol.* 1996;35(2):220–222.

130. Olsen EA, Bergfeld WF, Cotsarelis G, et al. Summary of North American Hair Research Society (NAHRS)—sponsored Workshop on Cicatricial Alopecia, Duke University Medical Center, February 10 and 11, 2001. *J Am Acad Dermatol.* 2003;48(1):103–110.

131. Nguyen JV, Hudacek K, Whitten JA, Rubin AI, Seykora JT. The HoVert technique: a novel method for the sectioning of alopecia biopsies. *J Cutan Pathol.* 2011;38(5):401–406.

132. Elston D. The "Tyler technique" for alopecia biopsies. *J Cutan Pathol.* 2012;39(2):306.

133. Sperling LC. Hair anatomy for the clinician. *J Am Acad Dermatol.* 1991;25:1–17.

134. Childs JM, Sperling LC. Histopathology of scarring and nonscarring hair loss. *Dermatol Clin.* 2013;31(1):43–56.

135. Milner Y, Sudnik J, Filippi M, Kizoulis M, Kashgarian M, Stenn K. Exogen, shedding phase of the hair growth cycle: characterization of a mouse model. *J Invest Dermatol.* 2002;119(3):639–644.

136. Rebora A, Guarrera M. Kenogen: a new phase of the hair cycle? *Dermatology.* 2002;205(2):108–110.

137. Solomon AR, Templeton SF. Alopecia. In: Farmer ER, Hood AF, eds. *Pathology of the Skin.* 2nd ed. McGraw-Hill; 2000.

138. Sperling LC. Evaluation of hair loss. *Curr Probl Dermatol.* 1996;8:97–136.

139. Whiting DA. Diagnostic and predictive value of horizontal sections of scalp biopsy specimens in male pattern androgenetic alopecia. *J Am Acad Dermatol.* 1993;28:755.

140. Sperling LL, Lupton GP. Histopathology of non-scarring alopecia. *J Cutan Pathol.* 1995;22:97.

141. Horenstein MG, Bacheler CJ. Follicular density and ratios in scarring and nonscarring alopecia. *Am J Dermatopathol.* 2013;35(8):818–826. doi:10.1097/DAD.0b013e3182827fc7

142. Sperling LC. Hair density in African Americans. *Arch Dermatol.* 1999;135(6):656–658.

143. Sperling L, Cowper S, Knopp E. *An Atlas of Hair Pathology with Clinical Correlations.* Informa Healthcare; 2012.

144. Lee HJ, Ha SJ, Lee JH, Kim JW, Kim HO, Whiting DA. Hair counts from scalp biopsy specimens in Asians. *J Am Acad Dermatol.* 2002;46(2):218–221.

145. Whiting DA. Possible mechanisms of miniaturization during androgenetic alopecia or pattern hair loss. *J Am Acad Dermatol.* 2001;45(3):S81–S86.

146. Eudy G, Solomon AR. The histopathology of noncicatricial alopecia. *Semin Cutan Med Surg.* 2006;25(1):35–40.

147. Stefanato CM. Histopathology of alopecia: a clinicopathological approach to diagnosis. *Histopathology.* 2010;56(1):24–38.

148. Chartier MB, Hoss DM, Grant-Kels JM. Approach to the adult female patient with diffuse nonscarring alopecia. *J Am Acad Dermatol.* 2002;47(6):809–818.

149. Werner B, Mulinari-Brenner F. Clinical and histological challenge in the differential diagnosis of diffuse alopecia: female androgenetic alopecia, telogen effluvium and alopecia areata—part I. *An Bras Dermatol.* 2012;87(5):742–747.

150. Gilhar A, Etzioni A, Paus R. Alopecia areata. *N Engl J Med.* 2012;366(16):1515–1525.

151. Alkhalifah A. Alopecia areata update. *Dermatol Clin.* 2013;31(1):93–108.

152. Madani S, Shapiro J. Alopecia areata update. *J Am Acad Dermatol.* 2000;42(4):549–566.

153. Headington JT, Mitchell A, Swanson N. New histopathologic findings in alopecia areata studied in transverse section. *J Invest Dermatol.* 1981;76:325.

154. Ihm CW, Hong SS, Mun JH, Kim HU. Histopathological pictures of the initial changes of the hair bulbs in alopecia areata. *Am J Dermatopathol.* 2004;26(3):249–253.

155. Peckham SJ, Sloan SB, Elston DM. Histologic features of alopecia areata other than peribulbar lymphocytic infiltrates. *J Am Acad Dermatol.* 2011;65(3):615–620.

156. Hanly AJ, Jorda M, Badiavas E, Valencia I, Elgart GW. Postoperative pressure-induced alopecia: report of a case and discussion of the role of apoptosis in non-scarring alopecia. *J Cutan Pathol.* 1999;26(7):357–361.

157. Whiting DA. Histopathology of alopecia areata in horizontal sections of scalp biopsies. *J Invest Dermatol.* 1995;104(5):27S–28S.

158. Abell E, Gruber HM. A histopathologic reappraisal of alopecia areata. *J Cutan Pathol.* 1987;14:347.

159. Whiting DA. Histopathologic features of alopecia areata: a new look. *Arch Dermatol.* 2003;139:1555.

160. Elston DM, McCollough ML, Bergfeld WF, Liranzo MO, Heibel M. Eosinophils in fibrous tracts and near hair bulbs: a helpful diagnostic feature of alopecia areata. *J Am Acad Dermatol.* 1997;37(1):101–106.

161. Muller CS, El Shabrawi-Caelen L. "Follicular Swiss cheese" pattern—another histopathologic clue to alopecia areata. *J Cutan Pathol.* 2011;38(2):185–189.

162. Tosti A, Whiting D, Iorizzo M, et al. The role of scalp dermoscopy in the diagnosis of alopecia areata incognita. *J Am Acad Dermatol.* 2008;59(1):64–67.

163. Norris D. Alopecia areata: current state of knowledge. *J Am Acad Dermatol.* 2004;51(1, suppl):S16–S17.

164. Kalish RS, Gilhar A. Alopecia areata: autoimmunity—the evidence is compelling. *J Investig Dermatol Symp Proc.* 2003;8(2):164–167.

165. Strazzulla LC, Wang EHC, Avila L, et al. Alopecia areata: disease characteristics, clinical evaluation, and new perspectives on pathogenesis. *J Am Acad Dermatol.* 2018;78(1):1–12. doi:10.1016/j.jaad.2017.04.1141

166. McElwee KJ, Hoffmann R. Alopecia areata—animal models. *Clin Exp Dermatol.* 2002;27(5):410–417.

167. Sundberg JP, Cordy WR, King LE. Alopecia areata in aging C3H/HeJ mice. *J Invest Dermatol.* 1994;102:847–856.

168. Michie HJ, Jahoda CAB, Oliver RF, Johnson BE. The DEBR rat: an animal model of human alopecia areata. *Br J Dermatol.* 1991;125:94–100.

169. Smyth JR Jr, McNeil M. Alopecia areata and universalis in the Smyth chicken model for spontaneous autoimmune vitiligo. *J Invest Dermatol.* 1999;4(3):211–215.

170. Duvic M, Nelson A, de Andrade M. The genetics of alopecia areata. *Clin Dermatol.* 2001;19(2):135–139.

171. Shellow WV, Edwards JE, Koo JY. Profile of alopecia areata: a questionnaire analysis of patient and family. *Int J Dermatol.* 1992;31:186–189.

172. Scerri L, Pace JL. Identical twins with identical alopecia areata. *J Am Acad Dermatol.* 1992;27:766–767.

173. Pratt CH, King LE Jr, Messenger AG, Christiano AM, Sundberg JP. Alopecia areata. *Nat Rev Dis Primers.* 2017;3:17011. doi:10.1038/nrdp.2017.11

174. Tobin DJ, Hann SK, Song MS, Bystryn JC. Hair follicle structures targeted by antibodies in patients with alopecia areata. *Arch Dermatol.* 1997;133(1):57–61.

175. Tobin DJ, Orentreich N, Fenton DA, Bystryn JC. Antibodies to hair follicles in alopecia areata. *J Invest Dermatol.* 1994;102:166–171.

176. Gilhar A, Landau M, Assy B, Shalaginov R, Serafimovich S, Kalish RS. Mediation of alopecia areata by cooperation between CD4+ and CD8+ T lymphocytes: transfer to human scalp explants on Prkdc(scid) mice. *Arch Dermatol.* 2002;138(7):916–922.

177. Paus R. Immunology of the hair follicle. In: Bos JD, ed. *The Skin Immune System.* CRC Press; 1997:377–398.

178. Paus R, Ito N, Takigawa M, Ito T. The hair follicle and immune privilege. *J Investig Dermatol Symp Proc.* 2003;8(2):188–194.

179. Hordinsky M, Kennedy W, Wendelschafer-Crabb G, Lewis S. Structure and function of cutaneous nerves in alopecia areata. *J Invest Dermatol.* 1995;104(suppl):28S–29S.

180. Lee JYY, Hsu ML. Alopecia syphilitica, a simulator of alopecia areata: histopathology and differential diagnosis. *J Cutan Pathol.* 1991;18:87.

181. Afanasiev OK, Zhang CZ, Ruhoy SM. TNF-inhibitor associated psoriatic alopecia: diagnostic utility of sebaceous lobule atrophy. *J Cutan Pathol.* 2017;44(6):563–569. doi:10.1111/cup.12932

182. Nuss MA, Carlisle D, Hall M, Yerneni SC, Kovach R. Trichotillomania: a review and case report. *Cutis.* 2003;72(3):191–196.

183. Walsh KH, McDougle CJ. Trichotillomania: presentation, etiology, diagnosis and therapy. *Am J Clin Dermatol.* 2001;2(5):327–333.

184. Hautmann G, Hercogova J, Lotti T. Trichotillomania. *J Am Acad Dermatol.* 2002;46(6):807–821; quiz 822–826.

185. Grant JE, Chamberlain SR. Trichotillomania. *Am J Psychiatry.* 2016;173(9):868–874.

186. Du Toit PL, van Kradenburg J, Niehaus DJ, Stein DJ. Characteristics and phenomenology of hair-pulling: an exploration of subtypes. *Compr Psychiatry.* 2001;42(3):247–256.

187. Royer MC, Sperling LC. Splitting hairs: the "hamburger sign" in trichotillomania. *J Cutan Pathol.* 2006;33(suppl 2):63–64.

188. Elston DM. What's new in the histologic evaluation of alopecia and hair-related disorders? *Dermatol Clin.* 2012;30(4):685–694, vii.

189. Muller SA. Trichotillomania: a histopathologic study in sixty-six patients. *J Am Acad Dermatol.* 1990;23:56.

190. Kaur H, Chavan BS, Raj L. Management of trichotillomania. *Indian J Psychiatry.* 2005;47(4):235–237.

191. Olsen EA. Androgenetic alopecia. In: Olsen EA, ed. *Disorders of Hair Growth.* McGraw-Hill; 2003.

192. Fox GN, Stausmire JM, Mehregan DR. Traction folliculitis: an underreported entity. *Cutis.* 2007;79(1):26–30.

193. Billero V, Miteva M. Traction alopecia: the root of the problem. *Clin Cosmet Investig Dermatol.* 2018;11:149–159. doi:10.2147/CCID.S137296

194. Hwang SM, Lee WS, Choi EH, Lee SH, Ahn SK. Nurse's cap alopecia. *Int J Dermatol.* 1999;38(3):187–191.

195. Akingbola CO, Vyas J. Traction alopecia: a neglected entity in 2017. *Indian J Dermatol Venereol Leprol.* 2017;83(6):644–649. doi:10.4103/ijdvl.IJDVL_553_16

196. Grossman KL, Kvedar JC. Anagen hair loss. In: Olsen EA, ed. *Disorders of Hair Growth.* McGraw-Hill; 2003.

197. Daneshpazhooh M, Mahmoudi HR, Rezakhani S, et al. Loss of normal anagen hair in pemphigus vulgaris. *Clin Exp Dermatol.* 2015;40(5):485–488.

198. Delmonte S, Semino MT, Parodi A, Rebora A. Normal anagen effluvium: a sign of pemphigus vulgaris. *Br J Dermatol.* 2000;142(6):1244–1245.

199. Kligman AM. Pathologic dynamics of human hair loss, I: telogen effluvium. *Arch Dermatol.* 1961;83:175.

200. Headington JT. Telogen effluvium. *Arch Dermatol.* 1993;129:356.

201. Fiedler VC, Hafeez A. Diffuse alopecia: telogen hair loss. In: Olsen E, ed. *Disorders of Hair Growth.* McGraw-Hill; 2003.

202. Tosti A, Piraccini BM, van Neste DJ. Telogen effluvium after allergic contact dermatitis of the scalp. *Arch Dermatol.* 2001;137(2):187–190.

203. Whiting DA. Chronic telogen effluvium: increased scalp hair shedding in middle-aged women. *J Am Acad Dermatol.* 1996;35(6):899–906.

204. Whiting DA. Chronic telogen effluvium. *Dermatol Clin.* 1996;14(4):723–731.

205. Sinclair R. Chronic telogen effluvium: a study of 5 patients over 7 years. *J Am Acad Dermatol.* 2005;52(2, suppl 1):12–16.

206. Thai KE, Sinclair RD. Chronic telogen effluvium in a man. *J Am Acad Dermatol.* 2002;47(4):605–607.

207. Bittencourt C, Ferraro DA, Soares TC, Moraes AM, Cintra ML. Chronic telogen effluvium and female pattern hair loss are separate and distinct forms of alopecia: a histomorphometric and immunohistochemical analysis. *Clin Exp Dermatol.* 2014;39(8):868–873. doi:10.1111/ced.12406

208. Sinclair R, Jolley D, Mallari R, Magee J. The reliability of horizontally sectioned scalp biopsies in the diagnosis of chronic diffuse telogen hair loss in women. *J Am Acad Dermatol.* 2004;51(2):189–199.

209. Chien Yin GO, Siong-See JL, Wang ECE. Telogen effluvium—a review of the science and current obstacles. *J Dermatol Sci.* 2021;101(3):156–163. doi:10.1016/j.jdermsci.2021.01.007

210. Pierard-Franchimont C, Pierard GE. Teloptosis, a turning point in hair shedding biorhythms. *Dermatology.* 2001;203(2):115–117.

211. Birch MP, Lalla SC, Messenger AG. Female pattern hair loss. *Clin Exp Dermatol.* 2002;27(5):383–388.

212. Olsen EA. Female pattern hair loss. *J Am Acad Dermatol.* 2001;45(3):S70–S80.

213. Hoffmann R, Happle R. Current understanding of androgenetic alopecia. Part II: clinical aspects and treatment. *Eur J Dermatol.* 2000;10(5):410–417.

214. Rocahel MC, Ackerman AB. Common baldness an inflammatory disease? *Dermatopathol Pract Concept.* 1999;5(4):319–322.

215. Ellis JA, Harrap SB. The genetics of androgenetic alopecia. *Clin Dermatol.* 2001;19(2):149–154.

216. Sperling LC, Winton GB. The transverse anatomy of androgenetic alopecia. *J Dermatol Surg Oncol.* 1990;16:1127.

217. Headington JT, Novak E. Clinical and histologic studies of male pattern baldness treated with topical minoxidil. *Curr Ther Res.* 1984;36:1098.

218. Whiting DA. Diagnostic and predictive value of horizontal sections of scalp biopsies in male pattern androgenetic alopecia. *J Cutan Pathol.* 1990;17:325.

219. Hoss D, Berke A, Murphy M, Kerr P, Grant-Kels J. Acid-fast (Ziehl-Neelsen) staining facilitates follicular counting in horizontally-sectioned scalp biopsies. *J Cutan Pathol.* 2005; 32:93.

220. Torkamani N, Rufaut NW, Jones L, Sinclair R. Destruction of the arrector pili muscle and fat infiltration in androgenic alopecia. *Br J Dermatol.* 2014;170(6):1291–1298. doi:10.1111/bjd.12921

221. Paus R, Cotsarelis G. The biology of hair follicles. *N Engl J Med.* 1999;341(7):491–497.

222. Jaworsky C, Kligman AM, Murphy GF. Characterization of inflammatory infiltrates in male pattern alopecia: implications for pathogenesis. *Br J Dermatol.* 1992;127:239–246.

223. Olsen EA. Female pattern hair loss and its relationship to permanent/cicatricial alopecia: a new perspective. *J Investig Dermatol Symp Proc.* 2005;10(3):217–221.

224. Abell E. Pathology of male pattern alopecia. *Arch Dermatol.* 1984;120:1607.

225. Kligman AM. The comparative histopathology of male-pattern baldness and senescent baldness. *Clin Dermatol.* 1988;6:108.

226. Deloche C, de Lacharriere O, Misciali C, et al. Histological features of peripilar signs associated with androgenetic alopecia. *Arch Dermatol Res.* 2004;295(10):422–428.

227. Oliveira I, Messenger AG. The hair follicle: a paradoxical androgen target organ. *Horm Res.* 2000;54(5–6):243–250.

228. Trueb RM. Molecular mechanisms of androgenetic alopecia. *Exp Gerontol.* 2002;37(8–9):981–990.

229. Sawaya ME, Price VH. Different levels of 5alpha-reductase type I and II, aromatase, and androgen receptor in hair follicles of women and men with androgenetic alopecia. *J Invest Dermatol.* 1997;109(3):296–300.

230. Bayne EK, Flanagan J, Einstein M, et al. Immunohistochemical localization of types 1 and 2 5alpha-reductase in human scalp. *Br J Dermatol.* 1999;141(3):481–491.

231. Hoffmann R, Rot A, Niiyama S, Billich A. Steroid sulfatase in the human hair follicle concentrates in the dermal papilla. *J Invest Dermatol.* 2001;117(6):1342–1348.

232. Happle R, Hoffmann R. Absence of male-pattern baldness in men with X-linked recessive ichthyosis? A hypothesis to be challenged. *Dermatology.* 1999;198(3):231–232.

233. Randall VA, Hibberts NA, Hamada K. A comparison of the culture and growth of dermal papilla cells from hair follicles from non-balding and balding (androgenetic alopecia) scalp. *Br J Dermatol.* 1996;134(3):437–444.

234. Whiting DA. Chronic telogen effluvium: increased scalp hair shedding in middle-aged women [comment]. *J Am Acad Dermatol.* 1997;37(6):1021.

235. Millikan LE. Androgenetic alopecia: the role of inflammation and Demodex. *Int J Dermatol.* 2001;40(7):475–476.

236. Tan E, Martinka M, Ball N, Shapiro J. Primary cicatricial alopecias: clinicopathology of 112 cases. *J Am Acad Dermatol.* 2004;50(1):25–32.

237. Sperling LC, Cowper SE. The histopathology of primary cicatricial alopecia. *Semin Cutan Med Surg.* 2006;25(1):41–50.

238. Sellheyer K, Bergfeld WF. Histopathologic evaluation of alopecias. *Am J Dermatopathol.* 2006;28(3):236–259.

239. Bolduc C, Sperling LC, Shapiro J. Primary cicatricial alopecia: other lymphocytic primary cicatricial alopecias and neutrophilic and mixed primary cicatricial alopecias. *J Am Acad Dermatol.* 2016;75(6):1101–1117.

240. Olsen E, Stenn K, Bergfeld W, et al. Update on cicatricial alopecia [erratum appears in *J Investig Dermatol Symp Proc.* 2004;123(4):805]. *J Investig Dermatol Symp Proc.* 2003;8(1):18–19.

241. Harries MJ, Paus R. The pathogenesis of primary cicatricial alopecias. *Am J Pathol.* 2010;177(5):2152–2162.

242. Sperling LC, Solomon AR, Whiting DA. A new look at scarring alopecia [comment]. *Arch Dermatol.* 2000;136(2):235–242.

243. Modly CE, Wood CM, Burnett JW. Evaluation of alopecia: a new algorithm. *Cutis.* 1989;43:148–152.

244. Elston DM, Bergfeld WF. Cicatricial alopecia (and other causes of permanent alopecia). In: Olsen EA, ed. *Disorders of Hair Growth.* McGraw-Hill; 2003.

245. Tan T, Guitart J, Gerami P, Yazdan P. Elastic staining in differentiating between follicular streamers and follicular scars in horizontal scalp biopsy sections. *Am J Dermatopathol.* 2018;40(4):254–258.

246. Tan TL, Doytcheva K, Guitart J, Gerami P, Yazdan P. Dilation of multiple eccrine ducts as a highly specific marker for cicatricial alopecia. *Am J Dermatopathol.* 2019;41(12):871–878. doi:10.1097/DAD.0000000000001396

247. Doytcheva K, Tan T, Guitart J, Gerami P, Yazdan P. Naked hair shafts as a marker of cicatricial alopecia. *Am J Dermatopathol.* 2018;40(7):498–501. doi:10.1097/DAD.0000000000001075

248. Elston DM, McCollough ML, Warschaw KE, Bergfeld WF. Elastic tissue in scars and alopecia. *J Cutan Pathol.* 2000;27(3):147–152.

249. Fung M, Sharon V, Ratnarathorn M, Konia TH, Barr KL, Mirmirani P. Elastin staining patterns in primary cicatricial alopecia. *J Am Acad Dermatol.* 2013;69(5):776–782.

250. Elston CA, Kazlouskaya V, Elston DM. Elastic staining versus fluorescent and polarized microscopy in the diagnosis of alopecia. *J Am Acad Dermatol.* 2013;69(2):288–293.

251. Elston DM. Demodex mites as a cause of human disease [comment]. *Cutis.* 2005;76(5):294–296.

252. Mirmirani P, Willey A, Headington JT, Stenn K, McCalmont TH, Price VH. Primary cicatricial alopecia: histopathologic findings do not distinguish clinical variants. *J Am Acad Dermatol.* 2005;52(4):637–643.

253. Headington JT. Cicatricial alopecia. *Dermatol Clin.* 1996;14(4):773–782.

254. Halley-Stott RP, Adeola HA, Khumalo NP. Destruction of the stem cell niche, pathogenesis and promising treatment targets for primary scarring alopecias. *Stem Cell Rev Rep.* 2020;16(6):1105–1120. doi:10.1007/s12015-020-09985-6

255. Stenn KS, Sundberg JP, Sperling LC. Hair follicle biology, the sebaceous gland, and scarring alopecias. *Arch Dermatol.* 1999;135:973–974.

256. Stenn KS. Insights from the asebia mouse: a molecular sebaceous gland defect leading to cicatricial alopecia. *J Cutan Pathol.* 2001;28(9):445–447.

257. Ramos-e-Silva M, Pirmez R. Disorders of hair growth and the pilosebaceous unit: facts and controversies. *Clin Dermatol.* 2013;31(6):759–763. doi:10.1016/j.clindermatol.2013.06.003

258. Salim A, Dawber R. A multiparametric approach is essential to define different clinicopathological entities within pseudopelade of Brocq. *Br J Dermatol.* 2003;148(6):1271; author reply 1271–1272.

259. Braun-Falco O, Imai S, Schmoeckel C, Steger O, Bergner T. Pseudopelade of Brocq. *Dermatologica.* 1986;172:18.

260. Sullivan JR, Kossard S. Acquired scalp alopecia, part I: a review. *Australas J Dermatol.* 1998;39(4):207–219; quiz 220–221.

261. Alzolibani AA, Kang H, Otberg N, Shapiro J. Pseudopelade of Brocq. *Dermatol Ther.* 2008;21(4):257–263.

262. Elston DM, Bergfeld WF. Pseudopelade of Brocq. In: Olsen EA, ed. *Disorders of Hair Growth.* McGraw-Hill; 2003.

263. Brocq L. Alopecia. *J Cutan Vener Dis.* 1885;3:49–50.

264. Brocq L, Lenglet E, Ayrignac J. Recherches sur l'alopecie atrophiante, variete pseudopelade. *Ann Dermatol Syphilol (France).* 1905;6(1):209.

265. Dawber R. What is pseudopelade? *Clin Exp Dermatol.* 1992;17:305–306.

266. Pinkus H. Differential patterns of elastic fibers in scarring and non-scarring alopecias. *J Cutan Pathol.* 1978;5:93.

267. Braun-Falco O, Bergner T, Heilgemeir GP. Pseudopelade Brocq-krankheitsbild oder krankheitsentität. *Hautarzt.* 1989;40:77.

268. Degos R, Rabut R, Duperrat B, et al. L'etat pseudopeladique. *Ann Dermatol Syphilol (France).* 1954;81:5.

269. Amato L, Mei S, Massi D, et al. Cicatricial alopecia; a dermatopathologic and immunopathologic study of 33 patients (pseudopelade of Brocq is not a specific clinico-pathologic entity). *Int J Dermatol.* 2002;41(1):8–15.

270. Silvers DN, Katz BE, Young AW. Pseudopelade of Brocq is lichen planopilaris: report of four cases that support this nosology. *Cutis.* 1993;51:99–105.

271. Pierard-Franchimont C, Pierard GE. Massive lymphocyte-mediated apoptosis during the early stage of pseudopelade. *Dermatologica.* 1986;172:254.

272. Otberg N, Wu WY, McElwee KJ, Shapiro J. Diagnosis and management of primary cicatricial alopecia: part I. *Skinmed.* 2008;7(1):19–26.

273. Shah SK, Alexis AF. Central centrifugal cicatricial alopecia: retrospective chart review. *J Cutan Med Surg.* 2010;14(5):212–222.

274. Olsen EA, Callender V, Sperling L, et al. Central scalp alopecia photographic scale in African American women. *Dermatol Ther.* 2008;21(4):264–267.

275. Horenstein MG, Simon J. Investigation of the hair follicle inner root sheath in scarring and non-scarring alopecia. *J Cutan Pathol.* 2007;34(10):762–768.

276. Sperling LC. Premature desquamation of the inner root sheath is still a useful concept! *J Cutan Pathol.* 2007;34(10):809–810.

277. Tan T, Guitart J, Gerami P, Yazdan P. Premature desquamation of the inner root sheath in noninflamed hair follicles as a specific marker for central centrifugal cicatricial alopecia. *Am J Dermatopathol.* 2019;41(5):350–354.

278. Fernandez-Flores A. Use of Giemsa staining in the evaluation of central centrifugal cicatricial alopecia. *J Cutan Pathol.* 2020;47(5):496–499.

279. Dina Y, Borhan W, Erdag G, et al. Preservation of sebaceous glands and peroxisome proliferator-activated receptor gamma expression in central centrifugal cicatricial alopecia. *J Am Acad Dermatol.* 2021;85(2):489–490.

280. Roche FC, Fischer AS, Williams D, Ogunleye T, Seykora JT, Taylor SC. Central centrifugal cicatricial alopecia: histologic progression correlates with advancing age. *J Am Acad Dermatol.* 2022;86(1):178–179.

281. Flamm A, Moshiri AS, Roche F, et al. Characterization of the inflammatory features of central centrifugal cicatricial alopecia. *J Cutan Pathol.* 2020;47(6):530–534. doi:10.1111/cup.13666

282. Sperling LC, Hussey S, Wang JA, Darling T. Cytokeratin 15 expression in central, centrifugal, cicatricial alopecia: new observations in normal and diseased hair follicles. *J Cutan Pathol.* 2011;38(5):407–414.

283. Sperling LC, Sau P. The follicular degeneration syndrome in black patients: "hot comb alopecia" revisited and revised. *Arch Dermatol.* 1992;128:68–74.

284. Gathers RC, Lim HW. Central centrifugal cicatricial alopecia: past, present, and future. *J Am Acad Dermatol.* 2009;60(4):660–668.

285. Olsen EA, Callender V, McMichael A, et al. Central hair loss in African American women: incidence and potential risk factors. *J Am Acad Dermatol.* 2011;64(2):245–252.

286. Kyei A, Bergfeld WF, Piliang M, Summers P. Medical and environmental risk factors for the development of central centrifugal cicatricial alopecia: a population study. *Arch Dermatol.* 2011;147(8):909–914.

287. Malki L, Sarig O, Romano MT, et al. Variant *PADI3* in central centrifugal cicatricial alopecia. *N Engl J Med.* 2019;380(9): 833–841.

288. Aguh C, Dina Y, Talbot CC Jr, Garza L. Fibroproliferative genes are preferentially expressed in central centrifugal cicatricial alopecia. *J Am Acad Dermatol.* 2018;79(5):904–912.e1.

289. Subash J, Alexander T, Beamer V, McMichael A. A proposed mechanism for central centrifugal cicatricial alopecia. *Exp Dermatol.* 2020;29(2):190–195.

290. LoPresti P, Papa C, Kligman A. Hot comb alopecia. *Arch Dermatol.* 1968;98:234.

291. Summers P, Kyei A, Bergfeld W. Central centrifugal cicatricial alopecia—an approach to diagnosis and management. *Int J Dermatol.* 2011;50(12):1457–1464.

292. Lawson CN, Bakayoko A, Callender VD. Central centrifugal cicatricial alopecia: challenges and treatments. *Dermatol Clin.* 2021;39(3):389–405.

293. Whiting DA, Olsen EA. Central centrifugal cicatricial alopecia. *Dermatol Ther.* 2008;21(4):268–278.

294. Templeton SF, Solomon AR. Scarring alopecia: a classification based upon microscopic criteria. *J Cutan Pathol.* 1994;21:97.

295. Annessi G. Tufted folliculitis of the scalp: a distinctive clinicohistological variant of folliculitis decalvans. *Br J Dermatol.* 1999;140(5):975–976.

296. Karakuzu A, Erdem T, Aktas A, Atasoy M, Gulec AI. A case of folliculitis decalvans involving the beard, face and nape. *J Dermatol.* 2001;28(6):329–331.

297. Elston DM, Bergfeld WF. Erosive pustular dermatosis and folliculitis decalvans. In: Olsen EA, ed. *Disorders of Hair Growth.* McGraw-Hill; 2003.

298. Powell JJ, Dawber RPR, Gatter K. Folliculitis decalvans including tufted folliculitis: clinical, histological and therapeutic findings. *Br J Dermatol.* 1999;140:328–333.

299. Matard B, Cavelier-Balloy B, Reygagne P. Epidermal psoriasiform hyperplasia, an unrecognized sign of folliculitis decalvans: a histological study of 26 patients. *J Cutan Pathol.* 2017;44(4): 352–357.

300. Bohnett MC, Kolivras A, Thompson AA, Thompson CT. Epidermal thickness is useful in distinguishing lichen planopilaris from neutrophil-poor/lymphocyte-predominant folliculitis decalvans. *J Cutan Pathol.* 2021;48(6):816–818.

301. Brooke RCC, Griffiths CEM. Folliculitis decalvans. *Clin Exp Dermatol.* 2001;26:120–122.

302. Samrao A, Mirmirani P. Gram-negative infections in patients with folliculitis decalvans: a subset of patients requiring alternative treatment. *Dermatol Online J.* 2020;26(2):13030/qt6nw2h5rh

303. Wu WY, Otberg N, McElwee KJ, Shapiro J. Diagnosis and management of primary cicatricial alopecia: part II. *Skinmed.* 2008;7(2):78–83.

304. Otberg N, Kang H, Alzolibani AA, Shapiro J. Folliculitis decalvans. *Dermatol Ther.* 2008;21(4):238–244.

305. Bunagan MJ, Banka N, Shapiro J. Retrospective review of folliculitis decalvans in 23 patients with course and treatment analysis of long-standing cases. *J Cutan Med Surg.* 2015;19(1):45–49. doi:10.2310/7750.2014.13218

306. Powell J, Dawber RP. Folliculitis decalvans and tufted folliculitis are specific infective diseases that may lead to scarring, but are not a subset of central centrifugal scarring alopecia. *Arch Dermatol.* 2001;137(3):373–374.

307. Elston DM. Tufted folliculitis. *J Cutan Pathol.* 2011;38(7):595–596.

308. Fernandes JC, Correia TM, Azevedo F, Mesquita-Guimarães J. Tufted hair folliculitis after scalp injury. *Cutis.* 2001;67(3): 243–245.

309. Petroni-Rosi V, Kruni A, Mijuskovi M, Vesić S. Tufted hair folliculitis: a pattern of scarring alopecia? *J Am Acad Dermatol.* 1999;41(1):112–114.

310. Kasuya A, Ito T, Hanai S, Phadungsaksawasdi P, Tokura Y. A steric structure of tufted hair folliculitis. *J Dermatol Sci.* 2020;97(1): 83–85.

311. Dalziel KL, Telfer NR, Wilson CL, Dawber RP. Tufted folliculitis: a specific bacterial disease? *Am J Dermatopathol.* 1990;12: 37–41.

312. Pincus LB, Price VH, McCalmont TH. The amount counts: distinguishing neutrophil-mediated and lymphocyte-mediated cicatricial alopecia by compound follicles. *J Cutan Pathol.* 2011;38(1):1–4.

313. Cevasco NC, Bergfeld WF, Remzi BK, de Knott HR. A case-series of 29 patients with lichen planopilaris: the Cleveland Clinic Foundation experience on evaluation, diagnosis, and treatment. *J Am Acad Dermatol.* 2007;57(1):47–53.

314. Bolduc C, Sperling LC, Shapiro J. Primary cicatricial alopecia: lymphocytic primary cicatricial alopecias, including chronic cutaneous lupus erythematosus, lichen planopilaris, frontal fibrosing alopecia, and Graham-Little syndrome. *J Am Acad Dermatol.* 2016;75(6):1081–1099. doi:10.1016/j.jaad.2014.09.058

315. Tandon YK, Somani N, Cevasco NC, Bergfeld WF. A histologic review of 27 patients with lichen planopilaris. *J Am Acad Dermatol.* 2008;59(1):91–98.

316. Mobini N, Tam S, Kamino H. Possible role of the bulge region in the pathogenesis of inflammatory scarring alopecia: lichen planopilaris as the prototype. *J Cutan Pathol.* 2005;32(10): 675–679.

317. Lanoue J, Yanofsky VR, Mercer SE, Phelps RG. The use of anti-keratin 903 antibodies to visualize colloid bodies and diagnose lichen planopilaris. *Am J Dermatopathol.* 2016;38(5): 353–358.

318. Kossard S. Postmenopausal frontal fibrosing alopecia: scarring alopecia in a pattern distribution. *Arch Dermatol.* 1994;130: 770–774.

319. Kossard S, Lee MS, Wilkinson B. Postmenopausal frontal fibrosing alopecia: a frontal variant of lichen planopilaris. *J Am Acad Dermatol.* 1997;36(1):59–66.

320. Tosti A, Piraccini BM, Iorizzo M, Misciali C. Frontal fibrosing alopecia in postmenopausal women. *J Am Acad Dermatol.* 2005;52(1):55–60.

321. Kerkemeyer KLS, Eisman S, Bhoyrul B, Pinczewski J, Sinclair RD. Frontal fibrosing alopecia. *Clin Dermatol.* 2021;39(2): 183–193. doi:10.1016/j.clindermatol.2020.10.007

322. Chew AL, Bashir SJ, Wain EM, Fenton DA, Stefanato CM. Expanding the spectrum of frontal fibrosing alopecia: a unifying concept. *J Am Acad Dermatol.* 2010;63(4):653–660.

323. Miteva M, Camacho I, Romanelli P, Tosti A. Acute hair loss on the limbs in frontal fibrosing alopecia: a clinicopathological study of two cases. *Br J Dermatol.* 2010;163(2):426–428.

324. Fernandez-Flores A, Manjón JA. Histopathology of keratotic papules of the limbs in frontal fibrosing alopecia. *J Cutan Pathol.* 2016;43(5):468–471.

325. Donati A, Molina L, Doche I, Valente NS, Romiti R. Facial papules in frontal fibrosing alopecia: evidence of vellus follicle involvement. *Arch Dermatol.* 2011;147(12):1424–1427.

326. Miteva M, Tosti A. The follicular triad: a pathological clue to the diagnosis of early frontal fibrosing alopecia. *Br J Dermatol.* 2012;166(2):440–442.

327. Wong D, Goldberg LJ. The depth of inflammation in frontal fibrosing alopecia and lichen planopilaris: a potential distinguishing feature. *J Am Acad Dermatol.* 2017;76(6):1183–1184.

328. Gálvez-Canseco A, Sperling L. Lichen planopilaris and frontal fibrosing alopecia cannot be differentiated by histopathology. *J Cutan Pathol.* 2018;45(5):313–317.

329. Zinkernagel MS, Trueb RM. Fibrosing alopecia in a pattern distribution: patterned lichen planopilaris or androgenetic alopecia with a lichenoid tissue reaction pattern? *Arch Dermatol.* 2000;136(2):205–211.

330. Griggs J, Trüeb RM, Gavazzoni Dias MFR, Hordinsky M, Tosti A. Fibrosing alopecia in a pattern distribution. *J Am Acad Dermatol.* 2021;85(6):1557–1564. doi:10.1016/j.jaad.2019.12.056

331. Olsen EA. Female pattern hair loss and its relationship to permanent/cicatricial alopecia: a new perspective. *J Investig Dermatol Symp Proc.* 2005;10(3):217–221.

332. Fergie B, Khaira G, Howard V, de Zwaan S. Diffuse scarring alopecia in a female pattern hair loss distribution. *Australas J Dermatol.* 2018;59(1):e43–e46. doi:10.1111/ajd.12557

333. Baibergenova A, Donovan J. Lichen planopilaris: update on pathogenesis and treatment. *Skinmed.* 2013;11(3):161–165.

334. Habashi-Daniel A, Roberts JL, Desai N, Thompson CT. Absence of catagen/telogen phase and loss of cytokeratin 15 expression in hair follicles in lichen planopilaris. *J Am Acad Dermatol.* 2014;71(5):969–972.

335. Garcovich S, Manco S, Zampetti A, et al. Onset of lichen planopilaris during treatment with etanercept. *Br J Dermatol.* 2008;158(5):1161–1163.

336. Fening K, Parekh V, McKay K. CD123 immunohistochemistry for plasmacytoid dendritic cells is useful in the diagnosis of scarring alopecia. *J Cutan Pathol.* 2016;43(8):643–648.

337. Nasiri S, Bidari Zerehpoosh F, Abdollahimajd F, Younespour S, Esmaili Azad M. A comparative immunohistochemical study of epidermal and dermal/perifollicular Langerhans cell concentration in discoid lupus erythematosus and lichen planopilaris: a cross-sectional study. *Lupus.* 2018;27(14):2200–2205.

338. Assouly P, Reygagne P. Lichen planopilaris: update on diagnosis and treatment. *Semin Cutan Med Surg.* 2009;28(1):3–10.

339. Shuster S. Psoriatic alopecia. *Br J Dermatol.* 1972;87(1):73–77.

340. Headington JT, Gupta AK, Goldfarb MT, et al. A morphometric and histologic study of the scalp in psoriasis: paradoxical sebaceous gland atrophy and decreased hair shaft diameters without alopecia. *Arch Dermatol.* 1989;125(5):639–642.

341. Bardazzi F, Fanti PA, Orlandi C, Chieregato C, Misciali C. Psoriatic scarring alopecia: observations in four patients. *Int J Dermatol.* 1999;38(10):765–768.

342. George SM, Taylor MR, Farrant PB. Psoriatic alopecia. *Clin Exp Dermatol.* 2015;40(7):717–721.

343. Runne U, Kroneisen-Wiersma P. Psoriatic alopecia: acute and chronic hair loss in 47 patients with scalp psoriasis [erratum appears in *Dermatology.* 1993;187(3):232]. *Dermatology.* 1992;185(2):82–87.

344. Runne U, Kroneisen P. Psoriatic alopecia manifestation, course and therapy in 34 patients. *Z Hautkr.* 1989;64(4):302–314.

345. Osorio F, Magro F, Lisboa C, et al. Anti-TNF-alpha induced psoriasiform eruptions with severe scalp involvement and alopecia: report of five cases and review of the literature. *Dermatology.* 2012;225(2):163–167.

346. Doyle LA, Sperling LC, Baksh S, et al. Psoriatic alopecia/alopecia areata-like reactions secondary to anti-tumor necrosis factor-α therapy: a novel cause of noncicatricial alopecia. *Am J Dermatopathol.* 2011;33(2):161–166.

347. Silva CY, Brown KL, Kurban AK, Mahalingam M. Psoriatic alopecia—fact or fiction? A clinicohistopathologic reappraisal. *Indian J Dermatol Venereol Leprol.* 2012;78(5):611–619.

348. Torres F. Androgenetic, diffuse and senescent alopecia in men: practical evaluation and management. *Curr Probl Dermatol.* 2015;47:33–44.

349. Fernandez-Flores A, Saeb-Lima M, Cassarino DS. Histopathology of aging of the hair follicle. *J Cutan Pathol.* 2019;46(7):508–519. doi:10.1111/cup.13467

350. Trüeb RM. Chemotherapy-induced hair loss. *Skin Therapy Lett.* 2010;15(7):5–7.

351. Tallon B, Blanchard E, Goldberg LJ. Permanent chemotherapy-induced alopecia: case report and review of the literature. *J Am Acad Dermatol.* 2010;63(2):333–336. doi:10.1016/j.jaad.2009.06.063

352. Miteva M, Misciali C, Fanti PA, Vincenzi C, Romanelli P, Tosti A. Permanent alopecia after systemic chemotherapy: a clinicopathological study of 10 cases. *Am J Dermatopathol.* 2011;33(4):345–350. doi:10.1097/DAD.0b013e3181fcfc25

353. Baker BW, Wilson CL, Davis AL, et al. Busulphan/cyclophosphamide conditioning for bone marrow transplantation may lead to failure of hair regrowth. *Bone Marrow Transplant.* 1991;7(1):43–47.

354. Palamaras I, Misciali C, Vincenzi C, Robles WS, Tosti A. Permanent chemotherapy-induced alopecia: a review. *J Am Acad Dermatol.* 2011;64(3):604–606.

355. Rubio-Gonzalez B, Juhász M, Fortman J, Mesinkovska NA. Pathogenesis and treatment options for chemotherapy-induced alopecia: a systematic review. *Int J Dermatol.* 2018;57(12):1417–1424.

356. Novice T, Novice M, Shapiro J, Lo Sicco K. Chemotherapy-induced alopecia—a potentially preventable side effect with scalp cooling. *J Am Acad Dermatol.* 2020;82(2):e57–e59. doi:10.1016/j.jaad.2019.09.059

357. Yang X, Thai KE. Treatment of permanent chemotherapy-induced alopecia with low dose oral minoxidil. *Australas J Dermatol.* 2016;57(4):e130–e132.

358. Yeager CE, Olsen EA. Treatment of chemotherapy-induced alopecia. *Dermatol Ther.* 2011;24(4):432–442. doi:10.1111/j.1529-8019.2011.01430.x

359. Cappel JA, Ioffreda MD, Kirby JS. JAAD grand rounds quiz. Fixed focal alopecia for 20 years. *J Am Acad Dermatol.* 2011;65(5):1071–1072.

360. Starace M, Carpanese MA, Abbenante D, Bruni F, Piraccini BM, Alessandrini A. Atypical presentation of congenital triangular alopecia: a case series in Italy. *Dermatol Pract Concept.* 2020;10(4):e2020122.

361. Yamazaki M, Irisawa R, Tsuboi R. Temporal triangular alopecia and a review of 52 past cases. *J Dermatol.* 2010;37(4):360–362. doi:10.1111/j.1346-8138.2010.00817.x

362. Trakimas CA, Sperling LC. Temporal triangular alopecia acquired in adulthood. *J Am Acad Dermatol.* 1999;40(5, pt 2):842–844.

363. Trakimas C, Sperling LC, Skelton HG 3rd, Smith KJ, Buker JL. Clinical and histologic findings in temporal triangular alopecia. *J Am Acad Dermatol.* 1994;31(2, pt 1):205–209.

364. Silva CY, Lenzy YM, Goldberg LJ. Temporal triangular alopecia with decreased follicular density. *J Cutan Pathol.* 2010;37(5):597–599.

365. Bang CY, Byun JW, Kang MJ, et al. Successful treatment of temporal triangular alopecia with topical minoxidil. *Ann Dermatol.* 2013;25(3):387–388.

366. Yasar S, Gunes P, Serdar ZA, et al. Clinical and pathological features of 31 cases of lipedematous scalp and lipedematous alopecia. *Eur J Dermatol.* 2011;21(4):520–528.

367. Chen E, Patel R, Pavlidakey P, Huang CC. Presentation, diagnosis, and management options of lipedematous alopecia. *JAAD Case Rep.* 2018;5(1):108–109.

368. Coskey RJ, Fosnaugh RP, Fine G. Lipedematous alopecia. *Arch Dermatol.* 1961;84:619–622.

369. Kane KS, Kwan T, Baden HP, Bigby M. Women with new-onset boggy scalp. *Arch Dermatol.* 1998;134:499.

370. Bridges AG, von Kuster LC, Estes SA. Lipedematous alopecia. *Cutis.* 2000;64(4):199–202.

371. Hong JY, Li K, Hong CK. Lipedematous alopecia in an Asian woman: is it an advanced stage of lipedematous scalp? *Ann Dermatol.* 2018;30(6):701–703.

372. Martin JM, Monteagudo C, Montesinos E, Guijarro J, Llombart B, Jordá E. Lipedematous scalp and lipedematous alopecia: a clinical and histologic analysis of 3 cases. *J Am Acad Dermatol.* 2005;52(1):152–156.

373. Piraccini BM, Voudouris S, Pazzaglia M, Rech G, Vicenzi C, Tosti A. Lipedematous alopecia of the scalp. *Dermatol Online J.* 2006;12(2):6.

374. High WA, Hoang MP. Lipedematous alopecia: an unusual sequela of discoid lupus, or other co-conspirators at work? *J Am Acad Dermatol.* 2005;53(2, suppl 1):S157–S161.

375. Garn MS, Selby S, Young R. Scalp thickness and fat-loss theory of balding. *Arch Dermatol Syph.* 1954;70:601–608.

376. Ikejima A, Yamashits M, Ikeda S, Ogawa H. A case of lipedematous alopecia occurring in a male patient. *Dermatol.* 2000;210(2):168–170.

377. Scheufler O, Kania NM, Heinrichs CM, Exner K. Hyperplasia of the subcutaneous adipose tissue is the primary histopathologic abnormality in lipedematous scalp. *Am J Dermatopathol.* 2003;25(3):248–252.

378. Fair KP, Knoell KA, Patterson JW, Rudd RJ, Greer KE. Lipedematous alopecia: a clinicopathologic, histologic and ultrastructural study. *J Cutan Pathol.* 2000;27(1):49–53.

379. Gonzalez-Guerra E, Haro R, Angulo J, Del Carmen Fariña M, Martín L, Requena L. Lipedematous alopecia: an uncommon clinicopathologic variant of nonscarring but permanent alopecia. *Int J Dermatol.* 2008;47(6):605–609.

380. Damste J, Prakken JR. Atrichia with papular lesions: a variant of congenital ectodermal dysplasia. *Dermatologica.* 1954; 108:114–117.

381. Kanzler MH, Rasmussen JE. Atrichia with papular lesions. *Arch Dermatol.* 1986;122:565–567.

382. Henn W, Zlotogorski A, Lam H, Martinez-Mir A, Zaun H, Christiano AM. Atrichia with papular lesions resulting from compound heterozygous mutations in the hairless gene: a lesson for differential diagnosis of alopecia universalis. *J Am Acad Dermatol.* 2002;47:519–523.

383. Bergman R, Schein-Goldshmid R, Hochberg Z, Ben-Izhak O, Sprecher E. The alopecias associated with vitamin D-dependent rickets type IIA and with hairless gene mutations: a comparative clinical, histologic, and immunohistochemical study. *Arch Dermatol.* 2005;141(3):343–351.

384. Rocha VB, Michalany N, Valente NYS, Pereira LB, Donati A. Atrichia with papular lesions: importance of histology at an early disease stage. *Skin Appendage Disord.* 2018;4(3):129–130.

385. Ahmad M, ul Haque MF, Brancolini V, et al. Alopecia universalis associated with a mutation in the human hairless gene. *Science.* 1998;279:720–724.

386. Miller J, Djabali K, Chen T, et al. Atrichia caused by mutations in the vitamin D receptor gene is a phenocopy of generalized atrichia caused by mutations in the hairless gene. *J Invest Dermatol.* 2001;117:612–617.

387. Liu L, Kim H, Casta A, Kobayashi Y, Shapiro LS, Christiano AM. Hairless is a histone H3K9 demethylase. *FASEB J.* 2014;28(4):1534–1542.

388. Wenzel FG, Horn TD. Nonneoplastic disorders of the eccrine glands. *J Am Acad Dermatol.* 1998;38(1):1–17.

389. Beatty CJ, Ghareeb ER. Neutrophilic eccrine hidradenitis. *N Engl J Med.* 2021;385(6):e19.

390. Takai T, Matsunaga A. A case of neutrophilic eccrine hidradenitis associated with streptococcal infectious endocarditis. *Dermatology.* 2006;212(2):203–205.

391. Antonovich DD, Berke A, Grant-Kels JM, Fung M. Infectious eccrine hidradenitis caused by Nocardia. *J Am Acad Dermatol.* 2004;50(2):315–318.

392. Smith KJ, Skelton HG, James WD, Holland TT, Lupton GP, Angritt P. Neutrophilic eccrine hidradenitis in HIV-infected patients. *J Am Acad Dermatol.* 1990;23:945–947.

393. Bassas-Vila J, Fernández-Figueras MT, Romaní J, Ferrándiz C. Infectious eccrine hidradenitis: a report of 3 cases and a review of the literature [in English, Spanish]. *Actas Dermosifiliogr.* 2014;105(2):e7–e12.

394. Bachmeyer C, Chaibi P, Aractingi S. Neutrophilic eccrine hidradenitis induced by granulocyte colony-stimulating factor. *Br J Dermatol.* 1998;139(2):354–355.

395. Herms F, Franck N, Kramkimel N, et al. Neutrophilic eccrine hidradenitis in two patients treated with BRAF inhibitors: a new cutaneous adverse event. *Br J Dermatol.* 2017;176(6):1645–1648.

396. Roustan G, Salas C, Cabrera R, Simón A. Neutrophilic eccrine hidradenitis unassociated with chemotherapy in a patient with acute myelogenous leukemia. *Int J Dermatol.* 2001;40(2):144–147.

397. Naimer SA, Zvulunov A, Ben-Amitai D, Landau M. Plantar hidradenitis in children induced by exposure to wet footwear. *Pediatr Emerg Care.* 2000;16(3):182–183.

398. Stahr BJ, Cooper PH, Caputo RV. Idiopathic plantar hidradenitis occurring primarily in children. *J Cutan Pathol.* 1994;21:289–296.

399. Ben-Amitai D, Hodak E, Landau M, Metzker A, Feinmesser M, David M. Idiopathic palmoplantar eccrine hidradenitis in children. *Eur J Pediatr.* 2001;160(3):189–191.

400. Rabinowitz LG, Cintra ML, Hood AF, Esterly NB. Recurrent palmoplantar hidradenitis in children. *Arch Dermatol.* 1995;131(7):817–820.

401. Simon M, Cremer H, von den Driesch P. Idiopathic recurrent palmplantar hidradenitis in children. *Arch Dermatol.* 1998;134:76–79.

402. Fiorillo L, Zucker M, Sawyer D, Lin AN. The *Pseudomonas* hot-foot syndrome. *N Engl J Med.* 2001;345:335–338.

403. Zvulunov A, Trattner A, Naimer S. *Pseudomonas* hot–foot syndrome. *N Engl J Med.* 2001;345(22):1643–1644.

404. Belot V, Perrinaud A, Corven C, de Muret A, Lorette G, Machet L. Adult idiopathic neutrophilic eccrine hidradenitis treated with colchicine [in French]. *Presse Med.* 2006;35(10, pt 1):1475–1478.

405. Shelley WB, Levy EJ. Apocrine sweat retention in man. II: Fox-Fordyce disease (apocrine miliaria). *Arch Dermatol.* 1956; 73:38.

406. Salloum A, Bouferraa Y, Bazzi N, et al. Pathophysiology, clinical findings, and management of Fox-Fordyce disease: a systematic review. *J Cosmet Dermatol.* 2021.

407. Helm TN, Chen PW. Fox-Fordyce disease. *Cutis.* 2002;69(5):335–342.

408. Ghislain PD, van Der Endt JD, Delescluse J. Itchy papules of the axillae. *Arch Dermatol.* 2002;138(2):259–264.

409. Boer A. Patterns histopathologic of Fox-Fordyce disease. *Am J Dermatopathol.* 2004;26(6):482–492.

410. Vega-Memije ME, Pérez-Rojas DO, Boeta-Ángeles L, Valdés-Landrum P. Fox-Fordyce disease: report of two cases with perifollicular xanthomatosis on histological image. *An Bras Dermatol.* 2018;93(4): 562–565.

411. Stashower ME, Krivda SJ, Turiansky GW. Fox-Fordyce disease: diagnosis with transverse histologic sections. *J Am Acad Dermatol.* 2000;42(1):89–91.

412. Kamada A, Saga K, Jimbow K. Apoeccrine sweat duct obstruction as a cause for Fox-Fordyce disease. *J Am Acad Dermatol.* 2003;48(3):453–455.

413. Bernad I, Gil P, Lera JM, Giménez de Azcárate A, Irarrazaval I, Idoate MÁ. Fox Fordyce disease as a secondary effect of laser hair removal. *J Cosmet Laser Ther.* 2014;16(3):141–143.

414. Kossard S, Dwyer P. Axillary perifollicular xanthomatosis resembling Fox-Fordyce disease. *Australas J Dermatol.* 2004;45(2):146–148.

415. Boer A. Axillary perifollicular xanthomatosis resembling Fox-Fordyce disease. *Australas J Dermatol.* 2004;45(4):238.

416. Cox NH. Posterior auricular chondrodermatitis nodularis. *Clin Exp Dermatol.* 2002;27(4):324–327.

417. Bal A, Rashid Z, Shamma HN. Chondrodermatitis nodularis nasi: a case report of a rare variant of chondrodermatitis nodularis helicis. *Am J Dermatopathol.* 2021.

418. Kasitinon SY, Vandergriff T. Chondrodermatitis nodularis nasi. *J Cutan Pathol.* 2020;47(11):1046–1049.

419. Goette DK. Chondrodermatitis nodularis chronica helicis: a perforating necrobiotic granuloma. *J Am Acad Dermatol.* 1980;2:148.

420. Cribier B, Scrivener Y, Peltre B. Neural hyperplasia in chondrodermatitis nodularis chronica helicis. *J Am Acad Dermatol.* 2006;55(5):844–848.

421. Magro CM, Frambach GE, Crowson AN. Chondrodermatitis nodularis helicis as a marker of internal disease associated with microvascular injury [erratum appears in *J Cutan Pathol.* 2005;32(9):646]. *J Cutan Pathol.* 2005;32(5):329–333.

422. Elgart ML. Cell phone chondrodermatitis. *Arch Dermatol.* 2000;136(12):1568.

423. Upile T, Patel NN, Jerjes W, Singh NU, Sandison A, Michaels L. Advances in the understanding of chondrodermatitis nodularis chronica helices: the perichondrial vasculitis theory. *Clin Otolaryngol.* 2009;34(2):147–150.

424. Salah H, Urso B, Khachemoune A. Review of the etiopathogenesis and management options of chondrodermatitis nodularis chronica helicis. *Cureus.* 2018;10(3):e2367. doi:10.7759/cureus.2367

425. Travelute CR. Self-adhering foam: a simple method for pressure relief during sleep in patients with chondrodermatitis nodularis helicis. *Dermatol Surg.* 2013;39(2):317–319.

426. Rapini RP, Warner NB. Relapsing polychondritis. *Clin Dermatol.* 2006;24(6):482–485.

427. Letko E, Zafirakis P, Baltatzis S, Voudouri A, Livir-Rallatos C, Foster CS. Relapsing polychondritis: a clinical review. *Semin Arthritis Rheum.* 2002;31(6):384–395.

428. Enright H, Miller W. Autoimmune phenomena in patients with myelodysplastic syndromes. *Leuk Lymphoma.* 1997;24(5–6):483–489.

429. Yanagi T, Matsumura T, Kamekura R, Sasaki N, Hashino S. Relapsing polychondritis and malignant lymphoma: is polychondritis paraneoplastic? *Arch Dermatol.* 2007;143(1):89–90.

430. Bochtler T, Hensel M, Lorenz HM, Ho AD, Mahlknecht U. Chronic lymphocytic leukaemia and concomitant relapsing polychondritis: a report on one treatment for the combined manifestation of two diseases. *Rheumatol.* 2005;44(9):1199.

431. Frances C, el Rassi R, Laporte JL, Rybojad M, Papo T, Piette JC. Dermatologic manifestations of relapsing polychondritis: a study of 200 cases at a single center. *Medicine.* 2001;80(3):173–179.

432. Kim MK, Park KS, Min JK, Cho CS, Kim HY. A case of polychondritis in a patient with Behcet's disease. *Korean J Intern Med.* 2005;20(4):339–342.

433. Imai H, Motegi M, Mizuki N, et al. Mouth and genital ulcers with inflamed cartilage (MAGIC syndrome): a case report and literature review. *Am J Med Sci.* 1997;314(5):330–332.

434. Handrock K, Gross W. Relapsing polychondritis as a secondary phenomenon of primary systemic vasculitis. *Ann Rheum Dis.* 1993;52:895.

435. McAdam LP, O'Hanlan MA, Bluestone R, Pearson CM. Relapsing polychondritis: prospective study of 23 patients and a review of the literature. *Medicine (Baltimore).* 1976;55:193.

436. Disdier P, Andrac L, Swiader L, et al. Cutaneous panniculitis and relapsing polychondritis: two cases. *Dermatology.* 1996;193(3):266–268.

437. Bernard P, Bedane C, Delrous JL, Catanzano G, Bonnetblanc JM. Erythema elevatum diutinum in a patient with relapsing polychondritis. *J Am Acad Dermatol.* 1992;26:312.

438. Valenzuela R, Cooperrider PA, Gogate P, Deodhar SD, Bergfeld WF. Relapsing polychondritis. *Hum Pathol.* 1980;11:19.

439. Thompson LD. Relapsing polychondritis. *Ear Nose Throat J.* 2002;81(10):705.

440. Terato K, Shimozuru Y, Katayama K, et al. Specificity of antibodies to type II collagen in rheumatoid arthritis. *Arthritis Rheum.* 1990;33:1493.

441. Zeuner M, Straub RH, Rauh G, Albert ED, Schölmerich J, Lang B. Relapsing polychondritis: clinical and immunogenetic analysis of 62 patients. *J Rheumatol.* 1997;24(1):96–101.

442. Lahmer T, Treiber M, von Werder A, et al. Relapsing polychondritis: an autoimmune disease with many faces. *Autoimmun Rev.* 2010;9(8):540–546.

443. Lim CM, Goh YH, Chao SS, Lynne L. Pseudocyst of the auricle. *Laryngoscope.* 2002;112(11):2033–2036.

444. Kopera D, Soyer HP, Smolle J, Kerl H. "Pseudocyst of the auricle", othematoma and otoseroma: three faces of the same coin? *Eur J Dermatol.* 2000;10(6):451–454.

445. Lim CM, Goh YH, Chao SS, Lim LH, Lim L. Pseudocyst of the auricle: a histologic perspective. *Laryngoscope.* 2004;114(7):1281–1284.

446. Miyamoto H, Okajima M, Takahashi I. Lactate dehydrogenase isozymes in and intralesional steroid injection therapy for pseudocyst of the auricle. *Int J Dermatol.* 2001;40(6):380–384.

447. Yamamoto T, Yokoyama A, Umeda T. Cytokine profile of bilateral pseudocyst of the auricle. *Acta Dermatol Venereol.* 1996;76:92.

Inflammatory Diseases of the Nail

Chapter

19

ADAM I. RUBIN

INTRODUCTION

An understanding of the normal anatomy and histology of the nail unit precedes an understanding of the pathology that may occur there (see Chapter 3). Inflammatory pathologic processes in the nail unit may affect one or multiple areas of the different anatomic areas of the nail unit, including the matrix, nail bed, hyponychium, and nail folds. Changes in the nail plate can occur secondarily to inflammation in other areas of the nail unit. A basic understanding of where pathologic processes affect the nail unit and the corresponding clinical signs will guide the practitioner in choosing a site of biopsy. As with dermatoses affecting other areas of the skin, understanding the location and type of pathology leads to more effective diagnosis and treatment.

Because of the unique anatomy of the nail unit, there are a limited number of possible reaction patterns to inflammatory processes. These reaction patterns may have features different from those seen in the skin. Because the nail unit produces a product, the nail plate, some inflammatory processes of the nail matrix may lead to irreversible damage, resulting in an abnormal or absent plate, much akin to processes affecting the hair unit that lead to scarring alopecia. On the other hand, processes affecting the nail bed and hyponychium that do not affect the formation of the plate may affect its shape or ability to adhere to the nail bed. The nail bed responds to injury by becoming metaplastic, that is, by switching from onycholemmal keratinization (without keratohyalin granules) to epidermoid keratinization. It becomes hyperplastic, showing hyperkeratosis, parakeratosis, and hypergranulosis. Spongiosis and exudative scale crust are common with a variety of nail unit inflammatory processes. Inflammatory diseases affecting the nail folds can alter the texture of the nail plate. For example, when the ventral surface of the proximal nail fold is affected, inflammation of the cuticle and alterations of the dorsal surface of the nail plate may be seen. Atopic dermatitis and contact dermatitis of the fingers may affect both the proximal and the lateral nail folds.

BIOPSY OF THE NAIL UNIT

Biopsy of the nail unit is recommended in many cases when the diagnosis of an inflammatory disorder is in doubt or when definitive histopathologic diagnosis is needed before beginning therapy. The highest yield in obtaining helpful information from a nail unit biopsy for inflammatory disorders is to target the biopsy site as it relates to the clinical signs manifested in the nail. For example, the best likelihood of obtaining useful information when onychorrhexis (longitudinal striations in the nail plate) is observed is to sample the nail matrix. Although the changes are observed in the nail plate, it is the matrix anatomic area of the nail unit that produces the nail plate (and associated abnormalities of it), so this is the area that should be biopsied to evaluate those specific changes. Another example would be the evaluation of onycholysis (separation of the nail plate from the nail bed). In this case, the nail bed is the best target to evaluate the clinical changes, as the nail bed is the anatomic site where responsible changes are likely to be found (1). In general, before performing a soft tissue biopsy of the nail unit, it is reasonable to have nail clippings examined histopathologically. This will help evaluate the presence of onychomycosis, and examination of the nail plate is also helpful for the evaluation of a number of other processes affecting the nail unit (2).

Nail matrix biopsy is best performed after reflecting back the proximal nail fold. The nail plate may remain intact or may be avulsed before the procedure to obtain matrix tissue. A 3-mm punch biopsy from the distal matrix for the evaluation of nail unit inflammatory disorders has a low risk of postoperative nail dystrophy. Care should be taken to avoid taking the specimen from the proximal matrix, because this nail unit component creates the dorsal aspect of the nail plate, and a scar in this area has a high risk of resulting in a permanent and obvious postprocedure nail dystrophy. One should avoid biopsying very deeply in the proximal matrix area, because it is possible to damage the tendon of the extensor digitorum communis, which inserts into the proximal dorsal portion of the terminal phalanx. Transection of this tendon will result in a drop deformity of the distal phalanx.

The nail bed may be sampled using a punch biopsy through the nail plate down to the periosteum. Depending on the degree of onycholysis affecting the selected nail unit, some nail plates may be required to be clipped away for good surgical access to the biopsy site. Longitudinal incisional biopsies may also be done. In this procedure, en bloc removal of the lateral nail fold, matrix, bed, and hyponychium is performed at a lateral aspect of the nail unit (3). This procedure is excellent for defining inflammatory disease processes of the nail unit. In general, the punch technique is satisfactory for the diagnosis of nail unit inflammatory dermatoses most of the time (4,5). However, a lateral longitudinal excision can be very valuable if the nail changes are difficult to diagnose, because this method allows simultaneous examination of multiple anatomic areas of the nail unit by the dermatopathologist.

The proximal nail fold region may be sampled by a punch biopsy, shave biopsy, transverse excisional biopsy, as well as other methods.

Several elegant surgical techniques have been published that allow for partial and selective nail avulsion before biopsy of the soft tissue of the nail unit (6). Removing only that portion of the nail plate necessary to access the area of interest in the nail unit not only simplifies the procedure but also allows for quicker recovery time for the patient and lowers the risk of postoperative complications.

ECZEMATOUS DERMATITIS

Clinical Summary. Most forms of eczematous dermatitis affect the nail unit, atopic dermatitis being the most common. Contact dermatitis secondary to nail cosmetics or occupational exposure may affect all areas of the nail unit. Nail plate changes usually result from matrix or proximal nail fold involvement. Onycholysis may be secondary to nail bed involvement, which begins distally at the hyponychium and spreads inward to involve the nail bed. Secondary chronic paronychia may occur. The biopsy should be focused on the site of involvement, usually the nail bed or nail matrix.

Histopathology. The histopathologic changes include spongiosis and exocytosis of mononuclear cells and an acanthotic epidermis. Staining for fungal organisms should be performed to rule out onychomycosis.

Pathogenesis. The pathogenesis of eczematous dermatitis affecting the nail unit will depend on the underlying factors, many of which are possible. Irritant dermatitis is possible from extensive exposure of the fingers to water. Contact allergies to nail cosmetics can also be a culprit.

Differential Diagnosis. The clinical differential diagnosis could include other inflammatory dermatoses affecting the nail unit, including nail unit psoriasis and nail unit lichen planus. The histopathologic features between these entities are usually distinctive.

Principles of Management: The most effective method of treating eczematous dermatitis affecting the nail unit is behavior modification. Protecting the hands with gloves in moist environments and avoiding allergic or irritant chemicals will be effective in the long term. Topical steroids may reduce inflammation during a flare, and emollition is essential to prevent recurrences and improve symptoms.

NAIL UNIT PSORIASIS

Clinical Summary. Nail involvement in psoriasis may occur in up to 50% of patients. Nail changes may occur in up to 80% of patients with psoriatic arthritis. In 10% of patients with psoriasis, nail involvement may be the only manifestation. Psoriasis is limited to the nails without any other skin involvement in 1% to 5% of cases (7). The severity of nail unit psoriasis can be measured with the NAPSI (Nail Psoriasis Severity Index) score (8), as well as the mNAPSI (Modified Nail Psoriasis Severity Index) score (9). If patients present with nail unit psoriasis, it is important to ask about joint pains, because there is a positive correlation between the presence of nail unit psoriasis and psoriatic arthritis. MRI imaging has demonstrated nail involvement in patients with psoriatic arthritis, even in those without clinically evident nail changes (10). Nail changes noted on MRI are more marked in patients with increased NAPSI scores (11). Related imaging work has implicated nail unit psoriasis as the main lesion for the development of distal phalanx damage and subsequent distal interphalangeal (DIP) joint arthritis (12). Nail unit psoriasis and psoriatic arthritis can also be associated with enthesitis (inflammation at the tendon and ligament attachments), because the nail unit is connected to the DIP joint by the extensor tendon and collateral ligament (13–16).

Psoriasis may involve any part of the nail unit, including the matrix, nail bed, hyponychium, and nail folds. Psoriatic involvement of the proximal nail matrix causes clinical pitting and roughening of the surface of the nail plate. Involvement of the mid- and distal matrix leads to clinical leukonychia (white discoloration of the nail). The "oil drop" sign of psoriatic nails (Fig. 19-1) is a reddish-brown discoloration of the nail bed and hyponychium. It represents an early, acute focus of psoriasis involving the nail bed or nail matrix. Psoriasis affecting the nail bed and hyponychium can cause onycholysis (separation of the nail plate from the nail bed), which causes the nail plate to appear white. Well-developed psoriasis of the nail bed leads to subungual hyperkeratosis and exudate, which lift the nail plate off the bed (17,18).

Histopathology. Sections should be stained with hematoxylin and eosin and also with periodic acid–Schiff (PAS) stain or silver methenamine stain to evaluate for fungal infection. Because psoriasis and onychomycosis share many clinical and histopathologic features, employing a fungal stain is essential in the evaluation of suspected nail unit psoriasis. It is important to remember that a patient with nail unit psoriasis may also develop onychomycosis. Treatment of the onychomycosis may unmask the underlying nail unit psoriasis.

The nail plate can show foci of parakeratosis on the surface of it, which, when shed, leave pits on the plate. With psoriatic leukonychia, foci of parakeratosis are located in the deeper portions of the plate. Nail clippings in psoriasis may demonstrate subungual hyperkeratosis, serous lakes, bacteria, neutrophils, and collections of hemorrhage (19).

The oil drop sign is histopathologically characterized by hyperkeratosis and parakeratosis, with collections of neutrophils in the stratum corneum representing a Munro microabscess and spongiform pustules in the granular layer. The nail unit epithelium may show hypergranulosis, with focal hypogranulosis. There is an elongation of the dermal papillae with dilatation and proliferation of capillaries surrounded by lymphocytes, histiocytes, and occasional neutrophils.

Distal nail onycholysis shows a similar histology and therefore has a similar histogenesis. The split in psoriatic onycholysis occurs between the locations of neutrophils and parakeratotic foci within the plate and the underlying hyponychium. The yellow leading edge of onycholytic nail correlates with the presence of neutrophils in the nail plate keratin.

The changes of well-developed nail unit psoriasis of the distal nail unit with subungual hyperkeratosis will show the nail bed epithelium with psoriasiform acanthosis, elongated rete ridges, and capillary proliferation. Neutrophils may be present in the superficial epidermis and within the keratin.

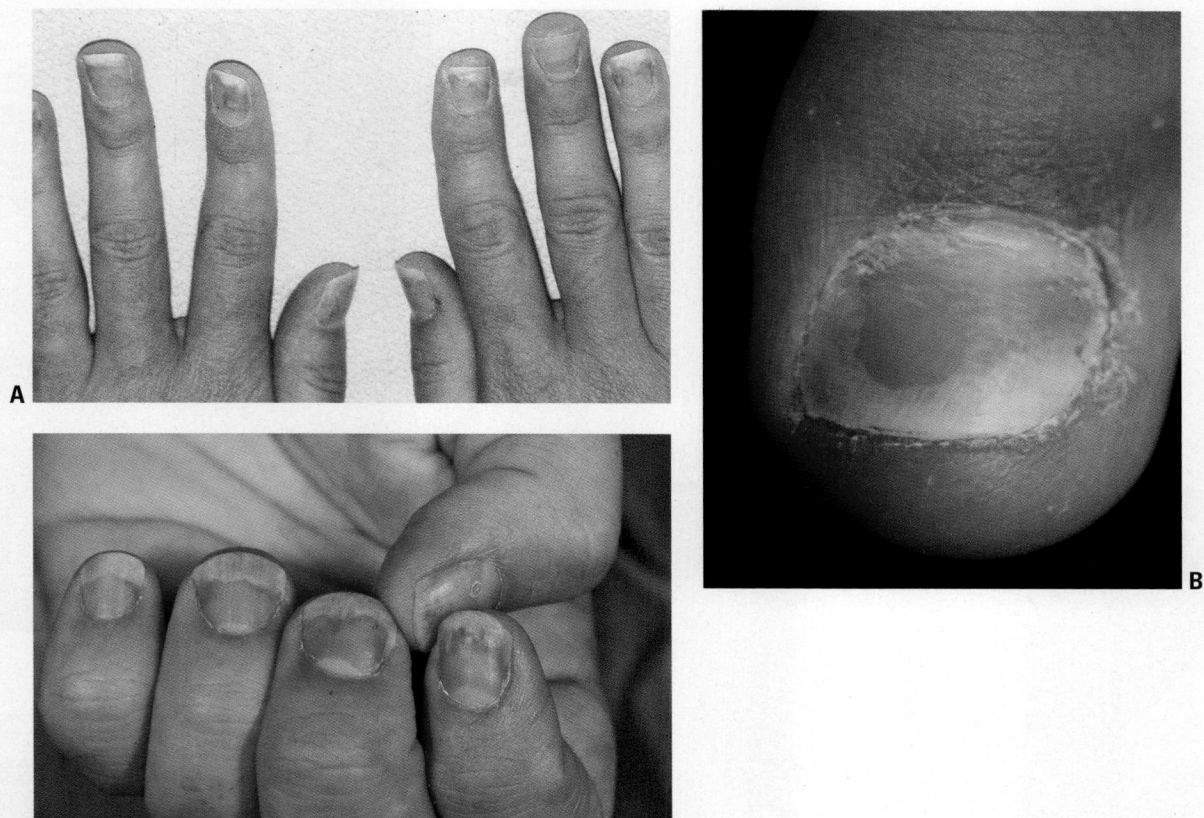

Figure 19-1 Nail unit psoriasis. **A:** Onycholysis and the oil drop sign are seen in the distal nail plate. **B:** Onycholysis seen on the great toenail in a patient with nail unit psoriasis. The nail bed biopsy from this nail is seen in Figure 19-2C–E. **C:** Typical features of nail unit psoriasis are seen in this image. There is onycholysis associated with an erythematous rim at the periphery of some of the nails, splinter hemorrhages, and a few pits.

Late or chronically traumatized psoriatic nails may develop features of lichen simplex chronicus, including marked compact orthokeratosis, hypergranulosis, and fibrosis of the papillary dermis, characterized by vertical streaks of coarse collagen fibers. Histopathologic features of nail unit psoriasis are presented in Figure 19-2.

Pathogenesis. The pathogenesis of nail unit psoriasis is the same as that of psoriasis affecting other areas of the skin. For a complete discussion, see Chapter 7.

Differential Diagnosis. The main clinical differential diagnosis of nail unit psoriasis is onychomycosis, given the common overlapping clinical features of nail plate thickening, subungual hyperkeratosis, and onycholysis. A nail clipping sent for histopathology is an efficient way to distinguish between these two entities. It is important to perform the nail clipping as proximally as possible to the free edge of the nail plate to obtain a sample with the highest likelihood of identifying the fungus. Nail plate changes seen with eczematous dermatitis affecting the nail unit can also mimic nail unit psoriasis occasionally.

Principles of Management: These are exciting times for the treatment of nail unit psoriasis. The selection of an appropriate therapy will depend on what anatomic areas of the nail unit are affected. Intralesional steroid works well for pitting, surface ridging, and thickening of the nail plate, as well as for subungual hyperkeratosis and onycholysis (20). Areas of onycholysis can have a good response to topical therapies such as topical retinoids, vitamin D analogs, anthralin, tacrolimus, and topical steroids (18,20–23). New information supporting the use of the 595-nm pulsed dye laser for the treatment of nail unit psoriasis is available (24). There are emerging data on the usefulness of topical indigo naturalis oil extract for nail unit psoriasis (25–27). Systemic therapies directed at treating cutaneous psoriasis and/or psoriatic arthritis will also improve the nails, including the new biologic medications, cyclosporine, methotrexate, and acitretin (17,18,20,23,28). In recent years, treatment options with biologic medications for nail unit psoriasis have been rapidly evolving. Treatment is considered based on the extent of disease and the presence or absence of concurrent psoriatic arthritis (9). First-line therapies include intralesional steroid injection, topical steroids, topical vitamin D analogs, and combination medication of vitamin D analogs in combination with topical steroids. The PDE-4 inhibitor apremilast and the biologics of infliximab, etanercept, adalimumab, golimumab, ustekinumab, secukinumab, ixekizumab, as well as others, have been shown to be effective in the treatment of nail unit psoriasis (9). Even though all these choices are possible, it is also important to remember that simple strategies of good nail care will also help control and alleviate nail unit psoriasis. These maneuvers include taking good care to protect the nails and keeping them short to avoid a Koebner phenomenon with a long nail plate acting as a lever and causing trauma at the nail plate–nail bed junction (20,23). All patients with nail psoriasis warrant an evaluation for psoriatic arthritis, which, if present, generally requires systemic therapy to manage.

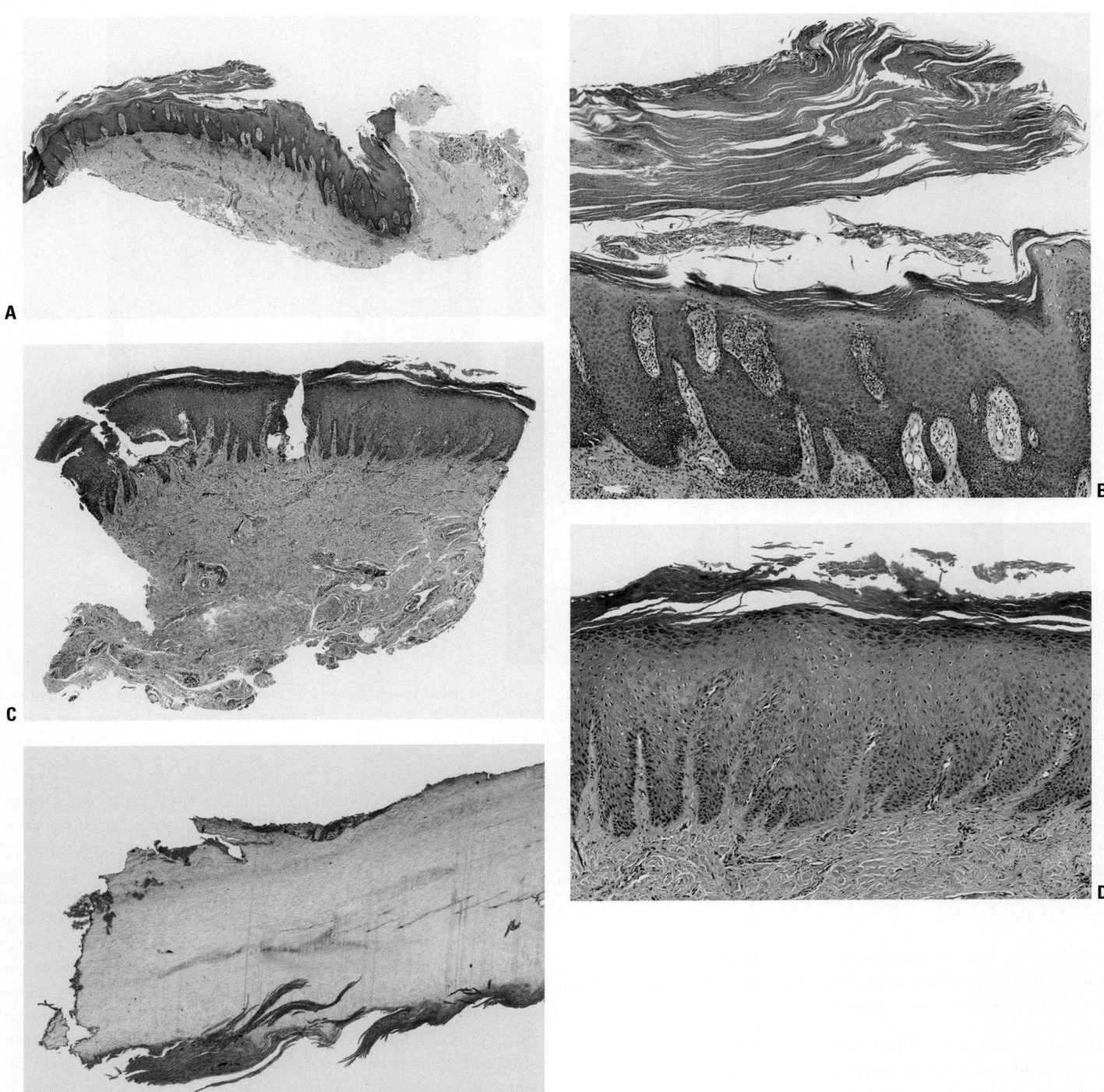

Figure 19-2 Nail unit psoriasis. **A:** This longitudinal excisional specimen includes the cul de sac, matrix epithelium, and part of the nail bed epithelium. Psoriasiform epidermal hyperplasia is seen. **B:** This medium-power view of the matrix epithelium shows epithelial hyperplasia, hypogranulosis, and neutrophils within areas of overlying parakeratosis. **C:** This punch biopsy of the nail bed shows features that can be seen in nail unit psoriasis affecting that anatomic area of the nail unit. There is psoriasiform epidermal hyperplasia with hypergranulosis and papillomatosis. Tortuous vessels are seen in the papillary dermis. **D:** Medium-power view of this same specimen described in C. **E:** The nail plate that was overlying the nail bed specimen seen in C. Note the neutrophils in an area of parakeratosis at the ventral aspect of the nail plate. The nail that was biopsied is seen in Figure 19-1B.

NAIL UNIT LICHEN PLANUS

Clinical Summary. The incidence of nail involvement occurring in association with disseminated lichen planus ranges from 1% to 10%. A study of 316 pediatric patients with a mean age of 10.28 years affected by lichen planus found the nails to be affected in 13.9% (29). In this pediatric study, 90.9% of patients with nail unit lichen planus had lichen planus at other sites (29). Lichen planus may develop in the absence of cutaneous involvement and is most common in the fifth and sixth decades of life. Fingernails are more commonly affected than toenails. Lichen planus may involve the nail matrix, nail bed, hyponychium, and nail folds. Examination and understanding of the pathogenesis of clinical changes will aid the clinician in determining where to sample the nail unit.

Involvement of the proximal nail matrix results in onychorrhexis (longitudinal grooves and ridges of the nail plate) (Fig. 19-3). If nail unit lichen planus is treated early in its course, the changes may be reversible. However, as with other skin appendages, such as hair, if the process progresses, fibrosis and scarring may result, leading to permanent deformity. If there is scarring of the nail unit from lichen planus, anonychia (total loss of the nail plate) can result. A classic clinical feature of nail unit lichen planus is the development of a pterygium, which is caused by scarring and connection of the proximal nail fold to the nail bed. The resulting and remaining nail plate resembles angel's wings.

If the nail matrix is involved diffusely, onychoschizia (lamellar changes with fragility and brittleness) results. Matrix involvement by lichen planus can also present clinically as trachyonychia (rough nails), red lunulae, erythronychia, and atrophy of the nail unit (30). Occasionally, lichen planus of the nail bed alone may occur and can manifest clinically as onycholysis. Papular lesions of lichen planus may occur in various locations of the nail bed and lead to focal atrophy. As a result, the overlying nail plate will be focally dimpled or spooned (koilonychia). Nail bed lichen planus lesions can also manifest clinically with hyperkeratosis (30). In some cases, complete shedding of the nail plate owing to diffuse nail bed involvement may occur. Hyperpigmentation of the nail (melanonychia) may result with nail unit lichen planus.

A study demonstrated a potential link between metals found in dental materials and the course of nail unit lichen planus (31). Six out of 10 patch test-positive nail unit lichen planus patients improved with the removal of the metal-containing dental materials or discontinuation of systemic disodium cromoglycate. Causative metals in the dental materials were found in biopsies of the nail tissues.

Idiopathic atrophy of the nails is a form of nail lichen planus seen exclusively in children and presents with diffuse and rapid destruction of the nails over a few months (32).

Lichen planus limited to the nail units, also known as isolated nail lichen planus (30), can be difficult to diagnose clinically, and in these cases a biopsy is extremely useful. Often, patients with this form of lichen planus have been treated with antifungal agents without success before being referred for evaluation. A large study of 67 cases of isolated nail lichen planus demonstrated an average age of 47, a male predominance (64%), and involvement of the fingernails in 94% of the cases and of the toenails in 53.73% of the cases (30). Only four of the patients had isolated nail lichen planus of the toenails only. In this study, 120 biopsy specimens were taken, and in 90% of the specimens, pathologic features of lichen planus were identified, confirming the utility of nail unit biopsy to confirm the diagnosis (30).

Histopathology. As in lichen planus of the skin, hyperkeratosis, hypergranulosis, acanthosis, vacuolar degeneration, necrotic keratinocytes, civatte bodies, and a bandlike infiltrate of lymphocytes and histiocytes at the dermal–epidermal junction accompanied by melanophages can be seen (Fig. 19-4). The hypergranulosis tends to be less wedge shaped than in other parts of the skin. From personal experience, the intensity of the inflammation in nail unit lichen planus is less than that seen in other areas of the skin. Accordingly, from personal experience, other histopathologic features typical of a lichenoid dermatitis are not as intense, such as the number of dyskeratotic keratinocytes and the degree of vacuolar degeneration. It is unusual, but the inflammation affecting the nail matrix may have a plasma cell predominance (33). A recent study, which is the largest study of the histopathology of nail unit lichen planus to date, comprised 45 patients with nail unit lichen planus, which included 25 punch biopsy specimens from the nail

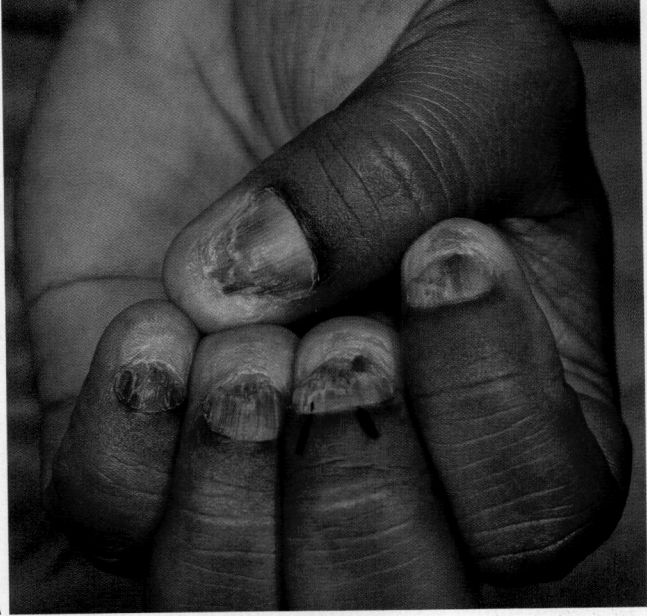
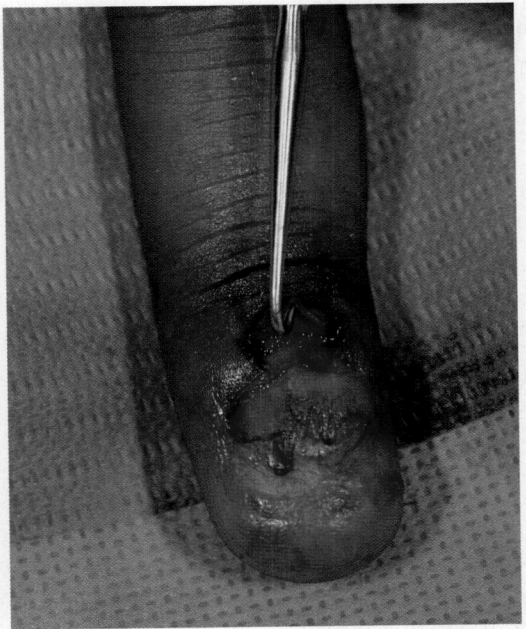

Figure 19-3 **A:** Typical features of nail unit lichen planus. There is onychorrhexis (longitudinal striations of the nail plate) and atrophy of the distal nail bed. The black ink lines mark the sites for incisions to obtain the matrix biopsy, seen in Figure 19-4. **B:** The nail matrix biopsy was obtained by reclining the proximal nail fold after incisions were made in it. The skin hook holds the reclined proximal nail fold away from the matrix biopsy site.

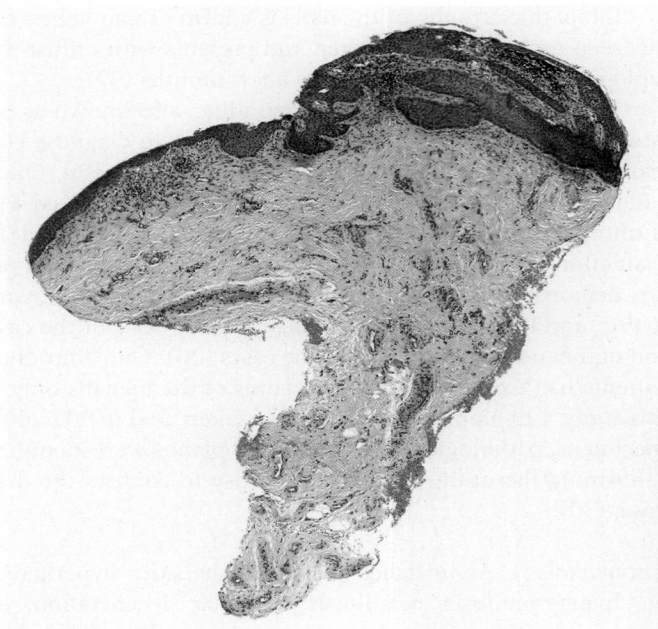
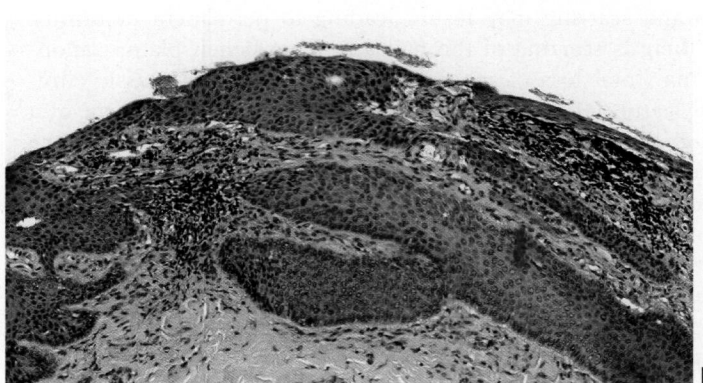

Figure 19-4 Biopsy of the nail matrix demonstrating features of nail unit lichen planus. **A:** Low-power view of this nail matrix punch biopsy shows a bandlike lymphocytic infiltrate that abuts the epithelium. **B:** Medium-power view shows some vacuolar change at the basal layer of the epithelium. This specimen is taken from one of the nails seen in Figure 19-3A. A part of the surgical procedure is seen in Figure 19-3B.

bed and 25 punch biopsy specimens from the nail matrix, and confirmed the usefulness of the punch biopsy method in establishing the diagnosis histopathologically (34). In this study, the histopathology showed that about half of the specimens demonstrated hypergranulosis of the nail matrix and nail bed epithelium and that there were lower percentages of saw-tooth acanthosis (44%) and lichenoid inflammation (24%). Features of focal parakeratosis, spongiosis, serum inclusions, pigment incontinence, and colloid bodies were observed with a lower frequency. These authors also defined a novel feature they observed in one-third of the nail unit lichen planus cases, the "frayed nail plate," which was found to correlate clinically with nail plate thinning. The authors defined the "frayed nail plate" as "a histopathological feature seen as separation of individual orthokeratotic onychocytes of the nail plate like a thinned or worn-out fabric where individual fibers are separating from each other." This study focused on nail unit lichen planus, so it is unknown at this time if the "frayed nail plate" may be found in other dermatoses affecting the nail unit (35).

Pathogenesis. The pathogenesis of nail unit lichen planus is the same as that of lichen planus affecting other areas of the skin. For a complete discussion, see Chapter 7.

Differential Diagnosis. The clinical differential diagnosis for nail unit lichen planus includes other inflammatory dermatoses affecting the nail unit, such as eczematous dermatitis and psoriasis. Graft-versus-host disease (GVHD) affecting the nail unit should also be considered in the clinical differential diagnosis. In a study that included 14 patients with chronic cutaneous GVHD, longitudinal ridging was the most frequently observed nail change, and roughness of the nail plate was the second most frequently observed finding. Other overlapping clinical findings between nail unit GVHD and nail unit lichen planus that were noted in the study include fragility, pterygium formation, onychoatrophy, and onycholysis (36). Examination of the other areas of the skin surface can be helpful if typical lesions of other dermatoses are present. Making the diagnosis can be difficult if the changes are limited to the nails. The histopathologic features are distinct from other inflammatory dermatoses affecting the nail unit when fully developed.

Principles of Management: Nail unit lichen planus can be difficult to treat. The therapeutic modality should be chosen based on what anatomic area of the nail unit is affected. For example, onychorrhexis is caused by inflammation affecting the matrix; so appropriately directed intralesional steroids to this area are helpful (37). Conversely, if onycholysis is present, topical steroids can be applied directly to the nail bed. Topical tacrolimus has also been reported to be effective (38). If many nails are affected, systemic steroids can be employed, and literature exists supporting both oral and intramuscular delivery routes (39). Case reports have demonstrated the effectiveness of the biologic medication etanercept, the oral retinoid alitretinoin, and the combination of the topical retinoid tazarotene and the topical steroid clobetasol for the treatment of nail unit lichen planus (40–42). Given the association between lichen planus and hepatitis C, patients with nail unit lichen planus may warrant evaluation for hepatitis C and should be referred to a hepatologist if evidence of infection is found. Recently, an expert consensus group provided recommendations for treatment of the classical form of nail unit lichen planus, including both tiered recommendations for systemic therapies and multiple methods of intralesional steroid injections (43). Therapeutic considerations are determined primarily by the number of nails affected as well as by the degree of severity of the affected nails. First-line therapy includes intralesional and intramuscular triamcinolone acetonide. Secondary therapies include the oral retinoids acitretin and alitretinoin (not available in the United States). Tertiary therapies include the immunosuppressants azathioprine, cyclosporine, and mycophenolate mofetil.

INFECTION

Onychomycosis

Clinical Summary. Fungal infection of the nails is the most common nail disorder, accounting for up to 50% of nail disorders. Onychomycosis is present in 2% to 14% of the general population, rising to 50% in adults older than 70 years (44). A study in Brazil showed 28.3% of 7,852 patients examined were clinically diagnosed with onychomycosis (45). Medical conditions associated with an increased incidence of onychomycosis include diabetes, peripheral vascular disease, HIV infection, immunosuppression, obesity, smoking, a family history of onychomycosis, and increased age (46),(47). Although onychomycosis is not a life-threatening disorder, it can affect the quality of life (48).

The main types of onychomycosis include distal lateral subungual onychomycosis, proximal subungual onychomycosis, white superficial onychomycosis, total dystrophic onychomycosis, and candidal onychomycosis. Dermatophytes, mainly *Trichophyton rubrum* and *T. mentagrophytes*, are the most common fungi causing onychomycosis, accounting for 90% of fungal infections (49). Nondermatophyte molds, mainly *Scopulariopsis brevicaulis*, *Fusarium* sp., *Aspergillus* sp., *Scytalidium dimidiatum*, and *Acremonium* sp., account for 10% of infections worldwide (50). Ninety percent of toenail infections are caused by dermatophytes of *Trichophyton*, *Microsporum*, and *Epidermophyton* spp. Fungal staining with either PAS or Grocott methenamine silver (GMS) should be performed to evaluate for fungal infection on all nail biopsies because of the overlapping features seen in inflammatory dermatoses involving the nail. Additionally, it is possible for concurrent onychomycosis to be associated with a primary nail inflammatory disorder.

Distal lateral subungual onychomycosis (Fig. 19-5) is the most common form of onychomycosis and is usually caused by *T. rubrum*. The fungus initially invades the hyponychium and lateral nail folds, causing yellowing, onycholysis, and eventual

subungual hyperkeratosis. In proximal subungual onychomycosis, infection initially involves the area of the proximal nail fold. Proximal subungual onychomycosis is rare in the general population but is more common in immunocompromised patients. It was originally reported in patients affected with HIV. In these patients, proximal white subungual onychomycosis is caused by *T. rubrum*. On the other hand, superficial white onychomycosis is most often caused by *T. mentagrophytes* and nondermatophyte molds, and the fungi are located on the superficial nail plate only. *Candida* onychomycosis is rare and affects immunosuppressed patients. It may involve the nail plate and nail bed in patients with chronic mucocutaneous candidiasis and in HIV-infected patients (Fig. 19-6). Endonyx onychomycosis is usually caused by *T. soudanense* (not found in the United States) and presents without onycholysis and subungual hyperkeratosis (44,51).

An onychomycosis severity index has been published that grades the severity of onychomycosis by three measures: the area of onychomycosis involvement, the proximity of infection to the matrix, and the fungal burden with a dermatophytoma or subungual hyperkeratosis (44,52). Poor prognostic factors for onychomycosis responding to therapy include the presence of immunosuppression, older age, poor peripheral circulation, poorly controlled diabetes, subungual hyperkeratosis greater than 2 mm, significant lateral disease, the presence of dermatophytoma, more than 50% nail involvement, slow rate of nail growth, severe onycholysis, matrix involvement, total dystrophic onychomycosis, as well as the onychomycosis caused by nondermatophyte molds, yeasts, and mixed infections (49,52–54).

Histopathology. PAS- or GMS-stained sections will reveal fungal organisms that are usually located in the lower layers of the nail plate near the nail bed epidermis. A PAS or GMS stain performed on a nail biopsy, clippings of infected nail plate, or scrapings of subungual debris will yield a diagnosis of onychomycosis more quickly than will a fungal culture, but it will not identify the organism (Fig. 19-7). Another disadvantage of histopathology for the diagnosis of onychomycosis is that it is not possible to determine whether the fungus present is alive or dead. The nail bed epidermis shows acanthosis, spongiosis, and exocytosis of lymphocytes and histiocytes. A dermatophytoma is a dense collection of fungal elements, which can be noted histopathologically. It is important for dermatopathologists to

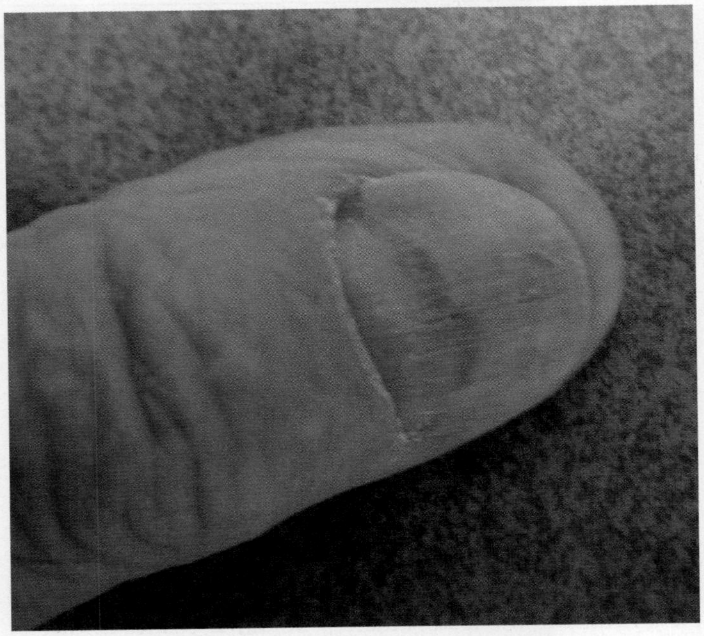

Figure 19-5 Onychomycosis of the nail. Distal subungual onychomycosis is seen in the thumb nail.

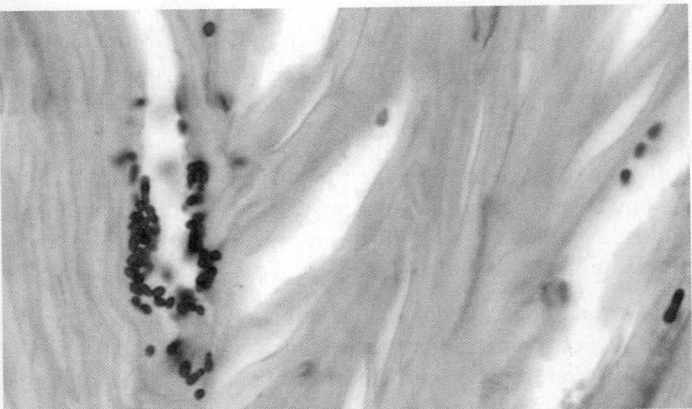

Figure 19-6 Candidiasis of the nail plate. Nail clippings showing budding yeast culture proven to be *Candida parapsilosis*.

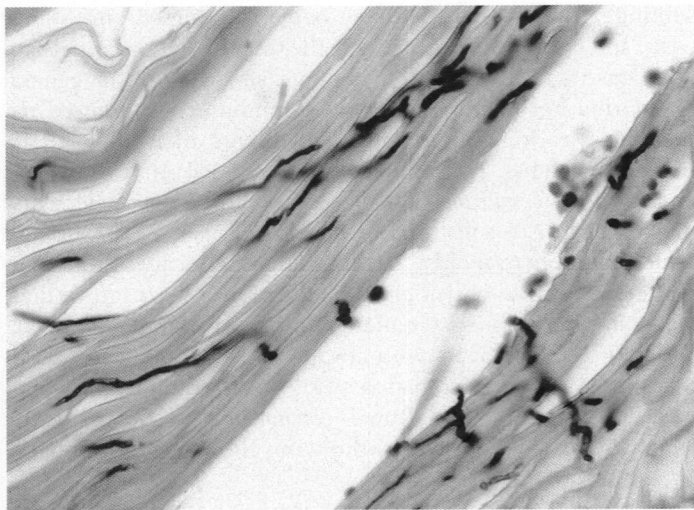

Figure 19-7 Onychomycosis of the nail plate. Nail clippings stained by periodic acid–Schiff with diastase showing septate hyphal elements culture proven to be *Trichophyton* sp. within the nail plate keratin.

alert the submitting physician of this entity if encountered, because physical removal of the dermatophytoma may be needed to clear the infection (55). Dermatophytomas can prevent the penetration of oral and topical medications and thus impair their effectiveness because of the production of a biofilm (56). Histopathology with PAS staining has the highest sensitivity in the detection of onychomycosis, compared with fungal culture and direct microscopy. In a recent study with 631 nail samples, the sensitivity was 82% with histology (including PAS staining), followed by a sensitivity of 53% with fungal culture, and a sensitivity of 48% with direct microscopy (57).

The slide quality of nail clipping specimens is improved by pretreatment with NaOH, which results in reduced tissue folding and fragmentation, improved ease of tissue cutting, and improved adherence of the tissue to the glass slides (58). Fungal elements are routinely detected on hematoxylin and eosin-stained sections with the use of fluorescence microscopy. This method could be useful if the cost of performing a special staining is a factor or if the tissue is exhausted and not available for special staining (59).

Comparison of the superiority of PAS or GMS stains for the detection of fungi in nail specimens is controversial in the scientific literature (60–62). However, PAS staining is generally technically easier to perform in the laboratory, and GMS staining can be easier to interpret with the contrast between the fungi and the background staining (62). Overall, it appears that PAS and GMS staining identify fungi with equal ability, but PAS staining is more cost-efficient, and may therefore be considered the preferred method (60,62).

Pathogenesis. As noted earlier, the most common causes of onychomycosis are the dermatophyte fungi. Nondermatophyte molds, as well as mixed infections, are occurring more commonly and can be difficult to treat.

Differential Diagnosis. The main clinical differential diagnosis for onychomycosis is nail unit psoriasis because of some of the overlapping features, including onycholysis and subungual hyperkeratosis. Other conditions that should be considered in the differential diagnosis of onychomycosis include nail unit lichen planus, onychogryphosis, traumatic onychodystrophy, pachyonychia congenita, yellow nail syndrome, and idiopathic onycholysis (44).

Principles of Management: Treatment choice for onychomycosis depends on a variety of factors, including the severity of disease, number of nails affected, age of the patient, causative organism, and cost. In adults, the standard therapy for dermatophyte onychomycosis is the antifungal medication terbinafine, which is fungicidal. Other oral antifungal options include itraconazole or fluconazole (63) (not FDA approved for this indication). If a nondermatophyte mold is the cause of onychomycosis, antifungal therapy should be tailored to the causative organism (50). Topical antifungal therapy can be effective in nails with less severity. It has been shown to be effective in children with onychomycosis (64). Topical therapies can also be considered for patients who are unwilling or unable to use oral antifungal drugs. Efinaconazole is a topical medication that has shown mycologic and complete cure rates similar to those seen with oral itraconazole (44). Efinaconazole has also been shown recently to have successfully treated dermatophytomas in 19 patients (65). Topical amphotericin B may be helpful for the therapy of nondermatophyte mold onychomycosis (66). For patients who may not be able to tolerate oral therapy, topical photodynamic therapy is an option (46). There has been substantial interest in the use of laser devices for the treatment of onychomycosis. In 2012, some Nd:YAG 1,064-nm laser devices were approved by the FDA for the "temporary increase of clear nail in onychomycosis" (67). However, only limited clinical trials exist for these laser devices, and it is not possible to compare their efficacy with that of the commonly used oral and topical antifungal medications used for onychomycosis (67). A recent systematic review of randomized controlled trials of laser monotherapy for dermatophyte onychomycosis of the great toenail concluded that the effectiveness of lasers as a therapeutic intervention of dermatophyte toenail onychomycosis is limited based on complete, mycologic, and clinical cure rates (68).

BULLOUS DISEASES

Several vesiculobullous diseases may affect the nail unit. Some of these dermatoses that may affect the nail unit are described here. For a complete description of the disorder, the reader is directed to the corresponding chapters elsewhere in the text (Chapters 6 and 9).

Darier Disease (Darier–White Disease)

In Darier disease, nail changes usually occur in association with other clinical findings. Rarely, involvement may be limited to the nail unit alone. Nail changes may occur in the proximal nail fold, matrix, nail bed, and hyponychium. The proximal nail fold may show keratotic papules that are histologically similar to those of acrokeratosis verruciformis of Hopf. However, in addition to papillary epidermal hyperplasia, focal areas of suprabasilar acantholysis may be seen.

Involvement of the nail matrix in Darier–White disease is usually located in the distal lunula and manifests clinically as a white longitudinal streak. Histologically, this leukonychia is secondary to foci of persistent parakeratosis in the lower nail plate related to the histopathology of Darier–White disease of the distal matrix. The features seen are suprabasilar acantholysis, with the formation of corps ronds and grains.

The nail bed and hyponychium are commonly involved in Darier–White disease. Involvement may be mild, leading to red and white longitudinal streaks. More severe involvement leads to wedge-shaped, distal, subungual keratosis, accompanied by nail fragility. In time, the nail plate may become markedly thickened. The nail bed epithelium becomes hyperplastic with parakeratosis between the nail bed and nail plate. Suprabasilar clefts are absent in the nail bed. An interesting finding is the presence of atypical keratinocytes in the nail bed epidermis, many of which may be multinucleated (69,70).

Pemphigus

Nail involvement in pemphigus vulgaris is present in about one-third of patients and may affect the proximal and lateral nail folds, leading to chronic paronychia (the most common finding) and superficial nail plate changes (71–73). Nail lesions often relapse shortly before recurrence or exacerbation of generalized disease (71,73,74). Involvement of the matrix causes onychomadesis (proximal separation of the nail plate). Nail matrix damage can also result in other nail plate changes, including onychoschizia, ridging, pitting, and trachyonychia (71,72). Severe nail dystrophy, discoloration of the nail plate, and destruction of the nail plate may occur (71,74). Subungual blisters can result in onycholysis, which may be hemorrhagic (73), a feature that might be correlated with a poor prognosis (75). A recent study of nail involvement with pemphigus demonstrated that the main clinical changes were paronychia and dystrophy. Destruction of the nail apparatus was seen in patients with pemphigus vegetans. The presence of ungual involvement was correlated with the severity of pemphigus, particularly with severe oral disease (76). Biopsy of the involved nail fold reveals suprabasilar acantholysis and positive direct immunofluorescence with immunoglobulin G (IgG) and C3 in the intercellular spaces of the epidermis. The paronychia seen with pemphigus vulgaris has specific histopathologic features, including suprabasal acantholysis without spongiosis or exocytosis (71). Pemphigus foliaceus may also affect the nail unit.

Pemphigoid

Bullous and cicatricial pemphigoid have been reported to uncommonly involve the nail unit. The nail folds are most commonly affected, but both the matrix and the nail bed may also be affected (71). Reported clinical signs include paronychia, onychomadesis, nail scarring with atrophy, total loss of the nails, and pterygium formation (71,77,78).

Epidermolysis Bullosa

Epidermolysis bullosa, in many of its manifestations, affects the nail unit. Early nail dystrophy and early nail loss are correlated with the severity of epidermolysis bullosa, especially with junctional epidermolysis bullosa and recessive dystrophic epidermolysis bullosa (79). Nails may also be the first area of the body to be affected by a form of epidermolysis bullosa. In severe cases of epidermolysis bullosa simplex, the nails may show onycholysis, onychomadesis, thickened nails, or onychogryphosis (79). Most forms of junctional epidermolysis bullosa can show severe nail dystrophy and anonychia (79). In the forms of dystrophic epidermolysis bullosa, the nail changes can be mild or severe. There is a subtype of nails-only dominant dystrophic epidermolysis bullosa where nail changes are the only feature (79). Nail changes common to both junctional epidermolysis bullosa and dystrophic epidermolysis bullosa include pachyonychia, dystrophic nails, nail atrophy, and anonychia (79). Loss of the nails has been described in epidermolysis bullosa acquisita (72,80).

CONNECTIVE TISSUE DISEASE

The nail unit is affected by most types of connective tissue disease, primarily in the microvasculature of the proximal nail fold. *In vivo* capillary microscopy reveals dilated capillary loops with adjacent hemorrhage and avascularity. This pattern is present in 80% to 95% of patients with progressive systemic sclerosis. However, an identical clinical pattern may be seen in patients with dermatomyositis, other connective tissue diseases, and idiopathic Raynaud phenomenon. A crescent-shaped biopsy of the proximal nail fold reveals deposits of eosinophilic PAS-positive material in the keratin of the cuticle. These deposits tend to be more extensive in patients with connective tissue disease and in patients with more severe *in vivo* capillary microscopy abnormalities. Direct immunofluorescence can also be performed on a proximal nail fold biopsy, revealing vascular deposits in connective tissue disease.

Pterygium inversum unguis (PIU) is a nail disorder, about half the cases of which are associated with an underlying connective tissue disease, including scleroderma and systemic lupus erythematosus. Clinically, there is a forward extension of the hyponychium that is adherent to the ventral aspect (underside) of the nail plate. The normal distal groove of the nail is no longer present. There is a visible subungual keratotic thickening between the hyponychium and the ventral nail plate. The usual symptom in patients is pain or bleeding while clipping the nails. Fingernails are more often affected than toenails, and women are more often affected than men (81).

Familial, congenital, and idiopathic cases of PIU have also been reported. There have been reports of PIU associated with other causes unrelated to connective tissue disease, such as an acrylate allergy, formaldehyde-containing hardeners, stroke, and subungual exostosis. A study of 17 women showed the development of PIU secondary to the use of gel nail polish, after 2 to 5 years of gel polish application. All but two of the patients experienced resolution of the PIU a few weeks after switching from gel nail polish to regular nail polish manicures (82). Screening for a potential underlying systemic disorder is prudent. Because PIU may be the presenting sign of a systemic disorder that may fully develop subsequently, patient follow-up is important.

There have only been a few descriptions of the histopathology of PIU. One case showed marked hyperkeratosis that extended up to and firmly affixed to an unremarkable nail plate. The nail bed showed minimal acanthosis, and the vasculature was normal (83). Another study demonstrated the presence of a highly eosinophilic keratinized substance that contained pale and nucleated corneocytes attached to the distal and visceral nail plate. This material was also present in the free edge of the nail plate. There was also a markedly eosinophilic whorled keratinized substance in the horny layer of the fingertip (84). It has been suggested that the pathogenesis of PIU relates to an abnormality in the regulation of the production of the horny layer by the nail isthmus (anatomic area located between the most distal part of the nail bed and the hyponychium) (84,85).

Treatment of PIU is difficult, and topical therapies, including keratolytics and topical steroids, have not shown good results. A report showed a good response with a topical lacquer that includes hydroxypropyl chitosan, horsetail extract, and methylsulfonylmethane. Therapy for an underlying disorder could improve PIU.

ACKNOWLEDGMENTS

The author wishes to acknowledge Dr. Thomas D. Griffin for his contributions to prior versions of this chapter.

REFERENCES

1. Hinshaw MA, Rubin A. Inflammatory diseases of the nail unit. *Semin Cutan Med Surg.* 2015;34(2):109–116.
2. Stephen S, Tosti A, Rubin AI. Diagnostic applications of nail clippings. *Dermatol Clin.* 2015;33(2):289–301.
3. Jellinek NJ, Rubin AI. Lateral longitudinal excision of the nail unit. *Dermatol Surg.* 2011;37(12):1781–1785.
4. Kharghoria G, Grover C, Bhattacharya SN, Sharma S. Histopathological evaluation of nail lichen planus: a cross-sectional study. *J Cutan Pathol.* 2021;48(1):11–17.
5. Hur K, Han B, Lim SS, Mun JH. Histopathologic findings of idiopathic trachyonychia: an analysis of 30 adult patients. *J Cutan Pathol.* 2021;48(3):396–402.
6. Collins SC, Cordova K, Jellinek NJ. Alternatives to complete nail plate avulsion. *J Am Acad Dermatol.* 2008;59(4):619–626.
7. Baran R. The burden of nail psoriasis: an introduction. *Dermatology.* 2010;221(suppl 1):1–5.
8. Rich P, Scher RK. Nail Psoriasis Severity Index: a useful tool for evaluation of nail psoriasis. *J Am Acad Dermatol.* 2003;49(2):206–212.
9. Rigopoulos D, Baran R, Chiheb S, et al. Recommendations for the definition, evaluation, and treatment of nail psoriasis in adult patients with no or mild skin psoriasis: a dermatologist and nail expert group consensus. *J Am Acad Dermatol.* 2019;81(1):228–240.
10. Soscia E, Sirignano C, Catalano O, et al. New developments in magnetic resonance imaging of the nail unit. *J Rheumatol Suppl.* 2012;89:49–53.
11. Soscia E, Scarpa R, Cimmino MA, et al. Magnetic resonance imaging of nail unit in psoriatic arthritis. *J Rheumatol Suppl.* 2009;83:42–45.
12. Scarpa R, Soscia E, Peluso R, et al. Nail and distal interphalangeal joint in psoriatic arthritis. *J Rheumatol.* 2006;33(7):1315–1319.
13. McGonagle D. Enthesitis: an autoinflammatory lesion linking nail and joint involvement in psoriatic disease. *J Eur Acad Dermatol Venereol.* 2009;23(suppl 1):9–13.
14. McGonagle DG, Helliwell P, Veale D. Enthesitis in psoriatic disease. *Dermatology.* 2012;225(2):100–109.
15. McGonagle D, Tan AL, Benjamin M. The nail as a musculoskeletal appendage—implications for an improved understanding of the link between psoriasis and arthritis. *Dermatology.* 2009;218(2):97–102.
16. Ash ZR, Tinazzi I, Gallego CC, et al. Psoriasis patients with nail disease have a greater magnitude of underlying systemic subclinical enthesopathy than those with normal nails. *Ann Rheum Dis.* 2012;71(4):553–556.
17. Radtke MA, Beikert FC, Augustin M. Nail psoriasis—a treatment challenge. *J Dtsch Dermatol Ges.* 2013;11(3):203–219; quiz 220.
18. Tan ES, Chong WS, Tey HL. Nail psoriasis: a review. *Am J Clin Dermatol.* 2012;13(6):375–388.
19. Werner B, Fonseca GP, Seidel G. Microscopic nail clipping findings in patients with psoriasis. *Am J Dermatopathol.* 2015;37(6):429–439.
20. de Berker D. Management of psoriatic nail disease. *Semin Cutan Med Surg.* 2009;28(1):39–43.
21. De Simone C, Maiorino A, Tassone F, et al. Tacrolimus 0.1% ointment in nail psoriasis: a randomized controlled open-label study. *J Eur Acad Dermatol Venereol.* 2013;27(8):1003–1006.
22. Edwards F, de Berker D. Nail psoriasis: clinical presentation and best practice recommendations. *Drugs.* 2009;69(17):2351–2361.
23. Oram Y, Akkaya AD. Treatment of nail psoriasis: common concepts and new trends. *Dermatol Res Pract.* 2013;2013:180496.
24. Treewittayapoom C, Singvahanont P, Chanprapaph K, et al. The effect of different pulse durations in the treatment of nail psoriasis with 595-nm pulsed dye laser: a randomized, double-blind, intrapatient left-to-right study. *J Am Acad Dermatol.* 2012;66(5):807–812.
25. Liang CY, Lin TY, Lin YK. Successful treatment of pediatric nail psoriasis with periodic pustular eruption using topical indigo naturalis oil extract. *Pediatr Dermatol.* 2013;30(1):117–119.
26. Lin YK. Indigo naturalis oil extract drops in the treatment of moderate to severe nail psoriasis: a small case series. *Arch Dermatol.* 2011;147(5):627–629.
27. Lin YK, See LC, Chang YC, et al. Treatment of psoriatic nails with indigo naturalis oil extract: a non-controlled pilot study. *Dermatology.* 2011;223(3):239–243.
28. Ricceri F, Pescitelli L, Tripo L, et al. Treatment of severe nail psoriasis with acitretin: an impressive therapeutic result. *Dermatol Ther.* 2013;26(1):77–78.
29. Pandhi D, Singal A, Bhattacharya SN. Lichen planus in childhood: a series of 316 patients. *Pediatr Dermatol.* 2014;31(1):59–67.
30. Goettmann S, Zaraa I, Moulonguet I. Nail lichen planus: epidemiological, clinical, pathological, therapeutic and prognosis study of 67 cases. *J Eur Acad Dermatol Venereol.* 2012;26(10):1304–1309.
31. Nishizawa A, Satoh T, Yokozeki H. Close association between metal allergy and nail lichen planus: detection of causative metals in nail lesions. *J Eur Acad Dermatol Venereol.* 2013;27(2):e231–e234.
32. Tosti A, Piraccini BM, Cambiaghi S, et al. Nail lichen planus in children: clinical features, response to treatment, and long-term follow-up. *Arch Dermatol.* 2001;137(8):1027–1032.
33. Hall R, Wartman D, Jellinek N, et al. Lichen planus of the nail matrix with predominant plasma cell infiltrate. *J Cutan Pathol.* 2008;35(suppl 1):14–16.
34. Kharghoria G, Grover C, Bhattacharya SN, Sharma S. Histopathological evaluation of nail lichen planus: a cross-sectional study. *J Cutan Pathol.* 2021;48(1):11–17.
35. Rubin AI. The "frayed nail plate" and further detailed analysis of the histopathologic features of nail unit lichen planus. *J Cutan Pathol.* 2021;48(1):6–7.
36. Sanli H, Arat M, Oskay T, et al. Evaluation of nail involvement in patients with chronic cutaneous graft versus host disease: a single-center study from Turkey. *Int J Dermatol.* 2004;43(3):176–180.
37. Brauns B, Stahl M, Schon MP, et al. Intralesional steroid injection alleviates nail lichen planus. *Int J Dermatol.* 2011;50(5):626–627.
38. Ujiie H, Shibaki A, Akiyama M, et al. Successful treatment of nail lichen planus with topical tacrolimus. *Acta Derm Venereol.* 2010;90(2):218–219.
39. Dehesa L, Tosti A. Treatment of inflammatory nail disorders. *Dermatol Ther.* 2012;25(6):525–534.
40. Irla N, Schneiter T, Haneke E, et al. Nail lichen planus: successful treatment with etanercept. *Case Rep Dermatol.* 2010;2(3):173–176.
41. Pinter A, Patzold S, Kaufmann R. Lichen planus of nails—successful treatment with Alitretinoin. *J Dtsch Dermatol Ges.* 2011;9(12):1033–1034.
42. Prevost NM, English JC III. Palliative treatment of fingernail lichen planus. *J Drugs Dermatol.* 2007;6(2):202–204.
43. Iorizzo M, Tosti A, Starace M, et al. Isolated nail lichen planus: an expert consensus on treatment of the classical form. *J Am Acad Dermatol.* 2020;83(6):1717–1723.

44. Elewski BE, Rich P, Tosti A, et al. Onchomycosis: an overview. *J Drugs Dermatol*. 2013;12(7):s96–s103.

45. Di Chiacchio N, Suarez MV, Madeira CL, et al. An observational and descriptive study of the epidemiology of and therapeutic approach to onychomycosis in dermatology offices in Brazil. *An Bras Dermatol*. 2013;88(suppl 1):3–11.

46. Gupta A, Simpson F. Device-based therapies for onychomycosis treatment. *Skin Therapy Lett*. 2012;17(9):4–9.

47. Gupta AK, Ryder JE, Summerbell RC. Onychomycosis: classification and diagnosis. *J Drugs Dermatol*. 2004;3(1):51–56.

48. Milobratovic D, Jankovic S, Vukicevic J, et al. Quality of life in patients with toenail onychomycosis. *Mycoses*. 2013;56(5):543–551.

49. Shemer A. Update: medical treatment of onychomycosis. *Dermatol Ther*. 2012;25(6):582–593.

50. Gupta AK, Drummond-Main C, Cooper EA, et al. Systematic review of nondermatophyte mold onychomycosis: diagnosis, clinical types, epidemiology, and treatment. *J Am Acad Dermatol*. 2012;66(3):494–502.

51. Hay RJ, Baran R. Onychomycosis: a proposed revision of the clinical classification. *J Am Acad Dermatol*. 2011;65(6):1219–1227.

52. Carney C, Tosti A, Daniel R, et al. A new classification system for grading the severity of onychomycosis: Onychomycosis Severity Index. *Arch Dermatol*. 2011;147(11):1277–1282.

53. Grover C, Khurana A. An update on treatment of onychomycosis. *Mycoses*. 2012;55(6):541–551.

54. Shemer A, Scher R, Farhi R, et al. Why there is a wide difference in the clinical and mycological results in different onychomycosis clinical studies. *J Eur Acad Dermatol Venereol* 2013;27(3):e434–e435.

55. Bennett D, Rubin AI. Dermatophytoma: a clinicopathologic entity important for dermatologists and dermatopathologists to identify. *Int J Dermatol*. 2013;52(10):1285–1287.

56. Burkhart CN, Burkhart CG, Gupta AK. Dermatophytoma: recalcitrance to treatment because of existence of fungal biofilm. *J Am Acad Dermatol*. 2002;47(4):629–631.

57. Wilsmann-Theis D, Sareika F, Bieber T, et al. New reasons for histopathological nail-clipping examination in the diagnosis of onychomycosis. *J Eur Acad Dermatol Venereol*. 2011;25(2):235–237.

58. Nazarian RM, Due B, Deshpande A, et al. An improved method of surgical pathology testing for onychomycosis. *J Am Acad Dermatol*. 2012;66(4):655–660.

59. Idriss MH, Khalil A, Elston D. The diagnostic value of fungal fluorescence in onychomycosis. *J Cutan Pathol*. 2013;40(4):385–390.

60. Barak O, Asarch A, Horn T. PAS is optimal for diagnosing onychomycosis. *J Cutan Pathol*. 2010;37(10):1038–1040.

61. D'Hue Z, Perkins SM, Billings SD. GMS is superior to PAS for diagnosis of onychomycosis. *J Cutan Pathol*. 2008;35(8):745–747.

62. Reza Kermanshahi T, Rhatigan R. Comparison between PAS and GMS stains for the diagnosis of onychomycosis. *J Cutan Pathol*. 2010;37(10):1041–1044.

63. Gupta AK, Drummond-Main C, Paquet M. Evidence-based optimal fluconazole dosing regimen for onychomycosis treatment. *J Dermatolog Treat*. 2013;24(1):75–80.

64. Friedlander SF, Chan YC, Chan YH, et al. Onychomycosis does not always require systemic treatment for cure: a trial using topical therapy. *Pediatr Dermatol*. 2013;30(3):316–322.

65. Wang C, Cantrell W, Canavan T, Elewski B. Successful treatment of dermatophytomas in 19 patients using efinaconazole 10% solution. *Skin Appendage Disord*. 2019;5(5):304–308.

66. Lurati M, Baudraz-Rosselet F, Vernez M, et al. Efficacious treatment of non-dermatophyte mould onychomycosis with topical amphotericin B. *Dermatology*. 2011;223(4):289–292.

67. Gupta AK, Simpson F. Newly approved laser systems for onychomycosis. *J Am Podiatr Med Assoc*. 2012;102(5):428–430.

68. Gupta AK, Venkataraman M, Quinlan EM. Efficacy of lasers for the management of dermatophyte toenail onychomycosis. *J Am Podiatr Med Assoc*. 2021:20–236.

69. Baran R. The red nail—always benign? *Actas Dermosifiliogr*. 2009;100(suppl 1):106–113.

70. Cohen PR. Longitudinal erythronychia: individual or multiple linear red bands of the nail plate: a review of clinical features and associated conditions. *Am J Clin Dermatol*. 2011;12(4):217–231.

71. Tosti A, Andre M, Murrell DF. Nail involvement in autoimmune bullous disorders. *Dermatol Clin*. 2011;29(3):511–513, xi.

72. Habibi M, Mortazavi H, Shadianloo S, et al. Nail changes in pemphigus vulgaris. *Int J Dermatol*. 2008;47(11):1141–1144.

73. Lee HE, Wong WR, Lee MC, et al. Acute paronychia heralding the exacerbation of pemphigus vulgaris. *Int J Clin Pract*. 2004;58(12):1174–1176.

74. Kolivras A, Gheeraert P, Andre J. Nail destruction in pemphigus vulgaris. *Dermatology*. 2003;206(4):351–352.

75. Reich A, Wisnicka B, Szepietowski JC. Haemorrhagic nails in pemphigus vulgaris. *Acta Derm Venereol*. 2008;88(5):542.

76. Baghad B, Chiheb S. Nail involvement during pemphigus. *Skin Appendage Disord*. 2019;5(6):362–365.

77. Gualco F, Cozzani E, Parodi A. Bullous pemphigoid with nail loss. *Int J Dermatol*. 2005;44(11):967–968.

78. Tomita M, Tanei R, Hamada Y, et al. A case of localized pemphigoid with loss of toenails. *Dermatology*. 2002;204(2):155.

79. Tosti A, de Farias DC, Murrell DF. Nail involvement in epidermolysis bullosa. *Dermatol Clin*. 2010;28(1):153–157.

80. Meissner C, Hoefeld-Fegeler M, Vetter R, et al. Severe acral contractures and nail loss in a patient with mechano-bullous epidermolysis bullosa acquisita. *Eur J Dermatol*. 2010;20(4):543–544.

81. Marinho Falcao Gondim R, Bezerra da Trindade Neto P, Baran R. Pterygium inversum unguis: report of an extensive case with good therapeutic response to hydroxypropyl chitosan and review of the literature. *J Drugs Dermatol*. 2013;12(3):344–346.

82. Cervantes J, Sanchez M, Eber AE, Perper M, Tosti A. Pterygium inversum unguis secondary to gel polish. *J Eur Acad Dermatol Venereol*. 2018;32(1):160–163.

83. Vadmal M, Reyter I, Oshtory S, et al. Pterygium inversum unguis associated with stroke. *J Am Acad Dermatol*. 2005;53(3):501–503.

84. Oiso N, Narita T, Tsuruta D, et al. Pterygium inversum unguis: aberrantly regulated keratinization in the nail isthmus. *Clin Exp Dermatol*. 2009;34(7):e514–e515.

85. Oiso N, Kurokawa I, Kawada A. Nail isthmus: a distinct region of the nail apparatus. *Dermatol Res Pract*. 2012;2012:925023.

Chapter 20

Inflammatory Diseases of the Subcutaneous Fat: Panniculitis

MAXWELL A. FUNG AND LUIS REQUENA

INTRODUCTION

The principles of a pattern-based approach to the histologic diagnosis of inflammatory diseases of the subcutaneous fat (panniculitis) follow those of other inflammatory diseases but with several unique considerations. Following the teachings of Hermann Pinkus, Wallace Clark, and others, the septal versus lobular patterns in panniculitis were formally established more than 40 years ago in A. Bernard Ackerman's *Histologic Diagnosis of Inflammatory Skin Disease* (1). Although these patterns are easy to grasp conceptually, they have remained notoriously difficult to apply to cases encountered in clinical practice. Ackerman himself stated "… it may be impossible to make a decisive judgment as to whether the process is predominantly septal or lobular" (1). Indeed, panniculitis has reputation to be one of the most difficult subjects in dermatopathology, the "ugly duckling" of dermatopathology and "source of considerable confusion and often cause of diagnostic difficulty to clinicians and pathologists alike" (2,3). With the exception of erythema nodosum, ulceration may occur in nearly any form of panniculitis but is perhaps most characteristic of infection. A recently proposed classification emphasized ulcerating (e.g., infection, erythema induratum) versus nonulcerating (e.g., erythema nodosum) panniculitis (4). In this chapter, our own experiences are combined with those published by others to offer a review of panniculitis that we hope will be suitable for educating physicians as well as a reference source for the practicing diagnostic dermatopathologist.

A pattern-based histologic classification for panniculitis is presented in Table 20-1. It is noted that other classifications of panniculitis recognize a "mixed" septal and lobular group, but in our view the members of this group have proved inconsistent and seemingly arbitrary. Actually, all cases of panniculitis combine some element of septal and lobular alteration, exemplifying the fact that attempts to classify human disease, especially those founded on a single methodology (e.g., histology), are imperfect. In practice, assessing the *predominant* or *most commonly encountered* pattern readily accomplishes the critical first step in the diagnostic assessment of panniculitis. As shown in the classification, assessment of pattern at scanning magnification is followed by assessment for vasculitis, adipocyte necrosis, inflammatory cell types (e.g., eosinophilic, lymphocytic [5], neutrophilic [6]), and other features requiring microscopic examination at higher magnification.

Not all of the disease entities in Table 20-1 are presented in detail in this chapter, and many are reviewed elsewhere

Table 20-1
Classification of Panniculitis

I. Mostly septal pattern—with vasculitis
  A. Polyarteritis nodosa
  B. Superficial migratory thrombophlebitis
  C. Subcutaneous involvement by small vessel leukocytoclastic vasculitis
    1. ANCA-associated vasculitis
      a. Granulomatosis with polyangiitis (Wegener)
      b. Eosinophilic granulomatosis with polyangiitis (Churg–Strauss)
      c. Microscopic polyangiitis
    2. Immune complex
      a. Cryoglobulinemia, IgA vasculitis (Henoch–Schönlein), urticarial vasculitis, etc.

II. Mostly septal pattern—no vasculitis
  A. Erythema nodosum
  B. Subcutaneous involvement by palisaded granulomatous dermatitis
    1. Deep/subcutaneous granuloma annulare
    2. Necrobiosis lipoidica
    3. Necrobiotic xanthogranuloma
    4. Rheumatoid nodule
  C. Sclerosing disorders
    1. Morphea profunda
    2. Systemic scleroderma
    3. Eosinophilic fasciitis (Schulman syndrome)
    4. Nephrogenic systemic fibrosis

III. Mostly lobular pattern—with vasculitis
  A. Erythema induratum/nodular vasculitis
  B. Lupus erythematosus profundus (lupus panniculitis)
  C. Dermatomyositis
  D. Crohn disease
  E. Behcet syndrome

IV. Mostly lobular pattern—no vasculitis
  A. Neutrophilic +/− granulomatous
    1. Reaction to ruptured infundibular follicular cyst
    2. Lipodermatosclerosis (sclerosing panniculitis)
    3. Infectious panniculitis

(continued)

Table 20-1

Classification of Panniculitis (*continued*)

    4. Pancreatic panniculitis

    5. α-1-antitrypsin deficiency panniculitis

  B. Lymphocytic

    1. Lupus panniculitis (lupus profundus)

    2. Dermatomyositis

  C. Granulomatous/histiocytic

    1. Erythema induratum (nodular vasculitis)

    2. Traumatic panniculitis

    3. Factitial panniculitis

    4. Sclerosing postirradiation panniculitis

    5. Lipoatrophic panniculitis of the ankles

    6. Subcutaneous fat necrosis of the newborn

    7. Sclerema neonatorum

    8. Gout

    9. Oxalosis

    10. Calciphylaxis

    11. Cold panniculitis

    12. Poststeroid panniculitis

    13. Cytophagic histiocytic panniculitis

  D. Eosinophilic panniculitis

  E. Neutrophilic panniculitis

  F. Drug-induced panniculitis

V. Loss of fat

  A. Lipoatrophy and lipodystrophy

  B. Lipedema

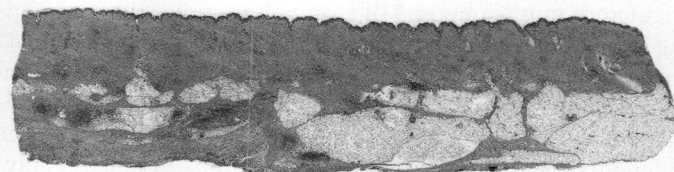

Figure 20-1 Incisional biopsy for panniculitis.

in this text: small vessel leukocytoclastic vasculitis (Chapter 8), connective tissue diseases and sclerosing disorders (Chapter 10), and noninfectious granulomatous disorders (Chapter 14).

As for most inflammatory skin disorders, it is especially true for panniculitis that a composite assessment of all available clinical, laboratory, and histopathologic features may be required to achieve the correct diagnosis (7). Diagnostic difficulties in panniculitis are many, with one or more of the following factors often combining to handicap the interpretation of a case:

1. *Insufficient sampling.* The ideal specimen for assessment of panniculitis is a full-thickness incisional biopsy, sectioned longitudinally (Fig. 20-1). However, panniculitis often presents on the legs of adults, where poor wound healing is a risk. The surgeon can minimize the risk by obtaining a narrow incisional biopsy (e.g., 1 cm in length but only a few millimeters wide), oriented vertically with respect to anatomic position, thereby minimizing wound edge tension and disruption of lymphatic drainage. Practically speaking, trephine (punch) biopsies are often obtained. Although it is possible to make the diagnosis from a trephine biopsy specimen, the likelihood of a nondiagnostic biopsy increases; not uncommonly, biopsies lack subcutis entirely. If subcutis is not grossly identified intraoperatively, the surgeon may

consider applying the biopsy instrument a second time to the wound base to obtain additional deep tissue. Unless other clinical considerations prevail, anything less than a 4-mm trephine biopsy is not advised.

2. *Limited range of clinical features.* When panniculitis presents without overlying epidermal or dermal changes, the clinical morphology is typically nonspecific: smooth, tender, erythematous nodules, most commonly on the lower extremities. The location or distribution of lesions can be helpful, especially when combined with other clinical features.

3. *Limited range and specificity of histopathologic features.* Even with good sampling, nondiagnostic biopsies in panniculitis are relatively common. Part of this may be attributable to sampling of late or resolving panniculitis, especially lobular patterns of panniculitis that commonly eventuate in nonspecific lipophagic necrosis. In contrast, the late stage of septal panniculitis may often still be specifically diagnosed (erythema nodosum, morphea profunda), and some lobular disorders (lupus profundus, pancreatic panniculitis) can also be diagnostic in their end stage. Best practices include consideration of step sections and assessment of clinical features and disease stage before rendering a nonspecific interpretation. "Diagnoses" such as eosinophilic panniculitis, neutrophilic panniculitis, or lipomembranous (membranocystic) panniculitis represent descriptions of recognized reaction patterns, each with a differential diagnosis, not specific entities. The inherent challenges represented by panniculitis are illustrated by the existence of variants of panniculitis generally no longer recognized as authentic (e.g., Weber–Christian and Rothmann–Makai variants), as well as the difficulty in distinguishing some cases of lupus profundus and cytophagic histiocytic panniculitis from subcutaneous T-cell lymphoma.

ANATOMY OF THE SUBCUTIS

The subcutis may be divided into lobules composed of mostly adipocytes (lipocytes), collagenous septa surrounding and demarcating each fat lobule, and associated vessels and nerves. The septa are contiguous with the overlying reticular dermis and with underlying fascia. The superficial subcutis contains appendageal structures, including the glands of eccrine and apocrine units and the bulbar portion of terminal anagen hair follicles. Adipocytes often surround these structures in a periappendageal distribution.

The septa contain the arteries, veins, lymphatics, and nerves that supply the plexus of vessels within the lobules as well as the overlying dermis. Each fat lobule is approximately 1 cm in diameter and may be subdivided into microlobules (each ~1 mm in diameter) supplied by (and defined as) a discrete circulatory unit, composed of a central arteriole and surrounding capillaries and postcapillary venules. This is a "terminal" configuration in that there is no collateral supply between adjacent microlobules. This unique anatomy accounts for diagnostically relevant features that are best exemplified in the differential diagnosis of two forms of vasculitis, cutaneous polyarteritis nodosa and erythema induratum (see appropriate sections). Lymphatic drainage originates in the overlying dermis, passing through the septa, where they accept venous drainage *en route* to regional lymph nodes (1,8).

Histology of the Adipocyte

Adipocytes differentiate from mesenchymal stem cells and form a closely regulated metabolic reserve capable of fat synthesis and fat storage, containing primarily neutral lipids and triglycerides. Mature adipocytes are large cells (100 μm) composed of a single fat vacuole that appears as an empty clear space in formalin-fixed sections. A small round/ovoid or spindled basophilic nucleus without discernible nuclear features is present along the border of the cell, creating a signet ring appearance. Immunohistochemical stains for S100 and vimentin highlight adipocytes in formalin-fixed specimens. In contrast, adipophilin stains multivacuolated lipid-containing cells such as sebocytes and foamy histiocytes but is negative in adipocytes (9,10). Oil Red O directly highlights cytoplasmic lipid within adipocytes in cryopreserved tissue.

Types of Adipocyte Necrosis in Panniculitis

The spectrum of appearances of necrotic adipocytes is distinct from other necrotic cells that generally exhibit nuclear pyknosis and condensed eosinophilic cytoplasm. Histologically distinct forms of fat necrosis encountered in panniculitis include lipophagic, hyaline, microcystic, lipomembranous/pseudomembranous/membranocystic, and pancreatic/enzymatic, as summarized in Table 20-2 and Figure 20-2 (8,11). Overall, the type of fat necrosis confers a limited degree of diagnostic specificity, with lipophagic and lipomembranous necrosis being the least specific, and hyaline and pancreatic/enzymatic types of necrosis perhaps being most specific (though not pathognomonic for any single disorder). Lipomembranous

fat necrosis exhibits a particularly distinctive appearance with distorted, cystic spaces lined by a thin eosinophilic layer, called a lipomembrane, which has fine, feathery, and often arabesque projections into the cystic cavity (Fig. 20-2D). These lipomembranes are highlighted by periodic acid–Schiff (PAS), lysozyme, and CD68, suggesting a contribution of these enzymes from the histiocytes in the production of lipomembranous necrosis; late or older lesions are only weakly positive or negative for CD68 and lysozyme (12). Lipomembranous and microcystic fat necrosis generally occur concomitantly; some authors reserve the term membranocystic fat necrosis to encompass their combined presence (13).

Systemic Interactions with Subcutaneous Fat

Subcutaneous fat has evolved as an important energy storage system with both endocrine effects and a role in local as well as systemic inflammation levels. Fat metabolism is set to store energy when food is abundant and to release energy when food is scarce. Although it also serves for cushioning and maintenance of body temperature, pathologic changes in the adipose tissue can have effects on the general metabolic state, with particular relevance for common disorders such as obesity, Type 2 diabetes mellitus, atherosclerosis, dyslipidemia, heart disease, and metabolic syndrome, as well as severe forms of lipodystrophy. As such, the subcutaneous fat may be regarded as a distinct organ from an endocrine perspective.

The cytokine hormone leptin is adipocyte-derived ("adipokine") and functions as a long-term appetite suppressant, with levels that correlate with the size and number of fat cells. Leptin inhibits the hypothalamus at centers that increase hunger and feeding activity. Children with a genetic block in the hypothalamus that prevents a response to high blood leptin levels have excessive eating, massive obesity, and significant comorbidities, including hypertension and accelerated atherosclerosis. Insulin levels are increased in the blood of such infants, and muscular movement activity levels are low. In common obesity in adult humans, leptin levels are high in the blood, but decreased hypothalamic sensitivity to leptin prevents a response to synthetic leptin administration. Leptin interaction with the normal hypothalamus can also influence the level of thyroid hormone, decrease reproductive activity, and interfere with inflammatory

Table 20-2

Distinctive Forms of Adipocyte Necrosis in Panniculitis (Fig. 20-2) (8,11)

Type	Description	Major Differential Diagnosis/Comments
Lipophagic	Lipophages (foamy macrophages)	Traumatic, lipodermatosclerosis Late stage of any panniculitis
Liquefactive	Granular, amphophilic	α-1-Antitrypsin deficiency, pancreatic
Enzymatic	Ghost adipocytes, calcification	Pancreatic, infection
Hyaline	Eosinophilic, glassy, hyaline, homogeneous	Lupus profundus, dermatomyositis, subcutaneous panniculitis-like T-cell lymphoma
Lipomembranous (membranocystic, pseudomembranous)	Eosinophilic or amphophilic, arabesque, crenulated cyst lining	Lipodermatosclerosis, traumatic Late stage of any lobular panniculitis
Microcystic	Fat vacuoles of varying sizes (microcysts, macrocysts), arises in setting of lipomembranous necrosis	Lipodermatosclerosis, traumatic Late stage of any lobular panniculitis
Ischemic	Adipocyte pallor	Erythema induratum, calciphylaxis
Basophilic	Granular, basophilic, neutrophils	Infection, pancreatic

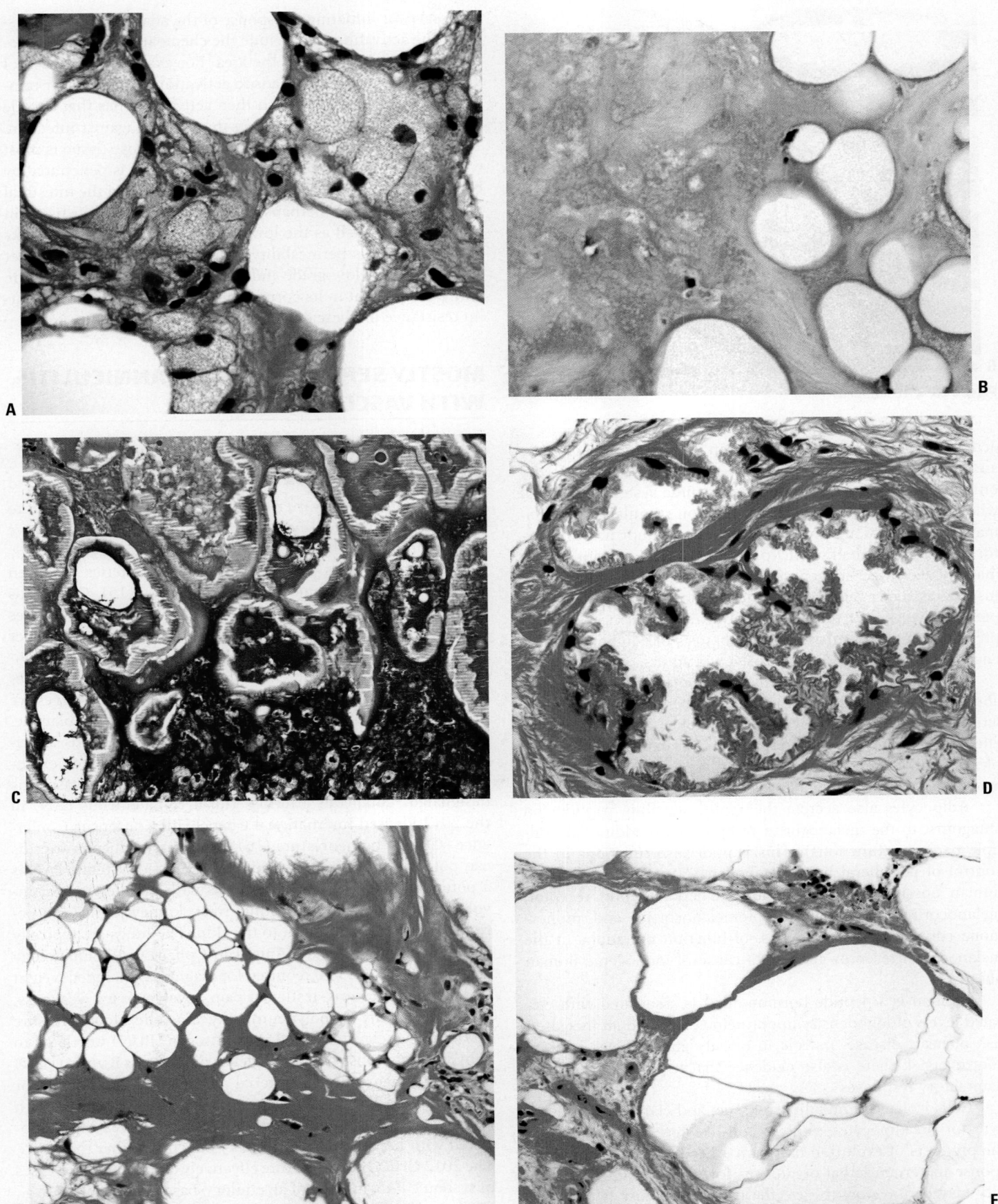

Figure 20-2 The histologic spectrum of adipocyte necrosis. A: Lipophagic. B: Hyaline. C: Enzymatic. D: Lipomembranous. E: Microcystic. F: Ischemic. G: Basophilic.

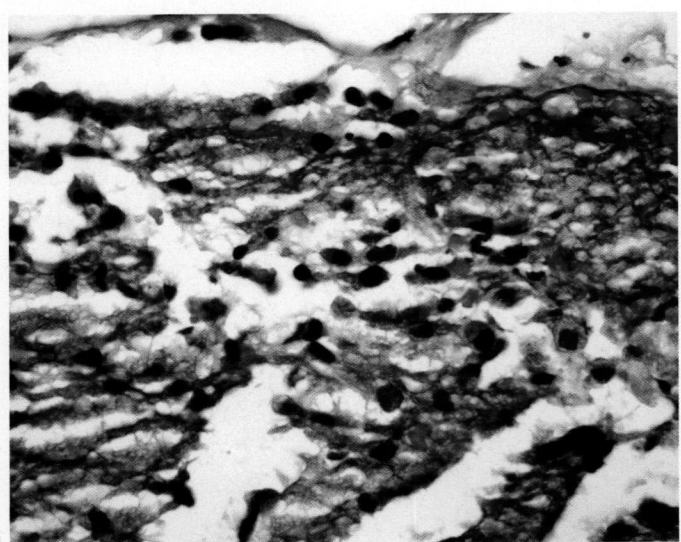

G

Figure 20-2 (*continued*)

activity and immune function. Leptin derived from adipocytes and preadipocytes has been shown to have regulatory activity on Toll-like receptors of the innate immune system. Studies of whole adipose tissue have shown that, on stimulation, inflammatory mediators are produced, including tumor necrosis factor (TNF)-α, interleukin (IL)-6, and IL-10. TNF-α regulates fat mass by decreased lipogenesis, increased lipolysis, induction of insulin resistance, and can initiate apoptosis in adipocytes and preadipocytes. IL-6 increases lipolysis. The balance between preadipocyte differentiation and apoptosis of adipocytes influences the number of adipocytes, even in adults.

Adiponectin plays a role in the suppression of metabolic abnormalities associated with diabetes, obesity, atherosclerosis, fatty liver, and metabolic syndrome. Adiponectin exerts central effects promoting weight reduction and therefore acts in complementary or synergistic fashion with leptin. Obesity is associated with downregulated adiponectin levels.

Adipocytes also secrete the agouti signaling peptide (an antagonist to the melanocortin receptor, with additional multiple paracrine functions). This peptide also functions in the control of peripheral lipid metabolism. Causes of monogenic human obesity include mutations in leptin, leptin receptor, melanocortin-4 receptor, proopiomelanocortin, and prohormone convertase 1/3 (14). Loss-of-function mutations in the melanocortin receptor gene are a cause of monogenic human obesity.

Resistin is a peptide hormone that is associated with elevated levels of low-density lipoprotein (LDL) and an increased risk of heart disease. Its role in obesity and diabetes is more controversial; there is also evidence that it plays a role in inflammatory responses.

Cells isolated from adipose tissue, and classified as adipocytes or preadipocytes, express Toll-like receptors, which are the products of evolution based on a need for a very rapid response to certain lethal organisms, for which adaptive immunity may be too slow to save the patient. At least 10 Toll-like receptors have been identified in humans recognizing different repetitive sequences on the surfaces of bacteria, including mycobacteria, and viruses. Activation of Toll-like receptors can stimulate the production of proinflammatory cytokines and chemokines and the expression of costimulatory molecules

necessary for initiating a response of the adaptive immune system. The activation can include the chemoattraction of neutrophils and macrophages to the area. For example, activation of Toll-like receptor TLR-4 leads to activation of the nuclear transcription factor NFkB, which then activates genes that encode for proteins that are involved in the defense against infection. The need for a rapid response system in adipose tissue is most easily understood in the mesenteric fat, which is penetrated by bacterial antigens that filter in from small leaks in the intestinal permeability barrier. Perhaps such reactivity in adipose tissue in other regions, such as the lower legs, has evolved from breaks in the cutaneous permeability barrier, for example in the feet and toes. Also, low-grade inflammation in the adipose tissue may be important in its correlation with the syndrome of insulin resistance in obese diabetic patients.

MOSTLY SEPTAL PATTERN PANNICULITIS, WITH VASCULITIS

See Table 20-1.

Polyarteritis Nodosa

Clinical Summary. Polyarteritis nodosa (PAN) is a term used to describe antineutrophil cytoplasmic antibody (ANCA)–negative neutrophilic vasculitis centered on medium-sized arteries, which in some cases will involve the small arteries (between 100 and 1,000 μm diameter) of the subcutis (15). Cutaneous involvement is characterized by painful subcutaneous nodules and ulcers, arising singly or clustered, typically on the lower extremities bilaterally, especially the legs (Fig. 20-3). Peripheral gangrene may ensue. The combined presence of nodules with livedo reticularis or retiform purpura is highly suggestive of PAN. Milder presentations may resemble atrophie blanche. Most patients with histologically classic subcutaneous arteritis have a favorable prognosis, with disease largely or exclusively confined to the skin, that is, a single-organ vasculitis designated "cutaneous arteritis" (formerly cutaneous PAN) in the 2012 Revised International Chapel Hill Consensus Conference (CHCC) nomenclature (16). However, cutaneous arteritis can potentially become systemic PAN. Classic systemic PAN is a potentially fatal systemic vasculitis with predilection for involvement of the gastrointestinal tract, kidney joints, and peripheral nerves, in addition to the skin. The lungs are typically spared. The original 1990 American College of Rheumatology criteria for PAN (≥3/10 required for diagnosis) included weight loss, livedo reticularis, testicular pain, myalgia or leg weakness, mononeuropathy or polyneuropathy, diastolic blood pressure >90 mm Hg, elevated blood urea nitrogen (BUN) unrelated to dehydration or obstruction, evidence of hepatitis B virus (HBV) infection, aneurysms or arterial occlusions, and small- or medium-sized arteritis containing neutrophils. However, with the advent of HBV vaccination, PAN became increasingly associated with hepatitis C virus (HCV) infection rather than HBV. The 2012 CHCC nomenclature effectively eliminated most cases of systemic PAN in favor of an etiology-base nomenclature, e.g., HBV- and HCV-associated vasculitis, minocycline-associated vasculitis (17), lupus vasculitis, and rheumatoid vasculitis (18).

Histopathology. The histologic hallmark of PAN is a neutrophilic leukocytoclastic vasculitis involving small arteries (i.e., arteritis) of the subcutaneous septa (Fig. 20-3B). Neutrophils,

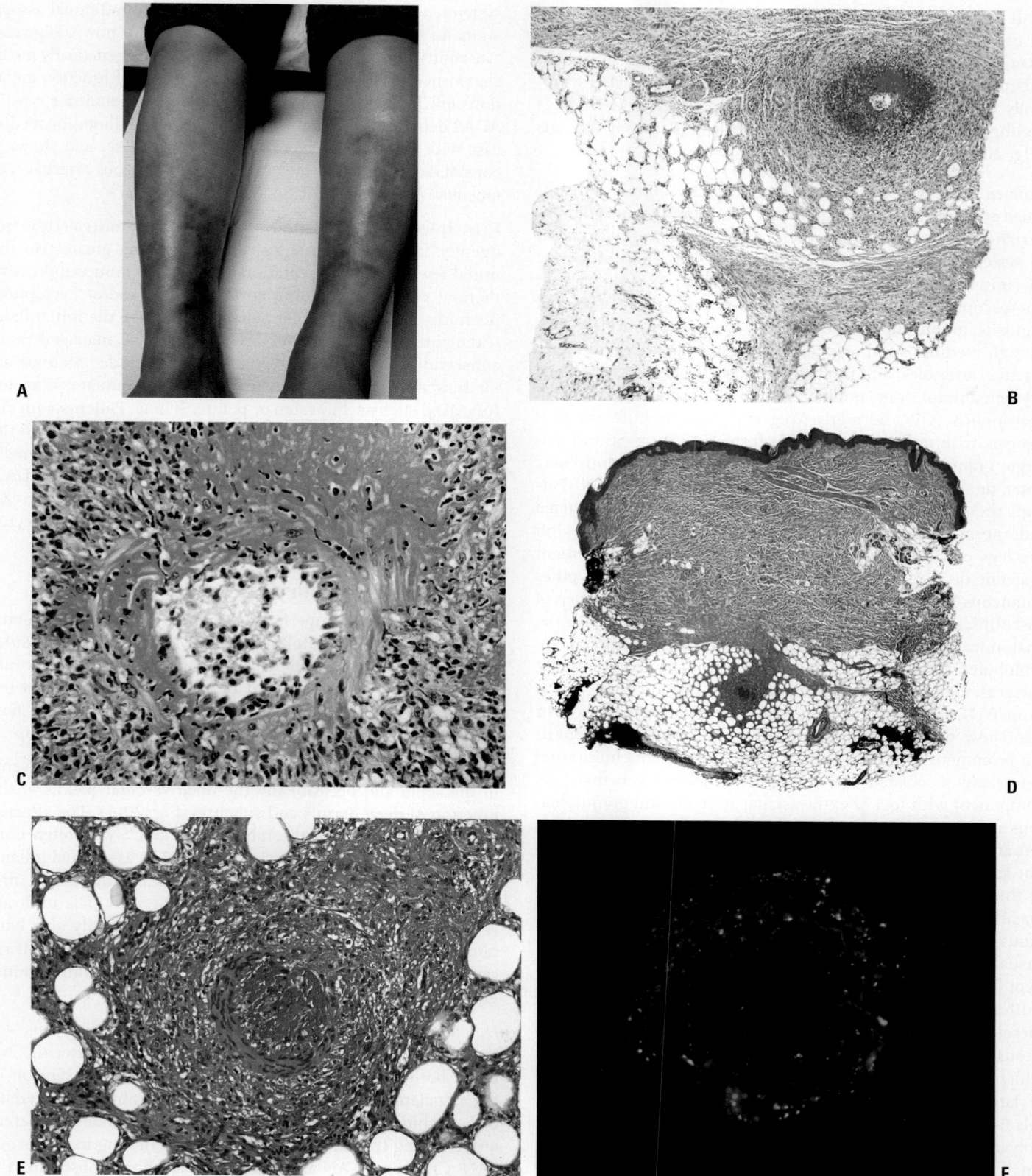

Figure 20-3 Cutaneous polyarteritis nodosa (cutaneous arteritis). **A:** Erythematous papules and nodules on the leg. **B:** Arteritis, with limited extension of the inflammatory infiltrate beyond the affected artery. **C:** Neutrophils and fibrin within and around the walls of a small subcutaneous artery. **D, E:** In later stages, the infiltrate is mostly lymphocytic. **F:** Granular deposition of C3 within the wall of a small artery (direct immunofluorescence).

leukocytoclastic nuclear debris (nuclear "dust"), extravasated erythrocytes, and fibrin aggregate within and around the affected artery. There is typically relatively minimal extravascular extension of the inflammatory infiltrate into surrounding subcutaneous fat lobules. In the late stage, neutrophils may be

sparse or absent, producing the histologic appearance of lymphocytic vasculitis (Fig. 20-3D). Sparse eosinophils and granulomatous changes are not expected but do not exclude the diagnosis. The artery may be obscured by the vasculitic process, but the typical round cross-sectional profile of an artery, with internal elastic lamina and compact muscular wall, may be discerned. Superficial biopsies may reveal only nonspecific tissue ischemia such as loss of nuclear staining and secondary subepidermal clefting. Direct immunofluorescence (DIF) typically demonstrates granular deposition of IgG, IgM, and C3 highlighting the walls of arteries in the deep dermis or subcutis (Fig. 20-3F).

Differential Diagnosis. Clinical correlation is required to distinguish systemic PAN from cutaneous PAN. However, it is our experience, as well as that of others, that cutaneous involvement in systemic PAN usually shows small vessel leukocytoclastic vasculitis (centered on postcapillary venules) as is the case in microscopic polyangiitis, whereas true arteritis is the usual and requisite finding in cutaneous PAN (cutaneous arteritis). Although medium-sized arteries are targeted, smaller and larger arteries, arterioles, and rarely veins may also be affected. Thus, erythema induratum (nodular vasculitis), granulomatosis with polyangiitis (GPA; formerly Wegener), eosinophilic granulomatosis with polyangiitis (EGPA; formerly Churg–Strauss, allergic granulomatosis), and superficial thrombophlebitis may enter the differential diagnosis of a skin biopsy of PAN. Perhaps the most common differential diagnosis is with erythema induratum, because both disorders present with nodules on the legs of adult women, usually without overt concomitant systemic disease. In contrast to the septal arteritis that typifies cutaneous PAN (cutaneous arteritis), the common presence of vasculitis involving centrilobular venules (combined with the anatomically "terminal" configuration of vessels within fat microlobules) in erythema induratum accounts for the prominent extravascular inflammation and necrosis that distinguishes it from PAN. GPA and EGPA typically involve small vessels or else show extravascular granulomatous changes. Eosinophils are prominent in EGPA. The vasculitis of erythema induratum is typically associated with a substantial lobular subcutaneous component with foci of extravascular necrosis and granulomatous inflammation. Superficial thrombophlebitis affects veins, not arteries; this distinction is discussed in greater detail later, but an occluding fibrin thrombus is a consistent feature only of thrombophlebitis. Lymphocytic thrombophilic arteritis and macular lymphocytic arteritis have been regarded as synonymous terms to describe patients with nonulcerating livedoid (usually macular) lesions, lymphocytic vasculitis with prominent fibrin vascular cuffs, and a benign clinical course (19–21); Authorities have both favored and challenged the view that these cases are within the mild end of the spectrum of cutaneous arteritis (cutaneous PAN) (a view we concur with), in which case the absence of neutrophils is attributable to a late or latent stage of the pathologic process (22–26). Small vessels (arterioles, capillaries, venules) are targeted in microscopic polyangiitis (formerly microscopic polyarteritis), resulting in small vessel leukocytoclastic vasculitis. Clinically, microscopic polyangiitis affects the kidney (necrotizing glomerulonephritis) and lung (capillaritis) and is associated with circulating ANCA.

Pathogenesis. PAN is characterized by transmural inflammation centered on medium-sized arteries with focal/segmental predilection for arterial bifurcations and branch points. As with all forms of vasculitis, immune complex deposition plays a key role, likely a cross-reaction against one or more antigens derived from antecedent infectious, inflammatory, or neoplastic systemic triggers. However, the 2012 CHCC nomenclature has essentially rendered

systemic PAN a rare idiopathic disorder, with traditional associations in systemic PAN such as HBC and HCV now designated "vasculitis associated with probable etiology." A genetically mediated form of PAN has been associated with loss-of-function mutations in *CECR1*, the gene encoding adenosine deaminase type 2. ADA2 deficiency is an autosomal recessive, childhood-onset disease with features similar to those of classic PAN and showing considerable variability in severity, from cutaneous arteritis (cutaneous PAN) to systemic PAN vasculopathy (27).

Principles of Management: Systemic PAN, untreated, is frequently fatal, the highest risk of death being greatest in the initial few years of presentation. Systemic immunosuppressive therapy, typically including corticosteroids and/or cyclophosphamide, has allowed most patients to survive the initial flare. Cutaneous PAN (cutaneous arteritis) may be managed more conservatively; treatment possibilities include prednisone, methotrexate, aspirin, nonsteroid anti-inflammatory agents (NSAIDs) such as ibuprofen or pentoxifylline. Patients with cutaneous PAN should be monitored longitudinally, although the risk of progression to systemic PAN appears to be exceptionally low. Screening for *CECR1* mutations, the gene encoding ADA2, may be considered for patients with treatment refractory vasculitis, cases of familial vasculitis, or screening of unaffected siblings of index cases (28).

Superficial Migratory Thrombophlebitis

Clinical Summary. Superficial (migratory) thrombophlebitis usually presents as painful induration or subcutaneous nodules on the lower extremity but occasionally on the arms and trunk. Linear cord-like or branching patterns of induration may be felt along the course of the inflamed vein. As lesions resolve, new nodules may erupt and superimposed purpura may develop.

Histopathology. Superficial thrombophlebitis affects large veins in the septa and occasionally the deep vascular plexus at the junction of deep dermis and subcutis (Fig. 20-4). The affected vein has an occluding thrombus and a thick wall often containing slender smooth muscle fascicles. The associated inflammatory infiltrate extends between the muscle bundles and only minimally into the tissue surrounding the vein. The infiltrate is initially composed of neutrophils and eventually also lymphocytes and macrophages, including sparse giant cells. If recanalization of the lumen of the vein takes place, intraluminal granulomas with giant cells can be found.

Differential Diagnosis. The main differential diagnosis for thrombophlebitis is cutaneous PAN (cutaneous arteritis) because both exhibit septal vasculitis with limited extension of the associated inflammatory infiltrate. Thrombus characteristically occludes the lumen of veins in thrombophlebitis, whereas an occluding thrombus is a more variable finding in cutaneous PAN. Cutaneous PAN affects arteries with fibrin, obscuring the region of the internal elastic lamina, often producing a targetoid eosinophilic fibrin ring. Arteries contain a compact muscular wall, whereas veins of the lower extremities contain thin smooth muscle fascicles demarcated by thin elastic fibers and an inconspicuous internal elastic lamina (Fig. 20-4C).

Pathogenesis. Recurrent migratory thrombophlebitis is usually associated with an underlying hypercoagulable state, for which the differential diagnosis is extensive. Primary hypercoagulable states include antiphospholipid antibodies (anticardiolipin,

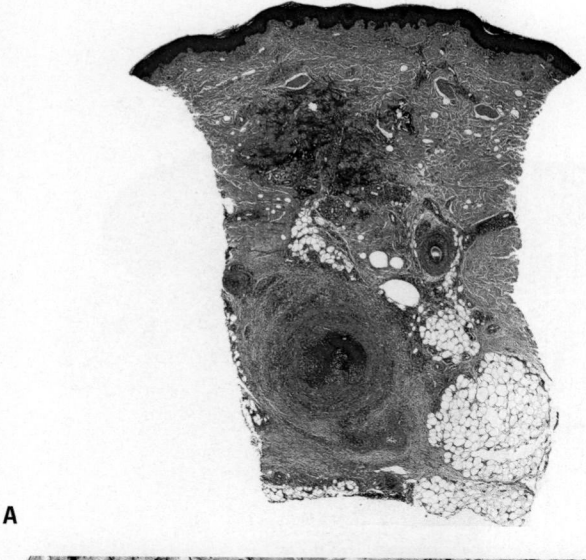

A

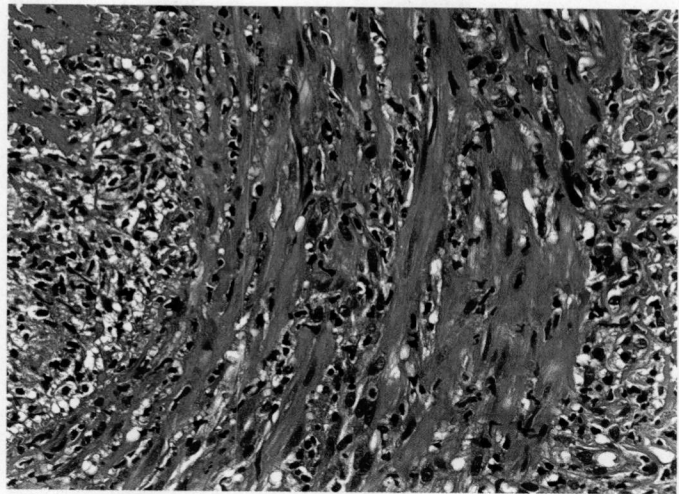

B

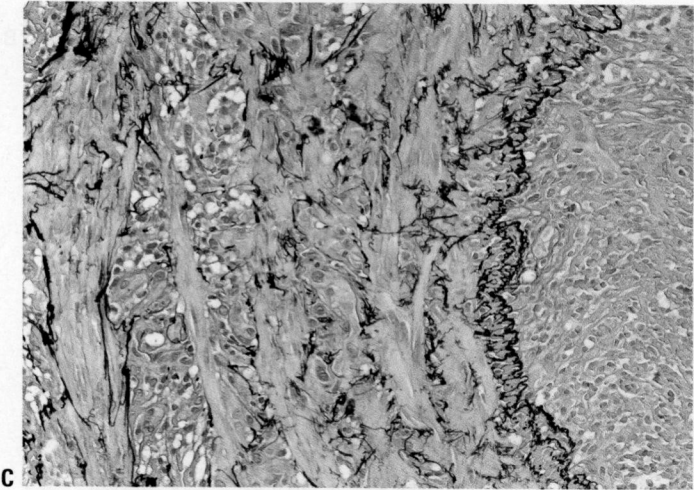

C

Figure 20-4 Superficial thrombophlebitis. **A:** Vasculitis affecting a subcutaneous muscular walled vein. The lumen is occluded by fibrin. **B:** A mixed infiltrate of neutrophils, lymphocytes, and histiocytes is present between fascicles of smooth muscle in the vessel wall. **C:** Elastic tissue staining demonstrates that this muscular walled vessel is a vein, characterized by thin delicate elastic fibers surrounding thin smooth muscle fascicles. Arteries have a more compact muscular wall and more prominent internal elastic lamina.

lupus anticoagulant), deficiencies of protein C, protein S, antithrombin III, heparin cofactor II, factor XII, tissue plasminogen activator, or factor V Leiden. Secondary hypercoagulable states include varicosity-associated stasis, paraneoplastic (Trousseau syndrome), pregnancy, oral contraceptive use, sepsis, intravenous injection or catheterization, and HIV-associated immune reconstitution inflammatory syndrome (IRIS) (29), among others. Acute superficial thrombophlebitis of the breast is known as Mondor disease (30).

Principles of Management: Management is focused on identifying and correcting any underlying predisposition and prevention of complications such as deep venous thrombosis. Simple remedies may include elevation, bed rest, compressive therapy, hot compresses, and possibly heparin, as well as analgesics (31,32).

MOSTLY SEPTAL PATTERN PANNICULITIS, WITHOUT VASCULITIS

See Table 20-1.

Erythema Nodosum

Clinical Summary. Erythema nodosum (EN) is an acute, self-limited reaction pattern consisting of several nonulcerating,

tender, erythematous minimally elevated 1- to 10-cm nodules or plaques. EN occurs in adults and children and has a predilection for involvement of the anterior legs (shins) (Fig. 20-5A). Posterior leg (calf) involvement may occur but generally does not predominate over pretibial involvement. Less common sites include the thighs, upper extremities, neck, and face. Distribution of lesions in EN is bilateral and basically symmetric. Crops or individual lesions last days to weeks, often leaving a bruise, but without atrophy or scar. EN may be accompanied by fever, malaise, headache, leukocytosis, conjunctivitis, and arthralgia. EN presenting with hilar adenopathy and arthritis (particularly around the ankles) is typical of sarcoid-associated Lofgren syndrome. The list of infectious, other inflammatory, and neoplastic systemic diseases that can present with EN is extensive and particularly notable for streptococcal pharyngitis, *Yersinia*, *Salmonella*, or *Shigella* enterocolitis, deep fungal infections in certain endemic locales, sarcoid, inflammatory bowel disease, and hematologic malignancy. Medications, particularly those containing estrogens, may also induce EN.

The rare chronic variant of EN is known as *erythema nodosum migrans*, as well as *chronic EN* and historically as *subacute nodular migratory panniculitis* (Vilanova and Piñol). The duration may be from a few months to a few years. EN migrans has a predilection for older women and presents with one or a few

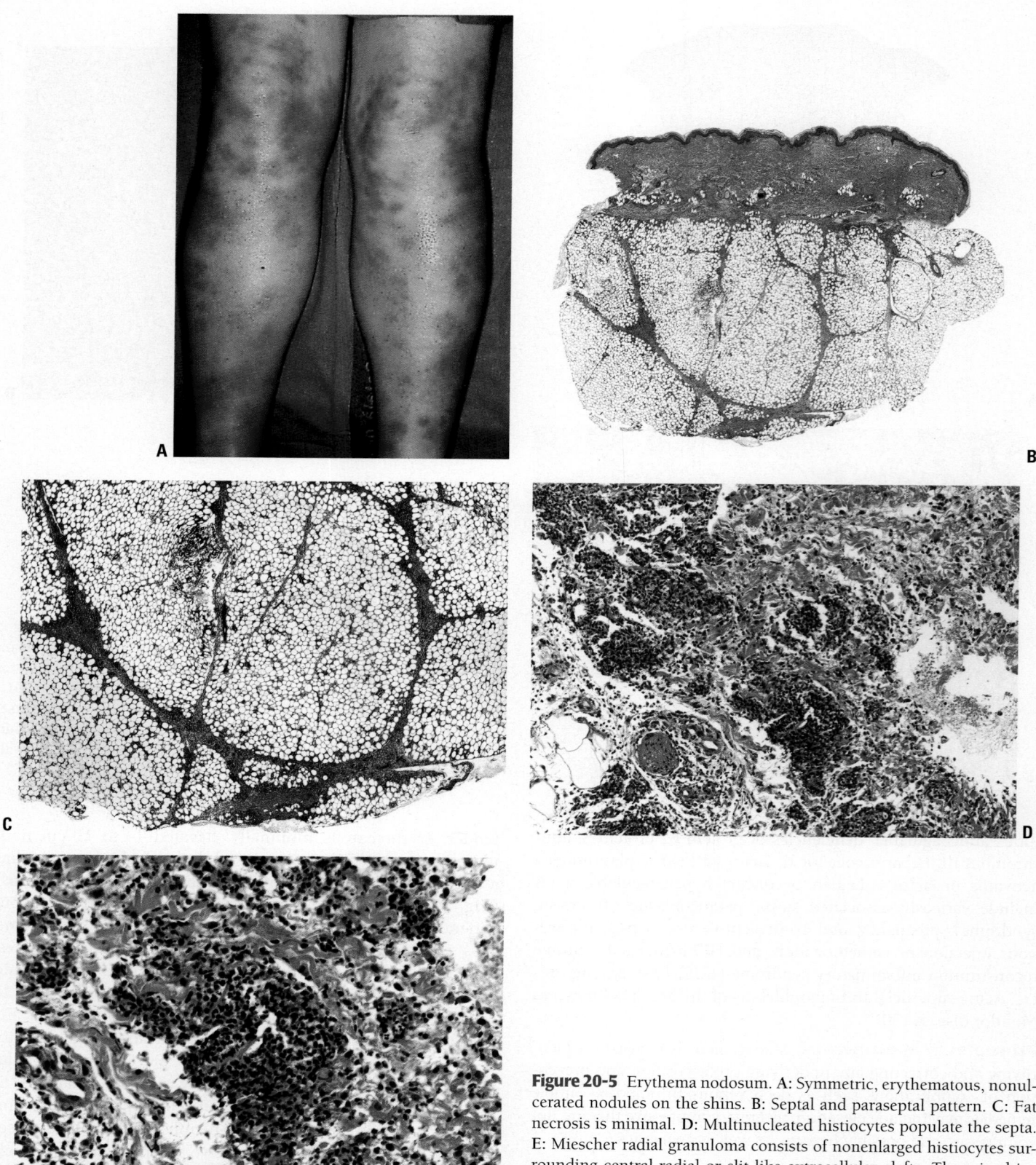

Figure 20-5 Erythema nodosum. **A:** Symmetric, erythematous, nonulcerated nodules on the shins. **B:** Septal and paraseptal pattern. **C:** Fat necrosis is minimal. **D:** Multinucleated histiocytes populate the septa. **E:** Miescher radial granuloma consists of nonenlarged histiocytes surrounding central radial or slit-like extracellular clefts. The mixed infiltrate in erythema nodosum also contains lymphocytes, neutrophils, and eosinophils.

asymptomatic or minimally tender lesions, most typically unilateral, on the lower leg (or else asymmetric if bilateral). Subcutaneous nodules may expand centrifugally and coalesce to form annular plaques with central clearing. Compared to classic acute EN, constitutional symptoms are minimal or absent. EN migrans is also not typically associated with systemic disease, although rare cases of EN migrans have been reported in association with hepatitis B infection (33) and acne fulminans with hepatomegaly.

Histopathology. EN is the prototype for septal panniculitis (Fig. 20-5B). The changes in EN are generally confined to the subcutis; there is no expected epidermal involvement, and the dermis usually exhibits only a sparse, nonspecific perivascular lymphocytic infiltrate. In early EN, there is edema of the subcutaneous septa associated with a mixed infiltrate of lymphocytes, neutrophils, and eosinophils. The inflammation tends to be centered on the junction of septa and lobules with limited extension into the periphery of the fat lobules, creating a paraseptal pattern. Fat necrosis in the form of lipophages and lipomembranous or microcystic alteration is usually minimal relative to the density of the inflammatory infiltrate compared to most forms of panniculitis (Fig. 20-5C). Miescher radial granuloma (MRG) is a sensitive and specific attribute of EN. MRG is most specifically defined as a collection of nonenlarged histiocytes forming a central radial or slit-like extracellular cleft, usually accompanied by mature neutrophils in early lesions (Fig. 20-5E). In fact, some of these "nonenlarged histiocytes" have been shown via immunohistochemistry for myeloperoxidase to be immature neutrophils, akin to those seen in histiocytoid Sweet syndrome (LR, personal observation). Large multinucleated histiocytes, sometimes containing intracytoplasmic radial clefts, are a feature of late-stage EN and have been postulated to be derived from MRG, but are not MRG as strictly defined (34). Some authors have postulated that the histiocytes in MRG are centered on a small blood vessel; however, MRG studied to date have been negative by immunohistochemistry for vascular-lymphatic (CD31) and lymphatic (podoplanin) markers and negative for evidence of vascular structures using electron microscopy. Vasculitis is an unexpected but rarely documented feature that has been observed in clinically and histologically confirmed cases of EN, particularly acute lesions (35,36). The late stage of acute EN shows widened fibrotic septa with septal and paraseptal inflammation; neutrophils are typically absent and histiocytes more prominent. Increased vascularization is also characteristic; sometimes, the appearances are indistinguishable from granulation tissue involving the interface between the septa and the fat lobule. Granulomas, if present, are often loosely formed and contain multinucleated giant cells, either foreign body (irregular distribution of nuclei) or Langhans (peripheral nuclei) type. Rarely, sarcoidal granulomas may occur in small numbers in the septa. End-stage lesions exhibit widened fibrotic septa with sparse inflammatory cells, although multinucleated histiocytes typically predominate. In EN migrans, the histologic findings resemble those of the late-stage classic EN, with variably thickened fibrotic septa, capillary prominence, and multinucleated histiocytes.

Differential Diagnosis. The histopathologic features of EN are usually characteristic. MRGs are fairly specific but have rarely been documented in Sweet syndrome (37), Behcet disease, necrobiosis lipoidica, erythema induratum (nodular vasculitis), and nephrogenic systemic fibrosis (38). Necrotizing vasculitis would be exceptional but does not exclude EN, pending clinical correlation and follow-up, because vasculitis has rarely been documented in initial biopsies of proven classic EN (35). Another rare consideration is subcutaneous Sweet syndrome, which often occurs in a setting of myeloid disorders and may exhibit a septal pattern with neutrophils mimicking early EN (39). Infection should be considered if neutrophils are present. DIF studies are not required; results are usually negative unless vasculitis is present.

Pathogenesis. EN may be regarded as a clinically and histologically distinct reaction pattern that is shared by numerous antecedent triggers or disease associations. Causes may be divided into the following categories: infections with bacteria, mycobacteria, fungi, or protozoa; viral diseases; malignancies; medications; and miscellaneous conditions. In approximately 50% of cases, there is no cause identified. MRG often contains neutrophils and represents a common feature of EN that may rarely be encountered in another cutaneous reaction pattern, Sweet syndrome (acute febrile neutrophilic dermatosis) (37).

Principles of Management: Treatment primarily includes identification and management of the underlying trigger, especially if infectious (40). The index of suspicion for deep fungal infections in endemic regions (e.g., coccidioidomycosis in the Southwestern United States, histoplasmosis in the Ohio River Valley) should be higher if the patient traveled in these endemic areas. Infection should be reasonably excluded before initiating immunosuppressive therapy, which may consist of prednisone or cyclosporine. For inflammatory bowel disease–associated EN, TNF inhibitors (e.g., infliximab, adalimumab) may concomitantly improve the underlying condition. Symptomatic therapy may include reduced activity, mild compressive therapy, NSAIDs (e.g., celecoxib, ibuprofen, indomethacin, naproxen), colchicine, saturated solution of potassium iodide (SSKI), or hydroxychloroquine (41). A thorough medication review is suggested, and given the association of EN with female hormones, patients may warrant pregnancy testing before initiating therapy, because many of the therapeutic options may be teratogenic.

Subcutaneous Involvement by Granulomatous Dermatitis

Many forms of granulomatous dermatitis may occasionally extend into the subcutis from the overlying dermis or, more rarely, present primarily in the subcutis. Subcutaneous granuloma annulare (GA) is typical in young children and has a predilection for the scalp in addition to the distal extremities (Fig. 20-6). As a rule, the histologic appearance of subcutaneous GA is a palisaded necrobiotic granuloma; even with an interstitial pattern of GA in the dermis, the pattern can "shift" to palisaded granulomas with extension into the subcutis septa. Necrobiosis lipoidica (Fig. 20-7), necrobiotic xanthogranuloma, rheumatoid nodule (Fig. 20-8), and sarcoid are reviewed primarily in Chapter 14. If involving primarily the subcutis, the lesions may exhibit minimal or no erythema. Prominent fibrosis surrounding sarcoidal granulomas has been documented as a distinctive feature in subcutaneous sarcoid (42,43). In contrast to subcutaneous GA, subcutaneous sarcoid often exhibits a lobular rather than septal pattern (Fig. 20-9).

Subcutaneous Involvement by Sclerosing Disorders

Many disorders characterized by dermal sclerosis may extend into the subcutis or, in some cases, present primarily in the subcutis. Subcutaneous involvement is septal, in continuity with the collagenous reticular dermis. These include morphea profunda, systemic scleroderma, chronic sclerodermoid graft-versus-host disease, and nephrogenic systemic fibrosis and are discussed in detail elsewhere in this textbook (Fig. 20-10). Of note, the toxic oil syndrome that occurred in Spain in the early 1980s was attributed to the sale of industrial oil (colza/rapeseed oil) as cooking oil and, in its late stage, showed a clinical and pathologic picture very similar to systemic scleroderma.

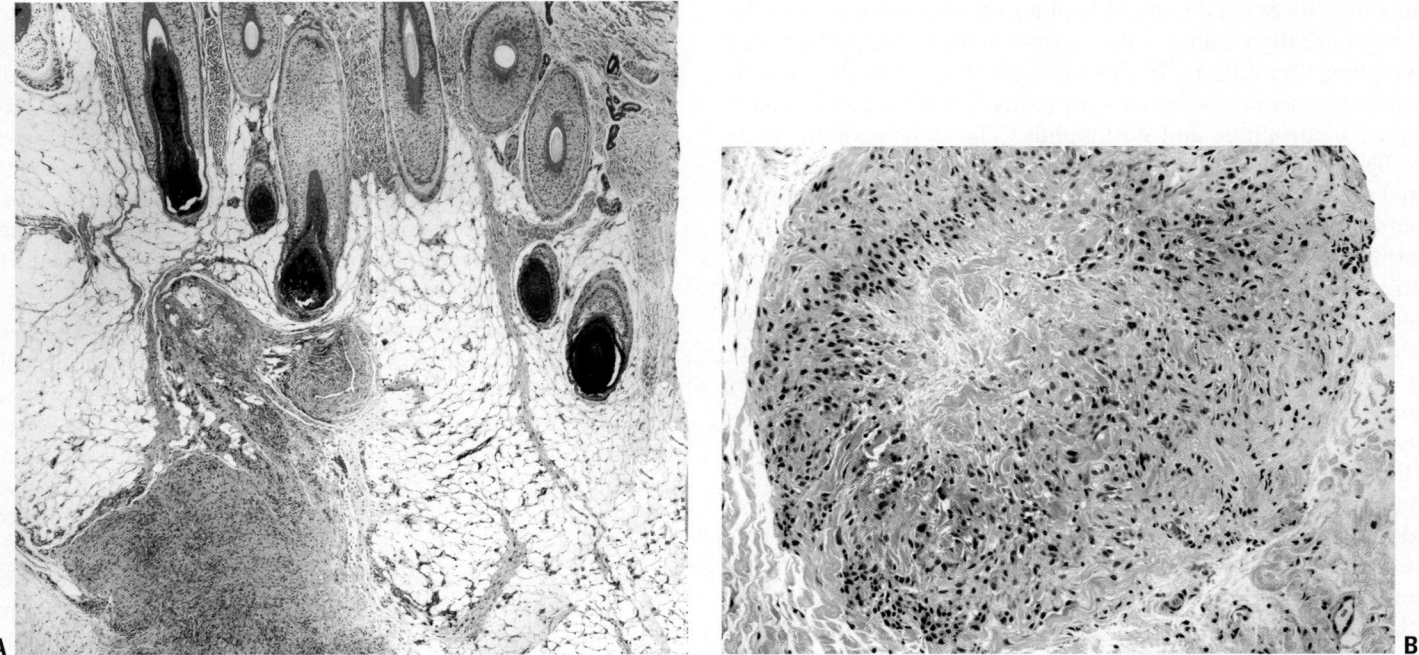

Figure 20-6 Subcutaneous granuloma annulare. **A:** The scalp is commonly affected. **B:** Palisaded granuloma with central interstitial mucin.

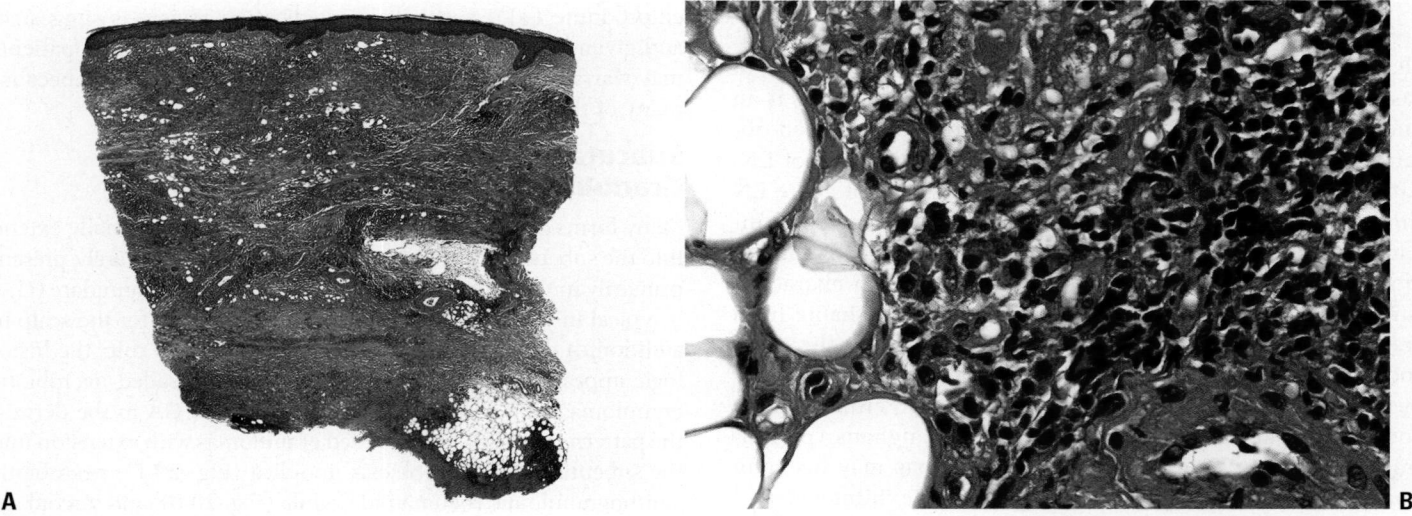

Figure 20-7 Necrobiosis lipoidica. **A:** Granulomatous dermatitis in the dermis and subcutis. **B:** Subcutaneous granulomas are associated with plasma cells.

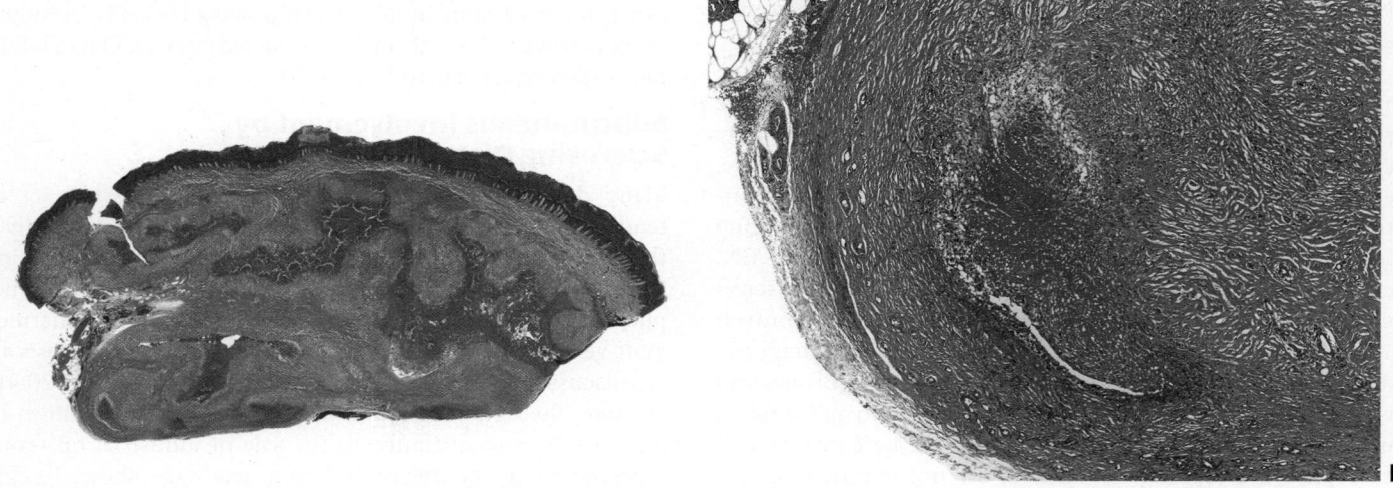

Figure 20-8 Rheumatoid nodule. **A:** Large, irregular, confluent palisaded granulomas with subcutaneous involvement. **B:** Subcutaneous palisaded granuloma with central fibrin.

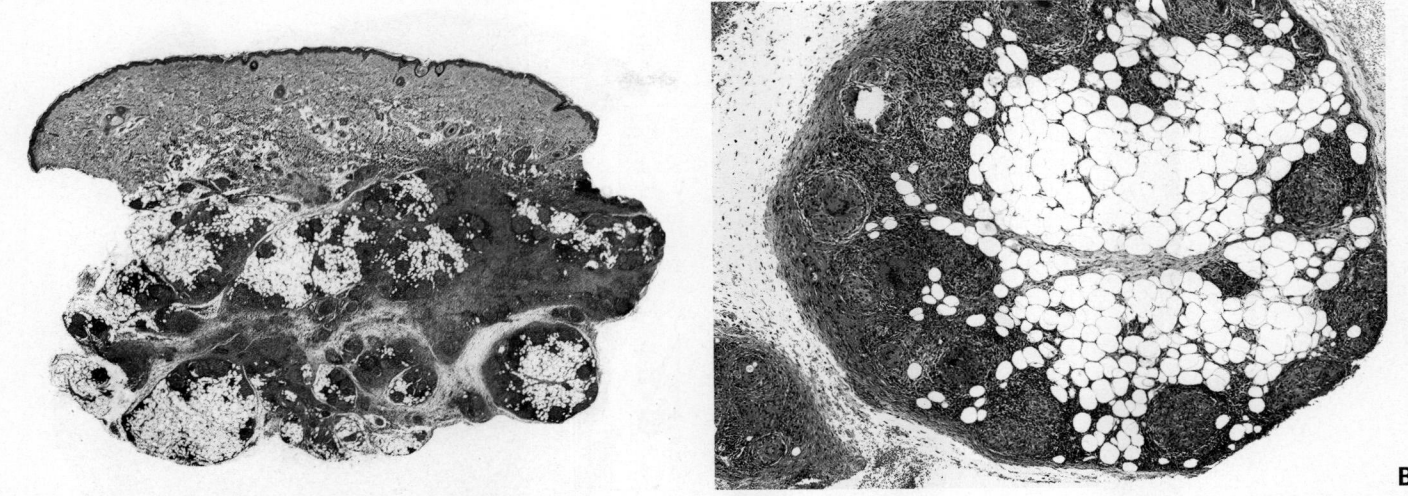

Figure 20-9 Subcutaneous sarcoid. A: Lobular and septal involvement by sarcoidal granulomas. B: Involvement can be mostly lobular. Fibrosis surrounds the granulomas.

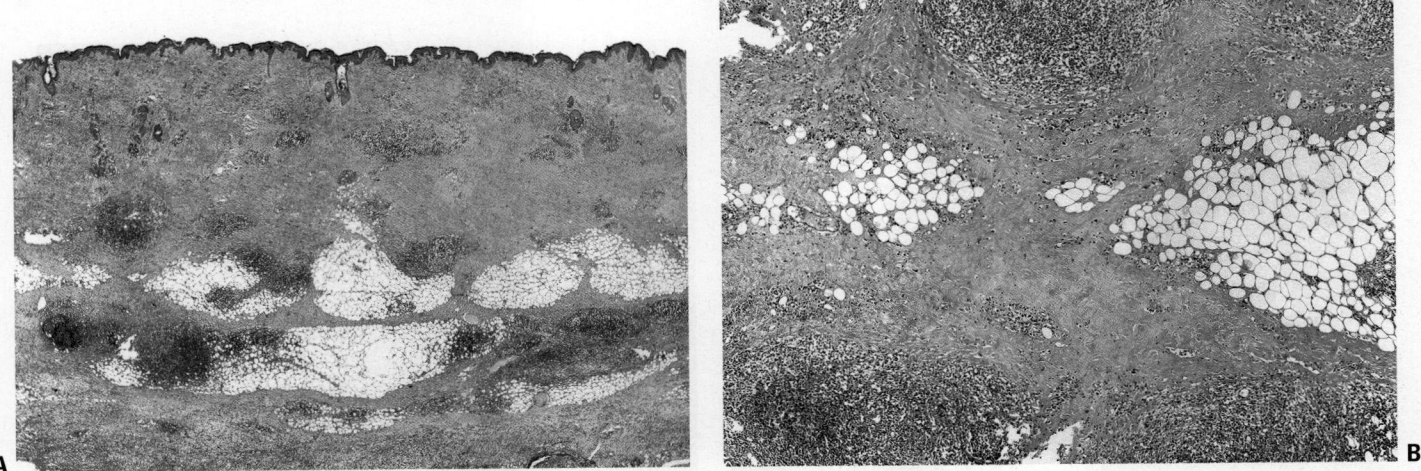

Figure 20-10 Morphea profunda. A: Dermal sclerosis with associated subcutaneous involvement. B: Widened sclerotic septa.

MOSTLY LOBULAR PATTERN PANNICULITIS, WITH VASCULITIS

See Table 20-1.

Erythema Induratum (Nodular Vasculitis)

Clinical Summary. Historically, multiple terms have been employed to describe this clinically and histologically distinct form of panniculitis. In 1855, Bazin introduced the term "erythema induratum" (EI) to describe nodules arising on the legs of adult women, which he classified as benign "scrofulids" (as a descriptive term, not a form of tuberculosis). The association with pulmonary tuberculosis and classification of EI as one form of Darier tuberculids came decades later; as of this writing, such cases are still often classified as EI of Bazin or Bazin EI (44,45). Subsequently, other cases accepted to be clinically and histologically identical to EI but without associated tuberculosis were documented under various designations, including EI of Whitfield and "nodular vasculitis" (46). The terms EI of Bazin and nodular vasculitis may be used interchangeably(41,47),

although others reserve the diagnosis of EI for cases associated with tuberculosis and nodular vasculitis for the remainder (3,48,49). For efficiency in describing clinical and histologic features, EI will herein be regarded as synonymous with nodular vasculitis. Clinically, EI usually occurs in young or middle-aged women with firm, violaceous nodules and plaques with predilection for the posterior legs (calves). Only rare cases in children have been reported. Involvement of the shins, thighs, feet, buttocks, and forearms has also been documented. Initial lesions are typically painless, with variable progression to ulceration, pain, tenderness, and secondary scarring, hyperpigmentation, and atrophy (Fig. 20-11A). Lesions often occur in recurrent crops (sometimes precipitated by the onset of cold weather). Constitutional symptoms are usually absent.

Histopathology. In contrast to the septal pattern of EN, EI is a lobular or mixed lobular and septal panniculitis with vasculitis (Fig. 20-11B). In some sections, the appearances may be that of lobular panniculitis without vasculitis. The absence of vasculitis within one or, exceptionally, multiple biopsies despite deeper level sections does not exclude EI if the context is otherwise

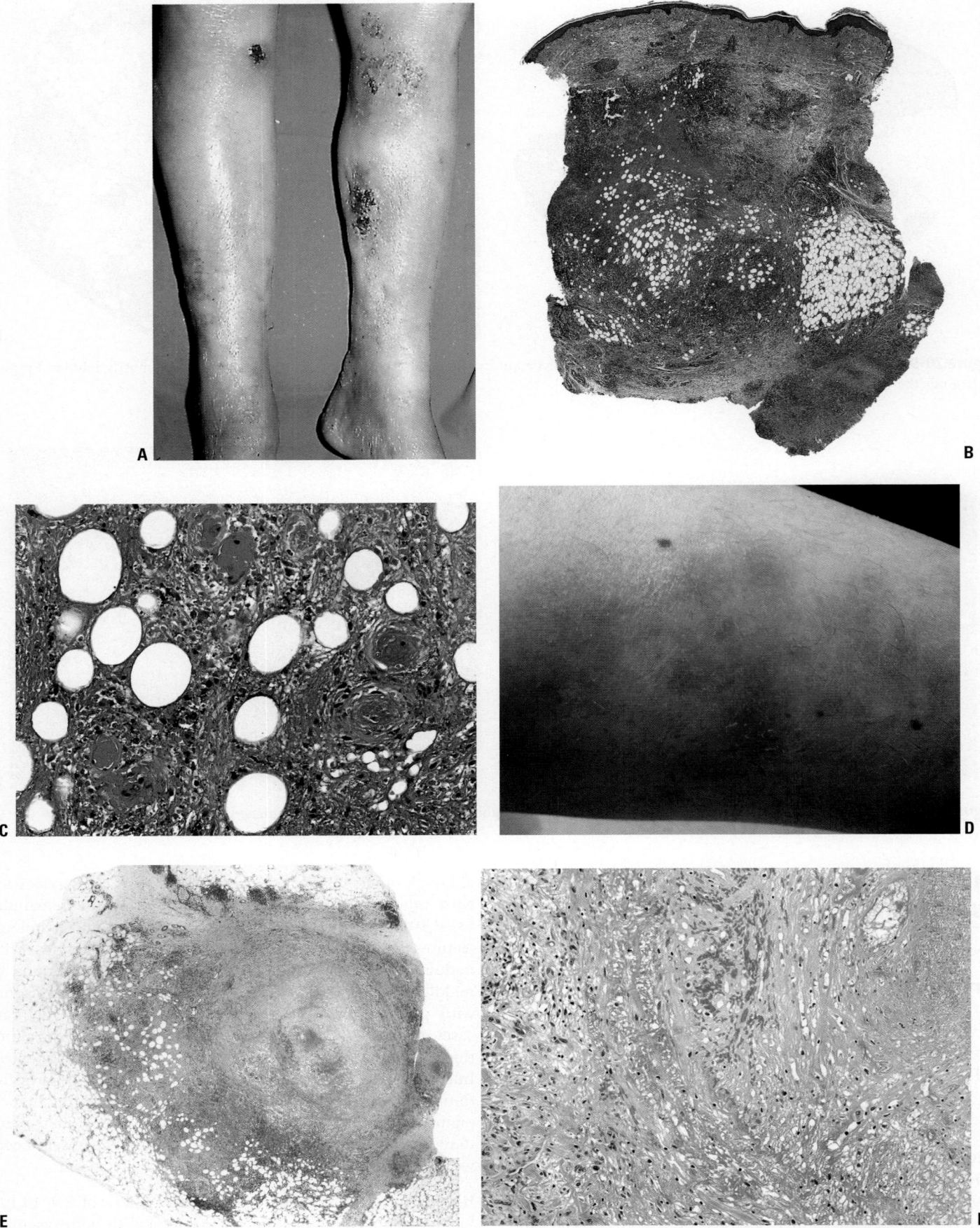

Figure 20-11 Erythema induratum (nodular vasculitis). **A:** Ulcerated nodules with predilection for the posterior leg (calf) region. **B:** Mostly lobular pattern. **C:** Vasculitis affecting venules with extensive lobular panniculitis with necrosis. **D:** A 38-year-old woman with nonulcerated plaques on the calf. There was no evidence of tuberculosis. **D, E:** In this case, a septal artery or vein is obliterated. **F:** Neutrophils may be absent in the late stage of vasculitis.

consistent. The lobular lymphohistiocytic panniculitis of EI additionally contains numerous neutrophils in early lesions, and granulomatous inflammation with foamy histiocytes, epithelioid histiocytes, Langhans-type multinucleated histiocytes variably form epithelioid or tuberculoid granulomas, plasma cells, and septal fibrosis in established lesions. Overt lipophagic and ischemic fat necrosis, and usually eosinophilic necrosis (coagulative, caseous, fibrinous), is a hallmark of all stages of EI. Sparse eosinophils may be present.

Since the first edition of *Histopathology of the Skin*, Lever recognized that vasculitis in EI may involve both small and medium vessels and both arteries and veins (50). Although some authorities have considered arteritis to be a hallmark of EI (1), a comprehensive analysis of more than 100 cases demonstrated that necrotizing vasculitis in EI is present in both early and fully developed lesions and most commonly involves centrilobular venules (Fig. 20-11C), followed in frequency by septal veins and/or septal arteries (with or without centrilobular venulitis) (Fig. 20-11E) (47). It should be noted that the walls of veins in the lower extremities are relatively muscular and appear to have been misinterpreted as arteries in some published cases. Also, in many instances, affected vessels in EI exhibit an appearance of lymphocytic vasculitis; however, primary neutrophilic vasculitis has been documented in EI (51), and EI has been classified as a neutrophilic vasculitis (52).

Differential Diagnosis. A classic clinical presentation of EI with crusted nodules on the posterior legs of a woman can be very helpful. Microscopically, the presence of lobular panniculitis with prominent fat necrosis favors EI over EN, even without demonstrated vasculitis. The presence of prominent lobular panniculitis also favors EI over cutaneous PAN or thrombophlebitis, because the inflammatory infiltrate in the latter disorders is confined to the vicinity of affected vessels. Stated another way, the degree of involvement of the fat lobule is a helpful clue, because in cutaneous PAN the fat lobule is spared or only minimally involved, whereas in EI there is extensive involvement of the center of the fat lobule with prominent ischemic necrosis of the adipocytes. It is the centrilobular venulitis (combined with the anatomically "terminal" configuration of vessels within fat microlobules) that accounts for the prominent extravascular inflammation and necrosis that distinguishes it from PAN. Moreover, the spectrum of vasculitis in EI is broad, whereas vasculitis in PAN is generally restricted to arteries, and in thrombophlebitis, to the veins. Elastic tissue stains may be helpful for distinguishing small arteries affected by polyarteritis from small veins affected by thrombophlebitis. However, the distinction between arteries and veins can be challenging when the inflammation destroys the elastic fibers or when the elastic tissue is increased in the walls of veins owing to venous hypertension and stasis in the lower legs. In the differential diagnosis of neutrophilic panniculitis without vasculitis, infection, factitial panniculitis, pancreatic panniculitis, or α-1-antitrypsin deficiency panniculitis, and subcutaneous Sweet syndrome may be considered.

Pathogenesis. EI may be regarded as a subcutaneous vasculitic reaction pattern most commonly triggered by tuberculosis, that is, a tuberculid (and designated nodular vasculitis if the trigger is not tuberculosis). Classic criteria for a tuberculid include nonlesional evidence of tuberculosis, absence of lesional organisms by histochemical stains or culture, and resolution of the tuberculid with antituberculous treatment. A century later, polymerase chain reaction (PCR) techniques have demonstrated evidence of *M. tuberculosis* in EI, with a sensitivity ranging from 0 to over

75% in different case series (53–56), depending at least in part on technical factors (57). Prominent lobular fat necrosis in EI is attributable to centrilobular venulitis–associated ischemia. Nodular vasculitis may be idiopathic but has been associated with Crohn disease, ulcerative colitis (58), rheumatoid arthritis, bacterial (*Nocardia, Pseudomonas, Chlamydophila pneumoniae* [59]), fungal (*Fusarium*), mycobacterial (*M. avium* [60], *M. chelonae* [61], *M. Monacense* [62]), and viral hepatitis (Hepatitis B [47], Hepatitis C) (63,64). Rare association with medication such as TNF inhibitors (certolizumab pegol [65], etanercept [66]), propylthiouracil, and chemotherapy (67) have been reported.

Principles of Management: Treatment of EI ideally addresses the underlying cause. Tuberculosis or other infection must be addressed and reasonably excluded in each case; this may entail tuberculin skin testing, interferon-γ release assays, PCR testing for *M. tuberculosis*, acid-fast and fungal staining, and lesional tissue culture. Symptomatic therapy is similar to that for EN and may include bed rest, elevation, compressive therapy, NSAIDs, SSKI, and systemic immunosuppressive therapy [41].

Crohn Disease

Clinical Summary. The spectrum of cutaneous involvement by Crohn disease (CD) includes contiguous oral or perianal CD, metastatic CD, associated reactions such as EN or pyoderma gangrenosum, and a neutrophilic granulomatous lobular panniculitis. The panniculitis presents clinically similar to EN, with tender erythematous nodules on the extensor lower extremities, including the thigh and leg (68,69). Associated constitutional symptoms are variable. Concurrent perianal CD was documented in one patient (70).

Histopathology. In contrast to EN, a predominantly lobular pattern with neutrophils and poorly defined noncaseating granulomas, including rare foci reminiscent of MRG, have been documented in fewer than a dozen cases reported to date (70). Septal edema has been documented. Changes in the overlying dermis include nonspecific perivascular lymphohistiocytic infiltrates (68), leukocytoclastic or granulomatous vasculitis, and lymphocytic eccrine hidradenitis (69). Cases with granulomatous phlebitis have been classified as erythema induratum–associated CD (71).

Differential Diagnosis. Clinical correlation is required. As for any predominantly neutrophilic infiltrate, infection must be reasonably excluded. If vasculitis is present, erythema induratum may be considered.

Pathogenesis. Some authorities consider CD-associated panniculitis within the spectrum of metastatic CD. Crowson and colleagues searched for intracellular consensus bacterial 16S rRNA and found no evidence of bacteria by this methodology in cutaneous lesions associated with CD, in contrast to their presence in the gastrointestinal tract (69).

Principles of Management: In a few cases documented to date, spontaneous resolution may occur. In some cases, treatment of CD may improve panniculitis.

Behcet Disease

Clinical Summary. Behcet disease (BD) is a multisystem autoinflammatory disorder classified as a variable vessel vasculitis (72). BD is characterized by recurrent oral and genital aphthous ulcers, a range of specific cutaneous manifestations including EN-like nodules corresponding to lobular panniculitis with vasculitis, and neutrophilic dermatoses (Sweet syndrome, pyoderma gangrenosum), and acral and facial acneiform (nonfollicular sterile pustules). In typical cases, BD initially presents with oral aphthae (sometimes the sole manifestation for years) with variable but potentially dramatic progression to other cutaneous manifestations and extracutaneous involvement. Severe cases may be fatal, often because of severe neurologic complications (aseptic meningitis, dural thrombosis) or a ruptured aneurysm. The EN-like nodules usually involve the anterior legs and are clinically indistinguishable from EN. The arms, face, neck, and buttock may also be involved. Lesions are usually self-limited, usually resolving within a couple of weeks. Nonspecific associations in BD include *bona fide* EN and superficial thrombophlebitis.

Histopathology. Despite the EN-like clinical appearances, the panniculitis of BD (herein referred to as "BD panniculitis") is primarily a vasculitis with secondary panniculitis in a lobular, mixed septal/lobular, or, least commonly, septal pattern. Vasculitis can be demonstrated in many, but not all, biopsies; may be lymphocytic or leukocytoclastic (neutrophilic); and may involve veins, arteries, or arterioles (73). The extravascular inflammatory infiltrate is mixed, with neutrophils, lymphocytes, histiocytes, and fat necrosis, including microcystic fat necrosis. Well-formed granulomas are not typical, but nodular aggregates of histiocytes and neutrophils consistent with MRGs have been documented. Overlying dermal perivascular lymphohistiocytic inflammation is typically present, with variable neutrophils and eosinophils (74,75).

Differential Diagnosis. Although a distinctive clinical presentation is very helpful, the EN-like clinical morphology is nonspecific. BD panniculitis may differ from erythema induratum (nodular vasculitis) only by a matter of degrees (73). Fat necrosis and granulomatous inflammation may be less prominent in BD panniculitis compared to erythema induratum. When arteritis is present, cutaneous polyarteritis must be considered (76). When phlebitis is present, superficial thrombophlebitis must be considered. The presence of associated lobular panniculitis or inflammation in the overlying dermis would favor BD over polyarteritis and thrombophlebitis.

Pathogenesis. Because BD panniculitis appears to be a primary vasculitis with secondary panniculitis, it likely represents one specific aspect of the variable vessel vasculitis that is the pathogenic signature of BD throughout all affected organ systems. In one study, immunohistochemical staining for adhesion molecules failed to distinguish BD panniculitis from EN (77). Although the cause of BD is unknown, genome-wide analysis has yielded potential candidate disease susceptibility genes, particularly HLA-B51 (78,79).

Principles of Management: Owing to its potentially fatal nature, early recognition and aggressive systemic immunosuppressive therapy is of paramount importance in the successful management of BD. Systemic corticosteroids, TNF inhibitors, colchicine, dapsone, and other agents may be employed (80).

MOSTLY LOBULAR PATTERN PANNICULITIS, WITHOUT VASCULITIS

See Table 20-1.

Lipodermatosclerosis

Clinical Summary. Sclerosing panniculitis, stasis panniculitis, and hypodermitis sclerodermiformis are synonymous designations. Patients with lipodermatosclerosis (LDS) are mostly adult women with preexisting venous stasis, many with elevated body mass index, who develop hyperpigmented, depressed, hard areas of skin on one or both lower legs (Fig. 20-12A) (81,82). Within the clinical classification for chronic venous disorders, LDS is designated class C4b (C6 is an active venous ulcer) (83). The sometimes-striking sclerosis between the calf and the ankle has been likened to an "inverted champagne bottle." Acute LDS (sometimes designated hypodermitis), especially if unilateral, presents as exquisitely tender erythema without induration or hyperpigmentation and may be clinically mistaken for bacterial cellulitis (82). The clinical presentation may be sufficiently distinctive to dispense with the need for biopsy. The possibility of poor wound healing is a valid concern.

Histopathology. The histopathologic features of acute or early LDS include sparse septal lymphohistiocytic infiltrates and foci of ischemic fat necrosis or hyalinization of the lobules (13,84). The more familiar appearance of fully developed lesions may be classified as mostly lobular or else mixed septal/lobular owing to widened, sclerotic septa (Fig. 20-12B). The normal architecture of the subcutaneous lobules may be markedly disrupted or completely destroyed, replaced by microcystic (includes microcysts and macrocysts) and lipomembranous (pseudomembranous) fat necrosis (Fig. 20-12D). Calcification and elastosis may be seen, sometimes combining to produce a moth-eaten appearance resembling the fragmented and calcified elastic fibers of pseudoxanthoma elasticum (PXE) (85); PXE-like fibers are positive for both von Kossa and Verhoeff van Gieson stains. Ossification has also been documented (86). Venous stasis changes are typically present in the overlying dermis; these include lobules of small slightly thick-walled vessels in concert with extravasated erythrocytes and hemosiderin (Fig. 20-12E). The hyperpigmentation in LDS is attributed to hemosiderin and melanin. Melanin may be increased in the epidermis and present within melanophages in LDS (87).

Differential Diagnosis. Clinical correlation is usually sufficient to establish the diagnosis of LDS. This is perhaps fortunate in view of the very nonspecific nature of some of the most commonly encountered and histologically distinctive features of LDS, if taken in isolation. The presence of lipomembranous fat necrosis should prompt consideration of LDS, but it can be seen in the late stage of numerous forms of panniculitis, including virtually any lobular panniculitis, as well as EN. Likewise, PXE-like elastosis has been documented in a wide variety of disorders, including calciphylaxis (uremic and nonuremic) (88,89), EN, GA, morphea profunda (85), and nephrogenic systemic fibrosis (90). Traumatic panniculitis may be histologically indistinguishable from LDS.

Pathogenesis. Venous insufficiency is considered the primary etiologic factor in LDS, and proposed mechanisms include impaired fibrinolysis and excessive protease activity secondary to trapping and activation within the microcirculation in areas of stasis, with resultant endothelial damage and formation of fibrin cuffs and fibrin microthrombi causing subcutaneous ischemia and fat necrosis (82). Other factors such as obesity or trauma may also contribute in some cases.

Principles of Management: Leg elevation and compressive therapy help control venous stasis. Symptomatic therapy may include topical steroids or capsaicin cream. Systemic treatment options include pentoxifylline and anabolic steroids (for fibrinolytic effects) (82).

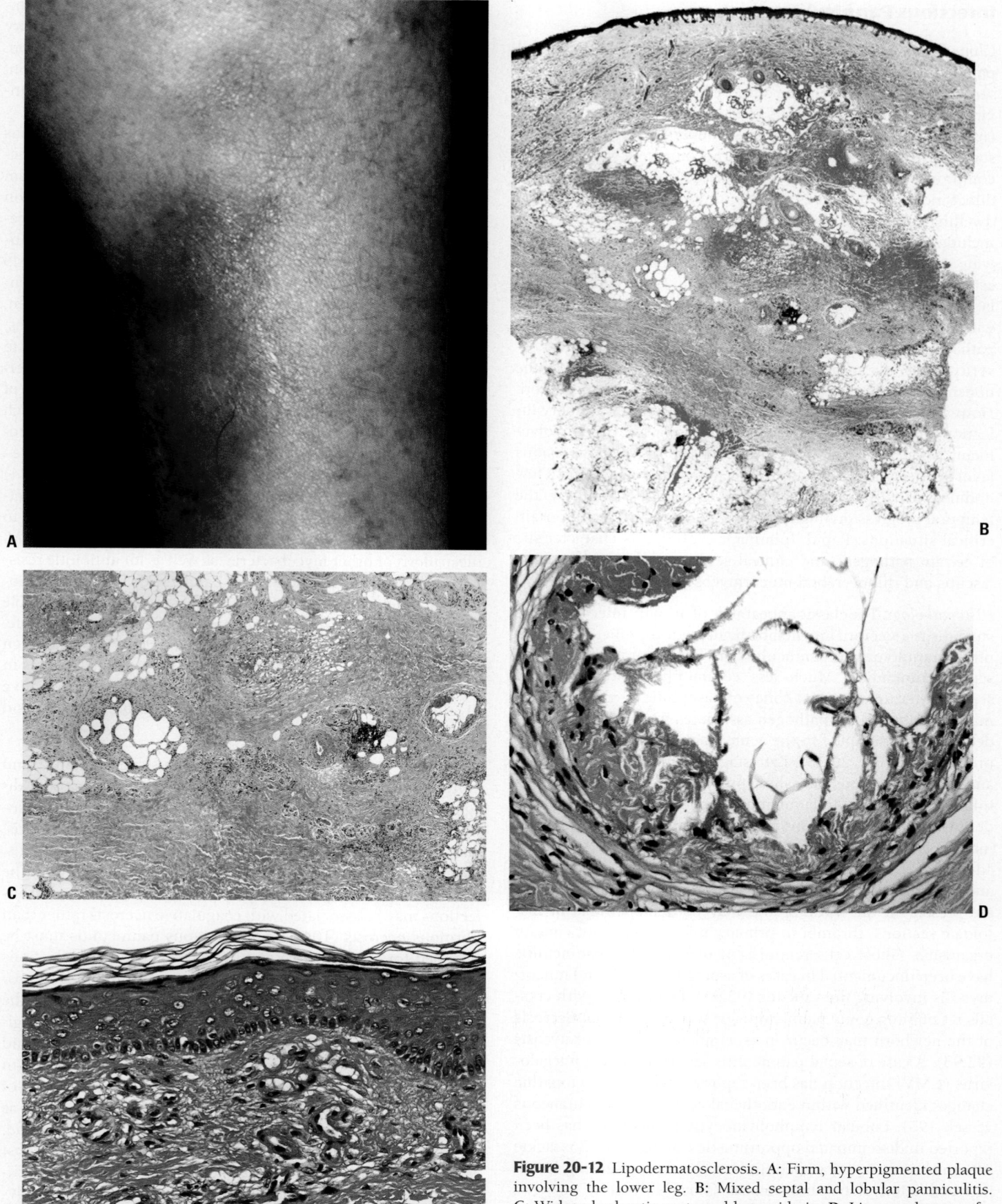

Figure 20-12 Lipodermatosclerosis. A: Firm, hyperpigmented plaque involving the lower leg. B: Mixed septal and lobular panniculitis. C: Widened sclerotic septa and hemosiderin. D: Lipomembranous fat necrosis. E: Venous stasis changes in the papillary dermis.

Infectious Panniculitis

Clinical Summary. Infection-induced (infectious or infective) panniculitis may display a relatively wide range of clinical presentations depending on one or more key factors, including the virulence of the pathogen, its mode of entry into the subcutis (primary cutaneous infection vs. secondary infection), and the status of the host response (immunocompetent vs. immunocompromised) (91). Primary cutaneous infection occurs via direct inoculation such as external trauma, injection, or an indwelling catheter with occlusive dressing. Secondary infection includes septicemia or spread from adjacent infected tissue. A wide variety of bacterial, mycobacterial, fungal, viral, and parasitic pathogens have been documented (see "Pathogenesis" later). Infections in immunocompromised hosts are associated with a wider spectrum of pathogens, including opportunistic pathogens but may not necessarily exhibit greater clinical severity. Generally speaking, the clinical morphology tends to be nonspecific, with erythema, and variable necrosis or ulceration. However, the distribution of lesions can be helpful: Primary infection tends to present as a solitary lesion or localized involvement, whereas numerous, widespread, and/or bilateral lesions favor septicemia. Rarely, septicemia may present as one or a few nodules, usually on the peripheral extremities. Similarly, the temporal progression might provide a diagnostic clue in certain critical situations: Rapid, fulminant evolution is characteristic of certain pathogens and clinical settings such as necrotizing fasciitis and rhinocerebral mucormycosis (92).

Histopathology. The classic appearance of primary infection of the subcutis is a necrotizing, hemorrhagic, neutrophilic, or neutrophilic granulomatous panniculitis in a lobular or mixed lobular/septal panniculitis. Much less commonly, a predominantly septal pattern may occur. Zones of basophilic necrosis are primarily attributable to pathogen-associated neutrophilic nuclear debris. When sampled in the acute stage, neutrophils typically predominate (Fig. 20-13). Late-stage or chronic mycobacterial and fungal infections may show predominantly granulomatous inflammation. The inflammation may involve the overlying dermis. In septicemia, features of "septic vasculitis" are present, including neutrophils, leukocytoclastic nuclear debris (nuclear "dust"), fibrin within and around subcutaneous vessel walls, and occluding fibrin thrombi. Whereas in septicemia organisms are present in the thrombi and may be demonstrable in histologic sections, thrombi in primary infections do not contain organisms. Ghost cells reminiscent of pancreatic panniculitis have been documented in cases of aspergillosis (93) and mucormycosis involving the subcutis (92,94). Panniculitis with crystals resembling gouty panniculitis or subcutaneous fat necrosis of the newborn may occur in aspergillosis and mucormycosis (92,93). A case of septal panniculitis secondary to cytomegalovirus (CMV) infection has been reported, with viral cytopathic changes identified within endothelial cells of the subcutaneous vessels (95). Lobular lymphohistiocytic panniculitis has been reported in disseminated opportunistic Enterovirus (Coxsackie A9) infection (96). Panniculitis may be the presenting lesion in reactivation of trypanosomiasis (Chagas disease) in organ transplant recipients (97).

Histochemical stains and, in select situations, immunohistochemical or molecular diagnostic tests are typically used to confirm the presence of infection. Among these, histochemical stains remain cost-effective, widely available, and highly specific for the presence of organisms. However, histochemical stains can be relatively insensitive among these ancillary diagnostic methods and do not permit unequivocal speciation. Thus, negative histochemical stains do not exclude infection, and culture of lesional tissue remains the practical gold standard for speciation and specific diagnosis.

Particularly in immunocompromised patients, organisms may be numerous. However, in many cases, multiple step sections may be required to identify organisms, and a rare organism may be present in a hematoxylin and eosin (H&E) step section rather than the special stain. Although easily missed if not specifically searched for, fungal pathogens can usually be identified in H&E sections and highlighted by PAS, PASD, or GMS histochemical stain. Gram stains are typically required to identify bacterial pathogens. Acid-fast stains (Fite, Ziehl–Neelsen, Kinyoun) are required to identify mycobacterial pathogens. Among the acid-fast stains, the Fite stain may be required to demonstrate *M. leprae*, which only rarely extends from the dermis into subcutis (98). In the past, an additional method of screening for mycobacteria as well as bacteria and fungi such as sporotrichosis in formalin-fixed tissue was immunohistochemical staining for polyclonal *M. bovis* (bacillus Calmette–Guérin [BCG]) (99,100); however, the antibody (clone B124) was subsequently purified and is now suitable only for detecting mycobacteria. PCR–based methods are also available to test formalin-fixed tissue for specific agents, for example, *M. tuberculosis* or other mycobacteria, as well as for antibiotic resistance patterns. Septal and lobular panniculitis have been documented in leishmaniasis; amastigotes, if searched for, are visible on H&E and may also be highlighted by Giemsa stain. Of note, a specific clone of anti-CD1a (MTB1, not clone 010) has been documented to specifically highlight *Leishmania* amastigotes in formalin-fixed tissue (but not decalcified) and may be positive in a limited number of cases without discernible pathogens on H&E (101–103).

Differential Diagnosis. Clinical correlation, special stains, and cultures are often invaluable in addressing the differential diagnosis of neutrophilic lobular and granulomatous panniculitis, which includes α-1-antitrypsin deficiency panniculitis, and panniculitis associated with CD or rheumatoid arthritis. Special stains for bacteria, mycobacteria, and fungi should be considered for any panniculitis with neutrophils. Bacterial infections may be associated with coagulative necrosis rather than fibrinous necrosis (104). Granulomatous panniculitis must be screened for mycobacteria and fungi. Mycobacterial infections may not induce granulomas, for example, in immunocompromised hosts where abscess formation is more likely, and the host response may be sparse and nonspecific. Necrosis originating in the subcutaneous septa with granulation tissue and giant cells, without caseation necrosis, has been described in panniculitis associated with *M. ulcerans* (91). The presence of small or medium vessel vasculitis may suggest septicemia, as has been documented in cases of panniculitis from *Nocardia*, *Pseudomonas*, and *Fusarium* (105). As noted previously, ghost cells reminiscent of pancreatic panniculitis have been documented in cases of aspergillosis (93) and mucormycosis involving the subcutis (92).

Pathogenesis. Bacteria include *Staphylococcus aureus*, *Streptococcus pyogenes*, *Pseudomonas* sp, *Nocardia* sp, *Klebsiella*, and *Brucella*. Most reported cases of mycobacterial panniculitis

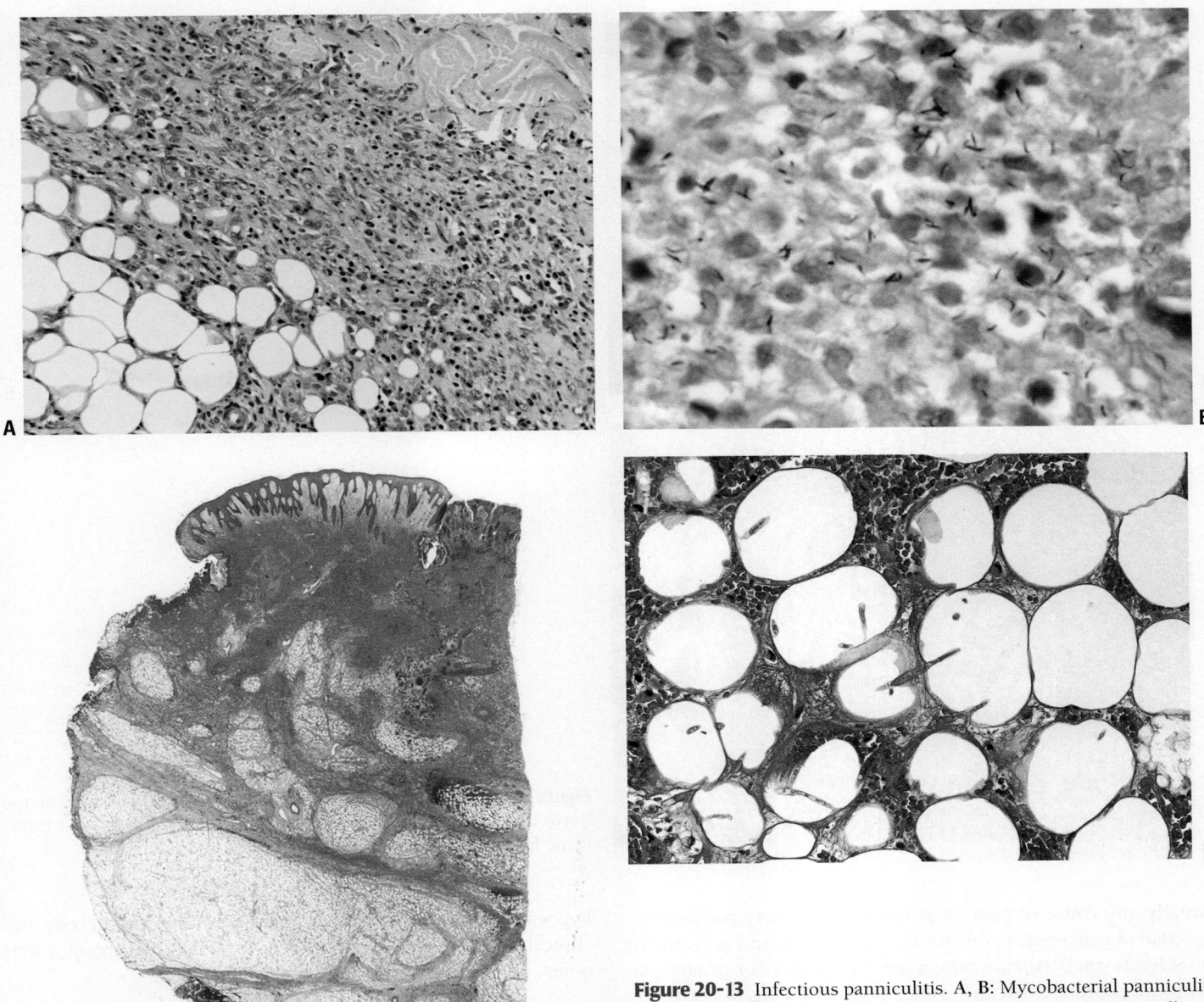

Figure 20-13 Infectious panniculitis. **A, B:** Mycobacterial panniculitis with neutrophils and acid-fast bacilli on AFB stain. **C, D:** *Aspergillus* sp. Mixed septal and lobular pattern with prominent hemorrhage. Infections in immunocompromised hosts may exhibit numerous organisms and sparse inflammatory host response.

have been nontuberculous, including *Mycobacterium chelonae*, *M. fortuitum*, *M. avium intracellulare complex*, *M. ulcerans*, *M. kansasii*, *M. malmoense*, *M. abscessus*, and, less commonly, *M. tuberculosis* or *M. leprae*. Disseminated fungal infections may be caused by *Candida* sp, *Aspergillus* sp (Fig. 20-13C), *Fusarium* sp, and *Histoplasma*. Among subcutaneous mycoses, sporotrichosis, eumycotic mycetoma, and chromomycosis are probably most common, but, essentially, any subcutaneous mycosis would typically induce panniculitis. Extracellular lipases produced by *Aspergillus* sp. and the Mucoraceae family of fungi appear to account for the ghost adipocytes seen in panniculitis caused by these organisms (92).

Principles of Management: Systemic antibiotics are indicated for infectious panniculitis. Selection of antibiotics should be guided by cultures and sensitivities whenever possible. Broad-spectrum coverage is indicated if cultures are not available. Coverage for methicillin-resistant *Staph. aureus* (MRSA) and dual coverage for *P. aeruginosa* are standard when those

organisms are suspected. Multiagent regimens have been established for mycobacterial infections (104).

Pancreatic Panniculitis

Clinical Summary. Pancreatic panniculitis arises in the setting of pancreatic insufficiency and presents as multiple nodules on the distal lower extremities (Fig. 20-14A). The knees, pretibial, and ankle regions are most commonly affected. The thighs, buttocks, abdomen, arms, elbows, and scalp may also be involved. In mild, self-limited cases, the nodules may be painless. In more severe or chronic cases, the nodules are tender and may discharge sterile, oily brown fluid through fistulae. Pancreatic panniculitis was first documented by Chiari in the late 19th century and in the English literature in 1961 by Szymanski and Bluefarb, who reported on five cases, four (including two fatal cases) in association with chronic pancreatitis, and one associated with pancreatic carcinoma. Pancreatitis associated with alcohol intake or gallstones may represent the most common clinical settings, but

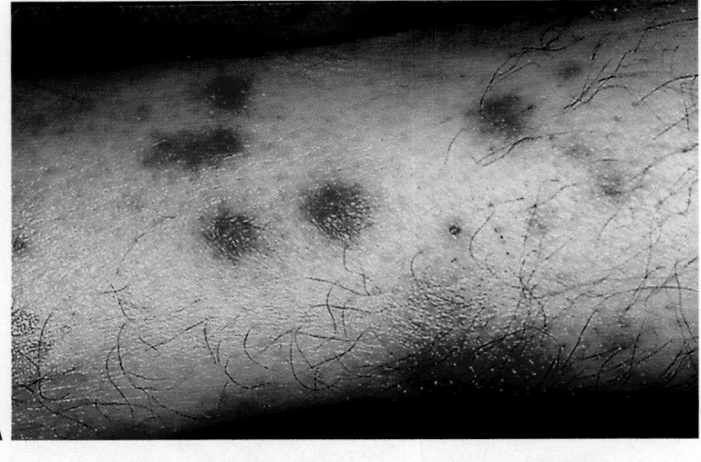

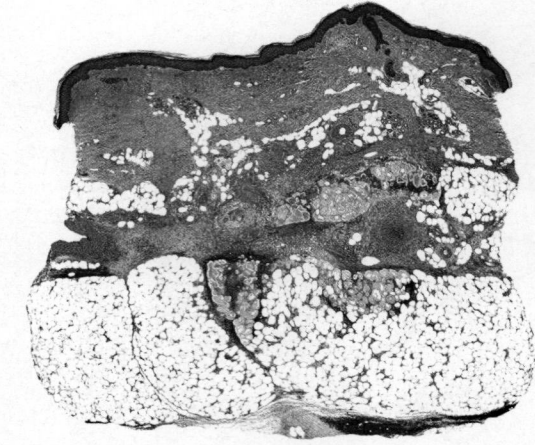

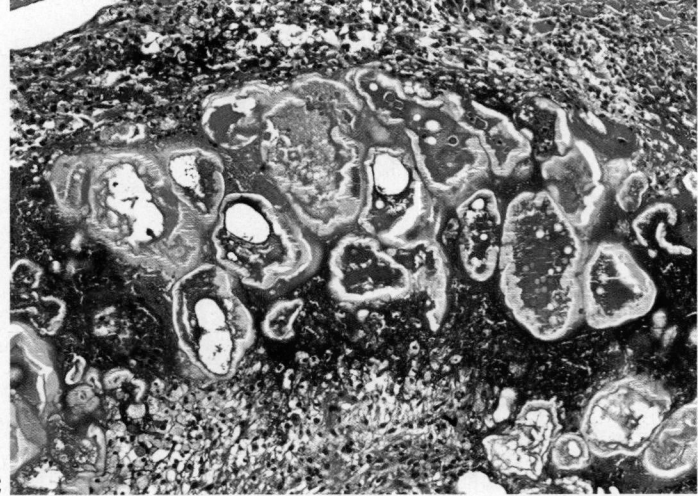

Figure 20-14 Pancreatic panniculitis. **A:** Erythematous nodules on the lower legs. **B:** Mostly lobular panniculitis with neutrophils. **C:** Enzymatic fat necrosis includes ghost adipocytes and calcification.

virtually any cause of pancreatic insufficiency may predispose. The triad of pancreatic panniculitis, eosinophilia, and polyarthritis (Schmid triad) is reportedly associated with poor prognosis, and some postulate that the arthritis occurs owing to periarticular fat-pad panniculitic degeneration. In addition to acute and chronic pancreatitis and certain forms of pancreatic carcinoma (mostly, acinar cell carcinoma and, less commonly, acinar cell cystadenocarcinoma [106], adenosquamous carcinoma [107], islet cell endocrine carcinoma [108], neuroendocrine tumors of pancreatic or adrenal origin [109,110], or papillary intraductal mucinous neoplasm [111]), pancreatic panniculitis has also been associated with pancreatic pseudocyst, pancreas divisum (in one case associated with an intraductal carcinoid tumor [112]), sulindac therapy, therapy for hepatitis C (113), allograft pancreatitis (114), hepatic carcinoma (115), HIV-associated hemophagocytic syndrome, lupus pancreatitis, carcinoembryonic antigen and MUC1 anticancer vaccine therapy for pancreatic cancer (116), and pancreatitis associated with acute fatty liver of pregnancy and HELLP syndrome (hemolysis, elevated liver enzymes, low platelets) (117). Associated arthropathy has been attributed to the effects of pancreatic enzymes that have traveled parenterally to periarticular adipose tissue (118). The same fat necrosis may also occur in internal organs, including the pancreas itself, surrounding fat tissue, and in the fat of the omentum, mesentery, pericardial and perirenal regions, as well as in the mediastinum and bone marrow. Calcium precipitation with the released fatty acids can be extensive enough to produce life-threatening

hypocalcemia. The cutaneous manifestation can precede the clinical onset of pancreatic disease, especially pancreatic carcinoma, by several months (119).

Histopathology. The histologic appearance of pancreatic panniculitis is characteristic in most instances. The pattern is typically lobular with neutrophils and contains a nearly pathognomonic form of adipocyte necrosis known as enzymatic fat necrosis (Fig. 20-14B). Enzymatic fat necrosis consists of distinctive ghost-like, enlarged fat cells having thick, faintly stained cell peripheries and loss of basophilic nuclear staining. Calcification forms basophilic granules in the cytoplasm of the necrotic fat cells and sometimes forms lamellar deposits around individual fat cells or patchy basophilic deposits at the periphery of the fat necrosis (Fig. 20-14C). A polymorphous infiltrate surrounds the foci of fat necrosis with mostly neutrophils, as well as lymphocytes, macrophages, lipophages, and foreign-body giant cells. Eosinophils are variable. There can be extensive hemorrhage, but vasculitis is usually absent. In early lesions, biopsies may show only a nonspecific necrotizing panniculitis with a neutrophilic inflammatory response. In very early lesions, a mostly septal pattern with lymphocytes, eosinophils, and "occasional" neutrophils has been described (120). Older lesions contain macrophages, lipophages, lymphocytes, and fibroblasts, with fibrosis and hemosiderin deposition.

Differential Diagnosis. Enzymatic fat necrosis (i.e., the combined presence of ghost adipocytes with calcification) is so distinctive that it may be regarded as indicative of pancreatic panniculitis unless proved otherwise. However, lipases are also produced by *Aspergillus* sp. and the *Mucoraceae* family of fungi, accounting for the ghost adipocytes seen in infectious panniculitis caused by these organisms (92,93). Numerous organisms accompany the ghost adipocytes in these cases. In the early stage of pancreatic panniculitis, nonspecific neutrophilic infiltrates may evoke a differential diagnosis of α-1 antitrypsin (AAT) deficiency, infectious panniculitis, or other causes of neutrophilic lobular panniculitis. Basophilic DNA debris from neutrophil nuclei must be distinguished from calcium deposits. Von Kossa stains for calcium phosphate are positive on the calcium deposits and negative on necrotic nuclei. The fat necrosis with calcification caused by subcutaneous interferon-β injections may resemble that of pancreatic panniculitis; in addition to this unique clinical context, classic ghost adipocytes have not been documented, and concomitant lipoatrophy, vascular thrombosis, and dermal mucinosis have been described (121).

Pathogenesis. It has been generally accepted for decades, without unequivocal proof, that enzymatic fat necrosis results from damaged and/or neoplastic pancreatic acinar cells that release lipase, phospholipase, trypsin, and amylase into the surrounding tissues and vascular-lymphatic circulation, resulting in hydrolysis of neutral fat to form glycerol and free fatty acids (i.e., saponification) in all affected organ systems. Free fatty acids released by the lipolysis combine with calcium to form soapy basophilic deposits. Local changes in vascular permeability attributable to trauma or other circulating enzymes, such as trypsin or phospholipase A2, might allow pancreatic lipase to enter the cytoplasm of the adipocytes. Lipase has been demonstrated immunohistochemically in a lesion of pancreatic panniculitis. Serum values for amylase and lipase are usually elevated transiently. Amylase levels may peak a few days after the appearance of panniculitis but, overall, correlate poorly with the time course of the panniculitis (108). Enzymatic damage to the integrity of the vascular wall can produce extensive hemorrhage. However, it is not clear how pancreatic proenzymes become activated or why most patients with pancreatic insufficiency do not develop pancreatic panniculitis. Evidence in support of an immune-mediated mechanism is virtually nonexistent; moreover, immunosuppressive therapy has no role in the management of pancreatic panniculitis.

Principles of Management: Treatment of pancreatic panniculitis depends primarily on the identification and management of the underlying cause. Surgical excision, or metastasectomy, can achieve clinical remission (122). The somatostatin analog, octreotide, which reduces pancreatic enzyme output, has been reported to be beneficial in some cases but not others (123,124). NSAIDs, corticosteroids, or other immunosuppressive therapies have no demonstrated benefit.

α1-Antitrypsin Deficiency Panniculitis

Clinical Summary. Panniculitis associated with deficiency of the serine protease inhibitor, AAT presents as subcutaneous nodules in a manner somewhat similar to the nodules of pancreatic panniculitis (125). Most lesions arise on the lower extremities, especially the proximal extremities; less commonly, the upper extremities, trunk, and face may be affected. Skin lesions can often be precipitated by trauma. Early or mild lesions may resemble cellulitis. Chronic or recurrent nodules can drain oily yellow fluid derived from the enzymatic breakdown of the fibrous tissue and fat (Fig. 20-15A) (126). The ulcerated lesions eventuate in atrophic scars. Among more than 120 alleles of the *SERPINA1* gene that encodes AAT, at the locus 14q32.1, only the severest minority subset is associated with mutations that produce sufficient deficiency of AAT to produce clinical symptoms. Liver disease is often the presenting problem, including hepatomegaly, neonatal cholestatic jaundice, and cirrhosis in children. AAT deficiency in the lung leads to the unopposed release of neutrophil elastase, which produces panacinar emphysema, involving the destruction of bronchioles, alveolar ducts, and alveoli (127). The pulmonary disease usually becomes evident in young to middle-aged adults, a process that is accelerated in tobacco users. Panniculitis can be the presenting sign in AAT deficiency. Onset is typically between the ages of 30 to 60 years, but AAT has been reported in all age groups.

Histopathology. AAT deficiency panniculitis usually shows a mostly lobular or mixed septal and lobular pattern with a predominantly neutrophilic infiltrate, without epidermal involvement. Less commonly, the neutrophilic infiltrate may be mostly septal (Fig. 20-15B). Sterile neutrophilic abscesses surround and isolate fat lobules, sometimes creating an appearance of "floating" lobules. Secondary leukocytoclastic or lymphocytic

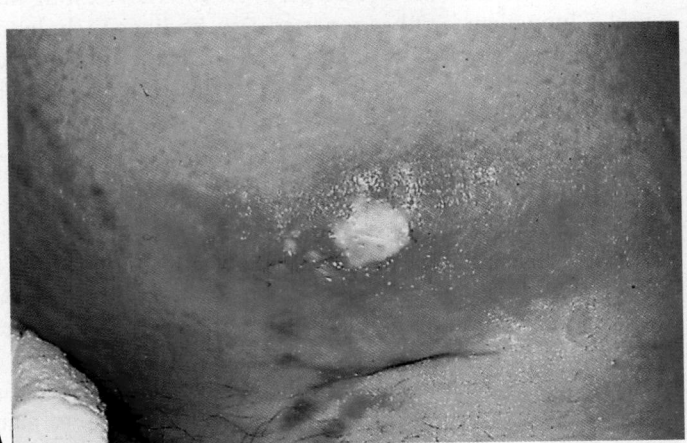
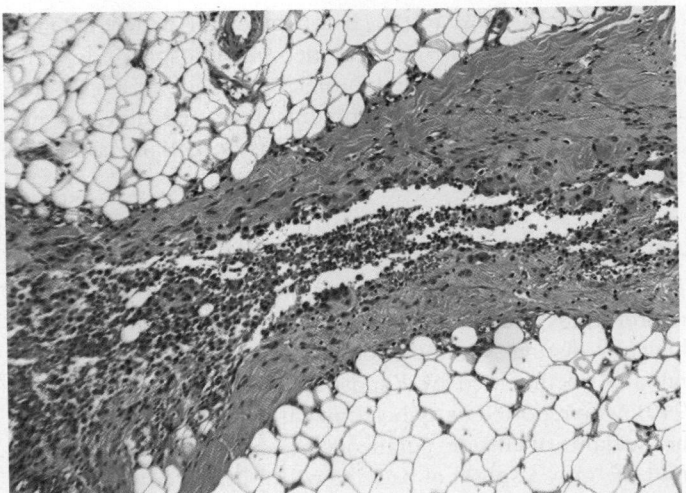

A   **B**

Figure 20-15 α-1-Antitrypsin deficiency panniculitis. A: Ulcerated, erythematous plaque. B: Neutrophilic abscess in the septa.

vasculitis may be present. Late lesions have an infiltrate of macrophages and lymphocytes with fibrosis and lipophages. The macrophages can exhibit cytophagic activity, ingesting neutrophil fragments and extravasated erythrocytes. Geller and Su reported interstitial neutrophils in the reticular dermis and subcutaneous lobules and septa as a subtle clue to the diagnosis of AAT deficiency panniculitis based on a single case report (128). (In the absence of additional data, this attribute is regarded as nonspecific as an isolated attribute; its utility as a diagnostic clue might be clinically relevant in the appropriate clinical context.) Microscopically, the panniculitis can be patchy with necrotic foci alternating with the uninvolved fat lobules.

Differential Diagnosis. The histopathologic changes in AAT deficiency panniculitis are not pathognomonic but are distinctive enough to typically enter the histologic differential diagnosis. Testing for serum AAT levels can be diagnostic. Serum AAT levels below the lower limit of normal (usually < 20 μmol/L) should be referred for PCR or isoelectric focusing for allelic analysis. Short of positive diagnostic confirmation, when neutrophils are prominent and ulceration present, the differential diagnosis includes infectious panniculitis, pancreatic panniculitis or pyoderma gangrenosum (as a diagnosis of exclusion), and possibly erythema induratum if lesions are confined to the extremities. Infection must be reasonably excluded by tissue staining and/or tissue cultures. Ghost cells have not been documented in AAT deficiency panniculitis. If cytophagic changes are present, cytophagic histiocytic panniculitis (which may represent an indolent form of primary cutaneous subcutaneous panniculitis-like T-cell lymphoma [SPTCL] with reactive cytophagic histiocytes) should be considered. The prominence of neutrophils in AAT deficiency is in contrast to the lymphocyte predominance in cytophagic histiocytic panniculitis.

Pathogenesis. The clinical manifestations may reflect quantitative and/or qualitative deficiencies of AAT. Proposed mechanisms of tissue damage include primarily the lack of inhibition of membrane-bound serine proteases (e.g., elastase) owing to functional AAT deficiency, as well as the predominantly neutrophilic infiltrate (neutrophils have a high content of serine proteases), complement cascade activation, loss of AAT function attributable to oxidation by neutrophil myeloperoxidase, and AAT polymer deposition within lesional and nonlesional tissue (129).

Principles of Management: Historically, AAT deficiency may be refractory to treatment. Colchicine, cyclophosphamide, dapsone, doxycycline (130), fenoprofen, intravenous augmentation therapy with AAT, methylprednisolone, nafcillin, plasma exchange, and liver transplantation are potentially available therapeutic modalities (131–133).

Lupus Erythematosus Panniculitis

Clinical Summary. Lupus erythematosus panniculitis (LEP; lupus profundus, Kaposi–Irgang disease) is a clinically and histologically distinct variant of chronic cutaneous LE. LEP was originally documented by Kaposi (1883) and later by Irgang (1940), who reported its association with discoid LE (134). Like other variants of chronic cutaneous LE, such as discoid LE and tumid LE, only a subset of patients with LEP have systemic LE. However, many patients with LEP also have discoid LE. In contrast to most forms of panniculitis, the legs are not predisposed to developing LEP. Tender nodules and plaques tend to involve

the face, trunk, breast (lupus mastitis), buttocks, and proximal upper and lower extremities, particularly their lateral aspects (Fig. 20-16A). LEP in children is relatively rare but tends to involve the face. Linear and annular lupus panniculitis of the scalp represents a distinct clinical subset (135). A chronic, relapsing clinical course is the norm. Lesions may be solitary or may occur in crops and may be triggered or exacerbated by trauma, including injection or biopsy. Multiple areas may be involved, although widely disseminated disease is unusual. Associated overlying epidermal and dermal changes are clinically and histologically appreciated in about half to two-thirds of cases, characterized clinically by erythema, follicular plugging, scale, dyspigmentation (i.e., peripheral hyperpigmentation and central hypopigmentation or depigmentation), telangiectasia, atrophy, scarring, or ulceration, that is, superimposed changes of discoid LE. The end stage of lesions without epidermal and dermal changes may clinically resemble lipoatrophy, with pauci-inflammatory dell-shaped depressions remaining, itself a clinical clue to the diagnosis.

Histopathology. LEP is the prototypical lobular lymphocytic panniculitis (Fig. 20-16B). The small lymphocytic infiltrate is moderately dense in active lesions but may be sparse in "burnt out" lesions that exhibit more prominent hyaline fat necrosis and septa widened by sclerosis. Associated changes include reactive lymphoid follicles and lymphocytic vasculitis with lymphocytic nuclear "dust" (nuclear debris). Hyaline fat necrosis is specifically associated with LEP and is characterized by a hyalinized, glassy, homogeneous eosinophilic appearance with loss of nuclear staining surrounding residual empty round fat vacuoles (Fig. 20-16C). Lipomembranous fat necrosis has also been documented. Overlying epidermal and dermal changes of LE are often present: atrophic interface changes, moderately dense superficial and deep dermal perivascular and periadnexal (including perieccrine) lymphocytic infiltrates with plasma cells, increased interstitial mucin in the reticular dermis, and hyalinization of the papillary dermis. Calcification is often present in established lesions. Although eosinophils are rare or absent in most forms of cutaneous LE, eosinophils may be present in LEP. Peters and Su regarded plasma cells and eosinophils as minor criteria for the diagnosis of LEP (136). Neutrophils have also been rarely documented, including a case of mixed septal and lobular panniculitis with neutrophils within lymphoid follicles and widened fibrotic septa; this case also exhibited neutrophils within the overlying dermal perivascular infiltrate (137). To the extent that concomitant discoid LE is present, DIF testing may reveal a lupus band. Other reported DIF findings include immune globulin deposition along the dermal epidermal junction and deep dermis (138) or subcutis and IgG highlighting the periphery of adipocytes (139).

Differential Diagnosis. The distinction between LEP and exceptionally rare instances of panniculitis attributable to dermatomyositis requires clinical correlation (140). Erythema induratum may exhibit eosinophilic hyaline-like fat necrosis in concert with lymphocytic vasculitis but characteristically contains prominent granulomatous inflammation as well as neutrophils. The septal sclerosis in LEP may closely resemble that of morphea profunda; however, morphea spares the fat lobule that is invariably involved in LEP. Injection site reactions to glatiramer acetate may resemble LEP (141), although other cases present as lipophagic granulomatous panniculitis with eosinophils and neutrophils (142).

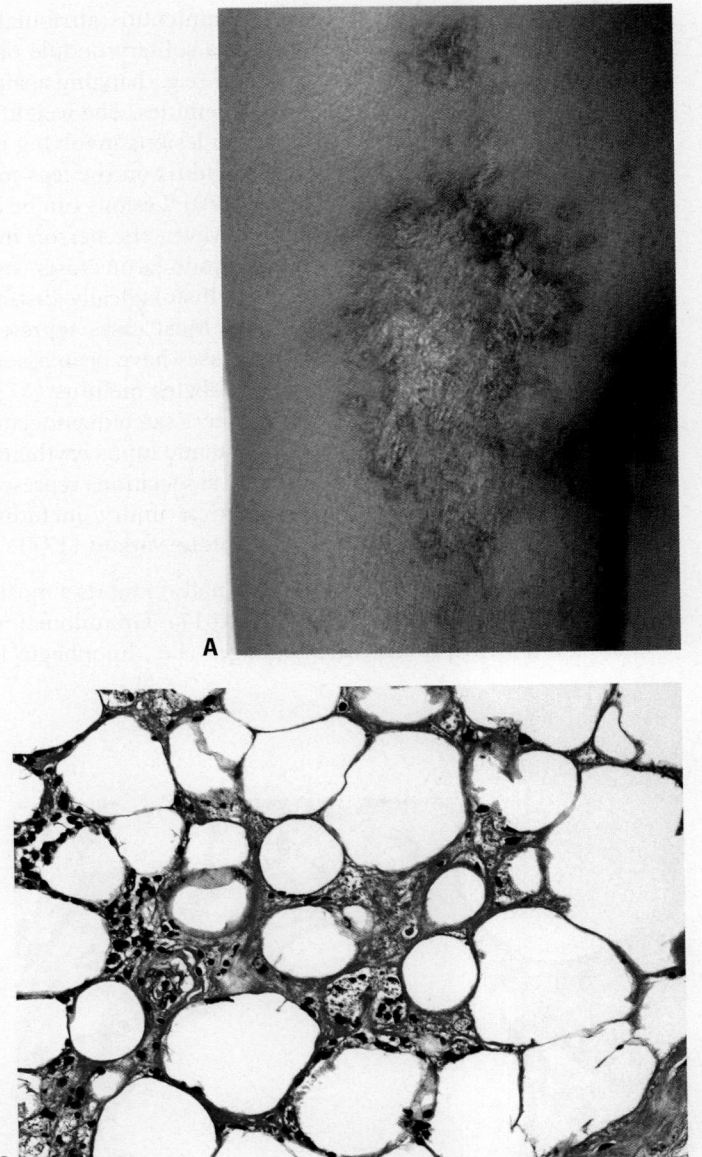

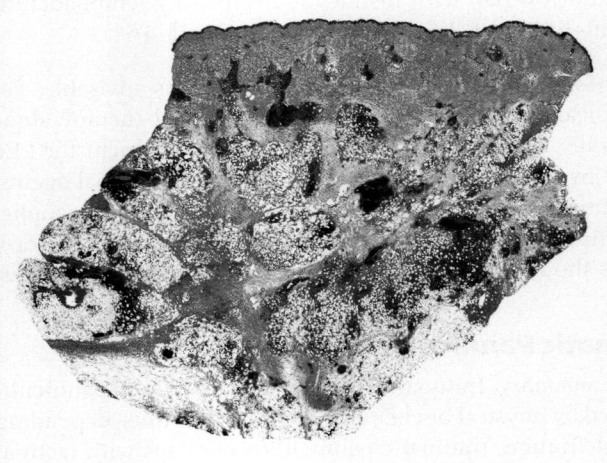

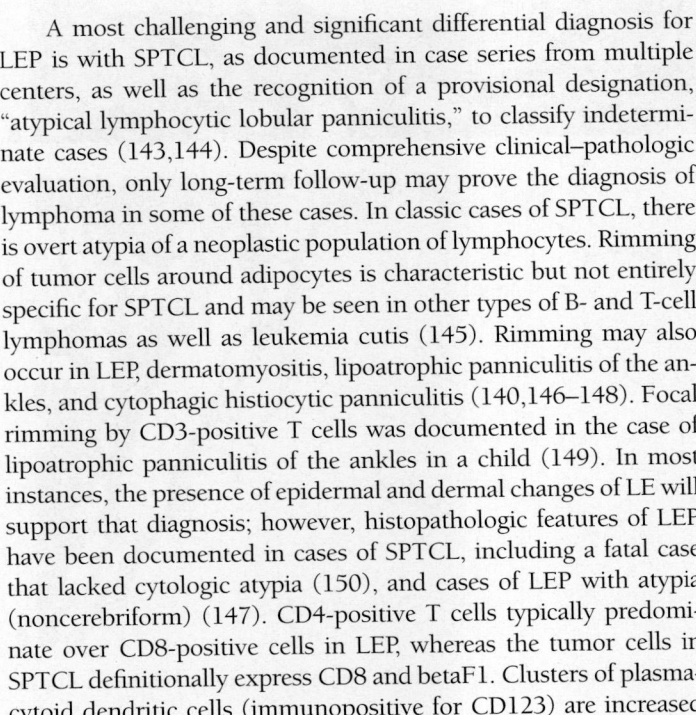

Figure 20-16 Lupus erythematosus panniculitis. **A:** Indurated subcutaneous plaque with postinflammatory hyper- and hypopigmentation on the lateral thigh. **B:** Lobular lymphocytic panniculitis with overlying perivascular and periadnexal dermatitis. **C:** Hyaline fat necrosis.

A most challenging and significant differential diagnosis for LEP is with SPTCL, as documented in case series from multiple centers, as well as the recognition of a provisional designation, "atypical lymphocytic lobular panniculitis," to classify indeterminate cases (143,144). Despite comprehensive clinical–pathologic evaluation, only long-term follow-up may prove the diagnosis of lymphoma in some of these cases. In classic cases of SPTCL, there is overt atypia of a neoplastic population of lymphocytes. Rimming of tumor cells around adipocytes is characteristic but not entirely specific for SPTCL and may be seen in other types of B- and T-cell lymphomas as well as leukemia cutis (145). Rimming may also occur in LEP, dermatomyositis, lipoatrophic panniculitis of the ankles, and cytophagic histiocytic panniculitis (140,146–148). Focal rimming by CD3-positive T cells was documented in the case of lipoatrophic panniculitis of the ankles in a child (149). In most instances, the presence of epidermal and dermal changes of LE will support that diagnosis; however, histopathologic features of LEP have been documented in cases of SPTCL, including a fatal case that lacked cytologic atypia (150), and cases of LEP with atypia (noncerebriform) (147). CD4-positive T cells typically predominate over CD8-positive cells in LEP, whereas the tumor cells in SPTCL definitionally express CD8 and betaF1. Clusters of plasmacytoid dendritic cells (immunopositive for CD123) are increased in LEP compared to SPTCL; their presence in the papillary dermis correlates with the presence of interface dermatitis (151). The proliferation index (measured by Ki-67) in LEP is usually low, in contrast to a high proliferative index in SPTCL. Clonal rearrangement of the T-cell receptor gene by PCR may be demonstrable in SPTCL but not LEP. SPTCL associated with hemophagocytic lymphohistiocytosis (HLH)/macrophage activation syndrome represents an aggressive subset that has been associated with mutations in HAVCR2 that abrogate its immune checkpoint protein product, TIM-3, resulting in a proinflammatory state (152–155). Other types of lymphoma, including gamma/delta lymphoma, primary cutaneous CD30 anaplastic large cell lymphoma, and primary cutaneous B cell lymphomas, may also show a clinical and/or histopathologic appearance of panniculitis.

Pathogenesis. LE is a classical autoimmune disease that is recognized to be a complex, multifactorial disorder with genetic and environmental predispositions. The pathogenesis of cutaneous LE has been specifically associated with certain genetic variations as well as environmental triggers, the best characterized of which is ultraviolet radiation (156,157). Specific investigations into the pathogenesis of LEP have been limited to date. However, reports of increased interferon and interferon-inducible factors such as CD123 positive plasmacytoid dendritic cells (158,159), human myxovirus resistance protein 1(MxA), and IL-17 in cutaneous LE appear to be applicable to LEP (160–162). LEP has also been associated with interferon-β injections in a patient with multiple sclerosis (163). Association and/or overlap with histiocytic necrotizing lymphadenitis (Kikuchi–Fujimoto disease) has been reported (164).

Principles of Management: Sun protection is advisable. Potent topical steroids are often used, but topical therapy alone is generally inadequate. Systemic agents for treatment for LEP include hydroxychloroquine and alternate antimalarial agents, thalidomide, systemic corticosteroids, azathioprine, mycophenolate mofetil, cyclophosphamide, and cyclosporine (165,166). Patients should be evaluated for systemic lupus erythematosus.

Traumatic Panniculitis

Clinical Summary. Traumatic panniculitis can refer to panniculitis caused by physical or chemical agents (167); thus, depending on the definition, traumatic panniculitis overlaps with factitial panniculitis as well as cold panniculitis, which are addressed

separately in this chapter. Traumatic panniculitis attributable to physical trauma typically presents as a solitary nodule on a trauma-prone site such as the shin, thigh (e.g., banging against a desk or chair), or elsewhere on the extremities. The weight of excess tissue itself has been attributed to lesions involving the breast and panniculus. Traumatic panniculitis on the legs may be associated with hypertrichosis (168–170). Lesions can be induced by airbag deployment (171). However, the person may not recall trauma to the area. Nodular cystic fat necrosis (mobile encapsulated lipoma) represents a histologically distinct variant of traumatic panniculitis (172). Most cases represent an isolated finding, but rarely reported cases have been associated with systemic disease, including diabetes mellitus (173), scleroderma (174), Heerfordt syndrome (sarcoid-associated uveitis and facial nerve palsy) (175), systemic lupus erythematosus (176), and EN. Whether these rare associations represent chance occurrences is unknown. Electrical injury, including from electroacupuncture, represents a unique variant (177).

Histopathology. Traumatic panniculitis usually exhibits a mostly lobular or mixed lobular pattern (Fig. 20-17). Granulomatous inflammation with prominent lipophages (i.e., lipophagic fat

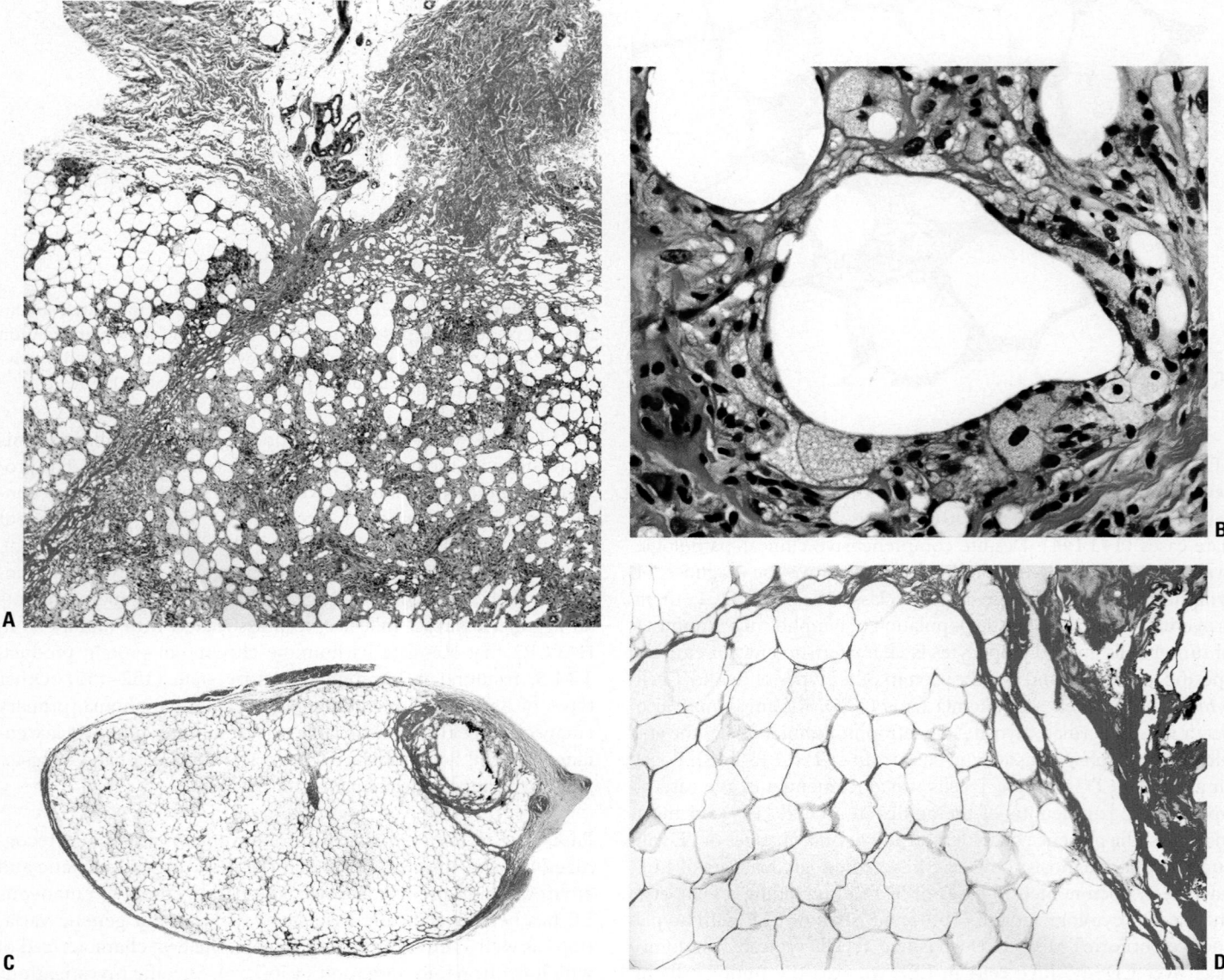

Figure 20-17 Traumatic panniculitis. A: Mostly lobular panniculitis. B: Prominent lipophages. C: Nodular cystic fat necrosis exhibits a fibrous sclerotic capsule. D: Loss of adipocyte nuclei in nodular cystic fat necrosis.

necrosis) is typical, and lipomembranous fat necrosis, microcystic fat necrosis, dystrophic calcification, and ossification may also be present. Septal fibrosis develops in established lesions. Extravasated erythrocytes and hemosiderin are often present. In nodular cystic fat necrosis, the lesion is enclosed within a fibrous sclerotic capsule (Fig. 20-17C), with characteristic loss of adipocyte nuclei amid minimal to absent inflammation and relatively minimal disruption of the size and shape of the adipocyte vacuoles (Fig. 20-17D). Lipomembranous and microcystic fat necrosis, calcification, and ossification may be present in nodular cystic fat necrosis (178). Necrotic adipocytes and associated vessels may rarely resemble parasite parts.

Differential Diagnosis. Although a positive clinical history of trauma strongly supports a diagnosis of traumatic panniculitis, the absence of a history of trauma does not exclude it. The presence of venous stasis changes suggests LDS, which can exhibit all of the histopathologic features of traumatic panniculitis. The presence of hemosiderin confirms the presence of lesional hemorrhage, as opposed to technical artifact from the biopsy procedure (which often produces prominent extravasated erythrocytes at the base of the specimen). Rarely, degenerated erythrocytes may form large vacuoles containing smaller eosinophilic bodies (myospherulosis, spherulocytosis) or empty vacuoles (lipogranuloma) (179); some of these cases are attributable to topically applied ointments, in which case they may be classified as forms of factitial panniculitis.

Pathogenesis. Traumatic disruption of adipocytes and associated vessels accounts for the nonspecific fat necrosis and hemosiderin in traumatic panniculitis. Mechanistic studies have not specifically been reported for traumatic panniculitis. Postsurgical lipophagic panniculitis is a potential model for the study of traumatic panniculitis (180). Nodular cystic fat necrosis has been attributed to rapid vascular insufficiency in response to trauma (181).

Principles of Management: For small nodules, the biopsy can be both diagnostic and therapeutic. Treatment for traumatic panniculitis is primarily supportive, and the condition is usually self-limited (167).

Factitial Panniculitis

Clinical Summary. Depending on the definition, factitial panniculitis may be viewed as a subset of traumatic panniculitis but is defined here as panniculitis caused by direct injection of chemical substances rather than physical trauma. The term "factitial" implies a deliberate human action, although the intent is not necessarily to cause a lesion or disease. Thus, iatrogenic causes, as well as those motivated by secondary gain or associated with psychiatric disease are included (182). Factitial panniculitis usually presents as subcutaneous nodules at the sites of injection with variable erythema, tenderness, ulceration, and scarring. Clinical correlation can clinch the diagnosis, but in cases of secondary gain or psychiatric disorders, the answer may not be forthcoming even on repeated direct inquiry of the patient (183,184). In such cases, the number of lesions is small, and the distribution is typically confined to areas accessible to self-injection by the patient (a rare exception might be a child suffering from Munchausen syndrome by proxy). Any unusual distribution of lesions that does not fit any other known disorder may evoke suspicion. Intramuscular injections

are typically administered by health care providers to the shoulder or buttock. Injections of cosmetic fillers may involve the face, breasts, or penis. Rarely, topically applied ointments have been attributed to some cases of subcutaneous myospherulosis (spherulocytosis), characterized by the formation of large vacuoles containing smaller eosinophilic bodies.

Histopathology. Consistent with the wide variety of substances that may be injected, the histopathologic spectrum of factitial panniculitis is broad. Acute reactions to injected substances typically induce a mostly lobular neutrophilic panniculitis with variable necrosis and abscess formation. Insoluble, chronically retained substances will induce granulomatous inflammation. Oily substances such as liquid silicone, vegetable oils, or paraffin are removed during tissue processing and are therefore negative on polarized microscopy but produce a distinctive "Swiss cheese" appearance with pseudocystic empty vacuoles associated with foamy histiocytes and multinucleated histiocytes. The histologic appearances of the various cosmetic soft tissue fillers are varied but can be distinctive, and most are intentionally placed into the subcutis (185–187). Birefringent materials highlighted by polarized light include poly-L-lactic acid (Sculptra, New-Fill), silicone (impurities), polytetrafluoroethylene (Teflon), and E-polytetrafluoroethylene (Gortex). Nonbirefringent materials include calcium hydroxylapatite (Radiesse), polyvinylpyrrolidone-silicone suspension (Bioplastique), polymethacrylate microspheres suspended in carboxymethylcellulose and calcium gluconate (Metacrill), hyaluronic acid (Restylane, Hylaform, Captique), acrylic hydrogel particles in hyaluronic acid (DermaLive/DermaDeep), polyacrylamide (Aquamid), and paraffin. In one rare case that represented a suicide attempt, factitial panniculitis presented as an eosinophilic panniculitis (see the following section) (188).

Differential Diagnosis. In the absence of identifying the injected material, the histologic appearances are nonspecific, with mostly lobular panniculitis with neutrophils in the acute stage and a lobular or mixed pattern with granulomatous inflammation and variable fibrosis in the chronic stage. Infectious panniculitis must be reasonably excluded. A negative exam on polarized microscopy fails to confirm but does not exclude a foreign body. Conversely, the presence of a foreign body does not necessarily exclude other disorders, for example, sarcoid (189).

Pathogenesis. Iatrogenic causes include injections of meperidine, phytonadione (vitamin K_1), procaine povidone, gold salts, glatiramer acetate (141,142), opiates (meperidine, pentazocine, methadone), and vaccinations for tetanus, hepatitis, or cancer therapy. Self-injected substances can be bizarre, including sesame oil (190), milk, urine, or feces.

Principles of Management: Discontinuation of the offending agent is curative, but, for reasons noted previously, the causative agent can be very difficult to identify and remove. Granulomatous reactions against soft tissue fillers may be managed with intralesional corticosteroid injections. Endermology (a form of therapeutic massage) has been reported (191).

Cold Panniculitis

Clinical Summary. Cold panniculitis presents as slightly erythematous nontender subcutaneous nodules within a few days of cold exposure. Cold weather induces lesions on the chin of children, as originally reported by Hochsinger in 1902 (192,193). Distinctive sites of involvement include bilateral or unilateral involvement of the scrotum of prepubertal males and "popsicle panniculitis" on the cheeks of infants or young children who suck popsicles (ice lollies, ice pops) or ice (194). Cold panniculitis has developed on the neck and upper back after ice therapy for supraventricular tachycardia (195). Equestrian cold panniculitis involves the lateral thighs of female equestrians, cyclists, or motorcyclists, although some cases actually represent or overlap with perniosis (chilblains). With the appropriate clinical history, a potentially traumatic or disfiguring biopsy can often be avoided in cold panniculitis.

Histopathology. In cold panniculitis, inflammatory infiltrates are centered on the deep dermal vessels at the interface of the reticular dermis and subcutis with variable, sometimes patchy, involvement of the subcutaneous lobules. Blood vessels may exhibit thickened "fluffy edema" of their walls. Vasculitis is not a feature. Mucin deposition has been reported (192). In early lesions, neutrophils may be present, joined by lymphocytes and histiocytes in fully developed lesions. Eosinophils may be present (195).

Differential Diagnosis. The presence of a sparse inflammatory infiltrate centered on the junction of the reticular dermis might prompt consideration of inflammatory morphea. Denser infiltrates involving subcutaneous lobules might evoke consideration of lupus profundus or tumid lupus erythematosus; however, plasma cells are usually present in inflammatory morphea and lupus. The inflammatory infiltrates in cold panniculitis may overlap with the deep dermal perivascular and periadnexal lymphocytic infiltrates of perniosis.

Pathogenesis. The subcutaneous fat of children is more sensitive to cold injury than that of older children and adults; this is attributable to their greater saturated fat content (palmitic acid, stearic acid) that predisposes to fat crystallization at relatively higher temperatures compared to adult fat. Nearly a century ago, Lemež demonstrated that, in most or all newborn infants, the application of an ice cube to the skin for 50 seconds produced cold panniculitis. By 9 months of age, such cold sensitivity is rare (194). Although infants and young children are physiologically most susceptible, severe cold exposure or a predisposing disorder such as cryofibrinogenemia may facilitate the development of cold panniculitis in adults. Despite the common denominator of increased saturated fat in cold

panniculitis and subcutaneous fat necrosis of the newborn, their clinical and histopathologic differences suggest different pathomechanisms, with cold panniculitis bearing overlap with perniosis. For example, nodules arising on the lateral thighs of equestrians may exhibit overlapping features between perniosis and cold panniculitis; ischemia and wind chill from typically tight-fitting and poorly insulated riding pants have been implicated in these cases. A case of popsicle panniculitis that arose during systemic corticosteroid therapy has been reported, supporting the assumption that the immune system does not play a critical role in this disorder (196).

Principles of Management: If the source of cold exposure is removed, nodules of cold panniculitis resolve over several days or weeks without active treatment.

Postirradiation Pseudosclerodermatous Panniculitis

Clinical Summary. Postirradiation pseudosclerodermatous panniculitis (PIPP, also known as sclerosing postirradiation panniculitis) usually occurs in women with a history of megavoltage radiation for breast cancer (197). Clinical onset is localized to the irradiated area and manifests several months to several years (up to 17 years has been documented) following radiation therapy (198). PIPP is likely underreported, as lesions tend to be asymptomatic; biopsy is typically indicated to rule out late metastasis. The clinical morphology is a firm nodule or indurated plaque; focal ulceration may occur. Other than the breast, any irradiated site may be involved; a case involving the inguinal region has been documented (199). Another case was associated with bronchiolitis obliterans (200).

Histopathology. PIPP displays a mixed or mostly lobular pattern of panniculitis with a lobular lymphohistiocytic infiltrate with ischemic and lipophagic fat necrosis and associated septal eosinophilic sclerosis (Fig. 20-18). Plasma cells are typically present. Rare eosinophils may be present (198). Radiation vasculopathy is also characteristic, with fibrosis and hyalinization of vessel walls, without frank vasculitis.

Differential Diagnosis. The combined presence of septal sclerosis, lobular fat necrosis, and radiation vasculopathy is distinctive

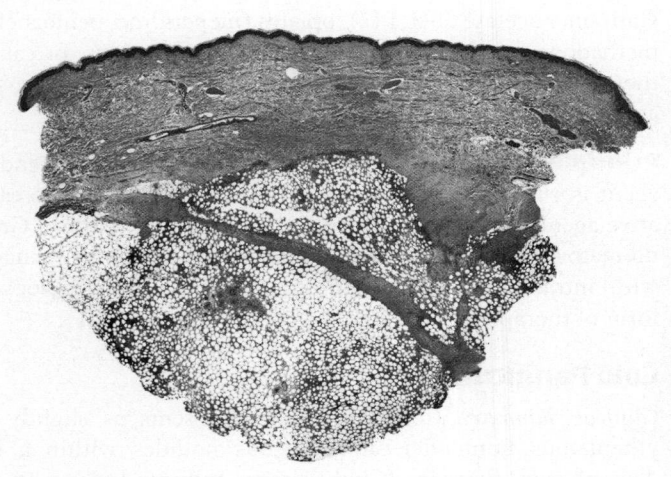
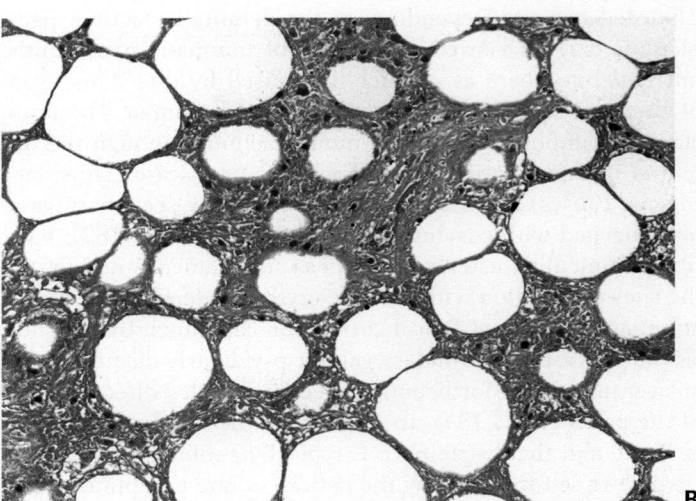

Figure 20-18 Postirradiation pseudosclerodermatous panniculitis. A: Mostly lobular pattern with septal sclerosis. B: Ischemic fat necrosis.

enough that the diagnosis of PIPP may be suspected on histologic grounds alone. If the history of irradiation is not known, the sclerosis may evoke consideration of a sclerosing disorder such as morphea profunda or late-stage lupus profundus. However, associated necrosis in the fat lobules is not a feature of primary sclerosing disorders such as morphea profunda. In lupus profundus, the lobular necrosis is of the hyaline type rather than lipophagic and ischemic and is often associated with many lymphocytes rather than histiocytes.

Pathogenesis. In PIPP, radiation vasculopathy likely contributes to subcutaneous ischemia, which results in secondary necrosis of the fat lobules. Septal sclerosis is directly attributable to the effects of megavoltage radiation therapy, analogous to the dermal changes of chronic radiation dermatitis.

Principles of Management: Given a clinical concern for late metastasis, reassurance is typically all that is necessary. Specific therapy for PIPP has not been reported to date.

Lipoatrophic Panniculitis of the Ankles

Clinical Summary. Lipoatrophic panniculitis of the ankles (LPA) is a rare childhood form of panniculitis. LPA was initially reported in 1970 by Shelley and Izumi as a form of partial lipodystrophy they designated annular atrophy of the ankles (201). Other cases have been reported as lipoatrophy of the ankles, lipoatrophic panniculitis (202), and annular LPA (203). LPA may occur after trauma to the ankles. Clinically, LPA presents as erythematous plaques with an annular scaly border, eventuating in permanent lipoatrophy. As indicated by many of these terms, a strong predilection for involvement of the ankle region has been observed. Involvement may extend to the dorsal feet and lower legs, soles, upper extremities, and trunk. Recurrent attacks of painful lesions may be associated with constitutional symptoms (204). A case clinically resembling eosinophilic fasciitis has been reported (205).

Histopathology. In the early inflammatory stage, LPA is mostly lobular panniculitis, with prominent lipophages accompanied by reactive lymphocytes (Fig. 20-19). Early lesions may show mostly lymphocytes, but neutrophils and immature myeloid cells (myeloperoxidase positive) may also be prominent in early lesions, with histiocytes (CD68 positive), including lipophages surrounding necrotic adipocytes present in later lesions (149,204). The epidermis is usually unremarkable, and the dermis may exhibit a mild dermal perivascular lymphocytic infiltrate. Mild lymphocytic atypia (without karyorrhectic nuclear debris) has been reported involving medium-sized vessels of the subcutaneous septa. Focal rimming of CD3-positive lymphocytes or neutrophils has also been documented. In this case, the proliferative activity was relatively high (up to 60% by MIB-1 immunohistochemical staining); reassuring features included a mixed population of CD4- and CD8-positive T lymphocytes without loss of CD7 staining amid few B cells, no cytotoxic or natural killer phenotype or evidence of Epstein Barr virus and no evidence of a clonal T-cell receptor gene rearrangement (149).

Differential Diagnosis. The combined age of onset and anatomic distribution should evoke consideration of LPA, especially if the lesions are known to be annular. The main pitfalls are probably lack of awareness of the entity or insufficient clinical information to facilitate suspicion of LPA. Based on histology alone, the mostly lobular pattern with prominent lipophages (lipophagic panniculitis) is relatively nonspecific and may suggest a differential diagnosis of traumatic panniculitis. Neutrophils are usually not prominent in LPA, but if neutrophils are focally present, the histologic differential diagnosis includes AAT deficiency panniculitis or factitial panniculitis. The presence of rimming of adipocytes by lymphocytes should evoke consideration of SPTCL, which can affect children but does not specifically favor the ankles and which exhibits a CD8 positive phenotype. Rimming has also rarely been documented in

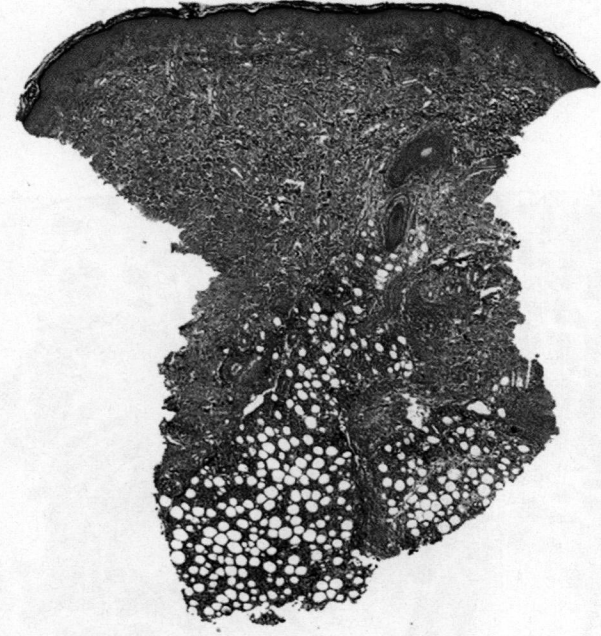

A

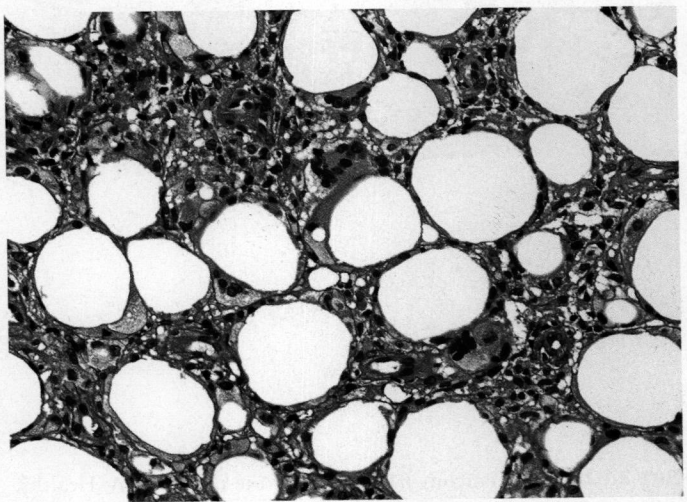

B

Figure 20-19 Lipoatrophic panniculitis of the ankles. A: Lobular panniculitis with lymphocytes and histiocytes, including prominent lipophages. B: Lipophagic fat necrosis.

lupus profundus, but involvement of the ankles is even less typical of lupus profundus. Cytophagocytosis may be seen in panniculitis-like lymphoma, cytophagic histiocytic panniculitis, lupus profundus, and AAT deficiency panniculitis but has not been documented in LPA.

Pathogenesis. The cause of LPA is unknown, but an autoimmune or autoinflammatory etiology has been suspected. Some patients have concomitant autoimmune disease or autoimmune serologies (203,206–208). Cases characterized by repeated attacks of painful lesions accompanied by malaise, arthralgia, and lesional immunopositivity for STAT1 support a possible autoinflammatory etiology (204).

Principles of Management: In most cases, residual lipoatrophy improves over time. At the case report level, prednisone, dapsone, hydroxychloroquine, methotrexate, and azathioprine-based therapies have been reported, among others (149,202).

Subcutaneous Fat Necrosis of the Newborn

Clinical Summary. In subcutaneous fat necrosis of the newborn, indurated, erythematous to violaceous nodules and plaques appear a few days to a week after birth (Fig. 20-20A). Subcutaneous fat necrosis of the newborn may occur in premature or full-term infants, often after a complicated forceps delivery, cesarean section, or other factors that might contribute to

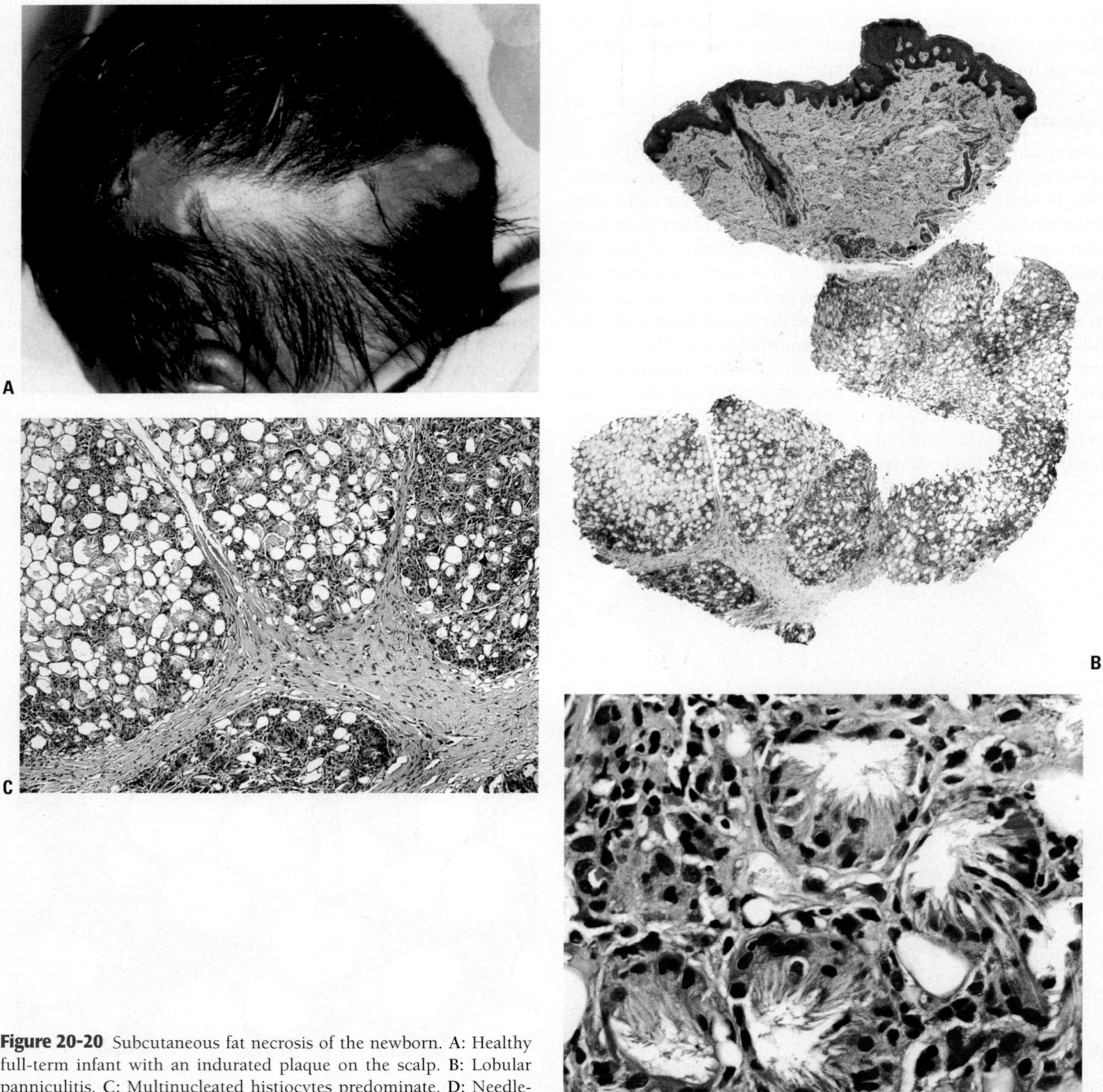

Figure 20-20 Subcutaneous fat necrosis of the newborn. **A:** Healthy full-term infant with an indurated plaque on the scalp. **B:** Lobular panniculitis. **C:** Multinucleated histiocytes predominate. **D:** Needle-shaped clefts within the cytoplasm of multinucleated histiocytes.

hypoxia and/or hypothermia, including extensive fat necrosis following passive or whole-body cooling (209), for example, induced hypothermia used in cardiac surgery or to treat hypoxic ischemic encephalopathy (210). The nodules typically resolve spontaneously after a few weeks or months. Lesions may rarely discharge caseous material. At the opposite extreme, in one case the skin nodules were subtle enough to be missed on initial physical exam (211). Most newborns are otherwise healthy, but hypercalcemia may occur in approximately one-third of cases, usually within one or a few months from the onset of skin nodules, rarely with fatal outcomes (212). Nephrocalcinosis persisting several years after resolution of the skin nodules has been reported (213). Thrombocytopenia, hypertriglyceridemia, and hypoglycemia may also occur. In contrast to cold panniculitis, histologic confirmation is generally required; the diagnosis has also been established using touch prep and fine needle aspiration techniques (214,215).

Histopathology. Subcutaneous fat necrosis of the newborn is characterized by a mostly lobular infiltrate of macrophages, with distinctive foreign-body type giant cells containing crystalline fat, which after tissue processing appears as empty needle-shaped clefts, classically in radial array, emanating from a peripheral point or central nidus within the cytoplasm (Fig. 20-20D). The crystals are present within histiocytes and adipocytes. In frozen sections, these clefts contain birefringent fat crystals. Scattered foci of calcification may be present within the necrotic fat. Extensive necrosis may be associated with large calcium deposits that require several years to be reabsorbed. The periphery of the cytoplasm of the multinucleated giant cells may be laced with distinctive fine eosinophilic granules (216). A mixed inflammatory infiltrate with eosinophils and/or neutrophils may be present, including neutrophilic microabscesses in early lesions. Cystic follicular plugging with folliculocentric pseudocarcinomatous hyperplasia has been reported (217).

Differential Diagnosis. The differential diagnosis for these distinctive radial clefts includes sclerema neonatorum and poststeroid panniculitis. Compared to subcutaneous fat necrosis of the newborn, sclerema neonatorum typically lacks inflammation, necrosis, and calcification, with radial clefts largely confined to adipocytes rather than histiocytes. Traumatic or factitial panniculitis lacks the crystals in the fat. Clinical correlation is of great value for resolving this differential diagnosis and is required to distinguish subcutaneous fat necrosis from poststeroid panniculitis. Similar nonbirefringent crystal artifact may be seen in the formalin-fixed lesions of gouty panniculitis, which typically exhibits a prominent palisaded granulomatous reaction. Crystals in aspergillus- and mucormycosis-associated panniculitis are birefringent in formalin-fixed specimens (92). Radial needle-shaped clefts within adipocytes have been documented in a case of gemcitabine-associated livedoid microangiopathy (218).

Pathogenesis. The high degree of saturated fatty acids and triglycerides in newborns raises the crystallization temperature or melting point of the fat tissue, accounting for the fatty crystals that produce the needle-shaped clefts. Historically, these fatty crystals were called "margarine crystals" and were subclassified into small, patternless, microsized crystals (A crystals) and large crystals arranged in rosettes (B crystals). Small amounts of these crystals have been documented in normal infants. Subsequent damage to adipocytes containing B crystals has been associated with the granulomatous inflammation characteristic of subcutaneous fat

necrosis of the newborn. Electron microscopic examination shows that the phagocytosis of fat crystals starts with the invasion of fat cells by cytoplasmic projections of macrophages. Subsequently, fat crystals are seen within the cytoplasm of macrophages and of foreign-body type giant cells, which result from the fusion of the macrophages. Brown fat may be involved (219). The distinctive eosinophilic granules appear to be from degranulated eosinophils (216,220). What triggers the development of subcutaneous fat necrosis in only certain newborns is unknown. It is generally assumed that factors contributing to hypoxia and/or hypothermia predispose to the development of this disorder.

Principles of Management: Most cases of subcutaneous fat necrosis resolve spontaneously. Severe cases are potentially fatal and require close symptomatic support, including pamidronate for hypercalcemia, which might reduce the risk of nephrocalcinosis (221,222).

Sclerema Neonatorum

Clinical Summary. In most countries, sclerema neonatorum is an exceptionally rare disorder that preferentially affects premature infants, characterized by diffuse, rapidly progressive, nonpitting hardening of the subcutaneous fat in the first few days of life, with a frequently fatal outcome. Only acral sites and genitalia may be spared. It is currently most commonly encountered in less developed countries. Patients often present with vomiting, diarrhea, and/or sepsis. Identified risk factors include poor feeding, jaundice, and bacterial sepsis (223–225). The skin seems wax-like, tight, cold, and indurated. Death typically supervenes in a few weeks if untreated. On autopsy, the subcutis is greatly thickened and hardened: "lard-like" (226). Infants with sclerema neonatorum are typically cyanotic at birth, have difficulty maintaining their body temperature, and have a major debilitating illness such as meconium aspiration. Older literature classifies subcutaneous fat necrosis of the newborn as one of two subsets of sclerema neonatorum, the other being the fulminant presentation retaining that designation, described here.

Histopathology. In sclerema neonatorum, the subcutaneous tissue owes its thickening to the increase in the size of the fat cells and to the presence of wide, intersecting fibrous bands (Fig. 20-21A). The lipid crystals inside the fat cells produce rosettes of fine needle-like clefts after lipid extraction in routine processing, albeit not as prominent as in subcutaneous fat necrosis of the newborn, reflecting a relatively greater content of A crystals (see later) (Fig. 20-21B). As in subcutaneous fat necrosis of the newborn, in frozen sections the birefringent crystals are not extracted. Classically, there is a minimal to absent inflammatory reaction or necrosis, and no epidermal or dermal involvement; only sparse neutrophils, eosinophils, and histiocytes, including multinucleated histiocytes, have been documented.

Differential Diagnosis. The histologic differential diagnosis typically includes subcutaneous fat necrosis of the newborn and poststeroid panniculitis. Clinical correlation is invaluable for resolving this differential diagnosis. Histologically, the presence of a histiocytic component with needle-like clefts presents within histiocytes and fat necrosis is against sclerema neonatorum. Clinical correlation is required to distinguish between subcutaneous fat necrosis of the newborn and poststeroid panniculitis. Radial needle-shaped clefts within adipocytes have been reported in association with gemcitabine-associated livedoid microangiopathy (218).

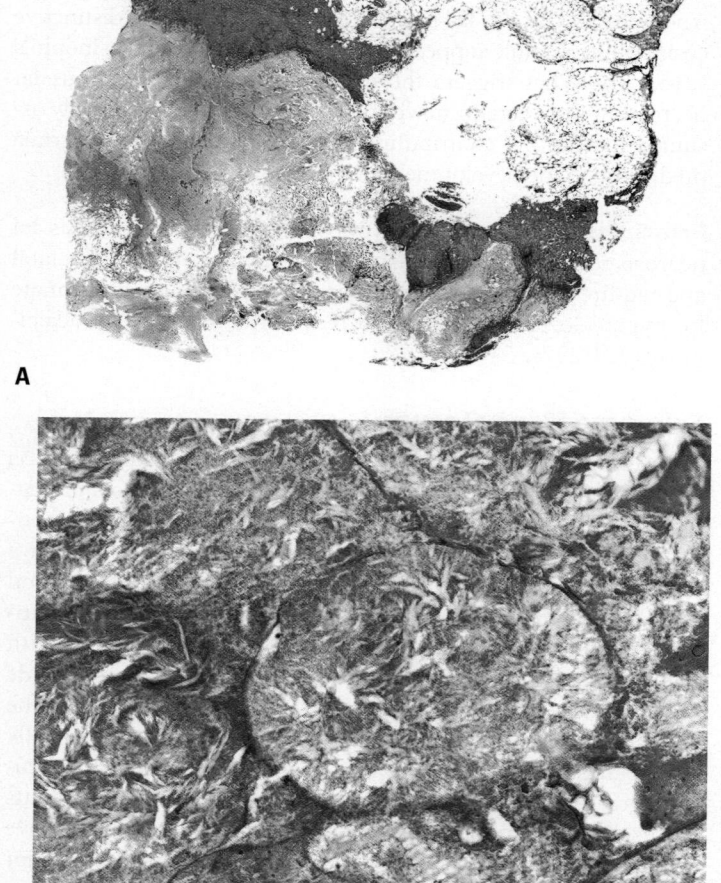

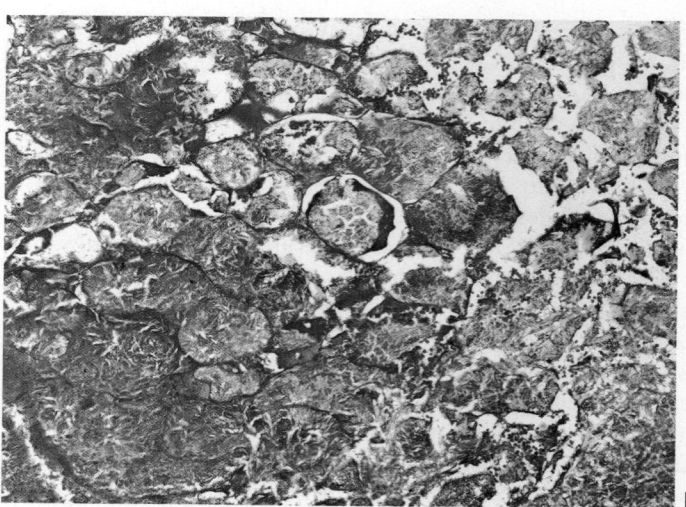

Figure 20-21 Sclerema neonatorum. **A:** Septal and lobular panniculitis with widened fibrotic septa. **B:** The fat lobules are replaced by enlarged adipocytes filled with crystallized fat. **C:** Needle-shaped clefts admixed with patternless microsized fat crystals.

Pathogenesis. As in subcutaneous fat necrosis of the newborn and many cases of cold panniculitis, the higher degree of saturation of the lipids in newborns raises the crystallization temperature of the fat and produces greater susceptibility to cold injury. In sclerema neonatorum, the changes seen in subcutaneous fat necrosis of the newborn seem to be significantly amplified so that the neutral fat (triglyceride) crystallizes at room temperature. In contrast to the B crystals associated with subcutaneous fat necrosis of the newborn, excessive accumulation of A crystals (small microsized) has been implicated in sclerema neonatorum why sclerema neonatorum occurs in certain cases is, however, unknown. In addition to prematurity, sepsis or other serious general illness is typically present in sclerema patients. Various theories related to defects in fat metabolism, inherent abnormality of the adipocytes or supporting connective tissue, or underlying severe systemic toxicity have been proposed (227). The identification of altered lipid peroxidation (increased blood lipid peroxidation, diminished superoxide dismutase activity) suggests the possibility that free radicals may play a role in the pathogenesis of sclerema neonatorum.

Principles of Management: It is tempting to believe that the use of thermally controlled incubators for premature infants might be associated with the fact that sclerema neonatorum is exceptionally rare in developed encounters. However, after-the-fact

warming of the body has no demonstrated benefit. Management includes aggressive therapy for underlying systemic diseases such as sepsis, and otherwise is essentially supportive, including warming and emollients. Exchange transfusion therapy in patients with sclerema and sepsis has been reported, but efficacy has not been established; moreover, reported cases were diagnosed clinically, without histologic confirmation. Intravenous immunoglobulin has been employed (228).

Poststeroid Panniculitis

Clinical Summary. Poststeroid panniculitis is an increasingly rare disorder that usually affects children within days or weeks of the discontinuation or rapid withdrawal of systemic corticosteroid therapy. Poststeroid panniculitis usually presents as symmetric erythematous indurated 0.5- to 4-cm nodules or plaques on the face, typically the cheeks. The jawline, arms, trunk, and lower extremities may also be involved. Most lesions are characteristically located in areas in which new fat deposition is induced by steroid treatment such as the face and posterior neck. Indeed, patients often have concomitant cutaneous evidence of systemic corticosteroid therapy, including a Cushingoid facies and/or buffalo hump. The lesions are usually both pruritic and tender. In a rare adult case, lesions on the arms and legs were reportedly painless (229). Urticarial appearances have been documented, as well as one lesion with a small overlying vesicle.

New nodules may arise while earlier ones resolve (sometimes with a bluish hue), but poststeroid panniculitis ultimately resolves without scarring or dyspigmentation. In reported cases with severe lesions that prompted reinstitution of prednisone therapy, dramatic improvement ensued. Underlying conditions requiring systemic corticosteroid therapy appear to be diverse and unrelated, including rheumatic fever and leukemia in the original series (230), brain stem glioma, hepatic encephalopathy, nephrotic syndrome, and Sjogren syndrome (229).

Histopathology. Poststeroid panniculitis is a mostly lobular panniculitis with lymphocytes and histiocytes, including lipophages. Neutrophils are usually present in both early and established lesions (231). The most distinctive finding in established lesions is radially arranged needle-shaped clefts within adipocytes and histiocytes. These clefts may not be present in biopsies of lesions that have been present only for a few days. The epidermis and dermis are uninvolved.

Differential Diagnosis. Clinical correlation is required (and usually sufficient) to distinguish poststeroid panniculitis from subcutaneous fat necrosis of the newborn and sclerema neonatorum. Although all of these disorders affect children, the age of onset and associated clinical and laboratory features are distinctive in each disorder.

Pathogenesis. As noted previously, lesions are often located in areas where new fat deposition is induced by corticosteroid therapy such as the face and posterior neck. Although the precise mechanisms are unknown, it has been suggested that corticosteroid withdrawal might cause abnormal lipid metabolism, which increases the saturated fatty acid content and saturated:unsaturated fatty acid ratio in these areas, resulting in changes essentially akin to those implicated in subcutaneous fat necrosis of the newborn.

Principles of Management: No treatment is generally required for poststeroid panniculitis. As noted previously, severe cases that prompted reinstitution of prednisone therapy were associated with improvement of this condition.

Calciphylaxis

Clinical Summary. Calciphylaxis (calcific uremic arteriolopathy, vascular calcification–cutaneous necrosis syndrome) nearly always occurs in patients with end-stage renal disease and/or hyperparathyroidism who develop indurated, erythematous, cold nodules and plaques with extensive dry gangrene (eschar) (Fig. 20-22A) (232,233). Plaques are often localized at sites of subcutaneous injection such as the thighs and abdomen, but the lower legs are often involved as well. Cases involving the penis and vulva have been reported (234–237). Calciphylaxis develops in less than 5% of patients on hemodialysis for end-stage renal disease and is characterized by acute onset of painful, violaceous livedo-like plaques that acutely progress to large zones of tissue necrosis, eschar, and often death (233). The classic presentation is acute, but more insidious subacute evolution ("protracted calciphylaxis") has also been documented (238).

Histopathology. Vascular calcification in calciphylaxis usually involves the tunica media and may involve the tunica intima and adluminal surfaces of small or medium-sized arteries, as well as the walls of arterioles, veins, and capillaries in the subcutis (Fig. 20-22B). Fibrointimal calcification of small arteries may also occur in the subcutaneous fat. Calcification of

capillaries and eccrine glands might represent sensitive diagnostic clues; however, the specificity of these findings is less certain, as small vessel calcification may also present in patients with chronic kidney disease without clinical evidence of calciphylaxis (239,240). Epidermal, follicular, and perineural calcification have also been reported. Extravascular calcification may additionally occur within the subcutaneous fat lobules and potentially obscure primary vascular involvement. PXE-like calcification of fragmented elastic fibers may occur (88,241). Vascular calcification with concomitant vascular thrombosis and/or diffuse dermal angiomatosis appears to be more specific for calciphylaxis (242,243). Occluding fibrin thrombi and endovascular fibrosis induce ischemic necrosis of the subcutaneous fat and overlying dermis and epidermis, with loss of nuclear staining, often with sparse neutrophils and secondary subepidermal clefting (Fig. 20-22D). In some cases, the H&E appearances are of a subcutaneous small vessel thrombosis (vasculopathy) without overt calcification on H&E; in a subset of these cases, subtle calcification can be demonstrated using additional special stains (von Kossa, Alizarin red) (244) (Fig. 20-22E, F).

Differential Diagnosis. When calciphylaxis is clinically suspected in the appropriate setting (e.g., end-stage renal disease), the presence of vascular calcification with secondary ischemic necrosis is diagnostic. However, a wide variety of cutaneous and systemic disorders, both inflammatory and neoplastic, may exhibit calcinosis cutis with vascular involvement. "Metastatic calcification" has been defined as the deposition of calcium in normal tissues associated with elevated calcium or phosphate levels. Thus, calciphylaxis may be regarded as a unique subset of metastatic calcification in most cases. When end-stage renal disease is absent and/or calciphylaxis is not clinically suspected, the differential diagnosis for nonspecific vascular calcification is broad, including rare cases of AIDS; antiphospholipid antibody syndrome; CD; EN; erythema induratum (nodular vasculitis); lupus; rheumatoid arthritis with splenomegaly and leukopenia (Felty syndrome) or associated with chronic corticosteroid and methotrexate therapy; polyneuropathy, organomegaly, endocrinopathy, monoclonal gammopathy, and skin changes (POEMS) syndrome; protein S deficiency (245); sarcoid; and traumatic ulceration; as well as calcium heparin or calcium nadroparin injection sites and in the setting of alcoholic cirrhosis and malignancies (metastatic breast carcinoma, cholangiocarcinoma, chronic myelomonocytic leukemia, melanoma, osteosclerotic myeloma) (246,247). Incidental background vascular calcification may be attributable to atherosclerosis, including fibrointimal calcification of arterioles and calcification of the tunica media of small- or medium-sized arteries (Mönckeberg medial calcific sclerosis) (248) or phleboliths (intravascular calcified thrombi) and has also been regarded as an epiphenomenon when present in injection sites, LDS, erythema induratum, leukocytoclastic vasculitis, traumatic ulcers, and scars (245). The presence of renal failure and vascular calcification in primary oxalosis may mimic calciphylaxis. Although there can be associated calcification in oxalosis, the oxalate deposits appear as needle-shaped or rectangular birefringent crystals in formalin-fixed tissue. In newborns, subcutaneous calcifications can result from subcutaneous fat necrosis of the newborn. In adults, the differential diagnosis also includes a prior episode of pancreatic fat necrosis or traumatic panniculitis. PXE-like calcification may be seen in a variety of disorders, including

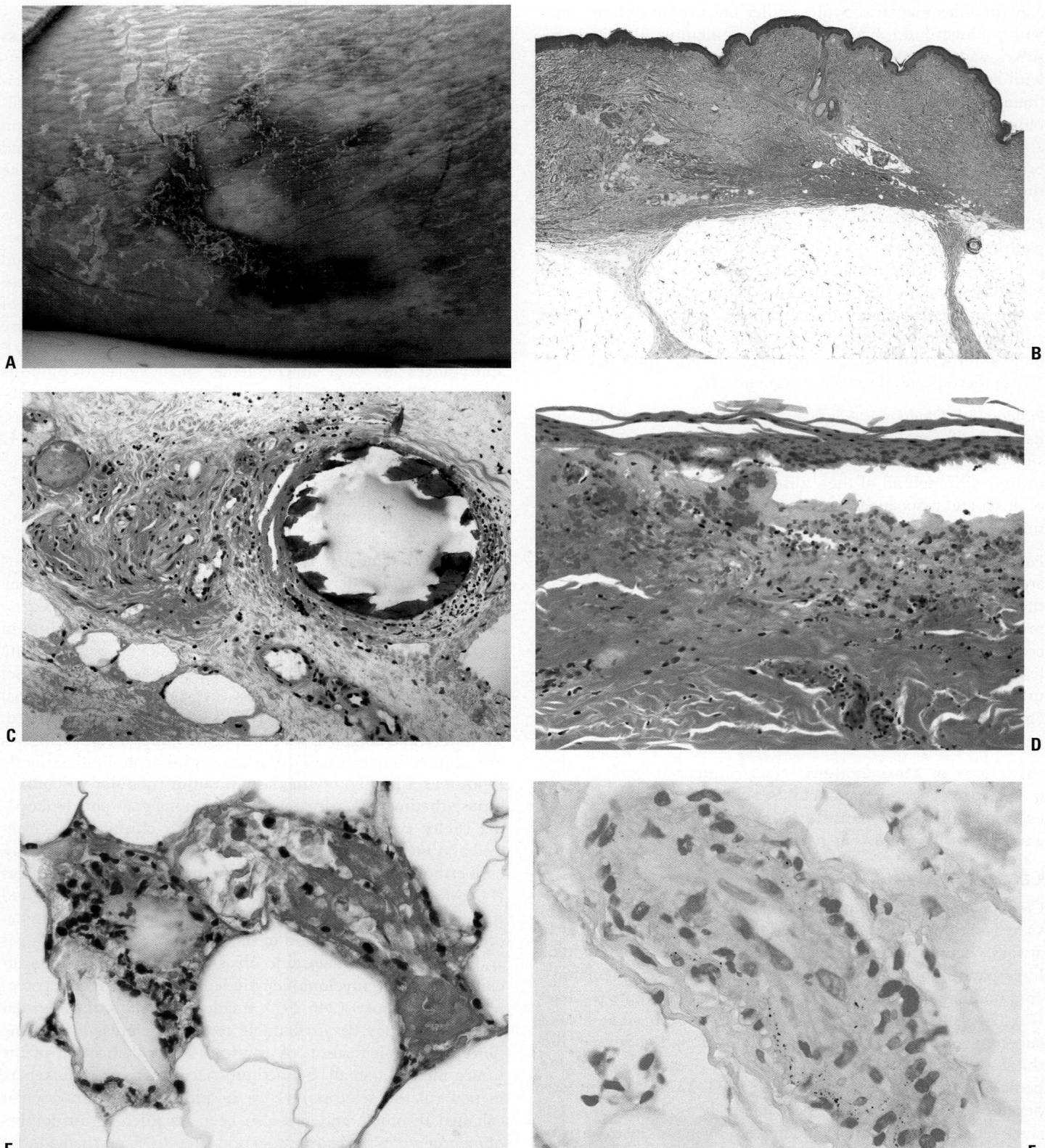

Figure 20-22 Calciphylaxis. A: Escharotic, ecchymotic plaque on the thigh of a patient with end stage renal disease. B: Incisional biopsy facilitates the identification of focal subcutaneous vascular calcification. C: Calcified arteriole with sparse neutrophils and ischemic fat necrosis. D: Secondary subepidermal cleft secondary to ischemic necrosis. E, F: Serial recut sections demonstrate a capillary microthrombus without overt calcification on H&E but with subtle calcification of the vessel wall demonstrable on Von Kossa stain.

nephrogenic systemic fibrosis (90), LDS (86), EN, GA, morphea profunda (85). In the differential diagnosis of vasculopathy, compared to most forms of thrombogenic vasculopathy, vessel involvement in calciphylaxis tends to be localized to the subcutaneous, with predominantly ischemic changes in the overlying dermis and epidermis (249).

Pathogenesis. Calciphylaxis is characterized by the acute precipitation of calcium phosphate in vessel walls. Serum calcium and/or phosphate levels, often expressed as an elevated calcium phosphate product, are elevated in many but not all cases, indicating that these are merely surrogate markers of the pathologic process. Although hypercalcemia and hyperphosphatemia associated with renal insufficiency and secondary hyperparathyroidism are implicated in the vast majority of cases, calcium precipitation can be induced locally by injections of an anticoagulant drug such as calcium heparinate or by infusions containing excess phosphate. Matrix Gla protein (MGP) is a vitamin K–dependent inhibitor of vascular calcification that is normally present in arterial walls; data from a rat model demonstrate that supratherapeutic warfarin (coumadin; a vitamin K antagonist) levels predispose to vascular calcification and that dietary vitamin K can reduce susceptibility to vascular calcification (250,251). Other mediators of vascular calcification such as high phosphate-induced bone morphogenic protein 2 (BMP-2) are inhibited by vitamin K–dependent carboxylation of MGP. Human studies have demonstrated upregulation of BMP-2, increased expression of inactive (uncarboxylated) MGP, and intraluminal exfoliation of CD31-positive endothelial cells in calciphylaxis (252). Increased expression of osteopontin has also been documented in both calcified subcutaneous vessels and "mineral poor" examples of calciphylaxis (253).

Principles of Management: Treatment of calciphylaxis is optimized by early diagnosis and an interdisciplinary, multimodality approach (254). Although some investigators have advised against biopsy of early (nonulcerated) lesions (255), this has not been our experience or practice, because diagnostic features are frequently identified in adequate specimens from early lesions (233). Initial priority should focus on management of underlying disease, control of calcium and phosphorus levels, and trigger agent cessation (e.g., warfarin, calcium-based phosphate binders, possibly corticosteroids). Bisphosphonates, antibiotics, chemical or surgical parathyroid hormone optimization with medications or parathyroidectomy, and surgical debridement may also play a role. Sodium thiosulfate appears to be beneficial in both uremic and nonuremic calciphylaxis (256). Intravenous administration of sodium thiosulfate is usual; intraperitoneal and intralesional sodium thiosulfate have also been reported (257). As previously suggested, vitamin K supplementation and other manipulations directed against osteogenesis-associated markers relevant for vascular calcification may represent future therapeutic options (250–252). Hyperbaric oxygen therapy may be attempted as an adjunctive measure.

Cytophagic Histiocytic Panniculitis

Clinical Summary. Cytophagic histiocytic panniculitis (CHP) is a rare, often indolent but potentially fatal panniculitis first reported by Winkelmann and colleagues in the early 1980s (148,258). CHP is defined by the histologic hallmark of hemophagocytosis in lesional subcutis; in some cases, hemophagocytosis also occurs in bone marrow, lymph nodes, spleen, and/or liver. Subcutaneous

nodules or plaques in CHP may be solitary, clustered, or more generalized, and individual or crops of lesions may regress after weeks or months. Lesions may appear flesh colored, erythematous, or violaceous, or hyperpigmented, and may ulcerate. Involvement of the extremities is most common, but the buttock, trunk (including the breast), shoulders, neck, face, and mucosal (oral, anal, vaginal) have also been documented. Signs and symptoms of systemic hemophagocytosis are most ominous and may include fever or other constitutional symptoms (malaise, weight loss, night sweats, chills, arthralgia, myalgia), gastrointestinal (nausea, vomiting, abdominal pain, hepatosplenomegaly), neurologic (headaches, mental status changes, seizure, coma), pulmonary symptoms (cough, dyspnea, chest pain), or pancytopenia. In cases with systemic symptoms, hemophagocytosis occurring in the bone marrow and other organ systems is associated with death resulting from a hemorrhagic diathesis caused by depletion of blood coagulation factors. In CHP, cytophagic macrophages can deplete nearly all bone marrow elements. Some patients have a more rapidly progressive course with death within 1 to 2 years. A second subset of patients exhibits a waxing and waning but ultimately fatal course over several years. In contrast, systemic symptoms tend to be minimal or absent in cases of CHP exhibiting an indolent course. Patients in this third subset experience a waxing and waning course but tend to respond to therapy and do not die from CHP (259). Most reported cases have been in adults; however, pediatric cases have been increasingly recognized. One pediatric case was documented following H1N1 vaccination (260).

Histopathology. CHP is a mostly lobular or mixed septal and lobular panniculitis with dermal and subcutaneous aggregates of macrophages in a mixed inflammatory background of neutrophils, eosinophils, and plasma cells in varying proportions, hemorrhage, and necrosis (Fig. 20-23A). The eosinophilic necrosis may be extensive or absent. The nuclear size and shape of the macrophages are within the range seen in benign inflammatory disorders. Some of the macrophages contain cellular and nuclear fragments of erythrocytes and/or leukocytes and sometimes platelets within their cytoplasm and have been called "bean bag" histiocytic cells (Fig. 20-23B) (258). Bean bag cells tend to be most prominent within the septa and edematous stroma and do not form discrete granulomas but, rather, appear as aggregates that may exhibit a syncytial appearance. In some cases, lymphocytes infiltrate medium-sized blood vessel walls. Over time, the cellular composition may remain stable or evolve toward a histiocyte—or lymphocyte—predominance (148). Rimming of atypical lymphocytes may be seen (Fig. 20-23C). Dermal perivascular and periadnexal histiocytes may be present. Cytophagic macrophages may be present in the bone marrow, liver, spleen, lymph nodes, myocardium, lungs, gastrointestinal tract, and mesentery.

Differential Diagnosis. Whereas the presence of bean bag cells should prompt primary consideration of both CHP and subcutaneous panniculitis-like T-cell or gamma/delta lymphoma, cases lacking bean bag cells or lymphocytic atypia may be indistinguishable from the late stage of many forms of lobular panniculitis. Conversely, benign cytophagic histiocytes (bean bag cells) may also be seen in AAT deficiency panniculitis, ruptured cysts, infections, albeit usually as a minor feature. Bean bag cells can resemble the emperipolesis that typifies Rosai–Dorfman disease (sinus histiocytosis with massive lymphadenopathy). In emperipolesis,

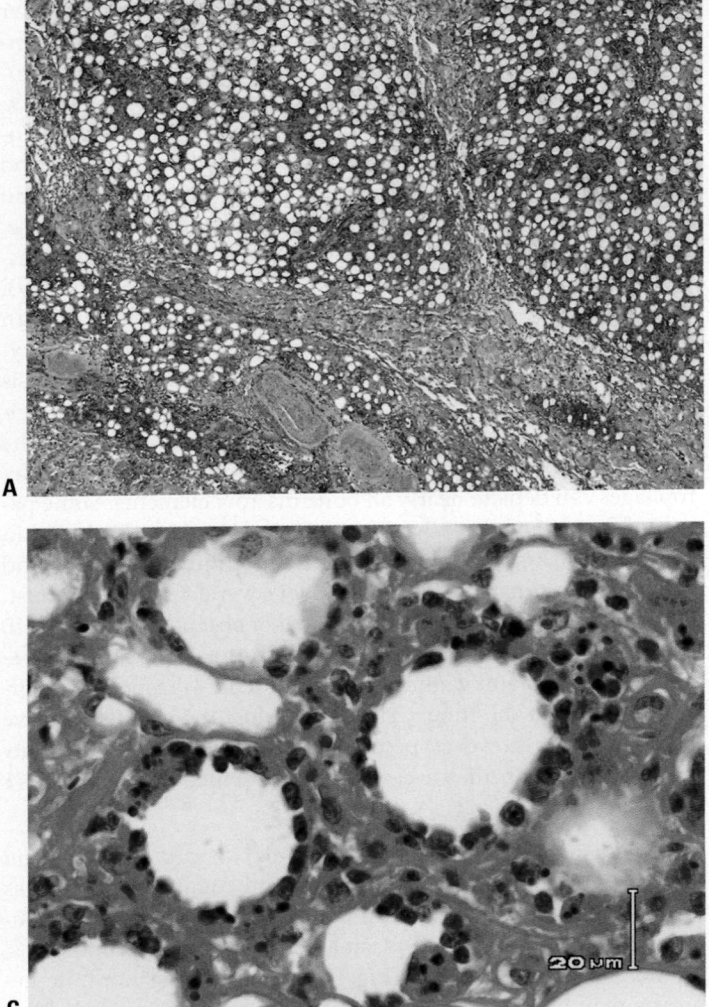

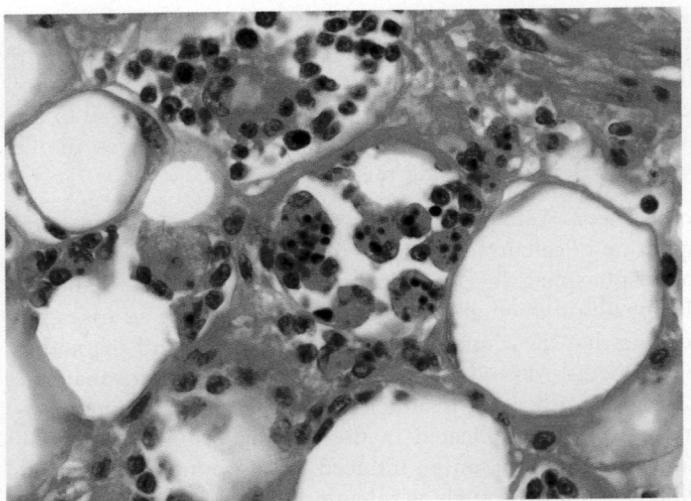

Figure 20-23 Cytophagic histiocytic panniculitis. **A:** Lobular infiltrate of histiocytes and lymphocytes. **B:** Cytophagic histiocytes that have engulfed lymphocytes and erythrocytes to form "bean bag" histiocytes. **C:** Distinctive rings or rosettes ("rimming") of atypical lymphocytes around adipocytes suggest the possibility of panniculitis-like T-cell lymphoma.

only intact cells, rather than cell fragments or nuclear debris, are present within the cytoplasm of the histiocyte. Hemophagocytic syndrome (HLH) includes a variety of primary familial and secondary acquired conditions (e.g., virus- and autoimmune-associated, including macrophage activation syndrome) that generally do not present with panniculitis. However, fatal CHP has been reported in children with primary/familial hemophagocytic lymphohistiocytosis (FHL) associated with a perforin gene mutation (one of several genes associated with FHL) (261).

Pathogenesis. The recognition of hemophagocytosis in both CHP and subcutaneous variants of T-cell lymphoma has led to the prevailing theory that CHP results from abnormal cytokine secretion by reactive or malignant T cells that stimulate macrophages to engage in hemophagocytosis, a histologic hallmark of HLH (262). The variants of primary cutaneous lymphoma associated with CHP (or potentially evolve from or are impossible to distinguish from CHP in certain cases) include gamma delta lymphoma, SPTCL (263), and extranasal NK/T-cell lymphoma (264). As of this writing, HAVCR2-associated TIM-3 deficiency has not been specifically linked to CHP. The documentation of a perforin gene mutation in a fatal pediatric case exhibiting both FHL and CHP suggests that if mutation analysis is performed on additional CHP cases, more cases of CHP harboring FHL-associated mutations may be revealed (261).

Principles of Management: Assuming T-cell lymphoma has been excluded (and continues to be excluded over time), management of any underlying disease triggers is paramount. However, this alone may not be enough to halt the progression of systemic hemophagocytosis. Systemic immunosuppressive and immunomodulating agents for CHP include prednisone, cyclosporine, azathioprine, chemotherapeutic regimens, and the interleukin receptor 1 antagonist, anakinra (148). The use of cyclosporine has been particularly advocated in pediatric cases (265). Tacrolimus might be effective in cases where cyclosporine fails (266).

Eosinophilic Panniculitis

Eosinophilic panniculitis is a histologic reaction pattern, not a specific clinical or clinical–pathologic entity. The term was first coined in 1985 to describe a case that exhibited overlapping features with eosinophilic cellulitis (Wells syndrome) (267). Lacking a characteristic clinical setting or any defined minimal histologic criteria, it is not surprising that examples of eosinophilic panniculitis have been reported in a wide variety of unrelated localized and systemic disorders. These include EN, leukocytoclastic vasculitis, arthropod bites, reactions to self-injected substances (188), medications (apomorphine [268]), and subcutaneous hypersensitivity reactions associated with parasitic infections, including gnathostomiasis (nodular migratory eosinophilic panniculitis) attributable to consumption of raw fish (mostly freshwater but also ceviche) (269), recurrent parotitis, coronavirus disease 2019 (COVID-19) (270), HIV (271), and autologous fat grafting (272). As such, there is no typical clinical presentation. Microscopically, associated eosinophilic spongiosis and/or dermal eosinophilia with or without flame figures have been reported. The pattern is usually lobular, although anticancer vaccine injection site reactions, specifically gangliosides for melanoma, and carcinoembryonic antigen and MUC1 for pancreatic cancer may show a mostly septal panniculitis with numerous eosinophils (186).

Neutrophilic Panniculitis

Like eosinophilic panniculitis, neutrophilic panniculitis is also a histologic reaction pattern, not a specific clinical or clinicopathologic entity (6,273). The term was employed in 2004 to classify a case associated with myelodysplasia, following prior case reports of neutrophilic panniculitis in this setting (274,275). BCR-ABL1-negative atypical chronic myeloid leukemia has also been associated. Infection, noniatrogenic causes of acute factitial panniculitis, or early pancreatic panniculitis or α-antitrypsin deficiency panniculitis should be reasonably excluded. If nuclear dust is prominent, subcutaneous Sweet syndrome (273) or a nondiagnostic sampling of vasculitis may be considered. Neutrophilic panniculitis has documented in patients receiving the BRAF inhibitors, vemurafenib, for metastatic melanoma or dabrafenib for glioblastoma (276–278). Other medications include granulocyte colony-stimulating factor (GCSF), filgrastim, and pegfilgrastim (most cases are classified as subcutaneous Sweet syndrome in the literature [279]), IL-2 (186), all-*trans*-retinoic acid for leukemia (280), and azacitidine for myelodysplasia (281). Associated granulomas are present in the neutrophilic panniculitis associated with CD (70).

Drug-Induced Panniculitis

Medications can induce reactions that resemble nearly every recognizable pattern of inflammatory skin disease, including panniculitis. Moreover, the same medication can induce different reactions in different hosts, and different medications can produce the identical relatively nonspecific histologic reaction. In some cases, the differences may be attributable to the age of the lesion. For example, most reactions to granulocyte-monocyte-colony-stimulating factor (GMCSF) or IL-2 produce a neutrophilic lobular panniculitis; however, persistent reactions exhibit a lymphohistiocytic lobular panniculitis (282). Pembrolizumab-induced lobular lymphohistiocytic panniculitis has been reported (283). As discussed in the preceding sections, medications often induce a histologic profile of eosinophilic panniculitis, neutrophilic panniculitis, traumatic or factitial panniculitis, or vasculitis, as well as rare cases associated with pancreatic panniculitis or resembling lupus profundus.

LOSS OF FAT

See Table 20-1.

Lipoatrophy and Lipodystrophy

Clinical Summary. The terms lipoatrophy and lipodystrophy have been variably and inconsistently defined in the literature. Some have employed a context-specific clinically oriented definition, defining lipodystrophy as fat redistribution in contrast to the loss of subcutaneous fat in lipoatrophy (284). Others have used the term lipoatrophy when the condition is localized, using lipodystrophy when the process is more extensive or diffuse loss of subcutaneous fat (285). From a pathologic perspective, *lipoatrophy* has been defined by dermatopathologists as loss of subcutaneous fat attributable to an inflammatory process, whereas *lipodystrophy* is loss of subcutaneous fat without evidence of inflammation (181). However, the pathologic process, as defined previously, does not always match the disease name, and both inflammatory (panniculitic) and noninflammatory (involutional) examples of disorders classified under either heading have been documented. For example, a review of one clinical subset, acquired generalized lipodystrophy, documents both inflammatory and noninflammatory cases (286). Moreover, lesions of lipoatrophy and lipodystrophy often exhibit a similar clinical appearance, and, histologically, both disorders involve loss of subcutaneous fat tissue. Ultimately, the two terms are prone to be used interchangeably from time to time, only perpetuating the confusion (287). Perhaps this reflects our inability to consistently and accurately determine whether previous inflammation existed, a lack of histologic data in many cases, and inherent limitations in the current classification scheme for this group of rare disorders.

Lipoatrophy is an acquired disorder that is usually localized. Lipoatrophy can be subdivided into primary idiopathic cases and lipoatrophy secondary to a wide variety of antecedent triggers, including blunt trauma, tight clothing, medication injections, infection, malignancy, or preceding panniculitis. Documented sites include the upper arm, thigh, calf, foot and ankle, buttock, and abdomen (Fig. 20-24A) (288). Lesions may be annular or semicircular in shape (289); LPA region in children is a particularly distinctive clinicopathologic entity that typically exhibits an annular configuration and was discussed separately earlier (149). More diffuse presentations of lipoatrophy are less common; a case of diffuse idiopathic lower limb lipoatrophy was recently reported (290).

Lipodystrophy may be genetic (congenital) or acquired and partial or generalized in extent. Of the many different forms of lipodystrophy, highly active antiretroviral therapy (HAART)–associated lipodystrophy is perhaps the most commonly encountered and distinctive form of lipodystrophy in countries where HAART therapy is widely available. HAART-associated lipodystrophy is characterized by fat redistribution with loss of subcutaneous fat on the face and extremities and increased central fat deposition that can manifest as a double chin, "buffalo hump," and increased visceral fat. More than one dozen forms of partial and generalized genetic lipodystrophy have been documented (287). One recently described form of genetic lipodystrophy occurs in CANDLE syndrome (chronic atypical neutrophilic dermatosis with lipodystrophy and elevated temperature), characterized by recurrent annular plaques and lipodystrophy of the face and body (291). Both acquired partial lipodystrophy and acquired generalized lipodystrophy (Lawrence syndrome) may be associated with autoimmune or other diseases (286). Most lipodystrophic syndromes predispose to metabolic complications seen in obesity, including insulin resistance, hepatic steatosis, diabetes mellitus, and dyslipidemia (292). Generalized lipodystrophy has been reported in association with pembrolizumab (293).

Histopathology. The histologic appearances of lipoatrophy and lipodystrophy can be described together but will vary depending

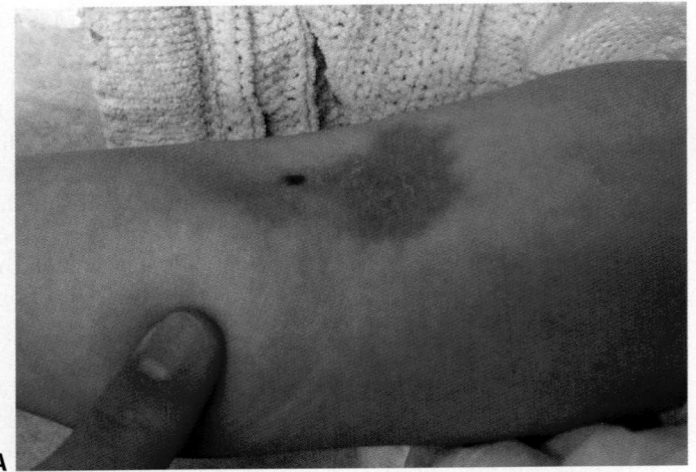

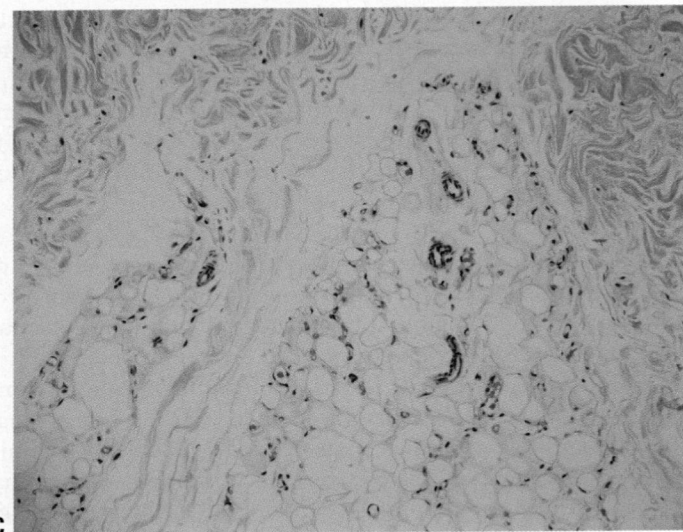

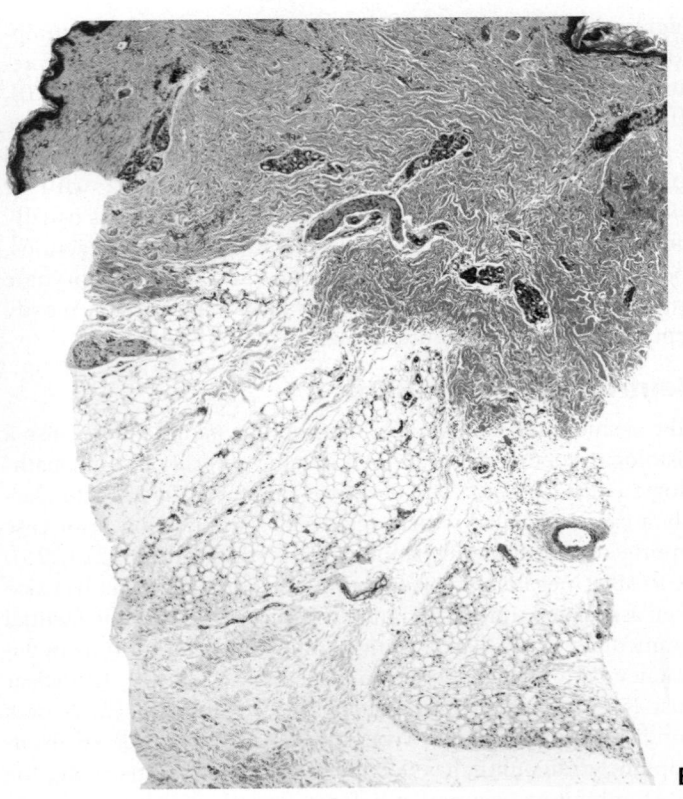

Figure 20-24 Localized lipoatrophy. **A:** Localized depression on the thigh. **B:** Shrunk, retracted fat lobules. **C:** Shrunken, retracted adipocytes with mucin and prominent capillaries.

on the stage of the disease and whether panniculitis is present. In early inflammatory lesions, the appearances may be that of a nonspecific lobular lymphohistiocytic panniculitis. The involutional changes in well-developed (i.e., fully involuted) noninflammatory lesions are most distinctive, exhibiting shrunken fat lobules with retraction of whole fat lobules from the surrounding collagenous septa (Fig. 20-24A). Within each affected fat lobule, individual lipocytes are shrunken and retracted from one another, and residual capillaries appear relatively prominent, reminiscent of embryonic fat tissue (so-called "reversal of embryogenesis") (Fig. 20-24B). In localized lipoatrophy associated with corticosteroid injections, the associated proliferation of vessels may impart an angiomatous appearance to the fat lobule (181). Space between shrunken adipocytes is replaced by a pale eosinophilic or myxoid stroma. In the inflammatory type of lipoatrophy, these involutional changes may be obscured by a mostly lobular or mixed septal and lobular infiltrate of lymphocytes, plasma cells, and histiocytes, often including lipophages, eosinophilic necrosis, and mild septal fibrosis. The end stage of lipodystrophy is total loss of the subcutaneous fat, resulting in dermis directly abutting fascia, without inflammation.

Pathogenesis. A normal amount of adipose tissue appears to be critical for optimal lipid and energy metabolism, as both obesity and lipodystrophy predispose to the metabolic

complications of diabetes, hepatic steatosis, and dyslipidemia. In lipodystrophy, the extent of fat loss is directly proportional to the severity of insulin resistance and dyslipidemia (292). Adipose tissue in adult mammals is under complex hormonal control. Insulin receptors on the surface of the fat cells inhibit lipolysis and stimulate lipogenesis. This contributes to increased fat deposition, whereas stimulation of β-adrenergic receptor sites on the plasma membrane of fat cells increases lipolysis. Glucagon can also increase lipolysis. Although the fat cells themselves in the subcutis receive no direct innervation, innervation of the small blood vessels of the fat may produce noradrenergic stimuli for lipolysis. It has been suggested that accelerated lipolysis and defective lipid storage are relevant in lipodystrophy and lipodystrophy-associated dyslipidemia (292). Among the many genetic lipodystrophies, a variety of mutations have been identified, many of which have identified roles in adipogenesis, adipocyte differentiation, adipocyte death, or lipid metabolisms (287). As one example, CIDEC, an inhibitor of lipolysis, has been implicated in familial partial lipodystrophy (294). In HAART-associated lipodystrophy, loss of fat tissue appears to be a direct effect of ART, whereas redistribution and fat gain are attributable to treatment of HIV infection (284). Endoplasmic reticulum stress (which can induce apoptosis) and impaired autophagy have been implicated (295).

Principles of Management: There are no proven effective treatments for most forms of lipoatrophy and lipodystrophy. Localized lipoatrophy can spontaneously resolve, so it is not established whether topical or oral corticosteroids possess efficacy. Autologous fat transfer and injectable fillers such as poly-L-lactic acid are effective for localized lipoatrophy HAART therapy–associated lipodystrophy (296). Leptin is an adipocyte-derived hormone that is deficient in severe lipodystrophy syndromes; recombinant leptin therapy is available.

Lipedema

Clinical Summary. Lipedema is an entity that is poorly recognized by dermatologists and pathologists but more prominent in the literature of surgeons and radiologists and was first described in 1940 by Allen and Hines (297,298). Lipedema is characterized by an abrupt thickening of the subcutaneous fat, initially presenting as a ring of soft, nonpitting and nonuniform edema of the legs just above the ankle, sometimes extending in painless, bilateral, and symmetric fashion to involve the thighs, buttocks, and hips of adult women. The feet are spared. The appearance of the affected legs has been likened to an Egyptian column, Michelin tire, pantaloon, or stovepipe, among other comparisons (297,299). Lipedema may be associated with secondary lymphedema (lipolymphedema) but is distinct from primary lymphedema. Like lymphedema, insidious gradual onset is typical. In contrast to lymphedema, in lipedema there is no reduction with bed rest. Thus, the diagnosis is primarily clinical. Patients tend to be misdiagnosed with lymphedema. A case of lipedema associated with multiple lipomas has been reported (300). A second form of lipedema presents as circumscribed thickening of the scalp with associated alopecia in women. Lesions have a doughy consistency and associated localized headache and burning sensations (301). The subcutis is two to three times the normal thickness (302).

Histopathology. The gross appearance of the fat in lipedema is unremarkable, lacking the fibrosis or lymph drainage typical of lymphedema. Microscopically, lipedema is characterized by increased interspaces between fat cells, without dilation of blood vessels or evident dilation of lymphatic spaces, without increased mucin on Alcian blue or colloidal iron stains, and without much inflammation. Aside from the increased thickness of the tissue, microscopically the subcutis may appear essentially normal (303). In some cases, trauma to these protuberant masses can result in deep depressions in the lesions, which correspond histologically to zones of loose fibrous tissue that lack fat cells, and have slight amounts of hemosiderin in macrophages. Mast cells may be slightly increased. There is no atypia of the adipocyte nuclei.

Similarly, in lipedematous alopecia, the subcutis is markedly thickened. Subcutaneous edema and dilated lymphatics have been noted, with variable mononuclear cell inflammation and preserved elastic fibers (301). The normal septal and lobular architecture of the fat may be disrupted with absence of the septa (304). Scant perivascular and perifollicular lymphocytes and eosinophils may be present (302). Overlying hyperkeratosis may be present. Diffuse loss of follicles with replacement by fibrous tracts has been documented (304). In other cases, hair follicle density has been reported normal, but reduced follicular density is to be expected when clinical alopecia is present.

Differential Diagnosis. In the rare biopsied case, clinical correlation is generally sufficient to establish the diagnosis. The histologic differential diagnosis for localized lipedema includes lipoma; a patient with both disorders has been reported (300). The lack of a delicate capsule makes lipedema different from lipoma. With edema or mucinous change, lymphedema, scleredema adultorum, or scleromyxedema might be considered. The lack of increased mucin on Alcian blue stains separates lipedema from scleredema, scleromyxedema, or myxoid lipoma.

Pathogenesis. Lipedema has been regarded as a type of lipodystrophy. Microaneurysms of the lymphatic vessels have been identified in lipedema, but their significance is unknown (305). Lipedema is different from cellulite, which produces a diffuse *peau d'orange* pebbly appearance to the skin of the thighs and buttocks regions of women. The cellular basis of cellulite is extension of adipose tissue from the subcutis up into the reticular dermis and not edema of the fat lobules. The anatomic construction of the border between reticular dermis and subcutis is more densely collagenous in males than in females, predisposing women to the development of cellulite. To date, lipedema of the scalp has been reported nearly exclusively in Egyptian and African American women. Compression of the scalp may play a role because all of the patients from Egypt wore a mandril (301).

Principles of Management: Conservative management of lipedema focuses on lymphatic massage therapy and compressive therapy (306). Suction-assisted lipectomy has also been reported (307).

ACKNOWLEDGMENTS

N. Scott McNutt, Abelardo Moreno, and Félix Contreras, for providing the foundation of the earlier edition's chapter.
J. Andrew Carlson and Ko-Ron Chen, for helpful references and comments.

REFERENCES

1. Ackerman AB. *Histologic Diagnosis of Inflammatory Skin Diseases.* 1st ed. *Lea & Febriger;* 1978.
2. Requena L, Yus ES. Panniculitis. Part I. Mostly septal panniculitis. *J Am Acad Dermatol.* 2001;45(2):163–183; quiz 184–166.
3. McKee PH, Calonje E, Brenn T, Lazar A. *McKee's Pathology of the Skin: With Clinical Correlations.* 4th ed. Elsevier Saunders; 2012.
4. Shavit E, Marzano AV, Alavi A. Ulcerative versus non-ulcerative panniculitis: is it time for a novel clinical approach to panniculitis? *Int J Dermatol.* 2021;60(4):407–417.
5. Shiau CJ, Abi Daoud MS, Wong SM, Crawford RI. Lymphocytic panniculitis: an algorithmic approach to lymphocytes in subcutaneous tissue. *J Clin Pathol.* 2015;68(12):954–962.
6. Llamas-Velasco M, Fraga J, Sanchez-Schmidt JM, et al. Neutrophilic infiltrates in panniculitis: comprehensive review and diagnostic algorithm proposal. *Am J Dermatopathol.* 2020;42(10):717–730.
7. Borroni G, Giorgini C, Tomasini C, Brazzelli V. How to make a specific diagnosis of panniculitis on clinical grounds alone: an integrated pathway of general criteria and specific findings. *G Ital Dermatol Venereol.* 2013;148(4):325–333.
8. Segura S, Requena L. Anatomy and histology of normal subcutaneous fat, necrosis of adipocytes, and classification of the panniculitides. *Dermatol Clin.* 2008;26(4):419–424, v.

9. Muthusamy K, Halbert G, Roberts F. Immunohistochemical staining for adipophilin, perilipin and TIP47. *J Clin Pathol.* 2006;59(11):1166–1170.

10. Ostler DA, Prieto VG, Reed JA, Deavers MT, Lazar AJ, Ivan D. Adipophilin expression in sebaceous tumors and other cutaneous lesions with clear cell histology: an immunohistochemical study of 117 cases. *Mod Pathol.* 2010;23(4):567–573.

11. Diaz Cascajo C, Borghi S, Weyers W. Panniculitis: definition of terms and diagnostic strategy. *Am J Dermatopathol.* 2000;22(6):530–549.

12. Diaz-Cascajo C, Borghi S. Subcutaneous pseudomembranous fat necrosis: new observations. *J Cutan Pathol.* 2002;29(1):5–10.

13. Huang TM, Lee JY. Lipodermatosclerosis: a clinicopathologic study of 17 cases and differential diagnosis from erythema nodosum. *J Cutan Pathol.* 2009;36(4):453–460.

14. Ranadive SA, Vaisse C. Lessons from extreme human obesity: monogenic disorders. *Endocrinol Metab Clin North Am.* 2008;37(3):733–751, x.

15. Chen KR. Histopathology of cutaneous vasculitis. In: Amezcua-Guerra LM, ed. *Advances in the Diagnosis and Treatment of Vasculitis.* InTech; 2011:19–56.

16. Morgan AJ, Schwartz RA. Cutaneous polyarteritis nodosa: a comprehensive review. *Int J Dermatol.* 2010;49(7):750–756.

17. Culver B, Itkin A, Pischel K. Case report and review of minocycline-induced cutaneous polyarteritis nodosa. *Arthritis Rheum.* 2005;53(3):468–470.

18. Jennette JC, Falk RJ, Bacon PA, et al. 2012 revised International Chapel Hill Consensus Conference Nomenclature of Vasculitides. *Arthritis Rheum.* 2013;65(1):1–11.

19. Lee JS, Kossard S, McGrath MA. Lymphocytic thrombophilic arteritis: a newly described medium-sized vessel arteritis of the skin. *Arch Dermatol.* 2008;144(9):1175–1182.

20. Saleh Z, Mutasim DF. Macular lymphocytic arteritis: a unique benign cutaneous arteritis, mediated by lymphocytes and appearing as macules. *J Cutan Pathol.* 2009;36(12):1269–1274.

21. Kossard S, Lee JS, McGrath MA. Macular lymphocytic arteritis. *J Cutan Pathol.* 2010;37(10):1114–1115.

22. Al-Daraji W, Gregory AN, Carlson JA. "Macular arteritis": a latent form of cutaneous polyarteritis nodosa? *Am J Dermatopathol.* 2008;30(2):145–149.

23. Llamas-Velasco M, Garcia-Martin P, Sanchez-Perez J, Sotomayor E, Fraga J, Garcia-Diez A. Macular lymphocytic arteritis: first clinical presentation with ulcers. *J Cutan Pathol.* 2013;40(4):424–427.

24. Macarenco RS, Galan A, Simoni PM, et al. Cutaneous lymphocytic thrombophilic (macular) arteritis: a distinct entity or an indolent (reparative) stage of cutaneous polyarteritis nodosa? Report of 2 cases of cutaneous arteritis and review of the literature. *Am J Dermatopathol.* 2013;35(2):213–219.

25. Kelly RI, Wee E, Balta S, Williams RA. Lymphocytic thrombophilic arteritis and cutaneous polyarteritis nodosa: clinicopathologic comparison with blinded histologic assessment. *J Am Acad Dermatol.* 2020;83(2):501–508.

26. Buffiere-Morgado A, Battistella M, Vignon-Pennamen MD, et al. Relationship between cutaneous polyarteritis nodosa (cPAN) and macular lymphocytic arteritis (MLA): blinded histologic assessment of 35 cPAN cases. *J Am Acad Dermatol.* 2015;73(6):1013–1020.

27. Navon Elkan P, Pierce SB, Segel R, et al. Mutant adenosine deaminase 2 in a polyarteritis nodosa vasculopathy. *N Engl J Med.* 2014;370(10):921–931.

28. Nanthapisal S, Murphy C, Omoyinmi E, et al. Deficiency of adenosine deaminase type 2: a description of phenotype and genotype in fifteen cases. *Arthritis Rheumatol.* 2016;68(9):2314–2322.

29. Alcaraz I, Revelles JM, Camacho D, et al. Superficial thrombophlebitis: a new clinical manifestation of the immune reconstitution inflammatory syndrome in a patient with HIV infection. *Am J Dermatopathol.* 2010;32(8):846–849.

30. Salemis NS, Merkouris S, Kimpouri K. Mondor's disease of the breast. A retrospective review. *Breast Dis.* 2011;33(3):103–107.

31. Di Nisio M, Wichers IM, Middeldorp S. Treatment for superficial thrombophlebitis of the leg. *Cochrane Database Syst Rev.* 2013;(4):CD004982.

32. Lee JT, Kalani MA. Treating superficial venous thrombophlebitis. *J Natl Compr Canc Netw.* 2008;6(8):760–765.

33. Lazaridou E, Apalla Z, Patsatsi A, Trigoni A, Ioannides D. Erythema nodosum migrans in a male patient with hepatitis B infection. *Clin Exp Dermatol.* 2009;34(4):497–499.

34. Sanchez Yus E, Sanz Vico MD, de Diego V. Miescher's radial granuloma. A characteristic marker of erythema nodosum. *Am J Dermatopathol.* 1989;11(5):434–442.

35. Thurber S, Kohler S. Histopathologic spectrum of erythema nodosum. *J Cutan Pathol.* 2006;33(1):18–26.

36. Wilk M, Zelger BG, Hayani K, Zelger B. Erythema nodosum, early stage-A subcutaneous variant of leukocytoclastic vasculitis? Clinicopathological correlation in a series of 13 patients. *Am J Dermatopathol.* 2020;42(5):329–336.

37. LeBoit PE. From Sweet to Miescher and back again. *Am J Dermatopathol.* 2006;28(4):381–383.

38. Naylor E, Hu S, Robinson-Bostom L. Nephrogenic systemic fibrosis with septal panniculitis mimicking erythema nodosum. *J Am Acad Dermatol.* 2008;58(1):149–150.

39. Chan MP, Duncan LM, Nazarian RM. Subcutaneous Sweet syndrome in the setting of myeloid disorders: a case series and review of the literature. *J Am Acad Dermatol.* 2013;68(6):1006–1015.

40. Perez-Garza DM, Chavez-Alvarez S, Ocampo-Candiani J, Gomez-Flores M. Erythema nodosum: a practical approach and diagnostic algorithm. *Am J Clin Dermatol.* 2021;22(3):367–378.

41. Gilchrist H, Patterson JW. Erythema nodosum and erythema induratum (nodular vasculitis): diagnosis and management. *Dermatol Ther.* 2010;23(4):320–327.

42. Resnik KS. The findings do not conform precisely: fibrosing sarcoidal expressions of panniculitis as example. *Am J Dermatopathol.* 2004;26(2):156–161.

43. Resnik KS. Subcutaneous sarcoidosis histopathologically manifested as fibrosing granulomatous panniculitis. *J Am Acad Dermatol.* 2006;55(5):918–919.

44. Sharon V, Goodarzi H, Chambers CJ, Fung MA, Armstrong AW. Erythema induratum of Bazin. *Dermatol Online J.* 2010;16(4):1.

45. Mascaro JM, Jr., Baselga E. Erythema induratum of Bazin. *Dermatol Clin.* 2008;26(4):439–445, v.

46. Montgomery H, O'Leary PA, Barker NW. Nodular vascular diseases of the legs: erythema induratum and allied conditions. *JAMA.* 1945;128:335–341.

47. Segura S, Pujol RM, Trindade F, Requena L. Vasculitis in erythema induratum of Bazin: a histopathologic study of 101 biopsy specimens from 86 patients. *J Am Acad Dermatol.* 2008;59(5):839–851.

48. Halpern AV, Heymann WR. Bacterial diseases. In: Bolognia JL, Jorizzo JL, Rapini RP, eds. *Dermatology.* 2nd ed. Mosby Elsevier; 2008:1118.

49. James WD, Berger TG, Elston DM. *Andrews' Diseases of the Skin: Clinical Dermatology.* 10th ed. Saunders Elsevier; 2006.

50. Lever WF. *Histopathology of the Skin.* 1st ed. J.B. Lippincott Company; 1949.

51. Schneider JW, Jordaan HF. The histopathologic spectrum of erythema induratum of Bazin. *Am J Dermatopathol.* 1997;19(4):323–333.

52. Carlson JA, Chen KR. Cutaneous vasculitis update: neutrophilic muscular vessel and eosinophilic, granulomatous, and lymphocytic vasculitis syndromes. *Am J Dermatopathol.* 2007;29(1):32–43.

53. Schneider JW, Jordaan HF, Geiger DH, Victor T, Van Helden PD, Rossouw DJ. Erythema induratum of Bazin. A clinicopathological study of 20 cases and detection of *Mycobacterium tuberculosis* DNA in skin lesions by polymerase chain reaction. *Am J Dermatopathol.* 1995;17(4):350–356.

54. Chen YH, Yan JJ, Chao SC, Lee JY. Erythema induratum: a clinicopathologic and polymerase chain reaction study. *J Formos Med Assoc.* 2001;100(4):244–249.

55. Baselga E, Margall N, Barnadas MA, Coll P, de Moragas JM. Detection of *Mycobacterium tuberculosis* DNA in lobular granulomatous panniculitis (erythema induratum-nodular vasculitis). *Arch Dermatol.* 1997;133(4):457–462.

56. Bayer-Garner IB, Cox MD, Scott MA, Smoller BR. Mycobacteria other than *Mycobacterium tuberculosis* are not present in erythema induratum/nodular vasculitis: a case series and literature review of the clinical and histologic findings. *J Cutan Pathol.* 2005;32(3):220–226.

57. Wang TC, Tzen CY, Su HY. Erythema induratum associated with tuberculous lymphadenitis: analysis of a case using polymerase chain reactions with different primer pairs to differentiate bacille Calmette-Guerin (BCG) from virulent strains of *Mycobacterium tuberculosis* complex. *J Dermatol.* 2000;27(11):717–723.

58. Pozdnyakova O, Garg A, Mahalingam M. Nodular vasculitis—a novel cutaneous manifestation of autoimmune colitis. *J Cutan Pathol.* 2008;35(3):315–319.

59. Sakuma H, Niiyama S, Amoh Y, Katsuoka K. *Chlamydophila pneumoniae* infection induced nodular vasculitis. *Case Rep Dermatol.* 2011;3(3):263–267.

60. Hattori M, Shimizu A, Hisada T, Fukumoto T, Ishikawa O. Erythema induratum in a patient with pulmonary *Mycobacterium avium* infection. *Acta Derm Venereol.* 2016;96(5):705–706.

61. Campbell SM, Winkelmann RR, Sammons DL. Erythema induratum caused by *Mycobacterium chelonei* in an immunocompetent patient. *J Clin Aesthet Dermatol.* 2013;6(5):38–40.

62. Romero JJ, Herrera P, Cartelle M, Barba P, Tello S, Zurita J. Panniculitis caused by *Mycobacterium monacense* mimicking erythema induratum: a case in Ecuador. *New Microbes New Infect.* 2016;10:112–115.

63. Fernandes SS, Carvalho J, Leite S, et al. Erythema induratum and chronic hepatitis C infection. *J Clin Virol.* 2009;44(4):333–336.

64. Gimenez-Garcia R, Sanchez-Ramon S, Sanchez-Antolin G, Velasco Fernandez C. Red fingers syndrome and recurrent panniculitis in a patient with chronic hepatitis C. *J Eur Acad Dermatol Venereol.* 2003;17(6):692–694.

65. Baba N, Takashima W, Tokuriki A, Ameshima S, Hasegawa M. Erythema induratum of Bazin which occurred after tumor necrosis factor antagonist therapy. *J Dermatol.* 2017;44(5):e87–e88.

66. Park SB, Chang IK, Im M, et al. Nodular vasculitis that developed during etanercept (enbrel) treatment in a patient with psoriasis. *Ann Dermatol.* 2015;27(5):605–607.

67. Vena GA, Apruzzi D, Vestita M, et al. Recurrence of erythema induratum of Bazin in a patient under chemotherapy for breast cancer. *New Microbiol.* 2011;34(3):331–333.

68. Yosipovitch G, Hodak E, Feinmesser M, David M. Acute Crohn's colitis with lobular panniculitis—metastatic Crohn's? *J Eur Acad Dermatol Venereol.* 2000;14(5):405–406.

69. Crowson AN, Nuovo GJ, Mihm MC Jr, Magro C. Cutaneous manifestations of Crohn's disease, its spectrum, and its pathogenesis: intracellular consensus bacterial 16S rRNA is associated with the gastrointestinal but not the cutaneous manifestations of Crohn's disease. *Hum Pathol.* 2003;34(11):1185–1192.

70. Ogawa Y, Aoki R, Harada K, et al. Neutrophilic panniculitis with non-caseating granulomas in a Crohn's disease patient. *Eur J Dermatol.* 2012;22(3):404–405.

71. Misago N, Narisawa Y. Erythema induratum (nodular vasculitis) associated with Crohn's disease: a rare type of metastatic Crohn's disease. *Am J Dermatopathol.* 2012;34(3):325–329.

72. Jennette JC. L17. What can we expect from the revised Chapel Hill consensus conference nomenclature of vasculitis? *Presse Med.* 2013;42(4, pt 2):550–555.

73. Demirkesen C, Tuzuner N, Mat C, et al. Clinicopathologic evaluation of nodular cutaneous lesions of Behcet syndrome. *Am J Clin Pathol.* 2001;116(3):341–346.

74. Kim B, LeBoit PE. Histopathologic features of erythema nodosum—like lesions in Behcet disease: a comparison with erythema nodosum focusing on the role of vasculitis. *Am J Dermatopathol.* 2000;22(5):379–390.

75. Babacan T, Onat AM, Pehlivan Y, Comez G, Tutar E. A case of the Behcet's disease diagnosed by the panniculits after mesotherapy. *Rheumatol Int.* 2010;30(12):1657–1659.

76. Azuma N, Natsuaki M, Yamanishi K, et al. Cutaneous necrotizing vasculitis in a patient with Behcet's disease; mimicking polyarteritis nodosa [in Japanese]. *Nihon Rinsho Meneki Gakkai Kaishi.* 2010;33(3):149–153.

77. Demirkesen C, Tuzuner N, Senocak M, et al. Comparative study of adhesion molecule expression in nodular lesions of Behcet syndrome and other forms of panniculitis. *Am J Clin Pathol.* 2008;130(1):28–33.

78. Horie Y, Meguro A, Kitaichi N, et al. Replication of a microsatellite genome-wide association study of Behcet's disease in a Korean population. *Rheumatology (Oxford).* 2012;51(6):983–986.

79. Lee YH, Choi SJ, Ji JD, Song GG. Genome-wide pathway analysis of a genome-wide association study on psoriasis and Behcet's disease. *Mol Biol Rep.* 2012;39(5):5953–5959.

80. Dalvi SR, Yildirim R, Yazici Y. Behcet's Syndrome. *Drugs.* 2012;72(17):2223–2241.

81. Bruce AJ, Bennett DD, Lohse CM, Rooke TW, Davis MD. Lipodermatosclerosis: review of cases evaluated at Mayo Clinic. *J Am Acad Dermatol.* 2002;46(2):187–192.

82. Miteva M, Romanelli P, Kirsner RS. Lipodermatosclerosis. *Dermatol Ther.* 2010;23(4):375–388.

83. Eklof B, Rutherford RB, Bergan JJ, et al. Revision of the CEAP classification for chronic venous disorders: consensus statement. *J Vasc Surg.* 2004;40(6):1248–1252.

84. Jorizzo JL, White WL, Zanolli MD, Greer KE, Solomon AR, Jetton RL. Sclerosing panniculitis. A clinicopathologic assessment. *Arch Dermatol.* 1991;127(4):554–558.

85. Bowen AR, Gotting C, LeBoit PE, McCalmont TH. Pseudoxanthoma elasticum-like fibers in the inflamed skin of patients without pseudoxanthoma elasticum. *J Cutan Pathol.* 2007;34(10):777–781.

86. Walsh SN, Santa Cruz DJ. Lipodermatosclerosis: a clinicopathological study of 25 cases. *J Am Acad Dermatol.* 2010;62(6):1005–1012.

87. Caggiati A, Rosi C, Franceschini M, Innocenzi D. The nature of skin pigmentations in chronic venous insufficiency: a preliminary report. *Eur J Vasc Endovasc Surg.* 2008;35(1):111–118.

88. Nikko AP, Dunningan M, Cockerell CJ. Calciphylaxis with histologic changes of pseudoxanthoma elasticum. *Am J Dermatopathol.* 1996;18(4):396–399.

89. Fernandez KH, Liu V, Swick BL. Nonuremic calciphylaxis associated with histologic changes of pseudoxanthoma elasticum. *Am J Dermatopathol.* 2013;35(1):106–108.

90. Lewis KG, Lester BW, Pan TD, Robinson-Bostom L. Nephrogenic fibrosing dermopathy and calciphylaxis with pseudoxanthoma elasticum-like changes. *J Cutan Pathol.* 2006;33(10):695–700.

91. Delgado-Jimenez Y, Fraga J, Garcia-Diez A. Infective panniculitis. *Dermatol Clin.* 2008;26(4):471–480, vi.

92. Requena L, Sitthinamsuwan P, Santonja C, et al. Cutaneous and mucosal mucormycosis mimicking pancreatic panniculitis and gouty panniculitis. *J Am Acad Dermatol.* 2012;66(6):975–984.

93. Colmenero I, Alonso-Sanz M, Casco F, Hernandez-Martin A, Torrelo A. Cutaneous aspergillosis mimicking pancreatic and gouty panniculitis. *J Am Acad Dermatol.* 2012;67(4):789–791.

94. Garrido PM, Pimenta R, Viana I, Kutzner H, Filipe P, Soares-Almeida L. Cutaneous mucormycosis mimicking pancreatic panniculitis. *J Cutan Pathol.* 2021;48(8):1007–1009.

95. Ballestero-Diez M, Alvarez-Ruiz SB, Aragues Montanes M, Fraga J. Septal panniculitis associated with cytomegalovirus infection. *Histopathology.* 2005;46(6):720–722.

96. Tekin B, Boire N, Shah K, Hanson J, Bridges AG. Viral panniculitis in a patient with disseminated opportunistic Enterovirus infection. *J Cutan Pathol.* 2021;48(3):434–438.

97. Souza BCE, Ang PL, Cerulli FG, Ponce JJ, Tyring SK, Oliveira W. Reactivation of Chagas disease in organ transplant recipients: panniculitis as the only skin manifestation in a three case series. *Australas J Dermatol.* 2021;62(2):231–232.

98. Alvarez-Ruiz SB, Delgado-Jimenez Y, Aragues M, Fraga J, Garcia-Diez A. Subcutaneous lepromas as leprosy-type presentation. *J Eur Acad Dermatol Venereol.* 2006;20(3):344–345.

99. Kutzner H, Argenyi ZB, Requena L, Rutten A, Hugel H. A new application of BCG antibody for rapid screening of various tissue microorganisms. *J Am Acad Dermatol.* 1998;38(1):56–60.

100. Byrd J, Mehregan DR, Mehregan DA. Utility of anti-bacillus Calmette-Guerin antibodies as a screen for organisms in sporotrichoid infections. *J Am Acad Dermatol.* 2001;44(2):261–264.

101. McCalmont TH. Caveat emptor. *J Cutan Pathol.* 2012;39(5):479–480.

102. Karram S, Loya A, Hamam H, Habib RH, Khalifeh I. Transepidermal elimination in cutaneous leishmaniasis: a multiregional study. *J Cutan Pathol.* 2012;39(4):406–412.

103. Dias-Polak D, Geffen Y, Ben-Izhak O, Bergman R. The role of histopathology and immunohistochemistry in the diagnosis of cutaneous leishmaniasis without "discernible" Leishman-Donovan bodies. *Am J Dermatopathol.* 2017;39(12):890–895.

104. Morrison LK, Rapini R, Willison CB, Tyring S. Infection and panniculitis. *Dermatol Ther.* 2010;23(4):328–340.

105. Patterson JW, Brown PC, Broecker AH. Infection-induced panniculitis. *J Cutan Pathol.* 1989;16(4):183–193.

106. Beltraminelli HS, Buechner SA, Hausermann P. Pancreatic panniculitis in a patient with an acinar cell cystadenocarcinoma of the pancreas. *Dermatology.* 2004;208(3):265–267.

107. Ariga H, Yonezaki S, Kashimura J, Takayashiki N. Pancreatic panniculitis in a patient with pancreatic adenosquamous carcinoma. *Clin J Gastroenterol.* 2021;14(1):382–385.

108. Garcia-Romero D, Vanaclocha F. Pancreatic panniculitis. *Dermatol Clin.* 2008;26(4):465–470, vi.

109. Guanziroli E, Colombo A, Coggi A, Gianotti R, Marzano AV. Pancreatic panniculitis: the "bright" side of the moon in solid cancer patients. *BMC Gastroenterol.* 2018;18(1):1.

110. Kasamatsu H, Oyama N, Hasegawa M, et al. Fatal case of pancreatic panniculitis caused by occult neuroendocrine tumor in the corresponding organ: a case report and review of the published work. *J Dermatol.* 2021;48(2):237–241.

111. Yamashita Y, Joshita S, Ito T, Maruyama M, Wada S, Umemura T. A case report of pancreatic panniculitis due to acute pancreatitis with intraductal papillary mucinous neoplasm. *BMC Gastroenterol.* 2020;20(1):286.

112. Outtas O, Barthet M, De Troyer J, Franck F, Garcia S. Pancreatic panniculitis with intraductal carcinoid tumor of the pancreas divisum [in French]. *Ann Dermatol Venereol.* 2004;131(5):466–469.

113. Pfaundler N, Kessebohm K, Blum R, Stieger M, Stickel F. Adding pancreatic panniculitis to the panel of skin lesions associated with triple therapy of chronic hepatitis C. *Liver Int.* 2013;33(4):648–649.

114. Pike JL, Rice JC, Sanchez RL, Kelly EB, Kelly BC. Pancreatic panniculitis associated with allograft pancreatitis and rejection in a simultaneous pancreas-kidney transplant recipient. *Am J Transplant.* 2006;6(10):2502–2505.

115. Corazza M, Salmi R, Strumia R. Pancreatic panniculitis as a first sign of liver carcinoma. *Acta Derm Venereol.* 2003;83(3):230–231.

116. Kaufman HL, Harandi A, Watson MC, et al. Panniculitis after vaccination against CEA and MUC1 in a patient with pancreatic cancer. *Lancet Oncol.* 2005;6(1):62–63.

117. Kirkland EB, Sachdev R, Kim J, Peng D. Early pancreatic panniculitis associated with HELLP syndrome and acute fatty liver of pregnancy. *J Cutan Pathol.* 2011;38(10):814–817.

118. Borowicz J, Morrison M, Hogan D, Miller R. Subcutaneous fat necrosis/panniculitis and polyarthritis associated with acinar cell carcinoma of the pancreas: a rare presentation of pancreatitis, panniculitis and polyarthritis syndrome. *J Drugs Dermatol.* 2010;9(9):1145–1150.

119. Rongioletti F, Caputo V. Pancreatic panniculitis. *G Ital Dermatol Venereol.* 2013;148(4):419–425.

120. Ball NJ, Adams SP, Marx LH, Enta T. Possible origin of pancreatic fat necrosis as a septal panniculitis. *J Am Acad Dermatol.* 1996;34(2, pt 2):362–364.

121. Ball NJ, Cowan BJ, Hashimoto SA. Lobular panniculitis at the site of subcutaneous interferon beta injections for the treatment of multiple sclerosis can histologically mimic pancreatic panniculitis. A study of 12 cases. *J Cutan Pathol.* 2009;36(3):331–337.

122. Banfill KE, Oliphant TJ, Prasad KR. Resolution of pancreatic panniculitis following metastasectomy. *Clin Exp Dermatol.* 2012;37(4):440–441.

123. Preiss JC, Faiss S, Loddenkemper C, Zeitz M, Duchmann R. Pancreatic panniculitis in an 88-year-old man with neuroendocrine carcinoma. *Digestion.* 2002;66(3):193–196.

124. Dauendorffer JN, Ingen-Housz-Oro S, Levy P, Weber N, Fiszenson-Albala F, Sigal-Grinberg M. Pancreatic panniculitis revealing a pancreaticportal fistula and portal thrombosis [in French]. *Ann Dermatol Venereol.* 2007;134(3, pt 1):249–252.

125. Lyon MJ. Metabolic panniculitis: alpha-1 antitrypsin deficiency panniculitis and pancreatic panniculitis. *Dermatol Ther.* 2010;23(4):368–374.

126. McBean J, Sable A, Maude J, Robinson-Bostom L. Alpha1-antitrypsin deficiency panniculitis. *Cutis.* 2003;71(3):205–209.

127. Geraminejad P, DeBloom JR 2nd, Walling HW, Sontheimer RD, VanBeek M. Alpha-1-antitrypsin associated panniculitis: the MS variant. *J Am Acad Dermatol.* 2004;51(4):645–655.

128. Geller JD, Su WP. A subtle clue to the histopathologic diagnosis of early alpha 1-antitrypsin deficiency panniculitis. *J Am Acad Dermatol.* 1994;31(2, pt 1):241–245.

129. Gross B, Grebe M, Wencker M, Stoller JK, Bjursten LM, Janciauskiene S. New Findings in PiZZ alpha1-antitrypsin deficiency-related panniculitis. Demonstration of skin polymers and high dosing requirements of intravenous augmentation therapy. *Dermatology.* 2009;218(4):370–375.

130. Chng WJ, Henderson CA. Suppurative panniculitis associated with alpha 1-antitrypsin deficiency (PiSZ phenotype) treated with doxycycline. *Br J Dermatol.* 2001;144(6):1282–1283.

131. Olson JM, Moore EC, Valasek MA, Williams LH, Vary JC. Panniculitis in alpha-1 antitrypsin deficiency treated with enzyme replacement. *J Am Acad Dermatol.* 2012;66(4):e139–141.

132. Al-Niaimi F, Lyon C. Severe ulcerative panniculitis caused by alpha 1-antitrypsin deficiency: remission induced and maintained with intravenous alpha 1-antitrypsin. *J Am Acad Dermatol.* 2011;65(1):227–229.

133. Franciosi AN, Ralph J, O'Farrell NJ, et al. Alpha-1 antitrypsin deficiency associated panniculitis. *J Am Acad Dermatol.* 2021. doi: 10.1016/j.jaad.2021.01.074

134. Irgang S. Lupus erythematosus profundus. Report of an example with clinical resemblance to Darier-Roussy sarcoid. *Arch Dermatol Syphilol.* 1940;42:97–108.

135. Udompanich S, Chanprapaph K, Suchonwanit P. Linear and annular lupus panniculitis of the scalp: case report with emphasis on trichoscopic findings and review of the literature. *Case Rep Dermatol.* 2019;11(2):157–165.

136. Peters MS, Su WP. Lupus erythematosus panniculitis. *Med Clin North Am.* 1989;73(5):1113–1126.

137. Brinster NK, Nunley J, Pariser R, Horvath B. Nonbullous neutrophilic lupus erythematosus: a newly recognized variant of cutaneous lupus erythematosus. *J Am Acad Dermatol.* 2012;66(1):92–97.

138. Ng PP, Tan SH, Tan T. Lupus erythematosus panniculitis: a clinicopathologic study. *Int J Dermatol.* 2002;41(8):488–490.

139. McNutt NS, Fung MA. More about panniculitis and lymphoma. *J Cutan Pathol*. 2004;31(4):297–299.

140. Santos-Briz A, Calle A, Linos K, et al. Dermatomyositis panniculitis: a clinicopathological and immunohistochemical study of 18 cases. *J Eur Acad Dermatol Venereol*. 2018;32(8):1352–1359.

141. Ball NJ, Cowan BJ, Moore GR, Hashimoto SA. Lobular panniculitis at the site of glatiramer acetate injections for the treatment of relapsing-remitting multiple sclerosis. A report of two cases. *J Cutan Pathol*. 2008;35(4):407–410.

142. Soares Almeida LM, Requena L, Kutzner H, Angulo J, de Sa J, Pignatelli J. Localized panniculitis secondary to subcutaneous glatiramer acetate injections for the treatment of multiple sclerosis: a clinicopathologic and immunohistochemical study. *J Am Acad Dermatol*. 2006;55(6):968–974.

143. Magro CM, Crowson AN, Byrd JC, Soleymani AD, Shendrik I. Atypical lymphocytic lobular panniculitis. *J Cutan Pathol*. 2004;31(4):300–306.

144. Magro CM, Schaefer JT, Morrison C, Porcu P. Atypical lymphocytic lobular panniculitis: a clonal subcutaneous T-cell dyscrasia. *J Cutan Pathol*. 2008;35(10):947–954.

145. Lozzi GP, Massone C, Citarella L, Kerl H, Cerroni L. Rimming of adipocytes by neoplastic lymphocytes: a histopathologic feature not restricted to subcutaneous T-cell lymphoma. *Am J Dermatopathol*. 2006;28(1):9–12.

146. Massone C, Kodama K, Salmhofer W, et al. Lupus erythematosus panniculitis (lupus profundus): clinical, histopathological, and molecular analysis of nine cases. *J Cutan Pathol*. 2005;32(6):396–404.

147. Magro CM, Crowson AN, Kovatich AJ, Burns F. Lupus profundus, indeterminate lymphocytic lobular panniculitis and subcutaneous T-cell lymphoma: a spectrum of subcuticular T-cell lymphoid dyscrasia. *J Cutan Pathol*. 2001;28(5):235–247.

148. Aronson IK, Worobec SM. Cytophagic histiocytic panniculitis and hemophagocytic lymphohistiocytosis: an overview. *Dermatol Ther*. 2010;23(4):389–402.

149. Santonja C, Gonzalo I, Feito M, Beato-Merino M, Requena L. Lipoatrophic panniculitis of the ankles in childhood: differential diagnosis with subcutaneous panniculitis-like T-cell lymphoma. *Am J Dermatopathol*. 2012;34(3):295–300.

150. Ma L, Bandarchi B, Glusac EJ. Fatal subcutaneous panniculitis-like T-cell lymphoma with interface change and dermal mucin, a dead ringer for lupus erythematosus. *J Cutan Pathol*. 2005;32(5):360–365.

151. Liau JY, Chuang SS, Chu CY, Ku WH, Tsai JH, Shih TF. The presence of clusters of plasmacytoid dendritic cells is a helpful feature for differentiating lupus panniculitis from subcutaneous panniculitis-like T-cell lymphoma. *Histopathology*. 2013;62(7):1057–1066.

152. Gayden T, Sepulveda FE, Khuong-Quang DA, et al. Germline HAVCR2 mutations altering TIM-3 characterize subcutaneous panniculitis-like T cell lymphomas with hemophagocytic lymphohistiocytic syndrome. *Nat Genet*. 2018;50(12):1650–1657.

153. Chaweephisal P, Sosothikul D, Polprasert C, Wananukul S, Seksarn P. Subcutaneous panniculitis-like T-cell lymphoma (SPTCL) with hemophagocytic lymphohistiocytosis (HLH) syndrome in children and its essential role of HAVCR2 gene mutation analysis. *J Pediatr Hematol Oncol*. 2021;43(1):e80–e84.

154. Polprasert C, Takeuchi Y, Kakiuchi N, et al. Frequent germline mutations of HAVCR2 in sporadic subcutaneous panniculitis-like T-cell lymphoma. *Blood Adv*. 2019;3(4):588–595.

155. Wegehaupt O, Gross M, Wehr C, et al. TIM-3 deficiency presenting with two clonally unrelated episodes of mesenteric and subcutaneous panniculitis-like T-cell lymphoma and hemophagocytic lymphohistiocytosis. *Pediatr Blood Cancer*. 2020;67(6):e28302.

156. Oke V, Wahren-Herlenius M. Cutaneous lupus erythematosus: clinical aspects and molecular pathogenesis. *J Intern Med*. 2013;273(6):544–554.

157. Yu C, Chang C, Zhang J. Immunologic and genetic considerations of cutaneous lupus erythematosus: a comprehensive review. *J Autoimmun*. 2013;41:34–45.

158. McNiff JM, Kaplan DH. Plasmacytoid dendritic cells are present in cutaneous dermatomyositis lesions in a pattern distinct from lupus erythematosus. *J Cutan Pathol*. 2008;35(5):452–456.

159. Tomasini D, Mentzel T, Hantschke M, et al. Plasmacytoid dendritic cells: an overview of their presence and distribution in different inflammatory skin diseases, with special emphasis on Jessner's lymphocytic infiltrate of the skin and cutaneous lupus erythematosus. *J Cutan Pathol*. 2010;37(11):1132–1139.

160. Oh SH, Roh HJ, Kwon JE, et al. Expression of interleukin-17 is correlated with interferon-alpha expression in cutaneous lesions of lupus erythematosus. *Clin Exp Dermatol*. 2011;36(5):512–520.

161. Wang X, Magro CM. Human myxovirus resistance protein 1 (MxA) as a useful marker in the differential diagnosis of subcutaneous lymphoma vs. lupus erythematosus profundus. *Eur J Dermatol*. 2012;22(5):629–633.

162. Wenzel J, Zahn S, Mikus S, Wiechert A, Bieber T, Tuting T. The expression pattern of interferon-inducible proteins reflects the characteristic histological distribution of infiltrating immune cells in different cutaneous lupus erythematosus subsets. *Br J Dermatol*. 2007;157(4):752–757.

163. Gono T, Matsuda M, Shimojima Y, Kaneko K, Murata H, Ikeda S. Lupus erythematosus profundus (lupus panniculitis) induced by interferon-beta in a multiple sclerosis patient. *J Clin Neurosci*. 2007;14(10):997–1000.

164. Pham AK, Castillo SA, Barton DT, et al. Kikuchi-Fujimoto disease preceded by lupus erythematosus panniculitis: do these findings together herald the onset of systemic lupus erythematosus? *Dermatol Online J*. 2020;26(8).

165. Braunstein I, Werth VP. Update on management of connective tissue panniculitides. *Dermatol Ther*. 2012;25(2):173–182.

166. Fraga J, Garcia-Diez A. Lupus erythematosus panniculitis. *Dermatol Clin*. 2008;26(4):453–463, vi.

167. Moreno A, Marcoval J, Peyri J. Traumatic panniculitis. *Dermatol Clin*. 2008;26(4):481–483, vii.

168. Lee DJ, Kim YC. Traumatic panniculitis with hypertrichosis. *Eur J Dermatol*. 2011;21(2):258–259.

169. Lee JH, Jung KE, Kim HS, Kim HO, Park YM, Lee JY. Traumatic panniculitis with localized hypertrichosis: two new cases and considerations. *J Dermatol*. 2013;40(2):139–141.

170. Ploydaeng M, Rojhirunsakool S, Suchonwanit P. Localized hypertrichosis with traumatic panniculitis: a case report and literature review. *Case Rep Dermatol*. 2019;11(2):180–186.

171. Wong JJ, Greenberg RD. Upper extremity nodules—quiz case. *Arch Dermatol*. 2004;140(2):231–236.

172. Hurt MA, Santa Cruz DJ. Nodular-cystic fat necrosis. A reevaluation of the so-called mobile encapsulated lipoma. *J Am Acad Dermatol*. 1989;21(3, pt 1):493–498.

173. Kubota Y, Nakai K, Moriue T, et al. Nodular cystic fat necrosis in a patient with diabetes mellitus. *J Dermatol*. 2009;36(6):353–354.

174. Toritsugi M, Yamamoto T, Nishioka K. Nodular cystic fat necrosis with systemic sclerosis. *Eur J Dermatol*. 2004;14(5):353–355.

175. Ueda N, Satoh T, Yamamoto T, Yokozeki H. Nodular cystic fat necrosis in Heerfordt's syndrome. *J Eur Acad Dermatol Venereol*. 2007;21(5):708–709.

176. Demitsu T, Yoneda K, Iida E, et al. A case of nodular cystic fat necrosis with systemic lupus erythematosus presenting the multiple subcutaneous nodules on the extremities. *J Eur Acad Dermatol Venereol*. 2008;22(7):885–886.

177. Jeong KH, Lee MH. Two cases of factitial panniculitis induced by electroacupuncture. *Clin Exp Dermatol*. 2009;34(5):e170–173.

178. Hanami Y, Hiraiwa T, Yamamoto T. Nodular cystic fat necrosis with calcification and metaplastic ossification. *Am J Dermatopathol*. 2012;34(7):782–784.

179. Park KY, Choi SY, Seo SJ, Hong CK. Posttraumatic lipogranuloma on the lower leg. *J Dermatol.* 2013;40(2):141–142.

180. Grassi S, Rosso R, Tomasini C, Pezzini C, Merlino M, Borroni G. Post-surgical lipophagic panniculitis: a specific model of traumatic panniculitis and new histopathological findings. *G Ital Dermatol Venereol.* 2013;148(4):435–441.

181. Requena L, Sanchez Yus E. Panniculitis. Part II. Mostly lobular panniculitis. *J Am Acad Dermatol.* 2001;45(3):325–361; quiz 362–324.

182. Sanmartin O, Requena C, Requena L. Factitial panniculitis. *Dermatol Clin.* 2008;26(4):519–527, viii.

183. Falagas ME, Christopoulou M, Rosmarakis ES, Vlastou C. Munchausen's syndrome presenting as severe panniculitis. *Int J Clin Pract.* 2004;58(7):720–722.

184. Boyd AS. Revision: cutaneous Munchausen syndrome: clinical and histopathologic features. *J Cutan Pathol.* 2014;41(4):333–336.

185. Dadzie OE, Mahalingam M, Parada M, El Helou T, Philips T, Bhawan J. Adverse cutaneous reactions to soft tissue fillers—a review of the histological features. *J Cutan Pathol.* 2008;35(6):536–548.

186. Requena L, Cerroni L, Kutzner H. Histopathologic patterns associated with external agents. *Dermatol Clin.* 2012;30(4):731–748, vii.

187. Requena L, Requena C, Christensen L, Zimmermann US, Kutzner H, Cerroni L. Adverse reactions to injectable soft tissue fillers. *J Am Acad Dermatol.* 2011;64(1):1–34; quiz 35–36.

188. Gomez Rodriguez N, Ortiz-Rey JA, de la Fuente Buceta A, Ibanez Ruan J. [Auto-induced eosinophilic panniculitis: a diagnostic dilemma]. *An Med Interna.* 2001;18(12):635–637.

189. Diez Morrondo C, Palmou Fontana N, Lema Gontad JM, et al. Facticial panniculitis and Lofgren's syndrome: a case. *Reumatol Clin.* 2012;8(6):368–371.

190. Georgieva J, Assaf C, Steinhoff M, Treudler R, Orfanos CE, Geilen CC. Bodybuilder oleoma. *Br J Dermatol.* 2003;149(6):1289–1290.

191. Rubio Fernandez D, Rodriguez Del Canto C, Marcos Galan V, et al. Contribution of endermology to improving indurations and panniculitis/lipoatrophy at glatiramer acetate injection site. *Adv Ther.* 2012;29(3):267–275.

192. Quesada-Cortes A, Campos-Munoz L, Diaz-Diaz RM, Casado-Jimenez M. Cold panniculitis. *Dermatol Clin.* 2008;26(4):485–489, vii.

193. Hochsinger C. Über eine akute kongelative Zellgewebsverhärtung in der Submentalregion bei Kindern. *Mschr Kinderheilk.* 1902;1:323–327.

194. Epstein EH Jr, Oren ME. Popsicle panniculitis. *N Engl J Med.* 1970;282(17):966–967.

195. Bolotin D, Duffy KL, Petronic-Rosic V, Rhee CJ, Myers PJ, Stein SL. Cold panniculitis following ice therapy for cardiac arrhythmia. *Pediatr Dermatol.* 2011;28(2):192–194.

196. Huang FW, Berk DR, Bayliss SJ. Popsicle panniculitis in a 5-month-old child on systemic prednisolone therapy. *Pediatr Dermatol.* 2008;25(4):502–503.

197. Requena L, Ferrandiz C. Sclerosing postirradiation panniculitis. *Dermatol Clin.* 2008;26(4):505–508, vii–viii.

198. Pielasinski U, Machan S, Camacho D, et al. Postirradiation pseudosclerodermatous panniculitis: three new cases with additional histopathologic features supporting the radiotherapy etiology. *Am J Dermatopathol.* 2013;35(1):129–134.

199. Carrasco L, Moreno C, Pastor MA, et al. Postirradiation pseudosclerodermatous panniculitis. *Am J Dermatopathol.* 2001;23(4):283–287.

200. Dalle S, Skowron F, Ronger-Savle S, Balme B, Thomas L. Pseudosclerodermatous panniculitis after irradiation and bronchiolitis obliterans organizing pneumonia: simultaneous onset suggesting a common origin. *Dermatology.* 2004;209(2):138–141.

201. Shelley WB, Izumi AK. Annular atrophy of the ankles. A case of partial lipodystrophy. *Arch Dermatol.* 1970;102(3):326–329.

202. Shen LY, Edmonson MB, Williams GP, Gottam CC, Hinshaw MA, Teng JM. Lipoatrophic panniculitis: case report and review of the literature. *Arch Dermatol.* 2010;146(8):877–881.

203. Corredera C, Iglesias M, Hernandez-Martin A, Colmenero I, Dilme E, Torrelo A. Annular lipoatrophic panniculitis of the ankles. *Pediatr Dermatol.* 2011;28(2):146–148.

204. Torrelo A, Noguera-Morel L, Hernandez-Martin A, et al. Recurrent lipoatrophic panniculitis of children. *J Eur Acad Dermatol Venereol.* 2017;31(3):536–543.

205. Comstock JR, Buhalog B, Peebles JK, Hinshaw MA, Co DO, Arkin LM. Lipoatrophic panniculitis in an adolescent. *Pediatr Dermatol.* 2020;37(3):572–573.

206. Martinez A, Malone M, Hoeger P, Palmer R, Harper JI. Lipoatrophic panniculitis and chromosome 10 abnormality. *Br J Dermatol.* 2000;142(5):1034–1039.

207. Dimson OG, Esterly NB. Annular lipoatrophy of the ankles. *J Am Acad Dermatol.* 2006;54(2, suppl):S40–42.

208. Kerns MJ, Stinehelfer S, Mutasim DF, Zalla MJ. Annular lipoatrophy of the ankles: case report and review of the literature. *Pediatr Dermatol.* 2011;28(2):142–145.

209. Calisici E, Oncel MY, Degirmencioglu H, et al. A neonate with subcutaneous fat necrosis after passive cooling: does polycythemia have an effect? *Case Rep Pediatr.* 2013;2013:254089.

210. Akcay A, Akar M, Oncel MY, et al. Hypercalcemia due to subcutaneous fat necrosis in a newborn after total body cooling. *Pediatr Dermatol.* 2013;30(1):120–123.

211. Alaoui K, Abourazzak S, Oulmaati A, Hida M, Bouharrou A. An unusual complication of subcutaneous fat necrosis of the newborn. *BMJ Case Rep.* 2011;2011. doi:10.1136/bcr.12.2010.3569

212. Mitra S, Dove J, Somisetty SK. Subcutaneous fat necrosis in newborn-an unusual case and review of literature. *Eur J Pediatr.* 2011;170(9):1107–1110.

213. Canpolat N, Ozdil M, Kurugoglu S, Caliskan S, Sever L. Nephrocalcinosis as a complication of subcutaneous fat necrosis of the newborn. *Turk J Pediatr.* 2012;54(6):667–670.

214. Schubert PT, Razack R, Vermaak A, Jordaan HF. Fine-needle aspiration cytology of subcutaneous fat necrosis of the newborn: the cytology spectrum with review of the literature. *Diagn Cytopathol.* 2012;40(3):245–247.

215. Lund JJ, Xia L, Kerr S, Stratman EJ, Patten SF. The utility of a touch preparation in the diagnosis of fluctuant subcutaneous fat necrosis of the newborn. *Pediatr Dermatol.* 2009;26(2):241–243.

216. Tajirian A, Ross R, Zeikus P, Robinson-Bostom L. Subcutaneous fat necrosis of the newborn with eosinophilic granules. *J Cutan Pathol.* 2007;34(7):588–590.

217. Kannenberg SMH, Jordaan HF, Visser WI, Ahmed F, Bezuidenhout AF. Report of 2 novel presentations of subcutaneous fat necrosis of the newborn. *Dermatopathology (Basel).* 2019;6(2):147–152.

218. Mir-Bonafe JM, Roman-Curto C, Santos-Briz A, Canueto J, Fernandez-Lopez E, Unamuno P. Gemcitabine-associated livedoid thrombotic microangiopathy with associated sclerema neonatorum-like microscopic changes. *J Cutan Pathol.* 2012;39(7):707–711.

219. Ichimiya H, Arakawa S, Sato T, et al. Involvement of brown adipose tissue in subcutaneous fat necrosis of the newborn. *Dermatology.* 2011;223(3):207–210.

220. Farinelli P, Gattoni M, Delrosso G, et al. Eosinophilic granules in subcutaneous fat necrosis of the newborn: what do they mean? *J Cutan Pathol.* 2008;35(11):1073–1074.

221. Lombardi G, Cabano R, Bollani L, Del Forno C, Stronati M. Effectiveness of pamidronate in severe neonatal hypercalcemia caused by subcutaneous fat necrosis: a case report. *Eur J Pediatr.* 2009;168(5):625–627.

222. Alos N, Eugene D, Fillion M, Powell J, Kokta V, Chabot G. Pamidronate: treatment for severe hypercalcemia in neonatal subcutaneous fat necrosis. *Horm Res.* 2006;65(6):289–294.

223. Zeb A, Rosenberg RE, Ahmed NU, et al. Risk factors for sclerema neonatorum in preterm neonates in Bangladesh. *Pediatr Infect Dis J.* 2009;28(5):435–438.

224. Chisti MJ, Ahmed T, Faruque AS, Saha S, Salam MA, Islam S. Factors associated with sclerema in infants with diarrhoeal disease: a matched case-control study. *Acta Paediatr.* 2009;98(5):873–878.

225. Chisti MJ, Saha S, Roy CN, et al. Predictors of mortality in infants with sclerema presenting to the Centre for Diarrhoeal Disease, Dhaka. *Ann Trop Paediatr.* 2009;29(1):45–50.

226. Kellum RE, Ray TL, Brown GR. Sclerema neonatorum. Report of a case and analysis of subcutaneous and epidermal-dermal lipids by chromatographic methods. *Arch Dermatol.* 1968;97(4):372–380.

227. Zeb A, Darmstadt GL. Sclerema neonatorum: a review of nomenclature, clinical presentation, histological features, differential diagnoses and management. *J Perinatol.* 2008;28(7):453–460.

228. Buster KJ, Burford HN, Stewart FA, Sellheyer K, Hughey LC. Sclerema neonatorum treated with intravenous immunoglobulin: a case report and review of treatments. *Cutis.* 2013;92:83–87.

229. Marovt M, Miljkovic J. Post-steroid panniculitis in an adult. *Acta Dermatovenerol Alp Panonica Adriat.* 2012;21(4):77–78.

230. Smith RT, Good RA. Sequelae of prednisone treatment of acute rheumatic fever. *Clin Res Proc.* 1956;4:156.

231. Kwon EJ, Emanuel PO, Gribetz CH, Mudgil AV, Phelps RG. Post-steroid panniculitis. *J Cutan Pathol.* 2007;34(suppl 1):64–67.

232. Dahl PR, Winkelmann RK, Connolly SM. The vascular calcification-cutaneous necrosis syndrome. *J Am Acad Dermatol.* 1995;33(1):53–58.

233. Essary LR, Wick MR. Cutaneous calciphylaxis. An underrecognized clinicopathologic entity. *Am J Clin Pathol.* 2000;113(2):280–287.

234. Muscat M, Brincat M, Degaetano J, Vassallo J, Calleja-Agius J. An unusual site for calciphylaxis: a case report. *Gynecol Endocrinol.* 2013;29(2):91–92.

235. Karpman E, Das S, Kurzrock EA. Penile calciphylaxis: analysis of risk factors and mortality. *J Urol.* 2003;169(6):2206–2209.

236. Kumar V, Patel N. Calcific uremic arteriolopathy of the penis. *Vasc Med.* 2013;18(4):239.

237. Barbera V, Di Lullo L, Gorini A, et al. Penile calciphylaxis in end stage renal disease. *Case Rep Urol.* 2013;2013:968916.

238. Doctoroff A, Purcell SM, Harris J, Griffin TD. Protracted calciphylaxis, Part I. *Cutis.* 2003;71(6):473–475.

239. Ellis CL, O'Neill WC. Questionable specificity of histologic findings in calcific uremic arteriolopathy. *Kidney Int.* 2018;94(2):390–395.

240. Chaudet KM, Dutta P, Nigwekar SU, Nazarian RM. Calciphylaxis-associated cutaneous vascular calcification in noncalciphylaxis patients. *Am J Dermatopathol.* 2020;42(8):557–563.

241. Penn LA, Brinster N. Calciphylaxis with pseudoxanthoma elasticum-like changes: a case series. *J Cutan Pathol.* 2018;45(2):118–121.

242. McMullen ER, Harms PW, Lowe L, Fullen DR, Chan MP. Clinicopathologic features and calcium deposition patterns in calciphylaxis: comparison with gangrene, peripheral artery disease, chronic stasis, and thrombotic vasculopathy. *Am J Surg Pathol.* 2019;43(9):1273–1281.

243. Nathoo RK, Harb JN, Auerbach J, Guo R, Vincek V, Motaparthi K. Pseudoxanthoma elasticum-like changes in nonuremic calciphylaxis: case series and brief review of a helpful diagnostic clue. *J Cutan Pathol.* 2017;44(12):1064–1069.

244. Bahrani E, Perkins IU, North JP. Diagnosing calciphylaxis: a review with emphasis on histopathology. *Am J Dermatopathol.* 2020;42(7):471–480.

245. Dauden E, Onate MJ. Calciphylaxis. *Dermatol Clin.* 2008;26(4):557–568, ix.

246. Campanelli A, Kaya G, Masouye I, Borradori L. Calcifying panniculitis following subcutaneous injections of nadroparin-calcium in a patient with osteomalacia. *Br J Dermatol.* 2005;153(3):657–660.

247. Eich D, Scharffetter-Kochanek K, Weihrauch J, Krieg T, Hunzelmann N. Calcinosis of the cutis and subcutis: an unusual non-immunologic adverse reaction to subcutaneous injections of low-molecular-weight calcium-containing heparins. *J Am Acad Dermatol.* 2004;50(2):210–214.

248. Micheletti RG, Fishbein GA, Currier JS, Fishbein MC. Monckeberg sclerosis revisited: a clarification of the histologic definition of Monckeberg sclerosis. *Arch Pathol Lab Med.* 2008;132(1):43–47.

249. Magro CM, Simman R, Jackson S. Calciphylaxis: a review. *J Am Col Certif Wound Spec.* 2010;2(4):66–72.

250. McCabe KM, Booth SL, Fu X, et al. Dietary vitamin K and therapeutic warfarin alter the susceptibility to vascular calcification in experimental chronic kidney disease. *Kidney Int.* 2013;83(5):835–844.

251. Schurgers LJ. Vitamin K: key vitamin in controlling vascular calcification in chronic kidney disease. *Kidney Int.* 2013;83(5):782–784.

252. Kramann R, Brandenburg VM, Schurgers LJ, et al. Novel insights into osteogenesis and matrix remodelling associated with calcific uraemic arteriolopathy. *Nephrol Dial Transplant.* 2013;28(4):856–868.

253. Magro CM, Momtahen S, Hagen JW. Osteopontin expression in biopsies of calciphylaxis. *Eur J Dermatol.* 2015;25(1):20–25.

254. Baldwin C, Farah M, Leung M, et al. Multi-intervention management of calciphylaxis: a report of 7 cases. *Am J Kidney Dis.* 2011;58(6):988–991.

255. Latus J, Kimmel M, Ott G, Ting E, Alscher MD, Braun N. Early stages of calciphylaxis: are skin biopsies the answer? *Case Rep Dermatol.* 2011;3(3):201–205.

256. Ning MS, Dahir KM, Castellanos EH, McGirt LY. Sodium thiosulfate in the treatment of non-uremic calciphylaxis. *J Dermatol.* 2013;40(8):649–652.

257. Strazzula L, Nigwekar SU, Steele D, et al. Intralesional sodium thiosulfate for the treatment of calciphylaxis. *JAMA Dermatol.* 2013;149:946–949.

258. Winkelmann RK, Bowie EJ. Hemorrhagic diathesis associated with benign histiocytic, cytophagic panniculitis and systemic histiocytosis. *Arch Intern Med.* 1980;140(11):1460–1463.

259. White JW Jr, Winkelmann RK. Cytophagic histiocytic panniculitis is not always fatal. *J Cutan Pathol.* 1989;16(3):137–144.

260. Pauwels C, Livideanu CB, Maza A, Lamant L, Paul C. Cytophagic histiocytic panniculitis after H1N1 vaccination: a case report and review of the cutaneous side effects of influenza vaccines. *Dermatology.* 2011;222(3):217–220.

261. Chen RL, Hsu YH, Ueda I, et al. Cytophagic histiocytic panniculitis with fatal haemophagocytic lymphohistiocytosis in a paediatric patient with perforin gene mutation. *J Clin Pathol.* 2007;60(10):1168–1169.

262. Hytiroglou P, Phelps RG, Wattenberg DJ, Strauchen JA. Histiocytic cytophagic panniculitis: molecular evidence for a clonal T-cell disorder. *J Am Acad Dermatol.* 1992;27(2, pt 2):333–336.

263. Willemze R, Jansen PM, Cerroni L, et al. Subcutaneous panniculitis-like T-cell lymphoma: definition, classification, and prognostic factors: an EORTC Cutaneous Lymphoma Group Study of 83 cases. *Blood.* 2008;111(2):838–845.

264. Abe Y, Muta K, Ohshima K, et al. Subcutaneous panniculitis by Epstein-Barr virus-infected natural killer (NK) cell proliferation terminating in aggressive subcutaneous NK cell lymphoma. *Am J Hematol.* 2000;64(3):221–225.

265. Bader-Meunier B, Fraitag S, Janssen C, et al. Clonal cytophagic histiocytic panniculitis in children may be cured by cyclosporine a. *Pediatrics.* 2013;132(2):e545–549.

266. Miyabe Y, Murata Y, Baba Y, Ito E, Nagasaka K. Successful treatment of cyclosporine-A-resistant cytophagic histiocytic panniculitis with tacrolimus. *Mod Rheumatol.* 2011;21(5):553–556.

267. Burket JM, Burket BJ. Eosinophilic panniculitis. *J Am Acad Dermatol.* 1985;12(1, pt 2):161–164.

268. Pot C, Oppliger R, Castillo V, Coeytaux A, Hauser C, Burkhard PR. Apomorphine-induced eosinophilic panniculitis and hypereosinophilia in Parkinson disease. *Neurology.* 2005;64(2):392–393.

269. Bravo FG. Emerging infections: mimickers of common patterns seen in dermatopathology. *Mod Pathol.* 2020;33(suppl 1):118–127.

270. Leis-Dosil VM, Saez Vicente A, Lorido-Cortes MM. Eosinophilic panniculitis associated with COVID-19. *Actas Dermosifiliogr.* 2020;111(9):804–805.

271. Ustuner P, Dilek N, Saral Y, Dilek AR, Bedir R. Eosinophilic panniculitis presenting with Kaposi's sarcoma-like plaques in a patient who is human immunodeficiency virus positive: a case report. *J Med Case Rep.* 2012;6(1):387.

272. Logunova V, Bridges AG. Subcutaneous mixed lobular and septal panniculitis with numerous eosinophils associated with autologous fat grafting: expanding the differential diagnosis of eosinophilic panniculitis. *J Cutan Pathol.* 2020;47(3):305–307.

273. Guhl G, Garcia-Diez A. Subcutaneous sweet syndrome. *Dermatol Clin.* 2008;26(4):541–551, viii–ix.

274. Suzuki Y, Kuroda K, Kojima T, Fujita M, Iseki T, Shinkai H. Unusual cutaneous manifestations of myelodysplastic syndrome. *Br J Dermatol.* 1995;133(3):483–486.

275. Matsumura Y, Tanabe H, Wada Y, Ohta K, Okamoto H, Imamura S. Neutrophilic panniculitis associated with myelodysplastic syndromes. *Br J Dermatol.* 1997;136(1):142–144.

276. Monfort JB, Pages C, Schneider P, et al. Vemurafenib-induced neutrophilic panniculitis. *Melanoma Res.* 2012;22(5):399–401.

277. Kim GH, Levy A, Compoginis G. Neutrophilic panniculitis developing after treatment of metastatic melanoma with vemurafenib. *J Cutan Pathol.* 2013;40(7):667–669.

278. Young TK, Gutierrez D, Criscito MC, Kim RH, Lakdawala N, Oza VS. Dabrafenib-induced neutrophilic panniculitis in a child undergoing dual BRAF-MEK inhibitor therapy for glioblastoma multiforme. *Pediatr Dermatol.* 2020;37(6):1185–1186.

279. Llamas-Velasco M, Garcia-Martin P, Sanchez-Perez J, Fraga J, Garcia-Diez A. Sweet's syndrome with subcutaneous involvement associated with pegfilgrastim treatment: first reported case. *J Cutan Pathol.* 2013;40(1):46–49.

280. Jagdeo J, Campbell R, Long T, Muglia J, Telang G, Robinson-Bostom L. Sweet's syndrome–like neutrophilic lobular panniculitis associated with all-trans-retinoic acid chemotherapy in a patient with acute promyelocytic leukemia. *J Am Acad Dermatol.* 2007;56(4):690–693.

281. Kim IH, Youn JH, Shin SH, et al. Neutrophilic panniculitis following azacitidine treatment for myelodysplastic syndromes. *Leuk Res.* 2012;36(7):e146–148.

282. Assmann K, Nashan D, Grabbe S, Luger TA, Metze D. [Persistent inflammatory reaction at the injection site of Il-2 with lymphoma-like inflammatory infiltrates]. *Hautarzt.* 2002;53(8):554–557.

283. Peterman CM, Robinson-Bostom L, Paek SY. Pembrolizumab-induced lobular panniculitis in the setting of metastatic melanoma. *Cutis.* 2020;105(1):E22–E23.

284. de Waal R, Cohen K, Maartens G. Systematic review of antiretroviral-associated lipodystrophy: lipoatrophy, but not central fat gain, is an antiretroviral adverse drug reaction. *PLoS One.* 2013;8(5):e63623.

285. McNutt NS, Moreno A, Contreras F. Inflammatory diseases of the subcutaneous fat. In: Elder DE, ed. *Lever's Histopathology of the Skin.* 10th ed. Wolters Kluwer; 2004:509–538.

286. Misra A, Garg A. Clinical features and metabolic derangements in acquired generalized lipodystrophy: case reports and review of the literature. *Medicine (Baltimore).* 2003;82(2):129–146.

287. Garg A. Clinical review#: Lipodystrophies: genetic and acquired body fat disorders. *J Clin Endocrinol Metab.* 2011;96(11):3313–3325.

288. Dahl PR, Zalla MJ, Winkelmann RK. Localized involutional lipoatrophy: a clinicopathologic study of 16 patients. *J Am Acad Dermatol.* 1996;35(4):523–528.

289. Rongioletti F, Rebora A. Annular and semicircular lipoatrophies. Report of three cases and review of the literature. *J Am Acad Dermatol.* 1989;20(3):433–436.

290. Camacho D, Pielasinski U, Revelles JM, et al. Diffuse lower limb lipoatrophy. *J Cutan Pathol.* 2011;38(3):270–274.

291. Torrelo A, Patel S, Colmenero I, et al. Chronic atypical neutrophilic dermatosis with lipodystrophy and elevated temperature (CANDLE) syndrome. *J Am Acad Dermatol.* 2010;62(3):489–495.

292. Simha V, Garg A. Lipodystrophy: lessons in lipid and energy metabolism. *Curr Opin Lipidol.* 2006;17(2):162–169.

293. Bedrose S, Turin CG, Lavis VR, Kim ST, Thosani SN. A case of acquired generalized lipodystrophy associated with pembrolizumab in a patient with metastatic malignant melanoma. *AACE Clin Case Rep.* 2020;6(1):e40–e45.

294. Rubio-Cabezas O, Puri V, Murano I, et al. Partial lipodystrophy and insulin resistant diabetes in a patient with a homozygous nonsense mutation in CIDEC. *EMBO Mol Med.* 2009;1(5):280–287.

295. Zha BS, Wan X, Zhang X, et al. HIV protease inhibitors disrupt lipid metabolism by activating endoplasmic reticulum stress and inhibiting autophagy activity in adipocytes. *PLoS One.* 2013;8(3):e59514.

296. Shuck J, Iorio ML, Hung R, Davison SP. Autologous fat grafting and injectable dermal fillers for human immunodeficiency virus-associated facial lipodystrophy: a comparison of safety, efficacy, and long-term treatment outcomes. *Plast Reconstr Surg.* 2013;131(3):499–506.

297. Fife CE, Maus EA, Carter MJ. Lipedema: a frequently misdiagnosed and misunderstood fatty deposition syndrome. *Adv Skin Wound Care.* 2010;23(2):81–92; quiz 93–94.

298. Allen EU, Hines EAJ. Lipedema of the legs. A syndrome characterized by fat legs and orthostatic edema. *Proc Staff Meet Mayo Clin.* 1940;15:184–187.

299. Bilancini S, Lucchi M, Tucci S. [Lipedema: clinical and diagnostic criteria]. *Angiologia.* 1990;42(4):133–137.

300. Pascucci A, Lynch PJ. Lipedema with multiple lipomas. *Dermatol Online J.* 2010;16(9):4.

301. El Darouti MA, Marzouk SA, Mashaly HM, et al. Lipedema and lipedematous alopecia: report of 10 new cases. *Eur J Dermatol.* 2007;17(4):351–352.

302. Fair KP, Knoell KA, Patterson JW, Rudd RJ, Greer KE. Lipedematous alopecia: a clinicopathologic, histologic and ultrastructural study. *J Cutan Pathol.* 2000;27(1):49–53.

303. Rudkin GH, Miller TA. Lipedema: a clinical entity distinct from lymphedema. *Plast Reconstr Surg.* 1994;94(6):841–847; discussion 848–849.

304. Gonzalez-Guerra E, Haro R, Angulo J, Del Carmen Farina M, Martin L, Requena L. Lipedematous alopecia: an uncommon clinicopathologic variant of nonscarring but permanent alopecia. *Int J Dermatol.* 2008;47(6):605–609.

305. Amann-Vesti BR, Franzeck UK, Bollinger A. Microlymphatic aneurysms in patients with lipedema. *Lymphology.* 2001;34(4):170–175.

306. Wagner S. Lymphedema and lipedema—an overview of conservative treatment. *Vasa.* 2011;40(4):271–279.

307. Peled AW, Slavin SA, Brorson H. Long-term outcome after surgical treatment of lipedema. *Ann Plast Surg.* 2012;68(3):303–307.

Bacterial Diseases

ALVARO C. LAGA

INTRODUCTION

A wide range of bacteria, including mycobacteria and rickett-siae, affect the skin and subcutis. In the ensuing descriptions of the histopathology of most of the cutaneous bacterial infections that may be encountered by the diagnostic pathologists, reference is also made to some epidemiology, clinical features, and pathophysiology. Within a given disease pattern, there is variation in both the histologic features and the organisms that cause the disease, especially in the setting of immunosuppression. Thus, in most cases, correlating skin findings with culture or molecular techniques is warranted to arrive at the best diagnosis for patient benefit. The pathogenesis of the skin lesions is multifactorial, including the following:

- Toxin production
- Pyogenic and granulation tissue chemoattractants
- Immunopathology (complement activation and cell-mediated immunity)
- Vasculitis

DISEASES CAUSED BY *STAPHYLOCOCCUS* AND *STREPTOCOCCUS*

Impetigo

Two types of impetigo occur: impetigo contagiosa, or nonbullous impetigo, usually caused by *Staphylococcus aureus* or group A streptococci; and bullous impetigo, caused by *S. aureus*, which may also cause the staphylococcal scalded-skin syndrome (1).

Impetigo Contagiosa

Clinical Summary. Impetigo contagiosa, also known as impetigo simplex or nonbullous impetigo, is primarily an endemic disease of preschool-age children that may occur in epidemics but may also affect adults, particularly immunocompromised hosts (2). Very early lesions consist of vesicopustules that rupture quickly and are followed by heavy, golden-yellow crusts. Lesions are most frequently located on the head and neck, followed by the upper extremity, and trunk and lower extremities (3). Acute glomerulonephritis of the postinfectious variety can follow this presentation. Ecthyma is essentially chronic, ulcerated impetigo contagiosa, often with a thick crust. It occurs chiefly below the knees as multiple crusted ulcers. Skin cultures are nearly always positive for group A streptococci. In addition, coagulase-positive staphylococci as secondary invaders can frequently be cultured from lesions (4).

Histopathology. Biopsies from early lesions of impetigo characteristically show a subcorneal pustule. The vesicopustule arises in the upper layers of the epidermis and may show cleavage above, within, or immediately below the granular layer. It contains numerous neutrophils (Fig. 21-1). Not infrequently, a few acantholytic cells can be observed at the floor of the vesicopustule. Occasionally, gram-positive cocci can also be found within the vesicopustule, both within neutrophils and extracellularly (5). In ecthyma, a nonspecific ulcer is observed with numerous neutrophils both in the dermis and in the serous exudate at the floor of the ulcer.

The stratum malpighii underlying the bulla is spongiotic, and neutrophils can often be seen migrating through it. The upper dermis contains a moderately severe inflammatory infiltrate of neutrophils and lymphoid cells.

At a later stage, when the vesicle has ruptured, the horny layer is absent, and a crust composed of serous exudate and the nuclear debris of neutrophils may be seen covering the stratum malpighii.

Pathogenesis. Group A streptococci, either alone or in association with *S. aureus,* are the most common bacterial causes of impetigo (6). Cultures of such lesions are vital in order to identify methicillin-resistant *S. aureus* (MRSA) as the causal agent versus other antibiotic-susceptible skin and environmental flora.

Differential Diagnosis. Histologic differentiation of impetigo contagiosa from subcorneal pustular dermatosis, pemphigus foliaceus, and immunoglobulin A (IgA) pemphigus can be difficult. However, only impetigo shows gram-positive cocci in the bulla cavity on routine Gram staining. In addition, pemphigus foliaceus usually shows fewer neutrophils, more acantholytic cells, and occasionally some dyskeratotic granular cells.

Bullous Impetigo and Staphylococcal Scalded-Skin Syndrome

Clinical Summary. Staphylococcus aureus may produce bullous impetigo and staphylococcal scalded-skin syndrome.

Bullous impetigo occurs mainly in newborns, infants, and young children (7,8). It is characterized by vesicles that rapidly progress to flaccid bullae with little or no surrounding erythema. The contents of the bullae are initially clear but may progress to turbid. There is often a distinctive honey-colored dried serous crust over inflamed skin. Bullous impetigo may spread and become generalized; so clinical distinction from staphylococcal scalded-skin syndrome may be impossible (9). An important difference, however, is that cultures from intact bullae of bullous impetigo, unlike those of the staphylococcal scalded-skin syndrome, grow phage group II *S. aureus*.

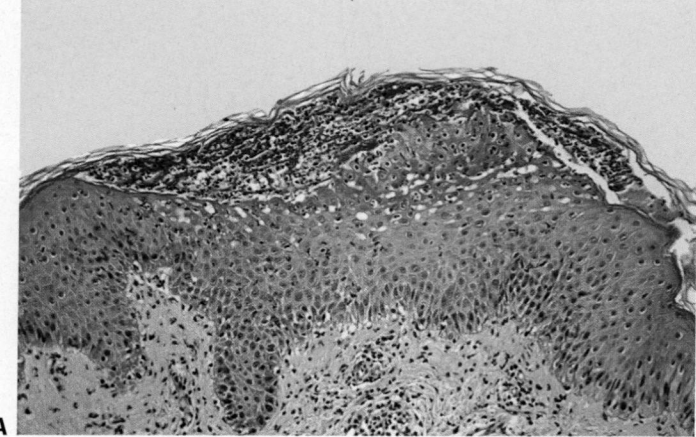

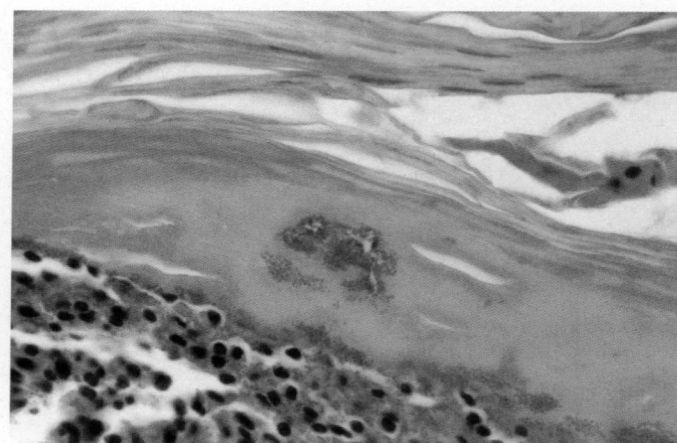

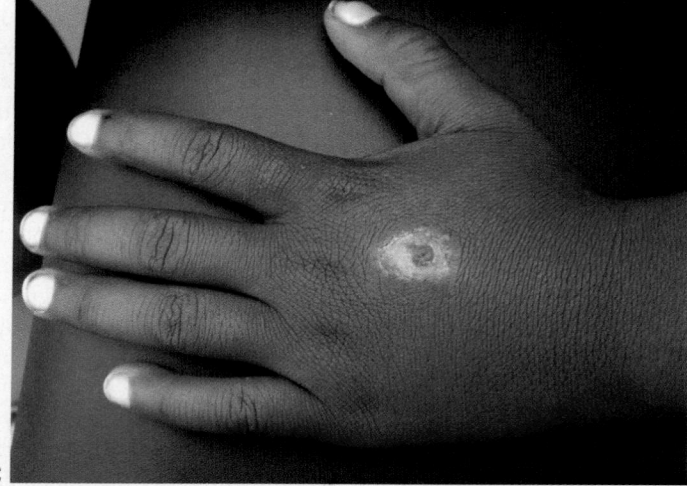

Figure 21-1 Impetigo contagiosa. **A:** In this relatively early lesion, neutrophils are seen in the upper epidermis, forming a subclone pustule. There is a superficial mixed infiltrate within the dermis. **B:** On closer inspection, neutrophils and bacterial colonies are found within the stratum corneum. **C:** Yellow crusted vesiculopustules on the back of the hand of a child. (**C:** Courtesy of C. Kovarik.)

Staphylococcal scalded-skin syndrome, first described more than 100 years ago and known as Ritter disease, occurs largely in the newborn and in children younger than 5 years. It rarely occurs in adults or in older children (10–12) except in the presence of severe underlying disease such as renal insufficiency, which leads to decreased toxin clearance (13).

The disease begins abruptly with diffuse erythema and fever, usually 48 hours after birth. Large, flaccid bullae filled with clear fluid form and rupture almost immediately. Large sheets of superficial epidermis separate and exfoliate. The disease runs an acute course and is fatal in more than 4% of all cases in children (14). Most fatalities occur in neonates with generalized lesions. In contrast, in the rare cases of staphylococcal scalded-skin syndrome occurring in adults, the prognosis is much worse, with a mortality rate exceeding 50%. Death is usually related to the coexistent disease or to immunosuppressive therapy given for it. Both bullous impetigo and staphylococcal scalded-skin syndrome are transmissible and can cause epidemics in nurseries, where they may occur together (15).

The absence of *S. aureus* from the bullae of staphylococcal scalded-skin syndrome results from the fact that these staphylococci are present at a distant focus. Usually, the distant focus is extracutaneous and consists of a purulent conjunctivitis, rhinitis, or pharyngitis. Rarely, the distant focus consists of a cutaneous infection or a septicemia.

Histopathology. In both bullous impetigo and staphylococcal scalded-skin syndrome, the cleavage plane of the bulla, like that in impetigo contagiosa, lies in the uppermost epidermis either below or, less commonly, within the granular layer (Fig. 21-2). A few acantholytic cells are often seen adjoining the cleavage plane. However, in contrast to impetigo contagiosa, there are few or no inflammatory cells within the bulla cavity. In bullous impetigo, the upper dermis may show a polymorphous infiltrate, whereas in the staphylococcal scalded-skin syndrome, the dermis is usually free of inflammation.

Pathogenesis. The causative epidermolysins are the exfoliative toxins (ETs) produced by *S. aureus*. There are many strains of these serine protease enzymes. Their target is desmoglein 1, a desmosomal glycoprotein, which has a role in cell-to-cell adhesion in the superficial epidermis (16).

Electron microscopy shows that the cleavage plane of lesions in humans as well as in mice is at the interface between the spinous and granular layers, with some upward extension into the lower granular layer. Splitting occurs without damage to adjacent acantholytic keratinocytes. ET appears to act primarily on the intercellular substance because in studies carried out on newborn mice, the intercellular spaces widen and microvilli form before the desmosomes separate within their interdesmosomal contact zone (17).

Differential Diagnosis. Staphylococcal scalded-skin syndrome and toxic epidermal necrolysis of Lyell type show clinically extensive detachment of the epidermis and may thus clinically resemble one another. This has resulted in confusion in the past; at one time, both diseases were referred to as *Lyell disease* or

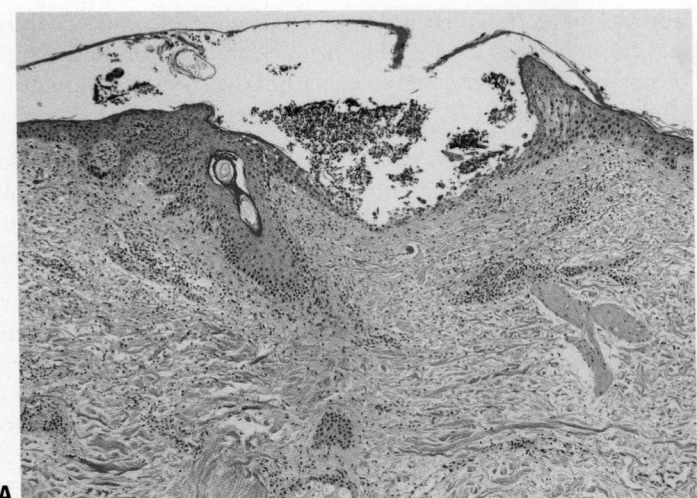
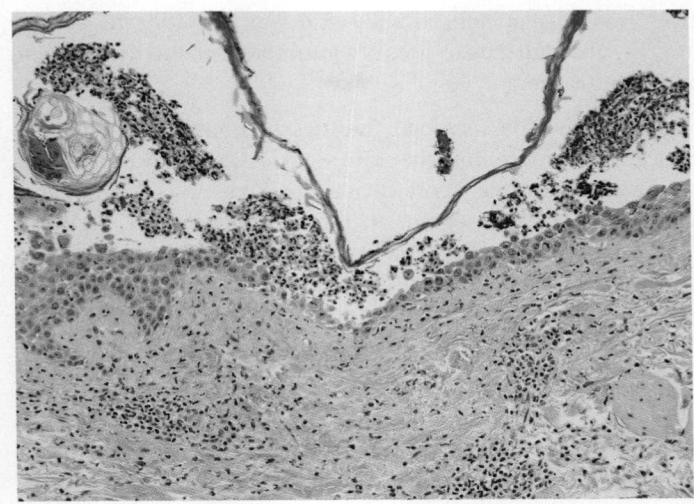

Figure 21-2 Bullous impetigo. **A:** Subcorneal pustular infiltrate is characteristic of bullous impetigo. **B:** Notice the prominent neutrophilic infiltrate and relative absence of dyskeratotic cells, which is helpful in distinguishing it from pemphigus follicaceous.

toxic epidermal necrolysis. As the target of staphylococcal toxin is desmoglein 1, clinically the epidermal split in this condition is superficial, leaving pink intact epidermis under superficially peeling skin, as opposed to toxic epidermal necrolysis, wherein the entire epidermis is diseased and detached, leaving moist, inflamed, raw dermis visible under the denuded areas. Similarly, staphylococcal scalded-skin syndrome should not affect the mucosa, whereas Stevens–Johnson syndrome and toxic epidermal necrolysis almost always do. Additionally, the two diseases can be easily differentiated histologically; in severe erythema multiforme/Stevens–Johnson syndrome, the entire, or nearly the entire, epidermis detaches itself, with considerable necrosis of the epidermal cells, whereas in staphylococcal scalded-skin syndrome, only the uppermost portion of the epidermis becomes detached, with relatively slight damage to the underlying epidermal cells. This difference can be readily identified with frozen section analysis of denuded detached skin for rapid diagnosis.

Principles of Management: The major objectives of impetigo treatment (including bullous impetigo) are reducing the spread of infection and supporting the resolution of discomfort and cosmetic appearance. Oral antimicrobial therapy with activity against β-hemolytic streptococci and *S. aureus* for 7 days is usually sufficient. Topical therapy, such as mupirocin ointment, may be administered in cases with a limited number of lesions without bullae. Handwashing is important for reducing the spread in children (18). Staphylococcal toxic shock syndrome (TSS) requires aggressive multidisciplinary care with supportive care and often parenteral antibiotics.

Methicillin-Resistant *S. aureus* (MRSA)

Clinical Summary. Originally described shortly after the introduction of methicillin in 1961, the prevalence of MRSA has increased in both health care and community settings. MRSA skin infections are currently classified as health care-associated (HA-MRSA) or community-associated (CA-MRSA), based on the presence or absence of health care exposure. Evolving epidemiologic observations suggest that there is no clear distinction between these two categories because patients can develop MRSA colonization in one realm and develop signs

and symptoms of infection in the other. HA-MRSA infections have been observed with increasing frequency in patients in community settings, and, similarly, infection by "community-associated" strains has become more common among patients in hospital settings. Moreover, studies suggest that CA-MRSA strains may be replacing traditional hospital-acquired strains. However, there are important clinical and molecular epidemiologic differences that merit consideration (19). Infection caused by CA-MRSA is considered to represent a worldwide epidemic, often presenting as a skin and soft tissue infection in young, otherwise healthy individuals. Athletes, certain ethnic populations, children, homeless persons, homosexual men, household members of infected people, HIV-infected patients, intravenous drug abusers, military personnel, newborns, pregnant and postpartum women, tattoo recipients, and urban dwellers of lower socioeconomic status in crowded living conditions are said to be at increased risk of developing CA-MRSA infection. A recent study conducted in primary care clinics in Texas found CA-MRSA to be the predominant pathogen implicated in skin and soft tissue infections in the ambulatory setting (20). Colonization by *S. aureus* in patients whose skin barrier is disrupted represents a potential reservoir for CA-MRSA. In addition, infection-associated risk factors are absent in many individuals who develop cutaneous CA-MRSA infection. The most common presentations of CA-MRSA infection are abscess, cellulitis, or both, not uncommonly misinterpreted by the patient as insect bites. Other manifestations of cutaneous CA-MRSA infection are impetigo, folliculitis, and paronychia.

Hospital-associated MRSA is defined as MRSA infection that occurs 48 hours or later following hospitalization or infection occurring outside of the hospital within 12 months of exposure to health care (e.g., surgery). It is often more virulent than CA-MRSA. Patients may be at risk for developing not just skin and soft tissue infections but bacteremia, sepsis, and seeding of internal devices, hardware, heart valves, and joints. Risk factors for HA-MRSA infection include prolonged hospitalization, antibiotic use, admission to intensive care, and hemodialysis, among others. Many hospitals routinely screen all patients admitted to identify carriers and enact strict contact isolation to limit the spread of MRSA through the hospital. This form of

MRSA may display substantially different antibiotic resistance patterns, and cultures to identify antibiotic sensitivities are essential to treatment.

Histopathology. The histologic findings are nonspecific, and correlation with microbiologic cultures is essential to establish a diagnosis of certitude. Prominent dermal edema and lymphatic dilatation may be observed. A diffuse inflammatory infiltrate around blood vessels, predominantly of polymorphonuclear neutrophils, may be present. Granulation tissue with a mononuclear infiltrate of lymphocytes and histiocytes is seen in later stages. A Gram stain may reveal abundant cocci in florid infections.

Pathogenesis. Methicillin resistance is encoded by the *mecA* gene on the staphylococcal chromosome cassette (SCCmec), encoding PBP-2a, a penicillin-binding protein that allows the microorganism to grow and divide in the presence of methicillin or other β-lactam antibiotics. By 2004, six major clones of MRSA had emerged worldwide, labeled SCCmecI–VI. Dissemination of resistance is mediated by horizontal transfer of the *mecA* gene (19).

Principles of Management: Incision and drainage of abscesses, systemic antibacterial therapy, and adjunctive topical antibacterial treatment are the essential components of management of CA-MRSA skin infections. The spread of cutaneous CA-MRSA infection can potentially be prevented by a combination of personal, environmental, and health care measures directed at eliminating the causes of acquisition and transmission of the bacteria (19). Patients may be chronic carriers, and staph eradication may be necessary with antimicrobial bathing, intranasal, perineal, and subungual topical antistaph antibiotics, and sometimes courses of combination oral antibiotics to reduce the carrier state. It is important for clinicians to be aware of MRSA resistance patterns in their community, to choose appropriate empiric antibiotics, and to tailor therapy based on culture data. For HA-MRSA, patients often require IV antibiotics and may need an infectious disease specialist to assist in selecting medications and determining therapeutic duration.

BLASTOMYCOSIS-LIKE PYODERMA (PYODERMA VEGETANS)

Clinical Summary. Two entirely different diseases have been described under the term *pyoderma vegetans* or *pyodermite végétante of Hallopeau.* One disease, now referred to as *pemphigus vegetans of Hallopeau,* shows the typical intercellular immunofluorescence of the pemphigus group on direct immunofluorescence testing. The other disease represents a vegetating tissue reaction, possibly secondary to bacterial infection (21). In order to emphasize the difference between it and pemphigus vegetans of Hallopeau, it is preferable to refer to this disease as *blastomycosis-like pyoderma* rather than as *pyoderma vegetans* (22).

Blastomycosis-like pyoderma shows one or multiple large, verrucous, vegetating plaques with scattered pustules and elevated borders. The plaques show considerable resemblance to those observed in fungal blastomycosis. The location of the plaques varies considerably from case to case, but predominant involvement of sun-damaged skin was documented in the latest and largest case series (21). In some instances, the face and legs are affected; in others, it is the intertriginous areas. Some authors have observed an association with ulcerative colitis, but no infectious etiology has been established in these cases, which have been rendered to be within the spectrum of neutrophilic dermatoses (23).

Histopathology. The two major features of blastomycosis-like pyoderma are pseudocarcinomatous hyperplasia and multiple abscesses in the dermis as well as in the hyperplastic epidermis. The abscesses are composed of neutrophils in some cases and of eosinophils in others.

Pathogenesis. Bacteria, most commonly *S. aureus,* can be found regularly in blastomycosis-like pyoderma; however, the presence of several different strains and the variable response of patients to antibiotic therapy suggest that the bacteria are secondary invaders, although they may be responsible for the vegetating tissue reaction. A deficiency in cellular immunity (24) and a decrease in the chemotactic activity of the neutrophils have also been observed.

Differential Diagnosis. In cases with largely eosinophils in the abscesses, pemphigus vegetans must be excluded by direct immunofluorescence. If there is marked pseudocarcinomatous hyperplasia, multiple biopsies may be necessary for differentiation from true squamous cell carcinoma.

Principles of Management: There is no standardized treatment plan available for pyoderma vegetans. Antimicrobial therapy has been used, with variable results. Alternatives include curettage and topical application of aluminum subacetate soaks. Attention to underlying systemic illness should also be considered (21).

ERYSIPELAS

Clinical Summary. Erysipelas, once termed *St. Anthony's fire,* is an acute superficial cellulitis of the skin caused by β-hemolytic streptococci. It is characterized by the presence of a well-demarcated, slightly indurated, dusky red patch or thin plaque with an advancing, palpable border. In some patients, erysipelas tends to recur periodically in the same areas. Recent data suggests a significant association between several single nucleotide polymorphisms (SNPs) in the promoter of the *AGTR1* gene (angiotensin II receptor type I) and susceptibility to erysipelas in humans (25). In the early antibiotic era, the incidence of erysipelas appeared to be on the decline, and most cases occurred on the face. More recently, however, there appears to have been an increase in the incidence, and facial sites are now less common, whereas erysipelas of the legs is predominant. Potential complications in patients with poor resistance or after inadequate therapy may include abscess formation, spreading necrosis of the soft tissue, infrequently necrotizing fasciitis, and septicemia (26). Nephritic and cardiac complications are rare because erysipelas is usually produced by nonnephritogenic and nonrheumatogenic strains of streptococci.

Histopathology. The findings are nonspecific, and the diagnosis relies on clinical and microbiologic culture correlation. The dermis shows marked edema and dilatation of the lymphatics and capillaries. There is a diffuse infiltrate, composed chiefly of neutrophils, that extends throughout the dermis and occasionally into the subcutaneous fat. It shows a loose arrangement around dilated blood and lymph vessels (Fig. 21-3). If sections

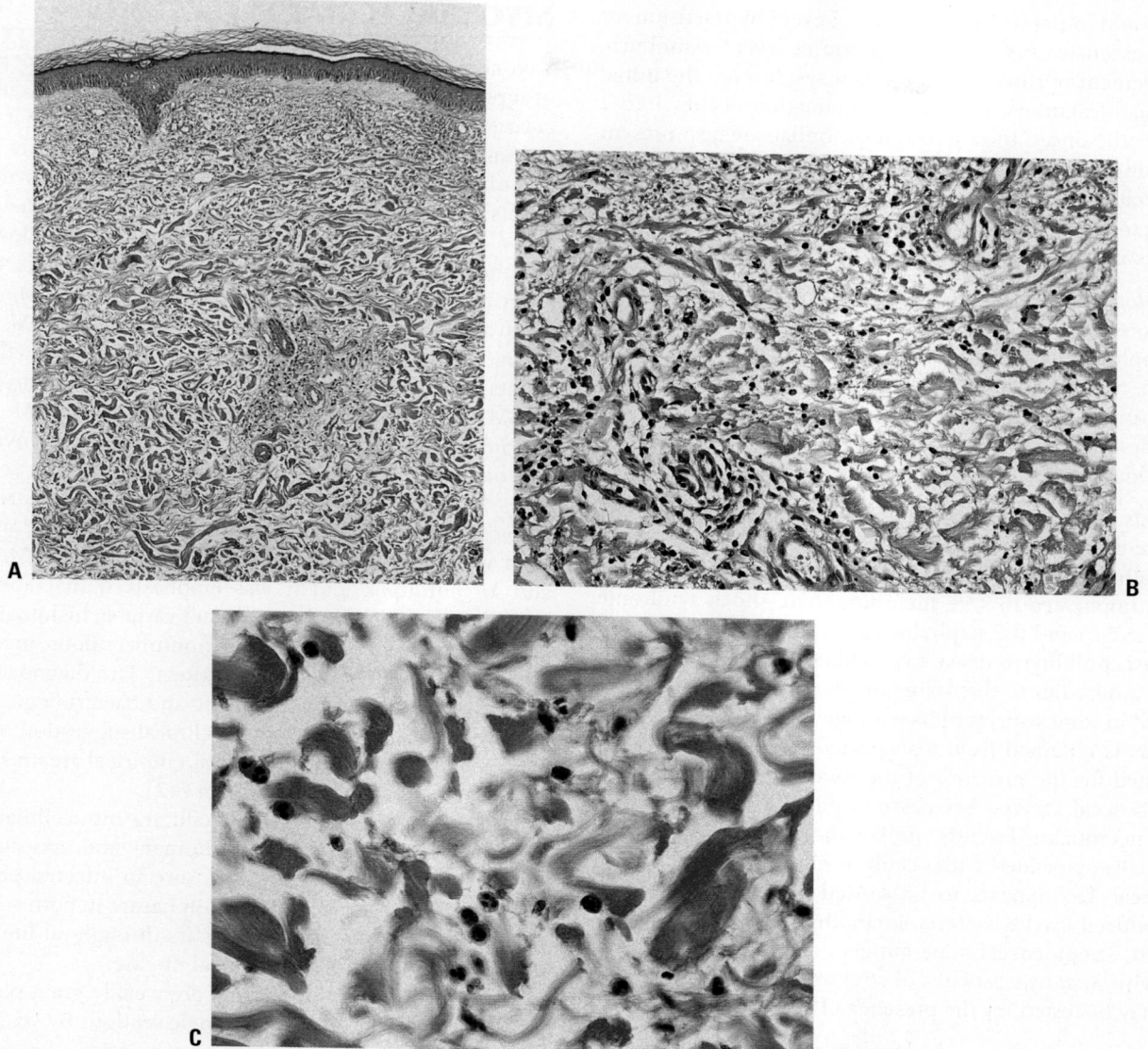

Figure 21-3 Cellulitis/erysipelas. **A:** There is interstitial edema and an infiltrate of neutrophils, which may be subtle at scanning magnification. **B:** Interstitial edema and neutrophils. **C:** Neutrophils among collagen bundles. The differential diagnosis for these images would include Sweet syndrome. Demonstration of organisms by Gram stain and/or culture, and clinicopathologic correlation, are important to establish the diagnosis. (From Elder DE, Elenitsas R, Rubin AI, et al, eds. *Atlas of Dermatopathology*. Wolters Kluwer; 2021.)

are stained with the Giemsa or Gram stain, streptococci are found in the tissue and within lymphatics. In cases of recurring erysipelas, the lymph vessels of the dermis and subcutaneous tissue show fibrotic thickening of their walls with partial or complete occlusion of the lumen.

Pathogenesis. Erysipelas and cellulitis are infections that develop as a result of bacterial entry via breaches in the skin barrier. Most cases are caused by β-hemolytic streptococci (groups A, B, C, G, and F) and *S. aureus*, including MRSA. Gram-negative aerobic bacilli are isolated in a minority of cases. Less common pathogens include *Haemophilus influenzae* (buccal cellulitis), clostridia and non–spore-forming anaerobes (crepitant cellulitis), pneumococcus, and meningococcus.

Principles of Management: Patients with classic manifestations of erysipelas are best treated with parenteral antimicrobial therapy, with ceftriaxone or cephazolin being choices with appropriate coverage. Patients with mild infection or after improvement with parenteral therapy may be treated with oral

β-lactam antimicrobials. Supportive measures such as elevation of affected area and treatment of underlying predisposing conditions should be included. Exacerbation of erythema after initiation of antimicrobial therapy may be observed because of pathogen destruction and enzymatic release and should not be mistaken for failure to respond (26).

TOXIC SHOCK SYNDROME

TSS is a fulminant illness usually caused by group A β-hemolytic *Streptococcus* and certain toxin-producing strains of *S. aureus* (27).

Clinical Summary. In the initial report in 1978, the disease was described in a series of seven children (28). Although many subsequent cases have been associated with the use of superabsorbent vaginal tampons by menstruating women, additional reported settings for TSS have included surgical wound infections of the skin (29), empyema, fasciitis, osteomyelitis, peritonsillar abscesses, and other infections (30). Fever, hypotension or shock, an extensive rash resembling scarlet fever or sunburn, and involvement of three or more organ systems are the initial defining manifestations, whereas desquamation occurs 1 to 2 weeks after the onset. In rare instances, bullae are also present (31). In addition, there may be conjunctivitis and oropharyngitis. Internal organs may be affected by toxic encephalopathy, thrombocytopenia, renal failure, or hepatic damage. Mortality has been estimated at 5% to 10% (32).

Histopathology. The histologic findings are nonspecific. A superficial perivascular and interstitial mixed-cell infiltrate containing neutrophils and sometimes eosinophils, foci of spongiosis containing neutrophils, and scattered necrotic keratinocytes that sometimes are arranged in clusters within the epidermis has been described (33). If bullae are present, they are subepidermal in location.

Pathogenesis. Even though in rare cases *S. aureus* bacteremia occurs, the cause of staphylococcal TSS is a toxin that is produced locally at the site of a toxigenic infection. Several toxins have been implicated in TSS, including toxic shock syndrome toxin 1 (TSST-1) and the staphylococcal enterotoxins B, C, and F (34). Susceptibility to disease correlates with the absence of protective antibodies to the toxin, and cytokine activation may be involved in some aspects of its pathogenesis. If a pure culture of *S. aureus* is obtained from a suspected patient, the bacteria can be tested for the presence of the toxin to confirm diagnosis. Streptococcal TSS has been associated with bacteremia and extensive necrotizing fasciitis, unlike the staphylococcal syndrome usually associated with occult or minor focal infections. Streptococcal TSS appears to be caused also by a variety of toxins produced by the bacteria, including pyrogenic exotoxin A and/or B, streptococcal superantigen, and mitogenic factor (35). As with *S. aureus*, isolates of streptococci from suspected patients may be tested for the presence of specific toxins (36).

Differential Diagnosis. A petechial rash mimicking meningococcemia is a rare manifestation of streptococcal TSS. Bacteremia is uncommon in staphylococcal TSS, in contrast to streptococcal TSS. In patients with fulminant presentations and suspicion for a possible skin infection, consideration should be given as to whether the patient may have necrotizing fasciitis, which represents both a medical and surgical emergency and requires immediate intervention.

Principles of Management: The mainstay of therapy for staphylococcal TSS is supportive with fluid replacement, which may be extensive at times to maintain perfusion in the setting of hypotension. Vasopressors may also be required. Foreign material should be sought after and removed if present (i.e., tampons, contraceptive sponges). Although it is not clear whether antibiotics alter the course of acute TSS, most patients receive broad IV antibiotics during their acute illness. Notably, antistaphylococcal antibiotic therapy is required to eradicate organisms and prevent recurrences (37). Streptococcal TSS requires aggressive, combined antibiotics, with patients often receiving third-generation cephalosporins, clindamycin (which may impair bacterial ribosomal protein production and theoretically reduce toxin formation), and vancomycin to cover for the possibility of resistant staphylococcal infections. Intravenous immunoglobulin (IVIg) is controversial and has been variably used to decrease the inflammatory response.

MYCOBACTERIAL INFECTIONS

Taxonomically, the mycobacteria are divided into two major groups: the rapid growers and the slow growers in culture. *Mycobacterium leprae* lies outside this scheme because it cannot be cultured *in vitro*. Within each group, the species are organized in subgroups according to certain culture (growth requirements) and biochemical characteristics. Among the infections to be considered in this chapter, the important slow growers are the *M. tuberculosis* complex, including Bacille Calmette–Guérin (BCG); the *M. avium* complex, including *M. avium* and *M. avium-intracellulare*; the *M. kansasii* complex; *M. marinum*; *M. ulcerans*; and mycobacteria with special growth requirements, such as *M. haemophilum*. Rapid-growing mycobacteria (RGM) include three clinically relevant species: *M. fortuitum*, *M. chelonae*, and *M. abscessus* (38). Many other mycobacteria can occasionally cause skin lesions (39–41). In a series of 25 cases from Israel, there were 16 cases with *M. marinum*, 3 of atypical *Mycobacterium* without species identification, and one each with *M. chelonae*, *M. xenopi*, *M. abscessus*, *M. gordonae*, and *M. fortuitum*, and it was emphasized that absence of a pathognomonic clinical picture and variable histologic findings often delay diagnosis of these nontuberculous mycobacteria (NTM)-induced cutaneous infections. The diagnosis of NTM should be confirmed by histologic and bacteriologic studies of tissue cultures. However, strong clinical suggestion of *M. marinum* infection may warrant initial empirical treatment to prevent progression to deep infection (42).

Tuberculosis and leprosy bacilli are intracellular parasites that are found in the tissues of humans and occasionally animals. Transmission requires exposure to infected people. The other mycobacteria are abundant in nature in both soil and water, and exposure to infection occurs throughout life, although usually without significant clinical disease.

Mycobacteria are bacilli that are weakly gram positive and are classically identified in histologic sections by stains that exploit their resistance to decoloration by acid—that is, acid-fast bacilli. All mycobacteria apart from the leprosy bacillus have been historically reported to stain well by the standard Ziehl–Neelsen technique. However, likely owing to widespread adoption of automated staining, the sensitivity of the Ziehl–Neelsen technique has decreased significantly as compared with the Fite-Faraco stain or mycobacterial immunohistochemistry (43). We and others routinely use and recommend the modified acid-fast stains (Fite-Faraco and Nocardia) and immunohistochemistry over the standard Ziehl–Neelsen. At a minimum, the reader and/or frequent user of these techniques would be well served by running a comparative study of these stains in their laboratory to know what to expect.

LEPROSY

Clinical Summary. Leprosy, also known as Hansen disease, is a chronic granulomatous infection caused by *M. leprae* and that predominantly affects the skin and peripheral nerves. The disease is endemic in many tropical and subtropical countries but is declining in prevalence as a result of multidrug therapy. The Indian subcontinent, Southeast Asia, sub-Saharan countries in Africa, and Brazil comprise the areas most affected at present (44,45). The mode of transmission of leprosy is unknown, but the transmissibility is thought to be low. The mechanism is probably inhalation of bacilli, which may be excreted from the nasal passages of a multibacillary patient or possibly implanted from organisms in the soil. High numbers of bacilli of *M. leprae* have been documented in the nasal mucosa of infected patients (100 million bacilli), and bacterial load in the nose has been proposed to correlate with immune response in leprosy patients (46). Direct person-to-person infection by means of the skin occurs rarely if at all. After inhalation, it is likely that bacilli pass through the blood to peripheral and cutaneous nerves, where infection and host reaction commence.

Immunopathologic Spectrum of Leprosy

The sequence of disease pathogenesis is complex, very chronic, and depends on host–mycobacteria immunologic interactions. The leprosy bacillus is nontoxic, and clinicopathologic manifestations are the result of immunopathology and/or the progressive accumulation of infected cells. Leprosy is the best example of a disease showing an immunopathologic spectrum whereby the host immune reaction to the infective agent ranges from apparently none to marked, with a consequent range of clinicopathologic manifestations (47,48). Tuberculoid leprosy indicates a high cellular immune response (i.e., T cells and macrophage activation) and few bacilli in tissues; at the opposite pole, lepromatous leprosy indicates an absent cellular immune response to *M. leprae* antigens, with no macrophage activation and abundant bacilli in tissues. The spectrum of leprosy is a continuum, and patients may move in either direction according to host response and treatment. The standard delineation follows that of Ridley and Jopling, with categories defined along the spectrum by a combination of clinical, microbiologic, histopathologic, and immunologic indices: TT (tuberculoid), BT (borderline tuberculoid), BB (midborderline), BL (borderline lepromatous), and LL (lepromatous). The term *borderline* is used to denote patterns that share some features of both tuberculoid and lepromatous leprosy (45,47).

TT and LL patients are stable, the former often self-healing and the latter remaining heavily infected unless given appropriate chemotherapy. Patients presenting at the BT point will

often downgrade toward BL leprosy in the absence of treatment. The central point of the spectrum (BB) is the most unstable, with most patients downgrading to LL if not treated. The term *indeterminate leprosy* is used to describe patients presenting with very early leprosy lesions that cannot be categorized along the immunopathologic spectrum and having the potential to self-heal or evolve into TT, BL, or LL leprosy.

It is likely that in endemic zones, a high proportion of people are infected by *M. leprae* but either have full immunity and no disease or have developed one or a few lesions that have self-healed without significant morbidity. The progression of infection and disease is summarized in Figure 21-4. Patients with determined leprosy are most numerous at the BT and LL points of the spectrum.

Staining of *Mycobacterium Leprae* Bacilli

The classic method for demonstrating leprosy bacilli in lesions is a modified Ziehl–Neelsen stain, where the degree of acid and alcohol removal of carbol fuchsin is less than in the methods used for identifying other mycobacteria. The Fite-Faraco method is the most used (48). Methenamine silver stains are also useful in detecting fragmented acid-fast bacilli. The sensitivity of detection of acid-fast bacilli by histologic means remains poor because about 1,000 bacilli per cubic centimeter of tissue must be present in order to detect one bacillus in a section. For lesions where bacilli are scanty, it is recommended that at least six sections be examined before declaring them negative (49). The standard enumeration of leprosy bacilli in lesions—the bacterial index (BI)—follows Ridley's logarithmic scale (which applies to both skin biopsies and slit skin smears).

- BI = 0: no bacilli observed
- BI = 1: 1 to 10 bacilli in 10 to 100 high-power fields (hpf, oil immersion)
- BI = 2: 1 to 10 bacilli in 1 to 10 hpf
- BI = 3: 1 to 10 bacilli per hpf
- BI = 4: 10 to 100 bacilli per hpf
- BI = 5: 100 to 1,000 bacilli per hpf
- BI = 6: >1,000 bacilli per hpf

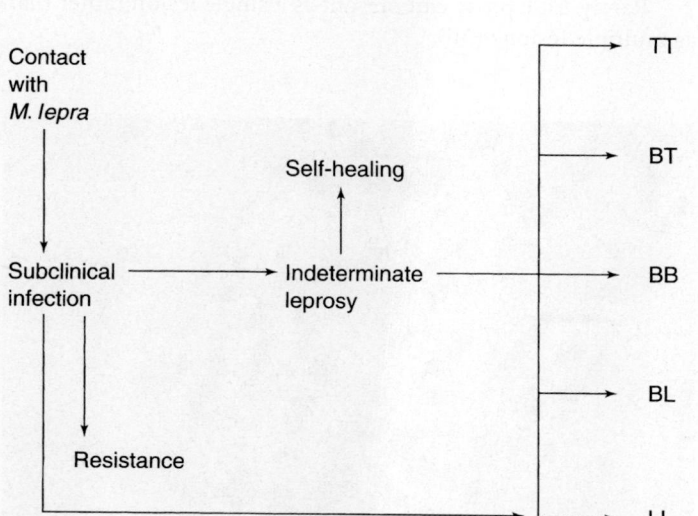
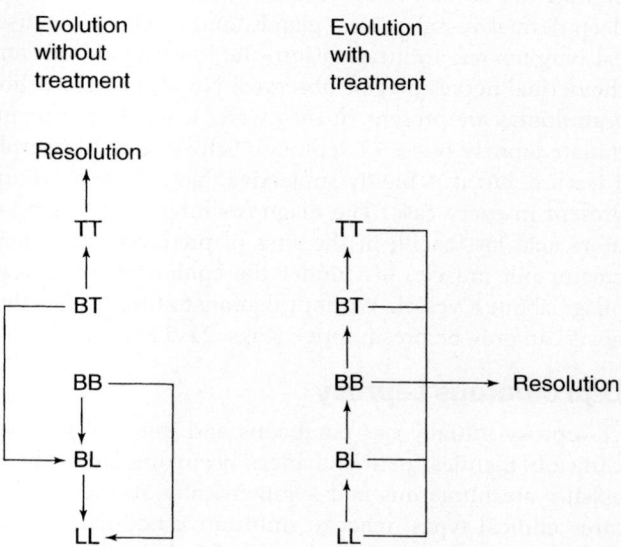

Figure 21-4 Leprosy. The sequence of events that may follow infection with *M. leprae*. (BB, midborderline; BL, borderline lepromatous; BT, borderline tuberculoid; LL, lepromatous; TT, tuberculoid.)

Solid-staining bacilli indicate that the organisms are capable of multiplication. Fragmented (beaded) and granular acid-fast bacilli indicate that they are dead. In 1998, the World Health Organization's (WHO) Expert Committee on Leprosy determined that therapy could be initiated before smear tests or skin biopsy was performed. Consequently, a rapid means of classification for worldwide application was established on the basis of the number of skin lesions. Patients with five or fewer skin lesions are termed *paucibacillary*, whereas patients with six or more skin lesions are termed *multibacillary* (45,50,51). This system has been criticized for misclassifying multibacillary patients as paucibacillary, with negative repercussions given that treatment for the paucibacillary form is only 6 months—compared with 12 for multibacillary (45,51).

Immunocytochemical methods for demonstrating mycobacterial antigens have a limited role. The most frequently used is a polyclonal anti-BCG antibody (52). In untreated lesions, it will not detect small numbers of bacilli if ordinary histochemical methods have proved negative. However, immunocytochemistry does have a role in demonstrating the presence of leprosy antigen after the bacilli have fragmented, been partly digested by macrophage enzymes, and lost their acid-fast staining quality.

Clinical Pathology of Leprosy

For general discussions of clinical leprosy and leprosy pathology, the reader is referred to Job (53) and Britton and Lockwood (45).

Early, Indeterminate Leprosy

Many patients present with obvious or advanced skin and peripheral nerve lesions (the latter are primarily nerve enlargement and the consequences of anesthesia). These patients have "determined leprosy." However, the earliest detectable skin lesion comprises one or a few hypopigmented macules with variable loss of sensation anywhere on the body. This is known as indeterminate leprosy, and it usually progresses to one of the major types of leprosy.

Histopathology. There is mild lymphocytic and macrophage accumulation around neurovascular bundles, the superficial and deep dermal vessels, sweat glands, and erector pili muscle; focal lymphocytic infiltration into the lower epidermis and into the dermal nerves may be observed. No formed epithelioid cell granulomas are present (if they were, it would not be indeterminate leprosy but a TT leprosy). Schwann cell hyperplasia is a feature, but it is highly subjective. Not all these features are present in every case. The diagnosis hinges on finding one or more acid-fast bacilli in the sites of predilection: in nerve, in erector pili muscle, just under the epidermis, or in a macrophage about a vessel. Without demonstrating bacilli, the diagnosis can only be presumptive (Figs. 21-5 and 21-6).

Lepromatous Leprosy

LL leprosy initially has cutaneous and mucosal lesions, with clinically manifest neural changes occurring later. The lesions usually are numerous and symmetrically arranged. There are three clinical types: macular, infiltrative-nodular, and diffuse. In the macular type, numerous ill-defined, confluent, either hypopigmented or erythematous macules are observed. They are frequently slightly infiltrated. The infiltrative-nodular type, the classical and most common variety, may develop from the macular type or arise as such. It is characterized by papules, nodules,

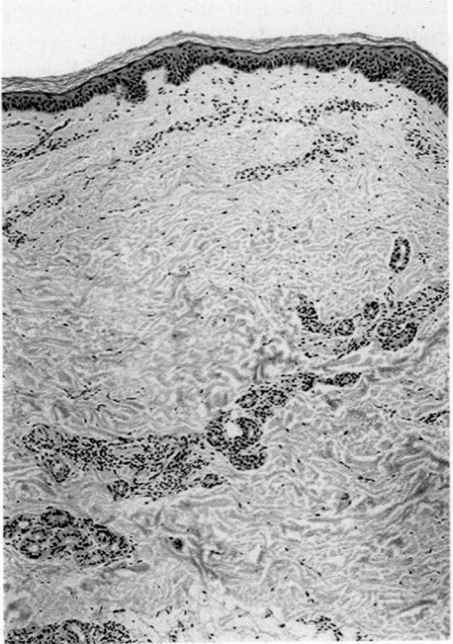

Figure 21-5 Indeterminate leprosy. Slight pandermal perineurovascular and periappendageal chronic inflammation (H&E stain).

and diffuse infiltrates that are often dull red. Involvement of the eyebrows and forehead often results in leonine facies, with loss of eyebrows and eyelashes. The lesions themselves are not notably hypoesthetic, although through involvement of the large peripheral nerves, disturbances of sensation and nerve paralyses develop. The nerves that are most commonly involved are the ulnar, radial, and common peroneal nerves.

The diffuse type of leprosy, called *Lucio leprosy*, which is most common in Mexico and Central America, shows diffuse infiltration of the skin without nodules. This infiltration may be quite inconspicuous except for the alopecia of the eyebrows and eyelashes it produces. Acral, symmetric anesthesia is generally present (54).

A distinctive variant of LL leprosy, the histoid type, first described in 1963 (55), is characterized by the occurrence of well-demarcated cutaneous and subcutaneous nodules resembling dermatofibromas.

Rarely, LL leprosy can present as a single lesion rather than as multiple lesions (56).

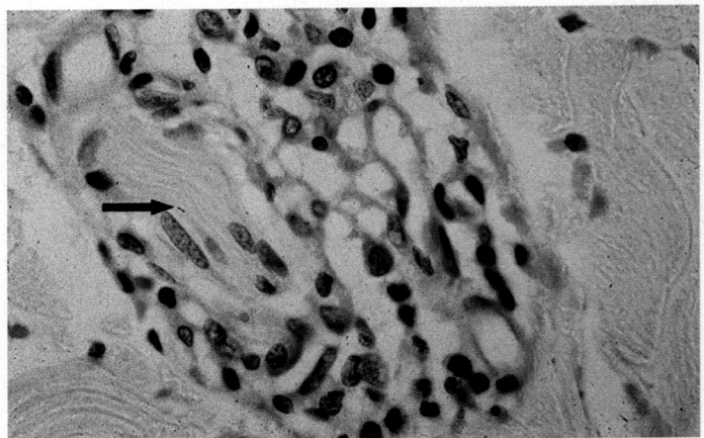

Figure 21-6 Indeterminate leprosy. High-power view of a small dermal nerve with surrounding lymphocytes and an intraneural acid-fast bacillus (*arrow*). There is no granuloma formation (Wade-Fite stain).

Histopathology. LL leprosy, in the usual macular or infiltrative-nodular lesions, exhibits an extensive cellular infiltrate that is almost invariably separated from the flattened epidermis by a narrow grenz zone of normal collagen (Figs. 21-7 and 21-8). The macular lesions show a mild-to-moderate, superficial and deep, perivascular and periadnexal infiltrate of foamy histiocytes. The infiltrate may cause the destruction of the cutaneous appendages and extends into the subcutaneous fat. In florid lesions, the macrophages have abundant eosinophilic cytoplasm and contain a mixed population of solid and fragmented bacilli (BI = 4 or 5) (Fig. 21-5). The bacilli, on Wade-Fite staining, can be seen to measure about 5.0 by 0.5 μm and, if solid, may be packed like cigars. Bacilli are commonly observed in endothelial cells as well (Fig. 21-9). There is no macrophage activation to form epithelioid cell granulomas. Lymphocyte infiltration is not prominent, but there may be many plasma cells.

In time, and with antimycobacterial chemotherapy, degenerate bacilli accumulate in the macrophages—the so-called lepra cells or Virchow cells—which then have foamy or vacuolated cytoplasm (Fig. 21-10). They resemble xanthoma cells and, on staining with fat stains, are shown to contain lipid—largely neutral fat and phospholipids—rather than cholesterol. The Wade-Fite stain reveals that the bacilli are fragmented or granular and, especially in very chronic lesions, disposed in large basophilic clumps called *globi*. In LL leprosy, in contrast to TT leprosy, the nerves in the skin may contain considerable numbers of leprosy bacilli but remain well preserved for a long time and slowly become fibrotic.

When LL leprosy is treated, the bacilli die rapidly and become fragmented within weeks or months. However, it can take several years for the bacterial debris to be cleared by host macrophages. The *M. leprae* antigen may persist even longer and can be demonstrated by immunocytochemical stains (Wade-Fite or silver) even when no bacilli are evident (Fig. 21-11).

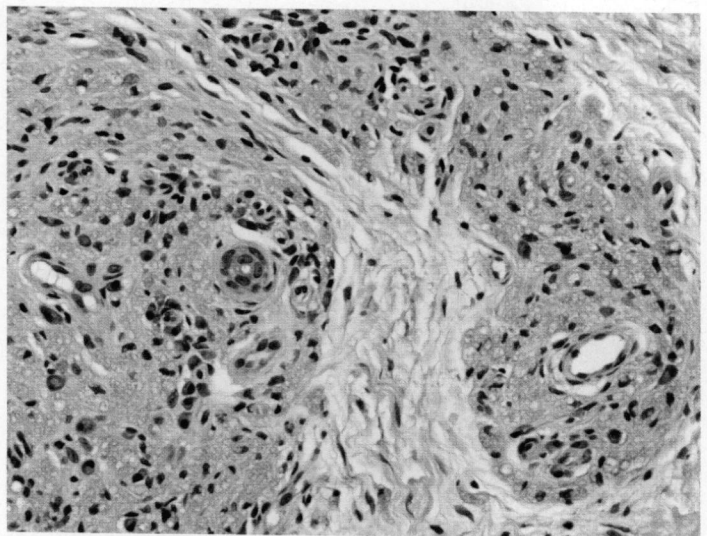

Figure 21-7 Lepromatous leprosy. Skin in multibacillary leprosy with a mass of macrophages in the dermis (no granuloma formation) (H&E stain).

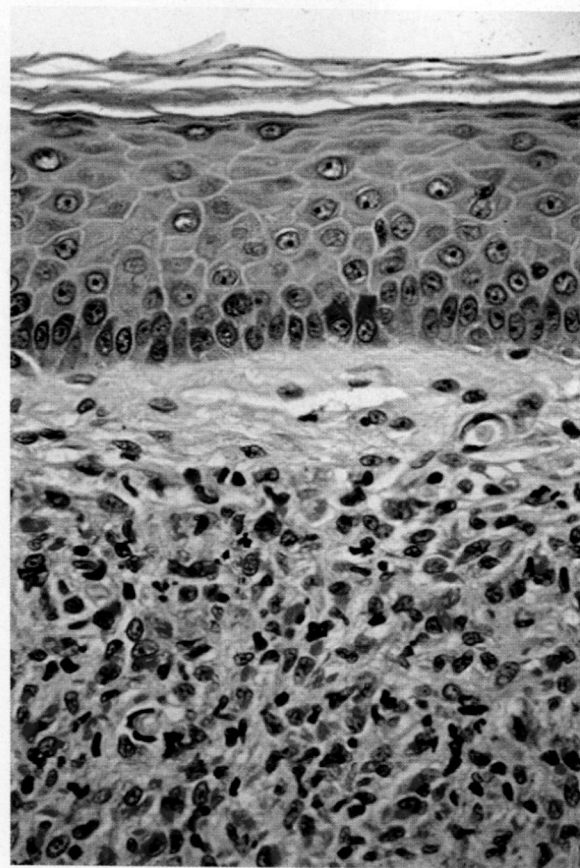

Figure 21-8 Lepromatous leprosy. Acid-fast bacilli, mostly solid, in large numbers (Fite-Faraco stain).

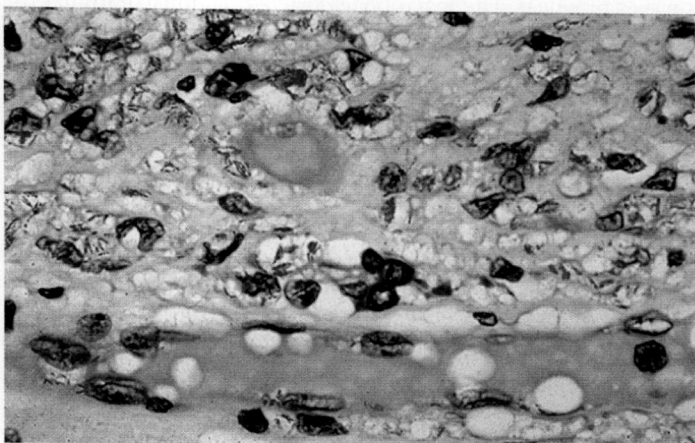

Figure 21-9 Lepromatous leprosy. Macrophages and endothelial cells of the capillary contain solid acid-fast bacilli (Wade-Fite stain).

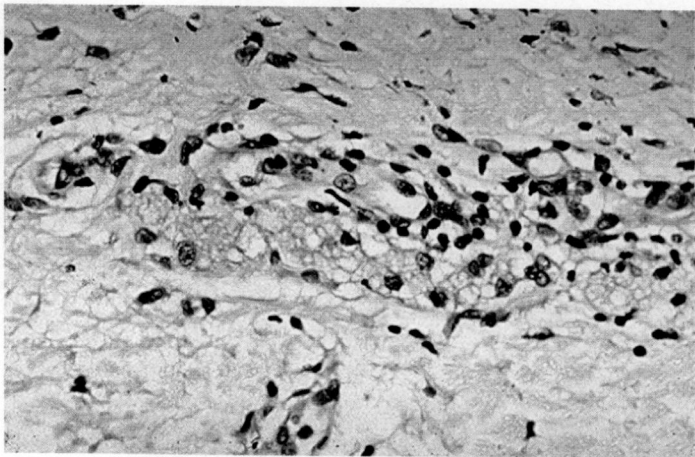

Figure 21-10 Lepromatous leprosy. Old, treated lesion, with large foamy macrophages and no identifiable bacilli (Wade-Fite stain).

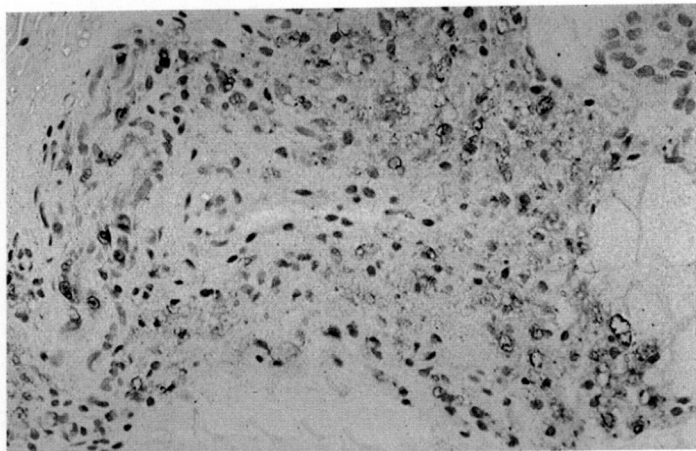

Figure 21-11 Lepromatous leprosy. Old, treated lesion; foamy macrophages remain but no acid-fast bacilli visible. However, an antimycobacterial immunocytochemical stain reveals persistent leprosy antigen (anti-BCG stain).

The histopathology of Lucio (diffuse) leprosy is similar but with a characteristic heavy bacillary infiltrate of the small blood vessels in the skin (54).

Histoid Leprosy

Histoid leprosy shows the highest loads of bacilli (frequently, the BI is 6), and the majority are solid staining and arranged in clumps like sheaves of wheat. The macrophage reaction is unusual in that the cells frequently become spindle shaped and oriented in a storiform pattern, similar to those of a fibrous histiocytoma (Fig. 21-12). The epidermis may be stretched over such dermal expansile nodules.

Borderline Lepromatous Leprosy

The lesions of BL leprosy are less numerous and less symmetrical than LL lesions and often display some central dimples.

Histopathology. The important difference between LL and BL leprosy histology is that in BL, the lymphocytes are more prominent, and there is a tendency for some activation of macrophages to form poorly to moderately defined granulomas. Perineural fibroblast proliferation, forming an "onion skin" in

cross section, is typical. Foamy cells are not prominent, and globi do not usually accumulate; the BI ranges from 4 to 5.

Midborderline Leprosy

In BB leprosy, the skin lesions are irregularly dispersed and shaped erythematous plaques with punched-out centers. There may be small satellite lesions. Edema is prominent in the lesions.

Histopathology. In BB leprosy, the macrophages are uniformly activated to epithelioid cells but are not focalized into distinct granulomas, and lymphocytes are scanty. There are no Langhans giant cells. The BI ranges from 3 to 4. Dermal edema is prominent between the inflammatory cells.

Borderline Tuberculoid Leprosy

In BT leprosy, the lesions are asymmetrical and may be scanty. They are dry, hairless plaques with central hypopigmentation. Nerve enlargement is usually found, and the lesions are usually anesthetic.

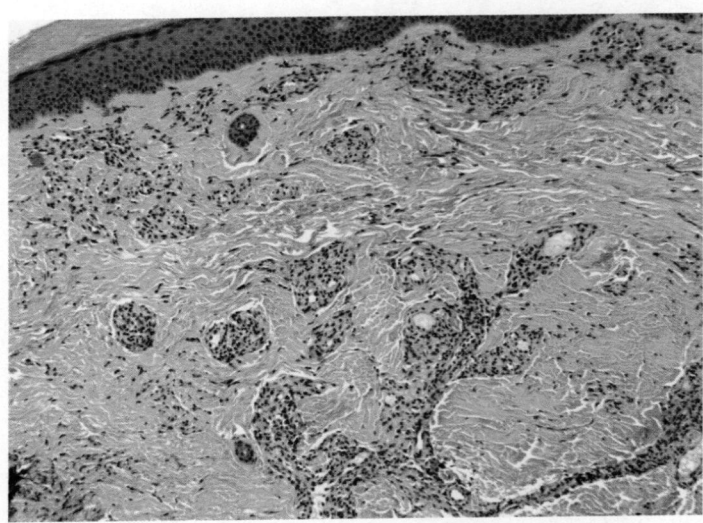

Figure 21-13 Tuberculoid leprosy. A typical lesion, showing pandermal perineurovascular granulomas and lymphocytes (H&E stain).

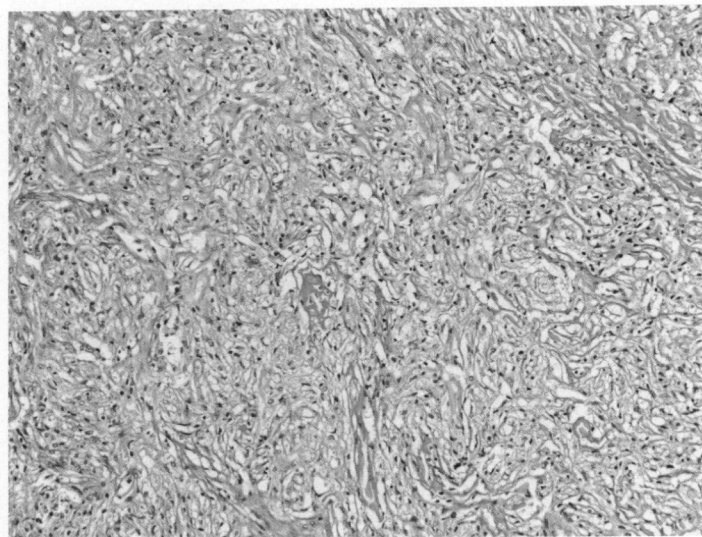

Figure 21-12 Lepromatous leprosy. A histoid lesion, with spindle cell proliferation of macrophages, resembling a storiform tumor. The acid-fast bacillus stain showed larger numbers of bacilli (H&E stain).

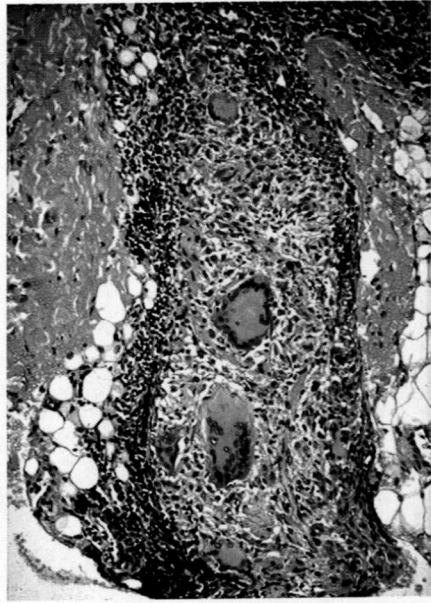

Figure 21-14 Tuberculoid leprosy. Granulomatous neuritis; dense lymphocytosis surrounding and eroding into the deep dermal nerve with giant cells (H&E stain).

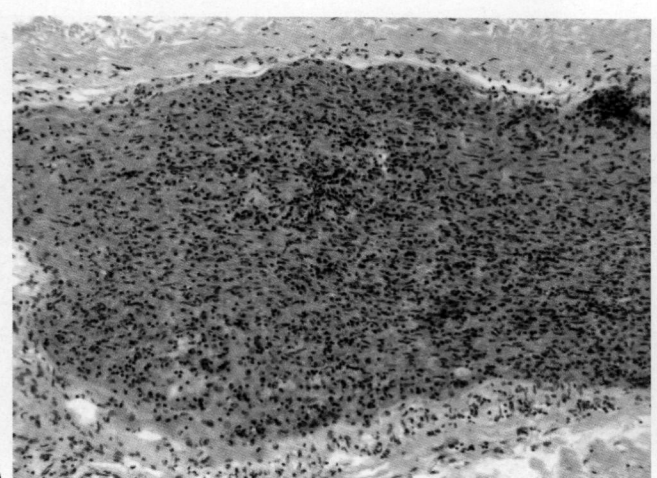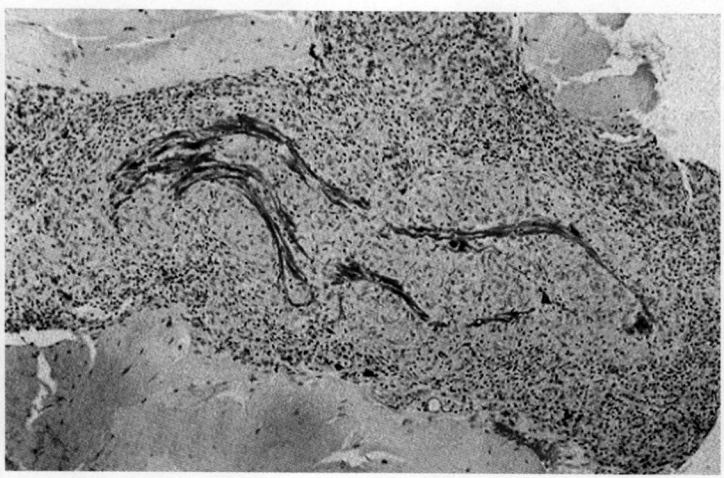

Figure 21-15 Tuberculoid leprosy. **A:** Typical endoneuritis with granulomas eroding into the nerve (H&E stain). **B:** Granulomatous neuritis; granulomas within the dermal nerve disrupting the Schwann cells and axons (S-100 immunoperoxidase stain).

Histopathology. Granulomas with peripheral lymphocytes follow the neurovascular bundles and infiltrate sweat glands and erector pili muscles. Langhans giant cells are variable in number and are not large. Granulomas along the superficial vascular plexus are frequent, but they do not infiltrate up into the epidermis. Nerve erosion and obliteration are typical (Figs. 21-13 to 21-15). Acid-fast bacilli are scanty (BI ranges from 0 to 2) and most readily found in the Schwann cells of nerves. Immunocytochemical staining for S-100 protein often demonstrates the perineural and intraneural granuloma well (Fig. 21-15B).

Tuberculoid Leprosy

The skin lesions of TT leprosy are scanty, dry, erythematous, hypopigmented papules or plaques with sharply defined edges. Anesthesia is prominent (except on the face). The number of lesions ranges from one to five. Thickened local peripheral nerves may be found. The lesions heal rapidly on chemotherapy.

Histopathology. Primary TT leprosy has large epithelioid cells arranged in compact granulomas along with neurovascular bundles, with dense peripheral lymphocyte accumulation. Langhans giant cells are typically absent. Dermal nerves may be absent (obliterated) or surrounded and eroded by dense lymphocyte cuffs. Acid-fast bacilli are rarely found, even in nerves. A second pattern of TT leprosy is found in certain reactional states (see p. 660).

Leprosy Reactions

Leprosy reactions are classified into two main types (1 and 2). A third reaction is specific to Lucio multibacillary leprosy (57,58).

Type 1 Reactions

Because the immunopathologic spectrum of leprosy is a continuum, patients may move along it in both directions. Should such shifts be rapid, they induce an inflammatory reaction with edema that results in enlargement of lesions with more erythema (Fig. 21-16).

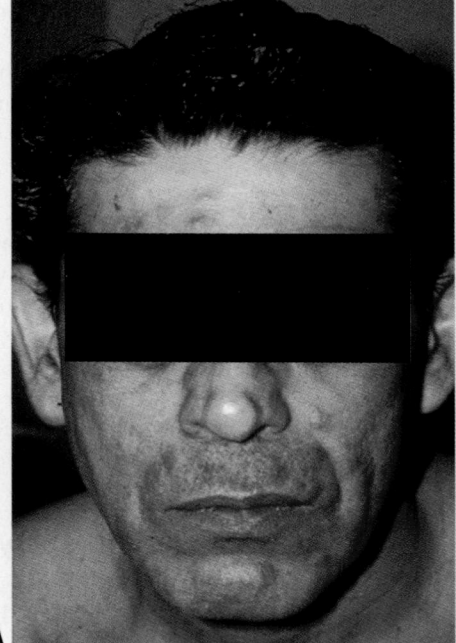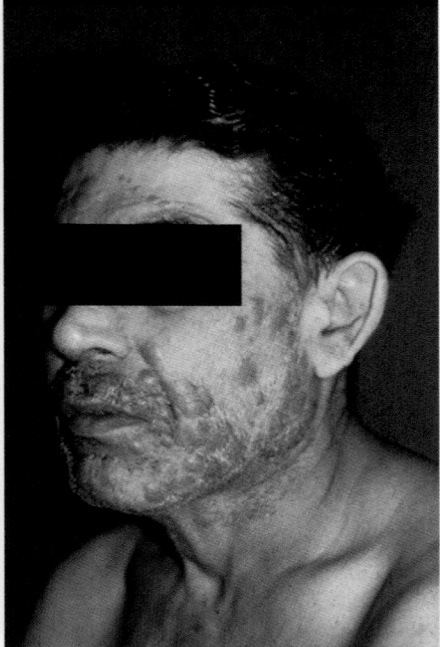

Figure 21-16 Leprosy reversal reaction. **A:** Pretreatment BL leprosy. **B:** Three months posttreatment, with enlargement of the skin lesions caused by increased inflammation.

Shifts toward the tuberculoid pole are called *upgrading* or *reversal reactions*; shifts toward the lepromatous pole are termed *downgrading reactions*. Both are aspects of delayed hypersensitivity, or type 1, leprosy reactions. TT patients are stable. BT patients may downgrade without treatment. Multibacillary patients, particularly those at the BL point, frequently upgrade on chemotherapy, and about one-quarter of them will exhibit significant reactions. BB patients are most unstable and will move either way depending on therapy, often with reactions. The most important aspect of type 1 reactions is not the skin but the condition of the peripheral nerves, in which a similar inflammatory process is going on; reaction induces increased intraneural inflammation and edema, which is damaging. At worst, there is caseous necrosis of large peripheral nerves resulting from upgrading reactions.

Histopathology. The histopathology of type 1 reactions is nonspecific. The morphologic changes, as described next, are difficult to evaluate, likely not reproducible, and insensitive. Therefore, the diagnosis must be made on clinical grounds alone. The distinction between upgrading and downgrading reactions is difficult to make and may require serial examinations. Typically, there is edema within and about the granulomas and proliferation of fibrocytes in the dermis. In upgrading reactions, the granuloma becomes more epithelioid and activated, and Langhans giant cells are larger (Fig. 21-17); there may be erosion of granulomas into the lower epidermis, and there may be fibrinoid necrosis within granulomas and even within dermal nerves. In downgrading reactions, necrosis is much less common, and over time the density of bacilli increases. Multibacillary leprosy patients who upgrade on therapy show old foamy macrophages and degenerate bacilli admixed with newly developing epithelioid cell granulomas (59).

Type 2 Reaction: Erythema Nodosum Leprosum

Erythema nodosum leprosum (ENL) occurs most commonly in LL leprosy and less frequently in BL leprosy. It may be observed not only in patients under treatment but also in untreated patients. Clinically, ENL manifests with tender red plaques and nodules, together with areas of erythema, and occasionally purpura and vesicles are also observed. Ulceration and erythema multiforme-like lesions, however, are rare. The eruption is widespread and accompanied by fever, malaise, arthralgia, and leukocytosis. New lesions appear for only a few days in some cases

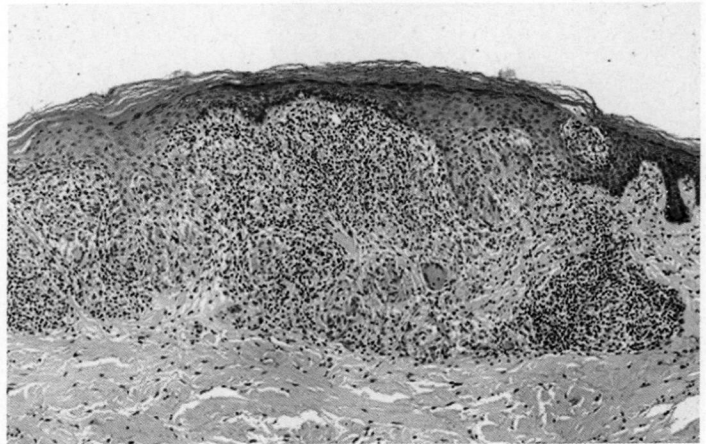

Figure 21-17 Leprosy: type 1 reaction (delayed hypersensitivity). Granulomatous erosion of the epidermis; this feature is not usually encountered in nonreacting leprosy (H&E stain).

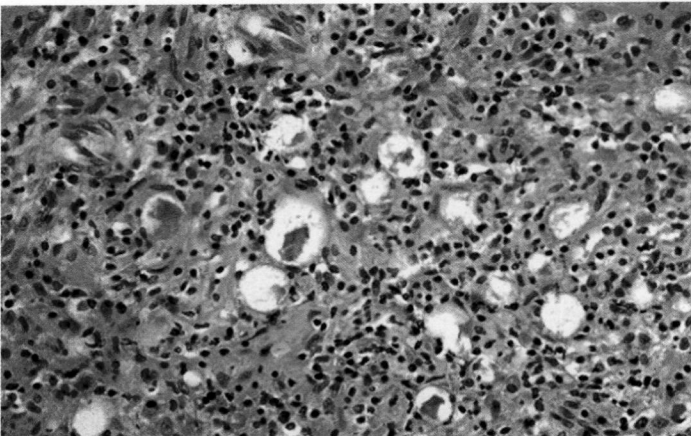

Figure 21-18 Leprosy: erythema nodosum leprosum (type 2 reaction). Macrophages with vacuoles and globi and a polymorphonuclear cell infiltrate (H&E stain).

but for weeks and even years in others. This is the only type of reactional leprosy that responds to treatment with thalidomide, although the range of treatment options has greatly expanded.

Histopathology. In ENL, the lesions are foci of neutrophilic inflammation superimposed on chronic multibacillary leprosy (Fig. 21-18). Polymorph neutrophils may be scanty or so abundant as to form a dermal abscess with ulceration (60). Whereas foamy macrophages containing fragmented bacilli are usual, in some patients no bacilli remain, and macrophages have a granular pink hue on Wade-Fite staining, indicating mycobacterial debris. An antimycobacterial immunocytochemical stain (e.g., anti-BCG) will indicate abundant antigen. A necrotizing vasculitis affecting arterioles, venules, and capillaries occurs in some cases of ENL; these patients may have superficial ulceration.

Lucio Reaction

The Lucio reaction occurs exclusively in diffuse LL leprosy, in which it is a fairly common complication. It usually occurs in patients who have received either no treatment or inadequate treatment. In contrast to ENL, fever, tenderness, and leukocytosis are absent. The lesions consist of barely palpable, hemorrhagic, sharply marginated, irregular plaques. They develop into crusted lesions and, particularly on the legs, into ulcers. There may be repeated attacks or continuous appearance of new lesions for years. They are thought to result from immune complex deposition.

Histopathology. In the Lucio reaction, vascular changes are critical (48). Endothelial proliferation leading to lumenal obliteration is observed in association with thrombosis in the medium-sized vessels of the dermis and subcutis. There is a sparse, largely mononuclear infiltrate. Dense aggregates of acid-fast bacilli are found in the walls and the endothelium of normal-appearing vessels as well as in vessels with proliferative changes (Fig. 21-19). Ischemic necrosis, brought on by the vascular occlusion, leads to hemorrhagic infarcts and results in crusted erosions or frank ulcers.

Electron Microscopy of Leprosy

Under electron microscopy, *M. leprae* can be seen to consist of an electron-dense cytoplasm lined by a trilaminal plasma membrane. Outside of this membrane lies the bacterial cell wall surrounded by a radiolucent area, the waxy coating typical of

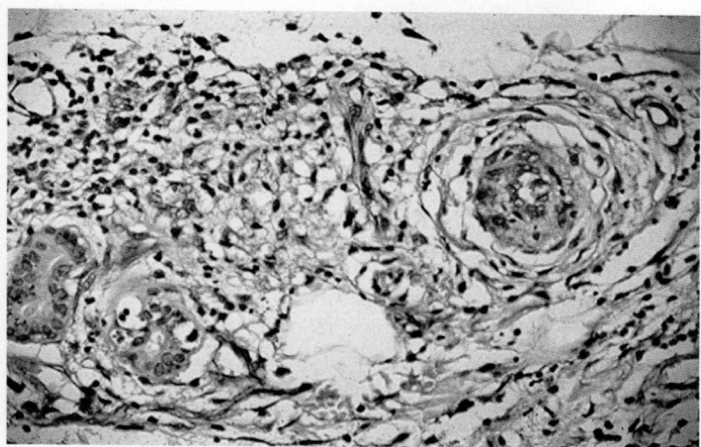

Figure 21-19 Leprosy, Lucio reaction. Dermal vessels showing endarteritis obliterans and abundant bacilli within endothelial cells (Wade-Fite stain).

mycobacteria (43). Lepra bacilli are found in the skin, predominantly in macrophages and in Schwann cells.

Pathogenesis of Leprosy

With respect to immunologic reactivity, patients with LL leprosy have a defect in cell-mediated immune responses to the lepra bacilli, which therefore cannot be eradicated from the body spontaneously (45,61,62). The primary defect lies in the T lymphocytes, which can be stimulated only slightly or not at all to react against the lepra bacilli and thus do not adequately activate macrophages to destroy phagocytosed bacilli. This defect is specific for *M. leprae* because patients with LL leprosy show normal immunologic responses to antigens other than lepromin in both *in vivo* and *in vitro* testing.

The specific inability of T lymphocytes obtained from patients with LL leprosy to react against lepromin is shown by the fact that when these lymphocytes are incubated with lepromin, they show little or no production of macrophage migration-inhibiting factor (MIF). In contrast, the lymphocytes of patients with TT leprosy produce significant amounts of MIF on exposure to lepromin. One modern view is that in tuberculoid patients, exposure to leprosy antigens results in a predominant T-helper 1 (T_H1) cytokine secretion profile, which results in macrophage activation. Conversely, in lepromatous patients, the cytokine profile (T_H2) inhibits cell-mediated immunity and promotes humoral immunity, which does not contribute to host defense (61,63). In reversal reactions, there is an increase in the lymphocyte response to lepromin during the reaction and a decrease during the postreaction phase.

Analysis of T-cell subsets in lesions has shown that in TT leprosy, with its high degree of resistance to the leprosy bacilli, the T-helper lymphocytes are distributed evenly throughout the epithelioid cell aggregates and that the suppressor T lymphocytes are restricted to the peripheries of the granulomas. In LL leprosy, both helper and suppressor T lymphocytes are distributed diffusely throughout the lesions (64). It is noteworthy that the distribution of helper and suppressor T cells in TT leprosy is similar to that observed in sarcoidosis.

In patients with either ENL or the Lucio reaction, deposits of IgG and the third component of complement (C3), as well as circulating immune complexes, have been found in the vessel walls of the dermal lesions. This suggests that both reactions are mediated by immune complexes (Gell and Coombs type III reaction) (52).

The lepromin skin test, or Mitsuda test, consists of the intradermal injection of a preparation of *M. leprae* derived from autoclaved infected human tissue. A positive reaction consists of the formation of a nodule measuring 5 mm in diameter or more after 2 to 4 weeks. On histologic examination, the nodule shows an epithelioid cell granuloma. The reaction is positive only in the high-resistance (TT and BT tuberculoid) forms of the disease. In indeterminate leprosy, it may be positive or negative. The test reveals the inability of patients at the lepromatous end of the spectrum to react to the injection of *M. leprae* with an epithelioid cell granuloma, and its main value is therefore as a marker of specific cell-mediated immunity to this organism. Because HIV induces a generalized immunosuppressive state, a wide range of intracellular infectious agents normally controlled by the T-cell/macrophage system may proliferate to cause significant disease. Accordingly, it was expected that leprosy might become more prevalent in HIV and leprosy coendemic areas and that individual patients might downgrade toward lepromatous disease as their HIV disease progressed. However, epidemiologic studies have shown no effect of HIV infection on the incidence of leprosy in properly controlled studies (65,66), nor has a change in the proportions of tuberculoid versus lepromatous patients been noted (67). The only clinicopathologic difference between HIV-infected and noninfected leprosy patients that is suggested is an increased likelihood of HIV-positive patients undergoing type 1 upgrading reactions (67,68).

Histopathologic Differential Diagnosis

The leprosy bacillus cannot yet be grown *in vitro*. TT (granulomatous) leprosy needs to be distinguished from the many other granulomatous dermatitides. The presence of acid-fast bacilli in nerves is conclusive proof of leprosy, as is the demonstration of an intraneural granuloma. The S-100 stain may highlight this phenomenon (69), although in practice, if the diagnosis is in doubt after investigation with ordinary stains, this immunocytochemical method is not usually diagnostic either. In leprosy, naked granulomas are found only in BB leprosy, and acid-fast bacilli will be found in the lesions. Sarcoidosis may rarely cause granulomas to form within peripheral nerves and has rarely been reported to mimic leprosy (70). The general vertical perineurovascular distribution of granulomatous inflammation and involvement of sweat glands in TT leprosy are helpful. The presence or absence of plasma cells or of intraepidermal lymphocytes is not helpful. Unlike other mycobacterial skin infections such as tuberculosis, and unlike granulomatous leishmaniasis, the epidermis in TT leprosy is usually flat and nonhyperplastic. Late secondary and tertiary cutaneous syphilis is characterized by epithelioid and giant cell granulomas in the dermis, not directly involving nerves, and the epithelium is usually hyperplastic. Intragranuloma necrosis (fibrinoid or caseating) occurs in leprosy in type 1 reactions, sometimes spontaneously; this can be confused with necrobiotic lesions such as granuloma annulare. Necrosis within a nerve that is granulomatous is diagnostic of leprosy.

Early, indeterminate leprosy overlaps with many nonspecific dermatitides manifesting perineurovascular lymphocytic infiltrates. Finding bacilli in a nerve, under the epidermis, in erector pili muscle, or in macrophages is critical to make the diagnosis. In the absence of bacilli and the presence of a pandermal infiltrate, leprosy can only be suspected. Problems may arise from contaminant mycobacteria in staining solutions and in the water baths used for floating out sections. Such organisms are usually above the plane of the section, overlap the cell nuclei, and usually stain darker than *M. leprae*. The use of polymerase chain reaction (PCR) for identifying paucibacillary leprosy in skin sections has been greatly improved (71), but it is used mainly in research, and clinical testing is not widely available.

Ultimately, there are a proportion of suspect paucibacillary leprosy lesions for which the histopathologist cannot make a firm diagnosis either way, and intra- and interobserver variation may be considerable (72).

LL leprosy infiltrates can resemble xanthoma, although the cytoplasmic granularity is coarser in the latter disease. The presence of acid-fast bacilli is obviously important, and in long-treated lesions that may cause confusion, antimycobacterial immunocytochemistry is helpful. ENL may be overlooked because it is a combined chronic and acute inflammatory infiltrate, but once thought of, the presence of bacilli or antigen is diagnostic. Certain other mycobacterioses in immunosuppressed patients, such as *M. avium* complex, may produce histoid-like multibacillary lesions (73) (see Figs. 21-30 to 21-32); however, nerves are not involved in this infection.

Principles of Management

Multidrug therapy is essential to prevent development of resistance. Common regimens include dapsone plus rifampin for TT leprosy, and clofazimine may be added to these for LL leprosy, for 6 and 12 months, respectively. Treatment algorithms depend somewhat on the burden of disease, and all patients with a diagnosis of leprosy should be treated in conjunction with an infectious disease specialist. Neuritis and immunologic reactions may be treated with corticosteroids with or without other anti-inflammatory agents. Type 1 reactions may be observed in HIV patients after initiation of antiretroviral therapy. The response to treatment appears to be comparable among HIV-positive and HIV-negative individuals (51).

TUBERCULOSIS

Tuberculosis remains a dominant public health problem in resource-poor countries and has reemerged in the remaining countries around the world owing to a global resurgence. Factors leading to the increased incidence of tuberculosis include immigration from endemic countries (particularly in Asia and Africa), increased movement of refugees, the HIV pandemic, and poverty (74). As a result, cutaneous tuberculosis remains a clinical and diagnostic problem (75,76). It is estimated that cutaneous tuberculosis accounts for a small proportion of all tuberculosis infections (1% to 2%), but given the high prevalence of tuberculosis in some areas, the absolute number of cases is not insignificant (77).

Infection of the skin and subcutis by *M. tuberculosis* occurs by three routes: (a) by direct inoculation into the skin (causing a primary chancre or tuberculosis verrucosa cutis [TVC] or tuberculosis cutis orificialis lesions); (b) by hematogenous spread from an internal lesion (causing lupus vulgaris, miliary tuberculosis, and tuberculous gumma lesions); and (c) from an underlying tuberculous lymph node by direct extension

(causing scrofuloderma). For descriptive purposes, these different tuberculous dermatitides are delineated (a modified "Beyt classification" is used) (40). But in clinical practice, many cases do not readily fit into these clinical and histologic categories (41,78,79). Scrofuloderma and lupus vulgaris appear to be the most common forms (77). In a study of cutaneous manifestations associated with tuberculosis in a pediatric population from India, with histopathologic evaluation, there was a large spectrum of clinical patterns. The different patterns seen were scrofuloderma (37%), lichen scrofulosorum (33%), lupus vulgaris (21%), TVC (4%), papulonecrotic tuberculid (4%), and erythema nodosum (3%). Systemic associations were seen in 53%, namely tuberculosis lymphadenitis (30%), pulmonary tuberculosis (13%), abdominal tuberculosis (6%), and tuberculosis arthritis (6%) (80).

The basic reaction of human tissues to tuberculous bacilli is a sequence, first of acute nonspecific inflammation, during which the bacilli multiply and cannot be phagocytosed and killed by neutrophil polymorphs. Macrophages then phagocytose the organisms, but their efficacy in killing them depends crucially on enhanced activation. T-cell–mediated immunity to tuberculous antigens induces secretion of cytokines that recruit and activate macrophages, which become epithelioid cells. Some will fuse to form giant cells, the typical form of which in tuberculosis is the Langhans giant cell with the nuclei arranged around the periphery of the cytoplasm. As delayed hypersensitivity increases, there is caseation necrosis within the granuloma, caseation being a homogeneous eosinophilic infarct-like necrotic process whereby the macrophages die. It is probably mediated by cytokines (such as tumor necrosis factor [TNF]) and the macrophage proteases. This necrotic process inactivates or kills many of the mycobacteria in the lesion but does not eliminate them (81,82).

The necrotic granuloma is thus typical of tuberculosis and other mycobacterial infections, but it is not specific, being seen in numerous other infections that involve this type of cell-mediated immunity (e.g., histoplasmosis, syphilis, and leishmaniasis).

M. tuberculosis is an obligate aerobe and thrives at a pO_2 of 140 mm Hg, which is near the pO_2 of atmospheric air. This is why in conditions like scrofuloderma, where the lesion is exposed to the outside air, bacterial growth, and consequent detection on smears and sections, is much higher than in other forms of cutaneous tuberculosis.

The determinants of what happens in tuberculosis infection therefore include the virulence of the organism (tuberculosis is more virulent than most of the nontuberculosis mycobacteria), the size of the inoculum, the route of infection, and the immune status of the patient. It is evident that if cell-mediated immunity is impaired, the T-cell/macrophage system will not operate to contain the infection. The resulting pathology is generally less granulomatous (fewer activated macrophages) and has a higher density of mycobacteria. Such conditions are HIV infection with its sequel to AIDS, steroid therapy, and cytotoxic drugs. The concept of bacterial load in cutaneous tuberculosis has been proposed (analogously to that described for *M. leprae* in Hansen disease). Accordingly, cutaneous tuberculosis can be subclassified into multibacillary forms (primary inoculation tuberculosis, scrofuloderma, tuberculosis periorificialis, acute miliary tuberculosis, and gumma) and paucibacillary forms (TVC, occasional forms of lupus vulgaris, papulonecrotic tuberculid, erythema induratum of Bazin, and lichen scrofulosorum) (77).

Multibacillary Forms

In the multibacillary forms of tuberculosis, numerous mycobacteria can be frequently demonstrated using the Ziehl–Neelsen technique and are more readily cultured (83).

Primary Tuberculosis

Clinical Summary. Primary infection with tuberculosis occurs only rarely on the skin. Children or adults may acquire it following minor trauma or contact with infected material—as a result, for instance, of mouth-to-mouth artificial respiration (84), inoculation during an autopsy (85), needle-stick injury (86), or inoculation during tattooing (87). Not surprisingly, this form of cutaneous tuberculosis is frequent in health care and laboratory personnel. Affected children are usually infected through exposure to a household member or caregiver with active pulmonary tuberculosis. The most commonly affected sites are face, hands, and feet. In countries where tuberculosis is endemic, such as India, some patients develop primary (or more often secondary) infection on the soles of the feet, from walking barefoot over expectorated tuberculosis. Primary gingivitis, granulomatous paronychia, and penile chancre are considered variants of this form. The primary lesion is typically a papule or nodule that eventually ulcerates (77). Usually, the fully developed cutaneous lesion arises within 2 to 4 weeks after the inoculation. It consists of an asymptomatic crust-covered ulcer referred to as *tuberculous chancre.* The regional lymph nodes become enlarged and tender and may suppurate and produce draining sinuses.

Histopathology. The histologic development of the lesion is very much like that observed in experimental cutaneous inoculation of the guinea pig. In the earliest phase, the histologic picture is that of an acute neutrophilic reaction, with areas of necrosis resulting in ulceration. Numerous tubercle bacilli are present, particularly in the areas of necrosis (85). After 2 weeks, monocytes and macrophages predominate. Three to 6 weeks after onset, epithelioid cells and giant cell granulomas develop, followed by caseation necrosis within the granuloma (Fig. 21-20). In time, the necrosis lessens, and the number of tubercle bacilli

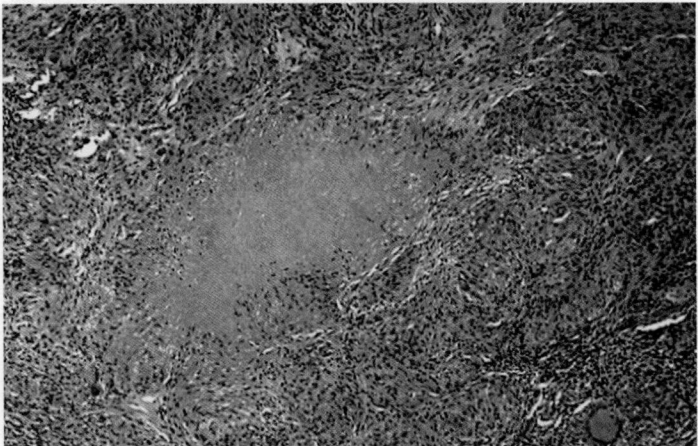

Figure 21-20 Tuberculosis. A prosector's wart following inoculation of the finger from a tuberculous cadaver. There is central caseation necrosis with dense macrophage and lymphocyte surround (H&E stain).

decreases until it is so greatly reduced that the bacilli may be impossible to demonstrate in histologic sections. Simultaneous with the decrease in the number of tubercle bacilli in the lesion, the tuberculin test with purified protein derivative (PPD), previously negative, becomes positive. The draining lymph nodes receive tubercle bacilli and enlarge through developing caseating granulomas, parallel to a primary infection in the lung. Of note, primary cutaneous tuberculosis only rarely evolves into disseminated disease.

Scrofuloderma

Clinical Summary. Scrofuloderma is the most common form of cutaneous tuberculosis in developing countries, and some series from Europe. It represents a direct extension to the skin of an underlying tuberculous infection present most commonly in a lymph node, and less commonly in joints or a bone. The lesion first manifests itself as a blue-red, painless swelling that breaks open and then forms an ulcer with irregular, undermined, blue borders. The ulcer is frequently surrounded by keloidal cicatricial tissue. The axillae, neck, chest wall, and inguinal region are most affected. Patients typically have active pulmonary or pleural tuberculosis (77).

Histopathology. The center of the lesion usually exhibits nonspecific changes, such as abscess formation or ulceration. In the deeper portions and at the periphery of the lesion, if the biopsy specimen is adequate, tuberculoid granulomas with a considerable amount of necrosis and a pronounced inflammatory reaction are usually seen. Often, the number of tubercle bacilli is sufficient for them to be found in acid-fast stained histologic sections. The PPD is typically strongly positive.

Tuberculosis Cutis Orificialis

Clinical Summary. This form of cutaneous tuberculosis is rare. The lesions of tuberculosis cutis orificialis (periorificial tuberculosis) are shallow, painful ulcers (in contrast to mucocutaneous leishmaniasis and rhinoscleroma, which are typically nonpainful) with a granulating base occurring singly or in small numbers on or near the mucosal orifices of patients with advanced internal tuberculosis. The infection has spread by direct contamination from an internal lesion that is excreting bacilli. Most patients have a low degree of immunity. The ulcers, which are often very tender, may occur inside the mouth, on the lips, around the anus, or on the perineum (88). Anal lesions must be differentiated from malignancy. In the case of genitourinary tuberculosis, ulcers may occur on the vulva.

Histopathology. The histologic picture may show merely an ulcer surrounded by a nonspecific inflammatory infiltrate. In most instances, tuberculoid granulomas with pronounced necrosis are found deep in the dermis. Tubercle bacilli are usually readily demonstrated in the sections, even when the histologic appearance is nonspecific.

Acute Miliary Tuberculosis

Clinical Summary. Involvement of the skin with miliary tuberculosis is rare in the immunocompetent, occurring mostly in children and adolescents and only occasionally in adults. Usually, internal involvement is widespread as a result of hematogenous dissemination, and the cutaneous eruption is generalized, consisting of erythematous papules and pustules 2 to 5 mm in diameter (89). The tuberculin test is generally negative. The disease has a high fatality rate.

However, a milder form of hematogenous dissemination of tubercle bacilli exists in neonates born of tuberculous mothers. This form shows limited visceral involvement and only a few scattered erythematous papules with central crusts (90).

Histopathology. In severe cases, the center of the papule shows a microabscess containing neutrophils, cellular debris, and numerous tubercle bacilli. This is surrounded by a zone of macrophages with occasional giant cells. In the milder form, the histologic picture in the skin is similar, except that the Ziehl–Neelsen stain is negative for acid-fast organisms.

Tuberculous Gumma

Clinical Summary. Tuberculous gummas are cold abscesses typically occurring on the trunk or extremities of patients with no involvement of the underlying tissue. They are thought to represent hematogenous infection of the skin from an internal lesion that remains latent, and under the appropriate conditions (malnutrition, immunosuppression) may result in a large dermal or subcutaneous nodule that is necrotic and that ultimately ulcerates the epidermis.

Histopathology. Most of the lesion is caseation necrosis with a rim of epithelioid cells and giant cells (Figs. 21-21 and 21-22). Acid-fast bacilli are scanty but usually demonstrable on histologic sections.

Paucibacillary Forms

In the paucibacillary forms, mycobacteria may be difficult or impossible to detect using the Ziehl–Neelsen technique and are less readily cultured (83).

Tuberculosis Verrucosa Cutis

Clinical Summary. TVC represents an inoculated exogenous infection of the skin in persons with a degree of immunity—that is, previous exposure to tuberculosis. In TVC, a single, painless verrucous plaque with an inflammatory border and showing gradual peripheral extension is usually observed. The verrucous surface exhibits fissures from which pus can often be expressed. The most common sites are the hands and, in children, the knees, buttocks, thighs, and feet.

Histopathology. The characteristic histologic picture is that of pseudocarcinomatous squamous hyperplasia with marked hyperkeratosis and acanthosis. Beneath the epidermis, there is often a

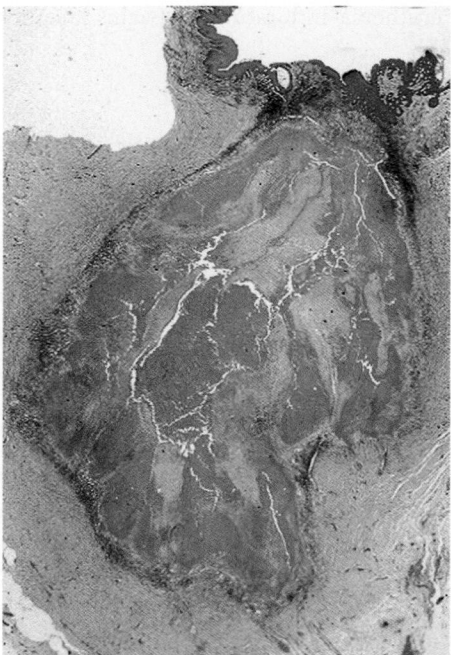

Figure 21-22 Tuberculosis. A tuberculoma-like appearance with much caseation necrosis in the dermis (H&E stain).

mixed lymphohistiocytic infiltrate with an occasional sprinkling of neutrophils. This may have a lichenoid appearance. Abscess formation may be observed in the upper dermis or within downward extensions of the epidermis. In the mid-dermis or upper dermis, tuberculoid granulomas are usually present, although multiple step sections often need to be cut before a granuloma is found (Fig. 21-23). Identification of tuberculous bacilli and/or their isolation from culture is the exception rather than the rule. Lesions tend to chronicity but may remain sensitive to antituberculous treatment, which may function as a diagnostic aid (77).

Lupus Vulgaris

Clinical Summary. Lupus, which translates into "wolf" in Latin, was initially used to refer to any ulcerative lesion resembling a wolf bite. In 1808, Willan used the word lupus for the first time to describe the late stages of facial cutaneous tuberculosis in his

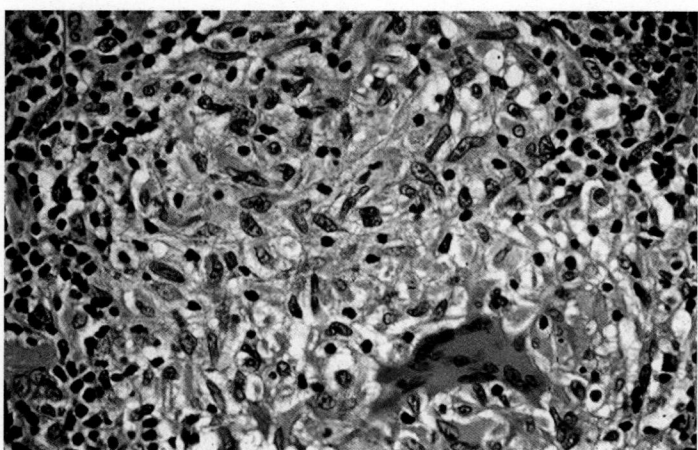

Figure 21-21 Lupus vulgaris. Same lesion as in Figure 21-25, showing an epithelioid cell granuloma and Langhans giant cell (H&E stain).

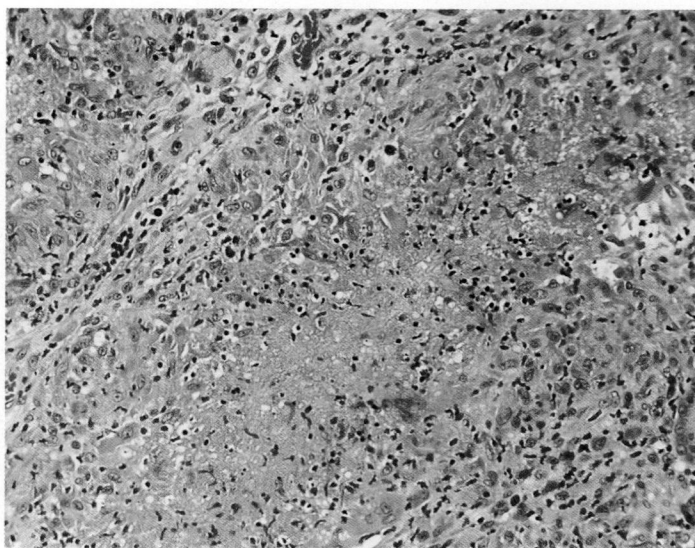

Figure 21-23 Tuberculosis. An epithelioid cell granuloma and caseation (H&E stain).

book "On Cutaneous Diseases." Lupus vulgaris is the most common form of cutaneous tuberculosis in India and Pakistan, and it used to be the predominant form encountered in Europe. The lesions of lupus vulgaris are usually found on the face. The skin of and around the nose is frequently involved (91). The primary lesion consists of one or a few well-demarcated, reddish-brown patches containing deep-seated nodules, each about 1 mm in diameter, known as "lupomes." If the blood is pressed out of the skin with a glass slide (diascopy), these nodules stand out clearly as yellow-brown macules, referred to, because of their color, as *apple-jelly nodules*. The characteristic fully developed lesion is a slowly enlarging plaque with a slightly elevated, verruciform border and central atrophy. It is a characteristic feature of lupus vulgaris that new lesions may appear in areas of atrophy, particularly after temporal immunosuppression. Superficial ulceration or verrucous thickening of the skin occurs occasionally. Squamous cell carcinoma develops at the margins of ulcers in rare instances.

Histopathology. Tuberculoid granulomas composed of epithelioid cells and giant cells are present. Caseation necrosis within the tubercles is slight or absent (92). Although the giant cells are usually of the Langhans type, with peripheral arrangement of the nuclei, some can be of the foreign body type, with irregular arrangement of the nuclei. There is an associated infiltrate of lymphocytes (Figs. 21-24 and 21-25). Sometimes, this may be

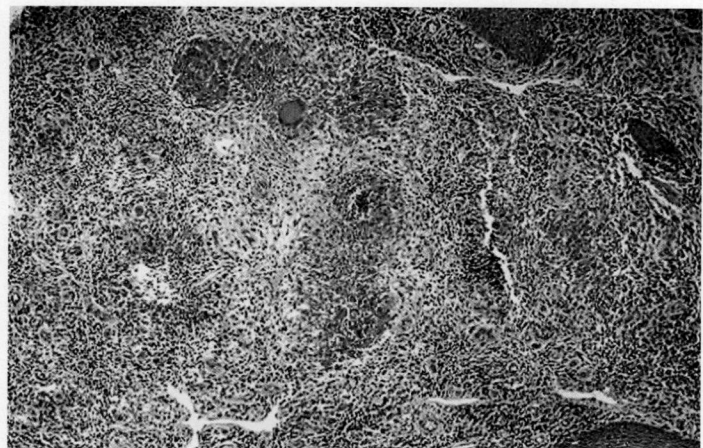

Figure 21-24 Tuberculosis. Epithelioid cell granulomas with central acute inflammation ("mixed" granuloma). Scanty acid-fast bacilli were seen in this case (H&E stain).

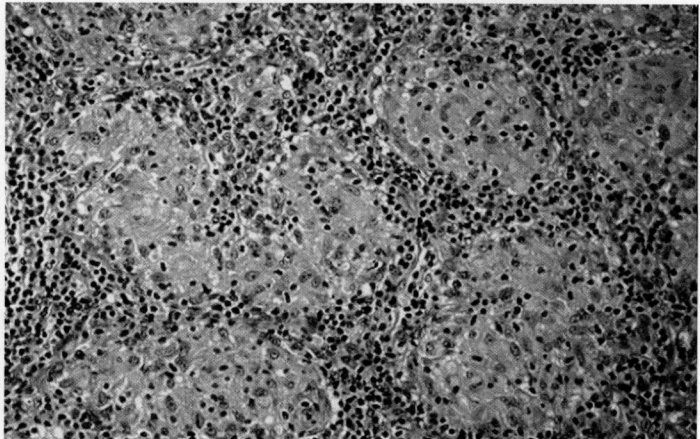

Figure 21-25 Lupus vulgaris. Near-confluent nonnecrotizing epithelioid cell granulomas in the dermis (H&E stain).

so prominent that the granulomatous component is obscured. This is often seen in TVC-like lesions. Tuberculoid granulomas cause destruction of the cutaneous appendages. In areas of healing, extensive fibrosis may be present.

Secondary changes in the epidermis are common. The epidermis may undergo atrophy and subsequent destruction, causing ulceration, or it may become hyperplastic, showing acanthosis, hyperkeratosis, and papillomatosis. At the margins of ulcers, pseudoepitheliomatous hyperplasia often exists. Unless a deep biopsy is done in such cases, only the epithelial hyperplasia and a nonspecific inflammation may be seen, and the diagnosis may be missed. In rare instances, squamous cell carcinoma supervenes (93).

Tubercle bacilli are present in such small numbers that they can very rarely be demonstrated by staining methods or mycobacterial culture. Single case reports and small series have suggested that PCR detection of mycobacterial DNA is more often positive (94). However, the difference in sensitivity when comparing PCR with histopathologic sections stained with the Ziehl–Neelsen technique was only marginal in the largest series (79.4% vs. 73.5%, respectively) and not statistically significant (95). In some instances of lupus vulgaris, when an old focus of primary infection cannot be detected, a positive tuberculin test and the response to antituberculous therapy must suffice as proof of a tuberculous etiology.

Pathogenesis. Lupus vulgaris is a form of secondary or reactivation tuberculosis developing in previously infected and sensitized persons. Hypersensitivity to PPD tuberculin is high. Although the mode of infection is often not apparent, the disease rarely seems to be the result of an exogenous reinfection of the skin; it usually results from hematogenous spread from an old, reactivated focus in the lung or from lymphatic extension from a tuberculous cervical lymphadenitis (40).

Tuberculids

The *tuberculids*, a term first proposed in 1896 (96), is traditionally used to denote three entities: papulonecrotic tuberculid, lichen scrofulosorum, and erythema induratum of Bazin (Bazin disease, nodular vasculitis; see Chapters 8 and 20). More recently, the term nodular tuberculid has been proposed for a rare subset of patients with nonulcerating nodules in the lower extremities, in whom the histopathologic changes are in the dermis and the subcutaneous fat, thus representing a hybrid between papulonecrotic tuberculid and erythema induratum of Bazin (97,98).

Tuberculids are thought to represent a cutaneous immunologic reaction in patients with tuberculosis, often occult, elsewhere in the body. The most common sites of infection are lymph nodes (99). By definition, stains for acid-fast bacilli and culture for mycobacteria are negative; delayed hypersensitivity skin tests for tuberculosis are positive, and the lesions heal on antituberculous therapy. Recently, using the PCR technique, mycobacterial DNA has been identified in some lesions (100). There is controversy as to whether tuberculids represent immunologic reactions to degenerate dead bacilli or antigenic fragments thereof that have been deposited in the skin and subcutis or true paucibacillary infections where bacilli are extremely difficult to detect (77).

Papulonecrotic Tuberculid

Clinical Summary. Papular necrotic tuberculid (papulonecrotic tuberculid) is believed to represent a paucibacillary form of hematogenous spread of tuberculosis. Primary lesions consist of 1- to 5-mm erythematous papules with an umbilicated necrotic center that usually develop on the extensor region of the limbs in a symmetrical distribution (101). The lower abdomen, trunk, buttocks, and earlobes can also be affected. The ulcers heal, leaving varioliform, depressed scars. Children and young adults with active tuberculosis elsewhere are most commonly affected. Recurrences may be observed until treated. Occasionally, they may develop into lupus vulgaris.

Histopathology. Vascular involvement is observed in early lesions. It may consist of a leukocytoclastic vasculitis or a lymphocytic vasculitis. In either case, it is associated with fibrinoid necrosis and thrombotic occlusion of individual vessels (102). Subsequently, a wedge-shaped area of necrosis forms, with its broad base toward the epidermis (101) (Figs. 21-26 and 21-27). As this wedge is gradually cast off, epithelioid and giant cells gather around its periphery, although focal granuloma formation is poor. Follicular necrosis or suppuration may occur, although diffuse acute inflammatory cells are infrequent. Ziehl–Neelsen stains are, of course, negative.

Differential Diagnosis. Numerous conditions may be confused clinically or histopathologically with papulonecrotic tuberculids. They include pityriasis lichenoides et varioliformis acuta, syphilides, miliary tuberculosis, sarcoidosis, perforating granuloma annulare, and suppurative folliculitis (101).

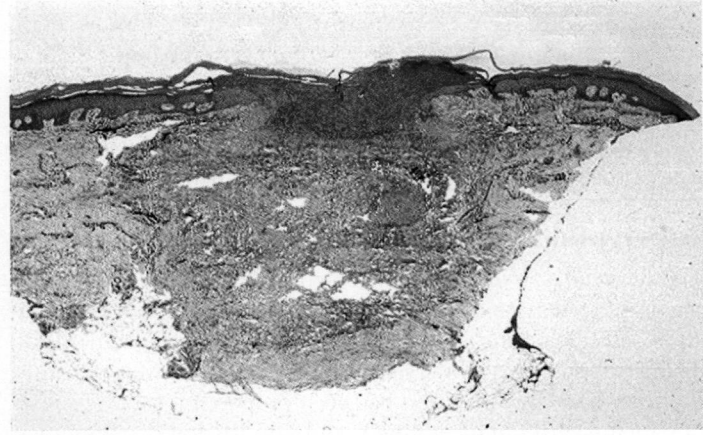

Figure 21-26 Papulonecrotic tuberculid. Wedge-shaped infarction of the dermis and epidermis caused by vasculitis (H&E stain).

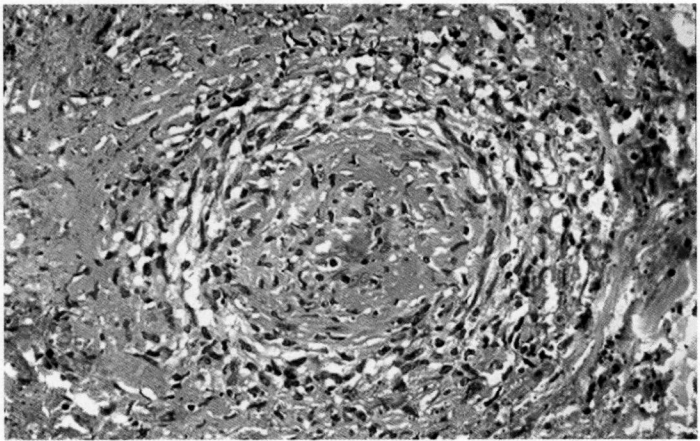

Figure 21-27 Papulonecrotic tuberculid. Necrotizing vasculitis of a dermal artery with granulomatous surround (H&E stain).

Lichen Scrofulosorum

Clinical Summary. Lichen scrofulosorum consists of yellow or brown follicular or parafollicular lichenoid papules, 0.5 to 3.0 mm in diameter, on the trunk. The papules are commonly grouped in clusters and most commonly affect the trunk. Most patients are children and adolescents with pulmonary tuberculosis, but up to one-third of patients may not have an obvious focus. They heal without scarring.

Histopathology. Superficial dermal granulomas are observed, usually in the vicinity of hair follicles or sweat ducts. The granulomas are composed of epithelioid cells, with some Langhans giant cells and a narrow margin of lymphoid cells at the periphery (Fig. 21-28). Generally, caseation necrosis is absent. Replacement of hair follicles by granulomas, in part or completely, is a characteristic feature of lichen scrofulosorum.

Differential Diagnosis. Distinction of lichen scrofulosorum from sarcoidosis may occasionally be impossible on histologic grounds alone. Lichen spinulosus, lichen nitidus, keratosis pilaris, pityriasis rubra pilaris are also in the differential diagnosis. Lichen scrofulosorum has been described after BCG vaccination and in association with *M. avium* infections (103).

Pathogenesis. The pathogenesis of tuberculids is still unclear. Tubercle bacilli are absent in tuberculids, either because they have arrived hematogenously in fragmented form or because they have been destroyed at the sites of the tuberculids by immunologic mechanisms. Mycobacterial DNA is, however, demonstrable in many cases (100,104). The reaction in the papulonecrotic tuberculid consists of an Arthus reaction with vasculitis followed by a delayed hypersensitivity response with granuloma formation. In the case of lichen scrofulosorum, there is only a delayed hypersensitivity reaction, resulting in granuloma formation (98).

Tuberculid-type reactions are also described with nontuberculosis mycobacteria (*M. bovis* and *M. avium*) (105,106).

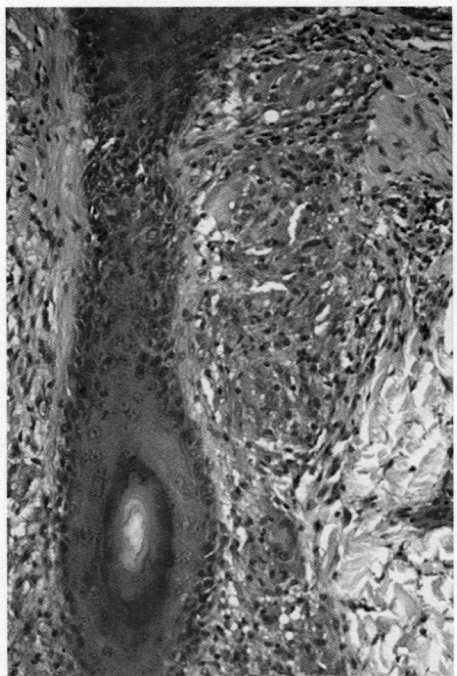

Figure 21-28 Lichen scrofulosorum. Nonnecrotizing epithelioid cell granulomas alongside a hair shaft (H&E stain).

Differential Diagnosis of Cutaneous Tuberculosis

Because tuberculosis can produce such a wide variety of inflammatory reactions—nonnecrotic granulomas, necrotic granulomas, nonspecific acute inflammation, and epithelial hyperplasia—it is not surprising that many other lesions have similar histologic appearances. These other entities include sarcoidosis, mycoses, leishmaniasis, nontuberculosis mycobacterioses and leprosy, syphilis, foreign body implantation reactions, Wegener granulomatosis, and rosacea.

Sarcoidosis usually has little lymphocytic reaction around the granulomas, unlike most forms of granulomatous tuberculosis. When necrosis occurs in a sarcoid granuloma, it is usually fibrinoid in type rather than caseating. A thorough search for acid-fast bacilli, a search for fungal infection with periodic acid–Schiff (PAS) and Grocott stains, and the use of polarizing light to exclude foreign material are obviously important in arriving at a diagnosis. Clinical data and the result of a tuberculin test are also significant. Culture of a lesion should establish the diagnosis in most cases. In a recent review, the utility of a PCR test versus other laboratory tests was studied in 37 skin biopsies from patients with different variants of cutaneous tuberculosis. The PCR test showed the maximum positivity of 79%, followed by histopathology (73%), BACTEC culture (47%), Lowenstein–Jensen (LJ) media culture (29%), and smear examination (6%). Using culture as the gold standard, the sensitivity and specificity of PCR testing were 95.2% and 100.0%, respectively. The mean times to a positive result in different tests were more than 24 hours for smear examination, 1 day for the PCR test, and 23 to 38 days for different culture methods, demonstrating that PCR is a rapid and sensitive test for diagnosis of cutaneous tuberculosis using skin biopsy samples, but not significantly better than histopathology (P > .05) (95). The best use of PCR, in the opinion of these authors, is as follows: In the setting of a positive acid-fast stain for mycobacteria, PCR is the best tool to rapidly determine a species, yet a negative PCR result does not exclude the existing histologic diagnosis.

Principles of Management of Cutaneous Tuberculosis

Treatment of cutaneous tuberculosis is the same as for systemic tuberculosis. Multidrug therapy is the mainstay of treatment. An initial bactericidal regimen (quadruple therapy) administered over 8 weeks to induce rapid reduction of mycobacterial burden is followed by a longer-term (usually 4 more months) treatment phase to eradicate the remaining bacteria. Patient overall health, comorbidities, and mycobacterial resistance patterns influence the choice of a specific regimen. A clinical response should be expected between 4 and 6 weeks after initiation of therapy. Failure to respond should raise suspicion of a mistaken diagnosis and then of drug resistance (77). Culture with sensitivity testing is paramount to adequate therapy. Plastic reconstructive surgery may be necessary in patients with destructive lesions of lupus vulgaris.

INFECTIONS WITH NONTUBERCULOSIS MYCOBACTERIA

Among the nontuberculosis, nonleprosy mycobacterial infections of the skin, those caused by *M. marinum* are the most common among immunocompetent people (107). Unlike *M. tuberculosis*, which is transmitted from person to person, nontuberculosis mycobacteria are abundant in nature, in soil and water, and contact is frequent in most zones of the world (39,108).

These skin infections may be acquired by direct inoculation into the skin or by hematogenous spread from a visceral focus. Increased use of immunosuppression in medicine (e.g., for transplantation and cancer chemotherapy) and the pandemic of HIV/AIDS have resulted in many more mycobacterial skin infections. The cell-mediated immune system is a major defense against such organisms and is affected or destroyed during the course of these immunosuppressive conditions. The clinical and histopathologic patterns are also altered, with organisms being found in greater density than in immunocompetent persons.

The histopathologic picture in nontuberculosis mycobacterioses is just as variable as the clinical picture and may present nonspecific acute and chronic inflammation, suppuration and abscess formation, or tuberculoid granulomas with or without caseation (78,109). In some instances, both tissue reactions occur concurrently. The presence or absence of acid-fast bacilli depends on the tissue reaction. In suppurative lesions, numerous acid-fast (and gram positive) bacilli can often be found.

Infection with *Mycobacterium kansasii*

Clinical Summary. M. kansasii is usually a lymph node and pulmonary infection; skin lesions are unusual. Implantation causes a chronic cutaneous nodule and sometimes ulceration (39). The lesions are often crusted. There may be sporotrichoid lymphatic spread of lesions up the extremity (105). In immunocompromised patients, such as those with HIV infection, there may be multiple visceral lesions (lung and bone) with hematogenous dissemination to skin.

Histopathology. The skin lesions are acute abscesses with large numbers of acid-fast bacilli (Fig. 21-29).

Infection with *Mycobacterium avium-intracellulare*

Clinical Summary. M. avium complex infection is a common cause of cervical lymph node mycobacteriosis in normal children and of pulmonary disease in previously damaged lungs (39). Prior to the HIV pandemic, skin infections were rare, with hematogenously borne lesions in skin and subcutis observed in patients usually with immunosuppressing diseases (40).

Severely immunocompromised patients, such as those with HIV infection, have a very high prevalence of M. avium-intracellulare bacteremia (110), and many show one or more cutaneous papules and nodules (111,112). Therapy with steroids and the new biologics also predisposes to skin lesions.

Histopathology. The histology may be granulomatous or mixed acute and chronic inflammatory, as with tuberculosis (39). Sometimes, there is a histology resembling that of LL leprosy (Figs. 21-30 to 21-32). Macrophages contain large numbers of bacilli without necrosis, and a spindle cell transformation of macrophages, forming a histoid-like lesion (as in leprosy), can occur (73,113).

Infection with *Mycobacterium marinum*

Clinical Summary. Infections with M. marinum can be contracted through minor abrasions incurred while bathing in swimming pools or in ocean or lake water or while cleaning home aquariums (114). Infected swimming pools have caused epidemics,

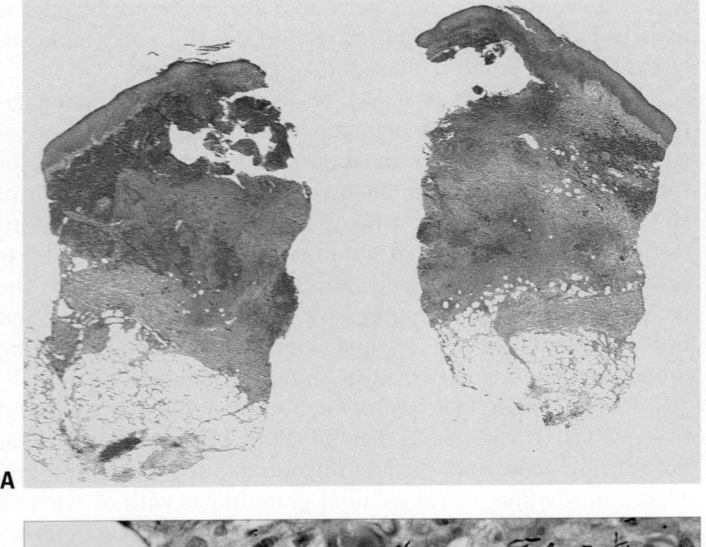

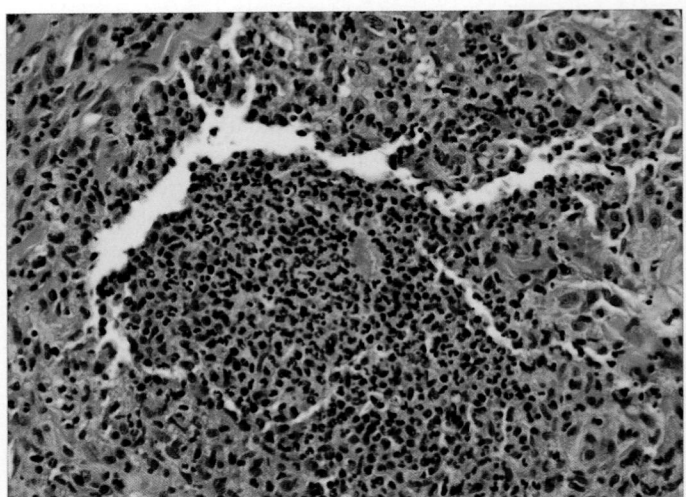

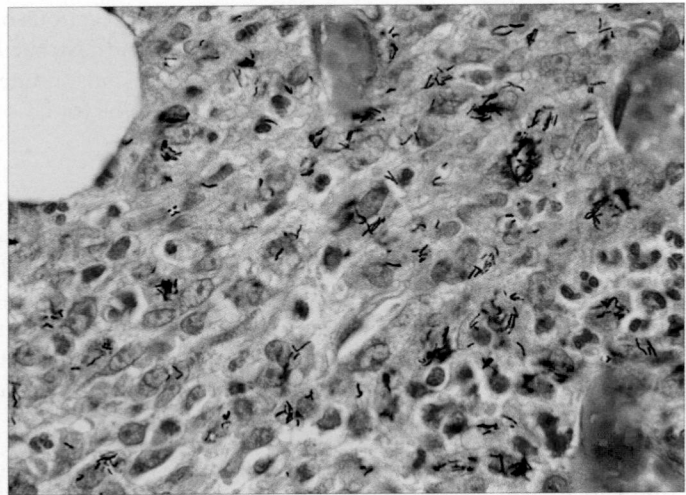

Figure 21-29 *Mycobacterium kansasii* infection. **A:** A superficial dermal abscess cavity with surrounding prominent inflammatory infiltrate is seen on scanning magnification (H&E stain). **B:** A predominantly neutrophilic infiltrate without granulomatous inflammation may be seen occasionally with *M. kansasii* and is characteristic of nontuberculous rapid growers (H&E stain). **C:** Abundant elongated acid-fast bacilli typical of *M. kansasii* were present (Ziehl–Neelsen stain).

the largest of which affected 290 persons (115), as have infected nail salons. The period of incubation is usually about 3 weeks but may be longer (107).

Clinically, most of the lesions caused by *M. marinum* are solitary and consist of indolent, dusky red, hyperkeratotic, papillomatous papules, nodules, or plaques. Superficial ulceration

is occasionally observed. The fingers, knees, elbows, and feet are most affected. In some instances, satellite papules arise, and ascending sporotrichoid spread occurs (116). Lesions may form at different sites in the case of multiple injuries. Although spontaneous healing usually takes place within a year, the lesions persist in some patients for many years. A few HIV-associated

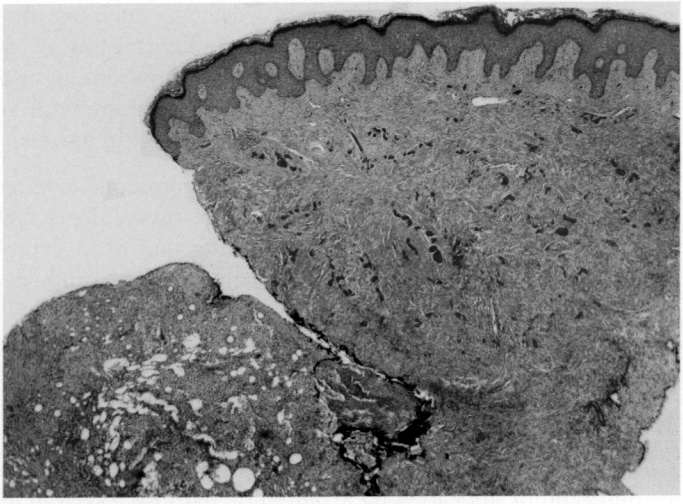

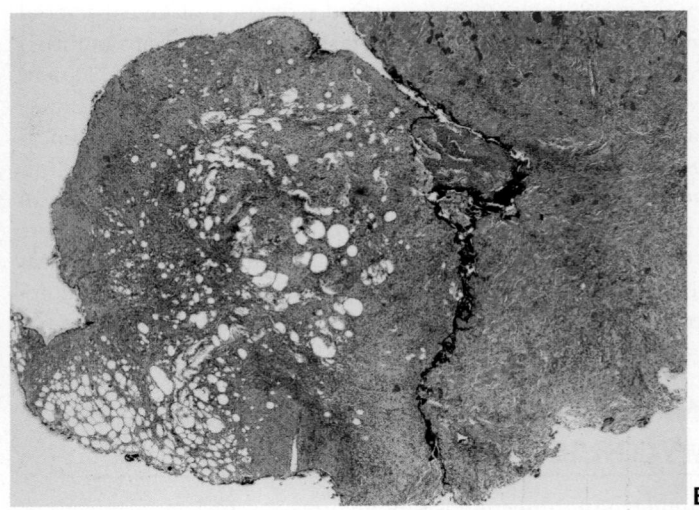

Figure 21-30 *Mycobacterium avium* complex infection. **A** and **B:** Deep dermal and subcutaneous abscess in immunocompromised patient (H&E stain).

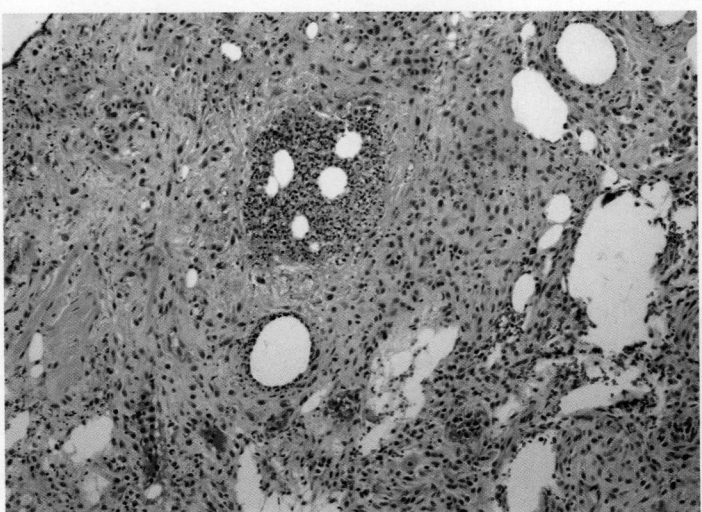

Figure 21-31 *Mycobacterium avium* complex infection. Same lesion as in Figure 21-30. Suppurative inflammation with pseudocyst formation, characteristic of rapid growers, is illustrated here (H&E stain).

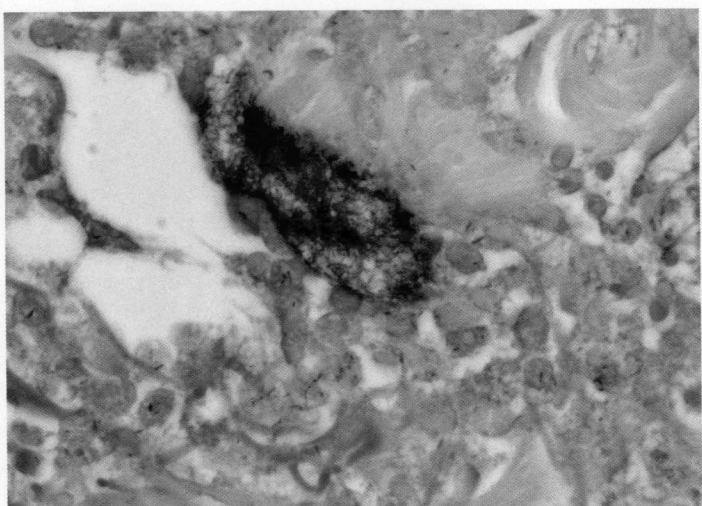

Figure 21-32 *Mycobacterium avium* complex infection. Same lesion as in Figure 21-30, showing abundant acid-fast bacilli within a pseudocyst (Ziehl–Neelsen stain).

cases have been reported (117). Fatal disseminated *M. marinum* infection is rare (118).

Histopathology. Early lesions, no more than 2 or 3 months old, show a nonspecific inflammatory infiltrate composed of neutrophils, monocytes, and macrophages. In lesions about 4 months old, a few multinucleated giant cells and a few small epithelioid cell granulomas are usually present, and in lesions 6 months old or older, typical tubercles or tuberculoid structures may be seen (119). Areas of necrosis are only occasionally present in the centers of the granulomas. The epidermis often shows marked hyperkeratosis with an acute inflammatory infiltrate and ulceration (Fig. 21-33).

Acid-fast and gram-positive bacilli can usually be identified in histologic sections of early lesions that show a nonspecific inflammatory infiltrate. In contrast, tuberculoid granulomas generally no longer show acid-fast organisms unless areas of central necrosis are present. Although primary lesions usually require a few months for the formation of tuberculoid granulomas, the

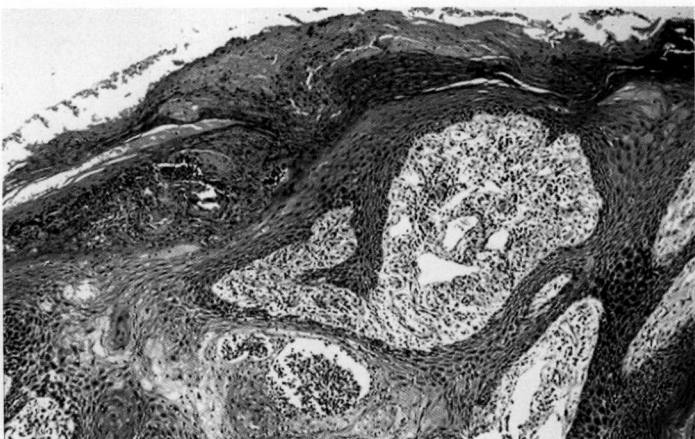

Figure 21-33 *Mycobacterium marinum* infection. A marked pseudoepitheliomatous epidermal hyperplasia, with acute inflammatory foci within the epidermis (H&E stain).

sporotrichoid nodules that arise later show tuberculoid granulomas and a lack of acid-fast bacilli even when they have been present for only a few weeks.

Differential Diagnosis. The granulomatous reaction produced by *M. marinum* is similar to that observed in TVC or lupus vulgaris. The pattern of pseudoepitheliomatous hyperplasia with granulomas and polymorphonuclear neutrophil infiltrate is also seen in several cutaneous mycoses (e.g., sporotrichosis and chromoblastomycosis); so fungal stains need to be examined alongside Ziehl–Neelsen stains. For definitive identification, culture may be necessary.

Buruli Ulcer (*Mycobacterium Ulcerans*)

Clinical Summary. Buruli ulcer, an infection caused by a nontuberculosis mycobacterium, *M. ulcerans*, is endemic in West and Central Africa, Central America, and South Australia (120–122). The organism is now identified in nature, near inland water and rivers, and is directly implanted or follows an aquatic insect bite. The infection commences as a palpable cutaneous nodule. In some cases, this may heal but more usually progresses to ulceration of the skin with extensive undermining of the epidermis and extension of the necrosis down to fascia and even bone (123). These painless ulcers are usually located on the extremities and buttocks, but trunk and facial ulcers also occur.

Histopathology. The infection begins as a subcutaneous nodule exhibiting "ghost" ischemic-type dermal collagen and fat necrosis with deposition of fibrin and hematoxyphilic material, likely attributable, at least in part, to extracellular clumps of mycobacteria. Ulceration proceeds as the epidermis loses its vascular supply. Ziehl–Neelsen stains reveal vast numbers of acid-fast bacilli in the necrotic fat (Figs. 21-34 to 21-36); their distribution is often irregular. A variable degree of neutrophil infiltration and thrombosis of vessels are also observed. In time, a nonspecific granulation tissue or a granulomatous reaction commences from the depth and sides of the ulcer; healing and reepithelialization take place with considerable scarring. Acid-fast bacilli decline rapidly in number during healing (121,124). The histopathologic case definition for Buruli ulcer, useful for research studies, is (a) the typical pattern of infarctive necrosis of deep dermal collagen and fat and (ideally, but

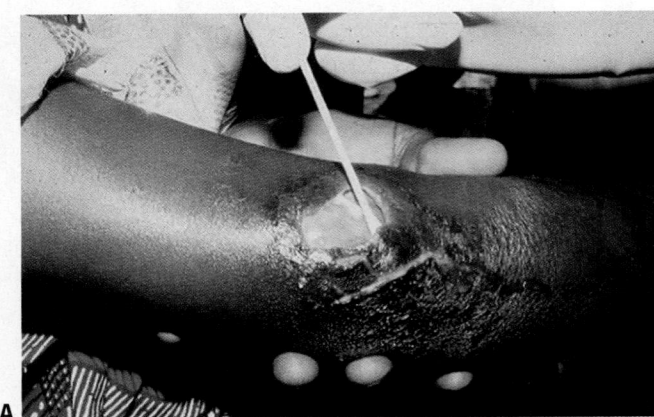

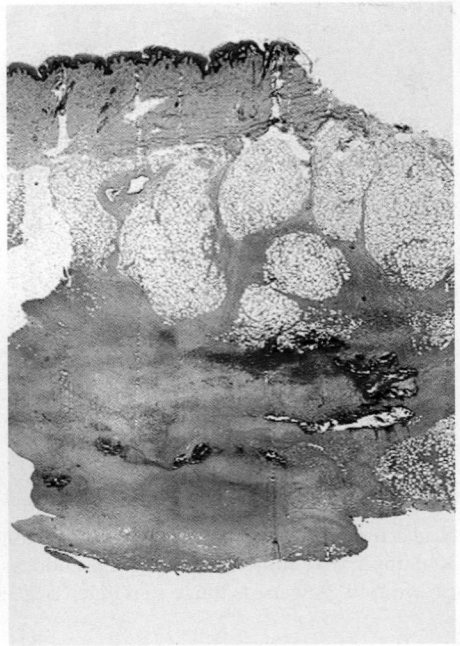

Figure 21-34 Buruli ulcer (*M. ulcerans* infection). **A:** An evolving ulcer with undermined edge. **B:** Early, preulcerating lesion, with deep dermal and subcutaneous fat necrosis (H&E stain).

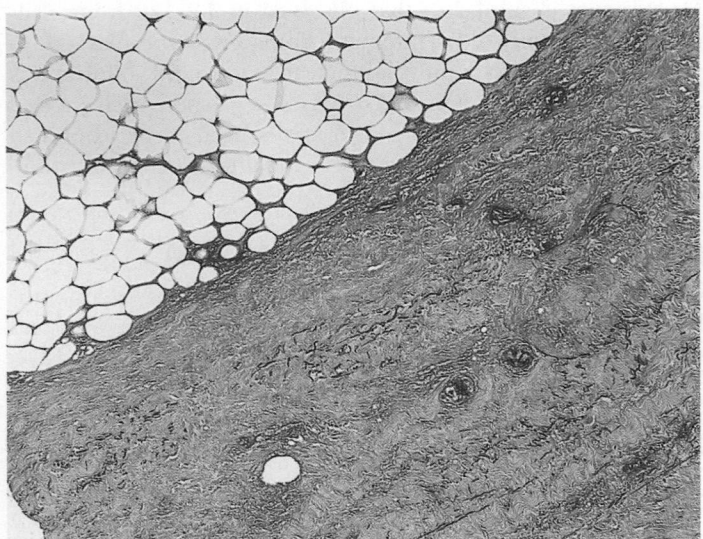

Figure 21-35 Buruli ulcer. The ischemic-type fat and collagen necrosis without cellular reaction; the hematoxyphilic clusters are mycobacteria (H&E stain).

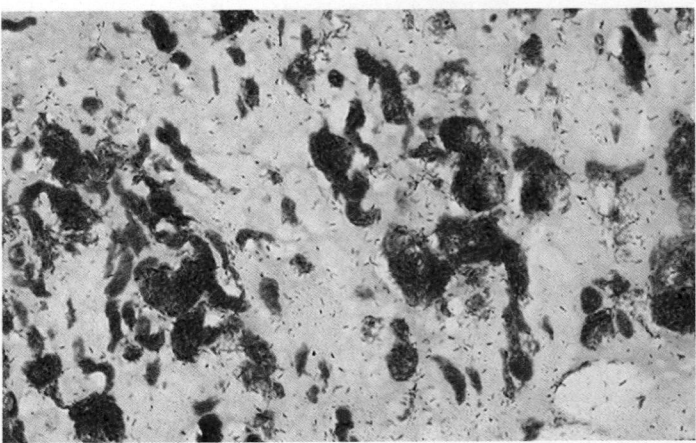

Figure 21-36 Buruli ulcer. Clumps of acid-fast bacilli within the fat necrosis (Ziehl–Neelsen stain).

not always, found in limited samples) (b) nearby clusters of acid-fast bacilli.

Pathogenesis. The widespread necrosis of subcutaneous tissue is caused by a toxin secreted by *M. ulcerans*, a pathogenesis unique to this species of mycobacteria. It is polyketide mycolactone, and strain and geographical differences in mycolactone virulence are already described (the disease is less severe in Australia than in central Africa, related to different mycolactone strains). This toxin causes necrosis when inoculated into guinea pig skin and into macrophages in tissue culture (120). Like *M. marinum*, *M. ulcerans* shows optimal cultural growth at 30°C to 33°C. Comparative genomic studies suggest that *M. ulcerans* evolved from *M. marinum* (125).

PCR technology has been used to track the distribution of *M. ulcerans* in Buruli ulcer lesions and to compare the mycobacterial burden with histopathologic changes (126). Although peaks of mycobacterial DNA and histopathologically recognized acid-fast bacilli in the necrotic base of the ulcers marked the position of the primary infection focus, mycobacterial DNA (and sometime microcolonies) was also present in samples from the periphery of the ulcers and occasionally from macroscopically and histologically healthy-looking excised tissue margins and in sites where satellite lesions were developing. Even when granulomas provided evidence for the development of cell-mediated immunity, development of satellite lesions by contiguous spreading was not completely prevented.

Healing of Buruli ulcer coincides with the development of delayed hypersensitivity to the mycobacterium, possibly contingent on the cessation of mycolactone production. In a recent study, expression of cytokines was correlated with the inflammatory response evaluated by histopathology (127). All of the cases showed extensive necrosis and chronic inflammation. The most important feature correlating with chronicity was considered to be the presence or absence of granulomas coexisting with a mixed proinflammatory/anti-inflammatory cytokine balance. Granulomas were absent from relatively early ulcerative lesions, which contained more bacilli and little interferon (IFN)-γ, suggesting that at this stage of the disease strong suppression of the protective cellular immune response facilitates proliferation of bacilli. When granulomas were present, significantly higher expression of IFN-γ was seen as well as lower bacillary counts.

Other Nontuberculosis Mycobacterioses

Infections in the skin and subcutis caused by the rapid growers *M. chelonae*, *M. fortuitum*, and *M. abscessus* are associated with medical injections through unsterile contaminated needles and cannulas and may occur postoperatively following invasive surgical procedures (39,120,128). Sporotrichoid spread can occur with *M. chelonae* (129). Patients with purulent surgical sites or sites of catheter placement that fail to respond to traditional antibacterial therapies should prompt consideration and evaluation for atypical mycobacterial infections. These may present with a variety of clinical morphologies, including multiple interconnected draining sinus tracts, orange-red plaques which may ulcerate, and erythema and pustules arising in and around sites of iatrogenic manipulation. The inflammatory reaction is usually a mixed acute (neutrophilic) and chronic (granulomatous) response, with acid-fast bacilli visible on sections (39) (Figs. 21-37 and 21-38). Localized and disseminated *M. haemophilum* (a slow-growing acid-fast bacillus) infection is reported in patients with HIV and other causes of immunosuppression (130–132).

BCG is the most commonly used vaccine, yet it rarely results in significant cutaneous lesions. Persisting ulcerating lesions may be observed. Histologically, these lesions are caseating granulomas in the dermis, as seen in tuberculosis, but acid-fast bacilli are rarely observed. In immunocompromised patients, there may be generalized cutaneous nodules, and histology shows abundant bacilli, poorly formed bacilli, and variable or no necrosis (133). BCG is used therapeutically to treat certain malignancies, generally some bladder cancers, but has also been used to treat melanoma. Intradermal BCG injections

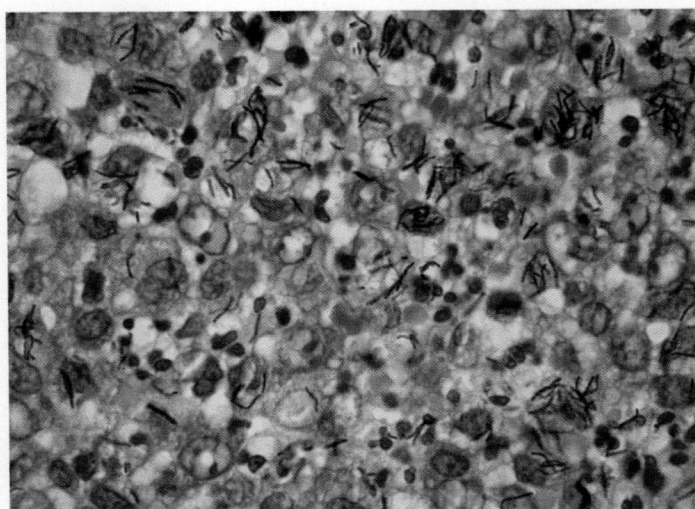

Figure 21-38 *Mycobacterium fortuitum* injection abscess. Same lesion as in Figure 21-37. Numerous clusters of acid-fast bacilli (Ziehl–Neelsen stain).

in melanoma therapy may lead to both local and distant granulomatous reactions, including "Id reactions" similar to the tuberculides.

Principles of Management of Nontuberculous Mycobacterial Infections

Data on the optimal management of extrapulmonary nontuberculous mycobacterial infection are lacking. Pharmacologic therapy with at least two active agents after susceptibility testing should be pursued because of development of resistance. Wide surgical excision of the sort that would be used to approach a malignant tumor with the goal of "clean margins" is recommended in serious skin and soft tissue infections. Early surgical intervention when there is soft tissue and bone involvement in addition to cutaneous disease may be limb sparing. Surgical excision has been the main form of treatment for infections with *M. ulcerans* (Buruli ulcer); however, some studies in West Africa have shown that rifampin and streptomycin for 2 months may be curative and is the current regimen recommended by the WHO. Consultation with a mycobacterial specialist when available is recommended (134). *M. marinum* infection is one of the more common cutaneous nontuberculous mycobacterial infections and may respond to empiric therapy with minocycline, trimethoprim–sulfamethoxazole, and/or clarithromycin, often used in combinations. Notably, most nontuberculous mycobacterial infections are slow growing, and it is best to wait for bacterial cultures to identify the causative organism and perform susceptibility testing so that appropriate combination therapy may be selected.

CUTANEOUS MANIFESTATIONS OF BACTEREMIA AND VASCULAR INFECTIONS

Acute Septicemia

There are several types of acute fulminating septicemia that have cutaneous manifestations of diagnostic significance. They are those caused by *Neisseria meningitidis*, *Pseudomonas aeruginosa*, *Vibrio vulnificus*, and *Capnocytophaga canimorsus*.

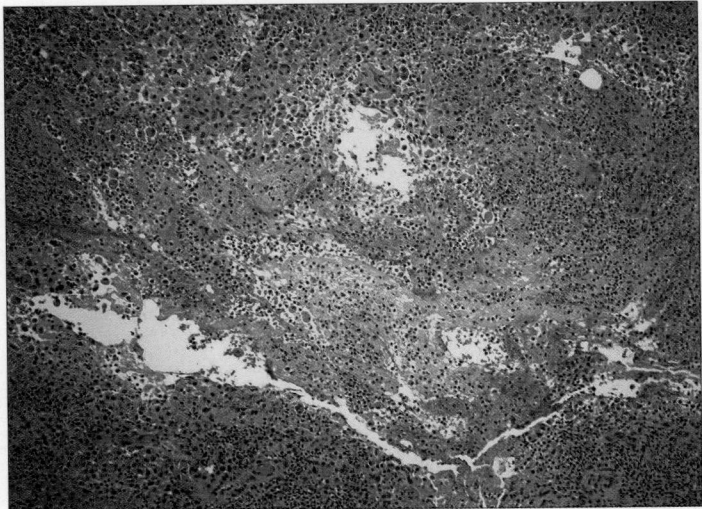

Figure 21-37 *Mycobacterium fortuitum* abscess. Dermal suppurative and histiocytic inflammation (H&E stain).

Acute Meningococcemia

Clinical Summary. Fulminant septicemic infections with *N. meningitidis* exhibit extensive purpura consisting of both petechiae and ecchymoses (purpura fulminans), often with striking confluent patches of purpura. The centers of the petechiae may show small pustules. In addition, shock, cyanosis, and severe consumption coagulopathy occur (135). Without treatment, death may result within 12 to 24 hours. On autopsy, extensive hemorrhaging is found in many internal organs, especially the lungs, kidneys, and adrenals.

On rare occasions, acute septicemia with purpura can be produced by other organisms such as *Streptococcus pneumoniae* or *S. aureus* (136).

Histopathology. The cutaneous petechiae and ecchymoses show, in many dermal vessels, thrombi composed predominantly of fibrin (Fig. 21-39). In addition, there may be an acute vasculitis with considerable damage to the vascular walls, resulting in large and small areas of hemorrhaging into the tissue. Neutrophils and nuclear dust are present within and around the damaged vessels. In most instances, many meningococci can be demonstrated in the luminal thrombi, within vessel walls, and around vessels as gram-negative diplococci. They are present in the cytoplasm of endothelial cells and neutrophils and also extracellularly. Intraepidermal and subepidermal pustules filled with neutrophils may also be observed (137).

Pathogenesis. Paradoxically, *N. meningitidis* is a saprophytic organism commonly inhabiting the human nasopharynx. Only in a small proportion of colonized subjects do the bacteria enter the bloodstream and cause septicemia or meningitis. The reasons why only some individuals are affected remain unclear, but human genetic polymorphisms are likely important in determining outcome, particularly with respect to the risk of purpura fulminans (138). The primary pathogenic mechanism involves endothelial invasion. *N. meningitidis* adheres to endothelial cells through interaction between type IV pili and an unknown adhesion receptor. Following adhesion, type IV pili mediate organization of a specific cytoplasmic molecular complex known as cortical plaques. The formation of cortical plaques promotes the opening of cell–cell junctions, allowing transmigration of bacteria through the endothelium (139). In the past, vascular collapse and death were attributed to massive bilateral hemorrhaging into the adrenal glands and were known as the *Waterhouse–Friderichsen*

syndrome. However, it was then learned that death can occur without significant damage to the adrenals. Therefore, it was assumed that the generalized hemorrhagic diathesis was caused by the consumptive depletion of plasma clotting factors and the resulting disseminated intravascular coagulation (140). It seems likely, however, that there are two distinct pathophysiologic mechanisms operating in acute meningococcemia (135). First, a shock-like terminal phase is associated with the development of widespread thrombosis of the pulmonary microcirculation. These thrombi, which are caused by meningococcal toxins, are composed of leukocytes and fibrin and often also contain meningococci. They produce severe cor pulmonale, which cannot be prevented by treatment with heparin. Similar microthrombi are found also in the skin, spleen, heart, and liver. Second, a meningococcal endotoxin produces disseminated intravascular coagulation, resulting in thrombi composed of only fibrin. These thrombi are found in the capillaries of the adrenal cortex and the kidneys and may cause hemorrhagic infarction of the adrenal glands and renal cortical necrosis. This secondary phase of the disease can be modified with heparin therapy, but its control does not improve survival, because the adrenal and renal lesions are not immediately life threatening, in contrast to the pulmonary lesions, which result in shock and death.

Differential Diagnosis. Other causes of consumptive coagulopathy (e.g., disseminated intravascular coagulation) such as sepsis, malignancy, and obstetric complications produce a similar clinical picture and histologic findings and should be considered.

Principles of Management: Early recognition and treatment markedly improves outcome in meningococcal septicemia. Therefore, meningococcal infection should be considered in the differential diagnosis of any patient with abrupt onset febrile illness and petechiae or meningeal signs. Pretreatment blood cultures are considered sufficient to initiate antibiotic therapy and should not be delayed while waiting for a lumbar puncture. Third-generation cephalosporins (e.g., cefotaxime or ceftriaxone) may be used to treat suspected or culture-proven meningococcal infection prior to susceptibility testing (141).

Pseudomonas Septicemia (Ecthyma Gangrenosum)

Clinical Summary. The classic and diagnostic cutaneous lesions of *P. aeruginosa* or *Burkholderia cepacia* septicemia are referred

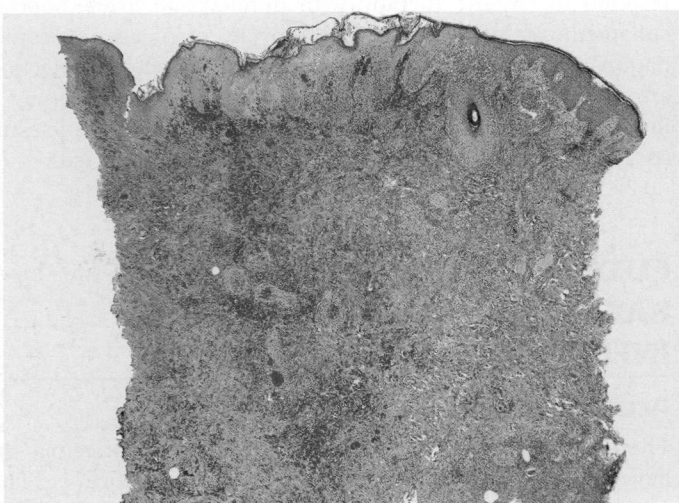

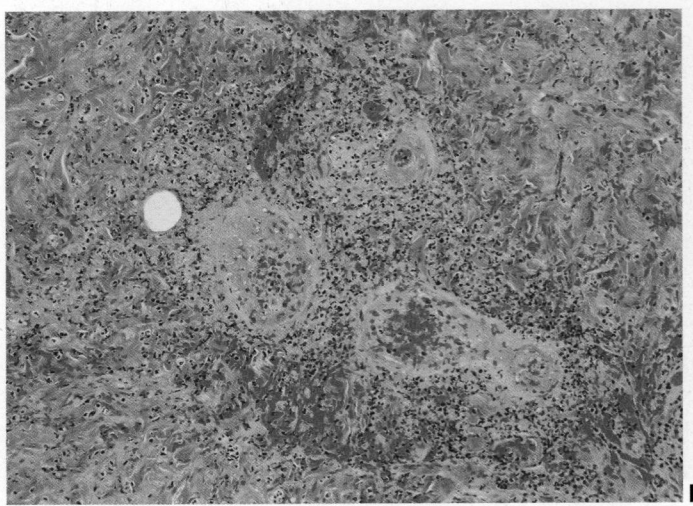

Figure 21-39 Acute meningococcemia. **A:** Epidermal ischemic necrosis in purpura fulminans. **B:** Fibrin thrombi are present throughout dermal vessels (H&E stain).

to as *ecthyma gangrenosum*. Ecthyma gangrenosum has recently been described in association with other gram-negative rods, MRSA, and candidemia, and has since been accepted to occur in the setting of any form of fulminant bacteremia where skin seeding occurs. *Pseudomonas* septicemia usually occurs in debilitated, leukemic, or severely burned patients, particularly after they have received treatment with several antibiotics. The cutaneous lesions may be single but are usually multiple. They consist of angulated ecchymotic patches that can develop hemorrhagic bullae and evolve into larger, punched-out ulcers (about 1 cm in diameter) that have hemorrhagic borders (142). In Tzanck smears prepared from the bases of the lesions, gram-negative rods can be identified, confirming the diagnosis. In rare instances of *Pseudomonas* septicemia, multiple large, indurated, subcutaneous nodules are observed in addition to the cutaneous ulcers (143,144).

Occasionally, lesions of ecthyma gangrenosum have been observed in immunocompromised patients without bacteremia; these cases have better prognoses (145). These lesions are believed to occur by direct skin inoculation and infection, rather than from hematogenous dissemination and septicemia.

Histopathology. The characteristic findings of ecthyma gangrenosum are epidermal necrosis, frequently in the form of a well-demarcated zone of infarction with extensive hemorrhage. There is a mixed inflammatory infiltrate composed of neutrophils, lymphocytes, and histiocytes. The causative organism, often gram-negative bacilli, may be detected in the dermis, or within the wall of venules. There is often a pauci-inflammatory response that is out of proportion to the large numbers of microorganisms in the skin. Secondary vasculitis with fibrin thrombi may also be found (146) (Fig. 21-40).

The subcutaneous nodules are the result of cellulitis caused by the presence of large numbers of *Pseudomonas* bacilli (143).

Differential Diagnosis. It is important to recognize that although characteristic, ecthyma gangrenosum is not pathognomonic of *P. aeruginosa* bacteremia and has been documented with other infections.

Principles of Management: Treatment with two antipseudomonal antibiotics from different classes (one being an aminoglycoside, unless precluded by nephrotoxicity) to which the isolate is susceptible is the recommended treatment in patients with neutropenia or sepsis (147); often, severely compromised hosts will receive empiric antibiotic therapy for other potential etiologic agents, including gram-positive bacteria and yeasts/fungi.

Vibrio vulnificus Septicemia

Clinical Summary. *V. vulnificus* infections occur in coastal regions of the United States. Raw seafood consumption, particularly raw oysters, or wounds acquired in marine environments can cause the infection. *V. vulnificus* is a virulent pathogen, producing significant morbidity and, unless treated, mortality, especially in patients with cirrhosis of the liver.

Striking skin lesions are an early sign of septicemic infection. Indurated plaques show blue discoloration, vesicles, and bullae. Large ulcers may develop (148). *V. vulnificus* may also cause necrotizing fasciitis (149).

Histopathology. Noninflammatory bullae form as the result of dermal necrosis, which is caused by the extracellular toxin produced by the bacterium. Clusters of bacteria may be seen in dermal vessels without associated dermal infiltrate (150).

Pathogenesis. *V. vulnificus* is a gram-negative rod that is motile by means of a single polar flagellum. It can be isolated from the blood and bullae of patients with this infection. *V. vulnificus* has three major virulence factors: (a) an antiphagocytic polysaccharide capsule that provides protection against phagocytosis; (b) the RtxA toxin, which induces significant reactive oxygen species generation, leading to cell death in intestinal epithelium; and (c) iron availability and iron acquisition systems, which help promote bacterial growth and replication.

Principles of Management: As with other potentially fatal infections, early recognition and management in an intensive care unit with prompt initiation of antimicrobial therapy appears to improve outcome. Based on apparent synergism between cefotaxime and minocycline on *in vitro* and *in vivo* studies in mice, this combination has been proposed as a regime for treating patients with severe wound infections or septicemia attributable to *V. vulnificus*. A potential alternative is levofloxacin (151).

Capnocytophaga canimorsus Septicemia

Clinical Summary. *C. canimorsus* is a gram-negative rod, a habitual member of dog's mouth flora. It was discovered in 1976 in patients with severe infections after bites, scratches, or simply licks from a dog (152). It is now recognized as the principal pathogen in humans after dog bites, and it most commonly causes sepsis, frequently accompanied by intravascular consumptive coagulopathy manifested as purpura fulminans and associated septic shock. *C. canimorsus* is a rare cause of infections in humans, with an estimated incidence of approximately 0.5 per million inhabitants per year in northern Europe. Immune deficiency, such as from asplenia, and history of alcohol abuse have been identified as important risk factors. According to a report by Janda et al. (153) on a large series of 56 patients, the most reported symptoms were fever (85%), diarrhea or abdominal pain (21%), vomiting (18%), headache (18%), confusion (12%), and myalgia or malaise (<10%). It has been reported that up to 50% of individuals affected by *C. canimorsus* septicemia develop purpura fulminans, and, therefore, *C. canimorsus* should always be considered as a potential causative agent in this context (154).

It is important to note that a recent history of a dog bite proper cannot always be elicited, but close contact with dogs is usually documented. In cases with cellulitis secondary to dog bite, *C. canimorsus* can be recovered from blood but typically not from wounds. *C. canimorsus* can be difficult to identify, with only 5 of 18 (28%) *C. canimorsus* strains correctly identified to genus and species in isolates forwarded to a reference laboratory (153). Recently, the use of amplification and 16S rRNA sequencing by PCR has proved increasingly useful for identifying slow-growing, fastidious bacteria, and it is reliable in distinguishing *C. cynodegmi*, which is phenotypically similar to *C. canimorsus*. The differential diagnosis, clinically and histopathologically, includes meningococcemia and *V. vulnificus* septicemia.

Histopathology. The presence of rod-shaped intracellular bacterial forms on the peripheral blood smear has been reported in numerous cases of purpura fulminans secondary to *C. canimorsus* (155–157). The findings on skin biopsy are those of consumptive coagulopathy/purpura fulminans and are thus nonspecific. There are scattered fibrin thrombin associated with prominent vascular congestion and extravasated red blood cells (Fig. 21-41). Prominent dyskeratosis within the epidermis and incipient necrosis of eccrine glands may also be seen. Gram stain is usually negative.

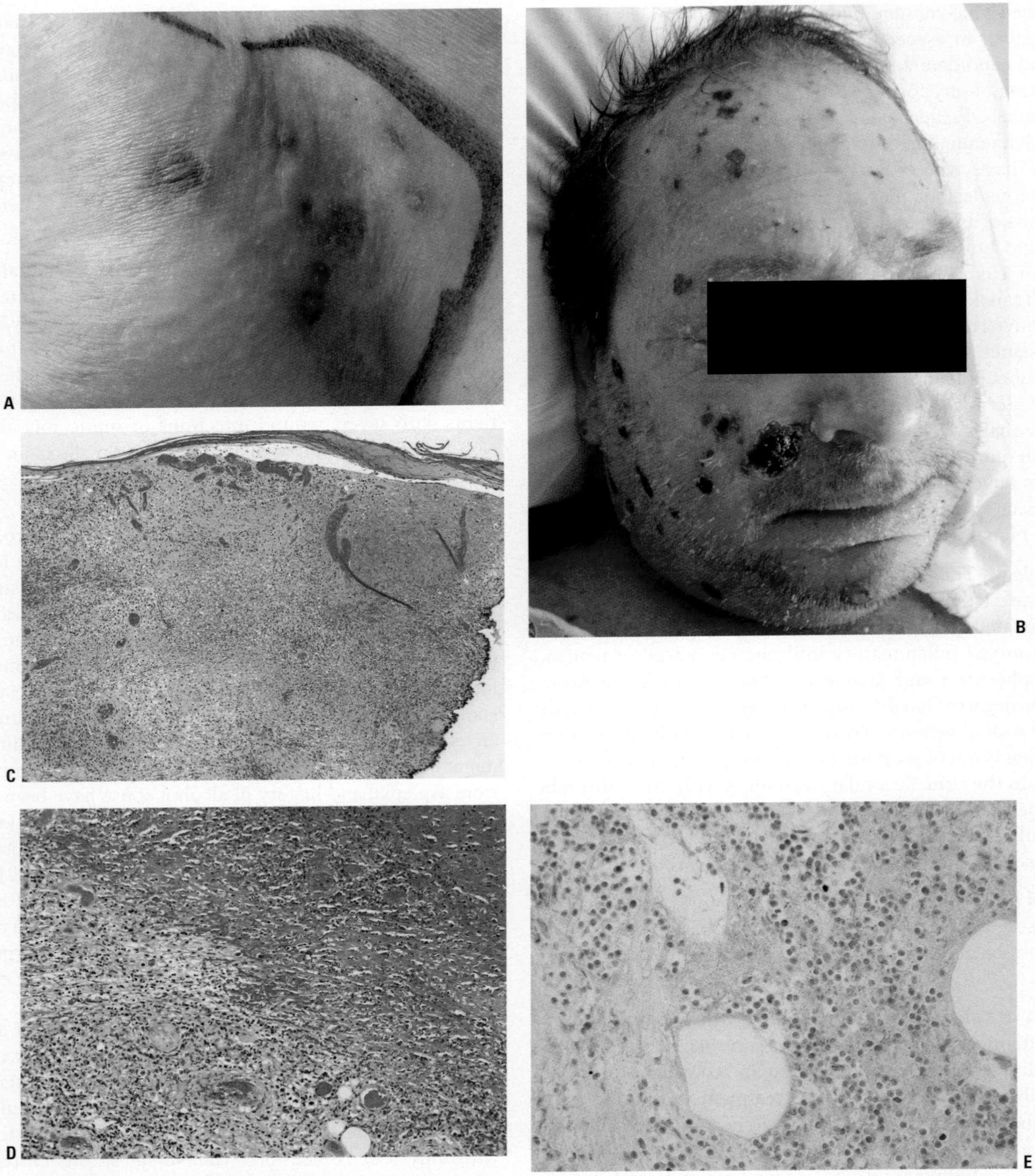

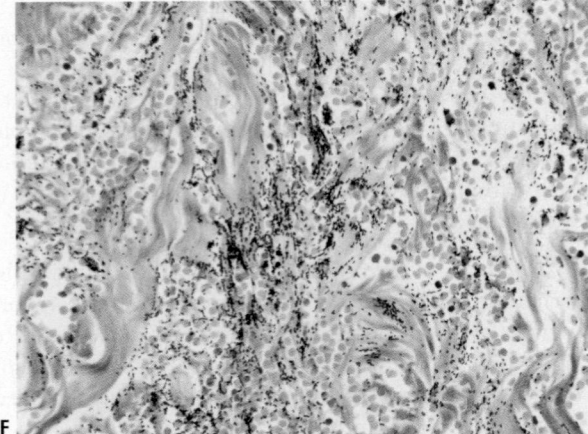

Figure 21-40 Ecthyma gangrenosum (*Pseudomonas* septice-mia). **A:** Early lesions typically present as erythematous to violaceous, painless macules with an erythematous halo that become indurated, as illustrated here in the axillary region of an elderly patient. **B:** The lesions then become gangrenous and show a characteristic black eschar. **C:** Scanning magnifi-cation shows well-demarcated ischemic epidermal infarction. **D:** Fibrin thrombi are characteristic. **E:** Gram-negative rods can be identified within the inflammatory debris, which were isolated as *Pseudomonas* sp. by culture (H&E stain **C** and **D**). **F:** Same lesion as in **E**. The gram-negative rods are more read-ily in a Warthin–Starry Stained section. (**E:** Brown–Hopps stain; **F:** Warthin–Starry stain; **A** and **B:** Courtesy of Drs. Car-men Castilla and Arash Mostaghimi, Brigham and Women's Hospital and Harvard Medical School, Boston, MA.)

Pathogenesis. *C. canimorsus* can evade complement fixation and phagocytosis by human granulocytes and macrophages. Whole bacteria are poor agonists of Toll-like receptor 4 (TLR-4), which results in lack of the proinflammatory cytokine response by macrophages. Additional important pathogenetic events include deglycosylation of human IgG and endotoxic shock induced by lipopolysaccharide, a potent endotoxin (152).

Differential Diagnosis. Meningococcemia and other causes of purpura fulminans should also be considered because they produce identical clinical and histologic pictures.

Principles of Management: Antimicrobial treatment with β-lactam/β-lactamase inhibitors and carbapenems are usually active against *C. canimorsus* (152–155).

Chronic Septicemia

Meningococcemia and gonococcemia can occur in association with a chronic intermittent, benign eruption.

Chronic Meningococcemia

Clinical Summary. In patients with partial immunity to *N. meningitidis*, an infection with this organism produces chronic meningococcemia. This disease is characterized by recurrent attacks of fever, each lasting about 12 hours, associated with migratory joint pains and a papular and petechial eruption. Positive blood cultures are obtained during the febrile attacks.

Histopathology. The cutaneous lesions of chronic meningococcemia, in contrast to those of acute meningococcemia, show no bacteria and no vascular thrombosis or necrosis. Instead, a perivascular infiltrate composed largely of lymphoid cells and only a few neutrophils is observed in papular lesions (158,159). In petechial lesions, in addition to a limited area of perivascular hemorrhage, a fairly high percentage of neutrophils and fibrinoid material in the walls of the vessels may be found; thus, the histologic picture resembles that of a leukocytoclastic vasculitis (Fig. 21-42). The presence of meningococci may be difficult to demonstrate.

Differential Diagnosis. Chronic meningococcemia cannot be distinguished from chronic gonococcemia except by isolation of the causative organism.

Principles of Management: Penicillin G remains the antimicrobial of choice, when the isolate is susceptible. Third-generation cephalosporins are the alternative of choice (160).

Chronic Gonococcemia

Clinical Summary. Patients with chronic gonococcemia, also referred to as *disseminated gonococcal infection* (161), like those with chronic meningococcemia, have intermittent attacks of fever and polyarthralgia. The cutaneous lesions of the two diseases are also similar, except that those of chronic gonococcemia are few and have a predominantly acral distribution. In contrast to chronic meningococcemia, there are often, in addition to papules and petechiae, vesicopustules with hemorrhagic halos and, rarely, hemorrhagic bullae, sometimes concentrated over joints. Blood cultures are often positive for *Neisseria gonorrhoeae* but only during attacks of fever. A search for gonococci should also be made in possible sites of primary infection.

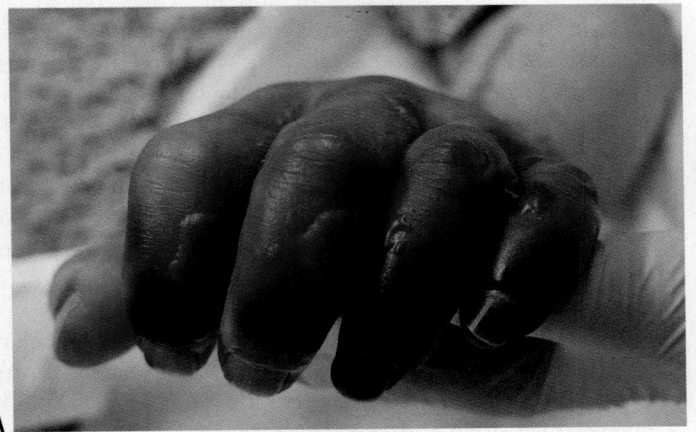

A

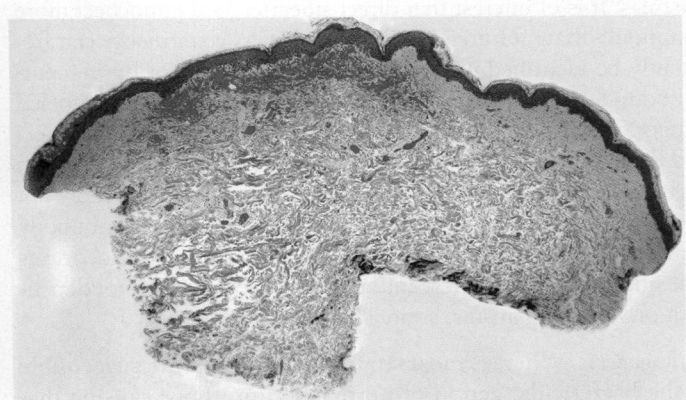

B

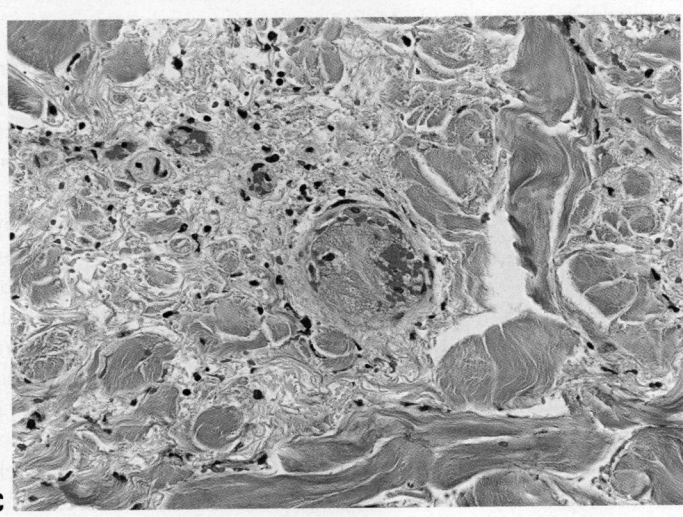

C

Figure 21-41 *Capnocytophaga canimorsus* sepsis. **A:** Purpura fulminans with characteristic acral involvement is a common presentation of this rare but deadly infection. **B:** Scanning magnification shows vascular congestion and hemorrhage in the superficial dermis. **C:** Incipient fibrin thrombi in microvasculature are seen, indistinguishable from other thrombotic coagulopathies. The Gram stains performed on these sections proved negative; *C. canimorsus* was eventually identified by PCR performed at the Centers for Disease Control, Atlanta, Georgia. (**A:** Courtesy of Dr. Ryan Sells, Brigham and Women's Hospital and Harvard Medical School, Boston, MA.)

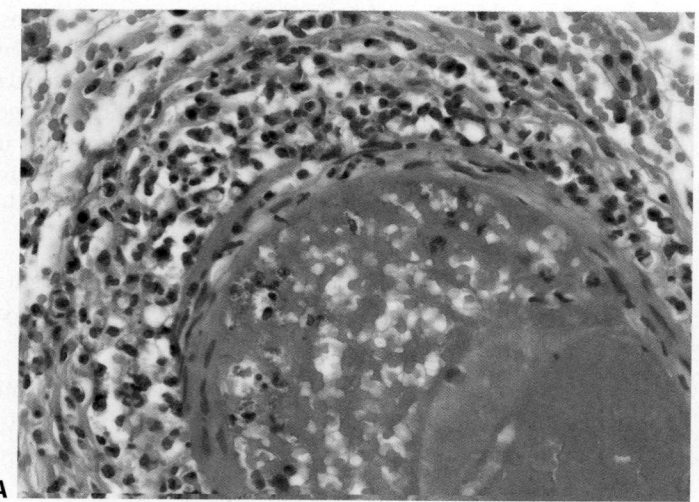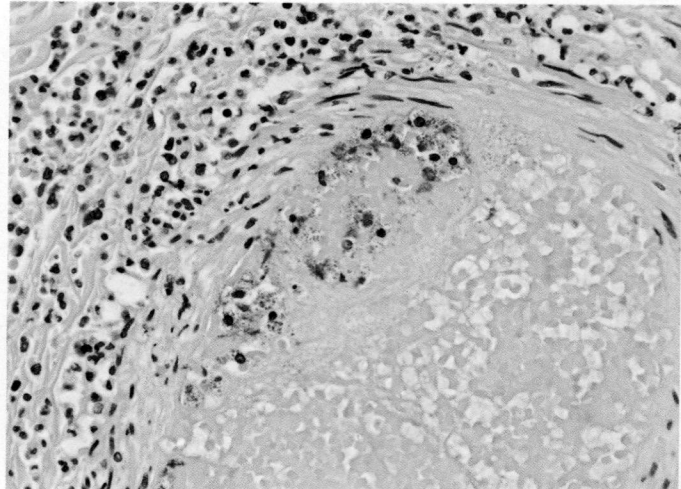

Figure 21-42 Meningococcal sepsis. **A:** Skin vasculitis. Inflamed dermal vessel. **B:** Skin vasculitis. Brown–Hopps Gram stain showing gram-negative cocci in the monocytes and within the vessel wall.

Histopathology. The capillaries in the upper dermis and mid-dermis are surrounded by an infiltrate of neutrophils and a variable admixture of mononuclear cells and red cells. There is often nuclear dust, as in leukocytoclastic vasculitis. Fibrinoid material may be present in the walls of some vessels and fibrin thrombi in some lumina (137). Pustular lesions are usually observed in intraepidermal locations with neutrophils both within them and in the underlying dermis (162). Bullae are subepidermal in location (163).

Gram-negative diplococci are observed in tissue sections only on rare occasions in the walls of blood vessels (164). They are found more readily in direct smears of pus from freshly opened pustules. It is of interest that direct smears reveal gonococci more commonly than cultures (165). However, *N. gonorrhoeae* can frequently be identified in tissue sections by the use of fluorescent-antibody techniques (166). For this purpose, fluorescein-labeled antigonococcus globulin is used. Diplococci, as well as single cocci and disintegrated antigenic material, are then observed, largely in perivascular locations. The reason that direct smears are more apt to show diplococci than cultures and that the fluorescent-antibody technique is particularly effective in demonstrating gonococci is that smears and the fluorescent-antibody technique are not dependent on living organisms, as are cultures.

Pathogenesis. Whereas most strains of gonococci are susceptible to the bactericidal action of normal serum, those causing disseminated gonococcal infection are resistant (161).

Differential Diagnosis. As stated previously, chronic meningococcemia cannot be distinguished from chronic gonococcemia except by isolation of the causative organism.

Principles of Management: Parenteral therapy with ceftriaxone is the preferred initial treatment for disseminated gonococcal infection. Alternative regimens include cefotaxime or ceftizoxime. Azithromycin or doxycycline should be administered concomitantly to cover for potential *C. trachomatis* coinfection (167). Patients should undergo HIV testing, and consideration should be given for further sexually transmitted disease (STD) evaluations.

RICKETTSIAL INFECTIONS

Clinical Summary. Rickettsial infections are acquired by tick bites, the natural reservoir being infected animals. Rocky Mountain spotted fever is caused by *Rickettsia rickettsii*, a small,

pleomorphic coccobacillus that is an obligate intracellular parasite. Contrary to what its name suggests, the disease is encountered mostly in the southeastern United States and has been acquired even within New York City (168,169). Boutonneuse fever (Mediterranean spotted fever) is caused by *Rickettsia conorii* and is widespread in Africa too.

In *R. rickettsii* infection, after an incubation period of 1 to 2 weeks, chills and fever develop, and a few days later, a rash appears that begins on the extremities and spreads to the trunk. At first, the lesions are macular to papular but become purpuric within 2 to 3 days. There may be only petechiae, but in fatal cases widespread ecchymoses are common. Gangrene may result from small-vessel occlusion (170). Because the diagnosis may not be made in the beginning and the course may be rapid, mortality exceeds 10%, despite the effectiveness of antibiotics such as doxycycline if given in time. Whenever a diagnosis of Rocky Mountain spotted fever is suspected, a search should be made for an eschar indicating the site of a tick bite. A hemorrhagic crust 8 to 10 mm in diameter surrounded by an erythematous ring may be found. Studies have shown that in up to 20% of cases there are no obvious skin lesions (171,172).

In boutonneuse fever, characteristic "tache noire" eschars develop. The histopathology is similar in both infections. A recent study found a rickettsial protein in serum (RC0497) to be a potential sensitive and specific marker for acute rickettsial spotted rickettsioses (173).

Histopathology. In the advanced lesion, there is dermal and epidermal necrosis. The small vessels of the dermis and of the subcutaneous fat exhibit a necrotizing vasculitis with a perivascular infiltrate consisting mostly of lymphocytes and macrophages (Figs. 21-43 and 21-44). There is extravasation of erythrocytes. As a result of injury to the endothelial cells, luminal thrombosis and microinfarcts occur. The causative organism, which measures 0.3 by 1.0 μm, is too small to be visible by light microscopy using ordinary stains. However, rickettsial antigen can be identified in sections of skin lesions by immunohistochemistry (172), and PCR on skin samples is specific. Coccoid and bacillary forms are observed in endothelial cells in association with perivascular lymphocytic infiltration. Electron microscopic examination of the tick bite site demonstrates rickettsial organisms within the cytoplasm and the nuclei of endothelial cells. These organisms appear as electron-dense, round

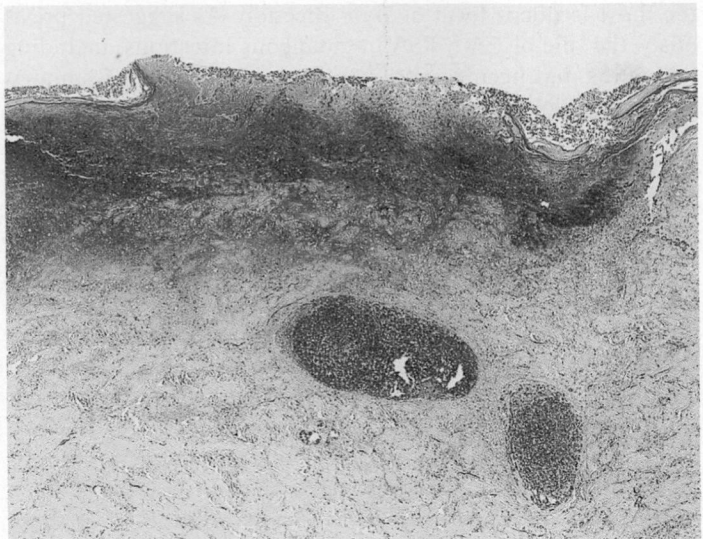

Figure 21-43 *Rickettsia conorii* infection. Typical eschar necrosis of superficial dermis and epithelium (H&E stain).

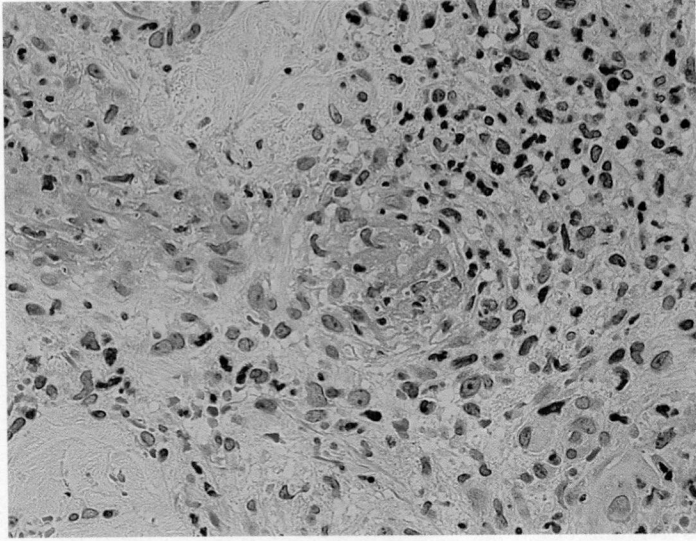

Figure 21-44 *Rickettsia conorii* infection. Dermal arteriole with arteritis and fibrin thrombosis (H&E stain).

or oval structures surrounded by an electron-lucent halo. The entire organism is bounded by a limiting cell wall. The organisms range in size from 0.3 to 0.5 μm in greatest diameter.

Principles of Management: The treatment of all the so-called "spotted fever group" rickettsiae is doxycycline. Given the high mortality associated with this severe disease, doxycycline is generally the drug of choice even in populations where tetracycline-class antibiotics are normally avoided. Supportive therapy may be necessary in those with severe disease (174).

PATTERNS OF DISEASE OF THE HAIR FOLLICLES

Folliculitis

Folliculitis may involve the superficial, middle, or deep portion of the hair follicle and may be caused by a variety of etiologies, not all infectious. The common staphylococcal superficial folliculitis is the prototype (Figs. 21-45 to 21-47) and is perhaps

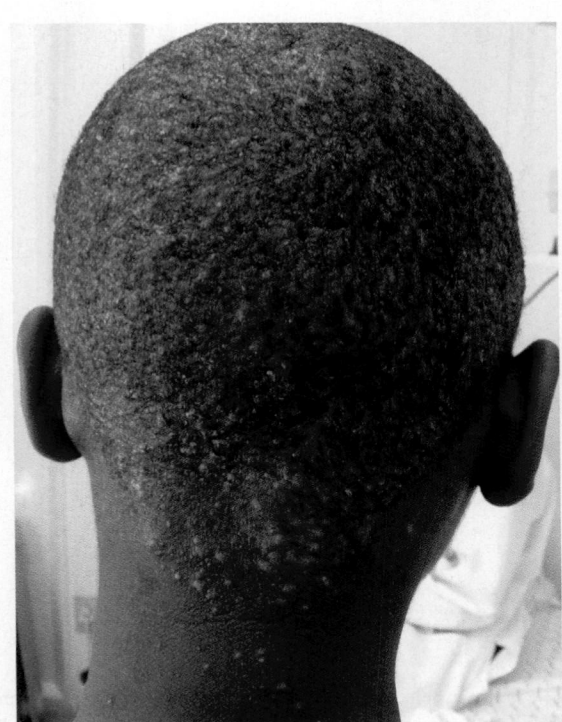

Figure 21-45 Acute folliculitis. Multiple follicular pustules on the scalp. Gram-positive cocci were demonstrated in the exudate. (Image courtesy of C. Kovarik.)

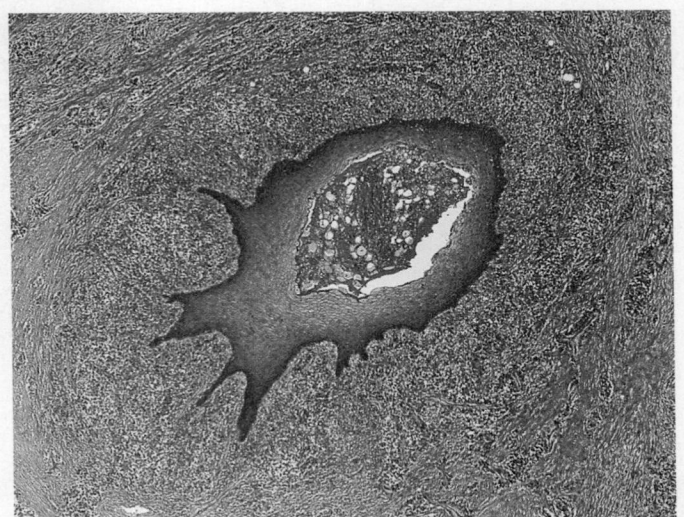

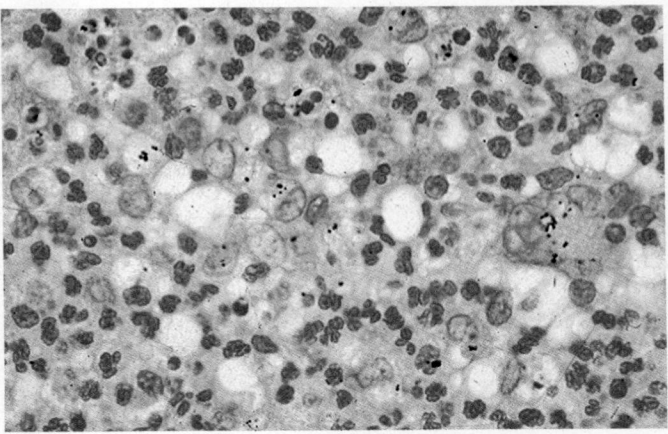

Figure 21-46 Acute folliculitis. **A:** Hair shaft with early internal inflammation and perifolliculitis (H&E stain). **B:** Gram-positive cocci visible in the inflammation (Gram stain).

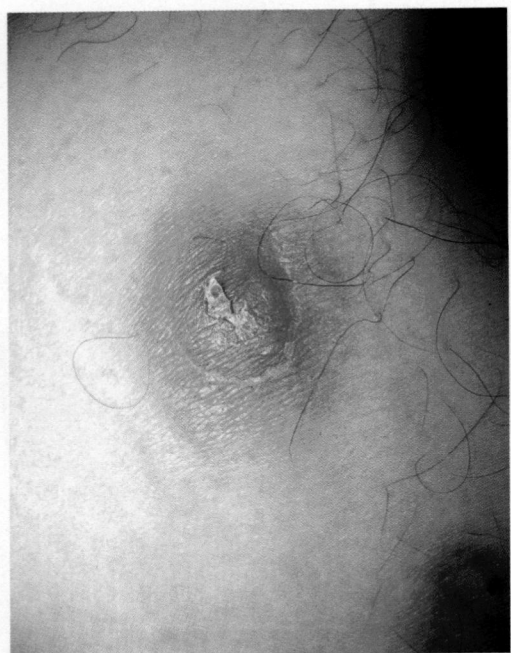

Figure 21-47 Furuncle. A deep-seated cutaneous tender, *red*, perifollicular swelling with a superficial scale, which may terminate in the discharge of pus. (Image courtesy of R. Lee.)

the most frequent form of skin infection. As suggested previously, the role of CA-MRSA in cutaneous infections, including folliculitis, has been recently emphasized. Table 21-1 summarizes the follicle-specific diseases of skin.

Follicular Occlusion Triad (Hidradenitis Suppurativa, Acne Conglobata, and Perifolliculitis Capitis Abscedens Et Suffodiens)

Clinical Summary. Hidradenitis suppurativa, acne conglobata, and perifolliculitis capitis abscedens et suffodiens, the three diseases included in the follicular occlusion triad, have similar pathogeneses and similar histopathologic findings. Quite frequently, two of the three diseases, and occasionally all three, are encountered in the same patient (182). All three diseases represent a chronic, recurrent, deep-seated folliculitis resulting in abscesses, followed by the formation of sinus tracts and scarring. Although the primary etiology of these conditions is not bacterial, they are discussed in this chapter because the differential diagnosis includes the deep bacterial folliculitides.

In *hidradenitis suppurativa*, the axillary and anogenital regions are affected. Acute and chronic forms can be distinguished (183). The acute form exhibits red, tender nodules that become fluctuant and heal after discharging pus. In the chronic form,

Table 21-1
Clinicopathologic Spectrum of Follicle-Centered Infectious Diseases

Disease	Organisms	Clinical	Histology
Impetigo of Bockhart (acute superficial)	Staphylococci	Eruption of small pustules, many of which are pierced by hairs	Subcorneal pustule at opening of a hair follicle; upper portion of the hair follicle with inflammatory infiltrate (neutrophils)
Pseudomonas folliculitis (acute) (175–177)	Pseudomonads (gram-negative rods in tissue, culture required for definitive diagnosis)	Pruritic macules, papules, and follicular pustules after heated swimming pools, whirlpools, or hot tubs use (onset 8–48 h after exposure, resolution spontaneously within 7–10 d)	Distension and disruption of a hair follicle; pilar canal with neutrophils; perifolliculitis, disrupted epithelium of the hair follicle
Furuncle (acute deep) (Fig. 21-47) (178)	Staphylococci (gram-positive cocci)	Tender, red, perifollicular swelling terminating in the discharge of pus and of a necrotic plug	Perifollicular necrosis containing fibrinoid material and many neutrophils; large abscess
Acne varioliformis/acne necrotica (chronic superficial) (179)	Staphylococci and *Propionibacterium*	Recurrent, small, indolent, follicular papules on the forehead and scalp undergo central necrosis and usually heal with small, pitted scars	Marked perifollicular lymphocytic infiltrate with exocytosis of lymphocytes into the external root sheath; necrosis of hair follicle and perifollicular epidermis; late lesions have central cores of necrotic tissue.
Folliculitis barbae (chronic deep)	Staphylococci	Follicular papules and pustules; erythema, crusting, and boggy infiltration of the skin; ± abscesses; scarring and permanent hair loss	Perifollicular infiltrate of neutrophils, lymphocytes cells, histiocytes, and plasma cells; perifollicular abscess with destruction of hair and follicles; chronic granulation tissue (plasma cells, lymphocytes, fibroblasts); foreign body giant cells around hair/keratin; fibrosis with healing

Table 21-1

Clinicopathologic Spectrum of Follicle-Centered Infectious Diseases (*continued*)

Disease	Organisms	Clinical	Histology
Folliculitis decalvans (*chronic deep*) (180)	Staphylococci? Role of bacteria unclear	Scalp with bald, atrophic areas with follicular pustules at peripheries; beard, pubic regions, axillae, eyebrows, and eyelashes may be involved; atrophic areas spread peripherally.	Perifollicular infiltrate of neutrophils, lymphocytes cells, histiocytes, and plasma cells; perifollicular abscess with destruction of hair and follicles; chronic granulation tissue (plasma cells, lymphocytes, fibroblasts); foreign body giant cells around hair/keratin; fibrosis with healing
Folliculitis keloidalis nuchae (*chronic deep*)	Unclear	Male, nape of the neck with hypertrophic scarring; early = follicular papules, pustules, and possibly abscesses; replaced gradually by indurated fibrous nodules	Chronic folliculitis with numerous thick bundles of sclerotic collagen
Pseudofolliculitis barbae (181)	Keratin polymorphisms; noninfectious	Occurs in men with curly hair, especially blacks, who shave closely; follicular papules and pustules resembling bacterial folliculitis, but no comedones are observed	Foreign body inflammatory reaction surrounding an ingrown beard hair; growing hair causes invagination = intradermal microabscess; severe inflammatory reaction with downgrowth (attempted epithelial sheathing) with abscess formation within the pseudofollicle and a foreign body giant cell reaction

deep-seated abscesses lead to the discharge of pus through sinus tracts. Severe scarring results (184).

Acne conglobata, an entity different from acne vulgaris, occurs mainly on the back, buttocks, and chest and only rarely on the face or the extremities. In addition to comedones, fluctuant nodules discharging pus or a mucoid material occur as well as deep-seated abscesses that discharge through interconnecting sinus tracts.

In *perifolliculitis capitis abscedens et suffodiens*, nodules and abscesses as described for acne conglobata occur in the scalp.

Pilonidal sinus is often considered to be a part of this group of disorders ("follicular occlusion tetrad"). Its pathogenesis appears to be similar, and it is often present in patients with one or more of the other members of the group.

Histopathology. Early lesions in all three diseases of the follicular occlusion triad show follicular hyperkeratosis with plugging and dilatation of the follicle. The follicular epithelium may proliferate or be destroyed (Figs. 21-48 and 21-49). At first, there is little inflammation, but eventually a perifolliculitis develops with an extensive infiltrate composed of neutrophils, lymphocytes, and histiocytes. Abscess formation results and leads to the destruction, first, of the pilosebaceous structures and, later, also of the other cutaneous appendages. Apocrine glands in hidradenitis suppurativa of the axillae or groin regions may be secondarily involved by the inflammatory process. In response to this destruction, granulation tissue containing lymphoid and plasma cells, and foreign body giant cells related to fragments of keratin and to embedded hairs, infiltrates the area near the remnants of hair follicles. As the abscesses extend deeper into the subcutaneous tissue, draining sinus tracts develop that are lined with epidermis. In areas of healing, extensive fibrosis may be observed (182).

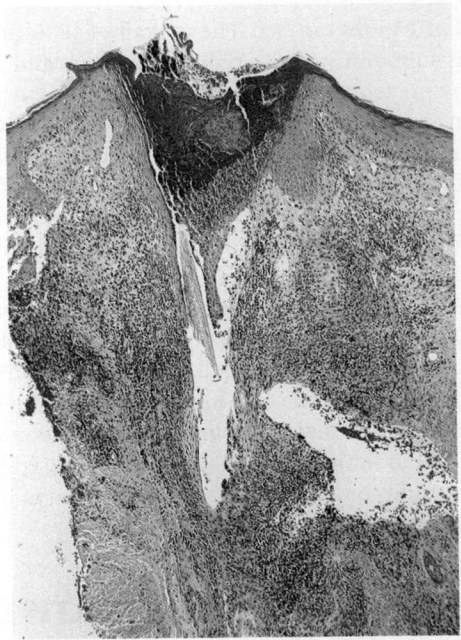

Figure 21-48 Follicular occlusion disorder. Dissecting cellulitis of the scalp, low power. Early lesions may show follicular plugging with acute perifollicular inflammation. Eventually, the follicle is destroyed and replaced by dense mixed inflammation. The appearances are indistinguishable from hidradenitis suppurativa (H&E stain).

Pathogenesis. The common initiating event in the three diseases of the follicular occlusion triad appears to be follicular hyperkeratosis leading to retention of follicular products. Thus, the designation *hidradenitis suppurativa* is a misnomer, because

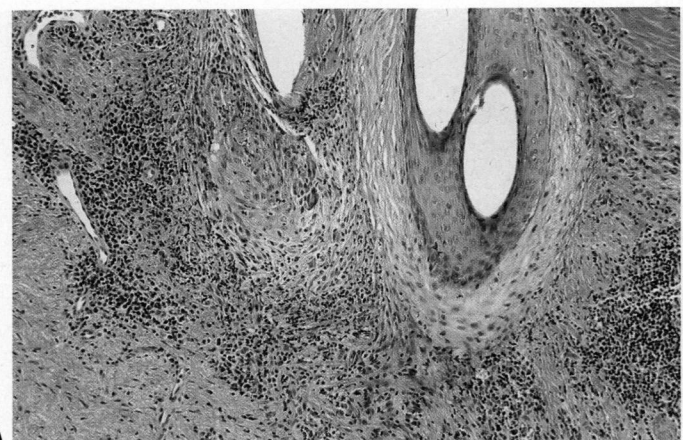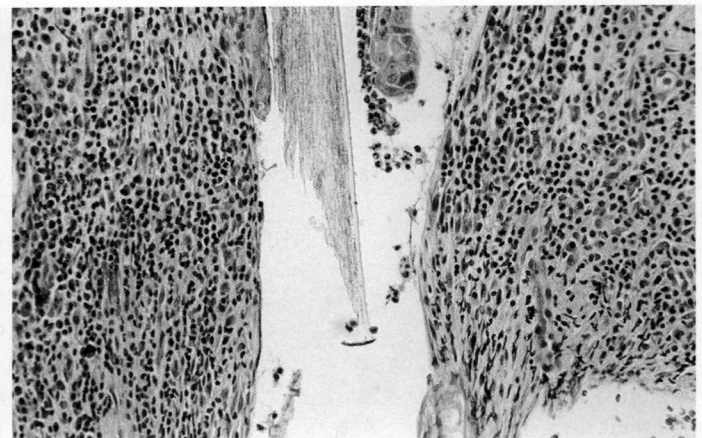

A   B

Figure 21-49 Follicular occlusion disorder. **A:** Dissecting cellulitis of the scalp, medium power. Perifollicular fibrosis ensues and is accompanied by granulomatous inflammation in reaction to follicular contents. Advanced lesions may show sinus tract formation. **B:** Dissecting cellulitis of the scalp, high power. The follicular epithelium is almost completely destroyed, leaving a hair shaft exposed to the dermis and a mixed infiltrate of neutrophils, lymphocytes, histiocytes, and plasma cells (H&E stain).

involvement of apocrine as well as of eccrine glands represents a secondary phenomenon and is the result of the extension of the inflammatory process into deep structures.

It appears doubtful that the diseases comprising the follicular occlusion triad are caused primarily by bacterial infection, because cultures from unopened abscesses are often negative (185).

The beneficial effect of the internal administration of corticosteroid suggests that the three diseases represent antigen–antibody reactions resulting in tissue breakdown. Defects in cell-mediated immunity exist in some patients with hidradenitis suppurativa.

Principles of Management: The overall goals of treatment of hidradenitis suppurativa are to reduce the extent and progression of disease by preventing the formation of new lesions, to remove chronic sinuses, and to limit cicatrix formation. However, there are no definitive guidelines to do so. General measures include avoidance of skin trauma, daily gentle cleansing of affected areas to reduce occurrence of secondary infection, and weight management. Topical clindamycin may be used in mild disease. Tetracyclines are considered first-line antibiotic therapy in patients with more advanced disease (inflammatory nodules, sinus tracts, or scarring). Clindamycin and rifampin is an option for patients who fail to respond to conventional therapy. TNF inhibitors may offer therapeutic benefit in some cases, particularly with weight-based dosing. Spironolactone, dapsone, and systemic retinoids have been used in limited cases. Surgery can be used for treating individual nodules or sinus tracts. Wide excision is reserved for patients with severe, advanced disease (186).

DISEASE PATTERNS WITH MULTIPLE BACTERIAL ORIGINS

Necrotizing Fasciitis

Clinical Summary. Necrotizing fasciitis is a severe, potentially fatal bacterial infection of the subcutaneous tissues. It may present following surgical intervention, minor trauma, apparently insignificant skin abrasions, or chronic wound. Although it was first recognized to be caused by group A β-hemolytic streptococci, recent studies suggest that it can be caused by a range of organisms with polymicrobial infection in a significant

proportion of cases. The lower extremities are most commonly affected, and diabetes mellitus and immunosuppression have been proposed as important susceptibility factors.

The clinical manifestations include rapidly spreading erythema, swelling, and pain (187). However, the erythema is ill-defined and progresses to painless ulceration and necrosis along fascial planes. There is often severe pain and clinical signs of sepsis far out of proportion to the visible skin manifestations. The Laboratory Risk Indicator for Necrotizing Fasciitis (LRINEC) scoring system was devised to help assess the likelihood of an infection being necrotizing fasciitis (Table 21-2). A score of 5 or lower indicates low risk (<50% chance that the infection is necrotizing fasciitis); a score of 6 to 7 indicates intermediate risk (50% to 75% risk); and 8 or more indicates a high risk (>75%) that the infection is necrotizing fasciitis (188). Whereas erysipelas involves the more superficial layers of the skin, necrotizing fasciitis extends more deeply into the subcutaneous tissues (189).

The list of implicated pathogens in necrotizing fasciitis is much more extensive. In addition to group A streptococci, possible etiologic agents include *S. aureus* and, less frequently, *Streptococcus pneumoniae*, *H. influenzae*, and (rarely) a laundry list of other organisms, including vibrios (*vulnificus*, *parahaemolyticus*), gram-negative bacteria such as pseudomonas,

Table 21-2		
Laboratory Risk Indicator for Necrotizing Fasciitis		
Parameter	Range	Score
C-reactive protein	>150 mg/L	4
White cell count	<15/mm^3	0
	15–25/mm^3	1
	>25/mm^3	2
Hemoglobin	>13.5 g/dL	1
	<11 g/dL	2
Sodium	<135 mmol/L	2
Creatinine	>141 mmol/L	2
Glucose	>10 mmol/L	1

aeromonas, clostridia, and other anaerobes, legionella, *Erysipelothrix rhusiopathiae*, and *Helicobacter cinaedi*. Minor trauma is frequently a predisposing factor, and there is a significant association with chicken pox in children (190). In these and other patients with necrotizing fasciitis owing to group A streptococci, there may be onset of shock and organ failure, which are manifestations of the streptococcal TSS. Unless treated by wide surgical debridement, necrotizing fasciitis is often fatal (191). Probing of the subcutaneous tissue discloses extensive undermining and a serosanguineous exudate (192).

Histopathology. The histologic picture is dependent on location with clinically evident areas characterized by necrosis and variable acute and chronic inflammation, whereas the leading edge may show only bacteria in a subtly necrotic fascia (Figs. 21-50 and 21-51) (193). Clumps of bacteria are usually present (Fig. 21-52). Often, there is thrombosis of blood vessels as the result of damage to vessel walls from the inflammatory process. The key feature in distinguishing necrotizing fasciitis from a less threatening superficial cellulitis is the location of the

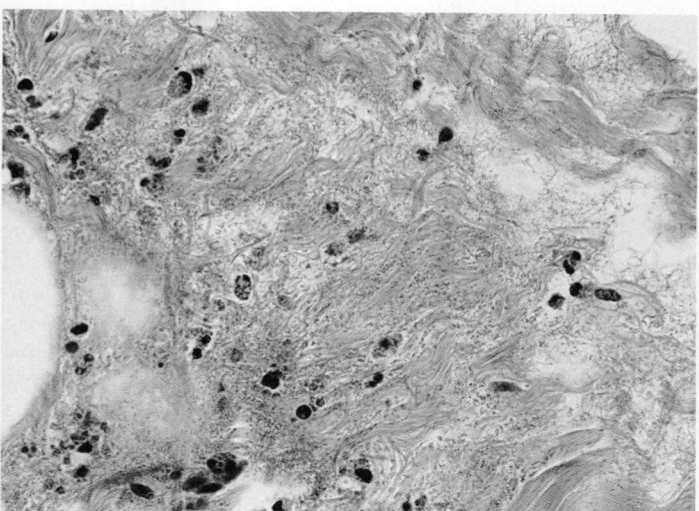

Figure 21-52 Necrotizing fasciitis. Close inspection reveals abundant bacillary bacterial forms, which in this florid case are readily identifiable on H&E stain.

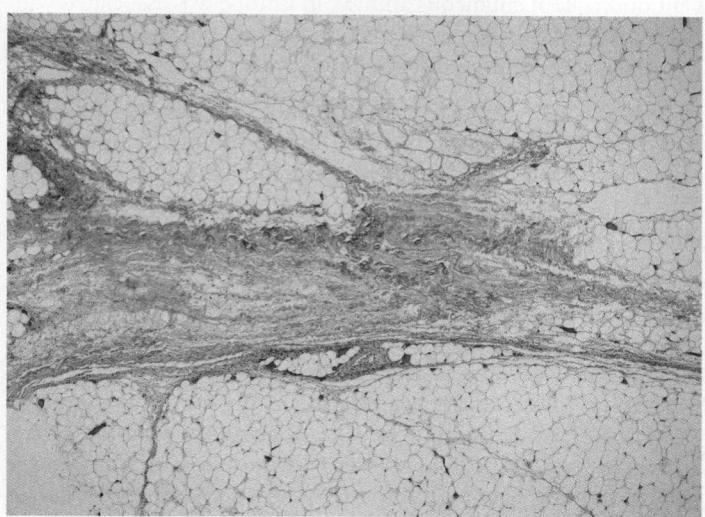

Figure 21-50 Necrotizing fasciitis. Septal necrosis is evident in the subcutis (H&E stain).

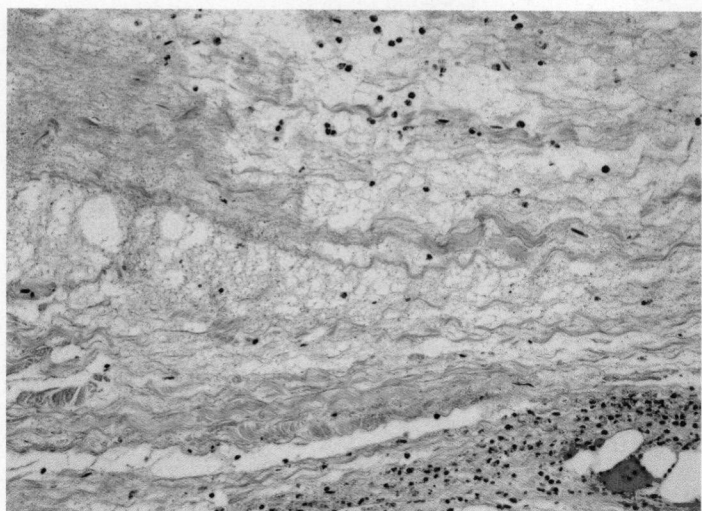

Figure 21-51 Necrotizing fasciitis. There is abundant basophilic debris; note the relative absence of inflammatory cells (H&E stain).

inflammation. In the former, the inflammation involves the subcutaneous fat, fascia, and muscle in addition to the dermis. A biopsy may be submitted at the time of surgical debridement for frozen section examination. In an appropriate setting, the presence of edema and neutrophils in these deep locations supports the diagnosis; frank necrosis may not be demonstrable, and bacteria are frequently not evident in an initial biopsy. Although routinely performed, a recent systematic study found frozen sections to be unreliable for the diagnosis of necrotizing soft tissue infections and thus likely of limited clinical utility (194). Clinicopathologic correlation is of vital importance, and the diagnosis should not be dismissed even if histopathologic findings are subtle in an initial biopsy, if the clinical setting is appropriate.

Differential Diagnosis. Viral and parasitic myositis, pyomyositis, clostridial cellulitis, and gas gangrene are in the differential diagnosis. Microbiologic identification or isolation of an organism may be the only way to distinguish them.

Principles of Management: Treatment comprises early and aggressive surgical exploration and debridement in conjunction with broad spectrum antimicrobial pharmacotherapy and hemodynamic support. Surgical debridement to bacteria-free margins, perhaps with judicious use of frozen section support, is key. Indications for surgery include severe pain, toxicity, fever, and elevated creatine kinase, with or without radiologic evidence of fasciitis. It should be noted that antibiotic therapy alone without debridement is associated with a high mortality rate approaching 100%. Antibiotic regimens include a carbapenem or β-lactam/β-lactamase inhibitor plus clindamycin, but should be tailored to Gram stain, culture, and/or sensitivity results when available (195).

Malakoplakia

Malakoplakia is a rare, chronic inflammatory disorder that may affect various organs, most commonly the urinary tract and the gastrointestinal tract (196). In rare instances, it involves the skin, particularly the vulva and perianal region (197,198). The lesions are thought to be an unusual granulomatous response to bacterial infection, the result of an inability of macrophages to phagocytose bacteria adequately. The most common organism grown in cultures of tissue material is *Escherichia coli* (199), but in some instances, other bacteria such as *S. aureus*, *Rhodococcus equi*, and nontuberculosis mycobacteria (200) are cultured. Some patients with lesions of malakoplakia have altered immune responsiveness as a result of carcinoma, autoimmune systemic diseases such as systemic lupus erythematosus, or immunosuppressive therapy for lymphoma or for renal transplantation (201).

Clinical Summary. Cutaneous malakoplakia lesions are chronic and may be associated with internal lesions. The appearance of the cutaneous lesions is nonspecific and variable. Most commonly, a fluctuant area, a draining abscess, draining sinuses, or an ulcer is observed; however, in some patients, a solitary, tender nodule or a cluster of tender papules is observed. The cutaneous disease is benign and self-limited.

Histopathology. There are sheets of large histiocytes containing fine, eosinophilic granules in their cytoplasm. In addition to the granules, many of them contain ovoid or round basophilic inclusions, referred to as *Michaelis–Gutmann bodies*, that vary in size from 5 to 15 µm (70) (Fig. 21-53). These bodies either are homogeneous or have a "target" appearance by showing concentric laminations. The infiltrate may also contain lymphocytes, plasma cells, and polymorphs.

The Michaelis–Gutmann inclusion bodies and the cytoplasmic granules are periodic acid–Schiff (PAS)-positive, diastase resistant, and Alcian blue positive. In addition, the Michaelis–Gutmann bodies stain with the von Kossa stain for calcium and contain small amounts of iron, which may be demonstrated by Perl stain. With the Gram stain, gram-negative bacteria may be seen in some of the histiocytes, and in the rare case caused by mycobacteria, Ziehl–Neelsen stain reveals the organisms (202).

Pathogenesis. Electron microscopic examination reveals that the cytoplasm of the granular cells contains numerous phagolysosomes corresponding to the PAS-positive granules. Some phagolysosomes contain lamellae in a concentric arrangement (198). The Michaelis–Gutmann bodies develop within phagolysosomes by the progressive deposition of electron-dense calcific material on the whorled or concentric lamellae until they are ultimately completely calcified. Bacteria may be observed in the cytoplasm of the granular cells and in various stages of digestion within phagolysosomes (200).

Malakoplakia represents an acquired defect in the lysosomal killing and digestion of phagocytized bacteria. Deficiencies of β-glucuronidase and of 3′,5′-guanosine monophosphate dehydrogenase have been documented (199–203).

Principles of Management: Antimicrobials that concentrate in macrophages have been associated with high response rates (e.g., fluoroquinolones, trimethoprim–sulfamethoxazole). Pharmacotherapy directed against *E. coli*, in combination with surgery, provides the best chance of cure. Discontinuation of immunosuppressive therapy is usually needed to treat malakoplakia effectively (196).

Injection Abscesses

Clinical Summary. The pandemic of injection drug abuse has resulted in numerous patients presenting with dermal and subcutaneous abscesses from the use of contaminated syringes and needles. Similar abscesses have also been frequently noted in health care settings, where injection solutions may also be contaminated (204). Numerous bacterial and mycobacterial species may be found on culture, including staphylococci and streptococci. A recent epidemic in the United Kingdom involved *Clostridium perfringens* and *Clostridium novyi* infections (205). As mentioned previously, a recent outbreak of cutaneous anthrax in Europe was associated with heroin use. These infections may progress to necrotizing fasciitis, myositis, bacteremia, and septic shock with fatalities.

Histopathology. A standard panel of Gram, silver stain (e.g., Grocott), and Ziehl–Neelsen is useful in identifying the organisms, although culture is required for specific diagnosis (Fig. 21-54). The histopathology is not usually specific. Acute inflammation, edema, and tissue necrosis are usual. In chronic lesions, much granulation tissue, fibrosis, and sinuses develop. In mycobacterial injection lesions, there may also be granulomas.

Principles of Management: Incision and drainage is required for treatment of skin abscesses. The obtained material should be sent for culture and susceptibility testing for optimal antimicrobial therapy. Although the role of ancillary antibiotic therapy in the treatment of abscesses is uncertain, empiric therapy should include agents with activity against MRSA in areas of high prevalence. First-choice regimens for gram-negative and anaerobic pathogens include piperacillin–tazobactam or ceftriaxone plus metronidazole. Alternative empiric regimens include a combination of a fluoroquinolone plus metronidazole or a monotherapy with a carbapenem (206).

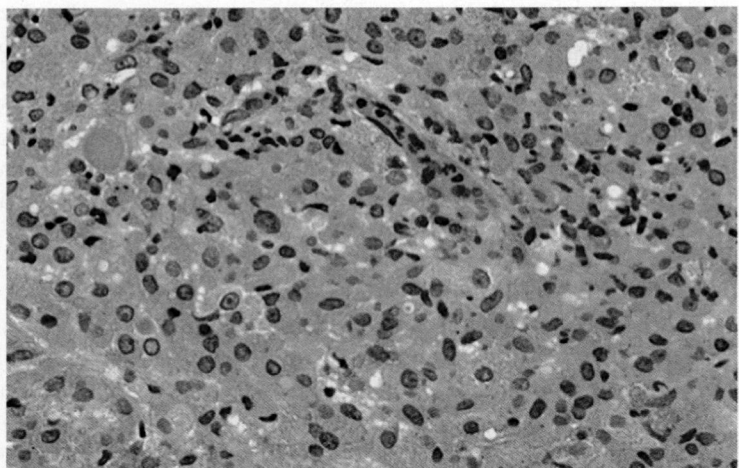
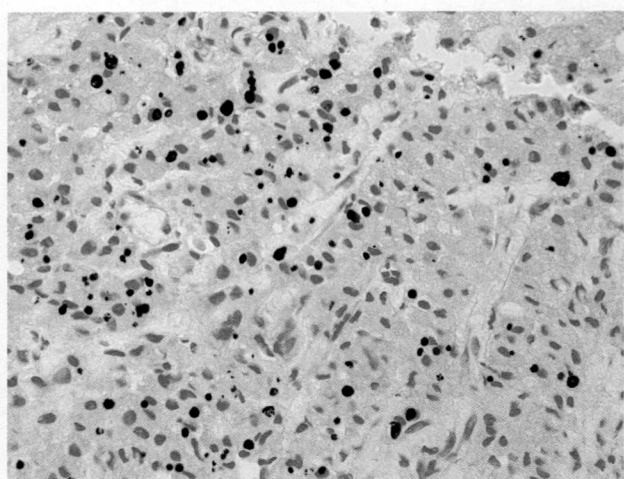

Figure 21-53 **A:** Malakoplakia. Sheets of macrophages with eosinophilic cytoplasm; several in the center contain Michaelis–Gutmann inclusion bodies (H&E stain). **B:** Michaelis–Gutmann inclusion bodies are highlighted by the Von Kossa stain for calcium salts.

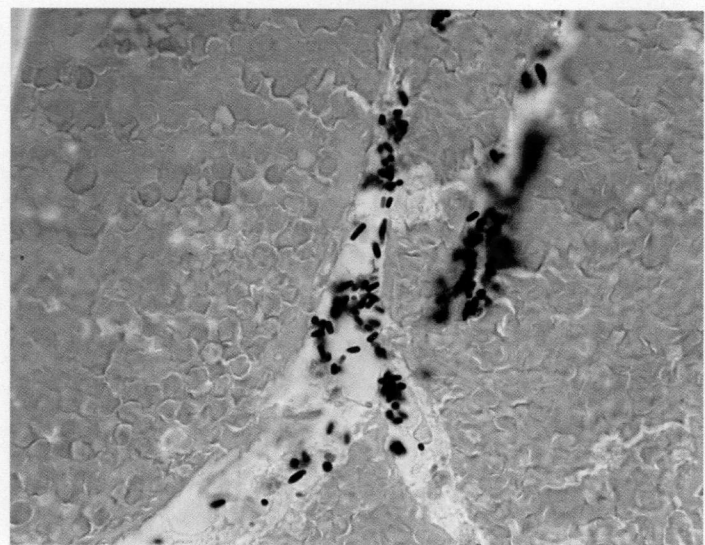

Figure 21-54 Clostridium perfringens injection abscess. Cluster of wide gram-positive rods, typical of *Clostridium* sp. (Gram stain).

Botryomycosis

Botryomycosis, despite its name, is not a fungal infection but a chronic suppurative infection of skin (and other organs such as lungs and meninges) in which pyogenic bacteria form granules similar to those seen in mycetoma (207). Although immunosuppressed patients, including those with HIV infection, may acquire botryomycosis (208), most patients have no known immune defect.

Clinical Summary. The skin lesions are local nodules, ulcers, or sinuses communicating with deep abscesses. They occur mainly on the extremities (209).

Histopathology. The dermal inflammation is predominantly that of neutrophil polymorph abscesses with surrounding granulation tissue and fibrosis (Fig. 21-55). Within the abscesses are granules (grains) shaped like a bunch of grapes; hence the name of the disease (Fig. 21-56). The grains may vary from 20 μm to

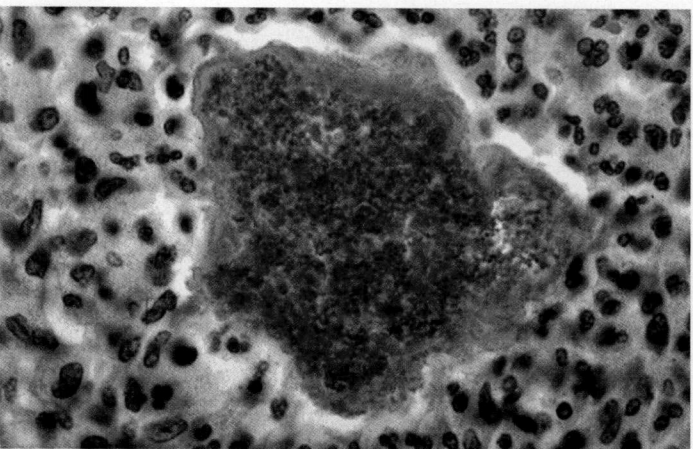

Figure 21-56 Botryomycosis. An abscess within which is a basophilic bacterial clump with an eosinophilic surrounding HS reaction (H&E stain, high power).

2 mm in diameter. They are composed of closely aggregated nonfilamentous bacteria with a peripheral, radial deposition of intensely eosinophilic material—a Hoeppli–Splendore (HS) reaction. The bacteria are usually *S. aureus*, but streptococci and certain gram-negative bacilli such as *Proteus*, *Pseudomonas*, and *E. coli* are sometimes found. Gram stains delineate these broad categories of infection, although sometimes the organisms in gram-positive infections are degenerate and lose their gram-positive staining reaction (Fig. 21-57). The HS reaction material comprises antibody and fibrin.

The overlying epithelium often exhibits pseudoepitheliomatous hyperplasia. Transepithelial elimination of grains may be observed (as with mycetoma) (210).

Pathogenesis. Local implantation of infection may be a factor in some cases, with persistence of a foreign body. Bacteremia is documented in many patients; however, in others, the lesions appear *de novo*. The characteristic formation of the peribacterial HS reaction probably prevents phagocytosis and intracellular killing of the bacteria, leading to chronicity.

Principles of Management: Treatment of cutaneous disease is based on antibiotic therapy and surgical debridement. Antimicrobial therapy alone may be sufficient for patients with superficial disease if a pathogen has been identified and malignancy

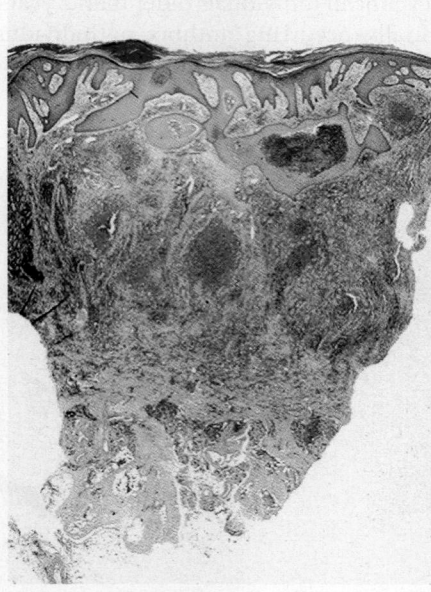

Figure 21-55 Botryomycosis. There are pseudoepitheliomatous hyperplasia and small abscesses in the dermis containing clumps of bacteria (H&E stain).

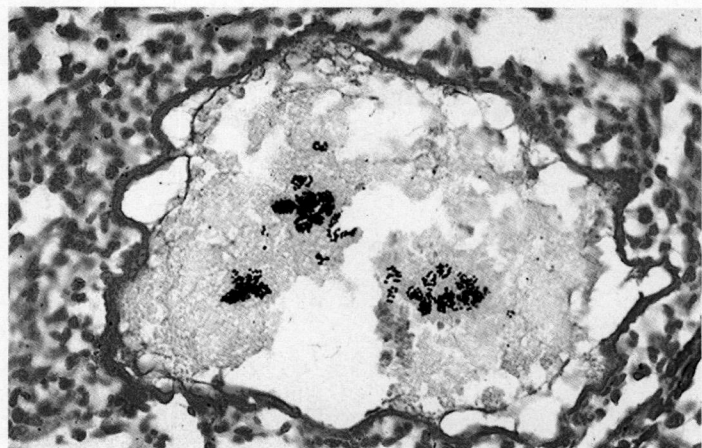

Figure 21-57 Botryomycosis. A staphylococcal lesion showing gram-positive cocci (the majority are degenerate and nonstaining) (Gram stain).

has been excluded. Trimethoprim–sulfamethoxazole, or oral clindamycin, can be used for gram-positive infections, including with *S. aureus*. For pseudomonal infections, ceftazidime, ciprofloxacin, aztreonam, or imipenem can be used (211,212).

AGENTS OF BIOTERRORISM

Anthrax

Anthrax, caused by the spore-forming *Bacillus anthracis*, is enzootic in many countries (213). It occurs occasionally among workers in tanneries and wool-scouring mills through the handling of infected hides, wool, or hair imported from Asia. After the 2001 bioterrorism attack in the United States, and the outbreak of anthrax infections in heroin users in Europe in 2009 and 2010, the clinical relevance and awareness of anthrax has increased. *B. anthracis* is a gram-positive rod that may remain viable in soil as a spore for decades.

Clinical Summary. In cutaneous anthrax, the lesion starts as a papule. The papule enlarges and a hemorrhagic pustule forms (214). After the pustule has ruptured, a thick, black eschar covers the area. Marked erythema and edema surround the lesion. Characteristically, pain is slight or absent.

Histopathology. At the site of the eschar, the epidermis is destroyed and the ulcerated surface is covered with necrotic tissue. There is marked edema of the dermis. Vasculitis, hemorrhage, and variable acute and chronic inflammatory infiltrate are observed (Figs. 21-58 and 21-59).

Anthrax bacilli are present in large numbers and can be recognized in sections stained with the Gram stain. The bacillus is large, rod shaped, encapsulated, gram positive, 6 to 10 μm long, and 1 to 2 μm thick. Anthrax bacilli are found particularly in the necrotic tissue toward the surface of the ulcer but also in the dermis (Fig. 21-60). Phagocytosis of the bacilli by either neutrophils or histiocytes is absent.

Pathogenesis. Invasion through the skin may occur via two mechanisms. Spores of *B. anthracis* appear to be capable of invading hair follicles and germinating. The microorganism can also gain access through skin abrasions. Unlike infection by the gastrointestinal or pulmonary routes, spore germination in skin does not

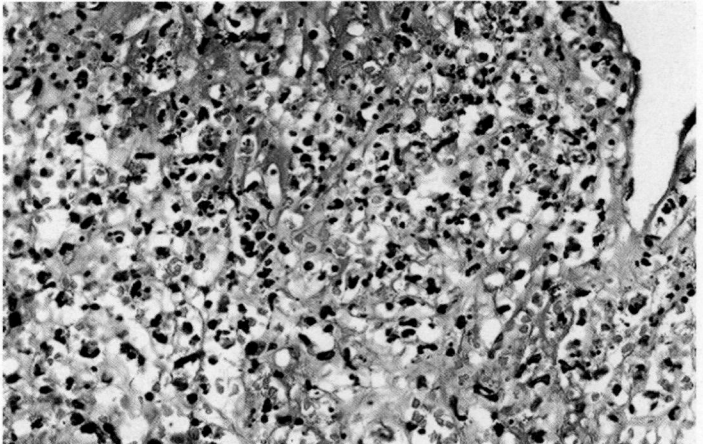

Figure 21-59 Anthrax. Acute inflammation and dermal edema (H&E stain).

appear to be associated with immune cell involvement. Animal products such as meat or hides from infected animals act as reservoirs for human contagion. Germination from spore to vegetative forms occurs within host macrophages. After germination, it appears that three factors are crucial to the pathogenesis of anthrax: (a) a capsule, (b) the production of two toxins (lethal toxin and edema toxin), and (c) the bacterial ability to reach high concentrations in infected hosts. The capsule resists phagocytosis and is only weakly immunogenic. The lethal toxin is a zinc metalloprotease that selectively inactivates MAP-kinases 1 to 4 and 6 and 7, leading to inhibition of intracellular signaling. Lethal toxin stimulates the release of TNF-α and interleukin 1β—which is thought to contribute to the sudden death that occurs in animals with high bacteremia. Edema factor is a calmodulin-dependent adenyl cyclase that increases intracellular cyclic adenosine monophosphate (cAMP) to very high levels, resulting in edema, inhibition of neutrophil function, and hindrance of production of TNF and interleukin 6 by monocytes (215,216).

Principles of Management: Localized, uncomplicated and naturally occurring anthrax may be treated with oral ciprofloxacin or doxycycline in individuals older than 2 years. For severe cases of naturally occurring anthrax or individuals younger than 2 years, intravenous ciprofloxacin or doxycycline are

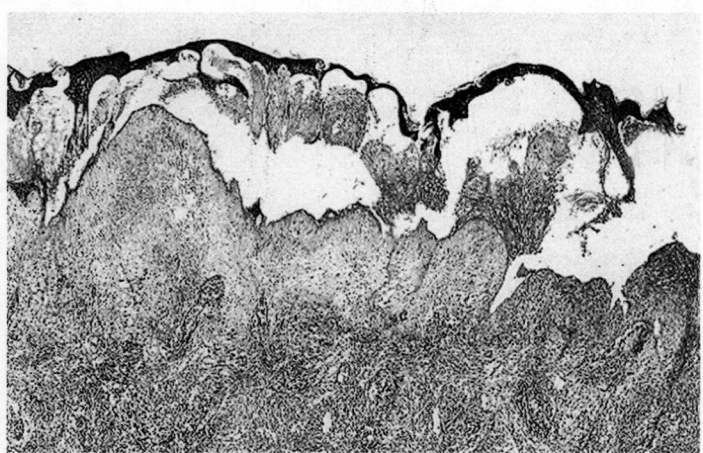

Figure 21-58 Anthrax. Acute lesion with epidermal necrosis and pandermal inflammation (H&E stain).

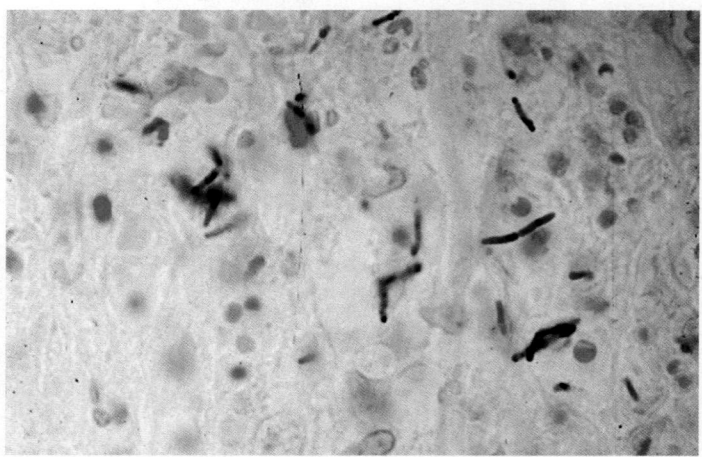

Figure 21-60 Anthrax. Numerous gram-positive thick bacilli within the acute inflammation (Gram stain).

recommended. Patients with bioterrorism-related cutaneous anthrax are at risk for inhalation anthrax owing to probable aerosol exposure. Therefore, antimicrobial therapy should be administered for 60 days to maximize postexposure prophylaxis against inhalational anthrax (217).

Tularemia

Clinical Summary. Tularemia is caused by *Francisella tularensis*, a small, gram-negative, pleomorphic coccobacillus. Tularemia occurs mainly in the northern hemisphere, with most cases reported in Scandinavia, northern America, Japan, and Russia. Two strains have been delineated on the basis of virulence: *F. tularensis* subsp. *tularensis* (also known as type A or nearctica) and subsp. *holarctica* (also known as type B or palearctica). Strains of *F. tularensis* subsp. *tularensis* are regarded as most virulent for humans and are found in North America and Europe. Strains of subsp. *holarctica* are found mainly in North America and Eurasia and are less virulent. The disease is usually acquired by humans through direct contact with rodents, but it may be transmitted from rodents to humans by insects, such as mosquitoes, ticks, or deer flies (218). The disease often occurs in small epidemics. There are two types: ulceroglandular (the more common type) and typhoidal. These disease types reflect differences in the route of entry of the bacterium into the body fundamentally. In ulceroglandular tularemia, usually owing to a bite from an arthropod vector, there is a vigorous inflammatory reaction, and the patient's prognosis is generally good even without treatment. Mortality from ulceroglandular tularemia is estimated to be less than 3%. In the typhoidal form, characterized by an acute course and septicemia, there are few localizing signs, pneumonia is more common, and the mortality rate is 30% to 60%.

In the ulceroglandular type, one or several painful ulcers occur as primary lesions at the site of infection, usually on the hands. Tender subcutaneous nodes may form along the lymph vessels that drain the primary lesion or lesions. There is considerable swelling of the regional lymph nodes, and the infection is associated with marked constitutional symptoms. Healing of the lesions takes place in 2 to 5 weeks (219,220).

Histopathology. At its base, the primary ulcer shows a nonspecific inflammatory infiltrate associated with a granulomatous reaction. In some cases, only a moderate number of epithelioid cells and a few giant cells are observed. In others, however, large, well-developed tuberculoid granulomas are apparent. These granulomas may show central necrosis with the presence of nuclear dust. Late lesions may show epithelioid cell tubercles that have no central necrosis and are surrounded by only a slightly inflammatory reaction, and their appearance may thus resemble that of sarcoidosis (221).

The tender nodes that may be found along lymph vessels show multiple granulomas deep in the dermis and extending into the subcutaneous tissue. The central zones of necrosis in the granulomas may attain a much greater size than in the primary ulcer. Similarly, the regional lymph nodes show multiple granulomas with centrally located abscess necrosis or caseous necrosis (218–222).

Principles of Management: Although spontaneous resolution in the absence of specific treatment has been documented, antimicrobial therapy should be administered in patients with suspected or confirmed tularemia. Streptomycin and gentamicin,

tetracyclines, chloramphenicol, and fluoroquinolones are efficacious in treating tularemia. Streptomycin is the drug of choice for all forms of tularemia except meningitis. Gentamicin is an acceptable alternative and may be administered intravenously (223).

SEXUALLY TRANSMITTED INFECTIONS

Although each infectious entity will be discussed separately, it is essential that practitioners recognize that patients with one sexually transmitted infection (STI) are at risk for others and that coinfection is common. Often, the suggested therapy for one disease includes empiric treatment for other likely coinfections. All patients should be offered screening for HIV infection and counseling about safe sex practices, and often these infections are reportable. Sexual partners should be identified, screened, and/or treated when appropriate.

Chancroid

Clinical Summary. Chancroid, caused by the gram-negative facultative anaerobic coccobacillus *Haemophilus ducreyi*, is a STD leading to one or several ulcers, chiefly in the genital region. It is nowadays exceedingly rare in the United States and globally largely owing to the introduction of syndromic management of STIs in the late 1990s to curb the HIV pandemic (224,225). The ulcers exhibit little if any induration and are often deep and purulent and have ragged undermined borders. They are usually tender. Inguinal lymphadenitis, either unilateral or bilateral, occurs in up to 50% of cases and unless treated often results in an inguinal abscess. Chancroid used to be endemic in some countries of Africa, Asia and the Caribbean, where it accounted for up to 50% of genital ulcers. Since the 1990s, multiple studies have documented the decline in incidence and even the disappearance of chancroid in countries where it was previously endemic. This is thought to be the result of increased use of condoms and/or reduction in the number of exposed sexual partners, with consequent rapid reduction of the reproductive rate (R_0) of this STI. Of interest, multiple reports have documented *H. ducreyi* as the causative agent of chronic limb ulcers in children and adults in recent years, particularly in Africa and the Pacific region. The *H. ducreyi* strains isolated from cutaneous ulcers are almost identical to the class I strains that cause chancroid and are believed to be a subpopulation that diverged from them approximately 0.2 million years ago (225).

Histopathology. The histologic changes observed beneath the ulcer consist of three zones overlying each other and show characteristic vascular changes (224,225) (Fig. 21-61). The surface zone at the floor of the ulcer is rather narrow and consists of neutrophils, fibrin, erythrocytes, and necrotic tissue. The next zone is wide and contains many newly formed blood vessels showing marked proliferation of their endothelial cells. As a result of the endothelial proliferation, the lumina of the vessels are often occluded, leading to thrombosis. In addition, there are degenerative changes in the walls of the vessels. The deep zone is composed of a dense infiltrate of plasma cells and lymphoid cells.

Demonstration of bacilli in tissue sections stained with Giemsa stain or Gram stain is occasionally possible (Fig. 21-62). The bacilli are most apt to be found between the cells of the surface zone (226). However, in smears of serous exudate obtained

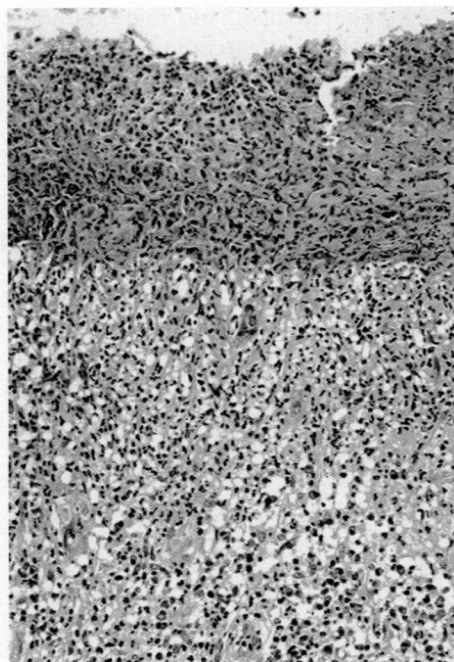

Figure 21-61 Chancroid. Three-zone pattern of ulcer and inflammation: superficial necrotic zone, underlying granulation tissue, and deeper fibrosis with plasma cells (H&E stain).

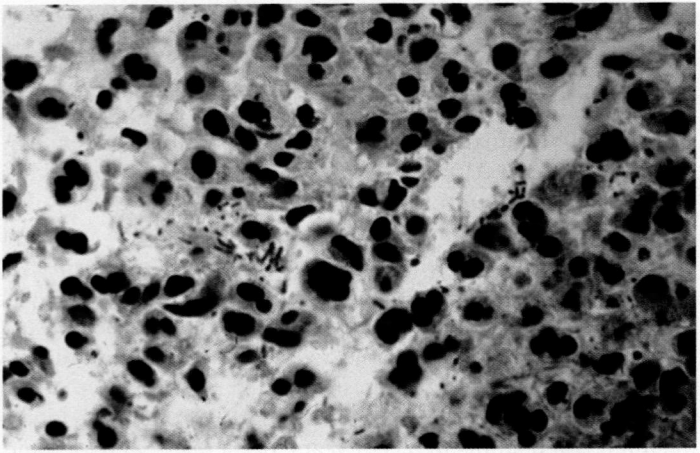

Figure 21-62 Chancroid. Bacilli (in the superficial zone) lying in parallel chains (Giemsa stain).

from the undermined edge of the ulcer, the bacilli can usually be seen on staining with the Giemsa or Gram stain. *H. ducreyi* is a fine, short, gram-negative coccobacillus, measuring about 1.5 by 0.2 μm, often arranged in parallel chains. It should be noted that ulcer material stain by the Gram method has a poor sensitivity and specificity and should not be used as a diagnostic test. *In situ* hybridization and multiplex PCR have higher sensitivity to detect *H. ducreyi* but are not widely available (227). Electron microscopy reveals that the bacilli are extracellular and thus rarely visible in phagosomes of macrophages (228).

The diagnosis of chancroid may be confirmed by culture on selective blood-enriched agar, but DNA amplification using multiple primers is considered more sensitive and the diagnostic test of choice when available (229). Chancroid may clinically resemble donovanosis by showing nontender or only slightly tender, indurated ulcers without undermined margins. On the other hand, particularly in the presence of several

lesions, herpes simplex has to be excluded, although in herpes simplex the ulcerations are usually not as deep as those in chancroid and tend to be exquisitely tender (230).

Pathogenesis. After trauma and micro abrasion of the skin, the microorganism penetrates the epidermis. A high inoculum is required for infection, on the order of 10,000 microorganisms. The main virulence determinants of *H. ducreyi* are superoxide dismutase, which is thought to increase survival and persistence of the organism within the host, and hemolysin, which promotes ulcer formation and invasion of epithelial cells. This latter determinant has immunogenic properties that make hemolysin a candidate for vaccine development (225).

Differential Diagnosis. As stated previously, the differential diagnosis is that of genital ulcer, including genital herpes, syphilis, chancroid, and granuloma inguinale.

Principles of Management: Directly observed single-dose therapy is highly desirable. Azithromycin, ceftriaxone, or ciprofloxacin is effective. When empiric therapy is administered, patients should also be treated for possible coinfection with *T. pallidum* resulting from frequent coinfection (231).

Granuloma Inguinale (Donovanosis)

Clinical Summary. Granuloma inguinale, also called *donovanosis*, is an STD caused by *Calymmatobacterium granulomatis*, also known as *Klebsiella granulomatis*, although controversy exists as to whether the latter is the same bacterium or only a highly related one (232,233). The organism is a gram-negative short bacillus, about 2 to 3 μm long, with bipolar staining. The disease is endemic, but relatively uncommon, in the tropics (234).

Granuloma inguinale occurs in the genital or perianal region either as a single lesion or as several lesions (235). The lesions consist of ulcers filled with exuberant granulation tissue that bleeds easily (the characteristic beefy appearance). The borders of the ulcers are elevated and often have serpiginous outlines. Because the lesions spread by peripheral extension, they may attain a large size. In some instances, ulceration leads to mutilation resulting from destruction of tissue (236). In others, excessive granulation tissue causes vegetating lesions. Occasionally, squamous cell carcinoma supervenes (237). Local lymphadenopathy occurs through secondary infection of ulcerated skin. Donovanosis presenting as polyps of the external auditory canal has been reported in two infants (4 and 6 months of age) born via vaginal delivery to infected mothers (238).

Histopathology. At the edge of the ulcer, the epidermis exhibits acanthosis that may reach the proportions of pseudocarcinomatous hyperplasia. Present in the dermis is a dense infiltrate that is composed predominantly of histiocytes and plasma cells (Fig. 21-63). Scattered throughout this infiltrate are small abscesses composed of neutrophils. The number of lymphoid cells is conspicuously small (239).

The macrophages, which may be large, have a typical vacuolated appearance; these vacuoles contain bacilli and comprise the so-called Donovan bodies. *C. granulomatis* does not stain with hematoxylin and eosin (H&E) but is well delineated by the Warthin–Starry method as short bacilli, either singly or in clumps (226–239) (Fig. 21-64). Giemsa stain shows bipolar condensations of stain. Electron microscopy reveals that the bacteria reside in phagosomes (240).

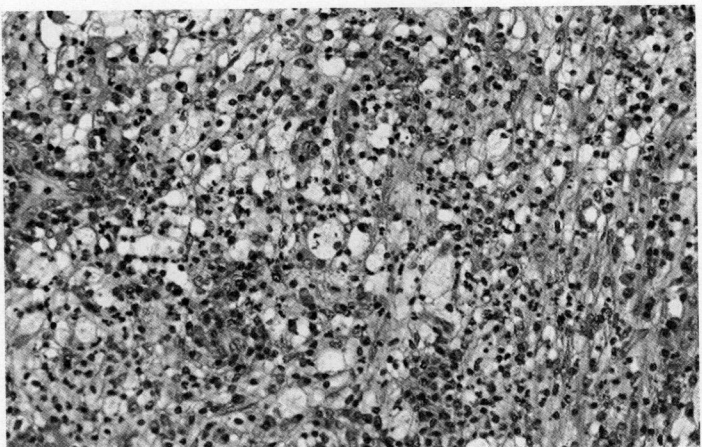

Figure 21-63 Donovanosis. Acute inflammation intermixed with foamy macrophages (H&E stain).

Differential Diagnosis. Overdiagnosis of carcinoma is possible because of pseudocarcinomatous epithelial hyperplasia. The inflammatory pattern is similar to that observed in rhinoscleroma.

Principles of Management: Doxycycline is considered as the preferred agent for the treatment of granuloma inguinale. An aminoglycoside may be added if there is no clinical improvement within the first few days after initiation of therapy. Pregnant women should be treated with erythromycin. Alternative active agents include azithromycin, ciprofloxacin, and trimethoprim–sulfamethoxazole (241).

Lymphogranuloma Venereum

Clinical Summary. Lymphogranuloma venereum (LGV) is an STD caused by *Chlamydia trachomatis* (CT) genovars L1, L2, and L3, with the L2 genovars being the most common in the United States and Europe (242). Chlamydiae are obligate intracellular parasites with a unique biphasic life cycle.

The incubation period of LGV varies from 3 to 30 days but averages 7 days. The primary lesion is a small erosion or papule 5 to 8 mm in size. This lesion heals within a few days and may pass unnoticed. Within 1 to 2 weeks after the appearance of the primary lesion, enlargement of the inguinal lymph nodes begins. Inguinal lymphadenopathy occurs in most men infected with this disease but in only some women. The involved inguinal lymph nodes are firm at first but subsequently develop

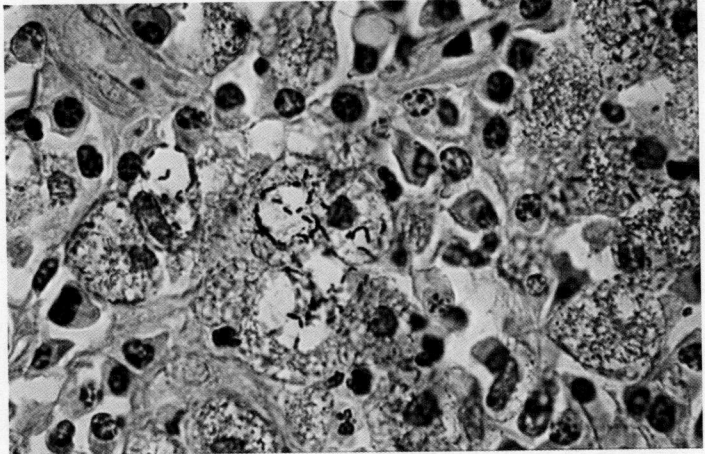

Figure 21-64 Donovanosis. Silver-positive bacilli within macrophages (Warthin–Starry stain).

multiple areas of suppuration, resulting in draining sinuses. The lymphadenopathy usually subsides within 2 to 3 months. Rarely, elephantiasis of the penis and scrotum or chronic penile ulcerations arise as a late complication (242).

In women in whom the infection begins in the lower portion of the vagina, drainage is to the iliac and anorectal lymph nodes rather than to the inguinal lymph nodes, which may result in proctitis (236). Rectal stricture and perineal ulcerations are fairly common late complications in these women. Lymph stasis may lead to marked vulvar edema, referred to as *esthiomene*. Proctitis and rectal stricture also occur in homosexual men (243).

Histopathology. The changes in the initial papule are nonspecific. There is ulceration and a nonspecific granulation tissue. In the lymph nodes, stellate abscesses with surrounding epithelioid cells and macrophage giant cells represent the characteristic lesion. A similar pathology is seen in cat scratch disease nodes. Ordinary histologic stains do not demonstrate the infecting organisms in skin or node. Early identification of the CT genovars that cause LGV is best accomplished by real-time PCR using commercially available assays and is important for adequate treatment (244).

Chlamydiae undergo a developmental cycle and, as can be seen by electron microscopy, occur in two forms: elementary body and initial body (245). The elementary body is adapted to an extracellular environment and is infective for other cells. It measures about 0.3 µm in diameter and consists of a round, electron-dense inner body surrounded by an electron-lucid halo and a membrane. After entering a host cell by means of phagocytosis, it develops into a metabolically active initial body 0.5 to 1.0 µm in diameter. Multiplication takes place by division of the nucleus. This division results in two elementary bodies, which, on leaving the host cell, can infect other cells.

Principles of Management: Antimicrobial therapy with doxycycline is the recommended treatment for granuloma inguinale, with erythromycin as a second-line choice. Buboes may require needle aspiration or incision and drainage to avoid rupture with consequent scarring and sinus formation (246).

ORGANISM-SPECIFIC PATTERNS IN SKIN INFECTIONS

Rhinoscleroma

Rhinoscleroma is a chronic, infectious but only mildly contagious disease caused by *Klebsiella rhinoscleromatis*, a gram-negative bacillus.

Clinical Summary. The nose, pharynx, larynx, trachea, and, occasionally, also the skin of the upper lip are distorted and infiltrated with hard, granulomatous masses. The disorder always begins in the nose. Although formerly endemic in Central Europe, it is now encountered mainly in Central America and Africa (247–249). Clinically and pathologically, rhinoscleroma can be subclassified into three stages: catarrhal, proliferative, and fibrotic. In the catarrhal stage, foul-smelling, purulent nasal discharge, and nasal obstruction are present. The proliferative stage is characterized by epistaxis, nasal deformity, hoarseness, anosmia, and epiphora. Red-blue, rubbery granulomatous lesions are present. Increased deformity and stenosis are noted during the fibrotic stage.

Histopathology. The characteristic histologic findings correspond to the proliferative stage of the disease. The cellular infiltrate is a chronic granulation tissue with abundant plasma cells and Mikulicz cells. Polymorphs may be present (but they cannot kill the bacteria). Russell bodies (plasma cells with retained globules of immunoglobulins) are frequently observed. The characteristic cell is the Mikulicz cell, a large histiocyte measuring from 10 to 100 μm in diameter (Fig. 21-65). It has a pale, vacuolated cytoplasm. Within the cytoplasm of the Mikulicz cells, one finds many bacilli (Fig. 21-66). They can be seen faintly in sections stained with H&E but are better visualized with the Giemsa stain or a Warthin–Starry silver stain (250). They are also stained red by the PAS technique. They are gram-negative rods that measure 2 to 3 μm in length and appear round or ovoid in cross section (248,251).

In long-standing lesions, marked fibrosis is present. The mucosal epithelium overlying the cellular infiltrate often exhibits hyperplasia, which may be so pronounced as to give rise to a mistaken diagnosis of squamous cell carcinoma.

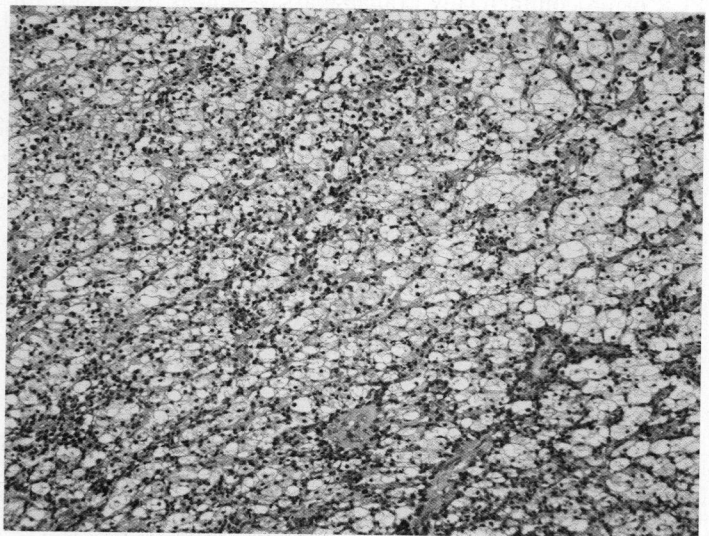

Figure 21-65 Rhinoscleroma. Foamy macrophages (Mikulicz cells) and plasma cells; the bacilli are faintly visible within the macrophages (H&E stain).

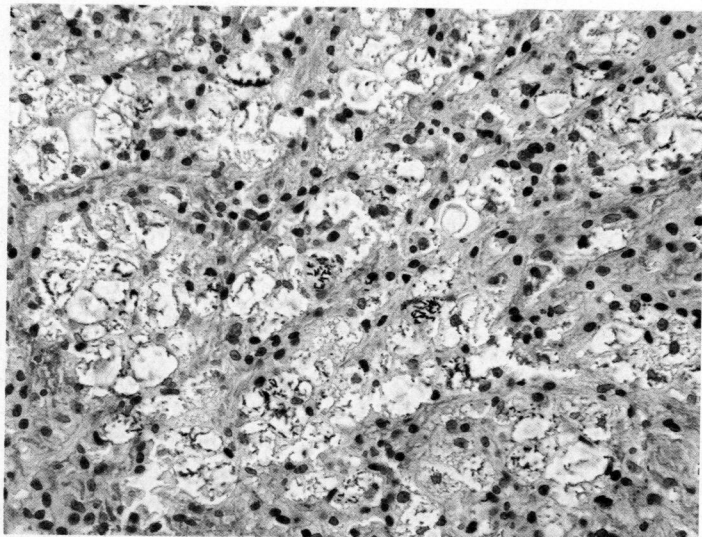

Figure 21-66 Rhinoscleroma. Bacilli within the macrophages (Warthin–Starry stain).

Electron microscopy reveals numerous phagosome vacuoles of varying size within the Mikulicz cells. Some vacuoles contain one or a few bacilli up to 4 μm in length. They are surrounded by a characteristic coat of finely granular, filamentous material arranged in a radial fashion. This coating material contains mucopolysaccharides and is responsible for the positive PAS reaction of the bacteria (249).

Differential Diagnosis. The histopathology of rhinoscleroma is essentially similar to that of donovanosis (granuloma inguinale). Foamy, vacuolated macrophages are also observed in many other chronic inflammatory conditions (e.g., leprosy, chronic staphylococcal abscess, mycoses, and leishmaniasis), but special stains and associated clinicopathologic features usually enable their distinction. Plasma cells and Russell bodies, similarly, correlate with chronicity in many diverse infections, such as treponematoses, amebiasis, leishmaniasis, and tuberculosis.

Principles of Management: Treatment should include long-term antimicrobial therapy and surgical intervention in patients with symptoms of obstruction. Third-generation cephalosporins plus clindamycin have been used successfully. Sclerotic lesions respond well to ciprofloxacin (251).

Bartonelloses

Cat Scratch Disease

Clinical Summary. Bartonella henselae (previously *Rochalimaea henselae*) causes cat scratch disease, and the organism is carried in the blood and oral cavities of cats (252). Cutaneous and lymph node involvement is most common in children. The skin lesion develops 2 to 4 days after a scratch or bite from an infected cat. Notably, the pathogen may also enter through prior trauma during innocuous contact with infected cats. The lesion may be macular, papular, or nodular, usually on the arm or hand. Two to 3 weeks later, a large, tender swelling of a group of lymph nodes develops in the drainage area of the scratch. The cat scratch heals in a normal fashion, but the affected lymph nodes become fluctuant as a result of suppuration. The average duration of lymph node enlargement is 2 months (253,254).

Histopathology. The primary papules at the site of the scratch show one or several acellular areas of necrosis in the dermis. These areas are of various shapes, including round, triangular, and stellate. Surrounding them are several layers of histiocytic and epithelioid cells, with the innermost layer exhibiting a palisading arrangement. A few giant cells may be present. The periphery of the epithelioid cell reaction is surrounded by a zone of lymphoid cells.

The reaction in the lymph nodes is similar to that observed in the skin, except that the central areas of necrosis in the epithelioid cell granulomas undergo abscess formation. Macrophage giant cells are also present. As the abscesses enlarge, they become confluent.

The delicate, pleomorphic, gram-negative bacilli can be demonstrated with the Warthin–Starry silver impregnation stain peripheral to the necrosis of involved lymph nodes and in the skin at the primary site of inoculation. Serodiagnostic tests are available. One study found the best diagnostic yield when observing at least two of the following criteria including *B. henselae* detection by PCR analysis: serologic, epidemiologic, or histologic evidence compatible with cat scratch disease (255).

Electron microscopic examination reveals that the bacteria are invariably extracellular and form small clusters. They are 0.8 to 1.5 μm long and 0.3 to 0.5 μm wide, with homogeneous bacterial walls (256).

Principles of Management: There is controversy with respect to the best course of action for cat scratch disease in immunocompetent individuals. Some experts recommend not treating patients with mild-to-moderate illness. Others suggest antimicrobial therapy with azithromycin. Alternatives for patients that cannot tolerate azithromycin include clarithromycin, rifampin, trimethoprim–sulfamethoxazole, and ciprofloxacin (257).

Bacillary Angiomatosis

Clinical Summary. Bacillary angiomatosis is a relatively new disease, first described in 1983 (258) as a skin or disseminated infection in patients immunosuppressed by HIV infection. It is also rarely encountered in patients with other immunocompromising conditions such as transplantation and even in immunocompetent people (259). The causative agents are gram-negative bacilli: *Bartonella quintana* and *B. henselae* (260). The pathology is similar to that of the late cutaneous stage of bartonellosis, caused by *B. bacilliformis* (261). As with cat scratch disease, exposure to cats is a major risk factor for acquiring this infection (262).

The skin lesions are reddish or brown papules on any part of the body, usually in large numbers, that resemble Kaposi sarcoma. They may also present as subcutaneous lumps without skin involvement (263,264).

Histopathology. The epidermis may be flat or hyperplastic. In the dermis, there are single or multinodular proliferations of capillaries accompanied by an inflammatory infiltrate that includes variable numbers of neutrophil polymorphs and mononuclear cells as well as edema. Leukocytoclasia is frequently observed (264). Characteristic of bacillary angiomatosis are extracellular deposits of palely hematoxyphilic granular material (Fig. 21-67). Warthin–Starry staining reveals these deposits to be dense masses of short bacilli (Fig. 21-68). The Grocott–Gomori methenamine silver method also demonstrates the argyrophilic bacilli. These bacilli may also be delineated by modified Gram stains such as the Brown–Hopps stain.

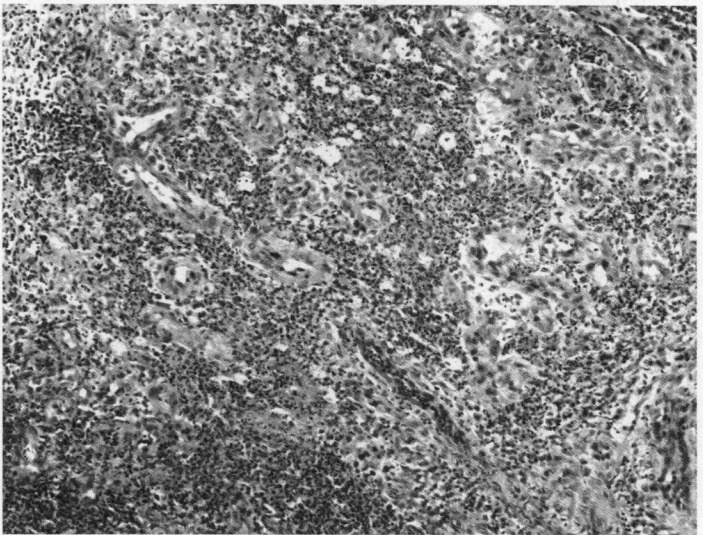

Figure 21-67 Bacillary angiomatosis. Dermis shows vascular proliferation and leukocytoclasia (H&E stain).

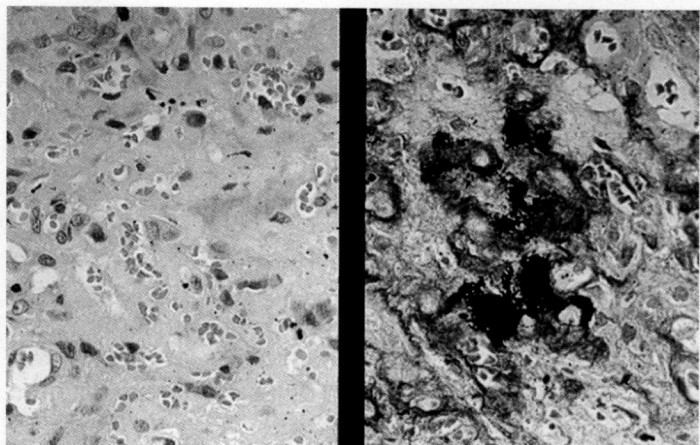

Figure 21-68 Bacillary angiomatosis. **Left:** Clumps and smudges of basophilic extracellular material—the bacteria (H&E stain). **Right:** Silver-positive bacilli (Warthin–Starry stain).

Differential Diagnosis. The major differential diagnoses are Kaposi sarcoma, pyogenic granuloma, and epithelioid hemangioma (264). The presence of clumps of bacilli is obviously important. The capillary proliferation does not have the organized arborizing quality of that in pyogenic granuloma, but it can be difficult to make this distinction in partial samples or ulcerated lesions with secondary changes. A helpful clue is the presence of neutrophilic aggregates in the deeper aspects of the lesion, particularly if not ulcerated. Spindle cell proliferation and intracellular hyaline globules as seen in Kaposi sarcoma are not features of bacillary angiomatosis, and Kaposi sarcoma does not include polymorphs; however, the two conditions may be difficult to distinguish, and many pathologists have learned about bacillary angiomatosis from being informed that the lesions of "Kaposi sarcoma" disappeared on treatment with antibiotics. Epithelioid hemangioma has plumper (histiocytoid) endothelial cell proliferation and no acute inflammation.

Principles of Management: Despite the lack of randomized controlled trials to evaluate optimal treatment for *Bartonella* infections in HIV-positive individuals, it is generally accepted that patients respond well to prolonged courses of either erythromycin or doxycycline. Trimethroprim–sulfamethoxazole, ciprofloxacin, penicillins, and cephalosporins do not have reliable antimicrobial activity and are therefore not recommended. Primary prophylaxis is not recommended for *Bartonella* (265).

Verruga Peruana

Clinical Summary. Infection by *B. bacilliformis* is responsible for a spectrum of diseases given multiple names, including bartonellosis, Carrion disease, Oroya fever, and verruga peruana. The disease is endemic to the Andean regions of Peru and Ecuador and Colombia. Carrion disease is now emerging as a public health problem in Peru, where it has been increasingly recognized in young children. The disease is transmitted by the sandfly *Lutzomyia verrucarum*, and humans are the only known reservoir. Only the female sandfly transmits the disease, and the preferred habitats for this vector are narrow river gorges between 500 and 3,200 m above sea level. Linear decrease in incidence with age suggests acquired immunity after exposure. The disease tends to cluster in specific areas within a community, much like malaria and leishmaniasis, such that epidemiologists refer to the "20/80" rule; that is, 20% of households or individuals in a susceptible population account for 80% of disease burden.

Two distinct clinical phases have been described: an initial acute phase, characterized by hemolytic anemia, headache, pallor, myalgia, arthralgia, and fever (Oroya fever); and a late phase, which may occur anytime from 2 weeks to several years after clinical recovery from the initial phase characterized by a cutaneous eruption of papules or nodules in the head and distal extremities termed *verruga peruana*. This chronic phase may present without an antecedent acute phase. In fact, recent outbreaks of the disease have documented a biphasic course only in a minority of cases (5%), and evidence of one phase or the other in 14% and 17%, respectively. Of interest, a large proportion of individuals (75%) have antibodies against *B. bacilliformis*, suggesting that in most individuals it is a subclinical infection.

Three different presentations have been recognized in the eruptive phase. A miliary form is the most common, in which numerous 1 to 3 mm erythematous papules are characteristic. The mular form consists of sessile nodules or frank tumors, frequently eroded (Fig. 21-69A, B). The last is a diffuse form in which multiple subcutaneous nodules are present. The lesions tend to heal spontaneously, and recurrences are rare.

Histopathology. Verruga peruana characteristically shows a striking angioblastic proliferation, mimicking malignant neoplasms such as angiosarcoma and lymphoma (Fig. 21-69C–E). In contrast to pyogenic granuloma, no lobules separated by septa are present. Besides endothelial cells, there are numerous dermal dendrocytes and an inflammatory infiltrate with macrophages, lymphocytes, and plasma cells. *B. bacilliformis* organisms may be visualized in Warthin–Starry or Giemsa-stained sections (Fig. 21-69F). An immunocytochemical antibody has also been developed, but it is available only at referral centers such as the CDC. The microorganism may appear within intracellular inclusions or free organisms within the extracellular matrix. Miliary lesions are most superficial, typically situated in the papillary to mid reticular dermis, whereas mular lesions tend to extend into the subcutaneous fat and may involve fascia and muscle (266–269).

Pathogenesis. Bartonella infection of endothelium has been shown to induce endothelial proliferation through stimulation by angiopoietin 2. Of note, vascular endothelial growth factor (VEGF), primarily produced by angiosarcomas and not benign tumors (hemangiomas), was not induced in an experimental model of *B. bacilliformis* (270).

Differential Diagnosis. The lesions of verruga peruana can mimic those of bacillary angiomatosis, pyogenic granuloma, acquired hemangioma, Kaposi sarcoma, and other malignancies. In contrast to bacillary angiomatosis, demonstration of bacteria can be challenging in verruga peruana because they are usually dispersed and not in clumps, as seen frequently in bacillary angiomatosis.

Principles of Management: Treatment recommendations of the eruptive phase of bartonellosis (verruga peruana) are based on a retrospective series from Peru, where the disease is endemic. Rifampin is the antimicrobial of choice, followed by streptomycin as the best alternative. With optimal response to treatment, the cutaneous lesions usually resolve within 1

month. Although studies *in vitro* suggest there may be resistance to rifampin, there are no adequate clinical studies to recommend combination therapy (271).

Nocardiosis

Clinical Summary. Nocardia sp. are gram-positive, weakly acid-fast, filamentous, branching bacilli that are ubiquitous in the soil. The main species are *N. asteroides*, which is global in distribution, and *N. brasiliensis*, which is found mainly in the Americas (272,273).

N. asteroides is an opportunist agent, and immunocompromised patients, such as those with HIV infection (274,275) and organ transplant recipients, are liable to nocardiosis. Infection of the skin follows direct implantation from the environment, hematogenous spread from pulmonary infection, or direct spread through the chest wall from a lung lesion. The skin lesions include erythematous nodules, pustular ulcers, and sinuses. They may be single or multiple.

N. brasiliensis affects immunocompetent as well as immunosuppressed people. The primary and secondary skin lesions are similar to those of *N. asteroides*. Sporotrichoid spread up a limb, with lymphatic involvement, may occur (276). Both species may produce a chronic mycetoma-like lesion with much fibrosis and tissue destruction.

Histopathology. The bacteria induce a mixed acute abscess and granulomatous response in the skin, with fibrosis. Occasionally, the bacteria are clumped together with a surrounding HS reaction (see sections on Botryomycosis and Mycetoma [Chapter 23]). More often, they are more loosely dispersed and resemble *Actinomycosis* sp. H&E stains demonstrate the bacilli poorly. They are 1 μm in diameter, filamentous, branching, beaded, gram positive, Grocott silver positive, and usually weakly acid fast so that a modified Ziehl–Neelsen stain appropriate for leprosy bacilli stains them (Fig. 21-70). This latter feature assists in the distinction of *Nocardia* from *Actinomyces* and related bacilli; specific antisera with immunocytochemistry are also helpful (274), and culture is definitive. The shape of the organisms distinguishes them from mycobacteria. The Grocott silver method is the most sensitive screening stain for nocardiosis.

Principles of Management: Cutaneous infection in an immunocompetent host can be treated with monotherapy. Clinical isolates of *Nocardia* spp. are variably resistant to antimicrobials. Therefore, empiric coverage with two to three antibiotics is recommended for patients with severe infection (pulmonary disease, disseminated disease, central nervous system, and immunocompromise). Trimethoprim–sulfamethoxazole is recommended as first-line therapy (277).

Actinomycosis

Clinical Summary. A. israelii is a gram-positive, branching, filamentous bacterium. It resides as a commensal organism in the oral cavity and tonsillar crypts. The main clinicopathologic manifestations are cervicofacial, thoracic, and intestinal actinomycosis (278). In the first of these, skin lesions result from extension of suppuration from the oral mucosa through to the facial skin, with sinus formation and discharge of pus and sulfur granules (see later). Thoracic and intestinal infections may produce discharging sinuses onto the skin from infection tracking outward from lung and gut (279). On rare occasions, purely cutaneous actinomycotic infection occurs, and hematogenous

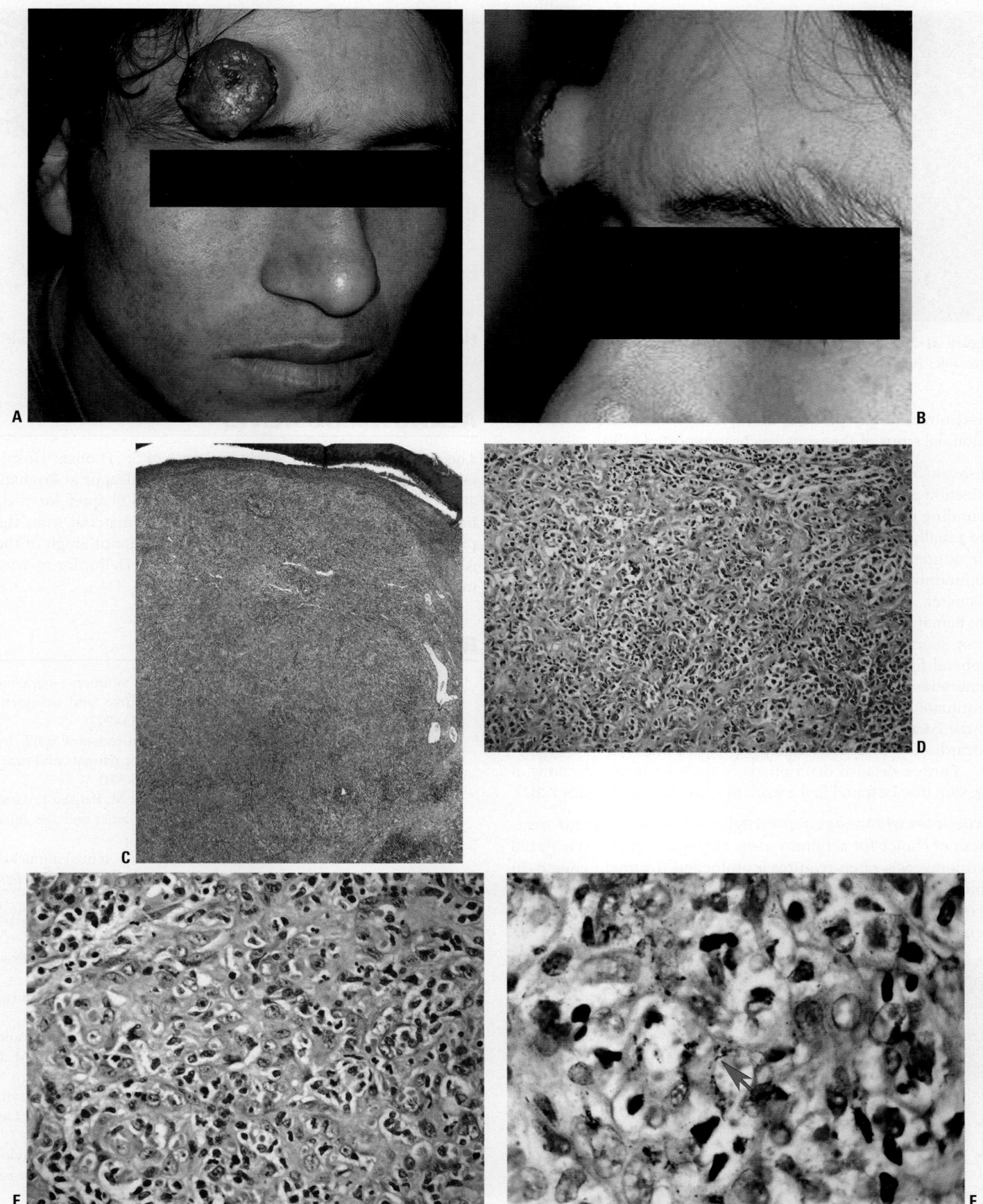

Figure 21-69 Verruga peruana. **A:** Large ulcerated tumor on the forehead of a young man, characteristic of the mular form of the disease. **B:** An epidermal collarette can be appreciated, consistent with rapid growth. **C:** On scanning magnification, an ulcerated, hypercellular mass is seen. **D:** Closer inspection reveals the vasoformative nature of the lesion. **E:** High-power view showing numerous vascular channels lined by large, atypical cells with prominent nucleoli, highly reminiscent of a malignant neoplasm. **F:** Rare, large bacillary forms (*arrow*) are diagnostic but difficult to document on tissue sections (Warthin–Starry stain). (Case courtesy of Dr. Cesar A. Chian, Universidad Peruana Cayetano Heredia, Lima, Peru.)

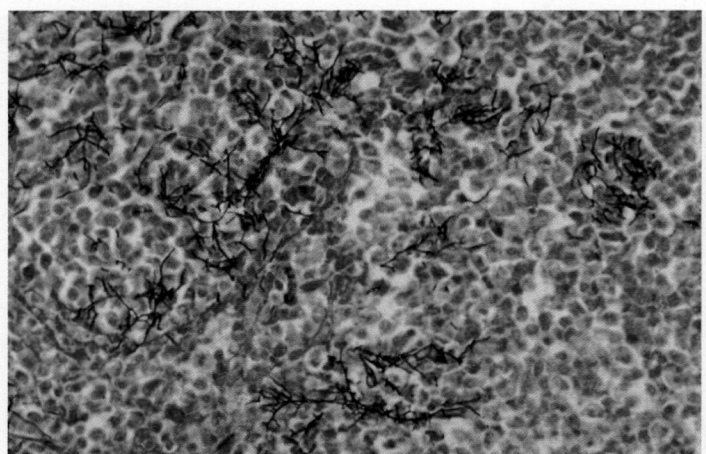

Figure 21-70 Nocardiosis. Fine, filamentous branching bacilli of *N. asteroides* (Grocott silver stain).

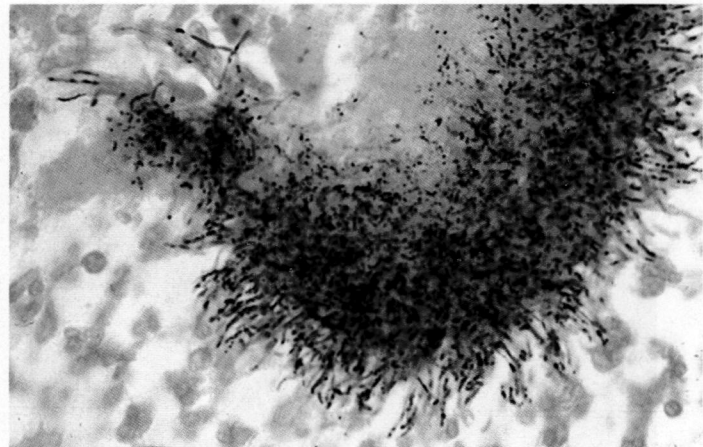

Figure 21-72 Actinomycosis. The edge of a grain, showing beaded gram-positive filaments (Gram stain).

dissemination can produce multiple skin sinuses. An infected pilonidal sinus of the penis has been reported (280).

Histopathology. The inflammatory reaction to actinomycotic infection is typically a chronic abscess with polymorphs, surrounding granulation tissue, and fibrosis (281). The organisms are usually tangled together in a matted colony, forming a granule or grain (like botryomycosis and mycetoma). These grains, commonly termed *sulfur granules*, may be 20 μm to 4 mm in diameter. The bacilli within are 1-μm-diameter filaments that are hematoxyphilic and gram positive (Figs. 21-71 and 21-72). They stain with the Grocott silver method. Often, only the peripheral filaments stain with the Gram method because of degeneration of the inner bacteria. The peripheral filaments often terminate in a club. An HS reaction may be found peripheral to the bacteria in the grain. The histologic differentiation from nocardiosis was discussed in the previous section.

Further detailed descriptions of these bacterial infections of the skin may be found in the work by Connor and Chandler (282).

Principles of Management: High-dose penicillin is the treatment of choice for actinomycosis. Management of cervicofacial actinomycosis often requires a prolonged treatment course. In complicated cases, surgical intervention may also be necessary. Tetracyclines are the best alternative for patients allergic to penicillin (283).

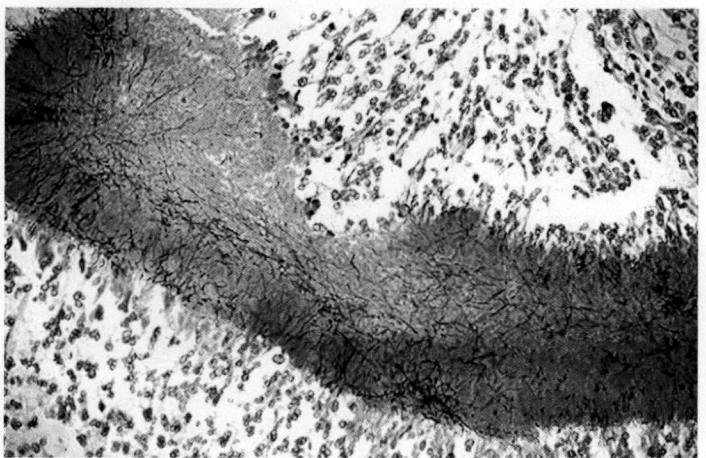

Figure 21-71 Actinomycosis. Part of a bacterial colony with hematoxyphilic filamentous bacteria (H&E stain).

ACKNOWLEDGMENTS

The author thanks Prof. Sebastien Lucas of St. Thomas' Hospital, London, and Danny Milner Jr., former colleague at Brigham and Women's Hospital and coauthor of this chapter for their help and generosity in allowing the use of material from the previous chapters. The editors thank Prof. Manoj Singh of the All India Institute of Medical Sciences, New Delhi, for reviewing the sections on mycobacterial diseases.

REFERENCES

1. Preda-Naumescu A, Elewski B, Mayo TT. Common cutaneous infections: patient presentation, clinical course, and treatment options. *Med Clin North Am.* 2021;105(4):783–797.
2. Cohen PR. Community-acquired methicillin-resistant *Staphylococcus aureus* skin infections: implications for patients and practitioners. *Am J Clin Dermatol.* 2007;8(5):529–570.
3. Kiriakis KP, Tadros A, Dimou A, Karamanou M, Banaka F, Alexoudi I. Case detection rates of impetigo by gender and age. *Infez Med.* 2012;20(2):105–107.
4. Orbuch DE, Kim RH, Cohen DE. Ecthyma: a potential mimicker of zoonotic infections in a returning traveler. *Int J Infect Dis.* 2014;29:178–180.
5. Wick MR. Bullous, pseudobullous, & pustular dermatoses. *Semin Diagn Pathol.* 2017;34(3):250–260.
6. Ibrahim F, Khan T, Pujalte GG. Bacterial skin infections. *Prim Care.* 2015;42(4):485–499.
7. Hartman-Adams H, Banvard C, Juckett G. Impetigo: diagnosis and treatment. *Am Fam Physician.* 2014;90(4):229–235.
8. Stanley JR, Amagai M. Pemphigus, bullous impetigo, and the staphylococcal scalded-skin syndrome. *N Eng J Med.* 2006;355(17):1800–1810.
9. Handler MZ, Schwartz RA. Staphylococcal scalded skin syndrome: diagnosis and management in children and adults. *J Eur Acad Dermatol Venereol.* 2014;28(11):1418–1423.
10. Mishra AK, Yadav P, Mishra A. A systematic review of staphylococcal scalded skin syndrome (SSSS): a rare and critical disease of neonates. *Open Microbiol J.* 2016;10:150–159.
11. Patel S, Caldwell JB, Lambert WC. Comparison of adult vs. paediatric inpatients with staphylococcal scalded skin syndrome: a retrospective database analysis. *Br J Dermatol.* 2021;184(4):767–769.
12. Suzuki R, Iwasaki S, Ito Y, et al. Adult staphylococcal scalded skin syndrome in a peritoneal dialysis patient. *Clin Exp Nephrol.* 2003;7(1):77–80.

13. Murray RJ. Recognition and management of *Staphylococcus aureus* toxin-mediated disease. *Intern Med J.* 2005;35(Suppl 2):S106–S119.

14. Ross A, Shoff HW. *Staphylococcal Scalded Skin Syndrome.* StatPearls Publishing; 2021.

15. Paranthaman K, Bentley A, Milne LM, et al. Nosocomial outbreak of staphylococcal scalded skin syndrome in neonates in England, December 2012 to March 2013. *Euro Surveill.* 2014;19(33):20880.

16. Ladhani S. Understanding the mechanism of action of the exfoliative toxin of *Staphylococcus aureus. FEMS Immunol Med Microbiol.* 2003;39(2):181–189.

17. Ladhani S, Joannou CL, Lochrie DP, Evans RW, Poston SM. Clinical, microbial, and biochemical aspects of the exfoliative toxins causing staphylococcal scalded-skin syndrome. *Clin Microbiol Rev.* 1999;12(2):224–242.

18. Baddour LM. Impetigo. In: Ofori AO, ed. *UpToDate.* UpToDate; 2021.

19. Anderson DJ. Epidemiology of methicillin-resistant *Staphylococcus aureus* infection in adults. In: Sexton DJ, ed. *UpToDate.* UpToDate; 2021.

20. Forcade NA, Parchman ML, Jorgensen JH, et al. Prevalence, severity, and treatment of community-acquired methicillin-resistant *Staphylococcus aureus* (CA-MRSA) skin and soft tissue infections in 10 medical clinics in Texas: a South Texas Ambulatory Research Network (STARNet) study. *J Am Board Fam Med.* 2011;24(5):543c550.

21. Scuderi S, O'Brien B, Robertson I, Weedon D. Heterogeneity of blastomycosis-like pyoderma: a selection of cases from the last 35 years. *Australas J Dermatol.* 2017;58(2):139–141.

22. Nguyen RT, Beardmore GL. Blastomycosis-like pyoderma: successful treatment with low-dose acitretin. *Australas J Dermatol.* 2005;46(2):97–100.

23. Gara S, Souissi A, Mokni M. Pyodermatitis pyostomatitis vegetans. *JAMA Dermatol.* 2020;156(3):335.

24. Guidry JA, Downing C, Tyring SK. Deep fungal infections, blastomycosis-like pyoderma, and granulomatous sexually transmitted infections. *Dermatol Clin.* 2015;33(3):595–607.

25. Hannula-Jouppi K, Massinen S, Siljander T, et al. Genetic susceptibility to non-necrotizing erysipelas/cellulitis. *PLoS One.* 2013;8(2):e56225.

26. Bonnetblanc JM, Bedane C. Erysipelas: recognition and management. *Am J Clin Dermatol.* 2003;4(3):157–163.

27. Burnham JP, Kollef MH. Understanding toxic shock syndrome. *Intensive Care Med.* 2015;41(9):1707–1710.

28. Todd J, Fishaut M, Kapral F, Welch T. Toxic shock syndrome caused by phage group I *Staphylococci. Lancet.* 1978;2(8100):1116–1118.

29. Andrey DO, Ferry T, Siegenthaler N, et al. Unusual staphylococcal toxic shock syndrome presenting as scarlet-like fever. *New Microbes New Infect.* 2015;8:10–13.

30. Descloux E, Perpoint T, Ferry T, et al. One in five mortality in non-menstrual toxic shock syndrome versus no mortality in menstrual cases in a balanced French series of 55 cases. *Eur J Clin Microbiol Infect Dis.* 2008;27(1):37–43.

31. Young K, Luni FK, Yoon Y. Toxic shock syndrome: an unusual organism. *Am J Med Sci.* 2016;352(1):86–90.

32. Wilkins AL, Steer AC, Smeesters PR, Curtis N. Toxic shock syndrome—the seven Rs of management and treatment. *J Infect Dis.* 2017;74(Suppl 1):S147–S152.

33. Hurwitz RM, Ackerman AB. Cutaneous pathology of the toxic shock syndrome. *Am J Dermatopathol.* 1985;7(6):563–578.

34. Low DE. Toxic shock syndrome: major advances in pathogenesis, but not treatment. *Crit Care Clin.* 2013;29(3):651–675.

35. Shumba P, Mairpady SS, Siemens N. The role of streptococcal and staphylococcal exotoxins and proteases in human necrotizing soft tissue infections. *Toxins (Basel).* 2019;11(6):332.

36. Cook A, Janse S, Watson JR, Erdem G. Manifestations of toxic shock syndrome in children, Columbus, Ohio, USA, 2010-2017. *Emerg Infect Dis.* 2020;26(6):1077–1083.

37. Chu VH. Staphylococcal toxic shock syndrome. In: Post TW, ed. *UpToDate.* UpToDate; 2021.

38. Griffith DE. Rapidly growing mycobacterial infections: *Mycobacteria abscessus, chelonae,* and *fortuitum.* In: Post TW, ed. *UpToDate.* UpToDate; 2021.

39. Larsen MH, Lacourciere K, Parker TM, et al. The many hosts of mycobacteria 8 (MHM8): a conference report. *Tuberculosis (Edinb).* 2020;121:101914.

40. Kromer C, Fabri M, Schlapbach C, et al. Diagnosis of mycobacterial skin infections. *J Dtsch Dermatol Ges.* 2019;17(9):889–893.

41. Franco-Paredes C, Marcos LA. Henao-Martinez A, et al. Cutaneous mycobacterial infections. *Clin Microbiol Rev.* 2019;32(1):e000069-18.

42. Dodiuk-Gad R, Dyachenko P, Ziv M, et al. Nontuberculous mycobacterial infections of the skin: a retrospective study of 25 cases. *J Am Acad Dermatol.* 2007;57(3):413–420.

43. Crothers JW, Laga AC, Solomon IH. Clinical performance of mycobacterial immunohistochemistry in anatomic pathology specimens. *Am J Clin Pathol.* 2021;155(1):97–105.

44. Declercq E. Guide to eliminating leprosy as a public health problem. *Lepr Rev.* 2001;72(1):106–107.

45. Britton WJ, Lockwood DNJ. Leprosy. *Lancet.* 2004;363(9416):1209–1219.

46. Naves Mde M, Ribeiro FA, Patrocinio LG, Patrocinio JA, Fleury RN, Goulart IM. Bacterial load in the nose and its correlation to the immune response in leprosy patients. *Lepr Rev.* 2013;84(1):85–91.

47. Ridley DS, Jopling WH. Classification of leprosy according to immunity: a five-group system. *Int J Lepr.* 1966;34(3):255–273.

48. Ridley DS. Histological classification and the immunological spectrum of leprosy. *Bull World Health Organ.* 1974;51(5):451–465.

49. Lowy L. Processing of biopsies for leprosy bacilli. *J Med Lab Technol.* 1956;13(8):558–560.

50. van Brakel WH, de Soldenhoff R, McDougall AC. The allocation of leprosy patients into paucibacillary and multibacillary groups for multidrug therapy, taking into account the number of body areas affected by skin, or skin and nerve lesions. *Lepr Rev.* 1992;63(3):231–246.

51. Eichelmann K, González SE, Salas-Alanis JC, Ocampo-Candiani J. Leprosy. An update: definition, pathogenesis, classification, diagnosis, and treatment. *Actas Dermosifiliogr.* 2013;104(7):554–563.

52. Ridley MJ, Ridley DS. The immunopathology of erythema nodosum leprosum: the role of extravascular complexes. *Lepr Rev.* 1983;54(2):95–107.

53. Job CK. Pathology of leprosy. In: Hastings RC, ed. *Leprosy.* Churchill Livingstone; 1994:193.

54. Jurado F, Rodriguez O, Novales J, Navarrete G, Rodriguez M. Lucio's leprosy: a clinical and therapeutic challenge. *Clin Dermatol.* 2015;33(1):66–78.

55. Bartos G, Shering R, Combs A, Rivlin D. Treatment of histoid leprosy: a lack of consensus. *Int J Dermatol.* 2020;59(10):1264–1269.

56. Ranjan Kar B, Belliapa PR, Ebenezer G, Job CK. Single lesion borderline lepromatous leprosy. *Int J Lepr Other Mycobact Dis.* 2004;72(1):45–47.

57. Geluk A. Correlates of immune exacerbations in leprosy. *Semin Immunol.* 2018;39:111–118.

58. Maymone MBC, Venkatesh S, Laughter M, et al. Leprosy: treatment and management of complications. *J Am Acad Dermatol.* 2020;83(1):17–30.

59. Lockwood DNJ, Lucas SB, Desikan KV, Ebenezer G, Suneetha S, Nicholls P. The histological diagnosis of leprosy type 1 reactions: identification of key variables and an analysis of the process of histological diagnosis. *J Clin Pathol.* 2008;61(5):595–600.

60. Bhat RM, Vaidya TP. What is new in the pathogenesis and management of erythema nodosum leprosum. *Indian Dermatol Online J.* 2020;11(4):482–492.

61. Nath I, Saini C, Valluri VL. Immunology of leprosy and diagnostic challenges. *Clin Dermatol.* 2015;33(1):90–98.

62. Mi Z, Liu H, Zhang F. Advances in the immunology and genetics of leprosy. *Front Immunol.* 2020;11:567.

63. Salgame P, Abrams JS, Clayberger C, et al. Differing lymphokine profiles of functional subsets of human CD4 and CD8 T cell clones. *Science.* 1991;254(5029):279–282.

64. Ma F, Hughes TK, Teles RMB, et al. The cellular architecture of the antimicrobial response network in human leprosy granulomas. *Nat Immunol.* 2021;22(7):839–850.

65. Mssone C, Talhari C, Ribeiro-Rodrigues R, et al. Leprosy and HIV coinfection: a critical approach. *Expert Rev Anti Infect Ther.* 2011;9(6):701–710.

66. Lockwood DNJ, Lambert SM. Human immunodeficiency virus and leprosy: an update. *Dermatol Clin.* 2011;29(1):125–128.

67. Gebre S, Saunderson P, Messele T, Bypass P. The effect of HIV status on the clinical picture of leprosy: a prospective study in Ethiopia. *Lep Rev.* 2000;71(3):338–343.

68. Pires CA, Juca Neto FO, de Albuquerque NC, Macedo GA, Batista Kde N, Xavier MB. Leprosy reactions in patients coinfected with HIV: clinical aspects and outcomes in two comparative cohorts in the amazon region, Brazil. *PLoS Negl Trop Dis.* 2015;9(6):e00003818.

69. Fleury RN, Bacchi CE. S-100 protein and immunoperoxidase technique as an aid in the histopathologic diagnosis of leprosy. *Int J Lepr.* 1987;55(2):338–344.

70. Kazi R, Kazlouskaya V, Ho J, Karunamurthy A. Sarcoidosis with cutaneous perineural granulomas and neurological manifestations: a potential mimicker of leprosy. *J Cutan Pathol.* 2020;47(7):625–627.

71. Manta FSN, Leal-Calvo T, Moreira SJM, et al. Ultra-sensitive detection of *Mycobacterium leprae*: DNA extraction and PCR assays. *PLoS Negl Trop Dis.* 2020;14(5):e0008325.

72. Fine PEM, Job CK, Lucas SB, Meyers WM, Pönnighaus JM, Sterne JA. The extent, origin and implications of observer variation in the histopathological diagnosis of leprosy. *Int J Lepr Other Mycobact Dis.* 1993;61(2):270–282.

73. Perrin C. A patient with acquired immunodeficiency syndrome (AIDS) and a cutaneous *Mycobacterium avium* intracellulare infection mimicking histoid leprosy. *Am J Dermatopathol.* 2007;29:(4):422.

74. World Health Organization. *Fact sheet: tuberculosis.* https://www.who.int/news-room/fact-sheets/detail/tuberculosis

75. Charifa A, Mangat R, Oakley AM. *Cutaneous Tuberculosis.* StatPearls Publishing; 2021.

76. Barbagallo J, Tager P, Ingleton R, Hirsch RJ, Weinberg JM. Cutaneous tuberculosis: diagnosis and treatment. *Am J Clin Dermatol.* 2002;3(5):319–328.

77. Bravo FG, Gotuzzo E. Cutaneous tuberculosis. *Clin Dermatol.* 2007;25(2):173–180.

78. Chen Q, Chen W, Hao F. Cutaneous tuberculosis: a great imitator. *Clin Dermatol.* 2019;37(3):192–199.

79. Dias MF, Bernardes Filho F, Quaresma MV, Nascimento LV, Nery JA, Azulay DR. Update on cutaneous tuberculosis. *An Bras Dermatol.* 2014;89(6):925–938.

80. Vashisht P, Sahoo B, Khurana N, et al. Cutaneous tuberculosis in children and adolescents: a clinicohistological study. *J Eur Acad Dermatol Venereol.* 2007;21(1):40–47.

81. Hunter RL. The pathogenesis of tuberculosis: the early infiltrate of post-primary (adult pulmonary) tuberculosis: a distinct disease entity. *Front Immunol.* 2018;9:2108.

82. Hunter RL. Tuberculosis as a three-act play: a new paradigm for the pathogenesis of pulmonary tuberculosis. *Tuberculosis (Edinb).* 2016;97:8–17.

83. Tigoulet F, Fournier V, Caumes E. Formes cliniques de la tuberculose cutanée [Clinical forms of the cutaneous tuberculosis] [in French]. *Bull Soc Pathol Exot.* 2003;96(5):362–367.

84. Helman KM, Muschenheim C. Primary cutaneous tuberculosis resulting from mouth-to-mouth respiration. *N Engl J Med.* 1965;273(19):1035–1036.

85. Goette DK, Jacobson KW, Doty RD. Primary inoculation tuberculosis of the skin. *Arch Dermatol.* 1978;114(4):567–569.

86. Kramer F, Sasse SA, Simms JC, Leedom JM. Primary cutaneous tuberculosis after a needle-stick injury from a patient with AIDS and undiagnosed tuberculosis. *Ann Intern Med.* 1993;119(7 Pt 1):594–595.

87. Semaan R, Traboulsi R, Kanj S. Primary *Mycobacterium tuberculosis* complex cutaneous infection: report of two cases and literature review. *Int J Infect Dis.* 2008;12(5):472–477.

88. Mansfield BS. Pieton K. Tuberculosis cutis orificialis. *Open Forum Infect Dis.* 2019;6(10):ofz428.

89. Del Giudice P, Bernard E, Perrin C, et al. Unusual cutaneous manifestations of miliary tuberculosis. *Clin Infect Dis.* 2000;30(1):201–204.

90. Li C, Liu L, Tao Y. Diagnosis and treatment of congenital tuberculosis: a systematic review of 92 cases. *Orphanet J Rare Dis.* 2019;14(1):131.

91. Halle A, Lombart F, Chaby G, Bendamman M, Lok C, Hamdad F. An erythemato-papular and nodular lesion on the earlobe. *Clin Infect Dis.* 2020;71(8):1969–1972.

92. Kaul S, Jakhar D, Mehta S, Singal A. Cutaneous tuberculosis. Part II: Complications, diagnostic workup, histopathological features, and treatment. *J Am Acad Dermatol.* 2022;S0190-9622(22)00203-1. doi: 10.1016/j.jaad.2021.12.064.

93. Motswaledi MH, Doman C. Lupus vulgaris with squamous cell carcinoma. *J Cutan Pathol.* 2007;34(12):939–941.

94. Tan SH, Tan HH, Sun YJ, Goh CL. Clinical utility of polymerase chain reaction in the detection of *Mycobacterium tuberculosis* in different types of cutaneous tuberculosis and tuberculids. *Ann Acad Med Singap.* 2001;30(1):3–10.

95. Negi SS, Basir SF, Gupta S, Pasha ST, Khare S, Lal S. Comparative study of PCR, smear examination and culture for diagnosis of cutaneous tuberculosis. *J Commun Dis.* 2005;37(2):83–92.

96. Darier MJ. Des "tuberculides" cutanees. *Arch Dermatol Syph.* 1896;7:1431.

97. Jordaan HF, Schneider JW, Abdulla EA. Nodular tuberculid: a report of four patients. *Pediatr Dermatol.* 2000;17(3):183–188.

98. Friedman PC, Husain S, Grossman ME. Nodular tuberculid in a patient with HIV. *J Am Acad Dermatol.* 2005;53(2 Suppl 1):S154–S156.

99. Breathnach SM, Black MM. Atypical tuberculide (acne scrofulosorum) secondary to tuberculous lymphadenitis. *Clin Exp Dermatol.* 1981;6(3):339–344.

100. Maldonado-Bernal C, Ramos-Garibay A, Rios-Sarabia N, et al. Nested polymerase chain reaction and cutaneous tuberculosis. *Am J Dermatopathol.* 2019;41(6):428–435.

101. Jordaan HF, van Niekerk DJ, Louw M. Papulonecrotic tuberculid: a clinical, histopathological and immunohistochemical study of 15 patients. *Am J Dermatopathol.* 1994;16(5):474–485.

102. Wilson-Jones E, Winkelmann RK. Papulonecrotic tuberculid: a neglected disease in Western countries. *J Am Acad Dermatol.* 1986;14:815–826.

103. Tobita R, Sumikawa Y, Imaoka K, et al. Lichen scrofulosorum caused by pulmonary *Mycobacterium avium* complex (MAC) infection. *Eur J Dermatol.* 2011;21(4):619–620.

104. Degitz K, Steidl M, Thomas P, Plewig G, Volkenandt M. Aetiology of tuberculids. *Lancet.* 1993;341(88839):239–240.

105. Urso B, Georgesen C, Harp J. Papulonecrotic tuberculid secondary to *Mycobacterium avium* complex. *Cutis.* 2019;104(5):E11–E13.

106. Williams JT, Pulitzer DR, DeVillez RL. Papulonecrotic tuberculid secondary to disseminated *Mycobacterium avium* complex. *Int J Dermatol.* 1994;33(2):109–112.

107. Brown BA, Wallace RJ. Infections due to non-tuberculous mycobacteria. In: Mandell GL, Bennett JE, Dolin R, eds. *Principles and Practice of Infectious Diseases.* 5th ed. Churchill Livingstone; 2000:2630–2636.

108. Nogueira LB, Garcia CN, Costa MSCD, Moraes MB, Kurizky PS, Gomes CM. Non-tuberculous cutaneous mycobacterioses. *An Bras Dermatol.* 2021;96(5):527–538.

109. Franco-Paredes C, Chastain DB, Allen L, Henao-Martinez AF. Overview of cutaneous mycobacterial infections. *Curr Trop Med Rep.* 2018;5(4):228–232.

110. Chiang CH, Lee GH, Chiang TH, Tang PU, Fang CT. Disseminated *Mycobacterium avium* complex infection as a differential diagnosis of tuberculosis in HIV patients. *Int J Tuberc Lung Dis.* 2020;24(9):922–927.

111. Havlir DV, Ellner JJ. *Mycobacterium avium* complex. In: Mandell GL, Bennett JE, Dolin R, eds. *Principles and Practice of Infectious Diseases.* 5th ed. Churchill Livingstone; 2000:2616–2629.

112. Ricotta EE, Adjemian J, Blakney RA, Lai YL, Kadri SS, Prevots DR. Extrapulmonary nontuberculous mycobacteria infections in hospitalized patients. *Emerg Infect Dis.* 2021;27(3):845–852.

113. Boyd AS, Robbins J. Cutaneous *Mycobacterium avium* intracellulare infection in an HIV+ patient mimicking histoid leprosy. *Am J Dermatopathol.* 2005;27(1):39–41.

114. Akram SM, Aboobacker S. *Mycobacterium marinum.* StatPearls Publishing; 2021.

115. Philpott JA, Woodburne AR, Philpott OS, Schaefer WB, Mollohan CS. Swimming pool granuloma. *Arch Dermatol.* 1963;88:158–162.

116. Costecu Strachinaru DI, Vanbrabant P, Stinga P, Strachinaru M, Soentjens P. Diagnosis of *Mycobacterium marinum* infection with Sporotrichoid Pattern. *Acta Derm Venereol.* 2021;101(3):adv00414.

117. Seneviratne K, Herieka E. A rifampicin-resistant *Mycobacterium marinum* infection in a newly diagnosed HIV-1 individual. *Int J STD AIDS.* 2013;24(1):75–77.

118. Tchornobay AM, Claudy AL, Perrot JL, Lévigne V, Denis M. Fatal disseminated *Mycobacterium* infection. *Int J Dermatol.* 1992;31(4):286–287.

119. Travis WD, Travis LB, Roberts GD, Su DW, Weiland LW. The histopathologic spectrum in *Mycobacterium marinum* infection. *Arch Pathol Lab Med.* 1985;109(12):1109–1113.

120. Van der Werf T, Stinear T, Stienstra Y, van der Graaf WT, Small PL. Mycolactones and *Mycobacterium ulcerans* disease. *Lancet.* 2003;362(9389):1062–1064.

121. Heyman J. Out of Africa: observations on the histopathology of *Mycobacterium ulcerans. J Clin Pathol.* 1993;46(1):5–9.

122. Millogo A, Zingue D, Bouam A, Godreuil S, Drancourt M, Hammoudi N. Confirming autochthonous Buruli ulcer cases in Burkina Faso, West Africa. *Am J Trop Med Hyg.* 2021;105(3):627–629.

123. Walsh DS, Dela Cruz Eduardo C, Abalos RM, et al. Clinical and histologic features of skin lesions in a cynomolgus monkey experimentally infected with *Mycobacterium ulcerans* (Buruli ulcer) by intradermal inoculation. *Am J Trop Med Hyg.* 2007;76(1):132–134.

124. Hayman J, McQueen A. The pathology of *Mycobacterium ulcerans* infection. *Pathology.* 1983;17:594–600.

125. Doig KD, Holt KE, Fyfe JA, et al. On the origin of *Mycobacterium ulcerans*, the causative agent of Buruli ulcer. *BMC Genomics.* 2012;13:258.

126. Rondini S, Horsfield C, Mensah-Quainoo E, Junghanss T, Lucas S, Pluschke G. Contiguous spread of *Mycobacterium ulcerans* in Buruli ulcer lesions analysed by histopathology and real-time PCR quantification of mycobacterial DNA. *J Pathol.* 2006;208(1):119–128.

127. Kiszewski AE, Becerril E, Aguilar LD, et al. The local immune response in ulcerative lesions of Buruli disease. *Clin Exp Immunol.* 2006;143(3):445–451.

128. Brown-Elliott BA, Philley JV. Rapidly growing mycobacteria. *Microbiol Spectr.* 2017;5(1). doi:10.1128/microbiolspec.TNMI7-0027-2016

129. Akram SM, Rathish B, Saleh D. *Mycobacterium cheloneae.* StatPearls Publishing; 2021.

130. Lindeboom JA, Bruijinesteijn van Coppenraet LES, van Soolingen D, Prins JM, Kuijper EJ. Clinical manifestations, diagnosis, and treatment of *Mycobacterium haemophilum* infections. *Clin Microbiol Rev.* 2011;24(4):701–717.

131. Camselle D, Hernandez J, Frances A, Montenegro T, Canas F, Borrego L. Infección cutánea esporotricoide por *Mycobacterium haemophilum* en un paciente con sida [Sporotrichoid cutaneous infection by *Mycobacterium haemophilum* in an AIDS patient]. *Actas Dermosifilogr.* 2007;98(3):188–193.

132. Kristjansson M, Bieluch VM, Byeff PD. *Mycobacterium haemophilum* infection in immunocompromised patients: case report and review of the literature. *Rev Infect Dis.* 1991;13(5):906–910.

133. Bernatowska EA, Wolska-Kusnierz B, Pac M, et al. Disseminated Bacillus Calmette-Guérin infection and immunodeficiency. *Emerg Infect Dis.* 2007;13(5):799–801. doi:10.3201/eid1305.060865

134. Kasperbauer S, Huitt G. Management of extrapulmonary mycobacterial infections. *Semin Respir Crit Care Med.* 2013;34(1):143–150.

135. Lécuyer H, Borgel D, Nassif X, Coureuil M. Pathogenesis of meningococcal purpura fulminans. *Pathog Dis.* 2017;75(3):ftx027. doi:10.1093/femspd/ftx027

136. Alvarez EF, Olarte KE, Ramesh MS. Purpura fulminans secondary to *Streptococcus pneumoniae* meningitis. *Case Rep Infect Dis.* 2012;2012:508503.

137. Shapiro L, Teisch JA, Brownstein MH. Dermatohistopathology of chronic gonococcal sepsis. *Arch Dermatol.* 1973;107(3):403–406.

138. Brouwer MC, de Gans J, Heckenberg SG, Zwinderman AH, van der Poll T, van de Beek D. Host genetic susceptibility to pneumococcal and meningococcal disease: a systematic review and meta-analysis. *Lancet Infect Dis.* 2009;9(1):31–44.

139. Coureuil M, Join-Lambert O, Lécuyer H, Bourdoulous S, Marullo S, Nassif X. Pathogenesis of meningococcemia. *Cold Spring Harb Perspect Med.* 2013;3(6):a012393.

140. Binder A, Endler G, Müller M, Mannhalter C, Zenz W. European meningococcal study group. 4G4G genotype of the plasminogen activator inhibitor-1 promoter polymorphism associates with disseminated intravascular coagulation in children with systemic meningococcemia. *J Thromb Haemost.* 2007;5(10):2049–2054. doi:10.1111/j.1538-7836.2007.02724.x

141. Apicella M. Treatment and prevention of meningococcal infection. In: Mitty J, ed. *UpToDate.* UpToDate; 2021.

142. Shah M, Crane JS. *Ecthyma Gangrenosum.* StatPearls Publishing; 2021. https://www.ncbi.nlm.nih.gov/books/NBK534777/

143. Schlossberg D. Multiple erythematous nodules as a manifestation of *Pseudomonas aeruginosa* septicemia. *Arch Dermatol.* 1980;116(4):446–447.

144. Bazel J, Grossman ME. Subcutaneous nodules in pseudomonas sepsis. *Am J Med.* 1986;80(3):528–529.

145. Hamed, A, Niehaus, AG, Bosshardt Hughes, O, Jakharia, N. Ecthyma gangrenosum without bacteremia in a 54-year-old woman with heart transplant. *Transpl Infect Dis.* 2020;22(4):e13319. doi:10.1111/tid.13319

146. Aygencel G, Dizbay M, Sahin G. Burkholderia cepacia as a cause of ecthyma gangrenosum-like lesion. *Infection.* 2008;36(3):271–273. doi:10.1007/s15010-007-6357-8

147. Kanj SS, Sexton DJ. Principles of antimicrobial therapy of *Pseudomonas aeruginosa* infections. In: Bloom A, ed. *UpToDate.* UpToDate; 2021.

148. Yun NR, Kim DM. *Vibrio vulnificus* infection: a persistent threat to public health. *Korean J Intern Med.* 2018;33(6):1070–1078. doi:10.3904/kjim.2018.159

149. Chao WN, Tsai SJ, Tsai CF, et al. The laboratory risk indicator for necrotizing fasciitis score for discernment of necrotizing fasciitis originated from *Vibrio vulnificus* infections. *J Trauma Acute Care Surg.* 2012;73(6):1576–1582.

150. Tyring SK, Lee PC. Hemorrhagic bullae associated with *Vibrio vulnificus* septicemia. *Arch Dermatol.* 1986;122(7):818–820.

151. Glenn Morris J. *Vibrio vulnificus* infections. In: Bloom A, ed. *UpToDate.* UpToDate; 2021.

152. Ittig S, Lindner B, Stenta M, et al. The lipopolysaccharide from *Capnocytophaga canimorsus* reveals an unexpected role

of the core-oligosaccharide in MD-2 binding. *PLoS Pathog.* 2012;8(5):e1002667.

153. Janda JM, Graves MH, Lindquist D, Probert WS. Diagnosing capnocytophaga canimorsus infections. *Emerg Infect Dis.* 2006;12(2):340–342.

154. Christiansen CB, Berg RM, Plovsing RR, Møller K. Two cases of infectious purpura fulminans and septic shock caused by *Capnocytophaga canimorsus* transmitted from dogs. *Scand J Infect Dis.* 2012;44(8):635–639.

155. Eefting M, Paardenkooper T. *Capnocytophaga canimorsus* sepsis. *Blood.* 2010;116(9):1396.

156. Wald K, Martinez A, Moll S. *Capnocytophaga canimorsus* infection with fulminant sepsis in an asplenic patient: diagnosis by review of peripheral blood smear. *Am J Hematol.* 2008;83(11):879.

157. Butler T. *Capnocytophaga canimorsus*: an emerging cause of sepsis, meningitis, and post-splenectomy infection after dog bites. *Eur J Clin Microbiol Infect Dis.* 2015;34(7):1271–1280. doi:10.1007/s10096-015-2360-7

158. Ognibene AJ, Ditto MR. Chronic meningococcemia. *Arch Intern Med.* 1964;114:29–32.

159. Dupin N, Lecuyer H, Carlotti A, et al. Chronic meningococcemia cutaneous lesions involve meningococcal perivascular invasion through the remodeling of endothelial barriers. *Clin Infect Dis.* 2012;54(8):1162–1165. doi:10.1093/cid/cis120

160. Apicella M. Clinical manifestations of meningococcal infection. In: Mitty J, ed. *UpToDate.* UpToDate; 2021.

161. Schoolnik GK, Buchanan TM, Holmes KK. Gonococci causing disseminated gonococcal infection are resistant to the bactericidal action of normal human sera. *J Clin Invest.* 1976;58(5):1163–1173.

162. Björnberg A. Benign gonococcal sepsis. *Acta Derm Venereol (Stockh).* 1970;50(4):313–316.

163. Ackerman AB. Hemorrhagic bullae in gonococcemia. *N Engl J Med.* 1970;282(14):793–794.

164. Ackerman AB, Miller RC, Shapiro L. Gonococcemia and its cutaneous manifestations. *Arch Dermatol.* 1965;91:227–232.

165. Abu-Nassar H, Fred HL, Yow EM. Cutaneous manifestations of gonococcemia. *Arch Intern Med.* 1963;112:731–737.

166. Jain S, Win HN, Chalam V, Yee L. Disseminated gonococcal infection presenting as vasculitis: a case report. *J Clin Pathol.* 2007;60(1):90–91. doi:10.1136/jcp.2005.034546

167. Klausner JD. Disseminated gonococcal infection. In: Bloom A, ed. *UpToDate.* UpToDate; 2021.

168. Salgo MP, Telzak EE, Currie B, et al. A focus of Rocky Mountain spotted fever within New York City. *N Engl J Med.* 1985;318(21):1345–1348.

169. Walker DH, Raoult D. *Rickettsia rickettsii* and other spotted fever group rickettsiae. In: Mandell GL, Bennett JE, Dolin R, eds. *Principles and Practice of Infectious Disease.* 5th ed. Churchill Livingstone; 2000:2035–2041.

170. Kirkland KB, Marcom P, Sexton DJ, Dumler JS, Walker DH. Rocky Mountain spotted fever complicated by gangrene: report of six cases and review. *Clin Infect Dis.* 1993;16(5):629–634.

171. Jay R, Armstrong PA. Clinical characteristics of Rocky Mountain spotted fever in the United States: a literature review. *J Vector Borne Dis.* 2020;57(2):114–120. doi:10.4103/0972-9062.310863

172. Kao GF, Evancho CD, Ioffe O, Lowitt MH, Dumler JS. Cutaneous histopathology of Rocky Mountain spotted fever. *J Cutan Pathol.* 1997;24(10):604–610. doi:10.1111/j.1600-0560.1997.tb01091.x

173. Zhao Y, Fang R, Zhang J, et al. Quantitative proteomics of the endothelial secretome identifies RC0497 as diagnostic of acute rickettsial spotted fever infections. *Am J Pathol.* 2020;190(2):306–322. doi:10.1016/j.ajpath.2019.10.007

174. Sexton DJ, McClaiin M. Other spotted fever group rickettsial infections. In: Mitty J, ed. *UpToDate.* UpToDate; 2013.

175. Yu Y, Cheng AS, Wang L, Dunne WM, Bayliss SJ. Hot tub folliculitis or hot hand-foot syndrome caused by *Pseudomonas aeruginosa. J Am Acad Dermatol.* 2007;57(4):596–600. doi:10.1016/j.jaad.2007.04.004

176. Fiorillo L, Zucker M, Sawyer D, Lin AN. The pseudomonas hot-foot syndrome. *N Engl J Med.* 2001;345(5):335–338. doi:10.1056/NEJM200108023450504

177. González-Padilla M, Jurado R, Rodríguez Martín AM, Torre-Cisneros J. Foliculitis del jacuzzi: descripción de un brote de 6 casos [Whirlpool folliculitis: 6 cases outbreak report] [in Spanish]. *Med Clin (Barc).* 2014;142(2):87–88. doi:10.1016/j.medcli.2013.07.006

178. Pinkus H. Furuncle. *J Cutan Pathol.* 1979;6:517.

179. Pitney LK, O'Brien B, Pitney MJ. Acne necrotica (necrotizing lymphocytic folliculitis): an enigmatic and under-recognised dermatosis. *Australas J Dermatol.* 2018;59(1):e53–e58. doi:10.1111/ajd.12592

180. Moreno-Arrones OM, Campo RD, Saceda-Corralo D, et al. Folliculitis decalvans microbiological signature is specific for disease clinical phenotype. *J Am Acad Dermatol.* 2021;85(5):1355–1357. doi:10.1016/j.jaad.2020.10.073

181. Strauss JS, Kligman AM. Pseudofolliculitis of the beard. *Arch Dermatol.* 1956;74(5):533–542.

182. Hyland CH, Kheir SM. Follicular occlusion disease with elimination of abnormal elastic tissue. *Arch Dermatol.* 1980;116(8):925–928.

183. Dvorak VC, Root RK, MacGregor RR. Host-defensive mechanisms in hidradenitis suppurative. *Arch Dermatol.* 1977;113(4):450–453.

184. Brunsting HA. Hidradenitis suppurativa: abscess of the apocrine sweat glands. *Arch Dermatol Syphiligr.* 1939;39:108.

185. Preda-Naumescu A, Ahmed HN, Mayo TT, Yusuf N. Hidradenitis suppurativa: pathogenesis, clinical presentation, epidemiology, and comorbid associations. *Int J Dermatol.* 2021;60(11):e449–e458. doi:10.1111/ijd.15579

186. Ingram JR. Hidradenitis suppurativa: management. In: Ofori AO, ed. *UpToDate.* UpToDate; 2021.

187. Swain RA, Hatcher JC, Azadian BS, Soni N, De Souza B. A five-year review of necrotising fasciitis in a tertiary referral unit. *Ann R Coll Surg Engl.* 2013;95(1):57–60.

188. Wong CH, Khin LW, Heng KS, Tan KC, Low CO. The LRINEC (Laboratory Risk Indicator for Necrotizing Fasciitis) score: a tool for distinguishing necrotizing fasciitis from other soft tissue infections. *Crit Care Med.* 2004;32(7):1535–1541.

189. Bisno AL, Stevens DL. Streptococcal infections of skin and soft tissues. *N Engl J Med.* 1996;334(4):240–245.

190. Laupland KB, Davies HD, Low DE, Schwartz B, Green K, McGeer A. Invasive group A streptococcal disease in children in association with varicella-zoster virus infection. *Pediatrics.* 2000;105(5):E60.

191. Stevens DL, Bryant AE, Goldstein EJ. Necrotizing soft tissue infections. *Infect Dis Clin North Am.* 2021;35(1):135–155. doi:10.1016/j.idc.2020.10.004

192. Koehn GS. Necrotizing fasciitis. *Arch Dermatol.* 1978;114(4):581–583.

193. Hidalgo-Grass C, Dan-Goor M, Maly A, et al. Effect of a bacterial pheromone peptide on host chemokine degradation in group A streptococcal necrotising soft-tissue infections. *Lancet.* 2004;363(9410):696–703.

194. Solomon IH, Borscheid R, Laga AC, Askari R, Granter SR. Frozen sections are unreliable for the diagnosis of necrotizing soft tissue infections. *Mod Pathol.* 2018;31(4):546–552. doi:10.1038/modpathol.2017.173

195. Stevens DL, Baddour LM. Necrotizing soft tissue infections. In: Baron EL, ed. *UpToDate.* UpToDate; 2021.

196. Kwan E, Riley CA, Robinson CA. *Malakoplakia.* StatPearls Publishing; 2021.

197. McClure J. Malakoplakia. *J Pathol.* 1983;140:275.

198. Kohl SK, Hans CP. Cutaneous malakoplakia. *Arch Pathol Lab Med.* 2008;132(1):113–117. doi:10.5858/2008-132-113-CM

199. Abou NI, Pombejara C, Sagawa A, et al. Malakoplakia: evidence for monocyte lysosomal abnormality correctable by cholinergic agonist in vitro and in vivo. *N Engl J Med.* 1973;297(26):1413–1419.

200. Wick MR. Granulomatous & histiocytic dermatitides. *Semin Diagn Pathol*. 2017;34(3):301–311. doi:10.1053/j.semdp.2016.12.003

201. Leão CA, Duarte MI, Gamba C, et al. Malakoplakia after renal transplantation in the current era of immunosuppressive therapy: case report and literature review. *Transpl Infect Dis*. 2012;14(6):E137–E141. doi:10.1111/tid.12012

202. Gliddon T, Proudmore K. Cutaneous malakoplakia. *N Engl J Med*. 2019;380(6):580. doi:10.1056/NEJMicm1809037

203. Jung YS, Chung DY, Kim EJ, Cho NH. Ultrastructural evidence of the evolutional process in malakoplakia. *Histol Histopathol*. 2020;35(2):177–184. doi:10.14670/HH-18-150

204. Rodriguez G, Ortegon M, Camargo D, Orozco LC. Iatrogenic *Mycobacterium abscessus* infection: histopathology of 71 patients. *Br J Dermatol*. 1997;137(2):214–218.

205. Ebright JR, Peiper B. Skin and soft tissue infections in injection drug users. *Infect Dis Clin North Am*. 2002;16(3):697–712.

206. Spelman D, Baddour LM. Celluitis and skin abscess: epidemiology, microbiology, clinical manifestations, and diagnosis. In: Baron EL, ed. *UpToDate*. UpToDate; 2021.

207. Neafie RC, Marty AM. Unusual infections in humans. *Clin Microbiol Rev*. 1993;6(1):34–56. doi:10.1128/CMR.6.1.34

208. Toth IR, Kazal HL. Botryomycosis in acquired immunodeficiency syndrome. *Arch Pathol Lab Med*. 1987;111(3):246–249.

209. Sirka CS, Dash G, Pradhan S, Naik S, Rout AN, Sahu K. Cutaneous botryomycosis in immunocompetent patients: a case series. *Indian Dermatol Online J*. 2019;10(3):311–315. doi:10.4103/idoj.IDOJ_370_18

210. Goette DK. Transepithelial elimination in botryomycosis. *Int J Dermatol*. 1981;20(3):198–200.

211. Lalani T, Murray JC. Botryomycosis. In: Baron EL, ed. *UpToDate*. UpToDate; 2021.

212. Pradhan S, Sirka CS, Panda M, Baisakh M. Cutaneous botryomycosis treated successfully with injectable ceftriaxone sodium in an immunocompetent child. *Indian J Dermatol Venereol Leprol*. 2018;84(4):485–487. doi:10.4103/ijdvl.IJDVL_927_17

213. Chateau A, Van der Verren SE, Remaut H, Fioravanti A. The bacillus anthracis cell envelope: composition, physiological role, and clinical relevance. *Microorganisms*. 2020;8(12):1864. doi:10.3390/microorganisms8121864

214. Breathnach AF, Turnbull PCB, Eykyn SJ, et al. A labourer with a spot on his chest. *Lancet*. 1996;347(8994):96.

215. Swartz MN. Recognition and management of anthrax—an update. *N Engl J Med*. 2001;345(22):1621–1626.

216. Friedlander AM. Tackling anthrax. *Nature*. 2001;414(6860):160–161.

217. Wilson KH. Treatment of anthrax. In: Bloom A, ed. *UpToDate*. UpToDate; 2021.

218. McLendon MK, Apicella MA, Allen LA. Francisella tularensis: taxonomy, genetics, and immunopathogenesis of a potential agent of biowarfare. *Annu Rev Microbiol*. 2006;60:167–185. doi:10.1146/annurev.micro.60.080805.142126

219. Ellis J, Oyston PC, Green M, Titball RW. Tularemia. *Clin Microbiol Rev*. 2002;15(4):631–646. doi:10.1128/CMR.15.4.631-646.2002

220. Myers SA, Sexton DJ. Dermatologic manifestations of arthropod-borne diseases. *Infect Dis Clin North Am*. 1994;8(3):689–712.

221. Aquino LL, Wu JJ. Cutaneous manifestations of category A bioweapons. *J Am Acad Dermatol*. 2011;65(6):1213.e1–1213.e15. doi:10.1016/j.jaad.2010.08.040

222. Treat JR, Hess SD, McGowan KL, Yan AC, Kovarik CL. Ulceroglandular tularemia. *Pediatr Dermatol*. 2011;28(3):318–320. doi:10.1111/j.1525-1470.2010.01204.x

223. Penn RL. Clinical manifestations, diagnosis, and treatment of tularemia. In: Bloom A, ed. *UpToDate*. UpToDate; 2021.

224. Lewis DA. Chancroid: clinical manifestations, diagnosis, and management. *Sex Transm Infect*. 2003;79(1):68–71. doi:10.1136/sti.79.1.68

225. Lewis DA, Mitjà O. *Haemophilus ducreyi*: from sexually transmitted infection to skin ulcer pathogen. *Curr Opin Infect Dis*. 2016;29(1):52–57. doi:10.1097/QCO.0000000000000226

226. Freinkel AL. Histological aspects of sexually transmitted genital lesions. *Histopathology*. 1987;11(8):819–831.

227. Lewis DA. Diagnostic tests for chancroid. *Sex Transm Infect*. 2000;76(2):137–141. doi:10.1136/sti.76.2.137

228. Marsch WC, Haas N, Stuttgen G. Ultrastructural detection of *Haemophilus ducreyi* in biopsies of chancroid. *Arch Dermatol Res*. 1978;263(2):153–157.

229. Lewis DA. Epidemiology, clinical features, diagnosis and treatment of *Haemophilus ducreyi*—a disappearing pathogen? *Expert Rev Anti Infect Ther*. 2014;12(6):687–696. doi:10.1586/14787210.2014.892414

230. Maliyar K, Mufti A, Syed M, et al. Genital ulcer disease: a review of pathogenesis and clinical features. *J Cutan Med Surg*. 2019;23(6):624–634. doi:10.1177/1203475419858955

231. Hicks CB. Chancroid. In: Mitty J, ed. *UpToDate*. UpToDate; 2021.

232. Ballard RC. *Calymmatobacterium granulomatis*. Donovanosis, granuloma inguinale. In: Mandell GL, Bennett JE, Dolin R, eds. *Principles and Practice of Infectious Disease*. 5th ed. Churchill Livingstone; 2000:2457–2458.

233. O'Farrell N. Donovanosis. *Sex Transm Infect*. 2002;78(6):452–457. doi:10.1136/sti.78.6.452

234. O'Farrell N, Moi H. 2016 European guideline on donovanosis. *Int J STD AIDS*. 2016;27(8):605–607. doi:10.1177/0956462416633626

235. Lucas SB. Tropical pathology of the female genital tract and ovaries. In: Fox H, ed. *Haines and Taylor Obstetrical and Gynaecological Pathology*. 5th ed. Churchill Livingstone; 2003:1133–1156.

236. Spagnolo DV, Coburn PR, Cream JJ, Azadian BS. Extragenital granuloma inguinale (donovanosis) diagnosed in the United Kingdom: a clinical, histological, and electron microscopical study. *J Clin Pathol*. 1984;37(8):945–949.

237. Arora AK, Kumaran MS, Narang T, Saikia UN, Handa S. Donovanosis and squamous cell carcinoma: the relationship conundrum! *Int J STD AIDS*. 2017;28(4):411–414. doi:10.1177/0956462416665996

238. Ramdial PK, Sing Y, Ramburan A, et al. Infantile donovanosis presenting as external auditory canal polyps: a diagnostic trap. *Am J Dermatopathol*. 2012;34(8):818–821.

239. Hart CA, Rao SK. Donovanosis. *J Med Microbiol*. 1999;48(8):707–709. doi:10.1099/00222615-48-8-707

240. Davis CM, Collins C. Granuloma inguinale: an ultrastructural study of *Calymmatobacterium granulomatis*. *J Invest Dermatol*. 1969;53:315–321.

241. Tuddenham S, Ghane, KG. Approach to the patient with genital ulcers. In: Mitty J, ed. *UpToDate*. UpToDate; 2021.

242. Jones RE, Batteiger BE. *Chlamydia trachomatis*. In: Mandell GL, Bennett JE, Dolin R, eds. *Principles and Practice of Infectious Disease*. 5th ed. Churchill Livingstone; 2000:1989–2003.

243. Martin-Iguacel R, Llibre JM, Nielsen H, et al. Lymphogranuloma venereum proctocolitis: a silent endemic disease in men who have sex with men in industrialised countries. *Eur J Clin Microbiol Infect Dis*. 2010;29(8):917–925. doi:10.1007/s10096-010-0959-2

244. Bernal-Martínez S, García Sánchez E, Sivianes N, Padilla L, Martin-Mazuelos E. Evaluation of 2 commercial assays for the detection of lymphogranuloma venereum in rectal samples. *Sex Transm Dis*. 2020;47(3):162–164. doi:10.1097/OLQ.0000000000001120

245. Ciccarese G, Drago F, Rebora A, Parodi A. Updates on lymphogranuloma venereum. *J Eur Acad Dermatol Venereol*. 2021;35(8):1606–1607. doi:10.1111/jdv.17468

246. Hamill M. Lymphogranuloma venereum. In: Mitty J, ed. *UpToDate*. UpToDate; 2021.

247. Umphress B, Raparia K. Rhinoscleroma. *Arch Pathol Lab Med*. 2018;142(12):1533–1536. doi:10.5858/arpa.2018-0073-RA

248. Meyer PR, Shum TK, Becker TS, Taylor CR. Scleroma (rhinoscleroma): a histologic immunohistochemical study with bacteriologic correlates. *Arch Pathol Lab Med.* 1983;107(7):377–383.

249. Elwany S, Fattah HA, Mandour Z, Ismail AS, Abdelnabi M. A myriad of scleroma presentations: the usual and unusual. *Head Neck Pathol.* 2020;14(3):588–592. doi:10.1007/s12105-019-01075-5

250. Corelli B, Almeida AS, Sonego F, et al. Rhinoscleroma pathogenesis: the type K3 capsule of *Klebsiella rhinoscleromatis* is a virulence factor not involved in Mikulicz cells formation. *PLoS Negl Trop Dis.* 2018;12(1):e0006201. doi:10.1371/journal.pntd.0006201

251. Tan SL, Neoh CY, Tan HH. Rhinoscleroma: a case series. *Singapore Med J.* 2012;53(2):e24–e27.

252. Nelson CA, Saha S, Mead PS. Cat-scratch disease in the United States, 2005–2013. *Emerg Infect Dis.* 2016;22(10):1741–1746. doi:10.3201/eid2210.160115

253. Tay SY, Freeman K, Baird R. Clinical manifestations associated with *Bartonella henselae* infection in a tropical region. *Am J Trop Med Hyg.* 2021;104(1):198–206. doi:10.4269/ajtmh.20-0088

254. Lins KA, Drummond MR, Velho PENF. Cutaneous manifestations of bartonellosis. *An Bras Dermatol.* 2019;94(5):594–602. doi:10.1016/j.abd.2019.09.024

255. Hansmann Y, DeMartino S, Piémont Y, et al. Diagnosis of cat scratch disease with detection of *Bartonella henselae* by PCR: a study of patients with lymph node enlargement. *J Clin Microbiol.* 2005;43(8):3800–3806. doi:10.1128/JCM.43.8.3800-3806.2005

256. Kudo E, Sakaki A, Sumitomo M, et al. An epidemiological and ultrastructural study of lymphadenitis caused by Warthin-Starry positive bacteria. *Virchows Arch A Pathol Anat Histopathol.* 1988;412(6):563–572.

257. Spach DH, Kaplan SL. Treatment of cat scratch disease. In: Mitty J, ed. *UpToDate.* UpToDate; 2021.

258. Stoler MH, Bonfiglio TA, Steigbigel RT, Pereira M. An atypical subcutaneous infection associated with AIDS. *Am J Clin Pathol.* 1983;80(5):714–718.

259. Luciani L, El Baroudi Y, Prudent E, Raoult D, Fournier PE. *Bartonella* infections diagnosed in the French reference center, 2014-2019, and focus on infections in the immunocompromised. *Eur J Clin Microbiol Infect Dis.* 2021;40(11):2407–2410. doi:10.1007/s10096-021-04244-z

260. Chian CA, Arrese JE, Peirrard GE. Skin manifestations of *Bartonella* infections. *Int J Dermatol.* 2002;41(8):461–466.

261. Cottell SL, Noskin GA. Bacillary angiomatosis: clinical and histologic features, diagnosis and treatment. *Arch Intern Med.* 1994;154(5):524–528.

262. Koehler JE, Sanchez MA, Garrido CS, et al. Molecular epidemiology of *Bartonella* infections in patients with bacillary angiomatosis-peliosis. *N Engl J Med.* 1997;337(26):1876–1883. doi:10.1056/NEJM199712253372603

263. Schinella RA, Greco MA. Bacillary angiomatosis presenting as a soft-tissue tumour without skin involvement. *Hum Pathol.* 1990;21(5):567–569.

264. LeBoit PE, Berger TG, Egbert BM, et al. Bacillary angiomatosis: the histopathology and differential diagnosis of a pseudoneoplastic infection in patients with HIV disease. *Am J Surg Pathol.* 1989;13(11):909–920.

265. Spach DH. Diagnosis, treatment, and prevention of *Bartonella* infections in HIV-infected patients. In: Mitty J, ed. *UpToDate.* UpToDate; 2021.

266. Maguiña C, Guerra H, Ventosilla P. Bartonellosis. *Clin Dermatol.* 2009;27(3):271–280. doi:10.1016/j.clindermatol.2008.10.006

267. Maco V, Maguiña C, Tirado A, Maco V, Vidal JE. Carrion's disease (*Bartonellosis bacilliformis*) confirmed by histopathology in the high forest of Peru. *Rev Inst Med Trop Sao Paulo.* 2004;46(3):171–174.

268. Huarcaya E, Maguiña C, Torres R, Rupay J, Fuentes L. Bartonellosis (Carrion's disease) in the pediatric population of Peru: an overview and update. *Braz J Infect Dis.* 2004;8(5):331–339.

269. Minnick MF, Anderson BE, Lima A, Battisti JM, Lawyer PG, Birtles RJ. Oroya fever and verruga peruana: bartonelloses unique to South America. *PLoS Negl Trop Dis.* 2014;8(7):e2919. doi:10.1371/journal.pntd.0002919

270. Cerimele F, Brown LF, Bravo F, Ihler GM, Kouadio P, Arbiser JL. Infectious angiogenesis: *Bartonella bacilliformis* infection results in endothelial production of angiopoietin-2 and epidermal production of vascular endothelial growth factor. *Am J Pathol.* 2003;163(4):1321–1327.

271. Spach DH. Bartonellosis: oroya fever and verruga peruana. In: Baron EL, ed. *UpToDate.* UpToDate; 2021.

272. Brown-Elliott BA, Brown JM, Conville PS, Wallace RJ Jr. Clinical and laboratory features of the *Nocardia* spp. based on current molecular taxonomy. *Clin Microbiol Rev.* 2006;19(2):259–282. doi:10.1128/CMR.19.2.259-282.2006

273. Hemmersbach-Miller M, Catania J, Saullo JL. Updates on nocardia skin and soft tissue infections in solid organ transplantation. *Curr Infect Dis Rep.* 2019;21(8):27. doi:10.1007/s11908-019-0684-7

274. Lucas SB, Hounnou A, Peacock CS, Beaumel A, Kadio A, De Cock KM. Nocardiosis in HIV-positive patients: an autopsy study in West Africa. *Tuber Lung Dis.* 1994;75(4):301–307.

275. Uttamchandari RB, Daikos GL, Reyes RR, et al. Nocardiosis in 30 patients with advanced human immunodeficiency virus infection: clinical features and outcome. *Clin Infect Dis.* 1994;18(3):348–353.

276. Ramos-E-Silva M, Lopes RS, Trope BM. Cutaneous nocardiosis: a great imitator. *Clin Dermatol.* 2020;38(2):152–159. doi:10.1016/j.clindermatol.2019.10.009

277. Spelman D. Treatment of nocardiosis. In: Mitty J, ed. *UpToDate.* UpToDate; 2021.

278. Russo TA. Agents of actinomycosis. In: Mandell GL, Bennett JE, Dolin R, eds. *Principles and Practice of Infectious Diseases.* 5th ed. Churchill Livingstone; 2000:2645–2654.

279. Könönen E, Wade WG. Actinomyces and related organisms in human infections. *Clin Microbiol Rev.* 2015;28(2):419–442. doi:10.1128/CMR.00100-14

280. Rashid AM, Williams RM, Parry D, et al. Actinomycosis associated with a pilonidal sinus of the penis. *J Urol.* 1992;148:405–406.

281. Behberhani MJ, Heeley JD, Jordan HV. Comparative histopathology of lesions produced by *Actinomyces israelii*, *Actinomyces naeslundii*, and *Actinomyces viscosus* in mice. *Am J Pathol.* 1983;110(3):267–274.

282. Connor DH, Chandler FW. Actinomycosis. In: Connor DH, Chandler FW, eds. *Pathology of Infectious Diseases.* Vol I, Pt III (Bacterial Infections). Appleton and Lange; 1996.

283. Sharkawy AA, Chow AW. Cervicofacial actinomycosis. In: Bogorodskaya M, ed. *UpToDate.* UpToDate; 2021.

Spirochete Infections (Treponemal and Other Spirochete Diseases)

Chapter **22**

A. NEIL CROWSON, ERICA S. KUMAR, CYNTHIA MAGRO, AND
MARTIN C. MIHM JR.

INTRODUCTION

The venereal and nonvenereal treponemal diseases are caused by motile bacteria of the family Spirochaetaceae, which also includes the genera *Borrelia* and *Leptospira*. Accurate recognition of spirochetal infections requires the correlation of a given patient's travel and medical histories with a detailed knowledge of the clinical and histologic expression of each pathogen. The pathogenic treponemes resemble each other in dark-field and biopsy preparations—being coiled, silver-staining organisms 6 to 20 μm by 0.10 to 0.18 μm—and have a high degree of DNA sequence homology (1,2). A single genetic difference in the 5′ and 3′ flanking regions of the 15-kD lipoprotein gene *tpp15* was described for venereal and nonvenereal treponematoses in one study (3), evidence suggesting that these organisms evolved from a common ancestor to cause different diseases (4,5). Size and sequence heterogeneity is demonstrated by other treponeme genes, such as those controlling the expression of the TprK antigen, a target of opsonizing antibodies that is important for host immune protection, a variance in which may play a role in the evasion of host response (6,7). The uncultivable pathogenic nonvenereal *Treponema pallidum* subspecies include *T. pallidum* subsp. *pertenue*, *T. pallidum* subsp. *endemicum*, and *T. carateum*, which cause yaws, bejel, and pinta, respectively. Oral treponemes may be important in the causation of periodontitis (8–10).

VENEREAL SYPHILIS

Clinical Summary. Acquired syphilis, caused by *T. pallidum*, has afflicted humanity since at least the 15th century (11). Although it was a major cause of morbidity and mortality in the early 20th century, public health programs and the advent of penicillin so reduced its incidence in the First World countries by mid-century that many physicians became unfamiliar with its signs and symptoms (1). The rate of syphilis infection continues to increase despite these medical advances. The World Health Organization (WHO) estimates that 5.6 million new cases of syphilis occurred worldwide among adolescents and adults between the ages of 15 and 49 years in 2012. The estimated prevalence of the disease was 18 million at this time, with a global prevalence of 0.5% among females and 0.5% among males aged 15 to 49 years (12). Syphilis rates are reported to have risen by 300% since 2000 in many Western countries (13). In 2018, the rate of syphilis was reported as 10.8 cases per 100,000 in

the United States, representing a 14.9% increase from 2017 (9.4 cases per 100,000) and a 71.4% increase compared with the cases in 2014 (6.3 cases per 100,000) (14). In 2017, the rate of reported primary and secondary syphilis cases in the United States among men (16.9 cases per 100,000 males) was higher than the rate among women (2.3 cases per 100,000). This trend was reflected in almost every region of the country (15). According to the data from the Regional Medical Laboratory in Tulsa, Oklahoma, the seropositivity rate in our tested population has increased by 225% from 2017 to 2020 (see Table 22-1). The rise in the rate of reported primary and secondary syphilis cases is largely attributable to increased cases among men, particularly men who have sex with men (MSM); however, cases among men who have sex with women (MSW) and cases among women have increased substantially as well. The increase in syphilis among women has been accompanied by a concurrent increase in congenital syphilis (16).

Despite efforts to eliminate syphilis in higher-income countries, there continue to be large increases in infection in certain populations, partly owing to budget reductions in public health programs and control efforts. In low- and middle-income countries, syphilis has remained endemic (17).

T. pallidum, of which there are three antigenically similar subspecies (18), is generally spread through contact between infectious lesions and disrupted epithelium at sites of minor trauma incurred during sexual intercourse. The transmission rate is between 10% and 60%. Early lesions reflect a delayed-hypersensitivity response to the organism, although some bacteria escape, in part owing to integral outer membrane proteins

Table 22-1					
Serologic Testing for Syphilis at Regional Medical Laboratory (RML), Tulsa, Oklahoma, 2017–2021					
RML Serologic Syphilis Results					
2017–2021 (Annualized)					
	2017	2018	2019	2020	2021
No. pts tested	26,219	27,749	26,337	25,729	27,282
Positive pts	269	297	425	598	732
% Inc previous yr		10%	43%	41%	22%
% Reactive pts	1.03%	1.20%	1.61%	2.32%	2.68%

Courtesy of Dr. Gerald C. Miller, Director of Microbiology and Immunology, Regional Medical Laboratory, Tulsa, OK.

699

that may render the treponeme invisible to the immune system (19). The result in untreated hosts is persistent infectivity over the course of decades.

The staging of syphilis should include an evaluation of the patient history, physical exam, and laboratory data (13).

Primary syphilis is defined by a skin lesion, or chancre, in which organisms are identified; it typically arises 21 days after exposure at the inoculation site and is classically a painless, brown-red, indurated, round papule, nodule, or plaque 1 to 2 cm in diameter. Lesions may be multiple or ulcerative, and the regional lymph nodes may be enlarged. One-third of the lesions are extragenital (13).

Secondary syphilis results from the hematogenous dissemination of organisms, characterized by widespread clinical signs accompanied by constitutional symptoms inclusive of fever, malaise, and generalized lymphadenopathy. Symptoms may appear 2 weeks to 6 months after exposure and can be concurrent with or up to 6 weeks after the appearance of a chancre (13). A generalized eruption comprises brown-red macules and papules, papulosquamous lesions resembling guttate psoriasis, and, rarely, pustules (20). Lesions may be follicular based, annular, or serpiginous, particularly in recurrent attacks of secondary syphilis. Other skin signs include alopecia and condylomata lata, the latter comprising broad, raised, gray, confluent papular lesions arising in anogenital areas, pitted hyperkeratotic palmoplantar papules termed "syphilis cornee," and, in rare severe cases, ulcerating lesions that define "lues maligna." Some patients develop shallow, painless ulcers in the mucosae.

Meningovascular syphilis is usually seen in tertiary syphilis after 7 to 12 years of disease (21) but can occur in the secondary stage and be symptomatic; usually, it manifests as basilar meningitis and can be associated with cranial nerve palsies (22). Acute transverse myelitis (23), glomerulonephritis, and self-limited hepatitis are other uncommon manifestations.

Primary- and secondary-stage lesions may resolve without therapy or go unnoticed by the patient, who then passes into a latent phase. This may be subdivided into early and late stages, an arbitrary distinction that may help to guide the therapeutic approach. The Centers for Disease Control (CDC) bases the distinction of the early (infectious) latent stage from the late (noninfectious) latent stage on whether the duration of the infection is less or more than 1 year, respectively. WHO uses a 2-year period to make this distinction. After a variable latent period, the patient enters the *tertiary stage*.

Without treatment, 14% to 40% of people with syphilis progress to the tertiary stage (defined by irreversible damage to any organ) (13). *Tertiary syphilis* comprises gummatous skin and mucosal lesions ("benign tertiary syphilis"), cardiovascular manifestations, and neurologic manifestations. The skin lesions may be solitary or multiple and can be divided into superficial nodular and deep gummatous types. The nodular type has a smooth, atrophic center with a raised, serpiginous border. The gummatous lesions present as subcutaneous swellings that ulcerate (24).

Congenital syphilis, on the rise since the mid-1980s (25), is a diagnosis rendered when organisms are identified in dark-field, immunofluorescent, or conventionally stained tissues or smears of lesional skin, placenta, or umbilical cord (26). A presumptive case is an infant born to a mother with inadequately treated syphilis at the time of delivery or when an infant or child with a reactive treponemal test for syphilis exhibits evidence of congenital syphilis by virtue of physical or long-bone radiologic examination, a reactive cerebrospinal fluid (CSF), Venereal Disease Research Laboratory (VDRL) test, an elevated CSF protein or white blood cell count of unknown cause, or quantitative treponemal titers four times higher than the mother's at the time of birth (26). Clinical signs include rhinitis, chancres, or a maculopapular desquamative rash (25). Transplacental infection occurs in more than 50% of infants born to mothers with primary or secondary syphilis, roughly 40% of those born to mothers in the early latent stage, and only 10% of those born to mothers with late latent infections (26).

Histopathology. The two fundamental pathologic changes in syphilis are (a) swelling and proliferation of endothelial cells and (b) a perivascular infiltrate of lymphoid cells and often of plasma cells. In late secondary and tertiary syphilis, there are also granulomatous infiltrates comprising epithelioid histiocytes and giant cells. Newborns with congenital syphilis at autopsy have shown multiorgan involvement by an angioinvasive CD68+ mononuclear cell infiltrate that imparts an "onion-skin" morphology to the involved vessels with numerous demonstrable spirochetes (27).

Primary Syphilis

The epidermis at the periphery of the syphilitic chancre reveals changes comparable to those observed in the lesions of secondary syphilis, namely, acanthosis, spongiosis, and exocytosis of lymphocytes and neutrophils. Toward the center, the epidermis becomes thinned, edematous, and permeated by inflammatory cells. In the center, the epidermis may be absent. The papillary dermis is edematous. A dense perivascular and interstitial lymphohistiocytic and plasmacellular infiltrate spans the entire thickness of the dermis (Fig. 22-1); the lymphocytes are principally of T-helper phenotype. Neutrophils are often admixed. Endarteritis obliterans characterized by endothelial swelling and mural edema is observed (Fig. 22-2).

By silver staining with the Levaditi or the Warthin–Starry stain, immunohistochemical, or immunofluorescent techniques, spirochetes are usually identified along the dermal–epidermal junction and within and around blood vessels. If seen in their full length, which is rare, spirochetes generally show 8 to 12 spiral convolutions, each measuring from 1 to

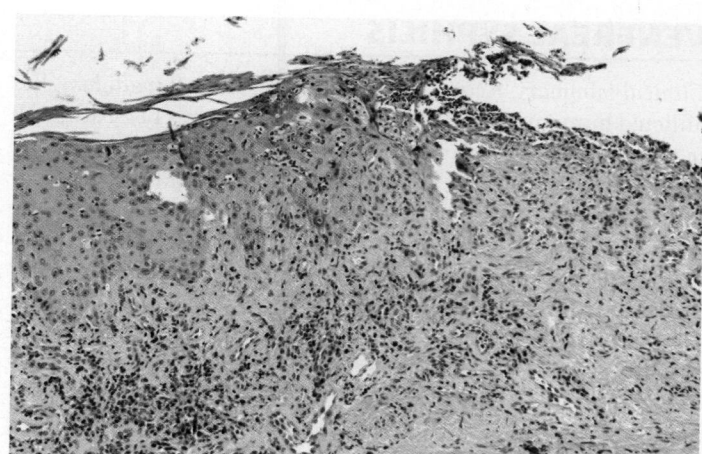

Figure 22-1 Primary syphilitic chancre. The epithelium is eroded and the corium contains a dense, plasma cell-rich infiltrate. There is neovascularization, with secondary necrotizing vasculitic changes manifested by mural fibrin deposition.

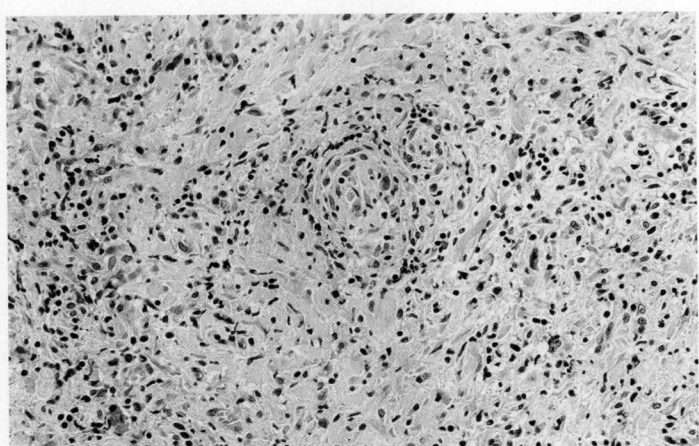

Figure 22-2 Primary syphilitic chancre. There is endarteritis obliterans manifested by endothelial cell swelling, endothelial hyperplasia, and expansion of vessel walls by edema and a lymphohistiocytic infiltrate with resultant lumenal attenuation. A diffuse extravascular plasma cell-rich infiltrate is present.

1.2 μm in length (Fig. 22-3A). It should be remembered that silver also stains melanin and reticulum fibers. Differentiation may cause some difficulties but should be possible based on the fact that the melanin in the dendritic processes of melanocytes has a granular appearance, the granules being thicker and more heavily stained than *T. pallidum* (28). Reticulin fibers, although wavy, do not exhibit a spiral appearance. Immunohistochemistry is more sensitive than the Warthin–Starry or Steiner silver staining techniques (71% vs. 41% sensitive) (Fig. 22-3B) (29). Serologic correlation is prudent; in addition to conventional serology, emerging point-of-care tests for rapid screening for syphilis on serum samples have a sensitivity of 75% to 90% and a specificity of 90% to 99%, whereas those for whole blood are both less sensitive and less specific (30).

Histologic examination of enlarged regional lymph nodes in primary syphilis most commonly reveals a chronic inflammatory infiltrate containing many plasma cells with endothelial hyperplasia and follicular hyperplasia. Spirochetes are numerous and can nearly always be identified with stains. In some cases, nonnecrotizing granulomas resembling those of sarcoidosis are found in the lymph nodes (31).

Histogenesis. T. pallidum can be demonstrated by histochemistry or by immunohistochemistry. The latter comprises immunofluorescent methods in frozen (32) or fresh specimens and immunoperoxidase methods employable in fixed tissues (33). By electron microscopy, the organism can be seen in both intra- and extracellular dispositions in the epidermis and dermis (34) and within keratinocyte nuclei (35), fibroblasts (35,36), nerve fibers (37), blood vessel endothelia, and the lumina of lymphatic channels (35). Phagocytic vacuoles of macrophages and neutrophils may contain organisms (38), as may the cytoplasm of plasma cells. Ultrastructurally, the organism is 8 to 16 μm in length with regular spirals, a wavelength of 0.9 μm with an amplitude of 0.2 μm, and a cytoplasmic body 0.13 μm in diameter with tapering ends, all enveloped by a 7-nm trilaminar cytoplasmic membrane (39). The organisms attach to host cells by means of acorn-shaped nosepieces. The contractile motility of the spirochete is mediated by three or four axial filaments that course the length of the cytoplasmic body (40). A paraplastic membrane surrounds these axial filaments in young organisms but is replaced by an electron-dense amorphous substance produced by the host cell as an immunologic response in older spirochetes (37).

Differential Diagnosis. Lesions of chancroid are the most difficult to differentiate clinically from a syphilitic chancre. The characteristic histopathology of chancroid is one of dense lymphohistiocytic infiltrates with a paucity of plasma cells and a granulomatous vasculitis. An epidermal reaction pattern similar to the syphilitic chancre is observed, namely, psoriasiform epidermal hyperplasia and spongiform pustulation. A Giemsa or Alcian blue stain reveals coccobacillary forms between keratinocytes and along the dermal–epidermal junction. The infiltrate is composed mainly of T-helper lymphocytes and histiocytes including Langerhans cells (41).

Secondary Syphilis

Clinical Summary. There is considerable histologic overlap among the various clinical forms of secondary syphilis, such as the macular, papular, and papulosquamous types (42). Nevertheless, epidermal changes are least pronounced in the macular type and most pronounced in papulosquamous lesions.

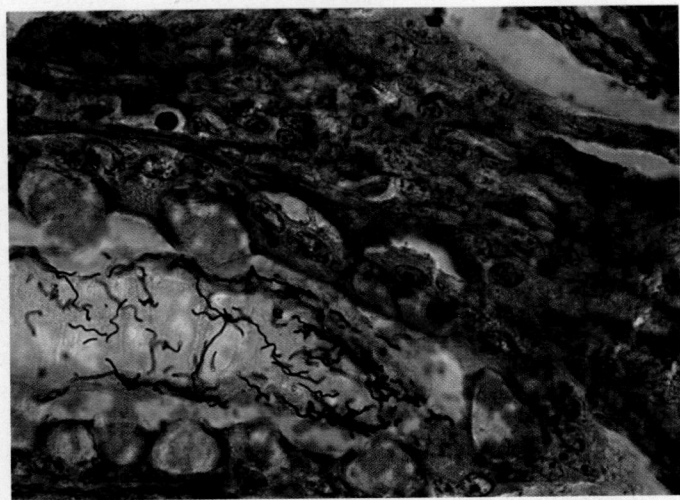
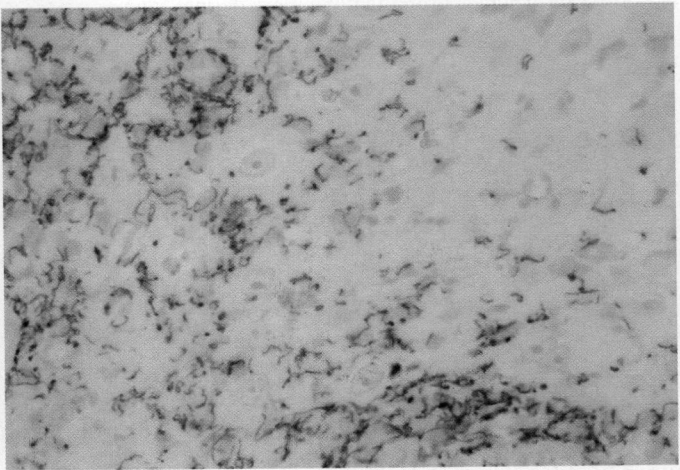

Figure 22-3 A: Treponeme morphology. A silver stain reveals numerous elongate, coiled spirochetes ranging in length from 8 to 12 μm. B: Immunohistochemistry highlights spirochetes in the epithelium of this mucosal biopsy from an ulcerated lesion of syphilis.

Biopsies generally reveal psoriasiform hyperplasia, often with spongiosis and basilar vacuolar alteration, often with edema of the papillary dermis (Fig. 22-4). Exocytosis of lymphocytes, spongiform pustulation, and parakeratosis also may be observed (28,42). The parakeratosis may be patchy or broad, with or without intracorneal neutrophilic abscesses. Although lesions may mimic psoriasis, attenuation of the suprapapillary plate is uncommon. Scattered necrotic keratinocytes may be observed. Ulceration is not a feature of macular, papular, or papulosquamous lesions of secondary syphilis. The dermal changes include marked papillary dermal edema and a perivascular and/or periadnexal infiltrate that may be lymphocyte predominant, lymphohistiocytic, histiocytic predominant, or frankly granulomatous; is of greatest intensity in the papillary dermis; and extends as loose perivascular aggregates into the reticular dermis. Obscuration of the superficial vasculature and lichenoid morphology is observed in some cases, and a cell-poor infiltrate is seen in others. In a few cases, when the infiltrate is heavy, atypical nuclei may be present and may then suggest the possibility of mycosis fungoides (43) or non-Hodgkin lymphoma. Neutrophils may permeate the eccrine coil to produce a neutrophilic eccrine hidradenitis or manifest as a neutrophil-imbued scale crust (Fig. 22-5) (28). Granulomatous inflammation is almost invariable in lesions of greater than 4 months' duration and may be present in some cases of early syphilis (44). A plasma cell component is usually present but is inconspicuous or absent in 25% of the cases (Fig. 22-6) (42). Eosinophils are not usually observed. Vascular changes such as endothelial swelling and mural edema accompany the angiocentric infiltrates in half of the cases (42). Necrotizing vascular injury is distinctly unusual. A confirmatory stain is recommended in all cases that are suspected of being secondary syphilis. A silver stain may show spirochetes in about one-third of the cases of secondary syphilis, mainly within the epidermis and less commonly around the blood vessels of the superficial plexus. In some instances, the silver stain is positive even when a dark-field examination of the patient's lesions is negative (28). By the immunofluorescent technique, essentially all cases are found to be positive. A phenotypic analysis of the infiltrate reveals a lymphoid populace composed mainly of T cells with an equal proportion of cytotoxic and T-helper cells.

There are several histologic variants of secondary syphilis—namely, condylomata lata, syphilitic alopecia, pustular lesions (Fig. 22-5), syphilis cornee, and lues maligna. Lesions of condylomata lata show all of the aforementioned changes observed in macular, papular, and papulosquamous lesions, but more florid epithelial hyperplasia and intraepithelial microabscess formation are observed (2). A Warthin–Starry stain shows numerous treponemes (37).

Biopsies of syphilitic alopecia may demonstrate a superficial and deep perivascular and perifollicular lymphocytic and plasmacellular infiltrate that permeates the outer root sheath epithelium with a concomitant perifollicular fibrosing reaction (28). An involutional tendency characterized by increased numbers of telogen hairs is observed. A concomitant necrotizing pustular follicular reaction may also be seen (20).

An unusual variant of secondary syphilis is lues maligna (45,46), an ulcerative form characterized by severe thrombotic endarteritis obliterans involving vessels at the dermal–subcutaneous junction with resultant ischemic necrosis. A concomitant dense plasmacellular infiltrate with a variable admixture of histiocytes may be observed. Defective cell-mediated immunity may play an integral role in the pathogenesis of lues maligna, particularly in cases in which vascular alterations are minimal (47,48). Several cases of lues maligna arising in the setting of HIV disease have been described, with the involvement of the oral cavity as the principal manifestation. A case of secondary syphilis resembling bullous pemphigoid by both light microscopy and immunofluorescent studies has been reported (49).

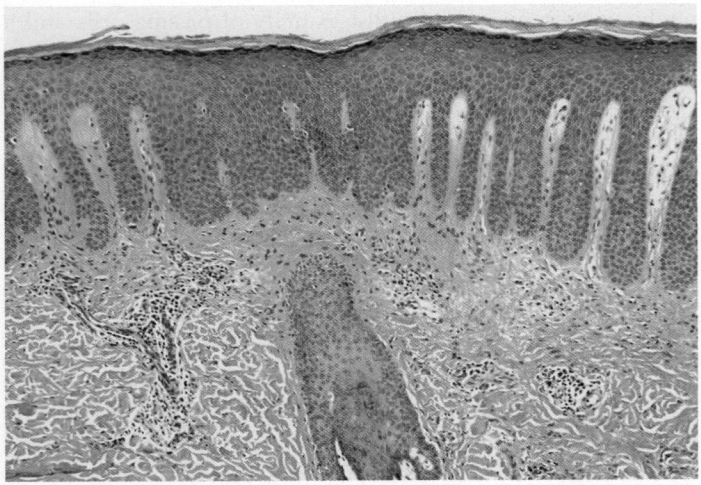

Figure 22-4 Secondary syphilis. There is striking psoriasiform hyperplasia of an epidermis surmounted by an orthohyperkeratotic and parakeratotic scale. There is prominent papillary dermal edema.

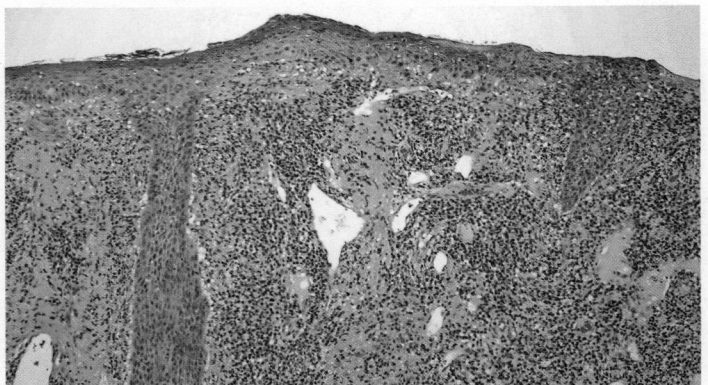

Figure 22-5 Secondary syphilis. There is psoriasiform epidermal hyperplasia with basilar vacuolopathy and lymphocytic interface dermatitis. The epidermis is surmounted by a parakeratotic scale rich in neutrophils.

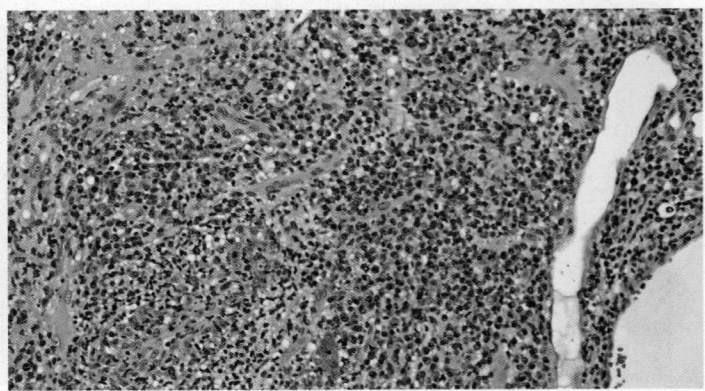

Figure 22-6 Secondary syphilis. A dense, lymphocytic, and often plasma cell-rich infiltrate surrounds the cutaneous vessels of the dermis.

Syphilis cornee/keratoderma punctatum associated with secondary syphilis manifests an epidermal invagination containing a horny plug composed of laminated layers of parakeratotic cells with loss of the granular cell layer and thinning of the stratum spinosum (50). A moderately dense perivascular plasmacellular infiltrate with concomitant capillary wall thickening involves the cutaneous vasculature.

In the rare pustular lesions of secondary syphilis, a necrotizing pustular follicular reaction accompanied by noncaseating granulomata and a perivascular lymphoplasmacellular infiltrate typically characterizes the histopathology (20). A pustular psoriasiform process with an absent granular cell layer and a strikingly thickened cornified layer laced with neutrophils may be seen (Fig. 22-5); if the clinical correlate is rugose or elephantine skin thickening, the designation *rupial syphilis* may be applied (20).

In addition to small, sarcoidal granulomata in papular lesions of early secondary syphilis, late secondary syphilis may show extensive lymphoplasmacellular and histiocytic infiltrates resembling nodular tertiary syphilis (51). Conversely, lesions of early tertiary syphilis may lack granulomata (52).

Although often nonspecific, the hepatitis of secondary syphilis may produce a granulomatous or cholestatic morphology on liver biopsy; hepatic necrosis and spirochetes may also be observed (53). Syphilis is a cause of reversible nephritic syndrome (54); kidney lesions of secondary syphilis show proliferative changes in the glomeruli (55).

Histogenesis. The renal changes in secondary syphilis relate to immune complexes containing treponemal antigen. Not only has direct immunofluorescence shown granular deposits of immunoglobulin and complement along the glomerular basement membrane (55,56), but indirect immunofluorescence antibody studies using rabbit treponemal antibody and sheep anti-rabbit globulin conjugate have demonstrated treponemal antigen in the glomerular deposits (55).

Differential Diagnosis. The differential diagnosis of lesions of secondary syphilis includes other causes of lichenoid dermatitis, including lichen planus, a lichenoid hypersensitivity reaction, pityriasis lichenoides and connective tissue disease, sarcoidosis, psoriasis, and psoriasiform drug eruptions (28). Prominent spongiosis, suprabasilar dyskeratosis, a mid- and deep perivascular component, and the presence of plasma cells are not histologic features of lichen planus or psoriasis (57). Although a mid-dermal perivascular infiltrate, keratinocyte necrosis, and prominent lymphocytic exocytosis are present in pityriasis lichenoides, the infiltrate is purely mononuclear in nature, and neither spongiform pustulation nor plasmacellular infiltration is observed (58). Although lichenoid hypersensitivity reactions and psoriasiform drug reactions may also demonstrate a perivascular infiltrate of plasma cells, tissue eosinophilia is typically observed as well.

Tertiary Syphilis

Tertiary syphilis is categorized into nodular tertiary syphilis confined to the skin; benign gummatous syphilis principally affecting the skin, bone, and liver; cardiovascular syphilis; syphilitic hepatic cirrhosis; and neurosyphilis. In the first variant, the granulomas are small and may be absent in rare cases (52). The granulomatous process is limited to the dermis, with scattered islands of epithelioid cells admixed with a few multinucleated giant cells, lymphocytes, and plasma cells.

As a rule, necrosis is not conspicuous. The vessels may show endothelial swelling (48).

In benign gummatous syphilis, the main pathology, irrespective of the organ involved, is one of granulomatous inflammation with central zones of acellular necrosis. In cutaneous lesions, the blood vessels throughout the dermis and subcutaneous fat exhibit endarteritis obliterans along with angiocentric plasmacellular infiltrates of variable density involving the dermis and subcutaneous fat.

In cardiovascular syphilis, elastic tissue fragmentation and reduplication with neovascularization and fibrosis of main arteries occur. Neurosyphilis includes an asymptomatic form—meningovascular syphilis—and parenchymatous syphilis, which is divided into generalized paresis of the insane and tabes dorsalis (59). In meningovascular syphilis, an inflammatory endarteritis involves the leptomeningeal vessels. In generalized paresis of the insane, gliosis with ventricular dilation is observed; spirochetes are identified in the cortex in 50% of the cases. In tabes dorsalis, there is demyelination of the posterior columns of the spinal cord, atrophy of the posterior spinal roots, and lymphoplasmacellular leptomeningitis (21,59).

Serology and Testing

According to the CDC, dark-field examinations and molecular tests for detecting *T. pallidum* directly from lesion exudates or tissues are the definitive methods for diagnosing early syphilis and congenital syphilis. Certain laboratories provide locally developed and validated polymerase chain reaction (PCR) tests for detecting *T. pallidum* DNA. A presumptive diagnosis of syphilis requires the use of two laboratory serologic tests: a nontreponemal test (i.e., VDRL or rapid plasma reagin [RPR] test) and a treponemal test (i.e., the *T. pallidum* passive particle agglutination [TP-PA] assay, various enzyme immunoassays [EIAs], chemiluminescence immunoassays [CIAs] and immunoblots, or rapid treponemal assays). It is stated that the use of only one type of serologic test (nontreponemal or treponemal) is insufficient for diagnosis and can result in false-negative results among persons tested during primary syphilis and in false-positive results among persons without syphilis or with previously treated syphilis (60).

Principles of Management: Antibiotic therapy is the mainstay of management.

NONVENEREAL TREPONEMATOSES

Yaws (Frambesia Tropica)

Clinical Summary. Yaws is caused by *T. pallidum* subsp. *pertenue*, which is indistinguishable microscopically from *T. pallidum* subsp. *pallidum* but has been shown to be distinctive by virtue of the substitution of a single nucleotide coding for a 19-kD polypeptide demonstrable by Southern blot analysis (61). Other molecular methodologies confirm distinctive DNA sequences (2,4). The bacterium causes a chronic relapsing treponematosis comprising highly contagious primary and secondary cutaneous lesions and noncontagious tertiary destructive bone lesions (62).

Yaws is spread by casual contact between primary or secondary lesions and abraded skin. Children are particularly afflicted; 75% to 80% of people infected are under 15 years of age (63,64). The sites of involvement include buttocks, legs, and feet. Unlike syphilis, yaws does not manifest transplacental spread to neonates (4). A positive side effect of yaws infection may be the production of antiphosphorylcholine antibodies that may be cardioprotective because they inhibit atherogenesis (65).

Yaws is prevalent in moist, warm, typically tropical climates. Interestingly, the highest incidence of yaws appears to occur in those tropical areas that experience heavy rainfall, and the number of cases (new cases and reinfections) tends to increase during the rainy seasons in these areas (62). There are at least 12 yaws-endemic countries generally recognized (62). Because reporting of yaws to WHO has not been mandatory since 1990, the data availability is somewhat limited (66). As of 2002, it was estimated that 2.5 million people were affected globally (67), and in some locations the disease appeared resurgent as late as 2010 (68). From 2008 to 2012, more than 300,000 new cases were reported to WHO (62). In 2018, 80,472 suspected cases were reported to WHO (888 of these were confirmed by the Dual Path Platform/DPP® Syphilis Screen and Confirm Assay) (63).

Primary Yaws

The initial primary-stage lesion, or "mother yaw," begins as an erythematous papule roughly 21 days postinoculation, which enlarges peripherally to form a 1- to 5-cm nodule surrounded by satellite pustules covered by an amber crust. A red crusted appearance prompted German physicians to give the appellation "frambesia," derived from the word "framboise," meaning raspberry in French, to the disease (69). Lesions may heal as pitted, hypopigmented scars. Fever, arthralgia, and lymphadenopathy may coexist.

Secondary Yaws

Similar constitutional symptoms weeks to months later may herald progression to the secondary stage, characterized by the involvement of skin, bones, joints, and/or CSF. *Skin lesions* resemble the "mother yaw" but tend to be smaller and more numerous, hence the designation "daughter yaws." Periorificial lesions may mimic venereal syphilis. A circinate appearance ("tinea yaws") may be observed, as may a morbilliform eruption and/or condylomatous vegetations involving the axillae and groins. Macular, hyperkeratotic, and papillomatous lesions may be present on palmoplantar surfaces and may cause the patient to walk with a painful, crablike gait ("crab yaws"). Papillomatous nail-fold lesions may give rise to "pianic onychia." Relapsing cutaneous disease occurs up to 5 years later, tending to involve periorificial and periaxillary or sites. A lifelong noninfectious latent state may then eventuate. *Bone lesions* consist of painful, sometimes palpable, periosteal thickening of arms and legs, occasionally accompanied by soft tissue swellings around the involved small bones of the hands and feet (70).

Tertiary Yaws

Roughly 10% of the cases progress to *tertiary yaws*, the skin manifestations of which comprise subcutaneous abscesses, ulcers that may coalesce to form serpiginous tracts, keloids, keratoderma, and palmoplantar hyperkeratosis. The bone and joint lesions of this stage include osteomyelitis, hypertrophic, or gummatous periostitis, and chronic tibial osteitis, which may lead to "saber shin" deformities. Bilateral hypertrophy of the nasal processes of the maxilla produces the rare but characteristic "goundou," which obstructs the nasal passages and, if not treated with early antibiotic therapy, may require surgery. Another otorhinolaryngologic complication is "gangosa," characterized by nasal septal or palatal perforation. Although neurologic and ophthalmologic involvement is not a universally accepted phenomenon, reports of macular atrophy and culture-positive aqueous humor suggest that yaws may exhibit neuroophthalmologic manifestations similar to those of venereal syphilis. A less virulent form of the disease, observed in lower-prevalence areas, is termed "attenuated yaws," the cutaneous manifestations of which comprise greasy gray lesions in the skin folds.

Histopathology. Primary lesions show acanthosis, papillomatosis, spongiosis, and neutrophilic exocytosis with intraepidermal microabscess formation. A heavy, diffuse, dermal infiltrate of plasma cells, lymphocytes, histiocytes, and granulocytes is observed; unlike the case in syphilis, blood vessels manifest little or no endothelial proliferation (Figs. 22-7 and 22-8) (71).

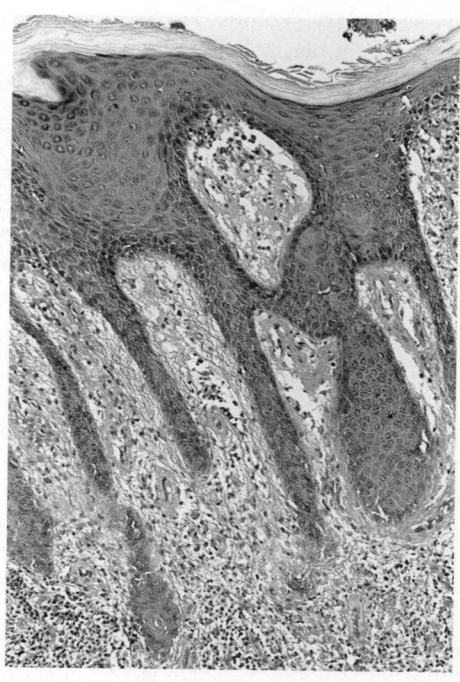

Figure 22-7 Yaws, the primary lesion. The biopsy shows a psoriasiform hyperplasia of the epidermis, accompanied by slight spongiosis and an intense lymphohistiocytic and plasmacellular infiltrate in the subjacent corium.

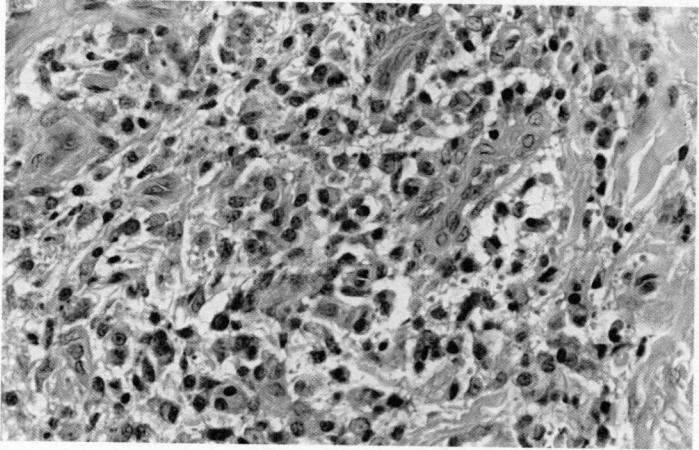

Figure 22-8 Yaws, the primary lesion. The biopsy shows an intense angiocentric lymphohistiocytic and plasmacellular infiltrate without the characteristic endarteritis obliterans vascular alterations observed in syphilis.

Secondary lesions show the same histologic appearance, resembling condylomata lata in their epidermal changes but differing by virtue of the dermal infiltrate being in a diffuse, as opposed to a perivascular, disposition. The ulcerative lesions of *tertiary yaws* greatly resemble those observed in late syphilis in histologic appearance (71). The spirochetes can be demonstrated in primary and secondary lesions by dark-field examination. Silver stains and immunohistochemical stains demonstrate numerous organisms between keratinocytes (70). Unlike *T. pallidum*, which is found in both epidermis and dermis, *T. pertenue* is almost entirely epidermotropic (71).

Differential Diagnosis. The distinction between yaws and syphilis is based on clinical features; although the location of the organism in a skin biopsy may be helpful, no histologic feature or laboratory test absolutely distinguishes the two diseases (70,72).

Principles of Management: Antibiotics are the mainstay of therapy for yaws. Widespread use of azithromycin in endemic areas has been proposed to control yaws with an ultimate view to global eradication (73). A single oral dose of azithromycin has been shown to be as effective as an intramuscular penicillin injection (74). Treatment failures occur in as many as 17% of treated patients (75), however.

Pinta

Clinical Summary. Unique among the treponematoses, pinta, caused by *T. carateum*, demonstrates only skin manifestations (76). The disorder is endemic to Central America and restricted to the Western Hemisphere. It affects no age group preferentially, although the peak age group is reported as 15 to 30 years (77). It is the mildest of the treponematoses, with hypopigmentation being the only significant sequela. The incidence of pinta is declining precipitously for unknown reasons. Transmission appears to be from lesion to skin, classically between family members; the ritualistic whipping of diseased adults and unaffected youths is the putative mode of transmission in one aboriginal tribe in the Amazon Basin (76).

The *primary lesion* is characterized by an erythematous papule surrounded by a halo and occurs 1 to 8 weeks postinoculation. By direct extension or through fusion of satellite lesions, the primary site may grow to a diameter of 12 cm, forming an ill-defined erythematous plaque on the legs or other exposed sites. In infants, the primary lesion classically occurs at the sites where the baby was held most closely to the affected mother. The *secondary lesions*, or "pintids," manifest months after inoculation as small, erythematous, scaly papules that coalesce to form psoriasiform plaques. Both primary and secondary lesions are highly infectious. In the tertiary stage, hypopigmented macules are present over bony prominences such as wrists, ankles, and elbows. Symmetric areas of achromia alternating with areas of normal or hyperpigmented skin may result in a mottled appearance. Atrophy and/or hyperkeratosis may be present. The tertiary lesions are not considered to be infectious. Skin lesions are often accompanied by regional lymphadenopathy (77). An attenuated variant is not described.

Histopathology. *Primary* and *secondary* lesions show a similar morphology—namely, acanthosis with spongiosis and a sparse dermal infiltrate of lymphocytes, plasma cells, and neutrophils disposed about dilated blood vessels (78). Endothelial swelling in the dermal vasculature is inconspicuous (79). Lichenoid inflammation may be present, accompanied by hyperkeratosis, hypergranulosis, basal layer vacuolopathy, and pigmentary incontinence. Increased numbers of Langerhans cells are present in the epidermis (80). Lesions of the *tertiary stage* are hyperpigmented, characterized by a large number of melanophages within the dermis, or depigmented, manifesting complete absence of epidermal melanin. Both lesions show epidermal atrophy and perivascular lymphocytic infiltrates. Organisms are present in all but late, long-standing lesions (69).

Histogenesis. Electron microscopy reveals absent melanocytes in depigmented lesions of tertiary or late pinta (80).

Endemic Syphilis (Bejel)

Clinical Summary. Primary-stage skin lesions are rare and are characterized by erythematous papules or ulcers of the oropharyngeal mucosa or the skin of the nipple of an uninfected mother nursing an infected infant. Unlike yaws, endemic syphilis, caused by *T. pallidum* subsp. *endemicum*, is largely confined to the arid climates of the Arabian Peninsula and the southern border of the Sahara Desert (76), whose seminomadic populations term the disease "bejel." Children 2 to 15 years of age constitute the principal reservoir. Although the mode of infection has not been extensively studied, it is thought that infection occurs by skin-to-skin contact or by means of fomites such as communal pipes or drinking vessels (69).

Primary-stage skin lesions are rare and are characterized by erythematous papules or ulcers of the oropharyngeal mucosa or the skin of the nipple of an uninfected mother nursing an infected infant.

More commonly, the initial manifestation is the presence of *secondary-stage* lesions, characteristically multiple, shallow, rather painless ulcers involving lips, buccal mucosa, tongue, fauces, or tonsils. Such lesions may be accompanied by hoarseness owing to treponemal laryngitis and/or regional lymphadenopathy. Condylomata lata involving the axillae and anogenital regions are also observed. Rarely, the secondary stage manifests as erythematous, crusted papules, macules, or an annular papulosquamous eruption, which may be accompanied by generalized lymphadenopathy or periostitis.

The *tertiary stage* comprises gummatous lesions of the nasopharynx, larynx, skin, and bone, which may progress to ulcers that heal as depigmented, sometimes geographic, scars with peripheral hyperpigmentation. Bone and joint involvement may manifest as tibial periostitis, which mimics that of yaws, or as mutilating lesions involving the nasal septum and palate. Ophthalmologic involvement comprises uveitis, chorioretinitis, choroiditis, and optic atrophy; *T. pallidum* has been cultured from intraocular fluid.

Histopathology. Although the pathology of early lesions of endemic syphilis is not well characterized, late lesions are said to show parakeratosis, acanthosis, spongiosis, pigmentary incontinence, and a dermal lymphohistiocytic and plasma cell infiltrate. Blood vessels demonstrate limited or no endothelial proliferation (69).

Lyme Disease

Clinical Summary. First described in patients from Lyme, Connecticut, in 1975 (81), Lyme disease, transmitted by *Ixodes* ticks, is a systemic spirochetosis caused by *Borrelia burgdorferi* sensu stricto, *B. afzelii*, *B. garinii*, and, in some cases in Europe, by *B. lusitaniae*, *B. bissettii,* and *B. spielmanii* (82). Mice, rabbits, and lizards serve as principal reservoirs in the United States, with the other animals including birds serving this role in Europe. Anywhere from 10% to 70% of *Ixodes* ticks in endemic areas carry the spirochete (82). Although the disease in the index cases manifested as inflammatory arthritis and central nervous system and cardiac symptoms (83) preceded by cutaneous erythema, manifestations may be protean and perplexing to the clinician. Lyme disease is the most common vector-borne disease in the United States, with roughly 20,000 new cases in 2005 (84). The incidence and geographic distribution of Lyme disease is increasing owing to human travel habits and changing habitats of the vector (85), which may partly be explained by climate change (82). Males are predominantly affected, with a bimodal age peak: children aged 5 to 14 years and adults aged 60 to 65 years; most cases occur between June and August (84). Recurrences after appropriate antimicrobial therapy have been reported; it appears that most represent second tick bite inoculations as opposed to relapses (86).

Although the tick *Ixodes dammini* is the prototypic vector (87), other species of ticks from the genus *Ixodes* can also be infected—namely, *I. ricinus* (88), *I. pacificus*, and *I. scapularis* (89–91). Lyme disease has been reported in 43 states, Europe, Canada, Africa, and Asia (89). Infection by multiple different bacterial species transmitted by the same infected tick may occur. Coinfection of ticks and of humans by *Ehrlichia chaffeensis*, the etiologic agent of human granulocytic ehrlichiosis, and by *B. burgdorferi* is demonstrable in areas where the two diseases are endemic (92–96). Babesiosis is another tick-borne infection that can be coexpressed with Lyme disease (94,97). Although it seems counterintuitive, one model suggests that certain animals, such as the lizard *Eumeces fasciatus* (the five-lined skink), can act as dilutional hosts, whereby reservoir incompetence can act to reduce vector infection prevalence and the associated risk of human infection (98).

There are three phases of Lyme disease. In stage I of the disease, hematogenous dissemination from lesions of erythema chronicum migrans to other organs may occur, the effects of which are usually self-limited (99) and include orchitis, splenomegaly, lymphadenopathy, and mild pneumonitis. The two main systems involved in stage II are neural and cardiac (99). The triad of meningitis, cranial neuritis, and radiculoneuritis is characteristic for neural involvement (100); Lyme cerebritis may also occur, and alteration of mental status may be the only initial clinical manifestation (101). Cardiac involvement manifests mainly as tachycardia and heart blocks, the basis of which is epi- and transmyocarditis. A biopsy of myocardium may show interstitial lymphoplasmacellular infiltrates, with a bandlike endocardial disposition said to be characteristic. A nonneutrophilic myocardial vasculitis has been described. Chronic disease at organ sites where spirochetes persist, most commonly the skin and nervous system in Europe and the musculoskeletal system in North America, constitutes stage III. Lyme arthritis and synovitis are characterized by a migratory oligoarthritis usually involving the knee joint, with the shoulder, wrist, temporomandibular, and ankle joints involved in some cases. Rarely reported is the involvement of other sites such as metatarsal heads with edema and soft tissue swelling (102).

Erythema Chronicum Migrans

Clinical Summary. Erythema chronicum migrans (89) is the distinctive, albeit not pathognomonic, gyrate erythema that manifests at the site of a primary tick inoculation (103) and appears to occur in roughly half of the cases of Lyme disease only (84). In the absence of a rash, the diagnosis depends on the demonstration of an antibody response to *B. burgdorferi* in an appropriate clinical setting (104). Unfortunately, patients who are immunosuppressed, such as those with underlying lymphoproliferative diseases, may never mount a detectable antibody response (105). Patients are frequently unaware of the often-painless tick bite (106). The lesion starts as an area of scaly erythema or a distinct red papule within 3 to 30 days after the tick bite, before spreading centrifugally with central clearing after a few weeks, occasionally reaching a diameter of 25 cm (107). The clinical presentation may be atypical by virtue of purpuric, vesicular, or linear lesions. The average lesional duration is 10 weeks in the European variant and 4 weeks in the American variant; in some cases, the lesions persist for as long as 12 months. Females are affected more frequently in the European variant than in the American variant. The lesions may be solitary or multiple, the latter reflecting hematogenous dissemination of the spirochete, which may be accompanied by fever, fatigue, headaches, cough, and arthralgias. Distinguishing erythema migrans from the rash of Southern tick-associated rash illness (STARI), or Masters disease, vectored by the lone star tick, is challenging (108,109).

Histopathology. An intense superficial and deep angiocentric, neurotropic, and eccrinotropic infiltrate predominated by lymphocytes with a variable admixture of plasma cells and eosinophils is the principal histopathology (Fig. 22-9). Plasma cells have been identified most frequently in the peripheries of lesions of erythema chronicum migrans, whereas eosinophils are identified in the centers of the lesions (110). Not infrequently, these florid dermal alterations are accompanied by eczematous epithelial alterations or an interface injury pattern (103), and some cases exhibit edema of blood vessels with transmural

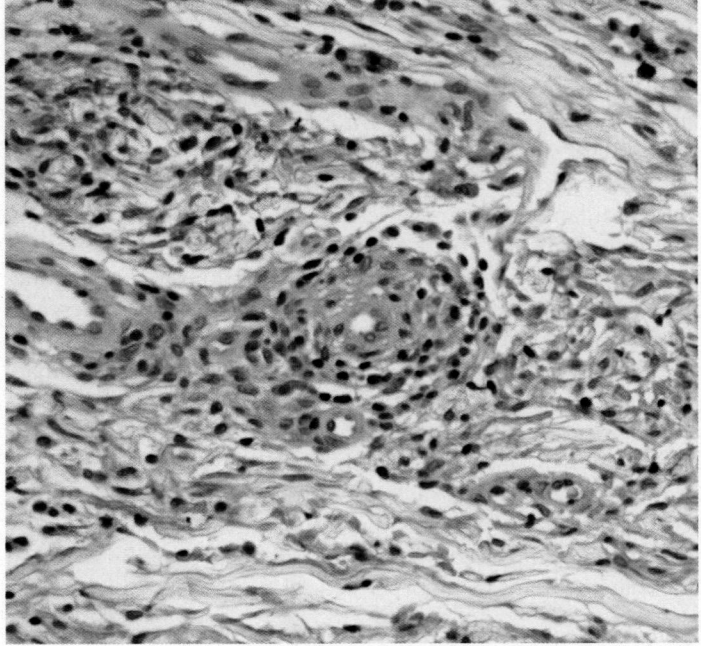

Figure 22-9 Erythema chronicum migrans. The central nidus at the inoculation site demonstrates a necrotizing granulomatous vasculitis, whereas the periphery is predominated by an angiocentric lymphohistiocytic vasculopathy, shown here.

migration of lymphocytes, histiocytes and occasionally plasma cells (Fig. 22-9), granulomatous neuritis or vasculitis with luminal thrombosis (personal observation), and interstitial infiltration of the reticular dermis with a concomitant incipient sclerosing reaction. Interstitial granulomatous dermatitis mimicking granuloma annulare has been reported (111). A Warthin–Starry stain may be positive; one study demonstrated spirochetes by this technique in 41% of the cases, with approximately one to two spirochetes, measuring 10 to 25 µm by 0.2 to 0.3 µm, per section (110). Spirochetes have been identified primarily from the advancing border of the lesion. There are a few labs that have developed Lyme disease immunohistochemistry; however, the treponemal immunostains also cross-react with *Borrelia* infection (112,113).

Differential Diagnosis. The differential diagnosis includes causes of delayed hypersensitivity in which potential antigenic stimuli include other forms of arthropod assaults, drugs, and contactants. A similar distribution of the dermal infiltrate is observed in connective tissue diseases; however, the presence of tissue eosinophilia along with concomitant eczematous changes is not a feature of the latter. Differentiation from erythema annulare centrifugum may be impossible.

Dermal Atrophying and Sclerosing Lesions as Manifestations of Lyme Disease: Acrodermatitis Chronica Atrophicans

Clinical Summary. First described in 1883 in Germany and subsequently named by Herxheimer in 1902 (114), acrodermatitis chronica atrophicans usually begins as a diffuse or localized erythema on one extremity with the underlying dermis having a doughy consistency. After several months, the lesions become atrophic. The skin is frequently so thin that vessels and the subcutaneous tissue can be easily visualized (115). Appendageal structures disappear, resulting in hair loss and decreased sweat and sebum production. The lesions are located mainly on the upper and lower extremities, frequently around joints, and spare the palms, soles, face, and trunk (115). Sclerosis may predominate in late-stage lesions and take several distinct forms: pseudosclerodermatous plaques over the dorsa of the feet; dense, fibrotic linear bands over ulnar and tibial areas; or localized fibromas overlying joint surfaces (114). Antibodies against *B. burgdorferi* are present in 100% of cases. Patients frequently have an elevated erythrocyte sedimentation rate and hypergammaglobulinemia. Either at the peripheries of lesions or distant from them, anetoderma, lymphocytoma, and morphea have also been described (115).

Histopathology. Within a few months to a year, the epidermis appears atrophic with loss of the rete ridges. There is granular layer diminution, and the epidermis is surmounted by a hyperkeratotic scale. In one study, a sparse interface dermatitis characterized by lymphocyte tagging along the dermal–epidermal junction, as well as basal layer cytolysis, was seen in 41% of cases (Fig. 22-10) (116), resulting in variable postinflammatory pigmentary alterations ranging from leukoderma to hyperpigmentation (114). The papillary dermis appears edematous, with a Grenz zone of collagen fibers oriented parallel to the epidermis ranging from a few strands to a wide zone (117), with subsequent eosinophilic homogenization. A bandlike lymphocytic infiltrate is found in the mid- and upper dermis and, in some cases, may produce a lichenoid morphology, obscuring the dermal–epidermal junction. Occasionally, it extends throughout the cutis and subcutis (116). The infiltrate is predominantly in an

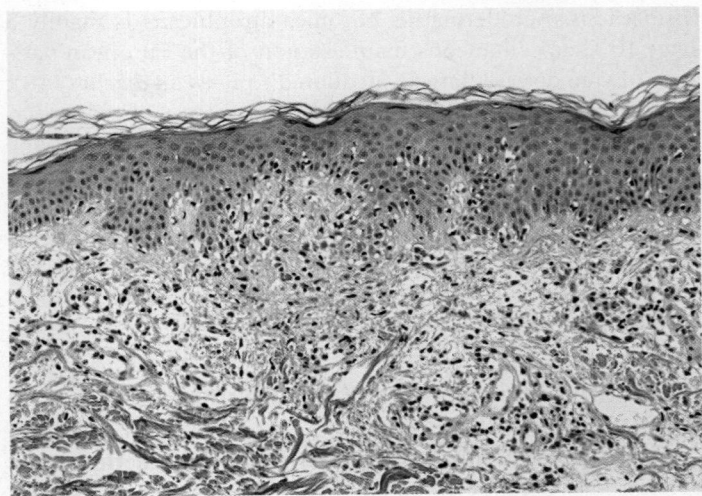

Figure 22-10 Acrodermatitis chronica atrophicans. The epidermis shows basket-weave orthokeratosis with a sparse interface dermatitis with lymphocyte tagging along the dermal–epidermal junction. The papillary dermis is edematous and the reticular dermal collagen fibers exhibit an orientation parallel to the epidermis. A concomitant interstitial lymphohistiocytic infiltrate is found in intimate apposition to the attenuated collagen fibers. This is an incipient or evolving lesion; atrophy follows with loss of the retiform pattern.

angiocentric, eccrinotropic, and folliculotropic disposition and comprises mainly lymphocytes and histiocytes with scattered eosinophils, neutrophils, and plasma cells. The vessels amid the superficial infiltrate appear destroyed (116). Within the infiltrate, there is piecemeal fragmentation of collagen and elastic tissue is lacking. Beneath the infiltrate, disorganization and destruction of the collagen, along with hyperplasia, fragmentation, and basophilia of the elastic fibers, are observed. An end-stage lesion exhibits a characteristic constellation of epidermal atrophy, large dilated dermal vessels, and an attenuated dermis composed of damaged and degenerated collagen and elastic fibers with fatty atrophy (lipoid phanerosis). The collagen may appear homogenized and hypereosinophilic and may resemble morphea (Fig. 22-11). There is ultimately marked atrophy of adnexa with periadnexal fibrosis.

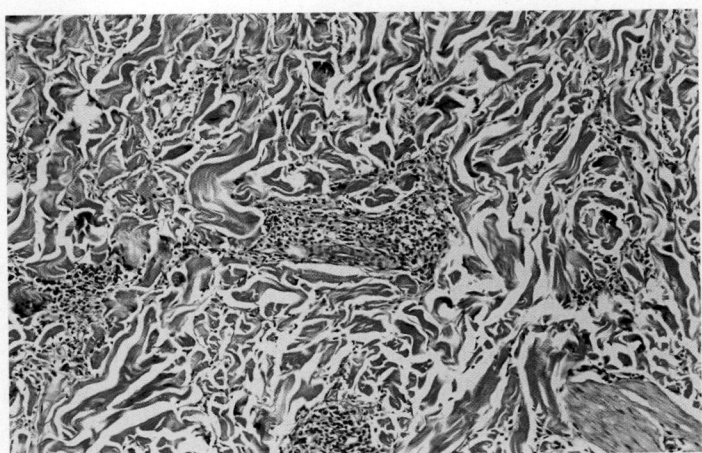

Figure 22-11 *Borrelia burgdorferi*-associated morphea. The dermis exhibits a sclerodermoid tissue reaction characterized by widened hypereosinophilic collagen fibers with loss of the normal fibrillar architecture and an interstitial lymphohistiocytic infiltrate in close apposition to the altered collagen fibers. Special stains reveal spirochetal forms amid the inflammatory infiltrate.

Histogenesis. Acrodermatitis chronica atrophicans is mainly a stage III (late) cutaneous manifestation of the European variant of Lyme disease, largely attributed to *Borrelia afzelii* (118); the major vector is *I. ricinus* (114) and, hence, the distribution of the lesion is worldwide, with Middle Europe being the epicenter. Most North American cases occur in European immigrants; *I. ricinus* is not indigenous to North America (114). Immunophenotyping reveals that most of the lymphocytes are of T-cell phenotype and that the elastic fibers express HLA-DR (116), suggesting a role for cell-mediated immunity in lesional development.

Other Atrophying and Sclerosing Disorders Associated with Lyme Disease

Clinical Summary. Atrophoderma of Pasini and Pierini, facial hemiatrophy of Parry–Romberg, lichen sclerosus et atrophicus, eosinophilic fasciitis, and morphea (Fig. 22-11) are among the atrophying and sclerosing disorders of connective tissue that have been associated with *B. burgdorferi* infection based on the positive serology for *B. burgdorferi* in patients with these conditions, the isolation of spirochetal organisms in cultures of the respective skin lesions, and/or their identification in histologic sections (89,90,117,119). In addition, acrodermatitis chronica atrophicans and morphea may coexist in the same patient. A possible etiologic basis of the sclerosis in all five entities—either as the inciting event (in morphea and eosinophilic fasciitis) or as an end-stage phenomenon (in atrophoderma, facial hemiatrophy, and lichen sclerosus)—may relate to increased production of interleukin 1 mediated by the *B. burgdorferi* spirochete, resulting in enhanced fibroblast production. Only progressive facial hemiatrophy will be considered further; all of the conditions are covered elsewhere in this book (see Chapter 10).

Facial hemiatrophy is an apposite term for an atrophying condition of the skin, subcutaneous fat, muscle, and bone involving either one division of the trigeminal nerve or half of the face. Occasionally, the entire ipsilateral side of the body may be affected, or the atrophy may first manifest on the trunk or extremities.

Histopathology. A sclerodermoid tissue reaction mimicking morphea is observed, including the presence of adnexal atrophy and subcutaneous fibrosis. The muscles are atrophic, with loss of striations, edema, and vacuolation. Ocular and neurologic complications including iritis, keratitis, optic nerve atrophy, trigeminal neuralgia, and facial palsy may occur (89).

Principles of Management: The mainstay of therapy remains doxycycline, amoxicillin, cefuroxime, or ceftriaxone (120). When neuroborreliosis supervenes, doxycycline is less likely to be used and alternative antibiotics gain prominence (120).

Borrelial Lymphocytoma Cutis

Clinical Summary. Lymphocytoma cutis is a benign cutaneous lymphoid hyperplasia first described by Spiegler before the end of the 19th century and subsequently named lymphocytoma cutis in 1921 by Kaufmann-Wolff. Various triggering factors have been isolated, such as drugs, contactants, and infections, suggesting that an excessive immune response to antigen may be its etiologic basis. The *B. burgdorferi* spirochete transmitted by *I. ricinus* has been implicated among the infectious agents. Evidence supportive of a spirochetal etiology of some cases of lymphocytoma cutis includes the identification of spirochete-like structures in mercury- and silver-stained sections of skin biopsies from patients with lymphocytoma cutis in whom increased serum titers of antibodies against *Borrelia* spirochetes are observed (121). The term *borrelioma* has been coined to describe such lesions. Lymphocytoma cutis in association with *B. burgdorferi* infection has the same clinical appearance as lesions arising in other settings—namely, as isolated or multiple violaceous, firm nodules and infiltrative plaques (89). Sites of predilection for the solitary lesions are the earlobes, nipples, and genital area. It is hypothesized that these sites may reflect a predilection for areas of lower body temperature, where disseminated *Borrelia* prefer to remain (122,123).

Lesions of lymphocytoma cutis may occur at sites of erythema chronicum migrans or in patients with stage II Lyme disease. Jessner lymphocytic infiltrate of skin is considered by some authors to be a form of lymphocytoma cutis and was reported in one patient whose biopsy showed spirochetes (89).

Histopathology. Skin biopsies show a polyclonal lymphocytic infiltrate involving the dermis and subcutis, with a predominance of CD20-positive B cells (124). There are often superficial and deep angiocentric, neurotropic, and eccrinotropic lymphocytic infiltrates, often accompanied by plasma cells and eosinophils, the former at the periphery and the latter in the center of lesions (110). The dermal alterations may be accompanied by epidermal spongiosis, and some cases show edema of blood vessels, transmural migration of lymphocytes and plasma cells, granulomatous vasculitis with luminal thrombosis, lymphohistiocytic neuritis, and interstitial reticular dermal infiltrates with a sclerosing reaction. Germinal centers may be observed (123). A florid inflammatory cell infiltrate with granulomatous vasculitis and neuritis is seen at the tick bite punctum, whereas a biopsy taken within 1 cm of the edge shows a pauci-inflammatory process with only sparse mononuclear cells, no eosinophils or plasma cells, and a vasculopathy comprising endothelial swelling, hyperplasia and mural edema accompanied by mucinosis (125). Biopsies taken between the center and edge show superficial and deep perivascular lymphocytic, plasmacellular, and eosinophilic infiltrates with variable eczematous alterations. Although spirochetes have been identified in the lesional border in only 40% of cases (110), most patients manifest elevated immunoglobulin M antibody titers (90), and one therefore relies heavily on serology to make the diagnosis. Others hold that the diagnosis at this stage is largely a clinical one owing to the incidence of false-positive and false-negative results (126); the sensitivity and specificity of confirmatory molecular tests are not optimal, and the culture is insensitive (127). The background high seropositivity rates in healthy patients in endemic and nonendemic areas have prompted a two-tiered approach through which seropositive patients undergo a subsequent and more specific Western blot analysis (128,129). Meta-analysis of molecular methods shows that assays of skin and synovial fluid have the highest sensitivities and specificities; plasma and CSF assays are less accurate (127). Quantitative PCR of erythema chronicum migrans lesions shows positivity in up to 80% of cases, with the mean number of spirochetes in a 2-mm biopsy specimen ranging from 10 to 11,000; larger numbers of spirochetes correlate with smaller lesions and a shorter duration of skin symptomatology (130). Molecular tests for Lyme disease should be reserved as confirmatory tools for cases in which the index of suspicion is high (127,131).

Alpha-Gal Syndrome

A recently recognized complication of a bite from the Lone Star tick is termed the alpha-gal syndrome, characterized by an allergic reaction as a late sequela of inoculation by the tick proboscis of a sugar molecule termed alpha-gal into the skin. This sugar molecule prompts an immunologic reaction in a susceptible individual, whereby an allergic reaction ranging from mild symptomatology to a potentially life-threatening anaphylactic response occurs following the ingestion of red meats such as beef, lamb, or pork. The culprit ticks include the Lone Star tick *Amblyomma americanum* and the American dog tick *Dermacentor variabilis* but not the other common tick species found in the American Southwest (132) whose mouthparts appear to lack the sugar moiety that provokes the immunologic response.

Differential Diagnosis. The clinical differential diagnosis encompasses other forms of annular erythema (133). Other causes of lymphocytoma cutis should be considered, such as drug therapy (134) or other infections (e.g., herpetic or mycobacterial). Well-differentiated lymphocytic lymphoma and chronic lymphocytic leukemia (CLL) should be excluded because both may mimic the diffuse type of lymphocytoma cutis; as the immune response mounted to the spirochetes in patients with underlying CLL comprises CD5/CD20$^+$ lymphocytes, the phenotype and histology may mimic cutaneous marginal zone B-cell leukemia (135). When eosinophils and plasma cells are present and when there are germinal centers, the distinction from other forms of lymphoma is less challenging.

Other arthropod assaults, drug hypersensitivity, contact reactions, and connective tissue diseases such as lupus erythematosus, scleroderma, morphea, Sjögren syndrome, mixed connective tissue disease, and relapsing polychondritis can mimic Lyme disease. Tissue eosinophilia and epidermal changes help to discriminate Lyme disease from connective tissue disease, but differentiation from erythema annulare centrifugum is more problematic. Tissue necrosis at the primary inoculation site of Lyme disease can mimic a brown recluse spider bite (136).

Histogenesis. Most ticks become infected with *B. burgdorferi* by feeding on small animals such as the white-footed mouse. *B. burgdorferi* is a long, narrow spirochete with flagella (137). It has at least 30 different proteins, including two major outer-surface proteins—Osp A and Osp B—which elicit antibody responses late in the course of the disease (137). It has been suggested that phagocytosis of the spirochete by macrophages leads to two different mechanisms of degradation: a phagolysosomal process—which may lead to major histocompatibility complex (MHC) class II-restricted antigen processing—and cytosolic degradation, which leads to MHC class I-restricted antigen presentation. This disparity may in part explain the variable immunologic aspects of Lyme disease (138).

Principles of Management: Antibiotic therapy, in particular, oral doxycycline, is the mainstay of treatment, although other first-line antibiotics include amoxicillin and cefuroxime axetil (139).

REFERENCES

1. Hook EW, Marra CM. Acquired syphilis in adults. *N Engl J Med.* 1992;326:1060.
2. Stamm LV, Greene SR, Bergen HL, Hardham JM, Barnes NY. Identification and sequence analysis of *Treponema pallidum tprJ*, a member of a polymorphic multigene family. *FEMS Microbiol Lett.* 1998;169:155.
3. Centurion-Lara A, Castro C, Castillo R, Shaffer JM, Van Voorhis WC, Lukehart SA. The flanking region sequence of the 15kDa lipoprotein gene differentiate pathogenic treponemes. *J Infect Dis.* 1998;177:1036.
4. Wicher K, Wicher V, Abbruscato F, Baughn RE. *Treponema pallidum* subsp. *pertenue* displays pathogenetic properties different from those of *T. pallidum* subsp. *pallidum*. *Infect Immunol.* 2000;68:3219.
5. Smajs D, Norris SJ, Weinstock GM. Genetic diversity in *Treponema pallidum*: implications for pathogenesis, evolution and molecular diagnostics of syphilis and yaws. *Infect Genet Evol.* 2012;12:191.
6. Centurion-Lara A, Godornes C, Castro C, Van Voorhis WC, Lukehart SA. The *tprK* gene is heterogeneous among *Treponema pallidum* strains and has multiple alleles. *Infect Immun.* 2000;68:824.
7. Hanicova K, Mukherjee P, Ogden G, et al. Multilocus sequence typing of *Borrelia Burgdorferi* suggests existence of lineages with differential pathogenic properties in humans. *PLoS One.* 2013;8:e73066.
8. Brissette CA, Simonson LG, Lukehart SA. Resistance to human beta-defensins is common among oral treponemes. *Oral Microbiol Immunol.* 2004;19:403.
9. Rôcas IN, Siqueira JR Jr. Occurrence of two newly named oral treponemes—*Treponema parvum* and *Treponema putidum*—in primary endodontic infections. *Oral Microbiol Immunol.* 2005;20:372.
10. Moter A, Riep B, Haban V, et al. Molecular epidemiology of oral treponemes in patients with periodontitis and in periodontitis-resistant subjects. *J Clin Microbiol.* 2006;44:3078.
11. Sparling PF. Natural history of syphilis. In: Homes KK, Mardh PA, Sparling PF, et al, eds. *Sexually Transmitted Diseases.* 2nd ed. McGraw-Hill; 1990:213.
12. World Health Organization. *WHO Guidelines for the Treatment of Treponema pallidum (Syphilis).* 2016. https://apps.who.int/iris/bitstream/handle/10665/249572/9789241549806-eng.pdf?sequence=1
13. O'Byrne P, MacPherson P. Syphilis. *BMJ.* 2019;365:l4159.
14. Centers for Disease Control and Prevention. 2017. Syphilis. https://www.cdc.gov/std/stats18/syphilis.htm
15. Centers for Disease Control and Prevention. 2017. Syphilis. https://www.cdc.gov/std/stats18/syphilis.htm#:~:text=The%20total%20number%20of%20reported,cases)%20(Table%201)
16. Centers for Disease Control and Prevention. 2018. Syphilis. https://www.cdc.gov/std/stats18/syphilis.htm
17. Kojima N, Klausner JD. An update on the global epidemiology of syphilis. *Curr Epidemiol Rep.* 2018;5(1):24–38.
18. Centurion-Lara A, Molini BJ, Godornes C, et al. Molecular differentiation of *Treponema pallidum* subspecies. *J Clin Microbiol.* 2006;44:3377.
19. Lafond RE, Lukehart SA. Biological basis for syphilis. *Clin Microbiol Rev.* 2006;19:29.
20. Noppakun N, Dinerart SM, Solomon AR. Pustular secondary syphilis. *Int J Dermatol.* 1987;26:112.
21. Stockli HR. Neurosyphilis heute. *Dermatologica.* 1982;165:232.
22. Moskovitz BL, Klimek JJ, Goldman RL, Fiumara NJ, Quintiliani R. Meningovascular syphilis after "appropriate" treatment of primary syphilis. *Arch Intern Med.* 1982;142:139.
23. Janier M, Pertuiset EF, Poisson M, et al. Manifestations précoces de la syphilis neuro-méningée. *Ann Dermatol Venereol (Stockholm).* 1985;112:133.
24. Tanabe JL, Huntley AC. Granulomatous tertiary syphilis. *J Am Acad Dermatol.* 1986;15:341.
25. Johnson PC, Farnie MA. Testing for syphilis. *Dermatol Clin.* 1994;12:9.
26. Sanchez PJ. Congenital syphilis. *Adv Pediatr Infect Dis.* 1992;7:161.
27. Guarner J, Greer PW, Bartlett J, et al. Congenital syphilis in a newborn: an immunopathologic study. *Mod Pathol.* 1999;12:82.

28. Jeerapaet P, Ackerman AS. Histologic patterns of secondary syphilis. *Arch Dermatol*. 1973;107:373.

29. Hoang MP, High WA, Molberg KH. Secondary syphilis: a histologic and immunohistochemical evaluation. *J Cutan Pathol*. 2004;31(9):595–599.

30. Jafari Y, Peeling RW, Shivkumar S, Claessens C, Joseph L, Pai NP. Are *Treponema pallidum* specific rapid and point-of-care tests for syphilis accurate enough for screening in resource limited settings? Evidence from a meta-analysis. *PLoS One*. 2013;8:e54695.

31. Hartsock RJ, Halling LW, King FM. Luetic lymphadenitis. *Am J Clin Pathol*. 1970;53:304.

32. Yobs AR, Brown L, Hunter EF. Fluorescent antibody technique in early syphilis. *Arch Pathol*. 1964;77:220.

33. Beckett JR, Bigbee JW. Immunoperoxidase localization of *Treponema pallidum*. *Arch Pathol*. 1979;103:135.

34. Metz J, Metz G. Elektronenmikroskopischer nachweis von *Treponema pallidum* in hauteffloreszenzen der unbehandelten lues I und II. *Arch Dermatol Forsch*. 1972;243:241.

35. Sykes JA, Miller JN, Kalan AJ. *Treponema pallidum* within cells of a primary chancre from a human female. *Br J Vener Dis*. 1974;50:40.

36. Wecke J, Bartunek J, Stuttgen G. *Treponema pallidum* in early syphilitic lesions in humans during high-dosage penicillin therapy: an electron microscopical study. *Arch Dermatol Res*. 1976;257:1.

37. Poulsen A, Kobayasi T, Secher L, Weismann K. *Treponema pallidum* in macular and papular secondary syphilis skin eruptions. *Acta Dermatol Venereol (Stockholm)*. 1986;66:251.

38. Azar RH, Pham TD, Kurban AK. An electron microscopic study of a syphilitic chancre. *Arch Pathol*. 1970;90:143.

39. Poulsen A, Kobayasi T, Secher L, Weismann K. The ultrastructure of *Treponema pallidum* isolated from human chancres. *Acta Dermatol Venereol (Stockholm)*. 1985;65:367.

40. Klingmuller G, Ishibashi Y, Radke K. Der elektronenmikroskopische Aufbau des *Treponema pallidum*. *Arch Klin Exp Dermatol*. 1968;233:197.

41. Magro CM, Crowson AN, Alfa M, et al. A comparative histomorphological analysis of chancroid in seronegative and HIV positive African patients. *Hum Pathol*. 1996;27:1066.

42. Abell E, Marks R, Wilson JE. Secondary syphilis. A clinicopathological review. *Br J Dermatol*. 1975;93:53.

43. Cochran RIE, Thomson J, Fleming KA, Strong AM. Histology simulating reticulosis in secondary syphilis. *Br J Dermatol*. 1976;95:251.

44. Kahn LE, Gordon W. Sarcoid-like granulomas in secondary syphilis. *Arch Pathol*. 1971;92:334.

45. Fisher DA, Chang LW, Tuffanelli DL. Lues maligna. *Arch Dermatol*. 1979;99:70.

46. Degos R, Touraine R, Collart P, et al. Syphilis maligne précoce d'evolution mortelle (avec examen anatomique). *Bull Soc Fr Dermatol Syphiligr*. 1970;77:10.

47. Adam W, Korting GW. Lues maligna. *Arch Klin Exp Dermatol*. 1960;210:14.

48. Petrozzi JW, Lockshin NA, Berger RI. Malignant syphilis. *Arch Dermatol*. 1974;109:387.

49. Lawrence T, Saxe N. Bullous secondary syphilis. *Clin Exp Dermatol*. 1992;17:44.

50. Kerdel-Vegas F, Kopf AW, Tolmach JA. Keratoderma punctatum syphiliticum: report of a case. *Br J Dermatol*. 1954;66:449.

51. Lantis LR, Petrozzi JW, Hurley HJ. Sarcoid granuloma in secondary syphilis. *Arch Dermatol*. 1969;99:748.

52. Matsuda-John SS, McElgunn PST, Ellis CN. Nodular late syphilis. *J Am Acad Dermatol*. 1983;9:269.

53. Longstreth P, Hoke AQ, McElroy C. Hepatitis and bone destruction as uncommon manifestations of early syphilis. *Arch Dermatol*. 1976;112:1451.

54. Handoko ML, Duijvestein M, Scheepstra CG, de Fijter CW. Syphilis: a reversible cause of nephritic syndrome. *BMJ Case Rep*. 2013;8:2013.

55. Tourville DR, Byrd LR, Kim DU, et al. Treponemal antigen in immunopathogenesis of syphilitic glomerulonephritis. *Am J Pathol*. 1976;82:479.

56. Bansal RC, Cohn H, Fani K, Lynfield YL. Nephrotic syndrome and granulomatous hepatitis. *Arch Dermatol*. 1978;114:1228.

57. Magro CM, Crowson AN. The clinical and histological features of pityriasis rubra pilaris: a comparative analysis with psoriasis. *J Cutan Pathol*. 1997;24:416.

58. Magro CM, Morrison C, Kovatich A, Burns F. Pityriasis lichenoides is a cutaneous T-cell dyscrasia: a clinical, genotypic, and phenotypic study. *Hum Pathol*. 2002;33:788.

59. Luxon LM. Neurosyphilis (review). *Int J Dermatol*. 1980;19:310.

60. Centers for Disease Control and Prevention. Sexually Transmitted Infections Treatment Guidelines, 2021: Syphilis. 2021. https://www.cdc.gov/std/treatment-guidelines/syphilis.htm

61. Noordhoek GT, Hermans PWM, Paul AN, Schouls LM, van der Sluis JJ, van Embden JD. *Treponema pallidum* subspecies *pallidum* (Nichols) and *Treponema pallidum* subspecies *pertenue* (CDC 2575) differ in at least one nucleotide: comparison of two homologous antigens. *Microb Pathog*. 1989;6:29.

62. Kazadi WM, Asiedu KB, Agana N, Mitjà O. Epidemiology of yaws: an update. *Clin Epidemiol*. 2014;6:119–128.

63. World Health Organization. *Yaws*. 2019. https://www.who.int/news-room/fact-sheets/detail/yaws

64. Engelkens HJH, Judanarso J, Oranje AP, et al. Endemic treponematoses: part 1. Yaws. *Int J Dermatol*. 1992;30:77.

65. Agmon-Levin N, Bat-sheva PK, Barzilai O, et al. Antitreponemal antibodies leading to autoantibody production and protection from atherosclerosis in Kitavans from Papua New Guinea. *Ann N Y Acad Sci*. 2009;1173:675.

66. World Health Organization. *Yaws Eradication*. 2012. https://www.ncbi.nlm.nih.gov/pmc/articles/PMC3979691/

67. Antal GM, Lukehart SA, Meheus AZ. The endemic treponematoses. *Microbes Infect*. 2002;4:83.

68. Fegan D, Glennon MJ, Thami Y, Pakoa G. Resurgence of yaws in Tannu, Vanuatu: time for a new approach? *Trop Doct*. 2010;40:68.

69. Giacani L, Lukehart SA. The endemic treponematoses. *Clin Microbiol Rev*. 2014;27(1):89–115.

70. Marks M, Lebari D, Solomon AW, Higgins SP. Yaws. *Int J STD AIDS*. 2015;26(10):696–703.

71. Hasselmann CM. Comparative studies on the histopathology of syphilis, yaws and pinta. *Br J Vener Dis*. 1957;33:5.

72. Greene CA, Harman RRM. Yaws truly: a survey of patients indexed under "Yaws" and a review of the clinical and laboratory problems of diagnosis. *Clin Exp Dermatol*. 1986;11:41.

73. Mitja O, Bassat Q. Developments in therapy and diagnosis of yaws and future prospects. *Expert Rev Anti Infect Ther*. 2013;11(10):1115–1121.

74. Mitja O, Hays R, Ipai A, et al. Single-dose azithromycin versus benzathine benzylpenicillin for treatment of yaws in children in Papua New Guinea: an open-label, non-inferiority, randomized trial. *Lancet*. 2012;379:342.

75. Mitja O, Hays R, Ipai A, et al. Outcome predictors in treatment of yaws. *Emerg Infect Dis*. 2011;17:1083.

76. Engelkens HJH, Niemel PLA, van der Sluis JL, Meheus A, Stolz E. Endemic treponematoses: part II. Pinta and endemic syphilis. *Int J Dermatol*. 1991;30:231.

77. Hook EW III. Endemic treponematoses. In: Bennett JE. Dolan R, Blaser MJ, eds. *Mandell, Douglas, and Bennett's Principles and Practice of Infectious Diseases*. 8th ed. W.B. Saunders; 2015:2710–2713.

78. Pardo-Castello V, Pinta FI. *Arch Dermatol Syph*. 1942;45:843.

79. Hasselmann CM. Studien uber die histopathologie von pinta, frambosie und syphilis. *Arch Klin Exp Dermatol*. 1955;201:1.

80. Rodriguez HA, Albores-Saavedra J, Lozano MM, Smith M, Feder W. Langerhans' cells in late pinta. *Arch Pathol.* 1971;91:302.

81. Steere AC, Grodzicki RL, Kornblatt AN, et al. The spirochetal etiology of Lyme disease. *N Engl J Med.* 1983;308:733.

82. Bhate C, Schwartz RA. Lyme disease. Part 1: advances and perspectives. *J Am Acad Dermatol.* 2011;64:619.

83. Steere AC, Malawista SE, Snydman DR, et al. Lyme arthritis: an epidemic of oligoarticular arthritis in children and adults in three Connecticut communities. *Arthritis Rheum.* 1977;20:7.

84. Kudish K, Sleavin W, Hathcock L. Lyme disease trends: Delaware, 2000–2004. *Del Med J.* 2007;79:51.

85. Vasuvedan B, Chatterjee M. Lyme borreliosis and the skin. *Indian J Dermatol.* 2013;58:167.

86. Krause PJ, Foley DT, Burke GS, et al. Reinfection and relapse in early Lyme disease. *Am J Trop Med Hyg.* 2006;75:1090.

87. Benach JL, Bosler EM, Hanrahan JP, et al. Spirochetes isolated from the blood of two patients with Lyme disease. *N Engl J Med.* 1983;308:740.

88. Barbour AB, Tessier SL, Todd WJ. Lyme disease spirochetes in Ixodid tick spirochetes share a common surface antigenic determinant defined by a monoclonal antibody. *Infect Immun.* 1983;41:795.

89. Abele DC, Anders KH. The many faces and phases of borreliosis. I: Lyme disease. *J Am Acad Dermatol.* 1990;23:167.

90. Asbrink E, Hovmark A. Cutaneous manifestations in *Ixodes*-borne *Borrelia* spirochetosis. *Int J Dermatol.* 1987;26:215.

91. Lebech AM. Polymerase chain reaction in diagnosis of *Borrelia burgdorferi* infections and studies on taxonomic classification. *APMIS Suppl.* 2002;105:1.

92. Christova I, Schouls L, van de Pol I, et al. High prevalence of granulocytic Ehrlichiae and *Borrelia burgdorferi sensu lato* in *Ixodes ricinus* ticks from Bulgaria. *J Clin Microbiol.* 2001;39:4172.

93. Cao WC, Zhao QM, Zhang PH, et al. Granulocytic Ehrlichiae in *Ixodes persulcatus* ticks from an areas in China where Lyme disease is endemic. *J Clin Microbiol.* 2000;38:4208.

94. Hilton E, deVoit J, Benach JL, et al. Seroprevalence and seroconversion for tick-borne diseases in a high-risk population in the northeast United States. *Am J Med.* 1999;106:404.

95. Bakken JS, Dumler JS. Human granulocytic ehrlichiosis. *Clin Infect Dis.* 2002;31:554.

96. Wormser GP, Horowitz HW, Nowakowski J, et al. Positive Lyme disease serology in patients with clinical and laboratory evidence of human granulocytic ehrlichiosis. *Am J Clin Pathol.* 1997;107:142.

97. Krause PJ, MacKay K, Thompson CA, et al. Disease-specific diagnosis of coinfecting tickborne zoonoses: babesiosis, human granulocytic ehrlichiosis, and Lyme disease. *Clin Infect Dis.* 2002;34:1184.

98. Giery ST, Ostfeld RS. The role of lizards in the ecology of Lyme disease in two endemic zones of the northeastern United States. *J Parasitol.* 2007;93:511.

99. Sigel LH, Curran AS. Lyme disease: a multifocal worldwide disease. *Ann Rev Public Health.* 1991;12:85.

100. Pachner AR, Steiner I. Lyme neuroborreliosis: infection, immunity, and inflammation. *Lancet Neurol.* 2007;6:544.

101. Chabria SB, Lawrason J. Altered mental status, an unusual manifestation of early disseminated Lyme disease: a case report. *J Med Case Rep.* 2007;1:62.

102. Endres S, Quante M. Oedema of the metatarsal heads II-IV and forefoot pain as an unusual manifestation of Lyme disease: a case report. *J Med Case Rep.* 2007;1:44.

103. Wilson TC, Legler A, Madison KC, Fairley JA, Swick BL. Erythema migrans: a spectrum of histopathologic changes. *Am J Dermatopathol.* 2012;34:834.

104. Gomes-Solecki MJ, Meirelles L, Glass J, Dattwyler RJ. Epitope length, genospecies dependency, and serum panel effect in the

IR6 enzyme-linked immunosorbent assay for detection of antibodies to *Borrelia burgdorferi. Clin Vaccine Immunol.* 2007;14:875.

105. Harrer T, Geissdörfer W, Schoerner C, Lang E, Helm G. Seronegative Lyme neuroborreliosis in a patient on treatment for chronic lymphatic leukemia. *Infection.* 2007;35:110.

106. Tibbles CD, Edlow JA. Does this patient have erythema migrans? *JAMA.* 2007;297:2617.

107. Cote J. Lyme disease. *Int J Dermatol.* 1991;30:500.

108. Blanton L, Keith B, Brzezinski W. Southern tick-associated rash illness: erythema migrans is not always Lyme disease. *South Med J.* 2008;101:759.

109. Masters EJ, Grigery CH, Masters RW. STARI, or Masters disease: lone star tick-vectored Lyme-like illness. *Infect Dis Clin North Am.* 2008;22:361.

110. Berger BW. Erythema chronicum migrans of Lyme disease. *Arch Dermatol.* 1984;120:1017.

111. Eisendle K, Zelger B. The expanding spectrum of cutaneous borreliosis. *G Ital Dermatol Venereol.* 2009;144:157.

112. Oliai BR. Immunohistochemistry in the diagnosis of Lyme disease. *The Focus-Immunohistochemistry.* 2007 July. http://www.ihcworld.com/_newsletter/2007/2007_07_lyme_disease_lowres.pdf

113. Neogenomics.com. *Spirochete | NeoGenomics Laboratories* [online]. 2021. Accessed April 21, 2021. https://neogenomics.com/test-menu/spirochete

114. Burgdorf WHS, Woret WI, Schultes O. Acrodermatitis chronica atrophicans. *Int J Dermatol.* 1979;18:595.

115. Kaufman L, Gruber BL, Phillips ME, Benach JL. Late cutaneous Lyme disease: acrodermatitis chronica atrophicans. *Am J Med.* 1989;86:828.

116. Aberer E, Klade H, Hobisch G. A clinical, histological, and immunohistochemical comparison of acrodermatitis chronica atrophicans and morphea. *Am J Dermatopathol.* 1991;13:334.

117. Aberer E, Klade H, Stanek G, Gebhart W. *Borrelia burgdorferi* and different types of morphea. *Dermatologica.* 1991;182:145.

118. Brandt FC, Ertas B, Falk TM, Metze D, Böer-Auer A. Histopathology and immunophenotype of acrodermatitis chronica atrophicans correlated with ospA and ospC genotypes of Borrelia species. *J Cutan Pathol.* 2015;42(10):674–692. doi: 10.1111/cup.12550

119. Aberer E, Stanek G, Ertl M, Neumann R. Evidence for spirochetal origin of circumscribed scleroderma (morphea). *Acta Dermatol Venereol (Stockholm).* 1987;67:225.

120. Bhate C, Schwartz RA. Lyme disease. Part II: management and prevention. *J Am Acad Dermatol.* 2011;64:639.

121. Hovmark A, Asbrink E, Olsson I. The spirochetal etiology of lymphadenosis benign cutis solitaria. *Acta Dermatol Venereol (Stockholm).* 1986;66:479.

122. Kandhari R, Kandhari S, Jain S. Borrelial lymphocytoma cutis: a diagnostic dilemma. *Indian J Dermatol.* 2014;59(6):595–597.

123. Colli C, Leinweber B, Müllegger R, Chott A, Kerl H, Cerroni L. Borrelia burgdorferi-associated lymphocytoma cutis: clinicopathologic, immunophenotypic, and molecular study of 106 cases. *J Cutan Pathol.* 2004;31(3):232–240.

124. Maraspin V, Klevišar MN, Ružić-Sabljić E, Lusa L, Strle F. Borrelial lymphocytoma in adult patients. *Clin Infect Dis.* 2016;63(7):914–921.

125. Shulman KJ, Melski JW, Reed KD, et al. The characteristic histologic features of erythema chronicum migrans [abstract]. *Lab Invest.* 1996;74:46A.

126. Edlow JA. Erythema migrans. *Med Clin North Am.* 2002;86:239.

127. Dumler JS. Molecular diagnosis of Lyme disease: review and meta-analysis. *Mol Diagn.* 2001;6:1.

128. Bunikis J, Barbour AG. Laboratory testing for suspected Lyme disease. *Med Clin North Am.* 2002;86:311.

129. Pinto DS. Cardiac manifestations of Lyme disease. *Med Clin North Am.* 2002;86:285.

130. Liveris D, Wang G, Girao G, et al. Quantitative detection of *Borrelia burgdorferi* in 2-millimeter skin samples of erythema

chronicum migrans lesions: correlation of results with clinical and laboratory findings. *J Clin Microbiol.* 2002;40:1249.

131. Huppertz HI, Bartmann P, Heinenger U, et al. Rational diagnostic strategies for Lyme borreliosis in children and adolescents: recommendations by the Committee for Infectious Diseases and Vaccinations of the German Academy for Pediatrics and Adolescent Health. *Eur J Pediatr.* 2012;171:1619.

132. Crispell G, Commins S, Archer-Hartman SA, et al. Discovery of alpha-gal-containing antigens in North American tick species believed to induce red meat allergy. *Front Immunol.* 2019;10:1056.

133. Grau RH, Allen PS, Cornelison RL Jr. Erythema migrans and the differential diagnosis of annular erythema. *J Okla State Med Assoc.* 2002;95:257.

134. Magro CM, Crowson AN. Drug-induced immune dysregulation as a cause of atypical cutaneous lymphoid infiltrates: a hypothesis. *Hum Pathol.* 1996;27:125.

135. Kash N, Fink-Puches R, Cerroni L. Cutaneous manifestations of B-cell chronic lymphocytic leukemia associated with *Borrellia burgdoferi* infection showing a marginal zone B-cell lymphoma-like infiltrate. *Am J Dermatopathol.* 2011;33:712.

136. Oosterhoudt KC, Zaoutis T, Zorc JJ. Lyme disease masquerading as brown recluse spider bite. *Ann Emerg Med.* 2002;39:558.

137. Jantausch BA. Lyme disease, Rocky Mountain spotted fever, ehrlichiosis: emerging and established challenges for the clinician. *Ann Allergy.* 1994;73:4.

138. Rittig MG, Haupl T, Krause A, Kressel M, Groscurth P, Burmester GR. *Borrelia burgdorferi*–induced ultrastructural alterations in human phagocytes: a clue to pathogenicity? *J Pathol.* 1994;173:269.

139. Mullegger RR, Glatz M. Skin manifestations of lyme borreliosis: diagnosis and management. *Am J Clin Dermatol.* 2008; 9:355.

Chapter 23

Fungal Diseases

MOLLY A. HINSHAW AND B. JACK LONGLEY

OVERVIEW

Fungi are eukaryotic protists that are distinguished from plants by their lack of chlorophyll (1). The Greek word *mycoses* means "fungus" and was first penned by R. Virchow in 1856 to describe infections by this group of organisms. In the past, bacterial infections, lymphoma, and other disorders have also been termed *mycoses* despite a lack of relation to fungi (2). Actinomycosis, botryomycosis, and erythrasma are examples of bacterial diseases that have historically been discussed with fungal diseases. These entities are covered in Chapter 21. Protothecosis is a cutaneous infection by algae of the genus *Prototheca* and will continue to be included in this chapter because there is no separate chapter for infections by algae.

The number of recognized fungal infections is growing as the number of diagnostic tests performed increases with increases in the worldwide population under medical care. Furthermore, with more atypical infections being identified in both immunocompetent and immunosuppressed patients and an increase in the availability of specific and sensitive molecular tests, the recognition of additional species of medically important fungi has accelerated and the nomenclature and classification of fungal species are in flux. For instance, a recent survey listed over 20 new and 15 revised fungal taxa identified from human clinical material during the two-year period from 2018 to 2019 alone (3). These include new species in well-known human-pathogenic fungal genera—such as *Alternaria*, *Aspergillus*, *Curvularia*, and *Fusarium*—and three new dermatophyte relatives, *Arthroderma chilionensis*, *Nannizzia perplicata*, and *Trichophyton indotineae*. In addition to standard techniques such as culture and histopathologic identification, molecular techniques including sequencing of 18S ribosomal RNA, restriction fragment length polymorphism (RFLP) analysis, polymerase chain reaction (PCR), and directed or global genome sequencing show great promise for more accurate classification and identification of fungi, including cryptic organisms. However, many of the currently reported studies use customized in-house assays, so their usefulness is hampered in part because they are biased by their choice of targets. Thus, some organisms may not be detected, and it is likely that nomenclature and classification may ultimately depend on whole-genome sequencing or other nonbiased techniques.

To combat unnecessary nomenclatural instability, groups established by the International Commission on the Taxonomy of Fungi (ICTF) and the Nomenclature Committee for Fungi (NCF) propose lists of retained (protected) and rejected names for key species/genera, with only definitive changes being ratified. For new names and classifications to be accepted, the International Code of Nomenclature for algae, fungi, and plants (ICN) requires that all such taxa are registered in recognized online repositories, such as MycoBank (http://www.mycobank.org/) and Index Fungorum (http://www.indexfungorum.org), both of which provide invaluable summaries of recent changes in nomenclature for fungi of medical importance. Regardless, novel fungal taxa and proposals to reassign or rename existing taxa are published continually in a wide range of scientific journals, and there is currently no single comprehensive source that clinicians, microbiologists, and mycologists can consult for all proposed nomenclatural changes. In this chapter, we will use common clinically recognized nomenclature. Many of the revised names have been widely adopted without further discussion. However, the acceptance of new names for common human pathogens may take time; so, when indicated, we will also include new and current names together.

Defining terminology in fungal diseases aids comprehension and diagnostic consistency (Table 23-1). *Hyphae* are elongated filamentous forms of fungi that usually form an intertwining mass called a *mycelium*. Septate hyphae give rise to arthrospores by asexual reproduction. Frequently, rounded, boxlike, or short cylindrical arthrospores can be identified. *Yeasts* are single-celled, usually rounded fungi that reproduce by budding (blastospore formation). Yeast cells and their progeny may adhere to one another and form chains or *pseudohyphae* that may also form mycelia; thus, they may be difficult to distinguish from true hyphae by light microscopy. *Dematiaceous fungi* are fungi that bear melanin-like pigments in their walls. *Tinea* is a clinical term that describes superficial fungal infections of the skin; it is usually modified with an anatomic or other term to describe the location or color of the infection. The *dermatophytes* are fungi that were originally classified by Sabouraud (2) and redefined by Emmons (4), including the three genera *Microsporum*, *Trichophyton*, and *Epidermophyton*. Therefore, *dermatophytosis* is not an appropriate histologic diagnostic term unless a definite assignment of an organism to one of these three genera of dermatophytes can be made. *Dermatomycosis* refers to any fungal infection of the skin and may be caused by dermatophytes, yeast, or other fungi, including those that do not usually cause cutaneous disease.

The primary cutaneous fungal pathogens can be separated into two groups: those that tend to cause superficial infections and those that cause deep infections. A third group of cutaneous fungal pathogens are those that usually cause systemic

Table 23-1
Terminology of Fungi

Term	Definition	Example
Dermatophyte	Imperfect fungi	*Trichophyton, Microsporum, Epidermophyton*
Dermatomycosis	Any fungal infection of the skin caused by dermatophytes, yeast, or other fungi, including those that do not usually cause disease	
Mold	Filamentous structural morphology of fungus	Dermatophytes, chromomycosis
Arthrospores	Asexual fungal spore formed by hyphal segmentation	Dermatophytes
Hyphae	Elongated filamentous forms of fungi	Dermatophytes
Mycelium	Intertwining mass of hyphae	
Yeast	Round-to-oval fungal forms that reproduce by budding or blastogenesis	*Candida, Cryptococcus, Malassezia*
Blastoconidia	Daughter cells of parent yeast	
Pseudohyphae	Chains of yeastlike cells that resemble hyphae	*Candida* spp.
Dematiaceous fungi	Mold or yeast with melanin pigment in their walls	Phaeohyphomycosis, chromomycosis
Sporangia	Spherule containing endospores	*Coccidioides immitis*
Sporangioblasts	Another term for endospores	*Rhinosporidium seeberi*
Grains	Dense accumulations (microcolonies) of fungi or bacteria	Eumycetoma
Tinea	Clinical term to describe superficial fungal infections of the skin	Faciei, cruris, pedis, manus
Dimorphic	Fungus that grows in more than one form (mold, yeast, sclerotic body, sulfur grains, spherules with endospores, etc.)	Histoplasmosis, coccidioidomycosis, blastomycosis, paracoccidioidomycosis

disease and only secondarily involve the skin. The basic pattern of cutaneous infection is relatively uniform within each of these three groups. The degree of inflammatory response to these three categories of fungal infection, however, varies based on a number of factors, particularly the host immune status. For example, infections with organisms causing superficial dermatomycoses, such as the dermatophytes, *Candida* spp., *Malassezia* (*Pityrosporum*) *furfur*, and *Cladosporium* (*Exophiala* or *Phaeoannellomyces*) *werneckii*, are generally characterized by hyphae or pseudohyphae and, sometimes, yeast cells in the keratin layer of the epidermis and in follicles. The variable intensity of the tissue reaction in the epidermis and follicular epithelium ranges from almost no response to a very mild focal spongiosis to a more exuberant or chronic spongiotic-psoriasiform pattern. Superficial fungal infections may provoke a superficial lymphocytic or a mixed dermal inflammatory infiltrate. Organisms causing superficial dermatomycosis are not found in the dermis except in the case of follicular rupture.

Deep cutaneous fungal infections typically show a mixed dermal inflammatory cell infiltrate that is often associated with pseudocarcinomatous hyperplasia and occasionally with dermal fibrosis. Primary cutaneous aspergillosis, chromomycosis, phaeohyphomycosis, eumycetoma, rhinosporidiosis, and lobomycosis are examples of fungi that infect the deeper cutaneous tissues.

Incidental cutaneous infections by fungi that usually primarily involve other organs, such as blastomycosis or coccidioidomycosis, typically show a pattern similar to that seen with the deep primary cutaneous fungi: a mixed dermal infiltrate with multinucleated giant cells associated with pseudoepitheliomatous hyperplasia. However, a few organisms such as *Histoplasma* and *Loboa loboi* are more likely to be associated with epidermal thinning than with hyperplasia. Other systemic fungal infections show characteristic tissue reaction patterns. For example, disseminated candidiasis has prominent microabscess formation, cryptococcosis has a gelatinous or granulomatous reaction pattern, and zygomycosis and aspergillosis have a tendency for vascular invasion and infarction.

Multiple special stains highlight certain fungal elements. These techniques can be helpful especially when the overall histologic pattern is suspicious for a fungal infection but fungi are not apparent on hematoxylin and eosin (H&E)-stained sections. The periodic acid–Schiff (PAS) reaction stains fungi red and can be used with diastase, i.e., periodic acid–Schiff–diastase (PAS-D), which clears the tissue of glycogen granules that may be mistaken for fungal spores. Fungi stain positively with PAS-D because their walls contain cellulose and chitin, both of which are rich in neutral polysaccharides and diastase resistant. Gomori methenamine silver (GMS) nitrate stains fungi black and is also useful but may be hard to interpret in tissue containing melanin pigment, which also stains black. Giemsa, Gram, Fontana–Masson, mucicarmine, Alcian blue, India ink, and acid-fast stains also highlight various fungal elements in other primary or secondary cutaneous fungal infections.

DERMATOPHYTOSIS

Dermatophytes are a group of molds that invade and consume keratin by generating proteases (5,6). They originally came from the soil, where they lived on keratinaceous debris, but ultimately were picked up by animals and humans to become the pathogens known today.

Three genera of imperfect fungi constitute the dermatophytes: *Epidermophyton, Microsporum,* and *Trichophyton.* More than 40 species exist, although many are not pathogenic to humans. Dermatophytes may be grouped according to their natural habitat as anthropophilic, zoophilic, and geophilic, with the primary reservoirs of infection in humans, animals, and soil, respectively (5). Fungi in all three categories may cause human infections. In immunocompetent hosts, the dermatophytes cause only superficial infections of the epidermis, hair, and nails. *Epidermophyton* spp., as the name suggests, infect mainly the epidermis, although occasionally the nails are involved. *Microsporum* spp. infect the epidermis and hair, whereas *Trichophyton* spp. may infect the epidermis, hair, and nails.

Clinical Summary. Fungal infections of seven anatomical regions are commonly recognized: tinea capitis (including tinea favosa or favus of the scalp), tinea faciei, tinea barbae, tinea corporis (including tinea imbricata), tinea cruris, tinea manus, tinea pedis, and tinea unguium (Table 23-2).

Tinea capitis is dermatophytosis of the skin and hair of the scalp. Clinically, scale crust and hairs that are broken off either at the level of the scalp or slightly above it are often seen. In the United States, *Trichophyton tonsurans* is the most common pathogen of this anatomic site. Because *T. tonsurans* invades the hair shaft (endothrix infection), infection presents as broken-off hairs (black-dot ringworm), which in some patients has an associated marked inflammatory reaction. Favus is a severe tinea capitis usually caused by *T. schoenleinii,* although a similar clinical picture may occasionally be seen with other fungi. Favus affects mainly the scalp, where it produces inflammation with the formation of perifollicular hyperkeratotic crusts called *scutula.* Destruction of the hair occurs relatively late in the infection, and lesions may heal, with scarring and permanent alopecia. Clinically, both *Microsporum canis* and *Microsporum audouinii* show a band of bright green fluorescence in the hair under a Wood light, but because *Microsporum canis* is zoophilic, it causes a greater inflammatory response than

Microsporum audouinii, which is anthropophilic. *Trichophyton* spp. do not fluoresce in a Wood light except for *T. schoenleinii,* which shows subtle pale green fluorescence along the length of the hair. A severe inflammatory boggy scalp plaque, called *kerion celsi,* may result from infection with zoophilic dermatophytes such as *Microsporum canis* and is often accompanied by posterior cervical lymphadenopathy. *Tinea faciei* is a fungal infection of the glabrous skin of the face characterized by a persistent eruption of red macules, papules, and patches, the latter of which may show an arcuate border. It is caused usually by *T. rubrum* and occasionally by *T. mentagrophytes* or *T. tonsurans* (7).

Tinea barbae is a fungal infection limited to the coarse hair-bearing beard and mustache areas of men. Tinea barbae is usually caused by *T. verrucosum* (sometimes called cattle ringworm because of its source) but may also be caused by *T. mentagrophytes.* Both *T. mentagrophytes* and *T. verrucosum* are zoophilic and typically cause a kerion-like, boggy, nodular inflammatory infiltration (8,9).

Tinea corporis is a dermatophytosis of glabrous skin most commonly caused by *T. rubrum,* followed by *Microsporum canis* and *T. mentagrophytes.* In the cases caused by *T. rubrum,* large erythematous patches with central clearing and an arcuate or polycyclic scaly border are seen. Infections with *Microsporum canis* are more inflammatory, and annular lesions may have a raised papulovesicular borders. *T. mentagrophytes* typically produces a few annular lesions with little or no central clearing. *T. verrucosum* may occasionally cause tinea corporis, appearing as grouped follicular pustules referred to as *agminate folliculitis* (8). The term *Majocchi granuloma* describes a nodular granulomatous perifolliculitis caused by rupture of an infected follicle, typically of the lower extremity. Majocchi granuloma is commonly caused by *T. rubrum* and is often associated with tinea pedis and/or onychomycosis. Majocchi granuloma may develop when superficial dermatophyte infections are inappropriately treated with topical steroids, allowing easier spread of the fungal organism down the hair follicle.

Tinea cruris presents as sharply demarcated erythematous patches or thin plaques in the groin, sometimes including the perineal, perianal regions, or scrotum. It is usually caused by *T. rubrum* and occasionally by *T. mentagrophytes* or *Epidermophyton floccosum.*

Tinea of the feet and hands (tinea pedis and manuum) are the most common forms of dermatophyte infection and are usually caused by *T. rubrum, E. floccosum,* and *T. mentagrophytes.* Tinea pedis may present clinically as interdigital maceration or plantar (i.e., "moccasin" scale) or vesiculobullous lesions. *T. rubrum* is anthropophilic and causes relatively noninflammatory scaling on the plantar feet. Infections with *T. mentagrophytes* tend to cause inflammatory, vesiculobullous tinea pedis.

Tinea unguium specifically refers to a dermatophyte infection of the nail, whereas onychomycosis is a nail infection owing to any fungi, including dermatophytes, *Candida,* or a nondermatophyte (10). Up to 90% of mycotic toenail infections and 50% of fingernail infections are caused by dermatophytes, but yeasts (especially *Candida albicans*) and nondermatophyte molds are also implicated (10). Criteria for diagnosing nondermatophyte onychomycosis include (a) the presence of hyphae in the infected subungual debris, (b) the persistent failure to culture recognized dermatophytes, and (c) positive cultures of a nondermatophyte (10,11).

Table 23-2
Common Causal Dermatophytes by Anatomic Regions

Clinical Diagnosis	Causal Organisms
Tinea capitis	*T. tonsurans* (black dot), *T. violaceum* (black dot), *T. schoenlenii* (favus), *M. canis*
Tinea faciei	*T. verrucosum, T. mentagrophytes, T. rubrum*
Tinea corporis	*T. rubrum, T. mentagrophytes, E. floccosum, T. concentricum*
Tinea manus	*T. rubrum*
Tinea pedis	*T. rubrum, T. mentagrophytes, E. floccosum*
Tinea unguium	*T. rubrum, T. mentagrophytes* (vesicobullous), *E. floccosum*

The four clinical types of onychomycosis include distal and lateral subungual onychomycosis (DLSO), superficial white onychomycosis (SWO), proximal subungual onychomycosis (PSO), and *Candida* infections of the nail. In general, hyperkeratosis and onycholysis are common clinical presentations of onychomycosis. DLSO is the most common form found in all patients, including those with HIV, and is caused by dermatophytes, usually *T. rubrum* (12). SWO is caused primarily by *T. mentagrophytes* and is more commonly seen in patients with HIV. PSO is typically caused by *T. rubrum* and is rare in the general population but can be a presenting sign of HIV. PSO in AIDS is often caused by *T. mentagrophytes* (13). *Candida* nail infections present as paronychia, hyperkeratosis, or onycholysis. Nondermatophytes implicated in onychomycosis include *Candida* spp., *Scytalidium* (*Hendersonula*), and *Aspergillus* (most commonly *Aspergillus niger*). Fungi thought to be contaminants in nail cultures in all but the immunosuppressed include *Cladosporium, Alternaria, Fusarium, Acremonium,* and *Scopulariopsis* (14). There is considerable controversy about the clinical significance of nondermatophyte fungi in nail cultures when a dermatophyte is also identified on culture. Molecular techniques such as sequencing of 18S ribosomal RNA, RFLP analysis, PCR, and genome sequencing are leading to an improved understanding of the epidemiology and pathogenesis of dermatophytes and other fungi such as Candida species, but they are not in general use owing to the higher cost and limited clinical availability of these more advanced techniques (15).

Histopathology. In *tinea capitis* and *tinea barbae*, infection of follicles usually starts with the colonization of the stratum corneum of the perifollicular epidermis (Fig. 23-1). Hyphae extend down the follicle and invade the hair, penetrating the cuticle first in the subcuticular portion of the cortex, just under the hair surface, and then more deeply in the hair cortex, extending to the upper limit of the zone of keratinization. Rounded and boxlike arthrospores may be found within the hair shaft in *endothrix* infections (*T. tonsurans or violaceum*) or penetrating the surface of the hair shaft and forming a sheath around it in *ectothrix* infections. Although hyphae invade the shafts in both types of infections, they may not be evident in a hair plucked from an endothrix infection because the more superficial hyphae rapidly break up into arthrospores and destroy the keratin of the hair shaft. When plucked, the weakened shaft typically breaks at a relatively superficial point so that only the arthrospores are seen. The dermis, which rarely contains fungi, shows a perifollicular mononuclear cell infiltrate of varying intensity. If there has been follicular disruption, multinucleated giant cells and neutrophils may be present in the dermis. In kerion celsi, there is a pronounced inflammatory tissue reaction to the zoophilic fungi with follicular pustule formation, interfollicular neutrophilic infiltration, and an intense chronic inflammatory infiltrate surrounding the hair follicles.

In *tinea of the glabrous skin*, which includes tinea faciei, tinea corporis, tinea cruris, and tinea of the feet and hands, fungi occur only in the horny layers of the epidermis and do not invade hairs and hair follicles. Two exceptions to this are *T. rubrum* and *T. verrucosum*, both of which may invade hairs and hair follicles, causing a subsequent perifolliculitis.

The number of fungi seen in the horny layer varies greatly but may be so small that they may be challenging to find even when treated with the PAS reaction or stained with GMS (16). Occasionally, they are present in sufficient numbers that they can be recognized as faintly basophilic, refractile structures, even in sections stained with H&E (Fig. 23-2). Their identification in H&E-stained sections may be aided by lowering the microscope condenser, which enhances the refractility of the fungal elements. In infections with *Microsporum* or *Trichophyton*, only hyphae are seen, and in infections with *E. floccosum*, chains of spores are present. If fungi are present in the horny layer, they are usually "sandwiched" between two zones of cornified cells, the upper being orthokeratotic and the lower consisting partially of parakeratotic cells. This "sandwich sign" should prompt the performance of a stain for fungi for verification. The presence of neutrophils in the stratum corneum is another valuable diagnostic clue (17). In the absence of demonstrable fungi, the histologic picture of fungal infections of the glabrous skin is not diagnostic. Depending on the degree of reaction of the skin to the presence of fungi, the histologic features are those of an acute, subacute, or chronic spongiotic dermatitis (see Chapter 9).

On staining with the PAS reaction or GMS, nodular perifolliculitis or Majocchi granuloma, caused by *T. rubrum*, shows numerous hyphae and spores within hair follicles and variably in the associated suppurative and granulomatous dermal inflammatory infiltrate. Although the spores present within hairs

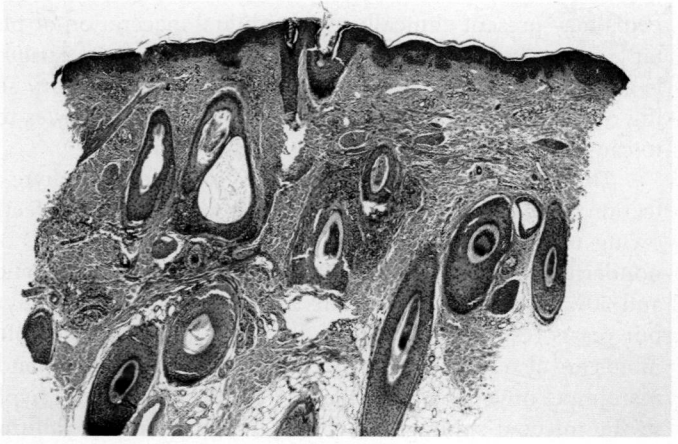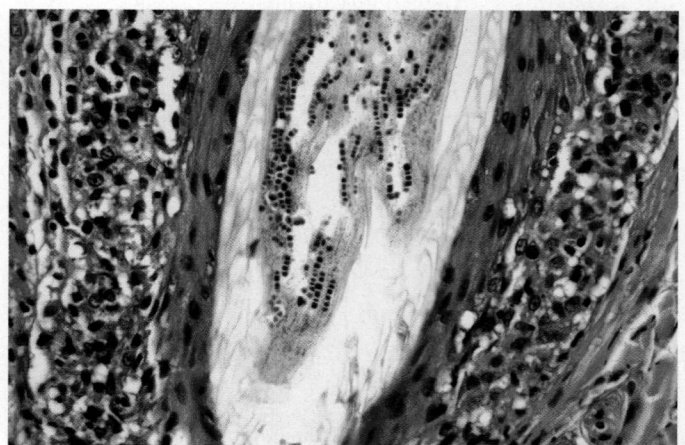

Figure 23-1 Tinea capitis. A: H&E stain shows arthrospores and hyphal elements in most follicles. A lymphohistiocytic, perifollicular infiltrate is present. B: H&E stain shows arthrospores in endothrix infection. (H&E, hematoxylin and eosin.)

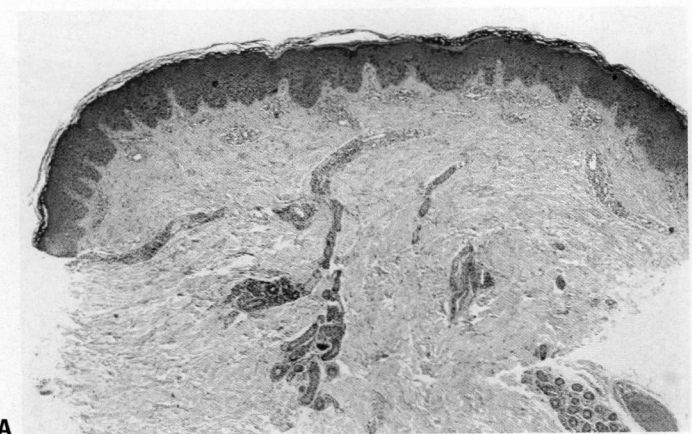
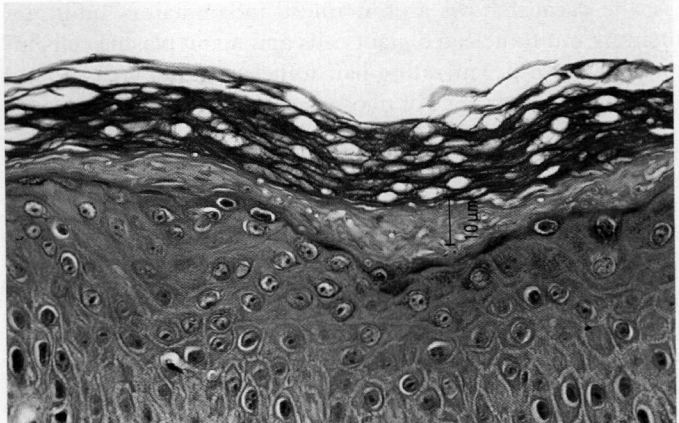

Figure 23-2 Tinea corporis. **A:** H&E stain shows a superficial perivascular, predominantly lymphoid infiltrate with mild psoriasiform epidermal hyperplasia and compact hyperkeratosis. **B:** Cross sections of refractile hyphae are visible as clear spaces in parakeratotic stratum corneum (H&E stain). (H&E, hematoxylin and eosin.)

or hair follicles measure about 2 μm in diameter, those located in the dermis, especially within multinucleated giant cells, may be larger—measuring up to 6 μm (16).

The agminate folliculitis caused by *T. verrucosum* (*faviforme*) shows hyphae and spores within hairs and hair follicles in PAS-stained sections (10). However, the dermis around the hair follicles contains no fungi. Depending on the severity and stage of the inflammatory reaction, either an acute or a chronic inflammatory infiltrate is predominant around the hair follicles in the dermis. In well-established lesions, the inflammatory infiltrate contains many plasma cells, microabscesses, and small aggregates of foreign-body giant cells (8).

In *tinea unguium*, histologic evaluation of the nail plate and subungual debris is potentially the method of choice for diagnosis. The organisms may be difficult or impossible to visualize in routine H&E sections because the dermatophytes are in a category of "hyaline" fungi whose staining does not contrast with that of the background keratin. Although a microscopic examination of potassium hydroxide mounts or cultures of nail fragments often establishes a diagnosis of onychomycosis, false-negative results may occur owing to inadequate sampling, often because the subungual debris containing fungus has not been sampled. Nail clippings or nail biopsy taken by punch technique or scalpel under local anesthesia will often reveal the fungi on PAS-stained sections (17). By far, *T. rubrum* is the most common causal fungus; occasionally, *T. mentagrophytes* is present.

Routine histologic examination of the nail plate with PAS staining is a simple, rapid, and sensitive test for fungal elements (18). Three histologic patterns are common in nail plate specimens of onychomycosis (19–21). In superficial infections, mycelial elements, best visualized with PAS or GMS, are seen on the outer layers of the nail plate. The second histologic pattern is PAS-positive slender, uniform mycelial elements invading the undersurface of the nail plate often occurring in the clinical setting of onycholysis (Fig. 23-3). The third common histologic pattern is seen in *Candida* infections, where hyphal forms are seen on the undersurface of the nail plate; this will be discussed in a later section (see p. 719). Biopsies of nail bed or nail fold epithelium may reveal psoriasiform hyperplasia, spongiosis, and hyperkeratosis, simulating a primary inflammatory disorder as opposed to an infectious one making the identification of fungal elements critical to the correct diagnosis.

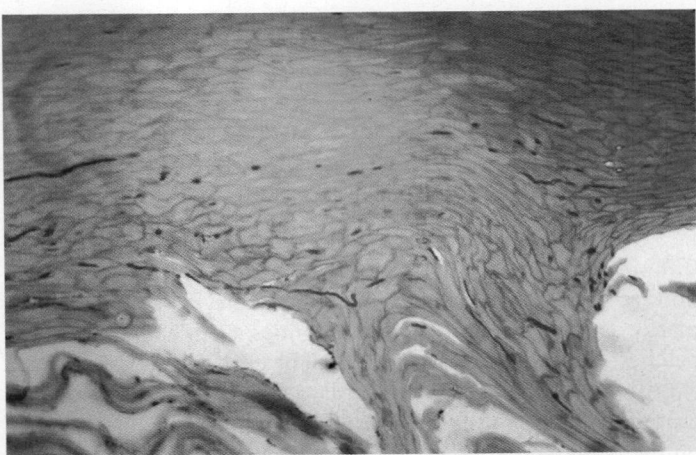

Figure 23-3 Tinea unguium. Slender, uniform mycelial elements can be seen within this parakeratotic nail plate (PAS stain). (PAS, periodic acid–Schiff.)

PCR amplification of DNA from nail plate biopsies is commercially available for the diagnosis of onychomycosis. PCR is very sensitive and the results are available within a day, but ubiquitous contaminant fungi may cause false-positive results, meaning that fungal cultures or histologic confirmation of hyphal or yeast forms within the nail plate and/or subungual debris might still be needed to confirm true infection (22).

Pathogenesis. Debate exists regarding the factors that predispose individuals to onychomycosis. Trauma is thought to facilitate the entry of fungus into the nail. Epidemiologic data suggest that genetic predisposition plays a role and that the incidence increases with age, but other factors such as humidity, local trauma, and common living/bathing sites have been variably significant predictors (23).

In *favus*, mainly hyphae and only a few spores of *T. schoenleinii* are present in the stratum corneum of the epidermis around and within hairs. The scutula (see p. 715) consist of compact keratin as well as parakeratotic cells, exudate, and inflammatory cells intermingled with segmented hyphae and spores that are well preserved at the periphery but appear degenerated and granular in the center of the scutula. In active areas, the dermis shows a pronounced inflammatory infiltrate containing multinucleated giant cells and many plasma cells in association with degenerating hair follicles. In old areas, there is fibrosis and an absence of pilosebaceous structures.

Principles of Management: Treatment of infections with dermatophytes is guided by the extent of involvement, specifically the depth of involvement in the skin and the total body surface area affected. Topical therapy is first line for superficial infections of localized areas, typically scaly macules and/or patches. Onychomycosis is difficult to treat and typically requires systemic therapy except in cases of SWO or limited nail involvement—in which case, topical therapy may be reasonably attempted. In the histologic setting of Majocchi granuloma, systemic therapy is typically first line. As always, therapy is individualized based on comorbidities, concomitant medications being taken by the patient, as well as the patient's willingness to agree to the risks of systemic therapy.

DISEASES CAUSED BY MALASSEZIA FURFUR

Malassezia is a genus of lipophilic yeast that causes two forms of dermatoses: pityriasis versicolor and *Malassezia* (*Pityrosporum*) folliculitis (24,25). The frequently used term *tinea versicolor* is not accurate, because *Malassezia* are not dermatophytes.

Clinical Summary. In pityriasis versicolor, multiple round-to-oval pink-to-light brown patches with fine white scale are seen primarily on the trunk and upper extremities. Gentle scraping of the patches will induce the scale that can be examined for spores and short hyphae. *Malassezia* (*Pityrosporum*) folliculitis is a pruritic eruption of 2- to 4-mm acneiform follicular papules and pustules on the trunk and arms of otherwise healthy hosts (25). In addition to these two diseases, *Malassezia* has been found in lesions of seborrheic dermatitis, atopic dermatitis, neonatal cephalic pustulosis, and confluent and reticulated papillomatosis of Gougerot and Carteaud (26–29). Seborrheic dermatitis, for example, has been reported to respond to antifungal therapy and has been associated with heavy colonization by *Malassezia furfur*. However, these observations and their interpretation are controversial, and it has not been definitively established that *Malassezia furfur* contributes to the pathogenesis of seborrheic dermatitis (26,28,29). Molecular classification has been reported for the evaluation of Malassezia (Pityrosporum) infections but they are not in general use for diagnosis (30).

Histopathology. In contrast to other fungal infections of the glabrous skin, the horny layer in lesions of *pityriasis (tinea) versicolor* contains abundant fungi, which can often be visualized in sections stained with H&E as faintly basophilic structures. *Malassezia* (*Pityrosporum*) is present as a combination of both hyphae and spores (Fig. 23-4), the light microscopic appearance of which is often referred to as *spaghetti and meatballs*. The inflammatory response in pityriasis versicolor is usually minimal, although there may occasionally be slight hyperkeratosis (29), slight spongiosis, or a minimal superficial perivascular lymphocytic infiltrate.

Pathogenesis. The names *Malassezia furfur*, *Pityrosporum orbiculare*, and *Pityrosporum ovale* are often used interchangeably, probably because these are identical in culture (30). *In vivo*,

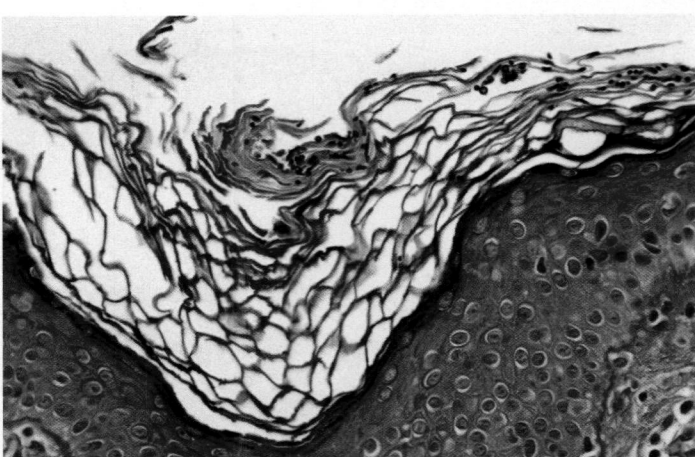

Figure 23-4 Pityriasis (tinea) versicolor. A slightly hyperkeratotic stratum corneum contains numerous hyphae and spores (H&E stain). (H&E, hematoxylin and eosin.)

Malassezia furfur becomes dimorphous by forming numerous true septate hyphae in addition to spores. The organism then becomes pathogenic (31,32).

Several theories exist to explain the characteristic clinical pigmentary alterations in pityriasis versicolor, although none have been convincingly proven. Hypopigmentation may be caused by filtering of ultraviolet light by the organism, a block in melanosome transfer to keratinocytes, or the inhibition of melanin synthesis by azelaic acid or lipoxygenase produced by *Malassezia* (31–33). Hyperpigmentation is thought by some to be secondary to inflammation, hyperkeratosis, or greater numbers of organisms in the skin.

Principles of Management: Pityrosporum versicolor is an infection at the level of the cornified layer and, therefore, easily reached by topical therapy. However, the extensive body surface area often involved means that oral therapy may be preferred. Regardless of the treatment utilized, it is important to educate the patient regarding the high risk of recurrence. One frequently utilized method for limiting recurrence is periodic washing with an antifungal shampoo.

Malassezia (Pityrosporum) Folliculitis

The involved pilosebaceous follicles show hyperkeratosis with dilatation resulting from plugging of the infundibulum with keratinous material. Inflammatory cells are present both within and around the follicular infundibulum. In some instances, the follicular epithelium is disrupted with the development of a peri-infundibular abscess (34) (Fig. 23-5). PAS-stained sections show PAS-positive, diastase-resistant, spherical-to-oval, singly budding yeast organisms that are 2 to 4 μm in diameter. They are located predominantly within the infundibulum and at the dilated orifice of the follicular lumen but are occasionally observed also in the perifollicular dermis.

Histogenesis. It has been assumed that *Malassezia* organisms cause hyperkeratosis in the follicular ostium, thereby preventing the normal flow of sebum and causing follicular, acne-like lesions.

Principles of Management: Treatment of pityrosporum folliculitis generally requires oral therapy with an azole antifungal. The dermal depth of involvement of this infection means topical therapy is less likely to be effective.

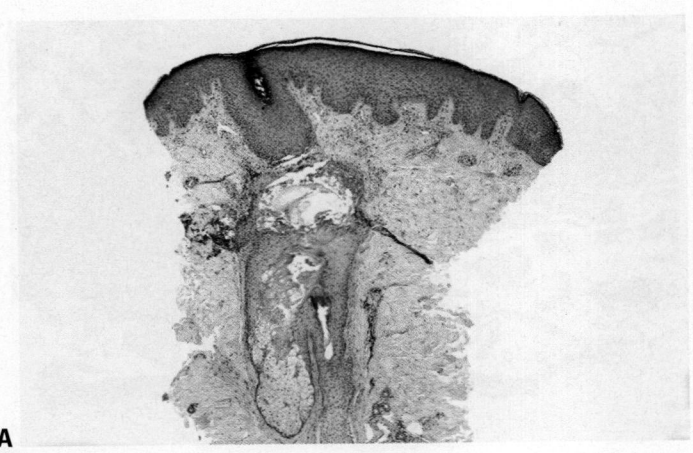
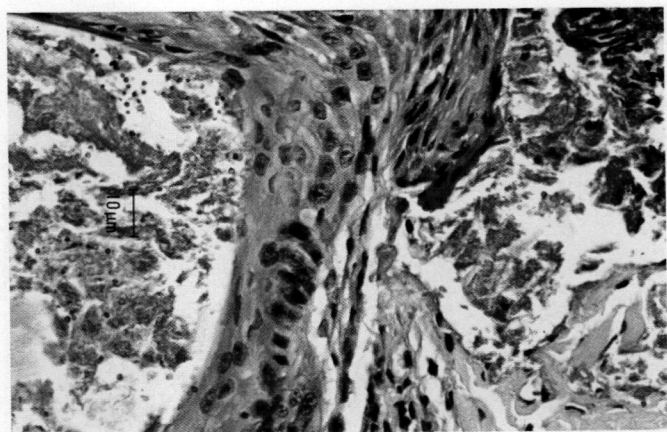

Figure 23-5 Malassezia (Pityrosporum) folliculitis. A: A plugged and ruptured follicle contains numerous round yeast forms (H&E stain). B: H&E staining shows round and budding yeast forms in follicle and surrounding dermis. (H&E, hematoxylin and eosin.)

CANDIDIASIS

Candida albicans is a dimorphous fungus growing in both yeast and filamentous forms on the skin. It exists in a commensal relationship with man. Molecular techniques such as sequencing of 18S ribosomal RNA, RFLP analysis, PCR, and genome sequencing are leading to an improved understanding of the epidemiology and pathogenesis of Candida and other fungi, but they are not in general use owing to higher cost and limited clinical availability of these more advanced techniques (35).

The spectrum of infection may be divided into four groups: acute mucocutaneous candidiasis, chronic mucocutaneous candidiasis (CMC), disseminated candidiasis, and *Candida* onychomycosis.

Acute Mucocutaneous Candidiasis

Clinical Summary. Acute mucocutaneous candidiasis is the benign, self-limited form of candidiasis and is caused by environmental changes that are local, as in hot, humid conditions, or that are systemic, as in antibiotic or corticosteroid therapy. Clinical variants of acute mucocutaneous candidiasis include erosio interdigitalis blastomycetica, *Candida* vaginitis, paronychia, *Candida* intertrigo, and thrush. Intertriginous lesions show erythematous, often-eroded patches and thin plaques often with peripheral erythematous macules and papules, the so-called satellite lesions. *Candida* infection of the mucous membranes is characterized by tender erythematous patches or white plaques that reveal a glistening, erythematous undersurface when scraped.

Candida infection is associated with specific host and environmental factors. *Candida* is the most common pathogen in patients who have had a solid organ transplant, and candidiasis tends to occur within the first 6 months after transplant. Age (infancy, old age), antibiotic use, malignancy, chemotherapy, endocrinopathies (diabetes, Cushing syndrome), and disorders of immunity, including HIV/AIDS, are risk factors for *Candida* infection (36). More effective treatment of AIDS has led to a decline in the incidence of clinically apparent candidiasis in these patients.

Congenital cutaneous candidiasis is a result of ascending intrauterine infection from vaginal candidiasis. There are widely scattered macules, papulovesicles, and pustules at birth or in a few days thereafter. *Neonatal candidiasis*, on the other hand, manifests as oral candidiasis or diaper dermatitis after the first week of life and is acquired during passage through the birth canal (37).

Histopathology. Cutaneous and mucous membrane *Candida* infections show similar features. If the primary lesion is a vesicle or pustule, it is usually subcorneal as in impetigo (Fig. 23-6A, B). In some instances, the pustules have a spongiform appearance, similar to the spongiform pustules of Kogoj seen in pustular psoriasis (see Chapter 7).

The fungal organisms are present, usually in small amounts only, in the stratum corneum. They are predominantly pseudohyphae and ovoid spores, with some of the latter in the budding stage. These septate pseudohyphae show branching at a 90-degree angle and measure 2 to 4 μm in diameter. The pseudohyphae tend to be constricted at their septa and to have septa at their branch points (38,39). The ovoid spores vary from 3 to 6 μm in size (Table 23-3).

Pathogenesis. By electron microscopy, the majority of the mycelia and spores are situated inside the cells of the stratum corneum, many of which are parakeratotic (40).

Principles of Management: Treatment of acute mucocutaneous candidiasis involves topical therapy with nystatin or treatment with topical or oral azole antifungal therapy. Attention should also be directed at minimizing factors that predispose the patient to recurrent infection. Patients who have recurrent disease may benefit from maintenance, preventative therapy.

Chronic Mucocutaneous Candidiasis

Clinical Summary. CMC is a heterogeneous group of conditions in which patients have chronic and recurrent candidal infections of the skin, nails, and mucous membranes. CMC may be inherited as an autosomal dominant or recessive condition. It may also be owing to endocrinopathies or immunodeficiency. By definition, systemic involvement does not occur in CMC (41). The individual lesions of CMC are similar clinically and histologically to those seen in acute mucocutaneous candidiasis and must be distinguished by their clinical course (41). The exception is seen in CMC beginning in childhood when a rare clinical variant called *Candida granuloma* may develop. Candida granuloma presents clinically as numerous hyperkeratotic, crusted plaques on the face and scalp but occasionally elsewhere (42).

Currently, the most common type of CMC is probably seen in patients with AIDS who often have recurrent candidal infections of the mouth and perianal area. Oral candidiasis may occur as an

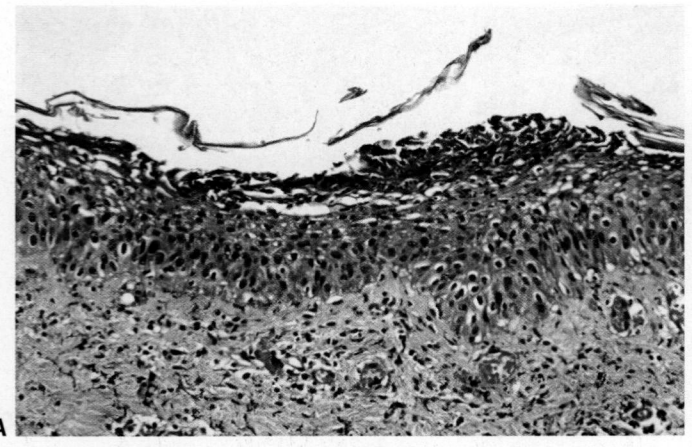

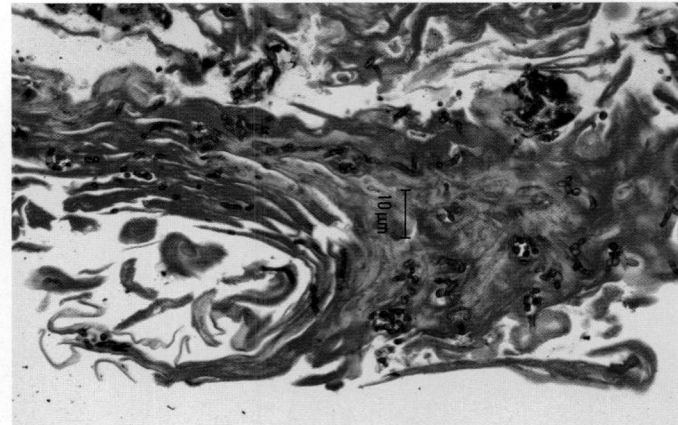

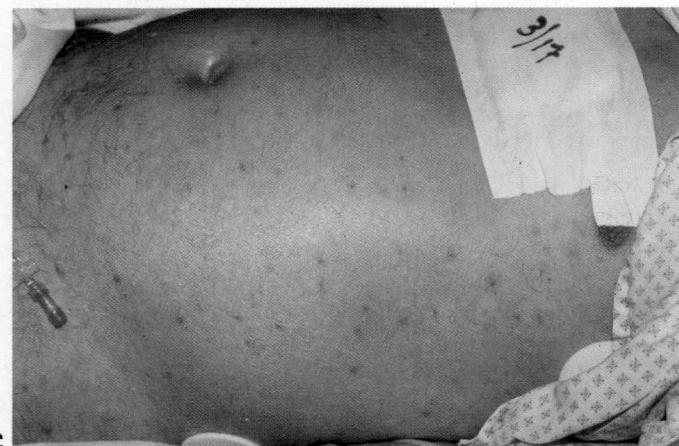

Figure 23-6 Candidiasis. **A:** H&E staining shows a subcorneal pustule with an underlying mixed dermal infiltrate. **B:** GMS staining shows pseudohyphae and ovoid yeast in hyperkeratotic stratum corneum. **C:** Erythematous to violaceous papulonodules of disseminated candidiasis in a patient with leukemia. (GMS, Gomori methenamine silver; H&E, hematoxylin and eosin.)

Table 23-3

Histologic Appearance of Tissue and Fungi in Superficial Dermatomycoses

Disease	Histologic Appearance	Fungal Size and Morphology
Dermatophytosis	Minimal to spongiotic-psoriasiform, pustular, or folliculitis pattern with mixed dermal infiltrate	Refractile, 1- to 2-µm septate hyaline hyphae in stratum corneum, occasional chains of spores
Pityriasis (tinea) versicolor	Slight hyperkeratosis	2- to 8-µm round spores, 2- to 3-µm-thick, short, sometimes curved, hyphae
Mallassezia (Pityrosporum) folliculitis	Plugged, sometimes ruptured follicle with follicular and perifollicular mixed infiltrate	2- to 8-µm round spores within the follicle, rarely in perifollicular tissue; usually, no hyphae
Candidiasis	Spongiotic or subcorneal pustular dermatitis with mixed dermal infiltrate; erosions may be present.	3- to 6-µm round-to-oval, sometimes budding, spores, 2- to 4-µm-thick pseudohyphae

early sign of immunosuppression, before other symptoms have appeared (41), and if persistent may be an indication of esophageal candidiasis (43). In addition, *Candida* organisms are frequently observed on the surface of lesions of oral hairy leukoplakia, which is a viral leukoplakia caused by Epstein–Barr virus, perhaps in combination with human papillomavirus (44) (see Chapter 25).

Histopathology. The histologic findings are identical with those of acute mucocutaneous candidiasis, except in cases of candidal granuloma. *Candidal granuloma* shows pronounced epidermal papillomatosis and hyperkeratosis and a dense infiltrate in the dermis composed of lymphoid cells, neutrophils, plasma cells, and multinucleated giant cells. The infiltrate may extend into

the subcutis. *Candida albicans* usually is present only in the stratum corneum. In some instances, however, fungal elements are found within hairs, viable epidermis, and dermis also.

Principles of Management: The heterogeneous nature of immunodeficiencies in patients with CMC has in common the inability of their cellular immunity to manage *Candida*. Therefore, medical management directed toward eradication of the infection, typically with a triazole antifungal such as fluconazole, must be followed by systemic maintenance therapy.

Disseminated Candidiasis

Clinical Summary. *Candida* is the fourth leading cause of hospital-acquired bloodstream infection in the United States, but cutaneous involvement is only seen in 13% of cases (45). It primarily affects those with impaired host-defense mechanisms, particularly those with hematologic malignancies. *Candida albicans* accounts for just over half of the cases of *Candida* fungemia, and *Candida glabrata* ranks number two, with the incidence of the latter increasing directly with age (45–49). Cutaneous lesions of disseminated candidiasis are erythematous or violaceous papulonodules with central clearing that measure 0.5 to 1.0 cm in diameter (Fig. 23-6C). The triad of fever, rash, and diffuse muscle tenderness in an immunocompromised host is presumptive for disseminated candidiasis. However, the clinical diagnosis may be delayed because patients often present with nonspecific symptoms and current methods for diagnosing candidemia rely on blood cultures that require several days. In addition, the speciation of *Candida* by culture is problematic given that all yeast cultures that form germ tubes and chlamydospores are by generalization designated *Candida albicans* in many labs. Thus, a skin biopsy may be critical to the early diagnosis of disseminated candidiasis. Because the diffuse muscle tenderness is caused by the infiltration of muscle tissue by yeast organisms, biopsy of a tender muscle may also aid in establishing the diagnosis of disseminated candidiasis (47–49).

Histopathology. Histologic examination reveals one or several aggregates of hyphae and spores focally within the dermis, often at sites of vascular damage and generally visible only in sections stained with the PAS reaction or GMS. Some of the spores, which are 3 to 6 μm in diameter, show budding. The aggregates of hyphae and spores may lie in an area of leukocytoclastic vasculitis, within a microabscess, or in an area of only mild inflammation. The aggregates of *Candida* often are small, and step sections through the biopsy specimen may be necessary to find them. The epidermis is usually unaffected.

Principles of Management: Candidemia, particularly in the neutropenic patient, is a life-threatening infection with risks of multiorgan failure and death. Treatment is a medical emergency requiring prompt systemic antifungal therapy and supportive measures. Certain species of *Candida* may exhibit resistance to standard first-line systemic antifungal agents and may require alternative agents; consultation with an infectious disease specialist is suggested to determine the appropriate therapy and duration of treatment.

Candida Onychomycosis

Clinical Summary. Candida onychomycosis is a form of nail infection characterized by separation of the nail plate from the nail bed. Paronychia and loss of the proximal nail fold are not uncommon in *Candida* infections of the nail unit.

Histopathology. Candida commonly causes onycholysis but distinguishes itself histologically from the dermatophytes by its lack of nail plate invasion (18). Yeast forms may be seen along the undersurface of the nail plate. *Candida* may mimic the psoriasiform changes and inflammatory response of onychomycosis caused by dermatophytes. *Candida* spp. occur as ovoid yeasts that measure 3 to 6 μm in diameter and as pseudohyphae that measure 2 to 4 μm in diameter. These pseudohyphae may appear thick and bulbous and have an irregular caliber compared with the smooth, thin, and regular hyphae of dermatophytes.

Principles of Management: The treatment of Candida onychomycosis is difficult, and consideration of treatment relies on an accurate diagnosis. In general, the diagnosis of onychomycosis by accurate diagnosis. In general, the diagnosis of onychomycosis by nondermatophytes requires nail culture of the same nondermatophyte at two separate periods in time, lack of dermatophyte on culture, and visualization of the fungus affecting the nail plate either by potassium hydroxide (KOH) or by light microscopy after PAS stain. The diagnosis should be certain before treatment with an oral azole antifungal is considered, particularly because contaminant yeast and molds are not uncommon in nail plate cultures, systemic antifungal medications have potentially serious side effects, and the risk of recurrent nail infection is significant. As an alternative or adjunct to medical therapy, if the nail is thickened and problematic, it may be chemically and/or manually thinned.

ASPERGILLOSIS

Aspergillus spp. are ubiquitous in the environment. Humans are constantly exposed to and frequently colonized by these organisms, although they rarely cause disease (50,51). Molecular techniques are available for the rapid diagnosis of Aspergillus (34).

Clinical Summary. Severe, invasive aspergillosis typically involves the lungs and is usually seen only in immunocompromised hosts, particularly those with neutropenia, hematologic malignancy, or a history of chronic corticosteroid or antibiotic therapy (50). Indeed, in neutropenic patients with hematologic malignancy, *Aspergillus* infection has overtaken candidal infections as the most frequent fungal infection in some populations. *Aspergillus fumigatus* is the most common cause of both colonization and invasive aspergillosis, followed in frequency by *A. flavus* and *A. niger* (51). Cutaneous aspergillosis may occur as a primary infection or may be secondary to disseminated aspergillosis (Table 23-4). The lesions of primary cutaneous aspergillosis are usually found at an intravenous infusion site: either at the actual access site or where the unit has been secured with a colonized board or tape (52,53). There may be one or more macules, papules, plaques, or hemorrhagic bullae that may rapidly progress into necrotic ulcers with a heavy black surface eschar (54) (Fig. 23-7A). In immunocompromised patients, dissemination may follow and is often fatal if untreated with amphotericin B, itraconazole, or caspofungin (50). In addition, *Aspergillus* may colonize burn or surgical wounds and subsequently invade viable tissue. Patients with AIDS may develop primary cutaneous infection, but dissemination is not typical unless they have one or more of the previously mentioned risk factors (50,54,55). Umbilicated papules clinically resembling lesions of molluscum contagiosum, or "dermatophyte-like" involvement of follicles, have been described in AIDS-related cases (55). Secondary cutaneous aspergillosis, usually associated with invasive lung disease, shows multiple scattered lesions as a result of embolic hematogenous spread and has a poor prognosis (50). Disseminated aspergillosis often manifests as angulated purpura with central areas of dusky necrosis, generally distally owing to hematogenous spread.

Histopathology. Unlike most deep cutaneous fungal infections, pseudocarcinomatous epidermal hyperplasia is not characteristic of cutaneous aspergillosis. In the more serious primary forms and in the secondary disseminated form, numerous *Aspergillus* hyphae are seen in the dermis (Fig. 23-7B, C). Hyphae may be seen in H&E-stained sections, but PAS or silver methenamine staining may be required. The hyphae, which measure 2 to 4 μm in diameter (50), are often arranged in a radiate fashion, are septate, and show branching at an acute angle. Spores are absent. Hyphae may

Table 23-4

Histologic Appearance of Tissue and Fungi in Deep and Secondary Dermatomycoses

Disease	Histologic Appearance	Fungal Size and Morphology
Aspergillosis	Primary infection: granulomatous infiltrate. Immunocompromised host (primary and secondary infection): angioinvasion, ischemic necrosis, and hemorrhage	2- to 4-μm septate hyphae with dichotomous branching at 45-degree angle
Zygomycosis (mucormycosis, phycomycosis)	Angioinvasion with thrombosis and infarction, necrosis, and variable, mild, neutrophilic infiltrate	7- to 30-μm hyphae with branching at irregular angles and intervals; variably thin, often collapsed or twisted walls
Subcutaneous phaeohyphomycosis (phaeohyphomycotic cyst)	Deep, coalescing, suppurative granulomatous foci surrounded by fibrous capsule	Loosely arranged, septate, occasionally branching pigmented hyphae varying from 2 to 25 μm in diameter
Alternariosis	Pseudocarcinomatous epithelial hyperplasia with intraepidermal microabscesses and suppurative granulomatous dermal infiltrate	5- to 7-μm septate hyphae with variable branching and brown pigmentation; 3–10-μm round-to-oval spores, often with double contours
North American blastomycosis	Pseudocarcinomatous epithelial hyperplasia with intraepidermal microabscesses; suppurative granulomatous dermal infiltrate with giant cells	8- to 15-μm thick-walled spores with single broad-based buds
Paracoccidioidomycosis	Like North American blastomycosis	6- to 20-μm spores with narrow-necked, single or multiple buds; "Mariner's wheels" up to 60 μm in diameter
Lobomycosis	Atrophic epidermis with dermal macrophage and giant cell infiltrate; unstained organisms give sievelike appearance to dermis.	9- to 10-μm "lemon-shaped" spores with single budding, often in chains
Chromoblastomycosis	Like North American blastomycosis	6- to 12-μm thick-walled, dark brown spores, often in clusters. Some cells possess cross walls.
Coccidioidomycosis	Primary inoculation: mixed dermal infiltrate with granulocytes, lymphocytes, and occasional histiocytic giant cells. Systemic: like North American blastomycosis, but granulomas may be more tuberculoid in nature.	10- to 80-μm thick-walled spores with granular cytoplasm; the larger spores contain endospores.
Cryptococcosis	Cryptococcosis "gelatinous reaction" with many spores; "granulomatous reaction" with fewer spores.	4- to 12-μm spore with wide capsule in "gelatinous reaction"; 2- to 4-μm spore in "granulomatous reaction"
Histoplasmosis var. *capsulatum*	Suppurative granulomatous infiltrate in ulcerative skin lesions, neutrophils and eosinophils in oral lesions; histiocytes contain variable numbers of organisms.	2- to 4-μm round, narrow-necked budding spores with clear halo (pseudocapsule) in the cytoplasm of large histiocytes
var. *duboisii* (African)	Granulomatous dermal infiltrate with focal suppuration	8- to 5-μm ovoid spores in macrophages and free in tissue
Sporotrichosis	Cutaneous lesions: epidermal hyperplasia with intraepidermal abscesses, suppurative granulomatous dermal infiltrate, occasional asteroid bodies; subcutaneous nodules: central zone of neutrophils surrounded by zones of epithelioid macrophages and round cells	4- to 6-μm round-to-oval spores
Eumycetoma	Abscess in granulation tissue, fibrosis, and sinus tracts	0.5- to 2.0-mm sulfur granules composed of 4–5-μm-thick septate hyphae
Rhinosporidiosis	Hyperplastic epithelium with papillomatosis, deep invagination with pseudocysts, and "Swiss cheese" corium	7- to 12-μm spores, sporangia up to 300 μm

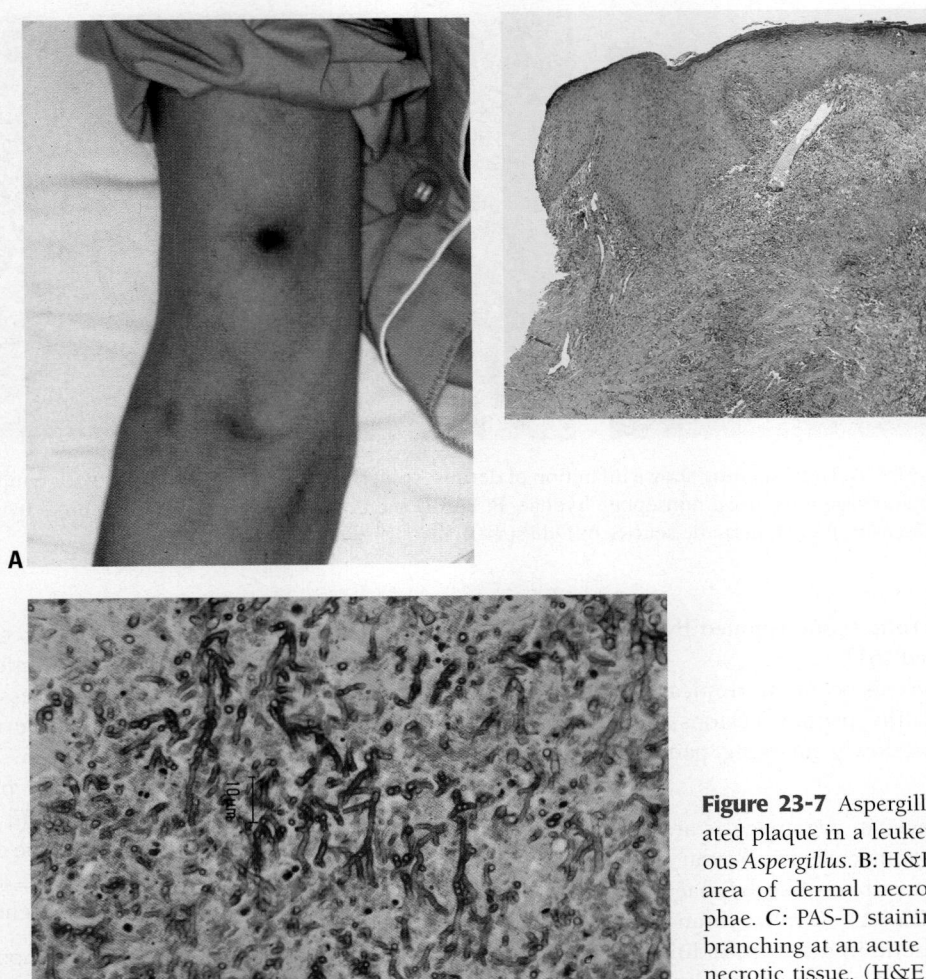

Figure 23-7 Aspergillosis. **A:** Necrotic ulcerated plaque in a leukemic patient with cutaneous *Aspergillus*. **B:** H&E staining shows a central area of dermal necrosis with branching hyphae. **C:** PAS-D staining shows septate hyphae branching at an acute angle in a background of necrotic tissue. (H&E, hematoxylin and eosin; PAS-D, periodic acid–Schiff–diastase.)

be seen invading blood vessels and may be seen around areas of ischemic necrosis with variable amounts of mixed inflammation. In general, it is best to report organisms identified in tissue without making definitive diagnoses based on histologic appearance alone because there is considerable overlap among disparate organisms. Confirmatory diagnosis by culture is standard clinical practice.

In patients with primary cutaneous or subcutaneous aspergillosis who are otherwise in good health, the number of hyphae present is relatively small and there is an associated granulomatous reaction.

Principles of Management: The treatment of secondary cutaneous aspergillus is a medical emergency and requires systemic antifungal therapy, debridement as necessary, and supportive measures. Primary cutaneous aspergillus requires systemic antifungal therapy and, often, debridement of the necrotic tissue.

ZYGOMYCOSIS (MUCORMYCOSIS, PHYCOMYCOSIS)

Zygomycosis describes infections by ubiquitous molds of two orders: Mucorales and Entomophthorales. The term *mucormycoses* describes infection with *Rhizopus* or *Mucor*, the two most medically significant genera of the order Mucorales (56,57).

Clinical Summary. Zygomycotic infections are aggressive and often occur in ketotic diabetics, but infections may also be seen in other settings such as burns, iatrogenic immunosuppression, chronic renal failure, hematopoietic malignancy, and AIDS (56). Widespread use of voriconazole prophylaxis in patients with hematopoietic malignancy may be contributing to increased incidence of zygomycotic infections in that population. Entomophthoraceae may cause chronic cutaneous and subcutaneous infections in otherwise healthy hosts.

Cutaneous zygomycosis occurs by implantation of fungi or by hematogenous dissemination. Three main forms exist: rhinocerebral, primary cutaneous, and chronic subcutaneous zygomycosis. Rhinocerebral zygomycosis is a fulminant infection of the paranasal sinuses that quickly spreads to contiguous structures such as the skin, nose, orbit, and brain (56,57). Clinical findings include nasal discharge, swelling, mucocutaneous ulceration, and eschar formation.

Primary cutaneous zygomycosis may occur following burns, major trauma, or minor trauma in immunosuppressed patients or those with diabetes (56–64). It has also been reported after the use of infected tape (57,61). Individual lesions occur early as pustules or blisters that soon ulcerate and form eschars. Depending on the host status, the ulcers either heal or lead to fatal systemic spread. These molds may cause acute, rapidly developing, often lethal infections of immunocompromised patients. Cutaneous lesions may also be seen as a result of embolization and infarction in patients with systemic zygomycosis. The lesions may begin as erythematous macules or nodules that blister and ulcerate (57). A "bull's-eye" lesion of

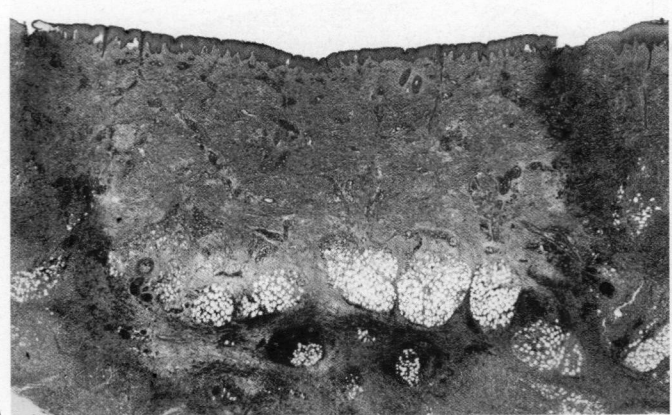
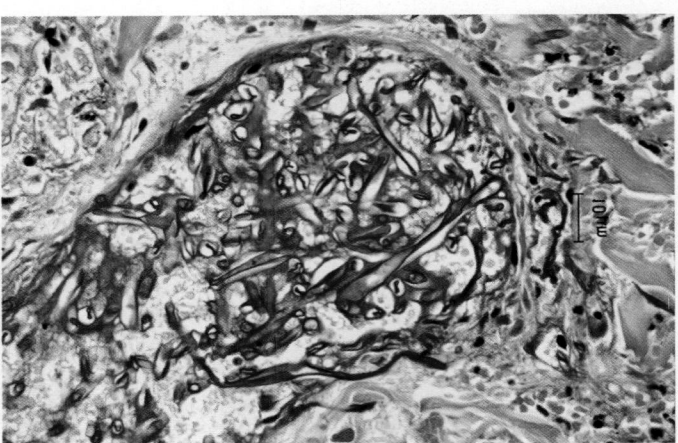

Figure 23-8 Zygomycosis (mucormycosis). **A:** H&E staining shows infarction of dermis, epidermis, and subcutaneous fat with lymphohistiocytic and neutrophilic infiltrate as well as angioinvasion by broad nonseptate hyphae. **B:** PAS-D staining shows irregularly branching, twisted, and collapsed hyphae. (H&E, hematoxylin and eosin; PAS-D, periodic acid–Schiff–diastase.)

progressive rings of advancing necrotic tissue rimmed by violaecous erythema has been described (61).

Chronic subcutaneous zygomycosis occurs in tropical and subtropical areas in otherwise healthy people. Lesions most commonly occur on the face and are slowly enlarging, painless, firm swellings in the dermis (58).

Histopathology. The histologic changes in zygomycosis are primarily dermal. The hallmark of zygomycosis is vascular invasion by very large, long, nonseptate ribbon-like hyphae with thrombosis and infarction (Fig. 23-8A). Hyphae branch at 90-degree angles and may also be found in the surrounding tissue (58,59). The hyphae are thin walled, so they may be twisted or collapsed and often appear ring-shaped or oval in cross or tangential sections (Fig. 23-8B). They are often easily located even in routinely stained sections because of their very large size, up to 30 µm in diameter, although they may be better visualized in PAS- or GMS-stained sections.

Principles of Management: Treatment of Zygomycosis requires surgical debridement, systemic antifungal therapy, often with high-dose amphotericin B, and sometimes combination of systemic antifungal agents, along with the minimization of predisposing factors.

SUBCUTANEOUS PHAEOHYPHOMYCOSIS

Phaeohyphomycosis is a subcutaneous or systemic infection caused by dematiaceous, mycelia-forming fungi (63,64). This is a histopathologic definition of a disease process that can be caused by many different organisms and can have different clinical presentations. *Bipolaris, Phialophora, Alternaria,* and *Exophiala* are fungi responsible for phaeohyphomycosis (65,66). Phaeohyphomycosis has been labeled a "chromic mycosis" in the past but is distinct from chromomycosis, which is characterized by pigmented spores without hyphal forms. In the interest of completeness, it is worth mentioning that eumycetoma is a clinical term that describes chronic subcutaneous infection by fungi, including dermatiaceous fungi, ultimately resulting in the destruction of adjacent soft tissue and other anatomic structures. Although advances in molecular techniques are promising, they have still not replaced histology and culture as primary diagnostic tools in the evaluation of phaeohyphomycosis.

Clinical Summary. Phaeohyphomycetes often infect people who are not overtly immunosuppressed. However, immunosuppression does increase the risk of infection with less commonly pathogenic phaeohyphomycetes such as *Alternaria infectoria* and increases the risk for disseminated disease (67,68).

Subcutaneous phaeohyphomycosis typically presents as a solitary abscess or nodule on the extremity of an adult male. A history of trauma or a splinter can sometimes be elicited. The other major clinical forms of phaeohyphomycosis are infection of the paranasal sinuses and central nervous system.

Histopathology. Lesions of subcutaneous phaeohyphomycosis start as small, often stellate foci of suppurative granulomatous inflammation. The area of inflammation gradually enlarges and usually forms a single large cavity of pus, with an associated granulomatous reaction and a surrounding fibrous capsule, the so-called phaeohyphomycotic cyst (69,70) (Fig. 23-9A). The organisms are found within the cavity and at its edge, often within histiocytes (Fig. 23-9B). The hyphae often have irregularly placed branches and show constrictions around their septae that may cause them to resemble pseudohyphae or yeast forms, but true yeast forms are rare. Mycelia, if present, are more loosely arranged than the compact masses of hyphae seen in eumycetoma. Pigmentation is not always obvious and may be highlighted using the Fontana–Masson stain (65). Diligent search may identify an associated splinter.

Pathogenesis. The subcutaneous cystic type of phaeohyphomycosis is usually caused by *Phialophora gougerotii* (formerly called *Sporotrichum gougerotii*) (67,68). Less commonly, it is due to *Exophiala (Fonsecaea, Wangiella) dermatitidis.* Melanin is directly involved in the virulence of phaeohyphomycetes (65,71–73). Melanin is able to scavenge free radicals used by phagocytic cells to kill fungi, and melanin may also bind the hydrolytic enzymes used by phagocytic cells to lyse fungal cell membranes. Strains of these fungi that lack pigment demonstrate reduced virulence in mouse models (74–76). Non-dematiaceous strains have decreased resistance to fungicidal effects of the phagolysosome (65,70). These factors may also help to explain the virulence of phaeohyphomycetes in immunocompetent patients.

Differential Diagnosis. The organisms of phaeohyphomycosis can be distinguished from *Aspergillus* spp. because the latter have hyphae with relatively uniform diameter and regular dichotomous branching. Furthermore, disseminated aspergillosis

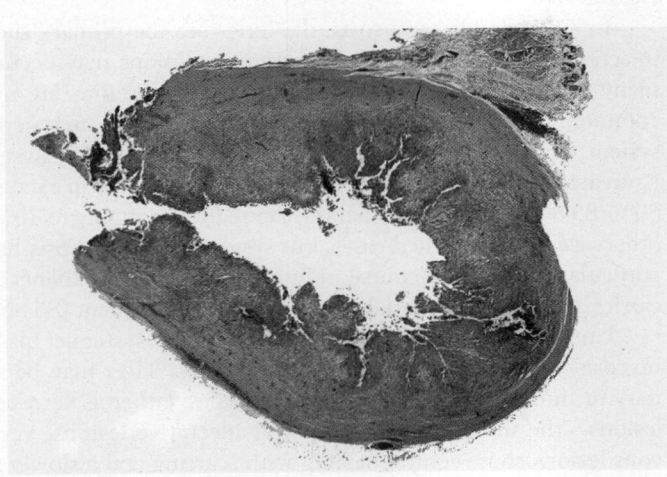
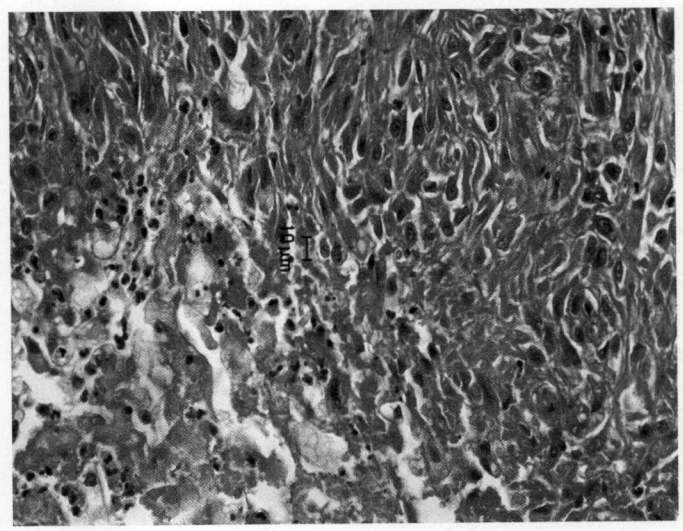

Figure 23-9 Phaeohyphomycosis. A: H&E staining shows a pseudocyst with a large central cavity and a fibrous capsule. B: H&E staining shows pigmented hyphal forms at the edge of cavity. (H&E, hematoxylin and eosin.)

is associated with vascular invasion, ischemic necrosis, and relatively less inflammation.

Principles of Management: Surgical debridement is necessary for the eradication of most infections with phaeohyphomycoses. In addition to surgical debridement, management includes systemic antifungal therapy with an azole such as posaconazole, and in life-threatening infections, amphotericin B.

CUTANEOUS ALTERNARIOSIS

Because the hyphae of *Alternaria* spp. are pigmented, alternariosis may also be considered a phaeohyphomycosis. Confirmation of *Alternariosis* with an in-house PCR assay has been reported, but molecular tests are not commonly used for primary diagnosis (72).

Clinical Summary. Alternaria spp. commonly colonize human skin but are generally nonpathogenic for humans. Cutaneous alternariosis may occur following trauma; by colonization of a preexisting lesion or rarely by hematologic spread, most commonly from pulmonary infection caused by inhalation of the organism (74–79). Patients with cutaneous alternariosis are often debilitated, immunocompromised, or receiving immunosuppressive therapy (79). Despite the increasing prevalence of

HIV infection, the disease is rare in patients with AIDS. Morphologically, the lesions of cutaneous alternariosis are so variable as to be nonspecific and include crusted ulcers, verrucous or granulomatous, and multilocular lesions and subcutaneous nodules (79).

Histopathology. Although fungi are found mainly in the deeper layers of the dermis and in the subcutaneous region in the hematogenous and the traumatogenic forms, they are localized predominantly in the epidermis in cases in which *Alternaria* colonizes preexisting lesions. The dermis shows a suppurative granulomatous reaction associated with variable pseudocarcinomatous epidermal hyperplasia and ulceration. Organisms may be present both as broad, branching, brown septate hyphae, 5 to 7 μm thick (Fig. 23-10), and as large, round-to-oval, often doubly contoured spores measuring 3 to 10 μm in diameter (79). The spores may be seen both lying free in the tissue and within macrophages and giant cells. There may be intraepidermal microabscesses with hyphae in the stratum corneum and stratum spinosum. The hyphae and spores stain deeply with PAS or silver methenamine.

Principles of Management: Management typically includes surgical debridement and medical management with an azole such as itraconazole.

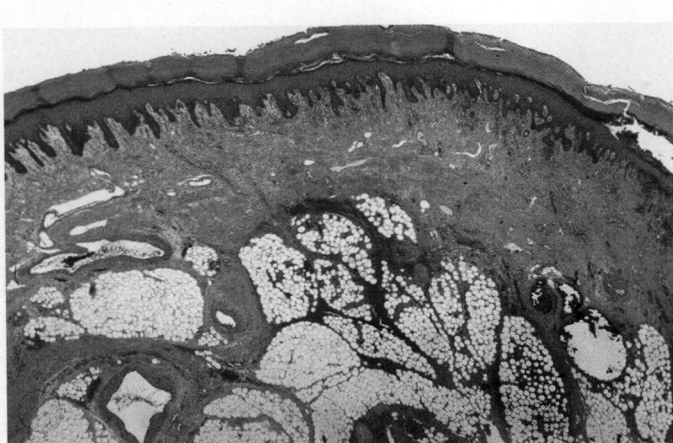
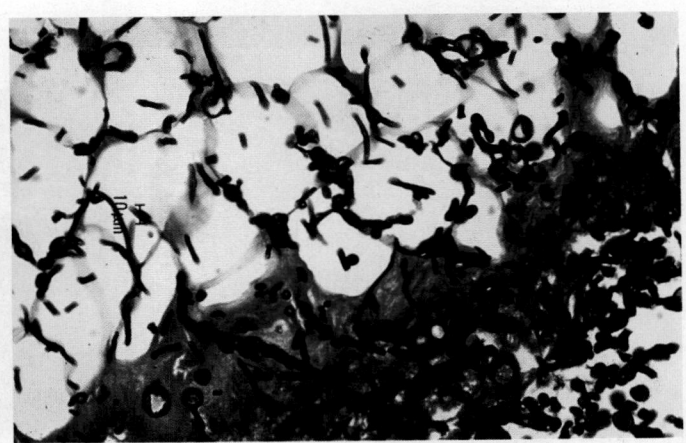

Figure 23-10 Alternariosis. A: H&E staining shows a mixed inflammatory infiltrate in the deep dermis and subcutaneous fat. B: GMS staining shows broad, branching hyphae. (GMS, Gomori methenamine silver; H&E, hematoxylin and eosin.)

NORTH AMERICAN BLASTOMYCOSIS

Clinical Summary. North American blastomycosis, caused by *Blastomyces dermatitidis,* occurs in three forms: primary cutaneous inoculation blastomycosis, pulmonary blastomycosis, and systemic blastomycosis (80–82).

Primary cutaneous inoculation blastomycosis is very rare and occurs almost exclusively as a laboratory or autopsy room infection. It starts at the site of injury on a hand or wrist as an indurated, ulcerated, chancriform solitary lesion. Lymphangitis and lymphadenitis may develop in the affected arm. Small nodules may be present along the involved lymph vessel. Spontaneous healing takes place within a few weeks or months (82–84).

Pulmonary blastomycosis, the usual route of acquisition of the infection, may be asymptomatic or may produce mild to moderately severe, acute pulmonary signs, such as fever, chest pain, cough, and hemoptysis. The pulmonary lesions either resolve or progress to chronic pulmonary blastomycosis with cavity formation. In rare instances, acute pulmonary blastomycosis is accompanied by erythema nodosum (82). Occasionally, however, cutaneous lesions are the only clinical manifestation after pulmonary infection. This phenomenon of a benign systemic disease presenting with cutaneous lesions may also be seen rarely after infection with coccidioidomycosis, cryptococcosis, histoplasmosis, and sporotrichosis. In the benign systemic form of blastomycosis with only cutaneous lesions, the lesions usually are on the face and are of the verrucous type.

In systemic blastomycosis, the lungs are the primary site of infection. Granulomatous and suppurative lesions may occur in many different organs; but aside from the lungs, they are most commonly found in the skin, followed by the bones, male genital system, oral and nasal mucosa, and the central nervous system. Untreated systemic blastomycosis has a mortality rate in excess of 80% (83,84). Antimycotic therapy can reduce mortality to 10% in otherwise uncomplicated cases, but systemic blastomycosis has a particularly aggressive course in immunosuppressed patients and carries at least a 30% mortality rate even with treatment (85,86).

Cutaneous lesions are very common in systemic blastomycosis, occurring in about 70% of patients. They may be solitary or numerous. They occur in two types: either as verrucous lesions—the more common type—or ulcerative lesions. Verrucous lesions show central healing with scarring and a slowly advancing, raised, verrucous border that is beset by a large number of pustules or small, crusted abscesses. Ulcerative lesions begin as pustules and rapidly develop into ulcers with a granulating base. In addition, subcutaneous abscesses may occur; they usually develop as an extension of bone lesions. Lesions of the oral or nasal mucosa may present either as ulcers or heaped-up masses of friable tissue. In some instances, they are contiguous with cutaneous lesions (87,88). An unusual early cutaneous manifestation of systemic blastomycosis is a pustular eruption that may be widespread (87) or largely acral in distribution (88) (Fig. 23-11A).

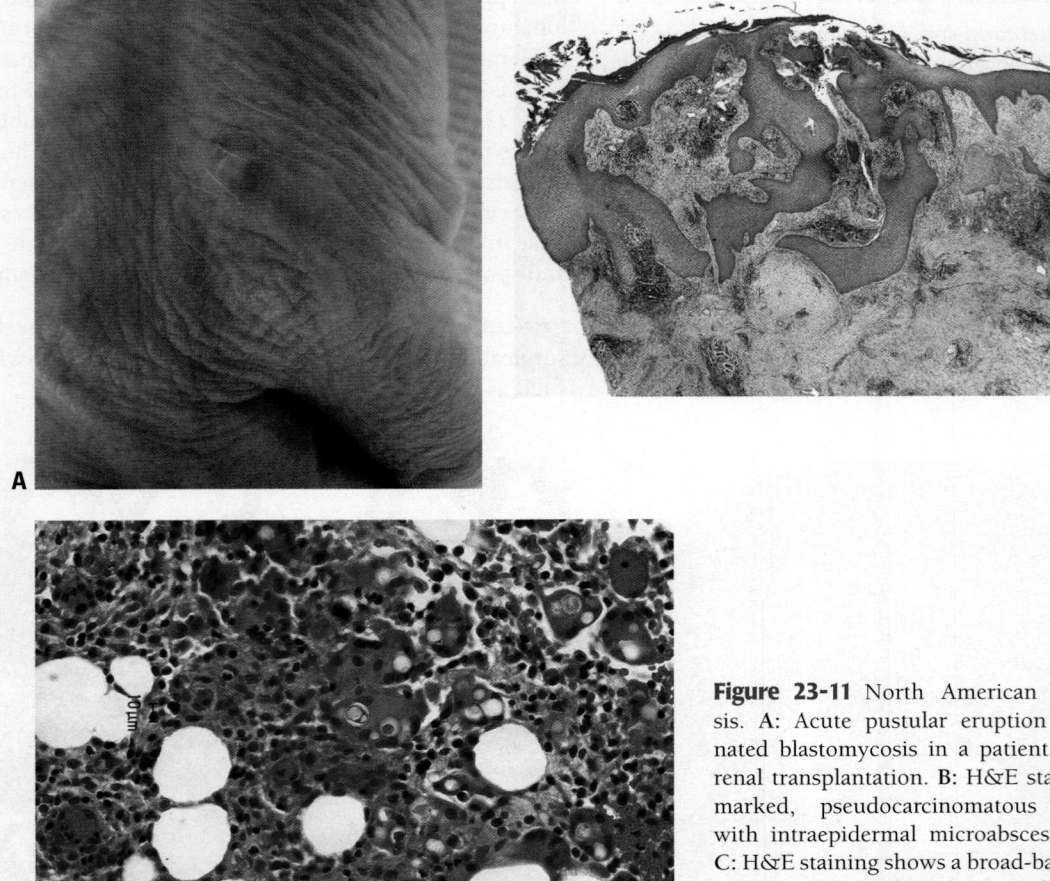

Figure 23-11 North American blastomycosis. **A:** Acute pustular eruption of disseminated blastomycosis in a patient with recent renal transplantation. **B:** H&E staining shows marked, pseudocarcinomatous hyperplasia with intraepidermal microabscess formation. **C:** H&E staining shows a broad-based budding spore in multinucleated giant cell. (H&E, hematoxylin and eosin.)

Histopathology. Early lesions of blastomycosis demonstrate a dermal inflammatory infiltrate of polymorphonuclear leukocytes with numerous organisms. After a few weeks, occasional giant cells may be seen. Later, a verrucous histologic pattern with pseudocarcinomatous hyperplasia is characteristic (Fig. 23-11B). The regional lymph nodes show a granulomatous reaction with numerous giant cells, in which the organisms are predominantly located.

A biopsy from the active border of a verrucous lesion will best demonstrate diagnostic histopathology. There is a considerable downward proliferation of the epidermis, often amounting to pseudocarcinomatous hyperplasia. Intraepidermal abscesses often are present. Occasionally, multinucleated giant cells are completely enclosed by the proliferating epidermis. The dermis is permeated by a polymorphous infiltrate. Neutrophils usually are present in large numbers and form small abscesses (83,84). Multinucleated giant cells are scattered throughout the dermis. Usually, they lie alone and not within groups of epithelioid cells. Occasionally, there are tuberculoid formations, although without evidence of caseation necrosis. In ulcerative lesions, the dermal changes are the same as in the verrucous lesions, but the epidermis is absent.

The spores of *B. dermatitidis* are found in histologic sections often only after a diligent search, usually among clusters of neutrophils or within giant cells (Fig. 23-11C). One or several spores may lie within a giant cell, where they are easily spotted even in H&E-stained sections. Unstained, the spores resemble small, round holes punched out of the cytoplasm of the giant cells. On high magnification, the spores are seen to have a thick wall, which gives them a double-contoured appearance. They measure 8 to 15 μm in diameter (average, 10 μm). Occasionally, spores show a single broad-based bud. As in most fungal infections, organisms are better visualized in sections stained with the PAS reaction or with methenamine silver than in routinely stained sections.

Pathogenesis. The diagnosis of *B. dermatitidis* is based on finding physical evidence of the organism because reliable serologic tests are not available and clinical examinations are nonspecific. Fine-needle aspiration or wet prep of wound fluid fixed in 95% alcohol and stained with the Papanicolaou stain is a rapid means to find diagnostic broad-based budding forms (89,90). Also of great value is the demonstration of the spores of *B. dermatitidis* in tissue sections either by direct immunofluorescence (91) or by immunoperoxidase (92). The required antiserum is prepared in rabbits with pure cultures of fungi and is conjugated either with fluorescein isothiocyanate or with horseradish peroxidase. The antiserum can be applied to fresh as well as to formalin-fixed, paraffin-embedded tissue sections. Prior staining with H&E does not interfere with the procedure.

Corresponding antisera are valuable also for the demonstration of the spores of *Sporothrix schenckii*, *Cryptococcus neoformans*, *Candida albicans*, *Candida tropicalis*, *Candida krusei*, *Aspergillus*, and *Histoplasma capsulatum* (93).

Differential Diagnosis. The verrucous lesions of systemic blastomycosis must be differentiated from other deep fungal infections, tuberculosis verrucosa cutis, halogenodermas, and squamous cell carcinoma. Mucicarmine staining, which highlights the capsule of *Cryptococcus neoformans*, allows its differentiation from the spores of *B. dermatitidis*, and the narrow-necked budding forms of *H. capsulatum* can be distinguished from the broader-based buds of *B. dermatitidis* without

special stains. Tuberculosis verrucosa cutis shows no spores in the tissue, the number of neutrophils is smaller, and areas of caseation necrosis are usually present. Halogenodermas may be difficult to differentiate from a deep fungal infection without obvious organisms, but the presence of intraepidermal abscesses, a mixed dermal inflammatory infiltrate, and multinucleated giant cells is usually sufficient to rule out squamous cell carcinoma. Keratoacanthoma shares morphologic features with blastomycosis, including a verrucous architecture and intraepidermal abscesses. However, keratoacanthoma has a high degree of keratinization, a glassy appearance of the keratinocyte cytoplasms, and an abrupt transition between the lesion and adjacent uninvolved epidermis.

Principles of Management: Evaluation of the extent of systemic involvement including the lungs is mandatory. Treatment is based on the extent of involvement and includes systemic antifungal therapy.

PARACOCCIDIOIDOMYCOSIS

Paracoccidioidomycosis, also called *South American blastomycosis* because it occurs almost exclusively in South and Central America, is a chronic granulomatous disease caused by *Paracoccidioides brasiliensis* (94–97). Although the diagnosis of *Paracoccidioides* infection can often be made clinically, laboratory tests are necessary for confirmation. The classic "marine's wheel" seen in histologic sections or cultures is pathognomonic in the proper clinical context, but molecular diagnostic tests are increasingly complementing standard assays in routine practice. Recently, taxonomic changes driven by whole-genome sequencing of *Paracoccidioides* have highlighted the need for a better definition of species boundaries to better ascertain *Paracoccidioides* taxonomy and to help identify cryptic agents. On the other hand, several PCR-based methods can detect polymorphisms in *Paracoccidioides* DNA and thus support limited species identification (98).

Clinical Summary. *Paracoccidioides brasiliensis* almost always gains entrance into the human body through inhalation and infects the lungs, where there is a subclinical infection that is not easily recognized. The typical patient with clinical disease is an adult male with an indolent, slowly progressive course. The first clinical manifestation is usually lesions in the oropharynx and on the gingivae. The lesions in the mouth begin as papules and nodules that then ulcerate. Subsequently, extensive granulomatous, ulcerated lesions develop in the mouth, nose, larynx, and pharynx. Extensive cervical lymphadenopathy develops, with suppuration of some of the lymph nodes. The oral lesions may extend to the neighboring skin, with the formation of similar granulomatous, ulcerated lesions around the mouth and nose (80,81).

Through both lymphatic and hematogenous spread, the disease may subsequently involve lymph nodes, both subcutaneous and visceral, and the lower gastrointestinal tract. In cases with wide dissemination, the lungs are clinically involved, presenting a picture greatly resembling chronic pulmonary tuberculosis (94,95). Adrenal insufficiency owing to destruction of the adrenal glands, uncommon in other systemic mycoses except histoplasmosis, is not infrequent (92). Rarely, widely scattered cutaneous lesions resulting from hematogenous spread are observed during the stage of dissemination. The lesions may be papular, pustular, nodular, papillomatous, or ulcerated (96,97).

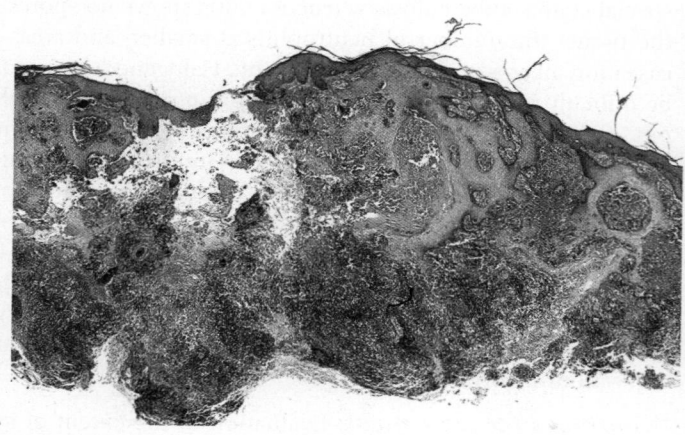
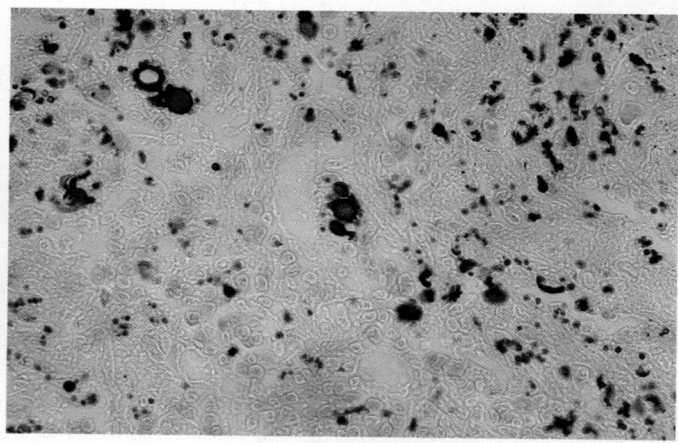

Figure 23-12 Paracoccidioidomycosis. **A:** H&E staining shows marked pseudocarcinomatous epidermal hyperplasia with microabscess formation and a mixed dermal infiltrate. **B:** GMS staining shows variably-sized yeast, some with multiple buds. (GMS, Gomori methenamine silver; H&E, hematoxylin and eosin.)

The disease develops and disseminates more rapidly in children and is then termed the *subacute progressive juvenile form* (94). Although experience is limited, it appears that there is little effect on the course of paracoccidioidomycosis in early HIV infection but that HIV patients with severe immunosuppression are at risk for a more fulminant course (99).

Histopathology. Examination of cutaneous or mucosal lesions reveals a granulomatous infiltrate showing epithelioid and giant cells in association with an acute inflammatory infiltrate and abscess formation (97,100). Spores may lie within giant cells or free in the infiltrate, especially in the abscesses. They are best demonstrated with the PAS reaction or methenamine silver. Pseudoepitheliomatous hyperplasia may be marked (Fig. 23-12A).

Many of the spores present in the tissue show only single, usually narrow-based buds or no buds at all. In the rare spores with multiple budding, peripheral buds are distributed over the whole surface of the ball-shaped fungus cell (Fig. 23-12B). Because of the protrusion of the peripheral buds, such yeast cells in cross sections have the appearance of a marine pilot's wheel. Whereas nonbudding or singly budding spores measure 6 to 20 µm in diameter, spores with multiple budding may measure up to 60 µm in size.

Differential Diagnosis. B. dermatitidis and *Cryptococcus neoformans* may be difficult to distinguish from *Paracoccidioides* when only single budding organisms are seen. North American blastomycosis is distinguished by its thick refractile wall and broad-based blastospores. The capsule of *Cryptococcus neoformans* stains with mucicarmine and is thus specifically identified.

Principles of Management: Paracoccidioidomycosis is the only endemic infection for which sulfa drugs are a therapeutic option. Treatment should continue until clinical and mycologic responses are noted. Amphotericin B and azole antifungals are also therapeutic options. Patients are often malnourished and/or anemic and correction of these predisposing factors should be prioritized.

LACAZIOSIS

Clinical Summary. Lacaziosis, formerly called lobomycosis, is a zoonotic mycosis caused by *Lacazia loboi* (101–103). *Lacazia loboi* may infect humans and dolphins; it is endemic in the

countries on the Atlantic and Indian oceans and in the Pacific Ocean of the Japanese coast. Lacaziosis is an extremely indolent fungal infection characterized by asymptomatic, usually smooth, nodular lesions that resemble keloids on the ear, face, or extremity. The lesions may coalesce to form plaques but generally are limited to one area. Although the lesions persist, the condition is limited to the skin, except for occasional involvement of a regional lymph node (97,101). The infection, which is probably caused by a minor local injury, occurs sporadically in the South American tropics and Panama (102). *Lacazia loboi* may infect humans and dolphins; it is endemic in the countries on the Atlantic and the Indian Ocean and in the Pacific Ocean of the Japanese coast (103). Molecular diagnostic studies are very uncommon.

Histopathology. The dermis shows an extensive infiltrate of macrophages and large giant cells separated from a usually atrophic epidermis by a grenz zone. Scattered lymphocytes and plasma cells are present, but neutrophils are not typically present. Numerous fungus spores lie both within these cells and outside of them, and because the fungus does not stain with H&E, there may be so many unstained areas that the section may have a sievelike appearance (Fig. 23-13).

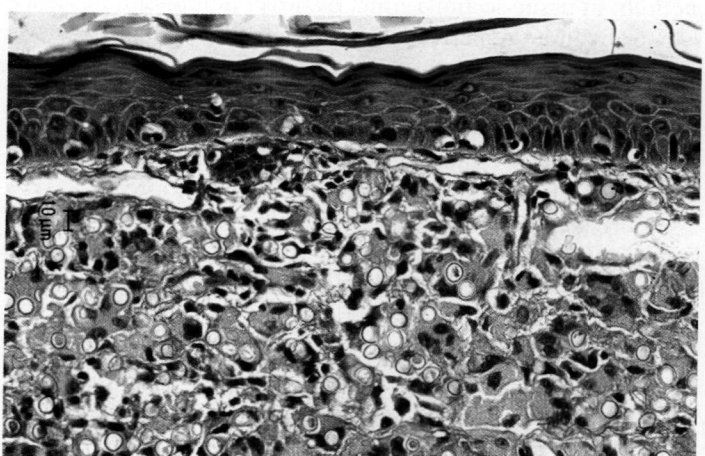

Figure 23-13 Lacaziosis (formally lobomycosis). A diffuse dermal infiltrate of multinucleated giant cells containing spores is present beneath a flattened epidermis (H&E stain). (H&E, hematoxylin and eosin.)

On staining with the PAS reaction or methenamine silver, the fungus spores average 10 μm in diameter. They possess a thick capsule, about 1 μm in thickness, with a tip that gives the organisms a distinctive "lemon-like" appearance. The spores occasionally show single budding (98) and often form single chains joined together by small, tubular bridges (101).

Pathogenesis. The macrophages contain abundant PAS-positive granular material that appears to consist of fragments of fungal capsules, indicating that the host macrophages are unable to digest the glycoproteins in the capsules (101–104).

Principles of Management: Surgical debridement is a mandatory component of treatment. Medical therapy has a limited role, though an azole such as itraconazole may be used as an adjunct, particularly in cases where the disease is more than localized.

CHROMOMYCOSIS

Chromomycosis is a slowly progressive cutaneous mycosis caused by pigmented (dematiaceous) fungi that occur as round, nonbudding forms in tissue sections (105). Inasmuch as budding is absent, the designation chromo*blasto*mycosis is somewhat inappropriate. In the past, the related term *chromomycosis* has also been used for cutaneous infections as well as for subcutaneous and cerebral infections by dematiaceous fungi in which hyphal forms almost always predominate. These two latter types of infections are clinically and histologically distinct and usually are classified as phaeohyphomycoses. Molecular studies are required to precisely identify pigmented fungi because phenotypic characteristics of these fungi are poorly informative (106). Partial ribosomal DNA large-subunit sequences are sufficiently conserved to show relationships at the ordinal or family level.

Chromomycosis is most often caused by one of seven closely related species: *Phialophora verrucosa, Fonsecaea pedrosoi, Fonsecaea compactum, Exophiala (Fonsecaea, Wangiella) jeanselmei, Exophiala spinifera, Rhinocladiella aquaspersa,* and *Cladosporium carrionii* may each produce chromomycosis (107). These fungi are saprophytes and thus can be found growing in soil, decaying vegetation, or rotten wood in subtropical and tropical countries.

Clinical Summary. The primary lesion is thought to develop as a result of traumatic implantation of the fungus into the skin (108). The cutaneous lesions generally arise on the lower extremities and are variably pruritic, papular, nodular, verrucous, or plaquelike lesions. Although some of the lesions heal with scarring, new ones may appear in the vicinity as a result of spreading of the fungus along superficial lymphatic vessels or autoinoculation (105,109). Lymphatic disruption with elephantiasis may occur.

Hematogenous dissemination may cause extensive cutaneous lesions, but it is a rare event, even in immunocompromised persons, and the disease is not as aggressive as other systemic fungal infections that secondarily involve the skin (109–111).

Histopathology. Cutaneous chromomycosis resembles North American blastomycosis, in that both demonstrate a lichenoid–granulomatous inflammatory pattern. In chromomycosis, there is pseudocarcinomatous epidermal hyperplasia and an extensive dermal infiltrate composed of many epithelioid histiocytes (105). Other components of the infiltrate include multinucleated giant cells; small abscesses and clusters of neutrophils; and variable numbers of lymphocytes, plasma cells, and eosinophils. Tuberculoid formations may be present, but caseation necrosis is absent.

Fungi are found within giant cells as well as free in the tissue, especially in the abscesses. They appear as conspicuous, dark brown, thick-walled, ovoid, or spherical spores varying in sizes from 6 to 12 μm that are likened to "copper pennies" and that may lie either singly or in chains or clusters (Fig. 23-14). Because of their brown pigmentation, the spores can be seen easily without the use of special stains. Reproduction is by intracellular wall formation and septation, not by budding, and cross walls can be seen in some of the spores. In cases demonstrating marked hyperplasia of the epidermis, fungal spores can be seen within microabscesses or giant cells, as in North American blastomycosis. Transepidermal elimination of fungal spores may be observed, resulting in clinically visible black dots (112,113).

Pathogenesis. Although percutaneous inoculation of the fungus is widely accepted as the mode of infection, the fact that the cutaneous manifestations show no chancriform syndrome

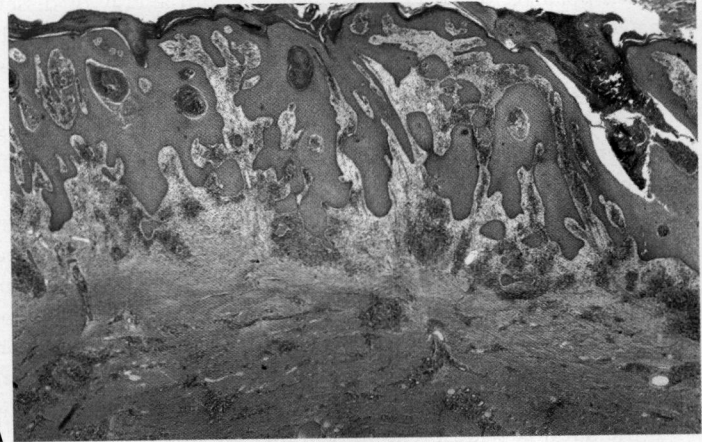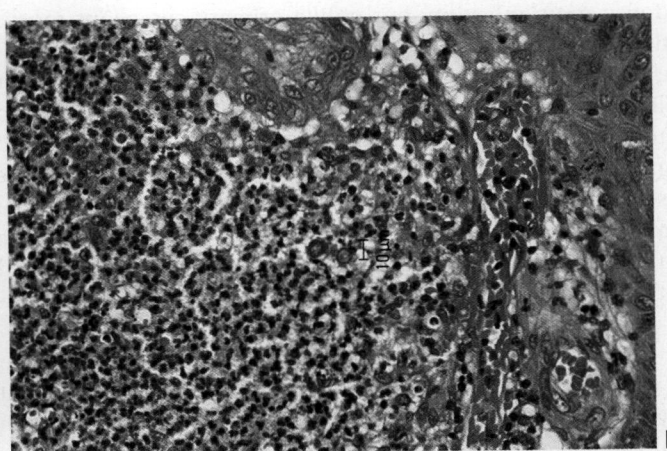

Figure 23-14 Chromoblastomycosis. **A:** H&E staining shows pseudocarcinomatosiss epidermal hyperplasia with microabscess formation and a mixed inflammatory infiltrate. **B:** Pigmented spores (adjacent to scale marker) resembling "copper pennies" are surrounded by a neutrophilic infiltrate (H&E stain). (H&E, hematoxylin and eosin.)

but rather a granulomatous infiltrate resembling that of North American blastomycosis suggests that the cutaneous lesions of chromomycosis may arise by hematogenous dissemination from a silent primary pulmonary focus. Although this view is supported by occasional reports of hematogenous dissemination and by the observation of multiple areas of calcification in the chest x-ray film of a patient with chromomycosis (109), convincing evidence is lacking. In support of the concept that cutaneous inoculation causes cutaneous chromomycosis, pigmented fungal elements are not infrequently found on embedded wood splinters associated with a foreign-body reaction, and have been found in direct contact with the surrounding dermis in two patients (110,111), one of whom developed classic cutaneous chromomycosis caused by *F. pedrosoi* after trauma with a tree branch containing the same organisms.

Principles of Management: Most cases of chromomycosis are chronic, indolent infections and eradication may be difficult even with prolonged therapy. A multiagent approach including surgical debridement, physical agents such as cryotherapy and systemic antifungal therapy may therefore be employed, although no one strategy is standard or universally effective.

COCCIDIOIDOMYCOSIS

Coccidioidomycosis, also known as *valley fever*, is caused by the dimorphic fungus *Coccidioides immitis* (114,115).

Clinical Summary. Like blastomycosis, coccidioidomycosis occurs in three forms: primary cutaneous inoculation coccidioidomycosis, pulmonary coccidioidomycosis, and systemic coccidioidomycosis. This soil-dwelling organism is endemic in the southwestern United States, especially in the San Joaquin and Sacramento valleys, southern Arizona, and Mexico (114,115). The vast majority of infections with *Coccidioidomycosis* result from inhalation of the aerosolized arthrospores. Approximately 60% of those infected are asymptomatic, and of the symptomatic patients, 90% to 99% experience only mild flulike symptoms.

Primary cutaneous inoculation coccidioidomycosis is very rare. In a few instances—as in primary cutaneous inoculation blastomycosis—it has occurred as a laboratory or an autopsy room infection; but unlike primary cutaneous inoculation blastomycosis, it has also been found as a naturally occurring infection through injuries by contaminated thorns or splinters (116–119). A tender, ulcerated nodule forms within 1 to 3 weeks at the site of inoculation and may enlarge into a granulomatous, ulcerated plaque. This is followed, as in the case of accidental inoculation with *B. dermatitidis*, by regional lymphangitis and lymphadenitis. Healing usually takes place within a few months, but meningitis developed in one reported patient, requiring prolonged intrathecal treatment with amphotericin B (114).

Pulmonary coccidioidomycosis is the most common form of the infection; epidemiologic skin test studies suggest that between 30% and 90% of the population in the southwestern United States have been infected (118–120). The fungus is resident in the soil of these arid or semiarid areas, and arthrospores are inhaled by the host when the soil is disturbed. Most immunocompetent infected individuals are asymptomatic, although about 40% will develop transient symptoms of an acute respiratory infection. The development of erythema nodosum is not uncommon, and most individuals recover without serious sequelae. In 2% to 8% of cases, however, the pulmonary lesions progress to chronic disease with cavity formation before finally healing.

Systemic coccidioidomycosis follows the primary pulmonary infection in only about 1 in 10,000 cases in otherwise immunocompetent whites. However, Mexicans are about 5 times, blacks 25 times, and Filipinos 175 times more likely to acquire systemic disease than whites, which has a mortality rate of about 50% when untreated (114). Studies of this difference have focused on human leukocyte antigen (HLA) genes, which produce molecules responsible for antigen presentation to T cells, the portion of the immune system important in the elimination of fungi. Some studies have shown HLA subtypes A9 and B5 as well as ABO blood group B to be associated with disseminated coccidioidomycosis, and each occurs with greater frequency in blacks and Filipinos than in whites. The risk of dissemination and a fatal outcome is also greater in HIV-infected patients, particularly those with AIDS (121–123). Disseminated coccidioidomycosis may occasionally represent the first manifestation of AIDS. Immunosuppressive therapy may cause activation of a latent pulmonary infection of coccidioidomycosis. Dissemination of the infection after iatrogenic immunosuppression is frequently explosive and may be fatal. Therefore, all patients with a history of travel or residence in endemic areas should receive a coccidioidin skin test and have a chest roentgenogram before immunosuppressive therapy is initiated. In systemic coccidioidomycosis, many organs, especially the meninges, lungs, bones, and lymph nodes, may be involved (124). Coccidioidal fungemia often occurs in severe, acute forms of systemic coccidioidomycosis and is associated with a high mortality (121,124,125).

The coccidioidin skin test, which consists of the intradermal injection of 0.1 mL of a 1:100 dilution of coccidioidin, is of value in diagnosing early infection. The test result changes from negative to positive within a few weeks of the primary pulmonary infection, even before a blood test would be positive. Patients with erythema multiforme or nodose lesions are exquisitely sensitive to coccidioidin, and even higher dilutions have been recommended for use in such cases (125). The test is helpful when positive; however, those patients with anergy or disseminated disease tend to have a persistently negative skin test (114). Histopathology and tissue culture are still the leading diagnostic methods for cutaneous coccidioidomycosis; but molecular techniques such as PCR targeting 18S rDNA in fixed tissue and *in situ* by hybridization with labeled nucleic acid probes are increasingly being used to differentiate between species (114).

Cutaneous lesions occur in 15% to 20% of cases of systemic coccidioidomycosis. They may consist of verrucous papules, nodules, or plaques, or of subcutaneous abscesses, which may break through the skin to form draining sinuses. One or a few cutaneous nodules or plaques may occasionally be the only clinical manifestation of systemic coccidioidomycosis, heralding a relatively good prognosis (123,124). A rare manifestation is the sudden widespread appearance of small pustules on an erythematous base (125), just as described in North American blastomycosis.

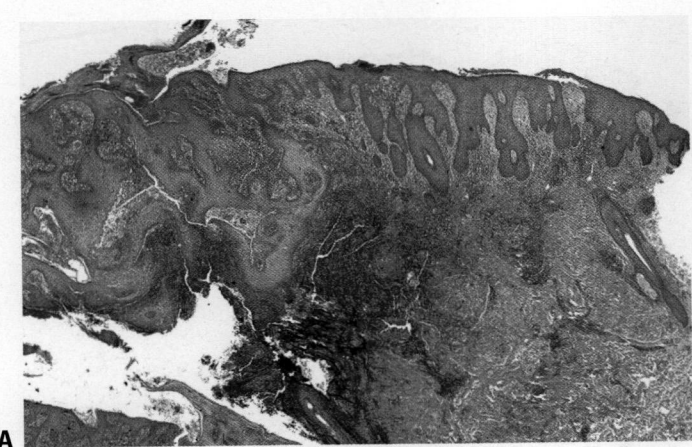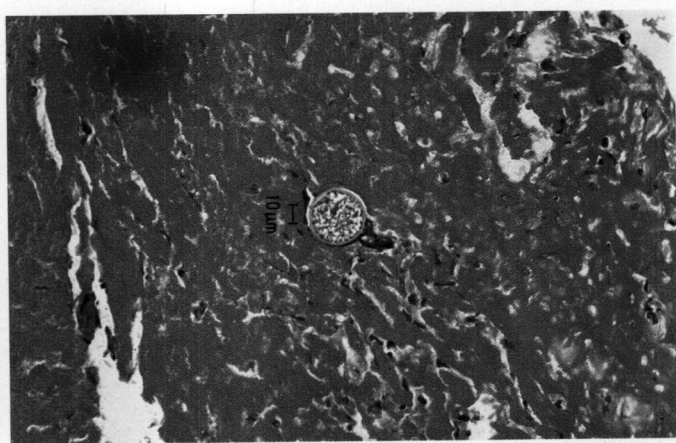

Figure 23-15 Coccidioidomycosis. **A:** The low-power pattern is similar to that of North American blastomycosis with pseudocarcinomatous epidermal hyperplasia and a mixed inflammatory infiltrate (H&E stain). **B:** A large, round, thick-walled spore with granular cytoplasm is present in a background of necrotic tissue (H&E stain). (H&E, hematoxylin and eosin.)

Histopathology. In primary cutaneous inoculation coccidioidomycosis, a dense dermal inflammatory infiltrate of neutrophils, eosinophils, lymphoid cells, and plasma cells with an occasional giant cell can be observed. Small abscesses may be seen. Spores, and in some cases also hyphae, are present. The regional lymph nodes show a well-developed granulomatous reaction consisting of epithelioid and giant cells. Spores are found within and outside the giant cells.

The verrucous nodules and plaques of the skin in systemic coccidioidomycosis histologically resemble those of North American blastomycosis (Fig. 23-15A). However, they show less of a tendency toward abscess formation, and caseation necrosis may occur. The causative organisms are found as spores, free in the tissue and within multinucleated giant cells, and, as a rule, in large numbers.

The subcutaneous abscesses show a central area of necrosis surrounded by a granulomatous infiltrate that is tuberculoid in type and composed of lymphoid cells, plasma cells, epithelioid cells, and some giant cells. Numerous spores are present extracellularly as well as intracellularly in the giant cells. The pustules seen in a few cases show the presence of spores within them. The nodose skin lesions occurring in primary pulmonary coccidioidomycosis have the same histologic appearance as those in idiopathic erythema nodosum (126,127).

The spores of *Coccidioides immitis* vary in size from 10 to 80 μm (Fig. 23-15B), with the average size being about 40 μm. Thus, the fungi of *Coccidioides* are much larger than those of *Blastomyces*, *Cryptococcus*, and *Phialophora*. The spores are round and thick-walled and have a granular cytoplasm. Multiplication takes place by the formation of endospores, which may be seen lying inside the larger spores. The endospores are released into the tissue by rupture of the spore wall. Endospores may measure up to 10 μm in diameter.

Principles of Management: Management of infection includes defining the extent of the infection and host factors that may predispose to severe infection. Patients with acute pulmonary infection in the absence of risk factors for complications may only require periodic assessment to ensure resolution. In contrast, patients with extensive disease and/or immunosuppression or other predisposing factors require systemic antifungal therapy (usually azoles), surgical debridement, or a combination of both.

CRYPTOCOCCOSIS

Cryptococcosis is an infection caused by the yeast *Cryptococcus neoformans*, which occurs throughout much of the world.

Clinical Summary. Cryptococcus neoformans is found in the excreta of birds, mainly pigeons and chickens, and in soil contaminated by them. The yeast is spread by aerosol, and transient colonization of the respiratory tract and skin of humans is not rare (128). Primary cutaneous (inoculation) cryptococcosis is extremely rare (129). The organism generally enters the body through the respiratory tract, where it can cause symptomatic or asymptomatic infection, either of which may be followed by hematogenous spread (130,131). Although the clinical disease occurs in some apparently normal individuals, it usually develops in immunocompromised hosts—especially those with AIDS (132,133) (Fig. 23-16A)—in patients taking corticosteroids (132,133), and in patients with hematopoietic malignancies (134,135) or sarcoidosis (135–137).

Meningitis is the most common clinical manifestation of systemic infection. Symptom onset is insidious. Patients report a dull headache, most commonly with little fever until late in the disease. Other signs of meningeal irritation such as nuchal rigidity are absent. In addition, there may be osseous lesions and involvement of the kidneys and prostate. Cutaneous lesions are found in 10% to 15% of the cases of systemic cryptococcosis (138). In rare instances, lesions of the oral mucosa also occur (134). Without adequate treatment, mortality with the systemic form is 70% to 80%; untreated cerebromeningeal cryptococcosis is almost invariably fatal. Cryptococcemia is an extremely grave prognostic sign (130,138).

In some instances of systemic cryptococcosis, central nervous system involvement is not seen, and there are only one or a few lesions in the skin, lymph nodes, bones, or eyes. In cases in which only cutaneous lesions are present, the disease may take a benign course, ending with healing of the lesions, even without treatment (139,140). However, cutaneous lesions may be the presenting sign of systemic cryptococcosis and may be followed by wide dissemination of the disease with a fatal ending (130,138).

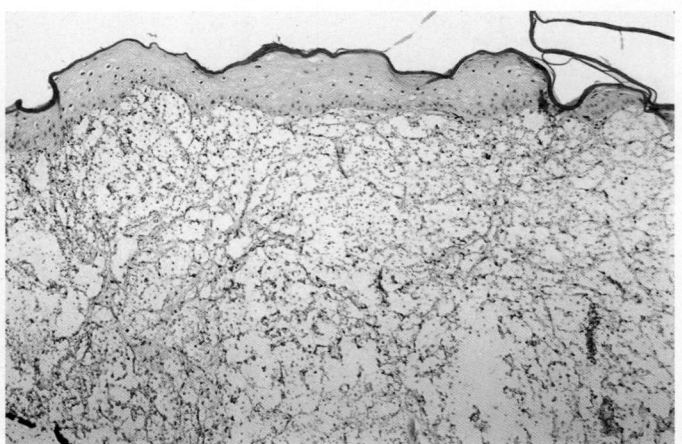

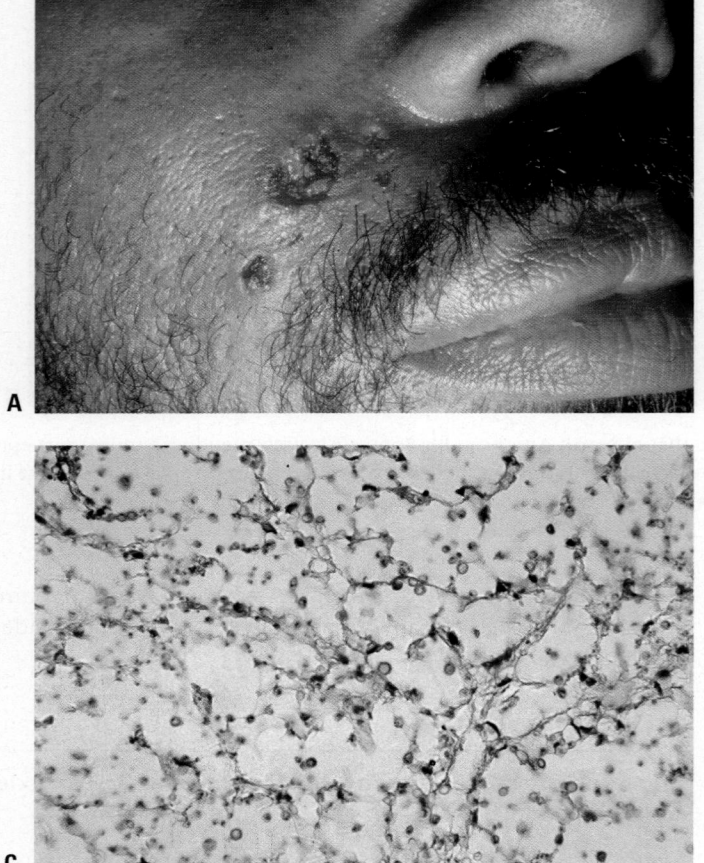

Figure 23-16 Cryptococcosis. **A:** Ulcerated papules and plaques of crytococcal infection in an HIV-positive male. **B:** H&E staining shows spores surrounded by wide capsules with relatively little inflammatory reaction. **C:** Spores, but not their capsules, can be visualized in routine stained sections (H&E stain). (H&E, hematoxylin and eosin.)

Cutaneous lesions are variable and may consist of papules, pustules, herpetiform vesicles, nodules, infiltrated plaques, subcutaneous swellings or abscesses, or ulcers (141). Lesions resembling those of molluscum contagiosum (umbilicated papules), Kaposi sarcoma, or acne have been described in patients with AIDS (142–144) (Fig. 23-16A). In infections limited to the skin, generally only one or possibly two lesions are present; but in cases with widespread systemic infection, there are often multiple cutaneous lesions (132,141).

Cryptococcal cellulitis is a variant form that may occasionally be limited to the skin. This form has an abrupt onset and spreads rapidly. There may be multiple sites of involvement. It is seen only in markedly immunosuppressed hosts, especially in renal transplant patients (145).

Histopathology. Two types of histologic reaction to infection with *Cryptococcus neoformans* may occur in the skin as well as elsewhere: gelatinous and granulomatous. Both types may be seen in the same skin lesion (130,133). Gelatinous lesions show numerous organisms in aggregates and only very little tissue reaction (Fig. 23-16B). In contrast, granulomatous lesions show a pronounced tissue reaction consisting of histiocytes, giant cells, lymphoid cells, and fibroblasts. Areas of necrosis may also be seen, and the organisms are present in a much smaller number than in gelatinous lesions, found mainly within giant cells and histiocytes or occasionally free in the tissue (146).

Cryptococcus neoformans, a round-to-ovoid spore, measures 4 to 12 μm in diameter in the gelatinous reaction but often only 2 to 4 μm in the granulomatous reaction (146) (Fig. 23-16C). The spore stains with the PAS reaction or methenamine silver

and shows a dark brown or black color with the Fontana–Masson stain, which completely disappears with melanin bleach (147). Like *B. dermatitidis*, it multiplies by budding. In the gelatinous reaction pattern, a broad capsule surrounds the fungus, and there is very little infiltration of inflammatory cells. The capsule does not stain with H&E or the PAS reaction; but because of the presence of acid mucopolysaccharides, it stains metachromatically purple with methylene blue, blue with Alcian blue (148), and red with mucicarmine. When the Alcian blue stain and PAS reaction are combined, the yeast cell stains red and the surrounding capsule blue. However, when the yeast cells do not form a capsule, an intense granulomatous inflammatory reaction of histiocytes, giant cells, lymphocytes, and fibroblasts is elicited (147). Diagnosis in these cases may be supported by Fontana–Masson staining, which stains the yeast cell wall brown (148).

Cryptococcal cellulitis shows nonspecific acute and chronic inflammation in which cryptococcal organisms can be demonstrated with the PAS and mucicarmine stains (145). PCR on skin biopsies, combined with laser capture microdissection, is a particularly sensitive but uncommon technique that has been used to confirm *Cryptococcus neoformans* infections (145).

Pathogenesis. Cryptococcus neoformans is inhaled as a relatively small, nonencapsulated organism measuring approximately 3 μm in diameter. Under favorable nutrient conditions in the human host, the size of the organism increases up to 12 μm, and a wide gelatinous capsule forms. The lack of a tissue reaction to encapsulated *Cryptococcus neoformans* is best explained by the fact that the thick capsule prevents contact of the organism with the host tissue and thus inhibits phagocytosis of the organism (146). Failure of the organism to form a capsule is probably the result of a defect in one of its metabolic pathways (147,148).

On electron microscopy, the mucinous capsule of *Cryptococcus neoformans* is seen to consist of radially arranged fibrillary material, with the fibrils intertwining and having a beaded appearance (149).

Ever since cases of cryptococcosis with only one or a few cutaneous lesions have been described, some authors have assumed that a purely cutaneous form of cryptococcosis produced by cutaneous inoculation exists (150). However, the fact that purely cutaneous lesions show no chancriform syndrome with regional lymphadenopathy speaks against the theory of primary inoculation of the skin (132). It has been recommended that all cases seeming to be purely cutaneous cryptococcosis should be considered potentially disseminated (150). Cultural studies should include the spinal fluid, sputum, prostatic fluid, and urine to rule out disseminated disease (151,152). Of note, there are multiple reports of cross-reactivity of *Cryptococcus* with unrelated fungi with the use of agglutination kits (153,154). Confirmation of a positive capsular antigen test with a second test helps to limit false positives.

Differential Diagnosis. In the granulomatous type of reaction, *Cryptococcus neoformans* may have no capsule, may be small with an average diameter of only 3 µm, and is found largely within macrophages and giant cells. Histologic differentiation from *B. dermatitidis* (which also reproduces by budding), *H. capsulatum*, and other fungi may then be difficult. However, only *Cryptococcus neoformans* stains deep brown or black with the Fontana–Masson stain (147,148).

Principles of Management: Treatment of Cryptococcal infection is a challenge with little recent drug development or definitive studies. However, if the patient's underlying disorder such as malignancy or HIV infection can be managed, then the infection can be controlled in the majority of patients with antifungal therapy tailored to their immune status and extent of involvement (155).

HISTOPLASMOSIS

Histoplasmosis is found throughout the world, but the largest endemic focus is in the central eastern United States, especially the Ohio and lower Mississippi river valleys (156).

Clinical Summary. Around 85% to 90% of the population in endemic areas have positive skin tests for histoplasmin. It has been estimated that 40 million people have had pulmonary infection with *H. capsulatum* and that there are 200,000 new cases annually in the United States (154,156).

Like blastomycosis and coccidioidomycosis, histoplasmosis may occur in three forms: primary cutaneous inoculation histoplasmosis, primary pulmonary histoplasmosis caused by inhalation, and disseminated histoplasmosis.

Primary cutaneous inoculation histoplasmosis, a very rare event, is benign and self-limited in duration. It generally occurs as a laboratory infection and presents as a chancriform syndrome, with a nodule or ulcer at the site of inoculation and associated lymphangitis and lymphadenitis (157–159).

Primary pulmonary histoplasmosis, the common form of infection, is usually asymptomatic, although acute pulmonary histoplasmosis with symptoms resembling those of influenza may develop in a minority of patients. Chronic pulmonary histoplasmosis usually occurs in patients with preexisting lung disease and may result in the formation of cavities. It develops in about 1 in 2,000 infections; resembles pulmonary tuberculosis in its symptoms; and may end fatally unless treated. Reactivation of pulmonary histoplasmosis following treatment with infliximab has been reported and should be considered when fever and pulmonary symptoms develop in these patients (160).

Before the advent of HIV, disseminated histoplasmosis developed in only 1 in 50,000 infections (161) and was usually found in infants, patients with lymphoma, or those receiving immunosuppressive treatment (161,162). Although not as frequent in the general AIDS population as coccidioidomycosis and cryptococcosis, disseminated histoplasmosis can be the most frequent opportunistic infection in AIDS patients living in highly endemic areas (163–166).

Disseminated histoplasmosis presents a variable clinical picture, depending on the degree of parasitization. Cases with severe degrees of parasitization (acute disseminated disease) occur principally in infants and immunosuppressed patients and may be fatal. There is often high, persistent fever and extensive involvement of the reticuloendothelial system with hepatosplenomegaly; anemia, leukocytopenia, and thrombocytopenia may also be seen. Cases with moderate degrees of parasitization (subacute disseminated disease) occur in both adults and infants, who if adequately treated may survive. Fever, hepatosplenomegaly, and bone marrow depression are mild or moderate. Adrenal involvement leading to adrenal insufficiency, as well as gastrointestinal ulceration, meningitis, and endocarditis, are common. Cases with mild degrees of parasitization (chronic disseminated disease) are associated with destructive focal lesions in a number of organs and occur almost exclusively in adults. There may or may not be fever, hepatosplenomegaly, bone marrow depression, adrenal insufficiency, meningitis, or endocarditis. In the chronic disseminated form, the response to treatment generally is good (167). If no cutaneous or oral lesions are present, the most useful diagnostic method is a bone marrow biopsy and occasionally biopsy of the liver or a palpable lymph node as well (168).

Cutaneous lesions occur in only 6% of patients with disseminated histoplasmosis but may rarely be the presenting sign (166–168). Cutaneous lesions occur in a wide variety of forms, none of which can be said to be characteristic. Most commonly, they consist of primary ulcers, often with annular, heaped-up borders (169,170). They may also consist of papules, nodules, or large plaquelike lesions. Papules may umbilicate, causing a resemblance to lesions of molluscum contagiosum (171). Lesions may be purpuric or crusted or may develop pustular caps and ulcerate (172). There may be tender, red nodules owing to panniculitis (173). A rare cutaneous manifestation is a generalized pruritic erythroderma (174). In addition, there may be a number of nonspecific cutaneous manifestations associated with histoplasmosis, including erythema nodosum and erythema multiforme.

In contrast to the rarity of cutaneous lesions, lesions of the oral mucosa occur in about half of all cases of disseminated histoplasmosis and are not infrequently the presenting sign of the disease (169,170). Lesions of the oral mucosa often start as painless papular swellings and usually ulcerate. The contiguous skin may also be involved. Biopsy of a mucosal or cutaneous lesion may be the most rapid method of arriving at a specific diagnosis of disseminated histoplasmosis and may allow for the rapid institution of lifesaving therapy as culture may require up to a 4-week incubation period (175). Diagnosis of histoplasmosis by detection of the internal transcribed spacer region of the fungal rRNA gene from a paraffin-embedded skin sample, from a dog, has been reported, but equivalent studies in human histoplasmosis have not been described (176).

Histopathology. The diagnostic feature in all types of cutaneous histoplasmosis is the presence of tiny 2- to 4-μm spores within the cytoplasm of macrophages and variably within giant cells (170,177). The spores of *H. capsulatum* are visualized in sections stained with H&E, Gram, or Giemsa (Fig. 23-17). They appear as round or oval bodies surrounded by a clear space that was originally interpreted as a capsule, giving rise to the name *H. capsulatum*. The spores, not including the clear space surrounding them, measure 2 to 4 μm in diameter. Silver impregnation stains and electron microscopic studies show that *H. capsulatum* does not possess a capsule and that the inner portion of the clear space represents the cell wall of the fungus and the clear space itself is filled with granular material that separates the cell wall of the fungus from the cytoplasm of the macrophage (176). On electron microscopy, it can be seen that each spore of *H. capsulatum*, including its halo, is located within a phagosome that is lined by a trilaminar membrane (176).

In acute disseminated histoplasmosis, lesions consist mostly of heavily parasitized histiocytes with relatively little surrounding tissue reaction. Cutaneous lesions in the chronic form of the disease tend to be composed of better-differentiated macrophages with fewer organisms (167). A suppurative granulomatous pattern may develop, especially in ulcerated lesions. There may be foci of necrosis, and giant cells may also be present. Although well-developed tubercles are characteristic of pulmonary histoplasmosis, they are unusual in the skin. Oral lesions, especially when ulcerated, may show a more mixed infiltrate with neutrophils and eosinophils.

Pathogenesis. H. capsulatum is a dimorphous fungus that grows in culture at temperatures below 35°C and on natural substrates in the soil as a mycelial fungus elaborating macroaleuriospores (8 to 16 μm) and microaleuriospores (2 to 5 μm). When inhaled, the latter sprout and transform into small budding yeasts that are 2 to 5 μm in diameter. In cultures at a temperature of 37°C, the organism also grows in the yeastlike form (177).

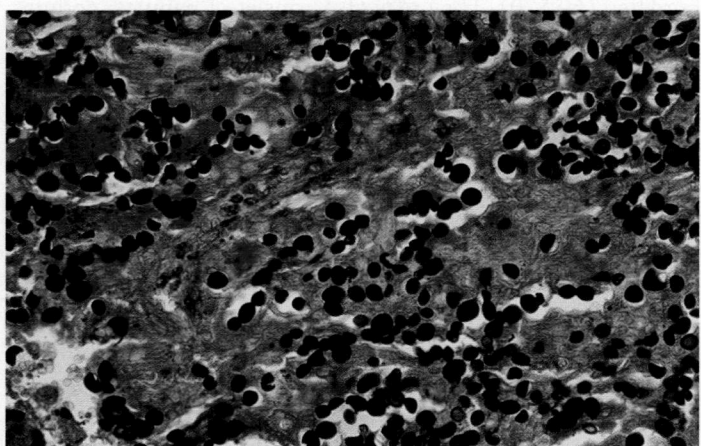

Figure 23-17 Histoplasmosis. Large spores of *H. capsulatum* var. *duboisii* are seen extracellularly and in giant cells (GMS stain). (GMS, Gomori methenamine silver.)

Differential Diagnosis. The histologic appearance of histoplasmosis, characterized by the presence of parasitized macrophages within a chronic inflammatory infiltrate, is much like that of rhinoscleroma, granuloma inguinale, and cutaneous leishmaniasis. *H. capsulatum* is the only pathogen to parasitize macrophages that stains with the usual fungal stains, such as the PAS reaction and methenamine silver. *Histoplasmosis* does not possess a true capsule and can thus be distinguished from *Cryptococcus neoformans*, particularly when the latter is noted to stain black with the Fontana–Masson stain.

Principles of Management: Certain forms of histoplasmosis cause life-threatening illness whereas others cause no symptoms or self-limited illnesses. Therefore, antifungal treatment depends on the extent of active involvement and patient's immune status. Prophylaxis of histoplasmosis is recommended for some immunosuppressed patients, particularly those living in endemic areas.

African Histoplasmosis

In addition to classical histoplasmosis caused by *H. capsulatum*, there is a form of histoplasmosis that is caused by *H. capsulatum* var. *duboisii* and that has been called *African histoplasmosis* because it occurs almost exclusively in Central Africa (178).

Clinical Summary. The portal of entry is not known. It usually occurs as a relatively indolent form involving the skin as well as the subcutaneous tissue, bones, and lymph nodes (178,179). This organism relatively rarely causes a disseminated form of disease that involves many internal organs and may be fatal, thus resembling more classical disseminated histoplasmosis (180).

The cutaneous lesions may be one, a few, or many. They consist of papules, nodules, and plaques that often ulcerate (181). There may be large, subcutaneous granulomas that develop into fluctuant, nontender abscesses (177). Purulent bone lesions may result in draining sinus tracts extending through the skin (178).

Histopathology. The cutaneous lesions show a dense, mixed cellular infiltrate containing numerous giant cells and scattered histiocytes, lymphocytes, and plasma cells. There are focal aggregates of neutrophils forming small abscesses (181). Numerous yeast cells, 8 to 15 μm in diameter, are present mainly in the giant cells and also in histiocytes and extracellularly (178).

Pathogenesis. Despite the fact that African histoplasmosis differs in its clinical character and in the size of the organism from classic histoplasmosis, it is clear that *H. capsulatum* and *Histoplasma duboisii* are variants of the same species, since after prolonged *in vitro* growth at 37°C, the small yeast cells of *H. capsulatum* can assume the same size as those of *H. duboisii* (178).

Principles of Management: Medical management is with antifungal therapy. Reports of HIV-infected individuals, including some with disseminated infection, are emerging. Outcomes have been favorable in a minority of patients.

SPOROTRICHOSIS

Surveys with the sporotrichin skin test show a positive reaction in up to 10% of the population in certain areas, suggesting that many infections with *S. schenckii* are minor or asymptomatic and not recognized clinically (182,183).

Clinical Summary. Clinical sporotrichosis usually occurs as one of two primary cutaneous forms, either the fixed cutaneous or the lymphocutaneous form. Both result from direct inoculation at a site of minor trauma. Although the infection may rarely disseminate from either form by autoinoculation to other skin sites or by hematogenous spread (184–186), systemic sporotrichosis more commonly follows pulmonary infection. Development of systemic sporotrichosis, although rare, occurs particularly in persons with a depressed immune response, such as patients with lymphoma or persons receiving long-term systemic corticosteroids. *S. schenckii* is not a common opportunist in HIV-infected individuals, but disseminated sporotrichosis has been seen in a few patients with AIDS (187).

The lymphocutaneous form of sporotrichosis starts with a painless papule that grows into an ulcer, usually on a finger or hand. Subsequently, a chain of asymptomatic nodules appears along the lymph vessel draining the area ("sporotrichoid spread"). These lymphatic nodules may undergo suppuration with subsequent ulceration.

In the fixed cutaneous form, a solitary plaque or occasionally a group of lesions is seen, most commonly on an arm or the face. It may show superficial crusting or a verrucous surface (188–190). There is no tendency toward lymphatic spread.

Systemic sporotrichosis may be unifocal or multifocal and usually develops subsequent to pulmonary infection. Unifocal systemic sporotrichosis may affect the lungs, a single joint or symmetric joints, the genitourinary tract, or—in rare cases—the brain (191). Chronic pulmonary sporotrichosis resembles pulmonary tuberculosis (192). Multifocal systemic sporotrichosis nearly always shows widely scattered cutaneous lesions, which start as nodules or as subcutaneous abscesses and undergo ulceration. In addition, involvement of the lungs (186) or of several joints of the extremities is usually observed. The predilection of *S. schenckii* for cooler parts of the body, such as the skin, lungs, and joints of the extremities, has been attributed to the fact that the organism grows best at temperatures less than 37°C. The gold standard for diagnosis of sporotrichosis is culture. However, serologic, histopathologic, and molecular approaches have been recently adopted as auxiliary tools to confirm the diagnosis (193–196).

Histopathology. Early primary cutaneous lesions of sporotrichosis usually show a nonspecific inflammatory infiltrate composed of neutrophils, lymphoid cells, plasma cells, and histiocytes (193). Longer-standing, clinically verrucous lesions show a hyperplastic epidermis with small, intraepidermal, and dermal lymphoplasmacytic infiltrate with small abscesses, eosinophils, giant cells, and small granulomas often associated with asteroid bodies (189,193). Later, through coalescence, a characteristic arrangement of the infiltrate in three zones may develop. These include a central "suppurative" zone composed of neutrophils; surrounding it, a "tuberculoid" zone with epithelioid cells and multinucleated histiocytes; and peripheral to it, a "round cell" zone of lymphoid cells and plasma cells.

The lymphatic nodules of lymphocutaneous sporotrichosis and the cutaneous nodules of multifocal systemic sporotrichosis at first show scattered granulomas within an inflammatory infiltrate predominantly in the deep dermis and subcutaneous fat (189,194). These enlarge and coalesce to form irregularly shaped suppurative granulomata and, eventually, a large abscess surrounded by zones of histiocytes and lymphocytes as described for primary lesions (189).

In many instances, it is not possible to recognize the causative organisms of *S. schenckii* in tissue sections, particularly in the two common forms: the lymphocutaneous and fixed cutaneous. This seems to be true especially in cases of sporotrichosis reported from the United States (195) and Europe (194). In these areas, negative findings are common even with diastase digestion of glycogen granules prior to staining of sections with the PAS reaction. Staining with methenamine silver has not increased the frequency of positive findings (194). Even in cases with positive findings, numerous sections often have to be examined before one or a few organisms are visualized. Immunohistochemical staining using primary antibodies directed against *S. schenckii* may increase the percentage of cases in which the organism can be demonstrated to 83%, more than double that achieved with ordinary histochemical methods (196). In addition, there are apparently significant geographic differences, since in a series of cutaneous sporotrichosis reported from Japan, 98% of the cases showed spores in tissue sections on staining with the PAS reaction (197). If present, the spores of *S. schenckii* appear as round-to-oval bodies 4 to 6 μm in diameter that stain more strongly at the periphery than in the center (194) (Fig. 23-18). Single or occasionally multiple buds are present. In some instances, small, cigar-shaped bodies up to 8 μm long are also present (185,193).

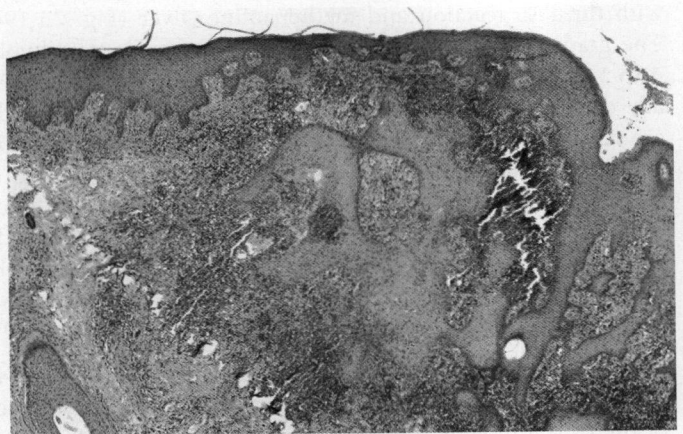
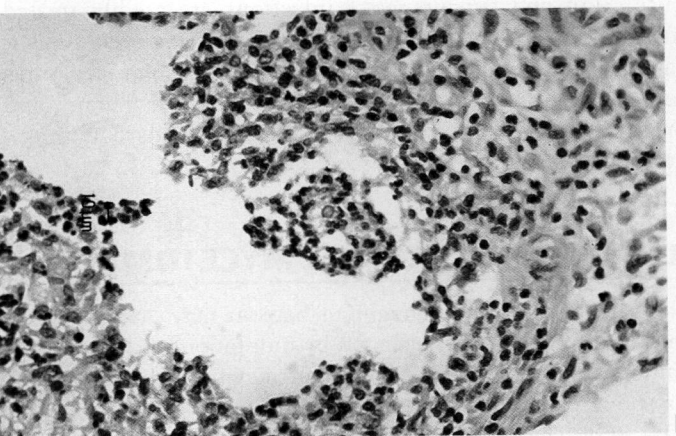

Figure 23-18 Sporotrichosis. **A:** H&E staining shows pseudocarcinomatous epidermal hyperplasia with microabscess formation. **B:** PAS-D staining shows a round spore, staining more darkly at the periphery than centrally, surrounded by a neutrophilic infiltrate. (H&E, hematoxylin and eosin; PAS-D, periodic acid–Schiff–diastase.)

In only very few cases can clumps of branching, nonseptate hyphae be demonstrated (195,197).

Asteroid bodies may be seen in sporotrichosis, as well as in a number of other infectious processes, and sarcoidosis. Asteroid bodies are visible in sections stained with H&E, and in sporotrichosis consist of a central spore 5 to 10 μm in diameter surrounded by radiating elongations of a homogeneous eosinophilic material. The phenomenon of radiating eosinophilic material found around infectious agents, described in sporotrichosis by Splendore (198) and in schistosomiasis by Hoeppli (199) and known as the *Splendore–Hoeppli phenomenon*, has been thought to represent the deposition of antigen–antibody complexes and debris from host inflammatory cells (200). Measurements of the greatest diameter of asteroid bodies in sporotrichosis vary from 7 to 25 μm, with a mean of 20 μm (189). Asteroid bodies have been observed in only a few cases of sporotrichosis occurring in the United States, and it may be difficult to demonstrate the central spore. However, asteroid bodies are found frequently in cases of sporotrichosis from South Africa, Japan, and Australia, with an incidence varying from 39% to 65% (201).

Pathogenesis. S. schenckii occurs throughout the world and is commonly contracted through exposure to vegetal matter, often a splinter or thorn as from a rosebush, although transmission by insects and animals has been reported (202). In nearly all cases of sporotrichosis, even in those without demonstrable fungi in the tissue, *S. schenckii* can be grown easily on Sabouraud medium. The fungus is dimorphic: At room temperature, it grows in a mycelial form with conidiophores bearing conidia as a "bouquet" at the tip; at 37°C, it grows as a yeast (195). At 39°C, there is no growth, a fact that has led to the use of local thermotherapy (194,197).

Differential Diagnosis. If the fungus is not found in sections, a diagnosis of sporotrichosis can only be suspected; however, it can be excluded in dubious cases by a negative cutaneous sporotrichin test, which is almost always positive except in cases of disseminated disease (194). The subcutaneous abscesses of tularemia and of infections with *Mycobacterium marinum* may have the same histologic appearance as that of the cutaneous and subcutaneous nodules and abscesses of sporotrichosis and must be excluded.

Principles of Management: Spontaneous resolution of sporotrichosis is rare and antifungal therapy is necessary in the majority of patients. Dissemination is uncommon except in the immunosuppressed and in those with a history of alcohol abuse. Skin and subcutaneous infections are readily treated with antifungal therapy such as itraconazole. However, disseminated infections involving viscera or osteoarticular structures are a therapeutic challenge even with antifungal therapy, and some require lifelong suppressive therapy, particularly if immunosuppression cannot be reversed.

EUMYCETOMA (FUNGAL MYCETOMA)

A number of fungi and filamentous bacteria may cause an indolent local infection, characterized by induration associated with draining sinuses. These diverse agents may have clinically identical presentations that have been collectively called *mycetoma* (203–205). The term *actinomycetoma* refers to such infections when filamentous bacteria cause them; they are discussed further in Chapter 21. *Eumycetoma*, however, is caused by a group of true fungi with thick septate hyphae, including *Petriellidium boydii*

(*Allescheria boydii* and *Pseudallescheria boydii*), *Madurella grisea*, and *Madurella mycetomatis* (204). Although much more common in tropical regions, eumycetoma is seen occasionally in the United States, where the most common cause is *Pseudallescheria boydii* (205). Differentiation between actinomycetoma and eumycetoma is important, because they respond to different treatments. Most *Madurella* species are phenotypically and clinically similar but differ in their response to antifungal drugs, so specific identification is required for optimal management of *Madurella* infections. Owing to the lack of sporulation or other *in vitro* phenotypic characteristics, morphologic assays have limited diagnostic value. However, novel multiplex real-time PCR using biopsies from eumycetoma-suspected patients yielded accurate diagnosis with specific identification of the causative species in three hours, confirming the usefulness of this approach (206).

Clinical Summary. Eumycetoma is a persistent, invariably progressive local infection without a tendency for systemic spread. There is no obvious association with immunosuppression. The infection starts as a subcutaneous nodule(s) usually on the foot at a site of trauma; in the past, these infections were not uncommon in the Madras region of India, and thus the term *Madura foot* has been used synonymously with mycetoma (204). The nodules eventuate in abscesses and draining sinuses (Fig. 23-19A). Gradually, the muscles and tendons are damaged and osteomyelitis develops. Grossly visible "sulfur granules" or "grains," which are tightly knit clusters of organisms, are discharged from the draining sinuses. These granules are black in cases of eumycetoma caused by the dematiaceous fungi *Madurella grisea* and *Madurella mycetomatis*, whereas they are colorless in eumycetoma caused by *Pseudallescheria boydii* (207).

Histopathology. Histologic examination of the indurated skin shows extensive granulation tissue containing abscesses that may lead into sinuses. The granulation tissue is nonspecific in appearance. In the early phase of the disease, the tissue surrounding the abscesses is composed of lymphoid cells, plasma cells, histiocytes, and fibroblasts, whereas in the late phase, fibroblasts may predominate. The diagnosis can be established only by finding the "sulfur granules" (Fig. 23-19B). Because they occur almost exclusively in abscesses or sinuses, an area containing purulent material should be chosen as the site for biopsy.

Most granules measure between 0.5 and 2.0 mm in diameter and are thus large enough to be visible macroscopically (208). The granules of both eumycetoma and actinomycetoma stain with the PAS reaction and methenamine silver (Fig. 23-19C). The granules of eumycetoma are composed of septate hyphae 4 to 5 μm thick, whereas the granules of actinomycetoma usually consist of fine, branching filaments or bacillary forms that are only about 1 μm thick. A Gram stain aids in differentiating bacterial from fungal causes of mycetoma; the filaments of actinomycetoma are gram positive, whereas the hyphae in grains of eumycetoma are gram negative (209,210). The study of discharged granules crushed on a slide and stained with lactophenol blue also allows differentiation between the thin filaments of actinomycetoma and the thicker hyphae of eumycetoma (209).

Principles of Management: Treatment is difficult and includes surgical debridement and antifungal therapy. Recovery of the causal organism allows identification of the species and perhaps susceptibility testing. No randomized controlled trials of treatment of eumycetoma exist, and treatment is guided by infectious disease expert opinions.

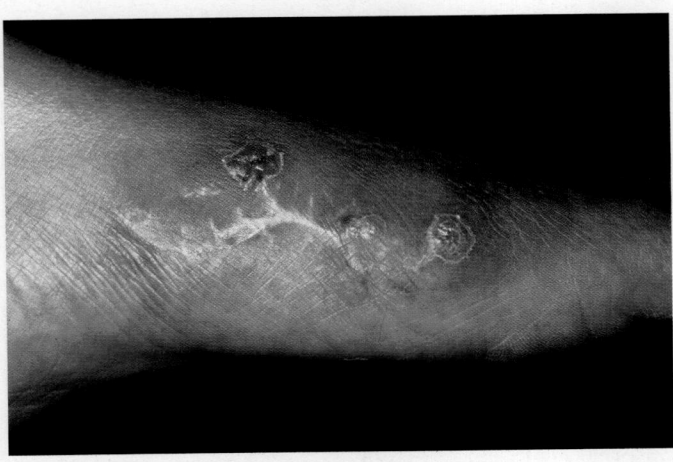
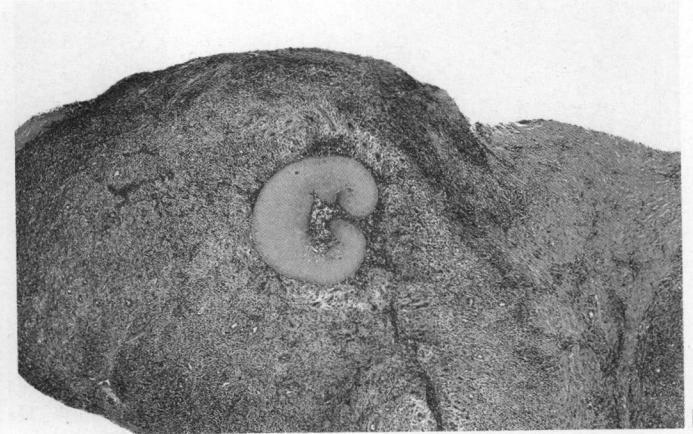

Figure 23-19 Eumycetoma. **A:** Ulcerated, indurated plaque of eumycotic mycetoma on the foot. **B:** H&E staining shows a "sulfur granule" in a purulent area of granulation tissue. (H&E, hematoxylin and eosin.)

RHINOSPORIDIOSIS

Rhinosporidiosis is a chronic infection that is caused by *Rhinosporidium seeberi*.

Clinical Summary. Rhinosporidiosis typically involves mucosal surfaces, most frequently the nasal mucosa, and may involve contiguous skin. This disease is seen primarily in India and Ceylon, but a number of cases have been seen in South America and a few in the United States (211).

The mode of transmission is not known. Lesions start as an often pruritic papule, which grows into an erythematous polypoid mass that may cause obstruction of the nose and nasopharynx. Small cysts and pseudocysts develop and may discharge a combination of mucus, pus, and organisms, creating tiny white dots and giving lesions a characteristic strawberry-like appearance. Lesions of the ocular mucosa tend to be flatter, and skin lesions have a warty shape (212). Involvement of the genital mucosa has also been reported (211). Dissemination of the organism is extremely rare (212).

Histopathology. The epithelium is hyperplastic with papillomatosis and deep invaginations, some of which form pseudocysts (Fig. 23-20A). Numerous globular cysts of varying shape, representing sporangia in different stages of development, give the corium a distinctive "Swiss cheese" appearance. There is a surrounding dense, mixed inflammatory infiltrate with lymphocytes and histiocytes, including occasional giant cells, plasma cells, neutrophils, and eosinophils.

R. seeberi is a large, endosporulating organism with a distinctive morphology that can usually be recognized in H&E-stained sections (Fig. 23-20B). Sporangia develop from individual spores about the size of an erythrocyte (213). The spores develop into small uninucleate cysts that enlarge and develop a chitinous, eosinophilic wall. With increasing size, nuclear divisions lead to the development of up to 16,000 spores in a sporangium. These distinctive structures may be 300 μm in diameter. Rupture of the cyst or release of the spores through a pore in the cyst wall results in individual spores into the surrounding tissue. The organisms stain with the PAS reaction at all stages, but GMS and mucicarmine stains are not effective for organisms less than 100 μm in diameter.

Differential Diagnosis. The different clinical presentations of coccidioidomycosis and the smaller size of the spherical coccidioidal sporangia (<60 μm in diameter) allow for an easy distinction of that disease from rhinosporidiosis.

Principles of Management: The treatment of choice for rhinosporidiosis is surgical debridement. Disseminated disease is rare.

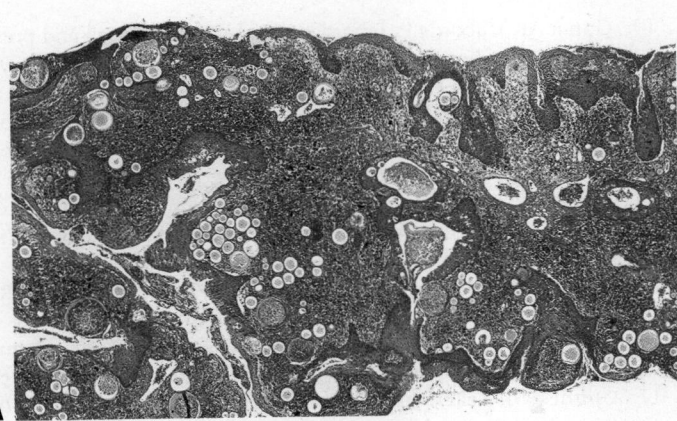
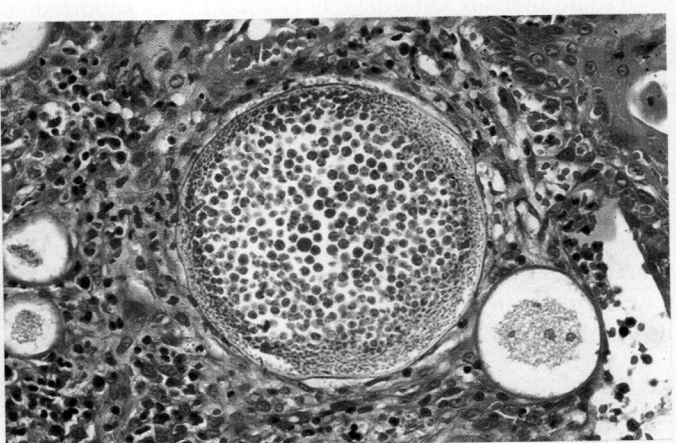

Figure 23-20 Rhinosporidiosis. **A:** H&E staining shows marked papillomatosis and deep invaginations of the nasal mucosa. **B:** A sporangium contains many individual spores (H&E stain). (H&E, hematoxylin and eosin.)

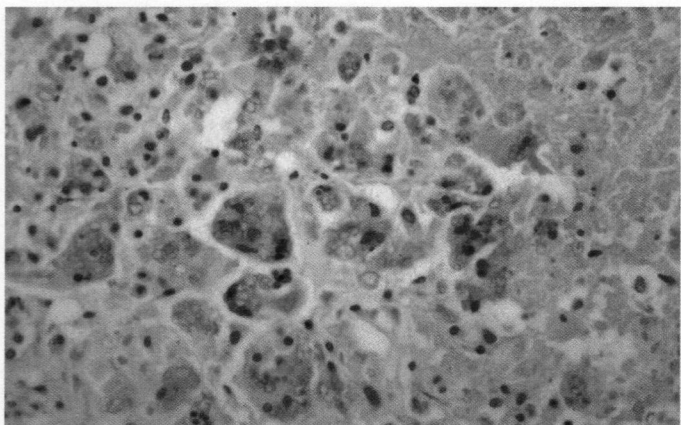
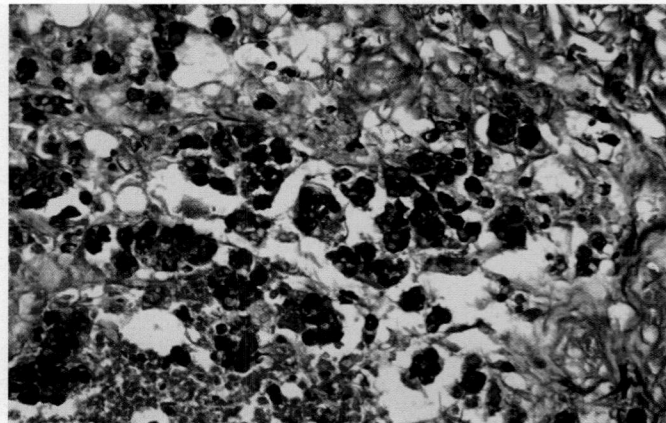

Figure 23-21 Protothecosis. **A:** H&E staining shows individual cells and clusters of organisms within giant cells. **B:** The morula-like clusters in multinucleated giant cells are highlighted by silver impregnation (GMS stain). (GMS, Gomori methenamine silver; H&E, hematoxylin and eosin.)

CUTANEOUS PROTOTHECOSIS

Prototheca is a genus of algae that causes cutaneous infections in humans (214,215). A discussion of *Prototheca* is included in this chapter because it may be isolated on Sabouraud medium, it has traditionally been discussed in mycology texts, and this text has no separate chapter for diseases caused by algae.

Clinical Summary. Although there is one report of cutaneous infection in a patient also infected with HIV, cutaneous protothecosis usually occurs in otherwise healthy persons following trauma and wound contamination with water (215). Lesions develop very slowly and may be single or multiple papules, plaques, or nodules with smooth, verrucous, or ulcerated surfaces (216–218).

Histopathology. The histologic appearance, like the clinical appearance, is not characteristic; so, the diagnosis depends on the finding of the organisms. Usually, there is a mixed inflammatory infiltrate with areas of necrosis and fairly numerous giant cells (Fig. 23-21). In sections stained with H&E, the organisms stain faintly or not at all. On staining with PAS or silver methenamine, however, the organisms stain well and are seen both within giant cells and free in the tissue (217).

Individual organisms are spherical and measure 6 to 10 μm in diameter. However, as a result of septation, many contain endospores and then are considerably larger. Further subdivision of daughter cells within the parent cell leads to the formation of "sporangia" containing as many as 50 cells lying clustered together as morula-like structures (216). Ultimately, such a sporangium breaks down into individual organisms.

Pathogenesis. Prototheca is a genus of saprophytic, achloric (nonpigmented) algae. These organisms reproduce asexually by way of internal septation, producing autospores identical to the parent cell. *Prototheca* forms creamy, yeastlike colonies on Sabouraud medium between 25°C and 37°C. These colonies become visible within 48 hours (215–218).

Principles of Management: Protothecosis is rarely self-healing. Treatment includes surgical debridement and systemic antifungal therapy. Dissemination and subsequent death from infection may occur in those with stem cell or solid organ transplant.

REFERENCES

1. Kirk PM, Cannon PF, David JC, Stalpers JA. *Ainsworth & Biby's Dictionary of the Fungi*. 9th ed. CABI Publishing; 2001.
2. Sabouraud R. *Les Teignes*. Masson et Cie; 1910.
3. Borman AM and Johnson AM. Name changes for fungi of medical importance, 2018 to 2019. *J Clin Microbiol*. 2021;59(2): e01811–e01820.
4. Emmons CW. Dermatophytes: natural groupings based on the form of spores and accessory organs. *Arch Dermatol Syphilol*. 1934;30:337.
5. Gnat S, Lagowski D, Nowakiewicz A, Zięba P. Phenotypic characterization of enzymatic activity of clinical dermatophyte isolates from animals with and without skin lesions and humans. *J Appl Micro*. 2018; 125:700–709.
6. Lesher JL. *An Atlas of Microbiology of the Skin*. Parthenon Publishing Group; 2000.
7. Weitzman I, Summerbell RC. The dermatophytes. *Clin Microbiol Rev*. 1995;8(2):240–259.
8. Pravda DJ, Pugliese MM. Tinea faciei. *Arch Dermatol*. 1978;114:250.
9. Birt AR, Wilt JC. Mycology, bacteriology, and histopathology of suppurative ring-worm. *Arch Dermatol*. 1954;69:441.
10. Kreijkamp-Kaspers S, Hawke K, Guo L, et al. *Oral Antifungal Medication for Toenail Onychomycosis (Review)*. The Cochrane Collaboration John Wiley & Sons, Ltd; 2017.
11. Ellis DH, Watson AB, Marley JE, Williams TG. Non-dermatophytes in onychomycosis of the toenails. *Br J Dermatol*. 1997;136: 490–493.
12. Zaias N. *The Nail in Health and Disease*. 2nd ed. Appleton & Lange; 1990.
13. Gupta AK, Taborda P, Taborda V, et al. Epidemiology and prevalence of onychomycosis in HIV-positive individuals. *Intern J Dermatol*. 2000;39:746–753.
14. Garcia HP, DeLucas R, Gonzalez J, et al. Toenail onychomycosis in patients with acquired immune deficiency syndrome: treatment with terbinafine. *Br J Dermatol*. 1997;137:577–580.
15. Enoch DA, Yang H, Aliyu SH, Micallef C. The changing epidemiology of invasive fungal infections. *Methods Mol Biol*. 2017;1508:17–65. doi: 10.1007/978-1-4939-6515-1_2
16. Gupta AK, Jain HC, Lynde CW, Watteel GN, Summerbell RC. Prevalence and epidemiology of unsuspected onychomycosis in patients visiting dermatologists' offices in Ontario, Canada—a multicenter survey of 2001 patients. *Int J Dermatol*. 1997;36:783–787.
17. Gottlieb GJ, Ackerman AB. The "sandwich sign" of dermatophytosis. *Am J Dermatopathol*. 1986;8:347.
18. Mikhail GR. *Trichophyton rubrum* granuloma. *Int J Dermatol*. 1970;9:41.

19. Scher RK, Ackerman AB. The value of nail biopsy for demonstrating fungi not demonstrable by microbiologic techniques. *Am J Dermatopathol.* 1980;2:55.

20. Longley BJ, Scher RK. Anatomy and growth of the normal nail. In: McKee PH, Calonje E, Grantner SR, eds. *Pathology of the Skin.* 3rd ed. Mosby; 2005.

21. Machler BC, Kirsner RS, Elgart GW. Routine histologic examination for the diagnosis of onychomycosis: an evaluation of sensitivity and specificity. *Cutis.* 1998;61:217–219.

22. Hafirassou AZ, Valero C, Gassem, N, Mihoubi I, Buitrago MJ. Usefulness of techniques based on real time PCR for the identification of onychomycosis-causing species. *Mycoses.* 2017; 60:638–644.

23. Tosti A, Piraccini BM, Mariani R, Stinchi C, Buttasi C. Are local and systemic conditions important for the development of onychomycosis? *Eur J Dermatol.* 1998;1:41–44.

24. Ashbee HR, Evans EGV. Immunology of diseases associated with Malessezia species. *Clin Microbiol Rev.* 2002;15:21–57.

25. Bäck O, Faergemann J, Hörnqvist R. *Pityrosporum* folliculitis: a common disease of the young and middle-aged. *J Am Acad Dermatol.* 1985;12:56.

26. Broberg A, Faergemann J. Infantile seborrhoeic dermatitis and *Pityrosporum ovale. Br J Dermatol.* 1989;120:359–362.

27. Sugita T, Takashima M, Shinoda T, et al. New yeast species, Malassezia dermati, isolated from patients with atopic dermatitis. *J Clin Microbiol.* 2002;40:1363–1367.

28. Heng MCY, Henderson CL, Barker DC, Haberfelde G. Correlation of *Pityrosporum ovale* density with clinical severity of seborrheic dermatitis as assessed by a simplified technique. *J Am Acad Dermatol.* 1990;23:82.

29. Leyden JJ, McGinley KJ, Kligman AM. Role of microorganisms in dandruff. *Arch Dermatol.* 1976;112:333.

30. Elshabrawy WO, Saudy N, Sallam M. Molecular and phenotypic identification and speciation of Malassezia yeasts isolated from Egyptian patients with pityriasis versicolor. *J Clin Diagn Res.* 2017;11(8):DC12–DC17. doi: 10.7860/JCDR/2017/27747.10416

31. Nazzaro-Porro M, Passi S, Picardo M, Mercantini R, Breathnach AS. Lipoxygenase activity of *Pityrosporum* in vitro and in vivo. *J Invest Dermatol.* 1986;87:108–112.

32. Galadari I, el Komy M, Mousa A, Hashimoto K, Mehregan AH. Tinea versicolor: histologic and ultrastructural investigation of pigmentary changes. *Int J Dermatol.* 1992;31:253.

33. Porro MN, Passi S, Caprilli F, Mercantini R. Induction of hyphae in cultures of *Pityrosporum* by cholesterol and cholesterol esters. *J Invest Dermatol.* 1977;69:531.

34. Potter BS, Burgoon CFJ, Johnson WC. *Pityrosporum* folliculitis: report of seven cases and review of the *Pityrosporum* organism relative to cutaneous disease. *Arch Dermatol.* 1973;107:388.

35. Bretagne S, Costa JM. Towards a molecular diagnosis of invasive aspergillosis and disseminated candidosis. *FEMS Immunol Med Microbiol.* 2005;45(3):361–368. doi: 10.1016/j.femsim.2005.05.012

36. Jautova J, Baloghova J, Dorko E, et al. Cutaneous candidosis in immunosuppressed patients. *Folia Microbiol.* 2001;46:359–360.

37. Chapel TA, Gagliardi C, Nichols W. Congenital cutaneous candidiasis. *J Am Acad Dermatol.* 1982;6:926.

38. Jautova J, Viragova S, Ondrasovic M, Holoda E. Incidence of Candida species from human skin and nails: a survey. *Folia Microbiol.* 2001;46:333–337.

39. Kwon-Chung KJ, Bennett JE. Candidiasis. In: Kwong-Chung KJ, Bennett JE, eds. *Medical Mycology.* Lea & Febiger; 1992:280.

40. Scherwitz C. Ultrastructure of human cutaneous candidiasis. *J Invest Dermatol.* 1982;78:200.

41. Kirkpatrick CH. Chronic mucocutaneous candidiasis. *J Am Acad Dermatol.* 1994;31:S14.

42. Kugelman TP, Cripps DJ, Harrell ER Jr. *Candida* granuloma with epidermophytosis: report of a case and review of the literature. *Arch Dermatol.* 1963;88:150.

43. Tavitian A, Raufman J-P, Rosenthal LE. Oral candidiasis as a marker for esophageal candidiasis in the acquired immunodeficiency syndrome. *Ann Intern Med.* 1986;104:54.

44. Conant MA. Hairy leukoplakia: a new disease of the oral mucosa. *Arch Dermatol.* 1987;123:585.

45. Edmond MB, Wallace SE, McClish DK, Pfaller MA, Jones RN, Wenzel RP. Nosocomial bloodstream infections in United States hospitals: a three-year analysis. *Clin Infect Dis.* 1999;29:239–244.

46. Kao AS, Brandt ME, Pruitt WR, et al. The epidemiology of candidemia in two United States cities: results of a population-based active surveillance. *Clin Infect Dis.* 1999;29:1164–1170.

47. Jacobs MI, Magid MS, Jarowski CI. Disseminated candidiasis: newer approaches to early recognition and treatment. *Arch Dermatol.* 1980;116:1277.

48. Kressel B, Szewczyk C, Tuazon CU. Early clinical recognition of disseminated candidiasis by muscle and skin biopsy. *Arch Int Med.* 1978;138:429.

49. Grossman ME, Silvers DN, Walther RR. Cutaneous manifestations of disseminated candidiasis. *J Am Acad Dermatol.* 1980; 2:111.

50. Kontoyiannis DP, Bodey GP. Invasive aspergillosis in 2002: an update. *J Clin Microbiol Infect Dis.* 2002;21:161–172.

51. Perusquía-Ortiz AM, Vázquez-González D, Bonifaz A. Opportunistic filamentous mycoses: aspergillosis, mucormycosis, phaeohyphomycosis and hyalohyphomycosis. *J Dtsch Dermatol Ges.* 2012;10(9):611–621.

52. Allo MD, Miller J, Townsend T, Tan C. Primary cutaneous aspergillosis associated with Hickman intravenous catheters. *N Engl J Med.* 1987;317:1105.

53. Hunt SJ, Nagi C, Gross KG, Wong DS, Mathews WC. Primary cutaneous aspergillosis near central venous catheters in patients with the acquired immunodeficiency syndrome. *Arch Dermatol.* 1992;128:1229.

54. Findlay GH, Roux HF, Simson IW. Skin manifestations in disseminated aspergillosis. *Br J Dermatol.* 1971;85:94.

55. Pursell KJ, Telzak EE, Armstrong D. *Aspergillus* species colonization and invasive disease in patients with AIDS. *Clin Infect Dis.* 1992;14:141.

56. Kwon-Chung KJ, Bennett JE. Mucormycosis. In: Kwon-Chung KJ, Bennett JE, eds. *Medical Mycology.* Lea & Febiger; 1992:524.

57. Adam RD, Hunter G, DiTomasso J, Comerci G Jr. Mucormycosis: emerging prominence of cutaneous infections. *Clin Infect Dis.* 1994;19:67.

58. Hammond DE, Winkelmann RK. Cutaneous phycomycosis: report of three cases with identification of *Rhizopus. Arch Dermatol.* 1979;115:990.

59. Gartenberg G, Bottone EJ, Keusch GT, Weitzman I. Hospital-acquired mucormycosis (*Rhizopus rhizopodiformis*) of skin and subcutaneous tissue. *N Engl J Med.* 1978;299:1115.

60. Meyer RD, Kaplan MH, Ong M, Armstrong D. Cutaneous lesions in disseminated mucormycosis. *JAMA.* 1973;225:737.

61. Grossman ME. Bull's-eye cutaneous infarct of zygomycosis: a bedside diagnosis confirmed by touch preparation [review]. *J Am Acad Dermatol.* 2004;51(6):996–1001.

62. Rabin ER, Lundberg GD, Mitchell ET. Mucormycosis in severely burned patients: report of two cases with extensive destruction of the face and nasal cavity. *N Engl J Med.* 1961;264:1286.

63. Ajello L. The gamut of human infections caused by dematiaceous fungi. *Jpn J Med Mycol.* 1981;22:1.

64. Fothergill AW. Identification of dematiaceous fungi and their role in human disease. *Clin Infect Dis.* 1996;22(suppl 2):S179–S184.

65. Pec J, Palencarova E, Plank L, et al. Phaeohyphomycosis due to Alternaria spp. and Phaeosclera dermatioides: a histopathological study. *Mycoses.* 1996;39:217–221.

66. McGinnis MR. Chromoblastomycosis and phaeohyphomycosis: new concepts, diagnosis, and mycology. *J Am Acad Dermatol.* 1983;8:1.

67. Gerdsen R, Uerlich M, De Hoog GS, Bieber T, Horré R. Sporotrichoid phaeohyphomycosis due to *Alternaria infectoria*. *Br J Dermatol*. 2001;145:484–486.

68. Revankar SG, Patterson JE, Sutton DA, Pullen R, Rinaldi MG. Disseminated phaeohyphomycosis: review of an emerging mycosis. *Clin Infect Dis*. 2002;34:467–476.

69. Ziefer A, Connor DH. Phaeomycotic cyst: a clinicopathologic study of twenty-five patients. *Am J Trop Med Hyg*. 1980;29:901.

70. Greer KE, Gross GP, Cooper PH, Harding SA. Cystic chromomycosis due to Wangiella dermatitidis. *Arch Dermatol*. 1979;115:1433.

71. Jacobson ES. Pathogenic roles for fungal melanins. *Clin Microbiol Rev*. 2000;13:708–713.

72. Feng B, Wang X, Hauser M, et al. Molecular cloning and characterization of WdPKS1, a gene involved in dihydroxynaphthalene melanin biosynthesis and virulence in Wangiella (Exophiala) dermatitidis. *Infect Immun*. 2001;69:1781–1794.

73. Schnitzler N, Peltroche-Llacsahuanga H, Bestier N, Zündorf J, Lütticken R, Haase G. Effect of melanin and carotenoids of Exophilia (Wangiella) dermatitis on phagocytosis, oxidative burst, and killing by human neutrophils. *Infect Immun*. 1999;67:94–101.

74. Kwon-Chung KJ, Bennett JE. Phaeohyphomycosis. In: Kwon-Chung KJ, Bennett JE, eds. *Medical Mycology*. Lea & Febiger; 1992:620.

75. Pedersen NB, Mardh PA, Hallberg T, Jonsson N. Cutaneous alternariosis. *Br J Dermatol*. 1976;94:201.

76. Mitchell AJ, Solomon AR, Beneke ES, Anderson TF. Subcutaneous alternariosis. *J Am Acad Dermatol*. 1983;8:673.

77. Male O, Pehamberger H. Sekundäre kutanmykosen durch alternariaarten. *Hautarzt*. 1986;37:94.

78. Chevrant-Breton J, Boisseau-Lebreuil M, Fréour E, Guiguen G, Launois B, Guelfi J. Les alternarioses cutanées humaines: a propos de 3 cas. Revue de la littérature. *Ann Dermatol Venereol*. 1981;108:653.

79. Bourlond A, Alexandre G. Dermal alternariosis in a kidney transplant recipient. *Dermatologica*. 1984;168:152.

80. Lemos LB, Guo M, Baliga M. Blastomycosis: organ involvement and etiologic diagnosis. A review of 123 patients from Mississippi. *Ann Diagn Pathol*. 2000;4(6):391–406.

81. Larson DM, Eckman MR, Alber RL, Goldschmidt VG. Primary cutaneous (inoculation) blastomycosis: an occupational hazard to pathologists. *Am J Clin Pathol*. 1983;79:253.

82. Miller DD, Davies SF, Sarosi GA. Erythema nodosum and blastomycosis. *Arch Int Med*. 1982;142:1839.

83. Klapman MH, Superfon NP, Solomon LM. North American blastomycosis. *Arch Dermatol*. 1970;101:653.

84. Witorsch P, Utz JP. North American blastomycosis: a study of 40 patients. *Medicine (Baltimore)*. 1968;47:169.

85. Witzig RS, Hoadley DJ, Greer DL, Abriola KP, Hernandez RL. Blastomycosis and human immunodeficiency virus: three new cases and review. *South Med J*. 1994;87:715.

86. Pappas PG, Threlkeld MG, Bedsole GD, Cleveland KO, Gelfand MS, Dismukes WE. Blastomycosis in immunocompromised patients. *Medicine (Baltimore)*. 1993;72:311.

87. Hashimoto K, Kaplan RJ, Daman LA, Stuart JM, Bernhardt H. Pustular blastomycosis. *Int J Dermatol*. 1977;16:277.

88. Henchy FP III, Daniel CR III, Omura EF, Kheir SM. North American blastomycosis: an unusual clinical manifestation. *Arch Dermatol*. 1982;118:287.

89. Desai AP, Pandit AA, Gupte PD. Cutaneous blastomycosis: report of a case with diagnosis by fine needle aspiration cytology. *Acta Cytologica*. 1997;41:1317–1319.

90. Sen SK, Talley P, Zua M. Blastomycosis: report of a case with noninvasive, rapid diagnosis of dermal lesions by the papanicolaou technique. *Acta Cytologica*. 1997;41:1399–1401.

91. Kaplan W, Kraft DE. Demonstration of pathogenic fungi in formalin-fixed tissues by immunofluorescence. *Am J Clin Pathol*. 1969;52:420.

92. Russell B, Beckett JH, Jacobs PH. Immunoperoxidase localization of *Sporothrix schenckii* and *Cryptococcus neoformans*. *Arch Dermatol*. 1979;115:433.

93. Moskowitz LB, Ganjei P, Ziegels-Weissman J, Cleary TJ, Penneys NS, Nadji M. Immunohistologic identification of fungi in systemic and cutaneous mycoses. *Arch Pathol Lab Med*. 1986;110:433.

94. Londero AT, Ramos CD. Paracoccidioidomycosis: a clinical and mycologic study of forty-one cases observed in Santa Maria, RS, Brazil. *Am J Med*. 1972;52:771.

95. Salfelder K, Doehnert G, Doehnert H-R. Paracoccidioidomycosis: anatomic study with complete autopsies. *Virchows Arch*. 1969;348:51.

96. Murray HW, Littman ML, Roberts RB. Disseminated paracoccidioidomycosis (South American blastomycosis) in the United States. *Am J Med*. 1974;56:209.

97. Hirsh BC, Johnson WC. Pathology of granulomatous diseases: mixed inflammatory granulomas. *Int J Dermatol*. 1984;23:585–598.

98. Pinheiro BG, Hahn RC, Camargo ZP, Rodrigues AM. Molecular tools for detection and identification of *Paracoccidioides* species: current status and future perspectives. *J Fungi (Basel)*. 2020;6(4):293. doi: 10.3390/jof6040293

99. Bakos L, Kronfeld M, Hampe S, Castro I, Zampese M. Disseminated paracoccidioidomycosis with skin lesions in a patient with acquired immunodeficiency syndrome. *J Am Acad Dermatol*. 1989;20:854.

100. Götz H. Klinische und experimentelle studien über das granuloma paracoccidioides. *Arch Dermatol Syphiligr*. 1954;198:507.

101. Azulay RD, Carneiro JA, Da Graça M, Cunha S, Reis LT. Keloidal blastomycosis (Lobo's disease) with lymphatic involvement: a case report. *Int J Dermatol*. 1976;15:40.

102. Tapia A, Torres-Calcindo A, Arosemena R. Keloidal blastomycosis (Lobo's disease) in Panama. *Int J Dermatol*. 1978;17:572.

103. Burns RA, Roy JS, Woods C, Padhye AA, Warnock DW. Report of the first human case of lobomycosis in the United States. *J Clin Microbiol*. 2000;38(3):1283–1285.

104. Bhawan J, Bain RW, Purtilo DT, et al. Lobomycosis: an electron-microscopic, histochemical and immunologic study. *J Cutan Pathol*. 1976;3:5.

105. Milam CP, Fenske NA. Chromoblastomycosis. *Dermatol Clin*. 1989;7(2):219–225.

106. Abliz P, Fukushima K, Takizawa K, Nishimura K. Identification of pathogenic dematiaceous fungi and related taxa based on large subunit ribosomal DNA D1/D2 domain sequence analysis, FEMS Immunology & Medical Microbiology. 2004;40(1):41–49.

107. Krzyściak PM, Pindycka-Piaszczyńska M, Piaszczyński M. Chromoblastomycosis. *Postepy Dermatol Alergol*. 2014;31(5):310–321. doi:10.5114/pdia.2014.40949

108. Tschen JA, Knox JM, McGavran MH, Duncan WC. Chromomycosis: the association of fungal elements and wood splinters. *Arch Dermatol*. 1984;120:107.

109. Bansal AS, Prabhakar P. Chromomycosis: a twenty-year analysis of histologically confirmed cases in Jamaica. *Trop Geogr Med*. 1987;41:222–226.

110. Azulay RD, Serruya J. Hematogenous dissemination in chromoblastomycosis. *Arch Dermatol*. 1967;95:57.

111. Wackym PA, Gray GF Jr, Richie RE, Gregg CR. Cutaneous chromomycosis in renal transplant recipients: successful management in two cases. *Arch Intern Med*. 1985;145:1036.

112. Batres E, Wolf JE Jr, Rudolph AH, Knox JM. Transepithelial elimination of cutaneous chromomycosis. *Arch Dermatol*. 1978;114:1231.

113. Goette DK, Robertson D. Transepithelial elimination in chromomycosis. *Arch Dermatol*. 1984;120:400.

114. Drutz DJ, Catanzaro A. Coccidioidomycosis: part I. *Am Rev Respir Dis*. 1978;117:559.

115. Drutz DJ, Catanzaro A. Coccidioidomycosis: part II. *Am Rev Respir Dis*. 1978;117:727.

116. Trimble JR, Doucette J. Primary cutaneous coccidioidomycosis: report of a case of a laboratory infection. *Arch Dermatol.* 1956;74:405.

117. Carroll GF, Haley LD, Brown JM. Primary cutaneous coccidioidomycosis. *Arch Dermatol.* 1977;113:933.

118. Levan NE, Huntington RW Jr. Primary cutaneous coccidioidomycosis in agricultural workers. *Arch Dermatol.* 1965;92:215.

119. Winn WA. Primary cutaneous coccidioidomycosis: reevaluation of its potentiality based on study of three new cases. *Arch Dermatol.* 1965;92:221.

120. Dodge RR, Lebowitz MD, Barbee R, Burrows B. Estimates of *C. immitis* infection by skin test reactivity in an endemic community. *Am J Public Health.* 1985;75:863.

121. Medoff G, Kobayashi GS. Strategies in the treatment of systemic fungal infections. *N Engl J Med.* 1980;302:145.

122. Ampel NM, Dols CL, Galgiani JN. Coccidioidomycosis during human immunodeficiency virus infection: results of a prospective study in a coccidioidal endemic area. *Am J Med.* 1993;94:235.

123. Wheat J. Histoplasmosis and coccidioidomycosis in individuals with AIDS: a clinical review. *Infect Dis Clin North Am.* 1994;8:467.

124. Schwartz RA, Lamberts RJ. Isolated nodular cutaneous coccidioidomycosis: the initial manifestation of disseminated disease. *J Am Acad Dermatol.* 1981;4:38.

125. Bayer AS, Yoshikawa TT, Galpin JE, Guze LB. Unusual syndromes of coccidioidomycosis: diagnostic and therapeutic considerations. *Medicine (Baltimore).* 1976;55:131.

126. Kwon-Chung KJ, Bennett JE. Coccidioidomycosis. In: Kwon-Chung KJ, Bennett JE, eds. *Medical Mycology.* Lea & Febiger; 1992:356.

127. Winer LH. Histopathology of the nodose lesion of acute coccidioidomycosis. *Arch Dermatol Syphilol.* 1950;61:1010.

128. Randhawa HS, Paliwal DK. Occurrence and significance of *Cryptococcus neoformans* in the oropharynx and on the skin of a healthy human population. *J Clin Microbiol.* 1977;6:325.

129. Glaser JB, Garden A. Inoculation of cryptococcosis without transmission of the acquired immunodeficiency syndrome. *N Engl J Med.* 1985;313:266.

130. Ng WF, Loo KT. Cutaneous cryptococcosis—primary versus secondary disease: report of two cases with review of literature. *Am J Dermatopathol.* 1993;15:372.

131. Hajjeh RA, Brandt ME, Pinner RW. Emergence of cryptococcal disease: epidemiologic perspectives 100 years after its discovery. *Epidem Rev.* 1995;17:303–320.

132. Dismukes WE. Cryptococcal meningitis in patients with AIDS. *J Infect Dis.* 1988;157:624.

133. Schupbach CW, Wheeler CE Jr, Briggaman RA, Warner NA, Kanof EP. Cutaneous manifestations of disseminated cryptococcosis. *Arch Dermatol.* 1976;112:1734.

134. Chu AC, Hay RJ, MacDonald DM. Cutaneous cryptococcosis. *Br J Dermatol.* 1980;103:95.

135. Cawley EP, Grekin RH, Curtis AC. Torulosis: a review of the cutaneous and adjoining mucous membrane manifestations. *J Invest Dermatol.* 1950;14:327.

136. Frieden TR, Bia FJ, Heald PW, Eisen RN, Patterson TF, Edelson RL. Cutaneous cryptococcosis in a patient with cutaneous T cell lymphoma receiving therapy with photophoresis and methotrexate. *Clin Infect Dis.* 1993;17:776.

137. Diamond RD, Bennett JE. Prognostic factors in cryptococcal meningitis: a study of 111 cases. *Ann Intern Med.* 1974;80:176.

138. Pema K, Diaz J, Guerra LG, Nabhan D, Verghese A. Disseminated cutaneous cryptococcosis: comparison of clinical manifestations in the pre-AIDS and AIDS eras. *Arch Intern Med.* 1994;154:1032.

139. Perfect JR, Durack DT, Gallis HA. Cryptococcemia. *Medicine (Baltimore).* 1983;62:98.

140. Sussman EJ, McMahon F, Wright D, Friedman HM. Cutaneous cryptococcosis without evidence of systemic involvement. *J Am Acad Dermatol.* 1984;11:371.

141. Kaplan MH, Rosen PP, Armstrong D. Cryptococcosis in a cancer hospital: clinical and pathological correlates in forty-six patients. *Cancer.* 1977;39:2265.

142. Gordon PM, Ormerod AD, Harvey G, Atkinson P, Best PV. Cutaneous cryptococcal infection without immunodeficiency. *Clin Exp Dermatol.* 1993;19:181.

143. Penneys NS, Hicks B. Unusual cutaneous lesions associated with acquired immunodeficiency syndrome. *J Am Acad Dermatol.* 1985;13:845.

144. Manrique P, Mayo J, Alvarez JA, Ganchegui X, Zabalza I, Flores M. Polymorphous cutaneous cryptococcosis: nodular, herpes-like, and molluscum-like lesions in a patient with the acquired immunodeficiency syndrome. *J Am Acad Dermatol.* 1992;26:122.

145. Blauvelt A, Kerdel FA. Cutaneous cryptococcosis mimicking Kaposi's sarcoma as the initial manifestation of disseminated disease. *Int J Dermatol.* 1992;31:279.

146. Carlson KC, Mehlmauer M, Evans S, Chandrasoma P. Cryptococcal cellulitis in renal transplant recipients. *J Am Acad Dermatol.* 1987;17:469.

147. Gutierrez F, Fu YS, Lurie HI. Cryptococcosis histologically resembling histoplasmosis: a light and electron microscopical study. *Arch Pathol.* 1975;99:347.

148. Ro JY, Lee SS, Ayala AG. Advantage of Fontana-Masson stain in capsule-deficient cryptococcal infection. *Arch Pathol Lab Med.* 1987;111:53.

149. Collins DN, Oppenheim IA, Edwards MR. Cryptococcosis associated with systemic lupus erythematosus: light and electron microscopic observations on a morphologic variant. *Arch Pathol.* 1971;91:78.

150. Miura T, Akiba H, Saito N, Seiji M. Primary cutaneous cryptococcosis. *Dermatologica.* 1971;142:374.

151. Noble RC, Fajardo LF. Primary cutaneous cryptococcosis: review and morphologic study. *Am J Clin Pathol.* 1972;57:13.

152. Sarosi GA, Silberfarb PM, Tosh FE. Cutaneous cryptococcosis: a sentinel of disseminated disease. *Arch Dermatol.* 1971;104:1.

153. Ruchel R. False-positive reaction of a Cryptococcus antigen test owing to Pseudallescheria mycosis. *Mycoses.* 1994;37:69.

154. Hamilton JR, Noble A, Denning DW, Stevens DA. Performance of cryptococcal antigen latex agglutination kits on serum and cerebrospinal fluid specimens of AIDS patients before and after pronase treatment. *J Clin Microbiol.* 1991;29:333–339.

155. Ruiter M, Ensink GJ. Acute primary cutaneous cryptococcosis. *Dermatologica.* 1964;128:185.

156. Kwon-Chung KJ, Bennett JE. Histoplasmosis. In: Kwon-Chung KJ, Bennett JE, eds. *Medical Mycology.* Lea & Febiger; 1992:464.

157. U.S. National Communicable Disease Center. Morbidity and mortality weekly report annual supplement: summary. 1968. *MMWR.* 1969:17.

158. Tosh FE, Balhuizen J, Yates JL, Brasher CA. Primary cutaneous histoplasmosis. *Arch Intern Med.* 1964;114:118.

159. Tesh RB, Schneidau JD Jr. Primary cutaneous histoplasmosis. *N Engl J Med.* 1966;275:597.

160. Nakelchik M, Mangino JE. Reactivation of histoplasmosis after treatment with infliximab. *Am J Med.* 2002;112:78.

161. Goodwin RA Jr, Owens FT, Snell JD, et al. Chronic pulmonary histoplasmosis. *Medicine (Baltimore).* 1976;15:413–452.

162. Ende N, Pizzolato P, Ziskind J. Hodgkin's disease associated with histoplasmosis. *Cancer.* 1952;5:763.

163. Kauffman CA, Israel KS, Smith JW, White AC, Schwarz J, Brooks GF. Histoplasmosis in immunosuppressed patients. *Am J Med.* 1978;64:923.

164. Bonner JR, Alexander WJ, Dismukes WE, et al. Disseminated histoplasmosis in patients with the acquired immune deficiency syndrome. *Arch Intern Med.* 1984;144:2178.

165. Wheat LJ. Histoplasmosis in Indianapolis. *Clin Infect Dis.* 1992;14:S91.

166. Neubauer MA, Bodensteiner DC. Disseminated histoplasmosis in patients with AIDS. *South Med J.* 1992;85:1166.

167. Goodwin RA Jr, Shapiro JL, Thurman GH, Thurman SS, Des Prez RM. Disseminated histoplasmosis: clinical and pathologic correlations. *Medicine (Baltimore).* 1980;59:1.

168. Studdard J, Sneed WF, Taylor MR Jr, Campbell GD. Cutaneous histoplasmosis. *Am Rev Respir Dis.* 1976;113:689.

169. Curtis AC, Grekin JN. Histoplasmosis: a review of the cutaneous and adjacent mucous membrane manifestations with a report of three cases. *JAMA.* 1947;134:1217.

170. Miller HE, Keddie FM, Johnstone HG, et al. Histoplasmosis: cutaneous and mucomembranous lesions, mycologic and pathologic observations. *Arch Dermatol Syphilol.* 1947;56:715.

171. Chanda JJ, Callen JP. Isolated nodular cutaneous histoplasmosis: the initial manifestation of recurrent disseminated disease. *Arch Dermatol.* 1978;114:1197.

172. Barton EN, Ince RWE, Patrick AL, et al. Cutaneous histoplasmosis in the acquired immune deficiency syndrome: a report of three cases from Trinidad. *Trop Geogr Med.* 1988;40:153.

173. Abildgaard WH Jr, Hargrove RH, Kalivas J. *Histoplasma* panniculitis. *Arch Dermatol.* 1985;121:914.

174. Samovitz M, Dillon TK. Disseminated histoplasmosis presenting as exfoliative erythroderma. *Arch Dermatol.* 1970;101:216.

175. Zarabi CM, Thomas R, Adesokan A. Diagnosis of systemic histoplasmosis in patients with AIDS. *South Med J.* 1992;85:1171.

176. Ueda Y, Sano A, Tamura M, et al. Diagnosis of histoplasmosis by detection of the internal transcribed spacer region of fungal rRNA gene from a paraffin-embedded skin sample from a dog in Japan. *Vet Microbiol.* 2003;94(3):219–24.

177. Rippon JW. *Medical Mycology.* Saunders; 1974.

178. Nethercott JR, Schachter RK, Givan KF, Ryder DE. Histoplasmosis due to *Histoplasma capsulatum* var *duboisii* in a Canadian immigrant. *Arch Dermatol.* 1978;114:595.

179. Lucas AO. Cutaneous manifestations of African histoplasmosis. *Br J Dermatol.* 1970;82:435.

180. Williams AO, Lawson EA, Lucas AO. African histoplasmosis due to *Histoplasma duboisii. Arch Pathol.* 1971;92:306.

181. Flegel H, Kaben U, Westphal H-J. Afrikanische histoplasmose. *Hautarzt.* 1980;31:50.

182. Schneidau JD Jr, Lamar LM, Hairston MA Jr. Cutaneous hypersensitivity to sporotrichin in Louisiana. *JAMA.* 1964;188:371.

183. Ingrish FM, Schneidau JD Jr. Cutaneous hypersensitivity to sporotrichin in Maricopa county, Arizona. *J Invest Dermatol.* 1967;49:146.

184. Urabe H, Honbo S. Sporotrichosis. *Int J Dermatol.* 1986;25:255.

185. Shelley WB, Sica PA Jr. Disseminate sporotrichosis of skin and bone cured with 5-fluorocytosine: photosensitivity as a complication. *J Am Acad Dermatol.* 1983;8:229.

186. Smith PW, Loomis GW, Luckasen JL, Osterholm RK. Disseminated cutaneous sporotrichosis: three illustrated cases. *Arch Dermatol.* 1981;117:143.

187. Shaw JC, Levinson W, Montanaro A. Sporotrichosis in the acquired immunodeficiency syndrome. *J Am Acad Dermatol.* 1989;21:1145.

188. Dellatorre DL, Lattanand A, Buckley HR, Urbach F. Fixed cutaneous sporotrichosis of the face: successful treatment of a case and review of the literature. *J Am Acad Dermatol.* 1982;6:97.

189. Lurie HI. Histopathology of sporotrichosis: notes on the nature of the asteroid body. *Arch Pathol.* 1963;75:421.

190. Carr RD, Storkan MA, Wilson JW, Swatek FE. Extensive verrucous sporotrichosis of long duration: report of a case resembling cutaneous blastomycosis. *Arch Dermatol.* 1964;89:124.

191. Wilson DE, Mann JJ, Bennett JE, Utz JP. Clinical features of extracutaneous sporotrichosis. *Medicine (Baltimore).* 1967;46:265.

192. Baum GL, Donnerberg RL, Stewart D, Mulligan WJ, Putnam LR. Pulmonary sporotrichosis. *N Engl J Med.* 1969;280:410.

193. Fetter BF. Human cutaneous sporotrichosis due to *Sporotrichum schenckii:* technique for demonstration of organisms in tissues. *Arch Pathol.* 1961;71:416.

194. Male O. Diagnostische und therapeutische probleme bei der kutanen sporotrichose. *Z Hautkr.* 1974;49:505.

195. Segal RJ, Jacobs PH. Sporotrichosis. *Int J Dermatol.* 1979;18:639.

196. Marques MEA, Coelho KIR, Sotto MN, Bacchi CE. Comparison between histochemical and immunohistochemical methods for diagnosis of sporotrichosis. *J Clin Pathol.* 1992;45:1089.

197. Kariya H, Iwatsu T. Statistical survey of 100 cases of sporotrichosis. *J Dermatol.* 1979;6:211.

198. Splendore A. Sobre a cultura d'uma nova especiale de cogumello pathogenico (sporotrichose de Splendore). *Revista de Sociedade Scientifa de São Paulo.* 1908;3:62.

199. Hoeppli R. Histological observations in experimental schistosomiasis Japonica. *Chin Med J.* 1932;46:1179.

200. Hiruma M, Kawada A, Ishibashi A. Ultrastructure of asteroid bodies in sporotrichosis. *Mycoses.* 1991;34:103.

201. Auld JC, Beardsmore GL. Sporotrichosis in Queensland: a review of 37 cases at the Royal Brisbane Hospital. *Australas J Dermatol.* 1979;20:14.

202. Reed KD, Moore FM, Geiger GE, Stemper ME. Zoonotic transmission of sporotrichosis: case report and review. *Clin Infect Dis.* 1993;16:384.

203. Palestine RF, Rogers RS III. Diagnosis and treatment of mycetoma. *J Am Acad Dermatol.* 1982;6:107.

204. Hay RJ, MacKenzie DWR. Mycetoma (Madura foot) in the United Kingdom: a survey of forty-four cases. *Clin Exp Dermatol.* 1983;8:553.

205. Green WO Jr, Adams TE. Mycetoma in the United States: a review and report of seven additional cases. *Am J Clin Pathol.* 1964;42:75.

206. Arastehfar A, Lim W, Daneshnia F, et al. Madurella real-time PCR, a novel approach for eumycetoma diagnosis. *PLoS Negl Trop Dis.* 2020;14(1):e0007845. doi: 10.1371/journal.pntd.0007845

207. Butz WC, Ajello L. Black grain mycetoma: a case due to *Madurella grisea. Arch Dermatol.* 1971;104:197.

208. Taralakshmi VV, Pankajalakshmi VV, Arumugam S, Subramanian S. Mycetoma caused by *Madurella mycetomii* in Madras. *Australas J Dermatol.* 1978;19:125.

209. Barnetson RSC, Milne LJR. Mycetoma. *Br J Dermatol.* 1978; 99:227.

210. Zaias N, Taplin D, Rebell G. Mycetoma. *Arch Dermatol.* 1969; 99:215.

211. Karunaratne WAE. *Rhinosporidiosis in Man.* Athlone Press of the University of London; 1964.

212. Kwon-Chung KJ, Bennett JE. Rhinosporidiosis. In: Kwon-Chung KJ, Bennett JE, eds. *Medical Mycology.* Lea & Febiger; 1992:695.

213. Rajam RV, Viswanathan GS, Rao A, et al. Rhinosporidiosis: a study with report of a fatal case of systemic dissemination. *Indian J Surg.* 1955;17:269.

214. Venezio FR, Lavoo E, Williams JE, et al. Progressive cutaneous protothecosis. *Am J Clin Pathol.* 1982;77:485.

215. Woolrich A, Koestenblatt E, Don P, Szaniawski W. Cutaneous protothecosis and AIDS. *J Am Acad Dermatol.* 1994;31:920.

216. Mayhall CG, Miller CW, Eisen AZ, Kobayashi GS, Medoff G. Cutaneous protothecosis: successful treatment with amphotericin B. *Arch Dermatol.* 1976;112:1749.

217. Nabai H, Mehregan AH. Cutaneous protothecosis: report of a case from Iran. *J Cutan Pathol.* 1974;1:180.

218. Wolfe ID, Sacks HG, Samorodin CS, et al. Cutaneous protothecosis in a patient receiving immunosuppressive therapy. *Arch Dermatol.* 1976;112:829.

Protozoan Diseases and Parasitic Infestations

ALVARO C. LAGA

Chapter

24

INTRODUCTION

The increase in international travel has brought diseases to North America and Europe that were once thought of as being confined to tropical countries. Furthermore, human immunodeficiency virus (HIV) infection and the increase in iatrogenic immunosuppression for the treatment of cancer and autoinflammatory diseases have become important cofactors in acquiring diseases that are otherwise rare in the developed world. Immigrants from and travelers to Asia, Africa, and South America represent another contingent of patients afflicted by diseases that are not frequent in the United States and Western Europe.

LEISHMANIASIS

Clinical Summary. Leishmania is an intracellular protozoan in the order Trypanosomatida. This organism exists in tissue as an aflagellate amastigote inside macrophages. It is transmitted by the phlebotomine sandfly (*Phlebotomus, Lutzomia,* and *Psychodopygus*) (1). With several notable exceptions, humans are incidental hosts, with other mammals acting as the reservoirs (2,3). Although there is debate on the classification of the diverse presentations of *Leishmania*, in general, they are categorized into three major groups: cutaneous leishmaniasis (CL), mucocutaneous leishmaniasis (ML), and visceral leishmaniasis (VL). Multiple other classification systems have been proposed (4,5). According to the World Health Organization, six countries have greater than 90% of the CL burden (Afghanistan, Iran, Brazil, Saudi Arabia, Syria, and Peru), and it is endemic in 98 countries and territories. Five countries harbor more than 90% of VL (India, Bangladesh, Nepal, Sudan, and Brazil), and three countries harbor more than 90% of ML (Bolivia, Brazil, and Peru). Classically, the subtypes of *Leishmania* were grouped according to their region of origin, vector of transmission, and the type of disease caused (6,7). *Leishmania* is most commonly spread through sandflies of the genus *Phlebotomus* in the Old World (Asia, Africa, and the Mediterranean) and of the genus *Lutzomyia* in the New World (Caribbean, Central America, and South America). However, with the advent of polymerase chain reaction (PCR) analysis, the concept of only certain species causing a particular clinical presentation of *Leishmania* has been called into question (7–10).

Approximately 1.5 million cases of CL are reported yearly. Acute lesions typically present as a papule or nodule that over a period of 1 to 3 months progresses to an ulcer (Fig. 24-1).

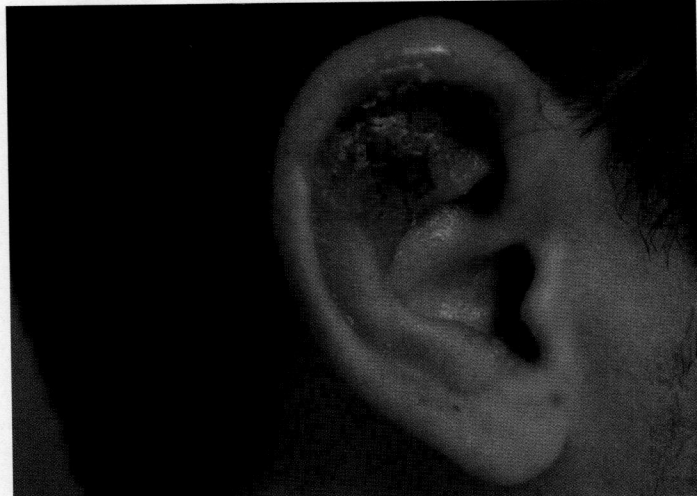

Figure 24-1 Acute cutaneous leishmaniasis. Ulceration with crust on the ear of a returning traveler from Costa Rica. (Photo courtesy of Dr. Misha Rosenbach, University of Pennsylvania, Philadelphia, PA.)

Localized CL tends to heal with time, leaving behind dyspigmentation and scar, but it can persist as a chronic condition. Lesions can be localized or disseminated (11). There is also a diffuse (pseudolepromatous) form that presents with progressive infiltrated plaques developing around the site of inoculation with symmetric progression and can be confused with lepromatous leprosy (Fig. 24-2). Although there is some confusing use of the terms "disseminate" and "diffuse" in the literature, it has been noted that disseminated leishmaniasis is differentiated from the diffuse form by the classic lepromatous leprosy–like presentation of the latter and the presence of subcutaneous nodules in the former (4). A recidivous or lupoid form describes the recurrence of leishmaniasis at the edge of the healed scar from primary CL (12–15). Several specialized regional forms of CL have been described, such as "chiclero ulcers" on the external ear caused by *L. mexicana* and "pian-bois" with sporotrichoid lesions caused by *L. guyanensis*. Atypical forms include unusual locations such as periungual, palms, soles, lips, eyelids, and genitals as well as unusual clinical morphologies such as zosteriform, eczematoid, erysipeloid, verrucoid, and psoriasiform (16–27). A case of discoid lupus erythematosus presenting in the scar of healed CL as an isotopic response has been reported (28).

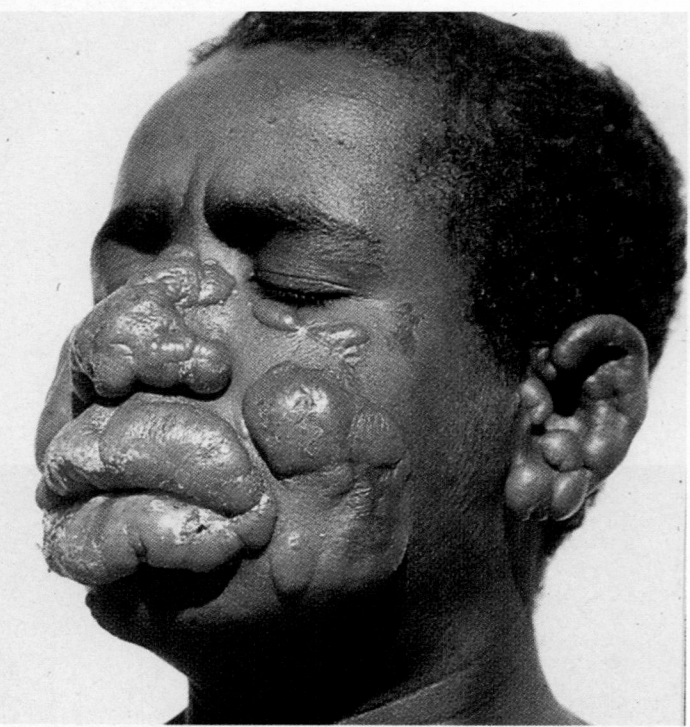

Figure 24-2 Diffuse acute cutaneous leishmaniasis. Ethiopian patient with pseudolepromatous appearance. (Reprinted by permission from Springer: Schaller KF. Protozoan dermatoses. In: Schaller KF, ed. *Colour Atlas of Tropical Dermatology and Venerology*. Springer; 1994:113. Copyright © 1994 Springer-Verlag Berlin Heidelberg.)

ML, also known as espundia, is a disease almost exclusively of South America and is rare in the United States (29,30). It constitutes approximately 5% of cases of New World leishmaniasis. It is primarily caused by *L. braziliensis* and *L. panamensis* (31). Patients present with ML several months to years after developing CL. However, cases of CL presenting synchronously with ML have been reported (32,33). ML presents with chronic nasal congestion, nasal bleeding, ulceration, and septal granulomas. In addition to the nasal mucosa, it has been described to involve the lips, palate, mouth, pharynx, larynx, and middle ear (34–37). It is an aggressive form of leishmaniasis, often leading to destruction of the nasopharynx tissue.

VL, also known as kala azar, causes over 50,000 deaths a year according to the WHO. It is characterized by undulating fevers, weight loss, hepatosplenomegaly, lymphadenopathy, and cytopenias (38). Except in patients with HIV, it rarely has cutaneous findings outside of the skin darkening and an erythematous malar rash seen on the Indian subcontinent. Patients with HIV may display a variety of cutaneous findings, including a spindle cell pseudotumor, colonization of a Kaposi sarcoma tumor, and coinfection at the site of herpes zoster infection (39–42). A bone marrow smear is the reference method for diagnosing VL; the condition can be confirmed through additional molecular tests. Serology is sometimes used in regions where a bone marrow smear is not available. Patients with resolved kala azar may develop cutaneous lesions in a form of leishmaniasis termed *post–kala azar dermal leishmaniasis* (PKDL). PKDL is primarily associated with *L. donovani*. These patients present with hypopigmented macules that progress to flesh-colored or erythematous papules and nodules. This form may be confused with lepromatous leprosy. PKDL can be differentiated from the diffuse cutaneous form of CL by the history of

previously treated or resolved VL in PKDL patients. PKDL has been a manifestation of the immune reconstitution inflammatory syndrome (IRIS) in patients with HIV upon the initiation of highly active antiretroviral therapy (HAART) and in transplant patients (43,44).

Cases of leishmaniasis are increasing. This is thought to be a result of global climate change, increased range of the phlebotomine sandflies, increased international travel, armed conflicts, the worldwide HIV epidemic, and increased iatrogenic immunosuppression (45). Transmission of leishmaniasis has been reported through blood transfusion (46). HIV is clearly a predisposition to more severe and atypical cases of *Leishmania*. Several cases of *Leishmania* presenting in patients undergoing treatment with TNF inhibitors have been reported (47–49).

A variety of ancillary testing is available for leishmaniasis, however; most tests described below are not widely available and only performed at specialized centers and research laboratories. Intradermal testing for *Leishmania* (Montenegro test) is available in some parts of the world. *Leishmania* can be cultured on Novy–MacNeal–Nicolle media or by animal inoculation. Organisms can be identified through isoenzyme analysis or other molecular methods. Identification of the causative species has become easier with the introduction of PCR testing (50). PCR is especially useful in cases of CL and ML where the overall number of organisms may be low. This testing can be done on fresh tissue as well as formalin-fixed, paraffin-embedded tissue. One of the most sensitive PCR methods targets the minicircle kinetoplast DNA (kDNA) (51,52).

Histopathology. All of the different species of *Leishmania* present with an identical morphology on microscopic examination. Careful examination of a biopsy with identification of characteristic amastigotes is usually sufficient for a diagnosis of leishmaniasis generic. Culture, isoenzyme analysis, and PCR (performed free of cost at the Centers for Disease Control, Atlanta, GA) are needed for identification at the species level. Amastigotes are 2 to 4 µm in size and round to oval in shape. They are notable for their nucleus and kinetoplast. The kinetoplast is a rod-shaped organelle that contains extranuclear DNA in maxi- and minicircles. Organisms are generally found within tissue macrophages but can be found extracellularly, especially in cases with high organism numbers. In the histiocyte, the organisms often stud the inner membrane in a "marquee" pattern. Amastigotes can be highlighted on Giemsa staining where the cytoplasm stains light blue and the nucleus and kinetoplast stain pink-red or violet. They do not stain with Grocott methenamine silver stain or Periodic acid–Schiff stain, which is helpful in distinguishing them from small intracellular yeasts (e.g., histoplasma) by the casual observer.

In CL, there is a dense mixed dermal inflammatory infiltrate predominantly of histiocytes, lymphocytes, and plasma cells (Fig. 24-3). Giant cells and eosinophils may also be seen, and neutrophils are noted once ulceration has occurred. Parasitized histiocytes are appreciable within the inflammation (Fig. 24-4A, B) (53–55). In early lesions, there may be overlying acanthosis or atrophy. In later lesions, ulceration and pseudoepitheliomatous hyperplasia may develop, and organisms may be difficult to find due to decreased numbers. In such instances, a high index of suspicion, good clinical history, and careful histopathologic examination are essential to avoid misclassification as squamous cell carcinoma. There is an increase in the number of tuberculoid granulomas, but perineural involvement and

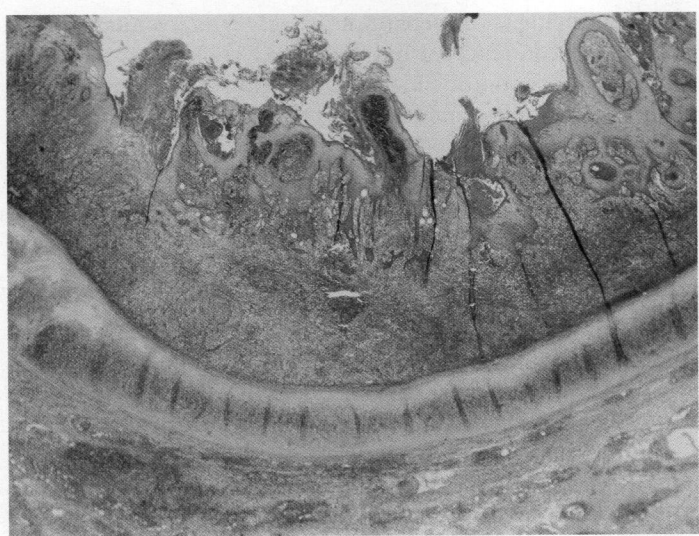

Figure 24-3 Leishmaniasis. Scanning magnification (×20) shows pseudocarcinomatous epidermal hyperplasia and a dense lymphohistiocytic infiltrate.

caseating necrosis are rarely seen (56,57). Tuberculoid granulomas are prominent in recidivous or lupoid disease.

The histopathologic features of ML are similar to the early and late stages of CL. Sangueza et al. (58) subdivide the histologic features into edematous, granulomatous, and necrotizing granulomatous stages. Suppuration and necrosis may be seen more frequently than in CL (58). Fibrosis can be seen in the dermis in long-standing lesions.

Cutaneous lesions in VL are rare. These lesions are characterized by a perivascular lymphohistiocytic infiltrate with parasitized histiocytes (59). Parasites have been noted in the eccrine glands, colonizing a tumor of Kaposi sarcoma and forming a spindle cell pseudotumor in other cases (39–41). There are few reports on the histopathology of PKDL. In a large case series looking at the dermal nodules in PKDL, there was an atrophic epidermis, prominent follicular plugging, a dense lymphohistiocytic inflammatory infiltrate, and collagen alteration (60). The authors of this case series highlight the importance of a negative Fite stain to rule out lepromatous leprosy. Similar

findings of a dense lymphohistiocytic infiltrate in the dermal nodules and a superficial perivascular infiltrate in the macular hypopigmented lesions have been reported by other groups (61–64).

Pathogenesis. As noted earlier, leishmaniasis is dependent not only on the type of *Leishmania* spp. but also on the host. Amastigotes disrupt macrophage activation, which leads to their persistence (65). Studies in mouse models of *Leishmania* and in humans have shown the importance of HLA and components of the cytokine and chemokine pathway in infection (66,67). Classically, resistance to disease progression has been associated with a Th1 response and susceptibility with a Th2 response. This is likely a much more complex issue with important contributions from Th17 and regulatory T cells (68).

Differential Diagnosis. The main differential is with the other infections that parasitize macrophages: histoplasmosis, *Klebsiella granulomatosis* (granuloma inguinale), *K. rhinoscleromatis* (rhinoscleroma), and penicilliosis. Special stains and the identification of the kinetoplast are most helpful in identifying *Leishmania. Leishmania* lacks the capsule seen in *Histoplasma capsulatum.* As lesions become more granulomatous, the differential diagnosis shifts to including other granulomatous conditions such as tuberculosis, sarcoidosis, and granulomatous rosacea. PCR may be helpful in identifying the correct diagnosis, especially in these cases.

Principles of Management: Treatment depends on the host, the parasite, and the form of leishmaniasis infection. Expert advice in planning the best treatment regimen is advised. Systemic therapies with good reports of effect include miltefosine, liposomal amphotericin B, conventional amphotericin B, and pentavalent antimony (sodium stibogluconate). Secondary agents include paromomycin, azole family antifungals, and pentamidine (69). Treatments for localized disease include cryotherapy, heat therapy, topical paromomycin, and intralesional sodium stibogluconate (70). ML and VL are always treated. CL is treated to hasten resolution, reduce scarring, decrease the chance of recurrence, and attempt to prevent mucosal disease; in general, patients in the United States with CL will receive therapy (69). Patients should be made aware of the chance of treatment failure and, despite satisfactory clinical response, the chance for

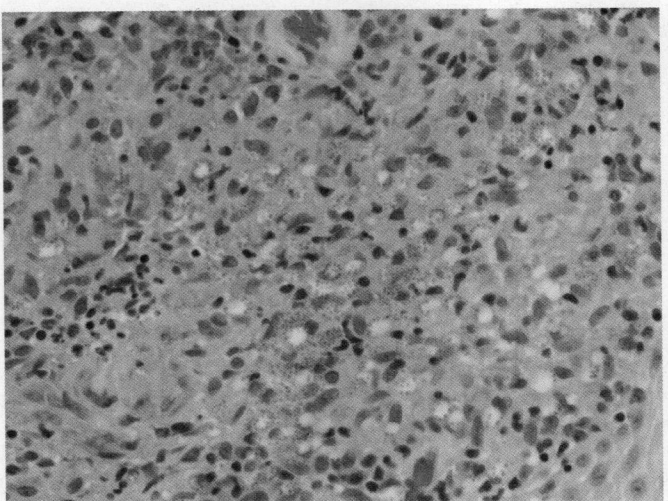
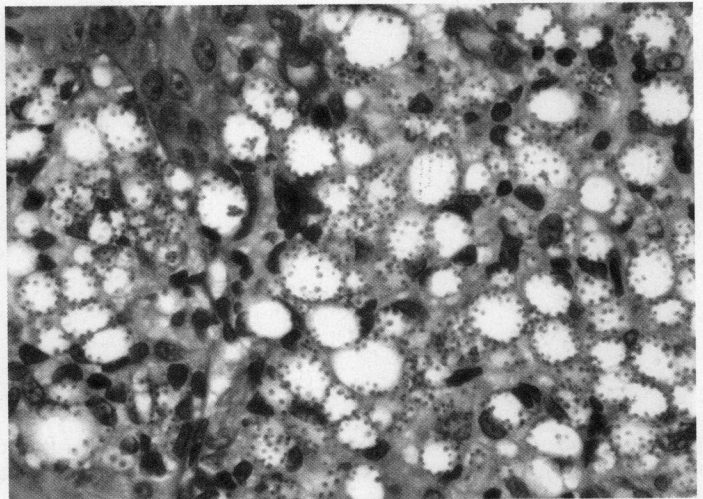

Figure 24-4 Leishmaniasis. A: Higher magnification of CL with mixed inflammatory infiltrate and parasitized histiocytes. B: Giemsa stain of CL with "marquee" sign of organisms lining the internal cell membrane of the histiocytes.

relapse and recurrence, including delayed relapse many months or even years after the initial infection.

AMEBIASIS

Clinical Summary. Human cutaneous amebiasis can be segregated into two main categories: infections caused by the parasitic *Entamoeba* spp. and infections caused by the free-living amebae (*Acanthamoeba*, *Naegleria fowleri*, and *Balamuthia mandrillaris*) (71). Amebae are single-cell organisms that exist in either the environmentally stable cyst form or the pathogenic trophozoite form. As opposed to free-living amebae that are considered facultative parasites of humans, *Entamoeba histolytica* is endemic in parts of Africa, Asia, and South America. It is reported to infect approximately 10% of the worldwide population although this number may be lower as molecular diagnostic techniques identify new subspecies of *Entamoeba*.

E. histolytica primarily infects the gastrointestinal tract. Cutaneous lesions typically result from either direct extension to the perianal and genital skin or through fistulas to the skin from underlying GI or hepatic abscesses. Primary cutaneous lesions have been reported but are rare (72). Typical lesions are painful and malodorous ulcers with a gray-white necrotic base (73). Perianal and genital lesions are often verrucous and may be mistaken for genital warts or squamous cell carcinomas (74). Venereal transmission has been reported. More advanced disease has been associated with HIV infection.

Free-living amebae are most commonly associated with devastating CNS infections. *Acanthamoeba* and *Balamuthia* cause granulomatous encephalitis and frequently present with cutaneous ulceronecrotic or suppurative nodules (Fig. 24-5A). *Naegleria* only causes meningoencephalitis, but no cutaneous lesions and thus will not be discussed further. *Acanthamoeba* is a causative organism of keratitis, especially in contact lens wearers (71). Chronic plaques and ulcers of the central facial region have been especially noted in *B. mandrillaris* infections in South America (75). Sporotrichoid spread has also been reported. HIV-positive and immunosuppressed patients have increased susceptibility (76,77). The skin involvement can be a result of direct inoculation or result from the underlying visceral disease.

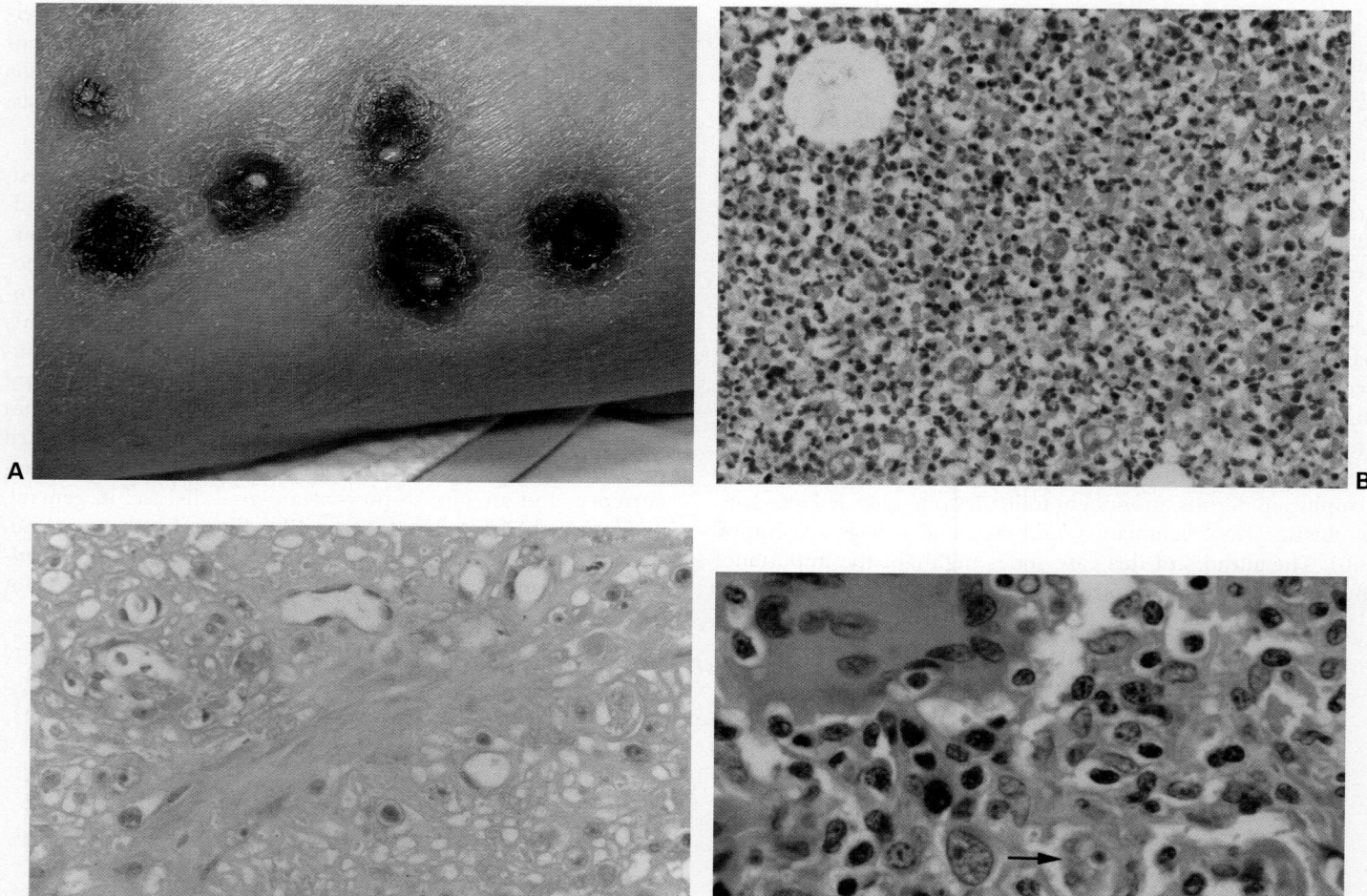

Figure 24-5 Acanthamebiasis. **A:** Ulceronecrotic nodules with purulent discharge are characteristic of cutaneous acanthamebiasis. **B:** The trophozoites are identified by their histiocytoid foamy cytoplasm with a central nucleus and prominent nucleolus-like karyosome within the inflammatory infiltrate. **C:** *Acanthamoeba* cysts show characteristic bilaminar wrinkled outer wall. **D:** The trophozoites of *Balamuthia mandrillaris* are very similar to those of *Acanthamoeba* but very difficult to find in sections in skin lesions of immunocompetent patients. The arrow points to an amebic trophozoite of *B. mandrillaris*.

Histopathology. Infections with *E. histolytica* demonstrate ulceration with necrosis and a mixed inflammatory infiltrate. Extravasated erythrocytes are often seen (78). *E. histolytica* is approximately 20 to 50 μm in size, round, and basophilic. There is an eccentrically placed nucleus and central karyosome. The nucleus is uniformly round and the karyosome resembles an enlarged nucleolus (79). Erythrocytes are commonly noted within the cytoplasm. PAS or Trichrome stain can be useful in contrasting the organism and ingested cells. As noted above, there may be pseudoepitheliomatous hyperplasia at the edge of the lesion or in place of the ulceration leading to confusion with verrucous carcinoma.

Free-living amebae tend to form a granulomatous infiltrate in the dermis and subcutaneous tissue. Granulomas are generally ill-defined but may be tuberculoid in appearance. There is often prominent necrosis and a surrounding lymphoplasmacytic infiltrate. Organisms can be identified within the necroinflammatory debris and near blood vessels. *Acanthamoeba* and *B. mandrillaris* are described as 8 to 40 μm and 50 to 60 μm in size in the trophozoite stage, respectively (71). *Acanthamoeba* trophozoites have a centrally placed nucleus and karyosome resembling a nucleolus, without erythrocytes or debris within the cytoplasm (Fig. 24-5B) (80). It should be noted that amoebic trophozoites are inconspicuous in tissue sections, have morphologic and tinctorial features similar to histiocytes, and may be easily overlooked. Free-living amoebic cysts stand out in tissue sections when present due to their well-delineated, irregular bilaminar (*Acanthamoeba*, Fig. 24-5C) or trilaminar (*Balamuthia*) cyst walls. Grocott silver or Periodic acid–Schiff stains highlight the wall of free-living amoebic cysts but not the trophozoites. Vasculitis is often appreciated, particularly in encephalitis (80). These organisms can be identified in the vessel walls in CNS disease suggesting that the organisms may directly contribute to the vasculitis. It is important to note that, in patients with AIDS or on immunosuppression, granulomas may not be present. Less commonly, these infections can present with ulceration and neutrophilic abscesses. Suppurative panniculitis has been described associated with *Acanthamoeba* (80–82). Ulceration with necrosis and surrounding pseudoepitheliomatous hyperplasia, similar to the ulcers seen in *E. histolytica* infection, can be seen in the cutaneous ulcers of *B. mandrillaris*. Distinction between *Acanthamoeba* spp. and *Balamuthia* by histopathology is practically not possible (Fig. 24-5D). Immunofluorescent and immunohistochemical stains exist but are generally only available at reference laboratories such as the Center for Disease Control and Prevention (Atlanta, GA, USA).

Differential Diagnosis. Because of the pseudoepitheliomatous hyperplasia seen in *E. histolytica*, it may be mistaken for verrucous carcinoma.

The granulomatous inflammation associated with free-living ameba is similar to that seen in other infectious processes, especially in leishmaniasis and mycobacterial infections, as well as other granulomatous conditions such as granulomatosis with polyangiitis (formerly Wegener), sarcoidosis, and lymphomas. Ameba may be mistaken for macrophages or fungal organisms if the distinctive eccentric nucleus and karyosome are not identified.

Principles of Management: Metronidazole is the treatment of choice for *E. histolytica* infections. Other options include diloxanide, tinidazole, and pentamidine. Numerous therapies

have been tried for free-living amebae but none have proved reliably effective. This may change with the introduction of miltefosine, which has been effective in the treatment of cases of *Acanthamoeba* and *Balamuthia* (83,84). Combination therapy with other agents such as amphotericin B, azithromycin, and rifampicin is recommended, but the response is low and the mortality high despite it (85).

SCABIES

Clinical Summary. Acarid mites produce several skin manifestations in humans, the most common one being scabies, which is caused by the eight-legged itch mite *Sarcoptes scabiei* var. *hominis*, also referred to as *S. scabiei*. Animal pathogenic mites can also affect the skin, although most commonly through bite reactions and not human infestation (1).

Burrows, which represent a tunnel through which a female mite travels just below the stratum corneum to lay her eggs, are the pathognomonic lesions of scabies and are found mostly in the florid, papulovesicular type infestation (Fig. 24-6A). They occur mainly on the palmar and lateral aspects of the fingers and toes, the interdigital spaces, the flexor surfaces of the wrists, the nipples of women, the genitals of men, and, to a lesser extent, the buttocks and axillae. Characteristically, the head is spared, except in infants, elderly, and immunocompromised (86). The burrows appear as fine, tortuous, grayish threads a few millimeters long. A vesicle may be visible near the blind end of the burrow. The mite, eggs, or feces (the latter also known as scybala) may be situated at the end of the burrow and are sometimes visible by dermatoscopy (87). Mites and their byproducts have also been easily identified using reflectance confocal microscopy in crusted scabies, and a relatively homogenous distribution has been noted in this condition over all body surfaces (88). Although pathognomonic, the burrow is not the most common lesion seen in scabies. Small, erythematous, often excoriated papules are more frequent (86).

In some patients, itching nodules persist for several months after successful treatment and therefore are named nodular scabies or persistent nodules. They are found most commonly on the scrotum and are believed to result from a prolonged response to persistent scabies antigens (89). In children, sometimes these nodules may grow so large they can be mistaken for infectious or malignant lesions.

In a third, rare variant called crusted scabies (formerly known as Norwegian scabies), innumerable mites are present. Patients with this variant typically have T-cell dysregulation/immunodeficiency (e.g., transplant patients) and show widespread erythema, hyperkeratosis, crusting, nail thickening, and subungual hyperkeratosis but no obvious burrows.

Histopathology. A definitive diagnosis of scabies can be made only by demonstration of the mite or its products (eggs or scybala). A very superficial epidermal biopsy or scraping of an early papule or, preferably, of an entire burrow may be carried out with a no. 15 scalpel blade (90). The specimen is placed on a glass slide, and a drop of immersion oil is placed on top of it for immediate evaluation at the dermatologist's office (Fig. 24-6B).

A biopsy for histopathologic analysis is not ideal because of its low sensitivity, except in crusted scabies. Occasionally, a burrow housing a scabetic mite is evident within the stratum corneum (91). Only the extreme, blind end of the burrow, where

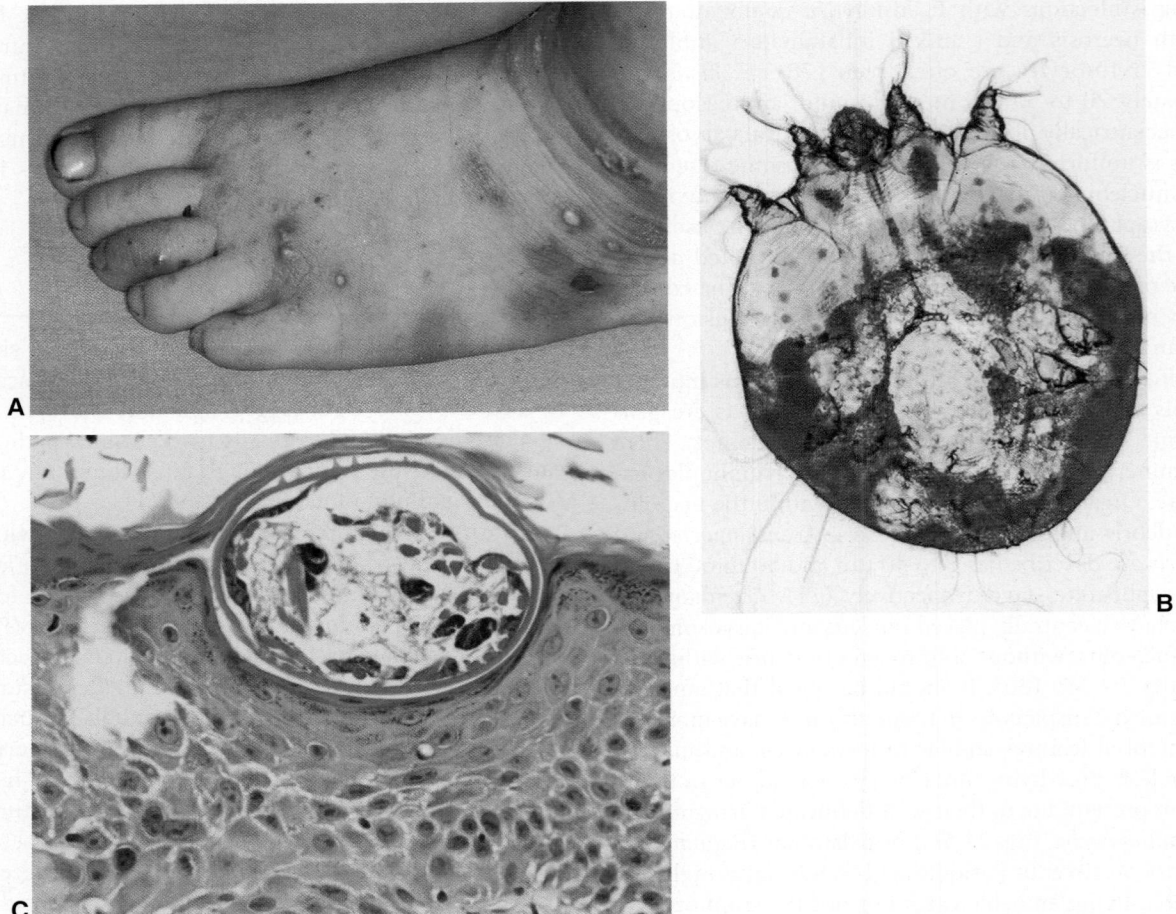

Figure 24-6 Scabies. **A:** Numerous pustules and papules are noted on the back of the foot and the toes of this infected child. **B:** Adult female mite found in skin scrapings. **C:** The female mite is located in the upper portion of the epidermis underneath the stratum corneum.

the female mite is situated, extends into the stratum malpighii (92). The mite has a rounded, dorsally convex body with characteristic cuticular spines and measures about 350 to 450 μm in length and 250 to 350 μm in width (Fig. 24-6C) (1). The presence of scabies can be made presumptively by the presence of pink pigtail-like structures, which are likely remnants of egg shells, within the intracorneal burrow (Fig. 24-7) (93). Polaroscopy may also be a helpful tool, given that attached and detached spines, as well as scybala, are polarizable (94).

In the papulovesicular form of scabies, spongiosis is present in the stratum malpighii near the mite to such an extent that formation of a vesicle is often the result. Even if no mite is found in the sections, the presence of eggs containing larvae, egg shells, or scybala within the stratum corneum is indicative of scabies (91,95). The dermal infiltrate in sections containing mites shows varying numbers of lymphocytes and eosinophils and is otherwise indistinguishable from other delayed-type hypersensitivity reactions. It takes approximately a month to mount a hypersensitivity response, which interestingly is thought to be triggered by the eggs and scybala and not the mite itself.

In nodular or persistent nodular scabies, there is a dense, chronic inflammatory, often pseudolymphomatous infiltrate in which many eosinophils may be present. Vasculitis is considered by some as being frequent (95) but by others as representing a rather uncommon event (89). These different findings may be related to the duration of the scabietic nodules and the

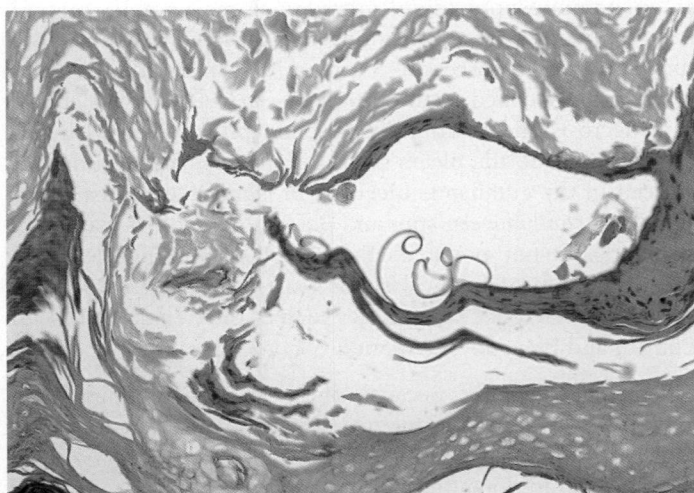

Figure 24-7 Scabies. Presence of scabies can be made presumptively by the presence of pink pigtail-like structures, which are likely remnants of egg shells.

timing of the biopsy (89). The nodules are rich in indeterminate cells, sometimes misleading to the diagnosis of Langerhans cell histiocytosis based on light microscopy and immunophenotyping alone (96). Atypical mononuclear, CD30$^+$ cells may be found (97), and in some instances, the nodules show, as in persistent arthropod bites or stings (see later discussion), a histologic picture resembling that of lymphoma (98). Viable mites are hardly ever found in the nodules. However, mite parts are seen in up to 22% of cases (89).

Other inflammatory patterns have been described in association with scabies infestation, including an interstitial histiocytic pattern mimicking granuloma annulare (99).

In crusted scabies, the thickened horny layer is riddled with innumerable mites, so that nearly every section shows several parasites (Fig. 24-8) (95).

Pathogenesis. Earlier scanning electron microscope studies revealed the keratinocytes around the burrow to be compacted, indicating that the mite physically forces its way in between the keratinocytes rather than chewing a passage (92). More recent studies, however, also using transmission electron microscopy, have found that the secretion of cytolytic substances by the mite is a contributing factor in advancing the parasite body through the skin in addition to mere compression (100). The cellular damage was greatest around the body, especially the mite capitulum.

Both cell-mediated and humoral immune responses are activated in scabies. The acute eczematoid reaction in the epidermis is indicative of cell-mediated hypersensitivity. A role for humoral hypersensitivity is suggested by the presence of immunoglobulin M and the third component of complement in vessel walls (89,101). Crusted scabies is observed generally in patients who are severely compromised in their immune responses, including those with leukemia, lymphoma, and the acquired immunodeficiency syndrome (102). Crusted scabies manifesting as an exuberant IRIS associated with HIV therapy has also been reported (103).

Principles of Management: The optimal treatment depends on the type of disease, the patient's age, and comorbidities. Topical medications, including permethrin 5% and malathion 0.5%, have proven excellent clinical success. In addition, oral ivermectin 200 µg/kg is a very effective treatment, particularly in patients with severe disease or crusted scabies. Combination therapy and repeated treatments are sometimes required in cases of extensive infestation or for immunocompromised hosts.

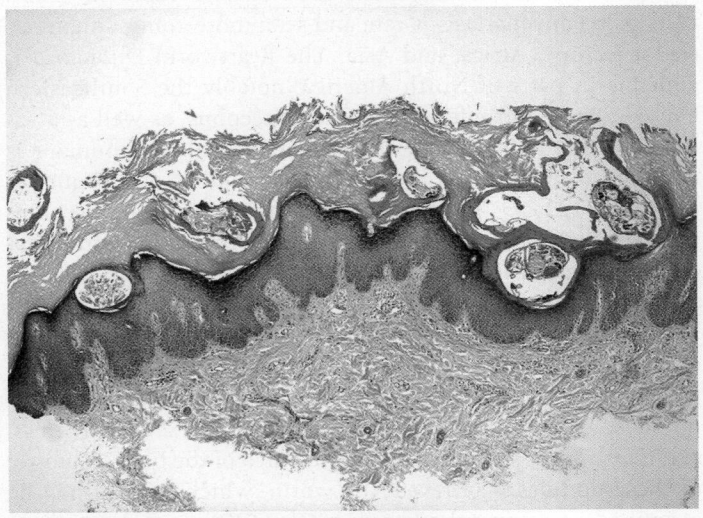

Figure 24-8 Crusted scabies. Thickened stratum corneum is riddled with numerous mites, so that nearly every section shows several parasites.

HOOKWORM-RELATED CUTANEOUS LARVA MIGRANS

Clinical Summary. Cutaneous larva migrans is caused by skin-penetrating larvae of nematodes, most commonly of the cat and dog hookworm *Ancylostoma braziliense*, *A. caninum*, *A. tubaeforme*, *Uncinaria stenocephala*, and *Bunostomum phlebotomum* (1,104–107). Other forms of cutaneous larva migrans are caused by human- and animal-type *Strongyloides* species and are then known as larva currens (see later discussion). *Gnathostomum spinigerum* does not belong to the hookworm family but to the group of spiruriids and can also evoke a deep cutaneous larva migrans-like eruption or migratory panniculitis (1).

Hookworm-related cutaneous larva migrans is the most common variant. The infestation occurs through contact with soil contaminated with the larvae. The exposed parts of the body, such as the feet, are most commonly involved, but any body part in direct contact with sand or soil may be affected. Creeping eruption represents the clinical manifestation of cutaneous larva migrans and is manifested by an irregularly linear, thin, raised, serpiginous burrow that is 2 to 3 mm wide (Fig. 24-9A). The larva and track may clinically be better visualized with the assistance of dermatoscopy or reflectance confocal microscopy (108). The larva moves a few millimeters per day. The eruption is self-limited because the causative species are zoonotic hookworms (not to be confused with the human hookworm *A. duodenale*) and humans represent accidental hosts, leaving the larva incapable of sexually maturing.

Histopathology. The visible track does not correlate with the exact location of the larva and represents an inflammatory response composed of lymphocytes admixed with many eosinophils in the epidermis and upper dermis (1,105,106). The parasite is found 1 to 2 cm ahead of the visible track within a burrow located in the upper layers of the epidermis (Fig. 24-9B) (109). The lesion, aside from the larva—which is often not observed in the biopsies, shows spongiosis and intraepidermal vesicles in which necrotic keratinocytes can be seen. Numerous eosinophils in the superficial and deep reticular dermis are also commonly observed. A specific subtype of hookworm-related cutaneous larva migrans, usually confined to the buttocks, is known as hookworm folliculitis (110). It is important to recognize this variant because the inflammation is typically perifollicular, the organisms are often deep within the follicles, and it is typically more difficult to treat (111).

Pathogenesis. The tissue penetration and the movements of the hookworm larvae within the epidermis are at least in part due to the active production and secretion of proteases by the parasite (112). However, with the exception of hookworm folliculitis, these enzymatic activities are typically not adequate to allow penetration into the dermis, and hence the nematode is located in the upper portion of the epidermis (113).

Principles of Management: Cutaneous larva migrans is often self-limited, but severe pruritus and risk of superficial infection may be reason for treatment. Oral thiabendazole or ivermectin may be used.

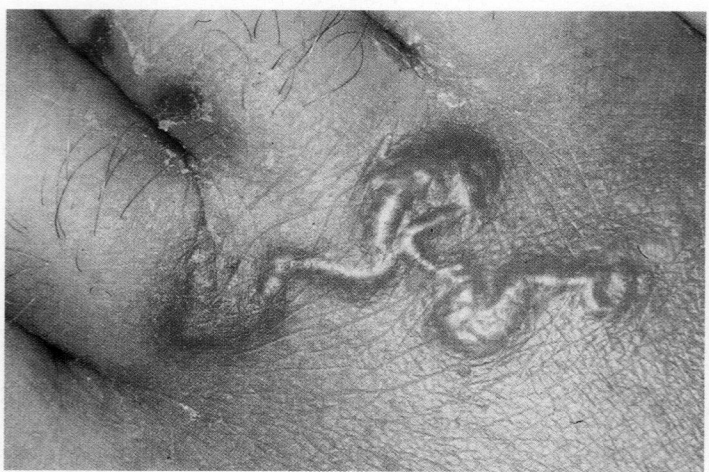 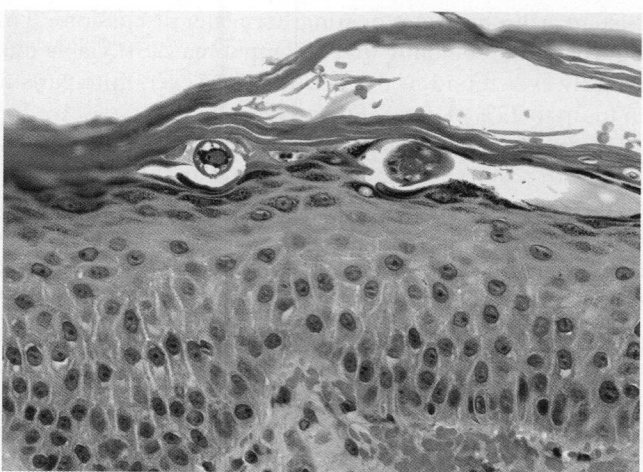

Figure 24-9 Cutaneous larva migrans. **A:** This curvilinear superficial burrow is the prototypical clinical manifestation. **B:** The organism is found underneath the stratum corneum in the upper portion of the stratum malpighii. (Specimen courtesy of Mandi Sachdeva, MD, and Rajiv Patel, MD, Cleveland Clinic Foundation, Cleveland, Ohio.)

STRONGYLOIDIASIS

Clinical Summary. Strongyloides stercoralis is a small intestinal nematode that is mainly endemic in the tropics and subtropics but is also found in the southeastern United States (especially eastern Kentucky, rural Tennessee, southern Virginia, and western North Carolina and South Carolina) (114). It is a geohelminth contracted by humans through cutaneous penetration of filariform larvae. A unique cycle includes traveling of the larvae via the venous system to the lungs, the patient coughing up and subsequently swallowing the larvae, and the parasite finding its final habitat in the small intestine (1). Three forms of strongyloidiasis can be delineated clinically: a not well-characterized acute form, a chronic form, and a disseminated form (114). The chronic type presents with gastrointestinal and pulmonary symptoms and the pathognomonic larva currens. The chronic form represents a linear or serpiginous urticarial tract moving at a rate of 5 to 15 cm/hour caused by rapidly migrating larvae and is a subtype of cutaneous larva migrans (see previous discussion). It is believed to derive from autoinoculation with intestinal larva in the perineal area. The disseminated variant of strongyloidiasis occurs in the setting of severe immunosuppression and is commonly fatal. Immunosuppressive therapy for autoimmune disease, iatrogenic immunosuppression for transplant patients, human T-cell lymphotropic virus (HTLV), and AIDS may predispose to disseminated infection (115). Patients with advanced hyperinfection present with a purpuric skin eruption (Fig. 24-10A), often located periumbilically (116,117). Other cutaneous manifestations of strongyloidiasis include chronic urticaria, prurigo nodularis, and lichen simplex chronicus (116–118).

Histopathology. The serpiginous urticarial lesions believed to represent the migrating path of larvae are consistently negative for organisms (116). In contrast to hookworm-associated cutaneous larva migrans, the migratory tracts of larva currens are not located in the epidermis but in the dermis (1). It is only in the disseminated variant of strongyloidiasis that organisms can be found. They occur in the form of filariform larvae, measuring from 9 to 15 μm in diameter, which can be seen at all levels of the dermis. These larvae are commonly associated with vascular damage producing purpura and petechiae, which are likely due to vascular damage by the filariform larvae migrating

through the vessel wall (Fig. 24-10B-D) (116,117,119,120). These changes often do not provoke a significant dermal inflammatory response, probably because these patients are severely immunocompromised (116,117,121) (Fig. 24-10A). Changes of leukocytoclastic vasculitis are also not noted (119–121). Eosinophil-rich granulomata around *Strongyloides* larvae are, however, occasionally described (114,120).

Principles of Management: Treatment of intestinal strongyloidiasis is highly successful with oral agents including thiabendazole, albendazole, or ivermectin. Systemic infection or infection in immunocompromised patients may require longer treatment and/or parenteral medication (115).

SUBCUTANEOUS DIROFILARIASIS

Clinical Summary. Dirofilariasis is a zoonotic infection caused by the heartworm of animals that serve as the definitive hosts. Humans are infected through mosquito bites and are terminal hosts as the worm cannot reach maturity in the human host. Human-to-human transmission has not been reported (122). Cutaneous dirofilariasis is rare and seen more commonly in areas of Europe, Africa, and Asia. The heartworm *Dirofilaria* is endemic in parts of North America, notably the Southeastern United States, and infects dogs, cats, raccoons, as well as a variety of other animals. Dirofilariasis in animals and humans is expected to increase as the range and number of mosquitoes increases (123). *D. immitis, D. repens,* and *D. tenuis* are the common species to cause disease in humans. Infections with *Dirofilaria* can result in subcutaneous nodules, pulmonary lesions, and ophthalmic lesions (124).

Subcutaneous nodules of dirofilariasis usually begin on an exposed area of skin where the mosquito bite occurs. An unusual aspect of these nodules is their description as migratory nodules, where one nodule will appear for 1 to 2 days, regress, and then appear soon after in another area of the body. A biopsy of these nodules may reveal the worm, which can be then be examined on a mineral oil preparation (125).

Histopathology. The organism is found in the center of an intense inflammatory response which forms the subcutaneous nodule. *Dirofilaria* can be identified by its thick laminated eosinophilic

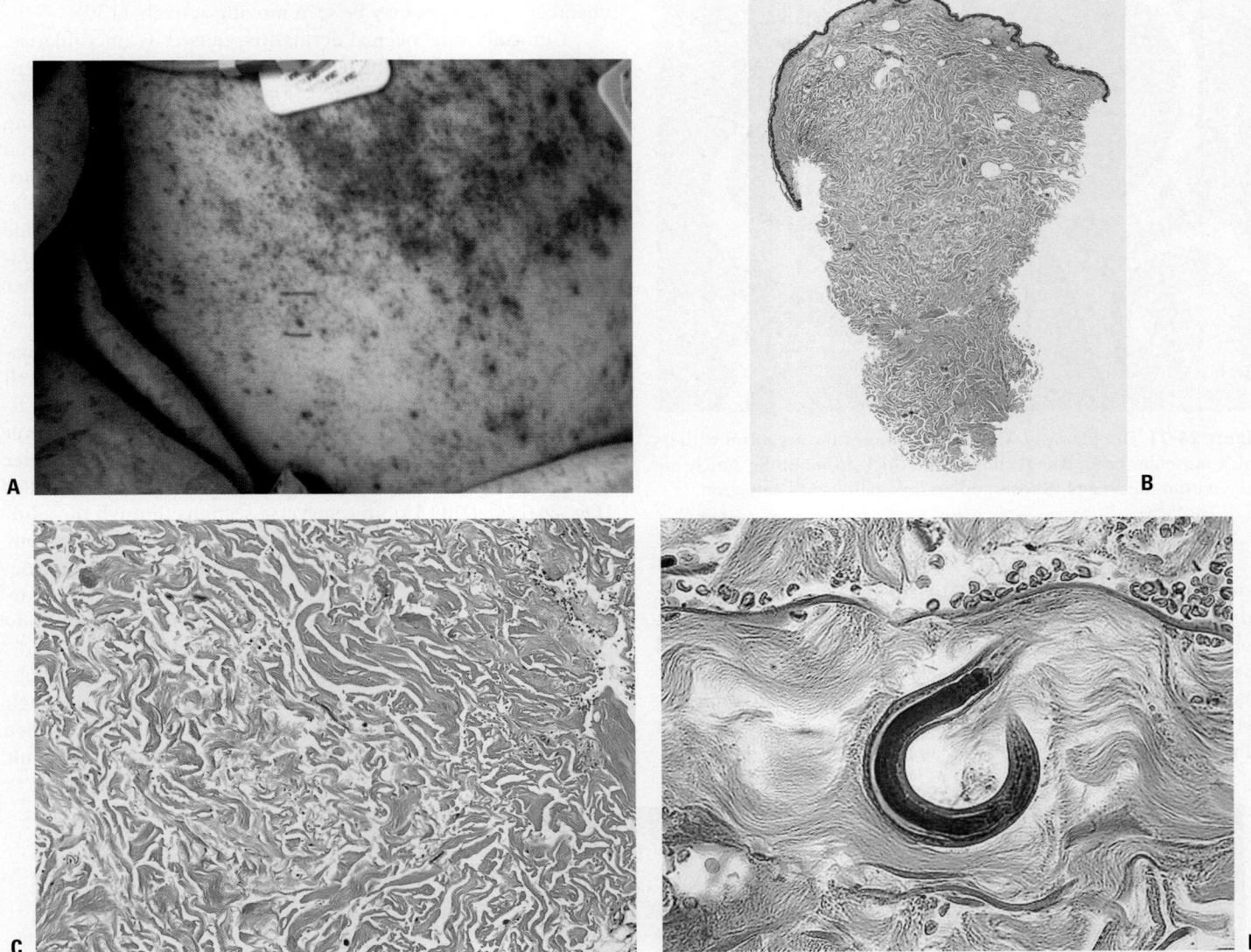

Figure 24-10 Strongyloidiasis. **A:** A purpuric eruption, shown here involving the abdomen, is characteristic of disseminated strongyloidiasis. **B:** On scanning magnification, the punch biopsy from the periumbilical purpuric eruption shows no obvious histopathologic changes. The patient died from disseminated strongyloidiasis. **C:** On medium-power magnification, extravasated erythrocytes are noted (upper right corner), and basophilic linear and round structures become apparent. **D:** On rare occasions, an entire nematode cut at the right angle is seen percolating between the collagen bundles. Note extravasated erythrocytes at the top of the micrograph. (**B, C:** Specimen courtesy of Arlene S. Rosenberg, MD, MetroHealth Medical Center, Cleveland, Ohio. **D:** Courtesy of Catherine M. Stefanato, MD, and Eduardo Calonje, MD, St. John's Institute of Dermatology, London, UK.)

cuticle, large lateral chords, and well-developed muscular layer (Fig. 24-11). It is usually solitary. The inflammatory response is primarily granulomatous with admixed neutrophils, eosinophils, histiocytes, and lymphocytes (126,127). It is important to cut multiple levels to identify the organism (124). *Dirofilaria* spp. are difficult to differentiate on histology alone. Molecular techniques may be helpful in speciation if required, but clinically not necessary.

Pathogenesis. *Dirofilaria* can be confirmed through PCR analysis on formalin-fixed paraffin-embedded tissue (128,129).

Differential Diagnosis. Subcutaneous dirofilariasis may clinically be confused with other benign and malignant dermal nodules (126). Histologically, *Dirofilaria* spp. can be confused with other onchocercids, notably *Onchocerca volvulus*. *Dirofilaria* has a thicker muscular layer than *O. volvulus* and is usually solitary as opposed to the multiple organisms seen in an onchocercoma.

Principles of Management: Treatment is with surgical excision of the subcutaneous nodule. Oral albendazole, oral ivermectin, and other antihelminthics are also given for possible systemic infection or incomplete excision (127).

ONCHOCERCIASIS

Clinical Summary. Onchocerciasis is common in certain regions of Central and South America as well as tropical Africa. It is transmitted by black flies of the genus *Simulium*, which breed in fast-flowing rivers. Through their probosces, the infective larvae of *O. volvulus*, a filarial nematode, enter the human skin. They mature to the adult stage in the subcutaneous tissue. The adult worms live in the deep dermis and subcutis and become clinically apparent as asymptomatic subcutaneous nodules called onchocercomas, of which there are usually only

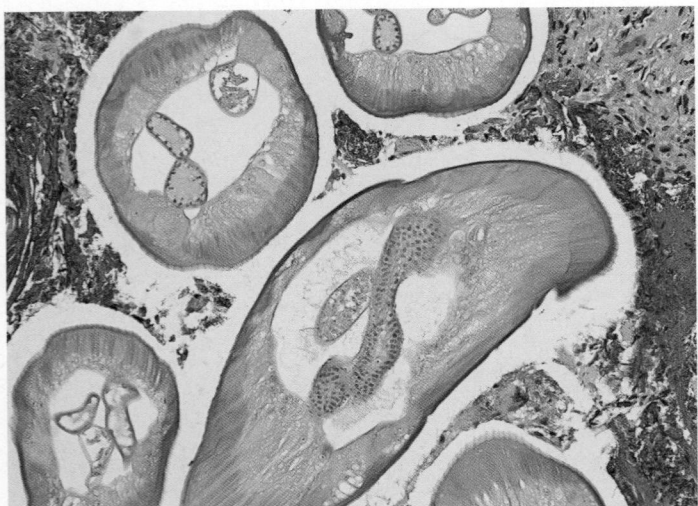

Figure 24-11 Dirofilariasis. Multiple sections of the organism with its thick muscular layer, lateral chords, and thick eosinophilic cuticle are seen within the area of fibrosis and granulomatous inflammation.

a few, ranging in size from 0.5 to 2.0 cm (Fig. 24-12A). The adult worms do not cause any harm; however, their progeny, consisting of millions of microfilariae, live in the dermis and the aqueous humor of the eyes, where they provoke inflammatory changes after several years. In the eyes, keratitis, iridocyclitis, chorioretinitis, and optic atrophy ultimately result in blindness, known in endemic areas as "river blindness" (130).

On slit-lamp examination, the microfilariae in the anterior chamber of the eyes may be seen moving actively (130).

Clinically, onchocercal dermatitis, caused by microfilariae, is characterized by itching, edema, lichenification, and pigmentary alteration ("leopard skin") (Fig. 24-12B) (131,132). Later, the skin becomes atrophic. A clinical classification and grading system of the cutaneous changes in onchocerciasis has been proposed but is not yet universally accepted (131). *O. volvulus*, like *Wuchereria bancrofti*, may also be a cause of lymphatic filariasis, in which massive numbers of microfilariae may occlude lymphatics and result in elephantiasis (133). Lymphadenopathy and so-called hanging groin (adenolymphocele) are other manifestations of the disease (133).

Histopathology. The onchocercomas show a chronic inflammatory infiltrate, including eosinophils and mast cells (134), as well as fibrosis at the periphery. Their centers consist of dense, fibrous tissue containing transverse and diagonal sections of adult worms measuring from 125 to 450 μm in transverse diameter and up to 500 mm in length for females and 42 mm for males (Fig. 24-12C, D) (133). In transverse sections through the adult female worm, a "double barrel"–shaped uterus with numerous microfilariae and a central gastrointestinal tube is characteristic. Some of them are alive at the time of biopsy. Dead worms are surrounded by an inflammatory reaction containing foreign-body giant cells. Microfilariae, which measure from 5 to 9 μm in diameter and from 220 to 360 μm in length, are occasionally observed within lymphatic vessels of the onchocercomas, through which they are disseminated in the skin (133). There is evidence that lymphatic and blood vascularization occurs around the adult

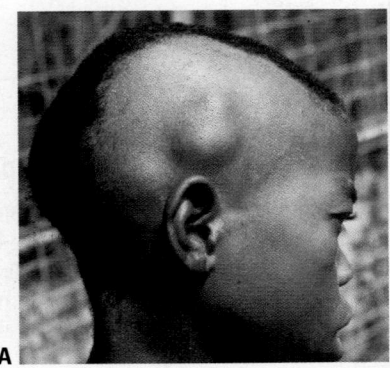

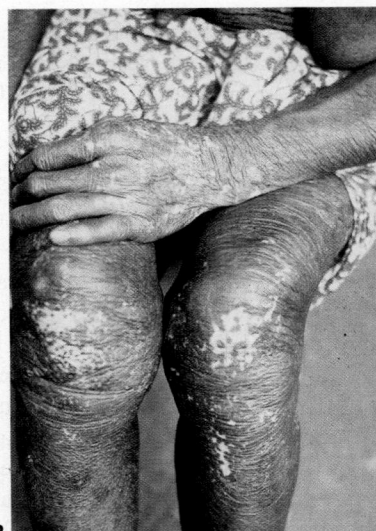

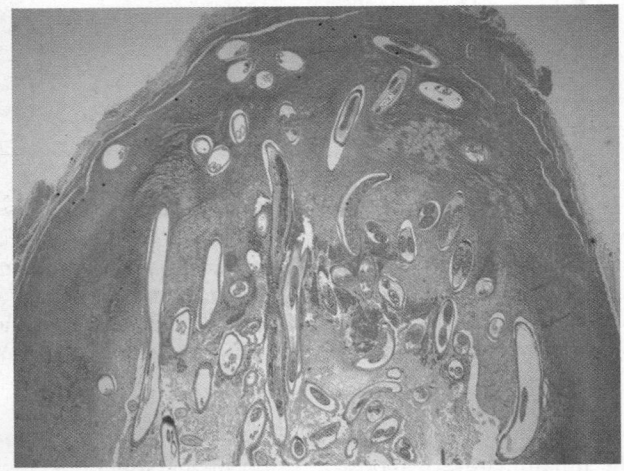

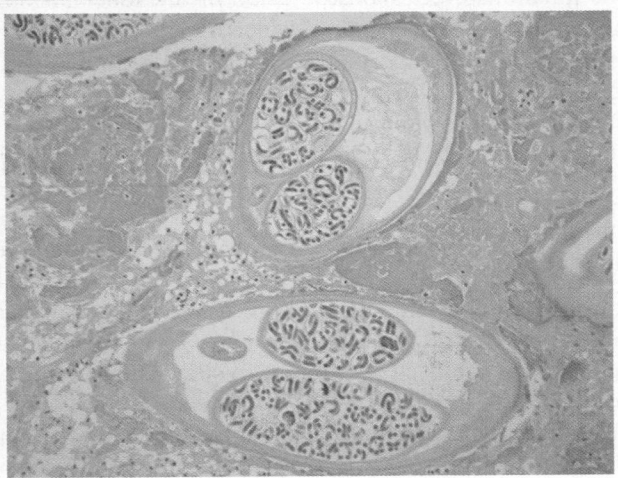

Figure 24-12 Onchocerciasis. **A:** African patient with onchocercoma on the head. **B:** African patient with oncocercal dermatitis. **C:** In an onchocercoma, multiple cross sections of the adult organism can be seen surrounded by dense fibrosis. **D:** On high magnification, the microfilariae within the female adult worm become obvious. When released by the female worm, the microfilariae evoke the changes seen in onchocercal dermatitis. (**A, B:** Reprinted by permission from Springer: Schaller KF. Helminthic dermatoses. In: Schaller KF, ed. *Colour Atlas of Tropical Dermatology and Venerology.* Springer; 1994:127. Copyright © 1994 Springer-Verlag Berlin Heidelberg.)

worms, which may be the result of the worms releasing angiogenic or lymphoangiogenic factors (135).

In early, untreated onchocercal dermatitis, many undulating microfilariae are present within the dermis, mainly close to the epidermis (132). Their number decreases greatly with time, and thus they may be difficult to find in old lesions. In early infections, reactive changes in the dermis are minimal, but in the course of years, chronic inflammatory cells including eosinophils accumulate around the vessels, and, ultimately, fibrosis of the dermis, especially perivascularly, results (132). Hyperorthokeratosis, parakeratosis, epidermal hyperplasia (in the late-stage flattening of the epidermis), tortuosity of dermal vessels, and pigment incontinence are other features of long-standing onchocercal dermatitis (132).

Pathogenesis. The slow development of the cutaneous and ocular changes suggests that microfilariae, as they gradually disintegrate, act as a source of foreign protein and that dermatitis and the various forms of eye involvement are the result of a coordinated response by the cellular and humoral immune system (132,133). While alive, microfilariae do not evoke a strong inflammatory response. Only when dying or dead, either during the natural course of their life span or therapeutically induced, do microfilariae produce a prominent inflammatory reaction, with eosinophils being essential in the process (132,133).

Principles of Management: Ivermectin is used for individual therapy, as well as through mass drug administration campaigns. Recently, doxycycline has also been used, given that it targets the symbiotic bacteria, *Wolbachia*, and has macrofilaricidal activity (136).

SCHISTOSOMIASIS

Clinical Summary. Schistosomiasis is caused by trematodes of the genus *Schistosoma* and affects 180 to 200 million people in over 70 countries, making it the most important trematode pathogenic to humans worldwide (137). It is acquired through exposure to skin-penetrating cercariae, a stage in the life cycle of the parasite. The cercariae emerge from a freshwater snail, which functions as an obligate intermediate host to the fluke. The cercariae burrow through the skin and migrate to venous plexuses, where they mature.

Three species of *Schistosoma* are pathogenic to humans. *Schistosoma mansoni* is common in the Caribbean islands and in northeastern South America; *S. japonicum* is found in Eastern Asia; and *S. haematobium* is common in the Middle East and in Africa. The usual habitats of *S. mansoni* are the portal circulation and mesenteric venules of the large intestines, with discharge of the eggs in the stool. The usual habitat of *S. japonicum* is the small gut, also resulting in discharge of the eggs with the stool. The usual habitats of *S. haematobium* are the pelvic and vesical venules, with the passage of the eggs with the urine. *S. mansoni* and *S. japonicum*, through granulomas and fibrosis in the liver, may cause cirrhosis with consequent portal hypertension and esophageal varices, and *S. haematobium*, through granulomas and fibrosis in the bladder, may lead to hematuria, hydronephrosis, and squamous cell carcinoma of the urinary bladder (138). In Africa, mixed infections with both *S. mansoni* and *S. haematobium* are not uncommon (139,140).

Pathogenesis. The cutaneous manifestations of schistosomiasis can be divided into three types, depending on the life cycle of the trematode (137,141).

Dermatitis schistosomica (swimmer's itch) is caused by the initial penetration of the skin by human or nonhuman cercariae and manifests as a pruritic maculopapular eruption usually lasting several hours, sometimes days, and, rarely, weeks, depending on previous sensitization. Cercariae of nonhuman *Schistosoma* species (usually avian species primarily affecting ducks or other water birds) can penetrate the skin but subsequently die. Dermatitis produced by anthropophilic *Schistosoma* ("duck itch") is milder than that caused by nonhuman species (137).

The second cutaneous manifestations of schistosomiasis, also transitory, are the *bilharzides* or *schistosomides*. Several weeks after penetration, the cercariae have matured into worms 15 to 25 mm in length. The female then releases thousands of eggs into the bloodstream. Their release may be accompanied by anaphylactoid reactions manifested by a combination of fever, urticaria, and sometimes purpura known in Japan as Katayama syndrome and in China as Yangtze fever (137,141).

A specific cutaneous involvement (known as bilharziasis cutanea tarda) represents the third cutaneous manifestation of schistosomiasis and is caused by ectopic deposition of eggs within the dermis when ova have become dislodged from their natural habitat in the venous circulation. Most commonly seen in *S. haematobium*, it is a rare event and presents as papular, verrucous, ulcerative, or granulomatous lesions usually of the genital or perianal skin (137,141,142). In rare instances, the thorax, abdomen, and, even less commonly, the face or scalp are involved (139,143,144).

Diagnosis is often made by clinical history, microscopy, and/or serology; however, molecular testing has recently been described. If the ova can be demonstrated on histologic examination, sequencing of the Schistosoma 28S rRNA can then be performed, after being extracted and amplified from paraffin-fixed tissue (145).

Histopathology. Bilharziasis cutanea tarda represents the main persistent cutaneous lesion of schistosomiasis. Its pathologic hallmark is a palisading, necrotizing granulomatous inflammation within the dermis consisting of histiocytes, lymphocytes, plasma cells, and rare multinucleated giant cells surrounding complete or degenerated schistosomal ova located in the central area of necrosis (Fig. 24-13A, B) (139,142,143). A predominant population of eosinophils as part of the inflammation is also described (142,144). In older lesions, the eggs are calcified and surrounded by fibrosis; the inflammatory infiltrate is sparse or absent (137). The overlying epidermis often reveals pseudocarcinomatous hyperplasia (142,143,146,147). Transepithelial elimination of the ova has been described (147).

The ova measure up to 180 μm in greatest dimension and possess a chitinous outer shell that can be readily identified by its ochre-yellow color on H&E-stained sections. The eggs stain positively with the PAS stain. However, it has been postulated that only *S. mansoni*, but not *S. haematobium* or *S. japonicum*, is acid fast-positive (139,143,144). The presence and position of a spine on the shell of the ova permit their classification, but this assessment is most reliable in ova and parasite preparations from stool or fresh lesions and unreliable in tissues, given that the angle of sectioning is, by necessity, fortuitous. *S. haematobium* ova have a spine in the apical position, which is tapered and fined that the prominent spine of *S. mansoni*, whereas the spine of *S. mansoni* ova is on the lateral aspect and more robust, and *S. japonicum* ova have no spine. In rare instances, one may also see adult worms within distended blood vessels in the dermis (Fig. 24-13C) (143).

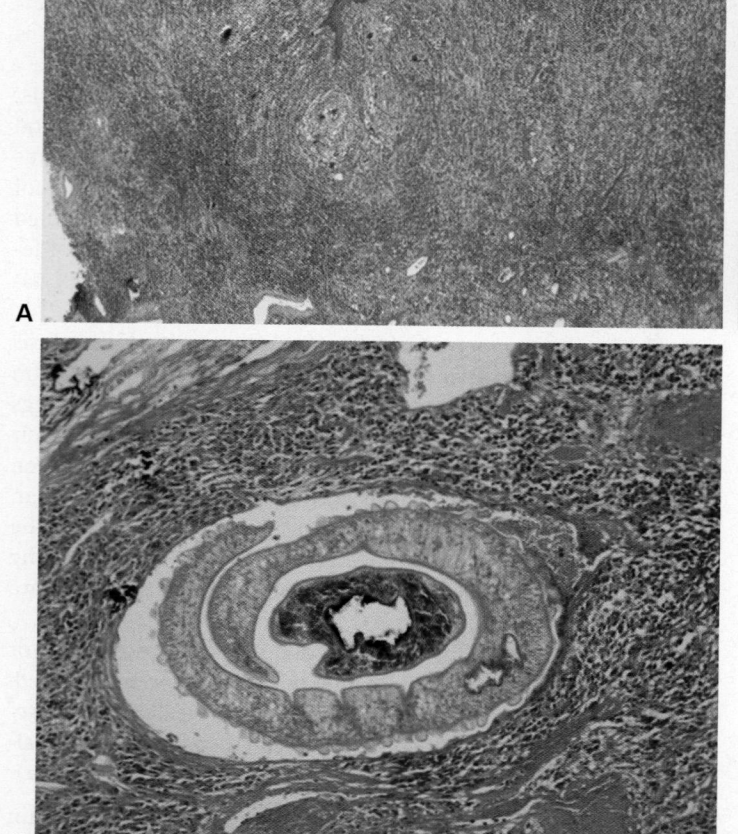

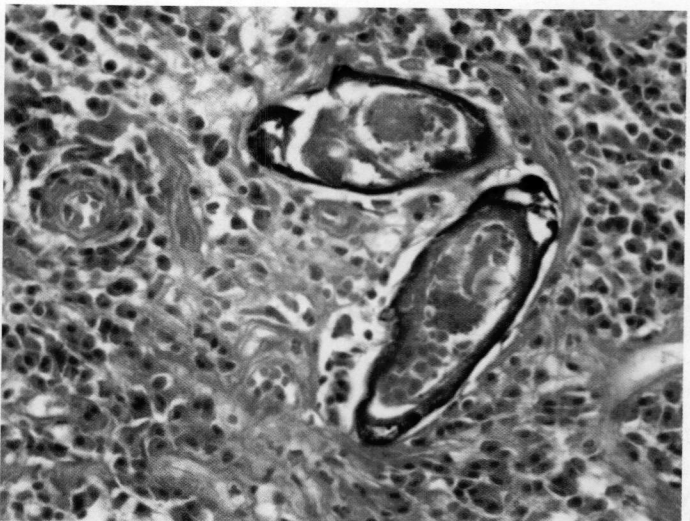

Figure 24-13 Schistosomiasis. **A:** In bilharziasis cutanea tarda, the schistosomal eggs provoke a granulomatous reaction within the dermis. **B:** The eggs of *S. mansoni* have a characteristic lateral spine. **C:** Rarely, the adult flukes may be present within dilated veins.

Pathogenesis. The eggs and larvae (miracidia) are said to release soluble substances that act as antigens sensitizing T lymphocytes. These, in turn, release lymphokines, leading to migration of macrophages and eosinophils and to granuloma formation (137).

Principles of Management: The drug of choice for treating all species of schistosomes is praziquantel. Depending on the stage and extent of the disease, corticosteroids may be given in addition. Large granulomas or tumors may require surgical intervention (148).

SUBCUTANEOUS CYSTICERCOSIS

Clinical Summary. Cysticercosis is caused by the larval stage of the pork tapeworm *Taenia solium.* Humans serve as definitive hosts for this globally distributed infection with estimates of more than 50 million people infected worldwide (149). Systemic disease can be acquired through ingestion of the eggs or through reverse peristalsis in individuals with taeniasis. The larva forms small 1- to 3-cm cysts in the subcutaneous tissue in cases with cutaneous involvement. Cysts may be solitary, multiple, or disseminated (150). There is a predilection for the upper trunk and extremities. The cysts can be seen on x-ray films,

ultrasound, and other imaging modalities (149). "Rice grain" calcification with long axes oriented along muscle fibers can be seen on plain films (151). The subcutaneous cysts are not symptomatic but should raise the concern for central nervous system disease that is present in approximately 50% of patients with subcutaneous cysticercosis, especially in patients with seizure activity (152).

Histopathology. There is a subcutaneous nodule with a thick fibrous capsule. Within the fibrous tissue, the cestode can be found as a cystic appearing cavity filled with clear fluid and best identified by detection of the cephalic segment with a scolex, suckers, and/or refractile hooks (Fig. 24-14). In the absence of a scolex, identification of a channel-rich matrix, cyst wall with a villous surface, and small ovoid calcific concretions known as calcareous bodies are helpful in determining at minimum that one is dealing with a cestode. Serial sections may be necessary to identify the protoscolex (153). Eosinophils are often found within the fibrous capsule. Caseating necrosis is absent (154). A mixed chronic inflammatory infiltrate with or without giant cells is noted in the surrounding tissue.

Differential Diagnosis. Clinically these cysts may be mistaken for more common benign cystic structures such as lipomas (155). Coenurosis, caused by the metacestode larvae of *Taenia*

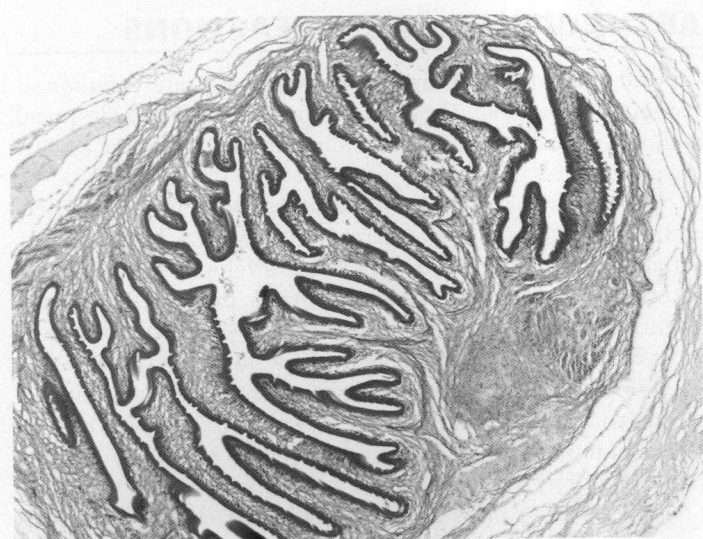

Figure 24-14 Subcutaneous cysticercosis. This cysticercus larva was found in a cavity within the subcutis surrounded by granulation tissue and necrotic debris. (Specimen courtesy of Dieter Krahl, MD, Institut für DermatoHistoPathologie, Heidelberg, Germany.)

multiceps, *T. serialis*, and *T. brauni* (zoonotic taenia of sheep, goats, and dogs), also presents with subcutaneous nodules clinically and histologically very similar to subcutaneous cysticerci. The distinction can be made by the identification of multiple protoscolices, characteristic of coenuri, in contrast to the single scolex of cysticercus. If no scolex is identified, sparganosis should be considered, caused by the plerocercoid larvae of *Spirometra* spp., cestodes that parasitize dogs and cats.

Principles of Management: Treatment is not necessary for cutaneous disease. Surgical excision can be performed for symptomatic lesions. For systemic disease, oral antiparasitics such as albendazole and praziquantel are used (149,150,152). Caution should be used when prescribing oral antiparasitics in patients with suspected neurocysticercosis due to the intense inflammatory response and resulting CNS damage.

MYIASIS

Clinical Summary. The order Diptera (having two wings) includes flies, gnats, and mosquitoes. When fly larvae inhabit the human body, the condition is called myiasis (from the Greek word for fly, *myia*). The distribution of myiasis is worldwide, with greater abundance of cases and causative species in the tropics.

The cutaneous manifestations of myiasis can be subdivided into three clinically recognized subcategories: wound myiasis, furuncular myiasis, and creeping myiasis (not to be mistaken with the creeping eruption caused by cutaneous larva migrans) (156–158).

In wound myiasis, which may be caused by many different fly species, including the common housefly *Musca domestica*, the fly larvae (maggots) are deposited on necrotic flesh.

Furuncular myiasis occurs mostly in the tropics and is caused in Africa by the tumbu fly *Cordylobia anthropophaga* and in the American tropics by the human botfly *Dermatobia hominis*. The latter has a unique life cycle. The female fly captures blood-sucking insects such as mosquitoes or other flies in the air and deposits a number of eggs on their abdomen. When these vectors come in contact with a human host, the *Dermatobia* larvae hatch due to a change in temperature and enter the skin, where they cause a furuncular lesion known as a "warble." The most common sites are exposed sites, including the scalp, face, and extremities (159). These furuncular lesions can enlarge to over 3 cm in diameter, and the host may experience pain and a sensation of movement. Dermatoscopy can be used to identify the posterior aspect of the larva and the breathing spiracles (160). Within 5 to 10 weeks, a third stage larva develops, leaves the human host through its breathing orifice, and falls to the ground to pupate in the soil.

In creeping myiasis, larvae of *Gasterophilus* species or *Hypoderma* species—flies parasitic to horses or cattle—burrow into the skin and cause a migratory pattern. In contrast to the creeping eruption seen in larva migrans, the movements are more restricted and proceed more slowly.

Histopathology. In wound myiasis, the larvae generally remain superficial, are usually alive, and can be recognized grossly at the time of biopsy (157). In furuncular myiasis, there is an intense mixed inflammatory infiltrate composed of neutrophils, eosinophils, lymphocytes, plasma cells, and Langerhans giant cells surrounding the cavity, which is occupied by the larva (Fig. 24-15A). The presence of curved, black spines in the integument is characteristic (Fig. 24-15B) (156,161,162). In creeping myiasis due to Hypoderma species, the inflammatory response is very minimal (157).

Pathogenesis. Both *Dermatobia hominis* and *Cordylobia anthropophaga* secrete a bacteriostatic fluid that prevents secondary bacterial infection of the larval cavity (156,163).

Principles of Management: The treatment includes expressing or surgically removing the larvae, although spontaneous

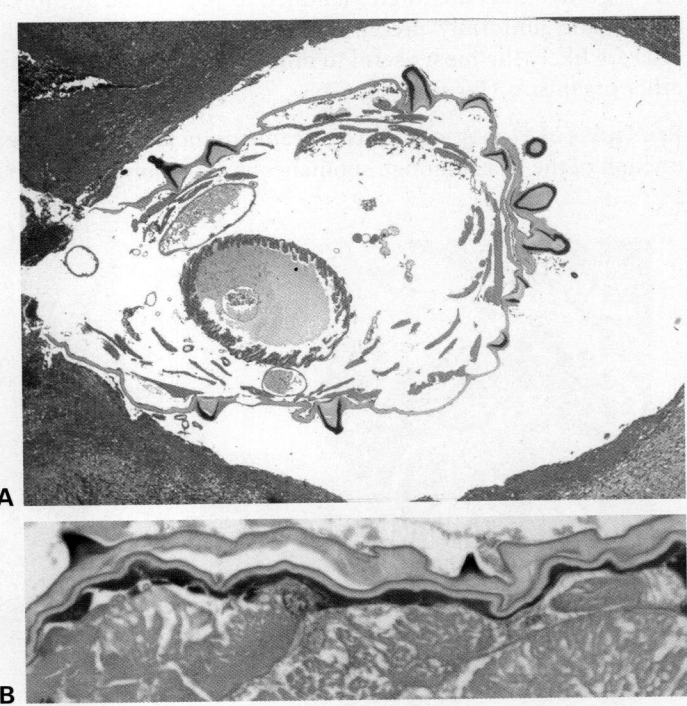

Figure 24-15 Myiasis. **A:** An intense inflammatory reaction surrounded this larva seen in a cystic cavity in a case of furuncular myiasis. **B:** The presence of slightly curved, black spines in the integument is characteristic of the these larvae.

extrusion may occur. The larvae may sometimes be forced to emerge by occluding the air-hole with thick emollients or submersion in water.

TUNGIASIS

Clinical Summary. Tungiasis is a cutaneous infestation by the gravid female sand flea *Tunga penetrans*, which is endemic in the Caribbean region, Central and South America, sub-Saharan Africa, and the Indian subcontinent (164,165).

Only the impregnated female fleas penetrate the skin. They burrow a cavity with the head turned toward the dermis, feeding on the host. The gravid female eliminates its eggs through an apical opening of the cavity to the outside, dies soon thereafter, and is sloughed from the skin, exhibiting a total life span of approximately 1 month (164).

The condition is most often acquired by walking barefoot. Characteristically, the lesions are located on the toes, the interdigital spaces, and the soles and heels. The lesions are initially asymptomatic, but they soon become inflammatory papules. A tender nodule with a central punctum ultimately develops, which may be 5 to 10 mm in diameter with a black-to-brown central tip representing the posterior end of the parasite. Dermatoscopy can be used for clinical verification through the visualization of the head of the parasite and the distended gravid abdomen (166).

Histopathology. The flea is located in the epidermis and upper dermis inside a cavity (Fig. 24-16A). The apical portion is surrounded by a hyperplastic epidermis. In the absence of bacterial superinfection, any perilesional inflammatory infiltrate is usually minimal and consists of lymphocytes, neutrophils, and eosinophils (164). Inside the cavity, an eosinophilic cuticle, yellowish-brown chitin, hypodermal layer, tracheal rings, and digestive tract are often identified as part of the arthropod (167). The uniformly present developing round eosinophilic eggs are likely the most useful to differentiate *T. penetrans* from other organisms (Fig. 24-16B (168).

Principles of Management: The treatment includes surgical extraction of the flea, although spontaneous extrusion may occur.

ARTHROPOD ASSAULT REACTIONS

Clinical Summary. Arthropod bites and stings are common afflictions in humans. They may induce localized, widespread, and/or systemic reactions, depending on the type of the assaulting species and the capacity of the body to react.

Most stings evoked by mosquitoes, bees, wasps, hornets, or bedbug bites are characterized initially by a localized urticarial reaction, often followed by the development of a papule and papulovesicle associated with intense pruritus. Frequently, a central punctum can be recognized. In more intense reactions, most commonly seen on the legs, the lesions may become bullous (Fig. 24-17A) (169). Typically, they resolve without sequelae within days. In rare cases, however, they may persist for weeks or months and are then referred to as a persistent arthropod assault reaction (170,171).

Bites by the brown recluse spider *Loxosceles reclusa* are common in the south central United States. Often painless initially, they are capable of inducing significant skin necrosis (necrotic arachnidism) (172).

Hypersensitivity to insect stings and bites, especially from fleas, gnats, mosquitoes, or bedbugs, may result in papular urticaria. It is characterized by grouped urticarial papules and papulovesicles which may be relatively widespread. Spontaneous resolution within several days is usual (173). The condition cannot be reliably distinguished from arthropod assaults of other types (174).

Histopathology. The classical histopathologic hallmark of an arthropod assault is a wedge-shaped, superficial and deep, perivascular, periadnexal, and interstitial inflammatory dermal infiltrate composed of lymphocytes and eosinophils, often in association with an overlying focus of spongiosis, sometimes evolving into a vesicle or even progressing to epidermal necrosis (Fig. 24-17B) (175). The presence of epidermal or eosinophilic spongiosis, with spongiosis of the infundibular epithelium and acrosyringia, can be an important clue (176). Another useful clue is the identification of altered interstitial tissue at low power. These changes may include narrowing of the spaces between collagen bundles and deposition of a loosely textured basophilic material between the bundles of collagen (177). The presence of homogenous intravascular eosinophilic deposits

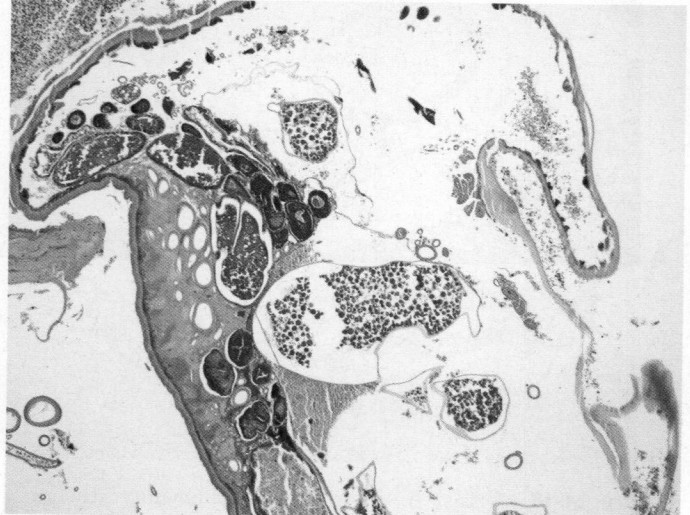
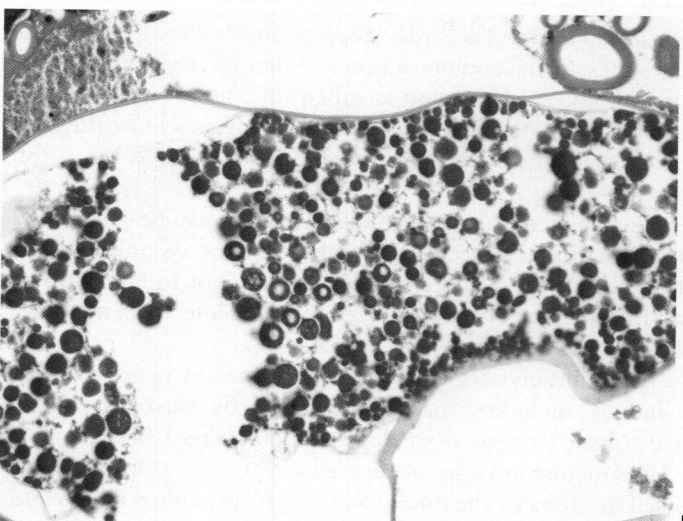

Figure 24-16 Tungiasis. **A:** On hematoxylin and eosin–stained section, the typical superficial intradermal location of the flea is noted. **B:** The round, eosinophilic developing eggs are characteristic.

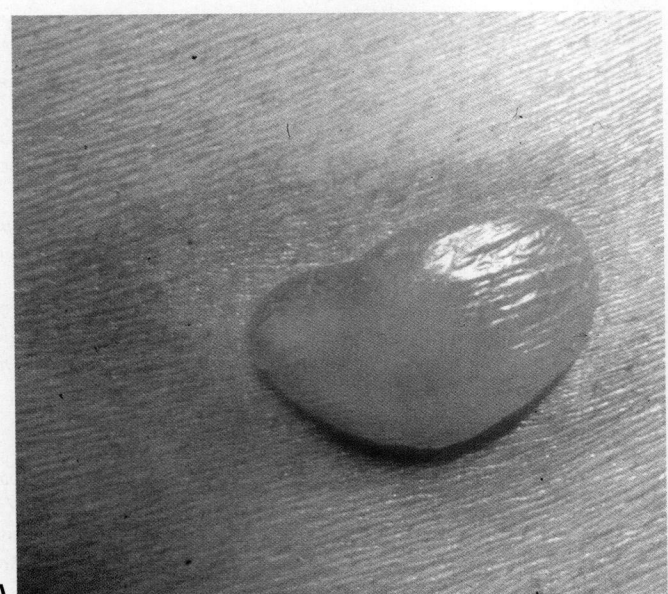
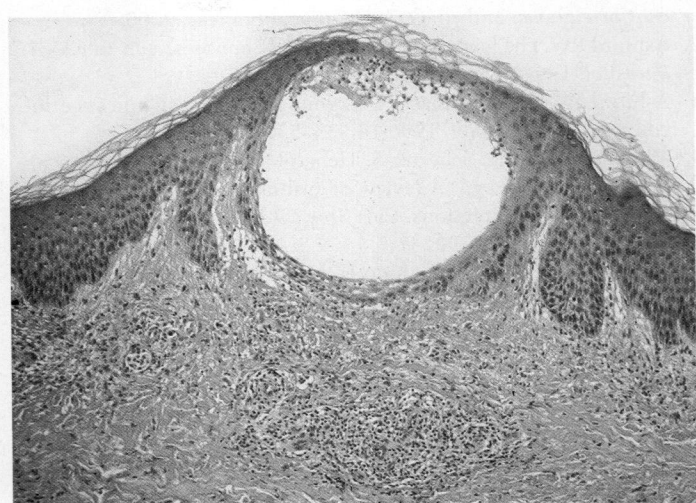

Figure 24-17 Arthropod assault reaction. **A:** Sometimes the clinical reaction to an arthropod assault is intense and results in a blister. **B:** On histologic sections, often an intraepidermal vesicle can be seen in the center of the arthropod assault.

has been described, primarily in tick-bite reactions, and may mimic the intravascular findings of cryoglobulinemia (178). Sweet syndrome–like reactions to bites have also been reported, with extensive papillary dermal edema, dense interstitial neutrophils, fibrin deposits, and no eosinophils noted (179).

Mosquito bites initially show mainly neutrophils, mostly vasculocentric, and later a predominantly mononuclear infiltrate of lymphocytes and plasma cells. Eosinophils are few or absent (180,181).

Bed bug bites manifest as an urticarial-like reaction, with dermal edema and a mixed dermal interstitial infiltrate. More exuberant bullous lesions may progress to demonstrate a neutrophil-rich leukocytoclastic vasculitis, which may evolve into a destructive necrotizing eosinophil-rich vasculitis (182).

Bites of the brown recluse spider initially show a neutrophilic perivasculitis with hemorrhage. Later, in cases of necrotic ulcers, arterial wall necrosis and an infiltrate containing many eosinophils may be present (183).

Some persistent arthropod assault reactions produce a dense lymphoid infiltrate, often with the formation of lymphoid follicles, which has to be differentiated from lymphoma (184). In contrast to lymphomas, the lymphoid follicles in persistent arthropod reactions frequently show germinal centers and do not show evidence of clonality. Large transformed, CD30+ lymphoid cells with hyperchromatic nuclei may also be found but do not represent a sign of malignancy (171). Extensive CD1a+ infiltrates of Langerhans cells have been described in the dermis in arthropod bite reactions and may be confused with Langerhans cell histiocytosis histologically (185).

Occasionally, parts of the sting apparatus may be retained within the dermis, inducing a chronic inflammatory response, often with associated eosinophils, accompanied by pseudocarcinomatous epidermal hyperplasia (186). Retention of the sting apparatus is more commonly seen in ticks (Fig. 24-18).

An entity known as "tick-bite alopecia" has been described, which is characterized clinically as an alopecic nodule at the site of the tick-bite reaction. Histologically, the lymphocytic infiltrate attacks the isthmus of the hair follicles, with associated

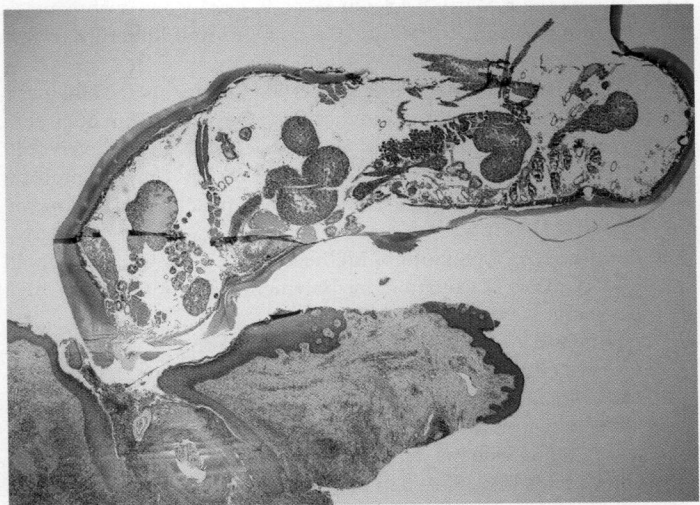

Figure 24-18 Tick-bite reaction. The tick is seen in cross section with its mouth parts extending into the superficial dermis.

hyperplasia of fibrous sheaths and only a destruction of the minority of hairs (187).

Pathogenesis. The primary toxin in the brown recluse envenomation is sphingomyelinase D, which interacts with the outer plasma membrane of erythrocytes, endothelial cells, and platelets. The severe skin necrosis seen in this spider bite is a consequence of vascular damage (188).

Principles of Management: Typical arthropod bite reactions are often self-limited, but the local reaction and pruritus may be managed with topical steroids and/or antihistamines.

ACKNOWLEDGMENTS

The author and editors are appreciative of Drs. Klaus Sellheyer, Eckart Haneke, Carrie Kovarik, and Casey Carlos' work on previous versions of this chapter in the earlier editions of the book.

REFERENCES

1. Guiterrez Y. *Diagnostic Pathology of Parasitic Infections with Clinical Correlations.* 2nd ed. Oxford University Press; 2000.
2. Ashford RW. The leishmaniases as model zoonoses. *Ann Trop Med Parasitol.* 1997;91:693–701.
3. Ashford RW. Leishmaniasis reservoirs and their significance in control. *Clin Dermatol.* 1996;14:523–532.
4. Mann S, Frasca K, Scherrer S, Henao-Martínez AF, Newman S, Ramanan P, Suarez JA. A review of leishmaniasis: current knowledge and future directions. *Curr Trop Med Rep.* 2021;8:1–12. doi: 10.1007/s40475-021-00232-7
5. Hashiguchi Y, Gomez EL, Kato H, Martini LR, Velez LN, Uezato H. Diffuse and disseminated cutaneous leishmaniasis: clinical cases experienced in Ecuador and a brief review. *Trop Med Health.* 2016;44:2. doi: 10.1186/s41182-016-0002-0
6. Pratt DM, David JR. Monoclonal antibodies that distinguish between New World species of Leishmania. *Nature.* 1981;291:581–583.
7. Antinori S, Schifanella L, Corbellino M. Leishmaniasis: new insights from an old and neglected disease. *Eur J Clin Microbiol Infect Dis.* 2012;31:109–118.
8. Gradoni L, Gramiccia M. Leishmania infantum tropism: strain genotype or host immune status? *Parasitol Today.* 1994;10:264–267.
9. del Giudice P, Marty P, Lacour JP, et al. Cutaneous leishmaniasis due to Leishmania infantum. Case reports and literature review. *Arch Dermatol.* 1998;134:193–198.
10. Gállego M, Pratlong F, Riera C, et al. Cutaneous leishmaniasis due to Leishmania infantum in the northeast of Spain: the isoenzymatic analysis of parasites. *Arch Dermatol.* 2001;137:667–668.
11. Ceyhan AM, Yildirim M, Basak PY, Akkaya VB. Unusual multifocal cutaneous leishmaniasis in a diabetic patient. *Eur J Dermatol.* 2009;19:514–515.
12. Momeni AZ, Yotsumoto S, Mehregan DR, et al. Chronic lupoid leishmaniasis. Evaluation by polymerase chain reaction. *Arch Dermatol.* 1996;132:198–202.
13. Bittencourt AL, Costa JM, Carvalho EM, Barral A. Leishmaniasis recidiva cutis in American cutaneous leishmaniasis. *Int J Dermatol.* 1993;32:802–805.
14. Landau M, Srebrnik A, Brenner S. Leishmaniasis recidivans mimicking lupus vulgaris. *Int J Dermatol.* 1996;35:572–573.
15. Gündüz K, Afsar S, Ayhan S, et al. Recidivans cutaneous leishmaniasis unresponsive to liposomal amphotericin B (AmBisome). *J Eur Acad Dermatol Venereol.* 2000;14:11–13.
16. Gomes CM, Morais OO, Leite AS, Soares KA, Motta Jde O, Sampaio RN. Periungual leishmaniasis. *An Bras Dermatol.* 2012;87:148–149.
17. Ceyhan AM, Basak PY, Yildirim M, Akkaya VB. A case of cutaneous leishmaniasis presenting as facial cellulitis. *J Dermatol.* 2010;37:565–567.
18. Ceyhan AM, Yildirim M, Basak PY, Akkaya VB, Erturan I. A case of erysipeloid cutaneous leishmaniasis: atypical and unusual clinical variant. *Am J Trop Med Hyg.* 2008;78:406–408.
19. Veraldi S, Bottini S, Currò N, Gianotti R. Leishmaniasis of the eyelid mimicking an infundibular cyst and review of the literature on ocular leishmaniasis. *Int J Infect Dis.* 2010;14(suppl 3):e230–e232.
20. Veraldi S, Bottini S, Persico MC, Lunardon L. Case report: Leishmaniasis of the upper lip. *Oral Surg Oral Med Oral Pathol Oral Radiol Endod.* 2007;104:659–661.
21. Veraldi S, Galloni C, Cremonesi R, Cavalli R. Psoriasiform cutaneous leishmaniasis. *Int J Dermatol.* 2006;45:129–130.
22. Veraldi S, Rigoni C, Gianotti R. Leishmaniasis of the lip. *Acta Derm Venereol.* 2002;82:469–470.
23. Omidian M, Mapar MA. Chronic zosteriform cutaneous leishmaniasis. *Indian J Dermatol Venereol Leprol.* 2006;72:41–42.
24. Bari A, Bari A, Ejaz A. Fissure leishmaniasis: a new variant of cutaneous leishmaniasis. *Dermatol Online J.* 2009;15:13.
25. Bari AU, Rahman SB. Many faces of cutaneous leishmaniasis. *Indian J Dermatol Venereol Leprol.* 2008;74:23–27.
26. Iftikhar N, Bari I, Ejaz A. Rare variants of cutaneous leishmaniasis: whitlow, paronychia, and sporotrichoid. *Int J Dermatol.* 2003;42:807–809.
27. Jafari AK, Akhyani M, Valikhani M, Ghodsi ZS, Barikbin B, Toosi S. Bilateral cutaneous leishmaniasis of upper eyelids: a case report. *Dermatol Online J.* 2006;12:20.
28. Bardazzi F, Giacomini F, Savoia F, Misciali C, Patrizi A. Discoid chronic lupus erythematosus at the site of a previously healed cutaneous leishmaniasis: an example of isotopic response. *Dermatol Ther.* 2010;23(suppl 2):S44–S446.
29. Murray HW, Berman JD, Davies CR, Saravia NG. Advances in leishmaniasis. *Lancet.* 2005;366:1561–1577.
30. den Boer M, Argaw D, Jannin J, Alvar J. Leishmaniasis impact and treatment access. *Clin Microbiol Infect.* 2011;17:1471–1477.
31. Amato VS, Tuon FF, Bacha HA, Neto VA, Nicodemo AC. Mucosal leishmaniasis. Current scenario and prospects for treatment. *Acta Trop.* 2008;105:1–9.
32. Lawn SD, Whetham J, Chiodini PL, et al. New world mucosal and cutaneous leishmaniasis: an emerging health problem among British travellers. *QJM.* 2004;97:781–788.
33. Harms G, Schonian G, Feldmeier H. Leishmaniasis in Germany. *Emerg Infect Dis.* 2003;9:872–875.
34. Casero R, Laconte L, Fraenza L, Iglesias N, Quinteros Greco C, Villablanca M. Recidivant laryngeal leishmaniasis: an unusual case in an immunocompetent patient treated with corticosteroids [in Spanish]. *Rev Argent Microbiol.* 2010;42:118–121.
35. Lessa HA, Carvalho EM, Marsden PD. Eustachian tube blockage with consequent middle ear infection in mucosal leishmaniasis. *Rev Soc Bras Med Trop.* 1994;27:103.
36. Motta AC, Arruda D, Souza CS, Foss NT. Disseminated mucocutaneous leishmaniasis resulting from chronic use of corticosteroid. *Int J Dermatol.* 2003;42:703–706.
37. Motta AC, Lopes MA, Ito FA, Carlos-Bregni R, de Almeida OP, Roselino AM. Oral leishmaniasis: a clinicopathological study of 11 cases. *Oral Dis.* 2007;13:335–340.
38. Herwaldt BL. Leishmaniasis. *Lancet.* 1999;354:1191–1199.
39. Perrin C, Michiels JF, Bernard E, Hofman P, Rosenthal E, Loubiere R. Cutaneous spindle–cell pseudotumors due to *Mycobacterium gordonae* and *Leishmania infantum.* An immunophenotypic study. *Am J Dermatopathol.* 1993;15:553–558.
40. Perrin C, Taillan B, Hofman P, Mondain V, Lefichoux Y, Michiels JF. Atypical cutaneous histological features of visceral leishmaniasis in acquired immunodeficiency syndrome. *Am J Dermatopathol.* 1995;17:145–150.
41. Taillan B, Marty P, Schneider S, et al. Visceral leishmaniasis involving a cutaneous Kaposi's sarcoma lesion and free areas of skin. *Eur J Med.* 1992;1:255.
42. Barrio J, Lecona M, Cosin J, Olalquiaga FJ, Hernanz JM, Soto J. Leishmania infection occurring in herpes zoster lesions in an HIV-positive patient. *Br J Dermatol.* 1996;134:164–166.
43. Antinori S, Longhi E, Bestetti G, et al. Post-kala-azar dermal leishmaniasis as an immune reconstitution inflammatory syndrome in a patient with acquired immune deficiency syndrome. *Br J Dermatol.* 2007;157:1032–1036.
44. Simon I, Wissing KM, Del Marmol V, et al. Recurrent leishmaniasis in kidney transplant recipients: report of 2 cases and systematic review of the literature. *Transpl Infect Dis.* 2011;13:397–406.
45. Pavli A, Maltezou HC. Leishmaniasis, an emerging infection in travelers. *Int J Infect Dis.* 2010;14:e1032–e1039.
46. Mestra L, Lopez L, Robledo SM, Muskus CE, Nicholls RS, Vélez ID. Transfusion-transmitted visceral leishmaniasis caused by leishmania (Leishmania) mexicana in an immunocompromised patient: a case report. *Transfusion.* 2011;51:1919–1923.

47. Mueller MC, Fleischmann E, Grunke M, Schewe S, Bogner JR, Löscher T. Relapsing cutaneous leishmaniasis in a patient with ankylosing spondylitis treated with infliximab. *Am J Trop Med Hyg.* 2009;81:52–54.

48. Cascio A, Iaria M, Iaria C. Leishmaniasis and biologic therapies for rheumatologic diseases. *Semin Arthritis Rheum.* 2010;40:e3–e5.

49. De Leonardis F, Govoni M, Lo Monaco A, Trotta F. Visceral leishmaniasis and anti-TNF-alpha therapy: case report and review of the literature. *Clin Exp Rheumatol.* 2009;27:503–506.

50. Andrade RV, Massone C, Lucena MN, et al. The use of polymerase chain reaction to confirm diagnosis in skin biopsies consistent with American tegumentary leishmaniasis at histopathology: a study of 90 cases. *An Bras Dermatol.* 2011;86:892–896.

51. Noyes HA, Chance ML, Croan DG, Ellis JT. Leishmania (sauroleishmania): a comment on classification. *Parasitol Today.* 1998;14:167.

52. de Bruijn MH, Barker DC. Diagnosis of New World leishmaniasis: specific detection of species of the Leishmania braziliensis complex by amplification of kinetoplast DNA. *Acta Trop.* 1992;52:45–58.

53. Andrade-Narvaez FJ, Medina-Peralta S, Vargas-Gonzalez A, Canto-Lara SB, Estrada-Parra S. The histopathology of cutaneous leishmaniasis due to Leishmania (Leishmania) mexicana in the Yucatan peninsula, Mexico. *Rev Inst Med Trop Sao Paulo.* 2005;47:191–194.

54. Botelho AC, Tafuri WL, Genaro O, Mayrink W. Histopathology of human American cutaneous leishmaniasis before and after treatment. *Rev Soc Bras Med Trop.* 1998;31:11–18.

55. Kurban AK, Malak JA, Farah FS, Chaglassian HT. Histopathology of cutaneous leishmaniasis. *Arch Dermatol.* 1966;93:396–401.

56. Peltier E, Wolkenstein P, Deniau M, Zafrani ES, Wechsler J. Caseous necrosis in cutaneous leishmaniasis. *J Clin Pathol.* 1996;49:517–519.

57. Satti MB, el-Hassan AM, al-Gindan Y, Osman MA, al-Sohaibani MO. Peripheral neural involvement in cutaneous leishmaniasis: a pathologic study of human and experimental animal lesions. *Int J Dermatol.* 1989;28:243–247.

58. Sangueza OP, Sangueza JM, Stiller MJ, Sangueza P. Mucocutaneous leishmaniasis: a clinicopathologic classification. *J Am Acad Dermatol.* 1993;28:927–932.

59. Postigo C, Llamas R, Zarco C, et al. Cutaneous lesions in patients with visceral leishmaniasis and HIV infection. *J Infect.* 1997;35:265–268.

60. Singh N, Ramesh V, Arora VK, Bhatia A, Kubba A, Ramam M. Nodular post-kala-azar dermal leishmaniasis: a distinct histopathological entity. *J Cutan Pathol.* 1998;25:95–99.

61. Mukherjee A, Ramesh V, Misra RS. Post-kala-azar dermal leishmaniasis: a light and electron microscopic study of 18 cases. *J Cutan Pathol.* 1993;20:320–325.

62. Ramesh V, Misra RS, Saxena U, Mukherjee A. Post-kala-azar dermal leishmaniasis: a clinical and therapeutic study. *Int J Dermatol.* 1993;32:272–275.

63. Ramesh V, Mukherjee A. Post-kala-azar dermal leishmaniasis. *Int J Dermatol.* 1995;34:85–91.

64. Ramesh V, Saxena U, Misra RS, Mukherjee A. Post-kala-azar dermal leishmaniasis: a case report strikingly resembling lepromatous leprosy. *Lepr Rev.* 1991;62:217–221.

65. Kane MM, Mosser DM. Leishmania parasites and their ploys to disrupt macrophage activation. *Curr Opin Hematol.* 2000;7:26–31.

66. Sakthianandeswaren A, Foote SJ, Handman E. The role of host genetics in leishmaniasis. *Trends Parasitol.* 2009;25:383–391.

67. Fakiola M, Strange A, Cordell HJ, et al. Common variants in the HLA-DRB1-HLA-DQA1 HLA class II region are associated with susceptibility to visceral leishmaniasis. *Nat Genet.* 2013;45:208–213.

68. Nylen S, Gautam S. Immunological perspectives of leishmaniasis. *J Glob Infect Dis.* 2010;2:135–146.

69. Murray HW. Leishmaniasis in the United States: treatment in 2012. *Am J Trop Med Hyg.* 2012;86:434–440.

70. Ben Salah A, Ben Messaoud N, Guedri E, et al. Topical paromomycin with or without gentamicin for cutaneous leishmaniasis. *N Engl J Med.* 2013;368:524–532.

71. Trabelsi H, Dendana F, Sellami A, et al. Pathogenic free-living amoebae: epidemiology and clinical review. *Pathol Biol (Paris).* 2012;60:399–405.

72. Parshad S, Grover PS, Sharma A, Verma DK, Sharma A. Primary cutaneous amoebiasis: case report with review of the literature. *Int J Dermatol.* 2002;41:676–680.

73. Fernandez-Diez J, Magana M, Magana ML. Cutaneous amebiasis: 50 years of experience. *Cutis.* 2012;90:310–314.

74. Majmudar B, Chaiken ML, Lee KU. Amebiasis of clitoris mimicking carcinoma. *JAMA.* 1976;236:1145–1146.

75. Bravo FG, Alvarez PJ, Gotuzzo E. *Balamuthia mandrillaris* infection of the skin and central nervous system: an emerging disease of concern to many specialties in medicine. *Curr Opin Infect Dis.* 2011;24:112–117.

76. May LP, Sidhu GS, Buchness MR. Diagnosis of Acanthamoeba infection by cutaneous manifestations in a man seropositive to HIV. *J Am Acad Dermatol.* 1992;26:352–355.

77. Paltiel M, Powell E, Lynch J, Baranowski B, Martins C. Disseminated cutaneous acanthamebiasis: a case report and review of the literature. *Cutis.* 2004;73:241–248.

78. Magaña M, Magaña ML, Alcántara A, Pérez-Martín MA. Histopathology of cutaneous amebiasis. *Am J Dermatopathol.* 2004;26:280–284.

79. Merad Y, Behague L, Valot S, et al. Epigastric cutaneous discharge: think amoebiasis. *Br J Dermatol.* 2020;183(5):e147. doi:10.1111/bjd.19246

80. Rosenberg AS, Morgan MB. Disseminated acanthamoebiasis presenting as lobular panniculitis with necrotizing vasculitis in a patient with AIDS. *J Cutan Pathol.* 2001;28:307–313.

81. Murakawa GJ, McCalmont T, Altman J, et al. Disseminated acanthamebiasis in patients with AIDS: a report of five cases and a review of the literature. *Arch Dermatol.* 1995;131:1291–1296.

82. Tan B, Weldon-Linne CM, Rhone DP, Penning CL, Visvesvara GS. Acanthamoeba infection presenting as skin lesions in patients with the acquired immunodeficiency syndrome. *Arch Pathol Lab Med.* 1993;117:1043–1046.

83. Martínez DY, Seas C, Bravo F, et al. Successful treatment of *Balamuthia mandrillaris* amoebic infection with extensive neurological and cutaneous involvement. *Clin Infect Dis.* 2010;51:e7–e11.

84. Aichelburg AC, Walochnik J, Assadian O, et al. Successful treatment of disseminated Acanthamoeba sp. infection with miltefosine. *Emerg Infect Dis.* 2008;14:1743–1746.

85. Kofman A, Guarner J. Infections caused by free-living amoebae. *J Clin Microbiol.* 2021;60:e0022821. doi:10.1128/JCM.00228-21

86. Thomas C, Coates SJ, Engelman D, Chosidow O, Chang AY. Ectoparasites: scabies. *J Am Acad Dermatol.* 2020;82(3):533–548. doi:10.1016/j.jaad.2019.05.109

87. Haliasos EC, Kerner M, Jaimes-Lopez N, et al. Dermoscopy for the pediatric dermatologist part I: dermoscopy of pediatric infectious and inflammatory skin lesions and hair disorders. *Pediatr Dermatol.* 2013;30(2):163–171.

88. Cinotti E, Perrot JL, Labeille B, et al. Reflectance confocal microscopy for quantification of Sarcoptes scabiei in Norwegian scabies. *J Eur Acad Dermatol Venereol.* 2013;27(2):e176–e178.

89. Liu HN, Sheu WJ, Chu TL. Scabietic nodules: a dermatopathologic and immunofluorescent study. *J Cutan Pathol.* 1992;19:124.

90. Martin WE, Wheeler CE Jr. Diagnosis of human scabies by epidermal shave biopsy. *J Am Acad Dermatol.* 1979;1:335.

91. Head ES, Macdonald EM, Ewert A, Apisarnthanarax P. Sarcoptes scabiei in histopathologic sections of skin in human scabies. *Arch Dermatol.* 1990;126:1475.

92. Shelley WB, Shelley ED. Scanning electron microscopy of the scabies burrow and its contents, with special reference to the Sarcoptes scabiei egg. *J Am Acad Dermatol.* 1983;9:673.

93. Reinig EF, Albertson D, Sarma D. Pink pigtail in a skin biopsy: what is your diagnosis? *Dermatol Online J.* 2011;17(1):12.

94. Foo CW, Florell SR, Bowen AR. Polarizable elements in scabies infestation: a clue to diagnosis. *J Cutan Pathol.* 2013;40(1):6–10.

95. Fernandez N, Torres A, Ackerman AB. Pathological findings in human scabies. *Arch Dermatol.* 1977;113:320.

96. Hashimoto K, Fujiwara K, Punwaney J, et al. Post-scabietic nodules: a lymphohistiocytic reaction rich in indeterminate cells. *J Dermatol.* 2000;27:181.

97. Gallardo F, Barranco C, Toll A, Pujol RM. CD30 antigen expression in cutaneous inflammatory infiltrates of scabies: a dynamic immunophenotypic pattern that should be distinguished from lymphomatoid papulosis. *J Cutan Pathol.* 2002;29:368.

98. Thomson J, Cochrane T, Cochran R, McQueen A. Histology simulating reticulosis in persistent nodular scabies. *Br J Dermatol.* 1974;90:421.

99. Piana S, Pizzigoni S, Tagliavini E, Serra S, Albertini G. Generalized granuloma annulare associated with scabies. *Am J Dermatopathol.* 2010;32(5):518–520.

100. Fimiani M, Mazzatenta C, Alessandrini C, Paccagnini E, Andreassi L. The behaviour of Sarcoptes scabiei var. hominis in human skin: an ultrastructural study. *J Submicrosc Cytol Pathol.* 1997;29:105.

101. Walton SF, Oprescu FI. Immunology of scabies and translational outcomes: identifying the missing links. *Curr Opin Infect Dis.* 2013;26(2):116–122. doi: 10.1097/QCO.0b013e32835eb8a6

102. Brites C, Weyll M, Pedroso C, Badaró R. Severe and Norwegian scabies are strongly associated with retroviral (HIV-1/HTLV-1) infection in Bahia, Brazil. *AIDS.* 2002;16:1292.

103. Fernández-Sánchez M, Saeb-Lima M, Alvarado-de la Barrera C, Reyes-Terán G. Crusted scabies-associated Immune reconstitution inflammatory syndrome. *BMC Infect Dis.* 2012;12:323.

104. Jelinek T, Maiwald H, Nothdurft HD, Löscher T. Cutaneous larva migrans in travelers: synopsis of histories, symptoms, and treatment of 98 patients. *Clin Infect Dis.* 1994;19:1062.

105. Gill N, Somayaji R, Vaughan S. Exploring tropical infections: a focus on cutaneous larva migrans. *Adv Skin Wound Care.* 2020;33(7):356–359. doi: 10.1097/01.ASW.0000662248.18996.b5

106. Caumes E, Danis M. From creeping eruption to hookworm-related cutaneous larva migrans. *Lancet Infect Dis.* 2004;4:659.

107. Purdy KS, Langley RG, Webb AN, Walsh N, Haldane D. Cutaneous larva migrans. *Lancet.* 2011;377(9781):1948.

108. Ramondetta A, Ribero S, Quaglino P, Broganelli P. In vivo observation of cutaneous larva migrans by fluorescence-advanced videodermatoscopy. *Emerg Infect Dis.* 2021;27(1):281–283. doi: 10.3201/eid2701.203137

109. Balfour E, Zalka A, Lazova R. Cutaneous larva migrans with parts of the larva in the epidermis. *Cutis.* 2002;69:368.

110. Caumes E, Ly F, Bricaire F. Cutaneous larva migrans with folliculitis: report of seven cases and review of the literature. *Br J Dermatol.* 2002;146:314.

111. Veraldi S, Persico MC, Francia C, Nazzaro G, Gianotti R. Follicular cutaneous larva migrans: a report of three cases and review of the literature. *Int J Dermatol.* 2013;52(3):327–330.

112. Hawdon JM, Jones BF, Perregaux MA, Hotez PJ. Ancylostoma caninum: metalloprotease release coincides with activation of infective larvae in vitro. *Exp Parasitol.* 1995;80:205.

113. Guimaraes LC, Silva JH, Saad K, Lopes ER, Meneses AC. Larva migrans within scalp sebaceous gland. *Rev Soc Bras Med Trop.* 1999;32:187.

114. Ly MN, Bethel SL, Usmani AS, Lambert DR. Cutaneous *Strongyloides stercoralis* infection: an unusual presentation. *J Am Acad Dermatol.* 2003;49(2 suppl):S157.

115. Basile A, Simzar S, Bentow J, et al. Disseminated *Strongyloides stercoralis*: hyperinfection during medical immunosuppression. *J Am Acad Dermatol.* 2010;63(5):896–902.

116. Von Kuster LC, Genta RM. Cutaneous manifestations of strongyloidiasis. *Arch Dermatol.* 1988;124:1826.

117. Chaudhary K, Smith RJ, Himelright IM, Baddour LM. Case report: purpura in disseminated strongyloidiasis. *Am J Med Sci.* 1994;308:186.

118. Jacob CI, Patten SF. *Strongyloides stercoralis* infection presenting as generalized prurigo nodularis and lichen simplex chronicus. *J Am Acad Dermatol.* 1999;41:357.

119. Purvis RS, Beightler EL, Diven DG, Sanchez RL, Tyring SK. Strongyloides hyperinfection presenting with petechiae and purpura. *Int J Dermatol.* 1992;31:169.

120. Kottkamp AC, Filardo TD, Holzman RS, Aguero-Rosenfeld M, Neumann HJ, Mehta SA. Prevalence of strongyloidiasis among cardiothoracic organ transplant candidates in a non-endemic region: a single-center experience with universal screening. *Transpl Infect Dis.* 2021;23:e13614. doi: 10.1111/tid.13614

121. Salluh JI, Bozza FA, Pinto TS, Toscano L, Weller PF, Soares M. Cutaneous periumbilical purpura in disseminated strongyloidiasis in cancer patients: a pathognomonic feature of potentially lethal disease? *Braz J Infect Dis.* 2005;9:419.

122. Simón F, Siles-Lucas M, Morchón R, et al. Human and animal dirofilariasis: the emergence of a zoonotic mosaic. *Clin Microbiol Rev.* 2012;25:507–544.

123. Simón F, Morchón R, González-Miguel J, Marcos-Atxutegi C, Siles-Lucas M. What is new about animal and human dirofilariosis? *Trends Parasitol.* 2009;25:404–409.

124. Joseph E, Matthai A, Abraham LK, Thomas S. Subcutaneous human dirofilariasis. *J Parasit Dis.* 2011;35:140–143.

125. Parks A, May J, Antonovich D, Maize J Jr. Migratory nodules caused by raccoon heartworms in an otherwise healthy adult male. *J Am Acad Dermatol.* 2011;64:e88–e89.

126. D'Amuri A, Senatore SA, Carlà TG, et al. Cutaneous dirofilariasis resulting in orchiectomy. *J Cutan Pathol.* 2012;39:304–305.

127. Böckle BC, Auer H, Mikuz G, Sepp NT. Danger lurks in the Mediterranean. *Lancet.* 2010;376:2040.

128. Stingl P. Onchocerciasis: developments in diagnosis, treatment and control. *Int J Dermatol.* 2009;48(4):393–396. doi: 10.1111/j.1365-4632.2009.03843.x

129. Hrc̆kova G, Kuchtová H, Miterpáková M, Ondriska F, Cibíček J, Kovacs S. Histological and molecular confirmation of the fourth human case caused by Dirofilaria repens in a new endemic region of Slovakia. *J Helminthol.* 2013;87:85–90.

130. Font RL, Guiterrez Y, Semba RD, et al. Ocular Onchocerciasis. In: Meyers WM, Neafie RC, Marty AM, et al., eds. *Pathology of Infectious Diseases.* Vol 1: Helminthiases. Armed Forces Institute of Pathology; 2000:307.

131. Murdoch ME, Hay RJ, Mackenzie CD, et al. A clinical classification and grading system of the cutaneous changes in onchocerciasis. *Br J Dermatol.* 1993;129:260.

132. Udall DN. Recent updates on onchocerciasis: diagnosis and treatment. *Clin Infect Dis.* 2007;44(1):53–60. doi: 10.1086/509325

133. Neafie RC, Marty AM, Duke BOL. Onchocerciasis. In: Meyers WM, Neafie RC, Marty AM, et al., eds. *Pathology of Infectious Diseases.* Vol. 1: Helminthiases. Armed Forces Institute of Pathology; 2000:287.

134. Fernandez-Flores A, Alija A. Cutaneous onchocerciasis: immunohistochemical detection of mast cell population. *Appl Immunohistochem Mol Morphol.* 2009;17(1):88–91.

135. Attout T, Hoerauf A, Dénécé G, et al. Lymphatic vascularisation and involvement of Lyve-1+ macrophages in the human onchocerca nodule. *PLoS One.* 2009;4(12):e8234.

136. Taylor MJ, Hoerauf A, Bockarie M. Lymphatic filariasis and onchocerciasis. *Lancet.* 2010;376(9747):1175–1185.

of specimens for viral culture is 4°C in a refrigerator or on wet ice. Most of the viruses are stable at this temperature for 3 to 5 days. If a specimen needs to be stored longer than 3 to 4 days, a −70°C freezer should be used, and the specimen should be transported on dry ice. With the development of molecular biology, PCR-based rapid viral detection assays have been developed and are used in clinical diagnostic laboratories.

HERPESVIRIDAE

The Herpesviridae are double-stranded DNA viruses with three subfamilies. Herpes virus infections of humans include herpes simplex virus (types 1 and 2), Varicellovirus, CMV, Roseolovirus (HHV-6), Epstein–Barr virus (Lymphocryptovirus), HHV-7, and HHV-8.

Herpes Simplex

Clinical Summary. Two immunologically distinct viruses can cause herpes simplex: herpes simplex virus type 1 (orofacial type) and herpes simplex virus type 2 (genital type), often referred to as HSV-1 and HSV-2, respectively (4). HSV is transmitted through the exchange of saliva, semen, cervical fluid, or vesicle fluid from active lesions. Primary infection with HSV-1 is often subclinical in childhood. In about 10% of the cases, acute gingivostomatitis occurs, usually in childhood and only rarely in early adult life. Primary infection may also occur in rare instances as a respiratory infection or Kaposi varicelliform eruption or keratoconjunctivitis or as a fatal visceral disease of the newborn. Recurrent HSV-1 infections occur most commonly on or near the vermilion border of the lips (herpes labialis—"cold sores," Fig. 25-1A). Recurrences may be triggered by sunlight, physical or emotional stress, immunosuppression, menses, hot or cold conditions, or by febrile illness (5). Besides the lips, any parts of the skin or oral mucosa can be affected by HSV-1. Herpes genitalis is one of the most common sexually transmitted diseases worldwide (Fig. 25-1B) (6). Seroconversion for HSV-2, the most common cause of genital herpes, rarely occurs before the onset of sexual activity. Occasionally, an infant contracts HSV-2 *in utero* or by direct contact in the birth canal (7). Even though most infections of the genitalia and adjoining skin are caused by HSV-2, some infections in this area are caused by

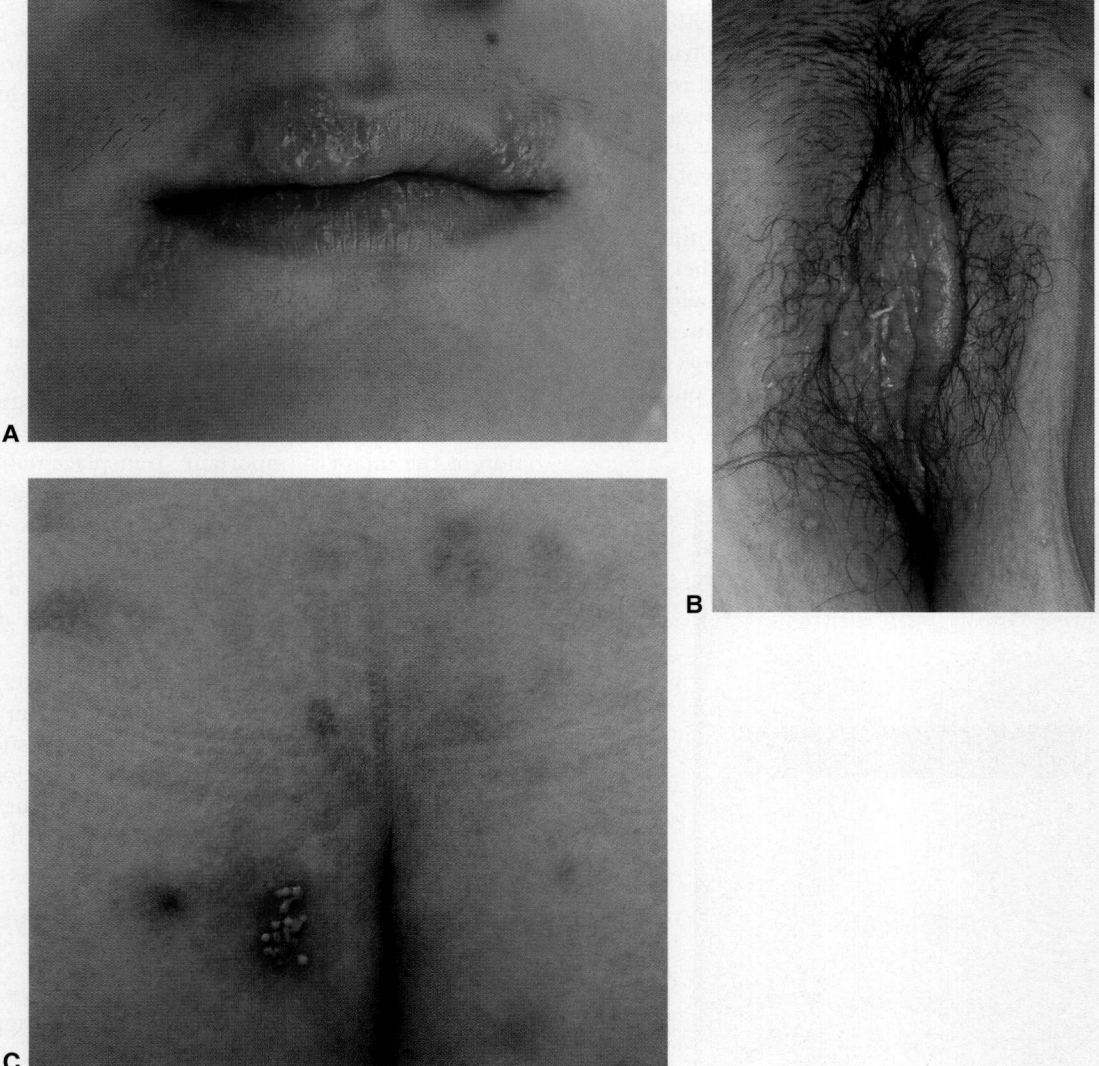

Figure 25-1 Herpes simplex. **A:** Recurrent HSV-1 infection showing grouped vesicles on an erythematous base, occurring most commonly on or near the vermilion border of the lips. **B:** Herpes simplex. HSV-2 infection showing grouped erosions and a few vesicles on the vulva. **C:** Grouped vesicles on the left buttock by HSV-2 infection.

HSV-1. Genital HSV-1 infections are less likely to recur than HSV-2 infections: the rate of recurrence was 14% for HSV-1 infections compared with 60% for HSV-2 infections (8). Only 10% to 25% of individuals who are HSV-2 seropositive report a history of genital herpes (9). Both primary and recurrent herpes simplex, in their earliest stages, show one or several groups of tiny clear vesicles on an edematous red base. If located on a mucous surface, the vesicles erode quickly, whereas if located on the skin they may become pustular before crusting. The lesions usually heal without scarring, except in cases where secondary bacterial infection occurs. The following are special forms of cutaneous herpes simplex: eczema herpeticum (Kaposi varicelliform eruption), herpetic folliculitis, and herpetic whitlow.

Eczema herpeticum is a potentially life-threatening herpetic infection of a preexisting skin disease (10). It occurs most commonly in patients with atopic eczema; however, it may also occur in other skin diseases such as seborrheic dermatitis, pityriasis rubra pilaris, pemphigus foliaceus, Darier disease, and post perioral dermabrasion (11). An extensive rash with small vesicles filled with yellow pus and high fever is the common presentation of eczema herpeticum (Fig. 25-2), which has been linked to increased interleukin (IL)-4 and decreased natural killer cells and IL-2 receptors in patients with atopic eczema (12,13). *Herpetic folliculitis* presents as painful, grouped erythematous, perifollicular vesicles that do not respond to antibacterial or antifungal agents, usually occurring in the bearded region and scalp (14). The characteristic vesiculofollicular lesions usually heal within a few weeks. *Herpetic whitlow* manifests as painful, deep-seated vesicles limited to the paronychial or volar aspects of the distal phalanx of a finger. Herpetic whitlow occurs largely in medical and dental personnel following minor injuries and may be caused by either HSV-1 or HSV-2 (15). Other forms of HSV infections include HSV keratoconjunctivitis, which is the leading cause of corneal blindness in the United States (3), and a rare necrotizing balanitis (16). Noncutaneous forms of herpes simplex infection include herpetic oropharyngitis, pneumonia, encephalitis, esophagitis, and proctitis.

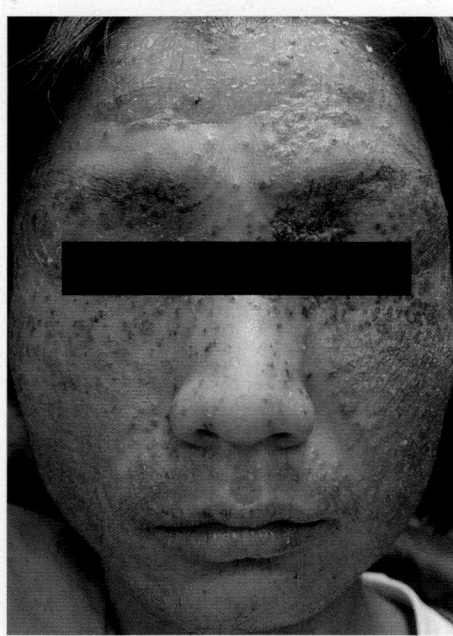

Figure 25-2 Eczema herpeticum. Extensive vesicles and crusts on the face. This lesion often occurs in atopic patients.

Herpes Simplex in Immunocompromised Hosts

Severe primary or secondary herpetic infection with systemic involvement may occur in immunocompromised patients. Coinfection with HSV and HIV frequently occurs, probably because they potentiate each other's transmission. About 70% of HIV-positive patients are seropositive for HSV-2 (17). Three forms of herpes simplex are characteristically found in children or adults with impairment of the cellular immune system. The most common of the three forms is *chronic ulcerative herpes simplex*, and the other two are *generalized acute mucocutaneous herpes simplex* and *systemic herpes simplex*.

Chronic ulcerative herpes simplex exhibits persistent ulcers and erosions (Fig. 25-3A), usually starting on the face or in the perineal region (18). Without treatment, gradual widespread extension is the rule. Some patients may develop chronic verrucous changes within and around the persistent ulcer, particularly in the presence of antiviral-resistant herpes infections. The infection may progress into systemic herpes simplex. *Generalized acute mucocutaneous herpes simplex* follows an initial localized vesicular eruption. Dissemination associated with fever takes place, suggestive of smallpox or varicella infection (19). *Systemic herpes simplex* usually follows oral or genital lesions of herpes simplex (Fig. 25-3B). Areas of necrosis, particularly in the liver, adrenals, pancreas, and brain, lead rapidly to death. In some patients, a few cutaneous lesions of herpes simplex also exist.

Congenital Herpes Simplex

Because almost 1% of patients in prenatal clinics have HSV-2 infections by culture of the vaginal cells and one-third of these have active lesions, there exists the potential of congenital herpes simplex infection. It is important, however, to distinguish primary HSV-2 infection of the mother from recurrent infection. In recurrent infection, the presence of neutralizing antibodies to HSV-2 results in a low rate of attack of the fetus (20). In maternal HSV-2 *primary infection*, the mode of infection of the infant is important. Transplacental infection of the fetus occurring during the first 8 weeks of gestation produces severe congenital malformations. If infection occurs at a later time, malformations are less severe and consist of growth and psychomotor retardation, microcephaly, and a widespread, recurrent vesicular eruption that can mimic a mechanobullous disorder.

Localized herpetic lesions several days after delivery are the initial manifestation if infection is acquired in the birth canal. In vertex deliveries, the scalp is a common site for the development of initial herpetic vesicles. It is rare for transplacental or neonatal infection to remain limited to the skin. It can be followed by systemic herpetic infection, such as encephalitis, hepatoadrenal necrosis, and pneumonia (7).

Herpes Simplex Associated with Erythema Multiforme

HSV is the most commonly identified etiologic agent in recurrent erythema multiforme (21). Molecular diagnostic methods, primarily the PCR, have been used to detect herpetic DNA in the skin lesions of recurrent erythema multiforme in both adults and children (22). The association is further supported by suppression of recurrent lesions in this group by therapy directed at HSV. These patients present clinically with herpetic

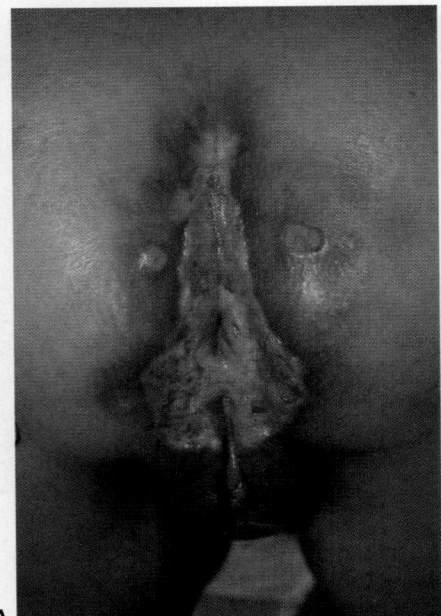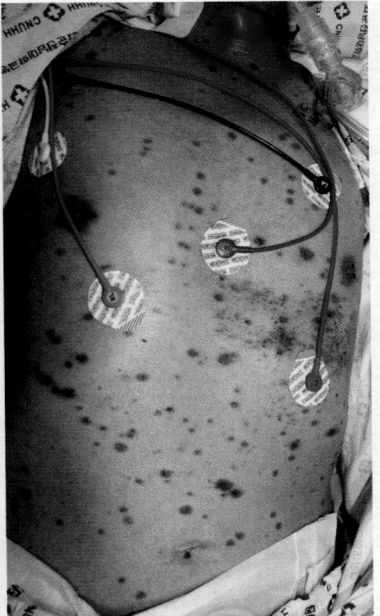

Figure 25-3 Herpes simplex in immunocompromised patients. **A:** Chronic ulcerative herpes simplex shows persistent ulcers and erosions. **B:** In an immunocompromised patient, herpes simplex infection can be generalized, manifesting as scattered necrotic erosive vesicles on the entire body.

outbreaks and target lesions symmetrically on acral sites, distant from the herpetic lesions themselves.

Histopathology of Herpes Simplex

The earliest changes of herpes simplex lesions include nuclear swelling of keratinocytes. With hematoxylin and eosin stains, these nuclei appear slate gray and homogeneous with margination of the nuclear chromatin (Fig. 25-4A). A few necrotic keratinocytes in the epidermis may also be seen. The changes usually begin along the basal layer keratinocytes and then involve the entire epidermis. Later, skin herpes simplex produces profound degeneration of keratinocytes, resulting in acantholysis and vesicle formation (Fig. 25-4B). Degeneration of epidermal keratinocytes occurs in two forms: ballooning degeneration and reticular degeneration. Ballooning degeneration is swelling of epidermal keratinocytes. Balloon cells have a homogeneous, eosinophilic cytoplasm. They may be multinucleated (Tzanck cells). Balloon cells lose their intercellular bridges and become separated from one another (secondary acantholysis), and unilocular vesicles result. Ballooning degeneration occurs mainly at the bases of viral vesicles so that the vesicle formed intraepidermally may ultimately be subepidermal. Ballooning degeneration can affect epithelial cells of hair follicles, sebaceous glands, and rarely eccrine duct cells (Fig. 25-4B). Reticular degeneration is the result of rupture of ballooning cells owing to progressive hydropic swelling of the epidermal cells. Reticular degeneration occurs in the upper portions and at the peripheries of viral vesicles. Reticular degeneration is not specific for viral vesicles, because it also occurs in the vesicles of contact dermatitis. Through coalescence of cells with reticular degeneration, a multilocular vesicle may result, the septa of which are formed by residual cell membrane. In older vesicles, the cellular walls disappear. The originally multilocular portions of the vesicle may become unilocular.

Inclusion bodies may be observed in the centers of enlarged, round nuclei of balloon cells. The inclusion bodies are eosinophilic and surrounded by a clear space or halo (Fig. 25-4C).

They measure from 3 to 8 μm in diameter. Most of the balloon cells at the floor of a vesicle exhibit characteristic homogeneous pale chromatin and nuclei molding without inclusion bodies (Fig. 25-4A). Neutrophils are often present within established vesicles. Neutrophils may be prominent in the lesions of herpetic whitlow. The upper dermis beneath viral vesicles contains an inflammatory infiltrate of variable density. In some cases of herpes simplex, vascular damage is present, showing necrosis of vessel walls, microthrombi, and hemorrhage subjacent to the vesicle (Fig. 25-5A, B). In addition, eosinophilic inclusions may be found in endothelial cells and fibroblasts. In later lesions, necrosis of epidermis is often present with abundant neutrophils (Fig. 25-5A). A dense mixed cell infiltrate in the upper dermis with ghosts of necrotic multinucleated acantholytic cells with slate gray nuclei may still be seen. As in all vesiculobullous diseases, an early lesion should be selected for biopsy; otherwise, secondary changes, especially invasion of inflammatory cells, may obscure the diagnostic features.

Herpetic involvement of hair follicle and pilosebaceous units is not uncommon in recurrent lesions (23). In fact, necrosis of a pilosebaceous unit is a clue to search for multinucleated cells with characteristic slate gray nuclei. In herpetic folliculitis, pilosebaceous involvement is a predominant feature. Rarely, the eccrine ducts and glands are involved by the virus. The histology of eczema herpeticum is similar to that of vesicles of herpes simplex, but usually with more dense neutrophilic infiltrates.

Chronic ulcerative herpes simplex may be difficult to recognize as being of viral genesis if the epidermis is absent. However, viral cytopathic changes may be observed in keratinocytes at the margin of the ulcer. Viral cultures or typing of HSV-1 and HSV-2 by direct immunofluorescence or immunoperoxidase technique can be used to prove the diagnosis. However, the most rapid and accurate method may be the use of molecular diagnostic methods such as the PCR (24).

Tzanck Smear. Cytologic examination of a Giemsa-stained smear taken from the floor of a freshly opened early vesicle is often useful. The presence of many balloon cells results from

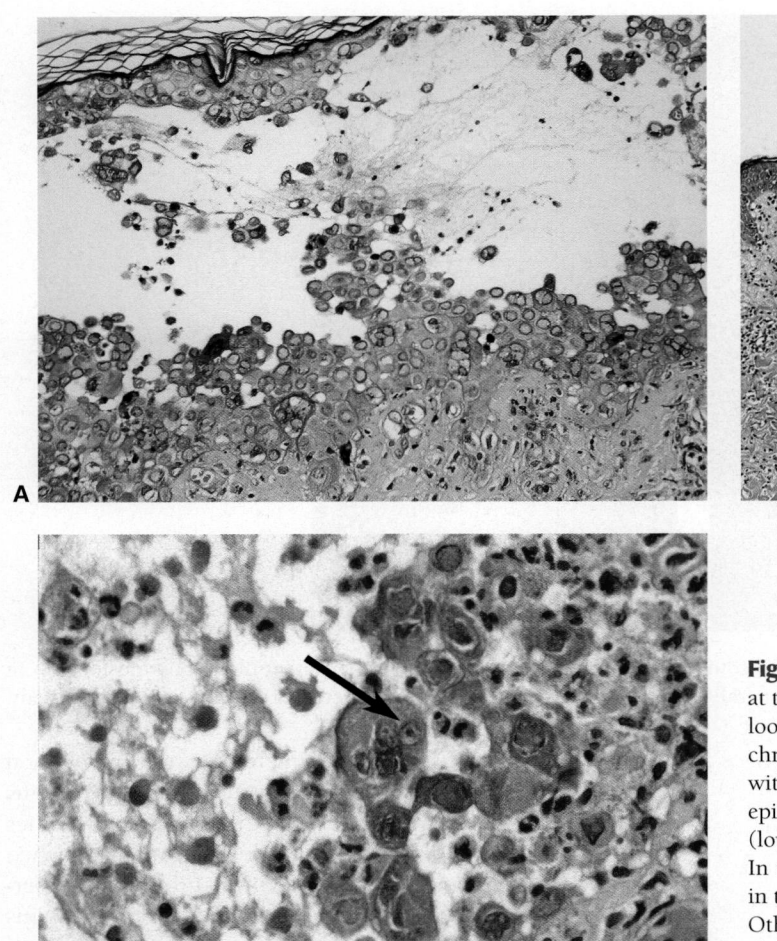

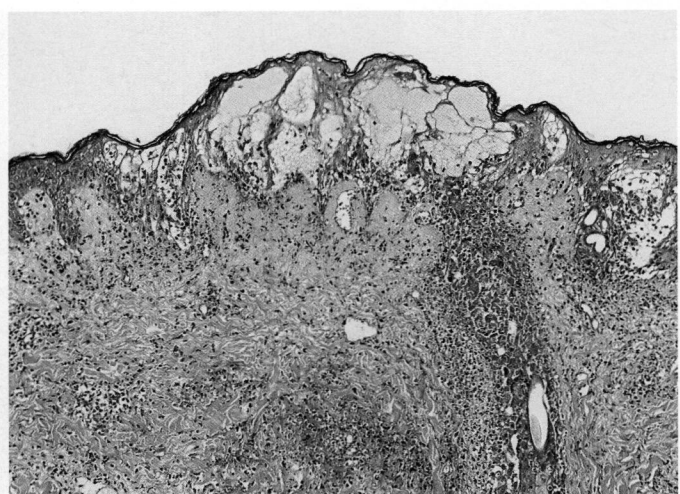

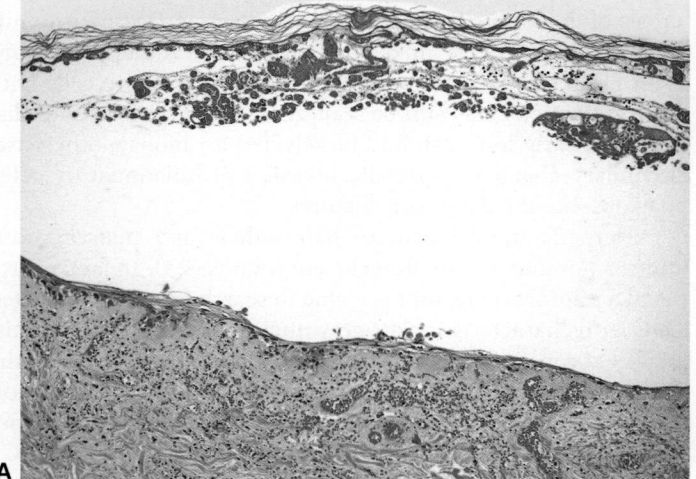

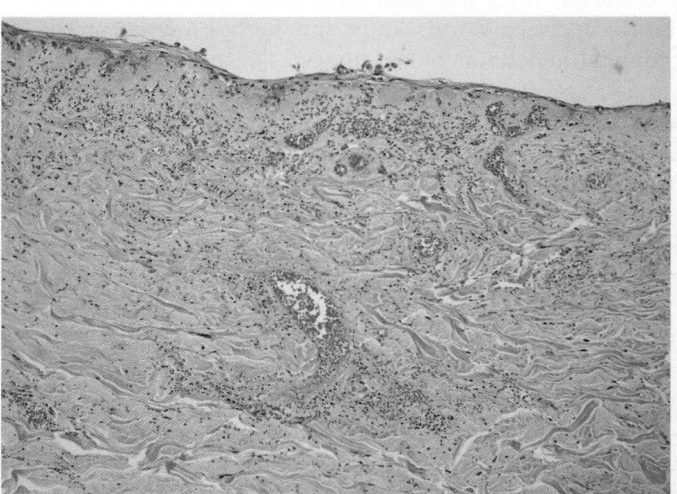

Figure 25-4 Herpes simplex. **A:** On high magnification, balloon cells at the floor of a vesicle are shown; these cells exhibit characteristic ballooning degeneration with steel gray nuclei with homogeneous pale chromatin and nuclei molding. **B:** An intraepidermal vesicular lesion with marked acantholysis and reticular degeneration of the cells at the epidermis. There are many necrotic cells in the follicular epithelium (low magnification). **C:** Balloon cells at the floor of a vesicle are shown. In the center, eosinophilic inclusion bodies surrounded by a halo lies in the nuclei of balloon cells (*arrow points to the intranuclear inclusion*). Other cells exhibit the more characteristic pattern of homogeneous pale chromatin without inclusion bodies.

Figure 25-5 Herpes simplex (biopsy from the patient of Fig. 25-3). **A:** There are marked epidermal necrotic cells appearing as ghost cells and hemorrhages and some inflammatory cells in the dermis at the later stage of herpes simplex infection. **B:** In the dermis, marked hemorrhages and vascular damages are seen, revealing fibrinoid necrosis on the vessel walls and prominent nuclear dust with many inflammatory cells around vessels.

the fact that the smear is taken from the floor of the blister, where ballooning degeneration is most pronounced (Fig. 25-6). Many acantholytic balloon cells with one or several nuclei may be seen in herpes simplex, varicella, and zoster. The Tzanck smear cannot distinguish among HSV-1, HSV-2, and VZV.

Histogenesis and Viral Identification. The HSV can be directly identified by culture, direct immunofluorescence testing, *in situ* hybridization, immunoperoxidase staining, or molecular diagnostic tests. The gold standard for diagnosis is a viral culture. For culture, material from the floor of a blister or other infected

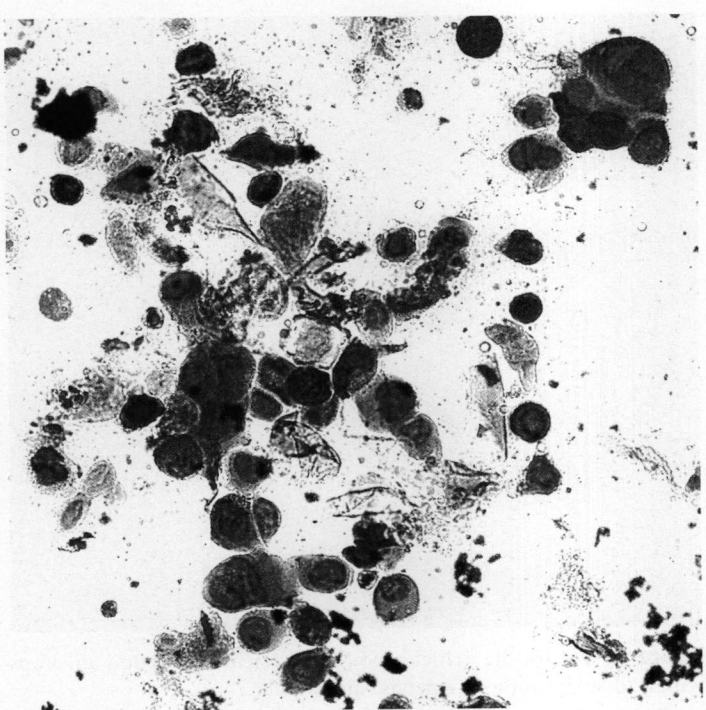

Figure 25-6 Tzanck Smear. A Tzanck smear from the floor of the vesicle of herpes simplex shows multinucleated giant cells and ballooning cells. There is also chromatin margination in the nuclei of infected cells (Wright–Giemsa stain).

material is inoculated onto HeLa cells, human amnion cells, or fibroblasts. The virus has cytopathic effects on the cultured cells. Direct immunofluorescence examination for the presence of the viral antigen in cells infected with HSV is then performed. Herpes simplex DNA can be extracted and amplified by PCR from stained or unstained Tzanck smears, crusts, fresh tissue, and paraffin sections of suspected lesions. With appropriate primers, each herpes-type virus can be specifically identified. Viral culture is particularly important in cases of chronic infection refractory to therapy, because viral culture is currently the gold standard for identifying resistance to antiviral medications.

For distinction between the two types of HSV, immunoperoxidase staining may be performed on sections of the lesions using monoclonal antibodies, one directed against HSV-1 and the other against HSV-2. *In situ* hybridization can also be used for visual demonstration of viral genomic material in tissue (25). For determination of the antibody titer in the patient's serum, a complement fixation reaction is usually used. The serologic test for HSV is useful to confirm HSV infection in persons with a questionable history of herpetic disease and in those who have unrecognized or subclinical infection so that they may be aware of their potential to transmit the virus.

On electron microscopy, the HSV is spherical. Its DNA-containing core measures approximately 40 nm in diameter. The virion has a diameter of about 100 nm and, together with its outer coat, measures around 135 nm (26). Ultrastructurally, the virion of herpes simplex is indistinguishable from that of varicella.

Differential Diagnosis. Viral vesicles produced by the HSV and by the VZV are identical. Furthermore, an incompletely developed case of herpes zoster can mimic herpes simplex infection, both clinically and histologically. In the context of immunosuppression, chronic cutaneous forms of both viruses exist, and

their specific identification may not be possible by clinical morphology or light microscopy. Molecular diagnostic methods are the quickest and most reliable way to separate and identify the specific viruses in these situations.

Eczema Herpeticum

Clinical Summary. Eczema herpeticum, also known as Kaposi varicelliform eruption, is a disseminated viral infection characterized by fever and clusters of itchy blisters or punched-out erosions. Most cases of eczema herpeticum are caused by HSV-1 or HSV-2, superimposed on a preexisting dermatosis (27), usually atopic dermatitis (28). Occasionally, seborrheic dermatitis or other dermatoses, such as Darier disease, benign familial pemphigus, pemphigus foliaceus, mycosis fungoides, Sézary syndrome, or ichthyosis vulgaris, provide the "soil" in which eczema herpeticum develops (11). Eczema herpeticum is better called Kaposi varicelliform eruption when a breakdown of the skin barrier is not attributable to eczema. Other viruses such as vaccinia virus, varicella-zoster, and Coxsackie A16 virus may also induce similar skin eruption.

Eczema herpeticum usually arises during the first episode of HSV infection but may also occur as a recurrent type of infection. A primary infection with HSV occurs in persons without circulating HSV antibodies. Most patients with the primary type of eczema herpeticum are infants and children. The recurrent type of eczema herpeticum occurs in patients with circulating HSV antibodies. The first attack of eczema herpeticum, whether of the primary or the recurrent type, may be the result of exogenous infection, whereas subsequent attacks may result from either reinfection or reactivation. The primary type of eczema herpeticum can be a serious disease with viremia and potential internal organ involvement resulting in death. In contrast, the recurrent type of eczema herpeticum generally shows no viremia and internal organ involvement except in immunologically compromised patients. Occasionally, secondary bacterial infection with subsequent septicemia may cause death. The mortality associated with eczema herpeticum is approximately 10%, with most fatalities occurring in infants and children with a primary type of herpetic infection and in adults with inadequate cellular immunity.

Clinically, all forms of eczema herpeticum and eczema vaccinatum look alike, but eczema vaccinatum has not been seen in modern practice because vaccinia virus has not been used, until recently, for smallpox prevention (29). Both show a more or less extensive eruption composed of vesicles and pustules that may be umbilicated. These vesicles and pustules occur chiefly in the areas of the preexisting dermatosis but also on normal skin. The face is usually severely affected and may be edematous. There may be fever and prostration.

Histopathology. Both eczema herpeticum and eczema vaccinatum show vesicles and pustules of the viral type. Even though the pustules exhibit only necrotic epidermis in their centers, one may still see reticular and ballooning degeneration at their peripheries. In eczema herpeticum, but not in eczema vaccinatum, multinucleated epithelial giant cells are often present.

Differential Diagnosis. Because eczema herpeticum and eczema vaccinatum look alike clinically, and the histologic similarity is great in the absence of inclusion bodies and of multinucleated epithelial cells, differentiation of the two diseases may have to depend on nonhistologic means, such as a history of possible exposure to the vaccinia virus. The most efficient and rapid means of identifying the viral agent is to use DNA amplification methods and appropriate probes.

Principles of Management: For all herpes simplex infections, the mainstay of treatment is antiviral medications. Generally, acyclovir, valacyclovir, or famciclovir is used as a first-line agent. Acyclovir is a nucleoside analog, a competitive inhibitor of the viral polymerase, and prematurely terminates viral DNA synthesis. Famciclovir and valaciclovir are prodrugs and are metabolized into active drugs in the body as penciclovir and acyclovir, respectively. Topical antiviral agents are used for HSV-1 and -2 infections. Immunosuppressed patients or those with widespread infection may benefit from parenteral administration. Once the vesicles develop and evolve into erosions, patients are at risk for secondary infection; meticulous skin care is essential to minimize scarring and prevent bacterial superinfection. Antiviral resistance may develop; second-line therapies include foscarnet, and, in some cases, cidofovir may be used. Immunosuppressed patients with chronic, verrucous resistant HSV may require either local or systemic cidofovir to achieve complete clearance (30,31).

Varicella and Herpes Zoster

Varicella (chickenpox) and herpes zoster (shingles) are produced by the same virus, the VZV. VZV is endemic in the population but becomes epidemic during late winter and early spring (32). Varicella results from contact of a nonimmune person with this virus, whereas herpes zoster occurs in persons who have had previous varicella, either clinically or subclinically. Herpes zoster is caused by reactivation of a latent infection in either a spinal or a cranial sensory ganglion. On reactivation, the virus spreads from the ganglion along the corresponding sensory nerve or nerves to the skin.

Varicella

Clinical Summary. In varicella, a generalized eruption develops after an incubation period of about 2 weeks. Varicella is primarily a disease of childhood; 90% of cases occur in children aged 14 years or younger (33). The transmission rate of acute varicella to susceptible household contacts is estimated to be as high as 80% to 90%, making it one of the most infectious viral diseases in humans. VZV is acquired from patients with primary varicella or herpes zoster through either direct contact with infected vesicular fluid or inhalation of aerosolized respiratory secretions. Recent experiments suggest that the VZV is lymphotropic, especially to T cells. After the initial viremia and a period of viral replication, a second, higher titer viremic phase results in widespread dissemination of the virus. The rash develops as VZV-infected mononuclear cells invade vascular endothelial cells, gaining access to cutaneous tissue. After the primary varicella infection resolves, the VZV enters a latent phase in the dorsal root ganglia (34). Pruritic rash of chickenpox, the hallmark of the disease, typically begins on the head and spreads to the trunk and, finally, the extremities; proximal involvement is greater than distal. The skin lesions of varicella begin as erythematous macules to small papules, which develop into vesicles (Fig. 25-7). In mild cases, most vesicles become crusted without changing into pustules. In severe cases, the vesicles may have slightly hemorrhagic bases ("dewdrops on rose petals"). New lesions continue to develop

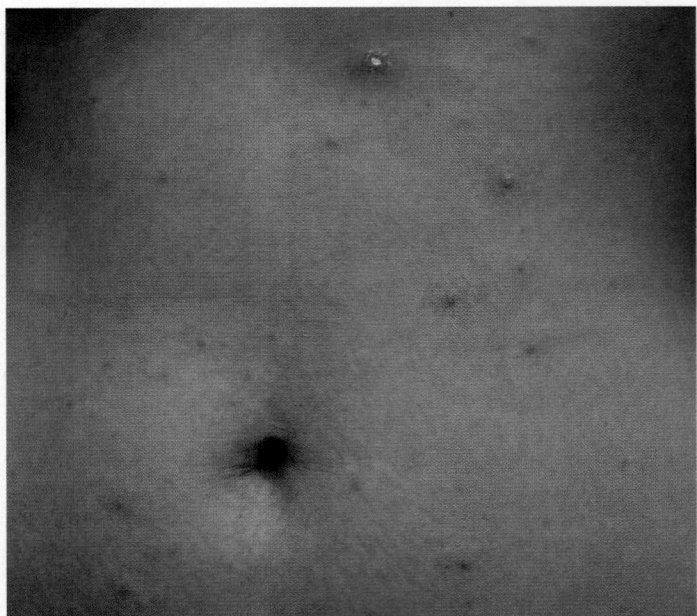

Figure 25-7 Varicella (chickenpox). A vesicular eruption in crops with a "dew drops on rose petals" appearance.

for several days, and so lesions in different stages, papules, vesicles, pustules, and crusted lesions can be observed. Because childhood varicella vaccination is now accepted practice, occasionally brief, attenuated courses of the disease may develop in previously vaccinated patients. Typically, varicella lesions heal without scarring as new epithelium forms at the base; however, hypopigmentation, skin pitting, and keloid formation may result, especially among darker-skinned individuals. Varicella in adults is generally associated with a greater number of skin lesions, more systemic complaints, and a higher risk of such serious complications as pneumonia, encephalitis, and death. Subclinical varicella, documented by increases in antibody titer after exposure to the virus, has been estimated to occur in as much as 5% of the population (35).

Three systemic complications can occur in varicella without the existence of immunosuppression: primary varicella pneumonia, Reye syndrome, and varicella of the fetus and newborn. Primary varicella pneumonia occurs in approximately 14% of adults with varicella and carries a significant mortality. Reye syndrome is an acute, severe, and usually fatal encephalopathy associated with fatty degeneration of the viscera, particularly of the liver. It follows mainly varicella but also other viral infections. The incidence of Reye syndrome declined soon after the report of the epidemiologic association of Reye syndrome and the ingestion of aspirin (36). Varicella in the first 20 weeks of pregnancy has a 2% risk of producing embryopathy or other congenital malformations (37). Maternal varicella late in pregnancy may be transmitted to the fetus transplacentally or may contaminate the baby during passage through the birth canal, resulting in neonatal varicella.

Varicella in Immunocompromised Hosts

In patients with impairment of the cellular immune system, continued viral replication may lead to a prolonged course and to dissemination to various organs, particularly the lungs and liver. Varicella pneumonia is not uncommon, even in children, and death may result from dissemination. VZV may cause particularly severe problems for patients with AIDS. There may be continuous dissemination of vesicular lesions, formation of chronic vegetative lesions, and large necrotic lesions (38).

Herpes Zoster

Clinical Summary. It is known that VZV establishes latency in ganglia following the primary infection causing varicella (chickenpox) and that the virus may reactivate after years of dormancy to produce herpes zoster (shingles). It is now widely accepted that the virus is mainly latent in neuronal cells, with only a small proportion of nonneuronal cells infected. The ganglia most often involved are those of the lumbar and thoracic nerves. When the virus is reactivated, newly synthesized viruses are transported along the sensory nerve and released into the skin. Trigger mechanisms include trauma, stress, old age, and immunosuppression. The incidence of herpes zoster (shingles) increases with age (39). Although herpes zoster occurs largely in adults, particularly in those of advanced age, about 5% of patients with herpes zoster are children under 15 years old. The course in children without immune defects is usually mild. The eruption in herpes zoster consists of vesicles grouped on inflammatory bases and arranged along the course of a sensory nerve (Fig. 25-8). The bases of the lesions are frequently hemorrhagic, and some may become necrotic and ulcerate. Not infrequently, there are a few scattered nondermatomal lesions, and rarely there is a generalized eruption, including mucosal lesions, indistinguishable from that of varicella. The most common places of involvement include the thoracolumbar (T3-L2) and facial (V1) dermatomes. Severe neuritis with acute pain, dysesthesia, and skin hypersensitivity is common and more severe in people older than 60 years and in immunocompromised patients. Zoster sine herpete, or "pain without the rash," is a rare presentation of herpes zoster; dermatomal pain is present with failure to develop a rash, likely because of neural inflammation and damage caused by viral reactivation. Zoster vaccines that may offer good protection are approved for patients age 50 and older. Herpes zoster during pregnancy is not as serious a problem as primary varicella during pregnancy; it does not result in serious morbidity or intrauterine VZV infection. Transplacental transmission of the virus does not occur

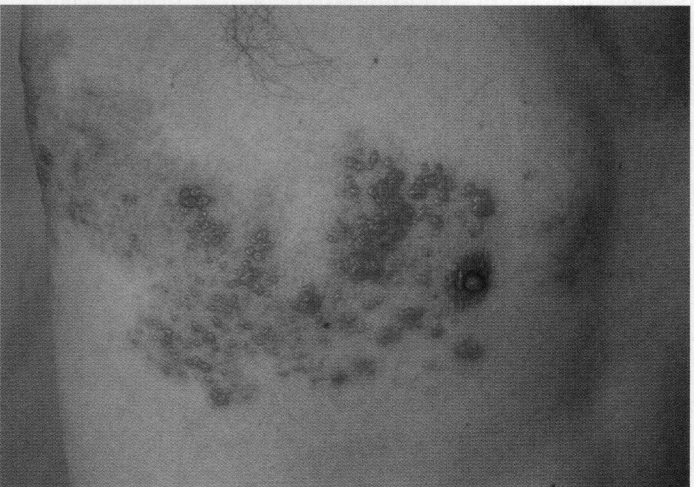

Figure 25-8 Herpes zoster (shingles). Vesicles with a characteristic dermatomal distribution on the right chest and back.

with maternal herpes zoster; preexisting normal immunity is thought to protect the fetus.

Herpes Zoster in Immunocompromised Hosts

Both the incidence and the severity of herpes zoster are greater in patients with impaired cellular immunity. The incidence of herpes zoster is particularly high in patients with advanced Hodgkin disease who are receiving chemotherapy or radiation and in persons infected with HIV. In the context of HIV infection, herpes zoster may fail to resolve, may disseminate, or may produce atypical vegetative and ulcerative lesions (40). Although patients with disseminated herpes zoster but without associated serious illness have good prognoses, patients with impaired cellular immunity may develop widespread, fatal systemic manifestations, such as pneumonia, gastroenteritis, or encephalitis.

Histopathology. Lesions of varicella and herpes zoster are histologically indistinguishable from those of herpes simplex (Fig. 25-4). Frequently, however, the degree of vessel damage, microthrombi, and hemorrhage are more pronounced in varicella and, particularly, in herpes zoster than in herpes simplex. Herpes zoster vasculitis may mimic giant-cell arteritis (41). In severe cases of varicella and in disseminated herpes zoster, eosinophilic inclusion bodies have also been observed in the dermis within the nuclei of capillary endothelial cells and of fibroblasts bordering the affected vessels. In contrast, in localized herpes zoster, in which the virus reaches the epidermis by way of the cutaneous nerves rather than the capillaries, inclusion bodies have been demonstrated within neurilemmal cells of the small nerves in the dermis underlying the vesicles. Immunohistochemical methods using specific monoclonal antibodies can be used to separate VZV from HSV. Using an antibody specific for an envelope glycoprotein, Nikkels and colleagues demonstrated VZV reactivity in sebaceous cells, endothelial cells, mononuclear phagocytes, and factor XIIIa–positive dendrocytes (42).

Tzanck Smear. Cytologic examination of the contents of vesicles is carried out for varicella and herpes zoster in the same way as for herpes simplex. It is a very useful diagnostic test, confirming the diagnosis in 80% to 100% of the cases, whereas viral cultures can provide such confirmation in only 60% to 64% (43).

Histogenesis and Viral Identification. Cultures remain the gold standard for virologic confirmation, and the virus can be cultured easily from vesicular fluid within 5 days of the onset of symptoms or before the crusting of lesions. However, culture is not very sensitive, and in contrast to herpes simplex, the VZV does not grow in ordinary tissue cultures but only in human fetal diploid kidney cells or human foreskin fibroblasts. Specific antibodies are available for serologic or immunohistochemical viral identification, and rapid qualitative PCR-based detection of VZV DNA in clinical specimens is also available in many laboratories. Electron microscopic examination of the cutaneous lesions of varicella and herpes zoster reveals virus particles in the capillary endothelium in varicella and sporadically in the axons of dermal nerves in herpes zoster. The HSV and the VZV are indistinguishable by electron microscopy.

Principles of Management: Varicella infection can be prevented or diminished by age-appropriate vaccine, either in childhood or at age 50 with the zoster vaccine. Once varicella infection occurs, the mainstay of treatment is antiviral medications and supportive pain relief. Generally, acyclovir or valacyclovir is used as a first-line agent. Systemic oral or intravenous antiviral treatments are required for the treatment of adult chickenpox and herpes zoster (44). Immunosuppressed patients or those with widespread infection may benefit from parenteral administration and should be evaluated for liver or lung involvement. Recently, herpes zoster vaccine has been shown to reduce the incidence of herpes zoster and postherpetic neuralgia in the older population (45). Patients with active varicella infection are contagious and should be advised to avoid pregnant and immunosuppressed people. Hospitalized patients with active zoster should be placed on contact isolation; patients with disseminated disease require airborne and contact isolation because the varicella virus can disseminate to the lungs and may be aerosolized.

CYTOMEGALOVIRUS

Clinical Summary. CMV is a herpes virus that is ubiquitous in human populations. It has been estimated that 1% of newborns are infected transplacentally, and about 5% more acquire the infection at birth. There is a steady increase with age in the number of individuals with antibodies in the serum, and this number jumps significantly in adolescence, presumably owing to transfer of virus through the oral route (46). CMV may also be sexually transmitted. Owing to its ability to remain latent in peripheral leukocytes, CMV can be transmitted via transfusion. Most individuals have a mild flulike episode on initial infection; however, the virus subsequently becomes latent and persists in many tissues in the body. In immunocompromised individuals, reactivation and involvement of almost any organ of the body can take place and produce a widespread, potentially fatal, systemic infection (47).

Skin manifestation of CMV infection is rare in immunocompetent persons. Cutaneous lesions reported in the immunocompromised patients vary greatly, from genital ulceration to ulceration of the oral cavity and chest, a more or less widespread maculopapular rash that may become purpuric, sharply punched-out ulcers, urticaria, vesiculobullous lesions, keratotic lesions, and epidermolysis (48). In the context of HIV infection, CMV-associated viral cytopathic changes can be observed as epiphenomena in skin biopsies in that they do not appear to be the primary pathogen in the specimen and the cause of the skin eruption.

Neonates with congenital CMV infection may exhibit the clinical picture of the "blueberry muffin baby" at delivery, which is manifested by petechiae and purpuric magenta-colored macules, papules, and plaques, as well as blueberry-colored ecchymoses. The hemorrhagic (purpuric) skin lesions are thought to reflect extramedullary hematopoiesis. Ultrastructural study demonstrates that complexes of red cells in various stages of maturation occur in the skin of these patients, similar to the erythroblastic islands in the bone marrow (49). Transplacental transfer of CMV is one of the causes of TORCH, a congenital infection caused by Toxoplasma, Rubella, CMV, or Herpesvirus, with extensive damage to the developing brain, chorioretinitis, and pneumonitis (50).

Histopathology. Dilated dermal vessels exhibit, among normal endothelial cells, large, irregularly shaped endothelial cells with large, hyperchromatic, basophilic, intranuclear inclusions that are around 10 μm in size, as well as small intracytoplasmic inclusions (around 3 μm in size; see Fig. 25-9). Some of the inclusions are surrounded by clear halos. A mixed inflammatory infiltrate with focal leukocytoclastic changes may also be present. In the context of HIV infection, other pathologic processes may also be present in the same tissue section.

Histogenesis and Viral Identification. CMV culture can be performed using human fibroblasts. PP65 is a CMV viral protein that is detectable in infected peripheral mononuclear cells, which is a sensitive method to estimate the systemic viral load (51). Immunohistochemical studies using monoclonal or polyclonal antibodies to CMV antigens can be used in paraffin-embedded sections to reveal viral proteins and confirm the presence of the virus. CMV DNA can also be amplified from skin biopsy specimens with PCR using specific primers for CMV or can be identified by *in situ* hybridization. Electron microscopy shows intranuclear viral particles approximately 110 nm in diameter. The virus greatly resembles that of herpes simplex.

Principles of Management: CMV infection in immunocompromised patients may be devastating. It is imperative for CMV to be detected early in its course to prevent mortality and is generally managed in conjunction with an infectious disease specialist; treatment usually revolves around ganciclovir. Ganciclovir, a deoxyguanosine analog, which is also a DNA polymerase inhibitor, is used for CMV infection as a monotherapy or in combination with immunoglobulin. Foscarnet and Cidofovir are approved for therapy for CMV retinitis in AIDS patients (52).

Epstein–Barr Virus

Clinical Summary. The Epstein–Barr virus (EBV) is thought to be responsible for many diseases such as IM, oral hairy leukoplakia, and cutaneous lymphoproliferative disorders, as well as Burkett lymphoma and nasopharyngeal carcinoma (53). Infection with the EBV develops first in the salivary gland. Large amounts of the virus are released in the saliva, enabling it to spread from one person to another. People infected with the EBV will retain it for life, and most are asymptomatic. It has been estimated that the virus infects almost everyone in developing countries and more than 80% of people in developed countries. Most people are infected with the virus during childhood and are usually not noticeably affected. On the other hand, people infected for the first time during or after adolescence (10% to 20% of people living in developed countries) have a 50% chance of developing IM. The main site of viral persistence is within latently infected lymphocytes, although infectious virus is also released into saliva from infected cells in the oropharynx (54).

IM is a self-limited manifestation of acute EBV infection. The transient rash that occurs quite commonly in patients with IM who have received antibiotic therapy is an erythematous, maculopapular eruption, usually located on the trunk and upper extremities. The palms, soles, and oral mucosa have also been reported to be occasionally involved. The pathogenesis of the rash is believed to be secondary to polyclonal B-cell activation, which occurs during EBV infection with the production of polyclonal antibodies that form immune complexes capable of fixing complement (55).

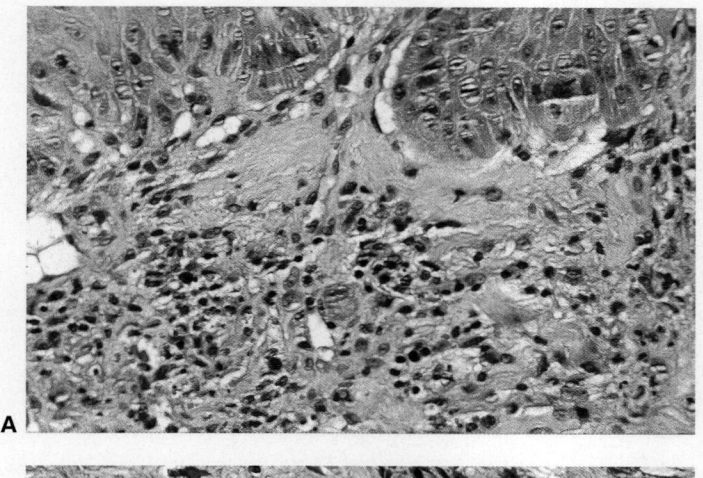

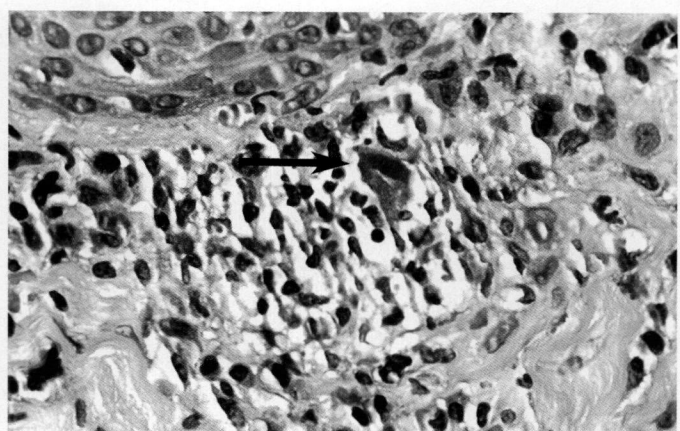

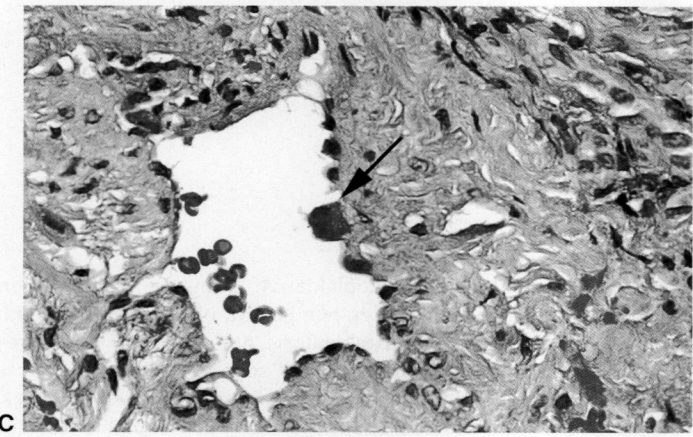

Figure 25-9 Cytomegalic inclusion disease. **A:** Scanning magnification shows superficial perivascular and diffuse inflammation with prominent vessels. Enlarged endothelial cells may be apparent at this magnification. **B:** On high magnification, one infected dermal cell in the center shows enlarged, hyperchromatic, basophilic, intranuclear inclusions. There is a mixed inflammatory infiltrate in the dermis. **C:** Dilated dermal vessel with large, irregularly shaped endothelial cells. The enlarged endothelial cells contain hyperchromatic, basophilic, intranuclear inclusions (*arrow points to an inclusion*). There may also be basophilic cytoplasmic inclusions.

Oral hairy leukoplakia is another manifestation of EBV infection that occurs in immunosuppressed HIV-positive and HIV-negative individuals. In HIV-positive individuals, it serves as an indicator of disease severity and rapid progression to AIDS. The presence of oral hairy leukoplakia in an individual should prompt the clinician to perform a thorough history-taking and investigation of immune status. These lesions characteristically resemble whitish patches with a verrucous or filiform irregular surface that cannot be scraped off and that are located primarily on the lateral surfaces of the tongue unilaterally or bilaterally. The condition is usually asymptomatic, but in some cases, a burning sensation can occur, which is most likely secondary to coinfection by Candida (56).

Lymphoproliferative disorders associated with EBV are well documented in the literature. Chronic active Epstein–Barr virus (CAEBV) disease is a rare disorder in which persons are unable to control infection with the virus. CAEBV often involves γδ T cells and NK cells. The disease is progressive, with markedly elevated levels of EBV DNA in the blood and infiltration of organs by EBV-positive lymphocytes. Patients often present with fever, lymphadenopathy, splenomegaly, EBV hepatitis, or pancytopenia. Chronic EBV infection has been associated with hydroa vacciniforme–like lymphoproliferative disorder (HV-LPD) (57). These patients have skin lesions on the face, extremities, or areas unexposed to the sun, including edema, blistering, ulceration, and scarring. The course is slowly progressive and relapsing. In addition, posttransplant lymphoproliferative disease, extranodal NK-/T-cell lymphoma, aggressive NK-cell leukemia, severe mosquito bite allergy, and chronic active EVB infection of T/NK type have been shown to be associated with EBV infection (58,59).

Histopathology. The histology of the macular lesion associated with IM is nonspecific and usually shows superficial perivascular lymphohistiocytic infiltrates. The histologic features that typify oral hairy leukoplakia include irregular epithelial hyperplasia with associated parakeratosis and acanthosis (Fig. 25-10A). Ballooning of keratinocytes occurs, and there are small, pyknotic nuclei with intranuclear inclusions and a clear perinuclear halo. The cytoplasm may adopt a ground-glass appearance (Fig. 25-10B). There is also a mild inflammatory infiltrate observed in the superficial dermis. Langerhans cells are noted to be absent in the epithelium. Hyphae of Candida are observed within the superficial epithelium of most patients with oral hairy leukoplakia and may play a role in the development of the epithelial hyperplasia observed in oral hairy leukoplakia. Leukocytoclastic vasculitis and neuropathy associated with chronic EBV infection have also been reported. EBV can be detected by *in situ* hybridization (Fig. 25-10C). Histopathology of HV-LPD shows an atypical lymphocytic infiltrate in the dermis and/or subcutaneous tissue. The lesions have a cytotoxic T/NK-cell immunophenotype (56).

Principles of Management: Patients with EBV infection generally require supportive care for acute disease; EBV-associated secondary processes require directed therapy, which will vary by disease type.

Human Herpesvirus-6, -7, and -8

Clinical Summary. Human herpesviruses 6, 7, and 8 may cause primary or chronic persistent infection or remain in a state of latency for many years until a decrease in the immunologic

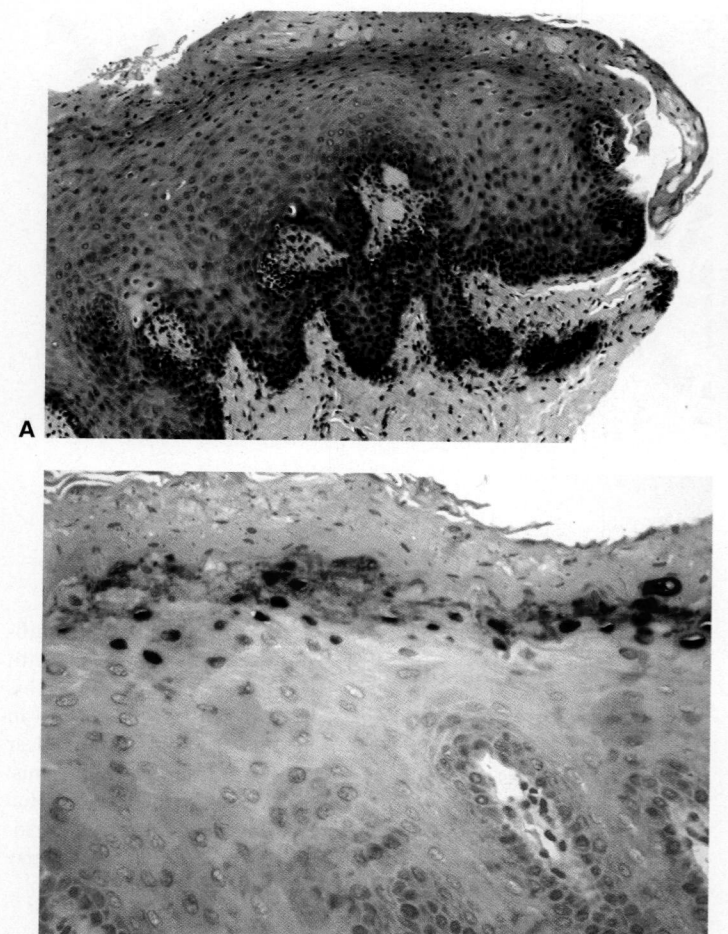

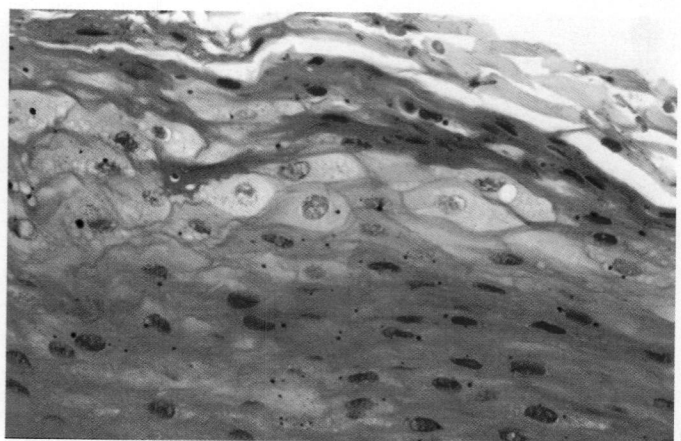

Figure 25-10 Oral hairy leukoplakia. **A:** Scanning magnification shows the characteristic complex rete pattern of lingual epithelium. There is hyperkeratosis and parakeratosis, and there may be neutrophils in the stratum corneum. Pallor of superficial keratinocytes is focally apparent. **B:** Detail of swollen, pale superficial keratinocytes, with open pale nuclei, but without specific viral cytopathic changes and scant inflammation in the superficial lamina propria. **C:** *In situ* hybridization shows EBV in the superficial keratinocytes.

state of the host leads to reactivation of infection. HHV-6 was first isolated in 1986 from patients with lymphoproliferative disorders and was classified into two variants: HHV-6A and HHV-6B. HHV-6B is the causative agent of exanthem subitum, also known as the sixth disease. Children start to be infected with HHV-6 at 6 months of age, and almost all have antibodies by 2 years of age. The transmission of HHV-6 is essentially by a salivary route (60). HHV-6 infects latently after the primary infection and reactivates especially under an immunosuppressive condition. Skin rash in the first month after allogeneic bone marrow transplant (61), generalized vesiculobullous eruptions after allogeneic bone marrow transplantation (62), papular-purpuric "gloves-and-socks" syndrome (63), Gianotti–Crosti syndrome (64), and a serious systemic reaction to a limited number of drugs called hypersensitivity syndrome have been associated with HHV-6 (65). Drug reaction with eosinophilia and systemic symptoms (DRESS) syndrome, also referred to as drug-induced hypersensitivity syndrome, has been reported to be associated with the reactivation of herpesviruses, especially HHV-6, although CMV, EBV, and HHV-7 are also implicated (66) (Fig. 25-11A). The cutaneous manifestations typically consist of an urticarial, maculopapular eruption and, in some instances, vesicles, bullae, pustules, purpura, target lesions, facial edema, cheilitis, and erythroderma. Some suggest that in genetically predisposed hosts, exposure to a drug triggers latent virus replication, and then the patient suffers from an exuberant host antiviral response, leading to the clinical phenotype of DRESS and some of the

delayed autoimmune sequela. Hematologic findings (eosinophilia, leukocytosis, etc.), and abnormal liver function tests may present. Visceral involvement (hepatitis, pneumonitis, myocarditis, pericarditis, nephritis, and colitis) is the major cause of morbidity and mortality in this syndrome. Sequential reactivations of several herpes viruses (HHV-6, HHV-7, EBV, and CMV) can be detected coincidentally with the clinical symptoms of drug hypersensitivity reactions. HHV-6 has also been detected in skin biopsy samples of patients with graft-versus-host disease, pityriasis rosea, and lymphoproliferative malignancies.

HHV-7, isolated from CD4+ T lymphocytes from the peripheral blood of a healthy individual, has been recognized as a new lymphotropic herpesvirus. Healthy adults frequently shed the virus into saliva, and children are infected at a young age but somewhat later than is the case with HHV-6. Latency is established in peripheral blood T cells, and a persistent infection in the salivary glands is believed to be the most likely mode of transmission. The primary infection with HHV-7 is linked to febrile illness with or without rash that resembles exanthema subitum. Pityriasis rosea is thought to be associated with HHV-7; however, the association is still controversial. Human herpesvirus 7, but not HHV-6, is currently a candidate for the etiology of lichen planus (LP). In skin biopsy specimens from 33 patients, cells infected by HHV-7 were identified more frequently in LP lesions than in skin without lesions or in psoriatic or healthy skin (67).

HHV-8 was first identified in tissue samples of patients with Kaposi sarcoma (KS) associated with AIDS in 1994.

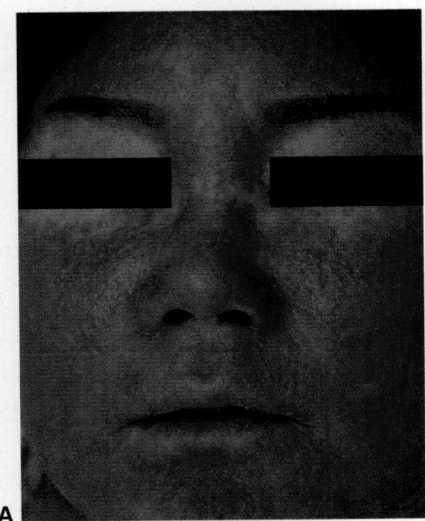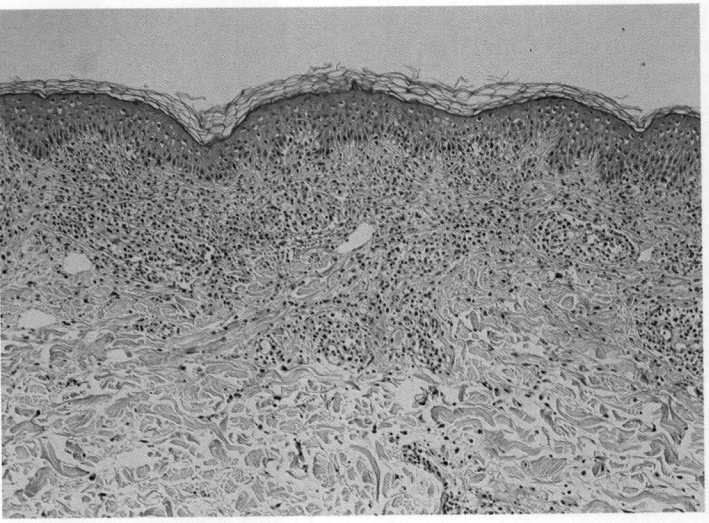

Figure 25-11 Drug reaction with eosinophilia and systemic symptoms (DRESS) syndrome. **A:** Tender erythematous swelling on the face. **B:** Skin biopsy shows dense mixed perivascular inflammation with red blood cells extravasation and a few eosinophils. Interface change is often present.

AIDS-associated KS commonly appear at the trunk, compared with classic KS, which arises on the lower extremity (Fig. 25-12). Serologic studies have demonstrated that, unlike other human herpesviruses, HHV-8 is not ubiquitous; instead, its infection rates parallel the incidence of KS in the region. HHV-8 spreads through exchange of saliva and other sexual activities. HHV-8 can be found in all types of KS, whether related to HIV or not. HHV-8 seems to resemble EBV in its possible transforming properties, and HHV-8 is clearly associated with KS, multicentric Castleman disease, and primary effusion lymphoma (68). There may be a synergistic relationship between the HIV-1 Tat protein and HHV-8 infection. Tat promotes the growth of the KS spindle cells. Like other herpesviruses, HHV-8 establishes latent and persistent infection. Only a minority of infected cells yield infectious viral particles, and their role in the development of KS and other associated diseases has not been clearly established. The presence of virus can be established in mononuclear cells of peripheral blood, endothelial cells, and spindle cells within skin lesions.

Histopathology. Exanthem subitum linked to HHV-6 infection is a form of superficial perivascular dermatitis with papillary dermal edema. Exocytosis of lymphocytes is often present. Inclusions similar to those in herpes simplex infection are not seen. DRESS is linked to HHV-6, HHV-7, EBV, and CMV reactivation. Interface dermatitis is commonly seen in DRESS (Fig. 25-11B). Eczematous, acute generalized exanthematous pustulosis–like and erythema multiforme–like patterns are also observed. The association of two or three of these patterns in a single biopsy was significantly more frequent in cases of DRESS than in nondrug-induced dermatoses. Histopathology of KS shows vascular spindle cell proliferation that is positive for HHV-8 in the dermis and is described in more detail in Chapter 34.

Principles of Management: Skin diseases caused by HHV-6 and HHV-7 only need symptomatic and supportive management, and there are currently no approved treatments for them (69).

POXVIRIDAE

The Poxviridae are double-stranded DNA viruses with two subfamilies and 11 genera. Poxvirus infections of humans include variola (smallpox), cowpox, vaccinia, molluscum contagiosum, paravaccinia (Milker nodule), and orf (ecthyma contagiosum).

Variola (Smallpox)

Clinical Summary. Smallpox was one of the most infectious and deadly diseases in the world, afflicting millions of people each year regardless of age, race, or socioeconomic status before it was eradicated in 1977 (70). There were two forms of smallpox: variola major and variola minor. Variola major had a case fatality rate of approximately 25%, whereas variola minor, a less virulent form, had a case fatality rate below 1%. Although the two forms caused diseases of different severity, they were indistinguishable from one another. Smallpox was spread through respiratory transmission of virus found in the oropharyngeal

Figure 25-12 Kaposi sarcoma associated with AIDS. Dark reddish to brownish plaques on the chest in an AIDS patient.

secretions of infected individuals. Penetration was usually through the respiratory tract and local lymph nodes, and then the virus entered the blood (primary viremia). Internal organs were infected; then the virus reentered the blood (secondary viremia) and spread to the skin. The onset of smallpox was acute, with fever, malaise, headaches, and backaches. The initial toxemia phase lasted 4 to 5 days. On about the third or fourth day, the characteristic rash appeared. First, it appeared on the buccal and pharyngeal mucosa, the face, and the forearms. Within a day, it spread to the trunk and lower limbs. The lesions of the rash began first as macules, which soon became papules, and then developed into pustular vesicles. The lesions usually protruded from the skin and were firm to touch. The lesions dried up and often became crusted by day 14. By the end of the third week, most crusts had fallen off, with the exception of the palms and the soles (71). This entire process took 3 to 4 weeks, and the areas affected by the rash could be permanently scarred. The rare hemorrhagic-type smallpox that appeared in immunocompromised individuals was associated with bleeding from the conjunctiva and mucous membranes, very severe toxemia, and early death, usually before the lesions of the skin had developed. Modified-type smallpox was seen in persons who had been vaccinated, usually many years earlier. In these cases, the skin lesions evolved quickly and were more variable in size.

Histopathology. There is prominent ballooning and reticular degeneration. Under light microscopy, aggregations of variola virus particles, called Guarnieri bodies, may be found in cytoplasm; occasional intranuclear inclusions can also be found. Similar changes can be seen in vaccinia, monkeypox, or cowpox.

Vaccinia

Clinical Summary. Vaccinia virus was used for smallpox vaccination via inoculation into the superficial layers of the skin of the upper arm. However, with the eradication of smallpox, routine vaccination with vaccinia virus ceased for many years but may soon become more common because of security concerns. Four to five days following vaccination with vaccinia virus, a papule appears at the site of vaccination. Two or 3 days later, the papular lesion becomes vesicular, growing until it reaches its maximum diameter on the 9th or 10th day. The lesion dries from the center outward, and the brown scab falls off after about 3 weeks, leaving a scar—a mark by which previous vaccines can be recognized (72). Complications of vaccination can occur but are very rare, including the following conditions: progressive vaccinia (vaccinia necrosum), which is a severe, potentially fatal illness characterized by progressive necrosis at the site of vaccination; eczema vaccinatum, which is similar to eczema herpeticum in patients with chronic eczema; generalized vaccinia, which is characterized by a vesicular rash that sometimes covers the entire body; and postvaccinal encephalitis, a neurologic complication in the most serious ones that occurred from vaccination with vaccinia virus (73). Other localized lesions such as keloid, dermatofibrosarcoma protuberans, and malignant fibrous histiocytoma have been reported at the site of inoculation. These complications are extremely rare.

Histopathology. The histologic changes are similar to those of herpes simplex and zoster and varicella. However, intracytoplasmic inclusions are seen in vaccinia, unlike in herpes infection.

Human Cowpox Infection

Clinical Summary. Despite its name, the reservoir hosts of cowpox virus are rodents, from which it can occasionally spread to cats, cows, humans, and zoo animals, including large cats and elephants. Infection in these animals is usually manifested as a single, small, crusted ulcer. Transmission to humans has traditionally occurred via contact with the infected teats of milking cows. However, currently, infection is seen more commonly among domestic cats, from which it can be transmitted to humans. Patients present with painful, hemorrhagic pustules or black eschars, usually on the hand or face, accompanied by edema, erythema, lymphadenopathy, and systemic involvement (74). Crusted lesions resembling anthrax and sporotrichoid infection have been reported.

Histopathology. The pathology of the skin lesions caused by cowpox virus is similar to that of smallpox, with prominent ballooning and reticular degeneration. However, there is greater epithelial thickening and less rapid cell necrosis. Early lesions of human cowpox infection show prominent reticular degeneration. Eosinophilic, intracytoplasmic inclusion bodies are present, a valuable feature in distinguishing poxvirus from herpesvirus infections. Under electron microscopic examination, the virus is rectangular and morphologically indistinguishable from the virus of variola.

Parapox Virus Infections (Milker Nodules and Orf)

Clinical Summary. Milker nodules, orf, and bovine papular stomatitis pox are clinically identical in humans and are induced by indistinguishable paravaccinia viruses. *Milker nodules* are acquired from udders infected with pseudocowpox or paravaccinia (parapox). This disease is called bovine papular stomatitis pox when the source of the infection is calves with oral sores contracted through sucking infected udders. *Orf* (ecthyma contagiosum) is acquired from infected sheep or goats with crusted lesions on the lips and in the mouth.

The most common presentation of orf is a circumscribed solitary nodule or papule on the fingers or hands (75). Milker nodules usually present with multiple lesions. After an incubation period of 3 to 7 days, parapox virus infections produce one to three (rarely more) painful lesions measuring 1 to 2 cm in diameter on the fingers or occasionally elsewhere as a result of autoinoculation. During a period of approximately 6 weeks, they pass through six clinical stages, each lasting about 1 week: (a) the maculopapular stage; (b) the target stage, during which the lesions have red centers, white rings, and red halos; (c) the acute weeping stage; (d) the nodular stage, which shows hard, nontender nodules; (e) the papillomatous stage, in which the nodules have irregular surfaces; and (f) the regressive stage, during which the lesions involute without scarring.

Histopathology. During the maculopapular and target stages, there is vacuolization of cells in the upper third of the stratum malpighii, leading to multilocular vesicles. Ballooning degeneration occurs, the affected keratinocytes rupture, and the resulting defects have a tendency to coalesce and to produce reticulated vesicles (Fig. 25-13A, B). Eosinophilic inclusion bodies are in the cytoplasm of vacuolated epidermal cells, a distinguishing feature from herpes virus infections (Fig. 25-13C). Intranuclear eosinophilic inclusion bodies are also present in

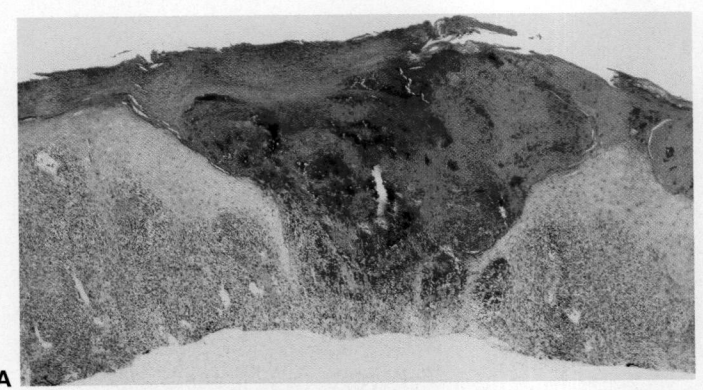

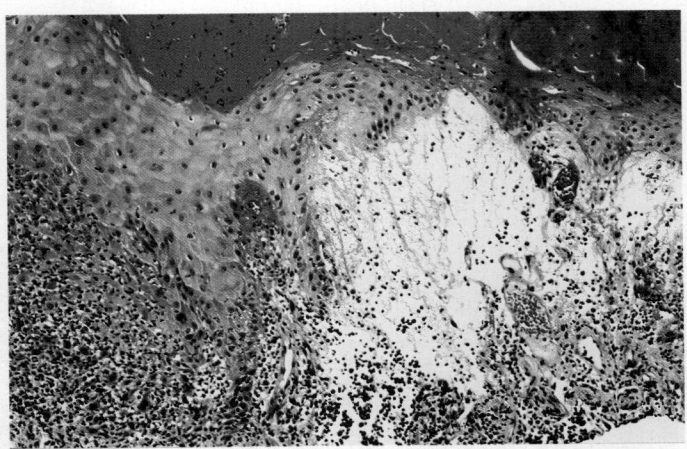

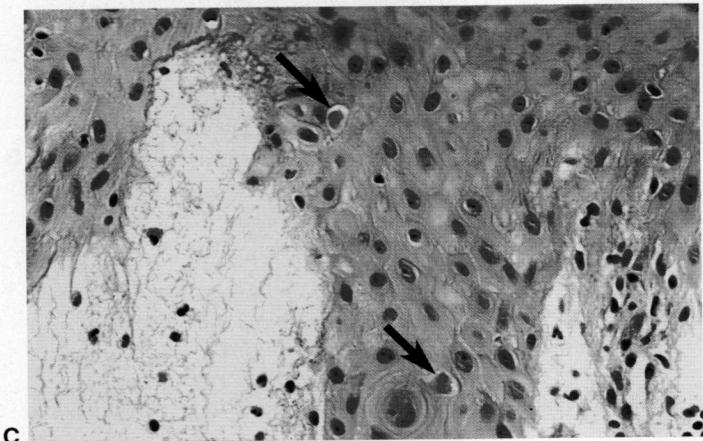

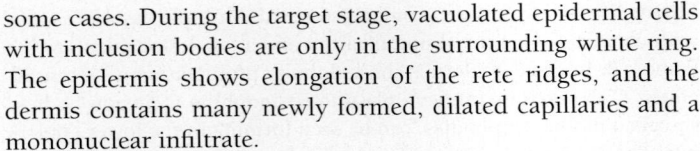

Figure 25-13 Orf. **A:** At scanning magnification, in the target stage, there is central hemorrhage and tissue necrosis with peripheral reticulated degeneration and dense inflammatory infiltrates. **B:** Reticulated vesicles (a characteristic feature of a viral infection affecting the epidermis) and the dermis contain many newly formed, dilated capillaries and a mononuclear infiltrate. **C:** Eosinophilic inclusion bodies in the cytoplasm of vacuolated epidermal cells (*arrow points to the inclusions*) distinguish orf from herpesvirus infections. Intranuclear eosinophilic inclusion bodies are also present in some cases.

some cases. During the target stage, vacuolated epidermal cells with inclusion bodies are only in the surrounding white ring. The epidermis shows elongation of the rete ridges, and the dermis contains many newly formed, dilated capillaries and a mononuclear infiltrate.

In the acute weeping stage, the epidermis is necrotic throughout. A massive infiltrate of mononuclear cells extends throughout the dermis. In some lesions, the mononuclear cell infiltrates may be comprised mainly of large, transformed lymphoblasts. Such lesions might be misdiagnosed as a lymphoid neoplasm, if careful attention is not given to the changes in the keratinocytes. A lichenoid reaction with a high percentage of histiocytes, a common response to viral infections of the skin, can also be seen. In the later stages, the epidermis shows acanthosis with fingerlike downward projections, and the dermis shows vasodilatation and chronic inflammation, followed by resolution. The histology of orf and milker nodule are identical.

Histogenesis and Viral Identification. In lesions less than 2 weeks old, the virus can be grown in tissue cultures of various cell types, including bovine or rhesus monkey kidney cells and human amnion cells or fibroblasts. In older lesions, one has to rely on serologic changes or on viral antigen demonstration in lesional material. Electron microscopy reveals that the parapox virus is cylindrical in shape and has convex ends. It consists of a dense DNA core surrounded by a less dense, wide capsid and by two narrow, electron-dense outer layers. On average, the virion measures 140 by 310 nm.

Principles of Management: Treatment of milker nodules and orf is symptomatic. Surgical drainage and excision are not necessary because the diseases are self-limited (76).

Molluscum Contagiosum

Clinical Summary. Molluscum contagiosum occurs worldwide. Although seen most commonly in children, it may be found in persons of all ages. The virus is transmitted by direct bodily contact, through minor abrasions, or indirectly via fomites. Among young adults, it is usually a sexually transmitted disease. The incubation period for this virus, as determined by human volunteers who underwent inoculation, ranges from 14 to 50 days.

Molluscum contagiosum may be found anywhere on the body but rarely occurs on the palms or soles. It consists of a variable number of small, discrete, waxy, skin-colored, umbilicated, dome-shaped papules, usually 2 to 5 mm in size (Fig. 25-14A). A papule of molluscum contagiosum may appear inflamed. In immunocompetent patients, the lesions involute spontaneously. During involution, there may be mild inflammation and tenderness.

Since 1980, there have been reports in the United States of greater severity of molluscum contagiosum in patients infected with HIV. In the setting of immunosuppression, molluscum contagiosum can attain considerable size and be widely disseminated. In immunocompromised patients, particularly those with AIDS, hundreds of lesions of molluscum contagiosum may be observed, showing little tendency toward involution. Furthermore, clinically normal skin in the vicinity of molluscum lesions in HIV-infected persons may be infected by molluscum virus (77). Infection with molluscum contagiosum produces little immunity, with reinfection being relatively common among immunocompromised individuals. In the context of AIDS, a variety of systemic fungal diseases, including cryptococcosis, histoplasmosis, and *Penicillium marneffei*, can disseminate and produce skin lesions that resemble molluscum contagiosum.

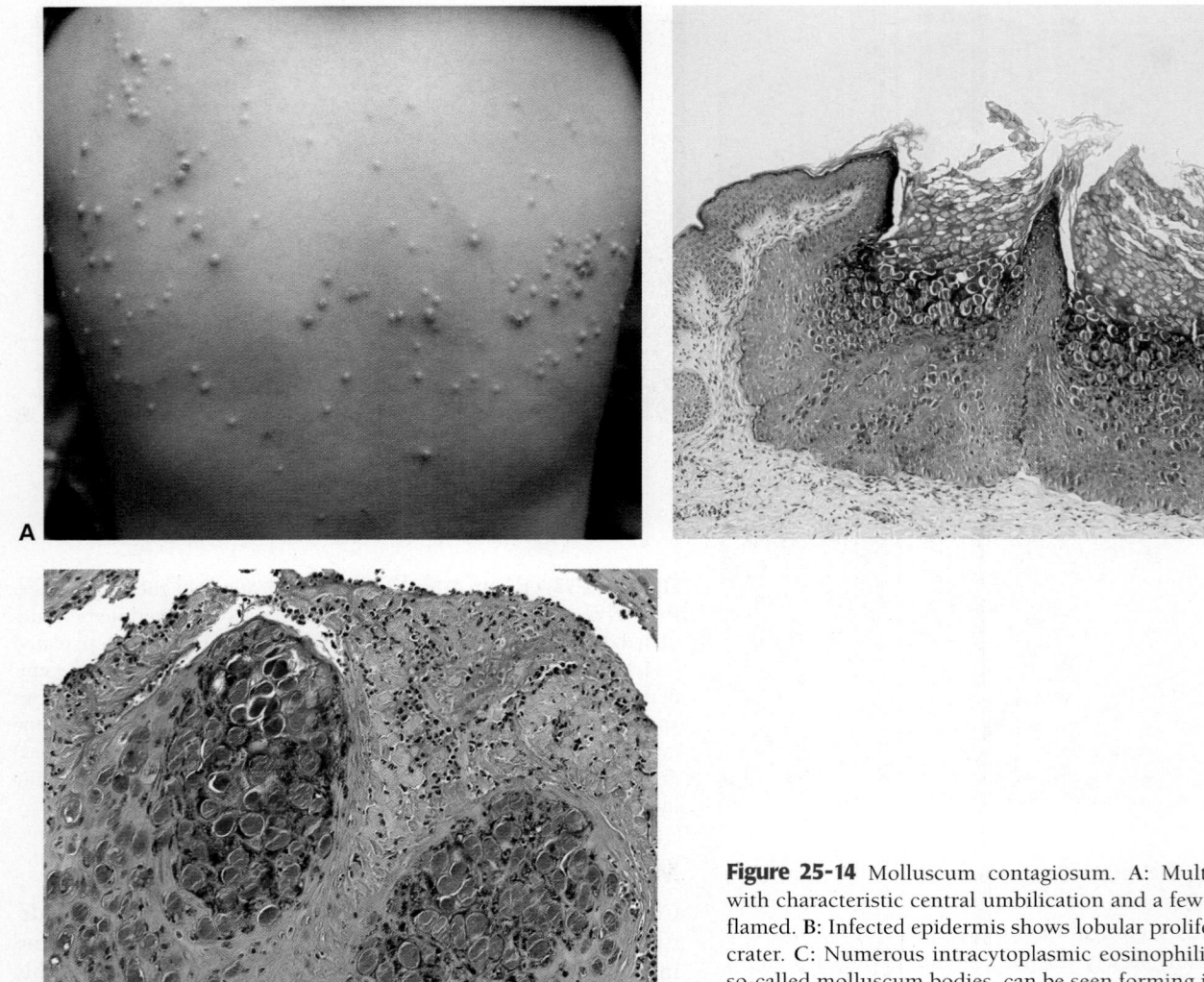

Figure 25-14 Molluscum contagiosum. **A:** Multiple lesions, some with characteristic central umbilication and a few lesions that are inflamed. **B:** Infected epidermis shows lobular proliferation with central crater. **C:** Numerous intracytoplasmic eosinophilic inclusion bodies, so-called molluscum bodies, can be seen forming in the lower epidermis. They increase in size as they move toward the surface.

Histopathology. In molluscum contagiosum, the epidermis is acanthotic. Infected epidermis shows lobular proliferation with a central crater (Fig. 25-14B). Many epidermal cells contain large, intracytoplasmic inclusion bodies—the so-called molluscum bodies (Fig. 25-14C). These bodies first appear as single, minute, ovoid eosinophilic structures in the lower cells of the stratum malpighii at a level one or two layers above the basal cell layer. The molluscum bodies increase in size as infected cells move toward the surface. The molluscum bodies in the upper layers of the epidermis displace and compress the nucleus so that it appears as a thin crescent at the periphery of the cell. At the level of the granular layer, the staining reaction of the molluscum bodies changes from eosinophilic to basophilic. In the horny layer, basophilic molluscum bodies measuring up to 35 μm in diameter lie enmeshed in a network of eosinophilic horny fibers. In the center of the lesion, the stratum corneum ultimately disintegrates, releasing the molluscum bodies. Thus, a central crater forms. Secondary infection and ulceration can occur.

The surrounding dermis shows little or no inflammatory reaction except in instances in which the lesion of molluscum contagiosum ruptures and discharges molluscum bodies and horny material into the dermis. During spontaneous involution, a mononuclear infiltrate may be observed in close apposition to the lesion infiltrating between the infected epidermal cells.

Electron microscopic examination reveals that the molluscum inclusion bodies contain, embedded in a protein matrix, large numbers of molluscum contagiosum viruses. The virus of molluscum contagiosum belongs to the poxvirus group. Like the viruses of variola, vaccinia, and cowpox, it is "brick shaped" and measures approximately 300 by 240 nm. The virus of molluscum contagiosum has not been grown in tissue culture. Molluscum contagiosum virus can be detected directly in tissue specimens using *in situ* hybridization (78).

Principles of Management: Molluscum contagiosum is benign and generally self-limiting; however, complications such as inflammation, pruritus, dermatitis, and secondary bacterial infections need to be treated. When therapy is needed for molluscum contagiosum, physical ablative methods, such as curettage, cryotherapy, lasers, and photodynamic therapy, are used. Podophyllotoxin cream (0.5%) is reliable as a home therapy for men but is not recommended for pregnant women because of presumed toxicity to the fetus. In addition, chemical agents such as 10% phenol or 100% trichloroacetic acid, 0.9% cantharidin, 12% salicylic acid gel, 10% benzoyl peroxide cream, 0.5% retinoic acid, and 5% to 10% potassium hydroxide solution may be used. Immune modulators, including 5% imiquimod cream, cimetidine, and diphencyprone, and antiviral agents such as cidofovir cream are tried. However, no evidence-based consensus has been reached as to the best treatment (79).

PAPILLOMAVIRIDAE

Human papillomaviruses (HPV) belong to the family Papillomaviridae. HPV are nonenveloped double-stranded DNA viruses. An infectious origin for skin warts was first recognized in 1891, and viral particles were isolated from human skin papillomatous lesions in 1949. Since then, over 80 fully sequenced HPV genotypes have been identified and 70 additional genotypes suggested through PCR analysis (80). The genetic heterogeneity is reflected in the differing clinical presentations of HPV infection. The cutaneous and mucosal manifestations of HPV infection include the common wart verruca vulgaris, the genital wart condyloma acuminatum, and less common entities, including epidermodysplasia verruciformis (EV) and oral focal epithelial hyperplasia (Heck disease). HPV is regarded as an oncogenic virus and is well known to be associated with cervical and anogenital cancers (81). HPV has also been implicated in oropharyngeal squamous cell carcinoma (82), lung cancer (83), esophageal cancer (84), and in nonmelanoma skin cancers (85), particularly in immunosuppressed patients (86). The specific viral genotypes show fairly good association with the different clinical presentations listed, although considerable overlap exists.

Verruca vulgaris: 1, 2, 4, 7, 49
Verruca plana: 3, 10, 28, 49
Palmoplantar wart: 1, 2, 3, 4, 27, 29, 57
Condyloma acuminatum (high cancer risk): 16, 18, 31, 33, 51
Focal epithelial hyperplasia (Heck disease): 13, 32
Bowenoid papulosis: 16, 18, 31, 33, 51
Butcher warts: 7
Epidermodysplasia verruciformis: 3, 5, 8–10, 12, 14, 17, 19–29, 36, 38, 47, 50
Laryngeal carcinoma: 30
Head and neck (oropharyngeal) squamous cell carcinoma: 16
Giant condyloma of Bushke and Loewenstein: 6
Cervical and vulvar dysplasia: 16, 18, 31, 33, 51

The association of particular HPV types with specific groups of warts, however, is not absolute. Definitive HPV typing can be obtained through DNA hybridization or amplification of HPV genomic material by the PCR. However, positive results cannot be considered definitive in predicting outcome. High-risk HPV types can be missed through sampling errors. In the end, close follow-up is important in the management of HPV infection, particularly when the patient has clinical exposure to potentially high-risk HPV types (87).

All HPV types target squamous epithelial cells, including metaplastic squamous epithelial cells in the uterine cervix. Entry of HPV into squamous epithelium results in three different types of infections: latent infection, in which there is no gross or microscopic evidence of disease; subclinical infection, in which colposcopy or microscopy reveals disease in the absence of clinical disease; and clinical disease. Early HPV genes are expressed in basal epithelial cells. Clinical and histologic evidence of HPV infection usually develops 1 to 8 months after initial exposure. Untreated, these lesions may regress spontaneously, persist as benign lesions, or progress to precancerous lesions and, eventually, cancer (88).

Verruca Vulgaris

Clinical Summary. Verruca vulgaris, the common wart, most commonly presents singly or in groups on the dorsal aspects of the fingers and hands as painless, circumscribed, firm elevated papules with papillomatous ("verrucous") hyperkeratotic surfaces (Fig. 25-15A). The palms and soles are less common sites and present at these sites as mosaic warts. Verruca vulgaris is rarely identified on the oral mucosa. The face and scalp are the most common sites for filiform warts, variants of verruca vulgaris that show threadlike, keratinous projections arising from horny bases.

Verrucae vulgaris are circumscribed, firm, elevated papules with papillomatous ("verrucous") hyperkeratotic surfaces. They occur singly or in groups. Generally, they are associated with little or no tenderness. New warts may form at sites of trauma (Koebner phenomenon). Verrucae vulgaris are often associated with HPV-2 but may be induced by HPV-1, -4, -7, and -49.

Histopathology. Verrucae vulgaris show acanthosis, papillomatosis, and hyperkeratosis (Fig. 25-15B). The rete ridges are elongated and, at the periphery of the verruca, are often bent inward so that they appear to point radially toward the center (arborization). The characteristic features that distinguish verruca vulgaris from other papillomas are foci of vacuolated cells, referred to as koilocytotic cells, vertical tiers of parakeratotic cells, and foci of clumped keratohyalin granules (Fig. 25-15C). These three changes are quite pronounced in young verrucae vulgaris and subtle or absent in older lesions. In such cases, a descriptive diagnosis such as "verrucous keratosis" may be rendered. The foci of koilocytes are located in the upper stratum malpighii and in the granular layer. The koilocytes possess small, round, deeply basophilic nuclei surrounded by a clear halo and pale-staining cytoplasm. These cells contain few or no keratohyalin granules, even when they are located in the granular layer. The vertical tiers (or columns) of parakeratotic cells are often located at the crests of papillomatous elevations of the rete malpighii overlying a focus of vacuolated cells. Compared with ordinary parakeratotic nuclei, the nuclei of the parakeratotic cells in verrucae vulgaris are larger and more deeply basophilic, and many of them appear rounded rather than elongated. Although no granular cells are seen overlying the papillomatous crests, they are increased in number and size in the intervening valleys and contain heavy, irregular clumps of keratohyalin granules. Dilated capillaries and small areas of hemorrhage may be seen in the thickened horny layer at the tip of the vertical tiers of parakeratotic cells (Fig. 25-15C). In filiform warts, the papillae are more elongated than in verrucae vulgaris (Fig. 25-15D).

Although warts are very common, especially in children and adolescents, defective cell-mediated immunity predisposes to the development of some types of warts. The frequency of warts in persons with renal transplants receiving immunosuppressive therapy is greater than that in the general population (89). In the context of HIV infection, a variety of papillomavirus infections have been reported. Eradication of cutaneous infection becomes increasingly difficult as the degree of immunosuppression becomes more profound.

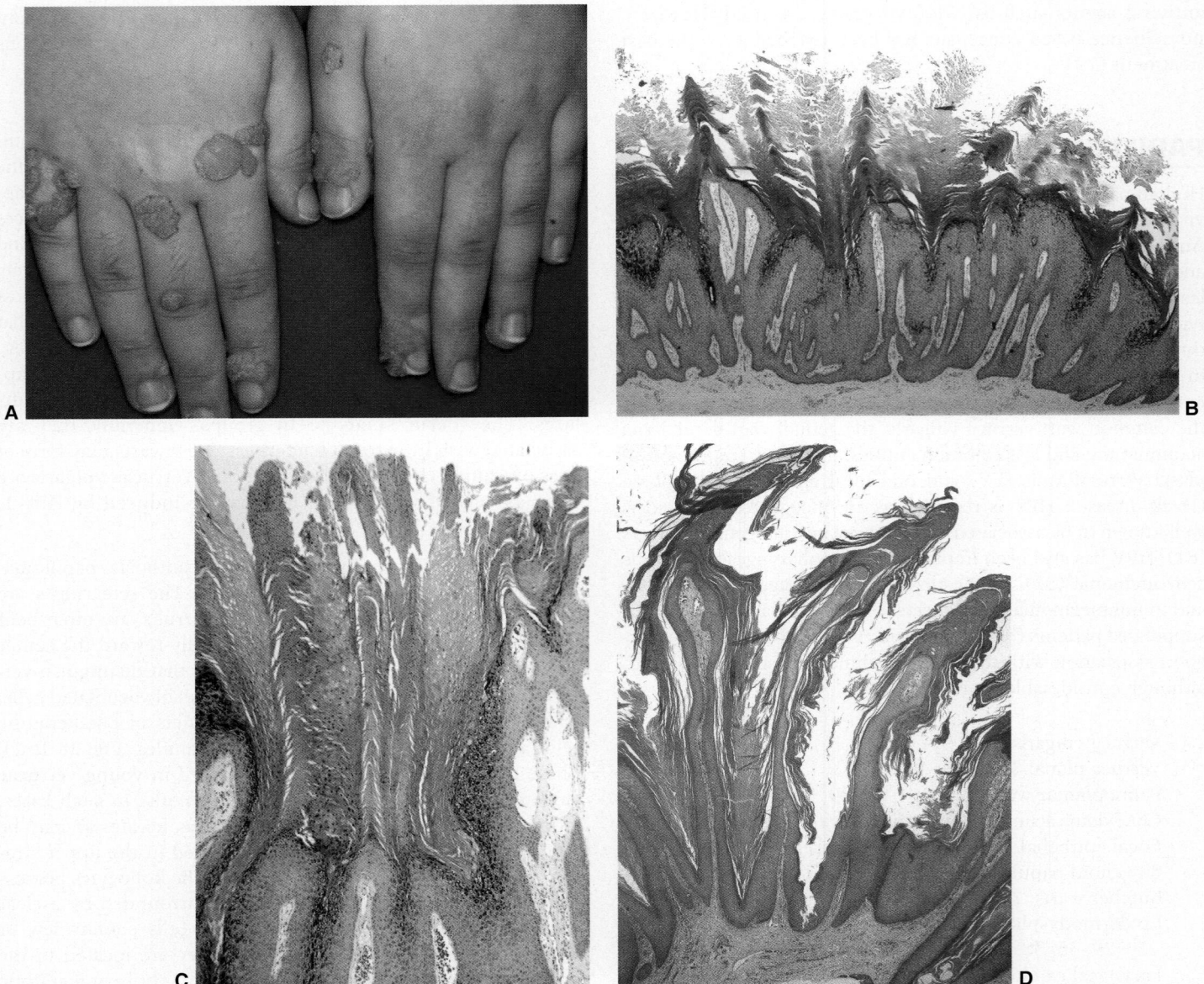

Figure 25-15 Verruca vulgaris. **A:** Multiple lesions most commonly seen on the hands and fingers. **B:** Low magnification. One observes hyperkeratosis, acanthosis, and papillomatosis. The rete ridges are elongated and bent inward at both margins, thus appearing to point radially to the center. **C:** High magnification. Groups of large, vacuolated cells lie in the upper stratum malpighii and in the granular layer. **D:** Verruca vulgaris of filiform type. There is marked papillomatosis.

Histogenesis and Viral Identification. No difference has been noted in electron microscopic appearance among the virus particles in the various types of HPV. However, the quantity varies with the different types. Frequently, virus particles are absent in verrucae vulgaris on electron microscopic examination. Negative results of electron microscopic examination do not exclude the presence of HPV. Viral antigens, such as papillomavirus common antigen, can be detected using immunohistochemistry, and HPV DNA can be amplified from lesions using PCR with appropriate primers. Viral genomic material can also be identified by *in situ* hybridization. Viral DNA replication occurs in proliferating basal cells, but structural capsid protein forms in the midepidermis, so mature HPV viral structures, if present, are observed only in the upper epidermis.

The virus particles are spherical bodies with a diameter of about 50 nm. Each particle consists of an electron-dense nucleoid with a stippled appearance surrounded by a less dense capsid. The wart virus replicates in the nucleus, where the viral particles are located as dense aggregates in a crystalloid

arrangement. Eosinophilic intranuclear bodies are very rare in verrucae vulgaris. The wart virus does not grow in tissue cultures and is not pathogenic for any animals.

Deep Palmoplantar Warts

Clinical Summary. Deep palmoplantar warts can be tender and occasionally swollen and red. Although they may be multiple, they do not coalesce, as do mosaic warts, which are verrucae vulgaris. Deep palmoplantar warts occur not only on the palms and soles but also on the lateral aspects and tips of the fingers and toes. Unlike superficial, mosaic-type palmoplantar warts, deep palmoplantar warts are usually covered with a thick callus (Fig. 25-16A). When the callus is removed with a scalpel, the wart becomes apparent.

A plantar wart associated with HPV-60 may appear as a nodule on the weight-bearing surface of the sole. The nodule is usually smooth with visible rete ridges but may become hyperkeratotic. HPV-60 infection is also associated with plantar epidermoid cyst.

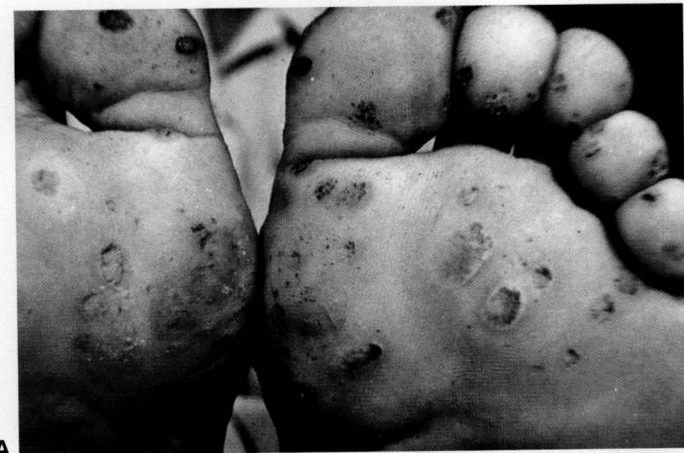

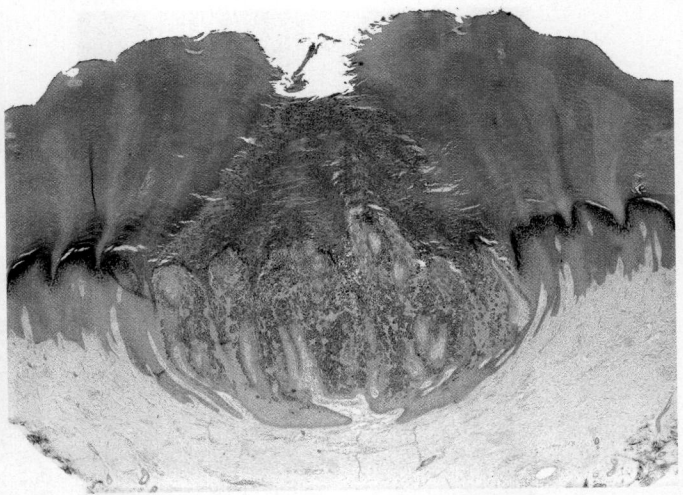

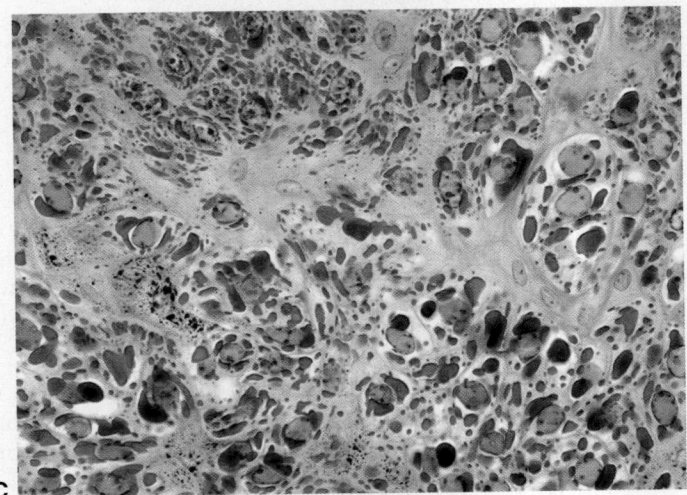

Figure 25-16 Palmoplantar wart (myrmecia). **A:** The lesions are flat with prominent hyperkeratosis on the sole. Vascular thromboses are seen in some lesions. **B:** Virally induced proliferation of keratinocytes results of the lesion. The elongated retia are displaced laterally, whereas their tips point to the center in the deep portion. The lesion is covered by thickened keratin, resulting in a tendency to grow inward rather than outward from the surface. **C:** The epidermal squamous cells contain polygonal, refractile-appearing, eosinophilic, cytoplasmic inclusions. Nuclei also contain round eosinophilic bodies.

If the lesion is incised, cheesy material may be expressed. A pigmented verrucous variant associated with HPV-65 and a whitish keratotic wart associated with HPV-63 has been reported.

Histopathology. Whereas superficial, mosaic-type palmoplantar warts have a histologic appearance analogous to that of verruca vulgaris and represent HPV-2 or HPV-4 infection, deep palmoplantar warts are commonly associated with HPV-1 infection but can also be seen with HPV-60, -63, and -65. These lesions, also known as myrmecia ("anthill") or inclusion warts, are characterized by abundant keratohyalin, which differs from normal keratohyalin by being eosinophilic. There is prominent hyperkeratosis. Starting in the lower epidermis, the cytoplasm of many cells contains numerous eosinophilic granules, which enlarge in the upper stratum malpighii and coalesce to form large, irregularly shaped, homogeneous "inclusion bodies." They either encase the vacuolated nucleus or are separated from it by perinuclear vacuolization. The nuclei in the stratum corneum persist, appearing as deeply basophilic round bodies surrounded by a wide, clear zone (Fig. 25-16B). In addition to the large intracytoplasmic eosinophilic inclusion bodies, some of the cells in the upper stratum malpighii with vacuolated nuclei contain a small intranuclear eosinophilic "inclusion body." It is round and of about the same size as the nucleolus, which, however, is basophilic (Fig. 25-16C). Regression of plantar warts is often associated with thrombosis of superficial vessels, hemorrhage, and necrosis of the epidermis.

Histogenesis and Viral Identification. Under electron microscopic examination, viral particles are first observed in the upper portion of the stratum malpighii within and around the nucleolus. Their number increases, and in cells just beneath the stratum corneum, nucleoli are no longer detected. In many instances, the material of the nucleus appears to be replaced entirely by virus particles except for a thin rim of chromatin closely applied to the nuclear membrane. The particles tend to be arranged in regular or crystalline formations. In the stratum corneum, no normal cell structures are recognizable, but there remain large, compact aggregates of virus particles surrounded by keratinous matter.

Verruca Plana

Clinical Summary. Verrucae planae are slightly elevated, flat, smooth papules. They may be hyperpigmented. Most commonly, the face and the dorsa of the hands are affected (Fig. 25-17A). In rare instances, there is extensive involvement, with lesions also on the extremities and trunk. If starting in childhood and occurring in several members of the family, such disseminate cases of verruca plana have been mistakenly held to be instances of EV, from which they differ by the absence of red, "tinea versicolor–like" patches and lack of malignant transformation of some of the exposed lesions.

Histopathology. Verrucae planae show hyperkeratosis and acanthosis but, unlike verrucae vulgaris, have no papillomatosis, but only slight elongation of the rete ridges, and no areas of parakeratosis. In the upper stratum malpighii, including the granular layer, there is diffuse vacuolization of the cells (Fig. 25-17B). Some of

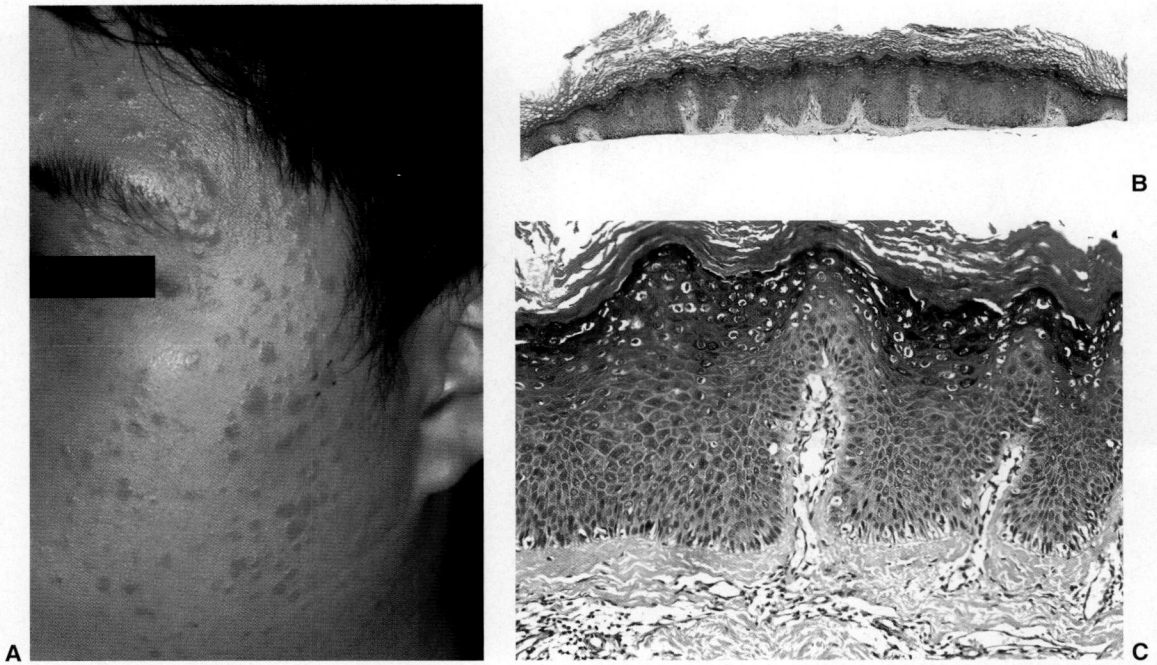

Figure 25-17 Verruca plana. A: Flat, smooth, flesh-colored papules, often on the face. B: One observes hyperkeratosis and acanthosis but no papillomatosis or parakeratosis. Numerous vacuolated cells lie in the upper stratum malpighii, including the granular layer. The horny layer has a pronounced basket-weave appearance resulting from the vacuolization of the horny cells. C: The nuclei of the vacuolated cells lie at the centers of the cells, presenting an owl's-eye appearance.

the vacuolated cells are enlarged to about twice their normal size. The nuclei of the vacuolated cells lie at the centers of the cells, and some of them appear deeply basophilic (Fig. 25-17C). The granular layer is uniformly thickened, and the stratum corneum has a pronounced basket-weave appearance resulting from vacuolization of the horny cells. The dermis appears normal. In spontaneously regressing warts, there is often a superficial lymphocytic infiltrate in the dermis with exocytosis and apoptosis of cells in the epidermis.

Histogenesis. Verrucae planae are induced by HPV-3 and HPV-10. Electron microscopic examination reveals marked cytoplasmic edema. The tonofilaments are dislodged to the periphery of the cell. The keratohyalin granules appear normal. Viral particles are numerous in the nuclei of vacuolated cells.

Epidermodysplasia Verruciformis

Clinical Summary. EV is an extremely rare genetic disease characterized by HPV infection with types not seen in otherwise healthy individuals. EV is sometimes referred to as "tree-man disease" or "tree-man syndrome." It usually begins in childhood and is characterized by a generalized infection by HPV, frequent association with cutaneous carcinomas, and abnormalities of cell-mediated immunity (90). Two forms of EV are recognized. One is induced by HPV-3 and HPV-10 and characterized by a persistent widespread eruption resembling verrucae planae with a tendency toward confluence into plaques (Fig. 25-18A). Some of the cases are familial. The second form is primarily related to HPV-5 and HPV-8. There is often a familial history with an autosomal recessive or X-linked recessive inheritance. The *EVER1* and *EVER2* genes have been identified as causative genetic mutations in patients with hereditary EV. In addition to the plane warts, irregularly outlined, slightly scaling macules of various shades of brown, red, and white, tinea versicolor–like lesions and seborrheic keratosis–like lesions have been noted (91).

The eruption usually begins in childhood. Development of Bowen disease (squamous cell carcinoma *in situ*) within lesions in exposed areas is a common occurrence, and invasive lesions of squamous cell carcinoma are occasionally found. Malignant transformation occurs in about 25% of patients with EV. The oncogenic potential is highest for HPV-5, followed by HPV-8. EV-like lesions can develop in solid organ transplant patients (92) and in HIV-infected persons (93).

Histopathology. The epidermal changes, although similar to those observed in verruca plana, often differ by being more pronounced and more extensive. Affected keratinocytes are swollen and irregularly shaped. They show abundant, blue-gray cytoplasm and contain numerous round, basophilic keratohyalin granules (Fig. 25-18B, C). A few dyskeratotic cells may be seen in the lower part of the epidermis. Although some nuclei appear pyknotic, others appear large, round, and empty owing to marginal distribution of the chromatin. In immunocompromised patients, EV often lacks the histologic features of verruca planae, a focally thickened granular layer is a marker for viral detection, and the risk of dysplasia in such lesions is much higher than in EV not associated with acquired immunosuppression (94).

Histogenesis. In EV skin lesions, many HPV types have been found, and in some individual patients, several types have been identified (95). Electron microscopic examination shows viral particles, often in a semicrystalline pattern, within nuclei located in the stratum granulosum. In contrast, the swollen cells in the stratum malpighii show virions in their nuclei in small aggregates only in some cases but none at all in others.

Viral particles are absent in lesions of Bowen disease or squamous cell carcinoma arising from EV, but rarely these can be observed in the upper layers of the epidermis overlying malignant lesions. However, HPV-5-specific DNA or HPV-8–specific DNA

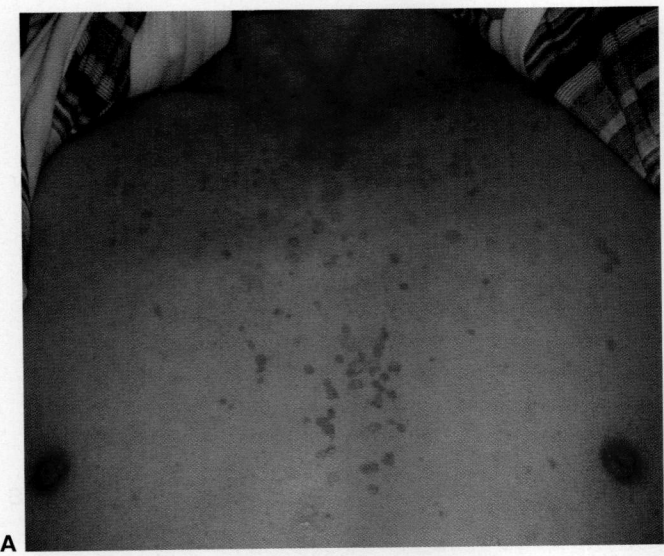

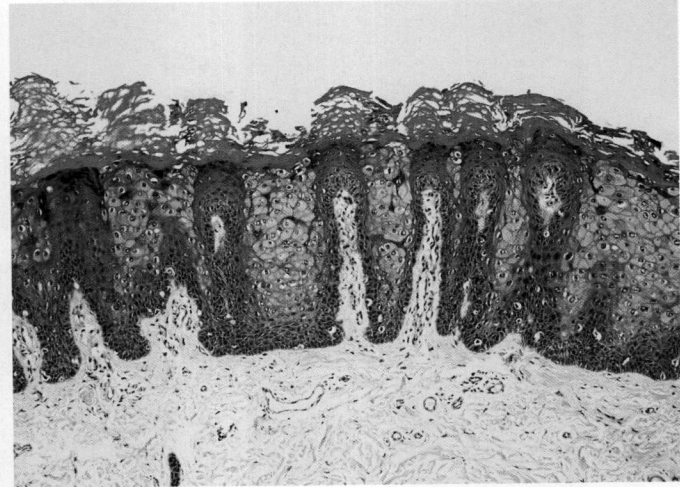

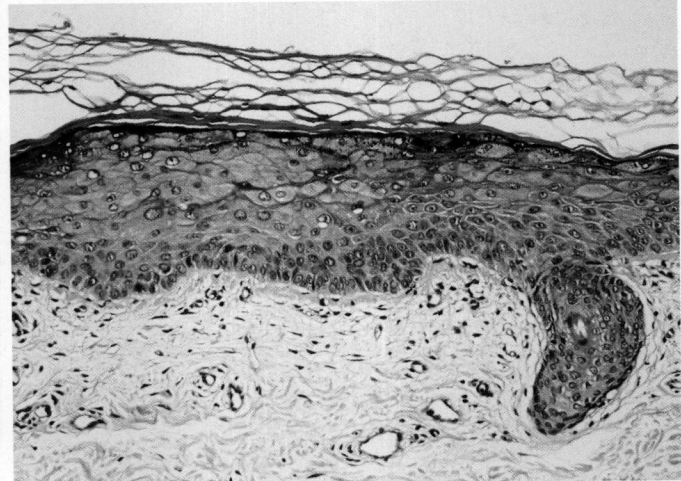

Figure 25-18 Epidermodysplasia verruciformis. **A:** Brownish-to-erythematous variable-sized flat macules on the chest and neck. **B:** The epidermis is hyperkeratotic and acanthotic. Vacuolated cells with swollen abundant blue-gray cytoplasm are present in the stratum malpighii and granular layer. **C:** Large affected keratinocytes have abundant blue-gray cytoplasm. Keratohyalin granules are prominent in the granular layer.

has been demonstrated on several occasions in squamous cell carcinomas arising in lesions of EV. The underlying defect in EV is not clear but may involve oncogene or immunologic dysfunction.

Condyloma Acuminatum

Clinical Summary. Condylomata acuminata, or anogenital warts, can occur on the penis, female genitals, and in the anal region. Condylomata acuminata may also involve the oral cavity. Condylomata acuminata are transmitted sexually, and HPV infection is one of the most common viral sexually transmitted diseases in the world, with an estimated 1% prevalence in the sexually active population in the United States. The estimated prevalence of HPV DNA or HPV antigens in young women may be as high as 10% to 11%. HPV DNA is detectable by PCR in more than 99.7% of cervical cancers, making HPV infection the most important risk factor in the development of this disease (96). Malignant progression is associated with infection by certain HPV types. Anogenital HPV types 6 and 11 rarely progress to invasive disease and are considered low risk. HPV types 16, 18, 31, 33, and 51 have been associated with both *in situ* and invasive processes of the male and female genital regions as well as the vagina and cervix in women. Additional types associated with malignancy include 35, 39, 42–45, 52, and 56. However, even with infection by high-risk

types, these lesions most often regress spontaneously, with no long-term adverse effects. Progression includes a spectrum from Bowen disease to squamous cell carcinoma, potentially with extension to metastasis.

Condylomata acuminata are usually found on the penis and around the anus in men. In women, frequent areas of infection include the vulva, vaginal introitus, perineal area, perianal area, and cervix. Lesions of the skin consist of fairly soft, verrucous papules that occasionally coalesce into cauliflower-like masses (Fig. 25-19A). Condylomas are flatter on mucosal surfaces.

Histopathology. In condyloma acuminatum, the stratum corneum is only slightly thickened. Lesions located on mucosal surfaces show parakeratosis. The stratum malpighii shows papillomatosis and considerable acanthosis, with thickening and elongation of the rete ridges. The elongated rete has a rounded surface contour rather than the pointed appearance seen in verrucae vulgaris. Mitotic figures may be present. Usually, invasive squamous cell carcinoma can be ruled out because the epithelial cells show an orderly arrangement and the border between the epithelial proliferations and the dermis is sharp (Fig. 25-19B). The most characteristic feature, important for the diagnosis, is the presence of areas in which the epithelial cells show distinct perinuclear vacuolization. These vacuolated epithelial cells are

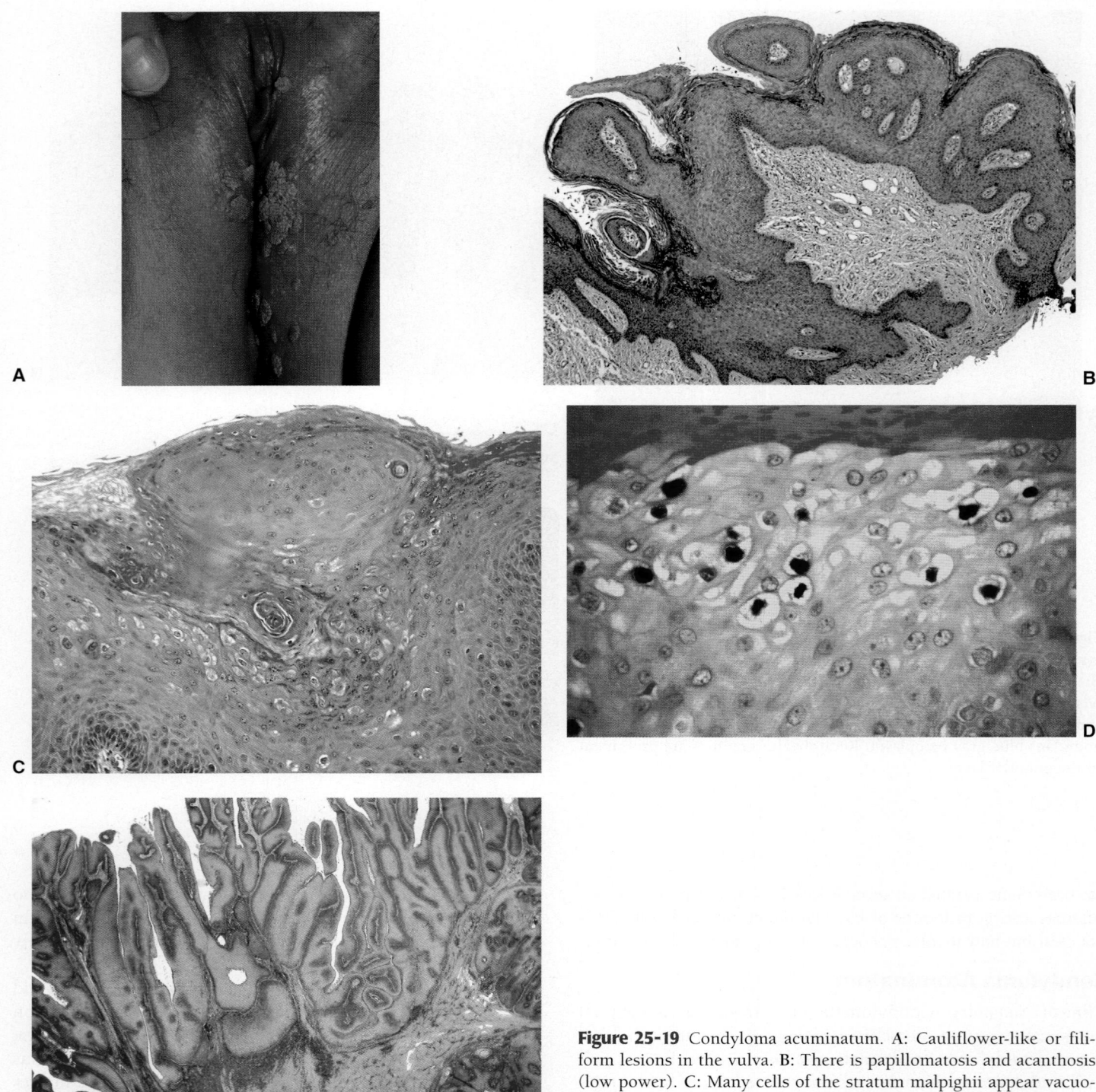

Figure 25-19 Condyloma acuminatum. **A:** Cauliflower-like or fili-form lesions in the vulva. **B:** There is papillomatosis and acanthosis (low power). **C:** Many cells of the stratum malpighii appear vacuo-lated and have round, hyperchromatic nuclei (high power). **D:** *In situ* hybridization shows HPV in the squamous cells. **E:** Giant condyloma acuminatum with marked acanthosis and more endophytic growth.

relatively large and possess hyperchromatic, round nuclei re-sembling the nuclei seen in the upper portion of the epidermis in verrucae vulgaris (Fig. 25-19C). It must be kept in mind, however, that vacuolization is a normal occurrence in the up-per portions of all mucosal surfaces, so that vacuolization in condylomata acuminata can be regarded as being possibly of viral genesis only if it extends into the deeper portions of the stratum malpighii. Koilocytotic ("raisin") nuclei, double nu-clei, and apoptotic keratinocytes may be present but are often less prominent than in uterine cervical lesions. Oral condyloma is difficult to separate from its mimics. The histologic features

significantly associated with oral condyloma were nonuniform perinuclear halos, often in association with epithelial crevices, and papillomatosis. HPV6 and HPV11 are detected in oral con-dylomata acuminata by *in situ* hybridization (97).

The diagnosis of HPV infection of the anogenital region can be complicated by the frequent absence of koilocytosis. HPV detection in lesions that depart from the typical mor-phology of condyloma can be achieved by *in situ* hybridization (Fig. 25-19D) or other molecular tests. In one study, HPV DNA—principally HPV6—was detected in 18 of 25 (72%) vulvar sebor-rheic keratoses, whereas 15% of nongenital seborrheic keratoses were positive for this virus. Therefore, most vulvar "seborrheic keratoses" may represent senescent condylomas (98). It has been shown that increased Ki-67 labeling in the upper two-thirds of the epithelial thickness detects anal HPV-related changes with a high degree of sensitivity and specificity, whereas increased p16/CDKN2A staining is strongly associated with high-grade squamous neoplasia (99).

Giant Condylomata Acuminata of Buschke and Loewenstein

Clinical Summary. The Buschke–Loewenstein tumor, also called giant condyloma acuminatum, is generally observed in males. The most frequent location is the glans penis and foreskin (where urethral fistulae may result), but they may occur also on the vulva and in the anal region. Clinically, it is a cauliflower-like tumor with resemblance to a large aggregate of condylomata acuminata, especially in the early stage. It is characterized by its large size with the propensity to ulcerate and infiltrate into deeper tissues, contrasting with a microscopically benign pattern. The hallmark of the disease is the high rate of recurrence (66%) and of malignant transformation (56%). Distant metastases are extremely rare. The overall mortality is 20%, all occurring in patients with recurrences (100).

Histopathology. The lesion shows a benign papillomatous growth characterized predominantly by epithelial hyperplasia, hyperacanthosis, and hyperkeratosis (Fig. 25-19E). Generally, vacuolization of keratinocytes is mild or absent, in contrast to condyloma acuminatum. There is tremendous proliferation of the epidermis with displacement of the underlying tissue, but the ratio of nucleus to cytoplasm is low. The invasive strands of tumor usually possess a well-developed basal cell layer. (For further discussion of verrucous carcinoma, see Chapter 29.)

Histogenesis. Papillomaviruses induce a variety of proliferative lesions in humans. Of the many types of HPV that have been identified, a subset that includes types 16, 18, 31, 33, and 51 is associated with anogenital cancers. These cancers develop from precursor lesions such as condylomata acuminata on the external genitalia, vaginal intraepithelial neoplasia in the vagina (VIN), cervical intraepithelial neoplasia on the cervix (CIN), and anal intraepithelial neoplasia of the anal mucosa (AIN). Viral production occurs in low-grade lesions that are only slightly altered in their pattern of differentiation from normal cells, but the concentration of mature virions in condylomata acuminata is low. The production of viral particles, genome amplification, capsid protein synthesis, and virion assembly is dependent on differentiation and is restricted to suprabasal cells. In more atypical lesions, viral DNA is usually found integrated into host chromosomes, and no viral production is noted. The viral DNA encodes nine overlapping genes: early (E1–E7) and late (L1–2). Early genes are involved in oncogenic transformation in high-risk HPV types, especially E6 and E7, which enable HPV to use cellular proteins for continued viral replication by arresting the process of keratinocyte differentiation and inactivation of cell cycle regulators such as p53 and retinoblastoma protein (Rb), thus providing the initial step in progression to malignancy (101).

BOWENOID PAPULOSIS OF THE GENITALIA

Clinical Summary. Bowenoid papuloses are small red papules of the genitalia. Some lesions are distinctly verrucous in appearance. The lesions are located in men on the glans and shaft of the penis and in women in the perineal and vulvar areas (Fig. 25-20A). Generally, the lesions are diagnosed clinically as genital warts, and the histologic finding of "Bowen disease" appears incongruous.

The lesions have a definite tendency toward spontaneous resolution; some lesions regress, but others may appear and in turn also regress. Still, in some patients, lesions have persisted for prolonged periods. In rare cases, invasive squamous cell carcinoma has been described as arising in a Bowenoid papule.

Some authors regard the disorder as benign and, in particular, as different from Bowen disease (55), but others have considered that Bowenoid papulosis represents a premalignant lesion with a high risk of cervical neoplasia both for female patients and for sexual partners of male patients. Invasive squamous cell carcinoma develops in a few cases, and it seems that women over 40 years old have the greatest risk.

Histopathology. Bowenoid papulosis shows the typical features of Bowen disease (see also Chapter 29). These features consist of full-thickness epidermal atypia with crowding and an irregular, "windblown" arrangement of the nuclei, many of which are large, hyperchromatic, and pleomorphic (Fig. 25-20B, C). Dyskeratotic and multinucleated keratinocytes are also present, as are atypical mitoses. The basement membrane is intact. True koilocytes are uncommon. Bowenoid papulosis may be histologically indistinguishable from vulvar intraepithelial neoplasia (VIN III), a term that is synonymous with squamous cell carcinoma *in situ* or Bowen disease. Some researchers believe that Bowenoid papulosis differs from Bowen disease by virtue of a lower degree of cytologic atypia. In a few instances, Bowenoid papulosis and condylomata acuminata have been found coexisting in the same patient.

Histogenesis. Bowenoid papulosis represents infection by HPV types associated with a high risk of malignancy evolution, such as HPV types 16, 18, 31, 33, and 51. As noted previously, these types elaborate oncoproteins that interfere with normal cellular homeostasis.

Differential Diagnosis. Bowenoid papulosis of the genitalia is in most instances differentiated from Bowen disease on the basis of clinical data, such as onset at an earlier average age, multiplicity of lesions, smaller size of lesions, verrucoid appearance of some lesions, and tendency toward spontaneous regression. Thus, Bowen disease or squamous cell carcinoma *in situ* (VIN III) cannot be ruled out by biopsy alone in most cases. Changes induced by the recent application of podophyllum resin need to be considered. The changes induced by podophyllum resin consist of necrotic keratinocytes and bizarre mitotic figures and are most pronounced during the first 72 hours after application.

VULVAR AND ANAL INTRAEPITHELIAL NEOPLASIA

Two pathways to squamous cell carcinoma are recognized in the vulva and anus; HPV-related and HPV-independent (102). Biopsies of these are not uncommonly submitted to dermatopathologists. Differentiated or simplex vulvar intraepithelial neoplasia (dVIN) has been identified as a precursor lesion for HPV-independent vulvar squamous cell carcinoma, which generally presents in an older age group. The Lower Anogenital Squamous

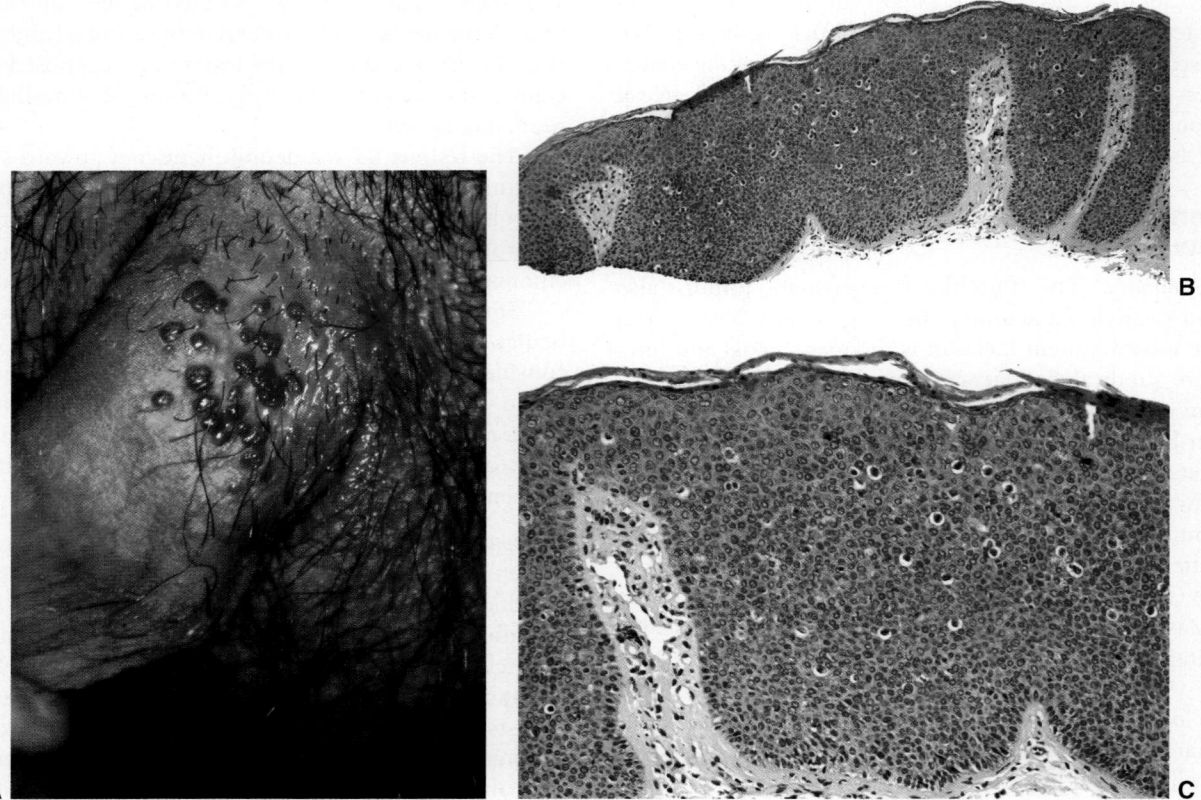

Figure 25-20 Bowenoid papulosis. **A:** Multiple brownish discrete papules in the genital region; occasionally, these papules can coalesce. **B:** The epithelium is irregularly thickened with disorderly maturation, which may impart a "windblown" look at scanning or intermediate magnification. **C:** The keratinocytic nuclei are crowded, and there is partial arrest of maturation. Mitoses are present above the basal layers, and the nuclei tend to be hyperchromatic and irregular, sometimes with nucleoli.

Terminology (LAST) Project has recommended unified terminology for all HPV-related squamous precursor lesions of the anogenital tract (including anus, perianus, vulva, penis, cervix, and vagina), with a two-tiered nomenclature system: low-grade squamous intraepithelial lesion (LSIL) and high-grade squamous intraepithelial lesion (HSIL) (103). LSIL can be further classified as "condyloma" or as "intraepithelial neoplasia 1" (-IN1; AIN1 when anal, VIN1 when vulvar). HSIL can be classified as IN2 (AIN2, VIN2) or IN3 (AIN3, VIN3), with the latter essentially synonymous with carcinoma *in situ*. In general, the diagnosis of condyloma is applied to well-differentiated, cytologically bland, papillary proliferations of squamous epithelium with viral cytopathic changes, which occur commonly in the perianal, penile, and vulvar regions (external anogenital areas), and are typically associated with low-risk HPV types 6 and 11. The diagnosis of LSIL (AIN1 or VIN1) is preferably applied to flat lesions, which are less common in the external genitalia compared with the cervix.

ORAL FOCAL EPITHELIAL HYPERPLASIA

Clinical Summary. A rare condition described in Native Americans, oral focal epithelial hyperplasia (Heck disease), has since been found to occur in many countries and races but most commonly among the Eskimos of Greenland. It primarily occurs in children, often in small endemic foci, but lesions may occur in young and middle-aged adults. There is no gender prediliction. Sites of greatest involvement include the labial, buccal, and lingual mucosa, but gingival and tonsillar lesions have also been reported.

There are numerous soft white papules 2 to 10 mm in diameter. Individual lesions are broad-based or slightly elevated as well as demarcated plaques. Papules and plaques are usually the color of normal mucosa but may be pale or, rarely, white. Most are discrete, but some are confluent. The lesions are asymptomatic. Although the disease is chronic, spontaneous remissions occur. Oral focal hyperplasia has been described in the context of HIV infection (104).

Histopathology. The oral epithelium shows acanthosis with thickening and elongation of the rete ridges. The thickened mucosa extends upward, not down into underlying connective tissues; hence, the lesional rete ridges are at the same depth as the adjacent normal rete ridges. The ridges themselves are widened, often confluent, and sometimes club shaped; they are not long and thin, as in psoriasis and other diseases. Throughout the epithelium, there are areas where the cells show marked vacuolization and stain only faintly. Vacuolization is most pronounced in the upper portion of the epithelium, but it may extend into the broadened rete ridges (Fig. 25-21).

Histogenesis. Electron microscopic examination reveals viral particles with the size of the HPV arranged in a crystalline pattern. HPV types 13 and 32 are typical for oral focal epithelial hyperplasia (105).

Differential Diagnosis. The histologic appearance of the affected oral epithelium in focal epithelial hyperplasia is identical to that of oral epithelial nevus, or white sponge nevus.

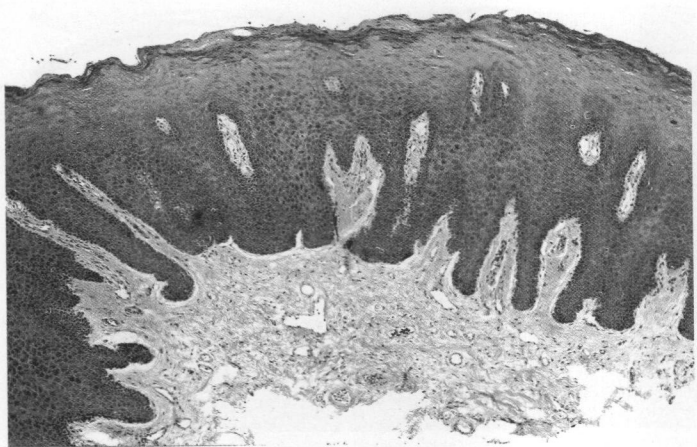

Figure 25-21 Oral focal epithelial hyperplasia. The oral epithelium shows acanthosis with thickening and elongation of the rete ridges. The ridges are widened, often confluent, and sometimes club shaped. Vacuolization is most pronounced in the upper portion of the epithelium.

Principles of Management of Papillomaviridae

There is no curative therapy for HPV infections. One review of meta-analysis and pooled analysis supported the use of salicylic acid as the first-line therapy for cutaneous warts, whereas cryotherapy, especially aggressive cryotherapy, should be considered as second-line therapy or as an alternative treatment. When these treatments fail, a third-line therapy such as bleomycin, dinitrochlorobenzene, and 5-fluorouracil can be considered (106). A wide range of therapies are in use with variable options for the treatment of genital warts. Topical agents, such as podophyllotoxin, 5% imiquimod cream, 3.75% imiquimod cream, 15% sinecatechins ointment, podophyllin, potent topical retinoids, and 5-fluorouracil are used. Destructive and surgical treatments include trichloroacetic acid, cryotherapy, electrosurgery, scissor excision, CO_2 laser, and photodynamic therapy. The treatment of choice varies somewhat by the lesion location, size, and host, and also by whether the HPV lesion has malignant potential. HPV can be oncogenic, particularly in immunosuppressed patients such as organ transplant recipients, in patients with HIV, and in patients with EV. Chronic, atypical, or large/extensive lesions should be evaluated for possible malignant degeneration. Some forms of HPV are sexually transmitted, and the presence of genital HPV should prompt evaluation for other STIs, such as HIV, and patients should inform their sexual partners to ensure they undergo appropriate screening. The USFDA approved HPV vaccines for the prevention of the diseases such as genital warts and cervical cancer caused by HPV types 6, 11, 16, and 18 (107). HPV vaccine is recommended for males and females ages 9 to 26.

PICORNAVIRIDAE

Picornaviridae consist of single-stranded RNA viruses that are 10 to 30 nm, naked, and icosahedral, and that contain only 4 to 6 genes. They are the smallest of RNA viruses and are very important in human disease. Picornaviridae infections of humans have been classified into five genera: enterovirus (polio), hepadnavirus (hepatitis A), cardiovirus (encephalomyocarditis), rhinovirus (common cold), and apthovirus (foot and mouth diseases). Picornaviridae infection is one of the most common

causes of viral exanthem. In addition to nonspecific findings, enterovirus infection also causes distinct syndromes such as hand–foot–mouth disease, herpangina, and hemorrhagic conjunctivitis (108).

Hand–Foot–Mouth Disease

Clinical Summary. Hand–foot–mouth disease is caused by a coxsackievirus, an enterovirus. In most instances, coxsackievirus type A16 has been isolated; only rarely has another type, such as A5 or A9, been found. Hand–foot–mouth disease occurs in small epidemics, affecting mainly children and having a mild course that usually lasts less than a week. More recently, cases of hand–foot–mouth disease have been reported in clusters of adults and may present with a more aggressive course, with fever, arthralgias, and widespread skin lesions (109). Transmission is mainly via fecal–oral contact and less commonly by respiratory droplets. Symptoms usually appear 3 to 5 days after exposure. After a 1- to 2-day mild prodrome of low-grade fever, sore throat, and malaise, small red macules present on the oral mucosa and progress to 1- to 3-mm small vesicles, where they evolve into small ulcers (110). Between 25% and 65% of patients may have the classic vesicular lesions on the hand and feet, which present as scattered small vesicles surrounded by an erythematous halo on the palms of the hands (Fig. 25-22A), the soles of the feet, and the ventral surfaces and sides of the fingers and toes (111). Similar lesions may develop on the rest of the skin.

Histopathology. Early vesicles are intraepidermal, whereas old vesicles may be subepidermal in location. There is pronounced reticular degeneration of the epidermis, resulting in multilocular vesiculation. In the deep layers of the epidermis, some ballooning degeneration may be found. Neither inclusion bodies nor multinucleated giant cells are present (see Fig. 25-22B, C).

Histogenesis and Diagnosis. Even though viral culture has been the gold standard, PCR has become the diagnostic test for rapid and accurate enterovirus infection. The sensitivity of PCR is almost double that of viral culture (112). Electron microscopic examination reveals that some keratinocytes contain within their cytoplasm aggregates of virus particles exhibiting a crystalloid pattern (113). The coxsackievirus can be cultured from stool and occasionally from skin vesicles. The virus grows well on human epithelial cell and monkey kidney cell cultures.

Principles of Management: The treatment of hand–foot–mouth disease is symptomatic and supportive care.

Hepatitis A Virus

The hepatitis A virus is a common cause of hepatitis worldwide. Spread of infection is through the fecal–oral route. Hepatitis A is endemic in developing countries, and most residents are exposed in childhood. In contrast, the adult population in developed countries demonstrates falling rates of exposure with improvements in hygiene and sanitation. Hepatitis A usually presents as fever, jaundice, and hepatomegaly. Extrahepatic manifestations are rarely found in hepatitis A viral infection. Urticaria and scarlatiniform eruption and rare cases of cutaneous vasculitis and cryoglobulinemia have been reported in the skin (114).

Principles of Management: The treatment of hepatitis A infection is symptomatic and supportive care.

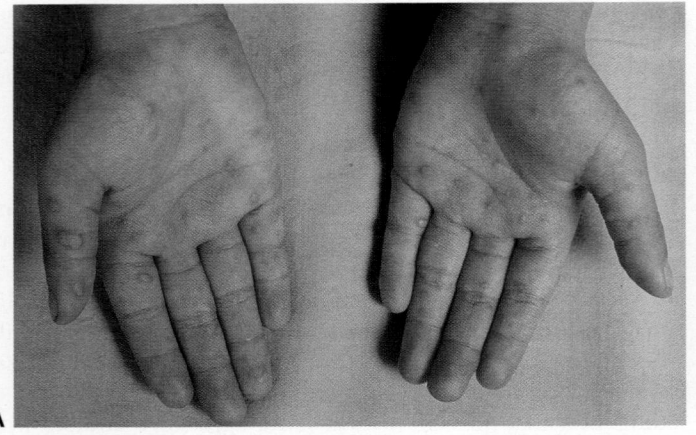

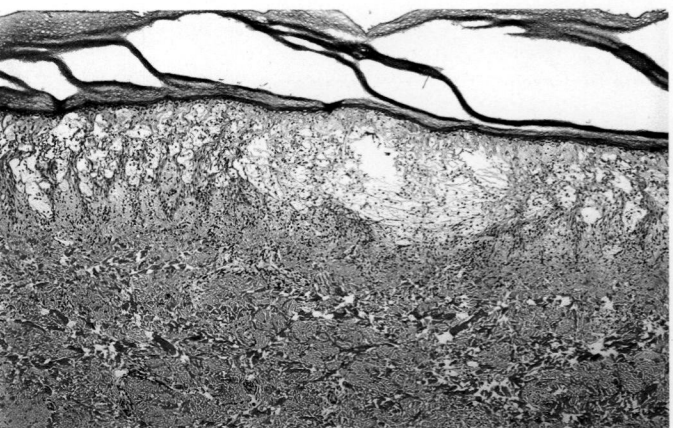

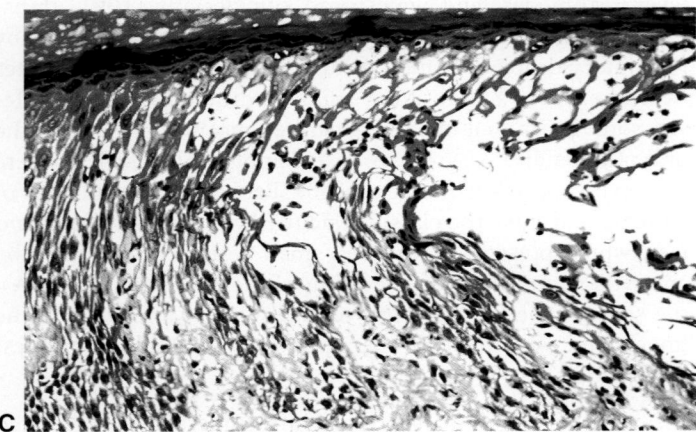

Figure 25-22 Hand–foot–mouth disease. **A:** Small vesicles on the palm of the hand with surrounding erythema. **B:** Scanning magnification shows intraepidermal vesicles with pronounced reticular degeneration. **C:** Pronounced reticular degeneration and balloon degeneration. Neither inclusion bodies nor multinucleated cells are present.

RETROVIRIDAE

Retroviridae are RNA retroviruses and are currently classified into seven genera, including HIV, the cause of AIDS, and human T-lymphotropic virus (HTLV).

Human Immunodeficiency Virus Infection

Clinical Summary. HIV infects predominantly CD4$^+$ cells, most notably T-helper cells, and leads to a profound alteration of immune system function that predisposes patients to numerous opportunistic infections, malignancies, and neurologic diseases, which may result in AIDS. The virus is spread almost exclusively through blood and semen.

Cutaneous findings in HIV disease are frequent and include viral, bacterial, fungal, and noninfectious etiologies (115). Some infections occur in clinically obscure forms because they do not have recognizable morphologic features. In addition, systemic infectious diseases can produce skin lesions, even though the classic organs of involvement for that agent may not include the skin. Dermatologic diseases common to the general population, such as seborrheic dermatitis, often have an increased prevalence or severity in these individuals (116). Several skin diseases occur nearly exclusively in HIV-infected individuals, such as oral hairy leukoplakia, bacillary angiomatosis, and KS.

HIV itself produces cutaneous findings shortly after exposure. In addition, gradual deterioration of the immune system renders HIV-infected patients susceptible to numerous cutaneous viral diseases, including herpesviruses, HPV, and molluscum contagiosum (117). Approximately 2 to 6 weeks following HIV exposure, patients may present with a transient illness related to HIV replication and host response. More than 50% of patients report symptoms of acute HIV infection: a macular or morbilliform rash usually involving the trunk is present in 40% to 80% of patients with acute HIV infection; oral ulcers may be a frequent finding in acute HIV seroconversion (118). Because the standard immunoassay and Western blot are often negative with acute infection, additional tests may be needed when there is a high index of suspicion, or patients should undergo both acute and convalescent titers. p24 antigen assay has fewer false positives and may be a more cost-effective way to diagnose primary HIV infection (119).

Pruritic papular eruption (PPE) is the most common cutaneous manifestation in HIV-infected patients. Opportunistic viral infections affecting the skin and mucous membranes are also common (38). *Herpetic infections* are one of the most important causes of opportunistic infections in patients with HIV and frequently include cutaneous manifestations. Unlike in the healthy individual, in which case the lesions are often self-limited, herpetic infections can cause significant chronic morbidity in the immunocompromised patients. As immune function declines, the herpetic lesions may become chronic and progress to painful ulceration. *Herpes zoster* may be complicated by repeated bouts, involvement of multiple dermatomes, and chronic verrucous zoster, and rarely, herpes zoster may disseminate. *CMV* infection is associated with CD4$^+$ cell counts of less than 100 and has a spectrum of presentations including pulmonary, ocular, gastrointestinal, and neurologic involvement, although CMV skin lesions are uncommon (120). Although most adults harbor EBV in the latent phase, *oral hairy leukoplakia* is a rare disorder found almost exclusively in HIV-infected individuals. Approximately 25% of HIV-infected individuals may be affected. White, verrucous, confluent plaques that are most commonly located on the lateral aspects of the tongue characterize oral hairy leukoplakia; these do not scrape off with a tongue depressor (121). EBV appears to be necessary for the production of this lesion, although HPV and Candida are also frequently present. The condition is a result of EBV infection of epithelial cells that leads to hyperkeratotic thickening. *Molluscum contagiosum* generally presents as CD4$^+$ counts fall below 100/mm^3. Although the lesions spontaneously resolve in immunocompetent hosts, the lesions are often extensive and progressive in HIV-infected individuals, who are also subject to so-called giant molluscum contagiosum, with lesions ranging from 1 to 6 cm in diameter (122).

Bacterial infections are also common in AIDS. *Staphylococcus aureus* is the most common cutaneous bacterial pathogen in HIV-seropositive patients. HIV-infected patients are also prone to streptococcal impetigo and axillary lymphadenitis. Another unique infectious disease first recognized in the context of HIV infection is *bacillary angiomatosis*. This is a systemic infectious disease caused by gram-negative *Bartonella henselae* or *B. quintana* (123). Patients may have palpable subcutaneous nodules, which may resemble KS or hemangioma but resolve with appropriate antibiotic therapy. The lesions are often painful, unlike those of KS. HIV-infected patients are susceptible to mycobacterial infections that can sometimes produce unusual skin manifestations. *Syphilis* is common in these individuals and often the presenting infection of HIV disease (124). *Secondary syphilis* assumes a variety of manifestations in HIV-infected patients, including oral erosions, nodules, papules, vesicles, hyperkeratotic plaques, and papulosquamous or maculopapular eruptions. Patients with HIV and syphilis coinfection may have initial negative RPR testing and sometimes require serial dilutions to detect a positive result, owing to the prozone phenomenon.

Patients with HIV are subject to fungal, protozoan, and arthropod infections that produce mucocutaneous findings. Oral candidiasis is often an early clinical manifestation of AIDS and in progressing may cause painful esophagitis. Other infections such as *Cryptococcus, Histoplasma, Coccidioidomycosis, tinea versicolor, phaeohyphomycosis, nocardiosis,* and *mucormycosis* are not uncommonly seen in these patients (125). *Scabies* mite is the most common parasitic infestation of HIV-infected individuals (126). Scabies is highly contagious in HIV-infected patients via direct contact. *Demodicidosis* involves the proliferation of Demodex mites within the pilosebaceous unit and is reported in association with HIV infection (127). *Disseminated acanthamebiasis* has been reported in these patients and often presents skin manifestations such as pustules, subcutaneous and deep dermal nodules, and ulcers, most often seen on the extremities and face.

Noninfectious cutaneous disorders are also common in HIV infection and can occur at all stages of the disease. An explosive episode of *psoriasis* or severe *seborrheic dermatitis* can be the presenting symptom of HIV disease. *Seborrheic dermatitis* is a common disease affecting 2% to 4% of the general population, but up to 85% of HIV-positive individuals experience seborrheic dermatitis at some time point during their diseases. It can be quite severe, with the severity correlating with the patient's clinical status and CD4 count (128). Less common areas such as the chest, back, axilla, and groin are often involved in HIV-seropositive patients. The histology of this eruption is similar to that of idiopathic seborrheic dermatitis, although

some feel that distinctive histologic patterns are present (129). Although the incidence of *psoriasis* in HIV disease is similar to that in the general population, it is often more severe and refractory to treatment and has a higher prevalence of psoriatic arthritis. Reactive arthritis (*Reiter syndrome*), characterized by arthritis, urethritis, and conjunctivitis, may be associated with psoriasis in HIV-infected individuals (130). As many as 30% of HIV-infected individuals experience *xerosis* or *acquired ichthyosis* with fine white scales and cracking skin without erythema, which may be diffuse or which may preferentially affect the anterior tibia, dorsal hand, and forearm (131). Whereas xerosis reveals minimal inflammation microscopically, acquired ichthyosis is histologically similar to ichthyosis vulgaris often with hyperkeratosis and diminished or absence of the granular cell layer. A nonspecific follicular eruption, named *eosinophilic pustular folliculitis*, is present in a significant number of patients with HIV infection (132). The eruption is chronic and pruritic. An interface dermatitis associated with HIV, observed in a series of 25 patients with AIDS, presents as a more or less widespread eruption of pink or red macules, papules, or plaques. It resembles and may represent a form of drug eruption or erythema multiforme (133).

Adverse cutaneous drug reactions are common in HIV-positive individuals, and they are prone to side effects associated with antimicrobial and antiviral medications (134). For example, after 1 to 2 weeks of trimethoprim–sulfamethoxazole treatment for *Pneumocystis carinii* infection, up to 50% to 60% of HIV-infected patients may develop a morbilliform rash. HIV-infected individuals also have higher rates of severe adverse drug reactions such as Stevens–Johnson syndrome/toxic epidermal necrolysis. HIV-infected individuals also have an increased incidence of photosensitivity reactions. *Chronic actinic dermatitis*, a rare photosensitivity reaction, is sometimes the presenting manifestation of HIV seropositivity (135). Patients with chronic HIV infection may also develop a more nonspecific photosensitivity and photodistributed lichenoid dermatitis. *Porphyria cutanea tarda (PCT)* is reported more frequently in HIV-infected individuals compared with the general population. Other lesions, such as pityriasis rubra pilaris, porokeratosis, yellow nail syndrome, alopecia, asteatosis, vasculitis, acrodermatitis enteropathica, and neutrophilic eccrine hidradenitis, have been reported.

KS is the most common AIDS-associated cancer in the United States. Over 95% of all KS lesions have been associated with HHV-8 (136). Skin lesions of KS typically present with asymptomatic reddish-purple patches that sometimes progress to raised plaques or nodules (Fig. 25-13). One-third of patients experience oral cavity lesions characterized by red-to-purple plaques or nodules. Other tumors such as melanoma (137), squamous, and basal cell carcinoma have been reported in these patients.

Histopathology. The histology of the acute exanthema of HIV infection is rather nonspecific, with a tight perivascular infiltrate of lymphocytes in the dermis. Epidermal changes are usually mild but may include spongiosis, vacuolar change, and/or keratinocyte apoptosis (138,139); or there may be nonspecific lymphocytic infiltrates with mild epidermal changes, primarily spongiosis (116).

The lesions of oral hairy leukoplakia show irregular keratin projections, parakeratosis, and acanthosis. A characteristic finding within the epithelium is vacuolar change of superficial keratinocytes (Fig. 25-11A–C). Candida organisms may be demonstrable. Seborrheic dermatitis in patients with AIDS may show nonspecific changes, including spotty keratinocytic necrosis, leukocytoclasia, and plasma cells in a superficial perivascular infiltrate (127). The papular eruption of AIDS may exhibit nonspecific perivascular eosinophils with mild folliculitis, although epithelioid cell granulomas have also been reported (140). The interface dermatitis shows, as the name implies, vacuolar alteration of the basal cell layer, scattered necrotic keratinocytes, and a superficial perivascular lymphohistiocytic infiltrate. The vacuolar alteration and number of necrotic keratinocytes tend to be more pronounced than in drug eruptions (131). The changes found are nonspecific but are suggestive of features described in graft-versus-host disease and become more prominent in late-stage disease. *Eosinophilic pustular folliculitis* shows folliculitis with transmigration of eosinophils into the follicular epithelium, mimicking the changes observed in Ofuji disease. However, in many cases, the histologic picture is less specific, showing only a polymorphous inflammatory response and mild folliculitis (137,141). *Cutaneous acanthamebiasis* shows both pustular and vasculitis changes; the microscopic identification of organisms is difficult because of the macrophage-like appearance of the microbes in routine sections (142). A periodic acid–Schiff (PAS) stain can be used to highlight the organisms.

Principles of Management of Retroviridae-Associated Skin Diseases

Management of retroviridae-associated skin diseases is similar to the management of the diseases listed previously that are not associated with retroviridae infection. Management of HIV infection is, of course, a key component of therapy and is beyond the scope of this book.

DISEASES CAUSED BY OTHER VIRUSES

Hepatitis B Virus

Clinical Summary and Histopathology. Hepatitis B virus (HBV) is a double-stranded DNA virus belonging to the hepadnavirus family. The virus is transmitted frequently through IV drug use, sexual activity, and mother-to-fetus transmission (143). During the acute phase, 15% of the patients will develop urticaria, fever, and malaise (144). Polyarteritis nodosum (PAN) is one of the more serious and common complications of HBV infection (145). About 2 out of 500 people with HBV develop PAN, but up to 50% of people with PAN test positive for HBsAg. Cutaneous involvement occurs in 10% to 20% of persons with PAN, which presents as palpable purpura that progresses to large ulcers. Tender, purple, subcutaneous nodules, as well as livedo vasculitis, can occur (146). There is fibrinoid necrosis of medium-size vessel wall, with a cellular infiltrate composed mainly of CD8+ T cells and macrophages. Depositions of immune complex, IgM, C3, and HBsAg in the vessel walls are observed.

Papular acrodermatitis of childhood (Gianotti–Crosti syndrome) occurs in children infected with HBV and is not common in adults (147). The clinical presentation includes a nonrelapsing erythematous papular eruption localized to the face and limbs (Fig. 25-23), with lymphadenopathy and acute

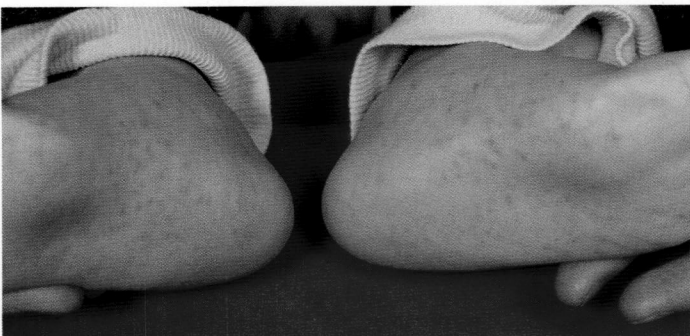

Figure 25-23 Papular acrodermatitis of childhood. Numerous erythematous papules on the feet of this boy.

hepatitis (mostly anicteric). The lesions do not affect mucosal surfaces. Papular acrodermatitis of childhood is common in southern Europe and Japan but rare in the United States. This condition can also be associated with CMV, EBV, respiratory syncytial virus, and enterovirus infection (148). The histology is characterized by a mixture of spongiotic and lichenoid dermatitis with a dense perivascular infiltrate.

Serum sickness–like syndrome is considered the most common dermatologic manifestation associated with HBV, which occurs in 20% to 30% of patients during the prodromal phase of the HBV infection. The skin manifestation includes urticaria, angioedema, and rashes. The urticaria lesions show erythrocyte extravasation, endothelial cell swelling, and various degrees of fibrinoid change of postcapillary venules (149). The pathology is induced by deposition of immune complexes, which are composed of HBsAg, IgG, IgM, and C3.

HBV has also been associated with mixed cryoglobulinemia (150); however, this is much less common than that associated with hepatitis C virus (HCV) infection. A recurrent papular rash on the trunk and extremities (151) and LP have been reported as complications of hepatitis B vaccination in both adults and children (152).

Hepatitis C Virus

Clinical Summary and Histopathology. HCV is a single-stranded RNA virus that belongs to Hepacivirus, the third genus of the Flaviviridae family. Individuals with exposure to blood or blood products are at risk for infection with HCV. The prevalence in the United States ranges from 0.5% to 2%. *Mixed cryoglobulinemia* is the most documented extrahepatic manifestation of HCV infection (153). It presents cutaneously as an inflammatory, palpable purpura that is usually confined to the lower extremities and that progresses to ulceration. It is established that most (80%) of what was previously known as essential mixed cryoglobulinemia is now known to be related to chronic HCV infection (154). Despite a high prevalence of HCV infection in patients with mixed cryoglobulinemia, only an estimated 13% to 54% of patients with chronic HCV will develop mixed cryoglobulinemia. It is believed that HCV–IgG and HCV–lipoprotein complexes may act as B-cell superantigens, inducing the synthesis of non–HCV-reactive IgM with rheumatoid factor–like activity that leads to immune complex formation. Because of the high prevalence of liver abnormalities seen in patients with mixed cryoglobulinemia, hepatotropic viruses should be ruled out as causative agents. Histologic features for mixed cryoglobulinemia are those of an acute vasculitis involving small and/or median-size dermal vessels. Intravascular hyaline deposits are generally not seen except in the areas beneath the ulcer.

LP is common in patients with HCV. The prevalence of HCV ranges from 16% to 55% and 0.17% to 4.8% in LP patients and control groups, respectively (155). The lesions of HCV-related LP are similar to those of classic LP. However, most reported HCV-related LP cases have oral involvement. Histologically, LP is characterized by a subepidermal, bandlike lymphohistiocytic infiltrate with interface change, sawtooth rete ridges, and pigmentary incontinence.

There is a high but variable prevalence of HCV infection in patients with PCT. The prevalence is higher in southern Europe (67% to 91%) and lower in northern Europe (8% to 10%). The prevalence in the United States is reported to be between 50% and 75% (156). In most cases, the HCV exposure and associated liver dysfunction precede the onset of PCT, suggesting that a viral infection can reveal a porphyrin metabolism defect in susceptible patients. Histologically, PCT is characterized by a cell-poor subepidermal bulla with increased PAS-positive diastase-resistant hyaline material in the vessel walls and basement membrane.

Other lesions associated with HCV infection include erythema multiforme and erythema nodosum (157), Henoch–Schönlein purpura (HSP) (158), Behçet syndrome (159), necrolytic acral erythema (160), PAN (161), prurigo nodularis (162), pyoderma gangrenosum (163), and urticarial vasculitis (164).

Principles of Management: The treatments of PAN and mixed cryoglobulinemia associated with HBV and HCV are the same as for nonvirus-related PAN and mixed cryoglobulinemia, but a combination with antiviral treatment is known to be more effective (165). However, antiviral treatments are controversial in most other skin manifestations associated with HBV and HCV infections, and they are treated in the same way as nonvirus-associated skin diseases (166).

Parvovirus B19

Clinical Summary and Histopathology. Parvovirus is a single-stranded DNA virus that belongs to the family Parvoviridae. Parvovirus B19 is the only parvovirus that clearly causes human disease (167). The virus is highly tropic for erythroid progenitor cells and is thus classified as an erythrovirus. The cellular receptor for B19 is a globoside, also known as blood group P antigen (38). Parvovirus infection is ubiquitous and occurs worldwide. Transmission of the virus occurs through the respiratory route in most cases. Two dermatologic conditions have been linked to Parvovirus B19 infection: *erythema infectiosum* and *papular-purpuric "gloves-and-socks" syndrome* (167,168). Infection may also result in nonspecific findings, such as reticular erythema, maculopapular eruptions, purpuric eruptions, palpable purpura, and angioedema. Other dermatologic entities, such as erythema multiforme (169), Gianotti–Crosti syndrome (170), and, recently, various vasculitic syndromes, including HSP, granulomatosis with eosinophilia (EGPA), and microscopic polyarteritis, have been linked to B19 infection (171).

The best-known dermatologic manifestation of parvovirus B19 is *erythema infectiosum.* This well-recognized exanthema is also called fifth disease, with a distinctive "slapped cheek" appearance (Fig. 25-24). The cause of parvovirus B19 rash is believed to be immunologically mediated, and the rash

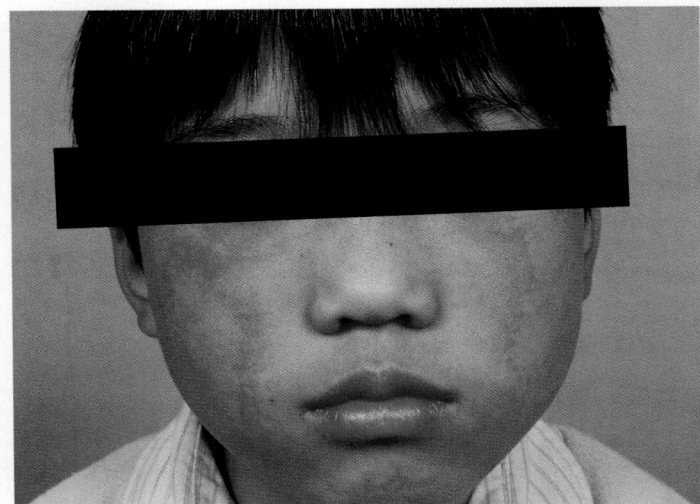

Figure 25-24 Erythema infectiosum (fifth disease). The lesion has a classic slapped cheek appearance. The bright red erythema appears abruptly over the cheeks and is marked by nasal, perioral, and periorbital sparing.

corresponds to the appearance of immunoglobulin M (IgM) in the serum. Papular-purpuric "gloves-and-socks" syndrome is also associated with parvovirus B19. It is mainly seen in young adults. Clinically, the rash consists of symmetric erythema and edema of the hands and feet, with gradual progression to petechiae and purpura. One of the clinical hallmarks of the rash is the sharp demarcation on the wrists and ankles. Resolution occurs within 1 to 2 weeks, with no permanent sequelae. However, in immunocompromised patients, papular-purpuric "gloves-and-socks" syndrome may lead to more serious complications, such as persistent anemia. The histology is not entirely specific. Most cases have revealed interstitial histiocytic infiltrates with piecemeal fragmentation of collagen and a mononuclear cell–predominant vascular injury pattern, showing dilated and irregular-shaped dermal vessels with swelling of endothelial cells. Mild-to-moderate perivascular infiltrates of mononuclear cells were noted (172).

Principles of Management: Parvovirus B19–associated dermatologic manifestations do not require specific treatment, and supportive treatment is the primary therapeutic modality (173).

Measles

Clinical Summary and Histopathology. Measles virus is a single-stranded RNA virus that belongs to the family Paramyxoviridae. Measles is an epidemic disease with a worldwide distribution. Measles virus is transmitted via respiratory secretions, predominantly as aerosols but also by direct contact. The symptoms usually last for 10 days and resolve without consequence. However, there is an increased risk of more severe diseases, such as severe pneumonitis or encephalitis, in immunocompromised individuals (174). Patients will often have diffuse erythematous macules and fine papules starting at the hairline and spreading downward, accompanied by fever, conjunctivitis, and bluish-white pinpoint spots on the inside of the mouth (Koplik spots). A biopsy of the rash shows nonspecific histologic change, with epidermal spongiosis and mild vesiculation with scattered degenerated keratinocytes (175). Biopsies from AIDS patients with measles show necrosis of clusters of keratinocytes in the upper spinous layer and granular layer of the epidermis, unlike in erythema multiforme, where the necrosis occurs in the basal layer keratinocytes. Multinucleated keratinocytes may or may not be prominent in the measles biopsy. Cytoplasmic swelling of the keratinocytes in the granular layer may be present even when multinucleated cells are sparse (176).

Principles of Management: The treatment of measles is supportive.

Rubella

Clinical Summary and Histopathology. Rubella is an enveloped, single-stranded RNA virus, a member of the family Togaviridae. Rubella, also known as German measles, is a viral exanthema of childhood that is generally subclinical and inconsequential. However, infection may be teratogenic when it occurs in pregnant women, especially in early pregnancy. Viremia occurs approximately 1 week before the rash; the rash is seen when circulating antibodies appear. The rash is maculopapular, erythematous, discrete, and pruritic. The face is usually the first area of devolvement, and then it spreads to the extremities. The entire body may be involved within 1 day. On the second day, there is clearing of the face, and the rash is commonly cleared by the third day. Histologically, the change is not specific, with a mild, perivascular lymphocytic infiltrate (177,178).

Principles of Management: The treatment of rubella is supportive.

Merkel Cell Polyomavirus

Clinical Summary and Histopathology. The Polyomaviridae family of viruses has three genera and 22 different species of polyomaviruses, all of which are nonenveloped, icosahedral viruses that contain a circular, double-stranded DNA genome of approximately 5,000 base pairs. In 2008, Feng et al. identified a novel polyomavirus whose DNA was clonally integrated into the tumor genome of Merkel cell carcinoma (MCC). This virus was termed the *Merkel cell polyomavirus* (MCV or MCPyV), and MCV was detected in 80% of MCC tumors (179). There are currently 11 identified human polyomaviruses, and MCPyV is the only human polyomavirus known as a causative agent of

a human malignancy (180). MCC is a highly malignant skin cancer and derives from Merkel cells in the epidermis. Merkel cells were first described as "touch cells" by Friedrich Sigmund Merkel in 1875; they are found in the basal layer of the epidermis, hair follicles, and certain mucosal tissues, and are most abundant in areas of the skin involved in the sensation of touch. MCC occurs commonly in older white men in the head and neck region (Fig. 25-25A), and the histopathology of MCC is that of one of the so-called small round blue cell tumors. MCPyV large T antigen can be detected using immunohistochemistry (Fig. 25-25B). Histology of MCC is described in detail in Chapter 37 (Tumors of Neural Tissue).

Viral-associated trichodysplasia of immunosuppression is a rare cutaneous eruption, characterized by shiny follicular papules affecting the central face clinically and involving abnormal anagen follicles with excessive inner root sheath differentiation histologically. The pathogenic virus of this disease has also been identified as a polyomavirus (181).

Principles of Management: Patients with MCC are usually first treated with surgery, and those with more advanced disease may receive adjuvant treatments such as radiation therapy and immunotherapy (182). PD-L1 and PD-1 checkpoint blockade immunotherapies have been approved for MCC. Viral-associated trichodysplasia may be treated by topical cidofovir (181).

SARS-CoV-2

Clinical Summary and Histopathology. Coronaviruses constitute the subfamily Orthocoronavirinae, in the family Coronaviridae, and realm Riboviria. They are enveloped viruses with a positive-sense single-stranded RNA genome and a nucleocapsid of helical symmetry. They have characteristic club-shaped spikes that project from their surface. Coronavirus disease 2019 (COVID-19) is a contagious disease caused by severe acute respiratory syndrome coronavirus 2 (SARS-CoV-2). Symptoms of COVID-19 are variable but often include fever, cough, headache, fatigue, breathing difficulties, and loss of smell and taste. Symptoms may begin 1 to 14 days after exposure to the virus. At least a third of people who are infected do not develop noticeable symptoms. SARS-CoV-2 causes multiple immune-related reactions at

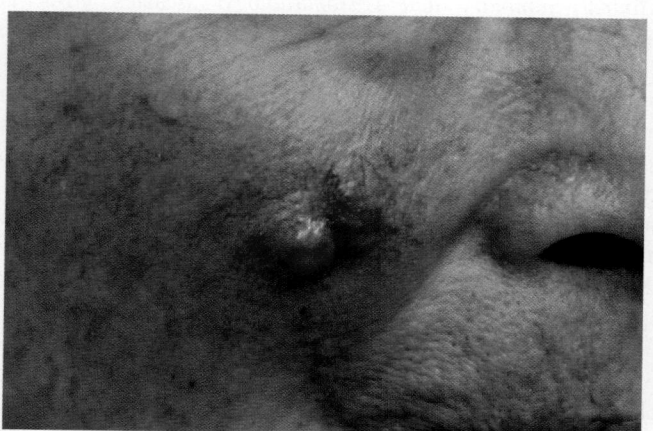
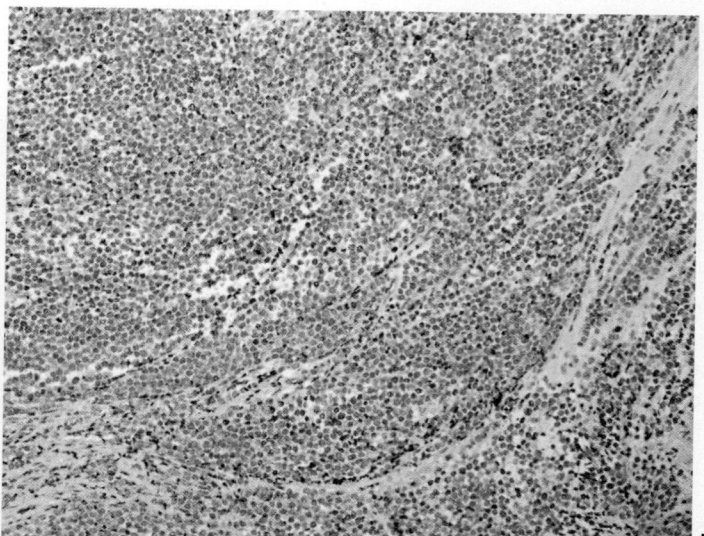

Figure 25-25 Merkel cell carcinoma. **A:** Erythematous nodules on the face. **B:** Anti–polyoma virus antibody T antigen stain shows diffuse nuclear positive pattern.

various stages of the disease with a wide variety of cutaneous presentations. It has been estimated that 8.8% of COVID-19 patients developed skin rash. A study by Casas et al. showed that cutaneous manifestations of COVID-19 may be classified as acral areas of erythema with vesicles or pustules (pseudo-chilblain) (19%), other vesicular eruptions (9%), urticarial lesions (19%), maculopapular eruptions (47%), and livedo or necrosis (6%). Among these, pseudo-chilblain and vesicular eruptions appear to be more specific for COVID-19 infection (183). Patients infected with SARS-CoV-2 who experience prolonged symptoms are said to have "long Covid," with studies reporting that 66% to 87% of these patients continued to have one or more COVID-19 symptoms 60 days after PCR positivity. Seven of the 103 cases (6.8%) with pseudo-chilblain had long COVID, and pseudo-chilblain lasted for more than 60 days (184).

Principles of Management: SARS-CoV-2–associated dermatosis does not require specific treatment. Virus-targeted therapies and supportive treatments are used for therapeutic modalities.

REFERENCES

1. Murray N, McMichael A. Antigen presentation in virus infection. *Curr Opin Immunol.* 1992;4:401.
2. Poranen MM, Daugelavicius R, Bamford DH. Common principles in viral entry. *Annu Rev Microbiol.* 2002;56:521.
3. Sieczkarski SB, Whittaker GR. Dissecting virus entry via endocytosis. *J Gen Virol.* 2002;83:1535.
4. Riley LE. Herpes simplex virus. *Semin Perinatol.* 1998;22:284.
5. Whitley RJ, Roizman B. Herpes simplex virus infections. *Lancet.* 2001;357:1513.
6. Nahmias AJ, Lee FK, Beckman-Nahmias S. Sero-epidemiological and -sociological patterns of herpes simplex virus infection in the world. *Scand J Infect Dis Suppl.* 1990;69:19.
7. Kohl S. Neonatal herpes simplex virus infection. *Clin Perinatol.* 1997;24:129.
8. Reeves WC, Corey L, Adams HG, Vontver LA, Holmes KK. Risk of recurrence after first episodes of genital herpes: relation to HSV type and antibody response. *N Engl J Med.* 1981;305:315.
9. Wald A, Zeh J, Selke S, et al. Reactivation of genital herpes simplex virus type 2 infection in asymptomatic seropositive persons. *N Engl J Med.* 2000;342:844.
10. Mackley CL, Adams DR, Anderson B, Miller JJ. Eczema herpeticum: a dermatologic emergency. *Dermatol Nurs.* 2002;14:307.
11. Yeung-Yue KA, Brentjens MH, Lee PC, Tyring SK. Herpes simplex viruses 1 and 2. *Dermatol Clin.* 2002;20:249.
12. Raychaudhuri SP, Raychaudhuri SK. Revisit to Kaposi's varicelliform eruption: role of IL-4. *Int J Dermatol.* 1995;34:854.
13. Goodyear HM, McLeish P, Randall S, et al. Immunological studies of herpes simplex virus infection in children with atopic eczema. *Br J Dermatol.* 1996;134:85.
14. Jang KA, Kim SH, Choi JH, Sung KJ, Moon KC, Koh JK. Viral folliculitis on the face. *Br J Dermatol.* 2000;142:555.
15. Giacobetti R. Herpetic whitlow. *Int J Dermatol.* 1979;18:55.
16. Powers RD, Rein MF, Hayden FG. Necrotizing balanitis due to herpes simplex type 1. *JAMA.* 1982;248:215.
17. Hook EW III, Cannon RO, Nahmias AJ, et al. Herpes simplex virus infection as a risk factor for human immunodeficiency virus infection in heterosexuals. *J Infect Dis.* 1992;165:251.
18. Salvini F, Carminati G, Pinzani R, Carrera C, Rancilio L, Plebani A. Chronic ulcerative herpes simplex virus infection in HIV-infected children. *AIDS Patient Care STDS.* 1997;11:421.
19. Lopyan L, Young AW Jr, Menegus M. Generalized acute mucocutaneous herpes simplex type 2 with fatal outcome. *Arch Dermatol.* 1977;113:816.
20. Prober CG, Hensleigh PA, Boucher FD, Yasukawa LL, Au DS, Arvin AM. Use of routine viral cultures at delivery to identify neonates exposed to herpes simplex virus. *N Engl J Med.* 1988;318:887.
21. Schofield JK, Tatnall FM, Leigh IM. Recurrent erythema multiforme: clinical features and treatment in a large series of patients. *Br J Dermatol.* 1993;128:542.
22. Darragh TM, Egbert BM, Berger TG, Yen TS. Identification of herpes simplex virus DNA in lesions of erythema multiforme by the polymerase chain reaction. *J Am Acad Dermatol.* 1991;24:23.
23. Weinberg JM, Mysliwiec A, Turiansky GW, Redfield R, James WD. Viral folliculitis: atypical presentations of herpes simplex, herpes zoster, and molluscum contagiosum. *Arch Dermatol.* 1997;133:983.
24. Nahass GT, Goldstein BA, Zhu WY, Serfling U, Penneys NS, Leonardi CL. Comparison of Tzanck smear, viral culture, and DNA diagnostic methods in detection of herpes simplex and varicella-zoster infection. *JAMA.* 1992;268:2541.
25. Wang JY, Montone KT. A rapid simple in situ hybridization method for herpes simplex virus employing a synthetic biotin-labeled oligonucleotide probe: a comparison with immunohistochemical methods for HSV detection. *J Clin Lab Anal.* 1994;8:105.
26. Morecki R, Becker NH. Human herpesvirus infection: its fine structure identification in paraffin-embedded tissue. *Arch Pathol.* 1968;86:292.
27. Mooney MA, Janniger CK, Schwartz RA. Kaposi's varicelliform eruption. *Cutis.* 1994;53:243.
28. Moss EM. Atopic dermatitis. *Pediatr Clin North Am.* 1978;25:225.
29. Moses AE, Cohen-Poradosu R. Images in clinical medicine: eczema vaccinatum—a timely reminder. *N Engl J Med.* 2002;346:1287.
30. Martinez CM, Luks-Golger DB. Cidofovir use in acyclovir-resistant herpes infection. *Ann Pharmacother.* 1997;31:1519–1521.
31. Castelo-Soccio L, Bernardin R, Stern J, Goldstein SA, Kovarik C. Successful treatment of acyclovir-resistant herpes simplex virus with intralesional cidofovir. *Arch Dermatol.* 2010;146:124–126.
32. Lin F, Hadler JL. Epidemiology of primary varicella and herpes zoster hospitalizations: the pre-varicella vaccine era. *J Infect Dis.* 2000;181:1897.
33. Preblud SR. Varicella: complications and costs. *Pediatrics.* 1986;78:728.
34. McCrary ML, Severson J, Tyring SK. Varicella zoster virus. *J Am Acad Dermatol.* 1999;41:1.
35. Pitel PA, McCormick KL, Fitzgerald E, Orson JM. Subclinical hepatic changes in varicella infection. *Pediatrics.* 1980;65:631.
36. Belay ED, Bresee JS, Holman RC, Khan AS, Shahriari A, Schonberger LB. Reye's syndrome in the United States from 1981 through 1997. *N Engl J Med.* 1999;340:1377–1382.
37. Pastuszak AL, Levy M, Schick B, et al. Outcome after maternal varicella infection in the first 20 weeks of pregnancy. *N Engl J Med.* 1994;330:901.
38. Gnann JW Jr. Varicella-zoster virus: atypical presentations and unusual complications. *J Infect Dis.* 2002;186(suppl 1):S91.
39. Schmader K. Herpes zoster in older adults. *Clin Infect Dis.* 2001;32:1481.
40. Garman ME, Tyring SK. The cutaneous manifestations of HIV infection. *Dermatol Clin.* 2002;20:193.
41. Al Abdulla NA, Rismondo V, Minkowski JS, Miller NR. Herpes zoster vasculitis presenting as giant cell arteritis with bilateral internuclear ophthalmoplegia. *Am J Ophthalmol.* 2002;134:912.
42. Nikkels AF, Debrus S, Sadzot-Delvaux C, et al. Comparative immunohistochemical study of herpes simplex and varicella-zoster infections. *Virchows Arch A Pathol Anat Histopathol.* 1993;422:121.
43. Solomon AR, Rasmussen JE, Weiss JS. A comparison of the Tzanck smear and viral isolation in varicella and herpes zoster. *Arch Dermatol.* 1986;122:282.
44. Zamora MR. DNA viruses (CMV, EBV, and the herpesviruses). *Semin Respir Crit Care Med.* 2011;32(4):454–470.

45. Izurieta HS, Wu X, Forshee R, et al. Recombinant Zoster Vaccine (Shingrix) real-world effectiveness in the first two years post-licensure. *Clin Infect Dis.* 2021;73(6):941–948. doi:10.1093/cid/ciab125

46. Khoshnevis M, Tyring SK. Cytomegalovirus infections. *Dermatol Clin.* 2002;20:291.

47. Vancikova Z, Dvorak P. Cytomegalovirus infection in immunocompetent and immunocompromised individuals—a review. *Curr Drug Targets Immune Endocr Metabol Disord.* 2001;1:179.

48. Lee JY. Cytomegalovirus infection involving the skin in immunocompromised hosts: a clinicopathologic study. *Am J Clin Pathol.* 1989;92:96.

49. Hodl S, Aubock L, Reiterer F, Soyer HP, Müller WD. Blueberry muffin baby: the pathogenesis of cutaneous extramedullary hematopoiesis [in German]. *Hautarzt.* 2001;52:1035.

50. Stegmann BJ, Carey JC. TORCH infections: toxoplasmosis, other (syphilis, varicella-zoster, parvovirus B19), rubella, cytomegalovirus (CMV), and herpes infections. *Curr Womens Health Rep.* 2002;2:253.

51. Arribas JR, Arrizabalaga J, Mallolas J, López-Cortés LF. Advances in the diagnosis and treatment of infections caused by herpesvirus and JC virus [in Spanish]. *Enferm Infecc Microbiol Clin.* 1998;16(suppl 1):11.

52. Wu JJ, Pang KR, Huang DB, Tyring SK. Advances in antiviral therapy. *Dermatol Clin.* 2005;23(2):313–322.

53. Iwatsuki K, Xu Z, Ohtsuka M, Kaneko F. Cutaneous lymphoproliferative disorders associated with Epstein-Barr virus infection: a clinical overview. *J Dermatol Sci.* 2000;22:181.

54. Steven NM. Epstein-Barr virus latent infection in vivo. *Rev Med Virol.* 1997;7:97.

55. Ikediobi NI, Tyring SK. Cutaneous manifestations of Epstein-Barr virus infection. *Dermatol Clin.* 2002;20:283.

56. Sangueza M, Plaza JA. Hydroa vacciniforme-like cutaneous T-cell lymphoma: clinicopathologic and immunohistochemical study of 12 cases. *J Am Acad Dermatol.* 2013;69:112–119.

57. Guo N, Chen Y, Wang Y, et al. Clinicopathological categorization of hydroa vacciniforme-like lymphoproliferative disorder: an analysis of prognostic implications and treatment based on 19 cases. *Diagn Pathol.* 2019;14:82.

58. Li S, Feng X, Li T, et al. Extranodal NK/T-cell lymphoma, nasal type: a report of 73 cases at MD Anderson Cancer Center. *Am J Surg Pathol.* 2013;37:14–23.

59. Kimura H, Fujiwara S. Overview of EBV-associated T/NK-cell lymphoproliferative diseases. *Front Pediatr.* 2019;6:417.

60. De Araujo T, Berman B, Weinstein A. Human herpesviruses 6 and 7. *Dermatol Clin.* 2002;20:301.

61. Yoshikawa T, Ihira M, Ohashi M, et al. Correlation between HHV-6 infection and skin rash after allogeneic bone marrow transplantation. *Bone Marrow Transplant.* 2001;28:77.

62. Yokote T, Muroi K, Kawano C, et al. Human herpesvirus-6-associated generalized vesiculobullous eruptions after allogeneic bone marrow transplantation. *Leuk Lymphoma.* 2002;43:927.

63. Ruzicka T, Kalka K, Diercks K, Schuppe HC. Papular-purpuric 'gloves and socks' syndrome associated with human herpesvirus 6 infection. *Arch Dermatol.* 1998;134:242.

64. Yasumoto S, Tsujita J, Imayama S, Hori Y. Case report: Gianotti-Crosti syndrome associated with human herpesvirus-6 infection. *J Dermatol.* 1996;23:499.

65. Fujino Y, Nakajima M, Inoue H, Kusuhara T, Yamada T. Human herpesvirus 6 encephalitis associated with hypersensitivity syndrome. *Ann Neurol.* 2002;51:771.

66. Husain Z, Reddy BY, Schwartz RA. DRESS syndrome: part I. Clinical perspectives. *J Am Acad Dermatol.* 2013;68:693.e1–e14.

67. Cacoub P, Musette P, Descamps V, et al. The DRESS syndrome: a literature review. *Am J Med.* 2011;124(7):588–597.

68. De Vries HJ, van Marle J, Teunissen MB, et al. Lichen planus is associated with human herpesvirus type 7 replication and infiltration of plasmacytoid dendritic cells. *Br J Dermatol.* 2006;154(2):361–364.

69. Wolz MM, Sciallis GF, Pittelkow MR. Human herpesviruses 6, 7, and 8 from a dermatologic perspective. *Mayo Clin Proc.* 2012;87(10):1004–1014.

70. Breman JG, Henderson DA. Diagnosis and management of smallpox. *N Engl J Med.* 2002;346:1300.

71. Klainer AS. Smallpox. *Clin Dermatol.* 1989;7:19.

72. Copeman PW, Banatvala JE. The skin and vaccination against smallpox. *Br J Dermatol.* 1971;84:169.

73. Goldstein JA, Neff JM, Lane JM, Koplan JP. Smallpox vaccination reactions, prophylaxis, and therapy of complications. *Pediatrics.* 1975;55:342.

74. Baxby D, Bennett M, Getty B. Human cowpox 1969-93: a review based on 54 cases. *Br J Dermatol.* 1994;131:598.

75. Leavell UW Jr, McNamara MJ, Muelling R, Talbert WM, Rucker RC, Dalton AJ. Orf. Report of 19 human cases with clinical and pathological observations. *JAMA.* 1968;203:657.

76. Georgiades G, Katsarou A, Dimitroqlou K. Human ORF (ecthyma contagiosum). *J Hand Surg Br.* 2005;30(4):409–411.

77. Smith KJ, Skelton HG III, Yeager J, James WD, Wagner KF. Molluscum contagiosum: ultrastructural evidence for its presence in skin adjacent to clinical lesions in patients infected with human immunodeficiency virus type 1: military medical consortium for applied retroviral research. *Arch Dermatol.* 1992;128:223.

78. Forghani B, Oshiro LS, Chan CS, et al. Direct detection of molluscum contagiosum virus in clinical specimens by in situ hybridization using biotinylated probe. *Mol Cell Probes.* 1992;6:67.

79. Chen X, Anstey AV, Bugert JJ. Molluscum contagiosum virus infection. *Lancet Infect Dis.* 2013;13(10):877–888.

80. Jenkins D. Diagnosing human papillomaviruses: recent advances. *Curr Opin Infect Dis.* 2001;14:53.

81. Crum CP. Contemporary theories of cervical carcinogenesis: the virus, the host, and the stem cell. *Mod Pathol.* 2000;13:243.

82. Mork J, Lie AK, Glattre E, et al. Human papillomavirus infection as a risk factor for squamous-cell carcinoma of the head and neck. *N Engl J Med.* 2001;344:1125.

83. Syrjanen KJ. HPV infections and lung cancer. *J Clin Pathol.* 2002;55:885.

84. Astori G, Merluzzi S, Arzese A, et al. Detection of human papillomavirus DNA and p53 gene mutations in esophageal cancer samples and adjacent normal mucosa. *Digestion.* 2001;64:9.

85. Jenson AB, Geyer S, Sundberg JP, Ghim S. Human papillomavirus and skin cancer. *J Investig Dermatol Symp Proc.* 2001;6:203.

86. Meyer T, Arndt R, Nindl I, Ulrich C, Christophers E, Stockfleth E. Association of human papillomavirus infections with cutaneous tumors in immunosuppressed patients. *Transpl Int.* 2003;16:146.

87. Rock B, Shah KV, Farmer ER. A morphologic, pathologic, and virologic study of anogenital warts in men. *Arch Dermatol.* 1992;128:495.

88. Brentjens MH, Yeung-Yue KA, Lee PC, Tyring SK. Human papillomavirus: a review. *Dermatol Clin.* 2002;20:315.

89. Leigh IM, Glover MT. Skin cancer and warts in immunosuppressed renal transplant recipients. *Recent Results Cancer Res.* 1995;139:69.

90. Pereira De Oliveira WR, Carrasco S, Neto CF, Rady P, Tyring SK. Nonspecific cell-mediated immunity in patients with epidermodysplasia verruciformis. *J Dermatol.* 2003;30:203.

91. Tomasini C, Aloi F, Pippione M. Seborrheic keratosis-like lesions in epidermodysplasia verruciformis. *J Cutan Pathol.* 1993;20:237.

92. Tieben LM, Berkhout RJ, Smits HL, et al. Detection of epidermodysplasia verruciformis-like human papillomavirus types in malignant and premalignant skin lesions of renal transplant recipients. *Br J Dermatol.* 1994;131:226.

93. Berger TG, Sawchuk WS, Leonardi C, Langenberg A, Tappero J, Leboit PE. Epidermodysplasia verruciformis-associated

papillomavirus infection complicating human immunodeficiency virus disease. *Br J Dermatol.* 1991;124:79.

94. Morrison C, Eliezri Y, Magro C, Nuovo GJ. The histologic spectrum of epidermodysplasia verruciformis in transplant and AIDS patients. *J Cutan Pathol.* 2002;29:480.

95. Nuovo GJ, Ishag M. The histologic spectrum of epidermodysplasia verruciformis. *Am J Surg Pathol.* 2000;24:1400.

96. Munoz N. Human papillomavirus and cancer: the epidemiological evidence. *J Clin Virol.* 2000;19:1.

97. Anderson KM, Perez-Montiel D, Miles L, Allen CM, Nuovo GJ. The histologic differentiation of oral condyloma acuminatum from its mimics. *Oral Surg Oral Med Oral Pathol Oral Radiol Endod.* 2003;96(4):420–428.

98. Bai H, Cviko A, Granter S, Yuan L, Betensky RA, Crum CP. Immunophenotypic and viral (human papillomavirus) correlates of vulvar seborrheic keratosis. *Hum Pathol.* 2003;34(6):559–564.

99. Pirog EC, Quint KD, Yantiss RK. P16/CDKN2A and Ki-67 enhance the detection of anal intraepithelial neoplasia and condyloma and correlate with human papillomavirus detection by polymerase chain reaction. *Am J Surg Pathol.* 2010;34(10):1449–1455.

100. Chu QD, Vezeridis MP, Libbey NP, Wanebo HJ. Giant condyloma acuminatum (Buschke-Lowenstein tumor) of the anorectal and perianal regions. Analysis of 42 cases. *Dis Colon Rectum.* 1994;37(9):950–957.

101. Munger K, Howley PM. Human papillomavirus immortalization and transformation functions. *Virus Res.* 2002;89:213.

102. Yang EJ, Kong CS, Longacre TA. Vulvar and anal intraepithelial neoplasia: terminology, diagnosis, and ancillary studies. *Adv Anat Pathol.* 2017;24(3):136–150.

103. Darragh TM, Colgan TJ, Cox JT, et al. The lower anogenital squamous terminology standardization project for HPV-associated lesions: background and consensus recommendations from the College of American Pathologists and the American Society for Colposcopy and Cervical Pathology. *Arch Pathol Lab Med.* 2012;136:1266–1297.

104. Viraben R, Aquilina C, Brousset P, Bazex J. Focal epithelial hyperplasia (Heck disease) associated with AIDS. *Dermatology.* 1996;193:261.

105. Henke RP, Guerin-Reverchon I, Milde-Langosch K, Koppang HS, Löning T. In situ detection of human papillomavirus types 13 and 32 in focal epithelial hyperplasia of the oral mucosa. *J Oral Pathol Med.* 1989;18:419.

106. Kwok CS, Holland R, Gibbs S. Efficacy of topical treatments for cutaneous warts: a meta-analysis and pooled analysis of randomized controlled trials. *Br J Dermatol.* 2011;165(2):233–246.

107. Yanofsky VR, Patel RV, Goldenberg G. Genital warts: a comprehensive review. *J Clin Aesthet Dermatol.* 2012;5(6):25–36.

108. Lopez-Sanchez AF, Guijarro-Guijarro B, Hernandez-Vallejo G. Human repercussions of foot and mouth disease and other similar viral diseases. *Med Oral.* 2003;8:26.

109. Ellis AW, Kennett ML, Lewis FA, Gust ID. Hand, foot and mouth disease: an outbreak with interesting virological features. *Pathology.* 1973;5:189.

110. Stewart CL, Chu EY, Introcaso CE, Schaffer A, James WD. Coxsackievirus A6-induced hand-foot-mouth disease. *JAMA Dermatol.* 2013;149(12):1419–1421.

111. Fields JP, Mihm MC Jr, Hellreich PD, Danoff SS. Hand, foot, and mouth disease. *Arch Dermatol.* 1969;99:243.

112. Tsao KC, Chang PY, Ning HC, et al. Use of molecular assay in diagnosis of hand, foot and mouth disease caused by enterovirus 71 or coxsackievirus A 16. *J Virol Methods.* 2002;102:9.

113. Haneke E. Electron microscopic demonstration of virus particles in hand, foot and mouth disease. *Dermatologica.* 1985;171:321.

114. Schiff ER. *Atypical clinical manifestations of hepatitis A. Vaccine.* 1992;10(suppl 1):S18.

115. Nunley JR. Cutaneous manifestations of HIV and HCV. *Dermatol Nurs.* 2000;12:163.

116. Kaplan MH, Sadick N, McNutt NS, Meltzer M, Sarngadharan MG, Pahwa S. Dermatologic findings and manifestations of acquired immunodeficiency syndrome (AIDS). *J Am Acad Dermatol.* 1987;16:485.

117. Costner M, Cockerell CJ. The changing spectrum of the cutaneous manifestations of HIV disease. *Arch Dermatol.* 1998;134:1290.

118. Hulsebosch HJ, Claessen FA, van Ginkel CJ, Kuiters GR, Goudsmit J, Lange JM. Human immunodeficiency virus exanthem. *J Am Acad Dermatol.* 1990;23:483.

119. Chandwani S, Moore T, Kaul A, Krasinski K, Borkowsky W. Early diagnosis of human immunodeficiency virus type 1-infected infants by plasma p24 antigen assay after immune complex dissociation. *Pediatr Infect Dis J.* 1993;12:96.

120. Cavert W. Viral infections in human immunodeficiency virus disease. *Med Clin North Am.* 1997;81:411.

121. Birnbaum W, Hodgson TA, Reichart PA, Sherson W, Nittayananta W, Axell TE. Prognostic significance of HIV-associated oral lesions and their relation to therapy. *Oral Dis.* 2002;8(suppl 2):110.

122. Williams LR, Webster G. Warts and molluscum contagiosum. *Clin Dermatol.* 1991;9:87.

123. Koehler JE, Tappero JW. Bacillary angiomatosis and bacillary peliosis in patients infected with human immunodeficiency virus. *Clin Infect Dis.* 1993;17:612.

124. Blocker ME, Levine WC, St Louis ME. HIV prevalence in patients with syphilis, United States. *Sex Transm Dis.* 2000;27:53.

125. Cohen PR, Grossman ME. Recognizing skin lesions of systemic fungal infections in patients with AIDS. *Am Fam Physician.* 1994;49:1627.

126. Czelusta A, Yen-Moore A, Van der SM, Carrasco D, Tyring SK. An overview of sexually transmitted diseases. Part III: sexually transmitted diseases in HIV-infected patients. *J Am Acad Dermatol.* 2000;43:409.

127. Patrizi A, Neri I, Chieregato C, Misciali M. Demodicidosis in immunocompetent young children: report of eight cases. *Dermatology.* 1997;195:239.

128. Lifson AR, Hessol NA, Buchbinder SP, Holmberg SD. The association of clinical conditions and serologic tests with CD4+ lymphocyte counts in HIV-infected subjects without AIDS. *AIDS.* 1991;5:1209.

129. Soeprono FF, Schinella RA, Cockerell CJ, Comite SL. Seborrheic-like dermatitis of acquired immunodeficiency syndrome: a clinicopathologic study. *J Am Acad Dermatol.* 1986;14:242.

130. Smith KJ, Skelton HG, Yeager J, et al. Cutaneous findings in HIV-1-positive patients: a 42-month prospective study: Military Medical Consortium for the Advancement of Retroviral Research (MMCARR). *J Am Acad Dermatol.* 1994;31:746.

131. Farthing CF, Staughton RC, Rowland Payne CM. Skin disease in homosexual patients with acquired immune deficiency syndrome (AIDS) and lesser forms of human T cell leukaemia virus (HTLV III) disease. *Clin Exp Dermatol.* 1985;10:3.

132. Buchness MR, Lim HW, Hatcher VA, Sanchez M, Soter NA. Eosinophilic pustular folliculitis in the acquired immunodeficiency syndrome: treatment with ultraviolet B phototherapy. *N Engl J Med.* 1988;318:1183.

133. Rico MJ, Kory WP, Gould EW, Penneys NS. Interface dermatitis in patients with the acquired immunodeficiency syndrome. *J Am Acad Dermatol.* 1987;16:1209.

134. Coopman SA, Stern RS. Cutaneous drug reactions in human immunodeficiency virus infection. *Arch Dermatol.* 1991;127:714.

135. Gregory N, DeLeo VA. Clinical manifestations of photosensitivity in patients with human immunodeficiency virus infection. *Arch Dermatol.* 1994;130:630.

136. Martinelli PT, Tyring SK. Human herpesvirus 8. *Dermatol Clin.* 2002;20:307.

137. McGregor JM, Newell M, Ross J, Kirkham N, McGibbon DH, Darley C. Cutaneous malignant melanoma and human

immunodeficiency virus (HIV) infection: a report of three cases. *Br J Dermatol.* 1992;126:516.

138. Smith KJ, Skelton HG III, Angritt P. Histopathologic features of HIV-associated skin disease. *Dermatol Clin.* 1991;9:551.

139. Hevia O, Jimenez-Acosta F, Ceballos PI, Gould EW, Penneys NS. Pruritic papular eruption of the acquired immunodeficiency syndrome: a clinicopathologic study. *J Am Acad Dermatol.* 1991;24:231.

140. Goodman DS, Teplitz ED, Wishner A, Klein RS, Burk PG, Hershenbaum E. Prevalence of cutaneous disease in patients with acquired immunodeficiency syndrome (AIDS) or AIDS-related complex. *J Am Acad Dermatol.* 1987;17:210.

141. Holmes RB, Martins C, Horn T. The histopathology of folliculitis in HIV-infected patients. *J Cutan Pathol.* 2002;29:93.

142. Murakawa GJ, McCalmont T, Altman J, et al. Disseminated acanthamebiasis in patients with AIDS. A report of five cases and a review of the literature. *Arch Dermatol.* 1995;131:1291.

143. Holland PV, Alter HJ. The clinical significance of hepatitis B virus antigens and antibodies. *Med Clin North Am.* 1975;59:849.

144. Befeler AS, Di Bisceglie AM. Hepatitis B. *Infect Dis Clin North Am.* 2000;14:617.

145. Willson RA. Extrahepatic manifestations of chronic viral hepatitis. *Am J Gastroenterol.* 1997;92:3.

146. Parsons ME, Russo GG, Millikan LE. Dermatologic disorders associated with viral hepatitis infections. *Int J Dermatol.* 1996;35:77.

147. Gianotti F. HBsAg and papular acrodermatitis of childhood. *N Engl J Med.* 1978;298:460.

148. Nelson JS, Stone MS. Update on selected viral exanthems. *Curr Opin Pediatr.* 2000;12:359.

149. Rosen LB, Rywlin AM, Resnick L. Hepatitis B surface antigen positive skin lesions: two case reports with an immunoperoxidase study. *Am J Dermatopathol.* 1985;7:507.

150. Gower RG, Sausker WF, Kohler PF, Thorne GE, McIntosh RM. Small vessel vasculitis caused by hepatitis B virus immune complexes: small vessel vasculitis and HBsAG. *J Allergy Clin Immunol.* 1978;62:222.

151. Pyrsopoulos NT, Reddy K. Extrahepatic manifestations of chronic viral hepatitis. *Curr Gastroenterol Rep.* 2001;3:71.

152. Limas C, Limas CJ. Lichen planus in children: a possible complication of hepatitis B vaccines. *Pediatr Dermatol.* 2002;19:204.

153. Jackson JM. Hepatitis C and the skin. *Dermatol Clin.* 2002;20:449.

154. Jones AM, Warken K, Tyring SK. The cutaneous manifestations of viral hepatitis. *Dermatol Clin.* 2002;20:233.

155. Pawlotsky JM, Dhumeaux D, Bagot M. Hepatitis C virus in dermatology a review. *Arch Dermatol.* 1995;131:1185.

156. Chuang TY, Brashear R, Lewis C. Porphyria cutanea tarda and hepatitis C virus: a case-control study and meta-analysis of the literature. *J Am Acad Dermatol.* 1999;41:31.

157. Calista D, Landi G. Lichen planus, erythema nodosum, and erythema multiforme in a patient with chronic hepatitis C. *Cutis.* 2001;67:454.

158. Madison DL, Allen E, Deodhar A, Morrison L. Henoch-Schonlein purpura: a possible complication of hepatitis C related liver cirrhosis. *Ann Rheum Dis.* 2002;61:281.

159. Akaogi J, Yotsuyanagi H, Sugata F, Matsuda T, Hino K. Hepatitis viral infection in Behcet's disease. *Hepatol Res.* 2000;17:126.

160. Khanna VJ, Shieh S, Benjamin J, et al. Necrolytic acral erythema associated with hepatitis C: effective treatment with interferon alfa and zinc. *Arch Dermatol.* 2000;136:755.

161. Cacoub P, Maisonobe T, Thibault V, et al. Systemic vasculitis in patients with hepatitis C. *J Rheumatol.* 2001;28:109.

162. Neri S, Raciti C, D'Angelo G, Ierna D, Bruno CM. Hyde's prurigo nodularis and chronic HCV hepatitis. *J Hepatol.* 1998;28:161.

163. Keane FM, MacFarlane CS, Munn SE, Higgins EM. Pyoderma gangrenosum and hepatitis C virus infection. *Br J Dermatol.* 1998;139:924.

164. Daoud MS, Gibson LE, Daoud S, el-Azhary RA. Chronic hepatitis C and skin diseases: a review. *Mayo Clin Proc.* 1995;70:559.

165. Zignego AL, Piluso A, Giannini C. HBV and HCV chronic infection: autoimmune manifestations and lymphoproliferation. *Autoimmun Rev.* 2008;8:107–111.

166. Berk DR, Mallory SB, Keeffe SB, Ahmed A. Dermatologic disorders associated with chronic hepatitis C: effect of interferon therapy. *Clin Gastroenterol Hepatol.* 2007;52:142–151.

167. Katta R. Parvovirus B19: a review. *Dermatol Clin.* 2002;20:333.

168. Grilli R, Izquierdo MJ, Farina MC, et al. Papular-purpuric "gloves and socks" syndrome: polymerase chain reaction demonstration of parvovirus B19 DNA in cutaneous lesions and sera. *J Am Acad Dermatol.* 1999;41:793.

169. Garcia-Tapia AM, Fernandez-Gutierrez dA, Giron JA, et al. Spectrum of parvovirus B19 infection: analysis of an outbreak of 43 cases in Cadiz, Spain. *Clin Infect Dis.* 1995;21:1424.

170. Boeck K, Mempel M, Schmidt T, Abeck D. Gianotti-Crosti syndrome: clinical, serologic, and therapeutic data from nine children. *Cutis.* 1998;62:271.

171. Cioc AM, Sedmak DD, Nuovo GJ, Dawood MR, Smart G, Magro CM. Parvovirus B19 associated adult Henoch Schonlein purpura. *J Cutan Pathol.* 2002;29:602.

172. Magro CM, Dawood MR, Crowson AN. The cutaneous manifestations of human parvovirus B19 infection. *Hum Pathol.* 2000;31:488.

173. Chakrabarty A, Beutner K. Therapy of other viral infections: herpes to hepatitis. *Dermatol Ther.* 2004;17:465–490.

174. Stalkup JR. A review of measles virus. *Dermatol Clin.* 2002;20:209.

175. Ackerman AB, Suringa DW. Multinucleate epidermal cells in measles. *Arch Dermatol.* 1971;103:180.

176. McNutt NS, Kindel S, Lugo J. Cutaneous manifestations of measles in AIDS. *J Cutan Pathol.* 1992;19:315.

177. Vander Straten MR, Tyring SK. Rubella. *Dermatol Clin.* 2002;20:225.

178. Cherry JD. Viral exanthems. *Dis Mon.* 1982;28:1.

179. Feng H, Shuda M, Chang Y, Moore PS. Clonal integration of a poluomavirus in human Merkel cell carcinoma. *Science* 2008;319:1096–1100.

180. Spurgeon ME, Lambert PF. Merkel cell polyomavirus: a newly discovered human virus with oncogenic potential. *Virology.* 2013;435:118–130.

181. Wanat KA, Holler PD, Dentchev T, et al. Viral-associated trichodysplasia: characterization of a novel polyomavirus infection with therapeutic insights. *Arch Dermatol.* 2012;148: 219–223.

182. PDQ Adult Treatment Editorial Board. *Merkel Cell Carcinoma Treatment (PDQ®): Health Professional Version. In PDQ Cancer Information Summaries [Internet].* National Cancer Institute (US); 2021.

183. Galván Casas C, Català A, Carretero Hernández G, et al. Classification of the cutaneous manifestations of COVID-19: a rapid prospective nationwide consensus study in Spain with 375 cases. *Br J Dermatol.* 2020;183(1):71–77.

184. McMahon DE, Gallman AE, Hruza GJ, et al. Long COVID in the skin: a registry analysis of COVID-19 dermatological duration. *Lancet Infect Dis.* 2021;21(3):313–314.

The Histiocytoses

MICHAEL WILK AND BERNHARD WILHELM HEINRICH ZELGER

INTRODUCTION

Histiocytoses cover a wide range of inflammatory as well as benign and malignant disorders unified only by being for the most part uncommon and poorly understood. The "X" in histiocytosis X, as originally proposed by Lichtenstein (1), was designed to reflect the unknown; even though we have drifted away from the designation, to some degree it still reflects the state of our knowledge. The word "histiocyte" itself is not particularly helpful. Loosely translated, it means a "cell of the tissue." The term histiocyte has been defined as a tissue macrophage or cell of the mononuclear phagocytic system; however, many of the diseases known as histiocytoses are not disorders of macrophages but instead involve dendritic cells or other lines of differentiation. Despite these misgivings, we retain the term histiocytosis, as have both textbooks (2) and reviews (3).

There are two major cell lines responsible for the spectrum of diseases considered as histiocytoses—macrophages and dendritic cells. They are noticeable in embryonic skin before the bone marrow starts to function (4,5). Both have common stem cell ancestors, which are located in the yolk sac and fetal liver (4). They are maintained in the tissue after birth via long life and self-renewal. Another pathway is the renewal of tissue-resident macrophages and Langerhans cells (LCs) by activation from bone marrow-derived precursors (e.g., monocytes or classic dendritic cell precursors) upon cell damage and inflammation. This, in the case of LCs, is characterized by take-up of antigens in the epidermis or mucosa and migration through the dermis to lymphatics and then lymph nodes where they present the processed antigens in association with major histocompatibility complex molecules to T cells (4). LCs seem to be capable of processing and presenting antigens already *in utero*. They move into the epidermis throughout life, unlike melanocytes—which do this only during embryogenesis (5).

Apart from LCs representing the dendritic cells of the multilayered squamous epithelium, there are further dendritic cells, especially classic dendritic cells, plasmacytoid dendritic cells, and monocyte-derived inflammatory dendritic cells, each of them having characteristic cell distributions and immunophenotypes. Their precise function in human disease is still being unraveled (4).

Histiocytoses, in actuality, comprise diseases from LCs, macrophages (with the capacity of phagocytosis) and monocytes—the latter being involved in the replenishment of the former during inflammation or the production of "inflammatory macrophages" (4).

The following markers are useful in identifying these groups of cells (Table 26-1):

1. There are a number of monoclonal antibodies available to identify macrophages; most are directed against CD68. Stains for CD14 and CD163 are also used. Both fascin and factor XIIIa also mark these cells but are less specific.
2. The LC as an antigen-processing dendritic cell is characterized by Birbeck granules, S100 protein, CD1a, and langerin (CD207) positivity. The more mature form having migrated to regional lymph nodes is the interdigitating dendritic cell (IDC), which lacks Birbeck granules, CD1a, and langerin.
3. A source of confusion is the indeterminate cell, whose vague name accurately reflects the current situation. No single definition is agreed upon; possibilities cited in the literature include the following:
   - A veiled cell, which is a LC migrating to the dermis.
   - A LC precursor (exactly the opposite of a veiled cell).
   - A cell with features of both a macrophage and a LC. There is marked overlap between the dermal dendritic cells and macrophages with potential for shifting markers even relatively late in development.

A number of cautions are in order. A diagnosis is rarely, if ever, based on the presence or absence of a single antigen but instead is based on the clinicopathologic picture. Both macrophages and dendritic cells go through a maturation process, and so their profiles may change. In addition, because monocytes and most dendritic cells arise from a similar bone marrow-derived stem cell, there are overlaps with macrophages expressing S100 proteins but not CD1a or langerin; similarly, dermal dendritic cells may express macrophage markers.

Histiocytic lesions can usually be diagnosed based on their light microscopic pattern and with a limited number of special stains (Table 26-2).

Table 26-1	
Markers for "Histiocytes"	
Cell Type	**Useful Marker**
Monocyte	CD14
Macrophage	CD14, CD68, CD163
Sinus histiocytosis macrophage	CD14, CD68, CD163, S-100 protein, fascin
Langerhans cell	CD1a, Langerin (CD207), S100 protein

Table 26-2

Simplified Approach to Histiocytic Lesions

	S100 Protein	CD1a or Langerin	CD68
LCD	+	+	-
RDD	+	-	+
JXG	-	-	+

JXG, juvenile xanthogranuloma; LCD, Langerhans cell disease; RDD, Rosai–Dorfman disease.

In recent years, a new classification of histiocytoses and neoplasms of the macrophage–dendritic cell lineages has emerged in the literature from the working group of the Histiocyte society (3). It is based on clinical, radiographic, pathologic, phenotypic, genetic, and/or molecular features (Table 26-3).

The basic histologic pattern created by macrophages is a granuloma. One variant is a xanthogranuloma (XG), which includes lipids as well as macrophages. In addition to the diseases

Table 26-3

Classification of the Five Groups of Histiocytoses

L Group

- LCH
- ICH
- ECD
- Mixed LCH/ECD

C Group

- Cutaneous non-Langerhans cell histiocytosis

XG family: JXG, AXG, GCRH, BCH, GEH, PNH

Non-XG family: cutaneous RDD, NXG

- Cutaneous non-Langerhans cell histiocytosis with significant system involvement

XG family: XD

Non-XG family: MRH

R Group

- Familial RDD
- Sporadic RDD: classic RDD, extranodal RDD, RDD with neoplasia or immune disease, unclassified

M Group

- Primary MH
- Secondary MH (hematologic neoplasia)

H Group

- Primary hemophagocytic lymphohistiocytosis: monogenic inherited conditions leading to HLH
- Secondary HLH (non-Mendelian)
- HLH of uncertain origin

AXG, adult xanthogranuloma; BCH, benign cephalic histiocytosis; ECD, Erdheim–Chester disease; GCRH, giant cell reticulohistiocytoma; GEH, generalized eruptive histiocytosis; HLH, hemophagocytic lymphohistiocytosis; ICH, histiocytosis of the indeterminate cell; JXG, juvenile xanthogranuloma; LCH, Langerhans cell histiocytosis; MH, malignant histiocytosis; MRH, multicentric reticulohistiocytosis; NXG, necrobiotic xanthogranuloma; PNH, progressive nodular histiocytosis; RDD, Rosai–Dorfman disease; XD, xanthoma disseminatum; XG, xanthogranuloma. Adapted from Emile et al. (3).

to be discussed in this chapter, a wide array of disorders can display similar histologic patterns. Most are discussed elsewhere in this book.

1. Metabolic disorders: In addition to hyperlipoproteinemias and other disorders of fat metabolism, which will be covered in this chapter, many lysosomal disorders and other storage diseases may feature cutaneous xanthomas or other infiltrates. The diagnosis of these latter disorders is not a practical question for the dermatopathologist, and they will not be further considered.

2. Infectious diseases: Tuberculosis, lepromatous leprosy, other mycobacterial infections, and leishmaniasis may produce granulomas.

3. Proliferations: Some lymphomas present with cutaneous granulomatous infiltrates; included in this group are Hodgkin lymphoma and some forms of T-cell lymphoma. Many diseases diagnosed in the past as histiocytic malignancies are lymphomas. Malignant fibrous histiocytoma and its more superficial cutaneous variant atypical fibroxanthoma are established diagnoses, but their line of differentiation remains controversial. Melanocytic lesions can be confused with macrophage disorders, both clinically and histologically. The red-brown color of XGs is similar to that of Spitz nevi. Touton giant cells can sometimes be confused with multinucleated rosette cells in melanocytic nevi.

4. Trauma: Most dermatofibromas and some verruciform xanthomas are the result of trauma, be it an insect bite, folliculitis, or another insult. Some xanthomas arise secondary to cutaneous damage from light or after marked inflammation. External objects—such as glass fragments, silica, and many others—may produce cutaneous granulomas, often of the sarcoidal type. A ruptured follicular cyst is also accompanied by a macrophage response.

5. Idiopathic: Unfortunately, most "histiocytic" diseases fit here, and there is little logic to what has been considered a macrophage disorder and what has been classified elsewhere. For example, granuloma annulare has a macrophage infiltrate but is considered a necrobiotic disorder with palisading granuloma. Both rheumatoid arthritis and sarcoidosis may feature infiltrates of macrophages in the skin and other organs; nonetheless, they are not considered "histiocytoses."

THE LANGERHANS GROUP (L GROUP)

Langerhans Cell Disease

Clinical Summary. The clinical spectrum of Langerhans cell disease (LCD) is broad, with skin involvement a common finding (6,7). Whereas LCD has been subdivided into several clinical types, overlaps are the rule, not the exception, and lumping appears more appropriate than splitting. Acute disseminated LCD (*Abt–Letterer–Siwe disease*) usually occurs in infants but can be seen in older children or adults. Most patients are seriously ill, around 10% of them having a fatal outcome. The most common manifestations are fever, anemia, thrombocytopenia, enlargement of the liver and spleen, and lymphadenopathy. In particular, patients with involvement of liver, spleen, or bone marrow carry a poor prognosis. Osteolytic lesions are uncommon except in the mastoid region of the temporal bone, resulting in a clinical picture of otitis media. Isolated pulmonary LCD is rare and typically occurs in adult smokers, but lung involvement can be seen in children with widespread disease, in whom it is a poor sign. LCD of the central nervous system can occur either as a central mass lesion (in the hypothalamic pituitary region leading to diabetes insipidus) or as a manifestation associated with progressive neurodegeneration (7).

Cutaneous lesions are found in about 80% of cases, often as a presenting sign. Numerous closely set, red-brown papules covered with scales or crusts may be accompanied by petechiae. This type of eruption may be extensive, involving particularly the scalp, face, and trunk, with a striking resemblance to seborrheic dermatitis. Cutaneous LCD is very pleomorphic; lesions may be vesicular, ulcerated, urticarial, or, rarely, xanthomatous. In the elderly, anogenital involvement is common and is often clinically misleading, causing a delay in diagnosis. If there is a diffuse cutaneous eruption, one must anticipate multiorgan involvement. Individual patients must be monitored closely because internal organ involvement may occur later in the course of the disease.

Congenital self-healing reticulohistiocytosis (CSHRH) (*Hashimoto–Pritzker disease*) (8) is another variant of LCD, not a distinct disorder. As the name implies, it usually has a favorable outcome. It is usually present at birth but may not appear until several days or weeks after delivery. Affected infants have scattered papules and nodules. Large nodules tend to become eroded or ulcerated. Usually, the number of lesions varies from several to a dozen; on rare occasions, numerous lesions are widely scattered over the entire skin. In about 25% of cases, a solitary nodule is present. The lesions begin to involute within 2 to 3 months and usually have completely regressed within 12 months. But the patients should be carefully followed up; relapses may occur, including bone involvement, and the occasional case may advance to acute disseminated disease (9,10). Although acute disseminated LCD may also be present at birth, it is rarely nodular.

In chronic multifocal LCD, diabetes insipidus, exophthalmos, and multiple defects of the bones, especially of the cranium, represent the classic triad of *Hand–Schüller–Christian disease*, a presentation of LCD usually affecting infants and less frequently older children and adolescents. Any one or even all three of the cardinal symptoms may be absent, and entirely different organs may be involved. For example, enlargement of the liver, spleen, lungs, or lymph nodes may be found. Osteolytic lesions of the long bones may result in spontaneous fractures. In Hand–Schüller–Christian disease, the diabetes insipidus is caused by granulomatous infiltration of the hypothalamus–pituitary axis; the exophthalmos, by retroorbital accumulations of granulomatous tissue; and the multiple defects in the skull by the osteolytic effect of granulomatous infiltrates. Cutaneous lesions occur in about one-third of the cases. Three types of skin lesions may be found. The most common are infiltrated nodules and plaques undergoing ulceration, especially in the axillae, the anogenital region, and the mouth. Next in frequency is an extensive eruption identical to that in Abt–Letterer–Siwe disease but usually less severe. Finally, in rare instances xanthomas are seen.

Chronic focal LCD or *eosinophilic granuloma* represents the fourth and least severe but most common variant, accounting for 70% to 80% of all pediatric LCDs usually affecting infants. The lesions are either solitary or few. Most common are

lesions of the bones, but the skin or the oral mucosa is occasionally involved, either with or without osseous lesions. Involvement of the jaw leading to a loose or floating tooth is a fairly typical occurrence. Although the lesions are usually chronic, some heal spontaneously, and simple surgery is generally curative. In rare instances, cases originally diagnosed as chronic focal disease may progress into multifocal or even disseminated diseases.

There are a number of unusual cutaneous manifestations of LCD. Mucosal involvement, such as of the lip, has been described (11). Nail changes are also seen and are generally associated with systemic involvement (12). There are cases where LCD is associated with juvenile xanthogranuloma (JXG) (13).

The clinical course and the prognosis of LCD are difficult to predict. The most important parameters in prognosis are those recommended for staging: the age of the patient, the number of organs involved, and the degree of organ dysfunction. Abnormalities of the bone marrow, spleen, liver, or lungs suggest a poor prognosis. Skin involvement alone correlates with a favorable outcome. Paradoxically, the presence of skin disease at birth (the nodules of CSHRH) is a good sign, but involvement before the age of 2 years (Letterer–Siwe disease) is a bad one. Histologic features correlate poorly with the outcome. In particular, adults with LCD are at risk for a variety of systemic neoplasms, including lymphomas, leukemias, and lung neoplasms, affecting around 30% of patients (14). In addition, they may experience secondary macrophage activation syndrome (MAS), also known as reactive hemophagocytic lymphohistiocytosis, which is usually fatal. In general, about 10% of patients with multifocal disease die, 30% undergo complete remission, and the remaining 60% embark upon a chronic, shifting course (15).

Histopathology. The histologic picture unites the many varied forms of LCD. The key to diagnosis is identifying the typical LCD cell in the appropriate surroundings. The cell has a distinct folded or lobulated, often kidney-shaped, nucleus. Nucleoli are not prominent, and the slightly eosinophilic cytoplasm is unremarkable. A variety of methods can be used to confirm the identity of such cells. For years, the gold standard has been to use electron microscopy to search for the typical Birbeck or LC granules. Today, S100 protein, CD1a, and langerin (CD207) can all be identified using paraffin-fixed tissue. Langerin is every bit as specific as Birbeck granules. In addition, the *BRAF p.V600E* mutation present in many cases of LCD can be detected immunohistochemically using the VE1 antibody (16).

Although Lever emphasized three kinds of histologic reactions in LCD—proliferative, granulomatous, and xanthomatous—only the first two are commonly seen. A relationship exists between the type of histologic reaction and the clinical type of disease. The visceral lesions seen in LCD show the same three types of reactions as the skin. In general, the proliferative reaction with its almost pure LC infiltrate is typical of acute disseminated LCD and the granulomatous reaction of chronic focal or multifocal LCD, as the name eosinophilic granuloma suggests. The xanthomatous reaction is seen in Hand–Schüller–Christian disease but primarily in other organs, especially the meninges and bones. Xanthomatous lesions in the skin are decidedly rare.

The proliferative reaction is encountered in the skin as petechiae, as well as almost translucent, hemorrhagic, or crusted papules. It is characterized by the presence of an extensive infiltrate of LCs. The infiltrate usually lies close to or involves the epidermis, resulting in ulceration and crusting (Fig. 26-1A). Large, kidney-shaped cells can be seen just below or even impinging on the epidermis (Fig. 26-1B–D). Staining for S100 protein, CD1a, or langerin (Fig. 26-1E) shows both the normal and abnormal LCs.

While CSHRH cannot be definitely separated from other lesions of LCD under the microscope, there are valuable clues. The nodules of CSHRH tend to show densely aggregated LCs, often with abundant eosinophilic cytoplasm (Fig. 26-1F) and eosinophils.

The granulomatous reaction is found most commonly in infiltrated plaques and nodules in the genital area, in the axillary region, or on the scalp, as well as in the soft tissue and

bone lesions. Extensive aggregates of LCs often extend deep into the dermis. Eosinophils are present in various quantities (Fig. 26-1F). Generally, they lie in clusters instead of being diffusely scattered and may develop into microabscesses. Irregularly shaped, multinucleated giant cells are occasionally seen. In addition, some neutrophils, lymphocytes, and plasma cells may be present. Frequently, extravasation of erythrocytes is found. The diversity of lesional cells being attracted by LCD cells may hide the latter, which often are in a minority.

The uncommon xanthomatous reaction reveals numerous foamy cells as well as varying numbers of LCs and some eosinophils in the dermis. Multinucleated giant cells are frequently present.

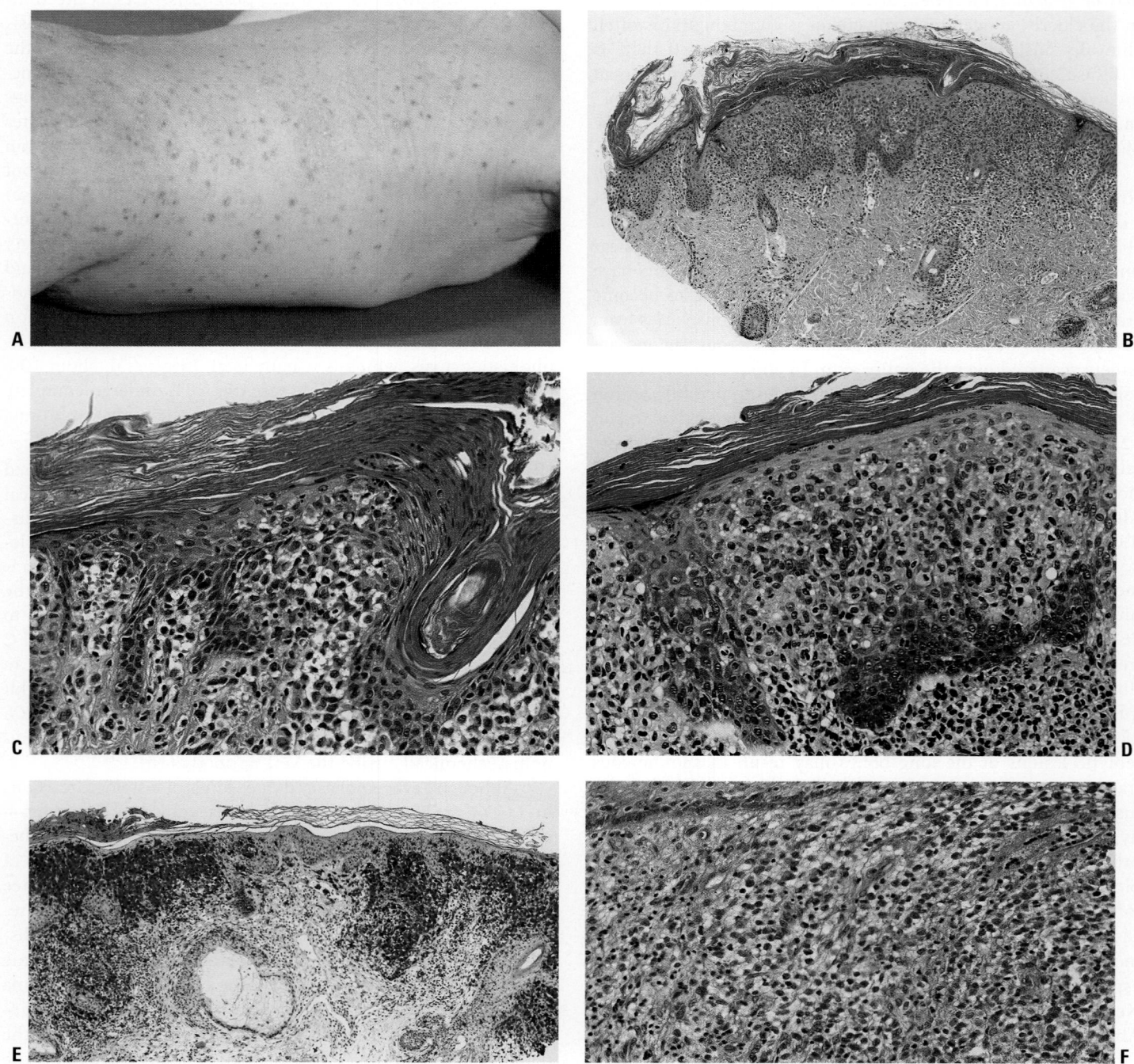

Figure 26-1 Langerhans cell (LC) disease. **A:** Widespread hemorrhagic papules with scale in an infant. **B:** Crusted papular lesion in an infant. A dense cellular infiltrate is seen beneath the crust. **C:** Higher magnification showing accumulations of LCs along the epidermal–dermal junction. **D:** Another lesion with extensive exocytosis of LCs. **E:** Staining with antilangerin identifies both normal epidermal LCs and the tumoral LCs. **F:** A deep, nodular cutaneous infiltrate rich in eosinophils with clusters of typical large LCs. (A: Courtesy of Wilfried Neuse, Düsseldorf, Germany.)

They are mainly of the foreign-body type but occasionally have the appearance of Touton giant cells. The S100 protein and CD1a staining is occasionally weak or mostly negative in the foamy cells.

Malignant LCD. Acute disseminated LCD can reasonably be argued to be a malignancy because it is progressive, destructive, and potentially fatal and shows clonality. Although some cases have been identified with marked cytologic atypia, including mitoses, and a poor clinical outcome, cellular morphology usually is a poor way to predict the course of LCD. The term Langerhans cell sarcoma has been applied to solitary or multiple cutaneous lesions with marked cellular atypia and increased mitotic rate (17,18). On occasion, soft tissue and nodal neoplasms have been found that stained only for LCD markers (19).

Pathogenesis. LCD is nowadays considered to represent a clonal expansion of myeloid precursors that differentiate into CD1a$^+$/CD207$^+$ in lesions and, thus, represent an inflammatory myeloid neoplasm (4,7). The neoplastic nature is supported by molecular biology having found recurrent *BRAFpV600E* mutations in about 50% of LCDs (20), correlating with high-risk disease. This mutation is not typically present in peripheral blood mononuclear cells in infants with skin-limited disease. A further 19% of patients harbor *MAP2K1* mutations (21–23). Other, more rare mutations including *ARAF, MAP3K1, PIK3CA, PICK1,* and *PIK3R2* have been identified as well (6,23).

Notably, LCD frequently does not behave like a malignant neoplasia, and spontaneous remissions occur, especially in the youngest patients presenting skin lesions at birth. Erdheim–Chester disease (ECD) exhibits similar molecular characteristics, which is reflected by an occasional association of both conditions which with respect to their dermatologic lesions look different (24). LCD has also been reported to occur together with lymphomas, indicating a clonal relationship. Although LCs and LCD cells share ultrastructural and immunohistologic characteristics (Birbeck granules, CD1a, Langerin-CD207), LCD cells are devoid of dendrites and do not have the capacity to migrate. In addition, LCD cells have been reported to have a different gene expression profile than do normal epidermal LCs, revealing the presence of a more immature myeloid precursor in the former (25).

Differential Diagnosis. The differential diagnosis for LCD varies with the histologic pattern. The most difficult situation is an early proliferative dermatitic lesion with little epidermotropism and few characteristic cells. Without adequate clinical background, it is easy to make the mistaken diagnosis of superficial perivascular or lichenoid dermatitis. One should keep LCD in mind in all biopsies of dermatitis from infants and freely employ the S100 protein stain for screening. When a nodule or tumor is present, the presence of eosinophils and the sheets of characteristic cells usually lead to the diagnosis. The cutaneous xanthomas are not distinctive, and whereas the foamy cells may stain weakly with S100 protein or CD1a, usually the surrounding infiltrate has enough positive cells to allow a diagnosis. Some cases of CSHRH may be clinically confused with the blueberry muffin syndrome, congenital leukemic infiltrates, or mast cell disease, but the microscopic picture provides clarity.

Principles of Management: Therapy is often not needed, as LCD has a tendency toward self-resolution. Treatment for purely cutaneous disease should not be aggressive. Solitary lesions can be excised. Topical corticosteroids are the first choice for cutaneous disease; alternatives include topical calcineurin inhibitors and topical nitrogen mustard as well as systemic methotrexate and thalidomide. All patients with systemic diseases should be considered for study protocols. The standard treatment is vincristine and prednisone, which is better tolerated by children than adults, in case supplemented by 6-mercaptopurine. The duration of therapy is 6 months for skin, bone, or lymph node involvement; patients with multisystemic, high-risk disease benefit from a prolonged 12 months maintenance treatment. For patients with low-risk disease, less toxic alternatives have been shown to be effective. The introduction of BRAF and MEK inhibitors provided promising results; however, the impact of these new therapeutic agents on overall survival rates must be awaited.

Indeterminate Cell Histiocytosis/Indeterminate Dendritic Cell Tumor

Clinical Summary. The diagnosis of indeterminate cell histiocytosis (ICH) was first proposed by Wood et al. (26) when they reassessed a previously reported case (27). Clinically, most patients are adults and show numerous frequently self-limiting, but sometimes persistent, red-brown papules or nodules on the trunk and extremities that may coalesce. The symptoms are almost always limited to the skin (28). A number of cases are paraneoplastic. The clinical presentation in itself is not distinctive, but the condition is also included in the World Health Organization (WHO) classification of skin tumors (29).

Histopathology. The histologic picture is quite variable. Most commonly, an infiltrate of vacuolated cells, most likely macrophages, intermingled with eosinophils, scattered giant cells, and foamy cells is found. The cells are positive for S100 protein and CD68 and show focal CD1a reactivity as well (30). In general, the infiltrates with S100 protein staining also tend to have eosinophils. A spindle cell variant has also been described (31). The other variation is a form of LCD without langerin positivity or Birbeck granules. Using these criteria, both cutaneous and nodal lesions have been reported (32,33). Our current approach is to try and classify the lesions as either LCD or XG and simultaneously investigate these patients for possible underlying hematologic malignancy.

Pathogenesis. Cases described as ICH have little to do with the several different cells described as indeterminate cells. We suspect that most cases are macrophage disorders—variants of XG in which the predominant cell is derived from an earlier or aberrant lineage (34). Other cases, such as those resembling CSHRH, are most likely variants on LCD. Some examples of ICH may be reactive; such infiltrates have been described in nodular scabies (35) and after pityriasis rosea (36). A *ETV3-NCOA2,* but inconsistent (28) gene fusion, has been detected in a number of cases (37). A few cases have been associated with a non-Hodgkin lymphoma (33,38), and recently, one patient with synchronous *NRAS p.G12V* mutated ICH and chronic myelomonocytic leukemia has been described (39). Future studies are necessary to reveal if ICH represents a distinct clinical disease.

Differential Diagnosis. The differential is usually some variant of XG, with all the other forms in the differential.

Principles of Management: There is no effective therapy.

Erdheim–Chester Disease

Clinical Summary. ECD is a rare macrophage disorder almost always seen in adult (mean age > 50 years) males more frequently than females, featuring osteosclerotic lesions of the long bones (in contrast to osteolytic lesions in LCD) associated with extraskeletal disease in 50% of cases (24,40,41). Rarely, children have been reported with the disease. Any organ can be infiltrated by ECD. Systemic involvement especially includes kidneys, lungs, and CNS, as well as retroperitoneum and diabetes insipidus, the latter often being the first clinical sign of the disease. Skin is the third most common such site involved in 30% of cases (42) and is the first manifestation of the disease in 20% of cases (42,43). Individuals most commonly present with lesions on the face, and some patients present with predominant skin disease (44), a presentation called asymptomatic or minimally symptomatic (45). Typical findings include xanthelasmas in particular and red-brown papules or nodules occasionally, suggesting JXG. Therefore, in patients with xanthelasmas, especially with more extensive presentation, a whole body examination should be performed. Patients with both LCD, ECD (46) or Rosai–Dorfman-like disease have been reported (47), and especially these may also suffer from myeloid neoplasms (48).

Histopathology. Owing to their long-standing character, the skin lesions are usually more fibrous than ordinary JXG and often have hemosiderin; Touton giant cells are found. The cells are positive for macrophage markers and occasionally S-100 protein with negativity for CD1a and langerin (CD207). However, patients with concomitant LCD may show features of both diseases in the same biopsy (48). In addition, biopsies from patients presenting with mutated *BRAF* stain positive for the anti-BRAF-p.V600E antibody VE1 (42). Unusual histologic features including neutrophilic infiltrates with microabscesses, dermatofibroma-like morphology, and dense perivascular lymphoid aggregates have been reported (49).

Pathogenesis. ECD is now considered to represent an inflammatory myeloid neoplasm (24,50). Using molecular biology techniques, *BRAF p.V600E* mutations have been found in 66% of cases as well as *MAP2K1, NRAS, KRAS, ARAF,* and *PIK3CA* mutations. Thus, the diagnosis of ECD is nowadays based on clinical/morphologic findings, histopathology, and molecular

features (24,50,51). This approach is especially important in order to exclude cases with disseminated disease of XG. In addition, it has been recommended to screen progressive cases of doubt for ALK expression after having considered and excluded ALK-positive anaplastic lymphoma (3).

Principles of Management: The outlook for patients with extraskeletal diseases is poor, with most dying within 3 to 5 years from cerebral, renal, cardiac, or pulmonary disease. The application of interferon alfa, anti-cytokine therapy, and—in severe cases—BRAF and MEK inhibitors have been shown to have benefit for the patient (24,50).

CUTANEOUS NON-LANGERHANS CELL HISTIOCYTOSES (C GROUP)

Xanthogranuloma Family

The XG family is the largest group of cutaneous histiocytic disorders. The source of XG cells is unclear; the two most likely candidates are macrophages and dendritic cells. Macrophages seem most promising based on CD68 and/or CD163 staining and their propensity for xanthomatous transformation (52). Another explanation is alternate activation of macrophages, leading to the expression of stabilin 1, a receptor that links exogenous signals to a variety of intracellular vesicular functions. Stabilin 1 can be identified by anti–MS-1 antibodies and seems to be a marker for cutaneous macrophage disorders, as compared to systemic ones (53). We use the term macrophages for the rest of this chapter, fully recognizing that it may be incorrect in some instances.

XGs contain cells with a wide variety of morphologic characteristics, including vacuolated (bright cytoplasm with moderate vacuoles), foamy (xanthomatized), spindle-shaped, scalloped (moderately eosinophilic cytoplasm with star-shaped tips), and oncocytic (epithelioid cells with homogeneously, strong eosinophilic cytoplasm) cells (Fig. 26-2). A classic XG contains a mixture of these different cell types, but there are

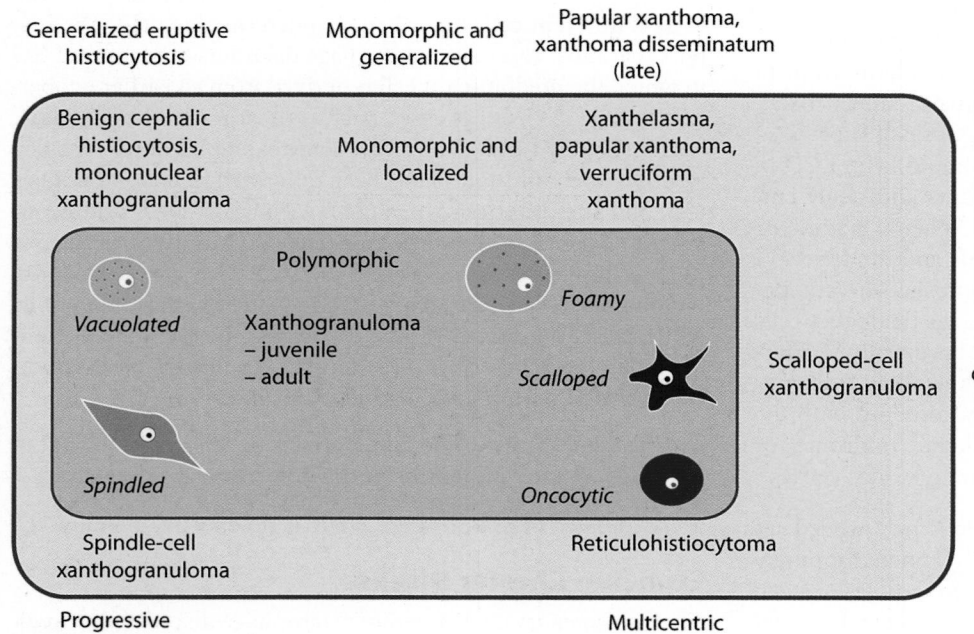

Figure 26-2 Unifying concept of the xanthogranuloma family. Within outer circle monomorphic and localized, outside the outer circle monomorphic and generalized entities are displayed.

some disorders in which one cell type predominates; these disorders may be further divided into solitary and multiple forms, as the diagram shows (54). Many lesions show two or three patterns, such as a combination of spindled and foamy areas. Incontinence of pigment and uptake by macrophages has been designated xanthosiderohistiocytosis but is not a specific disease, as it can be seen in all chronic forms. The early lesions dominated by nondistinctive vacuolated cells include benign cephalic histiocytosis (BCH) and generalized eruptive histiocytosis (GEH); these tend to regress, as do most JXGs in children. All the other lesions tend to be more permanent.

Polymorphic

Xanthogranuloma/Juvenile Xanthogranuloma

Clinical Summary. JXG is an inflammatory disorder in which one, several, or occasionally numerous red-to-yellow papules to nodules are present (Fig. 26-3A). Because the lesions are also seen in adults, JXG is admittedly an imperfect term. Because we have used XG to describe a type of lesion and family of disorders, we prefer to retain the designation JXG for these specific lesions (55).

The papules and nodules are usually 0.5 to 1.0 cm in diameter. Most lesions appear during the first year of life; 20% are present at birth and tend to occur on the head, upper body, and extremities. In children, the lesions may grow rapidly but almost always regress within 1 year and may occasionally take up to 3 to 5 years. Lesions in adults are not uncommon but are usually solitary and persistent. JXG may be clinically subdivided into several forms. The micronodular variant is most common; patients are infants with many papules and small nodules. Occasionally, a macronodular form is seen with only a few lesions, but these are often several centimeters in diameter. The solitary giant XG may be larger than 5 cm (56). Lichenoid papules (57), large plaques (58), or even destructive lesions such as with nasal involvement (the Cyrano sign) may be seen (59). There are also subcutaneous or deep JXG (60). As discussed above, JXG may develop in patients with LCD; this may represent a xanthogranulomatous response to the process of LCD.

A number of systemic complications are associated with JXG. Ocular involvement, including glaucoma and bleeding into the anterior chamber, is the most common; it occurs in less than 10% of young patients and is almost always unilateral (61). Oral lesions may occur. JXG has also been identified in many other organ systems, including the central nervous system, kidney, lungs, liver, testes, and pericardium. An association between JXG, café-au-lait macules, neurofibromatosis/von Recklinghausen disease, and juvenile chronic myelogenous leukemia (JCML) has been reported in around 20 cases (62,63). Although an association of neurofibromatosis and JCML may

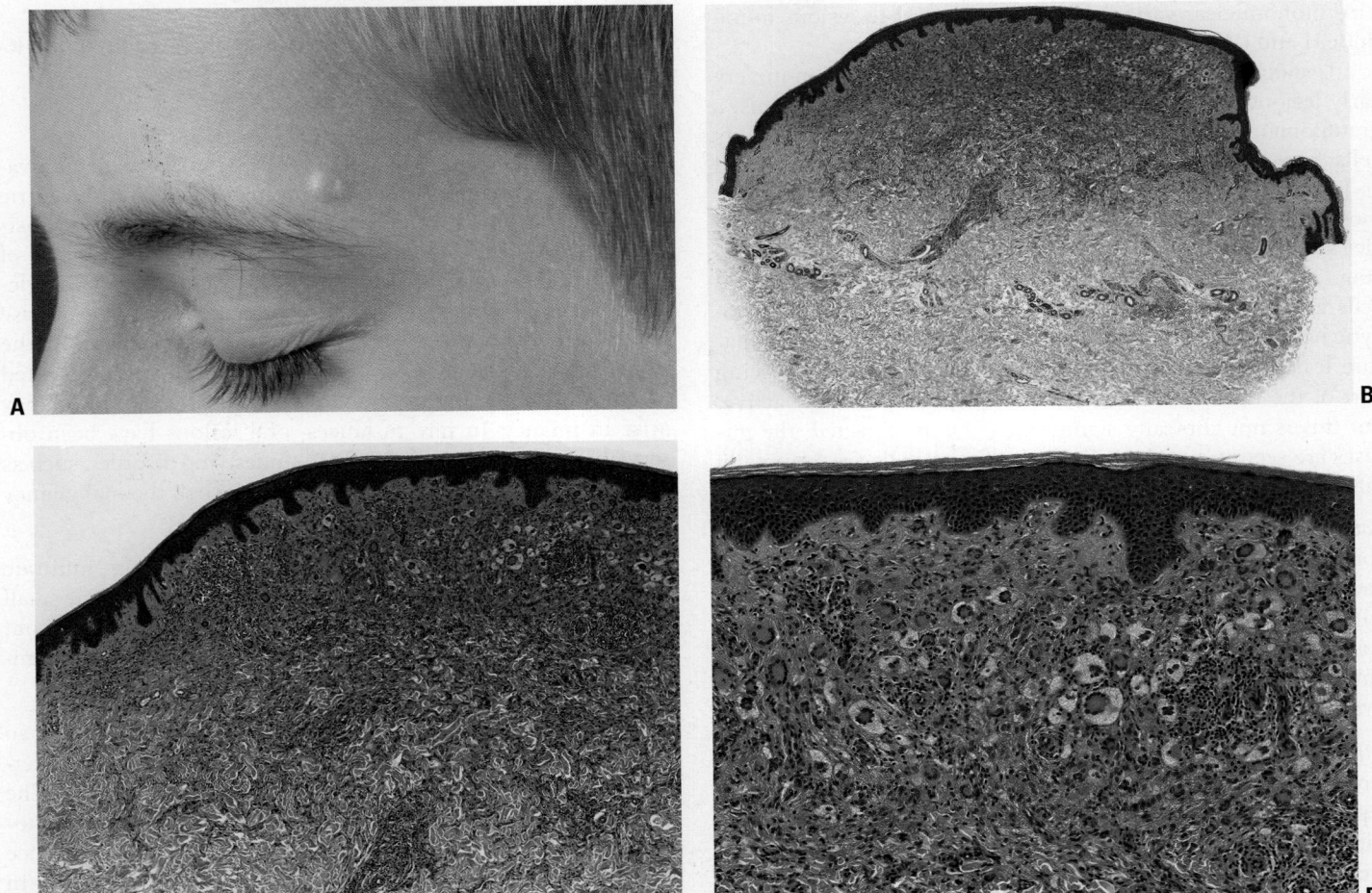

Figure 26-3 Juvenile xanthogranuloma. **A:** Yellow-brown nodule in a typical facial location in a child. **B:** Elevated nodule with epidermal collarette. At scanning magnification, giant cells already can be identified. **C:** Infiltrate rich in Touton giant cells; also note entrapment of collagen at periphery, just as seen in dermatofibroma. **D:** Numerous Touton giant cells at higher magnification; cytoplasm within the wreath of macrophages is eosinophilic in contrast to xanthomatized periphery. (**A:** Courtesy of Wilfried Neuse, Düsseldorf, Germany.)

occur and JCML may even be the presenting sign of the former, a "triple association" with JXG is likely a chance finding, because in clinical practice we and other referral centers of histiocytic disorders did not encounter this association in several decades of clinical experience with these entities (64,65).

In two large series, involving more than 300 patients in pediatric pathology referral centers, 5% of the patients had widespread systemic disease (66,67). These patients are at risk for infections and MAS, and some may die. Although some of these children present with cutaneous disease (68), most do not. It is neither necessary nor wise to raise the possibility of systemic involvement each time an infant or a child is seen with a solitary cutaneous JXG. XGs have also been associated with hematologic malignancies in adults (69) and following ionizing radiation (70). Adults with XGs and systemic problems may have ECD, as discussed on L Group within this chapter.

Histopathology. The typical JXG contains macrophages with a variety of cellular features. On low power, a well-circumscribed nodule, often exophytic and with an epidermal collarette, is found (Fig. 26-3B). Typically, many of the stylized morphologic variants of macrophages can be seen. There is usually a characteristic progression as the lesions mature. Early lesions may show large accumulations of vacuolated cells without significant lipid infiltration intermingled with only a few lymphocytes and eosinophils (Fig. 26-3C). When no foamy cells or giant cells are seen, the possibility of JXG is often overlooked. This mononuclear variant of JXG is identical to lesions found in BCH and GEH.

Usually, some degree of fat uptake is present, even in very early lesions, as manifested by pale cells. In mature lesions, a granulomatous infiltrate is usually present, containing foamy cells, foreign-body giant cells, and Touton giant cells as well as lymphocytes and eosinophils. The presence of giant cells, most of them Touton giant cells, showing a wreath of nuclei surrounded by foamy cytoplasm is quite typical for JXG (Fig. 26-3D) but not diagnostic, because wreath-shaped giant cells can be seen in other disorders, including some melanocytic nevi. Sometimes, Touton giant cells are absent even in mature lesions. Older, regressing lesions show fibrosis replacing part of the infiltrate. Occasional lesions are mitotically active, but this is not clinically significant (71); as expected, the mitoses are seen in non-foamy cells, as foamy cells are terminally differentiated and do not divide.

Pathogenesis. The cause of JXG is unknown. The cell of origin is controversial, as discussed previously. There are only very limited data about the genetic profile of JXG. Systemic JXG may present with multiple genomic alterations whereas solitary JXG usually has normal genomic profiles (55,72). Interestingly, the simultaneous occurrence of JXG has been reported in monozygotic twins (73).

Differential Diagnosis. The clinical differential diagnosis includes Spitz nevi, mastocytomas, and dermatofibromas. The typical histologic picture of JXG is unmistakable. The many variants lead to a baffling array of diagnostic possibilities, which are considered under the individual variants.

Principles of Management: Most lesions in children regress spontaneously; those in adults do not. Solitary or few lesions can be excised; re-excision is not needed if the margins are involved.

Monomorphic: Vacuolized
Benign Cephalic Histiocytosis

Clinical Summary. BCH is a self-healing eruption usually limited to the skin (74). The eruption usually starts during the first 3 years of life and is almost always on the face, although it may become generalized (Fig. 26-4A). The lesions consist of red-to-yellow papules, which after a few years become flat and pigmented and finally resolve (75). There are overlaps with multiple JXG (76). Systemic involvement is rare.

Histopathology. The infiltrate tends to be sparse and consists of macrophages with regularly shaped nuclei and sparse cytoplasm. Usually, there is a cohesive infiltrate of macrophages in the upper dermis. The cells tend to be large and have an eosinophilic cytoplasm. Foamy cells and epidermotropism are rare; eosinophils are often seen. Sometimes, the pattern is lichenoid; such cases are easily confused with LCD, but the nuclear changes seen in the latter are not present; crusting and ulceration are also uncommon (Fig. 26-4B, C).

Pathogenesis. The cause of BCH is unknown.

Differential Diagnosis. It is most important to exclude LCD because clinical distinction can on occasion be difficult and therefore, initially, clinical follow-up is advisory. Usually, however, the appearance is so distinctive that the diagnosis can be made with confidence. The microscopic findings are identical to GEH and early xanthoma disseminatum (XD).

Principles of Management: No treatment is required; the lesions invariably regress.

Generalized Eruptive Histiocytosis

Clinical Summary. GEH may represent the initial stage of a variety of macrophage disorders, including JXG, XD, multicentric reticulohistiocytosis, and progressive nodular histiocytosis (PNH) (77). Clinically, it is characterized by the presence of innumerable flesh-colored to red macules and papules that develop in crops and may involute spontaneously. The disease takes a variable course; it may persist, remit, or relapse. As the infiltrates regress, the lesions may evolve into hyperpigmented macules. Although most patients are adults, the condition may arise in infancy. In rare instances, oral lesions have been observed. There may be an associated underlying disorder, such as a malignancy; the eruption may improve when the malignancy is treated (78,79).

Histopathology. Histologic examination reveals an infiltrate composed of various types of macrophages; most often, small vacuolated cells are seen in a perivascular arrangement, but other morphologic variants may be represented or even dominate. Multinucleated giant cells are usually absent.

Pathogenesis. The etiology is unknown. These cells appear so rapidly that it is not surprising that they are often undifferentiated. Older lesions may show fibrosis or giant cells. The macrophages may in some cases appear in response to cytokines released by neoplasms; but, in general, their appearance remains unexplained. In a single case, a molecular fusion in *LMNA-NTRK1* has been observed (80). This fusion is nonspecific and its implication in GEH so far uncertain.

Differential Diagnosis. The sudden onset and the lack of foamy cells or giant cells should suggest the diagnosis, but cases

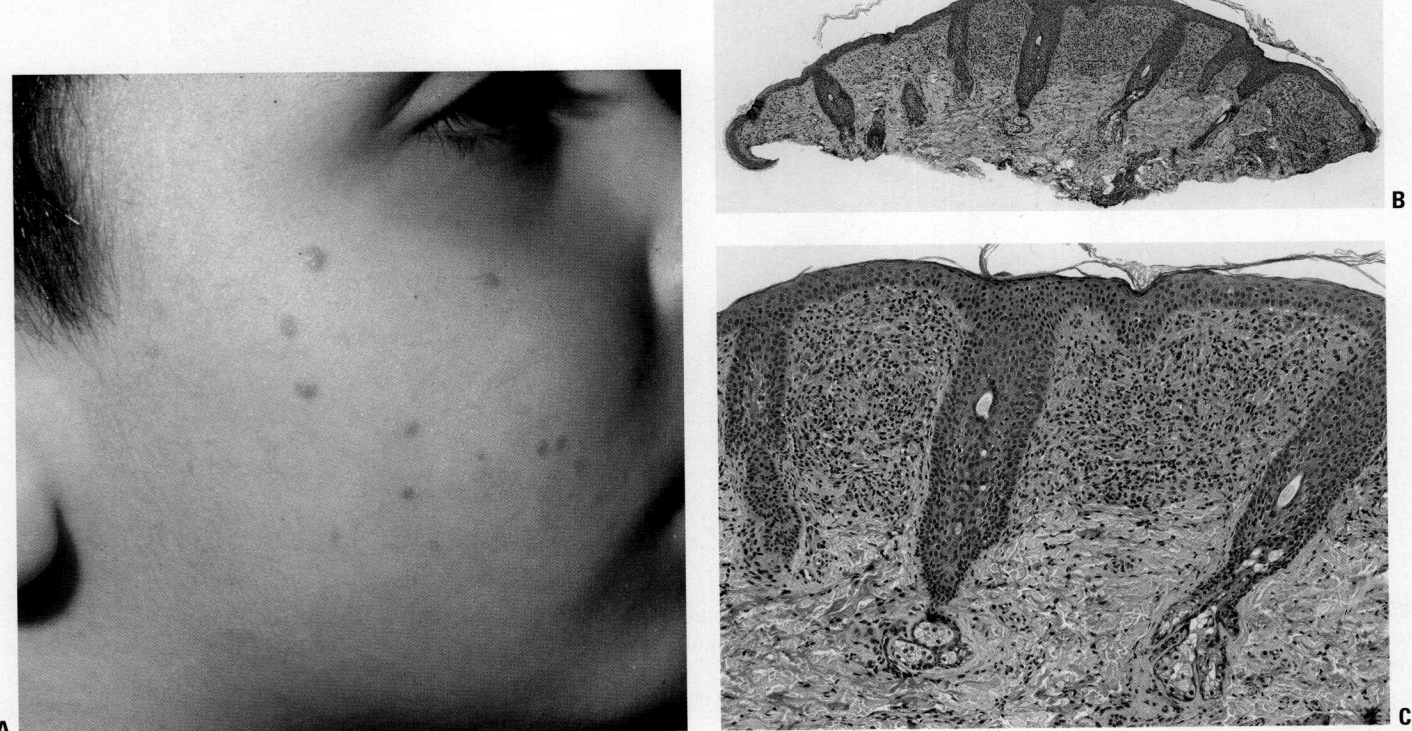

Figure 26-4 Benign cephalic histiocytosis. **A:** Young patient with several yellow-brown papules in a typical location on the cheek. **B:** A modest lichenoid infiltrate without foamy cells. **C:** The epidermis is normal. The macrophages are small and round. This histologic picture is not specific; it is the prototype of an early macrophage infiltrate as seen in eruptive histiocytoma, early juvenile xanthogranuloma, and benign cephalic histiocytosis.

associated with hyperlipidemia have to be excluded. Histologically, the lesions of BCH are identical in the early phase. We have seen an adult case with persistent, disseminated, partly agminated lesions histologically accompanied by multinucleate giant cells resembling multinucleate cell angiohistiocytoma. These findings indicate clinicopathologic overlap of these conditions (81).

Principles of Management: There is no effective treatment.

Monomorphic: Xanthomatized
Normolipemic Xanthomas
A wide number of disorders must be considered if xanthomas are identified in a normolipemic patient. They can arise because of the presence of the following:

1. Xanthelasmas are far and away the most common form of normolipemic xanthomas; but, they are generally included in the spectrum of lipid-related xanthomas and are therefore discussed in the section on xanthomas associated with lipid abnormalities.
2. Another source of excess is sterol (such as cholestanol in cerebrotendinous xanthomatosis or sitosterol in phytosterolemia). In both cases, tuberous and tendon xanthomas are most common, with marked amounts of extracellular lipids.
3. Lymphoproliferative disease (diffuse plane xanthomas and necrobiotic xanthogranuloma, for the latter, see section below on non-xanthogranuloma family).

In some instances, there is no lipoprotein abnormality or associated lymphoproliferative disease; many are idiopathic. In addition to those xanthomas in the xanthogranuloma family (XD and papular xanthoma [PX]) and rarely in LCD, one must

consider verruciform xanthoma, postinflammatory and posttraumatic xanthomas, and a variety of rare syndromes.

Verruciform Xanthoma
Clinical Summary. Verruciform xanthoma (VX) occurs most commonly in the oral cavity, where it was first described by Shafer (82). Lesions are typically solitary, asymptomatic hyperkeratotic papillomatous nodules. Most cases involve the gingival or alveolar mucosa, although other oral sites may be affected (83,84).

In addition, VX may occur in the skin in several settings (85,86). The most predictable situation is as part of a CHILD nevus, a type of epidermal nevus (congenital hemidysplasia with ichthyosiform erythroderma and limb defects; see Chapter 6). Idiopathic cutaneous VX is usually anogenital or perioral; trauma is probably the triggering agent. Similar changes have been seen in sun-damaged skin, sometimes associated with carcinoma *in situ*, but VX may also occur in association with benign keratinocytic lesions. In addition, VX has been reported secondary to a variety of inflammatory lesions, including viral warts, discoid lupus erythematosus, lichen planus, and bullous diseases, and following psoriasiform inflammation in HIV infections (87).

Histopathology. The low-power picture is that of a verruca, often leading to a mistaken diagnosis. There is marked elongation of the rete ridges extending to a uniform level in the dermis (Fig. 26-5A). Accompanying necrosis of keratinocytes is a frequent finding. An infiltrate of foamy cells is confined to the elongated dermal papillae located between the rete ridges (Fig. 26-5B). Sometimes, the xanthomatous cells may appear granular. The vessels in the papillae are also more prominent. The overlying

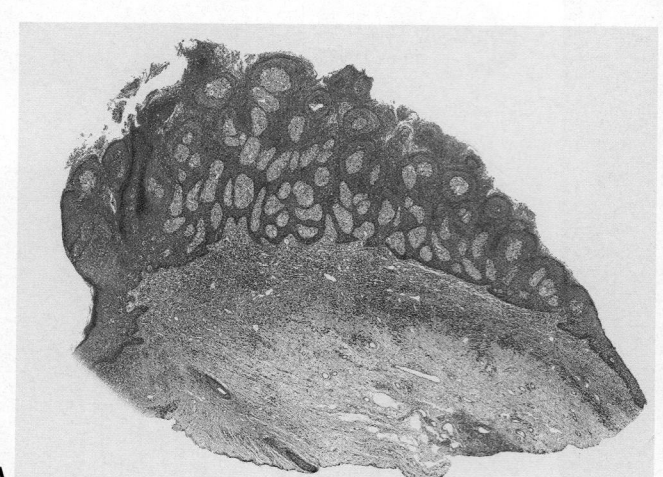
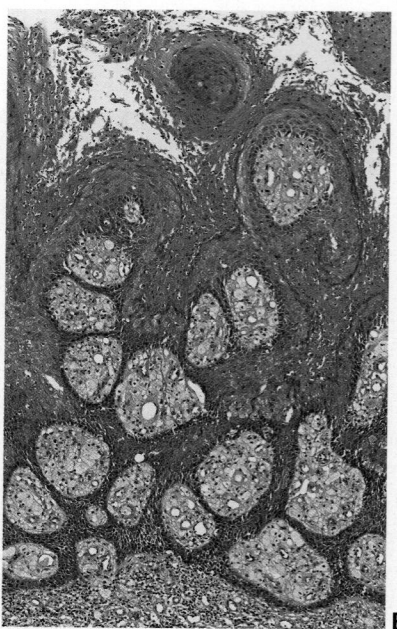

Figure 26-5 Verruciform xanthoma. **A:** Papilloma with marked elongation and thinning of the dermal papillae. There is prominent hyperkeratosis, with a modest lymphocytic infiltrate at the base. **B:** Higher magnification showing foamy cells in the papillae with polymorphonuclear leukocytes in the adjacent crust.

epithelium is parakeratotic, and candidal hyphae or bacteria may be found.

Pathogenesis. Trauma and inflammation are the two best-established triggers (87). Degenerating keratinocytes or perhaps even melanocytes are believed to be the source of the lipid material. The foamy cells are positive for macrophage markers. Although human papillomavirus has been searched for, it has not been unequivocally identified in more than a few scattered cases.

Principles of Management: Disturbing lesions can be excised.

Papular Xanthoma

Clinical Summary. PXs are small flesh-colored or yellow to red-brown papules. Patients present with one, several, or many papules (88). Although the lesions may be generalized, they have neither the distribution pattern of XD nor the confluence

of diffuse normolipemic plane xanthoma (DNPX). Plaques are not seen. The patients show no abnormalities of lipid metabolism. Most patients are adults, but occasional cases have been seen in children; in the latter, spontaneous remission is common. The oral mucosa may be involved. PXs are one of the two characteristic lesions of PNH.

Histopathology. Nodules containing foamy cells with numerous Touton giant cells are seen in the dermis. Extracellular lipids are not seen. Even when early lesions are biopsied, foamy cells predominate, with only a small component of mononuclear vacuolated macrophages or other cell types (Fig. 26-6A, B).

Pathogenesis. Why some macrophages become foamy in the presence of normal serum lipid levels is not known. Despite the early definition of PX as a macrophage disorder without a macrophage precursor phase, there must initially be macrophages

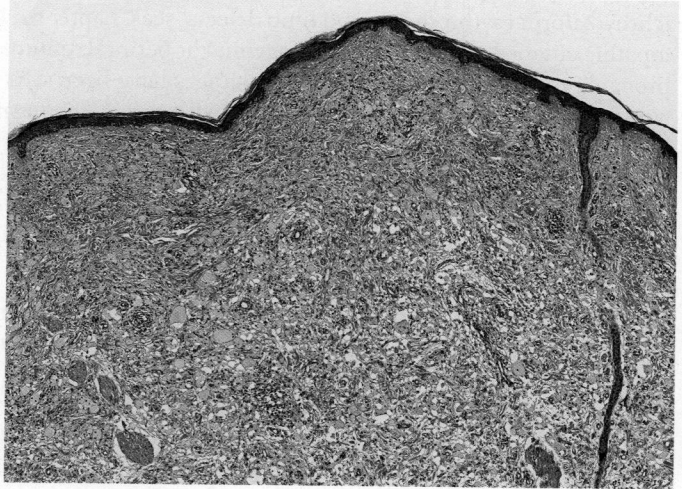
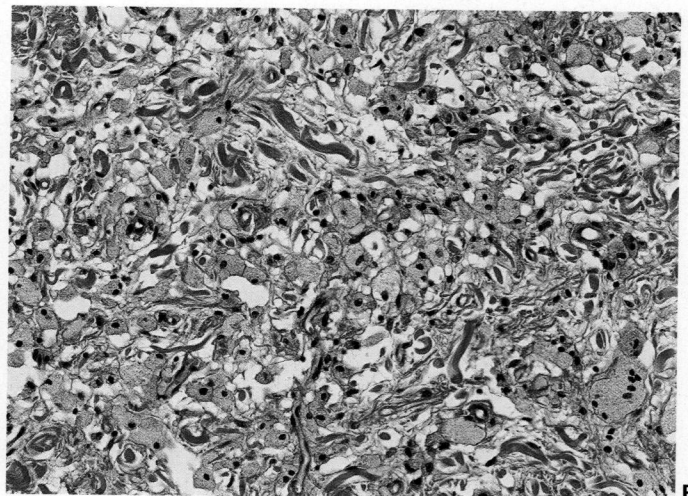

Figure 26-6 Papular xanthoma. **A:** Pale papule without epidermal reaction or clefting. **B:** Numerous foamy macrophages with typical granular cytoplasm. Extracellular lipids are not present.

that rapidly take lipids. PXs with neutrophils have been described in normolipemic patients with HIV infection (89).

Differential Diagnosis. Papules made up of predominantly foamy cells may also be associated with hyperlipidemia in which free lipids may be seen in the dermis, or be a paraneoplastic marker, as in DNPX. Solitary lesions may be mistaken clinically for dermatofibroma, Spitz nevus, and a variety of other benign proliferations.

Principles of Management: Solitary or few lesions can be excised.

Diffuse Normolipemic Plane Xanthoma

Clinical Summary. In DNPXs, another rare disorder, one observes papules, patches, or—most commonly—even larger diffuse areas of orange-yellow discoloration of the skin (90). Whereas the smaller lesions are distinct, the diffuse areas have a poorly defined border. The face, particularly the periorbital areas, and the upper trunk are sites of predilection. The disorder may mimic xanthelasmas initially but progresses to involve wide areas of the skin. The lesions usually persist indefinitely. By definition, the patient has no lipid abnormalities. Some cases of DNPX are associated with hematologic disorders (91), most commonly paraproteinemias, including multiple myeloma, benign monoclonal gammopathy (often immunoglobulin A), T-cell lymphoma, Castleman disease, and cryoglobulinemia. The skin disorder may precede the hematologic problem by many years. In children, the disease is uncommon but usually not associated with a hematologic disorder (92).

Generalized PX and eruptive normolipemic xanthomas are probably variations on the same theme; both have been reported in association with many of the conditions associated with DNPXs. In addition, DNPX has many features in common with necrobiotic xanthogranuloma, including the presence of large patches and plaques, periorbital involvement, and association with paraproteinemias.

Histopathology. Histologic examination reveals large sheets and clusters of foamy cells, diffusely scattered throughout the dermis, as well as singly and in small groups. In some areas, the foamy cells lie in thin streaks between collagen bundles, and occasionally a perivascular arrangement is noted. There may be an admixture of macrophages and lymphocytes; rarely, Touton giant cells are seen. Scattered foamy cells have been observed even in clinically normal skin.

Pathogenesis. The mechanism of xanthoma formation is unclear. Possible explanations include the secretion of cytokines or immunoglobulins by the underlying lymphocytic proliferation, which in turn could stimulate macrophages or alter lipoprotein activity. This theory fails to explain why the skin involvement so often occurs first. The immunohistochemical phenotyping of the macrophages has yielded variable results.

Differential Diagnosis. A single lesion cannot be distinguished from other small xanthomas. If marked necrobiosis or giant cell formation is present, necrobiotic xanthogranuloma should be considered.

Principles of Management: Solitary or few lesions can be excised; diffuse lesions are difficult to manage. Superficial destructive measures can be tried.

Xanthoma Disseminatum

Clinical Summary. XD is a rare but distinctive disorder featuring numerous widely disseminated but often closely set and even coalescing, round-to-oval, orange or yellow-brown papules,

and nodules (93,94). Lesions are found mainly on the flexor surfaces, such as the neck, axillae, antecubital fossae, groin, and perianal region. Peculiar target lesions may be seen. Often, there are lesions around the eyes. The mucous membranes are affected in 40% to 60% of cases. In addition to oral lesions, there may be pharyngeal and laryngeal involvement. Three patterns have been identified: the most typical is the persistent form; rarely, lesions may regress spontaneously; and, even more infrequently, in the progressive form there may be significant internal organ involvement. The largest review (93) suggests that most cases begin in childhood, where the diagnosis can be problematic, as, for example, in an infant with mucosal and pituitary lesions. We have only seen the disease in adults.

Diabetes insipidus is encountered in about 40% of cases but is usually less severe than that associated with LCD. Characteristically, internal lesions other than diabetes insipidus are absent. In a few instances, multiple osteolytic lesions—especially in the long bones—as well as internal organ involvement with lung and central nervous system infiltrates have been found.

Histopathology. In early lesions, scalloped macrophages dominate the histologic picture, with few foamy cells (Fig. 26-7A, B). Most well-developed lesions contain a mixture of scalloped cells, foamy cells, and inflammatory cells, as well as Touton and foreign-body giant cells (Fig. 26-7C) (95). Another rare feature is hemosiderin-laden macrophages in the upper dermis, also known as xanthosiderohistiocytosis.

Pathogenesis. Although in both XD and LCD, xanthomatous lesions and diabetes insipidus may occur, the two should not be confused. XD occurs in older patients, often has mucosal involvement, and only rarely involves bone. Finally, xanthomatous lesions are expected in XD and rare in LCD.

Principles of Management: There is no effective treatment. A variety of cytostatic agents have been employed but the disease usually progresses.

Xanthomas Associated with Lipid Abnormalities

Clinical Summary. Xanthomas associated with lipid abnormalities are not included in the new classification of histiocytoses but are discussed herein owing to their overlapping histologic findings. They are left as a separate category because they are generally viewed as such by both clinicians and pathologists. Xanthomas are a cutaneous clue to the possible presence of hyperlipidemia, defined as an elevated fasting cholesterol level of greater than 200 mg/dL or a triglyceride level of greater than 180 mg/dL. High-density lipoprotein (HDL) cholesterol is also measured and used to calculate the low-density lipoprotein (LDL) cholesterol level. The desirable LDL cholesterol level is less than 130 mg/dL. If abnormalities are detected, lipoprotein analysis is also usually performed. Hyperlipidemia may be unexpectedly identified during routine evaluations or searched for because of a family history of lipid abnormalities, cardiovascular disease, or the presence of one of its many secondary causes.

Once hyperlipidemia is identified, one must first exclude these secondary causes, which include diabetes mellitus, hypothyroidism, nephrotic syndrome, biliary disease, alcohol abuse, pancreatic disease, and a variety of medications, including estrogens, corticosteroids, and retinoids. In the 1960s, Frederickson classified the primary hyperlipidemias on the basis of their electrophoretic lipoprotein phenotype. He considered not just cholesterol and triglycerides but also the main

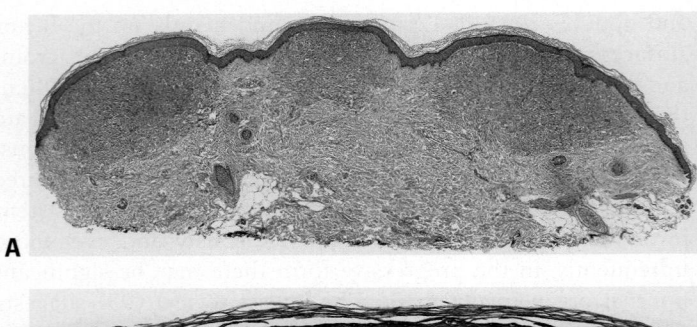

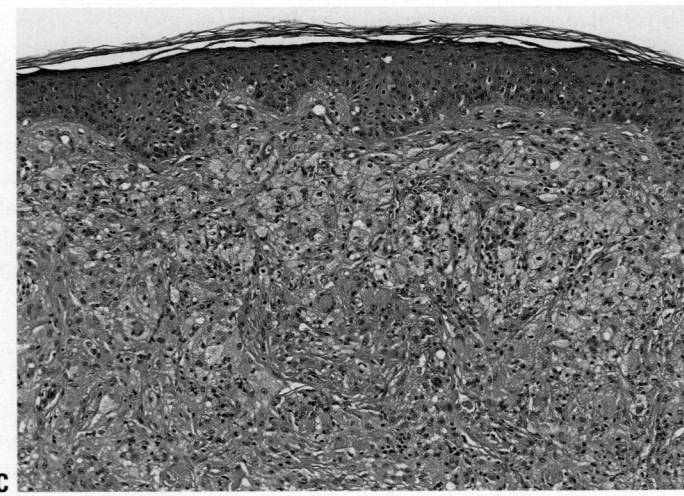

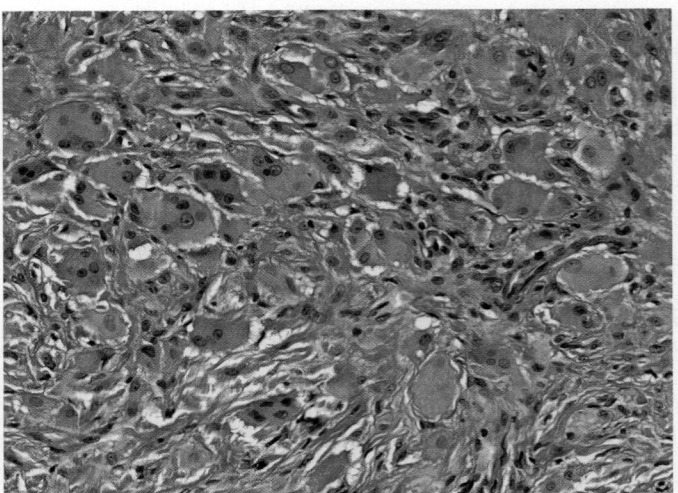

Figure 26-7 Xanthoma disseminatum. **A:** Early lesion with rather monomorphic infiltrates. **B:** Higher magnification, showing scalloped and oncocytic cells. **C:** Later lesion showing foam cells as well as occasional Touton giant cells.

lipoprotein classes in which they were transported throughout the body—chylomicrons, very low-density lipoproteins (VLDLs), LDLs, and HDLs. This traditional scheme is still used for a first diagnostic orientation, but often does not allow pathophysiologic classification of the lipoprotein disorder, which may require apoprotein analysis and genetic studies.

Most patients with lipoprotein abnormalities do not have xanthomas, but the presence of xanthomas and especially the identification of extracellular lipids on histologic examination of the lesion should alert the clinician to the need for an internal evaluation. The type of xanthoma is primarily a clinical diagnosis and may give clues about the exact lipid abnormality. With these limitations in mind, Table 26-4 gives a brief algorithmic approach to cutaneous xanthomas.

The *xanthomas* may clinically be divided into eruptive xanthomas, tuberous xanthomas, tendon xanthomas, plane xanthomas, and xanthelasmas. *Eruptive xanthomas* are almost always associated with chylomicronemia and are most commonly seen in secondary forms of hyperlipoproteinemia although primary variants occur. Eruptive xanthomas consist of small, soft, yellow papules with a predilection for the buttocks and the posterior aspects of the thighs (Fig. 26-8A). They come and go with fluctuations in the chylomicron level in the plasma. The lipid in these lesions is primarily triglycerides. Triglycerides are more rapidly metabolized than cholesterol. This may explain the more transient nature of eruptive xanthomas than other xanthomas.

Tuberous and tuberoeruptive xanthomas are found predominantly in cases with an increase in LDL and VLDL remnants. They are large nodes or plaques located most commonly on the elbows, knees, fingers, and buttocks, sometimes mimicking erythema elevatum et diutinum. Most of the lipid in these xanthomas is in the form of cholesterol.

Tendon xanthomas occur in patients with excessive plasma LDL levels, such as familial hypercholesterolemia and familial apolipoprotein B-100 protein defect, as well as in phytosterolemia

Table 26-4

Algorithm for Cutaneous Xanthomas

When an infiltrate with foamy cells is found:

1. Is extracellular lipid present?

If yes, marker for underlying hyperlipidemia

2. Check serum lipid levels

   a. If abnormal, diagnosis confirmed

   b. If normal, consider

      – XGs (PX, XD)

      – Noncholesterol lipid disorders (sitosterolemia, cholestanolemia)

      – Paraneoplastic disorders

      – Postinflammatory, posttraumatic lesions

      – Storage disorders and other rare syndromes

PX, papular xanthoma; XD, xanthoma disseminatum; XG, xanthogranuloma.

and cholestanolemia (cerebrotendinous xanthomatosis, caused by a mutation in *CYP27A1*). The Achilles tendons and the extensor tendons of the fingers are most frequently affected. They may occur together with tuberous xanthomas.

Plane xanthomas typically develop in skin folds and especially in the palmar creases, where they are diagnostic for dysbetalipoproteinemia. Diffuse plane xanthomas are typically seen as multiple grouped papules and poorly defined yellowish plaques in normolipemic patients, often with paraproteinemia, lymphoma, or leukemia. On the other hand, intertriginous plane xanthomas suggest homozygous familial hypercholesterolemia. The palmar xanthomas associated with cholestasis (primary biliary cirrhosis and biliary atresia) are plaque-like and tend to extend beyond the creases.

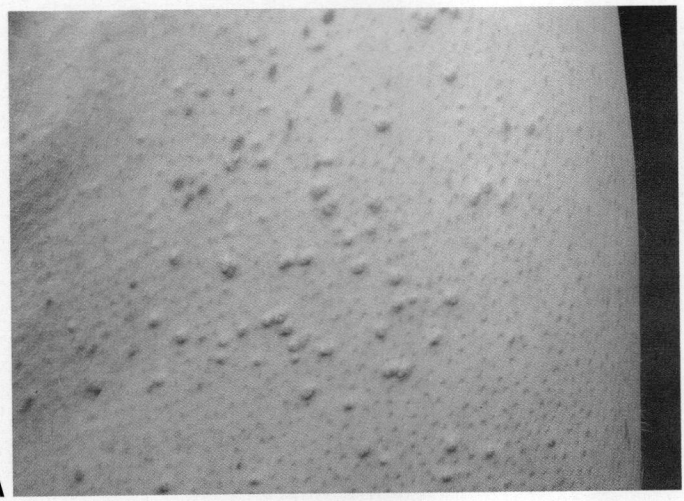

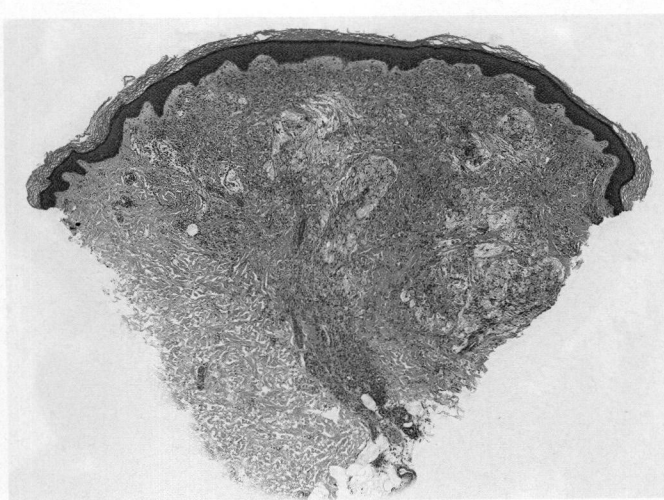

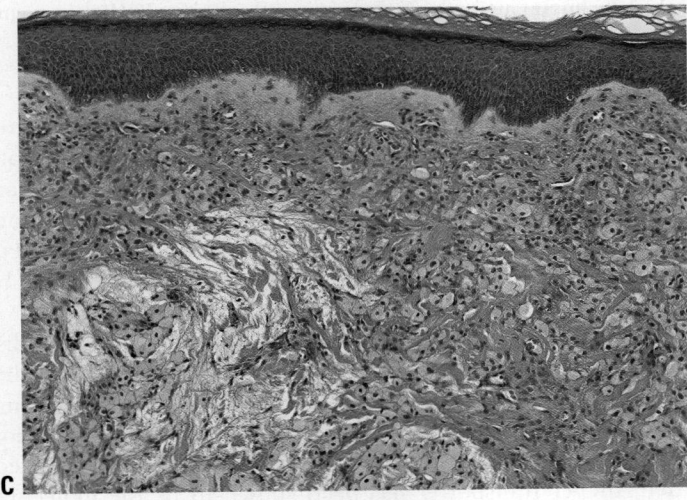

Figure 26-8 Eruptive xanthoma. **A:** Multiple suddenly-appearing red-yellow papules on the trunk. **B:** Pale areas containing foamy cells are dispersed throughout the dermis. **C:** At higher magnification, the extracellular lipids can be appreciated. They offer a reliable indication that this xanthoma is relatively recent in origin and is likely to be associated with a lipid abnormality. (**A:** Courtesy of Wilfried Neuse, Düsseldorf, Germany.)

Xanthelasmas consist of slightly raised, yellow, soft plaques on the eyelids. Although xanthelasmas are the commonest of the cutaneous xanthomas, they are also the least specific because they most frequently occur in persons with normal lipoprotein levels. We argue that xanthelasmas belong to the family of macrophage disorders because they rarely show extracellular lipids, frequently have giant cells, and do not typically disappear with appropriate lipid-lowering therapy.

Histopathology. The histologic appearance of xanthomas of the skin and the tendons is characterized by foamy cells, macrophages that have engulfed lipid droplets. Most of the xanthoma cells are mononuclear, but giant cells, especially of the Touton type with a wreath of nuclei, may be found. The most diagnostic finding suggesting that a xanthomatous lesion reflects an underlying lipid abnormality is the presence of free lipids that have not yet been taken up by macrophages. The lipid droplets can be better seen if frozen or formalin-fixed sections are stained with fat stains such as Scarlet red or Sudan red. There may be varying degrees of fibrosis, giant cells, and clefts, depending on the type and site of xanthoma sampled, but most are surprisingly similar. All xanthomas are characterized by a degree of fixation artifact. Formalin fixation and paraffin embedding remove lipids so that only their shadows are left behind. Larger extracellular deposits of cholesterol and other sterols leave behind clefts.

In the past, much emphasis was placed on the refractile nature of xanthomatous deposits. Frozen or formalin-fixed sections can be examined under polarized light. Cholesterol esters are doubly refractile, whereas other lipids are not. Thus, tendon and tuberous xanthomas tend to be doubly refractile, whereas other xanthomas are not. Chronic lesions are far more likely to show fibrosis.

Some differences exist in the histologic appearance of the various types of xanthoma. Eruptive xanthomas, when of recent origin, often show a considerable admixture of non-foamy cells, among them lymphocytes, vacuolated macrophages, and neutrophils, whereas the number of well-developed foamy cells may still be small (Fig. 26-8B). Because the rapid transport of lipid, especially triglycerides, into the tissue overwhelms the capacity of the macrophages, extracellular lipids are usually found (Fig. 26-8C). These pools of lipid surrounded by macrophages mimic granuloma annulare histologically. Fully developed eruptive xanthomas are rich in foamy cells. Some may show urate crystals, causing confusion with gout.

Tuberous xanthomas consist of large and small aggregates of foamy cells. In early lesions, there usually is a slight admixture of non foamy cells, among them lymphocytes, vacuolated macrophages, and neutrophils. In well-developed lesions, the infiltrate is composed almost entirely of foamy cells. Ultimately, collagen bundles replace many of these cells. Cholesterol clefts may be found (Fig. 26-9A, B). Tendon xanthomas are identical to tuberous xanthomas in histologic appearance but may be even larger and are often submitted without their overlying skin.

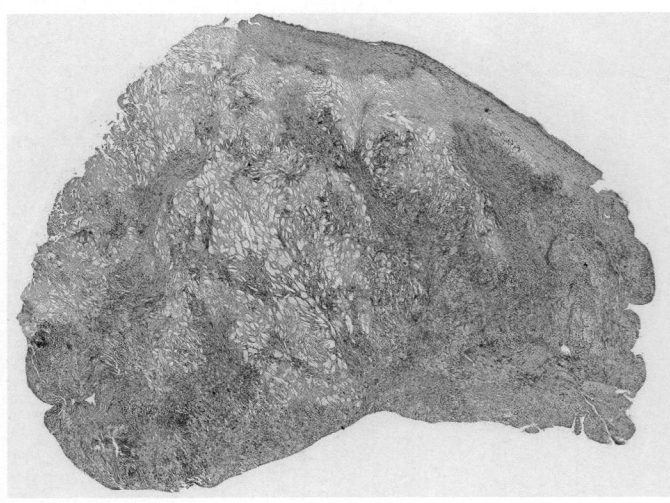
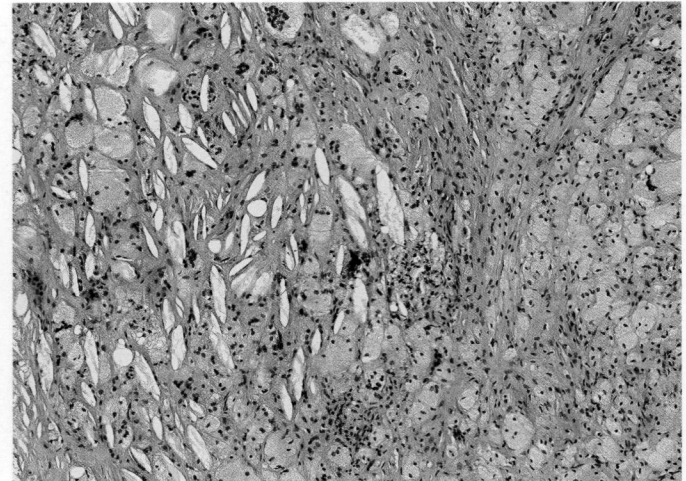

Figure 26-9 Tuberous xanthoma. A: Low-power view showing infiltrate with clefts impinging both on epidermis and subcutis. B: Higher magnification showing cholesterol clefts on left with foamy xanthoma cells on right.

Plane xanthomas should be suspected when the overlying epidermis is thickened with hyperkeratosis and a stratum lucidum, indicating a palmar location (Fig. 26-10A, B). Plane xanthomas from other sites have no unique features.

Xanthelasmas located on the eyelids differ from tuberous xanthomas by the fairly superficial location of the foamy cells and the nearly complete absence of fibrosis. Superficial striated muscles, vellus hairs, and a thinned epidermis all suggest location on the eyelid and serve as clues to their histologic diagnosis (Fig. 26-11A, B). Metastatic adenocarcinoma to the eyelids, most often of mammary origin, and primary adnexal carcinomas (sebaceous and signet ring) can be mistaken for xanthelasmas.

Pathogenesis. Whereas the pathogenesis of many forms of hyperlipidemia is well understood, the formation of xanthomas is a complex process of dysregulation of macrophage sterol flux. Elevated levels of cholesterol-rich LDL and VLDL remnants tend to predispose to xanthomas. Under physiologic conditions, about 80% of LDL cholesterol is taken up by specific LDL receptor-mediated endocytosis. The remaining LDL is removed from the circulation by the scavenger receptor pathways of macrophages. In familial hypercholesterolemia and familial dysbetalipoproteinemia, the accumulating LDL and VLDL remnants are predominantly scavenged by macrophages, a pathway without feedback regulation, leading to continuous cellular lipid accumulation and foamy cells. Thus, these xanthomas are caused by an increased load of altered sterol-rich lipoproteins.

On the other hand, xanthomas can also be caused by disturbed mechanisms of macrophage cholesterol reflux. Specific adenosine triphosphate (ATP)-binding cassette (ABC) transporters play the key role in macrophage sterol efflux, regulation of HDL metabolism, and reverse cholesterol transport. Defective ABCA1 transporter has been shown to be the molecular cause of Tangier disease and familial HDL deficiency. Thus, both overload of macrophages with altered and aged lipoproteins (increased scavenger pathway) and defective cholesterol efflux from macrophages (abnormal transporters) appear to play a crucial role in xanthoma formation.

Principles of Management: Many xanthomas improve or regress when the underlying hyperlipidemia is treated

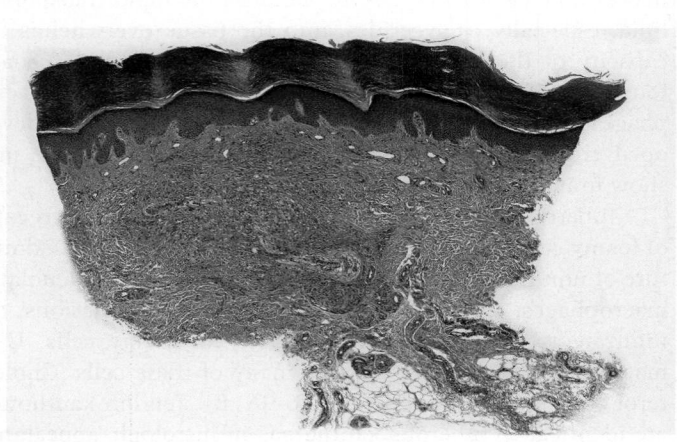
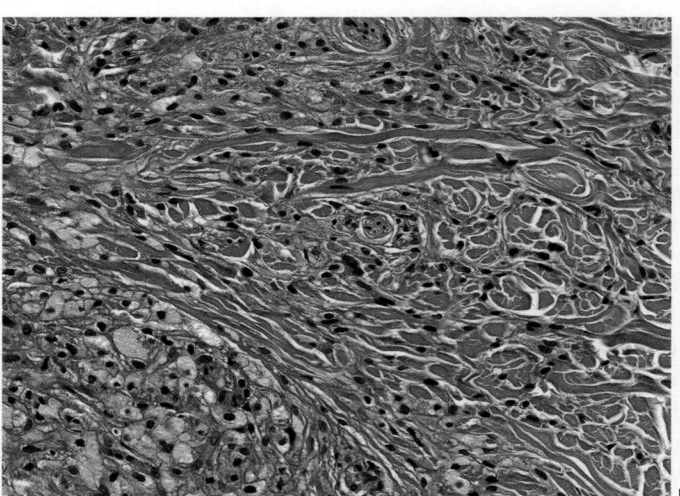

Figure 26-10 Plane xanthoma. A: Acral skin with dermis replaced by multiple pale bulbous infiltrates. B: At higher power, numerous foamy macrophages can be seen; in many, the nuclei are displaced to the cell periphery.

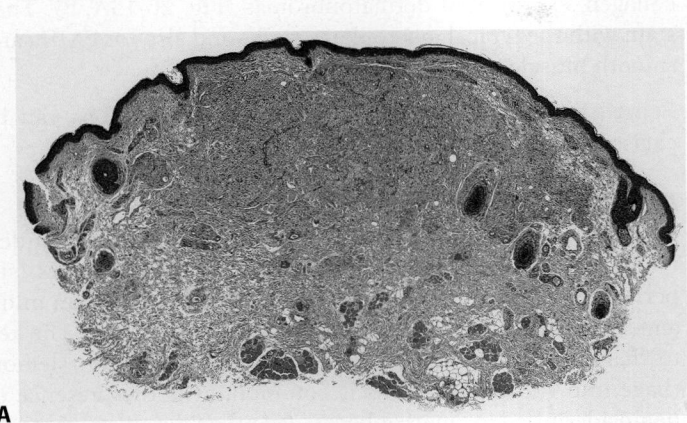

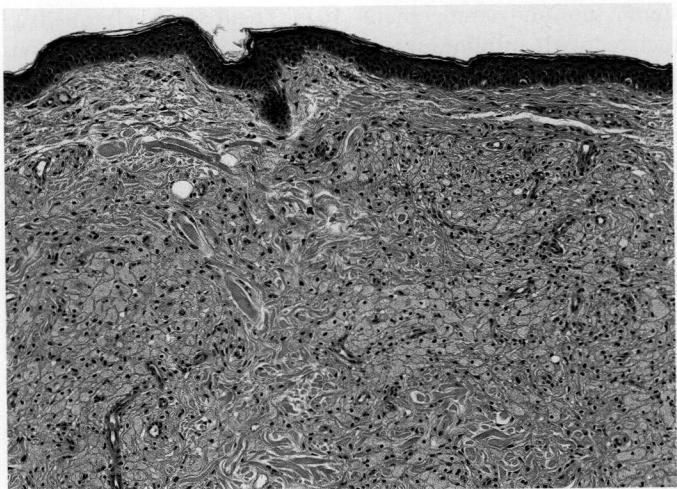

Figure 26-11 Xanthelasma. **A:** The thin epidermis and muscle fibers at the base are a clue to the eyelid location. **B:** Lobules of foamy cells in this location allow the specific diagnosis of xanthelasmas.

appropriately. Individual disturbing lesions can be excised or otherwise ablated.

Monomorphic: Scalloped Cell
Scalloped Cell Xanthogranuloma
Clinical Summary. Scalloped cell xanthogranuloma is not clinically distinct. We identified a number of lesions in which the predominant macrophage is scalloped, once we had become aware of this morphologic variant in XD and began searching for solitary lesions to fill in our unifying concept scheme (54,96). The lesions are typically on the head, neck, or back of young men and may be diagnosed as JXG or, less often, melanocytic nevus or basal cell carcinoma.

Histopathology. Although scalloped macrophages predominate (Fig. 26-7B), a mélange of other macrophage types may be found.

Principles of Management: Solitary or few lesions can be excised.

Monomorphic: Oncocytic
Reticulohistiocytoma, Reticulohistiocytosis, and Multicentric Reticulohistiocytosis
We divide what has also been called reticulohistiocytosis into giant cell reticulohistiocytoma (GCRH) with solitary as well as generalized variants and multicentric reticulohistiocytosis (MRH) (97). Both disorders occur almost exclusively in adults. The histologic picture is very similar in the two types, but everything else is different.

Clinical Summary. GCRH is simply a xanthogranuloma in which the oncocytic macrophages and giant cells predominate. It is never clinically unique but diagnosed as a JXG or dermatofibroma. The clinical features, distribution, and course are identical to those of JXG. In greater than 90% of cases, the lesion is single; but occasionally, multiple lesions are seen (98). Most patients with multiple cutaneous lesions show no sign of systemic involvement.

However, an association with acute myeloid leukemia has been reported (99) and in a recent review substantiated (100). A further subset of patients with multiple cutaneous lesions has been reported to present also with bone involvement, diabetes insipidus, and organomegaly different from MRH (101). It has recently been

proposed to classify these cases separately from GCRH and MRH (100).

In multicentric reticulohistiocytosis, a name first coined by Goltz and Laymon (102), the patients tend to be females, usually in the fifth or sixth decade of life, with widespread cutaneous involvement and a destructive arthritis (100,103,104). Papules or nodules ranging in size from a few millimeters and only exceptionally to several centimeters are most common on the extremities. Multiple papules on the face may coalesce, producing a leonine facies. Many small papules along the nail fold create the "coral bead sign." In about half of the patients, nodules are present also on the oral or nasal mucosa. Finally, about 25% also have xanthelasmas.

The polyarthritis may be mild or severe but is almost always present (97,100). The polyarthritis may precede the skin symptoms and can be mutilating, especially on the hands, through destruction of articular cartilage and subarticular bone. Some patients present with features mimicking dermatomyositis (105). In addition, there is an association with hyperlipidemia (30% to 50%), a variety of internal malignancies (15% to 30%), and autoimmune diseases (5% to 15%). The disease tends to wax and wane over many years.

Histopathology. The characteristic histologic feature in both GCRH and MRH is the presence of numerous multinucleate giant cells and oncocytic macrophages showing abundant eosinophilic, finely granular cytoplasm, often with a "ground glass" appearance (Fig. 26-12A, B). There may be subtle microscopic differences between solitary and multiple lesions (106). In older lesions, giant cells and fibrosis are more common.

The polyarthritis present in nearly all instances of MRH is caused by the same type of infiltrate as found in the cutaneous lesions. In early or mild cases, the granulomatous infiltrate is confined to the synovial membrane. Although similar infiltrates have been described in other organs, their clinical significance is unclear.

Pathogenesis. Ultrastructural examination shows abundant mitochondria and lysosomes, which correlate with the ground glass appearance. Similar changes are found in oncocytic thyroid and renal tumors. The cause of the solitary lesions is unknown, just as with JXG. Multicentric forms may be caused by a systemic immune derangement (107). The disease is frequently associated with autoimmune and neoplastic disorders. A subset of diffuse cutaneous (99), multisystem, non-arthropathic (101) as well as multicentric reticulohistiocytoses (108) seems to harbor different clonal molecular alterations. Whether there is an overlap in these latter single observations to other histiocytoses with molecular peculiarities remains to be definitely established. However, this recent research indicates that the etiology of reticulohistiocytosis may be more complex than previously considered.

Differential Diagnosis. It is futile to try and distinguish between a solitary GCRH and JXG. The two lesions are part of a spectrum, and overlaps occur. A single macrophage lesion with ground glass cytoplasm does not make the diagnosis of MRH, but instead, should simply be viewed as having the same clinical significance as JXG. The giant cells may show emperipolesis and thus be confused with Rosai–Dorfman disease (RDD). The clinical differential diagnosis of MRH is lengthy, but an excisional skin biopsy is quite helpful in pointing one in the right direction. Gout, rheumatoid arthritis, sarcoidosis, dermatomyositis, and even lepromatous leprosy may be considered.

Principles of Management: Solitary GCRH is cured by excision. For MRH, there is often no overall satisfactory treatment. In a number of cases, MRH improves upon remission of malignancy. Self-limiting courses may also occur.

Monomorphic: Spindle-Shaped
Spindle Cell Xanthogranuloma

Clinical Summary. Spindle cell xanthogranulomas are not clinically distinct (109). They are usually on the head or neck of young adults and identified as JXG or dermatofibromas. Deep spindle cell xanthogranulomas may cause puzzlement; in one case, a woman presented with cutaneous JXG and later developed spindle cell xanthogranuloma of the breast (110).

Histopathology. Under the microscope, they are even more likely to be misdiagnosed, usually as dermatofibromas or blue nevi.

Microscopically, they lack melanin and do not have reactive changes in the overlying epidermis or lateral entrapment of collagen so typical of dermatofibromas (Fig. 26-13A, B). They stain with the typical macrophage stains and also for FXIIIa and smooth muscle actin.

Principles of Management: Solitary or few lesions can be excised.

Progressive Nodular Histiocytosis

Clinical Summary. PNH is a rare, clinically distinct disorder. Patients typically have hundreds of lesions of two types: superficial xanthomatous papules and nodules 2 to 10 mm in diameter and deep fibrous tumors 1 to 3 cm in diameter. The key to diagnosis lies in these two distinct lesions (111). Hemorrhage into the larger lesions is common, as is the presence of hemosiderin-laden macrophages (xanthosiderohistiocytosis). Conjunctival, oral, or laryngeal lesions, as well as rare systemic lesions, may occur (112,113). Lesions rarely if ever regress. Familial or congenital cases have not been reported.

Histopathology. Two patterns can be recognized that correlate with the clinical lesions. The smaller papules are xanthomatous with foamy cells and occasional Touton giant cells; they are PXs (Fig. 26-6A, B). The larger nodules are spindle cell xanthogranulomas (Fig. 26-13A, B), which—aside from macrophage markers—may also express alpha smooth muscle actin and especially then may histologically be confused with dermatofibroma.; they can also have xanthomatous areas (Fig. 26-13C).

Differential Diagnosis. When the distinctive clinical picture is present, the diagnosis of PNH should be considered, but no harm is done if the patient is diagnosed with multiple JXG.

Principles of Management: The larger spindle cell lesions often become necrotic and painful, requiring excision.

Non-Xanthogranuloma Family

In the new classification of the Histiocyte Society, *cutaneous RDD* is assigned to the C Group but in this chapter is discussed within the R Group (section on RDD) owing to histologic

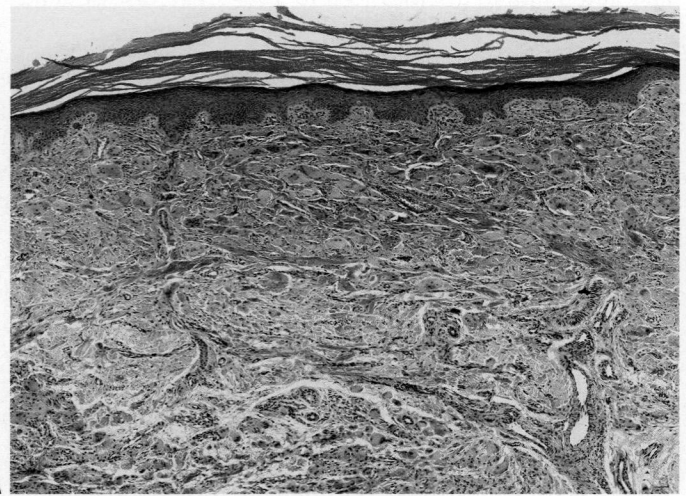
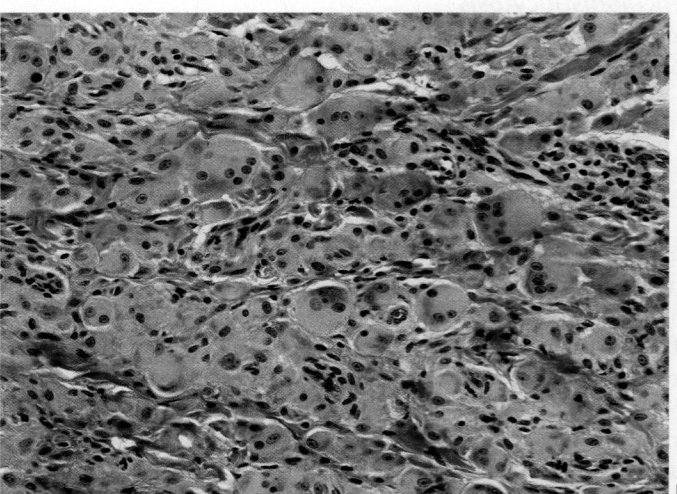

Figure 26-12 Multicentric reticulohistiocytosis. **A:** A diffuse dermal giant cell infiltrate with sparse inflammation and a thinned epidermis. **B:** Relatively clear giant cells with finely granular cytoplasm ("ground glass" appearance) replacing the upper dermis. The giant cells are large and irregular, containing many haphazardly arranged nuclei. These photomicrographs were made in 2013 from the original slide from one of Goltz and Laymon's patients reported in 1954 (102).

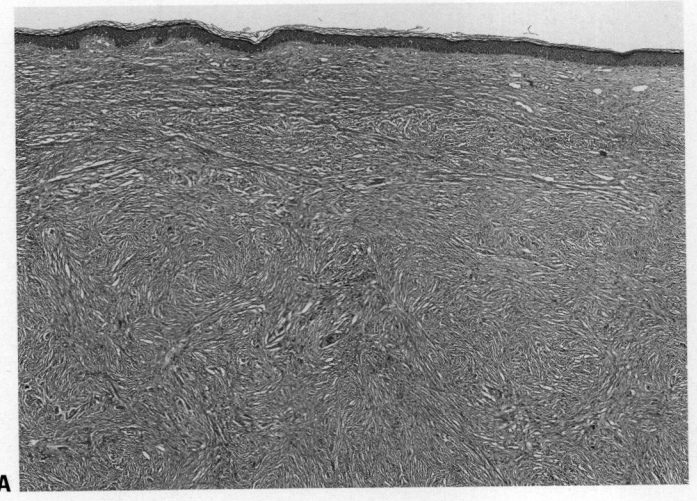

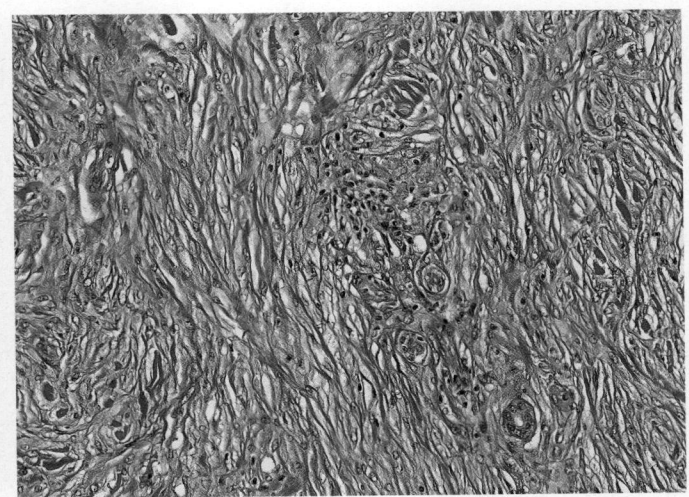

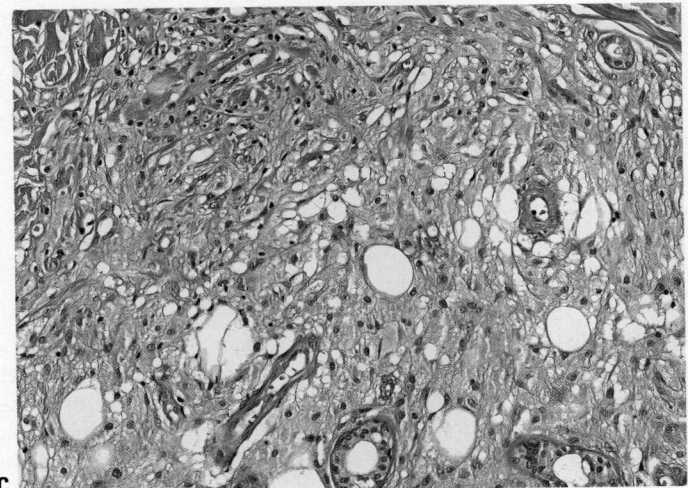

Figure 26-13 Spindle cell xanthogranuloma/progressive nodular histiocytosis. **A:** Dermal nodule with storiform pattern. No evidence of epidermal reaction. **B:** Spindled macrophages at higher magnification. **C:** Transition from spindled (upper left) to xanthomatous region.

similarities to the classic variant with systemic involvement. For the same reason, *MRH* is covered in the section on C Group.

Necrobiotic Xanthogranuloma with Paraproteinemia

Clinical Summary. Necrobiotic xanthogranuloma (NXG) with paraproteinemia was first described by Kossard and Winkelmann in 1980 (114). It can usually be recognized clinically and histologically (115–117), but may overlap with diffuse normolipemic plane xanthoma. NXG presents in adults and the elderly of either sex. Large, often yellowish, indurated plaques are found with atrophy, telangiectasia, and occasionally also ulceration. The most common location is periorbital. The skin of the thorax is also commonly affected. Mucosal affection may occur. Systemic disease includes cardiac myopathy with giant cell infiltrates and hematologic malignancies. Other organs such as lung, kidney, liver, and eye may also be involved.

Histopathology. The overall histopathologic findings are characteristic. Infiltrates containing macrophages, foamy cells, and often also an admixture of other inflammatory cells are present either as focal aggregates or as large, intersecting bands occupying the dermis and subcutaneous tissue (Fig. 26-14A). Typically, lymphoid follicles or aggregates are seen (Fig. 26-14B). The intervening tissue shows extensive necrobiosis (degeneration of collagen imparting unique staining characteristics). A further distinctive feature is the presence of numerous large giant cells, both of the Touton type with a peripheral rim of foamy

cytoplasm and of the foreign-body type (Fig. 26-14C). Cholesterol clefts are also common. Sometimes, all other features are present but no necrobiosis is found (118).

Pathogenesis. In most patients, serum protein electrophoresis shows an immunoglobulin G monoclonal gammopathy that usually consists of κ light chains. Bone marrow examination has revealed multiple myeloma, which may also develop in later stages of the disease. Cryoglobulinemia may also be present. Xanthomas seen in POEMS syndrome (polyneuropathy, organomegaly, endocrinopathy, M protein, and skin changes, which may include xanthomas and angiomas) may have a similar etiology. The cutaneous changes may not improve or even worsen as the underlying gammopathy is treated (119). One study has indicated the presence of spirochetes in the lesions (120).

Differential Diagnosis. Other necrobiotic disorders, especially necrobiosis lipoidica and subcutaneous granuloma annulare or rheumatoid nodule, may be considered. In necrobiotic xanthogranuloma, the necrobiosis is far more extensive and often occurs in broad bands, associated with extensive infiltrates of Touton giant cells, foamy macrophages, and lymphocytes. Vascular involvement is rare, but panniculitis is common. Thus, the cellularity and extent of necrobiosis usually serve as reliable clues, as does the usual periorbital location.

Principles of Management: Even when the underlying gammopathy is treated, the skin changes are scarcely influenced (121).

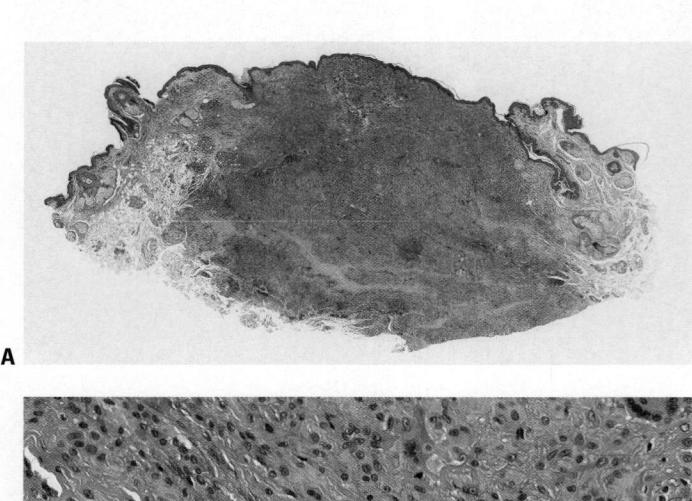

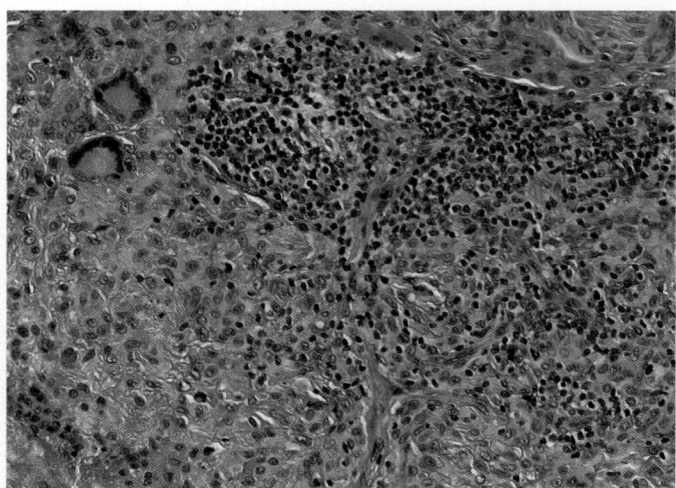

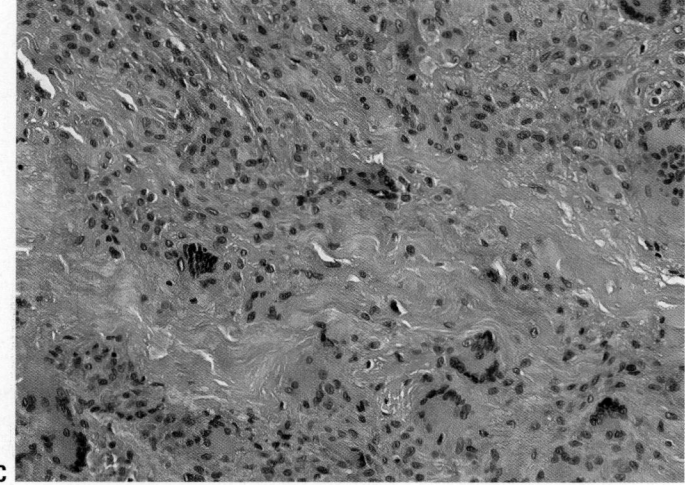

Figure 26-14 Necrobiotic xanthogranuloma: **A:** Low-power view showing a diffuse infiltrate with amorphous necrobiotic areas, cellular regions rich in giant cells, and a nodular lymphocytic infiltrate. **B:** Higher magnification, showing prominent lymphoid follicles and pale necrobiotic regions. **C:** Another view, showing numerous bizarre foreign-body and Touton giant cells and extensive necrobiosis.

ROSAI–DORFMAN DISEASE (R GROUP)

Clinical Summary. The term "sinus histiocytosis with massive lymphadenopathy" was first used by Rosai and Dorfman in 1969 (122), although Destombes had previously described the disorder in Africa (123). Massive cervical lymphadenopathy, usually bilateral and painless, is the most common manifestation accompanied by fever, night sweats, fatigue, and weight loss (124–126). The affected are predominantly children and young adults, more commonly males. RDD is an inflammatory disorder in spite of its propensity to form large masses and to disseminate to both nodal and extranodal sites. In most patients, the disease resolves spontaneously, others have persistent problems, and very few die. About 10% of patients with nodal disease show cutaneous involvement. The lesions are typically papules or nodules. The skin, nasal cavity, retro-orbital tissue, bone, and subcutaneous soft tissue are the most common sites of involvement when patients present with extranodal disease, which is seen in 43% of cases. Cutaneous RDD is most common in Asia and usually presents as solitary, rarely multiple lesions in adults, females more frequently than males. Patients tend to be older than those with classic nodal disease. Such individuals may represent a separate but closely related disorder because very few advance to nodal or systemic disease (127–131). Occasionally, a soft tissue lesion may present as a breast mass or panniculitis.

Histopathology. The skin lesions contain a polymorphous infiltrate in which lymphocytes and macrophages with clear cytoplasm are most prominent. The low-power view has been compared to that of a "lymph node in the skin" (Fig. 26-15A, B). Occasionally, the macrophages may be multinucleated or have a foamy cytoplasm. The hallmark histologic feature is emperipolesis of lymphocytes (Fig. 26-15C). Emperipolesis is allegedly slightly different from phagocytosis, in that the lymphocytes are taken up by macrophages but not attacked by digestive enzymes. Thus, they appear intact. We find this distinction somewhat theoretical. On occasion, red blood cells can also be taken up. Immunohistologically, these cells are positive for S100 protein, fascin, CD14, CD11c, CD68, and CD163 and negative for CD1a and langerin (CD207). There are also often IgG4-positive plasma cells, sometimes leading to deposits of crystalline immunoglobulins (132). It has been recommended in the current classification of histiocytosis to mention them in the histopathologic report possibly as a pointer toward the differential diagnosis of IgG4-related sclerosing disease (3). However, in isolation they are a nonspecific finding present in various inflammatory conditions. In the lymph nodes, the sinuses are greatly dilated and crowded with inflammatory cells, particularly macrophages. Here, they tend to have an abundant foamy cytoplasm and also to display emperipolesis.

Pathogenesis. The cells are unusual activated macrophages that are positive for CD68, other macrophage markers, and fascin but

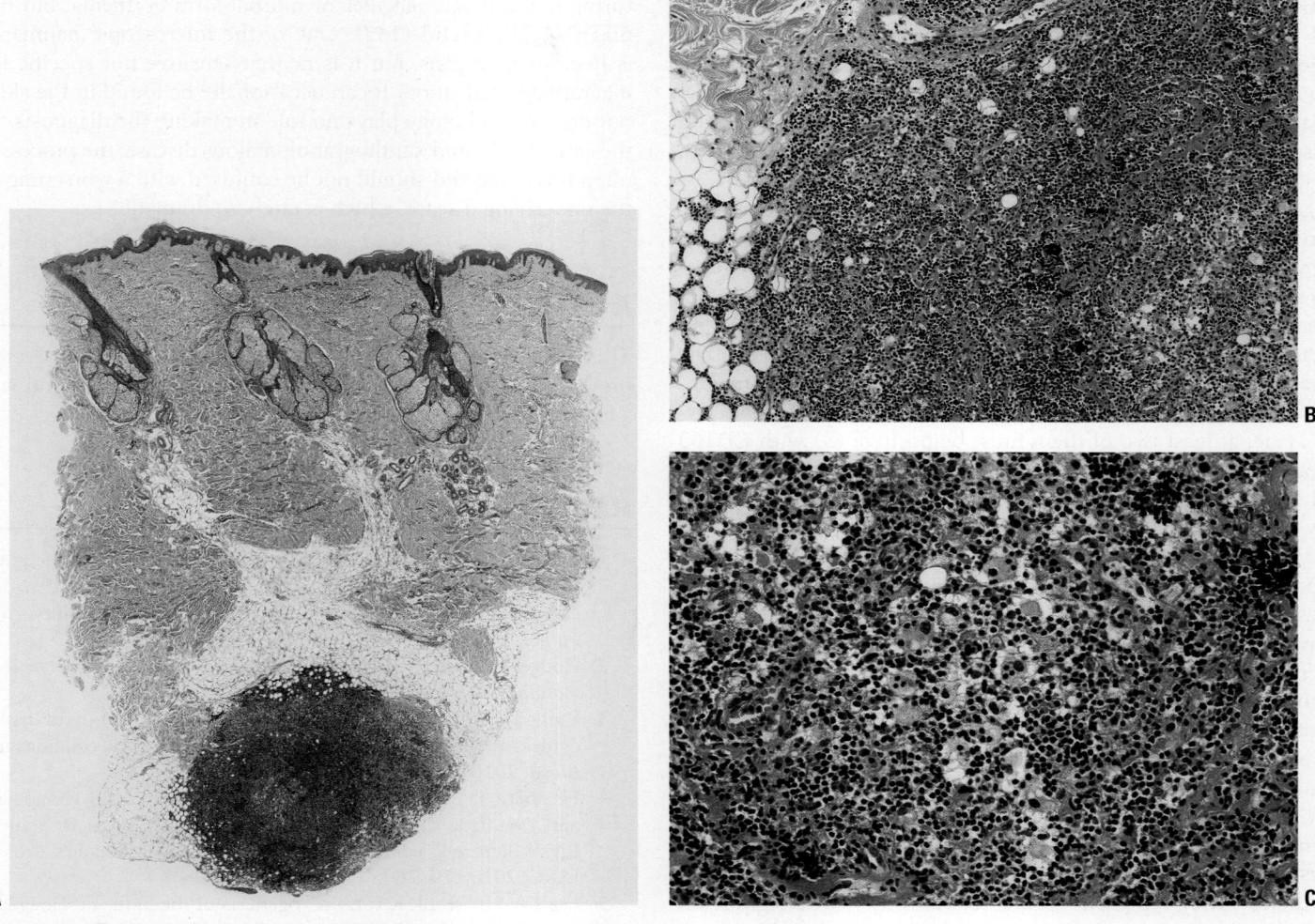

Figure 26-15 Sinus histiocytosis with massive lymphadenopathy. **A:** Subcutaneous nodular infiltrate ("lymph node in the skin") rich in pale-staining cells centrally. **B:** Typical pattern of pale sinusoidal macrophages admixed with darker-staining lymphocytes. **C:** Numerous large macrophages, several of which have ingested lymphocytes, demonstrating emperipolesis.

are also S100 protein positive. Over the years, a variety of viruses have been implicated as triggers, but none is firmly established. Molecular investigations on RDD have revealed kinase mutations in nodal and extranodal but not cutaneous disease (124–126). These include mutations in *ARAF, KRAS, NRAS,* and *MAP2K1* in around a third of cases, suggesting that a number of patients suffer from clonal disease. Familial RDD comprises individuals with germline mutations in *SLC29A3* encoding a nucleoside transporter (133) (histiocytosis-lymphadenopathy plus syndrome, also called Faisalabad histiocytosis, H syndrome, and pigmented hypertrichosis with insulin-dependent diabetes mellitus [PHID] syndrome) (124–126). Twenty percent of cases suffer from nodal and extranodal disease including the skin. The relation of these cases to ordinary RDD is unclear. Familial cases have also been observed as part of the autoimmune lymphoproliferative syndrome type IA (ALPS) caused by mutations in *TNFRSF6.* In this setting, 41% of cases have been documented to suffer from nodal disease, usually self-limiting.

Differential Diagnosis. The clinical differential diagnosis for lymphadenopathy is long, and the cutaneous lesions may be confused with sarcoidosis, xanthoma, xanthogranuloma, mastocytoma, and malignant infiltrates. The sinus histiocytes resemble the oncocytic macrophages of reticulohistiocytomas,

but the immunologic profile with marked S100 positivity usually facilitates separation.

Principles of Management: Solitary or few lesions can be excised. For classic RDD, there is no general recommendation of treatment; treatment must be adjusted to the individual circumstances. In most cases with uncomplicated disease, regular follow-up is recommended. Cases with multifocal, unresectable extranodal disease can be treated with a variety of immunomodulatory, antineoplastic, and targeted therapies, which in part are the subject of ongoing studies (125).

MALIGNANT HISTIOCYTOSIS (M GROUP)

Even though malignant lesions of macrophage lineage are rare, they are occasionally encountered in the skin. They are classified into primary and secondary malignant histiocytoses (MHs). Primary MH may present primarily in the skin (134) apart from other typically extranodal sites—such as gastrointestinal tract, soft tissue, and central nervous system (135). Solitary and multiple lesions may occur. Secondary MHs occur in association with another hematologic neoplasm, either from anaplastic progression with aberrant expression of histiocytic/DC markers or transdifferentiation (3). Various forms of lymphoma and leukemia have been reported to be involved. In fact, with the advent of immunohistochemistry and molecular biology, many cases of primary MH diagnosed as such in the past have been shown to represent T- or B-cell lymphomas. Other malignancies, especially of epithelial, melanocytic, and endothelial lineage, and also epithelioid sarcoma, must carefully be excluded as well with an appropriate panel of antibodies and molecular investigations. Histopathologically, MH in contrast to most cases of myeloid sarcomas is an anaplastic neoplasia. The lesions contain large cells with frequent mitoses and varying degrees of pleomorphism. Multinucleate giant cells, foamy cells, and spindle-shaped cells may be encountered. Erythrophagocytosis is absent or inconspicuous, whereas emperipolesis is even rarer. The diagnosis of MH must be supported by positivity for macrophage and dendritic cell markers, CD68, CD163, CD4, and lysozyme; at least two of them must be positive (3) with CD163 being an especially specific marker for the histiocytic lineage (136,137). Myeloid sarcomas representing tissue infiltration by monocytic leukemic cells usually express CD13, CD33, and myeloperoxidase aside from histiocytic markers (135). In MH, apart from *BRAF* mutation and chromosomal alteration suggesting relationship with hemopathy, more recent molecular investigations have revealed MAP kinase alterations reminiscent to those seen in LCD and ECD (135,138). In addition, a minor subset of histiocytic sarcomas may focally express S-100 protein or CD1a (139). Compared to LCD, however, MH generally harbors more frequent chromosomal alterations. Furthermore, in our experience, malignant cutaneous infiltrates with LC characteristics are extraordinary rare and, notably, neither tend to display prominent cytologic atypia/destructive growth histopathologically nor behave as biologically malignant. Nevertheless, they represent serious conditions with a significant number of deaths and are associated with leukemia and lymphoma in a number of cases. MH is an aggressive disease; only patients with solitary extranodal disease such as a single skin lesion are occasionally cured.

HEMOPHAGOCYTIC LYMPHOHISTIOCYTOSES (H GROUP)

The hemophagocytic lymphohistiocytosis (HLH) syndromes comprise a group of severe and often fatal syndromes best described as a form of hypercytokinemia and an accumulation of activated macrophages in various tissues with a resultant rapid uncontrolled systemic inflammatory response syndrome (SIRS), which generally feature fever, malaise, hepatosplenomegaly, jaundice, hyperferritinemia, and cytopenia (140). They may be *primarily* associated with Mendelian inherited conditions presenting in infants and only rarely in adults—with episodes triggered by infections and mutations in genes whose products are important in the NK/T-cell cytotoxic pathway (*PFR1, UNC13D, STX11* and *STXBP2*, and others) (3,141)—or occur at any age, *secondary* to infections (viral, bacterial, fungal, parasitic), malignancies (primarily hematopoietic), or rheumatic disorders. This latter subset of secondary HLH is often referred to as *macrophage activation syndrome*, which is most common in systemic-onset juvenile idiopathic arthritis, adult-onset Still disease, systemic lupus erythematosus, and vasculitis (142); but, it has also been reported in patients with LCD (143) and systemic xanthogranulomatous

disease (144). Cutaneous involvement is common, usually featuring hemorrhagic macules or morbilliform erythema, but not diagnostically useful (145). One of the microscopic hallmarks is hemophagocytosis, but it is neither sensitive nor specific for macrophage activation. It can occasionally be found in the skin, but dermatopathology plays no role in making the diagnosis. In the case of LCD and xanthogranulomatous disease, the process is often reversible and should not be confused with a worsening of the underlying disease, which is rarely so dramatic.

ACKNOWLEDGMENT

This chapter is dedicated to Walter H.C. Burgdorf, who covered previous editions of this chapter as the main/coauthor and was a close friend and mentor to one of us (B.Z.).

REFERENCES

1. Lichtenstein L, Histiocytosis X. Integration of eosinophilic granuloma, Letterer-Siwe disease and Hand-Schüller-Christian disease as related manifestations of a single nosologic entity. *Arch Pathol.* 1953;56:84–102.
2. Hoeger P, Kinsler V, Yan A, eds. *Harper's Textbook of Pediatric Dermatology.* 4th ed. Wiley Blackwell; 2020.
3. Emile J-F, Abla O, Fraitag S, et al. Revised classification of histiocytoses and neoplasms of the macrophage-dendritic cell lineages. *Blood.* 2016;127:2672–2681.
4. Facchetti F, Berti E., Jaffe ES, et al. Introduction to Histiocytic and Dendritic Cell Neoplasms. In: Elder DE, Massi D, Scolyer RA, Willemze R, eds. *WHO Classification of Skin Tumours.* 4th ed. IARC; 2018:279–280.
5. Lee LW, Holbrook KA. Embryogenesis of the Skin. In: Hoeger P, Kinsler V, Yan A, eds. *Harper's Textbook of Pediatric Dermatology.* 4th ed. Wiley Blackwell; 2020:1–35.
6. Facchetti F, Berti E. Langerhans Cell Histiocytosis. In: Elder DE, Massi D, Scolyer RA, Willemze R, eds. *WHO Classification of Skin Tumours.* 4th ed. IARC; 2018:281–282.
7. Rodriguez-Galindo C, Allen CE. Langerhans cell histiocytosis. *Blood.* 2020;135:1319–1331.
8. Hashimoto K, Pritzker MS. Electron microscopic study of reticulohistiocytoma. An unusual case of congenital, self-healing reticulohistiocytosis. *Arch Dermatol.* 1973;107:263–270.
9. Battistella M, Fraitag S, Teillac DH, Brousse N, de Prost Y, Bodemer C. Neonatal and early infantile cutaneous Langerhans cell histiocytosis: comparison of self-regressive and non-self-regressive forms. *Arch Dermatol.* 2010;146:149–156.
10. Kapur P, Erickson C, Rakheja D, Carder KR, Hoang MP. Congenital self-healing reticulohistiocytosis (Hashimoto-Pritzker disease): ten-year experience at Dallas Children's Medical Center. *J Am Acad Dermatol.* 2007;56:290–294.
11. Val-Bernal JF, Gonzalez-Vela MC, Sanchez-Santolino S, González-López MA. Localized eosinophilic (Langerhans' cell) granuloma of the lower lip. A lesion that may cause diagnostic error. *J Cutan Pathol.* 2009;36:1109–1113.
12. Mataix J, Betlloch I, Lucas-Costa A, Pérez-Crespo M, Moscardó-Guilleme C. Nail changes in Langerhans cell histiocytosis: a possible marker of multisystem disease. *Pediatr Dermatol.* 2008;25:247–251.
13. Tran DT, Wolgamot GM, Olerud J, Hurst S, Argenyi Z. An "eruptive" variant of juvenile xanthogranuloma associated with Langerhans cell histiocytosis. *J Cutan Pathol.* 2008;35(suppl 1):50–54.
14. Edelbroek JR, Vermeer MH, Jansen PM, et al. Langerhans cell histiocytosis first presenting in the skin in adults: frequent

association with a second haematological malignancy. *Br J Dermatol.* 2012;167:1287–1294.

15. Satter EK, High WA. Langerhans cell histiocytosis: a review of the current recommendations of the Histiocyte Society. *Pediatr Dermatol.* 2008;25:291–295.

16. Ritterhouse LL, Barletta JA. BRAF V600E mutation-specific antibody: a review. *Semin Diagn Pathol.* 2015;32:400–408.

17. Ferringer T, Banks PM, Metcalf JS. Langerhans cell sarcoma. *Am J Dermatopathol.* 2006;28:36–39.

18. Sagransky MJ, Deng AC, Magro CM. Primary cutaneous Langerhans cell sarcoma: a report of four cases and review of the literature. *Am J Dermatopathol.* 2013;35:196–204.

19. Pileri SA, Grogan TM, Harris NL, et al. Tumours of histiocytes and accessory dendritic cells: an immunohistochemical approach to classification from the International Lymphoma Study Group based on 61 cases. *Histopathology.* 2002;41:1–29.

20. Badalian-Very G, Vergilio J-A, Degar BA, et al. Recurrent BRAF mutations in Langerhans cell histiocytosis. *Blood.* 2010;116:1919–1923.

21. Brown NA, Furtado LV, Betz BL, et al. High prevalence of somatic MAP2K1 mutations in BRAFV600E-negative Langerhans cell histiocytosis. *Blood.* 2014;124:1655–1658.

22. Chakraborty R, Hampton OA, Shen X, et al. Mutually exclusive recurrent somatic mutations in MAP2K1 and BRAF support a central role for ERK activation in LCH pathogenesis. *Blood.* 2014;124:3007–3015.

23. Nelson DS, Quispel W, Badalian-Very G, et al. Somatic activating ARAF mutations in Langerhans cell histiocytosis. *Blood.* 2014;123:3152–3155.

24. Facchetti F, Zelger B, Berti E, et al. Erdheim-Chester Disease. In: Elder DE, Massi D, Scolyer RA, Willemze R, eds. *WHO Classification of Skin Tumours.* 4th ed. IARC; 2018:287–288.

25. Allen CE, Li L, Peters TL, et al. Cell-specific gene expression in Langerhans cell histiocytosis lesions reveals a distinct profile compared with epidermal Langerhans cells. *J Immunol.* 2010;184:4557–4567.

26. Wood GS, Hu CH, Beckstead JH, Turner RR, Winkelmann RK. The indeterminate cell proliferative disorder: report of a case manifesting as an unusual cutaneous histiocytosis. *J Dermatol Surg Oncol.* 1985;11:1111–1119.

27. Winkelmann RK, Hu CH, Kossard S. Response of nodular non-X histiocytosis to vinblastine. *Arch Dermatol.* 1982;118:913–917.

28. Davick JJ, Kim J, Wick MR, Gru AA. Indeterminate dendritic cell tumor: a report of two new cases lacking the ETV3-NCOA2 translocation and a literature review. *Am J Dermatopathol.* 2018;40:736–748.

29. Facchetti F, Berti E, Zelger B. Indeterminate Cell Histiocytosis/Indeterminate Dendritic Cell Tumour. In: Elder DE, Massi D, Scolyer RA, Willemze R, eds. *WHO Classification of Skin Tumours.* 4th ed. IARC; 2018:283.

30. Sidoroff A, Zelger B, Steiner H, Smith N. Indeterminate cell histiocytosis—a clinicopathological entity with features of both X- and non-X histiocytosis. *Br J Dermatol.* 1996;134:525–532.

31. Rosenberg AS, Morgan MB. Cutaneous indeterminate cell histiocytosis: a new spindle cell variant resembling dendritic cell sarcoma. *J Cutan Pathol.* 2001;28:531–537.

32. Deng A, Lee W, Pfau R, et al. Primary cutaneous Langerhans cell sarcoma without Birbeck granules: indeterminate cell sarcoma? *J Cutan Pathol.* 2008;35:849–854.

33. Rezk SA, Spagnolo DV, Brynes RK, Weiss LM. Indeterminate cell tumor: a rare dendritic neoplasm. *Am J Surg Pathol.* 2008;32:1868–1876.

34. Ratzinger G, Burgdorf WH, Metze D, Zelger BG, Zelger B. Indeterminate cell histiocytosis: fact or fiction? *J Cutan Pathol.* 2005;32:552–560.

35. Hashimoto K, Fujiwara K, Punwaney J, et al. Post-scabetic nodules: a lymphohistiocytic reaction rich in indeterminate cells. *J Dermatol.* 2000;27:181–194.

36. Wollenberg A, Burgdorf WH, Schaller M, Sander C. Long-lasting "christmas tree rash" in an adolescent: isotopic response of indeterminate cell histiocytosis in pityriasis rosea? *Acta Derm Venereol.* 2002;82:288–291.

37. Brown RA, Kwong BY, McCalmont TH, et al. ETV3-NCOA2 in indeterminate cell histiocytosis: clonal translocation supports sui generis. *Blood.* 2015;126:2344–2345.

38. Bettington A, Lai JK, Kennedy C. Indeterminate dendritic cell tumour presenting in a patient with follicular lymphoma. *Pathology.* 2011;43:372–375.

39. Kemps PG, Hebeda KM, Pals ST, et al. Spectrum of histiocytic neoplasms associated with diverse haematological malignancies bearing the same oncogenic mutation. *J Pathol Clin Res.* 2021;7:10–26.

40. Shamburek RD, Brewer HB Jr, Gochuico BR. Erdheim-Chester disease: a rare multisystem histiocytic disorder associated with interstitial lung disease. *Am J Med Sci.* 2001;321:66–75.

41. Skinner M, Briant M, Morgan MB. Erdheim-Chester disease: a histiocytic disorder more than skin deep. *Am J Dermatopathol.* 2011;33:e24–e26.

42. Chasset F, Barele S, Charlotte F, et al. Cutaneous manifestations of Erdheim-Chester disease (ECD): clinical, pathological, and molecular features in a monocentric series of 40 patients. *J Am Acad Dermatol.* 2016;74:513–520.

43. Estrada-Veras JI, O'Brien KJ, Boyd LC, et al. The clinical spectrum of Erdheim-Chester disease: an observational cohort study. *Blood Adv.* 2017;1:357–366.

44. Volpicelli ER, Doyle L, Annes JP, et al. Erdheim-Chester disease presenting with cutaneous involvement: a case report and literature review. *J Cutan Pathol.* 2011;38:280–285.

45. Diamond EL, Dagna L, Hyman DM, et al. Consensus guidelines for the diagnosis and clinical management of Erdheim-Chester disease. *Blood.* 2014;124:483–492.

46. Tsai JW, Tsou JH, Hung LY, Wu HB, Chang KC. Combined Erdheim-Chester disease and Langerhans cell histiocytosis of skin are both monoclonal: a rare case with human androgen-receptor gene analysis. *J Am Acad Dermatol.* 2010;63:284–291.

47. Razanamahery J, Diamond EL, Cohen-Aubart F, et al. Erdheim-Chester disease with concomitant Rosai-Dorfman like lesions: a distinct entity mainly driven by *MAP2K1. Haematologica.* 2020;105:e5–e8.

48. Papo M, Diamond EL, Cohen-Aubart F, et al. High prevalence of myeloid neoplasms in adults with non-Langerhans cell histiocytosis. *Blood.* 2017;130:1007–1013.

49. Ozkaya N, Rosenblum MK, Durham BH, et al. The histopathology of Erdheim-Chester disease: a comprehensive review of a molecularly characterized cohort. *Mod Pathol.* 2018;31:581–597.

50. Haroche J, Cohen-Aubart F, Amoura Z. Erdheim-Chester disease. *Blood.* 2020;135:1311–1318.

51. Haroche J, Charlotte F, Arnaud L, et al. High prevalence of BRAF V600E mutations in Erdheim-Chester disease but not in other non-Langerhans cell histiocytoses. *Blood.* 2012;120:2700–2703.

52. Zelger BW, Cerio R. Xanthogranuloma is the archetype of non-Langerhans cell histiocytoses. *Br J Dermatol.* 2001;145:369–371.

53. Kzhyshkowska J, Gratchev A, Goerdt S. Stabilin-1, a homeostatic scavenger receptor with multiple functions. *J Cell Mol Med.* 2006;10:635–649.

54. Zelger BW, Sidoroff A, Orchard G, Cerio R. Non-Langerhans cell histiocytoses. A new unifying concept. *Am J Dermatopathol.* 1996;18:490–504.

55. Facchetti F, Zelger B. Juvenile Xanthogranuloma. In: Elder DE, Massi D, Scolyer RA, Willemze R, eds. *WHO Classification of Skin Tumours.* 4th ed. IARC; 2018:285–286.

56. Zelger BG, Zelger B, Steiner H, Mikuz G. Solitary giant xanthogranuloma and benign cephalic histiocytosis—variants of juvenile xanthogranuloma. *Br J Dermatol.* 1995;133:598–604.

57. Torrelo A, Juarez A, Hernandez A, Colmenero I. Multiple lichenoid juvenile xanthogranuloma. *Pediatr Dermatol.* 2009;26:238–240.

58. Mowbray M, Schofield OM. Juvenile xanthogranuloma en plaque. *Pediatr Dermatol.* 2007;24:670–671.

59. Caputo R, Grimalt R, Gelmetti C, Cottoni F. Unusual aspects of juvenile xanthogranuloma. *J Am Acad Dermatol.* 1993;29(5, pt 2):868–870.

60. Sanchez Yus E, Requena L, Villegas C, Valle P. Subcutaneous juvenile xanthogranuloma. *J Cutan Pathol.* 1995;22:460–465.

61. Chang MW, Frieden IJ, Good W. The risk of intraocular juvenile xanthogranuloma: survey of current practices and assessment of risk. *J Am Acad Dermatol.* 1996;34:445–449.

62. Jans SRR, Schomerus E, Bygum A. Neurofibromatosis type 1 diagnosed in a child based on multiple juvenile xanthogranulomas and juvenile myelomonocytic leukemia. *Pediatr Dermatol.* 2015;32:e29–e32.

63. Zvulunov A, Barak Y, Metzker A. Juvenile xanthogranuloma, neurofibromatosis, and juvenile chronic myelogenous leukemia. World statistical analysis. *Arch Dermatol.* 1995;131:904–908.

64. Cambiaghi S, Restano L, Caputo R. Juvenile xanthogranuloma associated with neurofibromatosis 1: 14 patients without evidence of hematologic malignancies. *Pediatr Dermatol.* 2004;21:97–101.

65. Burgdorf WHC, Zelger B. JXG, NF1, and JMML: alphabet soup or a clinical issue? *Pediatr Dermatol.* 2004;21:174–176.

66. Dehner LP. Juvenile xanthogranulomas in the first two decades of life: a clinicopathologic study of 174 cases with cutaneous and extracutaneous manifestations. *Am J Surg Pathol.* 2003;27:579–593.

67. Janssen D, Harms D. Juvenile xanthogranuloma in childhood and adolescence: a clinicopathologic study of 129 patients from the Kiel pediatric tumor registry. *Am J Surg Pathol.* 2005;29:21–28.

68. Azorin D, Torrelo A, Lassaletta A, et al. Systemic juvenile xanthogranuloma with fatal outcome. *Pediatr Dermatol.* 2009;26:709–712.

69. Shoo BA, Shinkai K, McCalmont TH, Fox LP. Xanthogranulomas associated with hematologic malignancy in adulthood. *J Am Acad Dermatol.* 2008;59:488–493.

70. Cohen PR, Prieto VG. Radiation port xanthogranuloma: solitary xanthogranuloma occurring within the irradiated skin of a breast cancer patient-report and review of cutaneous neoplasms developing at the site of radiotherapy. *J Cutan Pathol.* 2010;37:891–894.

71. Ngendahayo P, de Saint Aubain N. Mitotically active xanthogranuloma: a case report with review of the literature. *Am J Dermatopathol.* 2012;34:e27–e30.

72. Paxton CN, O'Malley DP, Bellizi AM, et al. Genetic evaluation of juvenile xanthogranuloma: genomic abnormalities are uncommon in solitary lesions, advanced cases may show more complexity. *Mod Pathol.* 2017;30:1234–1240.

73. Chantorn R, Wisuthsarewong W, Aanpreung P, Sanpakit K, Manonukul J. Severe congenital systemic juvenile xanthogranuloma in monozygotic twins. *Pediatr Dermatol.* 2008;25:470–473.

74. Gianotti F, Caputo R, Ermacora E, Gianni E. Benign cephalic histiocytosis. *Arch Dermatol.* 1986;122:1038–1043.

75. Jih DM, Salcedo SL, Jaworsky C. Benign cephalic histiocytosis: a case report and review. *J Am Acad Dermatol.* 2002;47:908–913.

76. Sidwell RU, Francis N, Slater DN, Mayou SC. Is disseminated juvenile xanthogranulomatosis benign cephalic histiocytosis? *Pediatr Dermatol.* 2005;22:40–43.

77. Winkelmann RK, Muller SA. Generalized eruptive histiocytoma. *Arch Dermatol.* 1963;88:586–596.

78. Larson MJ, Bandel C, Eichhorn PJ, Cruz PD Jr. Concurrent development of eruptive xanthogranulomas and hematologic malignancy: two case reports. *J Am Acad Dermatol.* 2004;50:976–978.

79. Seward JL, Malone JC, Callen JP. Generalized eruptive histiocytosis. *J Am Acad Dermatol.* 2004;50:116–120.

80. Pinney SS, Jahan-Tigh RR, Chon S. Generalized eruptive histiocytosis associated with a novel fusion in LMNA-NTRK1. *Dermatol Online J.* 2016;22:13030/qt07d3f2xk.

81. Wilk M, Zelger BG, Zelger B. Generalized eruptive histiocytosis with features of multinucleate cell angiohistiocytoma. *Am J Dermatopathol.* 2016;38:470–472.

82. Shafer WG. Verruciform xanthoma. *Oral Surg Oral Med Oral Pathol.* 1971;31:784–789.

83. Shahrabi Farahani S, Treister NS, Khan Z, Woo SB. Oral verruciform xanthoma associated with chronic graft-versus-host disease: a report of five cases and a review of the literature. *Head Neck Pathol.* 2011;5:193–198.

84. de Andrade BAB, Agostini M, Pires FR, et al. Oral verruciform xanthoma: a clinicopathologic and immunohistochemical study of 20 cases. *J Cutan Pathol.* 2015;42:489–495.

85. Blankenship DW, Zech L, Mirzabeigi M, Venna S. Verruciform xanthoma of the upper-extremity in the absence of chronic skin disease or syndrome: a case report and review of the literature. *J Cutan Pathol.* 2013;40:745–752.

86. Mohsin SK, Lee MW, Amin MB, et al. Cutaneous verruciform xanthoma: a report of five cases investigating the etiology and nature of xanthomatous cells. *Am J Surg Pathol.* 1998;22:479–487.

87. Cumberland L, Dana A, Resh B, Fitzpatrick J, Goldenberg G. Verruciform xanthoma in the setting of cutaneous trauma and chronic inflammation: report of a patient and a brief review of the literature. *J Cutan Pathol.* 2010;37:895–900.

88. Breier F, Zelger B, Reiter H, Gschnait F, Zelger BW. Papular xanthoma: a clinicopathological study of 10 cases. *J Cutan Pathol.* 2002;29:200–206.

89. Smith KJ, Yeager J, Skelton HG. Histologically distinctive papular neutrophilic xanthomas in HIV-1 + patients. *Am J Surg Pathol.* 1997;21:545–549.

90. Altmann J, Winkelmann RK. Diffuse normolipemic plane xanthoma. *Arch Dermatol.* 1962;85:633–640.

91. Marcoval J, Moreno A, Bordas X, Gallardo F, Peyrí J. Diffuse plane xanthoma: clinicopathologic study of 8 cases. *J Am Acad Dermatol.* 1998;39:439–442.

92. Huang HY, Liang CW, Hu SL, Cheng CC. Normolipemic papuloeruptive xanthomatosis in a child. *Pediatr Dermatol.* 2009;26:360–362.

93. Caputo R, Veraldi S, Grimalt R, et al. The various clinical patterns of xanthoma disseminatum. Considerations on seven cases and review of the literature. *Dermatology.* 1995;190:19–24.

94. Park HY, Cho DH, Kang HC, Yun SJ. A case of xanthoma disseminatum with spontaneous resolution over 10 years: review of the literature on long-term follow-up. *Dermatology.* 2011;222:236–243.

95. Zelger B, Cerio R, Orchard G, Fritsch P, Wilson-Jones E. Histologic and immunohistochemical study comparing xanthoma disseminatum and histiocytosis X. *Arch Dermatol.* 1992;128:1207–1212.

96. Zelger BG, Orchard G, Rudolph P, Zelger B. Scalloped cell xanthogranuloma. *Histopathology.* 1998;32:368–374.

97. Berti E, Facchetti F, Zelger B. Reticulohistiocytosis. In: Elder DE, Massi D, Scolyer RA, Willemze R, eds. *WHO Classification of Skin Tumours.* 4th ed. IARC; 2018:289–290.

98. Miettinen M, Fetsch JF. Reticulohistiocytoma (solitary epithelioid histiocytoma): a clinicopathologic and immunohistochemical study of 44 cases. *Am J Surg Pathol.* 2006;30:521–528.

99. Fusco N, Bonometti A, Augello C, et al. Clonal reticulohistiocytosis of the skin and bone marrow associated with systemic mastocytosis and acute myeloid leukaemia. *Histopathology.* 2017;70:1000–1008.

100. Bonometti A, Berti E. Reticulohistiocytoses: a revision of the full spectrum. *J Eur Acad Dermatol Venereol.* 2020;34:1684–1694.

101. Bonometti A, Sacco G, De Juli E, et al. Multisystem non-arthropathic reticulohistiocytosis: problems and pitfalls in the differential diagnosis of multisystem non-Langerhans-cell histiocytosis. *J Eur Acad Dermatol Venereol.* 2019;33:e195–e198.

102. Goltz RW, Laymon CW. Multicentric reticulohistiocytosis of the skin and synovia. *Arch Dermatol.* 1954;69:717–730.

103. Luz FB, Kurizky PS, Ramos-e-Silva M. Reticulohistiocytosis. *Dermatol Clin.* 2007;25:625–632.

104. Tajirian AL, Malik MK, Robinson-Bostom L, Lally EV. Multicentric reticulohistiocytosis. *Clin Dermatol.* 2006;24:486–492.

105. Fett N, Liu RH. Multicentric reticulohistiocytosis with dermatomyositis-like features: a more common disease presentation than previously thought. *Dermatology*. 2011;222:102–108.

106. Zelger B, Cerio R, Soyer HP, Misch K, Orchard G, Wilson-Jones E. Reticulohistiocytoma and multicentric reticulohistiocytosis. Histopathologic and immunophenotypic distinct entities. *Am J Dermatopathol*. 1994;16:577–584.

107. Selmi C, Greenspan A, Huntley, Gershwin ME. Multicentric reticulohistiocytosis: a critical review. *Curr Rheumatol Rep*. 2015;17:511.

108. Murakami N, Sakai T, Arai E, et al. Targetable driver mutations in multicentric reticulohistiocytosis. *Haematologica*. 2020;105:e61–e64.

109. Zelger BW, Staudacher C, Orchard G, Wilson-Jones E, Burgdorf WH. Solitary and generalized variants of spindle cell xanthogranuloma (progressive nodular histiocytosis). *Histopathology*. 1995;27:11–19.

110. Shin SJ, Scamman W, Gopalan A, Rosen PP. Mammary presentation of adult-type "juvenile" xanthogranuloma. *Am J Surg Pathol*. 2005;29:827–831.

111. Burgdorf WH, Kusch SL, Nix TE Jr, Pitha J. Progressive nodular histiocytoma. *Arch Dermatol*. 1981;117:644–649.

112. Glavin FL, Chhatwall H, Karimi K. Progressive nodular histiocytosis: a case report with literature review, and discussion of differential diagnosis and classification. *J Cutan Pathol*. 2009;36:1286–1292.

113. Hilker O, Kovneristy A, Varga R, et al. Progressive nodular histiocytosis. *J Dtsch Dermatol Ges*. 2013;11:301–307.

114. Kossard S, Winkelmann RK. Necrobiotic xanthogranuloma with paraproteinemia. *J Am Acad Dermatol*. 1980;3:257–270.

115. Fernandez-Herrera J, Pedraz J. Necrobiotic xanthogranuloma. *Semin Cutan Med Surg*. 2007;26:108–113.

116. Flann S, Wain EM, Halpern S, Andrews V, Whittaker S. Necrobiotic xanthogranuloma with paraproteinaemia. *Clin Exp Dermatol*. 2006;31:248–251.

117. Wood AJ, Wagner MV, Abbott JJ, Gibson LE. Necrobiotic xanthogranuloma: a review of 17 cases with emphasis on clinical and pathologic correlation. *Arch Dermatol*. 2009;145:279–284.

118. Ferrara G, Palombi N, Lipizzi A, Zalaudek I, Argenziano G. Non-necrobiotic necrobiotic xanthogranuloma. *Am J Dermatopathol*. 2007;29:306–308.

119. Ziemer M, Wedding U, Sander CS, Elsner P. Necrobiotic xanthogranuloma-rapid progression under treatment with melphalan. *Eur J Dermatol*. 2005;15:363–365.

120. Zelger B, Eisendle K, Mensing C, Zelger B. Detection of spirochetal micro-organisms by focus-floating microscopy in necrobiotic xanthogranuloma. *J Am Acad Dermatol*. 2007;57:1026–1030.

121. Miguel D, Lukacs J, Illing T, Elsner P. Treatment of necrobiotic xanthogranuloma—a systematic review. *J Eur Acad Dermatol Venereol*. 2017;31:221–235.

122. Rosai J, Dorfman RF. Sinus histiocytosis with massive lymphadenopathy. A newly recognized benign clinicopathological entity. *Arch Pathol*. 1969;87:63–70.

123. Destombes P. Adénites avec surcharge lipidique, de l'enfant ou de l'adulte jeune, observées aux Antilles et au Mali. (Quatre observations) Adenitis with lipid excess, in children or young adults, seen in the Antilles and in Mali (4 cases) [in French]. *Bull Soc Pathol Exot Filiales*. 1965;58:1169–1175.

124. Bruce-Brand C, Schneider JW, Schubert P. Rosai-Dorfman disease: an overview. *J Clin Pathol*. 2020;73:697–705.

125. Abla O, Jacobson E, Picarsic J, et al. Consensus recommendations for the diagnosis and clinical management of Rosai-Dorfman-Destombes disease. *Blood*. 2018;131:2877–2890.

126. Facchetti F, Zelger B. Rosai-Dorfman Disease. In: Elder DE, Massi D, Scolyer RA, Willemze R, eds. *WHO Classification of Skin Tumours*. 4th ed. IARC; 2018:284.

127. Brenn T, Calonje E, Granter SR, et al. Cutaneous Rosai-Dorfman disease is a distinct clinical entity. *Am J Dermatopathol*. 2002;24:385–391.

128. Frater JL, Maddox JS, Obadiah JM, Hurley MY. Cutaneous Rosai-Dorfman disease: comprehensive review of cases reported in the medical literature since 1990 and presentation of an illustrative case. *J Cutan Med Surg*. 2006;10:281–290.

129. Kong YY, Kong JC, Shi DR, et al. Cutaneous Rosai-Dorfman disease: a clinical and histopathologic study of 25 cases in China. *Am J Surg Pathol*. 2007;31:341–350.

130. Lu CI, Kuo TT, Wong WR, Hong HS. Clinical and histopathologic spectrum of cutaneous Rosai-Dorfman disease in Taiwan. *J Am Acad Dermatol*. 2004;51:931–939.

131. Wang KH, Chen WY, Liu HN, Huang CC, Lee WR, Hu CH. Cutaneous Rosai-Dorfman disease: clinicopathological profiles, spectrum and evolution of 21 lesions in six patients. *Br J Dermatol*. 2006;154:277–286.

132. Kuo TT, Chen TC, Lee LY, Lu PH. IgG4-positive plasma cells in cutaneous Rosai-Dorfman disease: an additional immunohistochemical feature and possible relationship to IgG4-related sclerosing disease. *J Cutan Pathol*. 2009;36:1069–1073.

133. Colmenero I, Molho-Pessach V, Torrelo A, Zlotogorski A, Requena L. Emperipolesis: an additional common histopathologic finding in H syndrome and Rosai-Dorfman disease. *Am J Dermatopathol*. 2012;34:315–320.

134. Magro CM, Kazi N, Sisinger AE. Primary cutaneous histiocytic sarcoma: a report of five cases with primary cutaneous involvement and review of the literature. *Ann Diagn Pathol*. 2018;32:56–62.

135. Hung YP, Qian X. Histiocytic sarcoma. *Arch Pathol Lab Med*. 2020;144:650–654.

136. Vos JA, Abbondanzo SL, Barekman CL, Andriko JW, Miettinen M, Aguilera NS. Histiocytic sarcoma: a study of five cases including the histiocyte marker CD163. *Mod Pathol*. 2005;18:693–704.

137. Nguyen TT, Schwartz EJ, West RB, Warnke RA, Arber DA, Natkunam Y. Expression of CD163 (hemoglobin scavenger receptor) in normal tissues, lymphomas, carcinomas, and sarcomas is likely restricted to the monocyte/macrophage lineage. *Am J Surg Pathol*. 2005;29:617–624.

138. Shanmugam V, Sholl LM, Fletcher CD, Hornick JL. RAS/MAPK pathway activation defines a common molecular subtype of histiocytic sarcoma. *Mod Pathol*. 2018;31:551.

139. Hornick JL, Jaffe ES, Fletcher CDM. Extranodal histiocytic sarcoma: clinicopathologic analysis of 14 cases of a rare epithelioid malignancy. *Am J Surg Pathol*. 2004;28:1133–1144.

140. Rosado FG, Kim AS. Hemophagocytic lymphohistiocytosis: an update on diagnosis and pathogenesis. *Am J Clin Pathol*. 2013;139:713–727.

141. Canna SW, Marsh RA. Pediatric hemophagocytic lymphohistiocytosis. *Blood*. 2020;135:1332–1343.

142. Hayden A, Park, S, Giustini D, Lee AY, Chen LY. Hemophagocytic syndromes (HPSs) including hemophagocytic lymphohistiocytosis (HLH) in adults: a systematic scoping review. *Blood Rev*. 2016;30:411–420.

143. Favara BE, Jaffe R, Egeler RM. Macrophage activation and hemophagocytic syndrome in Langerhans cell histiocytosis: report of 30 cases. *Pediatr Dev Pathol*. 2002;5:130–140.

144. Hu WK, Gilliam AC, Wiersma SR, Dahms BB. Fatal congenital systemic juvenile xanthogranuloma with liver failure. *Pediatr Dev Pathol*. 2004;7:71–76.

145. Morrell DS, Pepping MA, Scott JP, Esterly NB, Drolet BA. Cutaneous manifestations of hemophagocytic lymphohistiocytosis. *Arch Dermatol*. 2002;138:1208–1212.

Chapter

27

Pigmentary Disorders of the Skin

LESLIE ROBINSON-BOSTOM, MARY CLARK, THINH CHAU, AND CARYN COBB

INTRODUCTION

This chapter considers a heterogeneous group of disorders that are associated with alterations in the intensity and patterns of pigmentation of the skin. Many of these disorders are genetic in nature, whereas other etiologies include inflammatory, degenerative, endocrine, toxic, and immunologic factors. Neoplastic and some other localized proliferations of melanocytes, which are also often associated with pigmentary alterations, are considered in Chapter 28.

CONGENITAL DIFFUSE MELANOSIS

Clinical Summary. Congenital diffuse melanosis, also termed *melanosis diffusa congenita* (1) or *generalized cutaneous melanosis* (2), is a rare genetic disease that usually appears at or shortly after birth and demonstrates progressive diffuse hyperpigmentation. A case with onset in adolescence has also been reported (3). The pigmentation is most intense on the abdomen and back and may be reticulate in the axillae and groin. Thin nails (2) and yellow-white hair (1) have been noted.

Histopathology. Increased melanization is seen in both the basilar and mid-epidermal keratinocytes, along with melanophages in the superficial dermis.

Pathogenesis. On electron microscopic examination, Braun-Falco and colleagues (1) noted increased numbers of single melanosomes in the keratinocytes, and Kint and associates (2) described dispersion of melanosomes throughout the keratinocyte cytoplasm.

Differential Diagnosis. Considerations include dyschromatosis universalis hereditaria, familial progressive hyperpigmentation, Riehl melanosis, and universal acquired melanosis (Carbon baby syndrome) (3).

Principles of Management: Symptomatic and cosmetic management could be considered.

RETICULATE PIGMENTARY ANOMALIES

Clinical Summary. A number of inherited pigmentary disorders are characterized by hypo- and hyperpigmented macules in a reticulate, retiform, or fishnet-like pattern. These disorders are unified by the presence of increased melanin within the epidermis and exclude postinflammatory pigmentary alterations and conditions displaying reticulation secondary to vascular phenomena, such as livedo reticularis. Clinically, the reticulate pigmentary disorders can be classified based on the distribution and extent of involvement (acral, flexural, localized, and generalized) (4).

Dyskeratosis congenita encompasses a spectrum of diseases classically characterized by an acquired reticulated brown hyperpigmentation, beginning in the first decade of life, which spreads across the face, neck, upper chest, and arms. Nail dystrophy, oral leukoplakia, and bone marrow failure are commonly seen (5,6). This syndrome demonstrates genetic and clinical heterogeneity (7). Other associated findings may include epiphora, pulmonary disease, extensive dental caries, short stature, and a predisposition to malignancy (5). Patients with dyskeratosis congenita are at an 11-fold increased risk of cancers of the upper aerodigestive tract, most of which (40%) are squamous cell carcinomas of the head and neck (6). These cancers may develop at a relatively young age (median age of squamous cell carcinoma is 29 to 37 years) (6).

Progressive cribriform and zosteriform hyperpigmentation begins in the second decade of life with tan cribriform macular hyperpigmentation of the lower half of the trunk or thighs in a dermatomal distribution (8). There are no associated internal abnormalities (9). Linear and whorled nevoid hypermelanosis (LWNH) has a similar clinical appearance, except the pigmentation appears within the first year of life and is present along the lines of Blaschko in diffuse streaks and swirls rather than localized hyperpigmented lesions (10).

Several entities are characterized by the presence of acral hyperpigmentation. *Acropigmentation symmetrica of Dohi* (dyschromatosis symmetrica hereditaria, reticulate acropigmentation of Dohi) is a progressive autosomal dominant disorder with an onset during childhood that appears as reticulate hyperpigmented and hypopigmented macules on the face and dorsa of the hands and feet, progressing to cover acral areas (11,12). *Reticulate acropigmentation of Kitamura* is an autosomal dominant disorder that presents as slightly depressed, well-demarcated hyperpigmented macules on the dorsal hands and feet that evolve to a reticulate pattern as the individual ages. There is progression to involve the flexor aspects of the wrists, the neck, knees, and elbows. Rarely, it can involve the palms and soles. There has been an association with palmar and plantar pits (11).

Reticulate acropigmentation of Kitamura (acropigmentatio reticularis) and *Dowling–Degos disease* (reticulate pigmented anomaly of the flexures) may appear together (11,13), supporting the concept that they are different expressions of one disorder. In Dowling–Degos disease, a dominantly inherited dermatosis, heavily pigmented macules are arranged in a reticulate pattern with a tendency to coalesce on flexural skin, including the axillae, lateral neck, inframammary and inguinal folds, antecubital and popliteal fossae, and intergluteal clefts. Other sites that may be involved include the genitalia, inner thighs, chest, face, and abdomen. Extensive areas of the skin may be affected. Pitted perioral scars, hyperpigmented comedones, hidradenitis suppurativa, multiple cysts and abscesses, keratoacanthomas, and squamous cell carcinoma have been associated (14). Rarely, hypopigmented lesions have been reported in patients with generalized Dowling–Degos disease (15). *Galli–Galli disease* is considered an acantholytic variant of Dowling–Degos disease, but they are clinically indistinguishable (16).

The *Naegeli–Franceschetti–Jadassohn syndrome* (Naegeli reticular pigmented dermatosis) and *dermatopathia pigmentosa reticularis* are autosomal dominant inherited disorders that share key clinical features, such as reticulate pigmentation of the skin, absence of dermatoglyphics, palmoplantar keratoderma, hypohidrosis, and other hair and nail abnormalities. Dermatopathia pigmentosa reticularis is distinguished from Naegeli–Franceschetti–Jadassohn syndrome by lifelong persistence of skin hyperpigmentation, hyperhidrosis, onychodystrophy, partial alopecia, and absence of dental anomalies (17).

Histopathology. Most of these conditions demonstrate hyperpigmentation of the basilar keratinocytes with either a normal or slightly increased number of melanocytes. Dyskeratosis congenita is characterized by occasional atrophy of the epidermis, mild interface vacuolization with melanophages in the upper dermis, and telangiectasias of superficial vessels (18). Reticulate acropigmentation of Kitamura and, to a greater degree, Dowling–Degos disease demonstrate digitated elongations of the hyperpigmented rete ridges with a tendency to spare the suprapapillary epithelium (Fig. 27-1A). In Dowling–Degos disease, these thin, branching, heavily pigmented downward proliferations also involve the infundibula of follicles; in some instances, horn cysts may be seen (14). Galli–Galli disease demonstrates similar thin, branching hyperpigmented rete ridges with foci of acantholysis (Fig. 27-1B) (16). Although there is no preceding inflammatory dermatosis in dermatopathia pigmentosa reticularis, clumps of melanin-laden melanophages are seen in the papillary dermis in a patchy distribution without overlying epidermal hyperpigmentation (19).

Pathogenesis. These conditions are thought to be inherited, although all of the genes responsible for their expression have not been definitively identified. Dyskeratosis congenita is a genetically heterogeneous disease of defective telomere maintenance that may demonstrate X-linked, autosomal recessive, or autosomal dominant patterns of inheritance (20). Defective genes include dyskerin, *TERC, TERT, NHP2, TIN2, TCAB1, C16orf57,* and *NOP10* (7). Dowling–Degos disease and *Galli–Galli disease* have been linked to mutations of the *keratin 5* gene (21,22). Dyschromatosis symmetrica hereditaria patients have mutations in genes involved in RNA editing (*ADAR1* [24] and *DSRAD*) (23–26). ADAR1 mutations are also identified in Aicardi–Goutières syndrome, which is a severe inflammatory disease in childhood that affects the brain and skin and has been rarely reported in a patient with associated dyschromatosis symmetrica hereditaria (11). Reticulate acropigmentation of Kitamura patients have mutations in ADAM10, KRT5, and POFUT1 (11). *Naegeli–Franceschetti–Jadassohn syndrome* and *dermatopathia pigmentosa reticularis* patients have mutations in keratin 14 (17).

Principles of Management: Treatment modalities include retinoids, bleaching agents, ultraviolet B (UVB) phototherapy, and azelaic acid. Ablative lasers have been shown to be effective in Dowling–Degos disease (27,28) and Galli–Galli disease (29).

LINEAR AND WHORLED NEVOID HYPERMELANOSIS

Clinical Summary. LWNH is a rare, occasionally familial disorder characterized by multiple hyperpigmented macules distributed in linear streaks and whorls following the lines of Blaschko (10,30). It appears within the first few weeks of life and progresses over 1 to 2 years before stabilization (31,32). The most common sites are trunk and extremities, and it usually spares the palms, soles, face, and mucosa. It can be associated with extracutaneous abnormalities including central nervous system (CNS) diseases, cardiac defects, psychomotor delay, deafness, brachydactyly, and hydrocephalus (33). A revised nomenclature has been proposed, grouping hypomelanosis of Ito and LWNH as a single entity (31,34).

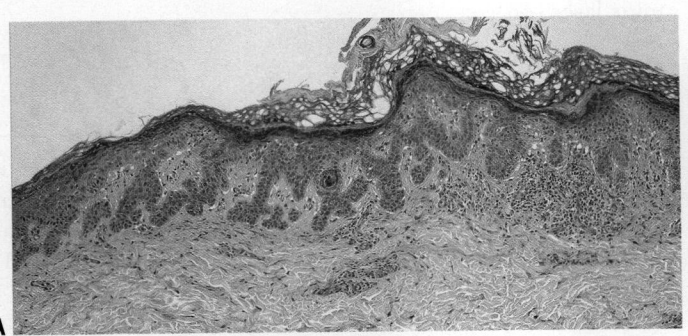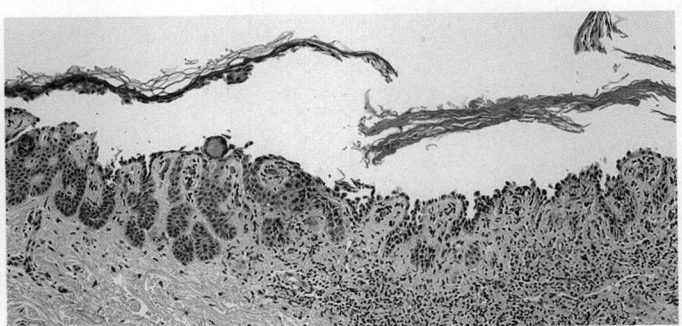

Figure 27-1 Dowling–Degos disease and Galli–Galli disease. **A:** Classic findings of Dowling–Degos disease include digitated elongations of hyperpigmented rete ridges sparing the suprapapillary epithelium. **B:** Galli–Galli disease showing similar thin-branching hyperpigmented rete ridges with foci of acantholysis.

Histopathology. There is hyperpigmentation of the basilar keratinocytes with prominent melanocytes and mild elongation of the rete ridges (30–32). Pigmentary incontinence with melanophages in the papillary dermis is variably present (32).

Pathogenesis. Somatic mosaicism, leading to proliferation and migration of two mixed populations of melanocytes with different potential for pigment production has been proposed as an explanation for this patterned hypermelanosis (30,32). Chromosomal abnormalities reported to date include trisomy 13 (35), mosaic trisomy 7 (36), 14, 18 (37), 20 (38) as well as X-chromosomal mosaicism (39).

Differential Diagnosis. Considerations include hypomelanosis of Ito (30), the third stage of incontinentia pigmenti, and epidermal nevus (30,32).

Principles of Management: No satisfactory treatment modalities are known. Chemical peels and laser treatments have been tried.

MELASMA

Clinical Summary. Melasma is an acquired, localized, usually symmetrical hyperpigmentation of the face, especially the forehead, malar areas, upper lip, and chin, occurring in women, particularly Fitzpatrick skin types III and IV (Fig. 27-2). It is often associated with pregnancy, exogenous hormones, and exposure to ultraviolet (UV) light. It has been shown that Wood's lamp examination may not be precise at predicting epidermal versus dermal pigment deposition (40). *In vivo* reflectance confocal microscopy has recently been used to define pigment presence and location in melasma (41,42).

Histopathology. An epidermal and a dermal type can be recognized, although frequently there is a combination of the two types. In the epidermal form, melanin deposition occurs mainly in the basal and suprabasal layers and the melanocytes are highly dendritic and full of pigment. In the dermal form, there is less prominent epidermal pigmentation with

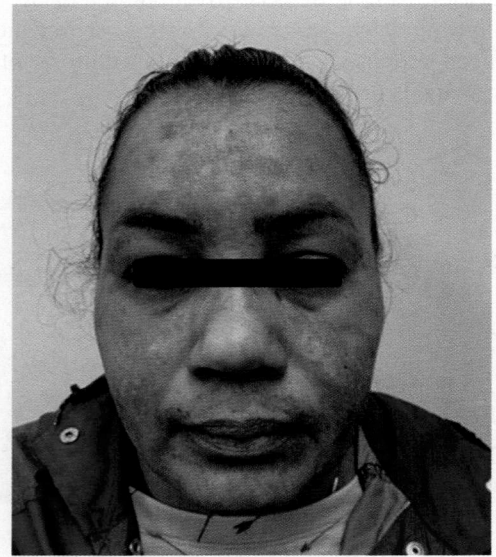

Figure 27-2 Melasma. There is symmetrical hyperpigmentation of the face.

superficial and deep dermal perivascular melanophages and free melanin deposits (43,44). Increased melanocyte activity has been suggested using Mel-5 immunostaining (45). Solar elastosis and telangiectasias may be present. Many studies have found increased vascularity in lesions of melasma compared to normal skin, in both the number and size of blood vessels in the dermis (46).

Pathogenesis. The pathogenesis of melasma is thought to include multiple factors, including genetic predisposition, hormonal imbalance, and visible and UV light exposure. UV-induced oxidative stress and subsequent DNA damage stimulate melanogenic activity through enhanced transfer of melanin from melanocytes to nearby keratinocytes and increased secretion of melanocyte-stimulating hormone by keratinocytes (46). Also, specific protection against shorter wavelengths of visible light (415 nm) may have an impact on melasma relapses. One study showed a larger increase in the Melasma Area and Severity Index (MASI) score using sunscreen with protection against only UVA/UVB compared with sun protection using a tinted sunscreen containing iron oxides (protective against ultraviolet A [UVA], UVB, and shorter wavelengths of visible light) (47). Newer studies show that the pathogenesis of melasma also involves aberrant angiogenesis and vasodilation of dermal blood vessels. UV radiation may stimulate the upregulation of proangiogenic proteins including the vascular endothelial growth factor (VEGF), fibroblast growth factor, and interleukin-8 (46). The exact link between hormones and melasma has not been fully elucidated, but hormone imbalances including pregnancy and oral contraceptive use are associated with increased melasma severity (40,46).

Differential Diagnosis. Considerations include postinflammatory hyperpigmentation, drug-induced hyperpigmentation, Addison disease, pigmented contact dermatitis, exogenous ochronosis, poikiloderma of Civatte, erythromelanosis follicularis faciei et colli, Hori nevus, and lichen planus pigmentosus.

Principles of Management: Treatment modalities include diligent sun protection (visible light and UV protection with tinted broad-spectrum sunscreens), topical bleaching agents containing hydroquinones, retinoids, corticosteroids (alone or in combination with retinoids and hydroquinones), azelaic acid, kojic acid, glycolic acid, and salicylic acid peels, ascorbic acid, dermabrasion, and resurfacing lasers (47,48). Newer treatments focus on addressing the vascular component of melasma, including tranexamic acid (oral and topical), and laser surgery including pulsed dye laser, QS-Nd:YAG laser, and copper bromide laser (46).

ADDISON DISEASE

Clinical Summary. Addison disease represents a hypofunction of the adrenal cortex and is characterized by progressive weakness, malaise, weight loss, hypotension, joint and back pain, and darkening of the skin and mucous membranes (49). The hyperpigmentation is generalized but most pronounced on sun-exposed skin, sites of friction, palmar creases, recent scars, and genital skin (49). Patchy oral mucosal pigmentation is often present (50). There can also be nail hyperpigmentation, mostly in the form of longitudinal melanonychia. In advanced cases, Addison disease can lack cutaneous hyperpigmentation, because destruction of melanocytes occurs as the disease progresses (50).

Histopathology. The histologic findings simulate the normal findings in patients with darker skin tones and are therefore not diagnostic. Increased amounts of melanin are seen in the basal keratinocytes and often in the keratinocytes in the upper spinous layer. The number of melanocytes is not increased. Variable numbers of melanophages may be seen in the papillary dermis (50). Other nonspecific findings that can be seen include acanthosis, hyperkeratosis, focal parakeratosis, spongiosis, and superficial perivascular lymphocytic inflammation (50).

Pathogenesis. Most commonly, Addison disease is the result of an autoimmune destruction of the adrenal glands, with subsequent inadequate production of cortisol and aldosterone. Addison disease is often associated with other autoimmune diseases, such as autoimmune glandular syndromes, insulin-dependent diabetes, vitiligo, and thyroid disease (49). The hyperpigmentation in Addison disease is caused by an increased release of melanocyte stimulating hormone (MSH) from the pituitary gland. Adrenocorticotropic hormone (ACTH) and MSH synthesis and secretion in the pituitary gland are linked. The increased production of ACTH and MSH in Addison disease is a compensatory, feedback-controlled response to low adrenal gland activity. The increase in production of ACTH then acts as an agonist of the melanocortin 1 receptor on the surface of melanocytes, stimulating the accumulation of eumelanin (50). Other causes of adrenal hypofunction include damage of adrenal glands by tuberculosis, metastatic carcinoma, and deep fungal infections. Autoimmune Addison disease is associated with certain MHC haplotypes such as DR3-DQ2 and DR4-DQ8 and gene mutations related to the regulation of T-cell–mediated autoimmunity (51,52).

Differential Diagnosis. Considerations include drug-induced hyperpigmentation, hemochromatosis, melasma, postinflammatory hyperpigmentation, pigmented contact dermatitis, and vitamin B_{12} deficiency (50).

Principles of Management: Treatment should focus on addressing the underlying hormonal deficiency.

POSTINFLAMMATORY PIGMENTARY ALTERATION

Clinical Summary. Pigment alteration in the skin from a preceding inflammatory disorder can produce clinical hypopigmentation, hyperpigmentation, or both. Processes that affect the dermal–epidermal interface such as fixed drug eruptions, lichen planus, benign lichenoid keratosis, and erythema multiforme are most commonly involved. Infections (pinta, syphilis, onchocerciasis) and cutaneous injuries from dermatologic procedures, irritants, and burns can also lead to pigment alterations (Fig. 27-3). In some individuals, the alteration can be dramatic, producing dark pigmentation resembling primary melanocytic lesions or marked hypopigmentation resembling vitiligo. Wood's light examination accentuates epidermal melanin and is useful as a clinical tool in defining the nature and extent of pigmentary alteration. Confocal laser microscopy may allow the evaluation of melanin content and distribution pattern of different hypomelanotic conditions (53).

Histopathology. Epidermal melanin shows increased clinical hyperpigmentation and decreased clinical hypopigmentation. In both clinical forms of pigmentary alteration, melanophages are present in the superficial dermis, along with a variably dense infiltrate of lymphohistiocytic inflammation around superficial blood vessels and in dermal papillae (54) (Fig. 27-3). Necrotic keratinocytes and coarse collagen bundles in the papillary dermis are occasionally seen (54).

Pathogenesis. Direct stimulation of melanocytes by inflammatory mediators such as IL-1, endothelin 1, and stem cell factor (55) as well as fibroblast-derived melanogenic growth factors have been proposed to play a role in postinflammatory hyperpigmentation (56).

Differential Diagnosis. The differential diagnosis includes vitiligo, idiopathic guttate hypomelanosis, progressive macular hypopigmentation, infections (tinea versicolor, leprosy, onchocerciasis, pinta), nevus depigmentosus, drug-induced hyperpigmentation, systemic diseases (Addison disease, hemochromatosis, hyperthyroidism, renal and hepatic failure, systemic lupus erythematosus, dermatomyositis), nutritional diseases (pellagra, malabsorption), ochronosis, and lymphoma.

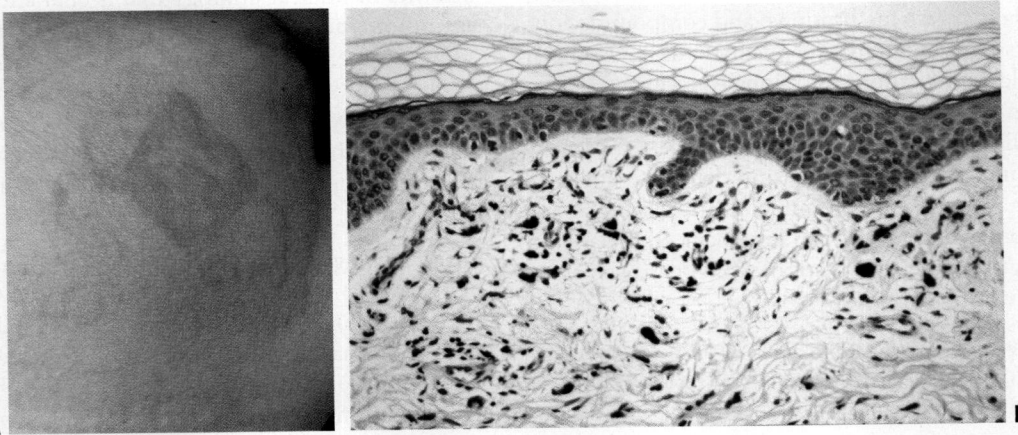

Figure 27-3 Postinflammatory hyperpigmentation. **A:** Clinical photo from postinflammatory pigmentation owing to adhesive in electrocardiogram (EKG) lead. **B:** Histology shows a normal epidermis with numerous melanophages in the papillary dermis and a mild perivascular lymphocytic infiltrate.

Principles of Management: Treatment should focus on addressing the underlying cause. In addition, for hyperpigmentation, bleaching creams containing hydroquinones, retinoids, topical corticosteroids, chemical peels, azelaic acid, laser treatment, and camouflage are recommended (57,58). For hypopigmentation, topical corticosteroids, topical calcineurin inhibitors, phototherapy, and skin grafts are recommended (59).

BERLOQUE DERMATITIS AND PHYTOPHOTODERMATITIS

Clinical Summary. Localized hyperpigmented patches produced by furocoumarin-containing oil of Bergamot found in perfumes have a distinctive clinical presentation. The patches assume drop-like shapes resembling pendants (French: *berloque*) and are usually located on the lateral neck or retroauricular areas. Contact with plants containing furocoumarins may also produce hyperpigmented patches and include lime, wild and cow parsnip, wild carrot, bergamot orange, and fig (60).

Histopathology. Features identical to postinflammatory hyperpigmentation are found, including increased epidermal melanin and melanophages in the superficial dermis. Variable chronic inflammation is present.

Differential Diagnosis. Considerations include postinflammatory hyperpigmentation.

Principles of Management: Treatment consists of avoidance of offending agents, topical corticosteroids, and bleaching agents.

CHEMICAL DEPIGMENTATION

Chemical leukoderma, or more recently termed chemical-induced vitiligo, is an acquired depigmentation resembling vitiligo caused by repeated exposure to agents that destroy melanocytes in genetically susceptible individuals. Hydroquinones, phenols, catechols as well as sulfhydryl compounds are the most common causes and are found in bleaching agents, adhesives, cosmetics, hair dyes, photographic processing materials, fabrics treated with azo dyes, and antioxidants used in rubber manufacturing (61–63). Depigmentation may also occur in body sites remote from chemical contact, presumably from systemic absorption or inhalation. Systemic medications (fluphenazine, chloroquine, and imatinib mesylate); optic medications; and compounds containing mercury, arsenic, and cinnamic aldehyde have also been reported to cause depigmentation. Additionally, localized depigmentation has been documented as a rare adverse effect of topical imiquimod in the setting of condyloma acuminata treatment (63-65). Systemic immunotherapy with interleukin-2, interferon-α-2, and—more recently—programmed death receptor-1 inhibitors pembrolizumab and nivolumab for advanced melanoma can also elicit vitiligo-like depigmentation, which has been associated with more favorable prognosis (66,67).

Histopathology. Features indistinguishable from vitiligo are found. Decreased to absent melanocytes are present with variable superficial perivascular lymphocytic infiltrate.

Differential Diagnosis. Considerations include vitiligo, infections (tinea versicolor, leprosy, onchocerciasis, pinta), genetic syndromes (piebaldism, hypomelanosis of Ito, tuberous

sclerosis, Waardenburg syndrome, Vogt–Koyanagi–Harada syndrome), postinflammatory hypopigmentation, nevus depigmentosus, idiopathic guttate hypomelanosis, and progressive macular hypomelanosis.

Principles of Management: Treatment consists of avoidance of offending agents and treatments used for vitiligo (see the section on Vitiligo).

IDIOPATHIC GUTTATE HYPOMELANOSIS

Clinical Summary. Idiopathic guttate hypomelanosis is a commonly acquired benign disorder of unknown etiology that produces few to numerous asymptomatic sharply circumscribed, 2- to 6-mm white macules. These lesions occur predominantly on the legs and forearms of persons over 30 years of age (68,69) (Fig. 27-4).

Histopathology. The lesional borders are sharply demarcated with a hypomelanotic epidermis featuring degenerated and reduced melanocytes, decreased melanosomes, and irregularly distributed melanin granules (70,71). Fontana–Masson stain shows sharp demarcation with abrupt loss of pigment whereas Melan-A and Sox10 stains reiterate decreased melanocyte density within the hypopigmented lesion (Fig. 27-4).

Pathogenesis. Under electron microscopy, the scattered residual melanocytes in lesional skin are round and less dendritic with fewer melanosomes that are incompletely melanized (72). Chronic sun exposure, trauma, autoimmunity, and genetic factors such as HLA-DQ3 have been proposed to contribute to disease pathogenesis.

Differential Diagnosis. The differential diagnosis includes postinflammatory hypopigmentation, progressive macular hypopigmentation, pityriasis versicolor, and vitiligo.

Principles of Management: Treatment modalities include topical calcineurin inhibitors (73), dermabrasion, cryotherapy (74), and lasers (75).

PROGRESSIVE MACULAR HYPOPIGMENTATION

Clinical Summary. Progressive macular hypopigmentation is a disorder of unclear etiology that is characterized by ill-defined, asymptomatic hypopigmented macules on the central trunk, sometimes extending to the neck and face predominantly in young adults (Fig. 27-5) (76). The lesions may be discrete or eventually become confluent and occur without previous inflammation or pathology (77). The lesional skin features pathognomonic follicular punctiform red-to-orange fluorescence under Wood's lamp (78).

Histopathology. Histologic features of lesional and nonlesional skin may be indistinguishable (Fig. 27-5). A subtle decrease in melanin content may be present in lesional skin, and staining with Fontana–Masson may demonstrate reduced basilar melanin (77,79). Electron microscopy studies found less dense pigmentation and fewer mature melanosomes in lesional skin compared with normal skin (80,81).

Pathogenesis. Different subtypes of *Cutibacterium acnes* have been suggested to play a role (82). *Cutibacterium acnes* has been

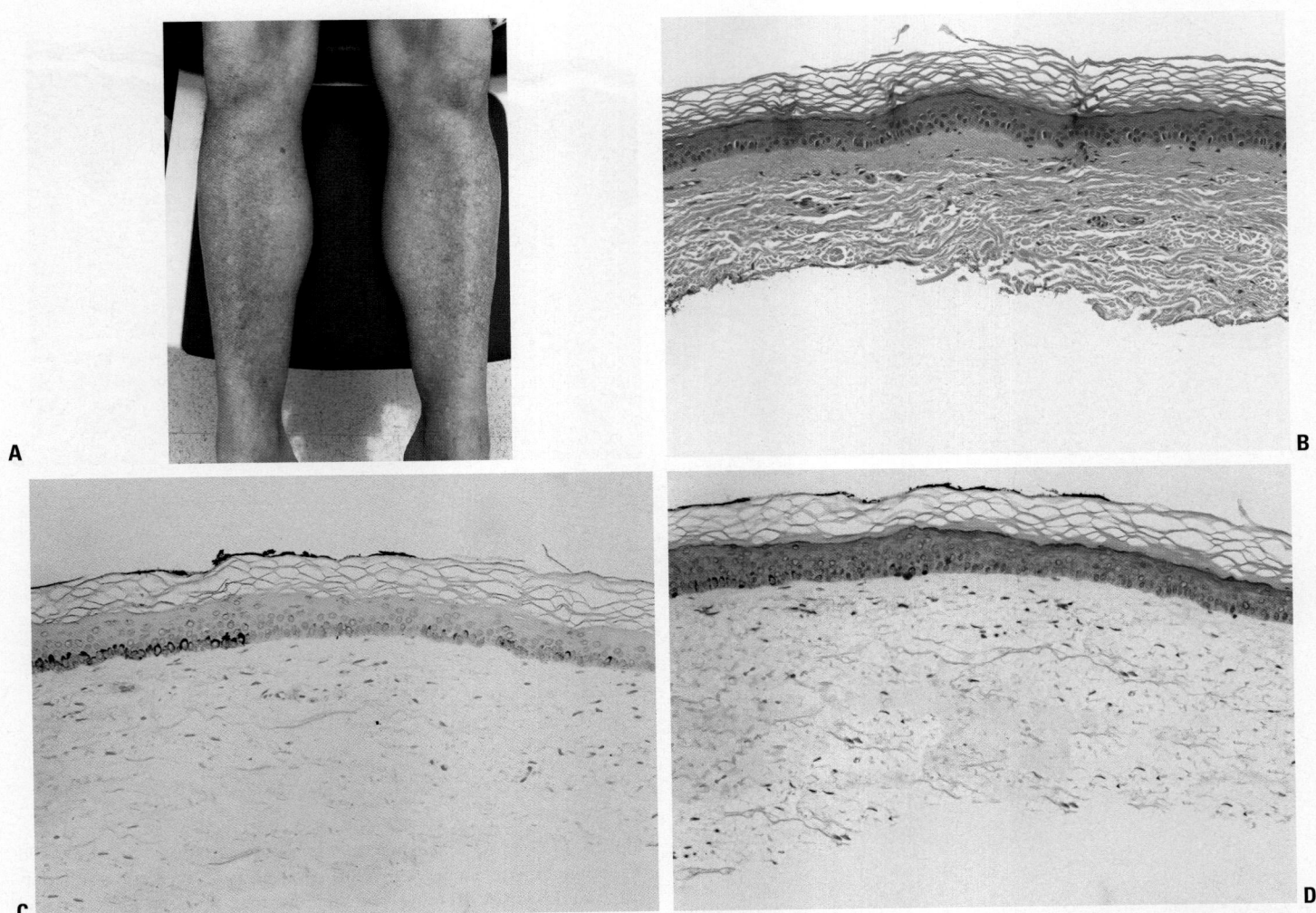

Figure 27-4 Idiopathic guttate hypomelanosis. **A:** Numerous sharply circumscribed white macules on the lower legs. **B:** Normal-appearing epidermis and dermis. **C:** Fontana–Masson showing sharp demarcation with abrupt loss of pigment. **D:** Sox10 showing decreased melanocytes within the hypopigmented lesion.

cultured and identified histologically in follicles of lesional skin but not follicles or interfollicular areas of healthy-looking adjacent skin. It has been proposed that the bacteria may interfere with melanogenesis in these skin lesions (79).

Differential Diagnosis. Considerations include idiopathic guttate hypomelanosis, postinflammatory hypopigmentation, pityriasis versicolor, vitiligo, and hypopigmented mycosis fungoides.

Principles of Management: Treatment consists of phototherapy (83), benzoyl peroxide, and clindamycin (84).

PSORALEN AND ULTRAVIOLET A-INDUCED PIGMENT ALTERATIONS

Clinical Summary. Psoralen and ultraviolet A (PUVA) therapy consists of the oral ingestion or topical application of a furocoumarin-containing psoralen compound followed by patient exposure to high-intensity UVA radiation in a controlled-light-box setting. Although previously widely used for treating psoriasis and cutaneous T-cell lymphoma as well as various other dermatoses including vitiligo, this treatment modality has sharply declined in usage owing to associated adverse effects as detailed in this section.

A spectrum of clinical and histologic changes is seen during and after PUVA therapy. Acutely, phototoxic erythema peaks at 48 to 72 hours. Hyperpigmentation (tanning) is delayed for several days and more pronounced and longer lasting than that induced by UVB exposure. Prolonged therapy leads to photoaging with cutaneous atrophy, fine wrinkling, mottled hyperpigmentation and hypopigmentation, telangiectasias, and loss of elasticity. Stellate lentigines or PUVA freckles often develop after prolonged therapy. Predisposing factors for developing PUVA lentigines include skin type, number of treatments, and sex (occurring more commonly in males than females). There is also a dose-dependent increase in the risk of melanoma and squamous cell carcinoma, especially in the genital areas (85).

Histopathology. The histologic changes of PUVA-induced acute phototoxicity are similar to a sunburn, with numerous apoptotic keratinocytes ("sunburn cells") scattered throughout the epidermis. Early in the therapeutic course, basilar melanocytes and mid-spinous keratinocytes become heavily melanized. Prolonged therapy leads to gradual flattening of the rete ridges, telangiectasias, increased papillary dermal acid mucopolysaccharide deposition, thinning and basophilic degeneration of elastic fibers, and hyperplasia and fragmentation of elastic fibers (86). Hyperpigmented skin without other clinical changes frequently demonstrates small foci of keratinocytic nuclear atypia

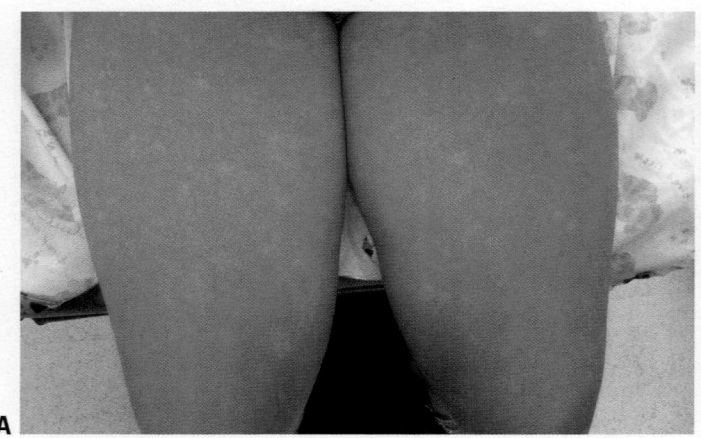

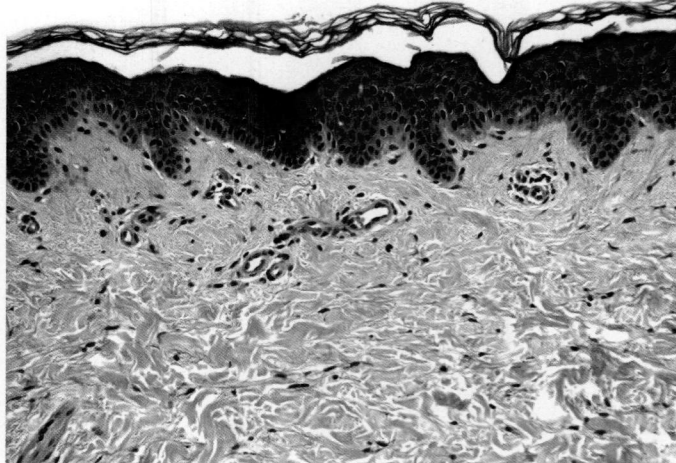

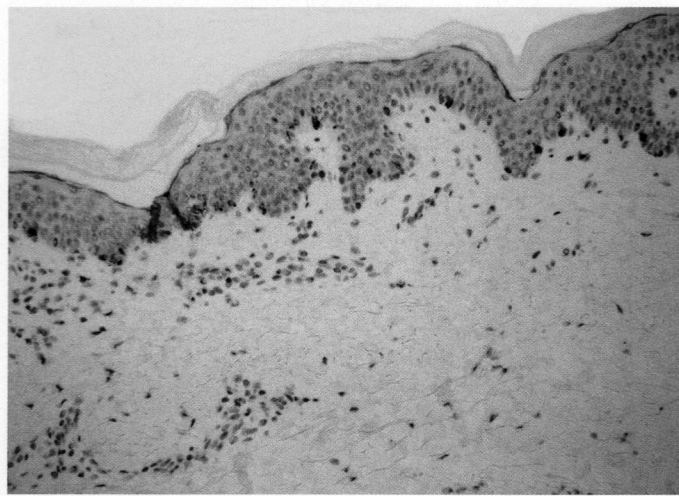

Figure 27-5 Progressive macular hypopigmentation. **A:** Ill-defined hypopigmented macules. **B:** Normal-appearing epidermis and dermis. **C:** Melan-A staining showing normal number of junctional melanocytes.

and loss of the normal maturation pattern (87). Actinic keratoses, Bowen disease, squamous cell carcinomas, and melanomas may develop. PUVA freckles or lentigines show increased melanocyte density and elongation of the rete ridges with focal melanocytic atypia (88).

Pathogenesis. On electron microscopy, melanosomes are diffusely distributed throughout the epidermis (89). There is basement membrane thickening with focal dissolution. Dermal elastic fibers appear homogenized and fragmented (90).

Differential Diagnosis. The differential diagnosis includes lentigo simplex, solar lentigo, and pigmented actinic keratosis.

Principles of Management: Discontinuation of PUVA therapy is usually recommended.

DRUG-INDUCED PIGMENTARY ALTERATIONS

Clinical Summary. Drug-induced pigmentary alterations are quite common and are discussed in greater detail in Chapter 11. Implicated agents include nonsteroidal anti-inflammatory drugs, antimalarials, tetracyclines, psychotropics including phenothiazines, antineoplastic agents including cytotoxics, heavy metals including gold, amiodarone, amitriptyline, imipramine, and clofazimine (91,92). A variety of pathogenic

mechanisms are seen, including increased melanin production leading to hyperpigmentation of basilar keratinocytes, vacuolar change at the dermal–epidermal junction with pigmentary incontinence and dermal melanophages, deposition of stable melanin–drug complexes, and deposition of the drug granules in macrophages or the dermal extracellular matrix. In addition, drugs may induce the synthesis of special pigments—such as lipofuscin—or damage blood vessels, leading to red blood cell extravasation and hemosiderophages (91,92). Clinical features vary from generalized hyperpigmentation to specific patterns attributed to individual drugs such as the flagellated streaks attributed to bleomycin (93).

Histopathology. Minocycline may cause three patterns of hyperpigmentation (94). The first pattern is a blue-black pigmentation of acne and other scars owing to black pigment deposition (highlighted with Prussian blue stain) in macrophages and dermal extracellular matrix. The second pattern consists of gray-blue pigmentation of the anterior legs and arms owing to the deposition of drug complexes and protein (highlighted with both Prussian blue and Fontana–Masson stains) extracellularly in the dermis, particularly around eccrine ducts and other adnexal structures. The third pattern consists of brown discoloration of sun-exposed sites owing to increased basilar keratinocytic melanin (highlighted with Fontana–Masson stain).

Antimalarial agents deposit yellow to dark-brown pigment granules in dermal macrophages and extracellularly (91). Both chloroquine and hydroxychloroquine bind melanin (95). Phenothiazines commonly deposit within dermal macrophages electron-dense granules composed of a drug metabolite and melanin, leading to progressive blue pigmentation on sun-exposed skin (96). Amiodarone may provoke a photoallergic reaction with blue-gray pigmentation owing to the deposition of lipofuscin granules in perivascular macrophages in the superficial dermis. These are accentuated by periodic acid–Schiff (PAS) staining. Lipofuscinosis may also be caused by antibiotics (91). Imipramine deposits dermal round golden-brown bodies in the extracellular dermis and within macrophages, which may represent abnormal drug metabolite–melanin complexes (97). Electron microscopy shows electron-rich granules within lysosomes and free in the dermis rich in copper and sulfur (98).

Chemotherapy agents commonly produce both generalized and localized hyperpigmentation of the basilar keratinocytes. Bleomycin, busulfan, doxorubicin, daunorubicin, fluorouracil, cyclophosphamide, and carmustine may also demonstrate melanophages in the superficial dermis (93). Globules of mercury have been found in dermal and subcutaneous abscesses after oral ingestion (99).

Differential Diagnosis. The differential diagnosis includes postinflammatory hyperpigmentation, phototoxic hyperpigmentation, systemic diseases (Addison disease, hemochromatosis, hyperthyroidism, renal and hepatic failure, systemic lupus erythematosus, dermatomyositis), nutritional diseases (pellagra, malabsorption), ochronosis, and lymphoma.

Principles of Management: Treatment modalities include discontinuation of the offending drug, sun protection, and laser therapy.

PIGMENTARY PRESENTATIONS OF CUTANEOUS AND SYSTEMIC DISEASES

Clinical Summary. A large number of cutaneous and systemic diseases present with changes in pigmentation. These diseases can be nutritional, autoimmune, metabolic, endocrine, neoplastic, or infectious in etiology. Some have localized versus generalized patterns of pigment change. Mycosis fungoides may present with hypopigmented (100) or hyperpigmented (101) lesions. The former, occurring in children and young adults with darker skin tones, is slowly progressive and often present for many years before being diagnosed. Sarcoidosis (102) may display hypopigmented skin lesions but usually demonstrates some degree of clinical induration. Darier (103) disease may also present with hypopigmentation. Although pigmented variants of basal cell carcinoma are not uncommon, pigmented Bowen disease (104), pigmented Paget disease (105), and depigmented extramammary Paget disease (106) can be difficult to recognize clinically. Skin metastases from breast carcinoma may be pigmented and can even simulate malignant melanoma (107). Furthermore, generalized hyperpigmentation may be the presenting sign of metastatic malignant melanoma and primary pituitary tumors.

Histopathology. The histologic changes are those of primary dermatoses. In hypopigmented mycosis fungoides, variable melanin pigmentation with hypochromic or achromic macules (100) and melanin incontinence are present (108) whereas hyperpigmented mycosis fungoides shows dermal infiltration

of atypical lymphocytes with nuclear enlargement, striking hyperchromasia, and abundant melanophages (101). Melanocytes are unaltered in hypopigmented sarcoidosis without appreciable changes in melanin (102). Decreased basilar melanin pigment is seen in hypopigmented Darier disease (103). Pigmented Bowen disease shows abundant melanin pigment in basal keratinocytes, highly dendritic melanocytes, and numerous melanophages (104). Pigmented Paget disease and pigmented epidermotropic metastatic breast carcinoma demonstrate dendritic melanocytes at the dermal–epidermal junction with variable cytoplasmic melanin of tumor cells (105). Normal numbers of melanocytes are present in depigmented extramammary Paget disease, but epidermal melanization is markedly reduced (106). In generalized hyperpigmentation from metastatic melanoma or endocrinopathy, variable epidermal pigment and melanophages are present.

Pathogenesis. Electron microscopy of hypopigmented mycosis fungoides shows melanocytic degeneration with abnormal melanogenesis, psoriasiform-type hyperplasia in the epidermis, vacuolar alteration of the dermoepidermal junction, and melanin incontinence in the papillary dermis (108). Giant melanosomes are seen in keratinocytes of the stratum spinosum in hyperpigmented mycosis fungoides (101). Fewer melanosomes are present within keratinocytes in hypopigmented sarcoidosis, and melanocytes feature variable degenerative changes (109).

Differential Diagnosis. Considerations include drug-induced hyperpigmentation.

Principles of Management: Treatment of primary dermatosis or systemic disease is recommended.

ALBINISM

Clinical Summary. Albinism is a heritable disorder, causing reduced to absent pigmentation of the skin, hair, and eyes. Albinism is typically diagnosed clinically and can present across a spectrum, ranging from depigmentation to complete loss of pigment in hair, skin, and eyes.

This condition was previously categorized based on the degree of tyrosinase activity and, as such, tyrosinase-positive or tyrosinase-negative classification. However, albinism is now classified based on the melanogenesis and melanosome transport genes affected. Presently, 19 genes have been associated with different presentations of albinism (110). *Ocular albinism* (OA) involving only the eyes is X-linked recessive whereas oculocutaneous albinism (OCA) affecting the eyes, hair, and skin is autosomal recessive.

There are seven types of OCA: OCA1 (type A and B), OCA2, OCA3, OCA4, OCA5, OCA6, and OCA7. OCA1A is the most severe form of albinism, and those affected have complete loss of melanin production throughout their life and are unable to repigment. Individuals with OCA have a defect in tyrosinase and, therefore, cannot oxidize tyrosine to dihydroxyphenylalanine (DOPA) as part of normal melanogenesis. Clinically, this presents as pale skin, fair or white hair, and eyes may vary from light brown to pale green to red, as light will reflect the blood vessels in the retina (110). OA involves the loss of pigment in the retina, with only type one classification, OA1. Affected individuals may also have nystagmus, delayed visual maturation, or decreased visual acuity (111).

Associated systemic disorders include platelet defect with mild bleeding diathesis, inflammatory bowel disease and/or pulmonary fibrosis, ceroid storage (Hermansky–Pudlak syndrome, Fig. 27-6), defects in immunity (Chédiak–Higashi and Griscelli syndromes), and microphthalmia, and intellectual disability (Cross syndrome). Photosensitivity and cutaneous malignancies, particularly squamous cell carcinoma, are frequent across all forms of albinism.

Prenatal diagnosis of OCA can be made by analysis for the tyrosinase gene in fetal cells obtained by chorionic villous sampling or amniocentesis (112).

Histopathology. Histologic examination of skin from patients with OCA shows the presence of basal melanocytes in the epidermis and hair bulb; however, Fontana–Masson stain fails to highlight melanin.

Hermansky–Pudlak syndrome is a disorder of prolonged bleeding and OCA in which lysosome-related organelles, such as melanosomes and platelet-dense granules, are dysfunctional. Giant melanosomes are seen in the epidermis along with melanophages in the dermis (113–115). This syndrome is diagnosed by the absence of platelet-dense granules under electron microscopy.

Pathogenesis. OCA is a disorder of melanin synthesis within the melanosome. Electron microscopic examination in OCA shows normally structured melanocytes in the epidermis; however, there is a reduction in the melanization of melanosomes (116). Melanosome transfer to keratinocytes is not altered.

The tyrosinase gene is located on chromosome 11q 14-21 on the P gene on chromosome 15q11.2 (111,117,118). Mutations to the tyrosinase gene lead to a range of clinical manifestations of albinism. Of the seven types of OCA, four subtypes, namely OCA1 (type A and B), OCA2, OCA3, and OCA4, are well classified. OCA1 is caused by decreased or absent tyrosinase genes, OCA2 by defective melanosomal transmembrane (P) protein gene, OCA3 by mutant tyrosine-related protein type 1 (TYRP1), and OCA4 by defective SLC45A2 gene (110,111). OCA5 is thought to be caused by a locus in the region of chromosome 4q24. OCA6 and OCA7 are caused by defects in SLC24A5 and C10orf11 genes, respectively (110). Additionally, for Hermansky–Pudlak syndrome, there are 10 human Hermansky–Pudlak genes that have been identified to encode one of the four protein complexes involved in the formation and trafficking of lysosome-related organelles (119).

Principles of Management: Treatment consists of sun avoidance, broad-spectrum sunscreen, frequent skin cancer screenings, and referral to ophthalmologist (120).

PIEBALDISM (PATTERNED LEUKODERMA)

Clinical Summary. Piebaldism is an autosomal dominant disorder characterized by irregularly shaped depigmented patches that are present at birth and associated in about 85% of cases with a white forelock arising from a depigmented area in the central forehead. Depigmentation has a predilection for ventral skin, that is, the central face, ventral chest, and abdomen. Small islands of hyperpigmentation, 1 to 5 mm in diameter, are usually present within the depigmented areas (Fig. 27-7). It is caused by a loss of function mutation in the KIT gene, which leads to aberrant migration of melanoblasts during embryogenesis (121). The condition was previously called *partial albinism*, but this term is no longer used because of the difference in pathogenesis between OCA and piebaldism.

Waardenburg syndrome is an autosomal dominant or recessive genetic disorder characterized by piebaldism, lateral displacement of the inner canthi of the eyes (dystopia canthorum), broad nasal root, heterochromia of the irides, and congenital deafness. About half of the affected individuals have a white forelock and approximately 12% have patches of depigmentation at birth.

Histopathology. The depigmented skin and hair usually have significantly reduced to no melanocytes owing to the aforementioned gene defects (122,123). Melanocytes are normal in number in the associated hyperpigmented areas (Fig. 27-7) (123). In some cases, white forelock epidermis may show a few melanocytes that are DOPA positive (124).

Pathogenesis. Electron microscopic examination of the depigmented skin usually reveals a complete absence of melanocytes (124). In some instances, an occasional melanocyte is seen with unmelanized ellipsoidal or spherical melanosomes. Electron microscopy of plucked forelock hair reveals the absence of melanin in the cortex, cuticle, and inner root sheath (124). The small hyperpigmented islands show many abnormal spherical, granular melanosomes.

A mutation of the *KIT* gene that encodes melanocytic migration into the hair follicle and epidermis during embryonic development has been implicated in piebaldism (121). In the Waardenburg syndrome, four subtypes have been described involving five transcription factors: Waardenburg syndrome (WS) 1, WS2, WS3, and WS4. There are six genes involved with the different subtypes, which include PAX-3 (encodes the paired box-3 transcription factor), MITF (microphthalmia-associated transcription factor), SOX-10 (encodes the Sry box 10 transcription factor), EDN3 (endothelin 3), EDNRB (endothelin receptor type B), and SNAI2 (snail homolog 2 transcription

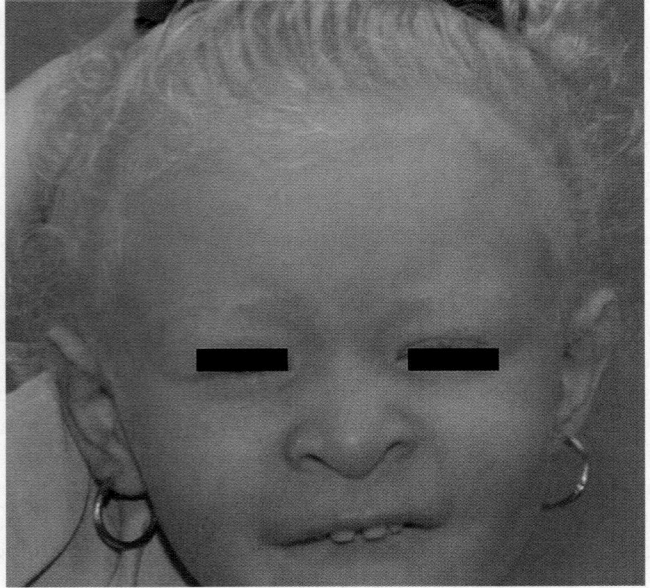

Figure 27-6 Hermansky–Pudlak disease. Clinical presentation of a patient with Hermansky–Pudlak disease, showing hypopigmentation of hair and skin.

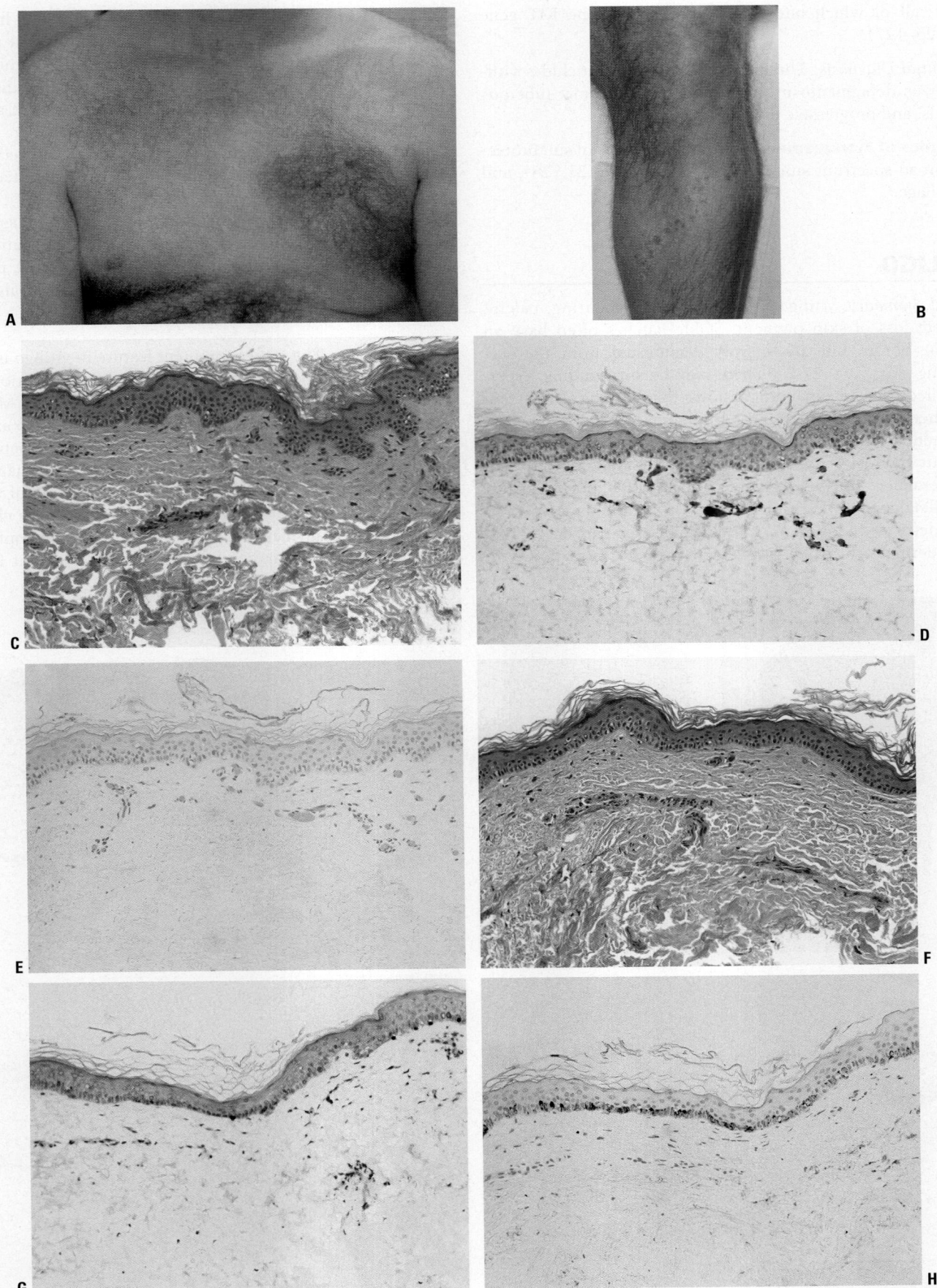

Figure 27-7 Piebaldism. **A, B:** Clinical presentation showing depigmented patches with islands of hyperpigmentation on chest and shin. **C–E:** Depigmented areas (**C**) showing loss of melanocytes on Sox10 stain (**D**) and loss of melanin pigment on Fontana–Masson stain (**E**). **F–H:** Associated area of hyperpigmentation in a patient with Piebaldism (**F**), showing normal numbers of melanocytes on Sox10 (**G**) and significantly increased melanin pigment on Fontana–Masson stain (**H**).

factor), all of which affect the expression of the KIT gene (114,125–127).

Differential Diagnosis. The differential diagnosis includes vitiligo, nevus depigmentosus, Waardenburg syndrome, tuberous sclerosis, and progressive macular hypomelanosis.

Principles of Management: Treatment consists of sun protection, broad-spectrum sunscreen, skin grafting (121,128), and camouflage.

VITILIGO

Clinical Summary. Vitiligo is an acquired, disfiguring, patchy, complete loss of skin pigment. Stable patches often have an irregular border but are sharply demarcated from the surrounding skin (Fig. 27-8). There may be surrounding hyperpigmented skin. In expanding lesions, there can be a slight rim of erythema at the border and a thin zone of transitory partial depigmentation (Fig. 27-9). Hairs in patches of vitiligo are often white (poliosis). The scalp and eyelashes are rarely affected. In generalized vitiligo, the face, upper trunk, dorsal hands, periorificial areas, and genitals are most commonly affected in a symmetrical distribution. Localized disease can occur as a linear, dermatomal patch (segmental vitiligo). Induction with

trauma (Koebner phenomenon) and association with halo nevi and metastatic melanoma occur with generalized but not segmental vitiligo. Vitiligo may be associated with autoimmune diseases including thyroiditis, pernicious anemia, Addison disease, diabetes, alopecia areata, and medications such as interferon, imiquimod, and BRAF inhibitors.

In *Vogt–Koyanagi–Harada syndrome*, a rare and very severe form of vitiligo, an aseptic meningitis is often the initial symptom, followed by uveitis, dysacousia, and vertigo (129). Patches of vitiligo involving the skin, and frequently the eyelashes and scalp, subsequently develop. There is often an association with alopecia areata. In addition, as previously mentioned, immune checkpoint inhibitors for advanced melanoma can also elicit vitiligo-like depigmentation (66,67).

Histopathology. The most prominent feature in vitiligo is the alteration of melanocytes at the dermal–epidermal junction. With silver stains or immunohistochemical stains such as Melan-A, Mart-1, or SOX-10, well-established lesions of vitiligo are completely devoid of melanocytes (Fig. 27-8). DOPA reaction was used in the past. Melanosomes in stage II/IV, or late stage, have been found to be present in the white/lesional skin of vitiligo. These late-stage melanosomes have been noted to be clumped together, forming melanin granules within the cytoplasm of basal and suprabasilar keratinocytes and are present even in

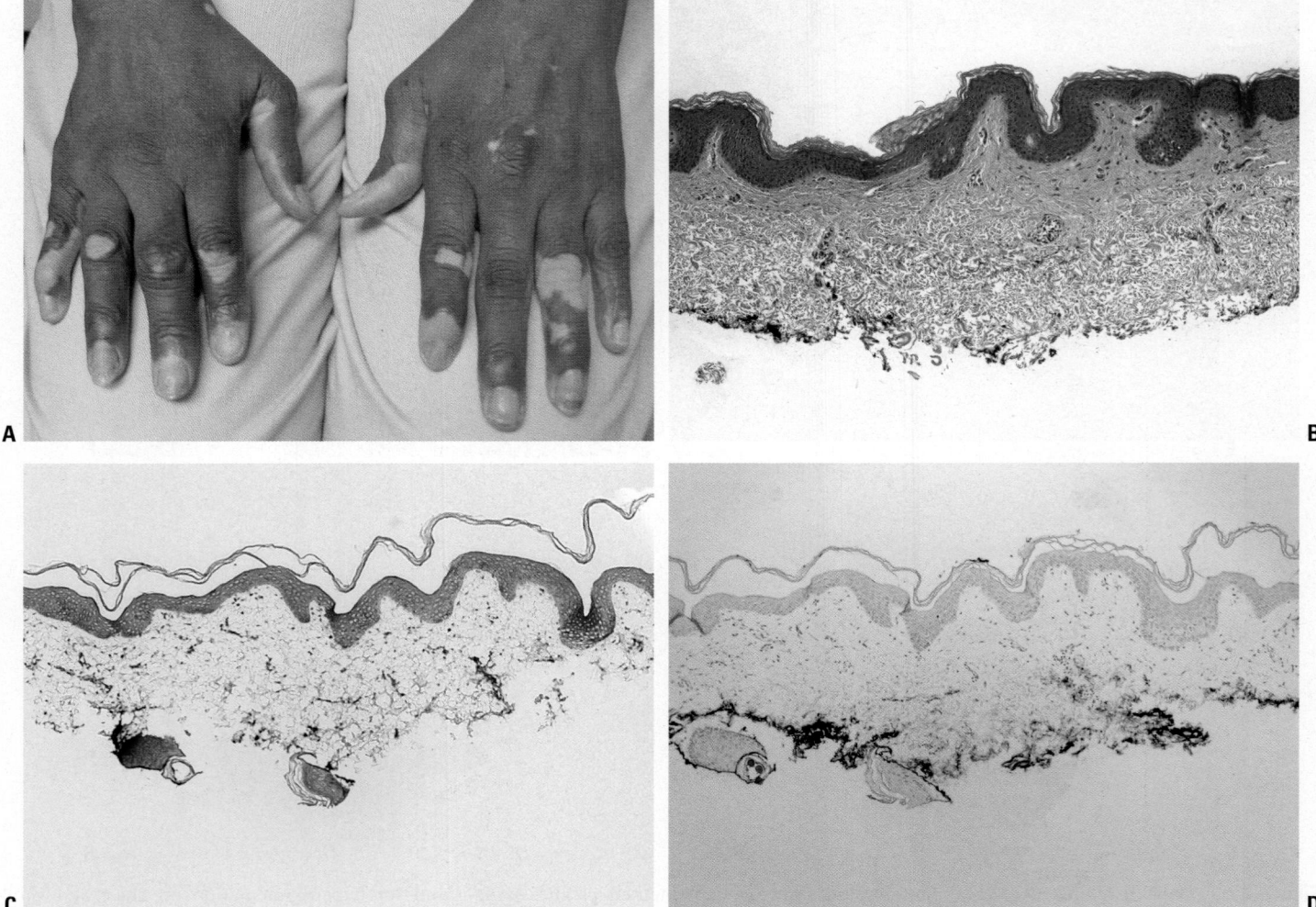

Figure 27-8 Vitiligo. A: Patchy loss of pigment in a patient with vitiligo. B: There is total loss of melanocytes in the depigmented skin. C: Sox10 stain showing loss of melanocytes. D: Fontana–Masson stain shows complete loss of melanin pigment.

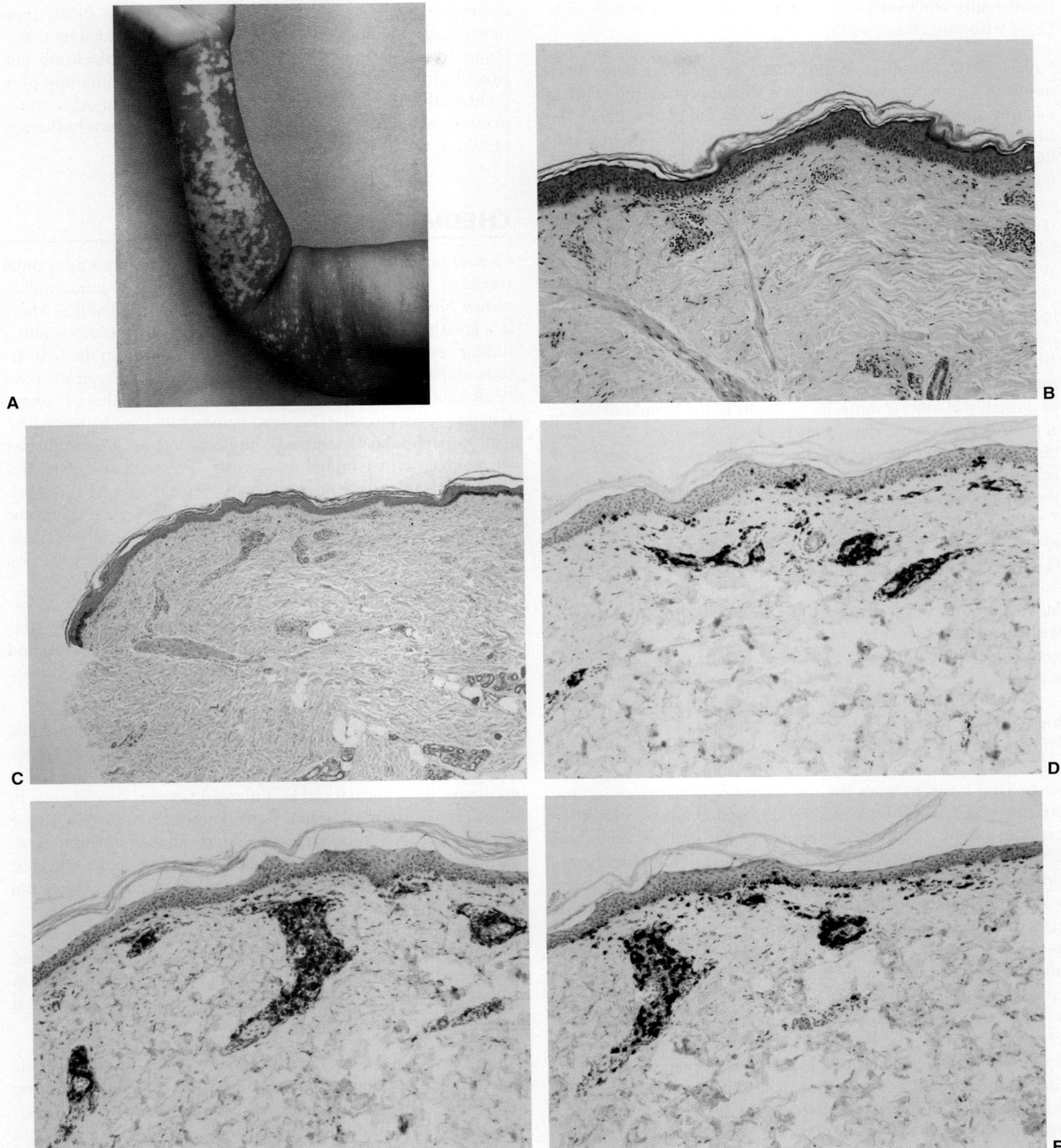

Figure 27-9 Inflammatory vitiligo. **A:** Clinical example of inflammatory vitiligo showing slightly raised sharply demarcated borders with depigmentation and hypopigmentation. **B:** Sections show focal vacuolar changes with increased lymphocytic inflammation, composed of primarily CD8-positive T lymphocytes. **C:** A Fontana–Masson stain showing abrupt loss of melanin staining (preserved staining focally at both edges). **D:** CD3 stain, highlighting T cells. **E:** CD4 stain. **F:** CD8 stain.

chronic disease (130). The periphery of expanding lesions, which are hypopigmented rather than completely depigmented, still shows few scattered melanocytes and some melanin granules in the basal layer. In the outer border of patches of vitiligo, melanocytes are often prominent and demonstrate long

dendritic processes filled with melanin granules. Early lesions show a superficial perivascular and occasionally lichenoid mononuclear cell infiltrate at the border. Focal areas of vacuolar change at the dermal–epidermal junction in association with a mild mononuclear cell infiltrate have been seen in the normal-appearing skin adjacent to vitiliginous areas, as well as those with progressive vitiligo (Fig. 27-9) (130).

Pathogenesis. Multiple immunologic mechanisms have been implicated in vitiligo pathogenesis. Melanocytes from vitiligo patients appear to be less able to tolerate cellular stress (131). Increased cellular stress from multiple causes can cause high production of melanin, which leads to increased misfolding of proteins (the so-called unfolded protein response) and subsequent activation of innate inflammation (131). Increased stress from UV radiation or chemicals can also lead to the generation of reactive oxygen species from mitochondrial metabolism (131,132). When the melanocytes become stressed, they release cytokines that activate innate immunity, which is thought to initiate vitiligo (129,131). Activation of the innate immune system involves natural killer cells and release of heat shock proteins (HSPs, specifically HSP70) and other cytokines (132). Once the innate immune system is activated, antigen-presenting cells are thought to present melanocyte antigens to T cells in the lymphoid tissue, activating them and initiating an adaptive response (129). Additionally, cytokines are released locally in the skin and activate T cells to directly kill melanocytes. Recent studies have shown that the presence of localized IL-15-induced tissue-resident memory T cells (TRM cells, which are cytotoxic to melanocytes) may explain the recurrent lesions of vitiligo in the same areas of the body (133). Autoimmunity in vitiligo patients is caused by increased numbers of melanocyte-specific cytotoxic CD8+ T cells in the blood and skin, and the degree of CD8+ T cells directly correlates with the disease severity (132,134,135). The melanocytic antigens targeted include gp100, MART1, tyrosinase, and tyrosinase-related proteins 1 and 2 (129).

Local release of interferon-gamma is involved in recruiting CD8+ T cells to the skin, through the chemokine CXCL10 and its receptor CXCR3 on the T cells. JAK1 and JAK2 are directly involved in interferon-gamma signaling, which activates STAT1 and induces the transcription of many genes, including CXCL10 (131,132,135). Increased expression of other cytokines is also reported in patients with vitiligo, including TNF-alpha, interleukin-6, and interleukin-7. Thus, there continues to be a role of biologics that block some of these pathways in the emerging treatments for vitiligo. CD4+ regulatory T cells are also involved in the prevention and control of disease, as patients with low levels of CD4+ T cells (such as those with immune polyendocrinopathy and X-linked syndrome) are at increased risk for vitiligo (129).

The "neural hypothesis" in the literature is based on the unilateral distribution of segmental vitiligo. However, there is insufficient evidence to support this hypothesis, as even segmental or "dermatomal" vitiligo appears mediated by autoimmunity, and does not usually follow a true dermatomal distribution (129). Somatic mosaicism is the theory that a single mutation in an embryonic melanocyte then differentiates into a functional melanocyte in the skin, resulting in a pattern of vitiligo that is distinct (neural crest derived), as seen in segmental vitiligo (129,131).

Differential Diagnosis. Considerations include chemical leukoderma/chemical-induced vitiligo, infections (tinea versicolor, leprosy, onchocerciasis, pinta), genetic syndromes (piebaldism, hypomelanosis of Ito, tuberous sclerosis, Waardenburg syndrome, Vogt–Koyanagi–Harada syndrome), postinflammatory hypopigmentation, nevus depigmentosus, idiopathic guttate hypomelanosis, and progressive macular hypomelanosis.

Principles of Management: Topical treatments (136) (corticosteroids, calcineurin inhibitors, vitamin D_3 analogs), systemic corticosteroids, JAK inhibitors such as tofacitinib and ruxolitinib (132,137,138), STAT inhibitors, phototherapy, photochemotherapy, laser therapy, skin grafting, melanocyte transplantation, camouflage, depigmentation, and psychotherapy (139) are usually recommended.

CHÉDIAK–HIGASHI SYNDROME

Clinical summary. Chédiak–Higashi syndrome is a rare autosomal recessive disorder characterized by variable OCA, immunodeficiency, bleeding diathesis, and neurological abnormalities. There is a greatly increased susceptibility to bacterial infections and a unique "accelerated phase," which leads to death in the first decade of life, and those who survive into adulthood typically have neurologic sequelae (140,141). The accelerated phase is manifested by fever, jaundice, hepatosplenomegaly, lymphadenopathy, pancytopenia, and widespread lymphohistiocytic organ infiltrates (hemophagocytic lymphohistiocytosis). Viruses, particularly Epstein–Barr virus, have been associated with triggering the accelerated phase. A diagnostic feature of Chédiak–Higashi syndrome is enlarged vesicles (lysosome-related organelles) in all cell types. These include lysosomes, melanosomes, platelet-dense granules, cytolytic granules, and many others (142).

Chédiak–Higashi syndrome is a subtype of OCA, and patients demonstrate fair skin with susceptibility to severe sunburn, silvery colored hair, and pale irides with photophobia and nystagmus. Severe and recurrent infections of the respiratory tract and skin are common.

Histopathology. Light microscopic features of skin sections show normal findings (143). Fontana–Masson stain shows sparse melanin granules, some of which are grouped and others that are larger than normal (143). Enlarged vesicles can be seen in all cell types, from lysosomes to melanosomes to platelet-dense granules (141). Similar large, irregularly shaped melanin granules are scattered in the upper dermis within melanophages. Hair shafts also demonstrate abnormal aggregates of melanin with giant melanosomes within the hair bulb (144).

The giant lysosomal granules can be demonstrated in peripheral blood, in skin (melanocytes or Langerhans cells), and other organs. A blood smear stained with Giemsa or Wright stain shows azurophilic granules present in all white blood cell lines but most prominent in neutrophils.

Pathogenesis. Within melanocytes, electron microscopy reveals giant, irregularly shaped melanosomes surrounded by a limiting membrane. They further increase in size by fusing with other giant particles. Within the giant melanosomes, a granular matrix and filaments showing periodicity and varying degrees of pigmentation are observed. The largest melanosomes show signs of degeneration, leading to the vacuolization and formation of residual bodies. In addition, normal melanosomes are present in melanocytes and are transferred to keratinocytes; however, they are packaged into abnormally large lysosomes. Similar abnormally large, membrane-bound lysosomes are found in the hair. The giant melanosomes in melanocytes and giant lysosomes in keratinocytes form because of defective membrane or microtubule function. Hypopigmentation occurs because the melanosomes within keratinocytes are concentrated within a relatively few large lysosomes rather than being dispersed throughout the cytoplasm.

The giant granules in the cytoplasm of white blood cells develop by the fusion of primary lysosomes with one another and with cytoplasmic material. Even though microorganisms are phagocytized into phagocytic vacuoles in a normal fashion, their intracellular killing is delayed because of the unavailability of primary lysosomes to discharge their bacterial enzymes into the phagocytic vacuoles. Also, cathepsin G, a potent antimicrobial protease in neutrophils, is absent in Chédiak–Higashi syndrome.

Mutations in the *CHS1/LYST* gene at 1q42.1 to 2 are associated with Chédiak–Higashi syndrome. *CHS1/LYST* encodes a protein that regulates lysosome-related organelle size and movement (114,141,145).

Differential Diagnosis. The differential diagnosis includes OCA type 2, Hermansky–Pudlak syndrome, chronic granulomatous disease, and Griscelli syndrome.

Principles of Management: Treatment consists of bone marrow transplant, chemotherapy, and sun protection (141).

ACKNOWLEDGMENTS

The authors thank Dr. Lionel Bercovitch and Dr. Erin O'Leary for Figure 27-5 and Dr. John Harris for Figure 27-9 and acknowledge the contributions of the authors of this chapter in previous editions: Flavia Fedeles, Carrie L. Kovarik, Richard L. Spielvogel, and Gary R. Kantor.

REFERENCES

1. Braun-Falco O, Burg G, Selzle D, Schmoeckel C. Diffuse congenital melanosis [in German]. *Hautarzt.* 1980;31(6):324–327.
2. Kint A, Oomen C, Geerts ML, Breuillard F. Congenital diffuse melanosis [in French]. *Ann Dermatol Venereol.* 1987;114(1):11–16.
3. Wang SY, Meng HM, Zhang L, Li L. A novel case of delayed congenital diffuse melanosis: immune dysfunction? *J Eur Acad Dermatol Venereol.* 2012;26(4):523–524.
4. Sardana K, Goel K, Chugh S. Reticulate pigmentary disorders. *Indian J Dermatol Venereol Leprol.* 2013;79(1):17–29.
5. Marrone A, Walne A, Dokal I. Dyskeratosis congenita: telomerase, telomeres and anticipation. *Curr Opin Genet Dev.* 2005;15(3):249–257.
6. Trott KE, Briddell JW, Corao-Uribe D, et al. Dyskeratosis congenita and oral cavity squamous cell carcinoma: report of a case and literature review. *J Pediatr Hematol Oncol.* 2019;41(6):501–503.
7. Dokal I. Dyskeratosis congenita. *Hematology Am Soc Hematol Educ Program.* 2011;2011:480–486.
8. Choi JC, Yang JH, Lee UH, Park HS, Chun DK. Progressive cribriform and zosteriform hyperpigmentation—the late onset linear and whorled nevoid hypermelanosis. *J Eur Acad Dermatol Venereol.* 2005;19(5):638–639.
9. Cho E, Cho SH, Lee JD. Progressive cribriform and zosteriform hyperpigmentation: a clinicopathologic study. *Int J Dermatol.* 2012;51(4):399–405.
10. Das A, Bandyopadhyay D, Mishra V, Gharami RC. Progressive cribriform and zosteriform hyperpigmentation. *Indian J Dermatol Venereol Leprol.* 2015;81(3):321.
11. Kono M, Akiyama M. Dyschromatosis symmetrica hereditaria and reticulate acropigmentation of Kitamura: an update. *J Dermatol Sci.* 2019;93(2):75–81.
12. Oyama M, Shimizu H, Ohata Y, Tajima S, Nishikawa T. Dyschromatosis symmetrica hereditaria (reticulate acropigmentation of Dohi): report of a Japanese family with the condition and a literature review of 185 cases. *Br J Dermatol.* 1999;140(3):491–496.
13. Al Hawsawi K, Al Aboud K, Alfadley A, Al Aboud D. Reticulate acropigmentation of Kitamura-Dowling Degos disease overlap: a case report. *Int J Dermatol.* 2002;41(8):518–520.
14. Kim YC, Davis MD, Schanbacher CF, Su WP. Dowling-Degos disease (reticulate pigmented anomaly of the flexures): a clinical and histopathologic study of 6 cases. *J Am Acad Dermatol.* 1999;40(3):462–467.
15. Pickup TL, Mutasim DF. Dowling-Degos disease presenting as hypopigmented macules. *J Am Acad Dermatol.* 2011;64(6):1224–1225.
16. El Shabrawi-Caelen L, Rutten A, Kerl H. The expanding spectrum of Galli-Galli disease. *J Am Acad Dermatol.* 2007;56(5, suppl):86–91.
17. Lugassy J, Itin P, Ishida-Yamamoto A, et al. Naegeli-Franceschetti-Jadassohn syndrome and dermatopathia pigmentosa reticularis: two allelic ectodermal dysplasias caused by dominant mutations in KRT14. *Am J Hum Genet.* 2006;79(4):724–730.
18. Costello MJ, Buncke CM. Dyskeratosis congenita. *AMA Arch Derm.* 1956;73(2):123–132.
19. Schnur RE, Heymann WR. Reticulate hyperpigmentation. *Semin Cutan Med Surg.* 1997;16(1):72–80.
20. Vulliamy T, Dokal I. Dyskeratosis congenita. *Semin Hematol.* 2006;43(3):157–166.
21. Liao H, Zhao Y, Baty DU, McGrath JA, Mellerio JE, McLean WH. A heterozygous frameshift mutation in the V1 domain of keratin 5 in a family with Dowling-Degos disease. *J Invest Dermatol.* 2007;127(2):298–300.
22. Betz RC, Planko L, Eigelshoven S, et al. Loss-of-function mutations in the keratin 5 gene lead to Dowling-Degos disease. *Am J Hum Genet.* 2006;78(3):510–519.
23. Kono M, Suganuma M, Akiyama M, Ito Y, Ujiie H, Morimoto K. Novel ADAR1 mutations including a single amino acid deletion in the deaminase domain underlie dyschromatosis symmetrica hereditaria in Japanese families. *Int J Dermatol.* 2014;53(3):e194–e196.
24. Lai ML, Yang LJ, Zhu XH, Li M. A novel mutation of the DSRAD gene in a Chinese family with dyschromatosis symmetrica hereditaria. *Genet Mol Res.* 2012;11(2):1731–1737.
25. Zhang JY, Chen XD, Zhang Z, et al. ADAR1 p150 isoform is involved in the pathogenesis of dyschromatosis symmetrica hereditaria. *Br J Dermatol.* 2013;169(3):637–644.
26. Zhang GL, Shi HJ, Shao MH, et al. Mutations in the ADAR1 gene in Chinese families with dyschromatosis symmetrica hereditaria. *Genet Mol Res.* 2013;12(3):2794–2799.
27. Yun JH, Kim JH, Choi JS, Roh JY, Lee JR. Treatment of Dowling-Degos disease with fractional Er:YAG laser. *J Cosmet Laser Ther.* 2013;15(6):336–339.
28. Wenzel G, Petrow W, Tappe K, Gerdsen R, Uerlich WP, Bieber T. Treatment of Dowling-Degos disease with Er:YAG-laser: results after 2.5 years. *Dermatol Surg.* 2003;29(11):1161–1162.
29. Voth H, Landsberg J, Reinhard G, et al. Efficacy of ablative laser treatment in Galli-Galli disease. *Arch Dermatol.* 2011;147(3):317–320.
30. Akiyama M, Aranami A, Sasaki Y, Ebihara T, Sugiura M. Familial linear and whorled nevoid hypermelanosis. *J Am Acad Dermatol.* 1994;30(5, pt 2):831–833.
31. Di Lernia V. Linear and whorled hypermelanosis. *Pediatr Dermatol.* 2007;24(3):205–210.
32. Menditta V, Sharma RC, Arya L, Sardana K. Linear and whorled nevoid hypermelanosis. *J Dermatol.* 2001;28(1):58–59.
33. Errichetti E, Pegolo E, Stinco, G. Linear and whorled nevoid hypermelanosis: a case report with dermoscopic findings. *Indian J Dermatol Venereol Leprol.* 2016;82:91–3.

34. Nehal KS, PeBenito R, Orlow SJ. Analysis of 54 cases of hypopigmentation and hyperpigmentation along the lines of Blaschko. *Arch Dermatol.* 1996;132(10):1167–1170.

35. Yuksel S, Savaci S, Bicak U, Yakinci C, Mizrak B. Linear and whorled nevoid hypermelanosis in trisomy 13. *Turk J Med Sci.* 2009;39(2):321–324.

36. Verghese S, Newlin A, Miller M, Burton BK. Mosaic trisomy 7 in a patient with pigmentary abnormalities. *Am J Med Genet.* 1999;87(5):371–374.

37. Komine M, Hino M, Shiina M, Kanazawa I, Soma Y, Tamaki K. Linear and whorled naevoid hypermelanosis: a case with systemic involvement and trisomy 18 mosaicism. *Br J Dermatol.* 2002;146(3):500–502.

38. Hartmann A, Hofmann UB, Hoehn H, Broecker EB, Hamm H. Postnatal confirmation of prenatally diagnosed trisomy 20 mosaicism in a patient with linear and whorled nevoid hypermelanosis. *Pediatr Dermatol.* 2004;21(6):636–641.

39. Taibjee SM, Bennett DC, Moss C. Abnormal pigmentation in hypomelanosis of Ito and pigmentary mosaicism: the role of pigmentary genes. *Br J Dermatol.* 2004;151(2):269–282.

40. Sheth VM, Pandya AG. Melasma: a comprehensive update. Part I. *J Am Acad Dermatol.* 2011;65(4):689–697; quiz 698.

41. Funasaka Y, Mayumi N, Asayama S, et al. In vivo reflectance confocal microscopy for skin imaging in melasma. *J Nippon Med Sch.* 2013;80(3):172–173.

42. Liu H, Lin Y, Nie X, et al. Histological classification of melasma with reflectance confocal microscopy: a pilot study in Chinese patients. *Skin Res Technol.* 2011;17(4):398–403.

43. Sanchez NP, Pathak MA, Sato S, Fitzpatrick TB, Sanchez JL, Mihm MC Jr. Melasma: a clinical, light microscopic, ultrastructural, and immunofluorescence study. *J Am Acad Dermatol.* 1981;4(6):698–710.

44. Kang WH, Yoon KH, Lee ES, et al. Melasma: histopathological characteristics in 56 Korean patients. *Br J Dermatol.* 2002; 146(2):228–237.

45. Grimes PE, Yamada N, Bhawan J. Light microscopic, immunohistochemical, and ultrastructural alterations in patients with melasma. *Am J Dermatopathol.* 2005;27(2):96–101.

46. Masub N, Nguyen J, Austin E, Jagdeo J. The vascular component of melasma: a systemic review of laboratory, diagnostic, and therapeutic evidence. *Dermatol Surg.* 2020;46(12):1642–1650.

47. Boukari F, Jourdan E, Fontas E, et al. Prevention of melasma relapses with sunscreen combining protection against UV and short wavelengths of visible light; a prospective randomized comparative trial. *J Am Acad Dermatol.* 2015;72(1):189–190.

48. Rivas S, Pandya AG. Treatment of melasma with topical agents, peels and lasers: an evidence-based review. *Am J Clin Dermatol.* 2013;14(5):359–376.

49. Nieman LK, Chanco Turner ML. Addison's disease. *Clin Dermatol.* 2006;24(4):276–280.

50. Fernandez-Flores A, Cassarino D. Histopathologic findings of cutaneous hyperpigmentation in Addison disease and immunostain of the melanocytic population. *Am J Dermatopathol.* 2017;39(12):924–927.

51. Husebye E, Lovas K. Pathogenesis of primary adrenal insufficiency. *Best Pract Res Clin Endocrinol Metab.* 2009;23(2):147–157.

52. Gombos Z, Hermann R, Kiviniemi M, et al. Analysis of extended human leukocyte antigen haplotype association with Addison's disease in three populations. *Eur J Endocrinol.* 2007;157(6): 757–761.

53. Xiang W, Xu A, Xu J, Bi Z, Shang Y, Ren Q. In vivo confocal laser scanning microscopy of hypopigmented macules: a preliminary comparison of confocal images in vitiligo, nevus depigmentosus and postinflammatory hypopigmentation. *Lasers Med Sci.* 2010;25(4):551–558.

54. Ackerman AB. *Histologic Diagnosis of Inflammatory Skin Diseases.* Lea & Febiger; 1978:178.

55. Ortonne JP, Bissett DL. Latest insights into skin hyperpigmentation. *J Investig Dermatol Symp Proc.* 2008;13(1):10–14.

56. Cardinali G, Kovacs D, Picardo M. Mechanisms underlying post-inflammatory hyperpigmentation: lessons from solar lentigo [in French]. *Ann Dermatol Venereol.* 2012;139(suppl 3):S96–S101.

57. Lynde CB, Kraft JN, Lynde CW. Topical treatments for melasma and postinflammatory hyperpigmentation. *Skin Ther Lett.* 2006;11(9):1–6.

58. Callender VD, St Surin-Lord S, Davis EC, Maclin M. Postinflammatory hyperpigmentation: etiologic and therapeutic considerations. *Am J Clin Dermatol.* 2011;12(2):87–99.

59. Vachiramon V, Thadanipon K. Postinflammatory hypopigmentation. *Clin Exp Dermatol.* 2011;36(7):708–714.

60. Stoner JG, Rasmussen JE. Plant dermatitis. *J Am Acad Dermatol.* 1983;9(1):1–15.

61. Boissy RE, Manga P. On the etiology of contact/occupational vitiligo. *Pigment Cell Res.* 2004;17(3):208–214.

62. Ghosh S, Mukhopadhyay S. Chemical leucoderma: a clinico-aetiological study of 864 cases in the perspective of a developing country. *Br J Dermatol.* 2009;160(1):40–47.

63. Harris JE. Chemical-induced vitiligo. *Dermatol Clin.* 2017;35(2): 151–161.

64. Al-Dujaili Z, Hsu S. Imiquimod-induced vitiligo. *Dermatol Online J.* 2007;13(2):10.

65. Kumar P, Dar L, Saldiwal S, et al. Intralesional injection of Mycobacterium w vaccine vs imiquimod, 5%, cream in patients with anogenital warts: a randomized clinical trial. *JAMA Dermatol.* 2014;150(10):1072–1078.

66. Hua C, Boussemart L, Mateus C, et al. Association of vitiligo with tumor response in patients with metastatic melanoma treated with pembrolizumab. *JAMA Dermatol.* 2016;152(1):45–51.

67. Nakamura Y, Tanaka R, Asami Y, et al. Correlation between vitiligo occurrence and clinical benefit in advanced melanoma patients treated with nivolumab: a multi-institutional retrospective study. *J Dermatol.* 2017;44(2):117–122.

68. Cummings KI, Cottel WI. Idiopathic guttate hypomelanosis. *Arch Dermatol.* 1966;93(2):184–186.

69. Shin MK, Jeong KH, Oh IH, Choe BK, Lee MH. Clinical features of idiopathic guttate hypomelanosis in 646 subjects and association with other aspects of photoaging. *Int J Dermatol.* 2011;50(7):798–805.

70. Ortonne JP, Perrot H. Idiopathic guttate hypomelanosis. Ultrastructural study. *Arch Dermatol.* 1980;116(6):664–668.

71. Kim SK, Kim EH, Kang HY, Lee ES, Sohn S, Kim YC. Comprehensive understanding of idiopathic guttate hypomelanosis: clinical and histopathological correlation. *Int J Dermatol.* 2010;49(2):162–166.

72. Ploysangam T, Dee-Ananlap S, Suvanprakorn P. Treatment of idiopathic guttate hypomelanosis with liquid nitrogen: light and electron microscopic studies. *J Am Acad Dermatol.* 1990;23(4, pt 1):681–684.

73. Rerknimitr P, Disphanurat W, Achariyakul M. Topical tacrolimus significantly promotes repigmentation in idiopathic guttate hypomelanosis: a double-blind, placebo-controlled study. *J Eur Acad Dermatol Venereol.* 2013;27(4):460–464.

74. Kumarasinghe SP. 3-5 second cryotherapy is effective in idiopathic guttate hypomelanosis. *J Dermatol.* 2004;31(5):437–439.

75. Goldust M, Mohebbipour A, Mirmohammadi R. Treatment of idiopathic guttate hypomelanosis with fractional carbon dioxide lasers. *J Cosmet Laser Ther.* 2013. doi: 10.3109/14764172 .2013.803369

76. Perman M, Sheth P, Lucky AW. Progressive macular hypomelanosis in a 16-year old. *Pediatr Dermatol.* 2008;25(1):63–65.

77. Kumarasinghe SPW, Tan SH, Thng S, Thamboo TP, Liang S, Lee YS. Progressive macular hypomelanosis in Singapore: a clinico-pathological study. *Int J Dermatol.* 2006;45(6):737–742.

78. Saleem MD, Oussedik E, Picardo M, Schoch JJ. Acquired disorders with hypopigmentation: a clinical approach to diagnosis and treatment. *J Am Acad Dermatol.* 2019;80(5):1233–1250.

79. Westerhof W, Relyveld GN, Kingswijk MM, de Man P, Menke HE. Propionibacterium acnes and the pathogenesis of progressive macular hypomelanosis. *Arch Dermatol.* 2004;140(2):210–214.

80. Wu XG, Xu AE, Song XZ, Zheng JH, Wang P, Shen H. Clinical, pathologic, and ultrastructural studies of progressive macular hypomelanosis. *Int J Dermatol.* 2010;49(10):1127–1132.

81. Relyveld GN, Dingemans KP, Menke HE, Bos JD, Westerhof W. Ultrastructural findings in progressive macular hypomelanosis indicate decreased melanin production. *J Eur Acad Dermatol Venereol.* 2008;22(5):568–574.

82. Relyveld GN, Westerhof W, Woudenberg J, et al. Progressive macular hypomelanosis is associated with a putative Propionibacterium species. *J Invest Dermatol.* 2010;130(4):1182–1184.

83. Kim MB, Kim GW, Cho HH, et al. Narrowband UVB treatment of progressive macular hypomelanosis. *J Am Acad Dermatol.* 2012;66(4):598–605.

84. Relyveld GN, Kingswijk MM, Reitsma JB, Menke HE, Bos JD, Westerhof W. Benzoyl peroxide/clindamycin/UVA is more effective than fluticasone/UVA in progressive macular hypomelanosis: a randomized study. *J Am Acad Dermatol.* 2006;55(5):836–843.

85. Richard EG. The science and (lost) art of psoralen plus UVA phototherapy. *Dermatol Clin.* 2020;38(1):11–23.

86. Bergfeld WF. Histopathologic changes in skin after photochemotherapy. *Cutis.* 1977;20(4):504–507.

87. Abel EA, Cox AJ, Farber EM. Epidermal dystrophy and actinic keratoses in psoriasis patients following oral psoralen photochemotherapy (PUVA). Follow-up study. *J Am Acad Dermatol.* 1982;7(3):333–340.

88. Rhodes AR, Harrist TJ, Day CL, Mihm MC Jr, Fitzpatrick TB, Sober AJ. Dysplastic melanocytic nevi in histologic association with 234 primary cutaneous melanomas. *J Am Acad Dermatol.* 1983;9(4):563–574.

89. Hashimoto K, Kohda H, Kumakiri M, Blender SL, Willis I. Psoralen-UVA-treated psoriatic lesions: ultrastructural changes. *Arch Dermatol.* 1978;114(5):711–722.

90. Zelickson AS, Mottaz JH, Zelickson BD, Muller SA. Elastic tissue changes in skin following PUVA therapy. *J Am Acad Dermatol.* 1980;3(2):186–192.

91. Crowson NA, Magro MC. The dermatopathology of drug eruptions. *Curr Probl Dermatol.* 2002;14(4):117–146.

92. Dereure O. Drug-induced skin pigmentation: epidemiology, diagnosis and treatment. *Am J Clin Dermatol.* 2001;2(4):253–262.

93. Weedon D. *Skin Pathology.* Churchill Livingstone; 1997.

94. Bowen AR, McCalmont TH. The histopathology of subcutaneous minocycline pigmentation. *J Am Acad Dermatol.* 2007;57(5):836–839.

95. Puri PK, Lountzis NI, Tyler W, Ferringer T. Hydroxychloroquine-induced hyperpigmentation: the staining pattern. *J Cutan Pathol.* 2008;35(12):1134–1137.

96. MacMorran WS, Krahn LE. Adverse cutaneous reactions to psychotropic drugs. *Psychosomatics.* 1997;38(5):413–422.

97. D'Agostino ML, Risser J, Robinson-Bostom L. Imipramine-induced hyperpigmentation: a case report and review of the literature. *J Cutan Pathol.* 2009;36(7):799–803.

98. Sicari MC, Lebwohl M, Baral J, Wexler P, Gordon RE, Phelps RG. Photoinduced dermal pigmentation in patients taking tricyclic antidepressants: histology, electron microscopy, and energy dispersive spectroscopy. *J Am Acad Dermatol.* 1999;40(2, pt 2):290–293.

99. Jun JB, Min PK, Kim DW, Chung SL, Lee KH. Cutaneous nodular reaction to oral mercury. *J Am Acad Dermatol.* 1997;37(1):131–133.

100. Amorim GM, Niemeyer-Corbellini JP, Quintella DC, Cuzzi T, Ramos-e-Silva M. Hypopigmented mycosis fungoides: a 20-case retrospective series. *Int J Dermatol.* 2018;57:306–312.

101. Erbil H, Sezer E, Koseoglu D, et al. Hyperpigmented mycosis fungoides: a case report. *J Eur Acad Dermatol Venereol.* 2007;21:977–1010.

102. Schmitt CE, Fabi SG, Kukreja T, Feinberg JS. Hypopigmented cutaneous sarcoidosis responsive to minocycline. *J Drugs Dermatol.* 2012;11(3):385–289.

103. Peterson CM, Lesher JL, Sangueza OP. A unique variant of Darier's disease. *Int J Dermatol.* 2001;40(4):278–280.

104. Krishnan R, Lewis A, Orengo IF, Rosen T. Pigmented Bowen's disease (squamous cell carcinoma in situ): a mimic of malignant melanoma. *Dermatol Surg.* 2001;27(7):673–674.

105. Requena L, Sangueza M, Sangueza OP, Kutzner H. Pigmented mammary Paget disease and pigmented epidermotropic metastases from breast carcinoma. *Am J Dermatopathol.* 2002;24(3):189–198.

106. Chen YH, Wong TW, Lee JY. Depigmented genital extramammary Paget's disease: a possible histogenetic link to Toker's clear cells and clear cell papulosis. *J Cutan Pathol.* 2001;28(2):105–108.

107. Hillianrd NJ, Huang C, Andea A. Pigmented extramammary Paget's disease of the axilla mimicking melanoma: a case report and review of the literature. *J Cutan Pathol.* 2009;36:995–1000.

108. Furlan FC, Sanches JA. Hypopigmented mycosis fungoides: a review of its clinical features and pathophysiology. *An Bras Dermatol.* 2013;88(6):954–960.

109. Clayton R, Breathnach A, Martin B, Feiwel M. Hypopigmented sarcoidosis in the negro: report of eight cases with ultrastructural observations. *Br J Dermatol.* 1977;96(2):119–125.

110. Marcon CR, Maia M. Albinism: epidemiology, genetics, cutaneous characterization, psychosocial factors. *An Bras Dermatol.* 2019;94:503–520.

111. Summers CG. Albinism: classification, clinical characteristics and recent findings. *Optomet Vision Sci.* 2009;86(6):659–662.

112. Hu H, Wang H, Jia Z, Xie Q. Prenatal genetic diagnosis for two Chinese families affected with oculocutaneous albinism type II [in Chinese]. *Chinese J Med Genet.* 2014;31(4):424–427.

113. Hurford MT, Sebastiano C. Hermansky-Pudlak syndrome: report of a case and review of the literature. *Int J Clin Exp Pathol.* 2008;1:550–554.

114. Tomita Y, Suzuki T. Genetics of pigmentary disorders. *Am J Med Genet C Semin Med Genet.* 2004;131C(1):75–81.

115. Wei AH, He X, Li W. Hypopigmentation in Hermansky-Pudlak syndrome. *J Dermatol.* 2013;40(5):325–329.

116. Hishida H, Electronmicroscopic studies of melanosomes in oculo-cutaneous albinismus [in Japanese]. *Nihon Hifuka Gakkai Zasshi.* 1973;83(3):119–132.

117. Wang X, Liu Y, Chen H, et al. LEF-1 regulates tyrosinase gene transcript in vitro. *PLoS One.* 2015;10(11):1–13.

118. Simeonov DR, Wang X, Wang C, et al. DNA variations in oculocutaneous albinism: an updated mutation list and current outstanding issues in molecular diagnostics. *Hum Mutat.* 2013;34(6):827–835.

119. Huizing M, Malicdan MC, Wang JA, et al. Hermansky-Pudlak syndrome: mutation update. *Hum Mutat.* 2020;41:535–580.

120. Gronskov K, Ek J, Brondum-Nielsen K. Oculocutaneous albinism. *Orphanet J Rare Dis.* 2007;2:43.

121. Oiso N, Fukai K, Kawada A, Suzuki T. Piebaldism. *J Dermatol.* 2013;40(5):330–335.

122. Saleem MD. Biology of human melanocyte development, Piebaldism and Waardenburg syndrome. *Ped Dermatol.* 2019;36:72–84.

123. Thomas I, Kihiczak GG, Fox MD, Janniger CK, Schwartz RA. Piebaldism: an update. *Int J Dermatol.* 2004;43(10):716–719.

124. Chang T, McGrae JD, Hashimoto K. Ultrastructural study of two patients with both piebaldism and neurofibromatosis 1. *Pediatr Dermatol.* 1993;10(3):224–234.

125. Yang T, Li X, Huang Q, et al. Double heterozygous mutations of MITF and PAX3 result in Waardenburg syndrome with increased penetrance in pigmentary defects. *Clin Genet.* 2013;83(1):78–82.

126. Zhang H, Luo H, Chen H, et al. Functional analysis of MITF gene mutations associated with Waardenburg syndrome type 2. *FEBS Lett.* 2012;586(23):4126–4131.

127. Hamadah I, Chisti M, Haider M, et al. A novel *KIT* mutation in a family with expanded syndrome of piebaldism. *JAAD Case Rep.* 2019;5:627–631.

128. Garg T, Khaitan BK, Manchanda Y. Autologous punch grafting for repigmentation in piebaldism. *J Dermatol.* 2003;30(11):849–850.

129. Rodrigues M, Ezzedine K, Hamzavi I, Pandya AG, Harris JE; Vitiligo Working Group. New discoveries in the pathogenesis and classification of vitiligo. *J Am Acad Dermatol.* 2017;77(1):1–13.

130. Tobin DJ, Swanson MM, Pittelkow MR, Peters EM, Schallreuter KU. Melanocytes are not absent in lesional skin of long duration vitiligo. *J Pathol.* 2000;191:407–416.

131. Katz EL, Harris JE. Translational research in vitiligo. *Front. Immunol.* 2021;12:624517.

132. Rashighi M, Harris JE. Vitiligo pathogenesis and emerging treatments. *Dermatol Clin.* 2017;35:257–265.

133. Fraczek A, Owczarczyk-Saczonek A, Placek W. The role of TRM cells in the pathogenesis of vitiligo: a review of the current state-of-the-art. *Int J Mol Sci.* 2020;21(10):3552.

134. Rashighi M, Harris JE. Interfering with the IFN-gamma/CXCL10 pathway to develop new targeted treatments for vitiligo. *Ann Transl Med.* 2015;3(21):343.

135. Craiglow BG, King BA. Tofacitinib citrate for the treatment of vitiligo: a pathogenesis-directed therapy. *JAMA Dermatol.* 2015;151(10):1110–1112.

136. Bacigalupi RM, Postolova A, Davis RS. Evidence-based, non-surgical treatments for vitiligo: a review. *Am J Clin Dermatol.* 2012;13(4):217–237.

137. Damsky W, King BA. JAK inhibitors in dermatology: the promise of a new drug class. *J Am Acad Dermatol.* 2017;76(4):736–744.

138. Petronelli M. Ruxolitinib cream NDA accepted for priority review by FDA. *Dermatol Tim.* 2021;42(4):30.

139. Felsten LM, Alikhan A, Petronic-Rosic V. Vitiligo: a comprehensive overview. Part II: Treatment options and approach to treatment. *J Am Acad Dermatol.* 2011;65(3):493–514.

140. Ajitkumar A, Yarrarapu ANS, Ramphul K. *Chediak Higashi Syndrome.* StatPearls; 2021.

141. Kaplan J, De Domenico I, Ward DM. Chediak-Higashi syndrome. *Curr Opin Hematol.* 2008;15(1):22–29.

142. De Chadarevian JP. Renal giant cytoplasmic inclusions in Chediak-Higashi syndrome: first ultrastructural demonstration in a human biopsy. *Ultrastruct Pathol.* 2011;35(4):172–175.

143. Carrillo-Farga J, Gutierrez-Palomera G, Ruiz-Maldonado R, Rondán A, Antuna S. Giant cytoplasmic granules in Langerhans cells of Chediak-Higashi syndrome. *Am J Dermatopathol.* 1990;12(1):81–87.

144. Veraitch O, Allison L, Vizcay-Barrena G, et al. Detailed hair shaft analysis in a man with delayed-onset Chediak-Higashi syndrome. *Br J Dermatol.* 2020;182:223–225.

145. Masliah-Planchon J, Darnige L, Bellucci S. Molecular determinants of platelet delta storage pool deficiencies: an update. *Br J Haematol.* 2013;160(1):5–11.

Melanocytic Tumors and Proliferations

DAVID E. ELDER, ROSALIE ELENITSAS, GEORGE F. MURPHY, AND
XIAOWEI XU

INTRODUCTION

Melanocytic tumors, especially malignant melanomas, are among the most important conditions that are encountered in dermatopathology. Although the term "melanoma" was once applied to benign as well as to malignant lesions, today it is used exclusively in reference to a malignant neoplasm of melanocytes that is the most common potentially lethal tumor of the skin, and its use is interchangeable with "malignant melanoma." The incidence of melanoma has risen rapidly over the last 50 or more years. The mortality rate, although substantial, has not increased at the same rate as incidence, suggesting that many lesions diagnosed as melanoma may not have had competence for systemic metastasis, which is the usual cause of death in melanoma patients. Thus, paradoxically and despite the substantial mortality, the cure rate for melanoma overall is high, in the range of 90% disease-free survival. The prognosis for melanoma varies greatly among lesions, depending on staging attributes, which will be discussed in this chapter. The incidence and mortality vary greatly around the globe, being highest in populations whose skin is susceptible to solar damage and who live in sunny locations or travel there for recreation or work, and have a cultural emphasis on tanning, including, especially, New Zealand, Australia, and Europe (1). Nevertheless, melanomas occur, at a lower rate, in all populations. The rise of tanning salons as a mechanism for skin darkening has also resulted in increased incidence of melanoma, particularly among young women (2).

PATHWAY CONCEPT OF MELANOMA DEVELOPMENT

Although all melanomas have the common definition of "a malignant tumor derived from melanocytes," they are not all the same. There is variation in epidemiology, etiology, pathogenesis, clinical and histologic morphology, and in genomic attributes of melanomas, which has led to the recent characterization of nine distinguishable "pathways to melanoma" (3,4). These pathways include not only the melanomas but also benign lesions that may progress to melanoma and that are therefore potential precursors, and it is also appropriate to discuss simulants of melanoma in this context. Among the benign lesions are fields of atypical melanocytic proliferation, "melanocytic nevi," and a subset of lesions with features that are intermediate between nevi and melanoma that has been provisionally termed

"melanocytomas." There is convincing evidence that nevi, melanocytomas, and melanomas are neoplasms derived from melanocytes, usually those residing in the epithelium of the skin and mucous membranes. Compared to melanocytes, nevus cells are able to form benign tumors that, once formed, are stable over time, whereas melanoma cells form malignant tumors characterized by (more or less) inexorable growth. Some salient characteristics of melanocytes, nevus cells, and melanoma cells are summarized in Table 28-1.

In general, nevus cells are distinguished from melanocytes in terms of their morphology, tending to lose the dendritic morphology of normal melanocytes, their relation to each other with nevus cells being defined by their propensity to lose the contact inhibition that keeps normal melanocytes separated, to form nests, and the presence of pigment, at least in superficially located nevus cells at an early point in their evolution. The pigment produced by melanocytes, in contrast, is typically transferred to basal keratinocytes soon after it is formed. The term "nevus" also refers, in general, to a hamartomatous malformation; however, the usual, common or banal melanocytic nevus is no longer considered to be a hamartoma but rather a neoplasm. Some other proliferations of melanocytes may be reactive, and a few may indeed be hamartomas. Nevi, in general, have importance in relation to melanoma as *potential precursors*, as *simulants of melanoma*, and as *markers of individuals at risk for developing melanoma*, whereas other melanocytic proliferations may be simulants of melanoma that do not necessarily have these properties. Because nevi are very much more common than melanomas in the general population, the risk

Table 28-1		
Melanocytes, Nevus Cells, and Melanoma Cells		
Melanocytes	**Nevus Cells**	**Melanoma Cells**
Contour is dendritic.	Contour is rounded or spindle shaped.	Contour is rounded or spindle shaped.
Cells are solitary.	Cells are arranged in clusters.	Cells are in clusters and large sheets.
Nuclei are small and regular.	Nuclei of most cells are small and regular.	Most nuclei are large, irregular, and hyperchromatic.
Mitoses are rare.	Mitoses are rare.	Mitoses are often present.

of progression of any one nevus to melanoma is exceedingly low. The diagnostic distinction between melanomas and other simulants, especially nevi, is the primary topic of this chapter.

The nine pathways to melanoma are listed in Table 28-2 (5). The lesions may in turn be classified into two different groups. In Group 1, an important element of the etiology and pathogenesis is ultraviolet light in the form of solar radiation. These lesions are characterized by "cumulative solar damage" (CSD), which, in practice, is estimated by the degree of solar elastosis in the skin (4), although there may exist individual variability in the threshold to form elastosis. This group of "CSD Melanomas" is in turn divided into "Low CSD" (also known as superficial spreading melanoma, SSM) and "High CSD" melanomas (lentigo maligna melanoma [LMM] and desmoplastic melanoma [DM]), which differ in terms of the pattern of sun exposure (acute–intermittent vs. chronic), and in their genomic landscape, as summarized in the tables.

Solar elastosis can be graded as has been defined as follows, all dependent on evaluation of a hematoxylin and eosin–stained section at a magnification of 20×. Grade 1 solar elastosis is represented by the finding of single elastic fibers that are barely perceptible in the reticular dermis at this magnification. In Grade 2, the fibers are present in bunches or fascicles and are readily recognizable. In Grade 3, there are globules of gray staining elastic material that have lost their fibrillary texture (6). The presence of solar elastosis, in general, correlates with other attributes of sun-damaged skin, including solar lentigines, solar keratoses, and an increased incidence of sun-related nonmelanoma skin cancers such as basal cell and squamous cell carcinomas (see the relevant chapters), in addition to melanomas, nevi, and fields of atypical melanocytic proliferation.

Although DM is relatively rare, the other sun-related melanomas, low and high CSD melanomas, are the most common forms of melanoma in the populations mentioned previously, constituting populations at high risk for melanoma and living in countries with a high incidence of melanoma. The other melanoma subtypes are much less common, in general, and their

---

Table 28-2

Pathways to Melanoma

Group 1. Lesions Associated with Cumulative Solar Damage (CSD) and Ultraviolet-Related Pathogenesis

Pathway I. Low CSD melanoma/superficial spreading melanoma

Pathway II. High CSD melanoma/lentigo maligna melanoma

Pathway III. Desmoplastic melanoma (high CSD)

Group 2. Lesions Not Associated with CSD or only Incidentally Associated

Pathway IV. Spitz melanoma

Pathway V. Acral melanoma

Pathway VI. Mucosal melanoma

Pathway VII. Melanoma arising in a congenital nevus

Pathway VIII. Melanoma arising in a blue nevus.

Group 3. Variable Pathways

Nodular melanoma

Based on Elder DE, Massi D, Scolyer RA, Willemze R. *WHO Classification of Skin Tumours.* 4th ed. IARC; 2018.

incidence is about the same throughout the world. Thus, these are the most common forms of melanoma in low-incidence countries, where the prevalence of the solar-related melanomas is very low; however, their absolute incidence is similar to that in the high-incidence countries. The precursor lesions of the various pathways probably follow a similar distribution.

Melanomas, like many other cancers, typically evolve through stages of tumor progression, commonly involving the stage of melanoma *in situ*, where the lesional cells are confined to the epidermis and have not acquired the ability to invade or survive in the dermis. Some superficially invasive melanomas have few cells in the dermis, but these have not acquired the capacity to proliferate and form a true tumor. Because these lesions had been observed clinically to expand centripetally along the radius of an imperfect circle near the skin surface, these have been called "radial growth phase" (RGP) melanomas. In histologic sections, these have a horizontal orientation, and the term "horizontal growth phase" has been suggested as a histologic correlate. With time, cells in the dermis of lesions of superficially invasive RGP melanoma may acquire the capacity to proliferate, exhibit mitotic activity, and to form a true tumor. This phase of progression has been termed the "vertical growth phase" (VGP) and also "tumorigenic melanoma." Melanomas that have a VGP but lack a preexisting histologically detectable RGP are termed "nodular melanomas." It is believed that nodular melanomas may evolve in any of the nine pathways and may therefore reflect the genomic landscape and other properties of the pathway from which they evolved.

PRINCIPLES OF MANAGEMENT OF PIGMENTED LESIONS

As has been demonstrated in a comprehensive study of accuracy and reproducibility, there is considerable discordance in the histologic diagnosis of melanoma, resulting in diagnostic uncertainty and complicating decision-making for appropriate treatment (7). This occurs because of complexity in the histologic continuum from benign to unequivocally malignant melanocytic lesions and is most pronounced in the gray zone between wholly benign and obviously malignant lesions (8). The difficulties are likely to be less pronounced within a single institution, where patterns of diagnostic terminology and communication have been established. Subjectively, this variation in terminology appears to be especially troublesome among institutions that adhere to different schools of thought. Between institutions, and especially when there is variation in expertise and experience, the level of disagreement can be high (9).

This lack of standardization is not unique to melanocytic pathology but affects other clinical fields. To improve precision in breast imaging, BI-RADS (Breast Imaging Reporting and Data System) was developed by U.S. Food and Drug Administration mandate and under the auspices of the American College of Radiology. This system standardizes results of mammogram interpretations and reports along a 5-point scale, with the objective of minimizing ambiguity regarding the necessity and type of therapeutic management (10). A similar system has been developed for the melanocytic tumor system, known as the MPATH-Dx (Melanocytic Pathology Assessment Tool and Hierarchy for Diagnosis) schema that comprises a Histology Reporting Form and a Diagnosis–Treatment Mapping Tool (11).

The terms used in the Histology Reporting Form are the "diagnoses" that are discussed in this and other reference texts and literature. The impact of variation in the exact form of words used for diagnosis in different classification systems is lessened when management implications are included as a primary outcome of the diagnostic process. The Mapping Tool is essentially a thesaurus that aims to encompass all of the terms in current use and maps these to one of five MPATH-Dx categories. These are intended to represent possible clinical approaches for the management of a lesion that is assumed for this purpose to be present at a specimen margin. The approaches are considered to be guidelines for consideration and not mandates. Where national guidelines exist, these should be followed. The guidelines vary according to the anticipated degree of aggressiveness believed to be associated with each diagnostic category, as follows (11):

MPATH-Dx Category 0: Incomplete study due to sampling and/or technical limitations. Clinical Outcome: Repeat testing or short-term follow-up.

MPATH-Dx Category 1: Benign lesions with essentially no probability of adverse consequences; for example, common (including mildly dysplastic) nevi, lentigines, and similar disorders. Clinical Outcome: No further treatment required.

MPATH-Dx Category 2: Lesions for which the probability of progressive disease is considered unlikely, but some risk of continued local proliferation and possible future adverse consequence cannot be ruled out; for instance, some examples of moderately dysplastic nevi, atypical Spitz tumors, deep-penetrating nevi, pigmented epithelioid melanocytomas (PEMs), cellular blue nevi, and others. Clinical Outcome: Consideration of narrow but complete excision (<5 mm).

MPATH-Dx Category 3: Lesions with a higher likelihood of local tumor progression and greater need for intervention; for example, melanoma in situ, most examples of severely dysplastic nevi. Clinical Outcome: Excision with at least 5 mm (but <1 cm) margins.

MPATH-Dx Category 4: Lesions with substantial risk for locoregional progression; for example, invasive melanoma, American Joint Committee on Cancer (AJCC) Stage T1a. Clinical Outcome: Follow national guidelines, for example, wide excision (≥1 cm margins).

MPATH-Dx Category 5: Lesions with greater risk for locoregional progression; for example, invasive melanoma, AJCC Stage T1b, or more. Clinical Outcome: Follow national guidelines, for example, wide excision (≥1 cm margins); consider sentinel node staging, possibly other adjuvant therapy.

Substantial health care resources are directed to the screening of populations considered to be at increased risk for melanoma, as in other neoplastic systems. Ambiguities in diagnostic reports are common, and there is a tendency to electively treat ambiguous lesions. Screening studies have led to a greater number of diagnoses of melanoma, without a concomitant increase in mortality, leading to suggestions that melanoma, like other cancers, is being overdiagnosed at a biologic level, even in cases where there is good agreement as to a given diagnosis (12). This is because there are presumably many cases that would never have progressed to clinical malignancy. Current technology does not provide the tools to distinguish the harmless lesions from those that would have progressed if not excised, although developing sophistication in genomic studies such as comparative genomic hybridization (CGH), fluorescence in situ hybridization (FISH), diagnostic gene expression profiling (GEP), or next-generation sequencing (NGS) and also in immunohistochemical markers, has the potential to improve this situation (13). Harm to patients can result not only from undertreatment but also from overtreatment of ambiguous disease in the forms of false fear of cancer, of morbidity from unnecessary treatment, and of misdirection of health care resources. These issues result not only from intrinsic limitations of the diagnostic processes but also as a response to medicolegal pressures and patient safety concerns. The MPATH-Dx Diagnostic–Treatment Mapping Tool may serve as an aid in reducing uncertainty and ambiguity in melanocytic lesion reporting and allowing for greater consistency in the management of pigmented lesions and also by facilitating the study of outcomes and resource allocation at the level of populations and health care systems (7).

PATHOLOGY OF FRECKLES AND LENTIGINES

Freckles (ephelides or ephelids) and lentigines (or lentigos) are clinically similar in that they both present as usually small macular hyperpigmented lesions. By definition, a freckle does not contain an obviously increased number of melanocytes; if this feature is present, the lesion should be termed a lentigo. In common parlance, it is not unusual for lesions that are actually lentigos to be referred to as freckles. Some freckles may be related to UV light, whereas others may represent a developmental phase, and some are components of a variety of heritable syndromes.

Freckles and Hyperpigmentations

These lesions, in general, are benign and not likely to be precursors of melanomas in most cases. Sometimes, they may present as clinically or histologically atypical simulants that need to be distinguished from melanomas. Some are related to sun exposure, whereas others are genodermatoses or idiopathic. Solar lentigines are often seen adjacent to LMMs; however, their potential precursor relationship remains uncertain.

By definition, a freckle (ephelid) is a small flat tan or brown lesion that histologically has increased pigment in keratinocytes but no increase in the number of melanocytes. Hyperpigmentations may be described as larger macular pigmented lesions that show increased melanin pigment in keratinocytes without melanocytic proliferation, or in the dermis in melanophages. Lentigines are macular hyperpigmentations that differ from freckles and hyperpigmentations in that the number of epidermal melanocytes is increased within the basal cell layer. However, in common parlance, the term "freckle" is often used to refer both to ephelides and to solar lentigines, as well as other forms of macular hyperpigmentations. Ephelides appear early in childhood and are associated with sun exposure, fair skin type, and red hair. Solar lentigines ("sunburn freckles") appear with age and are a sign of photodamage. These lesions are strong risk indicators for melanoma and nonmelanoma skin cancer. Sunburn freckles and also sun-related ephelides are strongly influenced by the melanocortin-1-receptor (MC1R) gene, which has been termed "the freckle gene" and is also associated with fair skin, red hair, and melanoma and nonmelanoma skin cancer. In a large case-control study, carriers of *MC1R* gene variants had a markedly increased risk of developing ephelides, whereas the risk of developing severe solar lentigines was moderately increased, suggesting that *MC1R* is a major gene controlling susceptibility to the development of both of these forms of macular hyperpigmentations (14). Natural variation at *MC1R* is a genetic risk factor for childhood/adolescent as well as for adult melanoma, possibly through a pigmentation-independent pathway, and the observed effect is stronger in melanoma patients aged less than 18 years (15).

Principles of Management of Freckles: Freckles generally do not require active therapy. As discussed previously, they are markers of skin at risk for development of melanoma, and as such they may play a part in a decision to offer skin surveillance. In other circumstances, such as Albright syndrome, freckles may have significance in diagnosis of a systemic condition.

Simple Ephelid (Freckle)

Clinical Summary. Freckles, or ephelides, are small, red-brown macules scattered over skin exposed to the sun. Exposure to the sun deepens the pigmentation of freckles, in contrast to lentigo simplex (see Lentigo Simplex p. 841), in which already deep pigment does not change. Ephelides, simple lentigines, and solar lentigines are difficult to distinguish from one another clinically and are considered together in most clinical and epidemiologic studies. Taken together, these lesions constitute a significant risk factor for the development of melanoma (16).

Histopathology. In freckles, there is hyperpigmentation of the basal cell layer, but in contrast to lentigines, there is no elongation of the rete ridges and, by traditional definition, no obvious increase in the concentration of melanocytes. However, in a quantitative study of lesions from children, melanocyte frequencies in freckles were significantly greater than in adjacent nonpigmented skin. Cellular atypia of melanocytes and reactivity of melanocytes for HMB-45 were noticed in some freckles (17). It is likely that freckles represent a hyperplastic and hyperactive response of melanocytes to UV light.

Histogenesis. On *electron microscopy,* the melanocytes within freckles are found to be essentially similar to those of darker skinned persons. Melanocytes of the surrounding epidermis of freckle-prone subjects, by contrast, show constitutionally few and minimally melanized melanosomes, many of which are rounded rather than elongated (18). Such rounded melanosomes (so-called pheomelanosomes) are characteristic of the lightly pigmented skin of individuals with red hair and/or blue eyes and a cutaneous phenotype that is prone to freckles. As noted previously, the tendency to develop freckles appears to be closely related to *MC1R* gene polymorphisms (14). In contrast to lentigines, which are more exclusively related to sun exposure, ephelides are much more associated with constitutional host factors such as fair skin and/or red hair, in addition to their induction on sun-exposed skin (19,20).

Melanotic Macules of Albright Syndrome

Clinical Summary. Albright syndrome is usually characterized by unilateral polyostotic fibrous dysplasia, precocious puberty in females, and melanotic patches. The patches are generally large in size and few in number; are located on only one side of the midline, often on the same side as the bone lesions; and have a jagged, irregular border resembling the "coast of Maine," in contrast to the smooth "coast of California" type of border of the *café au lait* patches of neurofibromatosis.

Histopathology. Except for hyperpigmentation of the basal layer, there is no other abnormality, and both the number and the size of the melanocytes are normal (21).

Differential Diagnosis. The melanotic macules of Albright syndrome only rarely show the "giant" melanin granules (macromelanosomes) that are commonly seen in some of the melanocytes and keratinocytes within the *café au lait* patches of neurofibromatosis. Histologically, the melanotic macules may be indistinguishable from ephelides without correlative clinical information (21).

Café au lait Patches (Spots)

Café au lait spots, like melanotic macules, are lesions also characterized by hyperpigmentation of basal keratinocytes without overt melanocytic proliferation. These are characteristic of neurofibromatosis, in which they are characteristically multiple (e.g., >5), in contrast to similar sporadic lesions that are usually isolated or few in number (22). The NF1 neurofibromatosis syndrome is caused by mutations in the NF1 gene that encodes the tumor suppressor, neurofibromin, which functions as a Ras-GTPase-activating protein, leading to overactivation of the Ras signaling pathway that functionally impacts both keratinocytes and melanocytes with regard to melanin synthesis and keratinocyte differentiation (23). Similar changes of progressive lentiginosis and multiple *café au lait* macules have been described as an unusual finding in Waardenburg syndrome related to PAX3 mutations (WS Type 1) (24).

Mucosal Melanotic Macules (Mucosal Lentigines)

These are discussed in the section on Mucosal Melanomas and Related Lesions.

Becker Melanosis

Clinical Summary. Becker melanosis, also called Becker pigmented hairy nevus, occurs most commonly as a large, unilateral patch showing hyperpigmentation and hypertrichosis on the shoulder, back, or chest of an adult male (25). However, in some instances, Becker melanosis affects areas other than the shoulder and chest. Also, it may be multiple and bilateral and may occasionally be found in women. The lesion commonly appears during the second decade of life. Usually, the patch is sharply but irregularly demarcated. Occasionally, however, the lesion presents as coalescing macules instead of a solitary patch.

In one report, nine cases of melanoma in association with Becker nevus were described (26). Five of these were on the same body site as the nevus. The few melanomas that have been described in association with Becker nevus have been of the superficial spreading type, originating in the epidermis (26). It remains to be determined whether these reports represent a greater incidence than chance would suggest.

The hairiness appears after the pigmentation, and, quite frequently, no hypertrichosis is seen. It is therefore possible that cases described as progressive cribriform and zosteriform hyperpigmentation represent a variant of Becker melanosis without hypertrichosis (27).

Of interest is the association of a pilar smooth muscle hamartoma with Becker melanosis. In such cases, the area of Becker melanosis may show slight papular perifollicular elevations or mild induration (28).

Histopathology. The epidermis shows slight acanthosis and irregular elongation and flattening with a tendency for fusion of the rete ridges. There is hyperpigmentation of the basal layer, and melanophages are seen in the upper dermis. The number of melanocytes is increased within the basal cell layer, as demonstrated using image analysis and staining with melanocyte markers, including S100 and MART-1. In the same study, androgen receptor expression was increased in the epidermis (29), suggesting a possible pathogenetic mechanism. The pilar structures may appear normal or increased in number.

An increase in smooth muscle fibers exists in nearly all cases, although it may be slight. In lesions with an associated smooth muscle hamartoma, irregularly arranged, thick bundles of smooth muscle are present in the dermis (28). The term Becker nevus syndrome has been proposed for a phenotype characterized by the presence of a particular type of organoid epithelial nevus showing hyperpigmentation, increased hairiness, hamartomatous augmentation of smooth muscle fibers (smooth muscle hamartoma), and other developmental defects such as ipsilateral hypoplasia of breast and skeletal anomalies including scoliosis, spina bifida occulta, or ipsilateral hypoplasia of a limb (30).

Principles of Management: These lesions may be biopsied if thought necessary to rule out melanoma.

Lentigines

Lentigines are macular hyperpigmentations in which the number of epidermal melanocytes is increased and there are no nests of melanocytes, as are present, by definition, in nevi. The term "lentigo" is derived from the Latin "lenz" meaning lens or lentil (31). Thus, the term in its original usage is clinical, referring to a small ovoid or lens-shaped pigmented spot. The term has come to be applied to larger pigmented lesions, especially those that recapitulate, to a greater or lesser extent, the histologic features of a lentigo simplex: basal proliferation of melanocytes arranged as single cells rather than in nests, typically, but not always, associated with elongation of the rete ridges. This pattern of melanocytic proliferation is termed "lentiginous." Lentiginous melanocytic proliferation is seen in the macules of solar lentigo and lentigo simplex and in the macular or plaque components of lentiginous junctional and compound nevi, of lentiginous dysplastic nevi, and of lentiginous melanomas, including lentigo maligna, acral, and mucosal lentiginous types.

Solar Lentigo (Actinic Lentigo)
Clinical Summary. Solar lentigines commonly occur as multiple lesions in areas exposed to the sun, such as the face and extensor surfaces of the forearms but most commonly on the dorsa of the hands. The lesions increase in number with age, in contrast to nevi that decline in number (32). Therefore, they have been referred to as senile lentigines. However, sun

exposure (especially sunburn), rather than age, is the eliciting factor (33). Thus, the lesions do not occur on sun-protected skin, even in the elderly. Solar lentigines are commonly seen in sun-exposed Caucasoids. They are not indurated, possess a uniform dark brown color, and have an irregular outline. They vary in diameter from minute to more than 1 cm and may coalesce. Solar lentigines, like ephelides, are risk markers for the development of melanoma (34) and are commonly numerous in the skin around melanomas, as seen in melanoma reexcision specimens. Lesions termed "sunburn freckles" by some overlap clinically and histologically with solar lentigines. They are blotchy macular areas of tan hyperpigmentation, often of the order of 1 cm in diameter, which often appear on the shoulders or other sun-exposed areas of a young person after a severe sunburn (35). Other potentially related lesions are intensely dark, perfectly macular reticulated lesions that have been called "reticulated lentigo" (36) or "ink-spot lentigo" (37).

Solar lentigines differ from ephelides in that they are more prevalent, increase in frequency and number with advancing age (ephelides tend to decline in number), and are most common on the trunk. They occur more frequently in males than in females, unlike ephelides, which are more evenly distributed and are not primarily related to sun exposure (19,20).

Solar lentigines and relatively flat seborrheic keratoses may resemble each other in clinical appearance, and both are commonly referred to as "liver spots" or "age spots." Seborrheic keratosis, in general, show more hyperkeratosis clinically. In contrast, lentigo maligna differs from solar lentigo in clinical appearance by its irregular distribution of pigment, often in a finely reticulated pattern, and by its greater asymmetry and border irregularity (p. 883).

Prolonged treatment with psoralen and ultraviolet light A (PUVA) can induce the formation of pigmented macules ("PUVA lentigines") in the irradiated areas. These are similar to solar lentigines, but their color is darker and their pigment more irregularly distributed (38).

Histopathology. A Japanese study described two patterns of solar lentigines on the skin of the face, both associated with hyperpigmentation of basal keratinocytes and an increased number of single basal melanocytes. In one pattern, there was a flattened epidermis with basal melanosis, and in the other pattern there was epidermal hyperplasia with elongated rete ridges composed of deeply pigmented basaloid cells (39). In the latter or "budding" pattern, the rete ridges are subtly or more significantly elongated. They either appear club shaped or are tortuous and show small, budlike extensions. The elongated rete ridges are composed, especially in their lower portion, of deeply pigmented basaloid cells intermingled with melanocytes, which are arranged mostly as single cells. Epidermal maturation may appear subtly perturbed in some lesions with associated keratinocyte enlargement. The melanocytes appear significantly increased in number in some cases but only slightly or not at all increased in others (Fig. 28-1). They possess a heightened capacity for melanin production, compared to the melanocytes of adjacent skin. In the upper dermis, there is elastosis and often scattered melanophages occasionally with a mild, perivascular lymphoid infiltrate. In the "flattened epidermis" pattern, there was a significantly thinner epidermis, more severe solar elastosis, and fewer Langerhans cells in the epidermis as compared with the budding group. In some lesions, the rete ridges

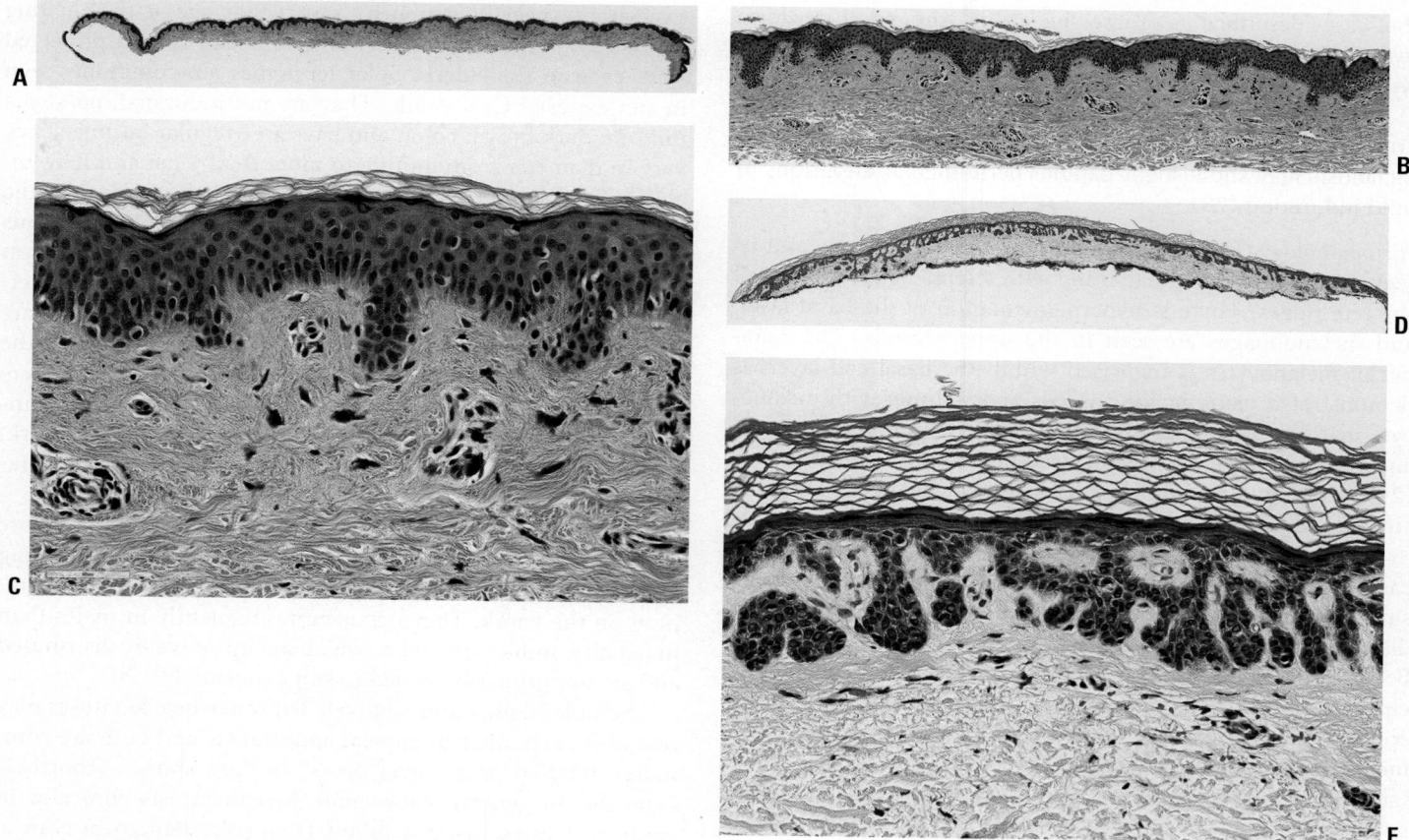

Figure 28-1 Actinic lentigo. **A:** Scanning magnification showing a localized area of elongated rete ridges in elastotic actinically damaged skin. **B:** Higher magnification shows basal hyperpigmentation and slight-to-moderate prominence of melanocytes, without contiguous proliferation. **C:** Sometimes, there is slight atypia of randomly scattered melanocytes (mild random atypia). **D:** Another example shows more prominent rete ridge changes across a broad extent. **E:** Actinic lentigines are characterized by some combination of hyperpigmentation of basal keratinocytes, elongation of rete ridges, and prominence of melanocytes, the latter not especially marked in this example.

are elongated to such an extent that strands of basaloid cells form anastomosing branches, resulting in a reticulated pattern closely resembling that seen in the reticulated pigmented type of seborrheic keratosis. However, unlike seborrheic keratoses, solar lentigines do not form horn cysts.

Elastosis within the superficial dermis is a marker for chronic solar damage (CSD), which is linked to the prevalence and distribution of solar lentigines and other sun-related conditions, including malignant melanoma. A system for the scoring of the degree of solar elastosis has been developed and validated. The following scoring system was used: CSD 0: absence of elastotic fibers visible at $200\times$ magnification; CSD 1: scattered elastotic fibers lying as individual units, not as bunches, between collagen bundles; CSD 2: densely scattered elastotic fibers distributed predominantly as bushels rather than individual units; CSD 3: amorphous deposits of blue-gray material with lost fiber texture (6). Solar elastosis is also discussed and illustrated in Chapters 12 and 15.

Solar lentigines differ histologically from ephelides, by definition, in having an increased number of epidermal melanocytes. However, in some lesions, the proliferation may be demonstrable only by formal counting (40). In contrast to lentigo simplex, lentiginous nevi, and lentiginous melanomas, the melanocytic proliferation is less contiguous and is non-nested. Often, a determining feature in differentiating a lentigo simplex from a solar lentigo is the presence of altered keratinocyte maturation in the latter.

PUVA-induced pigmented macules represent solar lentigines on the basis of irregular elongation of their rete ridges. They have an increased number of large melanocytes that may have slight nuclear atypia, which can be seen in the adjacent skin as well (41).

Large cell acanthoma, which presents as a slightly scaly tan macule on photodamaged skin, is identified histologically by having epidermal keratinocytes with nuclei roughly twice the size of adjacent keratinocytes but with minimal nuclear pleomorphism. There are clinical, histologic, and immunohistochemical overlapping characteristics with solar lentigo, suggesting that large cell acanthoma should be considered as a related condition (42,43). The lesions are distinguished from actinic keratoses by the lack of cytologic dysplasia (except for the nuclear enlargement) and the lack of parakeratosis.

In the *reticulated or "ink-spot" lentigo*, histologic evaluation, including electron microscopy and DOPA-incubated vertical sections, has demonstrated lentiginous hyperplasia of melanocytes in the epidermis, marked hyperpigmentation of the basal layer with "skip" areas that involved the rete ridges, and a minimal increase in the number of melanocytes (37). Dermal pigment incontinence is also often present.

Histogenesis. A microarray analysis of solar lentigines demonstrated upregulation of genes related to inflammation, fatty acid metabolism, and melanocytes and downregulation of cornified envelope-related genes; the authors suggest that solar lentigo may be induced by the mutagenic effect of repeated ultraviolet light exposures, leading to enhancement of melanin production along with decreased proliferation and differentiation of lesional keratinocytes on a background of chronic inflammation (44). In a skin model, it has been demonstrated that factors secreted by irradiated aged fibroblasts induce solar lentigo in pigmented reconstructed epidermis (45). It has been postulated that loss of epidermal melanin unit homeostasis with abnormal pigment retention in keratinocytes may be the primary disorder in solar lentigines (46).

Differential Diagnosis. In lentigo simplex (see below), the rete ridges are elongated, but, in contrast, the lesional melanocytes are more obviously increased in number and focally lie in contiguity with one another around the tips and sides of the rete but not between the rete. Lentigo maligna often shows flattening or absence of the rete ridges together with contiguous and continuous proliferation and uniform atypia of its melanocytes; like lentigo simplex, however, it may be associated with a dermal lymphocytic infiltrate. In solar lentigo, the rete are elongated, and the lesional melanocytes do not lie in contiguity with one another, even though they may be increased in number. There is minimal cytologic atypia and no pagetoid spread of melanocytes above the basal layer. In contrast to a pigmented actinic keratosis, there is no keratinocytic atypia and usually no parakeratosis.

Principles of Management: Lentigines generally do not require active therapy. As discussed previously, solar lentigines are markers of skin at risk for development of melanoma, and as such they may play a part in a decision to offer skin surveillance. Occasional lesions exhibit clinical atypia sufficient to prompt biopsy to rule out melanoma.

Lentigo Simplex and Related Lesions

Clinical Summary. Simple lentigines are macular hyperpigmentations in which the number of epidermal melanocytes is increased. In solar lentigines, as described previously, the cell bodies are separated from one another by those of keratinocytes, and the proliferation may be termed "noncontiguous." The proliferation may be described as "contiguous" if the cell bodies at least focally touch one another, as in lentigo simplex (and also in lentiginous nevi and in lentiginous melanomas).

Lentigo simplex most frequently arises in childhood, but it may appear at any age. Usually in lentigo simplex, there are only a few scattered lesions without predilection to areas of sun exposure. They are small, symmetrical, and well-circumscribed macules that are evenly pigmented but that vary individually from brown to black (Fig. 28-2A). They are not indurated and usually measure only a few millimeters in diameter. Clinically, a lentigo simplex is indistinguishable from a junctional nevus. Histologically, a lentigo simplex is characterized by proliferation of single cells along the basal layer of the tips and sides of elongated rete ridges, a pattern that is therefore termed "lentiginous" (Fig. 28-2B). The common form of lentigo simplex is thought to be an early stage of development of some junctional melanocytic nevi (47). Special forms of lentigo simplex include lentiginosis profusa, the multiple lentigines syndrome or LEOPARD syndrome, and speckled lentiginous nevus, also referred to as nevus spilus.

Lentiginosis profusa shows innumerable small, pigmented macules either from birth or childhood or early adulthood without any other abnormalities. The mucous membranes are spared, and there may be a family history. Some may be associated with a KIT mutation (48). Other cases may be part of the multiple lentigines syndrome with systemic abnormalities (see next paragraph) (49). Agminated or segmental lentigines have been defined as a circumscribed group of small pigmented macules arranged in a small or large group, often in a segmental pattern, each macule consisting of a lentiginous intraepidermal proliferation of melanocytes. Two types of segmentally arranged lentigines probably exist. The first has scattered light-brown lesions and may represent a type of mosaic NF1. Non-NF1 associated lesions have more densely packed, dark lesions (50).

The *speckled lentiginous nevus*, or *nevus spilus*, consists of a light-brown patch or band present from the time of birth that in childhood becomes dotted with small, dark brown macules and sometimes papules. Most appear to develop in early childhood (51). Papular nevus spilus coexisting with ipsilateral extracutaneous abnormalities involving peripheral nerves of the skin or

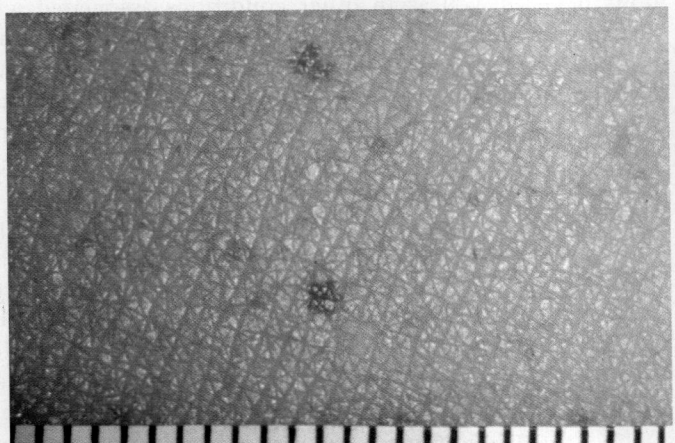
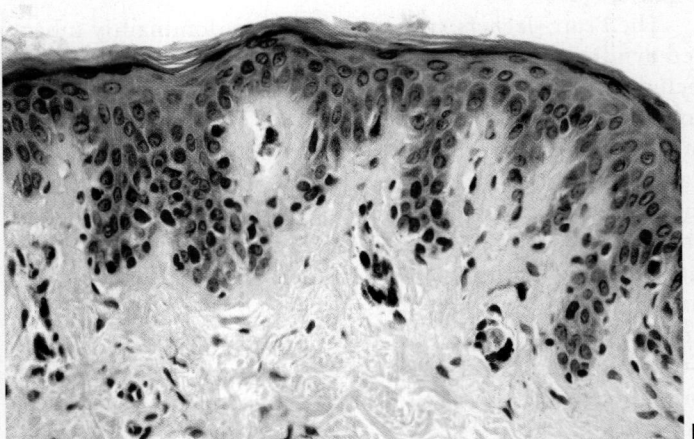

Figure 28-2 Lentigo simplex. A: Clinically, the lesions are small, usually less than 2 mm, fairly symmetrical and well circumscribed. It is not possible to distinguish clinically among ephelides, simple lentigines, and lentiginous junctional nevi. (Clinical photograph by Peter Wilson.) B: Melanocytes are present in contiguity near the tips and sides of elongated rete ridges, "lentiginous proliferation." There is no "continuous" proliferation between the rete. The presence of at least a single nest would define a lentiginous junctional nevus ("jentigo").

muscles is known as "papular nevus spilus (PNS) syndrome," a rare condition that can be considered to be part of a spectrum of mosaic RASopathies, including isolated PNS, isolated nevus sebaceus, PNS syndrome, Schimmelpenning syndrome, and phacomatosis pigmentokeratotica (52). The occurrence of melanoma in a nevus spilus has occasionally been reported (53), and also that of Spitz nevi, which may be associated with an activating *HRAS* mutation in both the Spitz and the background nevus (54).

The *multiple lentigines syndrome*, a dominant trait, is characterized by the presence of thousands of flat, dark brown macules on the skin but not on the mucosal surfaces. The lentigines appear in infancy and gradually increase in number over time. Although most macules vary from pinpoint dots to 5 mm in diameter, some dark spots are much larger, up to 5 cm in diameter. This rare syndrome, also known by the mnemonic *LEOPARD syndrome,* is now considered to be a variant of Noonan syndrome, caused by gain-of-function RAF1 mutations, or RASopathy syndromes. In addition to the lentigines (L), features may include electrocardiographic conduction defects (E), ocular hypertelorism (O), pulmonary stenosis (P), and abnormalities of the genitalia (A) consisting of gonadal or ovarian hypoplasia, retardation of growth (R), and neural deafness (D). Not all of these manifestations are present in every case. Cardiomyopathy is also often present and associated with significant morbidity (55).

Another syndrome associated with lentigines has been known under the acronyms *NAME* or *LAMB* or *myxoma* syndrome (lentiginous nevi, atrial and/or mucocutaneous myxomas, myxoid neurofibromas, ephelides, blue nevi). It has been proposed that these mnemonics be dropped because the particular features encompassed within this syndrome are unclear, and the term "cutaneous lentiginosis with atrial myxomas" is an adequate description of this syndrome (56). The *Carney complex*, a familial multitumoral syndrome, comprises spotty skin pigmentation (lentigines and blue nevi), myxomas (heart, skin, and breast), endocrine "overactivity" usually manifested by endocrine tumors (adrenal cortex, pituitary, testis, and thyroid), schwannomas, and two unusual pigmented tumors, epithelioid blue nevus (skin), and psammomatous melanotic schwannoma (involving skin, viscera, or nerve tissue). Carney complex has been linked to chromosome 2p16 and the *PRKAR1A* gene at 17q22–24 (57).

The *Peutz–Jeghers syndrome (PJS)* is a dominantly inherited syndrome that incurs an increased risk of malignancy, including benign ovarian sex cord tumors, calcifying Sertoli tumors of the testis, as well as cervical, breast, gastrointestinal, pancreatic, endometrial, and thyroid cancers. Diagnostic features of PJS include hamartomatous small intestinal polyps and mucosal hyperpigmentation, presenting characteristically as dark brown-blue macules, commonly found on the border of the lips, oral and bowel mucosa, and on skin involving the palms and soles, eyes, nares, and perianal region. Most cases have heterozygous mutations in the serine-threonine kinase STK11/LKB1 tumor suppressor gene located on chromosome 19p (58). These lesions are not commonly biopsied.

Histopathology of Lentigines. Lentigines, in general, show slight or moderate elongation of the rete ridges, an increase in the concentration of melanocytes in the basal layer, an increase in

the amount of melanin in both the melanocytes and the basal keratinocytes, and the presence of melanophages in the upper dermis (47). The melanocytes in the epidermis lie in focal contiguity with one another near the tips and sides of the elongated rete, but the proliferation is not continuous between the rete (Fig. 28-2B). There are no nests, by definition. In some instances, melanin is also seen in the upper layers of the epidermis, including the stratum corneum. A mild inflammatory infiltrate may be intermingled with the melanophages within the underlying papillary dermis. In lesions otherwise clinically characteristic of lentigo simplex, small nests of nevus cells are commonly seen at the epidermal–dermal junction, especially at the lowest pole of rete ridges. The lesions then combine features of a lentigo simplex and a junctional nevus, leading to their descriptive diagnosis as "jentigo" (59), lentigo with incipient junctional nevic nest formation, or "lentiginous junctional nevus." Because of the existence of these transitional forms, the lentigo simplex is regarded as a potential precursor of what may become a melanocytic nevus.

In *lentiginosis profusa* and the *multiple lentiginosis syndromes*, as a rule, the lesions are "pure" lentigines without the formation of nevus cell nests. In larger macules, however, there may be junctional nevus cell nests, and there may even be nevus cell nests in the upper dermis (60).

In *speckled lentiginous nevus*, or *nevus spilus*, the light-brown patch or band shows the histologic features of lentigo simplex. The speckled areas have junctional nests of nevus cells at the lowest pole of some of the rete ridges, diffuse lentiginous melanocytic proliferation, as well as dermal aggregates of nevus cells. Various types of nevi (e.g., junctional nevi, blue nevi, and Spitz nevi) may present in the same lesion over time, and histologic features of congenital melanocytic nevus (CMN) may be present within the spots, suggesting that these lesions may be considered as variants of congenital nevi (61).

In the lesions of PJS, the basal cell layer shows marked hyperpigmentation. Although the number of melanocytes may appear to be slightly increased, no increase has been found in DOPA-stained sections (62). The intestinal polyps appear to be hamartomas because glands are intermingled with smooth muscle bundles (58).

The presence of occasional giant melanin granules has been described in various forms of lentigines and lentiginous nevi, as well as in other conditions associated with hyperpigmentation, including the *café au lait* spots of neurofibromatosis and, less commonly, in *café au lait* spots without neurofibromatosis, and, on occasion, even in normal skin of healthy persons (63). Thus, they have no diagnostic specificity. Giant melanin granules vary in size from 1 to 6 μm. Because of their size and heavy melanization, the larger granules are readily recognized by light microscopy. Although seen largely within melanocytes, they also occur in keratinocytes and melanophages to which they have been transferred. On *electron microscopy*, the giant melanin granules have been termed macromelanosomes and are regarded as autolysosomes, referred to as "melanin macroglobules," that represent lysosome-mediated accumulation of melanosomes to form massive rounded to ellipsoid homogeneous membrane-bound melanized bodies (63).

Table 28-3 summarizes some of the salient clinical and histologic features observed in the various forms of hyperpigmentations and lentigines:

Table 28-3

Hyperpigmentations and Lentigines

	Clinical	Basal Layer	Melanocytes	Melanocytes Features
Ephelid	Sun-exposed skin; decrease with age; darker with exposure	Increased melanin	No increase by routine histology	HMB-45+; rounded melanosomes
Melanotic Macule Albright syndrome	Fibrous dysplasia, precocious puberty	Increased melanin	Normal in number and size	
Mucosal Lentigines	Lower lip, genital skin	Increased melanin	Appear normal to slightly increased	Mild acanthosis; pigment incontinence
Becker melanosis	Unilateral, hypertrichosis	Increased melanin	Increased	Elongation of rete; smooth muscle fibers in dermis
Solar lentigo	Sun-exposed skin; increase with age	Increased melanin	Appear normal to increased; no contiguity	Elongated rete; solar elastosis
Lentigo simplex	Early onset; not related to sun exposure	Increased melanin	Increased, in focal contiguity	Elongated rete
Lentiginosis profusa	Many lesions at birth or childhood	Increased melanin	Increased, in focal contiguity	Elongated rete; nevus nests in some lesions
Multiple lentiginosis syndromes (leopard, LAMB)	Many lesions; dominant trait	Increased melanin	Increased, in focal contiguity	Elongated rete; nevus nests in some lesions
Speckled lentiginous Nevus	Macule at birth, becomes speckled	Increased melanin	Increased, in focal contiguity	Elongated rete; nevus nests in speckled areas
Peutz–Jeghers lentigines	Perioral; dominant trait; GI polyps	Increased melanin (marked)	No increase by DOPA stain	

BENIGN MELANOCYTIC TUMORS IN SKIN WITH LOW CUMULATIVE SOLAR DAMAGE (LOW CSD)

Benign melanocytic tumors that occur in skin with low CSD represent the common melanoma pathway in which SSM ("low CSD melanoma") is the prototypic malignancy. These benign tumors, in general, are referred to as "melanocytic nevi" or simply "nevi." They range from wholly benign lesions that lack any evidence of atypia to atypical lesions that yet fall short of criteria for melanoma, for which the term "melanocytoma" was adopted in the 2018 WHO Classification of tumors of the skin (5).

Melanocytic Nevi

Although the term "nevus" may refer to a variety of hamartomatous and/or neoplastic lesions in the skin, the unqualified term in common usage and in this chapter refers to a *melanocytic nevus*, which is generally considered to be a benign neoplastic proliferation of melanocytes, leading to a localized pigmented or nonpigmented lesion usually less than 5 mm in diameter. In common use, the term "nevus" is often used alone. The proliferation is thought to occur first in the epidermis, when the lesion is a "junctional nevus." Nevus cells have the ability to migrate into the dermis, to form a "compound nevus," and may then lose their junctional component to become a "dermal nevus." There are many varieties of nevi; however, the common melanocytic nevus is the prototype and will be discussed next. These nevi typically occur in sun-exposed sites and are thought to be related to intermittent sun exposure. At the time of the initial development of most nevi, which occurs in childhood and adolescence, solar elastosis may be absent or present to a typically mild degree.

Common Melanocytic Nevus

Clinical Summary. Nevi vary considerably in their clinical appearance. In addition to the pathologic variants, which will be discussed separately, at least five clinical types may be recognized: (a) flat lesions, (b) slightly elevated lesions often with a raised center and a flat periphery, (c) papillomatous lesions, (d) dome-shaped lesions, and (e) pedunculated lesions (64). The first three types are always pigmented; the latter two may or may not be pigmented. Any of the elevated lesions may be surrounded by a flat periphery, or shoulder, within which changes of melanocytic dysplasia may be seen histologically ("nevus with dysplasia"). Dome-shaped lesions often contain several coarse hairs. Although exceptions occur, one can predict to a certain degree from the clinical appearance of a nevus whether on histologic examination it will prove to be a junctional nevus (confined to the epidermis), a compound nevus (epidermal and dermal), or a dermal nevus. Most small flat lesions represent either a lentigo simplex or a junctional nevus; flat lesions or lesions with a flat periphery 5 mm or more in diameter with irregular indefinite borders and pigment variegation are clinically dysplastic nevi, although if these changes are extreme, melanoma may need to be ruled out. Most slightly elevated lesions and some papillomatous lesions represent compound nevi (especially if they are pigmented), and most papillomatous lesions and nearly all dome-shaped and pedunculated lesions that are not pigmented represent intradermal nevi.

Melanocytic nevi are only rarely present at birth (see "Congenital Melanocytic Nevus," p. 909). Most nevi appear in childhood, adolescence, and early adulthood and become less numerous with age. It is uncertain whether this represents a phenomenon of loss of nevi through senescence and disappearance or a cohort effect relating to differing incidence rates of nevi through age cohorts (65); it seems likely that both mechanisms may apply (66). Exceptionally, nevi may occur episodically and, rarely, as widespread eruptive lesions (67–69). Occasionally, new nevi arise in midlife and rarely in later life, a phenomenon that should recommend scrutiny to rule out the possibility of an evolving melanoma. Except for occasional cosmetic significance as, for example, in giant congenital nevi (70), nevi are important only in relation to melanoma, for which they are risk markers, simulants, or potential precursors (34,47).

A general concept of clinical importance for melanocytic nevi is that, unlike melanomas that inexorably progress over time, nevi enlarge to a point, stabilize, and then involute, becoming less frequent in the elderly than in younger age groups (71). This clinical attribute is directly related to the importance of heightened suspicion that is aroused when a previously stable nevus undergoes change in size or pigmentation.

Histopathology. Melanocytic nevi are defined and recognized by the presence of nevus cells, which, even though they are melanocytes, differ from ordinary melanocytes in three morphologic attributes: they are arranged at least partially in clusters or "nests"; they have a tendency to appear round rather than have a dendritic cell shape; and they have a propensity to retain pigment in their cytoplasm rather than to transfer it to neighboring keratinocytes (72). Nevus cells vary considerably in appearance and are often not pigmented, and so they are frequently recognizable as nevus cells more by their arrangement in clusters or nests than by their cellular features. As a result of a characteristic shrinkage artifact, nevus cell nests often appear partially separated from their surrounding stroma and in some nevi, such as the spindle and epithelioid cell variant, from surrounding epithelium.

Although a histologic subdivision of nevi into junctional, compound, and intradermal nevi is generally accepted, these are believed to be transitional stages in the "life cycle" of nevi, from junctional to compound to intradermal and, finally, to involuting lesions. The concept of progression from a lentigo simplex to a junctional and then a compound nevus has been challenged by the finding that BRAF mutations are more common in compound and dermal than in junctional nevi and are not found in simple lentigines. However, it is possible that the BRAF mutations could develop as a later event in the pathogenesis of nevi, and also the diagnosis of lentigo simplex in this study did not require an increased number of melanocytes at the junction, suggesting the possibility of overlap with solar lentigo (73).

Lentigo Simplex. The lentigo simplex was described in the earlier section on Lentigo Simplex and Related Lesions (47) (p. 841). Histologically, these are small (usually <2 mm) and characterized by an increased number of melanocytes, present in focal contiguity with one another near the tips and sides of elongated rete ridges. This pattern, characteristic of lentigines, is therefore described as "lentiginous melanocytic proliferation." The lack of nests at the histologic level distinguishes the lentigo from a nevus, by definition. However, transitional forms between a simple lentigo and a lentiginous junctional nevus (a lentigo with a few nests) are commonly observed, and the two histologic "entities" are indistinguishable clinically, giving rise to the whimsical term "jentigo" (59). We prefer the term "lentiginous junctional nevus" for these very common lesions (36) (Fig. 28-3).

Junctional Nevus. In a junctional nevus, nevus cells may lie in well-circumscribed nests either entirely within the lower epidermis or bulging downward into the dermis but still in contact with the epidermis, perhaps in the process of "dropping off" to form a compound nevus. The nevus cells in these nests generally have a regular, rounded to cuboidal appearance, although

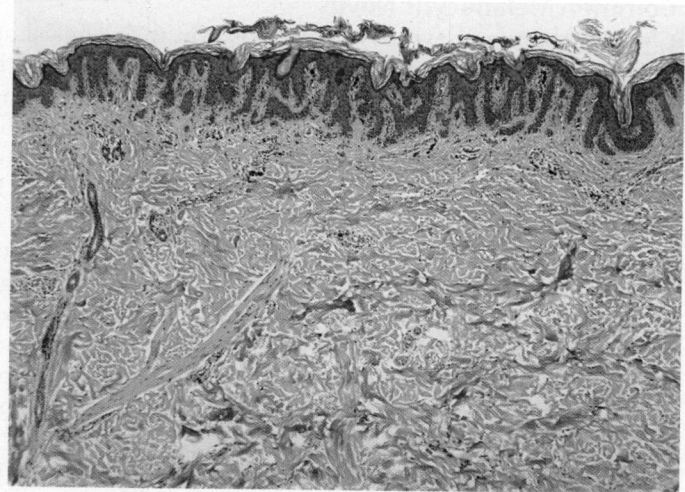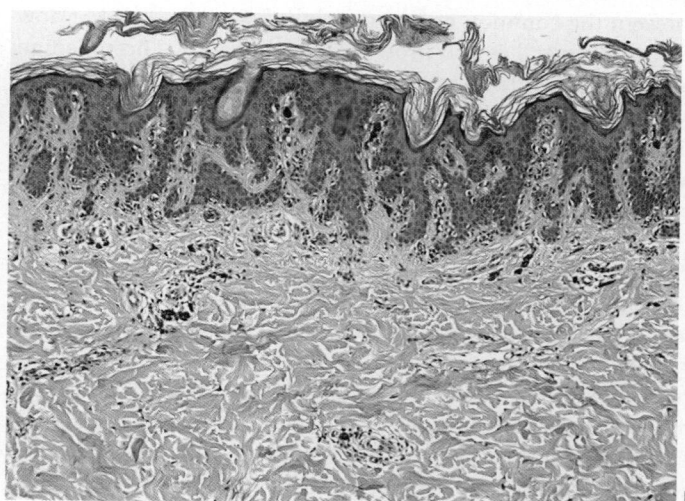

Figure 28-3 Lentiginous junctional nevus. **A:** Most examples are less than 4 mm, usually about 2 to 3 mm in diameter. A dermal component, if present in a lentiginous nevus, lies in the center of the lesion, and the epidermal component extends beyond its "shoulder." **B:** In the epidermis, single cells and nests of nevus are arranged near the dermal–epidermal junction near the tips and sides of elongated rete ridges (a "lentiginous" pattern). There is minimal or no atypia. There is no "continuous" proliferation of melanocytes in the suprapapillary regions of the epidermis between the rete ridges. These architectural features are repeated but exaggerated in dysplastic nevi, which, in addition, exhibit mild-to-moderate random cytologic atypia and more conspicuous stromal reactions.

they are occasionally spindle shaped. In addition, varying numbers of diffusely arranged single nevus cells are seen in the lowermost epidermis, especially in the basal cell layer. In many lesions, single cells are about as common as nests, focally recapitulating the histology of a simple lentigo. Such lesions in our practice are termed "lentiginous junctional nevi" (Fig. 28-3). Varying amounts of melanin granules are seen in the nevus cells. Some of the nevus cells, on immunostaining, show dendritic processes containing melanin granules, making them indistinguishable from melanocytes, but, in general, the degree of dendritic differentiation is markedly reduced. The nested and single melanocytes are arranged mainly at the tips and sides of rete ridges; "continuous" proliferation of single cells between the rete, confluence of nests, or pagetoid extension of cells into the suprabasal epidermal layers may be architectural indicators of dysplasia or evolving *in situ* melanoma.

Although nevus cells only occasionally penetrate into the upper layers of the epidermis ("pagetoid scatter"), aggregates of melanin granules may be seen in the stratum corneum in deeply pigmented junctional nevi. Often, the rete ridges are elongated as in lentigo simplex (p. 841), and single cells as well as nests of nevus cells are seen at the bases of the rete ridges. Not infrequently, as in lentigo simplex, the upper dermis contains an

infiltrate of melanophages and mononuclear cells. These lentiginous junctional nevi that combine features of lentigo simplex and junctional nevus are exceedingly common. Lesions with these features but larger than 5 mm clinically or 4 to 5 mm in a histologic section often prove to have cytologic atypia and to be dysplastic nevi (p. 855).

In children, some junctional nevi may show considerable cellularity with some degree of cellular enlargement, pleomorphism, and pagetoid cells above the basal layer. They may also have fine dusty melanin particles and a dense inflammatory infiltrate (74). Some of these lesions may represent Spitz nevi (p. 893) or dysplastic nevi (p. 855). Others may correlate with a tendency for ordinary junctional nevus cells to be enlarged, or epithelioid, in younger individuals (termed "age-related epithelioid cell change"). The small size of the lesion, the sharp lateral demarcation defined by discrete junctional nests, the lack of severe or uniform atypia and of mitoses, and the fact that in children melanomas are very rare are features that help in the distinction from melanoma. However, if the foregoing criteria are present, the diagnosis of melanoma should be considered, even in a child.

Compound Nevus. Clinically, a compound nevus is a pigmented papule (Fig. 28-4) or a plaque. In most nondysplastic

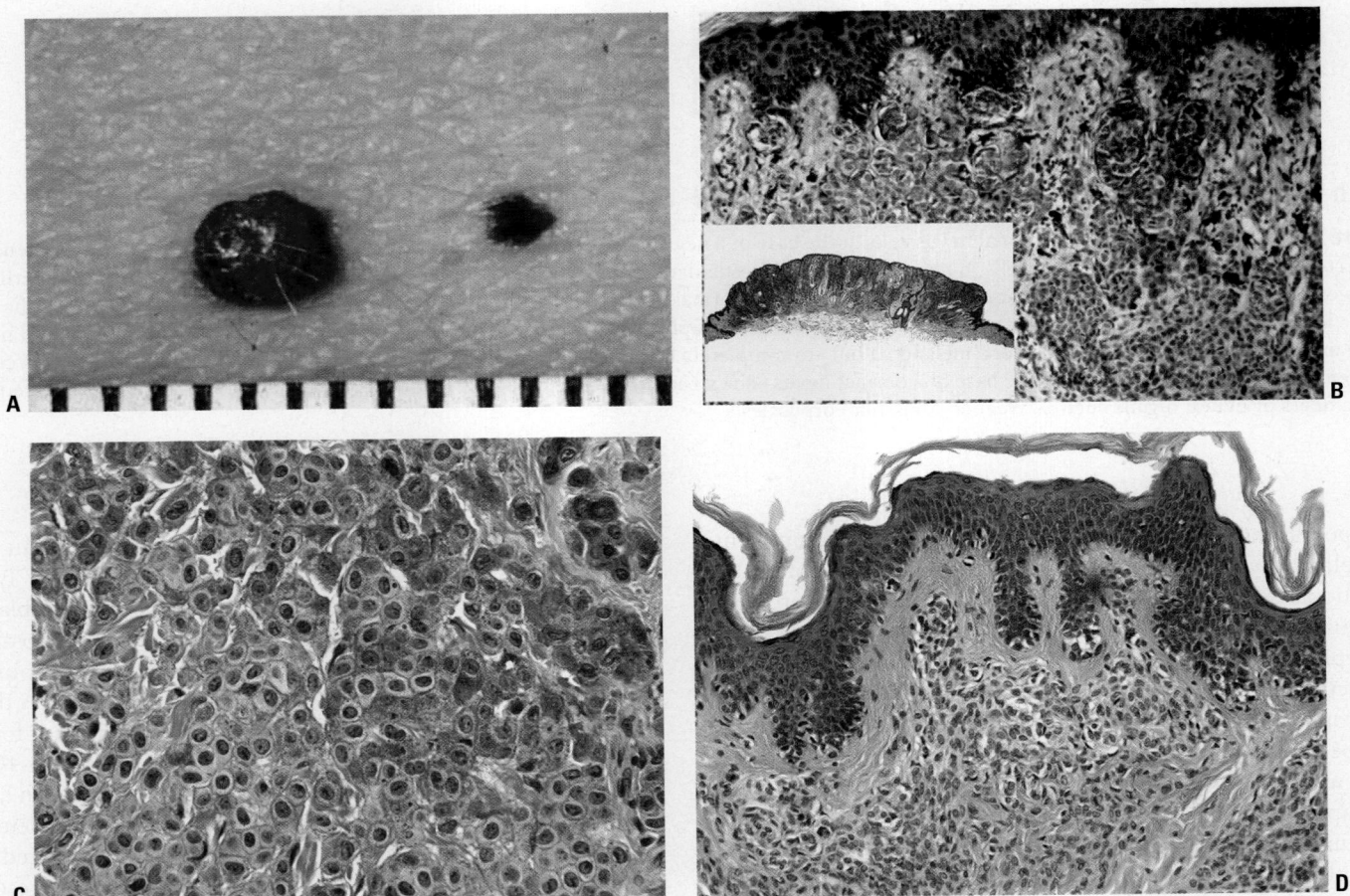

Figure 28-4 Compound nevi. **A:** Each lesion is a true papule without any adjacent macular component. The lesion on the right is a pigmented compound nevus. The lesion on the left has little pigment and is clinically a predominantly dermal nevus. **B:** Histologically, the lesion is a true papule without an adjacent junctional component (inset). Nests of nevus cells are present at the dermal–epidermal junction. It is believed that these nests become separated from the epidermis, to lie in the dermis, piling up on one another in an "accretive" pattern of growth, and resulting in gradual elevation of the epidermis above its original position to form the papule. Pigment is present mostly in junctional and superficial dermal nevus cells. **C:** Dermal nevus with type A nevus cells. The "type A" cells have visible cytoplasm that is in contact with that of neighboring nevus cells. The nuclei are small, without atypia or prominent nucleoli. There are no mitoses. **D:** Lentiginous compound nevus. In this, as in many nevi, nests are admixed with single cells in the junctional component, a lentiginous pattern. The cells in the dermis are small lymphocyte-like "Type B" cells.

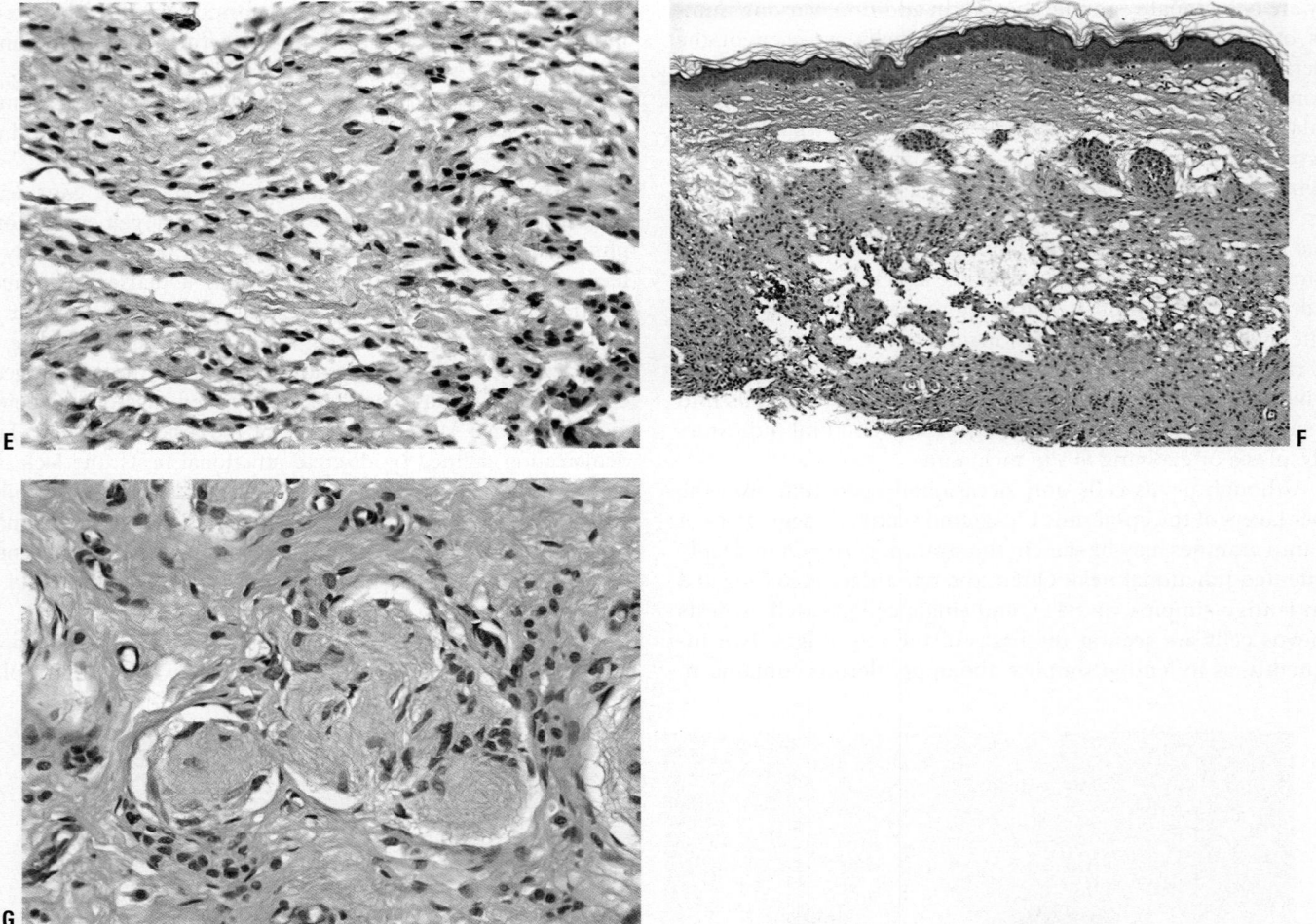

Figure 28-4 (*continued*) **E:** Type C dermal nevus cells at the base of a nevus. The cells at the base of a nevus tend to be spindle shaped and tend to have collagen between the individual cells. If they extend into the reticular dermis, they tend to "disperse" as individual cells among the superficial collagen fibers, a pattern that is also characteristic of Spitz nevi. **F:** Dermal nevus with "pseudo-lymphatic spaces." The type B nevus cells at the top of the lesion have small nuclei and scant cytoplasm, reminiscent of lymphocytes. The spaces are a common artifact in dermal or compound nevi. They may simulate lymphatic invasion of a melanoma but are completely benign. The cells at the base of the lesion are predominantly type C cells. **G:** Neurotized dermal nevus cells at the base of a dermal nevus. The structures at the base of a "neurotized" dermal nevus may be reminiscent of nerve fibers or neural organs such as Wagner–Meissner corpuscles.

compound nevi, there is no adjacent macular component. Histologically, a compound nevus possesses features of both a junctional and an intradermal nevus. Nevus cell nests are present in the epidermis, as well as appearing to "drop off" from the epidermis into the superficial dermis and in many lesions, the reticular dermis (Fig. 28-4B). This time-honored theory of "abtropfung" or dropping off of nevus cells proposed by Unna has been challenged by the finding that junctional nevi are at least as common in adults as in children (75). Nevus cells in the upper, middle, and lower dermis may present characteristic morphologic variations called types A, B, and C, respectively (76). Usually, the Type A nevus cells in the upper dermis are round to cuboidal, show abundant cytoplasm containing varying amounts of melanin granules, and tend to form nests. Type A cells with especially abundant cytoplasm, as may occur in children and young adults, may be termed "epithelioid cells" (Fig. 28-4C). Melanophages are occasionally seen in the surrounding stroma. The cells in the mid-dermis are usually type B cells; they are distinctly smaller than the type A cells, display less cytoplasm and less melanin, and generally lie in

well-defined aggregates or cords. They may to some extent resemble lymphoid cells ("lymphocyte-like") (Fig. 28-4D). Type C nevus cells in the lower dermis tend to resemble fibroblasts or Schwann cells in that they are usually elongated and possess a spindle-shaped nucleus. They often lie in strands and only rarely contain melanin (Fig. 28-4E). They may form spaces that can resemble lymphatic channels (Fig. 28-4F). Often, they form aggregates that resemble Meissner corpuscles (77) (Fig. 28-4G). The features of spindle cell and schwannian differentiation and Meissner corpuscle-like formations are referred to as "neurotization," and although all three stages are not encountered in most compound nevi, they are often considered to represent maturation, or, alternatively (and more likely) senescence (78). Occasional nevi have abnormal stratification within the deeper dermis of the otherwise benign type A nevus cells, resulting in the designation of "inverted type A nevus" (79). Some of these may represent combined nevi (see later section).

The decrease in cell size, melanization, and progression from nests to cords to more neuroid spindle cells with dermal descent seen in nevi is often referred to as maturation and is regarded as evidence of benignancy, because the size of the cells in a melanoma usually does not decrease with depth. The process of nevus cell maturation has alternatively been regarded as one of senescence or atrophy (78), likely driven by the tumor suppressor p16, which is activated in response to the effects of an overexpressed oncogene such as BRAF or *NRAS* in a phenomenon termed "oncogene-induced senescence" (80). In another study, it was found that the tumor suppressor p15, located near p16 on chromosome 9p21, is also expressed in nevi and lost in melanomas (81). Challenging the notion of oncogene-induced senescence, one comprehensive study showed that nevi lack a full complement of senescence markers, and they are capable of occasional, induced proliferation and transformation (82). If dermal nevus cells are confined to the papillary dermis, they often retain a discrete or "pushing" border that interfaces with the stroma. However, nevus cells that enter the reticular dermis tend to disperse among collagen fiber bundles as single cells or attenuated single files of cells. This pattern of infiltration of the dermis differs from that observed in most melanomas, where groups of cells tend to dissect and displace the collagen bundles in a more "expansive" pattern (83). Lesions where nevus cells extend into the lower reticular dermis and the subcutaneous fat or are located within nerves, hair follicles, sweat ducts, and sebaceous glands or budding into lymphatic spaces may be termed "congenital pattern nevi" because they share morphologic features with congenital nevi but are not necessarily present at birth (84) (p. 909).

Intradermal Melanocytic Nevus. Intradermal melanocytic nevi (or "dermal nevi") have essentially no junctional component. The upper dermis contains nests and cords of nevus cells. Multinucleated nevus cells may be seen, in which small nuclei lie either in a rosette-like arrangement or close together in the center of the cell. These nevus giant cells differ significantly in appearance from the irregularly and even bizarrely shaped giant cells that are seen frequently in Spitz nevus and occasionally also in melanoma. Likely as a result of shrinkage during tissue processing, clefts may form between some nests of nevus cells and the adjacent stroma, in some instances leaving a defect that simulates a lymphatic space and thus mimics lymphatic invasion (Fig. 28-4F) (85).

Whereas the nevus cell nests located in the upper dermis often contain a moderate amount of melanin (particularly type A cells), the types B and C nevus cells in the midportion and the lower dermis rarely contain melanin. Type C cells appear spindle shaped, are arranged in bundles, and are embedded in collagenous fibers having a loose, pale, wavy appearance similar to that of the fibers in a neurofibroma, resulting in a "neurotized nevus." Such formations have been referred to as neuroid tubes. In other areas, the nevus cells lie within concentrically arranged, loosely layered filamentous tissue, forming so-called nevic corpuscles that resemble Meissner tactile bodies (Fig. 28-4G). Neurotized nevus cells express the marker S100A6 protein, a form of S100 found in Schwann cells, supporting the hypothesis that maturation in these lesions recapitulates some features of Schwann cell differentiation (77). However, differences in the immunohistochemical profiles of neurofibromas and neurotized nevi have supported the concept that these neoplasms are histogenically distinct, despite their similar histologic appearance (see next paragraph) (86).

Occasional intradermal nevi are devoid of nevus cell nests in the upper dermis and contain only spindle-shaped nevus cells embedded in abundant, loosely arranged collagenous tissue. These nevi may be referred to as neural nevi. The differentiation from a solitary neurofibroma may be difficult in routinely stained sections, but distinction might be possible with an immunohistochemical technique employing myelin basic protein, which is positive only in neurofibroma (87) (see Histogenesis). Neurofibromas also tend to contain small nerve twigs and axons that can be highlighted with glial fibrillary acidic protein (GFAP) staining (86), a feature not typical of neurotized nevi. In addition, "melanocyte-specific markers" like Melan-A/MART-1, Sox10 and HMB-45, and others are usually positive in nevi but absent in neural cells and neurofibromas.

Some intradermal and, less commonly, compound nevi have overlying hyperkeratosis and papillomatosis, which may be associated with a lacelike, downward growth of epidermal strands and with horn cysts. Such nevi resemble seborrheic keratoses in their epidermal architecture. In other instances, large hair follicles are observed. Rupture of a large hair follicle may manifest itself clinically in an increase in the size of the nevus associated with an inflammatory reaction, leading to clinical suspicion of a melanoma. Histologic examination in such instances shows a partially destroyed epidermal follicular lining with a pronounced inflammatory infiltrate containing foreign-body giant cells as a reaction to the presence of keratin in the dermis. Occasionally, intradermal nevi contain scattered large fat cells within the aggregates of nevus cells. This could represent a regressive phenomenon in which fat cells replace involuting nevus cells, or, alternatively, adipocyte metaplasia within the stroma of the nevus.

Some dermal nevi, including variants of spindle and epithelioid cell nevi, induce marked deposition of thick, sometimes hyalinized collagen bundles. Such nevi are described as sclerosing variants. This change may occasionally confound diagnosis but is not of biologic significance.

Nevus with Mitoses. In occasional otherwise typical dermal nevi (or in the dermal component of compound nevi), rare mitoses are found in the dermis. This phenomenon has been described in children (74) and in association with pregnancy (88). In a comprehensive study, of 1,041 benign nevi, 82 (7.9%) contained one or more mitoses, most of which were in the papillary dermis of compound nevi. Only three cases contained three mitoses (89). If there are no other indicators of malignancy, we report these cases as "nevus with mitoses," and generally recommend complete excision. The possibility of nevoid melanoma (see section on Nevoid Melanoma, p. 892) should also be seriously considered in such lesions (90–92).

Histogenesis of Acquired Melanocytic Nevi. Although there are exceptions, most nevi appear in childhood, adolescence, and early adulthood, and, with advancing age, there is a progressive decrease in the number of nevi. It is unclear whether this represents loss of nevi with age or an effect of differing incidence of nevi in different age cohorts (93). The evolution and involution of nevi correlate with their histologic appearance. Junctional proliferation of nevus cells is present in almost every nevus in children but decreases with age. Intradermal nevi, by contrast, are most unusual in the first decade of life, and their proportion increases progressively with age. The incidence of fibrosis, fatty infiltration/metaplasia, and neuroid changes increases with age. Thus, the formation of cylindrical neuroid structures represents the end stage of differentiation and not a source of origin of intradermal nevi (94). In a large cross-sectional dermoscopic study, the globular pattern associated with compound nevi predominated in the youngest age group. By contrast, the reticular and/or homogeneous patterns associated with junctional nevi were increasingly observed in nevi from individuals older than 15 years, suggesting that there may be a different mechanism of nevogenesis in adults compared to children, likely involving cumulative effects of UV light (95).

Concerning the relationship between epidermal melanocytes and nevus cells, it would seem that the morphologic features by which nevus cells differ from melanocytes, such as the absence of dendrites as seen by light microscopy, their arrangement in cell nests, their larger size, and their tendency to retain pigment (72), are secondary adjustments of the cells. Immunohistochemical markers are similarly expressed between the two cell types. Thus, it seems established that nevus cells differ from Schwann cells and are benign neoplastic variants of melanocytes.

The molecular pathology of nevi is beginning to be understood. In a study of the BRAF oncogene, which had previously been found to be mutated in a high percentage of metastatic melanomas (96), mutations resulting in the V600E amino acid substitution were found in 68% of melanoma metastases, 80% of primary melanomas, and, unexpectedly, in 82% of nevi (97). Activating mutations of the oncogene NRAS (mutually exclusive with BRAF mutations) have also been described in melanoma-associated nevi and in congenital nevi (98,99). The BRAF mutations have been found to be clonal by sensitive genetic methods and also by using an antibody specific for the mutated gene, suggesting that these mutations are likely to be early events in melanocytic neoplasia (100). These data suggest that mutational activation of the RAS/RAF/MAPK mitogenic pathway in nevi is a critical step in the initiation of melanocytic neoplasia but alone is insufficient for melanoma tumorigenesis (97). High levels of the tumor suppressor protein p16 in benign nevi may represent the mechanism whereby the cell cycle remains regulated in nevi, even in the presence of activating oncogene mutations (80,101), and the closely related protein p15 may also be involved in this suppression (81). Of course, tumor progression in melanoma does not require an intermediate step through a nevus; progression can occur directly from a mutated melanocyte (or a field of mutated melanocytes) in otherwise clinically unremarkable sun-damaged skin. Bastian's group has recently proposed a mechanism for this based on the demonstration of a wide range of potentially activating mutations in individual melanocytes and in fields of melanocytes in sun-damaged skin. They have proposed that "strong" mutations, for example, BRAFV600E, may result in the development of a nevus with a small but finite risk of progression to melanoma, as discussed previously. Weaker mutations may reside in unremarkable-looking solitary melanocytes, which in some cases may develop a growth advantage and form a field, in either case having a finite risk of further progression owing to the acquisition of sequential genetic and epigenetic abnormalities (102–105).

Principles of Management of Nevi: Common nevi and related lesions generally do not require active therapy. Lesions are often excised for cosmetic reasons, and clinically atypical lesions are excised to rule out melanoma. An increased number of nevi, especially large nevi, is also a risk factor for future development of melanoma and may prompt consideration of surveillance. Except for congenital nevi in some instances, and some categories of atypical nevi that generally have more than one mutation (discussed in ensuing sections), most nevi are not generally managed as having a sufficient risk of progression that they should be excised to prevent the development of melanoma.

Nevi of Special Sites

There is apparent variation in the morphology of common nevi by site. In a study of Australian schoolchildren, gender differences in nevus density on the back and lower limbs were similar to gender differences for melanoma, with back lesions favoring males and lower extremity lesions favoring females. Small nevi (2–4 mm) were most concentrated on the arms, whereas large nevi (≥5 mm) occurred mostly on the posterior trunk, where they were related to age, male sex, and freckling. The findings were considered to support the hypothesis of site-specific differences in nevus proliferative potential (106). Nevi in certain locations may exhibit features that are unusual compared to the vast majority of common nevi on the trunk, limbs, or face and scalp (107–109).

Clinical Summary. "Special site nevi" have been best defined in acral locations (palmar and plantar, and subungual) and in genital skin. Nevi in skin flexural areas (ear lobe, axilla, umbilicus, inguinal creases, pubis, scrotum, and perianal area) may also have similar unusual features (110). More recently, the skin of the ears, the skin of the breast, and the skin of the scalp in adolescents have been added to this seemingly ever-expanding list of "special" sites (111–114). In general, the "special" features of the nevi may be seen in only a minority of the nevi from these sites; the other nevi are quite unremarkable. Nomenclature is not standardized—other names for nevi of special sites (NOSS) include atypical genital nevi (AGN), atypical melanocytic nevus of the genital type (AMNGT), melanocytic acral nevus with intraepithelial ascent of cells (MANIACs), acral-lentiginous nevus of plantar skin, atypical nevi of the scalp, flexural nevi, and special site nevi (108). In a study of nevi with mitoses, the highest incidence of mitoses among body sites was observed in special sites (10.9%), which included genitals, perineum, groin, and acral regions, perhaps supporting the notion that these nevi are more "active" than others (89).

General features of NOSS have been well summarized, as follows (108,109). The special sites include the embryonic milkline/flexural sites, genitalia, palms, soles, ear, and scalp. Not all nevi that occur in special sites are NOSS—at all special sites, stereotypical benign melanocytic nevi are the most prevalent diagnoses. NOSS are of importance because they may have histologic features in common with dysplastic nevi and melanoma, including large nest, dyshesive cells, and cytologic atypia. Mitotic activity is infrequent, however. NOSS of flexural/milkline skin, genitalia, and scalp tend to share similar histology—notably enlarged junctional nests with diminished cohesion of melanocytes. Ear and breast NOSS are generally more atypical than NOSS at other sites. Scalp and acral NOSS may have prominent pagetoid scatter. NOSS are thought to have a similar prognosis to stereotypical benign melanocytic nevi, but their long-term biologic behavior has not been definitively established. Surgical excision with clear margins, if technically feasible, is often recommended for NOSS.

Nevi of Acral Skin

These will be discussed in the section on acral melanomas and melanocytic proliferations (p. 905).

Nevi of Ear Skin

Sometimes considered to be an acral site, the ear differs in being heavily exposed to solar radiation in men, but not usually in women, and is the single most common site for melanoma in men after correction for unit area. Nevi of the ear may show somewhat similar features to acral nevi, although often with greater atypia (108). In one study, pagetoid spread, moderate-to-severe cytologic atypia, and prominent nucleoli were encountered in 50% to 60% of 21 auricular nevi. None of these cases showed mitoses or apoptotic melanocytes (113). In another study of 101 lesions, nests varied in size and shape and were located between rete ridges in most cases (as opposed to more normal localization at rete tips or sides), whereas in about 40% there was poor circumscription, lateral extension of the junctional component beyond the dermal component, and elongation of rete ridges with bridging (coalescence) between junctional nests. About 25% had uniformly large melanocytes with large vesicular nuclei without prominent nucleoli, and abundant pale, finely granular cytoplasm (112). These are features that could overlap considerably with dysplastic nevi or some melanomas. Features that tended to diminish concern for melanoma in these lesions included symmetry, lack of uniform nuclear pleomorphism, the absence of pagetoid scatter of melanocytes, and maturation of the dermal component in compound lesions. The lesions in this study did not exhibit a tendency to recur. Nevertheless, we would recommend complete excision for any lesion that exhibits these features to any significant degree, especially if they are present in sun-damaged skin of an older subject.

Nevi of Genital Skin

Clinical Summary. Clinically unremarkable nevi located on or near anogenital skin may present with histologic features that simulate some aspects of melanomas. The lesions have no clinical significance except the possibility of diagnostic error.

They have been termed "AMNGT" and are most often seen on the vulva of young (premenopausal) women but may also be detected on perineal and perianal skin (115,116). Similar lesions also occur uncommonly on the male genitalia (117). The lesions are often removed incidentally, for instance, during increased clinical surveillance during pregnancy. They are typically symmetrical papular lesions, usually less than 1 cm in diameter, and uniformly pigmented with discrete well-circumscribed borders. The atypical features appear to represent a histologic curiosity seen in a minority of vulvar nevi. In a comparative histologic study of vulvar and common nevi, most of the vulvar lesions were unremarkable. Vulvar nevi themselves are quite uncommon; in patients in a gynecology practice, the prevalence was only 2.3% (118). An interesting variant pattern of nevi has been described in association with lichen sclerosus et atrophicus, most commonly on skin of the vulva, perineum, or rarely elsewhere. These nevi had features in common with persistent ("recurrent") melanocytic nevi ("pseudomelanoma"; see section Recurrent Nevus, p. 853) and can mimic malignant melanoma. This "activated" melanocytic phenotype seen in lichen sclerosus–associated melanocytic nevi suggests a stromal-induced change (119). The clinical differential diagnosis for AGN also includes early "genital lentigines."

Histopathology. The scanning magnification impression is typically that of a small, well-circumscribed papular lesion composed of nevus cells arranged in clusters in the papillary dermis and arranged mainly in nests in the epidermis where the cells usually do not extend beyond the shoulder of the dermal component, as typically occurs in compound dysplastic nevi (Fig. 28-5). The epidermis is occasionally irregularly thickened, resulting in an asymmetrical silhouette. The nevus cells may be large, with prominent nucleoli and abundant cytoplasm containing finely divided ("dusty") melanin pigment. The nests tend to be variable in size, shape, and position, originating from the sides as well as the tips of rete and often oriented parallel to the surface and sometimes confluent. In a study of 56 lesions in 55 female patients with a median age of 26 years, the dominant histologic feature was a lentiginous and nested junctional

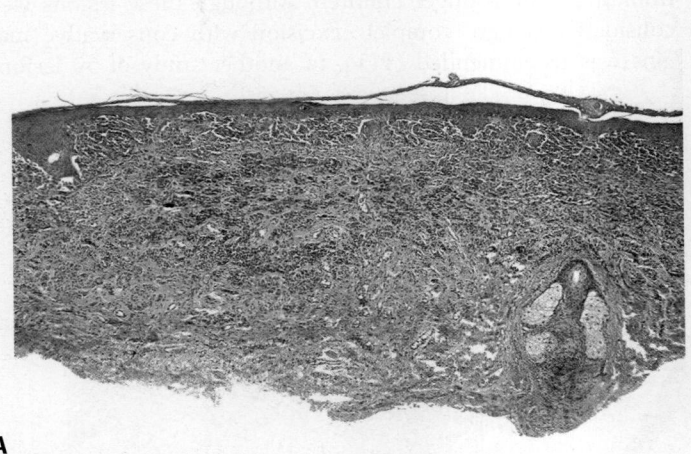

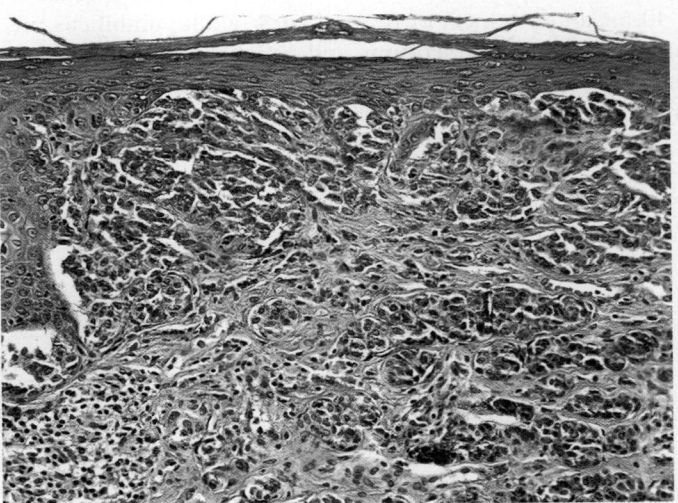

Figure 28-5 **A:** Nevus of genital skin. Nevi on genital skin may exhibit atypical features at high power but are usually relatively small and symmetrical and thus benign in their appearance at scanning magnification and also clinically. **B:** Atypical features in genital nevi may include nests that tend to be large and confluent, varying a good deal in size and shape, and include cells that tend to be large, with macronucleoli, and dyshesive from one another. Mitoses are rare or absent, and there is no adjacent *in situ* or microinvasive radial growth phase component.

component composed of prominent round or fusiform nests, often showing retraction artifact and/or cellular dyshesion (120). Cytologic atypia was mild in 11 cases (20%), moderate in 34 (60%), and severe in 11 (20%). Ten cases (18%) had focal pagetoid spread, generally to a low level of the epidermis. The atypical junctional melanocytic proliferation was associated with a large common dermal nevus component that was dominant in 26 cases (46%). Adnexal spread (46%) and nuclear atypia of melanocytes in the superficial dermis (39%) were relatively common, whereas dermal mitoses (7%) were uncommon, and maturation was present in all cases. A broad zone of dense eosinophilic fibrosis within the superficial dermis was a frequent finding (41%). Only one lesion recurred after the initial excision and was reexcised with no further consequences.

Some of the features seen in atypical vulvar nevi may arouse a suspicion of melanoma. However, the lesions are comparatively small and well circumscribed, without significant junctional proliferation of atypical melanocytes beyond the major dermal component, as is seen in most mucosal melanomas. Moreover, there is little or no pagetoid spread of single or nested melanocytes into the epidermis, there is no necrosis, and usually no ulcer, and, importantly, there is little or usually no mitotic activity in the dermis (121). Stromal patterns more characteristic of melanoma (diffuse fibroplasia) or dysplasia (concentric fibroplasia) are generally lacking in these lesions (116). The diagnosis of melanoma in vulvar skin should be made with caution (but is sometimes unavoidable) in a premenopausal woman. Occasional vulvar nevi do exhibit high-grade cytologic atypia; however, and because the biologic behavior of such lesions in young to middle-aged women has not been fully studied, it is prudent to modestly excise AGN in order to allow for their complete histologic evaluation and to minimize any potential for local persistence or recurrence in scar tissue, a situation that may prompt even more vexing diagnostic challenges.

Nevi of Flexural Sites and of Breast Skin

On the basis of histologic findings, it has been suggested that nevi in flexural sites may differ histologically from those at other sites, resembling, in general, the appearances of nevi of genital skin and potentially simulating melanoma. In a study of 40 melanocytic nevi of flexural sites (axilla, umbilicus, inguinal creases, pubis, scrotum, and perianal area), 22 of them had "a nested and dyshesive pattern" similar to the genital pattern nevi. This pattern was characterized by the confluence of

enlarged nests with variation in size, shape, and position at the dermoepidermal junction and by the diminished cohesion of melanocytes (110), particularly with regard to the perimeter of junctional nests as they incompletely interface with adjacent keratinocytes and thus produce crescentic cleftlike spaces. Because this category overlaps with nevi of anogenital skin, and given the vague concept of a skin fold as it relates to individual patients of various body types, the concept of the flexural nevus remains a work in progress.

Nevi of breast skin, on the other hand, may show similar features to all nevi occurring along the milkline (axilla to genital region), including intraepidermal melanocytes above the basal layer, melanocytic atypia, and dermal fibroplasia (114). Cytologic atypia is said to be somewhat greater than in other special site nevi (109), and thus lesions may resemble those typical of genital skin in young women that exhibit both cytologic as well as architectural atypia (see foregoing).

These changes in flexural and breast nevi, like those in other "special sites," should not be overinterpreted as indicative of melanoma; by the same token, authentic dysplastic nevi and melanomas may occur in these sites and should not be underdiagnosed (107). Accordingly, in significantly atypical breast and genital nevi, particularly in young women, we may render a diagnosis based on the histopathologic findings (e.g., lentiginous compound nevus with moderate-to-severe atypia of the junctional component), supplemented by a note indicating that such findings that are encountered in nevi at these sites and in this clinical setting may not have biologic significance as melanoma precursors or risk markers (although modest complete removal is prudent to permit complete histologic evaluation and to insure against local persistence or recurrence in scar tissue).

Nevi of Scalp Skin

In a study of 229 nevi of the scalp from all ages, about 10% of the nevi from adolescents had atypical cytologic and architectural aspects that included the presence of large bizarrely shaped nests scattered in a disorderly manner along the dermoepidermal junction with follicular involvement, pagetoid spread of cells above the junction, and a dyscohesive pattern of the melanocytes in the nests. Mild cytologic atypia was present but less significant (Fig. 28-6). These atypical features were not found in scalp nevi from adults or younger children. Although these lesions were considered benign, complete excision with conservative margins was recommended (111). In another study of 59 lesions,

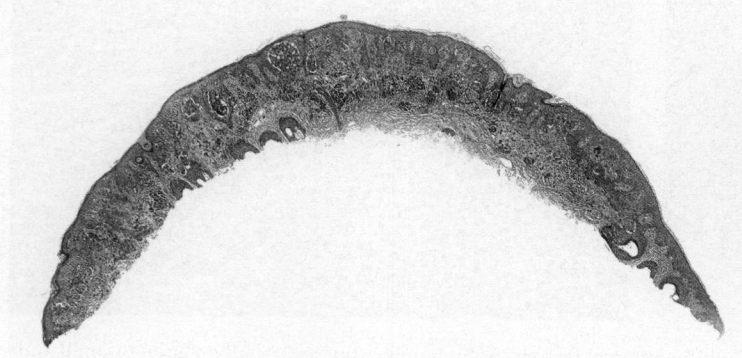
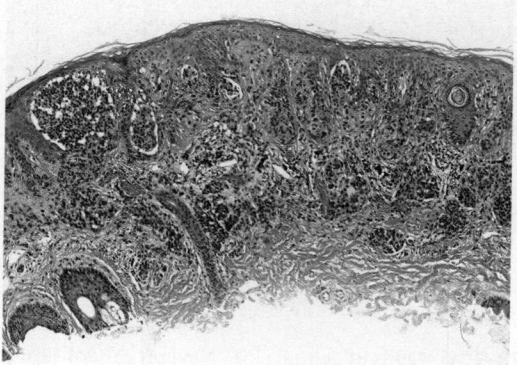

Figure 28-6 Nevus of special sites of the scalp. **A:** There is a broad lesion from the scalp of a 12-year-old boy. **B:** There is a prominent "large nested and dyshesive" pattern of the lesional cells in the epidermis, and there is evidence of maturation/senescence of the cells in the dermis.

the prototypical special site scalp nevus was considered to be one that contains poorly cohesive melanocytes arranged in large nests positioned both along the sides of rete and between rete ridges, containing random melanocytes with large nuclei and abundant pale cytoplasm, and exhibiting adnexocentricity and splaying of melanocytes through the reticular dermis. Overlapping features with dysplastic nevi including nests that bridge rete, lateral extension past the dermal component, and papillary dermal fibroplasia were also common to these lesions (122).

Special Site Nevi with Complicating Features

The aforementioned features of nevi from special sites may be additionally problematic when combined with age-related benign nevus cell enlargement (so-called epithelioid cell change that often occurs in the superficial component of nevi from children and younger adults), inflammation (as in halo-type regression), and trauma. Thus, just as it is important not to overlook true dysplasia in nevi, it is also imperative to consider components of atypia that may contribute to potential overdiagnosis of dysplasia or melanoma. Careful correlation of histologic changes with clinical parameters (age, halo-like changes, previous trauma, or biopsy) is of assistance in this regard.

Principles of Management of Special Site Nevi

Consideration of complete surgical excision is appropriate for all NOSS, to allow for complete pathologic examination, and minimize any chance of persistence, recurrence, or progression of the lesion (109). In selected cases, follow-up may be appropriate.

In most, if not all, of the studies of special site nevi, correlations with other clinicopathologic variables, including family history and the nature and characteristics of other melanocytic lesions present in these individuals, were not available. Melanoma and authentic dysplastic nevi may both occur in all or most of these sites, most often in adults and rarely in older children and adolescents. The descriptions of special site nevi in these various sites are helpful and should lead to a cautious approach to diagnosis of these lesions. In some cases, particularly in the distinction between a special site nevus and a dysplastic nevus or a melanoma, it is appropriate to express uncertainty. If there is uncertainty between a nevus of special sites and a dysplastic nevus, but no concern for melanoma, a term such as "compound or junctional nevus with atypical features" might be used. In a note, the differential diagnosis can be expressed.

An individual in whom such a lesion is diagnosed should likely be offered a complete skin exam, and a detailed family history should be taken. Especially if there are other clinically atypical nevi and/or a family or personal history of melanoma, periodic skin surveillance may be an appropriate consideration, whereas if the atypical lesion is an isolated phenomenon, it likely has no clinical significance except as a potential simulant of melanoma. In a case where the differential diagnosis includes melanoma, a term such as "superficial atypical melanocytic proliferation of uncertain significance (SAMPUS)" can be used if there are atypical cells in the dermis or "intraepidermal atypical melanocytic proliferation of uncertain significance (IAMPUS)" if the atypical proliferation is confined entirely to the epidermis (p. 875). Clinicians can then assess the level of uncertainty in determining their management recommendations.

Unusual and Reactive Nevi

Various subtypes of nevi have been described that, in general, are not important in the pathogenesis of melanoma but that may have unusual features that can cause diagnostic difficulty. Some of these may be reactive to stimuli such as trauma or UV light.

Halo Nevus

A halo nevus, also known as Sutton nevus or nevus depigmentosa centrifugum, represents a pigmented nevus surrounded by a depigmented zone, or halo (Fig. 28-7A).

Clinical Features. The nevus may be of almost any of the types described in the preceding sections, and a similar halo reaction may be seen rarely in relation to primary or metastatic melanoma. In the common type of halo nevus, which is characterized histologically by an inflammatory infiltrate and is therefore sometimes referred to as *inflammatory halo nevus*, the central nevus only rarely shows erythema or crusting; however, it undergoes involution in most instances, a process that may extend over a period of several years (123). The area of depigmentation has no clinical signs of inflammation, and even though it may persist for many months and even years, it ultimately repigments in most cases. Halo nevi tend to pass through several clinical stages or regression. The classic early lesion is a brown nevus with a surrounding usually symmetrical rim of vitiligo-like depigmentation. The central nevus may then lose its pigment and appear pink with a surrounding halo; the central papule may subsequently disappear, leading to a circular area of macular depigmentation, or the depigmented area may repigment, leaving no trace of its prior existence. In unusual lesions, darkening of the central nevus rather than lightening has been described (124). Most persons with halo nevi are children or young adults, and the back is the most common site. Not infrequently, halo nevi are multiple, occurring either simultaneously or successively.

Besides the more common inflammatory halo nevus with histologically apparent inflammation, there also are cases of *noninflammatory halo nevi* in which histologic examination shows no inflammatory infiltrate. In such instances, the nevus does not involute. In addition, there is the so-called *halo nevus phenomenon,* also referred to as *halo nevus without halo*. In these instances, the nevus shows histologic signs of inflammation analogous to a halo nevus but without presenting a halo clinically (125). Such nevi may or may not involute. An association with Turner syndrome has been described (126).

Histopathology. An inflammatory halo nevus in its early stage shows nests of nevus cells embedded in a dense inflammatory infiltrate in the upper dermis and at the epidermal–dermal junction (Fig. 28-7B–D). Later, scattered nevus cells tend to predominate over nests. Even when melanin is still present in the nevus cells, these cells often show evidence of damage to their nucleus and cytoplasm, and some frankly apoptotic nevus cells are commonly observed. Some cells, especially superficially, may have enlarged ovoid nucleoli, changes that may be regarded as a form of "reactive atypia, or alternatively a form of dysplastic atypia that has attracted immune surveillance" (125). Frank, severe high-grade nuclear atypia is not observed and if present should raise a consideration of melanoma. Importantly, the lesional cells tend to show evidence of "maturation," becoming smaller with descent from superficial to deep within the lesion. Nevus cell mitoses are rare and, if present, should prompt consideration of

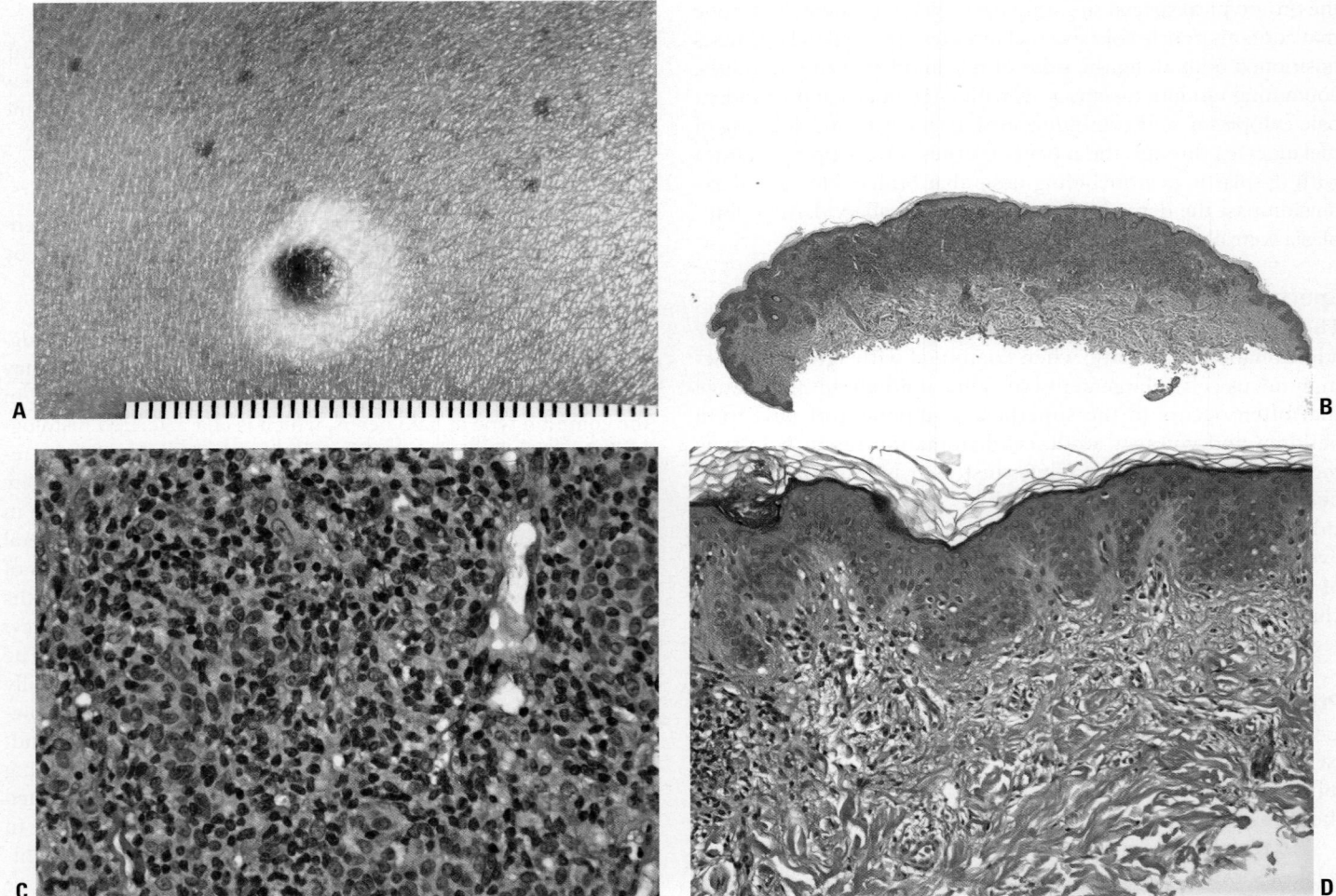

Figure 28-7 Halo nevus. **A:** The halo develops around a preexisting unremarkable compound nevus (clinical image). **B:** A dense infiltrative lymphocytic response blurs the silhouette of the lesional nevus cells in the dermis at scanning magnification. **C:** Small lymphocytes are diffusely placed among the dermal nevus cells, which may appear swollen and slightly atypical ("reactive" atypia). Severe or uniform atypia or mitotic activity should suggest the possibility of melanoma. **D:** At the periphery of the nevus, the halo is a region where pigment and melanocytes are reduced or absent, and there may be a subtle lymphocytic infiltrate at the dermal–epidermal junction, as here.

the possibility of melanoma. In this regard, it may be difficult to differentiate nevus cell mitoses from those attributable to the reactive mononuclear cells, a problem that can be lessened by use of a combined (dual) Mib-1 (Ki-67) and Melan-A/MART-1 stain. Most of the cells in the dense inflammatory infiltrate are lymphocytes. However, some of them are macrophages, in which varying amounts of melanin are contained. As the infiltrate invades the nevus cell nests, it is often difficult to distinguish between the lymphoid cells of the infiltrate and the type B nevus cells in the mid-dermis, because they, too, may have the appearance of lymphoid cells. Immunohistochemical studies using a specific marker such as Melan-A/MART1 may be very helpful in identifying the nevus cells in the infiltrate. The infiltrate tends to extend upward into the lower portion of the epidermis. In most instances, the infiltrate is characterized by dense cellular infiltration without vasodilatation or intercellular edema and by sharp demarcation along its lower border.

At a later stage, only a few, and finally no, distinct nevus cells can be identified. Gradually, after all nevus cells have disappeared, the inflammatory infiltrate subsides. Despite the clinical evidence of regression and the inflammatory infiltrate that consists predominantly of CD8 and also granzyme and perforin

positive T-cells (127), fibrosis is not a prominent feature (128). The inflammation is occasionally granulomatous (129).

Histogenesis. Both in halo nevi and in vitiligo, the depigmentation takes place through disappearance of the melanocytes. However, despite occasional patients who present with both lesions, halo nevus is likely not a form of vitiligo (130). The abundance of potential antigen-presenting cells and lymphocytes (including CD8 positive T-cells) in the regressing nevus at the site of depigmentation suggests that these cells participate in the destruction of nevus cells and melanocytes in the halo phenomenon (131). In an interesting study of the lymphoid elements infiltrating halo nevi, oligoclonal expansion of T-cells was observed in all patients, and in one patient T-cells using the same TCR beta chain were observed in distinct halo nevi, demonstrating a local expansion of common clones that are most likely activated by shared antigens within the nevi (132).

Differential Diagnosis. It can be difficult to differentiate early lesions of inflammatory halo nevus from a melanoma; both types of lesions may have a dense cellular infiltrate in the dermis, and, in halo nevi, the nevus cell nests, as a result of having been invaded by the cellular infiltrate, may appear atypical, which we consider to be "reactive." The danger of misinterpretation is greatest in halo nevi without a halo, the so-called halo nevus phenomenon. However, the inflammatory infiltrate in halo nevi is more pronounced than in melanoma and extends diffusely through the lesion, rather than being concentrated at the periphery as in most examples of tumorigenic melanoma. The diagnosis of melanoma rather than halo nevus is likely in a complex lesion that has an adjacent *in situ* or microinvasive component. Whether or not such an adjacent component is present, attributes of the nodule itself that should prompt consideration of melanoma include larger size, asymmetry, increased cellularity, lack of lesional cell maturation, uniform high-grade nuclear atypia, and mitotic activity. In the context of severe solar elastosis, fibrosis, vascular proliferation and ectasia, and marked rete ridge effacement, regressing melanoma should be considered (131).

If no identifiable nevus cells are present, the diagnosis of halo nevus may be suggested by the presence of melanophages in the dense cellular infiltrate and by the absence of melanin in the epidermis. However, one should also consider the possibility of a regressed basal or squamous cell lesion or a melanoma.

Principles of Management: Halo nevi and related lesions generally do not require active therapy. Lesions are often excised for cosmetic reasons, and to rule out melanoma, or, especially when multiple in an adolescent, they may be observed. A halo nevus is not a risk factor for future development of melanoma.

Meyerson Nevus

Halo dermatitis around a melanocytic nevus refers to a temporary inflammatory reaction surrounding a nevus (*Meyerson eczematous nevus*) (133,134). There is a papular compound nevus that becomes surrounded by an eczematous halo. Histologically, the epidermis adjacent to the nevus shows a symmetrical area of acanthosis, spongiosis, parakeratosis, and a dermal infiltrate of lymphocytes, histiocytes, and eosinophils. Immunohistochemical analysis reveals that the lymphocytes are CD3(+) with a predominance of CD4(+) cells, in comparison to CD8 (134). An analogous phenomenon of "nevocentric" erythema multiforme has also been described where cytotoxic/interface alterations predominate (135). Similar changes may be seen around atypical or dysplastic nevi (136) and also in relation to melanomas (137).

Balloon Cell Nevus

Balloon cell nevi are histologic curiosities that possess no clinical features by which they can be differentiated from other nevi. They are quite rare.

Histopathology. Balloon cells may be seen within the epidermis singly or in groups or may be absent from the epidermis. In the dermis, they lie arranged in lobules of varying size, often with an admixture of ordinary nevus cells and often with transitional forms between the ordinary and ballooned nevus cells (Fig. 28-8). The balloon cells may be multinucleated, and are considerably larger than ordinary nevus cells. Their nuclei are small, round, and usually centrally placed. Their cytoplasm appears empty, finely granular, or vacuolated, often with a few small melanin granules. There may be melanophages that are solidly packed with pigment. Stains for lipids, glycogen, and acid or neutral mucopolysaccharides are negative in the balloon cells. *Electron microscopic examination* reveals in balloon

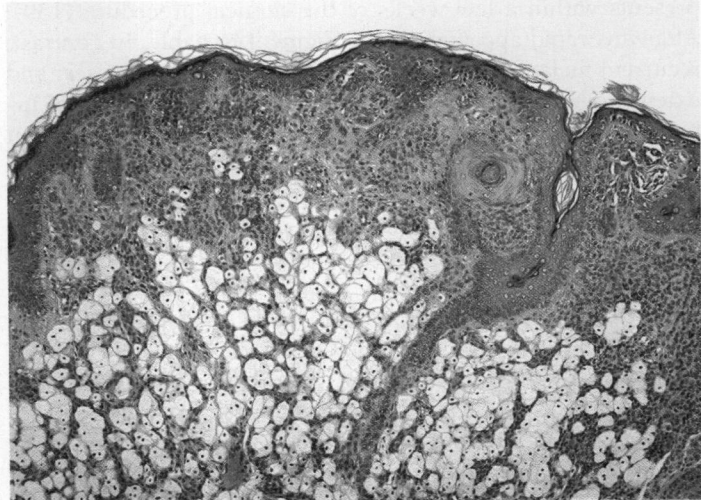

Figure 28-8 Balloon cell nevus. Large cells with pale cytoplasm are admixed with mature nevus cells. There is no high-grade atypia or mitotic activity.

cells numerous large vacuoles formed by enlargement and coalescence of degenerating melanosomes (138). Balloon cell nevus is differentiated from balloon cell melanoma by the usual criteria (p. 891), although the latter may occasionally be challenging when malignant nuclei are compressed within cells as a result of prominent balloon cell cytomorphology. The large adipocytes present in some intradermal nevi as a result of fatty infiltration or stromal metaplasia differ from balloon cells by routine histology by having a scalloped nucleus located at the periphery of the cell. In the differentiation from clear cell hidradenoma and other clear cell tumors, the absence of PAS-positive glycogen and keratin in balloon cell nevus might be helpful; balloon nevus cells also stain for S100 protein, and although eccrine neoplasms (and adipocytes) may also express this marker, the balloon cells will usually also be positive for Melan-A/MART-1 and negative for keratin markers.

Recurrent Nevus (Pseudomelanoma)

Recurrence of a nevus may show clinical hyperpigmentation, which on biopsy may show histologic changes suggestive of melanoma (139,140).

Clinical Features. Recurrence may follow incomplete removal of a nevus, particularly by a shave biopsy or electrodessication, or the nevus may apparently have been completely excised. A similar phenomenon has been described in relation to Spitz tumors (342). The term "persistent nevus" is sometimes used because it is considered that the clinical "recurrence" must have arisen from nevus cells that were not removed by the prior procedure. However, we have also considered the possibility that the "recurrent" pigmentation might be the result of a reactive hyperplasia and nevoid transformation of melanocytes in the epidermis above the healing biopsy site as a consequence of melanocyte growth factors known to be elaborated by scar tissue (e.g., c-kit ligand or fibroblast growth factors). In any event, at a clinical level, recurrence of apparently completely excised nevi is common. In a prospective follow-up study, 28% of all nevi and 41% of hairy nevi were reported to have recurred within 12 months after shave excision (141). The pigmentation in recurrent nevi is confined to the region of the scar and typically presents within a few weeks of the surgical procedure (139). After this rapid appearance, the pigment is stable. In contrast, recurrent melanoma does not respect the border of the scar and extends over time into the adjacent skin. Paradoxically, recurrent melanoma occurs more slowly, over months or years, but progresses inexorably.

Traumatized nevi ("irritated nevi") may be regarded as a special case of the recurrent nevus phenomenon. In a study of 92 patients with a history of trauma, and compatible histologic findings, histologic evidence of trauma was present (in order of frequency) in the form of parakeratosis, acanthosis, dermal telangiectasias, ulceration, melanin within the stratum corneum, dermal inflammation, granulation tissue, melanocytic apoptosis, and dermal fibrosis. Pagetoid spread of melanocytic cells limited to the site of trauma was observed in 20% of cases. One mitotic figure in a melanocyte was seen in three separate cases and was superficially located adjacent to the site of trauma. Melanocytic atypia was not a prominent feature with two cases having mild and one case having moderate atypia (142).

Histopathology. Although most recurrent nevi are not cytologically atypical, in a few instances they contain atypical melanocytes, both singly and in nests, arranged mainly along the epidermal–dermal junction, but occasionally also extending into the upper dermis and also into the epidermis in a pagetoid pattern

(Fig. 28-9). The junctional nests are often composed of pigmented epithelioid melanocytes forming irregular nests, possibly the result of their growth within an atrophic epidermal layer that interfaces with scar tissue. The rete ridge pattern may be preserved or effaced (140). Deep remnants of residual nevus may be seen in the reticular dermis beneath the scar (143). A lymphocytic infiltrate with melanophages may be seen in the upper dermis. The fibrosis of the scar may mimic and be mistaken for "regressive fibrosis" in a melanoma, especially in a superficial shave biopsy where the base of the scar cannot be visualized. Nevus cells in the dermis tend to show evidence of maturation, and the Ki-67 proliferation rate is low (144). Distinction from melanoma may be difficult without a pertinent history. However, the presence of scarlike fibrosis in the upper dermis where fibroblasts/myofibroblasts and collagen bundles lie parallel to the epidermal layer and of remnants of a melanocytic nevus beneath the zone of fibrosis, as well as the sharp demarcation of the melanocytic proliferation devoid of lateral extension beyond the scar, usually makes a correct diagnosis possible. As is true clinically, the recurrent nevus is confined to the epidermis above the scar, whereas recurrent melanoma may extend beyond the scar into the adjacent epidermis. However, persistent nevus, after a partial biopsy, may also involve skin adjacent to a scar. In this instance, ordinary criteria for the distinction between melanomas and nevi apply, as discussed later.

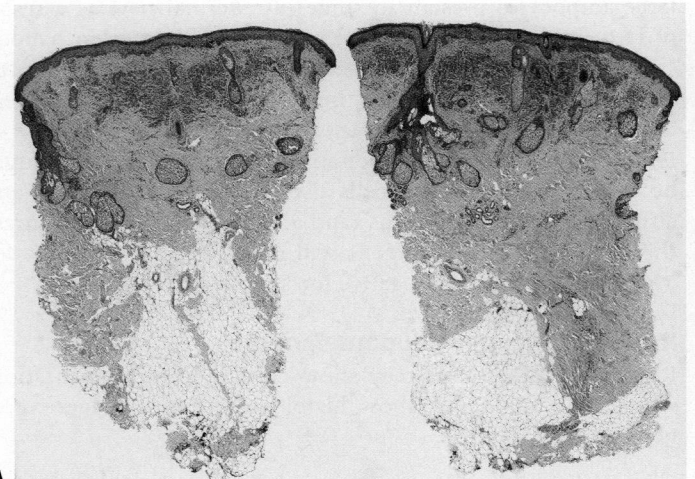

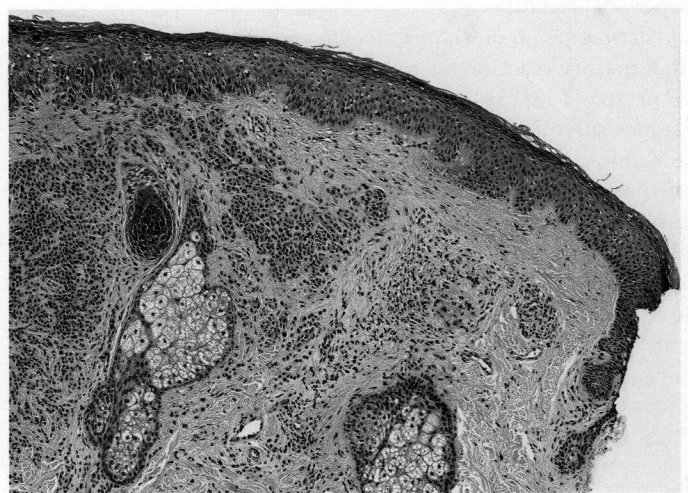

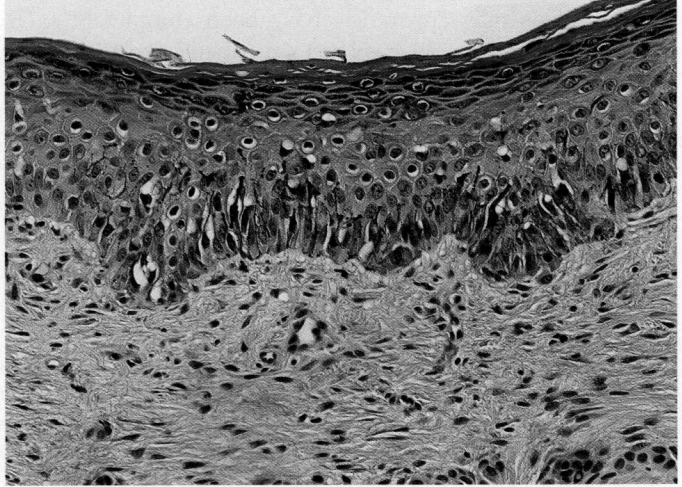

Figure 28-9 Recurrent and persistent melanocytic nevus. **A:** Recurrent pigmentation may occur after complete excision of a nevus or may occur in the scar of a partial removal, as in this example, where the pathology of the recurrent nevus is seen only above the scar, and residual dermal nevus cells of the persistent nevus are present beneath it. **B:** The proliferation in the epidermis does not extend beyond the peripheral extent of the biopsy scar. **C:** The cells of the recurrent nevus in the epidermis are variably enlarged, and they may be arranged with single cells predominating in foci and extending up into the epidermis in a pagetoid pattern, which is usually, as here, relatively subtle. Severe uniform atypia with extensive pagetoid proliferation should suggest the possibility of recurrent melanoma. The prior biopsy should be reviewed, if possible.

In any problematic case in which the diagnosis is in doubt, the original biopsy should be obtained for review. This is particularly important in view of the possibility that genuinely dysplastic primary lesions, after initial biopsy, may also exhibit recurrent nevus-type changes.

Histogenesis. The nevus cells in some recurrent lesions may originate from residual nevus cells located either at the periphery of the lesion or along the outer root sheath of hair follicles. Recurrences that follow complete excision may be attributable to activation of melanocytes, possibly related to a subclinical field of melanocytes with a lowered threshold for nevus cell transformation that surrounded the original lesion and as a consequence of melanocyte-stimulating factors, released during the healing response. The confinement of these reactive changes to the regenerating epidermis above the biopsy scar suggests that the process may be related to growth factors involved in wound healing. Some of these, such as fibroblast growth factors, c-kit ligand, and many others, are well known to be trophic for melanocytes *in vitro* (145).

It is important to note that while previous biopsy is the most common cause of the recurrent nevus phenomenon, trauma to a lesion, potentially unrecognized by the patient, may also produce similar changes. Accordingly, whenever traumatic scar formation is noted in the dermal component of a nevus with overlying abnormalities of atypical intraepidermal melanocytic proliferation (AIMP), this possibility should be considered.

Differential Diagnosis. The major differential is with regression or "regressive fibroplasia" in a melanoma (see also p. 930). In a recent study, 357 cases of recurrent nevus were compared with 34 cases of melanoma with regression. Four histologic patterns of epidermal changes above a dermal scar in recurrent nevus were identified. They are as follows: Type 1: Junctional melanocytic proliferation with effacement of the epidermal rete; Type 2: Compound melanocytic proliferation with effacement of rete; Type 3: Junctional melanocytic proliferation with retention of the rete; Type 4: Compound melanocytic proliferation with retention of the rete (140). In a comparative study including genomic analysis of hotspot *TERT* promoter mutations, these were more common in recurrent melanomas than in recurrent nevi, and the melanomas were more likely to have solar elastosis and to involve more months to recurrence (146). Of note, residual melanoma or nevus may be present in the epidermis and/or the dermis beyond the biopsy scar and should not be confused with the recurrent nevus phenomenon in which the atypical epidermal nevus cell population is confined to the epidermis above the scar.

Key to making this diagnosis is recognizing the distinction between a scar and local regression in a melanoma. A scar will generally have denser collagen and spindle cells that run parallel to the plane of the overlying atrophic epidermis, and, depending on its stage of evolution, there may be giant cells and increased vascularity running perpendicular to the epidermal plane, features that are not as likely to be seen in melanoma regression. Histologically, most recurrent nevi are readily identifiable; however, partial biopsies where the scar extends to the periphery of the specimen or cases without prior knowledge of the original biopsy can lead to misdiagnosis. Correlation with the clinical findings, which should be those of a recently recurrent pigmented lesion confined to the epidermis within an old

scar, actively seeking the history of a prior biopsy and reviewing it, if possible, and having a high index of suspicion help to establish the correct diagnosis.

Principles of Management: Recurrent nevi and related lesions generally do not require active therapy. Lesions are often excised for cosmetic reasons and to rule out melanoma. A recurrent nevus is not a risk factor for future development of melanoma.

Intermediate Lesions: Atypical or Dysplastic Nevi and Melanocytomas

There has long been recognition that some melanocytic tumors are "atypical" in the sense of having architectural and cytologic abnormalities that may also be seen, to a greater degree, in melanomas, leading to the concept that these lesions are "intermediate" between wholly benign lesions and melanomas. More recently, the term "melanocytoma," long used in a similar fashion in CNS lesions, has been applied to these cutaneous lesions in recognition of their intermediate status.

Dysplastic Nevus

Dysplastic nevi were first recognized as "large atypical nevi" (LAN) and then formally described under the designations of *B-K mole syndrome* or *Atypical Mole Syndrome* as multiple lesions occurring in patients with one or several melanomas and in some of their relatives (147,148). It soon became apparent that multiple moles, in addition to their familial occurrence, may occur as a sporadic phenomenon in patients with a predisposition to develop melanoma. This was referred to as the *dysplastic nevus syndrome* (149). Subsequently, cases of multiple dysplastic nevi without melanoma were reported (150). This was followed by the recognition that dysplastic nevi frequently occur as solitary lesions, and are quite common, being found in 5% to 20% of various populations, depending on the criteria used (151). Although the nature and number of moles appear to be under genetic control (152), dysplastic nevi do not constitute a single gene-related genetic syndrome, and in today's usage it is more appropriate, in our opinion, to simply characterize individuals as having dysplastic nevi, with an estimate of their number, degree of clinical and histopathologic atypia, and concurrence of a family history of melanoma, rather than as having a particular form of dysplastic nevus syndrome.

Clinical Summary. Dysplastic nevi, like nevi in general, are important as simulants, risk markers, and potential precursors of melanoma. Even though a substantial fraction of melanomas arise in a precursor nevus or in a field of lentiginous melanocytic dysplasia (153,154), most nevi, including dysplastic nevi, are stable or even involute throughout life, so they should not be managed as high-risk precursors unless histologic atypia is deemed to be significant (see later). The role of dysplastic nevi as simulants, important in the differential diagnosis of melanoma, will be the primary focus of this discussion. Dysplastic nevi have been reviewed from historical and management perspectives (155,156).

Dysplastic nevi may be located anywhere on the body but are found most commonly on the trunk. A suitable rigorous definition of a clinically dysplastic nevus (also known as a clinically atypical nevus) includes: (a) the presence of a macular component either as the entire lesion or surrounding a papular center; (b) large size, 5 mm or more; (c) irregular or ill-defined "fuzzy" border; and (d) irregular pigmentation within the lesion (Fig. 28-10A, B) (34,157). When defined in this manner, clinically recognized dysplastic nevi are a central risk factor for cutaneous melanoma; in a large case-control study, one clinically dysplastic nevus was associated with a 2-fold risk of melanoma, whereas 10 or more conferred a 12-fold increased risk (34). A meta-analysis of 46 studies concluded that a large number of common nevi were confirmed as an important risk factor with a substantially increased relative

risk of 6.9 associated with the presence of 101 to 120 compared to less than 15 nevi, whereas only 5 (vs. 0) atypical (dysplastic) nevi were associated with a comparable relative risk of 6.4 (158).

Histopathology. When dysplastic nevi were first described in association with melanoma, it was considered that dysplastic nevi, by definition, always contained cytologically atypical melanocytes (149). Later, it was argued by some that an abnormal

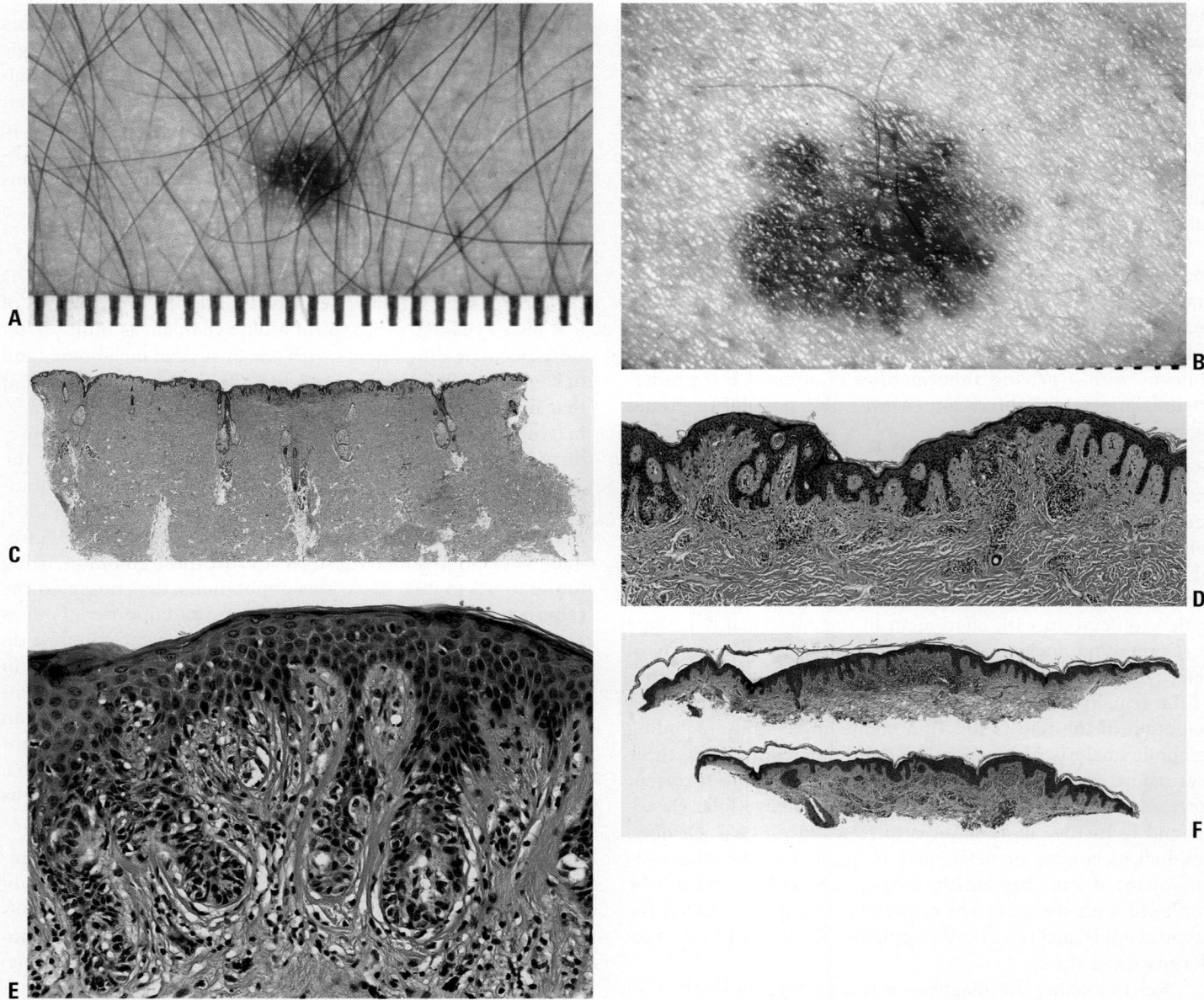

Figure 28-10 Dysplastic melanocytic nevus. **A:** Junctional dysplastic nevus. A lesion that meets minimal clinical criteria. The diameter is almost exactly 5 mm, the lesion is entirely flat, there is mild pigmentary variegation, and the border is ill-defined or "fuzzy." **B:** Compound dysplastic nevus. This lesion is relatively broad and quite irregular in outline, with variegated shades of tan and brown pigmentation. There is a papular compound portion near the center, and the periphery is flat, with an ill-defined "fuzzy" border in some areas but a more discrete border in others. This morphology overlaps with that of a radial growth phase melanoma of the superficial spreading type, and a lesion such as this should be considered carefully for excision to rule out a possible melanoma. **C:** Compound nevus with moderate dysplasia. At scanning magnification, the lesions are broad and symmetrical. If a dermal component is present, the epidermal component (which is always present, by definition) extends beyond its "shoulder," or (as in this case) the lesion is entirely junctional. **D:** In the junctional compartment of the nevus (the "shoulder" mentioned previously), the epidermal rete ridges are relatively uniformly elongated and delicate, and there are nests of lesional cells that tend to be oriented parallel to the surface and to bridge adjacent elongated rete. **E:** The lesional cell nuclei tend to be moderately enlarged compared to most banal type A nevus cells, and a few of them have irregular nuclei that are either hyperchromatic or have prominent nucleoli ("random" moderate cytologic atypia). **F:** Compound nevus with severe dysplasia. A broad junctional proliferation with elongated rete ridges and a dense lymphocytic infiltrate, in association with a dermal nevus component.

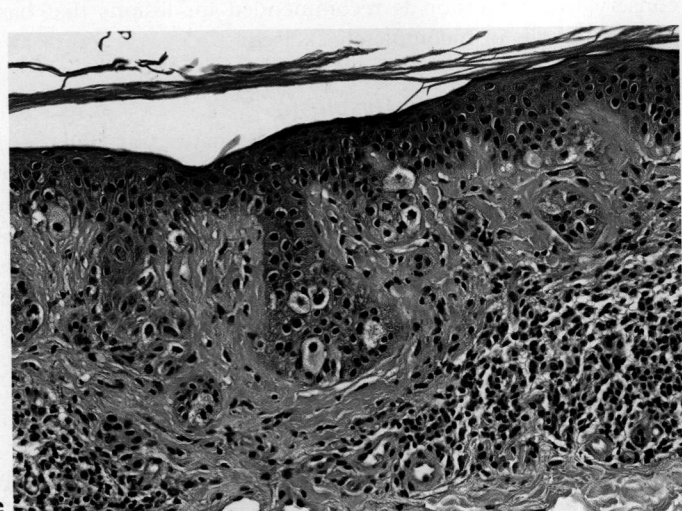
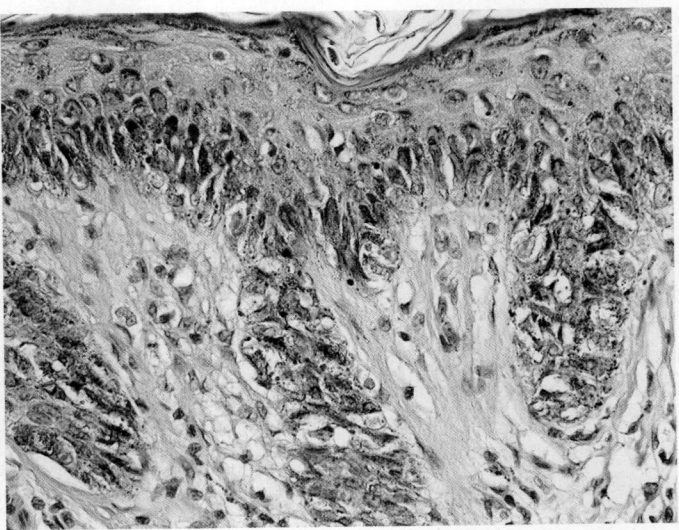

Figure 28-10 (*continued*) G: Large epithelioid melanocytes in the junctional component, some with moderate-to-severe nuclear atypia, in the form of enlargement, some irregularity, and hyperchromatism. Pagetoid scatter of these cells generally does not extend above the lower third. There is a bandlike lymphocytic infiltrate in the dermis. Diagnosis of "severe" dysplasia in this lesion is based on both architectural and cytologic criteria. H: Severe junctional melanocytic dysplasia with changes suggestive of evolving melanoma *in situ*. There is a tendency toward confluence and lack of definition of nests and to "continuous" extension of the proliferation in the suprapapillary plates between the rete. Cytologic atypia in the form of nuclear irregularity and the presence of nucleoli, although moderate in degree, is relatively uniform.

architectural pattern of lentiginous melanocytic growth was a sufficient criterion without requiring cytologic atypia (159). It was even stated that "most lentiginous compound nevi that are confined to the epidermis and the papillary dermis are dysplastic nevi" (159). Subsequently, the term "Clark nevus" was coined to encompass all nevi with lentiginous junctional components (either alone or adjacent to a dermal component), irrespective of lesional size or of the presence or absence of cytologic atypia (160). This inclusive definition would include very common small lentiginous junctional and compound nevi. Thus, the term "Clark nevus," as coined by Ackerman and Mihara, is not synonymous with the lesion originally described by Clark (149,161). Because of controversy regarding its use and definition, use of the term "dysplastic nevus" was discouraged by a National Institutes of Health (NIH) panel, which proposed the alternative term "nevus with architectural disorder and melanocytic atypia" (162). This clumsy moniker is currently used by a few dermatopathologists, whereas most favor the dysplastic nevus nomenclature (163). Specificity in distinguishing dysplastic from nondysplastic nevi is likely to be increased by the inclusion of size and cytologic atypia as criteria, as was done in the original reports by Clark et al. In our practice, small lesions or lesions with architectural features of dysplastic nevi but without cytologic atypia may be reported as "compound nevi" or as "lentiginous compound nevi," or the NIH descriptive terminology may be used. Although the archaic term "active junctional nevus" (164,165) might have some overlap with dysplastic nevus (and also with RGP melanoma), most dysplastic nevi are clinically stable or may involute over time (166), so they are not "active" in the sense of continuing growth.

Criteria for assessing melanocytic dysplasia may be summarized in two categories: *architectural features* and *cytologic features* (167). These features are correlated, albeit imperfectly (168) (Fig. 28-10).

In the *architectural pattern* of melanocytic dysplasia, either the lesions are entirely junctional or there is a prominent junctional component that is symmetrically or sometimes asymmetrically distributed at the "shoulders" or junctional edges that extend laterally beyond a central dermal component (if any) (Fig. 28-10C). At higher magnification, nested and lentiginous proliferation of nevus cells in the epidermis is the dominant feature in the junctional component. There is elongation of the rete ridges, and an increase in the number of junctional melanocytes, arranged in nests, with long axes tending to lie parallel to the epidermal surface. These nests tend to lie near the tips and sides of elongated rete ridges, as well as within interrete spaces and may form "bridges" via apparent fusion of nests between adjacent rete (Fig. 28-10D). There may be scattered single cells in lentiginous array as well, but these do not predominate, and there is no contiguous and continuous proliferation of single cells between the rete. The melanocytes in the junctional nests are frequently spindle shaped but may be large and epithelioid and have abundant cytoplasm with the fine, dusty (finely divided) melanin granules variety (Fig. 28-10E).

If the lesion is compound, nests of melanocytes in the papillary dermis show a uniform appearance and evidence of maturation with descent into the dermis, as seen in an ordinary compound nevus. In these compound dysplastic nevi, the intraepidermal component extends, by definition, beyond the lateral border of the dermal component, forming a "shoulder" to the lesion histologically and a "targetlike" or "fried-egg" pattern clinically. Pagetoid extension of melanocytes, if present, is absent or slight and limited to the lowermost layers. The nevus cells in the dermis are mature, and usually of the "type B" subtype. In some cases, they may extend into the upper reticular dermis (compound dysplastic nevus with congenital features).

Stromal responses are also of value in diagnosis of dysplastic nevi. A lymphoid inflammatory infiltrate, usually only of a mild or moderate degree and intermingled with melanophages, is present in the dermis beneath areas of junctional activity, and microvascular prominence or proliferation may also be present. The papillary dermis is also characteristically fibrotic, and, typically, lamellae of collagen encircle affected rete (concentric fibroplasia) and/or form stacked layers beneath dermal papillae (lamellar fibroplasia). This feature, although not in itself diagnostic, is of considerable assistance in recognizing dysplastic nevi in the context of the architectural and cytologic criteria discussed in this section. Diffuse fibroplasia with angiogenesis, in contrast, would be more characteristic of an RGP melanoma (169).

Cytologically, in addition to the lentiginous melanocytic hyperplasia, melanocytic nuclear atypia is required for the diagnosis. This atypia is characterized by irregularly shaped, large, hyperchromatic nuclei in some melanocytes. Careful studies by Rabkin (170) have provided quantification of the degree of cytologic atypia (see Table 28-4). Most atypical melanocytes lie singly or in small groups, and the atypia involves only a few of the lesional cells, constituting "random" cytologic atypia (Fig. 28-10E). Focal extension of atypical-appearing melanocytes into the lower spinous layer may be seen, but if this "pagetoid scatter" is prominent and includes the involvement of the stratum granulosum, the possibility that transformation into melanoma *in situ* may have occurred should be seriously considered. A borderline lesion may be a severely dysplastic nevus or an early SSM that is still *in situ* or microinvasive, and diagnostic equivocation may be appropriate in such borderline cases. Because such early evolving melanomas, even when microinvasive, are curable after simple excision (171,172), this distinction does not carry the implication of increased mortality, as long as the lesion is entirely removed. For lesions with severe dysplasia where the differential diagnosis includes the possibility of early melanoma, conservative reexcision is recommended for lesions that have been minimally or incompletely excised.

Grading of Melanocytic Dysplasia

Melanocytic dysplasia appears to be a quantitative trait, and several authors have produced guidelines for grading dysplasia. McNutt and his colleagues have published a detailed schema for grading lesions from nevi without atypia to melanoma, which includes cytologic atypia (nuclear size, nucleoli, chromatin clumping) and architectural features (circumscription, junctional extension, rete ridge distortion, concentric fibrosis, diffuse fibrosis, lymphocytes, upward migration, suprapapillary plate involvement, and dermal mitoses) (Table 28-4) (173). This schema has been correlated with biology in that patients with more atypia in their nevus biopsies are more likely to have had a primary melanoma.

Criteria for grading were developed more recently by Rabkin, who emphasized nuclear size as a potentially more quantifiable criterion and lesional size as an important marker (in addition to the number of lesions) of melanoma risk. In this scheme, cytologic atypia is graded on the highest degree of cytologic atypia present in three melanocytes/HPF for two or more adjacent HPF and/or the highest degree of cytologic atypia present in most melanocytes in two or more adjacent HPFs; it is graded as "moderate" (or low grade) if lesional nuclei are 1 to 1.5× the size of resting basal keratinocytes and "severe" (or high grade) if greater than 2× (170).

In our practice, we have found grading of dysplastic nevi to be facilitated by understanding of the cytomorphology of normal melanocytes that are restricted spatially to the basal cell layer of the epidermis and that contain uniformly round to ovoid nuclear contours with diffusely hyperchromatic nuclei that are smaller in diameter than that of an adjacent keratinocyte. Mild dysplasia is characterized by lentiginous and nested junctional proliferation of melanocytes that show random (nonuniform) nuclear enlargement (up to 1.5× that of an adjacent keratinocyte), nuclear contour angulation and irregularity, but with preservation of the normal nuclear hyperchromasia. Moderate atypia is heralded by random loss in some junctional melanocytes of diffuse nuclear hyperchromasia seen in normal or mildly dysplastic cells, with development of irregularly aggregated heterochromatin (vesicular chromatin), visible nucleoli, and enlargement of angulated and irregular nuclei to approximately 2× that of an adjacent keratinocyte. Severe atypia occurs along a continuum, with nuclear enlargement of such cells beyond 2× that of a basal keratinocyte, now with some architectural features that suggest early evolution in the direction of melanoma *in situ*, including foci of generally low-level (below the stratum granulosum) pagetoid spread, or short expanses of contiguous/continuous replacement of the basal cell layer. We find that this assists in defining those high-risk, diffusely moderately to severely atypical lesions for which modest complete excision should be considered.

In the 2018 World Health Organization (WHO) classification of skin tumors, 4th edition, new criteria for grading dysplastic nevi were presented, based largely on the work of Rabkin (170,174). It was considered that mildly dysplastic nevus is a diagnosis that is poorly reproducible and not associated with risk of melanoma and, therefore, that these lesions should be diagnosed as junctional or compound nevi but not as dysplastic nevi. Moderate dysplasia and severe dysplasia are proposed to be diagnosed as low- and high-grade dysplasia, respectively. Criteria for these distinctions are presented in Table 28-5.

Table 28-4

Criteria for Dysplastic Nevus Grading

Atypia	None	Mild	Mod	Severe	MM
Lateral circumscription	+++	++	+	+	+/−
Symmetry	+++	+++	+++	+/−	+/−
Junctional extension	+/−	+++	+++	+++	++++
Rete ridge distortion	+/−	+/−	++	+++	++++
Concentric fibrosis	+/−	+	++	+++	++++
Diffuse fibrosis	+/−	+/−	+/−	+/−	+++
Lymphocytes	+/−	+	++	+++	++++
Upward migration	+/−	+/−	+/−	+/−	++++
Suprapapillary plates involved	−	−	−	+/−	++++
Nuclear size	+	+	++	++	+++
Nucleoli	−	+/−	+/−	+++	++++
Chromatin clumping	−	−	+/−	++	++++
Dermal mitoses	−	−	−	−	+++

Source: Based on Arumi-Uria M, McNutt NS, Finnerty B. Grading of atypia in nevi: correlation with melanoma risk. *Mod Pathol.* 2003;16:764–771.

Table 28-5

Nuclear Features in Different Grades of Dysplasia

Former Grade	WHO Classification 2018	Nuclear Size vs. Resting Basal keratinocytes	Chromatin	Nuclear Size and Shape Variation	Nucleoli
Mild	Not a dysplastic nevus	1–1.5×	May be hyperchromatic	Minimal	Absent or small
Moderate	Low grade	1.5–2×	Hyperchromatic or dispersed	Present in a small minority of cells (random)	Small or absent
Severe	High grade	2× or more	Hyperchromatic, coarse granular, or peripherally condensed	Prominent in a larger minority of cells	Prominent, often lavender

Based on Xiong MY, Rabkin MS, Piepkorn MW, et al. Diameter of dysplastic nevi is a more robust biomarker of increased melanoma risk than degree of histologic dysplasia: a case-control study. *J Am Acad Dermatol.* 2014;71(6):1257–1258 (170) and Elder DE, Barnhill RL, Bastian BC, et al. Dysplastic naevi. In: Elder DE, Massi D, Scolyer RA, Willemze R, eds. *WHO Classification of Skin Tumours.* 4th ed. International Agency for Research on Cancer; 2018:82–86 (174).

In general, in our opinion, lesions that overlap with criteria for melanoma should be graded as severe dysplasia, with an indication, if appropriate, that evolving melanoma *in situ* cannot be ruled out (Fig. 28-10F). In cases of extreme doubt, a descriptive diagnosis such as "SAMPUS" or "IAMPUS" may be used, with a differential diagnosis and often with a recommendation for therapy (175). Such lesions should be managed by complete excision with, at a minimum, a clear margin of normal skin around the scar and any residual lesion. If melanoma *in situ* cannot be ruled out, current guidelines would recommend consideration of excision with a 5-mm margin.

The diagnosis of melanocytic dysplasia was found to be reproducible by international multidisciplinary groups that used agreed-upon criteria (176,177). In another study, including participants whose published criteria differed in their requirements for atypia and for a size criterion, it was concluded that the participating pathologists used different diagnostic criteria, but that their usage was consistent (178). It has been suggested that histologic criteria may be more specific when applied to larger lesions and that cytologic atypia may play a key role in the identification and significance of these lesions. Slight melanocytic atypia may be subtle and poorly reproducible and also may be of modest clinical significance. On the other hand, the diagnosis of higher grade dysplasia (severe dysplasia) is likely to be both more reproducible and of substantially greater biologic significance. These assumptions have been partially validated in the MPATH study that more closely resembled actual clinical practice, although the reproducibility was poor for all of the intermediate lesions, including T1a melanomas (7). In Piepkorn's recent case-control study (179), reviewed in more detail in the next section, any dysplasia beyond "mild" was associated with increased melanoma risk, suggesting that patients with moderate as well as severe dysplasia, but not mild dysplasia (in the absence of other risk factors), should be offered follow-up.

Significance of Dysplastic Nevi

This review has focused on the morphology of dysplastic nevi because of their important role as *simulants of melanoma* and, therefore, as lesions that are commonly considered in the differential diagnosis of melanoma. In addition, these lesions are occasionally precursors of melanoma. However, their major significance, other than in differential diagnosis, is as markers of increased risk for melanoma.

Dysplastic Nevi as Melanoma Precursors. Although melanomas in patients with dysplastic nevi may arise within a preexisting dysplastic nevus, most arise de novo. Histologic changes of an associated nevus, most often a dysplastic nevus or a superficial congenital pattern nevus, are seen at the periphery of melanomas in approximately 20% to 30% of cases (47,154), supporting the view that at least some cutaneous melanomas take origin in a dysplastic nevus. Even so, most dysplastic nevi, like other nevi, are clinically stable and will never evolve into melanomas (166,180). This paradox is explained by the fact that nevi, including dysplastic nevi, are vastly more common than melanomas in the general population and provides a rationale against indiscriminate excision of clinically stable dysplastic nevi for prophylaxis of melanoma.

It has been calculated that the risk of transformation of any given nevus to melanoma is very low indeed (180). However, significant dysplasia in nevi, especially severely dysplastic nevi, are a subset in which a higher transformation rate might be anticipated. In addition, because of overlapping criteria, it is possible that any given lesion with severely dysplastic features in one sampled region might have features diagnostic of melanoma in another region. In a study of 580 dysplastic nevi, 34% had a positive biopsy margin, increasing with grade of atypia. Only two reexcisions (1.6%) resulted in a clinically significant change in diagnosis, from biopsy-diagnosed moderately-to-severely dysplastic nevi before excision to melanoma *in situ* after excision (181). The local recurrence rate for mildly and moderately dysplastic nevi is very low, and the recurrences are typically benign (182,183). In a recent pigmented lesion clinic-based retrospective cohort study focusing on severely dysplastic nevi, the importance of excisional biopsy for concerning pigmented lesions was confirmed, as 9.7% of cases with positive biopsy margins were upstaged to melanoma on reexcision, compared with a single case (5.3%) with negative biopsy margins, and one local melanoma *in situ* recurrence was noted in a clinically observed group of cases with close or positive margins (184).

Dysplastic Nevi as Risk Markers. After the early descriptions of dysplastic nevi as markers of high risk for melanoma in hereditary melanoma kindreds, it was widely assumed that identification of individuals in the community at high risk for melanoma required biopsy of a nevus to "rule out dysplasia." Subsequent studies have shown that risk is best assessed by the clinical evaluation of the entire cutaneous phenotype, although biopsy can add useful information. The total number of nevi and the number of large nevi (34,185), light skin color, and high freckle density are all risk factors for development of melanoma, but in early studies the strongest single phenotypic risk factor was the presence and number of dysplastic nevi (34). Family history of melanoma is another significant risk factor (186), as is a personal history of prior melanoma (187,188), especially when multiple (186). In members of hereditary melanoma kindreds, the lifetime risk for melanoma approaches 100% in individuals who have clinically dysplastic nevi, corresponding to approximately 100-fold relative risk compared to the general population (187,188). In people without a family history of melanoma, the relative risk, as determined in multiple cohort and case-control studies from different geographic regions, is of the order of 3- to 10-fold, depending on the number of dysplastic (clinically atypical) nevi on their skin (34,158). Melanoma risk is related to ambient sun exposure, with the relative risk being higher in regions with a lower sun exposure, with more sunny environments increasing the number of nevi and perhaps diluting the risk (189). Pigmentary phenotype is also related to risk (189,190), as is the location of nevi, with truncal (i.e., intermittently sun-exposed nevi) having the highest risk (190). These data are based on clinical evaluation of nevi, which does not necessarily correlate well with histologic atypia (191). Even when a biopsy can be obtained, usually only one or two nevi are sampled, whereas clinical examination considers the whole phenotype.

Nevertheless, it is clear that histologic atypia in dysplastic nevi is associated with melanoma risk. In one early study, histologically verified clinically dysplastic nevi were associated with a relative risk of 4.6 for melanoma (192). In a multiobserver study where biopsies had been taken from 24 melanoma cases and 21 random controls, four of six observers (who had each used different criteria) found an increased prevalence of histologic dysplasia ranging up to a 3.5-fold increase in cases compared to controls (178). In an interesting study, Sagebiel and colleagues found that the degree of dysplasia in a nevus biopsy correlated with increasing age of the patient, with frank melanomas occupying the oldest age category (193). McNutt and colleagues in a very large single institution study have demonstrated a clear relationship between the degree of atypia in clinically atypical (dysplastic) nevi submitted for biopsy and the chance that a patient has had a melanoma, suggesting that the risk of melanoma is greater for persons who tend to make nevi with high-grade histologic atypia. In this study, the odds ratio as a measure of association between dysplastic nevi and personal history of melanoma was 4.08 for severe versus mild, 2.81 for severe versus moderate, and 1.45 for moderate versus mild dysplasia (173). Finally, this long-standing controversy seems to have been settled in a case-control study carried out by Piepkorn, who studied nevi from 80 melanoma cases and spouse controls and found that dysplastic nevi with moderate or severe histologic dysplasia were a risk factor for melanoma, with an adjusted risk ratio of 3.99 (179). In subsequent work, the reproducibility improved after agreement on criteria, while the role of lesional size as an independent risk factor was emphasized (170).

In the McNutt study, the risk of melanoma associated with mild histologic dysplasia could not be calculated but, by inspection of the data for risk of severe and moderate dysplasia, listed previously, would most likely be close to unity (i.e., a relative risk of 1). In the Piepkorn data, mild dysplasia was studied and was not associated with risk. These findings suggest that mild dysplasia in a nevus should be considered as a lesion that is relatively common and that has little or no clinical significance as a risk marker or a precursor. Moderate dysplasia is significant as a risk marker, whereas severe dysplasia is not only a risk marker but may also be a precursor of melanoma, and/or melanoma may be found focally within these lesions with such frequency that they should be completely excised.

Dysplastic Nevi as Intermediate Lesions of Tumor Progression. In keeping with their role as potential precursors and as simulants of melanoma, dysplastic nevi tend to occupy an intermediate position between nevi and melanomas in laboratory studies. In cell cycle proliferation marker studies, the reactivity of dysplastic nevi is intermediate, though closer to that of common nevi than of melanoma (194). Electron microscopic studies of dysplastic nevi demonstrated abnormal spherical and partially melanized melanosomes similar to those seen in SSMs (195). Although most *in situ* hybridization or immunohistochemical studies have shown profiles similar to common nevi, dysplastic nevi have reacted in an intermediate manner with some markers (196,197), while the reactivity with others has been more akin to that of melanomas (198) or ordinary nevi (199). Interesting studies have shown that the amount of red pheomelanin is greater in dysplastic nevi than in common nevi or normal skin (200). Because pheomelanin may be a generator of toxic free radicals after UV irradiation, this attribute may increase the risk of genetic mutations in these lesions that may contribute to continued tumor progression (201). Recently, differential expression of micro-RNAs in benign, dysplastic, and malignant melanocytic lesions was demonstrated, dysplastic nevi tending to occupy an intermediate position in terms of expression (202).

Genetic changes in nevi and dysplastic nevi have been cataloged. For example, loss of heterozygosity at the 9p locus (which contains the p16/*CDKN2A* tumor suppressor gene) was found in 64% of dysplastic nevi and 50% of benign nevi, whereas homozygous deletion of p16 was found in 29% of dysplastic nevi but never in benign nevi (203). In a recent study, exome sequencing revealed that dysplastic nevi harbored a substantially lower mutational load than melanomas (21 protein-changing mutations vs. >100) and that mutations in known progression genes for melanoma, including *CDKN2A*, *TP53*, *NF1*, *RAC1*, and *PTEN*, were not found among any melanocytic nevi sequenced (204). In addition, studies have demonstrated aberrations in DNA-repair pathways in dysplastic nevi (205), as well as microsatellite instability and loss of heterozygosity in melanomas and nevi, including dysplastic nevi (206–210), leading to the conclusion that "Dysplastic nevi might be defined as a monoclonal and genetically unstable, but limited, melanocytic proliferation that distinguishes this entity from the benign nevus and from malignant melanoma" (207). These findings are consistent with DNA-repair deficiency in patients with dysplastic nevi and tend to correlate with patient groups ordered according to increasing melanoma risk (210). In a seminal study of the genomic landscape of melanoma from Bastian's group, it was demonstrated that dysplastic nevi that are in contiguity with melanomas, and thus putative precursors of that melanoma, tend to have driver mutations other than

BRAFV600E, including non-V600E mutations of *BRAF* or of *NRAS*, *HRAS*, or *MAP2K1* (mutually exclusive), all members of the mitogen-activated protein (MAP) kinase pathway. In addition, these lesions all had a second mutation in a progression gene such as an activating *TERT* promoter mutation and hemizygous *CDKN2A* deletion (211).

Differential Diagnosis of Dysplastic Nevi

The major importance of biopsy in an individual with dysplastic nevi is to rule out the possibility of melanoma in a clinically problematic lesion. Key features in making this distinction are reviewed in Table 28-6. Generally speaking, a melanoma is broader than a dysplastic nevus, which is, by definition, greater than 4 mm in diameter and not often more than 10 mm. Dysplastic nevi generally have a more or less symmetrical architecture being in either entirely junctional or having a junctional component at the shoulders of a "head" formed by a compound component. In a dysplastic nevus, the rete ridges are generally uniformly elongated, narrow, and relatively delicate compared to an irregularly thickened and thinned epidermis often with effaced rete ridges in melanomas. Among the lesional cells, nests tend to predominate over single cells in the epidermis in dysplastic nevi, whereas single cells may predominate in melanomas. In a superficial spreading melanoma, there is often extensive and high-level pagetoid scatter into the epidermis, which would be a concerning feature in a nevus. The host response differs in that dysplastic nevi tend to have a patchy lymphocytic infiltrate with concentric and eosinophilic fibroplasia around elongated rete, whereas melanomas in the RGP tend to have a more bandlike lymphocytic infiltrate with diffuse fibroplasia that widens the papillary dermis. Cytologically, most cells are not atypical in a dysplastic nevus, whereas the converse is true in melanomas. Mitotic figures are rare or absent in nevi and present in about 1/3 of RGP melanomas in the junctional component with no mitoses, by definition, in the dermis. The dermal cells in the nevi have evidence of maturation to a smaller cell type and may disperse among upper reticular dermis collagen fibers, whereas those in a melanoma tend to resemble the cells in the epidermis.

A p16-Ki-67-HMB45 Immunohistochemistry Scoring System has demonstrated potential utility in the differentiation between nevi and melanomas. A Mart/Ki-67 double labeled stain would be a useful addition to this panel. The Ki-67 staining percentage in nevi is typically less than 5%, whereas staining in the 10% to 20% range could be regarded as borderline and concerning, and greater than 20% staining very concerning for melanoma. Staining for HMB45 in nevi is typically stratified with diminution of staining from superficial to deep, whereas, conversely, 100% of the cells should stain with Melan-A/Mart. Loss of p16 staining is concerning, especially when there is clonal loss. Sometimes, there is an abnormal pattern of staining with absence of nuclear staining, suggestive of a mutated, dysfunctional p16 protein (Fig. 28-11) (p. 900) (212).

Other conditions that enter the differential diagnosis of dysplastic nevi are of lesser importance than melanoma. However, one difference is that these conditions, in general, are not

---

Table 28-6

Dysplastic Nevus versus Radial Growth Phase Melanoma

Dysplastic Nevus	Radial Growth Phase Melanoma
Pattern Features	
May be <6 mm diameter, not often >10 mm	Usually >6 mm, often much >10 mm
Somewhat symmetrical	Often highly asymmetrical
Often symmetrically arranged about "shoulders" of a mature dermal nevus	If dermal nevus is present, it is often asymmetrically placed.
Uniformly elongated narrow, delicate rete ridges	Irregularly thickened epidermis, often with effaced rete ridges
No alteration of stratum corneum	May be hyperkeratotic
Nests predominate over single cells in the epidermis	Single cells predominate except in late lesions.
Little or no pagetoid spread of lesional cells into epidermis	Usually obvious pagetoid spread into epidermis, extending to stratum corneum
Patchy lymphocytic infiltrate in papillary dermis	Brisk bandlike infiltrate
No regression	Regression common
Last lesional cells at lateral border are often in a nest ("well circumscribed").	Last cells are often single and may be above the basal zone.
Cytologic Features	
Scattered atypical epithelioid cells with dusty melanin pigment, nucleoli, anisokaryosis ("random atypia")	Epithelioid cells with dusty pigment, nucleoli, anisokaryosis predominate ("uniform atypia")
Most cells are not atypical.	Most cells are atypical.
No mitoses in epidermis or dermis	Intraepidermal mitoses in about one-third of cases; no mitoses in dermis
Cells in dermis, if any, are smaller than those in epidermis ("maturation").	Cells in dermis are similar to those in epidermis.

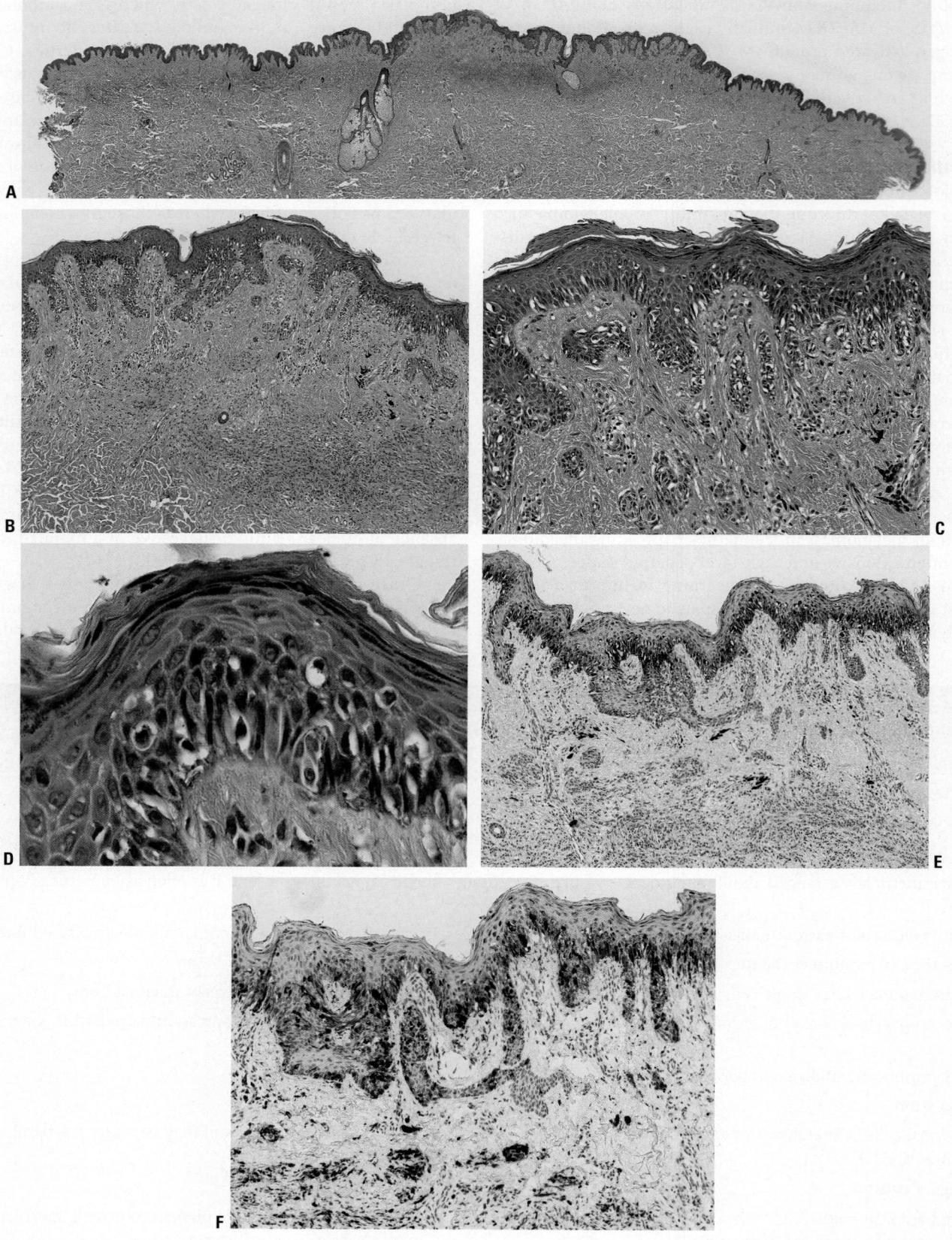

Figure 28-11 Compound nevus with severe dermal and epidermal dysplasia and focal changes initially concerning for melanoma, *in situ* and/or superficially invasive. **A:** A very broad, reasonably symmetrical lesion with junctional shoulders adjacent to a central compound portion. **B:** The junctional component has nests but also in some areas a preponderance of single cells. The dermal component is mature at the base; however, there are some atypical cells more superficially. **C:** The lesional cells have moderately to markedly enlarged nuclei, including in some nests in the superficial dermis. **D:** There is focally quite marked pagetoid scatter. **E:** Staining for HMB45 is reasonably well stratified with strong staining in the junctional component but with patchy weaker staining in some of the dermal cells. **F:** There is strong staining for p16 with nuclear and cytoplasmic staining in a partly "checker board" pattern (alternating groups of positive and negatively stained cells). There is no evidence of clonal loss. The KI-67 proliferation rate was minimal in the dermis (not shown).

strong risk markers for future melanoma risk. Conditions that need to be distinguished from dysplastic nevi have been discussed in previous sections and include some *junctional nevi* (p. 844), *special site nevi* (p. 848), and *pigmented spindle cell nevi* (p. 901). Also of lesser importance is the distinction between a dysplastic nevus and a junctional Spitz nevus (p. 883). The characteristic large spindle and/or epithelioid cells and the presence of Kamino bodies in the latter are important distinguishing features.

Lesions in which some features of dysplasia, generally relating to architecture, are observed but not judged to be diagnostic (or that fall below the threshold of diagnosis) may be reported as "lentiginous (junctional or compound) nevi" or "nevus with architectural disorder," with an interpretive note. Such a note may indicate that additional evaluation of the patient could be appropriate to assess melanoma risk and that periodic surveillance could be appropriate, especially if there are other clinically atypical (dysplastic) nevi or a family or personal history of melanoma (213–215).

Principles of Management of Dysplastic Nevi

The major role of biopsy and of histologic examination of nevi, including dysplastic nevi, is to rule out melanoma in a clinically suspicious or changing lesion. However, histologic atypia also correlates with a patient's risk of developing a melanoma in the future. Atypia is heterogeneous in these lesions (in contrast to the uniform atypia that characterizes most melanomas), and complete excisional biopsy is recommended (which can include shave or punch excisions as long as the entire lesion is included in the specimen).

In our practice, for purposes of classification of the lesion itself, we have long tended to distinguish between "mild to moderate" and lesions that at least focally show "severe" dysplasia (e.g., moderate to severe or severe). This approach has been codified in the 2018 WHO Classification of dysplastic nevi as either low grade or high grade, which should also result in reduced overuse of the term "dysplasia" in mildly atypical melanocytic lesions and, in addition, allow a less complicated approach to diagnosis and therapy (174).

Many lesions formerly interpreted as "mild dysplasia" are now considered to be junctional nevi (often well characterized as "lentiginous junctional nevi") and not to be dysplastic nevi. Lesions formerly classified as moderate dysplasia are classified in the WHO schema as low-grade dysplasia. Reexcision is not always needed for these lesions even if the margin is positive, at least when the patient is to be followed. In a high-risk clinical situation, 23% of patients with this diagnosis developed melanoma elsewhere on their skin but none at the lesional site. Prior melanoma was the factor most strongly associated with developing a melanoma at a separate site (odds ratio, 11.74), and, in addition, the findings suggested that the presence of two or more biopsied dysplastic nevi (one of which was moderately dysplastic) independently conferred twice the odds of developing a future melanoma at a separate site, suggesting that these patients, at least, should be offered formal surveillance (215). In patients having a single lesion and lacking any other risk factors for melanoma, it is likely, in our opinion, that this risk of future melanoma will be much lower, and it may be most judicious to offer a conservative but complete excision and recommend that the patient observe their skin, reporting for follow-up if any new lesions or "ugly ducklings" (lesions different from all other

nevi) develop. If there is clinically visible lesion remaining at the site of biopsy-proven moderate dysplasia, complete removal should be considered.

Severe or high-grade dysplasia shares sufficient characteristics with melanoma (Tables 28-4 to 28-6) to suggest that it should, in general, be managed as a lesion with potential for local recurrence, with complete excision and clear margins, or with careful expert follow-up (184,213). In a recent retrospective cohort study, 9.7% (6/66) of cases of severe dysplasia with positive biopsy margins and 5.3% (1/19) of those with negative biopsy margins were upstaged to melanoma or early melanoma on reexcision. One local melanoma *in situ* recurrence was noted in the clinically observed group of cases (1/26). These findings confirm the importance of excisional biopsy and/or complete excision for concerning pigmented lesions (184).

In patients with dysplastic nevi, periodic surveillance and evaluation of first-degree relatives may be indicated for early diagnosis of melanoma. This is especially so if the clinically dysplastic lesions are numerous and/or markedly atypical and in individuals who have a personal or family history of melanoma. There is evidence that surveillance and/or education of individuals at increased risk for melanoma can result in the diagnosis of melanomas in their early, curable stages (216,217). Guidelines for genetic counseling and genomic screening of patients with a family history of melanoma have been published; these vary according to the baseline incidence in different regions of the world (218).

Deep-Penetrating Nevus/Melanocytoma

This lesion, now considered to be in the "Low CSD," rather than the "Blue" pathway, is a distinctive entity that was originally described by Seab et al. in 1989 (219). In this first report of 70 cases from a referral center, many had previously been misdiagnosed histologically as melanomas. Similar lesions have also been described as plexiform spindle cell nevi (220). Deep-penetrating nevi (DPN) are regarded as intermediate lesions in tumor progression, for which the term "melanocytoma" has been applied (3). It has been demonstrated that these lesions result from combined activation of the MAP kinase pathway and beta-catenin or *APC*, which is a member of the WNT signaling pathway, and thus they have two mutations, one in each of these pathways (221). These lesions may present *de novo* in a pure form or may arise in combination with another nevus, usually a small congenital pattern nevus, as one of the most common forms of combined nevi (222).

Clinical Summary. In the first report, most of the lesions occurred in the second and third decades (range 3 to 63 years). The head, neck, and shoulder were the most frequent sites of involvement, with no occurrences on the hands or feet. The lesions ranged from 2 to 9 mm and were darkly pigmented papules and nodules, often diagnosed clinically as blue nevi or cellular blue nevi. In a mean follow-up of 7 years, none recurred or metastasized. Occasional recurrences, and a few instances of metastases, have since been described, mostly, if not entirely, confined to a category of lesions termed "borderline" or frank "plexiform melanomas," discussed further on (223,224). On cross section, the lesions typically extend at least halfway into the dermis, with a smooth, dome-shaped elevation of the epidermis. It is likely that many lesions termed "nevi with focal atypical epithelioid component" or "clonal" or "combined" nevi, and also "inverted type A nevi," all represent variants of

DPN, combined with other nevi (225). These distinctions are of potential importance in determining need for complete excision (see later), although the key distinction is from melanoma.

Histopathology. At scanning magnification, the lesions are circumscribed and pyramidal in shape, with a broad base abutting the epidermis, and an apex extending and pushing into or toward the fat (Fig. 28-12). Nests of nevus cells at the dermal–epidermal junction are usually present. The dermal component is comprised of loosely arranged nests or plexiform fascicles of large lightly pigmented spindle and epithelioid cells interspersed with melanophages. There is a tendency to form narrow spindle cells at the periphery of the nests, reminiscent of sustentacular cell differentiation. In many cases, there is an admixture of smaller, more conventional nevus cells. The lesional nests tend to surround skin appendages and to infiltrate the collagen at the periphery of the lesion. The cells do not tend to "mature" with descent into the dermis. Some lesions have a patchy mild lymphocytic infiltrate.

At higher magnification, nuclear pleomorphism may be striking in some lesions, with variation in size and shape, hyperchromasia, and nuclear pseudo inclusions. The atypia tends to be confined to randomly scattered cells rather than being "uniform" or present in most of the cells. Nucleoli are usually inconspicuous, although a few large eosinophilic nucleoli may be observed. Importantly, mitoses are absent or very rare, with no more than one or two in multiple sections of any given lesion. The cytoplasm is abundant and contains finely divided brown melanin pigment. The lesional cells react positively and diffusely for S-100 protein, Sox10, and HMB-45 antigen (the latter representing a distinct difference from common acquired nevi) and also for beta-catenin (Fig. 28-13). The constitutive activation and overexpression of beta-catenin mimics *WNT* signaling from keratinocytes and can account for both the larger cell size and the increased pigment that characterize DPN (221).

Some lesions in the general category of DPN have histologic features that overlap with those of melanomas, including a tendency to sheetlike rather than nested fascicular differentiation, the presence of more than a rare mitosis, and increasing degrees and greater uniformity of atypia. Some of these lesions have recurred locally, metastasized to regional nodes, or, in rare

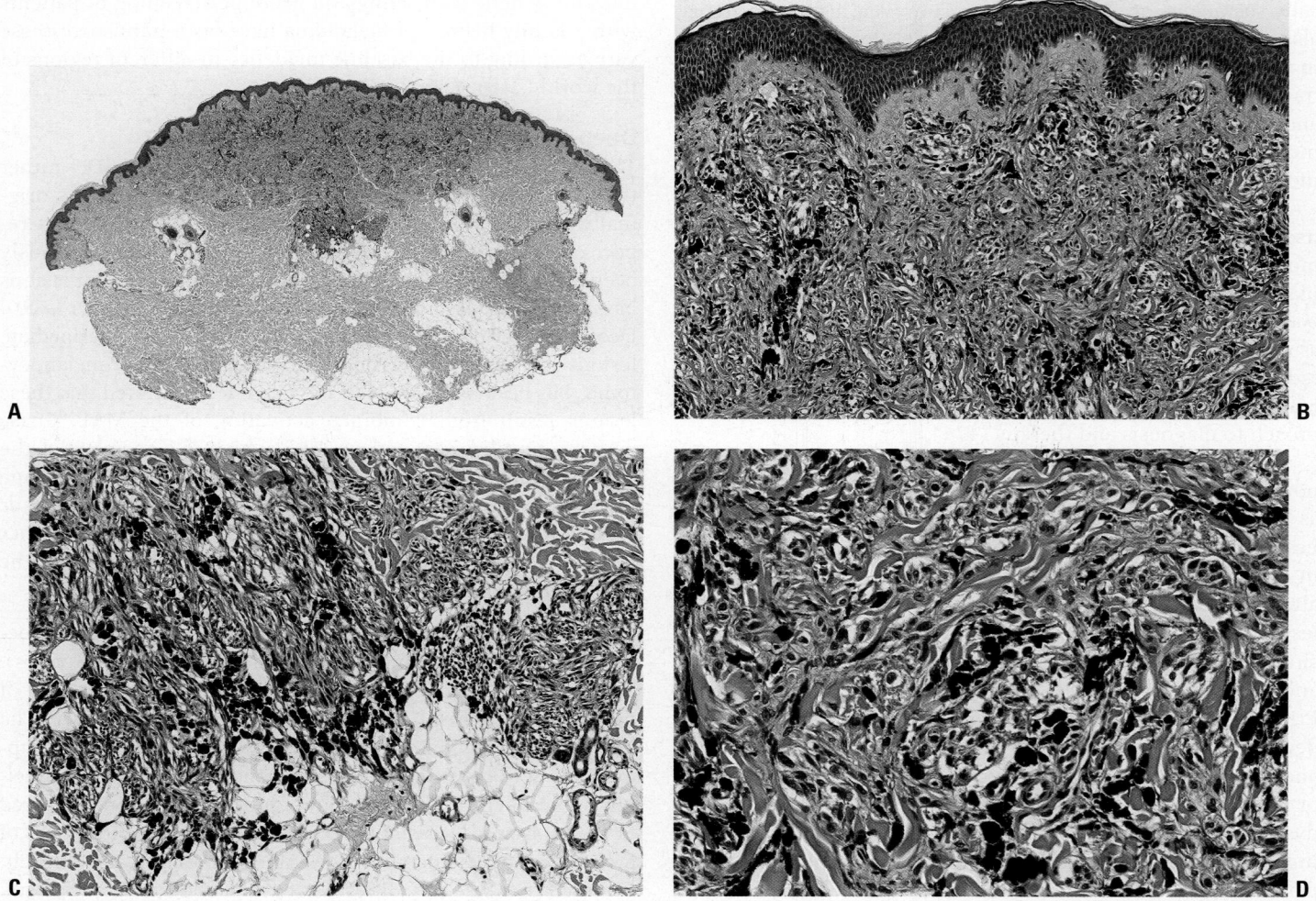

Figure 28-12 Deep-penetrating nevus. **A:** At scanning magnification, the lesion is pyramidal, with its base applied to the epidermis, and its apex in the reticular dermis. **B:** The lesional cells in the dermis are arranged in nests and plexiform fascicles. They may be heavily pigmented, and there may be scattered large, hyperchromatic, and pleomorphic nuclei, constituting "random" cytologic atypia. Mitoses are absent, or very rare. **C:** The lesions may span the reticular dermis and involve the subcutis. **D:** Scattered lesional cells may be enlarged, irregular, and hyperchromatic, constituting "random" cytologic atypia. There may be a suggestion of sustentacular cell differentiation at the periphery of some of the nests. Mitotic figures are absent in most lesions, or very rare.

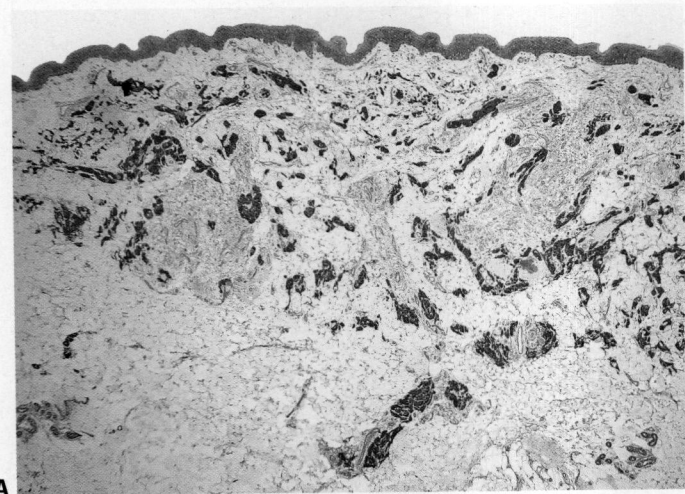
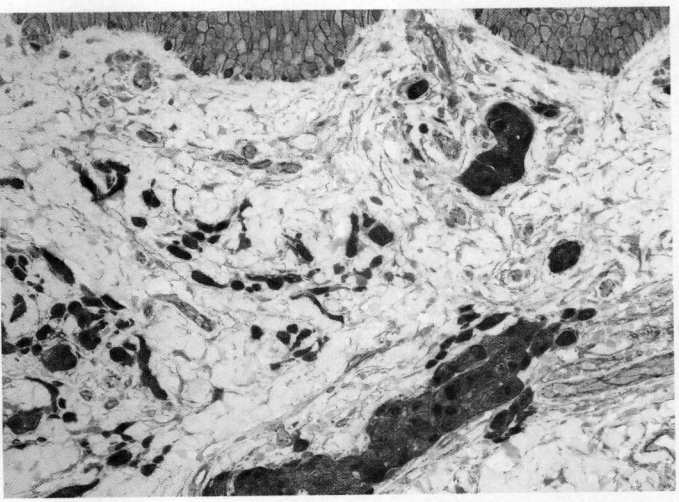

Figure 28-13 Deep-penetrating nevus stain for beta-catenin. **A:** There is a tumor comprised of plexiform fascicles extending with a pyramidal silhouette from the epidermis into the subcutis at the base. **B:** The lesional cells stain intensely for beta-catenin with nuclear as well as cytoplasmic staining. Note membrane staining in overlying keratinocytes.

cases, perhaps beyond. Such lesions have been placed into a category of "borderline melanocytic tumors" (226) or may be considered as "MELTUMP" (227). In DPN-like melanomas, copy number alterations and mutations in *TERT* promoter and p53 have been identified (221,228), in one case with a prominent UV signature (228). It may be pertinent that these lesions have had the less common *NRAS* or *MAP21K* (rather than *BRAF*) driver mutations.

Differential Diagnosis. DPN can be distinguished from *nodular melanoma* by architectural and cytologic features. Most bulky tumorigenic melanomas exhibit a more striking pattern of epidermal involvement with spread of atypical cells into the epidermis and often with ulceration. Melanomas are likely to be more broad than deep, while DPN tend to be vertically oriented, like Spitz nevi. Tumorigenic melanomas usually exhibit a more destructive pattern of infiltration, with displacement and compression of the stroma, and often with necrosis. Most also display marked nuclear atypia with frequent and often abnormal mitoses. A few nodular spindle cell melanomas have lower-grade nuclear atypia, and in these cases the presence of more than a few mitoses may be decisive. In this respect, a study found rates of expression of the cell cycle proliferation marker PCNA to be somewhat higher in DPN than in ordinary banal nevi but considerably lower than in melanomas (229).

Benign lesions that may show some tendency toward overlapping features with DPN include common and cellular blue nevi, as well as spindle and epithelioid cell nevi, and some clonal or combined nevi. Although DPN can usually be distinguished from these benign or low-grade lesions, the distinction from melanoma is of the greatest importance. Neural involvement may occur and is not an indicator of malignancy in these lesions. As previously indicated, some lesions termed "inverted type A nevi" likely represent the same entity as DPN (230).

Principles of Management: Although most DPN will have a benign clinical course, sufficient numbers have not been studied, in our opinion, to ensure this with certainty, and complete excision is recommended for such lesions (79,231). As with Spitz nevi, this approach also minimizes the possibility of local recurrence of a nevus variant with intrinsically unusual features in scar tissue, a situation at potential risk for overdiagnosis and overtreatment as outright melanoma.

Pigmented Epithelioid Melanocytoma

This heavily pigmented melanocytic tumor resembles lesions that were formerly termed animal-type melanoma as well as epithelioid blue nevi, as seen in Carney complex (232,233), and are also said to be impossible to distinguish from the epithelioid blue nevi seen in Carney complex (232,234). Mutations of the Protein Kinase CAMP-Dependent Type I Regulatory Subunit Alpha) (R1alpha) (coded by the *PRKAR1A* gene) are found in more than half of Carney patients. In an immunohistochemical study, R1alpha was lost in 8 epithelioid blue nevi from patients with Carney complex and in 28 of 34 PEMs but not in 297 other melanocytic tumors or in 5 equine melanomas. These data support the concept that PEM is a distinct melanocytic tumor that may occur in a sporadic setting and in the Carney complex and that it differs from melanomas in equine melanotic disease. Thus, the term animal-type melanoma is inappropriate. Loss of expression of R1alpha represents a useful diagnostic test to help distinguish PEM from lesions that may mimic it histologically (235).

Clinical Summary. This lesion affects males and females about equally, most commonly in the third decade, and over a wide age range, including young children and older adults. The lesions may present as a blue or black nodule, and the clinical impression may include seborrheic keratosis, congenital nevus, blue nevus, and melanoma. Multiple body sites may be affected, with extremities being the most common (232).

Histopathology. Histologically, there is a deep dermal nodule of heavily pigmented epithelioid and/or spindled melanocytes (Fig. 28-14), and some lesions occur in combination with other nevi. Ulceration may be present in occasional lesions, a finding generally not present in conventional epithelioid blue nevi. The characteristic cell type has abundant cytoplasm with variable pigment, and a large nucleus with pale chromatin, a regular ovoid nuclear membrane, and a prominent eosinophilic nucleolus (Fig. 28-14D). There is an admixture of (usually more

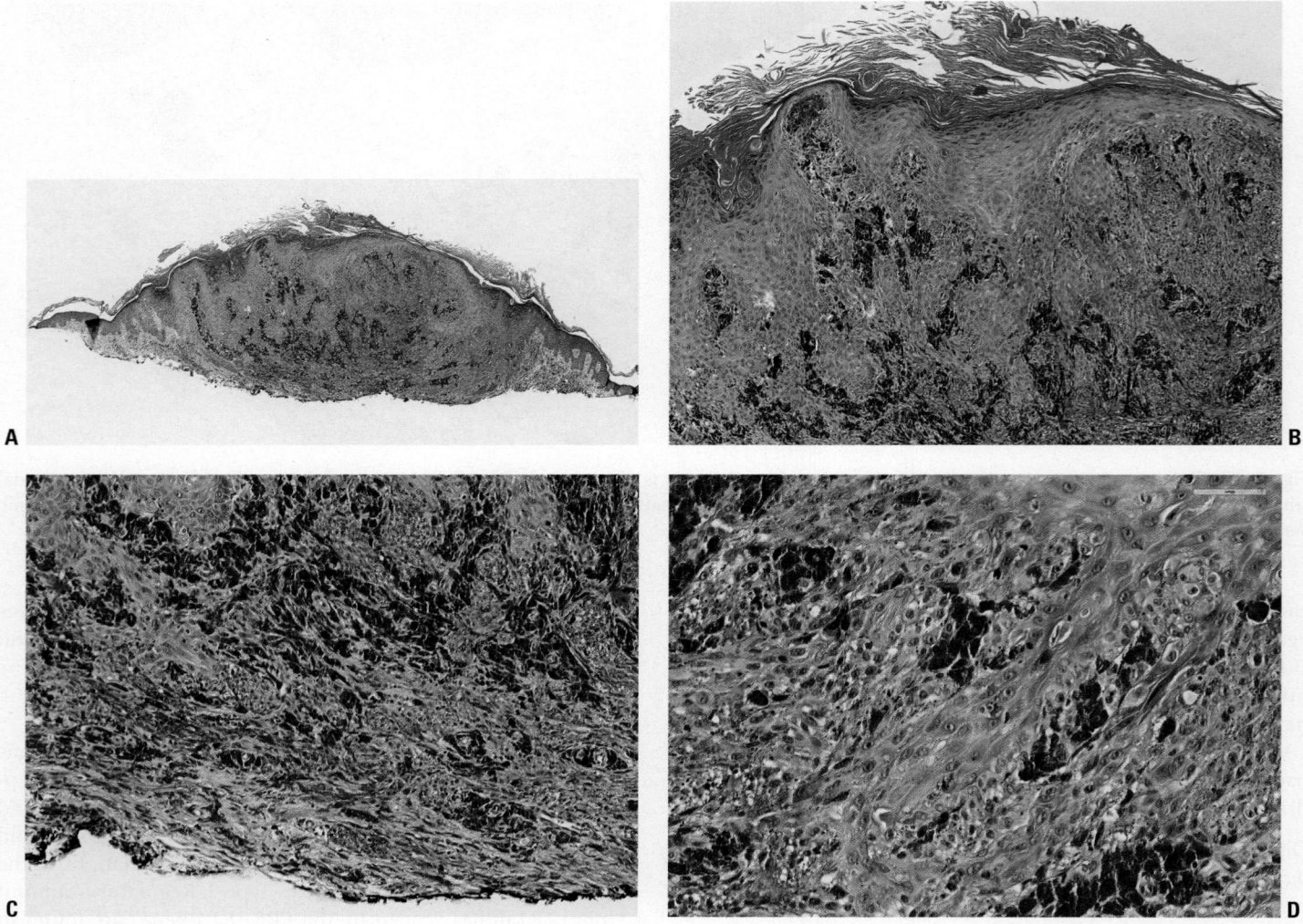

Figure 28-14 Pigmented epithelioid melanocytoma/PEM/epithelioid blue nevus. **A:** There is a heavily pigmented tumor extending from the epidermis into the reticular dermis. **B:** The epidermis is markedly hyperplastic. **C:** The lesional cells contain pigment, although to a lesser extent than in some examples of this condition. Mitoses are rare or absent. There is an admixture of melanophages. **D:** The lesional cells have characteristic cytology, with regular nuclei, pale chromatin, and prominent nucleoli. Mitoses are rare or absent.

heavily) pigmented melanophages. Although tumor cells may be quite bland and mitoses and necrosis inconspicuous or absent, regional lymph node involvement has been seen in 46% of cases studied. However, there have been no deaths. Similar lesions have been designated as "pigment synthesizing melanoma" (PSM) and regarded as a "low-grade" form of melanoma that may lack some of the signs of more aggressive melanomas of similar bulk, such as frequent mitoses, ulceration, and high-grade atypia (236). Metastases were not observed in the cases of epithelioid blue nevi seen in association with the Carney complex, which is a multiple neoplasia syndrome featuring cardiac, endocrine, cutaneous, and neural tumors, as well as a variety of pigmented lesions of the skin and mucosae, including lentigines, epithelioid blue nevi, and psammomatous melanocytic schwannoma (237).

Pigmented Epithelioid Melanoma/PRKAR1A-Inactivated Melanoma. The concept of melanocytoma implies that this group of lesions, with at least two mutations, may have a somewhat greater propensity to progress to melanoma than ordinary nevi, which have only a single mutation. A few lesions have been described that meet criteria for "PEM-like melanoma," or

"pigmented epithelioid melanoma." Cohen et al. described six cases of melanomas with inactivating mutations of *PRKAR1A*, terming them "*PRKAR1A*-inactivated melanomas." Collectively, these exhibited increased cellularity and mitotic activity, and one had a large area of necrosis. Melanocytes consistently outnumbered melanophages, a difference from usual PEM. Four of the six melanomas had *BRAF* V600E and *TERT* promoter mutations and chromosomal copy number changes typical of melanoma. Two tumors lacking *TERTp* mutations but with increased cellularity and p16 loss were classified as high-grade *PRKAR1A*-inactivated melanocytomas (233). In an archival search of 4,770 melanocytic neoplasms, Williams et al. found inactivating genomic abnormalities (GA) in *PRKAR1A* in 42 cases. Of these, 34 cases were melanoma, 6 were melanoma *in situ*, and 2 were melanocytomas. Among the melanomas, 94% had a pathogenic GA in *TERT* promoter, *CDKN2A*, or both; 50% were mutated in *BRAF* (10/17 *BRAF* V600E) 20% *NRAS*, 18% *NF1* and 18% were wild-type. Half of the melanomas with available histology had large epithelioid and dendritic melanocytes with prominent nucleoli, gray-blue cytoplasm, and abundant melanin pigment arranged in large confluent nests and fascicles, consistent with features described in PEM (238). In a similar case that we have seen, although lacking genomic classification, there was hypercellularity, with melanocytes focally outnumbering melanophages, a mitotic rate of 6 per mm^2, and loss of p16 protein by IHC. This lesion metastasized widely, including to bone and liver, and proved to be fatal in this young woman.

Principles of Management: These lesions should be completely excised. Sentinel node staging, although reasonable to consider, cannot be considered standard of care, because a positive sentinel node does not appear to be associated with a bad outcome in usual PEM (232). Well-documented "PEM-like melanomas" should likely be managed according to protocols for usual cutaneous melanoma.

BAP1 Inactivated Melanocytic Tumors (BIMT)

In 2011, Wiesner and colleagues described two families with a new autosomal dominant syndrome characterized by multiple, skin-colored, elevated melanocytic tumors (239). Differing from common acquired nevi, these neoplasms ranged from epithelioid nevi to atypical proliferations that had overlapping features with melanoma. Some affected individuals developed uveal or cutaneous melanomas. Segregating with this phenotype, they found inactivating germline mutations of *BRCA1*-associated protein (*BAP1*), a gene that encodes a ubiquitin carboxy-terminal hydrolase, with most of the atypical melanocytic neoplasms having lost the remaining wild-type allele through somatic alterations. In addition, *BAP1* mutations were identified in a subset of sporadic melanocytic neoplasms bearing histologic similarities to the familial tumors. Initially, the lesions were considered as a form of Spitz nevus/tumor (240). However, these lesions are now considered to be a discrete diagnostic entity, which has been described by a number of terms, including Wiesner nevus, nevoid melanoma-like melanocytic proliferation (NEMMP), *BAP1* mutant Spitz nevus, *BAP1* mutant nevoid melanoma, cutaneous BAPoma, and, more recently, cutaneous *BAP1 inactivated melanocytic tumor*, or BIMT (241), or BAP1-inactivated nevus/melanocytoma. The *BAP1* tumor predisposition syndrome was described by Haugh et al. in 215 patients, 28% of whom had uveal melanoma, 22% mesothelioma, 18% cutaneous melanoma, 17% cutaneous BIMTs, 9% renal cell carcinoma, and 14% basal cell carcinoma (242). Patients with a germline *BAP1* mutation develop cancers at an earlier age and often display cancer clustering, and they often have multiple cutaneous BIMTs.

Clinical Features. Clinically, the lesions are well-circumscribed, symmetrical, dome-shaped, or pedunculated red-brown papules with a shiny surface and an average diameter of about 5 mm (241). Most of the lesions seen in practice are sporadic and represent an isolated phenomenon, occurring in children or adults most commonly in the second or third decades. Patients with the germline syndrome may have many such lesions. When a BIMT is diagnosed, the patient should be evaluated for other similar lesions, especially when presenting in younger individuals.

Histopathology. There are two major histologic patterns. In one, lesions present as a *de novo* homogeneous nodule composed of large epithelioid cells. These cells have abundant eosinophilic glassy cytoplasm, with moderate nuclear variability and sometimes a prominent lymphocytic infiltrate. The mitotic rate is usually low. The morphology of the lesional cells has been

variously described as Spitzoid, as epithelioid (with larger or with smaller cells), or as having rhabdoid cytologic features. In the other presentation, the lesion presents as a form of *combined nevus*, with a nodule comprised of cells similar to those in the monophasic variant, associated with background nevus cells generally of the small congenital pattern type, being comprised of nevoid to epithelioid melanocytes that have evidence of maturation to a smaller cell type and disperse into reticular dermis collagen at the base (Fig. 28-15). The nodule may be dominant and may almost obscure the background nevus. These lesions likely account for most nevi/tumors formerly thought to represent combined Spitz and acquired/congenital pattern nevi (because the driver mutations are different in Spitz and acquired nevi, any such lesion would have to a true collision tumor, which must be very rare). It has been observed that tumors arising from germline mutation are more likely to demonstrate an extensive junctional component of BAP1-activated melanocytes (243).

Histogenesis. Although the tumors were at first considered to be in a category of Spitz tumors, they are now placed in the "low CSD" pathway of melanocytic tumors, because most of them have a *BRAFV600E* driver mutation, followed by loss of the tumor suppressor *BAP1* (244).

Differential Diagnosis. Although they may be quite Spitzoid in appearance, these lesions differ in several ways from Spitz nevi/tumors. The cytology is usually more purely epithelioid rather than spindle and/or epithelioid, and there are no Kamino bodies and typically no prominent clefting between nests and adjacent keratinocytes. This distinction may be of importance in cases where a germline mutation could be suspected. Lesions need to be distinguished from melanomas, which will usually have more prominent mitotic activity and may also show ulceration and necrosis. In addition, these lesions do not have an adjacent RGP/*in situ* component. Melanoma arising in a *BAP1*-inactivated melanocytic tumor can be recognized by usual criteria, including those mentioned in the previous sentence. Nodules similar to those seen in *BAP1*-inactivated may also be encountered that lack evidence for *BAP1* inactivation. These may be regarded as nonspecific cellular nodules. Their course is typically benign, although there have been cases that have recurred locally, sometimes with increased atypia, following incomplete excision (245). Of note, a case has been described in which there was a highly characteristic BIMT morphology with preserved *BAP1* expression, and additional investigation revealed a chromosome 3 loss with a deletion of one copy of BAP1 and with a possible functional disruption of the remaining allele, which did not alter its protein expression or nuclear localization as observed by IHC (246). Therefore, especially in an individual with other indicators of a possible germline syndrome who has an apparent BAP1 inactivated lesion but with retained expression, more sophisticated genomic investigation may be indicated.

Management. The lesions are best treated by complete excision because, by virtue of having at least two mutations, they are considered to be melanocytomas with a somewhat increased, although still low, risk of progression to melanoma (231). Although most cases encountered in practice are sporadic, the germline syndrome should be considered in any individual with two or more cutaneous BIMTs and/or a family history of

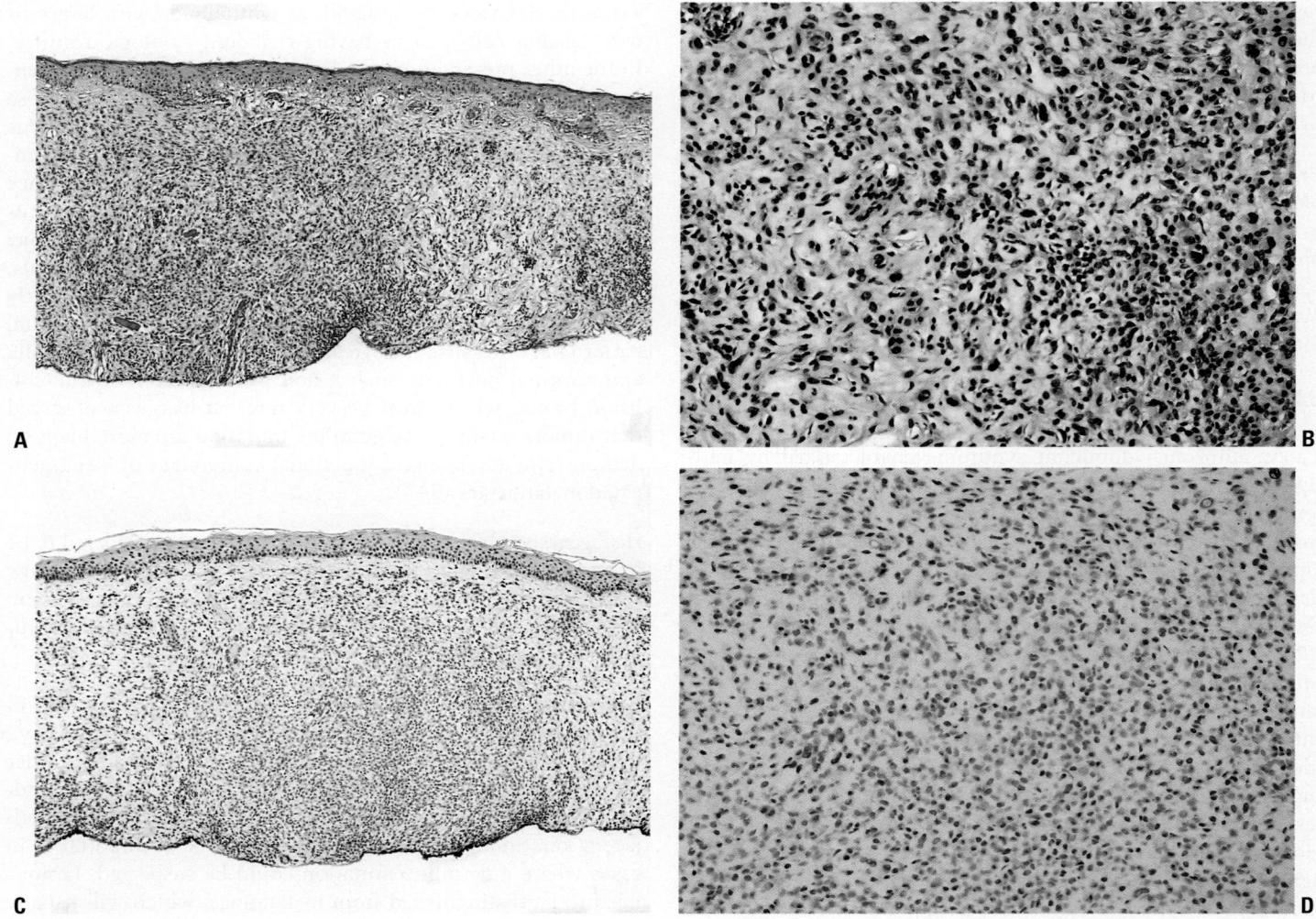

Figure 28-15 Combined BAP1 inactivated and congenital pattern nevus. A: In this case, there is a relatively ill-defined nodule within a background compound nevus. B: The nodule is comprised of larger cells, with moderately abundant epithelioid cytoplasm, blending with the background nevus cells at the bottom right corner. C, D: There is absence of staining for BAP1 in the cells of the nodule, with staining present in background nevus cells and in normal controls, including keratinocytes.

mesothelioma or cutaneous or uveal melanoma, and such patients should be referred for genetic counseling (243).

Combined Nevus/Melanocytoma

Introduction. Combined nevi contain two or more morphologically distinct melanocytic nevus components. Any combination could be envisaged, but, traditionally, combined nevi most often involve the common nevus component combined with a blue nevus, deep-penetrating nevus (DPM), or Spitz nevus component. Synonyms for combined nevi have included clonal nevus; melanocytic nevus with phenotypic heterogeneity; nevus with dermal epithelioid component; inverted type A nevus; nevus with atypical dermal nodules; combined *BAP1*-inactivated nevus; Wiesner nevus; *BAP1* deficient tumor; melanocytic *BAP1* mutated atypical intradermal tumor (247–249).

Clinical Features. Combined nevi are usually well-circumscribed papules with a diameter of less than 6 mm. They usually have two or more colors ranging from skin-colored reddish-pink or brown to black and blue. The exact morphology depends on the combination of nevic elements. Combined nevus with a blue nevus-like component or a DPM component will typically have a bluish-black focus within a background tan, dome-shaped

nevus. Combined BAP1-inactivated nevi are usually skin colored to red-pink, dome-shaped papules with a shiny surface, sometimes with a brown rim, which represents a background congenital pattern nevus. Patients sometimes report a sudden change in a long-standing nevus, likely representing the onset of the second component (247). The lesions most commonly occur on the head and neck, followed by the trunk and limbs. The conjunctiva is said to be a common site for combined nevi with a DPN component (222).

Histogenesis. Conceptually, a combined nevus could result from a collision between two different types of nevus, and this is most likely the mechanism whereby a common nevus is combined with a blue nevus because these lesions typically arise through disparate genomic pathways (3). It is possible that some might develop by divergent cellular differentiation triggered by genetic or environmental factors. More recently, it has been clearly demonstrated that combined nevi may arise by sequential acquisition of genomic alterations. Three such categories have been defined, namely, combined nevus, where ordinary nevus is associated with DPN; PEM; or *BAP1*-inactivated nevus (BIN) components. Typically, these second components arise in a preexisting small to intermediate banal nevus, often of the "congenital pattern" type. Most of these nevi are actually acquired rather than truly congenital, and they most commonly have a mutation or other genomic abnormality in *BRAFV600E*, or sometimes *NRAS*. Combined nevi with DPN features result from an activating genomic abnormality in beta-catenin or its pathway, those with a PEM component have an activating genomic abnormality in the pathway that includes *PRKAR1alpha*, and *BAP1*-inactivated nevi have lost expression of BAP1 in the clone that develops as a cellular nodule within the preexisting nevus that retains expression in the cells of the background nevus. It is likely that many lesions previously thought to represent combined nevi with a Spitz nevus component would be reclassified as BAP1-inactivated nevi today because these lesions arise through disparate pathways (3).

Histopathology. The histologic appearances vary with the combinations of nevus types. The most common form of combined nevi includes an ordinary nevocellular nevus combined with DPN (248). The combined nevus with a DPN component is comprised focally of spindled to epithelioid cells arranged in nests and plexiform fascicles, with an admixture of pigmented melanophages (Fig. 28-16). As is also true in PEM and *BAP1*-inactivated types of combined nevi, there may be evidence of blending between the two cell types, perhaps reflecting that the second cell type has arisen as a subclone of the first. These DPN components have likely been confused with blue nevi in the past. Combined nevi with blue nevus components might have a more stratified expression where ordinary nevic components are superficial to underlying blue nevus cells. These conditions (DPN, PEM, BIN, and also Spitz nevi and blue nevi are discussed further in their own sections).

Differential Diagnosis. The most important differential is with a nodular melanoma arising in a nevus (247,248). Distinguishing features in favor of a combined nevus include a generally younger age at presentation, a diameter of less than or equal to 6 mm, less than 1 mitosis per mm², low cellularity, "monomorphous" cytologic atypia, no ulceration or necrosis, little to no solar elastosis, and no pagetoid scatter or other patterns of melanoma *in situ*. Although the lesions are, by their nature, asymmetrical, each component of the lesion tends to have its own symmetry. Nodular melanoma arising in a nevus tends to

compress the adjacent nevus, whereas the cellular nodules in combined nevi tend not to have a growth advantage over the background nevus and not to compress it (247).

MALIGNANT MELANOMA

Most malignant melanomas arise in the epidermis, and these may be *in situ* (entirely within the epidermis) or may be invasive (extending from the epidermis into the dermis). Occasional invasive melanomas are entirely dermal at presentation. Invasive melanoma may be tumorigenic (VGP) or nontumorigenic (RGP). In the current WHO classification, CSD is an important classifier because it correlates with etiologic, pathogenic, and genomic differences among the melanomas (4). CSD is evaluated in terms of solar elastosis and graded on a scale of mild, moderate, to severe (3). The morphologic classification is based on CSD and the presence or absence and the subtypes of the RGP. Melanoma *in situ* and nontumorigenic invasive melanomas are divided into (a) superficial spreading (low CSD WHO 2018)), (b) lentigo maligna (high CSD), (c) acral-lentiginous, and (d) mucosal lentiginous types, the latter two of which are not associated with CSD. Tumorigenic melanoma may arise in relation to a preexisting nontumorigenic component of any of the foregoing types, in which case it is named accordingly. Alternatively, tumorigenic melanoma may arise *de novo*, without evidence of an adjacent *in situ* or microinvasive component at the time of detection, in which case it is termed (e) "nodular melanoma." Some, if not all, of these lesions probably arise initially via a nontumorigenic intraepidermal component that fails to develop or persist as the tumorigenic component evolves. Important variants of tumorigenic melanoma include (f) DM, a high CSD melanoma, and (g) neurotropic melanoma. Other unusual forms of tumorigenic melanoma will be discussed in later sections.

In a recent study from Australia, superficial spreading (57.2%), lentigo maligna (20.8%), and nodular (12.2%) were the most common histopathologic subtypes of melanoma (250). The relative incidence of LMM is lower in less sunny climates.

All major types of melanoma originate almost invariably from melanocytes at the epidermal–dermal junction. Although in the case of SSM the lesions are commonly associated with a preexisting

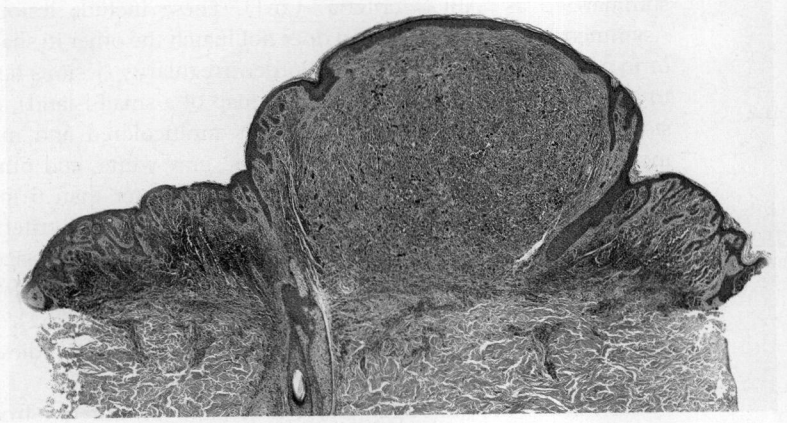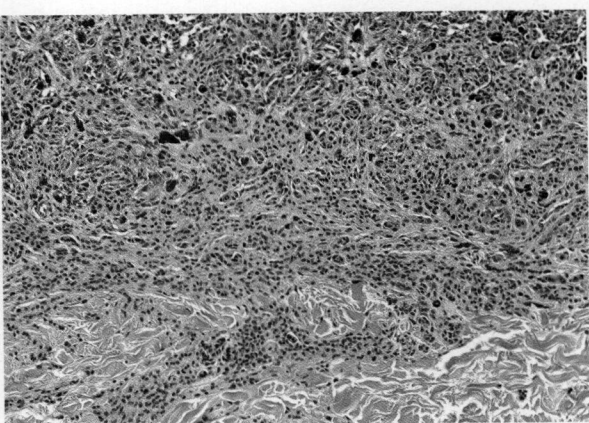

Figure 28-16 Combined nevus with deep-penetrating and congenital pattern nevus components. **A:** There is a plaquelike background nevus with a prominent nodular component, centrally placed in this example. **B:** The nodular component is comprised of pigmented cells with admixed melanophages, arranged in a plexiform pattern and tending to blend with the background nevus, which is comprised of small nevoid cells extending into the reticular dermis at the base. The DPN component is somewhat more cellular than average in this example; however, there is no extensive confluent proliferation, necrosis, mitotic activity, or other evidence of malignancy.

nevus, more than half of them arise either *de novo* from fields of precursor melanocytes or have completely supplanted the precursor nevus at the time of presentation. Most cutaneous melanomas are thought to be caused by sunlight exposure, either intermittent (sunburn episodes) in the more common SSMs, or chronic, in the LMMs. The cause of acral and mucosal melanomas is unknown.

Phases of Melanoma Progression in Relation to Classification

There are two major "phases" of melanoma development, which represent sequential stages of stepwise tumor progression (251). In the nontumorigenic *radial* or *horizontal growth phase*, the neoplastic melanocytes (melanoma cells) are confined to the epidermis (melanoma *in situ*) or to the epidermis and papillary dermis without evidence of proliferation in the dermis and without formation of an expansile tumor mass; such lesions constitute "microinvasive melanoma." This phase may be followed after varying lengths of time by the focal appearance of the mitogenic and/or tumorigenic *VGP*, which is a phase of dermal invasion with the capacity not only for cell survival but also for proliferation in the dermis and usually with expansile tumor formation. Thus, a fully evolved melanoma may have two major lesional "compartments": the nontumorigenic, *in situ*, or microinvasive RGP, in which there may have developed a contiguous tumorigenic VGP compartment. In addition, dermal and/or epidermal compartments of an associated nevus may be recognized in some melanomas. Variants of each of the major compartments have been described and are listed in Table 28-7 (251–254).

About 10% of melanomas in different series fall into "unclassified" or "other" categories (255). The fact that categorization of an individual case is occasionally difficult does not mean that classification of melanoma, after accounting for tumor thickness and site, is of no value, as has been argued by some (256). Even though in the tumorigenic stage, the prognosis is

similar for all four types of melanoma, depending largely on the depth of invasion, the epidemiology, age of onset and the pace of progression differ among the various forms (257). Furthermore, there are differences in the apparent etiology of the various forms of melanoma, as well as in their genomic landscapes (4).

In a study of phenotypic–genotypic correlations, attributes traditionally used in the classification of melanomas into the clinicopathologic subtypes mentioned previously correlated strongly with the mutation status of the tumors studied. An algorithm involving an initial separation based on melanoma cell nesting and scatter, followed by consideration of cell size and age-predicted BRAF mutation with an error estimate of 13%, demonstrated that parameters routinely available and traditionally used by practicing pathologists allow for good prediction of BRAF mutation status. It was concluded that this "strong association between genetic alterations and morphologic findings further supports the existence of biologically distinct melanoma types, and the use of genetic factors to develop and clarify improved clinically applicable classification systems" (258,259).

Finally, in our opinion, the separate description of the morphologic variants has nosologic and pedagogical value, facilitating accurate diagnosis by enabling the recognition of the variant patterns.

A classification of melanoma based on site/etiologic and genomic considerations was proposed by Bastian (445) and most recently developed in the 2018 *WHO Classification of Skin Tumors*, as recently summarized (4,244). In this schema, the major categories of nonocular melanomas are (a) melanomas on skin with lower CSD, broadly corresponding to SSM; (b) melanomas on skin with high CSD broadly corresponding to LMM; (c) Spitz melanoma; (d) acral melanomas; (e) mucosal melanomas; (f) melanomas occurring in congenital nevi; and (g) melanomas occurring in blue nevi (Table 28-2, p. 836).

Tumorigenic and Nontumorigenic Melanoma

In their nontumorigenic stage, melanomas tend to expand more or less inexorably along the radii of an imperfect circle, as viewed clinically. The clinically derived term "radial" growth has no intuitive histologic meaning, and the more visually meaningful (to histopathologists) histologic term "horizontal growth phase" has been suggested as an alternative (260).

Clinical Summary. The major clinical diagnostic criteria have been summarized as "ABCD criteria" (261). These include lesional Asymmetry (one-half of a lesion does not match the other in shape or in color distribution), lesional Border irregularity (lesions tend to have an indented coastline like the map of a small island), lesional Color variegation (the surface is multicolored and may include shades of tan, brown, blue-black, gray-white, and other variations), and lesional Diameter generally greater than 6 mm (though some melanomas are smaller) (Fig. 28-17). These criteria, although useful, are imperfect; recent guidelines have emphasized the value of the "ugly duckling" sign of the changing or different-looking mole in the practice of skin self-examination (262). In view of this, the letter E could be added to the criteria to indicate the "Evolving" nature of a changing melanocytic lesion.

Clinically, the tumorigenic VGP is qualitatively different from the plaquelike RGP. The tumor appears as an expanding papule within a previously indolent or slowly enlarging plaque lesion and grows in three dimensions in a balloon-like fashion to form a nodule (Fig. 28-17). Typically, the ABCD criteria do not apply to the tumor nodule itself, which is commonly symmetrical, with smooth borders. The color of the nodule is often quite uniform

---

Table 28-7
Classification of Melanoma Based on Growth Phase and Morphology
Radial Growth Phase (RGP)
Nontumorigenic Melanoma
In *Situ* or Microinvasive
Superficial spreading melanoma (SSM, low CSD* Melanoma)
Lentigo maligna melanoma (LMM, high CSD* melanoma)
Acral-lentiginous melanoma (ALM)
Unclassified radial growth phase (URGP)
Vertical Growth Phase (VGP)
Tumorigenic Melanoma
RGP Compartment Present (may be SSM, LMM, ALM, URGP)
Usual VGP
Desmoplastic VGP, many are also neurotropic
Neurotropic, not desmoplastic
VGP Present, No RGP Compartment
Nodular melanoma (NM)

*CSD, cumulative solar damage, assessed by the extent of solar elastosis.

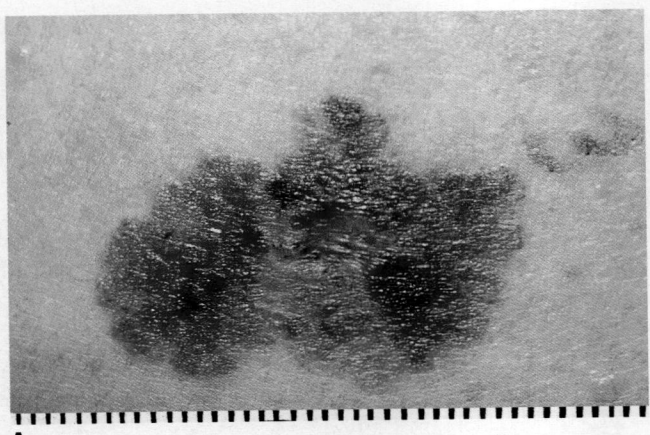

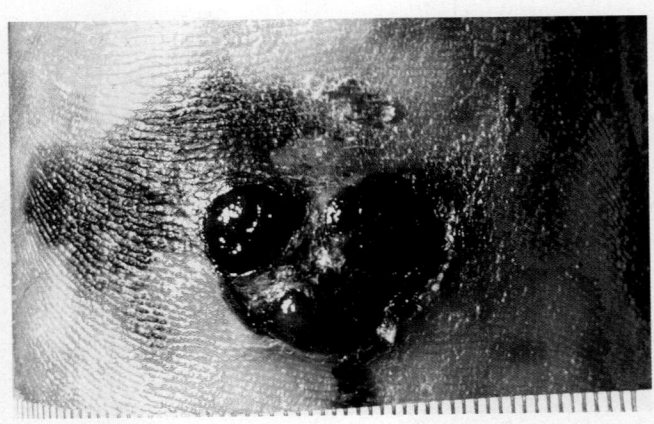

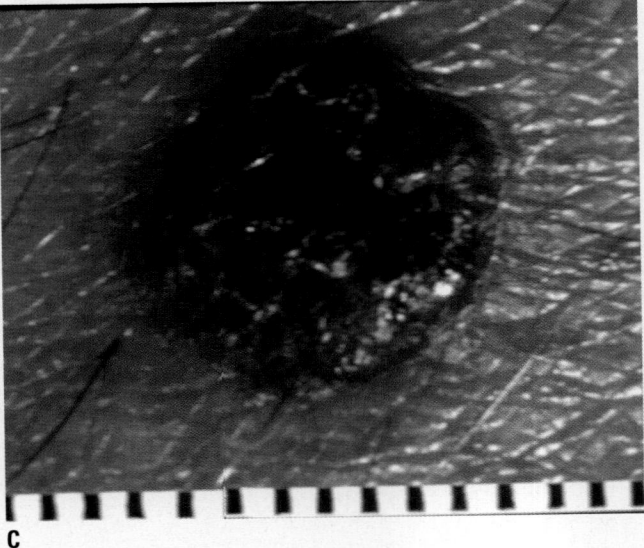

Figure 28-17 Clinical images of melanomas. **A:** Superficial spreading melanoma, nontumorigenic, radial growth phase (RGP) only (microinvasive), with focal regression. The lesion is large, asymmetric, with irregular border, and variegated colors, including reddish brown and focal areas of blue-black, as well as a focal grayish area of partial RGP regression (near the middle of the lesion). This morphology could overlap with that of the severely dysplastic nevus in Figure 28-10B. Each of these lesions is sufficiently atypical that it should be considered for excision for pathologic diagnosis. **B:** Acral-lentiginous melanoma, tumorigenic, with extensive RGP, partial regression of the RGP, and a bulky ulcerated tumorigenic vertical growth phase nodule (VGP). **C:** Nodular melanoma. The tumorigenic VGP nodule, lacking an adjacent RGP by definition, is relatively small, symmetrical, and uniform in color. The focally ulcerated surface may lead to presenting symptoms of bleeding and oozing, which are signs of a relatively advanced melanoma.

and may be pink rather than blue-black, and the diameter of the focus of VGP is often less than 6 mm, even in a quite high-risk lesion. For these reasons, clinical diagnosis of melanoma may be subtle in a nodular melanoma that lacks an adjacent nontumorigenic compartment, prompting the suggestion to add "EFG" to supplant Evolving (Elevated, Firm, and Growing for 1 month) to the widely used ABCD acronym to improve detection of this dangerous phase of melanoma progression (263) (Fig. 28-17C).

Histopathology. Histologically, most of the lesional cells in the nontumorigenic melanomas are located in the epidermis. Microinvasion is here defined as the presence of a few lesional cells in the papillary dermis, without "tumorigenic proliferation," which is defined elsewhere in this chapter. Microinvasive lesions are not specifically distinguishable from *in situ* melanomas on clinical grounds. These microinvasive and *in situ*, nontumorigenic melanomas lack competence for metastasis on complete excision; in a database of 624 clinical Stage I invasive melanoma cases followed 10 years or more, the 8-year survival rate from 161 microinvasive or *in situ* (pure RGP) melanomas was 100% ± 1%. In the same database, the patients with lesions having only RGP were 4.3 years younger than those additionally having VGP, consistent with the hypothesis that the RGP is antecedent to VGP, and relatively indolent (171,264).

The major histologic feature that distinguishes a tumorigenic melanoma is the capacity for proliferation of melanoma cells in the extracellular matrix of the dermis to form an expansile mass. In contrast, nontumorigenic melanoma cells may proliferate

inexorably in the epidermal compartment and may invade the dermis but do not proliferate there (Fig. 28-18). The lack of metastatic capacity in nontumorigenic melanomas may be explained by considering that cell proliferation in the extracellular matrix of a distant site is essential to the development of a metastasis. Thus, it is likely that a tumor that cannot proliferate in the matrix at its local site of origin would also not do so in a metastatic site. Operational definitions for tumorigenic and nontumorigenic melanoma and for RGP and VGP are as follows (172,264).

Tumorigenic Melanoma. A mass of melanoma cells is present in the dermis, defined as at least one cluster (nest) in the dermis that is larger than the largest intraepidermal cluster (indicative of a tumor with capacity for expansile growth in the dermis) (Fig. 28-18).

Nontumorigenic Melanoma. No mass of melanoma cells is present in the dermis (there is no cluster larger than the largest intraepidermal cluster) (Fig. 28-18C).

VGP. A lesion is classified as VGP if it is tumorigenic, or if there are any dermal mitoses even in the absence of architectural criteria for tumorigenic growth (i.e., mitogenic melanoma). The presence of any mitoses in the dermal component of the melanoma is indicative of a tumor with capacity for expansile growth in the dermis and defines the concept of typical VGP even in the absence of a frank tumor mass (Fig. 28-19).

RGP. A lesion is classified as radial growth phase only ("pure" RGP or "radial growth phase confined") if it is nontumorigenic and there

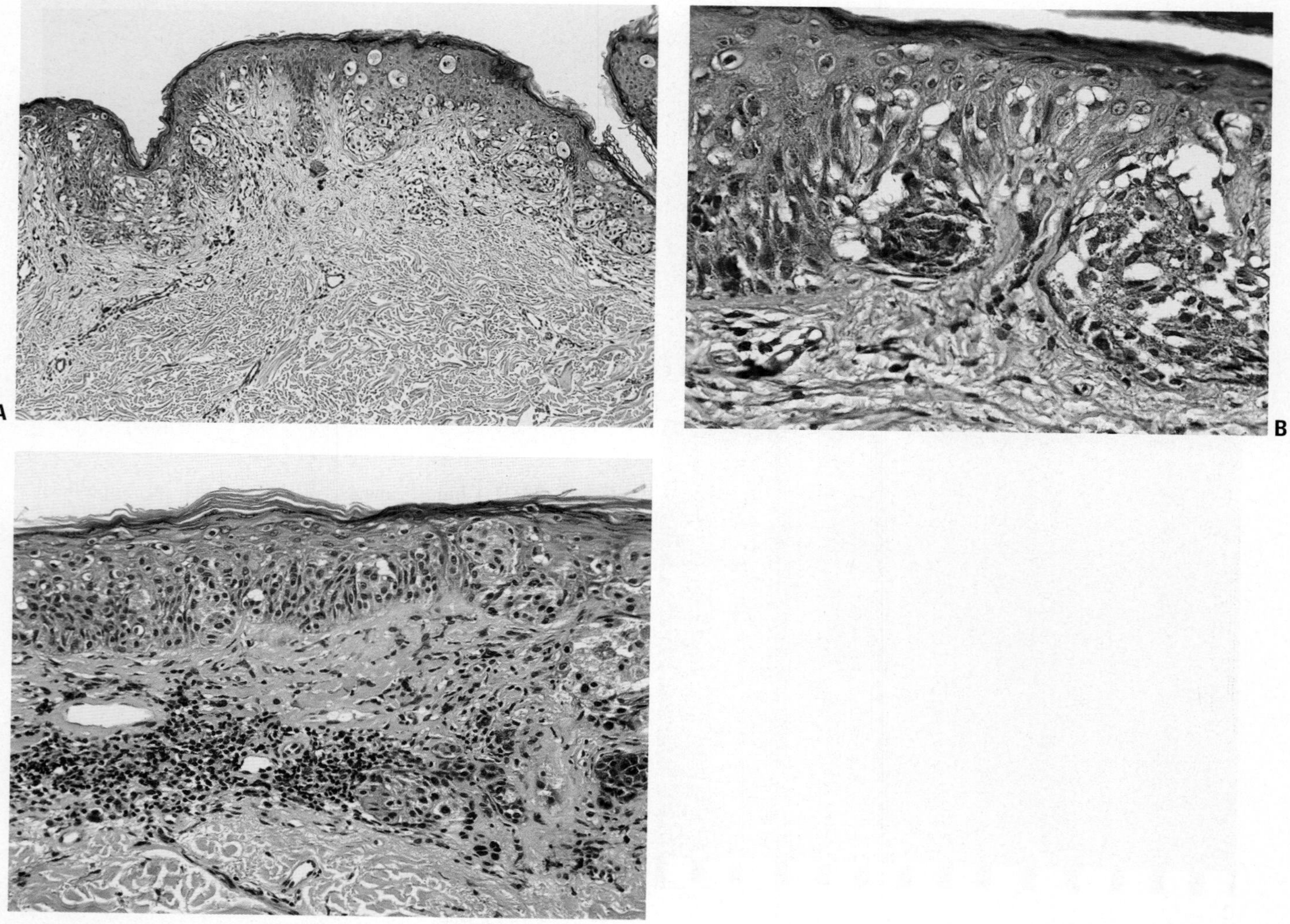

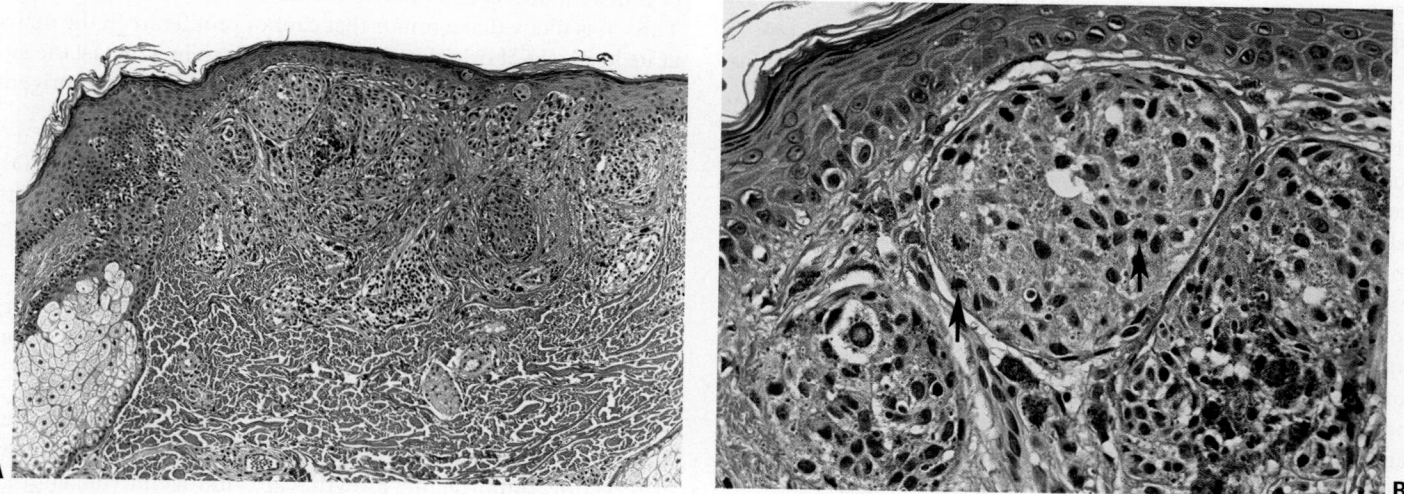

Figure 28-18 Superficial spreading melanoma, radial growth phase (RGP), invasive. **A:** At scanning magnification, there is a broad plaque that is asymmetrical in the distribution of the lesional cells and in that of the responding lymphocytes and keratinocytes. **B:** The lesional cells are uniformly atypical, and they tend to be arranged at least focally with single cells predominating and extending up into the epidermis in a pagetoid pattern. In this view, the basement membrane is intact (*in situ* RGP). **C:** In another portion of the lesion, there are scattered clusters of cells in the dermis that are smaller than the largest intraepidermal cluster, and there are no mitoses. These attributes define foci of "microinvasive" nontumorigenic melanoma (invasive RGP).

Figure 28-19 Melanoma with early tumorigenic vertical growth phase. **A:** This lesion is Clark level II because the papillary dermis is expanded but not quite filled by the proliferation. The Breslow thickness is approximately 0.5 mm. Several of the clusters of cells in the dermis are slightly larger than the largest clusters in the epidermis, indicative of tumorigenic proliferation in the dermis. The cells in the epidermis are smaller than those in the dermis, and they extend laterally as a predominantly *in situ* "radial growth phase compartment" in the primary melanoma. **B:** At high magnification, there is uniform atypia, and there are scattered lesional cell mitoses in the early vertical growth phase (*arrows*). The melanin pigment is finely divided or "dusty."

are no dermal mitoses. Alternatively, the RGP may be present as a "compartment" of a complex primary melanoma in which the above histologic criteria apply only to that portion of the melanoma adjacent to the VGP (Fig. 28-19). "Pure" RGP melanoma may be defined as "the absence of VGP in a primary melanoma" (Fig. 28-18C).

In some instances, a mass is formed in the dermal component of a melanoma by the "accretive" piling up of layers of cells often separated by collagen, in the absence of any single cluster of cells that is larger than the largest intraepidermal aggregate (Fig. 28-20). These lesions have been described as "variant VGP" by Reed (265) and are considered to be nontumorigenic. However, if any mitoses are present in such a lesion, it would meet the criteria for VGP defined earlier. The prognostic significance of variant VGP is uncertain. Most examples are thin, with a good prognosis, as judged by prognostic models. In our experience, rare instances of metastasis have been associated with the presence of variant VGP; however, the overall metastatic rate is exceedingly low, comparable to that associated with other nontumorigenic melanomas.

In contrast to variant VGP, tumorigenic VGP presents as an expansile mass, with mitotic activity (Fig. 28-21).

In a study conducted by the Pathology Panel of the Cancer Research Campaign in the United Kingdom, the level of agreement for recognition of VGP was "good," as judged by formal kappa analysis, and was improved after discussion of standardized criteria among members of the reviewing panel (266). Subsequently, two additional studies have confirmed this finding (267,268). The concept of VGP is of value, in our opinion, for a better understanding of the biology of melanoma. However, its prognostic significance is correlated with other attributes, especially Breslow thickness, and this attribute is not a part of current staging systems used for decision-making in melanoma management. Nevertheless, a recent large meta-analysis to examine predictors of sentinel lymph node biopsy (SLNB) positivity in patients with thin melanoma found that VGP had a strong association with lymph node positivity, superior to Breslow thickness, "providing support for its inclusion in standardized pathologic reporting" (269).

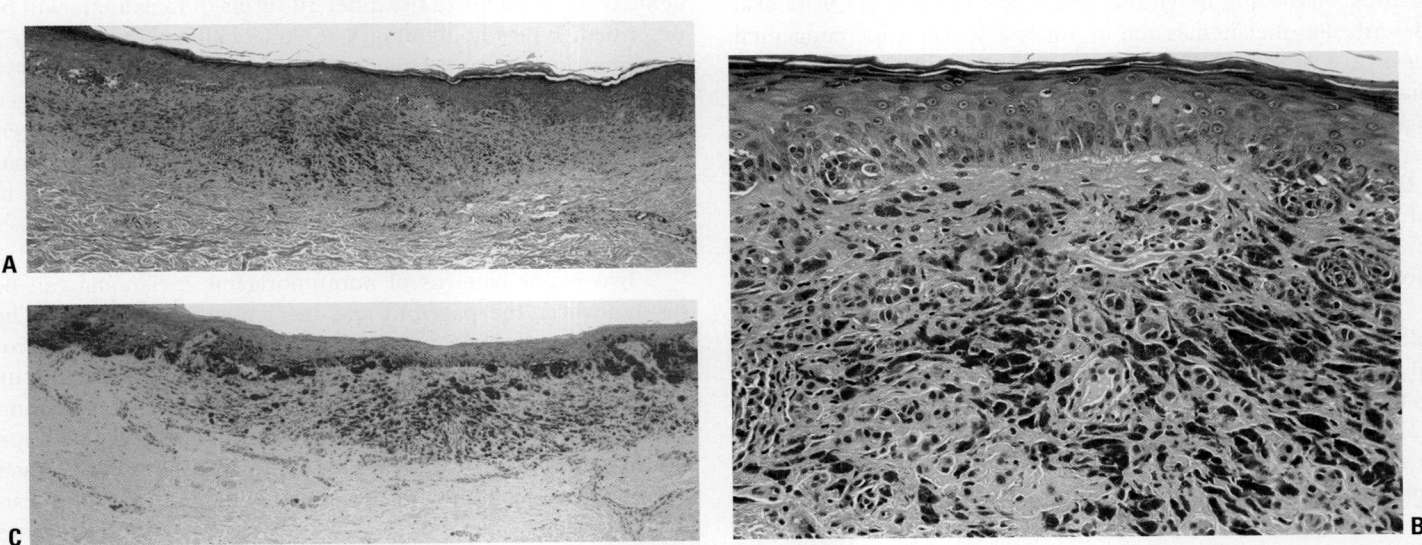

Figure 28-20 Melanoma with variant vertical growth phase ("accretive VGP"). **A:** There is a region in the center of the lesion where the papillary dermis is expanded by a small mass. **B:** The mass appears to have been formed by the accretive growth of numerous small nests, none of which are larger than the largest intraepidermal nests. **C:** A Melan-A stain graphically demonstrates the smaller nests in the dermis, and the larger nests in the epidermis.

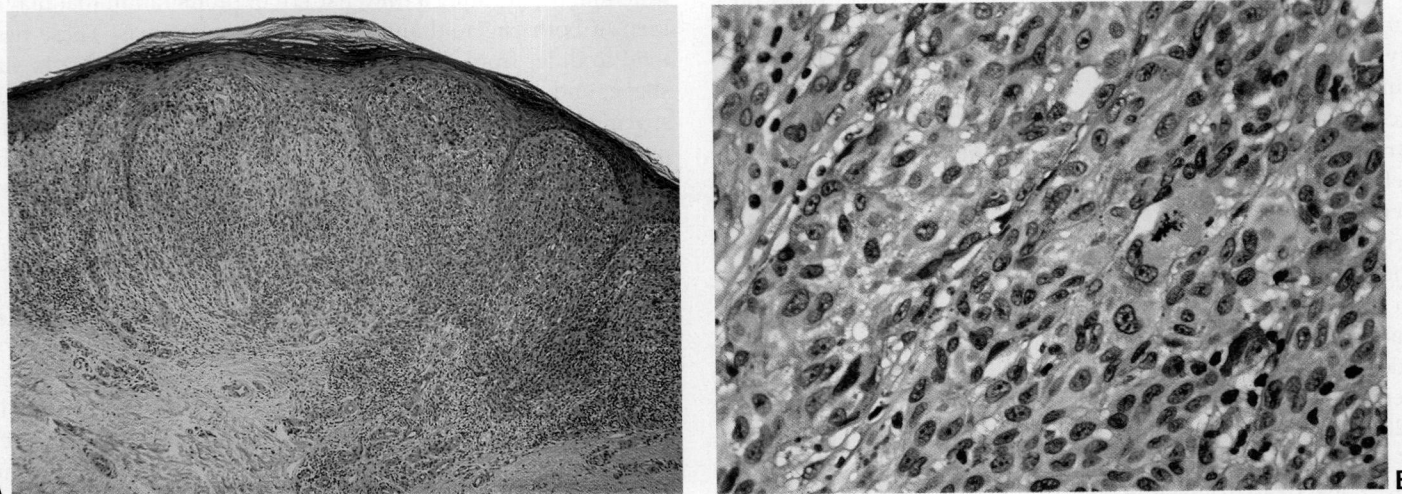

Figure 28-21 Malignant melanoma, tumorigenic. **A:** At scanning magnification, there is a bulky ulcerated tumor nodule, which is eccentrically placed in contiguity with a broad plaque, the nontumorigenic radial growth phase compartment (not shown, to the right of the image field). **B:** The tumorigenic nodule is composed of uniformly atypical mitotically active fully malignant melanocytes (melanoma cells).

Principles of Management for Melanoma

Management of melanoma has been codified in guidelines published in many different communities, including the National Comprehensive Cancer Network (NCCN) (270), discussed further beginning on p. 934.

Genomic Landscape of Melanoma

Knowledge of the molecular pathology of melanoma has expanded dramatically since the discovery, in 2001, of a high frequency of mutation of the oncogene *BRAF* in primary and metastatic melanomas (96), and the recognition that activation of the MAP kinase pathway was a common event in melanoma, mediated by mutated *BRAF* and also by autocrine growth factors (271). In one study, *BRAF* mutations resulting in the common activating pV600E amino acid substitution were found in 68% of melanoma metastases, 80% of primary melanomas, and, unexpectedly at that time, in 82% of nevi (97). In subsequent studies, the incidence has been generally lower, yet still substantial. Activating mutations of the oncogene *NRAS* were also described in melanomas and in tumor-associated and congenital nevi (272,273), and *KIT* mutations have been identified in a substantial subset of cases, especially mucosal, acral, and sun-damaged skin melanomas, mostly LMM (274). Mutations of *NF1* have been identified as the predominant driver mutation in DMs (275). A series of 37 cases with an activating in-frame deletion of *MAP2K1* was recently published, representing a novel form of MAP kinase pathway activation (276). These activating mutations tend to be mutually exclusive.

The list of oncogenes that are mutated in melanoma is rapidly expanding with the advent of NGS techniques. In one study of *BRAF/NRAS* wild-type tumors, targetable and potentially targetable mutations were spread over various signaling pathways (277). In addition to activating mutations of oncogenes, gene fusions are now beginning to be discovered as an alternative means of activation in melanoma (278,279).

Mutations in associated nevi were generally the same as in the primary melanomas (273). These data suggest that although mutational activation of the RAS/RAF/MAPK mitogenic pathway in nevi is a critical step in the initiation of melanocytic neoplasia, alone it is insufficient for melanoma tumorigenesis (99,280).

Tumor progression to melanoma from a nevus or other precursor state generally involves the loss of suppressor gene activity and also the activation of telomerase, which promotes cellular "immortality" (281). The *CDKN2A* tumor suppressor gene product p16 is highly expressed in most nevi (101), presumably restraining the proliferative pressure in these lesions despite the activating oncogene mutations in a phenomenon termed "oncogene-induced senescence" (80). Similar changes have been described in p14 and p15, additional tumor suppressors at or near the same locus, respectively (81,282). Loss of these suppressors in melanomas, in the context of activated mitogenic signaling pathways, represents an important mechanism of progression. In addition, the senescence pathway can be bypassed by multiple genes, including *CDK6*, even in the presence of functional p16 (283), so this is not a perfect marker for melanoma.

BAP1, mentioned earlier in the context of a subset of BAP1-inactivated melanocytic tumors (p. 867), is another example of a tumor suppressor lost in some melanomas, especially of the uveal tract and in the blue nevus–melanoma pathway (284).

In addition to mutations in the genome, epigenetic events are a topic of interest in melanoma (105,285,286). For example, loss of 5-hydroxymethyl cytosine (5-hmC) has been noted in patients' melanomas, and its reconstitution in animal models inhibited melanoma growth and development (105,285,286). Because epigenetic events (DNA methylation, histone modification) that may be associated with the melanoma phenotype and influence gene transcription are potentially reversible, this area is a current focus with respect to both new biomarkers and novel therapies.

The genomic landscape of melanoma has been recently discussed by Bastian et al., with respect to patterns that differ among the nine pathways to melanoma presented in the 2018 *WHO Classification of Skin Tumours* (244), and these patterns will be presented in the discussion of the individual pathways later in this chapter.

Nontumorigenic Melanoma (RGP)

In the sections that follow, the morphology of the nontumorigenic compartments of the different forms of melanoma will be described. Typically, about 85% to 90% of all melanomas have a nontumorigenic compartment, and about half of these also have a tumorigenic focus; about 10% to 15% of melanomas, termed "nodular melanomas," have a tumorigenic but no directly overlying *in situ* or invasive RGP compartment. Nodular melanomas contribute disproportionately to mortality from melanoma; in a population-based study, they accounted for 14% of the cases but 37% of the deaths (287).

Two major patterns of nontumorigenic melanoma can be distinguished: the pagetoid and the lentiginous patterns. The lentiginous pattern recapitulates that of focally contiguous proliferation of nevus cells in the simplest melanocytic neoplasm, the lentigo simplex. However, there is more uniform and complete contiguous basal replacement, and thus the proliferation is also continuous, at least in part, between adjacent rete ridges or often in association with effacement of the rete. Pagetoid scatter, graphically described as "buckshot scatter" of melanocytes within the epidermis, is the best known pattern of melanomas. However, many melanomas, including the lentiginous ones, are entirely or partly lacking in pagetoid proliferation, and pagetoid spread is not entirely specific for melanoma. In some melanomas, as in nevi, nests of melanocytes are present at the dermal–dermal junction, constituting a third pattern of proliferation that may be seen in both pagetoid and lentiginous melanomas. These nests tend to differ from those in nevi in being more variable in size, shape, and orientation, and with regard to their more irregular spacing along the junction (288). Pagetoid and nested patterns of proliferation tend to predominate in low CSD melanomas with a *BRAF* mutation, whereas lentiginous patterns are more prevalent in high CSD, *NRAS* mutated melanomas (258,259).

Differential Diagnosis of RGP Melanoma

The differential diagnosis differs somewhat among the different pathways of melanoma and is discussed in more detail in each section. Immunohistochemical studies have lately come to have considerable value in the distinction between RGP melanomas and benign simulants, including severely dysplastic nevi and pagetoid Spitz nevi/tumors. A p16-Ki-67-HMB45 Immunohistochemistry Scoring System has demonstrated potential utility in the differentiation between nevi and melanomas, as previously discussed in the Dysplastic Nevus Differential Diagnosis section (p. 861) (212). The cancer-testis antigen PRAME (preferentially expressed antigen in melanoma) also has value in making these distinctions (289), and so do molecular methods, including FISH (290) and diagnostic GEP (291).

Superficial Atypical Melanocytic Proliferation of Uncertain Significance

Even though histology is the "gold standard" for melanoma diagnosis, it is not always possible to make absolute distinctions among melanomas with a predominantly junctional component and their benign simulants, because of conflicting, uncertain, or unreliable criteria that do not always permit definition of breakpoints along the biologic continuum of lesion evolution. A common problem is the distinction between a severely dysplastic nevus and an early melanoma *in situ*, or an invasive but nontumorigenic melanoma, and this is especially difficult when one of the so-called special sites is involved (see p. 848). When the process is entirely *in situ*, the descriptive term "AIMP," or some similar variant, has commonly been used (292). When atypical cells are also present in the dermis, this term is obviously inappropriate, or at least incomplete, and for some of these lesions the descriptive term "superficial atypical melanocytic proliferation of uncertain significance," or "SAMPUS," may be appropriate when the differential diagnosis might include a T1a melanoma with an excellent prognosis after complete excision (175,293–295). For *in situ* lesions, the more traditional "AIMP" term can be used, or the lesions can be referred to as "IAMPUS" (175). In any event, these terms are descriptive, not definitive diagnoses, and should always be accompanied by a differential diagnosis. For example, for a problematic lesion of the skin of the breast, we might use the term "SAMPUS" and, in a note, express a differential diagnosis that is a nevus with severe dermal and epidermal dysplasia, a nontumorigenic melanoma, or an unusual presentation of a special site nevus. The first lesion could have significance as a marker of risk for melanoma, the second could have locally recurring but not metastatic potential, and the last could have no biologic significance at all for the patient. If melanoma is in the differential, we provide sufficient information for AJCC staging as a guide to therapy. If the lesion has a potential tumorigenic and/or mitogenic dermal component, and therefore some degree of competence for metastasis, the term "melanocytic tumor of uncertain malignant potential," or "MELTUMP," is used, as discussed in a later section (p. 880). Because the differential diagnosis of IAMPUS and SAMPUS includes melanoma *in situ* or a thin invasive melanoma, which could locally persist, recur, and grow inexorably, although without metastatic potential at the time of diagnosis, we recommend that such lesions be excised in a manner that insures against local persistence and recurrence. The dimensions of such a procedure could follow guidelines for melanoma *in situ* (5-mm margins), or T1a melanomas as the case may be, or at a minimum should be discussed with the patient and optimized according to patient and physician preferences. Of note, these terms are not used in their abbreviated form but are always written out fully in any given case and, as discussed previously, they are accompanied by a discussion of differential diagnosis and usually of potential management considerations.

As discussed in the preceding section, the use of modern genomic and immunohistochemical techniques can be expected to continually reduce the proportion of lesions in which clinically significant uncertainty remains an issue.

The Tumorigenic Compartment of Primary Malignant Melanoma (VGP)

The morphology of the variant forms of nontumorigenic melanoma has been briefly discussed previously and in sections following. A tumorigenic VGP may develop in association with any of these to form a "complex" primary melanoma. In such cases, the histology shows a tumorigenic compartment adjacent to or within the confines of a nontumorigenic compartment. Nodular melanoma differs from these complex melanomas in that it is a tumorigenic melanoma with no clinically or histologically evident adjacent nontumorigenic compartment (296), although such changes may occur directly overlying some lesions. The morphology of the "usual" or "common" forms of VGP will be described below under Common Tumorigenic Melanoma Including Nodular Melanoma.

Occasional melanomas exhibit variant patterns that may lead to diagnostic confusion because they are more characteristically seen in nonmelanocytic tumors. Several variants of melanoma deserve at least a brief description in the following sections: desmoplastic, neurotropic, polypoid, verrucous, balloon cell, signet cell, myxoid, "animal type," nevoid, and minimal deviation melanoma. Other variants that will not be described here include small cell, adenoid/papillary, pleomorphic (fibrohistiocytic) (297), melanomas with rhabdoid cytoplasmic features (298,299), and the rare bone-forming or "osteogenic" melanoma (300).

Common Tumorigenic Melanoma Including Nodular Melanoma

In contrast to nontumorigenic melanoma (RGP), where the proliferation of neoplastic melanocytes is largely or exclusively confined to the epidermis and forms a patch or plaque lesion, in a tumorigenic melanoma an expansile mass lesion is contiguously formed in the dermis, forming a nodule. Confusingly, the term "nodular melanoma" is reserved for those VGP melanomas that lack an adjacent RGP (nontumorigenic compartment), by convention, for three or more rete ridges. Nevertheless, this distinction has clinical as well as histologic significance, as discussed in the following sections.

Clinical Summary. Nodular melanoma, by definition, contains only tumorigenic vertical growth (sometimes associated with a precursor) and, because of this, has a poorer prognosis on average than SSM. However, when other risk factors such as thickness are controlled, the prognosis of nodular melanoma is similar to or only slightly worse than other forms of melanoma (301). Nodular melanomas occur in somewhat older patients than the common SSM and are relatively more frequent in men (296). A nodular melanoma starts as an elevated, variably pigmented papule that may increase in size rapidly to become a nodule and often undergoes ulceration.

The ABCD criteria reviewed earlier do not apply to nodular melanomas (302), which often present clinically as relatively small, symmetrical, and well-circumscribed papules or nodules (Fig. 28-19C). These may be conspicuously pigmented, oligomelanotic, or even amelanotic. The tumorigenic nodule that forms nodular melanoma does not differ clinically or histologically from that which may occur in relation to a preexisting nontumorigenic melanoma. Indeed, nodular melanomas may represent examples of "telescoped" tumor progression in which the antecedent radial phase has been so short-lived as to be unapparent or inconspicuous (303). The clinical importance of the nodular subtype has recently been emphasized; these lesions are more likely to present at a biologically advanced stage despite a comparatively short clinical history (263,287). The mutation profile of nodular melanoma is closer to that of SSM than to the other subtypes, in that *BRAF* or *NRAS* are commonly mutated, although it seems likely that nodular melanoma (NM) can occur in all of the pathways to melanoma (4).

Certain rare "*primary dermal melanomas*" comprised of cytologically malignant melanocytes and lacking an *in situ* component might also be considered in this category, although their prognosis is generally better (304).

Histopathology of Nodular Melanoma and Common VGP (Tumorigenic Melanoma)

Architectural Features. In a typical tumorigenic melanoma, there is confluent proliferation of neoplastic melanocytes in the dermis, forming a tumor mass that is larger (usually much larger) than the largest nest in the overlying epidermis. Asymmetry is often apparent at the cytologic level as variation in cell size,

shape, and pigmentation, and distribution of the host immune response, such that one-half of the lesion is not a mirror image of the other. However, the silhouette of the entire lesion may be quite symmetrical, especially in NM, which, by definition, lacks an adjacent nontumorigenic component (Fig. 28-22A). Conversely, if a nontumorigenic RGP compartment is present in association with a melanoma nodule, asymmetry is likely to be more apparent, at both clinical and histologic levels. The tumor mass is comprised of uniformly atypical cytologically fully malignant, mitotically active cells usually growing in confluent nests or in sheets (Fig. 28-22B). Usually, the tumor mass fills and expands the papillary dermis (Clark level III) or invades between or displaces coarse collagen fibers of the reticular dermis (level IV). Most level III melanomas and most melanomas greater than 0.75 mm in thickness are tumorigenic, whereas, conversely, most level II or "thin" melanomas have no cluster in the dermis that is larger than the largest intraepidermal aggregate and are therefore nontumorigenic. The epidermis is frequently ulcerated, or there is an adherent scale crust. It is often stretched and attenuated, with junctional melanoma cell

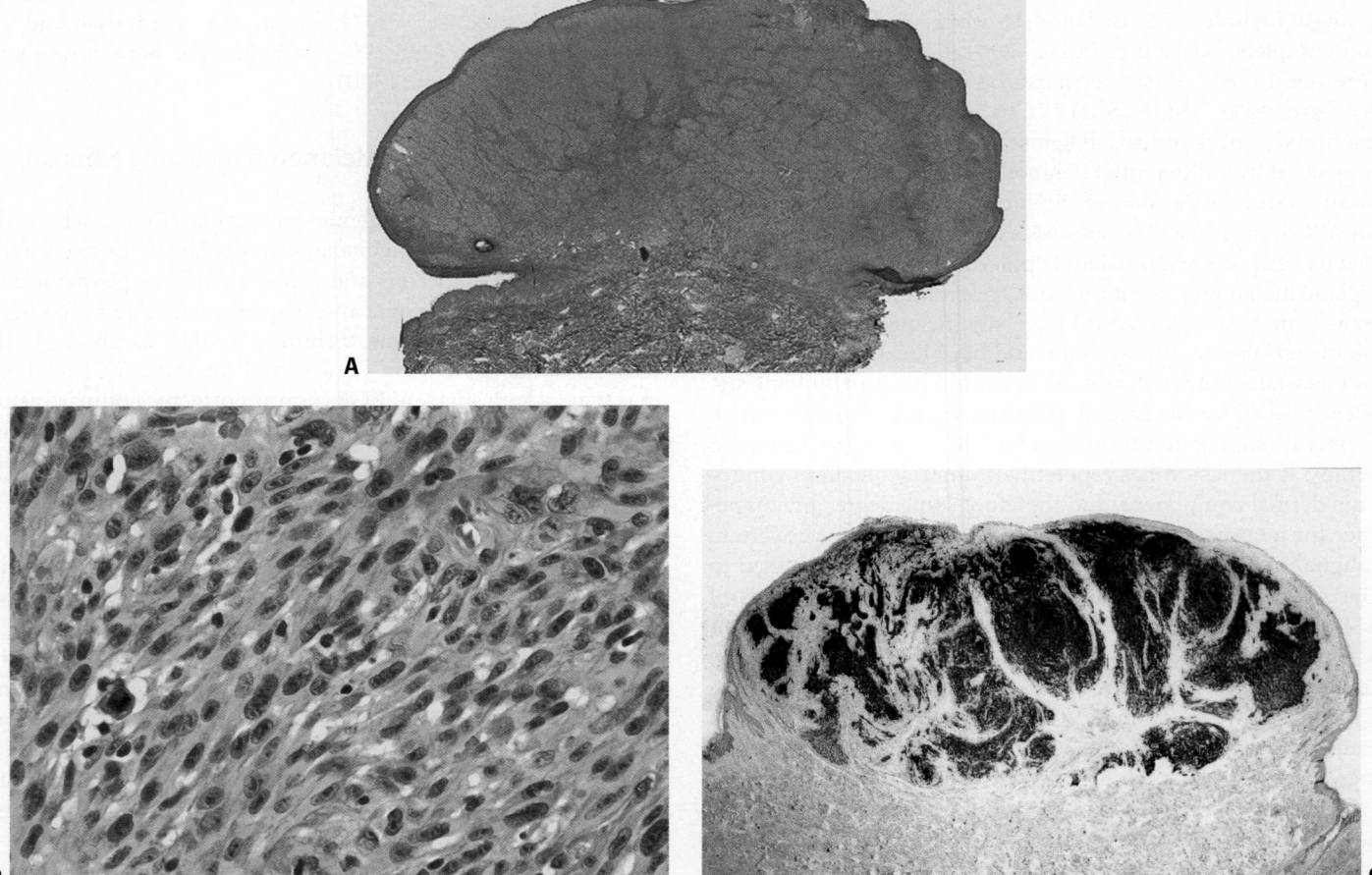

Figure 28-22 Tumorigenic melanoma, nodular type (vertical growth phase without radial growth phase). **A:** The nodules of tumorigenic melanomas tend to be symmetrical at scanning magnification, although there may be an uneven distribution of pigment and of the lymphocytic response within many of the lesions. When there is no adjacent nontumorigenic radial growth phase (RGP) component, as here, the lesion is termed "nodular melanoma." If an RGP component is present, the melanoma is classified according to the type of that compartment (e.g., "superficial spreading or acral-lentiginous") melanoma with tumorigenic vertical growth phase (VGP). **B:** The lesional cells of nodular melanoma exhibit severe uniform cytologic atypia, usually with readily evident mitoses. In any given high-power field such as this, the appearances are indistinguishable from those of a VGP associated with a superficial spreading, lentigo maligna, or acral-lentiginous melanoma, or from those of a metastasis (compare Figs. 28-21B, 28-22B, 28-53, and 28-60A). **C:** Nodular melanoma, S100 immunohistochemical stain. The brown reaction product in the lesional cells is striking, even at scanning magnification. Note the absence of S100 positive lesional cells in the adjacent skin.

aggregates appearing to "take bites" out of the adjacent epidermal layer in a phenomenon that usually does not occur in nevi and that has been termed "consumption of the epidermis" (305). Alternatively, the epidermis may be irregularly hyperplastic and even pseudoepitheliomatous, a pattern that has been termed "verrucous melanoma" (306).

Perhaps the best known single criterion for melanoma is the upward "pagetoid" extension of tumor cells into the epidermis overlying the melanoma. However, this "pagetoid scatter" (or "pagetoid spread" or "pagetoid melanocytosis" or "buckshot scatter") is not specific for melanoma (307). Although in NM, permeation of the epidermis with tumor cells may be absent or limited to that portion overlying the dermal tumor, lateral extension of melanoma cells in the epidermis, and in some lesions also in the papillary dermis beyond the confines of the dermal tumor, typifies the nontumorigenic compartment of complex primary melanomas (SSM, LMM, acral-lentiginous melanoma [ALM]). This phenomenon greatly aids in histologic recognition of these tumors; conversely, the recognition of NMs, which lack this adjacent component, may be difficult. For this reason, nodular melanoma may be difficult or impossible to distinguish from a metastatic melanoma in the skin, and when such a tumor is amelanotic, the distinction from other cutaneous neoplasms may be impossible without IHC.

Primary dermal melanoma, Cutaneous melanocytoma, and Clear cell sarcoma. *Primary dermal melanomas* are tumorigenic malignant melanocytic lesions (i.e., melanomas) that lack an adjacent or overlying junctional component. Several case series have been published (304,308–313). The lesions present as a solitary, usually well-circumscribed but nonencapsulated, tumorigenic deposit of melanoma in the dermis and/or subcutis. There is no evidence of overlying regression or ulceration. The lesions generally have sufficient cytologic atypia and mitotic activity to easily justify a diagnosis of melanoma, and the Breslow depth tends to be substantial. However, the survival rate is relatively high—in one series of 123 cases with a mean Breslow depth of 9.6 mm, the survival was 92% in a median 44-month follow-up (310). The differential diagnosis for primary dermal melanoma includes nodular or other tumorigenic melanomas with complete regression of the junctional component, metastasis from another site (which should be considered with imaging studies as appropriate), and a group of lesions called *cutaneous melanocytoma*, which tend to have a lower-grade cytology with lower mitotic rates and a favorable prognosis. The largest published collection of these cases has been associated with a CRTC1-TRIM11 driver fusion gene rearrangement (314). It is likely that some occurrences of primary dermal melanoma might fit into this category if subjected to appropriate genomic analysis. The prognosis, with limited follow-up, appears to be excellent. Another group of clear cell dermal tumors with melanocytic differentiation and an ACTIN-MITF translocation, again without evidence to date of aggressive behavior (315). *Clear cell sarcoma* should also be considered and can be identified by its characteristic nested or fascicular morphology of cells, often with clear cytoplasm and with tumor giant cells, and a fusion gene rearrangement involving *EWSR1* and *ATF1* or *CREB1* (316).

The amount of *inflammatory infiltrate* in tumorigenic melanomas varies. As a rule, early invasive and many in situ melanomas show a bandlike inflammatory infiltrate, often intermingled with melanophages, at the base of the tumor. In tumors that extend deep into the dermis, the inflammatory infiltrate is quite variable, but it is often only slight to moderate rather than pronounced. Lymphocytes extending among tumor cells are often associated with morphologic evidence of damage to individual tumor cells (apoptosis). These *tumor-infiltrating lymphocytes* (TIL) have been shown to have independent favorable prognostic significance (317,318). The infiltrate is a predominantly T cell response (319). TIL extracted from melanomas (mostly metastatic cases) may be cytotoxic and may be directed against immunogenic melanoma-associated antigens (320).

Cytologic Features. The tumor cells in the dermis have great variation in size and shape. However, two major types of cells can be recognized: an epithelioid and a spindle-shaped cell type. Many tumors show both types of cells, but usually one type predominates. Generally, the "lentiginous" forms of melanoma (e.g., LMM and ALM) tend to show a predominance of spindle-shaped cells in their invasive dermal components, whereas superficial spreading and NMs tend to be composed largely of epithelioid cells. The epithelioid type of cells tends to lie in alveolar or nested formations and the spindle-shaped type of cells in irregularly branching and fascicular formations. The nested formations of the epithelioid cells are surrounded by thin fibers of collagen containing a few fibroblasts. Tumors in which spindle cells predominate may resemble sarcomas or other spindle cell tumors but in most cases differ from them by the presence of junctional melanocytic activity and often by the presence of pigment at least focally in the neoplasm as well as in terms of immunohistochemical markers.

The uniformly atypical nuclei of the cells that constitute the tumor nodule are larger than those of melanocytes or nevus cells, with irregular nuclear membranes; hyperchromatic chromatin; and, often, prominent nucleoli that tend to be irregular in size, shape, and number. The atypia is considered by us to be "uniform" if more than 50% of the cells have these characteristics, but more often than not, all or most of the cells are atypical. In addition to this uniform moderate or severe cytologic atypia, there is also a diagnostically important failure of the melanocytes in the deeper layers of the dermis to decrease in size (absence of "maturation") (Fig. 28-19). This must not be confused, however, with the presence of an intradermal nevus beneath a melanoma, a fairly common feature (p. 925). Not uncommonly, melanoma cells will recapitulate nevic cell maturation ("pseudomaturation"), but in these instances the smaller cells at the base retain nuclear characteristics of malignant cells, and there will be cytologic "continuity" between these nevoid cells and the overlying larger and more atypical lesional cells.

Mitotic figures are present in the dermal compartment of about 85% of tumorigenic melanomas (317) (Fig. 28-21). Mitoses may also be seen in junctional lesional cells and in adjacent hyperplastic keratinocytes. The nuclei of these hyperplastic epidermal keratinocytes may be enlarged with prominent nucleoli, although they are not irregular or hyperchromatic. In contrast, mitotic figures are rarely seen in benign nevi other than Spitz nevi, and even in the latter lesions the rate is usually low or zero, with one potential exception being occasional nevi of pregnancy, and other benign "nevi with mitoses" which lack other compelling features of malignancy (321).

Differential Diagnosis. Considerable difficulty may at times be encountered in the differentiation of a NM from an atypical dermal or compound nevus. This distinction is particularly difficult to make when there is evidence of nevoid maturation, a lesser degree of cytologic atypia, and a low mitotic rate. This differential must also consider the "nevoid melanoma" variant, to be discussed in a following section (p. 892). When there is doubt, the uncertainty should be acknowledged and the differential diagnosis clearly indicated, so that appropriate therapeutic intervention can be planned. Incisional biopsies are a common source of interpretive difficulty, because full assessment of all features, especially size, circumscription, and symmetry, is often not possible. The site of melanocytic lesions that have been partially removed by shave or punch biopsy should be excised to assure complete removal if there is any doubt concerning the diagnosis.

The most important attributes that differentiate the tumorigenic VGP of melanoma from nevi include *asymmetry, lack of maturation* of lesional cells with descent into the dermis, *mitotic activity,* and *uniform cytologic atypia.* Apoptotic tumor cells, which often accompany mitotically active lesions, may also be of assistance. Ulceration and microscopic satellites may be helpful diagnostic features in advanced lesions.

Considerations in the important distinction between thin melanomas and dysplastic nevi are discussed in the section beginning on p. 861, and are presented in Table 28-6, p. 861. The most important differential diagnostic consideration for nodular melanoma is the Spitz nevus. The criteria for this distinction are presented in Table 28-8, and are discussed in the section beginning on p. 878.

In some instances, it may be difficult to recognize a highly undifferentiated melanoma as such. The specific identification of a tumor as melanoma depends on the detection of melanin, or on appropriate immunohistochemical reactivity for melanocytic lineage. The *amount of melanin* present varies greatly in melanomas. In some tumors, considerable melanin is found not only within the tumor cells but also within melanophages located in the stroma. In others, there may be no evidence of melanin in hematoxylin and eosin–stained stains. In the past, Fontana staining, DOPA staining, and electron microscopy were used in some difficult cases. However, in current practice, these methods have been almost entirely supplanted by immunohistochemical techniques.

Immunohistochemistry of Tumorigenic Melanoma (Primary and/or Metastatic). Most of the problems in distinguishing amelanotic or oligomelanotic tumorigenic melanomas from other tumors can be resolved by IHC using a panel of antibodies, including S100, Sox10, Melan-A/MART 1, and/or HMB-45, sometimes with keratin (low and intermediate molecular weight such as AE1/3) and LCA (322). On immunohistochemical testing, S100 protein is nearly always positive in melanoma. A keratin stain can be done in addition to staining for S100 protein to rule out not uncommon S100-positive carcinomas but is usually not necessary when more specific melanoma markers are also used. Sox10 is as sensitive as S100 for melanoma (323), and, like S100, it can stain some carcinomas (e.g., sweat gland tumors and some breast carcinomas), and most, if not all, benign melanocytic lesions (324). Keratin reactivity occurs in some melanomas, usually but not invariably in advanced metastatic disease (325,326). Reactivity of melanomas, mostly advanced metastatic cases, has been described with polyclonal but not monoclonal carcinoembryonic antigen (CEA), and occasional melanomas react with the epithelial marker EMA (327).

Table 28-8
Comparative Features of Spitz Nevi, Atypical Spitz Tumors, and Spitzoid/Spitz Melanomas

	Spitz Nevus (SN)	Atypical Spitz Tumor (AST)	Spitz or Spitzoid Melanomas
Clinical	Generally younger, small, symmetrical, pink plaque/nodule	Any age, often <40 yrs., larger plaque or nodule, usually symmetrical	Often >40 yrs, larger, asymmetrical nodule, variegated pigment, history of change
Histopathology	Small, symmetrical, maturation of dermal component, few mitoses	Larger, usually symmetrical, may be ulcerated, impaired maturation, 2–6 dermal mitoses/mm² (≥3 in adults)	Share attributes with SN and AST but, in addition, often very large, asymmetrical, often ulcerated, maturation lacking, mitoses > 6/mm², deep and/or marginal mitoses
Cytology	Large nuclei with regular nuclear membranes, pale chromatin, large nucleoli	May be increased pleomorphism (low grade)	May be severe pleomorphism, hyperchromatism (high grade)
IHC	HMB45, Ki-67 stratification, Ki-67 <5%, p16 usually expressed, PRAME usually negative	HMB45, Ki-67 stratification, Ki-67 5%–20%, p16 usually expressed, PRAME usually negative	HMB45, Ki-67 often with deep staining, Ki-67 >20%, p16 often lost, PRAME often diffusely positive
Genomic	Kinase fusions, or an activating *HRAS* mutation, isolated chromosomal gains	Kinase fusions, *PTEN* mutations, heterozygous or homozygous loss of 9p21, may have >1 chromosomal aberration	Kinase fusions (true Spitz melanoma) or *BRAF, NRAS*, or other activating mutation (Spitzoid melanomas). *PTEN* mutations, homozygous *CDKN2A* loss, activating *TERTp* mutations

Based on Barnhill RL, Bahrami A, Bastian BC, et al. Spitz melanoma. In: Elder DE, Massi D, Scolyer RA, Willemze R, eds. *WHO Classification of Skin Tumours.* 4th ed. IARC; 2018:108–110. Reprinted with permission from Dr. Raymond Barnhill.

Melanomas, unlike most carcinomas, express vimentin, an intermediate filament that is usually associated with mesenchymal tissues, and synaptophysin, GFAP, and neurofilament protein reactivity have also been described (326). Lymphomas are usually positive with LCA, while S100 and HMB-45 are negative. The anaplastic large cell type of non-Hodgkin lymphoma, which could present primarily in the skin, may be confused with melanoma, but these tumors are usually positive for the CD30 antigen as well as CD45 (328). Occasional examples of histiocytic tumors such as epithelioid histiocytomas or juvenile xanthogranulomas may be confused with nodular melanomas, especially when foam cells or Touton giant cells are inconspicuous. Melan-A and tyrosinase markers, along with CD68, CD163, and PU.1, are sensitive and specific in making this distinction.

Like S100 and Sox10, HMB-45 (gp100) is positive in many benign melanocytic tumors and is thus not specific for melanoma. Its sensitivity of about 70% overall is less than that of S100, for which the sensitivity is close to 100% but the specificity is lower (323). HMB-45 expression is generally negative in desmoplastic and, to a lesser extent, other spindle cell melanomas (329). The specificity of the HMB-45 antigen depends on the context in which it is used. Benign melanocytic lesions that may react with HMB-45 include the junctional component of most nevi and the dermal components of dysplastic nevi, blue nevi, cellular blue nevi, DPN, and Spitz nevi. Thus, HMB-45 cannot be used to distinguish benign from malignant melanocytic neoplasms, although a "top heavy" (stratified) staining pattern can be supportive of a benign diagnosis. In an interesting study using automated quantitative analysis, the ratio of nuclear to cytoplasmic labeling for HMB-45 was increased in the dermal component of nevi, resulting in a sensitivity of 0.92 and a specificity of 0.80 for distinguishing benign nevi from malignant melanomas (330). HMB-45 is also a component of a p16-Ki-67-HMB-45 IHC scoring system that has been presented as an ancillary diagnostic tool in the diagnosis of melanoma, because of its striking tendency to stratify in intensity of staining from superficial to deep in the dermal components of nevi but not melanomas (212).

If the diagnostic differential is between melanoma and carcinoma, lymphoma or sarcoma, the diagnostic specificity of a positive HMB-45 stain is very high, albeit not 100%. The most important group of nonmelanocytic tumors that stain with HMB-45 is the family of "perivascular epithelioid cell neoplasms" or "PEComas." These cells coexpress muscle and melanocytic markers and contain membrane-bound dense granules consistent with premelanosomes. The lesions tend to be comprised of clear to granular epithelioid and/or spindled cells arranged in nests and fascicles, with consistent arrangement around blood vessels. The tumors may be associated with tuberous sclerosis, or may be sporadic. The family of tumors includes angiomyolipoma, clear cell sugar tumor of the lung, lymphangioleiomyomatosis, and other very rare tumors, including clear cell tumors in skin and in subcutis (331). Although a typical staining pattern is for positive reactivity with SMA and HMB-45, with S100 negative, about one-third of cases can express S100, and also Melan-A and MITF, and about 20% of the cases are actin-negative, whereas 30% may express desmin (and some caldesmon) in addition to actin. Based primarily on nuclear grade and mitotic activity, PEComas can be characterized as "benign," "of uncertain malignant potential," or "malignant" (332).

Melan-A (MART-1), like gp100/HMB45, is an antigen initially recognized by T-cells in melanoma patients ("melanoma antigen recognized by T-cells") and, like HMB-45, is associated with the pigmentary apparatus. The sensitivity of this antigen is somewhat greater than HMB-45 and its specificity, although differing in details, is about the same. The Melan-A antibody labels reactive cases strongly and clearly but is less sensitive in spindle cell melanomas and usually negative in the spindle cells of DMs. It must also be noted that whereas Melan-A has more specificity than HMB-45 for detecting cells of melanocytic lineage, it also reacts strongly with normal melanocytes and with nevus cells so that it has no utility as a potential marker for malignancy. In addition, although Melan-A and MART-1 recognized the same antigen, the epitopes are presumably different, and Melan-A, but not MART-1, can react with adrenocortical tumor cells (333).

Other markers that have been studied include the cancer-testis antigens, including, especially, PRAME (see later) and (less so) the MAGE series of antigens, tyrosinase, and MITF. Xu et al. evaluated reactivity for alternative markers in 14 HMB-45 negative, nondesmoplastic melanomas. MITF was positive in 9, Melan-A in 9, tyrosinase in 6, and MAGE-1 in 11. In eight desmoplastic malignant melanomas, (DM) MAGE-1 was positive in three, and all other markers were negative. The five markers tested were negative in all but two schwannomas, one with focal melanocyte-specific transcription factor and the other with tyrosinase and weak MAGE-1 reactivity. It was concluded that MAGE-1, MITF, tyrosinase, and Melan-A may be useful markers in the diagnosis of malignant melanocytic lesions when HMB-45 is negative (334); however, these markers are now not often used because of the advent of Sox10. Sox10, as noted previously is also quite sensitive in melanomas, including spindle cell melanomas but, like S100, is not specific for melanoma (324).

In another study, a "pan-melanoma cocktail," composed of HMB-45, MART-1, and tyrosinase, labeled 98% of all melanomas but only 60% of DMs, all of which were positive for S100 (335). If a DM is labeled by these markers, it is typically only in the epithelioid component of a "mixed" desmoplastic melanoma (see p. 886). The pan-melanoma cocktail is more specific than S100 and is often useful as a complementary marker, except for DM, in which Sox10 is a valuable marker in addition to S100.

The lineage-related markers discussed previously provide little information as to the benign or malignant nature of a lesion. However, as emphasized, the pattern of staining with HMB-45 can be of some assistance—melanomas tend to have more diffuse staining, while staining in benign lesions tends to be "top heavy," no doubt reflecting a form of maturation or senescence (336). In addition, the S100 subunit S100A6 has been of some use in the distinction between Spitz tumors and melanomas, with a strong and diffuse staining pattern favoring the former (337). A variety of markers such as p53 (338), cyclin D (339), structures called "nuclear organizer regions" (340), and antibodies against the PHH3 histone involved in the mitotic apparatus (341) have been evaluated. The most useful of these is Ki-67 (Mib-1). In one study, a "high" Ki-67 labeling rate of 10% (based on counting several hundred cells) or more would favor a malignant diagnosis, whereas a "low" rate of 2% or less (especially zero reactivity) would favor a benign diagnosis (342). Using a "hot spot" methodology, the range favoring melanoma may be of the order of greater than 15% to 20%, whereas less than 10% would favor a nevus (343). In our experience, although we will often order Ki-67 to assess proliferative activity, most diagnostically equivocal tumors fall into the gray zone of Ki-67 reactivity between these cut points. Loss of the tumor suppressor marker p16 (and also p14 and p15), and homozygous loss of their locus on chromosome 9p21, has also been associated with aggressive outcomes in studies especially directed at Spitzoid lesions, but as a single marker it is less predictive than TERT promoter activation as detected by genomic sequencing. The combination of histology and p16-Ki-67-HMB45 IHC has been advocated as a first-line tool to diagnose a difficult melanocytic tumor, followed by cytogenetics analyses in cases of discrepancies between histology and IHC (344).

Finally, PRAME is now coming into wide use as a diagnostic immunohistochemical marker (289), and it will be interesting to see more studies of these markers used in combination. In the first comprehensive study of PRAME as a diagnostic marker in melanoma, diffuse nuclear immunoreactivity was found in 87% of 100 metastatic and 83.2% of 135 primary melanomas (although only 35% of DMs). Of 140 cutaneous melanocytic nevi, 86.4% were completely negative for PRAME, with immunoreactivity for PRAME, usually only in a few cells, seen in a few dysplastic nevi, common acquired nevi, traumatized/recurrent nevi, and Spitz nevi. In that study, diffuse (4+, i.e., >75% of cells reacting), PRAME positivity had a sensitivity of ~90% and a specificity of ~99% for unequivocal nonspindle cell melanomas (289). In a study of more difficult cases with many challenging lesions, the sensitivity of diffuse PRAME expression for melanoma was only 75%, with a specificity of 98.8%, whereas the overall agreement between PRAME IHC results and the final diagnostic interpretation was 92.7%. There is, therefore, a degree of subjectivity in the interpretation of results for this marker (Fig. 28-23).

This marker, used judiciously, can also be useful for margin assessment in melanoma *in situ* (289), for identification of melanoma-associated nevus cells (345), which could affect thickness measurement, and for distinguishing nodal nevi from melanoma (346), if needed in a difficult case.

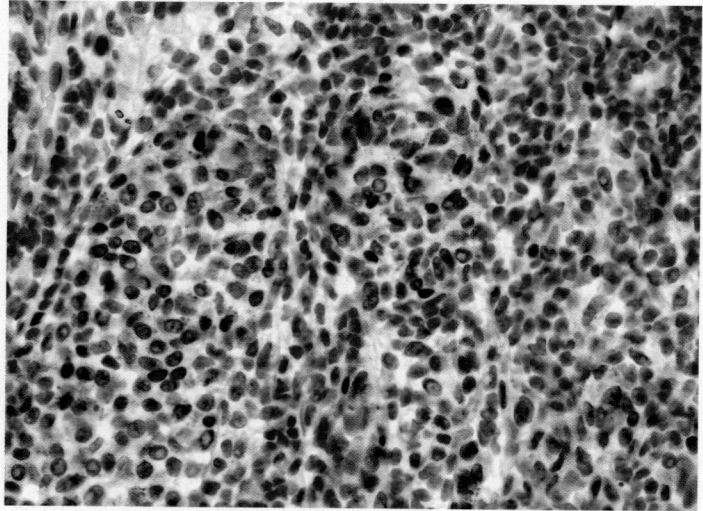

Figure 28-23 Melanocytic tumor of uncertain malignant potential stained with an antibody to PRAME. An atypical lesion, suspicious for nevoid melanoma, was stained for PRAME. This level of staining (< 75%), over the whole lesion, or the whole region of concern, would be insufficient for a definitive positive test interpretation.

Epigenetic biomarkers, especially loss 5-hmC, have also been shown to have potential utility in assessing melanocytic proliferations. For example, in addition to its loss in melanoma but not in nevi (105), 5-hmC IHC has proven to be useful in differentiating melanoma-associated nevus from melanoma pseudomaturation (347), in assessing degree of dysplasia in nevi (104), and in distinguishing nodal melanoma metastases from nevic cell rests (348).

Melanocytic Tumors of Uncertain Malignant Potential

This is a descriptive term for a heterogeneous group of melanocytic tumors that exhibit some features indicative of possible malignancy, such as nuclear atypia, macronucleoli, mitotic activity, necrosis, or ulceration, but in number or degree insufficient to justify a malignant diagnosis (175,349). Accordingly, they reflect the biologic reality that occasional melanocytic lesions that do not meet criteria for fully evolved melanoma cannot be predicted to be benign with 100% accuracy.

Histopathology. Tumors appropriately placed in this descriptive category may be quite bulky neoplasms of the order of several millimeters in diameter and thickness and composed of pigmented often spindle-shaped cells. The overall cellularity may be relatively low compared to fully malignant melanomas. There may be occasional mitoses, but not more than one or a few per section plane. Abnormal mitoses, if present, are usually indicative of frank malignancy. Focal areas of individual cell death may be present, but if there are areas of confluent geographic necrosis, or if an ulcer is present, a frankly malignant diagnosis is appropriate. There may be a few enlarged melanocytes in the epidermis; however, if there is an intraepidermal component that can be identified as an RGP of melanoma of any of the common types, a diagnosis of melanoma should be made.

Other examples include melanocytic tumors that superficially resemble ordinary nevus variants but that also include some (but not all) features associated with a malignant diagnosis. For example, a compound or dermal nevus with significant atypia within the dermal component, a Spitz nevus–like proliferation with some degree of asymmetry and deep mitotic activity, or a deep-penetrating nevus with unusual features could all be placed in this category. In general, uncertain malignant potential implies an intradermal architecture with some features of tumorigenic growth (and, hence, some overlap with VGP melanoma), as opposed to a SAMPUS that is devoid of a dermal tumorigenic component, thus having no metastatic potential (albeit with some potential to progress or recur on incomplete excision).

Differential Diagnosis. This descriptive diagnosis is one of exclusion, and the differential diagnosis includes specific neoplasms described elsewhere in this chapter, including atypical Spitz nevi/Spitz tumors, so-called minimal deviation melanomas, some DPN, cellular neurothekeoma (discussed in the chapter on neural tumors), atypical cellular blue nevi, and certain nevoid melanoma variants.

Some lesions that may be placed in this descriptive category (as has been discussed previously) are composed of tumoral intradermal proliferations of dendritic to epithelioid cells packed with abundant and coarsely divided pigment that may obscure the nucleus (350). Sometimes, these melanocytic cells are difficult to distinguish from melanophages. They are also reminiscent of dermal "melanophores" seen in some vertebrates, which may occasionally in animals give rise to malignant tumors resembling malignant blue nevi. Some of these lesions may have prominent epidermal involvement, with pagetoid spread of the heavily pigmented lesional cells into the epidermis, and a dermal component that is broader in the papillary than in the reticular dermis. These lesions, despite their unusual cytology, have architectural features that are relatively characteristic of melanoma. There is overlap between these lesions and the lesions termed PEMs, which in turn overlap with epithelioid blue nevi, (232) on the one hand, and "pigment synthesizing melanomas (PSMs)," on the other (236). Some related lesions, where criteria for malignancy are not deemed to have been fully met, may also be placed in the descriptive category of "uncertain malignant potential" (175). Yet other previously rare lesions are now seen more often in the era of immune therapy present as nodular clusters of authentic melanophages ("tumoral melanosis") (131). These lesions may be examples of complete regression of a pigmented VGP nodule, a very rare phenomenon that is quite different from the partial regression frequently observed in the RGP compartment of common melanomas.

Principles of Management for MELTUMPs: As was discussed in the 2015 NCCN guidelines (351), the existence of these "difficult" or "uncertain" cases, where diagnostic agreement is not likely to be achieved even among experienced observers, suggests a need for a practical means of dealing with these cases in the best interests of the patients. In this regard, two principles apply. First, lesions should be managed by means sufficient to provide adequate therapy for the most clinically significant entity in the differential diagnosis of an uncertain neoplasm, and, second, patients and their physicians deserve to know that their lesion cannot be diagnosed specifically with presently available means. A pathology report in such a case should not provide a false assurance of confidence in any given diagnosis. In these cases, we typically recommend management with the differential diagnosis of melanoma taken into consideration and provide microstaging attributes sufficient at least for AJCC staging of the lesion as melanoma. The dimensions of a reexcision procedure could follow guidelines for the AJCC stage of the "melanoma" or, at a minimum, should be discussed with the patient and include a margin of normal tissue around the scar and any residual lesion.

In addition, an SLN sampling procedure may be discussed with the patient. Sentinel lymph node sampling has been offered to patients with "atypical" or "uncertain" melanocytic tumors in a number of centers (352–356). Some of these cases have been found to be associated with lymph node metastases. In such circumstances, there may be a temptation to revise the diagnosis to "malignant melanoma." However, as previously discussed, there have been reports of lesions with characteristics of Spitz nevi that have metastasized to regional lymph nodes, sometimes followed by prolonged, perhaps indefinite, survival (357–361). Similar situations have been reported in relation to cellular blue nevi (362). Therefore, in a situation where a MELTUMP is found to be associated with regional lymph node metastases, we report the metastasis as "MELTUMP," where the word malignant refers to clinical course as a consequence of persistence and inexorable progression of disease, rather than simply the ability of a neoplasm to travel to a draining lymph node. We indicate that the biologic potential of this metastatic tumor remains uncertain. However, the prognosis is clearly more guarded in the presence of such metastases, and in these

circumstances, the possibility of adjuvant therapy may be taken into consideration, preferably after consultation with an expert tumor board.

As with SAMPUS, it can be expected that continuing advances in genomic and immunohistochemical diagnosis will reduce, but likely not eliminate, this category of "MELTUMPs."

Melanomas in Low CSD Skin

Low CSD skin is defined as skin with mild-to-moderate solar elastosis.

Superficial Spreading (Low CSD) Melanoma

SSM, also referred to as pagetoid melanoma (254), and most recently as "Low CSD melanoma" (4), is the most frequent form of melanoma (about 70% of all cases) and may therefore be regarded as the "common" or "prototypic" form of melanoma. The *in situ* component of these lesions has been described in the past as "precancerous melanosis," a term that dates back to, perhaps, the earliest description of melanoma by Dubreuilh in 1912 (363), "active junctional nevus" (165), or "atypical melanocytic hyperplasia" (364), whereas today the term "melanoma" *in situ*, superficial spreading type (or "low CSD") is preferred.

This is the prototypic lesion of Pathway I of the WHO 2018 Classification of Melanoma (4) (Table 28-2, p. 836) and was also called the "nevus-associated pathway" by Mishima.

Clinical Summary. The lesions of SSM, which occur in a relatively young to middle-aged patient population, may occur on exposed skin but are rather more commonly found on intermittently exposed skin and are rare on unexposed skin. Compared to LMM, SSM arises in patients with a higher density of benign nevi (365) and is more likely to be associated with a precursor nevus (366).

The lesions are slightly or more prominently elevated, with a palpable border and an irregular outline. There is often variation in color that includes not only tan, brown, and black, but also pink, blue, and gray. White or gray areas may be seen at sites of spontaneous regression (Fig. 28-19A). Microinvasion may be clinically unapparent, but the onset of tumorigenic vertical growth is indicated by the development of a papule, followed by nodularity and sometimes also ulceration, the latter usually being a late feature. In rare instances, the lesion has a verrucous surface in which case differentiation from a seborrheic keratosis may be difficult (367). In its early stage of development, SSM may be indistinguishable clinically from a dysplastic nevus. Although dermoscopy can improve clinical and histologic diagnostic specificity, histologic examination remains the "gold standard" for melanoma diagnosis and is necessary for accurate diagnosis (368).

Histopathology. Architectural features of importance in the diagnosis include the large diameter of the lesions (often 10 mm or greater), poor circumscription (the cells forming the edge of the lesion tending to be small, single, and scattered), and asymmetry (one-half of the lesion does not mirror the other half) (288). The epidermis is irregularly thickened and thinned, in contrast to the consistently elongated rete ridge pattern of a dysplastic nevus. Uniformly rounded, large melanocytes are scattered in a pagetoid pattern throughout the epidermis. The large cells lie predominantly in nests in the lower epidermis and singly in the upper epidermis. The nests tend to vary considerably in size and shape and focally to become confluent. Dermal melanophages and a dermal infiltrate are regularly present. The lymphocytic infiltrate may be patchy and perivascular, as in a dysplastic nevus, but is typically dense and bandlike, especially in invasive lesions (Fig. 28-18A). The presence of partial regression, seen as an area of absence of melanoma within a lesion, usually with fibroplasia, a lymphocytic infiltrate, vascular prominence and ectasia, and melanophages, is more often seen in RGP melanomas than in nevi. CSD manifested by moderate actinic elastosis often with actinic lentigines is usually present in the adjacent skin and differs from the usually severe CSD usually seen in the lentiginous melanomas.

The lesions termed "large nested melanoma" appear to represent a variant of low CSD/superficial spreading melanoma, in which the nesting pattern dominates over the pagetoid pattern, presenting as a row of cannonballs in the epidermis. They tend to occur in low CSD skin and may be associated with a nevus (369,370).

Cytologically, the lesional cells are rather uniform and have abundant cytoplasm containing varying amounts of melanin that often consists of small, "dusty" granules. They are almost entirely devoid of readily visible dendrites. The nuclei tend to be large and hyperchromatic, with irregular nuclear membranes and irregularly clumped chromatin (Fig. 28-18B). This "uniform cytologic atypia" is of considerable diagnostic importance and contrasts with the random atypia of dysplastic nevi.

When the lesion is *in situ,* the basement membrane is intact (as in the field seen in Fig. 28-18B), and there are no lesional cells in the dermis. In an invasive but nontumorigenic lesion (invasive RGP or "microinvasive" melanoma), cells similar to those in the epidermis are present in the dermis in the form of small nests, with no nests larger than those in the epidermis, and with no dermal mitoses (Fig. 28-18C). When tumorigenic VGP is present, there is at least one, or often more than one, cluster of cells in the dermis that is larger than the largest intraepidermal nest, and/or there may be lesional cell mitoses in the dermis (Fig. 28-19A, B).

In a semiquantitative study of microscopic attributes that were correlated with the WHO classification of a series of melanomas, the major factors that distinguished between SSM and LMM included higher values for circumscription, epidermal thickening, pagetoid scatter, nesting and pigment, and lower CSD for SSM. These attributes were found to be reproducible in a subsequent study (259).

On *electron microscopic examination,* melanosomes are present in great numbers in the large pagetoid tumor cells. Their shape is largely spheroid, rather than ellipsoid, as is the case for normal melanocytes and the tumor cells of lentigo maligna (371). They often also have other abnormalities, such as absence of cross-linkages of the filaments within the melanosomes. Melanization within the melanosomes is variable but often incomplete (372). This accounts for the finely divided "dusty" character of the pigment in the cells of many melanomas.

Pathogenesis. The lesions, which occur in a relatively young to middle-aged patient population, may occur on sun-exposed skin but are more commonly found on intermittently exposed skin and are rare on unexposed skin. There is a clear relationship between incidence and sun exposure (373). In contrast to lentigo maligna, SSM is thought to be associated with "acute–intermittent" rather than "chronic continuous" sun exposure, which is often

recreational rather than occupational (374). The most frequently involved sites are the upper back, especially in men, and the lower legs, especially in women. In an epidemiologic study of risk factors for LMM compared with SSM, a propensity to lentigines was a stronger predictor of LMM, whereas high nevus propensity was a stronger predictor of SSM. Skin cancer history was associated with LMM risk, whereas the number of lifetime sunburns was associated with SSM. Shared risk factors included the number of solar keratoses and sun-sensitive complexion, that is, light eye and hair colors, sunburn propensity, and freckling (375). These differences were encapsulated into the "divergent pathways" hypothesis of the epidemiology of melanoma (376), pathways that were simultaneously recognized at the molecular level in terms of BRAF versus *NRAS*-predominant driver mutations in the two pathways (377) and also that had been previously recognized as the "melanocytic and nevocytic" oncogenic pathways to melanoma of Mishima (371). As already mentioned, it is likely that most SSMs have mutually exclusive activating mutations of BRAF, less often than of *NRAS* or other oncogenes, whereas the latter are more common in LMM. In a genotype–phenotype correlation study, melanomas that had prominent nesting and pagetoid scatter of melanocytes, criteria similar to those for SSM, were more likely than other melanomas to be associated with BRAF mutations (258,259). These evolving genetic data will lead to the refinement of the clinicopathologic melanoma classification system in the future.

Differential Diagnosis. A junctional nevus differs from SSM in RGP by a lack of atypia in the tumor cells, particularly in their nuclei; by a lack of pagetoid upward extension of tumor cells; by the absence of a significant inflammatory infiltrate in the upper dermis; and often, but not always, by a sharper lateral demarcation (p. 844). Salient features in the important distinction from junctional melanocytic dysplasia have been reviewed (Table 28-6, p. 861) and include, at scanning magnification, larger size, asymmetry, an irregularly thickened and thinned epidermis, and a bandlike lymphocytic infiltrate in SSM. At higher power, indicators of melanoma include the presence of high-level and extensive pagetoid melanocytosis (large neoplastic cells scattered singly among benign keratinocytes), high-grade and/or uniform cytologic atypia, and lesional cell mitoses (the latter present in about one-third of cases) (Fig. 28-24).

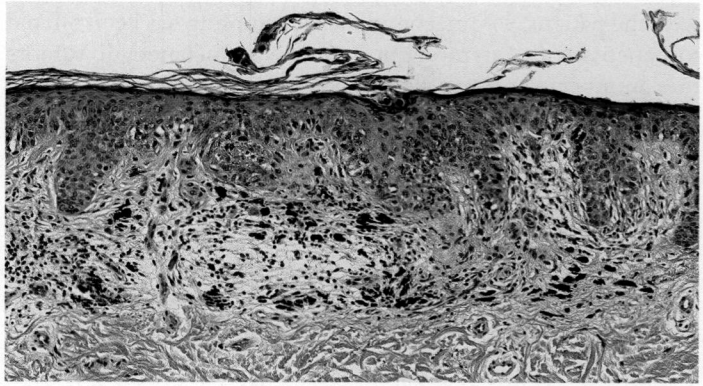

Figure 28-24 Classic superficial spreading melanoma. Features include high degrees of nesting, pagetoid scatter and pigment, in a low cumulative solar damage ("Low CSD"), low elastosis environment. There is a focal invasive, nontumorigenic, and nonmitogenic radial growth phase (invasive RGP), and there is also diffuse fibroplasia and a patchy but focally bandlike lymphocyte with scattered melanophages, all characteristic stromal features.

A junctional Spitz nevus, especially the uncommon "pagetoid Spitz nevus" variant, may closely simulate SSM. Distinguishing features in pagetoid Spitz nevus include generally smaller size, the presence of large spindle and/or epithelioid cells, the presence of Kamino bodies, and the lack of "consumption" or thinning of the epidermis above the lesion, as previously discussed (p. 896).

The so-called nevi of special sites, including flexural sites, ears, scalp, and breast may also simulate this form of melanoma, in particular, and these should be seriously considered when a biopsy from one of these sites is examined (see also p. 851).

Caution should be exercised when what at first appears to be melanoma *in situ* is restricted to the epidermis that overlies a surgical or traumatic scar, as this must be differentiated from the recurrent nevus phenomenon (see p. 853). Helpful features in recognition of recurrent nevus phenomenon include the precise spatial restriction of the atypical intraepidermal focus to the zone overlying (but not extending horizontally beyond) the scar, the presence of residual nevus cells, and generally less severe and uniform cytologic atypia. Whenever possible, it is important to also review the initial biopsy in such cases.

The differential diagnostic distinction from lentiginous melanomas is of less consequence, because the management is similar, although there may be differences that are primarily site related. In lentigo maligna, the epidermis is atrophic, and pagetoid melanocytosis and nesting are less prominent, and contiguous replacement of the basal cell layer by atypical melanocytes is the dominant pattern. Problematic cases can be reported as "malignant melanoma" (*in situ* or microinvasive, etc.) without designation as to the type.

When tumorigenic VGP is present, it does not differ consistently from that in any other form of melanoma, except for the adjacent RGP (Fig. 28-21). Epithelioid morphology and more abundant pigmentation are more likely to be seen in the SSM subset. Classification of such "complex tumorigenic" primary melanomas is based on the morphology of the RGP.

Among the nonmelanocytic neoplasms that must be differentiated from an SSM *in situ* are Paget disease and pagetoid examples of Bowen disease (squamous cell carcinoma *in situ*) and also Merkel cell tumors and sebaceous carcinomas. Paget disease (discussed in detail in Chapter 37) usually shows remnants of compressed basal cells beneath the tumor cells, whereas in SSM, the lesional cells extend to the basement membrane. In Paget disease, the tumor cells may stain positively for CEA and cytokeratin-7 and are negative for HMB-45 and Melan-A. S100 reactivity, although unusual, may occasionally be observed in Paget disease. Pagetoid Bowen disease (discussed in Chapter 29) shows, as a rule, a well-preserved basal cell layer, except in areas in which dermal invasion has taken place, and immunohistochemically the atypical cells stain positively with anti-keratin antibodies (e.g., AE1/AE3). They do not typically stain with S100 or with Melan-A or HMB-45. It should be noted that the cells of Paget disease and of Bowen disease may contain melanin pigment, because of transfer from reactive melanocytes in the adjacent skin, and it is conceivable that Melan-A/Mart1, tyrosinase, and HMB-45 staining could show some reactivity in such cases because these identify pigmentation-associated antigens. In a recent study based on morphology, crushing of basal keratinocytes and the presence of atypical cells in the stratum corneum and of large cells with amphophilic cytoplasm were significantly associated with Paget disease. Transition

between the atypical cells and surrounding keratinocytes was absent in all cases of melanoma *in situ* and in most Paget disease but was present in most cases of Bowen disease. Dyskeratotic cells were significantly associated with Bowen disease (378). Uncommonly, Merkel cell carcinoma and sebaceous carcinoma may have pagetoid cells in the epidermis, mimicking melanoma. IHC for melanocytic markers is negative in these lesions, and positive staining for relevant markers, for example, EMA, CK20, and CK7, respectively, is also useful (379).

Another pitfall in evaluating nonmelanocytic mimics of intraepidermal melanoma involves the variable tendency of keratinocytes within the uppermost epidermal layers to exhibit nuclear retraction presumably owing to nuclear shrinkage associated with biopsy or with tissue processing. These cells may produce in an otherwise benign or dysplastic melanocytic lesion the false appearance of true pagetoid spread, thus prompting consideration of a diagnosis of SSM. However, keratinocytes so altered are recognizable at high magnification as cells with nuclei surrounded by clear spaces (retraction clefts) that themselves are bordered by a rim of cytoplasm and joined by desmosomes, in contrast to pagetoid melanoma cells that lack desmosomes and whose nuclei are directly enveloped by relatively clear cytoplasm that may be surrounded by a thin clear mantle of retraction that separates the cell from adjacent keratinocytes.

Melanocytic Tumors in High CSD Skin

High CSD skin is defined as skin with severe solar elastosis.

Lentigo Maligna Melanoma (High CSD Melanoma, LMM)

LMM, previously referred to as melanosis circumscripta preblastomatosa of Dubreuilh (363) and also as melanotic freckle of Hutchinson (380) (or Hutchinson melanotic freckle, HMF, a term used currently in Australia for this condition), accounts for about 10% of melanomas, although likely higher than this in sun-susceptible populations in sunny climates (252). The term "lentigo maligna" (LM) may be regarded as synonymous with "lentigo maligna melanoma *in situ*" for most purposes. It is controversial whether LM should be regarded as a form of melanoma *in situ* in all cases or whether some cases should be regarded as precursor lesions (lentigo maligna) of *in situ* melanoma (melanoma *in situ*, lentigo maligna type) (381). In any case, these lesions, like other melanomas *in situ*, do not metastasize after complete excision, although they may persist and recur if not adequately excised.

This is the prototypic lesion of Pathway II of the WHO 2018 Classification of Melanoma (4) (Table 28-2, p. 836).

Clinical Summary. The lesions typically occur on the chronically exposed cutaneous surfaces of the elderly, most commonly on the face, and occasionally on the back, the forearms, or the lower legs. This form of melanoma tends to evolve slowly over many years, starting as an unevenly pigmented macule that gradually extends peripherally and may attain a diameter of several centimeters. It has an irregular border and, as long as it remains *in situ* or microinvasive, shows no induration. While extending in some areas, it may show spontaneous regression in others, resulting in irregular depigmented areas. The color varies from light brown to brown with minute dark brown or black flecks. Fine reticulated lines are usually also present and helpful in distinguishing the lesions from actinic lentigines. In contrast to SSM, the border is usually impalpable and indistinct, and some lesions are essentially amelanotic. For these reasons, the accurate clinical delineation of the border of an LMM can be problematic, and this not uncommonly results in unexpected positive or close margins in resection specimens. When a lesion of LM lacks melanin pigmentation, the clinical appearance may then resemble that of a solar keratosis or Bowen disease, or of an inflammatory patch, such as lupus erythematosus (382).

It has been suggested that the risk of progression from lentigo maligna melanoma in situ (LM) to invasive LMM may be about 5% (383), although some cases may progress rapidly (384), and a more recent estimate is higher, but still low, equating to an average time for LM to progress to LMM of 28.3 years (385). After adjustment for tumor thickness and other factors, LMM has the same prognosis as other forms of melanoma (386), although exceptions regarding metastatic potential may exist for certain variants (e.g., pure desmoplastic lesions). However, its demographics and associations differ from those of the most common form of melanoma, SSM. For example, patients with LMM have fewer nevi but more actinic keratoses than patients with SSM, consistent with a hypothesis of chronic sun exposure in the etiology of LMM (376). In addition, especially in older individuals, lesions that lack nesting and pagetoid scatter of melanocytes and with high solar elastosis, criteria similar to those described previously for LMM, are less likely to be associated with a BRAF mutation and more likely to have an NRAS mutation than when nesting and pagetoid growth are prominent, as in SSMs (258). In addition, mutations of the oncogene KIT are positively associated with melanomas in CSD skin (387). These evolving genetic data have been summarized and form a large part of the data driving the current WHO classification of melanoma (4).

Histopathology of Lentigo Maligna Melanoma

Architectural Features. In its earliest stage, LM may show at its periphery only hyperpigmentation with slight melanocytic proliferation, mainly in the basal cell layer. Toward the center of the lesion, there is a more pronounced increase in the concentration of basal melanocytes and some irregularity in their arrangement. Until there is contiguous and continuous proliferation of lesional melanocytes, these changes are not specific and may overlap with those of actinic lentigines. The epidermis is frequently flattened, in contrast to SSM, where it is irregularly thickened and thinned, or actinic lentigines, where there is elongation of the rete. This feature, although one of diagnostic importance, is less prominent than in SSM (Fig. 28-25). Noteworthy is the tendency of the basal layer of follicular infundibula to also be involved by the lentiginous proliferation of atypical melanocytes in LM.

Some nesting of melanocytes in the basal layer may be seen, but this is not usually pronounced until invasion of the dermis is developing. The atypical melanocytes within the nests usually retain their spindled shape and often "hang down" like rain droplets from the interface (296). Except in areas of nesting, the melanocytes tend to retain their dendritic processes. If the melanocytes are heavily melanized, some dendrites may be visible even in sections stained with hematoxylin–eosin; otherwise, these may also be visualized in immunostains.

The upper dermis, which invariably shows at least moderate and usually severe elastotic solar degeneration, contains numerous melanophages and, often, a rather pronounced, often bandlike, inflammatory infiltrate, although this may be minimal in predominantly in situ regions. Invasion may be demonstrable in these areas of dermal inflammation. Because invasion in an LMM (as in other melanomas) is a focal process, one should ensure that the specimen is adequately grossed and sectioned so as not to miss such areas. The presence or absence of tumorigenic VGP is recognized using criteria already presented (p. 875). The possibility of a desmoplastic VGP component (see later section) should be kept in mind because this may be a subtle finding. In case of doubt, an S100 or Sox10 stain can be crucial in demonstrating the lesion (329).

In some cases of LMM, the in situ component may show features overlapping with those of dysplastic nevi, including regions of nests predominating over single cells and bridging between adjacent rete ridges. Factors that help to distinguish these lesions include greater size, greater variability, and lesser symmetry, of architecture, and generally more severe and uniform atypia in LMM. Focal pagetoid scatter is often present, although the predominant intraepidermal architecture is lentiginous. There is usually severe actinic elastosis in the dermis. These changes have been described as LMMs with dysplastic nevus-like morphology (388). Somewhat similar lesions have been described as "lentiginous melanoma," in which cases the features tended to overlap with those of lentiginous nevi (389). The term "nevoid lentigo maligna" can be used to encompass these lesional patterns (390). As a general rule, we would advocate caution in making the diagnosis of a dysplastic nevus in skin with severe CSD. However, dysplastic nevi and atypical lentiginous nevi can occur in this setting.

Mitotic figures are uncommonly present in the epidermal compartment of LMM; if present in the dermis, they are indicative of VGP. When tumorigenic vertical growth supervenes, it is often of the spindle cell type, including the desmoplastic and neurotropic variants. Invasion in LMM may be extremely subtle, particularly when the involved cells exhibit desmoplastic or small cell (nevoid) features. Close attention to subtle yet uniform atypia, aided by immunohistochemical approaches (i.e., Sox10, S100, and Melan-A/MART-1 staining) to support melanocytic (e.g., vs. fibroblastic) lineage, may be helpful in such problematic lesions.

Identification of the in situ component of LMM can be difficult in melanoma reexcision specimens because the density of the cellularity declines toward the periphery of these lesions. Similar difficulty can be encountered in the diagnosis of subtle early lesions. Sox10 and Melan-A stains have been used to assist in this task, and, more recently, PRAME has been demonstrated to be a sensitive and specific marker. All of these stains need to be interpreted judiciously to avoid overinterpretation of atypical melanocytic proliferations that frequently occur in chronically sun-damaged skin (391).

Cytologic Summary. In fully evolved lesions of LM, the lesional melanocytes in the epidermis show a marked increase in concentration, bringing them in contiguity with one another, and their number in some areas exceeds that of the basal keratinocytes. Many of them are elongated and spindle shaped. Their nuclei appear atypical, being enlarged, hyperchromatic, and pleomorphic. However, the chromatin pattern is often not as open or "vesicular" as that seen in the more epithelioid cells of SSM in its radial phase of growth. Frequently, atypical melanocytes extend along the basal cell layer of hair follicles, often for a considerable distance, occasionally extending to the base of a

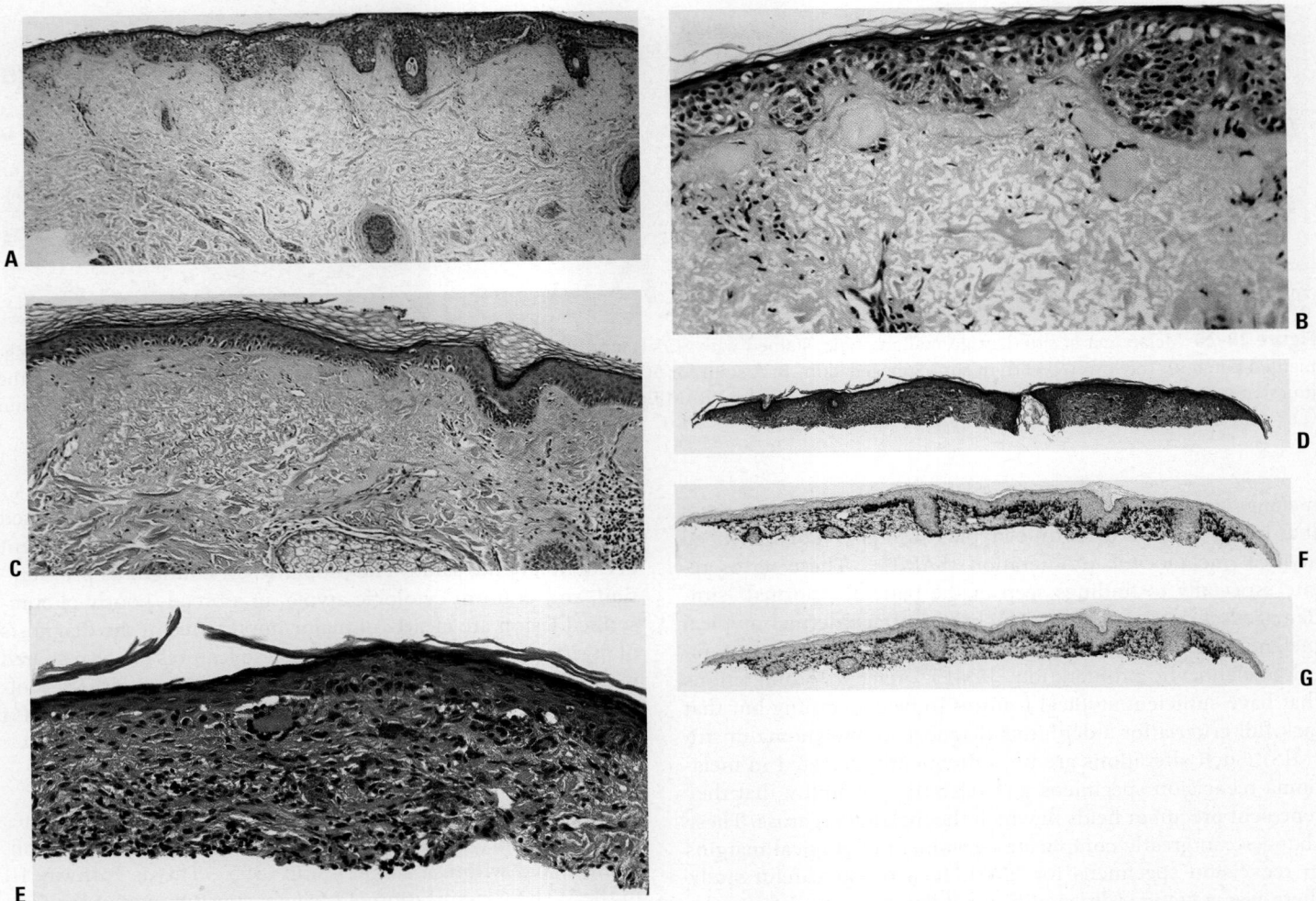

Figure 28-25 Lentigo maligna melanoma, *in situ*. **A:** At low magnification, the lesions are broad and asymmetrical in the distribution of lesional and host responding cells. **B:** The epidermis is atrophic, and there is usually severe actinic elastosis in the dermis. **C:** As in superficial spreading melanoma, the lesional cells exhibit moderate-to-severe uniform cytologic atypia. There is usually some evidence of pagetoid proliferation in lentigo maligna melanoma (LMM), especially near areas of invasion. However, especially at the periphery of the lesion, this is much less prominent, and the lesional cells are smaller than in superficial spreading melanoma. **D:** LMM, invasive. A broad, moderately to highly cellular lesion occurring in skin with severe chronic solar damage. **E:** Higher magnification demonstrates continuous basal proliferation of uniformly atypical melanocytes and a mixture of cells in the dermis, of uncertain lineage, including lymphocytes, histiocytes, and atypical spindle cells. **F:** A Melan-A stain demonstrates the continuous basal proliferation and also highlights many of the spindle cells in the dermis. **G:** An MITF stain (or Sox10 stain) can complement the Melan-A stain because the nuclear staining more clearly delineates the individual cells.

shave biopsy specimen. Usually, the proliferating melanocytes contain moderate melanin, and melanin is also present in keratinocytes. There is usually some upward pagetoid extension of atypical melanocytes, although this is generally only focal and high-level pagetoid spread into the stratum granulosum, as seen in SSM, is rare.

Pathogenesis. As an explanation for the somewhat distinctive behavior of LM, the theory was offered by Mishima that it is derived from spindle-shaped junctional melanocytes and thus represents a melanocyte-derived melanoma, in contrast to the SSM that is derived from rounded junctional nevus cells and can be regarded as a nevus cell–derived melanoma (371). The "pathway concept" of the pathogenesis supports this general idea, based on epidemiologic and genomic differences. However, the hypothesis does not consider the alternative possibility that both LM and SSM are derived from junctional melanocytes, although the genomic and epigenomic pathways involved in SSM involve a more nevoid intermediate in evolution to full malignancy. Although progression of LM is often slow, some

cases progress more rapidly, and complete excision of these lesions (rather than observation) is recommended to prevent the development of a more dangerous melanoma (392).

Differential Diagnosis of Lentigo Maligna. The major differential diagnostic considerations are between actinic lentigines with atypia, atypical lentiginous nevi, and dysplastic nevi. Actinic lentigines are defined by a variable combination of three features: elongated rete ridges, hyperpigmentation of basal keratinocytes, and prominence of melanocytes. Continuous proliferation of melanocytes is lacking, and, although there may be atypia, it is random rather than uniform. Staining with Melan-A/MART1 is useful in demonstrating confluent proliferation and is often combined with Sox10, a nuclear marker that may help to avoid any tendency for overcalling confluence caused by labeling of dendrites in a MART1 stain, and, more recently, PRAME (391) (Fig. 28-26).

It should also be remembered that some individuals with chronic sun damage may have diffuse, clinically covert, noncontiguous lentiginous proliferation of somewhat atypical

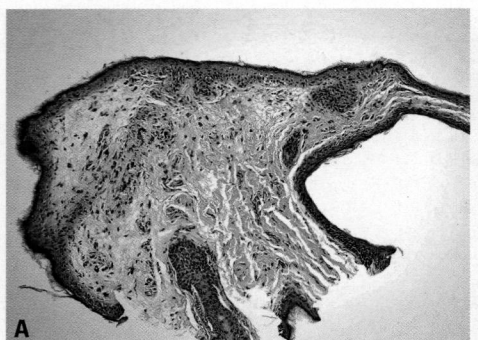 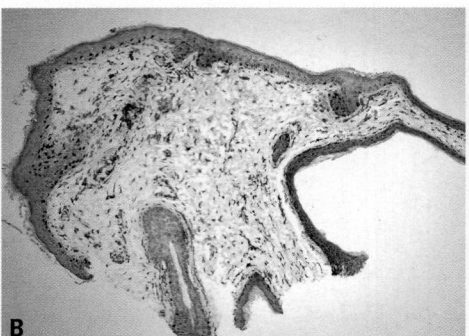 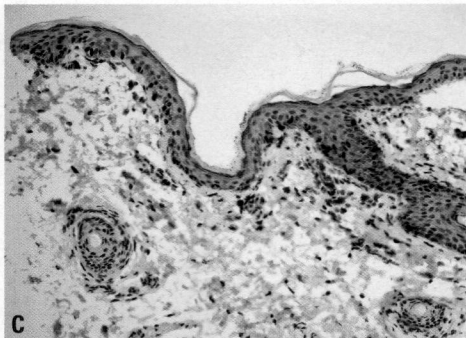

Figure 28-26 Melanoma *in situ*, lentigo maligna type, stained with SOX10 and PRAME. **A:** A small and challenging biopsy from a 2.4-cm pigmented patch on the lower eyelid, in sun-damaged skin. **B:** A stain for SOX10 protein demonstrates an increased number of melanocytes at the junction with focal upward scatter. **C:** The lesional cells stain for PRAME protein, demonstrating a similar distribution to that in the SOX10 stain (i.e., near 100% staining).

melanocytes within the epidermal basal cell layer, a process that has been termed "actinic atypia," and also "solar induced atypical melanocytic proliferation (SAMP)." These terms relate especially to findings seen in the patient's "normal" sun-damaged skin. Other terms, such as "intraepidermal atypical melanocytic proliferation" and "junctional lentiginous (atypical) melanocytic proliferation (JLMP)," refer to proliferations that have sufficient atypical features to be concerning but that lack full criteria for a definitive diagnosis of melanoma in situ (MIS). Such alterations are not infrequently detected in melanoma reexcision specimens and raise the possibility that they represent precursor fields in which the melanomas arose. These changes can greatly complicate assessment of surgical margins in reexcision specimens for LMM. In a recent careful study, there was a statistically significant difference found for melanocyte density, irregular melanocyte distribution, melanocyte clustering, follicular infundibular involvement, and nesting between JLMP and MIS. However, criteria such as nesting, epithelioid cells, and melanocyte clustering were seen in both sun-damaged skin and MIS. Of the criteria evaluated, melanocytic density was the most objective histologic criterion and did not overlap between the sun-damaged and JLMP/MIS groups (393). Correlation with clinical appearance may be helpful in determining the biologic significance of such low-grade atypical melanocytic hyperplasias.

LM with junctional nest formation may also be mistaken for a superficial dysplastic nevus, especially in a partial biopsy specimen, as discussed previously in the discussion of nevoid LM (388). It is important in such situations to note the greater breadth and asymmetry often with foci of atypical proliferation in an atrophic epidermis devoid of elongation of rete ridges; the uniform (rather than random) atypia of the lesional cells; and, if present, the presence of follicular extension by the atypical melanocytes in LM.

"Melanocytic pseudonests" that can be seen in interface and lichenoid inflammatory reactions can stain nonspecifically with Melan-A/MART1 and can mimic melanoma *in situ* of the LM type. In addition, true melanocytic nests have been described in lichenoid dermatitis yet not thought to be indicative of an atypical melanocytic proliferation. The revised terminology of "melanocytic nests arising in lichenoid inflammation" has been suggested to describe this pattern of benign melanocytic proliferation in a subset of lichenoid dermatoses. Clinicopathologic correlation is essential for avoiding diagnostic error in these cases (394).

The differential diagnosis with SSM has been discussed previously and is of less importance because the management is essentially the same. The properties of contiguous proliferation, and uniform cytologic atypia, in a broad, poorly circumscribed lesion are clearly of major importance in the diagnosis of *in situ* or microinvasive LMM. These features are also shared with SSM, whereas focal pagetoid melanocytosis, although often present, is less prominent in LM/LMM. By definition, LMM occurs in skin with high CSD (4).

Desmoplastic and Neurotropic Melanoma
Desmoplastic malignant melanomas (DM) present attributes of melanocytic, fibroblastic, and schwannian differentiation, often mixed within a single lesion (395). This is Pathway III in the WHO Classification of Melanocytic Tumours of the Skin (Table 28-2, p. 836).

Clinical Summary. The lesions occur on chronically sun-damaged skin, usually in elderly patients, most commonly on the head and neck (396). The lower lip is a relatively common site, sometimes in younger patients and often in association with neurotropism (397). In a large series of 280 cases of DM, the male-to-female ratio was 1.75:1 and the median patient age 61 years. The median tumor thickness was 2.5 mm, and 44% of cases were amelanotic. Five-year survival was 75%. Significant predictors of overall survival were a high mitotic rate and tumor thickness. All the DMs exceeded 1.5 mm in thickness and were Clark level IV or V. There was a significant increase in local recurrence when neurotropism was present. In this prospectively and expertly treated series of cases, the rate of local recurrence was not higher for DM than for other cutaneous melanomas (398). However, in meta-analysis of other series of cases, local recurrence was not uncommon (often owing to misdiagnosis), and was associated with a greater risk of progression to systemic disease (396).

DM in high CSD skin has among the highest tumor mutation burden rates of any cancer, with a prominent UV signature (275), and patients with advanced DM derive substantial clinical benefit from PD-1 or PD-L1 immune checkpoint blockade therapy (399). Distinct genetic alterations known to activate the *MAPK* and *PI3K* signaling cascades differ from those in other melanomas, affecting *NF1*, *CBL*, *ERBB2*, *MAP2K1*, *MAP3K1*, *BRAF*, *EGFR*, *PTPN11*, *MET*, *RAC1*, *SOS2*, *NRAS*, and *PIK3CA* (275). Inactivating mutations in NF1, which is a downregulator of *RAS*, have been found in 93% of DMM, compared to 20% in non-DM, and appear to be the most important "driver" of DM tumors (400).

Cases of DM not associated with CSD, often in relation to lentiginous melanomas, occur in acral/subungual (401) and mucosal sites (402). These are not likely to have the same UV signature, tumor mutation burden, and responsiveness to checkpoint immune therapy that characterize the high CSD DMM.

Histopathology. Desmoplasia is most often seen in a spindle cell VGP of LMM or acral or mucosal lentiginous melanoma. However, desmoplastic changes can be seen occasionally in tumors with rounded or undifferentiated melanoma cells. The collagen in DMs is arranged as delicate fibrils that extend between the tumor cells and separate them from one another. The relationship between tumor cells and stroma is thus similar to that seen in sarcomas, in contrast to most melanomas, where an epithelial pattern of collagen fibers surrounding groups or clusters of tumor cells may be demonstrated, for example, with a reticulin

stain. Interestingly, neurotized nevi may also show the pattern of individual cells surrounded by collagen that characterizes DMs, and the arrangement of the cells of DMs in "wavy" fiber bundles comprised of "S-shaped" or "serpentine" cells may also recall the "schwannian" patterns of neurofibromas, neurotized nevi, and malignant schwannomas.

In DM, scanning magnification usually demonstrates an alteration of the architecture of the dermis, which may be subtle or more prominent. Frequently, this alteration extends throughout the full thickness of the reticular dermis into the fat. Typically, nodular clusters of lymphocytes and occasional plasma cells are present in the tumor or at its periphery, serving as a valuable clue at scanning magnification (Fig. 28-27A). Of note, these aggregates have also been described in some desmoplastic nevi (403). At higher magnification, the melanoma cells are usually elongated and amelanotic and embedded in a markedly fibrotic stroma, often making it difficult to decide which are fibroblasts and which are melanoma cells. This problem is enhanced by the relative absence of nuclear atypia in many of the neoplastic

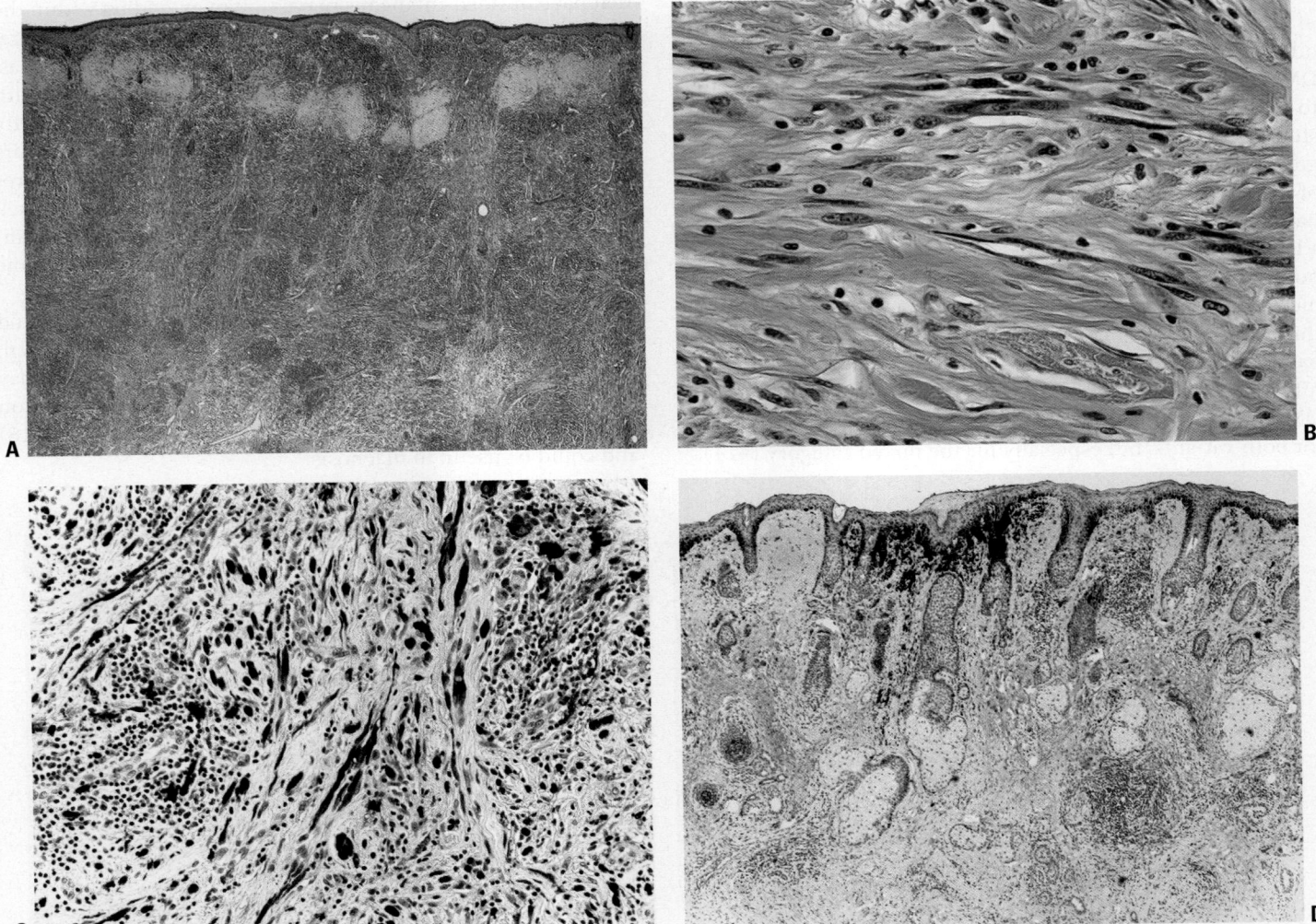

Figure 28-27 Desmoplastic melanoma. **A:** At scanning magnification, the architecture of the reticular dermis is altered by a cellular infiltrate including nodular clusters of lymphocytes, appearances that can simulate an inflammatory infiltrate. **B:** Atypical spindle cells arranged in loose fascicles extend into the deeper dermis and subcutis, beneath the epithelioid cell component. This subtle proliferation is easily overlooked, resulting in potential "undercalling" of the diagnosis and microstage. **C:** The spindle cells are S100 positive. S100 stain is of great value in delineating the boundaries of desmoplastic melanomas but should be interpreted cautiously because it is not specific for melanoma cells. **D:** An immunohistochemical study for Melan-A focally stains the *in situ* and superficial dermal epithelioid cell component of the melanoma. The deeper spindle cells are uniformly negative.

spindle cells, although close scrutiny will usually reveal cells with nuclear hyperchromasia and contour irregularities not typical of resting or activated benign mesenchymal cells (Fig. 28-27B). Because of the frequent absence of melanin, differentiation from a fibrohistiocytic or neural lesion may be difficult.

DMs have been shown to produce fibrogenic cytokines, neurotrophins, and neurotrophin receptors (such as p75NGFR), which together can account for their desmoplastic and neurotropic propensities (404,405). A rare lesion, termed "osteogenic desmoplastic melanoma," has been described and could be difficult to differentiate from an osteosarcoma (406). Aside from the diagnostic challenges posed by these differentiation patterns, such lesions may provide evidence of the inherent plasticity of a subpopulation of melanoma stem cells that drives the tumorigenic potential of advanced lesions.

By routine histology, DMs have been classified into two types: "pure" DMs that are characterized by predominant fibrosis, which extends between individual tumor cells, and "mixed" tumors, in which fibrosis is well developed only in parts of an otherwise nondesmoplastic (i.e., epithelioid) melanoma (Fig. 28-28A, B). The "pure" group had a better 5-year survival of 90% compared to 70% in the mixed tumors (407), and in another study, after adjustment for thickness, patients with pure DM had half the chance of melanoma-specific death compared to a comparison group of SSM patients (408). In a comparative study, expression of most markers was similar in the two subgroups; however, there was significantly increased expression of c-kit, and also of Ki-67, in the mixed subgroup, which also had a higher proliferative index than the pure group (409). In a large series of 252 patients who had sentinel node biopsy, the node positive rate was lower than in patients with conventional melanoma, and survival was related to node status and the thickness of the primary tumor (410). In another study of 205 patients, the overall rate of sentinel node involvement was significantly higher for mixed (24.6%) compared with pure (9.0%) DM, suggesting that sentinel node staging should be considered for both variants, but especially for the mixed category (411).

Although the reported survival rate for DM in the early literature was poor, this is likely because many of these cases had already recurred when the diagnosis was made. A report of a series of DMs that had been prospectively diagnosed and definitively treated at their initial presentation showed that the survival was no different than for usual forms of melanoma, when thickness, mitotic rate, host response, and other risk factors were controlled. Indeed, the probability of survival is relatively good for prospectively diagnosed and definitively treated DM, because despite the considerable thickness of many of these lesions, the prognostically important mitotic rate and lymphocytic responses are often favorable (412).

Neurotropic melanoma is often a variant of DM, occurring most commonly in the head and neck (398,413,414). There may be a propensity for involvement of the lower lip, and the lesions may initially present as a benign-appearing nodule (415). In a large series, 28% of DMs were also neurotropic, whereas 72% of neurotropic cases were desmoplastic. The incidence of neurotropism was 0.8% in nondesmoplastic melanomas (416).

Histologically, there are fascicles of spindle cell melanoma that have invaded cutaneous nerves, often extending within the fiber itself (endoneurial invasion) as opposed to the "perineural invasion" that is more characteristic of neurotropic carcinomas. The involvement of nerves may therefore be quite subtle, with the first clue being the impression of slight hypercellularity within a given nerve branch. The neurotropism usually occurs in association with a spindle cell vertical component with fibrosis (Fig. 28-29). However, some neurotropic melanomas lack these latter features of DM. Many of these are spindle cell tumorigenic melanomas of acral-lentiginous or LM type, but some are composed of epithelioid cells.

Desmoplastic and spindle cell melanomas, in general, tend to express a high level of p75 neurotrophin receptor antigen, as well as other neurotrophins and their receptors, which may contribute to the high predisposition for perineural extension in the desmoplastic subset of spindled melanomas (417,418) and could be useful in diagnosis.

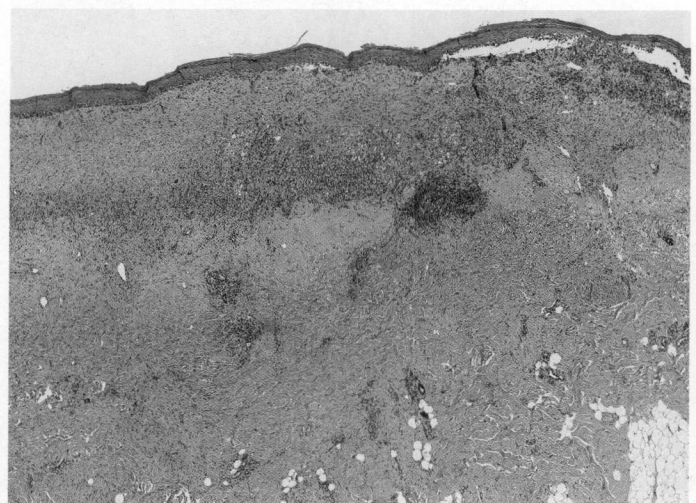
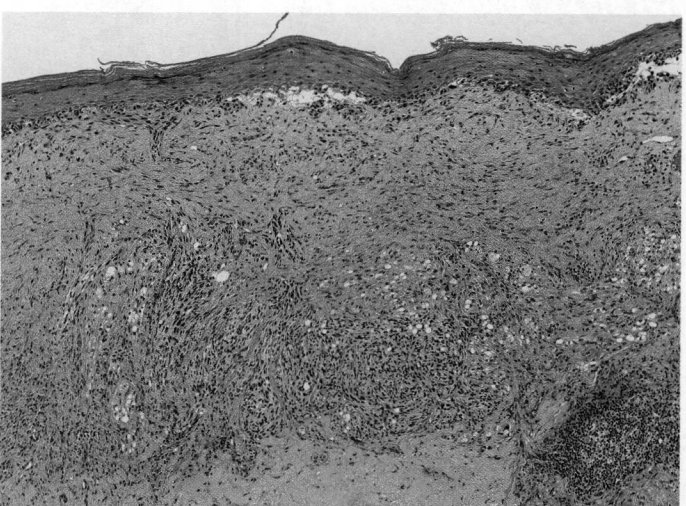

Figure 28-28 Desmoplastic melanoma, pure and spindle cell patterns, with Sox10 staining (see also Fig. 28-30). **A:** There is a tumor with an *in situ* and superficial invasive component comprised of epithelioid melanocytes (top right) and with a desmoplastic component that permeates the reticular dermis, extending all the way to the bottom left of the image and beyond. Note nodular clusters of lymphocytes scattered within the tumor, a low-power diagnostic flow. **B:** Pure desmoplastic melanoma in the top half of the image, with spindle cell (nondesmoplastic) melanoma above a region of severe solar elastosis near the bottom, and a nodular cluster of lymphocytes at the bottom right.

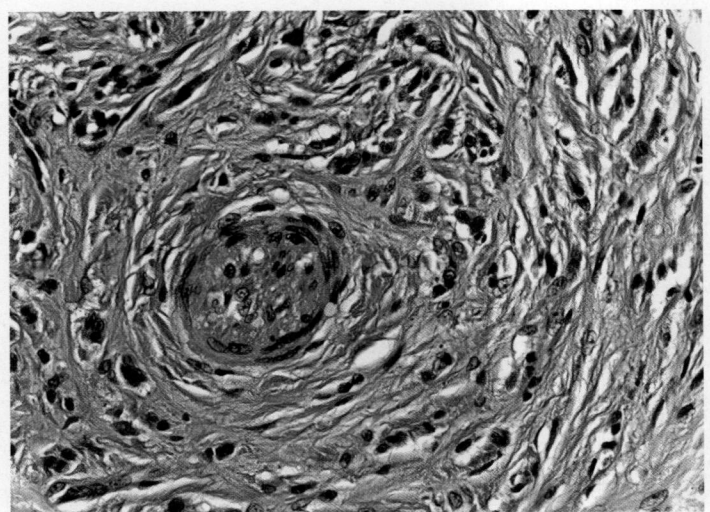

Figure 28-29 Neurotropism in a desmoplastic melanoma. A nerve in the center of the image contains atypical neoplastic spindle cells both in the nerve itself (endoneurial invasion) and in the perineurium (perineural invasion). The adjacent stroma contains neoplastic spindle cells separated by desmoplastic stroma.

Neurotropism in a primary melanoma is historically associated with increased risk for local recurrence, even after standard "definitive" therapy, and may also be associated with increased mortality (412); however, prospective expert diagnosis and management can lead to improved results, with clear surgical margins being of paramount importance (414). In the largest study to date, based on 671 prospectively diagnosed and expertly treated cases, it was found that that neurotropism, whether present in a desmoplastic or nondesmoplastic melanoma, did not confer any independent survival or recurrence risk or benefit after adjustment for known predictors of outcome, which included age, sex, thickness, stage, site, ulceration status, mitotic rate, and excision margin. These factors tended to be highly expressed, pointing to higher risk in the neurotropic melanomas. The neurotropic melanomas were nearly three times as likely to have a borderline pathologic margin of excision compared with control melanomas, increasing the likelihood of local and regional or distant recurrence fourfold and twofold, respectively. Neurotropic melanomas with borderline excision margins were responsive to adjuvant radiotherapy, potentially halving the risk of local recurrence (416) (Fig. 28-29).

Reexcision Specimens. Evaluation of reexcision specimens of desmoplastic and neurotropic melanomas can present considerable difficulties. It is important that these procedures encompass a margin of normal tissue around the scar, both for completeness of excision and because of the difficulty of excluding subtle melanoma involvement of the scar. In this regard, it is helpful to remember that residual melanoma is likely to present at the periphery of the scar and to infiltrate normal tissue adjacent to it. The specimens should be carefully coated with India ink or colored dyes, and the inked margin should be scrutinized for residual invasive melanoma and for subtle neurotropic involvement of small nerves. A clue to the presence of melanoma, both in nerves and in the stroma, is the presence of clusters of lymphocytes, which may sometimes almost completely obscure the tumor cells themselves. S100 staining can be useful, but it has been demonstrated that S100-positive cells may be present in

benign scars (419). However, persistent S100-positive spindle cell melanoma cells tend to occur in small clusters and fascicles, rather than as single cells as in scar tissue that often represent S100-positive dendritic cells of hematopoietic lineage. Additional markers are now available to assist in this difficult distinction, as discussed in the next section.

Immunohistochemistry. Desmoplastic and, to a somewhat lesser extent, other spindle cell melanomas tend to differ from the more common epithelioid cell melanomas in their immunohistochemical reactivity. Although S100 is almost always positive, the more specific markers such as HMB-45 and Melan-A/MART-1 are usually negative, except for occasional reactivity of a minor epithelioid cell component that is sometimes present in the epidermis or superficial dermal component of the neoplasm (Fig. 28-27D). In a study of 20 DMs, all were positive for S100 protein, whereas 7 were positive for MITF, 6 for HMB-45, and 11 for tyrosinase. Immunoreactivity for MITF was seen not only in melanocytes of normal skin but also in macrophages, lymphocytes, fibroblasts, Schwann cells, and smooth muscle cells at various sites and in tumors derived from these cell types (420). In another study, only 4 of 13 spindle cell and DMs (all positive with anti-S100 and negative with HMB-45) were immunoreactive with Melan-A/MART-1 (2 focally, 2 diffusely) (421). Thus, S100 reactivity is key in distinguishing these tumors from fibroblastic lesions. However, it is of no use in the distinction from neural tumors or from desmoplastic nevi. In contrast, Melan-A/MART-1 reactivity is usually present in desmoplastic nevi, including sclerotic blue nevi, and such reactivity may be very helpful in ruling out a DM in some such lesions (422), although this is not pathognomonic. Similarly, HMB-45 reactivity would also support a diagnosis of a deep spindle cell proliferation other than DM (e.g., a relatively amelanotic blue nevus).

Also, as indicated previously, the HMB-45, Melan-A, and tyrosinase antigens are usually not demonstrable in the spindle cell compartment of DMs but may be focally demonstrable in superficial dermal or *in situ* epithelioid melanocytes (Fig. 28-27D), especially in mixed cases. However, the markers SOX10, MITF, and p75NGF have been found to be useful in DM (Fig 28-30). In a comparative study, SOX10 was strongly expressed by DM and was less likely than S100 and MITF to be expressed by background fibrocytes and histiocytes within scars (423). In a study of spindle cell tumors that may mimic DM, SOX10 showed 100% sensitivity for DM and was negative in spindle cell carcinoma, atypical fibroxanthoma (AFX), and sarcomas. Similar to S100 protein, some malignant peripheral nerve sheath tumors (MPNSTs) showed scattered positivity but not how diffuse positivity seen in DM (424). However, reactivity of scattered individual cells for Sox10 has been described in DMs, representing a potential diagnostic pitfall (425,426). The nerve growth factor receptor p75NGFR labels DM cells with considerable sensitivity (427). However, this marker also labels cells in scars, thought to represent nerve twigs, Schwann cells, and/or reactive myofibroblasts (428) (Fig. 28-30).

Differential Diagnosis. It is, of course, very important to differentiate DM from benign conditions, including benign melanocytic and neural tumors, fibrous and fibrohistiocytic tumors, other spindle cell malignancies, and scars. Neurotized nevi and neurofibromas share serpentine spindle cell and wavy fiber bundle patterns of schwannian differentiation with DMs but lack an *in*

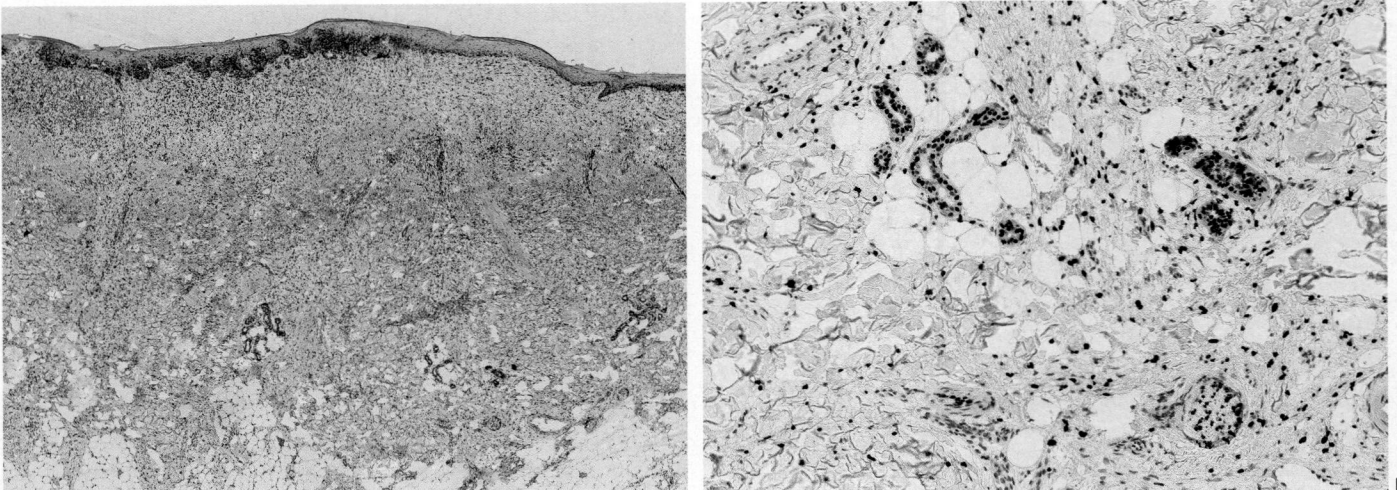

Figure 28-30 Sox10 staining in a desmoplastic melanoma. Same lesion as in Figure 28-28. **A:** There is strong Sox10 staining of a superficial/*in situ* component (*top center-left*) and there is subtle (at scanning magnification) nuclear staining of cells infiltrating through the reticular dermis and into the subcutis. **B:** High magnification from near the base of the tumor demonstrates infiltrating small cells (whose spindled cytoplasm is not apparent in this preparation), in this field ramifying around a sweat duct unit. Note positive Sox10 staining of sweat duct epithelium and of Schwann cells of a small cutaneous nerve (*bottom right*).

situ melanoma component and lack atypia and mitotic activity as well as lymphocytic infiltrates in the dermal component. According to a study by Harris et al., similarities between desmoplastic nevi and DMs included the presence of atypical cells and HMB-45 expression in the superficial portion of the lesions. The infrequent location on the head or neck, the absence of mitotic figures, a significantly lower number of Ki-67-reactive cells, and the presence of HMB-45 expression in the deep area of the lesions helped distinguish desmoplastic nevi from DM. The diagnosis of DM should be made with abundant caution if the dermal spindle cell component is positive for Melan-A (422). Fibrous tumors such as connective tissue nevi or cellular dermatofibromas can be distinguished by immunohistochemical studies, including negative S100 staining.

Misdiagnosis of DMs as one or another of the benign lesions listed previously is not uncommon, because attributes of malignancy such as anaplasia or frequent mitoses are often not prominent features of DMs. However, the large size and asymmetrical silhouette of many of these lesions differ from most benign lesions. As previously emphasized, an important and sometimes subtle clue to the diagnosis at low power is the frequent presence of a lymphocytic infiltrate, distributed as nodular aggregates of infiltrating lymphocytes throughout the tumor, which are not seen in neurofibromas, nevi, or most fibrohistiocytic lesions. Lymphocytes may also be clustered about nerves involved by tumor cells in neurotropic melanomas. Other helpful diagnostic attributes, which may not be readily evident unless sought because of a high index of suspicion, include the presence of an atypical intraepidermal melanocytic component, which may be subtle and not always diagnostic of frank melanoma, and usually the presence, on diligent search, of at least a few mitoses in the dermal component of the lesion.

Other considerations include low-grade malignancies such as fibromatoses and dermatofibrosarcoma protuberans, atypical smooth muscle neoplasms, and malignant lesions such as MPNSTs. The latter group of lesions may overlap biologically as well as morphologically, and their management is similar, namely, complete excision and follow-up. IHC staining for loss of H3K27me3 can be used as a marker for MPNST, although its sensitivity and specificity are not well characterized (429). Because spindle cell melanomas may be confused with other malignant spindle cell neoplasms (e.g., malignant tumors of neural cells, smooth muscle, fibrohistiocytic cells, and spindle cell variants of squamous cell carcinoma), particularly when careful search fails to reveal evidence of *in situ* growth, immunohistochemical screening by the panel approach is recommended in such instances.

Rarely, spindle cell melanomas may form vessel-like structures, and when such lesions occur on the scalp of elderly individuals, they produce confusion with angiosarcoma. Immunohistochemical identification of S100 protein (and SOX10) and exclusion of CD31 endothelial reactivity may be helpful in such instances (430).

The distinction from a neurogenic sarcoma may be very difficult or impossible in such cases where there is no pigment and there is no characteristic superficial RGP component (431). Some of these lesions might alternatively be regarded as superficial malignant epithelioid schwannomas. The prognostic implications are similar, whichever diagnostic term is used. When such a lesion is marked by strong and diffuse S100 positivity, we will usually render a diagnosis of DM, even in the absence of an *in situ* component or pigment.

Unusual Variants of Melanoma

Unusual variants of melanoma, in general, do not have independent prognostic implications, but an understanding of these variants may be useful in the accurate diagnosis of these lesions. Most of these variants might be placed in the Low CSD category (pathway), but some of them could be found in other categories as well.

Polypoid Melanoma

Also termed pedunculated melanoma, this term designates a melanoma that presents as a protruding nodule connected to the underlying skin by a pedicle or stalk, which can occasionally be quite long (432). The surface of the nodule is often eroded or ulcerated. Because these tumors are bulky, the prognosis is often poor but probably not worse than predicted by other risk factors (433). By convention, polypoid melanomas, even when the greatly expanded papillary dermis is not filled, are considered to represent level III invasion unless tumor cells extend into the reticular dermis (level IV).

On histologic examination, the nodule is filled with melanoma cells, whereas the underlying stalk or pedicle may be free of tumor cells; in other cases, the tumor may infiltrate the pedicle and the dermis adjacent to the pedicle. The lesions need to be distinguished from polypoid nevi by the usual criteria, including cytologic atypia, failure of maturation, and mitotic activity (434).

Verrucous Melanoma

These melanomas present as a markedly hyperkeratotic, tumorigenic nodule that may simulate a verruca, verrucous benign keratosis, or a verrucous carcinoma clinically (306,367,435). Histologically as well, the lesions are associated with marked acanthosis, hyperkeratosis, and verrucous hyperplasia of keratinocytes that may assume pseudoepitheliomatous proportions and raise a question of squamous cell carcinoma unless the underlying neoplastic melanocytes are appreciated (436). Some other lesions are misdiagnosed histologically as benign nevi or seborrheic keratoses (306), highlighting the potential importance of histologic sampling of changing or symptomatic nevic or keratosis-like lesions. "Verrucous" changes of adjacent keratinocytes are sometimes observed in the immediate vicinity of acral and, especially, subungual melanomas, which are often clinically mistaken for warts on initial presentation when pigment is not prominent. In such instances, an inadequate biopsy that does not include the underlying neoplasm could appear to be consistent with a wart.

Balloon Cell Melanoma

In addition to more characteristic melanoma cells of the epithelioid type, some melanomas contain aggregates of "balloon cells" (437). These balloon cells, characterized by their abundant, clear cytoplasm, may show relatively little nuclear atypia and may thus resemble those seen in a balloon cell nevus (p. 853). The clear cytoplasm is the result of vacuolar degenerative alterations affecting melanosomes and may expand the cytoplasm in a manner that compresses the nucleus, partially obscuring its size and cytologic features helpful in identifying a malignant phenotype. However, the overall architecture of the lesion and the presence of at least foci of detectable cytologic atypia, usually with mitotic activity, identify the tumor as a melanoma. IHC (Melan-A, HMB-45, and/or tyrosinase reactivity) may sometimes be required to distinguish the lesions from other clear cell or foamy tumors, such as renal cell carcinoma or xanthoma, respectively (438). GEP has been used to support the diagnosis (439).

Transitions from the melanoma cells to balloon cells are usually seen. The metastases of a balloon cell melanoma may or may not be composed largely of balloon cells, and balloon cell metastases have been described from a melanoma that did not contain them in the primary tumor (440). In addition, a metastatic balloon cell melanoma has been described in the absence of a known primary (441). Thus, this possibility should be considered in the differential diagnosis of metastatic clear cell tumors. The cells exhibit immunopathologic reactivity characteristic of melanoma.

Signet Cell Melanoma

Melanomas that contain prominent signet-ring cells may be confusing and must be distinguished from adenocarcinomas, tumors of vascular endothelium or adipose tissue, lymphomas, and epithelioid smooth muscle tumors (442,443). The signet cell morphology may be recognized in the primary tumors or only in metastatic sites. Similar cells may be seen in benign nevi, and a somewhat similar change may also occur as a result of freezing artifact (442). IHC may be used to confirm the diagnosis of a melanocytic lesion and rule out competing possibilities. In evaluating these results, it should be recognized that expression of both CEA (only seen using polyclonal antibodies) (444,445) and (mostly in metastases) keratin (mostly in metastases) (446) has been described in melanomas.

Myxoid Melanoma

A histologic pattern of prominent myxoid stroma has been described in some primary and metastatic melanomas (447,448). In addition, a myxoid clear cell sarcoma has been described (449). The differential diagnosis may be very broad, including lipoblastic, myoblastic, fibroblastic, neurogenic, or chondroblastic, and other melanocytic tumors with myxoid stroma (447,448). If the diagnosis is suspected, IHC can be performed to support the diagnosis. Fontana stain may reveal melanin pigment, and electron microscopy in a few cases has shown melanosomes.

Animal-Type Melanoma (Pigment Synthesizing Melanoma)

Rare tumors, comprised of asymmetric, predominantly dermal nodules of heavily pigmented cells that mimic melanocytic neoplasms, are seen in horses and laboratory animals (e.g., Sinclair swine) and have thus been termed animal-type melanomas (350,450). Behavior of these lesions is unpredictable. In two published series totaling 20 cases (236,350), the lesions were described as blue-black nodules with irregular borders from 1 to 4 cm in size, located on the scalp, lower extremities, back, and sacrum. Sections showed confluent dermal sheets of round or short spindle-shaped heavily melanized cells whose nuclei, where discernible, were large with irregularly thickened membranes; coarse and somewhat hyperchromatic chromatin; and prominent, often spiculated nucleoli. Mitoses were infrequent. In some cases, appreciation of nuclear detail obscured by the extensive cytoplasmic melanization has been facilitated by the use of a melanin bleach protocol. Four lesions had an epidermal component. One patient suffered metastases to regional lymph nodes, liver, and lungs with lethal effect, whereas all of the others were alive with variable follow-up, despite five of them with regional lymph node metastases, one with hepatic metastases, and three with local satellite metastases. In a study of 14 similar cases, the term "pigment synthesizing melanoma (PSM)" was suggested for these lesions, which were considered to be a distinctive, possibly low-grade form of melanoma (236). In addition, many lesions that had in the past been termed "animal melanomas" may be better classified today as PEM. However, some of these have had a fatal outcome (236), suggesting that usual criteria for malignancy should be applied in this category of cases, which would include increased mitotic activity, presence of sheetlike growth with increased density of lesional cells, and GAs such as loss of p16 (*CDKN2A*), *TERTp* mutation, and others (233,238).

Minimal Deviation Melanoma

Recognized by only some authors, this lesion is referred to as "borderline type" when it is limited to the papillary dermis and as "minimal deviation type" when it extends into the reticular dermis (451). These tumors are considered to exhibit less cytologic atypia than the common forms of melanoma, although the architectural characteristics of melanoma are usually present. Accordingly, they may be considered to show morphologic overlap between an atypical nevus and a melanoma with fully evolved anaplasia. The lesions in their vertical phase consist of uniformly expansile nodules, and the cells in the nodules tend to be arranged in uniform patterns. If the tumor cells are epithelioid in type, they may resemble cells of the ordinary acquired nevus. In the spindle cell variants, the tumor cells may resemble the cells of a Spitz nevus or, if pigmented or arranged in compact fascicles, a pigmented spindle cell nevus. Because of the resemblance to nevus cells, the term nevoid melanoma has also been used. However, nevoid melanoma (discussed in the next section) technically differs from most so-called borderline/minimal deviation melanomas by virtue of a more nevoid architecture, albeit formed by mitotically active cells. In one study, expression rates of the proliferation marker Ki-67 in borderline/minimal deviation melanomas were intermediate between those seen in nevi and those in SSMs (452). Even though recurrences, metastases, and death may occur, most minimal deviation melanomas are thought to be biologically not as aggressive as common melanomas. However, in our opinion and that of others, prognosis is probably more accurately predicted by multivariable prognostic models (453).

Nevoid Melanoma

Although related to minimal deviation melanoma, this term has been used somewhat differently. Nevoid melanomas are defined as lesions that, to a greater or lesser extent, mimic a benign nevus histologically, often with an emphasis on a nevoid architecture (in contrast to minimal deviation melanoma, where melanoma architecture tends to be preserved) (454,455). Usually, the resemblance is most apparent at scanning magnification, where lesions may appear symmetrical, nested, and devoid of radial growth, features that can lead to a missed diagnosis if sufficient attention is not paid to cytologic and subtle architectural features. Discriminating attributes include high cellularity with "sheetlike" growth, cellular atypia (albeit somewhat monotonous), mitoses, infiltration of adnexa, infiltrative growth in the deeper dermis, and incomplete or absent maturation (Fig. 28-31). Tumor thickness was the most important prognostic criterion (454). Nevoid melanomas are generally considered to have the same biologic potential as other melanomas with similar microstaging attributes. Key to the recognition of a nevoid melanoma is a high index of suspicion and the identification of mitotic activity and cytologic atypia in the dermal component of

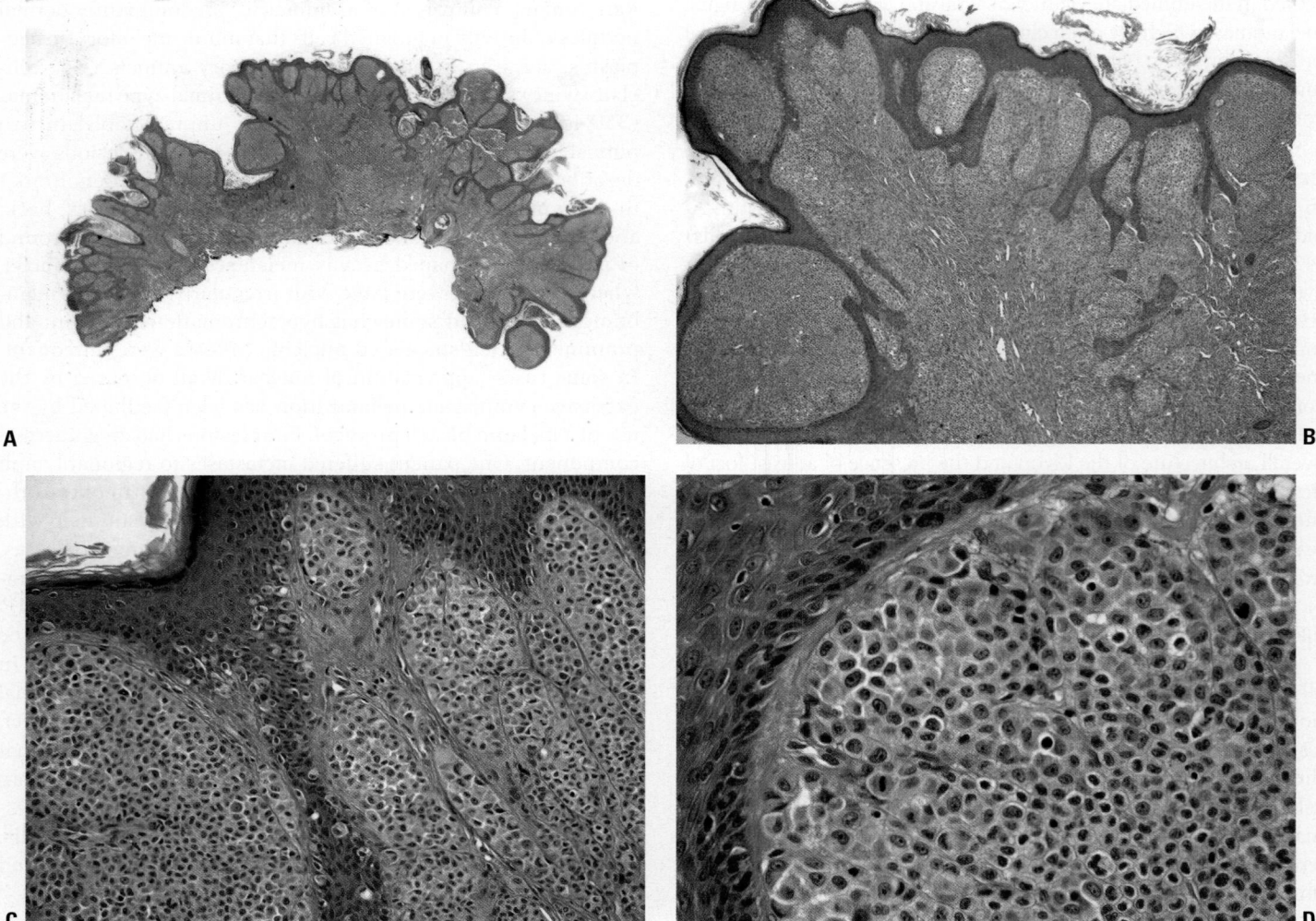

Figure 28-31 Nevoid melanoma. **A:** This lesion from the face of a 44-year-old man is an example of a category that has been termed "nevoid and verrucous melanoma." **B:** Although the resemblance to a nevus is close, the cellularity is greater with a tendency to expansion of the "verrucous" papillae. **C:** There may be subtle pagetoid proliferation in the epidermis; if this were more prominent, the melanoma would not be "nevoid." **D:** Mitotic figures in the dermal component are essential for the diagnosis.

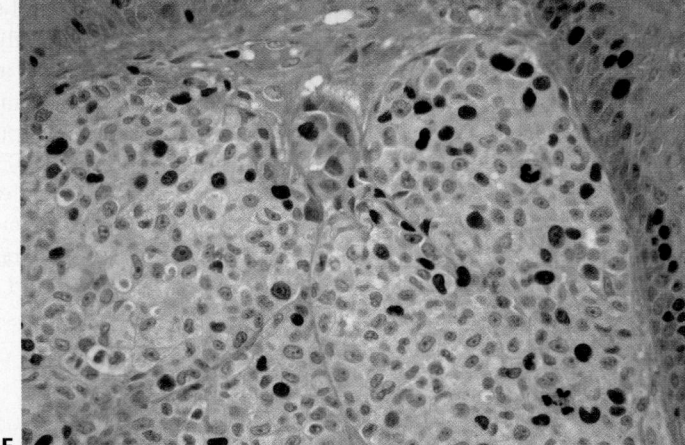

Figure 28-31 (*continued*) **E:** An elevated Ki-67 proliferation rate, as here, may also be of assistance in making the diagnosis.

the lesion. In a study of growth patterns in nevoid melanoma, it was found that patterns including confluence of dermal melanocytes with no intervening connective tissue and a "parallel theque pattern" (dermal chords/strands of melanocytes one or more cells thick and disposed as parallel arrays with ropy collagen fibers in between) could be helpful in suggesting the diagnosis at scanning magnification (456). Because epidermotropic melanoma metastases may also develop "nevoid" architectural and cytologic characteristic, this possibility must also be considered when rendering a diagnosis of nevoid melanoma, particularly when the epidermal component is inconspicuous or there are clinical parameters that would support this possibility.

According to McNutt, reactivity of the intradermal component for HMB-45 antigen, or for Ki-67 antigen, can show that the dermal cells have an activated and hyperproliferative phenotype and, in combination with histologic criteria, can help support a diagnosis of nevoid malignant melanoma (457). In a study using chromosomal FISH markers, all of 10 nevoid melanomas (4 of which had metastasized), but none of 10 mitotically active nevi, had copy number abnormalities (458). In more recent studies, nevoid melanomas have been studied genomically and have had marked differences compared to control mitotically active nevi ("nevi with mitoses"). In one study, 85% of 14 nevi from pregnant patients (of which 4 had mitoses) had staining of greater than 5% for p16, whereas 65% of 20 nevoid melanomas (65%) had staining of less than 5% (459). In another study of 18 cases, nevoid melanomas tended to have hotspot mutations in *NRAS* (75%) and also noncoding mutations and less frequent copy number alterations, whereas these were rare in 30 nevi with mitoses, most of which had driver BRAF mutations (92). In another study, deep/marginal mitoses, lack of maturation with depth, and pseudomaturation (characterized by diminution of cell volume but not nuclear size with depth) were significantly more common in 13 nevoid melanomas, whereas by IHC, complete loss of p16 was seen in 70% of these nevoid melanomas, and highly correlated with loss of the CDKN2A gene (chromosome 9p21), changes that were not seen in 12 nevi with mitoses (91).

The nevoid melanomas described previously have generally had a papulonodular and often papillomatous silhouette at scanning magnification. Recently, another category, termed "maturing naevoid melanoma," has been described (460). These have had a flat or slightly raised profile with an SSM-like junctional component maturing to a small nevoid cell type. The mitotic rate was generally low, and most expressed p16 and had a BRAF mutation.

None of these cases metastasized, despite a mean thickness of 0.9 mm, with a range of 0.4 to 3.0 mm. In our opinion, these lesions overlap considerably with a group of lesions that have been termed "nevi with regression-like fibrosis (NRLF)" (461), "sclerosing nevi with pseudomelanomatous features" (462), "Clark/dysplastic nevi with florid fibroplasia associated with pseudomelanomatous features" (463), and, more generally, "sclerosing melanocytic lesions" (464). Although some of these lesions may represent authentic melanomas, fatal cases have been very rare, if they occur at all, and we would not make a diagnosis of a maturing nevoid melanoma in the absence of compelling criteria.

MELANOCYTIC TUMORS NOT (OR INCIDENTALLY) ASSOCIATED WITH SUN EXPOSURE

In the 2018 "*WHO Classification of Skin Tumours*," an important classifier of the melanomas is the presence of solar elastosis as a marker of CSD, which in turn is a marker of solar exposure and susceptibility (5). Among populations with pale skin color that is susceptible to solar damage, the "CSD melanomas" predominate. In populations with more pigmented skin, these are relatively less common, and most melanomas are not attributable to sun exposure. These "no-CSD melanomas" include the very rare Spitz melanomas and also acral and mucosal melanomas and melanomas associated with congenital nevi and with blue nevi (and also ocular melanoma, not considered here).

Spitz Tumors

The Spitz melanoma pathway is Pathway IV in the 2018 WHO Classification of melanomas (465) (Table 28-2, p. 836). Although it is not clear whether the very rare Spitz melanomas progress from a precursor Spitz nevus or arise *de novo*, there is a very clear progression of phenotypic attributes in these lesions, from usual or typical *Spitz nevi (SN)* to *atypical Spitz tumors (AST)* or "*Spitz melanocytomas*" to *Spitz melanomas (SM)*.

Spitz Nevus

The Spitz nevus, named after Sophie Spitz, who first described it in 1948 (466), has also been known as *benign juvenile melanoma* (a term that is archaic and no longer used) and as *spindle and/or epithelioid cell nevus*.

Clinical Summary. The lesion was originally thought to occur largely in children, but it is now well recognized in young-to-early middle-aged or even older adults (467). Rarely, it is present at birth (468). Because of a degree of unpredictability in the behavior of a subset of cases, particularly when lesions occur in adults, the term "Spitz tumor" has been suggested as preferable to "nevus," except in the most typical cases, especially those in young children (469).

The lesion is usually solitary and encountered most commonly on the lower extremities and trunk and in children somewhat more frequently on the head and neck, but it can occur anywhere (470,471). In most instances, the lesion consists of a dome-shaped, hairless, pink nodule. SN tend to be smaller than most melanomas,

including Spitzoid melanomas, with a mean diameter of 7.6 compared to 10.5 mm, respectively, in one large study (470). The color is usually pink because of a paucity of melanin and in some lesions associated with vascularization of the stroma, leading to the clinical impression of a pyogenic granuloma, an angioma, or a dermal nevus. However, it may be tan and, in some cases, brown or even black. Ulceration is seen only rarely and in our experience most commonly in lesions from young children, perhaps because of excoriation. After an initial period of growth, most SN are stable.

In rare instances, multiple tumors are encountered. These may be either agminated (grouped) in one area or widely disseminated and sometimes eruptive (472) (Fig. 28-32); occasionally,

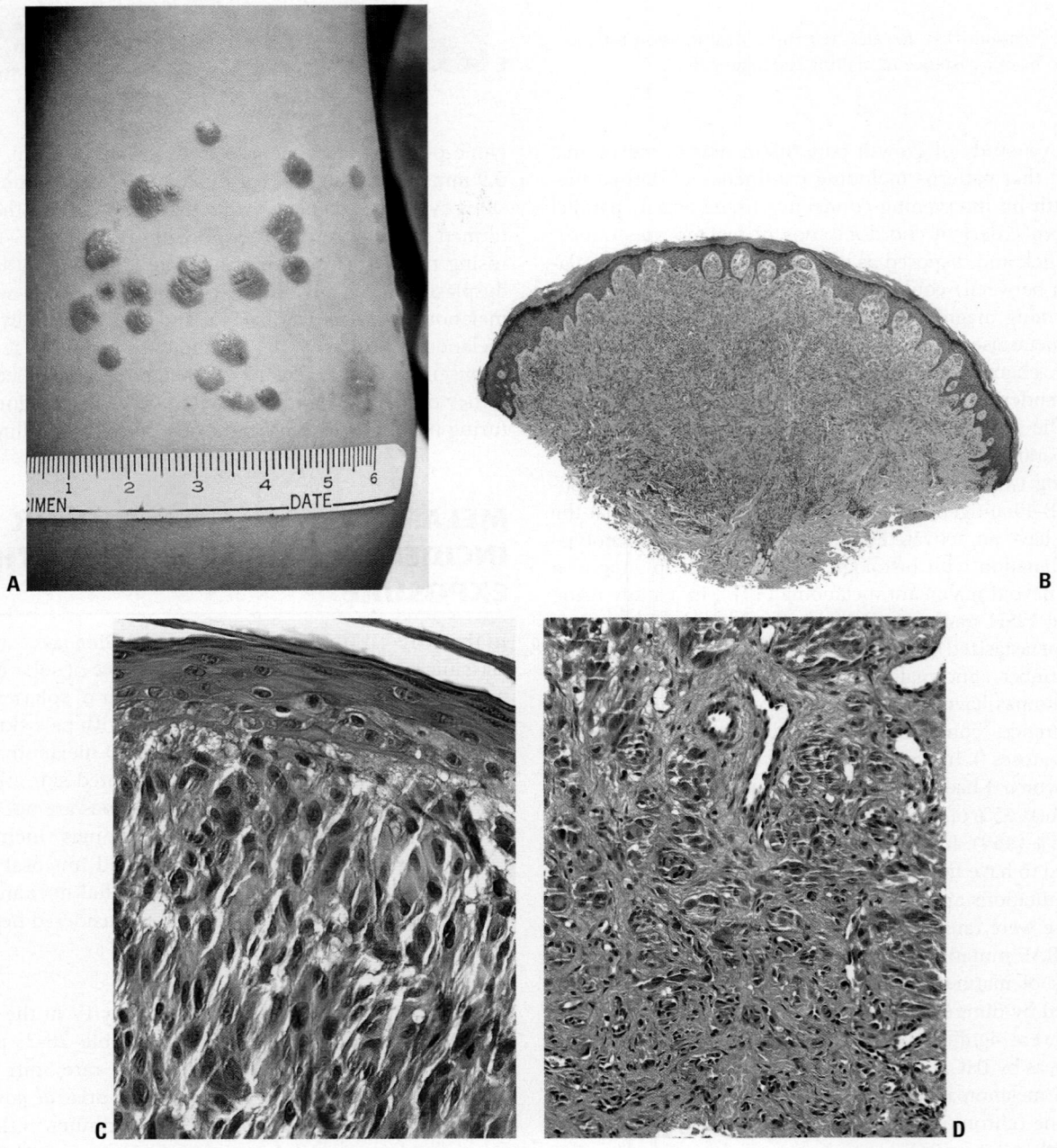

Figure 28-32 Spitz nevus. A: Agminated Spitz nevi. Most Spitz nevi are single lesions. In this example of agminated, or grouped Spitz nevi, each individual lesion is a characteristic Spitz nevus—relatively small, symmetrical, well-circumscribed tan papules. B: Spitz nevus. Most Spitz nevi are small, circumscribed, symmetrical papules, at scanning magnification and clinically. This lesion is somewhat larger than most examples. C: Spitz nevi are defined by the presence of large cells, with abundant amphophilic cytoplasm, which may be spindled or polygonal in shape ("large spindle and/or epithelioid melanocytes"). The nuclei in a given Spitz nevus are more homogeneous than in most melanomas, usually large but with open chromatin and smooth nuclear membranes, and with prominent nucleoli. D: "Maturation" from larger cells near the surface to smaller cells at the base is an important feature of Spitz nevi.

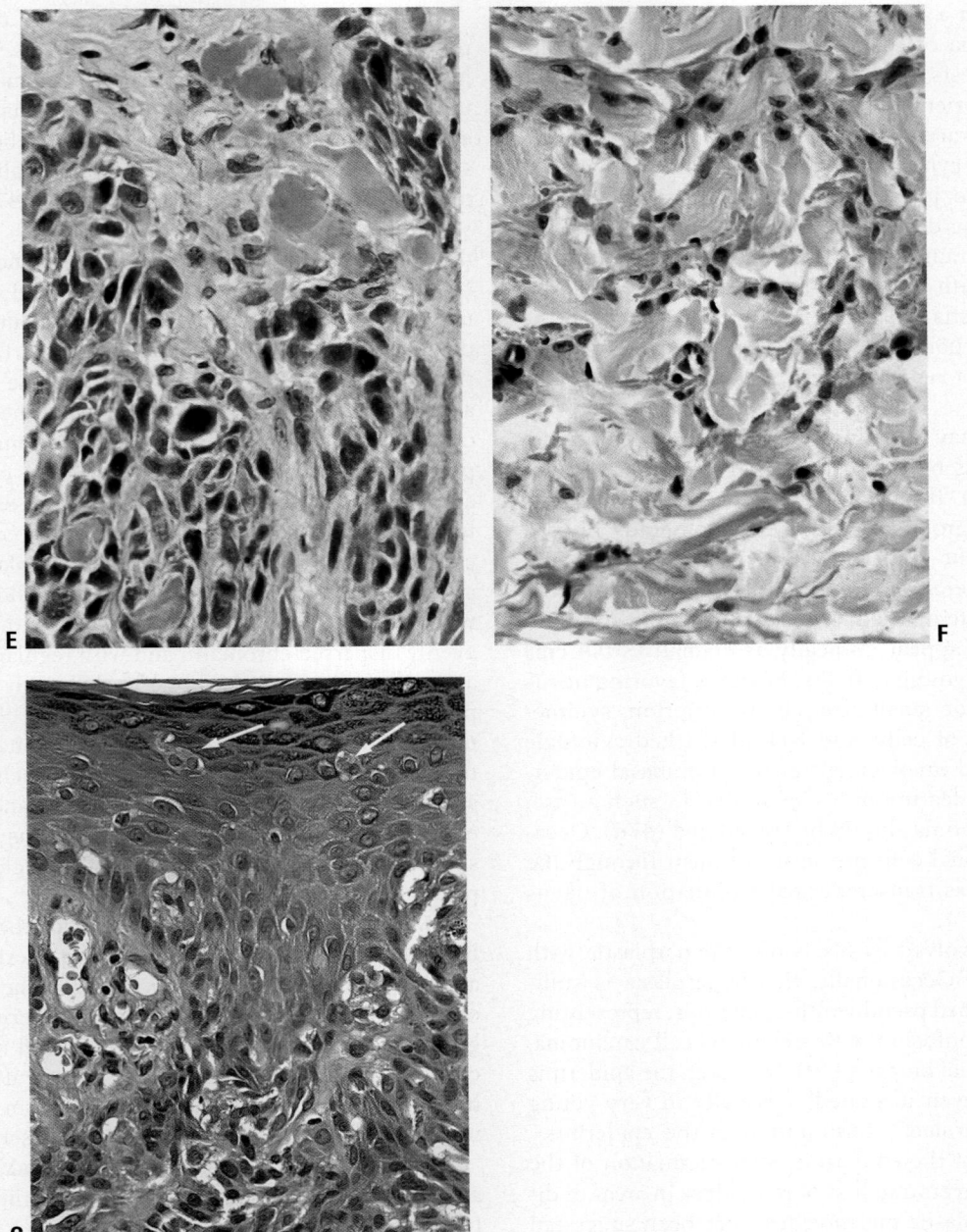

Figure 28-32 (*continued*) E: Spitz nevus with globoid eosinophilic bodies ("Kamino bodies"). Although not pathognomonic, these structures are highly characteristic of Spitz nevi. F: At the base of a Spitz nevus, the lesional cells become smaller and become "dispersed" among the reticular dermis collagen fibers. This is the same lesion as (D). Note the diminution in size ("maturation") of the lesional cells at the base. G: Pagetoid melanocytosis. Pagetoid extension of some cells of a Spitz nevus into the epidermis, as seen here (*arrows*), is not diagnostic of a melanoma if other attributes of melanoma are not observed. This pagetoid melanocytosis is not uncommon at least focally in lesions of young children.

they occur within a nevus spilus (473). A few lesions studied have had *HRAS* mutations, and a case with a novel fusion gene has been described, whereas the localization is thought to be the result of genetic mosaicism (474). The histopathologic findings can range from those of a classic Spitz nevus to an atypical Spitzoid neoplasm that may be difficult to distinguish from a Spitzoid melanoma. In a series of nine patients with this rare phenomenon of multiple SN, 53% of the excised lesions showed no atypical histopathologic features, and none had recurred after a reexcision (472).

Histopathology. Ackerman's term "nevus of large spindle and/or epithelioid cells" reflects the characteristic cytologic appearance that provides the essential definition for the lesion (467).

Because of the large size of the lesional cells, often with considerable nuclear and cytoplasmic pleomorphism, and the frequent presence of an inflammatory infiltrate, the histologic picture often resembles that of a NM. There is no doubt that before the recognition of SN as an entity, many cases were diagnosed as melanoma. Even today, differentiation from a melanoma can often be very difficult and occasionally even impossible. Features that aid in the distinction may be summarized as *architectural pattern* and *cytologic* features (Fig. 28-32).

In terms of their fundamental *architectural pattern,* SN resemble common nevi. They are usually compound, but they can be entirely dermal or junctional. They are small, symmetrical, and well circumscribed. It is somewhat unusual for the intraepidermal component to extend beyond the dermal component, and such a finding should prompt consideration of associated dysplasia or melanoma. The epidermal component is arranged in nests and fascicles often formed by spindle cells that tend to be oriented vertically and, although large, do not show significant variation in size and shape or tend to become confluent. The cytoarchitecture of spindle cells aligned in parallel within the junctional nests is characteristic and forms the basis for the descriptive terms of nests of cells that are considered to be "raining down" or that resemble "bunches of bananas." In SN with junctional activity, there are often artifactual semilunar clefts separating nests of nevus cells at the epidermal–dermal junction from adjacent and overlying epidermal cells. This feature is not very commonly seen in melanoma but is diagnostically useful.

Although there may be diffuse junctional activity, permeation of the epidermis by tumor cells (pagetoid melanocytosis) is relatively slight. If present, it usually consists of single nevus cells or small groups of cells and is generally limited to the lower half of the epidermis (Fig. 28-10G) (467). In a few SN, however, pagetoid migration of lesional cells into the epidermis may be quite marked, especially in young children. These "pagetoid SN" appear clinically as a small (<0.4 cm) pigmented macule in young patients. Features favoring nevus over melanoma include small size, circumscription, symmetry, even distribution of cells, and lack of marked cytologic atypia (475). Pagetoid involvement of the suprabasal epidermis is not a common feature of SN in adults; in such a case, the diagnosis of melanoma should be considered (476). Occasionally, nests of lesional cells are seen in transit through the epidermis, described as transepidermal elimination of nevus cells (477,478).

The epidermis involved by SN is often hyperplastic with elongated rete ridges. Occasionally, this hyperplasia is sufficiently florid to be termed pseudoepitheliomatous, representing a possible source of confusion with squamous cell carcinoma, especially in a superficial biopsy (479). However, the epidermis may be thinned and even ulcerated, especially in very young children. A pattern termed "consumption of the epidermis," defined as "thinning of the epidermis with attenuation of the basal and suprabasal layers and loss of rete ridges in areas of direct contact with neoplastic melanocytes," has been suggested as an additional criterion for differentiating melanoma from nevi. This feature is seen in many melanomas but is absent in most Spitz tumors (305). Found in fewer than half of the patients, diffuse edema, stromal hyalinization, and telangiectasia in the papillary dermis, if present, are of slight diagnostic importance. The edema may cause a loose arrangement of the nevus cell nests.

A useful, though not pathognomonic, cytologic criterion for SN is the presence within the epidermis of dull pink globules resembling colloid bodies in 60% to 80% of cases (480). They may form larger bodies through coalescence. These "Kamino bodies" are most commonly seen in the basal layer above the tips of dermal papillae (Fig. 28-10E). Similar appearing eosinophilic globules have been noted in the epidermis in as many as 12% of melanomas and 8% of ordinary nevi, in which they are, however, less conspicuous because they do not coalesce (481). Although often these bodies may resemble apoptotic cells, formal studies have found no evidence of active apoptosis and have related the eosinophilic material to hyalinized collagen or basement membrane–like material (482).

In a large and detailed study, most of the cases were composed of epithelioid and/or spindled cells, whereas additional histopathologic findings, in order of frequency, included maturation, a lymphocytic infiltrate, epidermal hyperplasia, presence of melanin, telangiectasias, Kamino bodies, desmoplastic stroma, mitosis, pagetoid spread, and hyalinization, the latter more frequent in adults than in children (471).

Important *cytologic features* of SN include especially the presence of large spindle cells and epithelioid cells (Fig. 28-32C). Spindle cells or epithelioid cells may predominate, or the two types of cells may be intermingled ("large spindle and/or epithelioid cells") (467). Apart from the shape of their cell bodies, the spindle cells and the epithelioid cells in any given Spitz nevus resemble one another in nuclear and in cytoplasmic texture, suggesting that they may represent dimorphic expression of a single cell type. The cells have abundant amphophilic cytoplasm that may contain scant, finely divided melanin pigment, although in most of the cells pigment is typically absent. On close inspection, the cytoplasm may sometimes appear finely and faintly vacuolated or show an amphophilic netlike character. The nuclei are large, with pale, delicate, and evenly dispersed chromatin and with regular, smooth, uniform, and delicate nuclear membranes, but with prominent eosinophilic or amphophilic nucleoli. The size of the lesional cells, more than any other feature, sets the Spitz nevus apart from the common nevus, and also from most melanomas. Bizarre giant cells may be seen both in melanoma and in SN, the difference being that in the latter they usually have regular nuclei of similar size, whereas in melanoma the nuclei are usually more pleomorphic.

Mitoses are absent in about half of the cases, and this is helpful in ruling out melanoma in these lesions. Usually, there are only a few mitoses, but occasionally they are quite numerous in the epidermal compartment. A dermal mitotic rate of greater than 2 mitoses per mm², abnormal mitoses, or mitoses close to the base of the dermal component (within the lower half of the dermal component) is unusual in SN (483) and may warrant a diagnosis of melanoma or a descriptive diagnosis of "melanocytic tumor of uncertain potential." Atypical mitoses are uncommon, and, if they are found, the lesion should be interpreted with great caution (483).

Of special importance is *maturation* of the cells with increasing depth, making them smaller and appear more like the cells of a common nevus (Fig. 28-32D–F). Also important is the *uniformity* of the lesional cells from one side of the lesion to the other: at any given level of the lesion from the epidermis to its base, the lesional cells look the same. Although large superficially, the cells at the base of most SN are small, and they tend to disperse delicately as single cells or files of single cells among reticular dermis collagen bundles. Involvement of the reticular dermis is highly characteristic of SN, and as they descend into this part of the dermis, the cells become dispersed as single cells, and some of them become separated from the apparent border of the lesion to form "outlier cells" (484) that can be revealed, for example, by a stain for Melan-A/Mart. Other benign nevi also tend to infiltrate in this way if they involve the reticular dermis (83). Melanomas, in contrast, tend to form solid tongues or fascicles of tumor cells that separate and displace the collagen bundles in the reticular dermis, without forming outlier cells. This is because melanoma cells that infiltrate as single cells tend to proliferate and thus appear as fascicles, whereas nevus cells tend not to do so.

Melanin pigment is in many instances completely or nearly absent in SN. In some cases, melanin is moderate or dense, and in these cases it is usually "top heavy" (471). Some of these "pigmented SN" are better classified as pigmented spindle cell nevi, related lesions that are discussed in the next section.

A *lymphocytic infiltrate* is found in many SN and may be quite dense. Its distribution can be bandlike, mainly at the base, as in some melanomas. Often, however, the infiltrate is patchy around blood vessels and is seen throughout the lesion (471). In a detailed study, inflammation with the presence of lymphocytic aggregates predominated in SN but was not pathognomonic for benignity, whereas strong and intense inflammation was suggestive of an underlying malignancy (485).

Desmoplastic Spitz Nevi. In some examples of SN (and also in some nevi with smaller cells that may not meet criteria for SN), diffuse fibrosis is present (486). These desmoplastic SN generally show no junctional activity, nesting, or pigmentation. The nevus cells are predominantly spindle shaped and compressed by a desmoplastic stroma. However, they differ from a dermatofibroma by the presence of epithelioid and often also multinucleated cells. DM (p. 920) often has an associated lentiginous *in situ* component, in contrast to the rarity of junctional activity in desmoplastic SN. Furthermore, DMs are almost invariably negative (in their spindle cell component) for the HMB-45 and Melan-A (MART-1) melanocytic markers, which, in contrast, are usually positive in SN (403,422). Some desmoplastic nevi have clusters of lymphocytes, a finding that can raise concern for DM; however, in a study of six such lesions, other features of melanoma were lacking, and the lesions all expressed Melan-A and the tumor suppressor p16, and had negative results by FISH testing for melanoma (403). In another study, all of 5 desmoplastic nevi strongly expressed for p16; however, 6 of 22 DMs were also diffusely positive, indicating that this is not a reliable marker for this distinction (487).

Hyalinizing Spitz Nevi. These are related lesions that present with spindle or epithelioid nevus cells embedded in a paucicellular hyalinized collagenous stroma. Some of these lesions have been mistaken histologically for metastatic carcinomas (471).

Angiomatoid Spitz Nevi. These lesions present histologically with large spindle and/or epithelioid cells placed among "angiomatoid" densely arranged, small blood vessels lined by plump endothelial cells embedded in a collagenous stroma. The Spitz nevus cells may be quite inconspicuous among the vessels in some cases. There have been no reported cases of recurrence or metastases (488,489).

Spitz Nevus of Special Sites. Occasionally, a Spitz nevus will involve a special site (e.g., acral). In such cases, it is important to recognize the retention of the basic architectural and cytologic features of a Spitz nevus (as described previously), albeit in the context of potentially confounding site-dependent architectural characteristics. The thigh has also been identified as a site of localization of atypical Spitzoid lesions, particularly in young women and distinguishable from pigmented spindle cell nevi or Reed (490). The ability to define such lesions as SN from the outset is critical to avoiding overdiagnosis where the perceived degree of cytologic atypia in the context of the site may lead to an erroneous diagnosis of melanoma.

Atypical Spitz Tumor

AST is a lesion that has morphologic (and, lately, immunophenotypic, chromosomal, and genomic) features that are intermediate between Spitz nevus and melanoma. Spatz, Calonje, and Barnhill provided a set of criteria for grading risk in AST, considering metastasizing cases in childhood. These criteria include diagnosis at age greater than 10 years, diameter of the lesion greater than 10 mm, presence of ulceration, involvement of the subcutaneous fat (level V), and mitotic activity of at least 6/mm^2 (469).

Immunophenotypic features of AST may include heterogeneous dermal expression of the differentiation marker HMB45, a high Ki-67 proliferation rate (>10%), and/or clonal loss of the tumor suppressor p16. Chromosomal aberrations may be demonstrated by FISH or CGH. GAs include, especially, TERT promoter mutation, which can potentially confer immortality on the lesional cells (231). Ruling out biologic malignancy, or guaranteeing benign behavior, is not always possible owing to overlapping phenotypes (Fig. 28-33). The diagnosis of "Spitz melanoma of childhood" has been proposed for well-studied lesions that are of a true Spitz lineage. However, the prognosis for these tumors, especially in young children, is excellent in the absence of compelling indicators of malignancy, and a designation as "atypical" or "uncertain" is preferable in our opinion to the use of the term "malignant melanoma," even when issued with a caveat. Sentinel node staging, although perhaps reasonable to consider, is not standard of care for these lesions.

As noted previously, it is not always possible to make an unequivocal distinction between a melanoma or a Spitz tumor/nevus, and in these doubtful cases we will often use the descriptive term "melanocytic (or Spitzoid) tumor of uncertain potential" (MELTUMP or STUMP) and provide a differential diagnosis, which might in cases of extreme doubt include microstaging attributes that would apply if the lesion were interpreted as a melanoma (175). Cerroni et al. studied 57 cases of Spitzoid MELTUMP with follow-up of at least 5 years. The only

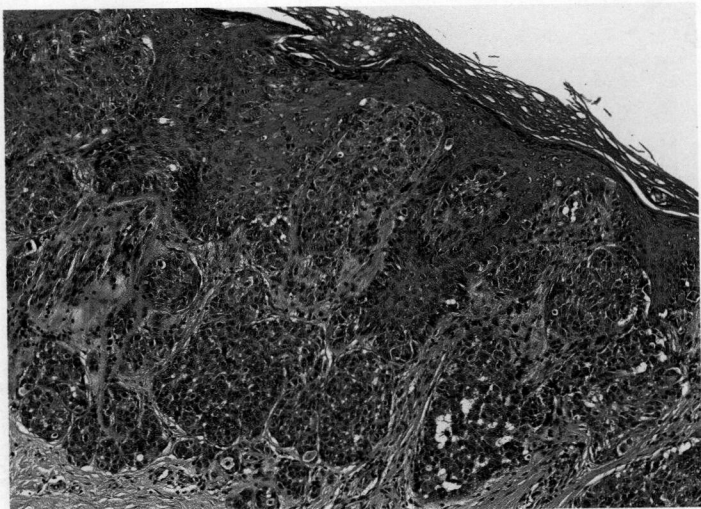

Figure 28-33 Atypical Spitzoid neoplasm in a 12-year-old child. This lesion has many Spitzoid features, with a low mitotic rate; however, multiple chromosomal abnormalities were demonstrated by comparative genomic hybridization. A sentinel node procedure contained a small deposit. There were no further events reported.

three histopathologic criteria that were statistically different between the groups of favorable and unfavorable cases were presence of mitoses, mitoses near the base, and an inflammatory reaction. It was considered that these lesions (MELTUMP) as a group exist and that they may be biologically different from conventional melanoma and benign melanocytic nevi. The controversial terminology reflects the uncertainty in classification and interpretation of these atypical melanocytic tumors (491).

Spitz Melanoma (Malignant Spitz Tumor) and Melanoma of Childhood

Malignant melanoma is a disease primarily of adults. The incidence of prepubertal melanoma is very low. In a few instances, it has occurred as multiple metastases resulting from transplacental transmission (492).

Otherwise, three patterns of childhood melanoma have been described (493). The genomic landscape of pediatric melanomas has been recently described in terms of these patterns (494).

The first of these patterns is cutaneous melanoma of adult type, usually in the low CSD category, discussed elsewhere in this chapter. Prognosis and outcomes in these lesions are determined by attributes similar to those in adults. The diagnosis of usual forms of melanoma is not different in children than

in adults, except that the threshold of significance for criteria such as pagetoid scatter and mitotic activity may be increased to some extent. Discussion with colleagues and consideration of referral to an experienced consultant would be reasonable in such a circumstance.

The second pattern is melanoma arising in a congenital nevus, which is the least rare cause of death from melanoma in childhood, and this will be discussed in a subsequent section (495) (p. 914).

The third pattern is that of Spitzoid melanomas, which have a histologic picture reminiscent of that seen in SN and AST and which may also be termed "Spitz-like" (493). In the 2018 WHO Classification of melanocytic tumors, a clear distinction has been made between true "Spitz melanomas," which have genomic attributes similar to those of SN and AST, and "Spitzoid melanomas," which have genomic attributes more characteristic of adult melanomas, usually those of low CSD skin, described in detail earlier in this chapter (465). In cases with unknown genomic status, the term "Spitzoid melanoma" is most appropriate (Fig. 38-34). Especially if metastasis occurs, genomic studies are important to characterize the lesion as either a Spitz or a non-Spitz melanoma, because it is possible that the prognosis may differ.

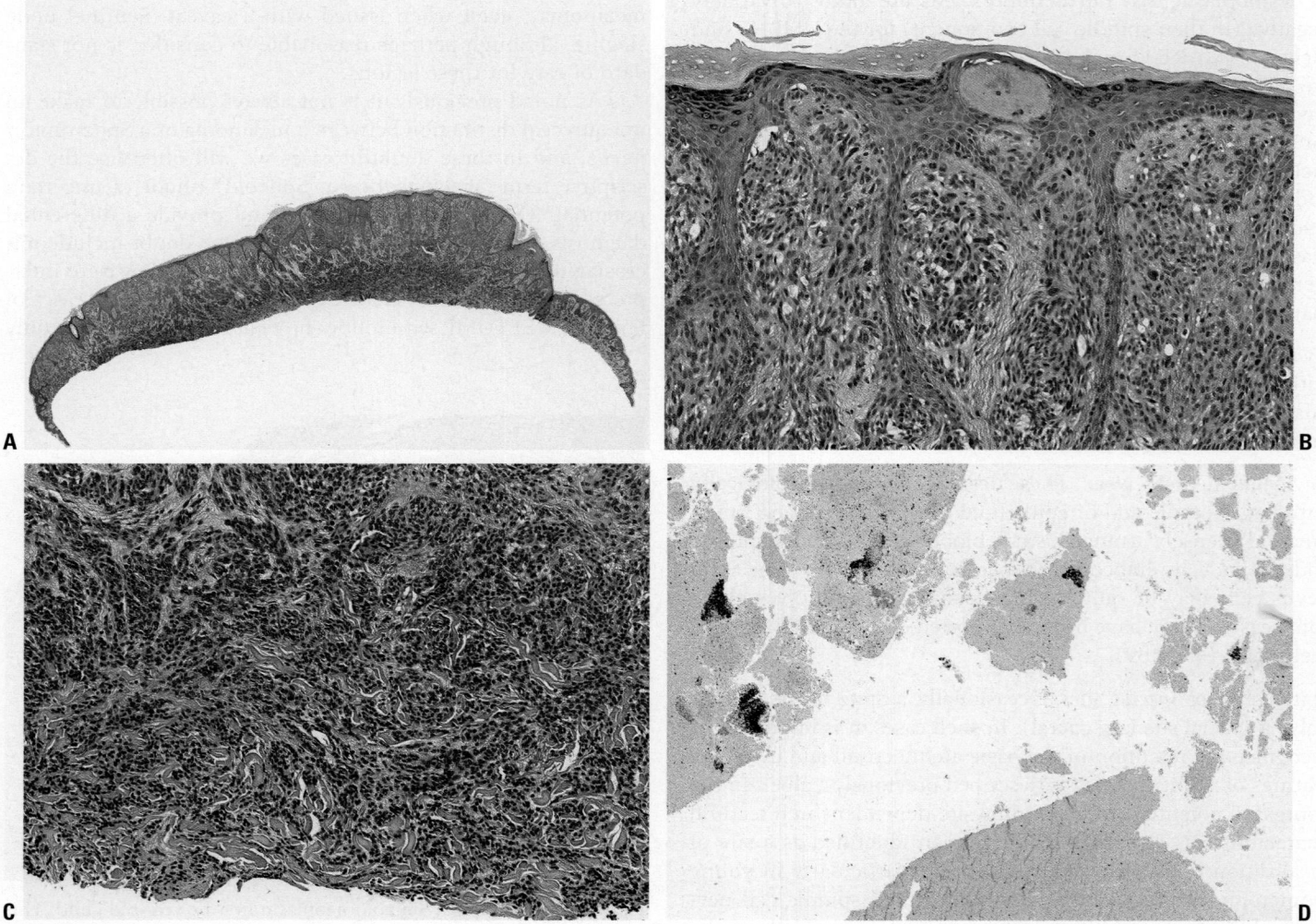

Figure 38-34 Spitzoid/spindle cell melanoma of childhood. **A:** An asymmetrical and very broad moderately to highly cellular neoplasm. **B:** The lesional cells are large spindle and/or epithelioid cells. Nuclear chromatin tends to be hyperchromatic, and there is considerable pleomorphism. The mitotic rate was 4 per mm². A well-developed Kamino body is present in the upper center. **C:** There is incomplete maturation at the base and failure of the lesional cells to disperse as single cells into the reticular dermis. **D:** Liver metastasis documented in this Melan-A stain. No further follow-up is available.

In some of the cases that have been diagnosed as Spitzoid melanoma (and in many AST as well), metastases occur that are limited to the regional lymph nodes, and the child survives after treatment (496). "Spitzoid melanoma" with a fatal outcome has very rarely been reported in children (497) and, slightly less rarely, in teenagers or preteens (494). Only a few of these have been characterized by full genomic studies as truly "Spitz melanomas" (494). These lesions have been considered by some to represent a special category of "Spitzoid melanomas of childhood," in which there may be a relatively high incidence of regional metastasis but a relatively low (but not zero) risk of more distant progression (496). However, it is not clear that melanomas with Spitzoid morphology but with genomic attributes characteristic of non-Spitz melanomas seen more often in adults (*BRAF* or *NRAS* mutations, etc.) will exhibit this more favorable behavior.

Lesions termed "Spitzoid melanomas" in adults are likely examples of melanomas in other pathways that have a Spitzoid phenotype, but an adult melanoma genomic profile, and likely a prognosis more characteristic of an adult melanoma.

In considering a diagnosis of a Spitz melanoma, the following attributes should be evaluated. These lesions may occur at any age, but often occur at greater than 40 years, and may present as an asymmetrical plaque or nodule with a history of continuing progressive change. The lesions are often greater than 1 cm in breadth and often ulcerated. Histologically, there may be irregular and confluent nesting, and there may be extensive pagetoid scatter. The epidermis may be effaced or "consumed." In the dermis, there may be lack of maturation of lesional cells, and often there are more than 6 mitoses per mm^2 with deep, marginal, and/or atypical mitoses. Cytologically, there may be high-grade atypia. By IHC deep staining is common with HMB45 and Ki-67, and there is often an elevated Ki-67 proliferation index (>20%). Reactivity for PRAME may be present. Expression of p16 may be diminished or absent. Molecular pathology is essential in determining whether the lesion is a true Spitz tumor, although this may not be necessary for management. *BRAF* and *NRAS* mutations are rare, and in a true Spitz tumor kinase fusions characteristic of other Spitz lesions are present, by definition. There may be homozygous loss of 9p21, and *TERT* promoter mutations are commonly present, especially in those lesions that will progress to a fatal outcome (465).

The clinical presentation of childhood melanoma may often not follow the traditional "ABCD" patterns, and an alternative acronym, Amelanotic, Color Uniformity, De novo, any Diameter, and Evolution, has been proposed (498). Some of these lesions may be best termed "melanocytic tumors of uncertain malignant potential," as criteria for reliable distinction between benign and malignant examples of these lesions are not always well defined.

The histogenesis, immunopathology and genomic landscape of Spitz lesions, including the distinction from SM, are extensively discussed in the next section, and the distinctions among SN, AST, and Spitz and Spitzoid melanomas are summarized in Table 28-8.

- SM are lesions with morphologic attributes and also with genomic characteristics of Spitz tumors, including either an *HRAS* activating mutation or one of an expanding list of gene fusions (mutually exclusive). Spitzoid melanomas have morphologic attributes of a Spitz lesion (e.g., large spindle and/or epithelioid cells) but have genomic attributes that are more characteristic of more usual forms of melanoma, such as a driver mutation of BRAF or *NRAS* or another less common mutant gene.

Histogenesis, Immunopathology and Genomic Landscape of Spitz Tumors

Biologic marker studies have shed little or no light on the mechanisms whereby SN appear to have the capacities for relatively rapid invasive and tumorigenic proliferation in the dermis but to lack the capacity for metastasis.

Genomic Landscape. The genetic basis of Spitz tumors is now quite well understood, and there are important differences compared to common nevi and to melanomas. In a seminal study by Bastian et al. using CGH and FISH, copy number increases often associated with oncogenic mutations involving the *HRAS* gene on chromosome 11p were found in about 10% of cases of Spitz tumors (499). The tumors with 11p copy number increases were larger, predominantly intradermal, had marked desmoplasia, characteristic cytologic features, and had an infiltrating growth pattern. *HRAS* activation by either mutation or copy number increase alone could explain several of the histologic features that overlap with those of melanoma. It has been speculated that *HRAS* activation in the absence of cooperating additional genetic alterations may drive the partially transformed melanocytes of these "atypical" SN into senescence or a stable growth arrest, likely as a result of p16 activation in a process termed "oncogene-induced senescence" (500). There are no data to suggest that SN with *HRAS* activation are at special risk for progression to melanoma; however, the biologic potential of these lesions is not completely understood.

A subset of Spitzoid tumors was found to be associated with loss of the tumor suppressor, *BAP1*, which is also associated with ocular melanoma. These *BRAF*-mutated, *BAP1*-negative tumors were primarily dermal and composed predominantly of epithelioid melanocytes with abundant amphophilic cytoplasm and well-defined cytoplasmic borders. Nuclei were commonly vesicular and exhibited substantial pleomorphism and conspicuous nucleoli (240). The lesions are commonly situated within a congenital pattern nevus in which *BAP1* expression is preserved, constituting a type of combined nevus. To date, the biologic behavior of these lesions has been benign. These lesions are now considered to represent a separate entity, BAP1 inactivated nevi, which are a member of Pathway 1, as *BRAF*-mutated lesions and not true SN, and are discussed elsewhere in this chapter (p. 867).

In general, with the exception of the few *HRAS*-mutated Spitz tumors already mentioned, mutations of traditional oncogenes are not demonstrated in these tumors. In a seminal study by Bastian's group, 20 benign SN and 8 AST, which had been selected for morphologic features inconsistent with *HRAS* or *BRAF*/*BAP1* mutations, were screened for mutations of known cancer-causing genes and for kinase fusion genes. Only a single case had a point mutation in *HRAS*, and no known alterations were found in other known oncogenes. Remarkably, genomic rearrangements were observed in 19 cases. These rearrangements fused the intact kinase domains of *ROS1* (36%), *ALK* (14%), *RET* (7%), *NTRK1* (7%), and *BRAF* (4%) to a wide range of predominantly novel 5′ partners, forming constitutively activated chimeric oncogenes (501). The list of fusions continues to expand, with *MAP3K8* and other fusions having been added, and likely more to follow (231). The fusions occurred in a mutually exclusive pattern and were more common in younger patients. These gene fusions found in two-thirds of Spitz tumors are likely to be useful as diagnostic markers and as potential therapeutic targets for those few tumors that may metastasize

(501). AST and SM differ from typical SN in terms of their acquisition of progression, such as *CDKN2A* loss, *TERT* promoter mutations, and other changes, to be discussed later and in previous sections.

Diagnostic and Prognostic Markers. Immunohistochemical and morphometric studies have shown differences between SN, AST, and melanomas, and some of these are now in common use. By IHC, SN react not only with differentiation markers for melanocytes such as S100 antigen but also with HMB-45 and Melan-A/MART-1, the first melanosomal antigen often expressed in proliferating melanocytic lesions (as well as melanoma), and other more specific markers of melanocytic lineage (502). SN tend to show a more orderly "top heavy" pattern of stratification of HMB-45 reactivity from superficial to deep compared to melanomas (503). Studies have demonstrated differences in S100A6 protein expression between SN and melanomas, although interpretation remained subjective (337,504). Like nevi and unlike most melanomas, SN show a tendency toward diminution of nuclear size and/or DNA content (505), as well as for reactivity with certain antigens, from the superficial to the deep portions of the nevus (503). This stratification may be regarded as an expression of maturation/senescence, which is diagnostically and undoubtedly also biologically important in the distinction between SN and melanomas.

Cell proliferation and cell cycle markers are important discriminators between benign, atypical, and malignant Spitzoid neoplasms. The simplest of these is the determination of mitotic rate. Studies by Crotty and colleagues demonstrated that the presence of abnormal mitoses, a dermal mitotic rate of greater than 2/mm^2, and mitotic figures within 0.25 mm of the deep border of the lesion favored a melanoma diagnosis (483). In studies primarily based in children, a cutoff of greater than 6/mm^2 for mitoses has been found more suitable (469). Using the proliferation marker Ki-67/Mib-1, Crotty's group found that the maximal (i.e., "hot spot") percentage of positive nuclei was about 10 in the Spitz tumors versus 32 in the melanomas studied, indicating quite good discrimination (343). Vollmer has emphasized the important interactions between age and proliferative activity, indicating from a meta-analysis of the literature that a Ki-67 proliferation rate of more than 10% favors a melanoma diagnosis and less than 2%, a Spitz nevus. Values between 2% and 10% yield various predictive values for Spitz nevus, depending on the *a priori* probability of this diagnosis based on age and other factors (i.e., clinical, histologic, and marker studies) (506).

The cell cycle and tumor suppression molecule p16 is an important marker for benign SN and for nevi in general. In a study of p16 expression in 6 Spitzoid malignant melanomas (i.e., lesions deemed to be melanomas with Spitzoid morphology but not confirmed genomically), compared to 18 SN and 12 compound nevi in children younger than 18 years, all of the childhood melanoma cases were associated with loss of p16, whereas all the Spitz and other benign nevi had strong positive nuclear and cytoplasmic expression of p16 (507). The tumor suppressor p15, located at the same locus, may have equal or even greater value for this purpose; however, it is not widely available in automated strainers (508). In a large study of Spitz and other nevi compared to melanomas, patterns of expression were distinguished, and it was found that the pattern of "Total p16 loss (single pattern or part of multiple patterns)" identified 61% of melanomas and no nevi (101).

Combining two of the most useful markers discussed previously, a combined p16-Ki-67-HMB45 score has had demonstrated utility in sorting benign from malignant Spitz tumors (509), and in our practice we often used these markers in developing a differential diagnosis, although we do not consider them to be pathognomonic.

In the last few years, CGH and FISH have been applied to series of cases of Spitzoid and other neoplasms. In a CGH study, a limited variety of copy number aberrations including gains of 11p and, much more rarely, 7q were seen in SN. Conversely, melanomas with Spitzoid features typically have multiple chromosomal copy number aberrations involving a variety of loci (510). Markers derived from CGH were used in a large study of 64 AST with 5 years of uneventful follow-up and 11 AST that had resulted in advanced locoregional disease, distant metastasis, or death. Gains in 6p25 or 11q13 and homozygous deletions in 9p21 had statistically significant association with aggressive clinical behavior with P-values of 0.02, 0.02, and less than 0.0001, respectively. In multivariate analysis, homozygous 9p21 deletion was highly associated with clinically aggressive behavior ($P < 0.0001$) and death caused by disease ($P = 0.003$) (511). In another study, of 31 Spitzoid lesions, 9p21 loss was present in the only fatal case of a Spitzoid melanoma (in a 41-year-old man), but 5 cases with 9p21 deletions by FISH were alive and well at follow-up intervals ranging from 6 to 135 months, indicating that 9p21 loss alone does not predict a fatal outcome (512).

The chromosomal locus 9p21 includes the site of the tumor suppressor gene p16, which is downregulated in essentially all melanomas by one means or another, including homozygous loss, as demonstrated in the FISH studies reviewed previously (511,512). In that study, increased mitotic rate and homozygous 9p21 loss were the only independent factors predicting mortality from Spitzoid lesions. Of note, this locus also includes two other important suppressor genes, p14 and p15. This finding reinforces the potential value of p16 (or p15) immunostaining in assessing Spitzoid tumors. If a p16 immunostain is positive, then 9p21 loss cannot have occurred, favoring a benign prognosis. If the p16 stain is negative, then FISH or CGH could be done, and if homozygous 9p21 loss is identified (and especially if there is also a *TERT* promoter mutation), the evidence suggests that management of the lesion as having the potential for systemic metastasis would be appropriate, while recognizing that the prognosis of Spitzoid melanomas is better than that for usual melanomas, and 9p21 loss alone does not predict a fatal outcome (512).

PRAME is an additional marker that can be helpful in the distinction between benign and malignant Spitz proliferations, especially when expression is diffuse (289,513–515). However, it has been demonstrated that benign SN and AST can infrequently express diffuse PRAME (513), and so this marker should be used in combination with other markers and attributes, as discussed previously.

Genomic sequencing can also add important prognostic information. In a series of AST and Spitzoid melanomas from 56 patients, the associations with metastatic disease of *TERT* promoter (TERT-p) mutations, homozygous CDKN2A deletion, homozygous *PTEN* deletion, various kinase fusions, *BRAF/NRAS* mutations, nodal status, and histopathologic parameters were studied. The presence of *TERT*-p mutations was the most significant predictor of hematogenous dissemination ($P < .0001$) among these variables. This finding suggests an important role for NGS in establishing the diagnosis of a Spitz melanoma (516). However, *TERT*-p mutation is not always associated with a fatal outcome in Spitz tumors, at least in the short term. In a study of 24 Spitz lesions, none (15/15) of the typical lesions but two of nine atypical Spitzoid tumors contained *TERT*-p mutation, and neither of these cases developed advanced disease in a 5.5-year follow-up (517).

Differential Diagnosis of Spitz Tumors

The distinction between Spitz nevi/tumors and common nevi is of importance in that complete excision is usually recommended for SN, unlike banal common nevi. Also, unlike dysplastic nevi, which may be indicators of an individual at increased risk for melanoma, a Spitz nevus diagnosis carries no such connotation. In cases of doubt in this regard, we add a note to the effect that the differential diagnosis may include a dysplastic nevus and recommend that the patient be evaluated for other risk factors, such as multiple dysplastic nevi, and a family or personal history of melanoma. Management can then be based on the patient's overall risk profile.

Occasional examples of histiocytic tumors such as epithelioid histiocytomas or juvenile xanthogranulomas may be confused with epithelioid SN or with melanomas, especially when foam cells or Touton giant cells are inconspicuous. Immunostains such as Melan-A/Mart and others can be used to establish the diagnosis of a melanocytic lesion, whereas histiocytic markers such as CD163 (preferred over CD68 because this can be positive in melanoma) and Factor XIIIa are likely to be positive in the histiocytic lesions (see Chapter 26) (518). Cellular neurothekeoma is another lesion that can strongly mimic a Spitz tumor or a melanoma. The distinction can be made by recognizing the complete absence of pigment and usually also of substantial cytologic atypia and mitotic activity and the characteristic profile of negative reactivity for S100, HMB-45, Melan-A/MART1, and EMA. Positive staining may be seen with CD63 (NKI/C3) (519) and S100A6 (520). These markers have limited specificity and should always be used as part of a panel (e.g., at a minimum with S100 and a cytokeratin marker).

The differential diagnosis with melanoma is, of course, of much greater importance. Differentiation of a Spitz nevus from a NM can be difficult and even impossible in some cases because all of the changes seen in the Spitz nevus may also be observed in melanoma. This differential has been discussed extensively previously. To summarize, Crotty and colleagues consider that the presence of symmetry, Kamino bodies, and uniformity of cell nests or sheets from side-to-side favor a Spitz nevus, whereas the presence of abnormal mitoses, a dermal mitotic rate of greater than $2/mm^2$, and mitotic figures within 0.25 mm of the deep border of the lesion favor a melanoma in an adult (483), while the cutoff of $2/mm^2$ for mitoses is more appropriate in a child (469). To this list we would add the characteristic dispersion pattern of single cells at the base, favoring a Spitz or other benign nevus, and also, when needed, immunohistochemical and genomic studies discussed in the previous section can be added (Table 28-9).

Approaches to Management of Spitz Tumors

Because of the difficulty of making an absolutely certain distinction from melanoma, it is, in our opinion, advisable as a precautionary measure that lesions diagnosed as Spitz tumors/nevi be excised completely, especially in persons at or beyond puberty, particularly because such lesions are usually small in size. Although the issue is debatable (359,521), exceptions to this general rule might include those lesions where there are cosmetic or other contraindications to excision and where the diagnosis of a benign Spitz nevus is certain despite the partial nature of the biopsy, as may be the case, for example, in lesions of children that lack any atypical features and where the margin involvement is minimal. However, one should never exclude a diagnosis of melanoma based on age alone, because melanomas may arise in children, although this is very rare (p. 898).

Although there are cases that had been diagnosed as instances of Spitz nevus or AST but later proved to be lethal melanomas, other such cases, including those that have been diagnosed as Spitzoid melanomas (i.e., melanomas with Spitzoid features but either not characterized genomically or having genomic characteristics of a more usual melanoma), have metastasized to regional lymph nodes but not beyond (496). These lesions, often large, ulcerated, deeply infiltrative, and mitotically active, can alternatively be signed out descriptively as "melanocytic tumors of uncertain malignant potential" (p. 880). Others regard these lesions as "Spitzoid melanomas (of childhood)", with most considering that the prognosis for these tumors may be better than expected for an ordinary melanoma with similar microstaging attributes (496). In a comprehensive review of AST, 56% of 541 patients had SLNB, and the results were positive in 39%, with 99% surviving in a mean follow-up interval of five years (361). This analysis indicates that a sentinel node procedure does not predict outcome even when positive in patients with AST and, therefore, that sentinel node staging cannot be considered standard of care for these lesions.

The diagnosis of a Spitz nevus/tumor depends on an assessment of multiple morphologic features, which have been summarized previously and in (Table 28-9). Given that so-called metastasizing Spitz nevi/tumors are frequently associated with at least medium- to long-term survival (361), it may be appropriate to regard the metastases as "metastatic melanocytic tumors of uncertain potential (metastatic MELTUMP)," rather than unqualified metastatic malignant melanoma. However, in most institutions, such individuals would be offered a consideration of adjuvant protocols for metastatic melanoma, preferably based on tumor board discussion.

Pigmented Spindle Cell Nevus (Reed Nevus)

This tumor, first described by Richard Reed in 1973 (365), may be regarded as a variant of the Spitz nevus (367), or as a distinctive clinicopathologic entity. The demonstration that most pigmented spindle cell nevi (PSCN) of Reed are the result of genomic fusions, with the most frequent and characteristic aberration being an NTRK3 fusion, tends to support the former interpretation (522). However, in our experience and that of others, most cases differ significantly from classical SN, but some present with overlapping features, indicative of a close relationship between the two entities. Although this distinction has no clinical significance in that each is a benign lesion, it is important to rule out melanoma, and this is facilitated by an understanding of the differences between these two common melanoma simulants.

Clinical Summary. The lesions are usually 3 to 6 mm in diameter, deeply pigmented, and either flat or slightly raised. Most patients are young adults, and the most common location is on the lower extremities. PSCN are uncommon after the age of 35. A classical presentation is that of a newly evolved black plaque on the thigh of a young woman. Because of the heavy pigment and the history of sudden appearance, a diagnosis of melanoma is

Table 28-9

Spitz Nevus/Tumor Versus Melanoma

Spitz Nevus/Tumor	Melanoma
Pattern Features	
Usually <6 mm diameter	Usually >6 mm
Usually symmetrical	Often but not always asymmetrical
Single attenuated cells between reticular dermis collagen bundles at base	Nests and fascicles rather than single cells in the reticular dermis
Epidermal hyperplasia, hyperkeratosis, and hypergranulosis may be prominent.	Epidermal reaction is often minimal: may be "consumption of the epidermis."
Usually little or no pagetoid spread of lesional cells into epidermis	Usually obvious pagetoid spread into epidermis
Epidermal component usually does not extend beyond the lateral border.	Lateral extension (radial growth phase) is common except in nodular melanoma.
Ovoid nests of lesional cells oriented perpendicular to epidermis	Nests variable in size, shape, and orientation
Discontinuous junctional proliferation	May be continuous proliferation
Little or no pigment	Often heavily pigmented or irregularly scattered pigmented cells within lesion
Small uniform nests in dermis at base	Larger variable nests at base
Cytologic Features	
Nuclear chromatin is open, with prominent nucleoli.	Nuclei may be hyperchromatic and clumped.
Nuclear membranes are regular.	Irregular nuclear membranes
Single and confluent eosinophilic globoid bodies in epidermis and superficial dermis	If present, globoid "Kamino" bodies are inconspicuous and usually single.
Mitoses absent or low mitotic rate	Mitoses rarely absent, rate often high
Atypical mitoses rare or absent	Atypical mitoses common
Mitoses rare in lower third of lesion	Mitoses common in lower third
Cells uniform from side to side	Greater tendency to cellular variability
Cells mature with descent to base.	Little or no maturation

often suspected clinically. In contrast, SN are usually submitted with a benign clinical diagnosis, such as an angioma or a dermal nevus. Like SN, the lesions are generally stable after a relatively sudden appearance and a short-lived period of growth.

Histopathology. The PSCN is characterized by its relatively small size and its symmetry, and by a proliferation of uniform, narrow, elongated, spindle-shaped, often heavily pigmented melanocytes at the dermal–epidermal junction (523). The nests of spindle cells are vertically oriented and tend to blend with adjacent keratinocytes rather than forming clefts, as in SN. Eosinophilic globules ("Kamino bodies") may be present (Fig. 28-35). The tumor cells often form bundles that are separated by elongated rete ridges. In the papillary dermis, the nevus cells lie in compact clusters, pushing the connective tissue aside. Numerous melanophages are characteristically diffusely present within the underlying papillary dermis. Involvement of the reticular dermis, common in SN, is unusual in PSCN. Some lesions show upward epidermal extension of junctional nests of melanocytes. Single-cell upward spread within the epidermis in a pagetoid pattern may be present but is usually not prominent. Hypopigmented examples have been described, having all the typical features of conventional PSCN but not containing abundant melanin (524).

Features that may lead to a diagnosis qualified as "atypical pigmented spindle cell nevus" include architectural abnormalities, including poor circumscription and pagetoid melanocytosis, significant cytologic atypia, or a prominent epithelioid cell component. There may also be considerable overlap with dysplastic nevi (523). The significance of these "atypical" variants appears to lie in their greater chance of being misdiagnosed as melanoma, because all reports of PSCN emphasize their benign behavior after excision.

Differential Diagnosis. The most important differential is with melanoma of the superficial spreading type. In contrast to these melanomas, PSCN are smaller and symmetrical and show sharply demarcated lateral margins. The tumor cells appear strikingly uniform "from side to side." If lesional cells of PSCN descend into the papillary dermis, they mature along nevus lines, in contrast to melanomas. Mitoses may be present in the epidermis in either lesion but are uncommon in the dermis in PSCN. Abnormal mitoses are exceedingly uncommon. Pagetoid melanocytosis is usually not prominent, and the spindle cell cytology differs from that of the epithelioid cells that predominate in most SSMs. LMMs may have spindle cells in their VGP component, but the epidermal component is usually comprised of smaller nevoid, albeit atypical, cells. Some PSCN may present

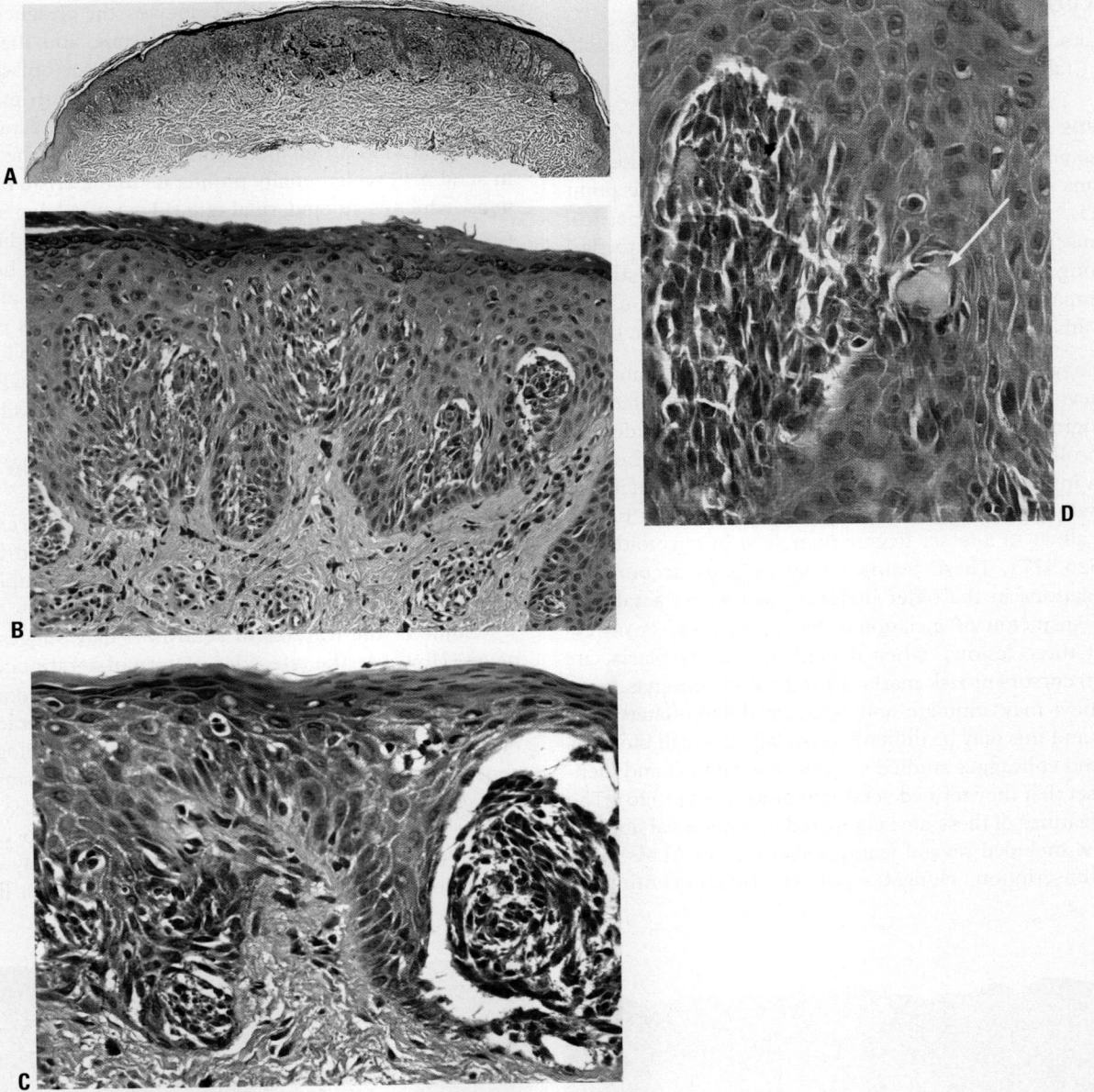

Figure 28-35 Pigmented spindle cell nevus. **A:** The typical configuration of this lesion is that of a small plaque whose breadth is considerably greater than its height. The lesional cells are typically junctional or confined to the epidermis and the papillary dermis. **B:** As in the classic Spitz nevus, the lesional cells are arranged in nests that tend to be vertically oriented. Unlike those of the Spitz nevus, the cells are narrow elongated spindle cells without epithelioid cells, and they contain abundant usually coarse melanin pigment. **C:** As in Spitz nevi, some (usually slight) degree of pagetoid melanocytosis is not unexpected. Mitoses may be numerous in the epidermis, but the lesional cells in the dermis tend to be mature, with few, if any, mitoses. Clefting artifact between the nests and the adjacent keratinocytes tends to be less prominent than in Spitz nevi but may be present, as here. **D:** Kamino body in a pigmented spindle cell nevus. This nevus has a prominent eosinophilic globoid "Kamino body" (*arrow*) in its epidermal compartment.

overlapping features with dysplastic nevi but can usually be distinguished on the basis of their irregularly thickened epidermis, their vertically oriented nests, and the uniformity of cell type, the absence of cytologic dysplasia, extent of underlying pigment incontinence in the dermis, and the absence of typical stromal alterations (e.g., lamellar fibrosis). In cases of extreme doubt, we may classify the lesions as SAMPUS and provide a differential diagnosis that includes atypical PSCN, dysplastic nevus, or unusual melanoma *in situ*. In the case of melanoma *in situ*, a reexcision procedure with 5-mm margins would be recommended; in the case of dysplastic nevus with low-grade atypia, we would recommend assessment of melanoma risk factors and perhaps follow-up, especially if the patients have other

clinically atypical nevi or a family or personal history of melanoma (175); and in the case of atypical PSCN, consideration of a modest reexcision would be appropriate. Some rare examples of lesions with larger expansile intradermal nodules may be difficult to distinguish from melanoma, and a descriptive diagnosis may be appropriate ("melanocytic tumor of uncertain potential," MELTUMP, p. 880).

Principles of Management: PSCN without atypia and related lesions generally do not require active therapy. Lesions are often excised for cosmetic reasons and to rule out melanoma. The presence of such a lesion is not a risk factor for future development of melanoma.

Melanocytic Tumors in Acral Skin

Acral tumors constitute Pathway V in the 2018 WHO Classification (4) (Table 28-2, p. 836).

Acral Nevus

Clinical Summary. Melanocytic nevi are present on the skin of the palms or soles in as much as 4% to 9% of the population (525). Clinically, they are usually small, symmetrical, well-circumscribed brown macules, with a tendency to dark ridging along dermatoglyphics that can be clinically striking and may impart a seemingly irregular border. They are usually stable and are more often junctional than are nevi of the trunk.

Histopathology. Acral nevi tend to be more cellular than most common nevi, and the nevus cells may be arranged in predominantly lentiginous rather than nested patterns in the epidermis. Pagetoid proliferation ("pagetoid melanocytosis") of lesional nevus cells in the epidermis above the basal layer, particularly more centrally within lesions, is relatively common in benign acral nevi, albeit to a lesser degree than seen in pagetoid melanomas (526,527). These features may perhaps account for recommendations in the older literature to remove acral nevi because of suspicion of melanoma. However, there is no evidence that these lesions, when devoid of true dysplasia, are common precursors or risk markers for acral melanomas.

Acral nevi may simulate and must be differentiated from melanoma, and this may be difficult, especially in small biopsies. Clemente and colleagues studied a series of acral nevi and identified a subset that they termed acral-lentiginous nevi (526). The distinctive features of these nevi compared to other acral nonlentiginous nevi included several features also seen in ALMs: poor lateral circumscription, elongation of rete ridges, continuous

junctional proliferation of melanocytes, the presence of scattered melanocytes within the upper epidermis, and the presence of junctional melanocytes with abundant pale cytoplasm and round to oval, sometimes hyperchromatic, nuclei with prominent nucleoli. Cytologic atypia is not marked in most acral nevi of the palms and soles. Compared to acral melanomas, the lesional cells in acral nevi preferentially proliferate in the crista profunda limitans, which is an epidermal rete ridge underlying a surface furrow. As a result, regular melanin columns are produced beneath these surface furrows, which, however, can only be seen when the specimen has been appropriately embedded and sectioned perpendicular to the dermatoglyphics (528). This phenomenon results in discrete and localized pulses of melanin within the acral scale, a feature not replicated in acral melanoma, where melanin transmitted into the stratum corneum is often broad, haphazard, and not well demarcated.

In compound acral nevi, the nevus cells in the dermis, unlike melanoma cells, mature to the lesional base. There is no high-grade uniform cytologic atypia, generally no extensive and high-level pagetoid scatter in the epidermis, and there are no mitoses (Fig. 28-36). There may be patchy lymphocytes and occasional melanophages in the dermis.

Some of the features of acral nevi may suggest dysplastic nevus. However, the rete ridge pattern of keratinocytes in most acral nevi does not show the uniform elongation with occasional accentuation of anastomosing rete that characterizes dysplastic nevi, bridging nests are uncommon, cytologic atypia is generally minimal or absent, and the complete array of stromal changes of dysplastic nevi are not observed in most acral nevi.

In case of doubt, it may be appropriate to evaluate the patient's other nevi, especially if there is a family or personal history of melanoma. An acral-lentiginous lesion that extends

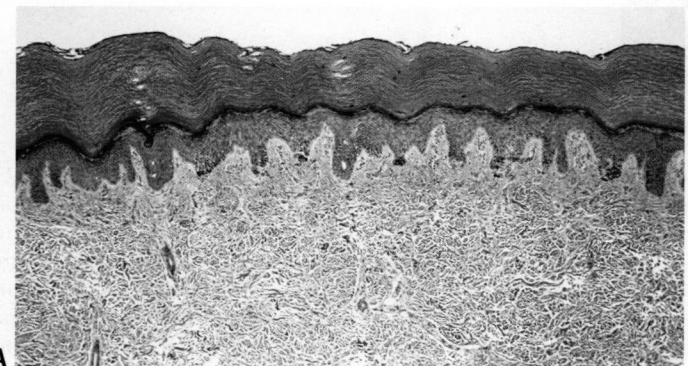

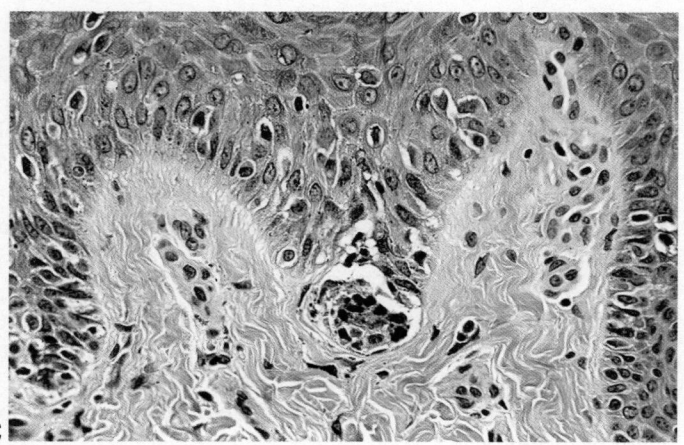

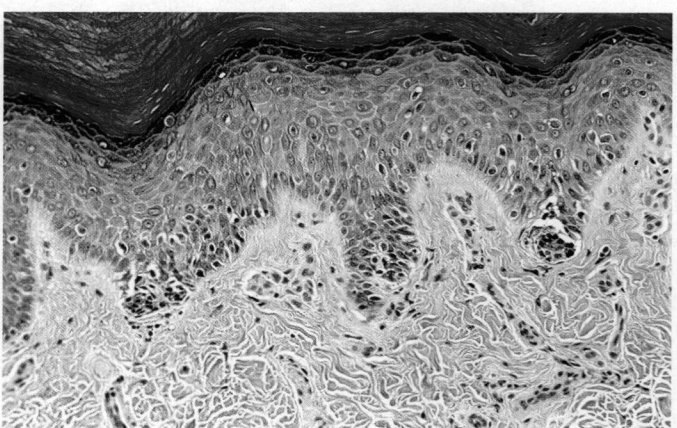

Figure 28-36 Acral-lentiginous nevus. **A:** The lesion is small, quite well circumscribed, and entirely contained within the biopsy specimen. **B:** Nests of nevoid to small epithelioid melanocytes predominate near the dermal–epidermal junction. They tend to be small, evenly spaced, and discrete. **C:** Although a few lesional cells may be present above the junction in a "pagetoid" pattern, there is no severe uniform atypia or mitotic activity, and there is no continuous proliferation of single cells between the nests.

to specimen borders should be evaluated carefully, and clinicopathologic correlation should be obtained to ensure that the specimen does not represent the periphery of a larger lesion. In such cases it may be judicious to recommend complete excision, to rule out additional pathology, and to preclude persistence or recurrence of the lesion. This is also recommended for any acral-type nevus, which, in addition to exhibiting site-related architectural features, also shows significant cytologic atypia. Finally, a nevus that is acral does not preclude the unusual possibility that it is also dysplastic, but this diagnosis must rely on the presence of cytologic and stromal criteria for dysplastic nevus in addition to those commonly encountered in nevi of acral sites.

Subungual Nevi and Melanonychias

Clinical Summary. Melanonychia striata (see also Chapter 19) refers to a pigmented band extending in the long axis of the nail, also known as longitudinal melanonychia (LMN). Such bands are common in Blacks and Asians and are therefore regarded as normal. However, the sudden appearance of LMN is cause for concern, often requiring a punch biopsy of the nail matrix (529). An exception is the melanonychia striata seen in the Laugier–Hunziker syndrome, which may affect one, several, or all fingernails in association with pigmented macules of the lips or the buccal mucosa. This type of melanonychia is always benign (530).

For carrying out the biopsy, longitudinal bilateral releasing incisions are made along the medial and lateral sides of the posterior nail fold. Next, the entire posterior nail fold is reflected proximally to expose and make visible the very end of the pigmented streak, which is usually within the matrix of the nail. Then the biopsy specimen is taken with a 3- or 4-mm punch through the nail plate and matrix down to the phalangeal bone (531).

Histopathology. Histologic examination in most instances shows only basal cell layer hyperpigmentation without an obvious increase in the number of melanocytes. Such lesions have been termed "melanotic macules" or "nail matrix activation," referring to an increased production of melanin with a normal number of melanocytes (531,532). In a study of 15 cases, 13 were melanotic macules, 1 case was a junctional nevus, another was tinea nigra (532). In other cases, an ALM, either *in situ* or invasive, may be found. The junctional or compound nevi tend to be of the lentiginous acral nevus pattern described previously. LMN may also be associated with pigmented Bowen disease and with subungual hemorrhage. Exclusion of a biologically significant lesion should involve adequate sampling of the nail matrix, and when there is doubt as to whether a proximal site of origin for the clinical lesion is included, additional sampling should be considered.

LMN in children is almost always benign: in a study of 35 cases, 17 were diagnosed as lentigines and 18 as naevi, among which 11 cases were categorized as lentigines/naevi with atypical melanocytic hyperplasia. Mild-to-moderate nuclear atypia, confluence of melanocytes, focal pagetoid spread, and periungual skin involvement were found in 25% to 40% of the cases, respectively; however, 13 cases tested by FISH showed no copy number aberration at the probed loci, and there were no biologic indicators of aggressive behavior (533). Subungual melanomas, though very rare, do occasionally occur in children;

for example, the diagnosis in a 13-year-old boy was supported by CGH findings and the development of a bulky regional node metastasis; however, the child was without disease 7 years later. This case was presented at a conference, and an expert panel (without knowledge of the lymph node metastasis) was split between the diagnosis of Spitz nevus and melanoma (534). Despite this problematic case, consideration of observation may be appropriate for children with LMN, especially in the preteen years (535).

Acral Melanoma (Acral-Lentiginous and Acral Nodular Melanoma)

Acral melanoma, by definition, occurs on the hairless skin of the palms and soles and in the ungual and periungual regions, the soles being the most common site (536).

Clinical Summary. Acral melanoma is uncommon in all ethnic groups, but it is the predominant form of melanoma in individuals with darker skin. In groups such as Asians, Hispanics, Polynesians, and Blacks, where the overall incidence of melanoma is low, most melanomas are of the acral type. However, the absolute incidence of acral melanoma in these groups is similar to that in Caucasians, who have a much higher incidence of melanoma overall (537). These considerations suggest that different etiologic factors, likely not involving sunlight, are operative in acral, but not in other sites. The survival rate of patients with acral melanomas in most series is relatively poor, especially in underserved populations (537). Although this is often because of their typically advanced microstage and/or clinicopathologic stage at diagnosis, acral melanoma had a survival inferior to that of extremity nonacral melanomas when matched for stage in one large study, perhaps reflecting different biology (538).

Most acral melanomas are of the acral-lentiginous type (ALM), originally described in 1977 (253), while some are pagetoid from the outset and may represent examples of "low CSD" melanoma (SSM) in acral skin. Pagetoid proliferation may be seen in the central, more advanced area of any ALM.

Nodular melanomas may also be seen in acral skin and may share genomic attributes with the ALM or, less often, with the SSM subtype (539).

Clinically, *in situ* or microinvasive ALM has uneven pigmentation with shades of brown, black and blue-black and an irregular, often indefinite border. The soles of the feet are most commonly involved, with a preference for more physically stressed sites, such as the center of the heels and inner forefoot, and along naturally occurring creases caused by long-term pressure on the soles (536). If the tumor is situated in the nail matrix, the nail and nail bed may show a longitudinal pigmented band, and the pigment may extend onto the nail fold (Hutchinson sign) which, however, is neither clinically nor histologically pathognomonic of subungual melanoma (540). Tumorigenic vertical growth may be heralded by the onset of a nodule, with the development of ulceration (Fig. 28-17B). However, some acral melanomas may be deeply invasive while remaining quite flat, because the thick stratum corneum seems to act as a barrier to exophytic growth.

Histopathology. ALM are termed "lentiginous" because the lesional cells tend to be single and located near the dermal–epidermal junction, especially at the periphery of the lesion (Fig. 28-37). However, some tumor cells can usually be found in the upper layers of the epidermis, especially near areas of

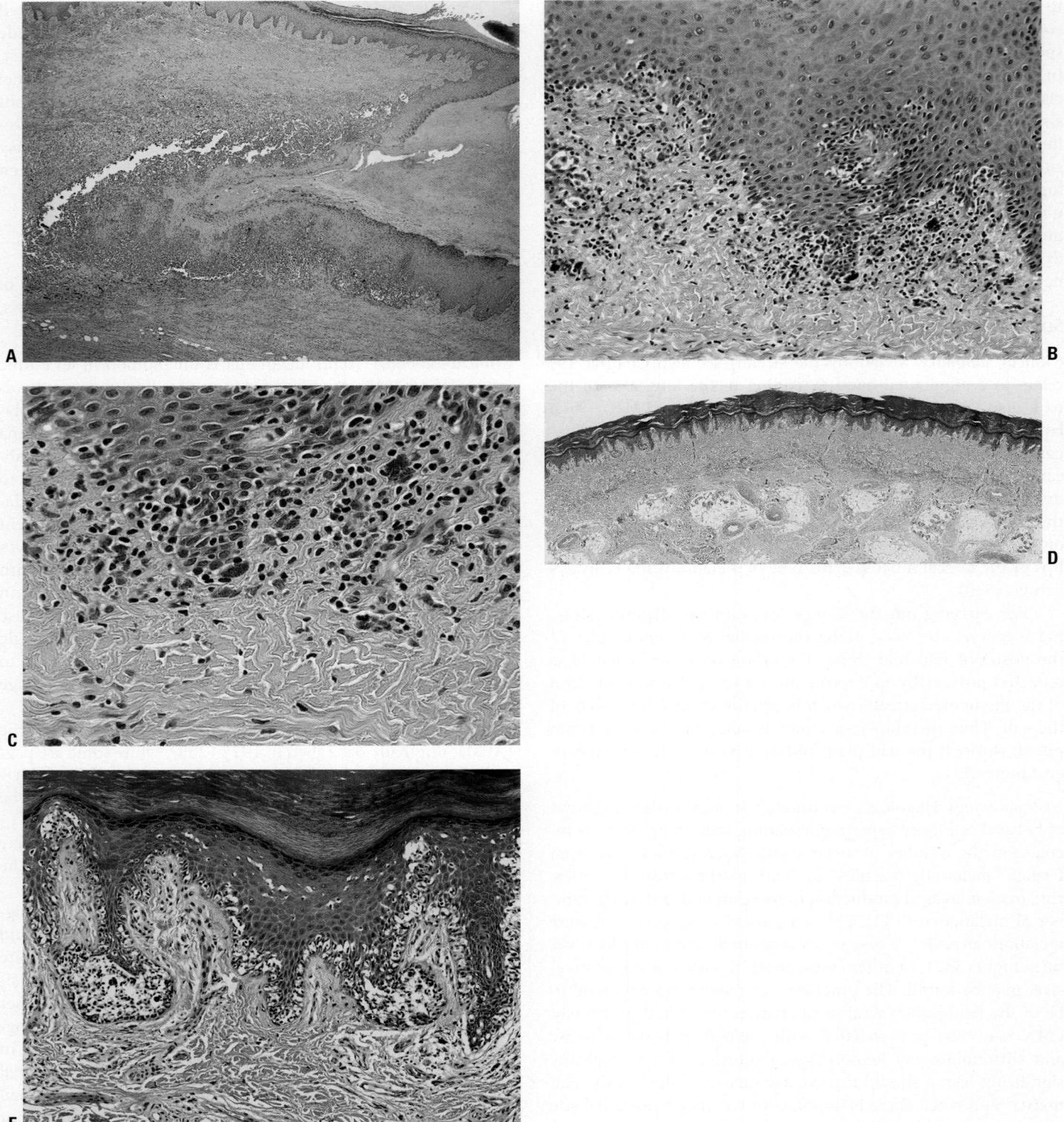

Figure 28-37 Acral-lentiginous melanoma, subungual (radial growth phase). A: At low magnification, a lichenoid lymphocytic infiltrate along the dermal–epidermal junction is the clue to the presence of the lesion. This feature may simulate an inflammatory condition. In this lesion, the process is seen to extend into the nail fold at the top of the image. B: As in lentigo maligna and other lentiginous melanocytic proliferations, the lesional cells in acral-lentiginous melanoma tend to be arranged as single cells near the dermal–epidermal junction ("lentiginous" pattern), especially at the periphery of the lesion. C: As in any melanoma, there is moderate-to-severe uniform cytologic atypia. Pagetoid melanocytosis may be present near the center of the lesion, but this is less prominent than in superficial spreading melanoma. When these features are less severe, the diagnosis may be subtle. Also, the neoplastic cells may be difficult to identify because of "masking" by the inflammatory infiltrate, as in this example. D: Acral melanoma, *in situ* portion of an invasive and tumorigenic lesion. The image shows a portion of a reexcision specimen, showing extensive proliferation of nested and single melanocytes along the dermal–epidermal junction, in acral skin. E: At higher magnification, in addition to nested proliferation that could simulate a dysplastic nevus, there is extensive continuous basal proliferation of uniformly atypical cells, with relatively limited pagetoid scatter into the epidermis, consistent with a "lentiginous" proliferation.

invasion in the center of the lesions, which could give rise to uncertainty and lack of agreement as to the histologic classification, while supporting the more important diagnosis of melanoma. The histologic picture differs from that of LM, because of irregular acanthosis, the lack of elastosis in the dermis, and the frequently dendritic character of the lesional cells in ALM. Early *in situ* or microinvasive lesions may show, especially at the periphery, a deceptively subtle histologic picture consisting of an increase in basal melanocytes and hyperpigmentation with only focal atypia of the melanocytes. However, in the center of the lesions, there is usually readily evident uniform, severe cytologic atypia. One important feature of noninvasive ALM is that malignant cells may colonize eccrine epithelium, sometimes down to the coil, thus potentially accounting for a deep recurrence of a lesion that was paradoxically in its *in situ* phase of progression. There may be a lichenoid lymphocytic infiltrate that may largely obscure the dermal–epidermal junction, and in some cases this may be so dense as to simulate an inflammatory process. In most of the lesions, both spindle-shaped and rounded, pagetoid tumor cells are seen, and, in many cases, pigmented dendritic cells are prominent. Pigmentation is often pronounced, resulting in the presence of melanophages in the upper dermis and of large and broad aggregates of melanin in the broad stratum corneum. As in LM, when tumorigenic VGP is present, it is often of the spindle cell type, and not uncommonly desmoplastic and/or neurotropic, and sometimes deeply invasive including into bone. In other instances, the invasive and tumorigenic cells in the dermis may be deceptively differentiated along nevoid lines (small cell invasion).

Histogenesis. Bastian et al. studied melanomas and nevi for copy number alterations by CGH and found that melanomas of the palms, soles, and subungual sites were distinguished by the presence of multiple gene amplifications, about 50% of which were found at the cyclin D1 locus. Such amplifications are significantly less frequent in other cutaneous melanoma types, and, if present, arise later in progression. The GAs in acral melanomas include distinctive complex copy number alterations, called tyfonas, which are "typhoons" of high-junction copy number events and fold-back inversions with hypermutated DNA near the junctional end points, that have been observed only in acral melanomas and dedifferentiated liposarcomas (541). Single basal melanocytes with similar gene amplifications have been identified in the histologically normal appearing skin immediately adjacent to a melanoma. These "field cells" appear to represent subtle melanoma *in situ*, or a precursor state, and might represent minimal residual disease that could potentially lead to local recurrences (542).

Acral (and also mucosal) melanomas have a markedly different genomic landscape from cutaneous melanoma, with a far lower mutation burden and a higher prevalence of large-scale structural variants. Significantly mutated genes in acral melanoma include *BRAF* (21%, less common than in low CSD melanomas), *NRAS* (28%), and also *KIT* (12%) (543,544). Other MAPK pathway activating alterations include fusions of *BRAF* (2.5%), *NTRK3* (2.5%), *ALK* (0.8%), and *PRKCA* (0.8%) (potentially targetable by available inhibitors), and inactivation of *NF1* (544). Some of these genetic changes have been correlated with morphology: in a study by Yun's group, *BRAF* mutation was associated with round epithelioid cells and *NRAS* and *NF1* mutations with bizarre cells. *NF1* and *GNAQ* mutations correlated with elongated and spindle cells with prominent

dendrites, whereas *KIT* mutations were common in amelanotic acral melanoma (545).

Differential Diagnosis of Acral Melanoma. The major consideration in the differential diagnosis of ALM is the benign acral-lentiginous nevus, discussed earlier. Features that distinguish this lesion from melanoma include smaller size, greater symmetry, lack of pagetoid lateral spread, absence of high-grade uniform atypia (not always present, however, in some melanomas), absence of mitotic activity, especially in the dermal component, and evidence of dermal nevocytic differentiation. In Japanese studies, the presence of melanin granules in the cornified layer detected as melanin columns regularly distributed under the surface furrows strongly suggests that the lesion is a benign acral nevus, whereas in melanomas the pigment pattern is more haphazard (528). In a difficult case, clinicopathologic correlation is essential, and the availability of high-quality clinical images can be decisive.

Genital and Mucosal Melanocytic Tumors

Acral tumors constitute Pathway V in the 2018 WHO Classification (4).

Mucosal Melanotic Macules and Lentigines

Nevi of genital skin usually resemble those of ordinary skin; however, a few have atypical features and are discussed in the section on Special Site Nevi (p. 848).

Clinical Summary. Mucosal melanotic macules present as a pigmented patch on a mucous membrane. Common locations include vermilion border of the lower lip, the oral cavity, the vulva, and, less often, the penis. These lesions may simulate melanoma clinically, but histologically there is no contiguous melanocytic proliferation and no significant atypia. Because there may be a slight increase in the number of melanocytes, although there is no nest formation, the term "genital lentiginosis" has been proposed for those lesions affecting genital paramucosae (546). The lesions may be synonymously referred to as "mucosal lentigo" or "mucosal melanotic macule."

In the common location on the vulva ("vulvar lentigo"), this process may appear quite alarming clinically, presenting as a broad, irregular, and asymmetric patch of brown to blue-black hyperpigmentation, often meeting the "ABCD" criteria for melanoma. Similar lesions may also be seen on penile skin (546). The lesions may be multicentric with alternating areas of normal and pigmented mucosa resembling areas of partial regression of a melanoma. The lesions are entirely macular, which would be unusual in an invasive melanoma.

The so-called "labial lentigo" (also known as "labial melanotic macule" or "labial melanosis"), a hyperpigmented macule of the lip, is quite similar to the lesions of genital skin. It is rarely biopsied because the clinical appearances are characteristic and do not suggest malignancy. These lesions are uniformly pigmented, light to dark brown, usually completely macular, and generally less than about 6 mm in diameter. These macules are biologically indolent (547).

Histopathology. On initial inspection, a biopsy specimen may appear normal. The findings include mild acanthosis, often without elongation of rete ridges, and hyperpigmentation of basal keratinocytes, often best recognized in comparison with surrounding epithelium, in association with scattered melanophages in the dermis (Fig. 28-38). In some cases, there is

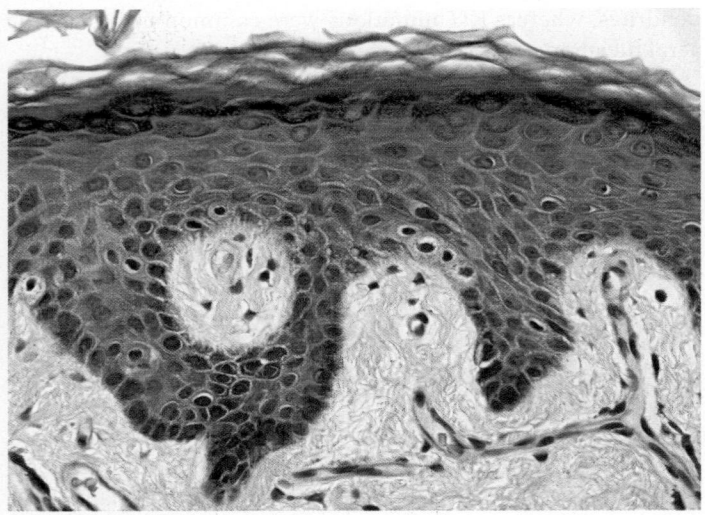

Figure 28-38 Mucosal lentigo of the penis (penile lentigo). In this clinically and histologically small lesion, there is increased pigmentation of basal keratinocytes with only slight prominence of melanocytes, without atypia.

lentiginous elongation of rete ridges (Fig. 28-39). Although melanocytes may be normal in number, in most instances they are slightly increased (546). Because of this slight increase in melanocyte number, the lesions are termed lentigines (as opposed to ephelides) by strict histologic criteria (546). In contrast to true melanocytic neoplasms (nevi or melanomas), the cell bodies of the lesional melanocytes are separated by those of keratinocytes, that is, there is no contiguous proliferation of melanocytes. Occasionally, especially in the penile and vulvar lesions, there are prominent dendrites of melanocytes ramifying among the hyperpigmented keratinocytes. There may be associated mild keratinocytic hyperplasia, and scattered melanophages in the papillary dermis, resulting from pigmentary incontinence, may account for the blue-black color and the pigmentary variegation that can simulate melanoma clinically.

Differential Diagnosis. The histologic distinction from RGP melanoma is easy because of the absence of neoplastic (contiguous)

melanocytic proliferation and cytologic atypia of melanocytes, although atypical and "borderline" examples are occasionally encountered and may be interpreted descriptively as SAMPUS, with a note addressing the differential diagnosis and perhaps treatment options.

Histogenesis. The process appears likely to be one of reactive hyperplasia with some features of postinflammatory hyperpigmentation, rather than a neoplasm. The phenomenon is benign with associated lesional growth stabilization over time.

Principles of Management: These lesions may need to be biopsied to rule out melanoma. If there is melanocytic atypia, complete excision and follow-up should be considered.

Mucosal Lentiginous Melanoma

Mucosal tumors constitute Pathway VI in the 2018 WHO Classification (4) (Table 28-2, p. 836).

After the skin and eyes, melanoma is most apt to arise in the juxtacutaneous mucous membranes, such as the oral mucosa, nose and nasal sinuses (548), vagina and vulvar mucosa and paramucosa (549), and anorectal mucosa (550). Mucosal melanomas are analogous to acral melanomas in histologic appearance and aggressiveness, leading to the use of the histologic term "mucosal lentiginous" melanoma (255). *KIT* mutation and/or amplification are found in 25% or more of these lesions (549) and may predict therapeutic responsiveness (551). In a comprehensive study of 67 tumors, there was a low point mutation burden and there were many structural variants, including recurrent rearrangements targeting *TERT, CDK4,* and *MDM2.* Potentially important mutated genes included *NRAS, BRAF, NF1, KIT, SF3B1, TP53, SPRED1, ATRX, HLA-A CHD8,* and *CTNNB1.* Some of these are familiar from cutaneous melanoma, whereas others are novel. *TERT* aberrations and *ATRX* mutations were associated with alterations in telomere length. These mutation profiles suggested potential susceptibility to *CDK4/6* and/or *MEK* inhibitors in many of the tumors (550,552).

Histopathology. The lesions are characterized by the RGP; when a VGP is present, it is likely to have attributes similar to those associated with other melanomas. Occasionally, the vertical growth is desmoplastic; however, the characteristic GAs of DM

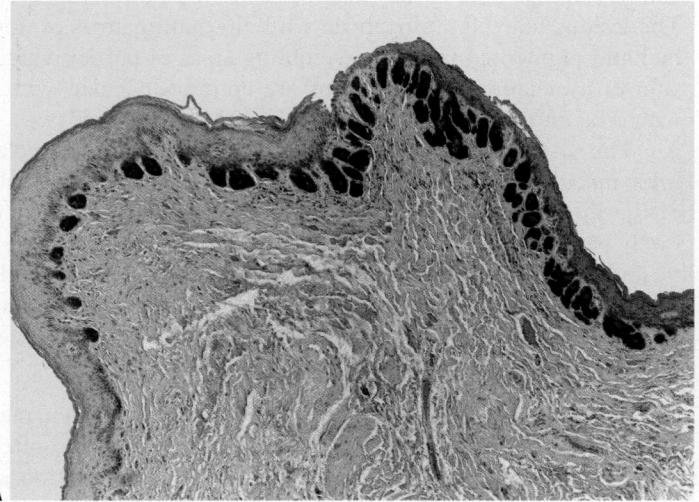

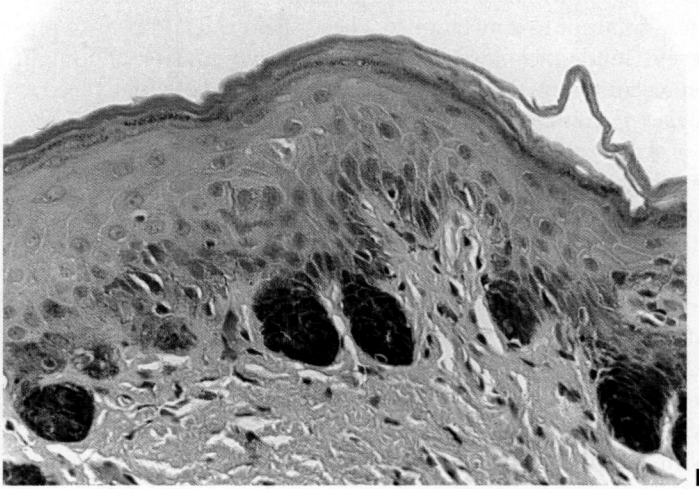

Figure 28-39 Mucosal lentigo of the vulva. A: In this instance, there is quite prominent elongation of rete ridges. B: There is no melanocytic atypia.

in high CSD skin are not present. The pattern of involvement in the RGP is most often lentiginous (Fig. 28-40), but prominent pagetoid pattern is sometimes encountered. In some lesions with pagetoid proliferation, a BRAF driver mutation has been demonstrated.

We generally provide prognostic attributes as for usual cutaneous melanomas as a guide to therapy. In the physiologic absence of a granular layer in a mucous membrane, we generally measure thickness from the top of the epithelium to the deepest invasive tumor cell; however, it is worth noting that Breslow thickness and its optimal ascertainment have not been adequately studied in mucosal melanomas.

Congenital Nevi and Melanocytic Tumors Arising in Them

Melanocytic tumors arising in congenital melanocytic nevi constitute Pathway VII in the 2018 WHO Classification of Melanocytic Tumors (5) (Table 28-2, p. 836).

Congenital Melanocytic Nevus

A CMN may be defined as a lesion present at birth and containing nevus cells.

Clinical Summary. Congenital nevi are found in about 1% to 2% of newborn infants (51,553), and, thus, although such lesions are rare when compared to the total number of all noncongenital nevi, their occurrence is a relatively common clinical event. In many instances, congenital nevi are larger than acquired nevi, measuring more than 1.5 cm in diameter. However, only a few are of considerable size. Those measuring more than 20 cm in greatest diameter are referred to as *giant CMN* (Fig. 28-41A) (554), and these have an incidence of approximately 1:250,000 births (555). Melanoma may arise in these lesions, and this is the most common (least rare) category of fatal melanoma in young children (Fig. 28-41B). *Nongiant CMN* are usually slightly raised and often pigmented, and they may show a moderate growth of hair. They may be classified as "small" (<1.5 cm in diameter) or "intermediate" (>1.5 and <20 cm, or

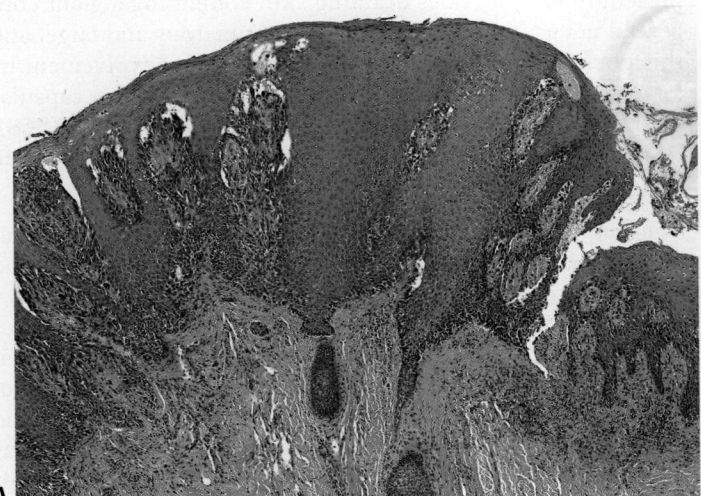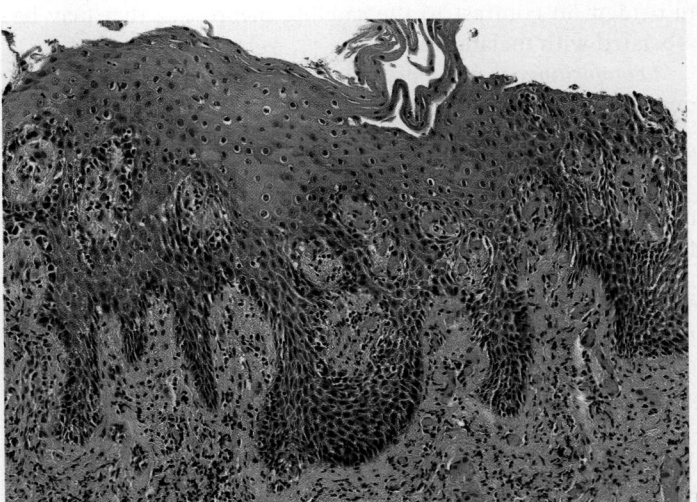

Figure 28-40 Melanoma *in situ* of the vulva. **A:** There is a broad lesion characterized by an increased number of uniformly atypical melanocytes, arranged in a lentiginous pattern mostly near the basal layers of the epidermis. There is some suprabasal scatter. **B:** At the periphery of the lesion, it is poorly circumscribed, with decreasing density of lesional cells that may present difficulties in identifying the exact periphery of the lesion.

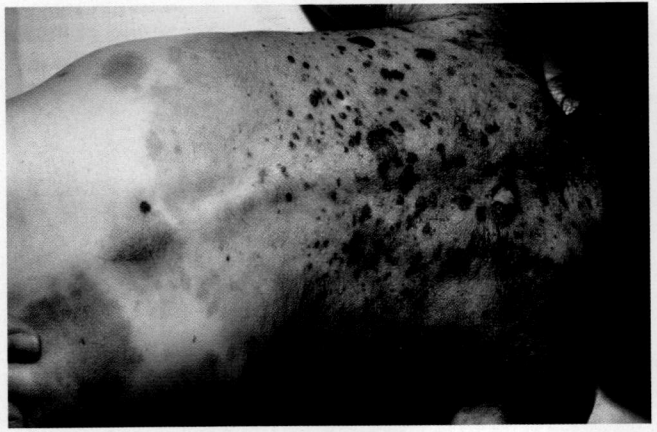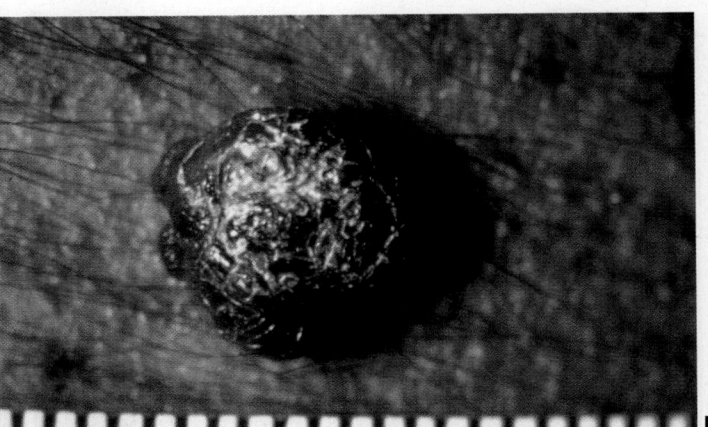

Figure 28-41 Giant congenital nevus, clinical. **A:** These lesions have also been called "garment nevi" because of their coverage of such large areas of skin. Focal areas of increased pigmentation, sometimes associated with palpable nodularity, are not uncommon in giant congenital nevi. Such foci should be followed carefully, and any lesions showing evidence of progressive changes should be excised to rule out melanoma. **B:** Melanoma in a giant congenital nevus. This nodule developed on the back of the patient illustrated in (A), at the age of 4 years. The patient died within about 2 years of metastatic melanoma.

amenable to local excision). Other potential classifiers in children include projected adult size (PAS), location, satellite nevus counts, and morphologic characteristics (color heterogeneity, rugosity, nodularity, and hypertrichosis) (556).

A number of variants have been described, such as the *cerebriform congenital nevus,* which presents as a skin-colored, convoluted mass (557); the *spotted grouped pigmented nevus,* also known as *congenital follicular melanocytic nevus,* comprised of closely set brown to black papules (558); the *congenital acral melanocytic nevus,* which consists of a blue-black patch on the sole or the distal portion of a finger clinically resembling an ALM (559); and the *desmoplastic hairless hypopigmented nevus,* which presents clinically as a hard, ligneous, progressively hypopigmented and alopecic giant congenital nevus and is characterized histologically by intense dermal fibrosis, scarce nevus cells, and hypertrophic or absent hair follicles (560,561). *Giant CMN* often have the distribution of a garment ("garment nevi"). They are usually deeply pigmented and are covered with a moderate growth of hair. Often, there are many scattered "satellite" lesions of a similar appearance (562,563). These satellite nevi are benign, in contrast to the satellite metastases that may be associated with melanomas.

Leptomeningeal melanocytosis can occur in patients with congenital nevi (see section on Leptomeningeal Melanocytosis).

Histopathology. Histopathologic studies have identified differences between true giant congenital nevi and small/intermediate nevi, in which there may or may not be a convincing history of true congenital onset (presence at birth) (564).

Giant Congenital Nevi. The histologic appearance of giant CMN differs dramatically from that of acquired nevi in terms of their greater size and depth and in the involvement of skin appendages and sometimes even deeper tissues (e.g., galea aponeurotica and cranial nerve extension in scalp lesions) (Fig. 28-42). In an early study, congenital nevi had three major diagnostic features that separated them from acquired nevi: (1) presence of nevus cells in the lower two-thirds of reticular dermis and often in the subcutis; (2) nevus cells disposed between collagen bundles singly and in files; and (3) nevus cells involving appendages, nerves, and vessels in the lower two-thirds of the reticular dermis or subcutis, especially nevus cells within sebaceous glands (565). These features apply mainly to giant and deep congenital nevi (in which the history of congenital onset is usually unequivocal) and are not specific or sensitive in small nevi (see next paragraph) (564). Cytologically, the cells of congenital nevi are similar to those of acquired nevi.

Often, these giant nevi are more complex than nongiant congenital nevi. Three patterns have been found within them: a compound or intradermal nevus, a "neural nevus," and a blue nevus pattern (566). In most instances, the compound or intradermal nevus component predominates, whereas in others the "neural nevus" component predominates. In the latter case, formations such as neuroid tubes and nevic corpuscles are present (p. 846). These areas may show considerable similarity to a neurofibroma. A component resembling a blue nevus or a cellular blue nevus (CBN) is found in some of the giant pigmented nevi, usually as a minor component. In rare instances, however, the entire congenital lesion consists of a giant blue nevus, often on the scalp (567). Nevus cells may be present in lymph nodes draining skin containing a giant congenital nevus; these deposits may be numerous and large, and this phenomenon should not be mistaken for involvement by a melanoma. In general, the nodal nevus cells lie in capsular or sinusoidal septal collagen, and the cells lack atypia (568). HMB45, Ki-67, p16, and PRAME staining could be helpful in difficult cases.

Nongiant (Small and Intermediate) CMN. Nongiant congenital nevi may have the same histologic appearance as acquired nevi or features of congenital nevi (Fig. 28-43) (84,569,570). Nongiant congenital nevi may be junctional, compound, or intradermal nevi, and their location in the dermis may be either superficial, which may include a junctional involvement, or superficial and deep (571). They may differ from acquired nevi by one or more features, as also seen in giant nevi: (a) presence of melanocytes, often in nests, around and within hair follicles, in sweat ducts and glands, in sebaceous glands, in or in intimate association with vessel walls, in arrector pili muscles, and in the perineurium of nerves; (b) extension of melanocytes

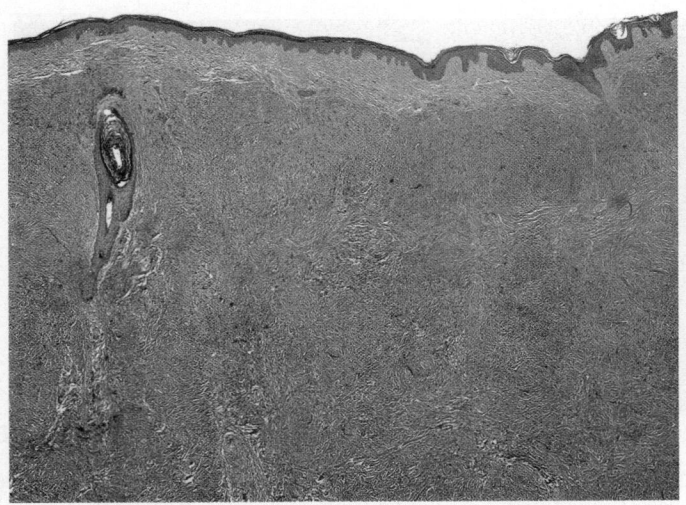
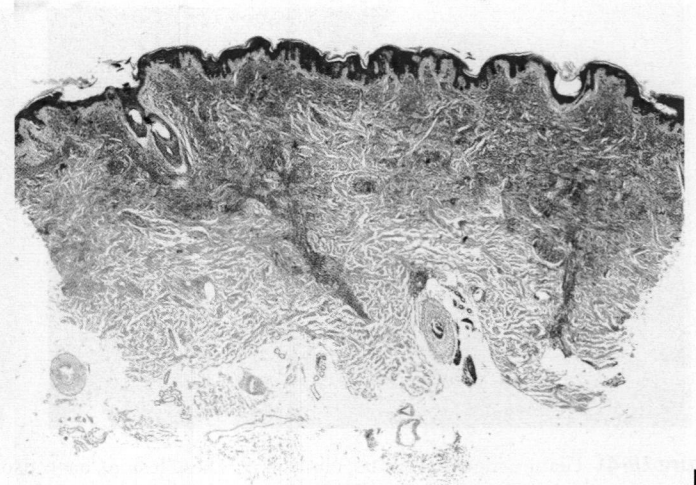

A   **B**

Figure 28-42 Giant congenital nevus, histopathology. **A:** This nevus is very broad (many centimeters, extending well beyond the borders of the image), and "deep," that is, the lesional cells extend from the epidermis through the reticular dermis and into the fat. **B:** In another giant congenital nevus, sheets of nevus cells are placed among reticular dermis collagen bundles. The dermal component of giant congenital nevi is often variably cellular, and, in addition to nevic differentiation, there may be evidence of schwannian or even heterotopic elements.

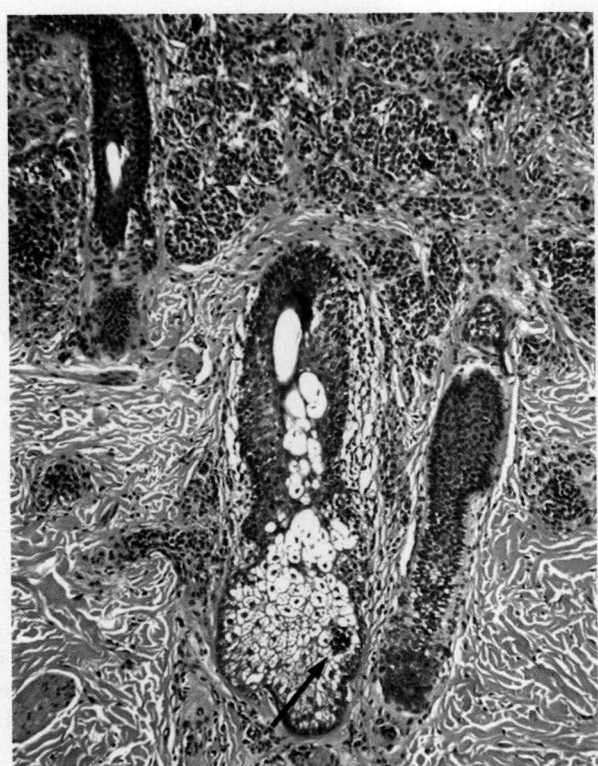

Figure 28-43 Compound nevus with congenital pattern features. Nevus cells extend around skin appendages and between fibers of the reticular dermis. The presence of nevus cells "within" skin appendages (as here in the sebaceous unit, see arrow) is a quite specific feature indicating true congenital onset of a nevus. The extension of nevus cells into the upper reticular dermis and around skin appendages is quite characteristic of congenital nevi. However, acquired nevi may also exhibit this "deep" pattern, and, conversely, congenital nevi are not always "deep."

between collagen bundles singly or in double rows; and (c) extension into the deepest reticular dermis and into the subcutis (Fig. 28-43) (565). However, these features in nongiant congenital nevi are neither sensitive nor specific for truly congenital origin of a nevus: a histologic study with comparison with clinical data found that 32 nevi with the histologic criteria of congenital nevi were actually acquired and that 179 nevi present at birth did not fulfill these criteria. Such studies are complicated by the possibility that some congenital nevi may be clinically covert at birth and thus regarded as acquired. In the case of deep and large (giant) congenital nevi, in contrast, the clinicopathologic correlation was 100% (564). Of note, however, many nongiant congenital nevi have none of these features. For example, some documented congenital nevi have been entirely junctional (571), whereas the likelihood of deep dermal involvement appears to increase with the size of the lesion (572) and is actually uncommon in lesions smaller than 3 cm (573). Conversely, the presence of most of the features mentioned previously has been documented in nevi that indubitably became clinically apparent after birth (and therefore called "tardive" or "congenital pattern" nevi) (574). Thus, nevi with the constellation of features described previously may be characterized as "nevi with congenital pattern features," but not all of these lesions are truly congenital in origin.

Among the special forms of nongiant congenital nevi, the *cerebriform congenital nevus* usually presents as an intradermal nevus with neuroid changes simulating those seen in neurofibroma (557). The lesions, called *spotted grouped pigmented nevi*, are also intradermal nevi. They are either eccrine centered or

follicle centered. If they are eccrine centered, each eccrine sweat duct is tightly enveloped by nevus cells, whereas hair follicles are only minimally involved (558). If they are follicle centered, nevus cell nests are found mainly around the hair follicles. In the *acral nevus of congenital origin,* the lesion may simulate melanoma clinically; however, the histologic appearance is characteristic of a congenital nevus (559). In the lesion called desmoplastic hairless hypopigmented nevus, there is intense dermal fibrosis, scarce nevus cells, and hypotrophic or absent hair follicles. Follow-up biopsies have documented the progressive nature of the fibrosis and nevus cell depletion (561).

In some CMN, changes are observed that may simulate a melanoma. In a study of 42 cases in patients with a mean age of 20 years, features that could simulate malignant melanoma in a congenital nevus included: (a) asymmetry and poor circumscription; (b) an increased number of single melanocytes that predominated over nests of melanocytes in some high-power fields; (c) single melanocytes not equidistant from one another; (d) presence of scattered single melanocytes above the dermoepidermal junction; and (e) confluence of nests of melanocytes, all features in common with some malignant melanomas (575). In our experience, such changes are generally slight in degree, and severe uniform cytologic atypia or frequent mitoses are not observed. However, occasionally a biopsy in a neonate may show disturbing cytologic and architectural atypia of junctional and/or dermal components; in our experience of several such cases, the lesions have subsequently undergone maturation and become indistinguishable from a benign congenital nevus. Therefore, a diagnosis of melanoma in a congenital nevus in a neonate should be made with great caution, and the presence of these histopathologic features alone should neither be interpreted as evidence for potential malignant behavior nor necessarily serve as grounds for further excision (576).

Histogenesis and Genomic Landscape. As is the case for common nevi, a dual origin of congenital nevi has been proposed and it seems likely that the dermal component of these lesions, at least, must be derived directly from neural crest precursors, rather than by a process of "abtropfung," or "dropping down" from the epidermis. Based on studies in aborted fetuses and stillbirths, it has recently been suggested that many clinically acquired nevi were actually formed in utero, like congenital nevi, and these have been termed "prenatal nevi" (577).

There is evidence that these lesions differ genetically from common nevi. As in other nevi, oncogenic mutations in *NRAS, BRAF,* and other potential driver genes have been described in individual congenital nevus lesions (578). It appears that most large and "true" congenital nevi have mutation of *NRAS,* in contrast to most acquired nevi that have mutated *BRAF.* In a comprehensive study of 21 large/giant CMN, mutational screening mutations were found in 76% of large/giant CMNs, with an *NRAS* mutation in 57%, and mutations in other genes such as *BRAF, KRAS, APC,* and *MET* in 14%. RNA fusion transcripts were found in two patients. Thus, large/giant CMN may result from a variety of GAs in addition to *NRAS* mutations, including point mutations and fusion transcripts (579).

In another contrast, most of the "congenital pattern" nevi that are actually acquired have BRAF mutations, likely related to sun exposure (578). The lesions appear to undergo oncogene-induced senescence, similar to acquired nevi (580). It remains to be seen whether such nevi have any special significance as risk markers or potential precursors of melanoma.

The pathogenesis of multiple CMN within the same subject has been explained in terms of *NRAS* mutant mosaicism. Kinsler et al. found consistent oncogenic mutations in codon

61 of *NRAS* in affected neurologic and cutaneous tissues of 12 out of 15 patients but not in normal tissues. All 11 nonmelanocytic and melanocytic CNS samples from 5 patients were mutation positive, despite *NRAS* rarely being reported as mutated in CNS tumors. These results suggest that single postzygotic *NRAS* mosaic mutations are responsible for multiple CMN and associated neurologic lesions in most cases (581).

In studies of cellular differentiation in giant congenital nevi using melanocytic and stem cell markers, Kinsler et al. identified two groups of cases: those with nevus cell nesting and those with only diffuse dermal infiltration. Samples from the nested lesions were significantly more likely to express melanocytic differentiation markers, the expression of which decreased significantly with depth. The stem cell markers were often coexpressed. The dermal lesions frequently coexisted with normal overlying melanocyte development, suggesting that these lesions likely develop from a cutaneous stem cell independent of, or remaining after, normal melanocytic migration and capable of some degree of melanocytic differentiation superficially (582).

Principles of Management of Congenital Nevi: Excision of giant congenital nevi is suggested by some groups; however, heroic surgical procedures are often required, and hence cosmetic improvement may be debatable. Because removal is not often complete and because of the risk of neurocutaneous melanosis, lifelong follow-up may be reasonable to consider even after efforts at surgical excision. In a registry-based study of 301 families, there was a high level of satisfaction with surgery in the patients who had small or intermediate facial lesions. This was significantly reduced with increasing lesion size. There was no evidence that surgery reduced the incidence of adverse clinical outcomes in childhood. The natural history of most untreated congenital nevi was to lighten spontaneously, whereas some treatments may cause adverse effects (583). On the basis of considerations like these, many groups opt for follow-up over surgical removal of these lesions.

The excision of all nongiant congenital nevi, where feasible, is often considered (584). The risk of melanoma in any given lesion is low and not limited to childhood. In an individual within only a single small or intermediate congenital nevus, excision may be a simpler choice than follow-up, or, alternatively, a patient could be given guidelines for self-examination/observation. The small "congenital pattern nevi" discussed earlier are probably best managed as for common acquired nevi, namely, by excision, to rule out melanoma only for lesions that are changing or otherwise atypical.

Cellular and/or Proliferative Nodules in Congenital Melanocytic Nevi

Clinical Features: Although melanomas may occur in the dermal component of congenital nevi, cellular and/or proliferative nodules (PNs) that develop in these nevi often do not behave in a clinically aggressive fashion (585). Such lesions may arise as one or more relatively small nodules that develop sometimes rapidly within a preexisting congenital nevus, particularly in infancy and early childhood.

Histopathology. The lesions present as a nodule of cells that are often larger than those in the background nevus and often more densely packed (Fig. 28-44). Mitotic figures may be present but are often absent. There is no high-grade cellular atypia as

a rule. In a clinical pathologic study of a cohort of 26 cases, with a mean of 5-year follow-up on 16 patients, the lesions had an invariably benign clinical course. The features that are useful in differentiating PN from melanoma include: (a) lack of high-grade uniform cellular atypia; (b) lack of necrosis within the nodule; (c) rarity of mitoses; (d) evidence of maturation in the form of blending or transitional forms between the cells in the nodule and the adjacent nevus cells; (e) lack of pagetoid spread into the overlying epidermis; and (f) no destructive expansile growth. Because of the frequent complete absence of mitoses in these lesions, we tend to use the term "cellular nodule" for these lesions, with a comment as to absence or degree of proliferation (e.g., "cellular and weakly proliferative nodule" for a lesion with few mitoses) (245). If the features that distinguish PN from melanoma are only partially represented, the descriptive diagnosis of "melanocytic tumor of uncertain potential" may be appropriate (p. 880).

Histogenesis and Molecular Testing. Potential ancillary tests in distinguishing between PN and melanoma in giant CMN include IHC, CGH, NGS, FISH, and GEP. Comprehensive studies of the validity of these tests are lacking. Perhaps the most useful test in a difficult case is CGH, although in our experience this is not needed in most lesions. By CGH, cases of cellular nodules in congenital nevi demonstrate chromosome loss with patterns that differ from the findings in frank melanomas, that is, numerical aberrations of whole chromosomes exclusively, compared to melanomas that had multiple cytogenetic aberrations in a pattern indistinguishable from that of melanomas not associated with congenital nevus. The CGH finding of frequent numerical chromosomal aberrations in atypical nodular proliferations arising in CMN is considered to identify these as clonal neoplasms with a genomic instability consistent with a mitotic spindle checkpoint defect (586). By NGS, most of these lesions have mutations of *NRAS* rather than BRAF, considered to be characteristic of lesions that develop in the absence of sun exposure; however, this information alone has no value in predicting behavior (578). In the case of a PN in a giant CMN with a normal CGH prolife, a GEP study was negative. Immunostaining for PRAME was also negative, and this test could have diagnostic value (587). Epigenetic methylation changes between PNs, and melanomas in giant CMN may be a useful diagnostic marker (588). Significant loss of H3K27me3, a regulator of chromatin remodeling-controlled transcription, was seen in 4 of 5 melanomas but not in any of 20 PNs in giant CMN (589). IHC for p16 and the 4-probe FISH melanoma analysis have been found not to be useful for distinguishing PN from childhood as opposed to adult-onset melanoma (590).

Melanoma and Other Tumors in Congenital Nevi

A variety of benign and malignant tumors can occur in congenital nevi, the most important of which is malignant melanoma. Melanoma in a congenital nevus is the most common cause of death from melanoma in young children (p. 914, Fig. 28-45, 46) (591–593). Although risk is highest in childhood, melanoma can occur at any age (594).

Clinical Summary. The pattern of occurrence of melanoma in giant congenital nevi was studied in a review of 34 patients who had primary cutaneous melanomas within their nevi; in 2 additional patients, melanoma developed at cutaneous sites other than within their nevi. All patients in whom melanoma

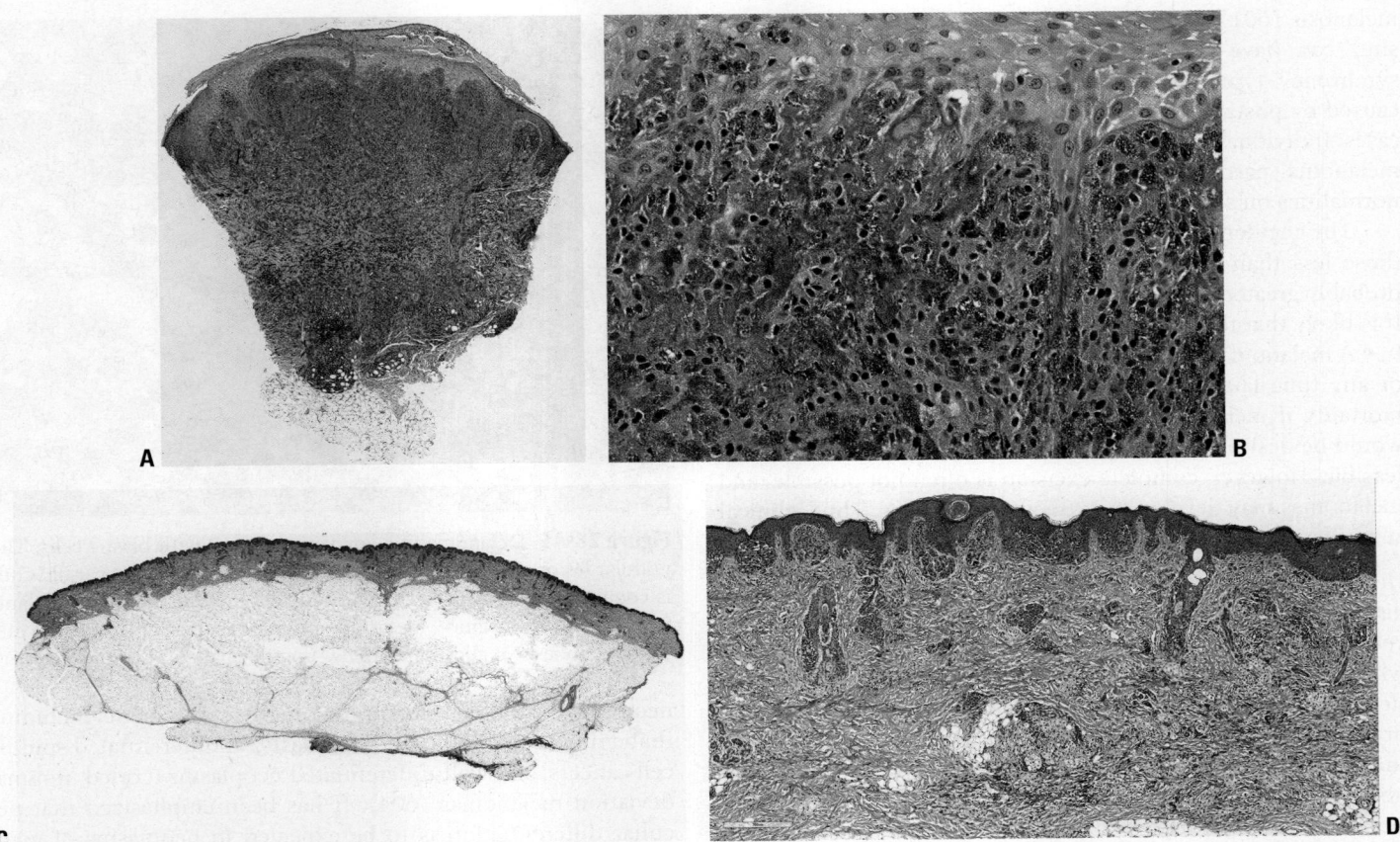

Figure 28-44 Atypical cellular and proliferative nodule in a large congenital nevus. **A:** This nodular lesion presented in a 2-month-old child with a large congenital pigmented nevus of the leg. **B:** The lesion extends to the epidermis, which is unusual; however, there is no well-developed *in situ* or junctional component. Few mitoses were focally present. There is some resemblance to a pigmented epithelioid melanocytoma; however, the characteristic nuclear changes (with prominent nucleoli and pale chromatin) are not observed. **C:** A complete excision of the lesional site was done. **D:** There is similar residual lesion in a congenital nevus background. There have been no reported adverse events in a period of more than 12 years.

developed within the nevi had nevi in axial locations; however, 91% of the nevi overall were axial. No melanoma was found that had arisen in any of the 26 nevi confined to the extremities. In addition, no melanoma was found that had arisen in thousands of satellite nevi (595). Melanoma can arise either in the skin or as a primary in the brain or rarely in other sites.

In a retrospective analysis, abnormal DNA content, aneuploidy, and abnormal cell cycle were found by flow cytometry in samples from giant congenital nevi from 6 patients with, but not from 28 patients without melanoma elsewhere in the nevus. It is possible that these phenomena could relate to risk of malignant transformation and provide a basis for risk assessment (596).

If a melanoma arises in a small or intermediate congenital nevus, it usually originates at the epidermal–dermal junction, and the appearances are those of an ordinary form of melanoma, usually of the superficial spreading or nodular types (p. 869). Most of the congenital nevi associated with such melanomas are small and superficial (597). Because of their much greater frequency (and despite their much lower individual risk), congenital pattern nevi are more frequently observed as precursors of melanoma than giant nevi (598). Melanoma in a giant congenital nevus, in contrast to nearly all other cutaneous melanomas, typically arises in the dermis or subcutis (594,599).

Melanomas in giant congenital nevi are frequently highly aggressive and often fatal (593); however, this does not apply to those in small congenital and congenital pattern nevi, in which the usual prognostic factors may apply.

Incidence of Melanoma in Congenital Nevi. In a comprehensive meta-analysis, 14 articles were chosen from a large literature database for further analysis. The frequency of melanomas ranged between 0.05% and 10.7% and was significantly higher in smaller studies. In a total of 6,571 patients with congenital nevi who were followed in various studies for a mean of 3.4 to 23.7 years, 46 patients (0.7%) developed 49 melanomas, a lower number than might have been expected, likely reflecting selection bias in published smaller studies. The mean age at diagnosis of melanoma was 15.5 years (median 7), indicative of a maximum risk in childhood and adolescence. By comparison with age-adjusted population-based data, the patients with congenital nevi carry an approximately 465-fold increased relative risk of developing melanoma during childhood and adolescence. Risk for melanomas was related to lesion size. Primary melanomas arose inside the nevi in 33 of 49 cases (67%). In seven cases (14%), metastatic melanoma with unknown primary was encountered; in four cases (8%), the melanoma developed at an extracutaneous site. One-third of the melanomas were fatal (600).

Of note, the majority of patients with congenital nevi, even large ones, will never develop melanoma. In a large registry study, increasing numbers of satellite lesions and larger lesional diameters were associated with melanoma and neurocutaneous melanosis (601). Multiple CMN (two or more, of any size or site) can have extracutaneous associations, termed "CMN syndrome," typically including craniofacial abnormalities and caused by postzygotic mosaicism for *NRAS* mutations in most cases. Individuals with multiple CMN have an increased risk of melanoma, particularly if there are congenital neurologic abnormalities on screening MRI in the first 6 months of life.

The incidence of melanoma in nongiant congenital nevi, those less than 20 cm in greatest diameter, is unknown but probably greater than that in a comparable area of normal skin. It is likely that the risk is related to lesion size (600).

A melanoma may be present at birth or may arise in infancy or any time later in life (Fig. 28-41B). Given the substantial mortality if melanoma develops, it is generally agreed that it would be desirable for giant melanocytic nevi to be excised, if feasible. However, complete excision is often not possible, and melanomas may develop in extracutaneous sites. Thus, clinical surveillance is considered to be an acceptable alternative.

Histopathology. In our experience, some of the melanomas in giant congenital nevi have been comprised of large epithelioid cells similar to those of many melanomas in adults (Fig. 28-45), whereas others have been comprised of undifferentiated "blastic" (or small round blue) cells resembling lymphoblasts with or without melanin (Fig. 28-46). Other patterns of malignancy that have been described in congenital nevi have included neoplasms with the appearance of a neurosarcoma (602); lesions that have been termed malignant blue nevus (603,604);

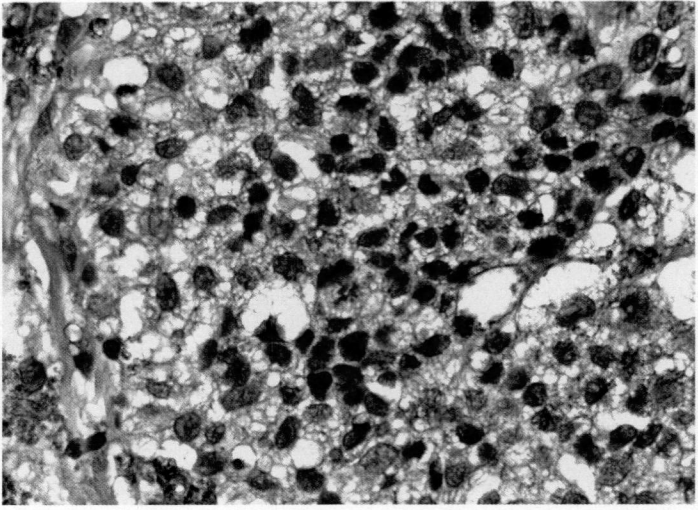

Figure 28-46 Melanoma in a congenital nevus, with blastic cells. This nodular lesion that developed in a congenital nevus of a 4-year-old child is comprised of "blastic" cells with nuclear molding and with melanin pigment in this instance. Metastatic tumor was present in three of four sentinel nodes. No additional follow-up information is available.

neoplasms with heterologous mesenchymal elements including rhabdomyoblasts (605) and lipoblasts; undifferentiated spindle cell cancers; and well-differentiated neoplasms termed minimal deviation melanomas (604). It has been emphasized that peculiar differentiation is to be expected in neoplasms of giant

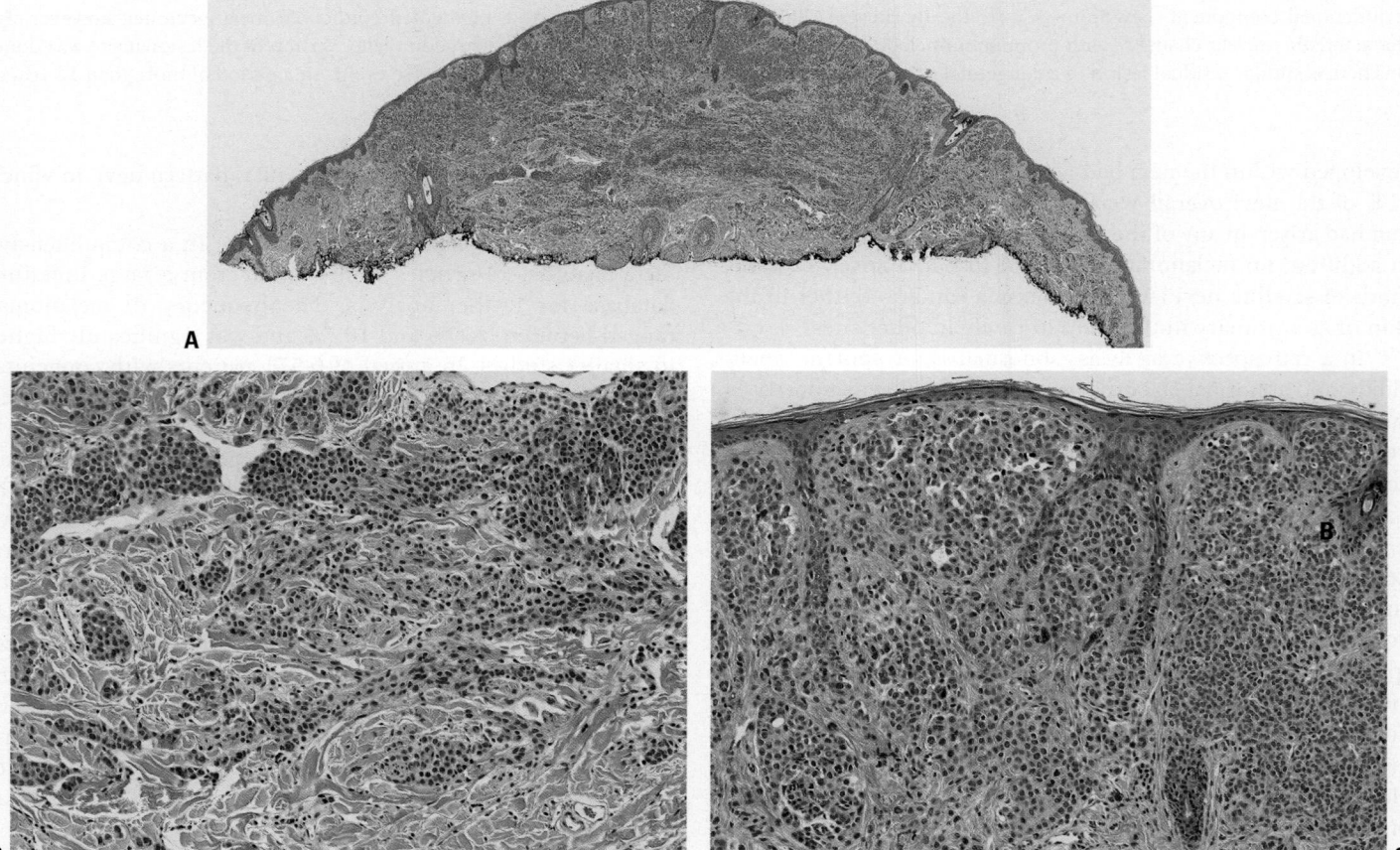

Figure 28-45 Melanoma in a large congenital nevus. A: A changing congenital lesion in a 12-month old child was excised. B: Near the base, the lesional cells are mature in the pattern of a congenital nevus, with cells splaying among collagen fibers of the reticular dermis and extending around skin appendages (sweat glands, upper right, and hair follicles elsewhere). C: Superficially, the lesion is more cellular, with large nuclei and with mitotic activity. This child developed disseminated metastatic melanoma and died 2 years after the first presentation.

congenital nevi and that alarmingly cellular neoplasms may not behave aggressively (604). Thus, pathology does not always readily predict outcome. This is especially true in our experience when apparent melanomas arise in the first few months of life. Modern molecular techniques may be of assistance in distinguishing among these cases.

Cytologic and architectural atypia may occasionally be seen in congenital pattern nevi, and criteria for the distinction of these lesions from melanoma are similar to those discussed in the differential diagnosis of dysplastic nevi and SSMs.

In a study of melanomas that had arisen in 48 "small" or intermediate CMN that measured less than 10 cm in diameter, only five of the nevi reached the lower-third of the dermis or subcutis and were classified as "deep type," whereas the remainder were limited to the upper two-thirds of the dermis ("superficial type"). All of the melanomas were of "epidermal" origin, and most were of the superficial spreading type (569). The age at diagnosis ranged from 18 to 79 years, and prepubertal melanomas were not observed in this series. Melanomas in small congenital nevi are typically of the usual superficial spreading type. In a large study, 40 of 190 cases of melanoma were associated with preexisting nevi; of these, 15 had congenital features with a largest diameter of 1.5 cm, that is, "small congenital pattern nevi." These 15 cases were melanomas of the superficial type with a mean tumor thickness lower than that of melanomas not associated with nevi (0.33 vs. 1.50). Thus, a relatively high percentage of melanomas were found to be associated with small congenital pattern nevi, indicating that these may be considered as potential melanoma precursors (606). However, the risk of progression of any given lesion is very low.

Molecular and Other Ancillary Techniques in Diagnosis of Melanoma in Congenital Nevi. As in other areas of pathology, molecular diagnostic techniques can be of assistance in supporting diagnosis of melanoma versus benign proliferations in congenital nevi, and these can potentially include immunohistochemical markers such as Ki-67 and p16 (p. 878), FISH, CGH, GEP, and NGS.

In a study that included five melanomas in congenital nevi in childhood, it was concluded that IHC and the 4-probe FISH melanoma analysis were not useful for distinguishing PN from childhood-onset melanoma as opposed to adult-onset melanoma (590).

NGS is most relevant in cases of metastatic melanoma. As in the nevi themselves, limited data suggest that mutations of *NRAS* are more common than those of *BRAF* in melanomas arising in giant congenital nevi. In one NGS study of a metastatic melanoma in a patient with a giant CMN, a *NRASQ61R* mutation was detected. In a comparative study of *NRAS* mutated cases, the most upregulated genes in *NRAS*-mutant melanoma were *PRAME* and *NES*, whereas downregulated genes in *NRAS*-mutant melanoma included the tumor suppressor genes *TP63*, *TP73*, *BCL6*, and *FBXW7* (607). Mutations of *BRAF* may be expected in the numerically more common melanomas that arise in small congenital pattern nevi, which are generally *BRAF*-mutated.

The pattern of progression genes may differ from that in ordinary melanomas. In one lesion studied with a large panel by NGS, there was a *TP53* mutation with a UV signature, coupled with a paradoxical overexpression of p16 (608). Another study also found retained expression of p16 in childhood-onset PNs and melanomas, whereas this was lost as expected in a comparison group of adult-onset melanomas (590).

In a study focusing on the important melanoma progression gene, telomerase (*TERT*), the more usually seen promoter activating mutations were not found in three melanomas in giant CMN, but rather this gene was found to be upregulated by a methylation-dependent mechanism, perhaps representing another unique aspect of this pathway of melanoma (609).

CGH is perhaps the most useful ancillary test in difficult cases. Melanomas in giant CMN have multiple chromosomal abnormalities similar to those found in other melanomas (586). In a study of 10 melanomas in giant CMN, histologic diagnosis was difficult in only 2 cases in which neither IHC nor FISH were helpful, whereas CGH demonstrated a high number of chromosomal aberrations, leading to a formal diagnosis (610).

Leptomeningeal Melanocytosis Associated with Giant Congenital Nevi

Leptomeningeal melanocytosis may be present, especially in cases in which the giant congenital nevus involves the posterior axis and in those with multiple "satellite" lesions (563). There may be not only epilepsy and mental retardation, but a primary leptomeningeal melanoma may also occur (566,611).

Histopathology. There is a diffuse infiltration of the leptomeninges with pigmented melanocytes. Also, the blood vessels entering the brain and spinal cord may be surrounded by melanocytes, and there may be areas of infiltration of the brain or spinal cord with melanocytes. Leptomeningeal melanoma can infiltrate the leptomeninges and form nodules that may enter the brain (594,611).

Histogenesis and Genomic Landscape. Meningeal melanosis associated with giant CMN (unlike that with nevus of Ota, which is likely to be G-protein related) appears to be related to a mosaic mutation of *NRAS*, and melanomas that arise in this condition are likely to be *NRAompS* mutated, similar to the lesions in the skin, based on limited data (612).

Melanocytic Tumors Arising in Blue Nevus and Related Lesions

The "blue" tumors constitute Pathway VIII in the 2018 WHO Classification (4) (Table 28-2, p. 836).

Blue nevi are proliferations of melanocytes that differ from usual nevi in that they tend to be located in the reticular dermis or deeper structures and to be heavily pigmented. The presence of melanin pigment in the reticular dermis and deeper imparts a blue coloration to the lesion clinically because of the Tyndall effect, whereby skin acts to preferentially scatter and transmit shorter wavelength blue light in response to deep-dermal melanin pigment. The spectrum of "blue lesions" includes dermal melanocytoses/hamartomas, blue nevi, cellular blue nevi, and melanomas arising in a blue nevus (MBN). These lesions had long been characterized together by traditional morphology, and, more recently, genomic analyses have demonstrated that they tend to be driven by mutations in a characteristic set of genes in the G-protein–coupled receptor pathway, which can drive progression in the MAP kinase pathway.

Dermal Melanocytoses and Hamartomas

It is important to distinguish dermal melanoses (implying only increase in dermal melanin pigment) caused by the presence of melanocytes in the dermis (melanocytoses) from those produced by the presence of melanin within nonmelanocytic cells (e.g., macrophages) within the dermis. Clinically, the two different processes may have very similar appearances. In this section, we consider the former condition. Dermal melanosis associated with metastatic melanoma is discussed in a later section of this chapter (p. 924), whereas inflammatory disorders associated with pigmentary alterations are discussed in Chapter 27.

Congenital Dermal Melanocytosis ("Mongolian Spot")

Clinical Summary: It has been recognized of late that the origin of the medical term "Mongolian Spot" dates back to an 18th century pseudoscientific and erroneous belief in the inferiority of all non-Caucasian racial groups (613). This lesion later came to be viewed as evidence for arrested evolutionary development among individuals of Asian descent, the "Mongolians" (614). This term should no longer be used.

The typical example of this lesion occurs in the sacrococcygeal region of an infant as a uniformly blue discoloration somewhat resembling a bruise. It consists of a noninfiltrated, round or ovoid, rather ill-defined patch of varying size, found more frequently in infants of Asian and African ethnicity. It is present at birth and usually disappears spontaneously within 3 to 4 years (615).

Occasionally, congenital dermal melanocytoses occur outside the lumbosacral region as aberrant Mongolian spots, such as on the middle or upper part of the back; they may then be multiple and bilateral and persist. Extensive congenital dermal melanocytoses may be seen in patients with bilateral nevus of Ota (616), and generalized and progressive forms may be associated with certain inborn errors of metabolism, including storage diseases and neurocristopathies (615).

Histopathology. In congenital dermal melanocytoses, the dermis contains in its lower half or two-thirds greatly elongated, slender, often slightly wavy dendritic cells containing melanin granules that are distributed within the dendrites, rendering them visible. These cells are present in a low concentration and lie widely scattered between the collagen bundles, and, like the involved collagen bundles, they generally lie parallel to the skin surface. No melanophages are seen.

Principles of Management: Education and reassurance are appropriate.

Nevi of Ota, Ito, and Hori; Dermal Melanocyte Hamartoma

Clinical Summary. Nevi of Ota and Ito and dermal melanocyte hamartoma are types of melanocytosis that differ from the congenital dermal melanocytoses by usually having a speckled rather than a uniform blue appearance and by showing a greater concentration of dermal melanocytes, with location in the upper rather than in the lower portion of the dermis. The importance of these lesions is primarily cosmetic and rarely also as potential precursors of melanoma, although the relative risk is unknown (617).

The nevus of Ota is most often a unilateral discoloration of the face composed of blue and brown, partially confluent macules. The periorbital region, temple, forehead, malar area, and nose are usually involved. Because of this usual distribution, Ota called the lesion "nevus fuscocaeruleus ophthalmomaxillaris." There is frequently also a patchy blue discoloration of the sclera of the ipsilateral eye and occasionally a similar discoloration of the conjunctiva, cornea, and retina. In some instances, the oral and nasal mucosa are similarly affected. In about 10% of the cases, the lesions of the nevus of Ota are bilateral rather than unilateral. They may be present at birth; they may also appear during the first year of life or during adolescence but only rarely in childhood. They have a tendency toward gradual enlargement. Malignant change in the cutaneous lesions of a nevus of Ota is extremely rare (617).

In the nevus of Ota, the involved areas of the skin show a brown to slate-blue uniform or mottled discoloration, usually without any induration. Occasionally, however, some areas are slightly raised. In some patients, discrete nodules varying in size from a few millimeters to a few centimeters and having the appearance of blue nevi are found within the areas of discoloration. Persistent congenital dermal melanocytoses are quite common in association with the nevus of Ota. Extensive congenital dermal melanocytoses are typically found in bilateral cases of nevus of Ota (9).

The nevus of Ito differs from the nevus of Ota by its location in the supraclavicular, scapular, and deltoid regions. It may occur alone or in association with an ipsilateral or bilateral nevus of Ota. Like the nevus of Ota, it has a mottled, macular appearance.

Nevus of Hori is a form of acquired dermal melanocytosis. It is also known as "acquired bilateral nevus of Ota-like macules" and "acquired symmetrical dermal melanocytosis" (618). The patients present with speckled blue-brown or gray macules that are located bilaterally in the malar region. Most of the reported cases have been seen in Asian women. Histology reveals dendritic pigmented melanocytes in the mid- and upper dermis. Electron microscopy has revealed a predominance of stage IV melanosomes and melanocyte dendrites encircling elastic fibers (619).

In the dermal melanocyte hamartoma, there may be a single, very extensive area of gray-blue pigmentation present from the time of birth, occurring in a dermatomal or segmental pattern, or there may be coalescing blue macules. Histologic examination reveals numerous dermal melanocytes described to occur in the upper half of the dermis. Very few cases have been reported (620).

Histopathology of Dermal Melanocytoses. The noninfiltrated areas of the nevus of Ota, as well as the nevi of Ito and Hori and the dermal melanocyte hamartoma, are comprised, like congenital dermal melanocytoses, of elongated, dendritic melanized cells scattered among the collagen bundles (621). The lesional cells are melanocytes, as judged by IHC and other supporting evidence. In these four forms of dermal melanocytosis, the melanocytes are generally more numerous and more superficially located than in congenital dermal melanocytoses. Although most of the dendritic melanocytes lie in the upper third of the reticular dermis, melanocytes may also occur in the papillary layer and may extend as far down as the subcutaneous tissue. Melanophages are seen in only few lesions. There is variation among Ota nevi according to the distribution of the dermal melanocytes from superficial to deep. This correlates to some extent with the color and location of the nevus (622).

Slightly raised and infiltrated areas have a larger number of elongated, dendritic melanocytes than do noninfiltrated areas, thus approaching the histologic picture of a blue nevus, and nodular areas are histologically indistinguishable from a blue nevus (615).

Malignant Melanoma Arising in Dermal Melanocytoses. Malignant changes, mostly involving nevus of Ota, have been reported in a handful of cases and may be cutaneous, orbital/uveal, or intracranial (617). In a 2015 review, 14 cases of cutaneous melanoma were described. One of these in a nevus of Ito had mutations of *GNAQ* and *BAP1*, similar to melanomas in blue nevi (MBN) and to ocular/uveal melanomas (623). The histologic appearance of the tumors may be similar to an MBN. These lesions are typically bulky, histologically fully malignant tumors, and their prognosis is poor. In a molecular study, progressive evaluation of melanoma was demonstrated in a nevus of Ota, with intermediate stages resembling CBN (624). In addition to melanoma, a benign or low-grade lesion, termed a melanocytoma of the meninges, may also occur (625). Two such cases have been reported to have *BRAFV600E* mutations (626).

Histogenesis of the Dermal Melanocytoses. The blue color of the dermal melanocytoses depends on the phenomenon whereby light passing through the skin is scattered as it strikes dark particles, such as melanin. Owing to this scattering phenomenon, termed the Tyndall effect, the colors of light that have a longer wavelength, such as red, orange, and yellow, tend to be less scattered and therefore continue to travel in a forward direction, but the colors of shorter wavelength, such as blue, indigo, and violet, are scattered to the side and backward to the skin surface. This phenomenon is also responsible for the distinctive color of blue nevi and of blood in veins.

In a study of 17 cases of nevus of Ota and 46 cases of uveal melanoma, activating mutations in the cell surface signaling G protein *GNAQ* were found in 6% and 46%, respectively, providing a genetic basis for the implication of nevus of Ota as a low-level risk factor and a rare potential precursor of uveal melanoma (627).

The finding of *GNAQ* (and no doubt other genes yet to be discovered) as a genetic link between nevi of Ota and melanomas that arise in them (and perhaps also in nevi of Ito and Hori and in the so-called dermal melanocyte hamartoma) suggests that these lesions are neoplastic, not hamartomatous or reactive. The congenital dermal melanocytosis is thought to be the result of the delayed disappearance of dermal melanocytes during embryogenesis, and as such it could perhaps be considered as a reactive or hamartomatous condition.

Principles of Management: Complete excision of the dermal melanocytoses is generally not possible. Laser therapy may be used for cosmesis. Consideration of periodic follow-up with imaging may be appropriate, especially for those lesions that involve the eye or the central nervous system.

Blue Nevi

Blue nevi are benign localized pigmented lesions that generally occur on the skin, although, occasionally, they may be observed in mucous membranes (628). On the skin, three types of benign blue nevi are recognized: the common blue nevus, the CBN, and the combined nevus with a blue nevus component. In addition, there are malignant blue nevi, discussed in a later section.

Histologically, the common feature of blue nevi is the presence of pigmented spindle and dendritic melanocytes in a focal area of the reticular dermis, associated (unlike the dermal melanocytoses) with alterations in the dermal collagen architecture. This deeply situated pigment differs from the pigment in acquired nevi that is typically superficial only, and accounts for the blue color of these lesions, due to the light-scattering Tyndall effect.

Common Blue Nevus

Clinical Summary. The common blue nevus occurs as a small, well-circumscribed, dome-shaped nodule of slate-blue or blue-black color (Fig. 28-47). The lesion rarely exceeds 1 cm in diameter. Common blue nevi are frequently found on or near the dorsa of the hands and feet, as well as on the scalp. Usually, there is only one lesion, but there may be several. A rare manifestation is the plaque type of blue nevus, which shows numerous macules and papules within a circumscribed area. This type of lesion may be present at birth or may become clinically apparent later in life (629,630). Malignant degeneration has been reported in the plaque type (631) but apparently not in the common blue nevus.

Histopathology. In the common blue nevus, the melanocytes have a similar appearance to those in congenital dermal melanocytoses and in the nevus of Ota, but they are typically larger, and their density is much greater. Greatly elongated, slender, often slightly wavy melanocytes with long, occasionally branching dendritic processes lie grouped in irregular bundles in the dermis (Fig. 28-47B–D). The bundles of cells may extend into the subcutaneous tissue or lie close to the epidermis. However, there is no junctional component. The greatly elongated melanocytes lie predominantly with their long axis parallel to the epidermis. Most of them are filled with numerous fine granules of melanin, often so completely that their nuclei cannot be visualized. The melanin granules also characteristically fill the long, often wavy, occasionally branching dendritic processes. Wavy fiber bundles similar to nerves may be present, indicative of schwannian differentiation (632). Occasionally, lesional cells are seen in the perineurium of authentic nerves, a finding that is not indicative of malignancy. Melanophages may be seen near the bundles of melanocytes but are usually not numerous or dense. The melanophages differ from the melanocytes by being more round to ovoid, by showing no dendritic processes, and by containing larger granules. The melanocytes of blue nevi are positive for S100, MITF, and HMB-45 (633) and also for Melan-A/MART and Sox10. The staining with HMB45 is uniform, rather than stratified, as in common nevi. The number of fibroblasts and the amount of collagen are generally increased in blue nevi, resulting in disruption of the normal architecture of the connective tissue. In some lesions, the collagen is unusually prominent, and these have been termed desmoplastic blue nevi (or desmoplastic cellular blue nevi) (422). Despite their name, the color of blue nevi varies with a variety of colors, including blue, hypochromic, black, and brown variants, correlating to some extent with the depth and density of the lesional cells and their melanization (634).

If melanocytes are relatively sparsely distributed and minimally pigmented, these lesions may be mistaken for a fibrohistiocytic lesion such as a dermatofibroma. A few blue nevi are hypopigmented or even amelanotic (634), requiring IHC for their confirmation, with HMB-45-positivity representing a most helpful adjunct. On occasion, and particularly in small biopsies, the differential of DM versus amelanotic blue nevus may be raised, and, again, HMB-45 positivity in the latter, but usually not in the former, is of assistance (635). In some cases, S100 and HMB45 staining may be weak or negative, and the use of other markers may then be considered (Immunohistochemistry, p. 878). Although blue nevi are usually strictly dermal, rare "compound blue nevi" have been described in which there are pigmented dendritic melanocytes in the epidermis near the dermal–epidermal junction, although most such lesions

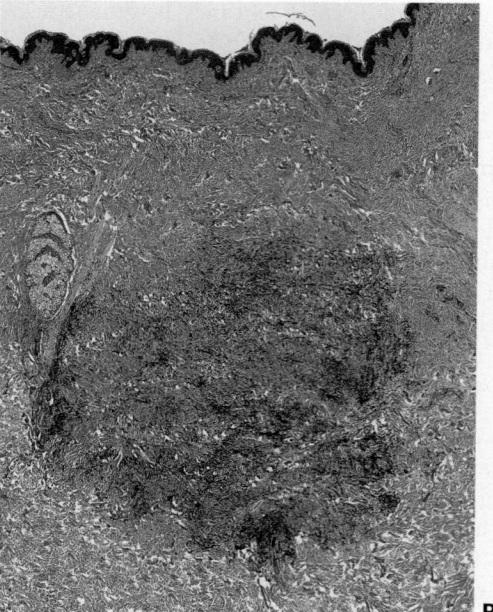

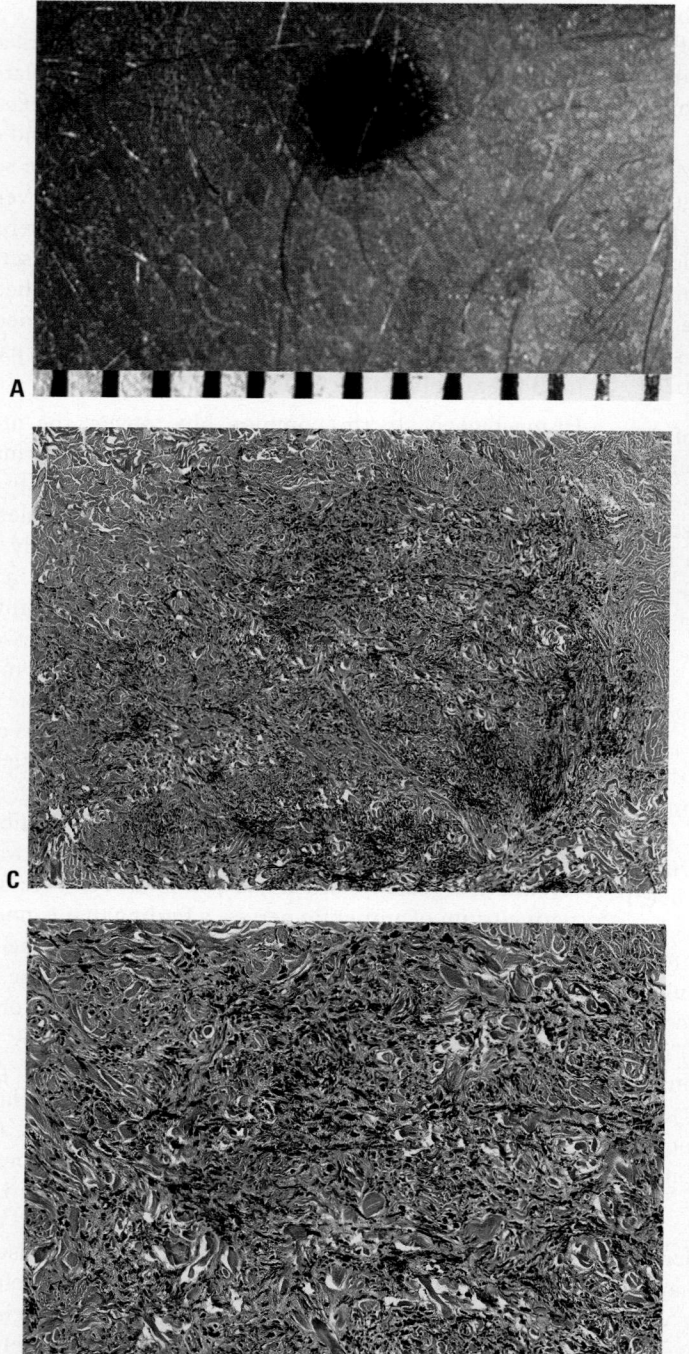

Figure 28-47 Blue nevus. **A:** A relatively small, well-circumscribed, slightly elevated blue-black pigmented lesion. **B:** Another somewhat more deep-seated lesion. Spindle-shaped or dendritic melanocytes are placed among reticular dermis collagen bundles, which are often slightly thickened. **C:** Unlike the cells of most common or congenital nevi that involve the reticular dermis, the cells of blue nevi are usually heavily pigmented, with coarsely divided melanin granules. **D:** Especially at the periphery of the lesion, the cells are arranged as single cells placed among collagen bundles, rather than sheets or fascicles.

would today likely be interpreted as pigmented melanocytomas (636). Junctional melanocytes may also be seen in the setting of "combined nevi"; however, today these are usually considered to represent a combination of a compound nevus with a second component, such as a DPN.

Principles of Management: Although not generally considered mandatory, consideration of complete excision of blue nevi is appropriate, especially if a lesion has been partially sampled or was clinically dynamic or atypical, or if there are histologically "cellular" areas or mitotic activity.

In one study, persistence and recurrence of blue nevi was discussed, demonstrating that blue nevi of all histologic types and combinations are capable of persistence with clinical recurrence. The persistence is usually histologically similar to the original but

in some cases is more "cellular" and/or atypical. Limited follow-up of these cases has not demonstrated frankly malignant behavior. Clinical recurrence may also be associated with malignancy of a blue nevus-like lesion, but this study demonstrates that tumor progression to malignancy is not necessarily the case. In the absence of necrosis en masse, marked cytologic atypia, and frequent mitotic figures, recurrence of a blue nevus or a CBN is likely to be a benign phenomenon (637). However, we would recommend complete excision and follow-up for such recurrent lesions.

Cellular Blue Nevus

Clinical Summary. The CBN consists of a blue nodule that is usually larger than the common blue nevus (638,639). It generally measures 1 to 3 cm in diameter, but it may be larger.

It shows either a smooth or an irregular surface. These lesions occur on the trunk or extremities, often involving the buttocks or the sacrococcygeal region. Although it is rare, malignant degeneration of cellular blue nevi can occur, representing the phenomenon of melanoma arising in a blue nevus (MBN) (640) (p. 920).

Histopathology. The profile of a CBN is often distinctive at scanning magnification, with a bulky, heavily pigmented cellular tumor often spanning the reticular dermis, and not associated with an overlying *in situ* melanoma (Fig. 28-48). In lesions that enter the subcutis, there is often a cellular nodule at the base, connected to the overlying tumor in a "dumbbell"

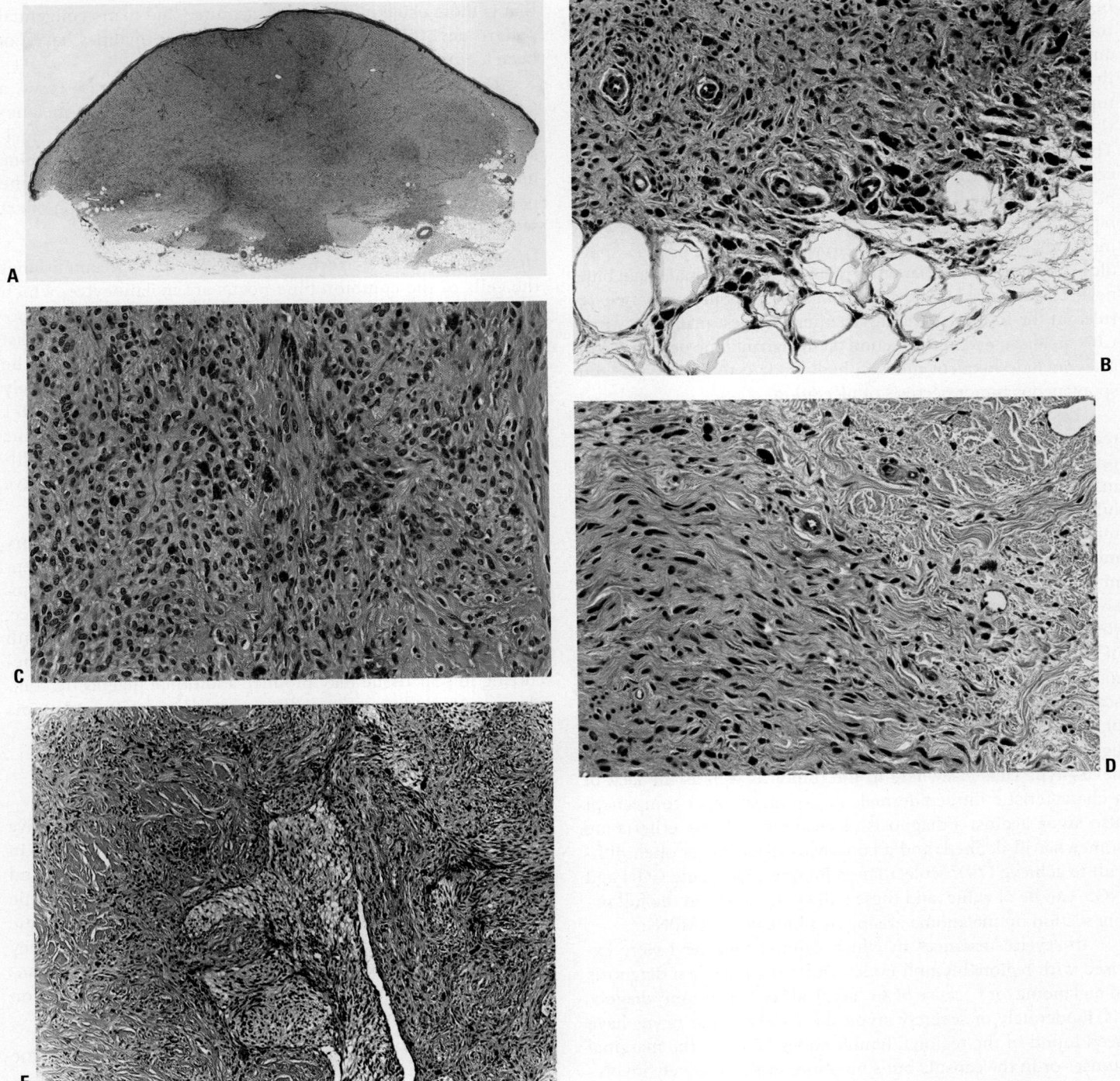

Figure 28-48 Cellular blue nevus. **A:** Usually broader at its surface than its base, the cellular blue nevus spans the reticular dermis, usually involving the superficial panniculus. Often, there is a region of increased cellularity that may form a bulbous expansion at the base. **B:** Spindle cells usually predominate in cellular blue nevi. They lie in contiguity with one another, unlike the cells of common blue nevi, most of which are separated from one another by collagen bundles. The lesional cells infiltrate into the panniculus at the tumor base. **C:** In the more "cellular" areas, there are sheets and nests of cuboidal cells with pale cytoplasm, often separated by spindle cells. Mitoses are very rare in most examples. **D:** Changes at the periphery may be indistinguishable from those of a common blue nevus, although often with minimal pigment as here. **E:** Another lesion showing a characteristic "mixed-biphasic" pattern is a distinctive feature of many cellular blue nevi, with ovoid islands of polygonal cells with somewhat clear cytoplasm alternating with spindle cells, the latter often pigmented.

pattern. Areas of deeply pigmented dendritic melanocytes, as also seen in the common type of blue nevus, are admixed with cellular islands composed of closely aggregated, rather large spindle-shaped or more epithelioid cells with ovoid nuclei and abundant pale cytoplasm often containing little or no melanin. Melanophages with abundant melanin may be present between the islands. Although pigment is usually prominent, amelanotic CBN have been described (635). Four histologic subtypes have been recognized: mixed biphasic; alveolar; fascicular, or neuronevoid (also known as the monophasic spindle cell type); and atypical CBN (362). In the common mixed-biphasic type, there are clusters of epithelioid cells with somewhat clear cytoplasm, between which there are fascicles of spindle cells (Fig. 28-48E). Pigment is usually more prominent in the latter. The alveolar type is characterized by rounded nests of clear spindle cells embedded in a matrix of dendritic and spindle-shaped, more heavily pigmented melanocytes similar to those of the mixed-biphasic pattern. The monophasic spindle cell type is somewhat more problematic and may overlap with PEMs (see p. 865), spindle cell tumorigenic melanomas (p. 886), and with malignant blue nevi. The absence of an overlying in situ component may help to rule out the former. Attributes that may suggest malignancy in a CBN are discussed in the section on malignant blue nevi (p. 928). They include frequent mitoses, high-grade cytologic atypia, and spontaneous tumor necrosis or ulceration.

Lesions termed "atypical" cellular blue nevi have become recognized as a variant of cellular blue nevi characterized by unusual features, including architectural atypia (infiltrative margin and/or asymmetry) and/or cytologic atypia (hypercellularity, nuclear pleomorphism, hyperchromasia, occasional mitotic figures, and/or subtle necrosis) (640,641). Although most of these lesions have a benign course, a few cellular blue nevi (not necessarily all "atypical") have been locally aggressive (642) or have metastasized at least to regional lymph nodes (643), and a guarded prognosis is appropriate in the presence of more than a few mitoses (see section on Melanocytic Tumors of Uncertain Malignant Potential, p. 880). The absence or scarcity of mitotic figures and the absence of areas of necrosis or of high-grade atypia are evidence against a diagnosis of malignant blue nevus, and the presence of areas of dendritic blue nevus–type cells elsewhere in the tumor as well as the lack of a characteristic intraepidermal (in situ melanoma) component also argue against a diagnosis of melanoma. These criteria are somewhat ill-defined, and a consensus diagnosis is often difficult to achieve (79). Molecular techniques, including CGH and NGS, can be of value, and these will be discussed in the following section on melanoma arising in a blue nevus (MBN).

In several instances in which cellular blue nevi were excised with regional lymph nodes under the mistaken diagnosis of melanoma, or because of an "atypical" or "uncertain" diagnosis, moderately or severely atypical cells of cellular nevus have been found in the regional lymph nodes, often in the marginal sinuses or in the capsule but sometimes more massively involving the node (643). It is sometimes assumed that these cells do not represent true metastases but were passively transported to the lymph nodes and lodged there as inert deposits. However, some examples of this phenomenon in our experience have shown high-grade uniform atypia, necrosis, and fairly numerous mitoses, apparently indicative of an active neoplasm. Some of these lesions may best be interpreted as "metastatic melanocytic tumors of uncertain malignant potential" ("metastatic

MELTUMP") (p. 881). The possibility that the primary tumor could be a melanoma mimicking a CBN ("MMCBN") should be considered (see next section) (284).

Genomic aspects of blue nevi and related lesions have been increasingly documented. Somatic mutations of the G protein signaling molecule GNAQ were found in 83% of 29 blue nevi, indicative of an alternative pathway to MAP kinase activation in these lesions, differing from the BRAF or NRAS activation that is more usual in commonly acquired and many congenital pattern nevi (627). Structural genomic abnormalities have not been identified in blue nevi.

Despite these negative genomic findings, in rare cases, a CBN is seen adjacent to an unequivocally malignant melanocytic proliferation. This phenomenon has been termed "melanoma arising in a cellular blue nevus" or "malignant blue nevus" and indicates that these lesions have some low but finite potential for progression and malignant transformation (next section).

Histogenesis of Blue Nevi. There is general agreement that the cells of the common blue nevus are melanocytes, which may show evidence of schwannian differentiation. This occasional resemblance to neural tumors had led in the past to suggestions of neural origin for blue nevi. However, the lesional cells of blue nevi and their variants react positively with antibodies to the S100, HMB-45, and Melan-A/MART-1 antigens, the latter two in this context being quite specific for melanocytic differentiation and also serving to help differentiate these lesions from DMs that are typically negative for these markers.

Principles of Management: Lesions in this general category should, at a minimum, be excised completely, not only to ensure that the lesion has been completely examined using histologic techniques but also to minimize any chance of persistence, recurrence, and progression to a more significant lesion. With regard to local persistence, it is of note that such lesions recurring in scar tissue may produce additional diagnostic complexities, including potentially increased risk for melanoma overdiagnosis.

Melanoma Arising in a Blue Nevus ("Malignant Blue Nevus")

Melanoma arising in a blue nevus (MBN) represents a distinctive "pathway" of melanoma characterized by specific mutations in G-protein alpha subunit genes such as GNAQ and GNA11, and is Pathway VIII in the 2018 WHO Classification of Melanocytic Tumors, also known as the "Blue Group." Because prognostic models specific to these entities have not been developed, they are often regarded as "blue nevus–like melanomas" and managed in the same way as any other melanoma variants, based on clinical and pathologic staging variables (644).

Clinical Summary. MBN is a rare tumor. It may arise in a blue or CBN (644–647), a giant congenital nevus (604), or in a nevus of Ota (617,648), or it may be malignant from the start as a melanoma mimicking a blue nevus (284,647). Malignant blue nevi may involve the dermis and may be ulcerated or may present as a deep-seated expansile mass. In some lesions that have been classified as malignant blue nevus, metastases occur that are limited to the regional lymph nodes, and the patient survives after removal of the tumor and the involved lymph nodes (645). There may be overlap in these cases with the

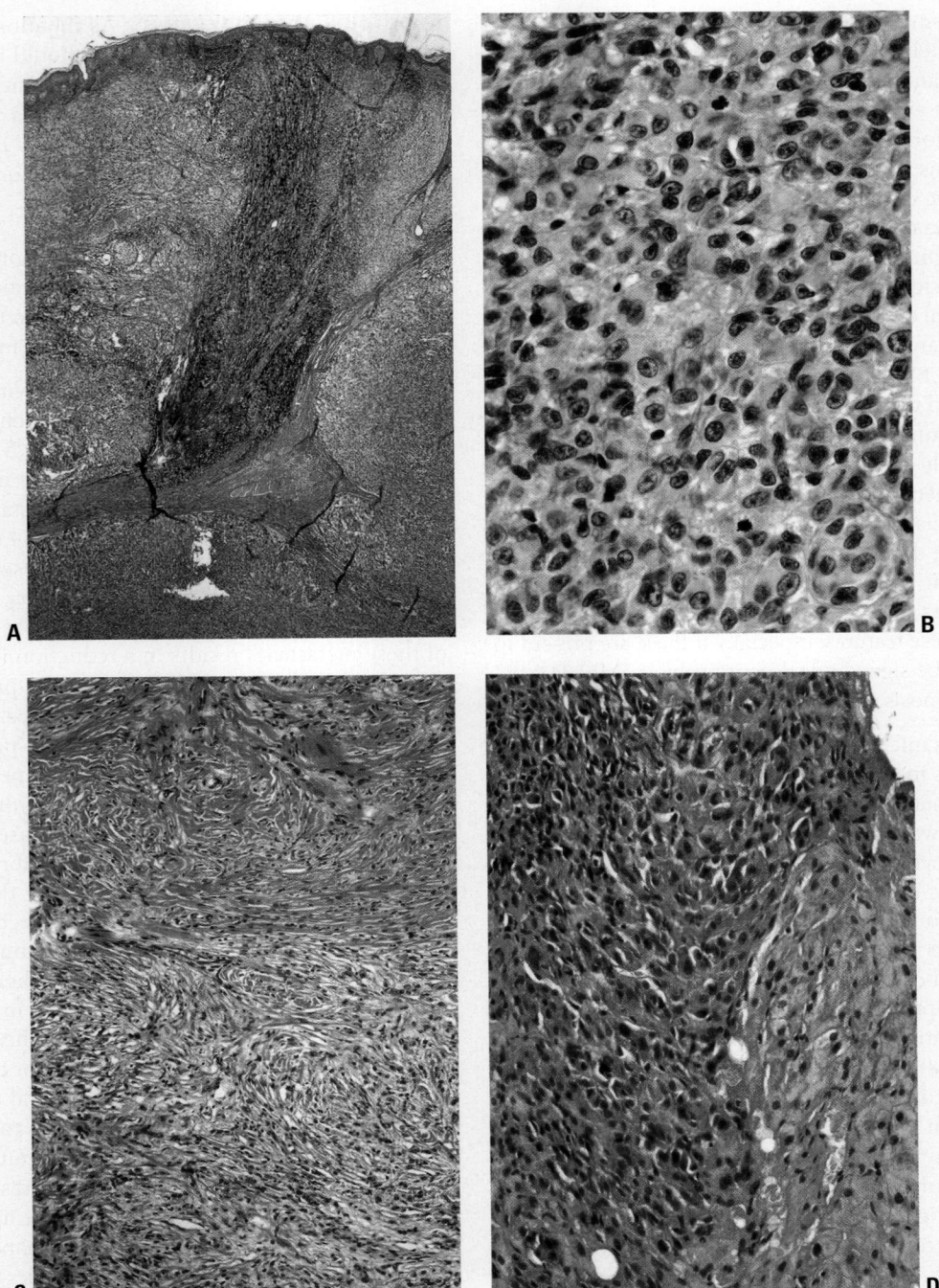

Figure 28-49 Melanoma in a blue nevus (Malignant blue nevus). **A:** A bulky melanocytic tumor with variegated patterns of architecture and pigmentation is present in the dermis, without an associated *in situ* component in the epidermis. **B:** An area of solid growth showing severe uniform atypia and frequent mitoses. **C:** An area of blue nevus–like pattern at the top, with a more cellular blue nevus–like pattern at the bottom. **D:** Liver metastasis from a malignant blue nevus. Neoplastic melanocytes (left) in liver tissue (right) from a needle biopsy.

phenomenon of cellular blue nevi with regional metastases. In other cases, however, death occurs as the result of widespread metastases (284,640). Reliable distinction between these two groups of cases is difficult but can be assisted by modern genomic techniques in selected situations.

Histopathology. Recognition of a lesion as a malignant blue nevus rather than a common melanoma, or a melanoma mimicking a CBN, is based on the absence of junctional activity and the presence of at least some bipolar benign tumor cells with branching dendritic processes typically containing melanin granules, representing a background component of blue

nevus or CBN (Fig. 28-49A–D). In some cases, pigment may be scant (649). Genomic sequencing is decisive, when a characteristic *GNA11* or *GNAQ* mutation is detected (284). Progression to melanoma is related to loss of the tumor suppressor *BAP1*, located on chromosome 3, which is often lost in MBN (as in ocular melanoma, which is closely related morphologically and genomically). BAP1 protein loss can be demonstrated by IHC (284), and chromosome 3 loss (along with additional less specific segmental chromosomal abnormalities) can be demonstrated by CGH (284,640,650).

In addition to showing the standard features of malignancy, such as asymmetry, large size, invasiveness of the tumor, atypia with hyperchromatism, pleomorphism, and irregularity of the nuclei, prominent nucleoli and presence of numerous and atypical mitoses, malignant blue nevi often have areas of necrosis and/or ulceration as evidence of their aggressive nature. The combination of uniform high-grade cytologic atypia, spontaneous tumor necrosis, and more than a few mitoses may be considered diagnostic of malignant blue nevus in a lesion with a characteristic associated blue nevus pattern (640,647). Such cases are easily recognized as fully malignant neoplasms.

Melanoma mimicking a CBN ("MMCBN") should be considered in the differential diagnosis of MBN. MMCBN, also named "blue nevus–like melanoma," is a lesion in which there is no benign blue nevus or CBN component. If there is such a component, the lesion would then be termed "melanoma arising in blue nevus (MBN)." The tumors themselves are identical morphologically and genomically (see later). The differential diagnosis of MMCBN includes metastatic melanoma mimicking BN, PEM, atypical DPN, and melanomas arising in these entities (284).

Some lesions that do not meet all of these criteria, for example, some lesions that have lacked necrosis, have metastasized (647). Atypical tumors with the overall appearance of CBN that show only some of these features, especially if these are present to a minor degree, may be signed out descriptively as "MELTUMP," with a differential diagnosis and a detailed description (see p. 880).

Histogenesis. Electron microscopic studies have shown the presence of melanosomes in the cells and a lack of cytoplasmic enclosures of unmyelinated axons, which would be seen if the tumor cells were Schwann cells. Thus, it is evident that the tumor cells are melanocytes. Mutation of the oncogenes *GNAQ* or *GNA11*, characteristic of blue nevi, CBN, and MBN, is a major point of difference from other forms of melanoma (284). Progression to melanoma is often related to loss of the tumor suppressor *BAP1*, located on chromosome 3, which is often lost in MBN (284). In a comprehensive study, most blue nevi had mutually exclusive activating mutations in *GNAQ* (53%) or *GNA11* (15%). In addition, rare *CYSLTR2* (1%) and *PLCB4* (1%) mutations were identified. *EIF1AX*, *SF3B1*, and *BAP1* mutations were also found, with *BAP1* and *SF3B1R625* mutations being present only in clearly malignant tumors. In data from a large cohort of skin melanomas, this genetic profile was also identified in tumors not originally diagnosed as MBN. The findings indicate that the genetic profile of coexistent *GNAQ* or *GNA11* mutations with *BAP1* or *SF3B1* mutations can aid the histopathologic diagnosis of MBN and distinguish blue nevus–like melanoma ("MMCBN") from cutaneous melanomas that arise in epidermal melanocytes (651).

Differential Diagnosis. MBN differs from conventional primary melanoma by the absence of junctional activity and by the presence of associated common and/or CBN. However, distinction of a malignant blue nevus from a metastatic melanoma can be difficult, because metastatic melanoma is occasionally found without a demonstrable primary melanoma. The primary melanoma may have involuted/regressed or may be located at an obscure internal site. The presence of benign dendritic cells indicative of an associated blue nevus or CBN component is then the most reliable criterion favoring a diagnosis of malignant blue nevus instead of a metastatic melanoma. In doubtful cases, the differential diagnosis of metastatic melanoma should be expressed, and a workup for another primary should be considered clinically.

Principles of Management: As mentioned previously, it has been suggested that these lesions should be regarded as "melanoma arising in a blue nevus" and that they should be managed in the same way as any other melanoma variants (644). However, they differ from usual melanomas in their characteristic driver mutations and in their lower tumor mutation burden.

Metastatic Melanoma

A metastasis is the result of discontinuous spread from a primary site, usually by lymphatic or blood vascular channels. Metastatic spread, uncommon in relation to thin melanomas, is quite common in tumors thicker than 2 mm.

Clinical Summary. Regional skin and lymph node metastases usually present earlier than hematogenous metastases. Although metastases tend to occur within 5 years after the onset of the disease, their appearance may be delayed, especially in "thin" melanomas (652,653). Late metastases, beyond 10 years, do occur, but they are relatively rare (654,655).

Clinically evident cutaneous metastases are arbitrarily called "satellites" if within 2 cm of the primary tumor or "in-transit metastases" if beyond this limit but still regional. The presence of these metastases results in a reduction in 10-year survival of about 20 percentage points (656). The prognosis for patients with distant metastatic disease in the past was very poor. In the 2009 AJCC 7th Edition, the 1-year prognosis for patients with distant metastases in skin, subcutaneous tissue or distant lymph nodes and a normal lactate dehydrogenase (LDH) was 62%; for those with visceral site metastases and a high LDH it was 33%, whereas the 10-year outlook for these was dismal at less than 1% (657). Nearly 10 years later, the prognosis is better as a result of modern targeted and, especially, immune checkpoint therapy (658); however, there remains a subset of patients whose tumors do not respond to these therapies and for whom there has been little if any improvement in their outlook.

In about 4% to 10% of the patients who present initially with metastases of melanoma, no primary tumor can be found. The sex ratio, age incidence, family history, survival rates, and patterns of recurrence and further metastases in these patients with unknown primary melanomas are consistent with an unnoticed cutaneous lesion as the site of origin for the metastatic disease (659). Although a primary tumor may in some instances be in an internal organ or perhaps secondary to malignant transformation of extracutaneous nevus cell rests (as in lymph node capsules), it seems likely that in most instances it was located in the skin and regressed spontaneously. In a study of 40 patients with unknown primary melanoma, patients with lymph node metastasis survived significantly longer than those diagnosed with lymph node metastasis concurrent with a known cutaneous primary melanoma. The prevalence of dysplastic nevi was intermediate between that reported among primary melanoma patients and that reported among population controls, suggesting the likelihood of a primary cutaneous origin for the metastatic melanoma (660). In some instances, there is a history of a spontaneously resolving pigmented lesion, and one may see at that site either a hypopigmented area or an irregular, flat, pigmented lesion, consistent with complete regression of a putative primary melanoma at that site (661).

In recent years, availability of targeted therapy and immunotherapy for melanoma, as for other cancers, has changed the landscape of metastatic disease and has very favorably impacted patient outcomes. In a pooled analysis of six adjuvant trials of these therapies, with a median follow-up time ranging from 20 to 54 months, excision of an enlarged node was performed after a few weeks' interval. A pathologic complete response (pCR) occurred in 40% of patients: 47% with targeted therapy and 33% with immunotherapy. The attainment of pCR correlated with improved relapse-free survival (RFS) (pCR 2-year 89% vs. no pCR 50%). The survival with immunotherapy was superior to that with targeted therapy; in patients with complete, near complete, or partial pathologic response with immunotherapy, very few relapses were seen, with a 2-year RFS of 96%, and, at the time of this writing, no patient had died from melanoma. It was considered likely that any degree of pathologic response (or immune cell infiltration) in the resection specimen will identify patients with long-term survival with neoadjuvant immunotherapy. It was considered that pathologic response should be an early surrogate end point for melanoma clinical trials and a new benchmark for their development and approval (662).

Histopathology. The histologic appearance of melanoma *metastases in the skin* resembles the tumorigenic VGP of a primary melanoma but usually differs from that of a primary melanoma by the absence of junctional activity and also often of an inflammatory infiltrate (Fig. 28-50). However, primary melanomas may occasionally fail to involve the epidermis and may also not have an inflammatory infiltrate, particularly when they are deeply invasive. However, significant lymphoid infiltrates may be seen in metastases of patients who have received immunotherapy, such as checkpoint blockade protocols. Furthermore, in occasional instances, even metastases exhibit prominent lymphocytic infiltrates (663) and can contact the overlying epidermis in a way that is suggestive of junctional activity, with nests of atypical melanocytes in the epidermis, and these cases may particularly resemble a primary NM (664). Some metastatic melanomas may have a nevoid phenotype (some epidermotropic metastases), and clinicopathologic correlation (e.g., follow-up) may be required to differentiate them from a primary nevoid melanoma or even from a nevus (665). In the latter situation, careful examination of specimen levels will generally reveal mitotic activity and apoptotic cells in true nevoid metastases, and other markers may also be of assistance, such as loss of HMB45 stratification, high

Ki-67 proliferation rate, loss of expression of p16, and expression of PRAME, in addition to possible genetic testing (664). In follow-up, additional metastases will usually develop in cases of metastatic melanoma, making the diagnosis clear at least in retrospect.

Microscopic satellites were originally defined as deposits of tumor more than 0.05 mm in diameter and separated from the primary mass by normal tissue, such as reticular dermis collagen (666). In the 8th edition of the AJCC staging system, a microsatellite is defined as "a microscopic cutaneous and/or subcutaneous metastasis adjacent to or deep to and completely discontinuous from a primary melanoma with unaffected stroma occupying the space between, identified on pathologic examination of the primary tumor site. Fibrous scarring and/or inflammation noted between an apparently separate nodule and the primary tumor (rather than normal stroma) may represent regression of the intervening tumor; if these findings are present, the nodule is considered to be an extension of the primary tumor and not a microsatellite" (656). Patients with microsatellites, so defined, have significantly worse prognosis; in a recent study, there was a 21% 5-year disease-free survival compared with 56% in a control group. Increasing distance of the microsatellite from the primary melanoma was found to adversely influence disease-free survival; however, number and size of microsatellites were not significant prognostic factors. The presence of microsatellites was the only factor that proved to be an independent predictor of sentinel node positivity in multivariate analysis. Microsatellites were significantly associated with more locoregional recurrences but not distant metastases (667). Satellites are rare in melanomas less than 2.0 mm in Breslow thickness (668).

Epidermotropic metastatic melanoma refers to a metastatic deposit that is initially localized to the papillary dermis and involves the overlying epidermis (Fig. 28-51). Most of these lesions occur in an extremity regional to a distal primary melanoma. Epidermotropic metastasis was originally characterized by (a) thinning of the epidermis by aggregates of atypical melanocytes within the dermis, (b) inward turning of the rete ridges at the periphery of the lesion, (c) usually no lateral extension of

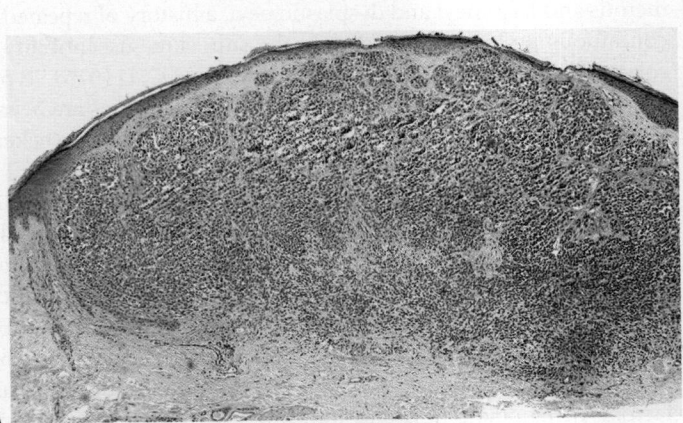
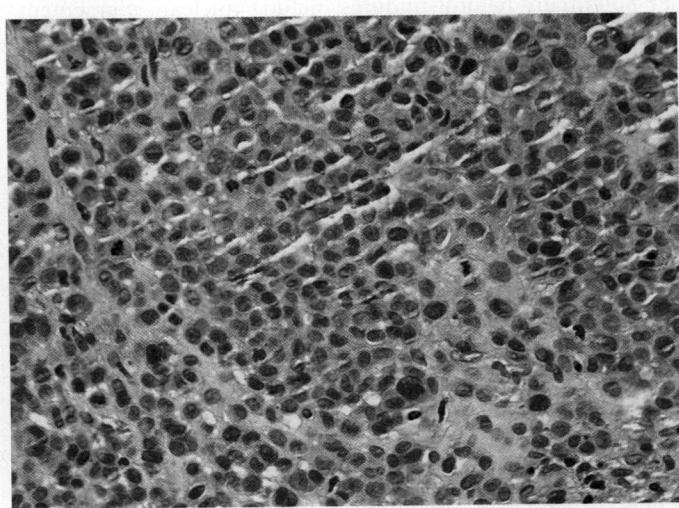

Figure 28-50 Dermal metastatic melanoma. **A:** Metastatic melanoma often presents as a fairly symmetrical cellular nodule in the reticular dermis or subcutis. The lesions are often quite small at the time they are excised and presented for an initial diagnosis of metastatic spread. **B:** Cytologically, the cells are uniformly atypical, as in tumorigenic primary melanomas (compare Figs. 28-21, 28-22, 28-50). Sometimes, especially in superficial or epidermotropic cutaneous metastases, atypia is deceptively minimal. The identification of mitotic activity, and of lymphatic invasion, may be very helpful in making the diagnosis.

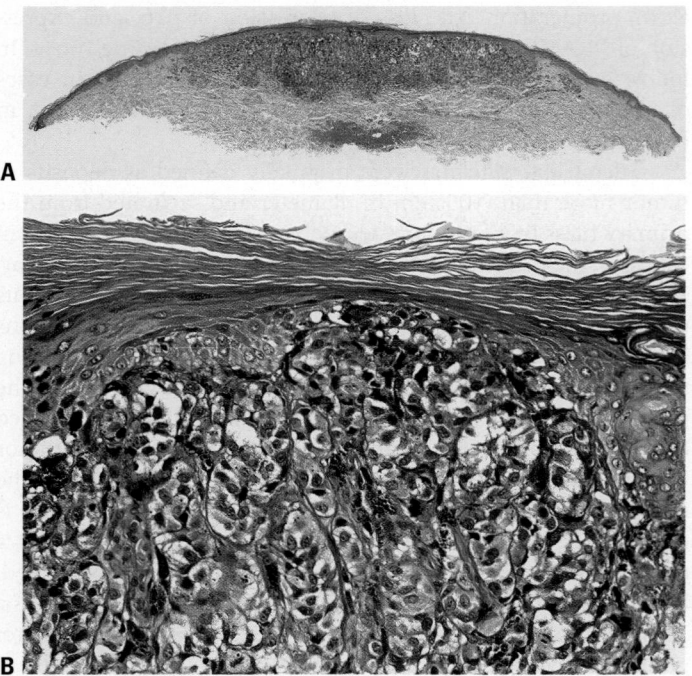

Figure 28-51 Epidermotropic metastatic melanoma. **A:** This lesion developed in the thigh several years after definitive therapy of a melanoma in the leg of a 72-year-old woman and closely simulates a primary melanoma. **B:** Usually, epidermotropic metastatic melanoma involves the epidermis only above the dermal component; however, exceptions to this rule have been described.

atypical melanocytes within the epidermis beyond the concentration of the metastasis in the dermis, and (d) easily detectable lymphatic invasion (669). However, this distinction can be very difficult at times, and cases have been reported in which there was lateral extension beyond the dermal component (664). In some other cases, the metastatic cells are small and nevoid, with few, if any, mitoses, and in these instances of *differentiated or nevoid epidermotropic metastatic melanoma* or "epidermotropic metastatic melanomas with maturation," the lesions can be mistaken for compound nevi. In addition to the aforementioned features, other potentially helpful findings include nuclear enlargement, hypercellular areas, architectural confluence, increased mitotic figures, increased Ki-67 and gp100 expression in both the superficial and deep portions, and more melanin (deep); however, the distinction often remains difficult (670). In a comprehensive histopathologic comparison of epidermotropic metastatic melanoma and primary NM, morphologic features in a multivariate logistic regression model that were highly predictive of primary NM included large tumor size (>10 mm), ulceration, prominent tumor-infiltrating plasma cells, lichenoid inflammation, and epidermal collarets (664).

Diffuse Melanosis in Metastatic Melanoma

This is a rare phenomenon that may be associated with widespread melanoma metastases (671). It is characterized by diffuse slate-blue discoloration of the entire skin, the conjunctivae, and the oral and pharyngeal mucous membranes, often with melanuria. Melanin granules have also been observed in blood smears within neutrophils and monocytes. Autopsy reveals a similar discoloration in the intima of the large arteries and of many visceral organs.

Histologically, numerous melanin granules may be seen located within macrophages throughout the dermis, especially around capillaries. In most instances, only melanophages have

been found. It is assumed that the melanin is produced by distant melanoma cells and then carried, likely as precursor molecules, by the blood to the skin, to be deposited within dermal melanophages (672). At autopsy, melanin phagocytosis may be seen in many organs, especially in the Kupffer cells of the liver and the cells lining the sinusoids of the lymph nodes, spleen, and adrenal glands.

Principles of Management of Metastatic Disease: Localized cutaneous and subcutaneous metastases of melanoma are typically excised, with clear margins as a goal. Excision specimens should be inked to facilitate margin assessment. Nonsurgical approaches, such as radiation therapy, are also available (673).

Resection to clear margins is also recommended for limited metastatic disease at other sites.

Disseminated disease is managed by systemic therapy. Currently available options have been greatly expanded recently and now include targeted therapy based on demonstration of specific oncogene mutations, such as Vemurafenib for mutated BRAF; immune response modifiers such as CTLA-4 and PD1 blockers, and traditional chemotherapy. Consensus statements from the NCCN are regularly updated to convey the state-of-the-art information (673).

Pathology departments in many institutions are involved in genetic testing for melanoma and other cancers, and anatomic pathologists with competence in melanocytic lesion pathology should be involved in the selection of tissue for genetic analysis (674).

Epidemiology, Prognosis, and Management of Melanoma

Phenotypic risk factors for the development of melanoma can offer clues to the etiology and pathogenesis of the disease. Prognostic factors can help predict the outcome of individual cases of melanoma based on experience from large groups of cases. These risk and prognostic factors have been identified through case-control studies and follow-up of cohorts of patients, often from high-risk melanoma clinics. Together, they can aid in developing evidence-based guidelines as to the most effective management strategies for melanoma patients.

Risk Factors for the Development of Melanomas

The major risk factors include age, family or personal history of prior melanoma, the presence of potential precursors such as numerous and large nevi and dysplastic nevi, a history of repeated or continuous prolonged exposure to the sun, skin susceptibility to solar damage, and the presence of indicators of CSD (675). Type I skin that burns easily and tans poorly is a risk factor, as are behavioral factors, such as living in a sunny climate, a history of weekend and vacation sun exposure, and a history of sunburn episodes. The presence of indicators of exposure to the sun, and of susceptibility to solar damage such as freckles and actinic skin changes, are also strongly associated with melanoma risk (p. 837) (16). Even more closely correlated with risk is the presence on the skin of potential precursors, including attributes of nevi such as the total number of banal nevi (p. 859), the presence and number of large nevi, and the presence of dysplastic nevi (p. 859) (158). Among these risk factors, melanocytic nevi and indicators of "acute, intermittent" sun exposure are more strongly related to superficial spreading and NM, whereas skin type, ethnic background, and measures of total accumulated exposure to the sun ("chronic, continuous sun exposure") are more strongly related to LMM. For these common cutaneous melanomas, the existence of two distinct biologic pathways of development has been postulated: a nevus-prone pathway initiated by early sun exposure and promoted by intermittent sun exposure and possibly host factors, and a chronic sun exposure pathway in sun-sensitive people (374).

Age is also a strong risk factor, operating in a continuously progressive fashion in LMM and perhaps also in acral and mucosal melanomas, in contrast to a more complex pattern for superficial and NM (676). Many of these factors are under genetic control, and a family history of melanoma constitutes another major risk factor, especially as the number of melanomas in a family increases. Only a relatively small proportion of these familial melanomas are attributable to the presence of a major high penetrance melanoma risk genes, such as *CDKN2A* (p16) or *CDK4*, both of which are tumor suppressors that act through the retinoblastoma (Rb) pathway (217). Other genes contributing to risk may have lower penetrance but may be present in more individuals in the population, thus accounting for a substantially higher proportion of cases (i.e., a higher "attributable risk"). Examples of such genes include the melanocortin receptor *MC1R*, which controls skin pigmentation (677), and DNA-repair genes. In general, genes that are associated with melanoma risk include those that are related to pigmentation, to nevus prevalence, to telomere maintenance, as well as other categories (675).

Preexisting Melanocytic Nevus and Nevus-Associated Melanoma

It is well known that melanomas can develop in association with congenital and congenital pattern nevi (p. 912) and in dysplastic nevi (p. 896, 900). In a histopathologic review of 667 consecutive cases of primary cutaneous melanoma, 148 melanomas with benign melanocytic nevus components (22.1%) were identified, among which 87 were acquired nevi, 80 of them dysplastic, and 57 were congenital pattern nevi, only one of them deep and therefore likely truly congenital (154). It has been proposed that there are two different types of nevus-associated melanoma (NAM): a melanoma that arises in the center of the mole and a melanoma that grows next to the mole, the first arising from a congenital or congenital pattern nevus and the second from a compound dysplastic acquired nevus (678). Histologically, remnants of a banal nevus are found in a substantial number of melanomas, of the order of about 10% to 35%, and evidence of associated melanocytic dysplasia may be seen in up to about 40% of these (47,154,678,679). Analysis has demonstrated that this relationship is likely to be nonrandom (680). Nevi are much more likely to be associated with melanomas of the SSM type rather than LMM (679).

Several studies have found that NAM differs from desmoplastic neurotropic melanoma (DNM) in important attributes, including thickness and body site differences (681), and in survival with NAM enjoying a significant survival advantage in some but not all studies (682). These differences are considered to support the concept of divergent pathways of development for common cutaneous melanomas, suggesting that DNM are different from NAM and that the differences are not simply a consequence of obliteration of nevus remnants in the DNM (681).

Remnants of a dysplastic nevus adjacent to an RGP melanoma (usually of the superficial spreading type) can be distinguished from the latter using the criteria presented in Table 28-6, p. 861. Remnants of a dermal component of a nevus deep to a melanoma can be distinguished from the melanoma cells by the following criteria (Fig. 28-52): (a) the dermal nevus cells

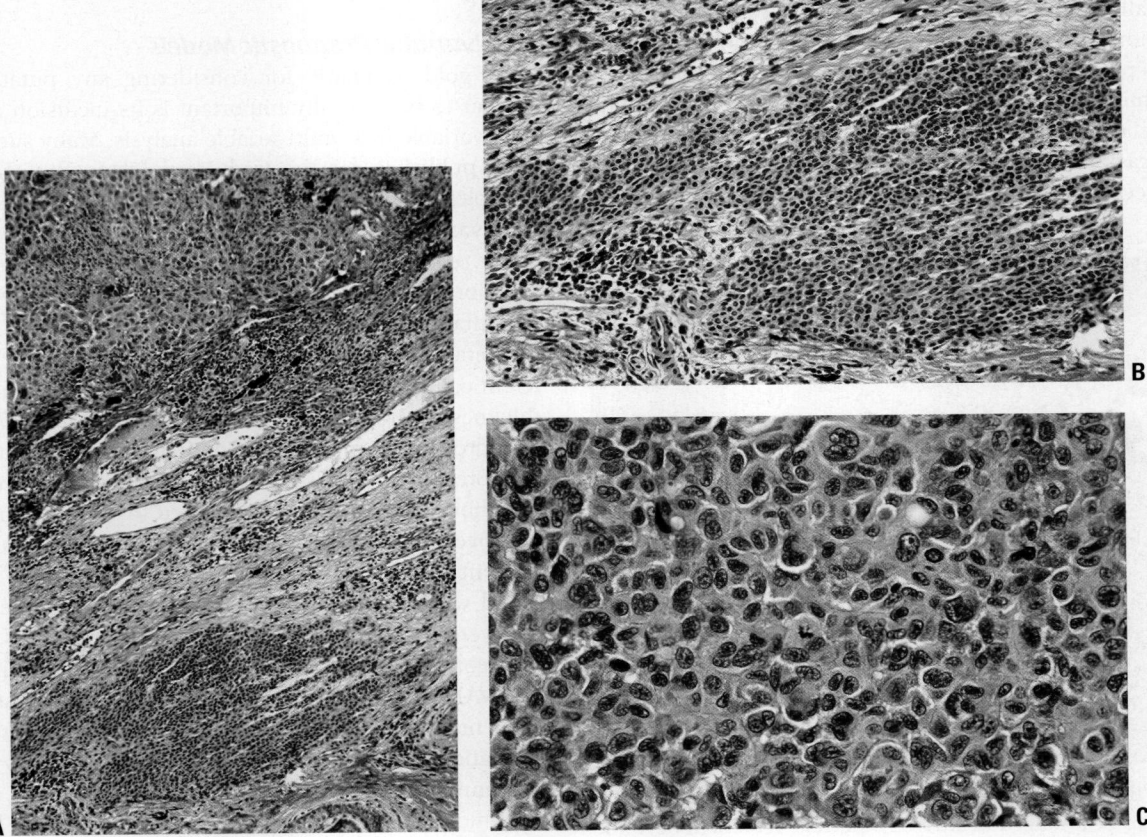

Figure 28-52 Nevus cells deep to a tumorigenic melanoma. **A:** A collection of smaller cells is present at the interface of the papillary and reticular dermis deep to a tumor of vertical growth phase melanoma. **B:** The nevus cells are smaller than the cells of the tumorigenic melanoma. **C:** The tumorigenic melanoma cells have large, hyperchromatic nuclei with irregularly clumped nuclear chromatin and with mitotic figures.

are smaller; (b) they are arranged in nests that tend to be uniform in size and shape; (c) there may be evidence of maturation from superficial to deep within the nevus but not the melanoma cell population; (d) there is no evidence of continuous differentiation from a more obviously malignant superficial component to the nevoid cells at the base of the tumor; (e) there is no high-grade atypia, and there are no mitoses in the dermal nevus cells; (f) nevus cells tend to disperse as single cells if they enter the reticular dermis, whereas melanoma cells tend to infiltrate as sheets or clusters (Fig. 28-53). This paradoxically less "invasive" pattern is related to the greater proliferative capacity of melanoma cells—invasion probably initially involves single cells that then proliferate to form the final pattern of sheets or fascicles in the reticular dermis. For the same reason, cutaneous metastases tend to be sharply demarcated, "expansive" lesions (83). Occasional examples of differentiated dermal melanoma cells may meet some of these criteria and thus present difficulties of interpretation (see section on Nevoid Melanoma).

In the seminal study of tumor progression at the molecular level by Shain et al. (293), cancer-relevant genes were assessed in 150 areas of 37 primary melanomas and their adjacent precursor lesions, which included unequivocally benign lesions (e.g., dermal nevi), intermediate lesions (e.g., dysplastic nevi), and intraepidermal or invasive melanomas (211). The nevi were characterized by driver mutations such as in *BRAF* or *NRAS*, and the associated melanomas had the same mutations, with the addition of GAs involved in progression such as *CDKN2A* loss and *TERT* activation. These results are consistent with a causal relationship for the development of melanoma within a preexistent associated nevus and also support the hypothesis that these genetic alterations play a necessary, but not sufficient, role in the development of at least some early melanomas, because they are found in histologically benign melanoma-associated nevi.

In addition to dysplastic nevi and banal dermal nevi, superficial and deep congenital pattern nevi are also commonly associated with melanomas (154,683). An exception to the general rule that melanoma arises at the epidermal–dermal border is observed occasionally in congenital nevi, in which a melanoma may arise deep in the dermis. However, these proliferations

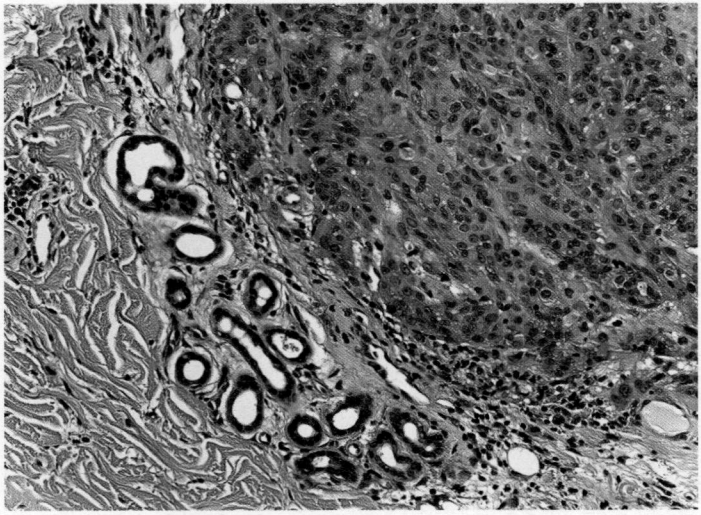

Figure 28-53 Infiltration of tumorigenic melanoma at base of lesion. The cells tend to be arranged in clusters or sheets. In benign nevi, the cells in the papillary dermis may be clustered, but when they enter the reticular dermis they tend to disperse as single cells (compare with Figure 28-4E and G).

should be distinguished from benign cellular/PNs that may occur in congenital nevi (245) (p. 912) and also from combined nevi that may present as a nodule in a nevus (247).

Multiple Primary Melanomas

People who have had a cutaneous melanoma are at risk for developing additional melanomas, which may be synchronous or nonsynchronous (684), with an incidence of approximately 5% in the first 10 years after diagnosis, a rate that has varied over time with a rising trend (685). The occurrence of multiple and familial melanomas has already been pointed out in relation to dysplastic nevi (p. 860). A prior melanoma is a strong risk factor for subsequent melanoma, as are dysplastic nevi, especially in young patients and in familial melanoma kindreds. In general, the additional primary melanomas are thinner and associated with lower risk than the first one (686). It is important to differentiate an additional melanoma from a metastatic melanoma, especially from an epidermotropic metastasis (p. 923), because the prognosis of an independent primary is likely to be much better than that of a metastasis. This may be difficult, however, because some epidermotropic metastases closely mimic primary melanomas, and, accordingly, correlation with clinical parameters (e.g., more than one lesion) may be critical in differentiating a second primary from a metastasis in such instances. Individuals with multiple primary melanomas have also been found to have a modestly increased incidence of a family history of melanoma, dysplastic nevi, and basal cell carcinoma, an earlier age of onset, and a relatively small incidence of *CDKN2A* mutations (687). Therefore, in addition to the multiple primary melanoma index case, other family members can benefit from screening and regular surveillance of their skin.

Multivariable Prognostic Models

The "gold standard" for considering any putative prognostic marker to be clinically important is its inclusion as an independent variable in a multivariable analysis. Many such studies have been published for the traditional histopathologic and clinical variables reviewed in the earlier sections. On the basis of these multivariable analyses, prognostic models have been published, either requiring the use of a calculator to determine a regression function or, more simply, using published tables to provide a quantitative probability estimate. In early studies, these models combined basic clinical and pathologic variables, including different combinations of age, gender, anatomic location, ulceration, thickness, growth phase, TIL, and regression (317,688–694). In one prognostic model, a combination of attributes, including age, Breslow thickness, ulceration, mitotic rate, regression, and lymphovascular invasion, were used to develop a nomogram that improved prediction of sentinel lymph node status (695). Subsequent modeling has incorporated expression of proteins associated with progression. In an analysis of 23 potential markers, five were selected, and a low-risk group of patients was identified by a combination of elevated levels of beta-catenin and nuclear p21WAF1, decreased levels of fibronectin, and distributions that favor nuclear concentration for p16INK4A but cytoplasmic concentration for ATF2 (696). Although these models may be useful in planning therapy, especially in the development and execution of clinical trials, thickness and ulceration are the factors in predominant use for planning of therapy for Stage I melanoma, as discussed in the next section. Prognostic modeling may be considered as a form of staging of the primary tumor ("microstaging").

Staging of Melanoma

The purpose of staging is to define subsets of cases with a similar prognosis for management and investigational purposes. The five-stage (0–IV) clinicopathologic staging system of the AJCC primarily considers aspects of the tumor (T), the presence and size of nodal metastases (N), and the presence and sites of distant metastases (M) to determine a stage based on all three attributes (TNM). The 5-year survival for newly diagnosed localized primary melanoma cases (Stages 0–II) is about 80% compared to 35% survival when lymph nodes are involved (Stage III). Using prognostic models discussed further on, subsets of cases with more or less favorable prognosis can be identified. When distant metastases are present, the survival at 5 years is of the order of 10%, in patients who do not have a favorable response to targeted or immune therapy (656).

TNM Staging System for Melanoma

The tumor–node–metastasis (TNM) system of tumor staging considers factors related to the primary tumor, to regional lymph nodes (and other regional soft tissues), and to distant metastases, resulting in a classification that is associated with the probability of survival and representing the basis of the AJCC staging protocols in wide use around the world (AJCC). The factors considered in the primary tumor (T) category include some of the microstaging attributes discussed previously. Thus, the TNM classification combines staging and microstaging information in a single format.

The latest AJCC staging system (8th edition) was presented in 2018 by Gershenwald et al. (697). Changes recommended for TNM and stage-grouping criteria included the use of a rounded single-digit number for Breslow thickness with a return to the original "Breslow number" of 0.76mm rounded to 0.8mm for the cutoff marking the lowest risk group, Stage T1a. This resulted in the loss of efficacy of mitogenicity, which had been used as a stage modifier in the 7th edition (657).

The staging system is based primarily on survival studies done in several collaborating institutions.

Pathologic staging includes microstaging of the primary melanoma and pathologic information about the regional lymph nodes after partial or complete lymphadenectomy. Pathologic stage Tis or stage T1a patients do not require pathologic evaluation of their lymph nodes. Clinical staging includes microstaging of the primary melanoma and clinical/radiologic evaluation for metastases. By convention, clinical staging should be used after complete excision of the primary melanoma, with clinical assessment for regional and distant metastases. The latest revision (2018) of the pathologic tumor (T) categories is presented in Table 28-10 and the stage groupings in Table 28-11.

In the 8th edition, the definitions of the N subcategories have been revised, with clinically occult nodes designated as N1a, N2a, or N3a, depending on the number of involved nodes, with clinically detected nodes as N1b, N2b, or N3b, and with the presence of microsatellites, satellites, or in-transit metastases categorized as N1c, N2c, or N3c. The N1 category is used when a single node is involved, N2 for two or three nodes, and N3 for four or more nodes (656).

For metastatic melanoma (M Category), anatomic sites of metastasis and LDH levels are used to assign patients to one of four M subcategories. Patients with distant metastasis to skin, subcutaneous tissue, muscle, or distant lymph nodes, regardless of serum LDH level, are categorized as M1a. Patients with metastasis to lung (with or without concurrent metastasis to

Table 28.10

Tumor (T) Classification for Primary Melanoma of the Skin

T Category	Thickness	Ulceration	10-year Survival
			(for cases with negative nodes)
TX (Thickness not assessable)	e.g., curettings	Not applicable	
T0 (Unknown/no primary tumor)	Cannot be assessed	Not applicable	
Tis (melanoma *in situ*)	No invasion	Not applicable	
T1	≤1 mm	Unknown or not specified	
T1a	<0.8 mm	Nonulcerated	99%
T1b	<0.8 mm or	Ulcerated	96%
	0.8–1.0 mm	Ulcerated or Nonulcerated	
T2	>1.0–2.0 mm	Unknown or not specified	
T2a	>1.0–2.0 mm	Nonulcerated	92%
T2b	>1.0–2.0 mm	Ulcerated	88%
T3	>2.0–4.0 mm	Unknown or not specified	
T3a	>2.0–4.0 mm	Nonulcerated	88%
T3b	>2.0–4.0 mm	Ulcerated	81%
T4	>4.0 mm	Unknown or not specified	
T4a	>4.0 mm	Nonulcerated	83%
T4b	>4.0 mm	Ulcerated	75%

Adapted with the permission of the American College of Surgeons. Gershenwald JE, Scolyer RA, Hess KR, et al. Melanoma of the skin. In: Amin MB, Edge SB, Greene FL, et al, eds. *AJCC Cancer Staging Manual*. 8th ed. Springer; 2017:563–585.

skin, subcutaneous tissue, muscle, or distant lymph nodes and regardless of serum LDH level) are categorized as M1b. Patients with metastases to any other visceral site(s), exclusive of the CNS, are designated as M1c, whereas patients with metastases to the CNS are designated as M1d (656).

Table 28.11

Stage Groupings and Survival Rates for Melanoma of the Skin

Pathologic Stage Group	T	N	M	10-Year Survival*
IA	T1a or T1b	N0	M0	98%
IB	T2a	N0	M0	94%
IIA	T2b or T3a	N0	M0	88%
IIB	T3b or T4a	N0	M0	82%
IIC	T4b	N0	M0	75%
IIIA	T1 or T2a	N1a or N2a	M0	88%
IIIB	T1 or T2a	N2c or N3	M0	77%
	T2b or T3a	N1a or N2b	M0	
IIIC	T1a-T3a	N2c or N3a	M0	60%
	T3b/T4a	Any N > 1	M0	
	T4b	N1a-N2c	M0	
IIID	T4B	N3A/B/C	M0	24%*
IV	Any T, Tis	Any N	M1	23% (5 yr*)

*Survival rates are in flux as effective therapies are developed and are likely greater than the quoted rates in the advanced subsets, especially for patients who respond to these therapies.

Adapted with the permission of the American College of Surgeons. Gershenwald JE, Scolyer RA, Hess KR, et al. Melanoma of the skin. In: Amin MB, Edge SB, Greene FL, et al, eds. *AJCC Cancer Staging Manual.* 8th ed. Springer; 2017:563–585.

Stage groupings are made up of a combination of the T stages, as listed in Table 28-10, with the N and M stages described previously. The TNM staging system differs from previously used, simple, primarily clinical staging systems (localized, regional, and metastatic disease) in that pathologic attributes of the primary neoplasm ("microstaging attributes") are considered in the definition of the first three stages of the "Stage Groups." Tumors in Stage Groups I and II are always nonmetastatic (Table 28-11). Stages I–III are modified by the presence or absence of ulceration in the primary tumor, even in the presence of nodal metastases. Stage IV is always metastatic beyond the region (656).

The TNM staging system incorporates clinical and pathologic attributes of the primary neoplasm ("microstaging attributes") in the definition of the "Stage Groups." Tumors in Stage Groups I and II are nonmetastatic, and Stage III is not associated with distant metastasis. Stage IV is always metastatic. Because these stages are different from those defined in other previously used staging systems, it is clear that the system in use (e.g., AJCC Stage X) should be clearly specified when staging is used as a basis for therapy or prognosis.

Given the complexity of current staging systems, which may be expected to increase in the future, nomograms have been developed to allow for risk assessment that could be used in individual cases, and online computer programs are under development. The European Organization for Research and Treatment of Cancer (EORTC) Melanoma Group proposed a prognostic model that was then validated in population-based data (698). This nomogram includes Breslow thickness, ulceration status, and anatomical location as parameters. Another nomogram, developed by the Melanoma Institute Australia, offers a prediction of the probability of sentinel involvement in patients with melanoma (699).

Pathology of Microstaging Attributes in Common Use

As discussed previously, the 2002 AJCC Staging System that is currently used worldwide incorporates several attributes of primary and metastatic melanomas, such as Breslow thickness, Clark levels of invasion, and the presence or absence of ulceration in the primary tumor. These and other attributes that may contribute to the assessment of prognosis are discussed in the following sections.

Breslow Thickness of the Tumor

Tumor thickness is the most important factor in predicting survival for Stage I patients. Breslow, in 1970, first measured tumor thickness objectively with a micrometer (700). The depth of invasion is measured from the top of the granular layer to the deepest extension of the tumor; in ulcerated lesions, measurement is from the ulcer base overlying the deepest point of invasion. In the initial report, metastasis did not occur in lesions less than 0.76 mm in greatest thickness. Since then, there have been reports of metastases from "thin" melanomas, though this continues to be rare and is often explained by the presence of VGP in the thin melanoma, characterized by tumorigenic and/or mitogenic proliferation in the dermis (701,702). A study by Gimotty et al. examined the factors associated with metastasis and death from Stage 1 melanoma in population-based data from the SEER registry (which did not include the attribute of VGP) and found that most deaths from thin melanomas occurred in the thickness category (selected by the computer algorithm) of greater than 0.78 mm, and in a few older patients, or patients with thinner Clark level III melanomas, suggesting the presence of VGP (172). The latest AJCC staging system uses a cutoff of 0.8 mm for low-risk disease (T1a), based in part on that and other studies, including those of Breslow, and so the "Breslow number" continues to have great validity and is used in the current NCCN guidelines as a cutoff above which sentinel node staging may be offered to patients with thin mitogenic melanoma (673).

In determining the depth of penetration, whether by level or by measurement, the following rules were suggested by Breslow and by Lever (703): (1) Melanocytes in junctional nests are not considered invasive, even though they may "push" into the papillary dermis; (2) if deep nests of melanoma cells arise from the epithelium of cutaneous appendages, they are not used in measurement from the surface; (3) a column of melanocytes extending from the lower border of the lesion into the deep dermis at nearly a right angle is not measured, because it is likely that the column arises from an appendage; this supposition can usually be verified by serial sections or keratin stains. In the latter circumstance, we may provide an estimate of tumor volume in the adventitial dermis of the follicle, including the extent of penetration into the surrounding skin; in all other cases, the measurement should be taken perpendicular to the skin surface (704) (Fig. 28-54).

Tumor Volume

Saldhana has recently offered a method of assessing the volume of tumor in the dermis as a prognostic attribute, presenting related concepts of "Breslow density," "calculated tumor area,"

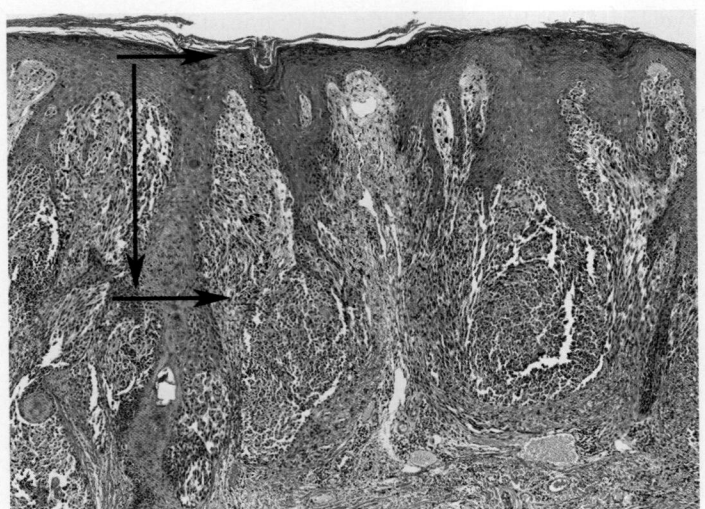

Figure 28-54 Extension of melanoma down a hair follicle. In a lentigo maligna melanoma, at right center, a hair follicle is largely replaced by melanoma cells, which are confined to the epidermis and adventitial dermis of the follicle. This melanoma is nontumorigenic. Invasive cells at the base of the follicle should not be used for thickness measurement. *Arrows* indicate where measurement should be taken perpendicularly from the top of the granular layer to the deepest invasive tumor cell.

and "invasion width," all of which depend on measuring the width of invasion in the dermis (705–707). In a multivariable analysis, the simple measurement of invasion width had significance independent of Breslow thickness, with ulceration, mitotic index also retaining significance. These studies, which await confirmation in large independent data sets, offer promise of improving the prediction of survival compared to current AJCC criteria (705).

Ulceration

Ulceration is defined by the loss of continuity of the epithelium over the surface of the tumor (Fig. 28-55). Evidence of a host reaction to the ulceration (fibrin extravasation, hemorrhage, inflammation, vascular proliferation, etc.) is also required, in

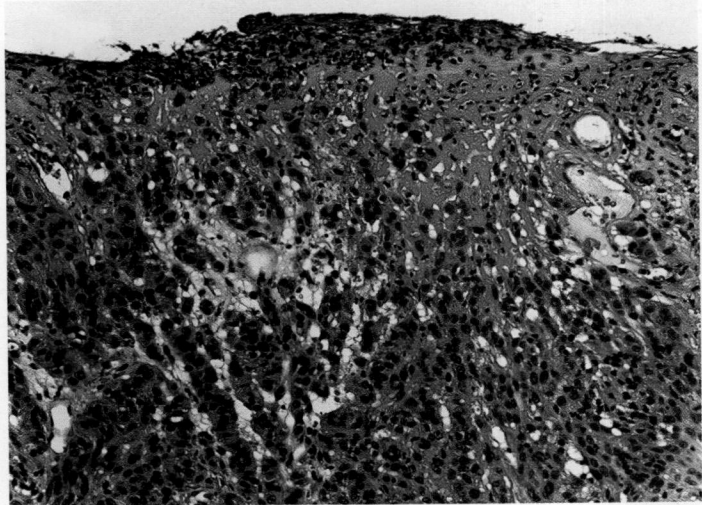

Figure 28-55 Ulcerated melanoma. An ulcer is defined as an area of loss of continuity of epithelium over the surface of the lesion, with evidence of a host reaction. The example here shows a neutrophilic and fibrinous exudate on the surface of the ulcer.

order to exclude epithelial loss caused by biopsy trauma (708). Even with a host response, it may be difficult or even impossible to determine whether ulceration is secondary to the tumor or a result of excoriation or environmental trauma, although excoriation often produces a small and discrete defect, whereas spontaneous ulceration caused by melanoma growth tends to be more substantial. Nonetheless, this attribute has prognostic significance in most multivariable analyses (656,698,709,710). Other studies, particularly those in which mitotic rate is an independent variable, have not identified ulceration as an independently significant prognostic attribute (317,711). Ulceration is a key substratifying variable in the latest AJCC staging system for melanoma (see Tables 28-10 and 28-11). In this system, the presence of an ulcerated primary is generally associated with survival approximately similar to that of a patient with a nonulcerated primary tumor in the next highest tumor thickness category (656). Interobserver agreement for ulceration has been found to be excellent (708,712). One source of occasional disagreement is the presence of a scale crust above a lesion that has a thin rim of remaining stratum corneum and therefore does not fully meet criteria for an ulcer. The prognostic significance, if any, of such "near ulcers" remains to be determined, and we discourage labeling such lesions as having incipient ulceration.

Mitotic Rate and Mitogenicity

Mitotic rate has been associated with prognosis in multiple studies (657,713–715), including the 7th edition AJCC model. However, other well-conducted, large studies have not identified this relationship in multivariable models (716). The differences among these studies may have to do with differences in the determination of mitotic rate or with interactions between mitotic rate and other variables such as ulceration. Areas where mitoses are counted should include those where they appear to be the highest (the "hot spot"). In the 1989 Clark prognostic model, developed and still in use in our institution, the prognosis is best when the mitotic rate is zero and worst when the rate is greater than 6 mitoses per square millimeter (317). The presence of mitoses may also be useful in identifying thin melanomas with a propensity to metastasize (Fig. 28-19B) (695,714). Interobserver agreement for tumor mitotic rate has been found to be excellent.

Guidelines for recording mitotic rate and mitogenicity have been presented (717). The mitotic rate should be determined by first scanning the sections for the region of maximal mitotic activity, the so-called "hot spot." Counting should proceed from this region, until an area of 1 mm² has been counted. In most microscopes, this represents approximately three or four high-power fields, and calibration of individual instruments should be done using an ocular micrometer (preferably a high-resolution etched glass calibration scale) to calculate the area of a high-power field for a 40× objective lens. The total number of mitoses in 1 mm² is the mitotic rate, expressed as a whole number. If the area of the lesion is smaller than 1 mm, the number of mitoses found in tumor cells is recorded as the mitotic rate, again as a whole number. Although it was mentioned in the first publication of the 2009 AJCC staging system, the term "less than 1" should not be used. This term has been used ambiguously, sometimes after applying a correction factor and sometimes to indicate that no mitotic activity was observed. The term "less than 1" is equated to "0" by most, if not all, tumor registrars. If no mitoses are observed, the mitotic rate is "0."

Critical to determining mitotic rate accurately is to (1) ensure that cells counted are confined to the dermis (not junctional); (2) establish that the cell counted is unequivocally a tumor cell (not an immune cell, endothelial cell, etc.); and (3) exclude potential mimics of cell mitosis (e.g., nuclear fragmentation caused by apoptosis).

Vertical Growth Phase

The morphology of VGP (i.e., the focal presence of tumorigenic or mitogenic growth of melanoma in the dermis) has already been presented (p. 871, Fig. 28-19). Here, we discuss its significance as a prognostic attribute in relatively thin melanomas with vertical growth and in level II melanomas ostensibly without vertical growth. In one series, metastases occurred in 2% of melanomas less than 0.76 mm thick. The cases that metastasized all had tumorigenic VGP. The rate of metastasis for tumorigenic melanomas less than 0.76 mm in thickness was 15%, whereas in nontumorigenic (RGP) melanoma of any thickness (most are <1 mm), the metastatic rate was zero (171,264). In rare instances of metastasizing thin melanomas, VGP is absent; most, if not all, of these cases in our experience and in the literature have had extensive partial or complete regression (see section on Regression later) (317). As already mentioned, reproducibility studies have been done for VGP in thin melanomas and have concluded that this determination can be reliably made by practicing pathologists (266,718). A study that investigated prognostic factors in metastasizing thin level II melanomas, concluded that VGP was the only statistically significant factor. It was proposed that growth phase evaluation should be added to the recommendations for melanoma histologic reporting, at least for level II SSMs (267). Even though VGP is the most common "explanation" for metastasizing thin melanoma, not all such lesions contain this feature (719). In a recent study of prognostic factors for sentinel node positivity in thin melanomas, VGP was strongly associated with positivity with an odds ratio of 4.3, which in the opinion of the authors provided support for its inclusion in standardized reporting (269).

Clark Levels of Invasion

Although tumor thickness is now considered to be the most important prognostic attribute, the levels of invasion defined by Clark (720) have prognostic value, at least in certain subsets of cases (172). They also have descriptive value. The different levels appear to reflect the sequential acquisition of new properties by evolving tumors and should be included in pathology reports, at least as an optional term (721). They are defined as follows, with survival rates for prospectively diagnosed and definitively treated clinical Stage I cases in parentheses (722).

Level I (100% 10-year disease-free survival): confinement of the melanoma cells to the epidermis and its appendages. These *in situ* melanomas (AJCC Stage 0) presumably lack the capacity to invade through a basement membrane. Level II: (96% survival). There is extension into the papillary dermis, with at most only a few melanoma cells extending to the interface between papillary and reticular dermis. These melanomas are "microinvasive," but lack the capacity to form tumors in all but a few cases. Almost all of the level II tumors that metastasize have a small tumorigenic papule (VGP), as previously defined (p. 916). In level III (86% survival), there is extension of the tumor cells throughout the papillary dermis, filling and sometimes expanding it and impinging on the reticular dermis without, however, invading it. These melanomas are thus showing competency for tumorigenic VGP in the papillary dermis, a loose mesenchyme that is specialized to support epithelium. Level IV (66% survival) tumors are not only invasive and tumorigenic but also have the capacity to invade the dense, sparsely vascular mesenchyme of the reticular dermis. Level V (53% survival) tumors invade the subcutaneous fat. Observer agreement for Clark level has been found to be fair to good (712).

Partial and Complete Regression of Melanoma

Partial regression is common in melanomas. Usually, it is observed in the nontumorigenic RGP compartment ("RGP regression"). Regression is defined as a focal area in which there is delicate, often edematous fibroplasia of the papillary dermis, often accompanied by proliferation of dilated blood vessels, and usually with a sprinkling of melanophages and lymphocytes, with melanoma present in the epidermis and/or papillary dermis to one or both sides, but not significantly within the area of regression (Fig 28-56). Fibrogenic cytokines have been demonstrated in these areas of regression (128).

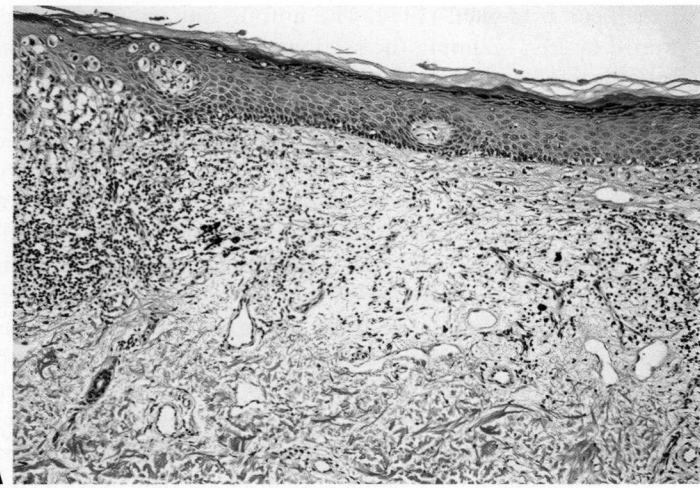
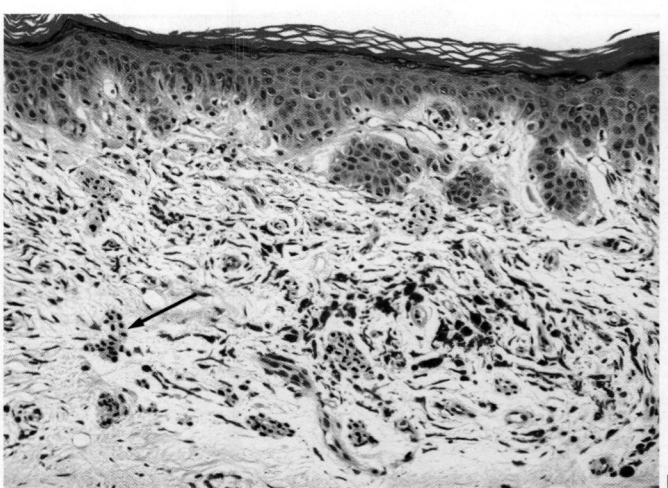

Figure 28-56 Partial regression of the radial growth phase. **A:** At left, there are melanoma cells in the epidermis and papillary dermis. To the right, there is fibrosis with lymphocytes and melanophages in the papillary dermis. **B:** In another area of partial radial growth phase regression, the papillary dermis is widened by fibroblasts with lymphocytes and melanophages. Remnants of a nevus are seen in the regressive fibroplasia (*arrow*), apparently unaffected by the regression process.

In a study of interobserver agreement, it was considered that histologic evidence of melanoma regression can be identified consistently if approached systematically, with agreement on explicitly defined criteria; however an attempt to define reproducible criteria for early, intermediate, and late regression was unsuccessful (723).

Paradoxically, partial regression of the RGP ("RGP regression") has been associated in some series with poorer prognosis (317,724,725), perhaps because a more significant dermal component had been present and had metastasized before it regressed or perhaps because RGP regression somehow favors VGP progression. In contrast, a meta-analysis of 10 studies, comprising 8,557 patients, found that those with histologic regression in their tumors had a lower relative risk of death than those without (726). Similarly, a large retrospective multisite study has recently found regression to be favorably associated with survival (727). However, the definition of regression used in that study differed from the one cited previously in that some cases had only partial, rather than complete, loss of melanoma in the regions diagnosed as regression (727).

In contrast to the apparent negative correlation of RGP regression with prognosis, TIL responses within the VGP, which may be considered as a potentially different form of immunologic regression ("VGP regression"), are associated with improved survival rates (317,728–730) (Fig. 28-57). Regression of the VGP has not been well described. Occasionally, one sees an area of fibrosis and melanophages apparently partially replacing a portion of a tumor nodule, and very infrequently, this process may proceed to completion, resulting in a collection of melanophages and other inflammatory cells in the dermis that could represent the residual evidence of a preexisting tumor nodule (131). This phenomenon has been aptly referred to as "tumoral melanosis" (Fig. 28-58) (731). Not all of these cases are caused by regression of a melanoma; pigmented basal cell carcinomas or other pigmented skin tumors may regress and produce similar findings (732).

Regression of metastases may occur in a similar manner to that of VGP regression, with similar morphologic findings. This may rarely occur spontaneously but is now being

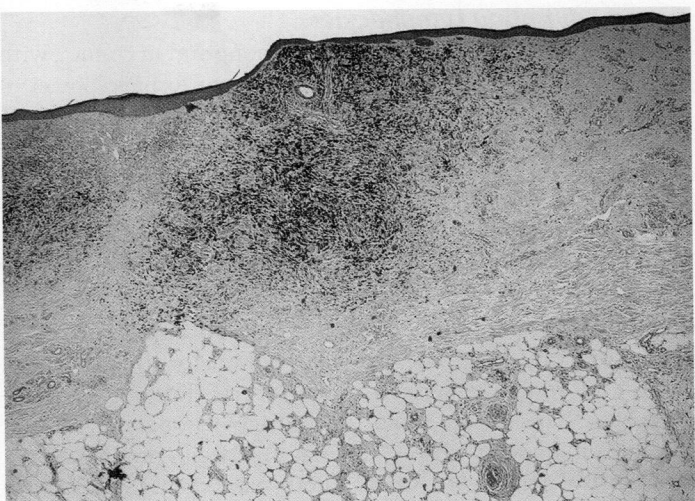

Figure 28-58 Tumoral melanosis. A localized collection of pigmented melanophages is present in the dermis, consistent with regression of a tumorigenic melanoma or of another pigmented tumor.

rather commonly seen in patients whose metastases respond to targeted or immune checkpoint inhibitor therapy. In a study of neoadjuvant targeted therapy against BRAFV600E, patients whose treated tumor showed any hyalinized fibrosis had longer survivals, whereas necrosis and/or immature/proliferative fibrosis correlated with shorter survival. Thus, the pattern, in addition to the mere presence of complete or partial pathologic response (pCR or pPR), correlates with outcome (733,734).

In occasional cases of metastatic melanoma with no obvious primary tumor (melanoma of unknown primary, MUP), clinical examination may reveal a hypopigmented or irregularly hyperpigmented atrophic patch in the skin of the nodal drainage region, consistent with a regressed primary melanoma, whereas others have no such stigmata (735). Some other cases of apparently regressed primary melanoma may present as clinically pigmented, variegated lesions, clinically suspicious for melanoma. Some of these have presented with concomitant metastases, but some, in our experience, have not been associated with metastasis. Although the diagnosis of melanoma cannot be made with certainty in these latter cases, we have seen at least one case in which metastatic melanoma developed after a period of follow-up. In the case of depigmented lesions, histologic examination shows telangiectasia and some pigmented macrophages in the papillary dermis, and in the case of still pigmented lesions an irregular band of melanophages and inflammatory cells in the upper part of the dermis. In some cases, serial sections may reveal a few melanoma cells in the dermis or in the subcutaneous tissue. It is presumed that in patients who present with metastatic melanoma without a clinically overt primary lesion, such completely regressed primary sites may be responsible, although they may evade detection. In such instances, it is important not to implicate other detectable melanocytic lesions (e.g., dysplastic nevi, melanoma *in situ*) as primary sources of metastasis by default.

Patients with MUP seem to have better outcomes compared to those with other stage matched melanomas, probably because of higher immunogenicity as a factor in the immunologically mediated primary site regression (735).

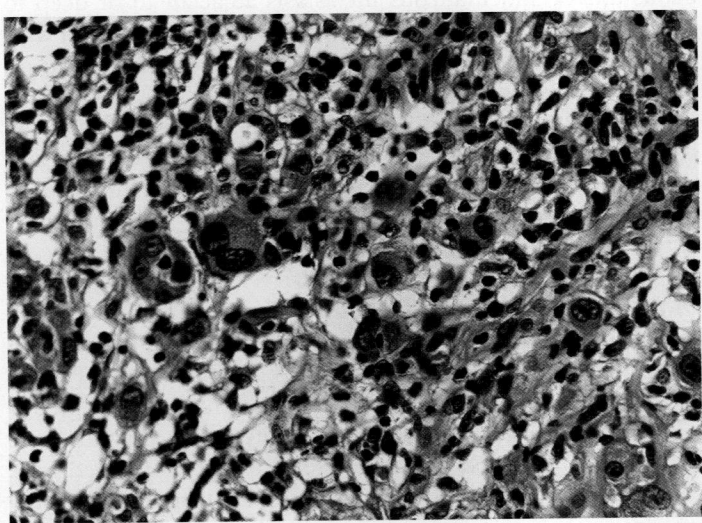

Figure 28-57 Tumor-infiltrating lymphocytes (TIL) at the base of the vertical growth phase of a primary melanoma. Lymphocytes that are "among" the tumor cells, often associated with evidence of apoptosis of the cells, are a favorable prognostic attribute.

Tumor-Infiltrating Lymphocytes

The presence of TIL that are actually among and in contact with the tumor cells of the VGP has been shown to have powerful independent prognostic significance. The lymphocytic infiltrate tends to diminish with increasing thickness of the primary melanoma and is usually scant in deeply invasive tumors (317,736) (Fig. 28-57). The histologic determination of the TIL response has been shown to be reproducible (737). The presence of a noninfiltrative lymphocytic infiltrate around the tumor, usually at its base, is not associated with prognosis (317). The presence of TIL in lymph node metastases is also associated with better survival (663). The prognosis is best for tumors with a "brisk" TIL response, defined as lymphocytes forming a continuous band beneath the tumor or diffusely throughout its substance. Tumors with "absent" TIL have the worst prognosis, and a "nonbrisk" response (discontinuous band) is associated with an intermediate prognosis (736). It has been demonstrated in large studies that the TIL response is a strong independent predictor of survival and/or SLN involvement (317,728–730). In a large population-based study, death as a result of melanoma was 30% less with nonbrisk TIL grade and 50% less with brisk TIL grade relative to TIL absence, adjusted for age, sex, site, and AJCC tumor stage (730). In a study of 655 cases from a single institution, TIL were measured by a simple estimation of the proportion of tumor cells in contact with lymphocytes, resulting in a percentage TIL score that was significant in multivariable analysis, including after adjustment for AJCC stage, reconfirming that higher amounts of TIL are associated with better prognosis and, in addition, demonstrating the value of a simplified numerical TIL scoring system (738).

TIL are clearly important in understanding the action of immune checkpoint inhibitors (ICI). In a comprehensive review of studies of biomarkers for response of melanoma patients to ICI, increased tumor-infiltrating CD8⁺ T-cells and decreased regulatory T-cells were correlated with response, in addition to mutational load, neoantigen load, and immune-related gene expression (739). Although the presence and distribution of TIL may have some descriptive and prognostic value, neither histologic attributes of the tumors nor testing for tumor or immune cell PD-L1 expression should be used at this time (2021) to guide clinical decision-making (673), except if indicated in a clinical trial.

Vascular or Lymphatic Invasion (LVI)

The presence of LVI frequently, although not invariably, has been found to correlate with survival in large series of cases studied by multivariable analysis (711) and also with sentinel node status (740,741). LVI generally implies the presence of tumor cells within blood or lymphatic vessels (Fig. 28-59); the sensitivity of detection is improved by double labeling of the vessel wall with either a pan endothelial marker such as CD31 or a specific lymphatic marker such as D-240 and of tumor cells with a specific marker such as Melan-A/Mart (740,741). Angiotropism, defined as cuffing of the external surface of vessels with tumor cells, also known as "extravascular migratory metastasis," has also been associated with aggressive behavior (742). Vascular invasion also appears to be a strong predictor of development of in-transit metastases in follow-up (743). Lymphovascular invasion may also be seen in metastases, and its presence should lead to a consideration of a metastasis simulating a primary, such as an epidermotropic metastatic melanoma (744).

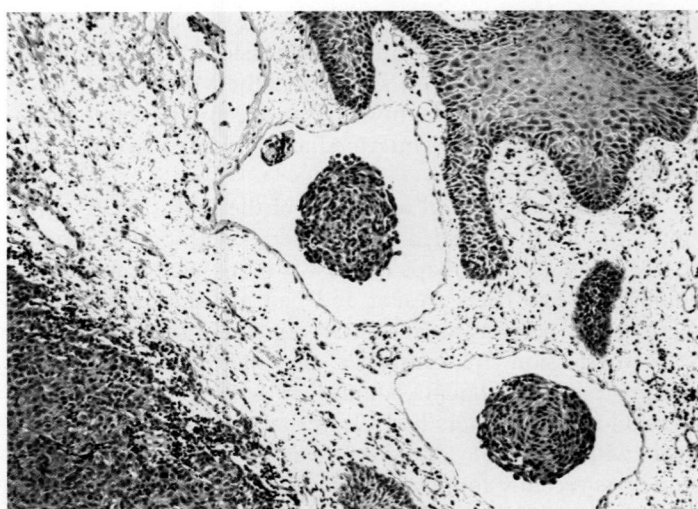

Figure 28-59 Lymphatic invasion. Although not often recognized, except in very thick tumors, lymphatic invasion is probably an adverse prognostic attribute.

Satellites

Satellites are defined as discontinuous foci of tumor (metastases) located within 2 cm of a primary melanoma (Fig. 28-60), whereas in-transit metastases are beyond 2 cm but still regional. Microscopic satellites are observed histologically in either the biopsy or the wide excision specimen. The presence of satellites and/or in transit metastases and/or microscopic satellites is a significant staging attribute in the current 8th edition AJCC staging system, defining a lesion as Nc and thus Stage III (656). In the seventh edition of the AJCC, these were defined as tumor nests, greater than 0.05 mm in diameter, in the reticular dermis, panniculus, or vessels beneath the principal invasive tumor mass but separated from it by at least 0.3 mm of normal tissue on the section in which the Breslow measurement was taken. In the current edition, this definition no longer applies (despite, in our opinion, providing useful conceptual guidelines), and a satellite is defined as "a microscopic cutaneous and/or subcutaneous metastasis adjacent to or deep to and completely discontinuous from a primary melanoma with unaffected stroma occupying the space between, identified on pathologic examination of the primary tumor site"; it is important not to confuse tumor islands that are still connected to the surface in other section planes with true satellites (656), and levels through a specimen block may sometimes facilitate determination of whether an apparent satellite is in reality attached to the VGP on three-dimensional reconstruction.

Other Clinicopathologic Prognostic Factors

In addition to thickness of the tumor, various other factors have been cited as influencing the prognosis of clinical Stage I melanoma, but many of them are directly related to thickness. In different clinicopathologic databases, multivariate analyses have led to prognostic models that differ somewhat in the predictive variables that are shown to have independent significance. Several features, however, have appeared in two or more of the studies.

Histogenetic Type. Among the histologic factors, the type of tumor, whether nodular (NM) or SSM, does not, in most studies,

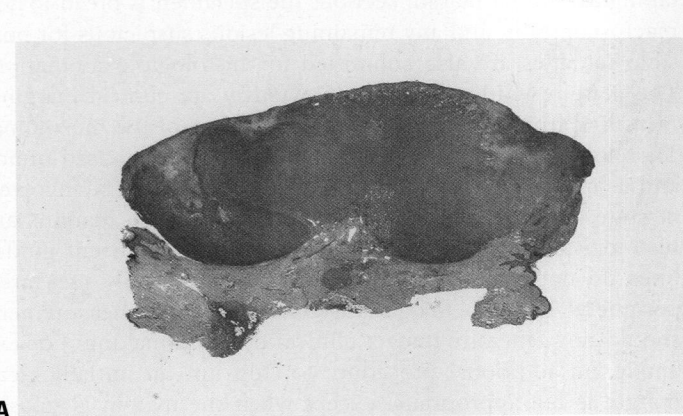
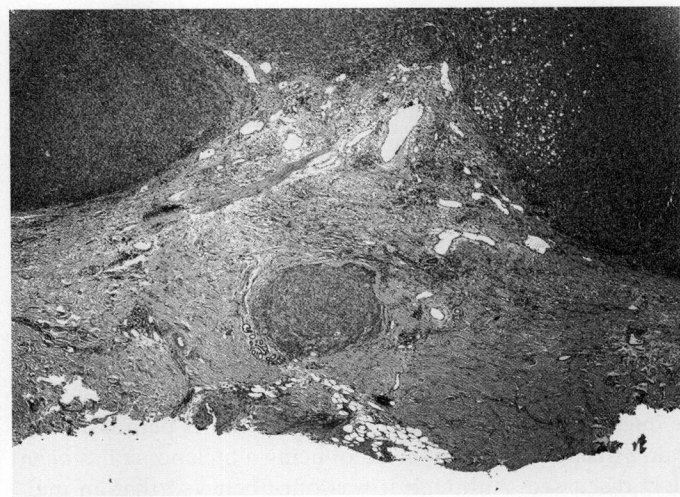

Figure 28-60 Microscopic satellite. **A:** Microscopic satellite present at the base of a bulky tumorigenic vertical growth phase melanoma. **B:** The satellite is located in the reticular dermis.

independently affect the prognosis as long as all other variables are matched (317,745). NM, on average, are thicker than SSM and thus have a worse prognosis overall. A large multicenter study recently concluded that NM is "a distinct melanoma subtype with a constellation of aggressive biologic characteristics that may confer worse prognosis." However, in a model stratified by regional metastasis, the differences were no longer statistically significant, likely because of offsetting factors in the model (745). Another large study recently found that NM was an independent risk factor for death in both a population-based SEER and in an institutional cohort, with hazard ratios of 1.6 and 1.5, respectively, controlling for thickness, ulceration, stage, and other variables. NM was associated with a higher rate of *NRAS* mutation, and high-throughput sequencing revealed NM-specific genomic alterations. It was concluded that "the data reveal distinct clinical and biologic differences between NM and SSM that support revisiting the prognostic and predictive impact of primary histology subtype in the management of cutaneous melanoma" (746).

The scarcity or absence of melanin in the tumor cells ("amelanotic melanoma"), indicative of poor differentiation, affects the prognosis adversely in some series but does so most likely because of correlations with advanced tumor stage, negative prognostic factors (such as deep tumor thickness and high mitotic rate), and/or perhaps potentially greater intrinsic aggressiveness (747).

As already discussed, differences among these "histogenetic types" appear to reside more in the areas of etiology and pathogenesis rather than prognosis or behavior. However, accumulating data are demonstrating that the underlying oncogenic genotype of the different clinicopathologic entities may vary in a more or less predictable manner, making assessment of characteristics of tumors that predict genotype profiles of relevance, as therapies directed against these oncogenes continue to be developed.

Lesional Location. In a number of multivariable studies, *location* of the tumor on the hair-bearing portions of the limbs has been found to be associated with a favorable prognosis, in contrast to location on the trunk, head, and neck or palms and soles (317,748). In one of these studies, lower trunk, thigh, lower leg, foot, lower arms, hands, and face were identified as intermediate sites, with the remaining sites representing higher risk (749). The posterior scalp has been emphasized as a high-risk site (748).

Gender and Age. There is general agreement that women have a better prognosis than men, owing partly, but not entirely, to the higher incidence in women of lesions on the extremities where the prognosis is favorable compared to the trunk and also to a more favorable mix of other prognostic factors (317,750). It also seems that females may enjoy some sort of protective response against metastases (750), possibly owing to higher immune signaling in younger female patients (751). The age of the patient has an adverse prognostic effect in most series (752), perhaps largely related to declining immune signaling (753).

Biologic Markers of Prognosis

Biologic markers derived from the study of the primary tumors or of host attributes may be expected to add to the precision of present prognostic models. The most consistently useful marker studied to date, both for diagnosis and for prognosis, appears to be the proliferation marker Mib-1 (Ki-67), which has been found to be significantly related to mortality risk in a number of studies (754–756). Other markers, in general, have not been studied in sufficiently large series of cases or have not been reproduced in other datasets, and no marker is in general use for this purpose.

Reproducibility of Staging Attributes

Although most of the individual microstaging attributes have been found to be reproducible in formal studies, agreement is nevertheless imperfect in the "real world." In a study of outside cases reviewed at a referral center, there was at least one alteration in 28% of the cases. Agreement for final diagnosis was 97%; for subtype, 92%; for Breslow thickness, 87%; for ulceration, satellites and LVI, 98%; and for microsatellites, mitotic rate, and growth phase, 99%. Despite these excellent agreement rates, a change in AJCC stage occurred in 7% of cases, with a change in management in 3%. It was concluded that the pathologic review had significant clinical implications for a small minority of cases (757). In another similar study based on the NCCN guidelines, 6% of patients had changes in their SLNB recommendations, and one of these had a positive node found on pathology. Changes in the T-stage were made in 10% of the cases, 4% of which also had changes in the recommended wide local excision margin (758). It was concluded by both these studies that internal pathology review should be an important component of care for melanoma patients at referral institutions.

Principles of Management for Melanoma

Management of melanoma has been codified in guidelines published in many different communities, including the NCCN (673), and is briefly discussed later.

Biopsy of Melanoma

The question of whether an incisional biopsy is permissible in a lesion that is highly suspected of being a melanoma has been widely discussed. Although it was once believed that an incisional biopsy might cause metastatic spread, this is no longer regarded as a primary concern; however, compete excisional biopsy is preferred to maximize the diagnostic and prognostic information that may be obtained. Because a correct diagnosis and accurate prognostic staging is more likely to be accomplished when the entire tumor can be studied, an excisional biopsy is advisable whenever feasible, and an incisional biopsy is indicated only in occasional instances, such as for very large lesions (721). If a tumorigenic VGP is present, it should be contained entirely within the biopsy, if possible. A shave biopsy or curetting is not optimal, because it may result in inadequate material for diagnosis; it may also make impossible a determination of the depth of penetration of the tumor, which is very important for prognosis and for planning of the extent of surgical procedures (see Prognosis, p. 924). Moreover, subsequent excision may show ulceration owing to the prior biopsy, a potential hazard in the rare instance when the excision is evaluated by one unaware of the previous procedure. Shave or punch biopsies that completely encompass the lesion are, of course, acceptable. However, a positive deep margin is commonly found in a shave biopsy, and this may compromise the ability to accurately diagnose and stage the lesion. Such positive deep margins should be characterized in the biopsy report with terminology such as "present at" or "broadly transected," because this correlates with the likelihood and extent of residual tumor in a reexcision and may also be used as a consideration in the recommendation for sentinel node staging (721).

Wide Local Excision

The purpose of "wide" local excision (WLE) for melanoma is to remove the primary tumor, including its RGP, and also to encompass as much as possible any field of satellite metastases in the region. Formerly, the margin of resection of the primary tumor was regarded by most authors as optimal at about 5 cm beyond the perimeter of the lesion. However, a much narrower margin is now acceptable (668). Current NCCN guidelines are for a clinically measured excision margin of 0.5 cm for *in situ*, 1.0 cm for melanomas with Breslow thickness less than 1 mm, 1 to 2 cm for melanomas greater than 1.0 to 2.0 mm, and 2.0 cm for melanomas greater than 2 mm in thickness (673,759). Others have considered lesser margins of 1.0 cm for Stage II or even for all invasive melanomas (759). This hypothesis is currently being tested in at least two randomized clinical trials.

In examining a resected WLE specimen for melanoma, we generally serially embed the area of the biopsy scar and sample the specimen margin with perpendicular sections. The specimen is first inked to identify the true margin surface. After taking the initial margin section, the specimen is bread-loafed macroscopically, and any remaining lesions suspicious for possible satellites are also submitted for histologic examination. The margin widths discussed previously are clinical margins, measured from the grossly visible periphery of the melanoma. Therefore, careful histologic examination of the excised tumor and its margins is mandatory, because margins may be involved in spite of a clinically normal appearance. When margins are histologically negative on the WLE specimen, current guidelines do not require reporting the microscopically measured peripheral or deep margin distances, and this measurement should not generally impact clinical decision-making. For example, an additional procedure to "top up" an initially clear margin is not appropriate, except when the margin is "close" (673). In our practice, we generally alert the clinician when the margin width is less than 0.1 cm (<1 mm) in a resection specimen. The dermis and subcutis should also be evaluated carefully (grossly and microscopically for the presence of satellites, which may have prognostic significance and which may occasionally be present at the margin). Satellites are rare in relation to thin tumors, but in one study they were detected in 22% of the reexcision specimens from melanomas greater than 2.25 mm in thickness (668). The presence of neurotropism should also be carefully sought and reported in melanoma resection specimens, especially, of course, if this neural invasion extends to the specimen margin.

According to current NCCN Guidelines, Mohs microscopically controlled surgery (MMS) is not generally recommended for primary treatment of invasive cutaneous melanoma. However, because data are lacking to guide surgical management in anatomically constrained areas, the NCCN Guidelines now indicate that MMS, and other surgical methods that provide comprehensive histologic assessment, such as staged excision with permanent sections for dermatopathology review ("Slow Mohs"), may be considered selectively for MIS (LM and acral-lentiginous types) and for minimally invasive (T1a) LM melanoma in anatomically constrained areas (673). Because satellites are vanishingly rare in this thickness subset, the dimensions of the local excision margin widths are presumably of less importance (and in any case are limited by the local constraints such as nearby vital organs). Practice standards vary among MMS practitioners; in the best hands, at least, excellent local control statistics have been achieved (760).

Therapeutic and Elective Lymph Node Dissection

According to current NCCN guidelines, a clinically positive lymph node in a patient with primary cutaneous melanoma should be biopsied, and if the node is histologically positive, a full regional node dissection should be done as a "therapeutic" procedure ("therapeutic regional lymph node dissection" [TRLND]) with curative intent and to gain local control (673). For clinically negative lymph nodes, the role of "elective regional lymph node dissection" (ERLND) has been supplanted by the sentinel node staging technique (see next section). Theoretically, regional nodes could be regarded as necessary filters that must be bypassed by all melanomas that metastasize systematically. However, it is clear that many melanomas also metastasize by the hematogenous route to distant organs without ever involving regional nodes or embark on both routes in tandem. Thus, lymph node involvement may in many cases be simply a marker of a melanoma that has already metastasized.

Melanoma patients with clinically detected (e.g., palpable) lymph node metastases ("macrometastases") are at increased risk for having distant metastases and are staged as "N1b, N2b, or N3b" subcategories. The number of involved lymph nodes and the depth of the tumor are important prognostic factors. If microsatellites, satellites, or in-transit metastases are present, patients are then assigned to an N "c" subcategory. In the AJCC 8th edition, it has been stipulated that melanoma cells in a lymphatic channel within or immediately adjacent to a lymph node should define that node as positive for staging purposes. The presence of matted nodes is defined as an N3 category. Curiously, the size of involved nodes is not independently related to survival. The presence of extranodal or extracapsular extension should be recorded as present or absent in all positive nodes. There is marked heterogeneity in prognosis among patients with Stage III regional node disease by N-category designation, ranging from 75% to 43% 10-year survival (656). The presence of brisk TIL in a lymph node metastasis is a favorable prognostic attribute and was associated in one study with a survival rate of 83%, compared to 29% in patients whose metastases lacked TIL. Multivariate analysis confirmed the prognostic value of TIL in predicting disease-free survival in patients with regional node metastases (663).

Selective Lymphadenectomy (SLN Dissection)

SLN was developed by Morton as a means of sampling regional lymph nodes while avoiding most of the complications of an elective dissection (761). The procedure is done for patients who are at risk for regional metastasis (generally T1b or higher stage) and do not have clinically positive nodes, and a histologically positive deposit of tumor in a clinically negative node is termed a "clinically occult" or "micrometastasis." The "sentinel" lymph node is identified by injections into the region of the melanoma of radioactive colloid and a vegetable dye ("blue dye"). The sentinel node is defined as the first in the regional lymph node basis to contain these markers ("hot and blue"). Studies have demonstrated that if the sentinel node is negative, the probability of metastases being found in the remainder of the lymph node basin is very low indeed. In early studies, the sentinel node was evaluated by frozen sections with rapid S100 staining (762). Currently, the standard procedure is to examine the node with paraffin H&E sections, with S100 as a sensitive marker, and with HMB-45 or Melan-A/Mart-1, as a more specific, though less sensitive, marker. Use of a "cocktail" of antibodies to MART-1, Melan-A, and tyrosinase has also been proposed and widely adopted (763), and Sox10 can also be used in place of S100 (323). In evaluating the S100 stain, reactive dendritic cells that are present in most sentinel nodes must be distinguished from metastatic melanoma deposits. Capsular nevic rests must also be distinguished (Fig. 28-61). These are located in capsular or trabecular collagen rather than in sinuses or intracapsular vessels, lack significant cytologic atypia, and stain (if needed) with S100, Melan-A, and p16, although usually not with Ki-67, PRAME, or HMB45, which are therefore useful as diagnostic markers to rule out an authentic melanoma deposit (346,764).

True melanoma micrometastases are often present as immunoreactive cells in the subcapsular sinuses and/or the lymph node parenchyma, generally with correlative detection of cytologically

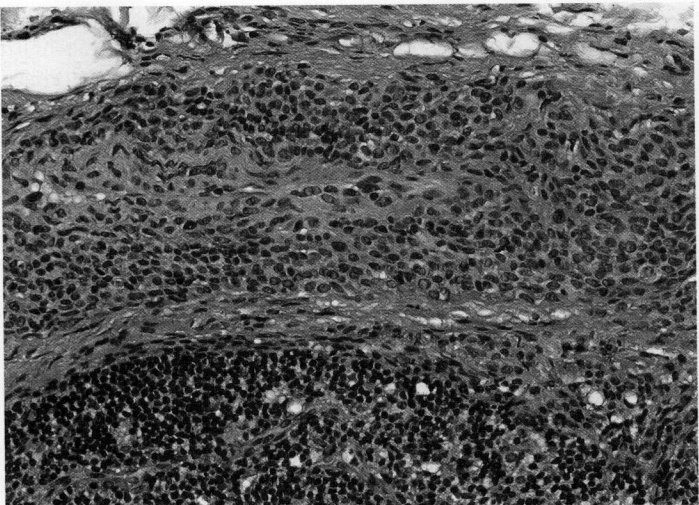

Figure 28-61 Capsular nevus in a sentinel node. Mature nevus cells are present in the capsule of the node.

malignant cells in corresponding H&E-stained sections (Fig. 28-62). Such deposits should be measured to provide some indication of tumor bulk, and if extension through the nodal capsule has occurred this feature should be noted. In situations where immunohistochemically suspicious cells are present but diligent attempts to confirm them as malignant cells in H&E sections fail, the findings should be reported descriptively, indicating that the features are suspicious but not conclusive. Often, isolated MART-1 or HMB-45-positive cells may be identified, usually as only one or two cells in the lymphoid parenchyma, and it may be unclear as to whether these represent true micrometastases. In one recent report, of a total of 821 patients who underwent an SLN biopsy, 57 (6.9%) had rare IHC-positive cells of undetermined clinical significance with no disease progression over a mean 59-month follow-up (765). In addition, these cells are morphologically incompatible with melanoma, having small nuclei and lacking pleomorphism, hyperchromatism, nucleoli, and mitoses (766). Moreover, not all MART-1/Melan-A-positive cells in lymph node parenchyma necessarily represent metastatic melanoma, as emphasized in a study where such cells were detected in lymph nodes of some nonmelanoma patients undergoing lymphadenectomy for breast cancer (767).

As before, it was stated that immunohistochemical detection of nodal metastases is acceptable, with no lower limit of size to designate N+ disease. The possible existence of a lower limit of size (such as submicroscopic micrometastases <0.1 mm) had been the subject of ongoing clinical trials and reports (768,769). In addition, in our opinion, and that of others, the pathologist should be convinced that the immunohistochemically positive cells are melanoma cells and not nevus cells, Schwann cells, or some artifact (766).

In the pathology report, the number of positive and negative SLNs examined should be recorded. When metastases are present, the greatest dimension of tumor size (in mm, measured to the nearest 0.1 mm using an ocular micrometer), location within the lymph node, and presence of extracapsular extension should be recorded. When multiple metastases are present, the single largest metastasis is measured, and the number and distribution of the metastases can be recorded descriptively (697).

Consideration of completion node dissection (CLND) was at one time recommended for all patients with a positive sentinel node. However, two prospective randomized studies have failed to find a better survival rate for patients with CLND than with observation alone. These patients with a positive SLNB are at higher risk for recurrence and should ideally followed with expert nodal basin ultrasound surveillance without completion lymph node dissection. The failure of CLND to improve survival suggests that a positive SLN acts as a risk marker rather than a necessary way station for metastases to spread from a primary site to the rest of the body. Immediate CLND in melanoma surgery is therefore no longer standard of care.

SLNB may thus be regarded as an important staging tool, but its impact on overall survival is unclear and likely limited to a few subsets, if any.

The Association of Directors of Anatomic and Surgical Pathology (ADASP) published guidelines for the processing of lymph nodes, including sentinel nodes submitted for evaluation of metastatic disease. It is recommended that small nodes be submitted in their entirety or that larger nodes be sectioned at 3- to 4-mm intervals and entirely submitted. Intraoperative examination should be limited to those cases where the procedure is likely to influence management (e.g., to confirm clinically and grossly positive nodes so that a complete node clearance can proceed). ADASP recommends that more than one section be performed on each sentinel node block. It is not clear how many sections and levels are optimal (770). Although the ADASP committee did not provide recommendations for immunostains, or even endorse this procedure unequivocally, in most centers it is currently the practice to perform Sox10 or S100 (more sensitive, less specific) and either HMB-45 or Melan-A (more specific, less sensitive) and/or PRAME (both reasonably sensitive and reasonably specific) staining on one profile from each block prepared from each submitted sentinel node (323,346,771).

Synoptic Pathology Report for Melanoma

Synoptic or structured pathology report formats have been proposed as a part of national guidelines in many countries (721,772,773). Attributes listed in these guidelines are generally separated into essential and optional elements as follows:

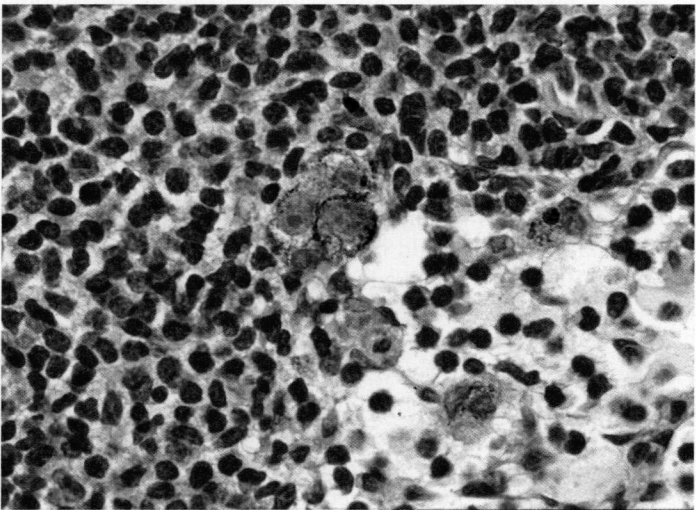

Figure 28-62 Small deposit of metastatic melanoma in a sentinel node. There is a small collection of cells in the lymph node parenchyma that are large, clustered in a group, have pigment consistent with melanin, and have prominent nucleoli, and (in this instance) contain pigment.

Essential elements: Anatomic site and laterality of the lesion, diagnosis of a primary melanoma, Breslow thickness, ulceration (optionally with diameter in mm), a statement about excision margins (e.g., excision complete, melanoma "present at" versus "broadly transected" or "close" to specimen base and/or peripheral margins, distinguishing *in situ* and invasive components and providing orientation when this has been defined by the surgeon). A measurement of the margin width is not required, and any such measurement should not be used to guide management except in the case of lesions that are "close," which may be regarded as a measured margin width of less than 1 mm, which should be reported as such.

Optional Elements: Dermal mitotic rate per mm2, LVI, neurotropism, DM component as a percentage of dermal invasive tumor, WHO classification (e.g., SSM, LMM, ALM, MLM, NM), TIL (e.g., brisk, nonbrisk, or absent), microscopic satellites, RGP regression (present or absent and an estimate of extent), associated nevus, solar elastosis.

REFERENCES

1. Karimkhani C, Green AC, Nijsten T, et al. The global burden of melanoma: results from global burden of disease study 2015. *Br J Dermatol.* 2017;177(1):134–140.
2. O'Sullivan DE, Brenner DR, Demers PA, Villeneuve PJ, Friedenreich CM, King WD. Indoor tanning and skin cancer in Canada: a meta-analysis and attributable burden estimation. *Cancer Epidemiol.* 2019;59:1–7.
3. Elder DE, Barnhill RL, Bastian BC, et al. Melanocytic tumour classification and the pathway concept of melanoma pathogenesis. In: Elder DE, Massi D, Scolyer RA, Willemze R, eds. *WHO Classification of Skin Tumours.* 4th ed. International Agency for Research on Cancer; 2018:66–71.
4. Elder DE, Bastian BC, Cree IA, Massi D, Scolyer RA. The 2018 World Health Organization classification of cutaneous, mucosal, and uveal melanoma: detailed analysis of 9 distinct subtypes defined by their evolutionary pathway. *Arch Pathol Lab Med.* 2020;144(4):500–522.
5. Elder DE, Massi D, Scolyer RA, Willemze R. *WHO Classification of Skin Tumours.* 4th ed. IARC; 2018.
6. Landi MT, Bauer J, Pfeiffer RM, et al. MC1R germline variants confer risk for BRAF-mutant melanoma. *Science.* 2006;313(5786):521–522.
7. Elmore JG, Barnhill RL, Elder DE, et al. Pathologists' diagnosis of invasive melanoma and melanocytic proliferations: observer accuracy and reproducibility study. *BMJ.* 2017;357:j2813.
8. Lott JP, Elmore JG, Zhao GA, et al. Evaluation of the Melanocytic Pathology Assessment Tool and Hierarchy for Diagnosis (MPATH-Dx) classification scheme for diagnosis of cutaneous melanocytic neoplasms: results from the International Melanoma Pathology Study Group. *J Am Acad Dermatol.* 2016;75(2):356–363.
9. Elder DE, Piepkorn MW, Barnhill RL, et al. Pathologist characteristics associated with accuracy and reproducibility of melanocytic skin lesion interpretation. *J Am Acad Dermatol.* 2018;79(1):52–59.e55.
10. Spak DA, Plaxco JS, Santiago L, Dryden MJ, Dogan BE. BI-RADS® fifth edition: a summary of changes. *Diagn Interv Imaging.* 2017;98(3):179–190.
11. Piepkorn MW, Barnhill RL, Elder DE, et al. The MPATH-Dx reporting schema for melanocytic proliferations and melanoma. *J Am Acad Dermatol.* 2014;70(1):131–141.
12. Welch HG, Mazer BL, Adamson AS. The rapid rise in cutaneous melanoma diagnoses. *N Engl J Med.* 2021;384(1):72–79.

13. Lee JJ, Lian CG. Molecular testing for cutaneous melanoma: an update and review. *Arch Pathol Lab Med.* 2019;143(7):811–820.
14. Bastiaens M, ter Huurne J, Gruis N, et al. The melanocortin-1-receptor gene is the major freckle gene. *Hum Mol Genet.* 2001;10(16):1701–1708.
15. Pellegrini C, Botta F, Massi D, et al. MC1R variants in childhood and adolescent melanoma: a retrospective pooled analysis of a multicentre cohort. *Lancet Child Adolesc Health.* 2019;3(5):332–342.
16. Bliss JM, Ford D, Swerdlow AJ, et al. Risk of cutaneous melanoma associated with pigmentation characteristics and freckling: systematic overview of 10 case-control studies. *Int J Cancer.* 1995;62:367–376.
17. Rhodes AR, Albert LS, Barnhill RL, Weinstock MA. Sun-induced freckles in children and young adults. A correlation of clinical and histopathologic features. *Cancer.* 1991;67(7):1990–2001.
18. Breathnach AS, Wyllie LM. Electron microscopy of melanocytes and melanosomes in freckled human epidermis. *J Invest Dermatol.* 1964;42:389–394.
19. Bastiaens M, Hoefnagel J, Westendorp R, Vermeer BJ, Bouwes Bavinck JN. Solar lentigines are strongly related to sun exposure in contrast to ephelides. *Pigment Cell Res.* 2004;17(3):225–229.
20. Bastiaens MT, Westendorp RG, Vermeer BJ, Bavinck JN. Ephelides are more related to pigmentary constitutional host factors than solar lentigines. *Pigment Cell Res.* 1999;12:316–322.
21. Benedict PH, Szabo G, Fitzpatrick TB, Sinesi SJ. Melanotic macules in Albright's syndrome and in neurofibromatosis. *JAMA.* 1968;205(9):618–626.
22. De Schepper S, Boucneau J, Vander HY, Messiaen L, Naeyaert JM, Lambert J. Cafe-au-lait spots in neurofibromatosis type 1 and in healthy control individuals: hyperpigmentation of a different kind? *Arch Dermatol Res.* 2006;297(10):439–449.
23. Peltonen S, Kallionpaa RA, Peltonen J. Neurofibromatosis type 1 (NF1) gene: beyond cafe au lait spots and dermal neurofibromas. *Exp Dermatol.* 2016;26(7):645–648.
24. Morice-Picard F, Letertre O, Lasseaux E, Cario-Andre M, Arveiler B, Taieb A. Lentiginosis and café-au-lait macules as part of the phenotypic spectrum of PAX3-related disorders. *Clin Exp Dermatol.* 2020;45(5):621–623.
25. Becker SW. Concurrent melanosis and hypertrichosis in distribution of nevus unius lateris. *Arch Dermatol Syph.* 1949;60:155–160.
26. Fehr B, Panizzon RG, Schnyder UW. Becker's nevus and malignant melanoma. *Dermatologica.* 1991;182:77–80.
27. Rower JM, Carr RD, Lowney ED. Progressive cribriform and zosteriform hyperpigmentation. *Arch Dermatol.* 1978;114(1):98–99.
28. Urbanek RW, Johnson WC. Smooth muscle hamartoma associated with Becker's nevus. *Arch Dermatol.* 1978;114(1):104–106.
29. Kim YJ, Han JH, Kang HY, Lee ES, Kim YC. Androgen receptor overexpression in Becker nevus: histopathologic and immunohistochemical analysis. *J Cutan Pathol.* 2008;35(12):1121–1126.
30. Happle R, Koopman RJ. Becker nevus syndrome. *Am J Med Genet.* 1997;68(3):357–361.
31. Taylor EJ. *Dorland's Illustrated Medical Dictionary.* 27th ed. W. B. Saunders; 1988.
32. Schafer T, Merkl J, Klemm E, Wichmann HE, Ring J. The epidemiology of nevi and signs of skin aging in the adult general population: results of the KORA-survey 2000. *J Invest Dermatol.* 2006;126(7):1490–1496.
33. Derancourt C, Bourdon-Lanoy E, Grob JJ, Guillaume JC, Bernard P, Bastuji-Garin S. Multiple large solar lentigos on the upper back as clinical markers of past severe sunburn: a case-control study. *Dermatology.* 2007;214(1):25–31.
34. Tucker MA, Halpern A, Holly EA, et al. Clinically recognized dysplastic nevi. A central risk factor for cutaneous melanoma. *JAMA.* 1997;277:1439–1444.
35. McLean DI, Gallagher RP. "Sunburn" freckles, cafe-au-lait macules, and other pigmented lesions of schoolchildren: the Vancouver Mole Study. *J Am Acad Dermatol.* 1995;32(4):565–570.
36. Elder DE, Murphy GF. Benign melanocytic tumors (nevi). In: Elder DE, Murphy GF, eds. *Melanocytic Tumors of the Skin.* Armed Forces Institute of Pathology; 1991:5–81.
37. Bolognia JL. Reticulated black solar lentigo ("ink spot" lentigo). *Arch Dermatol.* 1992;128:934–940.
38. Rhodes AR, Harrist TJ, Momtaz T. The PUVA-induced pigmented macule: a lentiginous proliferation of large, sometimes cytologically atypical, melanocytes. *J Am Acad Dermatol.* 1983;9(1):47–58.
39. Yonei N, Kaminaka C, Kimura A, Furukawa F, Yamamoto Y. Two patterns of solar lentigines: a histopathological analysis of 40 Japanese women. *J Dermatol.* 2012;39(10):829–832.
40. Andersen WK, Labadie RR, Bhawan J. Histopathology of solar lentigines of the face: a quantitative study. *J Am Acad Dermatol.* 1997;36(3 Pt. 1):444–447.
41. Abel EA, Reid H, Wood C, Hu CH. PUVA-induced melanocytic atypia: is it confined to PUVA lentigines? *J Am Acad Dermatol.* 1985;13(5 Pt. 1):761–768.
42. Mehregan DR, Hamzavi F, Brown K. Large cell acanthoma. *Int J Dermatol.* 2003;42(1):36–39.
43. Fraga GR, Amin SM. Large cell acanthoma: a variant of solar lentigo with cellular hypertrophy. *J Cutan Pathol.* 2014;41(9):733–739.
44. Aoki H, Moro O, Tagami H, Kishimoto J. Gene expression profiling analysis of solar lentigo in relation to immunohistochemical characteristics. *Br J Dermatol.* 2007;156(6):1214–1223.
45. Salducci M, Andre N, Guere C, et al. Factors secreted by irradiated aged fibroblasts induce solar lentigo in pigmented reconstructed epidermis. *Pigment Cell Melanoma Res.* 2014;27(3):502–504.
46. Cario-Andre M, Lepreux S, Pain C, Nizard C, Noblesse E, Taieb A. Perilesional vs. lesional skin changes in senile lentigo. *J Cutan Pathol.* 2004;31(6):441–447.
47. Clark WH Jr, Elder DE, Guerry D 4th, Epstein MN, Greene MH, Van Horn M. A study of tumor progression: the precursor lesions of superficial spreading and nodular melanoma. *Hum Pathol.* 1984;15(12):1147–1165.
48. Tran AK, Pearce A, López-Sánchez M, Pérez-Jurado LA, Barnett C. Novel KIT mutation presenting as marked lentiginosis. *Pediatr Dermatol.* 2019;36(6):922–925.
49. Que SK, Weston G, Suchecki J, Ricketts J. Pigmentary disorders of the eyes and skin. *Clin Dermatol.* 2015;33(2):147–158.
50. Torchia D. Melanocytic naevi clustered on normal background skin. *Clin Exp Dermatol.* 2015;40(3):231–237.
51. Rivers JK, MacLennan R, Kelly JW, et al. The eastern Australian childhood nevus study: prevalence of atypical nevi, congenital nevus-like nevi, and other pigmented lesions. *J Am Acad Dermatol.* 1995;32(6):957–963.
52. Torchia D, Happle R. Papular nevus spilus syndrome: old and new aspects of a mosaic RASopathy. *Eur J Dermatol.* 2019;29(1):2–5.
53. Brito MH, Dionisio CS, Fernandes CM, Ferreira JC, Rosa MJ, Garcia MM. Synchronous melanomas arising within nevus spilus. *An Bras Dermatol.* 2017;92(1):107–109.
54. Sarin KY, Sun BK, Bangs CD, et al. Activating HRAS mutation in agminated Spitz nevi arising in a nevus spilus. *JAMA Dermatol.* 2013;149(9):1077–1081.
55. Pandit B, Sarkozy A, Pennacchio LA, et al. Gain-of-function RAF1 mutations cause Noonan and LEOPARD syndromes with hypertrophic cardiomyopathy. *Nat Genet.* 2007;39(8):1007–1012.
56. Reed OM, Mellette JR, Fitzpatrick JE. Cutaneous lentiginosis with atrial myxomas. *J Am Acad Dermatol.* 1986;15(2 Pt. 2):398–402.
57. Stratakis CA. Carney complex: a familial lentiginosis predisposing to a variety of tumors. *Rev Endocr Metab Disord.* 2016;17(3):367–371.
58. Lodish MB, Stratakis CA. The differential diagnosis of familial lentiginosis syndromes. *Familial Cancer.* 2011;10(3):481–490.
59. Ackerman AB, Ragaz A. *The Lives of Lesions. Chronology in Dermatopathology.* Masson Publishing; 1984.

60. Selmanowitz VJ, Orentreich N, Felsenstein JM. Lentiginosis profusa syndrome (multiple lentigines syndrome). *Arch Dermatol.* 1971;104(4):393–401.

61. Schaffer JV, Orlow SJ, Lazova R, Bolognia JL. Speckled lentiginous nevus: within the spectrum of congenital melanocytic nevi. *Arch Dermatol.* 2001;137(2):172–178.

62. Yamada K, Matsukawa A, Hori Y, Kukita A. Ultrastructural studies on pigmented macules of Peutz-Jeghers syndrome. *J Dermatol.* 1981;8(5):367–377.

63. Horikoshi T, Jimbow K, Sugiyama S. Comparison of macromelanosomes and autophagic giant melanosome complexes in nevocellular nevi, lentigo simplex and malignant melanoma. *J Cutan Pathol.* 1982;9(5):329–339.

64. Lever WF, Schaumber-Lever G. *Histopathology of the Skin.* 7th ed. J.B. Lippincott; 1990.

65. Plasmeijer EI, Nguyen TM, Olsen CM, Janda M, Soyer HP, Green AC. The natural history of common melanocytic nevi: a systematic review of longitudinal studies in the general population. *J Invest Dermatol.* 2017;137(9):2017–2018.

66. Moreno S, Maiques O, Gatius S, et al. Descriptive study of naevus involution in a series of 74 patients with atypical naevus syndrome under SIAscopy digital follow-up. *J Eur Acad Dermatol Venereol.* 2020;34(6):1210–1217.

67. Shoji T, Cockerell CJ, Koff AB, Bhawan J. Eruptive melanocytic nevi after Stevens-Johnson syndrome. *J Am Acad Dermatol.* 1997;37:337–339.

68. Richert S, Bloom EJ, Flynn K, Seraly MP. Widespread eruptive dermal and atypical melanocytic nevi in association with chronic myelocytic leukemia: case report and review of the literature. *J Am Acad Dermatol.* 1996;35(2 Pt. 2):326–329.

69. Bovenschen HJ, Tjioe M, Vermaat H, et al. Induction of eruptive benign melanocytic naevi by immune suppressive agents, including biologicals. *Br J Dermatol.* 2006;154(5):880–884.

70. Kadhiravan T, Sharma SK. Images in clinical medicine. Giant congenital nevus. *N Engl J Med.* 2009;361(10):e15.

71. Zhong Y, Huang L, Chen Y, Yan T, Yang B, Man MQ. The efficacy of intense pulsed light for Becker's nevus: a retrospective analysis of 45 cases. *J Cosmet Dermatol.* 2021;20(2):466–471.

72. Whimster IW. Recurrent pigment cell naevi and their significance in the problem of endogenous carcinogenesis. *Ann Ital Dermatol Clin Sper.* 1965;19:168–191.

73. Hafner C, Stoehr R, van Oers JM, et al. The absence of BRAF, FGFR3, and PIK3CA mutations differentiates lentigo simplex from melanocytic nevus and solar lentigo. *J Invest Dermatol.* 2009;129(11):2730–2735.

74. Eng AM. Solitary small active junctional nevi in juvenile patients. *Arch Dermatol.* 1983;119(1):35–38.

75. Worret WI, Burgdorf WH. Which direction do nevus cells move? Abtropfung reexamined. *Am J Dermatopathol.* 1998;20:135–139.

76. Masson P. My conception of cellular nevi. *Cancer.* 1951;4:19–38.

77. Fullen DR, Reed JA, Finnerty B, McNutt NS. S100A6 preferentially labels type C nevus cells and nevic corpuscles: additional support for Schwannian differentiation of intradermal nevi. *J Cutan Pathol.* 2001;28(8):393–399.

78. Goovaerts G, Buyssens N. Nevus cell maturation or atrophy. *Am J Dermatopathol.* 1988;10:20–27.

79. Barnhill RL, Cerroni L, Cook M, et al. State of the art, nomenclature, and points of consensus and controversy concerning benign melanocytic lesions: outcome of an international workshop. *Adv Anat Pathol.* 2010;17(2):73–90.

80. Gray-Schopfer VC, Cheong SC, Chong H, et al. Cellular senescence in naevi and immortalisation in melanoma: a role for p16? *Br J Cancer.* 2006;95(4):496–505.

81. Taylor LA, O'Day C, Dentchev T, et al. p15 Expression differentiates nevus from melanoma. *Am J Pathol.* 2016;186(12):3094–3099.

82. Tran S, Rizos H. Human nevi lack distinguishing senescence traits. *Aging (Albany NY).* 2013;5(2):98–99.

83. Smolle J, Smolle-Juettner FM, Stettner H, Kerl H. Relationship of tumor cell motility and morphologic patterns. Part 1. Melanocytic skin tumors. *Am J Dermatopathol.* 1992;14(3):231–237.

84. Rhodes AR, Silverman RA, Harrist TJ, Melski JW. A histologic comparison of congenital and acquired nevomelanocytic nevi. *Arch Dermatol.* 1985;121:1266–1273.

85. Sagebiel RW. Histologic artifacts of benign pigmented nevi. *Arch Dermatol.* 1972;106:691–693.

86. Gray MH, Smoller BR, McNutt NS, Hsu A. Neurofibromas and neurotized melanocytic nevi are immunohistochemically distinct neoplasms. *Am J Dermatopathol.* 1990;12(3):234–241.

87. Penneys NS, Mogollon R, Kowalczyk A, Nadji M, Adachi K. A survey of cutaneous neural lesions for the presence of myelin basic protein. An immunohistochemical study. *Arch Dermatol.* 1984;120(2):210–213.

88. Foucar E, Bentley TJ, Laube DW, Rosai J. A histopathologic evaluation of nevocellular nevi in pregnancy. *Arch Dermatol.* 1985;121:350–354.

89. O'Rourke EA, Balzer B, Barry CI, Frishberg DP. Nevic mitoses: a review of 1041 cases. *Am J Dermatopathol.* 2013;35(1):30–33.

90. Zembowicz A, McCusker M, Chiarelli C, et al. Morphological analysis of nevoid melanoma: a study of 20 cases with a review of the literature. *Am J Dermatopathol.* 2001;23(3):167–175.

91. Mesbah Ardakani N, Singh S, Thomas C, et al. Mitotically active nevus and nevoid melanoma: a Clinicopathological and Molecular Study. *Am J Dermatopathol.* 2020;43(3):182–190.

92. Jackett LA, Colebatch AJ, Rawson RV, et al. Molecular profiling of noncoding mutations distinguishes nevoid melanomas from mitotically active nevi in pregnancy. *Am J Surg Pathol.* 2020;44(3):357–367.

93. Ribero S, Zugna D, Spector T, Bataille V. Natural history of naevi: a two-wave study. *Br J Dermatol.* 2020;184(2):289–295.

94. Maize JC, Foster G. Age-related changes in melanocytic naevi. *Clin Exp Dermatol.* 1979;4(1):49–58.

95. Zalaudek I, Grinschgl S, Argenziano G, et al. Age-related prevalence of dermoscopy patterns in acquired melanocytic naevi. *Br J Dermatol.* 2006;154(2):299–304.

96. Davies H, Bignell GR, Cox C, et al. Mutations of the BRAF gene in human cancer. *Nature.* 2002;417(6892):949–954.

97. Pollock PM, Harper UL, Hansen KS, et al. High frequency of BRAF mutations in nevi. *Nat Genet.* 2003;33(1):19–20.

98. Carr J, MacKie RM. Point mutations in the N-ras oncogene in malignant melanoma and congenital naevi. *Br J Dermatol.* 1994;131(1):72–77.

99. Papp T, Pemsel H, Zimmermann R, Bastrop R, Weiss DG, Schiffmann D. Mutational analysis of the N-ras, p53, p16INK4a, CDK4, and MC1R genes in human congenital melanocytic naevi. *J Med Genet.* 1999;36:610–614.

100. Yeh I, von DA, Bastian BC. Clonal BRAF mutations in melanocytic nevi and initiating role of BRAF in melanocytic neoplasia. *J Natl Cancer Inst.* 2013;105(12):917–919.

101. Oaxaca G, Billings SD, Ko JS. p16 Range of expression in dermal predominant benign epithelioid and spindled nevi and melanoma. *J Cutan Pathol.* 2020;47(9):815–823.

102. Tang J, Fewings E, Chang D, et al. The genomic landscapes of individual melanocytes from human skin. *Nature.* 2020;586(7830):600–605.

103. Lian CG, Murphy GF. The genetic evolution of melanoma. *N Engl J Med.* 2016;374(10):994–995.

104. Larson AR, Dresser KA, Zhan Q, et al. Loss of 5-hydroxymethylcytosine correlates with increasing morphologic dysplasia in melanocytic tumors. *Mod Pathol.* 2014;27(7):936–944.

105. Lian CG, Xu Y, Ceol C, et al. Loss of 5-hydroxymethylcytosine is an epigenetic hallmark of melanoma. *Cell.* 2012;150(6):1135–1146.

106. MacLennan R, Kelly JW, Rivers JK, Harrison SL. The Eastern Australian Childhood Nevus Study: site differences in density and size of melanocytic nevi in relation to latitude and phenotype. *J Am Acad Dermatol.* 2003;48(3):367–375.

107. Elder DE. Precursors to melanoma and their mimics: nevi of special sites. *Mod Pathol.* 2006;19(suppl 2):S4–S20.

108. Ahn CS, Guerra A, Sangueza OP. Melanocytic nevi of special sites. *Am J Dermatopathol.* 2016;38(12):867–881.

109. Mason AR, Mohr MR, Koch LH, Hood AF. Nevi of special sites. *Clin Lab Med.* 2011;31(2):229–242.

110. Rongioletti F, Ball RA, Marcus R, Barnhill RL. Histopathological features of flexural melanocytic nevi: a study of 40 cases. *J Cutan Pathol.* 2000;27(5):215–217.

111. Fabrizi G, Pagliarello C, Parente P, Massi G. Atypical nevi of the scalp in adolescents. *J Cutan Pathol.* 2007;34(5):365–369.

112. Lazova R, Lester B, Glusac EJ, Handerson T, McNiff J. The characteristic histopathologic features of nevi on and around the ear. *J Cutan Pathol.* 2005;32(1):40–44.

113. Saad AG, Patel S, Mutasim DF. Melanocytic nevi of the auricular region: histologic characteristics and diagnostic difficulties. *Am J Dermatopathol.* 2005;27(2):111–115.

114. Rongioletti F, Urso C, Batolo D, et al. Melanocytic nevi of the breast: a histologic case-control study. *J Cutan Pathol.* 2004;31(2):137–140.

115. Friedman RJ, Ackerman AB. Difficulties in the histologic diagnosis of melanocytic nevi on the vulvae of premenopausal women. In: Ackerman AB, ed. *Pathology of Malignant Melanoma.* Masson; 1981:119–127.

116. Clark WH Jr, Hood AF, Tucker MA, Jampel RM. Atypical melanocytic nevi of the genital type with a discussion of reciprocal parenchymal-stromal interactions in the biology of neoplasia. *Hum Pathol.* 1998;29(1 suppl 1):S1–S24.

117. Maize JC, Ackerman AB. *Pigmented Lesions of the Skin. Clinicopathologic Correlations.* Lea & Febiger; 1987.

118. Rock B, Hood AF, Rock JA. Prospective study of vulvar nevi. *J Am Acad Dermatol.* 1990;22:104–106.

119. Carlson JA, Mu XC, Slominski A, et al. Melanocytic proliferations associated with lichen sclerosus. *Arch Dermatol.* 2002;138(1):77–87.

120. Gleason BC, Hirsch MS, Nucci MR, et al. Atypical genital nevi: a clinicopathologic analysis of 56 cases. *Am J Surg Pathol.* 2008;32(1):51–57.

121. Christensen WN, Friedman KF, Woodruff JD, Hood AF. Histologic characteristics of vulval nevocellular nevi. *J Cutan Pathol.* 1987;14:87–91.

122. Fisher KR, Maize JC Jr, Maize JC Sr. Histologic features of scalp melanocytic nevi. *J Am Acad Dermatol.* 2013;68(3):466–472.

123. Aouthmany M, Weinstein M, Zirwas MJ, Brodell RT. The natural history of halo nevi: a retrospective case series. *J Am Acad Dermatol.* 2012;67(4):582–586.

124. Huynh PM, Lazova R, Bolognia JL. Unusual halo nevi—darkening rather than lightening of the central nevus. *Dermatology.* 2001;202(4):324–327.

125. Mooney MA, Barr RJ, Buxton MG. Halo nevus or halo phenomenon? A study of 142 cases. *J Cutan Pathol.* 1995;22(4):342–348.

126. Brazzelli V, Larizza D, Martinetti M, et al. Halo nevus, rather than vitiligo, is a typical dermatologic finding of turner's syndrome: clinical, genetic, and immunogenetic study in 72 patients. *J Am Acad Dermatol.* 2004;51(3):354–358.

127. Yang Y, Li S, Zhu G, et al. A similar local immune and oxidative stress phenotype in vitiligo and halo nevus. *J Dermatol Sci.* 2017;87(1):50–59.

128. Moretti S, Spallanzani A, Pinzi C, Prignano F, Fabbri P. Fibrosis in regressing melanoma versus nonfibrosis in halo nevus upon melanocyte disappearance: could it be related to a different cytokine microenvironment? *J Cutan Pathol.* 2007;34(4):301–308.

129. Denianke KS, Gottlieb GJ. Granulomatous inflammation in nevi undergoing regression (halo phenomenon): a report of 6 cases. *Am J Dermatopathol.* 2008;30(3):233–235.

130. de Vijlder HC, Westerhof W, Schreuder GM, de Lange P, Claas FH. Difference in pathogenesis between vitiligo vulgaris and halo nevi associated with vitiligo is supported by an HLA Association Study. *Pigment Cell Res.* 2004;17(3):270–274.

131. George EV, Kalen JE, Kapil JP, Motaparthi K. Comparison of the inflammatory infiltrates in tumoral melanosis, regressing nevi, and regressing melanoma. *Am J Dermatopathol.* 2019;41(7):480–487.

132. Musette P, Bachelez H, Flageul B, et al. Immune-mediated destruction of melanocytes in halo nevi is associated with the local expansion of a limited number of T cell clones. *J Immunol.* 1999;162:1789–1794.

133. Meyerson LB. A peculiar papulosquamous eruption involving pigmented nevi. *Arch Dermatol.* 1971;103(5):510–512.

134. Cook-Norris RH, Zic JA, Boyd AS. Meyerson's naevus: a clinical and histopathological study of 11 cases. *Australas J Dermatol.* 2008;49(4):191–195.

135. Pariser RJ. "Nevocentric" erythema multiforme. *J Am Acad Dermatol.* 1994;31:491–492.

136. Elenitsas R, Halpern AC. Eczematous halo reaction in atypical nevi. *J Am Acad Dermatol.* 1996;34:357–361.

137. Fernández-Sartorio C, Alós L, García-Herrera A, Ferrando J, Carrera C. Multiple primary melanoma with the Meyerson phenomenon in a young patient. *Melanoma Res.* 2019;29(3):325–327.

138. Hashimoto K, Bale GF. An electron microscopic study of balloon nevus cells. *Cancer.* 1972;30:530–540.

139. Kornberg R, Ackerman AB. Pseudomelanoma. Recurrent melanocytic nevus following partial surgical removal. *Arch Dermatol.* 1975;111:1588–1590.

140. King R, Hayzen BA, Page RN, Googe PB, Zeagler D, Mihm MC Jr. Recurrent nevus phenomenon: a clinicopathologic study of 357 cases and histologic comparison with melanoma with regression. *Mod Pathol.* 2009;22(5):611–617.

141. Bong JL, Perkins W. Shave excision of benign facial melanocytic naevi: a patient's satisfaction survey. *Dermatol Surg.* 2003;29(3):227–229.

142. Selim MA, Vollmer RT, Herman CM, Pham TT, Turner JW. Melanocytic nevi with nonsurgical trauma: a histopathologic study. *Am J Dermatopathol.* 2007;29(2):134–136.

143. Park HK, Leonard DD, Arrington JHI, Lund HZ. Recurrent melanocytic nevi: clinical and histologic review of 175 cases. *J Am Acad Dermatol.* 1987;17:285–292.

144. Hoang MP, Prieto VG, Burchette JL, Shea CR. Recurrent melanocytic nevus: a histologic and immunohistochemical evaluation. *J Cutan Pathol.* 2001;28(8):400–406.

145. Wang Y, Viennet C, Robin S, Berthon JY, He L, Humbert P. Precise role of dermal fibroblasts on melanocyte pigmentation. *J Dermatol Sci.* 2017;88(2):159–166.

146. Walton KE, Garfield EM, Zhang B, et al. The role of TERT promoter mutations in differentiating recurrent nevi from recurrent melanomas: a retrospective, case-control study. *J Am Acad Dermatol.* 2019;80(3):685–693.

147. Clark WHJ, Reimer RR, Greene MH, Ainsworth AA, Mastrangelo MJ. Origin of familial melanomas from heritable melanocytic lesions. "The B-K mole syndrome." *Arch Dermatol.* 1978;114:732–738.

148. Lynch HT, Frichot BCI, Lynch JF. Familial atypical multiple mole-melanoma syndrome. *J Med Genet.* 1978;15:352–356.

149. Elder DE, Goldman LI, Goldman SC, Greene MH, Clark WHJ. Dysplastic nevus syndrome: a phenotypic association of sporadic cutaneous melanoma. *Cancer.* 1980;46:1787–1794.

150. Rahbari H, Mehregan AH. Sporadic atypical mole syndrome. A report of five nonfamilial B-K mole syndrome-like cases and histopathologic findings. *Arch Dermatol.* 1981;117(6):329–331.

151. Goldstein AM, Tucker MA. Dysplastic nevi and melanoma. *Cancer Epidemiol Biomarkers Prev.* 2013;22(4):528–532.

152. Landi MT, Bishop DT, MacGregor S, et al. Genome-wide association meta-analyses combining multiple risk phenotypes provide insights into the genetic architecture of cutaneous melanoma susceptibility. *Nat Genet.* 2020;52(5):494–504.

153. Pampena R, Kyrgidis A, Lallas A, Moscarella E, Argenziano G, Longo C. A meta-analysis of nevus-associated melanoma: prevalence and practical implications. *J Am Acad Dermatol.* 2017;77(5):938–945.e4.

154. Kaddu S, Smolle J, Zenahlik P, Hofmann-Wellenhof R, Kerl H. Melanoma with benign melanocytic naevus components: reappraisal of clinicopathological features and prognosis. *Melanoma Res.* 2002;12(3):271–278.

155. Duffy K, Grossman D. The dysplastic nevus: from historical perspective to management in the modern era: part I. Historical, histologic, and clinical aspects. *J Am Acad Dermatol.* 2012;67(1):1. e1–16.

156. Duffy K, Grossman D. The dysplastic nevus: from historical perspective to management in the modern era: part II. Molecular aspects and clinical management. *J Am Acad Dermatol.* 2012;67(1):19.e1–12.

157. Tucker MA, Fraser MC, Goldstein AM, et al. A natural history of melanomas and dysplastic nevi: an atlas of lesions in melanoma-prone families. *Cancer.* 2002;94(12):3192–3209.

158. Gandini S, Sera F, Cattaruzza MS, et al. Meta-analysis of risk factors for cutaneous melanoma: I. Common and atypical naevi. *Eur J Cancer.* 2005;41(1):28–44.

159. Ackerman AB, Mihara I. Dysplasia, dysplastic melanocytes, dysplastic nevi, the dysplastic nevus syndrome, and the relation between dysplastic nevi and malignant melanomas. *Hum Pathol.* 1985;16:87–91.

160. Ackerman AB, Briggs PL, Bravo F. Dysplastic nevus, compound type vs. Clark's nevus, compound type. In: Ackerman AB, Briggs PL, Bravo F, eds. *Differential Diagnosis in Dermatopathology III.* 1st ed. Lea & Febiger; 1993:158–161.

161. Reimer RR, Clark WHJ, Greene MH, Ainsworth AM, Fraumeni JFJ. Precursor lesions in familial melanoma. A new genetic preneoplastic syndrome. *JAMA.* 1978;239:744–746.

162. National Institutes of Health Consensus Development Conference Statement on Diagnosis and Treatment of Early Melanoma, January 27–29, 1992. *Am J Dermatopathol.* 1993;15(1):34–43.

163. Shapiro M, Chren MM, Levy RM, et al. Variability in nomenclature used for nevi with architectural disorder and cytologic atypia (microscopically dysplastic nevi) by dermatologists and dermatopathologists. *J Cutan Pathol.* 2004;31(8):523–530.

164. Tucker SB, Horstmann JP, Hertel B, Aranha G, Rosai J. Activation of nevi in patients with malignant melanoma. *Cancer.* 1980;46:822–827.

165. Allen AC. A reorientation on the histogenesis and clinical significance of cutaneous nevi and melanomas. *Cancer.* 1949;2(1):28–56.

166. Halpern AC, Guerry D 4th, Elder DE, Trock B, Synnestvedt M, Humphreys T. Natural history of dysplastic nevi. *J Am Acad Dermatol.* 1993;29(1):51–57.

167. Elder DE. Dysplastic naevi: an update. *Histopathology.* 2010;56(1):112–120.

168. Shea CR, Vollmer RT, Prieto VG. Correlating architectural disorder and cytologic atypia in Clark (dysplastic) melanocytic nevi. *Hum Pathol.* 1999;30:500–505.

169. Clark WH Jr, Tucker MA, Goldstein AM. Parenchymal-stromal interactions in neoplasia—theoretical considerations and observations in melanocytic neoplasia. *Acta Oncol.* 1995;34:749–757.

170. Xiong MY, Rabkin MS, Piepkorn MW, et al. Diameter of dysplastic nevi is a more robust biomarker of increased melanoma risk than degree of histologic dysplasia: a case-control study. *J Am Acad Dermatol.* 2014;71(6):1257–1258.

171. Guerry D, 4th, Synnestvedt M, Elder DE, Schultz D. Lessons from tumor progression: the invasive radial growth phase of melanoma is common, incapable of metastasis, and indolent. *J Invest Dermatol.* 1993;100:342S–345S.

172. Gimotty PA, Elder DE, Fraker DL, et al. Identification of high-risk patients among those diagnosed with thin cutaneous melanomas. *J Clin Oncol.* 2007;25(9):1129–1134.

173. Arumi-Uria M, McNutt NS, Finnerty B. Grading of atypia in nevi: correlation with melanoma risk. *Mod Pathol.* 2003;16(8):764–771.

174. Elder DE, Barnhill RL, Bastian BC, et al. Dysplastic naevi. In: Elder DE, Massi D, Scolyer RA, Willemze R, eds. *WHO Classification of Skin Tumours.* 4th ed. International Agency for Research on Cancer; 2018:82–86.

175. Elder DE, Xu X. The approach to the patient with a difficult melanocytic lesion. *Pathology.* 2004;36(5):428–434.

176. Clemente C, Cochran AJ, Elder DE, et al. Histopathologic diagnosis of dysplastic nevi: concordance among pathologists convened by the World Health Organization Melanoma Programme. *Hum Pathol.* 1991;22(4):313–319.

177. De Wit PEJ, Van't Hof-Grootenboer B, Ruiter DJ, et al. Validity of the histopathological criteria used for diagnosing dysplastic naevi. An interobserver study by the pathology subgroup of the EORTC Malignant Melanoma Cooperative Group. *Eur J Cancer.* 1993;29A:831–839.

178. Piepkorn MW, Barnhill RL, Cannon-Albright LA, et al. A multiobserver, population-based analysis of histologic dysplasia in melanocytic nevi. *J Am Acad Dermatol.* 1994;30(5 Pt. 1):707–714.

179. Shors AR, Kim S, White E, et al. Dysplastic naevi with moderate to severe histological dysplasia: a risk factor for melanoma. *Br J Dermatol.* 2006;155(5):988–993.

180. Tsao H, Bevona C, Goggins W, Quinn T. The transformation rate of moles (melanocytic nevi) into cutaneous melanoma: a population-based estimate. *Arch Dermatol.* 2003;139(3):282–288.

181. Reddy KK, Farber MJ, Bhawan J, Geronemus RG, Rogers GS. Atypical (dysplastic) nevi: outcomes of surgical excision and association with melanoma. *JAMA Dermatol.* 2013;149(8):928–934.

182. Tallon B, Snow J. Low clinically significant rate of recurrence in benign nevi. *Am J Dermatopathol.* 2012;34(7):706–709.

183. Goodson AG, Florell SR, Boucher KM, Grossman D. Low rates of clinical recurrence after biopsy of benign to moderately dysplastic melanocytic nevi. *J Am Acad Dermatol.* 2010;62(4):591–596.

184. Fleming NH, Shaub AR, Bailey E, Swetter SM. Outcomes of surgical re-excision versus observation of severely dysplastic nevi: a single-institution, retrospective cohort study. *J Am Acad Dermatol.* 2020;82(1):238–240.

185. Holly EA, Kelly JW, Shpall SN, Chiu SH. Number of melanocytic nevi as a major risk factor for malignant melanoma. *J Am Acad Dermatol.* 1987;17(3):459–468.

186. McMeniman E, De'Ambrosis K, De'Ambrosis B. Risk factors in a cohort of patients with multiple primary melanoma. *Australas J Dermatol.* 2010;51(4):254–257.

187. Carey WP Jr, Thompson CJ, Synnestvedt M, et al. Dysplastic nevi as a melanoma risk factor in patients with familial melanoma. *Cancer.* 1994;74:3118–3125.

188. Greene M, Clark WHJ, Tucker MA, Kraemer KH, Elder DE, Fraser MC. High risk of malignant melanoma in melanoma-prone families with dysplastic nevi. *Ann Intern Med.* 1985;102:458–465.

189. Cust AE, Drummond M, Bishop DT, et al. Associations of pigmentary and naevus phenotype with melanoma risk in two populations with comparable ancestry but contrasting levels of ambient sun exposure. *J Eur Acad Dermatol Venereol.* 2019;33(10):1874–1885.

190. Rishpon A, Navarrete-Dechent C, Marghoob AA, et al. Melanoma risk stratification of individuals with a high-risk naevus phenotype—a pilot study. *Australas J Dermatol.* 2019;60(4):e292–e297.

191. Annessi G, Cattaruzza MS, Abeni D, et al. Correlation between clinical atypia and histologic dysplasia in acquired melanocytic nevi. *J Am Acad Dermatol.* 2001;45(1 Pt. 1):77–85.

192. Augustsson A, Stierner U, Rosdahl I, Suurkula M. Common and dysplastic naevi as risk factors for cutaneous malignant melanoma in a Swedish population. *Acta Derm Venereol.* 1991;71(6):518–524.

193. Sagebiel RW, Banda PW, Schneider JS, Crutcher WA. Age distribution and histologic patterns of dysplastic nevi. *J Am Acad Dermatol.* 1985;13:975–982.

194. Urso C, Bondi R, Balzi M, et al. Cell kinetics of melanocytes in common and dysplastic nevi and in primary and metastatic cutaneous melanoma. *Pathol Res Pract.* 1992;188(3):323–329.

195. Jimbow K, Horikoshi T, Takahashi H, Akutsu Y, Maeda K. Fine structural and immunohistochemical properties of dysplastic melanocytic nevi: comparison with malignant melanoma. *J Invest Dermatol.* 1989;92(5 suppl):304S–309S.

196. Hussein MR. Melanocytic dysplastic naevi occupy the middle ground between benign melanocytic naevi and cutaneous malignant melanomas: emerging clues. *J Clin Pathol.* 2005;58(5):453–456.

197. Elder DE, Rodeck U, Thurin J, et al. Antigenic profile of tumor progression stages in human melanocytic nevi and melanomas. *Cancer Res.* 1989;49:5091–5096.

198. Gao K, Dai DL, Martinka M, Li G. Prognostic significance of nuclear factor-{kappa}B p105/p50 in human melanoma and its role in cell migration. *Cancer Res.* 2006;66(17):8382–8388.

199. Ding Y, Prieto VG, Zhang PS, et al. Nuclear expression of the antiapoptotic protein survivin in malignant melanoma. *Cancer.* 2006;106(5):1123–1129.

200. Salopek TG, Yamada K, Ito S, Jimbow K. Dysplastic melanocytic nevi contain high levels of pheomelanin: quantitative comparison of pheomelanin/eumelanin levels between normal skin, common nevi, and dysplastic nevi. *Pigment Cell Res.* 1991;4(4):172–179.

201. Pavel S, van Nieuwpoort F, Van Der MH, et al. Disturbed melanin synthesis and chronic oxidative stress in dysplastic naevi. *Eur J Cancer.* 2004;40(9):1423–1430.

202. Quiohilag K, Caie P, Oniscu A, Brenn T, Harrison D. The differential expression of micro-RNAs 21, 200c, 204, 205, and 211 in benign, dysplastic and malignant melanocytic lesions and critical evaluation of their role as diagnostic biomarkers. *Virchows Arch.* 2020;477(1):121–130.

203. Tran TP, Titus-Ernstoff L, Perry AE, Ernstoff MS, Newsham IF. Alteration of chromosome 9p21 and/or p16 in benign and dysplastic nevi suggests a role in early melanoma progression (United States). *Cancer Causes Control.* 2002;13(7):675–682.

204. Melamed RD, Aydin IT, Rajan GS, et al. Genomic characterization of dysplastic nevi unveils implications for diagnosis of melanoma. *J Invest Dermatol.* 2017;137(4):905–909.

205. Korabiowska M, Brinck U, Kellner S, Droese M, Berger H. Relation between two independent DNA-repair pathways in different groups of naevi. *In Vivo.* 1999;13:243–245.

206. Palmieri G, Ascierto PA, Cossu A, et al. Assessment of genetic instability in melanocytic skin lesions through microsatellite analysis of benign naevi, dysplastic naevi, and primary melanomas and their metastases. *Melanoma Res.* 2003;13(2):167–170.

207. Rubben A, Bogdan I, Grussendorf-Conen EI, Burg G, Boni R. Loss of heterozygosity and microsatellite instability in acquired melanocytic nevi: towards a molecular definition of the dysplastic nevus. *Recent Results Cancer Res.* 2002;160:100–110.

208. Hussein MR, Wood GS. Microsatellite instability in human melanocytic skin tumors: an incidental finding or a pathogenetic mechanism? *J Cutan Pathol.* 2002;29(1):1–4.

209. Hussein MR, Sun M, Tuthill RJ, et al. Comprehensive analysis of 112 melanocytic skin lesions demonstrates microsatellite instability in melanomas and dysplastic nevi, but not in benign nevi. *J Cutan Pathol.* 2001;28(7):343–350.

210. Birindelli S, Tragni G, Bartoli C, et al. Detection of microsatellite alterations in the spectrum of melanocytic nevi in patients with or without individual or family history of melanoma. *Int J Cancer.* 2000;86:255–261.

211. Shain AH, Yeh I, Kovalyshyn I, et al. The genetic evolution of melanoma from precursor lesions. *N Engl J Med.* 2015;373(20):1926–1936.

212. Uguen A, Uguen M, Guibourg B, Talagas M, Marcorelles P, De Braekeleer M. The p16-Ki-67-HMB45 immunohistochemistry scoring system is highly concordant with the fluorescent in situ hybridization test to differentiate between melanocytic

213. Tripp JM, Kopf AW, Marghoob AA, Bart RS. Management of dysplastic nevi: a survey of fellows of the American Academy of Dermatology. *J Am Acad Dermatol.* 2002;46(5):674–682.

214. Tessiatore KM, Choi H, Kumar A, Patel NS. Survey analysis on the management of moderately dysplastic nevi among academic dermatologists across the United States. *J Am Acad Dermatol.* 2019;80(1):278–280.

215. Kim CC, Berry EG, Marchetti MA, et al. Risk of subsequent cutaneous melanoma in moderately dysplastic nevi excisionally biopsied but with positive histologic margins. *JAMA Dermatol.* 2018;154(12):1401–1408.

216. Masri GD, Clark WHJ, Guerry DI, Halpern A, Thompson CJ, Elder DE. Screening and surveillance of patients at high risk for malignant melanoma result in detection of earlier disease. *J Am Acad Dermatol.* 1990;22:1042–1048.

217. Tucker MA, Elder DE, Curry M, et al. Risks of melanoma and other cancers in melanoma-prone families over 4 decades. *J Invest Dermatol.* 2018;138(7):1620–1626.

218. Leachman SA, Carucci J, Kohlmann W, et al. Selection criteria for genetic assessment of patients with familial melanoma. *J Am Acad Dermatol.* 2009;61(4):677.e1–14.

219. Seab JAJ, Graham JH, Helwig EB. Deep penetrating nevus. *Am J Surg Pathol.* 1989;13:39–44.

220. Barnhill RL, Mihm MC Jr, Magro CM. Plexiform spindle cell naevus: a distinctive variant of plexiform melanocytic naevus. *Histopathology.* 1991;18(3):243–247.

221. Yeh I, Lang UE, Durieux E, et al. Combined activation of MAP kinase pathway and beta-catenin signaling cause deep penetrating nevi. *Nat Commun.* 2017;8(1):644.

222. Šekoranja D, Vergot K, Hawlina G, Pižem J. Combined deep penetrating nevi of the conjunctiva are relatively common lesions characterised by BRAFV600E mutation and activation of the beta catenin pathway: a clinicopathological analysis of 34 lesions. *Br J Ophthalmol.* 2020;104(7):1016–1021.

223. Magro CM, Crowson AN, Mihm MC Jr, Gupta K, Walker MJ, Solomon G. The dermal-based borderline melanocytic tumor: a categorical approach. *J Am Acad Dermatol.* 2010;62(3):469–479.

224. Cosgarea I, Griewank KG, Ungureanu L, Tamayo A, Siepmann T. Deep penetrating nevus and borderline-deep penetrating nevus: a literature review. *Front Oncol.* 2020;10:837.

225. High WA, Alanen KW, Golitz LE. Is melanocytic nevus with focal atypical epithelioid components (clonal nevus) a superficial variant of deep penetrating nevus? *J Am Acad Dermatol.* 2006;55(3):460–466.

226. Magro CM, Abraham RM, Guo R, et al. Deep penetrating nevus-like borderline tumors: a unique subset of ambiguous melanocytic tumors with malignant potential and normal cytogenetics. *Eur J Dermatol.* 2014;24(5):594–602.

227. Abraham RM, Ming ME, Elder DE, Xu X. An atypical melanocytic lesion without genomic abnormalities shows locoregional metastasis. *J Cutan Pathol.* 2012;39(1):21–24.

228. Isales MC, Khan AU, Zhang B, et al. Molecular analysis of atypical deep penetrating nevus progressing to melanoma. *J Cutan Pathol.* 2020;47(12):1150–1154.

229. Mehregan DR, Mehregan DA, Mehregan AH. Proliferating cell nuclear antigen staining in deep-penetrating nevi. *J Am Acad Dermatol.* 1995;33:685–687.

230. Dadras SS, Lu J, Zembowicz A, Flotte TJ, Mihm MC. Histological features and outcome of inverted type-A melanocytic nevi. *J Cutan Pathol.* 2018;45(4):254–262.

231. de la Fouchardiere A, Blokx W, van Kempen LC, et al. ESP, EORTC, and EURACAN Expert Opinion: practical recommendations for the pathological diagnosis and clinical management of intermediate melanocytic tumors and rare related melanoma variants. *Virchows Arch.* 2021;479(1):3–11.

232. Zembowicz A, Carney JA, Mihm MC. Pigmented epithelioid melanocytoma: a low-grade melanocytic tumor with metastatic potential indistinguishable from animal-type melanoma and epithelioid blue nevus. *Am J Surg Pathol.* 2004;28(1):31–40.

233. Cohen JN, Yeh I, Mully TW, LeBoit PE, McCalmont TH. Genomic and clinicopathologic characteristics of PRKAR1A-inactivated melanomas: toward genetic distinctions of animal-type melanoma/pigment synthesizing melanoma. *Am J Surg Pathol.* 2020;44(6):805–816.

234. Carney JA, Ferreiro JA. The epithelioid blue nevus. A multicentric familial tumor with important associations, including cardiac myxoma and psammomatous melanotic schwannoma. *Am J Surg Pathol.* 1996;20(3):259–272.

235. Zembowicz A, Knoepp SM, Bei T, et al. Loss of expression of protein kinase a regulatory subunit 1alpha in pigmented epithelioid melanocytoma but not in melanoma or other melanocytic lesions. *Am J Surg Pathol.* 2007;31(11):1764–1775.

236. Antony FC, Sanclemente G, Shaikh H, Trelles AS, Calonje E. Pigment synthesizing melanoma (so-called animal type melanoma): a clinicopathological study of 14 cases of a poorly known distinctive variant of melanoma. *Histopathology.* 2006;48(6):754–762.

237. Stratakis CA, Kirschner LS, Carney JA. Clinical and molecular features of the Carney complex: diagnostic criteria and recommendations for patient evaluation. *J Clin Endocrinol Metab.* 2001;86(9):4041–4046.

238. Williams EA, Shah N, Danziger N, et al. Clinical, histopathologic, and molecular profiles of PRKAR1A-inactivated melanocytic neoplasms. *J Am Acad Dermatol.* 2020;84(4):1069–1071.

239. Wiesner T, Obenauf AC, Murali R, et al. Germline mutations in BAP1 predispose to melanocytic tumors. *Nat Genet.* 2011;43(10):1018–1021.

240. Wiesner T, Murali R, Fried I, et al. A distinct subset of atypical Spitz tumors is characterized by BRAF mutation and loss of BAP1 expression. *Am J Surg Pathol.* 2012;36(6):818–830.

241. Zhang AJ, Rush PS, Tsao H, Duncan LM. BRCA1-associated protein (BAP1)-inactivated melanocytic tumors. *J Cutan Pathol.* 2019;46(12):965–972.

242. Haugh AM, Njauw CN, Bubley JA, et al. Genotypic and phenotypic features of BAP1 cancer syndrome: a report of 8 new families and review of cases in the literature. *JAMA Dermatol.* 2017;153(10):999–1006.

243. Garfield EM, Walton KE, Quan VL, et al. Histomorphologic spectrum of germline-related and sporadic BAP1-inactivated melanocytic tumors. *J Am Acad Dermatol.* 2018;79(3):525–534.

244. Bastian BC, de la Fouchardiere A, Elder DE, et al. Genomic landscape of melanoma. In: Elder DE, Massi D, Scolyer RA, Willemze R, eds. *WHO Classification of Skin Tumours.* 4th ed. IARC; 2018:72–75.

245. Xu X, Bellucci KS, Elenitsas R, Elder DE. Cellular nodules in congenital pattern nevi. *J Cutan Pathol.* 2004;31(2):153–159.

246. Linos K, Atkinson AE, Yan S, Tsongalis GJ, Lefferts JA. A case of molecularly confirmed BAP1 inactivated melanocytic tumor with retention of immunohistochemical expression: a confounding factor. *J Cutan Pathol.* 2020;47(5):485–489.

247. Wiesner T, Mihm MCJ, Scolyer RA. Combined naevus, including BAP1-inactivated naevus/melanocytoma. In: Elder DE, Massi D, Scolyer RA, Willemze R, eds. *WHO Classification of Skin Tumors.* 4th ed. IARC; 2018:99–101.

248. Scolyer RA, Zhuang L, Palmer AA, Thompson JF, McCarthy SW. Combined naevus: a benign lesion frequently misdiagnosed both clinically and pathologically as melanoma. *Pathology.* 2004;36(5):419–427.

249. Pulitzer DR, Martin PC, Cohen AP, Reed RJ. Histologic classification of the combined nevus: analysis of the variable expression of melanocytic nevi. *Am J Surg Pathol.* 1991;15:1111–1122.

250. Wee E, Wolfe R, McLean C, Kelly JW, Pan Y. The anatomic distribution of cutaneous melanoma: a detailed study of 5141 lesions. *Australas J Dermatol.* 2020;61(2):125–133.

251. Clark WHJ, From L, Bernardino EA, Mihm MCJ. The histogenesis and biologic behavior of primary human malignant melanomas of the skin. *Cancer Res.* 1969;29:705–727.

252. Clark WHJ, Mihm MCJ. Lentigo maligna and lentigo-maligna melanoma. *Am J Pathol.* 1969;55:39–67.

253. Arrington JH 3rd, Reed RJ, Ichinose H, Krementz ET. Plantar lentiginous melanoma: a distinctive variant of human cutaneous malignant melanoma. *Am J Surg Pathol.* 1977;1:131–143.

254. McGovern VJ. The classification of melanoma and its relationship with prognosis. *Pathology.* 1970;2(2):85–98.

255. McGovern VJ, Cochran AJ, Van der EEP, Little JH, MacLennan R. The classification of malignant melanoma, its histological reporting and registration: a revision of the 1972 Sydney classification. *Pathology.* 1986;18:12–21.

256. Ackerman AB. Malignant melanoma: a unifying concept. *Hum Pathol.* 1980;11(6):591–595.

257. Flotte TJ, Mihm MCJ. Melanoma: the art versus the science of dermatopathology. *Hum Pathol.* 1986;17:441–442.

258. Viros A, Fridlyand J, Bauer J, et al. Improving melanoma classification by integrating genetic and morphologic features. *PLoS Med.* 2008;5(6):e120.

259. Broekaert SM, Roy R, Okamoto I, et al. Genetic and morphologic features for melanoma classification. *Pigment Cell Melanoma Res.* 2010;23(6):763–770.

260. Bono A, Bartoli C, Baldi M, et al. Narrower surgical margins might be sufficient in invasive horizontal growth phase melanoma. *Tumori.* 2004;90(5):464–466.

261. Rigel DS, Friedman RJ. The rationale of the ABCDs of early melanoma. *J Am Acad Dermatol.* 1993;29:1060–1061.

262. Scope A, Dusza SW, Halpern AC, et al. The "ugly duckling" sign: agreement between observers. *Arch Dermatol.* 2008;144(1):58–64.

263. Mar V, Roberts H, Wolfe R, English DR, Kelly JW. Nodular melanoma: a distinct clinical entity and the largest contributor to melanoma deaths in Victoria, Australia. *J Am Acad Dermatol.* 2012;68(4):568–575.

264. Elder DE, Guerry DI, Epstein MN, et al. Invasive malignant melanomas lacking competence for metastasis. *Am J Dermatopathol.* 1984;6:55–62.

265. Reed RJ, Ichinose H, Clark WHJ, Mihm MCJ. Common and uncommon melanocytic nevi and borderline melanomas. *Semin Oncol.* 1975;2:119–147.

266. Cook MG, Clarke TJ, Humphreys S, et al. The evaluation of diagnostic and prognostic criteria and the terminology of thin cutaneous melanoma by the CRC Melanoma Pathology Panel. *Histopathology.* 1996;28:497–512.

267. Lefevre M, Vergier B, Balme B, et al. Relevance of vertical growth pattern in thin level II cutaneous superficial spreading melanomas. *Am J Surg Pathol.* 2003;27(6):717–724.

268. Meier F, Satyamoorthy K, Nesbit M, et al. Molecular events in melanoma development and progression. *Front Biosci.* 1998;3:D1005–D1010.

269. Appleton SE, Fadel Z, Williams JS, Bezuhly M. Vertical growth phase as a prognostic factor for sentinel lymph node positivity in thin melanomas: a systematic review and meta-analysis. *Plast Reconstr Surg.* 2018;141(6):1529–1540.

270. Coit DG, Thompson JA, Albertini MR, et al. Cutaneous melanoma, version 2.2019, NCCN Clinical Practice Guidelines in Oncology. *J Natl Compr Canc Netw.* 2019;17(4):367–402.

271. Satyamoorthy K, Li G, Gerrero MR, et al. Constitutive mitogen-activated protein kinase activation in melanoma is mediated by both BRAF mutations and autocrine growth factor stimulation. *Cancer Res.* 2003;63(4):756–759.

272. Omholt K, Karsberg S, Platz A, Kanter L, Ringborg U, Hansson J. Screening of N-ras Codon 61 mutations in paired primary and metastatic cutaneous melanomas: mutations occur early and persist throughout tumor progression. *Clin Cancer Res.* 2002;8(11):3468–3474.

273. Demunter A, Stas M, Degreef H, Wolf-Peeters C, Van den Oord JJ. Analysis of N-and k-ras mutations in the distinctive tumor progression phases of melanoma. *J Invest Dermatol.* 2001;117(6):1483–1489.

274. Beadling C, Jacobson-Dunlop E, Hodi FS, et al. KIT gene mutations and copy number in melanoma subtypes. *Clin Cancer Res.* 2008;14(21):6821–6828.

275. Shain AH, Garrido M, Botton T, et al. Exome sequencing of desmoplastic melanoma identifies recurrent NFKBIE promoter mutations and diverse activating mutations in the MAPK pathway. *Nat Genet.* 2015;47(10):1194–1199.

276. Williams EA, Montesion M, Shah N, et al. Melanoma with in-frame deletion of MAP2K1: a distinct molecular subtype of cutaneous melanoma mutually exclusive from BRAF, NRAS, and NF1 mutations. *Mod Pathol.* 2020;33(12):2397–2406.

277. Mar VJ, Wong SQ, Li J, et al. BRAF/NRAS wild-type melanomas have a high mutation load correlating with histological and molecular signatures of UV damage. *Clin Cancer Res.* 2013;19(7):4589–4598.

278. Turner J, Couts K, Sheren J, et al. Kinase gene fusions in defined subsets of melanoma. *Pigment Cell Melanoma Res.* 2017;30(1):53–62.

279. Williams EA, Shah N, Montesion M, et al. Melanomas with activating RAF1 fusions: clinical, histopathologic, and molecular profiles. *Mod Pathol.* 2020;33(8):1466–1474.

280. Papp T, Pemsel H, Rollwitz I, et al. Mutational analysis of N-ras, p53, CDKN2A (p16(INK4a)), p14(ARF), CDK4, and MC1R genes in human dysplastic melanocytic naevi. *J Med Genet.* 2003;40(2):E14.

281. Shaughnessy M, Njauw CN, Artomov M, Tsao H. Classifying melanoma by TERT promoter mutational status. *J Invest Dermatol.* 2020;140(2):390–394.e1.

282. Sargen MR, Cloutier JM, Sarin KY, et al. Biomarker discovery analysis: alterations in p14, p16, p53, and BAP1 expression in nevi, cutaneous melanoma, and metastatic melanoma. *Pigment Cell Melanoma Res.* 2019;32(3):474–478.

283. Lee WJ, Skalamera D, Dahmer-Heath M, et al. Genome-wide overexpression screen identifies genes able to bypass p16-mediated senescence in melanoma. *SLAS Discov.* 2017;22(3):298–308.

284. Costa S, Byrne M, Pissaloux D, et al. Melanomas associated with blue nevi or mimicking cellular blue nevi: clinical, pathologic, and molecular study of 11 cases displaying a high frequency of GNA11 mutations, BAP1 expression loss, and a predilection for the scalp. *Am J Surg Pathol.* 2016;40(3):368–377.

285. Venza M, Visalli M, Biondo C, et al. Epigenetic regulation of p14(ARF) and p16(INK4A) expression in cutaneous and uveal melanoma. *Biochim Biophys Acta.* 2015;1849(3):247–256.

286. Salgado C, Oosting J, Janssen B, Kumar R, Gruis N, van Doorn R. Genome-wide characterization of 5-hydroxymethylcytosine in melanoma reveals major differences with nevus. *Genes Chromosomes Cancer.* 2020;59(6):366–374.

287. Shaikh WR, Xiong M, Weinstock MA. The contribution of nodular subtype to melanoma mortality in the United States, 1978 to 2007. *Arch Dermatol.* 2012;148(1):30–36.

288. Price NM, Rywlin AM, Ackerman AB. Histologic criteria for the diagnosis of superficial spreading melanoma: formulated on the basis of proven metastatic lesions. *Cancer.* 1976;38:2434–2441.

289. Lezcano C, Jungbluth AA, Nehal KS, Hollmann TJ, Busam KJ. PRAME expression in melanocytic tumors. *Am J Surg Pathol.* 2018;42(11):1456–1465.

290. Gerami P, Li G, Pouryazdanparast P, et al. A highly specific and discriminatory FISH assay for distinguishing between benign and malignant melanocytic neoplasms. *Am J Surg Pathol.* 2012;36(6):808–817.

291. Clarke LE, Flake DD, Busam K, et al. An independent validation of a gene expression signature to differentiate malignant melanoma from benign melanocytic nevi. *Cancer.* 2017;123(4):617–628.

292. Zhang J, Miller CJ, Sobanko JF, Shin TM, Etzkorn JR. Frequency of and factors associated with positive or equivocal margins in conventional excision of atypical intraepidermal melanocytic proliferations (AIMP): a single academic institution cross-sectional study. *J Am Acad Dermatol.* 2016;75(4):688–695.

293. Roncati L, Piscioli F, Pusiol T. SAMPUS, MELTUMP and THIMUMP—diagnostic categories characterized by uncertain biological behavior. *Klin Onkol.* 2017;30(3):221–223.

294. Pusiol T, Piscioli F, Speziali L, Zorzi MG, Morichetti D, Roncati L. Clinical features, dermoscopic patterns, and histological diagnostic model for Melanocytic Tumors of Uncertain Malignant Potential (MELTUMP). *Acta Dermatovenerol Croat.* 2015;23(3):185–194.

295. Mooi WJ. "Lentiginous melanoma": full-fledged melanoma or melanoma precursor? *Adv Anat Pathol.* 2014;21(3):181–187.

296. Clark WHJ, Elder DE, Van Horn M. The biologic forms of malignant melanoma. *Hum Pathol.* 1986;5:443–450.

297. Nakhleh RE, Wick MR, Rocamora A, Swanson PE, Dehner LP. Morphologic diversity in malignant melanomas. *Am J Clin Pathol.* 1990;93:731–740.

298. Chang ES, Wick MR, Swanson PE, Dehner LP. Metastatic malignant melanoma with "rhabdoid" features. *Am J Clin Pathol.* 1994;102:426–431.

299. Ishida M, Iwai M, Yoshida K, Kagotani A, Okabe H. Rhabdoid melanoma: a case report with review of the literature. *Int J Clin Exp Pathol.* 2014;7(2):840–843.

300. Trevisan F, Tregnago AC, Lopes Pinto CA, et al. Osteogenic melanoma with desmin expression. *Am J Dermatopathol.* 2016;39(7):528–533.

301. Allais BS, Beatson M, Wang H, et al. Five-year survival in patients with nodular and superficial spreading melanomas in the US population. *J Am Acad Dermatol.* 2020;84(4):1015–1022.

302. Kelly JW, Chamberlain AJ, Staples MP, McAvoy B. Nodular melanoma. No longer as simple as ABC. *Aust Fam Physician.* 2003;32(9):706–709.

303. Heenan PJ, Holman CD. Nodular malignant melanoma: a distinct entity or a common end stage? *Am J Dermatopathol.* 1982;4:477–478.

304. Harris CG, Lo S, Ahmed T, et al. Primary dermal melanoma: clinical behaviour, prognosis and treatment. *Eur J Surg Oncol.* 2020;46(11):2131–2139.

305. Hantschke M, Bastian BC, LeBoit PE. Consumption of the epidermis: a diagnostic criterion for the differential diagnosis of melanoma and Spitz nevus. *Am J Surg Pathol.* 2004;28(12):1621–1625.

306. Blessing K, Evans AT, Al-Nafussi A. Verrucous naevoid and keratotic malignant melanoma: a clinico-pathological study of 20 cases. *Histopathology.* 1993;23:453–458.

307. Gerami P, Barnhill RL, Beilfuss BA, LeBoit P, Schneider P, Guitart J. Superficial melanocytic neoplasms with pagetoid melanocytosis: a study of interobserver concordance and correlation with FISH. *Am J Surg Pathol.* 2010;34(6):816–821.

308. Bowen GM, Chang AE, Lowe L, Hamilton T, Patel R, Johnson TM. Solitary melanoma confined to the dermal and/or subcutaneous tissue: evidence for revisiting the staging classification. *Arch Dermatol.* 2000;136(11):1397–1399.

309. Swetter SM, Ecker PM, Johnson DL, Harvell JD. Primary dermal melanoma: a distinct subtype of melanoma. *Arch Dermatol.* 2004;140(1):99–103.

310. Cassarino DS, Cabral ES, Kartha RV, Swetter SM. Primary dermal melanoma: distinct immunohistochemical findings and clinical outcome compared with nodular and metastatic melanoma. *Arch Dermatol.* 2008;144(1):49–56.

311. Sidiropoulos M, Obregon R, Cooper C, Sholl LM, Guitart J, Gerami P. Primary dermal melanoma: a unique subtype of melanoma to be distinguished from cutaneous metastatic melanoma: a clinical, histologic, and gene expression-profiling study. *J Am Acad Dermatol.* 2014;71(6):1083–1092.

312. Teow J, Chin O, Hanikeri M, Wood BA. Primary dermal melanoma: a West Australian cohort. *ANZ J Surg.* 2015;85(9):664–667.

313. Zamir H, Feinmesser M, Gutman H. Primary Dermal Melanoma (PDM): histological and Clinical Interdependence to Guide Therapy. *J Cutan Med Surg.* 2020;25(1):53–58.

314. Cellier L, Perron E, Pissaloux D, et al. Cutaneous melanocytoma with CRTC1-TRIM11 fusion: report of 5 cases resembling clear cell sarcoma. *Am J Surg Pathol.* 2018;42(3):382–391.

315. de la Fouchardiere A, Pissaloux D, Tirode F, Karanian M, Fletcher CDM, Hanna J. Clear cell tumor with melanocytic differentiation and ACTIN-MITF translocation: report of 7 cases of a novel entity. *Am J Surg Pathol.* 2021;45(7):962–968.

316. Hisaoka M, Ishida T, Kuo TT, et al. Clear cell sarcoma of soft tissue: a clinicopathologic, immunohistochemical, and molecular analysis of 33 cases. *Am J Surg Pathol.* 2008;32(3):452–460.

317. Clark WHJ, Elder DE, Guerry DI, et al. Model predicting survival in stage I melanoma based on tumor progression. *J Natl Cancer Inst.* 1989;81:1893–1904.

318. Mishra K, Barnhill RL, Paddock LE, Fine JA, Berwick M. Histopathologic variables differentially affect melanoma survival by age at diagnosis. *Pigment Cell Melanoma Res.* 2019;32(4):593–600.

319. Paschen A, Schadendorf D. The era of checkpoint inhibition: lessons learned from melanoma. *Recent Results Cancer Res.* 2020;214:169–187.

320. Roncati L, Palmieri B. Adoptive cell transfer (ACT) of autologous tumor-infiltrating lymphocytes (TILs) to treat malignant melanoma: the dawn of a chimeric antigen receptor T (CAR-T) cell therapy from autologous donor. *Int J Dermatol.* 2020;59(7):763–769.

321. Ruhoy SM, Kolker SE, Murry TC. Mitotic activity within dermal melanocytes of benign melanocytic nevi: a study of 100 cases with clinical follow-up. *Am J Dermatopathol.* 2011;33(2):167–172.

322. Ordonez NG. Value of melanocytic-associated immunohistochemical markers in the diagnosis of malignant melanoma: a review and update. *Hum Pathol.* 2013;45(2):191–205.

323. Szumera-Cieckiewicz A, Bosisio F, Teterycz P, et al. SOX10 is as specific as S100 protein in detecting metastases of melanoma in lymph nodes and is recommended for sentinel lymph node assessment. *Eur J Cancer.* 2020;137:175–182.

324. Mohamed A, Gonzalez RS, Lawson D, Wang J, Cohen C. SOX10 expression in malignant melanoma, carcinoma, and normal tissues. *Appl Immunohistochem Mol Morphol.* 2012;21(6):506–510.

325. Agaimy A, Specht K, Stoehr R, et al. Metastatic malignant melanoma with complete loss of differentiation markers (undifferentiated/dedifferentiated melanoma): analysis of 14 patients emphasizing phenotypic plasticity and the value of molecular testing as surrogate diagnostic marker. *Am J Surg Pathol.* 2016;40(2):181–191.

326. Romano RC, Carter JM, Folpe AL. Aberrant intermediate filament and synaptophysin expression is a frequent event in malignant melanoma: an immunohistochemical study of 73 cases. *Mod Pathol.* 2015;28(8):1033–1042.

327. Banerjee SS, Harris M. Morphological and immunophenotypic variations in malignant melanoma. *Histopathology.* 2000;36(5): 387–402.

328. Gru AA, Lu D. Concurrent malignant melanoma and cutaneous involvement by classical Hodgkin lymphoma (CHL) in a 63 year-old man. *Diagn Pathol.* 2013;8(1):135.

329. Plaza JA, Bonneau P, Prieto V, et al. Desmoplastic melanoma: an updated immunohistochemical analysis of 40 cases with a proposal for an additional panel of stains for diagnosis. *J Cutan Pathol.* 2016;43(4):313–323.

330. Rothberg BE, Moeder CB, Kluger H, et al. Nuclear to non-nuclear Pmel17/gp100 expression (HMB45 staining) as a discriminator between benign and malignant melanocytic lesions. *Mod Pathol.* 2008;21(9):1121–1129.

331. Walsh SN, Sanguéza OP. PEComas: a review with emphasis on cutaneous lesions. *Semin Diagn Pathol.* 2009;26(3):123–130.

332. Folpe AL, Mentzel T, Lehr HA, Fisher C, Balzer BL, Weiss SW. Perivascular epithelioid cell neoplasms of soft tissue and gynecologic origin: a clinicopathologic study of 26 cases and review of the literature. *Am J Surg Pathol.* 2005;29(12):1558–1575.

333. Ohsie SJ, Sarantopoulos GP, Cochran AJ, Binder SW. Immunohistochemical characteristics of melanoma. *J Cutan Pathol.* 2008;35(5):433–444.

334. Xu X, Chu AY, Pasha TL, Elder DE, Zhang PJ. Immunoprofile of MITF, tyrosinase, melan-A, and MAGE-1 in HMB45-negative melanomas. *Am J Surg Pathol.* 2002;26(1):82–87.

335. Orchard G. Evaluation of melanocytic neoplasms: application of a pan-melanoma antibody cocktail. *Br J Biomed Sci.* 2002;59(4):196–202.

336. Lazzaro B, Strassburg A. Tumor antigen expression in compound dysplastic nevi and superficial spreading melanoma defined by a panel of nevomelanoma monoclonal antibodies. *Hybridoma.* 1996;15(2):141–146.

337. Ribe A, McNutt NS. S100A6 protein expression is different in Spitz nevi and melanomas. *Mod Pathol.* 2003;16(5):505–511.

338. Chen H, Li Y, Long Y, et al. Increased p16 and p53 protein expression predicts poor prognosis in mucosal melanoma. *Oncotarget.* 2017;8(32):53226–53233.

339. Lopes Carapeto FC, Neves CA, Germano A, et al. Marker protein expression combined with expression heterogeneity is a powerful indicator of malignancy in acral lentiginous melanomas. *Am J Dermatopathol.* 2017;39(2):114–120.

340. Fogt F, Vortmeyer AO, Tahan SR. Nucleolar organizer regions (AgNOR) and Ki-67 immunoreactivity in cutaneous melanocytic lesions. *Am J Dermatopathol.* 1995;17(1):12–17.

341. Hale CS, Qian M, Ma MW, et al. Mitotic rate in melanoma: prognostic value of immunostaining and computer-assisted image analysis. *Am J Surg Pathol.* 2013;37(6):882–889.

342. Vollmer RT. Use of Bayes rule and MIB-1 proliferation index to discriminate Spitz nevus from malignant melanoma. *Am J Clin Pathol.* 2004;122(4):499–505.

343. Li LX, Crotty KA, McCarthy SW, Palmer AA, Kril JJ. A zonal comparison of MIB1-Ki67 immunoreactivity in benign and malignant melanocytic lesions. *Am J Dermatopathol.* 2000;22(6): 489–495.

344. Redon S, Guibourg B, Talagas M, Marcorelles P, Uguen A. A diagnostic algorithm combining immunohistochemistry and molecular cytogenetics to diagnose challenging melanocytic tumors. *Appl Immunohistochem Mol Morphol.* 2017;26(10): 714–720.

345. Lohman ME, Steen A, Grekin RC, North JP. The utility of PRAME staining in identifying malignant transformation of melanocytic nevi. *J Cutan Pathol.* 2021;48(7):856–862.

346. See SHC, Finkelman BS, Yeldandi AV. The diagnostic utility of PRAME and p16 in distinguishing nodal nevi from nodal metastatic melanoma. *Pathol Res Pract.* 2020;216(9):153105.

347. Lee JJ, Cook M, Mihm MC, et al. Loss of the epigenetic mark, 5-Hydroxymethylcytosine, correlates with small cell/nevoid subpopulations and assists in microstaging of human melanoma. *Oncotarget.* 2015;6(35):37995–38004.

348. Lee JJ, Granter SR, Laga AC, et al. 5-Hydroxymethylcytosine expression in metastatic melanoma versus nodal nevus in sentinel lymph node biopsies. *Mod Pathol.* 2014;28(2):218–229.

349. McGinnis KS, Lessin SR, Elder DE, et al. Pathology review of cases presenting to a multidisciplinary pigmented lesion clinic. *Arch Dermatol.* 2002;138(5):617–621.

350. Crowson AN, Magro CM, Mihm MC Jr. Malignant melanoma with prominent pigment synthesis: "animal type" melanoma—a clinical and histological study of six cases with a consideration of other melanocytic neoplasms with prominent pigment synthesis. *Hum Pathol.* 1999;30:543–550.

351. Swetter SM, Thompson JA, Albertini MR, et al. NCCN Guidelines® Insights: Melanoma: Cutaneous, Version 2.2021. *J Natl Compr Canc Netw.* 2021 Apr 1;19(4):364-376.

352. Urso C, Borgognoni L, Saieva C, et al. Sentinel lymph node biopsy in patients with "atypical Spitz tumors." A report on 12 cases. *Hum Pathol.* 2006;37(7):816–823.

353. Su LD, Fullen DR, Sondak VK, Johnson TM, Lowe L. Sentinel lymph node biopsy for patients with problematic spitzoid melanocytic lesions: a report on 18 patients. *Cancer.* 2003;97(2): 499–507.

354. Kelley SW, Cockerell CJ. Sentinel lymph node biopsy as an adjunct to management of histologically difficult to diagnose melanocytic lesions: a proposal. *J Am Acad Dermatol.* 2000;42:527–530.

355. Mihic-Probst D, Zhao J, Saremaslani P, Baer A, Komminoth P, Heitz PU. Spitzoid malignant melanoma with lymph-node metastasis. Is a copy-number loss on chromosome 6q a marker of malignancy? *Virchows Arch.* 2001;439(6):823–826.

356. Gamblin TC, Edington H, Kirkwood JM, Rao UN. Sentinel lymph node biopsy for atypical melanocytic lesions with Spitzoid features. *Ann Surg Oncol.* 2006;13(12):1664–1670.

357. Smith KJ, Barett TL, Skelton HG, Lupton GP, Graham JH. Spindle cell and epithelioid cell nevi with atypia and metastasis (malignant Spitz tumor). *Am J Surg Pathol.* 1989;13:931–939.

358. Busam KJ, Murali R, Pulitzer M, et al. Atypical spitzoid melanocytic tumors with positive sentinel lymph nodes in children and teenagers, and comparison with histologically unambiguous and lethal melanomas. *Am J Surg Pathol.* 2009;33(9):1386–1395.

359. Bartenstein DW, Fisher JM, Stamoulis C, et al. Clinical features and outcomes of spitzoid proliferations in children and adolescents. *Br J Dermatol.* 2019;181(2):366–372.

360. McCormack CJ, Conyers RK, Scolyer RA, et al. Atypical Spitzoid neoplasms: a review of potential markers of biological behavior including sentinel node biopsy. *Melanoma Res.* 2014;24(5):437–447.

361. Lallas A, Kyrgidis A, Ferrara G, et al. Atypical Spitz tumours and sentinel lymph node biopsy: a systematic review. *Lancet Oncol.* 2014;15(4):e178–e183.

362. Temple-Camp CR, Saxe N, King H. Benign and malignant cellular blue nevus. A clinicopathological study of 30 cases. *Am J Dermatopathol.* 1988;10(4):289–296.

363. Dubreuilh MW. De la melanose circonscrite precancereuse. *Ann Dermatol Syphiligr (Paris).* 1912;3:129.

364. Sagebiel RW. Histopathology of borderline and early malignant melanomas. *Am J Surg Pathol.* 1979;3:543–552.

365. Taylor NJ, Thomas NE, Anton-Culver H, et al. Nevus count associations with pigmentary phenotype, histopathological melanoma characteristics and survival from melanoma. *Int J Cancer.* 2016;139(6):1217–1222.

366. Bevona C, Goggins W, Quinn T, Fullerton J, Tsao H. Cutaneous melanomas associated with nevi. *Arch Dermatol.* 2003;139(12):1620–1624.

367. Steiner A, Konrad K, Pehamberger H, Wolff K. Verrucous malignant melanoma. *Arch Dermatol.* 1988;124:1534–1537.

368. Shi K, Compres E, Walton KE, et al. Incorporation of dermoscopy improves inter-observer agreement among dermatopathologists in histologic assessment of melanocytic neoplasms. *Arch Dermatol Res.* 2020;313(2):101–108.

369. Leecy TN, McQuillan P, Harvey NT, et al. Large nested melanoma: a clinicopathological, morphometric and cytogenetic study of 12 cases. *Pathology.* 2020;52(4):431–438.

370. Kutzner H, Metzler G, Argenyi Z, et al. Histological and genetic evidence for a variant of superficial spreading melanoma composed predominantly of large nests. *Mod Pathol.* 2012;25(6):838–845.

371. Mishima Y. Melanocytic and nevocytic malignant melanomas. Cellular and subcellular differentiation. *Cancer.* 1967;20:632–649.

372. Clark WHJ, Ainsworth AM, Bernardino EA, Yang CH Jr, Reed RJ. The developmental biology of primary human malignant melanomas. *Semin Oncol.* 1975;2:83–103.

373. Islami F, Sauer AG, Miller KD, et al. Cutaneous melanomas attributable to ultraviolet radiation exposure by state. *Int J Cancer.* 2020;147(5):1385–1390.

374. Shors AR, Kim S, White E, et al. Dysplastic naevi with moderate to severe histological dysplasia: a risk factor for melanoma. *Br J Dermatol.* 2006 Nov;155(5):988-93.

375. Kvaskoff M, Siskind V, Green AC. Risk factors for lentigo maligna melanoma compared with superficial spreading melanoma: a case-control study in Australia. *Arch Dermatol.* 2011;148(2):164–170.

376. Whiteman DC, Watt P, Purdie DM, Hughes MC, Hayward NK, Green AC. Melanocytic nevi, solar keratoses, and divergent pathways to cutaneous melanoma. *J Natl Cancer Inst.* 2003;95(11):806–812.

377. Maldonado JL, Fridlyand J, Patel H, et al. Determinants of BRAF mutations in primary melanomas. *J Natl Cancer Inst.* 2003;95(24):1878–1890.

378. Elbendary A, Xue R, Valdebran M, et al. Diagnostic criteria in intraepithelial pagetoid neoplasms: a histopathologic study and evaluation of select features in Paget disease, Bowen disease, and melanoma in situ. *Am J Dermatopathol.* 2017;39(6): 419–427.

379. D'Agostino M, Cinelli C, Willard R, Hofmann J, Jellinek N, Robinson-Bostom L. Epidermotropic Merkel cell carcinoma: a case series with histopathologic examination. *J Am Acad Dermatol.* 2010;62(3):463–468.

380. Hutchinson J. Senile freckles. *Arch Surg (London).* 1892;3:319.

381. Flotte TJ, Mihm MC Jr. Lentigo maligna and malignant melanoma in situ, lentigo maligna type. *Hum Pathol.* 1999;30:533–536.

382. Jaimes N, Braun RP, Thomas L, Marghoob AA. Clinical and dermoscopic characteristics of amelanotic melanomas that are not of the nodular subtype. *J Eur Acad Dermatol Venereol.* 2011;26(5):591–596.

383. Weinstock MA, Sober AJ. The risk of progression of lentigo maligna to lentigo maligna melanoma. *Br J Dermatol.* 1987;116: 303–310.

384. Michalik EE, Fitzpatrick TB, Sober AJ. Rapid progression of lentigo maligna to deeply invasive lentigo maligna melanoma. Report of two cases. *Arch Dermatol.* 1983;119(10):831–835.

385. Menzies SW, Liyanarachchi S, Coates E, et al. Estimated risk of progression of lentigo maligna to lentigo maligna melanoma. *Melanoma Res.* 2020;30(2):193–197.

386. Koh HK, Michalik E, Sober AJ, et al. Lentigo maligna melanoma has no better prognosis than other types of melanoma. *J Clin Oncol.* 1984;2:994–1001.

387. Gong HZ, Zheng HY, Li J. The clinical significance of KIT mutations in melanoma: a meta-analysis. *Melanoma Res.* 2018;28(4): 259–270.

388. Farrahi F, Egbert BM, Swetter SM. Histologic similarities between lentigo maligna and dysplastic nevus: importance of clinicopathologic distinction. *J Cutan Pathol.* 2005;32(6):405–412.

389. King R, Page RN, Googe PB, Mihm MC. Lentiginous melanoma: a histologic pattern of melanoma to be distinguished from lentiginous nevus. *Mod Pathol.* 2005;18(10):1397–1401.

390. Kossard S. Atypical lentiginous junctional naevi of the elderly and melanoma. *Australas J Dermatol.* 2002;43(2):93–101.

391. Gradecki SE, Valdes-Rodriguez R, Wick MR, Gru AA. PRAME immunohistochemistry as an adjunct for diagnosis and histological margin assessment in lentigo maligna. *Histopathology.* 2020;78(7):1000–1008.

392. Kelly JW. Following lentigo maligna may not prevent the development of life-threatening melanoma. *Arch Dermatol.* 1992;128(5): 657–660.

393. Speiser J, Tao J, Champlain A, et al. Is melanocyte density our last hope? Comparison of histologic features of photodamaged skin and melanoma in situ after staged surgical excision with concurrent scouting biopsies. *J Cutan Pathol.* 2019;46(8):555–562.

394. Chung HJ, Simkin AD, Bhawan J, Wolpowitz D. "Melanocytic nests arising in lichenoid inflammation": reappraisal of the terminology "melanocytic pseudonests." *Am J Dermatopathol.* 2015;37(12):940–943.

395. Conley J, Lattes R, Orr W. Desmoplastic malignant melanoma (a rare variant of spindle cell melanoma). *Cancer.* 1971;28:914–935.

396. Lens MB, Newton-Bishop JA, Boon AP. Desmoplastic malignant melanoma: a systematic review. *Br J Dermatol.* 2005;152(4): 673–678.

397. Hui JI, Linden KG, Barr RJ. Desmoplastic malignant melanoma of the lip: a report of 6 cases and review of the literature. *J Am Acad Dermatol.* 2002;47(6):863–868.

398. Quinn MJ, Crotty KA, Thompson JF, Coates AS, O'Brien CJ, McCarthy WH. Desmoplastic and desmoplastic neurotropic melanoma: experience with 280 patients [see comments]. *Cancer.* 1998;83:1128–1135.

399. Eroglu Z, Zaretsky JM, Hu-Lieskovan S, et al. High response rate to PD-1 blockade in desmoplastic melanomas. *Nature.* 2018;553(7688):347–350.

400. Wiesner T, Kiuru M, Scott SN, et al. NF1 mutations are common in desmoplastic melanoma. *Am J Surg Pathol.* 2015;39(10): 1357–1362.

401. Tan KB, Moncrieff M, Thompson JF, et al. Subungual melanoma: a study of 124 cases highlighting features of early lesions, potential pitfalls in diagnosis, and guidelines for histologic reporting. *Am J Surg Pathol.* 2007;31(12):1902–1912.

402. Prasad ML, Patel SG, Busam KJ. Primary mucosal desmoplastic melanoma of the head and neck. *Head Neck.* 2004;26(4):373–377.

403. Kiuru M, Patel RM, Busam KJ. Desmoplastic melanocytic nevi with lymphocytic aggregates. *J Cutan Pathol.* 2012;39(10):940–944.

404. Kubo M, Kikuchi K, Nashiro K, et al. Expression of fibrogenic cytokines in desmoplastic malignant melanoma. *Br J Dermatol.* 1998;139(2):192–197.

405. Frydenlund N, Leone DA, Mitchell B, et al. Neurotrophin receptors and perineural invasion in desmoplastic melanoma. *J Am Acad Dermatol.* 2015;72(5):851–858.

406. Emanuel PO, Idrees MT, Leytin A, Kwon EJ, Phelps RG. Aggressive osteogenic desmoplastic melanoma: a case report. *J Cutan Pathol.* 2007;34(5):423–426.

407. Hawkins WG, Busam KJ, Ben-Porat L, et al. Desmoplastic melanoma: a pathologically and clinically distinct form of cutaneous melanoma. *Ann Surg Oncol.* 2005;12(3):207–213.

408. Howard MD, Wee E, Wolfe R, McLean CA, Kelly JW, Pan Y. Differences between pure desmoplastic melanoma and superficial spreading melanoma in terms of survival, distribution and other clinicopathologic features. *J Eur Acad Dermatol Venereol.* 2019;33(10):1899–1906.

409. Miller DD, Emley A, Yang S, et al. Mixed versus pure variants of desmoplastic melanoma: a genetic and immunohistochemical appraisal. *Mod Pathol.* 2012;25(4):505–515.

410. Murali R, Shaw HM, Lai K, et al. Prognostic factors in cutaneous desmoplastic melanoma: a study of 252 patients. *Cancer.* 2010;116(17):4130–4138.

411. Han D, Zager JS, Yu D, et al. Desmoplastic melanoma: is there a role for sentinel lymph node biopsy? *Ann Surg Oncol.* 2013;20(7):2345–2351.

412. Baer SC, Schultz D, Synnestvedt M, Elder DE. Desmoplasia and neurotropism—prognostic variables in patients with stage I melanoma. *Cancer.* 1995;76:2242–2247.

413. Reed RJ, Leonard DD. Neurotropic melanoma. A variant of desmoplastic melanoma. *Am J Surg Pathol.* 1979;3:301–311.

414. Chen JY, Hruby G, Scolyer RA, et al. Desmoplastic neurotropic melanoma: a clinicopathologic analysis of 128 cases. *Cancer.* 2008;113(10):2770–2778.

415. Lin D, Kashani-Sabet M, McCalmont T, Singer MI. Neurotropic melanoma invading the inferior alveolar nerve. *J Am Acad Dermatol.* 2005;53(2 suppl 1):S120–S122.

416. Varey AHR, Goumas C, Hong AM, et al. Neurotropic melanoma: an analysis of the clinicopathological features, management strategies and survival outcomes for 671 patients treated at a tertiary referral center. *Mod Pathol.* 2017;30(11):1538–1550.

417. Iwamoto S, Burrows RC, Agoff SN, Piepkorn M, Bothwell M, Schmidt R. The p75 neurotrophin receptor, relative to other Schwann cell and melanoma markers, is abundantly expressed in spindled melanomas. *Am J Dermatopathol.* 2001;23(4):288–294.

418. Innominato PF, Libbrecht L, Van den Oord JJ. Expression of neurotrophins and their receptors in pigment cell lesions of the skin. *J Pathol.* 2001;194(1):95–100.

419. Chorny JA, Barr RJ. S100-positive spindle cells in scars: a diagnostic pitfall in the re-excision of desmoplastic melanoma. *Am J Dermatopathol.* 2002;24(4):309–312.

420. Busam KJ, Iversen K, Coplan KC, Jungbluth AA. Analysis of microphthalmia transcription factor expression in normal tissues and tumors, and comparison of its expression with S-100 protein, gp100, and tyrosinase in desmoplastic malignant melanoma. *Am J Surg Pathol.* 2001;25(2):197–204.

421. Busam KJ, Chen YT, Old LJ, et al. Expression of melan-A (MART1) in benign melanocytic nevi and primary cutaneous malignant melanoma. *Am J Surg Pathol.* 1998;22:976–982.

422. Kucher C, Zhang PJ, Pasha T, et al. Expression of Melan-A and Ki-67 in desmoplastic melanoma and desmoplastic nevi. *Am J Dermatopathol.* 2004;26(6):452–457.

423. Ramos-Herberth FI, Karamchandani J, Kim J, Dadras SS. SOX10 immunostaining distinguishes desmoplastic melanoma from excision scar. *J Cutan Pathol.* 2010;37(9):944–952.

424. Palla B, Su A, Binder S, Dry S. SOX10 expression distinguishes desmoplastic melanoma from its histologic mimics. *Am J Dermatopathol.* 2013;35(5):576–581.

425. Harvey NT, Acott NJ, Wood BA. Sox10-positive cells within scars: a potential diagnostic pitfall. *Am J Dermatopathol.* 2017;39(10): 791–793.

426. Jackett LA, McCarthy SW, Scolyer RA. SOX10 expression in cutaneous scars: a potential diagnostic pitfall in the evaluation of melanoma re-excision specimens. *Pathology.* 2016;48(6):626–628.

427. Lazova R, Tantcheva-Poor I, Sigal AC. P75 nerve growth factor receptor staining is superior to S100 in identifying spindle cell and desmoplastic melanoma. *J Am Acad Dermatol.* 2010;63(5):852–858.

428. Otaibi S, Jukic DM, Drogowski L, Bhawan J, Radfar A. NGFR (p75) expression in cutaneous scars; Further evidence for a potential pitfall in evaluation of reexcision scars of cutaneous neoplasms, in particular desmoplastic melanoma. *Am J Dermatopathol.* 2011;33(1):65–71.

429. Owosho AA, Estilo CL, Huryn JM, Chi P, Antonescu CR. A clinicopathologic study of head and neck malignant peripheral nerve sheath tumors. *Head Neck Pathol.* 2018;12(2):151–159.

430. Baron JA, Monzon F, Galaria N, Murphy GF. Angiomatoid melanoma: a novel pattern of differentiation in invasive periocular desmoplastic malignant melanoma. *Hum Pathol.* 2000;31(12):1520–1522.

431. Jain S, Allen PW. Desmoplastic malignant melanoma and its variants. A study of 45 cases. *Am J Surg Pathol.* 1989;13:358–373.

432. Kiene P, Petres-Dunsche C, Fölster-Holst R. Pigmented pedunculated malignant melanoma. A rare variant of nodular melanoma. *Br J Dermatol.* 1995;133:300–302.

433. Reed KM, Bronstein BR, Mihm MCJ, Sober AJ. Prognosis for polypoidal melanoma is determined by primary tumor thickness. *Cancer.* 1986;57:1201–1203.

434. Mesbah Ardakani N, Harvey NT, Wood BA. Polypoid compound melanocytic proliferations: a clinicopathological study. *Am J Dermatopathol.* 2019;41(8):578–584.

435. Pampena R, Lai M, Lombardi M, et al. Clinical and dermoscopic features associated with difficult-to-recognize variants of cutaneous melanoma: a systematic review. *JAMA Dermatol.* 2020;156(4):430–439.

436. Kamino H, Tam ST, Alvarez L. Malignant melanoma with pseudocarcinomatous hyperplasia—an entity that can simulate squamous cell carcinoma. A light-microscopic and immunohistochemical study of four cases. *Am J Dermatopathol.* 1990;12: 446–451.

437. Kao GF, Helwig EB, Graham JH. Balloon cell malignant melanoma of the skin: a clinicopathologic study of 34 cases with histochemical, immunohistochemical, and ultrastructural observations. *Cancer.* 1992;69:2942–2952.

438. Northcutt AD. Epidermotropic xanthoma mimicking balloon cell melanoma. *Am J Dermatopathol.* 2000;22:176–178.

439. Friedman BJ, Stoner R, Sahu J, Lee JB. Association of clinical, dermoscopic, and histopathologic findings with gene expression in patients with balloon cell melanoma. *JAMA Dermatol.* 2018;154(1):77–81.

440. Mowat A, Reid R, MacKie R. Balloon cell metastatic melanoma: an important differential in the diagnosis of clear cell tumours. *Histopathology.* 1994;24:469–472.

441. Baehner FL, Ng B, Sudilovsky D. Metastatic balloon cell melanoma: a case report. *Acta Cytol.* 2005;49(5):543–548.

442. Livolsi VA, Brooks JJ, Soslow R, Johnson BL, Elder DE. Signet cell melanocytic lesions. *Mod Pathol.* 1992;5:515–520.

443. Sheibani K, Battifora H. Signet-ring cell melanoma: a rare morphologic variant of malignant melanoma. *Am J Surg Pathol.* 1988;12:28–34.

444. Sanders DSA, Evans AT, Allen CA, et al. Classification of CEA-related positivity in primary and metastatic malignant melanoma. *J Pathol.* 1994;172:343–348.

445. Selby WL, Nance KV, Park HK. CEA immunoreactivity in metastatic malignant melanoma. *Mod Pathol.* 1992;5:415–419.

446. Safadi RA, Bader DH, Abdullah NI, Sughayer MA. Immunohistochemical expression of keratins 6, 7, 8, 14, 16, 18, 19, and MNF-116 pancytokeratin in primary and metastatic melanoma of the head and neck. *Oral Surg Oral Med Oral Pathol Oral Radiol.* 2016;121(5):510–519.

447. Hitchcock MG, McCalmont TH, White WL. Cutaneous melanoma with myxoid features: twelve cases with differential diagnosis. *Am J Surg Pathol.* 1999;23(12):1506–1513.

448. Bhuta S, Mirra JM, Cochran AJ. Myxoid malignant melanoma. A previously undescribed histologic pattern noted in metastatic lesions and a report of four cases. *Am J Surg Pathol.* 1986;10:203–211.

449. Kim YC, Vandersteen DP, Jung HG. Myxoid clear cell sarcoma. *Am J Dermatopathol.* 2005;27(1):51–55.

450. Levene A. Disseminated dermal melanocytosis terminating in melanoma. A human condition resembling equine melanotic disease. *Br J Dermatol.* 1979;101(2):197–205.

451. Muhlbauer JE, Margolis RJ, Mihm MCJ, Reed RJ. Minimal deviation melanoma: a histologic variant of cutaneous malignant melanoma in its vertical growth phase. *J Invest Dermatol.* 1983;80:63s–65s.

452. Chorny JA, Barr RJ, Kyshtoobayeva A, Jakowatz J, Reed RJ. Ki-67 and p53 expression in minimal deviation melanomas as compared with other nevomelanocytic lesions. *Mod Pathol.* 2003;16(6):525–529.

453. Stas M, Van den Oord JJ, Garmyn M, Degreef H, De W, I, Wolf-Peeters C. Minimal deviation and/or naevoid melanoma: is recognition worthwhile? A clinicopathological study of nine cases. *Melanoma Res.* 2000;10(4):371–380.

454. Schmoeckel C, Castro CE, Braun-Falco O. Nevoid malignant melanoma. *Arch Dermatol Res.* 1985;277:362–369.

455. Levene A. On the histological diagnosis and prognosis of malignant melanoma. *J Clin Pathol.* 1980;33:101–124.

456. Idriss MH, Rizwan L, Sferuzza A, Wasserman E, Kazlouskaya V, Elston DM. Nevoid melanoma: a study of 43 cases with emphasis on growth pattern. *J Am Acad Dermatol.* 2015;73(5):836–842.

457. McNutt NS. "Triggered trap": nevoid malignant melanoma. *Semin Diagn Pathol.* 1998;15:203–209.

458. Gerami P, Wass A, Mafee M, Fang Y, Pulitzer MP, Busam KJ. Fluorescence in situ hybridization for distinguishing nevoid melanomas from mitotically active nevi. *Am J Surg Pathol.* 2009;33(12):1783–1788.

459. Koh SS, Roehmholdt BF, Cassarino DS. Immunohistochemistry of p16 in nevi of pregnancy and nevoid melanomas. *J Cutan Pathol.* 2018;45(12):891–896.

460. Cook MG, Massi D, Blokx WAM, et al. New insights into naevoid melanomas: a clinicopathological reassessment. *Histopathology.* 2017;71(6):943–950.

461. Ferrara G, Giorgio CM, Zalaudek I, et al. Sclerosing nevus with pseudomelanomatous features (nevus with regression-like fibrosis): clinical and dermoscopic features of a recently characterized histopathologic entity. *Dermatology.* 2009;219(3):202–208.

462. Fabrizi G, Pennacchia I, Pagliarello C, Massi G. Sclerosing nevus with pseudomelanomatous features. *J Cutan Pathol.* 2008;35(11):995–1002.

463. Ko CJ, Bologna JL, Glusac EJ. "Clark/dysplastic" nevi with florid fibroplasia associated with pseudomelanomatous features. *J Am Acad Dermatol.* 2011;64(2):346–351.

464. Grcar-Kuzmanov B, Bostjancic E, Bandres JAC, Pizem J. Sclerosing melanocytic lesions (sclerosing melanomas with nevoid features and sclerosing nevi with pseudomelanomatous features)—an analysis of 90 lesions. *Radiol Oncol.* 2018;52(2):220–228.

465. Barnhill RL, Bahrami A, Bastian BC, et al. Spitz melanoma. In: Elder DE, Massi D, Scolyer RA, Willemze R, eds. *WHO Classification of Skin Tumours.* 4th ed. IARC; 2018:108–110.

466. Spitz S. Melanomas of childhood. *Am J Pathol.* 1948;24:591–609.

467. Paniago-Pereira C, Maize JC, Ackerman AB. Nevus of large spindle and/or epithelioid cells (Spitz's nevus). *Arch Dermatol.* 1978;114(12):1811–1823.

468. Harris MN, Hurwitz RM, Buckel LJ, Gray HR. Congenital spitz nevus. *Dermatol Surg.* 2000;26(10):931–935.

469. Spatz A, Calonje E, Handfield-Jones S, Barnhill RL. Spitz tumors in children: a grading system for risk stratification. *Arch Dermatol.* 1999;135(3):282–285.

470. Lott JP, Wititsuwannakul J, Lee JJ, et al. Clinical characteristics associated with Spitz nevi and Spitzoid malignant melanomas: the Yale University Spitzoid Neoplasm Repository experience, 1991 to 2008. *J Am Acad Dermatol.* 2014;71(6):1077–1082.

471. Requena C, Requena L, Kutzner H, Sanchez YE. Spitz nevus: a clinicopathological study of 349 cases. *Am J Dermatopathol.* 2009;31(2):107–116.

472. Zayour M, Bologna JL, Lazova R. Multiple Spitz nevi: a clinicopathologic study of 9 patients. *J Am Acad Dermatol.* 2012;67(3):451–458.

473. Porubsky C, Teer JK, Zhang Y, Deschaine M, Sondak VK, Messina JL. Genomic analysis of a case of agminated Spitz nevi and congenital-pattern nevi arising in extensive nevus spilus. *J Cutan Pathol.* 2018;45(2):180–183.

474. Goto K, Pissaloux D, Durand L, Tirode F, Guillot B, de la Fouchardière A. Novel three-way complex rearrangement of TRPM1-PUM1-LCK in a case of agminated Spitz nevi arising in a giant congenital hyperpigmented macule. *Pigment Cell Melanoma Res.* 2020;33(5):767–772.

475. Busam KJ, Barnhill RL. Pagetoid Spitz nevus. Intraepidermal Spitz tumor with prominent pagetoid spread. *Am J Surg Pathol.* 1995;19(9):1061–1067.

476. Merot Y, Frenk E. Spitz nevus (large spindle cell and/or epithelioid cell nevus). Age-related involvement of the suprabasal epidermis. *Virchows Arch A Pathol Anat Histopathol.* 1989;415(2):97–101.

477. Merot Y. Transepidermal elimination of nevus cells in spindle and epithelioid cell (Spitz) nevi. *Arch Dermatol.* 1988;124(9):1441–1442.

478. Kantor G, Wheeland RG. Transepidermal elimination of nevus cells. A possible mechanism of nevus involution. *Arch Dermatol.* 1987;123:1371–1374.

479. Scott G, Chen KTK, Rosai J. Pseudoepitheliomatous hyperplasia in Spitz nevi: a possible source of confusion with squamous cell carcinoma. *Arch Pathol Lab Med.* 1989;113:61–63.

480. Kamino H, Flotte TJ, Misheloff E, Alba Greco M, Ackerman AB. Eosinophilic globules in Spitz's nevi. New findings and a diagnostic sign. *Am J Dermatopathol.* 1979;1:319–324.

481. Arbuckle S, Weedon D. Eosinophilic globules in the Spitz nevus. *J Am Acad Dermatol.* 1982;7:324–327.

482. Wesselmann U, Becker LR, Brocker EB, LeBoit PE, Bastian BC. Eosinophilic globules in spitz nevi: no evidence for apoptosis. *Am J Dermatopathol.* 1998;20:551–554.

483. Crotty KA, Scolyer RA, Li L, Palmer AA, Wang L, McCarthy SW. Spitz naevus versus Spitzoid melanoma: when and how can they be distinguished? *Pathology.* 2002;34(1):6–12.

484. Weedon D, Little JH. Spindle and epithelioid cell nevi in children and adults. A review of 211 cases of the Spitz nevus. *Cancer.* 1977;40:217–225.

485. Hillen LM, Vandyck HLD, Leunissen DJG, et al. Integrative histopathological and immunophenotypical characterisation of the inflammatory microenvironment in spitzoid melanocytic neoplasms. *Histopathology.* 2020;78(4):607–626.

486. Barr RJ, Morales RV, Graham JH. Desmoplastic nevus: a distinct histologic variant of mixed spindle cell and epithelioid cell nevus. *Cancer.* 1980;46:557–564.

487. Blokhin E, Pulitzer M, Busam KJ. Immunohistochemical expression of p16 in desmoplastic melanoma. *J Cutan Pathol.* 2013;40(9):796–800.

488. Tetzlaff MT, Xu X, Elder DE, Elenitsas R. Angiomatoid Spitz nevus: a clinicopathological study of six cases and a review of the literature. *J Cutan Pathol.* 2009;36(4):471–476.

489. Diaz-Cascajo C, Borghi S, Weyers W. Angiomatoid Spitz nevus: a distinct variant of desmoplastic Spitz nevus with prominent vasculature. *Am J Dermatopathol.* 2000;22(2):135–139.

490. Buonaccorsi JN, Lynott J, Plaza JA. Atypical melanocytic lesions of the thigh with spitzoid and dysplastic features: a clinicopathologic study of 29 cases. *Ann Diagn Pathol.* 2013;17(3):265–269.

491. Cerroni L, Barnhill R, Elder D, et al. Melanocytic tumors of uncertain malignant potential: results of a tutorial held at the XXIX Symposium of the International Society of Dermatopathology in Graz, October 2008. *Am J Surg Pathol.* 2010;34(3):314–326.

492. Alexander A, Samlowski WE, Grossman D, et al. Metastatic melanoma in pregnancy: risk of transplacental metastases in the infant. *J Clin Oncol.* 2003;21(11):2179–2186.

493. Barnhill RL, Flotte TJ, Fleischli M, Perez-Atayde A. Cutaneous melanoma and atypical spitz tumors in childhood. *Cancer.* 1995;76:1833–1845.

494. Lu C, Zhang J, Nagahawatte P, et al. The genomic landscape of childhood and adolescent melanoma. *J Invest Dermatol.* 2015;135(3):816–823.

495. Oei W, Fledderus AC, Spuls PI, et al. Development of an international core domain set for medium, large and giant congenital melanocytic nevi as a first step towards a core outcome set for clinical practice and research. *Br J Dermatol.* 2020;185(2):371–379.

496. Merkel EA, Mohan LS, Shi K, Panah E, Zhang B, Gerami P. Paediatric melanoma: clinical update, genetic basis, and advances in diagnosis. *Lancet Child Adolesc Health.* 2019;3(9):646–654.

497. Massi D, Tomasini C, Senetta R, et al. Atypical Spitz tumors in patients younger than 18 years. *J Am Acad Dermatol.* 2015;72(1):37–46.

498. Cordoro KM, Gupta D, Frieden IJ, McCalmont T, Kashani-Sabet M. Pediatric melanoma: results of a large cohort study and proposal for modified ABCD detection criteria for children. *J Am Acad Dermatol.* 2013;68(6):913–925.

499. Bastian BC, LeBoit PE, Pinkel D. Mutations and copy number increase of HRAS in Spitz nevi with distinctive histopathological features. *Am J Pathol.* 2000;157(3):967–972.

500. Maldonado JL, Timmerman L, Fridlyand J, Bastian BC. Mechanisms of cell-cycle arrest in Spitz nevi with constitutive activation of the MAP-kinase pathway. *Am J Pathol.* 2004;164(5):1783–1787.

501. Wiesner T, He J, Yelensky R, et al. Kinase fusions are frequent in Spitz tumours and spitzoid melanomas. *Nat Commun.* 2014;5:3116.

502. Paradela S, Fonseca E, Pita S, et al. Spitzoid melanoma in children: clinicopathological study and application of immunohistochemistry as an adjunct diagnostic tool. *J Cutan Pathol.* 2008;36(7):740–752.

503. Lazzaro B, Rebers A, Herlyn M, Menrad A, Johnson B, Elder DE. Immunophenotyping of compound and Spitz nevi and vertical growth phase melanomas using a panel of monoclonal antibodies reactive in paraffin sections. *J Invest Dermatol.* 1993;100(3):313S–317S.

504. Puri PK, Ferringer TC, Tyler WB, Wilson ML, Kirchner HL, Elston DM. Statistical analysis of the concordance of immunohistochemical stains with the final diagnosis in Spitzoid Neoplasms. *Am J Dermatopathol.* 2011;33:72–77.

505. LeBoit PE, Van Fletcher H. A comparative study of Spitz nevus and nodular malignant melanoma using image analysis cytometry. *J Invest Dermatol.* 1987;88:753–757.

506. Vollmer RT. Patient age in Spitz nevus and malignant melanoma: implication of Bayes rule for differential diagnosis. *Am J Clin Pathol.* 2004;121(6):872–877.

507. Al DR, Agoumi M, Gagne I, McCuaig C, Powell J, Kokta V. p16 Expression: a marker of differentiation between childhood malignant melanomas and Spitz nevi. *J Am Acad Dermatol.* 2011;65(2):357–363.

508. Ma SA, O'Day CP, Dentchev T, et al. Expression of p15 in a spectrum of spitzoid melanocytic neoplasms. *J Cutan Pathol.* 2019;46(5):310–316.

509. Garola R, Singh V. Utility of p16-Ki-67-HMB45 score in sorting benign from malignant Spitz tumors. *Pathol Res Pract.* 2019;215(10):152550.

510. Ali L, Helm T, Cheney R, et al. Correlating array comparative genomic hybridization findings with histology and outcome in spitzoid melanocytic neoplasms. *Int J Clin Exp Pathol.* 2010;3(6):593–599.

511. Gerami P, Scolyer RA, Xu X, et al. Risk assessment for atypical spitzoid melanocytic neoplasms using FISH to identify chromosomal copy number aberrations. *Am J Surg Pathol.* 2013;37(5):676–684.

512. Cesinaro AM, Schirosi L, Bettelli S, Migaldi M, Maiorana A. Alterations of 9p21 analysed by FISH and MLPA distinguish atypical spitzoid melanocytic tumours from conventional Spitz's nevi but do not predict their biological behaviour. *Histopathology.* 2010;57(4):515–527.

513. Raghavan SS, Wang JY, Kwok S, Rieger KE, Novoa RA, Brown RA. PRAME expression in melanocytic proliferations with intermediate histopathologic or spitzoid features. *J Cutan Pathol.* 2020;47(12):1123–1131.

514. Muto Y, Fujimura T, Kambayashi Y, et al. Metastatic PRAME-expressing juvenile spitzoid melanoma on the buttock. *Case Rep Oncol.* 2020;13(3):1141–1144.

515. Jansen B, Hansen D, Moy R, Hanhan M, Yao Z. Gene expression analysis differentiates melanomas from spitz nevi. *J Drugs Dermatol.* 2018;17(5):574–576.

516. Lee S, Barnhill RL, Dummer R, et al. TERT promoter mutations are predictive of aggressive clinical behavior in patients with Spitzoid Melanocytic Neoplasms. *Sci Rep.* 2015;5:11200.

517. Requena C, Heidenreich B, Kumar R, Nagore E. TERT promoter mutations are not always associated with poor prognosis in atypical spitzoid tumors. *Pigment Cell Melanoma Res.* 2017;30(2):265–268.

518. Wick MR. Selected benign cutaneous lesions that may simulate melanoma histologically. *Semin Diagn Pathol.* 2016;33(4):174–190.

519. Jo VY, Fletcher CD. p63 Immunohistochemical staining is limited in soft tissue tumors. *Am J Clin Pathol.* 2011;136(5):762–766.

520. Plaza JA, Torres-Cabala C, Evans H, Diwan AH, Prieto VG. Immunohistochemical expression of S100A6 in cellular neurothekeoma: clinicopathologic and immunohistochemical analysis of 31 cases. *Am J Dermatopathol.* 2009;31(5):419–422.

521. Elder DE, Barnhill RL. The pink papules and plaques of Spitz. *Br J Dermatol.* 2019;181(2):235.

522. VandenBoom T, Quan VL, Zhang B, et al. Genomic fusions in pigmented spindle cell nevus of reed. *Am J Surg Pathol.* 2018;42(8):1042–1051.

523. Barnhill RL, Barnhill MA, Berwick M, Mihm MC Jr. The histologic spectrum of pigmented spindle cell nevus: a review of 120 cases with emphasis on atypical variants. *Hum Pathol.* 1991;22:52–58.

524. Requena C, Requena L, Sanchez-Yus E, et al. Hypopigmented Reed nevus. *J Cutan Pathol.* 2008;35(suppl 1):87–89.

525. MacKie RM, English J, Aitchison TC, Fitzsimons CP, Wilson P. The number and distribution of benign pigmented moles (melanocytic naevi) in a healthy British population. *Br J Dermatol.* 1985;113(2):167–174.

526. Clemente C, Zurrida S, Bartoli C, Bono A, Collini P, Rilke F. Acrallentiginous naevus of plantar skin. *Histopathology.* 1995;27:549–555.

527. Boyd AS, Rapini RP. Acral melanocytic neoplasms: a histologic analysis of 158 lesions. *J Am Acad Dermatol.* 1994;31:740–745.

528. Saida T, Koga H, Goto Y, Uhara H. Characteristic distribution of melanin columns in the cornified layer of acquired acral nevus: an important clue for histopathologic differentiation from early acral melanoma. *Am J Dermatopathol.* 2011;33(5):468–473.

529. Perrin C. Tumors of the nail unit. A review. Part I: acquired localized longitudinal melanonychia and erythronychia. *Am J Dermatopathol.* 2013;35(6):621–636.

530. Wang WM, Wang X, Duan N, Jiang HL, Huang XF. Laugier-Hunziker syndrome: a report of three cases and literature review. *Int J Oral Sci.* 2012;4(4):226–230.

531. Jellinek N. Nail matrix biopsy of longitudinal melanonychia: diagnostic algorithm including the matrix shave biopsy. *J Am Acad Dermatol.* 2007;56(5):803–810.

532. Husain S, Scher RK, Silvers DN, Ackerman AB. Melanotic macule of nail unit and its clinicopathologic spectrum. *J Am Acad Dermatol.* 2006;54(4):664–667.

533. Ren J, Ren M, Kong YY, Lv JJ, Cai X, Kong JC. Clinicopathological diversity and outcome of longitudinal melanonychia in children and adolescents: analysis of 35 cases identified by excision specimens. *Histopathology.* 2020;77(3):380–390.

534. Takata M, Maruo K, Kageshita T, et al. Two cases of unusual acral melanocytic tumors: illustration of molecular cytogenetics as a diagnostic tool. *Hum Pathol.* 2003;34(1):89–92.

535. Koga H, Yoshikawa S, Shinohara T, et al. Long-term follow-up of longitudinal melanonychia in children and adolescents using an objective discrimination index. *Acta Derm Venereol.* 2016;96(5):716–717.

536. Jung HJ, Kweon SS, Lee JB, Lee SC, Yun SJ. A clinicopathologic analysis of 177 acral melanomas in Koreans: relevance of spreading pattern and physical stress. *JAMA Dermatol.* 2013;149(11):1281–1288.

537. Huang K, Fan J, Misra S. Acral lentiginous melanoma: incidence and survival in the United States, 2006–2015, an analysis of the SEER registry. *J Surg Res.* 2020;251:329–339.

538. Bello DM, Chou JF, Panageas KS, et al. Prognosis of acral melanoma: a series of 281 patients. *Ann Surg Oncol.* 2013;20(11):3618–3625.

539. Dika E, Veronesi G, Altimari A, et al. BRAF, KIT, and NRAS mutations of acral melanoma in white patients. *Am J Clin Pathol.* 2020;153(5):664–671.

540. Baran LR, Ruben BS, Kechijian P, Thomas L. Non-melanoma Hutchinson's sign: a reappraisal of this important, remarkable melanoma simulant. *J Eur Acad Dermatol Venereol.* 2018;32(3):495–501.

541. Shain AH. Two trajectories to melanoma on the hands and feet. *JAMA Dermatol.* 2021;157(7):769–770.

542. Bastian BC, Kashani-Sabet M, Hamm H, et al. Gene amplifications characterize acral melanoma and permit the detection of occult tumor cells in the surrounding skin. *Cancer Res.* 2000;60:1968–1973.

543. Hayward NK, Wilmott JS, Waddell N, et al. Whole-genome landscapes of major melanoma subtypes. *Nature.* 2017;545(7653):175–180.

544. Yeh I, Jorgenson E, Shen L, et al. Targeted genomic profiling of acral melanoma. *J Natl Cancer Inst.* 2019;111(10):1068–1077.

545. Moon KR, Choi YD, Kim JM, et al. Genetic alterations in primary acral melanoma and acral melanocytic nevus in Korea: common mutated genes show distinct cytomorphological features. *J Invest Dermatol.* 2018;138(4):933–945.

546. Barnhill RL, Albert LS, Shama SK, Goldenhersh MA, Rhodes AR, Sober AJ. Genital lentiginosis: a clinical and histopathologic study. *J Am Acad Dermatol.* 1990;22:453–460.

547. Gupta G, Williams REA, MacKie RM. The labial melanotic macule: a review of 79 cases. *Br J Dermatol.* 1997;136:772–775.

548. Francisco AL, Furlan MV, Peresi PM, et al. Head and neck mucosal melanoma: clinicopathological analysis of 51 cases treated in a single cancer centre and review of the literature. *Int J Oral Maxillofac Surg.* 2016;45(2):135–140.

549. Zarei S, Voss JS, Jin L, et al. Mutational profile in vulvar, vaginal, and urethral melanomas: review of 37 cases with focus on primary tumor site. *Int J Gynecol Pathol.* 2020;39(6):587–594.

550. Vergara IA, Wilmott JS, Long GV, Scolyer RA. Genetic drivers of non-cutaneous melanomas: challenges and opportunities in a heterogeneous landscape. *Exp Dermatol.* 2021;31(1):13–30.

551. Hodi FS, Corless CL, Giobbie-Hurder A, et al. Imatinib for melanomas harboring mutationally activated or amplified KIT arising on mucosal, acral, and chronically sun-damaged skin. *J Clin Oncol.* 2013;31(26):3182–3190.

552. Newell F, Kong Y, Wilmott JS, et al. Whole-genome landscape of mucosal melanoma reveals diverse drivers and therapeutic targets. *Nat Commun.* 2019;10(1):3163.

553. Walton RG, Jacobs AH, Cox AJ. Pigmented lesions in newborn infants. *Br J Dermatol.* 1976;95:389–396.

554. Kopf AW, Bart RS, Hennessey P. Congenital nevocytic nevi and malignant melanomas. *J Am Acad Dermatol.* 1979;1:123–130.

555. Vourc'h-Jourdain M, Martin L, Barbarot S. Large congenital melanocytic nevi: therapeutic management and melanoma risk: a systematic review. *J Am Acad Dermatol.* 2012;68(3):493-8e1–14.

556. Price HN, O'Haver J, Marghoob A, Badger K, Etchevers H, Krengel S. Practical application of the new classification scheme for congenital melanocytic nevi. *Pediatr Dermatol.* 2015;32(1):23–27.

557. Fronek LF, Braunlich K, Farsi M, Miller RA. A rare case of cutis verticis gyrata with underlying cerebriform intradermal nevus. *Cureus.* 2019;11(12):e6499.

558. Sardana K, Arora P, Khurana N, Chugh S. "Congenital follicular melanocytic naevi": a more appropriate term for spotted grouped pigmented naevi. *Clin Exp Dermatol.* 2012;37(8):871–873.

559. Botet MV, Caro FR, Sanchez JL. Congenital acral melanocytic nevi clinically stimulating acral lentiginous melanoma. *J Am Acad Dermatol.* 1981;5(4):406–410.

560. Hassab-El-Naby HM, Sadek A, Amer HA, Esmat MM. Desmoplastic hairless hypopigmented nevus. *Cutis.* 2016;98(3):E1–E3.

561. Ruiz-Maldonado R, Orozco-Covarrubias L, Ridaura-Sanz C, Duran-McKinster C, Gutierrez DMSDO, Tamayo-Sanchez L. Desmoplastic hairless hypopigmented naevus: a variant of giant congenital melanocytic naevus. *Br J Dermatol.* 2003;148(6):1253–1257.

562. Kinsler V. Satellite lesions in congenital melanocytic nevi-time for a change of name. *Pediatr Dermatol.* 2011;28(2):212–213.

563. Marghoob AA, Dusza S, Oliveria S, Halpern AC. Number of satellite nevi as a correlate for neurocutaneous melanocytosis in patients with large congenital melanocytic nevi. *Arch Dermatol.* 2004;140(2):171–175.

564. Cribier BJ, Santinelli F, Grosshans E. Lack of clinical-pathological correlation in the diagnosis of congenital naevi. *Br J Dermatol.* 1999;141(6):1004–1009.

565. Mark GJ, Mihm MCJ, Liteplo MG, Reed RJ, Clark WHJ. Congenital melanocytic nevi of the small and garment type. Clinical, histologic, and ultrastructural studies. *Hum Pathol.* 1973;4:395–418.

566. Reed WB, Becker SW, Becker SWJ, Nickel WR. Giant pigmented nevi, melanoma, and leptomeningeal melanosis. *Arch Dermatol.* 1965;91:100–119.

567. Ribeiro CS, Serpa SS, Sousa MA, Jeunon T. Melanoma associated with congenital intermediate common blue nevus of the scalp—case report. *An Bras Dermatol.* 2016;91(4):514–516.

568. Bowen AR, Duffy KL, Clayton FC, Andtbacka RH, Florell SR. Benign melanocytic lymph node deposits in the setting of giant congenital melanocytic nevi: the large congenital nodal nevus. *J Cutan Pathol.* 2015;42(11):832–839.

569. Illig L, Weidner F, Hundeiker M, et al. Congenital nevi less than or equal to 10 cm as precursors to melanoma. 52 cases, a review, and a new conception. *Arch Dermatol.* 1985;121:1274–1281.

570. Wu M, Yu Q, Gao B, Sheng L, Li Q, Xie F. A large-scale collection of giant congenital melanocytic nevi: clinical and histopathological characteristics. *Exp Ther Med.* 2020;19(1):313–318.

571. Stenn KS, Arons M, Hurwitz S. Patterns of congenital nevocellular nevi. *J Am Acad Dermatol.* 1983;9:388–393.

572. Barnhill RL, Fleischli M. Histologic features of congenital melanocytic nevi in infants 1 year of age or younger. *J Am Acad Dermatol.* 1995;33(5 Pt. 1):780–785.

573. Everett MA. Histopathology of congenital pigmented nevi. *Am J Dermatopathol.* 1989;11:11–12.

574. Clemmensen OJ, Kroon S. The histology of "congenital features" in early acquired melanocytic nevi. *J Am Acad Dermatol.* 1988;19(4):742–746.

575. Hurwitz RM, Buckel LJ. Superficial congenital compound melanocytic nevus. Another pitfall in the diagnosis of malignant melanoma. *Dermatol Surg.* 1997;23(10):897–900.

576. Simons EA, Huang JT, Schmidt B. Congenital melanocytic nevi in young children: histopathologic features and clinical outcomes. *J Am Acad Dermatol.* 2017;76(5):941–947.

577. Cramer SF, Salgado CM, Reyes-Mugica M. The high multiplicity of prenatal (congenital type) nevi in adolescents and adults. *Pediatr Dev Pathol.* 2016;19(5):409–416.

578. Bauer J, Curtin JA, Pinkel D, Bastian BC. Congenital melanocytic nevi frequently harbor NRAS mutations but no BRAF mutations. *J Invest Dermatol.* 2007;127(1):179–182.

579. Martins da Silva V, Martinez-Barrios E, Tell-Martí G, et al. Genetic abnormalities in large to giant congenital nevi: beyond NRAS mutations. *J Invest Dermatol.* 2019;139(4):900–908.

580. Michaloglou C, Vredeveld LC, Soengas MS, et al. BRAFE600-associated senescence-like cell cycle arrest of human naevi. *Nature.* 2005;436(7051):720–724.

581. Kinsler VA, Thomas AC, Ishida M, et al. Multiple congenital melanocytic nevi and neurocutaneous melanosis are caused by postzygotic mutations in Codon 61 of NRAS. *J Invest Dermatol.* 2013;133(9):2229–2236.

582. Kinsler VA, Anderson G, Latimer B, et al. Immunohistochemical and ultrastructural features of congenital melanocytic naevus cells support a stem cell phenotype. *Br J Dermatol.* 2013;169(2):374–383.

583. Kinsler VA, Birley J, Atherton DJ. Great Ormond Street Hospital for children registry for congenital melanocytic naevi: prospective study 1988–2007. Part 2—evaluation of treatments. *Br J Dermatol.* 2009;160(2):387–392.

584. Berg P, Lindelof B. Congenital nevocytic nevi: follow-up of a Swedish birth register sample regarding etiologic factors, discomfort, and removal rate. *Pediatr Dermatol.* 2002;19(4):293–297.

585. Mancianti M-L, Clark WHJ, Hayes FA, Herlyn M. Malignant melanoma simulants arising in congenital melanocytic nevi do not show experimental evidence for a malignant phenotype. *Am J Pathol.* 1990;136:817–829.

586. Bastian BC, Xiong J, Frieden IJ, et al. Genetic changes in neoplasms arising in congenital melanocytic nevi: differences between nodular proliferations and melanomas. *Am J Pathol.* 2002;161(4):1163–1169.

587. Braunberger TL, Adelman M, Shwayder TA, Clarke LE, Friedman BJ. Proliferative nodule resembling angiomatoid Spitz tumor with degenerative atypia arising within a giant congenital nevus. *J Cutan Pathol.* 2020;47(12):1200–1204.

588. Pavlova O, Fraitag S, Hohl D. 5-Hydroxymethylcytosine expression in proliferative nodules arising within congenital nevi allows differentiation from malignant melanoma. *J Invest Dermatol.* 2016;136(12):2453–2461.

589. Busam KJ, Shah KN, Gerami P, Sitzman T, Jungbluth AA, Kinsler V. Reduced H3K27me3 expression is common in nodular melanomas of childhood associated with congenital melanocytic nevi but not in proliferative nodules. *Am J Surg Pathol.* 2017;41(3):396–404.

590. Vergier B, Laharanne E, Prochazkova-Carlotti M, et al. Proliferative nodules vs melanoma arising in giant congenital melanocytic nevi during childhood. *JAMA Dermatol.* 2016;152(10):1147–1151.

591. Marghoob AA, Schoenbach SP, Kopf AW, Orlow SJ, Nossa R, Bart RS. Large congenital melanocytic nevi and the risk for the development of malignant melanoma—a prospective study. *Arch Dermatol.* 1996;132:170–175.

592. Egan CL, Oliveria SA, Elenitsas R, Hanson J, Halpern AC. Cutaneous melanoma risk and phenotypic changes in large congenital nevi: a follow-up study of 46 patients. *J Am Acad Dermatol.* 1998;39:923–932.

593. Kinsler VA, O'Hare P, Bulstrode N, et al. Melanoma in congenital melanocytic naevi. *Br J Dermatol.* 2017;176(5):1131–1143.

594. Yun SJ, Kwon OS, Han JH, et al. Clinical characteristics and risk of melanoma development from giant congenital melanocytic naevi in Korea: a nationwide retrospective study. *Br J Dermatol.* 2012;166(1):115–123.

595. DeDavid M, Orlow SJ, Provost N, et al. A study of large congenital melanocytic nevi and associated malignant melanomas: review of cases in the New York University Registry and the world literature. *J Am Acad Dermatol.* 1997;36:409–416.

596. Alvarez-Mendoza A, Reyes-Esparza J, Ruiz-Maldonado R, Lopez-Corella E, Juarez-Herrera NC. Malignant melanoma in children and congenital melanocytic nevi: DNA content and cell cycle analysis by flow cytometry. *Pediatr Dev Pathol.* 2001;3(4):73–81.

597. Rhodes AR, Sober AJ, Day CL, et al. The malignant potential of small congenital nevocellular nevi. An estimate of association based on a histologic study of 234 primary cutaneous melanomas. *J Am Acad Dermatol.* 1982;6:230–241.

598. Caccavale S, Calabrese G, Mattiello E, et al. Cutaneous melanoma arising in congenital melanocytic nevus: a retrospective observational study. *Dermatology.* 2020:1–6.

599. Rhodes AR, Wood WC, Sober AJ, Mihm MCJ. Nonepidermal origin of malignant melanoma associated with a giant congenital nevocellular nevus. *Plast Reconstr Surg.* 1981;67:782–790.

600. Krengel S, Hauschild A, Schafer T. Melanoma risk in congenital melanocytic naevi: a systematic review. *Br J Dermatol.* 2006;155(1):1–8.

601. Hale EK, Stein J, Ben-Porat L, et al. Association of melanoma and neurocutaneous melanocytosis with large congenital melanocytic naevi—results from the NYU-LCMN registry. *Br J Dermatol.* 2005;152(3):512–517.

602. Weidner N, Flanders DJ, Jochimsen PR, Stamler FW. Neurosarcomatous malignant melanoma arising in a neuroid giant congenital melanocytic nevus. *Arch Dermatol.* 1985;121:1302–1306.

603. Furuya A, Namiki T, Takayama K, et al. Dermal melanoma arising in a congenital large plaque-type blue nevus. *J Dtsch Dermatol Ges.* 2017;15(8):842–844.

604. Hendrickson MR, Ross JC. Neoplasms arising in congenital giant nevi: morphologic study of seven cases and a review of the literature. *Am J Surg Pathol.* 1981;5(2):109–135.

605. Hoang MP, Sinkre P, Albores-Saavedra J. Rhabdomyosarcoma arising in a congenital melanocytic nevus. *Am J Dermatopathol.* 2002;24(1):26–29.

606. Betti R, Inselvini E, Vergani R, Crosti C. Small congenital nevi associated with melanoma: case reports and considerations. *J Dermatol.* 2000;27(9):583–590.

607. Chang LW, Iqbal R, Badal B, et al. Genomic analysis of metastatic melanoma in an adult with giant congenital melanocytic nevus. *Pigment Cell Melanoma Res.* 2020;33(4):633–636.

608. Ricci C, Ambrosi F, Grillini M, et al. Next-generation sequencing revealing TP53 mutation as potential genetic driver in dermal deep-seated melanoma arising in giant congenital nevus in adult patients: a unique case report and review of the literature. *J Cutan Pathol.* 2020;47(12):1164–1169.

609. Fan Y, Lee S, Wu G, et al. Telomerase expression by aberrant methylation of the TERT promoter in melanoma arising in giant congenital nevi. *J Invest Dermatol.* 2016;136(1):339–342.

610. Lacoste C, Avril MF, Frassati-Biaggi A, et al. Malignant melanoma arising in patients with a large congenital melanocytic naevus: retrospective study of 10 cases with cytogenetic analysis. *Acta Derm Venereol.* 2015;95(6):686–690.

611. Machado A, Nunes DBC, Carneiro FRO, Mendes AMD. Primary melanoma of leptomeninge in a patient with giant congenital melanocytic nevus. *An Bras Dermatol.* 2020;95(3):404–406.

612. Garrido MC, Maronas-Jimenez L, Morales-Raya C, Ruano Y, Rodriguez-Peralto JL. Acquisition of somatic NRAS mutations in central nervous system melanocytes: a predisposing risk factor to primary melanoma of the central nervous system, a frequently forgotten pitfall in congenital nevi. *Am J Dermatopathol.* 2018;40(7):506–510.

613. Zhong CS, Huang JT, Nambudiri VE. Revisiting the history of the "Mongolian spot": the background and implications of a medical term used today. *Pediatr Dermatol.* 2019;36(5):755–757.

614. Prose NS. Bringing an end to the "Mongolian Spot." *Pediatr Dermatol.* 2019;36(5):758.

615. Baykal C, Yılmaz Z, Sun GP, Büyükbabani N. The spectrum of benign dermal dendritic melanocytic proliferations. *J Eur Acad Dermatol Venereol.* 2019;33(6):1029–1041.

616. Kose O, Huseynov S, Demiriz M. Giant Mongolian macules with bilateral ocular involvement: case report and review. *Dermatology.* 2012;224(2):126–129.

617. Williams NM, Gurnani P, Labib A, Nuesi R, Nouri K. Melanoma in the setting of nevus of Ota: a review for dermatologists. *Int J Dermatol.* 2020;60(5):523–532.

618. Ee HL, Wong HC, Goh CL, Ang P. Characteristics of Hori naevus: a prospective analysis. *Br J Dermatol.* 2006;154(1):50–53.

619. Hori Y, Kawashima M, Oohara K, Kukita A. Acquired, bilateral nevus of Ota-like macules. *J Am Acad Dermatol.* 1984;10(6):961–964.

620. Pranteda G, Grieco T, Contini S, Bottoni U, Gomes V, Panasiti G. Dermal melanocyte hamartoma and hereditary motor and sensory neuropathy type 2A. *Acta Derm Venereol.* 2002;82(1):66–67.

621. Zembowicz A, Mihm MC. Dermal dendritic melanocytic proliferations: an update. *Histopathology.* 2004;45(5):433–451.

622. Rho NK, Kim WS, Lee DY, Yang JM, Lee ES, Lee JH. Histopathological parameters determining lesion colours in the naevus of Ota: a morphometric study using computer-assisted image analysis. *Br J Dermatol.* 2004;150(6):1148–1153.

623. Tse JY, Walls BE, Pomerantz H, et al. Melanoma arising in a nevus of Ito: novel genetic mutations and a review of the literature on cutaneous malignant transformation of dermal melanocytosis. *J Cutan Pathol.* 2016;43(1):57–63.

624. Gerami P, Pouryazdanparast P, Vemula S, Bastian BC. Molecular analysis of a case of nevus of ota showing progressive evolution to melanoma with intermediate stages resembling cellular blue nevus. *Am J Dermatopathol.* 2010;32(3):301–305.

625. Kuo KL, Lin CL, Wu CH, et al. Meningeal melanocytoma associated with nevus of Ota: analysis of twelve reported cases. *World Neurosurg.* 2019;127:e311–e320.

626. Munoz-Hidalgo L, Lopez-Gines C, Navarro L, et al. BRAF V600E mutation in two distinct meningeal melanocytomas associated with a nevus of Ota. *J Clin Oncol.* 2014;32(20):e72–e75.

627. van Raamsdonk CD, Bezrookove V, Green G, et al. Frequent somatic mutations of GNAQ in uveal melanoma and blue naevi. *Nature.* 2009;457(7229):599–602.

628. Buchner A, Leider AS, Merrell PW, Carpenter WM. Melanocytic nevi of the oral mucosa: a clinicopathologic study of 130 cases from northern California. *J Oral Pathol Med.* 1990;19(5):197–201.

629. Pittman JL, Fisher BK. Plaque-type blue nevus. *Arch Dermatol.* 1976;112(8):1127–1128.

630. Busam KJ, Woodruff JM, Erlandson RA, Brady MS. Large plaque-type blue nevus with subcutaneous cellular nodules. *Am J Surg Pathol.* 2000;24(1):92–99.

631. Yan L, Tognetti L, Nami N, et al. Melanoma arising from a plaque-type blue naevus with subcutaneous cellular nodules of the scalp. *Clin Exp Dermatol.* 2018;43(2):164–167.

632. Misago N. The relationship between melanocytes and peripheral nerve sheath cells (part II): blue nevus with peripheral nerve sheath differentiation. *Am J Dermatopathol.* 2000;22(3):230–236.

633. Xia J, Wang Y, Li F, et al. Expression of microphthalmia transcription factor, S100 protein, and HMB-45 in malignant melanoma and pigmented nevi. *Biomed Rep.* 2016;5(3):327–331.

634. Ferrara G, Soyer HP, Malvehy J, et al. The many faces of blue nevus: a clinicopathologic study. *J Cutan Pathol.* 2007;34(7):543–551.

635. Zembowicz A, Granter SR, McKee PH, Mihm MC. Amelanotic cellular blue nevus: a hypopigmented variant of the cellular blue nevus: clinicopathologic analysis of 20 cases. *Am J Surg Pathol.* 2002;26(11):1493–1500.

636. Ferrara G, Argenziano G, Zgavec B, et al. "Compound blue nevus": a reappraisal of "superficial blue nevus with prominent intraepidermal dendritic melanocytes" with emphasis on dermoscopic and histopathologic features. *J Am Acad Dermatol.* 2002;46(1):85–89.

637. Harvell JD, White WL. Persistent and recurrent blue nevi. *Am J Dermatopathol.* 1999;21(6):506–517.

638. Rodriguez HA, Ackerman LV. Cellular blue nevus. *Cancer.* 1968;21:393–405.

639. Gartmann H. Neuronaevus bleu Masson—cellular blue nevus Allen. *Arch Klin Exp Dermatol.* 1965;221:109–121.

640. Hung T, Argenyi Z, Erickson L, et al. Cellular blue nevomelanocytic lesions: analysis of clinical, histological, and outcome data in 37 cases. *Am J Dermatopathol.* 2016;38(7):499–503.

641. Avidor I, Kessler E. "Atypical" blue nevus—a benign variant of cellular blue nevus. Presentation of three cases. *Dermatologica.* 1977;154(1):39–44.

642. Marano SR, Brooks RA, Spetzler RF, Rekate HL. Giant congenital cellular blue nevus of the scalp of a newborn with an underlying skull defect and invasion of the dura mater. *Neurosurgery.* 1986;18(1):85–89.

643. Bui J, Ardakani NM, Tan I, Crocker A, Khattak MA, Wood BA. Metastatic cellular blue nevus: a rare case with metastasis beyond regional nodes. *Am J Dermatopathol.* 2017;39(8):618–621.

644. Martin RC, Murali R, Scolyer RA, Fitzgerald P, Colman MH, Thompson JF. So-called "malignant blue nevus": a clinicopathologic study of 23 patients. *Cancer.* 2009;115(13):2949–2955.

645. Loghavi S, Curry JL, Torres-Cabala CA, et al. Melanoma arising in association with blue nevus: a clinical and pathologic study of 24 cases and comprehensive review of the literature. *Mod Pathol.* 2014;27(11):1468–1478.

646. Murali R, McCarthy SW, Scolyer RA. Blue nevi and related lesions: a review highlighting atypical and newly described variants, distinguishing features and diagnostic pitfalls. *Adv Anat Pathol.* 2009;16(6):365–382.

647. Granter SR, McKee PH, Calonje E, Mihm MC, Busam K. Melanoma associated with blue nevus and melanoma mimicking cellular blue nevus: a clinicopathologic study of 10 cases on the spectrum of so-called "malignant blue nevus." *Am J Surg Pathol.* 2001;25(3):316–323.

648. Blundell AR, Moustafa D, Samore WR, Hawryluk EB. Fatal GNAQ-mutated CNS melanoma in an adolescent with nevus of Ota. *Pediatr Dermatol.* 2021;38(2):497–499.

649. Mishima Y. Cellular blue nevus. Melanogenic activity and malignant transformation. *Arch Dermatol.* 1970;101(1):104–110.

650. Held L, Eigentler TK, Metzler G, et al. Proliferative activity, chromosomal aberrations, and tumor-specific mutations in the differential diagnosis between blue nevi and melanoma. *Am J Pathol.* 2012;182(3):640–645.

651. Griewank KG, Muller H, Jackett LA, et al. SF3B1 and BAP1 mutations in blue nevus-like melanoma. *Mod Pathol.* 2017;30(7): 928–939.

652. Salama AK, de Rosa N, Scheri RP, et al. Hazard-rate analysis and patterns of recurrence in early stage melanoma: moving towards a rationally designed surveillance strategy. *PLoS One.* 2013;8(3):e57665.

653. Rogers GS, Kopf AW, Rigel DS, Friedman RJ, Levenstein M, Bart RS. Hazard-rate analysis in stage I malignant melanoma. *Arch Dermatol.* 1986;122:999–1002.

654. Osella-Abate S, Ribero S, Sanlorenzo M, et al. Risk factors related to late metastases in 1,372 melanoma patients disease free more than 10 years. *Int J Cancer.* 2015;136(10):2453–2457.

655. Schmid-Wendtner MH, Baumert J, Schmidt M, et al. Late metastases of cutaneous melanoma: an analysis of 31 patients. *J Am Acad Dermatol.* 2000;43(4):605–609.

656. Gershenwald JE, Scolyer RA, Hess KR, et al. Melanoma staging: evidence-based changes in the American Joint Committee on Cancer eighth edition cancer staging manual. *CA Cancer J Clin.* 2017;67(6):472–492.

657. Balch CM, Gershenwald JE, Soong SJ, et al. Final version of 2009 AJCC melanoma staging and classification. *J Clin Oncol.* 2009;27(36):6199–6206.

658. Uprety D, Bista A, Chennamadhavuni A, et al. Survival trends among patients with metastatic melanoma in the pretargeted and the post-targeted era: a US population-based study. *Melanoma Res.* 2018;28(1):56–60.

659. Song Y, Karakousis GC. Melanoma of unknown primary. *J Surg Oncol.* 2019;119(2):232–241.

660. Anbari KK, Schuchter LM, Bucky LP, et al. Melanoma of unknown primary site: presentation, treatment, and prognosis—a single institution study. University of Pennsylvania Pigmented Lesion Study Group. *Cancer.* 1997;79(9):1816–1821.

661. Khosravi H, Akabane AL, Alloo A, Nazarian RM, Boland GM. Metastatic melanoma with spontaneous complete regression of a thick primary lesion. *JAAD Case Rep.* 2016;2(6):439–441.

662. Menzies AM, Amaria RN, Rozeman EA, et al. Pathological response and survival with neoadjuvant therapy in melanoma: a pooled analysis from the International Neoadjuvant Melanoma Consortium (INMC). *Nat Med.* 2021;27(2):301–309.

663. Mihm MC Jr, Clemente CG, Cascinelli N. Tumor infiltrating lymphocytes in lymph node melanoma metastases: a histopathologic prognostic indicator and an expression of local immune response. *Lab Invest.* 1996;74:43–47.

664. Skala SL, Arps DP, Zhao L, et al. Comprehensive histopathological comparison of epidermotropic/dermal metastatic melanoma and primary nodular melanoma. *Histopathology.* 2018;72(3):472–480.

665. McNutt NS, Urmacher C, Hakimian J, Hoss DM, Lugo J. Nevoid malignant melanoma: morphologic patterns and immunohistochemical reactivity. *J Cutan Pathol.* 1995;22(6):502–517.

666. Harrist TJ, Rigel DS, Day CLJ, et al. "Microscopic satellites" are more highly associated with regional lymph node metastases than is primary melanoma thickness. *Cancer.* 1984;53:2183–2187.

667. Niebling MG, Haydu LE, Lo SN, et al. The prognostic significance of microsatellites in cutaneous melanoma. *Mod Pathol.* 2020;33(7):1369–1379.

668. Elder DE, Guerry DI, Heiberger RM, et al. Optimal resection margin for cutaneous malignant melanoma. *Plast Reconstr Surg.* 1983;71:66–72.

669. Kornberg R, Harris M, Ackerman AB. Epidermotropically metastatic malignant melanoma. Differentiating malignant melanoma metastatic to the epidermis from malignant melanoma primary in the epidermis. *Arch Dermatol.* 1978;114:67–69.

670. Ruhoy SM, Prieto VG, Eliason SL, Grichnik JM, Burchette JL Jr, Shea CR. Malignant melanoma with paradoxical maturation. *Am J Surg Pathol.* 2000;24(12):1600–1614.

671. Sebaratnam DF, Venugopal SS, Frew JW, et al. Diffuse melanosis cutis: a systematic review of the literature. *J Am Acad Dermatol.* 2012;68(3):482–488.

672. Adrian RM, Murphy GF, Sato S, Granstein RD, Fitzpatrick TB, Sober AJ. Diffuse melanosis secondary to metastatic malignant melanoma. Light and electron microscopic findings. *J Am Acad Dermatol.* 1981;5:308–318.

673. Swetter SM, Thompson JA, Albertini MR, et al. NCCN Guidelines(R) Insights: melanoma: cutaneous, Version 2.2021. *J Natl Compr Canc Netw.* 2021;19(4):364–376.

674. Zarabi SK, Azzato EM, Tu ZJ, et al. Targeted next generation sequencing (NGS) to classify melanocytic neoplasms. *J Cutan Pathol.* 2020;47(8):691–704.

675. Cust AE, Mishra K, Berwick M. Melanoma—role of the environment and genetics. *Photochem Photobiol Sci.* 2018;17(12): 1853–1860.

676. Elder DE. Skin cancer: melanoma and other specific nonmelanoma skin cancers. *Cancer.* 1995;75(suppl):245–256.

677. Kanetsky PA, Rebbeck TR, Hummer AJ, et al. Population-based study of natural variation in the melanocortin-1 receptor gene and melanoma. *Cancer Res.* 2006;66(18):9330–9337.

678. Vezzoni R, Conforti C, Vichi S, et al. Is there more than one road to nevus-associated melanoma? *Dermatol Pract Concept.* 2020;10(2):e2020028.

679. Gruber SB, Barnhill RL, Stenn KS, Roush GC. Nevomelanocytic proliferations in association with cutaneous malignant melanoma: a multivariate analysis. *J Am Acad Dermatol.* 1989;21:773–780.

680. Smolle J, Kaddu S, Kerl H. Non-random spatial association of melanoma and naevi—a morphometric analysis. *Melanoma Res.* 1999;9:407–412.

681. Dessinioti C, Geller AC, Stergiopoulou A, et al. A multicenter study of nevus-associated melanoma versus de novo melanoma, tumor thickness and body site differences. *Br J Dermatol.* 2021;185(1):101–109.

682. Lin WM, Luo S, Muzikansky A, et al. Outcome of patients with de novo versus nevus-associated melanoma. *J Am Acad Dermatol.* 2015;72(1):54–58.

683. Massi D, Bastian BC, LeBoit PE, Prieto VG, Xu X. Melanoma arising in giant congenital nevus. In: Elder DE, Massi D, Scolyer RA, Willemze R, eds. *WHO Classification of Skin Tumours.* 4th ed. IARC; 2018:132–133.

684. Xiong J, Su Y, Bing Z, Zhao B. Survival between synchronous and non-synchronous multiple primary cutaneous melanomas-a SEER database analysis. *PeerJ.* 2020;8:e8316.

685. Helgadottir H, Isaksson K, Fritz I, et al. Multiple primary melanoma incidence trends over five decades, a nation-wide population-based study. *J Natl Cancer Inst.* 2020;113(3):318–328.

686. Stam-Posthuma JJ, Duinen C, Scheffer E, Vink J, Bergman W. Multiple primary melanomas. *J Am Acad Dermatol.* 2001;44(1):22–27.

687. Blackwood MA, Holmes R, Synnestvedt M, et al. Multiple primary melanoma revisited. *Cancer.* 2002;94(8):2248–2255.

688. Schuchter L, Schultz DJ, Synnestvedt M, et al. A prognostic model for predicting 10-year survival in patients with primary melanoma. *Ann Intern Med.* 1996;125:369–375.

689. Leon P, Daly JM, Synnestvedt M, Schultz DJ, Elder DE, Clark WH Jr. The prognostic implications of microscopic satellites in patients with clinical stage I melanoma. *Arch Surg.* 1991;126(12): 1461–1468.

690. Slingluff CLJ, Vollmer R, Seigler HF. Stage II malignant melanoma: presentation of a prognostic model and an assessment of specific active immunotherapy in 1,273 patients. *J Surg Oncol.* 1988;39:139–147.

691. Blois MS, Sagebiel RW, Tuttle MS, Caldwell TM, Taylor HW. Judging prognosis in malignant melanoma of the skin. A problem of inference over small data sets. *Ann Surg.* 1983 Aug;198(2):200-6.

692. Day CLJ, Sober AJ, Kopf AW, et al. A prognostic model for clinical stage I melanoma of the upper extremity. The importance of anatomic subsites in predicting recurrent disease. *Ann Surg.* 1981;193:436–440.

693. Day CLJ, Sober AJ, Kopf AW, et al. A prognostic model for clinical stage I melanoma of the trunk location near the midline is not an independent risk factor for recurrent disease. *Am J Surg.* 1981;142:247–251.

694. Day CLJ, Sober AJ, Kopf AW, et al. A prognostic model for clinical stage I melanoma of the lower extremity. Location on foot as independent risk factor for recurrent disease. *Surgery.* 1981;89:599–603.

695. Maurichi A, Miceli R, Eriksson H, et al. Factors affecting sentinel node metastasis in Thin (T1) cutaneous melanomas: development and external validation of a predictive nomogram. *J Clin Oncol.* 2020;38(14):1591–1601.

696. Gould Rothberg BE, Bracken MB, Rimm DL. Tissue biomarkers for prognosis in cutaneous melanoma: a systematic review and meta-analysis. *J Natl Cancer Inst.* 2009;101(7):452–474.

697. Gershenwald JE, Scolyer RA. Melanoma staging: American Joint Committee on Cancer (AJCC) 8th edition and beyond. *Ann Surg Oncol.* 2018;25(8):2105–2110.

698. El Sharouni MA, Ahmed T, Witkamp AJ, et al. Predicting recurrence in patients with sentinel node-negative melanoma: validation of the EORTC nomogram using population-based data. *Br J Surg.* 2020;108(5):550–553.

699. Lo SN, Ma J, Scolyer RA, et al. Improved risk prediction calculator for sentinel node positivity in patients with melanoma: The Melanoma Institute Australia Nomogram. *J Clin Oncol.* 2020;38(24):2719–2727.

700. Breslow A. Thickness, cross-sectional areas and depth of invasion in the prognosis of cutaneous melanoma. *Ann Surg.* 1970;172:902–908.

701. Bedrosian I, Faries MB, Guerry D, et al. Incidence of sentinel node metastasis in patients with thin primary melanoma (< or = 1 mm) with vertical growth phase [see comments]. *Ann Surg Oncol.* 2000;7(4):262–267.

702. Gimotty PA, Guerry D, Ming ME, et al. Thin primary cutaneous malignant melanoma: a prognostic tree for 10-year metastasis is more accurate than American Joint Committee on Cancer staging. *J Clin Oncol.* 2004;22:3668–3676.

703. Lever WF, Schaumber-Lever G. Melanocytic tumors. In: Lever WF, Schaumber-Lever G, eds. *Histopathology of the Skin.* 7th ed.Lippincott; 2005, p. 792

704. Breslow A. Prognostic factors in the treatment of cutaneous melanoma. *J Cutan Pathol.* 1979;6:208–212.

705. Saldanha G, Khanna A, O'Riordan M, Bamford M. The width of invasion in malignant melanoma is a novel prognostic feature that accounts for outcome better than Breslow thickness. *Am J Surg Pathol.* 2020;44(11):1522–1527.

706. Saldanha G, Yarrow J, Elsheikh S, O'Riordan M, Uraiby H, Bamford M. Development and initial validation of calculated tumor area as a prognostic tool in cutaneous malignant melanoma. *JAMA Dermatol.* 2019;155(8):890–898.

707. Saldanha G, Yarrow J, Pancholi J, et al. Breslow density is a novel prognostic feature that adds value to melanoma staging. *Am J Surg Pathol.* 2018;42(6):715–725.

708. Spatz A, Cook MG, Elder DE, Piepkorn M, Ruiter DJ, Barnhill RL. Interobserver reproducibility of ulceration assessment in primary cutaneous melanomas. *Eur J Cancer.* 2003;39(13):1861–1865.

709. Balch CM, Wilkerson JA, Murad TM, Soong SJ, Ingalls AL, Maddox WA. The prognostic significance of ulceration of cutaneous melanoma. *Cancer.* 1980;45:3012–3017.

710. Masback A, Olsson H, Westerdahl J, Ingvar C, Jonsson N. Prognostic factors in invasive cutaneous malignant melanoma: a population-based study and review. *Melanoma Res.* 2001;11(5):435–445.

711. Namikawa K, Aung PP, Gershenwald JE, Milton DR, Prieto VG. Clinical impact of ulceration width, lymphovascular invasion, microscopic satellitosis, perineural invasion, and mitotic rate in patients undergoing sentinel lymph node biopsy for cutaneous melanoma: a retrospective observational study at a comprehensive cancer center. *Cancer Med.* 2018;7(3):583–593.

712. Scolyer RA, Shaw HM, Thompson JF, et al. Interobserver reproducibility of histopathologic prognostic variables in primary cutaneous melanomas. *Am J Surg Pathol.* 2003;27(12):1571–1576.

713. Larsen TE, Grude TH. A retrospective histological study of 669 cases of primary cutaneous malignant melanoma in clinical stage I. 2. The relation of cell type, pigmentation, atypia and mitotic count to histological type and prognosis. *Acta Pathol Microbiol Scand.* 1978;86A(6):513–522.

714. Skochdopole AJ, Kutlu OC, Engelhardt KE, Lancaster WP, Abbott AM, Camp ER. High mitotic rate predicts sentinel lymph node involvement in thin melanomas. *J Surg Res.* 2020;256:198–205.

715. Kesmodel SB, Karakousis GC, Botbyl JD, et al. Mitotic rate as a predictor of sentinel lymph nodepositivity in patients with thin melanomas. *Ann Surg Oncol.* 2005;12(6):449–458.

716. Cherpelis BS, Haddad F, Messina J, et al. Sentinel lymph node micrometastasis and other histologic factors that predict outcome in patients with thicker melanomas. *J Am Acad Dermatol.* 2001;44(5):762–766.

717. Gershenwald JE, Soong SJ, Balch CM. 2010 TNM staging system for cutaneous melanoma...and beyond. *Ann Surg Oncol.* 2010;17(6):1475–1477.

718. McDermott NC, Hayes DP, al-Sader MH, et al. Identification of vertical growth phase in malignant melanoma. A study of interobserver agreement. *Am J Clin Pathol.* 1998;110:753–757.

719. Cook MG, Spatz A, Brocker EB, Ruiter DJ. Identification of histological features associated with metastatic potential in thin (<1.0 mm) cutaneous melanoma with metastases. A study on behalf of the EORTC Melanoma Group. *J Pathol.* 2002;197(2):188–193.

720. Clark WHJ. A classification of malignant melanoma in man correlated with histogenesis and biologic behavior. In: Montagna W, Hu F, eds. *Advances in the Biology of the Skin Volume VIII.* Pergamon Press; 1967:621–647.

721. Swetter SM, Tsao H, Bichakjian CK, et al. Guidelines of care for the management of primary cutaneous melanoma. *J Am Acad Dermatol.* 2019;80(1):208–250.

722. Büttner P, Garbe C, Bertz J, et al. Primary cutaneous melanoma: optimized cutoff points of tumor thickness and importance of Clark's level for prognostic classification. *Cancer.* 1995;75:2499–2506.

723. Kang S, Barnhill RL, Mihm MCJ, Sober AJ. Histologic regression in malignant melanoma: an interobserver concordance study. *J Cutan Pathol.* 1993;20:126–129.

724. Sondergaard K, Hou Jensen K. Partial regression in thin primary cutaneous malignant melanomas clinical stage I. A study of 486 cases. *Virchows Arch A Pathol Anat Histopathol.* 1985;408:241–247.

725. Guitart J, Lowe L, Piepkorn M, et al. Histological characteristics of metastasizing thin melanomas: a case-control study of 43 cases. *Arch Dermatol.* 2002;138(5):603–608.

726. Gualano MR, Osella-Abate S, Scaioli G, et al. Prognostic role of histological regression in primary cutaneous melanoma: a systematic review and meta-analysis. *Br J Dermatol.* 2018;178(2):357–362.

727. El Sharouni MA, Aivazian K, Witkamp AJ, et al. Association of histologic regression with a favorable outcome in patients with stage 1 and stage 2 cutaneous melanoma. *JAMA Dermatol.* 2020;157(2):166–173.

728. Taylor RC, Patel A, Panageas KS, Busam KJ, Brady MS. Tumor-infiltrating lymphocytes predict sentinel lymph node positivity in patients with cutaneous melanoma. *J Clin Oncol.* 2007;25(7): 869–875.

729. Azimi F, Scolyer RA, Rumcheva P, et al. Tumor-infiltrating lymphocyte grade is an independent predictor of sentinel lymph node status and survival in patients with cutaneous melanoma. *J Clin Oncol.* 2012;30(21):2678–2683.

730. Thomas NE, Busam KJ, From L, et al. Tumor-infiltrating lymphocyte grade in primary melanomas is independently associated with melanoma-specific survival in the population-based genes, environment and melanoma study. *J Clin Oncol.* 2013; 31(33):4252–4259.

731. Barr RJ. The many faces of completely regressed malignant melanoma. In: LeBoit PE, ed. *Malignant Melanoma and Melanocytic Neoplasms.* Hanley & Belfus; 1994:359–370.

732. Flax SH, Skelton HG, Smith KJ, Lupton GP. Nodular melanosis due to epithelial neoplasms: a finding not restricted to regressed melanomas. *Am J Dermatopathol.* 1998;20:118–122.

733. Tetzlaff MT, Adhikari C, Lo S, et al. Histopathological features of complete pathological response predict recurrence-free survival following neoadjuvant targeted therapy for metastatic melanoma. *Ann Oncol.* 2020;31(11):1569–1579.

734. Tetzlaff MT, Messina JL, Stein JE, et al. Pathological assessment of resection specimens after neoadjuvant therapy for metastatic melanoma. *Ann Oncol.* 2018;29(8):1861–1868.

735. Boussios S, Rassy E, Samartzis E, et al. Melanoma of unknown primary: new perspectives for an old story. *Crit Rev Oncol Hematol.* 2020;158:103208.

736. Clemente CG, Mihm MG, Bufalino R, Zurrida S, Collini P, Cascinelli N. Prognostic value of tumor infiltrating lymphocytes in the vertical growth phase of primary cutaneous melanoma. *Cancer.* 1996;77:1303–1310.

737. Busam KJ, Antonescu CR, Marghoob AA, et al. Histologic classification of tumor-infiltrating lymphocytes in primary cutaneous malignant melanoma. A study of interobserver agreement. *Am J Clin Pathol.* 2001;115(6):856–860.

738. Saldanha G, Flatman K, Teo KW, Bamford M. A novel numerical scoring system for melanoma tumor-infiltrating lymphocytes has better prognostic value than standard scoring. *Am J Surg Pathol.* 2017;41(7):906–914.

739. Ouwerkerk W, van den Berg M, van der Niet S, Limpens J, Luiten RM. Biomarkers, measured during therapy, for response of melanoma patients to immune checkpoint inhibitors: a systematic review. *Melanoma Res.* 2019;29(5):453–464.

740. Moy AP, Mochel MC, Muzikansky A, Duncan LM, Kraft S. Lymphatic invasion predicts sentinel lymph node metastasis and adverse outcome in primary cutaneous melanoma. *J Cutan Pathol.* 2017;44(9):734–739.

741. Xu X, Chen L, Guerry D, et al. Lymphatic invasion is independently prognostic of metastasis in primary cutaneous melanoma. *Clin Cancer Res.* 2011;18(1):229–237.

742. Lugassy C, Zadran S, Bentolila LA, et al. Angiotropism, pericytic mimicry and extravascular migratory metastasis in melanoma: an alternative to intravascular cancer dissemination. *Cancer Microenviron.* 2014;7(3):139–152.

743. Borgstein PJ, Meijer S, Van Diest PJ. Are locoregional cutaneous metastases in melanoma predictable? *Ann Surg Oncol.* 1999;6:315–321.

744. Gerami P, Shea C, Stone MS. Angiotropism in epidermotropic metastatic melanoma: another clue to the diagnosis. *Am J Dermatopathol.* 2006;28(5):429–433.

745. Dessinioti C, Dimou N, Geller AC, et al. Distinct clinicopathological and prognostic features of thin nodular primary melanomas: an international study from 17 centers. *J Natl Cancer Inst.* 2019;111(12):1314–1322.

746. Lattanzi M, Lee Y, Simpson D, et al. Primary melanoma histologic subtype: impact on survival and response to therapy. *J Natl Cancer Inst.* 2018;111(2):180–188.

747. Gong HZ, Zheng HY, Li J. Amelanotic melanoma. *Melanoma Res.* 2019;29(3):221–230.

748. Howard MD, Wee E, Wolfe R, McLean CA, Kelly JW, Pan Y. Anatomic location of primary melanoma: survival differences and sun exposure. *J Am Acad Dermatol.* 2019;81(2):500–509.

749. Garbe C, Büttner P, Bertz J, et al. Primary cutaneous melanoma: prognostic classification of anatomic location. *Cancer.* 1995;75:2492–2498.

750. Stidham KR, Johnson JL, Seigler HF. Survival superiority of females with melanoma: a multivariate analysis of 6383 patients exploring the significance of gender in prognostic outcome. *Arch Surg.* 1994;129:316–324.

751. Farahi JM, Fazzari M, Braunberger T, et al. Gender differences in melanoma prognostic factors. *Dermatol Online J.* 2018;24(4):13030.

752. Scoggins CR, Ross MI, Reintgen DS, et al. Gender-related differences in outcome for melanoma patients. *Ann Surg.* 2006;243(5):693–700.

753. Kim YJ, Kim K, Lee KH, Kim J, Jung W. Immune expression signatures as candidate prognostic biomarkers of age and gender survival differences in cutaneous melanoma. *Sci Rep.* 2020;10(1):12322.

754. Al-Rohil RN, Curry JL, Torres-Cabala CA, et al. Proliferation indices correlate with diagnosis and metastasis in diagnostically challenging melanocytic tumors. *Hum Pathol.* 2016;53:73–81.

755. Lawrence NF, Hammond MR, Frederick DT, et al. Ki-67, p53, and p16 expression, and G691S RET polymorphism in desmoplastic melanoma (DM): a clinicopathologic analysis of predictors of outcome. *J Am Acad Dermatol.* 2016;75(3):595–602.

756. Gimotty PA, Van BP, Elder DE, et al. Biologic and prognostic significance of dermal Ki67 expression, mitoses, and tumorigenicity in thin invasive cutaneous melanoma. *J Clin Oncol.* 2005;23(31):8048–8056.

757. Bhoyrul B, Brent G, Elliott F, et al. Pathological review of primary cutaneous malignant melanoma by a specialist skin cancer multidisciplinary team improves patient care in the UK. *J Clin Pathol.* 2019;72(7):482–486.

758. Isom C, Hooks M, Kauffmann RM. Internal pathology review of invasive melanoma: an academic institution experience. *J Surg Res.* 2020;250:97–101.

759. Doepker MP, Thompson ZJ, Fisher KJ, et al. Is a wider margin (2 cm vs. 1 cm) for a 1.01–2.0 mm melanoma necessary? *Ann Surg Oncol.* 2016;23(7):2336–2342.

760. Etzkorn JR, Sobanko JF, Elenitsas R, et al. Low recurrence rates for in situ and invasive melanomas using Mohs micrographic surgery with melanoma antigen recognized by T cells 1 (MART-1) immunostaining: tissue processing methodology to optimize pathologic staging and margin assessment. *J Am Acad Dermatol.* 2015;72(5):840–850.

761. Morton DL, Thompson JF, Essner R, et al. Validation of the accuracy of intraoperative lymphatic mapping and sentinel lymphadenectomy for early-stage melanoma: a multicenter trial. Multicenter Selective Lymphadenectomy Trial Group. *Ann Surg.* 1999;230:453–463.

762. Morton DL, Wen D-R, Wong JH, et al. Technical details of intraoperative lymphatic mapping for early stage melanoma. *Arch Surg.* 1992;127:392–399.

763. Shidham VB, Qi D, Rao RN, et al. Improved immunohistochemical evaluation of micrometastases in sentinel lymph nodes of cutaneous melanoma with "MCW Melanoma Cocktail"—a mixture of monoclonal antibodies to MART-1, melan-A, and tyrosinase. *BMC Cancer.* 2003;3(1):15.

764. Piana S, Tagliavini E, Ragazzi M, et al. Lymph node melanocytic nevi: pathogenesis and differential diagnoses, with special reference to p16 reactivity. *Pathol Res Pract.* 2015;211(5):381–388.

765. LeBlanc RE, Barton DT, Li Z, et al. Small and isolated immunohistochemistry-positive cells in melanoma sentinel lymph nodes

are associated with disease-specific and recurrence-free survival comparable to that of sentinel lymph nodes negative for melanoma. *Am J Surg Pathol.* 2019;43(6):755–765.

766. Scolyer RA, Gershenwald JE, Thompson JF. Isolated imunohistochemistry-positive cells without morphologic characteristics of melanoma should not result in designation as a positive sentinel lymph node according to the AJCC 8th edition staging system. *Am J Surg Pathol.* 2019;43(10):1442–1444.

767. Yan S, Brennick JB. False-positive rate of the immunoperoxidase stains for MART1/MelanA in lymph nodes. *Am J Surg Pathol.* 2004;28(5):596–600.

768. van der Ploeg AP, van Akkooi AC, Haydu LE, et al. The prognostic significance of sentinel node tumour burden in melanoma patients: an international, multicenter study of 1539 sentinel node-positive melanoma patients. *Eur J Cancer.* 2014;50(1):111–120.

769. van der Ploeg AP, van Akkooi AC, Rutkowski P, et al. Prognosis in patients with sentinel node-positive melanoma is accurately

defined by the combined Rotterdam tumor load and dewar topography criteria. *J Clin Oncol.* 2011;29(16):2206–2214.

770. ADASP Committee. ADASP recommendations for the processing and reporting of lymph node specimens submitted for evaluation of metastatic disease. *Mod Pathol.* 2001;14:629–632.

771. Kucher C, Zhang PJ, Acs G, Roberts S, Xu X. Can Melan-A replace S-100 and HMB-45 in the evaluation of sentinel lymph nodes from patients with malignant melanoma? *Appl Immunohistochem Mol Morphol.* 2006;14(3):324–327.

772. Scolyer RA, Rawson RV, Gershenwald JE, Ferguson PM, Prieto VG. Melanoma pathology reporting and staging. *Mod Pathol.* 2020;33(suppl 1):15–24.

773. Tumino R, Minicozzi P, Frasca G, et al. Population-based method for investigating adherence to international recommendations for pathology reporting of primary cutaneous melanoma: results of a EUROCARE-5 high resolution study. *Cancer Epidemiol.* 2015;39(3):424–429.

Chapter 29

Tumors and Cysts of the Epidermis

NIGEL KIRKHAM, SU ENN LOW, AND KHADIJA ALJEFRI

CLASSIFICATION OF TUMORS OF THE EPIDERMIS

Epidermal tumors can be divided into tumors of the surface epidermis and tumors of the epidermal appendages. In each of the two classes, benign and malignant tumors occur.

Benign tumors in general are characterized by (a) a symmetric architecture and a circumscribed profile, (b) a tendency to differentiate along organized tissue lines, (c) uniformity in the appearance of the tumor cell nuclei, (d) architectural order in the arrangement of the tumor cell nuclei, (e) restraint in the rate of growth, and (f) absence of metastases.

Malignant tumors, in contrast, are characterized by (a) a less symmetric architecture and a poorly circumscribed profile; (b) a variable but, often, poorly differentiated phenotype; (c) atypicality in the appearance of the tumor cell nuclei, which show pleomorphism (i.e., great variability in size and shape), and anaplasia (i.e., hyperplasia and hyperchromasia); (d) architectural disorder in the arrangement of the tumor cell nuclei with loss of polarity; (e) rapid growth with the presence of mitoses, including atypical mitoses; and (f) potentiality to give rise to metastases.

Of the criteria of malignancy just cited, only the potentiality to give rise to metastases is decisive evidence for the malignancy of a tumor. For metastases to form, the tumor cells must possess a degree of autonomy that nonmalignant cells do not have. This autonomy enables malignant tumor cells to induce foreign tissue to furnish the necessary stroma in which they can multiply.

In addition to malignant tumors, one finds in the surface epidermis the so-called premalignant tumors, better regarded as tumors located largely *in situ*. Although cytologically malignant, they are biologically still benign. The World Health Organization (WHO) has classified tumors of the surface epidermis (1). Tumor staging by the TNM system is presently in its eighth edition (2).

PRINCIPLES OF MANAGEMENT: GENERAL

Tumors and cysts of the epidermis show a range of behaviors on the spectrum from benign cosmetic blemishes to true malignancies with capacity for regional and distant metastasis. In the majority of cases, treatment involves the removal of the primary lesion, most frequently using some form of surgical procedure ranging from shave excision, through punch excision or simple ellipse excision, to more extensive procedures. Treatment guidelines have been developed for the commoner entities described in this chapter: squamous cell carcinoma (SCC) and basal cell carcinoma (BCC), Bowen disease, as well as melanoma (3–7). Treatment success is related to the completeness and adequacy of the primary excision, although opinions vary on what constitutes an adequate surgical margin. There is a greater risk of local recurrence with some of the more aggressive or high-risk subtypes of tumors. Mohs micrographic surgery has become increasingly accepted as a way of achieving clear surgical excision margins, especially in the presence of tumors at difficult anatomic sites and tumors with high-risk features such as perineural invasion, so as to reduce the likelihood of locally recurrent disease (8,9), although this service is not always available (10). When the surgical margins are positive for tumor histologically, this does not necessarily imply that recurrence will always follow. Location, tumor size, histologic subtype, and clinical conditions of the patient must be considered when choosing the best treatment option (11).

LINEAR EPIDERMAL NEVUS

Clinical Summary. Linear epidermal nevi, or verrucous nevi, may be either localized or systematized.

In the *localized type*, which is present usually but not invariably at birth, only one linear lesion is present. It consists of closely set, papillomatous, hyperkeratotic papules. It may be located anywhere—on the head, trunk, or extremities. Being located on only one side of the patient, it is often referred to as *nevus unius lateris* (Figs. 29-1 and 29-2). In its configuration, the localized type of linear epidermal nevus resembles the inflammatory linear verrucous epidermal nevus (ILVEN), but the latter differs clinically by the presence of erythema and pruritus and histologically by the presence of inflammation and parakeratosis (12–14) (see Chapter 7).

In the *systematized type*, papillomatous hyperkeratotic papules in a linear configuration are present not just as one linear lesion, as in the localized type, but as many linear lesions. These linear lesions often show a parallel arrangement, particularly on the trunk. They may be limited to one side of the patient or may have a bilateral, symmetric distribution. The term *ichthyosis hystrix* is occasionally used, perhaps unnecessarily, for instances of extensive bilateral lesions.

Localized and, more commonly, systematized linear epidermal nevi may be associated with skeletal deformities and

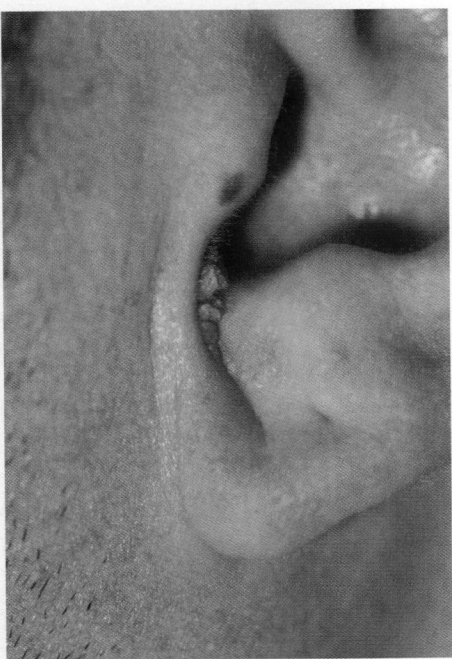

Figure 29-1 Epidermal nevus. The nevus lies in a fold of the external ear and has a papillary appearance.

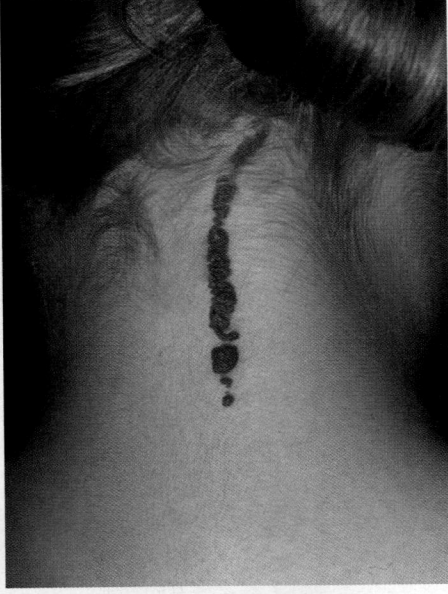

Figure 29-2 Linear epidermal nevus. This example is pigmented and lies in the midline, on the back of the neck.

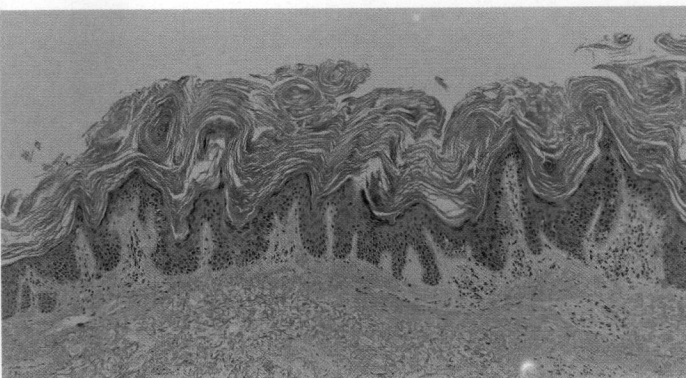

Figure 29-3 Epidermal nevus. The nevus shows a hyperkeratotic papillary appearance.

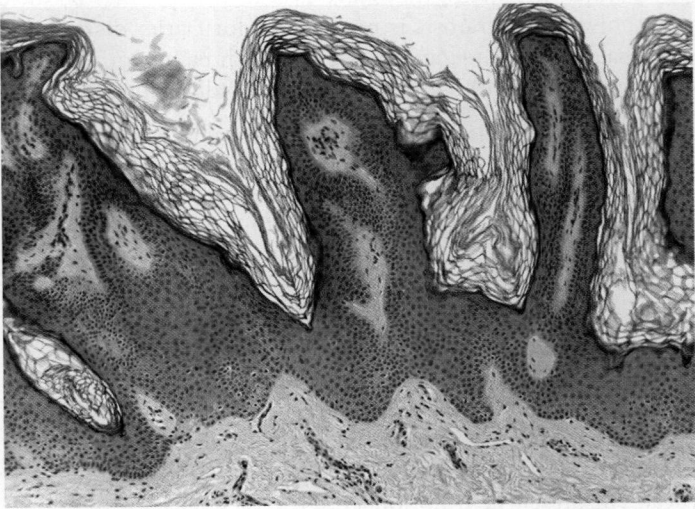

Figure 29-4 Epidermal nevus. The nevus shows orthokeratotic hyperkeratosis and flat-topped papillary projections.

central nervous system deficiencies, such as mental retardation, epilepsy, and neural deafness.

The presence of a BCC within a linear epidermal nevus has been observed occasionally, particularly on the head in cases in which the linear epidermal nevus has been associated with either a nevus sebaceous or a syringocystadenoma papilliferum (see Chapter 30). In areas other than the head, it is very rare. Similarly, the development of an SCC has been described only rarely; but in one instance, the SCC had metastasized to a regional lymph node.

Histopathology. Nearly all cases of the localized type of linear epidermal nevus and some cases of the systematized type show the histologic picture of a benign papilloma. One observes

considerable hyperkeratosis, papillomatosis, and acanthosis with elongation of the rete ridges resembling seborrheic keratosis (Figs. 29-3 and 29-4).

Occasionally in cases of the localized type, but quite frequently in cases of the systematized type—particularly those with a widespread distribution—one observes the rather striking histologic picture referred to either as *epidermolytic hyperkeratosis* or as *granular degeneration of the epidermis*. It is the same process that was first recognized in all cases of bullous congenital ichthyosiform erythroderma, a disorder that is often referred to as *epidermolytic hyperkeratosis* (see Chapter 6). It has since been found to occur in several other conditions as well (see the section on Isolated and Disseminated Epidermolytic Acanthoma).

The salient histologic features of epidermolytic hyperkeratosis are (a) perinuclear vacuolization of the cells in the stratum spinosum and in the stratum granulosum; (b) irregular cellular boundaries peripheral to the vacuolization; (c) an increased number of irregularly shaped, large keratohyalin granules; and (d) compact hyperkeratosis in the stratum corneum.

In some instances, histologic examination of unilateral linear lesions reveals features of acantholytic dyskeratosis as seen in Darier disease (Fig. 29-5) (see Chapter 6). In some patients, these linear lesions have been present since birth or infancy,

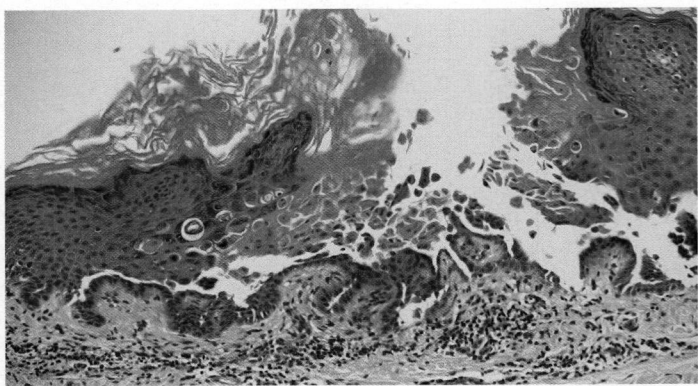

Figure 29-5 Unilateral linear epidermal nevus. The nevus shows suprabasal acantholysis of Darier disease type.

but in most instances, they have arisen in adult life. Because acantholytic dyskeratosis is not specific for Darier disease, the proposal has been made to designate such cases not as Darier disease but as acantholytic dyskeratotic epidermal nevus (15).

Differential Diagnosis. The histologic picture of a benign papilloma, as found in most cases of linear epidermal nevus, can also be seen in seborrheic keratosis, verruca vulgaris, and acanthosis nigricans. Even though these four conditions have hyperkeratosis and papillomatosis in common, they can be differentiated easily in typical cases; however, one is occasionally unable to make a diagnosis any more specific than benign papilloma or verrucous keratosis. Thus, in the following three situations, clinical data are required for differentiation from linear epidermal nevus: (a) the hyperkeratotic type of seborrheic keratosis, which is characterized by the absence of basaloid cells and horn cysts and instead shows upward extension of epidermis-lined papillae; (b) old verrucae vulgares, which no longer show vacuolization of epidermal cells or columns of parakeratosis (see Chapter 25); and (c) acanthosis nigricans showing more pronounced acanthosis and greater elongation of the rete ridges than usual (see Chapter 17).

NEVOID HYPERKERATOSIS OF NIPPLE AND AREOLA

Clinical Summary. Nevoid hyperkeratosis and papillomatosis of nipples and areola present as sharply demarcated papules and plaques, often appearing at puberty or during pregnancy and persisting unchanged. There are no associated systemic or dermatologic conditions. The main differential diagnosis is seborrheic keratosis (16,17).

Histopathology. There are papillomatous elongations of the epidermis with hyperkeratosis and areas of keratotic plugging. This condition represents a nevoid form of hyperkeratosis.

NEVUS COMEDONICUS

Clinical Summary. A nevus comedonicus consists of closely set, slightly elevated papules that have in their center a dark, firm, hyperkeratotic plug resembling a comedo. Nevus comedonicus, like linear epidermal nevus, usually has a linear configuration and occurs as a single lesion. In some instances, however, there are multiple bilateral linear lesions or lesions that are randomly

distributed rather than linear. Lesions may be present on the palms or soles in addition to other areas. Such cases may represent a combination of nevus comedonicus with a porokeratotic eccrine duct nevus (see the next section).

Histopathology. Each comedo is represented by a wide, deep invagination of the epidermis filled with keratin (Figs. 29-6 and 29-7). These invaginations resemble dilated hair follicles; in fact, as evidence that they actually represent rudimentary hair follicles, one occasionally finds in the lower portion of an invagination one or even several hair shafts. One or two small sebaceous gland lobules may also be seen opening into the lower pole of invaginations.

In several instances, the keratinocytes composing the follicular epithelial wall have shown the typical changes of epidermolytic hyperkeratosis (see the following section), indicative of a relationship of nevus comedonicus to systematized nevus verrucosus (see Chapter 30).

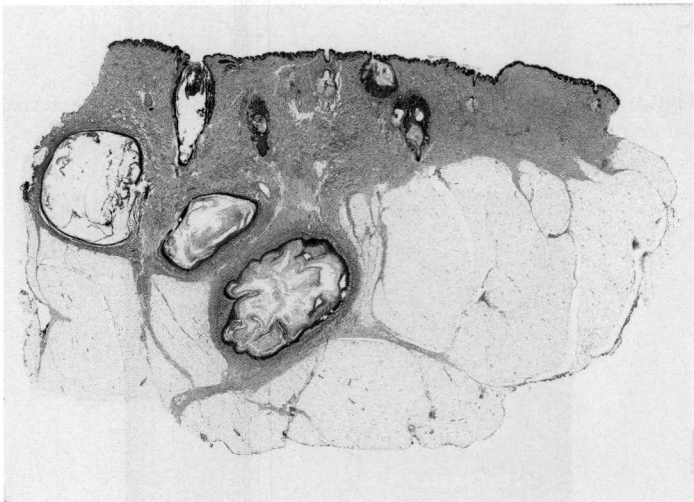

Figure 29-6 Nevus comedonicus. There is a deep invagination of the epidermis containing keratin, and there are several keratinous cysts in the dermis. This is a staged excision of a larger lesion (note a scar at the right of the image).

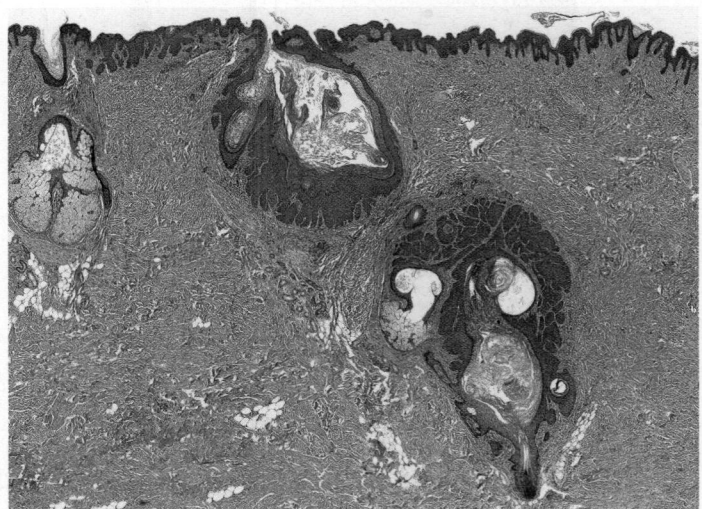

Figure 29-7 Nevus comedonicus. Two follicles from near the center of the specimen are dilated and filled with keratin. There is hamartomatous thickening of the epithelium of these follicles, and dermal papillae are elongated in the overlying epidermis.

POROKERATOTIC ECCRINE OSTIAL AND DERMAL DUCT NEVUS

Clinical Summary. Porokeratotic eccrine ostial and dermal duct nevus may be limited to a palm or to a sole but may be present on both hands and feet and elsewhere (18). It may involve not only eccrine ducts but also hair follicles on the hairy parts of the body.

Histopathology. In the porokeratotic eccrine duct nevus, each invagination consists of a dilated eccrine duct containing a parakeratotic plug. The absence of a granular layer at the base of the plug together with the presence of keratinocytes showing vacuolization of their cytoplasm results in a histologic picture resembling that of porokeratosis (see Chapter 6).

ISOLATED AND DISSEMINATED EPIDERMOLYTIC ACANTHOMA

Clinical Summary. Isolated epidermolytic acanthoma, histologically characterized by the presence of "epidermolytic hyperkeratosis," does not have a characteristic clinical appearance or location. Usually, it occurs as a solitary papillomatous lesion less than 1 cm in diameter. Occasionally, several lesions are seen in a localized area. One case has been described that was probably secondary to trauma.

Disseminated epidermolytic acanthoma occurs as numerous discrete, flat, brownish papules 2 to 6 mm in diameter, resembling seborrheic keratoses. The upper trunk, especially the back, is the site of predilection (19,20).

Histopathology. In addition to hyperkeratosis and papillomatosis, one observes pronounced epidermolytic hyperkeratosis, also referred to as *granular degeneration*, throughout the stratum malpighii, sparing only the basal layer, just as seen in linear epidermal nevi with epidermolytic changes. One observes both intracellular and intercellular edema of the epidermal cells and keratohyalin granules that are coarser than normal and extend to a greater depth in the stratum malpighii (21).

Differential Diagnosis. Myrmecia warts, caused by human papillomavirus type 1 (HPV-1), also show perinuclear vacuolization and an abundance of keratohyalin granules, representing a type of "granular degeneration" similar to that seen in epidermolytic hyperkeratosis. However, in myrmecia warts, the keratohyalin granules are eosinophilic and coalesce in the upper layers of the epidermis to form large, homogeneous, eosinophilic "inclusion bodies." In verrucae vulgares, usually caused by HPV-2, foci of vacuolated cells and clumped basophilic keratohyalin granules may be present, but these changes are limited to the upper layers of the epidermis. In addition, both myrmecia warts and verrucae vulgares show focal parakeratosis rather than orthokeratosis as seen in epidermolytic hyperkeratosis (see Chapter 25).

INCIDENTAL EPIDERMOLYTIC HYPERKERATOSIS

Clinical Summary. Epidermolytic hyperkeratosis is seen not only in isolated and disseminated epidermolytic hyperkeratosis (see previous section) but also as a *regular* finding in epidermolytic hyperkeratosis or bullous congenital ichthyosiform erythroderma (see Chapter 6) and in epidermolytic keratosis palmaris et plantaris and as an *occasional* finding in linear epidermal nevus and nevus comedonicus. In addition, epidermolytic hyperkeratosis may represent an *incidental* histologic finding in many different types of lesions including nevi, infundibular cysts, rosacea, and drug-induced acne (22–27). It has also been observed in normal oral mucosa adjacent to lesions of SCC and BCC.

Histopathology. Epidermolytic hyperkeratosis may be seen throughout an entire lesion of solar keratosis and in the entire lining of trichilemmal cyst. More commonly, however, the histologic features of epidermolytic hyperkeratosis are seen as a small focus, often limited to a single epidermal rete ridge, in such diverse lesions as sebaceous hyperplasia, intradermal nevus, hypertrophic scar, superficial BCC, seborrheic keratosis, the margin of an SCC, lichenoid amyloidosis, and granuloma annulare. In some instances, the process is limited to one or two intraepidermal sweat duct units. It is more frequently seen in dysplastic nevi than in ordinary melanocytic nevi.

ISOLATED AND DISSEMINATED ACANTHOLYTIC ACANTHOMA

Clinical Summary. This condition usually occurs as a solitary papule or small nodule, although there may be multiple lesions. No characteristic clinical appearance or location exists, although multiple lesions have been seen largely in the genital region and in organ transplant recipients (28–30).

Histopathology. Acantholysis is the most prominent feature. The pattern may resemble that of pemphigus vulgaris, pemphigus vegetans, pemphigus foliaceus, or benign familial pemphigus. Acantholysis may be combined with dyskeratosis, in which case, the histologic picture resembles that of Darier disease as a result of the presence of corps ronds and grains.

INCIDENTAL FOCAL ACANTHOLYTIC DYSKERATOSIS

Clinical Summary. Analogous to epidermolytic hyperkeratosis, acantholytic dyskeratosis is seen as a *regular* histologic feature in Darier disease (see Chapter 6), transient acantholytic dermatosis (Grover disease), and warty dyskeratoma. It is also an *occasional* finding in acantholytic dyskeratotic epidermal nevus, a variant of linear epidermal nevus. In addition, again like epidermolytic hyperkeratosis, focal acantholytic dyskeratosis is observed occasionally as an *incidental* histologic finding in a variety of lesions, including vascular nevi, discoid lupus erythematosus, rosacea, and trichofolliculoma (23,31–35).

Histopathology. Focal suprabasal clefts with overlying acantholytic and dyskeratotic cells, some of which have the appearance of corps ronds (Figs. 29-8 and 29-9), have been seen as a single focus in the epidermis overlying such diverse lesions as dermatofibroma, BCC, melanocytic nevus, and chondrodermatitis nodularis helicis, as well as in pityriasis rosea and acral lentiginous malignant melanoma.

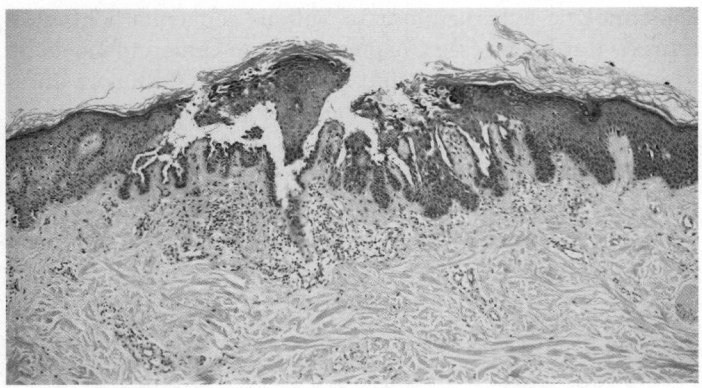

Figure 29-8 Incidental focal acantholytic dyskeratosis. Focally, within an excision biopsy of another lesion, there is suprabasal cleft with overlying dyskeratotic cells.

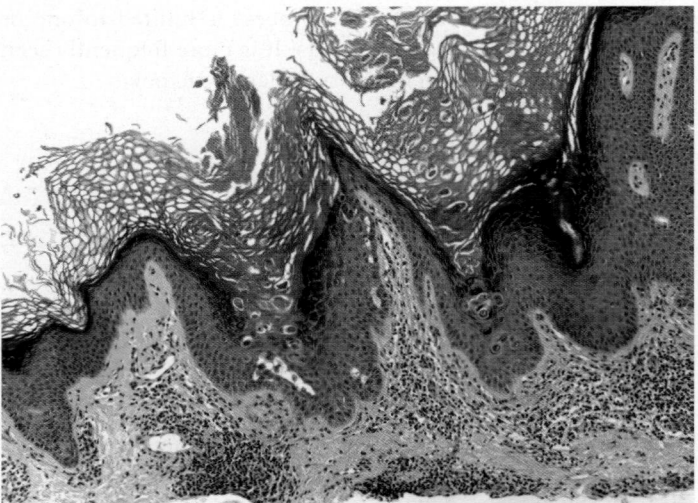

Figure 29-9 Incidental focal acantholytic dyskeratosis. Focally, within the biopsy, there is suprabasal cleft formation with overlying dyskeratotic cells.

ORAL WHITE SPONGE NEVUS

Clinical Summary. First described in 1935 (36), oral white sponge nevus is a benign autosomal dominant disorder that affects noncornifying stratified squamous epithelia (37). It may be present at birth or have its onset in infancy, childhood, or adolescence (38,39). Extensive areas of the oral mucosa and sometimes the entire oral mucosa have a thickened, folded, creamy white appearance. In some instances, the rectal mucosa, vagina, nasal mucosa, or esophagus is also involved. This distribution of lesions suggests that mutations in the epithelial keratins K14 and/or K13 may be responsible (40,41).

The oral lesions seen in pachyonychia congenita are both clinically and histologically indistinguishable from a white sponge nevus (see Chapter 6). Both leukoplakia and oral lichen planus are clinical differential diagnoses.

Histopathology. The oral epithelium shows hyperplasia with much more pronounced hydropic swelling of the epithelial cells than is normal for the oral mucosa. The swelling, though extensive, is focal. It extends into the rete ridges but spares the basal layer. The nuclei appear smaller than normal. The surface shows parakeratosis—as does the normal oral mucosa—and

only rarely are there small accumulations of keratohyalin granules.

Pathogenesis. On electron microscopic examination, large cytoplasmic areas of the epithelial cells appear optically empty or contain only faint granular material. Tonofilaments are limited to the perinuclear and peripheral areas. The intercellular areas show irregular dilation, and large, irregularly shaped vacuoles are present within the cytoplasm. A possibly fundamental disturbance is the presence of numerous intracellular Odland bodies or membrane-coating granules (see Chapter 3), which are not extruded into the intercellular spaces.

Differential Diagnosis. The histologic picture of oral white sponge nevus is identical to that seen in pachyonychia congenita (see the preceding text) and to that of oral focal epithelial hyperplasia and of leukoedema of the oral mucosa (see the following section).

Principles of Management: There is no standard treatment for this condition. Successful treatment with antifungals and antibiotics has been reported (42).

LEUKOEDEMA OF THE ORAL MUCOSA

Clinical Summary. Leukoedema is a common benign condition that is significantly more prevalent in Afro-Caribbean individuals and is characterized by a blue, gray, or white appearance of the oral mucosa, in particular the buccal mucosa (43). When pronounced, it shows a clinical and histologic resemblance to oral white sponge nevus. However, leukoedema differs from white sponge nevus by being patchy rather than diffuse, by having exacerbations and remissions and adult onset, and by not being inherited. The exact etiology of the condition is unknown, but it is thought to be caused by local irritation—such as tobacco smoking and khat chewing (44). Thorough clinical examination should differentiate leukoedema from leukoplakia, lichen planus, and oral white sponge nevus (45).

Histopathology. In leukoedema of the oral mucosa, as in oral white sponge nevus, the suprabasal epithelial cells show marked intracellular edema. The nuclei appear smaller than normal.

Principles of Management: No treatment is required for this benign condition.

LINGUA GEOGRAPHICA

Clinical Summary. Geographic tongue, also referred to as superficial migratory glossitis, is a common benign clinical condition of unknown etiology although it may be associated with adverse effects to dental materials (46). It typically presents on the dorsum of the tongue, showing irregularly shaped red patches surrounded by a whitish, raised border a few millimeters wide. It is common, affecting 2% to 3% of the population (47). It is usually asymptomatic, with local loss of filiform papillae, leading to the development of ulcer-like lesions that rapidly change color and size (48).

Histopathology. Whereas the dorsum of the tongue normally shows a granular and a horny layer, these layers are absent in the red patches of lingua geographica. Along the whitish border, the epithelium shows irregular thickening and infiltration of neutrophils. In its upper portion, the epithelium shows collections of neutrophils within the interstices of a sponge-like network formed by degenerated and thinned epithelial cells. The histologic picture thus shows Kogoj spongiform pustules, which are indistinguishable from those seen in pustular psoriasis.

Pathogenesis. The presence of spongiform pustules generally is regarded as diagnostic of pustular psoriasis and as almost specific for it (see Chapter 7), even though it rarely occurs in other pustules, such as those caused by *Candida albicans*. It has therefore been suggested that geographic tongue represents a localized form of pustular psoriasis. However, even though both pustular psoriasis and lingua geographica may show annular lesions on the tongue, pustular psoriasis of the mouth generally shows clinical evidence of pustules and is usually seen in other areas of the mouth also. It is therefore best to regard lingua geographica as a separate entity.

Principles of Management: Geographical tongue does not typically require any treatment. If it is associated with discomfort, corticosteroid ointments or rinses could be used.

SEBORRHEIC KERATOSIS

Clinical Summary. Seborrheic keratoses are very common: sometimes single but often multiple (49–51). They occur mainly on the trunk and face and also on the extremities, excluding palms and soles. They usually do not appear before middle age but are present in about 20% of the elderly. They are sharply demarcated, often brownish in color, and slightly raised, often appearing as though stuck on the surface of the skin (Figs. 29-10 and 29-11). Most have a verrucous surface, and a soft, friable consistency. Some have a smooth surface but characteristically show keratotic plugs, which can complicate dermoscopic assessment (52). Although most lesions measure only a few millimeters in diameter, some occasionally reach a size of several centimeters. Crusting and an inflammatory base are found if the lesion has been subjected to trauma. Occasionally, small examples are pedunculated, especially on the neck and upper chest, where they resemble soft fibromas (see Chapter 32). Frequent genetic mutations, most with ultraviolet (UV) signature, and

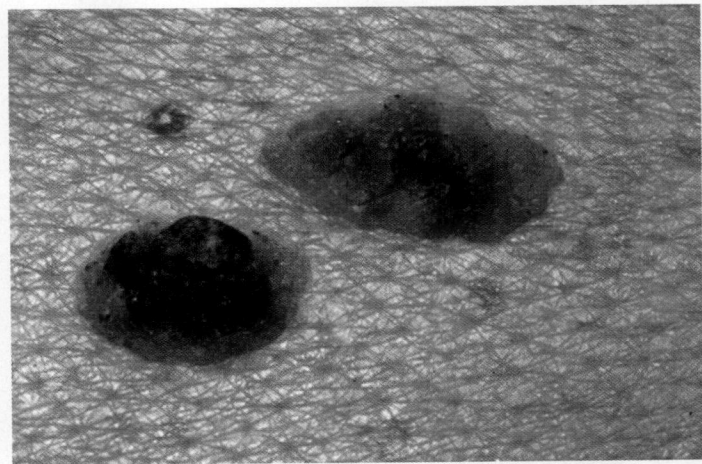

Figure 29-11 Seborrheic keratosis. Two keratoses lie close together and show variable pigmentation.

many involving known oncogenes or progression-related genes have been described in seborrheic keratoses, even though these lesions typically appear to be genetically stable (53). Malignant change is rare but has been reported in association with unusual clinical appearances to the seborrheic keratoses.

Histopathology. Seborrheic keratoses show a considerable variety of histologic appearances. Six types are generally recognized: irritated, adenoid or reticulated, plane, clonal, melanoacanthoma, inverted follicular keratosis, and benign squamous (Figs. 29-12 to 29-15). Often, more than one type is found in the same lesion.

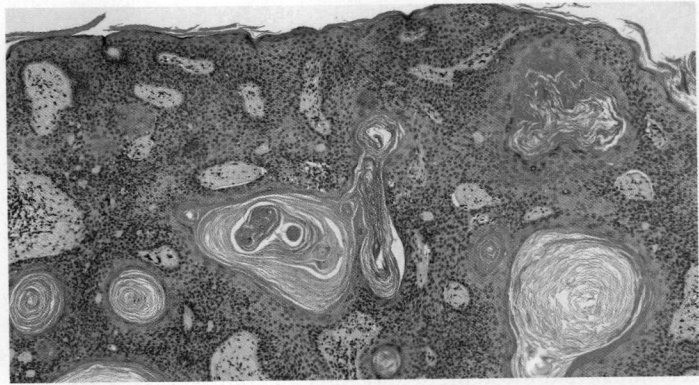

Figure 29-12 Seborrheic keratosis. Low magnification. The keratosis is composed of basaloid keratinocytes and contains several horn cysts.

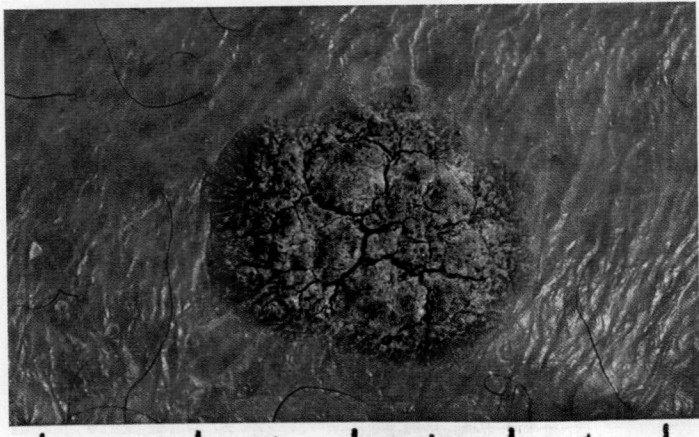

Figure 29-10 Seborrheic keratosis. The keratosis has a grayish waxy appearance.

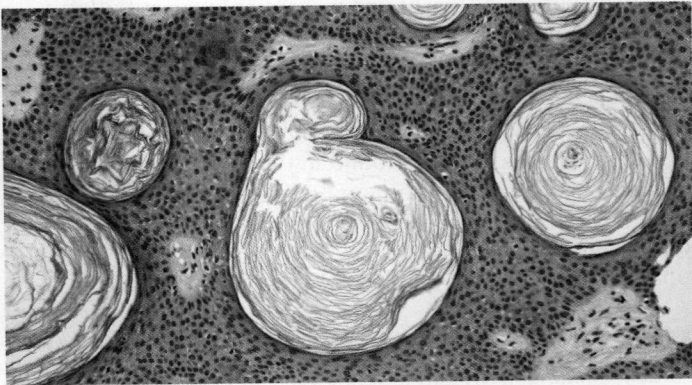

Figure 29-13 Seborrheic keratosis. High magnification. Most of the cells have a basaloid appearance, with interspersed horn cysts filled with keratin.

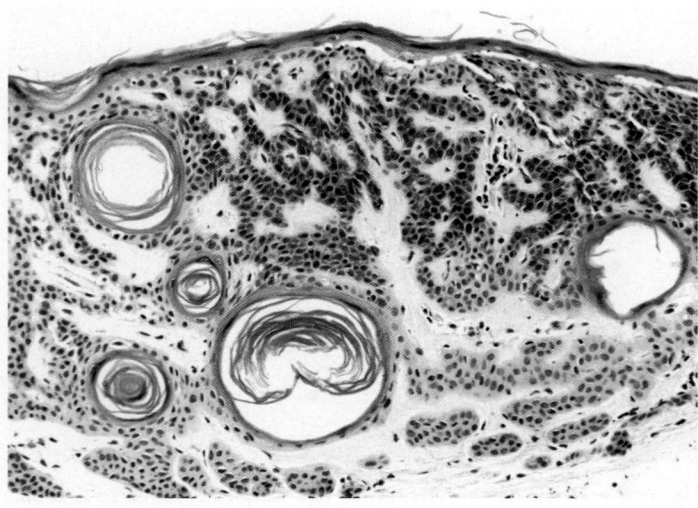

Figure 29-14 Pigmented seborrheic keratosis. Thin interwoven cords of basaloid cells show cytoplasmic melanin pigmentation and horn cysts.

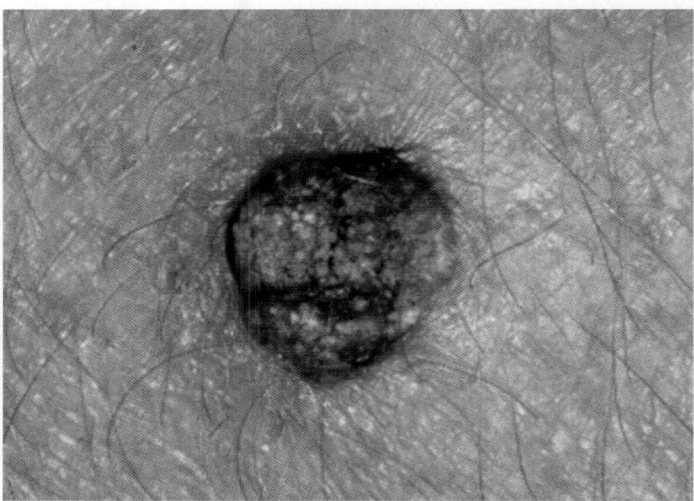

Figure 29-16 Irritated seborrheic keratosis. Showing inflammation of the adjacent skin.

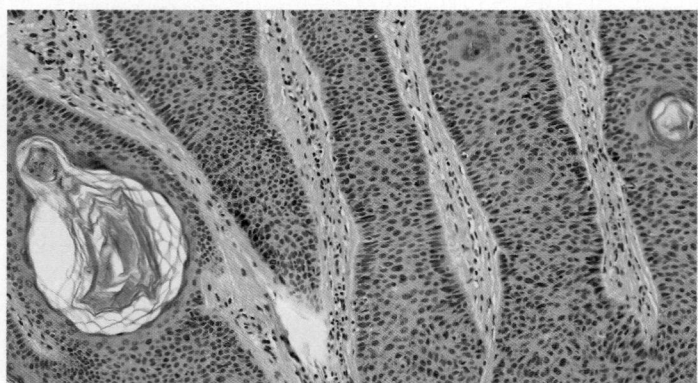

Figure 29-15 Pigmented seborrheic keratosis. Melanin is present in both basal cells and in basaloid cells within the lesion.

Differential diagnosis from Pagetoid Bowen disease can be made with high expression of Ki 67 and p16 favoring a diagnosis of Pagetoid Bowen disease (54). A desmoplastic variant may mimic an invasive malignant lesion (55). In addition, two clinical variants of seborrheic keratosis will be described—dermatosis papulosa nigra and stucco keratosis (Fig. 29-20).

All types of seborrheic keratosis have in common hyperkeratosis, acanthosis, and papillomatosis. The acanthosis in most instances is due entirely to upward extension of the tumor. Thus, the lower border of the tumor is even and generally lies on a straight line that may be drawn from the normal epidermis at one end of the tumor to the normal epidermis at the other end. Two types of cells are usually seen in the acanthotic epidermis: squamous cells and basaloid cells. The former have the appearance of squamous cells normally found in the epidermis; the basaloid cells are small and uniform in appearance and have a relatively large nucleus. In areas of slight intercellular edema, intercellular bridges can be easily recognized. Thus, they resemble the basal cells found normally in the basal layer of the epidermis.

Irritated Type and Inverted Follicular Keratosis

Clinical Summary. Irritated seborrheic keratosis will typically appear inflamed, with inflammation extending to involve the surrounding skin (Fig. 29-16).

Histopathology. Squamous cells typically outnumber basaloid cells. The characteristic feature is the presence of numerous whorls or eddies composed of eosinophilic, flattened squamous cells arranged in an onion-peel fashion, resembling poorly differentiated horn pearls (Fig. 29-17). These "squamous eddies" are easily differentiated from the horn pearls of SCC by their large number, small size, and circumscribed configuration. Irritated seborrheic keratoses, in addition, may show areas of downward proliferation breaking through the horizontal demarcation generally present in nonirritated seborrheic keratoses. Frequently, some of these proliferations are seen to originate from the walls of keratin-filled invaginations. Inflammation beneath irritated seborrheic keratoses usually is mild or absent, indicating that irritated seborrheic keratoses are different from inflamed seborrheic keratoses.

In a few instances, acantholysis has been observed within tumor nests composed of squamous cells. These acantholytic changes differ from those occurring in incidental focal

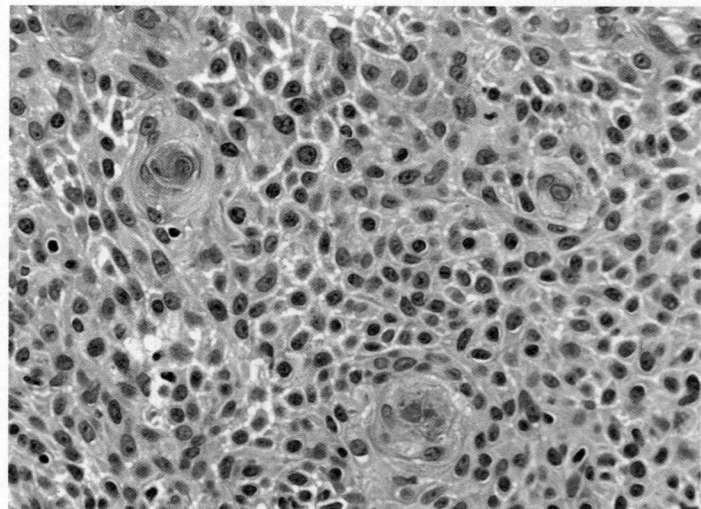

Figure 29-17 Inverted follicular keratosis. Squamous eddies are present, composed of whorls of squamous cells. There is no substantial cytologic atypia.

acantholytic dyskeratosis by not showing suprabasal location or dyskeratotic cells resembling corps ronds.

Pathogenesis. The formation of numerous squamous eddies is a result of the "activation" of resting basaloid cells into squamous cells. This unique and highly diagnostic feature of irritated or activated seborrheic keratoses, as well as their downward proliferation, is the result of irritation. This has been proved experimentally by the excision of seborrheic keratoses either after a previous biopsy or after irritation with croton oil.

The identical histologic picture as seen in irritated seborrheic keratosis has been described under the designations of *inverted follicular keratosis* and *follicular poroma*. As these terms indicate, the authors regard the keratin-filled invaginations as follicular infundibula and the proliferations arising from them as composed of cells of the follicular infundibulum. The follicular infundibulum consists of cells with the same type of keratinization as the surface epidermis, and there is evidence that seborrheic keratoses incorporate cells of the infundibular portion of the hair follicle and are partially derived from these cells. Seborrheic keratoses, like inverted follicular keratoses, occur exclusively on hair-bearing skin. Some seborrheic keratoses even contain aggregates of vellus hairs within the keratinous invaginations, an occurrence analogous to trichostasis spinulosa (see Chapter 18). Although some authors merely concede that irritated seborrheic keratoses and inverted follicular keratoses may be histologically indistinguishable, others regard the two disorders as identical. Because of their histologic similarity and particularly because of the highly specific appearance of the squamous eddies that occur in these two conditions, they are best regarded as identical.

Adenoid or Reticulated Type

In the adenoid or reticulated type of seborrheic keratosis, numerous thin tracts of epidermal cells extend from the epidermis and show branching and interweaving in the dermis. Many tracts are composed of only a double row of basaloid cells. Horn cysts and pseudo–horn cysts are absent in purely reticulated lesions; however, the reticulated type often also shows areas of the acanthotic type, and horn cysts and pseudo–horn cysts are commonly seen in these areas. The basaloid cells of the reticulated type of seborrheic keratosis usually show marked hyperpigmentation.

There is both clinical and histologic evidence of a close relationship between solar or senile lentigo senilis and the reticulated type of seborrheic keratosis. A lesion of solar lentigo may even become a reticulated seborrheic keratosis through exaggeration of the process of downward budding of pigmented basaloid cells (see Chapter 28).

Acanthotic Type

In the acanthotic type—the most common type of seborrheic keratosis—hyperkeratosis and papillomatosis often are slight, but the epidermis is greatly thickened. Although only narrow papillae are included in the thickened epidermis in some cases, one can see in other lesions a retiform pattern composed of thick, interwoven tracts of epithelial cells surrounding islands of connective tissue. Horny invaginations that on cross sections appear as pseudo–horn cysts are numerous. In addition, there are also true horn cysts, which—like the pseudo–horn cysts—show sudden and complete keratinization with only a very thin granular layer.

The true horn cysts begin as foci of orthokeratosis within the substance of the lesion. In time, they enlarge and are carried by the current of epidermal cells toward the surface of the lesion, where they unite with the invaginations of surface keratin. In the greatly thickened epidermis, basaloid cells usually outnumber squamous cells.

The amount of melanin in seborrheic keratoses of the acanthotic type is often greater than normal. Excess amounts of melanin are seen in about one-third of the specimens stained with hematoxylin–eosin; staining with silver reveals excess amounts in about two-thirds of the cases. In dopa-stained sections, melanocytes are limited to the dermal–epidermal junctional layer present at the base of the tumor and at the interfaces between the tumor tracts and the islands of dermal stroma. The word *dopa* is an abbreviation for 3,4-dioxyphenylalanin, a phenol which, when dissolved in an alkaline solution and exposed to air oxidizes spontaneously to a black substance resembling melanin, if not actually identical with it (56). The melanin, largely present in keratinocytes, is in most instances also limited to keratinocytes located at the dermal–epidermal junction. Only deeply pigmented lesions show melanin widely distributed throughout the tumor within basaloid cells.

A mononuclear inflammatory infiltrate is seen quite frequently in the dermis underlying a seborrheic keratosis. The inflammation may impinge on the tumor in a lichenoid or eczematous pattern. In the lichenoid pattern, a bandlike infiltrate is seen hugging the basal cell layer of the tumor. In the eczematous pattern, there is exocytosis leading to spongiosis. Squamous eddies, typical of irritated seborrheic keratoses, are only rarely seen in inflamed seborrheic keratoses.

The formation of an *in situ* carcinoma within an acanthotic seborrheic keratosis, the so-called bowenoid transformation, is seen occasionally. It seems to occur predominantly in lesions located in sun-exposed areas of the skin; so, sun damage may be a factor. In one reported case, a metastasis in a regional lymph node was found. On rare occasions, a BCC may form within an acanthotic seborrheic keratosis and may extend from there into the underlying dermis.

Pathogenesis. Electron microscopic examination has confirmed the light microscopic impression that the small basaloid cells seen in the acanthotic type of seborrheic keratosis are related to cells of the epidermal basal cell layer rather than to the basaloma cells of BCC. They possess a fair number of desmosomes and a moderate number of tonofilaments that differ from those present in cells of the epidermal basal cell layer only by showing less orientation.

Hyperkeratotic Type

In the hyperkeratotic type, also referred to as the digitate or serrated type, hyperkeratosis and papillomatosis are pronounced, whereas acanthosis is not very conspicuous. The numerous digitate upward extensions of epidermis-lined papillae often resemble church spires. The histologic picture then resembles that seen in acrokeratosis verruciformis of Hopf (see Chapter 6). The epidermis consists largely of squamous cells, although small aggregates of basaloid cells may be seen here and there. As a rule, no excess amounts of melanin are found.

Clonal Type

In the clonal, or nesting, type of seborrheic keratosis, well-defined nests of cells are located within the epidermis. In some instances, the nests resemble the foci of BCC because the nuclei appear small and dark-staining and intercellular bridges are seen in only a few areas (see Figs. 29-18 and 29-19). The histologic picture in such cases has been erroneously interpreted by some authors as

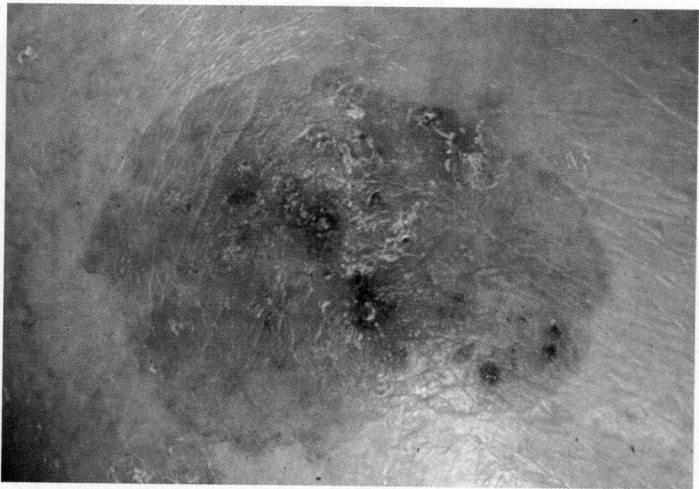

Figure 29-18 Clonal seborrheic keratosis. Showing focal variation in pigmentation.

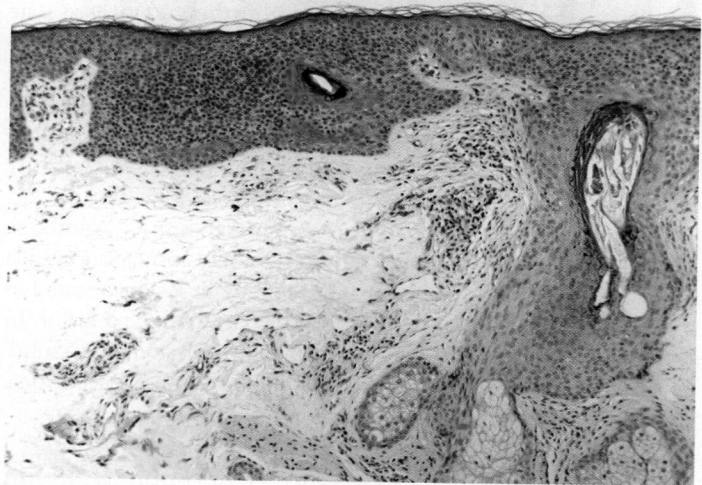

Figure 29-19 Clonal seborrheic keratosis. Showing foci of basaloid cells surrounded by more eosinophilic squamous cells.

representing an intraepidermal epithelioma of Borst–Jadassohn (see Chapter 30). In other instances of clonal seborrheic keratosis, the nests are composed of fairly large cells showing distinct intercellular bridges, with the nests separated from one another by strands of cells exhibiting small, dark nuclei.

Melanoacanthoma

This rather rare variant of pigmented seborrheic keratosis differs from the usual type of pigmented seborrheic keratosis by showing a marked increase in the concentration of melanocytes. Rather than being confined to the basal layer of the tumor lobules, many melanocytes are scattered throughout the tumor lobules. In some instances, well-defined islands of basaloid cells intermingled with many melanocytes are distributed through the tumor. The melanocytes are large and richly dendritic and contain variable amounts of melanin. The block in transfer of melanin from melanocytes to keratinocytes often is only partial, although in some instances nearly all the melanin is retained in the melanocytes. The lesions may be single or multiple (57,58).

It is important in the clinical differential diagnosis of cutaneous melanoma (59,60) and also in pigmented lesions presenting in oral mucosa (61,62).

Pathogenesis. Melanoacanthoma is a benign mixed tumor of melanocytes and keratinocytes.

Principles of Management: Treatment for asymptomatic seborrheic keratosis is largely carried out for cosmetic reasons. Symptomatic lesions are commonly removed by cryotherapy, curettage, or shave excision. Other methods for removal such as laser vaporization and electrodesiccation are also performed.

DERMATOSIS PAPULOSA NIGRA

Clinical Summary. Dermatosis papulosa nigra is a benign condition considered by some to be a type of seborrheic keratosis. It is found in about 35% of all adult blacks, often has its onset during adolescence, and has been described in a 3-year-old child. It also occurs among Asians, although the exact incidence is unknown. The lesions are located predominantly on the face—especially in the malar regions—but they may also occur on the neck and upper trunk. They usually consist of small, smooth, pigmented papules, except on the neck and trunk, where they may be pedunculated. Dermatosis papulosa nigra is likely to be genetically determined, with 40% to 50% of patients having a family history. It is thought to be due to a nevoid mutation of the hair follicle.

Histopathology. The lesions have the histologic appearance of seborrheic keratoses but are smaller. Most lesions are of the acanthotic type and show thick interwoven tracts of epithelial cells. The cells are largely squamous in appearance, with only a few basaloid cells. Horn cysts are quite common. An occasional lesion shows a reticulated pattern in which the tracts are composed of a double row of basaloid cells. Melanin pigmentation is pronounced in all lesions.

Principles of Management: Treatment for dermatosis papulosa nigra is usually carried out for cosmetic reasons. Hypopigmentation posttreatment is a concern, and it is advised to perform treatment on a small area of skin to begin with. Dermatosis papulosa nigra is commonly treated with snip excision, curettage, and light electrodesiccation (63).

STUCCO KERATOSIS

Clinical Summary. This entity was first described by Kocsard and Ofner in 1965 (64). Stucco keratoses are benign, small, gray-white seborrheic keratoses measuring 1 to 3 mm in diameter, located in symmetric arrangement on the distal portions of the extremities—especially the ankles (Fig. 29-20). They can easily be scraped off without any resultant bleeding.

The name stucco keratosis is derived from the "stuck-on" appearance of the lesions. No known cause has been found for their development, and they are not thought to be inherited genetically. However, DNA from HPV types 9, 16, 23b, DL322, and a variant of HPV 37 was detected with nested polymerase chain reaction analysis of lesional material from a 75-year-old man with extensive stucco keratoses (65). The finding of FGFR3 and PIK3CA mutations in stucco keratoses and lesions of dermatosis papulosis nigra supports the concept that both skin lesions are specific variants of seborrheic keratosis, sharing a common genetic background (66).

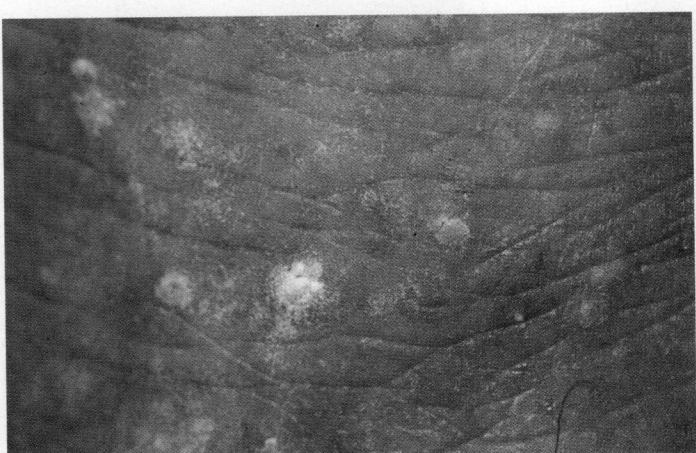

Figure 29-20 Stucco keratoses. Multiple small white, gray-white seborrheic keratoses.

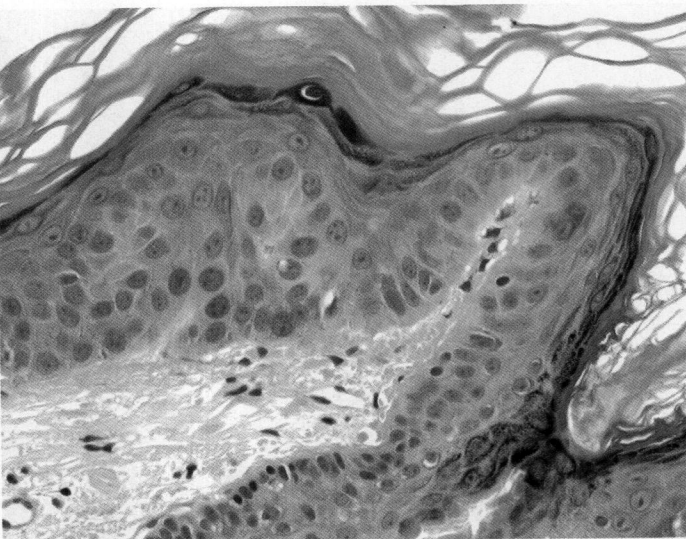

Figure 29-21 Large cell acanthoma. Keratinocytes are increased in size and arranged in a disorderly manner. The granular layer is present and there is no parakeratosis.

Histopathology. Stucco keratoses have the appearance of the hyperkeratotic type of seborrheic keratosis, showing the church-spire pattern of upward-extending papillae. Horn cysts and basaloid cells are usually absent.

Principles of Management: As for seborrheic keratosis, treatment is performed for cosmetic reasons. Destruction with cryotherapy, curettage, or simple excision can be used for removal.

LESER–TRÉLAT SIGN

Clinical Summary. The Leser–Trélat sign is characterized by the sudden appearance of numerous seborrheic keratoses in association with a malignant tumor. Although many reports concerning this sign have appeared in recent years and although its existence is accepted, it is not always easy to decide which cases should be included. In some instances, numerous seborrheic keratoses develop on inflamed skin, but this does not represent the Leser–Trélat sign. The Leser–Trélat sign has been interpreted as "an incomplete form of acanthosis nigricans" or as "potentially representing an early stage of acanthosis nigricans" (see Chapter 17).

Although the malignant tumor in 67% of the reported cases consisted of an abdominal adenocarcinoma, the remaining 33% included many different types of malignancies, including leukemia and mycosis fungoides (67–69).

Histopathology. The seborrheic keratoses in the Leser–Trélat sign are the same as other seborrheic keratoses. The hyperkeratotic form is indistinguishable from malignant acanthosis nigricans.

LARGE CELL ACANTHOMA

Clinical Summary. Large cell acanthoma occurs as a slightly hyperkeratotic, sharply demarcated patch, usually on the sun-exposed skin of the head or extremities. As a rule, it measures less than 1 cm in size. Generally, it is a solitary lesion; occasionally, multiple lesions are observed (70–72). It may also occur on the conjunctiva (73,74).

Histopathology. Within a well-demarcated area of the epidermis, the scattered large keratinocytes are about twice the normal size and have proportionally large nuclei. There may be a disordered arrangement of the keratinocytes (Fig. 29-21). Unlike in an actinic keratosis, there is no parakeratosis.

Pathogenesis. The lesion is aneuploid, with various stages of development, and is probably related to stucco keratosis.

Principles of Management: Destruction or excision is the option for the treatment of this benign entity.

CLEAR CELL ACANTHOMA

Clinical Summary. Clear cell acanthoma, a tumor that is clinically and histologically quite distinct, was first described in 1962 (75). It is not rare (76,77). Typically, the lesions are solitary and occur on the legs. Cases have also been reported on the nipple and areola (78–80) and on the palate (81) along with multiple eruptive examples (82). They are slowly growing, sharply delineated, red nodules or plaques 1 to 2 cm in diameter and are usually covered with a thin crust and exude some moisture. A collarette is often seen at the periphery. It has been said that the lesion appears stuck-on, like a seborrheic keratosis, and is vascular, like a granuloma pyogenicum (Fig. 29-22).

Histopathology. Within a sharply demarcated area of the epidermis, all epidermal cells, with the exception of cells of the basal cell layer, appear strikingly clear and slightly enlarged (Figs. 29-23 and 29-24). The nuclei of the clear epidermal cells appear normal. When staining is carried out with the periodic acid–Schiff (PAS) reaction, the presence of large amounts of glycogen is revealed within the cells.

Slight spongiosis is present between the clear cells. The rete ridges are elongated and may show intertwining. The surface shows parakeratosis with few or no granular cells. The acrosyringia and acrotrichia within the tumor retain their normal stainability. There is an absence of melanin within the tumor cells, but dendritic melanocytes containing melanin are occasionally seen interspersed between the clear cells.

A conspicuous feature in most lesions is the presence throughout the epidermis of numerous neutrophils, many of which show fragmentation of their nuclei (Fig. 29-24). The

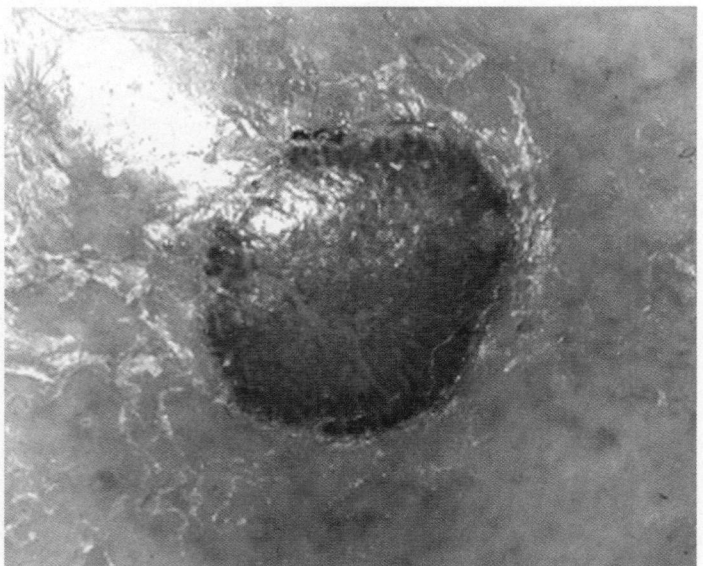

Figure 29-22 Clear cell acanthoma. A raised, sharply demarcated red patch.

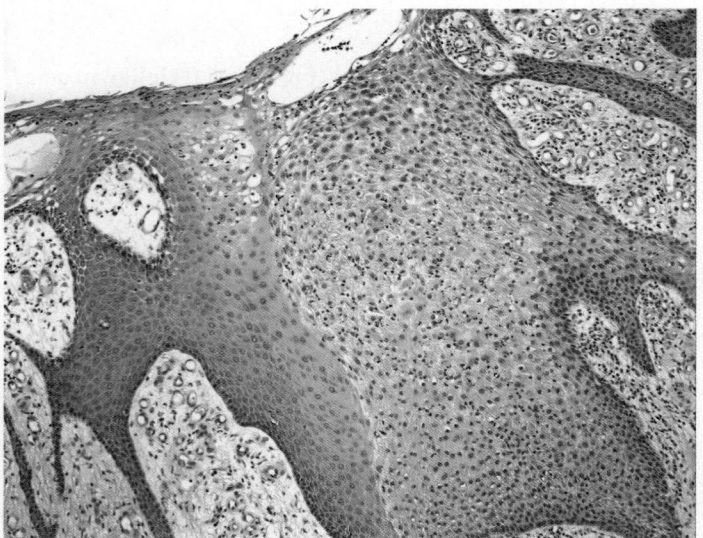

Figure 29-23 Clear cell acanthoma. The cells within the lesion appear pale by comparison with the adjacent normal epidermis.

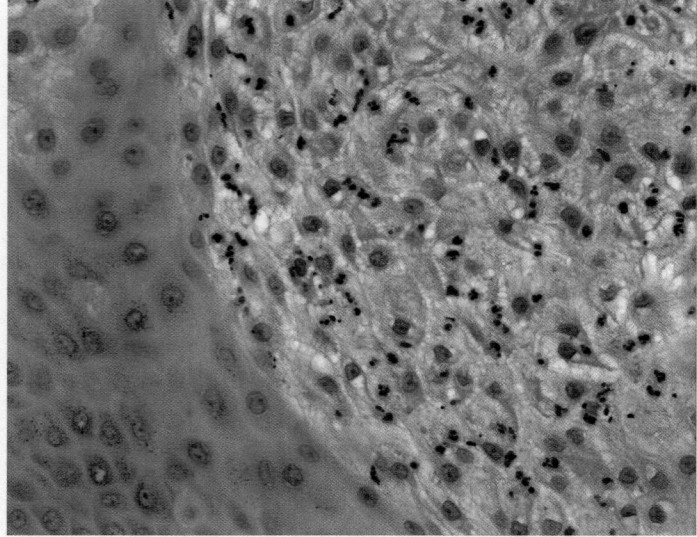

Figure 29-24 Clear cell acanthoma. High magnification. Neutrophils and nuclear dust are scattered through the clear cells of the lesion.

neutrophils often form microabscesses in the parakeratotic horny layer. Dilated capillaries are seen in the elongated papillae and often also in the dermis underlying the tumor. In addition, a mild to moderately severe cellular infiltrate composed largely of lymphoid cells is present in the dermis. Some clear cell acanthomas appear papillomatous; so they have the configuration of a seborrheic keratosis.

Beneath the tumor, some cases have shown hyperplasia of sweat ducts or syringoma-like proliferations.

Pathogenesis. On histochemical examination, phosphorylase is absent in clear cell acanthoma except for the basal cell layer. This enzyme is normally present in the epidermis and necessary for the degradation of glycogen.

Electron microscopy reveals glycogen granules in the tumor cells, except in the cells of the basal cell layer. In the lower portion of the tumor, the glycogen granules are seen largely around the nuclei. In the upper portion, however, the amount of glycogen is increased, and the granules are seen to infiltrate between the tonofilaments.

Although the melanocytes, including their dendrites, contain melanosomes, hardly any melanosomes are present within the tumor cells, indicating a blockage in the transfer of melanosomes from the melanocytes to the tumor cells.

Principles of Management: Simple destruction or excision is adequate for removal and lesions do not usually recur. A response to topical steroids has also been reported (78).

EPIDERMAL OR INFUNDIBULAR CYST

Clinical Summary. Epidermal cysts are slowly growing, elevated, round, firm, intradermal, or subcutaneous tumors that cease growing after having reached 1 to 5 cm in diameter. They occur most commonly on the face, scalp, neck, and trunk (Fig. 29-25). Although most epidermal cysts arise spontaneously in hair-bearing areas, occasionally they occur on the palms or soles or form as a result of trauma. Usually, a patient has only one or a few epidermal cysts, rarely many. In Gardner syndrome, however, numerous epidermal cysts occur, especially on the scalp and face (see Chapter 32).

Histopathology. Epidermal cysts have a wall composed of true epidermis, as seen on the skin surface and in the

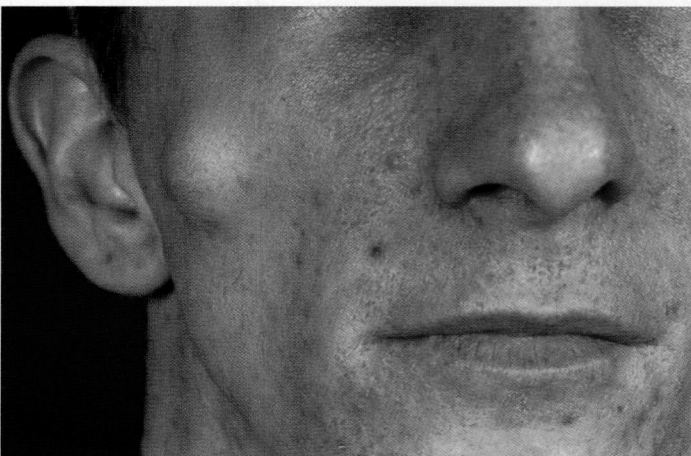

Figure 29-25 Epidermal cyst. The cyst distends the overlying skin of the cheek.

infundibulum of hair follicles, the infundibulum being the uppermost part of the hair follicle that extends down to the entry of the sebaceous duct. In young epidermal cysts, several layers of squamous and granular cells can usually be recognized (Fig. 29-26). In older epidermal cysts, the wall is often markedly atrophic, either in some areas or in the entire cyst, and may consist of only one or two rows of greatly flattened cells. The cyst is filled with horny material arranged in laminated layers. In sections stained with hematoxylin–eosin, melanocytes and melanin pigmentation of keratinocytes and melanophages can be seen only rarely in epidermal cysts of whites but frequently in epidermal cysts of those with darker skin such as Indians (83). Silver stains reveal that most of the melanin is located in the basal layer of the cyst lining, but some melanin is also seen in the contents of the cyst.

When an epidermal cyst ruptures and the contents of the cyst are released into the dermis, a considerable foreign-body reaction with numerous multinucleated giant cells results, forming a *keratin granuloma* (Figs. 29-27 to 29-29). The foreign-body reaction usually causes disintegration of the cyst wall. However, it may lead to a pseudocarcinomatous proliferation in the remnants of the cyst wall, simulating an SCC.

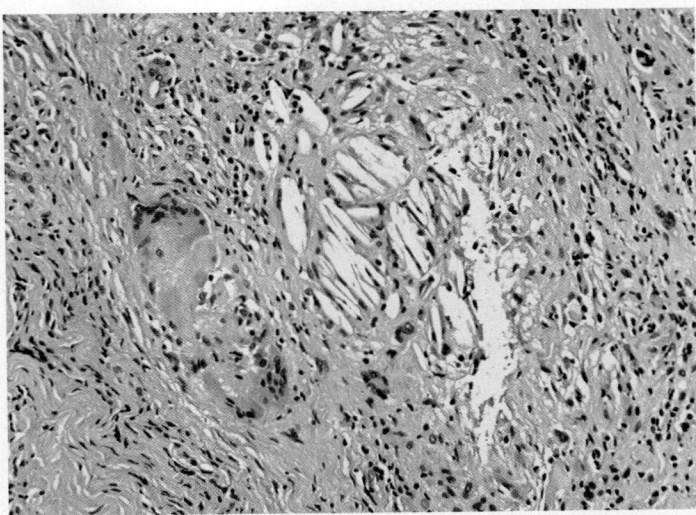

Figure 29-28 Keratin granuloma. At the edge of a partially ruptured cyst, cholesterol clefts form part of a keratin granuloma.

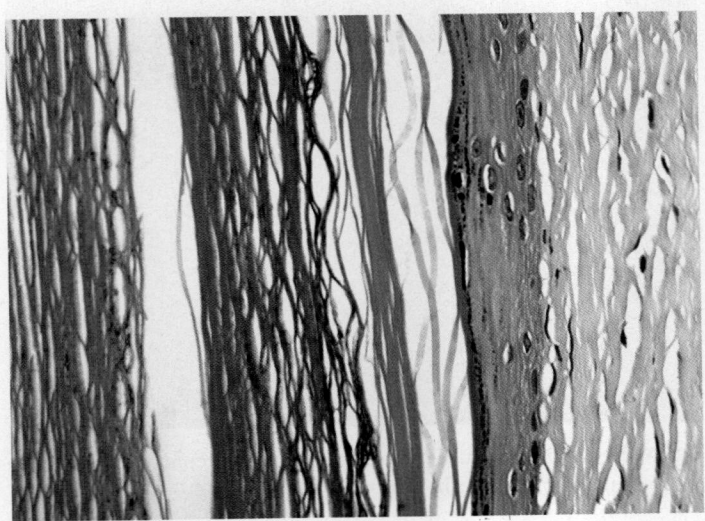

Figure 29-26 Epidermal cyst. The cyst is lined by stratified squamous epithelium with a granular layer. The cyst is filled with keratin flakes.

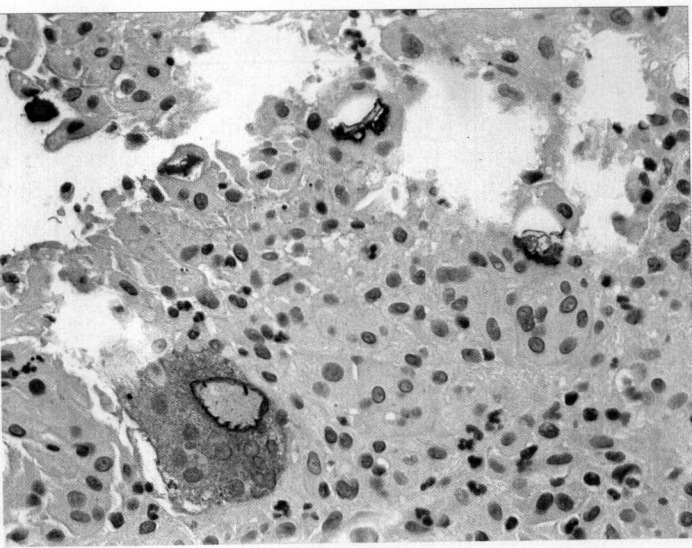

Figure 29-29 Keratin granuloma. Cytokeratin staining highlights keratin flakes in giant cells within a keratin granuloma.

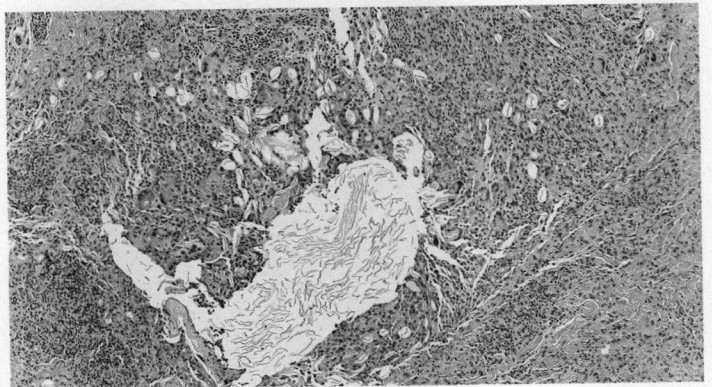

Figure 29-27 Ruptured epidermal cyst. The lining epithelium is lost and replaced by granulation tissue.

The development of a BCC, a lesion of Bowen disease, or an SCC in epidermal cysts is a rare event. In cases of SCC, the tumor is apt to be of low malignancy and does not metastasize. It is likely that some cases that were regarded in the past as malignant degeneration of epidermal cysts now are interpreted either as pseudocarcinomatous hyperplasia in a ruptured epidermal cyst or as proliferating trichilemmal tumor (see Chapter 30).

Pathogenesis. It is widely assumed that most spontaneously arising epidermal cysts are related to the follicular infundibulum, and may thus be regarded as a form of retention cyst. The occurrence of hybrid cysts with partially epidermal and partially trichilemmal lining favors this assumption. Epidermal cysts in nonfollicular regions, such as the palms or soles, and also many that occur at sites of prior trauma including surgical sites, probably form as a result of the traumatic implantation of epidermis into the dermis or subcutis. These less common epidermal cysts may be regarded as inclusion cyst for which the often used term "epidermal inclusion cyst" (EIC) may be appropriate, as an option.

HUMAN PAPILLOMAVIRUS–ASSOCIATED CYST (VERRUCOUS CYST)

Clinical Summary. These cysts are found most frequently on the soles of the feet but have also been reported on the scalp, face, back, and extremities. They may have the typical appearance of a cyst or possibly suggest dermatofibroma or BCC.

Histopathology. The cysts are lined by epidermal-type epithelium showing koilocytic changes and hypergranulosis, suggestive of verrucous change.

Pathogenesis. HPV has been demonstrated in the epithelium by molecular methods. It is unclear whether these cysts are traumatic implantations of verrucae or represent epidermal cysts with secondary HPV infection (84).

MILIA

Clinical Summary. Milia are multiple, superficially located, white, globoid, firm lesions generally only 1 to 2 mm in diameter. A distinction is made between primary milia, which arise spontaneously on the face in predisposed individuals, and secondary milia, which occur either in diseases associated with subepidermal bullae—such as bullous pemphigoid, dystrophic epidermolysis bullosa, and porphyria cutanea tarda—or after dermabrasion and other trauma.

Histopathology. *Primary milia* of the face are derived from the lowest portion of the infundibulum of vellus hairs at about the level of the sebaceous duct. The milia often are still connected with the vellus hair follicle by an epithelial pedicle. Primary milia are small cysts differing from epidermal cysts only in size. They are lined by a stratified epithelium a few cell layers thick and contain concentric lamellae of keratin.

Secondary milia have the same histologic appearance as primary milia. They may develop from any epithelial structure; on serial sections, may still show a connection to the parent structure—whether a hair follicle, sweat duct, sebaceous duct, or epidermis. Secondary milia that follow blistering arise in most instances from the eccrine sweat duct and very rarely from a hair follicle. In a certain percentage of cases, however, no connection is found with any skin appendage, suggesting that the milia have developed from aberrant epidermis. In milia derived from eccrine sweat ducts, the sweat ducts are frequently seen to enter the cyst wall at the bottom of the milium.

Pathogenesis. Primary milia of the face represent a keratinizing type of benign tumor. In contrast, secondary milia represent retention cysts caused by proliferative tendencies of the epithelium after injury.

Principles of Management: Milia are benign and can be left untreated. Surgical treatment is usually performed for cosmetic reasons. An incision with a cutting-edge needle and manual expression of the contents is an easy and cost-effective treatment. Treatments with electrodesiccation, laser, dermabrasion, and cryosurgery have been reported to be effective.

PILAR OR TRICHILEMMAL CYST

Clinical Summary. Pilar or trichilemmal cysts are clinically indistinguishable from epidermal cysts but differ from them in frequency and distribution. They are less common than epidermal cysts, constituting only about 25% of the combined material; about 90% occur on the scalp (Fig. 29-30). Pilar cysts often show an autosomal dominant inheritance pattern and are solitary in only 30% of the cases, with 10% of patients having more than 10 cysts. Furthermore, in contrast to epidermal cysts, pilar cysts are easily enucleated and appear as firm, smooth, white-walled cysts (Fig. 29-31).

Histopathology. The wall of trichilemmal cysts is composed of epithelial cells possessing no clearly visible intercellular bridges. The peripheral layer of cells shows a distinct palisade arrangement not seen in epidermal cysts. The epithelial cells close to the cystic cavity appear swollen and are filled with pale cytoplasm (Fig. 29-32). These swollen cells do not produce a granular layer but generally undergo abrupt keratinization, although nuclear remnants are occasionally retained in a few cells. The content of the cysts consists of homogeneous eosinophilic material.

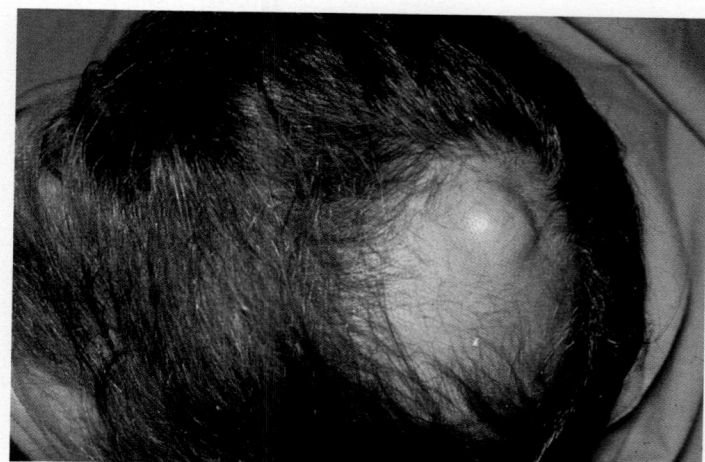

Figure 29-30 Pilar cyst. Clinically similar to an epidermal cyst, but more frequently seen on the scalp.

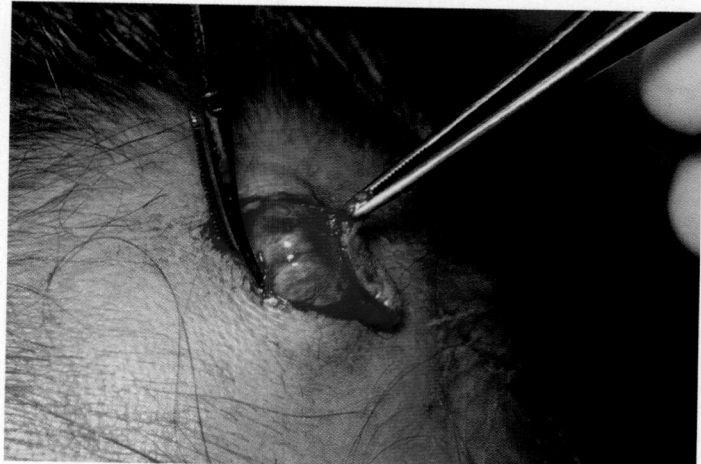

Figure 29-31 Pilar cyst. The cyst has a well-defined margin, as seen at the time of excision.

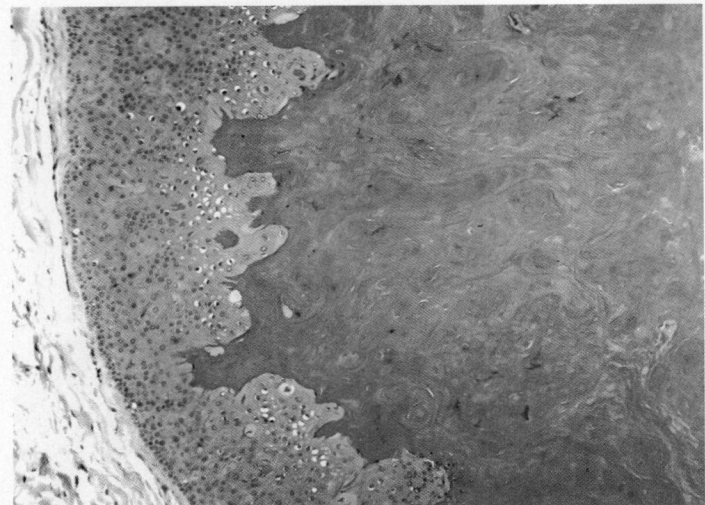

Figure 29-32 Pilar cyst. The cyst is lined by a squamous epithelium without a granular layer and with swelling of the cells close to the cyst cavity, filled with homogeneous keratin.

Whereas focal calcification of the cyst content does not occur in epidermal cysts, foci of calcification are seen in approximately one-fourth of trichilemmal cysts. A considerable foreign-body reaction results when the wall of a trichilemmal cyst ruptures, and the cyst may then undergo partial or complete disintegration.

Trichilemmal cysts frequently disclose small, acanthotic foci in their walls that are indistinguishable from solid areas, as seen in a proliferating trichilemmal cyst. The association of a trichilemmal cyst with tumor lobules of a proliferating trichilemmal cyst is also seen occasionally (see Chapter 30).

Pathogenesis. Pilar cysts were originally called sebaceous cysts. The name was changed when it became apparent that the keratinization in them is analogous to the keratinization that takes place in the outer root sheath of the hair follicle, or trichilemmal, which does not keratinize wherever it covers the inner root sheath, but keratinizes normally in two areas—the follicular isthmus of anagen hairs and the sac surrounding catagen and telogen hairs—because in these two regions the inner root sheath has disappeared. The follicular isthmus of anagen hairs is the short, middle portion of the hair follicle, extending upward from the attachment of the arrector pili muscle to the entrance of the sebaceous duct. At the lower end of the follicular isthmus, the inner root sheath sloughs off, exposing the outer root sheath, which, in its exposed portion, undergoes a specific type of homogeneous keratinization without the interposition of a granular layer. This type of trichilemmal keratinization also takes place in the sac surrounding catagen and telogen hairs because hairs in these stages have lost their inner root sheath. The differentiation toward hair keratin in trichilemmal cysts has been confirmed by immunohistochemical staining because they stain with antikeratin antibodies derived from human hair, in contrast to epidermal cysts, which stain with antikeratin antibodies obtained from human callus (85).

Differential Diagnosis. Even though both the pilar cyst and the proliferating trichilemmal cyst/tumor show trichilemmal types of keratinization and can occur together, one is essentially a cyst and the other essentially a solid, tumorlike proliferation. The latter is therefore discussed under the section on tumors with differentiation toward hair follicle components in Chapter 30.

STEATOCYSTOMA MULTIPLEX

Clinical Summary. Steatocystoma multiplex is inherited in an autosomal dominant pattern. One observes numerous small, rounded, moderately firm cystic nodules that are adherent to the overlying skin and usually measure 1 to 3 cm in diameter (Fig. 29-33). When punctured, the cysts discharge an oily or creamy fluid and, in some instances, also small hairs (19). They are found most commonly in the axillae, in the sternal region, and on the arms. Steatocystoma also occurs occasionally as a solitary, noninherited tumor in adults, where it is referred to as *steatocystoma simplex*. It may also occur in association with eruptive vellus hair cysts and trichofolliculoma (86).

Histopathology. The cysts have walls that are intricately folded with several layers of epithelial cells, although in atrophic areas only two or three layers of flat cells may be present. Elsewhere, there is a basal layer in palisade arrangement, above which are two or three layers of swollen cells without recognizable intercellular bridges. Central to these cells, there is a thick, homogeneous, eosinophilic horny layer that forms without an intervening granular layer. It protrudes irregularly into the lumen in a fashion simulating the decapitation secretion of apocrine glands (Fig. 29-34).

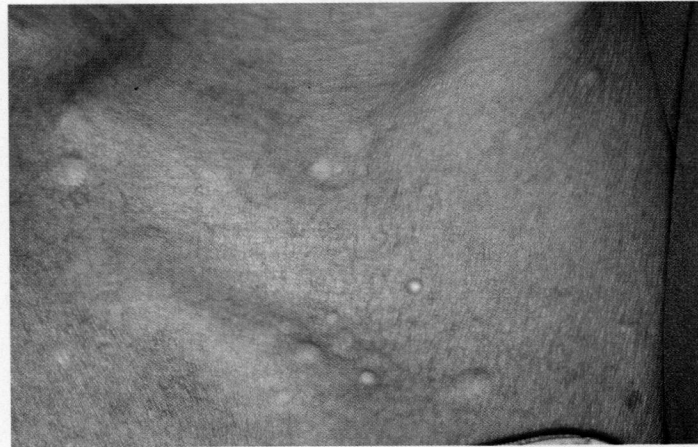

Figure 29-33 Steatocystoma multiplex. Multiple small rounded cysts are present in the axilla.

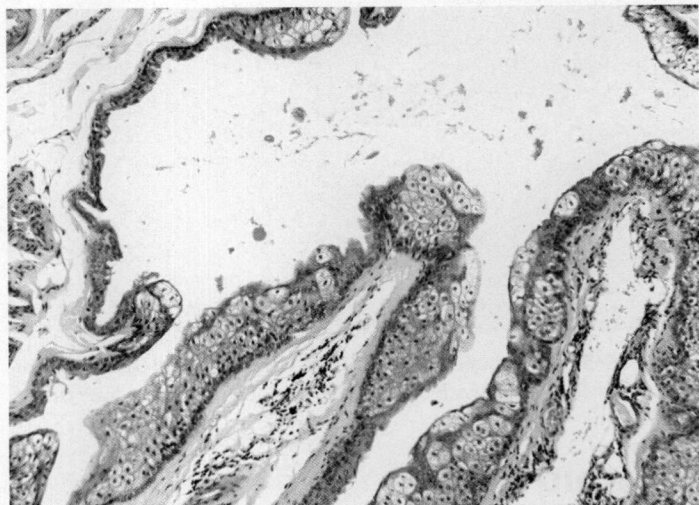

Figure 29-34 Steatocystoma multiplex. The cyst wall shows intricate folding. The lining stratified squamous epithelium has sebaceous gland lobules within and close to it.

A characteristic feature seen in most lesions of steato-cystoma is the presence of flattened sebaceous gland lobules either within or close to the cyst wall. In some cysts, invaginations resembling hair follicles extend from the cyst wall into the surrounding stroma, and in rare instances, true hair shafts are seen within them, indicating that the invaginations represent the outer root sheath of hairs. In a few cysts, the lumen contains clusters of hair, mainly of lanugo size but partially of intermediate character. When stained with the PAS reaction, the cells of the cyst wall are found to be rich in glycogen.

Pathogenesis. Electron microscopic examination has shown that the cyst wall consists of keratinizing cells. Nearest to the lumen, the cyst wall consists of several layers of flattened, very elongated horny cells interconnected by desmosomes.

It appears likely that differentiation in the cyst wall of steatocystoma multiplex is to a large extent in the direction of the sebaceous duct. The sebaceous duct and the outer root sheath are composed of similar cells, but undulation and thinning of the horny layer and the existence of sebaceous cells in the cyst wall are characteristic features of the sebaceous gland side of the sebaceous duct. Sebaceous duct cells—like outer root sheath cells—contain abundant glycogen and amylophosphorylase; keratinize without the interposition of keratohyalin granules; and, on electron microscopic examination, retain their desmosomes after keratinization.

Mutations in the Keratin 17 gene are implicated in the pathogenesis of these lesions (87,88).

PIGMENTED FOLLICULAR CYST

Clinical Summary. This is an uncommon pigmented lesion resembling a nevus.

Histopathology. The cyst wall consists of infundibular epidermis. The cyst contains, in addition to laminated keratin, numerous large pigmented hair shafts. One or two growing hair follicles are seen in the wall of the cyst (Fig. 29-35) (89,90)

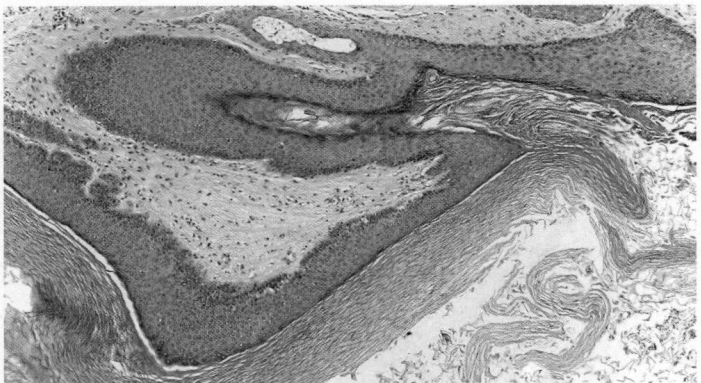

Figure 29-35 Pigmented follicular cyst. The cyst wall consists of infundibular epithelium with basal pigmentation and shallow rete ridges.

DERMOID CYST

Clinical Summary. Dermoid cysts are subcutaneous cysts that usually are present at birth. They occur most commonly on the head—mainly around the eyes—and occasionally on the neck.

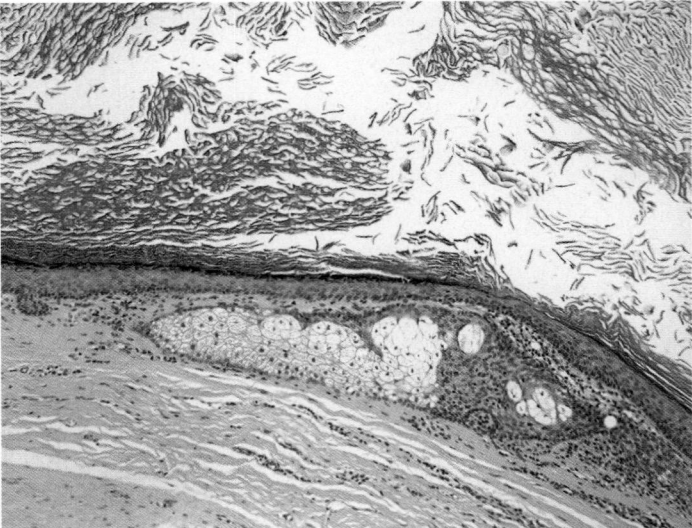

Figure 29-36 External angular dermoid cyst. The cyst is lined by stratified squamous epithelium, with adnexal structures in the wall.

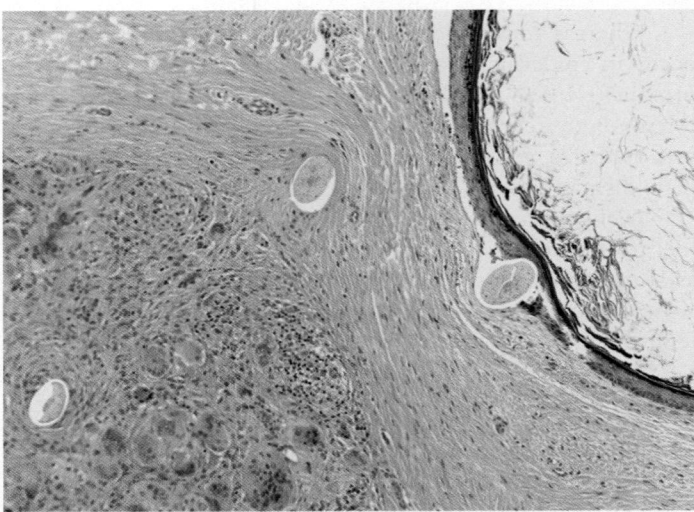

Figure 29-37 External angular dermoid cyst. In this example, the cyst has ruptured—producing an adjacent granuloma containing hair shafts derived from the cyst.

When located on the head, they are often adherent to the periosteum. Usually, they measure between 1 and 4 cm in diameter.

Histopathology. Dermoid cysts, in contrast to epidermal cysts, are lined by an epidermis that possesses various epidermal appendages that are usually fully matured (Figs. 29-36 and 29-37). Hair follicles containing hairs that project into the lumen of the cyst are often present. In addition, the dermis of dermoid cysts usually contains sebaceous glands—often eccrine glands—and, in about 20% of the cases, apocrine glands that have matured.

Pathogenesis. Dermoid cysts are a result of the sequestration of skin along the lines of embryonic closure.

BRONCHOGENIC AND THYROGLOSSAL DUCT CYSTS

Clinical Summary. Bronchogenic cysts are rare. They are small, solitary lesions seen most commonly in the skin or subcutaneous tissue just above the sternal notch. Rarely, they are located on

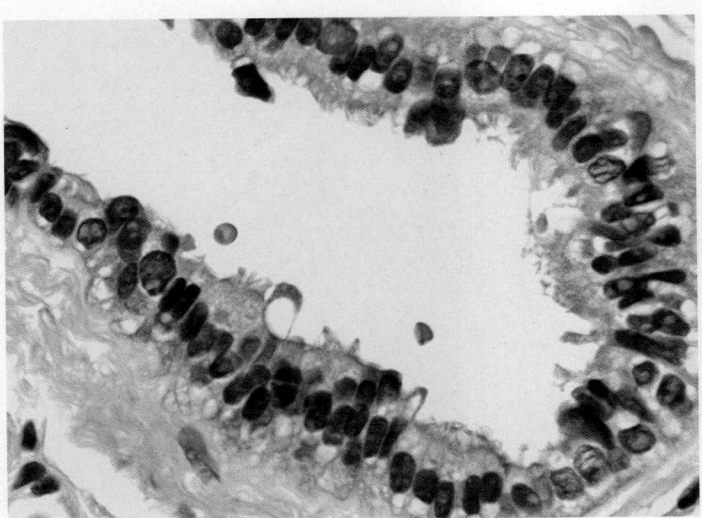

Figure 29-38 Bronchogenic cyst. High magnification. The lining epithelium is columnar with a ciliated surface.

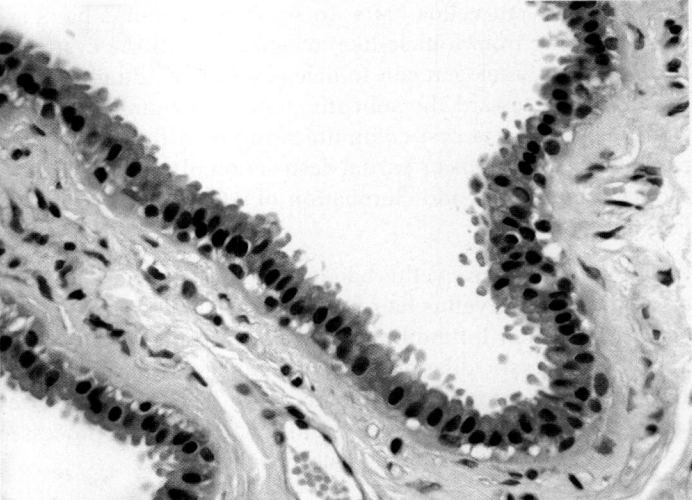

Figure 29-39 Apocrine cyst. In this small dermal cyst, the lining epithelium forms a single layer with apocrine snouting secretion.

the anterior aspect of the neck or on the chin. As a rule, they are discovered shortly after birth. They may show a draining sinus.

Thyroglossal duct cysts are clinically indistinguishable from bronchogenic cysts, except that they are usually located on the anterior aspect of the neck.

Histopathology. Bronchogenic cysts are lined by a mucosa consisting of ciliated pseudostratified columnar epithelium (Fig. 29-38). Goblet cells may be interspersed. The wall frequently contains smooth muscle and mucous glands but only rarely contains cartilage (91).

Thyroglossal duct cysts differ from bronchogenic cysts in that they do not contain smooth muscle and they frequently contain thyroid follicles (92).

Pathogenesis. On electron microscopy, the cilia show two central microtubules surrounded by nine paired microtubules (93).

CUTANEOUS CILIATED CYST

Clinical Summary. Cutaneous ciliated cysts are found very rarely in females as a single lesion, largely on the lower extremities, and even more rarely in males and on the back (20). They usually measure several centimeters in diameter. They are either unilocular or multilocular and are filled with clear or amber fluid. The finding of one on the perineum led the authors to suggest a primitive tailgut origin to this cyst, probably from the embryonic remnants of cloacal membrane (94).

Histopathology. Cutaneous ciliated cysts show numerous papillary projections lined by a simple cuboidal or columnar ciliated epithelium. Mucin-secreting cells are absent.

Pathogenesis. The epithelial lining of the cysts resembles that seen in the fallopian tube. On electron microscopy, the cilia show two central filaments encircled by nine pairs of filaments (93).

MEDIAN RAPHE CYST OF THE PENIS

Clinical Summary. Median raphe cysts of the penis usually occur in young adults. They are located on the ventral aspect of the penis, most commonly on the glans. They are solitary and measure only a few millimeters in diameter. However, they may

extend over several centimeters in a linear fashion. It seems that, in some instances, median raphe cysts have been erroneously reported as apocrine cystadenoma of the penis (95–97) (Fig. 29-39; see also Chapter 30).

Histopathology. The cysts are lined by pseudostratified columnar epithelium varying from one to four cells in thickness, mimicking the transitional epithelium of the urethra. Some of the epithelial cells have clear cytoplasm; mucin-containing cells are uncommon and a case lined by ciliated epithelium has been reported.

Pathogenesis. It is likely that median raphe cysts do not represent a defective closure of the median raphe but rather the anomalous budding and separation of urethral columnar epithelium from the urethra.

Principles of Management: This is a benign condition, and surgical treatment is considered only for symptomatic or cosmetic purposes.

ERUPTIVE VELLUS HAIR CYSTS

Clinical Summary. In eruptive vellus hair cysts, a condition first described in 1977 (98), asymptomatic follicular papules 1 to 2 mm in diameter occur, most commonly on the chest but in some instances elsewhere. Some of the papules have a crusted or umbilicated surface. The condition is usually seen in children and young adults but can develop at any age. Spontaneous clearing may take place in a few years. Autosomal dominant inheritance has been reported. Cytokeratin studies have shown that epidermoid cysts expressed cytokeratin 10 and eruptive vellus hair cysts expressed cytokeratin 17, whereas trichilemmal cysts and steatocystoma multiplex showed the expression of both cytokeratin 10 and cytokeratin 17, supporting the opinion that eruptive vellus hair cysts, which stained negative for cytokeratin 10, and steatocystoma multiplex are distinct entities and not variants of one disorder (99).

Histopathology. A cystic structure is usually seen in the mid-dermis lined by squamous epithelium. It contains laminated keratinous material and varying numbers of transversely and obliquely cut vellus hairs. In some cysts, vellus hairs are seen emerging from follicle-like invaginations of the cyst wall. In other cysts, a telogen hair follicle is seen extending from the lower surface toward the subcutis. Crusted or umbilicated lesions show either a cyst communicating with the surface and extruding its contents or partial destruction of a cyst by a granulomatous infiltrate and elimination of vellus hairs to the surface of the skin.

Pathogenesis. Eruptive vellus hair cysts represent a developmental abnormality of vellus hair follicles that predisposes them to occlusion at their infundibular level. This results in the retention of hairs, cystic dilation of the proximal part of the follicle, and secondary atrophy of the hair bulbs. There is a close relationship with steatocystoma multiplex (86). Both processes could be described as multiple pilosebaceous cysts.

WARTY DYSKERATOMA

Clinical Summary. Warty dyskeratoma, first described in 1957 (100), usually occurs as a solitary lesion, most commonly on the scalp, face, or neck, although a case with multiple lesions has been reported (101). It has also been reported in non–sun-exposed skin, including the oral mucosa, usually on the hard palate or an alveolar ridge (102). Although its clinical appearance is not always distinctive, it often occurs as a slightly elevated papule or nodule with a keratotic umbilicated center. The lesion, after having reached a certain size, persists indefinitely.

Histopathology. The center of the lesion is occupied by a large, cup-shaped invagination connected with the surface by a channel filled with keratinous material (Figs. 29-33 to 29-35). The large invagination contains numerous acantholytic, dyskeratotic cells in its upper portion. The lower portion of the invagination is occupied by numerous villi, that is, markedly elongated dermal papillae that are often lined with only a single layer of basal cells and project upward from the base of the cup-shaped invagination (Fig. 29-40). Typical corps ronds can usually be seen in the thickened granular layer lining the channel at the entrance to the invagination (Figs. 29-41 and 29-42).

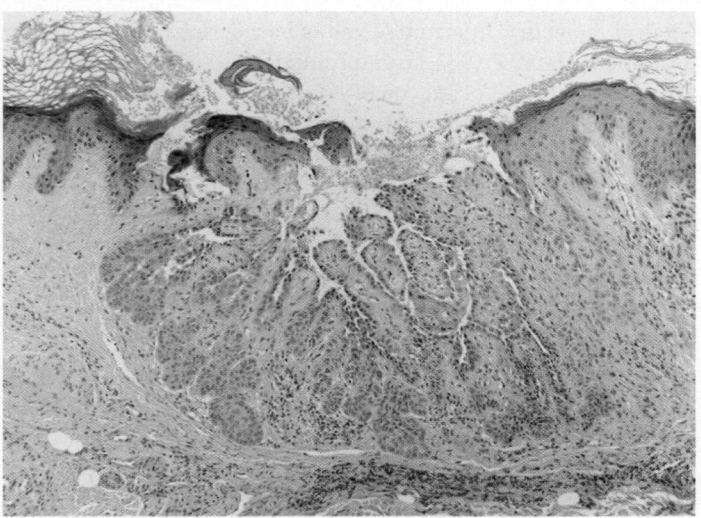

Figure 29-40 Warty dyskeratoma. Low magnification. A large invagination is connected to the surface by a channel.

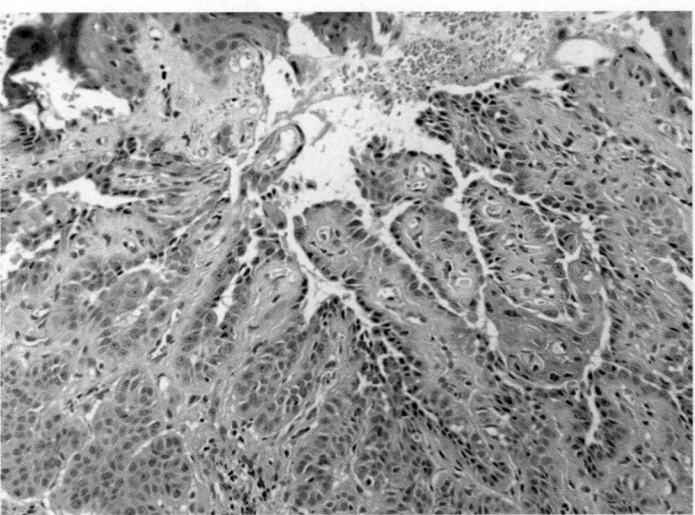

Figure 29-41 Warty dyskeratoma. The villi at the base of the invagination are covered with a single layer of cells. Acantholytic, dyskeratotic cells lie above the villi.

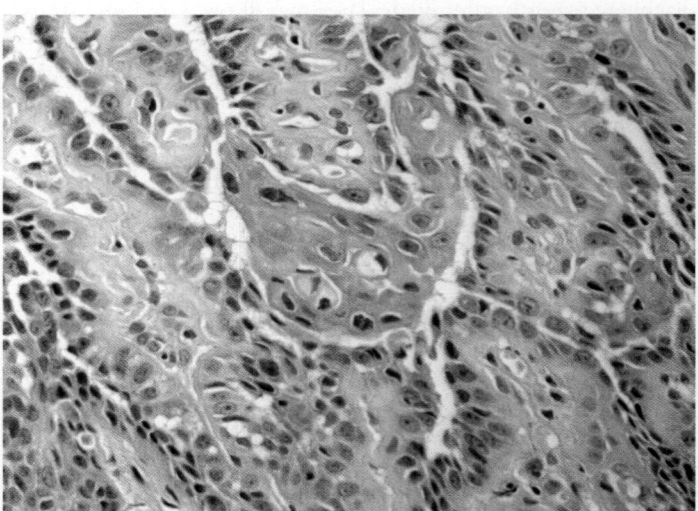

Figure 29-42 Warty dyskeratoma. High magnification. Acantholytic and dyskeratotic cells lie above the basal layer of epithelial cells.

Pathogenesis. The central cup-shaped invagination has been interpreted by several observers as a greatly dilated hair follicle because in early lesions a hair follicle or sebaceous gland is often connected with the invagination. Occasionally, two or three adjoining follicles seem to be involved. The fact, however, that warty dyskeratoma can arise on the oral mucosa indicates that, as in Darier disease, the dyskeratotic, acantholytic process is not always derived from a pilosebaceous structure.

Although attempts were made at first to correlate warty dyskeratoma with Darier disease, it is now generally agreed that warty dyskeratoma represents an entity—"a benign cutaneous tumor that resembles Darier disease microscopically." Indeed, it has been proposed that the entity should be regarded as a benign follicular adnexal neoplasm and designated as "follicular dyskeratoma" (101).

Principles of Management: This is a benign condition that does not require treatment. Surgical excision is performed for removal if desired or to obtain histologic diagnosis.

ACTINIC KERATOSIS (SOLAR KERATOSIS)

Clinical Summary. Solar keratoses are also known as actinic keratoses. The adjective *solar* is more specific because it refers to the sun as the cause, whereas the adjective *actinic* refers to a variety of rays. Even among the sun's rays, action spectrum evaluations indicate that the ultraviolet B (UVB) rays (290 to 320 nm) are the most damaging ("carcinogenic") rays, although ultraviolet A (UVA) rays (320 to 400 nm) can augment the damaging effects of UVB rays.

Actinic keratoses are usually seen as multiple lesions in the sun-exposed areas of the skin in persons in or past middle life who have fair complexions (Figs. 29-43 and 29-44). Excessive exposure to sunlight over many years and inadequate protection against it are the essential predisposing factors. Actinic keratoses are seen most commonly on the face and the dorsa of the hands and in the bald portions of the scalp in men.

Usually, the lesions measure less than 1 cm in diameter. They are erythematous; are often covered by adherent scales; and, except in their hypertrophic form, show little or no infiltration. Some actinic keratoses are pigmented and show peripheral spreading, making clinical differentiation from lentigo maligna difficult. Occasionally, lesions show marked hyperkeratosis and then have the clinical aspect of cutaneous horns. A lesion analogous to actinic keratosis occurs on the vermilion border of the lower lip as *solar cheilitis* and may show areas of erosion and hyperkeratosis.

Actinic keratosis and solar cheilitis can develop into an SCC. However, the incidence of this transformation is difficult to determine because the borderline between actinic keratosis and SCC is not clear-cut (see Histopathology). It has been estimated that in 20% of patients with actinic keratoses, SCC develops in one or more of the lesions. Usually, SCCs arising either in actinic keratoses or *de novo* in sun-damaged skin do not metastasize. The incidence of metastasis in different series varies from 0.5% to 3%. In carcinoma of the vermilion border of the lip, however, metastases have been found in 11% of the cases (103,104).

Histopathology. Actinic keratoses are keratinocytic dysplasias. This definition is preferable to their designation as precancerous because most of them never progress to invasive cancers. Biologically, the lesions are still benign; invasion into the dermis, if present at all, is limited to the most superficial portion, the papillary dermis (see *Differential Diagnosis*).

Five types of actinic keratosis can be recognized histologically: hypertrophic, atrophic, bowenoid, acantholytic, and pigmented (Figs. 29-45 to 29-53). Transitions and combinations

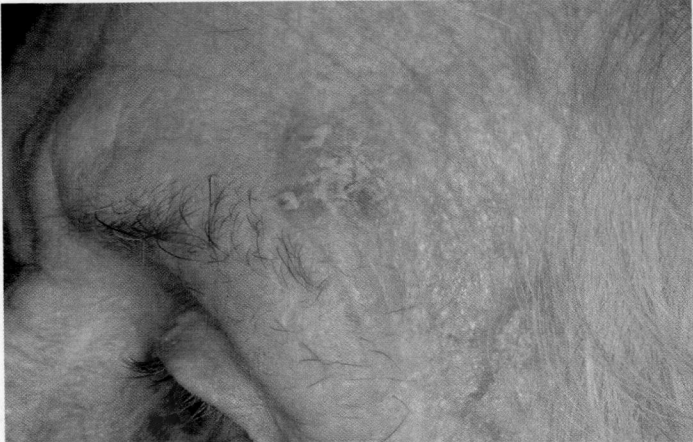

Figure 29-43 Actinic keratosis. The lesion on the forehead is crusted and erythematous.

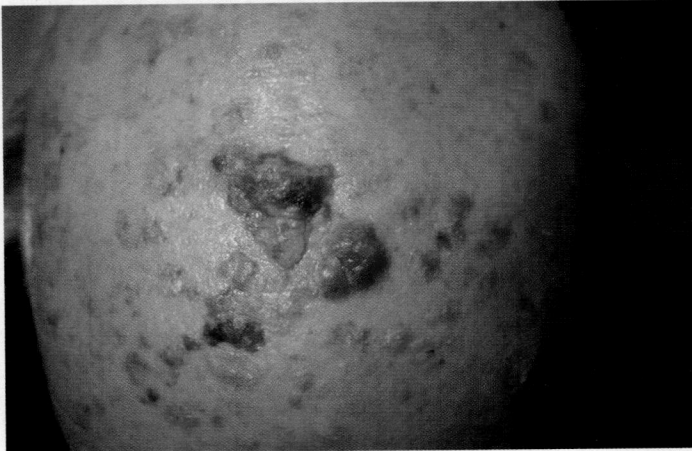

Figure 29-44 Actinic keratosis. Multiple lesions on this sun-damaged scalp.

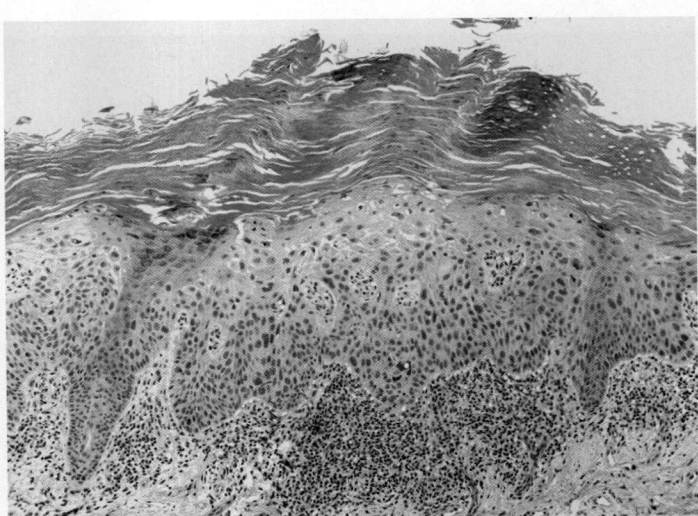

Figure 29-45 Actinic keratosis. Tall columns of parakeratotic keratin alternate with bands of orthokeratotic keratin, with moderate atypia of the underlying keratinocytes.

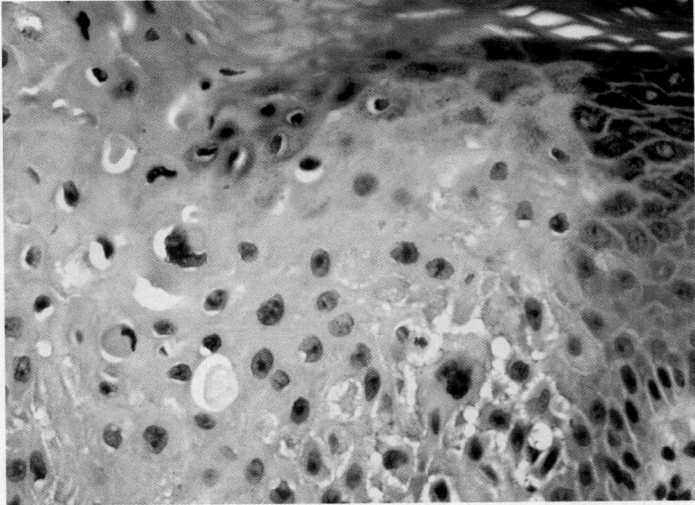

Figure 29-46 Actinic keratosis. Beneath a thick layer of parakeratotic keratin, the epidermis shows cytologic atypia.

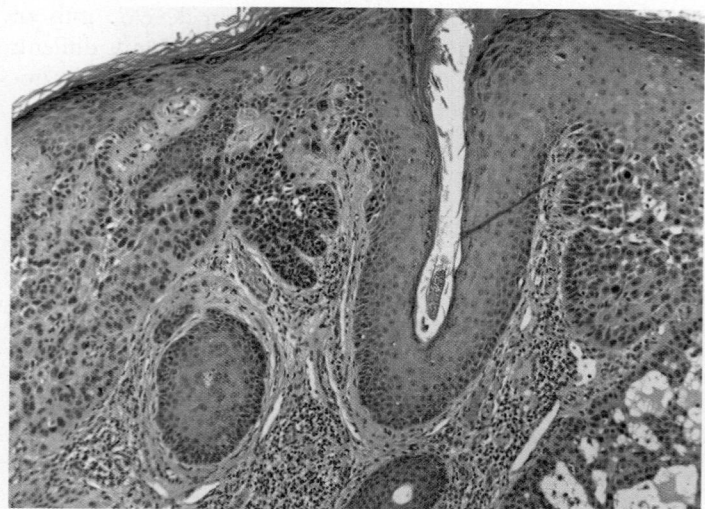

Figure 29-47 Actinic keratosis, hypertrophic type. The lesion shows hyperkeratosis and papillomatosis with prominent cytologic atypia. There is a moderate lymphocytic infiltrate in the underlying papillary dermis.

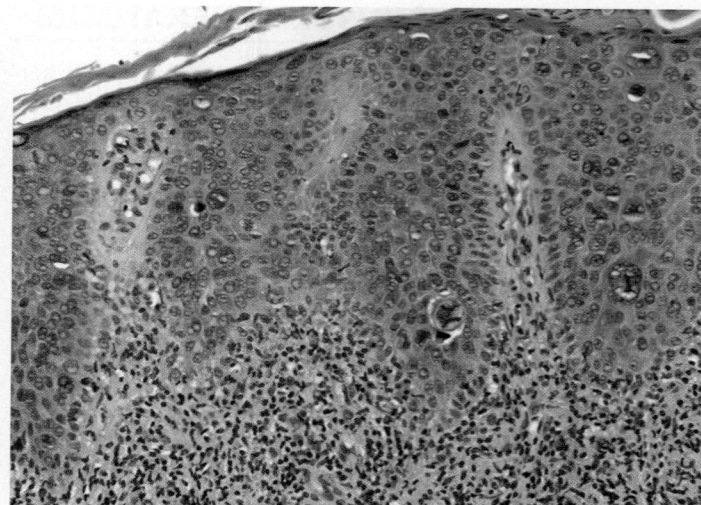

Figure 29-50 Bowenoid actinic keratosis. Medium magnification. Marked cellular and nuclear pleomorphism is present together with frequent and atypical mitoses in a Bowenoid actinic keratosis (squamous cell carcinoma *in situ*).

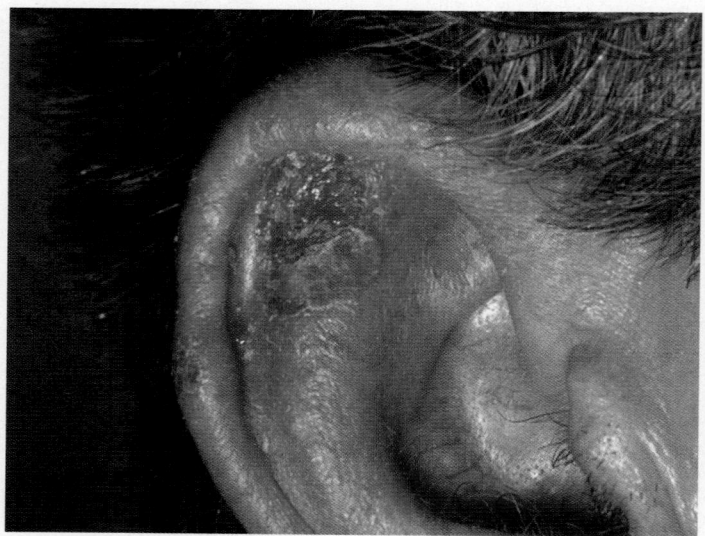

Figure 29-48 Bowenoid actinic keratosis. A crusted lesion on the ear helix.

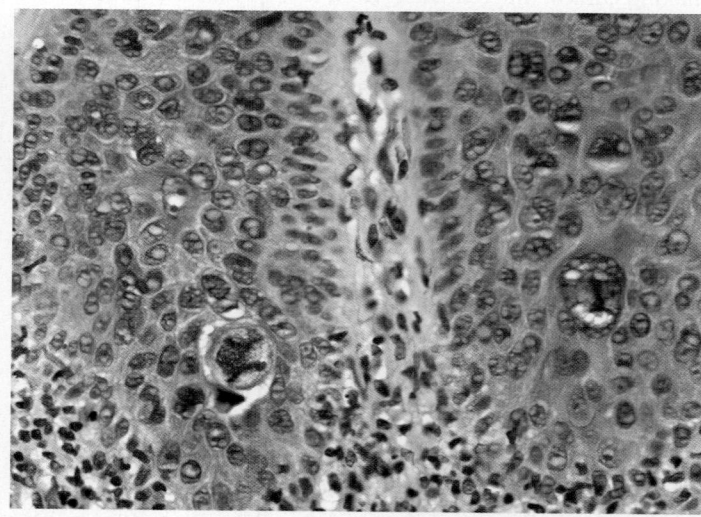

Figure 29-51 Bowenoid actinic keratosis. High magnification. Large atypical mitoses are prominent in this Bowenoid actinic keratosis.

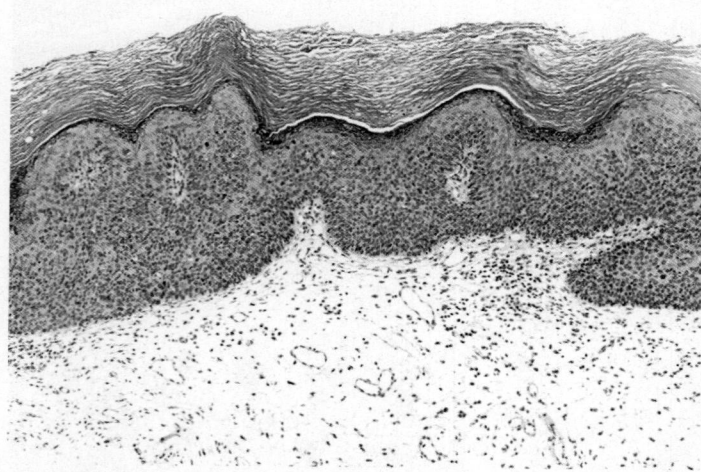

Figure 29-49 Bowenoid actinic keratosis. Low magnification. Beneath a thick layer of parakeratotic keratin, the epidermis shows cytologic atypia.

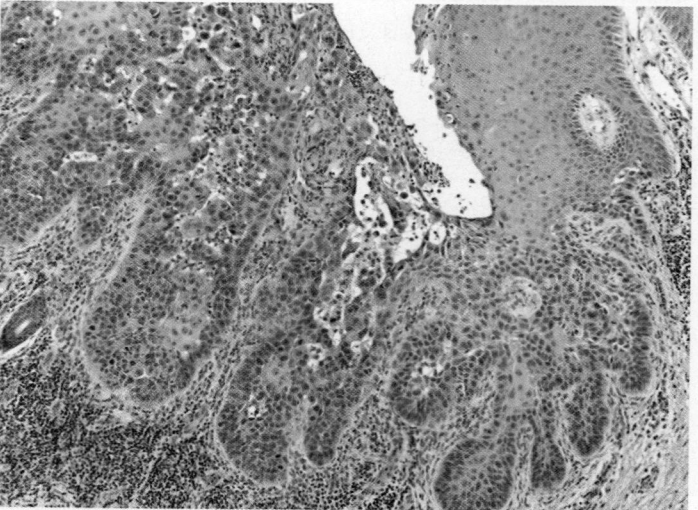

Figure 29-52 Actinic keratosis, acantholytic type. Low magnification. The epidermis is markedly hyperkeratotic. In the dermis, there is a dense lichenoid inflammatory infiltrate. The keratosis shows focal acantholytic change.

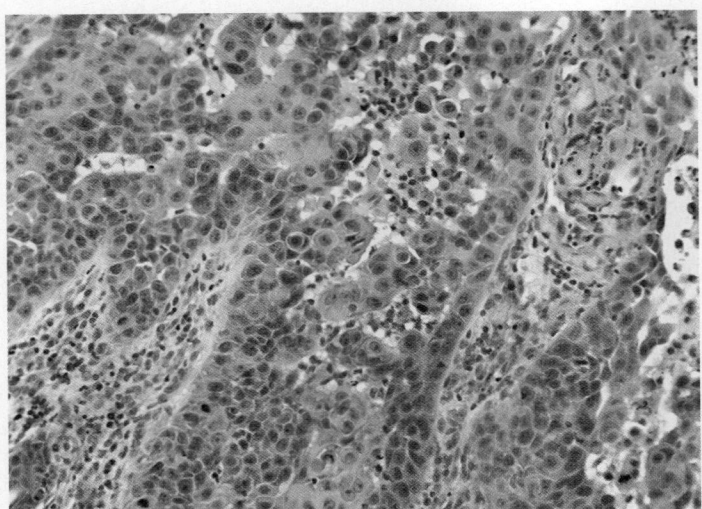

Figure 29-53 Actinic keratosis, acantholytic type. High magnification. Keratinocytes in the basal layer are crowded, with an increased nuclear-cytoplasmic ratio. They tend to become separated from one another and adopt a rounded configuration. This process of "secondary acantholysis" may in some instances result in the formation of pseudoglandular spaces that may mimic a glandular pattern of differentiation.

among these five types occur. In addition, many cutaneous horns histologic examination prove on to be actinic keratoses.

In the *hypertrophic type* of actinic keratosis, hyperkeratosis is pronounced and is usually intermingled with areas of parakeratosis. This variety of keratosis, sometimes referred to as *florid keratosis*, may easily be overdiagnosed as invasive SCC by the unwary. Mild or moderate papillomatosis may be present. The epidermis is thickened in most areas and shows irregular downward proliferation that is limited to the uppermost dermis and does not represent frank invasion (Fig. 29-40). A varying proportion of the keratinocytes in the stratum malpighii shows a loss of polarity and thus a disorderly arrangement. Some of these cells show pleomorphism and atypicality ("anaplasia") of their nuclei, which appear large, irregular, and hyperchromatic. Often, the nuclei in the basal layer are closely crowded together. Some of the cells in the midportion of the epidermis show premature keratinization, resulting in dyskeratotic cells or apoptotic bodies characterized by homogeneous, eosinophilic cytoplasm with or without a nucleus. In contrast to the epidermal keratinocytes, the cells of the hair follicles and eccrine ducts that penetrate the epidermis within actinic keratoses retain their normal appearance and keratinize normally. Occasionally, cells of the normal adnexal epithelium extend over the atypical cells of the epidermis in an umbrella-like fashion. In these cases, the keratin overlying the hyperplastic adnexal epithelium may be orthokeratotic, resulting in a characteristic pattern of alternating hyperkeratosis (over the dysplastic clone of cells) and orthokeratosis. In some cases, abnormal keratinocytes extend downward on the outside of the follicular infundibulum to the level of the sebaceous duct and, less commonly, along the eccrine duct.

A variant of the hypertrophic type of actinic keratosis is the lichenoid actinic keratosis, which demonstrates nuclear atypia, irregular acanthosis and hyperkeratosis, the presence of basal cell liquefaction, degeneration of the basal cell layer, and a bandlike "lichenoid" infiltrate in close apposition to the epidermis. Fairly numerous eosinophilic, homogeneous apoptotic bodies

are seen in the upper dermis as the so-called Civatte bodies. Aside from the presence of nuclear atypicality, there is considerable resemblance to lichen planus and benign lichenoid keratosis. An additional distinguishing feature may be the presence of plasma cells in the lichenoid infiltrate (see Chapter 7).

In rare instances of actinic keratosis of the hypertrophic type, in addition to finding anaplastic nuclei in the lower epidermis, one finds areas of epidermolytic hyperkeratosis in the upper epidermis. These changes are like those seen in bullous congenital ichthyosiform erythroderma, in linear epidermal nevus, and as incidental epidermolytic hyperkeratosis in a variety of lesions. In areas of epidermolytic hyperkeratosis, one observes clear spaces around the nuclei and a thickened granular layer with large, irregularly shaped keratohyalin granules in the upper epidermis. Epidermolytic hyperkeratosis may also occur in the lesions of solar cheilitis.

In the *atrophic type* of actinic keratosis, hyperkeratosis is usually slight. The epidermis is thinned and devoid of rete ridges. Atypicality of the cells is found predominantly in the basal cell layer, which consists of cells with large hyperchromatic nuclei that lie close together. The atypical basal layer may proliferate into the dermis as buds and ductlike structures. It may also surround—as cell mantles—the upper portion of pilosebaceous follicles and sweat ducts, the epithelium of which otherwise appears normal.

The *Bowenoid type* of actinic keratosis is histologically indistinguishable from Bowen disease and may indeed be better termed SCC *in situ* (SCCIS). As in Bowen disease, within the epidermis, there is considerable disorder in the arrangement of the nuclei, as well as clumping of nuclei and dyskeratosis (Figs. 29-48 to 29-51).

In the *acantholytic type* of actinic keratosis, immediately above the atypical cells composing the basal cell layer, there are clefts or lacunae similar to those seen in Darier disease (see Chapter 6). These clefts form as a result of anaplastic changes in the lowermost epidermis, resulting in dyskeratosis and loss of the intercellular bridges (Fig. 29-52). A few acantholytic cells may be present within the clefts (Fig. 29-53). Because the acantholysis is preceded by cellular changes, it is referred to as *secondary acantholysis*, in contrast to the primary acantholysis seen in the "acantholytic" diseases, such as pemphigus vulgaris and Darier disease. Above the acantholytic clefts, the epidermis shows varying degrees of atypicality but, generally, less atypicality than is seen in the basal cell layer. The anaplastic cells of the basal cell layer frequently show extensions into the upper dermis as buds or short, ductlike structures. Suprabasal acantholysis may also be seen around hair follicles and sweat ducts in the upper dermis. When atypia is full thickness or high grade, the term *acantholytic SCC in situ* may be applied.

In the *pigmented type* of actinic keratosis, excessive amounts of melanin are present, especially in the basal cell layer. In some cases, the atypical keratinocytes are well melanized. In others, almost all of the melanin is retained within the cell bodies and dendrites of the melanocytes, indicating some block in melanin transfer. Numerous melanophages are seen in most cases in the superficial dermis.

In all five types of actinic keratosis, the upper dermis usually shows a fairly dense, chronic inflammatory infiltrate composed predominantly of lymphoid cells but often also containing plasma cells. Solar cheilitis, more frequently than actinic keratosis of the skin, shows an inflammatory infiltrate in which plasma cells predominate. Although the upper dermis usually shows solar or basophilic degeneration, this may be absent in areas with a pronounced inflammatory reaction, probably because the inflammation has resulted in a regeneration of collagen.

In instances in which the histologic diagnosis is actinic keratosis but the clinical diagnosis is SCC, it is advisable to section more deeply into the block of tissue because progression into SCC may have taken place in another area. Because no sharp line of demarcation exists between the two conditions, it is not always possible to decide whether a lesion can still be regarded as actinic keratosis or should be classified as early SCC. Thus, some authors regard SCC as a lesion in which irregular aggregates of atypical keratinocytes are found in the papillary dermis, not in continuity with the overlying epidermis. Others call a lesion that does not extend downward to the level of the reticular dermis an actinic keratosis without qualification. This decision is rarely a vital one because early SCC arising in an actinic keratosis rarely causes metastases, although it may become deeply invasive and destructive through further growth. Because carcinomas arising in solar cheilitis have a significantly higher tendency to metastasize than carcinomas arising in actinic keratosis, and because invasion of the dermis in solar cheilitis may be focal, lesions of solar cheilitis require a thorough examination by means of step sections.

Pathogenesis. Because sun exposure is the main cause of actinic keratoses, their development is closely related to pale skin, sun exposure, and inadequate sun protection (105). There is evidence that actinic keratoses and/or SCCIS have a significant mutational burden that is largely analogous to that in cutaneous SCCs (cSCCs) as well as in the sun-exposed keratinocytes from which keratoses arise (106).

Differential Diagnosis. In actinic keratoses showing relatively slight atypicality, or anaplasia, of the tumor cells, diagnosis may be difficult. Thus, a hypertrophic actinic keratosis with a lichenoid inflammatory infiltrate may show a close histologic resemblance to the lesion known as *benign lichenoid keratosis*. In fact, this lesion was at one time believed to be a variant of actinic keratosis. Benign lichenoid keratosis differs from actinic keratosis by showing dissolution rather than atypicality of the basal cell layer, analogous to lichen planus (see Chapter 7).

An atrophic actinic keratosis may closely resemble lupus erythematosus because both types of lesions show flattening of the epidermis. Although lupus erythematosus shows vacuolization and actinic keratosis shows atypicality of the cells in the basal layer, these two changes are not always easily distinguished from one another. Therefore, other findings, such as follicular plugging and a patchy, periappendageal infiltrate in lupus erythematosus, are necessary for differentiation (see Chapter 10).

A pigmented actinic keratosis may resemble lentigo maligna, particularly if the melanin is seen largely within the melanocytes. Usually, however, lentigo maligna shows more flattening of the epidermis than pigmented actinic keratosis and, more importantly, a great increase in the number of melanocytes, together with atypicality in the melanocytes but not in the basal keratinocytes (see Chapter 28).

Principles of Management: There are several options available for treating actinic keratosis. The natural history of the lesions studied in the United Kingdom suggests that treatment is not always required on the basis of preventing progression to SCC (22). Nevertheless, many feel that the main reason for treatment is the prevention of SCC. Treatment options can be divided into topical and surgical. Topical treatment is in the form of immunomodulators such as 5-fluorouracil, imiquimod

5%, and diclofenac gel. No therapy or emollient is also a reasonable option for mild actinic keratoses. Application of sun blocks and screens for protection should always be recommended. Surgical options include cryosurgery, curettage, and surgical excision. Cryosurgery is reported to be effective in 75% of lesions when compared with photodynamic therapy (PDT). Although there are no studies of curettage and surgical excisions, they are of value in determining the exact histology of these lesions, especially unresponsive or atypical ones. PDT is also reported to be an effective treatment for actinic keratosis (107–110).

CUTANEOUS HORN

Clinical Summary. Cutaneous horn, or *cornu cutaneum*, is the clinical term for a circumscribed, conical, markedly hyperkeratotic lesion in which the height of the keratotic mass amounts to at least half of its largest diameter (Fig. 29-54). The term refers to a reaction pattern and not to a specific lesion.

Histopathology. On histologic examination, different types of lesions can be seen at the base of the conical hyperkeratosis of a cornu cutaneum. Most commonly, an actinic keratosis is encountered (Fig. 29-55). In some instances, a burn scar, filiform verruca,

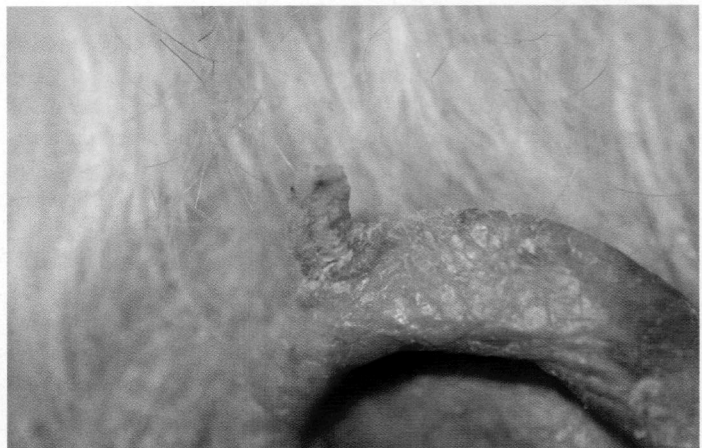

Figure 29-54 Cutaneous horn. The horn consists of a column of keratin arising on the sun-exposed skin of the ear.

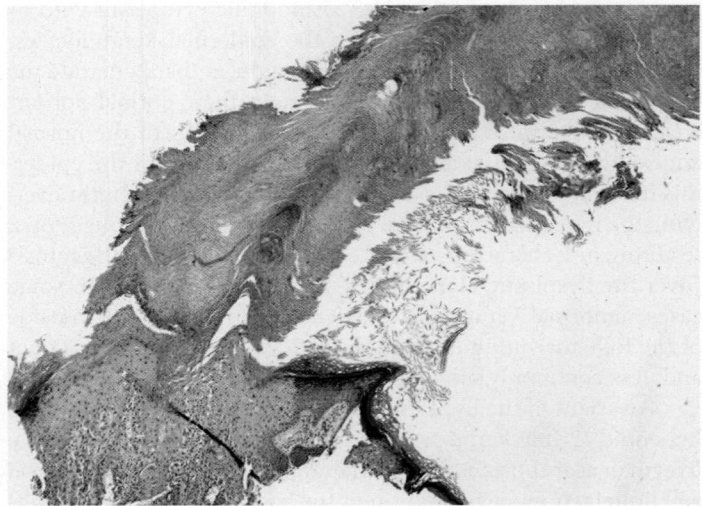

Figure 29-55 Cutaneous horn. The horn consists of a column of keratin arising in an actinic keratosis.

seborrheic keratosis, SCC, or verrucous carcinoma is found. On rare occasions, a trichilemmoma or a BCC is seen (111,112). For a description of trichilemmal horn, see Chapter 30.

ORAL LEUKOPLAKIA

Clinical Summary. The term *leukoplakia* was used in the past by dermatologists and gynecologists to designate white patches of the oral mucosa or the vulva that showed early, *in situ*, anaplastic changes; the term *leukokeratosis* was used for patches with a histologically benign appearance (113). However, leukoplakia has been redefined on the basis of the concept proposed by oral pathologists, and this concept has been accepted by the WHO (Fig. 29-56).

According to this concept, the term *leukoplakia* carries no histologic connotation and is used only as a clinical description. It is defined as a white patch or plaque that will not rub off and that cannot be characterized clinically or histologically as any specific disease (e.g., lichen planus, lupus erythematosus, candidiasis, and white sponge nevus). The reason for using the term *leukoplakia* as a purely clinical designation is that a distinction between benign leukoplakia and leukoplakia with dysplastic changes cannot be made on clinical grounds. It is therefore essential that all white plaques that either are idiopathic in origin or persist for 3 to 4 weeks after any existing irritation has been eliminated be examined histologically. In many cases of oral leukoplakia, either chemical irritation through tobacco use or mechanical irritation through dental stumps or ill-fitting dentures plays a role. Although the leukoplakia clears in some instances after the irritation has been removed, it persists in others. Leukoplakia is considered the most common premalignant condition of the oral cavity (114,115). Therefore, any leukoplakia that is growing or altering its appearance requires a repeat biopsy. Leukoplakia in low-risk sites such as the buccal mucosa and hard palate require regular clinical follow-up with the cessation of carcinogenic habits such as tobacco smoking. Leukoplakia with moderate or severe dysplasia requires complete surgical or ablative (CO_2 laser) removal and monitoring (116).

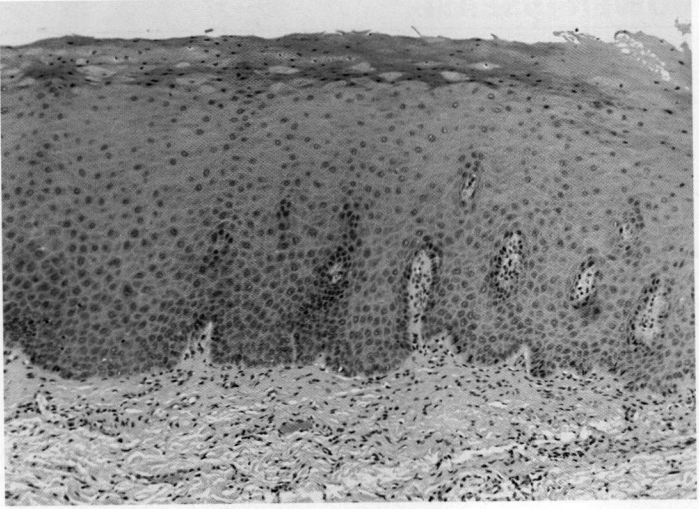

Figure 29-56 Oral leukoplakia. In this example, the squamous epithelium is hyperkeratotic and acanthotic but shows little evidence of dysplasia.

Clinically, lesions of leukoplakia on the oral mucosa consist of one or several white patches that may not be raised and that appear ill-defined. However, when elevated they appear sharply demarcated, with an irregular outline.

Erythroplakia of the oral mucosa consists of red, sharply delineated patches that vary greatly in size. Some of these lesions are sprinkled or intermingled with patches of leukoplakia, which are then referred to as *speckled erythroplakia* (117). Erythroplakia is a far less common condition than leukoplakia, where histologic changes show more advanced dysplastic changes than leukoplakia.

On examination by histology, scraping, or culture, both leukoplakia and erythroplakia frequently show *C. albicans* as a secondary invader, a finding that may give rise to an incorrect diagnosis of candidiasis. However, infection with *C. albicans* may cause oral lesions that are clinically indistinguishable from leukoplakia.

The analysis of oral leukoplakias and oral invasive carcinomas for HPV-related DNA has shown that a significant percentage of these lesions is reactive with papillomavirus antibodies, allowing the conclusion that they are induced by papillomaviruses, especially by HPV-11 and HPV-16 (see Chapter 25).

For a discussion of leukoplakia of the vulva, see page 981, and of oral hairy leukoplakia, see Chapter 25.

Histopathology. The whiteness of leukoplakia is the result of hydration of a thickened horny layer. On histologic examination, about 80% of the lesions of oral leukoplakia are found to be benign. Such lesions show hyperkeratotic or parakeratotic thickening of the horny layer, acanthosis, and a chronic inflammatory infiltrate (Fig. 29-49). Of the remaining 20% of the cases, 17% show varying degrees of dysplasia or *in situ* carcinoma and 3% show infiltrating SCC. Ultimate development of carcinoma has been observed in 7% to 13% of all cases of leukoplakia. Localization of the leukoplakia seems to play an important role in the presence of malignancy. Leukoplakias on the buccal mucosa were found to be benign in 96% of the cases, whereas on the floor of the mouth, only 32% of the leukoplakias were benign, and 31% showed a carcinoma *in situ* and 37% an invasive carcinoma.

In situ carcinoma, also referred to as precancerous leukoplakia, may have a similar histologic appearance to the hypertrophic type of actinic keratosis. Thus, the most important features observed within a moderately acanthotic epithelium are, first, pleomorphism and atypicality of the nuclei—which appear large, irregular, and hyperchromatic—and, second, loss of polarity, resulting in a disorderly arrangement of the cells. In some instances, one finds premature keratinization resulting in dyskeratotic cells in the midportion of the epithelium, crowding of nuclei in the basal cell layer, and irregular downward proliferations of the epithelium as additional features. There is considerable histologic, philosophical, and biologic overlap among lesions categorized as high-grade dysplasia and carcinoma *in situ* in oral as in other mucous membranes.

Erythroplakia of the oral mucosa, in contrast to leukoplakia, invariably shows nuclear atypicality. One observes *in situ* carcinoma in half of the cases and invasive carcinoma in the other half. The red appearance is explained by the absence of the normal surface covering of orthokeratin or parakeratin.

Differential Diagnosis. A decision as to whether *in situ* carcinoma exists in a leukoplakia can be difficult because some pleomorphism of nuclei and some loss of polarity of the cells can be seen occasionally in various inflammatory conditions also, including benign leukoplakia. In cases of doubt, step sections throughout the biopsy specimen are required, along with, possibly, an examination of additional biopsy specimens. The decision as to whether a leukoplakia is benign or low grade or is a high-grade dysplasia or a carcinoma *in situ* is of great importance. In comparison with SCC of the skin developing in an actinic keratosis, SCC of the oral mucosa developing in a leukoplakia with *in situ* carcinoma has a much greater tendency to metastasize.

Differentiation of leukoplakia from oral lichen planus may also cause difficulties both clinically and histologically. In lichen planus, no atypia is seen and there often is partial absence of basal cells. In addition, the prevalence of Langerhans cells in lesions of lichen planus may aid in the differentiation.

Principles of Management: It is not clear whether active treatment prevents the development of SCC. Therefore, lifelong close follow-up is recommended whether treatment is received or not. General advice to avoid aggravating factors such as tobacco smoking or chewing is important. Treatments include medical therapy such as retinoids and surgical interventions such as simple excision, CO_2 laser, and PDT. A biopsy of any changing lesion is highly recommended (118,119).

VERRUCOUS HYPERPLASIA, VERRUCOUS CARCINOMA OF THE ORAL MUCOSA

Clinical Summary. Verrucous hyperplasia of the oral mucosa consists of extensive verrucous, white patches that may arise as such or develop from lesions of leukoplakia. Verrucous hyperplasia and verrucous carcinoma are indistinguishable clinically. They may coexist, or verrucous carcinoma may develop from verrucous hyperplasia. In some instances, verrucous hyperplasia develops into frank SCC rather than into verrucous carcinoma (120,121). Exophytic verrucous hyperplasia may also occur on a background of submucous fibrosis, with histology required to distinguish between benign and malignant lesions in this context (122).

Verrucous carcinoma of the oral mucosa is also known as *oral florid papillomatosis*. Clinically, one observes white, cauliflower-like lesions that may involve large areas of the oral mucosa and that may gradually extend and coalesce. Extensive local tissue destruction may occur. However, metastases are rare, and if they occur, they remain limited to the regional lymph nodes.

Histopathology. Verrucous hyperplasia shows a hyperplastic epithelium with an upward extension of verrucous projections located predominantly superficial to the adjacent epithelium.

Verrucous carcinoma (oral florid papillomatosis) differs in its early stage from verrucous hyperplasia by showing, in addition to the surface verrucous projections, extension of the lesion into the underlying connective tissue. The downward extensions of the epithelium are round and club shaped and appear well demarcated from the surrounding stroma. Nuclear pleomorphism or hyperchromasia and the formation of horn pearls are absent.

The presence of lichenoid inflammation may mask the changes of dysplasia or invasive malignancy, possibly leading to an underdiagnosis of the malignancy (123,124).

Some lesions of verrucous carcinoma persist in this stage for many years, although ultimately they show—in the areas of deepest extension—a moderate loss of polarity, increased cytoplasmic basophilia, nuclear hyperchromasia, and frequent mitotic figures. These features, however, do not suffice for a diagnosis of SCC. Other lesions show sufficient nuclear atypicality and loss of polarity in the downward proliferations to indicate the presence of a well-differentiated SCC. In about 10% of the cases of verrucous carcinoma, transformation into a classic SCC takes place. (For a more detailed discussion of verrucous carcinoma, see p. 987.)

Principles of Management: Surgical excision is the treatment of choice for oral verrucous carcinoma. Achieving tumor-free excision margins is important to reduce recurrence rates. The presence of oral leukoplakia, submucosal fibrosis, and tumor location in the upper alveolar–palatal complex gives worse prognosis (125). Neck dissection is necessary in some cases.

EOSINOPHILIC ULCER OF THE TONGUE

Clinical Summary. Asymptomatic ulcers arise suddenly on the tongue. Spontaneous healing takes place within a few weeks (126). The appearances may masquerade as a malignant ulcer (127). Epstein Barr virus may play a role in the development of ulceration (128).

Histopathology. A dense cellular infiltrate is present at the base of the ulcer, extending through the submucosa into the striated muscle bundles of the tongue. Most of the cells are eosinophils, but there are also lymphocytes and histiocytes, with an occasional report of focal leukocytoclastic vasculitis.

Differential Diagnosis. This lesion differs from eosinophilic granuloma of histiocytosis X (see Chapter 26) clinically by its tendency to arise and heal rapidly and histologically by the smaller number and smaller size of the histiocytes.

Principles of Management: No specific treatment is required for this condition as the ulcer commonly resolves within a month. Analgesia may be required for symptomatic relief. Surgical excision and curettage have been described for removal.

BOWEN DISEASE

Clinical Summary. Bowen disease usually consists of a solitary lesion. It may occur on exposed or on unexposed skin. It may be caused on exposed skin by exposure to the sun and on unexposed skin by the ingestion of arsenic (see *Pathogenesis* and the section on Arsenical Keratosis and Carcinoma). Lesions of Bowen disease can form in lesions of epidermodysplasia verruciformis caused by HPV-5 (see Chapter 25). Not infrequently, the fingers, including the nail fold or nail bed, are involved.

Bowen disease manifests as a slowly enlarging erythematous patch of sharp but irregular outline showing little or no infiltration. Within the patch are generally areas of scaling and crusting (Fig. 29-57). Although Bowen disease may resemble a superficial BCC, it differs from it by the absence of a fine, pearly border and lack of a tendency to heal with central atrophy. Lesions of Bowen disease can occur on the glans penis, where they are referred to also as erythroplasia of Queyrat.

Bowenoid papulosis of the genitalia, because of its probable relationship to genital warts, is discussed in Chapter 25.

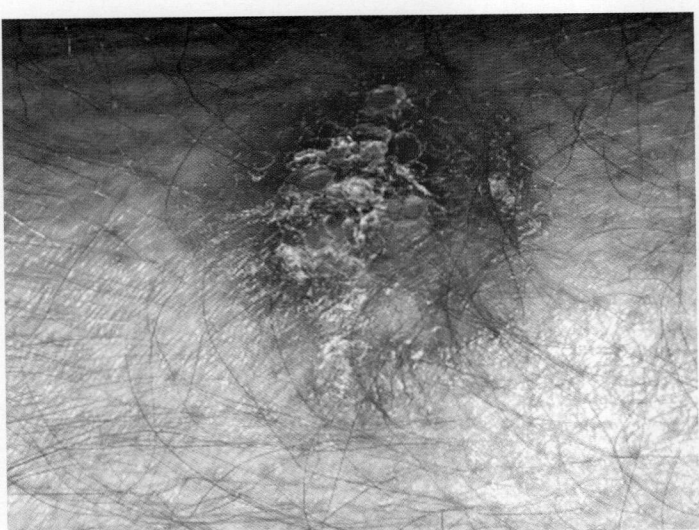

Figure 29-57 Bowen disease. The lesion is crusted and erythematous, with a poorly defined margin.

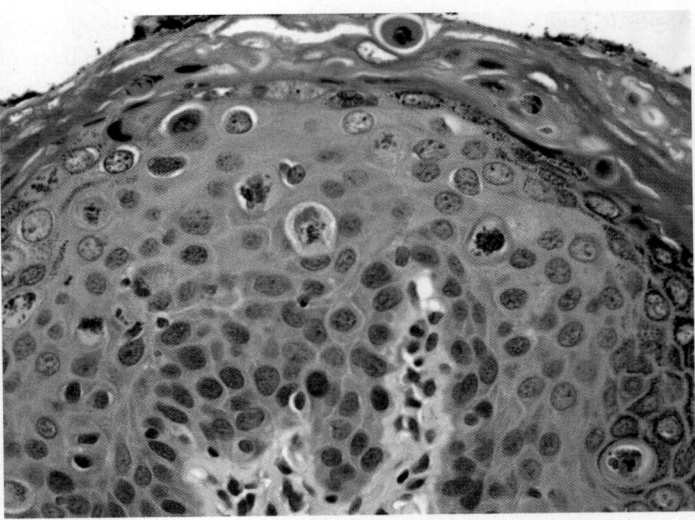

Figure 29-59 Bowen disease. Throughout the epidermis, the cells lie in disarray, with frequent large atypical mitoses.

Histopathology. Bowen disease is an intraepidermal SCC referred to also as SCC *in situ*. Thus, it biologically but not morphologically represents a *precancerous dermatosis*, under which designation it was described originally in 1912.

The epidermis shows acanthosis with the elongation and thickening of the rete ridges, often to such a degree that the papillae located between the rete ridges are reduced to thin strands. On the surface, there is usually parakeratosis with an associated loss of the granular layer. In a minority of cases, typically in female and younger patients, there is predominant orthokeratosis, with the retention of the granular cell layer (129). Throughout the epidermis, the cells lie in complete disorder, resulting in a "windblown" appearance (Figs. 29-58 and 29-59). Many cells appear highly atypical, showing large, hyperchromatic nuclei. Multinucleated epidermal cells containing clusters of nuclei are often present. The horny layer usually is thickened and consists largely of parakeratotic cells with atypical, hyperchromatic nuclei.

A common and rather characteristic feature is the presence of cells showing atypical individual cell keratinization. Such dyskeratotic cells are large and round and have a homogeneous, strongly eosinophilic cytoplasm and a hyperchromatic nucleus. The infiltrate of atypical cells in Bowen disease frequently extends into follicular infundibula and causes replacement of the follicular epithelium by atypical cells down to the entrance of the sebaceous duct.

Even though the marked atypicality of the epidermal cells includes the cells of the basal layer, the border between the epidermis and dermis everywhere appears sharp, and the basement membrane remains intact. The upper dermis usually shows a moderate amount of a chronic inflammatory infiltrate.

Immunohistochemical staining for Ki-67 and for p16 may show positive cells through the full thickness of the abnormal epidermis (Fig. 29-60) (130).

An occasional finding in Bowen disease is the vacuolization of cells, especially in the upper portion of the epidermis. In addition, in exceptional cases, multiple nests of atypical cells are scattered through a normal epidermis, sometimes with sparing of the basal cell layer, resulting in the histologic picture described as "intraepidermal epithelioma of Borst–Jadassohn" (see Chapter 30).

In a small percentage of cases of Bowen disease, an invasive SCC develops. The usual figure quoted is 3% to 5% (131). The highest incidence reported so far is 11% (132). On the

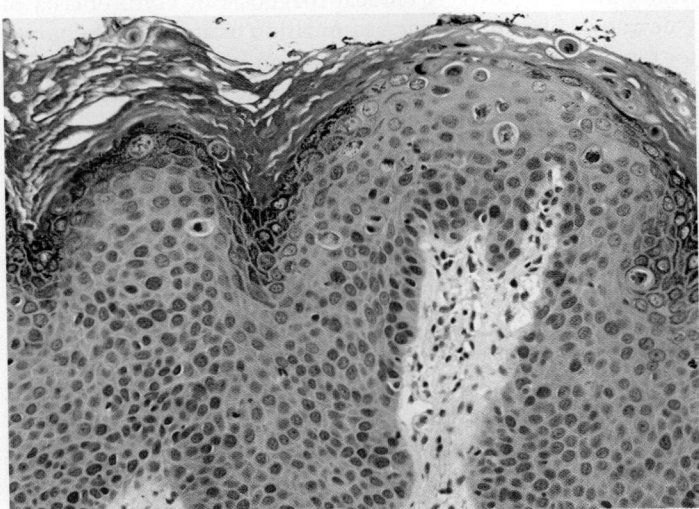

Figure 29-58 Bowen disease. The epidermis is irregularly thickened. The normal maturation pattern is effaced.

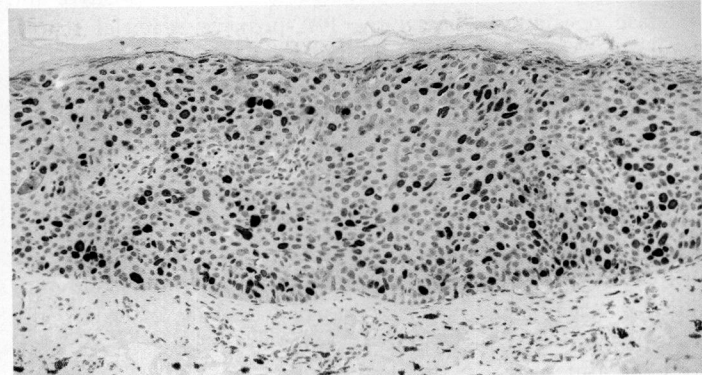

Figure 29-60 Ki-67 staining in Bowen disease. Positively stained nuclei are present at all levels in the epidermis.

opposite end is a statement that, in the vast majority of cases, Bowen disease remains a carcinoma *in situ* during the lives of those affected (133). If invasion happens, it usually takes place after many years' duration of the disease. The invasive tumor retains the cytologic characteristics of the intraepidermal tumor, and invasion may occur at first in only a limited area. To avoid missing such an area, it is advisable to examine representative sections throughout the entire tissue block. As soon as the invasion has taken place, the prognosis changes. So long as Bowen disease remains in its intraepidermal stage, metastases do not occur. However, once invasion of the dermis has occurred, there exists the possibility of regional and even visceral metastases (132). Spindle cell SCC has also been reported as developing in Bowen disease (134).

Pathogenesis. No agreement exists about the frequency with which visceral carcinoma develops in patients with Bowen disease. The first authors to point out an association between Bowen disease and visceral cancer found that of 35 patients with Bowen disease who were known to have died, 20 (57%) had an associated internal cancer (132). In a subsequent series, however, a significant increase in the incidence of associated internal cancer was observed only in patients in whom the lesions of Bowen disease were located in areas not exposed to the sun; in patients in whom the lesions were in exposed areas, the incidence of visceral cancer was low. Subsequent studies, with one exception, have not demonstrated a significantly increased risk of internal malignancy in patients with Bowen disease.

In a study of HPV involvement in Bowen disease, HPV was found in less than 50% of cases (129).

Differential Diagnosis. No histologic difference exists between bowenoid actinic keratosis and Bowen disease. They may differ merely in size, with the bowenoid actinic keratosis usually being smaller than Bowen disease.

In some cases of Bowen disease, there are single atypical cells scattered among benign keratinocytes in a pattern of "Pagetoid Bowen disease" or "Pagetoid SCC *in situ*" that must be differentiated from superficial spreading melanoma *in situ*, if necessary with the use of immunostaining for keratin markers and melanocytic markers such as S100 and/or Melan-A/MART-1 (see Chapter 28). Paget disease may similarly share with Bowen disease the presence of vacuolated cells in a "pagetoid" pattern, but, in contrast to Bowen disease, it shows no dyskeratosis. In addition, immunostaining for the aforementioned melanocytic markers and for carcinoembryonic antigen (CEA) and keratins may be used to aid in making this distinction, and furthermore the material contained in Paget cells is often PAS positive and diastase resistant, whereas the PAS-positive material that is sometimes present in the vacuolated cells of Bowen disease is glycogen and therefore diastase labile.

Another differential diagnosis is microclonal seborrheic keratosis, which will not typically show the same high expression of p16 and Ki-67 seen in Bowen disease (54).

Principles of Management: There are various therapeutic options available for the treatment of Bowen disease. The choice of treatment is usually influenced by multiple factors, including the patients' age group, comorbidities, size of lesion, site of lesion, number of lesions, recurrence of disease, availability of treatments, and, in some centers, the cost of treatment. Treatment options include nonsurgical and surgical treatments. Nonsurgical treatments include topical treatments with 5-fluorouracil and imiquimod creams, cryotherapy, and PDT. Surgical treatments include excision and curettage and cautery (5). There is also an argument for "no treatment" and observation rather than intervention in some cases with slowly progressive thin lesions on the lower leg of elderly patients where healing is poor. A Cochrane review assessing the effects of therapeutic interventions for cutaneous Bowen disease showed that there is very little good-quality research on the treatment of this disease and that there is lack of enough evidence available to provide guidance on choosing surgical over topical treatments or vice versa (135).

ERYTHROPLASIA OF QUEYRAT (BOWEN DISEASE OF THE GLANS PENIS, CARCINOMA *IN SITU*)

Clinical Summary. Erythroplasia of Queyrat is the term often used for carcinoma *in situ* located on the glans penis. Clinically and histologically, it is identical to Bowen disease, and this designation would seem preferable for simplicity's sake. The only reason for keeping the term *erythroplasia of Queyrat* alive is that it was introduced in 1911, 1 year before the description of Bowen disease (136).

Erythroplasia or Bowen disease of the glans penis is seen almost exclusively in uncircumcised men. It manifests itself as an asymptomatic, sharply demarcated, bright-red, shiny, very slightly infiltrated plaque on the glans penis or, less often, in the coronal sulcus or on the inner surface of the prepuce. Erythroplasia of Queyrat has been associated with HPV infections, in particular HPV types 8 and 16 (137). However, this proposed association remains controversial as one particular study failed to detect HPV DNA in lesional skin (138).

Histopathology. Erythroplasia of Queyrat of the glans penis has the same histologic appearance as Bowen disease. Progression into an invasive SCC has been observed in up to 30% of the patients, with metastases in about 20% of the patients with invasive erythroplasia. It thus has a greater tendency for invasion and metastasis than Bowen disease of the skin and other forms of Bowen disease of the penis.

Differential Diagnosis. A clinical diagnosis of erythroplasia of Queyrat requires histologic examination of an adequate biopsy for confirmation because differentiation from balanitis circumscripta plasmacellularis is not possible on a clinical basis.

Principles of Management: Consideration to offer a high cure rate while preserving the function and cosmesis is important. Treatment with topical immunomodulating agents such as imiquimod 5% is effective and is commonly used (139).

ZOON PLASMA CELL BALANITIS

Clinical Summary. A disorder first described by Zoon in 1952 (140), balanitis circumscripta plasmacellularis has the same clinical appearance as erythroplasia of Queyrat or Bowen disease of the glans penis (Fig. 29-61). In some instances, erosions with a tendency to bleed are present. Like erythroplasia, this disorder is seen almost exclusively in uncircumcised males (141). However, it is important to distinguish this entity from

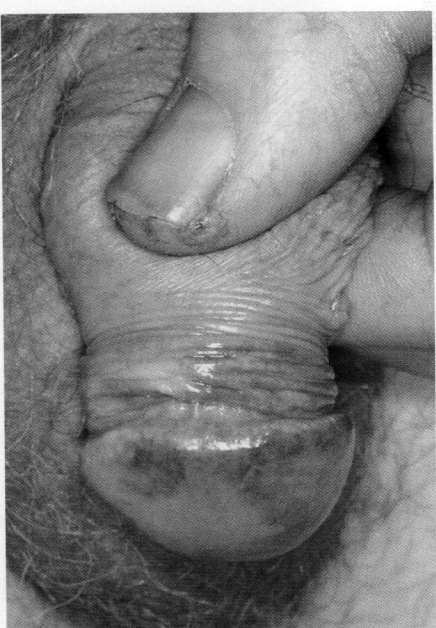

Figure 29-61 Zoon balanitis. Shiny, moist, erythematous, well-demarcated plaques on the glans penis of an uncircumcised male.

erythroplasia of Queyrat as Zoon balanitis is a benign condition, whereas erythroplasia is considered premalignant. On rare occasions, an analogous lesion referred to as *vulvitis circumscripta plasmacellularis* is observed on the vulva. The etiology of this condition is unknown but trauma, friction, heat, poor hygiene, and chronic infection with *Mycobacterium smegmatis* have been proposed. No link has been demonstrated between HPV and Zoon balanitis.

Histopathology. The epidermis appears thinned and often shows an absence of its upper layers. It may be partially detached as a result of subepidermal cleavage or even absent. If present, the epidermis often has a rather distinctive appearance; in addition to being thinned and flattened, it is composed of diamond- or lozenge-shaped, flattened keratinocytes that are separated from each other by uniform intercellular edema. Erythrocytes may be seen permeating the epidermis. In some cases, the keratinocytes appear degenerated or necrotic.

The upper dermis shows a bandlike infiltrate in which numerous plasma cells are often seen. In some cases, however, their number is only moderate or even small. In addition, the capillaries are dilated, and there may be extravasations of erythrocytes and deposits of hemosiderin.

Pathogenesis. It has been pointed out that plasma cells frequently predominate in the inflammatory response at mucocutaneous junctions in a variety of benign and malignant processes. Thus, the term *circumorificial plasmacytosis* was introduced for benign plasma cell infiltrates on the glans penis, vulva, and lips. However, the combination of histologic and clinical features seen in balanitis circumscripta plasmacellularis, and probably also in vulvitis circumscripta plasmacellularis, is unique and deserves recognition as an entity.

Principles of Management: Topical corticosteroids can be effective, especially with symptomatic relief; other medical therapy is generally ineffective. Circumcision almost always cures this disease.

VULVAR INTRAEPITHELIAL NEOPLASIA

Clinical Summary. The term leukoplakia of the vulva is purely a clinical designation, now usually replaced by vulvar intraepithelial neoplasia (VIN) and requiring histologic examination for clarification of the diagnosis, especially to decide whether atypicality of the epithelial cells exists. The clinical aspect of leukoplakia of the vulva is more variable than that of oral leukoplakia because it does not always consist only of white patches as in the mouth but may also have a papular or verrucous appearance (Fig. 29-62). The reason is that on the vulva, HPV infections can occur as flat or papular condylomas, often in association with similar lesions on the cervix. In addition, the condition previously described as bowenoid papulosis, in the presence of multiple, coalescing papules, may result in a verrucous aspect of the leukoplakia (see Chapter 25). A clear-cut histologic decision is often not possible unless adequate clinical data are available.

Further investigation of dysplastic lesions in the vulva has shown that there are two types of VIN (142). The first of these is *undifferentiated VIN*, which is associated with oncogenic HPV infection (HPV 16, 18, 31, and 33), occurs mainly in younger women, tends to be multicentric, and is of the undifferentiated or bowenoid type. This is probably what has previously been called bowenoid papulosis. The second type is *differentiated VIN*, which is not associated with HPV infection, typically occurs in older women, and is often unifocal. It is commonly associated with lichen sclerosus or squamous hyperplasia and carries a substantial risk of progression to invasive SCC.

Histopathology. Flat condylomas that may be associated with VIN show intracellular vacuolization that may result in a somewhat atypical appearance of the epithelium referred to as *koilocytotic atypia.* This may be difficult to differentiate from true atypia. In undifferentiated VIN, the changes are those of undifferentiated basaloid or bowenoid dysplasia. In differentiated VIN, the epithelium is thickened and parakeratotic with elongated and

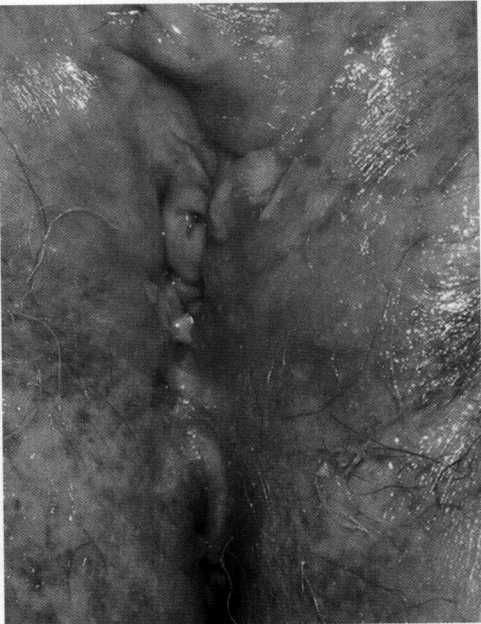

Figure 29-62 Vulvar intraepithelial neoplasia (VIN). The area of dysplasia shows white leukoplakia, with surrounding erythema.

anastomosing rete ridges. The characteristic feature is the presence of large basal or parabasal eosinophilic keratinocytes with abnormal vesicular nuclei and prominent intercellular bridges. Intraepithelial pearls may be present in the rete ridges. There is little or no atypia above the basal layer of the epidermis.

Principles of Management: The aim of treating VIN should be to remove the abnormal tissue to minimize the risk of developing invasive vulvar cancer while preserving vulvar anatomy and function. Treatment modalities include vulvectomy, wide local excision, laser ablation, laser excision, and topical treatment with imiquimod. Small lesions (<2 cm) with superficial invasion only (<1 mm) have negligible risk of lymph node metastasis, and therefore wide local excision with peripheral and deep free margins are sufficient. A meta-analysis of the effectiveness of medical treatment in VIN included four randomized controlled trials and concluded that imiquimod is an effective treatment, but further studies are required to assess the adverse effects (143). Long-term follow-up for these patients should be mandatory to allow prompt detection of an invasive disease.

Immunization with HPV vaccine has been shown to reduce the risk of developing VIN, cervical cancer, and genital warts, but further longitudinal studies are needed to assess its use in the prevention of progression to cancer (144).

ARSENICAL KERATOSIS AND CARCINOMA

Clinical Summary. Inorganic arsenic was a frequently used oral medication for a number of dermatoses until evidence accumulated in the 1930s that, besides its long-known tendency to form arsenical keratoses on the palms and soles, inorganic arsenic quite frequently causes carcinoma of the skin (145). In the 1950s, it became apparent that inorganic arsenic could cause visceral carcinoma. The most common form in which inorganic arsenic has been administered is Fowler solution containing 1% potassium arsenite (146).

Careless handling of industrial wastes can introduce arsenic into well water used for domestic consumption, resulting in "epidemic" occurrences of arsenical keratoses and cutaneous carcinomas (147–149).

Arsenical keratoses of the palms and soles, consisting of verrucous papules without surrounding inflammation, are a common manifestation of prolonged arsenic ingestion. Thus, in a follow-up study of 262 patients who had been taking Fowler solution for 6 to 26 years before this study, arsenical keratoses of the palms and soles were observed in 40% and arsenic-induced carcinomas of the skin in 8% (149,150). In a study from Taiwan, 80% of the 428 patients with arsenical carcinomas of the skin had arsenical keratoses of the palms and soles (151). The minimal latent period between the beginning of arsenic intake and the onset of arsenical keratoses of the palms and soles was 2.5 years, and the average latent period 6 years (150). In the presence of arsenic exposure, shorter telomere length predisposes individuals to an increased risk of BCC. The effect is synergistic in individuals with the highest arsenic exposure and the shortest telomeres (152).

Cutaneous carcinomas following arsenic ingestion are usually multiple, and about three-fourths of them are located on the trunk. They consist of erythematous, scaling, occasionally crusted patches that slowly increase in size. Carcinomas can also arise in arsenical keratoses of the palms and soles (150,151).

The average latency between the beginning of arsenic intake and the onset of carcinoma was 18 years, with a range from 3 to 40 years (153).

Visceral carcinoma can be caused by arsenic intake, but the actual incidence is difficult to determine because of the long latent period, which may vary from 13 to 50 years, with an average of 24 years (154). The most common locations appear to be bronchi and the genitourinary system. There are on record at least two incidences of prolonged arsenic intake in which lung cancer occurred in a high percentage of the patients: One report concerned vineyard workers exposed to an arsenic insecticide (155) and the other dealt with villagers exposed to arsenic-containing drinking water (156). In the latter series, the onset of pulmonary cancer started 30 years after the arsenic exposure.

Because Bowen disease is the most common cutaneous carcinoma produced by arsenic, the possibility of a relationship between Bowen disease and visceral carcinoma is of interest. This association, first pointed out in 1959 (132), appears to be greatest in those cases of Bowen disease in which the lesions are located in unexposed areas and thus are not caused by sun exposure. In one report, an association with internal carcinoma was found in about one-third of the cases (157). It was suggested that arsenic is the common denominator in such cases, causing both Bowen disease and internal carcinoma. However, subsequent studies showed no significant relationship between Bowen disease in covered areas and internal malignancy (158), or if such a relationship was found, no arsenic ingestion was found in most of the patients (159).

Histopathology. In arsenical keratoses of the palms and soles, one may find, in some instances, only hyperkeratosis and acanthosis without evidence of nuclear atypicality. However, when one cuts deeper into the tissue block, atypicality may become apparent. Whereas some arsenical keratoses show only mild nuclear atypicality, the findings in others are those of an SCCIS and are analogous to Bowen disease or an actinic keratosis. One observes disorder in the arrangement of the squamous cells and nuclear atypicalities, such as hyperchromasia, clumping, or dyskeratosis. Atrophy of the epidermis and basophilic degeneration of the upper dermis, as seen in some actinic keratoses, are absent in arsenical keratoses. Evidence of development into an invasive SCC may be seen in some arsenical keratoses.

The type of cutaneous carcinoma that follows arsenic ingestion can be either SCC or BCC, usually as multiple lesions. SCCs usually occur as *in situ* lesions analogous to Bowen disease and BCCs occur most commonly as superficial BCCs, although invasive SCCs and BCCs occur occasionally. Invasive tumors may arise *de novo* or may develop within preexisting lesions of Bowen disease or superficial BCC.

A matter of controversy has been whether arsenical carcinomas occur more commonly as lesions of Bowen disease or as superficial BCCs. For many years, it was accepted that lesions of Bowen disease were the usual reaction (160). However, whereas two publications stated that superficial BCCs are far more prevalent than lesions of Bowen disease (150,161), in two other publications, Bowen disease was found to be much more common (151,162). The most likely explanation for this discrepancy appears to be that, in many instances, lesions of Bowen disease have been misinterpreted as superficial BCC (162). The distinction can indeed be difficult; one author who found mainly superficial BCCs conceded that 25% of them showed "squamous metaplasia" (161), and another author proposed the concept of "combined forms" consisting of a "mixture of superficial basal cell carcinoma and intraepidermal carcinoma" (151). It appears likely that lesions designated as superficial BCC with squamous metaplasia or as combined forms represent lesions of Bowen disease. (For histologic descriptions of Bowen disease and superficial BCC, see later sections in this chapter, respectively.)

Pathogenesis. In vitro experiments concerning the effects of inorganic arsenic on human epidermal cells have shown that arsenic depresses premitotic DNA replication. Furthermore, incubation with inorganic arsenic and subsequent exposure of the cell cultures to ultraviolet light causes interruption of the enzymatic "dark repair mechanism" in the epidermal cells. Among other enzymes, arsenic seems to block DNA polymerase predominantly by attaching itself to sulfhydryl groups. The damaging effect of arsenic on DNA may explain its carcinogenic effect (163). Chinese proprietary medicines containing inorganic arsenic are also a potential risk factor, with a long latency period between exposure and the development of disease (164).

SQUAMOUS CELL CARCINOMA

Clinical Summary. cSCC may occur anywhere on the skin and on mucous membranes with squamous epithelium. It rarely arises from normal-appearing skin. Most commonly, it arises in sun-damaged skin, either as such or from an actinic keratosis (Figs. 29-63 and 29-64). Next to sun-damaged skin, SCCs arise most commonly in scars from burns and in stasis ulcers, termed *Marjolin ulcers* (165–167). Carcinomas arising in sun-damaged skin have a very low propensity to metastasize, the incidence amounting to only about 0.5% (168). This is in contrast to a metastatic rate of 2% to 3% for all patients with SCC of the skin, with death resulting in about three-fourths of the patients with metastases (169,170). Carcinomas of the lower lip, even though in most cases they are also induced by exposure to the sun, have a much higher incidence of metastasis, about 16%, with death occurring in about half of these patients as a result of metastases (171). In addition, the rate of metastases is higher

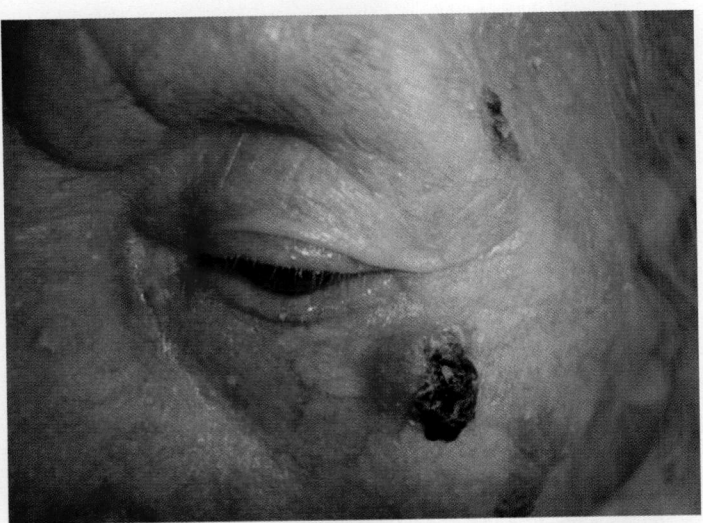

Figure 29-63 Squamous cell carcinoma. There is a hyperkeratotic horn on the surface of the tumor, which has a fleshy appearance around its base.

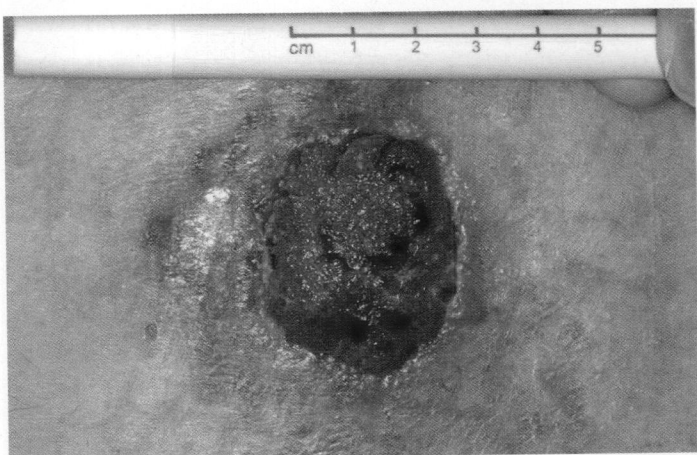

Figure 29-64 Squamous cell carcinoma. This unpigmented tumor has a fleshy surface.

in adenoid and mucin-producing SCCs of the skin than in the common type.

The diameter and thickness of cSCC are related to the likelihood of metastasis, which is most often seen in primary tumors with a diameter of at least 15 mm and a vertical tumor thickness of at least 2 mm. Decreasing degrees of differentiation, desmoplasia, and an inflammatory reaction including eosinophils and plasma cells are also more frequently seen in metastasizing tumors (172). The staging of cSCC is based on the lesion diameter, invasion depth, differentiation, and perineural invasion, the latter especially in nerves greater than 0.1 mm in diameter (173).

cSCCs that arise secondary to inflammatory and degenerative processes have a much higher rate of metastasis than those developing in sun-damaged skin (174,175). Thus, the rate of metastasis has been reported as 12%, with death caused by disease in 12.6% of SCCs arising in osteomyelitic sinuses (176) and 18% of carcinomas developing in burn scars (177). Furthermore, carcinomas arising from modified skin, such as the glans penis and the vulva, and from the oral mucosa have a rather high rate of metastasis unless recognized and adequately treated at an early stage.

The incidence of SCCs, like that of other malignant neoplasms, is significantly increased in immunosuppressed patients. In one study, 61% of patients developed nonmelanoma skin (NMSC), with the risk of SCC being 33% at 5 years and 62% at 10 years (178). A Fitzpatrick skin type III to VI was associated with a decreased risk of NMSC.

Clinically, SCC of the skin most commonly consists of a shallow ulcer surrounded by a wide, elevated, indurated border. Often, the ulcer is covered by a crust that conceals a red, granular base. Occasionally, raised, fungoid, verrucous lesions without ulceration occur. Multiprofessional guidelines for the management of patients with SCC have been published (179).

Four variants of SCC—basosquamous carcinoma, adenoid SCC, mucin-producing SCC, and verrucous carcinoma—are discussed later.

Histopathology. SCC of the skin is a true, invasive carcinoma of the surface epidermis. On histologic examination, one finds the tumor to consist of irregular masses of epidermal cells that proliferate downward into the dermis (Figs. 29-65 to 29-68). The invading tumor masses are composed in varying proportions of normal squamous cells and of atypical (anaplastic) squamous cells. The number of atypical squamous cells is higher in the

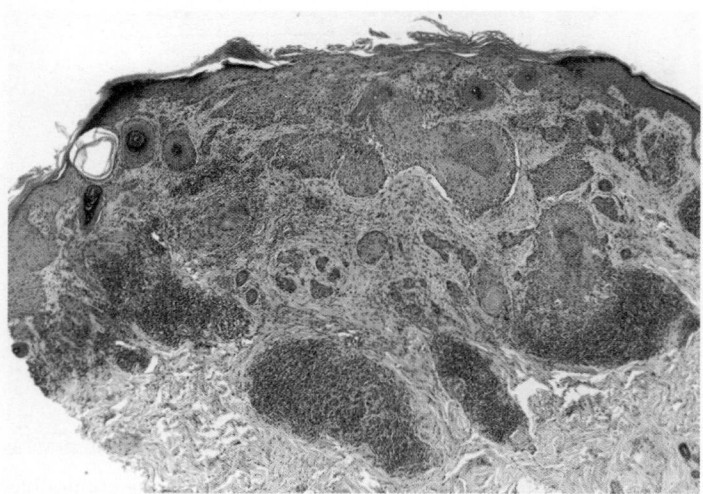

Figure 29-65 Squamous cell carcinoma arising in actinic keratosis. Low magnification. The epidermis shows features of an actinic keratosis. There is invasion of the dermis by epidermal masses. The dermis shows a marked inflammatory reaction.

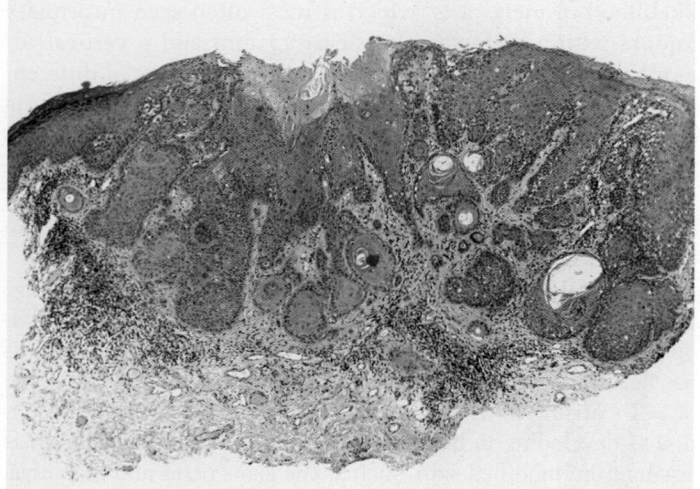

Figure 29-66 Squamous cell carcinoma, acantholytic type. In the deep part of the lesion, the invasive cell masses show much less keratinization than in a well-differentiated tumor.

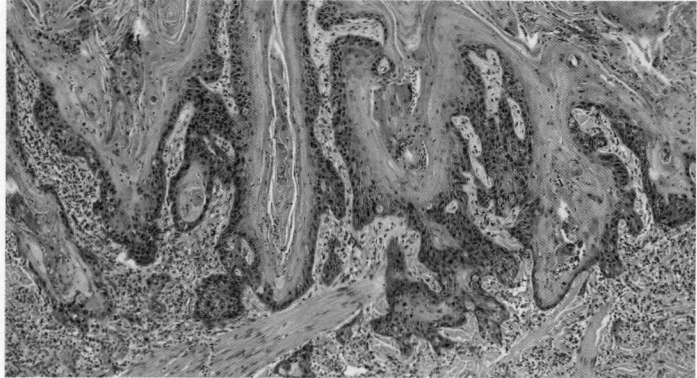

Figure 29-67 Invasive squamous cell carcinoma. This well-differentiated tumor on the face invades through muscle.

more poorly differentiated tumors. Atypicality of squamous cells expresses itself in such changes as great variation in the size and shape of the cells, hyperplasia and hyperchromasia of the nuclei, absence of intercellular bridges, keratinization of individual cells, and the presence of atypical mitotic figures.

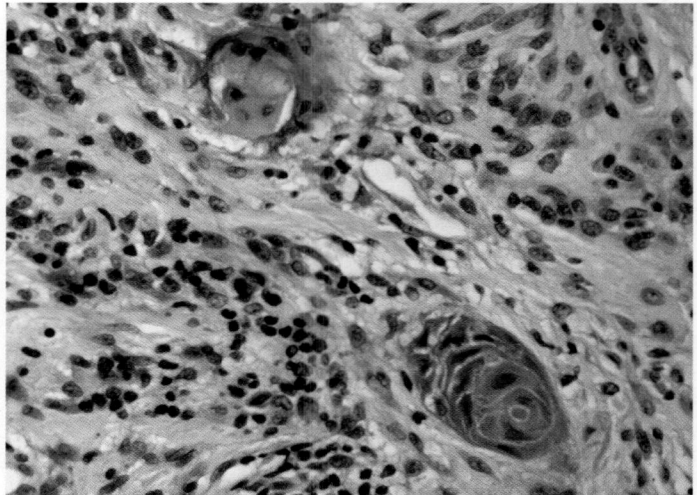

Figure 29-68 Squamous cell carcinoma. High magnification. Pleomorphic, hyperchromatic malignant squamous cells infiltrate the dermis.

Differentiation in SCC is in the direction of keratinization. Keratinization often takes place in the form of horn pearls (or keratin pearls), which are very characteristic structures composed of concentric layers of squamous cells showing gradually increasing keratinization toward the center. The center shows usually incomplete and only rarely complete keratinization. Keratohyalin granules within the horn pearls are sparse or absent. There have been attempts to produce grading systems for SCC, but classification into well-differentiated (Fig. 29-69), moderately differentiated (Fig. 29-70), and poorly differentiated (Fig. 29-71) carcinoma is the most widely adopted and reproducible way of describing the microscopic appearance of the tumors (1). Well-differentiated, moderately differentiated, and poorly differentiated SCCs are defined as carcinomas showing keratinization in more than 75%, in between 25% and 75% of the tumor, and in less than 25% of the tumor, respectively.

Marjolin ulcer is a term applied to tumors that arise at the periphery of a chronic ulcer or a scar. The scar may be caused by a remote burn or radiation, or there may be a chronic inflammatory process such as a draining osteomyelitis sinus. The tumors are often well differentiated and may arise in a

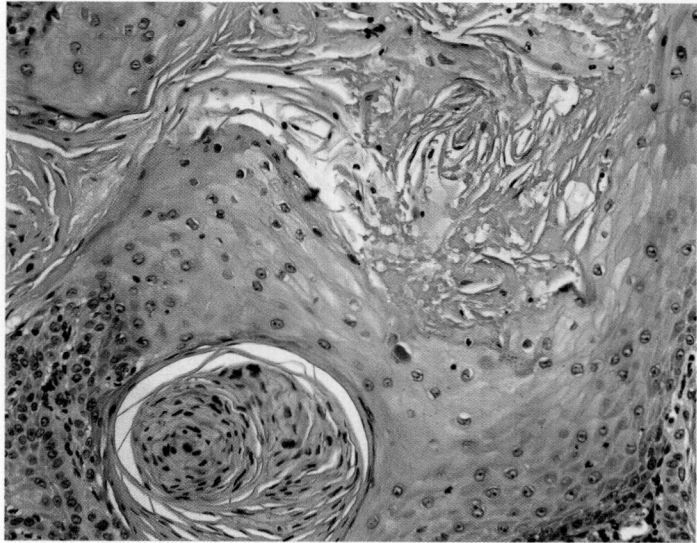

Figure 29-69 Squamous cell carcinoma, well differentiated. More than 75% of the tumor is keratinized.

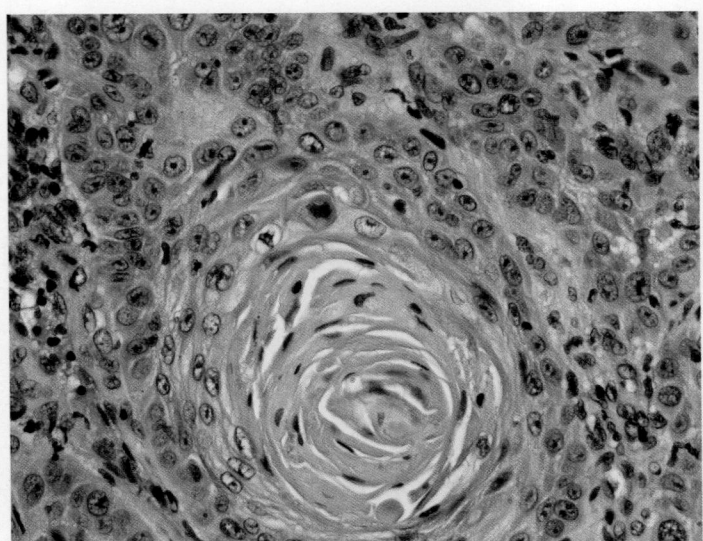

Figure 29-70 Squamous cell carcinoma, moderately differentiated. Between 25% and 75% of the tumor is keratinized.

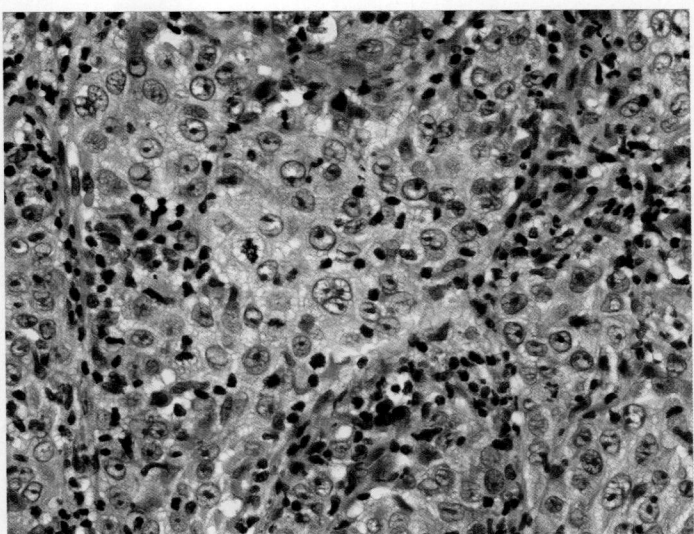

Figure 29-72 Lymphoepithelioma-like carcinoma. Shows similarities to poorly differentiated squamous cell carcinoma, but has a more syncytial appearance of tumor epithelial cells and a rich lymphocytic infiltrate.

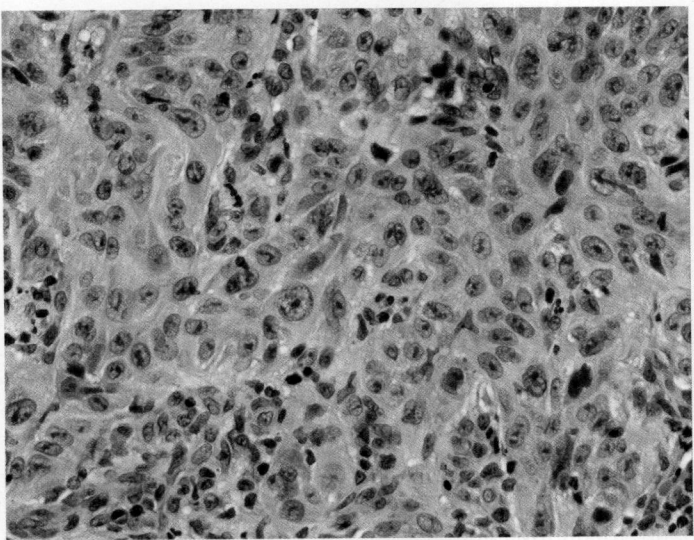

Figure 29-71 Squamous cell carcinoma, poorly differentiated. Less than 25% of the tumor is keratinized.

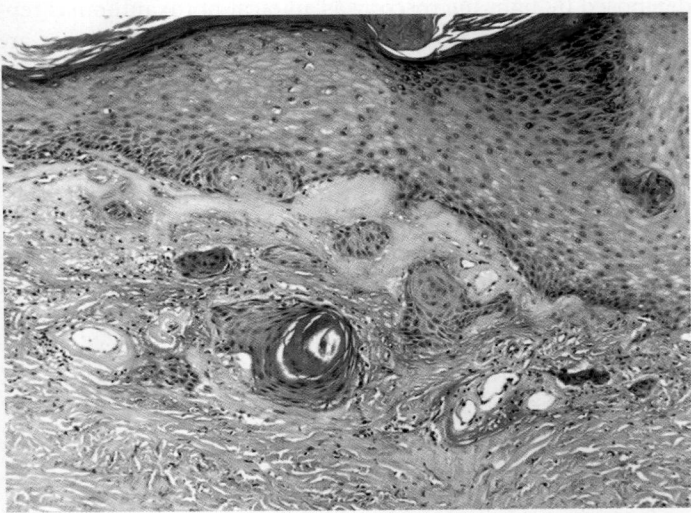

Figure 29-73 Postradiotherapy squamous cell carcinoma. This lesion, arising in an area treated many years previously with radiotherapy, shows a combination of invasive keratinizing squamous cell carcinoma and stromal damage secondary to radiotherapy.

background of pseudoepitheliomatous (pseudocarcinomatous) hyperplasia, making diagnosis difficult (see discussion on page 988) (Figs. 29-72 and 29-73).

Spindle cell SCC in particular may show a great resemblance to atypical fibroxanthoma. In some instances, spindle cell SCCs contain areas in which the cells either show intercellular bridges and beginning keratinization or show evidence of origin from the epidermis. In other cases, however, such areas cannot be detected. The spindle cells are intermingled with collagen and may be arranged in whorls. Not infrequently, pleomorphic giant cells are seen. In such instances, distinction from atypical fibroxanthoma may be difficult: Differential diagnosis by immunohistochemical examination is required (134) (see Pathogenesis).

Raised, verrucous lesions of SCC may show a considerable histologic resemblance to keratoacanthoma by having a central keratin-filled crater with peripheral buttresses. Keratoacanthomas typically do not extend into the dermis more deeply than

the sweat gland coils; so when a tumor invades into the dermis to a deeper level than this, it can be described with some confidence as carcinoma. There has been some reluctance among pathologists to even diagnose keratoacanthoma at all because of the view of some that the entity does not exist. A compromise position is to describe well-circumscribed and well-differentiated tumors as "well-differentiated, keratoacanthoma-like SCCs."

Pathogenesis. Most UV-associated cSCCs appear to progress through stepwise mutations in actinic keratoses or in fields of squamous dysplasia. Common mutations involve activating mutations in genes such as HRAS and KRAS, and inactivating mutations in suppressor genes such as TP53, NOTCH1, and NOTCH2 (173).

Electron microscopy of SCC, in comparison with normal epidermal squamous cells, shows a reduction in the number of desmosomes on the cell surface. In their place, microvilli extend into the widened intercellular spaces. Desmosomes can be seen within the cytoplasm of some of the tumor cells, either by themselves or attached to bundles of tonofilaments (180). Their intracytoplasmic location may be the result of either phagocytosis or invagination of the plasma membrane. However, it is not a specific finding for SCC; intracytoplasmic desmosomes can also be found in keratoacanthoma and Bowen disease as well as in several unrelated epidermal proliferations and even in normal keratinocytes. At the dermal–epidermal junction, the basement membrane shows sporadic discontinuities through which long cytoplasmic protrusions penetrate, indicating an invasion of the dermis by epidermal keratinocytes (181).

In early SCC, lymphocytes are often seen in close contact with tumor cells, some of which show degenerative changes such as disruption of the plasma membrane as well as fragmentation and subsequent release of organelles into the intercellular spaces. This can be interpreted as the cellular expression of an immune reaction against tumor cells (182).

The epithelial nature of the sarcoma-like cells in *spindle cell SCC* is supported by electron microscopic findings, which have shown that these cells contain tonofilaments and occasional desmosome-like structures (183,184). Electron microscopy (like immunohistochemistry) has also shown that structures diagnosed by light microscopy as atypical fibroxanthomas represent a heterogeneous group of neoplasms and that some are in actuality spindle cell SCCs (185,186).

Immunohistochemical methods are of considerable value in the differentiation of SCC from mesodermal tumors, such as atypical fibroxanthoma and malignant fibrous histiocytoma (pleomorphic sarcoma), and from malignant melanoma. For the identification of keratinocytes, primary antibodies directed against p63/p40, high-molecular-weight cytokeratins—such as cytokeratin 13, CK5/6, MNF116, and 34bE12—or a pancytokeratin marker may be used (173). In contrast, atypical fibroxanthoma and pleomorphic dermal sarcomas (PDSs) react with vimentin but not with keratin (see Chapter 32) and malignant melanoma with S100 protein, Sox10, and Melan-A/MART-1 (as well as with vimentin, see Chapter 28). CD10 is not a reliable marker for this distinction as it can be reactive in melanoma as well as in AFX/PDS. At times, even differentiation of an SCC from a lymphoma may be difficult, in which case a positive reaction with monoclonal antileukocyte antibody (LCA, CD45) would favor lymphoma (see Chapter 31). Immunohistochemistry using keratin markers may also be valuable in identifying tumor cells of an SCC in the midst of an inflammatory infiltrate and can, thus, aid in deciding whether the margins of an excised specimen are free of tumor cells. The immunohistochemical differential diagnosis of spindle cell neoplasms in the skin is discussed also in Chapters 4, 28, 32, and 34.

Differential Diagnosis. The diagnosis of SCC, although easily made in typical cases, may sometimes be difficult.

The differences between SCCIS and actinic keratosis lie in the degree as well as the type of changes. In both conditions, one finds atypicality of cells, with dyskeratosis of individual cells and downward proliferation of the epidermis. However, only in frank SCC is there invasion of the reticular dermis. No sharp line of demarcation exists between the two conditions, and not infrequently, on step sectioning for a lesion, the histologic appearance of actinic keratosis reveals one or several areas in which the changes have progressed to SCC.

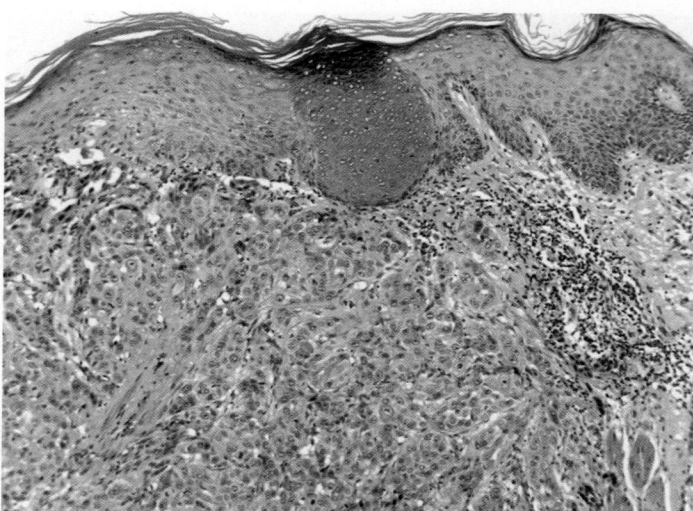

Figure 29-74 Metastatic squamous cell. A nodule of squamous cell carcinoma infiltrates the dermis beneath an epidermis devoid of dysplasia. This tumor was metastatic from a bronchial primary.

Metastatic SCC, for example, from another skin primary or from a mucous membrane or visceral primary, usually shows a greater degree of cytologic atypia, may be located deeper in the dermis or subcutis, and lacks an overlying *in situ* component (Fig. 29-74).

For discussions of differentiation of SCC from pseudocarcinomatous hyperplasia, see page 988; from keratoacanthoma, see page 1002; and from BCC, see page 989.

BASOSQUAMOUS CARCINOMA

Clinical Summary. The term *basosquamous carcinoma* is a confusing one (187). From the name alone, it is difficult to know whether this is a BCC with squamous differentiation, an SCC showing BCC, or something in between. There is a case for dispensing with the designation completely because a malignant squamous component is present, because examples of metastasis have been reported, and because reviews of SCCs have found areas of basal cell differentiation between 2% and 5% of cases. These tumors should be managed as an SCC, possibly using Mohs surgery to ensure clear excision margins (8,187–190).

Histopathology. The term *basosquamous carcinoma*, if it has any place in diagnosis at all, should be reserved for that small proportion of SCCs that show areas of basal cell differentiation in the upper dermal portion, often extending into the overlying epidermis. Ber EP4 has been advocated as an aid to differential diagnosis, being negative in pure SCC and showing strong cytoplasmic positivity in pure BCCs (see Fig. 29-78) (191,192). In basosquamous carcinoma, the basaloid component is highlighted by Ber EP4, but rather than strong cytoplasmic positivity, it typically shows strong membrane staining and weaker cytoplasmic positivity (Fig. 29-75) (192). Metatypical BCC—characterized by squamous differentiation in the advancing, invasive deep margin of the tumor—has a distinct appearance but may behave aggressively; so, it too should probably be considered to be a variant of SCC from the point of view of clinical management (see Fig. 29-105).

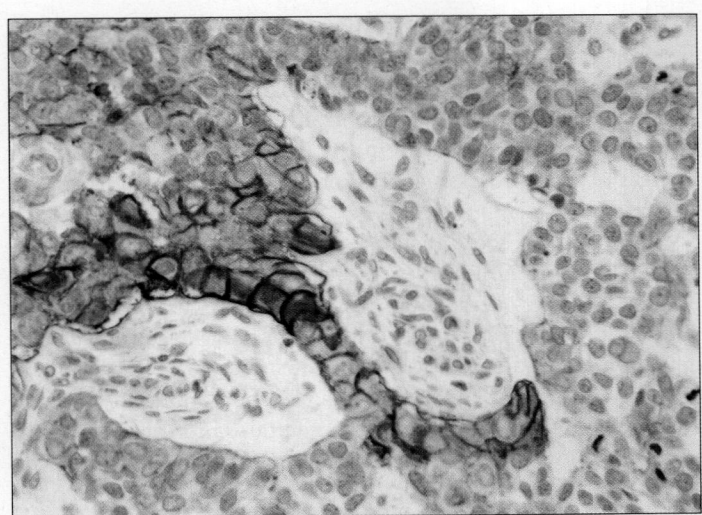

Figure 29-75 Basosquamous carcinoma. Ber-EP4 shows strong membrane positivity and weaker cytoplasmic positivity compared with the strong cytoplasmic positivity typical of basal cell carcinoma.

ACANTHOLYTIC (ADENOID) SQUAMOUS CELL CARCINOMA

Clinical Summary. As a result of dyskeratosis and subsequent acantholysis, SCCs occasionally show what may appear to be tubular and alveolar formations on histologic examination. Such lesions have been termed *adenoid* or *pseudoglandular* SCCs, but they are better termed *acantholytic*. Clinically, they are found almost exclusively in sun-damaged skin of elderly patients, especially on the face and ears (193).

On sun-exposed skin, acantholytic SCCs may arise as such or may develop from an actinic keratosis. In most instances, they do not differ in clinical appearance from the usual type of SCC and, thus, commonly show a central ulceration surrounded by a raised, indurated border. Occasionally, they greatly resemble a keratoacanthoma in clinical appearance. The incidence of metastases varies. In one series, it was only 2%, but in another series, 14% of the patients had fatal metastases, with tumor size greater than 15 mm correlating with the risk of an adverse outcome (172). A report from Queensland recorded no deaths, low perineural invasion, and low recurrence rates, suggesting that acantholytic SCC is a low-risk tumor (193).

Histopathology. The adenoid changes may be seen in only a portion of an SCC or throughout the lesion. Not infrequently, an actinic keratosis of the acantholytic type is seen overlying the lesion. There are tubular and alveolar lumina lined with one or several layers of epithelium (Figs. 29-59 and 29-60). In areas in which the lumina are lined with a single layer of epithelium, the epithelial cells resemble glandular cells; but in areas with several layers of epithelium, squamous and partially keratinized cells usually form the inner layers. The lumina are filled with desquamated acantholytic cells, many of which are partially or fully keratinized. In some cases, the eccrine ducts at the periphery of these tumors show signs of dilatation and proliferation. These ductal changes probably are induced by the surrounding inflammatory infiltrate.

Pathogenesis. These tumors represent SCCs of lobular growth in which there is considerable dyskeratosis with individual cell keratinization, resulting in acantholysis in the center of the lobular formations. This process is analogous to the suprabasal clefts seen in some

actinic keratoses (194). Acantholytic SCCs differ from sweat gland carcinomas (see Chapter 30), in which the single row of cuboidal cells lining the lumina consists of true glandular cells (195,196). In some instances, the latter tumors may be highly malignant.

MUCIN-PRODUCING SQUAMOUS CELL CARCINOMA

Clinical Summary. This rare variant of SCC has been reported only rarely under different designations, such as mucoepidermoid carcinoma and adenosquamous carcinoma of the skin. The latter designation may lead to confusion with adenoid SCC. It is probably a slow-growing neoplasm that should be differentiated from metastatic mucoepidermoid carcinoma (197–199).

Histopathology. A carcinoma located in the dermis with variable proportions of squamous differentiation and PAS-positive goblet cells may be seen. Occasionally, true glandular lumina are present. Some of the lumina resemble distorted eccrine ducts and stain positively for carcinoembryonic antigen. Immunohistochemistry shows positivity for cytokeratins (AE1AE3, 7, and 34βE12), epithelial membrane antigen (EMA), and p63, whereas cytokeratins 18 and 20 and gross cystic disease fluid protein (GCDFP15) are negative. The p63 positivity may help to differentiate primary and metastatic mucoepidermoid carcinoma in the skin (198).

Principles of Management of Squamous Cell Carcinoma

Multiple patient- and lesion-specific factors have to be taken into consideration in choosing a treatment modality for SCC. The goal of treatment is complete removal of the carcinoma. Surgical excision is the standard treatment for the majority of cSCCs. It allows full histologic examination of the tumor and the surgical margins (normal-appearing tissue around the tumor) (179). Mohs micrographic surgery is often superior to standard surgical excision because it provides higher cure and lower recurrence rates; it is especially recommended for recurrent and aggressive SCCs (200) and in problematical locations. There are some data on the successful use of curettage and cautery for SCCIS and small well-defined SCCs but not with larger tumors (201,202). Radiotherapy is used as an adjuvant treatment to surgical excision in aggressive or high-risk SCC. cSCC of the head and neck is associated with higher metastatic rate to parotid glands and cervical lymph nodes, and this scenario is associated with poor prognosis. Treatment with surgical excision, lymph node neck dissection, and radiation therapy is often used in these circumstances. Oral retinoids have been used as prophylaxis therapy to prevent the development of SCCs and other nonmelanoma skin cancers in high-risk patients such as transplant patients (203). Pembrolizumab as monotherapy for locally advanced cSCC that cannot be cured by surgery or radiotherapy was the subject of the KEYNOTE-629 trial (204) and was given U.S. Food and Drug Administration (FDA) approval for this indication following the second interim analysis of the trial.

VERRUCOUS CARCINOMA

Clinical Summary. Verrucous carcinoma, first described in 1948 by Lauren V Ackerman (205,206), is a clinicopathologic concept of an exophytic, low-grade, slow-growing, locally aggressive, well-differentiated SCC with minimal metastatic potential (207,208).

The diagnosis of verrucous carcinoma requires an evaluation of the clinical and microscopic appearance and biologic behavior of the neoplasm. It is a slowly growing, at first exophytic, verrucous, and fungating tumor that may ultimately penetrate deep into the tissue, reaching bones in some cases (Fig. 29-76). However, it causes regional metastases only very late, if at all. Because of its high degree of histologic differentiation, it is often not recognized as a carcinoma for a long time. Three major forms of verrucous carcinoma are recognized and classified according to their anatomic location, all of them occurring in areas of maceration.

Verrucous carcinoma of the oral cavity, also called oral florid papillomatosis, shows white, cauliflower-like lesions that may involve large areas of the oral mucosa.

Verrucous carcinoma of the genitoanal region, also called giant condylomata acuminatum of Buschke and Loewenstein, most commonly occurs on the glans penis and foreskin of uncircumcised males, where it consists of papillomatous proliferations. Ultimately, it may penetrate into the urethra. It may also occur on the vulva in females and in the anal region (Chapter 25).

Plantar verrucous carcinoma—also called carcinoma cuniculatum (from the Latin *cuniculus* meaning "rabbit warren" because of the multiple sinuses and crypts found in this tumor)—at first shows a striking resemblance to an intractable plantar wart. As the exophytic mass grows, it shows a great tendency toward deep, penetrating growth, resulting in numerous deep crypts filled with horny material and pus. The tumor ultimately penetrates the plantar fascia and may even destroy metatarsal bones and invade the skin of the dorsum of the foot.

The occurrence of verrucous carcinoma has been described occasionally in many other areas, such as the face, back, and axilla (209), as well as in preexisting lesions, such as chronic ulcers and draining sinuses of hidradenitis suppurativa. It has also been described in association with oral lichen planus (210,211).

Histopathology. For the diagnosis of verrucous carcinoma, a large, deep biopsy is essential. The superficial portions generally resemble a verruca by showing hyperkeratosis, parakeratosis, and acanthosis. The keratinocytes appear well differentiated, stain lightly with eosin, and possess a small nucleus. The tumor

invades with broad strands that often contain keratin-filled cysts in their center. There are large, bulbous, downward proliferations that compress the collagen bundles and push them aside. Thus, the tumor has been said to invade by "bulldozing rather than stabbing." Even in the deep portions of the tumor, nuclear atypia, individual cell keratinization, and horn pearls are absent.

However, in some instances—particularly in the oral cavity and occasionally also in the genitoanal region and on the plantar surface—verrucous carcinoma may ultimately show sufficient nuclear atypicality and loss of polarity to indicate the development of a true SCC. In rare instances, the development of regional lymph node metastases has been observed in verrucous carcinoma of the mouth, the genitals, and the soles of the feet. Radiation therapy has led, in some instances of oral verrucous carcinoma, to anaplastic transformation and extensive metastases.

Pathogenesis. The exact pathogenesis of verrucous carcinoma is unclear. However, HPV infection, chronic inflammation, and tobacco chewing have been described as possible factors (212,213). Although a viral cause of verrucous carcinoma has been suspected for a long time, the demonstration of viral particles by electron microscopy has been possible in only a few instances of verrucous carcinoma. Virus-like particles were demonstrated in 1 case of plantar verrucous carcinoma presumed to be associated with a plantar wart, in the superficial epithelium of 5 of 13 cases of plantar verrucous carcinoma, and in 1 case of verrucous carcinoma of the vagina. DNA hybridization has succeeded in proving an association of HPV with verrucous carcinoma in some but not all cases. HPV-6, and less frequently HPV-11 and HPV-16, has been found in Buschke–Loewenstein tumors of the external genitals in both sexes (214).

Principles of Management: Early and complete excision of verrucous carcinoma is advocated (215). Surgical excision especially with Mohs micrographic surgery is the treatment of choice. Excision with conventional margins of healthy tissue may be sufficient in small well-demarcated verrucous carcinomas. However, the main advantage of Mohs micrographic surgery is that it allows examining the margins that may be histologically but not clinically involved in verrucous carcinoma (216,217). Radiation therapy is generally blind to the histologic margins and has a far inferior cure rate to surgical excision. Therefore, the use of radiotherapy for primary verrucous carcinoma should only be restricted to elderly patients who cannot tolerate surgery. Other treatments such as bleomycin, 5-fluorouracil, cisplatin, methotrexate, CO_2 laser, and PDT have all been used and reported as case studies or series in the treatment of verrucous carcinoma (218).

PSEUDOCARCINOMATOUS HYPERPLASIA

Clinical Summary. Pseudocarcinomatous hyperplasia, or *pseudoepitheliomatous hyperplasia*, as it is often called, represents a considerable downward proliferation of the epidermis into the dermis. Clinically and histologically, this downward proliferation may suggest an SCC. It occurs occasionally (a) in chronic proliferative inflammatory processes—such as bromoderma, blastomycosis, blastomycosis-like pyoderma (pyoderma vegetans), or hidradenitis suppurativa—and (b) at the edges of chronic ulcers, as seen in but not limited to the following

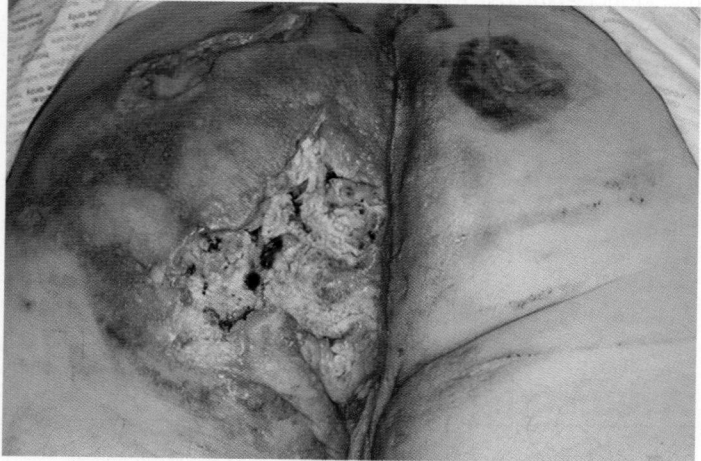

Figure 29-76 Verrucous carcinoma. There is extensive involvement mainly of the left buttock, with multiple exophytic, hyperkeratotic warty tumors.

conditions: after burns or in stasis dermatitis, pyoderma gangrenosum, BCC, lupus vulgaris, osteomyelitis, scrofuloderma, gumma, and granuloma inguinale. In addition, granular cell tumor is known to quite frequently evoke a pseudocarcinomatous hyperplasia.

Histopathology. Pseudocarcinomatous hyperplasia shows an epithelial hyperplasia that often closely resembles moderately- or well-differentiated SCC but on closer inspection is seen to involve adnexal epithelium, especially that of hair follicle infundibulum (219). Although SCCs may develop at the edges of chronic ulcers, it is likely that some cases that are regarded as such actually represent pseudocarcinomatous hyperplasia. Nevertheless, a lesion starting out as pseudocarcinomatous hyperplasia at the edge of an ulcer may eventually develop into an SCC and even metastasize.

The histologic picture of pseudocarcinomatous hyperplasia shows irregular invasion of the dermis by uneven, jagged, often sharply pointed epidermal cell masses and strands with horn pearl formation and, often, numerous mitotic figures (Figs. 29-77 and 29-78). These irregular proliferations of the epidermis may extend below the level of the sweat glands, where they appear in sections as isolated islands of the epidermal tissue. However, the squamous cells are usually well differentiated, and atypicalities—such as individual cell keratinization and nuclear hyperplasia and hyperchromasia—are minimal or absent. Furthermore, one often sees the invasion of the epithelial proliferations by leukocytes and disintegration of some of the epidermal cells in pseudocarcinomatous hyperplasia, findings that are usually absent in SCC. The dermis that is infiltrated by the epithelial strands in this condition is usually abnormal—inflamed and often necrotic, perhaps stimulating this unusual, atypical but reactive proliferation. It would be unusual to see an invasion of native, normal tissue. Nevertheless, even when all of these criteria are taken into account, it may still be difficult to differentiate SCC from pseudocarcinomatous hyperplasia by the study of just one histologic section. Multiple biopsies, sometimes over time, and detailed clinical data (including therapeutic responsiveness or resistance) may be necessary for differentiation.

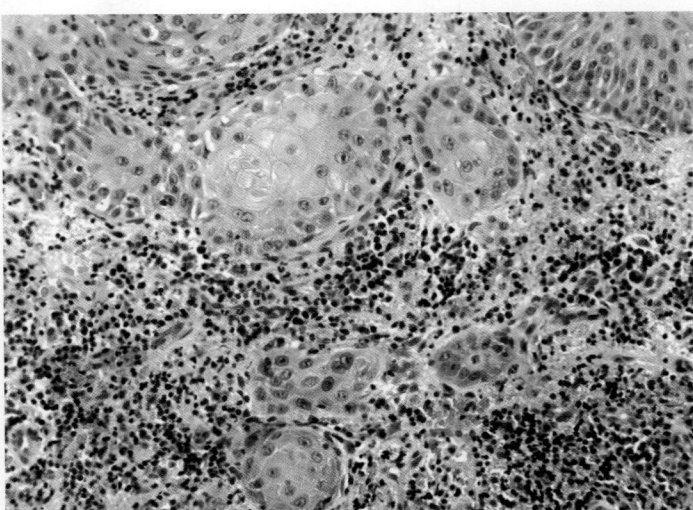

Figure 29-78 Pseudocarcinomatous hyperplasia. This curetting specimen shows a proliferative squamous lesion without substantial atypia and mimicking an invasive lesion. In this one field, the distinction would be almost impossible to make.

In every section in which a diagnosis of SCC is contemplated, it is worthwhile to study the inflammatory infiltrate for the possible presence of granulomas—as seen in tuberculosis and deep mycoses—or of intraepidermal abscesses—as seen in bromoderma, or even cutaneous T-cell lymphoma (220). If such evidence is found, one may be dealing with pseudocarcinomatous hyperplasia rather than SCC. In mucous membranes, and especially in the tongue, pseudoepitheliomatous hyperplasia of considerable degree and strongly simulating SCC may be seen above a granular cell tumor.

Differential Diagnosis. Differentiation of pseudocarcinomatous hyperplasia from verrucous carcinoma rarely causes difficulties because in verrucous carcinoma, there is verrucous upward proliferation and downward proliferation. In addition, verrucous carcinoma shows more pronounced keratinization in the downward extensions, which appear bulbous rather than sharply pointed.

BASAL CELL CARCINOMA

Clinical Summary. BCCs are nonmelanocytic epithelial tumors that are the most common type of skin cancer, and the majority have an excellent prognosis. If left untreated, they can grow, causing local destruction. BCCs are seen almost exclusively on hair-bearing skin, especially on the face. Except in the nevoid BCC syndrome (see p. 992), they rarely occur on the palms or on the soles (221,222).

BCCs usually occur as single lesions, although the occurrence of several lesions—either simultaneously or subsequently—is not infrequent. About 40% of patients who have had a BCC will have one or more BCCs within 10 years. BCCs generally occur in adults, although they may be seen in children also. However, there are three rare forms of BCC with early onset. In the linear, unilateral basal cell nevus, all lesions are present at birth. In the nevoid basal cell syndrome and the Bazex syndrome, some patients manifest lesions before puberty.

Predisposing Factors. Although BCCs may arise without apparent reason, there are several predisposing factors. The most

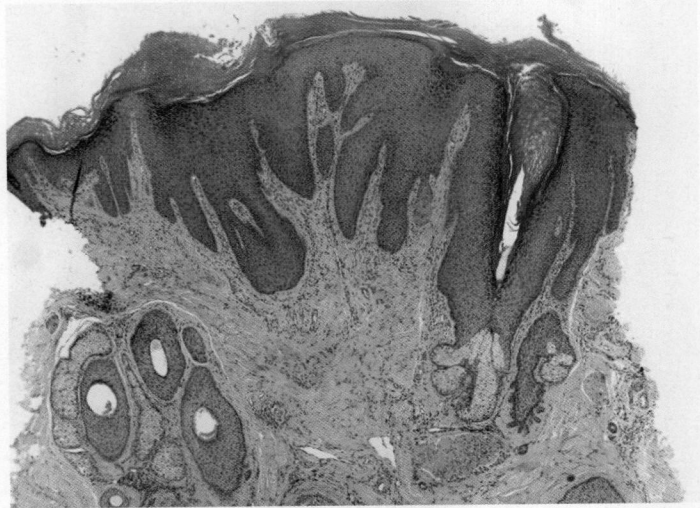

Figure 29-77 Lichen simplex chronicus. This punch biopsy specimen shows how epidermal hyperplasia can mainly involve hair follicles to produce a proliferative lesion mimicking an invasive process.

common is a light skin color in association with prolonged exposure to strong sunlight (223). The predisposing effect of sun exposure is particularly evident in patients with xeroderma pigmentosum, in whom both BCC and SCC are common (see Chapter 6). That prolonged sun exposure alone does not suffice to produce BCCs is suggested by their great rarity on the dorsa of hands and fingers. Additional factors that predispose a person to develop both BCC and SCC are large or numerous doses of x-rays and, less commonly, burn scars and other scars. In contrast, most carcinomas of the skin caused by the prolonged intake of inorganic arsenic are SCCs, which often, like Bowen disease, are located *in situ*. Occasionally, however, BCCs—particularly superficial BCCs—can result (151) (see the section on Arsenical Keratosis and Carcinoma).

Occurrence of Metastases. As a rule, BCCs do not metastasize. However, there are exceptions. The incidence of metastasis ranges from 0.01% in pathologic specimens to 0.028% in dermatologic patients (224) to 0.1% in patients from surgical centers (225). A review published in 1984 described 175 cases with histologically proven metastases (226).

The typical case history of a metastatic BCC is that of a large, ulcerated, locally invasive and destructive primary lesion that has recurred despite repeated surgical procedures or radiotherapy (227–229). However, massive size, ulceration, and history of multiple recurrences are not absolute prerequisites for metastasis (230). Most observers have found no specific histologic type of BCC that is more capable of metastasizing than others (231–233). In addition, as a rule, no evidence exists that the hosts' immunologic defenses are severely compromised (226). However, some authors assert that the metatypical or basosquamous type of BCC is the most likely to metastasize (234). This view would suggest that these variants should be better regarded as variants of SCC from the point of view of clinical management.

In contrast to metastatic SCC of the skin, which shows lymphogenic metastases to lymph nodes in 80% to 90% of cases, in metastatic BCC, hematogenic and lymphogenic spread show about an even distribution (226). Although about 50% of the patients with metastatic BCC have metastases to lymph nodes as their first site of spread, lungs and bones are also frequently the first sites of involvement. Metastases to the liver, other viscera, and the skin or subcutaneous tissues have occurred. However, these areas were usually involved only when at least one of the three major sites of metastasis was also affected (235). The average survival time after metastasis to the lungs, bones, or internal organs is about 10 months (236).

Pathogenesis. Although the exact mechanism of BCC formation is not understood, it is thought to be related to the pilosebaceous unit as BCCs usually occur on hair-bearing skin. The tumors normally arise from the epidermis and occasionally from the outer root sheath of a hair follicle. Notably, the gene most altered in BCC is the patched (PTCH) gene. Two-thirds of BCCs show loss of heterozygosity and/or truncating mutations in the PTCH gene. The Patched–Hedgehog intracellular signaling pathway plays a role in sporadic BCC development and also in the autosomal dominant nevoid BCC syndrome. During fetal development, the Patched–Hedgehog pathway influences the differentiation of various tissues. After embryogenesis, its function is the regulation of cell growth and differentiation. Loss of inhibition of this pathway is associated with malignancy

including BCC development (237,238). The Hedgehog gene encodes an extracellular protein that binds to a cell membrane receptor complex to start a cascade of cellular events leading to cell proliferation. There are three known human analogs. Sonic Hedgehog (SHH) protein is the most relevant to BCC. PTCH protein is the ligand-binding component of the Hedgehog receptor complex in the cell membrane. The third protein is Smoothened (SMO), which is responsible for transducing Hedgehog signaling to downstream genes, and this is mutated in around 20% of BCCs. The second most common mutation in BCCs are point mutations in the p53 tumor suppressor gene, where the vast majority of these mutations are missense mutations that carry a UV signature (239,240).

Vismodegib is an oral biologic treatment that has been licensed for use in metastatic BCC. It is designed to selectively inhibit abnormal signaling in the Hedgehog pathway. Vismodegib binds to and inhibits SMO (241,242). Metastatic tumors may also be sensitive to PD-1 blockade (243).

Clinical Appearance. Clinicopathologic subtypes of BCC include (a) superficial BCC, (b) nodular BCC, (c) micronodular BCC, (d) infiltrating BCC, (e) fibroepithelioma, and (f) infundibulocystic BCC. In addition, there are three clinical syndromes in which BCCs play an important part. They are (a) the nevoid BCC syndrome, (b) the linear unilateral basal cell nevus, and (c) the Bazex syndrome, showing follicular atrophoderma with multiple BCCs.

Superficial BCC consists of one or several erythematous, scaling, only slightly infiltrated patches that slowly increase in size by peripheral extension. The patches are often surrounded, at least in part, by a fine, threadlike, pearly border (Fig. 29-79). The patches usually show small areas of superficial ulceration and crusting. In addition, their center may show smooth, atrophic scarring. In contrast to the first three types of BCC, which are commonly situated on the face, superficial BCC occurs predominantly on the trunk.

Nodular BCC begins as a small, waxy nodule that often shows a few small telangiectatic vessels on its surface (Fig. 29-80). The nodule usually increases slowly in size and often undergoes central ulceration. A typical lesion then consists

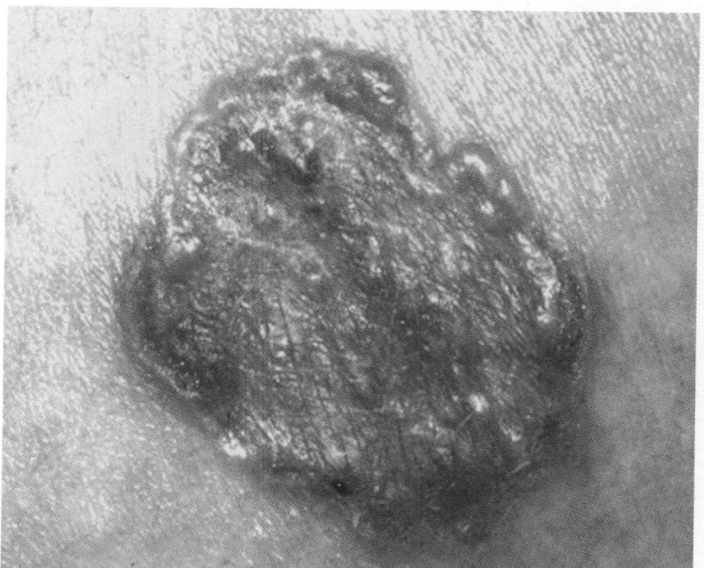

Figure 29-79 Superficial basal cell carcinoma. This tumor shows a well-demarcated edge.

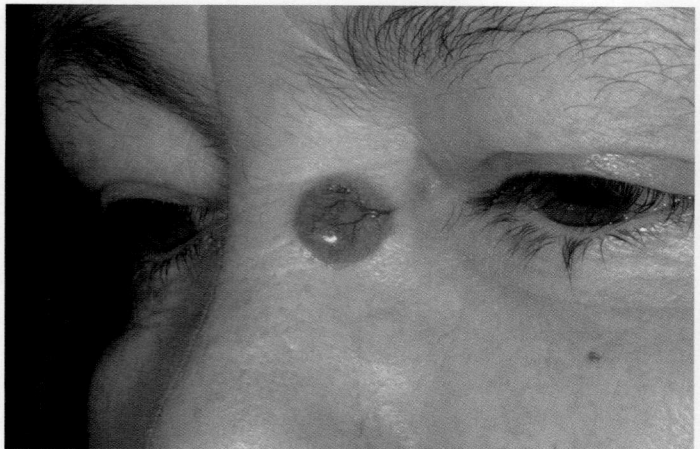

Figure 29-80 Nodular basal cell carcinoma. The lesion is well defined.

of a slowly enlarging ulcer surrounded by a pearly, rolled border. This represents the so-called rodent ulcer (Fig. 29-81).

Micronodular BCC is diagnosed histologically and may have a diffusely infiltrative growth pattern that extends for some distance beyond the clinically apparent margins of the tumor. This subtype is one of the "infiltrating" patterns of BCC that have been associated with a higher rate of local recurrence than other subtypes. The use of Mohs micrographic surgery has been advocated to ensure complete excision of the infiltrating component (Figs. 29-82 and 29-83).

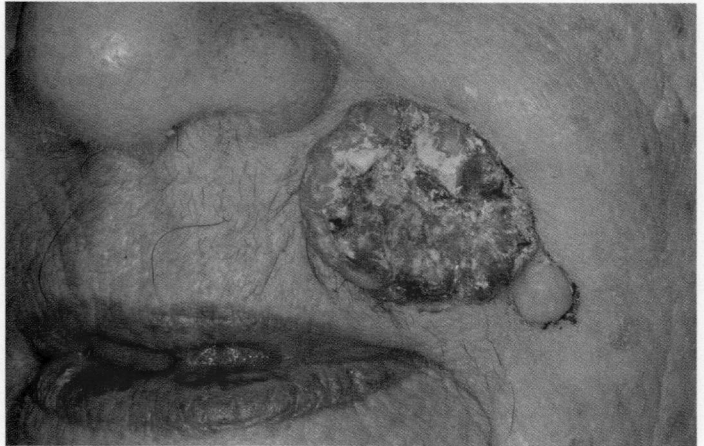

Figure 29-81 Basal cell carcinoma. This example has been neglected, producing a "rodent ulcer."

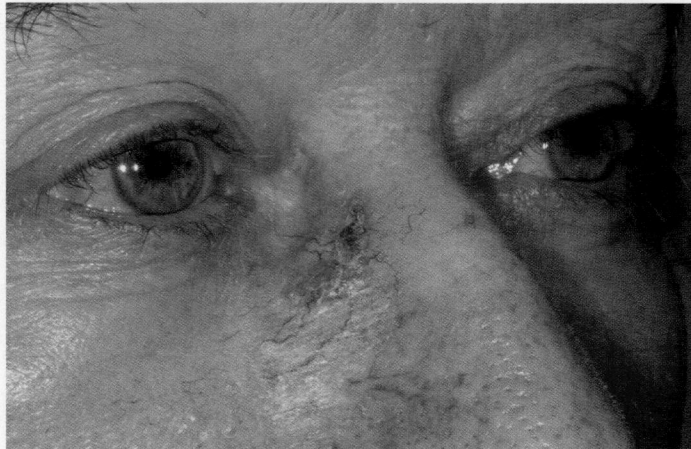

Figure 29-82 Micronodular basal cell carcinoma. The tumor has poorly defined clinical margins. An indication for Mohs micrographic surgery.

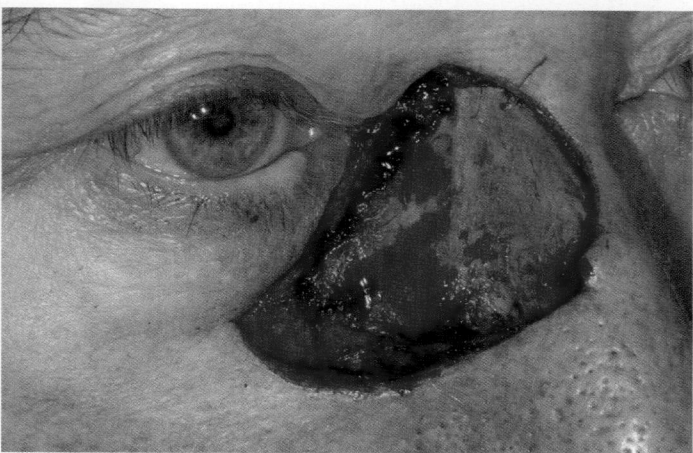

Figure 29-83 Micronodular basal cell carcinoma. An extensive resection was required, using Mohs micrographic surgery, to achieve clear surgical margins.

Most rodent ulcers possess a limited potential for growth; however, occasionally they can be infiltrative and aggressive and then can reach considerable size and invade deeply. On the face, they may destroy the eyes and nose (244), or they may penetrate the skull and invade the dura mater (245). Death may then ensue. (Such destructive BCCs are also seen occasionally in the nevoid BCC syndrome; see the following text.)

Pigmented BCC differs from the nodular type only by the brown pigmentation of the lesion.

Morphea-like or fibrosing BCC is another infiltrating subtype that manifests as a solitary, flat, or slightly depressed, indurated, yellowish plaque. The surface is smooth and shiny. The border is often ill-defined (Fig. 29-84). The overlying skin remains intact for a long time before ulceration finally occurs. The term arises from a clinical resemblance to localized scleroderma or morphea. The tumors, despite being deeply infiltrative, may be mistaken clinically for a lesion of morphea or for a scar.

Fibroepithelioma consists usually of only one but occasionally of several raised, moderately firm, slightly

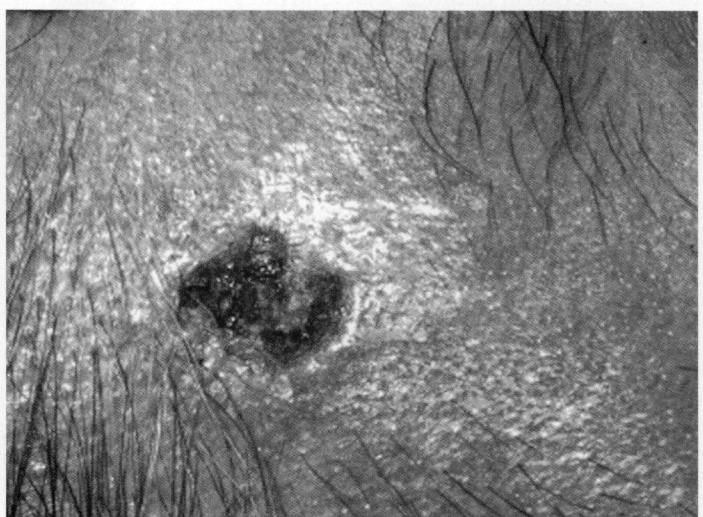

Figure 29-84 Basal cell carcinoma, morpheic. The central part of the tumor is clearly seen, but the margins are not well defined.

pedunculated nodules covered by smooth, slightly reddened skin. Clinically, they resemble fibromas. The most common location is the back.

The *nevoid BCC syndrome*, also known as Gorlin syndrome and Gorlin–Goltz syndrome, is an autosomal dominant condition caused by a mutation in the PTCH gene located on chromosome arm 9q (237,238). This condition has complete penetrance and variable expressivity, hence the variable phenotype. About one-third of cases are caused by a new mutation. The syndrome is a multisystem condition that affects the skin, bone, central nervous system, endocrine system, and genitourinary system. Clinically, small nodules appear between puberty and 35 years of age, and there may be hundreds or thousands of them (246). During the "nevoid" stage, the nodules slowly increase in number and size. They are haphazardly distributed over the face and body. During adulthood, many of the BCCs undergo ulceration, and later in life, the disease sometimes enters a "neoplastic" stage in which some of the BCCs, especially of the face, become invasive, destructive, and mutilating. Occasionally, even death occurs as a result of the invasion of an orbit and of the brain (247–249). There may also be metastases to the lung (247).

Half of the adult patients with the nevoid BCC syndrome show numerous palmar and plantar pits 1 to 3 mm in diameter. These pits usually develop during the second decade of life and represent formes frustes of BCC (see Histopathology) (250). In addition, epidermal cysts are quite common (251).

Most patients show multiple skeletal and central nervous system anomalies (248), among which are odontogenic keratocysts of the jaws, anomalies of the ribs, scoliosis, mental retardation, and calcification of the falx cerebri. In several reported cases, there were also cerebellar medulloblastomas (252) or fibrosarcomas of a mandible or maxilla (253). In the jaw cysts, an ameloblastoma may arise (254).

Multiple hereditary infundibulocystic BCCs have been described as a genodermatosis different from the nevoid BCC syndrome. The patients had multiple papular lesions, mostly located on the face, and none had palmar pits or jaw cysts (255).

The *linear unilateral basal cell nevus*, first described in 1985, is very rare and is defined by an extensive unilateral linear or zosteriform eruption that tends to grow preferentially in one direction with straight borders and with its length much greater than its width (3:1), usually present since birth, consisting of closely set nodules of BCC (256). They may be interspersed with comedones (257,258) and striae-like areas of atrophy (259). The lesions do not increase in size with aging of the patient. The majority of cases occur on the lower eyelid and the cheek, and the second most common site is the neck followed by the trunk and genital folds.

The *Bazex syndrome*, first described in 1966 (260), is dominantly inherited and shows as its main features (a) follicular atrophoderma characterized by widened follicular openings like "ice-pick marks" mainly on the extremities and (b) multiple, small BCCs on the face, usually arising first in adolescence or early adulthood (261), but occasionally in late childhood (262). In addition, there may be localized anhidrosis or generalized hypohidrosis, as well as congenital hypotrichosis on the scalp and elsewhere (262).

Histopathology. BCCs tend to share the common features of a predominant basal cell type, peripheral palisading of lesional cell nuclei, a specialized stroma, and clefting artifact between the epithelium and the stroma. In addition, there are variable degrees of cytologic atypia and mitotic activity; some degree of these latter changes is virtually always present (Figs. 29-85 to 29-107). In nodular BCC, nodular masses of basaloid cells are formed that extend into the dermis in relation to a delicate, specialized tumor stroma (Figs. 29-80 to 29-82). Cystic spaces may form as a result of tumor necrosis or cellular dyshesion. As a rule, the nuclei in BCCs have a rather uniform appearance. They usually show no pronounced variation in size or intensity of staining and no abnormal mitoses, even in the rare instances of BCC with metastases. In the exceptional cases of BCC in which one finds—interspersed among the usual cells of BCC—cells with large hyperchromatic nuclei, multiple nuclei, and bizarre "starburst" mitoses, the clinical course is not different from that of the usual BCC (49,251).

The connective tissue stroma proliferates with the tumor and is arranged in parallel bundles around the tumor masses so that a mutual relationship seems to exist between the parenchyma of the tumor and its stroma (263,264). The stroma adjacent to the tumor masses often shows numerous young

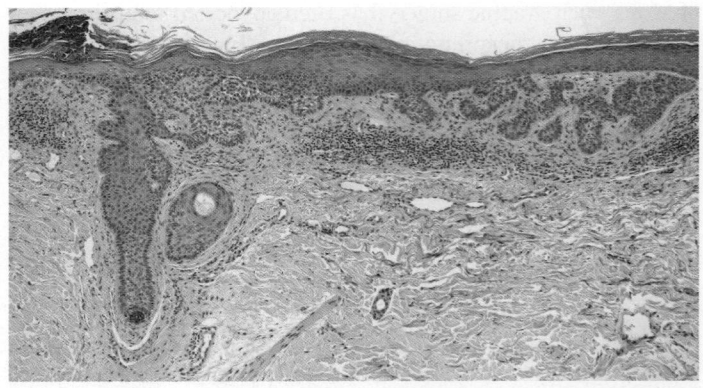

Figure 29-85 Superficial basal cell carcinoma. The tumor shows buds and irregular proliferations of tumor tissue attached to the undersurface of the epidermis.

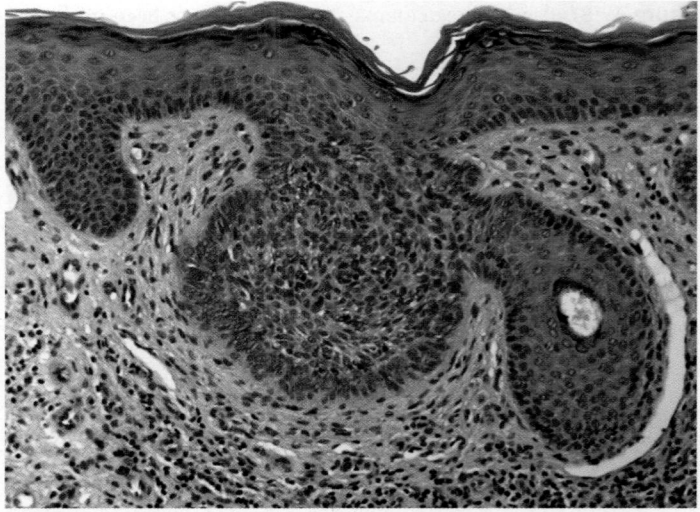

Figure 29-86 Superficial basal cell carcinoma. High magnification. The tumor shows a bud of cells in the bulge zone of a hair follicle similar to the primary epithelial germ buds in embryonal skin. A cleft is also present at the interface with the dermis.

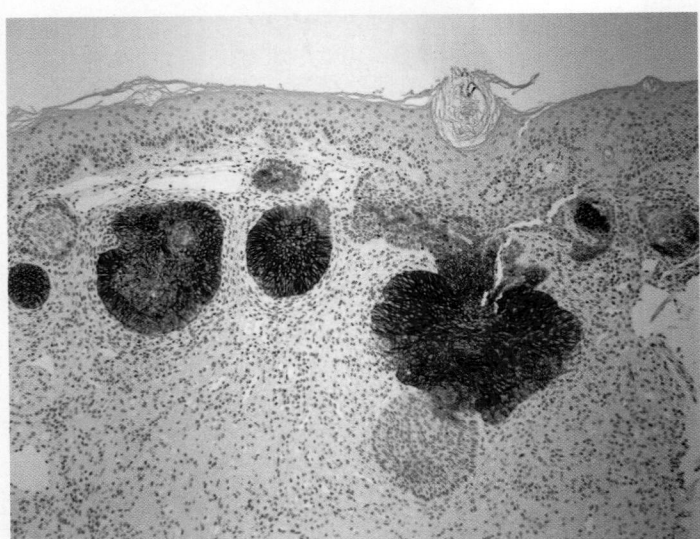

Figure 29-87 Superficial basal cell carcinoma. Ber EP4 staining highlights the tumor with normal epidermal structures unstained. The tumor shows strong cytoplasmic positivity in contrast to the membrane positivity typical of basosquamous carcinoma.

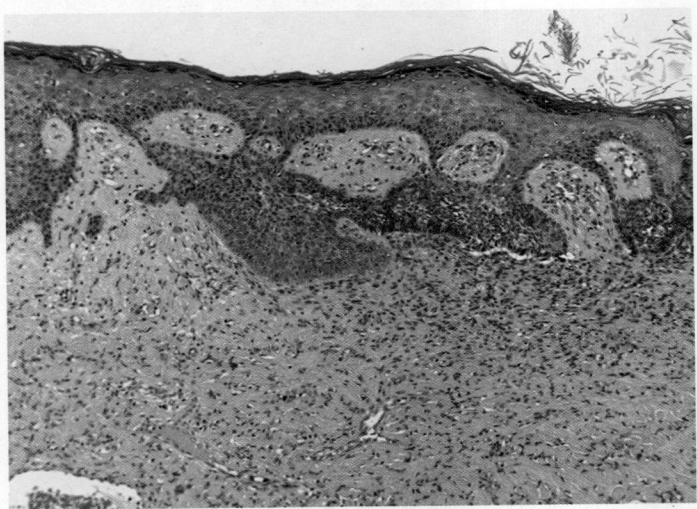

Figure 29-88 Dermatofibroma. There is a basal proliferation of basaloid cells mimicking the appearances of a superficial basal cell carcinoma.

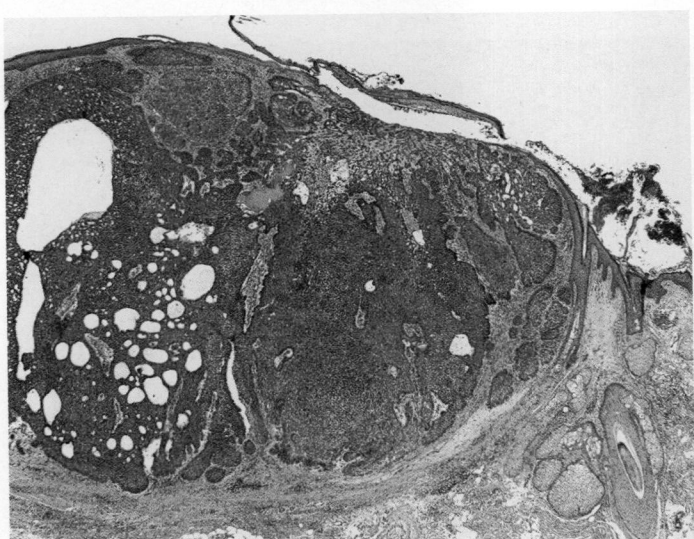

Figure 29-89 Basal cell carcinoma, nodular type. This excision specimen shows a nodular tumor with peripheral palisading, and a generally circumscribed border.

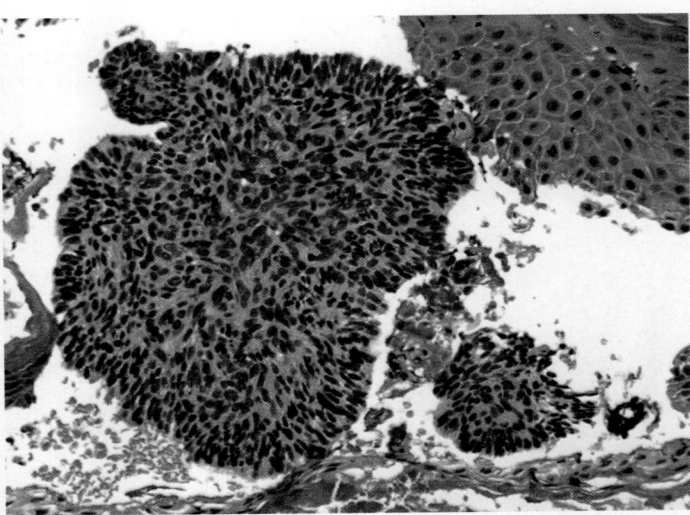

Figure 29-90 Basal cell carcinoma, nodular type. In this curetting specimen, nests of cells from a nodular basal cell carcinoma show peripheral palisading.

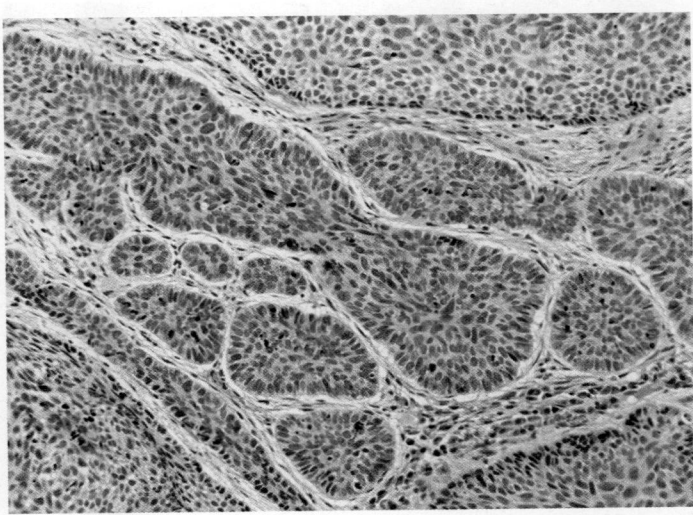

Figure 29-91 Nodular basal cell carcinoma. Medium magnification. The islands of tumor cells show peripheral palisading as well as mitotic and apoptotic figures.

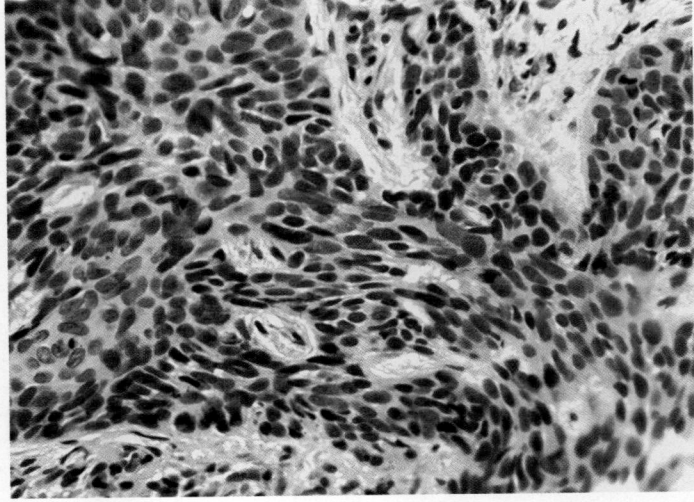

Figure 29-92 Basal cell carcinoma, solid type. High magnification. The basaloid tumor cells flow through the dermis with a variable degree of peripheral palisading.

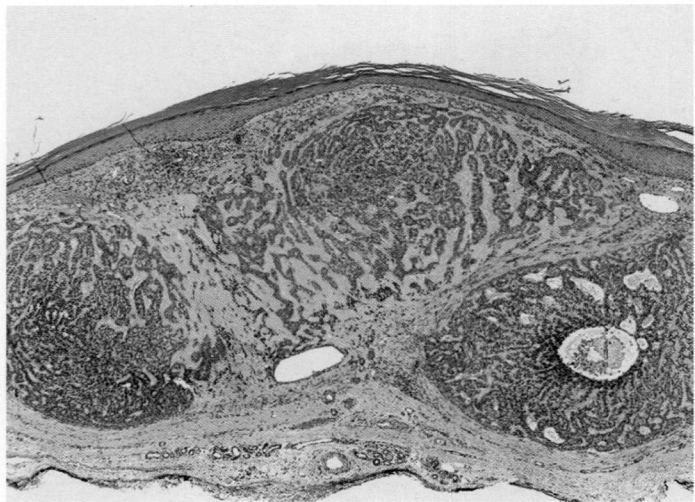

Figure 29-93 Adenoid basal cell carcinoma. Scanning magnification. The strands of epithelial cells form nodules with a lacelike pattern of cells within the nodules.

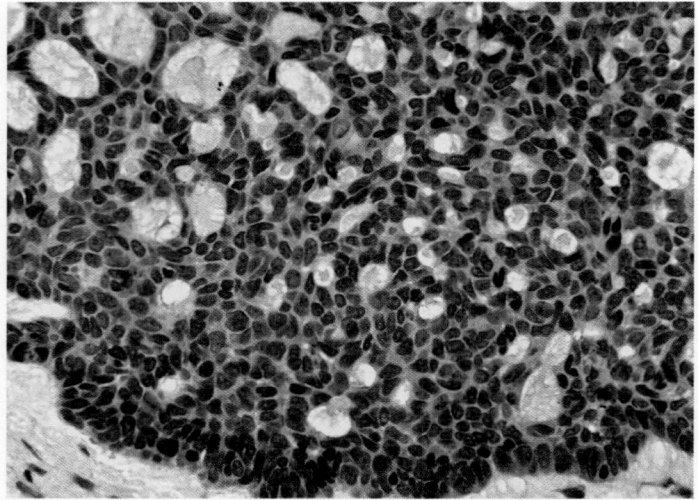

Figure 29-94 Adenoid basal cell carcinoma. Medium magnification. The strands of epithelial cells present a lacelike pattern. The stroma has a mucoid appearance.

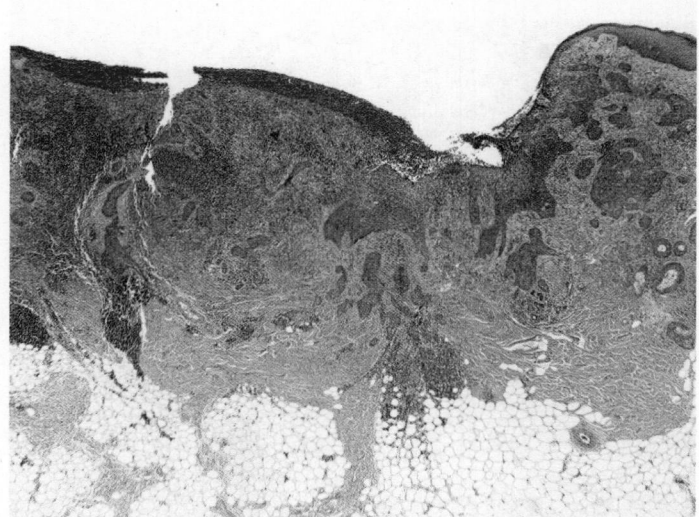

Figure 29-95 Micronodular basal cell carcinoma. The tumor is relatively symmetrical and circumscribed, but with a more infiltrative element at its base.

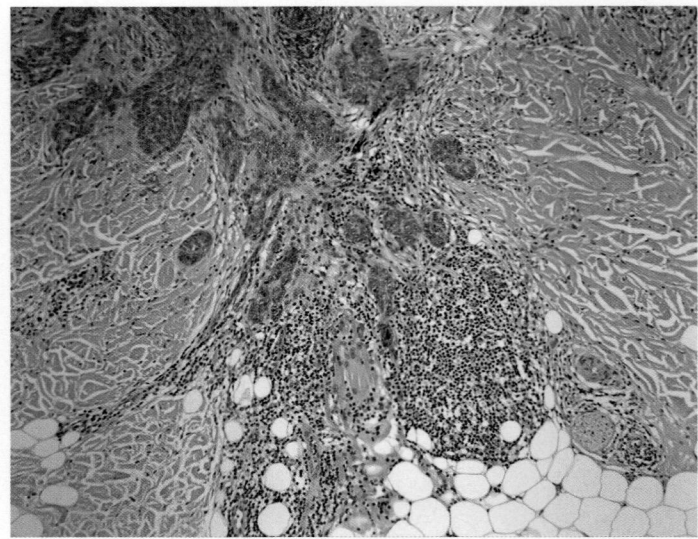

Figure 29-96 Micronodular basal cell carcinoma. Medium magnification. The infiltrative element at the base of the tumor extends through the full thickness of the dermis to the subcutis.

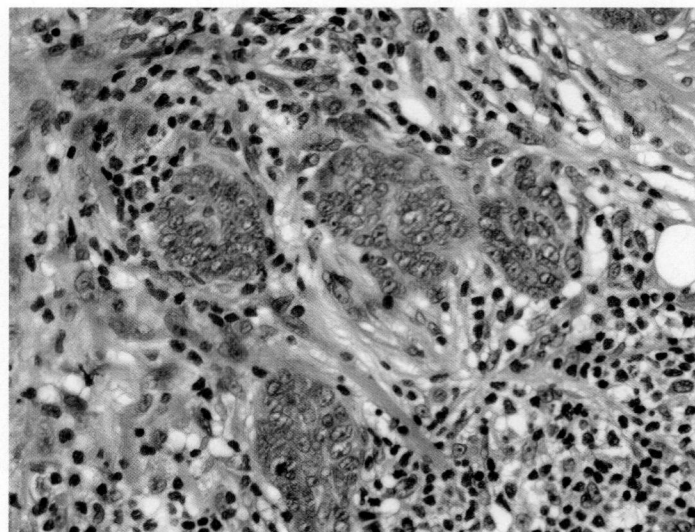

Figure 29-97 Micronodular basal cell carcinoma. High magnification. Micronodules of tumor infiltrate the deep dermis.

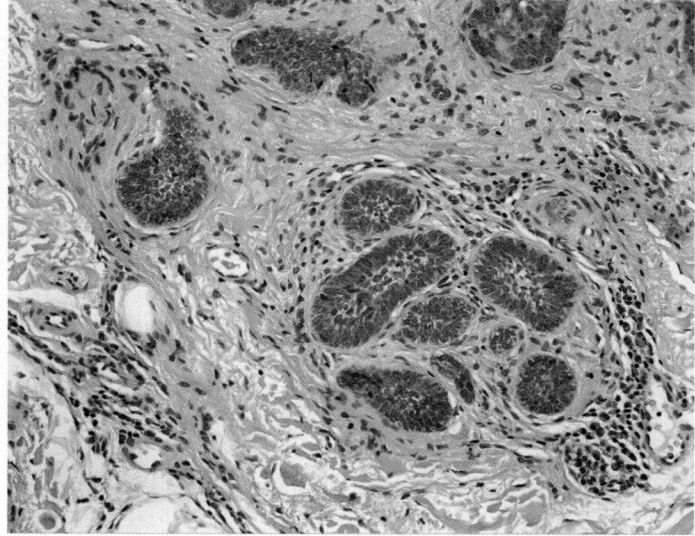

Figure 29-98 Micronodular basal cell carcinoma. High magnification. A less inflamed example showing micronodules of invasive basal cell carcinoma.

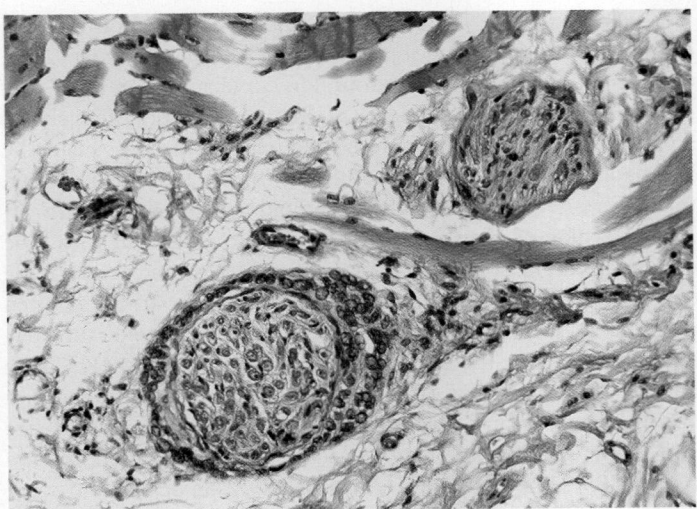

Figure 29-99 Micronodular basal cell carcinoma. High magnification. Tumor cells show perineural invasion close to the excision margin.

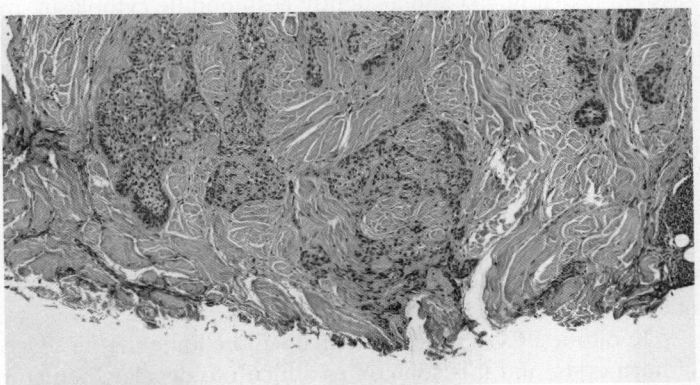

Figure 29-100 Micronodular basal cell carcinoma. Medium magnification. Invasive tumor extends to the surgical margin.

fibroblasts; in addition, it may appear mucinous (265,266). Frequently, there are areas of retraction of the stroma from tumor islands, resulting in peritumoral lacunae (Fig. 29-86). These lacunae once were regarded as a fixation artifact, but peritumoral lacunae can also be observed on cryostat sections. Immunostaining with antibodies to laminin, type IV collagen, and bullous pemphigoid has revealed the presence of laminin and type IV collagen on the stromal side of the lacunae, but bullous pemphigoid antigen is absent at the site of lacunae (267). Even though bullous pemphigoid antigen is diminished in other areas of BCC (268), it is likely that a loss of this antigen contributes to the formation of peritumoral lacunae (267). Because these lacunae are quite typical for some BCCs, their presence aids in the differentiation of BCC from other tumors, such as SCC. In addition, stromal or intratumor deposits of amyloid are found quite frequently (see Pathogenesis) (269). A mild inflammatory infiltrate is often seen in the stroma of nonulcerated BCCs but may be entirely lacking. If ulceration occurs, there usually is a rather pronounced inflammatory reaction.

From a histologic point of view, BCCs can be divided into two groups: undifferentiated and differentiated. Those of the latter group show a slight degree of differentiation toward the cutaneous appendages of hair, sebaceous glands, apocrine glands, or eccrine glands. A sharp dividing line between the two groups cannot be drawn because many undifferentiated BCCs show differentiation in some areas, and most differentiated BCCs show areas lacking differentiation. By correlating the clinical classification with the histologic classification, it can be stated that nodular BCC—as well as the lesions of the nevoid BCC syndrome, the linear unilateral basal cell nevus, and the Bazex syndrome—may show differentiation or no differentiation, but the other four types of BCC—pigmented BCC, fibrosing BCC, superficial BCC, and fibroepithelioma—usually show little or no differentiation (Figs. 29-103 and 29-104).

From a clinical point of view, it is probably more relevant to classify BCCs into those with a low risk of recurrence (nodular, nodulocystic, and fibroepithelioma of Pinkus) and those with a high risk of local recurrence (superficial, micronodular, infiltrative, morpheic, and metatypical). Except for superficial BCC, in which recurrence is common but usually remains superficial, these are all infiltrating patterns of BCC that may extend deep into the dermis and beyond. Of these, the *micronodular BCC* probably carries as high a risk of local recurrence as the others in the high-risk group (Figs. 29-95 to 29-102). They vary between symmetric, circumscribed examples and others that are asymmetric and infiltrate between collagen bundles. The risk of local recurrence may be related to the presence of perineural invasion (which may occur in other types of BCC as well; Fig. 29-99) and to the focal nature, owing to which the tumor may infiltrate deeply into the dermis to involve the excision margin (Fig. 29-100). Micronodular BCC is rarely seen without other forms of BCC differentiation. More typically, micronodular differentiation is seen toward the base of a tumor. When a BCC infiltrates deeply into the dermis or reaches the subcutis, micronodular differentiation may frequently be present in the deeper compartment of the tumor. There is an overlap of appearances between morpheic and micronodular BCCs. In deciding on the subtype with which one is dealing, the element representing more than 50% of the whole tumor should take precedence; however, it is important to identify an infiltrating component when it is present.

BCCs showing differentiation toward hair structures (Fig. 29-94) are called *keratotic*; toward sebaceous glands, *BCCs with sebaceous differentiation*; and toward tubular glands, *adenoid* BCCs (Figs. 29-84 and 29-85). A *signet ring cell* variant has also been described (270). In many differentiated BCCs, differentiation is directed toward more than one of these cutaneous appendages. For example, areas of keratinization may be found in a tumor that also shows adenoid structures. No difference exists in the rate of growth between undifferentiated and differentiated BCCs.

Infundibulocystic BCC is a lesion with follicular differentiation that presents as a relatively well-circumscribed basaloid neoplasm comprised of buds and cords of neoplastic cells arranged in an anastomosing pattern, with scant stroma. Some of the cords of cells contain tiny infundibular cysts filled by keratinizing cells, sometimes with melanin pigment. These lesions need to be distinguished from trichoepithelioma, basaloid follicular hamartoma, and folliculocentric basaloid proliferation. The distinction from basaloid follicular hamartoma may be especially difficult and it may be that there is biologic as well as morphologic overlap between these two conditions (Fig. 29-101) (255).

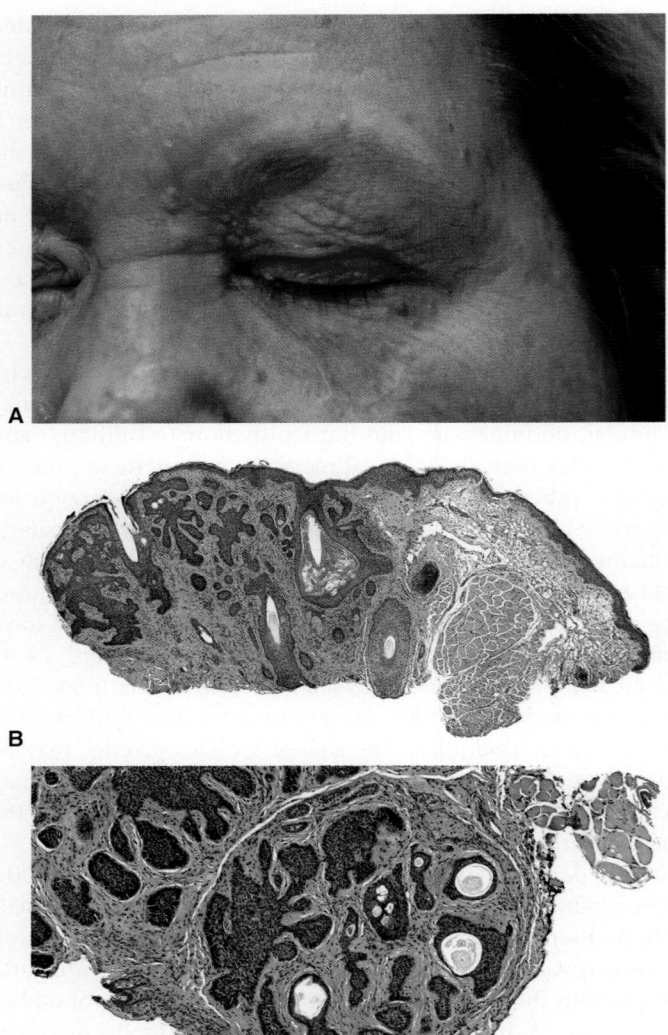

Figure 29-101 Infundibulocystic BCC. **A:** Multiple flesh-colored papules in a periorbital distribution and on the nose. **B, C:** Islands and anastomosing cords of basaloid cells are present in the dermis, with an epidermal connection. The surrounding stroma has increased dermal mucin. Some stromal retraction is observed. Follicular differentiation in the form of infundibular cysts is present within the tumor islands. (Images courtesy Emily Chu, MD.)

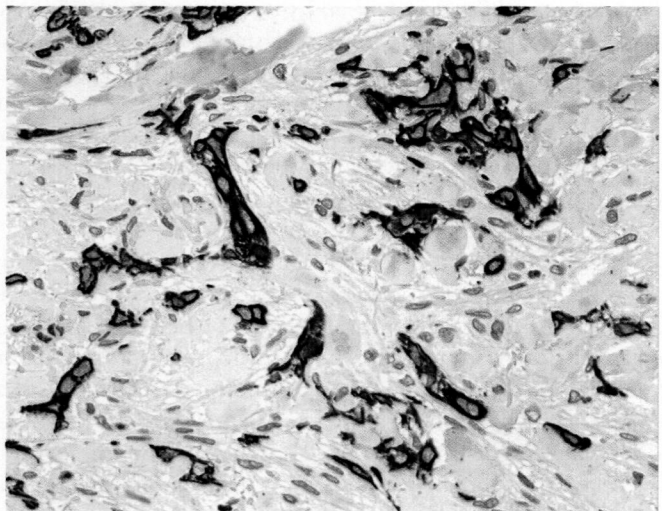

Figure 29-102 Basal cell carcinoma, morpheic. Basaloid cells, emphasized by cytokeratin staining, infiltrate the dermis within their specialized stroma.

In more than 90% of BCCs, a connection between tumor cell formations and the surface epidermis can be shown to exist (271). Occasionally, a tumor mass is found in contact with an outer root sheath. The peripheral cell layer of the tumor masses often shows a palisade arrangement, whereas the nuclei of the cells inside lie in a haphazard fashion. *BCCs* of the *infiltrative* type, also referred to as *aggressive* BCCs, show the basaloid cells predominantly arranged as elongated strands only a few layers thick and with little or no palisading of the peripheral cells. Such strands can invade deeply. The demarcation of the tumor from the stroma is often poor (272). Immunohistochemical staining for cytokeratin may aid in highlighting the infiltrating tumor cells (Fig. 29-91). There are cell aggregates that display an irregular, spiky configuration (273). The cells and their nuclei show great variations in size and shape (274). There may be foci of squamous differentiation (Fig. 29-95). The number of inflammatory cells depends to some degree on the extent of ulceration. There often is perineural infiltration (272), and, on the face, there may be invasion of bone (245).

Keratotic BCC shows parakeratotic cells and horn cysts in addition to undifferentiated cells. The parakeratotic cells possess elongated nuclei and a slightly eosinophilic cytoplasm, in contrast to the deeply basophilic cytoplasm of undifferentiated cells. The parakeratotic cells may lie in strands, in concentric whorls, or around the horn cysts. It is likely that they are cells with initial keratinization somewhat similar to the nucleated cells in the keratogenic zone of normal hair shafts. The horn cysts, which are composed of fully keratinized cells, represent attempts at hair shaft formation (275). Just as in the keratinization of the hair shaft, the horn cysts form without the interposition of granular cells. Some keratotic BCCs possess horn cysts of considerable size.

Keratotic BCC shares with trichoepithelioma the presence of horn cysts, and it is sometimes difficult to decide whether a lesion represents a keratotic BCC or a trichoepithelioma (see Chapter 30). Clinical data may be necessary for a decision to be reached. The horn cysts must not be confused with the horn pearls that occur in SCC (see *Differential Diagnosis*).

BCC with sebaceous differentiation shows essentially a BCC in which there are interspersed aggregates of sebaceous cells. A clear-cut separation from sebaceoma (sebaceous epithelioma) is at times impossible because transitions exist. Most examples of lesions believed to represent BCCs with sebaceous differentiation are probably actually sebaceomas (276).

Adenoid BCC shows formations suggesting tubular, glandlike structures. The cells are arranged in intertwining strands and radially around islands of connective tissue, resulting in a tumor with a lacelike pattern (Figs. 29-93 and 29-94). In rare instances, lumina may be surrounded by cells that have the appearance of secretory cells. The lumina may be filled with a colloidal substance or with an amorphous granular material, but definite evidence of secretory activity of the cells lining the lumina cannot be obtained, even with histochemical methods. Similarly, because of the low degree of differentiation of the cells, histochemical reactions that would indicate either apocrine or eccrine differentiation are negative (277). The tumor originally described as basal cell tumor with eccrine differentiation (278) is now regarded as an eccrine carcinoma and referred to as *syringoid eccrine carcinoma* (see Chapter 30).

Four uncommon histologic variants of BCC have been described: an adamantinoid type, a granular type, a clear cell type, and a type with matricial differentiation. *Adamantinoid BCC* shows a marked histologic resemblance to dental ameloblastoma or adamantinoma (279). One observes solid masses of basaloid cells with palisading at the periphery. Inside this layer, the cells show elongated nuclei and stellate cytoplasm stretched as thin, connecting bridges across empty spaces, as seen in adamantinoma. In *granular BCC*, some of the tumor cells have the usual appearance of basaloid cells, whereas others show a gradual transition to granular cells. The granular cells show, in their cytoplasm, numerous eosinophilic granules with a tendency to coalesce (280,281). The eosinophilic lysosome-like granules markedly resemble those seen in granular cell tumor (see Chapter 37). In the *clear cell BCC*, the clear cell pattern may occupy all or part of the tumor islands. The clear cells contain vacuoles of different sizes filled with glycogen (282). The vacuoles often cause peripheral displacement of the nucleus, giving the cells a signet ring appearance (283). In *BCC with matricial differentiation*, islands of shadow cells, as seen in pilomatricoma, are located within a BCC (284).

Although about 75% of BCCs are found by immunostaining to contain melanocytes and melanin is present in about 25% of them (285), large amounts of melanin are encountered only rarely (Fig. 29-96). The melanin is produced by benign melanocytes that colonize the tumor. These tumors are called *pigmented BCCs*.

Superficial BCC shows buds and irregular proliferations of tumor tissue attached to the undersurface of the epidermis (Figs. 29-85 to 29-87). The peripheral cell layer of the tumor formations often shows palisading. In most cases, there is little penetration into the dermis. The overlying epidermis usually shows atrophy. Fibroblasts, often in a fairly large number, are arranged around the tumor cell proliferations. In addition, a mild or moderate amount of a nonspecific chronic inflammatory infiltrate is present in the upper dermis.

In *fibroepithelioma*, first described by Pinkus in 1953 (263), long, thin, branching, anastomosing strands of BCC are embedded in a fibrous stroma (Figs. 29-103 and 29-104). Many of the strands show connections with the surface epidermis. Here and there, small groups of dark-staining cells showing a palisade arrangement of the peripheral cell layer may be seen along the epithelial strands, like buds on a branch. Usually, the tumor is quite superficial and is well demarcated at its lower border. Fibroepithelioma combines features of the intracanalicular fibroadenoma of the breast, the reticulated type of seborrheic

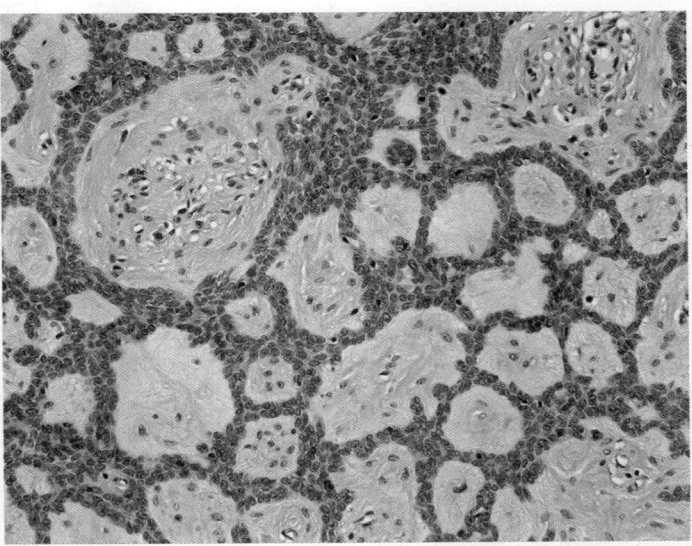

Figure 29-104 Fibroepithelioma of Pinkus (fibroepithelial basal cell carcinoma). Long, thin, branching, anastomosing strands of basal cell carcinoma are embedded in a fibrous stroma.

keratosis, and superficial BCC (263). Fibroepithelioma can change into an invasive and ulcerating BCC (285).

The multiple BCCs seen in the *nevoid BCC syndrome* present no features that distinguish them from ordinary BCC, even while they are still in the early nevoid stage and have not yet become invasive and destructive, as they may be later in the neoplastic stage (286). All of the diverse features of BCC, such as solid, adenoid, cystic, keratotic, superficial, and fibrosing formations, can be seen in the lesions of the nevoid BCC syndrome. Usually, a histologic distinction between the nevoid BCC syndrome (287) and typical trichoepithelioma is easy because keratotic cysts are more prominent in the latter. However, some lesions of trichoepithelioma show relatively few horn cysts. A histologic distinction in such cases may be impossible (288), and clinical data will be necessary (see Chapter 30).

The palmar and plantar pits are a result of the premature desquamation of most of the horny layer (286). On histologic examination, the epidermal rete ridges beneath the pits are found to be crowded with cells resembling those of BCC. Overlying these rete ridges is a markedly thinned granular layer topped by a very thin layer of loose keratin (250). In some patients, the pits actually show the presence of small BCCs at their base (289). In rare instances, one or several clinically visible BCCs arise on the palms or soles in patients with palmar and plantar pits (286,290,291).

The jaw cysts represent odontogenic keratocysts. They are lined by a festooned epithelium consisting of two to five layers of squamous cells that form keratin without the presence of a granular cell layer (292). Each jaw cyst may consist of either one large cyst or multiple microcysts (287). Some of the cutaneous cysts, instead of being epidermal cysts, have the appearance of the jaw cysts and are similar to those cysts seen in steatocystoma multiplex but without showing sebaceous lobules.

The BCCs in *linear unilateral basal cell nevus* have a variable histologic appearance. The tumor formations may be solid, adenoid, keratotic, or cystic (257,258). In addition, there may be areas resembling trichoepithelioma (263) or eccrine spiradenoma (293). The walls of the comedones show numerous buds of BCC extending into the surrounding dermis (257,259).

The BCCs encountered in the *Bazex syndrome* have a variable histologic appearance. Some of them are indistinguishable

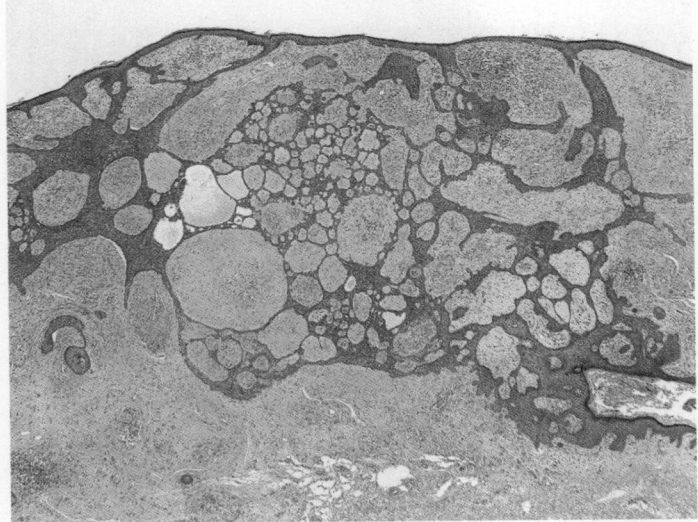

Figure 29-103 Fibroepithelioma of Pinkus (fibroepithelial basal cell carcinoma). The tumor has an elevated nodular appearance.

from trichoepithelioma (261,262). The areas of follicular atrophoderma show a dilated follicular ostium leading into a distorted and underdeveloped pilosebaceous unit (262).

The tumor described in 1926 by Jadassohn and regarded by him as an intraepidermal epithelioma analogous to the one previously reported by Borst has been referred to as *Borst–Jadassohn epithelioma.* For a long time, this tumor and similar tumors subsequently described were believed to be intraepidermal BCCs because the cells composing the intraepidermal islands are usually small and have a deeply basophilic cytoplasm (294). However, on careful examination, it became evident that the cells composing the intraepidermal islands in the presumed intraepidermal BCCs possess intercellular bridges and are seborrheic keratoses of the clonal type (295,296). The existence of an intraepidermal BCC is also unlikely because the close relationship that exists between tumor and stroma in BCC excludes the formation of intraepidermal nests, which would lack any contact with the stroma (297).

However, there are several types of tumors—some benign and some malignant—that on occasion show well-defined islands of cells within the epidermis that differ in their appearance from the surrounding epidermal cells (298). This is referred to as the *Jadassohn phenomenon.* Among the tumors that occasionally have an intraepidermal location are the following:

Clonal Seborrheic Keratosis. Some of these tumors show intraepidermal aggregates of basaloid cells suggestive of a BCC *in situ* (Figs. 29-18 and 29-19) (295), whereas others show intraepidermal islands of an irritated seborrheic keratosis simulating an SCCIS.

Bowen Disease. Occasionally, one observes clonal aggregates of Bowen disease within the epidermis (299). At a later stage, there may be dermal invasion (300).

Intraepidermal poroma is also referred to as *hidroacanthoma simplex* (see Chapter 30) (301,302).

Intraepidermal malignant eccrine poroma (303). In cases of intraepidermal metastases of malignant eccrine poroma, the tumor masses extend through the superficial lymphatics from the dermis into the epidermis (see Chapter 30) (304).

The concept of intraepidermal tumors also includes Paget disease of the breast, extramammary Paget disease (see Chapter 30), pagetoid SCC *in situ,* intraepidermal junction nevus (see Chapter 28), and melanoma *in situ* (see Chapter 28) (298).

Some authors have regarded the intraepidermal epithelioma of Jadassohn as a distinct entity that may invade the dermis and occasionally cause metastases (305). It has been postulated that this tumor arises from acrosyringium keratinocytes or pluripotential adnexal cells and represents an adnexal carcinoma (305).

The existence of *BCCs with features of SCC* was first postulated in 1922 (306). Two types of basosquamous carcinomas, referred to as *metatypical epitheliomas,* were recognized: a mixed and an intermediary type. The mixed type was described as showing focal keratinization consisting of pearls with a colloidal or parakeratotic center, and the intermediary type as showing two kinds of cells within a network of narrow strands, an outer row of dark-staining basal cells and an inner layer of cells appearing larger, lighter, and better defined than the basal cells and regarded as intermediate in character between basal and squamous cells.

Basosquamous carcinomas or metatypical epitheliomas are considered by some to represent a transition from BCC to SCC, or part of a continuum that extends from BCC at one extreme to SCC at the other (307). The incidence of basosquamous carcinomas among BCCs has been judged to be 3% (307), 8% (308), and even

12% (309). It has also been stated that basosquamous carcinomas show a greater tendency to metastasize than BCCs (237,307,309).

However, the existence of basosquamous carcinomas is questioned by many (264). It would seem that the entirely different genesis of SCC—a true anaplastic carcinoma of the epidermis—and BCC—a tumor composed of immature rather than anaplastic cells—makes the occurrence of transitional forms quite unlikely (see *Pathogenesis*). It can be assumed that the so-called mixed type of basal squamous cell carcinoma represents a keratotic BCC (Fig. 29-102) and that the intermediate type represents a BCC with differentiation into two types of cells (BCC with squamous differentiation). This form of differentiation is often seen deep into an area of ulceration. Other putative examples of basosquamous differentiation are better interpreted as *BCC with follicular differentiation* (Fig. 29-105). However, because these tumors may behave much more aggressively than typical BCCs, they should probably be regarded as variants of SCC (see the section on Basosquamous Carcinoma).

Mixed carcinoma shows an SCC contiguous to a BCC as a so-called collision tumor. It is likely that, in most instances, the SCC develops secondary to the BCC. As other chronic

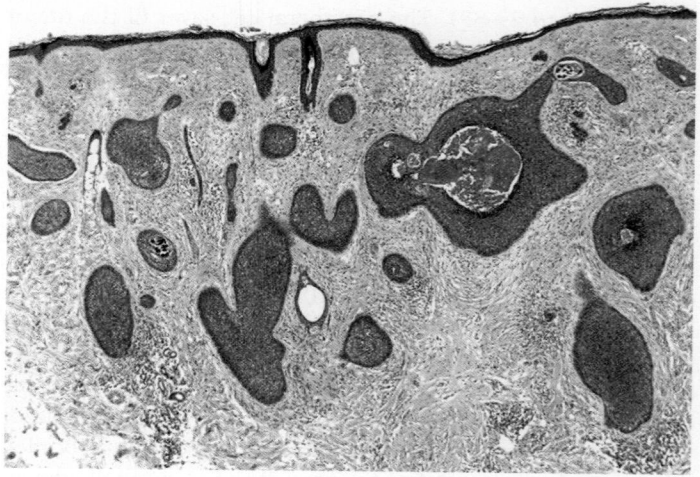

Figure 29-105 Basal cell carcinoma showing follicular differentiation. Epithelium and stroma form structures reminiscent of follicular germs, and there is formation of a horn cyst resembling a follicular structure.

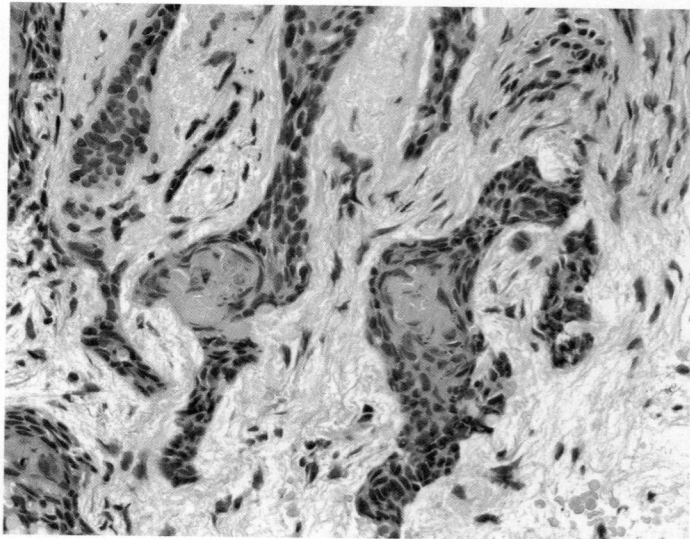

Figure 29-106 Basal cell carcinoma, infiltrative, metatypical. There is focal squamous differentiation within the infiltrating cords of basaloid cells.

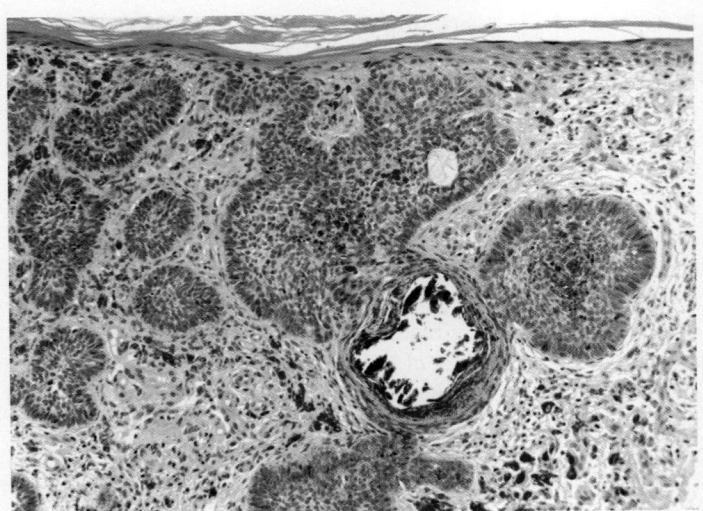

Figure 29-107 Pigmented basal cell carcinoma. Melanin pigment is present within solid islands of basal cell carcinoma and in macrophages between the islands of tumor cells.

ulcerative lesions, such as burns and stasis ulcers, BCC may stimulate the development of an SCC. Before making a diagnosis of mixed carcinoma, however, one must rule out the possibility of pseudocarcinomatous hyperplasia occurring in a BCC.

Pathogenesis of Basal Cell Carcinoma

When Krompecher described BCC in 1903, he regarded it as a carcinoma of the basal cells of the epidermis and that these tumors that show a tendency toward gland formation are imitating the potential of the basal cells to form cutaneous glands (310). According to Geschickter and Koehler, only those basal cells with a potential to develop into glandular cells give rise to BCC. They suggested the designation *appendage cell carcinoma* (311). Mallory thought that BCCs are carcinomas of hair matrix cells (312). In 1947, Foot expressed the view that BCCs are carcinomas that have developed from distorted primordia of dermal adnexa rather than from ordinary epidermal basal cells (275). He stated that the tumors imitate the embryonal development of one or all three types of adnexal primordia, that is, hair, sebaceous gland, and sweat gland.

The first author to express doubts that BCCs are carcinomas was Adamson; in 1914, he stated that BCCs are nevoid tumors originating "from latent embryonic foci aroused from their dormant state at a later period in life" (313). He believed that the latent embryonic foci are usually embryonic pilosebaceous follicles but occasionally embryonic sweat ducts. Several other authors reached similar conclusions, among them Wallace and Halpert, who stated in 1950 that they regarded BCCs as benign tumors arising from cells destined to form hair follicles (314). They proposed the term *trichoma* for them.

In 1948, Lever expressed his belief that BCCs are not carcinomas and are not derived from basal cells but rather are nevoid tumors, or hamartomas, derived from primary epithelial germ cells. In other words, BCCs originate from incompletely differentiated, immature cells and not from anaplastic cells (315). Although γ-glutamyl transpeptidase activity is observed in the atypical cells in SCC, Bowen disease, and actinic keratoses, no such activity is expressed in the cells of BCC (316). In this view, BCC represents the least differentiated of the appendage tumors.

It was originally assumed, analogous to Adamson's view, that the primary epithelial germ cells giving rise to BCC are in all instances embryonic cells that lie dormant until the onset of

neoplasia. Even though this view applies to the linear unilateral basal cell nevus, which is usually present from birth, it is likely that—as suggested by Pinkus—BCCs occurring later in life arise not from dormant embryonic primary epithelial germ cells but from pluripotential cells that form continuously during life and—like embryonic primary epithelial germ cells—have the potential of forming hair, sebaceous glands, and apocrine glands (263). The fact that BCCs may arise in sun-exposed areas and in areas of radiodermatitis supports this view. Their tendency for local invasion and tissue destruction, their capacity for local persistence and recurrence if not ablated, and their occasional capacity for metastasis support the concept that these lesions are carcinomas, albeit in most instances with little or no capacity for metastasis.

It is now widely accepted that disruption of the Hedgehog–Patched pathway is a key event in the development of basal cell cancer, providing additional support for the concept that BCCs are true neoplasms. In addition to PTCH gene alterations, p53 gene mutations are frequently present (317–325).

Pilar Differentiation. Differentiation in BCC is predominantly toward pilar keratin. The presence of citrulline in keratinized structures indicates that the origin of the keratin is the hair matrix because epidermal keratin contains no citrulline (326). Studies with monoclonal cytokeratin antibodies support the assumption of pilar differentiation in BCC. Thus, a cytokeratin antibody binding to the follicular epithelium but not to the interfollicular epidermis stains all cells of BCC (327). Furthermore, a monoclonal antibody against BCC keratin stains, in addition to the cells of BCC, all follicular cells below the isthmus portion of normal anagen hair follicles (328). These findings contribute to the general view that BCC should be regarded as a hair follicle tumor rather than an epidermal tumor.

Stromal Factor. The importance of stroma in the development of BCCs is borne out by the fact that autotransplants of BCCs survive only when they include connective tissue stroma (329). In addition, the rarity of BCCs on the palms and soles and the fact that the palmar and plantar pits of the nevoid BCC syndrome very rarely show a full-fledged BCC suggest that the palms and soles do not possess the stromal factor necessary for the formation of BCCs (330).

Lack of Autonomy. BCCs, when transplanted to the anterior chamber of the rabbit's eye together with their connective tissue stroma, fail to grow, in contrast to SCC (331). Furthermore, BCCs, in contrast to many human tumors, do not grow when transplanted subcutaneously to athymic nude mice. These observations suggest a lack of autonomy of the cells of at least some BCCs. Because the autonomy of tumor cells is a prerequisite for the formation of metastases and represents a characteristic feature of malignant tumors, the absence of autonomy in BCC is consistent with its inability to metastasize in most instances.

Site of Origin. The usual site of origin of BCC appears to be the surface epidermis. Alternatively, however, the tumor may originate from the outer root sheath of a hair follicle, and in the 2006 WHO classification, BCCs were classified with the skin adnexal tumors (332), though not so in the 2018 WHO Fourth Edition (1,333).

Of particular interest is the manner of growth of *superficial BCC*. Routine sectioning carried out perpendicular to the skin surface shows seemingly independent nests of BCC, suggestive, at times, of the growth of primary epithelial germs in the embryonic skin. Thus, it was at one time widely assumed that the peripheral extension seen in superficial BCC was based on a "multicentric" growth characterized by the formation of new buds of tumor tissue at the periphery. However, on the basis of findings in serial sections and in wax reconstructions of superficial BCCs, Madsen favored the theory of a "unicentric" origin (334,335). Madsen was able to show that the tumor strands are continuous but are attached to the undersurface of the epidermis only at intervals, like garlands. Madsen found not only in his wax reconstructions but also in sections cut parallel to the surface of the skin that individual tumor islands are interconnected. Oberste-Lehn (336), using a technique of separating the epidermis from the dermis by maceration, could not find such interconnections, but the possibility could not be excluded, as Madsen pointed out, that the interconnections had ruptured as a result of the maceration. It was subsequently shown, when trypsin was used for the separation of the epidermis from the dermis, that interconnections exist between tumor cell nests in superficial BCC. Similarly, three-dimensional reconstruction by means of serial horizontal microscopic sections and a special computer confirmed a unicentric origin (337).

Electron Microscopy. The predominant cell in undifferentiated BCC is characterized by a large nucleus, poorly developed desmosomes, and rather sparse tonofilaments. Thus, the tumor cells differ from normal epidermal basal cells. They resemble the cells of the undifferentiated hair matrix (338) or the immature basal cells of the embryonic epidermis, particularly those of the primary epithelial germ (339,340). In addition to the prevalent large, light cells, a few cells that are smaller, darker, and more irregularly shaped can be found (271,340). The darkness of the latter cells is because of the abundance of ribonucleoprotein particles in their cytoplasm. A well-developed basement membrane separates the tumor from the dermis (338). Processes from the tumor cells do not usually penetrate the basement membrane in BCC, in contrast to SCC, in which processes extend through a fragmented basement membrane into the stroma (341).

Keratinization is commonly observed by electron microscopy in BCC, especially in the keratotic type. In addition to well-developed desmosomes and many thick bundles of tonofilaments, dense clumps of homogeneous, dyskeratotic material are present in many keratinizing cells. A small number of keratohyalin granules are often seen. They probably represent trichohyaline granules, which occur in the process of keratinization of the inner root sheath and its cuticle (340).

Some BCCs show areas of adenoid differentiation in which cells are grouped around glandlike lumina. Such cells may show pronounced infolding of the plasma membrane at their lateral borders as seen normally in eccrine ductal cells (342).

In pigmented BCCs, most of the melanin is found within melanocytes of the tumor and in melanophages located in the connective tissue stroma. Although numerous melanosomes are present in the dendrites of the melanocytes, the tumor cells generally do not phagocytize the melanin-containing dendrites, resulting in a blockage of the transfer of melanin from melanocytes to the tumor cells (343,344). This is analogous to the blocked transfer from melanocytes to tumor cells in some pigmented seborrheic keratoses referred to as *melanoacanthoma*. Nevertheless, in occasional instances of pigmented BCC, some transfer of melanosomes to the tumor cells takes place. The tumor cells then contain melanosomes, which are located largely as melanosome complexes within lysosomes (340).

Presence of Amyloid. Cell proliferation in BCC is considerable. The experimentally determined cell-doubling time of 9 days, however, does not conform to the clinical observation that

BCC, as a rule, is a very slowly growing tumor (345). This suggests that there must be cell death. In addition to phagocytosis by neighboring tumor cells and macrophages, apoptosis of tumor cells also often takes place, with the transformation of these cells into colloid bodies and subsequently into amyloid (342,346). This conversion of epithelial cells into amyloid is analogous to that occurring in lichenoid and macular amyloidosis. Colloid bodies, demonstrable by direct immunofluorescence for immunoglobulin M, have been found in 89% of BCCs (342). Amyloid has been observed in the stroma and inside the tumor islands both by histochemistry and by electron microscopy in as many as 65% of BCCs. This amyloid shows positive staining with antikeratin antiserum, indicating that it is derived from tonofilaments (347). The fact that the amyloid is permanganate resistant indicates that it is not secondary amyloid (347). The presence of amyloid may contribute to an apparent lack of sensitivity to radiotherapy (348).

Differential Diagnosis of Basal Cell Carcinoma

Many diagnostic entities show morphologic and immunophenotypic overlap with BCC, including nonneoplastic processes, such as follicular induction over dermatofibroma; benign follicular tumors, such as trichoblastoma, trichoepithelioma, or basaloid follicular hamartoma; and malignant tumors, such as sebaceous carcinoma or Merkel cell carcinoma. Thus, misdiagnosis has significant potential to result in overtreatment or undertreatment (349).

Differentiation of BCC from SCC can sometimes be difficult; however, as a rule, differentiation is fairly easy. One of the best points of differentiation is that most cells of BCC stain deeply basophilic, whereas most cells of SCC, at least in low-grade lesions, have an eosinophilic tint owing to partial keratinization. The cells in high-grade SCC may appear basophilic because of the absence of keratinization. However, they differ from BCC by showing much greater atypicality of their nuclei and their mitotic figures. It is important to remember that keratinization is not a prerogative of SCC; it also occurs in BCC with differentiation toward hair structures (see the discussion on keratotic Basal Cell Carcinoma section). Keratinization in BCCs may be partial and then result in parakeratotic bands and whorls, or it may be complete and result in horn cysts. The keratinization seen in the horn cysts differs from that seen in the horn pearls of SCCs by being abrupt and complete rather than gradual and incomplete. The fairly common presence in BCC of areas of retraction of the tumor cell masses from the surrounding connective tissue also aids in the differentiation of this tumor from SCC, in which such areas of retraction are rarely found.

The differential diagnosis of BCC from trichoepithelioma is discussed in Chapter 30. Of particular importance is the differentiation of fibrosing BCC from desmoplastic trichoepithelioma. Both tumors have in common thin strands of small basaloid cells embedded in a dense, fibrous stroma, but desmoplastic trichoepithelioma also shows a considerable number of horn cysts. Many tumors in the past diagnosed as BCCs in children and teenagers could be reclassified as desmoplastic trichoepithelioma (350).

In making a biopsy diagnosis, it is important to have sections that adequately represent the lesion. It is curious that in punch biopsies, the initial sections may not show the tumor. Further sections should always be examined if the clinical diagnosis is one of BCC (351). There is also a limited evidence base to recommend the most effective and economical excision margins. It seems likely that a margin of 3 mm may be adequate in most cases, but in high-risk BCC this may be insufficient (352–355).

Principles of Management of Basal Cell Carcinomas

There are several effective ways to treat BCCs. To choose the appropriate treatment modality, an assessment of the individual patient and the tumor factors should be considered. These factors include the tumor size, tumor site (BCCs around the ears, nose, lips, and eyes pose a higher risk of recurrence), definition of clinical margins (poorly defined clinical margins pose a higher risk of recurrence), histologic features including those indicating aggressive behavior (perineural and perivascular involvement), failure of previous treatments, and immunosuppression. In general, treatment can be divided into surgical and nonsurgical methods. Recently, the oral biologic treatment, vismodigeb, has been licensed for use in metastatic disease (4).

Surgical treatments include excision with peripheral and deep margins and destructive methods. Surgical excision is a highly effective method for treating primary BCCs with a reported recurrence rate of less than 2% at 5 years (356). The optimum peripheral and deep excision margins of the tumor depend on the type and location of the BCC. The suggested clinical peripheral excision margin for a well-defined, small lesion (<20 mm) is 4 to 5 mm—this is reported to produce peripheral clearance rate in more than 95% of the cases (357,358). Morpheic and large BCCs require wider peripheral excision margins to maximize the chance of complete histologic clearance. Few data exist on the optimum deep excisional margin; for infiltrating carcinomas, excision of the underlying subcutaneous fat is often advisable.

Mohs micrographic surgery is a controlled, staged surgery that aims to remove all tumor calls while conserving as much normal tissue as possible. During the surgery, after each stage of tissue removal, the specimen is histologically examined using frozen sections while the patient waits. If the margins are not clear, a further stage of tissue removal is undertaken. Of all treatment modalities, Mohs micrographic surgery yields the highest cure rate. A review of studies published reports an overall 5-year cure rate of 99% for primary BCCs and 94.4% for recurrent BCCs (359,360).

Recurrent BCCs are more difficult to treat than primary BCCs. The currently available data show cure rates that are inferior to those of treated primary BCC. Recurrent lesions should be surgically excised with wider peripheral margins or ideally with Mohs micrographic surgery (359).

Destructive surgical methods include curettage and cautery, cryosurgery, and CO_2 laser therapy. Curettage and cautery is the second most common form of treatment after surgical excision. The success outcome of this treatment relies on the appropriate selection of the lesion as well as the operator's skill and experience. It is suitable for the treatment of low-risk lesions but contraindicated for high-risk facial lesions because it is associated with a high recurrence rate. A literature review reports a 5-year cure rate of selected primary BCCs of 92.3% (360). Liquid nitrogen cryosurgery is a good treatment for low-risk BCCs. It used extreme cold ($-50°C$ to $-60°C$) to cause deep destruction of tumor cells and surrounding tissue. Double freeze–thaw cycles are generally recommended. CO_2 laser therapy remains an uncommon form of treatment, with few published data on its use in comparison to other treatment modalities.

Nonsurgical methods are best used for low-risk BCCs or in patients who are unable to undergo surgical procedures. The treatments include topical immunotherapy with 5% imiquimod, 5-fluorouracil, PDT, and radiotherapy. 5% imiquimod is an immunomodulator that works through stimulating toll-like receptors. A few randomized controlled trials using 5% imiquimod against vehicle have reported its efficacy (78–80,361–363). The current approved regimen by the European Medicines Agency is application five times per week for 6 weeks. 5-Fluorouracil is only recommended for small superficial BCCs when other methods are impractical. It is thought to work by interfering with DNA synthesis through inhibiting the methylation of deoxyuridylic acid synthesis and subsequently cell proliferation. PDT is administered orally, parenterally, or topically; it localizes into tumor cells before activation by exposure to the light source. Its efficacy is low, and this treatment is frequently palliative. Radiotherapy is effective in the treatment of primary BCC, surgically recurrent BCC, and as adjuvant therapy. It is probably the treatment of choice for high-risk BCC in patients who are unwilling or unable to tolerate surgery (80,364).

Vismodigeb, as previously mentioned, is an oral biologic treatment that is licensed for use in metastatic BCC. It is designed to selectively inhibit abnormal signaling in the Hedgehog pathway (241,242).

EPIDERMAL TUMORS IN IMMUNOSUPPRESSED HOSTS

Clinical Summary. The widespread use of immunosuppressive therapy as part of organ transplantation and in the treatment of some immunologically mediated diseases has led to a new phenomenon of rapidly developing warts and epidermal tumors (365,366). There is a spectrum of squamous atypia ranging from typical viral warts through dysplastic or atypical warts to SCCs, which are often very poorly differentiated (Fig. 29-108). The SCCs have been shown to have similar proliferative potential to similar lesions in hosts with normal immune function (367), although they lack the host immune response that would normally be present (368). They also share the same early expression of keratin 17 seen in a number of epidermal hyperproliferative

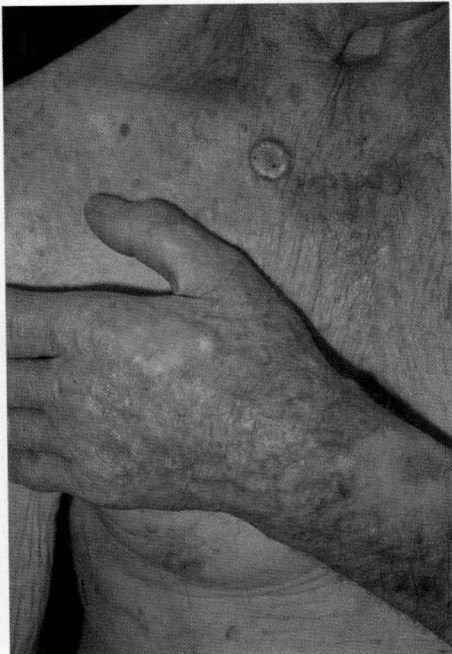

Figure 29-108 Squamous cell carcinoma in a renal transplant recipient. The patient has a carcinoma on the chest and multiple keratoses on the back of the hand and arm.

states (369). Mutations of p53 may play a part in the development of the tumors (370). Rapidly progressing multiple SCCs have also been reported in association with chronic myeloid leukemia (371). BCCs tend to show an infiltrative rather than a nodular growth pattern more frequently in immunosuppressed patients (372). Kaposi sarcoma can also present as a fulminant process after liver or kidney transplantation (373,374) and may recur with the introduction of cyclosporin A therapy (375). It has also been suggested that HIV-positive hosts have an increased risk of developing malignant melanoma (376).

KERATOACANTHOMA

Keratoacanthomas are common skin tumors that arise from the pilosebaceous unit and clinically and pathologically resemble SCCs. Two types of keratoacanthoma exist: solitary and multiple.

Solitary Keratoacanthoma

Clinical Summary. Solitary keratoacanthoma was first described in 1889 by Hutchinson as a "crateriform ulcer of the face," and since 1950 it has been recognized as an entity and differentiated from SCC, which it often resembles clinically and histologically (377–379). Solitary keratoacanthoma occurs in elderly persons usually as a single lesion; however, occasionally there are several lesions, or new lesions develop. The lesion consists of a firm, dome-shaped nodule 1.0 to 2.5 cm in diameter with a horn-filled crater in its center (Fig. 29-109). The sites of predilection are exposed areas, where about 95% of solitary keratoacanthomas occur, but they may occur on any hairy cutaneous site (380,381). They have not been reported on the palms, soles, or mucous surfaces, although, in rare instances, they occur subungually (see the following text). Keratoacanthomas located on the vermilion border of the lip probably arise from hair follicles in the adjacent skin (382). Keratoacanthomas usually reach their full size within 6 to 8 weeks and involute spontaneously, generally in less than 6 months. Healing takes place with a slightly depressed scar. In some instances, a keratoacanthoma increases in size for more than 2 months and takes up to 1 year to involute (381).

An increased incidence of keratoacanthoma is observed in immunosuppressed patients (383). In addition, keratoacanthomas commonly occur in the Muir–Torre syndrome of sebaceous neoplasms and keratoacanthomas associated with visceral

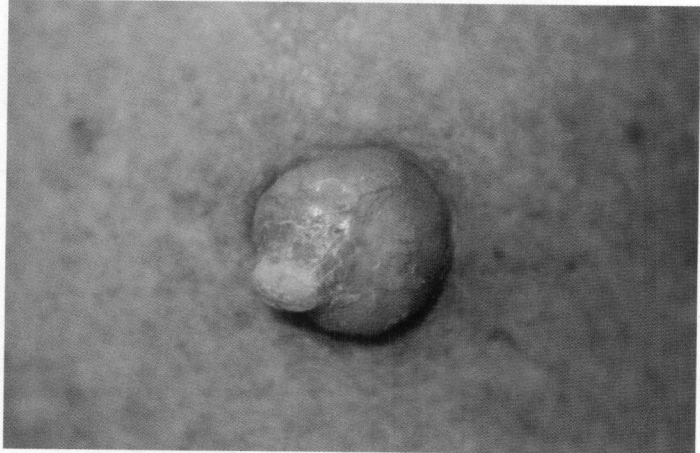

Figure 29-109 Keratoacanthoma. The lesion is symmetrical with keratin protruding from its center.

carcinomas (see Chapter 30). Keratoacanthomas may be the only type of cutaneous tumor present in this syndrome (384,385).

There are three rare clinical variants of solitary keratoacanthoma. In two forms—giant keratoacanthoma and keratoacanthoma centrifugum marginatum—the keratoacanthoma attains a large size. In *giant keratoacanthoma*, the growth rapidly reaches a size of 5 cm or more and may cause the destruction of underlying tissues. Nevertheless, spontaneous involution takes place after several months, often accompanied by the detachment of a large keratotic plaque. The most common sites are the nose (386,387) and the eyelids (381,388,389). In *keratoacanthoma centrifugum marginatum*, the lesion may reach a size of 20 cm in diameter. There is no tendency toward spontaneous involution; instead, there is peripheral extension with a raised, rolled border and atrophy in the center of the lesion. The most common locations are the dorsa of the hands (390,391) and the legs (392,393). The third rare variant is *subungual keratoacanthoma*, which shows a destructive crateriform lesion with keratotic excrescences under the distal portion of a fingernail. It fails to regress spontaneously, is tender, and, by roentgenogram, shows damage to the terminal phalanx by pressure erosion (394–396).

Claims have been made that keratoacanthoma can undergo transformation into an SCC either spontaneously (379,390) or as a result of immunosuppression. It appears more likely, however, that the SCC existed from the beginning in such instances (see *Differential Diagnosis*) (380,397).

Histopathology. The architecture of the lesion in a keratoacanthoma is as important to the diagnosis as the cellular characteristics. Therefore, if the lesion cannot be excised in its entirety, it is advisable that a fusiform specimen be excised for biopsy from the center of the lesion and that this specimen include the edge at least of one side and preferably of both sides of the lesion (398). A shave biopsy is inadvisable because the histologic changes at the base of the lesion are often of great importance in the differentiation from SCC. Frequently, a curettage specimen will be submitted, in which case clear distinction between keratoacanthoma and SCC may be impossible to achieve with confidence.

In the early proliferative stage, one observes a horn-filled invagination of the epidermis from which strands of epidermis protrude into the dermis. These strands are poorly demarcated from the surrounding stroma in many areas and may contain cells showing nuclear atypia (399), as well as many mitotic figures (400). Even atypical mitoses may be seen occasionally (401). Dyskeratotic cells, that is, cells showing individual cell keratinization, may also be seen in areas that otherwise do not show advanced keratinization. However, even at this early stage, some of the tumor areas show a fairly pronounced degree of keratinization, giving them an eosinophilic, glassy appearance. In the dermis, a rather pronounced inflammatory infiltrate is present (400). Perineural invasion is occasionally seen in the proliferative phase of keratoacanthoma and should not be over-interpreted as conclusive evidence of malignancy (402,403).

A fully developed lesion shows in its center a large, irregularly shaped crater filled with keratin (Fig. 29-110). The epidermis extends like a lip or a buttress over the sides of the crater. At the base of the crater, irregular epidermal proliferations extend both upward into the crater and downward from the base of the crater. These proliferations may still appear somewhat atypical, but less so than in the initial stage; the keratinization is extensive and fairly advanced, with only a thin shell of one or two layers of basophilic, nonkeratinized cells at

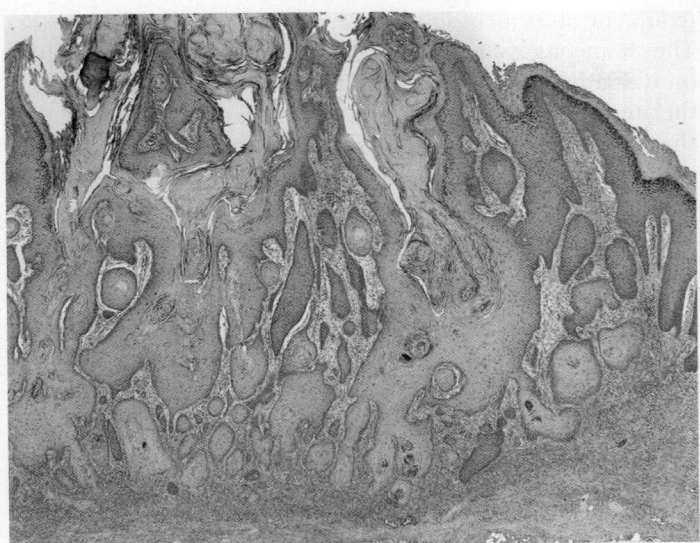

Figure 29-110 Keratoacanthoma. Low magnification. There is a central keratin-filled crater. On the right, the epidermis extends like a buttress over the side of the crater. Irregular epidermal proliferations extend downward from the base of the crater into the dermis.

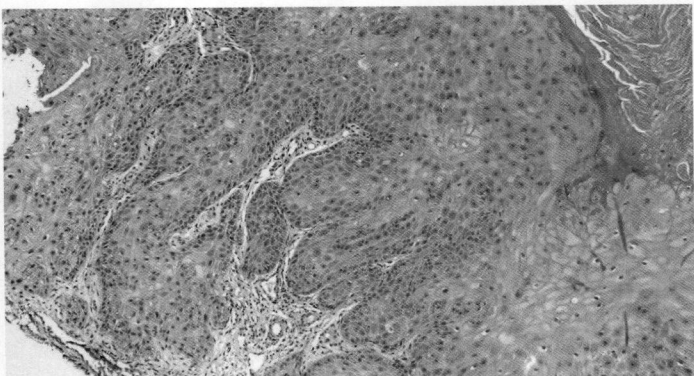

Figure 29-112 Keratoacanthoma. Medium magnification. The proliferation at the base resembles squamous cell carcinoma.

the periphery of the proliferations, whereas the cells within this shell appear eosinophilic and glassy as a result of keratinization (Fig. 29-111). There are many horn pearls, most of which show complete keratinization in their center. There are often prominent collections of neutrophils in relation to this keratin. The base of a fully developed keratoacanthoma appears regular and well demarcated and usually does not extend below the level of the sweat glands, in contrast to SCC, which frequently does. A rather dense inflammatory infiltrate is often present at the base of the lesion (Fig. 29-112) (380,404).

In the involuting stage, proliferation has ceased, and most cells at the base of the crater have undergone keratinization. There may be shrunken, eosinophilic cells analogous to colloid or Civatte bodies among the tumor cells located nearest to the stroma as well as in the stroma, suggesting that cell degeneration

followed by apoptosis contributes to the involution of the keratoacanthoma (393). Gradually, the crater flattens and finally disappears during healing.

Pathogenesis. It is generally agreed that the lesion starts with hyperplasia of the infundibulum of one or several adjoining hair follicles and with squamous metaplasia of the attached sebaceous glands (403). The application of cutaneous carcinogens to the skin of animals frequently produces, among other tumors, lesions with the histologic appearance of keratoacanthomas, and these tumors also have their origin in the infundibulum of one or several hair follicles (381).

The cause of keratoacanthoma is not known. The theory of a viral genesis has not been confirmed. The electron microscopic findings are largely nonspecific. However, keratoacanthomas, like SCCs and lesions of Bowen disease, often show the presence of fairly numerous intracytoplasmic desmosomes (406,407).

Differential Diagnosis. The differentiation of typical, mature lesions of keratoacanthoma from SCC generally is not difficult. In favor of a diagnosis of keratoacanthoma are the architecture of a crater surrounded by buttresses and the high degree of keratinization, which is manifested by the eosinophilic, glassy appearance of many of the cells. Clinical data are also of great value: A rapid development of an exophytic lesion showing a central, horn-filled crater speaks for keratoacanthoma rather than for SCC.

The greatest difficulties in the differentiation of a keratoacanthoma from an SCC are encountered in very early lesions because a horn-filled invagination may be seen in SCC, and cells with an atypical appearance may occur in a keratoacanthoma. Occasionally, an early keratoacanthoma shows a greater degree of nuclear atypia than do some SCCs (408). In addition, individual cell keratinization can occur in keratoacanthoma. On rare occasions, even adenoid formations caused by dyskeratosis and acantholysis can occur in keratoacanthoma (409). Thus, it was found on reclassification in one study that in only 81% of the cases of keratoacanthoma could a diagnosis of SCC be fully excluded, and that in only 86% of the cases of SCC could keratoacanthoma be ruled out with certainty. These findings explain why, on rare occasions, lesions classified as keratoacanthoma cause metastases (397). Great caution is indicated in the diagnosis of giant keratoacanthomas. Several cases diagnosed as such turned out to be SCCs either by metastasizing (410) or by deep invasion into the muscle (411). In addition, some keratoacanthomas can be locally destructive before involuting.

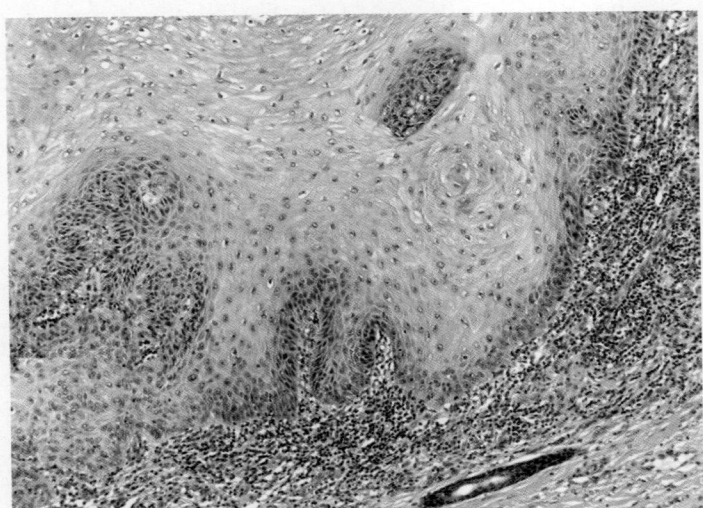

Figure 29-111 Keratoacanthoma. Medium magnification. The proliferation at the base resembles squamous cell carcinoma. However, there is more keratinization than is usual in squamous cell carcinoma, giving the tumor islands a glassy appearance. The lesion lies above the level of the sweat gland coils in the dermis.

Because it is widely agreed that SCCs can masquerade as keratoacanthomas clinically and histologically (380,412), it is best to err on the safe side in case of doubt and to proceed on the assumption that the lesion is an SCC. Where the tumor is well differentiated and has architectural features of keratoacanthoma, the term *keratoacanthoma-like SCC* can be used.

Attempts at differentiating between keratoacanthoma and SCC by histochemical or immunohistochemical methods have shown distinct differences in typical cases but not necessarily in borderline cases.

Multiple Keratoacanthoma

There are two classic variants of *multiple keratoacanthoma*: the multiple self-healing epitheliomas of the skin—or Ferguson-Smith type—and the eruptive keratoacanthomas, or Grzybowski type. Both variants are rare in comparison with solitary keratoacanthoma. In addition, keratoacanthoma-like tumors have been described in patients taking targeted therapy directed against the BRAF and perhaps other oncogenes (413).

In *multiple self-healing epitheliomas* of the skin, lesions begin to appear in childhood or adolescence on any part of the skin, including the palms and soles, but especially on the face and the extremities. Subungual lesions have also been described (395). Generally, there are no more than a dozen lesions at any one time (414). The lesions may reach the same size as solitary keratoacanthomas and after a few months heal with a depressed scar (415,416). In some cases, however, the lesions do not heal (379). In some patients, the condition is inherited (417,418).

In *eruptive keratoacanthoma*, lesions do not appear until adult life. Many hundreds of follicular papules are present, measuring from 2 to 3 mm in diameter (419,420). The oral mucosa and larynx may be involved (421,422).

Histopathology. The histologic appearance of the lesions of multiple self-healing epitheliomas of the skin is similar to that of solitary keratoacanthoma (414,416). More frequently than in solitary keratoacanthoma, the cutaneous proliferations in multiple self-healing epitheliomas of the skin are seen to be continuous with the follicular epithelium (419). The cutaneous lesions in eruptive keratoacanthoma show less crater formation than those in solitary keratoacanthoma. The mucosal lesions lack a crater and can easily be misinterpreted as SCC (421,422).

Pathogenesis. It appears likely that multiple keratoacanthoma basically represents the same condition as solitary keratoacanthoma and that predisposition or genetic factors are responsible for the greater number of lesions (423). In multiple—as in solitary—keratoacanthoma, lesions arising in hair-bearing parts of the skin have their onset in the upper portion of a hair follicle, whereas the site of origin of lesions arising on the palms, the soles, and the mucous membranes is not apparent (424).

Principles of Management: The primary treatment for keratoacanthoma is surgical excision with adequate margin (3 to 5 mm). This is necessary for adequate histologic evaluation and to distinguish it from invasive SCC.

PAGET DISEASE OF THE BREAST

Clinical Summary. Paget disease of the breast occurs almost exclusively in women. Only a few instances have been reported in men (425). Of interest is its occurrence in the male breast after treatment of a carcinoma of the prostate with estrogen (426). The cutaneous lesion in Paget disease of the breast begins either on the nipple or the areola of the breast and extends slowly to the surrounding skin. It is always unilateral and consists of a sharply defined, slightly infiltrated area of erythema showing scaling, oozing, and crusting. There may or may not be ulceration or retraction of the nipple. Benign inflammatory dermatoses, such as eczema, are differential diagnoses, and early detection of Paget disease and any underlying malignancy is required for prompt treatment.

The cutaneous lesion is nearly always associated with carcinoma of the breast, and in more than half of the patients, a mass can be felt on palpation of the breast. Metastases in the axillary lymph nodes were found by one group of investigators in about 67% of their patients with a palpable mass of the breast and in 33% of those without a palpable mass (427). This contrasts with the experience of others, who encountered no axillary metastases in the absence of a palpable mass of the breast (428).

A clinical picture indistinguishable from that of early Paget disease of the nipple may be seen in erosive adenomatosis of the nipple, a benign condition of the major nipple ducts (see Chapter 30).

The prognosis of Paget disease is related to the stage of disease; it appears to be similar to that of women with other types of breast cancer. Patients who have a palpable underlying breast lump at presentation have a survival rate of 38% to 40% at 5 years and of 22% to 33% at 10 years. The reported survival rate of patients without a palpable breast tumor ranges from 92% to 94% at 5 years and from 82% to 91% at 10 years.

Histopathology. In early lesions of Paget disease of the breast, the epidermis usually shows only a few scattered Paget cells. They are large, rounded cells that are devoid of intercellular bridges and contain a large nucleus and ample cytoplasm. The cytoplasm of these cells stains much lighter than that of the adjacent squamous cells (Fig. 29-113). As the number of Paget cells increases, they compress the squamous cells to such an extent that the latter may merely form a network, the meshes of which are filled with Paget cells lying singly and in groups. In particular, one often observes flattened basal cells lying between Paget cells and the underlying dermis.

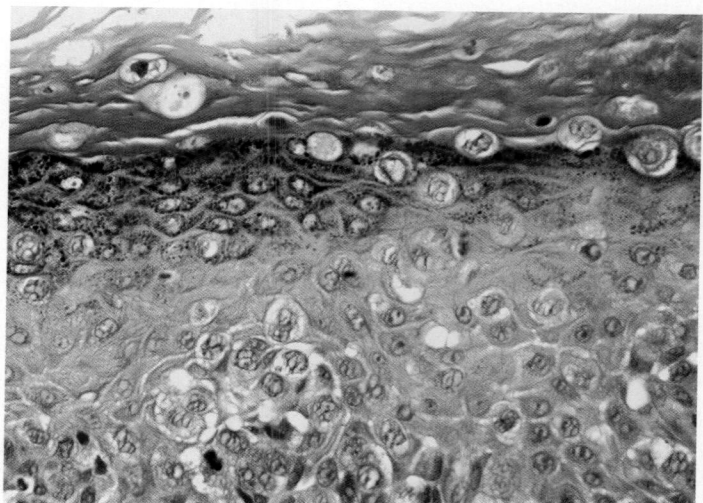

Figure 29-113 Paget disease. High magnification. Large rounded Paget cells with ample pale-staining cytoplasm, devoid of intercellular bridges, are scattered through the epidermis.

The dermis in Paget disease shows a moderately severe chronic inflammatory reaction. Although Paget cells do not invade the dermis from the epidermis, they may be seen extending from the epidermis into the epithelium of hair follicles (429).

Histologic examination of the mammary ducts and glands nearly always shows malignant changes in some of them. At first, the carcinoma is confined within the walls of the ducts and glands, but the tumor cells ultimately invade the connective tissue. From then on, lymphatic spread and metastases occur, just as in other types of mammary carcinoma. In mammary Paget disease, the malignant changes have their onset in the lactiferous ducts and from there extend into the epidermis, but there are rare instances in which the malignant cells are confined to the epidermis of the nipple or involve only the most distal portion of one lactiferous duct (430).

Pathogenesis. As long as *electron microscopic examination* constituted the major factor in analyzing the derivation or the direction of differentiation of the cells in Paget disease of the nipple, no clear decision could be reached whether the constituting cells were keratinocytes or glandular cells. The presence of desmosomes between neighboring Paget cells and between Paget cells and keratinocytes seemed to support a derivation from keratinocytes (431). On the other hand, scattered desmosomes are normally found connecting the cells of the lactiferous ducts (432), and wherever cytoplasmic processes of Paget cells lie in contact with the basal lamina, no hemidesmosomes are present—as they would be in the case of keratinocytes (432). Also, Paget cells can be found bordering small lumina in areas in which groups of Paget cells lie together (431–433).

Immunohistochemical studies have proved beyond any doubt the glandular derivation of the Paget cells of both mammary and extramammary Paget disease. Thus, CEA is regularly found in Paget cells. Whereas intervening keratinocytes and melanocytes do not stain, CEA is present in the cells of normal eccrine and apocrine glands (434). Furthermore, Paget cells express cytokeratins typical of glandular epithelia but do not react with antibodies to epidermal keratin (435). Paget cells often express cell markers that mimic those of the underlying breast carcinoma, including glandular epithelial cell markers (e.g., low-molecular-weight cytokeratins or cellular adhesion molecule CAM 5.2 that stains positive in 70% to 90% of the cases). Associated breast carcinomas are most commonly HER2 positive, with the luminal subtype being the most frequent (436).

Cytokeratin 7 is nearly a 100% sensitive marker for Paget disease; however, it is not a specific marker for Paget disease. As well as staining Paget cells, it may also stain intraepidermal Merkel cells and Toker cells; so, positive staining needs to be correlated with morphology when interpreting the appearances in a section (437). Cytokeratin 20, on the other hand, is negative in mammary Paget disease and positive in only 30% of cases in extramammary Paget disease.

A panel of Cytokeratin 7, GATA3, and HER2 will identify most cases, especially in those examples that are Cytokeratin7 negative (Figs. 29-114 to 29-116) (438).

The prevailing view is that most cases of mammary Paget disease originate from *in situ* or invasive ductal carcinoma. Both Paget cells and the underlying ductal carcinoma cells have been shown to be positive for the oncogene *HER2/neu.* Heregulin-α is thought to be a mobility factor that is produced and released by normal keratinocytes. Heregulin-α acts through the HER2/

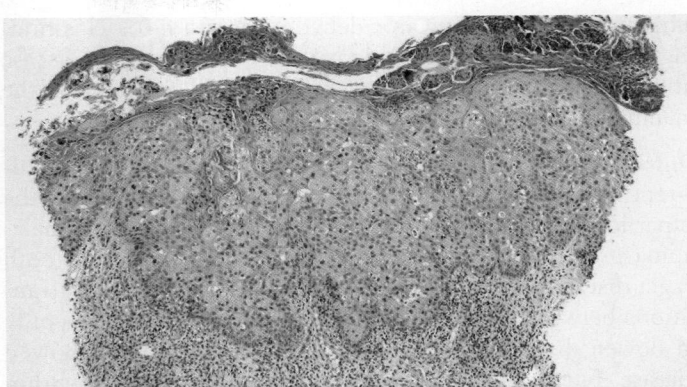

Figure 29-114 Paget disease. High magnification. Large rounded Paget cells with ample pale-staining cytoplasm consume the epidermis.

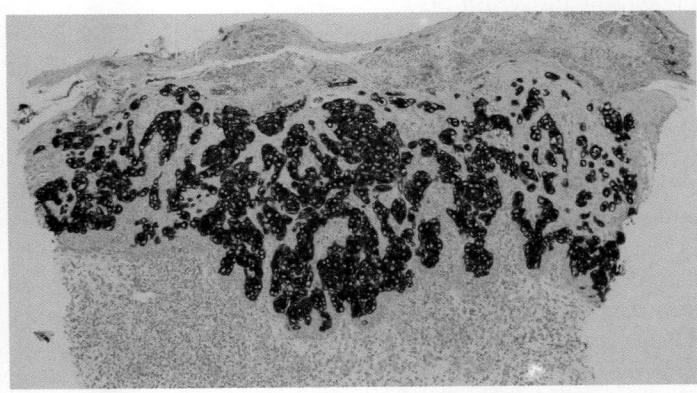

Figure 29-115 Paget disease. Cytokeratin 7-positive lesional cells infiltrate widely through the epidermis.

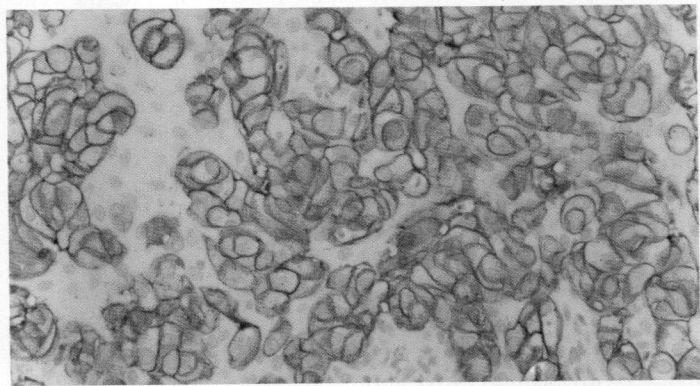

Figure 29-116 Paget disease. Her2–positive cells infiltrate the epidermis. This positivity is also likely to be present in any underlying breast tumor.

neu receptors on Paget cells forming a receptor complex on Paget cells, resulting in chemotaxis of the breast ductal cells and in turn migration and infiltration from the underlying ductal structures to the epidermis. This mobility factor is considered to play a significant role in the pathogenesis of Paget disease and explains, at least in part, the mechanism by which the Paget cells infiltrate and spread to the overlying epidermal layers of the nipple and adjacent areola (439).

Enzyme histochemistry in Paget disease of the breast has shown the presence of an apocrine enzymatic pattern in the intraepidermal Paget cells consisting of a strong reactivity for acid phosphatase and esterase and only a weakly positive reaction for aminopeptidase and succinic dehydrogenase (440). This finding suggests that the intraepidermal Paget cells in Paget disease of the breast are derived from mammary gland cells because the mammary gland represents a modified apocrine gland.

Differential Diagnosis. Paget disease of the breast must be differentiated from Bowen disease or pagetoid SCCIS and the superficial spreading or "Pagetoid" type of malignant melanoma *in situ.* Although vacuolated cells may occur in both Paget disease and Bowen disease, one observes clear-cut transitions between the vacuolated cells and epidermal cells only in Bowen disease. Furthermore, one may observe in Bowen disease, but not in Paget disease, clumping of nuclei within multinucleated epidermal cells and individual cell keratinization. In addition, the cells in Bowen disease do not contain CEA but react with prekeratin contained in rabbit antihuman prekeratin antiserum (441).

In the superficial spreading or Pagetoid type of malignant melanoma *in situ*—as in the epidermis of Paget disease of the breast—there are large, vacuolated cells scattered through the epidermis. The difficulty in distinguishing between the two types of cells may be increased by the fact that Paget cells occasionally also contain melanin. The most important points to remember in differentiating the two types of cells are as follows: (a) Paget cells are separated in many areas from the dermis by flattened basal cells, whereas melanoma cells border directly on the dermis. (b) Paget cells do not usually invade the dermis, whereas melanoma cells often do. (c) The tumor cells of malignant melanoma contain abundant cytoplasmic S-100 protein; but in tissues from Paget disease, S-100 protein is usually (not always) absent in the tumor cells, although it may be seen in myoepithelial cells, Langerhans cells, and Schwann cells of cutaneous nerves (442). (d) Finally, melanoma cells, unlike Paget cells, may be positive for the HMB-45 antigen, Melan-A, Sox10, and other melanocytic markers.

Principles of Management: The primary treatment for Paget disease is surgical and adjuvant treatment according to the nature and the stage of the underlying breast cancer. Modified radical mastectomy is considered the standard of care in the treatment of patients with mammary Paget disease (443,444). In some selected cases, it may be appropriate to offer conservative treatment with local excision of the nipple, wedge, or cone resection of the underlying breast, and radiation therapy. However, the recurrence rate is reported to be higher in those treated with a conservative approach in some studies (445,446).

EXTRAMAMMARY PAGET DISEASE

Clinical Summary. Extramammary Paget disease was recognized as an entity over a decade after Paget disease was first described. Both diseases show clinicopathologic similarities but show differences in their pathogenesis, association with underlying malignancy, and anatomic location. Paget disease is not a common disorder but should be considered in patients with a picture of chronic genital dermatitis (447). Extramammary Paget disease affects most commonly the vulva (142), less commonly the male genital area (448) or the perianal area, and, in exceptional cases, the axillae, the region of the ceruminal glands (449), or that of Moll glands (450). In cases with the involvement of axillae, the genital area may also be affected (451). Thus, extramammary

Paget disease involves areas in which apocrine glands are normally encountered. Only very few cases of an association between mammary and vulvar Paget disease have been described (452). Extramammary Paget disease may be a secondary event caused by extension of an adenocarcinoma of the rectum to the perianal region, of the cervix to the vulvar region (453), or of the urinary bladder to the urethra and glans penis (454) or to the groin (455). On the other hand, long-standing genital Paget disease can extend inward to the cervix and urinary tract (456). In perianal Paget disease, the underlying colorectal lesion may be an adenoma, with high-grade dysplasia or intramucosal adenocarcinoma (457). Primary Paget disease may also become invasive, with possible nodal metastasis (458).

In extramammary Paget disease, the clinical picture shows a slowly enlarging reddish patch with oozing and crusting. The patch resembles an eczematous lesion but has a sharp, irregular border. In extramammary Paget disease, in contrast to the mammary type, itching is common.

Histopathology. Extramammary Paget disease shares with Paget disease the presence of varying numbers of Paget cells within the epidermis. In some instances, the Paget cells are found to be limited to the epidermis. Frequently, Paget cells can also be identified within the epithelium of some hair follicles or eccrine sweat ducts (459). Such *in situ* malignancy associated with extramammary Paget disease has the same favorable prognosis as extramammary Paget disease limited to the epidermis. However, the prognosis is much more serious in cases in which the Paget cells have invaded the dermis from the epidermis (459,460) or from an underlying sweat gland carcinoma (461). In this respect, extramammary Paget disease differs from mammary Paget disease, in which an invasion of the dermis from the overlying epidermis does not occur (429). Glandular clusters with a central lumen, absent in mammary Paget disease, may be seen in the lower epidermis in extramammary Paget disease (459,462).

Immunohistochemical staining of both Paget and extramammary Paget disease is similar. The subtle differences that exist may indicate the different cell of origin in the two conditions (437). Typically in primary Paget disease, the Paget cells stain positively for cytokeratin 7, whereas in secondary cases the cells may be cytokeratin 20 positive (437).

In the case of "secondary" extramammary Paget disease, the process extends from a mucous-secreting adenocarcinoma of the rectum to the perianal skin (463,464), from a mucous-secreting endocervical carcinoma to the vulva (453), or from a transitional cell carcinoma of the urinary bladder with urethral extension (454,455). The prognosis in secondary extramammary Paget disease is poor.

The prognosis of "primary" extramammary Paget disease generally is better than that of mammary Paget disease. In two large, combined series of 123 patients with vulvar Paget disease, only 26 patients (21%) showed an underlying invasive carcinoma in the dermis at the time of operation (459,460). In the other 79%, the Paget cells were present only within the epidermis and the epithelium of the cutaneous appendages; so, the process was still *in situ.* Thus, one author observed only two examples of invasive sweat gland carcinoma among more than 100 cases of extramammary Paget disease (461), and another author reported none among 12 cases (435). However, the rate of local recurrence is high even after seemingly adequate excision. The reasons for this are that (a) the extent of histologically demonstrable disease is often far greater than that of the clinically visible lesion and (b) extramammary Paget disease, in contrast to mammary Paget disease, can arise multifocally even in clinically normal-appearing areas of the skin (465).

Pathogenesis. Earlier, the widely accepted view was that in primary extramammary Paget disease, the Paget cells in the epidermis are there as a result of an *in situ* upward extension of an *in situ* adenocarcinoma of sweat glands along eccrine or apocrine ducts (462,466). This view is analogous to the generally accepted views that secondary extramammary Paget disease represents an extension of a rectal, cervical, or urinary bladder adenocarcinoma and that the development of mammary Paget disease is an extension of an epidermotropic lactiferous duct carcinoma. The fact that an underlying *in situ* adenocarcinoma often could not be demonstrated was explained by the anatomic differences between the breast, which has only 20 large, conspicuous lactiferous ducts, and the genital skin, which has thousands of small apocrine and eccrine glands, making the location of the particular small gland involved by carcinoma technically difficult. Staining with antikeratin monoclonal antibodies indicated that an upward extension of an *in situ* adenocarcinoma derived from malignant secretory cells present within sweat ducts can occur (467).

Even though in some cases extramammary Paget disease is a result of the extension of an underlying apocrine or eccrine sweat gland carcinoma to the overlying epidermis, in most instances it has its origin within the epidermis (460). Careful subserial total sectioning of excised lesions of vulvar Paget disease showed that the lesions within the epidermis and its appendages have a multifocal origin (465). Another pertinent argument in favor of the independence of the epidermal foci from any appendageal foci is the observation that in cases with extensive epidermal lesions, the involvement of eccrine ducts and glands is often sparse and the involvement of apocrine ducts and glands almost invariably absent, even though some Paget cells form apocrine glandular structures in the epidermis (459). Even if there is continuity between the epidermal and the ductal foci, there is no certain way of determining whether the extension is in an upward or downward direction. However, the clinching argument in favor of the autonomy of the epidermal foci in primary extramammary Paget disease is the fact that, in contrast to mammary Paget disease, dermal invasion generally originates from the epidermis and not ductal or glandular structures (459,460).

In cases in which the extramammary Paget disease arises within the epidermis and extends from there at a later date into the adnexa and still later from the epidermis into the dermis, the question is, which cell gives rise to the Paget cell? Two possibilities have been suggested, although proof for either is lacking. The first is that the Paget cell arises within the poral portion of an apocrine duct (468). The second is that because the disease tends to occur in areas rich in apocrine glands and because there is in some cases unequivocal evidence of apocrine differentiation in the epidermis, intraepidermal Paget cells may be formed by pluripotential germinative cells within the epidermis that go awry trying to form apocrine structures (441,459,469,470).

Immunohistochemical studies indicate an apocrine genesis of extramammary Paget disease. It is true that CEA merely indicates that the extramammary Paget cells are glandular rather than epidermal cells and does not decide whether they are apocrine or eccrine (434,441). However, two immunoreactants for apocrine glands—GCDFP15 (471) and apocrine epithelial antigen (435)—have been shown to react with the Paget cells of extramammary Paget disease, providing evidence for an apocrine pattern of differentiation.

The majority of cases of mammary and extramammary Paget disease are cytokeratin 7 positive. Those few cases that are negative have been reported to be more commonly associated with the presence of an underlying malignancy. In contrast, cytokeratin 20 is found more frequently in cases of extramammary Paget disease with an underlying malignancy. The pattern of cytokeratin expression can therefore be used to predict the likelihood of the presence or absence of an associated internal malignancy (437).

For working up a tumor with intraepidermal atypia in a site of predilection for extramammary Paget disease (e.g., the groin, perineum, and axillae), a screening panel of immunohistochemical markers that can include melanocytic markers such as S100, Melan-A, HMB-45, high-molecular-weight cytokeratins such as 34βE12 or pankeratins such as AE1/3, MNF116 or OSCAR, CEA, and/or GATA3 as markers of glandular differentiation, low-molecular-weight cytokeratins such as Cam5.2 and/or CK7, CK20 for perianal disease, and p63 can be considered to fully characterize the lesion.

Differential Diagnosis. Extramammary Paget disease, see Paget Disease of the Breast section, must be differentiated from Bowen disease and especially from superficial spreading or pagetoid malignant melanoma *in situ* (see Paget Disease section and *Differential Diagnosis*).

Principles of Management: Surgical excision is the preferred treatment, in particular, Mohs micrographic surgery, where margin-controlled surgery is performed. Complete excision, even with Mohs, is a surgical challenge owing to the microscopic and multifocal nature of the disease. Nevertheless, recurrence rates after excisions of primary tumors with Mohs micrographic surgery are lower than with standard wide local excisions at 8% to 26% and 30% to 60%, respectively (447,472,473). When surgical excision is a challenge or contraindicated, topical treatments with 5-fluorouracil and 5% imiquimod cream have been described (474–476). Close follow-up every 3 months and for 2 years postsurgical excision is the standard. Thorough examination and investigations for underlying malignancy with clinical examination, imaging, and endoscopies are essential.

ACKNOWLEDGMENTS

We thank the late Prof. Neil Cox for Figures 29-1, 29-2, 29-11, 29-16, 29-18, 29-44, 29-48, 29-54, 29-57, 29-63, 29-79, 28-107, and 29-108; Dr. Phil Hampton for Figure 29-84; Dr. James Langtry for Figures 29-10, 29-29, 29-22, 29-25, 29-30, 29-31, 29-33, 29-43, 29-80, 29-81, 29-82, and 29-83; the late Dr. Janet McLelland for Figures 29-61 and 29-62; Dr. Tom Oliphant for Figure 29-64; and Dr. Akhtar Husain for Figure 29-71.

REFERENCES

1. Elder DE, Massi D, Scolyer RA, Willemze R, eds. *WHO Classification of Skin Tumours.* 4th ed. International Agency for Research on Cancer; 2018.

2. Keohane SG, Proby CM, Newlands C, et al. The new 8th edition of TNM staging and its implications for skin cancer: a review by the British Association of Dermatologists and the Royal College of Pathologists, U.K. *Br J Dermatol.* 2018;179(4):824–828.

3. Motley R, Kersey P, Lawrence C. Multiprofessional guidelines for the management of the patient with primary cutaneous squamous cell carcinoma. *Br J Dermatol.* 2002;146(1):18–25.

4. Telfer NR, Colver GB, Morton CA. Guidelines for the management of basal cell carcinoma. *Br J Dermatol.* 2008;159(1):35–48.

5. Cox NH, Eedy DJ, Morton CA. Guidelines for management of Bowen's disease: 2006 update. *Br J Dermatol.* 2007;156(1):11–21.

6. Marsden JR, Newton-Bishop JA, Burrows L, et al. Revised UK guidelines for the management of cutaneous melanoma 2010. *J Plast Reconstr Aesthet Surg.* 2010;63(9):1401–1419.

7. Keohane SG, Botting J, Budny PG, et al. British Association of Dermatologists guidelines for the management of people with cutaneous squamous cell carcinoma 2020. *Br J Dermatol.* 2021;184(3):401–414.

8. Leibovitch I, Huilgol SC, Selva D, Richards S, Paver R. Basosquamous carcinoma: treatment with Mohs micrographic surgery. *Cancer.* 2005;104(1):170–175.

9. Motley R, Arron S. Mohs micrographic surgery for cutaneous squamous cell carcinoma. *Br J Dermatol.* 2019;181(2):233–234.

10. Ferry AM, Sarrami SM, Hollier PC, Gerich CF, Thornton JF. Treatment of non-melanoma skin cancers in the absence of Mohs micrographic surgery. *Plast Reconstr Surg Glob Open.* 2020;8(12):e3300.

11. Fidelis MC, Stelini RF, Staffa LP, Moraes AM, Magalhães RF. Basal cell carcinoma with compromised margins: retrospective study of management, evolution, and prognosis. *An Bras Dermatol.* 2021;96(1):17–26.

12. Lee SH, Rogers M. Inflammatory linear verrucous epidermal naevi: a review of 23 cases. *Australas J Dermatol.* 2001;42(4):252–256.

13. Miteva LG, Dourmishev AL, Schwartz RA. Inflammatory linear verrucous epidermal nevus. *Cutis.* 2001;68(5):327–330.

14. Tanita K, Fujimura T, Sato Y, Lyu C, Aiba S. Widely spread unilateral inflammatory linear verrucous epidermal nevus (ILVEN). *Case Rep Dermatol.* 2018;10(2):170–175.

15. Lee CH, Hsiao CH, Chiu HC, Tsai TF. Acantholytic dyskeratotic epidermal nevus. *Indian J Dermatol Venereol Leprol.* 2011;77(2):253.

16. Baykal C, Buyukbabani N, Kavak A, Alper M. Nevoid hyperkeratosis of the nipple and areola: a distinct entity. *J Am Acad Dermatol.* 2002;46(3):414–418.

17. Higgins HW, Jenkins J, Horn TD, Kroumpouzos G. Pregnancy-associated hyperkeratosis of the nipple: a report of 25 cases. *JAMA Dermatol.* 2013;149(6):722–726.

18. Agulló-Pérez AD, Resano-Abarzuza M, Córdoba-Iturriagagoitia A, Yanguas-Bayona JI. Porokeratotic eccrine and hair follicle nevus: a report of two cases and review of the literature. *An Bras Dermatol.* 2017;92(5, suppl 1):121–125.

19. Hijazi MM, Succaria F, Ghosn S. Multiple localized epidermolytic acanthomas of the vulva associated with vulvar pruritus: a case report. *Am J Dermatopathol.* 2015;37(4):e49–52.

20. Moulonguet I, Serre M, Herskovitch D. [Multiple epidermolytic acanthomas of the genitalia]. *Ann Dermatol Venereol.* 2017;144(4):295–300.

21. Abbas O, Wieland CN, Goldberg LJ. Solitary epidermolytic acanthoma: a clinical and histopathological study. *J Eur Acad Dermatol Venereol.* 2011;25(2):175–180.

22. Mahaisavariya P, Cohen PR, Rapini RP. Incidental epidermolytic hyperkeratosis. *Am J Dermatopathol.* 1995;17(1):23–28.

23. Hutcheson AC, Nietert PJ, Maize JC. Incidental epidermolytic hyperkeratosis and focal acantholytic dyskeratosis in common acquired melanocytic nevi and atypical melanocytic lesions. *J Am Acad Dermatol.* 2004;50(3):388–390.

24. Conlin PA, Rapini RP. Epidermolytic hyperkeratosis associated with melanocytic nevi: a report of 53 cases. *Am J Dermatopathol.* 2002;24(1):23–25.

25. Chung HC, Lee JW, Bak H, Ahn SK. Incidental focal epidermolytic hyperkeratosis in rosacea. *J Dermatol.* 2017;44(6):722–723.

26. Steele CL, Shea CR, Petronic-Rosic V. Epidermolytic hyperkeratosis within infundibular cysts. *J Cutan Pathol.* 2007;34(4):360–362.

27. Gaertner EM. Incidental cutaneous reaction patterns: epidermolytic hyperkeratosis, acantholytic dyskeratosis, and Hailey-Hailey-like acantholysis: a potential marker of premalignant skin change. *J Skin Cancer.* 2011;2011:645743.

28. Goldenberg A, Lee RA, Cohen PR. Acantholytic dyskeratotic acanthoma: case report and review of the literature. *Dermatol Pract Concept.* 2014;4(3):25–30.

29. Bürgler C, Schlapbach C, Feldmeyer L, Haneke E. Multiple acantholytic dyskeratotic acanthomas in an organ transplant recipient. *JAAD Case Rep.* 2018;4(7):695–697.

30. Ko CJ, Barr RJ, Subtil A, McNiff JM. Acantholytic dyskeratotic acanthoma: a variant of a benign keratosis. *J Cutan Pathol.* 2008;35(3):298–301.

31. Kim HR, Lim SK, Lee HE, et al. Incidental focal acantholytic dyskeratosis in a patient with discoid lupus erythematosus: a possible role for SPCA1 in the pathogenesis of the disease. *Ann Dermatol.* 2017;29(5):655–657.

32. Park SY, Lee HJ, Shin JY, Ahn SK. Incidental focal acantholytic dyskeratosis in the setting of rosacea. *Ann Dermatol.* 2013;25(4):518–520.

33. Bogle MA, Cohen PR, Tschen JA. Trichofolliculoma with incidental focal acantholytic dyskeratosis. *South Med J.* 2004;97(8):773–775.

34. DiMaio DJ, Cohen PR. Incidental focal acantholytic dyskeratosis. *J Am Acad Dermatol.* 1998;38(2, pt 1):243–247.

35. Gambichler T, Rapp S, Sauermann K, Jansen T, Hoffmann K, Altmeyer P. Uncommon vascular naevi associated with focal acantholytic dyskeratosis. *Clin Exp Dermatol.* 2002;27(3):195–198.

36. Cannon AB. White sponge nevus of the mucosa: naevus spongiosus albus mucosae. *Arch Derm Syphilol.* 1935;31:365.

37. Sobhan M, Alirezaei P, Farshchian M, Eshghi G, Ghasemi Basir HR, Khezrian L. White sponge nevus: report of a case and review of the literature. *Acta Med Iran.* 2017;55(8):533–535.

38. Elfatoiki FZ, Capatas S, Skali HD, Hali F, Attar H, Chiheb S. Oral white sponge nevus: an exceptional differential diagnosis in childhood. *Case Rep Dermatol Med.* 2020;2020:9296768.

39. Kürklü E, Öztürk Ş, Cassidy AJ, et al. Clinical features and molecular genetic analysis in a Turkish family with oral white sponge nevus. *Med Oral Patol Oral Cir Bucal.* 2018;23(2):e144–e150.

40. Westin M, Rekabdar E, Blomstrand L, Klintberg P, Jontell M, Robledo-Sierra J. Mutations in the genes for keratin-4 and keratin-13 in Swedish patients with white sponge nevus. *J Oral Pathol Med.* 2018;47(2):152–157.

41. Terrinoni A, Rugg EL, Lane EB, et al. A novel mutation in the keratin 13 gene causing oral white sponge nevus. *J Dent Res.* 2001;80(3):919–923.

42. Cai W, Jiang B, Yu F, et al. Current approaches to the diagnosis and treatment of white sponge nevus. *Expert Rev Mol Med.* 2015;17:e9.

43. Martin JL. Leukoedema: a review of the literature. *J Natl Med Assoc.* 1992;84(11):938–940.

44. Gorsky M, Epstein JB, Levi H, Yarom N. Oral white lesions associated with chewing khat. *Tob Induc Dis.* 2004;2(3):145–150.

45. Huang BW, Lin CW, Lee YP, Chiang CP. Differential diagnosis between leukoedema and white spongy nevus. *J Dent Sci.* 2020;15(4):554–555.

46. Mittermüller P, Hiller KA, Schmalz G, Buchalla W. Five hundred patients reporting on adverse effects from dental materials: frequencies, complaints, symptoms, allergies. *Dent Mater.* 2018;34(12):1756–1768.

47. Neville BW, Damm DD, Allan CM. *Oral and Maxillofacial Pathology.* 2nd ed. WB Saunders; 2002.

48. Assimakopoulos D, Patrikakos G, Fotika C, Elisaf M. Benign migratory glossitis or geographic tongue: an enigmatic oral lesion. *Am J Med.* 2002;113(9):751–755.

49. Wollina U. Recent advances in managing and understanding seborrheic keratosis. *F1000Res.* 2019;8:F1000 Faculty Rev-1520.

50. Karadag AS, Parish LC. The status of the seborrheic keratosis. *Clin Dermatol.* 2018;36(2):275–277.

51. Jackson JM, Alexis A, Berman B, Berson DS, Taylor S, Weiss JS. Current understanding of seborrheic keratosis: prevalence, etiology, clinical presentation, diagnosis, and management. *J Drugs Dermatol.* 2015;14(10):1119–1125.

52. Minagawa A. Dermoscopy-pathology relationship in seborrheic keratosis. *J Dermatol.* 2017;44(5):518–524.

53. Heidenreich B, Denisova E, Rachakonda S, et al. Genetic alterations in seborrheic keratoses. *Oncotarget.* 2017;8(22):36639–36649.

54. Bahrani E, Sitthinamsuwan P, McCalmont TH, Pincus LB. Ki-67 and p16 immunostaining differentiates pagetoid Bowen disease from "microclonal" seborrheic keratosis. *Am J Clin Pathol.* 2019;151(6):551–560.

55. King R, Page RN, Googe PB. Desmoplastic seborrheic keratosis. *Am J Dermatopathol.* 2003;25(3):210–214.

56. Laidlaw GF. Melanoma studies. I. The dopa reaction in general pathology. *Am J Pathol.* 1932;8(5):477–490.

57. Jain S, Barman KD, Garg VK, Sharma S, Dewan S, Mahajan N. Multifocal cutaneous melanoacanthoma with ulceration: a case report with review of literature. *Indian J Dermatol Venereol Leprol.* 2011;77(6):699–702.

58. Yarom N, Hirshberg A, Buchner A. Solitary and multifocal oral melanoacanthoma. *Int J Dermatol.* 2007;46(12):1232–1236.

59. Gutierrez N, Erickson CP, Calame A, Sateesh BR, Cohen PR. Melanoacanthoma masquerading as melanoma: case reports and literature review. *Cureus.* 2019;11(6):e4998.

60. Rosebush MS, Briody AN, Cordell KG. Black and brown: non-neoplastic pigmentation of the oral mucosa. *Head Neck Pathol.* 2019;13(1):47–55.

61. Cantudo-Sanagustín E, Gutiérrez-Corrales A, Vigo-Martínez M, Serrera-Figallo M, Torres-Lagares D, Gutiérrez-Pérez JL. Pathogenesis and clinicohistopathological caractheristics of melanoacanthoma: a systematic review. *J Clin Exp Dent.* 2016;8(3):e327–e336.

62. Tandon A, Srivastava A, Jaiswal R, Bordoloi B. A rare case of oral melanoacanthoma. *J Oral Maxillofac Pathol.* 2018;22(3):410–412.

63. Lupo MP. Dermatosis papulosis nigra: treatment options. *J Drugs Dermatol.* 2007;6(1):29–30.

64. Kocsard E, Carter JJ. The papillomatous keratoses. The nature and differential diagnosis of stucco keratosis. *Australas J Dermatol.* 1971;12(2):80–88.

65. Stockfleth E, Rowert J, Arndt R, Christophers E, Meyer T. Detection of human papillomavirus and response to topical 5% imiquimod in a case of stucco keratosis. *Br J Dermatol.* 2000;143(4):846–850.

66. Hafner C, Landthaler M, Mentzel T, Vogt T. FGFR3 and PIK3CA mutations in stucco keratosis and dermatosis papulosa nigra. *Br J Dermatol.* 2010;162(3):508–512.

67. André R, Laffitte E, Abosaleh M, Cortès B, Toutous-Trellu L, Kaya G. Sign of Leser-Trélat and cutaneous T-cell lymphoma: a rare association. *Dermatopathology (Basel).* 2018;5(2):69–73.

68. Wick MR, Patterson JW. Cutaneous paraneoplastic syndromes. *Semin Diagn Pathol.* 2019;36(4):211–228.

69. Husain Z, Ho JK, Hantash BM. Sign and pseudo-sign of Leser-Trélat: case reports and a review of the literature. *J Drugs Dermatol.* 2013;12(5):e79–e87.

70. Mehregan DR, Hamzavi F, Brown K. Large cell acanthoma. *Int J Dermatol.* 2003;42(1):36–39.

71. Huther M, Cribier B. [Anatomoclinical study of large-cell acanthoma]. *Ann Dermatol Venereol.* 2016;143(2):118–123.

72. Fraga GR, Amin SM. Large cell acanthoma: a variant of solar lentigo with cellular hypertrophy. *J Cutan Pathol.* 2014;41(9):733–739.

73. Jakobiec FA, Mendoza PR, Colby KA. Clinicopathologic and immunohistochemical studies of conjunctival large cell acanthoma, epidermoid dysplasia, and squamous papilloma. *Am J Ophthalmol.* 2013;156(4):830–846.

74. Jakobiec FA, Cortes Barrantes P, Ma L, Mandeville J. Large cell acanthoma of the conjunctiva: clinicopathologic and immunohistochemical features. *Ocul Oncol Pathol.* 2019;5(5):312–318.

75. Degos R, Civatte J. Clear-cell acanthoma. Experience of 8 years. *Br J Dermatol.* 1970;83(2):248–254.

76. Usmani A, Qasim S. Clear cell acanthoma: a review of clinical and histologic variants. *Dermatopathology (Basel).* 2020;7(2):26–37.

77. Tempark T, Shwayder T. Clear cell acanthoma. *Clin Exp Dermatol.* 2012;37(8):831–837.

78. González-Guerra E, Rodriguez JR, Casado AF, Taboada AC, Toro JAC, Bran EL. Bilateral clear cell acanthoma of the areola and nipple: good response to topical corticosteroids. *An Bras Dermatol.* 2017;92(5, suppl 1):27–29.

79. Kuo KL, Lo CS, Lee LY, Yang CH, Kuo TT. Clear cell acanthoma (CCA)-like lesions of the nipple/areola: a clinicopathological study of 12 cases supporting a nonneoplastic eczematous disease. *J Am Acad Dermatol.* 2019;80(3):749–755.

80. Borda LJ, Mervis JS, Romanelli P, Lev-Tov H. Clear cell acanthoma on the areola. *Dermatol Online J.* 2018;24(7):13030/qt9q47d056.

81. Argyris PP, Ho D, Nelson AC, Koutlas IG. Pale (clear) cell acanthoma of the palate. *Head Neck Pathol.* 2020;14(2):535–541.

82. Zhou S, Qiao J, Bai J, et al. Multiple eruptive clear cell acanthoma. *Indian J Dermatol.* 2018;63(2):190–192.

83. Shet T, Desai S. Pigmented epidermal cysts. *Am J Dermatopathol.* 2001;23(5):477–481.

84. Hardin J, Gardner JM, Colome MI, Chevez-Barrios P. Verrucous cyst with melanocytic and sebaceous differentiation: a case report and review of the literature. *Arch Pathol Lab Med.* 2013;137(4):576–579.

85. Cotton DW, Kirkham N, Young BJ. Immunoperoxidase anti-keratin staining of epidermal and pilar cysts. *Br J Dermatol.* 1984;111(1):63–68.

86. Bridges AG, Erickson LA. Co-occurrence of steatocystoma multiplex, eruptive vellus hair cysts, and trichofolliculomas. *Cutis.* 2017;100(1):E23-e26.

87. Yang L, Zhang S, Wang G. Keratin 17 in disease pathogenesis: from cancer to dermatoses. *J Pathol.* 2019;247(2):158–165.

88. Zhang B, Sun L, Fu X, Yu G, Liu H, Zhang F. Mutation analysis of the KRT17 gene in steatocystoma multiplex and a brief literature review. *Clin Exp Dermatol.* 2020;45(1):132–134.

89. Sandoval R, Urbina F. Pigmented follicular cyst. *Br J Dermatol.* 1994;131(1):130–131.

90. Requena Caballero L, Sánchez Yus E. Pigmented follicular cyst. *J Am Acad Dermatol.* 1989;21(5 Pt 2):1073–1075.

91. Pinkus H. The pathogenesis of milia and benign tumors of the skin. *J Invest Dermatol.* 1956;26:10.

92. Ambiavagar PC, Rosen Y. Cutaneous ciliated cyst of the chin. Probable bronchogenic cyst. *Arch Dermatol.* 1979;115(7):895–896.

93. van der Putte SC, Toonstra J. Cutaneous "bronchogenic" cyst. *J Cutan Pathol.* 1985;12(5):404–409.

94. Sidoni A, Bucciarelli E. Ciliated cyst of the perineal skin. *Am J Dermatopathol.* 1997;19(1):93–96.

95. Syed MMA, Amatya B, Sitaula S. Median raphe cyst of the penis: a case report and review of the literature. *J Med Case Rep.* 2019;13(1):214.

96. Navalón-Monllor V, Ordoño-Saiz MV, Ordoño-Domínguez F, Sabater-Marco V, Pallás-Costa Y, Navalón-Verdejo P. Median raphe cysts in men. Presentation of our experience and literature review. *Actas Urol Esp.* 2017;41(3):205–209.

97. Navarro HP, Lopez PC, Ruiz JM, et al. Median raphe cyst. Report of two cases and literature review. *Arch Esp Urol.* 2009;62(7):585–589.

98. Esterly NB, Fretzin DF, Pinkus H. Eruptive vellus hair cysts. *Arch Dermatol.* 1977;113(4):500–503.

99. Torchia D, Vega J, Schachner LA. Eruptive vellus hair cysts: a systematic review. *Am J Clin Dermatol.* 2012;13(1):19–28.

100. Szymanski FJ. Warty dyskeratoma; a benign cutaneous tumor resembling Darier's disease microscopically. *AMA Arch Derm.* 1957;75(4):567–572.

101. Kaddu S, Dong H, Mayer G, Kerl H, Cerroni L. Warty dyskeratoma—"follicular dyskeratoma": analysis of clinicopathologic features of a distinctive follicular adnexal neoplasm. *J Am Acad Dermatol.* 2002;47(3):423–428.

102. Ghasemi Basir HR, Alirezaei P, Ebrahimi B, Khanali S. Oral warty dyskeratoma: an unusual presentation. *Dermatol Reports.* 2020;12(1):8236.

103. Reinehr CPH, Bakos RM. Actinic keratoses: review of clinical, dermoscopic, and therapeutic aspects. *An Bras Dermatol.* 2019;94(6):637–657.

104. Siegel JA, Korgavkar K, Weinstock MA. Current perspective on actinic keratosis: a review. *Br J Dermatol.* 2017;177(2):350–358.

105. Schwartz RA, Bridges TM, Butani AK, Ehrlich A. Actinic keratosis: an occupational and environmental disorder. *J Eur Acad Dermatol Venereol.* 2008;22(5):606–615.

106. Hedberg M, Seykora JT. Clarifying progress on the genomic landscape of actinic keratosis. *J Invest Dermatol.* 2021;141(7):1622–1624.

107. Fleming P, Zhou S, Bobotsis R, Lynde C. Comparison of the treatment guidelines for actinic keratosis: a critical appraisal and review. *J Cutan Med Surg.* 2017;21(5):408–417.

108. Szeimies RM, Karrer S, Radakovic-Fijan S, et al. Photodynamic therapy using topical methyl 5-aminolevulinate compared with cryotherapy for actinic keratosis: a prospective, randomized study. *J Am Acad Dermatol.* 2002;47(2):258–262.

109. Szeimies RM, Karrer S, Backer H. [Therapeutic options for epithelial skin tumors. Actinic keratoses, Bowen disease, squamous cell carcinoma, and basal cell carcinoma]. *Hautarzt.* 2005;56(5):430–440.

110. Freeman M, Vinciullo C, Francis D, et al. A comparison of photodynamic therapy using topical methyl aminolevulinate (Metvix) with single cycle cryotherapy in patients with actinic keratosis: a prospective, randomized study. *J Dermatolog Treat.* 2003;14(2):99–106.

111. Al-Zacko SM, Mohammad AS. Cutaneous horn arising from a burn scar: a case report and review of literature. *J Burn Care Res.* 2018;39(1):168–170.

112. Shahi S, Bhandari TR, Pantha T. Verrucous carcinoma in a giant cutaneous horn: a case report and literature review. *Case Rep Otolaryngol.* 2020;2020:7134789.

113. Loning T, Ikenberg H, Becker J, Gissmann L, Hoepfer I, zur Hausen H. Analysis of oral papillomas, leukoplakias, and invasive carcinomas for human papillomavirus type related DNA. *J Invest Dermatol.* 1985;84(5):417–420.

114. Lee JJ, Hong WK, Hittelman WN, et al. Predicting cancer development in oral leukoplakia: ten years of translational research. *Clin Cancer Res.* 2000;6(5):1702–1710.

115. Woo SB. Oral epithelial dysplasia and premalignancy. *Head Neck Pathol.* 2019;13(3):423–439.

116. van der Hem PS, Nauta JM, van der Wal JE, Roodenburg JL. The results of CO2 laser surgery in patients with oral leukoplakia: a 25 year follow up. *Oral Oncol.* 2005;41(1):31–37.

117. Shafer WG, Waldron CA. Erythroplakia of the oral cavity. *Cancer.* 1975;36(3):1021–1028.

118. Holmstrup P, Dabelsteen E. Oral leukoplakia-to treat or not to treat. *Oral Dis.* 2016;22(6):494–497.

119. van der Waal I. Potentially malignant disorders of the oral and oropharyngeal mucosa; terminology, classification and present concepts of management. *Oral Oncol.* 2009;45(4–5):317–323.

120. Müller S. Oral epithelial dysplasia, atypical verrucous lesions and oral potentially malignant disorders: focus on histopathology. *Oral Surg Oral Med Oral Pathol Oral Radiol.* 2018;125(6):591–602.

121. Akrish S, Eskander-Hashoul L, Rachmiel A, Ben-Izhak O. Clinicopathologic analysis of verrucous hyperplasia, verrucous carcinoma and squamous cell carcinoma as part of the clinicopathologic spectrum of oral proliferative verrucous leukoplakia: a literature review and analysis. *Pathol Res Pract.* 2019;215(12):152670.

122. Shah AM, Bansal S, Shirsat PM, Prasad P, Desai RS. Exophytic verrucous hyperplasia in oral submucous fibrosis: a single-center study. *J Oral Maxillofac Pathol.* 2019;23(3):393–399.

123. Davidova LA, Fitzpatrick SG, Bhattacharyya I, Cohen DM, Islam MN. Lichenoid characteristics in premalignant verrucous lesions and verrucous carcinoma of the oral cavity. *Head Neck Pathol.* 2019;13(4):573–579.

124. Müller S. Oral lichenoid lesions: distinguishing the benign from the deadly. *Mod Pathol.* 2017;30(s1):S54-s67.

125. Walvekar RR, Chaukar DA, Deshpande MS, et al. Verrucous carcinoma of the oral cavity: a clinical and pathological study of 101 cases. *Oral Oncol.* 2009;45(1):47–51.

126. Didona D, Paolino G, Donati M, Didona B, Calvieri S. Eosinophilic ulcer of the tongue—case report. *An Bras Dermatol.* 2015;90(3, suppl 1):88–90.

127. Sah K, Chandra S, Singh A, Singh S. Eosinophilic ulcer of the tongue masquerading as malignant ulcer: an unexplored distinct pathology. *J Oral Maxillofac Pathol.* 2017;21(2):321.

128. Abdel-Naser MB, Tsatsou F, Hippe S, et al. Oral eosinophilic ulcer, an Epstein-Barr virus-associated CD30+ lymphoproliferation? *Dermatology.* 2011;222(2):113–118.

129. Idriss MH, Misri R, Böer-Auer A. Orthokeratotic Bowen disease: a histopathologic, immunohistochemical and molecular study. *J Cutan Pathol.* 2016;43(1):24–31.

130. Riethdorf S, Neffen EF, Cviko A, Löning T, Crum CP, Riethdorf L. p16INK4A expression as biomarker for HPV 16-related vulvar neoplasias. *Hum Pathol.* 2004;35(12):1477–1483.

131. Kao GF. Carcinoma arising in Bowen's disease. *Arch Dermatol.* 1986;122(10):1124–1126.

132. Graham JH, Helwig EB. Bowen's disease and its relationship to systemic cancer. *AMA Arch Derm.* 1959;80(2):133–159.

133. Ackerman AB. Reply to Mascaro JM: bowenoid papulosis. *J Am Acad Dermatol.* 1981;4:608.

134. Kogame T, Tanimura H, Nakamaru S, Makimura K, Okamoto H, Kiyohara T. Spindle cell squamous cell carcinoma arising in Bowen's disease: case report and review of the published work. *J Dermatol.* 2017;44(9):1055–1058.

135. Bath-Hextall FJ, Matin RN, Wilkinson D, Leonardi-Bee J. Interventions for cutaneous Bowen's disease. *Cochrane Database Syst Rev.* 2013;6:CD007281.

136. Queyrat L. Erythroplasie du gland. *Bull Soc Fr Dermatol Syphiligr.* 1911;22:378.

137. Wieland U, Jurk S, Weissenborn S, Krieg T, Pfister H, Ritzkowsky A. Erythroplasia of Queyrat: coinfection with cutaneous carcinogenic human papillomavirus type 8 and genital papillomaviruses in a carcinoma in situ. *J Invest Dermatol.* 2000;115(3):396–401.

138. Nasca MR, Potenza MC, Alessi L, Paravizzini G, Micali G. Absence of PCR-detectable human papilloma virus in erythroplasia of Queyrat using a comparative control group. *Sex Transm Infect.* 2010;86(3):199–201.

139. Arlette JP. Treatment of Bowen's disease and erythroplasia of Queyrat. *Br J Dermatol.* 2003;149(suppl 66):43–49.

140. Zoon JJ. Chronic benign circumscript plasmocytic balanoposthitis. *Dermatologica.* 1952;105(1):1–7.

141. Mallon E, Hawkins D, Dinneen M, et al. Circumcision and genital dermatoses. *Arch Dermatol.* 2000;136(3):350–354.

142. Fox H, Wells M. Recent advances in the pathology of the vulva. *Histopathology.* 2003;42(3):209–216.

143. Pepas L, Kaushik S, Bryant A, Nordin A, Dickinson HO. Medical interventions for high grade vulval intraepithelial neoplasia. *Cochrane Database Syst Rev.* 2011(4):CD007924.

144. Bryan S, Barbara C, Thomas J, Olaitan A. HPV vaccine in the treatment of usual type vulval and vaginal intraepithelial neoplasia: a systematic review. *BMC Womens Health.* 2019;19(1):3.

145. Montgomery H. Arsenic as an etiologic agent in certain types of epithelioma. *Arch Derm Syphilol.* 1935;32:218.

146. Hinojosa JA, Williams CL, Vandergriff T, Le LQ. Arsenical keratosis secondary to Fowler solution. *JAAD Case Rep.* 2018;4(1):72–74.

147. Mazumder DN, Das GJ, Chakraborty AK, Chatterjee A, Das D, Chakraborti D. Environmental pollution and chronic arsenicosis in south Calcutta. *Bull World Health Organ.* 1992;70(4):481–485.

148. Das D, Chatterjee A, Mandal BK, Samanta G, Chakraborti D, Chanda B. Arsenic in ground water in six districts of West Bengal, India: the biggest arsenic calamity in the world. Part 2. Arsenic concentration in drinking water, hair, nails, urine, skin-scale and liver tissue (biopsy) of the affected people. *Analyst.* 1995;120(3):917–924.

149. Ruiz de Luzuriaga AM, Ahsan H, Shea CR. Arsenical keratoses in Bangladesh—update and prevention strategies. *Dermatol Clin.* 2011;29(1):45–51.

150. Fierz U. Follow-up studies of the side-effects of the treatment of skin diseases with inorganic arsenic. *Dermatologica.* 1965;131(1):41–58.

151. Yeh S. Skin cancer in chronic arsenicism. *Hum Pathol.* 1973;4(4):469–485.

152. Srinivas N, Rachakonda S, Hielscher T, et al. Telomere length, arsenic exposure and risk of basal cell carcinoma of skin. *Carcinogenesis.* 2019;40(6):715–723.

153. Neubauer O. Arsenical cancer; a review. *Br J Cancer.* 1947;1(2):192–251.

154. Sommers SC, McManus RG. Multiple arsenical cancers of skin and internal organs. *Cancer.* 1953;6(2):347–359.

155. Roth F. Chronic arsenic poisoning of Moselle vineyard-workers, with special reference to arsenic cancer. *Z Krebsforsch.* 1956;61(3):287–319.

156. Miki Y, Kawatsu T, Matsuda K, Machino H, Kubo K. Cutaneous and pulmonary cancers associated with Bowen's disease. *J Am Acad Dermatol.* 1982;6(1):26–31.

157. Peterka ES, Lynch FW, Goltz RW. An association between Bowen's disease and internal cancer. *Arch Dermatol.* 1961;84:623–629.

158. Andersen SL, Nielsen A, Reymann F. Relationship between Bowen disease and internal malignant tumors. *Arch Dermatol.* 1973;108(3):367–370.

159. Callen JP, Headington J. Bowen's and non-Bowen's squamous intraepidermal neoplasia of the skin. Relationship to internal malignancy. *Arch Dermatol.* 1980;116(4):422–426.

160. Montgomery H, Waisman M. Epithelioma attributable to arsenic. *J Invest Dermatol.* 1941;4:365.

161. Ehlers G. Clinical and histological studies on the problem of drug-induced arsenic tumors. *Z Haut Geschlechtskr.* 1968;43(18):763–774.

162. Hundeiker M, Petres J. Morphogenesis and variety of precancerous lesions induced by arsenic. *Arch Klin Exp Dermatol.* 1968;231(4):355–365.

163. Jung EG, Trachsel B. Molecular biology of arsenic carcinogenesis. *Arch Klin Exp Dermatol.* 1970;237(3):819–826.

164. Wong SS, Tan KC, Goh CL. Cutaneous manifestations of chronic arsenicism: review of seventeen cases. *J Am Acad Dermatol.* 1998;38(2, pt 1):179–185.

165. Bazaliński D, Przybek-Mita J, Barańska B, Więch P. Marjolin's ulcer in chronic wounds—review of available literature. *Contemp Oncol (Pozn).* 2017;21(3):197–202.

166. Chalya PL, Mabula JB, Rambau P, et al. Marjolin's ulcers at a university teaching hospital in Northwestern Tanzania: a retrospective review of 56 cases. *World J Surg Oncol.* 2012;10:38.

167. Xiang F, Song HP, Huang YS. Clinical features and treatment of 140 cases of Marjolin's ulcer at a major burn center in southwest China. *Exp Ther Med.* 2019;17(5):3403–3410.

168. Lund HZ. How often does squamous cell carcinoma of the skin metastasize? *Arch Dermatol.* 1965;92(6):635–637.

169. Moller R, Reymann F, Hou-Jensen K. Metastases in dermatological patients with squamous cell carcinoma. *Arch Dermatol.* 1979;115(6):703–705.

170. Epstein E, Epstein NN, Bragg K, Linden G. Metastases from squamous cell carcinomas of the skin. *Arch Dermatol.* 1968;97(3):245–251.

171. Frierson HF Jr, Cooper PH. Prognostic factors in squamous cell carcinoma of the lower lip. *Hum Pathol.* 1986;17(4):346–354.

172. Quaedvlieg PJ, Creytens DH, Epping GG, et al. Histopathological characteristics of metastasizing squamous cell carcinoma of the skin and lips. *Histopathology.* 2006;49(3):256–264.

173. Murphy GF BT, Cerio R, et al. Squamous cell carcinoma. In: Elder DE, Massi D, Scolyer RA, Willemze R, eds, *WHO Classification of Skin Tumours.* IARC; 2018.

174. Caruso G, Gerace E, Lorusso V, Cultrera R, Moretti L, Massari L. Squamous cell carcinoma in chronic osteomyelitis: a case report and review of the literature. *J Med Case Rep.* 2016;10:215.

175. Li Q, Cui H, Dong J, et al. Squamous cell carcinoma resulting from chronic osteomyelitis: a retrospective study of 8 cases. *Int J Clin Exp Pathol.* 2015;8(9):10178–10184.

176. Jiang N, Li SY, Zhang P, Yu B. Clinical characteristics, treatment, and prognosis of squamous cell carcinoma arising from extremity chronic osteomyelitis: a synthesis analysis of one hundred and seventy six reported cases. *Int Orthop.* 2020;44(11):2457–2471.

177. Arons MS, Lynch JB, Lewis SR, Blocker TG Jr. Scar tissue carcinoma. I. A clinical study with special reference to burn scar carcinoma. *Ann Surg.* 1965;161:170–188.

178. De Rosa N, Paddon VL, Liu Z, Glanville AR, Parsi K. Non-melanoma skin cancer frequency and risk factors in Australian heart and lung transplant recipients. *JAMA Dermatol.* 2019;155(6):716–719.

179. Keohane SG, Botting J, Budny PG, et al. Exton and on behalf of the British Association of Dermatologists' Clinical Standards Unit. British Association of Dermatologists guidelines for the management of the people with cutaneous squamous cell carcinoma 2020. *Br J Dermatol.* 2021;184:401–414.

180. Klingmuller G, Klehr HU, Ishibashi Y. Desmosomes in the cytoplasm of dedifferentiated keratinocytes of squamous cell carcinoma. *Arch Klin Exp Dermatol.* 1970;238(4):356–365.

181. Kobayasi T. Dermo-epidermal junction in invasive squamous cell carcinoma. An electron microscopic study. *Acta Derm Venereol.* 1969;49(5):445–457.

182. Boncinelli U, Fornieri C, Muscatello U. Relationship between leukocytes and tumor cells in pre-cancerous and cancerous lesions of the lip: a possible expression of immune reaction. *J Invest Dermatol.* 1978;71(6):407–411.

183. Manglani KS, Manaligod JR, Ray B. Spindle cell carcinoma of the glans penis: a light and electron microscopic study. *Cancer.* 1980;46(10):2266–2272.

184. Battifora H. Spindle cell carcinoma: ultrastructural evidence of squamous origin and collagen production by the tumor cells. *Cancer.* 1976;37(5):2275–2282.

185. Evans HL, Smith JL. Spindle cell squamous carcinomas and sarcoma-like tumors of the skin: a comparative study of 38 cases. *Cancer.* 1980;45(10):2687–2697.

186. Barr RJ, Wuerker RB, Graham JH. Ultrastructure of atypical fibroxanthoma. *Cancer.* 1977;40(2):736–743.

187. Costantino D, Lowe L, Brown DL. Basosquamous carcinoma-an under-recognized, high-risk cutaneous neoplasm: case study and review of the literature. *J Plast Reconstr Aesthet Surg.* 2006;59(4):424–428.

188. Archbald E, Garcia C. Letter: Re: Metastatic basosquamous carcinoma: report of two cases. *Dermatol Surg.* 2010;36(3):426–427.

189. Lopes de Faria J, Nunes PH. Basosquamous cell carcinoma of the skin with metastases. *Histopathology.* 1988;12(1):85–94.

190. Brantsch K, Sotlar K, Brod C, Breuninger H. Metastatic basosquamous carcinoma: report of two cases. *Dermatol Surg.* 2008;34(12):1738–1741.

191. Beer TW, Shepherd P, Theaker JM. Ber EP4 and epithelial membrane antigen aid distinction of basal cell, squamous cell and basosquamous carcinomas of the skin. *Histopathology.* 2000;37(3):218–223.

192. Kirkham N, Too JX. Ber EP4 in the differential diagnosis of non-melanoma skin cancer. *J Pathol.* 2013;231(s1):1–51.

193. Pyne JH, Myint E, Barr EM, Clark SP, David M, Na R. Acantholytic invasive squamous cell carcinoma: tumor diameter, invasion depth, grade of differentiation, surgical margins, perineural invasion, recurrence and death rate. *J Cutan Pathol.* 2017;44(4):320–327.

194. Muller SA, Wilhelmj CM Jr, Harrison EG Jr, Winkelmann RK. Adenoid squamous cell carcinoma (adenoacanthoma of lever). Report of seven cases and review. *Arch Dermatol.* 1964;89: 589–597.

195. Lasser A, Cornog JL, Morris JM. Adenoid squamous cell carcinoma of the vulva. *Cancer.* 1974;33(1):224–227.

196. Underwood JW, Adcock LL, Okagaki T. Adenosquamous carcinoma of skin appendages (adenoid squamous cell carcinoma, pseudoglandular squamous cell carcinoma, adenocanthoma of sweat gland of Lever) of the vulva: a clinical and ultrastructural study. *Cancer.* 1978;42(4):1851–1858.

197. Riedlinger WF, Hurley MY, Dehner LP, Lind AC. Mucoepidermoid carcinoma of the skin: a distinct entity from adenosquamous carcinoma: a case study with a review of the literature. *Am J Surg Pathol.* 2005;29(1):131–135.

198. Suárez-Peñaranda JM, Vieites B, Valeiras E, Varela-Duran J. Primary mucoepidermoid carcinoma of the skin expressing p63. *Am J Dermatopathol.* 2010;32(1):61–64.

199. Weidner N, Foucar E. Adenosquamous carcinoma of the skin. An aggressive mucin- and gland-forming squamous carcinoma. *Arch Dermatol.* 1985;121(6):775–779.

200. Holmkvist KA, Roenigk RK. Squamous cell carcinoma of the lip treated with Mohs micrographic surgery: outcome at 5 years. *J Am Acad Dermatol.* 1998;38(6, pt 1):960–966.

201. Rowe DE, Carroll RJ, Day CL Jr. Prognostic factors for local recurrence, metastasis, and survival rates in squamous cell carcinoma of the skin, ear, and lip. Implications for treatment modality selection. *J Am Acad Dermatol.* 1992;26(6):976–990.

202. de Graaf YG, Basdew VR, van Zwan-Kralt N, Willemze R, Bavinck JN. The occurrence of residual or recurrent squamous cell carcinomas in organ transplant recipients after curettage and electrodesiccation. *Br J Dermatol.* 2006;154(3):493–497.

203. Brewster AM, Lee JJ, Clayman GL, et al. Randomized trial of adjuvant 13-cis-retinoic acid and interferon alfa for patients with aggressive skin squamous cell carcinoma. *J Clin Oncol.* 2007;25(15): 1974–1978.

204. Grob JJ, Gonzalez R, Basset-Seguin N, et al. Pembrolizumab monotherapy for recurrent or metastatic cutaneous squamous cell carcinoma: a single-arm phase II Trial (KEYNOTE-629). *J Clin Oncol.* 2020;38(25):2916–2925.

205. Ackerman LV. Verrucous carcinoma of the oral cavity. *Surgery.* 1948;23(4):670–678.

206. Steffen C. The man behind the eponym: Lauren V. Ackerman and verrucous carcinoma of Ackerman. *Am J Dermatopathol.* 2004;26(4):334–341.

207. Wang N, Huang M, Lv H. Head and neck verrucous carcinoma: a population-based analysis of incidence, treatment, and prognosis. *Medicine (Baltimore).* 2020;99(2):e18660.

208. Schwartz RA. Verrucous carcinoma of the skin and mucosa. *J Am Acad Dermatol.* 1995;32(1):1–21; quiz 22–24.

209. Assaf C, Steinhoff M, Petrov I, et al. Verrucous carcinoma of the axilla: case report and review. *J Cutan Pathol.* 2004;31(2): 199–204.

210. Castano E, Lopez-Rios F, Alvarez-Fernandez JG, Rodriguez-Peralto JL, Iglesias L. Verrucous carcinoma in association with hypertrophic lichen planus. *Clin Exp Dermatol.* 1997;22(1):23–25.

211. Warshaw EM, Templeton SF, Washington CV. Verrucous carcinoma occurring in a lesion of oral lichen planus. *Cutis.* 2000;65(4):219–222.

212. Aroni K, Lazaris AC, Ioakim-Liossi A, Paraskevakou H, Davaris PS. Histological diagnosis of cutaneous "warty" carcinoma on a pre-existing HPV lesion. *Acta Derm Venereol.* 2000;80(4):294–296.

213. Mirbod SM, Ahing SI. Tobacco-associated lesions of the oral cavity: Part II. Malignant lesions. *J Can Dent Assoc.* 2000;66(6): 308–311.

214. Miyamoto T, Sasaoka R, Hagari Y, Mihara M. Association of cutaneous verrucous carcinoma with human papillomavirus type 16. *Br J Dermatol.* 1999;140(1):168–169.

215. Koch H, Kowatsch E, Hödl S, et al. Verrucous carcinoma of the skin: long-term follow-up results following surgical therapy. *Dermatol Surg.* 2004;30(8):1124–1130.

216. Padilla RS, Bailin PL, Howard WR, Dinner MI. Verrucous carcinoma of the skin and its management by Mohs' surgery. *Plast Reconstr Surg.* 1984;73(3):442–447.

217. Alkalay R, Alcalay J, Shiri J. Plantar verrucous carcinoma treated with Mohs micrographic surgery: a case report and literature review. *J Drugs Dermatol.* 2006;5(1):68–73.

218. Nikkels AF, Thirion L, Quatresooz P, Pierard GE. Photodynamic therapy for cutaneous verrucous carcinoma. *J Am Acad Dermatol.* 2007;57(3):516–519.

219. Grunwald MH, Lee JY, Ackerman AB. Pseudocarcinomatous hyperplasia. *Am J Dermatopathol.* 1988;10(2):95–103.

220. Jeunon T, Assoni A, Verdolin A. Pseudocarcinomatous hyperplasia, squamous cell carcinoma, and keratoacanthoma associated to lymphomas of the skin and external mucous membranes: a case report and literature review. *Am J Dermatopathol.* 2020;42(9):662–672.

221. Crowson AN. Basal cell carcinoma: biology, morphology and clinical implications. *Mod Pathol.* 2006;19(suppl 2):S127–S147.

222. Liersch J, Schaller J. [Basal cell carcinoma and rare form variants]. *Pathologe.* 2014;35(5):433–442.

223. Basset-Seguin N, Herms F. Update in the management of basal cell carcinoma. *Acta Derm Venereol.* 2020;100(11):adv00140.

224. Paver K, Poyzer K, Burry N, Deakin M. Letter: The incidence of basal cell carcinoma and their metastases in Australia and New Zealand. *Australas J Dermatol.* 1973;14(1):53.

225. Cotran RS. Metastasizing basal cell carcinomas. *Cancer.* 1961;14:1036–1040.

226. von Domarus H, Stevens PJ. Metastatic basal cell carcinoma. Report of five cases and review of 170 cases in the literature. *J Am Acad Dermatol.* 1984;10(6):1043–1060.

227. Amonette RA, Salasche SJ, Chesney TM, Clarendon CC, Dilawari RA. Metastatic basal-cell carcinoma. *J Dermatol Surg Oncol.* 1981;7(5):397–400.

228. Jones VS, Chandra S, Smile SR, Narasimhan R. A unique case of metastatic penile basal cell carcinoma. *Indian J Pathol Microbiol.* 2000;43(4):465–466.

229. Ribuffo D, Alfano C, Ferrazzoli PS, Scuderi N. Basal cell carcinoma of the penis and scrotum with cutaneous metastases. *Scand J Plast Reconstr Surg Hand Surg.* 2002;36(3):180–182.

230. Dzubow LM. Metastatic basal cell carcinoma originating in the supra-parotid region. *J Dermatol Surg Oncol.* 1986;12(12):1306–1308.

231. Assor D. Basal cell carcinoma with metastasis to bone. Report of two cases. *Cancer.* 1967;20(12):2125–2132.

232. Wermuth BM, Fajardo LF. Metastatic basal cell carcinoma. A review. *Arch Pathol.* 1970;90(5):458–462.

233. Soffer D, Kaplan H, Weshler Z. Meningeal carcinomatosis due to basal cell carcinoma. *Hum Pathol.* 1985;16(5):530–532.

234. Farmer ER, Helwig EB. Metastatic basal cell carcinoma: a clinico-pathologic study of seventeen cases. *Cancer.* 1980;46(4):748–757.

235. Mikhail GR, Nims LP, Kelly AP Jr, Ditmars DM Jr, Eyler WR. Metastatic basal cell carcinoma: review, pathogenesis, and report of two cases. *Arch Dermatol.* 1977;113(9):1261–1269.

236. Safai B, Good RA. Basal cell carcinoma with metastasis. Review of literature. *Arch Pathol Lab Med.* 1977;101(6):327–331.

237. Gorlin RJ. Nevoid basal cell carcinoma (Gorlin) syndrome. *Genet Med.* 2004;6(6):530–539.

238. Hahn H, Wicking C, Zaphiropoulous PG, et al. Mutations of the human homolog of Drosophila patched in the nevoid basal cell carcinoma syndrome. *Cell.* 1996;85(6):841–851.

239. Zhang H, Ping XL, Lee PK, et al. Role of PTCH and p53 genes in early-onset basal cell carcinoma. *Am J Pathol.* 2001;158(2):381–385.

240. Brash DE, Rudolph JA, Simon JA, et al. A role for sunlight in skin cancer: UV-induced p53 mutations in squamous cell carcinoma. *Proc Natl Acad Sci U S A.* 1991;88(22):10124–10128.

241. LoRusso PM, Rudin CM, Reddy JC, et al. Phase I trial of hedge-hog pathway inhibitor vismodegib (GDC-0449) in patients with refractory, locally advanced or metastatic solid tumors. *Clin Cancer Res.* 2011;17(8):2502–2511.

242. De Smaele E, Ferretti E, Gulino A. Vismodegib, a small-molecule inhibitor of the hedgehog pathway for the treatment of advanced cancers. *Curr Opin Investig Drugs.* 2010;11(6):707–718.

243. Falchook GS, Leidner R, Stankevich E, et al. Responses of metastatic basal cell and cutaneous squamous cell carcinomas to anti-PD1 monoclonal antibody REGN2810. *J Immunother Cancer.* 2016;4:70.

244. Dvoretzky I, Fisher BK, Haker O. Mutilating basal cell epithelioma. *Arch Dermatol.* 1978;114(2):239–240.

245. Gormley DE, Hirsch P. Aggressive basal cell carcinoma of the scalp. *Arch Dermatol.* 1978;114(5):782–783.

246. Gorlin RJ. Nevoid basal-cell carcinoma syndrome. *Medicine (Baltimore).* 1987;66(2):98–113.

247. Taylor WB, Anderson DE, Howell JB, Thurston CS. The nevoid basal cell carcinoma syndrome. Autopsy findings. *Arch Dermatol.* 1968;98(6):612–614.

248. Southwick GJ, Schwartz RA. The basal cell nevus syndrome: disasters occurring among a series of 36 patients. *Cancer.* 1979;44(6):2294–2305.

249. Berendes U. Clinical significance of the oncotic phase in the basal cell nevus syndrome. *Hautarzt.* 1971;22(6):261–263.

250. Howell JB, Mehregan AH. Pursuit of the pits in the nevoid basal cell carcinoma syndrome. *Arch Dermatol.* 1970;102(6):586–597.

251. Leppard BJ. Skin cysts in the basal cell naevus syndrome. *Clin Exp Dermatol.* 1983;8(6):603–612.

252. Hermans EH, Grosfeld JC, Spaas JA. The fifth phacomatosis. *Dermatologica.* 1965;130(6):446–476.

253. Reed JC. Nevoid basal cell carcinoma syndrome with associated fibrosarcoma of the maxilla. Report of a case. *Arch Dermatol.* 1968;97(3):304–306.

254. Happle R. Nevobasalioma and ameloblastoma. *Hautarzt.* 1973;24(7):290–294.

255. Requena L, Fariña MC, Robledo M, et al. Multiple hereditary infundibulocystic basal cell carcinomas: a genodermatosis different from nevoid basal cell carcinoma syndrome. *Arch Dermatol.* 1999;35(10):1227–1235.

256. Anderson TE, Best PV. Linear basal-cell naevus. *Br J Dermatol.* 1962;74:20–23.

257. Carney RG. Linear unilateral basal-cell nevus with comedones; report of a case. *AMA Arch Derm Syphilol.* 1952;65(4):471–476.

258. Horio T, Komura J. Linear unilateral basal cell nevus with comedo-like lesions. *Arch Dermatol.* 1978;114(1):95–97.

259. Bleiberg J, Brodkin RH. Linear unilateral basal cell nevus with comedones. *Arch Dermatol.* 1969;100(2):187–190.

260. Bazex A, Dupre A, Christol B. Follicular atrophoderma, baso-cellular proliferations and hypotrichosis. *Ann Dermatol Syphiligr (Paris).* 1966;93(3):241–254.

261. Viksnins P, Berlin A. Follicular atrophoderma and basal cell carcinomas: the Bazex syndrome. *Arch Dermatol.* 1977;113(7):948–951.

262. Plosila M, Kiistala R, Niemi KM. The Bazex syndrome: follicular atrophoderma with multiple basal cell carcinomas, hypotrichosis and hypohidrosis. *Clin Exp Dermatol.* 1981;6(1):31–41.

263. Pinkus H. Premalignant fibroepithelial tumors of skin. *AMA Arch Derm Syphilol.* 1953;67(6):598–615.

264. Pinkus H. Epithelial and fibroepithelial tumors. *Arch Dermatol.* 1965;91:24–37.

265. Fanger H, Barker BE. Histochemical studies of some keratotic and proliferating skin lesions. I. Metachromasia. *AMA Arch Pathol.* 1957;64(2):143–147.

266. Moore RD, Stevenson J, Schoenberg MD. The response of connective tissue associated with tumors of the skin. *Am J Clin Pathol.* 1960;34:125–130.

267. Merot Y, Faucher F, Didierjean L, Saurat JH. Loss of bullous pemphigoid antigen in peritumoral lacunas of basal cell carcinomas. *Acta Derm Venereol.* 1984;64(3):209–213.

268. Stanley JR, Beckwith JB, Fuller RP, Katz SI. A specific antigenic defect of the basement membrane is found in basal cell carcinoma but not in other epidermal tumors. *Cancer.* 1982;50(8):1486–1490.

269. Weedon D, Shand E. Amyloid in basal cell carcinomas. *Br J Dermatol.* 1979;101(2):141–146.

270. Aroni K, Lazaris AC, Nikolaou I, Saetta A, Kavantzas N, Davaris PS. Signet ring basal cell carcinoma. A case study emphasizing the differential diagnosis of neoplasms with signet ring cell formation. *Pathol Res Pract.* 2001;197(12):853–856.

271. Hundeiker M, Berger H. [On the morphogenesis of basaliomas]. *Arch Klin Exp Dermatol.* 1968;231(2):161–169.

272. Mehregan AH. Aggressive basal cell epithelioma on sunlight-protected skin. Report of eight cases, one with pulmonary and bone metastases. *Am J Dermatopathol.* 1983;5(3):221–229.

273. Jacobs GH, Rippey JJ, Altini M. Prediction of aggressive behavior in basal cell carcinoma. *Cancer.* 1982;49(3):533–537.

274. Lang PG Jr, Maize JC. Histologic evolution of recurrent basal cell carcinoma and treatment implications. *J Am Acad Dermatol.* 1986;14(2, pt 1):186–196.

275. Foot NC. Adnexal carcinoma of the skin. *Am J Pathol.* 1947;23(1):1–27.

276. Troy JL, Ackerman AB. Sebaceoma. A distinctive benign neoplasm of adnexal epithelium differentiating toward sebaceous cells. *Am J Dermatopathol.* 1984;6(1):7–13.

277. Wood MG, Pranich K, Beerman H. Investigation of possible apocrine gland component in basal cell epithelioma. *J Invest Dermatol.* 1958;30(6):273–279.

278. Freeman RG, Winkelmann RK. Basal cell tumor with eccrine differentiation (eccrine epithelioma). *Arch Dermatol.* 1969;100(2):234–242.

279. Lerchin E, Rahbari H. Adamantinoid basal cell epithelioma. A histological variant. *Arch Dermatol.* 1975;111(5):586–588.

280. Barr RJ, Graham JH. Granular cell basal cell carcinoma. A distinct histopathologic entity. *Arch Dermatol.* 1979;115(9):1064–1067.

281. Mrak RE, Baker GF. Granular cell basal cell carcinoma. *J Cutan Pathol.* 1987;14(1):37–42.

282. Barnadas MA, Freeman RG. Clear cell basal cell epithelioma: light and electron microscopic study of an unusual variant. *J Cutan Pathol.* 1988;15(1):1–7.

283. Cohen RE, Zaim MT. Signet-ring clear-cell basal cell carcinoma. *J Cutan Pathol.* 1988;15(3):183–187.

284. Aloi FG, Molinero A, Pippione M. Basal cell carcinoma with matrical differentiation. Matrical carcinoma. *Am J Dermatopathol.* 1988;10(6):509–513.

285. Degos R, Hewitt J. Premalignant fibroepithelial tumors of Pinkus and basal cell epithelioma; two new cases. *Ann Dermatol Syphiligr (Paris).* 1955;82(2):124–139.

286. Howell JB, Freeman RG. Structure and significance of the pits with their tumors in the nevoid basal cell carcinoma syndrome. *J Am Acad Dermatol.* 1980;2(3):224–238.

287. Mason JK, Helwig EB, Graham JH. Pathology of the nevoid basal cell carcinoma syndrome. *Arch Pathol.* 1965;79:401–408.

288. Jablonska S. Basalioma of nevoid origin (nevobasalioma or basal cell nevi). *Hautarzt.* 1961;12:147–157.

289. Holubar K, Matras H, Smalik AV. Multiple palmar basal cell epitheliomas in basal cell nevus syndrome. *Arch Dermatol.* 1970;101(6):679–682.

290. Ward WH. Naevoid basal celled carcinoma associated with a dyskeratosis of the palms and soles. A new entity. *Aust J Dermatol.* 1960;5:204–208.

291. Taylor WB, Wilkins JW Jr. Nevoid basal cell carcinoma of the palm. *Arch Dermatol.* 1970;102(6):654–655.

292. Barr RJ, Headley JL, Jensen JL, Howell JB. Cutaneous keratocysts of nevoid basal cell carcinoma syndrome. *J Am Acad Dermatol.* 1986;14(4):572–576.

293. Blanchard L, Hodge SJ, Owen LG. Linear eccrine nevus with comedones. *Arch Dermatol.* 1981;117(6):357–359.

294. Sims CF, Parker RL. Intraepidermal basal cell epithelioma. *Arch Derm Syphilol.* 1949;59(1):45–49.

295. Morales A, Hu F. Seborrheic verruca and intraepidermal basal cell epithelioma of Jadassohn. *Arch Dermatol.* 1965;91(4):342–344.

296. Steffen C, Ackerman AB. Intraepidermal epithelioma of Borst-Jadassohn. *Am J Dermatopathol.* 1985;7(1):5–24.

297. Holubar K, Wolff K. Intra-epidermal eccrine poroma: a histochemical and enzyme-histochemical study. *Cancer.* 1969;23(3):626–635.

298. Mehregan AH, Pinkus H. Intraepidermal epithelioma: a critical study. *Cancer.* 1964;17:609–636.

299. Okun MR, Blumental G. Basal cell epithelioma with giant cells and nuclear atypicality. *Arch Dermatol.* 1964;89:598–600.

300. Berger P, Baughman R. Intra-epidermal epithelioma. Report of case with invasion after many years. *Br J Dermatol.* 1974;90(3):343–349.

301. Coburn JG, Smith JL. Hidroacanthoma simplex; an assessment of a selected group of intraepidermal basal cell epitheliomata and of their malignant homologues. *Br J Dermatol.* 1956;68(12):400–418.

302. Mehregan AH, Levson DN. Hidroacanthoma simplex. A report of two cases. *Arch Dermatol.* 1969;100(3):303–305.

303. Bardach H. Hidroacanthoma simplex with in situ porocarcinoma. A case suggesting malignant transformation. *J Cutan Pathol.* 1978;5(5):236–248.

304. Pinkus H, Mehregan AH. Epidermotropic eccrine carcinoma. A case combining features of eccrine poroma and Paget's dermatosis. *Arch Dermatol.* 1963;88:597–606.

305. Graham JH, Johnson WC. *Dermal Pathology.* Harper & Row; 1972.

306. Darier J, Ferrand M. L'épithéliome pavimenteux mixte et intermédiaire. *Ann Dermatol Syphiligr (Paris).* 1955;82:124.

307. Borel DM. Cutaneous basosquamous carcinoma. Review of the literature and report of 35 cases. *Arch Pathol.* 1973;95(5):293–297.

308. Gertler W. Zur epithelverbundenheit der basaliome. *Dermatol Wochenschr.* 1965;151:673.

309. Montgomery H. Basal squamous cell epithelioma. *Arch Derm Syphilol.* 1928;82:124.

310. Krompecher E. *Der Basalzellenkrebs.* Gustav Fischer; 1903.

311. Geschickter CF, Koehler HP. Ectodermal tumors of the skin. *Am J Cancer.* 1935;23:804.

312. Mallory FB. Recent progress in the microscopic anatomy and differentiation of cancer. *J Am Med Assoc.* 1910;55:1513.

313. Adamson HG. On the nature of rodent ulcer: its relationship to epithelioma adenoides cysticum of Brooke and to other trichoepitheliomata of benign nevoid character; its distinction from malignant carcinoma. *Lancet.* 1914;i:810.

314. Wallace SA, Halpert B. Trichoma: tumor of hair anlage. *Arch Pathol (Chic).* 1950;50(2):199–208.

315. Lever WF. Pathogenesis of benign tumors of cutaneous appendages and of basal cell epithelioma. *Arch Derm Syphilol.* 1948;57(4):679–724.

316. Chiba M, Jimbow K. Expression of gamma-glutamyl transpeptidase in normal and neoplastic epithelial cells of human skin: a marker for distinguishing malignant epithelial tumours. *Br J Dermatol.* 1986;114(4):459–464.

317. Bale AE, Yu KP. The hedgehog pathway and basal cell carcinomas. *Hum Mol Genet.* 2001;10(7):757–762.

318. Bonifas JM, Pennypacker S, Chuang PT, et al. Activation of expression of hedgehog target genes in basal cell carcinomas. *J Invest Dermatol.* 2001;116(5):739–742.

319. Ling G, Ahmadian A, Persson A, et al. PATCHED and p53 gene alterations in sporadic and hereditary basal cell cancer. *Oncogene.* 2001;20(53):7770–7778.

320. Saldanha G. The Hedgehog signalling pathway and cancer. *J Pathol.* 2001;193(4):427–432.

321. Toftgard R. Hedgehog signalling in cancer. *Cell Mol Life Sci.* 2000;57(12):1720–1731.

322. Wicking C, McGlinn E. The role of hedgehog signalling in tumorigenesis. *Cancer Lett.* 2001;173(1):1–7.

323. Sardi I, Piazzini M, Palleschi G, et al. Molecular detection of microsatellite instability in basal cell carcinoma. *Oncol Rep.* 2000;7(5):1119–1122.

324. Tojo M, Kiyosawa H, Iwatsuki K, Kaneko F. Expression of a Sonic Hedgehog signal transducer, hedgehog-interacting protein, by human basal cell carcinoma. *Br J Dermatol.* 2002;146(1):69–73.

325. Zedan W, Robinson PA, Markham AF, High AS. Expression of the Sonic Hedgehog receptor "PATCHED" in basal cell carcinomas and odontogenic keratocysts. *J Pathol.* 2001;194(4):473–477.

326. Holmes EJ, Bennington JL, Haber SL. Citrulline-containing basal cell carcinomas. Differentiation toward hari structures with induction of dermal hair papillae. *Cancer.* 1968;22(3):663–670.

327. Kariniemi AL, Holthofer H, Vartio T, Virtanen I. Cellular differentiation of basal cell carcinoma studied with fluorescent lectins and cytokeratin antibodies. *J Cutan Pathol.* 1984;11(6):541–548.

328. Shimizu N, Ito M, Tazawa T, Katsuumi K, Sato Y. Anti-keratin monoclonal antibody against basal cell epithelioma keratin: BKN-1. *J Dermatol.* 1987;14(4):359–363.

329. Van Scott EJ, Reinertson RP. The modulating influence of stromal environment on epithelial cells studied in human autotransplants. *J Invest Dermatol.* 1961;36:109–131.

330. Covo JA. The pits in the nevoid basal cell carcinoma syndrome. *Arch Dermatol.* 1971;103(5):568–569.

331. Gerstein W. Transplantation of basal cell epithelioma to the rabbit. *Arch Dermatol.* 1963;88:834–836.

332. LeBoit PE, Burg G, Weedon D. *Pathology and Genetics of Skin Tumours.* IARC Press; 2006.

333. Messina J, Epstein EH Jr, Kossard S. Basal cell carcinoma. In: Elder DE, Massi D, Scolyer RA, Willemze R, eds., *WHO Classification of Skin Tumours.* 4th ed. IARC; 2018:26–34.

334. Madsen A. De l'épithélioma baso-cellulaire superficiel. *Acta Derm Venereol Suppl (Stockh).* 1941;7(22, suppl):1.

335. Madsen A. Studies on basal-cell epithelioma of the skin. The architecture, manner of growth, and histogenesis of the tumours. Whole tumours examined in serial sections cut parallel to the skin surface. *Acta Pathol Microbiol Scand.* 1965;(suppl 177):3–63.

336. Oberste-Lehn H. The histogenesis of basalioma. *Z Haut Geschlechtskr.* 1954;16(11):334–339.

337. Lang PG Jr, McKelvey AC, Nicholson JH. Three-dimensional reconstruction of the superficial multicentric basal cell carcinoma using serial sections and a computer. *Am J Dermatopathol.* 1987;9(3):198–203.

338. Zelickson AS. Electron microscope study of the basal cell epithelioma. *J Invest Dermatol.* 1962;39:183–187.

339. Kumakiri M, Hashimoto K. Ultrastructural resemblance of basal cell epithelioma to primary epithelial germ. *J Cutan Pathol.* 1978;5(2):53–67.

340. Lever WF, Hashimoto K. Electron microscopic and histochemical findings in basal cell epithelioma, squamous cell carcinoma and some appendage tumors. In: Jadassohn W, Schirren CG, eds. *Proceedings, XIIIth International Congress of Dermatology.* Vol 1. Springer-Verlag; 1968:3.

341. Cutler B, Posalaky Z, Katz HI. Cell processes in basal cell carcinoma. *J Cutan Pathol.* 1980;7(5):310–314.

342. Reidbord HE, Wechsler HL, Fisher ER. Ultrastructural study of basal cell carcinoma and its variants with comments on histogenesis. *Arch Dermatol.* 1971;104(2):132–140.

343. Zelickson AS. The pigmented basal cell epithelioma. *Arch Dermatol.* 1967;96(5):524–527.

344. Bleehen SS. Pigmented basal cell epithelioma. Light and electron microscopic studies on tumours and cell cultures. *Br J Dermatol.* 1975;93(4):361–370.

345. Weinstein GD, Frost P. Cell proliferation in human basal cell carcinoma. *Cancer Res.* 1970;30(3):724–728.

346. Hashimoto K, Kobayashi H. Histogenesis of amyloid in the skin. *Am J Dermatopathol.* 1980;2(2):165–171.

347. Masu S, Hosokawa M, Seiji M. Amyloid in localized cutaneous amyloidosis: immunofluorescence studies with anti-keratin antiserum especially concerning the difference between systemic and localized cutaneous amyloidosis. *Acta Derm Venereol.* 1981;61(5):381–384.

348. Cox NH, Nicoll JJ, Popple AW. Amyloid deposition in basal cell carcinoma: a cause of apparent lack of sensitivity to radiotherapy. *Clin Exp Dermatol.* 2001;26(6):499–500.

349. Stanoszek LM, Wang GY, Harms PW. Histologic mimics of basal cell carcinoma. *Arch Pathol Lab Med.* 2017;141(11):1490–1502.

350. Rahbari H, Mehregan AH. Basal cell epithelioma (carcinoma) in children and teenagers. *Cancer.* 1982;49(2):350–353.

351. Haupt HM, Stern JB, Dilaimy MS. Basal cell carcinoma: clues to its presence in histologic sections when the initial slide is nondiagnostic. *Am J Surg Pathol.* 2000;24(9):1291–1294.

352. Bisson MA, Dunkin CS, Suvarna SK, Griffiths RW. Do plastic surgeons resect basal cell carcinomas too widely? A prospective study comparing surgical and histological margins. *Br J Plast Surg.* 2002;55(4):293–297.

353. Dieu T, Macleod AM. Incomplete excision of basal cell carcinomas: a retrospective audit. *ANZ J Surg.* 2002;72(3):219–221.

354. Kumar P, Watson S, Brain AN, et al. Incomplete excision of basal cell carcinoma: a prospective multicentre audit. *Br J Plast Surg.* 2002;55(8):616–622.

355. Robinson JK, Fisher SG. Recurrent basal cell carcinoma after incomplete resection. *Arch Dermatol.* 2000;136(11):1318–1324.

356. Marchac D, Papadopoulos O, Duport G. Curative and aesthetic results of surgical treatment of 138 basal-cell carcinomas. *J Dermatol Surg Oncol.* 1982;8(5):379–387.

357. Wolf DJ, Zitelli JA. Surgical margins for basal cell carcinoma. *Arch Dermatol.* 1987;123(3):340–344.

358. Kimyai-Asadi A, Alam M, Goldberg LH, Peterson SR, Silapunt S, Jih MH. Efficacy of narrow-margin excision of well-demarcated primary facial basal cell carcinomas. *J Am Acad Dermatol.* 2005;53(3):464–468.

359. Rowe DE, Carroll RJ, Day CL Jr. Mohs surgery is the treatment of choice for recurrent (previously treated) basal cell carcinoma. *J Dermatol Surg Oncol.* 1989;15(4):424–431.

360. Rowe DE, Carroll RJ, Day CL Jr. Long-term recurrence rates in previously untreated (primary) basal cell carcinoma: implications for patient follow-up. *J Dermatol Surg Oncol.* 1989;15(3):315–328.

361. Marks R, Gebauer K, Shumack S, et al. Imiquimod 5% cream in the treatment of superficial basal cell carcinoma: results of a multicenter 6-week dose-response trial. *J Am Acad Dermatol.* 2001;44(5):807–813.

362. Geisse JK, Rich P, Pandya A, et al. Imiquimod 5% cream for the treatment of superficial basal cell carcinoma: a double-blind, randomized, vehicle-controlled study. *J Am Acad Dermatol.* 2002;47(3):390–398.

363. Geisse J, Caro I, Lindholm J, Golitz L, Stampone P, Owens M. Imiquimod 5% cream for the treatment of superficial basal cell carcinoma: results from two phase III, randomized, vehicle-controlled studies. *J Am Acad Dermatol.* 2004;50(5):722–733.

364. Caccialanza M, Piccinno R, Grammatica A. Radiotherapy of recurrent basal and squamous cell skin carcinomas: a study of 249 re-treated carcinomas in 229 patients. *Eur J Dermatol.* 2001;11(1):25–28.

365. Berg D, Otley CC. Skin cancer in organ transplant recipients: epidemiology, pathogenesis, and management. *J Am Acad Dermatol.* 2002;47(1):1–17.

366. Veness MJ, Quinn DI, Ong CS, et al. Aggressive cutaneous malignancies following cardiothoracic transplantation: the Australian experience. *Cancer.* 1999;85(8):1758–1764.

367. Hoyo E, Kanitakis J, Euvrard S, Thivolet J. Proliferation characteristics of cutaneous squamous cell carcinomas developing in organ graft recipients. Comparison with squamous cell carcinomas of nonimmunocompromised hosts by counting argyrophilic proteins associated with nucleolar organizer regions. *Arch Dermatol.* 1993;129(3):324–327.

368. Viac J, Chardonnet Y, Euvrard S, Chignol MC, Thivolet J. Langerhans cells, inflammation markers and human papillomavirus infections in benign and malignant epithelial tumors from transplant recipients. *J Dermatol.* 1992;19(2):67–77.

369. Proby CM, Churchill L, Purkis PE, Glover MT, Sexton CJ, Leigh IM. Keratin 17 expression as a marker for epithelial transformation in viral warts. *Am J Pathol.* 1993;143(6):1667–1678.

370. McGregor JM, Farthing A, Crook T, et al. Posttransplant skin cancer: a possible role for p53 gene mutation but not for oncogenic human papillomaviruses. *J Am Acad Dermatol.* 1994;30(5, pt 1):701–706.

371. Angeli-Besson C, Koeppel MC, Jacquet P, Andrac L, Sayag J. Multiple squamous-cell carcinomas of the scalp and chronic myeloid leukemia. *Dermatology.* 1995;191(4):321–322.

372. Oram Y, Orengo I, Griego RD, Rosen T, Thornby J. Histologic patterns of basal cell carcinoma based upon patient immunostatus. *Dermatol Surg.* 1995;21(7):611–614.

373. Hertzler G, Gordon SM, Piratzky J, Henderson JM, Gal AA. Case report: fulminant Kaposi's sarcoma after orthotopic liver transplantation. *Am J Med Sci.* 1995;309(5):278–281.

374. Abouna GM, Kumar MS, Samhan M. Kaposi's sarcoma in renal transplant recipients: a case report. *Transplant Sci.* 1994;4(1):20–21.

375. al-Sulaiman MH, Mousa DH, Dhar JM, al-Khader AA. Does regressed posttransplantation Kaposi's sarcoma recur following reintroduction of immunosuppression? *Am J Nephrol.* 1992;12(5):384–386.

376. McGregor JM, Newell M, Ross J, Kirkham N, McGibbon DH, Darley C. Cutaneous malignant melanoma and human immunodeficiency virus (HIV) infection: a report of three cases. *Br J Dermatol.* 1992;126(5):516–519.

377. Hutchinson J. The crateriform ulcer of the face: a form of epithelial cancer. *Trans Pathol Soc London.* 1889;40:275.

378. Musso L. Spontaneous resolution of a molluscum sebaceum. *Proc R Soc Med.* 1950;43(11):838–839.

379. Rook A, Whimster I. Keratoacanthoma—a thirty year retrospect. *Br J Dermatol.* 1979;100(1):41–47.

380. Ghadially FN. Keratoacanthoma. In: Fitzpatrick TB, Eisen AZ, Wolff K, eds. *Dermatology in General Medicine.* 2nd ed. McGraw-Hill; 1979:383.

381. Ghadially FN. The role of the hair follicle in the origin and evolution of some cutaneous neoplasms of man and experimental animals. *Cancer.* 1961;14:801–816.

382. Silberberg I, Kopf AW, Baer RL. Recurrent keratoacanthoma of the lip. *Arch Dermatol.* 1962;86:44–53.

383. Sullivan JJ, Colditz GA. Keratoacanthoma in a sub-tropical climate. *Australas J Dermatol.* 1979;20(1):34–40.

384. Muir EG, Bell AJ, Barlow KA. Multiple primary carcinomata of the colon, duodenum, and larynx associated with kerato-acanthomata of the face. *Br J Surg.* 1967;54(3):191–195.

385. Poleksic S. Keratoacanthoma and multiple carcinomas. *Br J Dermatol.* 1974;91(4):461–463.

386. Rapaport J. Giant keratoacanthoma of the nose. *Arch Dermatol.* 1975;111(1):73–75.

387. Bart RS, Popkin GL, Kopf AW, Gumport SL. Giant keratoacanthoma: a problem in diagnosis and management. *J Dermatol Surg.* 1975;1(2):49–55.

388. Kallos A. Giant keratoacanthoma. *AMA Arch Derm.* 1958;78(2):207–209.

389. Obermayer ME. Keratoakanthoma: its tissue destroying growth capacity. *Hautarzt.* 1964;15:628–630.

390. Belisario JC. Brief review of keratoacanthomas and description of keratoacanthoma centrifugum marginatum, another variety of keratoacanthoma. *Aust J Dermatol.* 1965;8(2):65–72.

391. Miedzinski F, Kozakiewicz J. Keratoacanthoma centrifugum—a special variety of keratoacanthoma. *Hautarzt.* 1962;13:348–352.

392. Weedon D, Wall D. Metastatic basal cell carcinoma. *Med J Aust.* 1975;2(5):177–179.

393. Heid E, Grosshans E, Lazrak B, Ben YD. Keratoacanthoma centrifugum marginatum. *Ann Dermatol Venereol.* 1979;106(4):367–370.

394. Macaulay WL. Subungual keratoacanthoma. *Arch Dermatol.* 1976;112(7):1004–1005.

395. Stoll DM, Ackerman AB. Subungual keratoacanthoma. *Am J Dermatopathol.* 1980;2(3):265–271.

396. Keeney GL, Banks PM, Linscheid RL. Subungual keratoacanthoma. Report of a case and review of the literature. *Arch Dermatol.* 1988;124(7):1074–1076.

397. Kern WH, McCray MK. The histopathologic differentiation of keratoacanthoma and squamous cell carcinoma of the skin. *J Cutan Pathol.* 1980;7(5):318–325.

398. Popkin GL, Brodie SJ, Hyman AB, Andrade R, Kopf AW. A technique of biopsy recommended for keratoacanthomas. *Arch Dermatol.* 1966;94(2):191–193.

399. Wade TR, Ackerman AB. The many faces of keratoacanthomas. *J Dermatol Surg Oncol.* 1978;4(7):498–501.

400. De Moragas JM, Montgomery H, McDonald JR. Keratoacanthoma versus squamous-cell carcinoma. *AMA Arch Derm.* 1958;77(4):390–395.

401. Giltman LI. Tripolar mitosis in a keratoacanthoma. *Acta Derm Venereol.* 1981;61(4):362–363.

402. Janecka IP, Wolff M, Crikelair GF, Cosman B. Aggressive histological features of keratoacanthoma. *J Cutan Pathol.* 1977;4(6):342–348.

403. Lapins NA, Helwig EB. Perineural invasion by keratoacanthoma. *Arch Dermatol.* 1980;116(7):791–793.

404. Levy EJ, Cahn MM, Shaffer B, Beerman H. Keratoacanthoma. *J Am Med Assoc.* 1954;155(6):562–564.

405. Calnan CD, Haber H. Molluscum sebaceum. *J Pathol Bacteriol.* 1955;69(1–2):61–66.

406. Takaki Y, Masutani M, Kawada A. Electron microscopic study of keratoacanthoma. *Acta Derm Venereol.* 1971;51(1):21–26.

407. von Bulow M, Klingmuller G. Electron microscopical studies on keratoacanthoma. Occurrence of intracytoplasmic desmosomes. *Arch Dermatol Forsch.* 1971;241(3):292–304.

408. Chalet MD, Connors RC, Ackerman AB. Squamous cell carcinoma vs. keratoacanthoma: criteria for histologic differentiation. *J Dermatol Surg.* 1975;1(1):16–17.

409. Stevanovic DV. Keratoacanthoma dyskeratoticum and segregans. *Arch Dermatol.* 1965;92(6):666–669.

410. Piscioli F, Boi S, Zumiani G, Cristofolini M. A gigantic, metastasizing keratoacanthoma. Report of a case and discussion on classification. *Am J Dermatopathol.* 1984;6(2):123–129.

411. Goldenhersh MA, Olsen TG. Invasive squamous cell carcinoma initially diagnosed as a giant keratoacanthoma. *J Am Acad Dermatol.* 1984;10(2, pt 2):372–378.

412. Nikolowski W. Keratoacanthoma. *Dermatol Monatsschr.* 1970;156(3):148–153.

413. Chu EY, Wanat KA, Miller CJ, et al. Diverse cutaneous side effects associated with BRAF inhibitor therapy: a clinicopathologic study. *J Am Acad Dermatol.* 2012;67(6):1265–1272.

414. Sullivan JJ, Donoghue MF, Kynaston B, McCaffrey JF. Multiple keratoacanthomas: report of four cases. *Australas J Dermatol.* 1980;21(1):16–24.

415. Ferguson Smith J. A case of multiple primary squamous-celled carcinomata of the skin in a young man with spontaneous healing. *Br J Dermatol.* 1934;46:267.

416. Tarnowski WM. Multiple keratoacanthomata. Response of a case to systemic chemotherapy. *Arch Dermatol.* 1966;94(1):74–80.

417. Hilker O, Winterscheidt M. Familial multiple keratoacanthomas. *Z Hautkr.* 1987;62(4):280–289.

418. Sommerville J, Milne JA. Familial primary self-healing squamous epithelioma of the skin (Ferguson Smith type). *Br J Dermatol.* 1950;62:485.

419. Grzybowski M. A case of peculiar generalized epithelial tumours of the skin. *Br J Dermatol.* 1950;62:310.

420. Sterry W, Steigleder GK, Pullmann H, Bauermeister K. Eruptive keratoacanthoma. *Hautarzt.* 1981;32(3):119–125.

421. Wright AL, Gawkrodger DJ, Branford WA, McLaren K, Hunter JA. Self-healing epitheliomata of Ferguson-Smith: cytogenetic and histological studies, and the therapeutic effect of etretinate. *Dermatologica.* 1988;176(1):22–28.

422. Winkelmann RK, Brown J. Generalized eruptive keratoacanthoma. Report of cases. *Arch Dermatol.* 1968;97(6):615–623.

423. Moffat JL, Rook A. Multiple self-healing epithelioma of Ferguson Smith type; report of a case of unilateral distribution. *AMA Arch Derm.* 1956;74(5):525–532.

424. Rossman RE, Freeman RG, KNOX JM. Multiple keratoacanthomas. A case study of the eruptive type with observations on pathogenesis. *Arch Dermatol.* 1964;89:374–381.

425. Lancer HA, Moschella SL. Paget's disease of the male breast. *J Am Acad Dermatol.* 1982;7(3):393–396.

426. Hadlich J, Goring HD, Linse R. Paget's disease in the male after estrogen therapy. *Dermatol Monatsschr.* 1981;167(5):305–308.

427. Ashikari R, Park K, Huvos AG, Urban JA. Paget's disease of the breast. *Cancer.* 1970;26(3):680–685.

428. Paone JF, Baker RR. Pathogenesis and treatment of Paget's disease of the breast. *Cancer.* 1981;48(3):825–829.

429. Orr JW, Parish DJ. The nature of the nipple changes in Paget's disease. *J Pathol Bacteriol.* 1962;84:201–208.

430. Lagios MD, Westdahl PR, Rose MR, Concannon S. Paget's disease of the nipple. Alternative management in cases without or with minimal extent of underlying breast carcinoma. *Cancer.* 1984;54(3):545–551.

431. Sagebiel RW. Ultrastructural observations on epidermal cells in Paget's disease of the breast. *Am J Pathol.* 1969;57(1):49–64.

432. Ebner H. On the ultrastructure of Paget's disease of the mamillae. *Z Haut Geschlechtskr.* 1969;44(9):297–304.

433. Caputo R, Califano A. Ultrastructural features of extramammary Paget's disease. *Arch Klin Exp Dermatol.* 1970;236(2):121–132.

434. Nadji M, Morales AR, Girtanner RE, Ziegels-Weissman J, Penneys NS. Paget's disease of the skin. A unifying concept of histogenesis. *Cancer.* 1982;50(10):2203–2206.

435. Kariniemi AL, Forsman L, Wahlstrom T, Vesterinen E, Andersson L. Expression of differentiation antigens in mammary and extramammary Paget's disease. *Br J Dermatol.* 1984;110(2):203–210.

436. Arafah M, Arain SA, Raddaoui EMS, Tulba A, Alkhawaja FH, Al Shedoukhy A. Molecular subtyping of mammary Paget's disease using immunohistochemistry. *Saudi Med J.* 2019;40(5):440–446.

437. Lloyd J, Flanagan AM. Mammary and extramammary Paget's disease. *J Clin Pathol.* 2000;53(10):742–749.

438. Arain SA, Arafah M, Said Raddaoui EM, Tulba A, Alkhawaja FH, Al Shedoukhy A. Immunohistochemistry of mammary Paget's

disease. Cytokeratin 7, GATA3, and HER2 are sensitive markers. *Saudi Med J*. 2020;41(3):232–237.

439. Schelfhout VR, Coene ED, Delaey B, Thys S, Page DL, De Potter CR. Pathogenesis of Paget's disease: epidermal heregulin-alpha, motility factor, and the HER receptor family. *J Natl Cancer Inst*. 2000;92(8):622–628.

440. Belcher RW. Extramammary Paget's disease. Enzyme histochemical and electron microscopic study. *Arch Pathol*. 1972;94(1):59–64.

441. Penneys NS, Nadji M, Morales A. Carcinoembryonic antigen in benign sweat gland tumors. *Arch Dermatol*. 1982;118(4):225–227.

442. Glasgow BJ, Wen DR, Al-Jitawi S, Cochran AJ. Antibody to S-100 protein aids the separation of pagetoid melanoma from mammary and extramammary Paget's disease. *J Cutan Pathol*. 1987;14(4):223–226.

443. Marcus E. The management of Paget's disease of the breast. *Curr Treat Options Oncol*. 2004;5(2):153–160.

444. Sakorafas GH, Blanchard K, Sarr MG, Farley DR. Paget's disease of the breast. *Cancer Treat Rev*. 2001;27(1):9–18.

445. Kawase K, Dimaio DJ, Tucker SL, et al. Paget's disease of the breast: there is a role for breast-conserving therapy. *Ann Surg Oncol*. 2005;12(5):391–397.

446. Siponen E, Hukkinen K, Heikkila P, Joensuu H, Leidenius M. Surgical treatment in Paget's disease of the breast. *Am J Surg*. 2010;200(2):241–246.

447. Kanitakis J. Mammary and extramammary Paget's disease. *J Eur Acad Dermatol Venereol*. 2007;581.

448. Murrell TW Jr, McMullan FH. Extramammary Paget's disease. A report of two cases. *Arch Dermatol*. 1962;85:600–613.

449. Fligiel Z, Kaneko M. Extramammary Paget's disease of the external ear canal in association with ceruminous gland carcinoma. A case report. *Cancer*. 1975;36(3):1072–1076.

450. Whorton CM, Patterson JB. Carcinoma of Moll's glands with extramammary Paget's disease of the eyelid. *Cancer*. 1955;8(5):1009–1015.

451. Duperrat B, Mascaro JM. Abdomino-scrotal Paget's disease (3d Report). Appearance of an apocrine epithelioma of the axilla and Paget's disease lesions on the subjacent axillary skin. *Bull Soc Fr Dermatol Syphiligr*. 1964;71:176–177.

452. Fetissoff F, Arbeille-Brassart B, Lansac J, Sam-Giao M, Granger M, Lorette G. Associated Paget's disease of the vulva and of the nipple in the same patient: pathology with ultrastructural study. *Ann Dermatol Venereol*. 1982;109(1):43–50.

453. McKee PH, Hertogs KT. Endocervical adenocarcinoma and vulval Paget's disease: a significant association. *Br J Dermatol*. 1980;103(4):443–448.

454. Metcalf JS, Lee RE, Maize JC. Epidermotropic urothelial carcinoma involving the glans penis. *Arch Dermatol*. 1985;121(4):532–534.

455. Ojeda VJ, Heenan PJ, Watson SH. Paget's disease of the groin associated with adenocarcinoma of the urinary bladder. *J Cutan Pathol*. 1987;14(4):227–231.

456. Powell FC, Bjornsson J, Doyle JA, Cooper AJ. Genital Paget's disease and urinary tract malignancy. *J Am Acad Dermatol*. 1985;13(1):84–90.

457. Hutchings D, Windon A, Assarzadegan N, Salimian KJ, Voltaggio L, Montgomery EA. Perianal Paget's disease as spread from non-invasive colorectal adenomas. *Histopathology*. 2021;78(2):276–280.

458. Zhao Y, Gong X, Li N, Zhu Q, Yu D, Jin X. Primary extramammary Paget's disease: a clinicopathological study of 28 cases. *Int J Clin Exp Pathol*. 2019;12(9):3426–3432.

459. Jones RE Jr, Austin C, Ackerman AB. Extramammary Paget's disease. A critical reexamination. *Am J Dermatopathol*. 1979;1(2):101–132.

460. Hart WR, Millman JB. Progression of intraepithelial Paget's disease of the vulva to invasive carcinoma. *Cancer*. 1977;40(5):2333–2337.

461. Wick MR, Goellner JR, Wolfe JT III, Su WP. Vulvar sweat gland carcinomas. *Arch Pathol Lab Med*. 1985;109(1):43–47.

462. Lee SC, Roth LM, Ehrlich C, Hall JA. Extramammary Paget's disease of the vulva. A clinicopathologic study of 13 cases. *Cancer*. 1977;39(6):2540–2549.

463. Yoell JH, Price WG. Paget's disease of the perineal skin with associated adenocarcinoma. *Arch Dermatol*. 1960;82:986–991.

464. Wood WS, Culling CF. Perianal Paget disease. Histochemical differentiation utilizing the borohydride-KOH-PAS reaction. *Arch Pathol*. 1975;99(8):442–445.

465. Gunn RA, Gallager HS. Vulvar Paget's disease: a topographic study. *Cancer*. 1980;46(3):590–594.

466. Koss LG, Brockunier A Jr. Ultrastructural aspects of Paget's disease of the vulva. *Arch Pathol*. 1969;87(6):592–600.

467. Tazawa T, Ito M, Fujiwara H, Shimizu N, Sato Y. Immunologic characteristics of keratins in extramammary Paget's disease. *Arch Dermatol*. 1988;124(7):1063–1068.

468. Pinkus H, Mehregan AH. *A Guide to Dermatopathology*. 3rd ed. Appleton-Century-Crofts; 1981:471.

469. Toker C. Glandular Paget's disease of the nipple. *Histopathology*. 2008;52(6):767.

470. Toker C. Some observations on Paget's disease of the nipple. *Cancer*. 1961;14:653–672.

471. Merot Y, Mazoujian G, Pinkus G, Momtaz T, Murphy GF. Extramammary Paget's disease of the perianal and perineal regions. Evidence of apocrine derivation. *Arch Dermatol*. 1985;121(6):750–752.

472. De MA, Checcucci V, Catalano C, et al. Vulvar Paget disease: a large single-centre experience on clinical presentation, surgical treatment, and long-term outcomes. *J Low Genit Tract Dis*. 2013;17(2):104–110.

473. Hendi A, Brodland DG, Zitelli JA. Extramammary Paget's disease: surgical treatment with Mohs micrographic surgery. *J Am Acad Dermatol*. 2004;51(5):767–773.

474. Beleznay KM, Levesque MA, Gill S. Response to 5-fluorouracil in metastatic extramammary Paget disease of the scrotum presenting as pancytopenia and back pain. *Curr Oncol*. 2009;16(5):81–83.

475. Ho SA, Aw DC. Extramammary Paget's disease treated with topical imiquimod 5% cream. *Dermatol Ther*. 2010;23(4):423–427.

476. Qian Z, Zeitoun NC, Shieh S, Helm T, Oseroff AR. Successful treatment of extramammary Paget's disease with imiquimod. *J Drugs Dermatol*. 2003;2(1):73–76.

Chapter 30

Tumors of the Epidermal Appendages

MATTHEW L. HEDBERG, MARGARET WAT, AND JOHN T. SEYKORA

CLASSIFICATION OF THE APPENDAGEAL TUMORS

Historically, appendageal tumors have been classified into four primary groups based on whether the histologic structures present resemble hair follicles, sebaceous glands, apocrine glands, or eccrine glands. This type of diagnostic nosology based on the microscopic attributes of appendageal structures has been useful for the classification of appendageal lesions.

However, in some cases, the diagnosis of appendageal neoplasms presents unique difficulties, in part related to the wide variety of tumors, the substantial frequency of one lesion exhibiting histologic features consisting of two or more appendageal types, and the complicated nomenclature (1–5). Histogenesis is a concept relating the histologic appearance of a tumor to the histology of the fully differentiated organ/structure from which the tumor "arose" ("cell of origin"). Today, the concepts describing appendageal tumorigenesis have been modified by new experimental data implicating the proliferation and differentiation of pluripotent and multipotent stem cells in the development of these tumors.

Appendageal tumors do not appear to be derived from mature (differentiated, postmitotic) cells; rather, these tumors originate from multipotent stem (undifferentiated) cells present in the epidermis or its appendageal structures (6,7). Such multipotent stem cells, when forming a tumor, may aberrantly express one or more types of appendageal differentiation in varying degrees; it is important to remember that multipotent stem cells that have acquired the neoplastic phenotype may express abnormal patterns of differentiation that are not restricted to one appendageal type. Taken together, these concepts predict that the histologic features of a tumor are related to the activation of molecular pathways utilized for forming the mature adnexal structure. The degree to which the eccrine, apocrine, sebaceous, and follicular differentiation programs are activated and recapitulated gives a tumor its histologic features. These concepts predict that appendageal tumors may imprecisely resemble their mature counterparts and that multiple lines of differentiation may be seen simultaneously in the same tumor (6,8). Given that tumor cell physiology differs from that of a postmitotic differentiating cell, it is remarkable that most adnexal neoplasms manifest predominantly one type of appendageal differentiation (Table 30-1).

Benign appendageal tumors in which there is a combination of follicular, eccrine, sebaceous, and/or apocrine differentiation, such as sebaceous units in association with either eccrine and/or apocrine elements, are occasionally a source of diagnostic confusion. Differentiation is probably influenced not only by the endogenous genetic potential of the stem cells giving rise to the tumor but also by exogenous stromal effects—such as regional vascularity and molecular attributes of the epidermis, basement membrane, dermis, or subcutis (7). In human skin, keratinocytes with markers of stem cells appear to reside in the "bulge" and basal layer of the epidermis (9). Cells with the capability of proliferating and differentiating along appendageal lines (progenitor cells) appear to traffic from this site to the basilar epidermis, the germinative layer of the sebaceous gland, and the hair follicle (6,8,10).

In addition to benign appendageal tumors, there are carcinomas of the epidermal appendages, which have the potential to metastasize. Three types of glandular carcinoma are recognized: carcinomas of sebaceous glands, eccrine glands, and apocrine glands. Other epithelial carcinomas exhibiting various types of follicular differentiation—such as pilomatrical carcinoma, malignant proliferating trichilemmal cyst, trichilemmal carcinoma, and trichoblastic carcinoma—have been reported (Table 30-1).

As noted, the histopathology of a tumor can often be interpreted by comparing it to the histology of skin appendages. For example, clear or pale cell change owing to cytoplasmic glycogen may recapitulate the acrosyringeal components in a nodular hidradenoma or the glycogenated follicular outer root sheath in a trichilemmoma. Cytoplasmic fat vacuoles that indent the nucleus are typical of sebaceous differentiation, which is seen in sebaceous glands, sebaceous adenomas, and sebaceous carcinomas. Many adnexal tumors contain a distinctive, eosinophilic hyaline stroma that is associated with epithelial elements. This stroma assists in differentiating many basaloid adnexal neoplasms from basal cell carcinoma (BCC). Eccrine tumors commonly exhibit a nearly acellular hyalinized eosinophilic stroma with dilated thin-walled vessels (e.g., nodular hidradenoma, eccrine poroma). Duct and tubule formation and focal keratinization occurring in eccrine tumors tend to differentiate them from renal cell or other metastatic clear cell carcinomas. Typically, immunohistochemistry has been of little value in definitively distinguishing the phenotypic patterns of adnexal neoplasms (11); however, with the identification of specific mutations in genes associated with appendageal neoplasms—for example, *CYLD1* in cylindromas (12)—further research on adnexal tumors using current technologies, especially next-generation sequencing and proteomic studies, may help identify molecular markers useful for classifying these lesions.

Table 30-1

Classification of Tumors of Epidermal Appendages

Lesion Type	Follicular Differentiation	Sebaceous Differentiation	Apocrine Differentiation	Eccrine Differentiation
Hyperplasias, hamartomas	Hair follicle nevus	Nevus sebaceous	Apocrine nevus	Eccrine nevus
	Dilated pore			
	Generalized hair follicle hamartoma	Sebaceous hyperplasia		
	Basaloid follicular hamartoma			
Benign neoplasms	Trichofolliculoma	Sebaceous adenoma	Apocrine hidrocystoma	Eccrine hidrocystoma
	Pilar sheath acanthoma	Sebaceoma	Hidroadenoma papilliferum	Syringoma
	Fibrofolliculoma		Syringocystadenoma papilliferum	Eccrine cylindroma
	Trichodiscoma			Eccrine poroma
	Trichoepithelioma			Eccrine syringofibroadenoma
	Trichoblastoma			
	Trichoadenoma		Erosive adenomatosis of the nipple	Mucinous syringometaplasia
	Pilomatricoma		Apocrine cylindroma	Eccrine spiradenoma
	Trichilemmoma			Papillary eccrine adenoma
	Tumor of follicular infundibulum			Nodular hidradenoma
				Chondroid syringoma
	Trichilemmal horn			
	Proliferating trichilemmal cyst			
Malignant neoplasms	Pilomatrix carcinoma	Sebaceous carcinoma	Malignant apocrine cylindroma	Porocarcinoma
	Malignant proliferating trichilemmal tumor			Malignant eccrine spiradenoma
	Trichilemmal carcinoma			Malignant nodular hidradenoma
	Trichoblastic carcinoma			
				Malignant chondroid syringoma
				Eccrine adenocarcinoma
				Microcystic adnexal carcinoma
				Aggressive digital papillary adenocarcinoma
				Adenoid cystic carcinoma
				Mucinous eccrine carcinoma
				Syringoid eccrine carcinoma
				Malignant eccrine cylindroma

Lesional histology evolves with time and in response to local effects. A trichilemmal cyst, possibly stimulated by inflammatory mediators, may, with time, transform into a proliferating trichilemmal cyst and ultimately into a solid pilar tumor of the scalp. It is almost certain that tumor progression, the "process whereby tumors go from bad to worse," also operates in appendageal tumors, as it does in most tumor types. From a clinical point of view, appendageal neoplasms should not always be regarded as precursors of malignancy.

Classification of Appendageal Tumors

The four primary groups of appendageal tumors with differentiation toward hair, sebaceous glands, apocrine glands, and eccrine glands can be divided, according to a gradient of decreasing differentiation, into three major subgroups: (a) hyperplasias, hamartomas, and cysts; (b) benign tumors; and (c) malignant tumors (Table 30-1). This classification is similar to the approach of the recent World Health Organization International Histological Classification of Tumours monograph (13).

Of the three subgroups of appendageal lesions, the hyperplasias, hamartomas, and cysts are composed of mature or nearly mature structures. The benign neoplasms, in general, show less complete differentiation than the hyperplasias; nonetheless, they exhibit well-developed, differentiated, or partially differentiated structures. The malignant neoplasms exhibit a lower degree of differentiation, and these lesions may lack differentiated cells or well-formed appendageal structures.

Although most of the appendageal tumors fit well into one of the entities listed in Table 30-1, tumors manifesting intermediate degrees of differentiation are occasionally encountered and may be difficult to classify (14).

Development of the Appendageal Tumors

Given that multipotent stem cells give rise to cutaneous appendageal structures and that stem cells are present in the skin, it is likely that appendageal tumors arise from stem cells that possess the potential for differentiating into tumors that manifest hair, sebaceous gland, eccrine gland, or apocrine structures (6). Appendageal tumors associated with genetic syndromes—such as multiple cylindromas, multiple trichoepitheliomas, and the nevoid BCC syndrome—are probably derived from abnormal multipotent stem cells that are genetically predisposed to proliferate and form tumors with altered appendageal structures. This scenario of tumor formation is likely to apply to sporadic occurrences of the same appendageal tumors. In some instances, multipotent stem cells may manifest more than one differentiation pattern, as seen most commonly on the scalp, where a syringocystadenoma may exhibit three different lines of appendageal differentiation.

Terminology

The terms *nevus, hamartoma,* and *carcinoma* used in the classification of the appendageal tumors require definition.

The term *nevus* is used in the literature in two different ways, referring (a) to a tumor composed of nevomelanocytes (nevocellular nevus, melanocytic nevus, pigmented nevus) or (b) to a lesion that is usually present at birth and is composed of mature or nearly mature structures—such as hair follicle nevus, nevus sebaceous, eccrine nevus, nevus verrucosus, and nevus flammeus. To avoid confusion, it is advisable to use the term *nevus* with a qualifying adjective and to assume that *nevus*

without a qualifying adjective designates a tumor composed of melanocytic nevus cells.

The term *hamartoma* is appropriate for those nevi that have no melanocytic nevus cells and, like congenital hyperplasias, are composed of mature or nearly mature structures. *Hamartoma*, derived from the Greek word *hamartanein* (to fail, to err), was chosen as the designation for "tumor-like malformations showing a faulty mixture of the normal components of the organ in which they occur" (15).

The term *epithelioma* has been used by many authors as a synonym for *carcinoma*. However, because the literal meaning of the word is "tumor of the epithelium," the term may be employed as a designation of benign as well as of malignant tumors of the epithelium, provided that a qualifying adjective is added (16). Because the term has been used for both benign and malignant neoplasms, it seems prudent to avoid its use except in a clearly defined context. The term *carcinoma* is used for malignant epithelial tumors, including those that are characterized by a tendency for continuous growth with local invasion and tissue destruction as well as those that may in addition have capacity for distant metastasis. We continue to use terms that are widely understood and utilized, not necessarily those that are above all semantic dissection (17).

TUMORS WITH DIFFERENTIATION TOWARD HAIR FOLLICLE COMPONENTS

Hair Follicle Nevus

Clinical Summary. This rare, small hamartoma presents as a small nodule on the face, often at birth. It has also been referred to as congenital vellus hamartoma (18–21). A few reported cases have raised the possibility of a novel neurocutaneous syndrome (22,23). Features of hair follicle nevus may be noted in porokeratotic adnexal ostial nevus (24–26). A mucinous variant of hair follicle nevus has also been reported (27).

Histopathology. There are focally increased vellus hair follicles, occasionally accompanied by a few small sebaceous glands. The lesion classically lacks the cartilage seen in accessory tragus and the central dilated pore seen in trichofolliculoma (Fig. 30-1) (18,28,29).

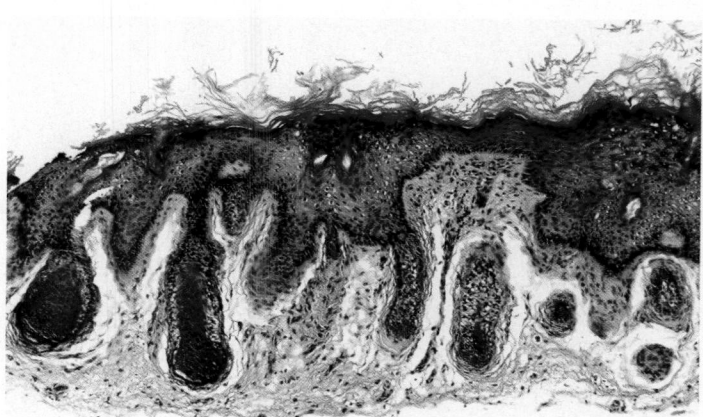

Figure 30-1 Hair follicle nevus. Increased numbers of small hair follicles are present in the dermis.

Differential Diagnosis. The small vellus hair follicles present in the central face resemble the hair follicles in a hair follicle nevus. Other entities to consider in the differential diagnosis include accessory tragus and hair follicle hamartoma (18,22,28,30). Some authors consider these entities to be on a spectrum of similar hamartomas (28,31).

Principles of Management: These lesions may be removed primarily for cosmetic reasons (18,19). There are no reports of these lesions behaving in a biologically aggressive manner.

Trichofolliculoma

Clinical Summary. Trichofolliculoma occurs in adults as a solitary lesion, usually on the face but occasionally on the scalp or neck also (32). More rarely, the lesions can be multiple and present on the extremities or genitalia (33). Trichofolliculoma consists of a small, skin-colored, dome-shaped nodule. Frequently, there is a central pore. If such a central pore is present, a wool-like tuft of immature, usually white hairs may be seen emerging from it, a highly diagnostic clinical feature (32).

Histopathology. On histologic examination, the dermis contains a cystic cavity lined by squamous epithelium; this cyst contains keratinized material and, frequently, fragments of hair shafts that are birefringent on polariscopic examination (Fig. 30-2) (34). In cases with a visible central pore, the cystic space is continuous with the surface epidermis, an indication that the lesion is analogous to an enlarged, distorted hair follicle. In some cases, multiple cystic spaces are present in the dermis. Radiating from the wall of these cysts are many small yet well-differentiated hair follicles (Fig. 30-3). Well-developed secondary hair follicles often show a hair papilla (Fig. 30-3). Furthermore, these follicles usually have an outer and an inner root sheath, the latter of which may contain eosinophilic trichohyaline granules and, located in the center, a small hair shaft (Fig. 30-3). These fine hairs are visualized best where the secondary hair follicles appear in cross sections. Small groups

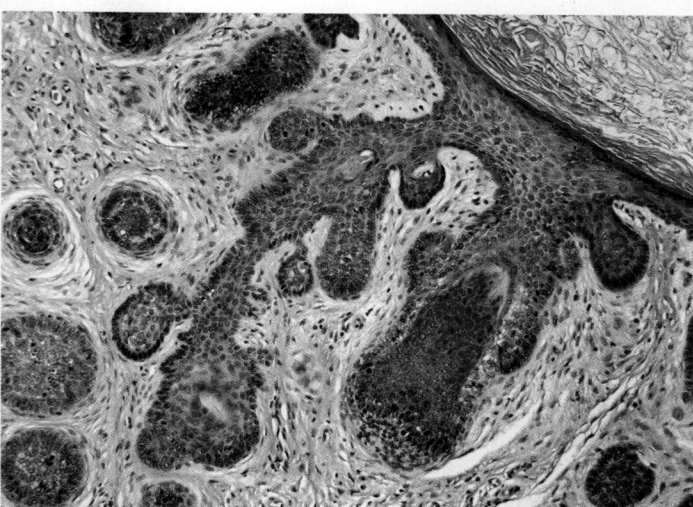

Figure 30-3 Trichofolliculoma. Emanating from the cyst wall are numerous small "secondary" hair follicles, some of which show, in addition to a hair and an outer root sheath, an inner root sheath with trichohyaline granules.

of sebaceous gland cells may be embedded in the walls of the secondary hair follicles (35).

In some of the more rudimentary secondary follicles, one observes a central horn cyst in place of a hair, as seen in trichoepithelioma also (36). Glycogen can be demonstrated in the outer root sheath of the secondary hair follicles, just as it is seen in mature hair follicles (34). The size of the secondary hair follicles can range in size from vellus to terminal hairs. Abnormal tertiary follicles have been identified in association with involuting secondary follicles (37).

Trichofolliculoma stains positively with CK16 and CK17, in the primary cystic structure and the secondary hair follicles, confirming outer root sheath differentiation. The basal layer of the primary follicle and the secondary follicle is positive for CK15, a marker for hair follicle stem cells (37). It is thought that the CK15-positive hair follicle stem cells proliferate to form abnormal secondary hair follicles, which do not mature properly (37). In all trichofolliculomas, epithelial strands interconnect the secondary hair follicles. Because these epithelial strands differentiate in the direction of the outer root sheath, the peripheral cell row is palisaded, and because of their glycogen content, the cells within the strands appear large and vacuolated (38).

The lesional stroma of trichofolliculoma is rich in CD34-positive fibroblastic cells; these cells are oriented in parallel bundles that encapsulate the epithelial proliferations in a manner resembling that of the normal fibrous root sheath (37). Rarely, S100-positive cells may be seen in the stromal component (37). The stroma of trichofolliculoma can also rarely have a striking myxoid appearance (39). Trichofolliculoma has been reported in association with angiomyxoma, BCC, and nevus lipomatosus superficialis (40–42).

Additional Studies. Experimental evidence suggests that trichofolliculomas undergo morphologic changes corresponding to the normal hair follicle cycle (43). Trichofolliculoma is thought to arise from a single dilated pore, which then differentiates toward the lower segment of the hair follicle via induction from the perifollicular stroma (44). Transgenic mice that overexpress a stabilized form of the β-catenin protein develop

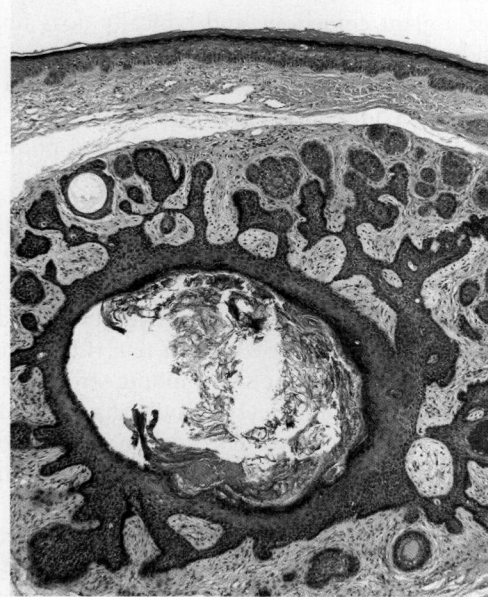

Figure 30-2 Trichofolliculoma. In the dermis, there is a keratin-filled cyst lined by squamous epithelium with associated follicular structures.

trichofolliculomas (45); therefore, increased signaling through the β-catenin pathway may play a role in the development of trichofolliculomas in humans. Transgenic mice with increased epidermal expression of the Noggin gene (*NOG*)—an inhibitor of bone-morphogenetic protein signaling—exhibit appendageal tumors resembling trichofolliculomas, likely via the Wnt and Shh signaling pathways (46–48).

Principles of Management: No treatment is necessary. For cosmetic reasons, these lesions are often treated by excision, electrodesiccation, or curettage. Complete removal is curative.

Folliculosebaceous Cystic Hamartoma

Clinical Summary. Folliculosebaceous cystic hamartoma exhibits many features of a trichofolliculoma. Although the two lesions may have similar pathogenesis through disordered epithelial–mesenchymal interactions, some believe that folliculosebaceous cystic hamartoma does not arise from trichofolliculoma (49,50).

Histopathology. The folliculosebaceous cystic hamartoma consists of a folliculosebaceous proliferation with a cyst-like infundibular dilation and a mesenchymal stroma with variable fibroplasia. It typically manifests more prominent sebaceous differentiation and a more prominent surrounding stroma (Figs. 30-4 and 30-5) (51). The folliculosebaceous cystic hamartoma may have rare focal follicular differentiation, but it typically lacks the secondary and tertiary hair follicles seen in trichofolliculoma and sebaceous trichofolliculoma (44,50).

Sebaceous Trichofolliculoma

Clinical Summary. Sebaceous trichofolliculoma shares features of folliculosebaceous cystic hamartoma and trichofolliculoma (50). It occurs in anatomic regions rich in sebaceous follicles, such as the nose. This tumor exhibits a centrally depressed, fistula-like opening from which terminal hairs and vellus hairs protrude (52).

Histopathology. There is a rather large, irregularly shaped, centrally located cavity lined by squamous epithelium. Many radially arranged pilosebaceous follicles connect to the

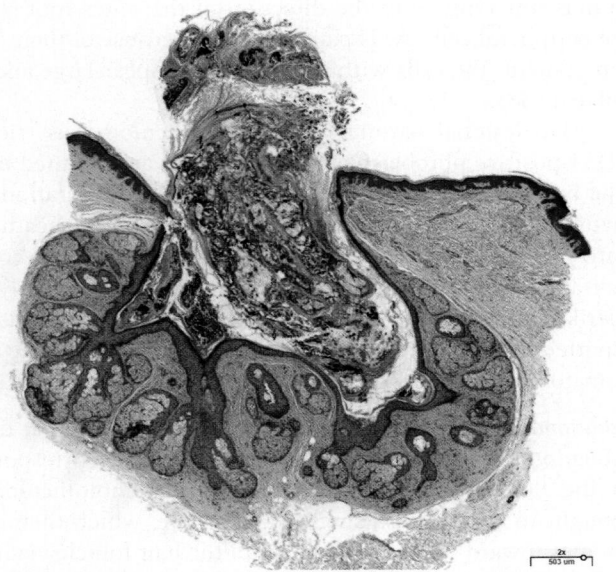

Figure 30-4 Folliculosebaceous cystic hamartoma. There is a cyst-like infundibular dilation with sebaceous differentiation.

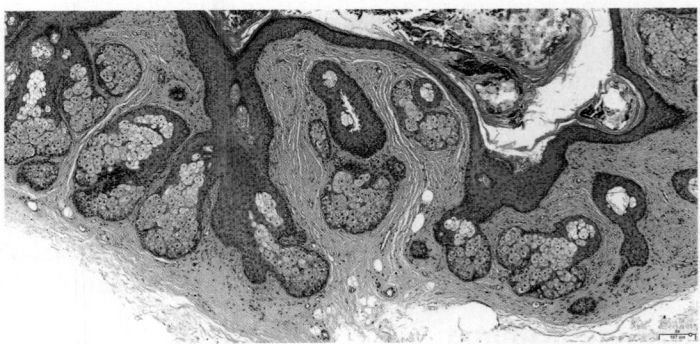

Figure 30-5 Folliculosebaceous cystic hamartoma. Prominent mature sebaceous units and a mesenchymal stroma with fibroplasia.

cavity. These follicles contain sebaceous ducts and numerous well-differentiated, large sebaceous lobules, as well as hair follicles containing partially terminal and partially vellus hairs (52).

Differential Diagnosis. Unlike folliculosebaceous cystic hamartoma, which presents as a solitary papule or nodule, sebaceous trichofolliculoma clinically presents with a central porelike opening that exhibits protruding hairs. Histopathologically, folliculosebaceous cystic hamartoma is additionally characterized by stromal mesenchymal prominence, a finding not seen in the previously reported cases of sebaceous trichofolliculoma (53).

Principles of Management: These benign lesions do not require removal unless there are symptomatic or cosmetic reasons to do so. Simple excisions have been used to treat these lesions.

Dilated Pore and Pilar Sheath Acanthomas

Clinical Summary. Dilated pore and pilar sheath acanthomas clinically share with trichofolliculoma and sebaceous trichofolliculoma the presence of a central pore and, histologically, the presence of a large cystic space that is continuous with the surface epidermis, lined by squamous epithelium, and filled with keratinous material.

The dilated pore, described in 1954 by Winer, occurs on the face, usually as a solitary lesion and predominantly in adult males (54). It can also occur on the eyelid (55). It has the appearance of a giant comedone and typically does not possess palpable induration (54).

The pilar sheath acanthoma is usually found on the skin of the upper lip of adults. It is seen elsewhere on the face only rarely (56). It occurs as a solitary skin-colored nodule with a central porelike opening (57).

Histopathology. The dilated pore differentiates toward the infundibulum both architecturally and cytologically (58). It shows a markedly dilated pilar infundibulum lined by an epidermis that is atrophic near the ostium but hypertrophic deeper in the cystic cavity, where it shows many rete ridges and irregular thin proliferations into the surrounding stroma (Figs. 30-6 and 30-7). The keratin-filled cystic cavity may extend into the subcutaneous fat. In the lower portion, small sebaceous gland lobules and vellus hair follicles may be attached to the lining epithelium (54).

The *pilar sheath acanthoma* differs from the dilated pore by showing a larger, irregularly branching cystic cavity. In place of thin proliferations, as seen in the dilated pore, numerous lobulated masses of cells radiate from the wall of the cystic cavity into the dermis and the subcutaneous tissue (Fig. 30-8) (57).

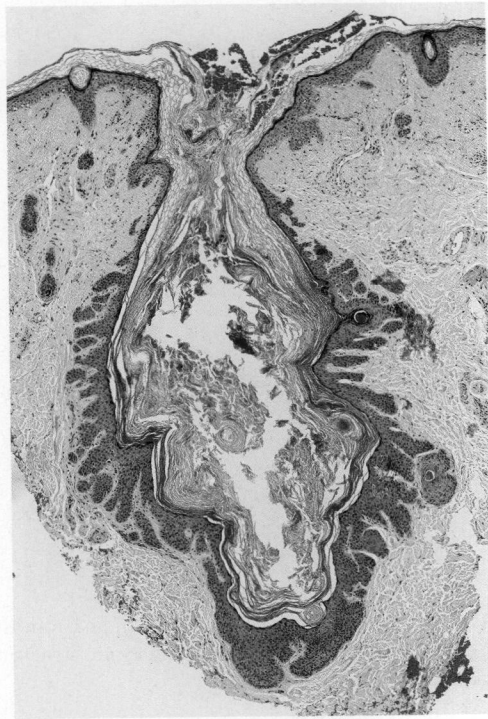

Figure 30-6 Dilated pore of Winer. An irregular cystic cavity containing keratin is present in the dermis.

The pilar sheath acanthoma can exhibit some features of the outer root sheath in that portions of the lesion may show peripheral palisading and contain varying amounts of glycogen (Fig. 30-9) (59). Abortive hair follicles may be seen, though no hair shafts should be seen in the central cystic cavity (56). It has been suggested that pilar sheath acanthomas can manifest differentiation of all components of the pilosebaceous unit.

Principles of Management: These lesions can be treated with simple excision.

Fibrofolliculoma and Trichodiscoma

Clinical Summary. Fibrofolliculomas and trichodiscomas consist of 2 to 4 mm, yellow-white, smooth, dome-shaped lesions,

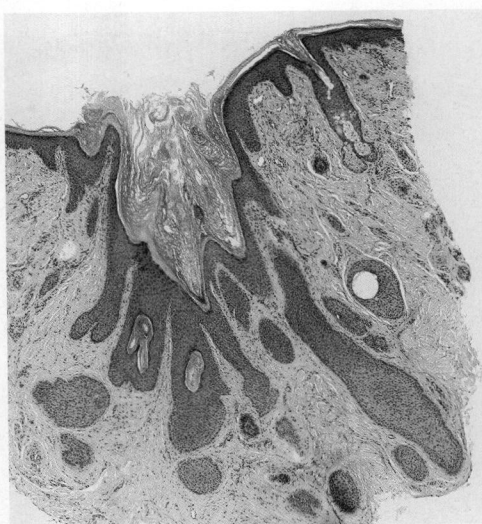

Figure 30-8 Pilar sheath acanthoma. Lobulated masses of cells extend from the cystic cavity into the surrounding dermis.

often on the face. Formerly, these lesions were considered separate entities, but they are now recognized as the same lesion and appear different based on the sectioning plane, anatomical site, and "age" of the lesion (60).

The lesions can be solitary or multiple. Multiple fibrofolliculomas have been described in association with kidney neoplasms, lung cysts, and spontaneous pneumothorax in Birt–Hogg–Dubé syndrome (61). In patients with the Birt–Hogg–Dubé syndrome, the lesions are numerous and mainly on the face and neck. Other less common mucocutaneous features of the Birt–Hogg–Dubé syndrome include multiple epidermal cysts, severe facial sebaceous hyperplasia, and oral papules (62). Multiple fibrofolliculomas may present outside of Birt–Hogg–Dubé as well. In a patient reported with a large connective tissue nevus, fibrofolliculomas were present in large numbers within as well as around the connective tissue nevus (63).

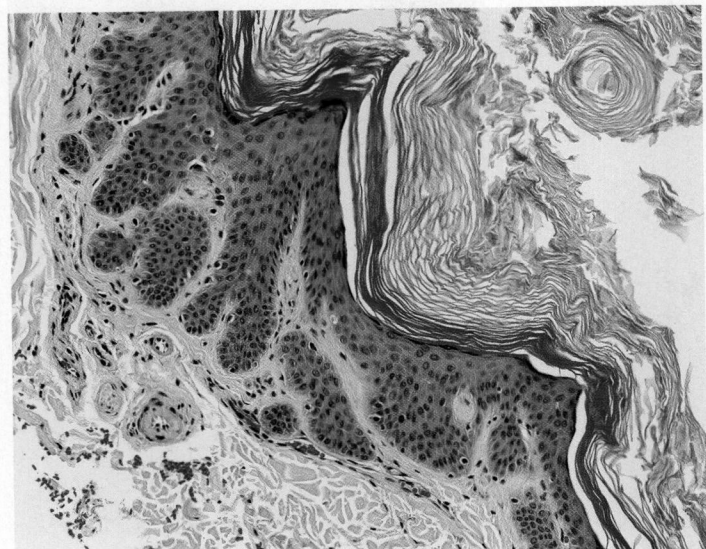

Figure 30-7 Dilated pore of Winer. Small projections of epithelial cells extend from the wall of the cyst into the surrounding dermis.

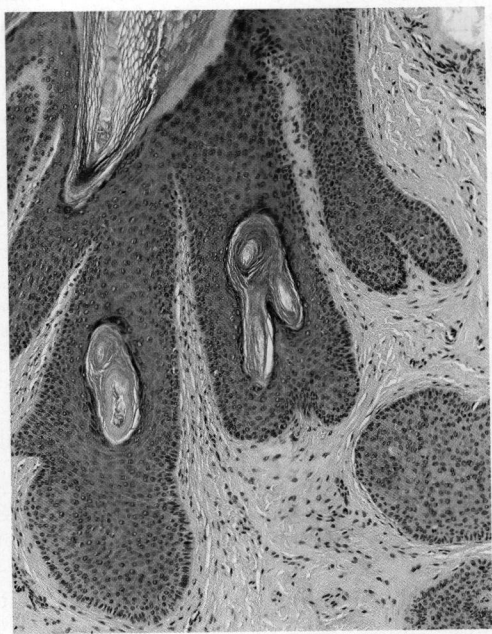

Figure 30-9 Pilar sheath acanthoma. The lobulated masses are comprised of bland cells resembling infundibular keratinocytes.

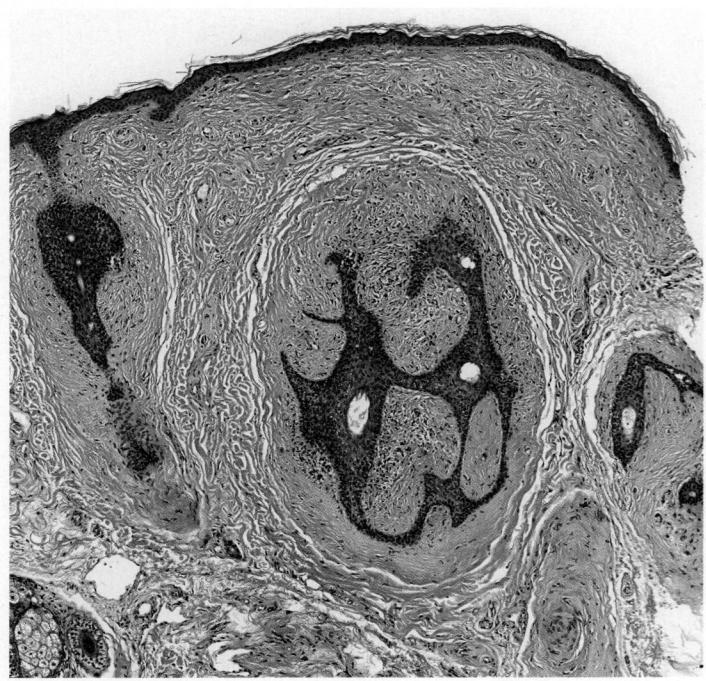

Figure 30-10 Fibrofolliculoma. In the dermis, there are distorted follicular structures associated with epithelial cords and a fibrous stroma.

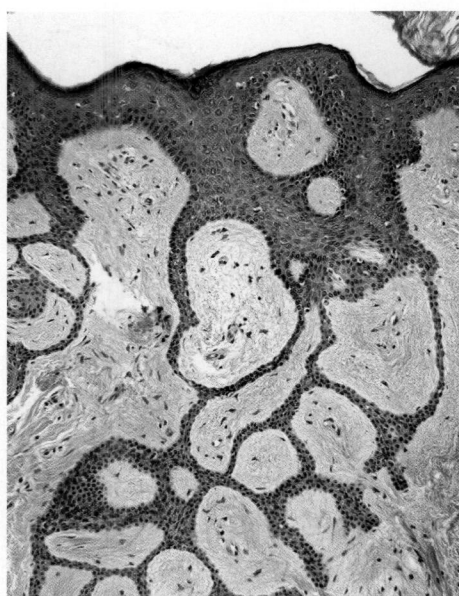

Figure 30-11 Fibrofolliculoma. Numerous thin, anastomosing bands of follicular epithelium extend from a central cystic structure into the bland fibrocellular stroma.

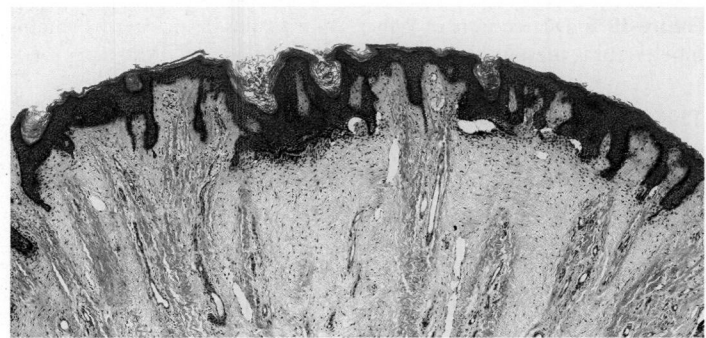

Figure 30-12 Trichodiscoma. Present in the dermis are areas of fine, fibrillar connective tissue.

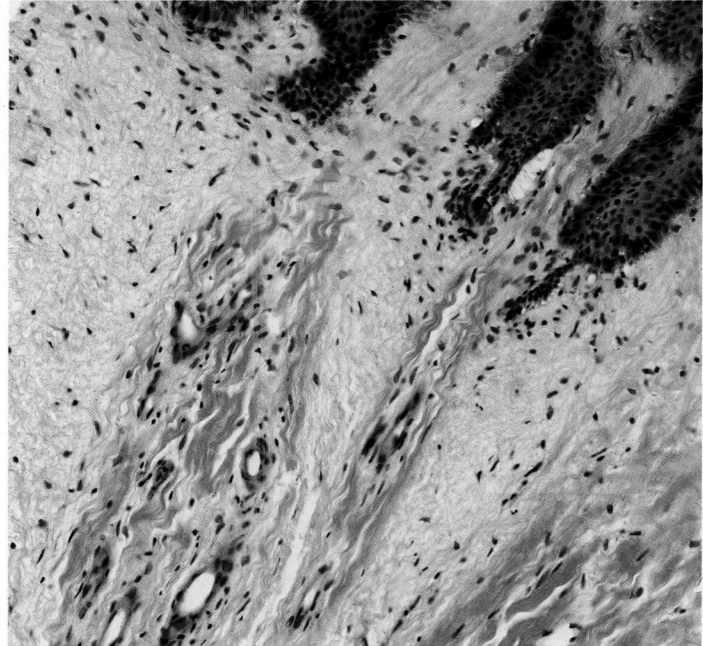

Figure 30-13 Trichodiscoma. The altered connective tissue exhibits ectatic vessels, a myxomatous appearance, increased numbers of mature fibrocytic cells, and basaloid follicular epidermal hyperplasia.

Besides occurring in association with multiple fibrofolliculomas, multiple trichodiscomas also occur without them, as small papules either widely disseminated or localized to one area (64,65). Familial multiple discoid fibromas, formerly familial multiple trichodiscomas, is a distinct syndrome unrelated to mutations in folliculin, whereby patients develop lesions around their pinnae at a young age, and lack the systemic features seen in Birt–Hogg–Dubé. Discoid fibromas lack the follicular epithelial features of fibrofolliculomas commonly seen in Birt–Hogg–Dubé (66,67).

Histopathology. *Fibrofolliculomas* exhibit a central distorted hair follicle that is surrounded by a mantle of basophilic, fibrous stroma (Fig. 30-10) (63,68). Numerous thin, anastomosing bands of follicular epithelium extend into this stroma (Fig. 30-11).

Trichodiscomas are seen in the dermis as an area of fine fibrillary connective tissue containing ectatic blood vessels (Figs. 30-12 and 30-13). Epithelial hyperplasia resembling follicular structures, including those seen in fibrofolliculomas, is often seen. A hair follicle is usually found at the margin of the lesion (63,68). Trichodiscomas have been regarded as hamartomas of the mesodermal component of hair disks (64). A symplastic variant of trichodiscoma with an increased number of spindled cells demonstrating multinucleation and "ancient change" has been reported (69).

Additional Studies. The immunophenotypic characteristics of syndromic-associated and sporadic types of fibrofolliculoma/trichodiscoma are identical and consist of perifollicular spindle cells that are positive for vimentin and CD34 and negative for factor XIII. These findings suggest that these lesions originate from the hair follicle mantle (70).

Birt–Hogg–Dubé syndrome is associated with mutations in the Folliculin (*FLCN*) gene on chromosome 17p. The *FLCN* gene product is believed to function as a tumor suppressor, which delays cell cycle progression through late S and

G2/M-phases (71). Aberrant *FLCN* expression may also directly impact adherens junctions, dysregulating the integrity of the epithelium (72).

Certain cases of Birt–Hogg–Dubé have been described with features overlapping with tuberous sclerosis, whereby patients develop renal angiomyolipomas as well as angiofibromas. Similarly, tuberous sclerosis patients have been reported with fibrofolliculomas (73). This phenotypic overlap is thought to occur owing to both folliculin and tuberous sclerosis complex proteins acting in a common pathway, the mammalian target of rapamycin (MTOR) (74,75).

Principles of Management: Although recurrence is common, multiple ablative therapies have been used—including excision, dermabrasion, laser therapy, and electrodesiccation.

Trichoepithelioma

Clinical Summary. Trichoepithelioma occurs either as a solitary lesion or multiple lesions. The name *trichoepithelioma* is preferred over others such as *epithelioma adenoides cysticum* and *multiple benign cystic epithelioma* because it is more indicative that the differentiation of this tumor is toward hair structures.

Multiple trichoepitheliomas are transmitted as an autosomal dominant trait (76). In most instances, the first lesions appear in childhood and gradually increase in number (77). Numerous rounded, skin-colored, firm papules and nodules usually between 2 and 8 mm in diameter are seen located mainly in the nasolabial folds and also the nose, forehead, and upper lip. Occasionally, lesions are also seen on the scalp, neck, and upper trunk.

Ulceration of the lesions occurs rarely and may indicate an occult malignancy. There have been a few cases of BCC arising in the setting of multiple trichoepitheliomas (78–81). Rarely, patients with multiple familial trichoepitheliomas can have malignant transformation of their lesions to trichoblastic carcinoma (82,83). Pigmented lesions, including malignant melanoma and blue nevus, have been described in association with trichoepitheliomas (84).

The simultaneous presence of trichoepithelioma and cylindroma, the latter of which is also dominantly inherited, has been observed repeatedly (see the section on Cylindroma).

Solitary trichoepithelioma occurs more commonly than multiple trichoepitheliomas (77). It is not inherited and consists of a firm, elevated, flesh-colored nodule, usually less than 2 cm in diameter. Its onset usually is in childhood or early adult life (85). Most commonly, the lesion is seen on the face, but it may occur elsewhere, including the vulva (86,87). The presence of a solitary trichoepithelioma and an apocrine adenoma within the same tumor has been reported (88). A solitary trichoepithelioma can also arise in the setting of a facial scar (89).

Giant solitary trichoepithelioma, measuring several centimeters in diameter, is a distinct variant of trichoepithelioma. It arises in later life and occurs most commonly on the thigh and in the perianal region but has been reported on the face also (90).

Histopathology. As a rule, multiple trichoepitheliomas are superficial dermal lesions. They appear well-circumscribed, small, and symmetric on histologic examination. Horn cysts are the most characteristic histologic feature, although they may be absent in some lesions. They consist of a fully keratinized center surrounded by basophilic cells that are similar in appearance

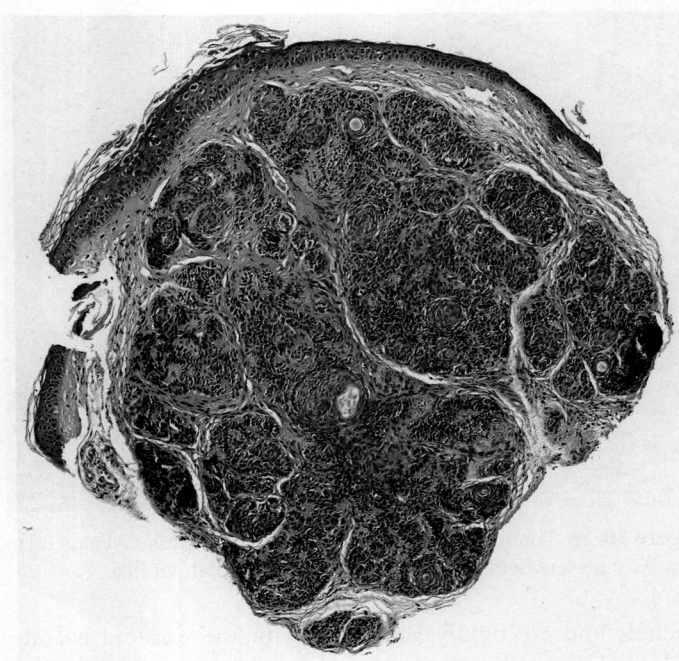

Figure 30-14 Trichoepithelioma. A dermal tumor with a prominent stroma, horn cysts of varying sizes, and basaloid epithelial formations.

to BCC cells, except they tend to lack high-grade atypia and mitoses, which may be prominent in some, but not all, carcinomas (Figs. 30-14 and 30-15). The keratinization is abrupt and complete, in the manner of so-called "trichilemmal" keratinization, as opposed to the horn pearls of squamous cell carcinoma. Quite frequently, one observes one or a few layers of cells with eosinophilic cytoplasm and large, oval, pale, vesicular nuclei situated between the basophilic cells and the horn cysts (77).

A second major component of multiple trichoepitheliomas are tumor islands composed of basophilic cells of the same appearance as epidermal or skin appendage basal cells, which are arranged usually in a lacelike or adenoid network but occasionally also as solid aggregates (Fig. 30-15). These tumor islands show peripheral palisading of their cells and are surrounded by a stroma with increased numbers of fibroblasts. The fibroblasts

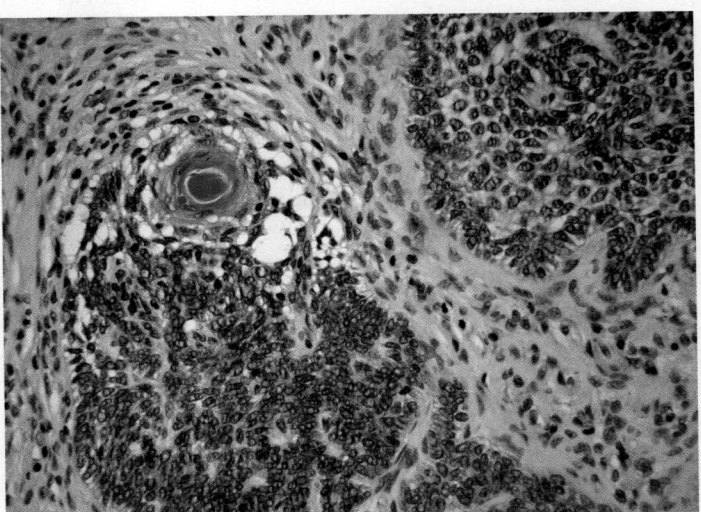

Figure 30-15 Trichoepithelioma. Fibroblasts encircle and are tightly associated with the basaloid epithelial islands, lacking the retraction artifact typical of basal cell carcinoma.

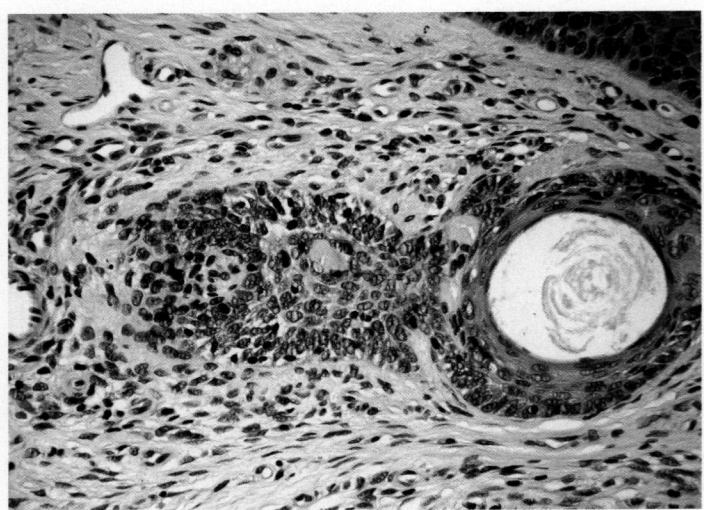

Figure 30-16 Trichoepithelioma. Some of the basophilic islands form papillary mesenchymal bodies resembling follicular papillae.

encircle and are tightly associated with the basaloid islands, lacking the retraction artifact typical of BCC (Fig. 30-15). Both the adenoid and the solid aggregates show invaginations, which contain numerous fibroblasts and resemble follicular papillae, also known as papillary mesenchymal bodies (Fig. 30-16) (91).

Additional findings, observed in some, but not all, trichoepitheliomas are the presence of a foreign-body giant cell reaction in the vicinity of ruptured horn cysts, calcium deposits—either within the foci of the foreign-body reaction or within intact horn cysts—and amyloid deposition (77,92). Occasionally, some lesions in patients with multiple trichoepitheliomas show relatively little differentiation toward hair structures. They contain only a few horn cysts, with many areas resembling BCC (77). Therefore, on a histologic basis, it may be difficult to definitively distinguish between multiple trichoepitheliomas and BCCs (see Differential Diagnosis).

Solitary trichoepithelioma often has a high degree of differentiation toward hair structures. Solitary lesions with relatively little differentiation toward hair structures could be classified as keratotic BCC. If a lesion is to qualify for the diagnosis of solitary trichoepithelioma, it should contain numerous horn cysts and abortive hair papillae and show only few areas with the appearance of BCC (85). Mitotic figures should be rare or absent, and the lesion should not be unduly large, asymmetric, or infiltrative.

Additional Studies. It is assumed that the basophilic cells surrounding horn cysts are similar to hair matrix cells and that the horn cysts represent attempts at hair shaft formation. The eosinophilic cells seen occasionally around horn cysts probably represent cells with initial keratinization and are similar to the nucleated cells seen in normal hair shafts at the keratogenous zone. An immunohistochemical analysis using a panel of monoclonal antikeratin antibodies suggests that trichoepitheliomas differentiate toward the outer root sheath (93). The expression of cytokeratin 15 in a subset of trichoepitheliomas suggests that these tumors contain cells that are related to hair follicle stem cells in the follicular bulge (94).

Numerous mutations in the *CYLD* gene, a deubiquitinating enzyme, have been identified in up to 88% of patients with Brooke–Spiegler syndrome (76). Brooke–Spiegler is characterized by the development of multiple adnexal cutaneous neoplasms including spiradenoma, cylindroma, spiradenocylindroma, and trichoepithelioma. Patients with multiple familial trichoepitheliomatosis, a phenotypic subtype of Brooke–Spiegler, also have *CYLD* mutations in 44% to 72% of cases (76,95–100).

The close relationship between trichoepithelioma and BCC has been explained on the theory that they have a common genesis from pluripotent cells, which, like primary epithelial germ cells, may develop toward hair structures (101). This hypothesis is supported by the fact that Patched gene (*PTCH1/2*) mutations are seen in both tumors (102). Additionally, BCC has been reported arising in a trichoepithelioma in a patient with known Brooke–Spiegler syndrome (81).

Differential Diagnosis. The difficulty of differentiating multiple trichoepitheliomas from keratotic BCC on histologic grounds has been pointed out. Diagnosis may be assisted by clinical data, such as the number and distribution of the lesions and the presence of hereditary transmission. The presence of well-formed horn cysts, papillary mesenchymal bodies, and lack of high-grade atypia and mitoses favor the diagnosis of trichoepithelioma (91). Other histologic features that favor BCC include the presence of myxoid stroma and stromal retraction or clefting around the basaloid islands (92).

Several immunohistochemical stains may be used to differentiate trichoepithelioma from BCC. A study of trichoepitheliomas and BCCs using a microarray found that the most reliable stains for distinguishing the two are CD10, cytokeratin 15, cytokeratin 20, and D2-40 (101). CD10 stains the stromal cells but not the epithelial cells in trichoepitheliomas, whereas in BCCs, CD10 is present in the epithelial cells and rarely in the stromal cells (103,104). CD10 was positive peripherally in BCC tumors in 60% and 30% showed central CD10 staining, whereas 22% showed stromal staining (105). Staining tumors for CK20 to identify Merkel cells, which are more common in trichoepitheliomas, may be also used (106). PHLDA1 (pleckstrin homology-like domain, family A, member 1) staining typically highlights trichoepitheliomas and is either negative or stains less than 25% of the cells in BCCs (107,108).

Androgen receptor (AR) immunohistochemical (IHC) staining may be absent in trichoepitheliomas, whereas BCCs may show patchy, focal nuclear staining. In one study, 59% of BCC cases were positive for AR and 41% were negative, whereas none of the trichoepitheliomas showed significant AR staining (105).

The differentiation of multiple trichoepitheliomas from the nevoid BCC syndrome on histologic grounds can be just as difficult. This diagnosis also requires clinical information. Although both diseases are dominantly inherited and have multiple lesions, the lesions in multiple trichoepitheliomas present mainly in the nasolabial fold, remain small, and hardly ever ulcerate, whereas the lesions in the nevoid BCC syndrome are haphazardly distributed and—especially in the late, "neoplastic" phase—can grow to a considerable size, ulcerate deeply, and show severely destructive growth. In addition, patients with the nevoid BCC syndrome almost invariably show multiple skeletal and central nervous system anomalies and frequently show multiple palmar and plantar pits (109).

Principles of Management: Solitary lesions are typically excised. Multiple lesions can be treated with cryotherapy, laser ablation, or dermabrasion.

Desmoplastic Trichoepithelioma

Clinical Summary. Desmoplastic trichoepithelioma (DTE), typically a sporadic lesion, has sufficient clinical and histologic characteristics to be regarded as a distinct variant of trichoepithelioma. The term *desmoplastic trichoepithelioma* appears preferable to the designation *sclerosing epithelial hamartoma* because it stresses the relationship of the lesion to solitary trichoepithelioma (110,111).

Clinically, the tumor almost always is located on the face, measures from 3 to 8 mm in diameter, and is markedly indurated. In many instances, there is a raised, annular border and a depressed nonulcerated center, causing the lesion to resemble granuloma annulare (110). Most commonly, the lesion appears in early adulthood, but it can also appear in the second decade of life (111). It is much more common in females than in males. Familial desmoplastic trichoepitheliomas have been reported infrequently (112,113).

Histopathology. The three characteristic histologic features are narrow strands of tumor cells, horn cysts, and a desmoplastic stroma (Figs. 30-17 and 30-18) (110). The tumor strands are usually one to three cells thick and are composed of small basaloid cells with prominent oval nuclei and scant cytoplasm. Usually, there are numerous horn cysts, which in some cases are large (114). Considerable amounts of densely collagenous stroma are present, forming an eosinophilic band around the strands of cells. Large aggregates of tumor cells are not seen. Foreign-body granulomas at the site of ruptured horn cysts and areas of calcification within some of the horn cysts are seen in many tumors (114).

Differential Diagnosis. The resemblance to microcystic adnexal (eccrine) carcinoma (MAC) and syringoma may be considerable, especially if a superficial specimen is taken for biopsy. Like desmoplastic trichoepithelioma, microcystic adnexal carcinoma has horn cysts, strands of basaloid cells, and a dense desmoplastic stroma. Histologic features such as skeletal muscle and subcutaneous tissue invasion, perineural invasion, ductal differentiation, and the presence of mitotic figures are significantly more frequent in microcystic adnexal carcinoma. CK19 is also more commonly positive in microcystic adnexal carcinoma (114).

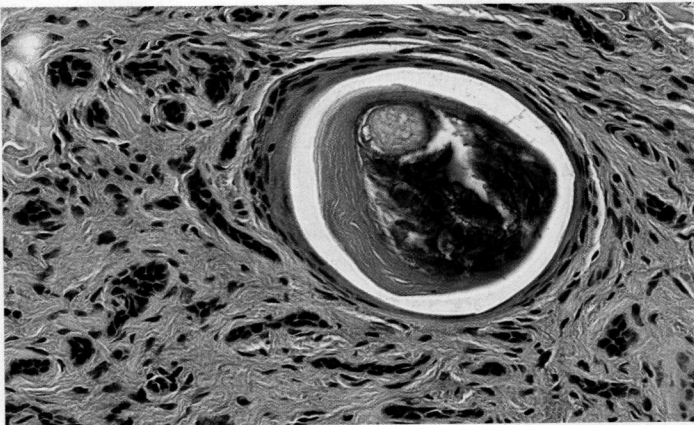

Figure 30-18 Desmoplastic trichoepithelioma. The strands of tumor cells are comprised of small basaloid cells and are usually one to three cells thick.

Features such as keratocysts, keratin granuloma, and calcification are more frequent in desmoplastic trichoepithelioma. It should be noted, however, that desmoplastic trichoepithelioma can rarely demonstrate perineural invasion (115,116).

The diagnosis of microcystic adnexal carcinoma should be considered in any tumor resembling a trichoepithelioma or a syringoma in which the lesional cells extend to the base of the specimen. Syringomas, which are usually periorbital, rarely have horn cysts, foreign-body granulomas, or calcification (110).

Desmoplastic trichoepithelioma may also resemble morpheaform (fibrosing) BCC. However, in morpheaform BCC, horn cysts are absent. Of value in ruling out BCC, especially the morpheaform form, are the absence of mitoses, individual cell necrosis, and mucinous stroma and the lack of foci of separation artifact of lesional epithelium and stroma (110). Signs of infundibular, follicular, or sebaceous differentiation, calcification, osteoma, association with a melanocytic nevus, and absence of solar elastosis below the lesion favor a diagnosis of desmoplastic trichoepithelioma over a morpheaform BCC (117).

Many immunohistochemical markers that may help differentiate desmoplastic trichoepithelioma and morpheaform BCC have been described. Desmoplastic trichoepithelioma is currently considered a follicular hamartoma mimicking the outer root sheath, based on strong p75NTR expression as seen in the later stages of hair follicle development. In contrast, morpheaform BCC generally lacks or is weakly positive for p75NTR expression and is more likely a primitive follicular lesion (118).

A recent study suggests that laminin (Ln)-γ 2, a chain of Ln-332, stains malignant sclerosing adnexal neoplasms compared to benign lesions, as the 26 DTEs in the study were negative for this marker (119). Matrix metalloproteinase stromelysin-3 (ST-3) expression has been demonstrated in morphea-like basal carcinomas but not desmoplastic trichoepitheliomas (120). The presence of Merkel cells by CK20 expression has been shown in desmoplastic trichoepitheliomas and not morphea-like BCCs (121). Combining AR and CK20 staining can significantly aid in diagnosis. The AR-negative, CK20-positive immunophenotype is sensitive (87%) and specific (100%) for desmoplastic trichoepithelioma whereas the AR-positive, CK20-negative immunophenotype is specific (100%) and moderately sensitive (61%) for morpheaform BCC (106,122). PHLDA1 is most commonly positive in desmoplastic trichoepithelioma and negative in morpheaform BCC, which can also aid in diagnosis (123).

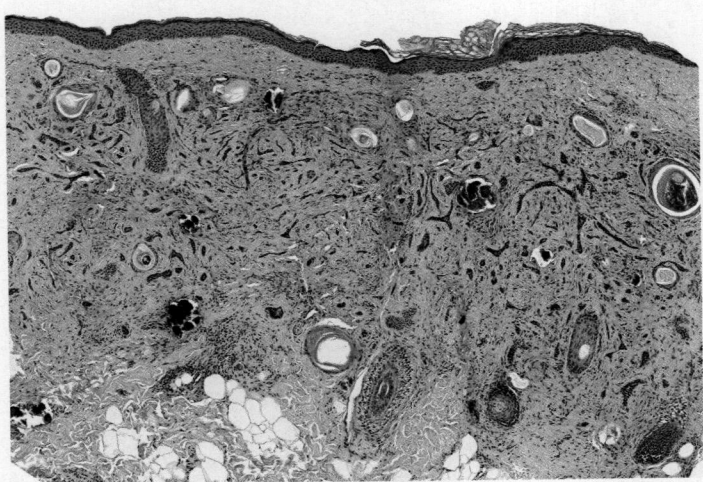

Figure 30-17 Desmoplastic trichoepithelioma. Horn cysts and narrow strands of epithelial cells are embedded in a fibrous stroma.

PHLDA1 can also be positive in microcystic adnexal carcinomas; an algorithm suggests using CK15 and CK19 as one approach to help distinguish DTE from MAC, with DTEs generally being CK15 positive and CK19 negative (123).

Fibroblast activation protein is expressed in peritumoral fibroblasts of morpheaform/infiltrative BCC but not in desmoplastic trichoepithelioma (124).

Finally, desmoplastic trichoepitheliomas are frequently positive for BerEP4; so, this marker cannot be used to distinguish them from BCCs (745).

Principles of Management: The treatment for these lesions parallels that for trichoepithelioma (p. 1026). Although desmoplastic trichoepitheliomas are considered to be indolent, their overlapping features with microcystic adnexal carcinoma, similarity to morpheaform BCC, and their own rare potential for malignant degeneration have been said to favor treatment with Mohs micrographic surgery upon diagnosis (125).

Trichoblastoma

Clinical Summary. Trichoblastomas are benign skin lesions that recapitulate some components of the developing hair follicle. They differ from trichoepitheliomas in their size, location, and lack of keratinizing cysts (126). Trichoblastomas are usually about 1 cm in size and most commonly occur on the scalp (Fig. 30-19) (127). Although usually solitary, multiple lesions have been described (128,129). As mentioned, these lesions are benign, though aggressive forms, termed trichoblastic carcinomas, may represent a type of BCC (130,131). Trichoblastomas and rare trichoblastic carcinomas have been reported to arise decades following radiation therapy (132).

Histopathology. Trichoblastomas consist of a proliferation of follicular germ cells manifested by a combination of various proportions of mesenchymal and epithelial cells. A spectrum of lesions is seen, depending on the proportions of mesenchymal and epithelial components. At one end of the spectrum is

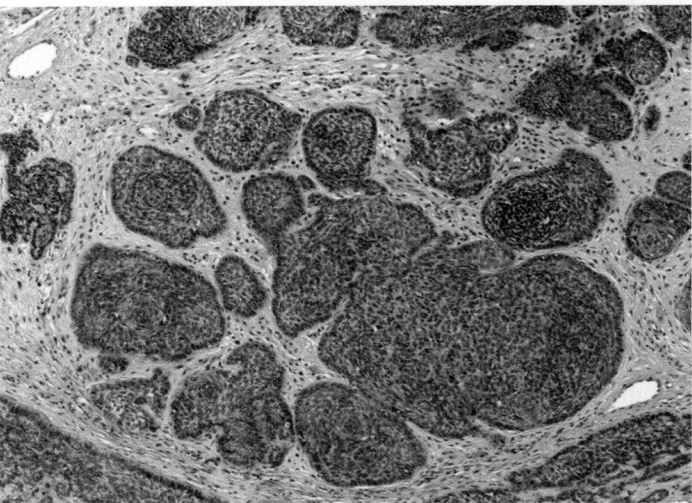

Figure 30-20 Trichoblastoma. Large islands of basaloid tumor cells are present in the dermis exhibiting peripheral palisading associated with a fibrous stroma.

the predominantly mesenchymal variant, termed the trichoblastic fibroma, and at the other end is the classic trichoblastoma composed predominantly of basaloid epithelial islands (127). The classic large lesion is comprised of islands of basaloid cells occupying the dermis with occasional extension into the subcutaneous fat (Fig. 30-20). These basaloid islands demonstrate peripheral palisading and a fibrocellular stroma similar to that surrounding follicles; mitotic activity can be seen (Fig. 30-21). There is no overlying epidermal connection. Less common variants have been described, including giant, clear cell, pigmented, cystic, giant melanotrichoblastoma, rippled-pattern trichoblastomas, and cutaneous lymphadenoma (129,133–140). Both neuroendocrine carcinoma and melanoma have been reported to occur within a trichoblastoma (141,142).

The trichoblastic fibroma variant displays small basaloid epithelial islands, exhibiting follicular differentiation, dispersed in a fibrotic stroma (Figs. 30-22 and 30-23). A rare trichoblastic sarcoma has been described as arising from a trichoblastic fibroma (143).

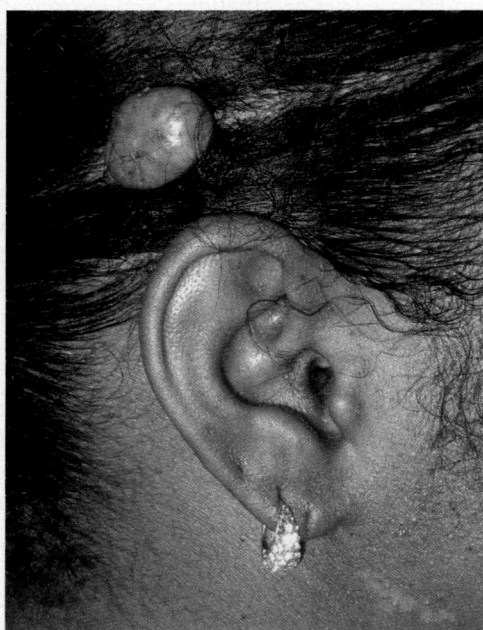

Figure 30-19 Trichoblastoma. A circumscribed, pigmented nodule is noted on the scalp.

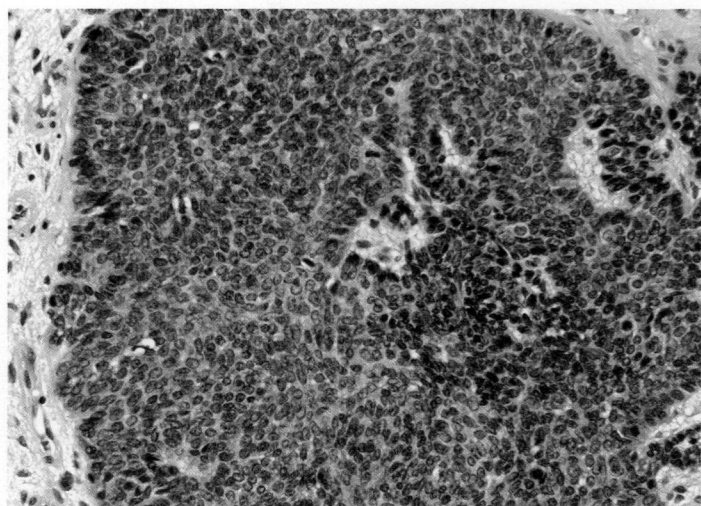

Figure 30-21 Trichoblastoma. Higher power showing epithelial structures reminiscent of follicular germs and occasional mitotic activity.

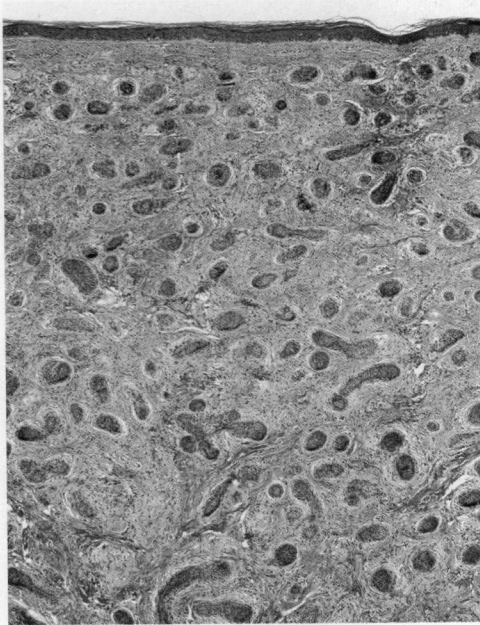

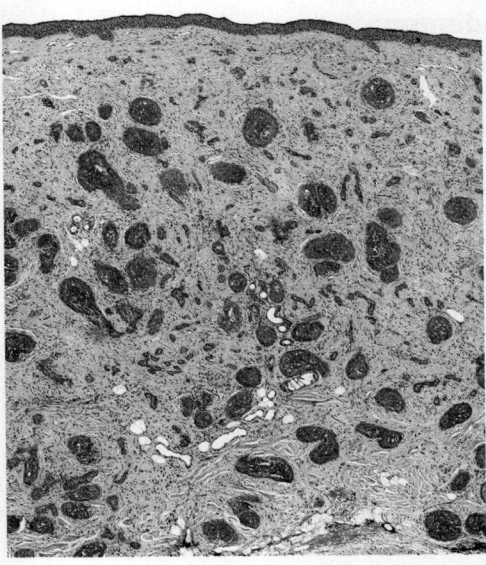

Figure 30-24 Trichoblastic carcinoma. A large dermal tumor comprised of irregular epithelial islands.

Figure 30-22 Trichoblastic fibroma. The lesion manifests small basaloid islands in a prominent fibrotic stroma.

Lesions that are infiltrative, exhibit cytologic atypia, and mitotic activity may be termed *trichoblastic carcinoma*, but these lesions may overlap with BCC (Figs. 30-24 and 30-25). Such problematic lesions may be signed out descriptively as *malignant adnexal neoplasm* with a description of the apparent differentiation. Criteria that may have value in distinguishing trichoblastomas from BCCs include the following: the presence in the former of symmetry, circumscription with smooth margins and "shelling out" of the normal tissue, and follicular and "racemiform" patterns of lesional cells, the lack of a clefting artifact between stroma and epithelium that is characteristic of BCC, the lack of stromal edema and lymphocytes, the formation of a delicate stroma reminiscent of that formed around immature hair follicles, and the lack of ulceration (144).

Immunohistochemical stains may help differentiate trichoblastoma from BCC. CK20 immunohistochemistry can help distinguish the two; CK20 highlights Merkel cells present in trichoblastomas, whereas these cells are rare or absent in BCCs (106).

Nestin is typically positive in the stromal cells of trichoblastomas, including those seen in nevus sebaceous, whereas the stromal cells in BCC are negative for nestin (145). PHLDA1 positivity can be used to distinguish clear cell trichoblastoma from clear cell BCC (146). Additionally, laminin-332 is most commonly negative in trichoblastoma and is consistently positive in all forms of BCC (147).

Additional Studies. The genetic basis for trichoblastomas is unclear. Genetic sequencing of sporadic trichoblastomas showed that classical *PTCH* mutations are not involved in their pathogenesis, unlike trichoepitheliomas and BCCs (148). Rarely, trichoblastomas may demonstrate mutations in the *CTNNB1* gene (149).

Principles of Management: This is a benign lesion that may be re-excised or removed by Mohs or other suitable techniques for cosmetic reasons or concern that any remaining lesion may transform into trichoblastic carcinoma.

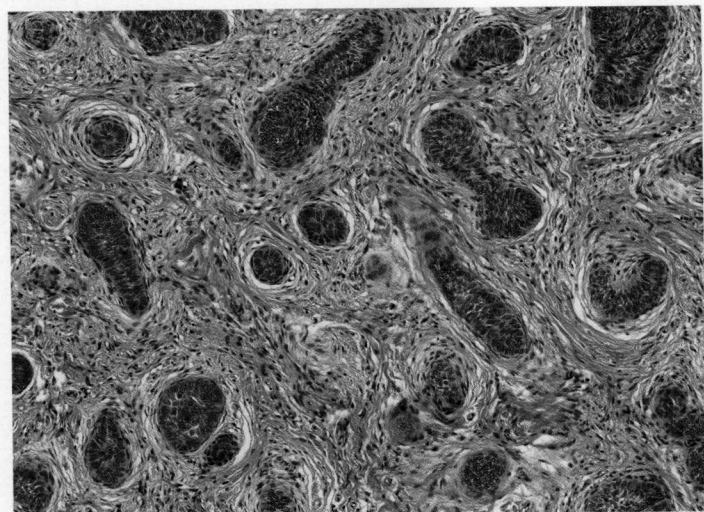

Figure 30-23 Trichoblastic fibroma. The epithelial–stromal structures mimic those of hair follicles.

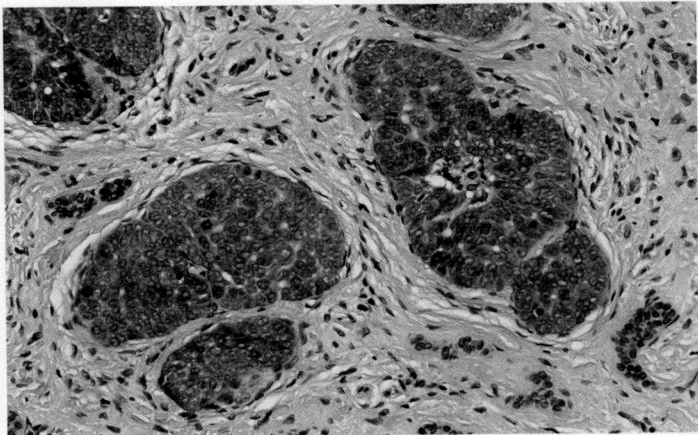

Figure 30-25 Trichoblastic carcinoma. Higher power demonstrates cytologic atypia, numerous mitoses, and a fibrocellular stroma.

Trichoadenoma

Clinical Summary. A rare, solitary tumor first described in 1958, trichoadenoma usually occurs on the face or buttocks as a solitary nodular lesion and varies from 3 to 15 mm in diameter (150,151). Other rare presentations of trichoadenoma exist in the nail bed and in the bony external auditory canal (152,153). It is more common in males and typically arises anytime during adult life (154). However, trichoadenomas can be congenital or appear in infancy (155,156). Trichoadenoma may clinically mimic BCC or sebaceous carcinoma (157).

Histopathology. Numerous horn cysts are present throughout the dermis (Fig. 30-26). They are surrounded by eosinophilic cells, which greatly resemble the eosinophilic cells that are often seen in trichoepithelioma located between the basophilic cells and the central horn cysts (Fig. 30-27). In some instances, a single layer of flattened granular cells is interpolated between the horn cysts and the surrounding eosinophilic cells (151,158). Some islands consist only of eosinophilic epithelial cells without central keratinization. Sparse intercellular bridges have been observed between the eosinophilic cells. Foci of foreign-body granuloma are present at the sites of ruptured horn cysts (150). A variant, termed verrucous trichoadenoma, which clinically resembles a seborrheic keratosis or a deep fungal granuloma has been described (159,160). Trichoadenoma has arisen within a melanocytic dermal nevus, mimicking malignant degeneration (161).

Additional Studies. In terms of morphologic differentiation, the trichoadenoma is situated between a trichofolliculoma and a trichoepithelioma (162). The general architecture of trichoadenoma resembles that of trichoepithelioma and thus suggests the development of immature hair structures. However, because the cyst wall consists of epidermoid cells and keratinization may take place with the formation of keratohyalin granules, it has been suggested that the tumor differentiates largely toward the infundibular portion of the pilosebaceous unit (151). In fact, the keratin expression pattern of trichoadenomas resembles that seen in follicular infundibula and the follicular bulge (163). Trichoadenoma and desmoplastic trichoepithelioma share some morphologic features; however, trichoadenoma is immunohistochemically distinct from desmoplastic trichoepithelioma in that it generally lacks positivity for BerEP4 (154).

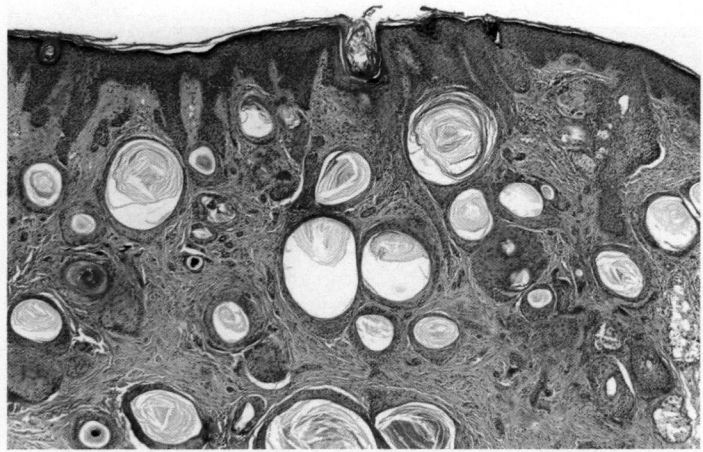

Figure 30-26 Trichoadenoma. Numerous horn cysts are present in the dermis.

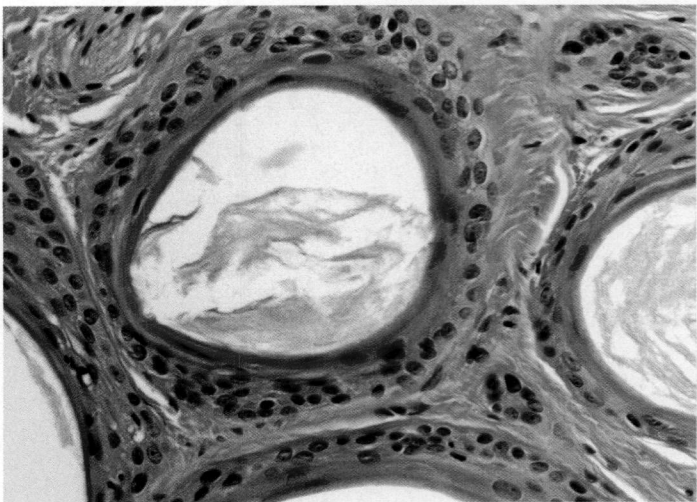

Figure 30-27 Trichoadenoma. The horn cysts are lined by eosinophilic cells and contain keratin.

Principles of Management: No treatment is necessary; however, these lesions can be excised for cosmetic reasons or if they become irritated.

Basaloid Follicular Hamartoma

Clinical Summary. The lesions of basaloid follicular hamartoma were originally described in *generalized hair follicle hamartoma*. This distinctive condition is characterized by progressive alopecia starting in adulthood; diffuse papules and plaques of the face; and an association with alopecia, myasthenia gravis, or systemic lupus erythematosus (164). Since the original description, generalized hair follicle hamartoma has been reclassified as one of several clinical settings in which basaloid follicular hamartoma occurs (165). Basaloid follicular hamartoma has a variable clinical appearance and can present as macules, patches, papules, or nodules, all with variable amounts of pigmentation (166).

Basaloid follicular hamartomas can be either solitary or multiple and can be congenital or acquired. The congenital forms include an autosomally dominantly inherited generalized variant associated with cystic fibrosis and diffuse alopecia, a localized linear and unilateral type, and a solitary plaque or nodule type (165,167,168). A form of congenital linear and unilateral basaloid follicular hamartoma associated with cerebral and ocular developmental abnormalities has been termed Happle–Tinschert syndrome (166,169,170). The acquired form is typically generalized and may have systemic associations such as myasthenia gravis and diffuse alopecia (164).

Histopathology. There is slight histologic variation in the basaloid follicular hamartomas found in different clinical contexts. In the context of generalized hair follicle hamartoma, the lesions within areas of alopecia without papules or plaques reveal more or less advanced replacement of the hair follicles by a lacelike network of basaloid cells with follicular differentiation resembling trichoepithelioma (171). The papules and plaques of the face show a complete lack of hair structures and extensive proliferations of basaloid cells embedded in a cellular stroma with the formation of horn cysts in some areas. The histologic appearance can be indistinguishable from that of trichoepithelioma (172).

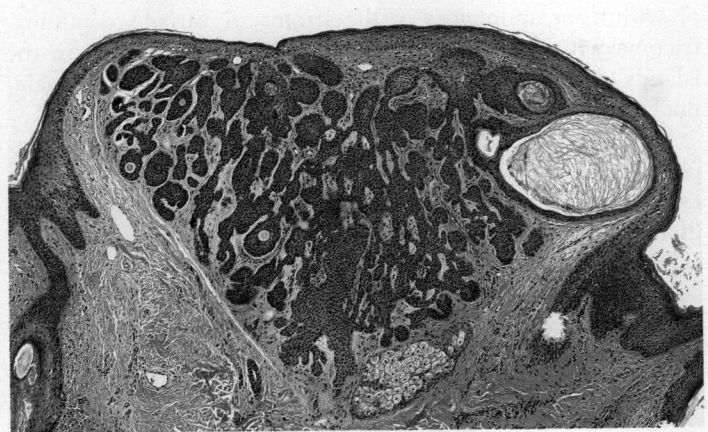

Figure 30-28 Basaloid follicular hamartoma. Present is a small, well-circumscribed lesion comprised of strands of epithelial cells with scattered cystic structures.

Basaloid follicular hamartomas seen in other clinical contexts tend to demonstrate strands and cords of small, basaloid cells emanating from the infundibular portion of the hair follicle (Figs. 30-28 and 30-29) (171). The tumor stroma is mildly fibrocellular. There is no significant clefting between tumor and stroma, and mitotic activity is rare (Fig. 30-29). These lesions may have a similar appearance to infundibulocystic BCC, but usually they can be distinguished on clinical and histologic grounds (173,174).

Differential Diagnosis. Mosaic forms of basal cell nevus syndrome (Gorlin), which are caused by *PTCH* mutations, may display basaloid follicular hamartomas but typically also contain adnexal tumors and BCC (169). *PTCH* mutations are typically absent in linear unilateral basaloid follicular hamartoma syndrome (170). In general, basaloid follicular hamartoma can be distinguished from BCC based on morphology and immunohistochemical studies. Basaloid follicular hamartoma is typically positive for CK20 highlighting Merkel cells, positive for CD34 in the stromal cells, and negative for AR and BER-EP4 (175).

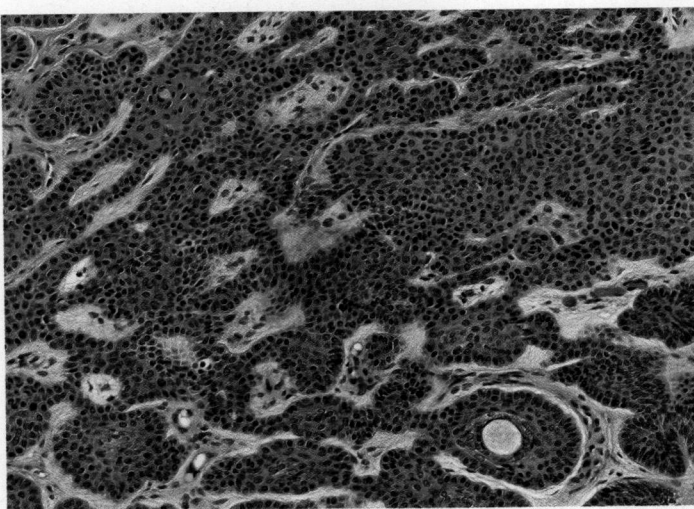

Figure 30-29 Basaloid follicular hamartoma. The lesion exhibits small basaloid cells lacking necrosis or mitotic activity. A mildly fibrocellular stroma is seen.

Additional Studies. Transgenic mice with increased epidermal expression of the Smoothened (*SMO*) gene demonstrate the activation of the Sonic Hedgehog signaling pathway and exhibit lesions similar to basaloid follicular hamartomas (176). Abnormalities in Patched signaling are associated with basaloid follicular hamartomas; however, they differ in intensity and distribution when compared with BCC (173).

Principles of Management: Typically, these lesions do not require excision except for cosmetic reasons. Lesions demonstrating recent growth may merit excision as BCC can occasionally develop in these lesions. Diffuse lesions have been treated with topical 5-aminolevulinic acid coupled with a filtered tungsten–halogen lamp (590 to 700 nm) or argon dye-pumped laser (177).

Pilomatricoma

Clinical Summary. Pilomatricoma (pilomatrixoma), or calcifying epithelioma of Malherbe, is a tumor with differentiation toward hair cells, particularly hair cortex cells. Pilomatricoma occurs usually as a solitary lesion; however, 5% of children with pilomatricomas will have multiple lesions (178). The head, neck, and upper extremities are the most common sites. Generally, the tumor varies in diameter from 0.5 to 3.0 cm, but it may be as large as 5 cm (179). The tumors may arise in persons of any age, but about 40% of them arise in children younger than 16 years of age, with a mean age at presentation of 32 years (180).

Pilomatricoma frequently presents as a firm, deep-seated nodule that is covered by normal skin. Occasionally, the tumor is more superficially located, causing a blue-red discoloration of the overlying skin, and can rarely protrude as a sharply demarcated, dark-red nodule.

Although solitary pilomatricoma is not hereditary, there are cases of familial occurrence with multiple lesions, most commonly associated with myotonic dystrophy. Additionally, multiple pilomatricomas and pilomatricoma-type changes can be seen in the epidermal cysts of Gardner syndrome (181). Less commonly, multiple pilomatricomas have been associated with sarcoidosis, skull dysostosis, Rubinstein–Taybi syndrome, Churg–Strauss syndrome, Turner syndrome, Soto syndrome, frontoparietal baldness, gliomatosis cerebri, and trisomy 9 (178). Unusual clinical variants include large, extruding, bullous, or perforating lesions; multiple eruptive cases; and familial cases (182,183).

Histopathology. The tumor is sharply demarcated and often surrounded by a connective tissue capsule (Fig. 30-30). It is usually located in the lower dermis and extends into the subcutaneous fat. Embedded in a rather cellular stroma are irregularly shaped islands of epithelial cells. As a rule, two types of cells—*basophilic cells* and *shadow cells*—compose the islands (Fig. 30-31) (184). In some tumors, however, basophilic cells are absent. The basophilic cells—which resemble cells of the hair matrix and are also known as matrical cells—possess round or elongated, deeply basophilic nuclei and scanty cytoplasm; so, the nuclei lie close together (Fig. 30-31). The cellular borders of the basophilic cells are often indistinct, so it appears as if the nuclei were embedded in a contiguous mass. The basophilic cells are arranged either on one side or along the periphery of the tumor islands. In some areas, the transition of basophilic cells into shadow cells is abrupt, whereas in others the transition is gradual. In areas of gradual transition, there are cells showing a gradual loss of nuclei and ultimately appearing as faintly eosinophilic, keratinized shadow

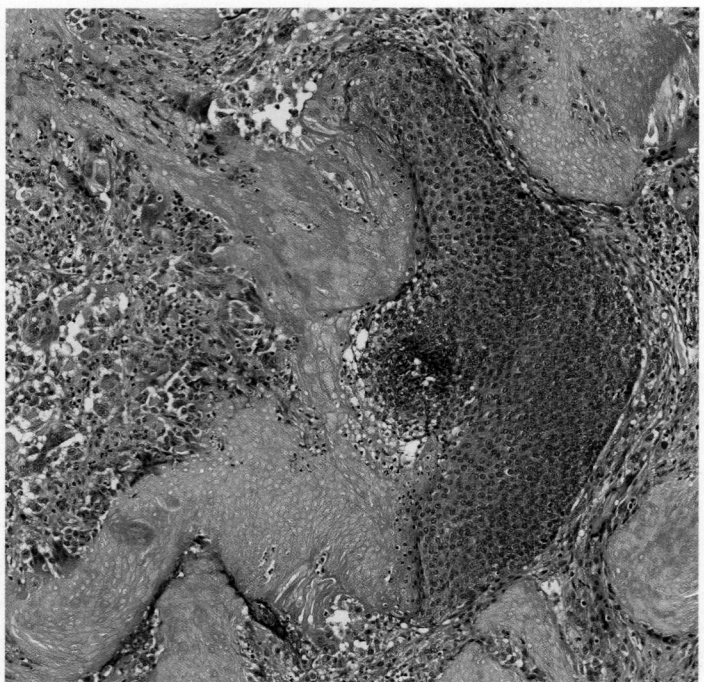

Figure 30-30 Pilomatricoma. The tumor is often well circumscribed and composed of epithelial islands embedded in a cellular stroma. Two types of cells comprise the islands: basophilic cells and shadow cells. The basophilic cells resemble hair matrix cells. The shadow cells show a central unstained shadow at the site of the lost nucleus. In the center of the field, one can see the transformation of basophilic cells into shadow cells.

cells. The shadow cells have a distinct border and possess a central unstained area as a shadow of the lost nucleus. In tumors of recent origin, numerous areas of basophilic cells are usually present. As the lesion ages, the number of basophilic cells decreases because of development into shadow cells, and in tumors of long-standing few or no basophilic cells remain (184).

In many tumors, small, round, eosinophilic centers of keratinization are seen within areas of basophilic cells or within aggregates of shadow cells. The keratinization within these centers is abrupt and complete (185). In some tumors, melanin is present, as can be expected in tumors with differentiation

toward hair bulbs. It is found most commonly in shadow cells or within melanophages of the stroma. A variant of pilomatricoma with numerous dendritic melanocytes located in the islands of basophilic cells has been described and termed melanocytic matricoma (186).

Calcium deposits are typically apparent as deeply basophilic collections in sections stained with hematoxylin–eosin. Using the von Kossa stain, these deposits are found in approximately 75% of tumors (187). Most of the tumors containing calcium are composed largely of shadow cells. The calcium is seen either as fine basophilic granules within the cytoplasm of the shadow cells or as large sheets of amorphous, basophilic material replacing the shadow cells. Occasionally, foci of calcification are seen in the stroma of the tumors. Areas of ossification are seen in 15% to 20% of the cases (188). Ossification takes place in the stroma next to areas of shadow cells, probably through metaplasia of fibroblasts into osteoblasts. Bone morphogenic protein-2 (BMP-2) has been shown in the cytoplasm of shadow cells but not in basophilic cells, indicating a possible role in bone formation (189). The stroma of pilomatricomas often shows a considerable foreign-body reaction containing many giant cells adjacent to the shadow cells (Fig. 30-32).

Additional Studies. Pilomatricoma was originally described in 1880 as calcified epithelioma of sebaceous glands; however, it was recognized in 1942 that the cells of the tumor differentiate in the direction of hair cortex cells, a finding that was subsequently confirmed by electron microscopic studies (190,191). On this basis, the designation *pilomatricoma* was suggested (188).

Several studies using immunohistochemistry and *in situ* hybridization with various cytokeratins and hair-specific keratins support the notion that pilomatricomas differentiate toward the components of normal hair shaft during their maturation process (192,193). Further investigations of keratin and filaggrin expression in pilomatricomas indicate that the tumor can differentiate toward not only the hair matrix and hair cortex but also follicular infundibulum, outer root sheath, and hair bulge. In pilomatricoma, basophilic cells, transitional cells, and shadow cells were negative for epithelial keratin and filaggrin

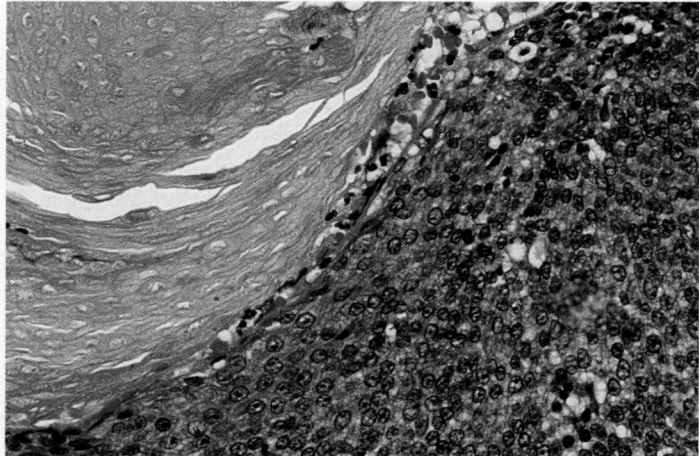

Figure 30-31 Pilomatricoma. The transformation of basaloid cells into shadow cells is associated with loss of nuclei.

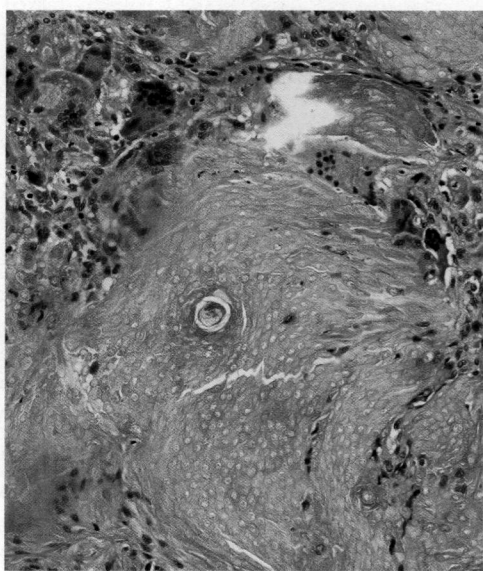

Figure 30-32 Pilomatricoma. The stroma often contains numerous multinucleated giant cells reacting to tumoral keratin.

antibodies as well as hair matrix and hair cortex keratins. However, the infundibular-like epithelium showed positivity for K1, K10 and filaggrin, and epithelium showing trichilemmal keratinization was positive for K14 and K16. Finally, K19 is distinctly positive in the hair bulge-like structure. This heterogeneity of keratin and filaggrin indicates that the differentiation of pilomatricoma is diversified (194).

Mutations in the gene for β-catenin (*CTNNB1*) have been described in pilomatricomas (149). The resulting mutation stabilizes the β-catenin protein, which translocates into the nucleus, where it activates gene transcription through members of the Lef/Tcf family (195).

Differential Diagnosis. The wall of trichilemmal cysts also contains basophilic cells, which gradually lose their nuclei and often undergo calcification as they keratinize. The peripheral layer of basophilic cells in trichilemmal cysts, however, shows a palisading pattern, whereas the basophilic cells of pilomatricoma do not. Furthermore, shadow cells characterized by a central unstained area at the site of the disintegrated nucleus are seen only in pilomatricomas and, exceptionally, in BCCs with foci of matrical differentiation (196). Pilomatricoma must also be differentiated from proliferating pilomatricoma (see below).

Principles of Management: Surgical excision is the treatment recommended.

Proliferating Pilomatricoma

Clinical Summary. Proliferating pilomatricoma is a rarely reported lesion, which usually presents as a solitary nodule measuring 1.5 to 5.5 cm on the head and neck. It may present with alopecia (197). It is most common in the elderly, with a mean age at presentation of 66 years (198). The tumors can recur locally after excision, but they have not been reported to metastasize (197,198).

Histology. Proliferating pilomatricoma demonstrates a large lobular proliferation of basaloid cells in association with small foci of eosinophilic shadow cells. The basaloid cells may show nuclear atypia and demonstrate a mitotic rate up to 15 mitoses per high-power field (197,198).

Differential Diagnosis. Proliferating pilomatricoma must be differentiated from pilomatricoma, which classically demonstrates larger areas of shadow cells and fewer basaloid cells. Pilomatricoma also lacks the high number of mitotic figures and atypia. Proliferating pilomatricoma can also be differentiated from pilomatrix carcinoma based on symmetry, relatively small size, circumscription, and lack of numerous basaloid aggregates. It also lacks the lymphatic and perineural invasion seen in pilomatrix carcinoma. BCC with matrical differentiation is typically attached to the epidermis and demonstrates retraction between lobules and the stroma (198). Some have suggested that these lesions be designated "pilomatrical tumor of low malignant potential" (199). Whether these lesions represent a transition to pilomatrix carcinoma from a preexisting pilomatricoma is plausible but remains unclear.

Principles of Management: Surgical excision is the treatment recommended (200).

Pilomatrix Carcinoma

Clinical Summary. Pilomatrix carcinoma is the rare malignant counterpart of pilomatricoma. The lesions have a male predominance and occur in older patients. Some pilomatricomas show

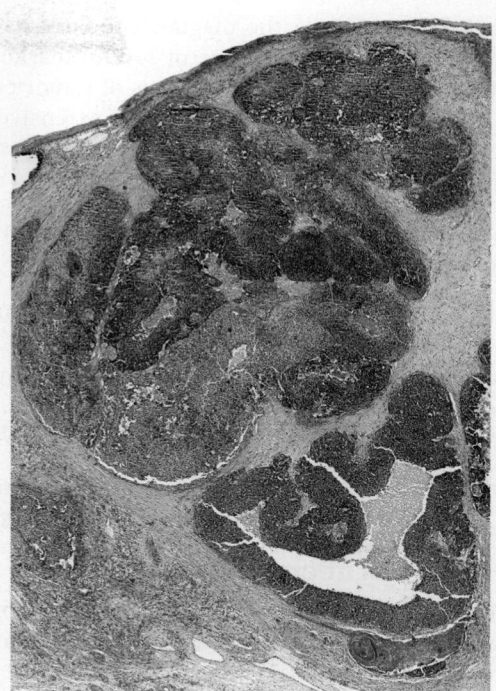

Figure 30-33 Pilomatrix carcinoma. There is a cellular, asymmetric, ulcerated tumor that infiltrates the dermis.

apparent transformation into carcinomas. Other cases are malignant from the onset. Pilomatrix carcinomas are not necessarily larger than pilomatricomas and may be mistaken clinically for an epidermoid cyst (201). The lesions recur locally in more than 60% of cases if not widely excised. The tumor may be more aggressive in the immunosuppressed (202). Pulmonary and bone metastases may occur in over 10% of cases, and life expectancy ranges from 3 months to 2 years from the diagnosis of metastatic disease (203). External beam radiotherapy may be useful as adjuvant treatment (204).

Histopathology. Pilomatrix carcinomas are asymmetric, cellular, infiltrative neoplasms (Fig. 30-33). Many areas, especially at the periphery of the tumor, show proliferations of large, anaplastic, hyperchromatic basophilic cells with numerous mitoses (Fig. 30-34). Toward the center of the tumor, there may be a transformation of basophilic cells into eosinophilic shadow cells of the type seen in benign pilomatricomas, or there may be large cystic centers containing necrotic debris (201). Features

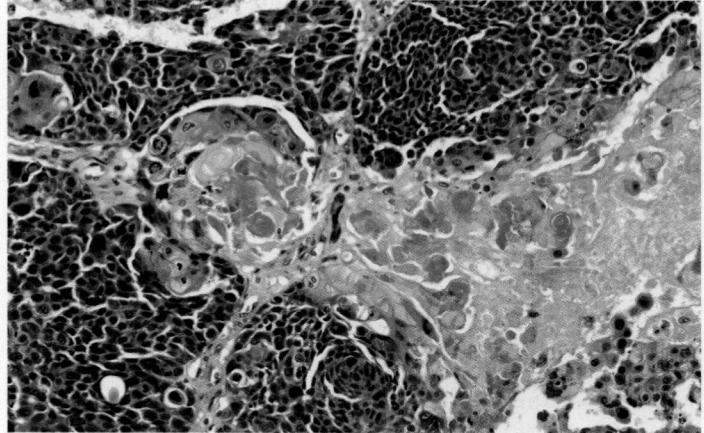

Figure 30-34 Pilomatrix carcinoma. Hyperchromatic, anaplastic cells exhibit mitotic activity and transition into shadow cells.

that are helpful in making the diagnosis include asymmetry and poor circumscription, presence of several markedly large and variably shaped basaloid aggregations of tumor cells, continuity of basaloid cells with the epidermis, extensive areas of necrosis en masse, infiltrative growth pattern, and presence of ulceration (205).

Differential Diagnosis. See the above text regarding proliferating pilomatricoma and pilomatricoma.

Additional Studies. Pilomatrix carcinoma has been found to express K5, K14, and K17, whereas pilomatricomas typically lack these keratins (206). In pilomatrix carcinomas, basaloid tumor cells demonstrate nuclear positivity with beta-catenin, and mutations in exon 3 of *CTNNB1* have been detected (149,207).

Principles of Management: Surgical excision with margins of 5 mm to 2 cm is the treatment recommended (205,208).

Proliferating Trichilemmal Tumor

Clinical Summary. The proliferating trichilemmal tumor, also referred to as proliferating trichilemmal cyst, or proliferating pilar cyst/tumor, is typically a single lesion; rarely, there are multiple lesions (209). About 85% of the cases occur on the scalp, with the residual 10% occurring mainly on the back. Lesions have been described in the vulva and other hair-bearing sites off the scalp (210). More than 80% of the patients are women, with a mean age of 62 years (range 21 to 88 years) (211).

Starting as a subcutaneous nodule suggestive of a wen, the tumor may grow into a large, elevated, lobulated mass that may undergo ulceration and, thus, may resemble a squamous cell carcinoma (212). The tumor may occur in association with one or even several trichilemmal cysts of the scalp (213). There is evidence that a proliferating trichilemmal tumor may develop from an ordinary trichilemmal cyst. However, the tumor may also give rise to one or several trichilemmal cysts, which may ultimately separate from it (214). In several instances, rapid enlargement of nodular scalp lesions has indicated malignant transformation (215,216).

Histopathology. The proliferating trichilemmal tumor is usually well demarcated from the surrounding tissue. It is composed of multiple, variably sized lobules of squamous epithelium, and the epithelial lining is typically thicker than that seen in pilar cysts (Fig. 30-35). Some of the lobules are surrounded by a vitreous layer and show palisading of their peripheral cell layer (214). Characteristically, the epithelium in the center of the lobules abruptly changes into eosinophilic amorphous keratin (Fig. 30-36). This amorphous keratin is of the same type as that seen in the cavity of ordinary trichilemmal cysts. In addition to showing trichilemmal keratinization, some proliferating trichilemmal tumors exhibit changes resembling the keratinization of the follicular infundibulum. These changes consist of epidermoid keratinization resulting in horn pearls, some of which resemble "squamous eddies" (211,217).

The tumor cells in many areas show some degree of nuclear atypia, as well as individual cell keratinization, which at first glance suggests a squamous cell carcinoma (Fig. 30-36). The tumor differs from a squamous cell carcinoma by a rather sharp demarcation from the surrounding stroma, as well as an abrupt mode of keratinization. Foci of calcification, although generally small, are often present in the areas of amorphous keratin (218). Some tumors show vacuolization or clear cell formation of some of the tumor cells as a result of glycogen storage (217).

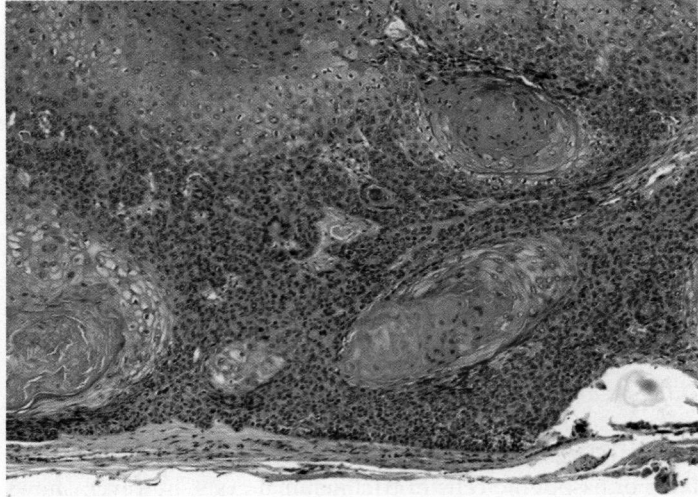

Figure 30-35 Proliferating trichilemmal cyst. The tumor is composed of irregularly shaped lobules of squamous epithelium undergoing an abrupt change into amorphous keratin. Central portions of the lobules demonstrate amorphous keratin.

Differential Diagnosis. In addition to its well-circumscribed nature, the presence of numerous, sharply demarcated areas of amorphous eosinophilic keratin in the center of tumor strands and lobules, and the absence of severe atypia and invasion of surrounding tissue, permits differentiation of proliferating trichilemmal tumor from its malignant counterpart and from squamous cell carcinoma. Regardless of the atypia or invasive properties, most proliferating trichilemmal tumors show positive staining with AE13 and AE14, monoclonal antibodies directed at pilar-type keratin polypeptides, whereas squamous cell carcinoma is consistently negative for these markers (211).

Additional Studies. Keratinization in proliferating trichilemmal tumors is of the same type as in ordinary trichilemmal tumors. Focal calcification is also seen in both lesions. Analogous to the outer root sheath, proliferating trichilemmal tumors show (a) an abrupt change of squamous epithelium into amorphous keratin;

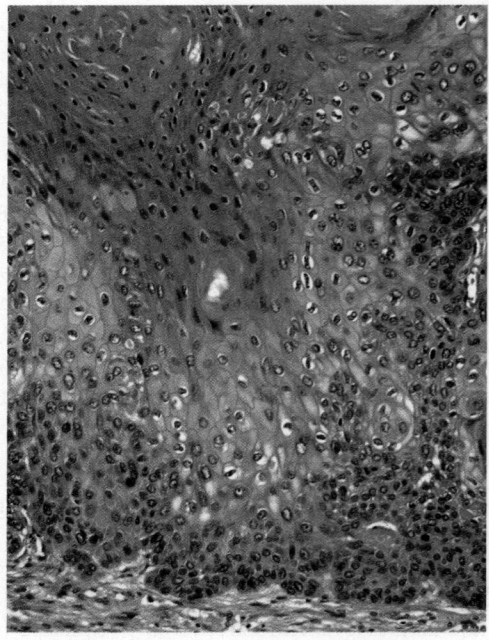

Figure 30-36 Proliferating trichilemmal cyst. Large, pale keratinocytes undergo abrupt keratinization without keratohyalin granules.

(b) vacuolated cells containing glycogen, like the cells of the outer root sheath; and (c) a prominent glassy layer of collagen surrounding some tumor formations (219). Owing to its close relationship with and potential transformation to a malignant proliferating trichilemmal tumor, treatment with wide local excision and close clinical follow-up are recommended (211,217,220).

Principles of Management: Complete excision with a margin of normal tissue is recommended; however, no standard has been determined regarding the margin size of the uninvolved tissue.

Malignant Proliferating Trichilemmal Tumor

Clinical Summary. Malignant transformation of proliferating trichilemmal tumors takes place more commonly than previously thought. They have recently been subclassified as low-grade or high-grade malignant proliferating trichilemmal tumors, based on their clinical and histologic features. Low-grade lesions tend to display local recurrence, whereas high-grade lesions are more likely to display regional metastases (211). Generalized metastases do occur and can be fatal (211,221). Overall, the local recurrence rate is reported at approximately 3% to 6%. Lymph node metastases occur in 1% to 2% of patients (211). Penetration of the tumor into cerebral sinuses has occurred, resulting in death (220,222).

Histopathology. Low-grade proliferating trichilemmal tumors demonstrate irregular infiltration of the surrounding dermis, a finding that should be absent in proliferating trichilemmal tumors. This growth pattern likely results in discontinuous foci in the dermis, which may be the root cause of frequent local recurrence after excision. Low-grade proliferating trichilemmal tumors lack the marked anaplasia seen in high-grade forms. High-grade proliferating trichilemmal tumors demonstrate marked cytologic atypia and significant anaplasia, likely giving them the ability to metastasize. Owing to these aggressive features, it may only be possible to distinguish high-grade proliferating trichilemmal tumors from squamous cell carcinoma by positive AE13 and AE14 staining (211).

Additional Studies. Unlike proliferating trichilemmal tumors, there is loss of CD34 expression in malignant proliferating trichilemmal tumors (223). DNA aneuploidy and a higher proliferation index have also been observed (223). Malignant proliferating trichilemmal tumors are on a spectrum with proliferating trichilemmal tumor (211,224). In addition, similar to squamous cell carcinomas, loss of heterozygosity at chromosome 17p and increased p53 immunoreactivity have been observed in malignant proliferating trichilemmal tumors (225,226).

Principles of Management: Owing to the chance of malignant transformation, all proliferating trichilemmal tumors should be treated with wide local excision and adequate follow-up (224). Radiotherapy and/or chemotherapy may be considered for lesions with high metastatic potential.

TRICHILEMMOMA

Trichilemmoma is a fairly common solitary tumor. In addition, multiple facial trichilemmomas are specifically associated with Cowden disease.

Solitary Trichilemmoma

Clinical Summary. Solitary trichilemmoma is generally a small tumor, 3 to 8 mm in diameter, occurring usually on the face (227). Occasionally, it measures several centimeters in diameter (228). It has no characteristic clinical appearance. In some instances, it is found at the base of a cutaneous horn (229).

Histopathology. One or several lobules are seen descending from the surface epidermis into the dermis. In some instances, the lobules are oriented about a central hair-containing follicle. A variable number of tumor cells have the appearance of clear cells because of their content of glycogen (Figs. 30-37 and 30-38). The periphery of the tumor lobules usually shows palisading of columnar cells and a distinct, often thickened basement membrane zone resembling the vitreous layer surrounding the lower portion of normal hair follicles (Fig. 30-38) (227). Paradoxically, trichilemmomas do not show the trichilemmal type of keratinization seen in trichilemmal cysts and proliferating trichilemmal cysts. Instead, at the surface, trichilemmomas display epidermoid keratinization, which is frequently pronounced, often associated with verrucous

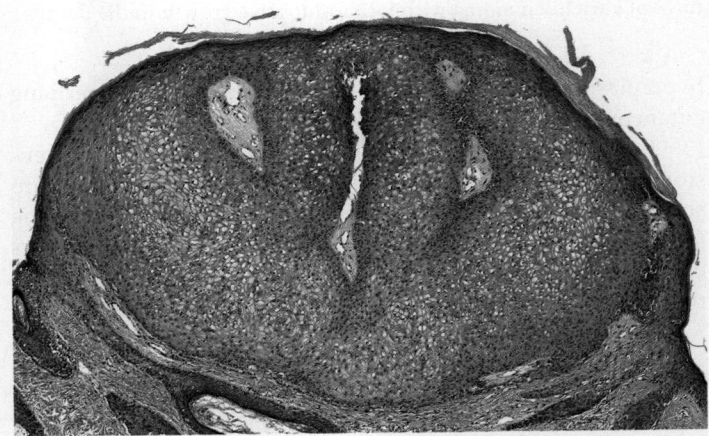

Figure 30-37 Trichilemmoma. The tumor shows verrucous hyperplasia with lobular formations extending into the superficial dermis. As a result of their differentiation toward outer root sheath cells, many cells appear clear.

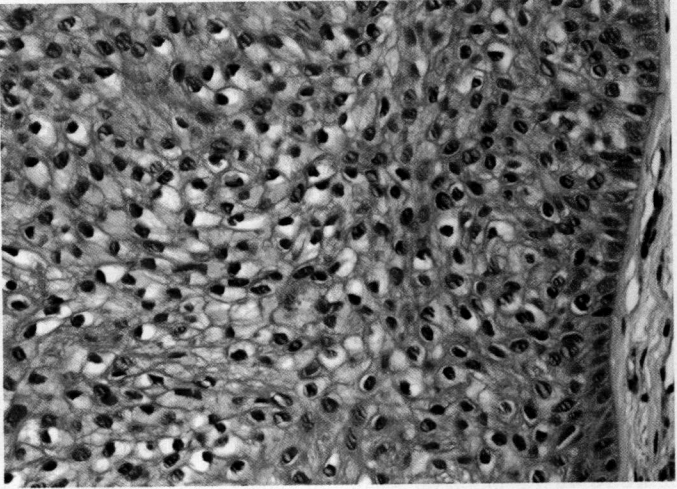

Figure 30-38 Trichilemmoma. Many cells demonstrate clear cytoplasm. The peripheral epithelial cells demonstrate palisading.

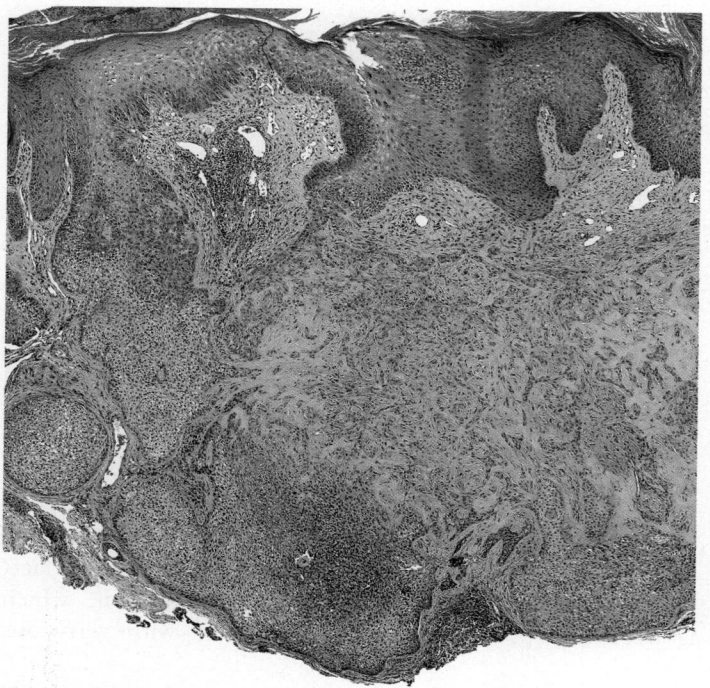

Figure 30-39 Desmoplastic trichilemmoma. The lesion exhibits features of a trichilemmoma with focal infiltrative growth in the dermis.

hyperplasia, and may even lead to the formation of an overlying cutaneous horn (230).

In *desmoplastic trichilemmoma*, there are irregular extensions of cells of the outer root sheath type that project into sclerotic collagen bundles and mimic invasive carcinoma (Figs. 30-39 and 30-40) (231). Superficially, the lesion shows changes of a trichilemmoma, a finding that aids in the distinction from an invasive carcinoma. In addition, unlike BCCs,

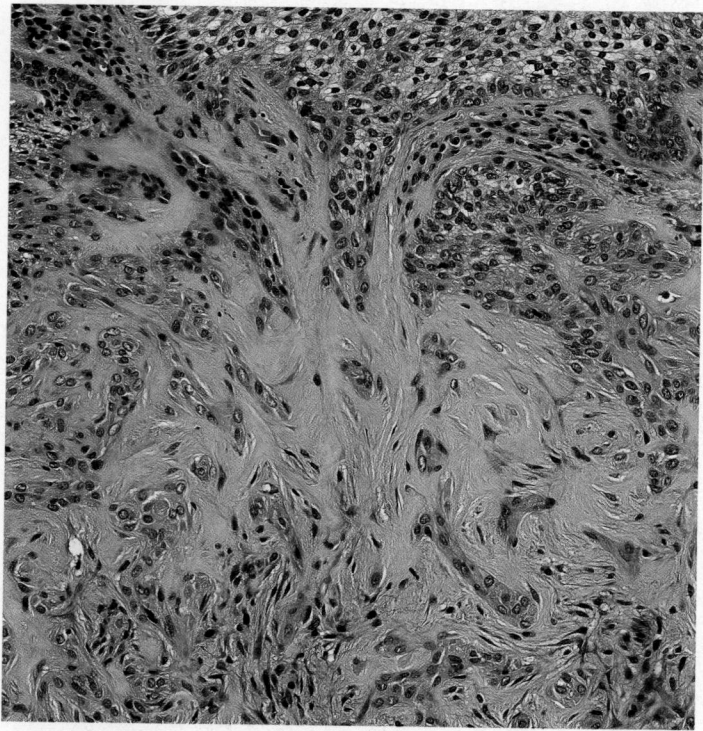

Figure 30-40 Desmoplastic trichilemmoma. Cords of bland epithelial cells infiltrate the dermis mimicking invasive carcinoma.

desmoplastic trichilemmomas stain with CD34 (232). Although desmoplastic trichilemmoma is a benign tumor, it may coexist with BCC, and therefore complete surgical excision with histologic confirmation of clear margins is recommended (233). As with most adnexal tumors, and in contrast with metastatic carcinomas to the skin, desmoplastic trichilemmoma is immunohistochemically positive for p63 and D2-40 (234).

Differential Diagnosis. In instances with relatively few clear cells and marked hypergranulosis and hyperkeratosis, differentiation from a verruca vulgaris may be difficult. A periodic acid–Schiff (PAS) stain for the demonstration of glycogen may aid in differentiating these two lesions. However, old verrucae—which often lack viral cytopathic changes—may acquire cytoplasmic glycogen and mimic many features of trichilemmoma. Trichilemmomas differ from ordinary verrucae by their lobulated rather than papillary (verrucous) configuration, their localization about follicular infundibula, the presence of basaloid palisading at the periphery of tumor lobules, and the presence of a thickened, hyalinized basement membrane that can be highlighted by a PAS stain. Molecular studies have not supported the notion that all trichilemmomas result from human papillomavirus infection (235,236).

Principles of Management: No treatment is required. For cosmetic reasons, lesions have been completely excised or ablated with carbon dioxide lasers.

Multiple Trichilemmomas in Cowden Syndrome

Clinical Summary. Cowden syndrome, or multiple hamartoma syndrome, is an autosomal dominant genodermatosis with distinctive mucocutaneous and systemic findings. The syndrome is characterized by multiple hamartomas in several organ systems including the skin, breast, thyroid, gastrointestinal tract, endometrium, and brain (237). The mucocutaneous lesions are a near-constant manifestation and include trichilemmomas, fibromas, oral papillomatoses, and acral and palmoplantar keratoses. The most frequent systemic findings include fibrocystic breast disease, breast fibroadenomas, thyroid adenomas, goiter, and intestinal polyposis. Individuals are at highest risk for the development of breast cancer, but other visceral malignancies, including thyroid and endometrial carcinomas, may occur (238). Rarely, certain Cowden syndrome patients develop immunosuppression with recurrent pyogenic and fungal skin infections, decreased total T- and B-cell counts, and an abnormal T-cell helper:suppressor ratio (237).

Multiple trichilemmomas are found in nearly all patients with Cowden disease, with most manifesting by the second or third decade of life. They are mostly limited to the face, where they are found mainly about the mouth, nose, and ears, but they can also occur in flexural sites (237). They consist of flesh-colored, pink, or brown papules that may resemble verrucae vulgaris (236). Multiple trichilemmomas precede the development of breast cancer and, thus, can identify women with a high risk of developing this cancer. Thus, the recognition of Cowden disease is important because of the high incidence and early development of breast cancer in women with this disease (239). In addition, there may be closely set oral papules, giving the lips, gingiva, and tongue a characteristic "cobblestone" appearance, as well as multiple small acral keratoses. Small hyperkeratotic papillomas are commonly found on the distal portions of the extremities (238).

The gene associated with Cowden disease was localized to chromosome 10q22-23 and subsequently identified as *PTEN* (phosphatase and tensin homolog deleted on chromosome 10) (240). Cowden syndrome is one of the *PTEN* hamartoma syndromes along with Lhermitte–Duclos disease (dysplastic cerebellar gangliocytoma) and Bannayan–Riley–Ruvalcaba syndrome (macrocephaly, lipomatosis, hemangiomatosis, and speckled penis) (241–243). *PTEN* encodes a dual-specificity phosphatase and is the major 3-phosphatase in the phosphoinositol-3-kinase pathway, which inactivates signals from (PI3K)/AKT kinases, an antiapoptotic pathway; therefore, a loss of *PTEN* function results in increased antiapoptotic signaling in the PI3K/AKT pathway (244). Mutational analysis has revealed germline mutations in the gene in multiple members of Cowden syndrome families (245,246).

Immunohistochemistry studies investigating trichilemmomas in Cowden syndrome show a loss of *PTEN* expression in most tumors. Although most solitary or spontaneous trichilemmomas in patients who do not meet clinical criteria for Cowden syndrome show normal *PTEN* expression, roughly 13% of these cases can show decreased *PTEN* expression. Therefore, a lack of PTEN staining in a trichilemmoma is not diagnostic for Cowden syndrome (247).

Histopathology. Multiple biopsy specimens may be needed to find the diagnostic histologic picture of trichilemmoma in the facial lesions. Thus, in one series, only 29 of 53 facial lesions showed findings diagnostic of trichilemmoma (230).

The oral lesions may show a fibromatous nodule composed of relatively acellular fibers patterned in whorls (sclerotic fibroma) or fibrovascular tissue with acanthosis (230). The extrafacial cutaneous lesions may resemble verruca vulgaris or acrokeratosis verruciformis (see Chapters 6 and 25). Some fibroma specimens show mild follicular hyperplasia as seen in trichilemmoma (237).

Differential Diagnosis. See *Differential Diagnosis* for solitary trichilemmoma.

Tumor of the Follicular Infundibulum

Clinical Summary. The tumor of the follicular infundibulum most commonly occurs as a solitary, flat, keratotic papule on the head and neck. It commonly presents as a plaque or more rarely as a hyper- or hypopigmented macule. Tumor of the follicular infundibulum may rarely present as multiple lesions; eruptive and widespread reticulated variants have also been described (248–250). There is a slight male predominance, and the average age at presentation is 67 years (ranging from 24 to 92 years) (248). Tumor of the follicular infundibulum presents in association with other primary lesions approximately 25% of the time. These lesions include BCC, actinic keratosis, squamous cell carcinoma, desmoplastic malignant melanoma, junctional melanocytic nevus, trichilemmoma, nevus sebaceous, and epidermal inclusion cyst (248,251). These associations have raised the possibility that the tumor of the follicular infundibulum represents a reactive process.

Histopathology. There is a plate-like growth of epithelial cells in the upper dermis extending parallel to the epidermis and showing multiple connections with the lower margin of the epidermis (Fig. 30-41). The peripheral cell layer of the tumor plate shows palisading, and the centrally located cells show a pale-staining cytoplasm as a result of their glycogen content;

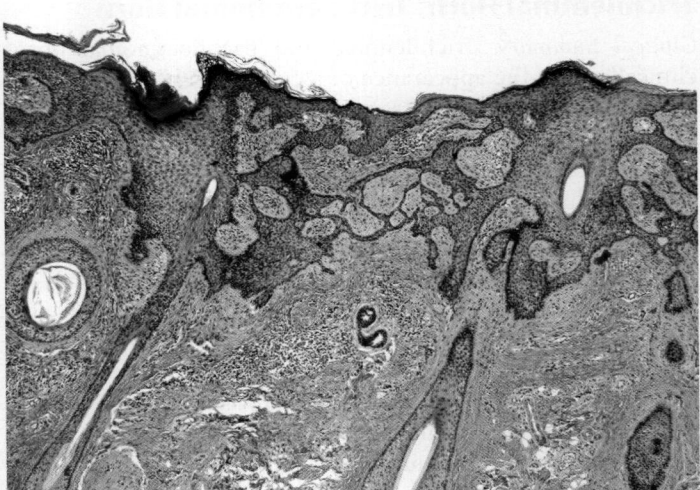

Figure 30-41 Tumor of the follicular infundibulum. A platelike growth of anastomosing epithelial cords extends parallel to the epidermis in the upper dermis and shows multiple connections with the epidermis.

small cysts resembling the follicular infundibulum are seen often (Fig. 30-42). Small hair follicles enter the tumor plate from below and lose their identity and then are no longer recognizable (252). Other common histologic features seen in the tumor of the follicular infundibulum include an eosinophilic cuticle, ductal differentiation, cornoid lamellae, and desmoplasia (248).

Differential Diagnosis. The plate-like growth with multiple connections to the epidermis resembles superficial BCC, which may also show peripheral palisading. Certain authors have suggested that tumor of the follicular infundibulum represents a form of BCC (253). However, atypia, necrosis, and mitotic activity are generally lacking in tumor of the follicular infundibulum (248). It is also negative for Ber-EP4 staining in contrast to BCC (254). The key histologic finding in tumor of the follicular infundibulum, as mentioned previously, is the presence of a plate-like growth of epithelium with multiple connections to the epidermis.

Principles of Management: Solitary lesions are treated by simple excision.

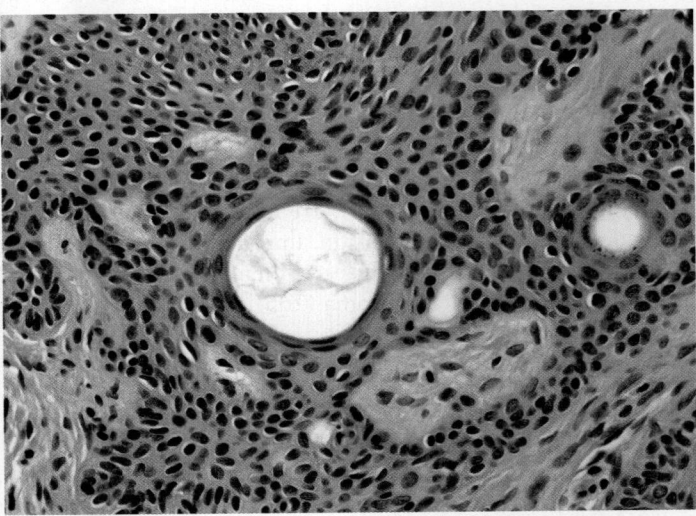

Figure 30-42 Tumor of the follicular infundibulum. Lesional cells demonstrate focal cytoplasmic clearing and horn cyst formation.

Trichilemmal Horn; Trichilemmomal Horn

Clinical Summary. Trichilemmal and trichilemmomal horns clinically have the appearance of a cutaneous horn, as seen in several other conditions (see Chapter 29). Both growths are solitary. The more common trichilemmal horn may be seen in many different areas; the trichilemmomal horn occurs on the face or scalp (229,255).

Histopathology. In a *trichilemmal horn*, trichilemmal keratinization occurs. At the base of the lesion, there is a prominent basement membrane zone, with palisading of the basal cell layer and a tendency of the viable epithelial cells to become large and pale staining. As trichilemmal cells, they keratinize without a granular layer (256). A seborrheic keratosis or verruca vulgaris with exuberant trichilemmal keratinization may mimic a trichilemmal horn (257). Immunohistochemical staining with CD34 has been shown, confirming an outer root sheath origin (258). A trichilemmal horn has been reported to arise within a burn scar (259).

In a *trichilemmomal horn*, a trichilemmoma is seen at the base of the lesion. At the surface, the trichilemmoma shows a cutaneous horn displaying epidermoid keratinization that is frequently pronounced, with a thick granular layer and massive hyperkeratosis (Fig. 30-39, top) (229).

Principles of Management: Solitary lesions can be treated by simple excision.

Trichilemmal Carcinoma

Clinical Summary. Trichilemmal carcinoma occurs largely on the face or ears as a slow-growing epidermal papule, indurated plaque, or nodule that may ulcerate (260). The pathogenesis is unclear; however, sun exposure has been proposed as a trigger. It can arise within other skin neoplasms, such as seborrheic keratosis (261). Unlike trichilemmomas, trichilemmal carcinoma is an unusual finding in Cowden disease (262). A case with neuroendocrine differentiation has been reported (263). Recurrence and metastases are uncommon, and the lesions are rarely locally aggressive.

Histopathology. This tumor is histologically invasive and consists of cytologically atypical clear cells resembling those of the outer root sheath (20). The lesional cells have abundant glycogenated clear cytoplasm. The lesional cells form solid, lobular, or trabecular growth patterns with foci of pilar-type keratinization and with peripheral palisading of cells with subnuclear vacuolization. Cytologic atypia is prominent, and there may be pagetoid spread of lesional cells into the epidermis, mimicking melanoma. The cells have hyperchromatic, pleomorphic, large nuclei. The cytoplasm contains glycogen, which is PAS positive and diastase sensitive (264). Trichilemmal carcinoma may rarely develop perineural invasion. Immunohistochemical positivity with CK17 distinguishes trichilemmomal carcinoma from invasive squamous cell carcinoma (265).

Differential Diagnosis. A trichilemmal carcinoma may resemble a trichilemmoma by showing a lobular architecture or may resemble a "tumor of the follicular infundibulum" by replacing the surface epidermis (264). Differentiation from other carcinomas with clear cell features such as squamous cell carcinoma, BCC, and sebaceous carcinoma may be difficult. Typical features of these carcinomas are usually seen adjacent to the clear cell component.

Additional Studies. The pathogenesis of trichilemmal carcinomas is unclear. The distribution of lesions suggests that sunlight may play a role. A few cases have been reported in association with a burn scar, irradiation, and xeroderma pigmentosum (260,266,267). Loss of *p53* has been shown in a trichilemmal carcinoma arising from a proliferating trichilemmal cyst (268). As with many skin adnexal carcinomas, trichilemmal carcinoma stains positively with D2-40, in contrast with metastatic adenocarcinomas (269).

Principles of Management: Conservative surgical excision with clear margins is normally curative; however, any recurrent tumor should be managed with wide excision or Mohs surgery (270).

TUMORS WITH SEBACEOUS DIFFERENTIATION

Nevus Sebaceus

Clinical Summary. Nevus sebaceus of Jadassohn is nearly always located on the scalp or the face as a single lesion and is present often at birth. In childhood, this lesion consists of a circumscribed, slightly raised, hairless plaque that is often linear in configuration, but it may be round or irregularly shaped. In puberty, the lesion becomes verrucous and nodular. Less commonly, nevus sebaceus consists of multiple extensive lesions found on the face, neck, or trunk. Usually, at least some of the lesions have a linear or Blaschkoid configuration (271). Giant forms of nevus sebaceus have also been described (272).

Certain patients with extensive nevus sebaceus may also develop epilepsy, mental retardation, other neurologic defects, or skeletal deformities, causing a neuroectodermal syndrome termed Schimmelpenning or nevus sebaceus syndrome (273). There is significant overlap with keratinocytic epidermal nevi and the epidermal nevus syndrome, and it is likely that these syndromes represent different phenotypes arising from mutations in *HRAS* and *KRAS* (see Chapter 6) (273,274).

The constellation of nevus sebaceus, central nervous system malformations, aplasia cutis congenita, limbal dermoid, and pigmented nevus together comprise the SCALP syndrome (sebaceous nevus syndrome, CNS malformations, aplasia cutis congenita, limbal dermoid, and pigmented nevus) (275). Occasionally, nevus sebaceus syndrome is associated with hypophosphatemic rickets. The pathogenesis of hypophosphatemia is unclear and has been attributed to increased levels of fibroblast growth factor-23 (276,277). There is also a rare hemimegalencephalic variant of the nevus sebaceus syndrome/epidermal nevus syndrome defined by severe epilepsy, mental retardation/developmental delay, ocular/visual involvement, and facial abnormalities (278).

Nevus sebaceus can also present with a speckled lentiginous nevus, skeletal, and neurologic abnormalities as part of a defined epidermal nevus syndrome termed phacomatosis pigmentokeratotica. Rarely, the cutaneous lesions may coexist without associated systemic abnormalities (279).

Histopathology. The sebaceous glands in nevus sebaceus follow the pattern of normal sebaceous glands during infancy, childhood, and adolescence. In the first few months of life, they are well developed. During the childhood or first stage, the sebaceous glands in nevus sebaceus may be underdeveloped and

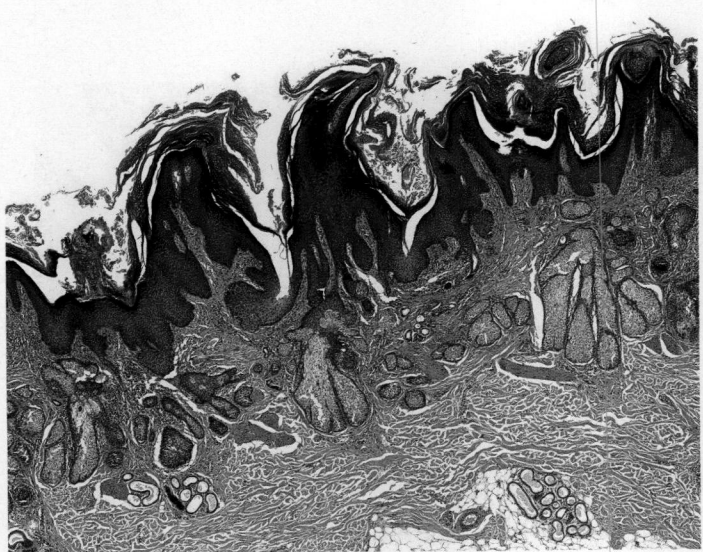

Figure 30-43 Nevus sebaceus. There is epidermal hyperplasia and papillomatosis. Dilated apocrine glands are present in the dermis, and anagen follicles are lacking.

greatly reduced in size and number (280,281). Thus, the diagnosis of nevus sebaceus may be missed. However, the presence of incompletely differentiated hair structures is typical of nevus sebaceus. There are often cords of undifferentiated cells resembling the embryonic stage of hair follicles (282). Some hair structures consist of dilated, keratin-filled infundibula showing multiple buds of undifferentiated cells (Fig. 30-43).

At puberty, or second stage, the lesion assumes its diagnostic histologic appearance. Large numbers of mature or nearly mature sebaceous glands and overlying papillomatous hyperplasia of the epidermis are seen. The hair structures remain small, except for occasional dilated infundibula. Ectopic apocrine glands develop in about two-thirds of the patients at puberty and sometimes at a younger age (Fig. 30-43). There are often buds of undifferentiated cells that resemble foci of BCC and represent malformed hair germs (Fig. 30-44). The apocrine glands are located deep in the dermis beneath the masses of sebaceous gland lobules (280,281).

In approximately 15% to 20% of nevus sebaceus in the third stage or adult stage, various types of appendageal tumors

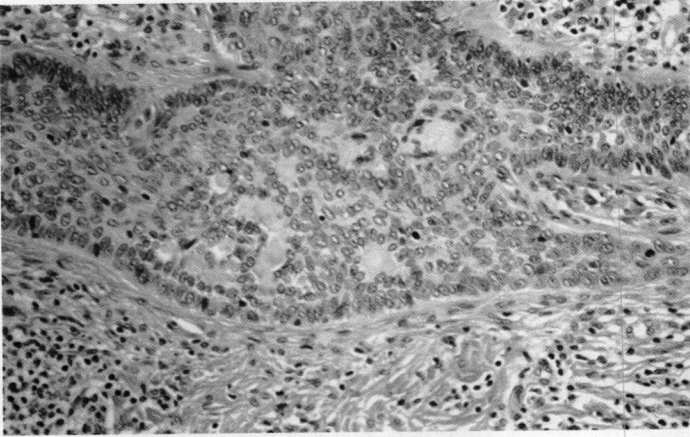

Figure 30-44 Nevus sebaceus. The basaloid epithelial proliferations often resemble basal cell carcinoma. However, the proliferations exhibit features of appendageal neoplasms as evidenced by the hyaline material within the lesion.

may develop. In two large case series, the most commonly associated appendageal tumors were basaloid neoplasms most consistent with trichoblastoma and syringocystadenoma papilliferum (SCAP) (Fig. 30-45) (280,281). Less commonly found benign appendageal tumors include nodular hidradenoma, syringoma, sebaceous epithelioma, chondroid syringoma, trichilemmoma, trichoadenoma, and cylindroma (282–286). Certain lesions of nevus sebaceus may contain several secondary neoplasms, and benign and malignant neoplasms may coexist in the same lesion (284,286).

Previously, it was believed that the basaloid neoplasms in nevus sebaceus represented BCC. However, this view was revised in several critical reviews stating that most of these BCCs actually represented trichoblastomas (280,281). The basaloid neoplasms that arise in nevus sebaceus may represent BCC or trichoblastoma, and it can be extremely difficult to differentiate them based on histologic grounds alone. Interestingly, the majority of basaloid tumors arising in nevus sebaceus are negative for PHLDA1, a follicular stem cell marker. PHLDA1 is generally positive in trichoepithelioma and trichoblastoma and negative in primary BCC. These findings indicate that many of the basaloid neoplasms may represent BCC rather than trichoblastoma (287). Further study of these lesions is necessary to fully define whether these represent BCC or trichoblastoma.

Basaloid epithelial proliferations resembling BCC are clinically evident in 5% to 7% of the cases of nevus sebaceus (288–290). In many instances, however, BCCs are found that are small, clinically not apparent, and show no aggressive growth pattern (290). It is not always possible to differentiate histologically between a BCC and the "basaloid proliferations" that arise in as many as half of all cases of nevus sebaceus (288). As original evidence that the BCC-like proliferations in many instances are not true BCCs, some proliferations contain Sudan-positive granules, as an indication of sebaceous differentiation, or glycogen, as an indication of pilar differentiation (291). Other proliferations show follicular differentiation with the formation of hair papillae and hair bulbs (292). Immunohistochemical studies with Ber-EP4, p53, Ki-67, bcl-2, CD34, and factor XIIIa support the concept that these basaloid proliferations represent areas of follicular differentiation rather than true BCC (289).

Rarely, malignant tumors other than BCC may arise within nevus sebaceus, including squamous cell carcinoma (293). Squamous cell carcinoma arising within a nevus sebaceus may be associated either with regional lymph node metastasis or with generalized metastases. Spindled cell squamous cell carcinoma within a nevus sebaceus has also been reported (286,294). Other malignant tumors include apocrine carcinomas, malignant eccrine poroma, keratoacanthoma, proliferating trichilemmal tumor, leiomyosarcoma, microcystic adnexal carcinoma, sebaceous carcinoma, and mucoepidermoid carcinoma (294–302). Additionally, primary skin adenocarcinoma arising in a nevus sebaceus with resulting metastases has been reported (303).

Additional Studies. Based on whole-exome sequencing, both keratinocytic epidermal nevi and sebaceus nevi are associated with activating *HRAS* p.Gly13Arg or *KRAS* p.Gly12Asp mutations (271,273). The mutations are likely to occur postzygotically and form a mosaic (274,304,305). Interestingly, both genital-type and epidermodysplasia verruciformis-type HPV DNA have been detected within nevus sebaceus, though the pathogenesis and implication of such infections are not clear (306).

Nevus sebaceus demonstrates differential cytokeratin expression based on the age of the patient. In the infant stage,

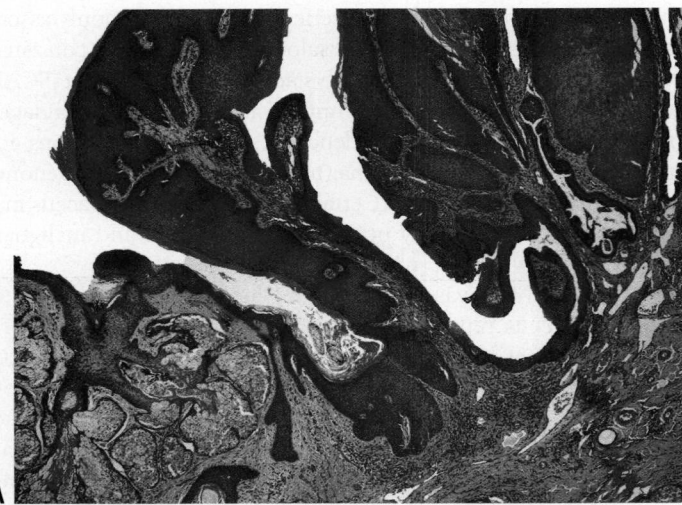
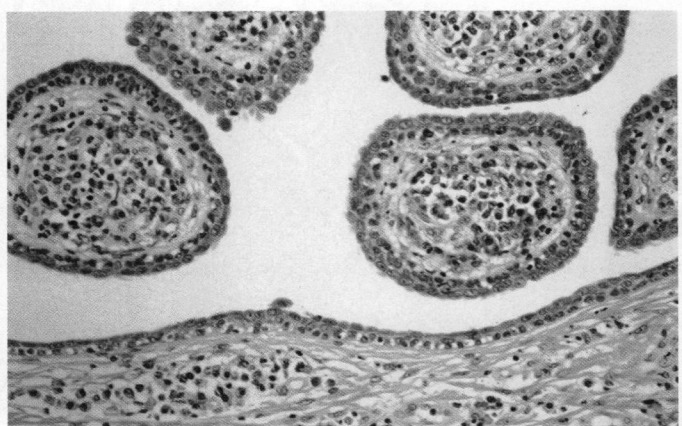

Figure 30-45 A, B: Nevus sebaceous with syringocystadenoma papilliferum. This nevus sebaceous (A) contains an associated syringocystadenoma papilliferum in the upper right-hand corner of the scanning magnification photomicrograph and the high magnification photomicrograph (B).

CK1 and CK10 are reduced, with increased CK14. In the adolescent stage, CK17 is additionally strongly expressed. In the adult stage, CK14, CK17, and CK19 were all expressed. Based on these findings, nevus sebaceus likely qualifies as a hamartomatous growth rather than a hyperproliferative one (307).

The frequent association of nevus sebaceus with other appendageal tumors and with apocrine glands suggests that nevus sebaceus is derived from an epithelial progenitor cell (308). Moreover, as has been reported in BCCs, the loss of heterozygosity of the human homolog of the *Drosophila* patched gene (*Ptch*) has been demonstrated in nevus sebaceus (309–311). This could partly explain the association of BCCs and other basaloid appendageal tumors with nevus sebaceus. However, a separate study of 11 lesions of nevus sebaceus found no demonstrable loss of heterozygosity. The reason for the discrepancy is uncertain; however, differences such as sampling during microdissection of other cell populations may account for this discrepancy (312).

Nevus sebaceus generally presents with marked alopecia as a result of lacking terminal hairs. Sebocytes within nevus sebaceus show an increase in the expression of hair growth–suppressing bioactive factors, including FGF-5, and a decrease in the expression of hair growth–stimulating factors, which may result in the decrease of terminal hairs within the lesion (313).

Principles of Management: Nonsurgical approaches include photodynamic therapy with topical aminolevulinic acid. Given their low malignant potential, strict guidelines for the excision of nevus sebaceus have not been established. However, critical review has shown that most should be removed at some time in childhood, ideally before the onset of the expansion phase of the nevus sebaceus. Though there is no recommended time point for this procedure, ideally it is performed when the parent, child, and physician are in agreement with the treatment plan (314,315).

Given the risk of the associated malignant components, full-thickness surgical excision is recommended.

Sebaceous Hyperplasia

Clinical Summary. The lesions of sebaceous hyperplasia nearly always occur on the face, chiefly on the forehead and cheeks, in elderly persons. It has also been reported in the vulva, penis, and areola (316–321). It clinically presents as one or, more commonly, several elevated, small, soft, yellow, slightly umbilicated papules. The usual size is 2 to 3 mm in diameter. Rarely, sebaceous hyperplasia occurs in adolescence or young adulthood and even more rarely in prepubescent children (322,323). A neonatal, transient form of sebaceous hyperplasia is very common and lasts for the first few weeks of life (324). Apparent familial forms have also been reported (325). Medications, specifically cyclosporine, may induce sebaceous hyperplasia (326).

Histopathology. Most lesions consist of a single, enlarged sebaceous gland composed of numerous lobules grouped around a centrally located, wide sebaceous duct (Fig. 30-46). Its opening to the surface corresponds to the central umbilication of the lesion. Serial sections show that all sebaceous lobules grouped around the central duct are connected with that duct. Large lesions may consist of several enlarged sebaceous glands and contain several ducts, with sebaceous lobules grouped around each of them. Although some sebaceous gland lobules appear fully mature, others show more than one peripheral row of undifferentiated, germinative cells in which there are few or no lipid droplets (327).

Additional Studies. Labeling with tritiated thymidine has shown that the migration of sebocytes from the basal cell area to the

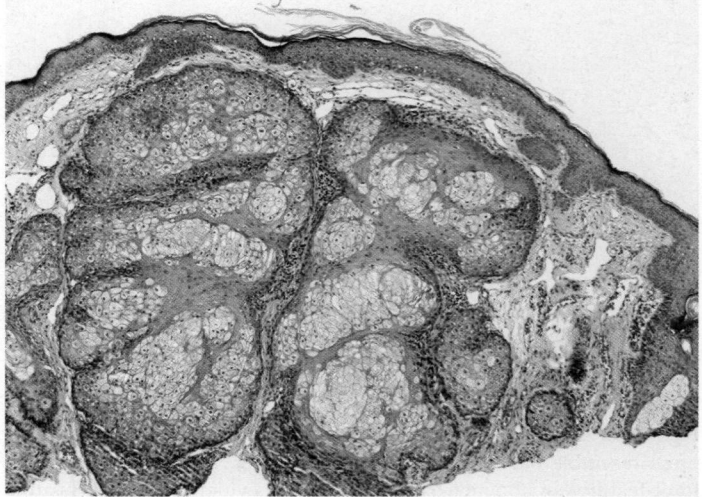

Figure 30-46 Sebaceous hyperplasia. The lesion consists of an enlarged sebaceous gland lying in close proximity to the epidermis.

center of the sebaceous lobules and into the sebaceous duct is distinctly slower in cases of sebaceous hyperplasia than in normal sebaceous glands (327). Microsatellite instability has been detected in very few cases of sebaceous hyperplasia as compared to other sebaceous neoplasms (see the section on Muir–Torre syndrome) (328,329).

Immunohistochemical staining for ARs has been shown to be fairly specific for sebaceous lesions as compared to BCCs, squamous cell carcinomas, and clear cell acanthomas (330). However, it is important to note that BCCs can stain positively for AR. Androgens affect sebaceous gland growth and differentiation, and sebocytes stain positively with AR (331). However, no increase in circulating androgens has been observed in patients with sebaceous hyperplasia (332). Sebaceous hyperplasia can occur after trauma, such as a burn, or overlying a dermatofibroma. This proliferation of sebocytes is thought to be caused by the upregulation of the EGF–EGFR signaling pathway and the Hedgehog–PTCH signaling pathway (333,334). Of note, sebaceous glands in sebaceous hyperplasia and many sebaceous neoplasms stain positively with D2-40 (335). In sebaceous hyperplasia and other sebaceous neoplasms, immunostaining for factor XIIIa and adipophilin may provide useful diagnostic information (336).

Differential Diagnosis. In rhinophyma, which also shows large sebaceous glands and ducts, there is no grapelike grouping of the sebaceous lobules around the ducts, and the lesion is not sharply demarcated. In nevus sebaceus, ductal structures are less apparent than in sebaceous hyperplasia and apocrine glands are often found beneath the sebaceous glands.

Occasionally, sebaceous hyperplasia may be difficult to distinguish from a sebaceous adenoma or other sebaceous tumors, and immunohistochemistry for α-methylacyl-CoA racemase (AMACR, P504S) may aid in diagnosis. AMACR is a protein that plays an important role in the mitochondrial and peroxisomal β-oxidation of branched-chain fatty acid and bile acid intermediates. Staining for AMACR is strongly positive in normal sebocytes and in sebaceous hyperplasia. AMACR shows decreasing positivity in more poorly differentiated sebaceous neoplasms, with sebaceous carcinoma showing little to no positive staining. Therefore, AMACR staining may be used to differentiate sebaceous neoplasms that are challenging to classify and to distinguish them from routine sebaceous gland hyperplasia (337).

Principles of Management: Treatment is not required. For cosmetic purposes, treatment options include photodynamic therapy, laser ablation, cryotherapy, cauterization, topical therapy with trichloroacetic acid, and excision.

FORDYCE SPOTS AND MONTGOMERY TUBERCLES

Clinical Summary. In Fordyce spots, groups of minute, yellow, globoid lesions are observed on the vermilion border of the lips, genital skin, or on the oral mucosa comprised of ectopic sebaceous glands. The incidence of this disorder increases with age, and 70% to 84% of elderly persons show such lesions (338). Montgomery tubercles are ectopic mature sebaceous glands located on the areola of the breast. Rarely, in adolescence, these can form cystic structures that drain nonmilky fluid from the areola. These tend to resolve without intervention (339).

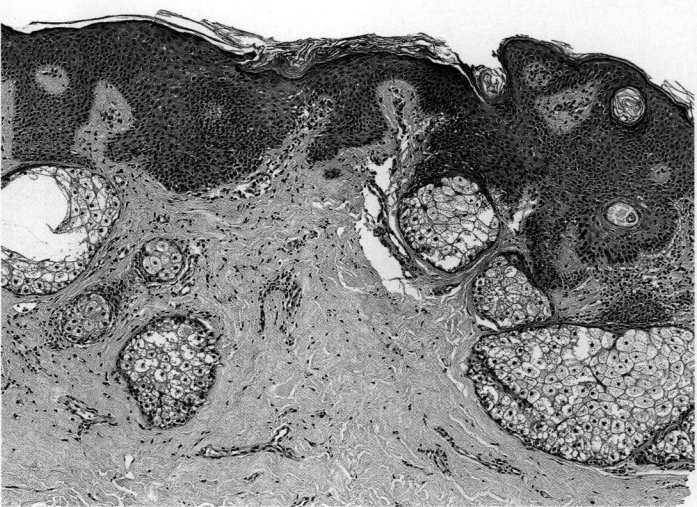

Figure 30-47 Montgomery tubercle. A mature sebaceous lobule in continuity with the epidermis is seen.

Histopathology. Each lesion consists of a group of small but mature sebaceous lobules situated around a small sebaceous duct leading to the surface epithelium (Fig. 30-47) (338). Because of the small size of the sebaceous duct, serial sections may be required to demonstrate its presence.

Additional Studies. There have been reports of unilateral Fordyce spots arising on the buccal mucosa in the setting of ipsilateral facial paralysis, suggesting that the sebaceous hyperplasia may be mediated by dysregulated neuroendocrine signaling (340).

Principles of Management: Treatment is not required. For cosmetic purposes, treatment options include photodynamic therapy, laser ablation, cauterization, and topical therapy with trichloroacetic acid or retinoids.

Sebaceous Adenoma

Clinical Summary. Sebaceous adenoma presents as a yellow, circumscribed nodule located on either the face or scalp. Rare intraoral and genital lesions have been described (341–343). Prior to 1968, sebaceous adenoma was regarded as a rare solitary tumor, and there were few publications about it (344). Since then, however, both solitary and multiple lesions have been well documented in patients with Muir–Torre syndrome (see the following text).

Histopathology. On histologic examination, sebaceous adenoma is sharply demarcated from the surrounding tissue. It is composed of incompletely differentiated sebaceous lobules that are irregular in size and shape (Fig. 30-48). Two types of cells are present in the lobules. There are undifferentiated basaloid cells at the periphery identical to those in normal sebaceous glands (Fig. 30-49). The central cells are mature sebocytes (Fig. 30-49). The distribution of basaloid and sebaceous cells within the lobules varies. Frequently, the proportion of mature sebaceous cells exceeds that of the surrounding basaloid cells (Fig. 30-49). Some lobules contain sebaceous cells mainly and thereby resemble mature sebaceous lobules. At most, the distribution of these two cell types occurs in approximately equal proportions. There often are transitional cells between the two types (345).

Fat stains, on properly preserved specimens, reveal the presence of lipid material in the sebaceous and transitional

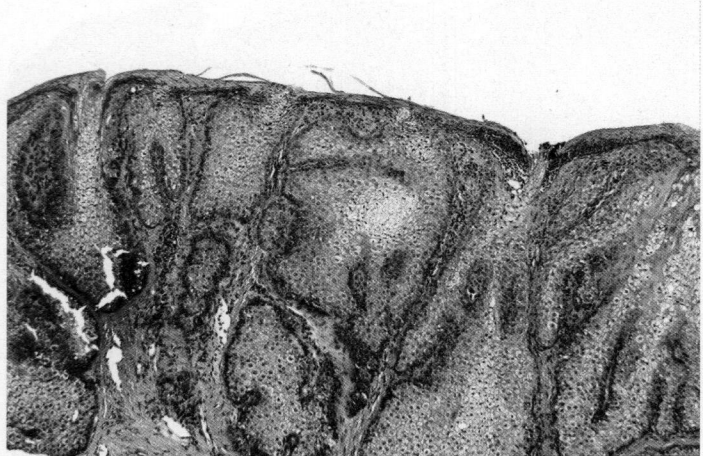

Figure 30-48 Sebaceous adenoma. The tumor is composed of enlarged sebaceous lobules of varying size and shape.

cells. Some large lobules contain cystic spaces in their center, formed by the disintegration of mature sebaceous cells. In addition, there may be foci of squamous epithelium with keratinization. These foci probably represent areas with differentiation toward cells of the infundibulum. Cystic sebaceous adenomas seem to occur exclusively in patients with Muir–Torre syndrome (346).

Differential Diagnosis. In terms of differentiation, sebaceous adenoma stands between sebaceous hyperplasia and sebaceous epithelioma (see the following text). In sebaceous hyperplasia, the sebaceous lobules are fully or nearly fully matured, and in sebaceous epithelioma, irregularly shaped cell masses predominate, and the percentage of tumor cells with mature sebaceous differentiation is less than 50%. Sebaceous adenoma and sebaceous epithelioma lack the marked nuclear atypia and pleomorphism that are seen in sebaceous carcinoma. Considerable mitotic activity in the basaloid regions, however, may be present in both sebaceous adenoma and epithelioma.

Principles of Management: Complete excision is curative.

Sebaceous Epithelioma

Clinical Summary. Clinically, sebaceous epithelioma (formerly sebaceoma) presents as a solitary, circumscribed nodule or an ill-defined plaque, often yellow in color (347). Most lesions are located on the face or scalp, though rare lesions have been described on the ear and eyelid (348–350). Sebaceus epithelioma may arise within a nevus sebaceus (284). Sebaceous epitheliomas may be multiple and can also occur in association with other sebaceous neoplasms and multiple visceral carcinomas in Muir–Torre syndrome (see the following text).

Histopathology. The histologic spectrum extends from that seen in sebaceous adenoma to lesions that may be difficult to distinguish from sebaceous carcinoma. Architecturally, a sebaceous epithelioma can range from a well-circumscribed nodule to irregularly shaped cell masses in the dermis. More than half of the cells are undifferentiated basaloid cells, but there are still significant aggregates of mature sebocytes and transitional cells (Figs. 30-50 and 30-51) (351). Disintegration of sebaceous cells may be present (347). Lesions verging on a sebaceous

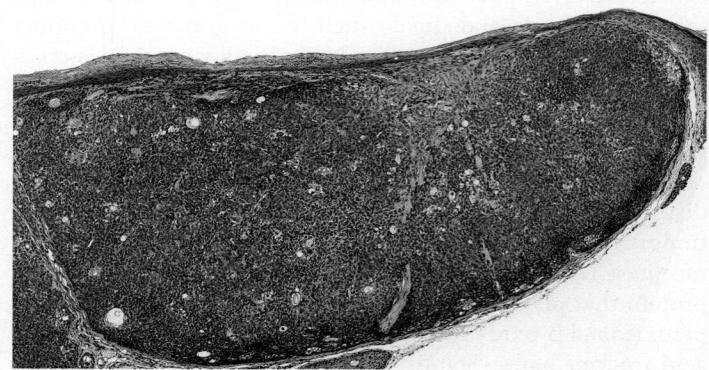

Figure 30-50 Sebaceous epithelioma. The tumor is a well-circumscribed nodule and comprised of basaloid epithelial cells. Scattered areas of clearer (sebaceous) cells are seen.

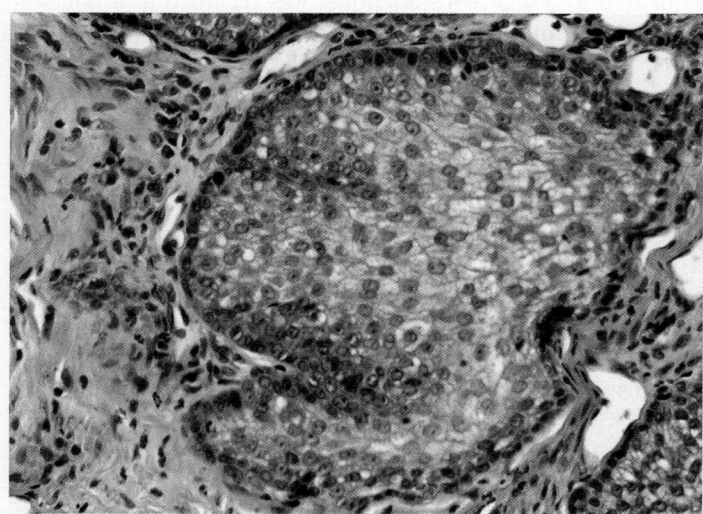

Figure 30-49 Sebaceous adenoma. In the lobules, two types of mature cells can be recognized: basaloid and sebaceous cells. However, sebaceous cells predominate. Cytologic atypia is not seen.

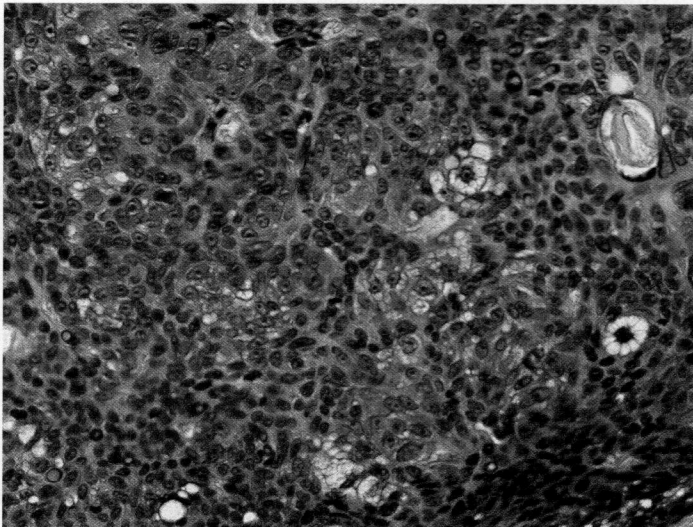

Figure 30-51 Sebaceous epithelioma. The majority of the lesion is composed of undifferentiated basaloid cells with islands of sebaceous cells and occasional sebaceous ducts.

carcinoma show some degree of irregularity in the arrangement of the cell masses (352). The upper part of a sebaceous epithelioma may rarely mimic a verruca or seborrheic keratosis (353). Rarely, sebaceous epitheliomas may demonstrate sebaceous and apocrine gland differentiation (354).

Differential Diagnosis. Criteria that may be of assistance in differentiating sebaceous adenoma from sebaceous epithelioma include the often greater size and depth of the latter and the lack of structures resembling normal sebaceous lobules. In contrast to sebaceous adenoma, nuclear atypia may be seen and mitoses may be numerous in sebaceous epithelioma (355).

The *rippled-pattern sebaceoma* is a variant of sebaceous epithelioma. It is more common in males and presents most frequently on the scalp (356). This variant exhibits a unique arrangement of small, monomorphous, cigar-shaped basaloid cells in linear rows parallel to one another, resembling Verocay bodies; this arrangement of cells produces the rippled pattern (Fig. 30-52). Scattered sebaceous cells and ducts are also typically seen (Fig. 30-53) (356).

Principles of Management: Complete excision is recommended.

Muir–Torre Syndrome

Clinical Summary. The Muir–Torre syndrome is defined by the combined occurrence of at least one sebaceous skin tumor and one internal malignancy in the same patient. Since 1967, when the first publication by Muir appeared concerning the coexistence of frequently multiple sebaceous tumors and usually multiple visceral carcinomas, scores of cases have been reported (357). Keratoacanthomas have also occurred in these patients, in some cases without sebaceous lesions, in association with visceral malignancies (358,359). Reticulated acanthoma with sebaceous differentiation may also be associated with the Muir–Torre syndrome (360). Cutaneous lesions vary in number from 1 to more than 100 lesions and can often precede the first manifestation of internal malignancy (361,362).

Colon carcinoma is the most common internal malignancy in Muir–Torre syndrome. The next most common malignancy is carcinoma of the genitourinary tract (including bladder, renal, pelvis, ovary, and uterus), followed by breast, head and neck, small intestinal, and lymphoma (362). Adenomatous colonic polyps are also common. Therefore, close surveillance for gastrointestinal and genitourinary malignancies in patients with sebaceous neoplasm is recommended (363). Glioblastoma multiforme also rarely occurs in Muir–Torre syndrome, overlapping with Turcot syndrome (364,365). Muir–Torre syndrome can be indolent and be unmasked by immunosuppression (366). Additionally, patients treated with localized radiation appear to be at risk for developing both further sebaceous carcinomas and soft tissue sarcomas within the radiation field (367,368).

Histopathology. Sebaceous adenomas are the most distinctive cutaneous markers of the Muir–Torre syndrome. They may be solid, cystic, or keratoacanthoma-like (345). Cystic sebaceous adenomas seem to occur exclusively in patients with Muir–Torre syndrome (346,369). Although ordinary keratoacanthomas occur in the Muir–Torre syndrome, often they have an accompanying sebaceous proliferation (370). Compared to adenomas, sebaceous epitheliomas have a reduced proportion of differentiated cells and are comprised predominantly of basaloid cells (Fig. 30-54).

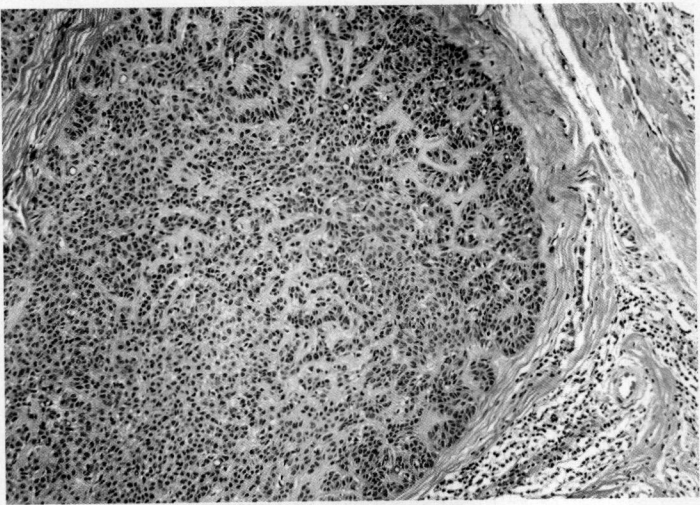

Figure 30-52 Rippled-pattern sebaceoma. Parallel arrangements of cells and nuclei are seen at low power.

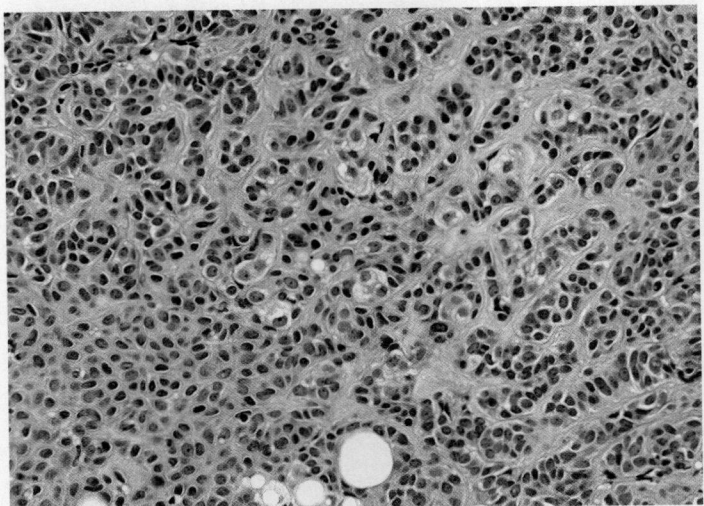

Figure 30-53 Rippled-pattern sebaceoma. The lesion is composed of undifferentiated basaloid cells with occasional sebaceous cells and sebaceous ducts.

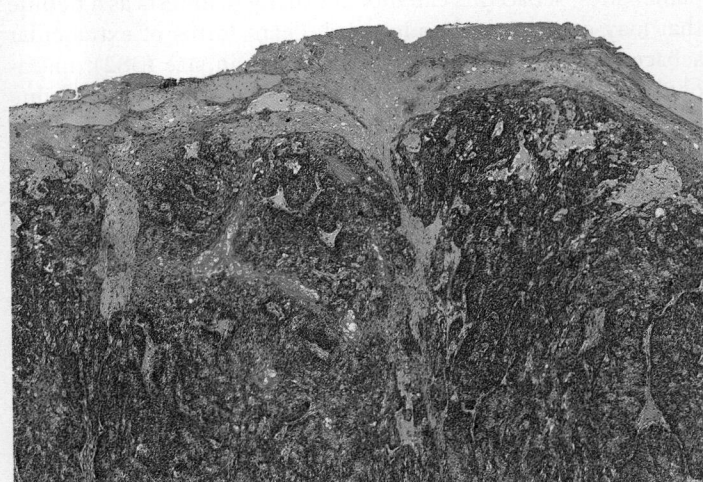

Figure 30-54 Sebaceous carcinoma. Irregular epithelial lobules are associated with epidermal ulceration and an infiltrative growth pattern in the dermis.

In addition to classic sebaceous adenomas, sebaceous epitheliomas, and BCCs with sebaceous differentiation, there are tumors that are difficult to classify. Therefore, sebaceous proliferations that lack a definitive diagnosis should raise suspicion for Muir–Torre syndrome (370). Sebaceous carcinomas also occur in Muir–Torre syndrome (361,371).

Additional Studies. Muir–Torre syndrome, when related to microsatellite instability, is a variant of hereditary nonpolyposis colorectal carcinoma syndrome (363). Microsatellite instability is identified in many patients with Muir–Torre syndrome, and nearly 90% have a germline mutation in the gene which encodes MSH-2. Approximately 10% have mutations in MLH-1 and even fewer patients have MSH-6 or PMS-2 mutations (372). Mutations in *MYH* gene have also been associated with Muir–Torre syndrome (373). The presence of microsatellite instability in sebaceous neoplasms is helpful in the detection of an underlying inherited DNA mismatch repair defect. Loss of MLH-1, PMS-2, MSH-2, and MSH-6 protein expression can be demonstrated by immunohistochemical staining and is warranted as a screening test for microsatellite instability and possible Muir–Torre syndrome (374,375).

Loss of expression of MLH1 and MSH2 is accompanied by loss of expression of PMS2 and MSH6, respectively (376). This is because MLH-1 forms an obligate heterodimer with PMS-2 and MSH-2 with MSH-6 (376). Another study suggests that a two-antibody approach (to MSH-6 and PMS-2) was as effective as a four-antibody approach, as initial screening for abnormal or equivocal mismatch repair protein expression (377).

In sebaceous neoplasms that do not demonstrate microsatellite instability, p53 overexpression may play a role (378).

Sebaceous Carcinoma

Clinical Summary. Sebaceous carcinomas have been traditionally classified into ocular and extraocular types. The ocular type most frequently occurs on the eyelids, typically originating from the meibomian glands and less commonly from the glands of Zeis. Extraocular sebaceous carcinoma has been reported most commonly on the head and neck; sometimes also on the vulva and penis; and rarely other locations (379,380). On the eyelids, sebaceous carcinoma may be easily mistaken for chronic blepharoconjunctivitis or a chalazion (381). On extraocular sites, sebaceous carcinoma usually manifests as a nodule that may or may not be ulcerated. Giant forms of extraocular sebaceous carcinoma can grow to 20 cm in size (382). Extraocular sebaceous carcinoma is highly associated with having another primary cancer. Sebaceous carcinoma occurs predominantly in elderly Caucasian patients; however, it can occur in adolescents (383). Ocular sebaceous carcinoma occurs equally between sexes; however, extraocular sebaceous carcinoma is more common in men. For unclear reasons, the incidence of extraocular sebaceous carcinoma appears to have increased over the past several decades (384).

Ocular sebaceous carcinomas quite frequently cause regional metastases. In addition, there may be orbital invasion; in 22% of the cases reported in one study, death resulted from visceral metastases (385). Though previously thought to be not aggressive, extraocular sebaceous carcinomas can widely metastasize and cause death just as frequently as ocular types (386). The sebaceous carcinomas that may be found among the multiple sebaceous neoplasms occurring in association with multiple visceral carcinomas in the Muir–Torre syndrome are less likely to metastasize (387). In some instances, a sebaceous carcinoma represents the only cutaneous manifestation of Muir–Torre syndrome (388).

Histopathology. The irregular lobular formations show great variations in the size of lobules (Fig. 30-54). Although many cells are undifferentiated, distinct sebaceous cells showing a foamy cytoplasm are present in the center of most lobules (Figs. 30-54 and 30-55). Many undifferentiated cells and sebaceous cells appear atypical, showing considerable nuclear and nucleolar pleomorphism (Fig. 30-55) (389). In addition, many of the undifferentiated cells have an eosinophilic cytoplasm, and when fat stains are used on frozen sections, the cells are found to contain fine lipid globules (381). Some of the large lobules show areas composed of atypical keratinizing cells, as seen in squamous cell carcinoma (352).

More than half of ocular sebaceous carcinomas show pagetoid spread of malignant cells either in the conjunctival epithelium, the epidermis of the lid skin, or both (385). These changes are seen very rarely in extraocular sebaceous carcinoma (390). The pagetoid cells contain no mucopolysaccharides, but they stain positively for fat with oil red O (385). Recognition of the pagetoid growth pattern in biopsy material can be essential to recognition of the existence of an underlying sebaceous carcinoma (391). Originally, sebaceous carcinoma was thought to occur strictly *de novo*; but, it can also arise from a sebaceous adenoma/epithelioma, and sebaceous carcinoma *in situ* can progress to an invasive carcinoma (392).

Additional Studies. Certain strains of human papillomavirus have been implicated in the pathogenesis of sebaceous carcinoma (393). Mutations in *TP53* have been seen in sebaceous carcinoma, and immunohistochemical staining for proliferating cell nuclear antigen and p53 seem to have some prognostic value (394,395). Interestingly, in sebaceous carcinomas that arise in nevus sebaceus, p53 overexpression is common, and these lesions are more indolent than *de novo* sebaceous carcinoma (396). c-Myc may also play a role in the development of sebaceous carcinoma. c-Myc can induce sebaceous gland differentiation, and dysregulation of c-Myc signaling through loss of AR or through aberrant p53 expression may result in lack of differentiation

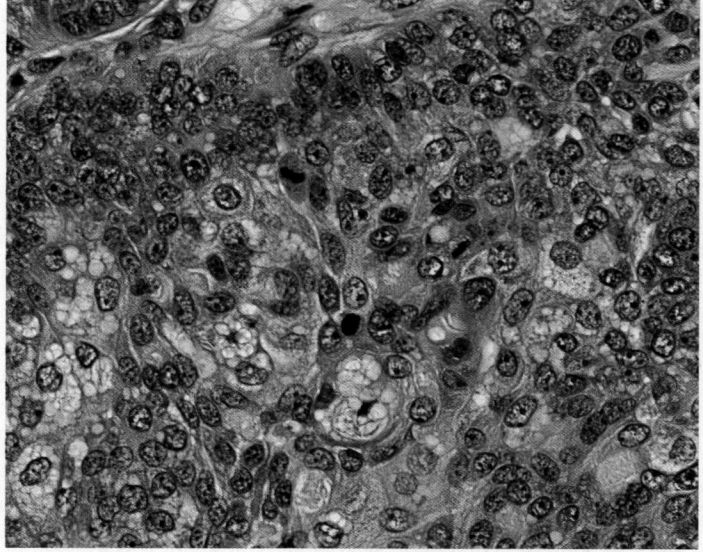

Figure 30-55 Sebaceous carcinoma. Lesional cells demonstrate marked cytologic atypia, mitotic activity, and focal sebaceous differentiation.

and progression to sebaceous carcinoma (397). Extraocular sebaceous carcinoma, when not associated with Muir–Torre syndrome, shows significantly increased *EGFR* expression, and may be effectively targeted with EGFR inhibitors (398).

In ocular sebaceous carcinoma, a higher expression of Shh, *ABCG2*, and Wnt is associated with a more aggressive course and increased rate of metastatic disease (399).

Differential Diagnosis. The tumor cells in sebaceous carcinoma are often large and squamoid in appearance or show basaloid differentiation with only inconspicuous lipidization. In the latter case, the tumor must be distinguished from BCCs with sebaceous differentiation; in the former case, the differential diagnosis includes squamous cell carcinomas with hydropic changes (400,401). Other malignant neoplasms with clear cells must also be considered, including metastatic lesions (386).

Sebaceous carcinomas do not show the typical changes seen in BCCs. Instead, the undifferentiated cells of sebaceous carcinoma show a more eosinophilic cytoplasm, greater cytologic atypia, and greater invasiveness (402). Clear cell squamous cell carcinoma usually shows evidence of keratinization in the form of dyskeratotic cells and squamous parakeratotic whorls. Using an immunohistochemical battery, including epithelial membrane antigen (EMA), anti–BCA-255 (BRST-1), and CAM 5.2 can be helpful in distinguishing sebaceous carcinoma from BCC and squamous cell carcinoma (403).

Clear cell malignant neoplasms do not show sebaceous differentiation. The cytoplasmic clearing is caused by glycogen accumulation, which causes the nuclei to be positioned eccentrically. In contrast, neoplastic cells with sebaceous differentiation show scalloped, centrally situated nuclei and microvacuolated cytoplasm secondary to lipid deposits. When sebaceous carcinoma is suspected or found at a frozen section, additional sections should be saved for fat stains. Sebaceous ductal differentiation consists of ductal structures lined by an eosinophilic corrugated cuticle similar to that of the normal sebaceous duct. Finally, metastases to the skin from malignant neoplasms composed of clear cells, namely, renal, breast, bladder, and prostatic carcinoma or melanoma, also may mimic sebaceous carcinoma. Histochemical and immunohistochemical methods can help in narrowing the differential diagnosis appropriately (403).

As in other malignant adnexal neoplasms, zones of necrosis, marked nuclear atypia, and abnormal mitotic figures are common in sebaceous carcinoma (Fig. 30-55). Pagetoid proliferation of tumor cells in the epidermis or conjunctiva may extend widely and confers a poorer prognosis. Other adverse prognostic attributes include multicentric involvement, poor differentiation (i.e., sparse lipid), necrosis, paucity of reactive lymphocytes, extensive local invasion, and vascular or bony invasion (395). Metastases first involve regional lymph nodes of the periauricular, submaxillary, and cervical chains. Visceral spread may occur and lead to death.

Differentiating sebaceous carcinoma from sebaceous epithelioma is sometimes challenging. Sebaceous carcinomas are larger, asymmetric, infiltrative, and poorly circumscribed, whereas sebaceous epitheliomas may extend into the subcutis but are circumscribed and symmetric. Carcinomas may ulcerate the epidermis, and there may be extensive necrosis ("necrosis en masse"). The ratio of differentiated (vacuolated) to undifferentiated (nonvacuolated) sebocytes varies but tends to be higher in sebaceous epitheliomas. Nuclear atypia is often striking, and mitotic figures are numerous and sometimes atypical

in carcinomas. Sebaceous epitheliomas, in contrast, lack striking nuclear atypia but may have few or many mitoses (355). In Muir–Torre syndrome and in transplant patients, borderline sebaceous neoplasms that have features of sebaceous carcinoma may occur, making a distinction even more challenging (404).

Principles of Management: Treatment is aimed at completely removing the tumor by surgery; wide surgical margins are recommended. Evaluation of lymph node involvement is needed. If widespread involvement of the eyelids is found, exenteration may be necessary.

TUMORS WITH APOCRINE DIFFERENTIATION

Apocrine Nevus

Clinical Summary. Large numbers of mature apocrine glands are frequently present in lesions of nevus sebaceus and SCAP. However, pure apocrine nevus is a rare tumor. Apocrine nevi have presented as papules, facial nodules, and, most frequently, soft tissue masses of the axillae (405–409).

Histopathology. These lesions consist of increased numbers of apocrine glands, usually situated in the reticular dermis with occasional extension into subcutaneous tissue (405–413).

Immunohistochemistry. Studies demonstrate positive staining for carcinoembryonic antigen, gross cystic disease fluid protein, EMA, low–molecular-weight keratins, MUC1, and MUC5AC (409,412–414). Lesions are typically negative for S100 and high–molecular-weight keratins.

Principles of Management: Apocrine nevi are benign and treatment is not required.

Apocrine Hidrocystoma

Clinical Summary. Apocrine hidrocystoma occurs usually as a solitary, translucent cystic nodule (405,406,408–413,415–417). The term "apocrine cystadenoma" has also been used to describe these lesions (416). Lesional diameter usually ranges from 1 to 15 mm; however, "giant" lesions, measuring 20 mm, have been described (418). Frequently, the lesions have a bluish hue and can resemble a blue nevus (Fig. 30-56). The usual location of apocrine hidrocystoma is on the face, but it is

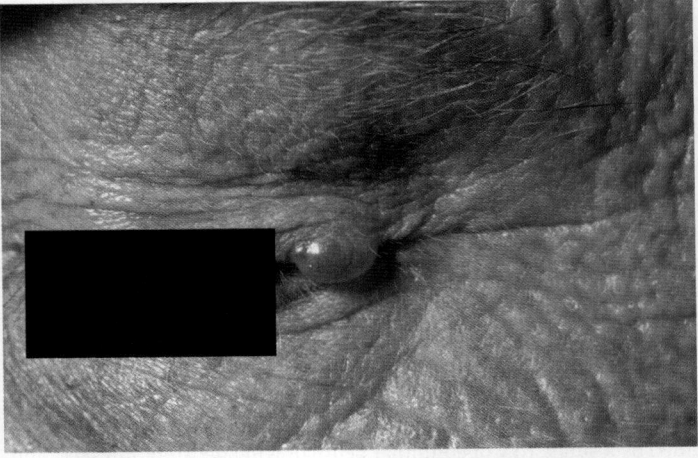

Figure 30-56 Apocrine hidrocystoma. A translucent cystic lesion with a bluish hue is noted.

occasionally seen on the ears, scalp, chest, shoulders, or vulva (415,419–424). Multiple apocrine hidrocystomas are rare and typically encountered in the setting of Goltz–Gorlin syndrome and Schopf–Schultz–Passarge syndrome (425–427). Lesions rarely occur on the penis and most often represent misdiagnosed median raphe cysts (see Chapter 29) (420,428).

The blue color in some of the cysts is not fully explained. Lipofuscin deposition has been associated with variation in the color tone, resulting in a phenomenon analogous to the Tyndall effect caused by the scattering of light in a colloidal mixture with the reflection of blue light (424,426,429).

Histopathology. The dermis contains one or several large cystic spaces into which papillary projections often extend (Fig. 30-57). The inner surface of the cyst and the papillary projections are lined by a row of columnar secretory cells of variable height showing "decapitation" secretion indicative of apocrine secretion (Fig. 30-58). Peripheral to the layer of secretory cells are elongated myoepithelial cells, their long axes running parallel to the cyst wall (424). In some cases, one finds superficially located lumina lined by a double layer of ductal epithelium in addition to the cysts lined by secretory cells (416).

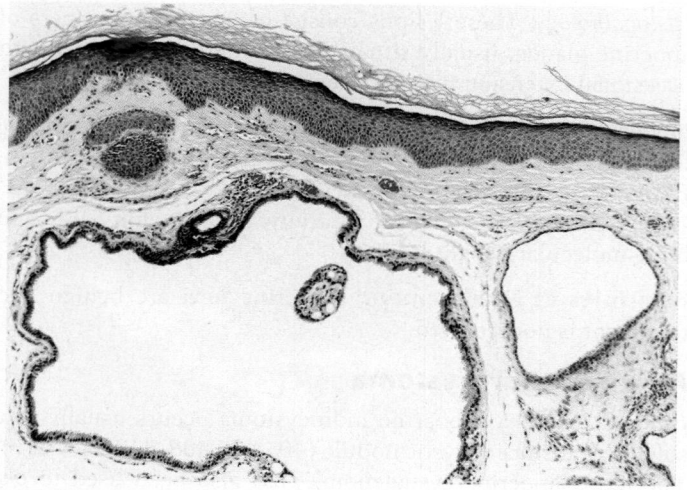

Figure 30-57 Apocrine hidrocystoma. The dermis contains a multiloculated cystic lesion lined by epithelial cells with occasional papillary projections.

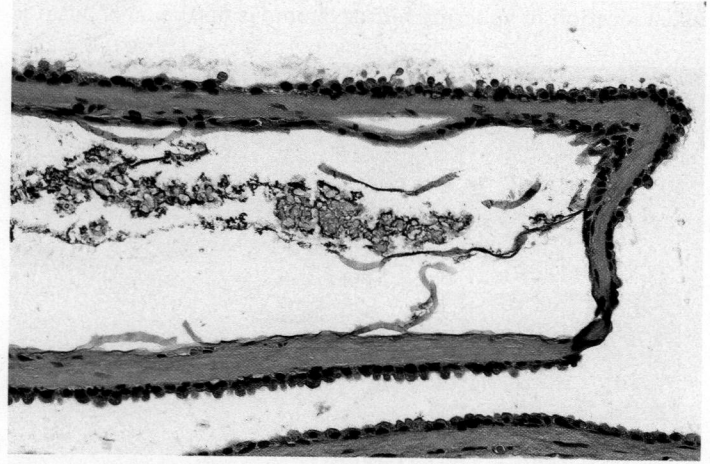

Figure 30-58 Apocrine hidrocystoma (cystadenoma). The cyst is lined by a single row of columnar cells showing decapitation secretion. Peripheral to the row of secretory cells are elongated myoepithelial cells.

Additional Studies. The apocrine nature of the secretion of the luminal cells has been demonstrated by the presence of numerous large PAS-positive, diastase-resistant granules in the secretory cells and by electron microscopy. Electron microscopic examination shows abundant secretory granules of moderate density and uniform internal structure in the secretory cells of apocrine hidrocystoma, particularly in their luminal portion, and evidence of apocrine secretion (430–432). Polarizable calcium oxalate crystals have been reported, though the frequency of this feature is unknown owing to the fact that processing may compromise the deposits (433). Apocrine hidrocystomas stain positively for S100 A2 protein and CK14 (434).

The apocrine hidrocystoma can be regarded as a cystic adenoma rather than as a retention cyst because the secretory cells do not appear flattened—as in a retention cyst—and because papillary projections can extend into the lumen of the cystic spaces (416).

Differential Diagnosis. Eccrine hidrocystomas, which are lined by ductal cells, differ from apocrine hidrocystomas by the absence of decapitation secretion. However, those portions of an apocrine hidrocystoma in which the cystic spaces are lined by ductal epithelium have the same appearance as the cystic spaces in eccrine hidrocystomas, except that the latter usually are unilocular and apocrine hidrocystomas are often multilocular. Median raphe cysts of the penis, which have been mistakenly reported as apocrine hidrocystomas, show a pseudostratified columnar cyst wall without evidence of decapitation secretion or myoepithelial cells (420).

Principles of Management: Lesions can be incised and drained. Electrosurgical destruction of the cyst wall is recommended to prevent recurrence. Multiple lesions can be treated with a carbon dioxide laser.

Hidradenoma Papilliferum

Clinical Summary. Hidradenoma papilliferum usually occurs in women, on the labia majora or in the perineal or perianal region (435–438). In males, it has been reported as a perineal or arm lesion (439,440). Occurrences on the upper eyelid and in the external ear canal have been reported (441,442). The tumor is covered by normal skin and measures only a few millimeters in diameter; some have been shown to grow in response to hormone stimulation (443). Malignant changes have been reported in hidradenoma papilliferum, as aggressive adenosquamous or squamous cell carcinomas (444,445).

Histopathology. The tumor represents an adenoma with apocrine differentiation (446). It is located in the dermis, is well circumscribed, is surrounded by a fibrous capsule, and lacks a connection with the overlying epidermis (Fig. 30-59). Within the tumor, one observes tubular and cystic structures (Fig. 30-60). Papillary folds project into the cystic spaces. The lumina are lined occasionally with only a single row of columnar cells—which show an oval, pale-staining nucleus located near the base, a faintly eosinophilic cytoplasm, and active decapitation secretion as seen in the secretory cells of apocrine glands (Fig. 30-60) (446). Usually, the lumina are surrounded by a double layer of cells consisting of an inner layer of secretory cells and an outer layer of small cuboidal cells with deeply basophilic nuclei that are myoepithelial cells (Fig. 30-60) (447).

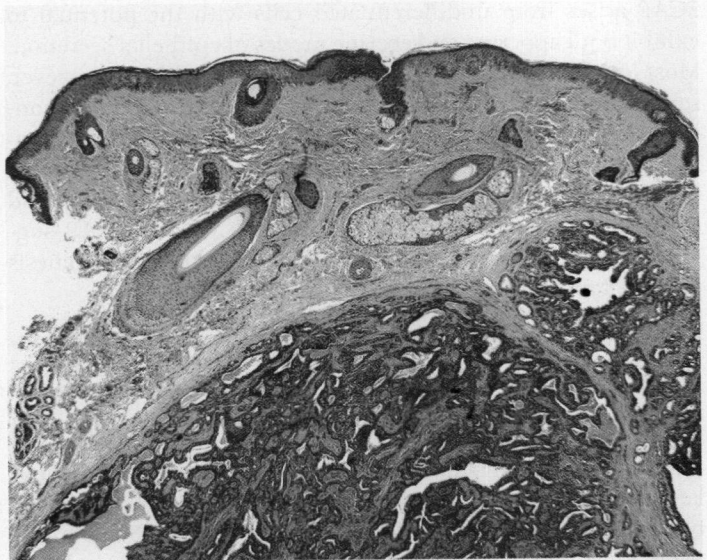

Figure 30-59 Hidradenoma papilliferum. The tumor consists of a well-circumscribed dermal nodule with scattered cystic and branching spaces.

Additional Studies. Apocrine differentiation in hidradenoma papilliferum has been established by histochemical, enzyme histochemical, and electron microscopic examinations.

Histochemically, the luminal cells contain many large, PAS-positive, diastase-resistant granules as seen in the secretory cells of apocrine glands. In addition, the luminal cells are positive for SOX-10, DOG-1, nonspecific esterase and acid phosphatase, the so-called apocrine enzymes, and negative for phosphorylase, a typical eccrine enzyme. Furthermore, the outer row of cells stains positive for alkaline phosphatase, as myoepithelial cells typically do (446,448,449).

Electron microscopic examination demonstrates two features of the luminal cells that are regarded as characteristic of apocrine secretory cells. First, numerous membrane-limited, secretory granules that are of varying size and density and that contain lipid droplets are present in the apical portion of these cells. Second, as evidence of decapitation secretion, portions of apical cytoplasm containing large secretory granules are released into the lumen (447). The peripheral layer of cells contains numerous myofilaments. Molecular analyses of lesions have demonstrated the presence of HPV-16, 31, 33, 53, and 56 DNA in these lesions (450,451).

Genetic studies have shown the PI3K/AKT signaling pathway to be highly altered in hidradenoma papilliferum. One cohort demonstrated hotspot-activating mutations in PIK3CA or AKT1 in 5/12 tumors and mutations in at least one gene known to be involved in PI3K/AKT signaling in all 7 nonhotspot tumors (452).

Principles of Management: Simple excision is curative in most cases.

Syringocystadenoma Papilliferum

Clinical Summary. SCAP occurs most commonly on the scalp or the face; however, in about one-fourth of the cases, it is seen elsewhere (453–456). It is usually first noted at birth or in early childhood and presents as a papule or several papules in a linear arrangement or as a plaque. The lesion increases in size at puberty, becoming papillomatous and often crusted (457). On the scalp, SCAP frequently arises around puberty within a nevus sebaceus that has been present since birth.

Histopathology. The epidermis shows varying degrees of papillomatosis. One or several cystic invaginations extend downward from the epidermis (Fig. 30-61). The upper portion of the invaginations and, in some instances, large segments of the cystic invaginations are lined by squamous, keratinizing cells similar to those of the surface epidermis (458). In the lower portion of the cystic invaginations, numerous papillary projections extend into the lumina of the invaginations. The papillary projections and the lower portion of the invaginations are lined by glandular epithelium often consisting of two rows of cells (Fig. 30-62).

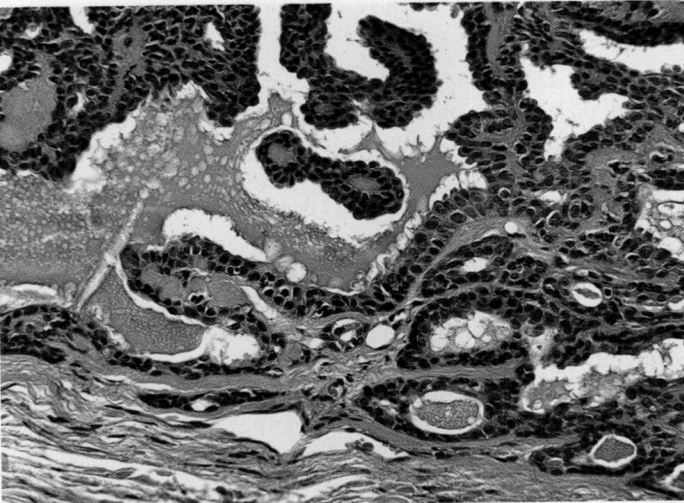

Figure 30-60 Hidradenoma papilliferum. Numerous papillary projections are seen within the lesion. The papillary folds are lined by one layer of high cylindrical cells, which show evidence of active "decapitation" secretion like that seen in apocrine glands. A basal layer of small cuboidal cells is also present.

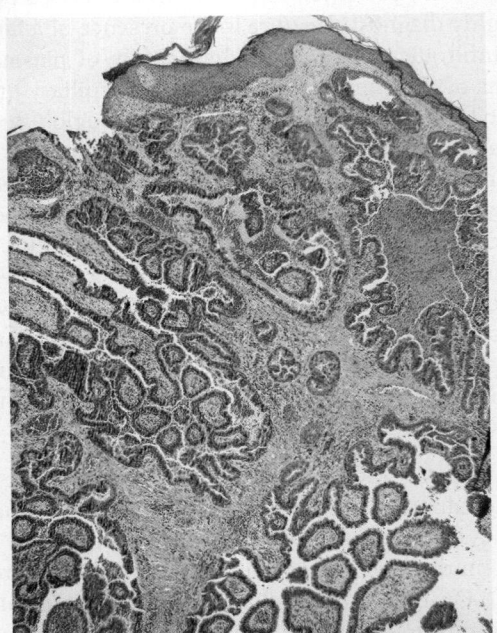

Figure 30-61 Syringocystadenoma papilliferum. The lesion exhibits a cystic invagination extending into the dermis, with numerous papillary projections.

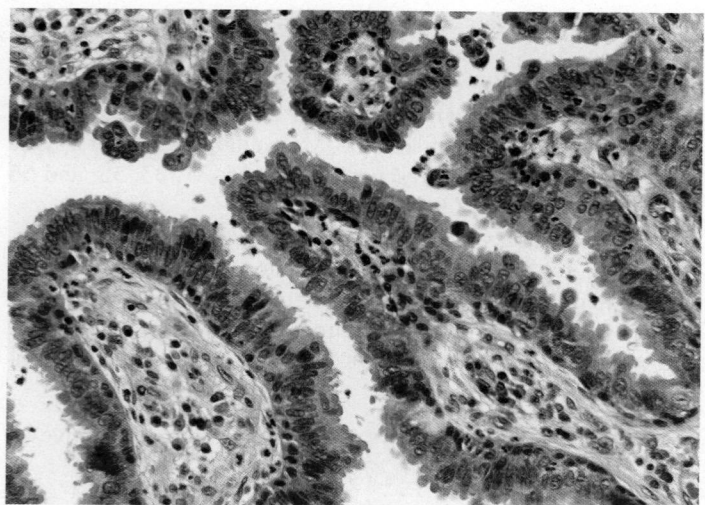

Figure 30-62 Syringocystadenoma papilliferum. The papillary projections are lined by two rows of cells. The luminal row of cells consists of columnar cells with evidence of active "decapitation" secretion. The outer row of cells consists of small cuboidal cells. Plasma cells are usually seen in the papillary core.

The luminal row of cells consists of high columnar cells with oval nuclei and faintly eosinophilic cytoplasm. Occasionally, some of these cells show active decapitation secretion, and cellular debris is found in the lumina (459). The outer row of cells consists of small cuboidal cells with round nuclei and scanty cytoplasm. In some areas, the cells of the luminal layer are arranged in multiple layers and form a lacelike pattern, resulting in multiple small, tubular lumina (455).

Beneath the cystic invaginations, deep in the dermis, one can find in many cases groups of tubular glands with large lumina. The cells lining the large lumina often show evidence of active decapitation secretion, indicating that they are apocrine glands (Fig. 30-62) (457). Connections of the apocrine glands deep in the dermis with the cystic invaginations in the upper dermis can be traced when step sections are carried out (14).

A highly diagnostic feature is the presence of a fairly dense cellular infiltrate composed predominantly of plasma cells in the stroma of this tumor, especially in the papillary projections (Fig. 30-62). These are typical of the immunoglobulin G (IgG) and immunoglobulin A (IgA) classes (460,461).

Frequently, there are malformed sebaceous glands and hair structures in the lesions of SCAP (457). In about one-third of the cases, SCAP is associated with a nevus sebaceus. In about 10% of the cases, a basaloid epithelial proliferation resembling BCC develops, but this is noted only in lesions that also exhibit a nevus sebaceous (455). A few instances of association with verrucous carcinoma as well as transition of a SCAP into an adenocarcinoma with regional lymph node metastases have been reported (462).

Additional Studies. SCAP can exhibit both apocrine and eccrine differentiation. For example, positive immunoreactivity for gross cystic disease fluid proteins 15 and 24 and zinc α-2 glycoprotein demonstrates evidence of apocrine differentiation (413,463). On the other hand, immunohistochemical analysis of cytokeratins in SCAP demonstrates similarities to eccrine poromas and the ductal component of eccrine glands (464). In addition, light and electron microscopic features of some lesions show evidence of eccrine differentiation (13). It is probable that

SCAP arises from undifferentiated cells with the potential to exhibit both apocrine and eccrine modes of epithelial secretion. Most lesions of SCAP exhibit apocrine differentiation; however, some demonstrate eccrine features (371). Studies have demonstrated *BRAF* (40% to 66.7%) and *HRAS* (7.7% to 26.1%) mutations, the presence of high-risk HPV DNA in select lesions in the anogenital area, and loss of heterozygosity for *Patched* and *CDKN2A*, a negative regulator of the cell cycle, in SCAP, suggesting that these molecules may play a role in the pathogenesis of these lesions (465,466).

Principles of Management: Complete excision is the treatment of choice.

Tubular Apocrine Adenoma

Clinical Summary. First described in 1972, additional cases of tubular apocrine adenoma have been reported (467–472). The tumor typically presents as a well-defined nodule that is located on the scalp. Most tumors are less than 2 cm in diameter, although one reported lesion located on the scalp measured 7 by 4 cm (469).

Histopathology. This tumor manifests numerous irregularly shaped tubular structures that are usually lined by two layers of epithelial cells (Fig. 30-63). The peripheral layer consists of cuboidal or flattened cells, and the luminal layer is composed of columnar cells (469). Some of the tubules have a dilated lumen with papillary projections extending into it (Fig. 30-63). Decapitation secretion of the luminal cells is seen in many areas. In addition, cellular fragments and eosinophilic granular debris are seen in some lumina. In some cases, tubular apocrine adenomas can arise in association with SCAP, and often the SCAP is situated in the superficial portion of the "combined" lesion (468,471,473). In cases with overlapping histopathologic features of SCAP and/or apocrine gland cysts, some authors have proposed the term tubulopapillary cystic adenoma with apocrine differentiation as unifying nomenclature (474).

Additional Studies. Electron microscopy has revealed secretory granules and evidence of apocrine-type decapitation secretion in the luminal cells (469,472). In contrast to hidradenoma papilliferum, the peripheral cell layer contains no myofilaments. Enzyme histochemistry is also consistent with apocrine differentiation (469).

Differential Diagnosis. In tubular apocrine adenomas with marked papillary proliferations, there may be some nuclear pleomorphism, which suggests sweat gland carcinoma or a metastatic adenocarcinoma. However, the presence of a peripheral layer of cuboidal or flattened cells is a feature favoring a benign lesion (470).

Tubular apocrine adenomas resemble papillary eccrine adenoma, and these two tumors were once regarded as identical (468). Genetic sequencing and IHC identified BRAF (60%, 9/15) and KRAS (22%, 2/9) mutations in TAA (475). Because of overlapping features in decapitation secretion, enzyme histochemistry, and in electron microscopy, the suggestion was made that they be referred to as *tubulopapillary hidradenoma*, with apocrine or eccrine differentiation (476). For a description of papillary eccrine adenomas, see page 1059. The term *tubulopapillary hidradenoma* may be considered to represent a spectrum of lesions that includes tubular apocrine adenoma and papillary eccrine adenoma, and these are also closely related to SCAP (477,478).

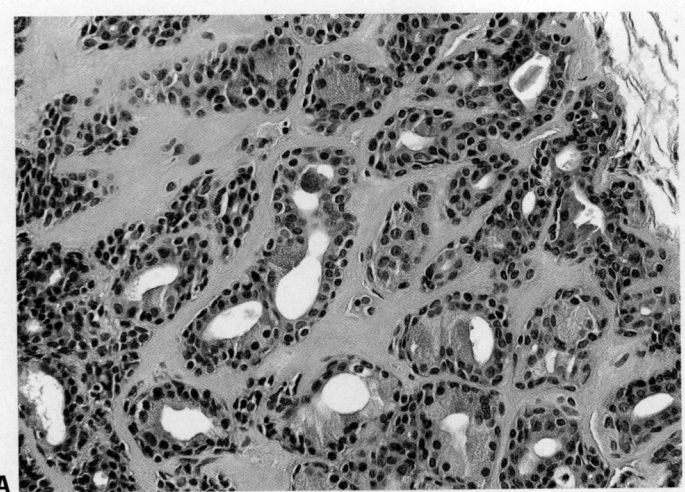
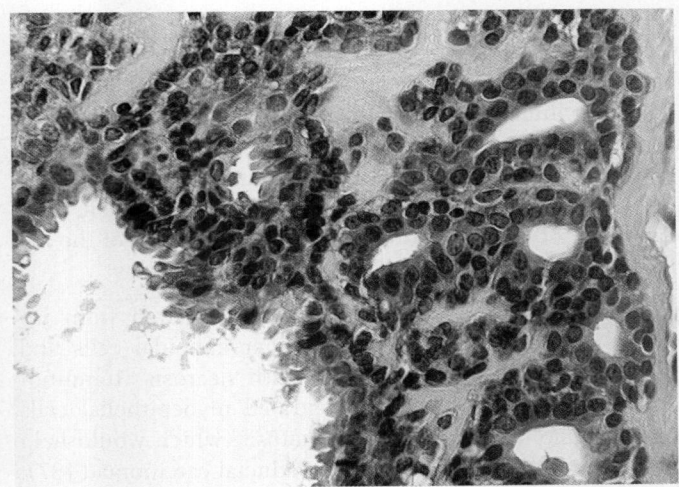

Figure 30-63 Tubular apocrine adenoma. **A:** There are numerous irregularly shaped tubular structures in the dermis. **B:** The tubules are usually lined by two layers of epithelial cells—an indicator of benignancy. The peripheral layer consists of cuboidal or flattened cells and the luminal layer is composed of columnar cells. Some of the tubules have a dilated lumen with papillary projections. Eosinophilic debris can be seen in the tubular lumens.

Principles of Management: Surgical excision is the treatment of choice. Mohs micrographic surgery has been used to treat some cases.

Apocrine Adenoma; Apocrine Fibroadenoma

Clinical Summary. Rare variants of apocrine adenomas can occur in apocrine areas, such as the axilla or the perianal region (479–481).

Histopathology. Apocrine lumina are readily recognized by the presence of decapitation secretion. In addition, there may be cystically dilated spaces (480,481). A stromal component resembling that in fibroadenomas of the breast has been described (479).

Principles of Management: These lesions are benign. Complete excision is the treatment of choice.

Erosive Adenomatosis of the Nipple

Clinical Summary. Erosive adenomatosis (papillary adenoma, florid papillomatosis) of the nipple (EAN) represents an adenoma of the major nipple ducts (482–485). In the early lesions, the nipple appears eroded and inflamed, often with a serous discharge. During this early erosive phase, clinical differentiation from Paget disease of the breast may be difficult. Later, the nipple shows nodular thickening; differentiation from Paget disease is then easier. Peak incidence for erosive adenomatosis is in the fifth decade of life; cases in girls as young as 8 years of age have been reported (486).

Histopathology. Extending downward from the epidermis are irregular, dilated tubular structures resembling those seen in tubular apocrine adenoma (Fig. 30-64) (485). These tubules are lined by a peripheral layer of cuboidal cells and a luminal

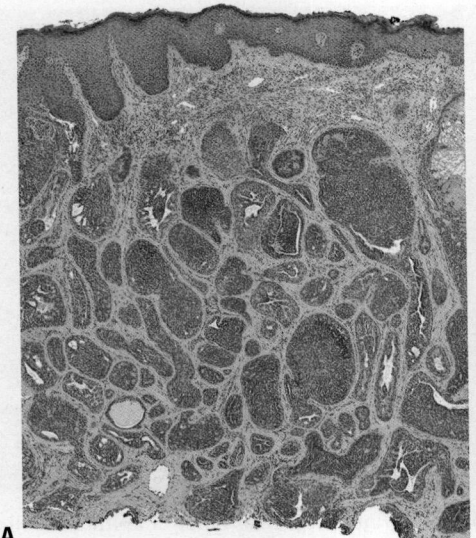
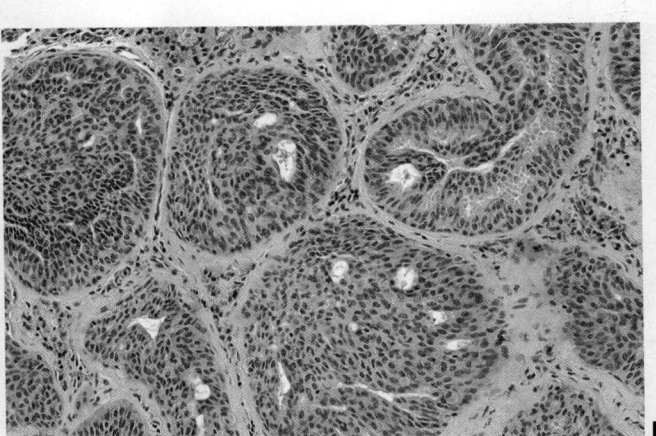

Figure 30-64 Erosive adenomatosis of the nipple. **A:** Dilated tubular structures are present at the dermal–epidermal junction and throughout the dermis. **B:** The dilated tubules are lined by a peripheral layer of cuboidal cells and a luminal layer of columnar cells that occasionally exhibit decapitation secretion. Other tubules exhibit a more solid proliferation resembling "papillomatosis" of mammary duct epithelium.

layer of columnar cells that occasionally demonstrate secretory projections at their luminal border (485). Some of the tubules demonstrate papillary proliferations of columnar cells that extend into the lumen; these proliferations may be so pronounced as to nearly fill the entire lumen. In other areas, detached, partially necrotic cells may be seen in the tubular lumina. In some lesions, considerable acanthosis of the epidermis is seen, with an extension of the squamous epithelium into some of the superficial ductal structures.

Differential Diagnosis. EAN must be differentiated from intraductal carcinoma, which shows larger cuboidal cells and uniform nuclear atypia, frequently with necrosis. Immunohistochemical studies have demonstrated myoepithelial cells within the lesions of erosive adenomatosis, which would help to differentiate these lesions from intraductal carcinoma (487). Hidradenoma papilliferum, in contrast to EAN, generally does not show connections of the tubular structures with the surface epidermis (488).

Principles of Management: EAN often recurs if not completely excised. Mohs micrographic surgery has been used to remove these lesions while minimizing tissue loss.

Cylindroma

Clinical Summary. Cylindroma occurs more often as a solitary lesion than as multiple lesions (489). Cases with multiple lesions are dominantly inherited and show numerous dome-shaped, smooth nodules of various sizes on the scalp. Occasionally, scattered nodules are also present on the face and, in rare instances, on the trunk and the extremities (490). The lesions begin to appear in early adulthood and increase in number and size throughout life. The tumors present as scalp nodules ranging in size from a few millimeters to several centimeters (Fig. 30-65). Nodules on the scalp may be present in such large numbers as to cover the entire scalp like a turban. For this reason, they are referred to occasionally as *turban tumors.*

The association of multiple lesions of cylindroma with multiple lesions of trichoepithelioma is quite common (489,491–494). In these cases, the lesions of the scalp are cylindromas, and those elsewhere are partially cylindromas and partially trichoepitheliomas. *CYLD* cutaneous syndrome (formerly Brooke–Spiegler syndrome) refers to a dominantly inherited disorder in which patients demonstrate multiple cylindromas,

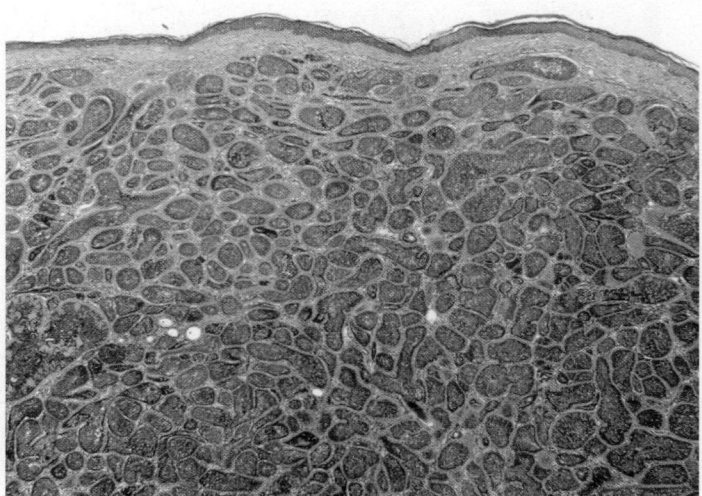

Figure 30-66 Cylindroma. The tumor is composed of irregularly shaped islands that fit together like pieces of a jigsaw puzzle. The islands are surrounded by a hyaline sheath.

spiradenomas, and trichoepitheliomas (491,494–497). In several instances, multiple cylindromas have been found in association with eccrine spiradenoma (489,498,499).

Sporadic, solitary cylindromas are not inherited but can harbor the same *CYLD* mutations; they appear in adulthood and occur either on the scalp or the face. Their histologic appearance is the same as that of multiple cylindromas (489).

Histopathology. Cylindromas represent a tumor that may manifest both apocrine and eccrine differentiation; however, features of apocrine differentiation usually predominate (489). The tumors of cylindroma are composed of numerous islands of epithelial cells. Varying considerably in size and shape and lying close together, separated often only by their hyaline sheath and a narrow band of collagen, the islands of epithelial cells seem to fit together like pieces of a jigsaw puzzle (Figs. 30-66 and 30-67). The hyaline sheath surrounding the tumor islands like a cylinder is quite variable in thickness. In addition, droplets

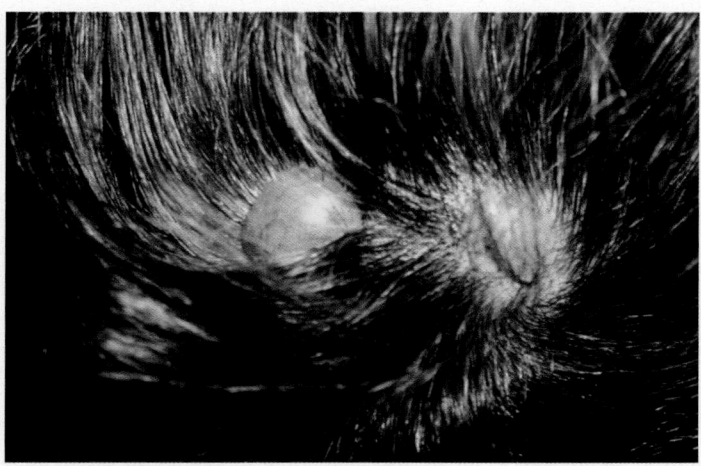

Figure 30-65 Cylindroma. The lesions typically present as scalp nodules.

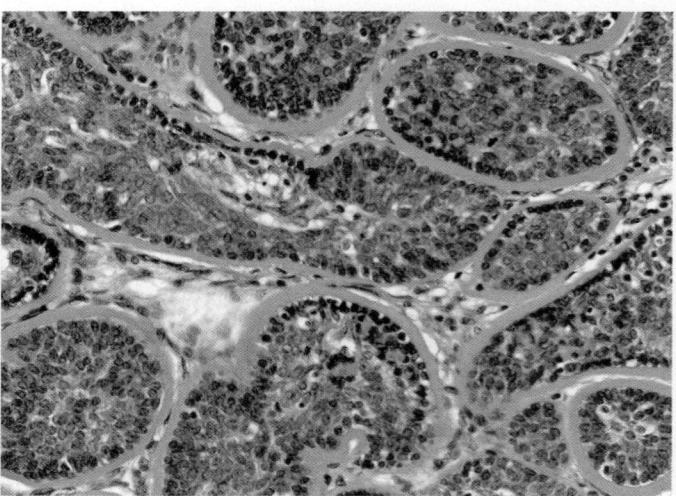

Figure 30-67 Cylindroma. Two types of epithelial cells comprise the islands: cells with small, dark nuclei representing undifferentiated cells and cells with large, pale nuclei representing cells with a certain degree of differentiation toward ductal or secretory cells. Droplets of hyaline material are seen in the islands.

of hyalin are present in many islands, and some islands consist largely of hyalin and contain only a few cells. The hyalin is PAS positive and diastase resistant (459).

Two types of cells constitute the islands: Cells with small, dark-staining nuclei are present predominantly at the periphery of the islands, often in a palisade arrangement, and cells with large, light-staining nuclei lie in the center of the islands (Fig. 30-67). In addition, tubular lumina are often present. In some cases, they are quite numerous, whereas in others only a few are found after a thorough search. The lumina are lined by cells that usually have the appearance of ductal cells (500). Occasionally, however, the luminal cells show active secretion, like the secretory cells of apocrine glands (14). Often, amorphous material is found within the lumina; it contains both neutral and acid mucopolysaccharides, as demonstrated by positive staining with the PAS reaction and Alcian blue (459).

Additional Studies. The ultrastructural and immunohistochemical features best fit differentiation toward the intradermal coiled duct region of eccrine sweat glands (501–503), with myoepithelial cell participation (504).

Electron microscopic examination, similar to examination by light microscopy, has revealed two major types of cells: undifferentiated basal cells with small, dark nuclei and differentiating cells with large, pale nuclei. Most of the differentiating cells still appear immature as "indeterminate cells," but some show a certain degree of differentiation toward secretory or ductal cells and are in part arranged around lumina (500,505,506).

Of interest, an early study of two large pedigrees led to the conclusion that cylindromas and trichoepitheliomas are different manifestations of the same disorder and not merely examples of genetic linkage (494). Genetic studies have identified a single gene, *CYLD1*, on 16q12-q13 as being altered in familial cylindromatosis syndrome (Brooke–Spiegler) (12). Loss of heterozygosity at the 16q12-q13 locus has been demonstrated in familial cylindromatosis and sporadic cylindromas (12). The CYLD1 gene has been cloned; the molecule contains cytoskeletal binding domains and domains similar to ubiquitin hydrolases (507). Frameshift mutations in the CYLD1 gene have also been associated with familial cylindromatosis (508). The various tumors associated with familial cylindromatosis may arise from different types of mutations in the CYLD1 gene; however, this has not been definitively demonstrated and evidence implicating other genes and pathways, such as MYB activation, has been identified (508,509). Recurrent mutations in epigenetic modifiers DNMT3A and BCOR have been identified in 29% of benign tumors from 13 patients from four multigenerational CYLD cutaneous syndrome families (510).

The thick hyaline band surrounding the tumor islands of cylindroma is composed mainly of an amorphous substance identical to the subepidermal lamina densa. It is connected with the tumor cells by half-desmosomes. Enmeshed in it are aggregated anchoring fibrils and thin collagen fibrils (13). This thick hyaline membrane and also the particles of hyaline present between the cells of the tumor islands react positively to staining with antibodies against type IV collagen and laminin, analogous to the subepidermal lamina densa. This hyaline is synthesized by the tumor cells and is similar to the deposits of basement membrane protein demonstrated in hyalinosis cutis et mucosae (511).

Principles of Management: Cylindromas are treated by surgical excisions. Electrodesiccation/curettage and cryotherapy have been used. Multiple tumors may require plastic surgery.

Malignant Cylindroma

Clinical Summary. Cylindromas rarely undergo malignant degeneration; however, a number of cases have been reported (512–518). In most of these patients, there were multiple cylindromas of the scalp, but in several cases, a single tumor was present (512–520). Usually, only one tumor was malignant, but in some cases, malignant progression had occurred in several tumors (521,522).

Death usually ensued through visceral metastases, but in a few patients, it occurred as a result of invasion of the skull with ensuing hemorrhage or meningitis.

Histopathology. Areas of malignant degeneration are characterized by islands of cells showing marked nuclear anaplasia and pleomorphism, many atypical mitotic figures, loss of the hyaline sheath, loss of palisading at the periphery, and invasion into the surrounding tissue.

Principles of Management: Surgical excision of the tumor is recommended. Mohs micrographic surgery has been used in some cases.

TUMORS WITH ECCRINE DIFFERENTIATION

Eccrine Nevus

Clinical Summary. Eccrine nevi are very rare. They may show a circumscribed area of hyperhidrosis (523,524), a solitary sweat-discharging pore (525), or papular lesions in a linear arrangement (526).

In the so-called eccrine angiomatous hamartoma, there may be one or several nodules (527) or a solitary large plaque (528). The lesions are generally present on an extremity at birth. Hyperhidrosis and/or pain may be apparent (529).

Histopathology. Eccrine nevi show an increase in the size of the eccrine coil or in both the size and the number of coils. In other cases, there is ductal hyperplasia consisting of thickening of the walls and dilation of the lumina. Some lesions also feature markedly increased mucin deposition in the dermis (530).

Eccrine angiomatous hamartomas usually lie in the deep dermis and contain increased numbers of eccrine structures and numerous capillary channels surrounding or intermingled with the eccrine structures (Figs. 30-68 and 30-69) (531). These hamartomas may also contain fatty tissue and pilar structures (532,533).

Principles of Management: Asymptomatic lesions require no treatment. Hyperhidrotic lesions may be treated with aluminum chloride, glycopyrrolate, botulinum toxin, or excision (534).

Eccrine Hidrocystoma

Clinical Summary. In this condition, solitary or multiple lesions may present on the face, usually on periorbital or malar skin (535). As in apocrine hidrocystoma, the lesion consists of a small, translucent, cystic nodule 1 to 3 mm in diameter, sometimes with a bluish hue. In some patients with numerous lesions, the number of cysts increases in warm weather (536). Graves disease has also been associated with multiple lesions

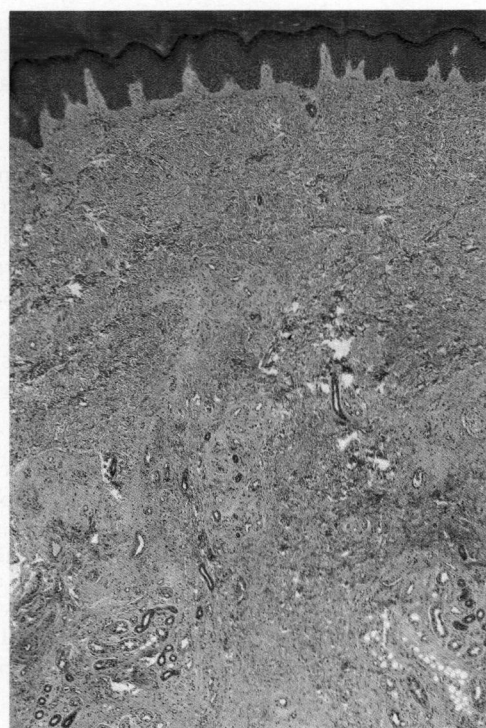

Figure 30-68 Eccrine angiomatous hamartoma. There is an increased number of eccrine structures and capillary channels in the deep dermis.

(537). The multiple variant may represent dilation and ectasia rather than a true neoplasm.

Histopathology. Eccrine hidrocystoma shows a single cystic cavity located in the dermis (Fig. 30-70). The cyst wall usually shows two layers of small, cuboidal epithelial cells (Fig. 30-71) (535). In some areas, only a single layer of flattened epithelial cells can be seen, their flattened nuclei extending parallel to the cyst wall. Small papillary projections extending into the cavity of the cyst are observed only rarely (537). Eccrine secretory tubules and ducts are often located below the cyst and in close approximation to it, and, on serial sections, one may find an eccrine duct leading into the cyst from below (505). However, typically no connection is found between the cyst and

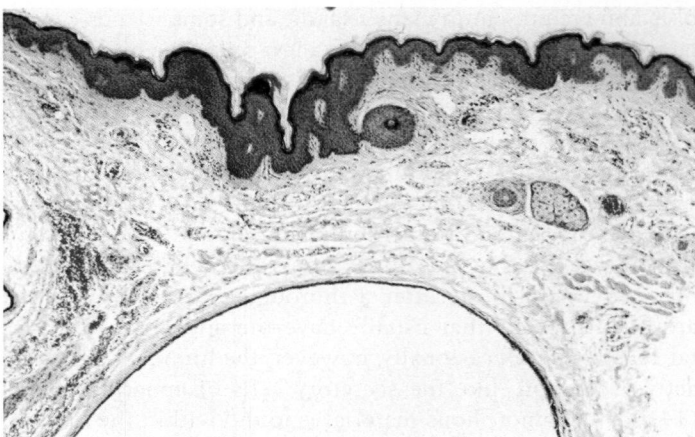

Figure 30-70 Eccrine hidrocystoma. A solitary cystic lesion is seen in the dermis.

the epidermis. Some controversy exists regarding the distinction between eccrine and apocrine hidrocystomas, with tumors previously thought to be eccrine hidrocystomas displaying apocrine features upon step sectioning (538), and most eyelid eccrine hidrocystomas displaying immunohistochemical staining more consistent with the apocrine secretory spiral (539).

Additional Studies. Electron microscopy of hidrocystomas has established that the cyst wall is composed of ductal cells, because the luminal cell membrane shows numerous microvilli and no secretory granules (540). Tonofilaments are seen in the luminal portion of the cells, and desmosomes connect the cells (541). It is likely that the obstruction of eccrine ducts leads to either temporary or permanent retention of sweat.

Differential Diagnosis. For a discussion of differentiation of eccrine from apocrine hidrocystoma, see page 1045.

Principles of Management: Eccrine hidrocystomas can be incised and drained; however, electrosurgical destruction of the cyst wall is often to prevent recurrence.

Syringoma

Clinical Summary. Based on histochemical and electron microscopic findings, syringoma represents an adenoma of intraepidermal eccrine ducts. It occurs predominantly in women at

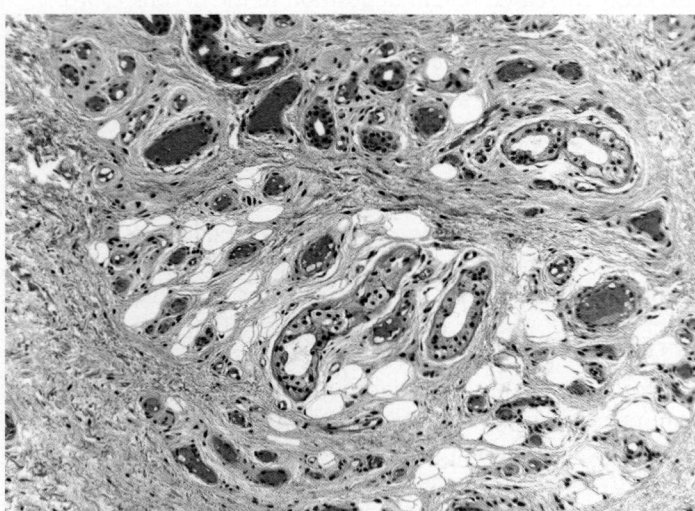

Figure 30-69 Eccrine angiomatous hamartoma. The eccrine coils and capillaries are associated with fatty tissue.

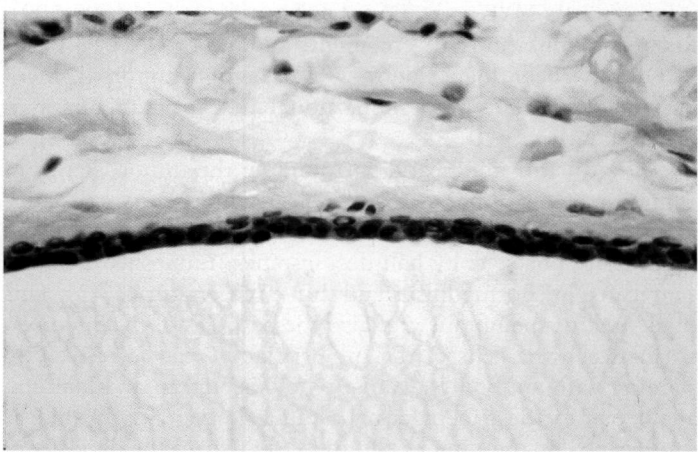

Figure 30-71 Eccrine hidrocystoma. The cyst is lined by a single layer of cuboidal epithelium.

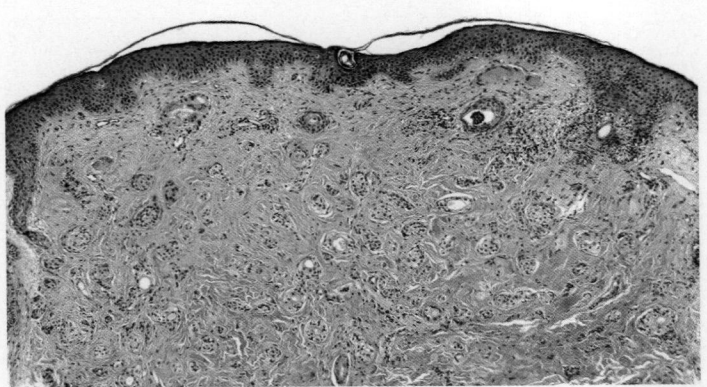

Figure 30-72 Syringoma. In the dermis, numerous tubular structures are embedded in a dense, collagenous stroma.

puberty or later in life. Although occasionally solitary, the lesions usually are multiple and may be present in great numbers. They are small, skin-colored, or slightly yellow, soft papules usually only 1 to 2 mm in diameter. In many patients, the lesions are limited to the lower eyelids. Other sites of predilection are the cheeks, thighs, axillae, abdomen, and vulva (542–545). In so-called eruptive hidradenoma or syringoma, the lesions arise in large numbers in successive crops on the anterior trunk of young persons (546), but more recent work has characterized some eruptive syringomas as likely reactive proliferations secondary to inflammation of the acrosyringium (547,548). A plaque-type variant can occur on the upper lip and may be clinically confused with a microcystic adnexal carcinoma (549). Infrequently, the lesions of syringoma show a unilateral, linear arrangement (550). In rare instances, occult syringomas of the scalp are associated with diffuse thinning of the hair (551) or with cicatricial alopecia.

Histopathology. Embedded in a fibrous stroma are numerous small ducts (Fig. 30-72), the walls of which are lined usually by two rows of epithelial cells (Fig. 30-73). In most instances, these cells are flat. Occasionally, the cells of the inner row appear vacuolated. The lumina of the ducts contain amorphous debris (Fig. 30-73). Some of the ducts possess small, comma-like tails

of epithelial cells, giving them the appearance of tadpoles. This "classic" feature, however, was only seen in 38.4% of syringomas in a large case series (n = 244) (552). In addition, there are solid strands of basophilic epithelial cells independent of the ducts.

Near the epidermis, there may be cystic ductal lumina filled with keratin and lined by cells containing keratohyalin granules (546). These keratin cysts resemble milia. Sometimes they rupture, producing a foreign-body reaction.

In rare instances, many of the tumor cells appear as clear cells secondary to glycogen accumulation (553). Typically, one observes only a few ductal structures and epithelial cords, with cell islands of irregular shape and size predominating. With the occasional exception of the peripheral cell layer, these islands are usually composed entirely of clear cells and have more cell layers than are generally seen in ordinary syringomas (Fig. 30-74) (554).

Additional Studies. Enzyme histochemical and electron microscopic studies have established syringoma as a tumor with differentiation toward intraepidermal eccrine sweat ducts (505,555). The enzyme pattern in the cells of syringoma shows a prevalence of eccrine enzymes such as succinic dehydrogenase, phosphorylase, and leucine aminopeptidase (556,557). In contrast to apocrine structures, syringomas react only weakly to lysosomal apocrine enzymes such as acid phosphatase and β-glucuronidase, except in a narrow, lysosome-rich periluminal zone (505,546). Sox10 and DOG1, which have been shown to have variable positivity in a variety of adnexal tumors, to date have been shown to be consistently negative in syringomas (558).

Electron microscopic examination reveals that the lumina of the ducts are lined not by secretory but by ductal cells showing numerous short microvilli, interconnecting desmosomes, a periluminal band of tonofilaments, and many lysosomes. In some tumor cells, intracytoplasmic cavities are formed by lysosomal action. The coalescence of several such intracytoplasmic cavities to form an intercellular lumen is the mode by which the ductal lumina are formed in syringoma; this is identical with the mode of formation of the embryonic and the regenerating intraepidermal eccrine ducts (546).

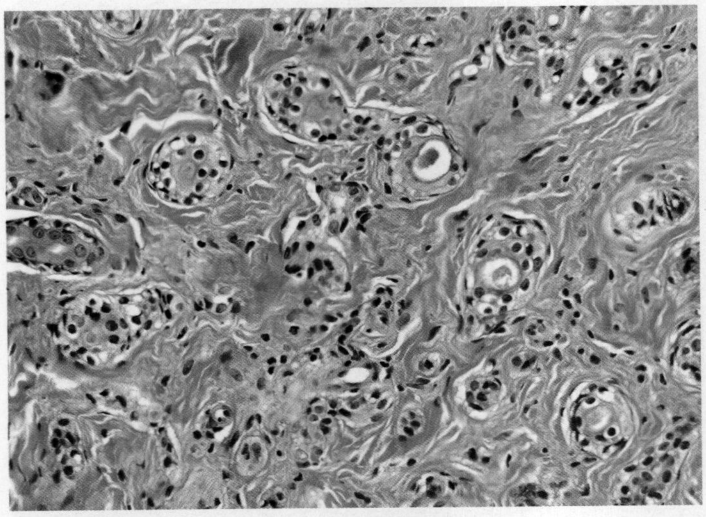

Figure 30-73 Syringoma. The walls of the ducts are predominantly lined by two rows of epithelial cells. Some ducts are lined by an eosinophilic cuticle, whereas others have comma-like tails. Granular eosinophilic material is seen in some ducts.

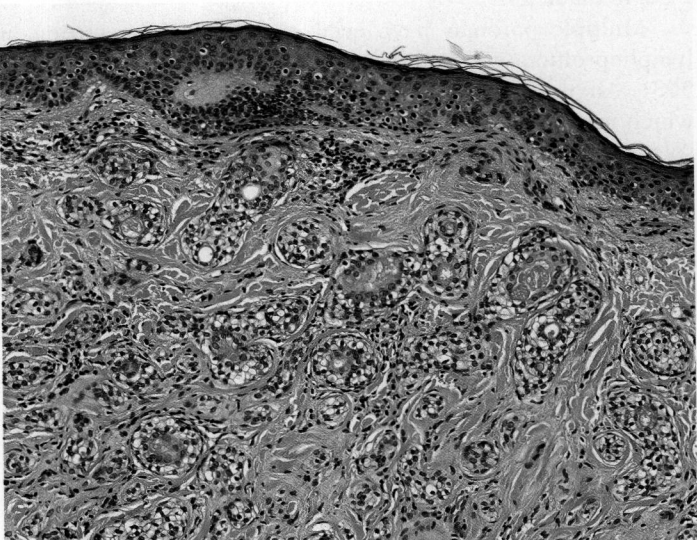

Figure 30-74 Clear cell syringoma. In this rare variant, the tumor islands consist largely of clear cells as a result of glycogen accumulation.

The finding of cystic ductal lumina filled with keratin near the epidermis is compatible with the natural keratinizing propensity of the luminal cells of the intraepidermal eccrine sweat duct toward the upper strata of the epidermis (546).

Differential Diagnosis. The solid strands of basophilic epithelial cells embedded in a fibrous stroma seen in some cases of syringoma have an appearance similar to that of the strands seen in fibrosing BCC. However, fibrosing BCC lacks ductal structures containing amorphous material. The horn cysts near the epidermis in syringoma resemble those occurring in trichoepithelioma, and their presence in syringoma was formerly misinterpreted as the occurrence of both types of tumors within the same lesion. Although trichoepithelioma (including desmoplastic trichoepithelioma) shows solid strands of basophilic epithelial cells and horn cysts, it lacks ductal structures. Syringoma can be distinguished from microcystic adnexal carcinoma by its smaller size, greater symmetry, superficial dermal location, lack of prominent horn cyst formation, and infrequent single-file strand formation. In addition, microcystic adnexal carcinoma, a much larger tumor than syringoma, extends into the subcutaneous tissue (559). The diagnosis of microcystic adnexal carcinoma should always be considered in any apparently syringomatous or trichoepitheliomatous neoplasm that extends to the base of a superficial biopsy.

Principles of Management: Syringoma is a benign lesion and does not require removal. For cosmetic purposes, lesions can be removed by excision or using a variety of ablative techniques including cryotherapy, laser ablation, trichloroacetic acid, and dermabrasion.

Eccrine Poroma

Clinical Summary. Initially described in 1956, eccrine poroma is a fairly common solitary tumor (560). In about two-thirds of the cases, it is found on the sole or the sides of the foot, occurring next in frequency on the hands and fingers (561). Eccrine poroma has also been observed in many other areas of the skin, such as the neck, chest, nose, and eyelid (562–565). Eccrine poroma generally arises in middle-aged persons. The tumor is most often asymptomatic, slightly raised or pedunculated, possesses a rather firm consistency, and usually measures less than 2 cm in diameter.

Multiple poromas have been observed in the setting of lymphoproliferative disorders and radiation exposure (566–568). An unusual clinical variant is *eccrine poromatosis*, in which more than 100 papules are observed on the palms and soles (569), with one report of widespread lesions in a diffuse distribution occurring in a patient with hidrotic ectodermal dysplasia (570).

Histopathology. In its typical form, eccrine poroma arises within the lower portion of the epidermis and it extends downward into the dermis as tumor masses that often consist of broad, anastomosing bands of epithelial cells (Fig. 30-75). The border between epidermis and tumor is readily apparent because of the distinctive appearance of the tumor cells. They are smaller than epidermal keratinocytes, with a uniform cuboidal appearance, a round, deeply basophilic nucleus, and intercellular bridges (Fig. 30-76). The lesional cells tend not to keratinize within the tumor, but they are able to keratinize on the surface of the tumor in instances in which the tumor has replaced the overlying epidermis. Although the border between tumor formations and

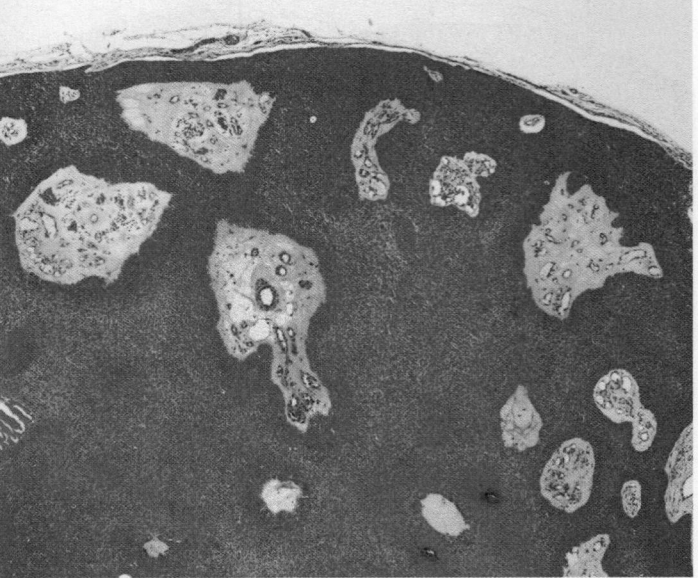

Figure 30-75 Eccrine poroma. The tumor consists of broad, anastomosing bands emanating from the epidermis.

the stroma is sharp, tumor cells located at the periphery show no palisading.

Characteristically, the tumor cells contain significant amounts of glycogen, which is associated with cytoplasmic clearing, usually in an uneven distribution (571). Melanocytes and melanin are often absent, although they may be present in tumors of individuals from various racial backgrounds (572–574).

In a majority of eccrine poromas, narrow ductal lumina and occasionally cystic spaces are found within the tumor bands (571). They are lined by an eosinophilic, PAS-positive, diastase-resistant cuticle similar to that lining eccrine sweat ducts.

Poromas can be situated entirely within the epidermis, where the lesion appears as a number of distinct cellular

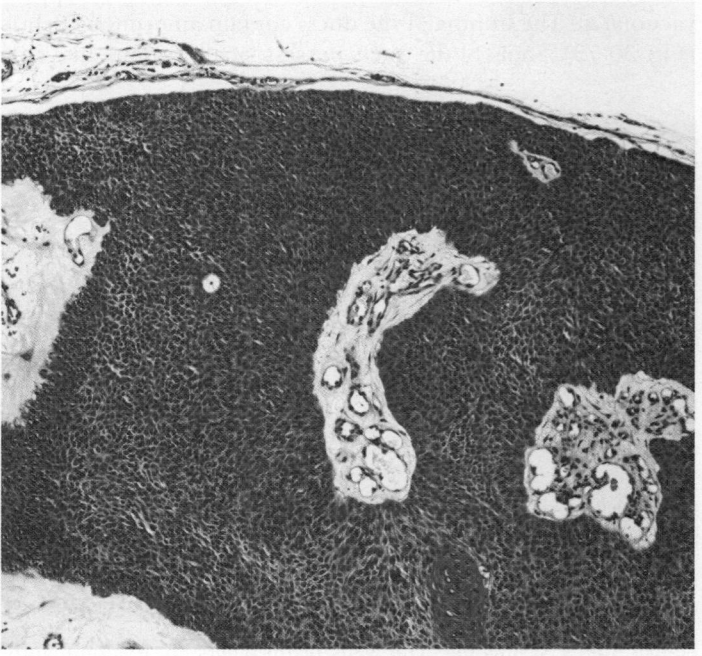

Figure 30-76 Eccrine poroma. The cells comprising the tumor have a uniformly small cuboidal appearance and are connected by intercellular bridges.

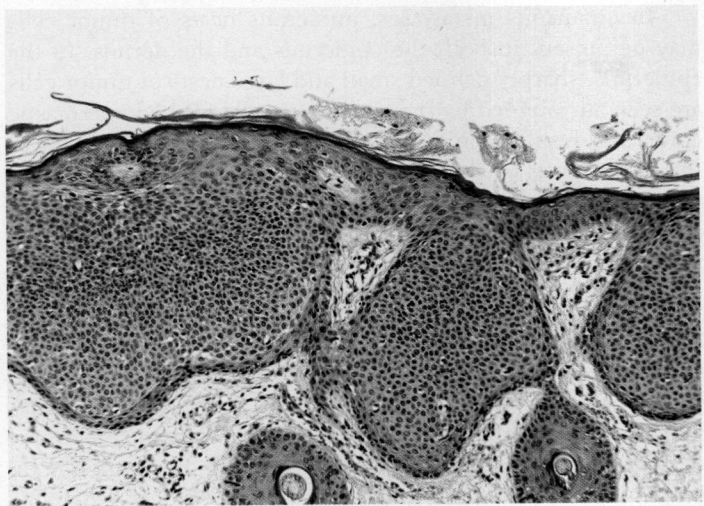

Figure 30-77 Hidroacanthoma simplex. There are discrete aggregates of poral cells in the epidermis, constituting one example of the so-called Borst–Jadassohn phenomenon of intraepithelial epitheliomas.

aggregates. Such intraepidermal poromas were first described under the designation *hidroacanthoma simplex*, about the same time at which poroma was first described (Fig. 30-77) (560,575). These lesions represent one example of the so-called Borst–Jadassohn phenomenon of intraepithelial epitheliomas. A few ductal lumina lined by an eosinophilic cuticle can often be seen within the intraepidermal islands (576). Eccrine poromas may also be located largely or entirely within the dermis, where they consist of variously shaped tumor islands containing ductal lumina; these lesions are referred to as *dermal duct tumors* (577).

Syringoacanthoma of Rahbari represents a clonal variant of eccrine poroma in which variously sized nests of small, deeply basophilic, ovoid, or cuboidal sweat duct–like cells are embedded within an acanthotic epidermis (578).

Additional Studies. Enzyme histochemical staining has shown the prevalence of eccrine enzymes in eccrine poromas, particularly phosphorylase and succinic dehydrogenase (579–581). Recurrent YAP1 translocations have been identified in eccrine poromas; translocation partners include NUTM1 and MAML2. YAP1 rearranged tumors may demonstrate loss of YAP1 C-terminus staining, and those harboring YAP1-NUTM1 fusions demonstrate NUT positivity by IHC (582,583).

Electron microscopic examination reveals that the tumor cells, except for the luminal cells, contain a moderate number of tonofilaments, are connected with each other by desmosomes, and appear identical to the cells that compose the outer layer of the intraepidermal eccrine duct (poral epithelial cells) (580). The luminal cells show a periluminal filamentous zone and, extending into the lumen, numerous tortuous microvilli coated with amorphous material that forms the eosinophilic cuticle seen by light microscopy. Some of the tumor cells may also exhibit features considered indicative of dermal duct differentiation (505,584).

Differential Diagnosis. Eccrine poroma must be differentiated from BCC and seborrheic keratosis. In BCC, the cells have no visible intercellular bridges, are more variable in size, often show peripheral palisading, and contain little or no glycogen. The cells of eccrine poroma greatly resemble the small basaloid

cells of seborrheic keratosis, especially because they possess clearly visible intercellular bridges. However, seborrheic keratoses have an even demarcation at their lower border; moreover, their cells have the potential to keratinize, and when they keratinize, they form pseudo–horn cysts. In addition, both BCC and seborrheic keratosis lack ductal lumina lined with an eosinophilic cuticle. Furthermore, these two types of tumors very rarely occur on the sole of the foot.

Principles of Management: Poromas are treated typically by complete excision.

Malignant Eccrine Poroma (Porocarcinoma)

Clinical Summary. Malignant eccrine poroma, or porocarcinoma, may arise *de novo* (585,586); however, it usually develops in a long-standing eccrine poroma (574,587–589). The tumor favors extremities, particularly legs and feet, usually in adults of either sex, but may occur on the face also. In some instances, the malignant eccrine poroma is localized, manifesting itself as a nodule, plaque, or ulcerated tumor (586,587,589,590); in other cases, there are multiple cutaneous metastases, which are usually associated with visceral metastases, resulting in death (574,588–590). The propensity to form multiple cutaneous metastases is an unusual feature of malignant eccrine poroma.

Histopathology. Malignant eccrine poroma may be seen associated with an eccrine poroma or hidroacanthoma simplex (587,589). In such cases, one observes areas composed of eccrine poroma cells with a benign appearance adjacent to areas of anaplastic cells. The malignant cells have large, hyperchromatic, irregularly shaped nuclei and may be multinucleated (Figs. 30-78 and 30-79) (589). Lesional cells are rich in glycogen (589).

In the primary tumor, the malignant cells may be limited to the epidermis or may extend into the dermis (Fig. 30-78). Some islands of tumor cells may lie free in the dermis. The epidermis often shows considerable acanthosis as a result of the proliferation of numerous well-defined tumor cell nests within it. Cystic

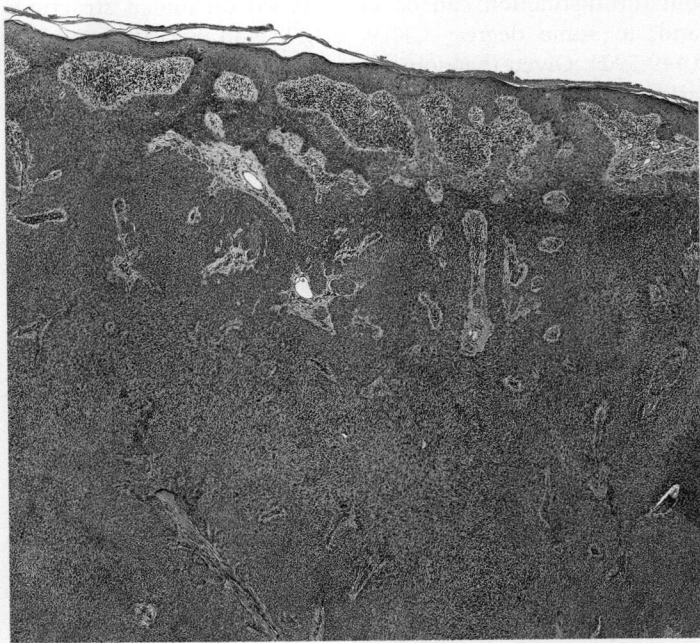

Figure 30-78 Porocarcinoma. Large islands of tumor cells are seen.

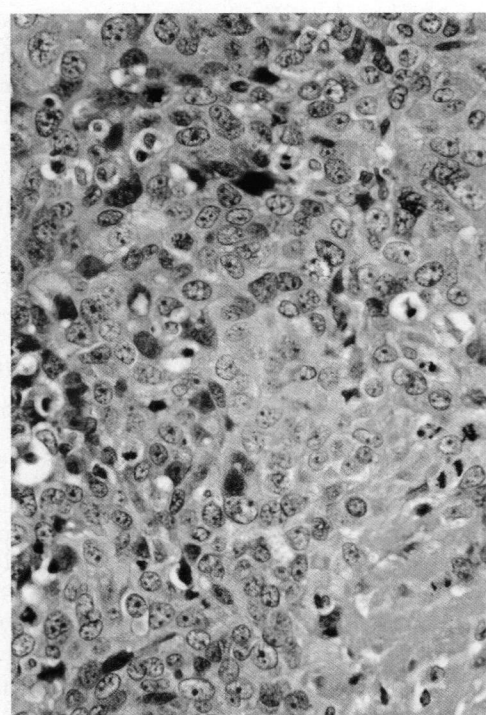

Figure 30-79 Porocarcinoma. Lesional cells demonstrate marked atypia, mitotic activity, and necrosis.

lumina may be seen within the epidermal and dermal tumor nests. The tumors are asymmetric, with cords and lobules of polygonal tumor cells, typically with a cribriform pattern. Nuclear atypia is evident, with frequent mitoses and necrosis (Fig. 30-79). Useful clues to eccrine differentiation include spiraling ductular structures, ducts lined by cuticular material, zones of cytoplasmic glycogenation, and also intraepidermal cells in discrete aggregates, often centered on acrosyringeal pores. The stroma may be fibrotic, hyalinized, highly myxoid, or frankly mucinous.

Differential diagnosis: Foci of squamous differentiation may resemble well-differentiated squamous cell carcinoma (591), but the distinction can be made based on ductal structures and, to some degree, CK19, c-KIT, and BerEP4 positivity (449,592). Given that some porocarcinomas display retraction artifact and focal BerEP4 positivity, the distinction from BCC can also be challenging with a partial biopsy (593). The same YAP1-NUTM1/MAML2 translocations identified in poromas are also seen in porocarcinomas, evidence of malignant transformation (582,583). Finally, porocarcinomas can also resemble metastatic adenocarcinoma, especially of mammary and lung origin (594). Ductal differentiation with the formation of a PAS-positive cuticle is evidence against a metastasis. P63 and D2-40 expression may also be helpful in differentiating primary adnexal tumors from metastases (234,269).

The term *ductal eccrine carcinoma* has been used to refer to tumors that may appear in the dermis as an infiltrative poroma (porocarcinoma) or as a moderately differentiated adenocarcinoma (595). About one-third of ductal eccrine carcinomas are fatal, usually because of distant metastasis (596).

Malignant eccrine poroma, analogous to its benign variant, can show a clonal ("intraepithelial epithelioma") pattern of its anaplastic acrosyringeal cells. The intraepidermal clones of such *malignant syringoacanthomas* may remain *in situ* or become invasive (578).

In cutaneous metastases, numerous nests of tumor cells may be present in both the epidermis and the dermis. In the epidermis, sharply defined small and large nests of tumor cells are seen surrounded by the squamous cells of the hyperplastic epidermis, resulting in a "pagetoid" pattern (574,585). Some of the tumor nests in the dermis are located within dilated lymphatic vessels, suggesting spread of the tumor in the lymphatics of the skin (585). From the lymphatics, the tumor cells invade the overlying epidermis because of the "epidermotropic" nature of the tumor cells.

Principles of Management: Porocarcinomas are treated by surgical excision, which is curative in about 80% of cases. Isolated reports of successful treatment with pembrolizumab; maxacalcitol and imiquimod; or paclitaxel, cetuximab, and radiotherapy have been reported (597–599). Sentinel lymph node biopsy is sometimes performed, but there are no data to demonstrate a positive impact on survival.

Eccrine Syringofibroadenoma

Clinical Summary. First described in 1963, this usually is a solitary, hyperkeratotic, nodular plaque, several centimeters in diameter, occurring on the extremities of elderly patients (600–602). Eccrine syringofibroadenoma and acrosyringeal nevi have many similarities, and some researchers consider them to be equivalent lesions (600–603). In one instance, a linear lesion has been reported to extend along a lower extremity (604). Eccrine syringofibroadenomatosis has been associated with inherited palmar-plantar keratodermas, including hidrotic ectodermal dysplasia and Schopf syndrome (605–608). Carcinomatous transformation of these lesions is rare but has been reported (609–611). Reactive syringofibroadenomatosis has also been reported occurring adjacent to squamous cell carcinomas and lesions of bullous pemphigoid, lichen planus, and trauma (612–615).

Histopathology. Slender, anastomosing epithelial cords of acrosyringeal cells—with or without formation of lumina—are embedded in a fibrovascular stroma (Figs. 30-80 and 30-81) (601). The net-like pattern of epithelial cells resembles that seen in fibroepithelioma (604). Lesions demonstrating prominent clear cell change have been described (611,616).

Additional Studies. Immunohistochemical studies and electron microscopy studies provide evidence for acrosyringeal differentiation in eccrine syringofibroadenomas (617–621).

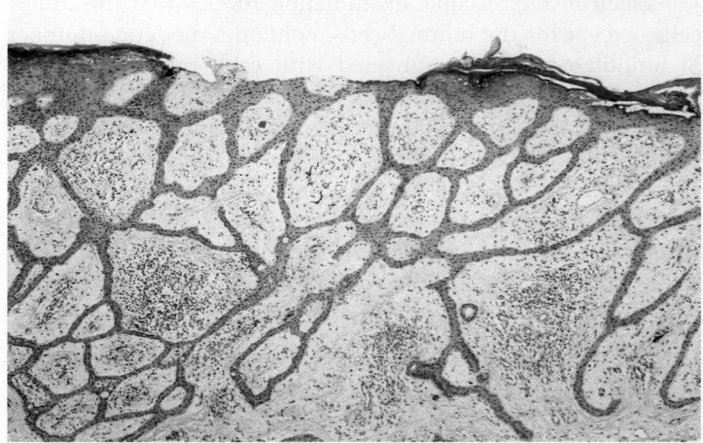

Figure 30-80 Eccrine syringofibroadenoma. The tumor is composed of thin, anastomosing epithelial cords associated with a fibrous stroma.

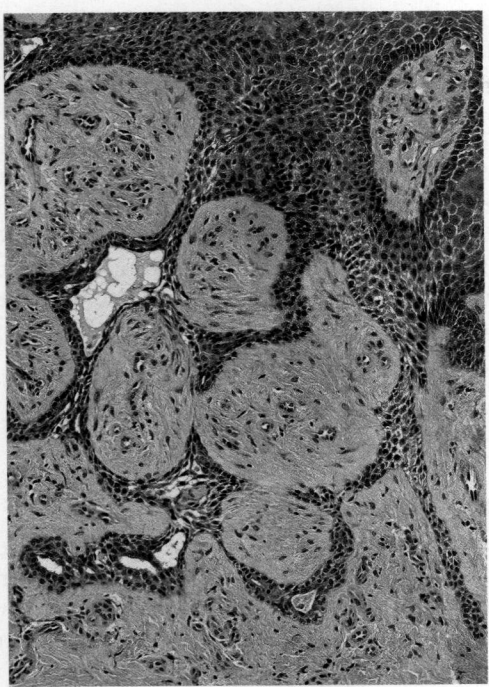

Figure 30-81 Eccrine syringofibroadenoma. The epithelial strands are comprised of mature acrosyringeal cells, which may form lumina and are embedded in a fibrovascular stroma.

Principles of Management: ESFAs have been treated with cryotherapy, radiotherapy, and flashlamp-pumped pulsed-dye lasers (622).

Mucinous Syringometaplasia

Clinical Summary. A rare condition first described in 1974, mucinous syringometaplasia occurs as a solitary lesion in two different forms: as a verrucous lesion in an acral location on the sole of a foot or a finger and as a plaque resembling a BCC in a more central location (623–625). With pressure, serous fluid can often be expressed (623).

Histopathology. An invagination lined by squamous epithelium extends into the dermis. One or several eccrine ducts lead into the invagination. They are lined in part by mucin-laden goblet cells (623). In addition, there may be mucinous metaplasia in the underlying eccrine coils (625,626). CEA and EMA may stain the luminal surfaces of the cells, and the goblet cells may stain with CAM 5.2 (627). The epithelial mucin is PAS positive and Alcian blue reactive, suggesting that it is sialomucin.

Principles of Management: Mucinous syringometaplasia is treated by complete excision.

Spiradenoma

Clinical Summary. Spiradenomas usually occur as solitary intradermal nodules measuring 1 to 2 cm in diameter. Occasionally, there are several lesions, and, rarely, there are numerous small nodules in a zosteriform pattern or large nodules, up to 5 cm, in a linear arrangement (628–631). In most instances, spiradenomas arise in early adulthood. Lesions can arise in a variety of locations, and the nodules are often tender and occasionally painful.

Histopathology. The tumor may consist of one large, sharply demarcated lobule, but more commonly, there are several lobules located in the dermis without connections to the epidermis (Fig. 30-82). The lobules are evenly and sharply demarcated

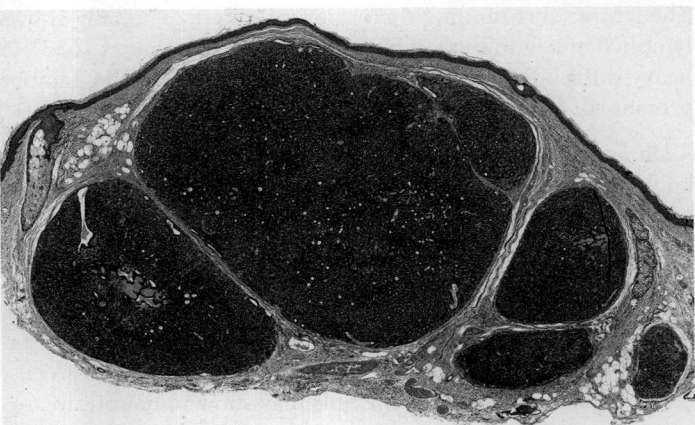

Figure 30-82 Eccrine spiradenoma. Well-circumscribed aggregates of blue tumor cells are seen in the dermis.

and may display a fibrous capsule (632). On low magnification, the tumor lobules often appear deeply basophilic because of the dense packing of nuclei.

On higher magnification, the epithelial cells within the tumor lobules are found to be arranged in intertwining cords (633,634). These cords may enclose small, irregularly shaped islands of edematous connective tissue (635). Two types of epithelial cells are present in the cords, both of which possess only scant amounts of cytoplasm (Fig. 30-83). The cells of the first type possess small, dark nuclei; they are generally located at the periphery of the cellular aggregates. The cells of the second type have large, pale nuclei; they are located in the center of the aggregates and may be arranged partially around small lumina observed in about half of the tumors (632). The lumina frequently contain small amounts of a granular, eosinophilic material that is PAS positive and diastase resistant (633). In the absence of lumina, the cells with pale nuclei may show a rosette arrangement. Glycogen is absent in the tumor cells or is present in insignificant amounts.

In some cases of spiradenoma, hyaline material is focally present in the stroma that surrounds the cords of tumor cells (Fig. 30-83). In addition, hyalin may be seen within some of the cords among the tumor cells as hyaline droplets (633).

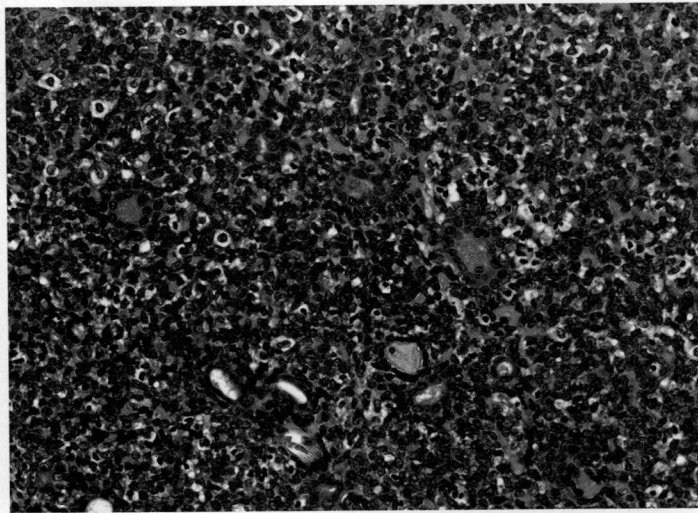

Figure 30-83 Eccrine spiradenoma. The epithelial cells are arranged in intertwining bands. Two types of cells can be seen. Cells with small, dark nuclei lie at the periphery of the bands; they represent undifferentiated cells. Cells with large, pale nuclei lie in the center of the bands and around small lumina. Collections of hyalinized material are seen.

The stroma surrounding the tumor lobules occasionally shows lymphedema with dilated blood vessels or lymphatics (633). A heavy diffuse lymphocytic infiltrate, mainly of T cells, may be present (636). Malignant progression can occur but is rare.

Additional Studies. Electron microscopic examination, similar to light microscopic examination, has shown two types of cells: undifferentiated basal cells with small, dark nuclei, and differentiating cells with large, pale nuclei. Most of the differentiating cells are immature ("indeterminate cells") and, in some tumors, may show no further differentiation (635). In most instances, however, there is some degree of differentiation toward intradermal eccrine ductal cells or toward eccrine secretory cells. Around the same lumen, some cells may show numerous microvilli and a well-developed periluminal zone of tonofilaments and thus resemble ductal cells, whereas other cells have only a few thin microvilli and thus resemble secretory cells (505,630). All secretory cells demonstrate features of serous cells (clear cells) (637). A few myoepithelial cells with typical myofilaments are present occasionally at the periphery of tubular structures (630).

Enzyme histochemical staining has revealed a prevalence of eccrine enzymes in spiradenoma, but the reactions are not as strong as in syringoma or eccrine poroma (630,635,638). A spiradenoma exhibits features of both the dermal duct and the secretory segment of the eccrine sweat gland, but the weakness and inconsistency of the enzyme histochemical reactions, the presence largely of undifferentiated and indeterminate cells, and the absence of dark mucous cells indicate a rather mild degree of differentiation. Immunohistochemical studies for cytokeratins demonstrate that the large, pale epithelial cells expressed keratins similar to those of luminal cells in the transitional portions between the secretory portions and the coiled ducts (639). The small, dark cells expressed cytokeratins similar to the basal cells in the transitional portions of the eccrine gland. Other findings, however, have cast doubt on the eccrine lineage of spiradenomas. Cylindromas, often classified as apocrine tumors, and spiradenomas appear to be closely related, and the same lesions may express features of both tumors (640). Some authors argue, based predominantly on CD200 positivity in spiradenomas and cylindromas, that both tumors are in fact of folliculosebaceous-apocrine unit origin, arising from the hair follicle bulge (641).

Spiradenomas and cylindromas also have very similar immunohistochemical and molecular profiles, and both can express apocrine markers on luminal cells (642). Spiradenomas also tend to arise in patients with Brooke–Spiegler syndrome, along with cylindromas and other tumors of folliculosebaceous and apocrine lineage (640). Several spiradenomas have also displayed clear decapitation secretion and immunohistochemical staining suggestive of apocrine differentiation (643). Recurrent, V1092A, somatic hotspot driver mutations in the α-kinase domain of ALPK1 have recently been identified in subsets of spiradenomas and their malignant counterparts and are mutually exclusive of CYLD mutations in these cases (644).

Principles of Management: The primary treatment for spiradenomas is complete excision.

Spiradenocarcinoma

Clinical Summary. Occasionally, malignant degeneration occurs in spiradenomas; usually, such lesions have been present for years (519,645,646). However, malignant transformation of spiradenomas has been reported in lesions with a clinical history as short as 7 months (646–648). Regional lymph node and distant metastases can occur (647,649,650). Notable clinical features may include pain and a history of enlargement in a previously stable lesion.

Histopathology. In malignant lesions, two distinct components typically are seen: benign eccrine spiradenoma and carcinomatous regions associated with areas of transitions (647,649). However, lesions consisting of well-demarcated zones of spiradenoma and spiradenocarcinoma have also been described (647). The carcinomatous lesion may display ductal formation, squamous differentiation, sarcomatous change, or no evidence of differentiation (647,649,651–655). Although mitoses may be seen in benign eccrine spiradenomas, malignant spiradenomas usually show a high mitotic rate (Fig. 30-84) (647,649). Other histologic features indicative of malignancy include the loss of two cell populations, increased nuclear-to-cytoplasmic ratio, hyperchromasia (Fig. 30-84) (647), and invasion into native tissue beyond the tumor stroma. Because the malignant changes may be focal in a benign spiradenoma, the malignancy may be missed if the specimen is inadequately sampled (656).

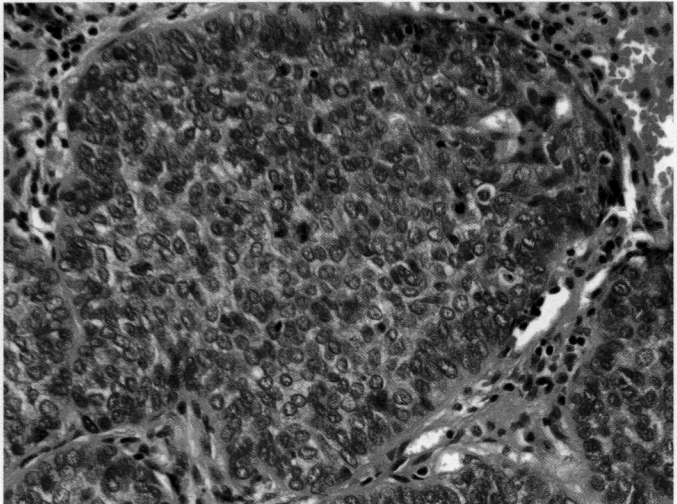
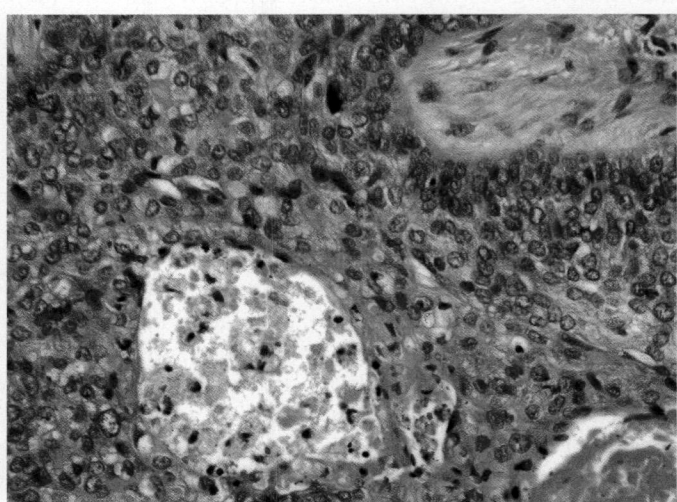

Figure 30-84 A, B: Spiradenocarcinoma. Lesional cells demonstrate marked atypia with a predominance of larger atypical cells. Cellular necrosis and mitotic activity are seen.

Principles of Management: The primary treatment for spiradenocarcinoma is complete excision. Metastasis can manifest years after complete removal (647).

Papillary Eccrine Adenoma

Clinical Summary. Papillary eccrine adenoma is a benign tumor that exhibits prominent eccrine differentiation and architectural features similar to tubular apocrine adenoma. First described in 1977, it occurs most commonly on the distal portions of the extremities as a small, solitary nodule (657).

Histopathology. As in tubular apocrine adenoma, the tumor comprises a well-circumscribed, symmetric collection of dilated, occasionally branching tubular structures lined by two layers of epithelial cells (Figs. 30-85 and 30-86). Papillary projections extend into the lumina (657). The ducts may contain amorphous eosinophilic material (Fig. 30-86) (658). However, evidence of decapitation secretion is lacking (659). Small microcysts representing dilated ducts may be present (659–662). The low-power impression may suggest a benign breast lesion, such as intraductal hyperplasia, especially when—as is characteristic—the tumor is located within the superficial and deep dermis and is not continuous with the overlying epidermis. Amorphous and granular eosinophilic secretions are present in many of the ducts, and occasionally there are small, keratin-filled cysts. Adenomatous

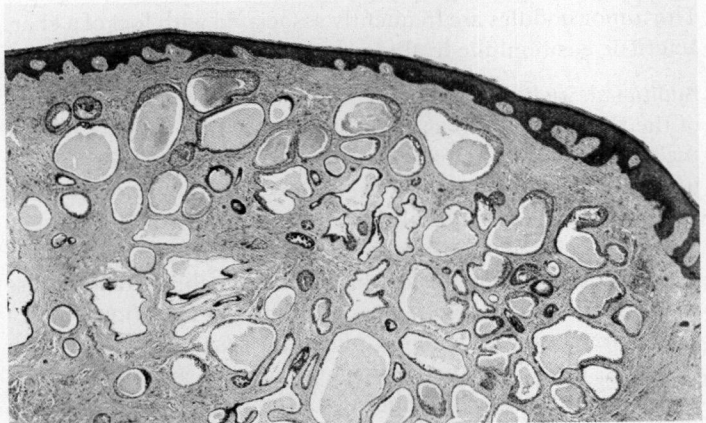

Figure 30-85 Papillary eccrine adenoma. The tumor is well circumscribed and symmetric and consists of dilated, occasionally branching tubular structures.

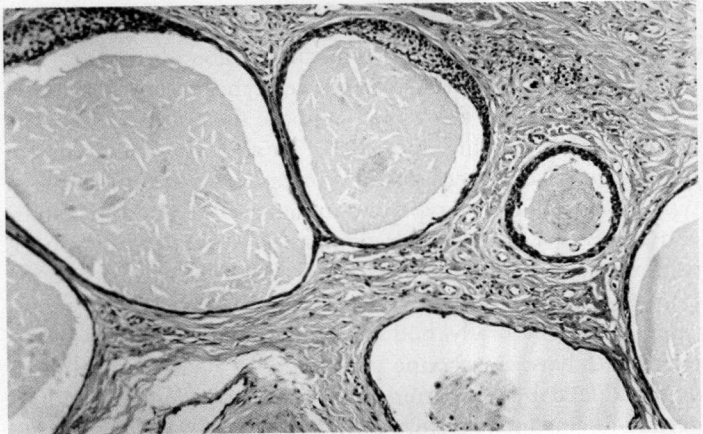

Figure 30-86 Papillary eccrine adenoma. The dilated tubular structures are lined by two layers of cells and contain amorphous eosinophilic material.

regions present variably spaced ducts and glands lined by one to several layers of cuboidal epithelium. The presence of a dense fibrovascular stromal tissue distinguishes this lesion from dermal endometriosis, which has a more cellular stroma. The tumor may recur locally but does not metastasize systemically.

Additional Studies. The amylophosphorylase reaction indicates that eccrine differentiation is prominent, but the reaction with acid phosphatase—an apocrine enzyme—shows practically no staining in the tumor (659). Immunoreactivity for S100 protein, carcinoembryonic antigen (CEA) and EMA is typically present, consistent with differentiation toward the secretory epithelium of sweat glands (658,661,662). Recurrent BRAFV600E mutations have been recently identified, as well (475).

Differential Diagnosis: Digital papillary adenocarcinomas can often be distinguished from eccrine papillary adenomas based on their greater cellularity and their cystic and nodular architecture, but some digital papillary adenocarcinomas may lack cytologic atypia.

Principles of Management: The primary treatment for papillary eccrine adenoma is complete excision.

Nodular Hidradenoma

Clinical Summary. Nodular hidradenoma is a fairly common cutaneous neoplasm that has been referred to as *clear cell myoepithelioma, clear cell hidradenoma, eccrine sweat gland adenoma of the clear cell type, solid cystic hidradenoma,* and *eccrine acrospiroma* (638,663–666). Nodular hidradenoma can arise in a variety of anatomic sites.

Nodular hidradenoma exhibits eccrine differentiation based on its enzyme histochemical and electron microscopic features (667). The tumor is usually solitary; however, on rare occasions, multiple lesions have been reported (667). The tumors present as intradermal nodules and in most instances measure between 0.5 and 2.0 cm in diameter, although they may sometimes be larger. They are usually covered by intact skin, but some tumors show superficial ulceration and discharge serous material (665). Although clinically the tumor only rarely gives the impression of being cystic, gross examination of the specimen often reveals the presence of cysts (664,666).

Histopathology. The tumor is well circumscribed and may appear encapsulated. It is composed of epithelial lobules located in the dermis, which may extend into the subcutaneous fat. Within the lobulated masses, tubular lumina of various sizes are often present (Figs. 30-87 and 30-88). However, such lumina may be absent or few in number, so that step sectioning is needed to find them. The tubular lumina in some instances are branched. There are often cystic spaces, which may be of considerable size and contain a faintly eosinophilic, homogeneous material (Fig. 30-87) (665). The tubular lumina are lined by cuboidal ductal cells or by columnar secretory cells. Occasionally, the secretory cells show active secretion suggestive of decapitation secretion (664,667). The wide cystic spaces are only rarely lined by a single row of luminal cells; more frequently, they are bordered by tumor cells that show no particular orientation and occasionally show degenerative changes (664). This suggests that the cystic spaces may result from tumor cell degeneration.

In solid portions of the tumor, two types of cells can be recognized (664,665,668,669). The proportion of these two types of cells varies considerably from tumor to tumor. One cell type

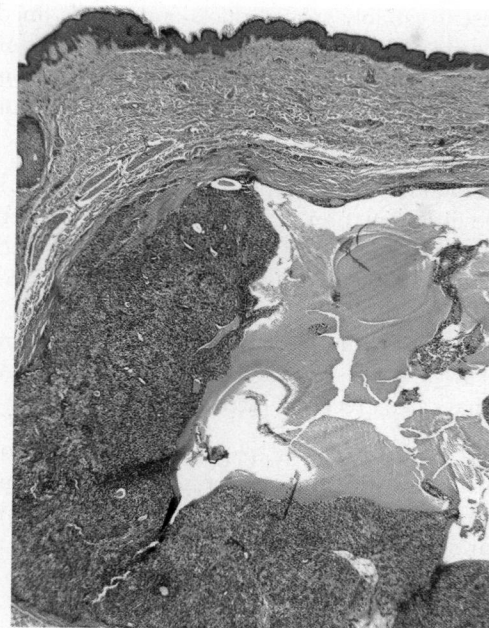

Figure 30-87 Nodular hidradenoma. Multiple lobules of lesional cells are present in the dermis. Focal cystic change is seen.

is polyhedral with a rounded nucleus and slightly basophilic cytoplasm. These cells may appear fusiform and show an elongated nucleus (Fig. 30-87). Another cell type is usually round and contains very clear cytoplasm, so the cell membrane is distinctly visible; the cell nucleus appears small and dark (Fig. 30-87). There are also cells with features of both varieties; these cells usually show a rather light, eosinophilic cytoplasm. The clear cells contain considerable amounts of glycogen, but they may show, in addition, significant amounts of PAS-positive, diastase-resistant material along their periphery (668). In some tumors, squamoid differentiation is seen, with the cells appearing large and polyhedral and showing eosinophilic cytoplasm (Fig. 30-88) (670). There even may be keratinizing cells with the formation of horn pearls (Fig. 30-88) (663,664). In other

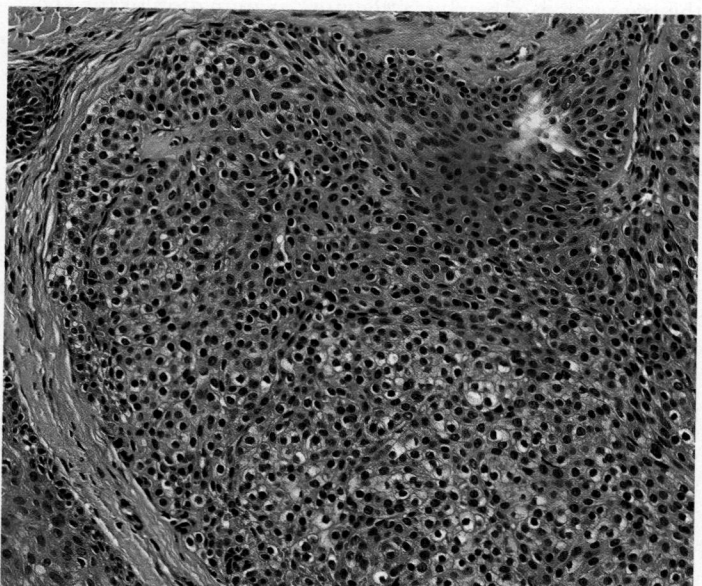

Figure 30-88 Nodular hidradenoma. The tumor comprises clear and polygonal cells, some of which appear fusiform. Foci of eosinophilic material and small ductal lumina are seen.

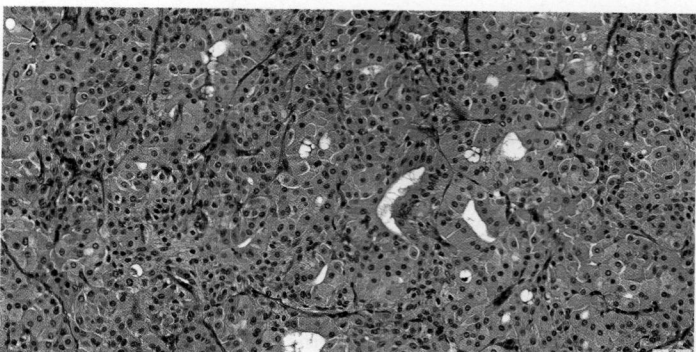

Figure 30-89 Nodular hidradenoma with oncocytic differentiation. Glands are lined by cells with a homogeneous eosinophilic cytoplasm, constituting "oncocytic" differentiation.

tumors, groups of squamous cells are arranged around small lumina that are lined with a well-defined eosinophilic cuticle and thus resemble the intraepidermal portion of the eccrine duct (666,668). Very rare variants with oncocytic differentiation have been reported (671) (Fig. 30-89), and mucinous cells may also be seen, sometimes forming glands.

In most cases, no connections of the tumor lobules with the surface epidermis are noted; however, in some instances, the tumor replaces the epidermis centrally and merges with the acanthotic epidermis at the periphery of the tumor (663,664,666) The tumor nodules are frequently associated with foci of a characteristic eosinophilic hyalinized stroma (Fig. 30-88).

Additional Studies. The polyhedral and fusiform cells, because of their location peripheral to the luminal cells and because of their shape, were originally regarded as cells exhibiting myoepithelial differentiation (664,667). However, the absence of alkaline phosphatase and, ultrastructurally, of myofilaments has disproved their relationship to myoepithelial cells.

Enzyme histochemical staining has established the presence in nodular hidradenoma of high concentrations of eccrine enzymes, particularly phosphorylase and respiratory enzymes, including succinic dehydrogenase and diphosphopyridine nucleotide diaphorase (669,671). Immunohistochemical reactivity for keratin, EMA, CEA, S100 protein, and vimentin is characteristic (672). A subset of (benign) clear cell hidradenomas has been found to express a t(11;19) *TORC1–MAML2* fusion protein also found in some salivary mucoepidermoid carcinomas (673).

Electron microscopy has demonstrated tonofilaments in the polyhedral and fusiform cells and an abundance of glycogen in the clear cells. These tumor cell types resemble those of eccrine poroma and those that compose the outer layers of the intraepidermal eccrine duct (669). In addition, four types of luminal cells can be recognized: a secretory type, dermal-ductal type, epidermal-ductal type, and immature type (669). It can be concluded that nodular hidradenoma shows differentiation toward intraepidermal and intradermal eccrine structures ranging from the poral epithelium to the secretory segment (663,669). Thus, ultrastructurally, nodular hidradenoma seems to be intermediate between eccrine poroma, with its largely intraepidermal ductal differentiation, and eccrine spiradenoma, with its dermal-ductal and secretory differentiation. From this point of view, the clear cells represent immature poral epithelial cells, and the horn-pearl formation can be regarded as the keratinization of poral epithelial cells.

Differential Diagnosis. Nodular hidradenoma shares with trichilemmoma the presence of clear cells rich in glycogen. Foci of keratinization may also be found in both. However, only nodular hidradenoma usually shows the presence of large cystic spaces and of tubular lumina, and only trichilemmoma shows peripheral palisading of its tumor cells. Spiradenomas may also present as dense dermal nodules; however, spiradenomas will lack large cystic spaces and will demonstrate hyalinized pink material, along with fewer ducts.

Although tumor nuclei may be hyperchromatic and there may be coarsely clumped chromatin, marked pleomorphism and frequent or atypical mitoses are not observed. If such changes are present, the tumor should be considered to have a potential for aggressive behavior. Zonal or diffuse patterns of necrosis also suggest malignancy, but the most important indicator of malignancy is an infiltrative, poorly circumscribed, and asymmetric perimeter.

Nodular hidradenomas may occasionally recur after local excision. Associated distortion and fibrosis may impede the diagnostic interpretation when the histology of the primary lesion is unknown or unavailable. Lesions that have frequent mitoses or nuclear atypia but lack clear evidence of asymmetric invasive growth may be termed atypical, and a re-excision to ensure their complete removal may be contemplated. There have been several cases of low-grade atypical hidradenomas that have metastasized to lymph nodes with subsequent indolent behavior following lymph node resection; the long-term natural history of these "benign metastases" is unknown (674).

Principles of Management: The primary treatment for nodular hidradenoma is complete excision.

Malignant Nodular Hidradenoma

Clinical Summary. Malignant nodular hidradenomas, also known as hidradenocarcinomas, are rare and usually malignant from their inception; however, malignant lesions may arise from benign nodular hidradenomas (674). Malignant nodular hidradenomas usually present as a solitary nodule on the head, trunk, or distal extremity. Most reported cases are in patients older than 50 years of age, though they may occur at any age. These lesions tend to metastasize, and they may cause death. Although there is insufficient evidence in the literature, the recurrence rate may be estimated at about 50% and distant metastases can occur to regional nodes, bone, viscera, and skin (674–676).

Histopathology. Whereas nodular hidradenomas are typically well-demarcated, malignant nodular hidradenomas are usually larger, asymmetric, and show an infiltrative growth pattern into the surrounding tissue (Fig. 30-90). In addition, there may be deep extension and angiolymphatic invasion (677). Mitoses are usually easily detected and some may be atypical. Tumor necrosis, areas of high cellularity, and focal or diffuse areas of marked cytologic atypia in which differentiated elements are unrecognizable are present in some examples (Fig. 30-91) (678). In these, the diagnosis of malignancy may be evident, but the recognition of adnexal origin and the precise subclassification may be problematic.

Here, the characteristic hyalinized stroma of hidradenomas may be of some assistance. In some instances, nuclear anaplasia may be only slight to moderate or even absent in both the primary tumor and the metastases (678). Nuclear anaplasia, if present, may be limited to the clear cells or found in both the polyhedral and the clear cells. Some tumors may contain other

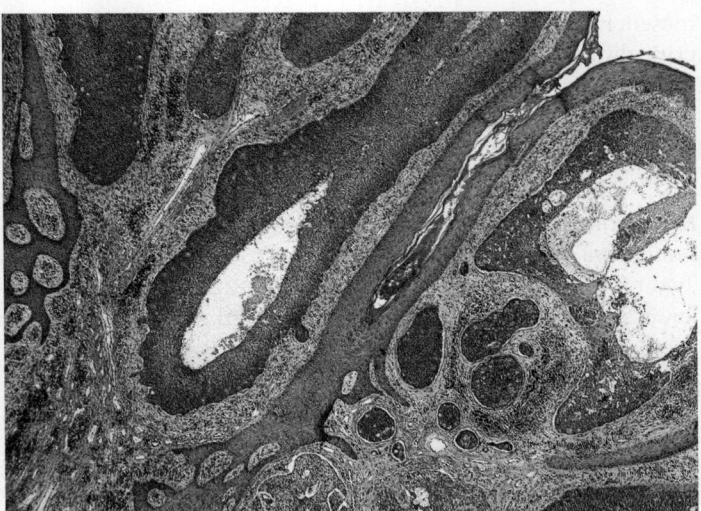

Figure 30-90 Hidradenocarcinoma. A large, cellular tumor with irregular, infiltrative borders is seen.

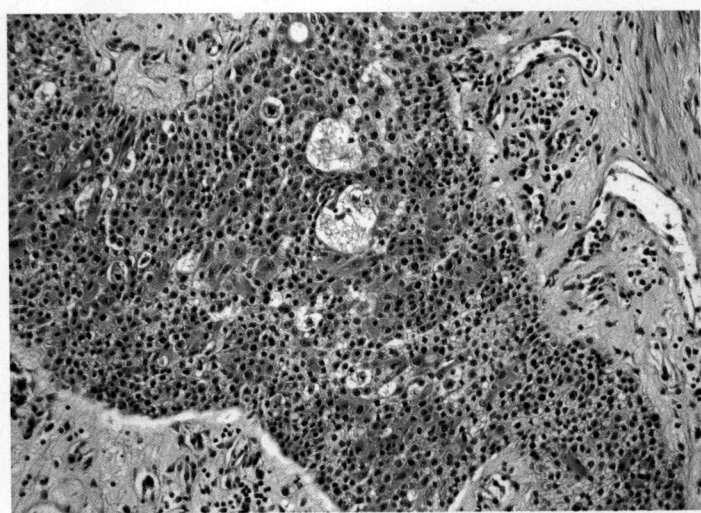

Figure 30-91 Hidradenocarcinoma. Sheets of atypical epithelial cells exhibit mitotic activity.

cell types, including epidermoid cells, mucinous cells, signet ring cells, and cells with high-grade sarcomatoid change (678). Hidradenocarcinomas typically stain with AE1/AE3, CK5, and CK6, with high Ki-67 expression helping to distinguish hidradenocarcinoma from atypical hidradenoma (679,680). Occasional tumors may demonstrate the (11;19) TORC1-MAML2 translocation seen in clear cell hidradenomas (678). Clear cell hidradenocarcinomas may be confused with metastatic clear cell carcinomas of the thyroid, lung, and kidney; TTF-1 may be helpful in differentiating hidradenocarcinoma from lung and thyroid carcinomas (681).

Principles of Management: The primary treatment for malignant nodular hidradenoma is radical surgical excision and selective lymph node dissection. The value of adjuvant radiotherapy and chemotherapy has not been confirmed (682).

Mixed Tumor of the Skin (Chondroid Syringoma)

Clinical Summary. The condition known by the term *chondroid syringoma*, introduced in 1961, is also known as *mixed tumor of the skin* because the tumor is epithelial, with associated mesenchymal changes, and may be of both eccrine and apocrine differentiation (683,684). Mixed tumors are firm intradermal or subcutaneous nodules. Although the overlying skin may be attached to the tumor, it otherwise appears normal. Mixed tumors occur most commonly on the head and neck (683,684). Their usual size is between 0.5 and 3.0 cm.

Histopathology. Histologically, this tumor can bear a marked resemblance to the pleomorphic adenoma of the salivary gland. Two types of mixed tumors can be recognized: one with tubular, cystic, partially branching lumina and the other with small, tubular lumina (683,684). The former type is much more common than the latter.

Chondroid syringoma with tubular, branching lumina shows marked variation in the size and shape of the tubular lumina; it also shows cystic dilation and branching (Figs. 30-92 and 30-93). Embedded in an abundant stroma, the tubular lumina are lined by two layers of epithelial cells: a luminal layer of cuboidal cells, and a peripheral layer of flattened cells (Fig. 30-93). Furthermore, there are large and small aggregates of epithelial cells without lumina, as well as single epithelial cells widely scattered through the stroma. It appears that cells from the peripheral cell layer of the tubular structures and from the solid aggregates proliferate into the stroma. In most instances, the tubular lumina contain small amounts of amorphous, eosinophilic material that is PAS positive and resistant to digestion with diastase. The tubular structures may be of both apocrine and eccrine differentiation (683–687).

The abundant stroma in many areas has a mucoid, faintly basophilic appearance and may change over time. Initially, delicate stellate, fibroblast-like cells and myoepithelial cells are suspended in the Alcian blue–positive, hyaluronidase-resistant myxoid stroma. These myoepithelial cells may be of varying morphologies, from clear cell to epithelioid to plasmacytoid (688,689). As a result of shrinkage of the mucoid substance, the fibroblasts and epithelial cells that are scattered through it are surrounded by a halo, so that they resemble the cells of cartilage (Fig. 30-93). The mucoid stroma stains with Alcian blue, mucicarmine, and aldehyde-fuchsin. The Alcian blue material

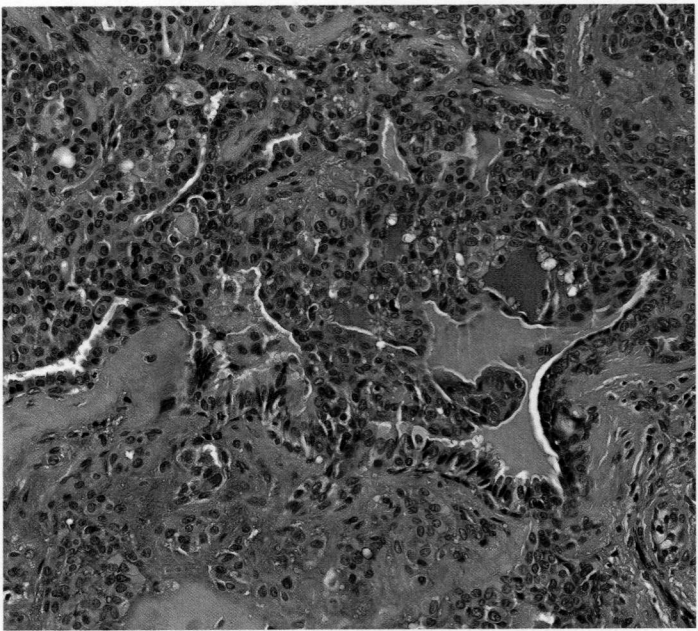

Figure 30-93 Chondroid syringoma. The tubular lumina are lined by two layers of cells: a luminal layer of cuboidal cells and a peripheral layer of flattened cells. Cells in the mucoid stroma have the appearance of chondrocytes.

is not appreciably decreased by predigestion with hyaluronidase (683). Furthermore, on staining with toluidine blue or the Giemsa stain, there is distinct metachromasia. Therefore, it can be concluded that the mucin consists largely of sulfated acid mucopolysaccharides or chondroitin sulfate. The stroma is histochemically similar to normal cartilage (683). In some lesions, there is complete synthesis of solid hyaline cartilage populated by cells in lacunae showing ultrastructural features of true chondrocytes and S100 positivity, with calcification and true bone formation as well (690–692). In a few areas, the stroma may appear homogeneous and eosinophilic, like hyaline, and is then PAS positive and diastase resistant (683,686). Stromal cells may acquire cytoplasmic lipid, resulting in a scattering of mature signet ring fat cells within the myxoid background. Mixed tumors of apocrine lineage may demonstrate foci of varied folliculosebaceous differentiation, ranging from infundibulocystic cells to follicular germ cells to sebocytes (689).

Chondroid syringoma with small, tubular lumina shows numerous small ducts, as well as small groups of epithelial cells and solitary epithelial cells scattered through a mucoid stroma (Fig. 30-94). The tubular lumina usually are lined by a single layer of flat epithelial cells, from which small, comma-like proliferations often extend into the stroma, resembling a syringoma (Fig. 30-95) (684). The mucoid stroma contains acid mucopolysaccharides that stain metachromatically with toluidine blue.

Additional Studies. By immunohistochemistry, the inner layer cells express cytokeratin, CEA, and EMA. The outer cell layer, when discernible, is positive for vimentin, S100 protein, neuron-specific enolase, calponin, and, occasionally, glial fibrillary acidic protein (687,693–696).

Electron microscopy demonstrates that both ductal and secretory lumina are present, with the secretory lumina lined by clear and dark cells as in eccrine secretory lumina (696). The myoepithelial cells composing the outer layer of the ductal

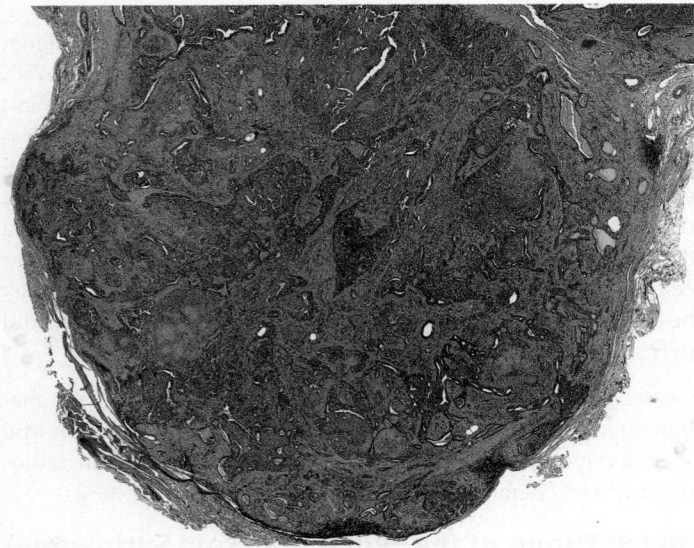

Figure 30-92 Chondroid syringoma. In the dermis, there is a nodular tumor comprised of branching tubular epithelial elements embedded in a basophilic stroma.

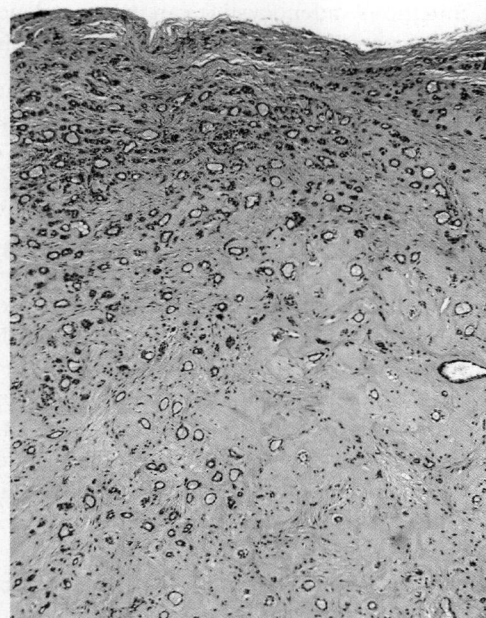

Figure 30-94 Chondroid syringoma, small tubular variant. In the dermis, there is a tumor comprised of nonbranching tubular epithelial elements embedded in an abundant stroma.

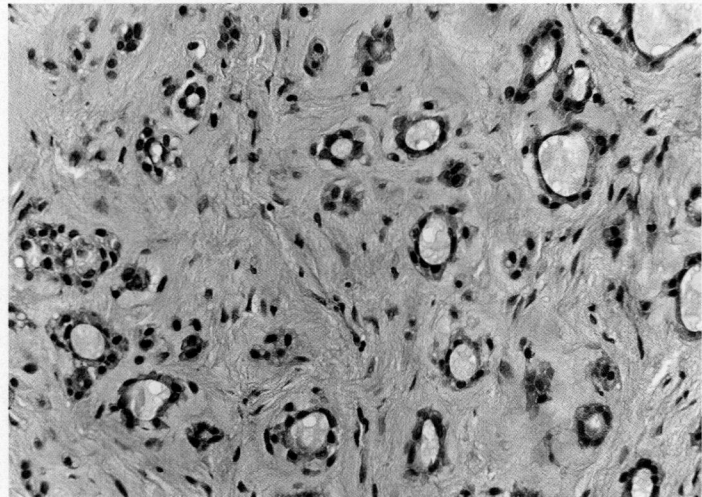

Figure 30-95 Chondroid syringoma, small tubular variant. The tubular lumina are lined by one or two layers of cells and are dispersed in the basophilic stroma.

structures contain numerous filaments and extend into the chondroid matrix, which they apparently produce (686).

Differential Diagnosis. Although most mixed tumors do not recur after surgical excision, seeding and regrowth of stromal and epithelial elements may occur, especially after an incomplete curettage. Lack of symmetry and an infiltrative pattern of growth are important features in distinguishing between benign mixed tumors and the rarely encountered malignant variant (697).

Principles of Management: The primary treatment for benign mixed tumor is complete excision.

Malignant Mixed Tumor (Malignant Chondroid Syringoma)

Clinical Summary. In most cases of malignant mixed tumor, anaplastic changes are present from the beginning (698). Rarely,

a mixed tumor of many years' duration suddenly undergoes malignant changes with widespread metastases (699,700). The degree of aggressive behavior varies with malignant chondroid syringomas. For example, there may be only a local recurrence, but some cases have shown bony invasion, regional lymph node metastases, or osseous metastasis (700). In several cases, fatal visceral metastases have occurred (699,701–703). When this tumor metastasizes, it generally does so as an adenocarcinoma, often losing the tendency to form chondroid stroma. These tumors occur in varied locations, including the extremities, trunk, and face.

Histopathology. Histologically, malignant chondroid syringoma is composed of epithelial structures with glandular differentiation and carcinomatous features embedded in a mucinous stroma with spindle mesenchymal cells and areas of chondroid differentiation (Figs. 30-96 to 30-98). Sheets of atypical cells

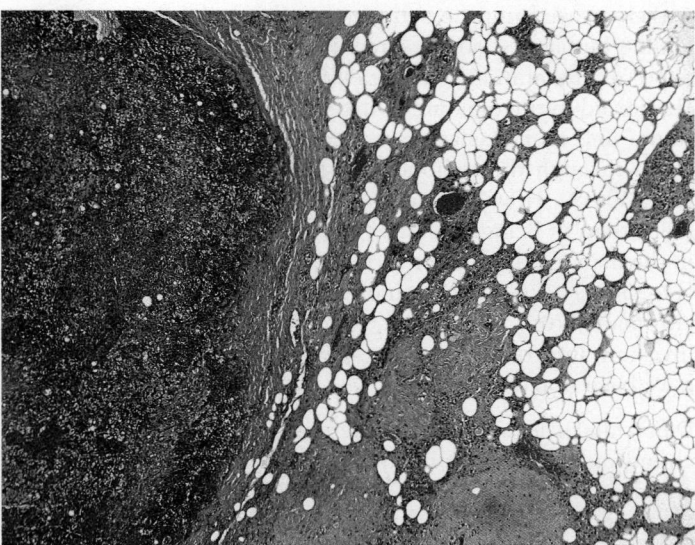

Figure 30-96 Malignant chondroid syringoma. An asymmetric cellular tumor is seen in the dermis and subcutis.

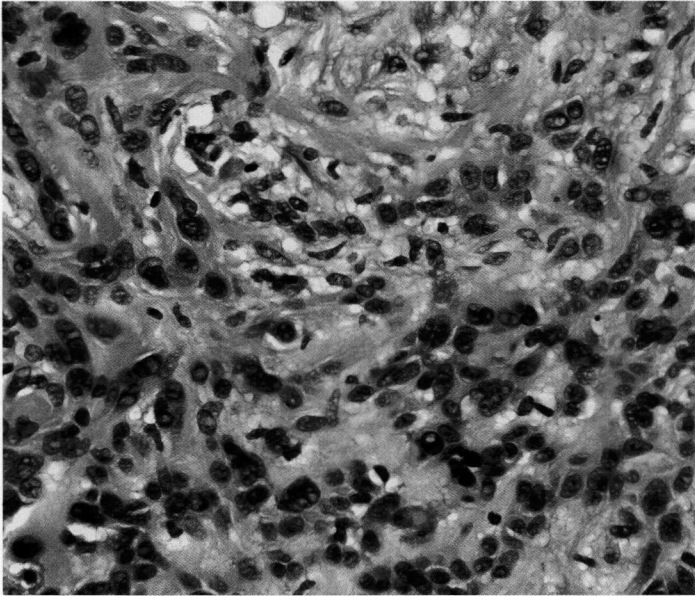

Figure 30-97 Malignant chondroid syringoma. Sheets of anaplastic cells are present.

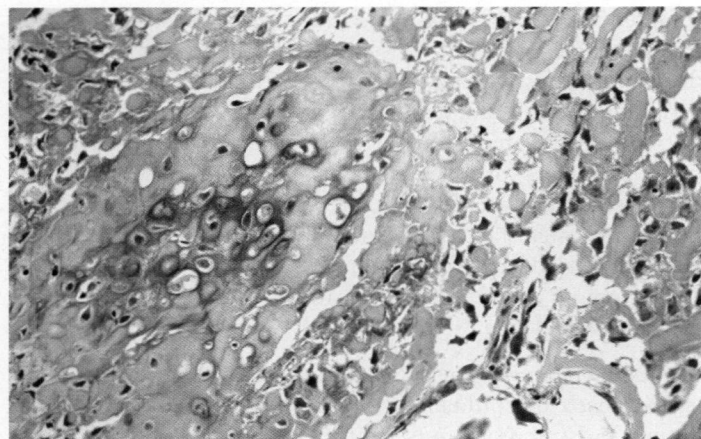

Figure 30-98 Malignant chondroid syringoma. Focally, cells embedded in a mucoid stroma reminiscent of chondroid syringoma are seen.

with increased mitotic activity can also be seen (Fig. 30-97). Unlike biphasic synovial sarcoma, in which both components express cytokeratins, only the epithelial structures of malignant chondroid syringoma are cytokeratin positive. The malignant tumor and its metastases are recognizable as chondroid syringoma through their chondroid stroma and tubular structures (Fig. 30-98). However, tubular differentiation is much less evident than in benign lesions (701). Most of the epithelial cells in the malignant tumor are arranged in irregular cords or sheets (Fig. 30-97) (704). The tumor cells appear atypical and hyperchromatic (705). In addition, an increased mitotic rate, vascular invasion, infiltration into the surrounding tissue, and necrosis have been noted (698).

Differential Diagnosis. The differential diagnosis of malignant chondroid syringomas includes mucinous carcinomas and adenoid cystic carcinomas. The former can be differentiated by the absence of ducts and thin septa between lakes of mucin, whereas the latter is distinguished by its cribriform appearance and frequent perineural invasion. Superficial biopsy has led to occasional misdiagnosis of malignant chondroid syringoma as BCC (706).

Principles of Management: The primary treatment for malignant mixed tumor is complete excision. These tumors have a significant incidence of metastasis.

CARCINOMAS OF APOCRINE AND ECCRINE GLANDS

Carcinomas exhibiting apocrine and eccrine differentiation can be classified in several different ways. One logical classification scheme distinguishes lesions based on whether the carcinoma may frequently evolve from a benign lesion. In reality, this group of tumors may derive either from a benign precursor through tumor progression or *de novo* as a malignant lesion. In this group are malignant cylindroma, malignant eccrine poroma, malignant eccrine spiradenoma, malignant nodular hidradenoma, and malignant chondroid syringoma, lesions that have already been discussed. The second group comprises apocrine and eccrine carcinomas that appear to have no benign precursor. In this group are carcinoma of apocrine glands, eccrine adenocarcinoma, syringoid eccrine carcinoma, microcystic adnexal

carcinoma, mucinous (adenocystic) carcinoma, adenoid cystic carcinoma, and aggressive digital papillary adenocarcinoma.

Principles of Management: These adnexal carcinomas are treated with complete excision. Mohs micrographic surgery has been used to treat these lesions and is useful in many cases.

CARCINOMAS OF APOCRINE GLANDS

Clinical Summary. Carcinomas of apocrine glands are rare tumors (480,707–711). These lesions occur primarily in the axillae and in other anatomic regions endowed with apocrine glands, including the anogenital region (480,708). Lesions can occur elsewhere on the skin (707,711). Apocrine carcinomas can also occur in the external auditory meatus, where ceruminous glands—which represent modified apocrine glands—are located (712,713). These tumors may involve the ear and preauricular skin (714).

Some cases of carcinoma of apocrine glands exhibit only local invasiveness, but other lesions metastasize to regional lymph nodes and may result in death from widespread metastases (480,708,711,715). In one population-based retrospective cohort study, the median survival was 51 months, with a disease-specific survival rate of 85% (715).

Histopathology. The histologic picture is that of an adenocarcinoma that may be well, moderately, or poorly differentiated.

In well-differentiated apocrine gland carcinomas, nuclear atypia and invasiveness are limited. Well-developed glandular lumina are present; these lumina may be cystic and show branching (480). The cytoplasm of the tumor cells is strongly eosinophilic. Evidence of decapitation secretion, typical of apocrine glands, is present, at least in some areas. In addition, the cytoplasm of the tumor cells contains PAS-positive, diastase-resistant granules and often contains iron-positive granules (480). Myoepithelial cells are seen rarely (711).

In moderately or poorly differentiated apocrine gland carcinomas, the apocrine histopathologic features may be difficult to assess, although even poorly differentiated tumors often demonstrate regions with prominent apocrine differentiation (480). The tumor may demonstrate ulceration and extension to the subcutis (716).

Additional Studies. Enzyme histochemical determinations are of value in establishing an apocrine genesis. Apocrine gland carcinomas show strong activity for apocrine enzymes—such as acid phosphatase, β-glucuronidase, and indoxyl acetate esterase—and low activity or absence of eccrine enzymes, such as phosphorylase and succinic dehydrogenase (707,711).

On immunohistochemical stains, tumor cells are almost always AR positive but exhibit mixed estrogen receptor and progesterone receptor positivity (716–718). Additionally, cells tend to be positive for CK 5/6 and GATA3, whereas they tend to be negative for adipophilin and HER2/neu (718). D2-40 staining is often positive, but unlike other primary adnexal tumors, cutaneous apocrine carcinomas may be p63 negative (375,718,719). CYFRA 21-1 has been proposed as a serum marker for disease and progression/recurrence (720).

Differential Diagnosis. Cutaneous apocrine carcinoma must be differentiated from metastatic apocrine carcinoma of the breast or primary apocrine carcinoma of the breast arising in ectopic breast tissue. Features that favor the diagnosis of a cutaneous apocrine carcinoma are the presence of neoplastic glands high in the dermis, normal apocrine glands near the tumor, and the presence of intracytoplasmic iron granules (480). Unlike cutaneous apocrine carcinomas, mammary apocrine carcinomas tend to be positive for adipophilin and may express strong positivity for mammaglobin and HER2/neu (718). One should note that both cutaneous and mammary apocrine carcinomas may be GATA3 and CK5/6 positive and p63 negative, creating a potential diagnostic pitfall (718,719).

Classic Type of Eccrine Adenocarcinoma

Clinical Summary. Few lesions of primary eccrine carcinoma possess a clinical appearance suggesting an eccrine malignancy. Although they may arise on the palms or on the soles, they more commonly arise elsewhere, particularly in the head and neck region (721–724). The classic type of eccrine gland adenocarcinoma has a high incidence of metastases. Of 68 patients followed for 5 years or more, 29 had regional lymph node metastases, and visceral metastases were present in 26 (722). More recent population-based studies demonstrate an 81% overall 5-year survival rate (725).

Histopathology. The histologic configuration in the classic type of eccrine gland adenocarcinoma varies from areas of fairly well-differentiated tubular structures to anaplastic cells in other areas, not recognizable by themselves as eccrine sweat gland structures (721–724). The tubular structures usually show only small lumina that are lined by either a single layer or a double layer of cells (721–724). In some areas, the lumina are lined by secretory cells, which appear large and vacuolated because of the presence of glycogen and which also often contain PAS-positive, diastase-resistant granules (726). Tumors frequently demonstrate a deep, infiltrative growth pattern and perineural invasion.

Additional Studies. Ductal cells may stain with EMA and CEA. A panel of immunohistochemical stains, including D2-40, p63, CK5/14/17, and mammoglobin may aid in differentiating eccrine carcinomas from metastatic breast carcinomas (727).

Differential Diagnosis. It is often difficult to differentiate the classic type of eccrine sweat gland carcinoma from a metastatic adenocarcinoma. Therefore, the diagnosis of metastatic adenocarcinoma should always be given serious consideration before a diagnosis of eccrine sweat gland carcinoma is decided on. Imaging studies may be of assistance in this regard.

A subset of eccrine carcinomas exhibit prominent squamoid differentiation, and may be misdiagnosed as squamous cell carcinomas (728,729). CD15 and CEA positivity may aid in the diagnosis (728).

Syringoid Eccrine Carcinoma

Clinical Summary. This tumor was originally referred to in 1969 as *basal cell tumor with eccrine differentiation* (730) and subsequently as *eccrine epithelioma* (731); the term *syringoid eccrine carcinoma* is preferable because the tumor differs from BCC in its cytologic and enzymatic patterns. It represents a relatively well-differentiated form of eccrine carcinoma (732). Although first reported as a deeply invasive and destructive tumor of the scalp (730), it also occurs in other locations, and metastases rarely occur (732).

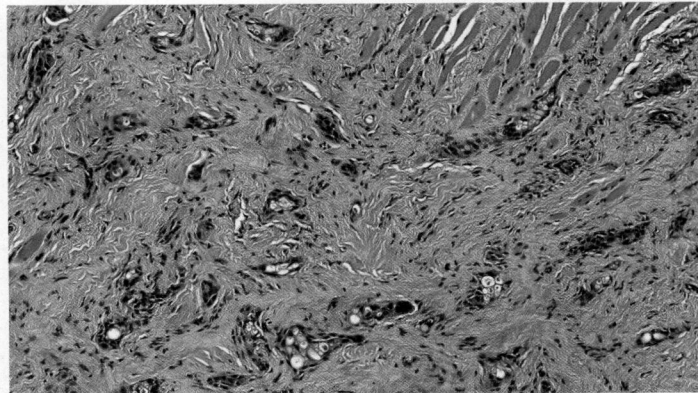

Figure 30-99 Syringoid eccrine carcinoma. An infiltrative tumor exhibiting ductal differentiation is identified.

Histopathology. Syringoid eccrine carcinoma resembles syringoma by showing ductal, cystic, and comma-like epithelial components and by containing eccrine enzymes such as phosphorylase and succinic dehydrogenase (Figs. 30-99 and 30-100) (730). It differs from syringoma by its cellularity, anaplasia, and deep infiltrative growth (Fig. 30-99). This uncommonly diagnosed tumor is probably related to the microcystic adnexal carcinoma. A clear cell variant of syringoid eccrine carcinoma has been described (733,734).

Additional Studies. Immunohistochemical analysis revealed that most tumor cells expressed simple epithelial cytokeratins (cytokeratins 7, 8, 18, 19), consistent with sweat gland secretory differentiation (735), along with EMA and CEA (736). Although the immunohistochemical pattern may resemble that of a primary cutaneous adenoid cystic carcinoma, syringoid eccrine carcinomas lack the mucinous stroma and cribriform architecture of these tumors.

Microcystic Adnexal Carcinoma

Clinical Summary. Microcystic adnexal carcinoma, or sclerosing sweat duct carcinoma, has been considered a sclerosing variant of ductal eccrine carcinoma (737,738). This tumor is most commonly seen on the skin of the upper lip, but occasionally also on the chin, nasolabial fold, or cheek (559,738). Rare cases of multiple primary microcystic adnexal carcinomas have been

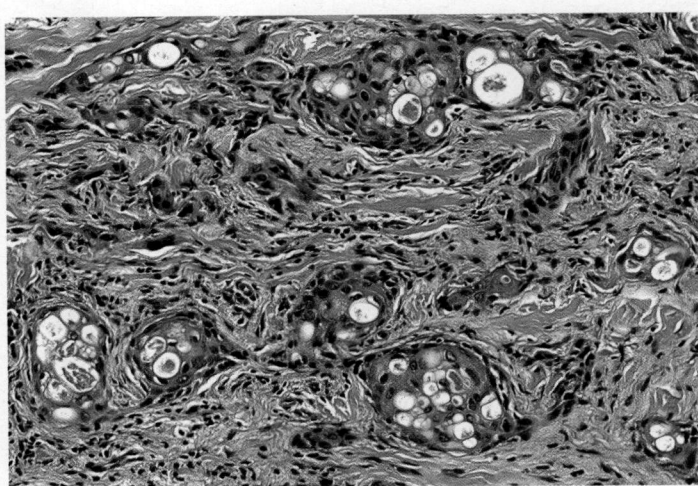

Figure 30-100 Syringoid eccrine carcinoma. Infiltrative epithelial elements resembling a syringoma are seen.

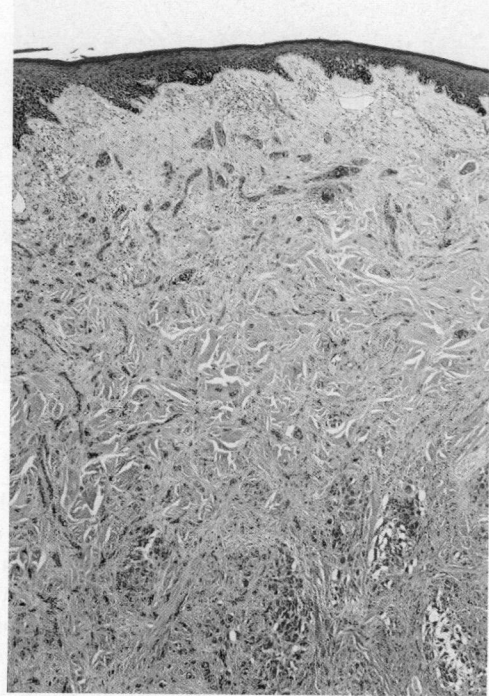

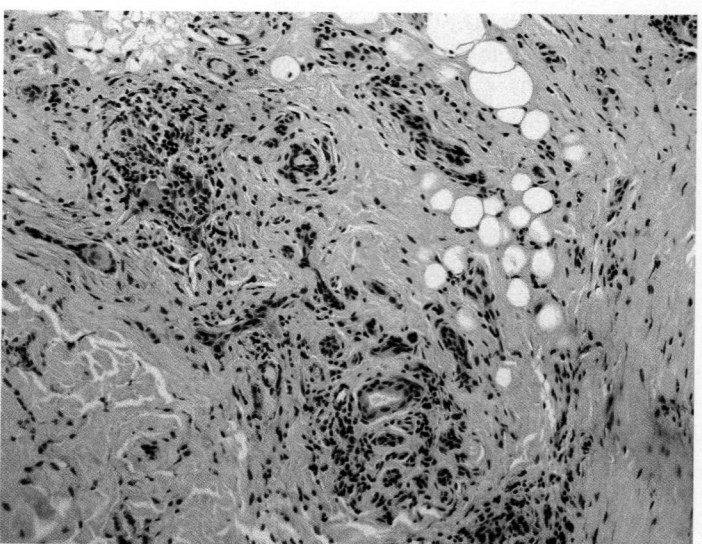

Figure 30-103 Microcystic adnexal carcinoma. In the deep dermis, cords of bland epithelial cells demonstrate focal ductal differentiation. A marked desmoplastic response is noted.

Figure 30-101 Microcystic adnexal carcinoma. There is a large, poorly circumscribed tumor comprised of epithelial cords invading deeply into the dermis.

reported (739). Microcystic adnexal carcinoma is a locally aggressive neoplasm that invades deeply. Local recurrence is common; however, metastases are quite rare, and patients appear to have a 5-year overall survival rate of 90% (725).

Histopathology. Microcystic adnexal carcinoma is a poorly circumscribed dermal tumor that may extend into the subcutis and skeletal muscle (Fig. 30-101). Continuity with the epidermis or follicular epithelium may be seen. Two components within a desmoplastic stroma may be evident. In some areas, basaloid keratinocytes are seen, some of which contain horn cysts and abortive hair follicles; in other areas, ducts and gland-like structures lined by a two-cell layer predominate (Figs. 30-102 and 30-103) (559). The tumor islands typically

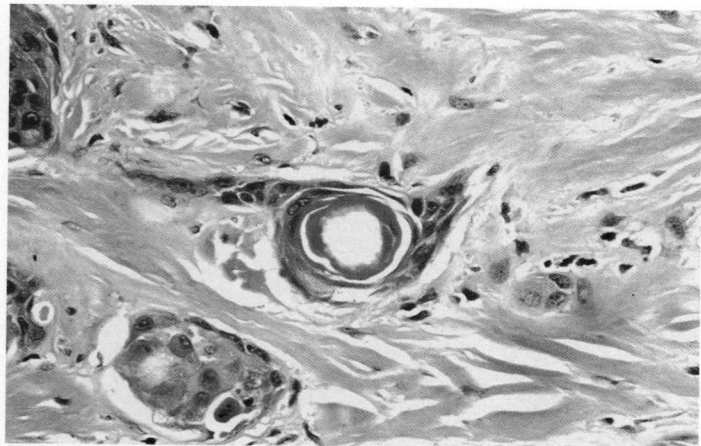

Figure 30-102 Microcystic adnexal carcinoma. Superficially, keratin-filled cystic glands are present and may be mistaken for the cysts of a trichoepithelioma, but the lesion invades deeply into the dermis.

reduce in size as the tumor extends deeper into the dermis. Cells with clear cytoplasm may be present, and sebaceous differentiation has been reported, raising the possibility of a folliculosebaceous origin (740,741). Cytologically, the cells are bland without significant atypia; mitoses are rare or absent. Perineural invasion may be seen, a feature that may account for the high recurrence rate, and the tumor cells may occasionally be surrounded by an eosinophilic infiltrate (742). Recently, a benign counterpart/precursor lesion called microcystic adnexal adenoma has been proposed by some authors, showing similar histopathologic findings but with a circumscribed border and, at most, mid-dermal depth of penetration (743).

Additional Studies. Immunoperoxidase staining for carcinoembryonic antigen stains the glandular structures but not the pilar structures (738). The presence of both pilar and eccrine structures allows differentiation from desmoplastic trichoepithelioma and syringoma. Lack of circumscription, deep dermal involvement, and perineural involvement all aid in diagnosis because the cytology mimics benign adnexal neoplasms. This diagnosis should always be considered and complete excision contemplated when a syringomatous or trichoepithelioma-like proliferation extends to the base of a biopsy, especially in an elderly patient. The Ln-γ 2 chain of laminin-332 has been proposed as a useful marker in differentiating between benign and malignant sclerosing adnexal neoplasms (119). Immunohistochemical studies have shown that CD23, CK15, and CK19 may help to distinguish microcytic adnexal carcinoma from desmoplastic trichoepithelioma (123,744). Morpheaform BCCs may also resemble microcystic adnexal carcinomas, but the presence of horn cysts and ducts and the absence of BerEP4 expression argue against a diagnosis of morpheaform BCC (123,745). Recent molecular studies show microcystic adnexal carcinomas to be molecularly heterogeneous tumors, most of which lack evidence of ultraviolet (UV) damage. Inactivated p53 or activated JAK/STAT signaling has been identified in a subset and may represent therapeutic targets (746).

Mucinous Eccrine Carcinoma

Clinical Summary. First described in 1971, mucinous eccrine carcinoma is a rather uncommon tumor occurring most often on the head and neck, especially on periorbital skin (747). It metastasizes to regional lymph nodes occasionally (748,749). Widespread metastases have been described only very rarely (750).

Histopathology. The histologic appearance of mucinous eccrine carcinoma is highly characteristic (751). The tumor is divided into numerous compartments by strands of fibrous tissue. In each compartment, abundant amounts of pale-staining mucin surround nests or cords of moderately anaplastic epithelial cells, some of which show a tubular lumen (Figs. 30-104 and 30-105) and myoepithelial cells (748,752). The mucin shows strongly positive reactions with both PAS and colloidal iron. The mucinous material is resistant to diastase and hyaluronidase but is sensitive to digestion with sialidase. The reaction with Alcian blue is positive at pH 2.5 but negative at pH 1.0 and pH 0.4, which indicates that the mucin is nonsulfated (753). It can be concluded that the mucin represents sialomucin, an epithelial mucin (748,752).

Additional Studies. Enzyme histochemical studies have revealed a prevalence of eccrine enzymes in these tumors (752). Electron microscopy has revealed two types of secretory cells in the tumor—dark and light—analogous to the two types normally encountered in eccrine coils. The sialomucin is secreted by the dark cells (754). Immunohistochemical results also suggest differentiation toward eccrine secretory coil (755). However, there have been several cases of mucinous carcinoma with decapitation secretion and secretory snouts, suggesting apocrine differentiation (747). Tumors usually stain with CK7, and occasionally exhibit ER, PR, and CK5/6 positivity (756).

Differential Diagnosis: It is important to differentiate this tumor from a metastatic mucinous adenocarcinoma, most commonly arising from the intestine or the breast (748). In both primary and metastatic mucinous adenocarcinoma, islands of tumor cells appear to be floating in lakes of mucin, but the tumor cells are more atypical in the metastatic type, and the atypical cells invade between collagen bundles at the margin of the nodule (757). Metastatic adenocarcinomas from the intestine are more likely to exhibit CK-20 positivity and a "dirty" necrosis, with nuclear debris, eosinophilic necrotic foci, and goblet cells (747). Given frequent CK7 and ER positivity, distinction from metastatic breast carcinoma can be very challenging, and exclusion of metastatic disease is often impossible by histology alone.

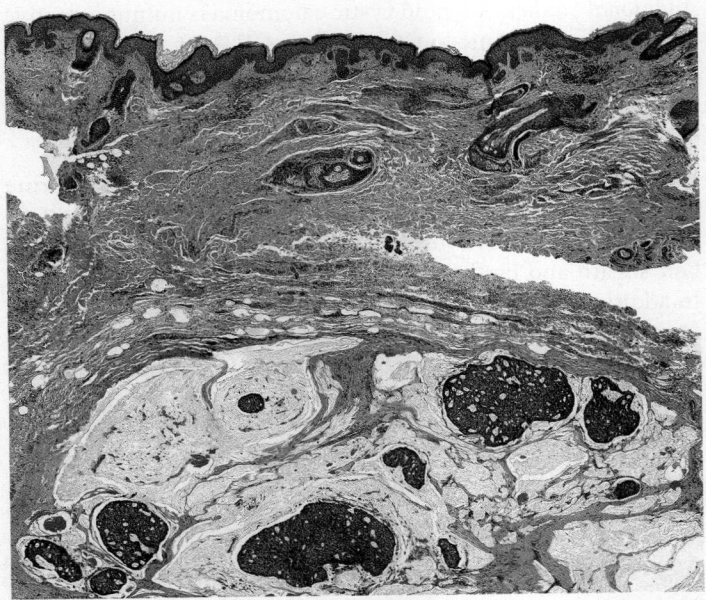

Figure 30-104 Mucinous eccrine adenocarcinoma. The tumor is divided into numerous compartments. In each compartment, abundant amounts of mucin surround small islets of tumor cells.

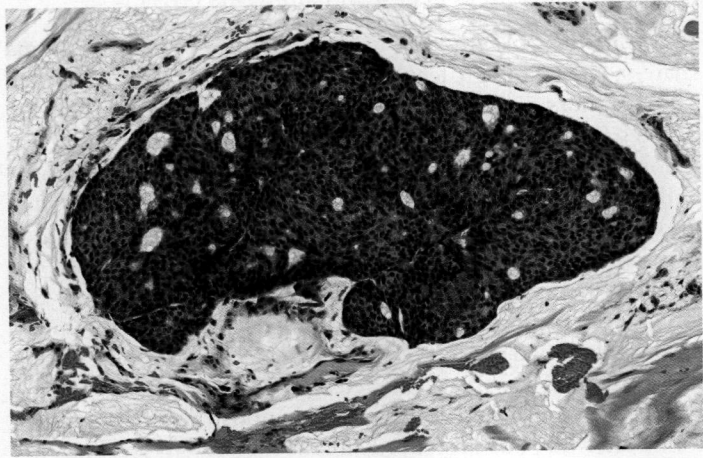

Figure 30-105 Mucinous eccrine adenocarcinoma. The islands of tumor cells show mild cytologic atypia and focal duct formation.

Endocrine Mucin-Producing Sweat Gland Carcinoma

Clinical Summary. A rare low-grade carcinoma usually occurring on periorbital skin, endocrine mucin-producing sweat gland carcinoma may be analogous to solid papillary carcinomas of the breast (758). It tends to occur in older women and often presents as a cyst or translucent nodule (759). There have been several reports of recurrence following incomplete surgical excision and one case with distant metastases (760–762).

Histopathology: These tumors are characterized by solid nodules with cystic and papillary areas. There are frequent fibrovascular bundles with surrounding pseudorosettes, and mucin can be found both within the cells and in the stroma. Cells are larger than those in eccrine ducts, with oval-to-round stippled nuclei, and may demonstrate peripheral palisading (759,763). These tumors may occur adjacent to cysts lined with atypical cells, perhaps providing evidence of an *in situ* component, and may also contain a component of "classic" mucinous carcinoma, with atypical cells floating in islands of mucin (759).

Additional Studies: Endocrine mucin-producing sweat gland carcinomas are at least focally positive for either synaptophysin or chromogranin and are often positive for neuron-specific enolase as well. They also stain with antibodies to estrogen or progesterone receptors, CK7, CAM 5.2, and EMA (759). A recent case series found diffuse IHC positivity for INSM1, BCL2, AR, RB1, and beta-catenin with focal positivity for MUC2, suggesting a conjunctival origin (764). The differential diagnosis includes hidradenomas, apocrine adenomas, malignant mixed tumors, and metastatic carcinoma, but partial biopsy of the cystic component may occasionally cause confusion with hidrocystoma (759,760,765).

Mucoepidermoid (Low-Grade Adenosquamous) Carcinoma

This tumor, which combines well-differentiated squamous and glandular epithelium, is histologically identical to that of salivary glands and may occur in the skin as a primary cutaneous malignancy (766–768) or as metastatic disease (769,770). Tumors are composed of a mixture of large, polygonal squamous cells, mucin-producing cells, and intermediate cells, with varying degrees of cystic architecture and cellular atypia. Partial or superficial biopsy may lead to confusion with benign cysts or mucinous syringometaplasia (770). Oncogenic CRTC1-MAML2 translocations resulting in p16-CDK4/6-RB pathway activity alterations have been identified in mucoepidermoid carcinomas (771).

Adenoid Cystic Carcinoma

Clinical Summary. This rare adnexal carcinoma was first described in 1975 (772). Metastases have been reported but are uncommon (773,774). Like its more aggressive counterpart in salivary and lacrimal glands, primary adenoid cystic carcinoma spreads in perineural spaces and therefore recurs in 20% to 46% of cases (773,775,776). It tends to occur on the head and neck and appears to be associated with a risk of subsequent hematologic malignancy (776).

Histopathology. Microscopic examination reveals lesions exhibiting an adenoid or cribriform pattern comprised of many small, epithelial islands (Fig. 30-106). Round spaces formed by malignant epithelial cells and containing amphophilic basement membrane–like material occur in the cribriform type and tubular variants (Fig. 30-107) (777). Through the accumulation of mucin, the adenoid spaces may be transformed into multiple cystic spaces lined by a flattened cuboidal epithelium. The adenoid and cystic spaces contain pale-staining mucin that in some cases is hyaluronidase sensitive but in others is resistant to hyaluronidase digestion and reacts with the Alcian blue stain at pH 2.5 and pH 0.5 (778,779). There is frequent perineural spread.

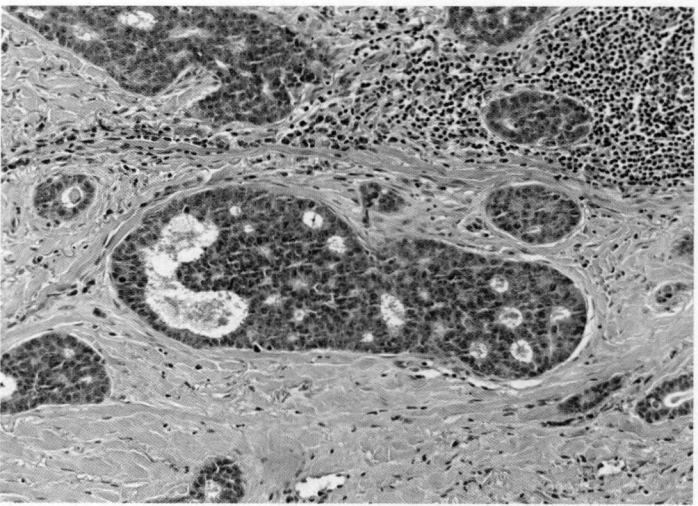

Figure 30-107 Adenoid cystic carcinoma of eccrine glands. Some epithelial islands demonstrate a cribriform pattern.

Additional Studies. Adenoid cystic carcinoma is immunoreactive for carcinoembryonic antigen, EMA, AE1/AE3, amylase, S100 protein, and CD117 (779,780). Seventy percent of adenoid cystic carcinoma exhibit translocations of MYBL1 and 90% demonstrate nuclear MYB staining (781,782).

Differential Diagnosis. Adenoid cystic carcinoma of eccrine glands must be distinguished from the adenoid type of BCC, from which it differs by lack of continuity with the epidermis or hair sheath and by the absence of peripheral palisading (778). In addition, the adenoid type of BCC shows negative reactions to carcinoembryonic antigen, amylase, and S100 protein (779). Cutaneous extension from a parotid tumor or scar recurrence should be ruled out in adjacent body sites. Adenoid cystic carcinomas may arise in the breast, lungs, and prostate. Rarely, cutaneous metastases from visceral tumors have been reported, and these are extremely difficult to differentiate from primary cutaneous tumors (774).

Aggressive Digital Papillary Adenocarcinoma

Clinical Summary. These tumors, originally described in 1987, occur on the fingers, toes, and adjacent skin of the palms and soles, especially in adult males, as a single, often cystic mass that rarely ulcerates but often invades soft tissue (783). Some lesions may present as persistent paronychia (784).

Histopathology. Aggressive digital papillary adenocarcinoma shares some histologic features with papillary eccrine adenoma. These tumors are usually cellular, dermal nodules with cystic cavities (Fig. 30-108). Characteristic histologic findings of this lesion include tubuloalveolar and ductal structures associated with papillary projections protruding into cystically dilated lumina (Figs. 30-109 and 30-110) (783). Macropapillae lined by atypical epithelial cells project into microcysts. These areas may merge with more cellular regions of moderately differentiated adenocarcinoma. Myoepithelial cells may be found around glandular structures even in aggressive tumors (784). p53 mutations have been characterized in several tumors (717). Overexpression of FGFR2 has been demonstrated by transcriptomic analyses, but overexpression at the protein level has not yet been definitively demonstrated by IHC (785,786). Mitotic activity and cytologic atypia are often present (Fig. 30-110).

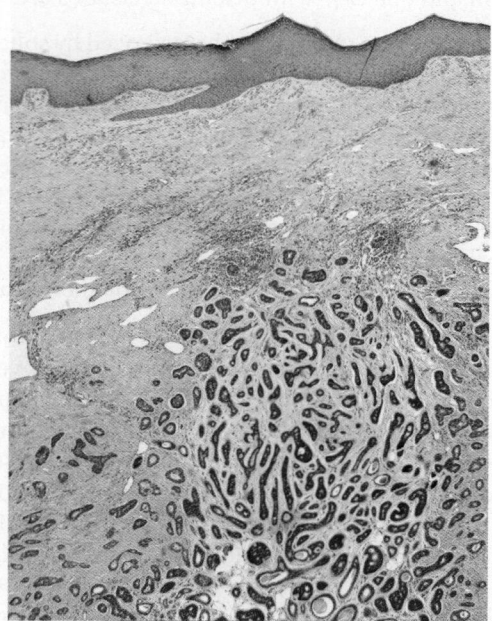

Figure 30-106 Adenoid cystic carcinoma of eccrine glands. A large cell mass shows an adenoid or cribriform pattern. In addition, many small, solid epithelial islands are present.

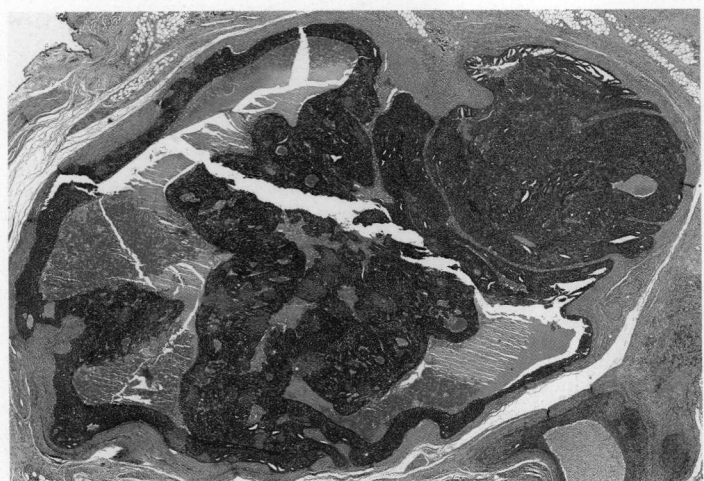

Figure 30-108 Digital papillary adenocarcinoma. A large, lobulated dermal tumor with focal cystic change is seen in the dermis of acral skin.

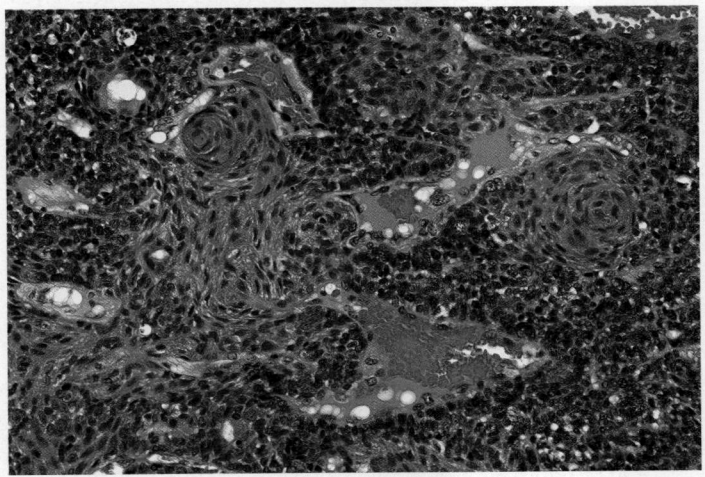

Figure 30-109 Digital papillary adenocarcinoma. Gland formation and focal squamoid differentiation are seen.

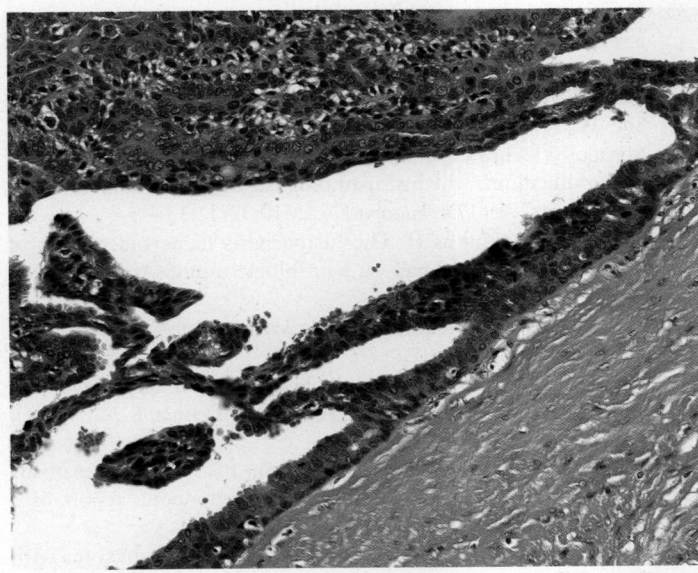

Figure 30-110 Digital papillary adenocarcinoma. Micropapillary structures are seen and mitotic activity is present.

The histologic differential diagnosis includes metastatic papillary carcinoma from breast, lung, thyroid, and ovary. Initially, a low-grade variant—"aggressive digital papillary adenoma"—was described that differed from adenocarcinoma based on the degree of pleomorphism, mitotic rate, and necrosis (783). However, subsequent studies suggest that histologic features alone cannot reliably predict clinical behavior, and, therefore, all lesions should be considered aggressive digital papillary adenocarcinomas (784,787,788). Metastases may occur as late as 20 years after presentation and most often involve regional lymph nodes and the lung (784).

Secretory Carcinoma

Clinical Summary. First described in 2009, secretory carcinoma of the skin is a rare adnexal carcinoma that is histopathologically identical to analogous neoplasms in the salivary gland and breast (789,790). There is a female predilection among the 26 reported cases thus far (1.9:1) and a wide age range (13 to 98 years [mean: 51.8]). The most common location is the axilla (n = 11) followed by the neck (n = 3), and lip (n = 3) (790). One axillary case was found to have a nodal metastasis, and this patient went on to have recurrent distant metastases to the lungs (791).

Histopathology. Secretory carcinomas are typically circumscribed, nonencapsulated, dermal tumors that may extend into the subcutis and typically lack an epidermal connection. The presence of ectopic salivary gland or breast tissue must be excluded as, if present, adnexal primacy must be questioned. The tumors are nodular aggregates of closely packed microcystic and tubular spaces comprised of bland oval, round, and cuboidal neoplastic cells with abundant, eosinophilic intraluminal secretions. Solid areas and pseudopapillae are often seen. Focal mucinous features, remnant eccrine/apocrine duct cells, hobnail cells, and blastoid cells are rare variants. The mitotic rate ranges from 0 to 4/mm². Lymphovascular and perineural invasion are exceedingly rare (Fig. 30-111) (789–791).

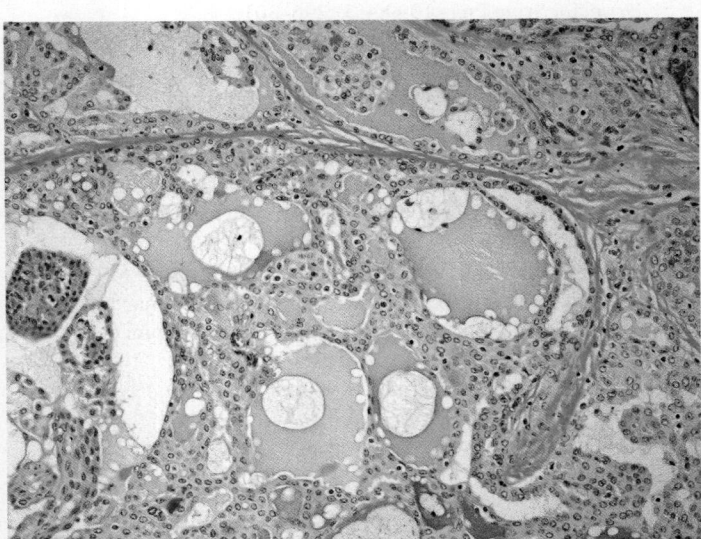

Figure 30-111 Secretory carcinoma. Closely packed microcystic and tubular spaces comprised of round and cuboidal neoplastic cells with bland nuclei and abundant, eosinophilic intraluminal secretions, case courtesy of Dr. Kohei Taniguchi.

Additional Studies. Tumor cells are positive for S-100 protein, mammaglobin, STAT5, GATA3, and NTRK. P63 can highlight myoepithelial cells, if present (B). ETV6-NTRK3 translocations have been identified in 23/26 reported cases, with one case harboring an NFIX-PKN1 translocation and another demonstrating heterozygous deletion of ETV6 in 25% of cells. Hence, as seen in the secretory carcinomas of other primary sites, ETV6 alterations are molecular hallmarks of cutaneous secretory carcinoma.

REFERENCES

1. Buchi ER, Peng Y, Eng AM, Tso MO. Eccrine acrospiroma of the eyelid with oncocytic, apocrine and sebaceous differentiation. Further evidence for pluripotentiality of the adnexal epithelia. *Eur J Ophthalmol.* 1991;1(4):187–193.
2. Massa MC, Medenica M. Cutaneous adnexal tumors and cysts: a review. Part I. Tumors with hair follicular and sebaceous glandular differentiation and cysts related to different parts of the hair follicle. *Pathol Annu.* 1985;20(pt 2):189–233.
3. Sanchez YE, Requena L, Simon P, Sanchez M. Complex adnexal tumor of the primary epithelial germ with distinct patterns of superficial epithelioma with sebaceous differentiation, immature trichoepithelioma, and apocrine adenocarcinoma. *Am J Dermatopathol.* 1992;14(3):245–252.
4. Weyers W, Nilles M, Eckert F, Schill WB. Spiradenomas in Brooke-Spiegler syndrome. *Am J Dermatopathol.* 1993;15(2):156–161.
5. Wong TY. Benign cutaneous adnexal tumors with combined folliculosebaceous, apocrine, and eccrine differentiation. Clinicopathologic and immunohistochemical study of eight cases [comment]. *Am J Dermatopathol.* 1996;18(2):165–171.
6. Oshima H, Rochat A, Kedzia C, Kobayashi K, Barrandon Y. Morphogenesis and renewal of hair follicles from adult multipotent stem cells. *Cell.* 2001;104(2):233–245.
7. Perez-Losada J, Balmain A. Stem-cell hierarchy in skin cancer. *Nat Rev Cancer.* 2003;3(6):434–443.
8. Lyle S, Christofidou-Solomidou M, Liu Y, Elder DE, Albelda S, Cotsarelis G. Human hair follicle bulge cells are biochemically distinct and possess an epithelial stem cell phenotype. *J Investig Dermatol Symp Proc.* 1999;4(3):296–301.
9. Plikus MV, Gay DL, Treffeisen E, Wang A, Supapannachart RJ, Cotsarelis G. Epithelial stem cells and implications for wound repair. *Semin Cell Dev Biol.* 2012;23(9):946–953.
10. Taylor G, Lehrer MS, Jensen PJ, Sun TT, Lavker RM. Involvement of follicular stem cells in forming not only the follicle but also the epidermis. *Cell.* 2000;102(4):451–461.
11. Penneys NS. Immunohistochemistry of adnexal neoplasms. *J Cutan Pathol.* 1984;11(5):357–364.
12. Biggs PJ, Chapman P, Lakhani SR, Burn J, Stratton MR. The cylindromatosis gene (cyld1) on chromosome 16q may be the only tumour suppressor gene involved in the development of cylindromas. *Oncogene.* 1996;12(6):1375–1377.
13. Heenan P, Elder DE Sobin LH. *Histologic Typing of Skin Tumors.* Vol 3. Springer; 1996.
14. Hashimoto K, Lever WF. *Appendage Tumors of the Skin.* Vol 47. Charles C Thomas; 1968.
15. Albrecht E. Uber hamartome. *Verh Dtsch Ges Pathol.* 1904;7:153.
16. Jadassohn J. Die benignen epitheliome. *Arch Derm Syphilol.* 1914;117:705.
17. Murphy GF, Elder DE. *Nonmelanocytic Tumors of the Skin.* Vol 1. Armed Forces Institute of Pathology; 1990.
18. Motegi S, Amano H, Tamura A, Ishikawa O. Hair follicle nevus in a 2-year old. *Pediatr Dermatol.* 2008;25(1):60–62.
19. Davis DA, Cohen PR. Hair follicle nevus: case report and review of the literature. *Pediatr Dermatol.* 1996;13(2):135–138.
20. Headington JT. Tumors of the hair follicle. A review. *Am J Pathol.* 1976;85(2):479–514.
21. Labandeira J, Peteiro C, Toribio J. Hair follicle nevus: case report and review. *Am J Dermatopathol.* 1996;18(1):90–93.
22. Germain M, Smith KJ. Hair follicle nevus in a distribution following Blaskho's lines. *J Am Acad Dermatol.* 2002;46(5 suppl):S125–S127.
23. Ikeda S, Kawada J, Yaguchi H, Ogawa H. A case of unilateral, systematized linear hair follicle nevi associated with epidermal nevus-like lesions. *Dermatology.* 2003;206(2):172–174.
24. Goddard DS, Rogers M, Frieden IJ, et al. Widespread porokeratotic adnexal ostial nevus: clinical features and proposal of a new name unifying porokeratotic eccrine ostial and dermal duct nevus and porokeratotic eccrine and hair follicle nevus. *J Am Acad Dermatol.* 2009;61(6):1060.e1061–1060.e1014.
25. Criscione V, Lachiewicz A, Robinson-Bostom L, Grenier N, Dill SW. Porokeratotic eccrine duct and hair follicle nevus (PEHFN) associated with keratitis-ichthyosis-deafness (KID) syndrome. *Pediatr Dermatol.* 2010;27(5):514–517.
26. Martorell-Calatayud A, Colmenero I, Hernandez-Martin A, Requena L, Torrelo A. Porokeratotic eccrine and hair follicle nevus. *Am J Dermatopathol.* 2010;32(5):529–530.
27. Tadini G, Boldrini MP, Brena M, Pezzani L, Marchesi L, Rongioletti F. Nevoid follicular mucinosis: a new type of hair follicle nevus. *J Cutan Pathol.* 2013;40(9):844–847.
28. Nagase K, Nagase K, Misago N, Narisawa Y. A preauricular hairy papule in an infant: hair follicle nevus closely similar to accessory tragus. *Arch Dermatol.* 2012;148(2):266–268.
29. Pippione M, Aloi F, Depaoli MA. Hair-follicle nevus. *Am J Dermatopathol.* 1984;6(3):245–247.
30. Ban M, Kamiya H, Yamada T, Kitajima Y. Hair follicle nevi and accessory tragi: variable quantity of adipose tissue in connective tissue framework. *Pediatr Dermatol.* 1997;14(6):433–436.
31. Asahina A, Mitomi H, Sakurai N, Fujita H. Multiple accessory tragi without cartilage: relationship with hair follicle naevi? *Acta Derm Venereol.* 2009;89(3):316–317.
32. Pinkus H, Sutton RL Jr. Trichofolliculoma. *Arch Dermatol.* 1965;91:46–49.
33. Choi CM, Lew BL, Sim WY. Multiple trichofolliculomas on unusual sites: a case report and review of the literature. *Int J Dermatol.* 2013;52(1):87–89.
34. Gray H, Helwig E. Trichofolliculoma. *Arch Dermatol.* 1962;86:619.
35. Hyman AB, Clayman SJ. Hair-follicle nevus; report of a case and a review of the literature concerning this lesion and some related conditions. *AMA Arch Derm.* 1957;75(5):678–684.
36. Sanderson K. Hair follicle nevus. *Trans St Johns Hosp Dermatol Soc.* 1961;47:154.
37. Misago N, Kimura T, Toda S, Mori T, Narisawa Y. A revaluation of trichofolliculoma: the histopathological and immunohistochemical features. *Am J Dermatopathol.* 2010;32(1):35–43.
38. Kligman AM, Pinkus H. The histogenesis of nevoid tumors of the skin. The folliculoma—a hair-follicle tumor. *Arch Dermatol.* 1960;81:922–930.
39. Lim P, Kossard S. Trichofolliculoma with mucinosis. *Am J Dermatopathol.* 2009;31(4):405–406.
40. Boran C, Parlak AH, Erkol H. Collision tumour of trichofolliculoma and basal cell carcinoma. *Australas J Dermatol.* 2007;48(2):127–129.
41. Bancalari E, Martinez-Sanchez D, Tardio JC. Nevus lipomatosus superficialis with a folliculosebaceous component: report of 2 cases. *Patholog Res Int.* 2011;2011:105973.
42. Perez TB, Saez AC, Fernandez PR. Superficial angiomyxoma with trichofolliculoma. *Ann Diagn Pathol.* 2008;12(5):375–377.
43. Schulz T, Hartschuh W. The trichofolliculoma undergoes changes corresponding to the regressing normal hair follicle in its cycle. *J Cutan Pathol.* 1998;25(7):341–353.

44. Wu YH. Folliculosebaceous cystic hamartoma or trichofolliculoma? A spectrum of hamartomatous changes inducted by perifollicular stroma in the follicular epithelium. *J Cutan Pathol.* 2008;35(9):843–848.

45. Gat U, DasGupta R, Degenstein L, Fuchs E. De novo hair follicle morphogenesis and hair tumors in mice expressing a truncated beta-catenin in skin. *Cell.* 1998;95(5):605–614.

46. Kan L, Liu Y, McGuire TL, Bonaguidi MA, Kessler JA. Inhibition of BMP signaling in P-cadherin positive hair progenitor cells leads to trichofolliculoma-like hair follicle neoplasias. *J Biomed Sci.* 2011;18:92.

47. Sharov AA, Mardaryev AN, Sharova TY, et al. Bone morphogenetic protein antagonist noggin promotes skin tumorigenesis via stimulation of the Wnt and Shh signaling pathways. *Am J Pathol.* 2009;175(3):1303–1314.

48. Sharov AA, Mardaryev AN, Sharova TY, et al. Bone morphogenetic protein antagonist noggin promotes skin tumorigenesis via stimulation of the Wnt and Shh signaling pathways. *Am J Pathol.* 2009; 175(3):1303–1314.

49. Cole P, Kaufman Y, Dishop M, Hatef DA, Hollier L. Giant, congenital folliculosebaceous cystic hamartoma: a case against a pathogenetic relationship with trichofolliculoma. *Am J Dermatopathol.* 2008;30(5):500–503.

50. Misago N, Kimura T, Toda S, Mori T, Narisawa Y. A revaluation of folliculosebaceous cystic hamartoma: the histopathological and immunohistochemical features. *Am J Dermatopathol.* 2010;32(2):154–161.

51. Schulz T, Hartschuh W. Folliculo-sebaceous cystic hamartoma is a trichofolliculoma at its very late stage. *J Cutan Pathol.* 1998;25(7):354–364.

52. Plewig G. Sebaceous trichofolliculoma. *J Cutan Pathol.* 1980; 7(6):394–403.

53. El-Darouty MA, Marzouk SA, Abdel-Halim MR, El-Komy MH, Mashaly HM. Folliculo-sebaceous cystic hamartoma. *Int J Dermatol.* 2001;40(7):454–457.

54. Winer L. The dilated pore, a trichoepithelioma. *J Invest Dermatol.* 1954;23(3):181–188.

55. Jakobiec FA, Bhat P, Sutula F. Winer's dilated pore of the eyelid. *Ophthalmic Plast Reconstr Surg.* 2009;25(5):411–413.

56. Bavikar RR, Gaopande V, Deshmukh SD. Postauricular pilar sheath acanthoma. *Int J Trichology.* 2011;3(1):39–40.

57. Mehregan AH, Brownstein MH. Pilar sheath acanthoma. *Arch Dermatol.* 1978;114(10):1495–1497.

58. Steffen C. Winer's dilated pore: the infundibuloma. *Am J Dermatopathol.* 2001;23(3):246–253.

59. Bhawan J. Pilar sheath acanthoma. A new benign follicular tumor. *J Cutan Pathol.* 1979;6(5):438–440.

60. Schulz T, Hartschuh W. Birt-Hogg-Dube syndrome and Hornstein-Knickenberg syndrome are the same. Different sectioning technique as the cause of different histology. *J Cutan Pathol.* 1999;26(1):55–61.

61. Toro JR, Wei MH, Glenn GM, et al. BHD mutations, clinical and molecular genetic investigations of Birt-Hogg-Dube syndrome: a new series of 50 families and a review of published reports. *J Med Genet.* 2008;45(6):321–331.

62. Kluger N, Giraud S, Coupier I, et al. Birt-Hogg-Dube syndrome: clinical and genetic studies of 10 French families. *Br J Dermatol.* 2010;162(3):527–537.

63. Weintraub R, Pinkus H. Multiple fibrofolliculomas (Birt-Hogg-Dube) associated with a large connective tissue nevus. *J Cutan Pathol.* 1977;4(6):289–299.

64. Pinkus H, Coskey R, Burgess GH. Trichodiscoma. A benign tumor related to haarscheibe (hair disk). *J Invest Dermatol.* 1974;63(2):212–218.

65. Grosshans E, Dungler T, Hanau D. Le trichodiscome de Pinkus. *Ann Dermatol Venereol.* 1981;108(11):837–846.

66. Starink TM, Houweling AC, van Doorn MB, et al. Familial multiple discoid fibromas: a look-alike of Birt-Hogg-Dube syndrome not linked to the FLCN locus. *J Am Acad Dermatol.* 2012;66(2):259.e251– 259.e259.

67. Wee JS, Chong H, Natkunarajah J, Mortimer PS, Moosa Y. Familial multiple discoid fibromas: unique histological features and therapeutic response to topical rapamycin. *Br J Dermatol.* 2013;169(1):177–180.

68. Birt AR, Hogg GR, Dube WJ. Hereditary multiple fibrofolliculomas with trichodiscomas and acrochordons. *Arch Dermatol.* 1977;113(12):1674–1677.

69. Battistella M, Van Eeckhout P, Cribier B. Symplastic trichodiscoma: a spindle-cell predominant variant of trichodiscoma with pseudosarcomatous/ancient features. *Am J Dermatopathol.* 2011;33(7):e81–e83.

70. Collins GL, Somach S, Morgan MB. Histomorphologic and immunophenotypic analysis of fibrofolliculomas and trichodiscomas in Birt-Hogg-Dube syndrome and sporadic disease. *J Cutan Pathol.* 2002;29(9):529–533.

71. Laviolette LA, Wilson J, Koller J, et al. Human folliculin delays cell cycle progression through late S and G2/M-phases: effect of phosphorylation and tumor associated mutations. *PLoS One.* 2013;8(7):e66775.

72. Medvetz DA, Khabibullin D, Hariharan V, et al. Folliculin, the product of the Birt-Hogg-Dube tumor suppressor gene, interacts with the adherens junction protein p0071 to regulate cell-cell adhesion. *PLoS One.* 2012;7(11):e47842.

73. Misago N, Narisawa Y. Fibrofolliculoma in a patient with tuberous sclerosis complex. *Clin Exp Dermatol.* 2009;34(8):892–894.

74. Byrne M, Mallipeddi R, Pichert G, Whittaker S. Birt-Hogg-Dube syndrome with a renal angiomyolipoma: further evidence of a relationship between Birt-Hogg-Dube syndrome and tuberous sclerosis complex. *Australas J Dermatol.* 2012;53(2):151–154.

75. Baba M, Hong SB, Sharma N, et al. Folliculin encoded by the BHD gene interacts with a binding protein, FNIP1, and AMPK, and is involved in AMPK and mTOR signaling. *Proc Natl Acad Sci U S A.* 2006;103(42):15552–15557.

76. Grossmann P, Vanecek T, Steiner P, et al. Novel and recurrent germline and somatic mutations in a cohort of 67 patients from 48 families with Brooke-Spiegler syndrome including the phenotypic variant of multiple familial trichoepitheliomas and correlation with the histopathologic findings in 379 biopsy specimens. *Am J Dermatopathol.* 2013;35(1):34–44.

77. Gray HR, Helwig EB. Epithelioma adenoides cysticum and solitary trichoepithelioma. *Arch Dermatol.* 1963;87:102–114.

78. Pariser RJ. Multiple hereditary trichoepitheliomas and basal cell carcinomas. *J Cutan Pathol.* 1986;13(2):111–117.

79. Johnson SC, Bennett RG. Occurrence of basal cell carcinoma among multiple trichoepitheliomas. *J Am Acad Dermatol.* 1993;28(2, pt 2):322–326.

80. Wallace ML, Smoller BR. Trichoepithelioma with an adjacent basal cell carcinoma, transformation or collision? *J Am Acad Dermatol.* 1997;37(2, pt 2):343–345.

81. Melly L, Lawton G, Rajan N. Basal cell carcinoma arising in association with trichoepithelioma in a case of Brooke-Spiegler syndrome with a novel genetic mutation in CYLD. *J Cutan Pathol.* 2012;39(10):977–978.

82. Kirby JS, Siebert Lucking SM, Billingsley EM. Trichoblastic carcinoma associated with multiple familial trichoepithelioma. *Dermatol Surg.* 2012;38(12):2018–2021.

83. Lee KH, Kim JE, Cho BK, Kim YC, Park CJ. Malignant transformation of multiple familial trichoepithelioma: case report and literature review. *Acta Derm Venereol.* 2008;88(1):43–46.

84. Martin R, Emanuel P. Combined cellular blue nevus and trichoepithelioma. *J Clin Aesthet Dermatol.* 2013;6(8):35–38.

85. Zeligman I. Solitary trichoepithelioma. *Arch Dermatol.* 1960;82: 35–40.

86. Baker GM, Selim MA, Hoang MP. Vulvar adnexal lesions: a 32-year, single-institution review from Massachusetts General Hospital. *Arch Pathol Lab Med.* 2013;137(9):1237–1246.

87. Heller J, Roche N, Hameed M. Trichoepithelioma of the vulva: report of a case and review of the literature. *J Low Genit Tract Dis.* 2009;13(3):186–187.

88. Muller-Hess S, Delacretaz J. [Trichoepithelioma with features of apocrine adenoma]. *Dermatologica.* 1973;146(3):170–176.

89. Yong LJ, Jin KD, Ho K, Sung-No J. Trichoepithelioma arising from facial scar tissue. *J Craniofac Surg.* 2013;24(3):e292–294.

90. Genc S, Sirin US, Arslan IB, et al. A giant solitary trichoepithelioma originating from the auricle. *Dermatol Surg.* 2012;38(9):1527–1528.

91. Brooke JD, Fitzpatrick JE, Golitz LE. Papillary mesenchymal bodies: a histologic finding useful in differentiating trichoepitheliomas from basal cell carcinomas. *J Am Acad Dermatol.* 1989;21(3, pt 1):523–528.

92. Bettencourt MS, Prieto VG, Shea CR. Trichoepithelioma: a 19-year clinicopathologic re-evaluation. *J Cutan Pathol.* 1999; 26(8):398–404.

93. Ohnishi T, Watanabe S. Immunohistochemical analysis of cytokeratin expression in various trichogenic tumors. *Am J Dermatopathol.* 1999;21(4):337–343.

94. Jih DM, Lyle S, Elenitsas R, Elder DE, Cotsarelis G. Cytokeratin 15 expression in trichoepitheliomas and a subset of basal cell carcinomas suggests they originate from hair follicle stem cells. *J Cutan Pathol.* 1999;26(3):113–118.

95. Espana A, Garcia-Amigot F, Aguado L, Garcia-Foncillas J. A novel missense mutation in the CYLD gene in a Spanish family with multiple familial trichoepithelioma. *Arch Dermatol.* 2007;143(9):1209–1210.

96. Young AL, Kellermayer R, Szigeti R, Teszas A, Azmi S, Celebi JT. CYLD mutations underlie Brooke-Spiegler, familial cylindromatosis, and multiple familial trichoepithelioma syndromes. *Clin Genet.* 2006;70(3):246–249.

97. Liang YH, Gao M, Sun LD, et al. Two novel CYLD gene mutations in Chinese families with trichoepithelioma and a literature review of 16 families with trichoepithelioma reported in China. *Br J Dermatol.* 2005;153(6):1213–1215.

98. Zheng G, Hu L, Huang W, et al. CYLD mutation causes multiple familial trichoepithelioma in three Chinese families. *Hum Mutat.* 2004;23(4):400.

99. Almeida S, Maillard C, Itin P, Hohl D, Huber M. Five new CYLD mutations in skin appendage tumors and evidence that aspartic acid 681 in CYLD is essential for deubiquitinase activity. *J Invest Dermatol.* 2008;128(3):587–593.

100. Zhao XY, Huang YJ, Liang YH, Huang L, Zhao Y, Zeng K. Multiple familial trichoepithelioma: report of a Chinese family not associated with a mutation in the CYLD gene and CYLD protein expression in the trichoepithelioma tumor tissue. *Int J Dermatol.* 2014;53(4):e279–e281.

101. Tebcherani AJ, de Andrade HF Jr, Sotto MN. Diagnostic utility of immunohistochemistry in distinguishing trichoepithelioma and basal cell carcinoma: evaluation using tissue microarray samples. *Mod Pathol.* 2012;25(10):1345–1353.

102. Vorechovsky I, Unden AB, Sandstedt B, Toftgard R, Stahle-Backdahl M. Trichoepitheliomas contain somatic mutations in the overexpressed PTCH gene: support for a gatekeeper mechanism in skin tumorigenesis. *Cancer Res.* 1997;57(21): 4677–4681.

103. Pham TT, Selim MA, Burchette JL Jr, Madden J, Turner J, Herman C. CD10 expression in trichoepithelioma and basal cell carcinoma. *J Cutan Pathol.* 2006;33(2):123–128.

104. Sari Aslani F, Akbarzadeh-Jahromi M, Jowkar F. Value of CD10 expression in differentiating cutaneous basal from squamous cell carcinomas and basal cell carcinoma from trichoepithelioma. *Iran J Med Sci.* 2013;38(2):100–106.

105. Astarci HM, Gurbuz GA, Sengul D, Hucumenoglu S, Kocer U, Ustun H. Significance of androgen receptor and CD10 expression in cutaneous basal cell carcinoma and trichoepithelioma. *Oncol Lett.* 2015;10(6):3466–3470.

106. Katona TM, Perkins SM, Billings SD. Does the panel of cytokeratin 20 and androgen receptor antibodies differentiate desmoplastic trichoepithelioma from morpheaform/infiltrative basal cell carcinoma? *J Cutan Pathol.* 2008;35(2):174–179.

107. Sellheyer K, Nelson P. Follicular stem cell marker PHLDA1 (TDAG51) is superior to cytokeratin-20 in differentiating between trichoepithelioma and basal cell carcinoma in small biopsy specimens. *J Cutan Pathol.* 2011;38(7):542–550.

108. Yeh I, McCalmont TH, LeBoit PE. Differential expression of PHLDA1 (TDAG51) in basal cell carcinoma and trichoepithelioma. *Br J Dermatol.* 2012;167(5):1106–1110.

109. Titinchi F, Nortje CJ, Parker ME, van Rensburg LJ. Nevoid basal cell carcinoma syndrome: a 40-year study in the South African population. *J Oral Pathol Med.* 2013;42(2):162–165.

110. Brownstein MH, Shapiro L. Desmoplastic trichoepithelioma. *Cancer.* 1977;40(6):2979–2986.

111. Macdonald DM, Jones EW, Marks R. Sclerosing epithelial hamartoma. *Clin Exp Dermatol.* 1977;2(2):153–160.

112. Dervan PA, O'Hegarty M, O'Loughlin S, Corrigan T. Solitary familial desmoplastic trichoepithelioma. A study by conventional and electron microscopy. *Am J Dermatopathol.* 1985;7(3):277–282.

113. Shapiro PE, Kopf AW. Familial multiple desmoplastic trichoepitheliomas. *Arch Dermatol.* 1991;127(1):83–87.

114. Tse JY, Nguyen AT, Le LP, Hoang MP. Microcystic adnexal carcinoma versus desmoplastic trichoepithelioma: a comparative study. *Am J Dermatopathol.* 2013;35(1):50–55.

115. Jedrych J, Leffell D, McNiff JM. Desmoplastic trichoepithelioma with perineural involvement: a series of seven cases. *J Cutan Pathol.* 2012;39(3):317–323.

116. McCalmont TH, Humberson C. Neurotropism in association with desmoplastic trichoepithelioma. *J Cutan Pathol.* 2012;39(3):312–314.

117. Costache M, Bresch M, Boer A. Desmoplastic trichoepithelioma versus morphoeic basal cell carcinoma: a critical reappraisal of histomorphological and immunohistochemical criteria for differentiation. *Histopathology.* 2008;52(7):865–876.

118. Krahl D, Sellheyer K. p75 Neurotrophin receptor differentiates between morphoeic basal cell carcinoma and desmoplastic trichoepithelioma: insights into the histogenesis of adnexal tumours based on embryology and hair follicle biology. *Br J Dermatol.* 2010;163(1):138–145.

119. Koga K, Anan T, Fukumoto T, Fujimoto M, Nabeshima K. Ln-gamma 2 chain of laminin-332 is a useful marker in differentiating between benign and malignant sclerosing adnexal neoplasms. *Histopathology.* 2020;76(2):318–324.

120. Thewes M, Worret WI, Engst R, Ring J. Stromelysin-3: a potent marker for histopathologic differentiation between desmoplastic trichoepithelioma and morphealike basal cell carcinoma. *Am J Dermatopathol.* 1998;20(2):140–142.

121. Hartschuh W, Schulz T. Merkel cells are integral constituents of desmoplastic trichoepithelioma: an immunohistochemical and electron microscopic study. *J Cutan Pathol.* 1995;22(5):413–421.

122. Arits AH, Van Marion AM, Lohman BG, et al. Differentiation between basal cell carcinoma and trichoepithelioma by immunohistochemical staining of the androgen receptor: an overview. *Eur J Dermatol.* 2011;21(6):870–873.

123. Sellheyer K, Nelson P, Kutzner H, Patel RM. The immunohistochemical differential diagnosis of microcystic adnexal carcinoma, desmoplastic trichoepithelioma and morpheaform basal cell carcinoma using BerEP4 and stem cell markers. *J Cutan Pathol.* 2013;40(4):363–370.

124. Abbas O, Richards JE, Mahalingam M. Fibroblast-activation protein: a single marker that confidently differentiates morpheaform/infiltrative basal cell carcinoma from desmoplastic trichoepithelioma. *Mod Pathol.* 2010;23(11):1535–1543.

125. Singh S, Rapini R, Schwartz M, Friedman-Musicante R, Friedman PM. Challenging the dogma of "watchful waiting" for

desmoplastic trichoepithelioma. *Dermatol Surg.* 2013;39(3, pt 1):483–486.

126. Gilks CB, Clement PB, Wood WS. Trichoblastic fibroma. A clinicopathologic study of three cases. *Am J Dermatopathol.* 1989;11(5):397–402.

127. Headington JT, French AJ. Primary neoplasms of the hair follicle. Histogenesis and classification. *Arch Dermatol.* 1962;86: 430–441.

128. Cohen C, Davis TS. Multiple trichogenic adnexal tumors. *Am J Dermatopathol.* 1986;8(3):241–246.

129. Wang L, Wang G, Yang L, Gao T. Multiple clear cell trichoblastoma. *J Cutan Pathol.* 2009;36(3):370–373.

130. Cowen EW, Helm KF, Billingsley EM. An unusually aggressive trichoblastoma [see comment]. *J Am Acad Dermatol.* 2000;42(2, pt 2):374–377.

131. Helm KF, Cowen EW, Billingsley EM, Ackerman AB. Trichoblastoma or trichoblastic carcinoma? [comment]. *J Am Acad Dermatol.* 2001;44(3):547.

132. Fazaa B, Cribier B, Zaraa I, et al. Low-dose X-ray depilatory treatment induces trichoblastic tumors of the scalp. *Dermatology.* 2007;215(4):301–307.

133. Diaz-Cascajo C, Borghi S, Rey-Lopez A, Carretero-Hernandez G. Cutaneous lymphadenoma. A peculiar variant of nodular trichoblastoma. *Am J Dermatopathol.* 1996;18(2):186–191.

134. Kanitakis J, Brutzkus A, Butnaru AC, Claudy A. Melanotrichoblastoma: immunohistochemical study of a variant of pigmented trichoblastoma. *Am J Dermatopathol.* 2002;24(6):498–501.

135. Yamamoto O, Hisaoka M, Yasuda H, Nishio D, Asahi M. A rippled-pattern trichoblastoma: an immunohistochemical study. *J Cutan Pathol.* 2000;27(9):460–465.

136. Tronnier M. Clear cell trichoblastoma in association with a nevus sebaceus. *Am J Dermatopathol.* 2001;23(2):143–145.

137. Requena L, Barat A. Giant trichoblastoma on the scalp. *Am J Dermatopathol.* 1993;15(5):497–502.

138. Juarez A, Rutten A, Kutzner H, Requena L. Cystic trichoblastoma (so-called trichoblastic infundibular cyst): a report of three new cases. *J Cutan Pathol.* 2012;39(6):631–636.

139. Kim DW, Lee JH, Kim I. Giant melanotrichoblastoma. *Am J Dermatopathol.* 2011;33(3):e37–e40.

140. Swick BL, Baum CL, Walling HW. Rippled-pattern trichoblastoma with apocrine differentiation arising in a nevus sebaceus: report of a case and review of the literature. *J Cutan Pathol.* 2009;36(11):1200–1205.

141. Battistella M, Durand L, Jouary T, Peltre B, Cribier B. Primary cutaneous neuroendocrine carcinoma within a cystic trichoblastoma: a nonfortuitous association? *Am J Dermatopathol.* 2011;33(4):383–387.

142. Juarez A, Diaz JL, Schaerer L, Kutzner H, Requena L. Trichoblastomelanoma. *Am J Dermatopathol.* 2013;35(7):e119–e123.

143. Rosso R, Lucioni M, Savio T, Borroni G. Trichoblastic sarcoma: a high-grade stromal tumor arising in trichoblastoma. *Am J Dermatopathol.* 2007;29(1):79–83.

144. Ackerman AB, de Viragh PA, Chonchitnant N, eds. Trichoblastoma: trichoepithelioma. In: *Tumors With Follicular Differentiation.* Vol 359. Lea & Febiger; 1993.

145. Misago N, Mori T, Narisawa Y. Nestin expression in stromal cells of trichoblastoma and basal cell carcinoma. *J Eur Acad Dermatol Venereol.* 2010;24(11):1354–1358.

146. Battistella M, Peltre B, Cribier B. PHLDA1, a follicular stem cell marker, differentiates clear-cell/granular-cell trichoblastoma and clear-cell/granular cell basal cell carcinoma: a case-control study, with first description of granular-cell trichoblastoma. *Am J Dermatopathol.* 2014;36:643–650.

147. Hamasaki H, Koga K, Hamasaki M, et al. Immunohistochemical analysis of laminin 5-gamma2 chain expression for differentiation of basal cell carcinoma from trichoblastoma. *Histopathology.* 2011;59(1):159–161.

148. Hafner C, Schmiemann V, Ruetten A, et al. PTCH mutations are not mainly involved in the pathogenesis of sporadic trichoblastomas. *Hum Pathol.* 2007;38(10):1496–1500.

149. Kazakov DV, Sima R, Vanecek T, et al. Mutations in exon 3 of the CTNNB1 gene (beta-catenin gene) in cutaneous adnexal tumors. *Am J Dermatopathol.* 2009;31(3):248–255.

150. Nikolowski W. Tricho-adenom (organoides follikel-hamartom). *Arch Klin Exp Dermatol.* 1958;207(1):34–45.

151. Rahbari H, Mehregan A, Pinkus H. Trichoadenoma of Nikolowski. *J Cutan Pathol.* 1977;4(2):90–98.

152. Matos TO, Linthicum FH Jr. Trichoadenoma of the external auditory canal. *Otol Neurotol.* 2011;32(9):e36–e37.

153. Miyazaki-Nakajima K, Hara H, Terui T. Subungual trichoadenoma showing differentiation toward follicular infundibulum. *J Dermatol.* 2011;38(11):1118–1121.

154. Shimanovich I, Krahl D, Rose C. Trichoadenoma of Nikolowski is a distinct neoplasm within the spectrum of follicular tumors. *J Am Acad Dermatol.* 2010;62(2):277–283.

155. Lee WS, Oh ST, Lee JY, Cho BK. Congenital trichoadenoma with an unusual clinical manifestation. *J Am Acad Dermatol.* 2007;57(5):905–906.

156. Lee JH, Kim YY, Yoon SY, Lee JD, Cho SH. Unusual presentation of trichoadenoma in an infant. *Acta Derm Venereol.* 2008;88(3):291–292.

157. Lever JF, Servat JJ, Nesi-Eloff F, Nesi FA. Trichoadenoma of an eyelid in an adult mimicking sebaceous cell carcinoma. *Ophthalmic Plast Reconstr Surg.* 2012;28(4):e101–e102.

158. Brownstein MH. Basaloid follicular hamartoma: solitary and multiple types. *J Am Acad Dermatol.* 1992;27(2, pt 1): 237–240.

159. Jaqueti G, Requena L, Sanchez Yus E. Verrucous trichoadenoma. *J Cutan Pathol.* 1989;16(3):145–148.

160. Arora S, Kaur J, Kaur H. Verrucous trichoadenoma—presenting as discharging sinus on face. *Indian Dermatol Online J.* 2013; 4(3):251–252.

161. Gonzalez-Vela MC, Val-Bernal JF, Garcia-Alberdi E, Gonzalez-Lopez MA, Fernandez-Llaca JH. Trichoadenoma associated with an intradermal melanocytic nevus: a combined malformation. *Am J Dermatopathol.* 2007;29(1):92–95.

162. Reibold R, Undeutsch W, Fleiner J. Das trichoadenom (Nikolowski) ubersicht von vier Jahrzehnten und sieben eigene Falle. *Hautarzt.* 1998;49(12):925–928.

163. Kurokawa I, Mizutani H, Nishijima S, Kato N, Yasui K, Tsubura A. Trichoadenoma: cytokeratin expression suggesting differentiation towards the follicular infundibulum and follicular bulge regions. *Br J Dermatol.* 2005;153(5):1084–1086.

164. Tsuru K, Ohashi A, Ueda M. A case of generalized hair follicle hamartoma associated with systemic lupus erythematosus. *J Dermatol.* 2004;31(7):573–576.

165. Lee MW, Choi JH, Moon KC, Koh JK. Linear basaloid follicular hamartoma on the Blaschko's line of the face. *Clin Exp Dermatol.* 2005;30(1):30–34.

166. Boccaletti V, Accorsi P, Pinelli L, et al. Congenital systematized basaloid follicular hamartoma with microphthalmia and hemimegalencephaly. *Pediatr Dermatol.* 2011;28(5):555–560.

167. Mascaro JM Jr, Ferrando J, Bombi JA, Lambruschini N, Mascaro JM. Congenital generalized follicular hamartoma associated with alopecia and cystic fibrosis in three siblings. *Arch Dermatol.* 1995;131(4):454–458.

168. Huang SH, Hsiao TF, Lee CC. Basaloid follicular hamartoma: a case report and review of the literature. *Kaohsiung J Med Sci.* 2012;28(1):57–60.

169. Happle R, Tinschert S. Segmentally arranged basaloid follicular hamartomas with osseous, dental and cerebral anomalies: a distinct syndrome. *Acta Derm Venereol.* 2008;88(4):382–387.

170. Itin PH. Happle-Tinschert syndrome. Segmentally arranged basaloid follicular hamartomas, linear atrophoderma with

hypo- and hyperpigmentation, enamel defects, ipsilateral hypertrichosis, and skeletal and cerebral anomalies. *Dermatology.* 2009;218(3):221–225.

171. Mehregan AH, Baker S. Basaloid follicular hamartoma: three cases with localized and systematized unilateral lesions. *J Cutan Pathol.* 1985;12(1):55–65.

172. Ridley CM, Smith N. Generalized hair follicle hamartoma associated with alopecia and myasthenia gravis: report of a second case. *Clin Exp Dermatol.* 1981;6(3):283–289.

173. Jih DM, Shapiro M, James WD, et al. Familial basaloid follicular hamartoma: lesional characterization and review of the literature. *Am J Dermatopathol.* 2003;25(2):130–137.

174. Walsh N, Ackerman AB. Basaloid follicular hamartoma: solitary and multiple types. *J Am Acad Dermatol.* 1993;29(1):125–129.

175. Jakobiec FA, Zakka FR, Kim N. Basaloid follicular hamartoma of the eyelid. *Ophthalmic Plast Reconstr Surg.* 2012;28(5): e127–e130.

176. Grachtchouk V, Grachtchouk M, Lowe L, et al. The magnitude of hedgehog signaling activity defines skin tumor phenotype. *EMBO J.* 2003;22(11):2741–2751.

177. Oseroff AR, Shieh S, Frawley NP, et al. Treatment of diffuse basal cell carcinomas and basaloid follicular hamartomas in nevoid basal cell carcinoma syndrome by wide-area 5-aminolevulinic acid photodynamic therapy. *Arch Dermatol.* 2005;141(1):60–67.

178. Hassan SF, Stephens E, Fallon SC, et al. Characterizing pilomatricomas in children: a single institution experience. *J Pediatr Surg.* 2013;48(7):1551–1556.

179. Souto MP, Matsushita Mde M, Matsushita Gde M, Souto LR. An unusual presentation of giant pilomatrixoma in an adult patient. *J Dermatol Case Rep.* 2013;7(2):56–59.

180. Abdeldayem M, Mekhail P, Farag M, et al. Patient profile and outcome of pilomatrixoma in district general hospital in United kingdom. *J Cutan Aesthet Surg.* 2013;6(2):107–110.

181. Trufant J, Kurz W, Frankel A, et al. Familial multiple pilomatrixomas as a presentation of attenuated adenomatosis polyposis coli. *J Cutan Pathol.* 2012;39(4):440–443.

182. Do JE, Noh S, Jee HJ, Oh SH. Familial multiple pilomatricomas showing clinical features of a giant mass without associated diseases. *Int J Dermatol.* 2013;52(2):250–252.

183. Bhushan P, Hussain SN. Bullous pilomatricoma: a stage in transition to secondary anetoderma? *Indian J Dermatol Venereol Leprol.* 2012;78(4):484–487.

184. Solanki P, Ramzy I, Durr N, Henkes D. Pilomatrixoma. Cytologic features with differential diagnostic considerations. *Arch Pathol Lab Med.* 1987;111(3):294–297.

185. Lever WF, Griesemer RD. Calcifying epithelioma of Malherbe; report of 15 cases, with comments on its differentiation from calcified epidermal cyst and on its histogenesis. *Arch Derm Syphilol.* 1949;59(5):506–518.

186. Ishida M, Okabe H. Pigmented pilomatricoma: an underrecognized variant. *Int J Clin Exp Pathol.* 2013;6(9):1890–1893.

187. Peterson WC Jr, Hult AM. Calcifying epithelioma of Malherbe. *Arch Dermatol.* 1964;90:404–410.

188. Forbis RJ, Helwig E. Pilomatrixoma (calcifying epithelioma). *Arch Dermatol.* 1961;83:606–618.

189. Kurokawa I, Kusumoto K, Bessho K, Okubo Y, Senzaki H, Tsubura A. Immunohistochemical expression of bone morphogenetic protein-2 in pilomatricoma. *Br J Dermatol.* 2000;143(4):754–758.

190. Turhan B, Krainer L. Bemerkungen über die sogenannten verkalkenden epitheliome der haut und ihre genese. *Dermatologica.* 1942;85:73.

191. Malherbe A, Chenantais J. Note sur l´épithéliome calcifié des glandes sebacées. *Prog Med.* 1880;8:826.

192. Cribier B, Peltre B, Langbein L, Winter H, Schweizer J, Grosshans E. Expression of type I hair keratins in follicular tumours. *Br J Dermatol.* 2001;144(5):977–982.

193. Cribier B, Scrivener Y, Grosshans E. Tumors arising in nevus sebaceus: a study of 596 cases. [see comment]. *J Am Acad Dermatol.* 2000;42(2, pt 1):263–268.

194. Kurokawa I, Yamanaka K, Senba Y, et al. Pilomatricoma can differentiate not only towards hair matrix and hair cortex, but also follicular infundibulum, outer root sheath and hair bulge. *Exp Dermatol.* 2009;18(8):734–737.

195. Behrens J, von Kries JP, Kuhl M, et al. Functional interaction of beta-catenin with the transcription factor LEF-1. *Nature.* 1996;382(6592):638–642.

196. Aloi FG, Molinero A, Pippione M. Basal cell carcinoma with matrical differentiation. Matrical carcinoma. *Am J Dermatopathol.* 1988;10(6):509–513.

197. Shirai M, Fujimoto N, Nakanishi G, Tanaka T. Proliferating type pilomatricoma presenting with alopecia. *Eur J Dermatol.* 2012;22(4):564–565.

198. Byun JW, Bang CY, Yang BH, et al. Proliferating pilomatricoma. *Am J Dermatopathol.* 2011;33(7):754–755.

199. Collina G, Filosa A, Requena L. Pilomatrical tumor of low malignant potential: a tumor between pilomatricoma and pilomatrical carcinoma. *Am J Dermatopathol.* 2021;43(2):146–148.

200. Kaddu S, Soyer HP, Wolf IH, Kerl H. Proliferating pilomatricoma. A histopathologic simulator of matrical carcinoma. *J Cutan Pathol.* 1997;24(4):228–234.

201. Cornejo KM, Deng A. Pilomatrix carcinoma: a case report and review of the literature. *Am J Dermatopathol.* 2013;35(3):389–394.

202. Agaiby S, Iyer K, Honda K, Mostow EN. Giant pilomatrix carcinoma in an immunosuppressed patient. *J Am Acad Dermatol.* 2011;65(2):e50–e51.

203. Autelitano L, Biglioli F, Migliori G, Colletti G. Pilomatrix carcinoma with visceral metastases: case report and review of the literature. *J Plast Reconstr Aesthet Surg.* 2009;62(12):e574–e577.

204. Aherne NJ, Fitzpatrick DA, Gibbons D, Collins CD, Armstrong JG. Recurrent malignant pilomatrixoma invading the cranial cavity: improved local control with adjuvant radiation. *J Med Imaging Radiat Oncol.* 2009;53(1):139–141.

205. Hardisson D, Linares MD, Cuevas-Santos J, Contreras F. Pilomatrix carcinoma: a clinicopathologic study of six cases and review of the literature [see comment]. *Am J Dermatopathol.* 2001;23(5):394–401.

206. Cribier B, Asch PH, Regnier C, Rio MC, Grosshans E. Expression of human hair keratin basic 1 in pilomatrixoma. A study of 128 cases. *Br J Dermatol.* 1999;140(4):600–604.

207. Nishioka M, Tanemura A, Yamanaka T, et al. Pilomatrix carcinoma arising from pilomatricoma after 10-year senescent period: immunohistochemical analysis. *J Dermatol.* 2010;37(8):735–739.

208. Lazar AJ, Calonje E, Grayson W, et al. Pilomatrix carcinomas contain mutations in CTNNB1, the gene encoding beta-catenin. *J Cutan Pathol.* 2005;32(2):148–157.

209. Satyaprakash AK, Sheehan DJ, Sangueza OP. Proliferating trichilemmal tumors: a review of the literature. *Dermatol Surg.* 2007;33(9):1102–1108.

210. Falleti J, Cuccuru A, Mignogna C. Proliferating trichilemmal cyst of the vulva. *Clin Exp Dermatol.* 2009;34(7):e459–e460.

211. Ye J, Nappi O, Swanson PE, Patterson JW, Wick MR. Proliferating pilar tumors: a clinicopathologic study of 76 cases with a proposal for definition of benign and malignant variants. *Am J Clin Pathol.* 2004;122(4):566–574.

212. Brownstein MH, Arluk DJ. Proliferating trichilemmal cyst: a simulant of squamous cell carcinoma. *Cancer.* 1981;48(5):1207–1214.

213. Holmes EJ. Tumors of lower hair sheath. Common histogenesis of certain so-called "sebaceous cysts," acanthomas and "sebaceous carcinomas". *Cancer.* 1968;21(2):234–248.

214. Hanau D, Grosshans E. Trichilemmal tumor undergoing specific keratinization: "keratinizing trichilemmoma". *J Cutan Pathol.* 1979;6(6):463–475.

215. Mehregan AH, Lee KC. Malignant proliferating trichilemmal tumors—report of three cases. *J Dermatol Surg Oncol.* 1987; 13(12):1339–1342.

216. Bronfenbrener R, Regan T, Lawrence N. Proliferating pilar tumor of the scalp. *Dermatol Surg.* 2012;38(8):1375–1377.

217. Sau P, Graham JH, Helwig EB. Proliferating epithelial cysts. Clinicopathological analysis of 96 cases. *J Cutan Pathol.* 1995;22(5):394–406.

218. Korting GW, Hoede N. [The so-called pilar tumor of the scalp]. *Arch Klin Exp Dermatol.* 1969;234(4):409–419.

219. Reed RJ, Lamar LM. Invasive hair matrix tumors of the scalp. Invasive pilomatrixoma. *Arch Dermatol.* 1966;94(3):310–316.

220. Harris T, Meyer E, Lubbe DE, Smit W, Walker C. Malignant proliferating trichilemmal tumor involving the sinuses. *Ear Nose Throat J.* 2011;90(7):E5–E8.

221. Amaral AL, Nascimento AG, Goellner JR. Proliferating pilar (trichilemmal) cyst. Report of two cases, one with carcinomatous transformation and one with distant metastases. *Arch Pathol Lab Med.* 1984;108(10):808–810.

222. Hodl S, Smolle J, Scharnagl E. [Importance of the proliferating trichilemmal cyst]. *Hautarzt.* 1984;35(12):640–644.

223. Herrero J, Monteagudo C, Ruiz A, Llombart-Bosch A. Malignant proliferating trichilemmal tumours: an histopathological and immunohistochemical study of three cases with DNA ploidy and morphometric evaluation. [see comment]. *Histopathology.* 1998;33(6):542–546.

224. Sau P, Graham JH, Helwig EB. Proliferating epithelial cysts. Clinicopathological analysis of 96 cases. *J Cutan Pathol.* 1995;22(5):394–406.

225. Fernandez-Figueras MT, Casalots A, Puig L, Llatjos R, Ferrandiz C, Ariza A. Proliferating trichilemmal tumour: p53 immunoreactivity in association with p27Kip1 over-expression indicates a low-grade carcinoma profile. *Histopathology.* 2001;38(5):454–457.

226. Takata M, Quinn AG, Hashimoto K, Rees JL. Low frequency of loss of heterozygosity at the nevoid basal cell carcinoma locus and other selected loci in appendageal tumors. *J Invest Dermatol.* 1996;106(5):1141–1144.

227. Brownstein MH, Shapiro L. Trichilemmoma. Analysis of 40 new cases. *Arch Dermatol.* 1973;107(6):866–869.

228. Mehregan AH, Medenica M, Whitney D, Kato I. A clear cell pilar sheath tumor of scalp: case report. *J Cutan Pathol.* 1988;15(6):380–384.

229. Brownstein MH, Shapiro EE. Trichilemmomal horn: cutaneous horn overlying trichilemmoma. *Clin Exp Dermatol.* 1979;4(1):59–63.

230. Brownstein MH, Mehregan AH, Bikowski JB, Lupulescu A, Patterson JC. The dermatopathology of Cowden's syndrome. *Br J Dermatol.* 1979;100(6):667–673.

231. Crowson AN, Magro CM. Basal cell carcinoma arising in association with desmoplastic trichilemmoma. *Am J Dermatopathol.* 1996;18(1):43–48.

232. Illueca C, Monteagudo C, Revert A, Llombart-Bosch A. Diagnostic value of CD34 immunostaining in desmoplastic trichilemmoma. *J Cutan Pathol.* 1998;25(8):435–439.

233. Afshar M, Lee RA, Jiang SI. Desmoplastic trichilemmoma—a report of successful treatment with Mohs micrographic surgery and a review and update of the literature. *Dermatol Surg.* 2012;38(11):1867–1871.

234. Plaza JA, Ortega PF, Stockman DL, Suster S. Value of p63 and podoplanin (D2-40) immunoreactivity in the distinction between primary cutaneous tumors and adenocarcinomas metastatic to the skin: a clinicopathologic and immunohistochemical study of 79 cases. *J Cutan Pathol.* 2010;37(4):403–410.

235. Leonardi CL, Zhu WY, Kinsey WH, Penneys NS. Trichilemmomas are not associated with human papillomavirus DNA. *J Cutan Pathol.* 1991;18(3):193–197.

236. Stierman S, Chen S, Nuovo G, Thomas J. Detection of human papillomavirus infection in trichilemmomas and verrucae using in situ hybridization. *J Cutan Pathol.* 2010;37(1):75–80.

237. Amer M, Mostafa FF, Attwa EM, Ibrahim S. Cowden's syndrome: a clinical, immunological, and histopathological study. *Int J Dermatol.* 2011;50(5):516–521.

238. Eng C. Will the real Cowden syndrome please stand up: revised diagnostic criteria. *J Med Genet.* 2000;37(11):828–830.

239. Agrawal S, Eng C. Differential expression of novel naturally occurring splice variants of PTEN and their functional consequences in Cowden syndrome and sporadic breast cancer. *Hum Mol Genet.* 2006;15(5):777–787.

240. Nelen MR, Padberg GW, Peeters EA, et al. Localization of the gene for Cowden disease to chromosome 10q22-23. *Nat Genet.* 1996;13(1):114–116.

241. Lima EU, Soares IC, Danilovic DL, Marui S. New mutation in the PTEN gene in a Brazilian patient with Cowden's syndrome. *Arq Bras Endocrinol Metabol.* 2012;56(8):592–596.

242. Zhou XP, Marsh DJ, Morrison CD, et al. Germline inactivation of PTEN and dysregulation of the phosphoinositol-3-kinase/Akt pathway cause human Lhermitte-Duclos disease in adults. *Am J Hum Genet.* 2003;73(5):1191–1198.

243. Pilarski R, Stephens JA, Noss R, Fisher JL, Prior TW. Predicting PTEN mutations: an evaluation of Cowden syndrome and Bannayan-Riley-Ruvalcaba syndrome clinical features. *J Med Genet.* 2011;48(8):505–512.

244. Waite KA, Eng C. Protean PTEN: form and function. *Am J Hum Genet.* 2002;70(4):829–844.

245. Liaw D, Marsh DJ, Li J, et al. Germline mutations of the PTEN gene in Cowden disease, an inherited breast and thyroid cancer syndrome. *Nat Genet.* 1997;16(1):64–67.

246. Nelen MR, van Staveren WC, Peeters EA, et al. Germline mutations in the PTEN/MMAC1 gene in patients with Cowden disease. *Hum Mol Genet.* 1997;6(8):1383–1387.

247. Jin M, Hampel H, Pilarski R, Zhou X, Peters S, Frankel WL. Phosphatase and tensin homolog immunohistochemical staining and clinical criteria for Cowden syndrome in patients with trichilemmoma or associated lesions. *Am J Dermatopathol.* 2013;35(6):637–640.

248. Abbas O, Mahalingam M. Tumor of the follicular infundibulum: an epidermal reaction pattern? *Am J Dermatopathol.* 2009;31(7):626–633.

249. Martin JE, Hsu MY, Wang LC. An unusual clinical presentation of multiple tumors of the follicular infundibulum. *J Am Acad Dermatol.* 2009;60(5):885–886.

250. Kolivras A, Moulonguet I, Ruben BS, Sass U, Cappelletti L, Andre J. Eruptive tumors of the follicular infundibulum presenting as hypopigmented macules on the buttocks of two Black African males. *J Cutan Pathol.* 2012;39(4):444–448.

251. MacGregor JL, Campanelli C, Friedman PC, Desciak E. Basal cell and squamous cell carcinoma occurring within a field of multiple tumors of the follicular infundibulum. *Dermatol Surg.* 2008;34(11):1567–1570.

252. Mehregan AH, Butler JD. A tumor of follicular infundibulum. Report of a case. *Arch Dermatol.* 1961;83:924–927.

253. Weyers W, Horster S, Diaz-Cascajo C. Tumor of follicular infundibulum is Basal cell carcinoma. *Am J Dermatopathol.* 2009;31(7):634–641.

254. Cardoso JC, Reis JP, Figueiredo P, Tellechea O. Infundibulomatosis: a case report with immunohistochemical study and literature review. *Dermatol Online J.* 2010;16(1):14.

255. Brownstein MH. Trichilemmal horn: cutaneous horn showing trichilemmal keratinization. *Br J Dermatol.* 1979;100(3):303–309.

256. Nakamura K. Two cases of trichilemmal-like horn. *Arch Dermatol.* 1984;120(3):386–387.

257. DiMaio DJ, Cohen PR. Trichilemmal horn: case presentation and literature review. *J Am Acad Dermatol.* 1998;39(2, pt 2):368–371.

258. Poblet E, Jimenez-Reyes J, Gonzalez-Herrada C, Granados R. Trichilemmal keratosis. A clinicopathologic and immunohistochemical study of two cases. *Am J Dermatopathol.* 1996;18(5):543–547.

259. Kudo M, Uchigasaki S, Baba S, Suzuki H. Trichilemmal horn on burn scar tissue. *Eur J Dermatol.* 2002;12(1):77–78.

260. Roismann M, Freitas RR, Ribeiro LC, Montenegro MF, Biasi LJ, Jung JE. Trichilemmal carcinoma: case report. *An Bras Dermatol.* 2011;86(5):991–994.

261. Oyama N, Kaneko F. Trichilemmal carcinoma arising in seborrheic keratosis: a case report and published work review. *J Dermatol.* 2008;35(12):782–785.

262. O'Hare AM, Cooper PH, Parlette HL 3rd. Trichilemmomal carcinoma in a patient with Cowden's disease (multiple hamartoma syndrome). *J Am Acad Dermatol.* 1997;36(6, pt 1):1021–1023.

263. Pozo L, Diaz-Cano SJ. Trichilemmal carcinoma with neuroendocrine differentiation. *Clin Exp Dermatol.* 2008;33(2):128–131.

264. ten Seldam RE. Tricholemmocarcinoma. *Australas J Dermatol.* 1977;18(2):62–72.

265. Allee JE, Cotsarelis G, Solky B, Cook JL. Multiply recurrent trichilemmal carcinoma with perineural invasion and cytokeratin 17 positivity. *Dermatol Surg.* 2003;29(8):886–889.

266. Mane DR, Kale AD, Hallikerimath S, Angadi P, Kotrashetti V. Trichilemmal carcinoma associated with xeroderma pigmentosa: report of a rare case. *J Oral Sci.* 2010;52(3):505–507.

267. Ko T, Tada H, Hatoko M, Muramatsu T, Shirai T. Trichilemmal carcinoma developing in a burn scar: a report of two cases. *J Dermatol.* 1996;23(7):463–468.

268. Takata M, Rehman I, Rees JL. A trichilemmal carcinoma arising from a proliferating trichilemmal cyst: the loss of the wild-type p53 is a critical event in malignant transformation [see comment]. *Hum Pathol.* 1998;29(2):193–195.

269. Liang H, Wu H, Giorgadze TA, et al. Podoplanin is a highly sensitive and specific marker to distinguish primary skin adnexal carcinomas from adenocarcinomas metastatic to skin. *Am J Surg Pathol.* 2007;31(2):304–310.

270. Kulahci Y, Oksuz S, Kucukodaci Z, Uygur F, Ulkur E. Multiple recurrence of trichilemmal carcinoma of the scalp in a young adult. *Dermatol Surg.* 2010;36(4):551–554.

271. Levinsohn JL, Tian LC, Boyden LM, et al. Whole-exome sequencing reveals somatic mutations in HRAS and KRAS, which cause nevus sebaceus. *J Invest Dermatol.* 2013;133(3): 827–830.

272. Chepla KJ, Gosain AK. Giant nevus sebaceus: definition, surgical techniques, and rationale for treatment. *Plast Reconstr Surg.* 2012;130(2):296e-304e.

273. Sun BK, Saggini A, Sarin KY, et al. Mosaic activating RAS mutations in nevus sebaceus and nevus sebaceus syndrome. *J Invest Dermatol.* 2013;133(3):824–827.

274. Happle R. Nevus sebaceus is a mosaic RASopathy. *J Invest Dermatol.* 2013;133(3):597–600.

275. Lam J, Dohil MA, Eichenfield LF, Cunningham BB. SCALP syndrome: sebaceous nevus syndrome, CNS malformations, aplasia cutis congenita, limbal dermoid, and pigmented nevus (giant congenital melanocytic nevus) with neurocutaneous melanosis: a distinct syndromic entity. *J Am Acad Dermatol.* 2008;58(5):884–888.

276. Sethi SK, Hari P, Bagga A. Elevated FGF-23 and parathormone in linear nevus sebaceous syndrome with resistant rickets. *Pediatr Nephrol.* 2010;25(8):1577–1578.

277. Narazaki R, Ihara K, Namba N, Matsuzaki H, Ozono K, Hara T. Linear nevus sebaceous syndrome with hypophosphatemic rickets with elevated FGF-23. *Pediatr Nephrol.* 2012;27(5):861–863.

278. Pavlidis E, Cantalupo G, Boria S, Cossu G, Pisani F. Hemimegalencephalic variant of epidermal nevus syndrome: case report and literature review. *Eur J Paediatr Neurol.* 2012;16(4):332–342.

279. Chantorn R, Shwayder T. Phacomatosis pigmentokeratotica: a further case without extracutaneous anomalies and review of the condition. *Pediatr Dermatol.* 2011;28(6):715–719.

280. Jaqueti G, Requena L, Sanchez YE. Trichoblastoma is the most common neoplasm developed in nevus sebaceus of Jadassohn: a clinicopathologic study of a series of 155 cases. *Am J Dermatopathol.* 2000;22(2):108–118.

281. Cribier B, Scrivener Y, Grosshans E. Tumors arising in nevus sebaceus: a study of 596 cases. *J Am Acad Dermatol.* 2000;42(2, pt 1):263–268.

282. Mehregan AH, Pinkus H. Life history of organoid nevi. Special reference to nevus sebaceus of Jadassohn. *Arch Dermatol.* 1965;91:574–588.

283. De D, Jain N, Kanwar AJ, Dogra S, Saikia UN. Cylindroma appearing in a pre-existing nevus sebaceous. *Int J Dermatol.* 2012;51(7):872–873.

284. Wang Y, Bu WB, Chen H, et al. Basal cell carcinoma, syringocystadenoma papilliferum, trichilemmoma, and sebaceoma arising within a nevus sebaceus associated with pigmented nevi. *Dermatol Surg.* 2011;37(12):1806–1810.

285. Rahbari H, Mehregan AH. Development of proliferating trichilemmal cyst in organoid nevus. Presentation of two cases. *J Am Acad Dermatol.* 1986;14(1):123–126.

286. Miller CJ, Ioffreda MD, Billingsley EM. Sebaceous carcinoma, basal cell carcinoma, trichoadenoma, trichoblastoma, and syringocystadenoma papilliferum arising within a nevus sebaceus. *Dermatol Surg.* 2004;30(12, pt 2):1546–1549.

287. Sellheyer K, Cribier B, Nelson P, Kutzner H, Rutten A. Basaloid tumors in nevus sebaceus revisited: the follicular stem cell marker PHLDA1 (TDAG51) indicates that most are basal cell carcinomas and not trichoblastomas. *J Cutan Pathol.* 2013;40(5):455–462.

288. Brownstein MH, Shapiro L. The pilosebaceous tumors. *Int J Dermatol.* 1977;16(5):340–352.

289. Barrett TL, Smith KJ, Williams J, Corner SW, Hodge JJ, Skelton HG. Immunohistochemical staining for Ber-EP4, p53, proliferating cell nuclear antigen, Ki-67, bcl-2, CD34, and factor XIIIa in nevus sebaceus. *Mod Pathol.* 1999;12(5):450–455.

290. Jones EW, Heyl T. Naevus sebaceus. A report of 140 cases with special regard to the development of secondary malignant tumours. *Br J Dermatol.* 1970;82(2):99–117.

291. Morioka S. The natural history of nevus sebaceus. *J Cutan Pathol.* 1985;12(3–4):200–213.

292. Alessi E, Wong SN, Advani HH, Ackerman AB. Nevus sebaceus is associated with unusual neoplasms. An atlas. *Am J Dermatopathol.* 1988;10(2):116–127.

293. Aguayo R, Pallares J, Casanova JM, et al. Squamous cell carcinoma developing in Jadassohn's sebaceous nevus: case report and review of the literature. *Dermatol Surg.* 2010;36(11): 1763–1768.

294. Wu ZW, Shi WM, Sun Y, Li XJ, Song J. Cutaneous spindle cell squamous cell carcinoma in nevus sebaceous. *Int J Dermatol.* 2010;49(12):1429–1431.

295. Domingo J, Helwig EB. Malignant neoplasms associated with nevus sebaceus of Jadassohn. *J Am Acad Dermatol.* 1979;1(6): 545–556.

296. Tarkhan II, Domingo J. Metastasizing eccrine porocarcinoma developing in a sebaceous nevus of Jadassohn. Report of a case. *Arch Dermatol.* 1985;121(3):413–415.

297. Kazakov DV, Calonje E, Zelger B, et al. Sebaceous carcinoma arising in nevus sebaceus of Jadassohn: a clinicopathological study of five cases. *Am J Dermatopathol.* 2007;29(3):242–248.

298. Lountzis N, Junkins-Hopkins J, Uberti-Benz M, Elenitsas R. Microcystic adnexal carcinoma arising within a nevus sebaceus. *Cutis.* 2007;80(4):352–356.

299. Manonukul J, Omeapinyan P, Vongjirad A. Mucoepidermoid (adenosquamous) carcinoma, trichoblastoma, trichilemmoma, sebaceous adenoma, tumor of follicular infundibulum and syringocystadenoma papilliferum arising within 2 persistent lesions of nevus sebaceous: report of a case. *Am J Dermatopathol.* 2009;31(7):658–663.

300. Premalata CS, Kumar RV, Malathi M, Shenoy AM, Nanjundappa N. Cutaneous leiomyosarcoma, trichoblastoma, and syringocystadenoma papilliferum arising from nevus sebaceus. *Int J Dermatol.* 2007;46(3):306–308.

301. Ujiie H, Kato N, Natsuga K, Tomita Y. Keratoacanthoma developing on nevus sebaceous in a child. *J Am Acad Dermatol.* 2007;56(2 suppl):S57–58.

302. Takeda H, Ikenaga S, Kaneko T, et al. Proliferating trichilemmal tumor developing in nevus sebaceous. *Eur J Dermatol.* 2010;20(5):664–665.

303. Kantrow SM, Ivan D, Williams MD, Prieto VG, Lazar AJ. Metastasizing adenocarcinoma and multiple neoplastic proliferations arising in a nevus sebaceus. *Am J Dermatopathol.* 2007;29(5):462–466.

304. Rijntjes-Jacobs EG, Lopriore E, Steggerda SJ, Kant SG, Walther FJ. Discordance for Schimmelpenning-Feuerstein-Mims syndrome in monochorionic twins supports the concept of a postzygotic mutation. *Am J Med Genet A.* 2010;152A(11):2816–2819.

305. Groesser L, Herschberger E, Sagrera A, et al. Phacomatosis pigmentokeratotica is caused by a postzygotic HRAS mutation in a multipotent progenitor cell. *J Invest Dermatol.* 2013;133(8):1998–2003.

306. Carlson JA, Cribier B, Nuovo G, Rohwedder A. Epidermodysplasia verruciformis-associated and genital-mucosal high-risk human papillomavirus DNA are prevalent in nevus sebaceus of Jadassohn. *J Am Acad Dermatol.* 2008;59(2):279–294.

307. Kurokawa I, Nishimura K, Yamanaka K, et al. Immunohistochemical study of cytokeratin expression in nevus sebaceous. *Int J Dermatol.* 2010;49(4):402–405.

308. Jones EW, Heyl T. Naevus sebaceus. A report of 140 cases with special regard to the development of secondary malignant tumours. *Br J Dermatol.* 1970;82(2):99–117.

309. Gailani MR, Stahle-Backdahl M, Leffell DJ, et al. The role of the human homologue of Drosophila patched in sporadic basal cell carcinomas [see comment]. *Nat Genet.* 1996;14(1):78–81.

310. Shen T, Park WS, Boni R, et al. Detection of loss of heterozygosity on chromosome 9q22.3 in microdissected sporadic basal cell carcinoma. *Hum Pathol.* 1999;30(3):284–287.

311. Xin H, Matt D, Qin JZ, Burg G, Boni R. The sebaceous nevus: a nevus with deletions of the PTCH gene. *Cancer Res.* 1999;59(8):1834–1836.

312. Takata M, Tojo M, Hatta N, Ohara K, Yamada M, Takehara K. No evidence of deregulated patched-hedgehog signaling pathway in trichoblastomas and other tumors arising within nevus sebaceous. *J Invest Dermatol.* 2001;117(6):1666–1670.

313. Lee WJ, Cha HW, Lim HJ, Lee SJ, Kim DW. The effect of sebocytes cultured from nevus sebaceus on hair growth. *Exp Dermatol.* 2012;21(10):796–798.

314. Rosen H, Schmidt B, Lam HP, Meara JG, Labow BI. Management of nevus sebaceus and the risk of Basal cell carcinoma: an 18-year review. *Pediatr Dermatol.* 2009;26(6):676–681.

315. Moody MN, Landau JM, Goldberg LH. Nevus sebaceous revisited. *Pediatr Dermatol.* 2012;29(1):15–23.

316. Ortiz-Rey JA, Martin-Jimenez A, Alvarez C, De La Fuente A. Sebaceous gland hyperplasia of the vulva. *Obstet Gynecol.* 2002;99(5, pt 2):919–921.

317. Rocamora A, Santonja C, Vives R, Varona C. Sebaceous gland hyperplasia of the vulva: a case report. *Obstet Gynecol.* 1986;68(3 suppl):63S–65S.

318. Carson HJ, Massa M, Reddy V. Sebaceous gland hyperplasia of the penis. *J Urol.* 1996;156(4):1441.

319. Belinchon I, Aguilar A, Tardio J, Gallego MA. Areolar sebaceous hyperplasia: a case report. *Cutis.* 1996;58(1):63–64.

320. Ju HY, Kim HS, Kim HO, Park YM. Sebaceous hyperplasia of the penile shaft. *J Eur Acad Dermatol Venereol.* 2009;23(4):443–444.

321. Krause W. Diseases of the male nipple and areola. *J Dtsch Dermatol Ges.* 2011;9(12):1004–1009.

322. Wang Q, Liu JM, Zhang YZ. Premature sebaceous hyperplasia in an adolescent boy. *Pediatr Dermatol.* 2011;28(2):198–200.

323. Oh ST, Kwon HJ. Premature sebaceous hyperplasia in a neonate. *Pediatr Dermatol.* 2007;24(4):443–445.

324. Kanada KN, Merin MR, Munden A, Friedlander SF. A prospective study of cutaneous findings in newborns in the United States: correlation with race, ethnicity, and gestational status using updated classification and nomenclature. *J Pediatr.* 2012;161(2):240–245.

325. Boonchai W, Leenutaphong V. Familial presenile sebaceous gland hyperplasia. *J Am Acad Dermatol.* 1997;36(1):120–122.

326. McDonald SK, Goh MS, Chong AH. Successful treatment of cyclosporine-induced sebaceous hyperplasia with oral isotretinoin in two renal transplant recipients. *Australas J Dermatol.* 2011;52(3):227–230.

327. Luderschmidt C, Plewig G. Circumscribed sebaceous gland hyperplasia: autoradiographic and histoplanimetric studies. *J Invest Dermatol.* 1978;70(4):207–209.

328. Kruse R, Rutten A, Schweiger N, et al. Frequency of microsatellite instability in unselected sebaceous gland neoplasias and hyperplasias. *J Invest Dermatol.* 2003;120(5):858–864.

329. Popnikolov NK, Gatalica Z, Colome-Grimmer MI, Sanchez RL. Loss of mismatch repair proteins in sebaceous gland tumors. *J Cutan Pathol.* 2003;30(3):178–184.

330. Bayer-Garner IB, Givens V, Smoller B. Immunohistochemical staining for androgen receptors: a sensitive marker of sebaceous differentiation. *Am J Dermatopathol.* 1999;21(5):426–431.

331. Zouboulis CC, Chen WC, Thornton MJ, Qin K, Rosenfield R. Sexual hormones in human skin. *Horm Metab Res.* 2007;39(2):85–95.

332. Tagliolatto S, Alchorne MM, Enokihara M. Sebaceous hyperplasia: a pilot study to correlate this skin disease with circulating androgen levels. *An Bras Dermatol.* 2011;86(5):917–923.

333. Yoneda K, Demitsu T, Matsuda Y, Kubota Y. Possible molecular pathogenesis for plate-like sebaceous hyperplasia overlying dermatofibroma. *Br J Dermatol.* 2008;158(4):840–842.

334. Yin Z, Xu J, Luo D, Zhang M. Sebaceous hyperplasia within epidermis after scald. *J Cutan Pathol.* 2012;39(1):75–77.

335. Gomaa AH, Yaar M, Bhawan J. Cutaneous immunoreactivity of D2-40 antibody beyond the lymphatics. *Am J Dermatopathol.* 2007;29(1):18–21.

336. Tjarks BJ, Pownell BR, Evans C, et al. Evaluation and comparison of staining patterns of factor XIIIa (AC-1A1), adipophilin and GATA3 in sebaceous neoplasia. *J Cutan Pathol.* 2018;45(1):1–7.

337. Halsey MA, Calder KB, Mathew R, Schlauder S, Morgan MB. Expression of alpha-methylacyl-CoA racemase (P504S) in sebaceous neoplasms. *J Cutan Pathol.* 2010;37(4):446–451.

338. Daley T. Pathology of intraoral sebaceous glands. *J Oral Pathol Med.* 1993;22(6):241–245.

339. Watkins F, Giacomantonio M, Salisbury S. Nipple discharge and breast lump related to Montgomery's tubercles in adolescent females. *J Pediatr Surg.* 1988;23(8):718–720.

340. Mansur AT, Aydingoz IE. Unilateral buccal fordyce spots with ipsilateral facial paralysis: a sign of neuro-sebaceous connection? *Acta Derm Venereol.* 2012;92(2):177–178.

341. Azevedo RS, Almeida OP, Netto JN, et al. Comparative clinicopathological study of intraoral sebaceous hyperplasia and sebaceous adenoma. *Oral Surg Oral Med Oral Pathol Oral Radiol Endod.* 2009;107(1):100–104.

342. Somashekara KG, Lakshmi S, Priya NS. A rare case of sebaceous adenoma of the palate, with literature review. *J Laryngol Otol.* 2011;125(7):750–752.

343. Terrell S, Wetter R, Fraga G, Kestenbaum T, Aires DJ. Penile sebaceous adenoma. *J Am Acad Dermatol.* 2007;57(2 suppl):S42–S43.

344. Essenhigh DM, Jones D, Rack JH. A sebaceous adenoma. Histological and chemical studies. *Br J Dermatol.* 1964;76:330–340.

345. Banse-Kupin L, Morales A, Barlow M. Torre's syndrome: report of two cases and review of the literature. *J Am Acad Dermatol.* 1984;10(5, pt 1):803–817.

346. Rutten A, Burgdorf W, Hugel H, et al. Cystic sebaceous tumors as marker lesions for the Muir-Torre syndrome: a histopathologic and molecular genetic study. *Am J Dermatopathol.* 1999;21(5):405–413.

347. Troy JL, Ackerman AB. Sebaceoma. A distinctive benign neoplasm of adnexal epithelium differentiating toward sebaceous cells. *Am J Dermatopathol.* 1984;6(1):7–13.

348. Yonekawa Y, Jakobiec FA, Zakka FR, Fay A. Sebaceoma of the eyelid. *Ophthalmology.* 2012;119(12):2645.e2641– 2645.e2644.

349. Jacobson JP, Weisstuch A, Hajdu C, Myssiorek D. Sebaceoma of the auricle. *J Laryngol Otol.* 2012;126(8):830–832.

350. El Demellawy D, Escott N, Salama S, Alowami S. Sebaceoma of the external ear canal: an unusual location. Case report and review of the literature. *J Cutan Pathol.* 2008;35(10):963–966.

351. Hori M, Egami K, Maejima K, Nishimoto K. Electron microscopic study of sebaceous epithelioma. *J Dermatol.* 1978;5(4):139–147.

352. Urban FH, Winkelmann RK. Sebaceous malignancy. *Arch Dermatol.* 1961;84:63–72.

353. Misago N, Mihara I, Ansai S, Narisawa Y. Sebaceoma and related neoplasms with sebaceous differentiation: a clinicopathologic study of 30 cases. *Am J Dermatopathol.* 2002;24(4):294–304.

354. Kazakov DV, Calonje E, Rutten A, Glatz K, Michal M. Cutaneous sebaceous neoplasms with a focal glandular pattern (seboapocrine lesions): a clinicopathological study of three cases. *Am J Dermatopathol.* 2007;29(4):359–364.

355. Steffen C, Ackerman AB. Sebaceoma. In: Steffen C, Ackerman AB, ed. *Neoplasms with Sebaceous Differentiation.* Lea & Febiger; 1994:385.

356. Ansai S, Kimura T. Rippled-pattern sebaceoma: a clinicopathological study. *Am J Dermatopathol.* 2009;31(4):364–366.

357. Muir EG, Bell AJ, Barlow KA. Multiple primary carcinomata of the colon, duodenum, and larynx associated with kerato-acanthomata of the face. *Br J Surg.* 1967;54(3):191–195.

358. Poleksic S. Keratoacanthoma and multiple carcinomas. *Br J Dermatol.* 1974;91(4):461–463.

359. Fathizadeh A, Medenica MM, Soltani K, Lorincz AL, Griem ML. Aggressive keratoacanthoma and internal malignant neoplasm. *Arch Dermatol.* 1982;118(2):112–114.

360. Shon W, Wolz MM, Newman CC, Bridges AG. Reticulated acanthoma with sebaceous differentiation: another sebaceous neoplasm associated with Muir-Torre syndrome? *Australas J Dermatol.* 2014;55(4):e71–e73.

361. Torre D. Multiple sebaceous tumors. *Arch Dermatol.* 1968;98(5):549–551.

362. Schwartz RA, Torre DP. The Muir-Torre syndrome: a 25-year retrospect. *J Am Acad Dermatol.* 1995;33(1):90–104.

363. Lee BA, Yu L, Ma L, Lind AC, Lu D. Sebaceous neoplasms with mismatch repair protein expressions and the frequency of co-existing visceral tumors. *J Am Acad Dermatol.* 2012;67(6):1228–1234.

364. Binder ZA, Johnson MW, Joshi A, et al. Glioblastoma multiforme in the Muir-Torre syndrome. *Clin Neurol Neurosurg.* 2011;113(5):411–415.

365. Grandhi R, Deibert CP, Pirris SM, Lembersky B, Mintz AH. Simultaneous Muir-Torre and Turcot's syndrome: a case report and review of the literature. *Surg Neurol Int.* 2013;4:52.

366. Landis MN, Davis CL, Bellus GA, Wolverton SE. Immunosuppression and sebaceous tumors: a confirmed diagnosis of Muir-Torre syndrome unmasked by immunosuppressive therapy. *J Am Acad Dermatol.* 2011;65(5):1054–1058.e1051.

367. Becker-Schiebe M, Hannig H, Hoffmann W, Donhuijsen K. Muir-Torre syndrome—an uncommon localization of sebaceous carcinomas following irradiation. *Acta Oncol.* 2012;51(2):265–268.

368. Yozu M, Symmans P, Dray M, et al. Muir-Torre syndrome-associated pleomorphic liposarcoma arising in a previous radiation field. *Virchows Arch.* 2013;462(3):355–360.

369. Abbott JJ, Hernandez-Rios P, Amirkhan RH, Hoang MP. Cystic sebaceous neoplasms in Muir-Torre syndrome. *Arch Pathol Lab Med.* 2003;127(5):614–617.

370. Burgdorf WH, Pitha J, Fahmy A. Muir-Torre syndrome. Histologic spectrum of sebaceous proliferations. *Am J Dermatopathol.* 1986;8(3):202–208.

371. Worret WI, Burgdorf WH, Fahmy A, Pitha J. [Torre-Muir syndrome. Sebaceous gland neoplasms, keratoacanthomas, multiple internal cancers and heredity]. *Hautarzt.* 1981;32(10):519–524.

372. Kacerovska D, Cerna K, Martinek P, et al. MSH6 mutation in a family affected by Muir-Torre syndrome. *Am J Dermatopathol.* 2012;34(6):648–652.

373. Guillen-Ponce C, Castillejo A, Barbera VM, et al. Biallelic MYH germline mutations as cause of Muir-Torre syndrome. *Fam Cancer.* 2010;9(2):151–154.

374. Abbas O, Mahalingam M. Cutaneous sebaceous neoplasms as markers of Muir-Torre syndrome: a diagnostic algorithm. *J Cutan Pathol.* 2009;36(6):613–619.

375. Fernandez-Flores A. Considerations on the performance of immunohistochemistry for mismatch repair gene proteins in cases of sebaceous neoplasms and keratoacanthomas with reference to Muir-Torre syndrome. *Am J Dermatopathol.* 2012;34(4):416–422.

376. Orta L, Klimstra DS, Qin J, et al. Towards identification of hereditary DNA mismatch repair deficiency: sebaceous neoplasm warrants routine immunohistochemical screening regardless of patient's age or other clinical characteristics. *Am J Surg Pathol.* 2009;33(6):934–944.

377. Mojtahed A, Schrijver I, Ford JM, Longacre TA, Pai RK. A two-antibody mismatch repair protein immunohistochemistry screening approach for colorectal carcinomas, skin sebaceous tumors, and gynecologic tract carcinomas. *Mod Pathol.* 2011;24(7):1004–1014.

378. Shalin SC, Sakharpe A, Lyle S, Lev D, Calonje E, Lazar AJ. p53 staining correlates with tumor type and location in sebaceous neoplasms. *Am J Dermatopathol.* 2012;34(2):129–135; quiz 136–138.

379. Escalonilla P, Grilli R, Canamero M, et al. Sebaceous carcinoma of the vulva. *Am J Dermatopathol.* 1999;21(5):468–472.

380. Oppenheim AR. Sebaceous carcinoma of the penis. *Arch Dermatol.* 1981;117(5):306–307.

381. Dixon RS, Mikhail GR, Slater HC. Sebaceous carcinoma of the eyelid. *J Am Acad Dermatol.* 1980;3(3):241–243.

382. Torres JS, Amorim AC, Hercules FM, Kac BK. Giant extraocular sebaceous carcinoma: case report and a brief review of a literature. *Dermatol Online J.* 2012;18(11):7.

383. Mirzamani N, Sundram UN. A case of sebaceous carcinoma diagnosed in an adolescent male. *J Cutan Pathol.* 2011;38(5):435–438.

384. Kuzel P, Metelitsa AI, Dover DC, Salopek TG. Epidemiology of sebaceous carcinoma in Alberta, Canada, from 1988 to 2007. *J Cutan Med Surg.* 2012;16(6):417–423.

385. Rao NA, Hidayat AA, McLean IW, Zimmerman LE. Sebaceous carcinomas of the ocular adnexa: a clinicopathologic study of 104 cases, with five-year follow-up data. *Hum Pathol.* 1982;13(2):113–122.

386. Moreno C, Jacyk WK, Judd MJ, Requena L. Highly aggressive extraocular sebaceous carcinoma. *Am J Dermatopathol.* 2001;23(5):450–455.

387. Leonard DD, Deaton WR Jr. Multiple sebaceous gland tumors and visceral carcinomas. *Arch Dermatol.* 1974;110(6):917–920.

388. Graham R, McKee P, McGibbon D, Heyderman E. Torre-Muir syndrome. An association with isolated sebaceous carcinoma. *Cancer.* 1985;55(12):2868–2873.

389. Rulon DB, Helwig EB. Cutaneous sebaceous neoplasms. *Cancer.* 1974;33(1):82–102.

390. Wick MR, Goellner JR, Wolfe JT 3rd, Su WP. Adnexal carcinomas of the skin. II. Extraocular sebaceous carcinomas. *Cancer.* 1985;56(5):1163–1172.

391. Russell WG, Page DL, Hough AJ, Rogers LW. Sebaceous carcinoma of meibomian gland origin. The diagnostic importance of pagetoid spread of neoplastic cells. *Am J Clin Pathol.* 1980;73(4):504–511.

392. Arits A, van Marion AM, Thissen CA, Kloos R, Kelleners-Smeets NW. Development and progression of a periorbital sebaceous gland carcinoma in situ. *Acta Derm Venereol*. 2010;90(5):529–530.

393. Hayashi N, Furihata M, Ohtsuki Y, Ueno H. Search for accumulation of p53 protein and detection of human papillomavirus genomes in sebaceous gland carcinoma of the eyelid. *Virchows Arch*. 1994;424(5):503–509.

394. Gonzalez-Fernandez F, Kaltreider SA, Patnaik BD, et al. Sebaceous carcinoma. Tumor progression through mutational inactivation of p53. *Ophthalmology*. 1998;105(3):497–506.

395. Hasebe T, Mukai K, Yamaguchi N, et al. Prognostic value of immunohistochemical staining for proliferating cell nuclear antigen, p53, and c-erbB-2 in sebaceous gland carcinoma and sweat gland carcinoma: comparison with histopathological parameter. *Mod Pathol*. 1994;7(1):37–43.

396. Izumi M, Tang X, Chiu CS, et al. Ten cases of sebaceous carcinoma arising in nevus sebaceus. *J Dermatol*. 2008;35(11):704–711.

397. Cottle DL, Kretzschmar K, Schweiger PJ, et al. c-MYC-induced sebaceous gland differentiation is controlled by an androgen receptor/p53 axis. *Cell Rep*. 2013;3(2):427–441.

398. Ivan D, Prieto VG, Esmaeli B, Wistuba II, Tang X, Lazar AJ. Epidermal growth factor receptor (EGFR) expression in periocular and extraocular sebaceous carcinoma. *J Cutan Pathol*. 2010;37(2):231–236.

399. Kim N, Kim JE, Choung HK, Lee MJ, Khwarg SI. Expression of Shh and Wnt signaling pathway proteins in eyelid sebaceous gland carcinoma: clinicopathologic study. *Invest Ophthalmol Vis Sci*. 2013;54(1):370–377.

400. Friedman KJ, Boudreau S, Farmer ER. Superficial epithelioma with sebaceous differentiation. *J Cutan Pathol*. 1987;14(4):193–197.

401. Kuo T. Clear cell carcinoma of the skin. A variant of the squamous cell carcinoma that simulates sebaceous carcinoma. *Am J Surg Pathol*. 1980;4(6):573–583.

402. Prioleau PG, Santa Cruz DJ. Sebaceous gland neoplasia. *J Cutan Pathol*. 1984;11(5):396–414.

403. Sinard JH. Immunohistochemical distinction of ocular sebaceous carcinoma from basal cell and squamous cell carcinoma. *Arch Ophthalmol*. 1999;117(6):776–783.

404. Kaminska EC, Iyengar V, Tsoukas M, Shea CR. Borderline sebaceous neoplasm in a renal transplant patient without Muir-Torre syndrome. *J Cutan Pathol*. 2013;40(3):336–340.

405. Ando K, Hashikawa Y, Nakashima M, Nakayama A, Ohashi M. Pure apocrine nevus. A study of light-microscopic and immunohistochemical features of a rare tumor. *Am J Dermatopathol*. 1991;13(1):71–76.

406. Civatte J, Tsoitis G, Preaux J. [Apocrine nevus. Study of 2 cases]. *Ann Dermatol Syphiligr (Paris)*. 1974;101(3):251–261.

407. Perez-Oliva N, del Pozo Hernando LJ, Tejerina JA, Quinones PA. [Apocrine nevus]. *Med Cutan Ibero Lat Am*. 1990;18(1):67–69.

408. Rabens SF, Naness JI, Gottlieb BF. Apocrine gland organic hamartoma (apocrine nevus). *Arch Dermatol*. 1976;112(4):520–522.

409. Schwartz RA, Rojas-Corona R, Lambert WC. The polymorphic apocrine nevus: a study of a unique tumor including carcinoembryonic antigen staining. *J Surg Oncol*. 1984;26(3):183–186.

410. Kim JH, Hur H, Lee CW, Kim YT. Apocrine nevus. *J Am Acad Dermatol*. 1988;18(3):579–581.

411. Mori O, Hachisuka H, Sasai Y. Apocrine nevus. *Int J Dermatol*. 1993;32(6):448–449.

412. Neill JS, Park HK. Apocrine nevus: light microscopic, immunohistochemical and ultrastructural studies of a case. *J Cutan Pathol*. 1993;20(1):79–83.

413. Mazoujian G. Immunohistochemistry of GCDFP-24 and zinc alpha2 glycoprotein in benign sweat gland tumors. *Am J Dermatopathol*. 1990;12(5):452–457.

414. Miyamoto T, Inoue S, Adachi K, Takada R. Differential expression of mucin core proteins and keratins in apocrine carcinoma, extramammary Paget's disease and apocrine nevus. *J Cutan Pathol*. 2009;36(5):529–534.

415. Benisch B, Peison B. Apocrine hidrocystoma of the shoulder. *Arch Dermatol*. 1977;113(1):71–72.

416. Mehregan AH. Apocrine cystadenoma; a clinicopathologic study with special reference to the pigmented variety. *Arch Dermatol*. 1964;90:274–279.

417. Mehregan AH, Rahbari H. Benign epithelial tumors of the skin. IV: Benign apocrine gland tumors. *Cutis*. 1978;21(1):53–56.

418. Schewach-Millet M, Trau H. Congenital papillated apocrine cystadenoma: a mixed form of hidrocystoma, hidradenoma papilliferum, and syringocystadenoma papilliferum. *J Am Acad Dermatol*. 1984;11(2, pt 2):374–376.

419. Adeloye A, Aghadiuno PU, Adesina MA, Ogunniyi J. A large apocrine hidrocystoma located over the thoracic spine in a Nigerian. *Cent Afr J Med*. 1987;33(3):74–76.

420. Asarch RG, Golitz LE, Sausker WF, Kreye GM. Median raphe cysts of the penis. *Arch Dermatol*. 1979;115(9):1084–1086.

421. De Fontaine S, Van Geertruyden J, Vandeweyer E. Apocrine hidrocystoma of the finger. *J Hand Surg*. 1998;23(2):281–282.

422. Glusac EJ, Hendrickson MS, Smoller BR. Apocrine cystadenoma of the vulva. *J Am Acad Dermatol*. 1994;31(3, pt 1):498–499.

423. Shields JA, Eagle RC Jr, Shields CL, de Potter P, Markowitz G. Apocrine hidrocystoma of the eyelid. *Arch Ophthal*. 1993;111(6):866–867.

424. Smith JD, Chernosky ME. Apocrine hidrocystoma (cystadenoma). *Arch Dermatol*. 1974;109(5):700–702.

425. Alessi E, Gianotti R, Coggi A. Multiple apocrine hidrocystomas of the eyelids. *Br J Dermatol*. 1997;137(4):642–645.

426. Kruse TV, Khan MA, Hassan MO. Multiple apocrine cystadenomas. *Br J Dermatol*. 1979;100(6):675–681.

427. Hafsi W, Badri T, Shah F. *Apocrine Hidrocystoma*. StatPearls; 2021.

428. Jo JW, Yang JW, Jeong DS. Apocrine hidrocystoma on the penis: report of a case and review of the previous cases. *Ann Dermatol*. 2019;31(4):442–445.

429. Kitamura S, Yanagi T, Imafuku K, Hata H, Shimizu H. Lipofuscin deposition causes the pigmentation of apocrine hidrocystoma. *J Dermatol*. 2018;45(1):91–94.

430. Gross BG. The fine structure of apocrine hidrocystoma. *Arch Dermatol*. 1965;92(6):706–712.

431. Hassan MO, Khan MA, Kruse TV. Apocrine cystadenoma. An ultrastructural study. *Arch Dermatol*. 1979;115(2):194–200.

432. Schaumburg-Lever G, Lever WF. Secretion from human apocrine glands: an electron microscopic study. *J Invest Dermatol*. 1975;64(1):38–41.

433. Johnson G, Gardner JM, Shalin SC. Polarizable crystals in apocrine sweat gland tumors: a series of 3 cases. *J Cutan Pathol*. 2017;44(8):698–702.

434. Zhu L, Okano S, Takahara M, et al. Expression of S100 protein family members in normal skin and sweat gland tumors. *J Dermatol Sci*. 2013;70(3):211–219.

435. Goette DK. Hidradenoma papilliferum. *J Am Acad Dermatol*. 1988;19(1, pt 1):133–135.

436. Ioannides G. Hidradenoma papilliferum. *Am J Obstet Gynecol*. 1966;94(6):849–853.

437. Virgili A, Marzola A, Corazza M. Vulvar hidradenoma papilliferum. A review of 10.5 years' experience. *J Reprod Med*. 2000;45(8):616–618.

438. Vortel V, Kraus Z, Andrys J. [Hidradenoma papilliferum vulvae]. *Cesk Gynekol*. 1972;37(1):58–59.

439. Loane J, Kealy WF, Mulcahy G. Perianal hidradenoma papilliferum occurring in a male: a case report. *Ir J Med Sci*. 1998;167(1):26–27.

440. Vang R, Cohen PR. Ectopic hidradenoma papilliferum: a case report and review of the literature. *J Am Acad Dermatol*. 1999;41(1):115–118.

441. Nissim F, Czernobilsky B, Ostfeld E. Hidradenoma papilliferum of the external auditory canal. *J Laryngol Otol.* 1981;95(8):843–848.

442. Santa Cruz DJ, Prioleau PG, Smith ME. Hidradenoma papilliferum of the eyelid. *Arch Dermatol.* 1981;117(1):55–56.

443. Olecki EJ, Scow JS. Hidradenoma papilliferum of the anus: a case report about the relationship between neoplasms of the mammary-like-glands and hormones. *Cureus.* 2021;13(2):e13061.

444. Bannatyne P, Elliott P, Russell P. Vulvar adenosquamous carcinoma arising in a hidradenoma papilliferum, with rapidly fatal outcome: case report. *Gynecol Oncol.* 1989;35(3):395–398.

445. Shenoy Y. Malignant perianal papillary hidradenoma. *Arch Dermatol.* 1961;83:965.

446. Meeker J, Neubecker R, Helwig E. Hidradenoma papilliferum. *Am J Clin Pathol.* 1962;37:182–195.

447. Hashimoto K. Hidradenoma papilliferum. An electron microscopic study. *Acta Derm Venereol.* 1973;53(1):22–30.

448. Cassarino DS, Su A, Robbins BA, Altree-Tacha D, Ra S. SOX10 immunohistochemistry in sweat ductal/glandular neoplasms. *J Cutan Pathol.* 2017;44(6):544–547.

449. Goto K. The role of DOG1 immunohistochemistry in dermatopathology. *J Cutan Pathol.* 2016;43(11):974–983.

450. Vazmitel M, Spagnolo DV, Nemcova J, Michal M, Kazakov DV. Hidradenoma papilliferum with a ductal carcinoma in situ component: case report and review of the literature. *Am J Dermatopathol.* 2008;30(4):392–394.

451. Kazakov DV, Mikyskova I, Kutzner H, et al. Hidradenoma papilliferum with oxyphilic metaplasia: a clinicopathological study of 18 cases, including detection of human papillomavirus. *Am J Dermatopathol.* 2005;27(2):102–110.

452. Pfarr N, Allgauer M, Steiger K, et al. Several genotypes, one phenotype: PIK3CA/AKT1 mutation-negative hidradenoma papilliferum show genetic lesions in other components of the signalling network. *Pathology.* 2019;51(4):362–368.

453. de Bliek JP, Starink TM. Multiple linear syringocystadenoma papilliferum. *J Eur Acad Dermatol Venereol.* 1999;12(1):74–76.

454. Goldberg NS, Esterly NB. Linear papules on the neck of a child. Syringocystadenoma papilliferum. *Arch Dermatol.* 1985;121(9):1198, 1201.

455. Helwig EB, Hackney VC. Syringadenoma papilliferum; lesions with and without naevus sebaceous and basal cell carcinoma. *AMA Arch Dermatol.* 1955;71(3):361–372.

456. Rostan SE, Waller JD. Syringocystadenoma papilliferum in an unusual location. Report of a case. *Arch Dermatol.* 1976;112(6):835–836.

457. Pinkus H. Life history of naevus syringadenomatosus papilliferus. *AMA Arch Dermatol Syphilol.* 1954;69(3):305–322.

458. Hashimoto K. Syringocystadenoma papilliferum. An electron microscopic study. *Arch Dermatol Forsch.* 1972;245(4):353–369.

459. Fusaro RM, Goltz RW. Histochemically demonstrable carbohydrates of appendageal tumors of the skin. *J Invest Dermatol.* 1962;38:137–142.

460. Mambo NC. Immunohistochemical study of the immunoglobulin classes of the plasma cells in papillary syringadenoma. *Virchows Arch A Pathol Anat Histol.* 1982;397(1):1–6.

461. Vanatta PR, Bangert JL, Freeman RG. Syringocystadenoma papilliferum. A plasmacytotropic tumor. *Am J Surg Pathol.* 1985;9(9):678–683.

462. Numata M, Hosoe S, Itoh N, Munakata Y, Hayashi S, Maruyama Y. Syringadenocarcinoma papilliferum. *J Cutan Pathol.* 1985;12(1):3–7.

463. Mazoujian G, Margolis R. Immunohistochemistry of gross cystic disease fluid protein (GCDFP-15) in 65 benign sweat gland tumors of the skin. *Am J Dermatopathol.* 1988;10(1):28–35.

464. Noda Y, Kumasa S, Higashiyama H, Mori M. Immunolocalization of keratin proteins in sweat gland tumours by the use of monoclonal antibody. *Pathol Res Pract.* 1988;183(3):284–291.

465. Boni R, Xin H, Hohl D, Panizzon R, Burg G. Syringocystadenoma papilliferum: a study of potential tumor suppressor genes. *Am J Dermatopathol.* 2001;23(2):87–89.

466. Konstantinova AM, Kyrpychova L, Nemcova J, et al. Syringocystadenoma papilliferum of the anogenital area and buttocks: a report of 16 cases, including human papillomavirus analysis and HRAS and BRAF V600 mutation studies. *Am J Dermatopathol.* 2019;41(4):281–285.

467. Burket JM, Zelickson AS. Tubular apocrine adenoma with perineural invasion. *J Am Acad Dermatol.* 1984;11(4, pt 1):639–642.

468. Civatte J, Belaich S, Lauret P. Adenome tubulaire apocrine (quatre cas). *Ann Dermatol Venereol.* 1979;106(8–9):665–669.

469. Landry M, Winkelmann RK. An unusual tubular apocrine adenoma. *Arch Dermatol.* 1972;105(6):869–879.

470. Okun MR, Finn R, Blumental G. Apocrine adenoma versus pocrine carcinoma. Report of two cases. *J Am Acad Dermatol.* 1980;2(4):322–326.

471. Toribio J, Zulaica A, Peteiro C. Tubular apocrine adenoma. *J Cutan Pathol.* 1987;14(2):114–117.

472. Umbert P, Winkelmann RK. Tubular apocrine adenoma. *J Cutan Pathol.* 1976;3(2):75–87.

473. Ansai S, Watanabe S, Aso K. A case of tubular apocrine adenoma with syringocystadenoma papilliferum. *J Cutan Pathol.* 1989;16(4):230–236.

474. Ansai SI, Anan T, Fukumoto T, Saeki H. Tubulopapillary cystic adenoma with apocrine differentiation: a unifying concept for syringocystadenoma papilliferum, apocrine gland cyst, and tubular papillary adenoma. *Am J Dermatopathol.* 2017;39(11):829–837.

475. Liau JY, Tsai JH, Huang WC, Lan J, Hong JB, Yuan CT. BRAF and KRAS mutations in tubular apocrine adenoma and papillary eccrine adenoma of the skin. *Hum Pathol.* 2018;73:59–65.

476. Falck VG, Jordaan HF. Papillary eccrine adenoma. A tubulopapillary hidradenoma with eccrine differentiation. *Am J Dermatopathol.* 1986;8(1):64–72.

477. Fox SB, Cotton DW. Tubular apocrine adenoma and papillary eccrine adenoma. Entities or unity? *Am J Dermatopathol.* 1992;14(2):149–154.

478. Ishiko A, Shimizu H, Inamoto N, Nakmura K. Is tubular apocrine adenoma a distinct clinical entity? *Am J Dermatopathol.* 1993;15(5):482–487.

479. Assor D, Davis JB. Multiple apocrine fibroadenomas of the anal skin. *Am J Clin Pathol.* 1977;68(3):397–399.

480. Warkel RL, Helwig EB. Apocrine gland adenoma and adenocarcinoma of the axilla. *Arch Dermatol.* 1978;114(2):198–203.

481. Weigand DA, Burgdorf WH. Perianal apocrine gland adenoma. *Arch Dermatol.* 1980;116(9):1051–1053.

482. Lewis HM, Ovitz ML, Golitz LE. Erosive adenomatosis of the nipple. *Arch Dermatol.* 1976;112(10):1427–1428.

483. Pratt-Thomas HR. Erosive adenomatosis of the nipple. *J S C Med Assoc.* 1968;64(2):37–40.

484. Smith EJ, Kron SD, Gross PR. Erosive adenomatosis of the nipple. *Arch Dermatol.* 1970;102(3):330–332.

485. Smith NP, Jones EW. Erosive adenomatosis of the nipple. *Clin Exp Dermatol.* 1977;2(1):79–84.

486. Albers SE, Barnard M, Thorner P, Krafchik BR. Erosive adenomatosis of the nipple in an eight-year-old girl. *J Am Acad Dermatol.* 1999;40(5, pt 2):834–837.

487. Diaz NM, Palmer JO, Wick MR. Erosive adenomatosis of the nipple: histology, immunohistology, and differential diagnosis. *Mod Pathol.* 1992;5(2):179–184.

488. Brownstein MH, Phelps RG, Magnin PH. Papillary adenoma of the nipple: analysis of fifteen new cases. *J Am Acad Dermatol.* 1985;12(4):707–715.

489. Crain RC, Helwig EB. Dermal cylindroma (dermal eccrine cylindroma). *Am J Clin Pathol.* 1961;35:504–515.

490. Baden H. Cylindromatosis simulating neurofibromatosis. *N Engl J Med.* 1962;267:296.

491. Gottschalk HR. Proceedings: dermal eccrine cylindroma, epithelioma adenoides cysticum of Brooke, and ecrine spiradenoma. *Arch Dermatol.* 1974;110(3):473–474.

492. Headington JT, Batsakis JG, Beals TF, Campbell TE, Simmons JL, Stone WD. Membranous basal cell adenoma of parotid gland, dermal cylindromas, and trichoepitheliomas. Comparative histochemistry and ultrastructure. *Cancer.* 1977;39(6):2460–2469.

493. Lausecker H. Beitrag zu den naevo-epitheliomen. *Arch Dermatol Syph.* 1952;194:639.

494. Welch JP, Wells RS, Kerr CB. Ancell-Spiegler cylindromas (turban tumours) and Brooke-Fordyce Trichoepitheliomas: evidence for a single genetic entity. *J Med Genet.* 1968;5(1):29–35.

495. Berberian BJ, Sulica VI, Kao GF. Familial multiple eccrine spiradenomas with cylindromatous features associated with epithelioma adenoides cysticum of Brooke. *Cutis.* 1990;46(1):46–50.

496. Burrows NP, Jones RR, Smith NP. The clinicopathological features of familial cylindromas and trichoepitheliomas (Brooke-Spiegler syndrome): a report of two families. *Clin Exp Dermatol.* 1992;17(5):332–336.

497. Delfino M, D'Anna F, Ianniello S, Donofrio V. Multiple hereditary trichoepithelioma and cylindroma (Brooke-Spiegler syndrome). *Dermatologica.* 1991;183(2):150–153.

498. Ferrandiz C, Campo E, Baumann E. Dermal cylindromas (turban tumour) and eccrine spiradenomas in a patient with membranous basal cell adenoma of the parotid gland. *J Cutan Pathol.* 1985;12(1):72–79.

499. Goette DK, McConnell MA, Fowler VR. Cylindroma and eccrine spiradenoma coexistent in the same lesion. *Arch Dermatol.* 1982;118(4):274–274.

500. Urbach F, Graham JH, Goldstein J, Munger BL. Dermal eccrine cylindroma: a histochemical, electron microscopic, and therapeutic (X-ray) study. *Arch Dermatol.* 1963;88:880–894.

501. Cotton DW, Braye SG. Dermal cylindromas originate from the eccrine sweat gland. *Br J Dermatol.* 1984;111(1):53–61.

502. Kallioinen M. Immunoelectron microscope demonstration of the basement membrane components laminin and type IV collagen in the dermal cylindroma. *J Pathol.* 1985;147(2):97–102.

503. Penneys NS, Kaiser M. Cylindroma expresses immunohistochemical markers linking it to eccrine coil. *J Cutan Pathol.* 1993;20(1):40–43.

504. Tellechea O, Reis JP, Ilheu O, Baptista AP. Dermal cylindroma. An immunohistochemical study of thirteen cases. *Am J Dermatopathol.* 1995;17(3):260–265.

505. Hashimoto K, Lever WF. Histogenesis of skin appendage tumors. *Arch Dermatol.* 1969;100(3):356–369.

506. Munger BL, Graham JH, Helwig EB. Ultrastructure and histochemical characteristics of dermal eccrine cylindroma (turban tumor). *J Invest Dermatol.* 1962;39:577–595.

507. Bignell GR, Warren W, Seal S, et al. Identification of the familial cylindromatosis tumour-suppressor gene. *Nat Genet.* 2000;25(2):160–165.

508. Gutierrez PP, Eggermann T, Holler D, et al. Phenotype diversity in familial cylindromatosis: a frameshift mutation in the tumor suppressor gene CYLD underlies different tumors of skin appendages. *J Invest Dermatol.* 2002;119(2):527–531.

509. Rajan N, Andersson MK, Sinclair N, et al. Overexpression of MYB drives proliferation of CYLD-defective cylindroma cells. *J Pathol.* 2016;239(2):197–205.

510. Davies HR, Hodgson K, Schwalbe E, et al. Epigenetic modifiers DNMT3A and BCOR are recurrently mutated in CYLD cutaneous syndrome. *Nat Commun.* 2019;10(1):4717.

511. Weber L, Wick G, Gebhart W, Krieg T, Timpl R. Basement membrane components outline the tumour islands in cylindroma. *Br J Dermatol.* 1984;111(1):45–51.

512. Bondeson L. Malignant dermal eccrine cylindroma. *Acta Dermato-Venereologica.* 1979;59(1):92–94.

513. Durani BK, Kurzen H, Jaeckel A, Kuner N, Naeher H, Hartschuh W. Malignant transformation of multiple dermal cylindromas. *Br J Dermatol.* 2001;145(4):653–656.

514. Gerretsen AL, van der Putte SC, Deenstra W, van Vloten WA. Cutaneous cylindroma with malignant transformation. *Cancer.* 1993;72(5):1618–1623.

515. Hammond DC, Grant KF, Simpson WD. Malignant degeneration of dermal cylindroma. *Ann Plast Surg.* 1990;24(2):176–178.

516. Lin PY, Fatteh SM, Lloyd KM. Malignant transformation in a solitary dermal cylindroma. *Arch Pathol Lab Med.* 1987;111(8):765–767.

517. Lotem M, Trattner A, Kahanovich S, Rotem A, Sandbank M. Multiple dermal cylindroma undergoing a malignant transformation. *Int J Dermatol.* 1992;31(9):642–644.

518. Ma A, Goldberg R, Medenica M, Lo JS. Malignant cylindroma of the scalp. *J Am Acad Dermatol.* 1991;25(5, pt 2):960–964.

519. Galadari E, Mehregan AH, Lee KC. Malignant transformation of eccrine tumors. *J Cutan Pathol.* 1987;14(1):15–22.

520. Urbanski SJ, From L, Abramowicz A, Joaquin A, Luk SC. Metamorphosis of dermal cylindroma: possible relation to malignant transformation. Case report of cutaneous cylindroma with direct intracranial invasion. *J Am Acad Dermatol.* 1985;12(1, pt 2):188–195.

521. Beideck MKA. Maligne entartung bei kutanen zylindromen. *Z Hautkr.* 1985;60:73.

522. Luger A. Das cylindrom der haut und seine maligne degeneration. *Arch Dermatol Syph.* 1949;188:155.

523. Goldstein N. Ephidrosis (local hyperhidrosis): nevus sudoriferus. *Arch Dermatol.* 1967;96:67.

524. Arnold H. Nevus seborrheicus et sudoriferus. *Arch Dermatol.* 1945;51:370.

525. Herzberg J. Ekkrines syringocystadenom. *Arch Klin Exp Dermatol.* 1962;214:600.

526. Imai S, Nitto H. Eccrine nevus with epidermal changes. *Dermatologica.* 1983;166(2):84–88.

527. Hyman AB, Harris H, Brownstein MH. Eccrine angiomatous hamartoma. *N Y State J Med.* 1968;68(21):2803–2806.

528. Zeller DJ, Goldman RL. Eccrine-pilar angiomatous hamartoma. Report of a unique case. *Dermatologica.* 1971;143(2):100–104.

529. Challa VR, Jona J. Eccrine angiomatous hamartoma: a rare skin lesion with diverse histological features. *Dermatologica.* 1977;155(4):206–209.

530. Tempark T, Shwayder T. Mucinous eccrine naevus: case report and review of the literature. *Clin Exp Dermatol.* 2013;38(1):1–4; quiz 5–6.

531. Sanmartin O, Botella R, Alegre V, Martinez A, Aliaga A. Congenital eccrine angiomatous hamartoma. *Am J Dermatopathol.* 1992;14(2):161–164.

532. Velasco JA, Almeida V. Eccrine-pilar angiomatous nevus. *Dermatologica.* 1988;177(5):317–322.

533. Donati P, Amantea A, Balus L. Eccrine angiomatous hamartoma: a lipomatous variant. *J Cutan Pathol.* 1989;16(4):227–229.

534. Dua J, Grabczynska S. Eccrine nevus affecting the forearm of an 11-year-old girl successfully controlled with topical glycopyrrolate. *Pediatr Dermatol.* 2014;31(5):611–612.

535. Smith JD, Chernosky ME. Hidrocystomas. *Arch Dermatol.* 1973;108(5):676–679.

536. Cordero A, Montes LF. Eccrine hidrocystoma. *J Cutan Pathol.* 1976;3:292.

537. Hassan MO, Khan MA. Ultrastructure of eccrine cystadenoma. A case report. *Arch Dermatol.* 1979;115(10):1217–1221.

538. Simon RS, Sanches YE. Does eccrine hidrocystoma exist? *J Cutan Pathol.* 1998;25(3):182–184.

539. Jakobiec FA, Zakka FR. A reappraisal of eyelid eccrine and apocrine hidrocystomas: microanatomic and immunohistochemical studies of 40 lesions. *Am J Ophthalmol.* 2011;151(2):358–374 e352.

540. Sperling LC, Sakas EL. Eccrine hidrocystomas. *J Am Acad Dermatol.* 1982;7(6):763–770.

541. Ebner H, Erlach E. Ekkrine hidrozystome. *Dermatol Wochenschr.* 1975;161(9):739–744.

542. Brown SM, Freeman RG. Syringoma limited to the vulva. *Arch Dermatol.* 1971;104(3):331.

543. Goyal S, Martins CR. Multiple syringomas on the abdomen, thighs, and groin. *Cutis.* 2000;66(4):259–262.

544. Lo JS, Dijkstra JW, Bergfeld WF. Syringomas on the penis. *Int J Dermatol.* 1990;29(4):309–310.

545. Thomas J, Majmudar B, Gorelkin L. Syringoma localized to the vulva. *Arch Dermatol.* 1979;115(1):95–96.

546. Hashimoto K, DiBella RJ, Borsuk GM, Lever WF. Eruptive hidradenoma and syringoma. Histological, histochemical, and electron microscopic studies. *Arch Dermatol.* 1967;96(5):500–519.

547. Guitart J, Rosenbaum MM, Requena L. "Eruptive syringoma": a misnomer for a reactive eccrine gland ductal proliferation? *J Cutan Pathol.* 2003;30(3):202–205.

548. Chandler WM, Bosenberg MW. Autoimmune acrosyringitis with ductal cysts: reclassification of case of eruptive syringoma. *J Cutan Pathol.* 2009;36(12):1312–1315.

549. Suwattee P, McClelland MC, Huiras EE, et al. Plaque-type syringoma: two cases misdiagnosed as microcystic adnexal carcinoma. *J Cutan Pathol.* 2008;35(6):570–574.

550. Yung CW, Soltani K, Bernstein JE, Lorincz AL. Unilateral linear nevoidal syringoma. *J Am Acad Dermatol.* 1981;4(4):412–416.

551. Shelley WB, Wood MG. Occult syringomas of scalp associated with progressive hair loss. *Arch Dermatol.* 1980;116(7):843–844.

552. Ciarloni L, Frouin E, Bodin F, Cribier B. Syringoma: a clinicopathological study of 244 cases. *Ann Dermatol Venereol.* 2016;143(8–9):521–528.

553. Headington JT, Koski J, Murphy PJ. Clear cell glycogenosis in multiple syringomas. Description and enzyme histochemistry. *Arch Dermatol.* 1972;106(3):353–356.

554. Feibelman CE, Maize JC. Clear-cell syringoma. A study by conventional and electron microscopy. *Am J Dermatopathol.* 1984;6(2):139–150.

555. Asai Y, Ishii M, Hamada T. Acral syringoma: electron microscopic studies on its origin. *Acta Dermato-Venereologica.* 1982;62(1):64–68.

556. Winkelmann RK, Muller SA. Sweat gland tumors. I. Histochemical studies. *Arch Dermatol.* 1964;89:827–831.

557. Mustakallio KK. Succinic dehydrogenase activity of syringomas. *Acta Derm Venereol.* 1959;39:318–323.

558. Lezcano C, Ho J, Seethala RR. Sox10 and DOG1 expression in primary adnexal tumors of the skin. *Am J Dermatopathol.* 2017;39(12):896–902.

559. Goldstein DJ, Barr RJ, Santa Cruz DJ. Microcystic adnexal carcinoma: a distinct clinicopathologic entity. *Cancer.* 1982;50(3):566–572.

560. Goldman P, Pinkus H, Rogin JR. Eccrine poroma; tumors exhibiting features of the epidermal sweat duct unit. *AMA Arch Derm.* 1956;74(5):511–521.

561. Hyman AB, Brownstein MH. Eccrine poroma. An analysis of forty-five new cases. *Dermatologica.* 1969;138(1):29–38.

562. Moore TO, Orman HL, Orman SK, Helm KF. Poromas of the head and neck. *J Am Acad Dermatol.* 2001;44(1):48–52.

563. Vu PP, Whitehead KJ, Sullivan TJ. Eccrine poroma of the eyelid. *Clin Exp Ophthalmol.* 2001;29(4):253–255.

564. Okun MA, Ansell HB. Eccrine poroma. *Arch Dermatol.* 1963;88:561.

565. Penneys NS, Ackerman AB, Indgin SN, Mandy SH. Eccrine poroma: two unusual variants. *Br J Dermatol.* 1970;82(6):613–615.

566. Mahlberg MJ, McGinnis KS, Draft KS, Fakharzadeh SS. Multiple eccrine poromas in the setting of total body irradiation and immunosuppression. *J Am Acad Dermatol.* 2006;55(2 suppl): S46–S49.

567. Kurokawa M, Amano M, Miyaguni H, et al. Eccrine poromas in a patient with mycosis fungoides treated with electron beam therapy. *Br J Dermatol.* 2001;145(5):830–833.

568. Fujii K, Aochi S, Takeshima C, et al. Eccrine poromatosis associated with polychemotherapy. *Acta Derm Venereol.* 2012;92(6):687–690.

569. Goldner R. Eccrine poromatosis. *Arch Dermatol.* 1970;101(5):606–608.

570. Wilkinson RD, Schopflocher P, Rozenfeld M. Hidrotic ectodermal dysplasia with diffuse eccrine poromatosis. *Arch Dermatol.* 1977;113(4):472–476.

571. Freeman RG, Knox JM, Spiller WF. Eccrine poroma. *Am J Clin Pathol.* 1961;36:444–450.

572. Yasuda T, Kawada A, Yoshida K. Eccrine poroma. A Japanese case showing melanin granules and melanocytes in the tumor. *Arch Dermatol.* 1964;90:428–431.

573. Knox J, Spiller W. Eccrine poroma. *Arch Dermatol.* 1958;77:726.

574. Krinitz K. Malignes itraepidermales ekkrines porom. *Z Haut Geschlechtskr.* 1972;47(1):9–17.

575. Coburn JG, Smith JL. Hidroacanthoma simplex. *Br J Dermatol.* 1956;68:400.

576. Mehregan AH, Levson DN. Hidroacanthoma simplex. A report of two cases. *Arch Dermatol.* 1969;100(3):303–305.

577. Winkelmann RM, McLeod WA. The dermal duct tumor. *Arch Dermatol.* 1966;94:50.

578. Rahbari H. Syringoacanthoma. Acanthotic lesion of the acrosyringium. *Arch Dermatol.* 1984;120(6):751–756.

579. Winkelmann RK, McLeod WA. The dermal duct tumor. *Arch Dermatol.* 1966;94(1):50–55.

580. Hashimoto KL, Lever WF. Eccrine poroma: histochemical and electron microscopic studies. *J Invest Dermatol.* 1964;43:237.

581. Sanderson KV, Ryan EA. The histochemistry of eccrine poroma. *Br J Dermatol.* 1963;75:86–88.

582. Prieto-Granada C, Morlote D, Pavlidakey P, et al. Poroid adnexal skin tumors with YAP1 fusions exhibit similar histopathologic features: a series of six YAP1-rearranged adnexal skin tumors. *J Cutan Pathol.* 2021;48:1139–1149.

583. Russell-Goldman E, Hornick JL, Hanna J. Utility of YAP1 and NUT immunohistochemistry in the diagnosis of porocarcinoma. *J Cutan Pathol.* 2021;48(3):403–410.

584. Hu CH, Marques AS, Winkelmann RK. Dermal duct tumor: a histochemical and electron microscopic study. *Arch Dermatol.* 1978;114(11):1659–1664.

585. Pinkus H, Mehregan AH. Epidermotropic eccrine carcinoma. A case combining features of eccrine poroma and Paget's dermatosis. *Arch Dermatol.* 1963;88:597–606.

586. Mishima Y, Morioka S. Oncogenic differentiation of the intraepidermal eccrine sweat duct: eccrine poroma, poroepithelioma and porocarcinoma. *Dermatologica.* 1969;138(4):238–250.

587. Bardach H. Hidroacanthoma simplex with in situ porocarcinoma. A case suggesting malignant transformation. *J Cutan Pathol.* 1978;5(5):236–248.

588. Gschnait F, Horn F, Lindlbauer R, Sponer D. Eccrine porocarcinoma. *J Cutan Pathol.* 1980;7(6):349–353.

589. Mohri S, Chika K, Saito I, Yagishita K. A case of porocarcinoma. *J Dermatol.* 1980;7(6):431–434.

590. Ishikawa K. Malignant hidroacanthoma simplex. *Arch Dermatol.* 1971;104:529.

591. Pena J, Suster S. Squamous differentiation in malignant eccrine poroma. *Am J Dermatopathol.* 1993;15(5):492–496.

592. Mahalingam M, Richards JE, Selim MA, Muzikansky A, Hoang MP. An immunohistochemical comparison of cytokeratin 7, cytokeratin 15, cytokeratin 19, CAM 5.2, carcinoembryonic antigen, and nestin in differentiating porocarcinoma from squamous cell carcinoma. *Hum Pathol.* 2012;43(8):1265–1272.

593. Afshar M, Deroide F, Robson A. BerEP4 is widely expressed in tumors of the sweat apparatus: a source of potential diagnostic error. *J Cutan Pathol.* 2013;40(2):259–264.

594. Cangelosi JJ, Nash JW, Prieto VG, Ivan D. Cutaneous adnexal tumor with an unusual presentation—discussion of a potential diagnostic pitfall. *Am J Dermatopathol.* 2009;31(3):278–281.

595. Urso C, Paglierani M, Bondi R. Histologic spectrum of carcinomas with eccrine ductal differentiation: sweat-gland ductal carcinomas. *Am J Dermatopathol.* 1993;15:435.

596. Kolde G, Macher E, Grundmann E. Metastasizing eccrine porocarcinoma. Report of two cases with fatal outcome. *Pathol Res Pract.* 1991;187(4):477–481.

597. Lee KA, Cioni M, Robson A, Bataille V. Metastatic porocarcinoma achieving complete radiological and clinical response with pembrolizumab. *BMJ Case Rep.* 2019;12(9):e228917.

598. Nagasawa T, Hirata A, Niiyama S, Enomoto Y, Fukuda H. Successful treatment of porocarcinoma with maxacalcitol and imiquimod. *Dermatol Ther.* 2019;32(2):e12830.

599. Godillot C, Boulinguez S, Riffaud L, et al. Complete response of a metastatic porocarcinoma treated with paclitaxel, cetuximab and radiotherapy. *Eur J Cancer.* 2018;90:142–145.

600. Weedon D, Lewis J. Acrosyringeal nevus. *J Cutan Pathol.* 1977;4(3):166–168.

601. Mehregan AH, Marufi M, Medenica M. Eccrine syringofibroadenoma (Mascaro). Report of two cases. *J Am Acad Dermatol.* 1985;13(3):433–436.

602. Mascaro J. Considérations sur les tumeurs fibroépithéliales: le syringofibroadénome eccrine. *Ann Dermatol Syphilgr.* 1963;90:143.

603. Weedon D. Eccrine syringofibroadenoma versus acrosyringeal nevus. *J Am Acad Dermatol.* 1987;16(3, pt 1):622–623.

604. Ogino A. Linear eccrine poroma. *Arch Dermatol.* 1976;112(6):841–844.

605. Gkolfinopoulos T, Ingen-Housz-Oro S, Cavelier-Balloy B, Blanchet-Bardon C. Syndrome de Schopf-Schulz-Passarge: 2 observations. *Dermatology.* 1997;195(4):309–310.

606. Simpson EL, Styles AR, Cockerell CJ. Eccrine syringofibroadenomatosis associated with hidrotic ectodermal dysplasia. *Br J Dermatol.* 1998;138(5):879–884.

607. Poonawalla T, Xia L, Patten S, Stratman EJ. Clouston syndrome and eccrine syringofibroadenomas. *Am J Dermatopathol.* 2009;31(2):157–161.

608. Starink TM. Eccrine syringofibroadenoma: multiple lesions representing a new cutaneous marker of the Schopf syndrome, and solitary nonhereditary tumors. *J Am Acad Dermatol.* 1997;36(4):569–576.

609. Bjarke T, Ternesten-Bratel A, Hedblad M, Rausing A. Carcinoma and eccrine syringofibroadenoma: a report of five cases. *J Cutan Pathol.* 2003;30(6):382–392.

610. Katane M, Akiyama M, Ohnishi T, Watanabe S, Matsuo I. Carcinomatous transformation of eccrine syringofibroadenoma. *J Cutan Pathol.* 2003;30(3):211–214.

611. Fretzin DF, Sloan JB, Beer K, Fretzin SA. Eccrine syringofibroadenoma. A clear-cell variant. *Am J Dermatopathol.* 1995;17(6):591–593.

612. Duffy KL, Bowen AR, Tristani-Firouzi P, Florell SR, Hadley ML. Eccrine syringofibroadenoma-like change adjacent to a squamous cell carcinoma: potential histologic pitfall in Mohs micrographic surgery. *Dermatol Surg.* 2009;35(3):519–522.

613. Schadt CR, Boyd AS. Eccrine syringofibroadenoma with co-existent squamous cell carcinoma. *J Cutan Pathol.* 2007;34(suppl 1):71–74.

614. French LE, Masgrau E, Chavaz P, Saurat JH. Eccrine syringofibroadenoma in a patient with erosive palmoplantar lichen planus. *Dermatology.* 1997;195(4):399–401.

615. Nomura K, Kogawa T, Hashimoto I, Katabira Y. Eccrine syringofibroadenomatous hyperplasia in a patient with bullous

616. Fouilloux B, Perrin C, Dutoit M, Cambazard F. Clear cell syringofibroadenoma (of Mascaro) of the nail. *Br J Dermatol.* 2001;144(3):625–627.

617. Kanitakis J, Zambruno G, Euvrard S, Hermier C, Thivolet J. Eccrine syringofibroadenoma. Immunohistological study of a new case. *Am J Dermatopathol.* 1987;9(1):37–40.

618. Ishida-Yamamoto A, Iizuka H, Eady RA. Filaggrin immunoreactive composite keratohyalin granules specific to acrosyringia and related tumours. *Acta Derm Venereol.* 1994;74(1):37–42.

619. Ohnishi T, Suzuki T, Watanabe S. Eccrine syringofibroadenoma. Report of a case and immunohistochemical study of keratin expression. *Br J Dermatol.* 1995;133(3):449–454.

620. Ishida-Yamamoto A, Iizuka H. Eccrine syringofibroadenoma (Mascaro). An ultrastructural and immunohistochemical study. *Am J Dermatopathol.* 1996;18(2):207–211.

621. Sueki H, Miller SJ, Dzubow LM, Murphy GF. Eccrine syringofibroadenoma (Mascaro): an ultrastructural study. *J Cutan Pathol.* 1992;19(3):232–239.

622. Morganti AG, Martone FR, Macchia G, et al. Eccrine syringofibroadenoma radiation treatment of an unusual presentation. *Dermatol Ther.* 2010;23(suppl 1):S20–S23.

623. King DT, Barr RJ. Syringometaplasia: mucinous and squamous variants. *J Cutan Pathol.* 1979;6(4):284–291.

624. Kwittken J. Muciparous epidermal tumor. *Arch Dermatol.* 1974;109(4):554–555.

625. Scully K, Assaad D. Mucinous syringometaplasia. *J Am Acad Dermatol.* 1984;11(3):503–508.

626. Mehregan AH. Mucinous syringometaplasia. *Arch Dermatol.* 1980;116(9):988–989.

627. Bergman R, David R, Friedman-Birnbaum R, Harth Y, Bassan L. Mucinous syringometaplasia. An immunohistochemical and ultrastructural study of a case. *Am J Dermatopathol.* 1996;18(5):521–526.

628. Shelley W, Wood MG. A zosteriform network of spiradenoma. *J Am Acad Dermatol.* 1980;2:59.

629. Munger BB, Berghorn BM, Helwig EB. A light and electron-microscopic study of a case of multiple eccrine spiradenoma. *J Invest Dermatol.* 1962;38:289.

630. Hashimoto K, Gross BG, Nelson RG, Lever WF. Eccrine spiradenoma. Histochemical and electron microscopic studies. *J Invest Dermatol.* 1966;46(4):347–365.

631. Tsur H, Lipskier E, Fisher BK. Multiple linear spiradenomas. *Plast Reconstr Surg.* 1981;68(1):100–102.

632. Mambo NC. Eccrine spiradenoma: clinical and pathologic study of 49 tumors. *J Cutan Pathol.* 1983;10(5):312–320.

633. Kersting D, Helwig EB. Eccrine spiradenoma. *Arch Dermatol Syph.* 1956;73:199.

634. Lever W. Myoepithelial sweat gland tumor: myoepithelioma. *Arch Dermatol Syph.* 1948;57:332.

635. Castro C, Winkelmann RK. Spiradenoma: histochemical and electron microscopic study. *Arch Dermatol.* 1974;109:40.

636. van den Oord JJ, De Wolf-Peeters C. Perivascular spaces in eccrine spiradenoma. A clue to its histological diagnosis. *Am J Dermatopathol.* 1995;17(3):266–270.

637. Hashimoto K, Kanzaki T. Appendage tumors of the skin: histogenesis and ultrastructure. *J Cutan Pathol.* 1984;11(5):365–381.

638. Winkelmann RK, Wolff K. Histochemistry of hidradenoma and eccrine spiradenoma. *J Invest Dermatol.* 1967;49(2):173–180.

639. Watanabe S, Hirose M, Sato S, Takahashi H. Immunohistochemical analysis of cytokeratin expression in eccrine spiradenoma: similarities to the transitional portions between secretory segments and coiled ducts of eccrine glands. *Br J Dermatol.* 1994;131(6):799–807.

640. Rajan N, Langtry JA, Ashworth A, et al. Tumor mapping in 2 large multigenerational families with CYLD mutations: implications for disease management and tumor induction. *Arch Dermatol.* 2009;145(11):1277–1284.

641. Sellheyer K. Spiradenoma and cylindroma originate from the hair follicle bulge and not from the eccrine sweat gland: an immunohistochemical study with CD200 and other stem cell markers. *J Cutan Pathol.* 2015;42(2):90–101.

642. Meybehm M, Fischer HP. Spiradenoma and dermal cylindroma: comparative immunohistochemical analysis and histogenetic considerations. *Am J Dermatopathol.* 1997;19(2):154–161.

643. Kazakov DV, Magro G, Kutzner H, et al. Spiradenoma and spiradenocylindroma with an adenomatous or atypical adenomatous component: a clinicopathological study of 6 cases. *Am J Dermatopathol.* 2008;30(5):436–441.

644. Rashid M, van der Horst M, Mentzel T, et al. ALPK1 hotspot mutation as a driver of human spiradenoma and spiradenocarcinoma. *Nat Commun.* 2019;10(1):2213.

645. Cooper PH, Frierson HF Jr, Morrison AG. Malignant transformation of eccrine spiradenoma. *Arch Dermatol.* 1985;121(11):1445–1448.

646. Wick MR, Swanson PE, Kaye VN, Pittelkow MR. Sweat gland carcinoma ex eccrine spiradenoma. *Am J Dermatopathol.* 1987;9(2):90–98.

647. Granter SR, Seeger K, Calonje E, Busam K, McKee PH. Malignant eccrine spiradenoma (spiradenocarcinoma): a clinicopathologic study of 12 cases. *Am J Dermatopathol.* 2000;22(2):97–103.

648. Dabska M. Malignant transformation of eccrine spiradenoma. *Pol Med J.* 1972;11(2):388–396.

649. Evans HL, Su D, Smith JL, Winkelmann RK. Carcinoma arising in eccrine spiradenoma. *Cancer.* 1979;43(5):1881–1884.

650. Andreoli MT, Itani KM. Malignant eccrine spiradenoma: a meta-analysis of reported cases. *Am J Surg.* 2011;201(5):695–699.

651. Herzberg A, Elenitsas R, Strohmeyer CR. Unusual case of early malignant transformation of spiradenoma. *Dermatol Surg Oncol.* 1995;21:1.

652. McKee PH, Fletcher CD, Stavrinos P, Pambakian H. Carcinosarcoma arising in eccrine spiradenoma. A clinicopathologic and immunohistochemical study of two cases. *Am J Dermatopathol.* 1990;12(4):335–343.

653. Saboorian MH, Kenny M, Ashfaq R, Albores-Saavedra J. Carcinosarcoma arising in eccrine spiradenoma of the breast. Report of a case and review of the literature. *Arch Pathol Lab Med.* 1996;120(5):501–504.

654. Itoh T, Yamamoto N, Tokunaga M. Malignant eccrine spiradenoma with smooth muscle cell differentiation: histological and immunohistochemical study. *Pathol Int.* 1996;46(11):887–893.

655. Kazakov DV, Zelger B, Rutten A, et al. Morphologic diversity of malignant neoplasms arising in preexisting spiradenoma, cylindroma, and spiradenocylindroma based on the study of 24 cases, sporadic or occurring in the setting of Brooke-Spiegler syndrome. *Am J Surg Pathol.* 2009;33(5):705–719.

656. Argenyi ZB, Nguyen AV, Balogh K, Sears JK, Whitaker DC. Malignant eccrine spiradenoma. A clinicopathologic study. *Am J Dermatopathol.* 1992;14(5):381–390.

657. Rulon DB, Helwig EB. Papillary eccrine adenoma. *Arch Dermatol.* 1977;113(5):596–598.

658. Urmacher C, Lieberman PH. Papillary eccrine adenoma. Light-microscopic, histochemical, and immunohistochemical studies. *Am J Dermatopathol.* 1987;9(3):243–249.

659. Falck VG, Jordaan HF. Papillary eccrine adenoma. A tubulopapillary hidradenoma with eccrine differentiation. *Am J Dermatopathol.* 1986;8(1):64–72.

660. Sexton M, Maize JC. Papillary eccrine adenoma. A light microscopic and immunohistochemical study. *J Am Acad Dermatol.* 1988;18(5, pt 1):1114–1120.

661. Megahed M, Holzle E. Papillary eccrine adenoma. A case report with immunohistochemical examination. *Am J Dermatopathol.* 1993;15(2):150–155.

662. Aloi F, Pich A. Papillary eccrine adenoma. A histopathological and immunohistochemical study. *Dermatologica.* 1991;182(1):47–51.

663. O'Hara J, Bensch K. Fine structure of eccrine sweat gland adenoma, clear cell type. *J Invest Dermatol.* 1967;49:261.

664. Lever W, Castleman B. Clear cell myoepithelioma of the skin. *Am J Pathol.* 1952;28:691.

665. Winkelmann RK, Wolff K. Solid-cystic hidradenoma of the skin. Clinical and histopathologic study. *Arch Dermatol.* 1968;97(6):651–661.

666. Johnson BL Jr, Helwig EB. Eccrine acrospiroma. A clinicopathologic study. *Cancer.* 1969;23(3):641–657.

667. Efskind J, Eker R. Myo-epitheliomas of the skin. *Acta Derm Venereol (Stockh).* 1954;34:279–283.

668. Kersting DW. Clear cell hidradenoma and hidradenocarcinoma. *Arch Dermatol.* 1963;87:323–333.

669. Hashimoto K, DiBella RJ, Lever WF. Clear cell hidradenoma. Histological, histochemical, and electron microscopic studies. *Arch Dermatol.* 1967;96(1):18–38.

670. Stanley RJ, Sanchez NP, Massa MC, Cooper AJ, Crotty CP, Winkelmann RK. Epidermoid hidradenoma. A clinicopathologic study. *J Cutan Pathol.* 1982;9(5):293–302.

671. Reddy SP, Chong K, Cassarino DS. A rare case of cutaneous oncocytic hidradenoma. *J Cutan Pathol.* 2017;44(3):289–291.

672. Haupt HM, Stern JB, Berlin SJ. Immunohistochemistry in the differential diagnosis of nodular hidradenoma and glomus tumor. *Am J Dermatopathol.* 1992;14(4):310–314.

673. Behboudi A, Winnes M, Gorunova L, et al. Clear cell hidradenoma of the skin—a third tumor type with a t(11;19)–associated TORC1-MAML2 gene fusion. *Genes Chromosomes Cancer.* 2005;43(2):202–205.

674. Mambo NC. The significance of atypical nuclear changes in benign eccrine acrospiromas: a clinical and pathological study of 18 cases. *J Cutan Pathol.* 1984;11(1):35–44.

675. Mehregan AH, Hashimoto K, Rahbari H. Eccrine adenocarcinoma. A clinicopathologic study of 35 cases. *Arch Dermatol.* 1983;119(2):104–114.

676. Keasbey L, Hadley G. Clear-cell hidradenoma: report of three cases with widespread metastases. *Cancer.* 1954;7:934.

677. Headington JT, Niederhuber JE, Beals TF. Malignant clear cell acrospiroma. *Cancer.* 1978;41(2):641–647.

678. Kazakov DV, Ivan D, Kutzner H, et al. Cutaneous hidradenocarcinoma: a clinicopathological, immunohistochemical, and molecular biologic study of 14 cases, including Her2/neu gene expression/amplification, TP53 gene mutation analysis, and t(11;19) translocation. *Am J Dermatopathol.* 2009;31(3):236–247.

679. Ko CJ, Cochran AJ, Eng W, Binder SW. Hidradenocarcinoma: a histological and immunohistochemical study. *J Cutan Pathol.* 2006;33(11):726–730.

680. Nazarian RM, Kapur P, Rakheja D, et al. Atypical and malignant hidradenomas: a histological and immunohistochemical study. *Mod Pathol.* 2009;22(4):600–610.

681. Obaidat NA, Alsaad KO, Ghazarian D. Skin adnexal neoplasms. Part 2: an approach to tumours of cutaneous sweat glands. *J Clin Pathol.* 2007;60(2):145–159.

682. Souvatzidis P, Sbano P, Mandato F, Fimiani M, Castelli A. Malignant nodular hidradenoma of the skin: report of seven cases. *J Eur Acad Dermatol Venereol.* 2008;22(5):549–554.

683. Hirsch P, Helwig EB. Chondroid syringoma. Mixed tumor of skin, salivary gland type. *Arch Dermatol.* 1961;84:835–847.

684. Headington J. Mixed tumors of skin: eccrine and apocrine types. *Arch Dermatol.* 1961;84:989–996.

685. Tsoitis G, Brisou B, Destombes P. Mummified cutaneous mixed tumor. *Arch Dermatol.* 1975;111(2):194–196.

686. Varela-Duran J, Diaz-Flores L, Varela-Nunez R. Ultrastructure of chondroid syringoma: role of the myoepithelial cell in the

development of the mixed tumor of the skin and soft tissues. *Cancer.* 1979;44(1):148–156.

687. Dominguez Iglesias F, Fresno Forcelledo F, Soler Sanchez T, Fernandez Garcia L, Herrero Zapatero A. Chondroid syringoma: a histological and immunohistochemical study of 15 cases. *Histopathology.* 1990;17(4):311–317.

688. Mentzel T, Requena L, Kaddu S, Soares de Aleida LM, Sangueza OP, Kutzner H. Cutaneous myoepithelial neoplasms: clinicopathologic and immunohistochemical study of 20 cases suggesting a continuous spectrum ranging from benign mixed tumor of the skin to cutaneous myoepithelioma and myoepithelial carcinoma. *J Cutan Pathol.* 2003;30(5):294–302.

689. Kazakov DV, Belousova IE, Bisceglia M, et al. Apocrine mixed tumor of the skin ("mixed tumor of the folliculosebaceous-apocrine complex"). Spectrum of differentiations and metaplastic changes in the epithelial, myoepithelial, and stromal components based on a histopathologic study of 244 cases. *J Am Acad Dermatol.* 2007;57(3):467–483.

690. Tirumalae R, Boer A. Calcification and ossification in eccrine mixed tumors: underrecognized feature and diagnostic pitfall. *Am J Dermatopathol.* 2009;31(8):772–777.

691. Jun HJ, Cho E, Cho SH, Lee JD. Chondroid syringoma with marked calcification. *Am J Dermatopathol.* 2012;34(8):e125–e127.

692. Awasthi R, Harmse D, Courtney D, Lyons CB. Benign mixed tumour of the skin with extensive ossification and marrow formation: a case report. *J Clin Pathol.* 2004;57(12):1329–1330.

693. Banerjee SS, Harris M, Eyden BP, Howell S, Wells S, Mainwaring AR. Chondroid syringoma with hyaline cell change. *Histopathology.* 1993;22(3):235–245.

694. Hassab-el-Naby HM, Tam S, White WL, Ackerman AB. Mixed tumors of the skin. A histological and immunohistochemical study. *Am J Dermatopathol.* 1989;11(5):413–428.

695. Kanitakis J, Zambruno G, Viac J, Panzini H, Thivolet J. Expression of neural-tissue markers (S-100 protein and Leu-7 antigen) by sweat gland tumors of the skin. An immunohistochemical study. *J Am Acad Dermatol.* 1987;17(2, pt 1):187–191.

696. Hernandez FJ. Mixed tumors of the skin of the salivary gland type: a light and electron microscopic study. *J Invest Dermatol.* 1976;66(1):49–52.

697. Trown K, Heenan PJ. Malignant mixed tumor of the skin (malignant chondroid syringoma). *Pathology.* 1994;26(3):237–243.

698. Harrist TJ, Aretz TH, Mihm MC Jr, Evans GW, Rodriquez FL. Cutaneous malignant mixed tumor. *Arch Dermatol.* 1981;117(11):719–724.

699. Shvili D, Rothem A. Fulminant metastasizing chondroid syringoma of the skin. *Am J Dermatopathol.* 1986;8(4):321–325.

700. Metzler G, Schaumburg-Lever G, Hornstein O, Rassner G. Malignant chondroid syringoma: immunohistopathology. *Am J Dermatopathol.* 1996;18(1):83–89.

701. Matz LR, McCully DJ, Stokes BA. Metastasizing chondroid syringoma: case report. *Pathology.* 1969;1(1):77–81.

702. Redono C, Rocamora A, Villoria F, Garcia M. Malignant mixed tumor of the skin: malignant chondroid syringoma. *Cancer.* 1982;49(8):1690–1696.

703. Ishimura E, Iwamoto H, Kobashi Y, Yamabe H, Ichijima K. Malignant chondroid syringoma. Report of a case with widespread metastasis and review of pertinent literature. *Cancer.* 1983;52(10):1966–1973.

704. Botha JB, Kahn LB. Aggressive chondroid syringoma. Report of a case in an unusual location and with local recurrence. *Arch Dermatol.* 1978;114(6):954–955.

705. Hilton JM, Blackwell JB. Metastasising chondroid syringoma. *J Pathol.* 1973;109(2):167–170.

706. Requena C, Brotons S, Sanmartin O, et al. Malignant chondroid syringoma of the face with bone invasion. *Am J Dermatopathol.* 2013;35(3):395–398.

707. Baes H, Suurmond D. Apocrine sweat gland carcinoma. Report of a case. *Br J Dermatol.* 1970;83(4):483–486.

708. Futrell JW, Krueger GR, Chretien PB, Ketcham AS. Multiple primary sweat gland carcinomas. *Cancer.* 1971;28(3):686–691.

709. Nishikawa Y, Tokusashi Y, Saito Y, Ogawa K, Miyokawa N, Katagiri M. A case of apocrine adenocarcinoma associated with hamartomatous apocrine gland hyperplasia of both axillae. *Am J Surg Pathol.* 1994;18(8):832–836.

710. Paties C, Taccagni GL, Papotti M, Valente G, Zangrandi A, Aloi F. Apocrine carcinoma of the skin. A clinicopathologic, immunocytochemical, and ultrastructural study. *Cancer.* 1993;71(2):375–381.

711. Sakamoto F, Ito M, Sato S, Sato Y. Basal cell tumor with apocrine differentiation: apocrine epithelioma. *J Am Acad Dermatol.* 1985;13(2, pt 2):355–363.

712. Michel RG, Woodard BH, Shelburne JD, Bossen EH. Ceruminous gland adenocarcinoma: a light and electron microscopic study. *Cancer.* 1978;41(2):545–553.

713. Neldner KH. Ceruminoma. *Arch Dermatol.* 1968;98(4):344–348.

714. Lynde CW, McLean DI, Wood WS. Tumors of ceruminous glands. *J Am Acad Dermatol.* 1984;11(5, pt 1):841–847.

715. Hollowell KL, Agle SC, Zervos EE, Fitzgerald TL. Cutaneous apocrine adenocarcinoma: defining epidemiology, outcomes, and optimal therapy for a rare neoplasm. *J Surg Oncol.* 2012;105(4):415–419.

716. Robson A, Lazar AJ, Ben Nagi J, et al. Primary cutaneous apocrine carcinoma: a clinico-pathologic analysis of 24 cases. *Am J Surg Pathol.* 2008;32(5):682–690.

717. Le LP, Dias-Santagata D, Pawlak AC, et al. Apocrine-eccrine carcinomas: molecular and immunohistochemical analyses. *PLoS One.* 2012;7(10):e47290.

718. Piris A, Peng Y, Boussahmain C, Essary LR, Gudewicz TM, Hoang MP. Cutaneous and mammary apocrine carcinomas have different immunoprofiles. *Hum Pathol.* 2014;45(2):320–326.

719. Mahalingam M, Nguyen LP, Richards JE, Muzikansky A, Hoang MP. The diagnostic utility of immunohistochemistry in distinguishing primary skin adnexal carcinomas from metastatic adenocarcinoma to skin: an immunohistochemical reappraisal using cytokeratin 15, nestin, p63, D2-40, and calretinin. *Mod Pathol.* 2010;23(5):713–719.

720. Fujioka M, Kato J, Sumikawa Y, Sato S, Sawada M, Uhara H. Cutaneous apocrine carcinoma with elevated serum cytokeratin 19 fragment 21-1 (CYFRA 21-1). *J Dermatol.* 2019;46(10):e387–e388.

721. Grant R. Sweat gland carcinoma with metastases. *JAMA.* 1960;173:490–492.

722. el-Domeiri AA, Brasfield RD, Huvos AG, Strong EW. Sweat gland carcinoma: a clinico-pathologic study of 83 patients. *Ann Surg.* 1971;173(2):270–274.

723. Swanson PE, Cherwitz DL, Neumann MP, Wick MR. Eccrine sweat gland carcinoma: an histologic and immunohistochemical study of 32 cases. *J Cutan Pathol.* 1987;14(2):65–86.

724. Teloh HA, Balkin RB, Grier JP. Metastasizing sweat-gland carcinoma; report of a case. *AMA Arch Derm.* 1957;76(1):80–86.

725. Avraham JB, Villines D, Maker VK, August C, Maker AV. Survival after resection of cutaneous adnexal carcinomas with eccrine differentiation: risk factors and trends in outcomes. *J Surg Oncol.* 2013;108(1):57–62.

726. Dave VK. Eccrine sweat gland carcinoma with metastases. *Br J Dermatol.* 1972;86(1):95–97.

727. Rollins-Raval M, Chivukula M, Tseng GC, Jukic D, Dabbs DJ. An immunohistochemical panel to differentiate metastatic breast carcinoma to skin from primary sweat gland carcinomas with a review of the literature. *Arch Pathol Lab Med.* 2011;135(8):975–983.

728. Chhibber V, Lyle S, Mahalingam M. Ductal eccrine carcinoma with squamous differentiation: apropos a case. *J Cutan Pathol.* 2007;34(6):503–507.

729. Terushkin E, Leffell DJ, Futoryan T, Cowper S, Lazova R. Squamoid eccrine ductal carcinoma: a case report and review of the literature. *Am J Dermatopathol.* 2010;32(3):287–292.

730. Freeman R, Winkelmann RK. Basal cell tumor with eccrine differentiation. *Arch Dermatol.* 1969;100:234.

731. Sanchez N, Winkelmann RK. Basal cell tumor with eccrine differentiation: eccrine epithelioma. *J Am Acad Dermatol.* 1982;6:514.

732. Mehregan AH, Hashimoto K, Rahbari H. Eccrine adenocarcinoma. A clinicopathologic study of 35 cases. *Arch Dermatol.* 1983;119(2):104–114.

733. Sanchez Yus E, Requena Caballero L, Garcia Salazar I, Coca Menchero S. Clear cell syringoid eccrine carcinoma. *Am J Dermatopathol.* 1987;9(3):225–231.

734. Ramos D, Monteagudo C, Carda C, Montesinos E, Ferrer J, Peydro-Olaya A. Clear cell syringoid carcinoma: an ultrastructural and immunohistochemical study. *Am J Dermatopathol.* 2000;22(1):60–64.

735. Ohnishi T, Kaneko S, Egi M, Takizawa H, Watanabe S. Syringoid eccrine carcinoma: report of a case with immunohistochemical analysis of cytokeratin expression. *Am J Dermatopathol.* 2002;24(5):409–413.

736. Sidiropoulos M, Sade S, Al-Habeeb A, Ghazarian D. Syringoid eccrine carcinoma: a clinicopathological and immunohistochemical study of four cases. *J Clin Pathol.* 2011;64(9):788–792.

737. Cooper PH. Sclerosing carcinomas of sweat ducts (microcystic adnexal carcinoma). *Arch Dermatol.* 1986;122(3):261–264.

738. Nickoloff BJ, Fleischmann HE, Carmel J, Wood CC, Roth RJ. Microcystic adnexal carcinoma. Immunohistologic observations suggesting dual (pilar and eccrine) differentiation. *Arch Dermatol.* 1986;122(3):290–294.

739. Page RN, Hanggi MC, King R, Googe PB. Multiple microcystic adnexal carcinomas. *Cutis.* 2007;79(4):299–303.

740. Nelson BR, Lowe L, Baker S, Johnson TM, LeBoit PE. Microcystic adnexal carcinoma of the skin. A reappraisal of the differentiation and differential diagnosis of an underrecognized neoplasm. *J Am Acad Dermatol.* 1993;29(5, pt 2):840–845.

741. Pujol RM, LeBoit PE, Su WP. Microcystic adnexal carcinoma with extensive sebaceous differentiation. *Am J Dermatopathol.* 1997;19(4):358–362.

742. McCalmont TH, Ye J. Eosinophils as a clue to the diagnosis of microcystic adnexal carcinoma. *J Cutan Pathol.* 2011;38(11):849, 850–852.

743. Torre-Castro J, Moya-Martinez C, Sangueza O, Requena L. Microcystic adnexal adenoma: the benign counterpart of microcystic adnexal carcinoma. *Am J Dermatopathol.* 2021;43(11):835–837.

744. Carvalho J, Fullen D, Lowe L, Su L, Ma L. The expression of CD23 in cutaneous non-lymphoid neoplasms. *J Cutan Pathol.* 2007;34(9):693–698.

745. Krahl D, Sellheyer K. Monoclonal antibody Ber-EP4 reliably discriminates between microcystic adnexal carcinoma and basal cell carcinoma. *J Cutan Pathol.* 2007;34(10):782–787. https://onlinelibrary.wiley.com/doi/10.1111/j.1600-0560.2006.00710.x

746. Chan MP, Plouffe KR, Liu CJ, et al. Next-generation sequencing implicates oncogenic roles for p53 and JAK/STAT signaling in microcystic adnexal carcinomas. *Mod Pathol.* 2020;33(6):1092–1103.

747. Kazakov DV, Suster S, LeBoit PE, et al. Mucinous carcinoma of the skin, primary, and secondary: a clinicopathologic study of 63 cases with emphasis on the morphologic spectrum of primary cutaneous forms: homologies with mucinous lesions in the breast. *Am J Surg Pathol.* 2005;29(6):764–782.

748. Mendoza S, Helwig EB. Mucinous (adenocystic) carcinoma of the skin. *Arch Dermatol.* 1971;103(1):68–78.

749. Santa-Cruz DJ, Meyers JH, Gnepp DR, Perez BM. Primary mucinous carcinoma of the skin. *Br J Dermatol.* 1978;98(6):645–653.

750. Yeung KY, Stinson JC. Mucinous (adenocystic) carcinoma of sweat glands with widespread metastasis. Case report with ultrastructural study. *Cancer.* 1977;39(6):2556–2562.

751. Snow SN, Reizner GT. Mucinous eccrine carcinoma of the eyelid. *Cancer.* 1992;70(8):2099–2104.

752. Headington JT. Primary mucinous carcinoma of skin: histochemistry and electron microscopy. *Cancer.* 1977;39(3):1055–1063.

753. Baandrup U, Søgaard H. Mucinous (adenocystic) carcinoma of the skin. *Dermatologica.* 1982;164:338.

754. Wright J, Font RL. Mucinous sweat gland adenocarcinoma of the eyelid. *Cancer.* 1979;44:1757.

755. Hein R, Kuhn A, Landthaler M, Krieg T, Eckert F. Cytokeratin expression in mucinous sweat gland carcinomas: an immunohistochemical analysis of four cases. *Br J Dermatol.* 1994;130(4):432–437.

756. Levy G, Finkelstein A, McNiff JM. Immunohistochemical techniques to compare primary vs. metastatic mucinous carcinoma of the skin. *J Cutan Pathol.* 2010;37(4):411–415.

757. Schmid U, Hardmeier T, Altmannsberger M, Balin AK. Mucinous carcinoma. *Histopathology.* 1992;21(2):161–165.

758. Flieder A, Koerner FC, Pilch BZ, Maluf HM. Endocrine mucin-producing sweat gland carcinoma: a cutaneous neoplasm analogous to solid papillary carcinoma of breast. *Am J Surg Pathol.* 1997;21(12):1501–1506.

759. Zembowicz A, Garcia CF, Tannous ZS, Mihm MC, Koerner F, Pilch BZ. Endocrine mucin-producing sweat gland carcinoma: twelve new cases suggest that it is a precursor of some invasive mucinous carcinomas. *Am J Surg Pathol.* 2005;29(10):1330–1339.

760. Emanuel PO, de Vinck D, Waldorf HA, Phelps RG. Recurrent endocrine mucin-producing sweat gland carcinoma. *Ann Diagn Pathol.* 2007;11(6):448–452.

761. Koike T, Mikami T, Maegawa J, Iwai T, Wada H, Yamanaka S. Recurrent endocrine mucin-producing sweat gland carcinoma in the eyelid. *Australas J Dermatol.* 2013;54(2):e46–e49.

762. Hadi R, Xu H, Barber BR, Shinohara MM, Moshiri AS. A case of endocrine mucin-producing sweat gland carcinoma with distant metastasis. *J Cutan Pathol.* 2021;48(7):937–942.

763. Dhaliwal CA, Torgersen A, Ross JJ, Ironside JW, Biswas A. Endocrine mucin-producing sweat gland carcinoma: report of two cases of an under-recognized malignant neoplasm and review of the literature. *Am J Dermatopathol.* 2013;35(1):117–124.

764. Mathew JG, Bowman AS, Saab J, Busam KJ, Nehal K, Pulitzer M. Next generation sequencing analysis suggests varied multistep mutational pathogenesis for endocrine mucin producing sweat gland carcinoma with comments on INSM1 and MUC2 suggesting a conjunctival origin. *J Am Acad Dermatol.* 2021. doi:10.1016/j.jaad.2020.11.073

765. Bulliard C, Murali R, Maloof A, Adams S. Endocrine mucin-producing sweat gland carcinoma: report of a case and review of the literature. *J Cutan Pathol.* 2006;33(12):812–816.

766. Landman G, Farmer ER. Primary cutaneous mucoepidermoid carcinoma: report of a case. *J Cutan Pathol.* 1991;18(1):56–59.

767. Wenig BL, Sciubba JJ, Goodman RS, Platt N. Primary cutaneous mucoepidermoid carcinoma of the anterior neck. *Laryngoscope.* 1983;93(4):464–467.

768. Friedman KJ. Low-grade primary cutaneous adenosquamous (mucoepidermoid) carcinoma. Report of a case and review of the literature. *Am J Dermatopathol.* 1989;11(1):43–50.

769. Abbas O, Reddy K, Demierre MF, Blanchard RA, Mahalingam M. Epidermotropic metastatic mucoepidermoid carcinoma. *Am J Dermatopathol.* 2010;32(5):505–508.

770. Lehmer LM, Ragsdale BD, Crawford RI, Bukachevsky R, Hannah LA. Mucoepidermoid carcinoma of the parotid presenting as periauricular cystic nodules: a series of four cases. *J Cutan Pathol.* 2012;39(7):712–717.

771. Chen Z, Ni W, Li JL, et al. The CRTC1-MAML2 fusion is the major oncogenic driver in mucoepidermoid carcinoma. *JCI Insight.* 2021;6(7):e139497.

772. Boggio R. Letter: adenoid cystic carcinoma of scalp. *Arch Dermatol.* 1975;111(6):793–794.

773. Seab JA, Graham JH. Primary cutaneous adenoid cystic carcinoma. *J Am Acad Dermatol.* 1987;17(1):113–118.

774. Rocas D, Asvesti C, Tsega A, Katafygiotis P, Kanitakis J. Primary adenoid cystic carcinoma of the skin metastatic to the lymph nodes: immunohistochemical study of a new case and literature review. *Am J Dermatopathol.* 2014;36(3):223–228.

775. Cooper PH, Adelson GL, Holthaus WH. Primary cutaneous adenoid cystic carcinoma. *Arch Dermatol.* 1984;120(6):774–777.

776. Dores GM, Huycke MM, Devesa SS, Garcia CA. Primary cutaneous adenoid cystic carcinoma in the United States: incidence, survival, and associated cancers, 1976 to 2005. *J Am Acad Dermatol.* 2010;63(1):71–78.

777. Fukai K, Ishii M, Kobayashi H, et al. Primary cutaneous adenoid cystic carcinoma: ultrastructural study and immunolocalization of types I, III, IV, V collagens and laminin. *J Cutan Pathol.* 1990;17(6):374–380.

778. Headington JT, Teears R, Niederhuber JE, Slinger RP. Primary adenoid cystic carcinoma of skin. *Arch Dermatol.* 1978; 114(3):421–424.

779. Wick MR, Swanson PE. Primary adenoid cystic carcinoma of the skin. A clinical, histological, and immunocytochemical comparison with adenoid cystic carcinoma of salivary glands and adenoid basal cell carcinoma. *Am J Dermatopathol.* 1986;8(1):2–13.

780. Ramakrishnan R, Chaudhry IH, Ramdial P, et al. Primary cutaneous adenoid cystic carcinoma: a clinicopathologic and immunohistochemical study of 27 cases. *Am J Surg Pathol.* 2013;37(10):1603–1611.

781. Goto K, Kajimoto K, Sugino T, et al. MYB translocations in both myoepithelial and ductoglandular epithelial cells in adenoid cystic carcinoma: a histopathologic and genetic reappraisal in six primary cutaneous cases. *Am J Dermatopathol.* 2021;43(4):278–283.

782. Pardal J, Sundram U, Selim MA, Hoang MP. GATA3 and MYB expression in cutaneous adnexal neoplasms. *Am J Dermatopathol.* 2017;39(4):279–286.

783. Kao GF, Helwig EB, Graham JH. Aggressive digital papillary adenoma and adenocarcinoma. A clinicopathological study of 57 patients, with histochemical, immunopathological, and ultrastructural observations. *J Cutan Pathol.* 1987;14(3):129–146.

784. Suchak R, Wang WL, Prieto VG, et al. Cutaneous digital papillary adenocarcinoma: a clinicopathologic study of 31 cases of a rare neoplasm with new observations. *Am J Surg Pathol.* 2012;36(12):1883–1891.

785. Surowy HM, Giesen AK, Otte J, et al. Gene expression profiling in aggressive digital papillary adenocarcinoma sheds light on the architecture of a rare sweat gland carcinoma. *Br J Dermatol.* 2019;180(5):1150–1160.

786. Satake K, Goto K, Sugino T, Sasaki Y, Yoshikawa S, Kiyohara Y. Limited immunoexpression of fibroblast growth factor receptor 2 (FGFR2) in digital papillary adenocarcinoma: comparison of FGFR2 immunohistochemistry between digital papillary adenocarcinoma, other sweat gland tumors and normal skin tissue. *J Dermatol.* 2021;48(2):e86–e87.

787. Duke WH, Sherrod TT, Lupton GP. Aggressive digital papillary adenocarcinoma (aggressive digital papillary adenoma and adenocarcinoma revisited). *Am J Surg Pathol.* 2000;24(6):775–784.

788. Jih DM, Elenitsas R, Vittorio CC, Berkowitz AR, Seykora JT. Aggressive digital papillary adenocarcinoma: a case report and review of the literature. *Am J Dermatopathol.* 2001;23(2):154–157.

789. Brandt SM, Swistel AJ, Rosen PP. Secretory carcinoma in the axilla: probable origin from axillary skin appendage glands in a young girl. *Am J Surg Pathol.* 2009;33(6):950–953.

790. Kastnerova L, Luzar B, Goto K, et al. Secretory carcinoma of the skin: report of 6 cases, including a case with a novel NFIX-PKN1 translocation. *Am J Surg Pathol.* 2019;43(8):1092–1098.

791. Taniguchi K, Yanai H, Kaji T, et al. Secretory carcinoma of the skin with lymph node metastases and recurrence in both lungs: a case report. *J Cutan Pathol.* 2021;48(8):1069–1074.

Chapter 31

Cutaneous Lymphomas and Leukemias

SAM SADIGH, GEORGE F. MURPHY, AND ELIZABETH A. MORGAN

INTRODUCTION

The subject of cutaneous lymphoma and leukemia has long been one of conceptual confusion and diagnostic challenge. Aside from the inherent difficulties in differentiating hyperplastic from neoplastic hematopoietic cells in skin, neoplastic infiltrates may be primary or secondary, and distinction between the two is critical given the considerable clinical implications. Moreover, some traditional didactic treatments of this issue too often provide information so abundant as to confound the overview necessary for a practical, confident, and accurate diagnostic approach to potential lymphoproliferative disorders of skin.

The classification system adapted to skin and used in this chapter is for the most part that of the most recent 2016 World Health Organization (WHO) Classification of Tumors of Haematopoietic and Lymphoid Tissues (1); it also incorporates the 2018 update of the WHO/European Organization for Research and Treatment of Cancer (EORTC) classification for primary cutaneous lymphomas (2). These distinct clinicopathologic entities offer pathologists, dermatologists, oncologists, and geneticists a universal system for cutaneous lymphoma/leukemia classification. In this regard, a synthesis of clinical, histopathologic, immunohistochemical, molecular, and/or cytogenetic features is often required to define individual disease entities.

Lymphoproliferative disorders of the skin fall into two major categories: primary cutaneous neoplasms and nodal-based or extranodal-based systemic lymphomas that may secondarily involve the skin. In some cases, these systemic lymphomas may initially present in the skin without evidence of systemic involvement at the time of diagnosis. Other hematopoietic neoplasms may secondarily involve cutaneous tissues such as those of the myeloid lineage or (rarely) classic Hodgkin lymphoma (CHL). The specific diseases that follow will thus be grouped according to the following schema in an attempt to encompass the broad array of hematolymphoid neoplasms with cutaneous manifestations (Table 31-1).

The approach to hematopoietic disorders in this chapter is in no small part indebted to the outstanding foundations that have been developed in previous editions of this text. In particular, the classification, images, and related commentary provided by LeBoit and McCalmont (3), Murphy and Schwarting (4), and Hsu and Murphy (5) were integral to the development of the present material and represent a major advance in the textural treatment of this difficult and ever-evolving topic.

CUTANEOUS HEMATOPOIETIC INFILTRATES: OVERVIEW AND GENERAL CONCEPTS

Hematopoietic Cell Lineage: Relevance to Cutaneous Immune Surveillance and Lineage Differentiation

One of the major functions of skin is protection against environmental hazards, including infectious organisms. Evolution has allowed the development of a highly effective two-tiered defense mechanism composed of a rapid "innate" and a sustained "adaptive" response. The innate immunity is mediated by macrophages, leukocytes, natural killer (NK) cells, γδ T cells, and dendritic cells, which detect nonspecific epitopes commonly shared by different pathogens (such as glycolipids, lipoproteins, peptidoglycans, and double-stranded RNA) and mount immediate responses. In contrast, the adaptive arm of the cutaneous immune system targets specific protein antigens in a major histocompatibility-restricted manner through effectors like αβ T and B cells. Most cutaneous lymphomas have putative lineage derivation from and perhaps biologic behavior attributable to the distinct cell populations of the immune system and their evolutionary stages of maturation. Malignant T cells and myeloid cells tend to recapitulate morphologic and antigenic features of cells undergoing intrathymic/postthymic and intraosseous maturation, respectively. Malignant B cells also have definite developmental relationships to normal B-cell ontogeny within bone marrow and lymphoid organs.

T- and B-Cell Infiltration Patterns

Although numerous exceptions exist, there are fundamental and often reproducible trends in the patterns produced when lymphocytes infiltrate the skin (Table 31-2) (6). This is based in part on differences in adhesive ligands between B and T cells, resulting in differential affinity for various compartments within the skin. Moreover, chemokinetic and chemotactic signals may influence the migration of various classes of lymphoid cells in different ways. The best example of this is the tendency for both benign and malignant T cells, but not B cells, to migrate into epithelial structures, including the epidermis and its adnexa. This results in the phenomena of "exocytosis" (generally used in benign settings) or "epidermotropism" (generally used in neoplastic settings) and "folliculotropism," accounting, respectively, for the tendency to identify T cells within the epidermal layer or follicular epithelium and often as a band of cells within

Table 31-1

Classification of Primary and Secondary Lymphomas/Leukemias of Skin

Primary Cutaneous Lymphomas

Mature B-cell lineage

Primary cutaneous marginal zone lymphoma

Primary cutaneous follicle center lymphoma

Primary cutaneous diffuse large B-cell lymphoma, leg type

EBV+ mucocutaneous ulcer

Mature T-/NK-cell lineage

Mycosis fungoides including variants/subtypes

Sézary syndrome

Primary cutaneous CD30+ T-cell lymphoproliferative disorders

    Lymphomatoid papulosis

    Primary cutaneous anaplastic large cell lymphoma

Subcutaneous panniculitis-like T-cell lymphoma

Primary cutaneous γδ T-cell lymphoma

Primary cutaneous CD8+ aggressive epidermotropic cytotoxic T-cell lymphoma (provisional)

Primary cutaneous acral CD8+ T-cell lymphoma (provisional)

Primary cutaneous CD4+ small/medium T-cell lymphoproliferative disorder (provisional)

Hydroa vacciniforme-like lymphoproliferative disorder

Cutaneous Involvement by Systemic Leukemias/Lymphomas

Myeloid lineage

Myeloid sarcoma

Chronic myelomonocytic leukemia

Plasmacytoid dendritic cell lineage

Blastic plasmacytoid dendritic cell neoplasm

B-cell lineage

B-lymphoblastic leukemia/lymphoma

Chronic lymphocytic leukemia/small lymphocytic lymphoma

Mantle cell lymphoma

Follicular lymphoma

Plasma cell neoplasm

Diffuse large B-cell lymphoma

Plasmablastic lymphoma

Intravascular large B-cell lymphoma

Lymphomatoid granulomatosis

T-/NK-cell lineage

T-lymphoblastic leukemia/lymphoma

Anaplastic large cell lymphoma

Angioimmunoblastic T-cell lymphoma

Adult T-cell leukemia/lymphoma

Extranodal NK/T-cell lymphoma, nasal type

Peripheral T-cell lymphoma, not otherwise specified

T-cell prolymphocytic leukemia

Classic Hodgkin lymphoma

Table 31-2

Comparison of T- and B-Cell 'Trafficking' Patterns

	T-Cell Patterns	B-Cell Patterns
Overall architecture	Band-like	Nodular
Pattern of the infiltrate	perivascular	Perivascular and interstitial
Epidermal involvement (exocytosis/ epidermotropism/ folliculotropism)	Present	Absent
Grenz zone	Absent	Present

the underlying papillary dermis (Fig. 31-1A). Occasionally, as is the case in epidermotropic phases of mycosis fungoides (MF), T cells may align along the basement membrane zone of the dermal–epidermal junction, a finding that may have a basis in expression by these cells of integrin receptors for the specific membrane components (7). This "T-cell pattern" of infiltration, however, is not invariable among T-cell malignancies, and epidermotropism may be blunted as tumors evolve and progress to more aggressive and poorly differentiated states. B cells, on the other hand, do not demonstrate the same affinity for the epidermis and adnexa, and seldom are these cells detected in significant numbers within the epidermis or papillary dermis. The sparing of the latter produces the characteristic "Grenz zone" of sparing beneath the epidermal layer seen in B-cell pattern infiltrates of the skin. Moreover, perhaps because of the innate proclivity of B cells to aggregate into follicular structures (germinal centers), B-cell infiltrates in the skin often (but not invariably) show a nodular architecture (Fig. 31-1B).

T- and B-cell patterns are potentially helpful in presumptive assignment of cell lineage, but they are not invariable, cannot be used as a reliable surrogate for immunohistochemical detection of lineage-related antigens, and do not permit separation of reactive from dysplastic and malignant populations. Although this latter distinction frequently depends on cytology, immunophenotype, and genotype, the architecture or "trafficking" patterns of hematopoietic cells in the skin may also provide insight into the biologic potential for aggressive behavior.

Abnormal Trafficking: Distinction from Inflammation

Skin is a lymphoid organ, and both the epidermal and dermal layers represent interactive immune systems that contribute to and partially regulate inflammatory cell trafficking (8,9). In both T- and B-cell responses in skin, circulating lymphocytes initially adhere to activated endothelium lining dermal postcapillary venules. Migration across the vessel wall results in perivascular or angiocentric dermatitis (Fig. 31-2A). If further migration is stunted, this exclusive angiocentric localization may produce a pattern suggestive of a specified number of differential diagnostic considerations based on correlation with clinical parameters (e.g., as in erythema chronicum migrans). Migration away from the vessel wall in other cases is presumably swift enough to permit papillary dermal accumulation of T cells and migration of T cells into the epidermis, in addition to persistent angiocentrism. However, activated T cells on an immunologic mission,

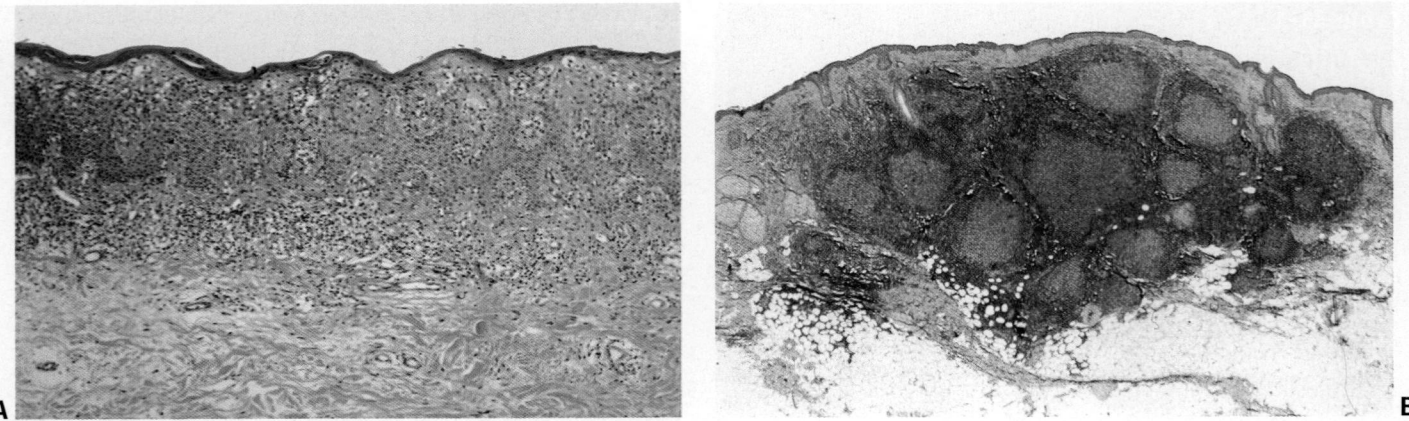

Figure 31-1 Patterns of T- and B-cell infiltration. **A:** T-cell pattern with infiltration of the overlying epidermis. **B:** B-cell pattern with Grenz zone and germinal center formation.

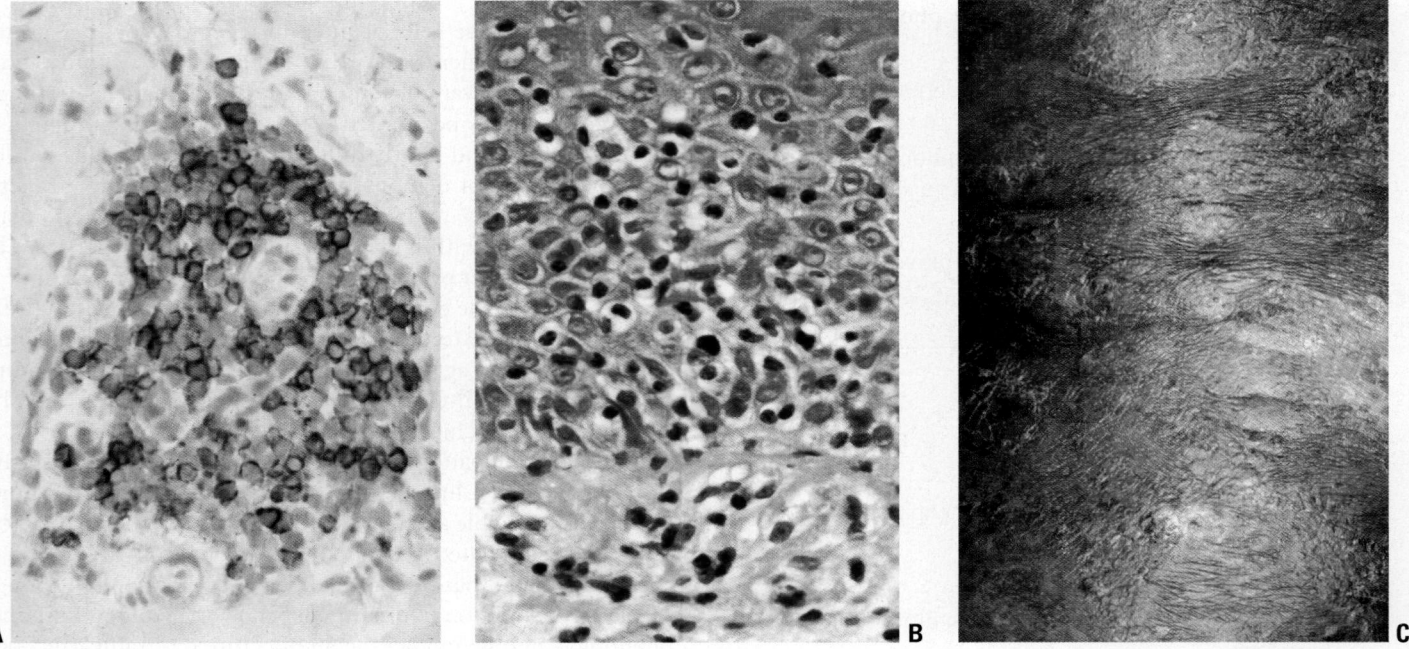

Figure 31-2 T-cell trafficking patterns. **A:** CD3 immunohistochemistry highlights angiocentric T cells. **B:** Abnormal epidermotropism into a "passive" epidermis. **C:** Scaling patches and plaques as a consequence of altered epidermal maturation associated with T-cell epidermotropism (MF).

as in the case of contact hypersensitivity, psoriasis, or cytotoxic dermatitis, generally alter the epidermis as they enter it, in part by way of the cytokines and growth factors that they produce. Thus, reactive T-cell exocytosis is often accompanied by epithelial spongiosis, acanthosis, or apoptosis. In the case of malignant epidermotropic T-cell infiltration, in contrast, the epidermis tends to be "passive," with T-cell infiltration resulting in permissive aggregation of variably atypical lymphocytes within the epidermis (Fig. 31-2B) and sometimes also or exclusively in adnexal epithelium. This infiltration is not generally associated with reactive epithelial alteration in the form of spongiosis or apoptosis but rather may be associated with epithelial injury in the form of localized mucinous degeneration, a potential contributing factor to the development of Pautrier microabscesses and follicular mucinosis that may accompany MF (10). Moreover, as the epidermis becomes more extensively infiltrated, impaired maturation often

manifests as clinical abnormalities in scale production. Hence, many T-cell lymphoproliferative disorders will show surface hyperkeratosis that in early stages may clinically mimic dermatitis (Fig. 31-2C).

Infiltration of the skin by reactive B cells often results in a perivascular accumulation of cells usually without significant involvement by the papillary dermis or epidermis, producing a Grenz zone of papillary dermal sparing and preservation of architecture. With persistence of antigenic stimulus, as may occur in the setting of some insect bite reactions attributable to intradermally injected antigen, nodular aggregates of B cells may form in the dermis, recapitulating germinal centers (Fig. 31-3A). Malignant B-cell infiltrates typically show a destructive relationship to preexisting structures. Accordingly, malignant B cells will frequently infiltrate in an interstitial pattern (vs. perivascular), resulting in splaying apart of collagen bundles and mesenchymal

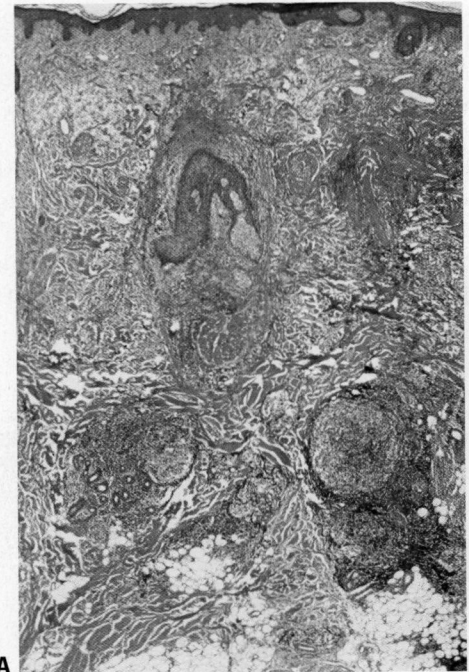
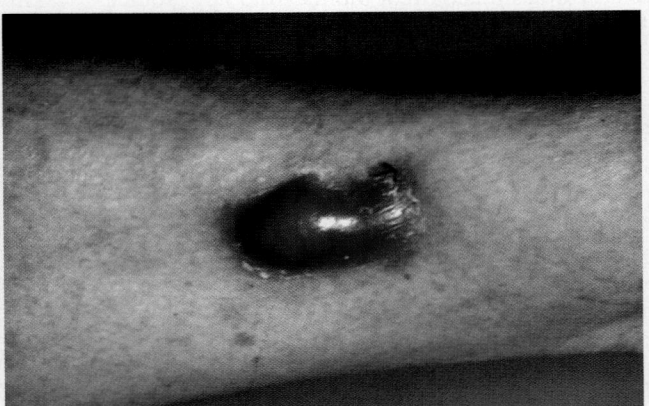

Figure 31-3 B-cell trafficking patterns. **A:** B-cell pattern showing nondestructive infiltration of superficial and deep dermis. **B:** Plum-colored nodule covered by thinned, glistening epidermis attributable to B-cell dermal infiltration.

cells (e.g., smooth muscle cells forming arrector pili muscles) within the reticular dermis. Moreover, nodular aggregations of malignant B cells tend to displace adnexal epithelium, resulting in their distortion and occasionally in their ischemic destruction in the process. Of note, malignant B cells may also form nodules vaguely reminiscent of germinal centers or even induce the formation of associated reactive B-cell infiltrates.

Circulating leukemia cells, like inflammatory cells, may show a perivascular pattern of infiltration on initial infiltration of skin. Although the cells avoid epithelial structures, they will evolve into a dermal interstitial pattern with time. Other nonmalignant conditions may show an interstitial architecture such as histiocytes in the setting of certain evolutionary stages of palisaded granulomatous dermatitis, lymphocytes in early inflammatory lesions of morphea, and myeloid cells in the setting of extramedullary hematopoiesis.

The tendency for progressive dermal infiltration with relative sparing of the epidermal layer in both B-cell and many leukemic malignancies results in clinical lesions that are red to plum colored and covered by thin, shiny (nonkeratotic) epidermal surfaces (Fig. 31-3B).

PRIMARY CUTANEOUS LYMPHOMAS

Mature B-Cell Lineage

Primary Cutaneous Marginal Zone Lymphoma

In the WHO classification system, marginal zone lymphomas (MZL) of the skin are grouped into the broader category of extranodal MZL of mucosa-associated lymphoid tissues, also known as MALT lymphoma (1). This category encompasses MALT lymphomas arising at all extranodal sites, including the gastrointestinal tract (most common), salivary gland, lung, head and neck, ocular adnexa, skin, thyroid, and breast. In the WHO–EORTC classification of primary cutaneous lymphomas,

skin lesions are distinctly categorized as primary cutaneous marginal zone B-cell lymphoma (PCMZL) (2). We will use the term "PCMZL" in this chapter. This category includes plasma cell–rich variants previously designated as primary cutaneous immunocytoma, follicular lymphoid hyperplasia with monotypic plasma cells, and extramedullary plasmacytoma of the skin in the absence of underlying multiple myeloma. Among primary cutaneous lymphomas, the frequency of PCMZL is approximately 9% (11). The diagnosis of PCMZL can be very challenging owing to nonspecific morphologic features, numerous admixed reactive lymphocytes, and lack of a diagnostic immunophenotype.

Clinical Summary. Typically, PCMZL manifests as single or multiple, clustered erythematous or violaceous papules, plaques, or nodules. The lesions occur most commonly on the trunk, upper extremities, or, less commonly, in the head and neck region. Of note, head and neck lesions in older patients may be a harbinger of an underlying nodal MZL and warrant systemic investigation (12). The male-to-female ratio is approximately 2:1 with a median age of occurrence of 55, although these lesions can also arise in children (13). Plasma cell–rich variants are more commonly associated with older patients and lower-extremity lesions. In endemic areas, plasma cell–rich cases of PCMZL may be associated with the tick-associated spirochete *Borrelia burgdorferi* (14–19). In general, PCMZL is an indolent form of lymphoma with a 5-year survival close to 100%. Following spontaneous regression or therapy, recurrence at the same or distant sites is observed in approximately 40% of patients but typically retains a low-grade morphology. Extracutaneous spread is rare. Very rare cases of transformation to diffuse large B-cell lymphoma (DLBCL) have been reported (20).

Histopathology. In PCMZL, the neoplastic lymphocytes form a nodular or diffuse dermal infiltrate, sparing the overlying epidermis (Fig. 31-4A, B). The infiltrate often surrounds reactive (nonneoplastic) lymphoid follicles, which may contain germinal centers (Fig. 31-5A, B). Unlike other extranodal MALT lymphomas, lymphoepithelial lesions are not a feature of PCMZL. The infiltrate may extend into the underlying subcutaneous tissue. The cells have small- to medium-sized nuclei with slightly irregular contours and inconspicuous nuclei and thus resemble centrocytes (Fig. 31-6A). The cytoplasm is pale; cells showing less cytoplasm resemble small lymphocytes, whereas those with more ample cytoplasm acquire a monocytoid appearance (Fig. 31-6B). Variable plasmacytic differentiation may also be present in the form of lymphoplasmacytoid cells or plasma cells (Fig. 31-7A), and in these cases Dutcher bodies (pale nuclear pseudoinclusions) or intracytoplasmic Russell bodies, both representing aggregated immunoglobulin, may be present and may suggest neoplasia, although they are nonspecific (Fig. 31-7B). Reactive plasma cells are often found at the periphery of the infiltrate. A minority population of centroblasts and immunoblasts, sometimes quite large in size, may also be observed. Many reactive T and B cells may be present and may outnumber the neoplastic B cells, confounding interpretation (21).

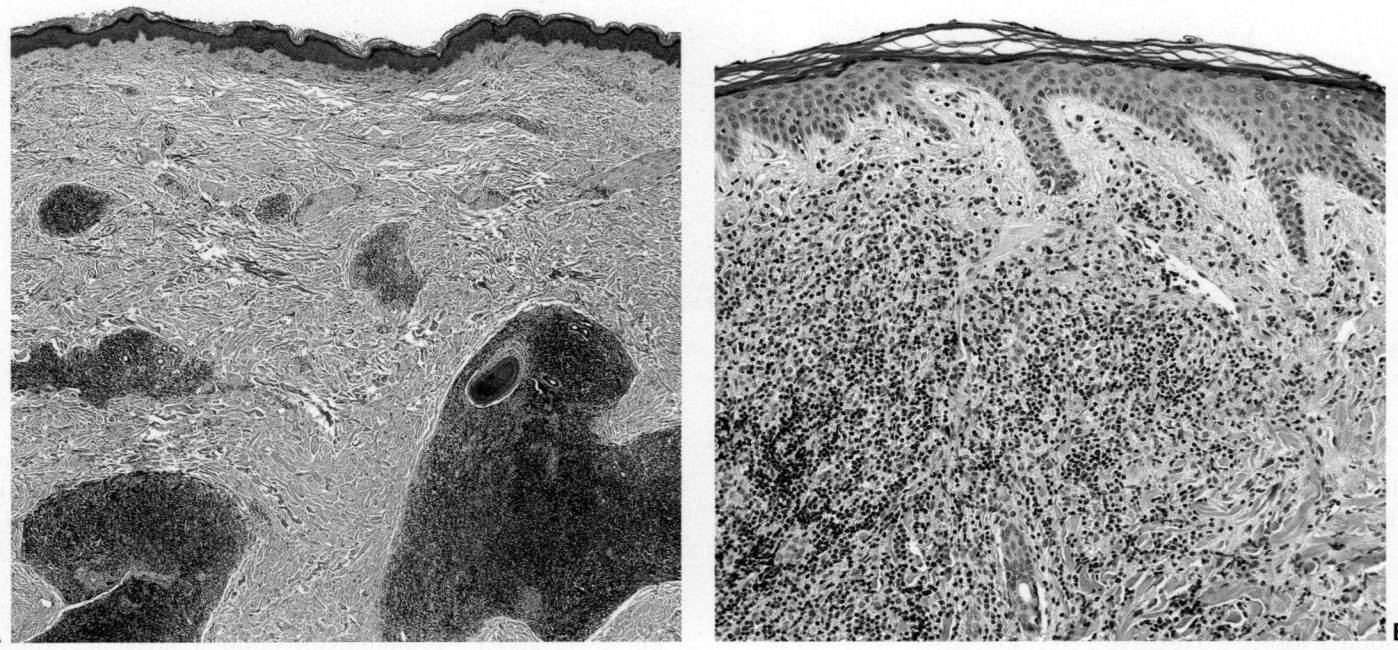

Figure 31-4 Primary cutaneous marginal zone lymphoma. **A:** Nodular infiltrate of neoplastic B cells forming dense, irregularly shaped aggregates in the reticular dermis. **B:** Diffuse dermal infiltrate of small-sized neoplastic B cells, separated from the overlying epidermis by a Grenz zone.

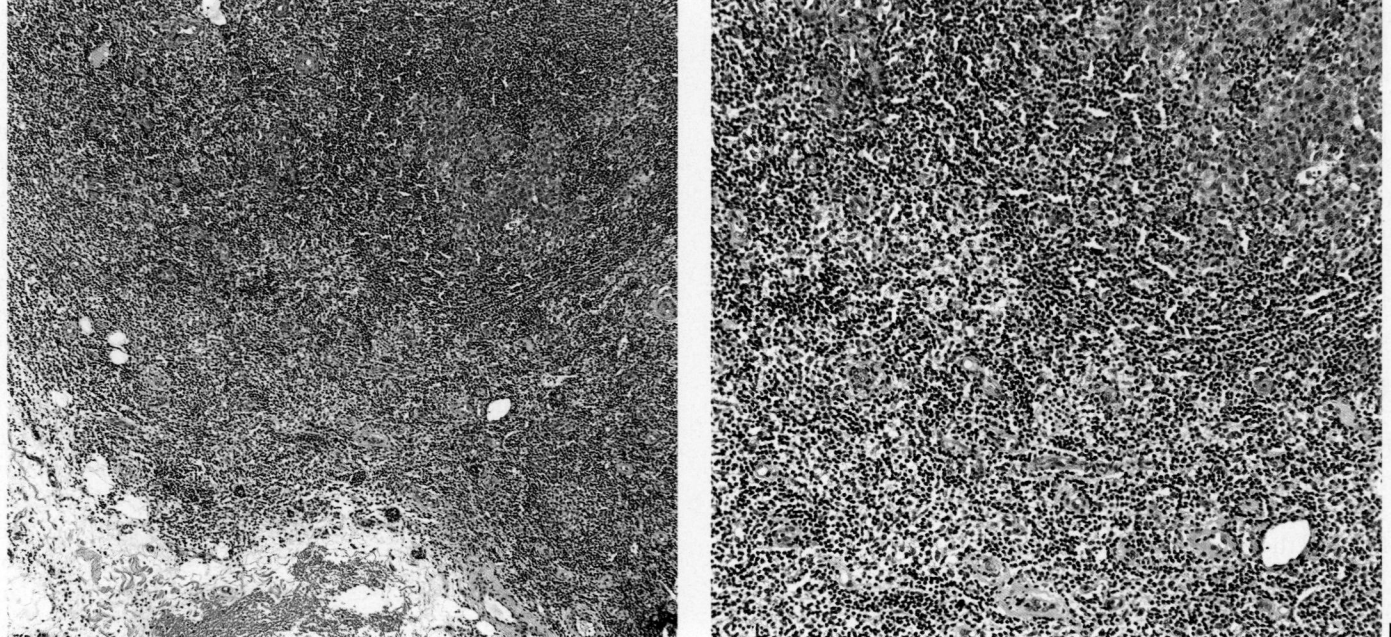

Figure 31-5 Primary cutaneous marginal zone lymphoma. **A:** Low-magnification view of a reactive germinal center and associated mantle zone surrounded by a neoplastic lymphoid infiltrate. **B:** Higher magnification showing the larger cells of the germinal center (upper right corner), the surrounding concentric layers of the mantle zone, and the interstitial neoplastic infiltrate.

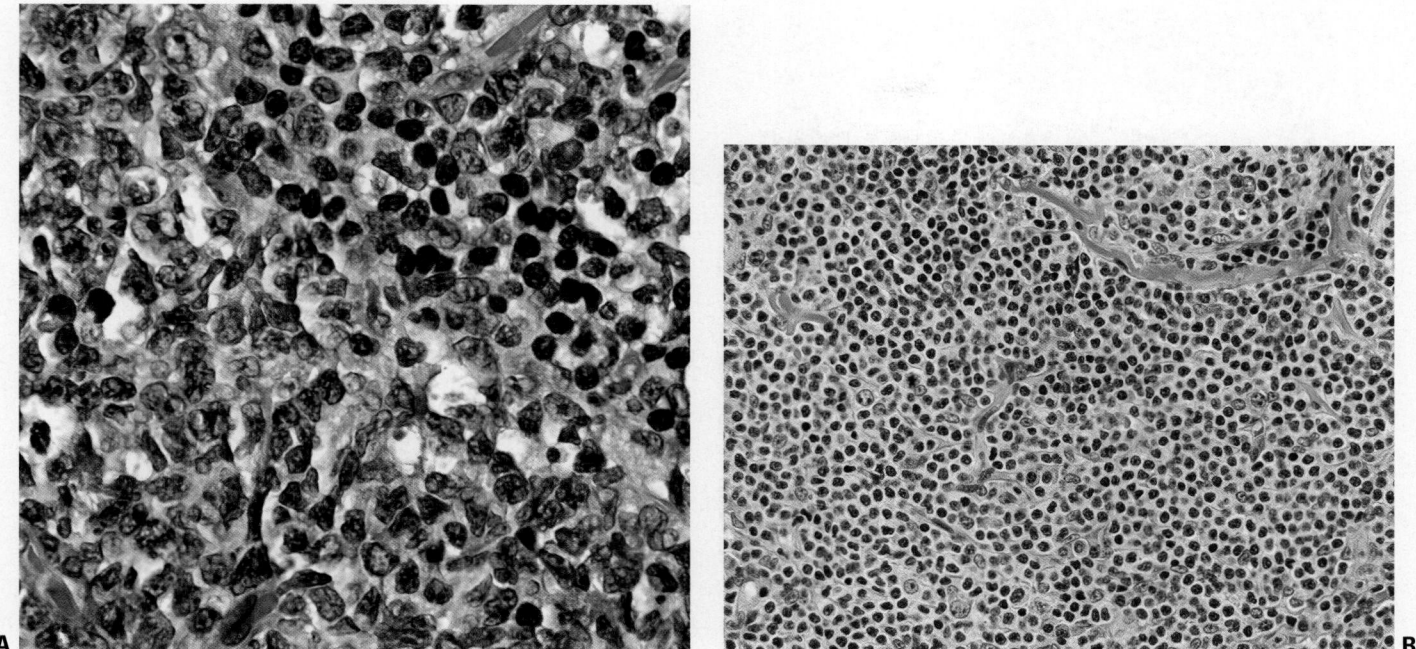

Figure 31-6 Primary cutaneous marginal zone lymphoma. **A:** The atypical neoplastic cells have irregular nuclear contours and slightly dispersed chromatin, compared to the admixed nonneoplastic lymphocytes with round nuclear contours and condensed chromatin (seen in the upper part of the field). **B:** Some proliferations are composed of cells with abundant clear cytoplasm, imparting a "monocytoid" appearance.

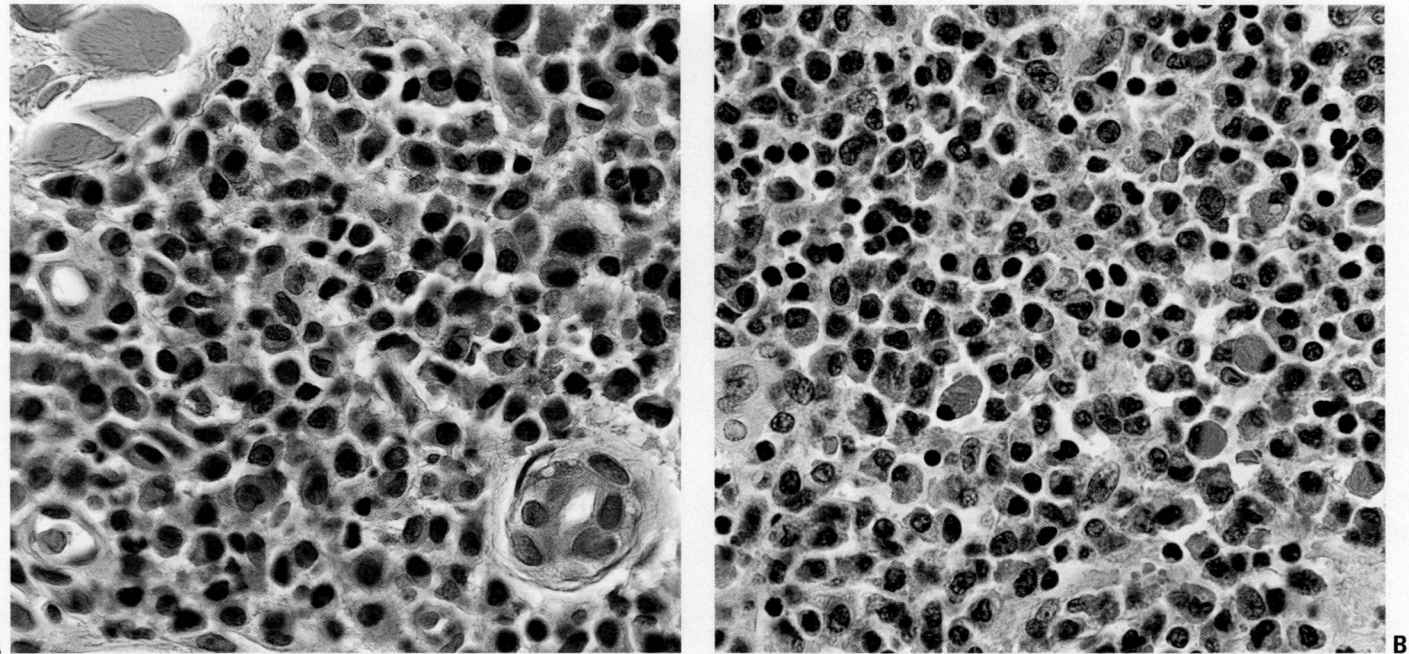

Figure 31-7 Primary cutaneous marginal zone lymphoma. **A:** Morphologic evidence of plasmacytoid differentiation as evidenced by the presence of eccentrically placed nuclei and, in some cells, a perinuclear clearing or "hof." **B:** Large, eosinophilic globules ("Russell bodies") are seen in the cytoplasm of some cells engorged with immunoglobulin.

Tumor cells show immunoglobulin light chain restriction. In the modern era, this is best documented by flow cytometry, although *in situ* hybridization for mRNA may be helpful if monotypic lymphoplasmacytoid forms or plasma cells are admixed. Importantly, *in situ* hybridization studies are only successful in cells with abundant cytoplasmic immunoglobulin mRNA (i.e., plasma cells or lymphoplasmacytoid cells). Flow cytometry may be falsely negative if the number of reactive B cells masks a minor clonal population; similarly, a reactive

plasma cell population may overshadow a neoplastic plasma cell infiltrate by *in situ* hybridization. The PCMZL B cells will be positive for CD20, but CD79a may be needed to pick up the lymphoplasmacytoid/plasma cell forms. Although a dense population of B cells at an extranodal site is a good clue that the infiltrate is neoplastic, no specific marker exists to confirm the diagnosis of PCMZL. The B cells express BCL2 and not CD5, CD10, and BCL6 (Fig. 31-8A–F). Unlike other MALT lymphomas, aberrant CD43 expression is not commonly found

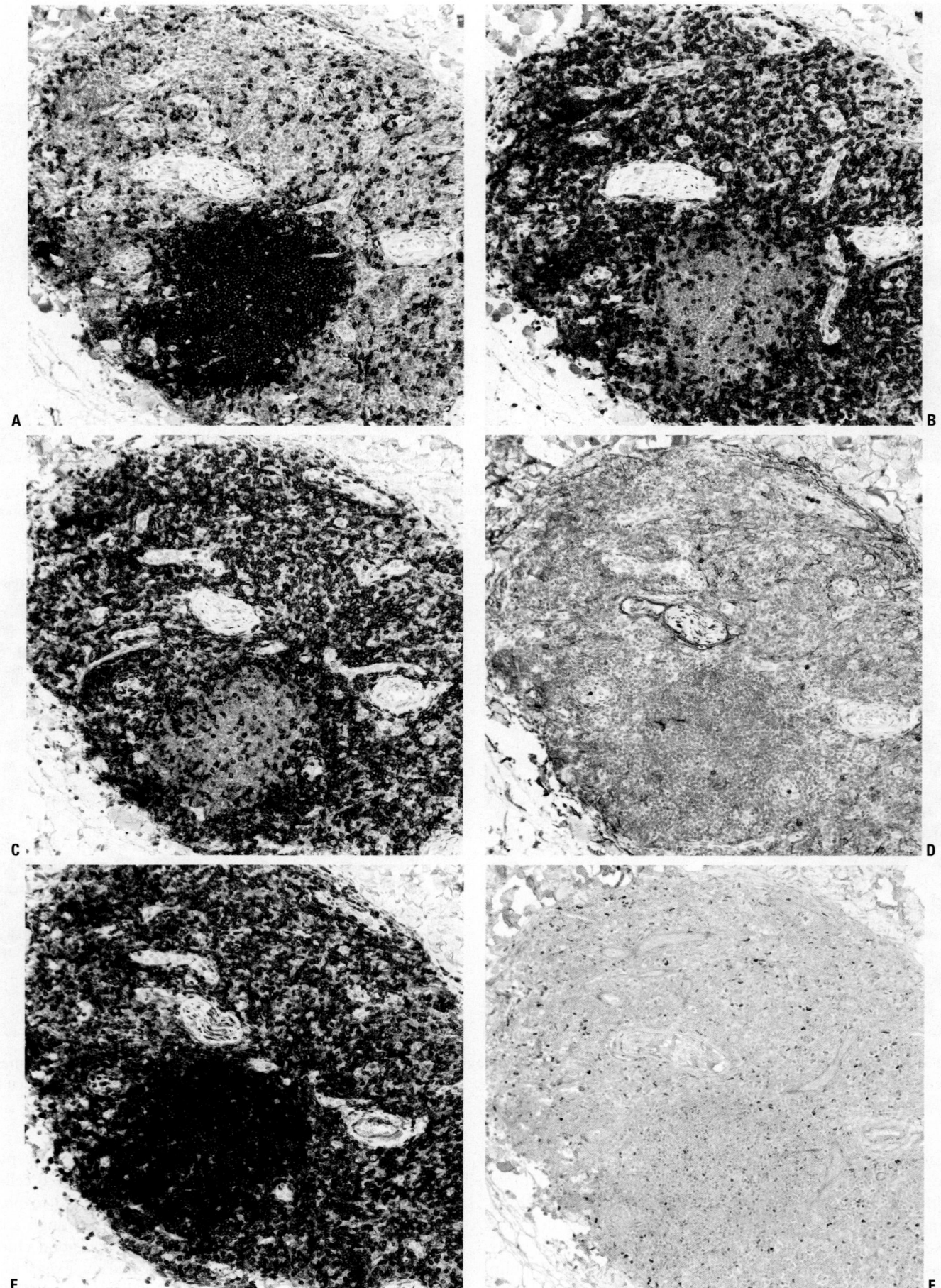

Figure 31-8 Primary cutaneous marginal zone lymphoma. Immunohistochemistry studies reveal an aggregate of CD20⁺ B cells (**A**), surrounded by reactive CD3⁺ T cells (**B**). The B cells do not express CD5 (**C**) or CD10 (**D**), do express BCL2 (**E**), and do not express BCL6 (**F**).

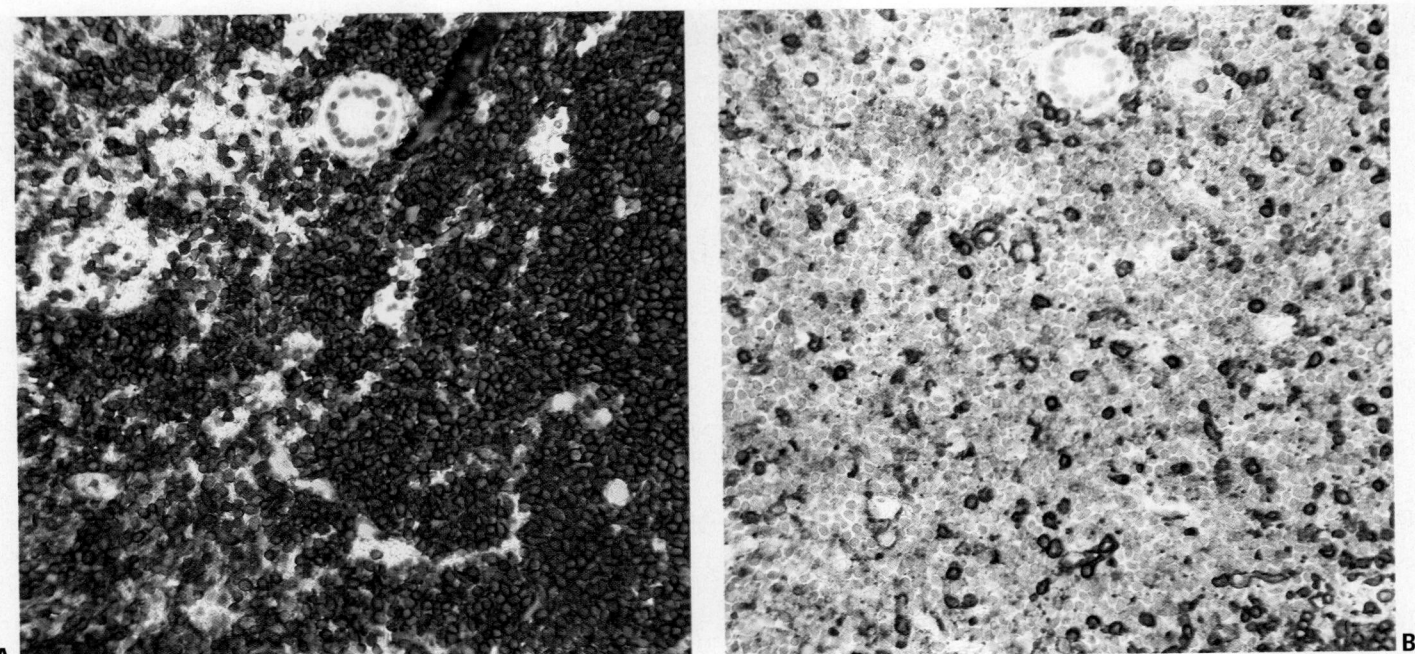

Figure 31-9 Primary cutaneous marginal zone lymphoma. CD43 is often aberrantly expressed in extranodal MALT lymphoma but not in PCMZL. Immunohistochemistry studies reveal that the CD20+ B cells (**A**) do not coexpress CD43 (**B**). The few admixed CD43+ cells seen in this field are reactive small T cells (strong staining) and macrophages (weak staining).

(Fig. 31-9A, B). CD21 will highlight disrupted follicular dendritic cell meshworks.

Recent studies have suggested that there are two distinct subtypes of PCMZL (21–23). The most common subtype contains B cells with evidence of immunoglobulin heavy chain class switching (IgG, or less commonly, IgA), with nearly half showing IgG4 heavy chain restriction; these cases often lack CXCR3 expression and are associated with a T-cell-predominant background enriched for T-helper type 2-like cytokines. This subtype may show monotypic plasma cells at the periphery of the infiltrate. The less common subtype is B-cell predominant, with expression of IgM and often CXCR3; these cases are more likely to involve the subcutis, with plasma cells diffusely scattered, and uniformly show follicular colonization. The IgM-positive cases share features with noncutaneous MZL and are often associated with extracutaneous disease.

Histogenesis. The cell of origin is speculated to be a post–germinal center marginal zone B cell. Immunoglobulin genes are clonally rearranged in approximately 85% of cases, although it is important to consider that clonal B-cell populations can also be detected in nonneoplastic proliferations (24). In addition, clonal rearrangements of the T-cell receptor (TCR) genes have been found in up to 35% of MALT lymphomas, including PCMZL (25). A minority of PCMZL cases demonstrate recurrent chromosomal abnormalities, including t(3;14)(p14.1;q32), t(14;18)(q32;q21), and t(11;18)(q21;q21), although none are specific for skin and have also been detected in MALT lymphomas occurring at other sites (26–32). The t(14;18) includes translocations between *IGH@* and *MALT1* as well as *IGH@* and *BCL2. FOXP1* on chromosome 3 partners with *IGH@* in the documented t(3;14) cases, although this is only seen in about 10% of PCMZL.

Differential Diagnosis. PCMZL may show overlapping features with both neoplastic and nonneoplastic cutaneous B-cell infiltrates (Table 31-3). PCMZL may sometimes lack a monocytoid

appearance and thus morphologically mimic secondary involvement by chronic lymphocytic leukemia/small lymphocytic lymphoma (CLL/SLL) or mantle cell lymphoma (MCL), but these can easily be distinguished by immunophenotyping. The neoplastic cells of PCMZL may sometimes colonize reactive follicles and/or contain increased numbers of centroblasts, raising the possibility of involvement by primary cutaneous follicle center lymphoma (PCFCL), although the expression of BCL6 and CD10 also outside of follicles would favor the neoplastic cells of PCFCL (33). Distinction of PCMZL from a benign reactive infiltrate secondary to injected antigen (arthropod bite) or drug may be very challenging, given the overlapping morphologic features and possibility of clonal immunoglobulin gene rearrangements in benign infiltrates. It may not be possible to distinguish between the two on histologic grounds, in which case correlation with clinical findings is essential. Although documentation of clonal plasma cells is a very helpful indicator of PCMZL, it is important to recognize that T-cell lymphomas such as angioimmunoblastic T-cell lymphoma (AITL) may be associated with clonal plasma cell populations (34). This may cause diagnostic difficulty in cases of PCMZL with a rich reactive T-cell infiltrate.

Principles of Management: The disease may spontaneously resolve, or otherwise typically responds well to a variety of therapeutic modalities, including radiation therapy, eradication of chronic antigenic stimulus in cases where infectious agents are implicated, and/or treatment with the anti-CD20 monoclonal antibody rituximab.

Primary Cutaneous Follicle Center Lymphoma

PCFCL is a neoplasm derived from follicular center B cells, including centrocytes (cleaved follicular center cells) and centroblasts (noncleaved follicular center cells). PCFCL accounts for approximately 10% of cases of cutaneous lymphoma (11) and typically follows an indolent clinical course.

Table 31-3

Differential Diagnosis of Cutaneous B-Cell Infiltrates

	Clonality*	Cytology	Architecture	B-Cell Immunohistochemistry					
				BCL2	BCL6	CD10	CD5	Cyclin D1	IRF4/ MUM1
Reactive									
B-CLH	Polyclonal	Small lymphocytes without atypia	Nodular or diffuse; reactive follicles†	(–) in follicles	(+) in follicles	(+) in follicles	(–)	(–)	(–)
Primary									
PCMZL	Clonal	Monocytoid morphology/ plasmacytic differentiation	Nodular or diffuse +/– reactive follicles†	Reactive follicles (–); infiltrate (+)	Reactive follicles (+); infiltrate (–)	Reactive follicles (+); infiltrate (–)	(–)	(–)	(–)
PCFCL	Clonal	Centrocytes, centroblasts	Follicular or diffuse	Often weak/ (–)	(+)	Follicular pattern often (+)	(–)	(–)	(–)
PCLBCL-LT	Clonal	Centroblasts, immunoblasts	Diffuse	(+)	(+)	(–)	(–)	(–)	(+)
EBV⁺ MCU	Subset clonal	Polymorphous	Circumscribed ulcer	Variable density of CD20⁺, EBV⁺ B cells; CD30+, CD15+/–, BCL6-, CD10-, MUM1+					
Secondary									
B-LBL	Clonal	Blasts	Diffuse	(+)	(–)	(+/–)	(–)	(–)	(-/+)
CLL/SLL	Clonal	Small lymphocytes with round nuclei	Variable; proliferation centers may be present	(+)	(–)	(–)	(+)	(–)	(-/+)
MCL	Clonal	Often blastoid	Diffuse	(+)	(–)	(–)	(+)	(+)	(-/+)
FL	Clonal	Centrocytes, centroblasts	Follicular or diffuse	(+)	(+)	(+)	(–)	(–)	(–)
DLBCL	Clonal	Centroblasts, immunoblasts	Diffuse	(+/–)	(+/–)	(+/–)	(–)	(–)	(+/–)
LYG	Clonal	Polymorphous	Angiodestructive	admixed CD20⁺, EBV⁺ B cells					

B-CLH, B-cell cutaneous lymphoid hyperplasia; PCMZL, primary cutaneous marginal zone lymphoma; PCFCL, primary cutaneous follicle center lymphoma; PCLBCL-LT, primary cutaneous diffuse large B-cell lymphoma, leg type; EBV⁺ MCU, EBV-positive mucocutaneous ulcer; B-LBL, B-lymphoblastic lymphoma; CLL/SLL, chronic lymphocytic leukemia/small lymphocytic lymphoma; MCL, mantle cell lymphoma; FL, follicular lymphoma; DLBCL, diffuse large B-cell lymphoma; LYG, lymphomatoid granulomatosis.

*The most common result is given; exceptions exists; in LYG, clonality most commonly detected in grades 2 and 3.
†Reactive follicles are characterized by germinal centers containing tingle-body macrophages and numerous mitoses, surrounded by well-formed mantle zones

Clinical Summary. PCFCL occurs primarily as one to several red- to plum-colored plaques, nodules, or tumors (Fig. 31-10A, B) often on the head or trunk of adults without sex prediction. PCFCL tends to remain localized in the skin and is often treated with radiation therapy (35). The prognosis of this disease is favorable (5-year survival >95%) despite variations in clinical or morphologic features (localized vs. multifocal disease at presentation; follicular or diffuse growth pattern; number of centroblasts) (11).

Histopathology. The lymphomatous infiltrates occur in the dermis without the involvement of the overlying epidermis. The neoplastic B cells can be arranged in small micronodular aggregates of neoplastic follicles (Fig. 31-11A) or in a diffuse pattern (Fig. 31-11B) or may show a combination of architectural patterns. The follicles are depolarized, are often devoid of mantle zones, and contain monomorphic neoplastic cells without

tingible-body macrophages, as occur in reactive germinal centers (36). Diffuse areas splay dermal fibers and may demonstrate associated sclerosis. The neoplastic infiltrate consists of medium- to large-sized centrocytes, which demonstrate angulated, folded, or twisted nuclear contours, inconspicuous nucleoli, and scant cytoplasm, as well as large centroblasts, which are transformed lymphocytes with round to oval nuclear contours, vesicular chromatin, and several visible nucleoli. The lesions are often predominantly composed of centrocytes, although an even admixture of centrocytes and centroblasts, or even a predominance of centroblasts, may be seen (Fig. 31-11C, D). Occasionally, the cells demonstrate a spindled morphology. Unlike nodal follicular lymphoma (FL), histologic grading of PCFCL is not performed, as the growth pattern and number of centroblasts do not appear to have prognostic relevance in the skin (37). However, tumors showing diffuse, monotonous sheets of centroblasts or immunoblasts are classified as

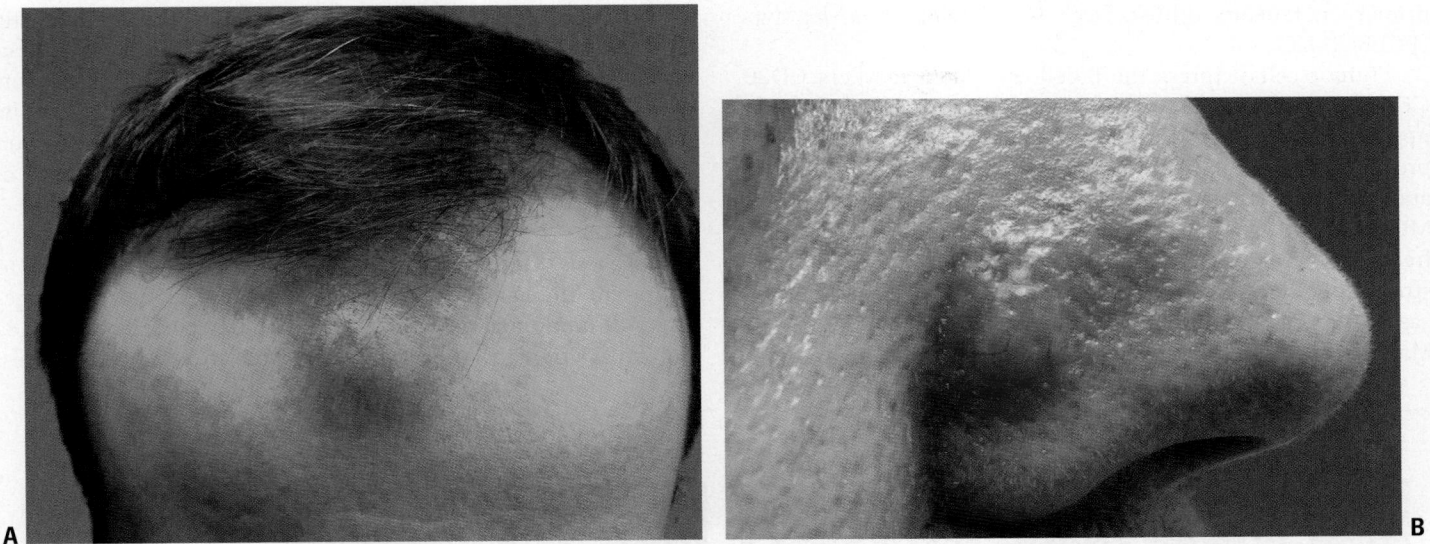

Figure 31-10 Primary cutaneous follicle center lymphoma. **A:** Erythematous tumor on the forehead. **B:** Small nodule with surrounding subtle papules on the nose. (Courtesy of Dr. Cecilia Larocca, Dana-Farber Cancer Institute, Boston, MA.)

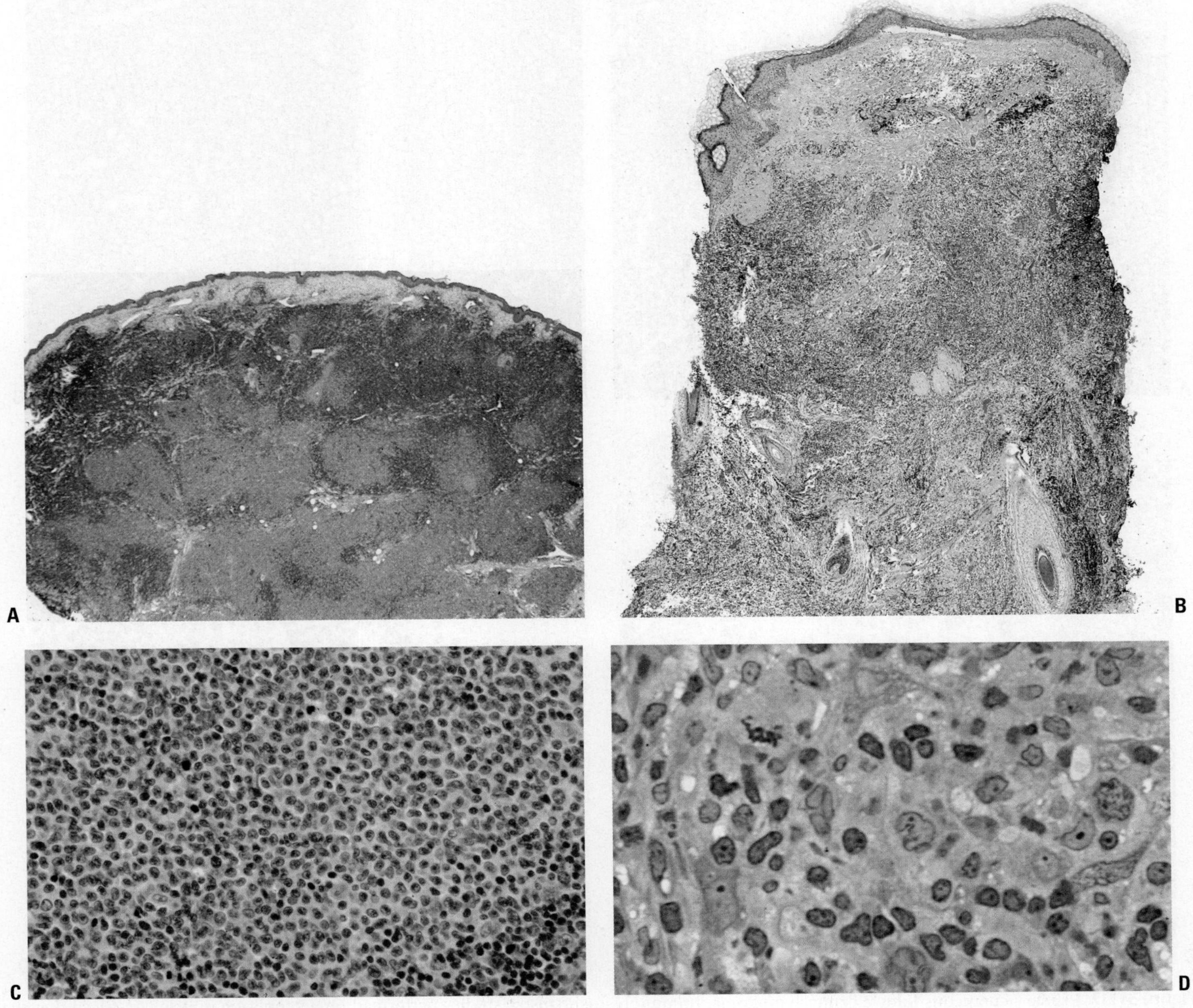

Figure 31-11 Primary cutaneous follicle center lymphoma. **A:** Scanning magnification showing coalescent nodules forming follicle-like architecture. **B:** Scanning magnification showing a diffuse infiltrative pattern. **C:** Higher magnification of malignant centrocytes and centroblasts. **D:** One-micron, toluidine blue–stained section showing cytologic features of centrocytes and centroblasts.

primary cutaneous diffuse large B-cell lymphoma, leg type (PCLBCL-LT).

Tumor cells express the B-cell-associated markers CD20, CD19, CD22, and CD79a but are usually negative for immunoglobulin. BCL6 expression is a constant feature; CD10 expression is more common in cases with a follicular architecture; and interferon regulatory factor-4/multiple myeloma-1 (IRF4/MUM1) staining is typically negative (Fig. 31-12A–F). BCL2 is frequently weak or negative in PCFCL (Fig. 31-12G), although strong, distinct expression has been described in a subset of cases, particularly those with follicular architecture (38–40). Markers of follicular dendritic cells (such as CD21 or CD35)

can be used to detect underlying, associated follicular dendritic cell meshworks in cases with at least partial follicular architecture (Fig. 31-12H). In cases with a diffuse pattern, these stains may highlight few residual follicular dendritic cells or may be completely negative (Fig. 31-13A–C). The Ki67 proliferation index may be high, particularly in diffuse cases composed of large centrocytes (41).

Histogenesis. Germinal center–derived B cells are believed to represent the cell of origin of PCFCL, and clonal rearrangement of immunoglobulin genes is often detected. The t(14;18) (q32;q21) translocation is detected only in a subset of cases,

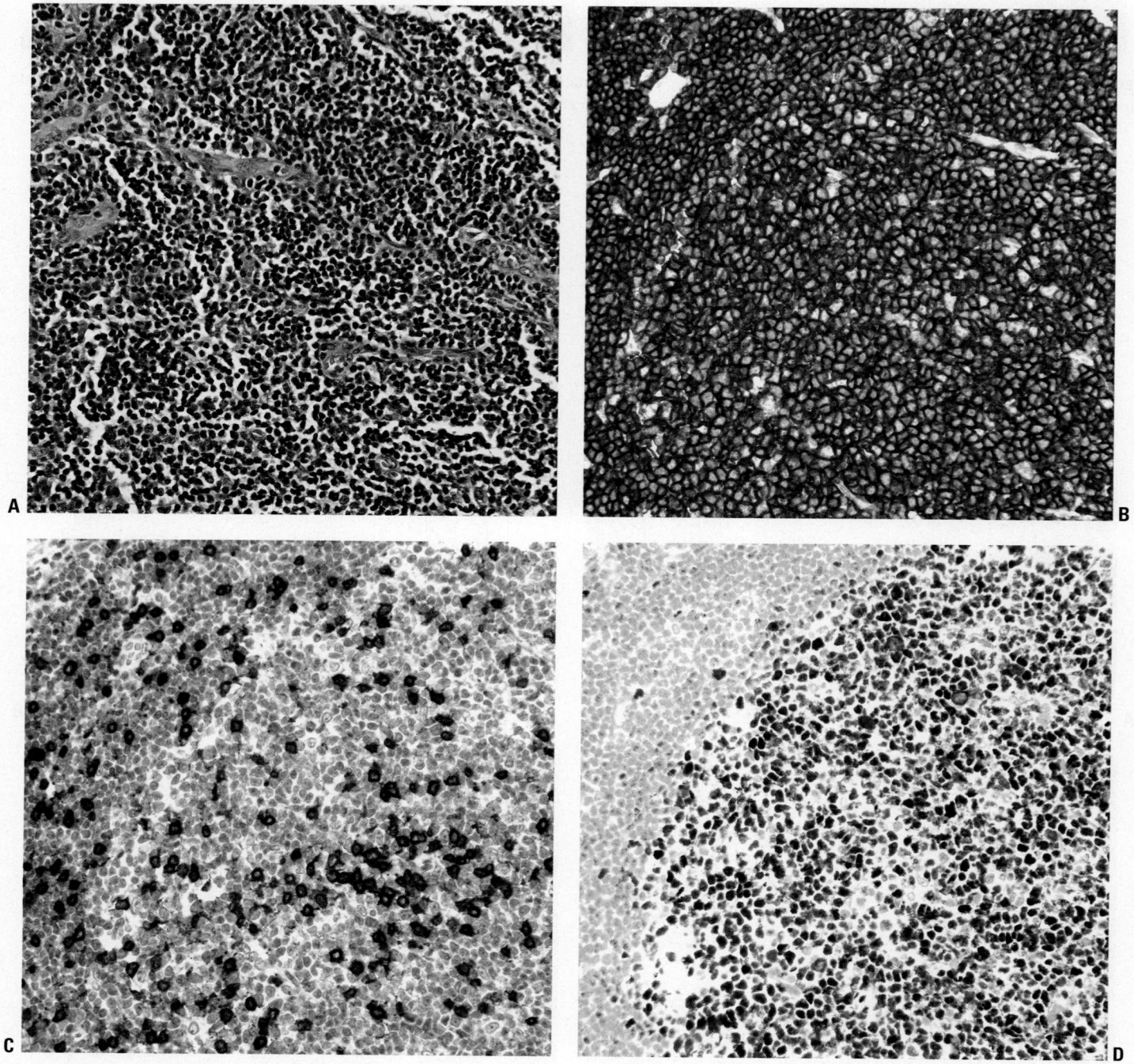

Figure 31-12 Primary cutaneous follicle center lymphoma. Immunohistochemistry studies performed on a neoplastic follicle (**A**) reveal that the follicles are composed of CD20+ B cells (**B**) and show few infiltrating reactive CD3+ T cells (**C**). The B cells commonly coexpress BCL6 (**D**)

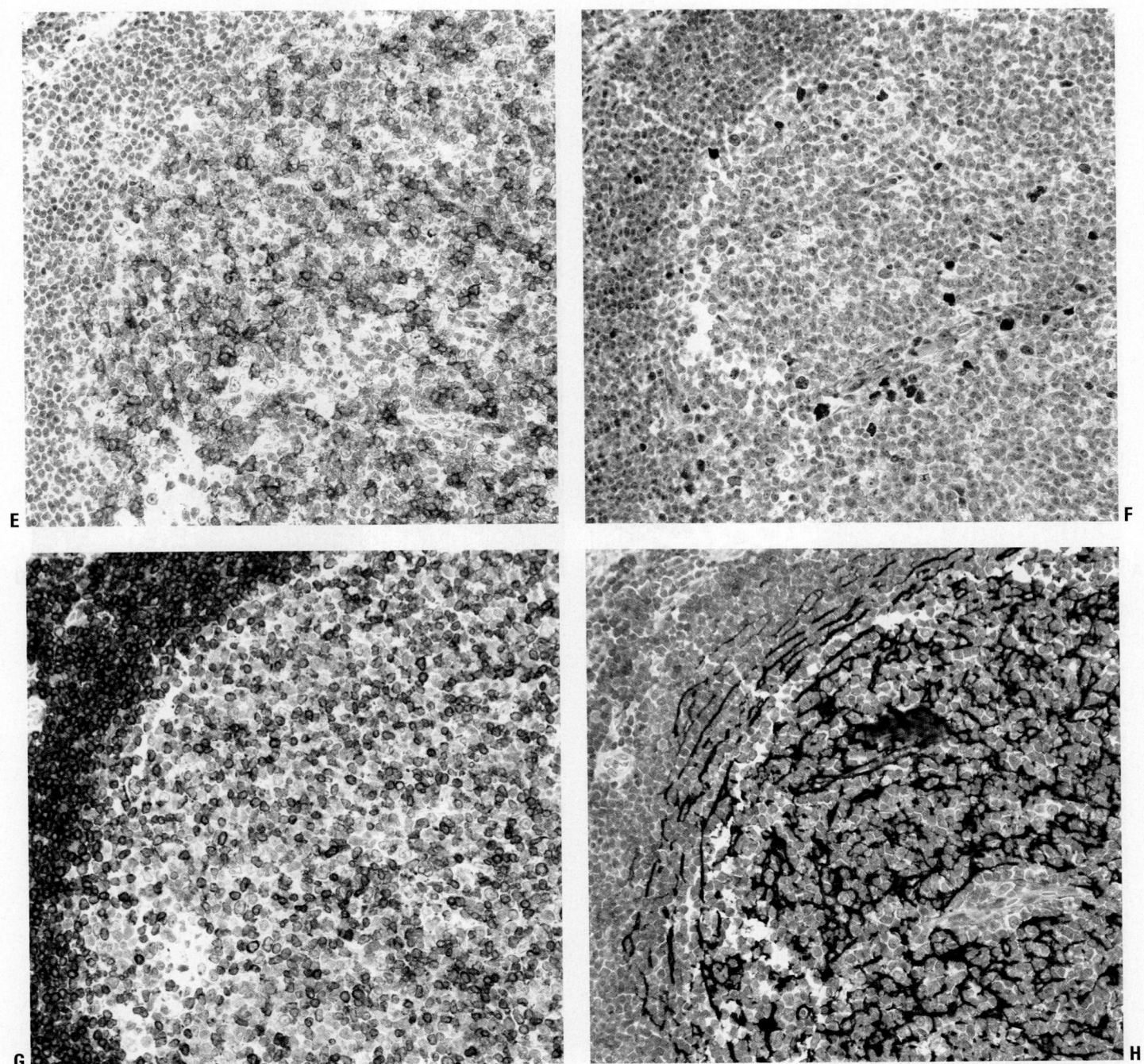

Figure 31-12 (*continued*) and CD10 (E) and are negative for IRF4/MUM1 (F). G: Weak, heterogeneous expression of BCL2 may be seen in the B-cell follicles. H: CD21 will highlight the underlying follicular dendritic cell meshworks.

apparently more consistently with fluorescence *in situ* hybridization (FISH)–based analysis compared to polymerase chain reaction (PCR) (40,42,43). Interestingly, BCL2 expression by immunohistochemistry can be detected in cases without an underlying t(14;18) (40). There is increasing recent evidence showing PCFCL harbor a distinctive genetic profile compared to systemic FL (44,45). PCFCL is highly enriched in *TNFRSF14* loss of function mutations and chromosome 1p36 copy number loss, but rarely contains mutations that are common in systemic FL, such as in chromatin-modifying genes *CREBBP* or *KMT2D*.

Differential Diagnosis. PCFCL may show overlapping features with both neoplastic and nonneoplastic cutaneous B-cell infiltrates (Table 31-3). Distinction from B-cell cutaneous lymphoid

hyperplasia (B-CLH), which may show similar clinical features, is necessary. The typical features of the reactive follicles in B-CLH (well-formed mantle zones, polarized germinal centers with tingible-body macrophages, and numerous mitotic figures) are morphologically distinct from the monomorphous follicles of PCFCL. In general, clonality studies will reveal a polyclonal B-cell population in B-CLH and a clonal B-cell population in PCFCL, although exceptions do exist, and therefore incorporation of morphologic and immunophenotypic findings is also needed. In addition, PCFCL must be differentiated from secondary cutaneous involvement by nodal-type FL. Although there are no absolute morphologic or immunophenotypic features that can reliably distinguish the two entities, strong immunoreactivity for both BCL2 and CD10 and/or detection of

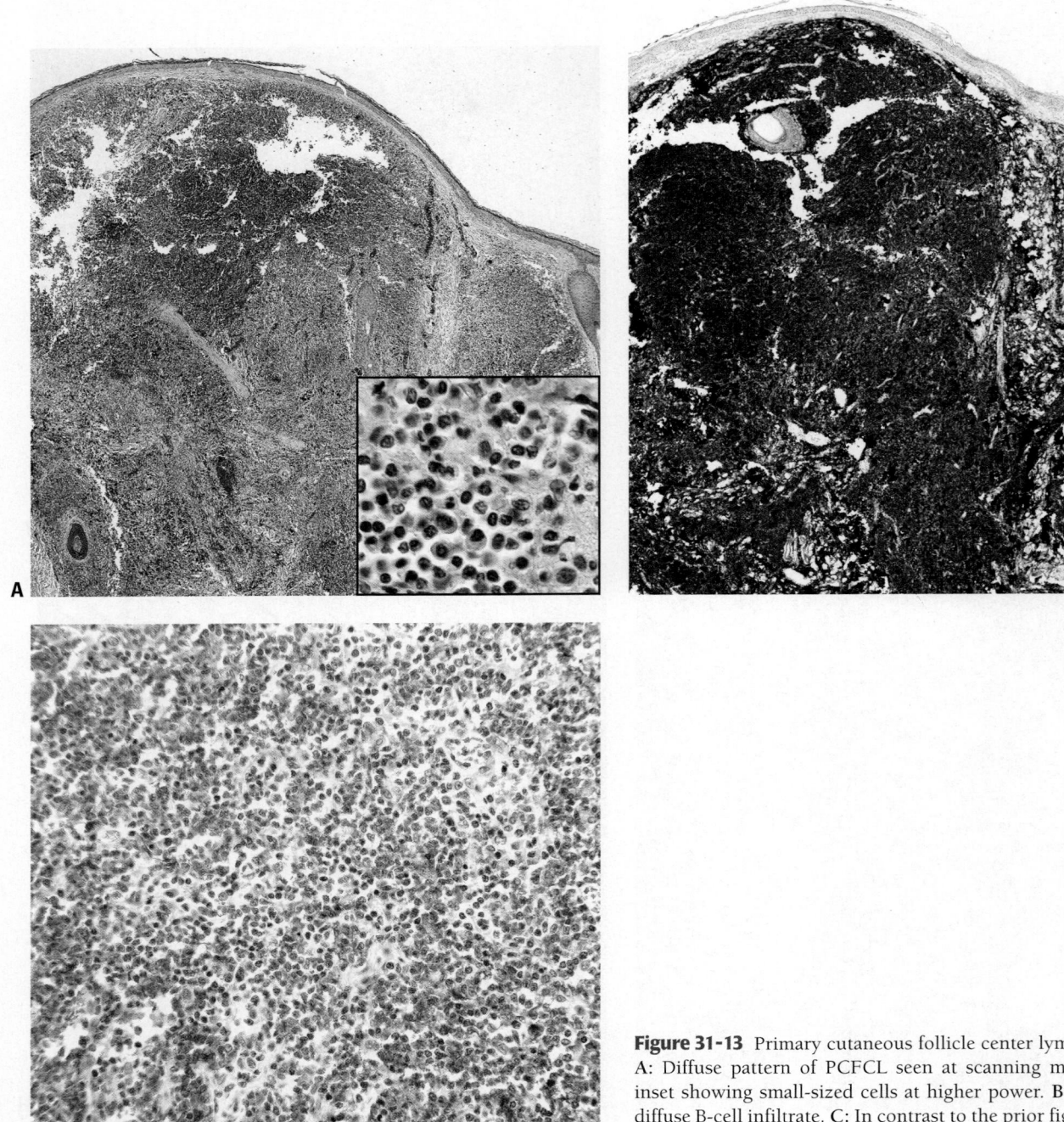

Figure 31-13 Primary cutaneous follicle center lymphoma (PCFCL). A: Diffuse pattern of PCFCL seen at scanning magnification, with inset showing small-sized cells at higher power. B: CD20 marks the diffuse B-cell infiltrate. C: In contrast to the prior figure, staining with CD21 reveals weak, nonspecific expression and does not highlight an underlying follicular dendritic cell meshwork.

t(14;18) raises the possibility of systemic FL. As discussed previously, there may be an emerging role for the genetic features of PCFCL aiding in its distinction from systemic FL. In any case lacking staging information, a differential diagnosis should be provided. Another potential diagnostic difficulty is the distinction between PCFCL and PCMZL demonstrating follicular colonization or associated reactive follicles. Assessing the immunophenotype of the interfollicular cells may help; PCFCL displays a $BCL2^{-/+}/CD10^{+/-}/BCL6^+$ phenotype, whereas PCMZL cells are $BCL2^+/CD10^-/BCL6^-$ (46). Finally, morphologic distinction between PCFCL with a purely diffuse pattern from PCLBCL-LT is difficult, especially in cases where centroblasts predominate in the PCFCL infiltrate. Immunohistochemical

profiling may be useful in this scenario, although it is essential to recognize that exceptions do exist. Both entities express BCL6, whereas CD10 is often negative in the latter. In addition, PCFCL may lack strong BCL2 reactivity and often lacks IRF4/MUM1 and forkhead box P1 (FoxP1) expression, all of which are strongly positive in PCLBCL-LT (47,48). Additionally, cytoplasmic expression of IgM (and less commonly also IgD) is frequently detected in PCLBCL-LT, whereas identification of either of these heavy chains is uncommon in PCFCL (49,50).

Principles of Management: PCFCL is typically an indolent disease, and solitary or localized lesions may be treated with radiation therapy or excision. Multifocal lesions may be treated with radiation, topical agents, or steroid injections. Systemic chemotherapy is rarely indicated. Cutaneous relapse is observed in approximately 30% of cases but does not portend a poorer prognosis (35). Of note, presentation on the leg does appear to have a less favorable prognosis and therefore also warrants close clinical management (47,51).

Primary Cutaneous Diffuse Large B-Cell Lymphoma, Leg Type

PCLBCL-LT is an aggressive primary cutaneous large B-cell lymphoma characterized by a diffuse, cutaneous infiltrate of immunoblasts or centroblasts in a sparse reactive background and strong immunoreactivity for IRF4/MUM1 and BCL2 (52,53).

Clinical Summary. PCLBCL-LT most commonly presents as solitary or multiple localized reddish-brown tumors or plaques (Fig. 31-14). Although the disease typically occurs on the leg, lesions with a similar morphology and phenotype can arise at any cutaneous site. Affected patients are usually elderly, with a female predominance. The overall prognosis is intermediate to poor, with a 5-year survival of 55% and a tendency to disseminate to extracutaneous sites. Ulceration, primary manifestation on the leg, or multiple lesions at presentation are associated with adverse prognosis (48,54,55).

Histopathology. PCLBCL-LT manifests as a dense, monotonous infiltrate of predominantly medium- to large-sized cells with round nuclear contours and prominent nucleoli (immunoblasts or centroblasts) (Fig. 31-15A, B). Frequent mitoses are seen, and reactive small lymphocytes are sparse. The infiltrate diffusely involves the dermis, obliterating the adnexa, and often extends into the underlying subcutaneous tissue. Focal epidermotropism with Pautrier-like microabscesses may be seen. The neoplastic cells strongly express IRF4/MUM1 and BCL2 but not CD10 (Fig. 31-16A–E). Most cases also express BCL6, a marker

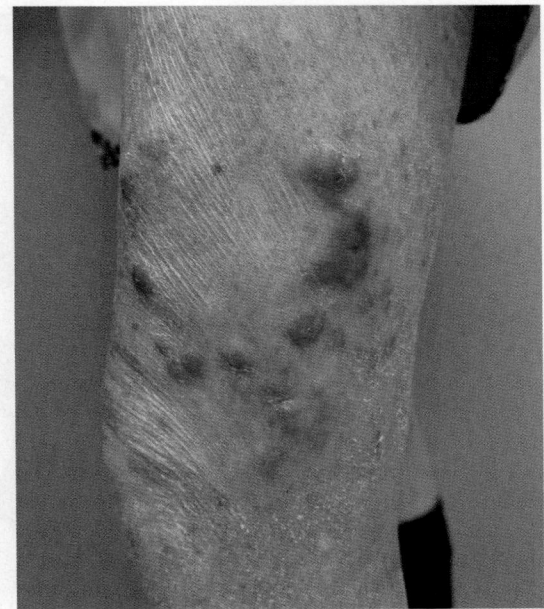

Figure 31-14 Primary cutaneous diffuse large B-cell lymphoma, leg type. Multiple erythematous tumors and plaques on the leg. (Courtesy of Dr. Nicole R. LeBoeuf, Dana-Farber Cancer Institute, Boston, MA.)

for B-cell germinal center differentiation, as well as IgM, or less commonly IgD (Fig. 31-17A,B) (49,50). Strong FoxP1 expression is also common. The Ki67 proliferation index is usually high (~ 70%) (47). CD30 expression may be detected, but this does not change the classification if the case otherwise meets morphologic and immunophenotypic criteria for this entity (56).

Histogenesis. PCLBCL-LT has a B-cell differentiation profile of post–germinal center (activated) B cells (57). Molecular profiling demonstrates a signature in PCLBCL-LT distinct from

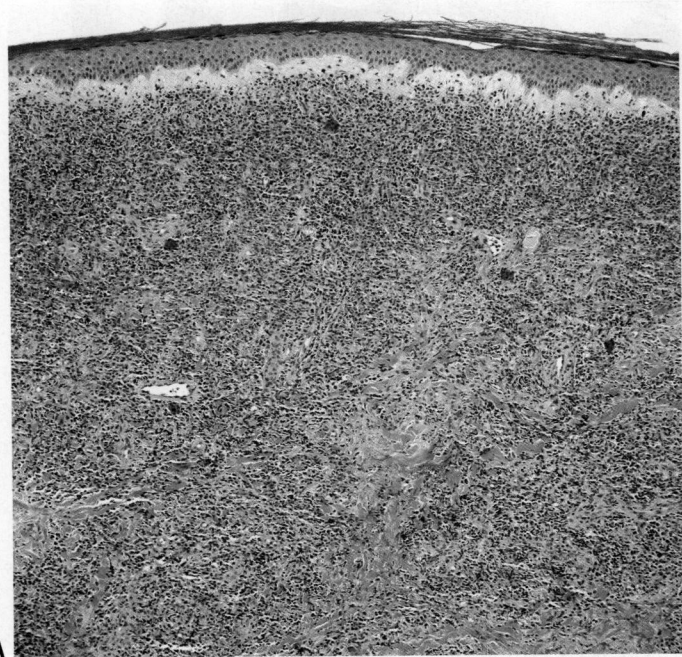

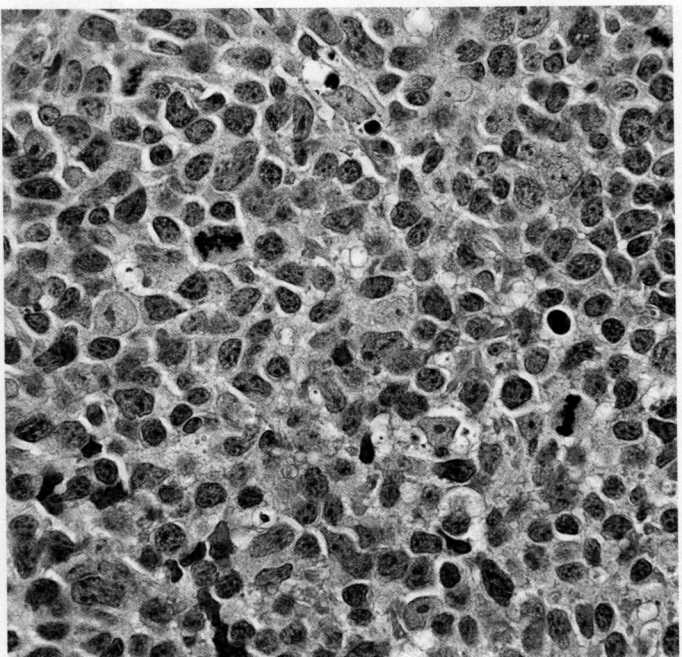

Figure 31-15 Primary cutaneous diffuse large B-cell lymphoma, leg type. **A:** Scanning magnification view shows a diffuse lymphoid infiltrate encompassing the entire dermis but separated from the overlying epidermis by a distinct Grenz zone. **B:** The neoplastic infiltrate is composed of large-sized cells with open chromatin and distinct nucleoli. Mitotic figures are abundant.

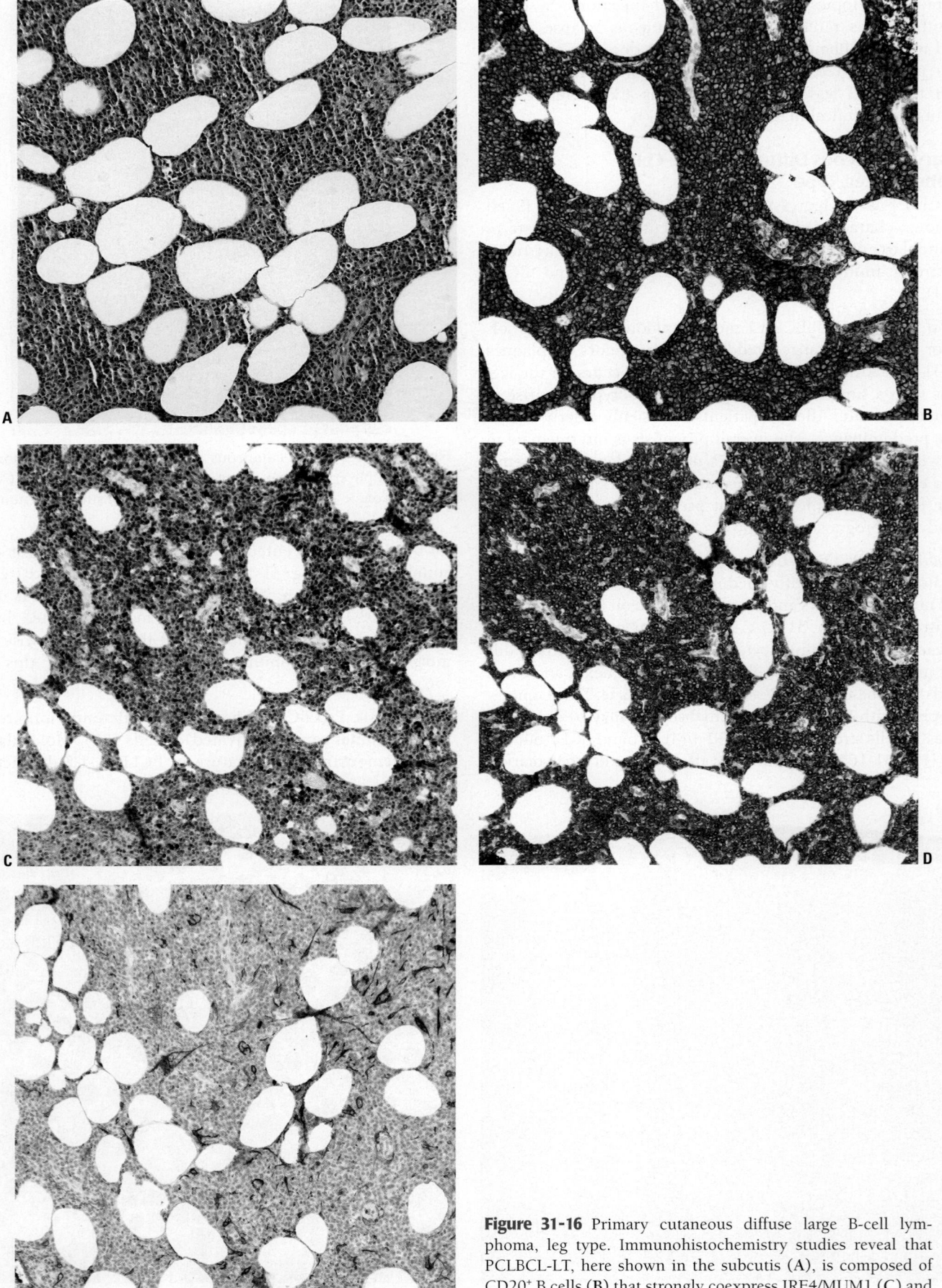

Figure 31-16 Primary cutaneous diffuse large B-cell lymphoma, leg type. Immunohistochemistry studies reveal that PCLBCL-LT, here shown in the subcutis (**A**), is composed of CD20⁺ B cells (**B**) that strongly coexpress IRF4/MUM1 (**C**) and BCL2 (**D**) and do not express CD10 (**E**).

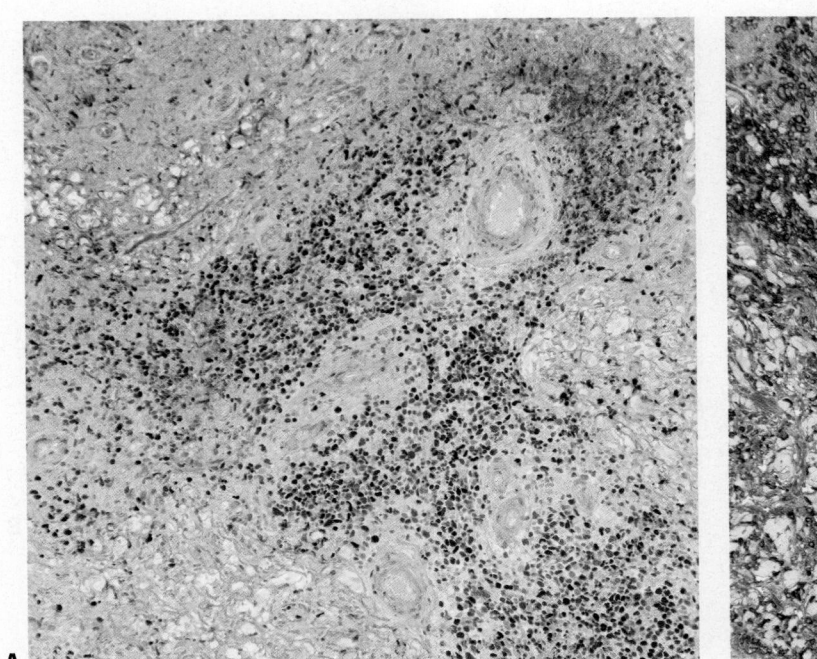
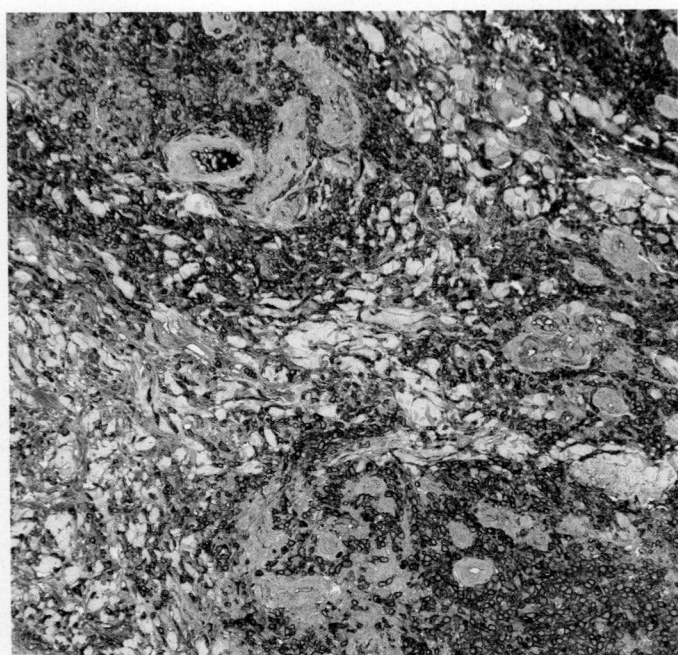

Figure 31-17 Primary cutaneous diffuse large B-cell lymphoma, leg type. Immunohistochemistry studies demonstrate strong expression of BCL6 (A) and IgM (B) in PCLBCL-LT.

other types of cutaneous B-cell lymphomas and most similar to the ABC subtype of systemic DLBCL (57–59); it also may resemble primary central nervous lymphomas and primary testicular lymphomas (60). The t(14;18) translocation involving IGH@ and BCL2 is not found in this entity. Unlike other cutaneous B-cell lymphomas that appear to be genetically unrelated to their nodal-based counterparts, cytogenetic studies of PCLBCL-LT have demonstrated frequent translocations similar to those in systemic DLBCL involving IGH@, MYC, and BCL6 loci (28), as well as the presence of the MYD88 oncogenic L265P mutation (61,62), or mutations in other genes activating the NF-kB pathway (60). Approximately 75% of cases exhibit inactivation of 9p21.3/CDKN2A via deletion or promoter hypermethylation, which is a poor prognostic indicator (59,63,64).

Differential Diagnosis. The differential diagnosis includes PCFCL, diffuse type, or systemic DLBCL secondarily involving the skin (Table 31-3). Cytomorphology may provide clues to the diagnosis (cleaved medium-sized centrocytes with inconspicuous nucleoli in PCFCL versus large, round centroblasts with prominent nucleoli in PCLBCL-LT). Occasionally, cases of PCFCL may exhibit an admixture of centrocytes and centroblasts or even predominance of centroblasts. In the latter scenarios, immunohistochemical profiling is paramount for diagnosis. In contrast to PCLBCL-LT, which strongly expresses BCL2, IRF4/MUM1, and IgM, PCFCL diffuse type is typically negative for these markers. Epstein–Barr virus (EBV)+ DLBCL, not otherwise specified (NOS), may involve the skin but is distinguished by positive *in situ* hybridization for EBV-encoded RNA (EBER), which is negative in PCLBCL-LT.

Principles of Management: Radiotherapy, systemic chemotherapy, and/or rituximab administration are mainstays of treatment. Regimens may need to be tailored to the underlying fitness of the patient given the frequent occurrence in elderly individuals.

EBV-Positive Mucocutaneous Ulcer

EBV+ mucocutaneous ulcer (MCU) is a newly recognized immunodeficiency-associated B-cell lymphoproliferative disorder manifesting as localized cutaneous or mucosal ulcerated lesions, typically with an indolent course (65).

Clinical Summary. EBV+ MCU occurs in the setting of advanced age–related immunosenescence or iatrogenic immunosuppression and presents as an isolated well-demarcated ulcerative lesion involving the skin, oropharyngeal mucosa, or gastrointestinal tract. In the former clinical scenario, the median age is more than 70 years. There is no systemic lymphadenopathy, hepatosplenomegaly, or bone marrow involvement. EBV+ MCU generally has a self-limited, indolent course and in the setting of medication-induced immunosuppression almost always shows resolution with reduction of immunosuppression, whereas age-related cases can wax and wane but do not show systemic progression (66).

Histopathology. The lesions are sharply circumscribed mucosal or cutaneous ulcers, containing a polymorphous infiltrate of lymphocytes and variably dense atypical large B cells, with either an immunoblastic morphology or with Hodgkin/Reed–Sternberg-like features (Fig. 31-18A, B). Frequent apoptotic cells are seen, and there can be a variable number of scattered plasma cells, histiocytes, and eosinophils. The infiltrate can focally involve vessel walls. Often, there is a rim of small lymphocytes at the base of the lesion, accentuating the sharp delineation (Fig. 31-18C). There can be pseudoepitheliomatous hyperplasia and reactive atypia in the adjacent surface epithelium. The atypical large B cells express PAX5, with variable CD20 (Fig. 31-18D, E), and are typically positive for CD30, with almost half of cases coexpressing CD15. They are usually positive for MUM1 and negative for CD10 and BCL6. In most cases, the atypical cells are positive for CD45 and show expression of B-cell nuclear transcription factors OCT-2 and BOB-1. The cells are positive by EBER *in situ* hybridization (Fig. 31-18F).

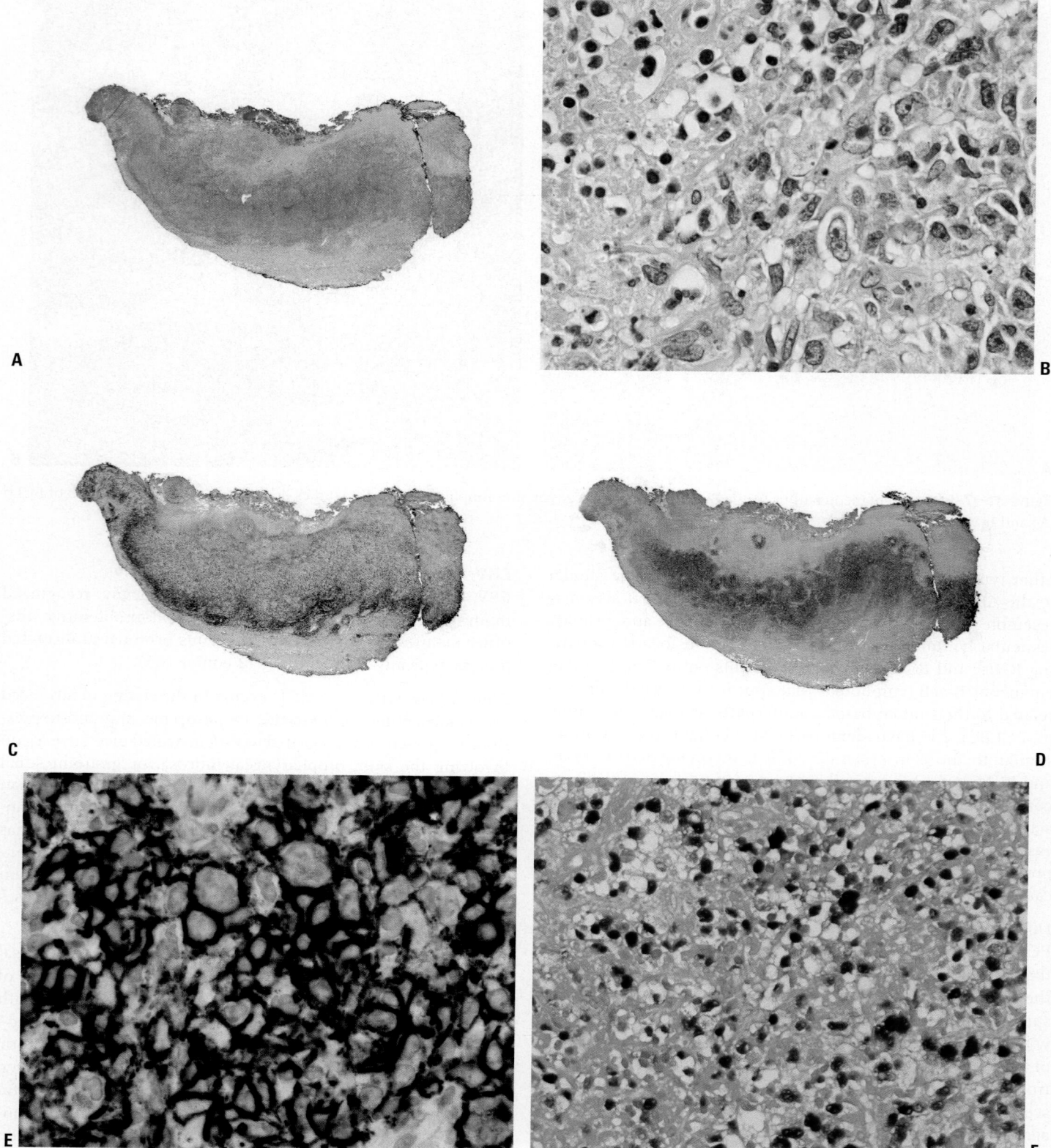

Figure 31-18 EBV+ mucocutaneous ulcer. **A:** Low-power histologic section of a sharply demarcated oral mucosal lesion shows a dense superficial infiltrate with surface ulceration. **B:** On high magnification, there is a polymorphous infiltrate of lymphocytes including atypical large cells, some of which have Hodgkin/Reed–Sternberg-like features, with adjacent apoptotic cells. **C:** There is a rim of CD3+ T cells at the periphery of the lesion. **D:** PAX5 demonstrates that most cells in the infiltrate are B cells. **E:** CD20 is positive in most lesional cells. **F:** These cells are positive for EBER *in situ* hybridization.

Histogenesis. EBV is implicated in the pathogenesis, occurring in the setting of immunosuppression or localized lapse in immuno-surveillance, with an altered T-cell response or diminished T-cell repertoire (65). Accordingly, monoclonal or oligoclonal patterns of TCR gene rearrangement can be seen. A subset of cases reveal clonal rearrangements of immunoglobulin genes (67,68).

Differential Diagnosis. The histology can overlap with EBV⁺ DLBCL. Helpful differential diagnostic features are the very well-demarcated and isolated nature of lesions in EBV⁺ MCU, and the frequent finding of a band of reactive lymphocytes at the periphery. However, histologic distinction can be difficult or impossible (66), and close clinical correlation to assess for other sites of disease is essential, because the two entities have very different therapeutic approaches and outcomes. The distinction with CHL also rests largely on the hallmark presentation of EBV⁺ MCU as an isolated, sharply demarcated, and ulcerated lesion and the exceptional rarity of primary presentation of CHL in the skin or mucosa. In addition, the atypical large cells in EBV⁺ MCU often express CD45 and have a more fully retained B-cell antigenic profile, and there is a more polymorphous spectrum of EBV⁺ cells. Presence of vasculopathic vessel involvement may raise the differential of lymphomatoid granulomatosis (LYG), a more aggressive systemic EBV⁺ lymphoproliferative disorder; the characteristic clinical presentation of EBV⁺ MCU and the absence of involvement of other organs, including lung, can aid in this distinction.

Principles of Management: In general, EBV⁺ MCU follows an indolent course, with some lesions spontaneously regressing and most patients showing improvement with discontinuation or reduction of immunosuppressants or with chemotherapy or radiation. Disease recurrences or progression have been rarely reported (69).

Mature T-/Natural Killer–Cell Lineage

Mycosis Fungoides

MF is the prototype of cutaneous T-cell lymphoma (CTCL) that typically begins as slowly progressive dermatitis-like patches and plaques that may evolve into nodules or tumors. Eventual systemic dissemination will occur in a subset of patients (70). The patch/plaque stage of the disease is the result of intraepidermal and superficial dermal infiltration by small- to medium-sized neoplastic T cells with characteristically

cerebriform nuclear contours. More advanced stages develop as a consequence of dermal or extracutaneous involvement by cytologically more atypical T cells. Diagnosis at early stages may be challenging solely on histologic grounds given the morphologic overlap with other (predominantly reactive) conditions and requires careful clinicopathologic correlation. The International Society for Cutaneous Lymphomas developed an integrative clinicopathologic diagnostic algorithm that may have utility in distinguishing suspected early MF from its mimics, although a subsequent validation study showed lack of specificity, and this remains an imperfect tool (71–73). Multiple biopsies at one time point, or periodically over time, may be necessary to establish the diagnosis. TCR gene rearrangements may or may not be present in MF, and reactive conditions may also show clonal TCR gene rearrangements, limiting the usefulness of this ancillary study in early-stage disease. However, demonstration of identical clones at different anatomic sites or over time will support a diagnosis of a neoplastic process.

Clinical Summary. MF is relatively rare, accounting for less than 1% of non-Hodgkin lymphomas. However, of lymphomas that arise primarily in skin, it is the most common, accounting for nearly 50% of cutaneous lymphomas (11). It is a disease predominantly of adults, with a male-to-female ratio of 2:1, although children are occasionally affected. MF has a plethora of clinicopathologic manifestations. Typical lesions initially present as large, erythematous scaling patches and plaques that may show arcuate or polycyclic configurations and are generally resistant to anti-inflammatory therapy (Fig. 31-19A). A number of distinct variants are described in the later sections. As the disease advances, larger plaques and nodules and even frank tumors will develop, often with associated ulceration (Fig. 31-19B), although patches and plaques are often still present at this stage. If extracutaneous spread occurs, the lymph nodes, spleen, liver, and lungs are often involved, in addition to the peripheral blood. Lymph node enlargement at such advanced stages must be differentiated from nodal hyperplasia resulting from chronic drainage of involved sites (dermatopathic lymphadenopathy), a condition that may also be seen in lymph nodes draining dermatitis. An erythrodermic manifestation may occur, but is uncommon, and must be differentiated from

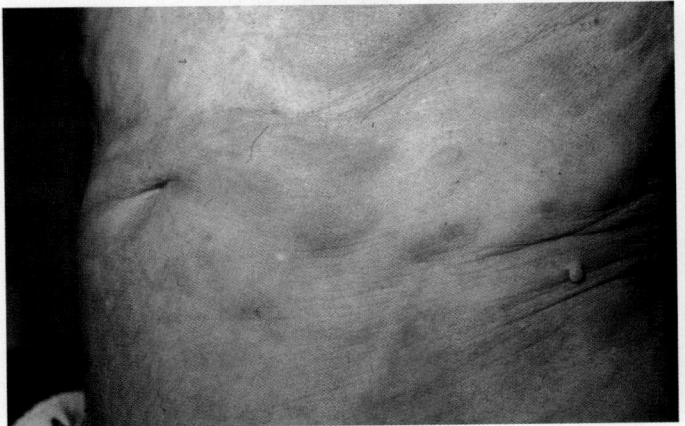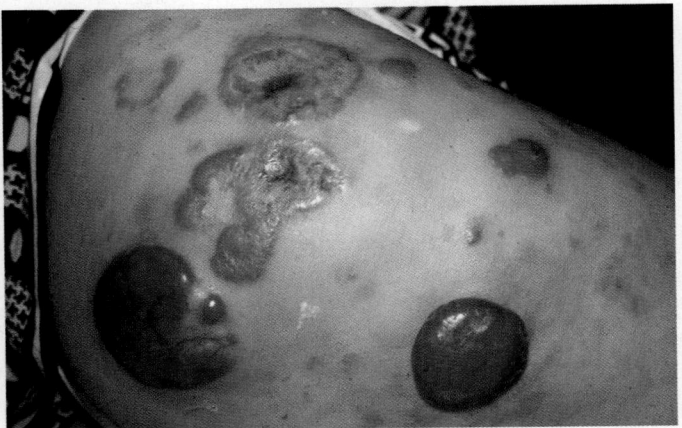

Figure 31-19 Mycosis fungoides: clinical features. **A:** Erythematous scaling patches and plaques of early disease. **B:** Plaques and nodules of advanced disease.

benign conditions that may also show erythrodermic phases, as well as Sézary syndrome (see later).

Clinical staging follows criteria uniquely developed for MF and also used for Sézary syndrome (SS) and incorporates evidence of histologic; immunophenotypic; and/or molecular involvement of cutaneous, nodal, and visceral sites as well as peripheral blood (74). Patients do not inevitably progress through all of the disease stages; in a large study, 71% of patients presented with early-stage disease, and disease progression occurred in 34% of patients (75). For those that do progress, higher stage is directly correlated with decreased survival. For example, patients with stage IA disease (limited patches, papules, and/or plaques covering <10% of the skin surface with or without low blood tumor burden) have a 10-year overall survival (OS) of 88%, those with stage IB (≥10% of the skin surface) have a 10-year OS of 70%, and those with one or more tumors (stage IIB) have a 10-year OS of 34% (76).

Histopathology. Cytologically, the neoplastic T cells in MF are small- to medium-sized lymphocytes that characteristically contain nuclei with dense heterochromatin and elaborately indented (cerebriform) nuclear contours that are often best appreciated by dynamic focusing through nuclei at high magnification (Fig. 31-20A, B). These cells may be difficult to differentiate from cytokine-activated T cells, although one helpful feature is the tendency for epidermotropic neoplastic T cells to predominantly or exclusively show cerebriform nuclear features and clear perinuclear halos.

The clinical manifestations of MF (patch, plaque, or tumor stage) roughly correlate with the microscopic appearance of the lesions. Early lesions of MF show a patchy bandlike lymphocytic infiltrate within the papillary dermis, often associated with coarse fibrosis (Fig. 31-21A, B). Frequently only a few of the atypical T cells are present in the dermis and are often obscured by a background of many small (reactive) T cells as well as admixed eosinophils, plasma cells, and histiocytes. This can make

the diagnosis of early-stage MF very challenging and indeed in some instances definitive diagnosis is not possible. Helpful clues for the diagnosis of MF include the linear accumulation of atypical lymphocytes along the basement membrane zone of the epidermis (a pattern frequently described as tagging) (Fig. 31-22A, B) or a single-cell pagetoid infiltrate of atypical lymphocytes into the epidermis (epidermotropism) (Fig. 31-22C). Lymphoid epidermotropism in MF, unlike lymphoid exocytosis in dermatitis, is generally not associated with significant epidermal spongiosis or evidence of cytotoxicity (basal cell layer vacuolization or apoptosis). Rather, the epithelium appears "passive," resulting in an accumulation of atypical lymphocytes within small lacunar spaces that separate them from seemingly permissive adjacent keratinocytes. Exceptions, of course, do exist, and infrequently marked spongiosis or an interface dermatitis may be seen in MF.

The presence of clustered epidermotropic atypical lymphocytes, known as Pautrier microabscesses (Fig. 31-22D), is uncommonly observed in early patch-stage MF but frequently encountered in plaque-stage disease. These intraepithelial aggregates of neoplastic T cells must be differentiated from similar aggregates of larger Langerhans cells, which also demonstrate irregular, frequently indented, nuclear profiles; these so-called Langerhans cell microgranulomas are commonly associated with dermatitis (Table 31-4) (9). In plaque-stage disease, the bandlike dermal infiltrate is denser than in patch stage, and the atypical T cells are abundant. An interstitial pattern may also be seen.

In more advanced stages, there is often loss of epidermotropism. The dermal infiltrate is characterized by a nodular to diffuse interstitial population of cytologically atypical T cells, which may extend into the subcutaneous tissues (Fig. 31-23A). These cells may retain the small/medium size of earlier stages (Fig. 31-23B) or may demonstrate transformation to large, highly atypical cells (large-cell transformation or LCT) (Fig. 31-23C). LCT is defined as large-sized cells with prominent

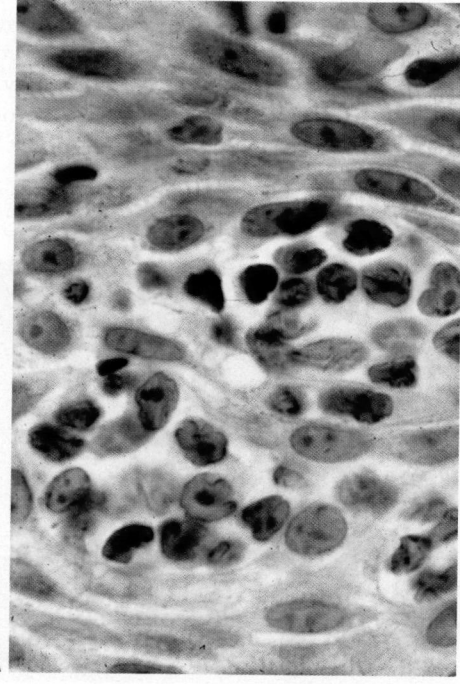
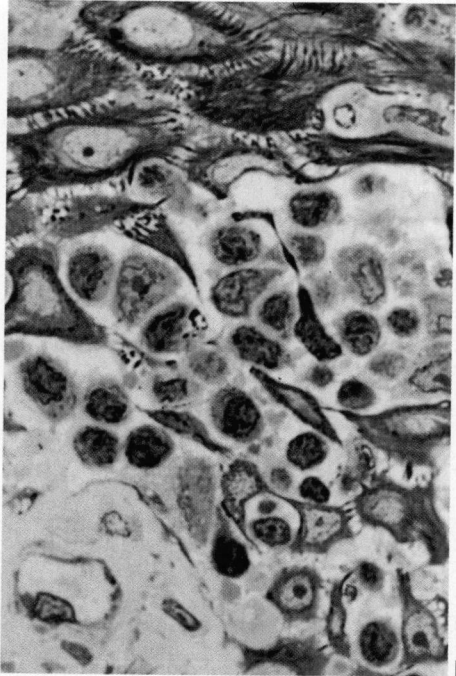

Figure 31-20 Mycosis fungoides: cytology. **A:** Oil immersion conventional microscopy of atypical lymphocytes within the epidermal layer. **B:** One-micron, toluidine blue–stained section of epidermotropic malignant lymphocytes showing characteristically infolded nuclear contours.

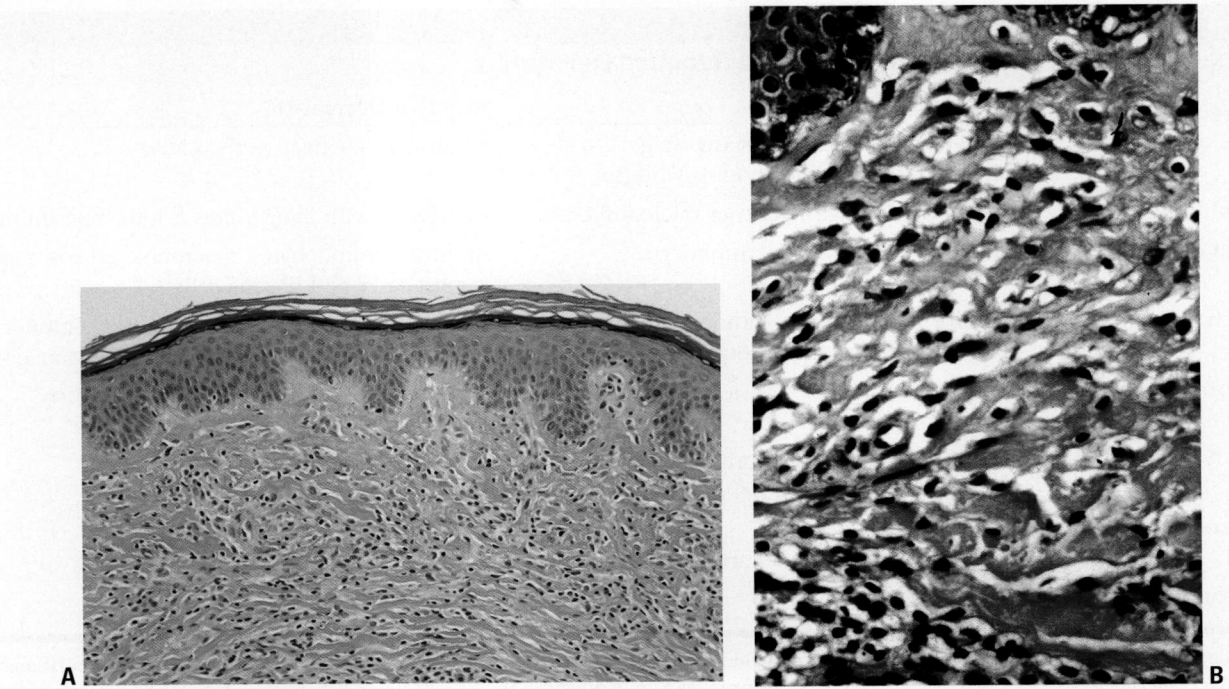

Figure 31-21 Mycosis fungoides: histologic features of early disease. A, B: Papillary dermal interstitial lymphoid infiltration associated with coarse fibrosis.

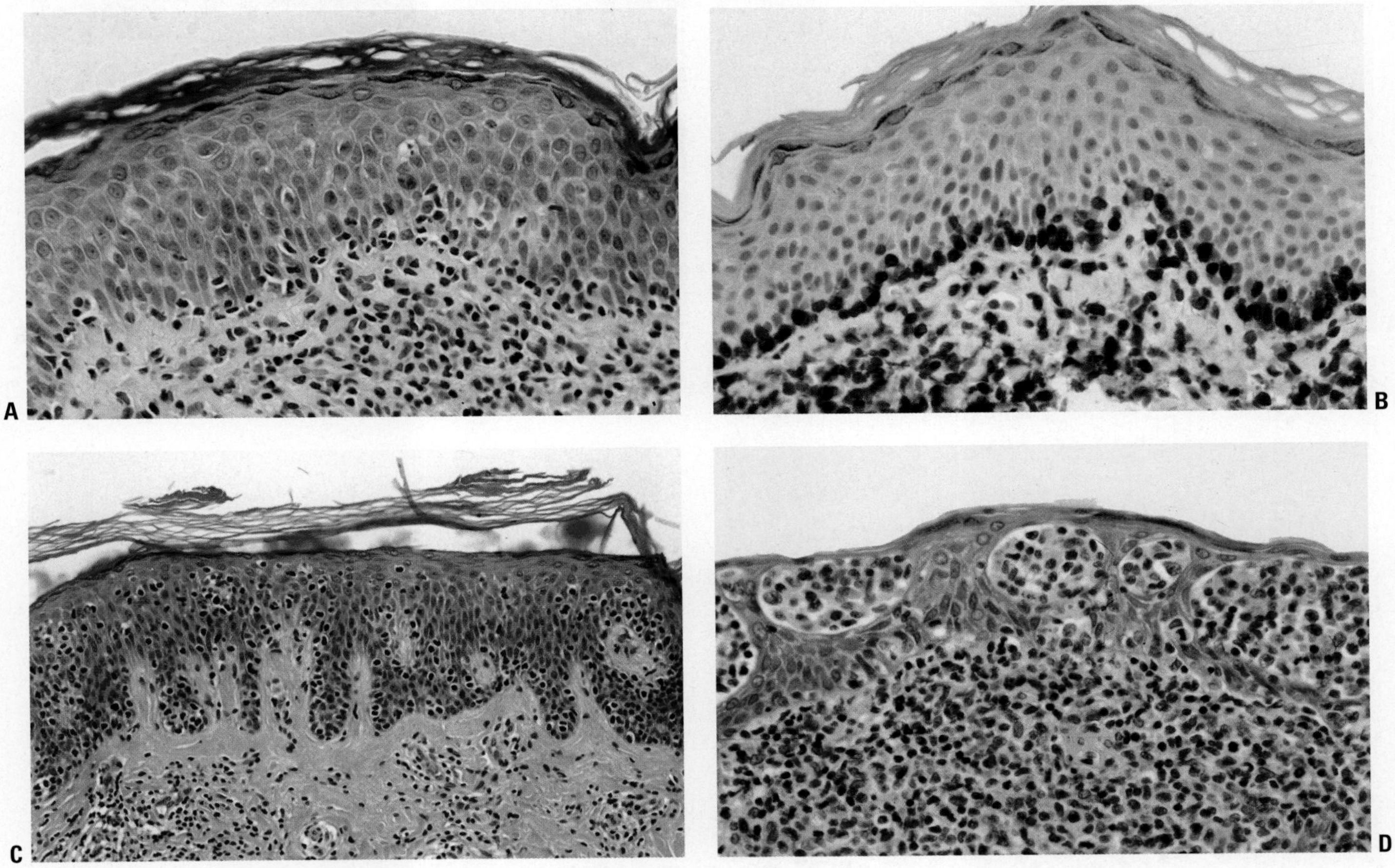

Figure 31-22 Mycosis fungoides: architectural patterns of epidermotropism. A: Papillary dermal interstitial infiltrate associated with linear aggregation of neoplastic lymphocytes along the dermal–epidermal junction. B: Adjacent section stained for CD4 emphasizing this linear pattern of early epidermotropism. C: Early plaque-stage disease with single-cell epidermotropism by atypical lymphocytes into a "passive" epidermal layer. D: Plaque-stage disease characterized by prominent clusters of atypical lymphocytes within the epidermis (Pautrier microabscesses).

Table 31-4		
Differential Findings in Mycosis Fungoides and Reactive Dermatitis		
	Mycosis Fungoides	**Reactive Dermatitis**
Architecture of infiltrate	Early/patch stage: patchy; plaque stage: lichenoid; tumor stage: nodular/diffuse	Superficial +/– deep perivascular
Pattern of infiltrate	Epidermotropism with Pautrier microabscesses	Exocytosis with Langerhans cell microgranulomas
Composition of infiltrate	Predominance of atypical lymphocytes	Admixed lymphocytes, macrophages, eosinophils, mast cells, and plasma cells
Epidermal changes	Psoriasiform hyperplasia without associated spongiosis or apoptotic keratinocytes	Associated spongiosis and apoptotic keratinocytes; psoriasiform hyperplasia seen in chronic disease
Papillary dermal changes	Coarse fibrosis	May be fibrotic if long-standing/previously traumatized
Cytology of lymphoid cells	Small to medium size; cerebriform hyperchromatic nuclei; perinuclear halos	Small size; round nuclei
Immunophenotyping of T cells	CD2$^{+/-}$, CD3^{+}, CD4^{+}, CD5$^{+/-}$, and CD8^{-} often with loss of CD7 (CD8^{+} variant less common)	Mixed CD4^{+} and CD8^{+}
TCR gene rearrangements	Clonal	polyclonal (rarely clonal)

Adapted from Song SX, Willemze R, Swerdlow SH, et al. Mycosis fungoides: report of the 2011 Society for Hematopathology/European Association for Haematopathology workshop. *Am J Clin Pathol* 2013;139(4):466–490. Reproduced by permission from American Society for Clinical Pathology and modified fromPimpinelli N, Olsen EA, Santucci M, et al. Defining early mycosis fungoides. *J Am Acad Dermatol* 2005;53(6):1053–1063. Copyright © 2005 American Academy of Dermatology, Inc. With permission.

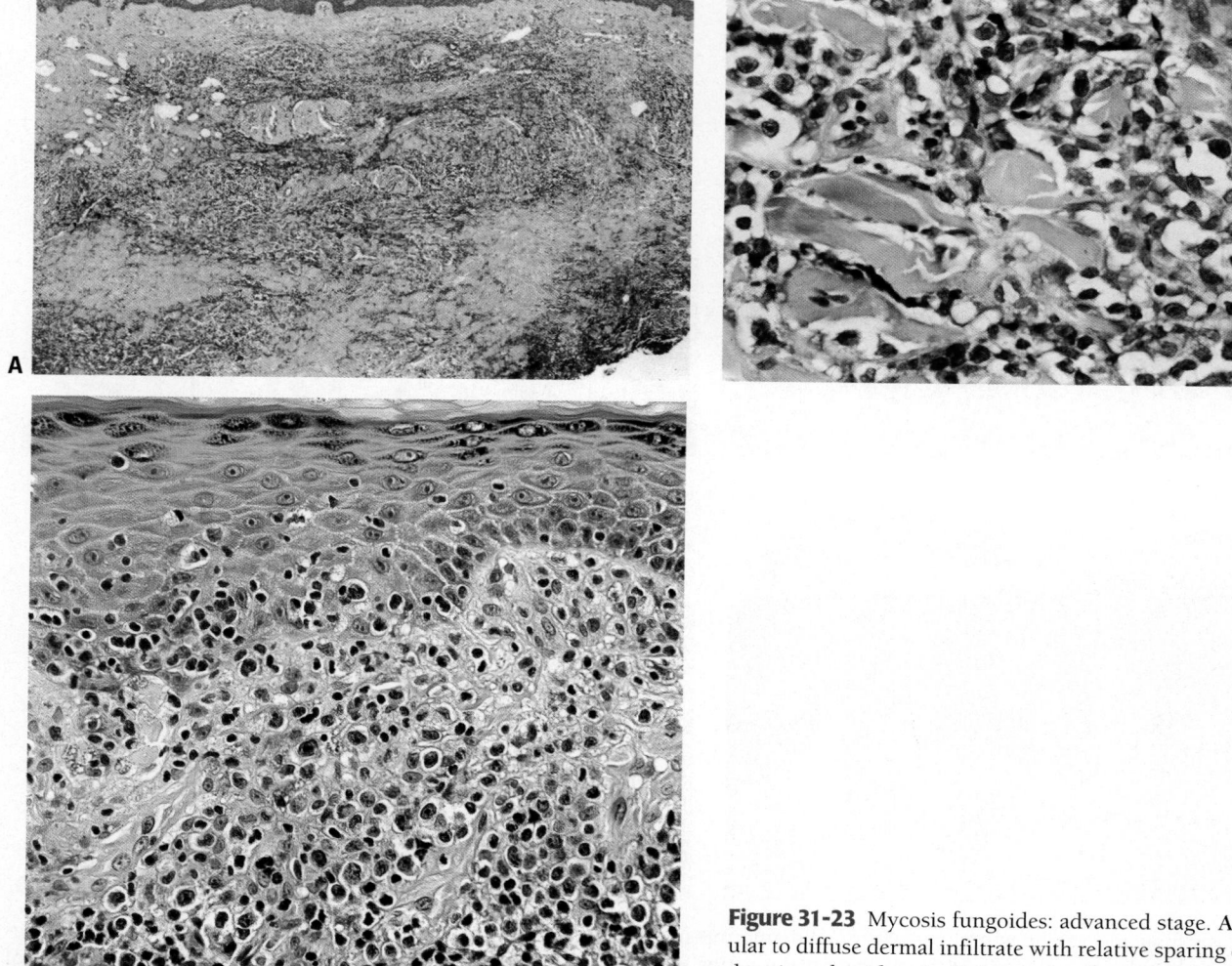

Figure 31-23 Mycosis fungoides: advanced stage. **A:** There is a nodular to diffuse dermal infiltrate with relative sparing of the superficial dermis and epidermis. **B:** In some cases, atypical lymphocytes retain the small/medium size of earlier stages. **C:** In other cases, transformation to large, highly atypical cells (large-cell transformation) occurs.

nucleoli, composing 25% or more of the dermal infiltrate or forming microscopic nodules (77), and is seen in greater than 50% of tumor-stage lesions (78). LCT is associated with the development of an aggressive biologic course (79), although a subset of cases may show more indolent behavior (80).

MF cells are most commonly αβ helper T cells with an immunophenotype of CD3⁺, CD4⁺, CD5⁺, and CD8⁻ (Fig. 31-24A–F), although a CD8⁺ αβ immunophenotype is occasionally observed. Lesions at all stages may show absence of CD7, although this finding in itself does not reliably permit differentiation of MF cells from reactive T cells. Loss of CD3, CD2, and/or CD5 expression in lesional T cells provides support for a neoplastic infiltrate, although this helpful sign is less common at early stages, where it is most often observed in the epidermotropic component, as is the preponderance of one or the other of CD4- or CD8-expressing T cells. Thus particularly

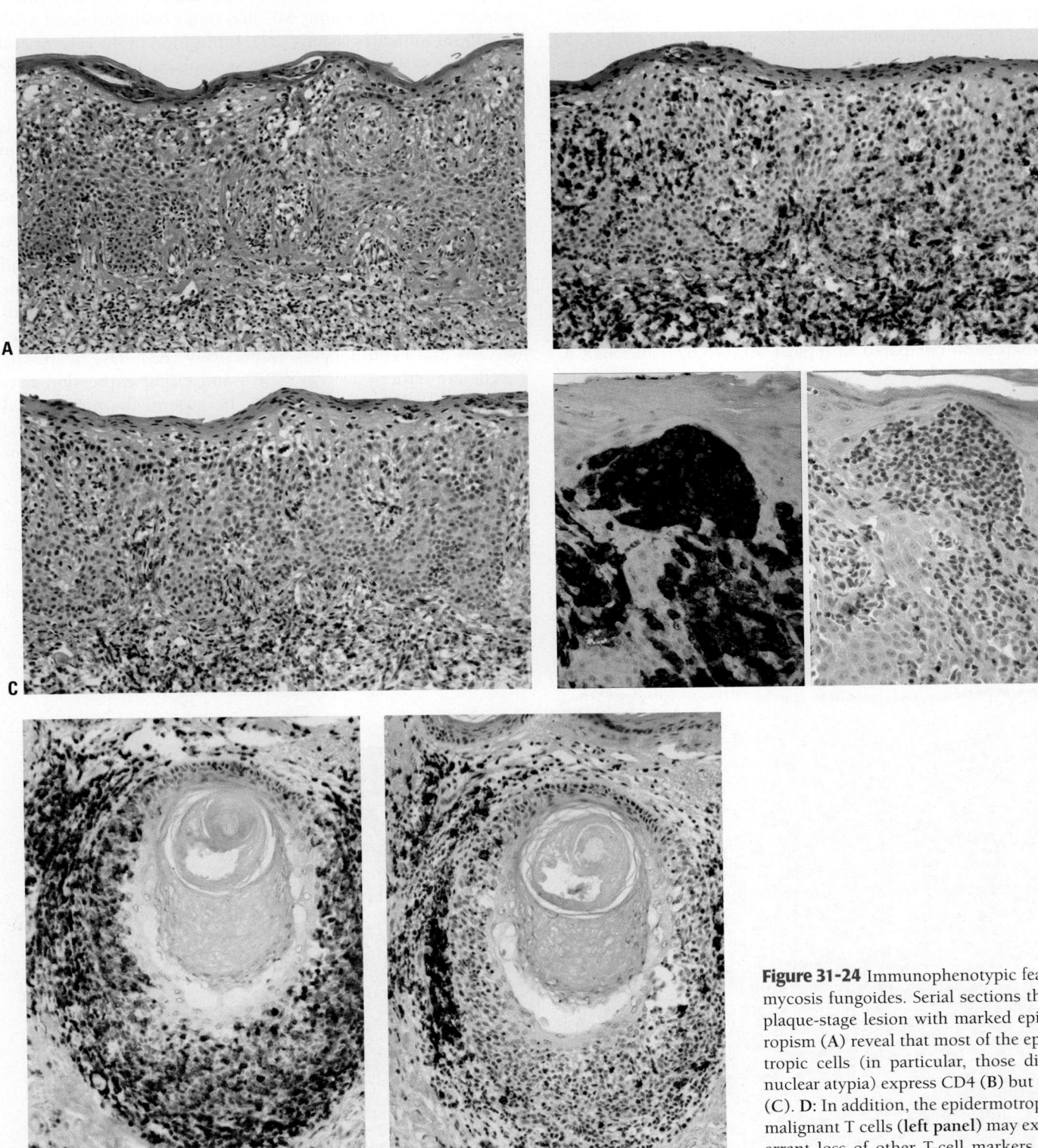

Figure 31-24 Immunophenotypic features of mycosis fungoides. Serial sections through a plaque-stage lesion with marked epidermotropism (**A**) reveal that most of the epidermotropic cells (in particular, those displaying nuclear atypia) express CD4 (**B**) but not CD8 (**C**). **D:** In addition, the epidermotropic CD4⁺ malignant T cells (**left panel**) may exhibit aberrant loss of other T-cell markers, such as CD7 (**right panel**). Similar findings are observed for folliculotropic T cells, which express CD4 (**E**) but not CD8 (**F**).

in early stages, careful evaluation of marker expression (or lack thereof) in the intraepidermal cells is necessary given the potentially confounding reactive T-cell infiltrate in the dermis. Cytotoxic markers (T-cell intracellular antigen [TIA-1], perforin, granzyme B) are negative in patch/plaque-stage disease, but subset expression may be detected at tumor stage (81). The skin-homing antigen cutaneous lymphocyte-associated antigen (CLA) is expressed in most cases. Although occasional CD30⁺ cells may be identified in the dermal infiltrates, this epitope is not expressed by most cells comprising the malignant clone. However, in advanced tumor-stage disease, especially with LCT, the cells may acquire CD30 expression (Fig. 31-25A, B). It is important to recognize that CD30 expression is not a prerequisite for the diagnosis of LCT, as not all cases of LCT demonstrate CD30 expression. Additionally, some data suggest that CD30⁺ cases of LCT in MF may portend a better prognosis than LCT cases that are negative for CD30 (80).

Apart from the classic MF described previously, there are a number of clinicopathologic variants and subtypes of MF. The clinically significant variants recognized by the 2016 WHO classification scheme (1) are the following:

Folliculotropic mycosis fungoides. A diagnosis of folliculotropic MF generally predicts poor survival and increased risk of disease progression compared to typical MF (75,82), although a subset of patients follow a more indolent course (83,84). Folliculotropic MF is characterized by infiltration of hair follicles by atypical T cells with minimal to absent epidermotropism, and thus the diagnosis may be overlooked when biopsies are too superficial. Often, but not always, there is associated follicular mucinosis secondary to intercellular mucin production by keratinocytes (85). These cells may eventually degenerate, potentially culminating in "alopecia mucinosa" (Fig. 31-26A–C). Other features include marked reactive lymphoid infiltrates, granulomatous reaction, abundant eosinophils

or plasma cells, or follicular cyst formation (86,87). Clinically, in addition to patchy alopecia, folliculotropic MF may manifest as follicular papules and plaques or comedones and can be associated with intense pruritus. This form of the disease may occur anywhere, although the skin of the face and the scalp as well as sun-exposed extremities are often involved. The deeper localization of the neoplastic infiltrate in folliculotropic MF may render reduced response to skin-targeted topical therapies. Although not formally included in this category, eccrine involvement by MF (syringotropic MF) has rarely been described, with or without follicular lesions (87). Infiltration of the eccrine coil may be associated with squamous metaplasia but not mucinosis (Fig. 31-26D).

Localized pagetoid reticulosis (Woringer–Kolopp disease). This is a rare form of MF characterized by robust epidermal infiltration of medium- to large-sized neoplastic T cells with abundant pale cytoplasm, often in the form of a solitary acral lesion where associated epidermal acanthosis and hyperkeratosis results in the clinical impression of a squamous proliferation such as a verruca, eczema, or squamous cell carcinoma. The pagetoid growth pattern of the neoplastic T cells may be attributable to their strong expression of adhesion molecules, in particular CLA and αEβ7, which facilitate interactions with endothelial cells and keratinocytes, respectively (88). The neoplastic T cells are either CD4⁺ or CD8⁺, and CD30 expression may be seen (89). Histopathologically, because of the pronounced epidermotropism, pagetoid reticulosis may mimic superficial spreading melanoma, pagetoid squamous carcinoma *in situ*, or extramammary Paget disease. However, diagnosis can be readily achieved on the basis of cytomorphologic and immunophenotypic features. Distinction of CD8⁺ pagetoid reticulosis from primary cutaneous acral CD8⁺ T-cell lymphoma relies on the higher degree of cytologic atypia and pagetoid pattern of involvement present in the former (90). The outcome of localized

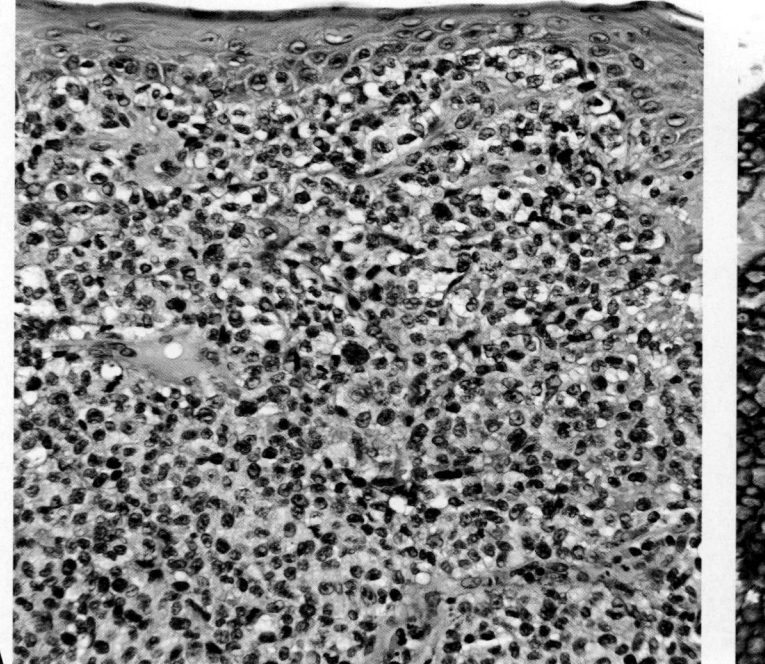
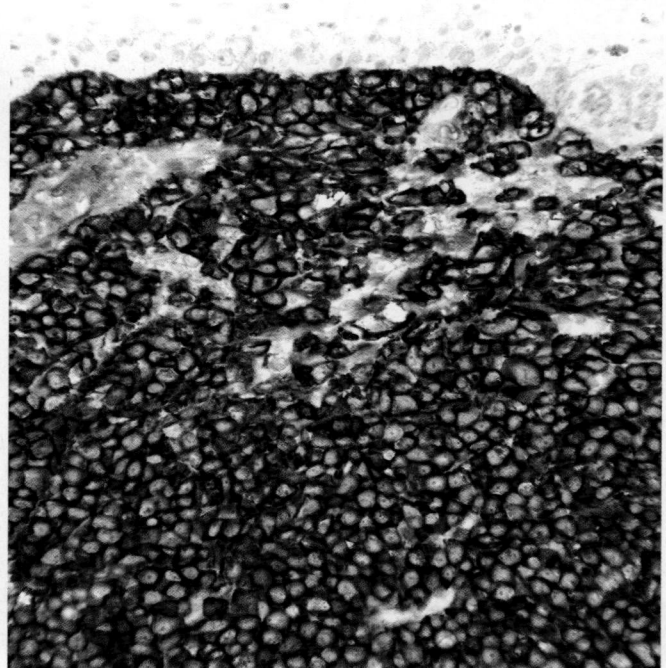

Figure 31-25 Mycosis fungoides with large-cell transformation. Immunohistochemistry studies reveal that the diffuse infiltrate of large, neoplastic cells (**A**) can acquire homogeneous, strong expression of CD30 (**B**).

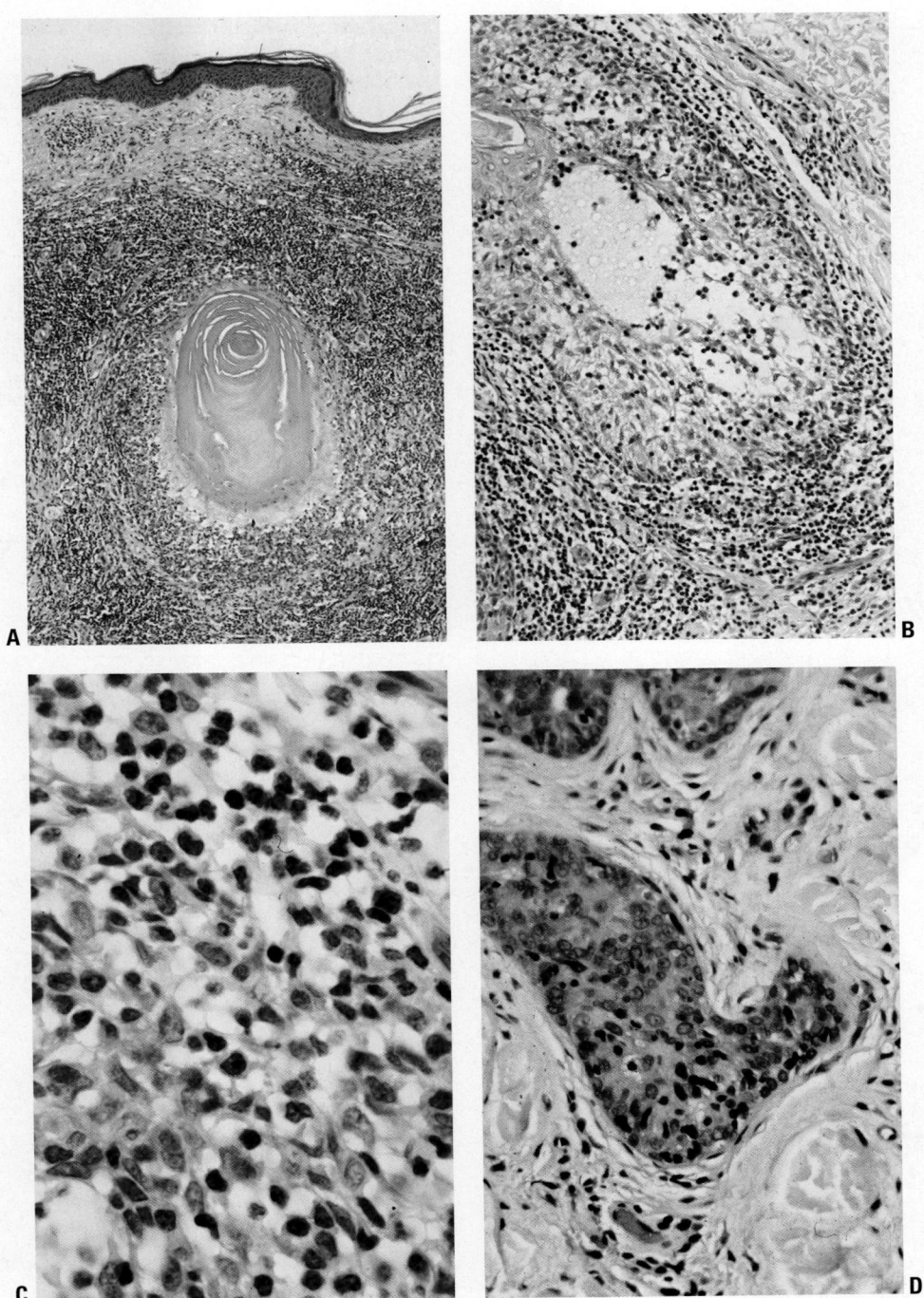

Figure 31-26 Adnexotropic mycosis fungoides. **A:** Infiltration is associated with architectural distortion and destruction of follicular structures. **B:** Follicular mucinosis characterized by pools of pale blue–staining mucin. **C:** Atypical T cells in a mucinous background. **D:** Eccrine involvement by atypical lymphocytes, associated with syringosquamous metaplasia.

pagetoid reticulosis is very good. Cases previously described as generalized pagetoid reticulosis (Ketron–Goodman disease) are distinct from this entity and represent, for the most part, examples of aggressive CD8+ T-cell lymphomas (cutaneous γδ T-cell lymphoma or primary cutaneous CD8+ aggressive epidermotropic cytotoxic T-cell lymphoma).

Granulomatous slack skin (GSS). This rare subtype is characterized by the presence of elastolytic granulomas that develop in association with a dermal lymphomatous component, which is typically dense and extends deep into the subcutis (Fig. 31-27A, B). Clinically, zones of skin with increased folding, redundancy, and decreased elasticity gradually develop, with preferential involvement of intertriginous sites, as a result of loss of elastic

fibers. Histologically, atypical T-cell infiltrates are intimately associated with noncaseating dermal granulomas formed by histiocytes and multinucleated giant cells (Fig. 31-27C) that may contain ingested elastic fibers (elastophagocytosis) or engulfed lymphocytes (lymphophagocytosis). These histologic features overlap with those seen in granulomatous MF, and distinction between the two entities is made on clinical grounds (91). In established lesions, there is marked reduction of elastic fibers (Fig. 31-27D). The disease demonstrates an indolent clinical course and may arise in association with preexisting MF or CHL.

In addition to those listed previously, other variants of MF have been described. Despite the presence of characteristic clinicopathologic features that permit segregation into distinct

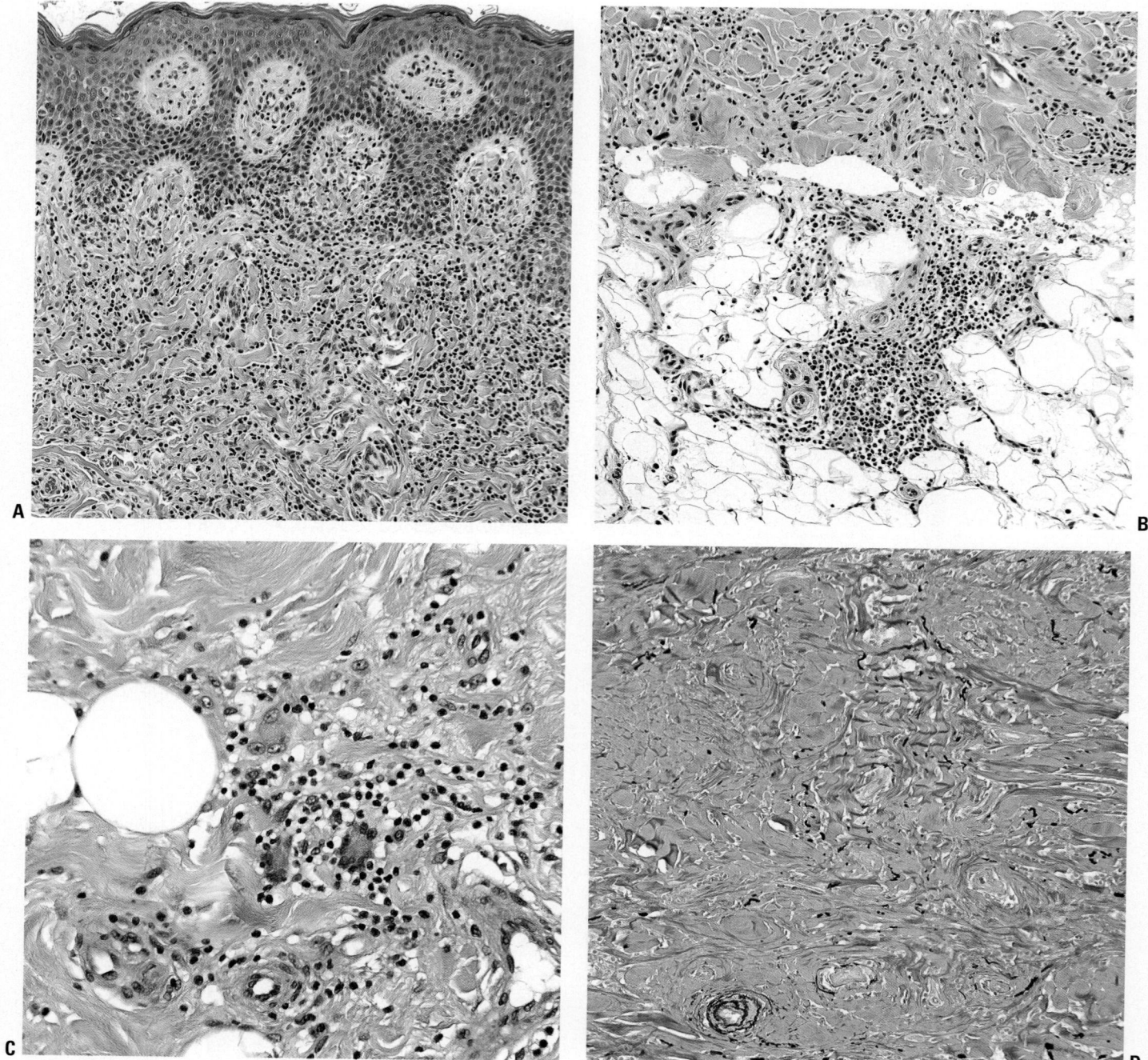

Figure 31-27 Granulomatous slack skin. The dermal lymphocytic infiltrate (A) extends into the underlying subcutis (B). C: Large, multinucleated giant cells are admixed among the lymphocytes and histiocytes. D: An elastin stain reveals a marked reduction of elastic fibers.

categories, these variants share a similar clinical course and prognosis with classical MF and thus do not have prognostic significance. Nonetheless, because of their clinical and histopathologic similarity to reactive dermatoses, diagnosis of these variants can be challenging, and familiarity with their clinical and histologic manifestations is necessary (92–94). A number of these variants are described in what follows.

Hypopigmented mycosis fungoides. This variant is predominantly seen in young patients with dark skin and demonstrates a good response to therapy though with frequent recurrences (95–97). The lesions appear as asymptomatic or slightly pruritic, hypopigmented patches that may or may not be accompanied by typical patches and plaques of classical MF. The underlying mechanisms leading to hypopigmentation have been a subject

of controversy. Some studies have found degenerative changes in melanocytes secondary to nonspecific cellular injuries, whereas others demonstrated impaired melanosome transfer to keratinocytes. In addition to prominent pigment incontinence, hypopigmented MF commonly demonstrates a CD8+ phenotype and shows prominent epidermotropism (Fig. 31-28A, B). Distinction from inflammatory lesions of vitiligo can be challenging and in some cases may be resolved only on long-term follow-up, although some have suggested that certain histologic features may distinguish the two entities (98).

Ichthyosiform mycosis fungoides. Another rare variant, ichthyosiform MF, presents with lesions that are pruritic and that form fishlike hyperkeratotic scales, often with excoriations. There may be accompanying comedo-like areas and/or follicular

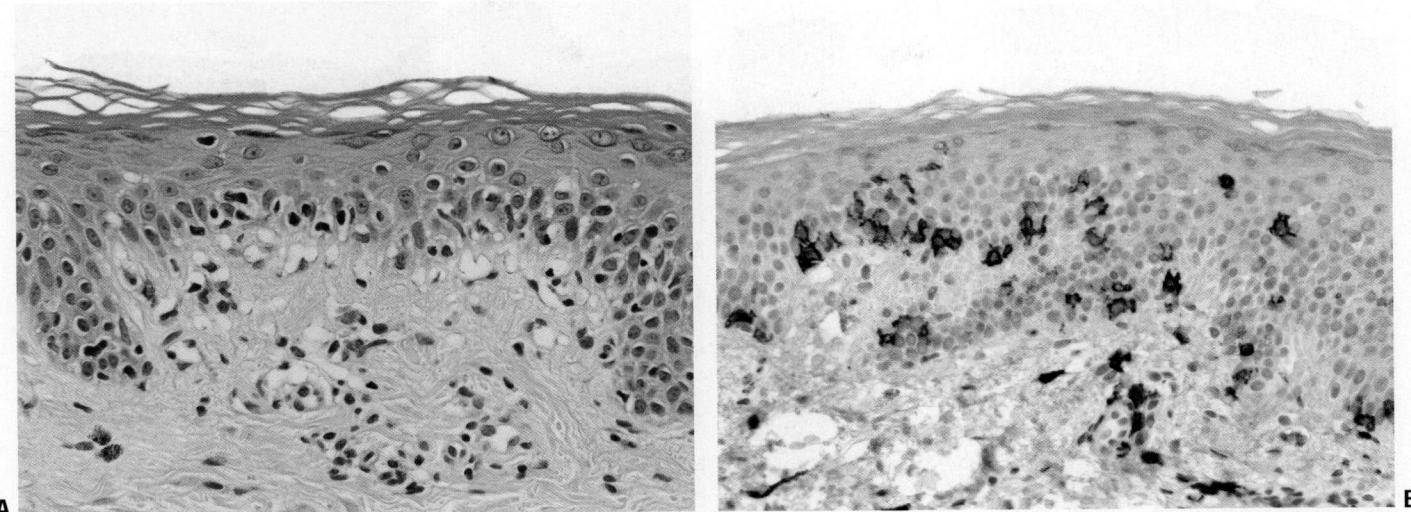

Figure 31-28 Hypopigmented mycosis fungoides. **A:** This variant is characterized by dermal pigment incontinence as well as the presence of an atypical T-cell infiltrate. **B:** CD8 highlights the atypical lymphocytes with single-cell epidermotropism.

keratotic papules. Microscopically, the ichthyosiform areas show typical features of MF with compact hyperorthokeratosis and hypergranulosis, whereas the follicular papules exhibit cystic dilatation of hair follicles with keratotic plugs and folliculotropic atypical lymphocytes (99).

Mycosis fungoides palmaris et plantaris. This variant defines cases where the MF lesions are limited to, predominantly affect, or initially present on the palms and/or soles (100). The lesions may present as annular hyperpigmented patches and plaques, vesicles, pustules, hyperkeratotic/verrucous plaques, psoriasiform plaques, ulceration, and/or nail dystrophy (101,102). Regardless of the associated variable secondary epidermal changes that may complicate the clinical differential and microscopic interpretation, the presence of histopathologic findings of classical MF and clonal rearrangement of the TCR genes will help in reaching the correct diagnosis.

Bullous (vesicular) mycosis fungoides. Bullous MF manifests clinically as blisters that may develop on normal skin or within typical plaques and tumors of MF. This variant is very rare but is of significant clinical relevance in terms of prognosis; approximately 50% of patients die within a year following the onset of blisters (103,104). In addition to common histologic features of classical MF, there is associated clefting, which may occur at different planes (subcorneal, intraepidermal, and subepidermal). Although the precise mechanism of the blister formation is not clear, it has been proposed that the subcorneal and intraepidermal separation may result from confluence of Pautrier microabscesses and that the subepidermal blister may be secondary to reduced keratinocyte adherence to the basement membrane in response to cytokines produced by the lymphoma cells (104). Unlike immunobullous disorders, immunofluorescence studies are consistently negative in bullous MF.

Pustular mycosis fungoides. Pustular MF presents as pustular eruptions that may be limited to the palmoplantar areas (MF palmaris et plantaris) or that may be generalized. Intraepidermal collections of atypical lymphocytes with neutrophils and eosinophils constitute the characteristic histopathologic findings (105).

Production of high levels of interleukin-8 by the lymphoma cells has been implicated in the formation of pustular lesions (106).

Granulomatous mycosis fungoides. Clinically, the lesions present as papules, plaques, and tumors that are not distinctive from classic cases (107). Histopathologically, granulomatous MF is characterized by the presence of typical MF as well as variable granulomatous inflammation, which may take the form of interstitial, tuberculoid/sarcoidal, or palisading granulomata reminiscent of granuloma annulare and/or necrobiosis lipoidica. Multinucleated giant cells, usually of the foreign-body type (although Langhans and Touton giant cells have been described as well) (Fig. 31-29A–C) with or without focal elastophagocytosis, may be seen (107,108). Special stains for microorganisms are useful in excluding concurrent infection in a patient with classical MF. Granulomatous MF can be differentiated from GSS clinically by the absence of bulky skin lesions. Lymphophagocytosis and elastophagocytosis are less common than in GSS (91). The diagnosis of granulomatous MF may be challenging, particularly when the granulomatous infiltrates mask or partially obliterate the neoplastic cells required for diagnosis. Accordingly, patients with persistent and therapy-refractory granulomatous dermatitis not associated with systemic comorbidities or infection should also be considered to potentially have this rare entity.

Histogenesis. The putative cell of origin in MF is believed to be a memory T cell that expresses the skin-homing molecule CLA. Studies have failed to define a single genetic pathway of lymphogenesis, suggesting that the disease is genetically heterogeneous. For example, a large meta-analysis of mRNA gene expression data in tumor-stage MF demonstrated that 718 genes were statistically significantly more highly expressed in MF compared to normal or inflamed skin (109). Oncogenic mutations in a number of pathways have been implicated in disease pathogenesis, including those involved in the regulation of apoptosis, cell-cycle progression, gene transcription, and cell signaling (110–112). Evidence suggests that classical MF is a neoplasm of resident memory T cells that normally reside in the skin, whereas SS is a *de novo* systemic lymphoproliferative disorder involving central memory T cells (113).

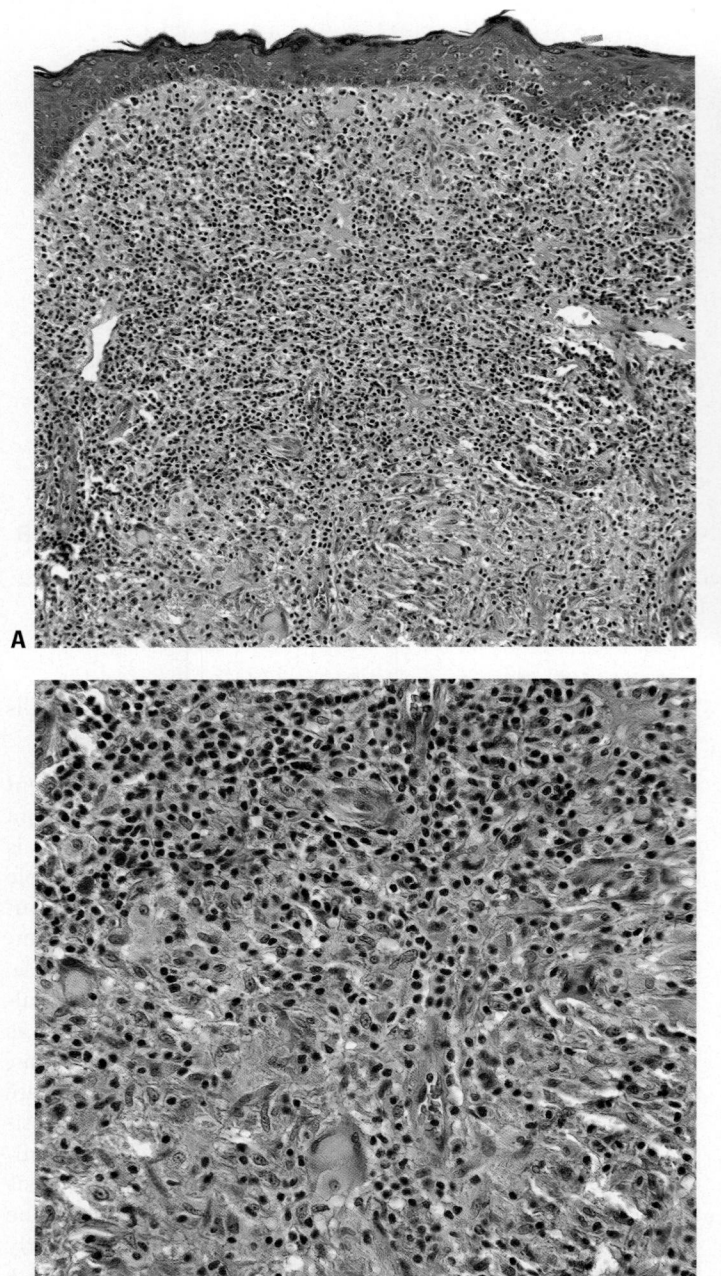

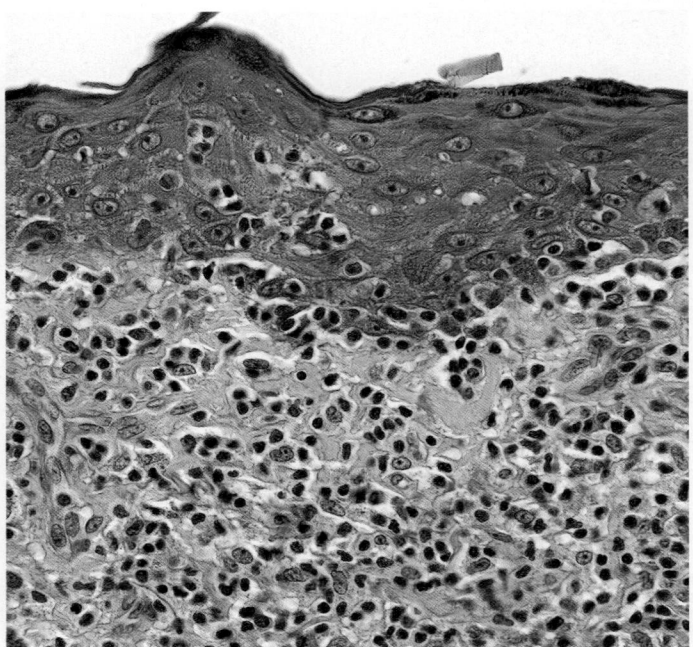

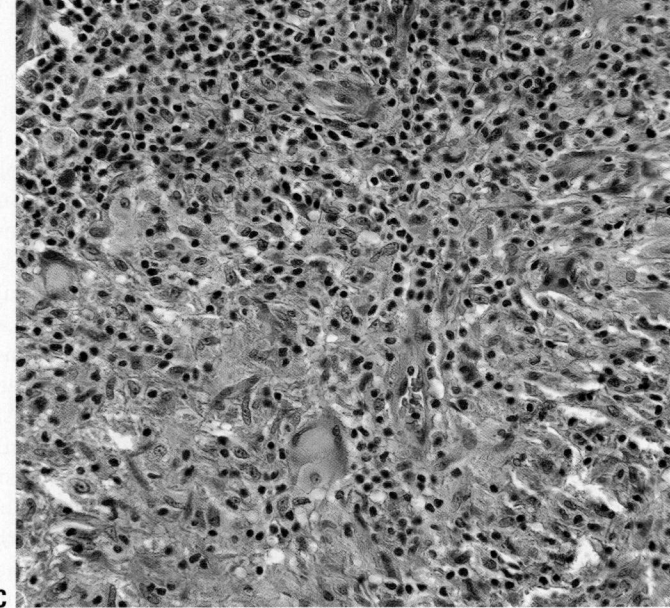

Figure 31-29 Granulomatous mycosis fungoides. High-power views of a biopsy from a patient with this variant (**A**) reveal epidermotropism of the atypical T cells (**B**) as well as multifocal giant cells admixed within the infiltrate (**C**).

Differential Diagnosis. The practical differential diagnosis of classical epidermotropic MF involves primarily reactive T-cell infiltrates with exocytosis or an abnormal papillary dermal interstitial homing pattern (Table 31-4). True dermatitis may show lymphoid exocytosis and development of Langerhans cell microgranulomas that may superficially resemble Pautrier microabscesses. However, the microgranulomas are generally associated with spongiosis or evidence of cytotoxic epidermal injury and CD1a positivity by immunohistochemistry (114). Adnexotropic lesions must be separated from forms of dermatitis centered primarily about hair follicles and sweat glands. The finding of uniformly atypical epitheliotropic lymphocytes and their tendency to be predominantly CD4+ by immunohistochemistry should assist in this differential. Careful clinical history is required to exclude the possibility of a drug-mediated skin eruption secondary to immune dysregulation that may be morphologically, immunophenotypically, and even genotypically difficult to differentiate from MF. Clearing of the skin lesions following discontinuation of the offending drugs or lack of correlation of TCR gene rearrangements among multifocal lesions is also helpful. Other common potential histologic mimickers of MF include persistent arthropod bite reaction, secondary syphilis, nodular scabies, actinic reticuloid, fungal infection, lichen sclerosus in the early inflammatory stage, lichen striatus, lichenoid keratosis, pigmented purpuric dermatitis, connective tissue disorders, inflamed vitiligo, and regressed melanoma (115). In addition to meticulous clinicopathologic correlation, the finding of cytologically atypical lymphocytes within epithelial niches devoid of reactive changes seen in immune-mediated phenomena (spongiosis, apoptosis) should always raise suspicion for a possible diagnosis of MF.

It is possible that very early evolutionary stages of MF involve a "dysplastic" phase in lymphocytic tumor progression. Such lesions may fulfill some, but not all, of the features required for a diagnosis of patch-stage disease, even when clinical findings strongly support this diagnosis. The authors generally refer to such lesions as being compatible with possible evolving T-cell dyscrasia and recommend close follow-up and interval biopsy sampling to assess disease evolution. Late-stage disease, where epithelial involvement is minimal to absent and cytologic features may be higher grade, must be distinguished from B-cell lymphomas involving the skin, particularly T-cell–rich types.

A well-described diagnostic dilemma is the distinction between MF and primary cutaneous CD30⁺ lymphoproliferative disorders, including lymphomatoid papulosis (LyP) or primary cutaneous anaplastic large cell lymphoma (cALCL). On pure histologic grounds, type B LyP mimics the bandlike infiltrate and epidermotropism of small- to medium-sized cells seen in MF, and type D LyP demonstrates striking epidermotropism that is morphologically similar to localized pagetoid reticulosis. Large, anaplastic CD30⁺ cells may be seen in both MF with LCT and cALCL, although a significant proportion of MF cases with LCT contain an admixture of large cells as well as small- to medium-sized cerebriform cells, which can also show folliculotropism (77,80). It cannot be overemphasized that incorporation of clinical history is essential for diagnosis. Rearrangements of 6p25.3 *IRF4/DUSP22* have been described in approximately a quarter of cALCL cases and rarely in transformed MF (116,117).

Principles of Management: MF is generally considered incurable, although many patients will show an indolent course. Treatment options are tailored to the stage of disease. Therapy for early-stage lesions includes topical agents (corticosteroids, chemotherapy, bexarotene), phototherapy (psoralen plus UV-A or UV-B radiation), systemic bexarotene, and/or radiotherapy. More advanced disease (high-stage or transformed), or nonresponsive early-stage disease, will require additional treatments such as systemic chemotherapy, extracorporeal photopheresis, interferon-α, and/or immunologic agents. Allogeneic stem cell transplant may also be considered for aggressive disease (76).

Sézary Syndrome
SS is a rare, aggressive disease classically characterized by a triad of generalized redness and scaling of the skin (erythroderma), lymphadenopathy, and the presence of clonally related neoplastic T cells in the skin, lymph nodes, and peripheral blood. Peripheral blood involvement requires ≥1,000/μL Sézary cells, a CD4:CD8 ratio greater than or equal to 10:1, or atypical CD4⁺ cells in the blood (CD4⁺CD7⁻ cells ≥40% or CD4⁺CD26⁻ cells ≥30%) (74,118). MF and SS are distinct entities with different postulated cells of origin (113) and underlying genetics (119). The term *Sézary syndrome* is restricted to cases without preceding MF lesions.

Clinical Summary. Patients generally present with diffuse skin erythema and lymphadenopathy. There may also be itching, hair loss, nail dystrophy, eye changes, and hyperkeratosis affecting the skin of the palms and soles. In addition to lymph node, skin, and blood involvement, malignant T cells may also infiltrate viscera in late stages, although bone marrow is often spared (120). The prognosis is poor, with a 5-year disease-specific survival of 36% (11). Of note, patients with an established diagnosis of MF who develop erythroderma are considered to have erythrodermic MF, not SS, although these cases can be grouped under the name of erythrodermic CTCL (121).

Histopathology. Affected skin may show changes similar to those of patch/plaque-stage MF, although the infiltrate is often sparse and epidermotropism less prominent (Fig. 31-30A). Similar to MF, the neoplastic T cells are generally CD4⁺ T cells that frequently show loss of CD7, although this marker alone may be of limited specificity. Other aberrant T-cell phenotypes are common, often with loss of T-cell markers such as CD2, CD3, and CD5; rare CD8⁺ variants have been described. One study suggested that the follicular helper T-cell marker programmed death-1 (PD-1) is differentially expressed in SS, with staining seen in greater than 50% of cells in 24 of 27 SS cases versus 8 of 60 MF cases (122). Involved lymph nodes are characterized by effacement of their architecture by infiltrates of atypical cells.

The peripheral blood contains atypical lymphocytes with cerebriform nuclear contours, historically called Lutzner cells and larger Sézary cells (Fig. 31-30B, C). However, neither these morphologic features nor evidence of a clonal T-cell population in the blood are sufficient evidence of SS, because atypical, cerebriform lymphocytes are also found in the peripheral blood of otherwise healthy individuals and those suffering from inflammatory skin conditions, and clonal T-cell populations can be detected in the peripheral blood of otherwise healthy elderly individuals or those with autoimmune disorders (121,123–125). Therefore, either the presence of an immunophenotypically aberrant T-cell population in the blood (as described above) or demonstration of an identical T-cell clone in both the blood and the skin is required for the diagnosis.

Histogenesis. In contrast to MF, where the neoplastic cell is considered to be a resident memory T cell, the putative cell of origin in SS is thought to be the central memory T cell, which expresses markers that promote lymph node homing and peripheral blood circulation (113), although the underlying etiology is unknown. Recent genomic studies have shown diverse and complex genetic alterations involving various cellular pathways in SS, although characteristic gene expression profiles have emerged (126–128).

Differential Diagnosis. SS must be differentiated from other dermatitic causes of erythroderma (e.g., atopic dermatitis, seborrheic dermatitis, pityriasis rubra pilaris, psoriasis, and drug reactions). This can be challenging solely on a morphologic basis because the histopathology of skin involvement in SS may be subtle, although an EORTC consensus study found the presence of increased atypical intraepidermal lymphocytes with Pautrier microabscesses, and expression of PD-1 or MUM1, to favor SS (129). Ultimately, demonstration of additional features such as peripheral blood involvement will be critical in pointing to a diagnosis of SS. Clinicopathologic correlation is needed to differentiate erythrodermic MF from SS. Patients with adult T-cell leukemia/lymphoma (ATLL) also have circulating atypical T cells and may present with skin lesions. However, the circulating lymphocytes tend to be polylobated (flowerlike) rather than cerebriform, and the cutaneous lesions manifest as multiple nodules rather than diffuse erythroderma.

Principles of Management: Treatment for erythrodermic CTCL is similar to advanced-stage MF, although extracorporeal photopheresis demonstrates superior efficacy in erythrodermic CTCL compared to MF (130–132).

Primary Cutaneous CD30-Positive T-Cell Lymphoproliferative Disorders
The entity of primary cutaneous CD30⁺ T-cell lymphoproliferative disorders encompasses a spectrum of diseases characterized

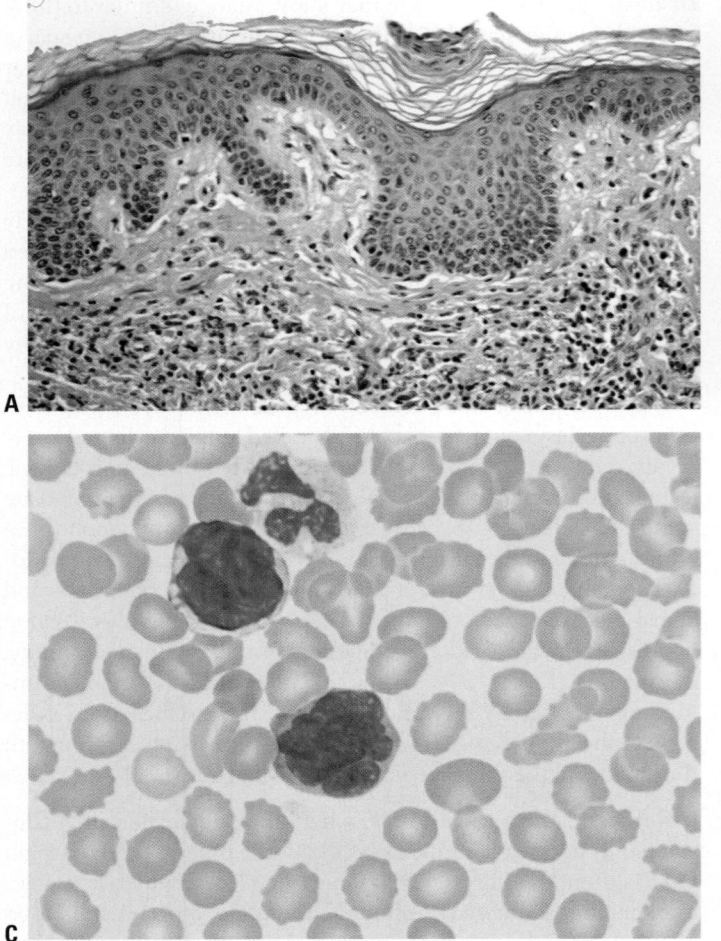

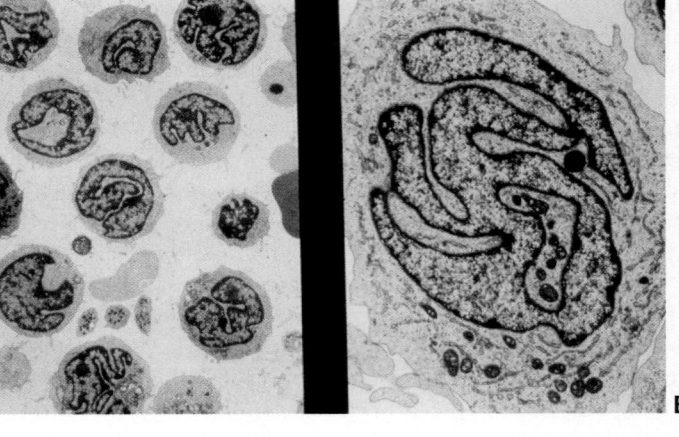

Figure 31-30 Sézary syndrome. **A:** There is a bandlike papillary dermal lymphoid infiltrate with minimal epidermotropism. **B:** Ultrastructural examination of peripheral blood buffy coat revealing numerous Sézary cells. **C:** High-magnification view of peripheral blood reveals the presence of atypical lymphocytes with lobulated ("cerebriform") nuclear contours (Wright stain).

by indolent clinical behavior and expression of CD30 and includes LyP and cALCL (133). Lesions that cannot be placed into one of these categories at initial diagnosis are considered borderline (1). Definitive diagnosis can be challenging on histologic grounds and requires careful clinical correlation.

Lymphomatoid Papulosis

Clinical Summary. LyP typically develops as generalized juicy red papules and nodules on the trunk and extremities that regress within weeks to several months (Fig. 31-31A, B), resulting in mild scarring (134). The papules or nodules are each usually less than 1 cm in diameter, and ulceration may occur. Lesions are often at different stages of development, resulting in a heterogeneous clinical appearance. The disease is typically chronic and can affect patients for months to years. LyP occurs most frequently in middle-aged adults (M:F 2–3:1), although it may also be seen in children. Five to 10 percent of cases may involve regional (draining) lymph nodes (135). A concurrent

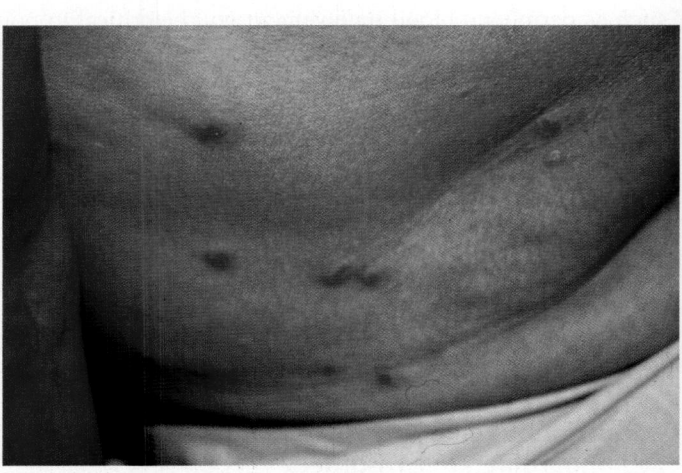

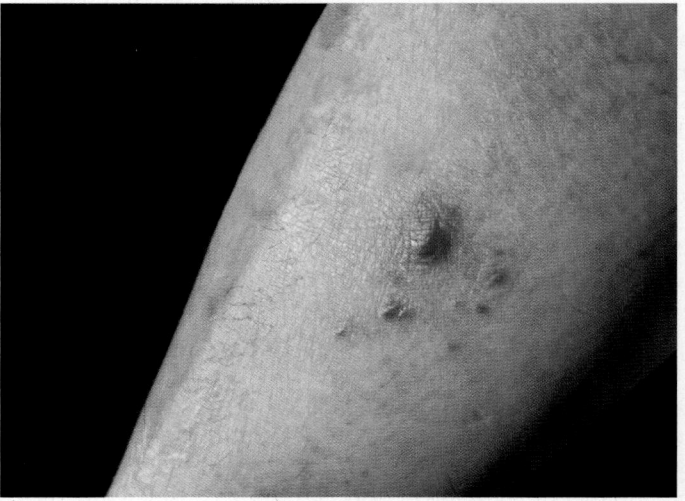

Figure 31-31 Lymphomatoid papulosis. Lesions clinically present as multiple, juicy red papules and nodules (A), with papules often showing regional clustering (B). (B: Courtesy of Dr. Cecilia Larocca, Dana-Farber Cancer Institute, Boston, MA.)

lymphoproliferative disorder such as CHL, cALCL, systemic ALCL, or MF may be present in up to 20% of cases (135–137). Although clonality can often be demonstrated in lesions of LyP, it is not clinically considered to be a malignant disorder.

Histopathology. LyP is characterized by a cutaneous infiltrate of large, atypical CD30+ cells, which typically have an immunoblastic or anaplastic cytology. There is an extremely broad histologic spectrum; multiple patterns have been described and may occur within the same patient. The most recent WHO–EORTC classification recognizes five histologic types as well as

a more recent molecularly defined subtype (11). LyP type A is the prototypical pattern typified by a wedge-shaped infiltrate extending from the superficial into the mid- and deep dermis (Fig. 31-32A). The infiltrate is composed of a marked inflammatory component (small lymphocytes, histiocytes, neutrophils, and eosinophils) as well as an admixed minority population of scattered or clustered atypical large lymphocytes, which can be Reed–Sternberg–like (Fig. 31-32B–D). Type B mimics MF with small- to medium-sized cerebriform cells forming a bandlike superficial dermal infiltrate and exhibiting epidermotropism. Type C lesions show a monotonous population of large cells,

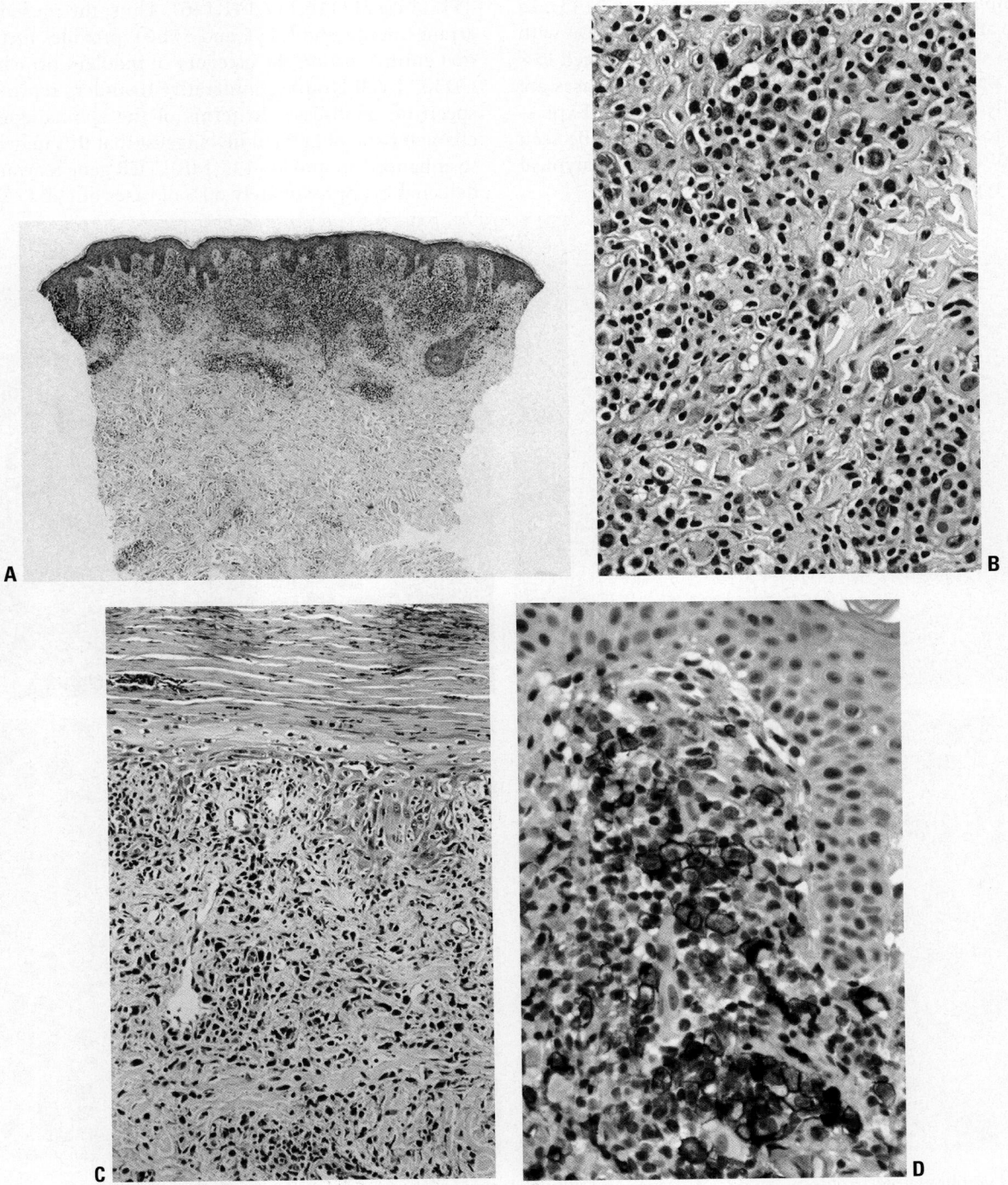

Figure 31-32 Lymphomatoid papulosis. A: Low power of localized infiltrate in superficial and middermis, forming what will become a wedge-shaped angiocentric architecture. B: Variably atypical lymphoid cells in the dermis. C: Epidermal infiltration with associated scale abnormalities and neutrophil infiltration. D: CD30+ cells are numerous within the superficial dermal component of the infiltrate.

with a sparse or minimal inflammatory component, and diffuse CD30 expression (Fig. 31-33A–D) similar to cALCL, but clinically behave like LyP, and hence their classification as such. Type D LyP recapitulates the striking epidermotropism of pagetoid reticulosis (Fig. 31-34A, B) and the cytotoxic immunophenotype of primary cutaneous CD8⁺ aggressive epidermotropic cytotoxic T-cell lymphoma (CD8⁺, TCR βF1⁺, and TIA-1⁺ and/or granzyme B⁺) (138–140), although the presence of strong, uniform CD30 expression (Fig. 31-34C, D) and the clinical picture support the diagnosis of LyP (141). More recently, type E LyP has been recognized as an angioinvasive variant characterized by ulcerative/necrotic lesions owing to an underlying angiocentric and angiodestructive infiltrate of small- to medium-sized atypical lymphocytes frequently expressing CD8 (142,143). In general, the atypical CD30⁺ cells show expression of CD4 with variable loss of CD2, CD3, or CD5, although pronounced loss of multiple pan-T antigens would be unusual. CD8⁺ cases are rare, typically seen in pediatric cases or types D and E. Expression of cytotoxic molecules (granzyme B, TIA-1) may be seen in the CD30⁺ cells (144). The small- to medium-sized atypical cells in LyP type B may or may not express CD30.

Histogenesis. The cell of origin is thought to be a skin-homing T cell. Until recently, recurrent genetic abnormalities had not been described in LyP, and no consistent chromosomal abnormalities defining the histopathologic type A through E patterns have been identified. However, a small series of spontaneously resolving, localized cutaneous lesions in elderly patients characterized by rearrangements of the *IRF4/DUSP22* locus on chromosome 6p25.3 has been reported (145). Although these cases did not fit perfectly into one of the five described LyP patterns, given the strong expression of CD30 and self-resolving course, they are now recognized as a new subtype of LyP (11). Previously, rearrangements at 6p25.3 were deemed to be a specific but insensitive indicator of cALCL, present in approximately 25% of cases (116,117,141,146). Thus, the presence of this rearrangement in both LyP and cALCL provides further evidence that entities within the category of indolent primary cutaneous CD30⁺ T-cell lymphoproliferative disorders represent a related spectrum of disease. In terms of the spontaneous resolution characteristic of LyP, studies suggest that this may be secondary to enhanced apoptosis (147,148). TCR gene rearrangements are detected in approximately 60% of cases of LyP (137).

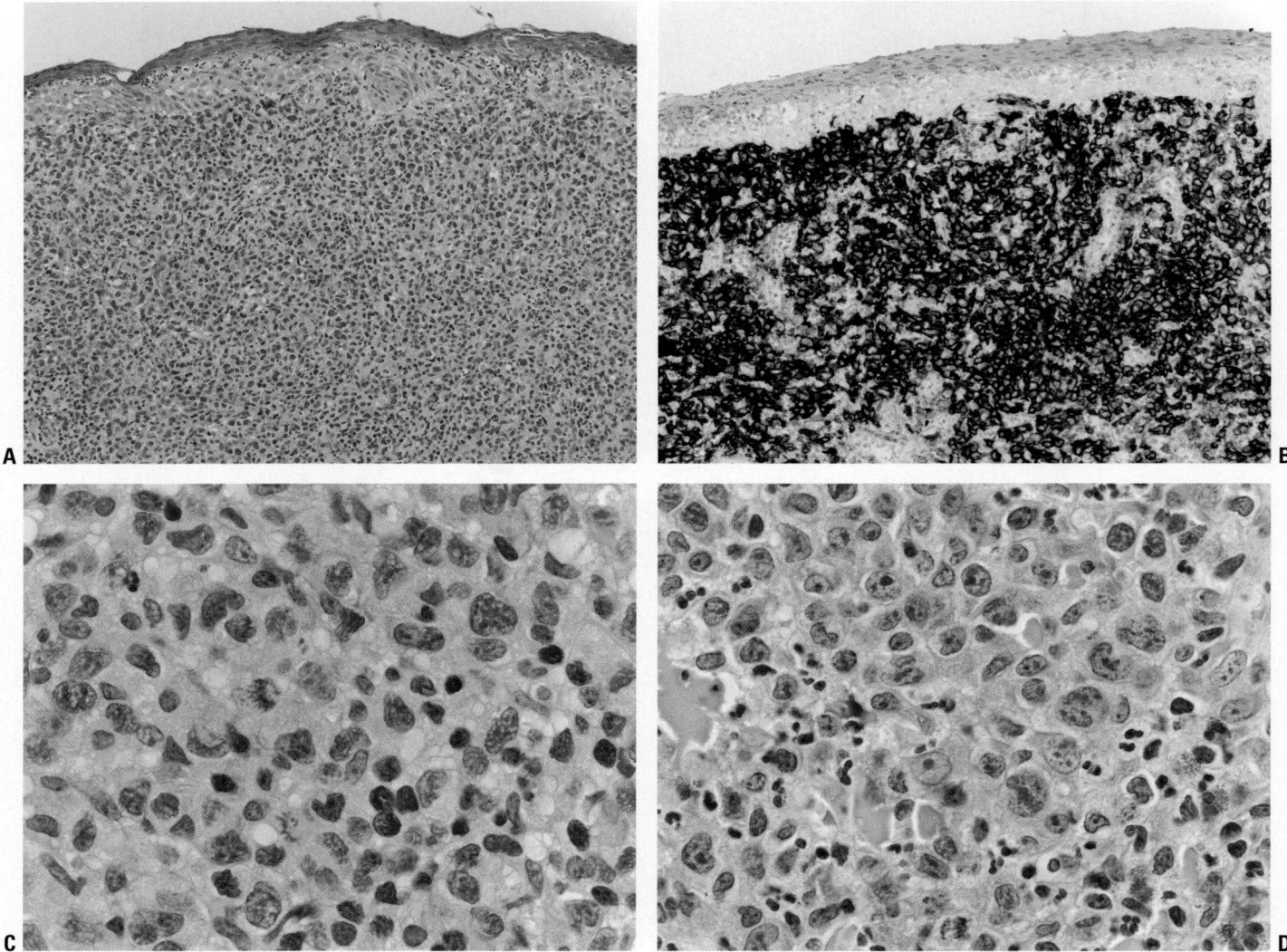

Figure 31-33 Lymphomatoid papulosis, type C. **A:** Dense and diffuse dermal infiltrate of atypical cells. **B:** There is diffuse positivity for CD30. **C:** High-magnification shows very large, pleomorphic cells with mitotic activity. **D:** A different case shows a similar predominance of large, pleomorphic cells and also includes a few background inflammatory cells. The morphologic features are indistinguishable from primary cutaneous anaplastic large cell lymphoma.

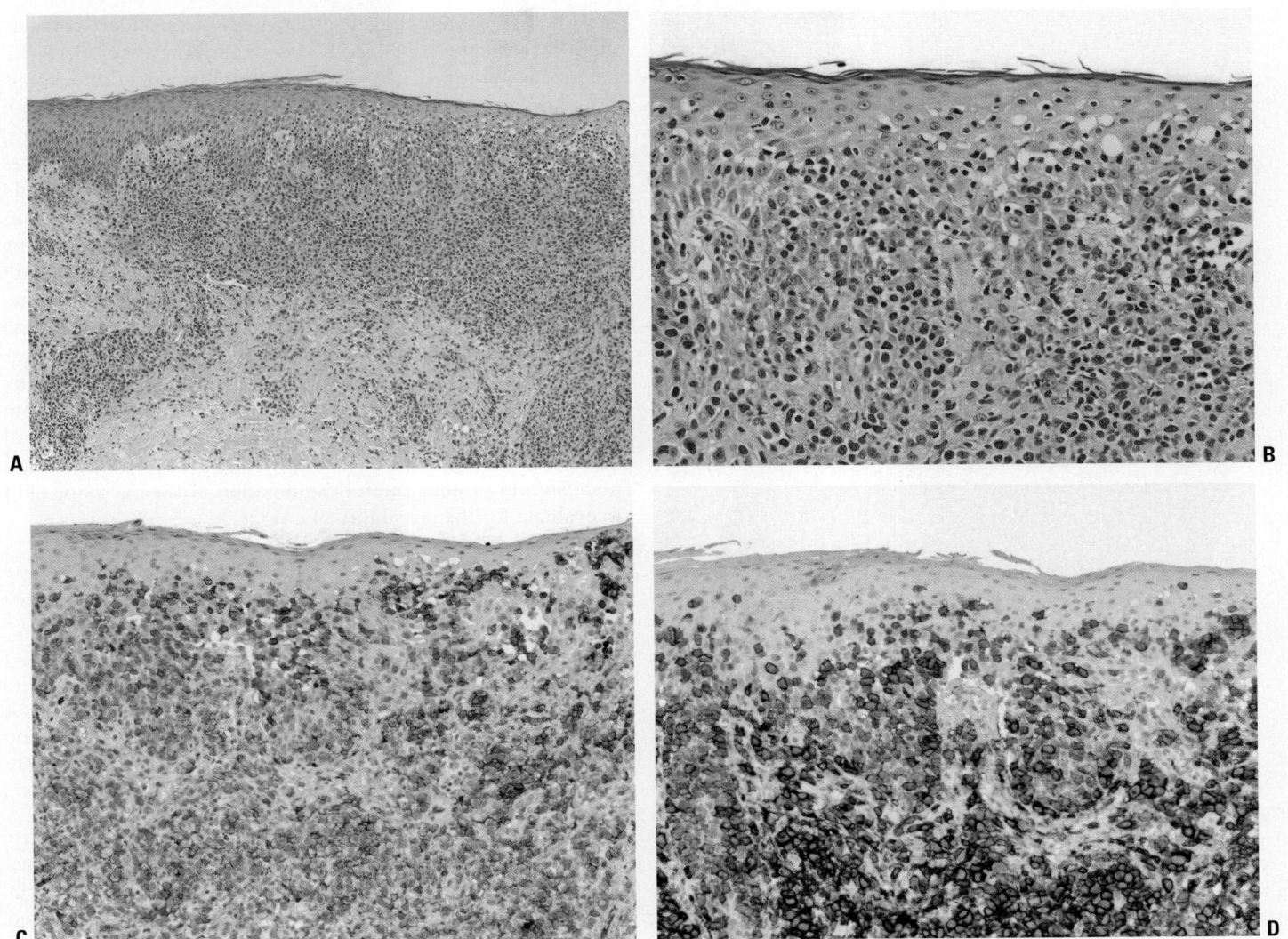

Figure 31-34 Lymphomatoid papulosis, type D. **A:** This variant exhibits a superficial infiltrate with marked epidermotropism. **B:** Closer inspection highlights further the striking epidermotropism with atypical lymphocytes. **C:** There is a predominance of CD8 staining. **D:** Strong, diffuse CD30 expression is seen.

Differential Diagnosis. In general, clinical correlation will be essential in distinguishing the various patterns of LyP from morphologically similar entities, as mentioned previously, as well as from transformed, CD30⁺ MF. Interestingly, rare cases have been reported in which MF and primary cutaneous CD30⁺ lymphoproliferative disorders coexist (135,149), and this may predict an improved prognosis compared to MF alone (75). Another entity to consider is pityriasis lichenoides et varioliformis acuta (PLEVA), which presents with papulonecrotic lesions; distinction may be particularly difficult in cases with numerous CD30⁺ cells (150). Other reactive, self-resolving conditions, including arthropod bites, drug eruptions, and viral infection (e.g., herpes simplex virus 1 and 2), should also be considered (151–153).

Principles of Management: LyP may not require any therapy, particularly in cases where the extent of disease is limited. Patients with disseminated or disruptive lesions may utilize phototherapy or low-dose methotrexate (133). Systemic chemotherapy will only provide short-term effectiveness and should not be used in this clinical setting. Long-term clinical follow-up is advised given the relationship of LyP with other lymphoproliferative disorders such as MF.

Primary Cutaneous Anaplastic Large Cell Lymphoma

Clinical Summary. Skin lesions of cALCL consist of one or more localized, rapidly growing, frequently ulcerated reddish-brown nodules (Fig. 31-35) or occasionally papules (135). Partial regression of untreated lesions may occur, but complete spontaneous resolution, as seen in LyP, is unusual. Multifocal disease is less common and may be associated with relapse following therapy. Nonetheless, cALCL is associated with an excellent prognosis with an estimated 5-year survival of greater than 90% (154). There may be involvement of regional, draining lymph nodes, but this does not affect prognosis (135). Extracutaneous dissemination occurs in approximately 10% of patients and may be more common in patients who present with multifocal disease (155).

Histopathology. cALCL is characterized by nodular or diffuse infiltrates of large, anaplastic cells that involve the dermis and occasionally the subcutis (Fig. 31-36A, B). Morphologically, biopsies of cALCL may closely resemble those of systemic ALCL with secondary skin involvement, although Reed–Sternberg–like cells and highly pleomorphic, multinucleated giant cells may be more numerous in the latter. The large, atypical cells should account for most of the infiltrate, although a

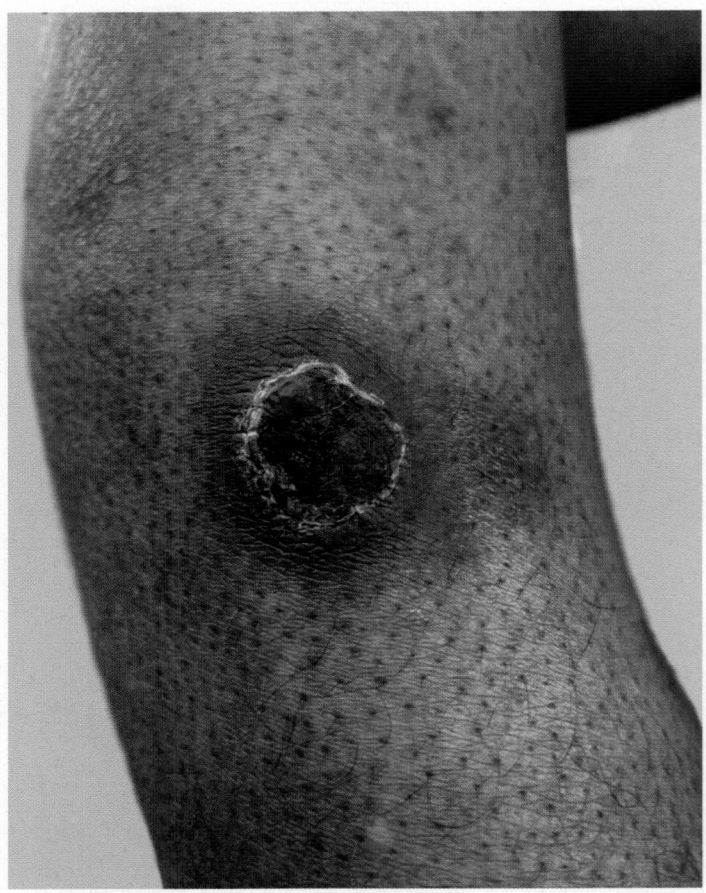

Figure 31-35 Primary cutaneous anaplastic large cell lymphoma. Solitary, large ulcerated plaque-like nodule on the arm, with surrounding erythema. (Courtesy of Dr. Cecilia Larocca, Dana-Farber Cancer Institute, Boston, MA.)

background of secondary inflammatory elements may be observed and occasionally eosinophilia is marked. Some cases exhibit areas of mucinous or myxoid-appearing stroma (Fig. 31-36C). Necrosis and/or angioinvasion may be seen. Marked epidermal hyperplasia, sometimes with keratoacanthoma-like features, epidermal invasion by atypical cells, and ulceration are often present. Greater than 75% of the infiltrate is, by definition, positive for CD30 (Fig. 31-36D). The cells are typically CD4$^+$ and frequently show expression of cytotoxic granule proteins (granzyme B, TIA-1) (144). Aberrant T-cell phenotypes with loss of CD2, CD3, CD5, and/or CD7 may be observed, and CD8 expression rather than CD4 expression may be seen. EMA and ALK1 are negative.

Histogenesis. All forms of primary cutaneous CD30$^+$ T-cell lymphoproliferative disorders are believed to be derived from an activated skin-homing T cell. Most cases of cALCL show clonal rearrangements of the TCR genes. In contrast to some cases of systemic ALCL, translocations involving the *ALK* (anaplastic lymphoma kinase) gene are not detected (156). Rearrangements at 6p25.3 involving the *IRF4/DUSP22* locus have been found to be present in approximately 25% of cALCL cases (116,117,141,146), although they have also been described in peripheral T-cell lymphomas (146) and a small subset of LyP cases (145). Recent whole-transcriptome sequencing identified a novel recurrent *NPM1-TYK2* gene fusion, leading to STAT signaling activation, in a subset of cALCL and LyP (157).

Differential Diagnosis. In general, demonstration of ALK1 expression in a cutaneous CD30$^+$ T-cell lymphoma with anaplastic morphology should suggest a diagnosis of secondary involvement by systemic ALCL, ALK$^+$. However, rare cases of CD30$^+$ cutaneous tumors with ALK1 immunohistochemical expression and/or *ALK* translocations arising in patients without evidence of systemic disease (even with long-term follow-up) have been described (141,158,159). Nonetheless, these cases are the exception and not the rule, and careful staging should always be performed in patients with CD30$^+$, ALK1$^+$ cutaneous tumors. Likewise, careful clinical correlation including staging is needed to distinguish cALCL from other CD30$^+$ tumors with considerably worse prognoses, including secondary cutaneous involvement by ALK1$^-$ systemic ALCL, LCT of MF, and other high-grade large-cell lymphomas that may also express CD30. Regional draining lymph nodes may be involved by cALCL, which may be morphologically indistinguishable from focal nodal involvement by CHL (160). Therefore, detection of CD30$^+$ cells with anaplastic morphology in an isolated lymph node should prompt careful examination of the overlying skin to evaluate for the possibility of cALCL.

Principles of Management: Surgical excision or radiotherapy may be utilized for localized lesions, whereas systemic chemotherapy may be needed in multifocal disease.

Subcutaneous Panniculitis-Like T-Cell Lymphoma

Subcutaneous panniculitis-like T-cell lymphoma (SPTCL) is a rare lymphoma that primarily infiltrates subcutaneous tissue and demonstrates an $\alpha\beta$ T-cell phenotype and is infrequently associated with a hemophagocytic syndrome (161).

Clinical Summary. SPTCL tends to show an equal gender distribution and occurs mainly in adults, although childhood cases have been reported (162). Affected individuals generally present with symptoms related to formation of solitary or generalized deeply seated, variably sized erythematous cutaneous nodules often involving the extremities and/or trunk. Ulceration is uncommon, and extracutaneous spread is rare. Approximately 60% of patients present with systemic symptoms such as fever, fatigue, and weight loss, and a smaller number (~ 20%) demonstrate evidence of a hemophagocytic syndrome. The disease has a protracted but indolent course with an overall 5-year survival of greater than 80% (163). Notably, the OS of patients without a hemophagocytic syndrome is 91% compared to only 46% when a hemophagocytic syndrome is present (161).

Histopathology. There is a diffuse, variably cellular infiltrate involving both septa and lobules within the subcutis (Fig. 31-37A), with relative sparing of the overlying dermis and epidermis. Given this distribution pattern, a large biopsy or excision is needed to evaluate for involvement when this disease is suspected. The infiltrate is composed of small- to medium-sized lymphocytes with visible cytoplasm admixed with fewer large transformed cells with hyperchromatic nuclei. Often, the initial biopsy, in which the more atypical elements are not well represented, may appear deceptively banal. Cells characteristically show peripheral alignment (rimming) around individual adipocytes, although this finding is nonspecific (Fig. 31-37B). Fat necrosis, karyorrhexis, and associated infiltration of reactive histiocytes may also be noted. Cellular necrosis, nuclear fragmentation, and vascular injury may all be observed. Although nonneoplastic small lymphocytes may be present, admixed plasma cells and eosinophils are not commonly observed. The malignant cells express a mature CD3$^+$, CD4$^-$, and CD8$^+$ T-cell

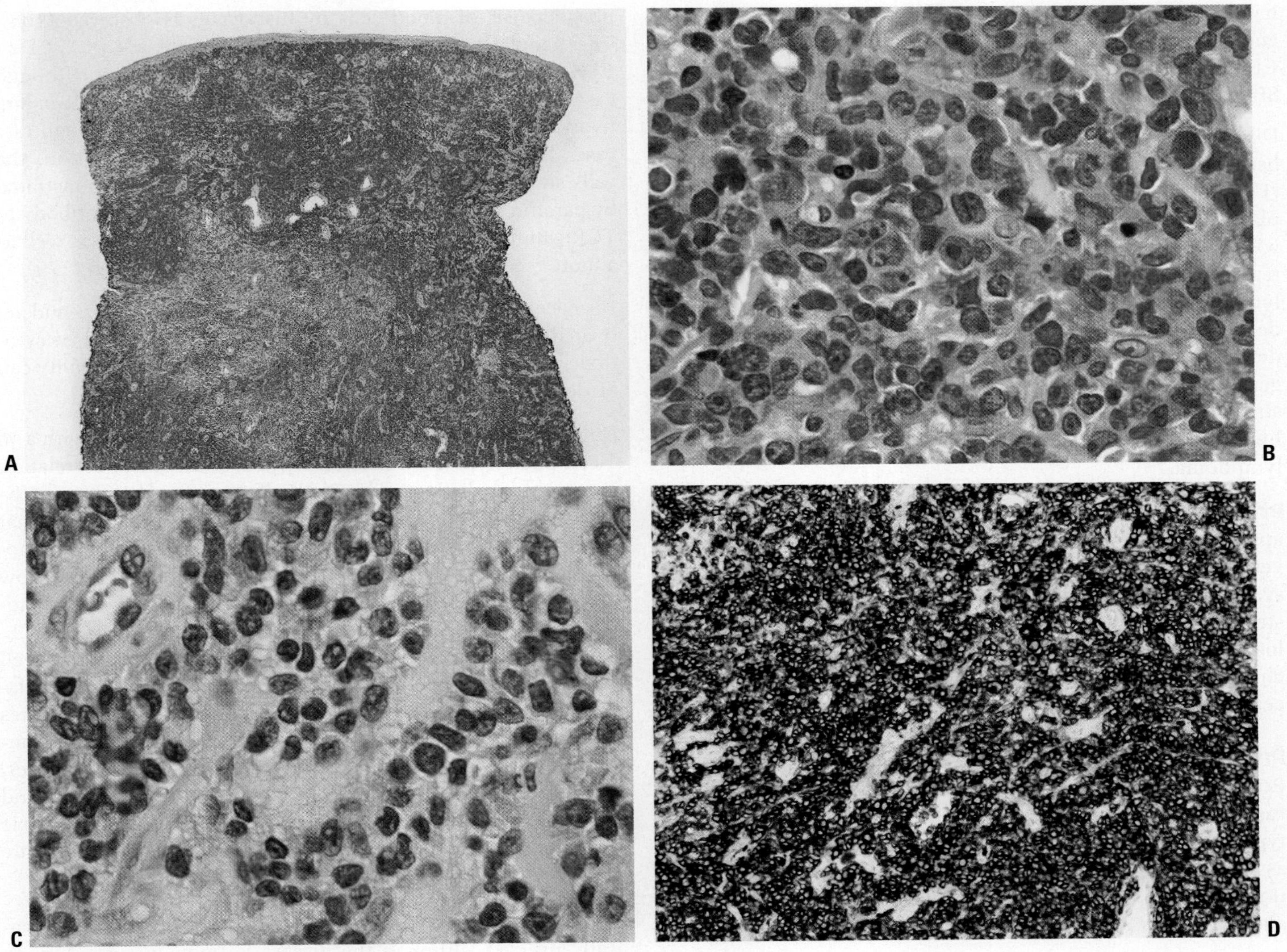

Figure 31-36 Primary cutaneous anaplastic large cell lymphoma. **A:** Tumoral infiltrate with dense, diffuse sheets of cells infiltrating the entire dermis. **B:** High magnification of the large, anaplastic lymphocytes. **C:** Areas exhibiting mucinous or myxoid-appearing stroma. **D:** Strong, uniform CD30 expression in the atypical lymphocytes.

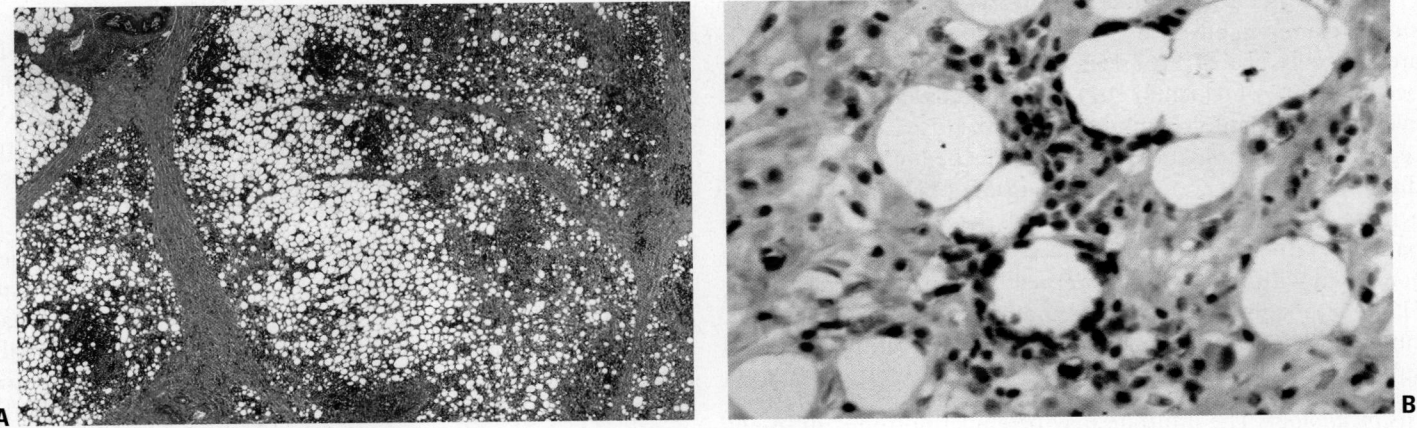

Figure 31-37 Subcutaneous panniculitis-like T-cell lymphoma. **A:** Lobular and septal pattern of subcutaneous infiltration. **B:** TIA-1 immunohistochemistry showing characteristic rimming around individual adipocytes.

phenotype. CD30 and CD56 staining are consistently negative. EBER *in situ* hybridization is also always negative. The cells, by definition, demonstrate an αβ T-cell phenotype, and use of antibodies to TCR βF1 and to the TCR gamma chain constant region or delta chain should be used in any suspected case of SPTCL to document the phenotype.

Histogenesis. In keeping with their presumed derivation from a cytotoxic T cell, the neoplastic T cells are also reactive for granzyme B, perforin, and TIA-1. Clonality can be demonstrated by TCR gene rearrangements. The mechanism underlying the association of hemophagocytic syndrome with SPTCL has not yet been fully determined. Recent whole-exome sequencing has shown that biallelic germline mutations in *HAVCR2*, a gene encoding TIM-3, an immune inhibitory receptor expressed on CD8+ T cells, confers high susceptibility to developing primary SPTCL (164).

Differential Diagnosis. SPTCL should be differentiated from benign panniculitis, such as lupus erythematosus panniculitis (LEP), which can have overlapping features. The presence of plasma cells, hyaline/myxoid changes, and lymphoid follicles with germinal centers and the lack of clonality in TCR gene rearrangement studies favor LEP (165). Extranodal NK/T-cell lymphoma, nasal type (ENKTCL), which frequently exhibits dermal in addition to subcutaneous involvement, is CD56+, demonstrates reactivity for EBER *in situ* hybridization, and generally does not show TCR gene rearrangements. Demonstration of a γδ T-cell phenotype excludes SPTCL and most likely indicates a diagnosis of primary cutaneous γδ T-cell lymphoma.

Principles of Management: A definitive consensus on therapy for SPTCL is yet to be determined. Depending on the severity of disease (including the presence of a hemophagocytic syndrome), possible treatments include the use of systemic steroids or other immunosuppressive therapies such as cyclosporine; radiation therapy for solitary lesions; or multiagent chemotherapy with or without autologous or allogeneic stem cell transplant.

Primary Cutaneous Gamma-Delta T-Cell Lymphoma

Primary cutaneous γδ T-cell lymphoma (PCGD-TCL) includes cases previously characterized as SPTCL with a γδ T-cell phenotype (166). The WHO–EORTC classification defines this entity as a cutaneous lymphoma originating from a clonal proliferation of mature, activated γδ T cells with a cytotoxic phenotype and a generally aggressive clinical behavior.

Clinical Summary. PCGD-TCL affects adults without gender predilection. Typical lesions include disseminated indurated plaques and ulcerated/necrotic nodules/tumors, most commonly on the extremities and trunk; scaly patches are infrequent (167). Systemic involvement of mucosal and other extranodal sites is common, but the lymph nodes, spleen, or bone marrow are generally spared (167,168). A hemophagocytic syndrome occurs in 50% of patients (161). The prognosis is disappointing even with systemic chemotherapy, with a 5-year OS of 11%, regardless of the presence or absence of a hemophagocytic syndrome (161). However, a distinct subset of patients has shown a more indolent course (169,170). It has been reported that patients with subcutaneous disease have a worse prognosis compared with those with epidermal or dermal infiltrates only (171), although no statistically significant difference in 2-year survival was seen in panniculitic or nonpanniculitic cases in a subsequent study (167).

Histopathology. The infiltrate may be epidermotropic, diffusely dermal, or panniculitic or show combinations of the above patterns either in one biopsy or in different specimens (Fig. 31-38A, B) (171,172). The cytomorphology is monomorphous, with variably sized cells displaying irregular to pleomorphic nuclei and coarsely clumped chromatin (Fig. 31-38C). Angioinvasion is common, although the presence of large areas of necrosis secondary to angiodestruction is not a typical feature. Subcutaneous involvement may show rimming of adipocytes, similar to SPTCL. In cases associated with hemophagocytic syndrome,

phagocytosis of blood cells by histiocytes is observed (168). The neoplastic cells commonly demonstrate a CD3+, CD2+, CD4−, CD5−, CD7+/−, CD8−, and CD56+ phenotype, although cases with CD8 expression are also seen (167). EBER *in situ* hybridization reactivity is generally not present, although rare cases have been described (167,173,174). By definition, the cells show a γδ T-cell phenotype, which can be demonstrated by paraffin section immunohistochemistry with an antibody to TCR gamma chain constant region (Fig. 31-39A, B), as well as a more recently available antibody to TCR delta chain (175).

Histogenesis. Given the postulated origin from a mature and activated cytotoxic γδ T cell, there is strong expression of cytotoxic proteins (TIA-1, granzyme B, and perforin). Clonality can be demonstrated by TCR gene rearrangement studies.

Differential Diagnosis. Rare cases of MF or LyP type D with a γδ T-cell phenotype have been described, and clinical correlation is needed for distinction (176). Differentiation between ENKTCL and PCGD-TCL can pose a particular problem given that both diseases share clinical, morphologic, and immunophenotypic features. In most cases, distinction is straightforward now that an antibody is available to demonstrate the γδ T-cell phenotype. Additionally, TCR gene rearrangements favor PCGD-TCL, whereas diffuse positivity for EBER *in situ* hybridization as well as large areas of necrosis associated with angiodestruction favors ENKTCL. However, cases showing overlapping features have been described (177), and indeed the two entities demonstrate similar genetic signatures (178). Therefore, in rare cases, definitive categorization may not be possible. Both SPTCL and primary cutaneous CD8+ aggressive epidermotropic cytotoxic T-cell lymphoma demonstrate an αβ T-cell phenotype and are generally CD56−.

Principles of Management: Systemic chemotherapy is typically utilized, although the disease is frequently resistant to treatment.

Primary Cutaneous CD8-Positive Aggressive Epidermotropic Cytotoxic T-cell Lymphoma (Provisional Entity)

This still provisional entity (herein referred to as PCCD8AC-TCL) is characterized by a proliferation of epidermotropic CD8+ cytotoxic T cells and an aggressive clinical course (179,180). Prior to the recognition of this category, patients with this tumor were classified as having generalized pagetoid reticulosis (Ketron–Goodman disease) or an aggressive MF.

Clinical Summary. Affected patients are typically middle-aged to elderly, with a median age of 54 years and a male-to-female ratio of 1.6:1.0 (180). Clinically, patients present with localized or disseminated eruptive papules, nodules, or tumors with central ulceration and necrosis or hyperkeratotic patches and plaques (180,181). Spread to other visceral sites, such as the lung, testis, central nervous system, and oral mucosa, has been documented, but nodal involvement is unusual (180). The clinical course is aggressive, with rapid progression and a median survival of 12 months (180).

Histopathology. PCCD8AC-TCL lesions are characterized by variably sized, pleomorphic T lymphocytes forming heterogeneous patterns including lichenoid, nodular, or diffuse infiltrates, commonly with marked epidermotropism (Fig. 31-40A, B). In advanced lesions, the epidermotropism may be less pronounced.

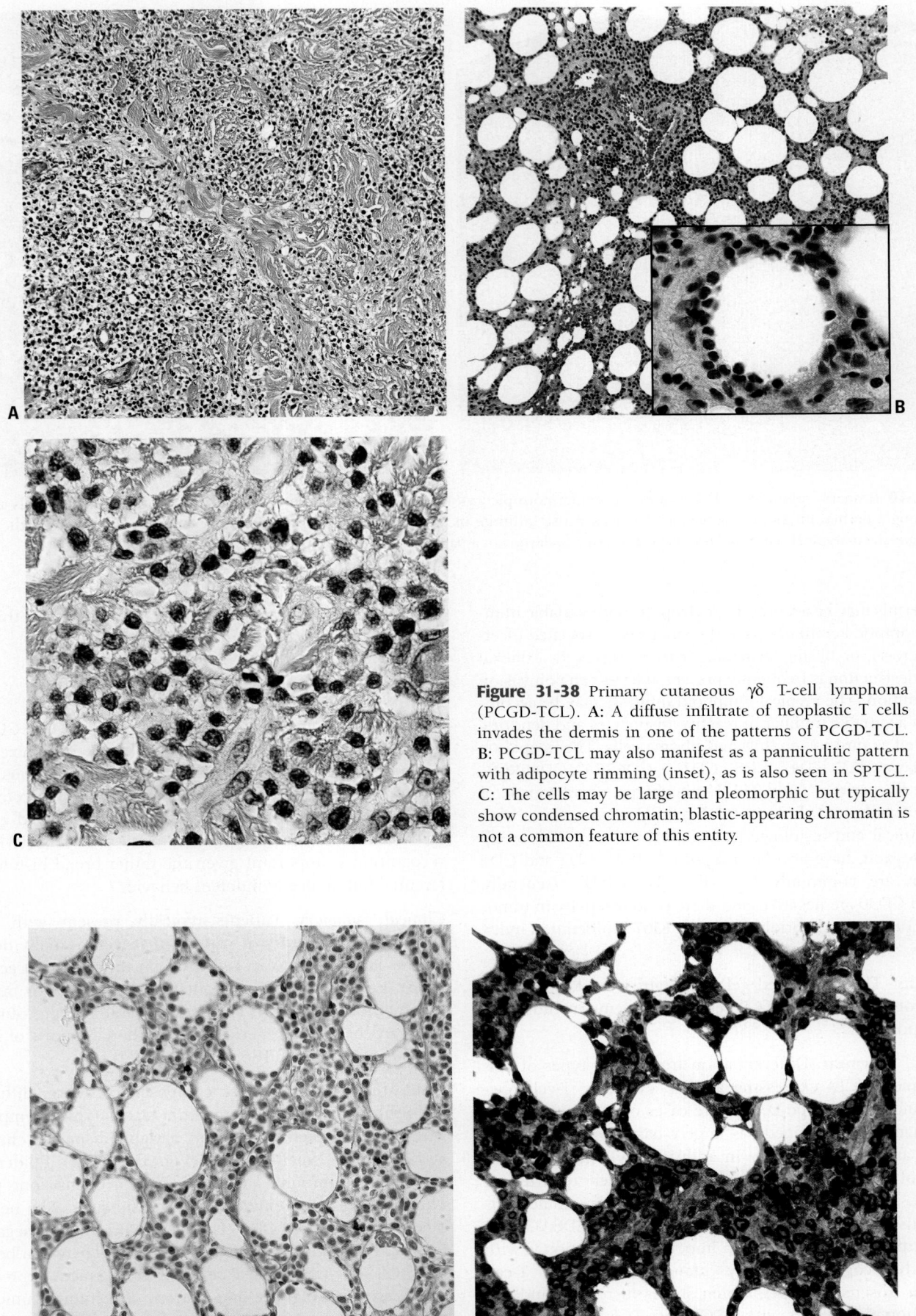

Figure 31-38 Primary cutaneous γδ T-cell lymphoma (PCGD-TCL). **A:** A diffuse infiltrate of neoplastic T cells invades the dermis in one of the patterns of PCGD-TCL. **B:** PCGD-TCL may also manifest as a panniculitic pattern with adipocyte rimming (inset), as is also seen in SPTCL. **C:** The cells may be large and pleomorphic but typically show condensed chromatin; blastic-appearing chromatin is not a common feature of this entity.

Figure 31-39 Primary cutaneous γδ T-cell lymphoma. **A:** Immunohistochemistry on paraffin sections using the TCR βF1 antibody demonstrates absence of reactivity in the infiltrate and highlights few admixed reactive T cells. **B:** Immunohistochemistry on paraffin sections using a monoclonal antibody to the TCR gamma chain constant region reveals strong reactivity within the infiltrate.

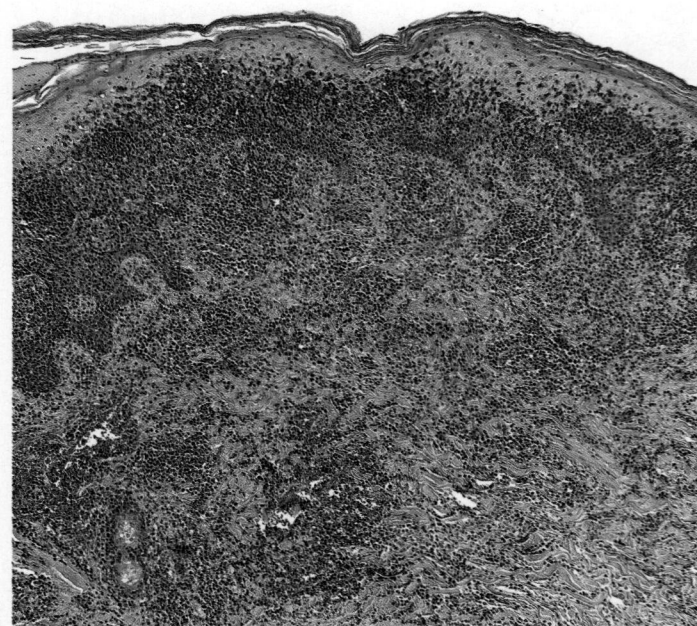
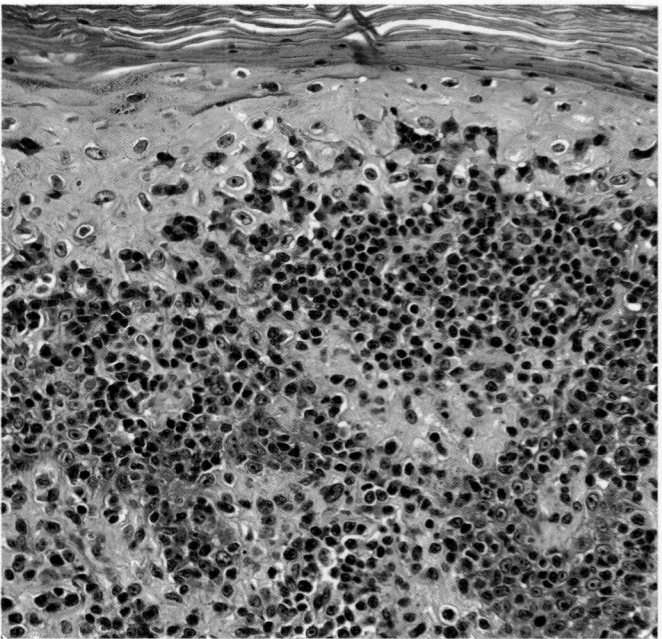

Figure 31-40 Primary cutaneous CD8⁺ aggressive epidermotropic cytotoxic T-cell lymphoma. **A:** Scanning magnification reveals neoplastic cells forming a dermal interstitial pattern as well as a dense infiltrate in the overlying epidermis. **B:** Higher magnification reveals the small- to intermediate-sized atypical lymphocytes permeating the epidermis in a pagetoid pattern.

The epidermis may be acanthotic or atrophic, with variable numbers of apoptotic keratinocytes and spongiosis. Associated ulceration, necrosis, or blister formation may be observed. Adnexal invasion/destruction is frequently present, whereas angioinvasion is less common. The atypical lymphoid infiltrate may be accompanied by a variable number of reactive histiocytes and dendritic cells as well as rare eosinophils and plasma cells. The neoplastic cells display a CD3⁺, CD4⁻, CD8⁺, CD7⁻/⁺, CD45RA⁺, CD45RO⁻, granzyme B⁺, perforin⁺, and TIA-1⁺ phenotype, characteristic of cytotoxic T cells, and show an αβ T-cell phenotype. Cases with similar clinical and histologic features, but lacking CD8 or αβ TCR expression, have also been reported (182). CD2 and CD5 expression are commonly lost (Fig. 31-41A–D). Generally, CD56 and CD30 are negative, and there is no reactivity in tumor cells for EBER *in situ* hybridization. The Ki67 proliferation index is high.

Histogenesis. The postulated cell of origin is a skin-homing, CD8⁺, cytotoxic αβ T cell. TCR gene rearrangement studies are typically positive.

Differential Diagnosis. Differentiation from other types of epidermotropic CTCLs expressing a CD8⁺ cytotoxic T-cell phenotype, such as LyP type D and rare cases of MF (particularly tumor stage or transformed), is largely based on clinical presentation and disease course. In addition, LyP will show expression of CD30, which has only rarely been reported in PCCD8AC-TCL (141). Although the clinical presentation is indistinguishable from PCGD-TCL, tumors of PCCD8AC-TCL are of an αβ T-cell phenotype. An important distinction is with the recently recognized primary cutaneous acral CD8⁺ T-cell lymphoma (discussed next), which shares histologic and immunophenotypic features with PCCD8AC-TCL but follows an indolent course and lacks the marked epidermotropism, frequent ulceration, and high Ki67 proliferation index characteristic of PCCD8AC-TCL.

Principles of Management: Given the rarity of this entity, treatment guidelines are not well established.

Primary Cutaneous Acral CD8-Positive T-Cell Lymphoma (Provisional Entity)

Primary cutaneous acral CD8⁺ T-cell lymphoma (PCACD8-TCL) is a newly described and provisional entity, recognized in the recent WHO–EORTC classification (11). These lesions are very rare and were initially reported as clinically indolent clonal proliferations of small- to medium-sized, nonactivated cytotoxic CD8⁺ T cells of the ear/face or at acral sites (183,184). Their recognition is important given the rather broad histologic differential but clinically indolent behavior.

Clinical Summary. Patients typically present with isolated slow-growing nodules or papules that were initially described on the ears but that can also arise on the face or at acral sites (185). Lesions are usually solitary, but bilateral or multifocal presentations can occur. There is an overall benign course, with only rare local recurrences, and exceptional reports of extracutaneous progression (186,187).

Histopathology. Tumors are composed of dense, diffuse dermal infiltrates of small- to medium-sized atypical lymphocytes with irregular nuclear contours, variably dispersed chromatin, and occasional small nucleoli (Fig. 31-42A, B). Epidermal involvement is minimal or absent, with a Grenz zone present. The infiltrate often extends into the subcutis. The neoplastic T cells express CD3, CD8, TIA-1, and βF1 and are negative for CD4, CD30, and CD56 (Fig. 31-42C, D). There can be loss of CD2, CD5, or CD7. The T cells exhibit frequent expression of CD68, with a Golgi dot–like pattern, a seemingly unique feature among cutaneous CD8⁺ lymphomas (188). There is variable expression of perforin and granzyme B in accordance with the nonactivated state. The Ki67 proliferation index is typically very low (<15%). The infiltrate can contain reactive B-cell

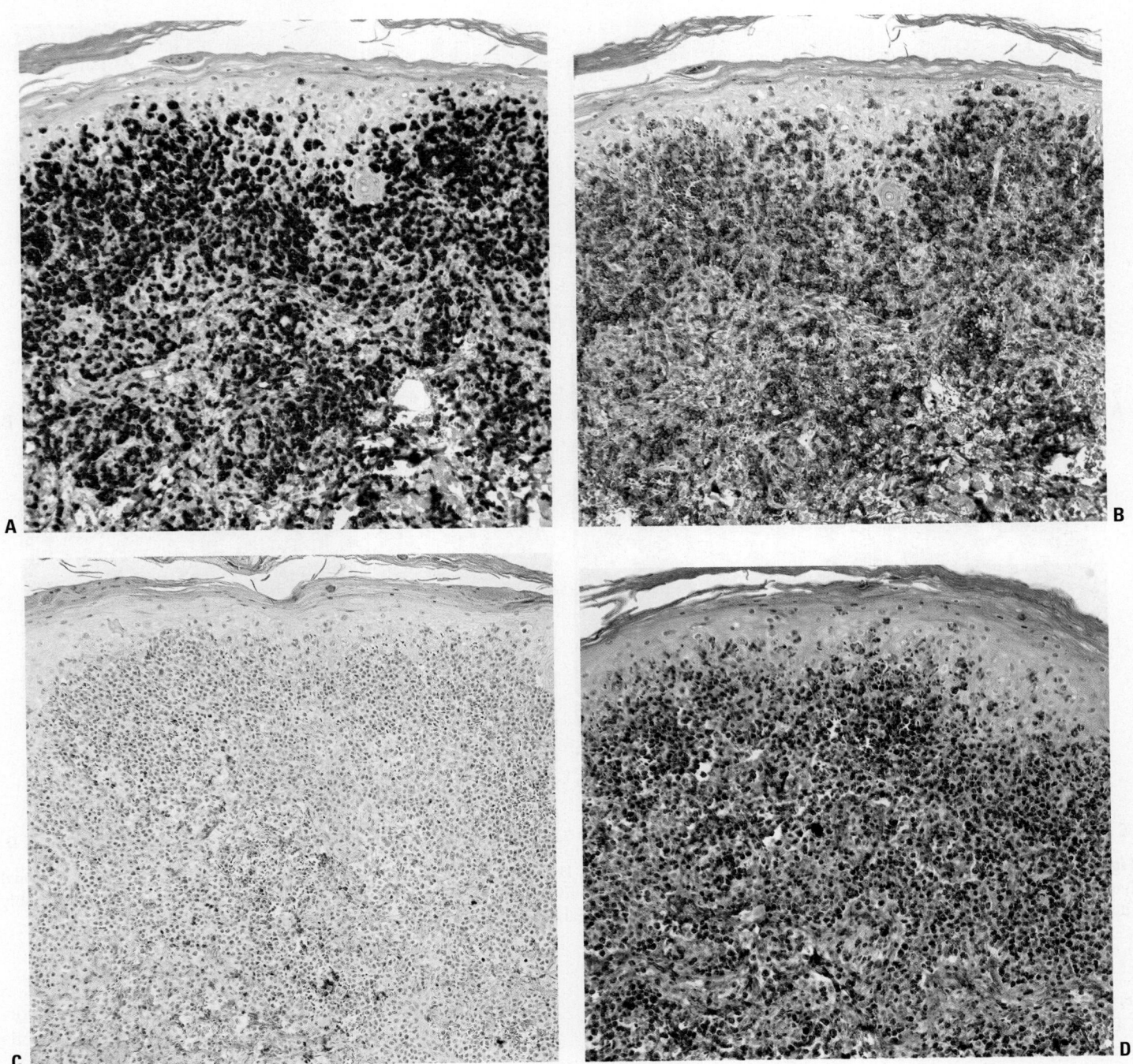

Figure 31-41 Primary cutaneous CD8⁺ aggressive epidermotropic cytotoxic T-cell lymphoma (PCCD8AC-TCL). Immunohistochemistry studies reveal the characteristic immunophenotype of PCCD8AC-TCL, including expression of CD3 (**A**), CD8 (**B**), loss of CD2, (**C**), and expression of the cytotoxic molecule perforin (**D**).

aggregates as well, although plasma cells, histiocytes, and eosinophils are rare.

Histogenesis. The postulated cell of origin is a skin-homing, non-activated cytotoxic αβ CD8⁺ T cell. The majority of reported cases have had clonal rearrangements of TCR gamma genes.

Differential Diagnosis. The diagnosis of PCACD8-TCL requires careful integration of clinical features, and the most important distinction would be from an aggressive CD8⁺ cutaneous lymphoma. In contrast to PCCD8AC-TCL, these lesions lack prominent epidermotropism, ulceration, or necrosis and do not follow an aggressive clinical course. The presentation and disease course are also important in distinguishing PCACD8-TCL

from rare cases of advanced CD8⁺ MF or type D LyP, although lack of CD30 expression will also be helpful.

Principles of Management: In general, these lesions resolve following excision or radiotherapy. Systemic dissemination does not occur, and there is no need for chemotherapy, although guidelines are not yet well established (189).

Primary Cutaneous CD4-Positive Small/Medium T-Cell Lymphoproliferative Disorder (Provisional Entity)

Primary cutaneous CD4⁺ small/medium T-cell lymphoproliferative disorder (PCSM-TLPD) is a provisional entity defined

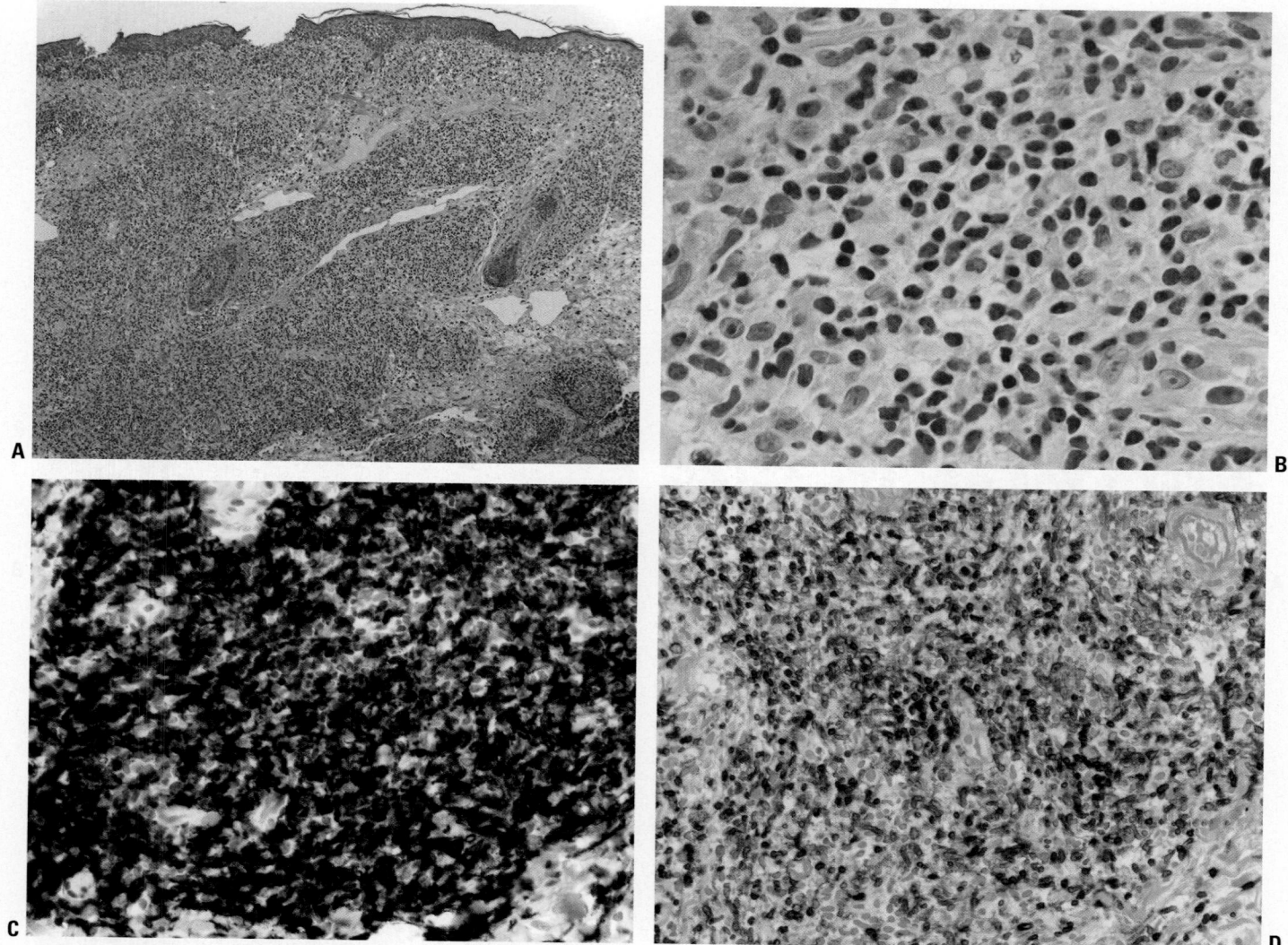

Figure 31-42 Primary cutaneous acral CD8-positive T-cell lymphoma. Histologic sections of a small nodule on the eyelid show a dense dermal lymphocytic infiltrate (A), which on high magnification reveals small- to medium-sized atypical lymphocytes with irregular nuclei and variably dispersed chromatin (B). **C:** Most lymphocytes are CD8⁺. **D:** The atypical cells are positive for TCR βF1.

as a cutaneous infiltrate of clonal small- to medium-sized, CD4⁺, pleomorphic T cells associated with a robust inflammatory component predominantly arising as an isolated lesion on the head or neck and showing a favorable clinical course. There are considerable overlapping clinical, morphologic, immunophenotypic, and genetic features between this entity and pseudo–T-cell lymphoma, with both showing a benign course (122,190), which led to a change to the more encompassing terminology of "lymphoproliferative disorder" in the 2016 WHO revision, in place of the prior "lymphoma" designation (1).

Clinical Summary. Patients are adults or elderly. The clinical lesions are often solitary plaque/nodules, or reddish papules, generally involving the upper half of the body (especially head and neck) without a history of patches or plaques to suggest MF. The prognosis is excellent, particularly in cases with a solitary lesion (122,191,192).

Histopathology. Typically, biopsies show a dense, diffuse, or nodular infiltrate of predominantly small- to medium-sized pleomorphic T cells filling the dermis and often extending into the upper subcutis (Fig. 31-43A). Epidermotropism may be seen

focally. The infiltrate contains fewer than 30% large pleomorphic cells (Fig. 31-43B), and abundant, small, reactive B cells and CD8⁺ T cells; histiocytes; and plasma cells are admixed. In some cases, multinucleated giant cells and/or granulomatous changes are present, and infiltration of adnexal structures (sweat glands, pilar units) is common (190). The neoplastic cells are of an αβ, helper T-cell phenotype and express CD3 and CD4 but not CD8 (Fig. 31-44A, B), TIA-1, granzyme B, or CD30. Pan-T-cell markers are lost in some cases (193). The proliferation index is generally less than 20% to 30% (190). The atypical CD4⁺ T cells express follicular T-cell markers PD-1 (Fig. 31-44C), BCL6, and CXCL13 but do not express CD10 (122,141,192).

Histogenesis. The cell of origin is thought to be a CD4⁺ skin-homing T cell of follicular helper T-cell phenotype. Clonality can be demonstrated by TCR gene rearrangement studies.

Differential Diagnosis. The prominent reactive B-cell infiltrate, along with the presence of admixed plasma cells, may erroneously suggest a diagnosis of PCMZL; immunophenotyping and perhaps even gene rearrangement studies may be needed for

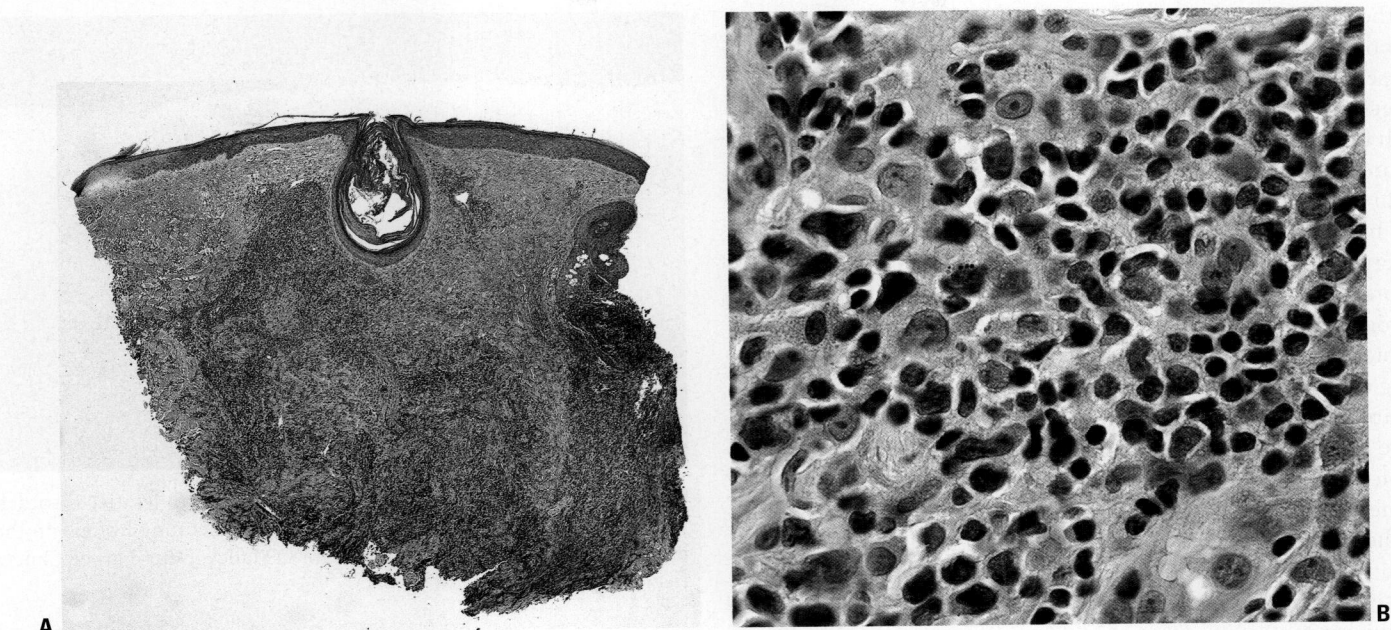

Figure 31-43 Primary cutaneous CD4⁺ small/medium T-cell lymphoproliferative disorder (PCSM-TLPD). **A:** Scanning magnification shows the typical dermal infiltration pattern of PCSM-TCL. **B:** Closer examination reveals an infiltrate of small- to intermediate-sized lymphocytes with irregular nuclear contours and condensed chromatin as well as a few admixed pleomorphic large cells with more dispersed chromatin and distinct nucleoli.

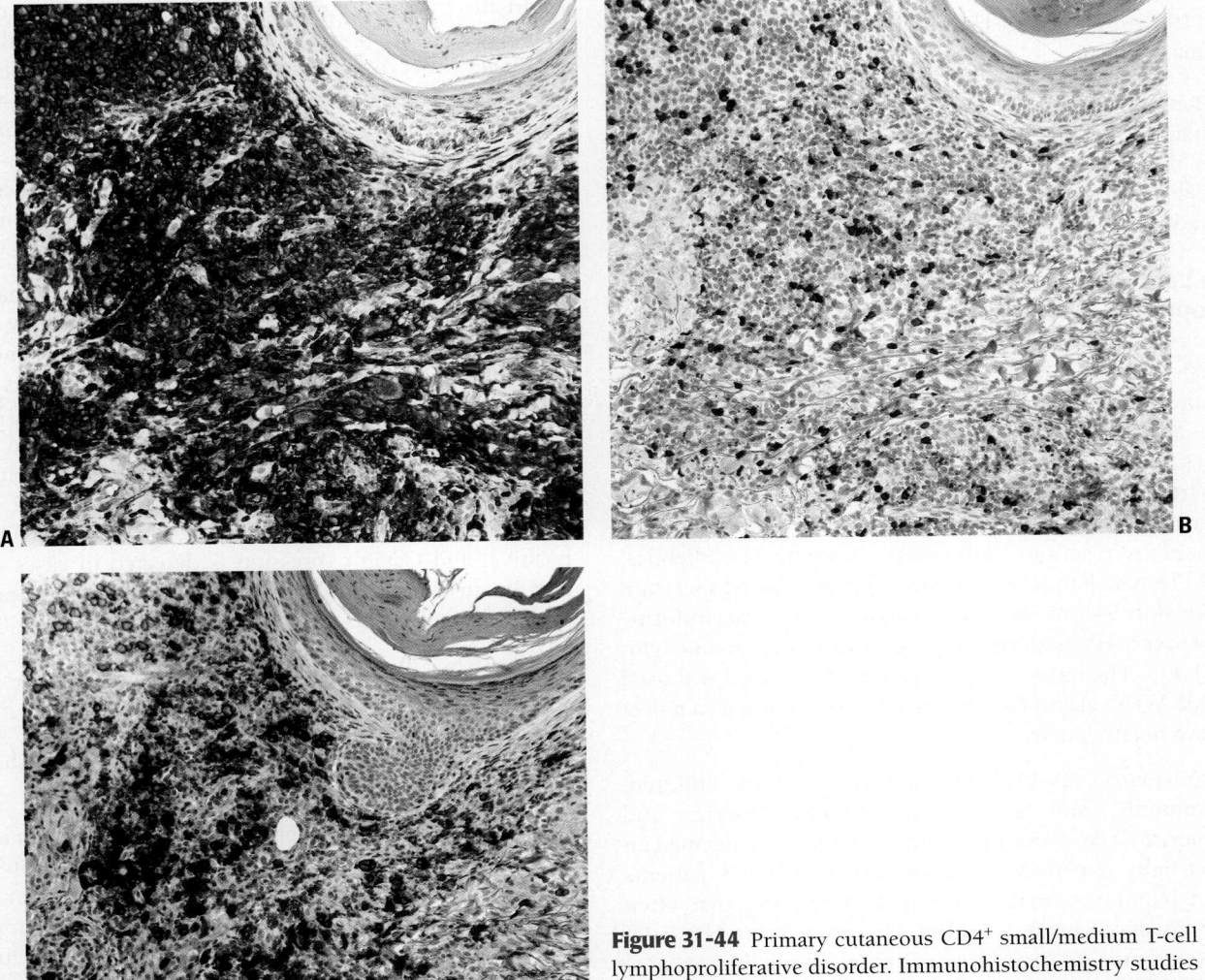

Figure 31-44 Primary cutaneous CD4⁺ small/medium T-cell lymphoproliferative disorder. Immunohistochemistry studies reveal that the infiltrate in PCSM-TCL is composed of CD4⁺ T cells (**A**), which do not express CD8 (**B**) and coexpress PD-1 (**C**). Interpretation may be challenging owing to the admixed histiocytes, which also express CD4 (as seen in **A**) and the presence of interspersed reactive CD8⁺ T cells (**B**).

further evaluation. Of note, a recent large series of PCSM-TLPD demonstrated the presence of *IGH* gene rearrangements in a subset of cases with increased B cells, leading to diagnostic challenges (194); however, a marked predominance of CD4+ T cells with follicular T-cell marker expression would be a helpful clue to prompt consideration of PCSM-TLPD. Because of morphologic and immunophenotypic overlap between this entity and MF, by definition, the diagnosis of PCSM-TLPD should only be entertained after exclusion of MF by clinical history. As alluded to previously, cutaneous pseudo–T-cell lymphoma was a term introduced in the 1990s to describe indolent lesions with an atypical bandlike infiltrate mimicking MF or a lymphomatoid drug eruption (often attributable to antiseizure medication). In addition, solitary lesions with a nodular or diffuse architecture were also included in this group, and these lesions were morphologically and immunophenotypically similar to those subsequently described as PCSM-TLPD (122,141). While initial studies using Southern blot analysis did not detect clonal TCR gene rearrangements in cutaneous pseudo–T-cell lymphoma, subsequent studies have shown the presence of clonal TCR gene rearrangements (122,141). Therefore, it is proposed that these entities fall within the same spectrum given the excellent prognosis particularly in patients with solitary lesions (122). Cases presenting with rapidly growing or disseminated lesions, and with greater than 30% large pleomorphic cells with a high Ki67 proliferation index, likely belong to another spectrum of disease (190,195) and may be best designated peripheral T-cell lymphoma, NOS.

Principles of Management: In general, it is recommended that solitary lesions be treated conservatively, including "watch and wait" because some may regress spontaneously (191), intralesional steroid injection, local excision, or in some cases localized radiotherapy.

Hydroa Vacciniforme–Like Lymphoproliferative Disorder

Hydroa vacciniforme–like lymphoproliferative disorder (HV-LPD) is a rare, chronic EBV+ cutaneous lymphoproliferative disorder of childhood characterized by a papulovesicular eruption, and a highly variable clinical course, that may progress with systemic symptoms. The updated WHO–EORTC classification recognizes a spectrum of cutaneous manifestations of chronic active EBV infection of T- and NK-cell types, including hypersensitivity reactions with severe mosquito bite allergies, and HV-LPD, which in turn now encompasses a broad spectrum of HV-like skin lesions, including classic hydroa vacciniforme (HV) and severe HV, with risk of progression to a systemic lymphoma (1,11). The term "HV-like lymphoma," which was used in the 2008 WHO classification, has now been revised to reflect this disease heterogeneity.

Clinical Summary. HV-LPD predominantly affects children, most commonly from Asia, Mexico, Central America, and South America (196–198). In classic HV, which was deemed an ultraviolet-light hypersensitivity condition, affected patients develop a papulovesicular eruption with scarring that often shows spontaneous remission (199). In more severe HV, cutaneous lesions may also manifest as indurated plaques or large tumors, which often develop ulceration (Fig. 31-45). In contrast to classic HV, lesions will arise on both sun-exposed and sun-protected areas. Patients often develop systemic symptoms such as fever, weight loss, hepatosplenomegaly, and

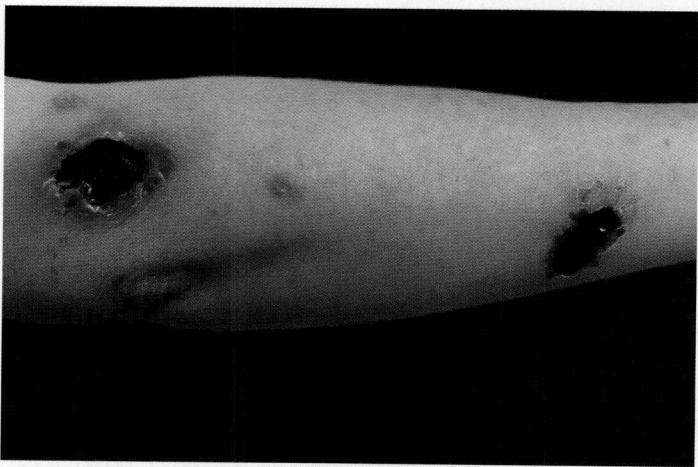

Figure 31-45 Hydroa vacciniforme–like lymphoproliferative disorder. This severe case exhibits indurated, necrotic ulcerating lesions on the back of the arm. (Courtesy of Dr. John O'Malley, Dana-Farber Cancer Institute, Boston, MA.)

lymphadenopathy, sometimes long after the initial cutaneous lesions appear (200). The lesions may eventually disseminate and manifest as a systemic lymphoma; however, no known clinical, morphologic, immunophenotypic, or molecular characteristics predict progression (201). A recent study of HV-LPD among Caucasian populations showed very rare incidence, with an earlier-onset disease but very indolent clinical course (202). An overlapping cutaneous manifestation of chronic active EBV infection is "severe mosquito bite allergy," wherein patients show hypersensitivity to insect bites, particularly mosquitoes, with intense local skin symptoms, followed by ulceration or scarring, and can exhibit some of the systemic symptoms of HV-LPD (203,204).

Histopathology. The lesions are characterized by variably dense infiltrates of atypical αβ or γδ T or, less commonly, NK cells. The lesional cells involve the dermis and may extend into the subcutis; overlying ulceration, necrosis, angiocentricity, and involvement of adnexal structures are common (Fig. 31-46A, B). The neoplastic cells are often small to medium-sized with only mild atypia, but severe cases include highly atypical, larger cells (Fig. 31-46C, D). The cells are positive for CD2, CD3, and CD8+/− with expression of cytotoxic molecules. CD30 is often positive, and CD56 expression is detected in cases characterized by an NK-cell infiltrate. *In situ* hybridization for EBER is positive (Fig. 31-46E, F).

Histogenesis. EBV likely plays a role in pathogenesis (205). Most cases have clonal TCR gene rearrangements, which is not necessarily related to severity of the disease (206,207), although those characterized by an NK-cell infiltrate will not show clonal TCR gene rearrangements.

Differential Diagnosis. Systemic EBV+ T-cell lymphoma of childhood is a fulminant disease with widespread involvement of visceral organs, lymph node, bone marrow, and skin. The histologic features can overlap with ENKTCL, and comprehensive immunophenotyping, with careful integration of clinical features and presentation, can help aid in the distinction.

Principles of Management: Reported outcomes are variable in this rare disorder, and treatment guidelines are not well established.

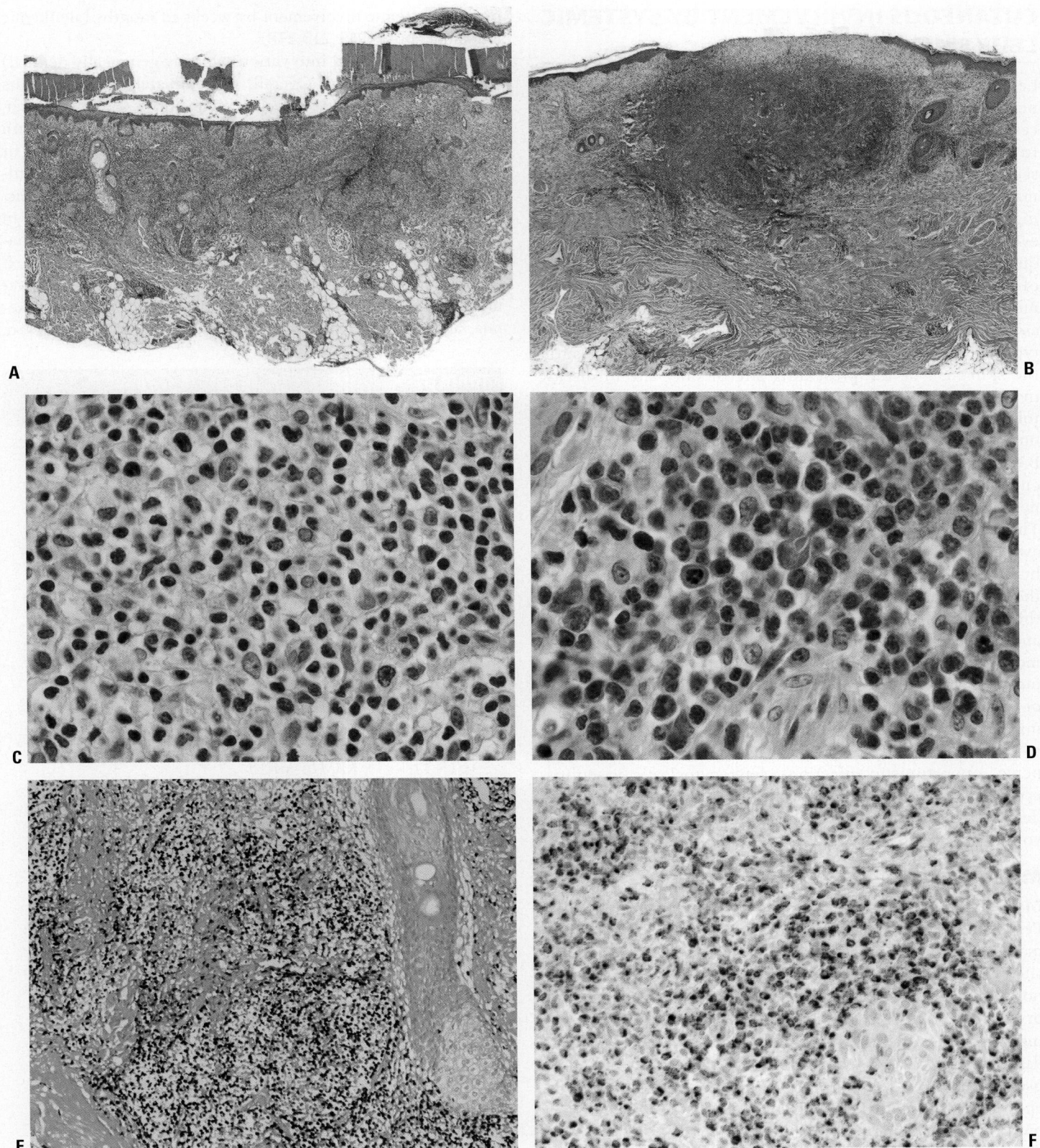

Figure 31-46 Hydroa vacciniforme–like lymphoproliferative disorder. **A:** Histologic sections of a blister-like papular lesion on the face, with a hemorrhagic crust, show a dermal infiltrate with periadnexal and perineural accentuation, extending to the subcutis. **B:** A more severe case exhibits ulceration and angiocentricity. The blister-like lesion exhibited small- to medium-sized lymphocytes with minimal atypia (**C**), whereas the more severe case showed larger, highly atypical and mitotically active neoplastic lymphocytes (**D**); this patient developed systemic lymphoma. **E:** The neoplastic cells are positive for EBER *in situ* hybridization. **F:** Granzyme B highlights the cytotoxic phenotype.

CUTANEOUS INVOLVEMENT BY SYSTEMIC LEUKEMIAS/LYMPHOMAS

Leukemia cutis is a nonspecific term used to indicate cutaneous involvement by a myeloid or lymphoid leukemic process, most commonly acute myeloid leukemia (AML) (208). In general, cutaneous lesions occur concomitantly with or secondary to bone marrow and/or peripheral blood involvement, although, occasionally, skin lesions can be the presenting sign of disease (aleukemic leukemia cutis). In these cases, evidence of systemic involvement typically emerges in subsequent weeks or months (209,210). In addition to the category of leukemia cutis, many lymphomatous processes that commonly arise in lymph nodes or other extranodal sites, such as FL or AITL, may involve the skin. Cutaneous disease is typically secondary to systemic involvement; less frequently, the skin may be the presenting site or only site of disease involvement. Within this category, there can be some histologic overlap between the primary cutaneous lymphomas outlined previously (specifically, the three primary cutaneous B-cell lymphomas as well as primary cALCL) and secondary cutaneous involvement by morphologically and immunophenotypically similar but clinically distinct systemic diseases. Therefore, it is critical for the practicing pathologist to be aware of the potential for secondary cutaneous involvement by systemic leukemic and lymphomatous processes, given the clinical implications. In this section, we review many of these entities with an emphasis on the clinical, morphologic, and immunophenotypic manifestations within the skin. A more detailed discussion of systemic leukemias and lymphomas is beyond the scope of this chapter. Of note, a number of nonneoplastic cutaneous conditions (leukemid reactions) may arise in patients with leukemia, such as pallor secondary to anemia, petechiae or purpura secondary to thrombocytopenia, opportunistic infections, leukocytoclastic vasculitis, erythema nodosum, erythema multiforme, and neutrophilic dermatoses. These entities are covered elsewhere in this volume.

Myeloid Lineage

Myeloid Sarcoma

Per the 2016 WHO classification, *myeloid sarcoma* is a tumor mass consisting of myeloid blasts occurring at any anatomic site outside of the bone marrow (extramedullary); older terminology includes *extramedullary myeloid cell tumor*, *granulocytic* or *monocytic sarcoma*, or *chloroma*. The most common extramedullary site in adults is the skin (211). Although the WHO definition indicates that the term myeloid sarcoma should be used for (usually) solitary masses with effacement of tissue architecture in the skin, we and others utilize the term cutaneous myeloid sarcoma (CMS) to represent (typically) clinically detectable cutaneous infiltrates of myeloid leukemic cells regardless of underlying architecture or anatomic pattern of involvement (212–214). CMS is most often associated with AML, although it may also represent acute leukemic progression from an underlying myelodysplastic syndrome or a myeloproliferative neoplasm (including blast crisis of chronic myeloid leukemia), or involvement by a myeloproliferative/myelodysplastic neoplasm (215–217). Although this most often occurs concomitant with or secondary to bone marrow involvement, or at relapse, in fewer than 10% of cases skin involvement may

precede systemic involvement by weeks to months (aleukemic leukemia cutis) (211,213,218).

AML is classified into various (mostly genetically defined) subtypes (Table 31-5). Overall, approximately 3% of patients with AML will develop cutaneous involvement (219). However, the incidence is higher (up to 30%) for patients with AML with monocytic differentiation (acute myelomonocytic leukemia or acute monoblastic/monocytic leukemia) (219,220), and, accordingly, acute myelomonocytic leukemia or acute monoblastic/monocytic leukemia are the most common AML subtypes in patients with CMS (214). AML with granulocytic differentiation (typically AML with or without maturation) is the next most frequent subtype seen in the skin. Cutaneous involvement by acute promyelocytic leukemia, acute erythroid leukemia, and acute megakaryoblastic leukemia is exceedingly rare

Table 31-5
WHO Classification of Acute Myeloid Leukemias
Acute myeloid leukemia with recurrent genetic abnormalities
Acute myeloid leukemia with t(8;21)(q22;q22.1); *RUNX1-RUNX1T1*
Acute myeloid leukemia with inv(16)(p13.1q22) or t(16;16) (p13.1;q22); *CBFB-MYH11*
Acute promyelocytic leukemia with *PML-RARA*
Acute myeloid leukemia with t(9;11)(p21.3;q23.3); *KMT2A-MLLT3* and variants
Acute myeloid leukemia with t(6;9)(p23;q34.1); *DEK-NUP214*
Acute myeloid leukemia with inv(3)(q21.3q26.2) or t(3;3) (q21.3;q26.2); *GATA2, MECOM*
Acute myeloid leukemia (megakaryoblastic) with t(1;22) (p13.3;q13.1); *RBM15-MKL1*
Acute myeloid leukemia with *BCR-ABL1* (provisional)
Acute myeloid leukemia with mutated *NPM1*
Acute myeloid leukemia with biallelic mutation of *CEBPA*
Acute myeloid leukemia with mutated *RUNX1* (provisional)
Acute myeloid leukemia with myelodysplasia-related changes
Therapy-related myeloid neoplasms
Acute myeloid leukemia, not otherwise specified
Acute myeloid leukemia with minimal differentiation
Acute myeloid leukemia without maturation
Acute myeloid leukemia with maturation
Acute myelomonocytic leukemia
Acute monoblastic and monocytic leukemia
Pure erythroid leukemia
Acute megakaryoblastic leukemia
Acute basophilic leukemia
Acute panmyelosis with myelofibrosis
Myeloid sarcoma
Myeloid proliferations related to Down syndrome

Data from Swerdlow SH, Campo E, Harris NL, et al. *WHO Classification of Tumours of Haematopoietic and Lymphoid Tissues, Revised 4th Edition.* IARC; 2017.

(221–223). Few cases of therapy-related myeloid neoplasms presenting in the skin have been reported (224).

Clinical Features. Cutaneous infiltrates may present as reddish-brown to purpuric patches, plaques, papules, or nodules (Fig. 31-47), infrequently with ulceration (225). Lesions may be solitary or, more commonly, multiple in a localized or generalized pattern (218). Any site may be involved (extremities, trunk, head, and neck), and some have observed that leukemic cells have a predilection for areas of prior or concurrent inflammation (226). Aleukemic leukemia cutis often presents as a generalized eruption (213). Cutaneous involvement can occur in a large subset (30%–92%) of infants with congenital AML and is associated with very high mortality; it characteristically manifests as disseminated gray-blue skin nodules (227,228).

Histopathology. Leukemic skin infiltration occurs in the dermis and often extends into the underlying subcutaneous tissue. The epidermis is spared and is typically separated from the region of dermal involvement by a Grenz zone. Architecturally, the infiltrate can be sparse to dense in an interstitial, perivascular/periadnexal, nodular, and/or diffuse pattern (Fig. 31-48A) (218). The cells may line up in a "single-file" fashion between bundles of collagen in the reticular dermis or may form concentric layers around vascular and adnexal structures (Fig. 31-48B, C). The neoplastic infiltrate is cytologically homogeneous and may demonstrate frequent mitotic figures, apoptotic bodies, and an admixed inflammatory infiltrate. The cytologic and immunophenotypic features may vary depending on the subtype of AML. In general, the cells are medium to large, with dispersed chromatin and small, variably distinct nucleoli (Fig. 31-48D). In AML with monocytic differentiation (acute myelomonocytic

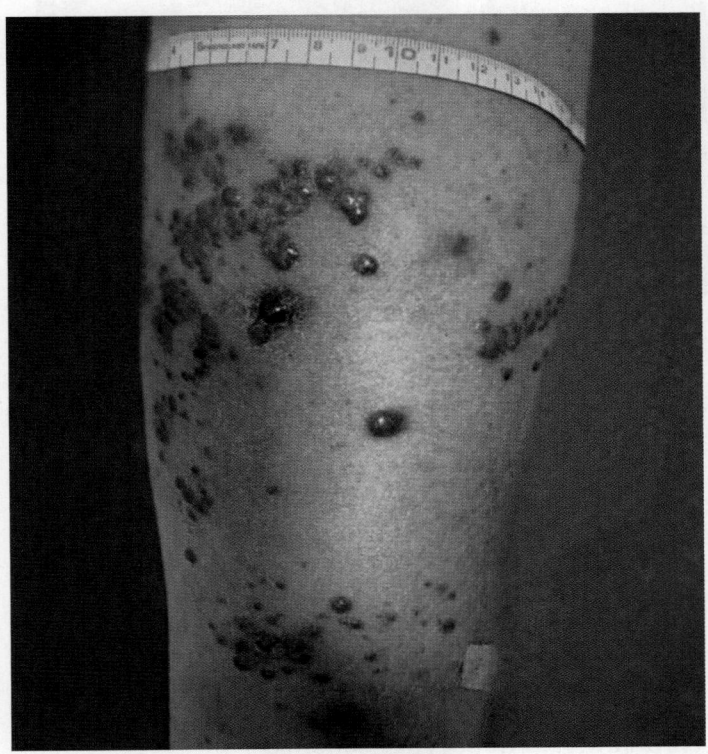

Figure 31-47 Cutaneous myeloid sarcoma in a patient with acute myeloid leukemia with monocytic differentiation. Multiple firm, erythematous papules and subcutaneous nodules are observed. (Courtesy of Mary E Gerard, PA-C, Dana-Farber Cancer Institute, Boston, MA.)

leukemia or acute monoblastic/monocytic leukemia), the cells are typically large in size, with folded to convoluted nuclear contours and moderate amounts of cytoplasm. AML with or without maturation generally demonstrates round to slightly irregular nuclear contours and medium-to-large cell size. Often, immunohistochemical studies are needed for diagnosis given the morphologic overlap with nonmyeloid leukemia cutis or nonneoplastic infiltrates. However, no single marker is consistently sensitive and specific, and a panel of markers along with incorporation of clinical and morphologic findings is required for diagnosis. Interestingly, cutaneous infiltrates are often negative for markers of immaturity CD34 and CD117 regardless of the underlying leukemic subtype or immunophenotype (214,218). Furthermore, CD117 will also highlight mast cells (strong staining), plasma cells, and a subset of T-LBL, which may confound interpretation (208). CD68 (KP-1 clone) is considered a highly sensitive marker (expressed in >95% of cases) and will mark cells with granulocytic or monocytic differentiation, although benign histiomonocytic cells also express CD68. Lysozyme behaves similarly. CD43 is highly sensitive but is also nonspecific, because it is also expressed in T cells and granulocytes. Myeloperoxidase and CD33 expression are detected in both granulocytic and monocytic infiltrates. CD14 is considered to be a relatively sensitive and specific indicator of monocytic differentiation (212). Approximately 20% of cases will express CD56, particularly in leukemia with monocytic differentiation (Fig. 31-49A–D). The Ki67 proliferation index is variable, most frequently less than 30% (218).

Histogenesis. It is postulated that cutaneous involvement arises owing to skin-homing properties of a subset of myeloid blasts, although the underlying molecular mechanisms are unknown (208). In cases of aleukemic leukemia cutis, it is uncertain whether the blasts originate in the skin or represent skin-homing cells from an otherwise undetectable systemic leukemic clone. Cytogenetic analysis of AML patients with cutaneous involvement has demonstrated an increased incidence of abnormalities on chromosome 8 compared to AML patients without leukemic involvement (214,219,229). Abnormalities involving the 11q23 locus have also been described in multiple series (212–214).

Differential Diagnosis. The differential diagnosis for CMS is broad. Cases with sparse involvement and monocytic differentiation can be difficult to distinguish from benign histiocytic infiltrates given the overlapping immunophenotype and frequent absence of markers of immaturity (CD34, CD117). In more robust infiltrates, morphologic diagnostic considerations include cutaneous involvement by other immature hematopoietic neoplasms (B- or T-cell lymphoblastic lymphoma or blastic plasmacytoid dendritic cell neoplasm [BPDCN]) as well as other hematopoietic and nonhematopoietic neoplasms (such as B- and T-cell non-Hodgkin lymphomas, poorly differentiated carcinoma or Merkel cell carcinoma, mastocytosis, melanoma, Ewing sarcoma, and Langerhans cell histiocytosis). Although a panel of immunohistochemical markers will differentiate most of these entities, distinction between CMS and BPDCN can be particularly challenging (see also section Blastic Plasmacytoid Dendritic Cell Neoplasm), particularly in cases of aleukemic leukemia cutis. Both entities express CD43. BPDCN typically expresses CD4 and CD56, but this can also be seen (albeit less frequently) in CMS with monocytic differentiation; alternatively, CMS frequently expresses CD68 and CD33, but this can

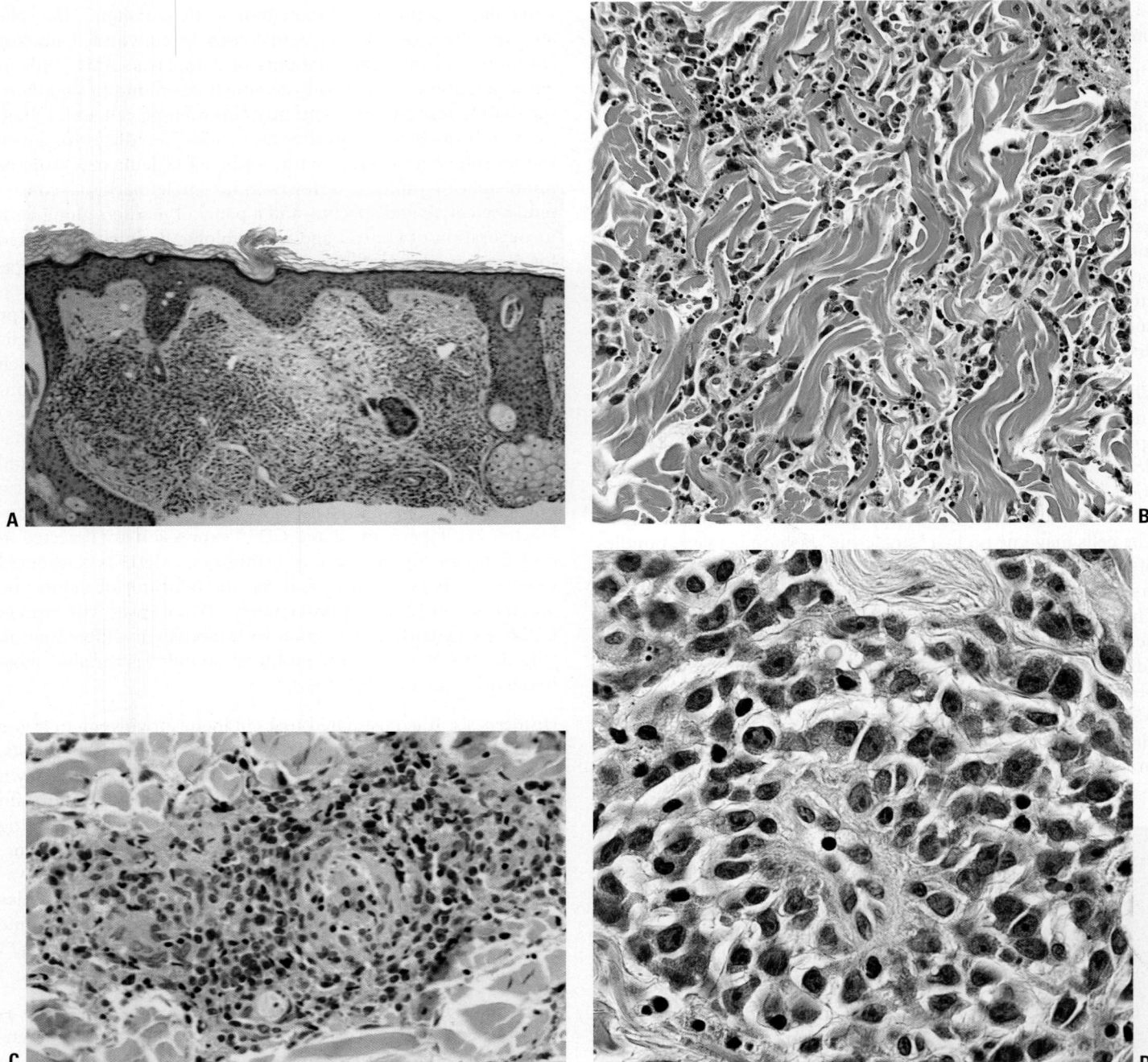

Figure 31-48 Cutaneous myeloid sarcoma. **A:** Mixed angiocentric and interstitial infiltration within dermis. **B:** Interstitial infiltrate of leukemic cells between dermal collagen bundles including "single-file" pattern. **C:** Perivascular infiltrate of cytologically monotonous and homogeneous myeloblasts. **D:** Higher magnification revealing the immature chromatin and distinct nucleoli of blast forms.

also be seen (albeit less frequently) in BPDCN. In general, BP-DCN will express CD4, CD56, CD123 (strong), and TCL-1 and lack myeloperoxidase, lysozyme, CD117, and CD34. Although CMS with monocytic differentiation may also lack myeloperoxidase, CD117, and CD34 expression, the presence of lysozyme reactivity and absence of strong CD123 and TCL-1 expression should support a diagnosis of CMS in most cases. An extensive panel of markers is often needed for confident diagnosis.

Principles of Management: In general, CMS is considered a marker of aggressive disease with a poor prognosis (214,215,225). Although a comparative study suggested that the outcome of patients with AML is not influenced by the presence or absence

of cutaneous involvement (219), a more recent large, matched-cohort study showed significantly decreased survival associated with CMS in AML patients (230). Patients with systemic leukemia and skin involvement are managed according to the underlying systemic leukemia. Aleukemic leukemia cutis is not well studied but is typically treated similarly to any myeloid sarcoma (231); in almost all cases, these patients will develop systemic involvement within weeks to months.

Chronic Myelomonocytic Leukemia
Chronic myelomonocytic leukemia (CMML) is a myelodysplastic/myeloproliferative (MDS/MPN) neoplasm defined by persistent peripheral blood monocytosis of greater than 1×10^9 cells/L,

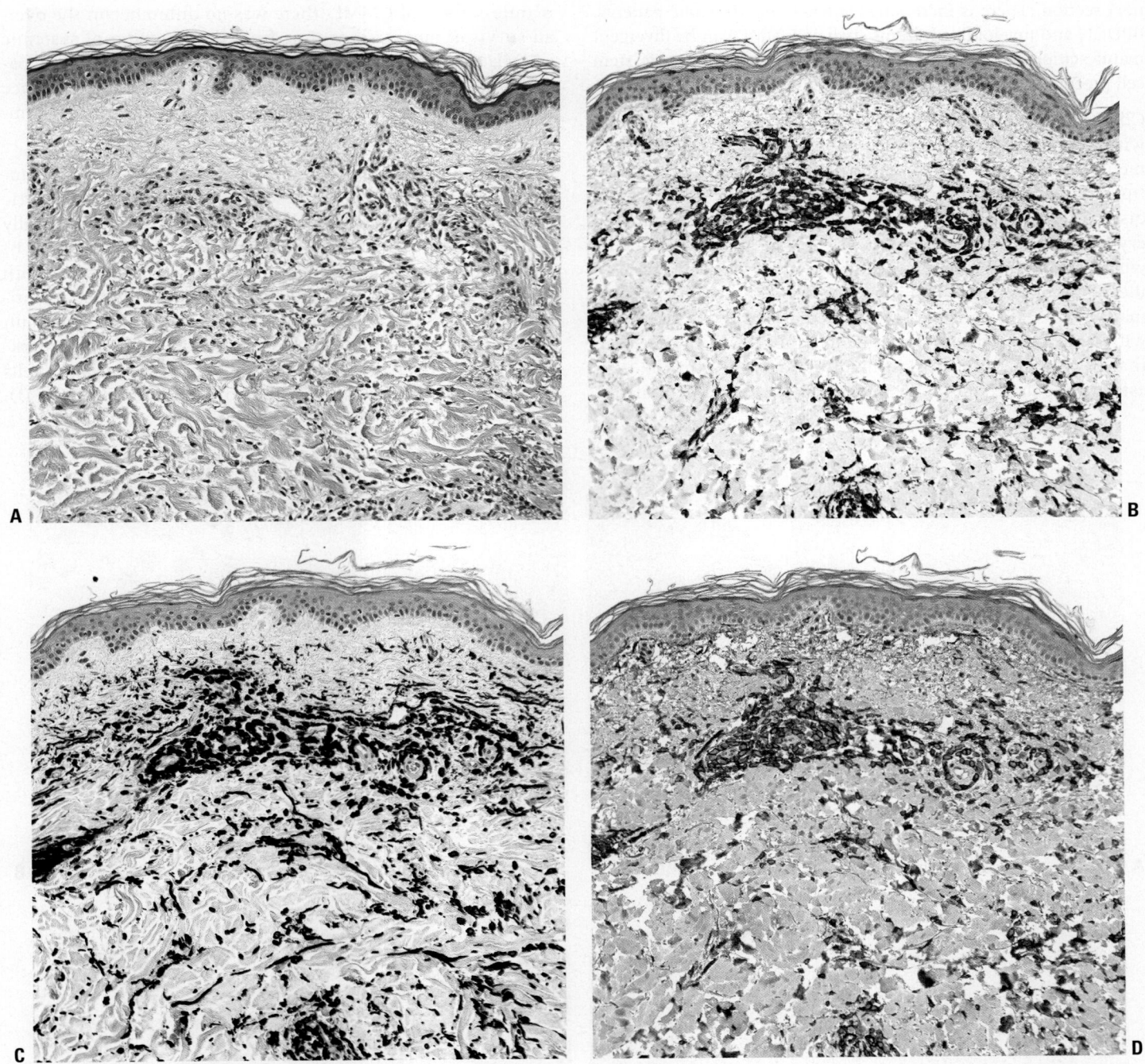

Figure 31-49 Cutaneous myeloid sarcoma. A: Superficial infiltrate of mononuclear cells appears deceptively bland. Immunohistochemical studies reveal that the infiltrate is composed of myeloid blasts, which express CD33 (**B**), lysozyme (**C**), and CD56 (**D**).

fewer than 20% blasts in peripheral blood or bone marrow, and morphologic evidence of myeloid dysplasia. Although CMML has both MDS and MPN features, and is classified by the WHO as an overlap entity, its presentation is often regarded as either a proliferative or dysplastic subtype, discriminated based on a WBC threshold of 13×10^9 cells/L (232,233). Diagnosis can be challenging and requires incorporation of clinical, morphologic, immunophenotypic, cytogenetic, and molecular findings as well as exclusion of other causes of peripheral monocytosis. Skin lesions arising concurrently with or subsequent to a diagnosis of CMML occur in less than 10% of patients with CMML and are often associated with or predictive of disease progression to AML (234). Although

distinct clinicopathologic groups have been previously proposed for categorizing skin lesions in CMML (235), there seems to be a spectrum of histopathologic features, with most cases exhibiting either infiltrates of myelomonocytic precursors and blasts or collections of mature plasmacytoid dendritic cells (PDCs), analogous to the development of mature PDC collections in association with nodal or marrow CMML, which is well described (236,237). More unusual manifestations can include tumors of indeterminate dendritic cell lineage (235,238), histiocytic proliferations (239), as well as a small subset of patients who develop skin lesions with clinical and pathologic features best classified as overt BPDCN, a distinct and aggressive hematologic malignancy discussed in the next section. There is increasing evidence that, in some patients, BPDCN and myeloid neoplasms such as CMML can be divergent manifestations of a common multipotential hematopoietic stem cell precursor (240,241).

Clinical Summary. Patients are typically older adults/elderly with a strong male predominance. Frank cutaneous involvement by myelomonocytic cells typically manifests as multiple erythematous papules or nodules in a wide anatomic distribution. Collections of mature PDCs form disseminated erythematous macules and papules that may be pruritic, whereas BPDCN presents as bruise-colored plaques and nodules. The development of skin lesions may herald transformation to AML, and the overall median survival of patients with CMML who develop cutaneous infiltrates is shorter than that of patients without skin involvement (234). In the largest series to date, among the patients with different cutaneous

manifestations of CMML, there was no difference in the overall survival, measured as time from development of systemic CMML to death/last follow-up, although progression of patients measured from the time of first skin lesion occurrence was slower in those with collections of mature PDCs compared to the other groups (235).

Histopathology. Skin lesions in CMML exhibit a broad histopathologic spectrum, as discussed previously. Myelomonocytic infiltrates contain mononuclear cells with characteristically folded or lobated nuclei and pale cytoplasm (Fig. 31-50A, B) and include variable numbers of immature blast forms with medium-to-large cell size and fine chromatin. Precise quantitation of blasts in these infiltrates can be exceptionally difficult (as they also often do not express immunohistochemical markers of immaturity); however, sheets of immature-appearing cells should be designated progression to CMS (Fig. 31-50C, D).

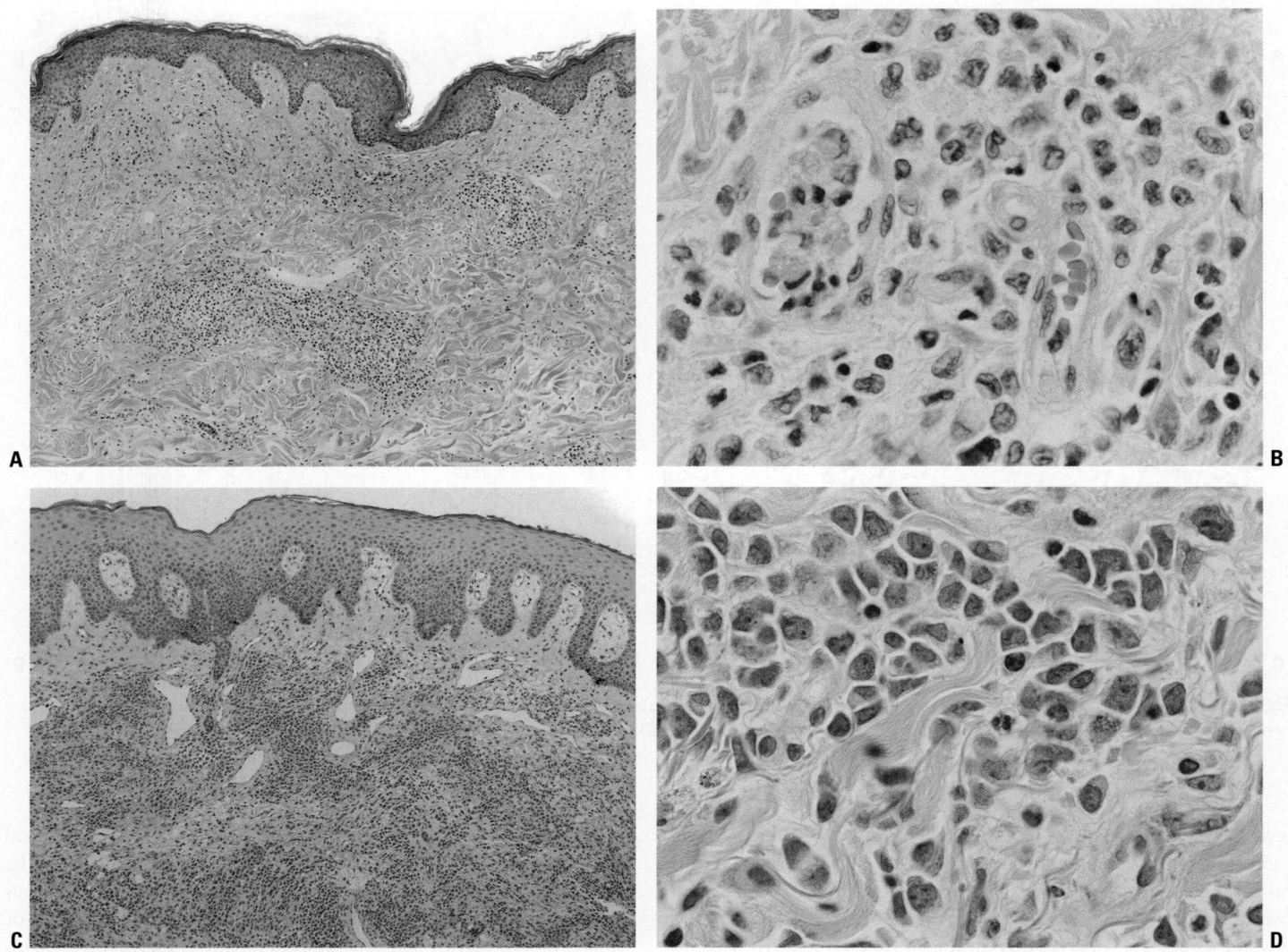

Figure 31-50 Chronic myelomonocytic leukemia (CMML) and progression to acute myeloid leukemia (AML). This patient with CMML had cutaneous involvement manifesting as superficial dermal, perivascular (**A**) infiltrates of myelomonocytic cells, many of which have characteristically folded or lobated nuclei with abundant pale cytoplasm (**B**) and show variably condensed chromatin. A different patient with CMML had skin lesions that showed an infiltrative, diffuse process (**C**) containing almost entirely immature-appearing cells with large, irregular nuclei, finely dispersed chromatin, and distinct nucleoli (**D**), which would histologically be in keeping with cutaneous myeloid sarcoma. Concurrent bone marrow examination showed AML.

Some lesions contain mature PDCs, which have a bland, mono-cyte-like appearance forming multiple dermal nodules with admixed inflammatory cells; the plasmacytoid features are difficult to discern on fixed tissue sections (Fig. 31-51A, B). Mature PDCs express CD4, CD123, TCL-1, BDCA-2/CD303, and granzyme B but not CD56, myeloperoxidase, or lysozyme and have a low Ki67 proliferation index (Fig. 31-51C–G). The morphologic and other features of BPDCN are described in the next section. Highly unusual skin manifestations of CMML include

dendritic cell or histiocytic proliferations that may be immuno-phenotypically distinct from the CMML but that share common clonal origins (242,243).

Histogenesis. The genetic basis for the development of these heterogeneous lesions within the skin of patients with CMML is uncertain. Postulated theories include a common progenitor cell or PDC differentiation of myelomonocytic cells (235).

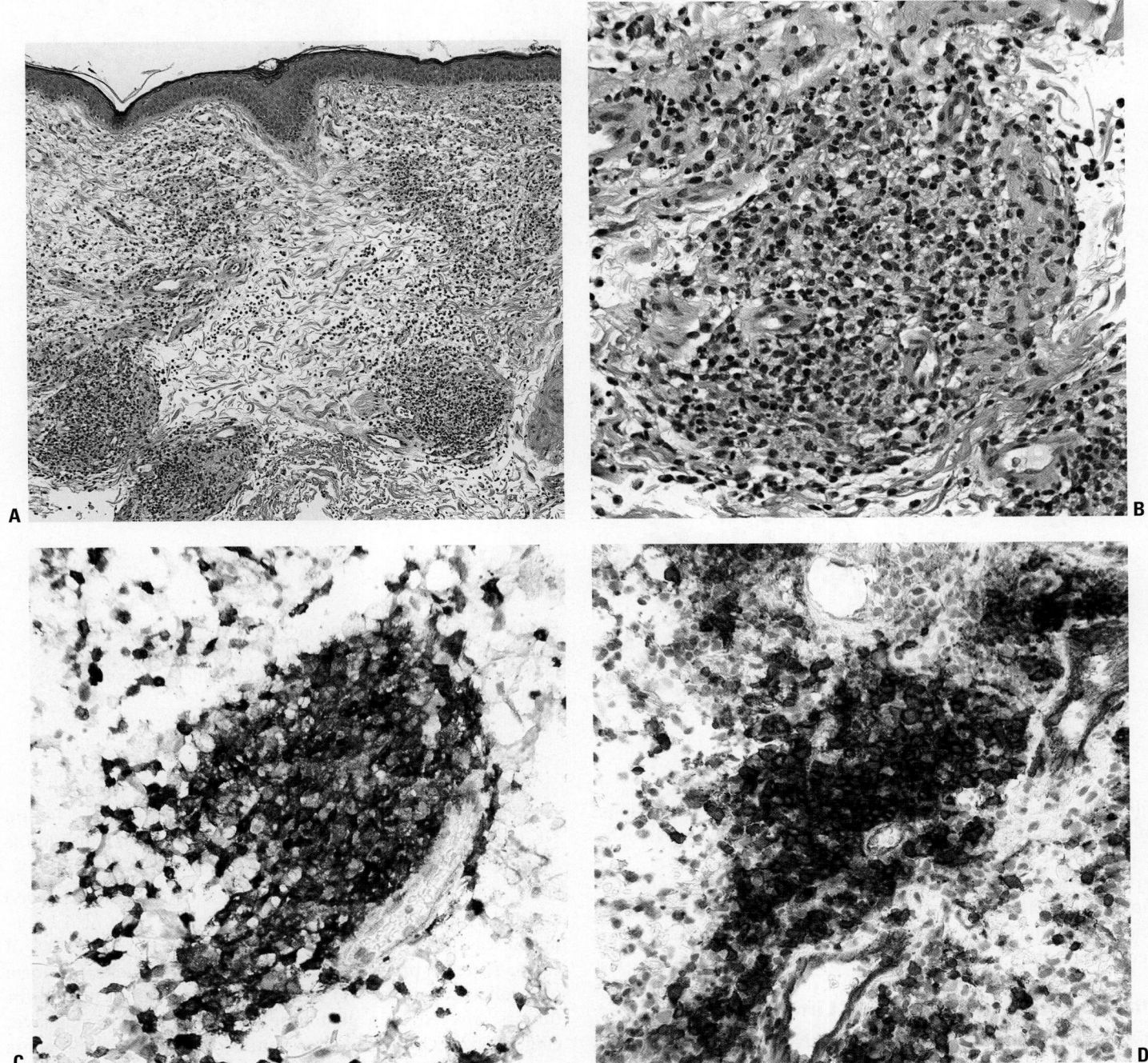

Figure 31-51 Collections of mature plasmacytoid dendritic cells (PDCs) in a patient with chronic myelomonocytic leukemia. **A:** The PDCs form multifocal nodules in the dermis. **B:** Higher magnification reveals bland cells with mature chromatin and moderate amounts of eosinophilic cyto-plasm. Immunohistochemical studies reveal that the PDCs express CD4 **(C)** and CD123 **(D)**

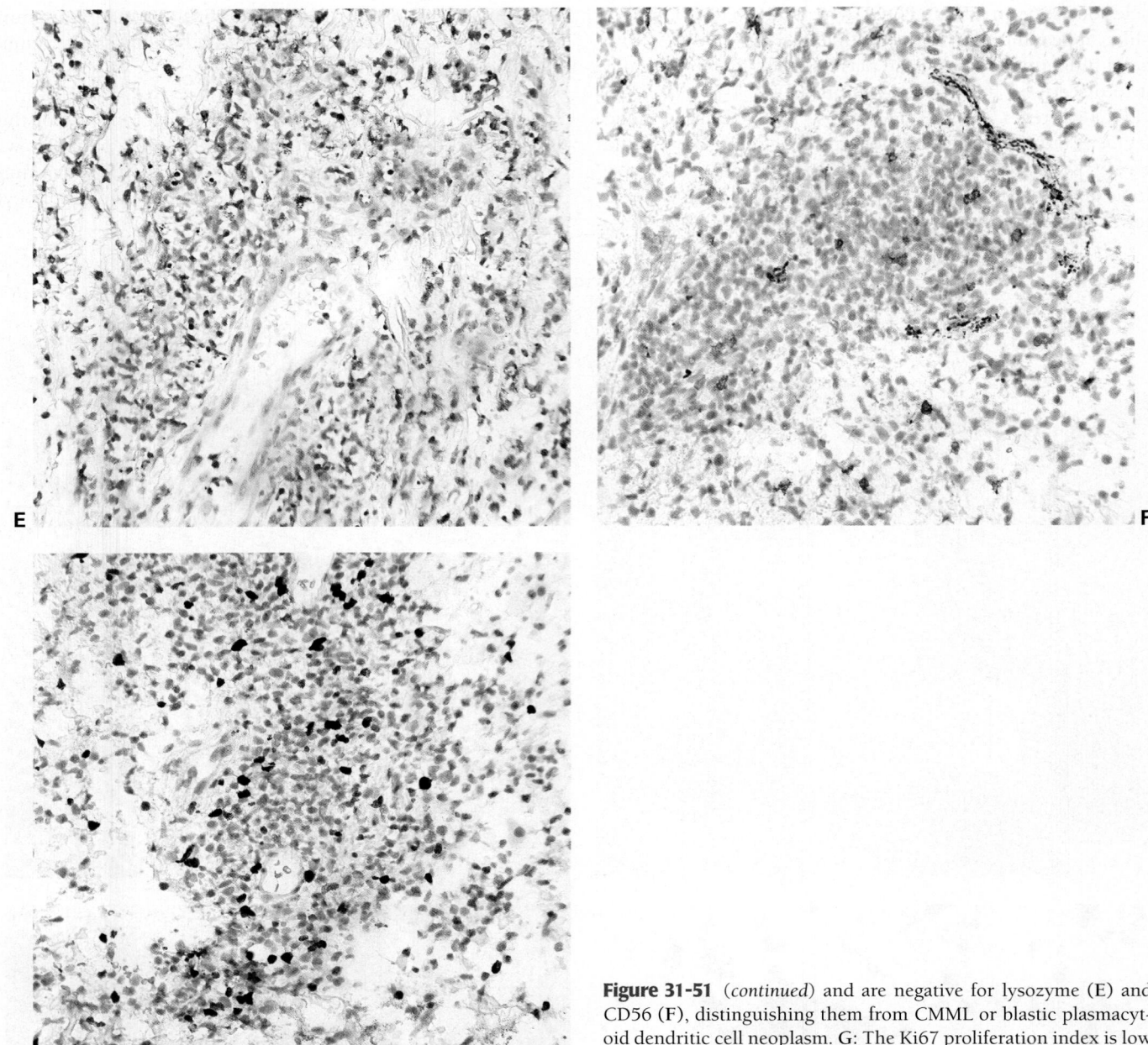

Figure 31-51 (*continued*) and are negative for lysozyme (**E**) and CD56 (**F**), distinguishing them from CMML or blastic plasmacytoid dendritic cell neoplasm. **G:** The Ki67 proliferation index is low (5%) in these collections.

Differential Diagnosis. Diagnostic considerations of skin lesions in patients with CMML include the entities outlined previously.

Principles of Management: Patients with cutaneous lesions in CMML are managed based on their systemic disease, and cutaneous progression to AML would also be treated accordingly.

Plasmacytoid Dendritic Cell Lineage

Blastic Plasmacytoid Dendritic Cell Neoplasm

BPDCN (previously known as *blastic NK-cell lymphoma* or *CD4+/CD56+ hematodermic neoplasm*, among other terms) is a rare, aggressive neoplasm that is derived from the precursor of PDCs (also called plasmacytoid monocytes) (244). Skin is typically involved at presentation, and systemic involvement occurs concurrently or subsequently. The neoplastic cells

characteristically coexpress CD4 and CD56 without B-, T-, and NK-cell or myeloid lineage-specific markers. The condition is rare, representing less than 1% of acute leukemia (244).

Clinical Summary. This neoplasm tends to affect middle-aged and elderly individuals, with a male:female ratio of 3:1. Pediatric cases have also been reported. In more than 80% of cases, patients present with skin lesions that take the form of localized or multifocal plum- or bruise-colored plaques or tumors covered by a glistening, attenuated epidermal layer (Fig. 31-52). Over weeks to months, systemic spread occurs involving bone marrow and/or peripheral blood, lymph node, spleen or liver, or other extramedullary locations (245,246). Cytopenias may develop, reflecting marrow involvement. Oral mucosal lesions are common. Although patients may respond to initial therapy, relapse is common, particularly in the adult population.

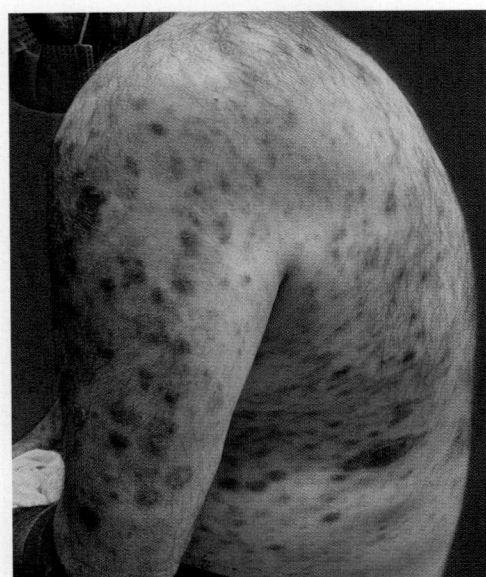

Figure 31-52 Blastic plasmacytoid dendritic cell neoplasm. Widespread involvement with numerous skin lesions appearing as plum- or bruise-colored plaques or tumors. (Courtesy of Dr. Andrew A. Lane, Dana-Farber Cancer Institute, Boston, MA.)

Histopathology. The dermis is diffusely infiltrated by a monotonous population of intermediate-sized cells with irregular nuclear contours; dispersed chromatin; and small, distinct nucleoli (Fig. 31-53A, B). There is sparing of the epidermis and extension into the subcutis. Zonal necrosis or angiocentric infiltration is uncommon. Extravasation of erythrocytes is frequently seen, corresponding to the bruiselike lesions clinically. The neoplastic cells lack B- and T-cell and myeloid lineage-specific antigens. The cells typically express CD4, CD56, CD123, TCL-1, and BDCA-2/CD303 as well as the nonspecific marker CD43; show variable expression of terminal deoxynucleotidyl transferase (TdT), CD7, CD22, CD33, and CD68; and are negative

for CD3, CD20, CD79a, CD34, CD117, myeloperoxidase, and lysozyme (Fig. 31-54A–F) (245,247–250). More recently, nuclear expression of TCF-4 by immunohistochemistry has been shown in PDCs and when used in conjunction with CD123 can be highly specific for PDC lineage, although it cannot distinguish reactive PDCs from BPDCN (251). Given the morphologic and immunophenotypic overlap with a number of entities (see Differential Diagnosis), an extensive panel of immunophenotyping is required for this diagnosis.

Histogenesis. BPDCN arises from a precursor of the PDC, a rare cell type in the peripheral blood that appears to be the primary source of interferon-α, and originates from a hematopoietic stem cell (252). Clonal rearrangement of the immunoglobulin or TCR genes is typically not detected, and EBER *in situ* hybridization is negative. Molecular and cytogenetic studies provide evidence for the unique classification of this entity. Although gene expression profiling and array-based comparative genomic hybridization studies demonstrate that BPDCN is genetically distinct from CMS (253), the expanding mutational spectrum in BPDCN shows common involvement of genes and pathways known to be important in myeloid lineage malignancies. The most recurrently mutated genes are *TET2* and *ASXL1*, with half of patients revealing recurrent mutations in epigenetic pathway genes, as well as transcriptional regulators and splicing factors (241,254). BPDCN may arise in patients with an underlying myelodysplastic syndrome, CMML, or as a therapy-related neoplasm (235,240,245,255). Alternatively, patients with BPDCN may develop acute myeloid or myelomonocytic leukemia, which may or may not arise from an underlying myelodysplastic syndrome (256,257). These findings further support the pathogenesis model of divergent clonal populations arising from a common hematopoietic cell of origin with multilineage potential (252,258).

Differential Diagnosis. Morphologically, the infiltrate seen in BPDCN is indistinguishable from myeloid or lymphoblastic

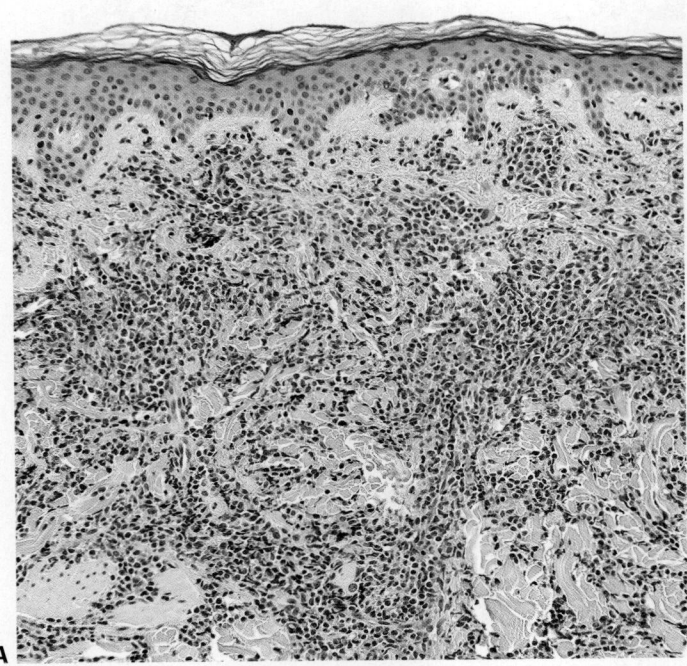

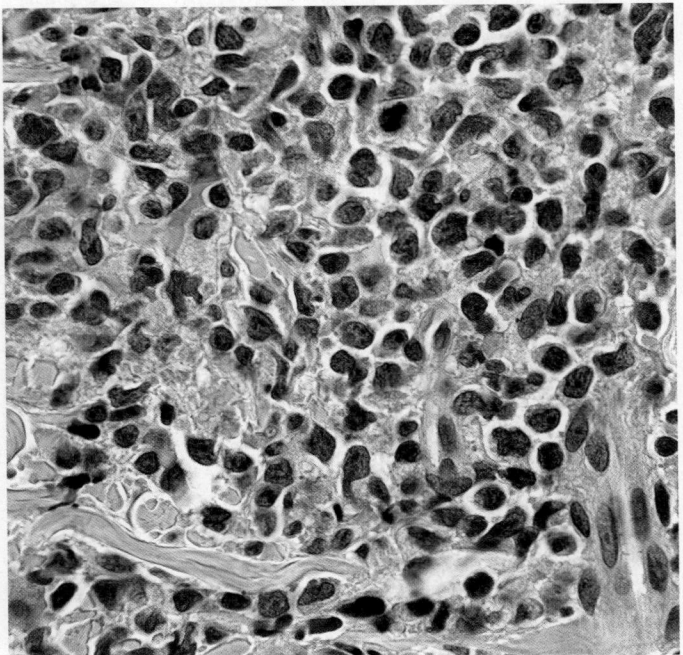

Figure 31-53 Blastic plasmacytoid dendritic cell neoplasm. **A:** The neoplastic cells form a diffuse interstitial infiltrate. **B:** Higher magnification reveals cells that are intermediate in size with irregular nuclear contours, slightly dispersed chromatin, and small distinct nucleoli.

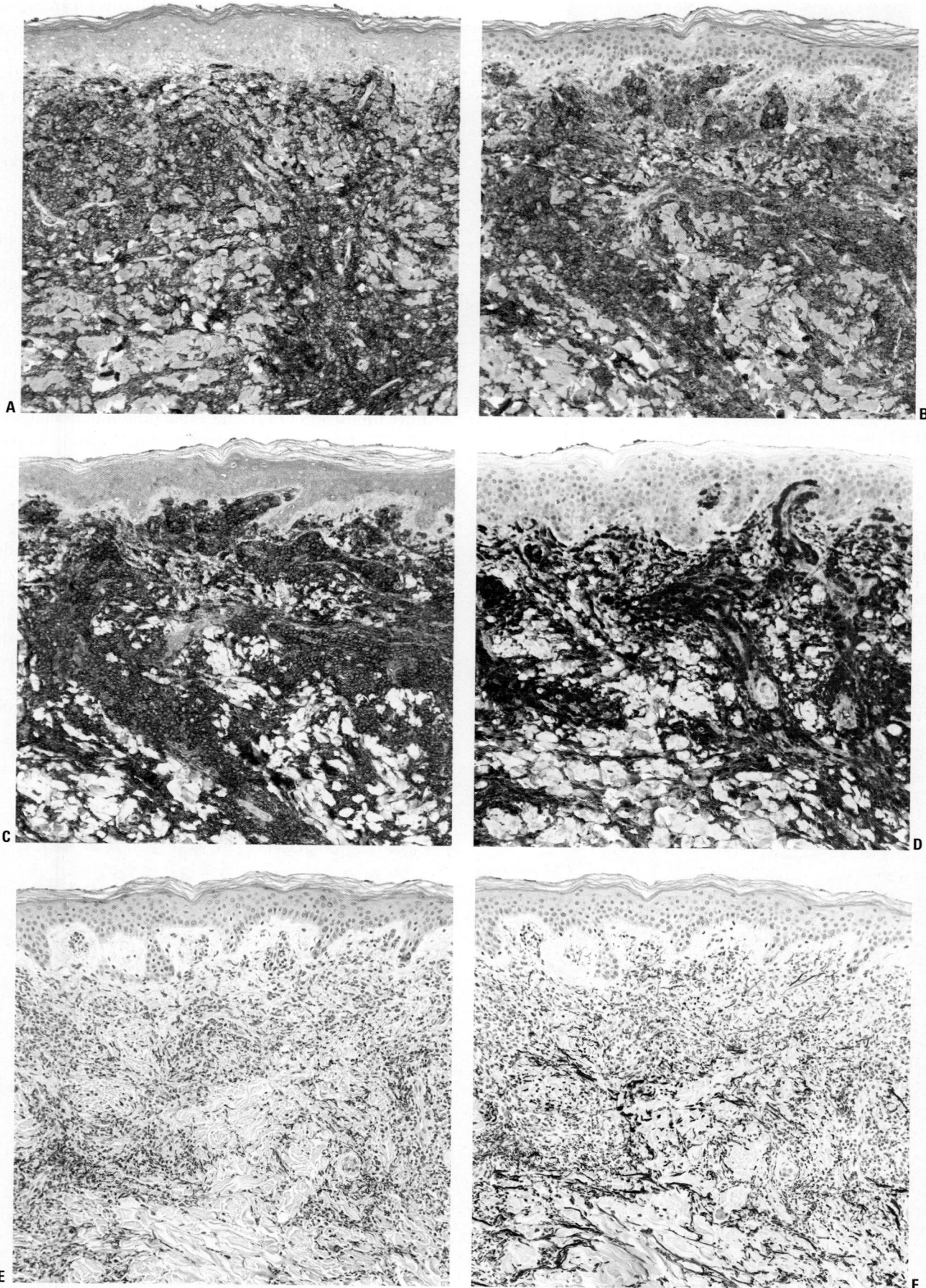

Figure 31-54 Blastic plasmacytoid dendritic cell neoplasm. Extensive immunophenotyping is often required for diagnosis, revealing the tumor cells to be CD4⁺ (A), CD56⁺ (B), CD123⁺ (C), TCL-1⁺ (D), myeloperoxidase⁻ (E), and lysozyme⁻ (F). Nonspecific staining with lysozyme is detected in stromal elements.

leukemia cutis. Although BPDCN often shows at least focal expression of TdT, lack of reactivity for CD3 and CD19 will distinguish BPDCN from T and B-lymphoblastic leukemia, respectively. Immunophenotypic overlap can be seen with CMS, particularly in cases showing monocytic differentiation and CD4 and CD56 expression. Absence of lysozyme expression and presence of strong CD123, TCL-1, or TCF-4 can assist in the diagnosis of BPDCN. Expression of CD4 and CD56, as well as angiocentricity (albeit infrequently seen in BPDCN) may suggest cutaneous involvement by ENKTCL, but BPDCN is negative by EBER *in situ* hybridization. Additionally, collections of nonneoplastic PCDs may be seen in cutaneous or nodal lesions associated with inflammatory, autoimmune, or neoplastic conditions (252). In contrast to BPDCN, reactive PCDs do not express CD56 or TdT, do express granzyme B, and show a low Ki67 proliferation index (259,260).

Principles of Management: Prognosis is poor with conventional chemotherapy, and allogeneic stem cell transplant following high-dose chemotherapy may provide some outcome improvement (261). Given that development of systemic disease occurs in almost every case, patients should be treated aggressively even if skin is the only detectable site of disease at presentation (252). More recently, targeted therapies for BPDCN using a CD123-directed cytotoxin have shown promise (262).

B-Cell Lineage

B-lymphoblastic Leukemia/Lymphoma

Precursor lymphoid neoplasms are high-grade malignancies derived from B-lymphoblasts or T-lymphoblasts. These entities may be classified as acute lymphoblastic leukemia (ALL; disease involving bone marrow and/or peripheral blood) or lymphoblastic lymphoma (LBL; disease involving nodal or extranodal sites). Both leukemic and lymphomatous involvement may be seen in the same patient. Although most cases presenting as ALL are derived from B-lymphoblasts, most cases presenting as LBL are derived from T-lymphoblasts. T-LBL typically involves lymph nodes or the mediastinum, whereas B-LBL has a propensity for bone and cutaneous sites (263).

Clinical Summary. B-LBL usually affects children and young adults who are younger than 35 years, with a male:female ratio of 1:1 (263). Skin lesions, if they occur, typically appear secondarily to or concomitant with B-ALL or nodal B-LBL (264,265). There are rare cases of patients who present with cutaneous B-LBL without evidence of disease elsewhere on concurrent staging (aleukemic leukemia cutis or primary cutaneous B-LBL); these patients are more likely to be female, sometimes with solitary head and neck lesions, and seem to show an excellent response to therapy (266–268), although one reported patient with primary cutaneous B-LBL developed posttherapy relapse with bone marrow involvement (269). In patients with a prior diagnosis of B-ALL, cutaneous involvement may be the first sign of relapse following therapy. The lesions take the form of solitary, less commonly multiple, erythematous papules and nodules. Some report a predilection for head and neck sites (especially in patients with limited cutaneous involvement) (264), although this has not been observed in other studies (270).

Histopathology. Skin involvement may be nodular or diffuse within the dermis, consisting of dense, homogeneous infiltration by mitotically active lymphoblasts with round to irregular nuclei containing finely stippled chromatin and small nucleoli (Fig. 31-55A, B). Cytoplasm is sparse and may be difficult to detect in routinely prepared tissue. The epidermis is spared, often separated from the region of dermal involvement by a Grenz zone. The infiltrate may extend into the subcutis. Further classification, including distinction between T- and B-cell lymphoblastic differentiation, requires immunohistochemical analysis. The neoplastic cells of B-LBL are typically positive for B-lineage markers CD19, CD79a, CD22, and PAX5, are often positive for CD10, and show variable expression of CD20 (Fig. 31-55C). The most consistent marker of immaturity is TdT (Fig. 31-55D), whereas CD34 and CD99 expression is variable. CD45, a common general marker for hematopoietic cells, can be deceptively weak to negative in lymphoblastic leukemia/lymphomas.

Histogenesis. The current WHO classification scheme groups both leukemic and lymphomatous manifestations into one entity, namely B-lymphoblastic leukemia/lymphoma, and further categorizes cases into B-lymphoblastic leukemia/lymphoma with recurrent genetic abnormalities and B-lymphoblastic leukemia/lymphoma (NOS) (Table 31-6). Some small series have suggested that B-LBL at any site may show an increased frequency of the high-hyperdiploidy ($\geq$50 chromosomes) genetic profile, whereas others have demonstrated the presence of additional chromosome 21 material but not characteristic B-ALL translocations such as t(9;22), t(1;19), and t(4;11) in B-LBL (271,272). In cutaneous cases specifically, *KMT2A* (formerly known as *MLL*) rearrangements appear to be enriched, with multiple cases documented in both adult and pediatric patients (273–275), whereas hyperdiploidy has only rarely been described (276). All tumors will demonstrate clonal immunoglobulin gene rearrangements.

Differential Diagnosis. Lesions must be differentiated from morphologically similar infiltrates of immature malignant cells (T-lymphoblasts, myeloblasts, blastic PDCs) by immunophenotyping. Occasionally, mitotically active B-LBL lesions in children may resemble the starry-sky pattern of Burkitt lymphoma, although Burkitt lymphoma will be negative for TdT and positive for BCL6. Lesions in adults may mimic the blastoid variant of MCL, which unlike B-LBL is positive for CD5 and cyclin D1 and negative for TdT (Table 31-3). Some carcinomas form diffuse infiltrates and demonstrate stippled chromatin, such as Merkel cell carcinoma or metastatic small cell carcinoma. These may morphologically mimic B-LBL but express keratins as well as neuroendocrine markers. In children, a significant diagnostic consideration is Ewing sarcoma. Importantly, both LBL (T or B) and Ewing sarcoma may express CD99, and therefore extensive immunophenotyping is required to elucidate the diagnosis (Fig. 31-56A–C).

Principles of Management: Patients with B-LBL are typically treated in the same manner as patients with B-ALL, namely systemic polychemotherapy with or without stem cell transplant (270).

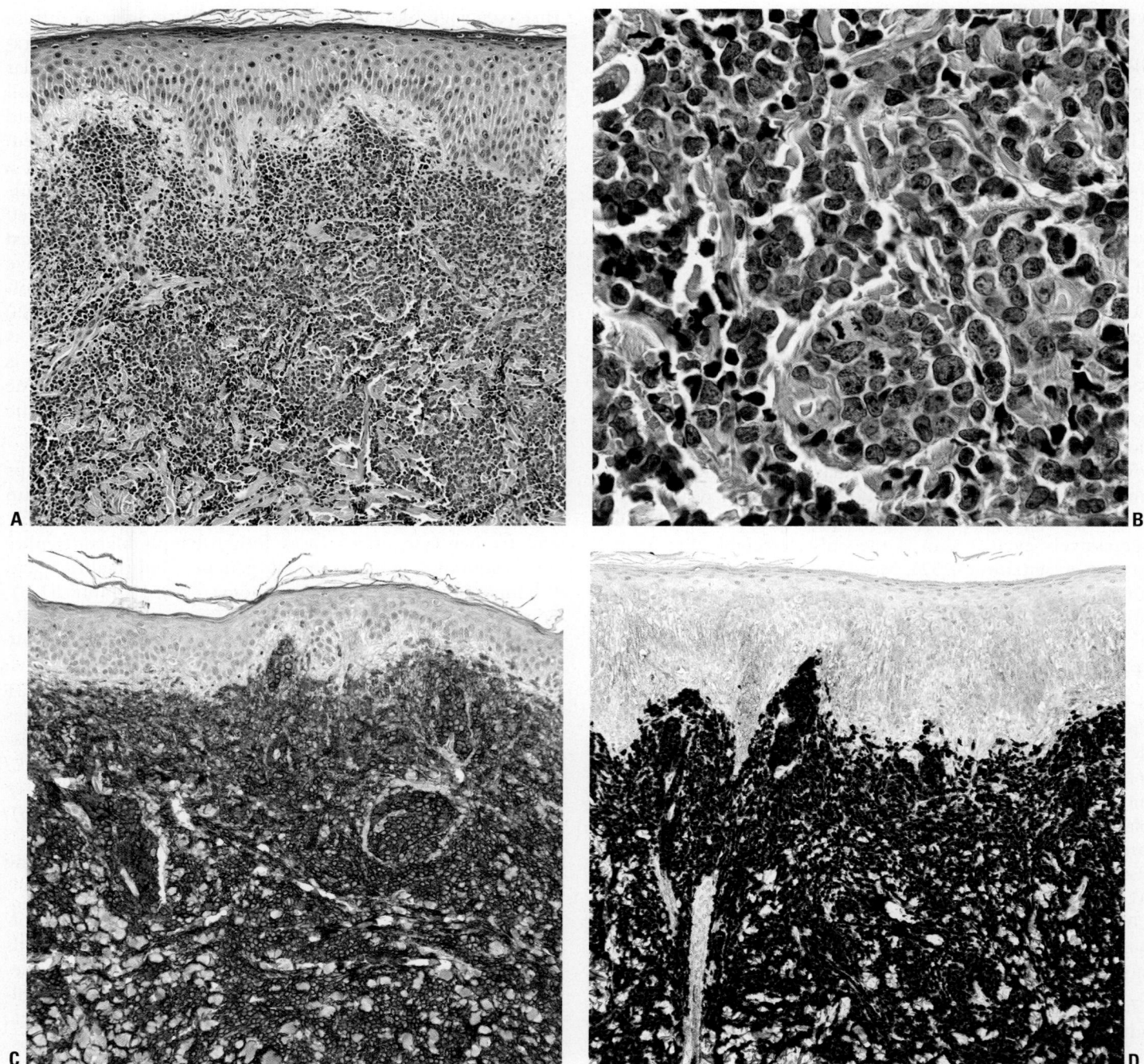

Figure 31-55 B-lymphoblastic lymphoma. **A:** Diffuse dermal infiltrate of lymphoblasts separated from the overlying epidermis by a Grenz zone. **B:** Higher magnification reveals a homogeneous infiltrate of lymphoblasts with round to irregular nuclei containing finely stippled chromatin and small nucleoli. Immunohistochemical studies reveal the lymphoblasts to be strongly positive for CD19 (**C**) and TdT (**D**).

Chronic Lymphocytic Leukemia/Small Lymphocytic Lymphoma

CLL/SLL is a B-cell lymphoma composed of small lymphocytes that may be present in the bone marrow and peripheral blood (CLL) and/or in tissues, particularly lymph nodes (SLL). CLL/SLL is the most common mature B-cell neoplasm to secondarily involve the skin, which occurs in 4% to 20% of patients with the disease and is considered a leukemia cutis (208). Patients with CLL/SLL may also demonstrate nonneoplastic cutaneous changes (leukemid reactions), including infection, vasculitis, purpura, generalized pruritus, exfoliative erythroderma, and paraneoplastic pemphigus (277), as well as an increased risk for non-CLL/SLL primary cutaneous lymphomas or nonhematologic cutaneous malignancies (278,279).

Clinical Summary. CLL/SLL generally affects older adults and shows a male:female ratio of 2:1. Leukemia cutis typically occurs in patients with established CLL/SLL; initial presentation

Table 31-6

WHO Classification of B-Lymphoblastic Leukemia/Lymphoma

B-lymphoblastic leukemia/lymphoma, not otherwise specified

B-lymphoblastic leukemia/lymphoma with recurrent genetic abnormalities

B-lymphoblastic leukemia/lymphoma with t(9;22) (q34.1;q11.2); *BCR-ABL1*

B-lymphoblastic leukemia/lymphoma with t(v;11q23.3); *KMT2A*-rearranged

B-lymphoblastic leukemia/lymphoma with t(12;21) (p13.2;q22.1); *ETV6-RUNX1 (TEL-AML1)*

B-lymphoblastic leukemia/lymphoma with hyperdiploidy

B-lymphoblastic leukemia/lymphoma with hypodiploidy

B-lymphoblastic leukemia/lymphoma with t(15;14) (q31.1;q32.1); *IL3-IGH*

B-lymphoblastic leukemia/lymphoma with t(1;19) (q23;p13.3); *TCF3-PBX1 (E2A-PBX1)*

B-lymphoblastic leukemia/lymphoma, *BCR-ABL1*-like

B-lymphoblastic leukemia/lymphoma with iAMP21

Data from Swerdlow SH, Campo E, Harris NL, et al. *WHO Classification of Tumours of Haematopoietic and Lymphoid Tissues, Revised 4th Edition.* IARC; 2017.

in the skin is less common (280,281). Cutaneous involvement may produce localized or disseminated erythematous papules, plaques, or nodules that may involve head and neck, trunk, and/or extremities. Occasionally skin infiltration can result in irregular thickening and furrowing, including on the face (generically called "facies leonina") (280). Leukemic cells may infiltrate areas of preexisting or active inflammation such as sites of herpes simplex or zoster or *B. burgdorferi* infection (282,283). Although not usually curable, the disease tends to run an indolent course, unless transformation to an aggressive large B-cell lymphoma supervenes. This phenomenon, known as Richter syndrome, occurs in approximately 3% to 10% of patients with CLL/SLL, and in some cases may manifest as solitary or multiple rapidly growing subcutaneous nodules or tumors (284,285). Patients with cutaneous Richter syndrome may or may not have a prior history of cutaneous involvement by CLL/SLL (286).

Histopathology. Skin involvement is often characterized by a variably dense periadnexal/perivascular infiltrate or a nodular/diffuse dermal infiltrate that extends into the underlying subcutaneous tissue (Fig. 31-57A, B) (280). Less frequently, a bandlike pattern may be seen in the upper dermis. As with B-cell pattern infiltrates, the epidermis and follicular epithelium is spared, and the papillary dermis is usually uninvolved, producing a typical Grenz zone. This infiltrate is composed of a uniform population of small lymphocytes demonstrating round nuclei, clumped chromatin, variably conspicuous nucleoli, and small amounts of cytoplasm (Fig. 31-57C). In lymph nodes and, occasionally, in other sites, proliferation centers containing a continuum of small to large lymphocytes, including

prolymphocytes and paraimmunoblasts, will produce a nodular pattern of regularly distributed pale-staining areas at scanning magnification. Richter syndrome is characterized by a diffuse infiltrate of large-sized immunoblasts and centroblasts.

Tumor cells express B-cell markers CD19, CD79a, and PAX5, as well as CD23 and LEF-1; demonstrate aberrant expression of T-cell markers CD5 and CD43; show weak expression of CD20; and do not show expression of CD10 and cyclin D1. In patients treated with anti-CD20 monoclonal antibodies, CD20 expression may be completely negative, and other B-cell markers are required to establish lineage. Light chain restriction is confined to surface immunoglobulin in CLL/SLL; thus, immunoglobulin restriction is best determined by flow cytometry and not fixed-section immunohistochemistry.

Histogenesis. Immunoglobulin genes are clonally rearranged, and this can be demonstrated by molecular analysis using PCR. Although there are no specific genetic markers in CLL/SLL, recurrent cytogenetic abnormalities include del(13q), del(11q), del(17p), del(6q), and trisomy 12 (287,288). Mutations in *TP53*, *NOTCH1*, *SF3B1*, and *ATM* can occur and confer adverse prognosis (289). The mutational status of the *IGH* gene variable region (*IGHV*) is an important prognostic marker; patients with high-level *IGHV* somatic hypermutation have a better prognosis than those lacking somatic hypermutation (290).

Differential Diagnosis. In certain cases, the small lymphocytes of CLL/SLL may show moderate irregularity of the nuclear contour, raising suspicion for MCL. The presence of proliferation centers containing prolymphocytes and paraimmunoblasts, along with positivity for CD23 and LEF-1 and absence of cyclin D1 and Sox11 immunoreactivity, will permit a diagnosis of CLL/SLL in such instances (Table 31-3). The perivascular pattern in CLL/SLL may result in confusion with forms of dermatitis characterized by a predominantly or exclusively angiocentric architecture of inflammatory cell infiltration. This differential would therefore include polymorphous light eruption, dermal forms of lupus erythematosus, certain dermal delayed hypersensitivity responses to drug or injected antigen, and the family of gyrate erythemas (e.g., erythema annulare centrifugum and erythema chronicum migrans). Although all of these conditions contain small lymphocytes, the cells of CLL/SLL tend to be more homogeneous at high magnification. Moreover, most forms of dermatitis are predominated by T cells, not B cells.

Principles of Management: Prognosis does not appear to be affected by cutaneous involvement unless there is evidence of Richter transformation, which predicts a poor clinical course. Patients with CLL/SLL leukemia cutis are treated according to their underlying systemic disorder.

Mantle Cell Lymphoma

MCL is a B-cell lymphoma composed of small- to medium-sized lymphocytes with irregular nuclear contours and usually behaves more aggressively than CLL/SLL. The most common site of involvement is the lymph node, although other hematopoietic organs (bone marrow, peripheral blood, spleen) may also be involved. Cutaneous involvement is rare.

Clinical Summary. This disease affects middle-aged and older individuals, with a male:female ratio of 2:1. Skin lesions, if they

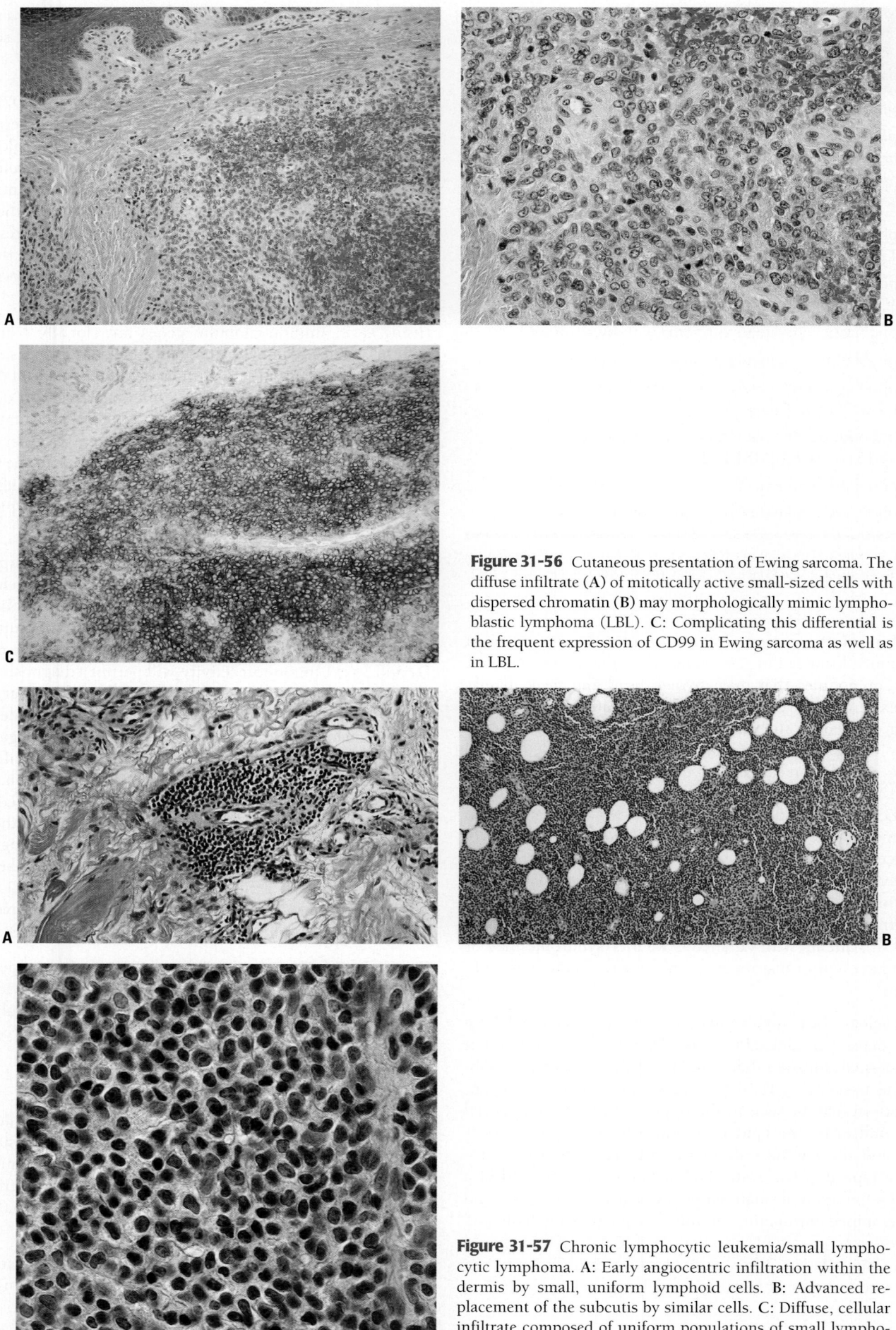

Figure 31-56 Cutaneous presentation of Ewing sarcoma. The diffuse infiltrate (**A**) of mitotically active small-sized cells with dispersed chromatin (**B**) may morphologically mimic lymphoblastic lymphoma (LBL). **C:** Complicating this differential is the frequent expression of CD99 in Ewing sarcoma as well as in LBL.

Figure 31-57 Chronic lymphocytic leukemia/small lymphocytic lymphoma. **A:** Early angiocentric infiltration within the dermis by small, uniform lymphoid cells. **B:** Advanced replacement of the subcutis by similar cells. **C:** Diffuse, cellular infiltrate composed of uniform populations of small lymphocytes containing rounded, hyperchromatic nuclei with inconspicuous nucleoli.

occur, are commonly solitary or multiple macules, nodules, or plaques (291).

Histopathology. Skin infiltration is characterized by a diffuse population of small- to medium-sized lymphocytes occupying the dermis and subcutis with sparing of the overlying epidermis (Fig. 31-58A). Proliferation centers, as detected at scanning magnification in CLL/SLL, are not seen. The cells have variably irregular nuclear contours, condensed chromatin, and indistinct nucleoli. MCL does not transform to a large-cell lymphoma but rather takes on a blastoid appearance or a pleomorphic appearance corresponding to more aggressive disease. In fact, biopsy of skin lesions will commonly show the blastoid variant, reflecting progression of disease (291,292). In these cases, the infiltrate is composed of medium-sized cells with blastlike (dispersed) chromatin and distinct nucleoli (Fig. 31-58B), and mitotic figures are frequent (at least 20 to 30 per 10 high-powered fields).

Tumor cells express B-cell markers CD19, CD20, CD79a, and PAX5; demonstrate aberrant expression of T-cell marker CD5 as well as expression of the nuclear proteins cyclin D1 and Sox11; and do not show expression of CD10 or CD23. In patients treated with anti-CD20 monoclonal antibodies, CD20 expression may be completely negative, and other B-cell markers are required to establish lineage. Light chain restriction is confined to surface immunoglobulin in MCL; thus, immunoglobulin restriction is best determined by flow cytometry and not fixed-section immunohistochemistry. The Ki67 proliferation index is routinely performed in samples of MCL because it provides prognostic information, and it is elevated in the blastoid variant.

Histogenesis. The tumor is believed to arise from a peripheral B cell of the inner mantle zone of the lymphoid follicle. The clonal nature of the process may be demonstrated via rearrangements of immunoglobulin genes. The cytogenetic hallmark of MCL is t(11;14)(q13;q32) with participation of the *CCND1* gene and the immunoglobulin heavy chain locus (293,294). Cyclin D1 is an important cell-cycle regulatory protein involved in restriction point control between the G1 and S phases. The genetic abnormality is detectable by conventional cytogenetics, FISH analysis, or PCR; overexpression of the gene product can also be readily assessed by immunohistochemical stains with antibodies directed against the nuclear cyclin D1 protein (295). A subset of MCL cases are negative for cyclin D1, may have rearrangements involving the cyclin D2 or D3 loci, and can be identified by immunohistochemical nuclear positivity for Sox11 (296,297).

Differential Diagnosis. MCL should be distinguished from other small-sized B-cell lymphoproliferative disorders involving the skin (Table 31-3). This is typically achieved by demonstrating coexpression of CD5 and cyclin D1 in cases of MCL. The blastoid variant of MCL will morphologically mimic leukemic infiltrates of LBL or CMS, and therefore immunohistochemistry, as outlined previously, is required for diagnosis.

Principles of Management: Patients with skin involvement by MCL are treated according to their underlying systemic disorder.

Follicular Lymphoma

FL is a B-cell lymphoma composed of admixed centrocytes and centroblasts and most commonly arises in lymph nodes. Involvement of other hematopoietic sites (bone marrow, spleen, peripheral blood) can also be detected. Infrequently, FL involves extranodal/extramedullary sites such as skin, gastrointestinal tract, ocular adnexa, breast, and testis. PCFCL (described previously) is a clinicopathologic entity distinct from FL, and differentiation between PCFCL and secondary cutaneous involvement by FL is critical given the divergent clinical implications (40).

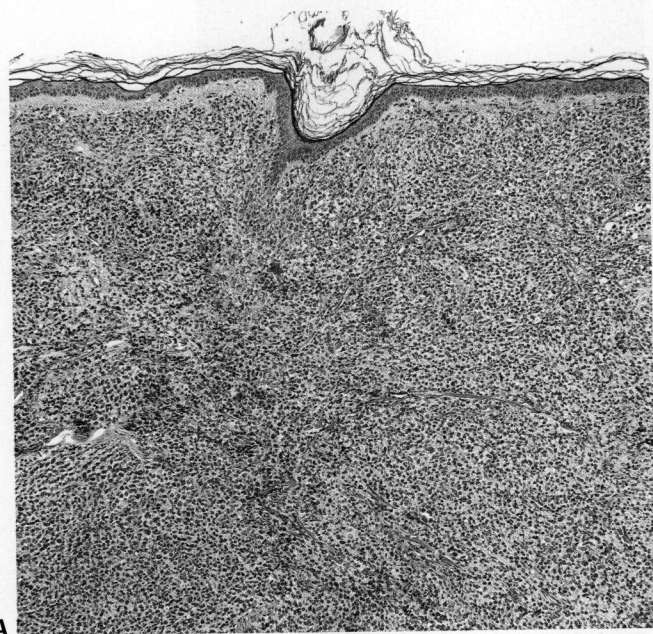
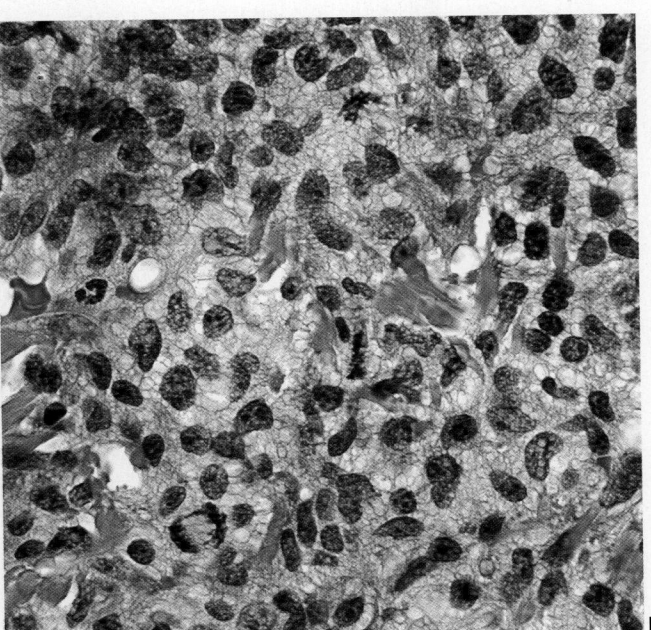

Figure 31-58 Mantle cell lymphoma. **A:** Diffuse population of small- to medium-sized lymphocytes filling the dermis with sparing of the overlying epidermis. **B:** Commonly, skin biopsies reveal morphologic evidence of the blastoid variant (mitotically active medium-sized cells with dispersed chromatin and distinct nucleoli), reflecting disease progression.

Clinical Summary. This type of lymphoma affects primarily older adults, with a median age in the sixth decade of life, and a male:female ratio of 1.2:1 (298). Of all cases of nodal FL, approximately 4% will show evidence of secondary skin involvement. Skin lesions typically occur concurrent with or following nodal involvement (40), with rare cases of disseminated FL initially manifesting with skin lesions (299). Head and neck is the most common location, and the lesions are often solitary. Relapse may occur in both cutaneous and extracutaneous sites.

Histopathology. Secondary cutaneous involvement by FL is characterized by a mid-dermal to subcutaneous nodular or diffuse infiltrate (299). The overlying epidermis is spared. At scanning magnification, the nodules may resemble germinal centers, but higher power examination reveals that the follicles are composed of admixed centrocytes and centroblasts without reactive features such as polarization, tingible-body macrophages, and numerous mitoses (Fig. 31-59A, B) (300). The follicles are surrounded by attenuated mantle zones. Some cases may be characterized by a more diffuse pattern with or without associated sclerosis. Although FL in nodal sites is graded on the basis of the architectural pattern(s) (nodular and/or diffuse) and the proportion of centrocytes and centroblasts, extranodal FL is typically not graded. However, diffuse sheets of centroblasts should not be classified as FL but instead are considered DL-BCL (see Diffuse Large B-Cell Lymphoma section).

FL is characterized by expression of B-cell markers (CD19, CD20, CD79a, PAX5), germinal center cell markers (CD10, BCL6), and aberrant expression of BCL2 (Fig. 31-59C). FL is negative for CD5, cyclin D1, and CD43. CD21 and CD23 will highlight the underlying follicular dendritic cell meshworks in cases with a follicular architecture.

Histogenesis. Germinal center B cells represent the cell of origin of FL. Clonal rearrangement of immunoglobulin genes is the rule, and cytogenetic abnormalities are almost always present,

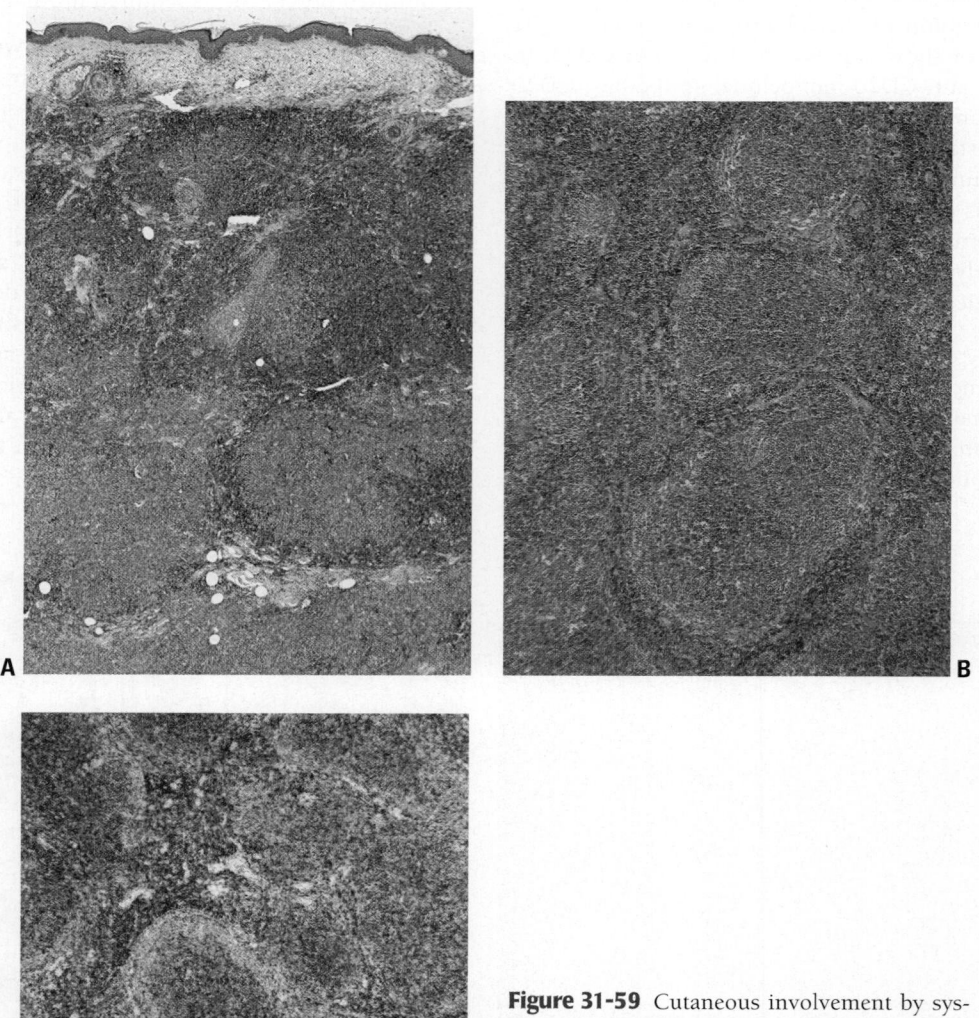

Figure 31-59 Cutaneous involvement by systemic follicular lymphoma. **A, B:** The dermis is replaced by nodules of neoplastic cells that superficially resemble germinal centers but show attenuated mantle zones and lack the "starry-sky" appearance of reactive germinal centers owing to the absence of tingible-body macrophages. **C:** Immunohistochemical studies reveal strong BCL2 expression in the follicles, which is characteristic of systemic FL but infrequent in PCFCL.

with the t(14;18)(q32;q21) rearrangement of the *BCL2* gene the most common (301,302). The BCL2 protein is situated on mitochondrial membranes and serves as an inhibitor of programmed cell death. Consequently, BCL2 expression in nodal FL appears to lend the tumor cells a distinct survival advantage when compared with their benign germinal center counterparts that undergo apoptosis.

Differential Diagnosis. Cutaneous involvement by nodal FL must be differentiated from B-CLH and other conditions associated with the formation of reactive follicles such as PCMZL (Table 31-3). The strong expression of BCL2 in FL, in particular, is very useful for distinguishing it from benign, reactive BCL2⁻ follicles. In addition, the morphologic features of secondary FL overlap with those of PCFCL, but distinction is critical given the divergent clinical courses. Both show a predilection for the head and neck region and show variably diffuse and/or nodular architectural patterns. Although there are no absolute morphologic or immunophenotypic features that can reliably distinguish the two entities, strong immunoreactivity for BCL2 and detection of t(14;18) is more suggestive of secondary involvement by FL (300). In any case lacking staging information, a differential diagnosis should be provided.

Principles of Management: Patients with skin involvement by FL are treated according to their underlying systemic disorder.

Plasma Cell Neoplasm

Plasma cell neoplasms are a group of disorders characterized by an expansion of clonal plasma cells. The clinicopathologic entities within the category of plasma cell neoplasm include monoclonal gammopathy of undetermined significance (MGUS), plasma cell myeloma (clinically called multiple myeloma), and plasmacytoma (extraosseous/extramedullary plasmacytoma or solitary plasmacytoma of bone). Cutaneous involvement by a plasma cell neoplasm is most commonly a secondary manifestation of systemic disease (multiple myeloma) and typically occurs in patients with late-stage disease and high tumor burden (303,304). Cutaneous disease may also reflect direct extension from an underlying bony lesion.

Clinical Summary. Most affected individuals are middle-aged to older males (male:female ratio is 2:1). Cutaneous lesions manifest as multiple erythematous or violaceous papules or nodules occurring over a wide anatomic distribution. Several cases of cutaneous tumors arising at an area of trauma (such as venous catheter access sites) have been reported (305). When cutaneous lesions occur in the setting of plasma cell myeloma, they typically signal advanced disease with a poor prognosis (303,306).

Histopathology. Histologic examination reveals a nodular or diffuse infiltrate involving the thickness of the dermis with extension into the underlying subcutaneous tissue (Fig. 31-60A). The epidermis is spared. The nodules are composed of cohesive aggregates of neoplastic plasma cells, while diffuse lesions tend to show an interstitial infiltrate of plasma cells that splay dermal collagen fibers. The infiltrate is composed of plasma cells that may demonstrate characteristic features (round, eccentrically placed nuclei; clumped chromatin; abundant amphophilic cytoplasm with a discernible hof) or that may show more pleomorphic or immature nuclei with prominent nucleoli (Fig. 31-60B). Bi- or multinucleation is common. The cytoplasm of the neoplastic plasma cells may contain a variety of inclusions usually related to abnormal accumulation of immunoglobulin, including round, eosinophilic (Russell) bodies. However, such cytoplasmic changes are not specific for neoplastic plasma cells and may also be seen in B-cell lymphomas with plasmacytic differentiation, or reactive proliferations. Rare cases of cutaneous plasma cell myeloma can have concurrent amyloid deposition (304). Immunohistochemical studies will demonstrate strong reactivity for CD138 in the plasma cells (with the epidermis serving as an internal positive control). Monotypic cytoplasmic immunoglobulin light chain restriction can easily be demonstrated by immunohistochemistry or *in situ* hybridization owing to the abundance of intracellular immunoglobulin. Aberrant CD56 expression is seen in approximately

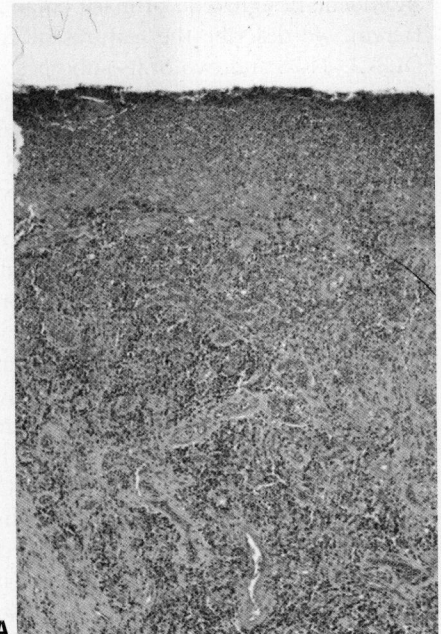
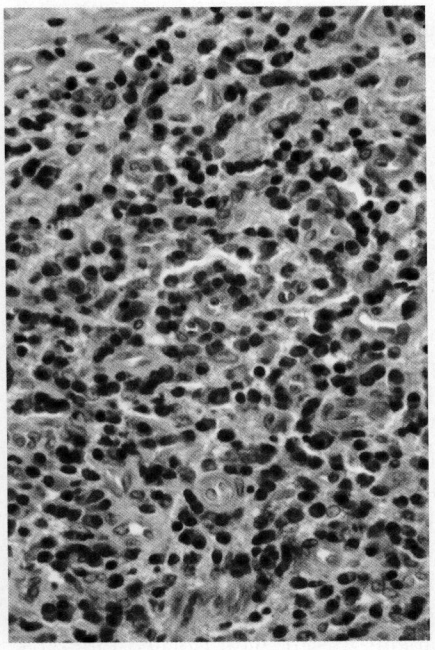

Figure 31-60 Plasma cell neoplasm. **A:** There is diffuse interstitial infiltration of the dermis associated with surface erosion. **B:** Higher magnification showing cellular infiltrate composed of plasma cells with characteristic eccentrically placed nuclei. Some cells show binucleation.

70% of cases of plasma cell myeloma, and its expression will support the neoplastic nature of the infiltrate. CD20, CD19, and CD45 are characteristically negative. Cutaneous cases of multiple myeloma appear enriched in immunoglobulin class A (IgA) and light chain deposition disease, with monoclonal immunoglobulin light chain deposits appearing as nonamyloid amorphous eosinophilic material (306,307).

Histogenesis. Clonal transformation of a peripheral plasma cell is the most likely cell of origin. Molecular studies generally reveal rearrangement of immunoglobulin genes. The molecular basis of plasma cells homing to the skin is not well understood, although it has been proposed that differential expression of adhesion molecules, and high *CCR10* expression, may promote migration toward cutaneous tissues (308). There is no apparent cytogenetic subtype of multiple myeloma with preferential involvement of skin (306).

Differential Diagnosis. Reactive, plasma cell–rich infiltrates may occur in the skin as part of an immune response, but reactive plasma cells will not show nuclear immaturity or pleomorphism and generally do not show monotypic immunoglobulin light chain restriction. Within the spectrum of neoplastic cutaneous lesions, the differential diagnosis includes PCMZL with marked plasmacytic differentiation, and correlation with clinical findings may be needed to distinguish the two entities.

Plasmablastic lymphoma is another B-cell lymphoma with plasmacytic differentiation, which may occur in the skin (309). Affected patients are typically immunosuppressed (HIV infection, posttransplant setting), and the disease has an aggressive course. The large, atypical cells often show plasmacytic differentiation and are CD138+ and frequently show light chain restriction; all of these features may raise the possibility of an anaplastic plasma cell myeloma. Although the presence of CD56 expression and absence of EBER *in situ* hybridization reactivity have traditionally been thought to support a diagnosis of plasma cell myeloma, occasional CD56 expression has been reported in plasmablastic lymphoma, as has EBV expression in plasma cell myeloma; therefore, clinical correlation is essential.

Principles of Management: Patients with skin involvement by a plasma cell neoplasm are treated according to their underlying systemic disorder. Localized radiotherapy may provide some debulking benefits (310).

Diffuse Large B-Cell Lymphoma

DLBCL is a neoplasm of large B cells characterized by diffuse tissue infiltration. Most cases of DLBCL fall into the category of "DLBCL, not otherwise specified," or DLBCL, NOS, although some cases show specific clinicopathologic features that permit more specific subtyping, namely T-cell/histiocyte-rich large B-cell lymphoma (THRLBCL), primary DLBCL of the central nervous system, PCLBCL-LT (as discussed in a prior section), and EBV+ DLBCL, NOS (Table 31-7). Other large B-cell lymphomas have also been grouped into categories on the basis of specific clinical, morphologic, immunophenotypic, and/or cytogenetic features (Table 31-7). DLBCL typically involves lymph nodes, although around one-third of DLBCL cases exhibit extranodal involvement. Of these, approximately 15% infiltrate skin or other soft tissue sites (311). Although this often represents spread from a systemic process, some patients present with isolated infiltrates of large B cells in the skin that do not fulfill clinicopathologic criteria for PCLBCL-LT (312). Such lesions were historically referred to as "primary cutaneous DLBCL, other" by the 2005

Table 31-7

WHO Classification of Large B-Cell Lymphomas

*Diffuse large B-cell lymphoma, not otherwise specified**

Other large B-cell lymphomas

T-cell/histiocyte-rich large B-cell lymphoma*

Primary diffuse large B-cell lymphoma of the central nervous system

Primary cutaneous diffuse large B-cell lymphoma, leg type*

EBV+ diffuse large B-cell lymphoma, NOS*

Diffuse large B-cell lymphoma associated with chronic inflammation

Lymphomatoid granulomatosis*

Large B-cell lymphoma with *IRF4* rearrangement

Primary mediastinal (thymic) large B-cell lymphoma

Intravascular large B-cell lymphoma*

ALK+ large B-cell lymphoma

Plasmablastic lymphoma*

HHV8-positive diffuse large B-cell lymphoma

Primary effusion lymphoma

High-grade B-cell lymphoma

High-grade B-cell lymphoma with *MYC* and *BCL2* and/or *BCL6* rearrangements

High-grade B-cell lymphoma, NOS

*Entities that most frequently show cutaneous involvement.
Data from Swerdlow SH, Campo E, Harris NL, et al. *WHO Classification of Tumours of Haematopoietic and Lymphoid Tissues, Revised 4th Edition.* Lyon, France: IARC; 2017.

WHO–EORTC classification scheme; however, the updated 2018 WHO–EORTC classification no longer contains this separate category, and rare cases of cutaneous large B-cell lymphomas that cannot be classified as PCLBCL-LT or other specified subtypes should be designated "primary cutaneous DLBCL, NOS" (11). Herein, we describe the features of cutaneous involvement by DLBCL, NOS and two of its subtypes, THRLBCL and EBV+ DLBCL, NOS. Three of the other large B-cell lymphomas that may show cutaneous involvement (plasmablastic lymphoma, intravascular large B-cell lymphoma, and lymphomatoid granulomatosis [LYG]) are described in the following sections.

Clinical Features. DLBCL may occur over a wide age range, including in children, although adult/elderly individuals are most often affected. In the skin, DLBCL forms red to purpuric papules, nodules, and infiltrated plaques. The lesions are often solitary with a predilection for the head and neck region or trunk. The outcome of DLBCL is variable given the range of clinical, histologic, and genetic features among patients. Nodal-based THRLBCL with or without cutaneous involvement is an aggressive disease, but rare cases of THRLBCL presenting only in the skin have followed a more indolent clinical course (313). EBV+ DLBCL, NOS was formerly designated EBV+ DLBCL of the elderly, and although it usually occurs in patients older than 50 years, a much wider age range of presentation has been shown (314). It frequently involves extranodal sites, including the skin with or without concurrent lymph node involvement, and is highly aggressive in elderly patients but shows a much more favorable prognosis in patients younger than 45 years (314).

Histopathology. Tissue infiltration in DLBCL generally results in local destruction and effacement of preexisting structures (Fig. 31-61A). Dermal infiltrates may be diffuse or nodular. Frequently, deep dermis is preferentially affected, producing a so-called bottom-heavy pattern. Cytologically, there is a uniform, monotonous population of large, transformed lymphoid cells resembling centroblasts or immunoblasts (Fig. 31-61B). These cells have scant cytoplasm, large nuclei with vesicular chromatin, and often prominent nucleoli. Immunohistochemistry will demonstrate a B-cell phenotype (expression of CD19, CD20, CD79a, and PAX5) and often a high Ki67 proliferation index (Fig. 31-61C, D). Variable expression of CD10, BCL2,

BCL6, and CD30 may be seen and will likely reflect the immunophenotype of the underlying systemic lymphoma. THRLBCL is morphologically characterized by a nodular to diffuse dermal infiltrate of few, scattered, large, atypical B cells in a background of numerous reactive T cells and histiocytes. The large B cells express pan-B-cell markers as well as BCL6 and IRF4/MUM1, show variable expression of BCL2 and EMA; and are negative for CD15, CD30, CD138, and EBER *in situ* hybridization.

EBV⁺ DLBCL, NOS results in effacement of the dermal architecture by either a polymorphous or large-cell infiltrate. The polymorphous infiltrate is characterized by atypical large cells in a mixed inflammatory background. By definition, the cells are

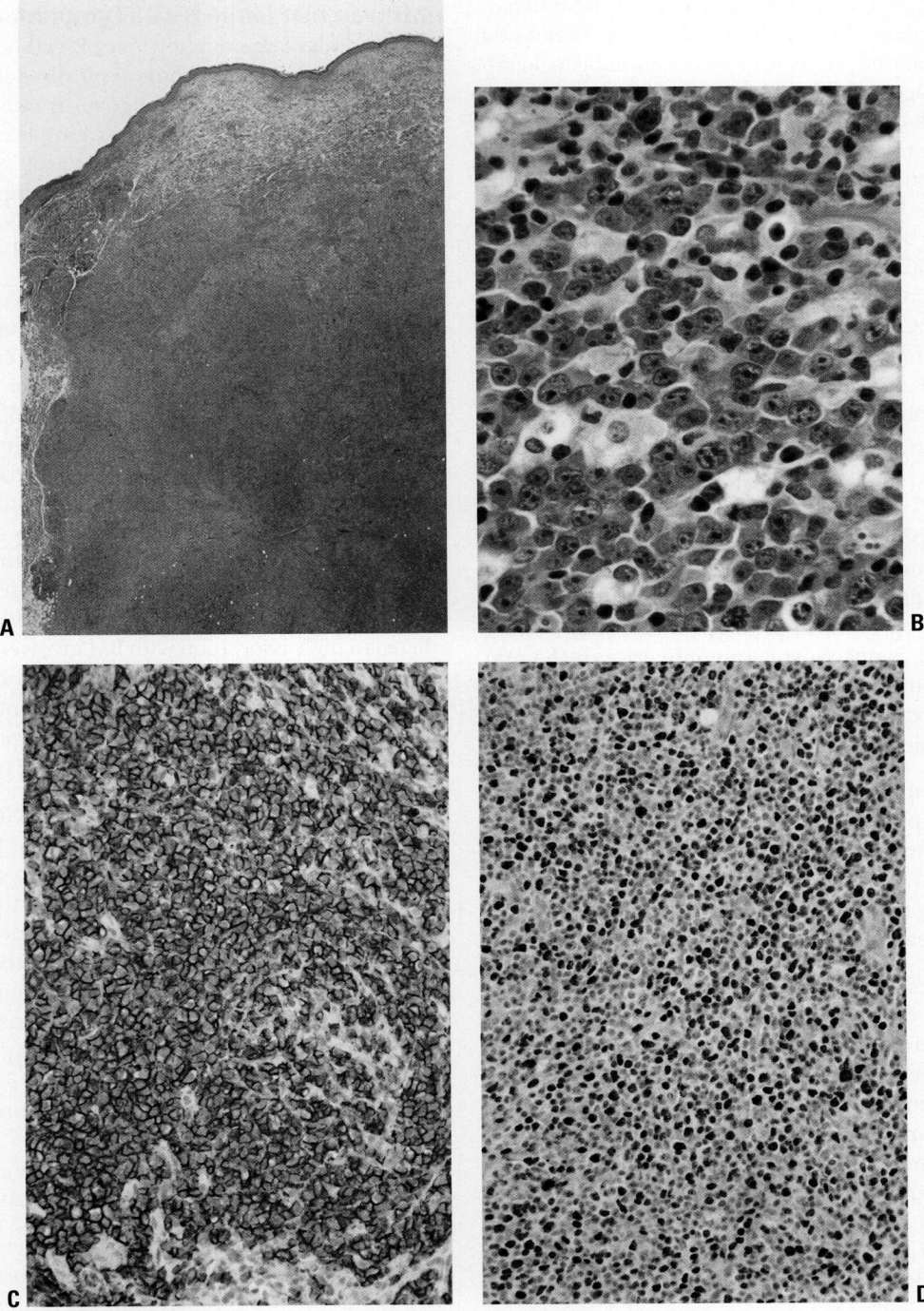

Figure 31-61 Diffuse large B-cell lymphoma. **A:** The dermis is diffusely effaced by a destructive infiltrate. **B:** High magnification showing an infiltrate composed of large, neoplastic lymphocytes. Immunohistochemistry shows the malignant cells to express CD20 (**C**) and demonstrates evidence of a high proliferative rate on the basis of Ki67 reactivity (**D**).

positive by EBER *in situ* hybridization. Although CD20 and CD79a are typically positive, CD20 expression may not be detected in cases with plasmablastic morphology. IRF4/MUM1 is strongly positive and CD30 expression is variable. These cases need to be distinguished from EBV⁺ MCU, which occurs in the setting of immunosuppression and often has a self-limited indolent course, and is defined as a solitary ulcerating lesion with large Hodgkin-like EBV⁺ B cells in a mixed inflammatory background. In contrast to EBV⁺ DLBCL, lesions of EBV⁺ MCU are very well demarcated and often show a band of reactive lymphocytes at the periphery (65).

Histogenesis. Immunoglobulin gene rearrangements are regularly encountered. EBV⁺ DLBCL, NOS is thought to arise secondary to immunosenescence.

Differential Diagnosis. Anaplastic lesions may raise the differential diagnosis of dermal involvement by anaplastic carcinoma and amelanotic melanoma, and in such cases, immunohistochemical screening for lineage-related markers (e.g., CD45, pan-B-cell antigens, cytokeratins, Melan A) is a useful initial point of departure for diagnostic evaluation. Once a B-cell lineage has been established, distinction of secondary involvement by a systemic DLBCL from PCLBCL-LT requires clinicopathologic correlation. Strong expression of both BCL2 and IRF4/MUM1 is most frequently seen in PCLBCL-LT (47). Unlike the blastoid variant of MCL, cells of DLBCL are typically negative for strong cyclin D1 expression. EBV⁺ DLBCL, NOS must be distinguished from other EBV⁺ B-cell lymphoproliferative disorders that may involve the skin, including EBV+ MCU (discussed previously), as well as plasmablastic lymphoma and LYG (see following sections).

Principles of Management: Therapy may be guided by the presence or absence of underlying systemic disease.

Plasmablastic Lymphoma

Plasmablastic lymphoma is an uncommon large B-cell lymphoma that arises in immunocompromised patients, often secondary to HIV infection but also in the posttransplant setting or in older patients. Lesions most commonly arise in the oral cavity (particularly in patients with HIV infection) and less frequently in other extranodal sites, including skin. Nodal involvement is uncommon.

Clinical Summary. Skin lesions typically occur as localized, single or multiple, asymptomatic red papules or nodules. In general, plasmablastic lymphoma has a poor prognosis, although patients with isolated skin lesions may demonstrate a better outcome compared to those with skin lesions secondary to underlying systemic disease (309).

Histopathology. The lesions are composed of diffuse dermal infiltrates of large-sized cells, which may resemble immunoblasts (round nuclear contours, vesicular chromatin, and prominent nucleoli) or may have a more plasmacytoid appearance with eccentrically placed nuclei. The overlying epidermis is spared. Admixed mitotic figures, apoptotic bodies, and tingible-body macrophages are commonly observed. The immunophenotype is similar to that of plasma cells, with expression of CD138 and IRF4/MUM1, and weak to no expression of B-cell markers CD20 and PAX5 or of CD45. EBER *in situ* hybridization is frequently positive. The Ki67 proliferation index is typically high.

Histogenesis. Immunoglobulin gene rearrangements will be detected in most cases. The postulated cell of origin is the plasmablast.

Differential Diagnosis. Secondary cutaneous involvement by a plasma cell neoplasm is a potential albeit rare diagnostic consideration. Given possible overlapping morphologic and immunophenotypic features, including occasional CD56 expression in plasmablastic lymphoma or EBV expression in plasma cell myeloma, careful clinical correlation is needed. Positivity by EBER *in situ* hybridization raises the possibility of EBV⁺ DLBCL, NOS, and clinicopathologic correlation may be needed for distinction, particularly in cases of EBV⁺ DLBCL, NOS with plasmablastic morphology.

Principles of Management: Treatment strategies include antiretroviral therapy for patients with HIV infection, reduction/cessation of immunosuppression in the posttransplant setting, systemic chemotherapy, and/or localized radiation therapy.

Intravascular Large B-Cell Lymphoma

Intravascular large (angiotropic) B-cell lymphoma is a rare and aggressive process that prototypically demonstrates intraluminal aggregation of large malignant B cells within vessels of involved tissues (315,316). It has long been postulated that the intravascular trapping of the neoplastic cells is associated with defects in homing receptors on the lymphoid cells and/or adhesion molecules on the endothelial cells. However, the precise mechanisms are still not fully elucidated.

Clinical Summary. Intravascular large B-cell lymphoma is a disease of adults. Because signs and symptoms relate primarily to vascular occlusion, clinical presentation is often highly variable and nonspecific, commonly with fever or neurologic symptoms at presentation (317,318). There is typically widely disseminated involvement of extranodal tissues, including the skin, lung, central nervous system, kidney, and adrenal glands. Rarely, skin is the only site of involvement. Skin lesions tend to be indurated, red/purple plaques and nodules, preferentially on the trunk or thighs. Telangiectasia and epidermal changes attributable to ischemia, including scaling and ulceration, may also be observed. Several series have shown that in Asian (particularly Japanese) patients, there is a high association with BM involvement and hemophagocytic lymphohistiocytosis with skin lesions less common, suggesting a distinct "hemophagocytic variant" (316,319,320). The prognosis of cases limited to the skin is reported to be superior to that of generalized involvement (321,322).

Histopathology. Involved vessels (particularly capillaries) are either entirely or partially occluded by populations of large, malignant-appearing lymphoid cells enmeshed in fibrin (Fig. 31-62A). In the case of the latter, these cells may adhere to inconspicuous and attenuated underlying endothelium, producing the false impression of endothelial atypia or malignancy (Fig. 31-62B). Cytologically, tumor cells contain large nuclei with vesicular chromatin patterns and prominent nucleoli. Confirmation of B-cell origin may be accomplished by immunohistochemistry for CD20 (Fig. 31-62C). IRF4/MUM1 and BCL2 are commonly positive. Coexpression of C-MYC and BCL2 confers a worse prognosis (323). There is variable expression of CD5, CD10, and BCL6. Rare cases of intravascular lymphoma with T-/NK-cell phenotype have been documented, but these are considered different entities (324).

Histogenesis. The malignant B cells are believed to have defective homing receptors, with expression of molecules enabling endothelial adhesion (such as CXCR3 and CXCR4), but lack factors critical for extravasation (such as CD29/beta 1 integrin,

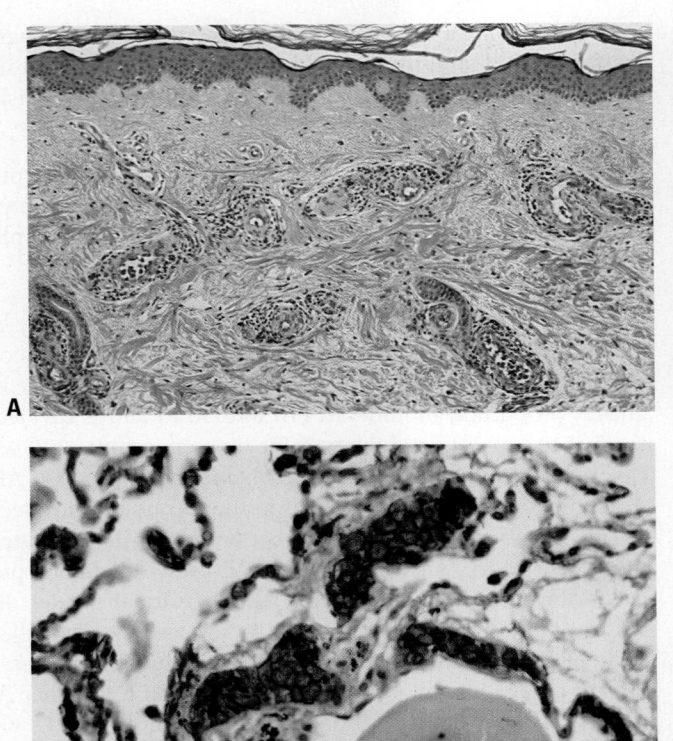

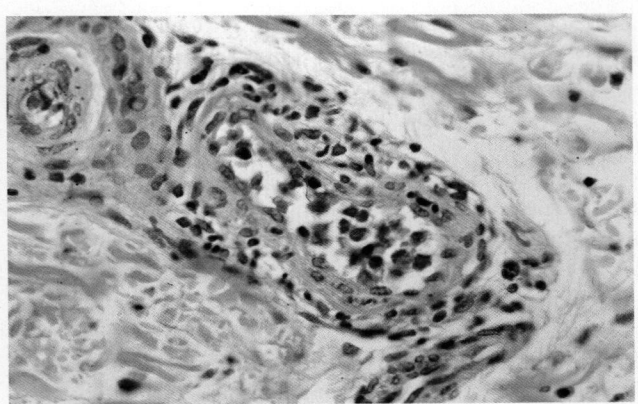

Figure 31-62 Intravascular large B-cell lymphoma. **A:** Superficial dermal vessels are partially occluded by hyperchromatic malignant cells. **B:** Higher magnification discloses malignant-appearing lymphocytes partially adherent to the endothelial surface of involved vessels. **C:** CD20 reactivity for malignant B cells within pulmonary vessels from a patient with diffuse extracutaneous involvement.

or CD54/ICAM1), resulting in their tendency for intravascular accumulation with impaired ability for diapedesis (325–327). Clonal rearrangements of immunoglobulin genes have been demonstrated (328), and a subset of cases have shown mutations in *MYD88* and/or *CD79B* genes (329).

Differential Diagnosis. Because lesions typically show malignant cells to be confined exclusively to vascular lumens, the primary differential diagnosis involves differentiation of these cells from malignant and reactive endothelium (e.g., angiosarcoma and diffuse dermal angiomatosis/reactive angioendotheliomatosis) (330). Differentiation from other intravascular malignant deposits (e.g., inflammatory carcinoma of the breast) may be confirmed by using lineage-related immunohistochemical markers.

Principles of Management: Intravascular large B-cell lymphoma is treated with systemic chemotherapy, historically with poor response, although earlier diagnosis and new regimens have improved the prognosis (331). Random skin biopsies have shown high diagnostic yield in patients presenting with suspicion for intravascular large B-cell lymphoma (332–334).

Lymphomatoid Granulomatosis
LYG is a rare and variably aggressive lymphoproliferative disorder characterized by angiocentric and angiodestructive infiltration of extranodal tissues, including the skin, by EBV⁺ B cells and reactive T cells (335,336).

Clinical Summary. Adult males are generally affected by LYG (male:female ratio of 2:1), although immunosuppressed children may also present with this disease. Although multiple organs may be involved, the lung is the most common, and if not infiltrated at time of presentation, it tends to be affected at some point during the natural evolution of the disease. Skin

involvement is quite common, being demonstrable in 25% to 50% of all cases. Skin lesions manifest variably as multiple red papules, plaques, or nodules, commonly on the trunk and extremities. Lymph node and spleen involvement are very rare (336–338).

Histopathology. Unlike most non-Hodgkin lymphomas, LYG shows an angiocentric and angiodestructive architecture and a polymorphous cytology (Fig. 31-63) (336,339). The infiltrates are composed of a variable number of large, EBV⁺ B cells in a prominent mixed inflammatory background (340). The B cells may resemble immunoblasts or may show more pleomorphic features. The infiltrating mononuclear cells show permeation and focal destruction and fibrinoid necrosis of vessel walls, and adjacent zones of ischemic necrosis may result. Occasional foci of epidermotropism may be observed in some lesions. The EBV⁺

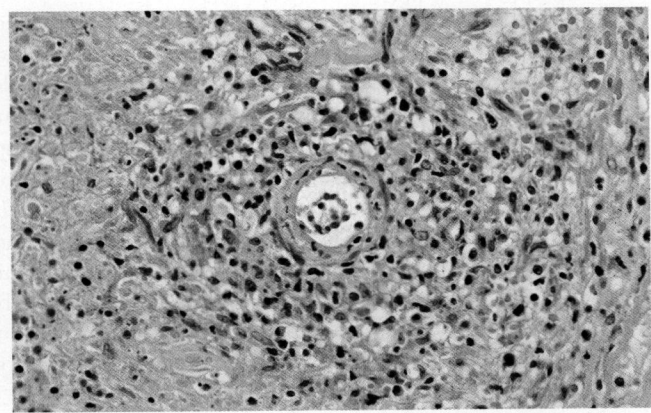

Figure 31-63 Lymphomatoid granulomatosis. Atypical lymphocytes have infiltrated and partially destroyed the involved vessel walls.

B cells are reactive for CD20, variably positive for CD30, and negative for CD15. The background lymphocytes are CD3⁺ T cells (CD4 > CD8). Grading of lesions (I–III) based on the proportion of EBV⁺ cells, extent of atypia, and necrosis may correlate with biologic behavior (336,339). Grade I lesions exhibit a polymorphous infiltrate, with minimal atypia, infrequent EBV⁺ cells (<5 per high-power field), and absent or focal necrosis. Grade II lesions contain more frequent EBV⁺ cells, usually between 5 and 20 per high-power field but can be focally higher. Grade III lesions have numerous EBV⁺ cells (>50 per high-power field); however, sheets of large B cells without a background inflammatory infiltrate are classified as EBV⁺ DLBCL, NOS.

Histogenesis. The underlying cause of LYG appears to be related to EBV-driven abnormal B-cell proliferation in the setting of immunodeficiency (341). Higher-grade lesions tend to show clonal rearrangement of immunoglobulin genes (336).

Differential Diagnosis. LYG must be differentiated from hematopoietic malignancies that may also show an angiodestructive growth pattern, such as ENKTCL (342). Identification of EBV⁺ cells that express CD20 is helpful in separating LYG from these entities. Occasional pleomorphic/multinucleated cells may raise the possibility of CHL, but classic Reed–Sternberg cells will not be present. EBV⁺ MCU can show vasculitic changes but is characteristically an isolated and sharply demarcated cutaneous or mucosal ulcer, without involvement of other organs or the lung.

Principles of Management: Prognosis is variable, depending on the extent of extracutaneous involvement and the overall grade. Therapeutic options include immune modulation and combination immunochemotherapy, the selection of which depends on the extent and grade of disease (341).

T-/NK-Cell Lineage

T-lymphoblastic Leukemia/Lymphoma

T-lymphoblastic leukemia (T-ALL)/lymphoblastic lymphoma (T-LBL) is a high-risk neoplasm that is derived from precursor T lymphocytes. T-LBL typically arises in the mediastinum or lymph nodes, and cutaneous involvement is rare.

Clinical Summary. Infiltration of the skin results in erythematous to hemorrhagic papules and nodules, or subcutaneous masses. Although T-LBL is more prevalent in children and young adults compared to older individuals, cutaneous T-LBL is more commonly seen in the adult population (265,266,343).

Histopathology. The dermis is preferentially involved by a diffuse interstitial infiltrate, with little or no epidermotropism, morphologically indistinguishable from B-LBL. Cytologically, the tumor cells are uniformly atypical, with scant cytoplasm and nuclei characterized by slightly irregular, sometimes grooved contours and moderately condensed to evenly dispersed chromatin patterns with small nucleoli. Occasionally, eosinophils will be present within the dermal infiltrate. The tumor cells are positive for TdT and may express CD1a, CD2, CD3, CD4, CD5, CD7, and/or CD8 to variable degrees. Of these, reactivity for cytoplasmic CD3 in combination with TdT and/or CD1a is the most specific indicator of T-LBL (208). Lineage ambiguity of these primitive cells may occur, however, as evidenced by occasional expression of the B-cell marker CD79a or myeloid marker CD33.

Histogenesis. The cell of origin is believed to be a precursor T lymphoblast. Clonal rearrangements of the TCR are typically detected.

Differential Diagnosis. The morphologic differential diagnosis includes B-LBL and its morphologic mimics, as outlined in the prior section. Immunohistochemistry will readily establish the hematopoietic and lineage characteristics of T-LBL.

Principles of Management: Patients with T-LBL are typically treated in the same manner as patients with T-ALL, namely systemic polychemotherapy with or without stem cell transplant.

Anaplastic Large-Cell Lymphoma

ALCL is a systemic T-cell neoplasm that is characterized by large, pleomorphic cells that strongly express CD30. ALCL accounts for approximately 3% of adult non-Hodgkin lymphomas and a greater proportion in children (10% to 30%) and is divided according to expression of the tyrosine kinase receptor ALK, which can be detected by immunohistochemistry (344,345). ALCL, ALK⁺ predominantly affects males in the second to third decades of life. These patients exhibit a better prognosis compared to those with ALCL, ALK-negative (ALCL, ALK⁻), which typically occurs in older individuals with relatively equal gender distribution. Both types of ALCL affect nodal and extranodal sites, particularly skin and also bone, soft tissue, lung, and liver. Secondary cutaneous involvement by systemic ALCL (either ALK⁺ or ALK⁻) must be differentiated from primary cALCL, which demonstrates a considerably better prognosis.

Clinical Summary. Patients often present at advanced stage with concomitant B symptoms including fever, weight loss, and night sweats. When skin is involved, the lesions range from papules to ulcerating tumors. Cutaneous involvement by systemic ALCL often portends a worse prognosis compared to cases without cutaneous involvement (135,346).

Histopathology. Secondary cutaneous involvement by ALCL typically manifests as a dermal nodule (Fig. 31-64A). The neoplastic cells are large with abundant cytoplasm and anaplastic nuclear features. Nuclei exhibit many shapes; they may be round to oval, reniform or horseshoe-shaped (so-called hallmark cells), or multinucleated (so-called wreath cells) or exhibit nuclear pseudoinclusions (so-called doughnut cells) (Fig. 31-64B, C). Sometimes, binucleate cells can be seen, resembling the Reed–Sternberg cells of CHL, and cases mimicking nodular sclerosis CHL have also been described (347). The chromatin pattern is generally finely aggregated, and nucleoli are variably prominent and usually multiple. A wide morphologic spectrum has been reported (348–350). Large cells may predominate (the common variant), or the large cells may be admixed with histiocytes (lymphohistiocytic variant) or with cytologically similar, albeit smaller, atypical lymphocytes (small-cell variant).

Most cases express T-cell antigens, and even those without T-cell antigen expression ("null-cell" phenotype) have evidence of T-cell lineage at a genomic level (351). Pan-T-cell maturation markers (e.g., CD3, CD5, and CD7) are frequently negative, and this is consistent with an aberrant T-cell phenotype. The cells show strong CD30 reactivity on the cell membrane and in association with the Golgi zone (Fig. 31-64D). In addition, most cases show positivity for cytotoxic-associated markers, including TIA-1, granzyme B, and/or perforin (352,353). ALK1 expression defines ALCL, ALK⁺ (Fig. 31-64E). Most of these cases are also positive for EMA, whereas cells of ALCL, ALK⁻ infrequently exhibit EMA expression.

Histogenesis. The presumed cell of origin for ALCL is a mature cytotoxic T cell. The majority of cases demonstrate clonal

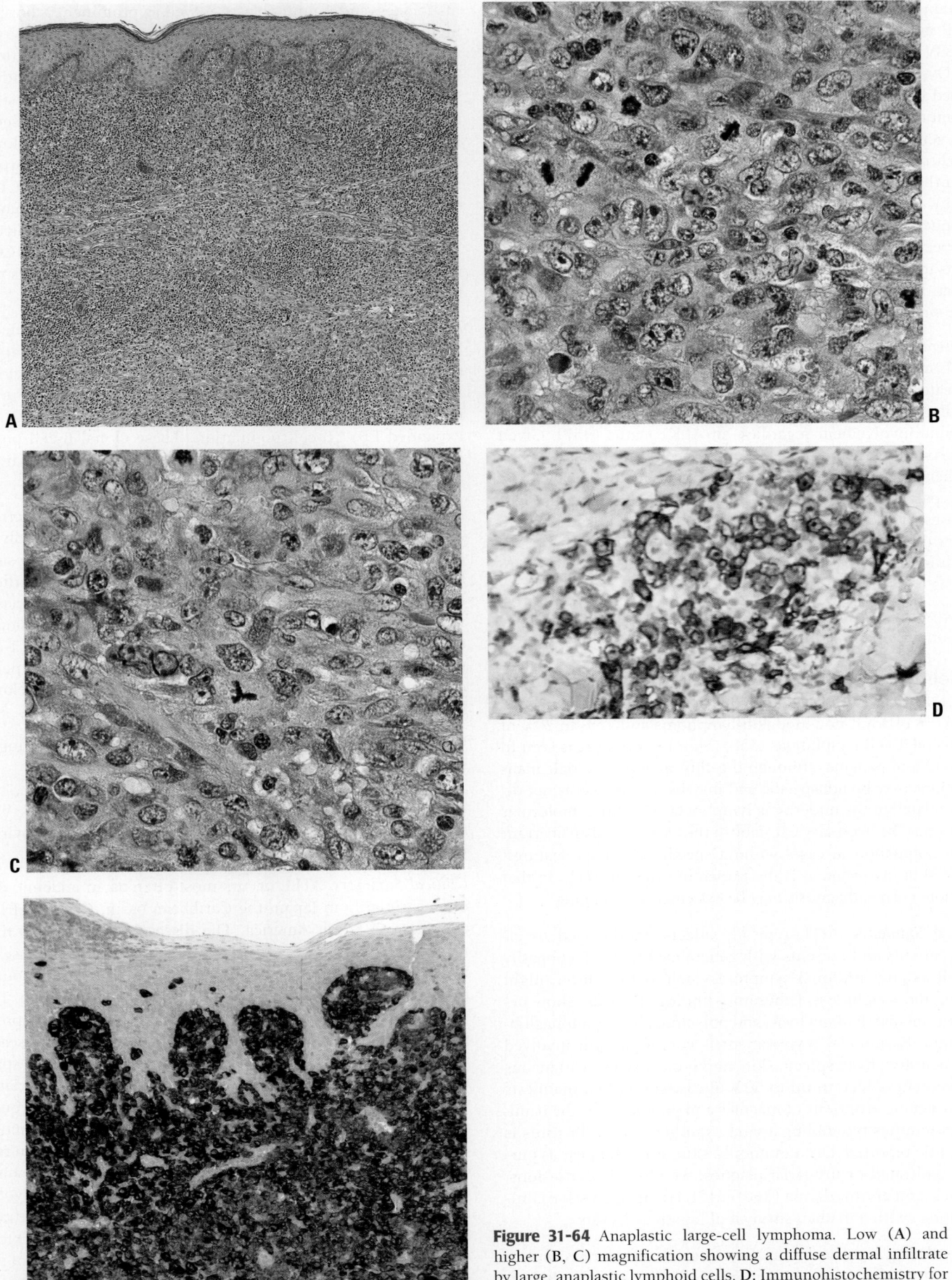

Figure 31-64 Anaplastic large-cell lymphoma. Low (**A**) and higher (**B, C**) magnification showing a diffuse dermal infiltrate by large, anaplastic lymphoid cells. **D:** Immunohistochemistry for CD30 shows very strong reactivity. **E:** Strong immunoreactivity to ALK1 in cutaneous spread of systemic ALCL, ALK⁺.

rearrangements of the TCR genes irrespective of expression of T-cell markers. Cases of ALCL are essentially always negative for EBV genomes, separating them from EBV$^+$ CHL (354).

Overexpression of the ALK protein in ALCL, ALK$^+$ is caused by alterations of the *ALK* gene at chromosome 2. Most commonly, t(2;5)(p23;q35) is seen with the participation of the *ALK* gene on chromosome 2 and nucleophosmin (*NPM*) gene on chromosome 5. However, breakpoints on chromosomes other than 5 can partner with the *ALK* gene. Classic t(2;5) leads to ALK protein overexpression, resulting in both cytoplasmic and nuclear staining with immunohistochemistry. ALCL, ALK$^-$ has been shown to contain 6p25.3 *IRF4/DUSP22* rearrangements in 30% of cases, and rearrangements of *TP63* in a smaller subset. *DUSP22*-rearranged ALCL has an improved prognosis, more similar to ALCL, ALK$^+$ (355,356).

Differential Diagnosis. Secondary cutaneous involvement by ALCL must be distinguished from primary cALCL (discussed in greater detail in the prior section on primary cALCL). In fact, any diagnosis of ALCL in the skin should prompt evaluation for systemic involvement regardless of ALK1 status (357). Given the strong expression of CD30 in the neoplastic cells of ALCL, another diagnostic consideration is cutaneous involvement by CHL, particularly when Reed–Sternberg–like cells are present. In cases of ALCL, ALK$^+$, expression of ALK1 is sufficient to render the correct diagnosis. Additionally, expression of PAX5, which is weakly expressed in the nuclei of true Reed–Stenberg cells, is not seen in ALCL (ALK$^+$ or ALK$^-$).

Principles of Management: Patients are treated according to their underlying systemic lymphoma.

Angioimmunoblastic T-Cell Lymphoma

AITL is a nodal T-cell lymphoma that accounts for approximately 1% to 2% of adult non-Hodgkin lymphoma and 15% to 20% of peripheral T-cell lymphomas (358). Skin involvement is seen in up to 50% of patients, although the clinical and histologic manifestations may be nonspecific and may be interpreted as not directly related to the underlying lymphoma. Therefore, molecular studies may be necessary to establish the existence of an aberrant clonal population in cases without specific histologic features. Rarely, skin involvement is the presenting sign of AITL. In that situation, correct diagnosis may be extremely challenging.

Clinical Summary. AITL typically affects middle-aged to elderly patients and presents with generalized lymphadenopathy as well as constitutional symptoms such as high fever, night sweats, and weight loss. Laboratory findings typically show hemolytic anemia, leukocytosis, and polyclonal hypergammaglobulinemia. Extranodal involvement is common, with involved sites including liver, spleen, skin, and bone marrow. Cutaneous involvement is seen in up to 50% of cases and often manifests as nonspecific eruptions of macules and papules over the trunk and extremities resembling a viral exanthem (359). Pruritus is frequently reported. Less commonly, skin lesions appear as purpura, infiltrated or urticarial plaques, papulovesicular lesions, nodules, and erythroderma (360). AITL has an aggressive clinical course, with a median survival of less than 3 years.

Histopathology. Involved lymph nodes show partial or complete architectural effacement with an interfollicular mixed polymorphous infiltrate of small- to medium-sized atypical lymphocytes with clear cytoplasm, plasma cells, eosinophils, epithelioid

histiocytes, and immunoblasts as well as prominent arborizing high-endothelial venules. Cutaneous lesions are generally subtle, and the morphologic features vary considerably. Patterns include a superficial perivascular lymphoid infiltrate with or without atypia; a dense superficial and deep perivascular atypical lymphoid infiltrate (Fig. 31-65A), often showing vascular hyperplasia; vasculitis (Fig. 31-65B); or necrotizing granulomas (359–361). The overlying epidermis is spared. When morphologically evident, the neoplastic infiltrate is composed of CD3$^+$/CD4$^+$ T cells, although frequent reactive CD8$^+$ T cells may be admixed (Fig. 31-65C). Coexpression of markers of follicular helper T-cell phenotype (CD10, PD-1, CXCL-13, BCL6, ICOS) is often seen in AITL (Fig. 31-65D). Scattered EBV$^+$ B cells may be present (Fig. 31-65E).

Histogenesis. TCR gene rearrangement studies of cutaneous lesions often display a clonal population identical to that detected in lymph nodes (360,362,363). Interestingly, clonal immunoglobulin gene rearrangements are detected in approximately a quarter of nodal AITL cases corresponding to the expanded EBV$^+$ B-cell population. These clonal B-cell populations may also be detected by molecular analysis in skin lesions of AITL (359).

Differential Diagnosis. Because of the subtle and wide spectrum of histopathologic manifestations, diagnosis of AITL involving the skin can be very challenging. The differential diagnosis is broad and includes inflammatory dermatoses with superficial or superficial and deep perivascular patterns, leukocytoclastic vasculitis, infection, sarcoidosis, and other primary granulomatous conditions. Use of immunohistochemistry to detect a T-cell population with expression of markers of follicular helper T cells in conjunction with molecular analysis comparing clones found in both skin and nodal sites may assist in diagnosis.

Principles of Management: Patients are treated according to their underlying systemic lymphoma.

Adult T-Cell Leukemia/Lymphoma

ATLL is a high-grade T-cell neoplasm caused by a retrovirus, human T-cell lymphotropic virus type 1 (HTLV-1).

Clinical Summary. ATLL occurs most often as an endemic disorder, primarily in Japan, the Caribbean basin, Central Africa, and parts of South America. The disease distribution is mirrored by the prevalence of HTLV-1 infection (364). The disease is also detected in populations in certain parts of the southeastern United States, where HTLV-1 seropositivity is high. The virus may be transmitted by blood and body fluids, and approximately 5% of infected patients develop an associated disease, including ATLL, HTLV-1-associated myelopathy/tropical spastic paraparesis (HAM/TSP), and infective dermatitis associated with HTLV-1 (IDH). Although infection often occurs at a young age, ATLL is a disease of adults (median age 55 years), reflecting a long latency period. The 2016 WHO classification system recognizes four subtypes: acute and chronic leukemic forms, smoldering form, and lymphomatous form. The disease may involve lymph nodes, peripheral blood, bone marrow, or other extranodal/extramedullary sites, and subtyping is based on the extent of disease and associated symptoms and signs. Regardless of the underlying subtype, patients frequently exhibit variable cutaneous manifestations, which range from multiple local to disseminated erythematous patches, papules, plaques, nodules, and

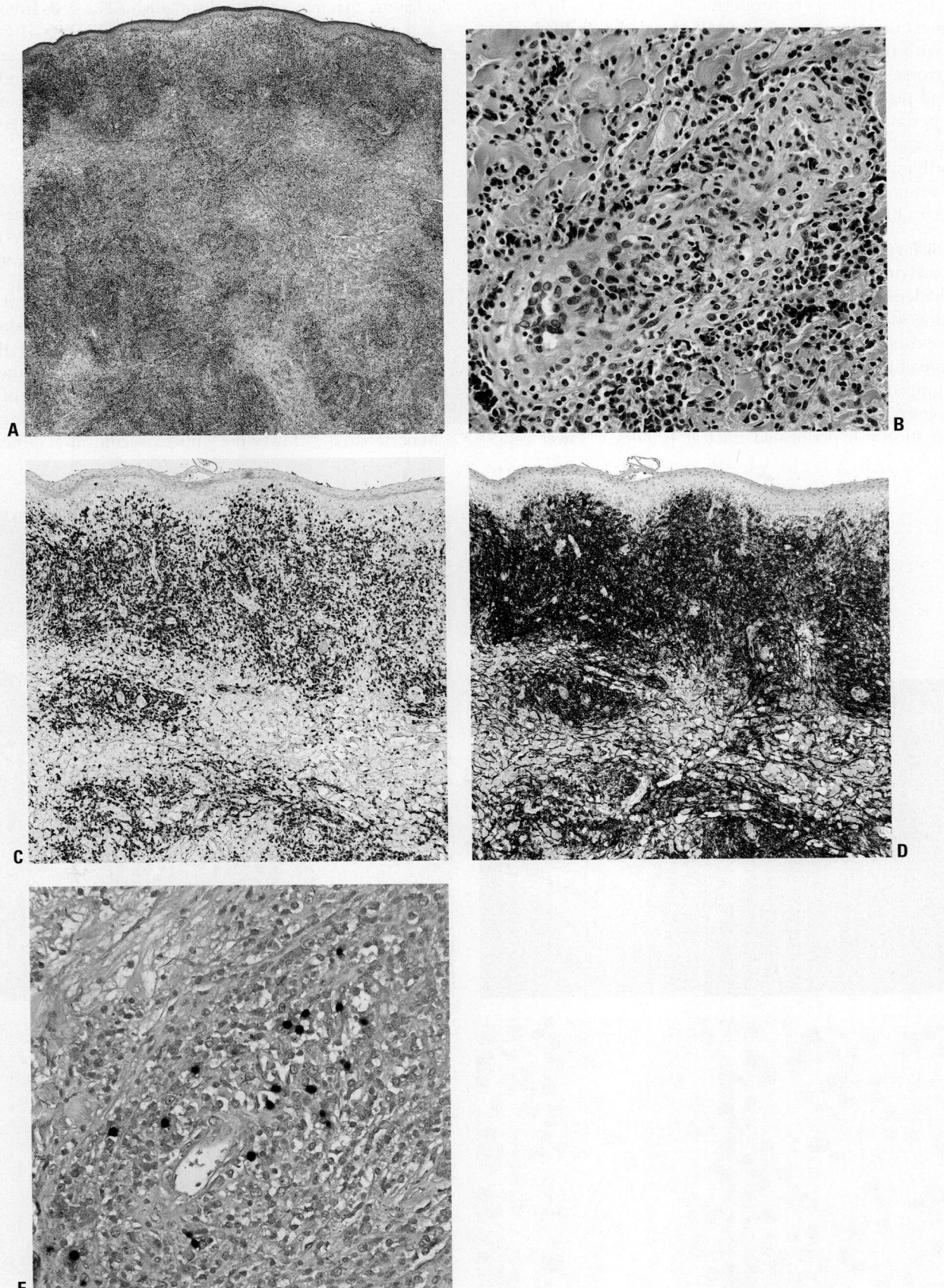

Figure 31-65 Angioimmunoblastic T-cell lymphoma. A: Dense superficial and deep perivascular atypical lymphoid infiltrate. B: Vasculitis. Immunohistochemical studies reveal that the CD3⁺ infiltrate (C) coexpresses CD10 (D). E: Admixed EBV⁺ B cells.

tumors to generalized erythroderma (Fig. 31-66A). In this way, the clinical presentation mimics MF. In general, individuals afflicted with the acute and lymphomatous types have a significantly worse prognosis, as do patients with the more recently described primary cutaneous tumoral ATLL, which lacks leukemic, nodal, or other lesions (364). The more indolent forms (chronic and smoldering) may evolve into the more aggressive acute or lymphomatous forms. The 4-year survival rates are 5% for the acute type, 5% to 7% for the lymphomatous type, 27% for the chronic type, and 63% for the smoldering type (365).

Histopathology. Skin lesions may show nodular to diffuse infiltrates of atypical lymphocytes and may exhibit papillary dermal involvement, epidermotropism, and/or Pautrier microabscess formation, mimicking MF (Fig. 31-66B). Cytologically, the neoplastic lymphocytes contain enlarged hyperchromatic nuclei with irregular, often convoluted nuclear profiles (Fig. 31-66C). Anaplastic cells with clumped nuclear chromatin and prominent nucleoli may also be observed. The peripheral blood contains atypical cells with characteristically hyperlobated nuclear profiles ("flower cells"),

a feature that may serve to distinguish ATLL cells from those of SS and systemically disseminated forms of MF (Fig. 31-66D). Tumor cells are CD4+ T cells that also express T-cell–associated antigens CD2, CD3, and CD5 but that generally lack CD7 and CD8. Rare cases that express CD8 but not CD4 or double-negative (CD4−/CD8−) cases may occur. Expression of CD25 and FoxP3 is also seen. Tumor cells may also express CD30.

Histogenesis. TCR gene rearrangements are present. Clonally integrated HTLV-1 is present, although additional genetic "hits" are needed for oncogenesis (366,367). The HTLV-1 transactivator, Tax, has been implicated as the viral oncoprotein (368).

Differential Diagnosis. The differential diagnosis primarily includes MF and SS, and distinction by histology alone may be impossible. Because most ATLL patients are not erythrodermic, this clinical feature may assist in differentiating the condition from SS. It should also be noted that the cytology of peripheral blood involvement in ATLL is distinctive, showing cells with hyperlobated, "flowerlike" nuclear contours rather than the

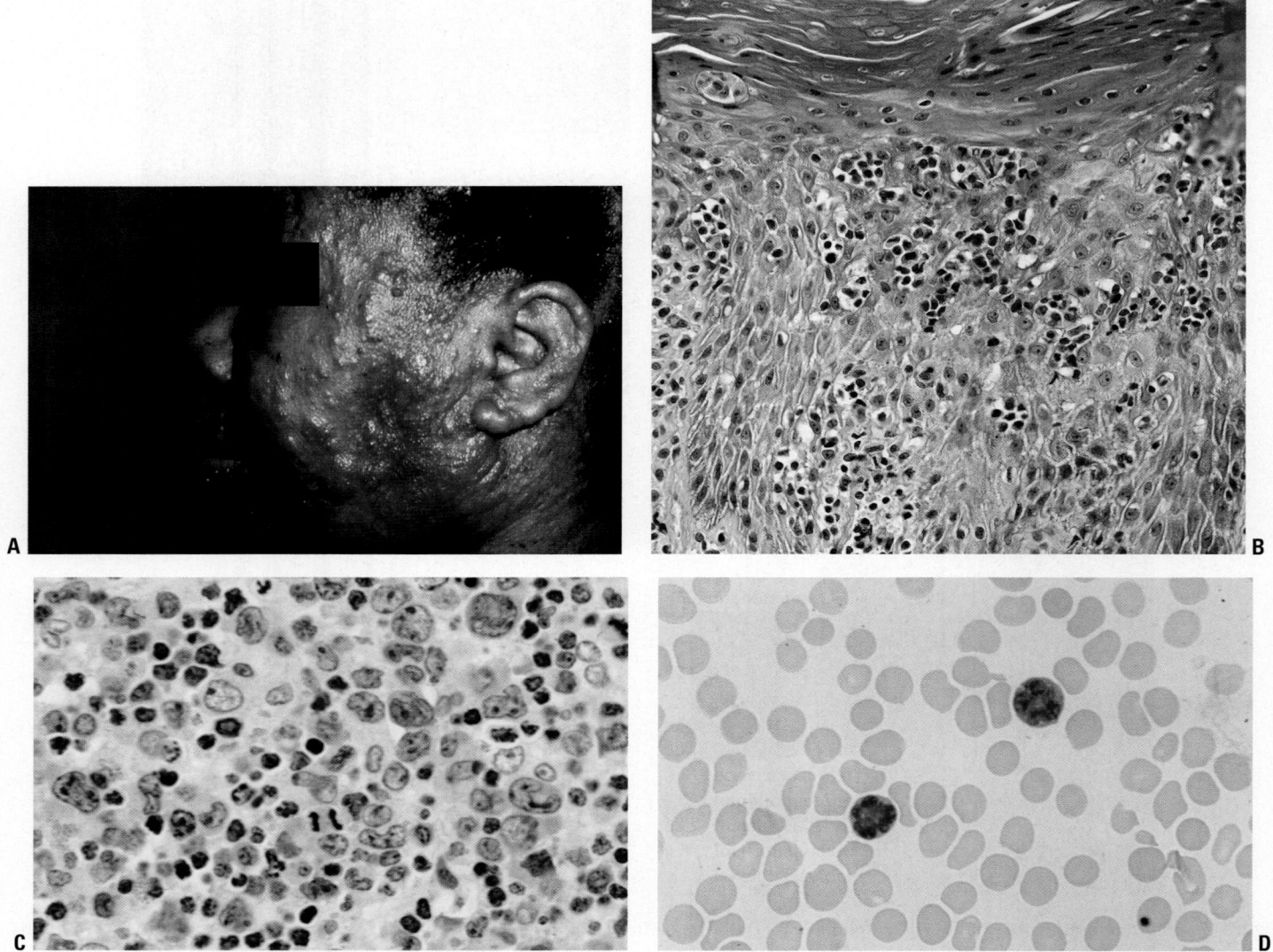

Figure 31-66 Adult T-cell leukemia/lymphoma. **A:** Clinical appearance, where multiple nodules explosively developed within several weeks in this patient with hypercalcemia. **B:** Epidermotropic atypical lymphocytes are indistinguishable by conventional paraffin histology from MF. **C:** Tissue infiltration by tumor cells with variably hyperchromatic and convoluted nuclear contours. **D:** Peripheral blood showing enlarged lymphoid cells with characteristically hyperlobated nuclear contours.

cerebriform nuclei of Sézary cells. In suspected cases of ATLL, HTLV-1 serology should be performed, although definitive diagnosis will ultimately depend on the demonstration of HTLV-1 gene integration within the malignant cells in skin or blood. Some of the anaplastic cases with CD30 expression may mimic ALCL, but ATLL does not demonstrate expression of the activated cytotoxic molecules perforin and granzyme B.

Principles of Management: Therapeutic interventions vary based on subtype and include antiretrovirals, monoclonal antibodies, chemotherapy, and allogeneic stem cell transplant (369).

Extranodal NK/T-Cell Lymphoma, Nasal Type
ENKTCL is an aggressive lymphoma characterized by angiocentric and angiodestructive infiltrates of EBV$^+$ malignant cells with an NK-cell or, rarely, a cytotoxic T-cell phenotype. The infiltrate often but not invariably involves tissues of the nasal cavity and may also be seen in extranodal/extranasal sites, including skin, soft tissue, gastrointestinal tract, and testis. Cutaneous involvement may be the primary manifestation of the disease ("primary cutaneous NK/T-cell lymphoma, nasal type") or may occur secondarily.

Clinical Summary. ENKTCL tends to affect adult males, with a geographical distribution showing concentration in Asia, Mexico, Central America, and South America. Cutaneous involvement manifests as rapidly growing reddish plaques or tumors, frequently with ulceration. Primary cutaneous involvement, defined as no evidence of extracutaneous disease on staging procedures, is typically followed by the development of clinically evident disease at extracutaneous sites (370). Regardless of whether the cutaneous involvement is primary or secondary, the disease follows a uniformly aggressive course (370,371).

Histopathology. The characteristic histopathology involves a diffuse, focally angiocentric, and angiodestructive dermal/subcutaneous infiltrate of variably sized, mitotically active lymphoid cells (Fig. 31-67A). Occasionally, focal epidermotropism is observed. Most commonly, cells are medium in size with irregular to elongated nuclei, coarse chromatin, inconspicuous nucleoli, and moderate quantities of pale cytoplasm (Fig. 31-67B). Some cases will show an admixture of reactive inflammatory cells, including activated lymphocytes, plasma cells, and eosinophils. Infiltration and fibrinoid necrosis of affected vessel walls, zones of coagulative necrosis, and apoptosis are characteristic findings (Fig. 31-67C). The epidermis or squamous epithelial mucosa may be ulcerated or, in some instances, may show florid pseudoepitheliomatous hyperplasia. The typical immunophenotype is surface CD3$^-$, cytoplasmic (ε chain) CD3$^+$, CD2$^+$, and CD56$^+$. Cytotoxic granule–associated proteins (TIA-1, granzyme B, perforin) are detected by immunohistochemistry, and reactivity for antibodies to CD4, CD5, CD8, CD16, CD57, TCR βF1, and the TCR gamma chain constant region is generally negative. EBER *in situ* hybridization should be used to document EBV positivity as immunohistochemical detection of latent membrane protein-1 (LMP-1) is inconsistent.

Histogenesis. The postulated cell of origin is the activated NK cell or, more rarely, the cytotoxic T cell. TCR and immunoglobulin genes are in the germline configuration in most cases. Frequent cytogenetic abnormalities have been detected, although a defining pathologic alteration has not been uncovered. There is a strong association with EBV, suggesting a possible causal role for this agent

(372). In rare CD56$^-$ cases, EBER *in situ* hybridization positivity and expression of cytotoxic proteins are required for diagnosis.

Differential Diagnosis. Some morphologic features of cutaneous ENKTCL overlap with those of other diseases; for example, focal epidermotropism may suggest MF, prominent subcutaneous involvement may suggest SPTCL, and angioinvasion may suggest PCGD-TCL or LYG. However, complete immunophenotyping should render the correct diagnosis in most cases. In addition, cases of tumor-stage MF may acquire a cytotoxic phenotype but will not be EBV$^+$. CD56 expression is not specific to ENKTCL and can also be seen in cutaneous involvement by BPDCN and, less commonly, myeloid sarcoma, primary cutaneous CD30+ T-cell lymphoproliferative disorders, MF, PCGD-TCL and peripheral T-cell lymphoma, not otherwise specified (PTCL, NOS).

Principles of Management: Localized nonnasal disease, or disseminated disease, requires systemic chemotherapy and, if feasible, directed radiotherapy (373).

Peripheral T-Cell Lymphoma, Not Otherwise Specified
PTCL, NOS is a heterogeneous group of nodal and extranodal T-cell neoplasms that do not meet the criteria for the other T-cell malignancies defined by the current classification scheme. In the skin, presentation is almost always secondary to systemic disease, although cutaneous lesions may be the first manifestation.

Clinical Summary. Most cases involve adults without gender predilection, although reports exist of children being affected. Clinical presentation generally involves constitutional symptoms and lymphadenopathy. Skin lesions may take the form of solitary, localized, or, more commonly, generalized eczematous plaques, nodules, or erythematous tumors; pruritus, peripheral eosinophilia, and hemophagocytic syndromes have also been described. The prognosis is poor; the 5-year survival rate ranges from 30% to 35%, even with standard chemotherapy (374).

Histopathology. Diffuse or nodular dermal and subcutaneous infiltrates with variable numbers of medium- to large-sized pleomorphic or immunoblast-like T cells are typical. Central ulceration may occur. Epidermotropism is generally mild or absent. Most cases show an aberrant CD4$^+$ T-cell phenotype with variable loss of pan-T-cell markers, such as CD5 and CD7.

Histogenesis. TCR genes are rearranged, but recurrent cytogenetic alterations are largely undefined given the heterogeneous nature of this entity.

Differential Diagnosis. Diagnosis of skin involvement by PTCL, NOS requires comprehensive clinical and immunophenotypic characterization to exclude involvement by any of the other primary or secondary CTCLs described herein.

Principles of Management: Patients are treated according to their underlying systemic lymphoma.

T-Cell Prolymphocytic Leukemia
T-cell prolymphocytic leukemia (T-PLL) is a relatively rare, aggressive neoplasm composed of T cells with a mature, postthymic phenotype. In addition to blood and bone marrow, sites of involvement include lymph nodes, liver, spleen, and skin (∼ 25% of cases) (375).

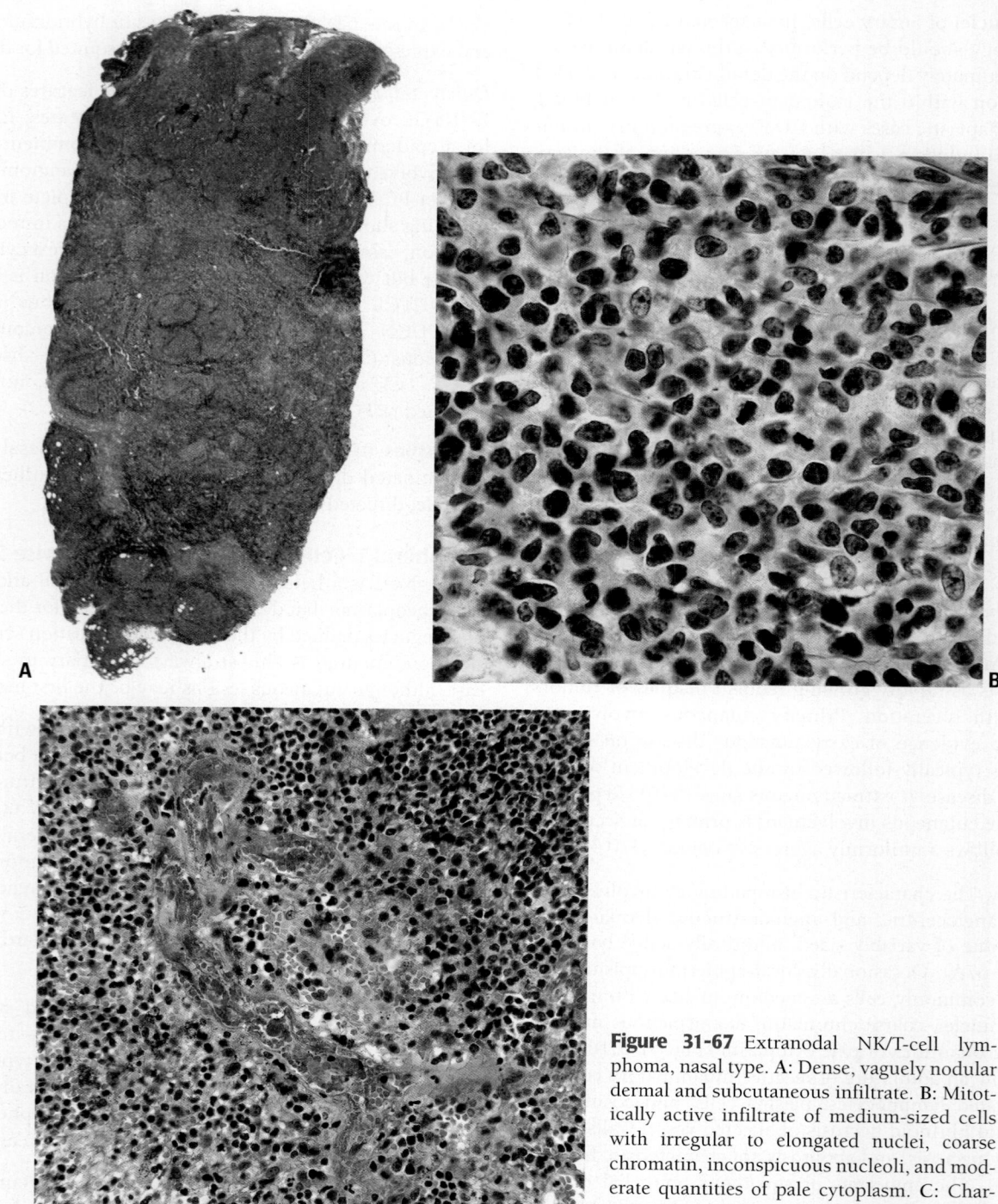

Figure 31-67 Extranodal NK/T-cell lymphoma, nasal type. **A:** Dense, vaguely nodular dermal and subcutaneous infiltrate. **B:** Mitotically active infiltrate of medium-sized cells with irregular to elongated nuclei, coarse chromatin, inconspicuous nucleoli, and moderate quantities of pale cytoplasm. **C:** Characteristic vascular infiltration and fibrinoid necrosis.

Clinical Summary. Most afflicted individuals are adults who present with generalized lymphadenopathy and enlargement of the spleen and liver. Anemia, thrombocytopenia, and atypical lymphocytosis (often >100 × 10⁹/L) are present; HTLV-1 serology is negative. Unlike SS, skin lesions are not erythrodermic but rather infiltrative. The leukemic infiltrates tend to form plaques and nodules that are variably erythematous to hemorrhagic in appearance.

Histopathology. Skin involvement takes the form of perivascular, periadnexal, or diffuse dermal infiltrates without epidermotropism (Fig. 31-68A). The cytologic details are best appreciated within the peripheral blood. The small- to intermediate-sized lymphoid cells exhibit round to irregular nuclear contours and frequently distinct nucleoli. Although the nuclear contours may sometimes be so irregular as to mimic the cerebriform contours of Sézary cells (375), the hallmark of T-PLL is the presence of cytoplasmic blebs (Fig. 31-68B). The neoplastic cells show intact expression of pan-T-cell antigens (CD2, CD5, and CD7) and often dim expression of surface CD3. The cells are frequently CD4⁺, although 25% of cases will show double positivity for CD4 and CD8, which is a helpful clue in the

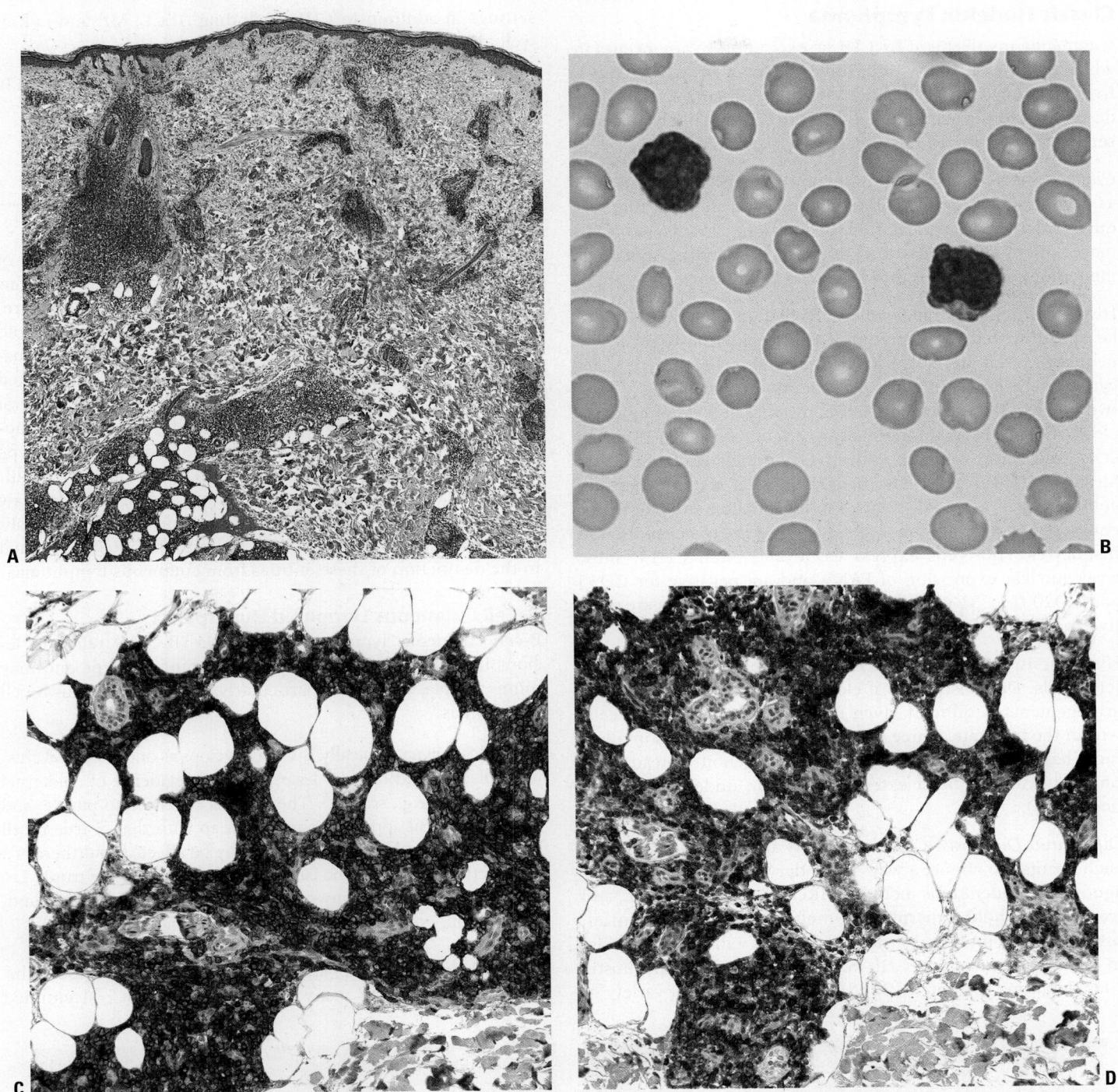

Figure 31-68 T-prolymphocytic leukemia. **A:** Perivascular dermal infiltrate without epidermotropism. **B:** Circulating cells exhibit round to irregular nuclear contours, distinct nucleoli, and cytoplasmic blebs. Immunohistochemistry studies demonstrate coexpression of CD4 (**C**) and CD8 (**D**) in 25% of cases, a feature essentially unique to this diagnosis among mature T-cell neoplasms.

distinction from other mature T-cell neoplasms (Fig. 31-68C, D). Exclusive CD8 expression is less common. Expression of the oncogene *TCL1* as detected by immunohistochemistry is also seen in cases of T-PLL.

Histogenesis. TCR genes are rearranged. Eighty percent of patients show inversion of chromosome 14 with breakpoints involving the long arm at q11 and q32 (376,377).

Differential Diagnosis. T-PLL must be differentiated from other forms of T-cell lymphoma showing skin involvement and a leukemic phase, such as SS, ATLL, and T-ALL. The clinical features

at presentation, absence of epidermotropism, absence of HTLV-1 positivity, characteristic cytoplasmic blebbing in peripheral blood smears, and coexpression of CD4 and CD8 (a feature virtually unique to T-PLL among mature T-cell neoplasms) should all assist in rendering a diagnosis of T-PLL. Unlike T-ALL, T-PLL cells do not express TdT, CD34, or CD1a (378).

Principles of Management: T-PLL is an aggressive disease that demonstrates a refractory response to conventional chemotherapy. Patients are often treated with the anti-CD52 antibody alemtuzumab, followed by autologous or allogeneic stem cell transplant.

Classic Hodgkin Lymphoma

Cutaneous involvement by CHL is exceedingly rare, occurs in advanced disease, and is indicative of a poor prognosis (379). Evidence suggests that the incidence is decreasing since its first description at the beginning of the 20th century, likely as a consequence of improved therapeutic interventions.

Clinical Summary. Cutaneous involvement by CHL manifests as asymptomatic erythematous papules and nodules that frequently demonstrate ulceration. In addition, patients with CHL may exhibit nonneoplastic skin lesions, including hyperpigmentation, urticaria, erythroderma, and alopecia.

Histopathology. Skin involvement by CHL manifests as a nodular or diffuse dermal infiltration without epidermotropism. The neoplastic cells are called Reed–Sternberg cells, and they are cytologically large in size with abundant cytoplasm and at least two nuclear lobes, each containing prominent eosinophilic nucleoli (Fig. 31-69A). Mononuclear variants are called Hodgkin cells, and these cells are collectively termed Hodgkin/Reed–Sternberg (HRS) cells. The neoplastic cells are the minority component of a mixed, nonneoplastic inflammatory infiltrate composed of small lymphocytes, plasma cells, eosinophils, and histiocytes. HRS cells express CD30 and often CD15, show weak nuclear expression of PAX5, and are negative for CD45 and CD20 (Fig. 31-69B). In some cases, the HRS cells are positive by EBER *in situ* hybridization.

Histogenesis. HRS cells are derived from mature germinal center B cells. Demonstration of clonal immunoglobulin gene rearrangements is difficult given the paucity of neoplastic cells within the infiltrate. Three mechanisms for cutaneous involvement have been proposed, namely, hematogenous spread, lymphatic spread, or direct extension from an underlying lymph node (379).

Differential Diagnosis. CHL only rarely involves the skin, and such events are almost always secondary to nodal disease. Diagnostic considerations include THRLBCL, DLBCL, ALCL, and reactive lymphoid hyperplasia. Careful correlation of clinical, histologic, and immunophenotypic features will generally assist in definitively excluding CHL from these differential diagnostic considerations. Of note, CD30+ cells may occur in a variety of settings in addition to CHL, including ALCL, MF, and LyP, as well as in reactive conditions (380).

Principles of Management: Patients are treated according to their underlying systemic lymphoma.

NONNEOPLASTIC PROLIFERATIONS

Cutaneous Lymphoid Hyperplasia

Critical to the consideration of B- and T-cell malignancies of the skin is an understanding of the patterns and compositions inherent to forms of cutaneous lymphoid hyperplasia. The term *pseudolymphoma* is often used to describe cutaneous lymphoid proliferations that are histologically similar to true lymphomatous infiltrates but are either idiopathic or etiologically related to drug exposure, infection, or other exogenous causes. Several classification systems have been proposed for pseudolymphomas, some of which argue that distinctions based on cell type are arbitrary (381). Herein, we will separately describe proliferations that are B-cell or T-cell predominant, in order to draw comparisons to the cutaneous lymphomas described previously. In all cases, careful incorporation of clinical findings is essential in the distinction of these entities from cutaneous lymphomas.

B-Cell Cutaneous Lymphoid Hyperplasia

B-cell cutaneous lymphoid hyperplasia (B-CLH) refers to lesions in which B cells are the predominant cell type and may mimic neoplastic entities, particularly primary cutaneous B-cell lymphomas.

Clinical Summary. Typically, B-CLH develops as one or several clustered plaques and nodular lesions without evidence of epidermal involvement (e.g., scaling). The color is often red to purple, and thus the clinical appearance may overlap with that of true B-cell lymphoma (Fig. 31-70A). Any site may be affected, but there is a predilection for skin of the face and scalp as well as the trunk. Lesions may persist for many months before resolution occurs, and, on occasion, evolution to lymphoma has been documented.

Histopathology. Infiltrates may show a nodular or diffuse architecture, and although many lesions will be most concentrated

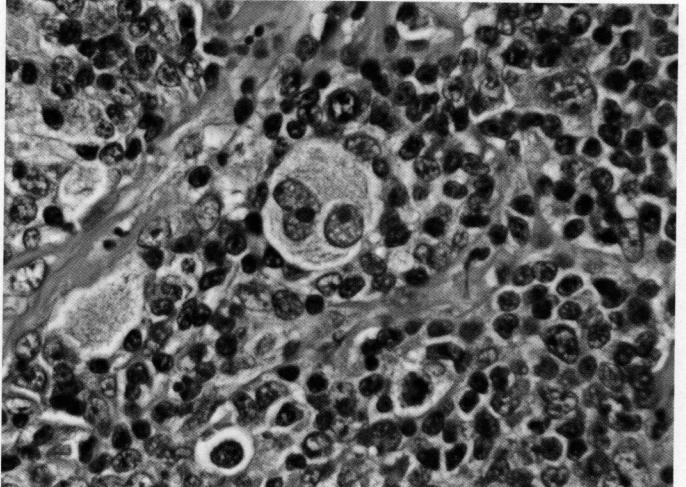

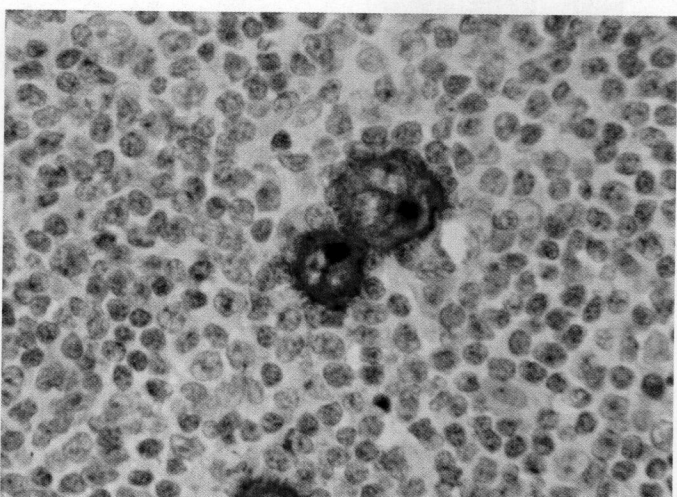

Figure 31-69 Classic Hodgkin lymphoma. CHL showing pleomorphic infiltrate and a characteristic Reed–Sternberg cell (**A**) that is reactive for the CD30 antigen (**B**).

in the more superficial dermal layers, equal or preferential involvement of the deeper dermis and subcutis may be seen (Fig. 31-70B, C). This "bottom-heavy" pattern of infiltration, which, by convention, has been associated with B-cell malignancies, does not reliably permit exclusion of B-CLH. Unlike true B-cell lymphoma, however, hyperplastic B-cell infiltrates generally do not exhibit a pattern of infiltration that destroys preexisting structures (e.g., vessels, adnexa). While hair follicles may be distorted and hyperplastic in certain cases where primary follicular pathology presumably incites the B-cell proliferative response (the so-called pseudolymphomatous folliculitis), this is distinct from secondary follicular injury that may be seen in the setting of true lymphoma.

The hallmark of B-CLH is the formation of true lymphoid follicles (Fig. 31-71A). These follicles contain a cytologic continuum of B-cell maturation and exhibit lymphocytes with small and large, cleaved and uncleaved nuclear contours (Fig. 31-71B, C), immunoblasts, and tingible-body macrophages. Mitotic figures and apoptotic cells may be numerous in follicles, showing florid evidence of immune activation (Fig. 31-71D). There tends to be aggregation of centroblasts

and tingible-body macrophages at one pole of the hyperplastic follicle and of centrocytes at the opposite pole, producing darker- and lighter-staining regions, respectively (polarization). Reactive follicles may show expanded mantle zones, whereas follicle-like structures formed in certain B-cell lymphomas tend to show thinned or absent mantle zones. Aberrant antigen expression (e.g., CD43 expression in CD20$^+$ B cells or BCL2 expression in germinal center B cells) is not present (382). Immunoglobulin heavy chain gene rearrangements are usually not present, although clonal proliferations within B-CLH have been described (383,384), and this feature alone should not be used to separate reactive from malignant infiltrates of B cells.

Histogenesis. The cause is often unknown, although persistent localized immune responses to injected or extruded antigens, as may occur with arthropod bite assaults, localized infection with the spirochete *B. burgdorferi*, or even in the context of follicular cyst rupture, have been implicated. Certain drugs may also result in B-cell as well as T-cell pattern cutaneous infiltrates that may mimic lymphoma both clinically and histologically (385).

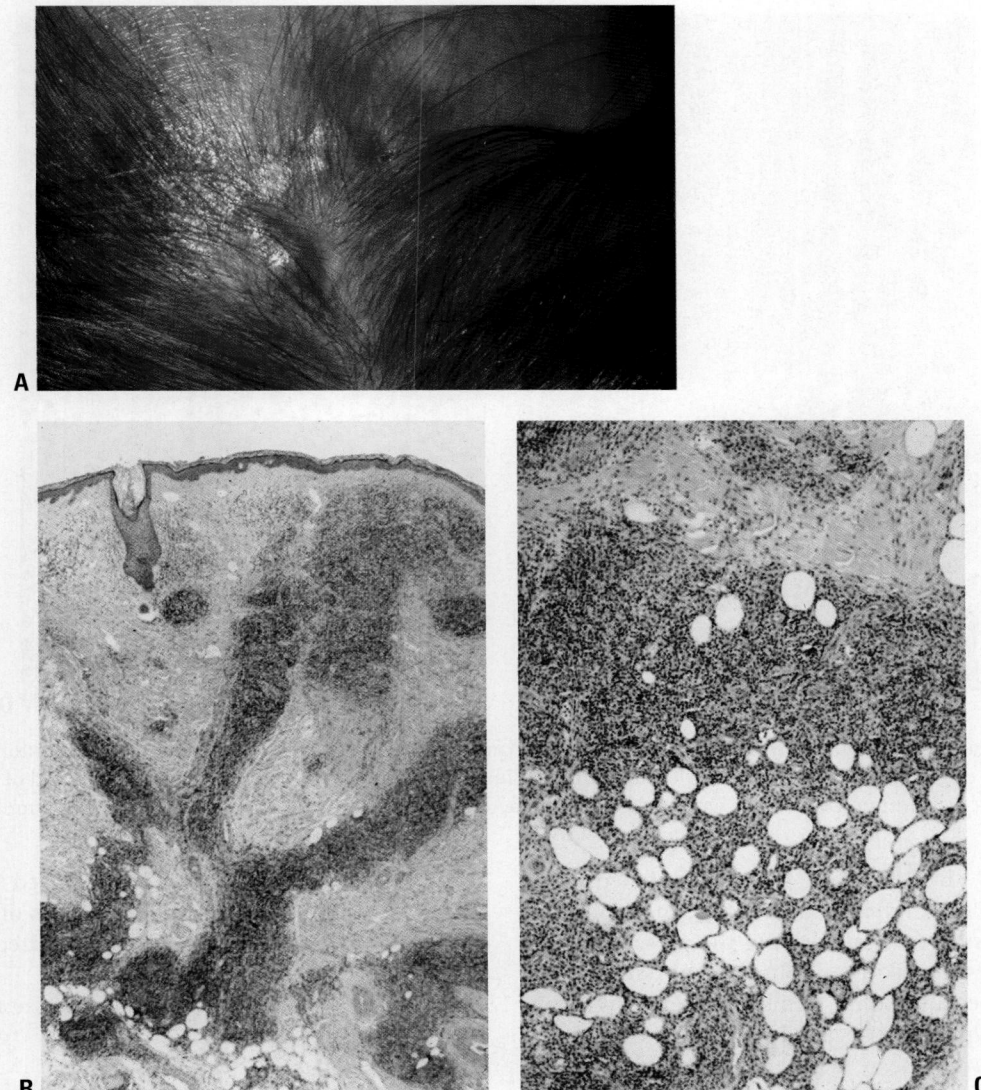

Figure 31-70 B-cell cutaneous lymphoid hyperplasia. **A:** Clinical lesions. **B:** Scanning magnification of dermal infiltrate. **C:** Involvement of deep dermis and subcutis.

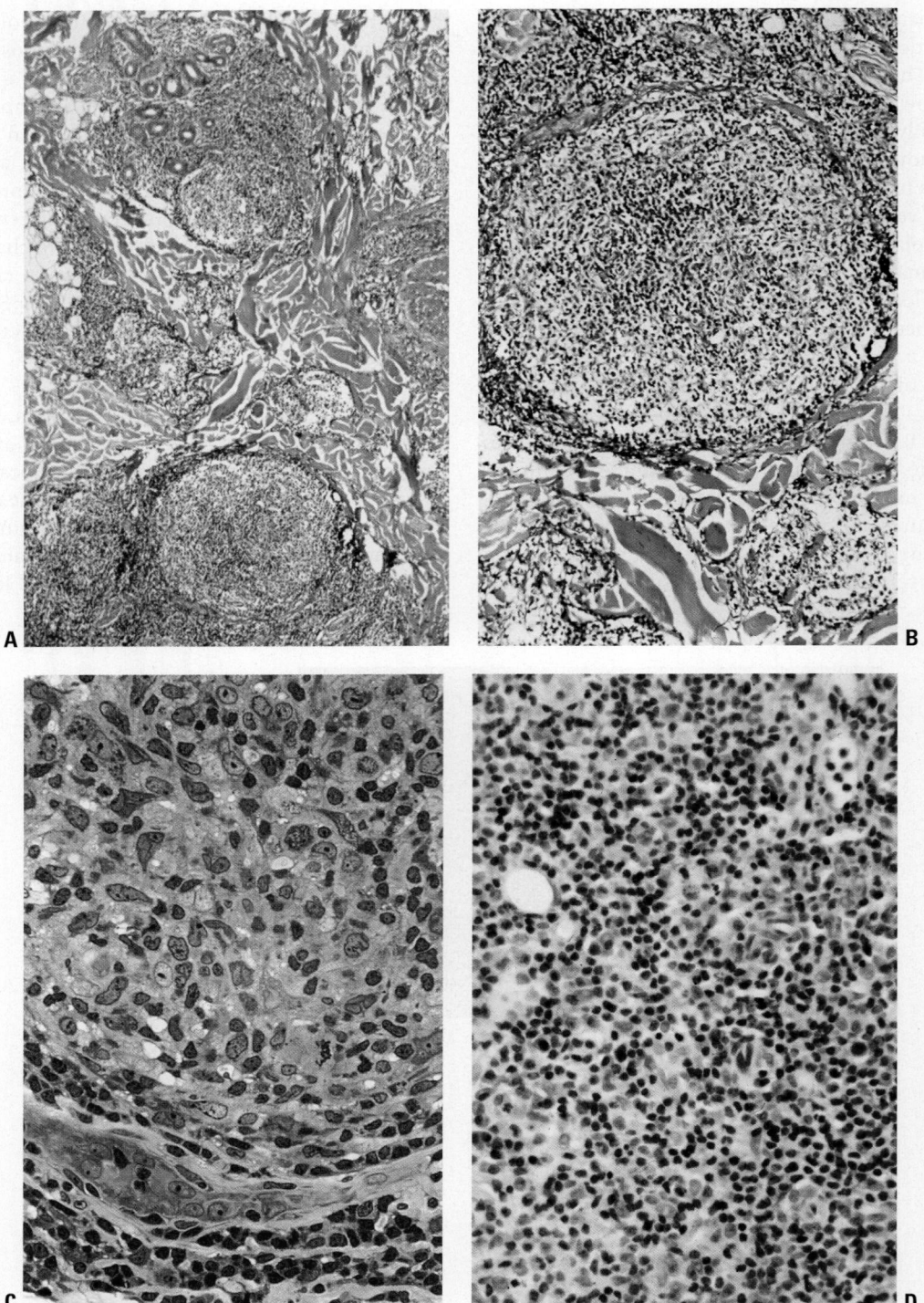

Figure 31-71 B-cell cutaneous lymphoid hyperplasia. **A:** Nodular dermal infiltration by lymphoid cells with formation of germinal centers. **B:** Higher magnification of germinal center. **C:** One-micron, toluidine blue–stained section of germinal center composed of admixture of lymphocytes in various stages of maturation. **D:** Reactive germinal center characterized by mitotically active follicular center lymphocytes.

Differential Diagnosis. B-CLH must be differentiated from PCFCL using morphologic, immunophenotypic, and molecular features. It is noteworthy that establishing the presence of reactive germinal centers in a skin infiltrate does not definitively exclude lymphoma because some forms of B-cell lymphoma such as PCMZL are typically associated with admixed reactive follicles. Moreover, as has been mentioned, patients with established B-CLH must be monitored over time in recognition of the fact that on occasion this presentation will be a harbinger of eventual development of a clonal B-cell malignancy (46).

Numerous eosinophils may be observed in association with some forms of B-CLH, including lesions of angiolymphoid hyperplasia with eosinophilia and its localized variants.

Principles of Management: Patients are treated according to their underlying condition.

T-Cell Cutaneous Lymphoid Hyperplasia

T-cell cutaneous lymphoid hyperplasia (T-CLH) refers to the occurrence of epidermotropic cutaneous immune responses composed of activated/proliferative T cells that produce a pattern that may mimic MF and its variants.

Clinical Summary. Because these conditions all share the feature of epitheliotropism, they—like various forms of MF—may be associated with the formation of scaling erythematous and variably indurated patches and plaques and, occasionally, with foci of alopecia. On occasion, subacute to chronic spongiotic or lichenoid dermatitis may be associated with lymphoid epidermotropism in the relative absence of intercellular edema or apoptosis, thus bringing to mind consideration of possible T-cell dyscrasia. Certain immune responses may also show a T-cell pattern in the setting of drug-induced immune dysregulation and therefore mimic T-cell dyscrasia or lymphoma.

Histopathology. Dermatitis with exocytosis in the relative absence of associated spongiosis or evidence of cytotoxic injury will generally show more typical findings on evaluation of deeper sections. Multiple biopsies may occasionally be required to better assess the sequential evolution of lesions and to identify stages where more characteristic inflammatory changes predominate. The finding of Langerhans cell microgranulomas (114) favors a reactive process, although care must be taken not to confuse these structures with true Pautrier microabscesses (Fig. 31-72A). Importantly, many examples of T-cell pattern lymphomatoid dermatitis will lack the uniform cytologic atypia within the epidermotropic component more characteristically seen in MF. An exception to this, however, are T-cell pattern reactive infiltrates occurring in patients with altered immune function, as may be seen in certain lymphomatoid drug eruptions (Fig. 31-72B) (385). In these settings, cytologically atypical epidermotropic infiltrates may closely mimic MF and may even show immunophenotypic (e.g., diminished CD7 expression) or genotypic (e.g., TCR gene rearrangements) abnormalities that are reversible on drug cessation (386).

Histogenesis. The histogenesis of T-cell pattern drug-induced lymphoid dyscrasia seems to relate to the concurrence of cutaneous hypersensitivity reactions caused by drugs that are themselves capable of inciting some level of immune dysregulation. These drugs include anticonvulsants, antidepressants, phenothiazines, calcium channel blockers, and angiotensin-converting enzyme inhibitors.

Differential Diagnosis. The primary differential diagnosis is the T-cell pattern immune response in the setting of immune dysregulation. Careful consideration of clinical factors, including duration of lesions, response to previous therapy, and potential relationship to drugs that influence lymphocyte function should be undertaken before definitively excluding a lymphomatoid drug eruption in the differential diagnosis of epidermotropic T-cell malignancies.

Principles of Management: Patients are treated according to their underlying condition.

Extramedullary Hematopoiesis

Extramedullary hematopoiesis refers to trilineage maturation of hematopoietic elements in tissues other than the bone marrow. In the skin, the process has been referred to as *dermal hematopoiesis*. Occasionally, extramedullary hematopoiesis is restricted to cells of erythroid lineage, a phenomenon termed *dermal erythropoiesis*, which may occur as compensatory erythropoiesis in neonates in association with the stress of various viral infections or hemoglobinopathies (387). In adults, this phenomenon is most commonly seen in the setting of a myeloproliferative neoplasm, and it has been proposed that this represents neoplastic involvement of the skin (388).

Clinical Summary. Lesions typically present as macules, papules, and, occasionally, nodules that have a dull blue-red hue. Dermal hematopoiesis in neonates tends to affect the head and neck (the so-called blueberry muffin rash). In adults, cutaneous extramedullary hematopoiesis manifests as firm, pink-purple, raised papules and nodules and frequently involves the trunk.

Histopathology. Poorly formed micronodules of pleomorphic cells are present in the dermis, and the pattern may initially mimic leukemia cutis or an unusual dermal inflammatory reaction. Maturing erythrocytes can be identified as clustered "colonies" of cells containing round basophilic nuclei rimmed by eosinophilic cytoplasm. Admixed myeloblasts, metamyelocytes, and characteristically large megakaryocytes containing prominently multilobated nuclei are often also present. These latter cells are reactive for CD61, a helpful marker in further confirming their lineage identity.

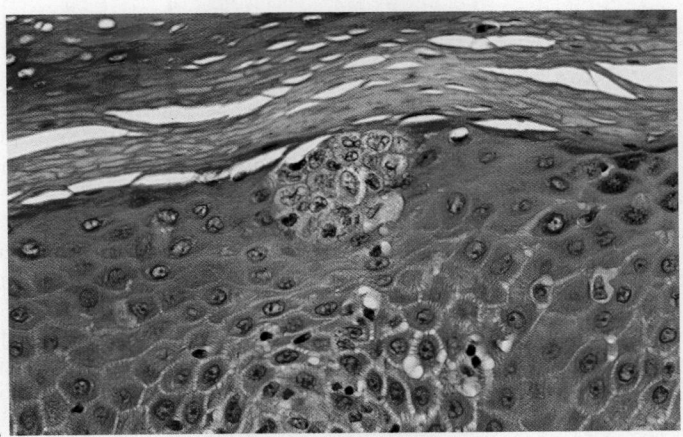
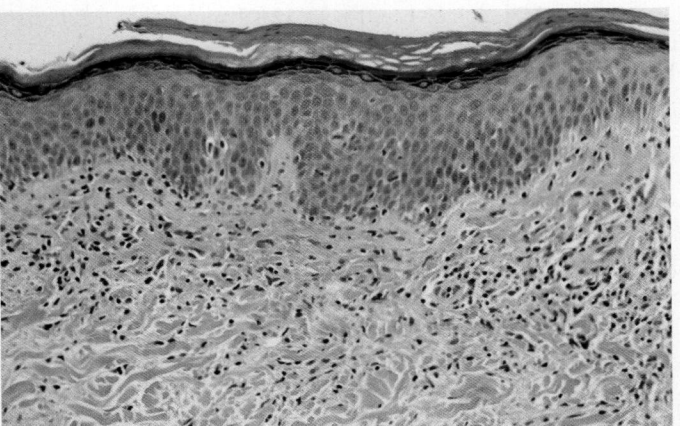

Figure 31-72 T-cell cutaneous lymphoid hyperplasia. A: Langerhans cell microgranuloma associated with T-cell immune response may mimic Pautrier microabscess. B: Lymphomatoid drug eruption, with papillary dermal interstitial and focally epidermotropic infiltrate of variably activated lymphocytes in a characteristic T-cell pattern.

Histogenesis. Although normal hematopoiesis occurs in the bone marrow, the occurrence of extramedullary hematopoiesis in the skin and other tissues underscores the fact that under certain conditions, extramedullary tissues contain the appropriate precursor cells and growth factors to serve as surrogates for the marrow microenvironment.

Differential Diagnosis. Extramedullary hematopoiesis in the skin must be distinguished from reactive and dysplastic polymorphous infiltrates that may contain large, atypical cells and from forms of leukemia cutis that harbor cells with primitive myeloid features. Clinical information may be helpful in determining whether patients have predisposing factors for this phenomenon. The morphologic identification of erythropoiesis and the presence of megakaryocytes, and further confirmation of the latter via immunohistochemistry for CD61, should assist in those rare circumstances when true extramedullary hematopoiesis is detected in the skin.

Principles of Management: Patients are treated according to their underlying condition.

REFERENCES

1. Swerdlow SH, Campo E, Harris NL, et al. *WHO Classification of Tumours of Haematopoietic and Lymphoid Tissues.* Rev. 4th ed. International Agency for Research on Cancer; 2017.
2. Elder D, Massi D, Scolyer R, Willemze R. *WHO Classification of Skin Tumors.* 4th ed. IARC Press; 2018.
3. LeBoit PE, McCalmont TH. Cutaneous lymphomas and leukemias. In: Elder DE, Elenitsas R, Jaworsky C, Johnson BL, eds. *Lever's Histopathology of the Skin.* 8th ed. Lippincott-Raven Publishers; 1995:805.
4. Murphy GF, Schwarting R. Cutaneous lymphomas and leukemias. In: Elder DE, Elenitsas R, Johnson BL, Murphy GF, eds. *Lever's Histopathology of the Skin.* 9th ed. Lippincott Williams & Wilkins; 2005:927.
5. Hsu MY, Murphy GF. Cutaneous lymphomas and leukemias. In: Elder DE, Elenitsas R, Johnson BL, Murphy GF, Xu X, eds. *Lever's Histopathology of the Skin.* 10th ed. Lippincott Williams & Wilkins; 2009:911.
6. Murphy GF, Mihm MC Jr. Benign, dysplastic and malignant lymphoid infiltrates of skin: an approach based on pattern analysis. In: Murphy GF, Mihm MC Jr, eds. *Lymphoproliferative Disorders of the Skin.* Butterworths; 1986:123.
7. Wayner EA, Gil SG, Murphy GF, Wilke MS, Carter WG. Epiligrin, a component of epithelial basement membranes, is an adhesive ligand for alpha 3 beta 1 positive T lymphocytes. *J Cell Biol.* 1993;121(5):1141.
8. Murphy GF, Liu V. The dermal immune system. In: Bos JD, ed. *The Skin Immune System (SIS): Cutaneous Immunology and Clinical Immunodermatology.* 2nd ed. CRC Press; 1997:347.
9. Murphy GF. The secret of "NIN": a novel neural immunological network potentially integral to immunologic function in human skin. In: Nickoloff BJ, ed. *Mast Cells, Macrophages and Dendritic Cells in Skin Disease.* CRC Press; 1993:227.
10. Nickoloff BJ. Epidermal mucinosis in mycosis fungoides. *J Am Acad Dermatol.* 1986;15(1):83.
11. Willemze R, Cerroni L, Kempf W, et al. The 2018 update of the WHO-EORTC classification for primary cutaneous lymphomas. *Blood.* 2019;133(16):1703–1714.
12. Gerami P, Wickless SC, Querfeld C, Rosen ST, Kuzel TM, Guitart J. Cutaneous involvement with marginal zone lymphoma. *J Am Acad Dermatol.* 2010;63(1):142.
13. Suarez AL, Pulitzer M, Horwitz S, Moskowitz A, Querfeld C, Myskowski PL. Primary cutaneous B-cell lymphomas: Part I.

Clinical features, diagnosis, and classification. *J Am Acad Dermatol.* 2013;69(3):329.e1.
14. Goodlad JR, Davidson MM, Hollowood K, et al. Primary cutaneous B-cell lymphoma and *Borrelia burgdorferi* infection in patients from the Highlands of Scotland. *Am J Surg Pathol.* 2000;24(9):1279–1285.
15. Slater DN. *Borrelia burgdorferi*-associated primary cutaneous B-cell lymphoma. *Histopathology.* 2001;38(1):73.
16. Wood GS, Kamath NV, Guitart J, et al. Absence of *Borrelia burgdorferi* DNA in cutaneous B-cell lymphomas from the United States. *J Cutan Pathol.* 2001;28(10):502.
17. Li C, Inagaki H, Kuo TT, Hu S, Okabe M, Eimoto T. Primary cutaneous marginal zone B-cell lymphoma: a molecular and clinicopathologic study of 24 Asian cases. *Am J Surg Pathol.* 2003;27(8):1061.
18. Goteri G, Ranaldi R, Simonetti O, et al. Clinicopathological features of primary cutaneous B-cell lymphomas from an academic regional hospital in central Italy: no evidence of *Borrelia burgdorferi* association. *Leuk Lymphoma.* 2007;48(11):2184.
19. Takino H, Li C, Hu S, et al. Primary cutaneous marginal zone B-cell lymphoma: a molecular and clinicopathological study of cases from Asia, Germany, and the United States. *Mod Pathol.* 2008;21(12):1517–1526.
20. Magro CM, Yang A, Fraga G. Blastic marginal zone lymphoma: a clinical and pathological study of 8 cases and review of the literature. *Am J Dermatopathol.* 2013;35(3):319.
21. Edinger JT, Kant JA, Swerdlow SH. Cutaneous marginal zone lymphomas have distinctive features and include 2 subsets. *Am J Surg Pathol.* 2010;34(12):1830.
22. van Maldegem F, van Dijk R, Wormhoudt TA, et al. The majority of cutaneous marginal zone B-cell lymphomas expresses class-switched immunoglobulins and develops in a T-helper type 2 inflammatory environment. *Blood.* 2008;112(8):3355–3361.
23. Carlsen ED, Swerdlow SH, Cook JR, Gibson SE. Class-switched primary cutaneous marginal zone lymphomas are frequently IgG4-positive and have features distinct from IgM-positive cases. *Am J Surg Pathol.* 2019;43(10):1403–1412.
24. Felcht M, Booken N, Stroebel P, Goerdt S, Klemke CD. The value of molecular diagnostics in primary cutaneous B-cell lymphomas in the context of clinical findings, histology, and immunohistochemistry. *J Am Acad Dermatol.* 2011;64(1):135.
25. Evans PA, Pott C, Groenen PJ, et al. Significantly improved PCR-based clonality testing in B-cell malignancies by use of multiple immunoglobulin gene targets. Report of the BIOMED-2 concerted action BHM4-CT98-3936. *Leukemia.* 2007;21(2):207.
26. Streubel B, Lamprecht A, Dierlamm J, et al. T(14;18)(q32;q21) involving IGH and MALT1 is a frequent chromosomal aberration in MALT lymphoma. *Blood.* 2003;101(6):2335.
27. Streubel B, Simonitsch-Klupp I, Mullauer L, et al. Variable frequencies of MALT lymphoma-associated genetic aberrations in MALT lymphomas of different sites. *Leukemia.* 2004;18(10):1722.
28. Hallermann C, Kaune KM, Gesk S, et al. Molecular cytogenetic analysis of chromosomal breakpoints in the IGH, MYC, BCL6, and MALT1 gene loci in primary cutaneous B-cell lymphomas. *J Invest Dermatol.* 2004;123(1):213.
29. Streubel B, Vinatzer U, Lamprecht A, Raderer M, Chott A. T(3;14)(p14.1;q32) involving IGH and FOXP1 is a novel recurrent chromosomal aberration in MALT lymphoma. *Leukemia.* 2005;19(4):652.
30. Schreuder MI, Hoefnagel JJ, Jansen PM, van Krieken JH, Willemze R, Hebeda KM. FISH analysis of MALT lymphoma-specific translocations and aneuploidy in primary cutaneous marginal zone lymphoma. *J Pathol.* 2005;205(3):302.
31. Wongchaowart NT, Kim B, Hsi ED, Swerdlow SH, Tubbs RR, Cook JR. t(14;18)(q32;q21) involving IGH and MALT1 is uncommon in cutaneous MALT lymphomas and primary cutaneous diffuse large B-cell lymphomas. *J Cutan Pathol.* 2006;33(4):286.

32. Palmedo G, Hantschke M, Rutten A, et al. Primary cutaneous marginal zone B-cell lymphoma may exhibit both the t(14;18)(q32;q21) IGH/BCL2 and the t(14;18)(q32;q21) IGH/MALT1 translocation: an indicator for clonal transformation towards higher-grade B-cell lymphoma? *Am J Dermatopathol.* 2007;29(3):231.

33. de Leval L, Harris NL, Longtine J, Ferry JA, Duncan LM. Cutaneous b-cell lymphomas of follicular and marginal zone types: use of Bcl-6, CD10, Bcl-2, and CD21 in differential diagnosis and classification. *Am J Surg Pathol.* 2001;25(6):732.

34. Bayerl MG, Hennessy J, Ehmann WC, Bagg A, Rosamilia L, Clarke LE. Multiple cutaneous monoclonal B-cell proliferations as harbingers of systemic angioimmunoblastic T-cell lymphoma. *J Cutan Pathol.* 2010;37(7):777.

35. Senff NJ, Noordijk EM, Kim YH, et al. European Organization for Research and Treatment of Cancer and International Society for Cutaneous Lymphoma consensus recommendations for the management of cutaneous B-cell lymphomas. *Blood.* 2008;112(5):1600.

36. Goodlad JR, Krajewski AS, Batstone PJ, et al. Primary cutaneous follicular lymphoma: a clinicopathologic and molecular study of 16 cases in support of a distinct entity. *Am J Surg Pathol.* 2002;26(6):733.

37. Swerdlow SH, Quintanilla-Martinez L, Willemze R, Kinney MC. Cutaneous B-cell lymphoproliferative disorders: report of the 2011 Society for Hematopathology/European Association for Haematopathology workshop. *Am J Clin Pathol.* 2013;139(4):515.

38. Aguilera NS, Tomaszewski MM, Moad JC, Bauer FA, Taubenberger JK, Abbondanzo SL. Cutaneous follicle center lymphoma: a clinicopathologic study of 19 cases. *Mod Pathol.* 2001;14(9):828.

39. Mirza I, Macpherson N, Paproski S, et al. Primary cutaneous follicular lymphoma: an assessment of clinical, histopathologic, immunophenotypic, and molecular features. *J Clin Oncol.* 2002;20(3):647.

40. Kim BK, Surti U, Pandya A, Cohen J, Rabkin MS, Swerdlow SH. Clinicopathologic, immunophenotypic, and molecular cytogenetic fluorescence in situ hybridization analysis of primary and secondary cutaneous follicular lymphomas. *Am J Surg Pathol.* 2005;29(1):69.

41. Gulia A, Saggini A, Wiesner T, et al. Clinicopathologic features of early lesions of primary cutaneous follicle center lymphoma, diffuse type: implications for early diagnosis and treatment. *J Am Acad Dermatol.* 2011;65(5):991.

42. Vergier B, Belaud-Rotureau MA, Benassy MN, et al. Neoplastic cells do not carry bcl2-JH rearrangements detected in a subset of primary cutaneous follicle center B-cell lymphomas. *Am J Surg Pathol.* 2004;28(6):748.

43. Streubel B, Scheucher B, Valencak J, et al. Molecular cytogenetic evidence of t(14;18)(IGH;BCL2) in a substantial proportion of primary cutaneous follicle center lymphomas. *Am J Surg Pathol.* 2006;30(4):529.

44. Barasch NJK, Liu YC, Ho J, et al. The molecular landscape and other distinctive features of primary cutaneous follicle center lymphoma. *Hum Pathol.* 2020;106:93–105.

45. Zhou XA, Yang J, Ringbloom KG, et al. Genomic landscape of cutaneous follicular lymphomas reveals 2 subgroups with clinically predictive molecular features. *Blood Adv.* 2021;5(3):649–661.

46. Leinweber B, Colli C, Chott A, Kerl H, Cerroni L. Differential diagnosis of cutaneous infiltrates of B lymphocytes with follicular growth pattern. *Am J Dermatopathol.* 2004;26(1):4.

47. Kodama K, Massone C, Chott A, Metze D, Kerl H, Cerroni L. Primary cutaneous large B-cell lymphomas: clinicopathologic features, classification, and prognostic factors in a large series of patients. *Blood.* 2005;106(7):2491.

48. Grange F, Beylot-Barry M, Courville P, et al. Primary cutaneous diffuse large B-cell lymphoma, leg type: clinicopathologic features and prognostic analysis in 60 cases. *Arch Dermatol.* 2007;143(9):1144.

49. Koens L, Vermeer MH, Willemze R, Jansen PM. IgM expression on paraffin sections distinguishes primary cutaneous large B-cell lymphoma, leg type from primary cutaneous follicle center lymphoma. *Am J Surg Pathol.* 2010;34(7):1043.

50. Demirkesen C, Tuzuner N, Esen T, Lebe B, Ozkal S. The expression of IgM is helpful in the differentiation of primary cutaneous diffuse large B cell lymphoma and follicle center lymphoma. *Leuk Res.* 2011;35(9):1269.

51. Senff NJ, Hoefnagel JJ, Neelis KJ, et al. Results of radiotherapy in 153 primary cutaneous B-Cell lymphomas classified according to the WHO-EORTC classification. *Arch Dermatol.* 2007;143(12):1520.

52. Santucci M, Pimpinelli N. Primary cutaneous B-cell lymphomas. Current concepts. I. *Haematologica.* 2004;89(11):1360.

53. Pimpinelli N, Santucci M, Giannotti B. Cutaneous B-cell lymphomas: facts and open issues. *J Eur Acad Dermatol Venereol.* 2004;18(2):126.

54. Zinzani PL, Quaglino P, Pimpinelli N, et al. Prognostic factors in primary cutaneous B-cell lymphoma: the Italian Study Group for Cutaneous Lymphomas. *J Clin Oncol.* 2006;24(9):1376.

55. Hallermann C, Niermann C, Fischer RJ, Schulze HJ. New prognostic relevant factors in primary cutaneous diffuse large B-cell lymphomas. *J Am Acad Dermatol.* 2007;56(4):588.

56. Herrera E, Gallardo M, Bosch R, Cabra B, Aneri V, Sanchez P. Primary cutaneous CD30 (Ki-1)-positive non-anaplastic B-cell lymphoma. *J Cutan Pathol.* 2002;29(3):181.

57. Hoefnagel JJ, Dijkman R, Basso K, et al. Distinct types of primary cutaneous large B-cell lymphoma identified by gene expression profiling. *Blood.* 2005;105(9):3671.

58. Dijkman R, Tensen CP, Buettner M, Niedobitek G, Willemze R, Vermeer MH. Primary cutaneous follicle center lymphoma and primary cutaneous large B-cell lymphoma, leg type, are both targeted by aberrant somatic hypermutation but demonstrate differential expression of AID. *Blood.* 2006;107(12):4926.

59. Dijkman R, Tensen CP, Jordanova ES, et al. Array-based comparative genomic hybridization analysis reveals recurrent chromosomal alterations and prognostic parameters in primary cutaneous large B-cell lymphoma. *J Clin Oncol.* 2006;24(2):296.

60. Zhou XA, Louissaint A Jr, Wenzel A, et al. Genomic analyses identify recurrent alterations in immune evasion genes in diffuse large B-cell lymphoma, leg type. *J Invest Dermatol.* 2018;138(11):2365–2376.

61. Pham-Ledard A, Cappellen D, Martinez F, Vergier B, Beylot-Barry M, Merlio JP. MYD88 somatic mutation is a genetic feature of primary cutaneous diffuse large B-cell lymphoma, leg type. *J Invest Dermatol.* 2012;132(8):2118.

62. Pham-Ledard A, Prochazkova-Carlotti M, Andrique L, et al. Multiple genetic alterations in primary cutaneous large B-cell lymphoma, leg type support a common lymphomagenesis with activated B-cell-like diffuse large B-cell lymphoma. *Modern Pathology.* 2014;27(3):402–411.

63. Belaud-Rotureau MA, Marietta V, Vergier B, et al. Inactivation of p16INK4a/CDKN2A gene may be a diagnostic feature of large B cell lymphoma leg type among cutaneous B cell lymphomas. *Virchows Arch.* 2008;452(6):607.

64. Senff NJ, Zoutman WH, Vermeer MH, et al. Fine-mapping chromosomal loss at 9p21: correlation with prognosis in primary cutaneous diffuse large B-cell lymphoma, leg type. *J Invest Dermatol.* 2009;129(5):1149.

65. Dojcinov SD, Venkataraman G, Raffeld M, Pittaluga S, Jaffe ES. EBV positive mucocutaneous ulcer—a study of 26 cases associated with various sources of immunosuppression. *Am J Surg Pathol.* 2010;34(3):405–417.

66. Ikeda T, Gion Y, Sakamoto M, et al. Clinicopathological analysis of 34 Japanese patients with EBV-positive mucocutaneous ulcer. *Mod Pathol.* 2020;33(12):2437–2448.

67. Di Napoli A, Giubettini M, Duranti E, et al. Iatrogenic EBV-positive lymphoproliferative disorder with features of EBV+ mucocutaneous ulcer: evidence for concomitant TCRγ/IGH rearrangements

in the Hodgkin-like neoplastic cells. *Virchows Arch.* 2011;458(5): 631–636.

68. Dojcinov SD, Venkataraman G, Pittaluga S, et al. Age-related EBV-associated lymphoproliferative disorders in the Western population: a spectrum of reactive lymphoid hyperplasia and lymphoma. *Blood.* 2011;117(18):4726–4735.

69. Ikeda T, Gion Y, Nishimura Y, Nishimura MF, Yoshino T, Sato Y. Epstein-Barr virus-positive mucocutaneous ulcer: a unique and curious disease entity. *Int J Mol Sci.* 2021;22(3):1053.

70. Kim YH, Liu HL, Mraz-Gernhard S, Varghese A, Hoppe RT. Long-term outcome of 525 patients with mycosis fungoides and Sezary syndrome: clinical prognostic factors and risk for disease progression. *Arch Dermatol.* 2003;139(7):857.

71. Pimpinelli N, Olsen EA, Santucci M, et al. Defining early mycosis fungoides. *J Am Acad Dermatol.* 2005;53(6):1053.

72. Ferrara G, Di Blasi A, Zalaudek I, Argenziano G, Cerroni L. Regarding the algorithm for the diagnosis of early mycosis fungoides proposed by the International Society for Cutaneous Lymphomas: suggestions from routine histopathology practice. *J Cutan Pathol.* 2008;35(6):549.

73. Vandergriff T, Nezafati KA, Susa J, et al. Defining early mycosis fungoides: validation of a diagnostic algorithm proposed by the International Society for Cutaneous Lymphomas. *J Cutan Pathol.* 2015;42(5):318–328.

74. Olsen E, Vonderheid E, Pimpinelli N, et al. Revisions to the staging and classification of mycosis fungoides and Sezary syndrome: a proposal of the International Society for Cutaneous Lymphomas (ISCL) and the cutaneous lymphoma task force of the European Organization of Research and Treatment of Cancer (EORTC). *Blood.* 2007;110(6):1713.

75. Agar NS, Wedgeworth E, Crichton S, et al. Survival outcomes and prognostic factors in mycosis fungoides/Sezary syndrome: validation of the revised International Society for Cutaneous Lymphomas/European Organisation for Research and Treatment of Cancer staging proposal. *J Clin Oncol.* 2010;28(31):4730.

76. Whittaker S, Hoppe R, Prince HM. How I treat mycosis fungoides and Sezary syndrome. *Blood.* 2016;127(25):3142–3153.

77. Kadin ME, Hughey LC, Wood GS. Large-cell transformation of mycosis fungoides-differential diagnosis with implications for clinical management: a consensus statement of the US Cutaneous Lymphoma Consortium. *J Am Acad Dermatol.* 2014;70(2):374–376.

78. Cerroni L, Rieger E, Hodl S, Kerl H. Clinicopathologic and immunologic features associated with transformation of mycosis fungoides to large-cell lymphoma. *Am J Surg Pathol.* 1992;16(6):543.

79. Vergier B, de Muret A, Beylot-Barry M, et al. Transformation of mycosis fungoides: clinicopathological and prognostic features of 45 cases. French Study Group of Cutaneious Lymphomas. *Blood.* 2000;95(7):2212.

80. Benner MF, Jansen PM, Vermeer MH, Willemze R. Prognostic factors in transformed mycosis fungoides: a retrospective analysis of 100 cases. *Blood.* 2012;119(7):1643.

81. Vermeer MH, Geelen FA, Kummer JA, Meijer CJ, Willemze R. Expression of cytotoxic proteins by neoplastic T cells in mycosis fungoides increases with progression from plaque stage to tumor stage disease. *Am J Pathol.* 1999;154(4):1203.

82. van Doorn R, Van Haselen CW, van Voorst Vader PC, et al. Mycosis fungoides: disease evolution and prognosis of 309 Dutch patients. *Arch Dermatol.* 2000;136(4):504.

83. van Santen S, Roach RE, van Doorn R, et al. Clinical staging and prognostic factors in folliculotropic mycosis fungoides. *JAMA Dermatol.* 2016;152(9):992–1000.

84. Hodak E, Amitay-Laish I, Atzmony L, et al. New insights into folliculotropic mycosis fungoides (FMF): a single-center experience. *J Am Acad Dermatol.* 2016;75(2):347–355.

85. van Doorn R, Scheffer E, Willemze R. Follicular mycosis fungoides, a distinct disease entity with or without associated follicular mucinosis: a clinicopathologic and follow-up study of 51 patients. *Arch Dermatol.* 2002;138(2):191.

86. Gerami P, Guitart J. The spectrum of histopathologic and immunohistochemical findings in folliculotropic mycosis fungoides. *Am J Surg Pathol.* 2007;31(9):1430.

87. Pileri A, Facchetti F, Rutten A, et al. Syringotropic mycosis fungoides: a rare variant of the disease with peculiar clinicopathologic features. *Am J Surg Pathol.* 2011;35(1):100.

88. Drillenburg P, Bronkhorst CM, van der Wal AC, Noorduyn LA, Hoekzema R, Pals ST. Expression of adhesion molecules in pagetoid reticulosis (Woringer-Kolopp disease). *Br J Dermatol.* 1997;136(4):613.

89. Haghighi B, Smoller BR, LeBoit PE, Warnke RA, Sander CA, Kohler S. Pagetoid reticulosis (Woringer-Kolopp disease): an immunophenotypic, molecular, and clinicopathologic study. *Mod Pathol.* 2000;13(5):502.

90. Sundram U. Cutaneous lymphoproliferative disorders: what's new in the revised 4th edition of the *World Health Organization (WHO) Classification of Lymphoid Neoplasms. Adv Anat Pathol.* 2019;26(2):93–113.

91. Kempf W, Ostheeren-Michaelis S, Paulli M, et al. Granulomatous mycosis fungoides and granulomatous slack skin: a multicenter study of the Cutaneous Lymphoma Histopathology Task Force Group of the European Organization for Research and Treatment of Cancer (EORTC). *Arch Dermatol.* 2008;144(12):1609.

92. Kazakov DV, Burg G, Kempf W. Clinicopathological spectrum of mycosis fungoides. *J Eur Acad Dermatol Venereol.* 2004;18(4):397.

93. Ahn CS, ALSayyah A, Sangüeza OP. Mycosis fungoides: an updated review of clinicopathologic variants. *Am J Dermatopathol.* 2014;36(12):933–948; quiz 49–51.

94. Willemze R. Mycosis fungoides variants-clinicopathologic features, differential diagnosis, and treatment. *Semin Cutan Med Surg.* 2018;37(1):11–17.

95. Akaraphanth R, Douglass MC, Lim HW. Hypopigmented mycosis fungoides: treatment and a 6(1/2)-year follow-up of 9 patients. *J Am Acad Dermatol.* 2000;42(1, pt 1):33.

96. Choe YB, Park KC, Cho KH. A case of hypopigmented mycosis fungoides. *J Dermatol.* 2000;27(8):543.

97. Castano E, Glick S, Wolgast L, et al. Hypopigmented mycosis fungoides in childhood and adolescence: a long-term retrospective study. *J Cutan Pathol.* 2013;40(11):924–934.

98. El-Darouti MA, Marzouk SA, Azzam O, et al. Vitiligo vs. hypopigmented mycosis fungoides (histopathological and immunohistochemical study, univariate analysis). *Eur J Dermatol.* 2006;16(1):17.

99. Marzano AV, Borghi A, Facchetti M, Alessi E. Ichthyosiform mycosis fungoides. *Dermatology.* 2002;204(2):124.

100. Resnik KS, Kantor GR, Lessin SR, et al. Mycosis fungoides palmaris et plantaris. *Arch Dermatol.* 1995;131(9):1052.

101. Nakai N, Hagura A, Yamazato S, Katoh N. Mycosis fungoides palmaris et plantaris successfully treated with radiotherapy: case report and mini-review of the published work. *J Dermatol.* 2014;41(1):63–67.

102. Spieth K, Grundmann-Kollmann M, Runne U, et al. Mycosis-fungoides-type cutaneous T cell lymphoma of the hands and soles: a variant causing delay in diagnosis and adequate treatment of patients with palmoplantar eczema. *Dermatology.* 2002;205(3):239.

103. McBride SR, Dahl MG, Slater DN, Sviland L. Vesicular mycosis fungoides. *Br J Dermatol.* 1998;138(1):141.

104. Bowman PH, Hogan DJ, Sanusi ID. Mycosis fungoides bullosa: report of a case and review of the literature. *J Am Acad Dermatol.* 2001;45(6):934.

105. Ackerman AB, Miller RC, Shapiro L. Pustular mycosis fungoides. *Arch Dermatol.* 1966;93(2):221.

106. Poszepczynska E, Martinvalet D, Bouloc A, et al. Erythrodermic cutaneous T-cell lymphoma with disseminated pustulosis. Production of high levels of interleukin-8 by tumour cells. *Br J Dermatol.* 2001;144(5):1073.

107. Fischer M, Wohlrab J, Audring TH, Sterry W, Marsch WC. Granulomatous mycosis fungoides. Report of two cases and review of the literature. *J Eur Acad Dermatol Venereol.* 2000;14(3):196.

108. Scarabello A, Leinweber B, Ardigo M, et al. Cutaneous lymphomas with prominent granulomatous reaction: a potential pitfall in the histopathologic diagnosis of cutaneous T-and B-cell lymphomas. *Am J Surg Pathol.* 2002;26(10):1259.

109. van Kester MS, Borg MK, Zoutman WH, et al. A meta-analysis of gene expression data identifies a molecular signature characteristic for tumor-stage mycosis fungoides. *J Invest Dermatol.* 2012;132(8):2050.

110. McGirt LY, Jia P, Baerenwald DA, et al. Whole-genome sequencing reveals oncogenic mutations in mycosis fungoides. *Blood.* 2015;126(4):508–519.

111. Ungewickell A, Bhaduri A, Rios E, et al. Genomic analysis of mycosis fungoides and Sezary syndrome identifies recurrent alterations in TNFR2. *Nat Genet.* 2015;47(9):1056–1060.

112. Choi J, Goh G, Walradt T, et al. Genomic landscape of cutaneous T cell lymphoma. *Nat Genet.* 2015;47(9):1011–1019.

113. Campbell JJ, Clark RA, Watanabe R, Kupper TS. Sezary syndrome and mycosis fungoides arise from distinct T-cell subsets: a biologic rationale for their distinct clinical behaviors. *Blood.* 2010;116(5):767.

114. Burkert KL, Huhn K, Menezes DW, Murphy GF. Langerhans cell microgranulomas (pseudo-Pautrier abscesses): morphologic diversity, diagnostic implications and pathogenetic mechanisms. *J Cutan Pathol.* 2002;29(9):511.

115. Reddy K, Bhawan J. Histologic mimickers of mycosis fungoides: a review. *J Cutan Pathol.* 2007;34(7):519.

116. Pham-Ledard A, Prochazkova-Carlotti M, Laharanne E, et al. IRF4 gene rearrangements define a subgroup of CD30-positive cutaneous T-cell lymphoma: a study of 54 cases. *J Invest Dermatol.* 2010;130(3):816.

117. Wada DA, Law ME, Hsi ED, et al. Specificity of IRF4 translocations for primary cutaneous anaplastic large cell lymphoma: a multicenter study of 204 skin biopsies. *Mod Pathol.* 2011;24(4):596.

118. Olsen EA, Whittaker S, Kim YH, et al. Clinical end points and response criteria in mycosis fungoides and Sezary syndrome: a consensus statement of the International Society for Cutaneous Lymphomas, the United States Cutaneous Lymphoma Consortium, and the Cutaneous Lymphoma Task Force of the European Organisation for Research and Treatment of Cancer. *J Clin Oncol.* 2011;29(18):2598.

119. van Doorn R, van Kester MS, Dijkman R, et al. Oncogenomic analysis of mycosis fungoides reveals major differences with Sezary syndrome. *Blood.* 2009;113(1):127.

120. Sibaud V, Beylot-Barry M, Thiebaut R, et al. Bone marrow histopathologic and molecular staging in epidermotropic T-cell lymphomas. *Am J Clin Pathol.* 2003;119(3):414.

121. Vonderheid EC, Bernengo MG, Burg G, et al. Update on erythrodermic cutaneous T-cell lymphoma: report of the International Society for Cutaneous Lymphomas. *J Am Acad Dermatol.* 2002;46(1):95.

122. Cetinozman F, Jansen PM, Willemze R. Expression of programmed death-1 in primary cutaneous CD4-positive small/medium-sized pleomorphic T-cell lymphoma, cutaneous pseudo-T-cell lymphoma, and other types of cutaneous T-cell lymphoma. *Am J Surg Pathol.* 2012;36(1):109.

123. Vonderheid EC, Pena J, Nowell P. Sezary cell counts in erythrodermic cutaneous T-cell lymphoma: implications for prognosis and staging. *Leuk Lymphoma.* 2006;47(9):1841.

124. Marie I, Cordel N, Lenormand B, et al. Clonal T cells in the blood of patients with systemic sclerosis. *Arch Dermatol.* 2005;141(1):88.

125. Morice WG, Katzmann JA, Pittelkow MR, el-Azhary RA, Gibson LE, Hanson CA. A comparison of morphologic features, flow cytometry, TCR-Vbeta analysis, and TCR-PCR in qualitative and quantitative assessment of peripheral blood involvement by Sezary syndrome. *Am J Clin Pathol.* 2006;125(3):364.

126. Michel L, Jean-Louis F, Begue E, Bensussan A, Bagot M. Use of PLS3, Twist, CD158k/KIR3DL2, and NKp46 gene expression combination for reliable Sezary syndrome diagnosis. *Blood.* 2013;121(8):1477–1478.

127. Boonk SE, Zoutman WH, Marie-Cardine A, et al. Evaluation of immunophenotypic and molecular biomarkers for Sezary syndrome using standard operating procedures: a multicenter study of 59 patients. *J Invest Dermatol.* 2016;136(7):1364–1372.

128. Elenitoba-Johnson KS, Wilcox R. A new molecular paradigm in mycosis fungoides and Sezary syndrome. *Semin Diagn Pathol.* 2017;34(1):15–21.

129. Klemke CD, Booken N, Weiss C, et al. Histopathological and immunophenotypical criteria for the diagnosis of Sezary syndrome in differentiation from other erythrodermic skin diseases: a European Organisation for Research and Treatment of Cancer (EORTC) Cutaneous Lymphoma Task Force Study of 97 cases. *Br J Dermatol.* 2015;173(1):93–105.

130. Oliven A, Shechter Y. Extracorporeal photopheresis: a review. *Blood Rev.* 2001;15(2):103.

131. Scarisbrick JJ, Taylor P, Holtick U, et al. U.K. consensus statement on the use of extracorporeal photopheresis for treatment of cutaneous T-cell lymphoma and chronic graft-versus-host disease. *Br J Dermatol.* 2008;158(4):659.

132. Dani T, Knobler R. Extracorporeal photoimmunotherapy-photopheresis. *Front Biosci (Landmark Ed).* 2009;14:4769.

133. Kempf W, Pfaltz K, Vermeer MH, et al. EORTC, ISCL, and US-CLC consensus recommendations for the treatment of primary cutaneous CD30-positive lymphoproliferative disorders: lymphomatoid papulosis and primary cutaneous anaplastic large-cell lymphoma. *Blood.* 2011;118(15):4024.

134. Macaulay WL. Lymphomatoid papulosis. A continuing self-healing eruption, clinically benign–histologically malignant. *Arch Dermatol.* 1968;97(1):23.

135. Bekkenk MW, Geelen FA, van Voorst Vader PC, et al. Primary and secondary cutaneous CD30(+) lymphoproliferative disorders: a report from the Dutch Cutaneous Lymphoma Group on the long-term follow-up data of 219 patients and guidelines for diagnosis and treatment. *Blood.* 2000;95(12):3653.

136. Kempf W. Cutaneous CD30-positive lymphoproliferative disorders. *Surg Pathol Clin.* 2014;7(2):203–228.

137. Kadin ME. Pathobiology of CD30+ cutaneous T-cell lymphomas. *J Cutan Pathol.* 2006;33(suppl 1):10.

138. Saggini A, Gulia A, Argenyi Z, et al. A variant of lymphomatoid papulosis simulating primary cutaneous aggressive epidermotropic CD8+ cytotoxic T-cell lymphoma. Description of 9 cases. *Am J Surg Pathol.* 2010;34(8):1168.

139. Cardoso J, Duhra P, Thway Y, Calonje E. Lymphomatoid papulosis type D: a newly described variant easily confused with cutaneous aggressive CD8-positive cytotoxic T-cell lymphoma. *Am J Dermatopathol.* 2012;34(7):762.

140. Bertolotti A, Pham-Ledard AL, Vergier B, Parrens M, Bedane C, Beylot-Barry M. Lymphomatoid papulosis type D: an aggressive histology for an indolent disease. *Br J Dermatol.* 2013;169(5):1157.

141. Quintanilla-Martinez L, Jansen PM, Kinney MC, Swerdlow SH, Willemze R. Non-mycosis fungoides cutaneous T-cell lymphomas: report of the 2011 Society for Hematopathology/European Association for Haematopathology workshop. *Am J Clin Pathol.* 2013;139(4):491.

142. Kempf W, Kazakov DV, Scharer L, et al. Angioinvasive lymphomatoid papulosis: a new variant simulating aggressive lymphomas. *Am J Surg Pathol.* 2013;37(1):1.

143. Sharaf MA, Romanelli P, Kirsner R, Miteva M. Angioinvasive lymphomatoid papulosis: another case of a newly described variant. *Am J Dermatopathol.* 2014;36(3):e75–e77.

144. Boulland ML, Wechsler J, Bagot M, Pulford K, Kanavaros P, Gaulard P. Primary CD30-positive cutaneous T-cell lymphomas

and lymphomatoid papulosis frequently express cytotoxic proteins. *Histopathology*. 2000;36(2):136.

145. Karai LJ, Kadin ME, Hsi ED, et al. Chromosomal rearrangements of 6p25.3 define a new subtype of lymphomatoid papulosis. *Am J Surg Pathol*. 2013;37(8):1173.

146. Feldman AL, Law M, Remstein ED, et al. Recurrent translocations involving the IRF4 oncogene locus in peripheral T-cell lymphomas. *Leukemia*. 2009;23(3):574.

147. Nevala H, Karenko L, Vakeva L, Ranki A. Proapoptotic and anti-apoptotic markers in cutaneous T-cell lymphoma skin infiltrates and lymphomatoid papulosis. *Br J Dermatol*. 2001;145(6):928.

148. Greisser J, Doebbeling U, Roos M, et al. Apoptosis in CD30-positive lymphoproliferative disorders of the skin. *Exp Dermatol*. 2005;14(5):380.

149. Gallardo F, Costa C, Bellosillo B, et al. Lymphomatoid papulosis associated with mycosis fungoides: clinicopathological and molecular studies of 12 cases. *Acta DermVenereol*. 2004;84(6):463.

150. Kempf W, Kazakov DV, Palmedo G, Fraitag S, Schaerer L, Kutzner H. Pityriasis lichenoides et varioliformis acuta with numerous CD30(+) cells: a variant mimicking lymphomatoid papulosis and other cutaneous lymphomas. A clinicopathologic, immunohistochemical, and molecular biological study of 13 cases. *Am J Surg Pathol*. 2012;36(7):1021.

151. Leinweber B, Kerl H, Cerroni L. Histopathologic features of cutaneous herpes virus infections (herpes simplex, herpes varicella/zoster): a broad spectrum of presentations with common pseudolymphomatous aspects. *Am J Surg Pathol*. 2006; 30(1):50.

152. Kempf W. CD30+ lymphoproliferative disorders: histopathology, differential diagnosis, new variants, and simulators. *J Cutan Pathol*. 2006;33(suppl 1):58.

153. Guitart J, Querfeld C. Cutaneous CD30 lymphoproliferative disorders and similar conditions: a clinical and pathologic prospective on a complex issue. *Semin Diagn Pathol*. 2009;26(3):131.

154. Benner MF, Willemze R. Applicability and prognostic value of the new TNM classification system in 135 patients with primary cutaneous anaplastic large cell lymphoma. *Arch Dermatol*. 2009;145(12):1399.

155. Liu HL, Hoppe RT, Kohler S, Harvell JD, Reddy S, Kim YH. CD30+ cutaneous lymphoproliferative disorders: the Stanford experience in lymphomatoid papulosis and primary cutaneous anaplastic large cell lymphoma. *J Am Acad Dermatol*. 2003;49(6):1049.

156. Herbst H, Sander C, Tronnier M, Kutzner H, Hugel H, Kaudewitz P. Absence of anaplastic lymphoma kinase (ALK) and Epstein-Barr virus gene products in primary cutaneous anaplastic large cell lymphoma and lymphomatoid papulosis. *Br J Dermatol*. 1997;137(5):680.

157. Velusamy T, Kiel MJ, Sahasrabuddhe AA, et al. A novel recurrent NPM1-TYK2 gene fusion in cutaneous CD30-positive lymphoproliferative disorders. *Blood*. 2014;124(25):3768–3771.

158. Sasaki K, Sugaya M, Fujita H, et al. A case of primary cutaneous anaplastic large cell lymphoma with variant anaplastic lymphoma kinase translocation. *Br J Dermatol*. 2004;150(6): 1202.

159. Oschlies I, Lisfeld J, Lamant L, et al. ALK-positive anaplastic large cell lymphoma limited to the skin: clinical, histopathological and molecular analysis of 6 pediatric cases. A report from the ALCL99 study. *Haematologica*. 2013;98(1):50.

160. Eberle FC, Song JY, Xi L, et al. Nodal involvement by cutaneous CD30-positive T-cell lymphoma mimicking classical Hodgkin lymphoma. *Am J Surg Pathol*. 2012;36(5):716.

161. Willemze R, Jansen PM, Cerroni L, et al. Subcutaneous panniculitis-like T-cell lymphoma: definition, classification, and prognostic factors: an EORTC Cutaneous Lymphoma Group Study of 83 cases. *Blood*. 2008;111(2):838.

162. Medhi K, Kumar R, Rishi A, Kumar L, Bakhshi S. Subcutaneous panniculitis like T-cell lymphoma with hemophagocytosis:

complete remission with BFM-90 protocol. *J Pediatr Hematol Oncol*. 2008;30(7):558.

163. Goyal A, Goyal K, Bohjanen K, Pearson D. Epidemiology of primary cutaneous γδ T-cell lymphoma and subcutaneous panniculitis-like T-cell lymphoma in the U.S.A. from 2006 to 2015: a surveillance, epidemiology, and end results-18 analysis. *Br J Dermatol*. 2019;181(4):848–850.

164. Polprasert C, Takeuchi Y, Kakiuchi N, et al. Frequent germline mutations of *HAVCR2* in sporadic subcutaneous panniculitis-like T-cell lymphoma. *Blood Adv*. 2019;3(4):588–595.

165. LeBlanc RE, Tavallaee M, Kim YH, Kim J. Useful parameters for distinguishing subcutaneous panniculitis-like T-cell lymphoma from lupus erythematosus panniculitis. *Am J Surg Pathol*. 2016;40(6):745–754.

166. Willemze R, Meijer CJ. Classification of cutaneous T-cell lymphoma: from Alibert to WHO-EORTC. *J Cutan Pathol*. 2006;33(suppl 1):18.

167. Guitart J, Weisenburger DD, Subtil A, et al. Cutaneous γδ T-cell lymphomas: a spectrum of presentations with overlap with other cytotoxic lymphomas. *Am J Surg Pathol*. 2012;36(11):1656.

168. Toro JR, Beaty M, Sorbara L, et al. Gamma delta T-cell lymphoma of the skin: a clinical, microscopic, and molecular study. *Arch Dermatol*. 2000;136(8):1024.

169. Endly DC, Weenig RH, Peters MS, Viswanatha DS, Comfere NI. Indolent course of cutaneous gamma-delta T-cell lymphoma. *J Cutan Pathol*. 2013;40(10):896.

170. Kempf W, Kazakov DV, Scheidegger PE, Schlaak M, Tantcheva-Poor I. Two cases of primary cutaneous lymphoma with a γ/δ+ phenotype and an indolent course: further evidence of heterogeneity of cutaneous γ/δ+ T-cell lymphomas. *Am J Dermatopathol*. 2014;36(7):570–577.

171. Toro JR, Liewehr DJ, Pabby N, et al. Gamma-delta T-cell phenotype is associated with significantly decreased survival in cutaneous T-cell lymphoma. *Blood*. 2003;101(9):3407.

172. Jaffe ES, Krenacs L, Raffeld M. Classification of cytotoxic T-cell and natural killer cell lymphomas. *Semin Hematol*. 2003;40(3):175.

173. Garcia-Herrera A, Song JY, Chuang SS, et al. Nonhepatosplenic γδ T-cell lymphomas represent a spectrum of aggressive cytotoxic T-cell lymphomas with a mainly extranodal presentation. *Am J Surg Pathol*. 2011;35(8):1214.

174. Caudron A, Bouaziz JD, Battistella M, et al. Two atypical cases of cutaneous gamma/delta T-cell lymphomas. *Dermatology*. 2011;222(4):297.

175. Jungbluth AA, Frosina D, Fayad M, et al. Immunohistochemical detection of γδ T lymphocytes in formalin-fixed paraffin-embedded tissues. *Appl Immunohistochem Mol Morphol*. 2019;27(8):581–583.

176. Rodriguez-Pinilla SM, Ortiz-Romero PL, Monsalvez V, et al. TCR-gamma expression in primary cutaneous T-cell lymphomas. *Am J Surg Pathol*. 2013;37(3):375.

177. Yu WW, Hsieh PP, Chuang SS. Cutaneous EBV-positive γδ T-cell lymphoma vs. extranodal NK/T-cell lymphoma: a case report and literature review. *J Cutan Pathol*. 2013;40(3):310.

178. Iqbal J, Weisenburger DD, Chowdhury A, et al. Natural killer cell lymphoma shares strikingly similar molecular features with a group of non-hepatosplenic γδ T-cell lymphoma and is highly sensitive to a novel aurora kinase A inhibitor in vitro. *Leukemia*. 2011;25(2):348.

179. Lu D, Patel KA, Duvic M, Jones D. Clinical and pathological spectrum of CD8-positive cutaneous T-cell lymphomas. *J Cutan Pathol*. 2002;29(8):465.

180. Robson A, Assaf C, Bagot M, et al. Aggressive epidermotropic cutaneous CD8+ lymphoma: a cutaneous lymphoma with distinct clinical and pathological features. Report of an EORTC Cutaneous Lymphoma Task Force Workshop. *Histopathology*. 2015;67(4):425–441.

181. Santucci M, Pimpinelli N, Massi D, et al. Cytotoxic/natural killer cell cutaneous lymphomas. Report of EORTC Cutaneous Lymphoma Task Force Workshop. *Cancer*. 2003;97(3):610.

182. Guitart J, Martinez-Escala ME, Subtil A, et al. Primary cutaneous aggressive epidermotropic cytotoxic T-cell lymphomas: reappraisal of a provisional entity in the 2016 WHO classification of cutaneous lymphomas. *Mod Pathol*. 2017;30(5):761–772.

183. Petrella T, Maubec E, Cornillet-Lefebvre P, et al. Indolent CD8-positive lymphoid proliferation of the ear: a distinct primary cutaneous T-cell lymphoma? *Am J Surg Pathol*. 2007;31(12):1887–1892.

184. Greenblatt D, Ally M, Child F, et al. Indolent CD8(+) lymphoid proliferation of acral sites: a clinicopathologic study of six patients with some atypical features. *J Cutan Pathol*. 2013;40(2):248–258.

185. Li JY, Guitart J, Pulitzer MP, et al. Multicenter case series of indolent small/medium-sized CD8+ lymphoid proliferations with predilection for the ear and face. *Am J Dermatopathol*. 2014;36(5):402–408.

186. Alberti-Violetti S, Fanoni D, Provasi M, Corti L, Venegoni L, Berti E. Primary cutaneous acral CD8 positive T-cell lymphoma with extra-cutaneous involvement: a long-standing case with an unexpected progression. *J Cutan Pathol*. 2017;44(11):964–968.

187. Tjahjono LA, Davis MDP, Witzig TE, Comfere NI. Primary cutaneous acral CD8+ T-cell lymphoma—a single center review of 3 cases and recent literature review. *Am J Dermatopathol*. 2019;41(9):644–648.

188. Wobser M, Roth S, Reinartz T, Rosenwald A, Goebeler M, Geissinger E. CD68 expression is a discriminative feature of indolent cutaneous CD8-positive lymphoid proliferation and distinguishes this lymphoma subtype from other CD8-positive cutaneous lymphomas. *Br J Dermatol*. 2015;172(6):1573–1580.

189. Kluk J, Kai A, Koch D, et al. Indolent CD8-positive lymphoid proliferation of acral sites: three further cases of a rare entity and an update on a unique patient. *J Cutan Pathol*. 2016;43(2):125–136.

190. Beltraminelli H, Leinweber B, Kerl H, Cerroni L. Primary cutaneous CD4+ small-/medium-sized pleomorphic T-cell lymphoma: a cutaneous nodular proliferation of pleomorphic T lymphocytes of undetermined significance? A study of 136 cases. *Am J Dermatopathol*. 2009;31(4):317.

191. Grogg KL, Jung S, Erickson LA, McClure RF, Dogan A. Primary cutaneous CD4-positive small/medium-sized pleomorphic T-cell lymphoma: a clonal T-cell lymphoproliferative disorder with indolent behavior. *Mod Pathol*. 2008;21(6):708.

192. Rodriguez Pinilla SM, Roncador G, Rodriguez-Peralto JL, et al. Primary cutaneous CD4+ small/medium-sized pleomorphic T-cell lymphoma expresses follicular T-cell markers. *Am J Surg Pathol*. 2009;33(1):81.

193. von den Driesch P, Coors EA. Localized cutaneous small to medium-sized pleomorphic T-cell lymphoma: a report of 3 cases stable for years. *J Am Acad Dermatol*. 2002;46(4):531.

194. Beltzung F, Ortonne N, Pelletier L, et al. Primary cutaneous CD4+ small/medium T-cell lymphoproliferative disorders: a clinical, pathologic, and molecular study of 60 cases presenting with a single lesion: a multicenter study of the French Cutaneous Lymphoma Study Group. *Am J Surg Pathol*. 2020;44(7):862–872.

195. Garcia-Herrera A, Colomo L, Camos M, et al. Primary cutaneous small/medium CD4+ T-cell lymphomas: a heterogeneous group of tumors with different clinicopathologic features and outcome. *J Clin Oncol*. 2008;26(20):3364.

196. Chen HH, Hsiao CH, Chiu HC. Hydroa vacciniforme-like primary cutaneous CD8-positive T-cell lymphoma. *Br J Dermatol*. 2002;147(3):587.

197. Xu Z, Lian S. Epstein-Barr virus-associated hydroa vacciniforme-like cutaneous lymphoma in seven Chinese children. *Pediatr Dermatol*. 2010;27(5):463–469.

198. Barrionuevo C, Anderson VM, Zevallos-Giampietri E, et al. Hydroa-like cutaneous T-cell lymphoma: a clinicopathologic and molecular genetic study of 16 pediatric cases from Peru. *Appl Immunohistochem Mol Morphol*. 2002;10(1):7–14.

199. Gupta G, Man I, Kemmett D. Hydroa vacciniforme: a clinical and follow-up study of 17 cases. *J Am Acad Dermatol*. 2000;42(2, pt 1):208–213.

200. Sangueza M, Plaza JA. Hydroa vacciniforme-like cutaneous T-cell lymphoma: clinicopathologic and immunohistochemical study of 12 cases. *J Am Acad Dermatol*. 2013;69(1):112–119.

201. Quintanilla-Martinez L, Ridaura C, Nagl F, et al. Hydroa vacciniforme-like lymphoma: a chronic EBV+ lymphoproliferative disorder with risk to develop a systemic lymphoma. *Blood*. 2013;122(18):3101.

202. Cohen JI, Manoli I, Dowdell K, et al. Hydroa vacciniforme-like lymphoproliferative disorder: an EBV disease with a low risk of systemic illness in whites. *Blood*. 2019;133(26):2753–2764.

203. Tokura Y, Ishihara S, Tagawa S, Seo N, Ohshima K, Takigawa M. Hypersensitivity to mosquito bites as the primary clinical manifestation of a juvenile type of Epstein-Barr virus-associated natural killer cell leukemia/lymphoma. *J Am Acad Dermatol*. 2001;45(4):569–578.

204. Kawa K, Okamura T, Yagi K, Takeuchi M, Nakayama M, Inoue M. Mosquito allergy and Epstein-Barr virus-associated T/natural killer-cell lymphoproliferative disease. *Blood*. 2001;98(10):3173–3174.

205. Iwatsuki K, Satoh M, Yamamoto T, et al. Pathogenic link between hydroa vacciniforme and Epstein-Barr virus-associated hematologic disorders. *Arch Dermatol*. 2006;142(5):587–595.

206. Cohen JI, Kimura H, Nakamura S, Ko YH, Jaffe ES. Epstein-Barr virus-associated lymphoproliferative disease in non-immunocompromised hosts: a status report and summary of an international meeting, 8–9 September 2008. *Ann Oncol*. 2009;20(9):1472.

207. Kimura H, Ito Y, Kawabe S, et al. EBV-associated T/NK-cell lymphoproliferative diseases in nonimmunocompromised hosts: prospective analysis of 108 cases. *Blood*. 2012;119(3):673.

208. Cho-Vega JH, Medeiros LJ, Prieto VG, Vega F. Leukemia cutis. *Am J Clin Pathol*. 2008;129(1):130.

209. Falini B, Lenze D, Hasserjian R, et al. Cytoplasmic mutated nucleophosmin (NPM) defines the molecular status of a significant fraction of myeloid sarcomas. *Leukemia*. 2007;21(7):1566–1570.

210. Tsimberidou AM, Kantarjian HM, Estey E, et al. Outcome in patients with nonleukemic granulocytic sarcoma treated with chemotherapy with or without radiotherapy. *Leukemia*. 2003;17(6):1100–1103.

211. Pileri SA, Ascani S, Cox MC, et al. Myeloid sarcoma: clinico-pathologic, phenotypic and cytogenetic analysis of 92 adult patients. *Leukemia*. 2007;21(2):340.

212. Amador-Ortiz C, Hurley MY, Ghahramani GK, et al. Use of classic and novel immunohistochemical markers in the diagnosis of cutaneous myeloid sarcoma. *J Cutan Pathol*. 2011;38(12):945.

213. Aboutalebi A, Korman JB, Sohani AR, et al. Aleukemic cutaneous myeloid sarcoma. *J Cutan Pathol*. 2013;40(12):996–1005.

214. Hurley MY, Ghahramani GK, Frisch S, et al. Cutaneous myeloid sarcoma: natural history and biology of an uncommon manifestation of acute myeloid leukemia. *Acta Derm Venereol*. 2013;93(3):319.

215. Chang YW, Lee CH, Tseng HC. Leukemia cutis in a medical center in southern Taiwan: a retrospective study of 42 patients. *J Formos Med Assoc*. 2021;120(1, pt 1):226–233.

216. Qi J, Zhang F, Liu Y, Yao J, Xu Y, He H. Extramedullary blast crisis of chronic myelogenous leukemia with a skin lesion: a case report and literature review. *Am J Dermatopathol*. 2021;43(6):450–453.

217. Patel LM, Maghari A, Schwartz RA, Kapila R, Morgan AJ, Lambert WC. Myeloid leukemia cutis in the setting of myelodysplastic syndrome: a crucial dermatological diagnosis. *Int J Dermatol*. 2012;51(4):383–388.

218. Benet C, Gomez A, Aguilar C, et al. Histologic and immunohistologic characterization of skin localization of myeloid disorders: a study of 173 cases. *Am J Clin Pathol*. 2011;135(2):278.

219. Agis H, Weltermann A, Fonatsch C, et al. A comparative study on demographic, hematological, and cytogenetic findings and prognosis in acute myeloid leukemia with and without leukemia cutis. *AnnHematol.* 2002;81(2):90.

220. Alexiev BA, Wang W, Ning Y, et al. Myeloid sarcomas: a histologic, immunohistochemical, and cytogenetic study. *Diagn Pathol.* 2007;2:42.

221. Obiorah IE, Ozdemirli M. Myeloid sarcoma with megakaryoblastic differentiation presenting as a breast mass. *Hematol Oncol Stem Cell Ther.* 2018;11(3):178–182.

222. Shvartsbeyn M, Pandey S, Mercer SE, Goldenberg G. Leukemia cutis presenting clinically as disseminated herpes zoster in a patient with unrecognized acute promyelocytic leukemia. *J Clin Aesthet Dermatol.* 2012;5(4):40.

223. Bachmeyer C, Buffet M, Moguelet P, Najman A, Aractingi S. Necrotic and ulcerated cutaneous and mucosal leukemia cutis in AML6. *Ann Hematol.* 2013;92(10):1431–1432.

224. Weinel S, Malone J, Jain D, Callen JP. Therapy-related leukaemia cutis: a review. *Australas J Dermatol.* 2008;49(4):187.

225. Li L, Wang Y, Lian CG, Hu N, Jin H, Liu Y. Clinical and pathological features of myeloid leukemia cutis. *An Bras Dermatol.* 2018;93(2):216–221.

226. Starnes AM, Kast DR, Lu K, Honda K. Leukemia cutis amidst a psoriatic flare: a case report. *Am J Dermatopathol.* 2012;34(3):292–294.

227. Torrelo A, Madero L, Mediero IG, Bano A, Zambrano A. Aleukemic congenital leukemia cutis. *Pediatr Dermatol.* 2004;21(4):458.

228. Green K, Tandon S, Ahmed M, et al. Congenital acute myeloid leukemia: challenges and lessons. A 15-year experience from the UK. *Leuk Lymphoma.* 2021;62(3):688–695.

229. Sen F, Zhang XX, Prieto VG, Shea CR, Qumsiyeh MB. Increased incidence of trisomy 8 in acute myeloid leukemia with skin infiltration (leukemia cutis). *Diagn Mol Pathol.* 2000;9(4):190.

230. Wang CX, Pusic I, Anadkat MJ. Association of leukemia cutis with survival in acute myeloid leukemia. *JAMA Dermatol.* 2019;155(7):826–832.

231. Bakst RL, Tallman MS, Douer D, Yahalom J. How I treat extramedullary acute myeloid leukemia. *Blood.* 2011;118(14):3785.

232. Ricci C, Fermo E, Corti S, et al. RAS mutations contribute to evolution of chronic myelomonocytic leukemia to the proliferative variant. *Clin Cancer Res.* 2010;16(8):2246–2256.

233. Cervera N, Itzykson R, Coppin E, et al. Gene mutations differently impact the prognosis of the myelodysplastic and myeloproliferative classes of chronic myelomonocytic leukemia. *Am J Hematol.* 2014;89(6):604–609.

234. Mathew RA, Bennett JM, Liu JJ, et al. Cutaneous manifestations in CMML: indication of disease acceleration or transformation to AML and review of the literature. *Leuk Res.* 2012;36(1):72.

235. Vitte F, Fabiani B, Benet C, et al. Specific skin lesions in chronic myelomonocytic leukemia: a spectrum of myelomonocytic and dendritic cell proliferations: a study of 42 cases. *Am J Surg Pathol.* 2012;36(9):1302.

236. Vermi W, Facchetti F, Rosati S, et al. Nodal and extranodal tumor-forming accumulation of plasmacytoid monocytes/interferon-producing cells associated with myeloid disorders. *Am J Surg Pathol.* 2004;28(5):585.

237. Orazi A, Chiu R, O'Malley DP, et al. Chronic myelomonocytic leukemia: the role of bone marrow biopsy immunohistology. *Mod Pathol.* 2006;19(12):1536.

238. Loghavi S, Curry JL, Garcia-Manero G, et al. Chronic myelomonocytic leukemia masquerading as cutaneous indeterminate dendritic cell tumor: expanding the spectrum of skin lesions in chronic myelomonocytic leukemia. *J Cutan Pathol.* 2017;44(12):1075–1079.

239. Li JJ, Talam S, Star P, Getta B. Atypical cutaneous histiocytic eruption in a patient with chronic myelomonocytic leukemia: a case report. *J Cutan Pathol.* 2021;48(5):680–688.

240. Luskin MR, Kim AS, Patel SS, Wright K, LeBoeuf NR, Lane AA. Evidence for separate transformation to acute myeloid leukemia and blastic plasmacytoid dendritic cell neoplasm from a shared ancestral hematopoietic clone. *Leuk Lymphoma.* 2020;61(9):2258–2261.

241. Sapienza MR, Abate F, Melle F, et al. Blastic plasmacytoid dendritic cell neoplasm: genomics mark epigenetic dysregulation as a primary therapeutic target. *Haematologica.* 2019;104(4):729–737.

242. Loghavi S, Khoury JD. Recent updates on chronic myelomonocytic leukemia. *Curr Hematol Malig Rep.* 2018;13(6):446–454.

243. Hebeda K, Boudova L, Beham-Schmid C, et al. Progression, transformation, and unusual manifestations of myelodysplastic syndromes and myelodysplastic-myeloproliferative neoplasms: lessons learned from the XIV European Bone Marrow Working Group Course 2019. *Ann Hematol.* 2021;100(1):117–133.

244. Jacob MC, Chaperot L, Mossuz P, et al. CD4+ CD56+ lineage negative malignancies: a new entity developed from malignant early plasmacytoid dendritic cells. *Haematologica.* 2003;88(8):941.

245. Pagano L, Valentini CG, Pulsoni A, et al. Blastic plasmacytoid dendritic cell neoplasm with leukemic presentation: an Italian multicenter study. *Haematologica.* 2013;98(2):239.

246. Taylor J, Haddadin M, Upadhyay VA, et al. Multicenter analysis of outcomes in blastic plasmacytoid dendritic cell neoplasm offers a pretargeted therapy benchmark. *Blood.* 2019;134(8):678–687.

247. Pileri SA, Grogan TM, Harris NL, et al. Tumours of histiocytes and accessory dendritic cells: an immunohistochemical approach to classification from the International Lymphoma Study Group based on 61 cases. *Histopathology.* 2002;41(1):1.

248. Cronin DM, George TI, Reichard KK, Sundram UN. Immunophenotypic analysis of myeloperoxidase-negative leukemia cutis and blastic plasmacytoid dendritic cell neoplasm. *Am J Clin Pathol.* 2012;137(3):367.

249. Reineks EZ, Osei ES, Rosenberg A, Auletta J, Meyerson HJ. CD22 expression on blastic plasmacytoid dendritic cell neoplasms and reactivity of anti-CD22 antibodies to peripheral blood dendritic cells. *Cytometry B Clin Cytom.* 2009;76(4):237–248.

250. Laribi K, Baugier de Materre A, Sobh M, et al. Blastic plasmacytoid dendritic cell neoplasms: results of an international survey on 398 adult patients. *Blood Adv.* 2020;4(19):4838–4848.

251. Sukswai N, Aung PP, Yin CC, et al. Dual expression of TCF4 and CD123 is highly sensitive and specific for blastic plasmacytoid dendritic cell neoplasm. *Am J Surg Pathol.* 2019;43(10):1429–1437.

252. Gera S, Dekmezian MS, Duvic M, Tschen JA, Vega F, Cho-Vega JH. Blastic plasmacytoid dendritic cell neoplasm: evolving insights in an aggressive hematopoietic malignancy with a predilection of skin involvement. *Am J Dermatopathol.* 2014;36(3):244–251.

253. Dijkman R, van Doorn R, Szuhai K, Willemze R, Vermeer MH, Tensen CP. Gene-expression profiling and array-based CGH classify CD4+CD56+ hematodermic neoplasm and cutaneous myelomonocytic leukemia as distinct disease entities. *Blood.* 2007;109(4):1720.

254. Menezes J, Acquadro F, Wiseman M, et al. Exome sequencing reveals novel and recurrent mutations with clinical impact in blastic plasmacytoid dendritic cell neoplasm. *Leukemia.* 2014;28(4):823–829.

255. Yun S, Chan O, Kerr D, et al. Survival outcomes in blastic plasmacytoid dendritic cell neoplasm by first-line treatment and stem cell transplant. *Blood Adv.* 2020;4(14):3435–3442.

256. Khoury JD, Medeiros LJ, Manning JT, Sulak LE, Bueso-Ramos C, Jones D. CD56(+) TdT(+) blastic natural killer cell tumor of the skin: a primitive systemic malignancy related to myelomonocytic leukemia. *Cancer.* 2002;94(9):2401.

257. Herling M, Jones D. CD4+/CD56+ hematodermic tumor: the features of an evolving entity and its relationship to dendritic cells. *Am J Clin Pathol.* 2007;127(5):687.

258. Sapienza MR, Pileri S. Molecular features of blastic plasmacytoid dendritic cell neoplasm: DNA mutations and epigenetics. *Hematol Oncol Clin North Am.* 2020;34(3):511–521.

259. Facchetti F, Vermi W, Santoro A, Vergoni F, Chilosi M, Doglioni C. Neoplasms derived from plasmacytoid monocytes/interferon-producing cells: variability of CD56 and granzyme B expression. *Am J Surg Pathol.* 2003;27(11):1489.

260. Jegalian AG, Facchetti F, Jaffe ES. Plasmacytoid dendritic cells: physiologic roles and pathologic states. *Adv Anat Pathol.* 2009;16(6):392.

261. Roos-Weil D, Dietrich S, Boumendil A, et al. Stem cell transplantation can provide durable disease control in blastic plasmacytoid dendritic cell neoplasm: a retrospective study from the European Group for Blood and Marrow Transplantation. *Blood.* 2013;121(3):440.

262. Pemmaraju N, Lane AA, Sweet KL, et al. Tagraxofusp in blastic plasmacytoid dendritic-cell neoplasm. *N Engl J Med.* 2019;380(17):1628–1637.

263. Lin P, Jones D, Dorfman DM, Medeiros LJ. Precursor B-cell lymphoblastic lymphoma: a predominantly extranodal tumor with low propensity for leukemic involvement. *Am J Surg Pathol.* 2000;24(11):1480.

264. Boccara O, Laloum-Grynberg E, Jeudy G, et al. Cutaneous B-cell lymphoblastic lymphoma in children: a rare diagnosis. *J Am Acad Dermatol.* 2012;66(1):51.

265. Bontoux C, De Masson A, Boccara O, et al. Outcome and clinicophenotypical features of acute lymphoblastic leukemia/lymphoblastic lymphoma with cutaneous involvement: a multicenter case series. *J Am Acad Dermatol.* 2020;83(4):1166–1170.

266. Vezzoli P, Novara F, Fanoni D, et al. Three cases of primary cutaneous lymphoblastic lymphoma: microarray-based comparative genomic hybridization and gene expression profiling studies with review of literature. *Leuk Lymphoma.* 2012;53(10):1978.

267. Song H, Todd P, Chiarle R, Billett AL, Gellis S. Primary cutaneous B-cell lymphoblastic lymphoma arising from a long-standing lesion in a child and review of the literature. *Pediatr Dermatol.* 2017;34(4):e182–e186.

268. Muljono A, Graf NS, Arbuckle S. Primary cutaneous lymphoblastic lymphoma in children: series of eight cases with review of the literature. *Pathology.* 2009;41(3):223–228.

269. Jouini R, Chabchoub I, Khanchel F, et al. Primary and isolated cutaneous precursor B-lymphoblastic lymphoma in an infant. *Pediatr Dermatol.* 2021;38(3):707–708.

270. Ducassou S, Ferlay C, Bergeron C, et al. Clinical presentation, evolution, and prognosis of precursor B-cell lymphoblastic lymphoma in trials LMT96, EORTC 58881, and EORTC 58951. *Br J Haematol.* 2011;152(4):441.

271. Maitra A, McKenna RW, Weinberg AG, Schneider NR, Kroft SH. Precursor B-cell lymphoblastic lymphoma. A study of nine cases lacking blood and bone marrow involvement and review of the literature. *Am J Clin Pathol.* 2001;115(6):868.

272. Schraders M, van Reijmersdal SV, Kamping EJ, et al. High-resolution genomic profiling of pediatric lymphoblastic lymphomas reveals subtle differences with pediatric acute lymphoblastic leukemias in the B-lineage. *Cancer Genet Cytogenet.* 2009;191(1):27.

273. Ahlmann M, Meyer C, Marschalek R, et al. Complex MLL rearrangement in non-infiltrated bone marrow in an infant with stage II precursor B-lymphoblastic lymphoma. *Eur J Haematol.* 2014;93(4):349–353.

274. Takachi T, Iwabuchi H, Imamura M, Imai C. Lymphoblastic lymphoma with mature b-cell immunophenotype and MLL-AF9 in a child. *Pediatr Blood Cancer.* 2011;57(7):1251–1252.

275. Kemps PG, Cleven AHG, van Wezel T, et al. B-cell lymphoblastic lymphoma with cutaneous involvement and a KMT2A gene rearrangement. *Am J Hematol.* 2020;95(11):1427–1429.

276. Shafer D, Wu H, Al-Saleem T, et al. Cutaneous precursor B-cell lymphoblastic lymphoma in 2 adult patients: clinicopathologic and molecular cytogenetic studies with a review of the literature. *Arch Dermatol.* 2008;144(9):1155.

277. Robak E, Robak T. Skin lesions in chronic lymphocytic leukemia. *Leuk Lymphoma.* 2007;48(5):855.

278. Agnew KL, Ruchlemer R, Catovsky D, Matutes E, Bunker CB. Cutaneous findings in chronic lymphocytic leukaemia. *Br J Dermatol.* 2004;150(6):1129–1135.

279. Liu YA, Finn AJ, Subtil A. Primary cutaneous lymphomas in patients with chronic lymphocytic leukemia/small lymphocytic lymphoma (CLL/SLL): a series of 12 cases. *J Cutan Pathol.* 2021;48(5):617–624.

280. Cerroni L, Zenahlik P, Hofler G, Kaddu S, Smolle J, Kerl H. Specific cutaneous infiltrates of B-cell chronic lymphocytic leukemia: a clinicopathologic and prognostic study of 42 patients. *Am J Surg Pathol.* 1996;20(8):1000.

281. Maughan C, Kolker S, Markus B, Young J. Leukemia cutis coexisting with dermatofibroma as the initial presentation of B-cell chronic lymphocytic leukemia/small lymphocytic lymphoma. *Am J Dermatopathol.* 2014;36(1):e14–e15.

282. Cerroni L, Hofler G, Back B, Wolf P, Maier G, Kerl H. Specific cutaneous infiltrates of B-cell chronic lymphocytic leukemia (B-CLL) at sites typical for *Borrelia burgdorferi* infection. *J Cutan Pathol.* 2002;29(3):142–147.

283. Ziemer M, Bornkessel A, Hahnfeld S, Weyers W. "Specific" cutaneous infiltrate of B-cell chronic lymphocytic leukemia at the site of a florid herpes simplex infection. *J Cutan Pathol.* 2005;32(8):581–584.

284. Yamazaki ML, Lum CA, Izumi AK. Primary cutaneous Richter syndrome: prognostic implications and review of the literature. *J Am Acad Dermatol.* 2009;60(1):157–161.

285. Yu L, Bandhlish A, Fullen DR, Su LD, Ma L. Cutaneous Richter syndrome: report of 3 cases from one institution. *J Am Acad Dermatol.* 2012;67(5):e187–e193.

286. Duong T, Grange F, Auffret N, et al. Cutaneous Richter's syndrome, prognosis, and clinical, histological and immunohistological patterns: report of four cases and review of the literature. *Dermatology.* 2010;220(3):226.

287. Döhner H, Stilgenbauer S, Benner A, et al. Genomic aberrations and survival in chronic lymphocytic leukemia. *N Engl J Med.* 2000;343(26):1910–1916.

288. Hallek M, Cheson BD, Catovsky D, et al. iwCLL guidelines for diagnosis, indications for treatment, response assessment, and supportive management of CLL. *Blood.* 2018;131(25):2745–2760.

289. Landau DA, Tausch E, Taylor-Weiner AN, et al. Mutations driving CLL and their evolution in progression and relapse. *Nature.* 2015;526(7574):525–530.

290. Seifert M, Sellmann L, Bloehdorn J, et al. Cellular origin and pathophysiology of chronic lymphocytic leukemia. *J Exp Med.* 2012;209(12):2183–2198.

291. Sen F, Medeiros LJ, Lu D, et al. Mantle cell lymphoma involving skin: cutaneous lesions may be the first manifestation of disease and tumors often have blastoid cytologic features. *Am J Surg Pathol.* 2002;26(10):1312.

292. Cao Q, Li Y, Lin H, Ke Z, Liu Y, Ye Z. Mantle cell lymphoma of blastoid variant with skin lesion and rapid progression: a case report and literature review. *Am J Dermatopathol.* 2013;35(8):851.

293. Gladkikh A, Potashnikova D, Korneva E, Khudoleeva O, Vorobjev I. Cyclin D1 expression in B-cell lymphomas. *Exp Hematol.* 2010;38(11):1047–1057.

294. Dreyling M, Kluin-Nelemans HC, Bea S, et al. Update on the molecular pathogenesis and clinical treatment of mantle cell lymphoma: report of the 11th annual conference of the European Mantle Cell Lymphoma Network. *Leuk Lymphoma.* 2013;54(4):699–707.

295. Athanasiou E, Kotoula V, Hytiroglou P, Kouidou S, Kaloutsi V, Papadimitriou CS. In situ hybridization and reverse transcription-polymerase chain reaction for cyclin D1 mRNA in the diagnosis

of mantle cell lymphoma in paraffin-embedded tissues. *Mod Pathol*. 2001;14(2):62–71.

296. Mozos A, Royo C, Hartmann E, et al. SOX11 expression is highly specific for mantle cell lymphoma and identifies the cyclin D1-negative subtype. *Haematologica*. 2009;94(11):1555–1562.

297. Salaverria I, Royo C, Carvajal-Cuenca A, et al. CCND2 rearrangements are the most frequent genetic events in cyclin D1(-) mantle cell lymphoma. *Blood*. 2013;121(8):1394–1402.

298. Cerhan JR. Epidemiology of follicular lymphoma. *Hematol Oncol Clin North Am*. 2020;34(4):631–646.

299. Franco R, Fernandez-Vazquez A, Mollejo M, et al. Cutaneous presentation of follicular lymphomas. *Mod Pathol*. 2001;14(9):913–919.

300. Servitje O, Climent F, Colomo L, et al. Primary cutaneous vs secondary cutaneous follicular lymphomas: a comparative study focused on BCL2, CD10, and t(14;18) expression. *J Cutan Pathol*. 2019;46(3):182–189.

301. Mohamed AN, Palutke M, Eisenberg L, Al-Katib A. Chromosomal analyses of 52 cases of follicular lymphoma with t(14;18), including blastic/blastoid variant. *Cancer Genet Cytogenet*. 2001;126(1):45–51.

302. Green MR, Gentles AJ, Nair RV, et al. Hierarchy in somatic mutations arising during genomic evolution and progression of follicular lymphoma. *Blood*. 2013;121(9):1604–1611.

303. Requena L, Kutzner H, Palmedo G, et al. Cutaneous involvement in multiple myeloma: a clinicopathologic, immunohistochemical, and cytogenetic study of 8 cases. *Arch Dermatol*. 2003;139(4):475.

304. Panse G, Subtil A, McNiff JM, et al. Cutaneous involvement in plasma cell myeloma. *Am J Clin Pathol*. 2021;155(1):106–116.

305. Gaba RC, Kenny JP, Gundavaram P, Katz JR, Escuadro LR, Gaitonde S. Subcutaneous plasmacytoma metastasis precipitated by tunneled central venous catheter insertion. *Case Rep Oncol*. 2011;4(2):315.

306. Jurczyszyn A, Olszewska-Szopa M, Hungria V, et al. Cutaneous involvement in multiple myeloma: a multi-institutional retrospective study of 53 patients. *Leuk Lymphoma*. 2016;57(9):2071–2076.

307. Hendricks C, Fernández Figueras MT, Liersch J, et al. Cutaneous light chain deposition disease: a report of 2 cases and review of the literature. *Am J Dermatopathol*. 2018;40(5):337–341.

308. Marchica V, Accardi F, Storti P, et al. Cutaneous localization in multiple myeloma in the context of bortezomib-based treatment: how do myeloma cells escape from the bone marrow to the skin? *Int J Hematol*. 2017;105(1):104–108.

309. Black CL, Foster-Smith E, Lewis ID, Faull RJ, Sidhu SK. Post-transplant plasmablastic lymphoma of the skin. *Australas J Dermatol*. 2013;54(4):277.

310. Nguyen SK, Dagnault A. Radiotherapy for multiple myeloma with skin involvement. *Curr Oncol*. 2010;17(5):74.

311. Castillo JJ, Winer ES, Olszewski AJ. Sites of extranodal involvement are prognostic in patients with diffuse large B-cell lymphoma in the rituximab era: an analysis of the surveillance, epidemiology and end results database. *Am J Hematol*. 2014;89(3):310–314.

312. Plaza JA, Kacerovska D, Stockman DL, et al. The histomorphologic spectrum of primary cutaneous diffuse large B-cell lymphoma: a study of 79 cases. *Am J Dermatopathol*. 2011;33(7):649.

313. Vezzoli P, Fiorani R, Girgenti V, et al. Cutaneous T-cell/histiocyte-rich B-cell lymphoma: a case report and review of the literature. *Dermatology*. 2011;222(3):225.

314. Nicolae A, Pittaluga S, Abdullah S, et al. EBV-positive large B-cell lymphomas in young patients: a nodal lymphoma with evidence for a tolerogenic immune environment. *Blood*. 2015;126(7): 863–872.

315. Eros N, Karolyi Z, Kovacs A, Takacs I, Radvanyi G, Kelenyi G. Intravascular B-cell lymphoma. *J Am Acad Dermatol*. 2002;47(5 suppl):S260.

316. Murase T, Yamaguchi M, Suzuki R, et al. Intravascular large B-cell lymphoma (IVLBCL): a clinicopathologic study of 96 cases with special reference to the immunophenotypic heterogeneity of CD5. *Blood*. 2007;109(2):478–485.

317. Brunet V, Marouan S, Routy JP, et al. Retrospective study of intravascular large B-cell lymphoma cases diagnosed in Quebec: a retrospective study of 29 case reports. *Medicine (Baltimore)*. 2017;96(5):e5985.

318. Matsue K, Abe Y, Narita K, et al. Diagnosis of intravascular large B cell lymphoma: novel insights into clinicopathological features from 42 patients at a single institution over 20 years. *Br J Haematol*. 2019;187(3):328–336.

319. Murase T, Nakamura S, Kawauchi K, et al. An Asian variant of intravascular large B-cell lymphoma: clinical, pathological and cytogenetic approaches to diffuse large B-cell lymphoma associated with haemophagocytic syndrome. *Br J Haematol*. 2000;111(3):826.

320. Hsieh MS, Yeh YC, Chou YH, Lin CW. Intravascular large B cell lymphoma in Taiwan: an Asian variant of non-germinal-center origin. *J Formos Med Assoc*. 2010;109(3):185–191.

321. Ferreri AJ, Campo E, Seymour JF, et al. Intravascular lymphoma: clinical presentation, natural history, management and prognostic factors in a series of 38 cases, with special emphasis on the "cutaneous variant". *Br J Haematol*. 2004;127(2):173.

322. Kong YY, Dai B, Sheng WQ, et al. Intravascular large B-cell lymphoma with cutaneous manifestations: a clinicopathologic, immunophenotypic and molecular study of three cases. *J Cutan Pathol*. 2009;36(8):865–870.

323. Boonsakan P, Iamsumang W, Chantrathammachart P, Chayavichitsilp P, Suchonwanit P, Rutnin S. Prognostic value of concurrent expression of C-MYC and BCL2 in intravascular large B-cell lymphoma: a 10-year retrospective study. *Biomed Res Int*. 2020;2020:1350820.

324. Cerroni L, Massone C, Kutzner H, Mentzel T, Umbert P, Kerl H. Intravascular large T-cell or NK-cell lymphoma: a rare variant of intravascular large cell lymphoma with frequent cytotoxic phenotype and association with Epstein-Barr virus infection. *Am J Surg Pathol*. 2008;32(6):891–898.

325. Ponzoni M, Arrigoni G, Gould VE, et al. Lack of CD 29 (beta1 integrin) and CD 54 (ICAM-1) adhesion molecules in intravascular lymphomatosis. *Hum Pathol*. 2000;31(2):220.

326. Kato M, Ohshima K, Mizuno M, et al. Analysis of CXCL9 and CXCR3 expression in a case of intravascular large B-cell lymphoma. *J Am Acad Dermatol*. 2009;61(5):888–891.

327. Nakajima S, Ohshima K, Kyogoku M, Miyachi Y, Kabashima K. A case of intravascular large B-cell lymphoma with atypical clinical manifestations and analysis of CXCL12 and CXCR4 expression. *Arch Dermatol*. 2010;146(6):686–687.

328. Kanda M, Suzumiya J, Ohshima K, et al. Analysis of the immunoglobulin heavy chain gene variable region of intravascular large B-cell lymphoma. *Virchows Arch*. 2001;439(4):540–546.

329. Schrader AMR, Jansen PM, Willemze R, et al. High prevalence of MYD88 and CD79B mutations in intravascular large B-cell lymphoma. *Blood*. 2018;131(18):2086–2089.

330. McMenamin ME, Fletcher CD. Reactive angioendotheliomatosis: a study of 15 cases demonstrating a wide clinicopathologic spectrum. *Am J Surg Pathol*. 2002;26(6):685.

331. Liu Z, Zhang Y, Zhu Y, Zhang W. Prognosis of intravascular large B cell lymphoma (IVLBCL): analysis of 182 patients from global case series. *Cancer Manag Res*. 2020;12:10531–10540.

332. Matsue K, Asada N, Odawara J, et al. Random skin biopsy and bone marrow biopsy for diagnosis of intravascular large B cell lymphoma. *Ann Hematol*. 2011;90(4):417–421.

333. Matsue K, Abe Y, Kitadate A, et al. Sensitivity and specificity of incisional random skin biopsy for diagnosis of intravascular large B-cell lymphoma. *Blood*. 2019;133(11):1257–1259.

334. Rozenbaum D, Tung J, Xue Y, Hoang MP, Kroshinsky D. Skin biopsy in the diagnosis of intravascular lymphoma: a retrospective diagnostic accuracy study. *J Am Acad Dermatol*. 2021;85(3): 665–670.

335. Culhaci N, Levi E, Sen S, Kacar F, Meteoglu I. Pulmonary lymphomatoid granulomatosis evolving to large cell lymphoma in the skin. *Pathol Oncol Res*. 2002;8(4):280.

336. Song JY, Pittaluga S, Dunleavy K, et al. Lymphomatoid granulomatosis—a single institute experience: pathologic findings and clinical correlations. *Am J Surg Pathol*. 2015;39(2):141–156.

337. Beaty MW, Toro J, Sorbara L, et al. Cutaneous lymphomatoid granulomatosis: correlation of clinical and biologic features. *Am J Surg Pathol*. 2001;25(9):1111–1120.

338. Kuriyama S, Majima Y, Egawa Y, Suzuki Y, Moriki T, Tokura Y. Cutaneous lymphomatoid granulomatosis with long-term absence of lung involvement. *J Dermatol*. 2019;46(2):e69–e70.

339. Katzenstein AL, Doxtader E, Narendra S. Lymphomatoid granulomatosis: insights gained over 4 decades. *Am J Surg Pathol*. 2010;34(12):e35–e48.

340. Colby TV. Current histological diagnosis of lymphomatoid granulomatosis. *Mod Pathol*. 2012;25(suppl 1):S39–S42.

341. Melani C, Jaffe ES, Wilson WH. Pathobiology and treatment of lymphomatoid granulomatosis, a rare EBV-driven disorder. *Blood*. 2020;135(16):1344–1352.

342. Goodlad JR. Epstein-Barr virus-associated lymphoproliferative disorders in the skin. *Surg Pathol Clin*. 2017;10(2):429–453.

343. Lee WJ, Moon HR, Won CH, et al. Precursor B-or T-lymphoblastic lymphoma presenting with cutaneous involvement: a series of 13 cases including 7 cases of cutaneous T-lymphoblastic lymphoma. *J Am Acad Dermatol*. 2014;70(2):318–325.

344. Stein H, Foss HD, Durkop H, et al. CD30(+) anaplastic large cell lymphoma: a review of its histopathologic, genetic, and clinical features. *Blood*. 2000;96(12):3681–3695.

345. Falini B, Mason DY. Proteins encoded by genes involved in chromosomal alterations in lymphoma and leukemia: clinical value of their detection by immunocytochemistry. *Blood*. 2002;99(2):409–426.

346. Sibon D, Fournier M, Briere J, et al. Long-term outcome of adults with systemic anaplastic large-cell lymphoma treated within the Groupe d'Etude des Lymphomes de l'Adulte trials. *J Clin Oncol*. 2012;30(32):3939–3946.

347. Vassallo J, Lamant L, Brugieres L, et al. ALK-positive anaplastic large cell lymphoma mimicking nodular sclerosis Hodgkin's lymphoma: report of 10 cases. *Am J Surg Pathol*. 2006;30(2):223–229.

348. Medeiros LJ, Elenitoba-Johnson KS. Anaplastic large cell lymphoma. *Am J Clin Pathol*. 2007;127(5):707–722.

349. Inghirami G, Pileri SA, European TCLSG. Anaplastic large-cell lymphoma. *Semin Diagn Pathol*. 2011;28(3):190–201.

350. King RL, Dao LN, McPhail ED, et al. Morphologic features of ALK-negative anaplastic large cell lymphomas with DUSP22 rearrangements. *Am J Surg Pathol*. 2016;40(1):36–43.

351. d'Amore ES, Menin A, Bonoldi E, et al. Anaplastic large cell lymphomas: a study of 75 pediatric patients. *Pediatr Dev Pathol*. 2007;10(3):181–191.

352. Doring C, Hansmann ML, Agostinelli C, et al. A novel immunohistochemical classifier to distinguish Hodgkin lymphoma from ALK anaplastic large cell lymphoma. *Mod Pathol*. 2014;27(10):1345–1354.

353. Vega F, Medeiros LJ. A suggested immunohistochemical algorithm for the classification of T-cell lymphomas involving lymph nodes. *Hum Pathol*. 2020;102:104–116.

354. Herling M, Rassidakis GZ, Jones D, Schmitt-Graeff A, Sarris AH, Medeiros LJ. Absence of Epstein-Barr virus in anaplastic large cell lymphoma: a study of 64 cases classified according to World Health Organization criteria. *Hum Pathol*. 2004;35(4):455–459.

355. Vasmatzis G, Johnson SH, Knudson RA, et al. Genome-wide analysis reveals recurrent structural abnormalities of TP63 and other p53-related genes in peripheral T-cell lymphomas. *Blood*. 2012;120(11):2280–2289.

356. Parrilla Castellar ER, Jaffe ES, Said JW, et al. ALK-negative anaplastic large cell lymphoma is a genetically heterogeneous disease with widely disparate clinical outcomes. *Blood*. 2014;124(9):1473–1480.

357. Yang S, Khera P, Wahlgren C, et al. Cutaneous anaplastic large-cell lymphoma should be evaluated for systemic involvement regardless of ALK-1 status: case reports and review of literature. *Am J Clin Dermatol*. 2011;12(3):203.

358. Rudiger T, Weisenburger DD, Anderson JR, et al. Peripheral T-cell lymphoma (excluding anaplastic large-cell lymphoma): results from the Non-Hodgkin's Lymphoma Classification Project. *Ann Oncol*. 2002;13(1):140.

359. Balaraman B, Conley JA, Sheinbein DM. Evaluation of cutaneous angioimmunoblastic T-cell lymphoma. *J Am Acad Dermatol*. 2011;65(4):855.

360. Martel P, Laroche L, Courville P, et al. Cutaneous involvement in patients with angioimmunoblastic lymphadenopathy with dysproteinemia: a clinical, immunohistological, and molecular analysis. *Arch Dermatol*. 2000;136(7):881.

361. Jayaraman AG, Cassarino D, Advani R, Kim YH, Tsai E, Kohler S. Cutaneous involvement by angioimmunoblastic T-cell lymphoma: a unique histologic presentation, mimicking an infectious etiology. *J Cutan Pathol*. 2006;33(suppl 2):6.

362. Mahendran R, Grant JW, Hoggarth CE, Burrows NP. Angioimmunoblastic T-cell lymphoma with cutaneous involvement. *J Eur Acad Dermatol Venereol*. 2001;15(6):589.

363. Murakami T, Ohtsuki M, Nakagawa H. Angioimmunoblastic lymphadenopathy-type peripheral T-cell lymphoma with cutaneous infiltration: report of a case and its gene expression profile. *Br J Dermatol*. 2001;144(4):878.

364. Cook LB, Fuji S, Hermine O, et al. Revised adult T-cell leukemia-lymphoma international consensus meeting report. *J Clin Oncol*. 2019;37(8):677–687.

365. Nicot C. Current views in HTLV-I-associated adult T-cell leukemia/lymphoma. *Am J Hematol*. 2005;78(3):232.

366. Ohshima K, Mukai Y, Shiraki H, Suzumiya J, Tashiro K, Kikuchi M. Clonal integration and expression of human T-cell lymphotropic virus type I in carriers detected by polymerase chain reaction and inverse PCR. *Am J Hematol*. 1997;54(4):306.

367. Ohshima K, Suzumiya J, Sato K, et al. Nodal T-cell lymphoma in an HTLV-I-endemic area: proviral HTLV-I DNA, histological classification and clinical evaluation. *Br J Haematol*. 1998;101(4):703.

368. Liu B, Liang MH, Kuo YL, et al. Human T-lymphotropic virus type 1 oncoprotein tax promotes unscheduled degradation of Pds1p/securin and Clb2p/cyclin B1 and causes chromosomal instability. *Mol Cell Biol*. 2003;23(15):5269.

369. Cook LB, Phillips AA. How I treat adult T-cell leukemia/lymphoma. *Blood*. 2021;137(4):459–470.

370. Assaf C, Gellrich S, Whittaker S, et al. CD56-positive haematological neoplasms of the skin: a multicentre study of the Cutaneous Lymphoma Project Group of the European Organisation for Research and Treatment of Cancer. *J Clin Pathol*. 2007;60(9):981–989.

371. Bekkenk MW, Jansen PM, Meijer CJ, Willemze R. CD56+ hematological neoplasms presenting in the skin: a retrospective analysis of 23 new cases and 130 cases from the literature. *Ann Oncol*. 2004;15(7):1097.

372. Chan JK, Yip TT, Tsang WY, et al. Detection of Epstein-Barr viral RNA in malignant lymphomas of the upper aerodigestive tract. *Am J Surg Pathol*. 1994;18(9):938.

373. Tse E, Kwong YL. How I treat NK/T-cell lymphomas. *Blood*. 2013;121(25):4997.

374. Savage KJ, Chhanabhai M, Gascoyne RD, Connors JM. Characterization of peripheral T-cell lymphomas in a single North American institution by the WHO classification. *Ann Oncol*. 2004;15(10):1467.

375. Staber PB, Herling M, Bellido M, et al. Consensus criteria for diagnosis, staging, and treatment response assessment of T-cell prolymphocytic leukemia. *Blood*. 2019;134(14):1132–1143.

376. Brito-Babapulle V, Catovsky D. Inversions and tandem translocations involving chromosome 14q11 and 14q32 in T-prolymphocytic leukemia and T-cell leukemias in patients with ataxia telangiectasia. *Cancer Genet Cytogenet*. 1991;55(1):1.

377. Maljaei SH, Brito-Babapulle V, Hiorns LR, Catovsky D. Abnormalities of chromosomes 8, 11, 14, and X in T-prolymphocytic

leukemia studied by fluorescence in situ hybridization. *Cancer Genet Cytogenet*. 1998;103(2):110.

378. Chen X, Cherian S. Immunophenotypic characterization of T-cell prolymphocytic leukemia. *Am J Clin Pathol*. 2013;140(5): 727.

379. Introcaso CE, Kantor J, Porter DL, Junkins-Hopkins JM. Cutaneous Hodgkin's disease. *J Am Acad Dermatol*. 2008;58(2):295.

380. Werner B, Massone C, Kerl H, Cerroni L. Large CD30-positive cells in benign, atypical lymphoid infiltrates of the skin. *J Cutan Pathol*. 2008;35(12):1100–1107.

381. Mitteldorf C, Kempf W. Cutaneous pseudolymphoma—a review on the spectrum and a proposal for a new classification. *J Cutan Pathol*. 2020;47(1):76–97.

382. Sarantopoulos GP, Palla B, Said J, et al. Mimics of cutaneous lymphoma: report of the 2011 Society for Hematopathology/European Association for Haematopathology workshop. *Am J Clin Pathol*. 2013;139(4):536.

383. Nihal M, Mikkola D, Horvath N, et al. Cutaneous lymphoid hyperplasia: a lymphoproliferative continuum with lymphomatous potential. *Hum Pathol*. 2003;34(6):617.

384. Böer A, Tirumalae R, Bresch M, Falk TM. Pseudoclonality in cutaneous pseudolymphomas: a pitfall in interpretation of rearrangement studies. *Br J Dermatol*. 2008;159(2):394–402.

385. Magro CM, Daniels BH, Crowson AN. Drug induced pseudolymphoma. *Semin Diagn Pathol*. 2018;35(4):247–259.

386. Magro CM, Crowson AN, Kovatich AJ, Burns F. Drug-induced reversible lymphoid dyscrasia: a clonal lymphomatoid dermatitis of memory and activated T cells. *Hum Pathol*. 2003;34(2):119.

387. Khalil S, Ariel Gru A, Saavedra AP. Cutaneous extramedullary haematopoiesis: implications in human disease and treatment. *Exp Dermatol*. 2019;28(11):1201–1209.

388. Fraga GR, Caughron SK. Cutaneous myelofibrosis with JAK2 V617F mutation: metastasis, not merely extramedullary hematopoiesis! *Am J Dermatopathol*. 2010;32(7):727.

Tumors of Fibrous Tissue Involving the Skin

TREVOR W. BEER, JOSEPH S. KATTAMPALLIL, AND PETER HEENAN

Chapter

32

CLASSIFICATION OF FIBROUS TISSUE AND RELATED TUMORS BY CLINICAL BEHAVIOR

The main importance of correctly identifying and classifying fibrohistiocytic and soft-tissue tumors lies in being able to predict their biologic potential and, hence, appropriate treatment and advice to patients. This has given rise to a system of classification based on expected clinical behavior (1–3). The principles of this system are used in this chapter and summarized in Table 32-1, although some lesions do not fall neatly into these recognized categories.

Most of the tumors described in this chapter can be diagnosed on the basis of histologic features in hematoxylin–eosin–stained sections. However, immunohistochemistry is essential at times (Tables 32-2 and 32-3). This should be used as an adjunct to standard histologic methods and clinical data. Additional techniques such as cytogenetics and electron microscopy can also be of value in categorizing some tumors. Some chromosomal aberrations frequently associated with some of the entities in this chapter are summarized in Table 32-4.

Table 32-1

Classification of Soft Tissue Tumors by Clinical Behavior (1–3)

Benign

Benign behavior is the rule, but in exceptional circumstances, tumors in this category may metastasize (e.g., fibrous histiocytoma, diffuse giant-cell tumor of tendon sheath).

Intermediate biologic potential

1. Locally aggressive

   Recurrence may occur with tissue infiltration and destruction, but metastases are not expected (e.g., abdominal desmoid tumor).

2. Rarely metastasizing

   A small proportion (<2%) of cases may metastasize, and these cannot be reliably predicted from histologic examination (e.g., plexiform fibrohistiocytic tumor, angiomatoid fibrous histiocytoma).

Malignant

Malignant behavior is to be anticipated.

The importance of clinicopathologic correlation cannot be overemphasized, particularly when dealing with partial biopsies. The possibility that a malignant lesion represents a metastasis must always be considered.

SO-CALLED FIBROHISTIOCYTIC TUMORS

The term "fibrohistiocytic" is somewhat controversial, and some of these lesions may be better regarded as of fibroblastic/myofibroblastic differentiation. Nevertheless, some of these tumors exhibit features suggesting histiocytic differentiation (e.g., foam cells, giant cells, and CD68 expression), while synthesizing collagen (suggesting fibroblastic differentiation). The term "fibrohistiocytic" has therefore been retained for these skin lesions.

Benign Fibrohistiocytic Tumors

These are tumors with little or no potential for metastasis. Nevertheless, there are rare exceptions such as cellular dermatofibroma (discussed in the next section). Some of these lesions can persist locally and may occasionally recur or progress. Local excision is considered adequate treatment for most (e.g., common dermatofibroma), the majority tending to regress even if only partially removed. For other lesions, complete excision is recommended.

Dermatofibroma (Fibrous Histiocytoma/Sclerosing Hemangioma)

Clinical Summary. Dermatofibromas (fibrous histiocytomas) are common skin tumors predominantly occurring on the extremities or trunk of young adults. They present as small, firm, solitary nodules that are often red to brown in color, owing to increased intraepidermal melanin or tumoral hemosiderin. This may suggest a melanocytic lesion clinically. Dermatofibromas are seen only rarely on the palms and soles (4) or digits (5) and are relatively uncommon on the face, where they are more likely to be of cellular type and recur (6,7). Multiple tumors occasionally occur, sometimes associated with immunosuppressive therapy (8), pregnancy (9,10), HIV infection (11), and after antiretroviral therapy (12). Although most lesions are usually only a few millimeters in diameter, they occasionally measure 2 to 3 cm. The cut surface is white to yellow or brown, depending on the proportions of fibrous tissue, lipid, and hemosiderin present (Fig. 32-1A). Dermatofibromas usually persist, although spontaneous involution has also been observed (13).

Table 32-2

Selected Immunohistochemical Stains as an Aid to the Diagnosis of Spindle-Cell Tumors of the Skin

EMA	Atypical Fibroxanthoma	Dermatofibrosarcoma Protuberans	Cellular Fibrous Histiocytoma (Dermatofibroma)	Spindle-Cell Squamous Cell Carcinoma	Desmoplastic Melanoma	Leiomyosarcoma
SOX10, S100	–	–	–	–	+	–
Desmin	–	–	–	–	–	+
CD34	Variable	+	Variable	–	–	Rare
Factor XIIIa	Variable	Rare	+	–	–	–
Cytokeratin	–	–	–	+	–	Rare
Epithelial Membrane Antigen	Rare	–	–	Variable	–	–
Smooth Muscle Actin	Often +	Variable	Variable	Rare	Variable	+

Note: Immunohistochemistry should always be used as an adjunct to routine histologic methods and clinical data.
–, negative; +, positive; EMA, epithelial membrane antigen.

Table 32-3

Recent Immunostains That May Aid in the Differential Diagnosis of Fibrous Tissue Tumors of the Skin

Stain	Tumor or Tissue	Comments
ERG	Normal and neoplastic endothelial cells (both blood vessel and lymphatic)	Stains some epithelioid sarcoma, Ewing sarcomas, and prostate adenocarcinomas
STAT 6	Solitary fibrous tumor	Stains some liposarcomas
INI1	*Loss* of staining in epithelioid sarcoma, malignant rhabdoid tumors	Loss of staining may be seen in epithelioid MPNST
TLE1	Synovial sarcoma	Intense, diffuse nuclear staining helps to distinguish from staining seen in other lesions such as PNST, solitary fibrous tumor, and some carcinomas

MPNST, malignant peripheral nerve sheath tumor; PNST, peripheral nerve sheath tumors.
Lin G, Doyle LA. An update on the application of newly described immunohistochemical markers in soft tissue pathology. *Arch Pathol Lab Med.* 2015;139:106–121.

Table 32-4

Selected Chromosomal Aberrations Associated With Entities in This Chapter (297,311,522,532)

Tumor	Chromosomal Abnormality	Gene(s)
Acral fibromyxoma	13q12 loss	RB1
Angiomatoid fibrous histiocytoma	t(12;22)	EWSR1-ATF
	t(2;22)	EWSR1-CREB1
	t(12;16)	FUS-ATF1 fusions (EWSR1-CREB1 is also seen in clear-cell sarcoma)
Collagenous fibroma (desmoplastic fibroblastoma)	t(2;11) translocation	FOSL1
	11q12 rearrangements	
Dermatofibrosarcoma protuberans and giant-cell fibroblastoma	t(17;22) and ring chromosomes in some tumors	COL1A1-PDGFB
Desmoid-type fibromatosis	3p	Beta-catenin CTNNB1
Epithelioid fibrous histiocytoma	2p23 rearrangements	ALK
Epithelioid sarcoma	22q	Inactivation SMARCB1 (INI)
Fibroma of tendon sheath	t(2;11) translocation	
Giant-cell tumor of tendon sheath	t(1;2)	COL6A3-CSF1
Inflammatory myofibroblastic tumor	t(2;5)	ALK
Nodular fasciitis	17p13	MHY6-USP6 gene fusion
Proliferative fasciitis/proliferative myositis	t(6;14)	FOS
	14q	
	Trisomy 2	
Solitary fibrous tumor	12q13 intrachromosomal inversion	NAB2-STAT6
Synovial sarcoma	t(X;18)	SYT–SSX fusion

Note: The frequency of these changes varies, and multiple different abnormalities may be present.

Histopathology. The epidermis is usually hyperplastic, with hyperpigmentation of the basal layer and elongation of the rete ridges, separated by a clear (Grenz) zone from the tumor in the dermis (Fig. 32-1B). This is composed of fibroblast-like spindle cells, histiocytes, and blood vessels in varying proportions (Fig. 32-1C–E). Foamy histiocytes and multinucleate giant cells containing lipid or hemosiderin are frequently present, sometimes in large numbers, forming xanthomatous aggregates. Prominent lipid accumulation is seen in the lipidized ("ankle-type") dermatofibroma. Capillaries may be plentiful in the stroma, giving the lesion an angiomatous appearance. When there is also associated sclerosis, such lesions have been referred to as "sclerosing hemangioma." Some dermatofibromas may be poorly cellular and subtle, with spindle cells extending between collagen bundles associated with apparent "rounding up" of collagen fibers. More cellular forms often exhibit a storiform pattern of interwoven, fascicled spindle cells. Tumors are typically poorly demarcated.

Significant hyperplasia of the overlying epidermis occurs in more than 80% of dermatofibromas (14) and assists in making the diagnosis and in distinguishing the atypical variant from atypical fibroxanthoma (AFX) (15). Hyperplasia usually consists of regular rete ridge elongation, often with hyperpigmentation of basal keratinocytes. In some cases, the changes resemble a seborrheic keratosis, and, occasionally, downgrowths show hair matrical differentiation (16). In up to 5% of dermatofibromas,

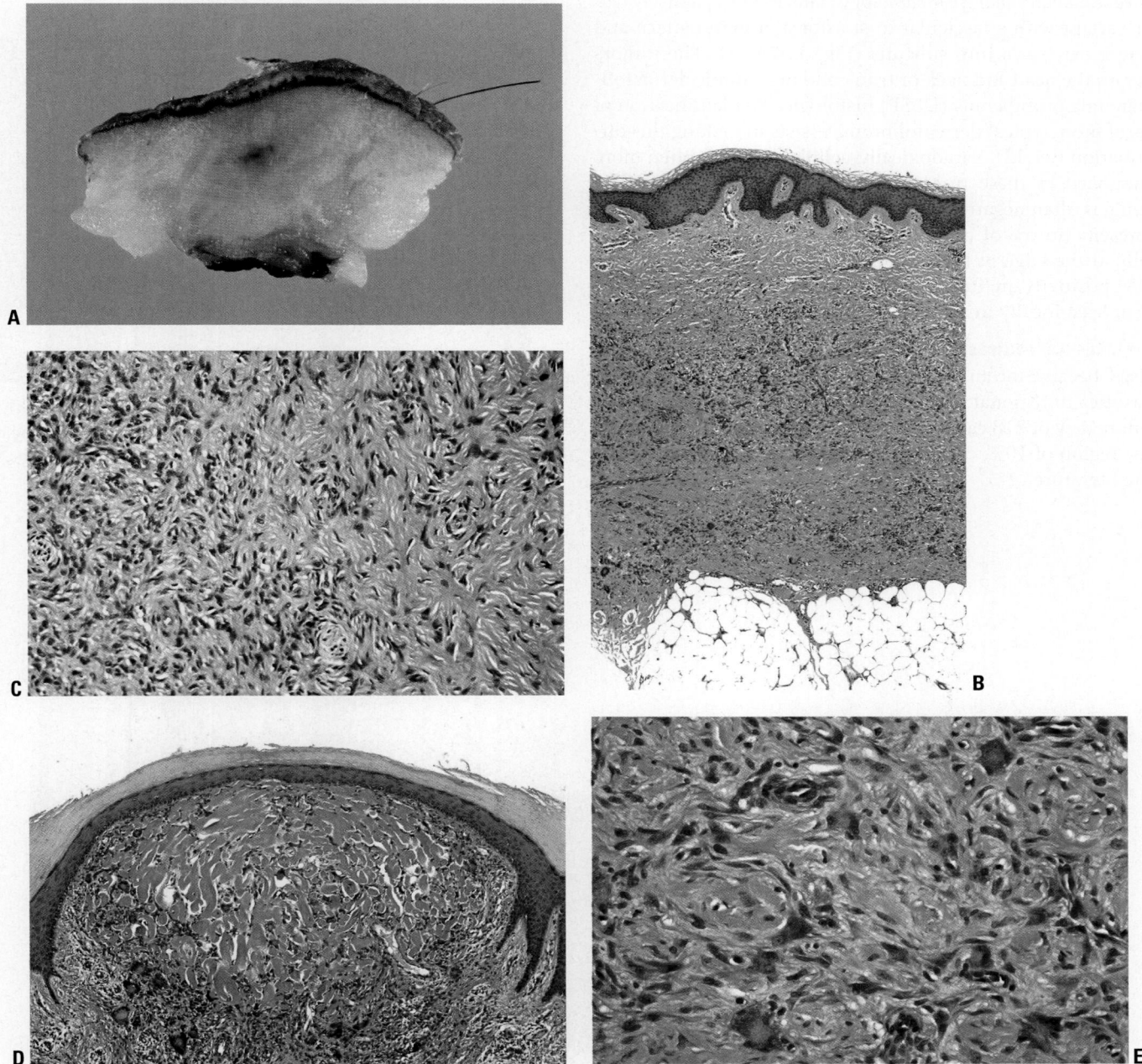

Figure 32-1 Dermatofibroma (fibrous histiocytoma). **A:** Gross specimen. A poorly circumscribed dermal lesion is present with epidermal hyperpigmentation and acanthosis. The tumor has a yellow cut surface with focal hemorrhage present centrally. **B:** The epidermis is hyperplastic and separated by a narrow Grenz zone from a moderately cellular spindle-cell tumor extending into the deep dermis. **C:** The tumor is composed of variably sized spindle cells with pale eosinophilic cytoplasm in a collagenous stroma. **D:** This dermatofibroma shows prominent hyalinization and pigmentation. **E:** Hemosiderin and multinucleated giant cells dominate in this zone of another dermatofibroma.

the downgrowths show areas that closely resemble superficial basal cell carcinoma (17). In rare instances, genuine invasive basal cell carcinoma development has been documented (18,19). Eight cases of dermatofibromas with included glands have been reported as adenodermatofibroma (20). It is unclear whether this represents glandular induction or included native glands, but it appears to be of no clinical significance.

Principles of Management: Local excision is considered adequate treatment, with most lesions tending to regress even if only partially removed. Complete excision of facial lesions has been recommended owing to their increased risk of recurrence (6).

Dermatofibroma Variants
Cellular Fibrous Histiocytoma (Dermatofibroma)
Clinical Summary and Histopathology. This is a rare, densely cellular variant with a fascicular-to-storiform growth pattern and frequent extension into subcutis (Fig. 32-2A, B). The tumors occur on the head and neck or trunk and may mimic dermatofibrosarcoma protuberans (DFSP) histologically. Identification of areas of more typical dermatofibroma assists in making this differentiation (21,22). Paradoxically, cellular atypia is often more pronounced in these tumors than in DFSP, and factor XIIIa staining is often negative (21,23). Areas of CD34 positivity may be present (in 6% of cases in one study) (23), but often only focally at the edge of the tumor. Foci of smooth muscle actin (SMA) positivity are frequent, and staining with desmin can be seen at least focally in up to 32% of cases (23,24).

Principles of Management: Complete surgical excision is advised because of an increased risk of recurrence, with rare metastases to regional nodes and the lung reported (21–26). A recent review of 218 cases suggests that the risk of recurrence is in the region of 10%, considerably less than previous estimates in the literature (27).

Aneurysmal Fibrous Histiocytoma
Histopathology. In these tumors, collections of capillaries, foci of hemorrhage, siderophages, and foamy macrophages surround cleft-like and cavernous blood-filled spaces in the center of the tumor. They are most frequently encountered on the limbs and may be several centimeters in size. The pseudovascular areas may dominate, simulating a vascular neoplasm, but intervening areas show more typical features of dermatofibroma (28–30) (Fig. 32-3). There is limited or no involvement of subcutis. To avoid confusion with angiomatoid fibrous histiocytoma (a tumor of intermediate malignancy; see later discussion), it has been suggested that these tumors should be referred to as "dermatofibroma with aneurysmal change" (31). One case has shown a t(12;19) translocation (32).

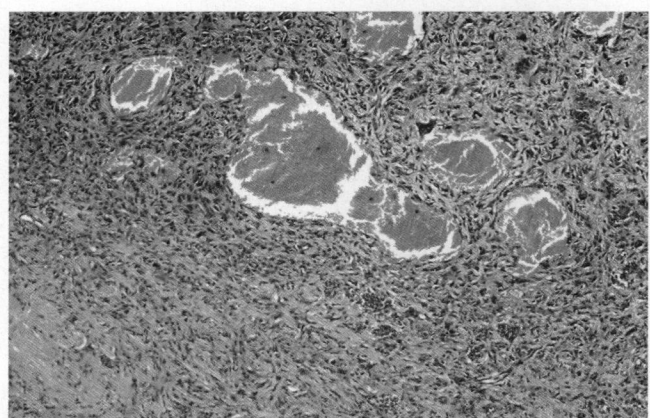

Figure 32-3 Aneurysmal fibrous histiocytoma (dermatofibroma). Dilated blood-filled spaces are prominent in this variant, with associated hemorrhage. Bland spindle cells and siderophages are seen in the surrounding tissue.

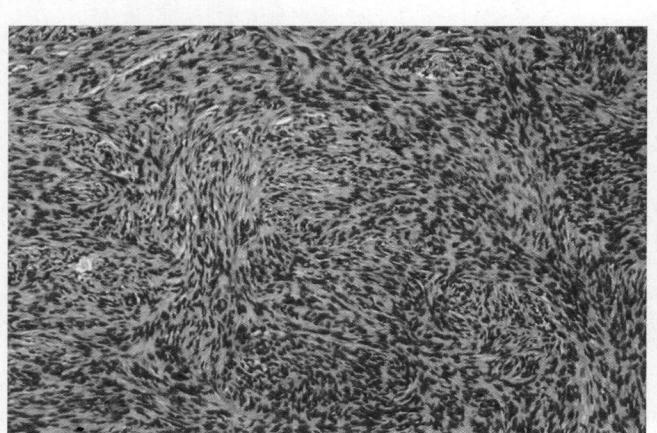

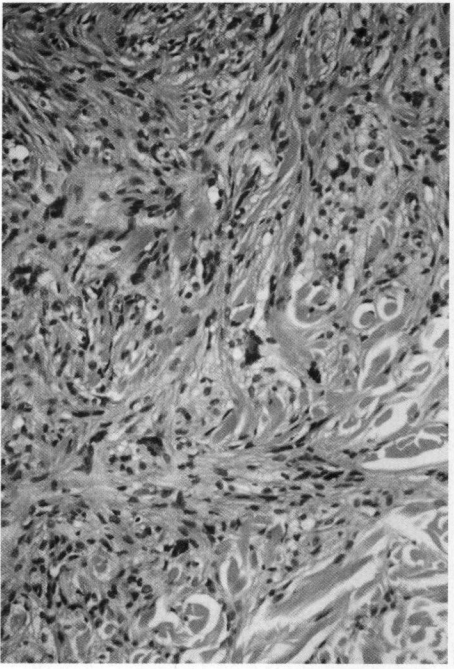

Figure 32-2 Cellular dermatofibroma (fibrous histiocytoma). **A:** The tumor consists of spindle cells arranged in densely cellular fascicles with storiform areas. **B:** At the border of the lesion, the spindle cells surround individual collagen bundles.

Principles of Management: Because a minority of lesions recur, complete excision is appropriate (24). Metastasis is exceptionally rare (33,34).

Atypical (Pseudosarcomatous) Fibrous Histiocytoma

Histopathology. Atypical cells are occasionally present in dermatofibroma, which may lead to misdiagnosis as AFX (35), and there is some overlap with cellular fibrous histiocytoma histologically. These tumors are usually small but occasionally reach 2.5 cm or greater in diameter (36). The atypical cells show enlarged, pleomorphic nuclei, sometimes referred to as "monster cells" (*dermatofibroma with monster cells*) (36,37). Mitoses of normal morphology may be evident in large numbers, and atypical mitotic figures have also been reported. Multinucleated giant cells with bizarre, large, hyperchromatic nuclei with little cytoplasm or irregular, vesicular nuclei with abundant foamy cytoplasm may also occur (Fig. 32-4A, B). Extension into superficial subcutis and focal necrosis may be seen. The presence of more usual appearing dermatofibroma in the background is very helpful to enable the correct diagnosis in these lesions (38). Variable staining for SMA and CD34 is reported, with often limited staining for factor XIIIa.

Principles of Management: Complete excision is required because of a significant risk of recurrence and very occasional metastases (38).

Epithelioid Fibrous Histiocytoma

Clinical Summary. This was originally thought to be a distinctive variant of dermatofibroma, although it is now generally considered to be a separate entity owing to its unique features and the presence of anaplastic lymphoma kinase (ALK) 2p23 rearrangements in the vast majority of cases (39–42). Epithelioid fibrous histiocytoma has also previously been described as epithelioid cell histiocytoma (43). Tumors most often present as solitary lesions in middle age, frequently on the lower limb (39).

Histopathology. Tumors form an exophytic nodule with an epidermal collarette resembling pyogenic granuloma, BAPoma, or intradermal Spitz nevus on low power (Fig. 32-5) (39,44,45). The lesions are often well circumscribed and composed of cells with abundant eosinophilic cytoplasm and occasional multinucleated forms. Areas of spindle cells may also be present or even

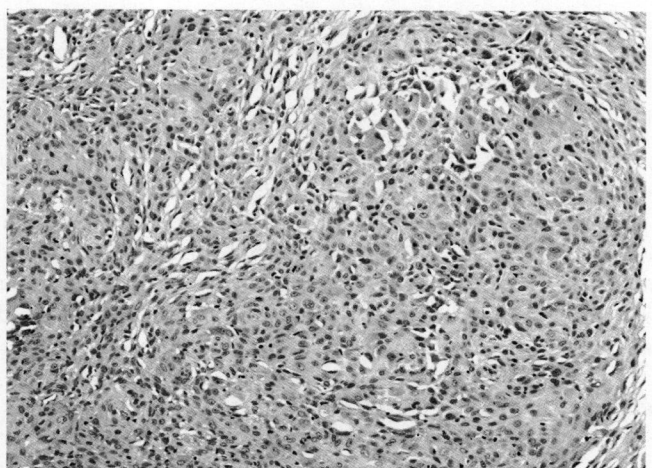

Figure 32-5 Epithelioid fibrous histiocytoma (dermatofibroma). The lesion shows sheets of epithelioid cells with eosinophilic cytoplasm. Differentiation from a melanocytic lesion such as a Spitz nevus may require immunohistochemistry in some cases.

dominate, with a complement of foamy macrophages in some cases (41). Immunohistochemistry may be required to differentiate the lesion from a melanocytic proliferation, for example. Tumors stain immunohistochemically similar to dermatofibromas, with, in addition, cytoplasmic or nuclear ALK staining as a consequence of ALK rearrangement, and there is epithelial membrane antigen (EMA) positivity in many cases (39).

Principles of Management: Local excision is considered adequate treatment, with no adverse clinical behavior reported to date.

Deep Fibrous Histiocytoma

Clinical Summary and Histopathology. This is a rare form that develops entirely within subcutaneous tissue, deep soft tissue, or parenchymal organs (46). Unlike typical dermatofibroma, deep fibrous histiocytoma tends to be well circumscribed, with a pseudocapsule and foci of hemorrhage consisting of monomorphic spindle cells resembling the cellular variant (47). Only one of seven cases recently studied cytogenetically showed a t(16;17) translocation, suggesting that this is a sporadic or rare

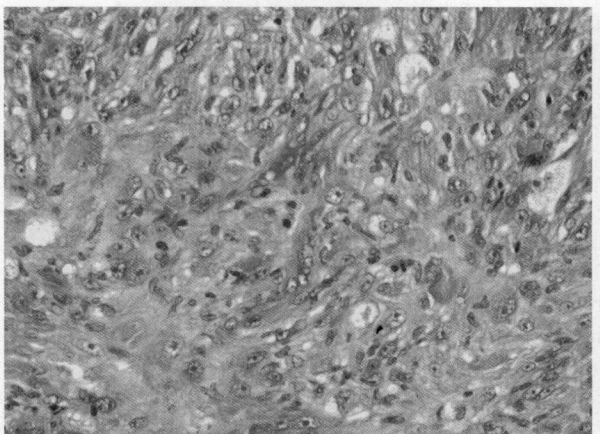
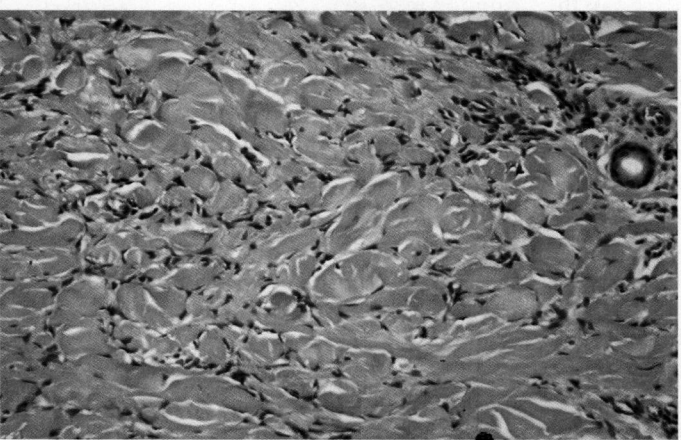

Figure 32-4 Atypical fibrous histiocytoma (dermatofibroma). **A:** This tumor shows histiocyte-like cells with enlarged and pleomorphic nuclei with prominent nucleoli. **B:** At the border of this tumor, the cells are arranged around individual collagen bundles in the pattern typical of the more usual form of dermatofibroma.

event in deep fibrous histiocytoma (48). In the largest series to date of 69 cases, 20% recurred, with metastasis in two cases (49). Both of the metastatic lesions were large tumors with a fatal outcome.

Principles of Management: Complete excision is indicated because of the risk of recurrence or, rarely, metastasis.

Other less common variants include clear-cell (50), granular cell (51), lipidized (52), myxoid (53), myofibroblastic (54), osteoclastic (55), keloidal (56), atrophic (57), and palisading forms (58). Rarely, bone formation is seen with osteoclast-like giant cells (59).

Neoplasm Versus Reactive Process

It has been suggested that dermatofibromas are reactive processes following minor trauma, such as an insect bite, leading to the term "nodular subepidermal fibrosis" (55), with some authorities regarding the lesions as fibrosing inflammatory processes, even in the presence of "monster cells" (36,60). The demonstration of clonality in some cases of dermatofibroma (48,61,62) and reports of metastasizing dermatofibroma (see later discussions), however, suggest a neoplastic nature in at least some forms. Analysis of X chromosome inactivation in 31 dermatofibromas showed a variable pattern, suggesting that the lesions are heterogeneous, with some being reactive and others possibly neoplastic in nature (63–66).

Pathogenesis. Enzyme histochemical, electron microscopic, and immunohistochemical studies have suggested histiocytic, myofibroblastic, and fibroblastic differentiation, possibly indicating a cell of primitive mesenchymal origin (67). The term *dermal dendrocytoma* was proposed owing to the presence of factor XIIIa (a marker of normal dermal dendrocytes) and the histiocytic marker MAC 387 (68,69). Other investigators believe that the factor XIIIa–positive cells are included reactive stromal cells, rather than tumor cells (67,70). Historical electron microscopic studies variously described fibrous histiocytomas as being composed of fibroblasts, histiocytes, and myofibroblasts (71–73).

Enzyme Histochemistry. The results of enzyme studies on dermatofibromas have shown variable reactions. Positive staining for lysozyme and α_1-antitrypsin has been interpreted as indicating histiocytic differentiation (74,75), whereas negative results for these enzymes have led to speculation that the fibroblastic and histiocyte-like cells in these tumors arise from primitive mesenchymal cells (76). The presence of HLA-DR antigens in the majority of cells in dermatofibromas has also been regarded as evidence in favor of a histiocytic origin (77).

Differential Diagnosis. Dermatofibromas must be distinguished from DFSP. Some distinguishing features are that dermatofibromas show overlying epidermal hyperplasia; a heterogeneous population of tumor cells, often with more pleomorphism; and extension of tumor cells at the edge of the lesion around individual hyalinized collagen bundles (78). Dermatofibromas (including cellular forms) tend to show higher mitotic counts than DFSP (79). Cellular fibrous histiocytoma may also extend into subcutis along the interlobular septa or in a bulging, expansile pattern rather than in the characteristic infiltrating honeycomb-like pattern of DFSP (22). DFSP is usually larger, often consisting of multiple nodules. Cellular fibrous histiocytoma may also be confused with leiomyosarcoma, but leiomyosarcomas have

plumper spindle cells, with eosinophilic cytoplasm and nuclei with rounded ends, and shows positive staining for desmin and α-SMA (67). It should be noted that some dermatofibromas may express CD34, particularly at the periphery of the lesion, and some DFSP may express factor XIIIa (80). This has led to the suggestion of a biologic spectrum between fibrous histiocytoma and DFSP, with coexistence of two different cell populations in indeterminate lesions (81). Tenascin (an extracellular matrix glycoprotein) expression has been demonstrated immunohistochemically at the dermoepidermal junction overlying fibrous histiocytomas but not DFSP (82,83).

Fibrous histiocytoma with aneurysmal change (*aneurysmal fibrous histiocytoma*) may be confused with neoplasms of vascular origin. Distinction can be made by demonstrating that factors VIII, CD31, and CD34 do not outline the pseudovascular spaces in fibrous histiocytoma, in contrast to true vascular lesions. Kaposi sarcoma shows slit-like spaces containing erythrocytes and a usually monomorphic CD34-positive spindle-cell population with HHV8 nuclear staining (67). *Angiomatoid fibrous histiocytoma* is distinguished by its presentation in a younger age group (sometimes with systemic symptoms), subcutaneous location and the presence of eosinophilic histiocytoid cells, a prominent lymphocytic infiltrate, and a thick pseudocapsule (84,85).

Epithelioid dermatofibroma (epithelioid cell histiocytoma) can resemble Spitz nevus and pyogenic granuloma clinically and histologically (45). The lesion differs from pyogenic granuloma by the presence of epithelioid cells between inconspicuous blood vessels, which are not arranged in lobules, with a less prominent inflammatory component and lack of protuberant endothelial cells. Intradermal Spitz nevus has a nested pattern superficially, and it often has spindle as well as epithelioid cells, intranuclear cytoplasmic inclusions, maturation with depth, and, frequently, Kamino bodies in the epidermis. Immunostaining of Spitz nevi reveals positivity for melanocyte markers with negative staining for factor XIIIa. ALK and EMA are frequently demonstrable immunohistochemically in epithelioid fibrous histiocytoma (39).

AFX differs from *atypical dermatofibroma* by being located on sun-exposed skin of the head and neck of elderly patients, frequent ulceration, severe cellular pleomorphism, numerous mitoses, including atypical forms, and the lack of a background of more usual dermatofibroma.

Metastasizing Fibrous Histiocytoma

Clinical Summary and Histopathology. Sporadic cases of metastasizing fibrous histiocytomas have been reported in the literature over the years (21,22,25,26), and in 2013, two significant series of cases were reported (34,86). In these two reports, a total of 22 cases of metastatic fibrous histiocytoma were described, which led to the death of eight of the patients. Factors associated with metastatic behavior tended to be large size; necrosis; prominent mitotic activity; and, in some cases, invasion of subcutis. Most of the original fibrous histiocytomas showed features of cellular, aneurysmal, or atypical variants. However, in some lesions, it is difficult to predict aggressive behavior from histologic features alone (26,86,87,88). Perineural invasion was reported in a cellular dermatofibroma that metastasized, suggesting that this could also be a risk factor for metastasis (89). Chromosomal aberrations identified by array-CGH (comparative genomic hybridization) may be of some value in identifying high-risk tumors (34), with metastasizing lesions showing greater chromosomal aberrations compared to atypical or cellular fibrous histiocytomas (90).

Principles of Management: Close follow-up is advised for tumors that show repeated or early recurrence (86). For metastatic disease, surgery, chemotherapy, and radiotherapy have all been used, but an optimum regime remains to be clarified (86).

Plaque-Like CD34-Positive Dermal Fibroma (Medallion-Like Dermal Dendrocyte Hamartoma)

Clinical Summary. This is a recently described and rare lesion that is often congenital and tends to occur on the neck, trunk, or extremities as an indurated plaque (91–93).

Histopathology. The epidermis is typically atrophic with an upper dermal proliferation of bland spindle-shaped cells that may show limited extension into subcutis (91–93). There may be an associated myxoid stroma with fine blood vessels. Mitotic activity is not a feature.

Pathogenesis. These lesions have been considered to be either hamartomatous or reactive in nature and not related to dermal dendrocytes (92). CD34 is strongly expressed and there may be some factor XIIIa positivity, but this varies, which is considered as evidence against a dermal dendrocytic origin.

Differential Diagnosis. S100 is negative, which aids in distinction from neurofibroma, and actin is not expressed, unlike in dermatomyofibroma. One of the principal differential diagnoses is congenital atrophic DFSP. The absence of a t(17;22) translocation aids in this distinction (92).

Principles of Management: Local excision is considered adequate treatment.

Giant-Cell Tumor of Tendon Sheath

Clinical Summary. Giant-cell tumor of tendon sheath occurs most commonly on the tendon sheath of young and middle-aged adults on the dorsum of the fingers, hands, and wrists. They can also be found on the feet and around the ankle and knee joints. Multiple lesions are very rare (94). Tumors are firm in consistency, with a yellowish-to-tan cut surface, and are from 1 to 3 cm in diameter. There is no tendency toward spontaneous involution. The tumor may erode the adjacent bone and, on rare occasions, may even extend into the overlying

skin (95,96). The lesions are benign, although they may recur in up to 30% of cases (97). Rates of recurrence as low as 5% have been reported when careful surgery is performed under magnification (98). Recurrences are cured by local reexcision (99). Although it has been suggested that this tumor is an inflammatory proliferation (100), it now appears more likely that the lesions are neoplastic with cytogenetic abnormalities identified in some cases, typically involving rearrangements of chromosome 1 (97,101).

Histopathology. The tumor consists of lobules of varied cellularity surrounded by a fibrous pseudocapsule (Fig. 32-6A). In cellular areas, most cells are macrophage-like mononuclear cells with folded, kidney-shaped or grooved, oval nuclei and abundant eosinophilic cytoplasm. There are variable numbers of foamy macrophages, which may be associated with cholesterol clefts and siderophages. Less cellular areas consist of spindle cells within a fibrous or hyalinized stroma (95,102). The characteristic osteoclast-like giant cells (103) are scattered through both the cellular and fibrous areas. Their cytoplasm is deeply eosinophilic with often large numbers of haphazardly distributed nuclei (Fig. 32-6B). Although mitotic figures are seen in a large proportion of cases and may be frequent (104), they are not atypical. There is no evidence that mitotic activity is related to metastasis, which is an extremely rare event, but it may be associated with an increased risk of recurrence (105).

Pathogenesis. Ultrastructural (103,106), enzyme (102), and immunohistochemical studies (102,107–109) have indicated variously that the cells may be related to synovial cells, monocytes, and osteoclasts. It should be noted that occasional dendritic cells may be desmin-positive, but these do not demonstrate other skeletal muscle markers such as myogenin (97).

Principles of Management: Local excision is indicated, with recurrence occurring in a proportion of cases that are incompletely excised.

Intermediate Biologic Potential (Locally Aggressive Fibrohistiocytic Tumors)

Lesions of intermediate biologic potential may be locally aggressive, with continued, destructive growth. These lesions only rarely metastasize. Complete excision, with careful consideration of optimal margin width, is recommended.

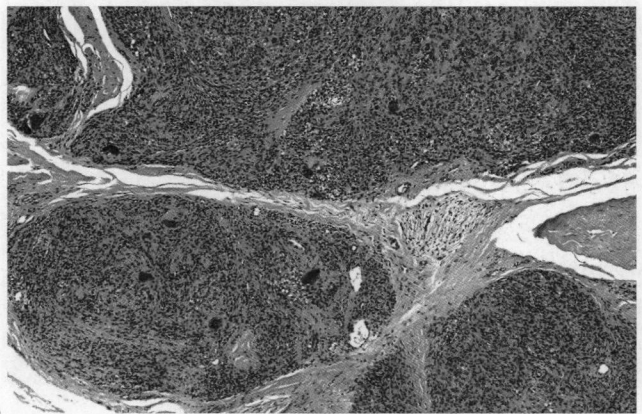
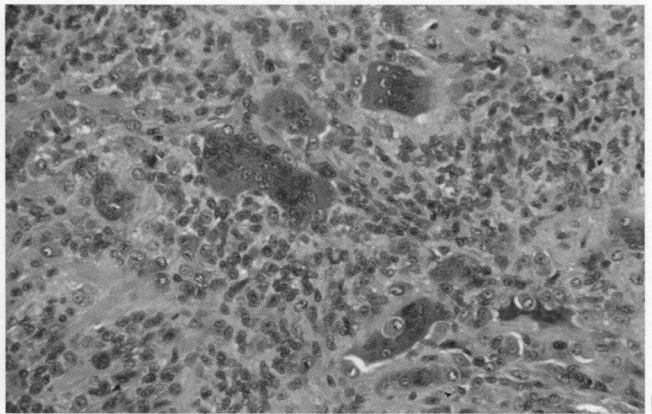

Figure 32-6 Giant-cell tumor of tendon sheath. **A:** The tumor is composed of circumscribed, densely cellular lobules surrounded by fibrous tissue. **B:** Giant cells with multiple nuclei, resembling osteoclasts, are scattered among plump epithelioid and spindle cells.

Dermatofibrosarcoma Protuberans

Clinical Summary. DFSP is a slowly growing, dermal spindle-cell neoplasm of intermediate malignancy, which has recently been comprehensively reviewed (110). It typically forms an indurated plaque on which multiple congested, firm nodules subsequently arise, sometimes with ulceration (Fig. 32-7A). The trunk and proximal limbs of young adults are most commonly affected, with occasional involvement of the head and neck or other sites (111,112). Presentation as an atrophic lesion is occasionally seen. A number of cases have been reported in childhood and, rarely, as congenital lesions (112–115). Local recurrence is common, and transformation to fibrosarcoma can occur, although metastasis is rare (116,117).

Histopathology. DFSP is composed of fascicles of densely packed, monomorphous spindle cells arranged in a storiform (mat-like) pattern. Lesions are poorly circumscribed, with diffuse infiltration of dermis and subcutis yielding a honeycomb pattern (Fig. 32-7B–D) (22). Infiltration into the underlying fascia and muscle occurs as a late event (117). Cytologically, the cells have a deceptively bland appearance, which can result in difficulty in defining the margin of the lesion. Mitotic activity is generally limited and typically less than 5 mitoses per 10 high-power fields are seen. Myxoid areas may occur, especially in recurrent tumors. Sometimes, there is a vascular component of fine anastomosing blood vessels with a "chicken-wire" appearance resembling myxoid liposarcoma (Fig. 32-8) (118).

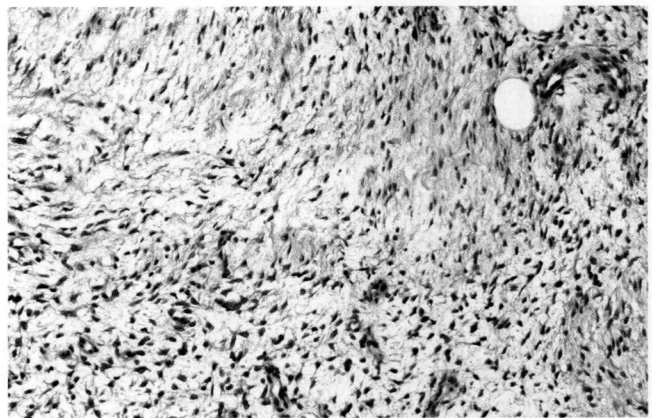

Figure 32-8 Myxoid dermatofibrosarcoma protuberans (DFSP). This DFSP shows a myxoid appearance as it extends into subcutis. Myxoid change is more common in recurrent tumors.

Pigmented DFSP is an extremely rare variant that has single or clustered pigmented melanosome-containing cells (which are S100, and HMB45 positive) the *Bednar tumor* (previously also known as storiform neurofibroma) (119–121). A number of congenital presentations of this tumor have been recorded (122).

Fibrosarcomatous areas are seen in a small proportion of DFSP, characterized by a fascicular or herringbone growth

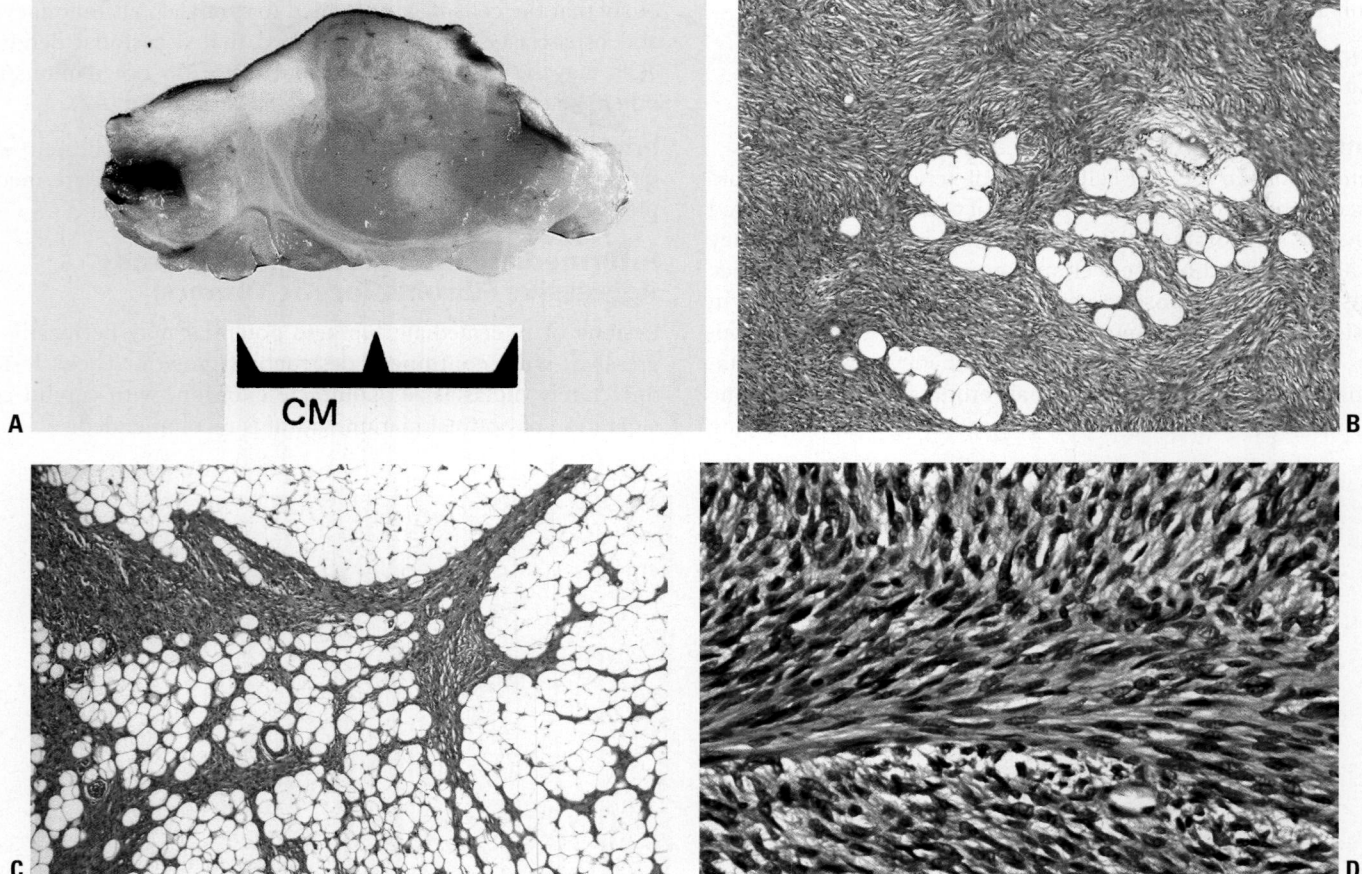

Figure 32-7 Dermatofibrosarcoma protuberans (DFSP). **A:** Gross specimen of a myxoid variant of DFSP. The lesion is better circumscribed than the more typical form of DFSP and forms a central nodule extending into subcutis, with lateral extension in the dermis showing a component of firmer white tissue. CM, centimeter. **B:** Densely packed spindle cells are present, arranged in a storiform pattern extending around fat cells. **C:** Strands of bland spindle cells infiltrate subcutis, producing a honeycomb-like pattern. **D:** This DFSP exhibits an area of fibrosarcomatous change.

pattern (123–125). This change carries an increased risk of metastasis and is associated with p53 mutation and increased proliferative activity (126,127). CD34 may be negative in areas of fibrosarcomatous change. Giant cells are rarely seen in otherwise typical DFSP but are characteristically prominent in the juvenile variant of DFSP, giant-cell fibroblastoma (see next section) (128–133).

Pathogenesis. Electron microscopic studies suggest that the tumor cells are fibroblasts because they show active synthesis of collagen in a well-developed endoplasmic reticulum (134,135). In some tumors, interrupted basement membrane–like material along the cell membrane suggested that the cells are modified fibroblasts with features of perineural and endoneurial cells (136). EMA expression in a few cases and consistent CD34 positivity raised the possibility of a perineural origin (137). Although DFSP is commonly regarded as a fibrohistiocytic tumor, immunohistochemical and ultrastructural evidence have also suggested a fibroblastic origin (118,138–140). In rare instances, particularly in fibrosarcomatous forms of DFSP, bundles of eosinophilic SMA-positive spindle cells are evident—in keeping with localized myofibroblastic or myoid differentiation. CD117 expression is typically absent in both DFSP and dermatofibroma (141).

Cytogenetic studies reveal a t(17;22) translocation in more than 90% of DFSP, leading to the formation of a ring chromosome in some tumors (142). The translocation involves the *COL1A1* gene on chromosome 17 and the platelet-derived growth factor B gene on chromosome 22. Although management is primarily surgical, high rates of clinical response have been achieved using imatinib, a tyrosine kinase inhibitor that affects platelet-derived growth factor beta receptors in unresectable or metastatic DFSP (143–145).

Differential Diagnosis. DFSP is generally characterized by more uniform spindle cells and a more prominent storiform pattern than that seen in dermatofibroma. Small biopsies may make the assessment of architecture impossible; so, caution is required in these cases. In contrast to cellular dermatofibroma, the epidermis overlying DFSP is usually attenuated or ulcerated rather than hyperplastic, and a clear (Grenz) zone between the epidermis and tumor may be absent. DFSP has a more infiltrative pattern of growth, in contrast to the well-demarcated bulging deep margin of cellular dermatofibroma, although this tumor may also extend into subcutis, predominantly along septa (22,78). CD34 staining is usually diffusely positive in DFSP and negative in most forms of dermatofibroma (146–148) (Fig. 32-9), but there is some overlap in CD34 expression (81). Some dermatofibromas exhibit a fairly characteristic pattern of peripheral "leading edge" CD34 staining, but with a conspicuous absence of staining centrally. Demonstration of tenascin at the dermoepidermal junction overlying dermatofibroma but not DFSP may help in the differential diagnosis (82,83). It has also been shown that dermatofibromas strongly express CD44 with only faint stromal hyaluronate, whereas DFSP shows reduced or absent CD44 and strong stromal hyaluronate deposition (149). Apolipoprotein D has been identified immunohistochemically in most DFSP but not in dermatofibromas (150). Neurofibroma expresses S100 protein, which is absent in DFSP, and shows other features of neural differentiation, without the dense, uniform cellularity of DFSP. Immunohistochemical staining for D2-40 has been reported as positive in dermatofibroma and negative in DFSP (151). In one study, Wilms Tumor 1 (WT1)

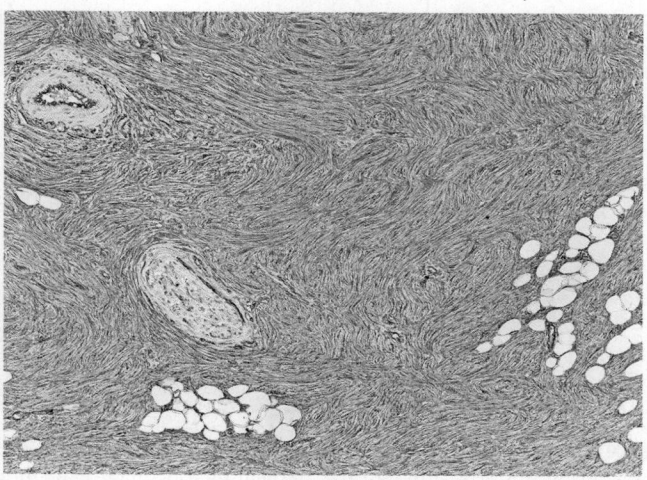

Figure 32-9 Dermatofibrosarcoma protuberans. Immunohistochemistry shows strong, uniform positivity for CD34. (Courtesy of Dr. E.-C. Jung, University of California, San Francisco, California.)

cytoplasmic positivity was evident in 95% of DFSP but not in dermatofibroma or other spindle-cell lesions tested, except for neurofibromas (152).

Principles of Management: A wide local excision with a 2-cm margin has been recommended because of the high risk of recurrence (144). Mohs surgery can be very effective, with low rates of recurrence (110,153–155), although in reexcisions, differentiating scar fibroblasts from residual tumor may be very difficult and require CD34 immunohistochemistry (IHC) on paraffin blocks (slow Mohs). Imatinib mesylate has been shown to be of some benefit in locally advanced or metastatic DFSP, as described earlier, despite the absence of stainable CD117 in DFSP (141,143–145). Tumors may be radiosensitive, but the role of radiotherapy remains to be fully established (144).

Giant-Cell Fibroblastoma

Clinical Summary. Giant-cell fibroblastoma represents a juvenile variant of DFSP and was first formally reported in 1989 (128). It is a rare tumor occurring mostly in children, with more than 75% of patients younger than 20 years (156). Lesions are solitary and most often sited on the trunk or thigh. Local recurrence after incomplete excision is common (157), but no metastases have been reported (158). Fibrosarcomatous change is very rare (156).

Histopathology. The proliferation is sited in the dermis and subcutis, usually with areas showing the honeycomb pattern typical of DFSP (Fig. 32-10A). In contrast, multinucleated giant cells line small clefts in the tissue (Fig. 32-10B), and foci of hemorrhage and perivascular lymphocytes may be seen (156). Zones of myxoid-to-hyalinized stroma are also present and often prominent. Electron microscopy suggests that the giant cells are not in fact multinucleated, but that the appearance represents multiple lobations of a single nucleus (128).

Pathogenesis. Ultrastructurally, the cells resemble fibroblasts. Immunohistochemistry shows CD34 positivity (including in the giant cells) with no staining for S100, SMA, or desmin (156,159).

The concept that giant-cell fibroblastoma is a variant of DFSP is supported by the coexistence of areas of both tumors in a single lesion in some instances, the same immunogenetic

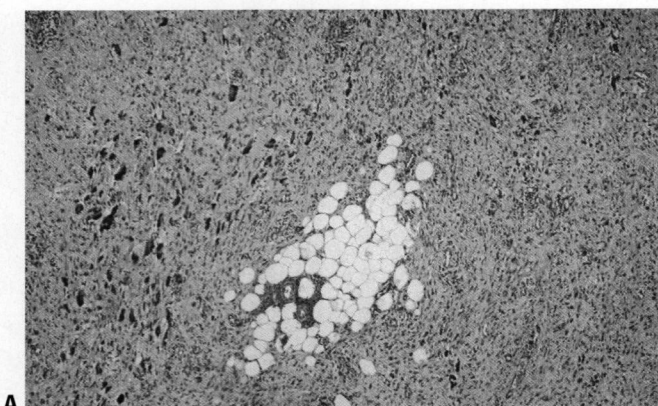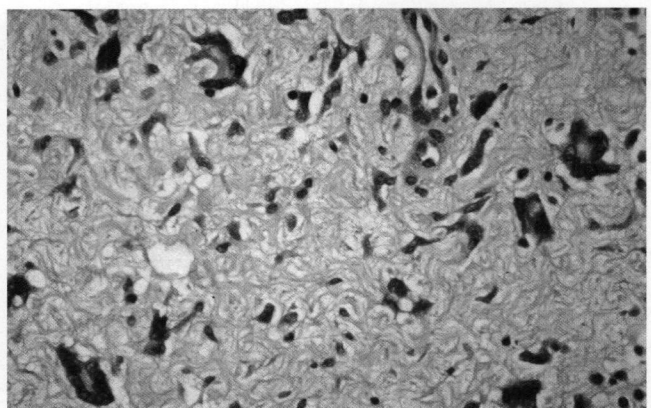

Figure 32-10 Giant-cell fibroblastoma. **A:** The growth pattern resembles that of dermatofibrosarcoma protuberans with infiltration of subcutaneous fat by uniform spindle cells, with numerous giant cells in addition. (Courtesy of Dr. I. Strungs, Adelaide Children's Hospital, Adelaide, Australia, and Dr. P. W. Allen, Flinders Medical Centre, Bedford Park, SA 5042, Australia.) **B:** Numerous multinucleated giant cells are present on high power, some with pleomorphic, multilobated nuclei.

and cytogenetic profile, and the recurrence of DFSP as giant-cell fibroblastoma and vice versa (128–133). As in DFSP, the translocation t(17;22), sometimes forming an extra ring chromosome, has been repeatedly identified (142,160), and responsiveness to imatinib in inoperable cases might therefore be anticipated (143).

The differential diagnosis includes fibrous hamartoma of infancy (see later discussions). Some distinguishing features are the patient's age, the presence of three "zones" in fibrous hamartoma, and its lack of multinucleated cells.

Principles of Management: Wide surgical excision is indicated, with recurrences frequent if excision is incomplete (157). Recurrences may have the appearance of a DFSP.

Intermediate Biologic Potential (Rarely Metastasizing Fibrohistiocytic Tumors)

These lesions commonly recur locally, but metastases to lymph nodes or viscera are only rarely seen.

Plexiform Fibrohistiocytic Tumor

Clinical Summary. Plexiform fibrohistiocytic tumor is a rare multinodular neoplasm of the dermis and subcutis composed of histiocyte-like cells, fibroblasts, and multinucleate giant cells in a plexiform pattern (161). This distinctive lesion occurs as a slowly growing mass, usually involving the arm of the young, especially females. Infants are occasionally affected (162). The lesion is of intermediate biologic potential, with local recurrence common but with only rare metastases to lymph nodes or viscera (163,164). No features predictive of recurrence or metastasis have been delineated.

Histopathology. A biphasic pattern is seen, with nodules of histiocytes surrounded by fascicles of spindle cells intersecting the stroma in a plexiform pattern. Osteoclast-like giant cells are identifiable in the majority of cases but not all (Fig. 32-11A) (165–167). The proportion of different cellular elements varies from case to case. Mitotic activity with mild nuclear atypia and pleomorphism may be present, but these are not reliable predictors of adverse behavior (164).

Pathogenesis. Ultrastructural and immunocytochemical studies have indicated histiocytic and myofibroblastic differentiation (163,168) in the different cellular components (Fig. 32-11B). No consistent genetic changes have been identified (169).

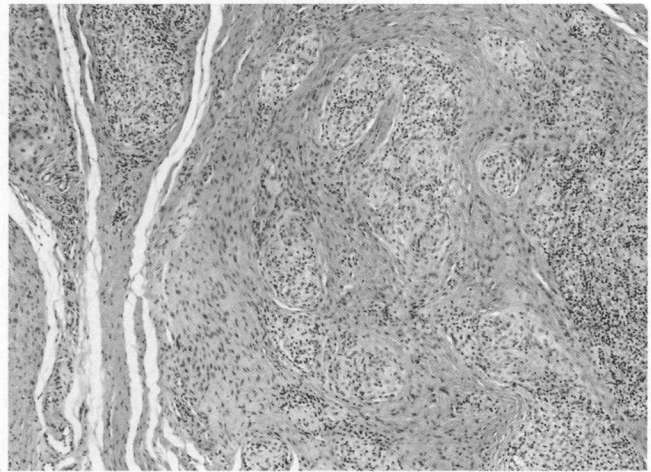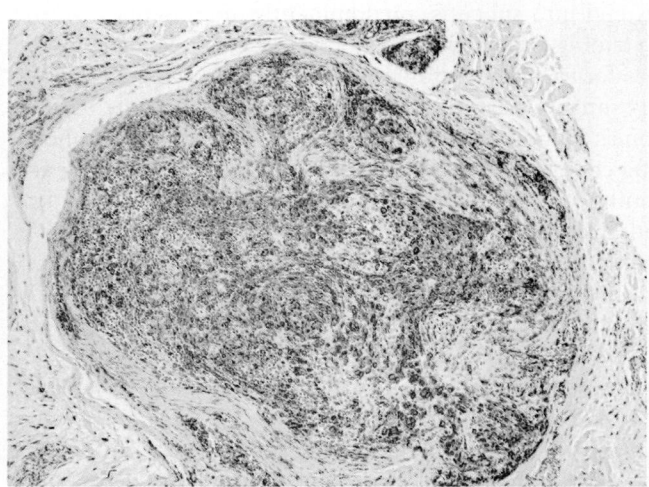

Figure 32-11 Plexiform fibrohistiocytic tumor. **A:** Pale, nodular groups of histiocyte-like cells are present between collagenous bands in the dermis and subcutis. **B:** Immunohistochemistry demonstrates that many of the pale cells are CD68-positive.

Differential Diagnosis. Cellular fibrous histiocytoma and dermatomyofibroma do not have the distinctive nodules of histiocytic-like cells of plexiform fibrohistiocytic tumor and tend to show a cohesive growth pattern. Fibromatoses and nodular fasciitis are usually more deeply situated and lack the characteristic plexiform architecture. Fibrous hamartoma of infancy has no histiocytic nodules or giant cells (157). Lesions can be mistaken for a granulomatous process. Distinction from neurothekeoma may be problematic, especially in tumors dominated by histiocytoid cells, and some have suggested that these lesions may be related (170). Both tumors tend to express CD10 and NKIC3 (171). A lack of identifiable MiTF and S100 staining in plexiform fibrohistiocytic tumors helps in this distinction (170–172). Most plexiform fibrohistiocytic tumors are CD68-positive, and actin is sometimes identifiable, in addition, with an absence of desmin staining (170–172).

Principles of Management: Surgical excision and clinical follow-up are indicated owing to the risk of local recurrence or metastasis. A recent literature review identified nodal metastasis in less than 3% of tumors, with lung metastasis in less than 2% (164).

Atypical Fibroxanthoma

Clinical Summary. AFX is characterized by a malignant histologic appearance but a generally benign course with only occasional recurrences and exceptionally rare metastases (173–175). Lesions are typically associated with actinic damage and tend to present on the head, neck, and in particular the ear of elderly patients (174). AFX usually forms a solitary nodule up to 2 cm in diameter, often with a short history of rapid growth.

Histopathology. The lesion forms a dermal tumor with, by definition, very minimal or no involvement of subcutis (176). AFXs are usually highly cellular, with marked and often striking pleomorphism and atypia of the constituent cells. Mitoses are readily identified with some atypical forms (Fig. 32-12A, B) (174,175,177). Most tumors are predominately composed of spindle cells, with areas of more epithelioid and histiocyte-like appearing forms also present. The cells may be arranged in disordered fascicles, surrounding but not destroying adnexal structures. An epidermal collarette is often seen, with ulceration

frequent. Scattered inflammatory cells are present, sometimes with focal hemorrhage. For tumors that infiltrate into the subcutis, the diagnosis of pleomorphic dermal sarcoma should be considered (see next section).

The spindle-cell *variant* of AFX consists exclusively of spindle cells with eosinophilic cytoplasm, vesicular nuclei, and prominent nucleoli arranged in fascicles. Some examples of this subtype have a somewhat more regular and bland cytologic appearance, and a plaque-like pattern of growth may be evident (Fig. 32-13A, B) (173,177). *Clear-cell AFX* is a rare variant composed of sheets of large cells with foamy cytoplasm and hyperchromatic, pleomorphic nuclei (Fig. 32-14) (178,179). *Granular cell, keloidal, myxoid,* and *sclerotic* variants have also been reported, and some tumors are pigmented owing to hemosiderin deposition (174,175,180–184).

Pathogenesis. Electron microscopic (185,186) and immunohistochemical (139,187) studies suggest that the progenitor cell is an undifferentiated mesenchymal cell capable of showing histiocytic, fibroblastic, and myofibroblastic differentiation. A role for UV induction is suggested by the presence of UV-associated cytogenetic changes in a number of studies (188–190).

Differential Diagnosis. Although the features of this tumor are often characteristic, it is essential to perform immunohistochemistry to exclude other malignancies, in particular melanoma, leiomyosarcoma, and poorly differentiated squamous cell carcinoma. The possibility of a metastasis should always be considered. In our laboratory, a broad panel of markers is applied, with an expected profile of negative staining for desmin, epithelial, and melanoma markers. Staining with Melan-A has been reported in a subset of cases, with absence of other melanoma markers including S100 (191). Positivity with CD68 is generally present (Fig. 32-15), with frequent SMA positivity, both of which are nonspecific. Negative staining for desmin helps to exclude leiomyosarcoma in cases of actin positivity. Although desmin positivity has been reported in AFX, such lesions might be better regarded as leiomyosarcoma, particularly if staining is extensive or intense (192). Vimentin, although expected to be positive, has little discriminatory value. CD10 is nearly always strongly and diffusely expressed in AFX. Although this marker has low specificity, being also seen (usually to a lesser degree) in some melanomas and carcinomas

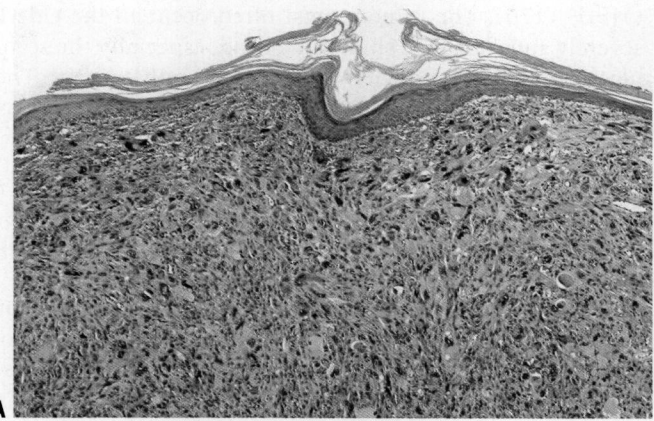 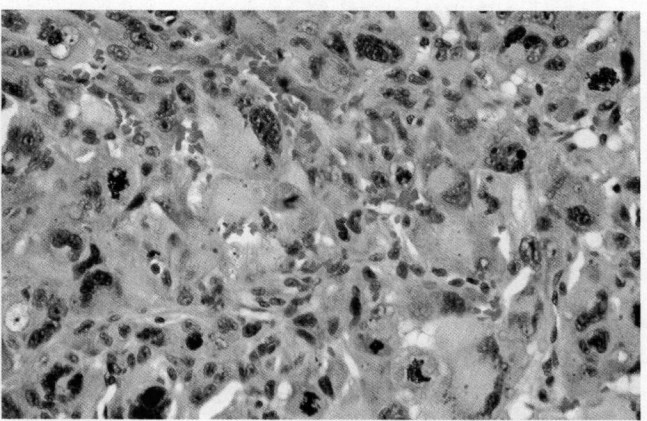

Figure 32-12 Atypical fibroxanthoma. **A:** The tumor is composed of a cellular mass of malignant cells that are unconnected to the epidermis. A lack of keratinization and pigmentation are clues to the diagnosis in these pleomorphic tumors, but immunohistochemistry is required in all cases for definitive diagnosis. **B:** Highly pleomorphic spindle cells are present with some multinucleated giant cells and scattered mitoses, including atypical forms.

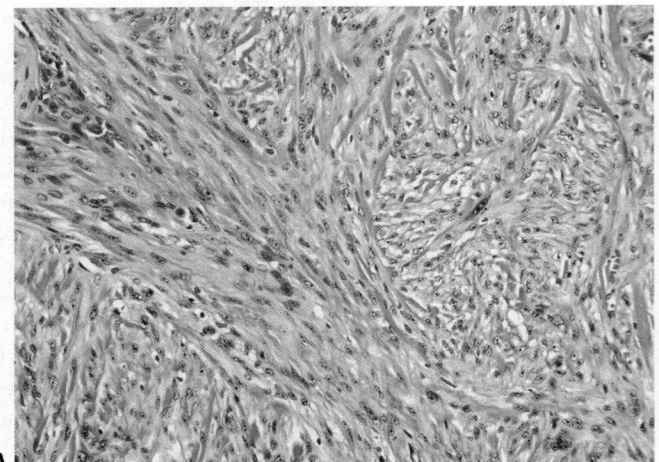
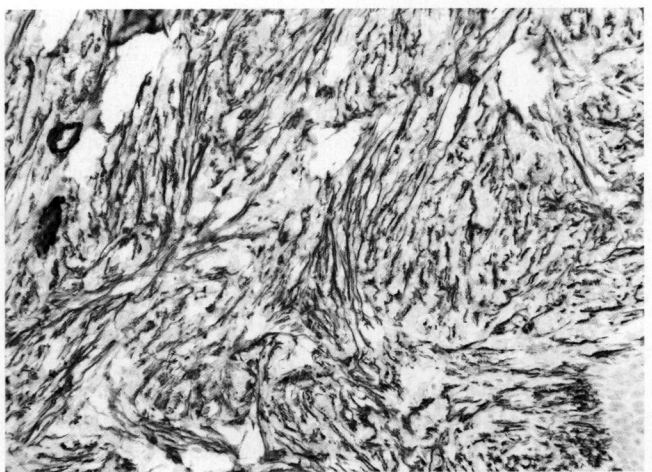

Figure 32-13 Spindle-cell atypical fibroxanthoma. **A:** Swathes of pleomorphic spindle cells are present, with some background collagen. Some tumors of this type show relatively monomorphic cytologic features. **B:** Immunohistochemistry demonstrates strong positivity in the cytoplasm of the spindle cells for smooth muscle actin. Desmin was negative (not shown).

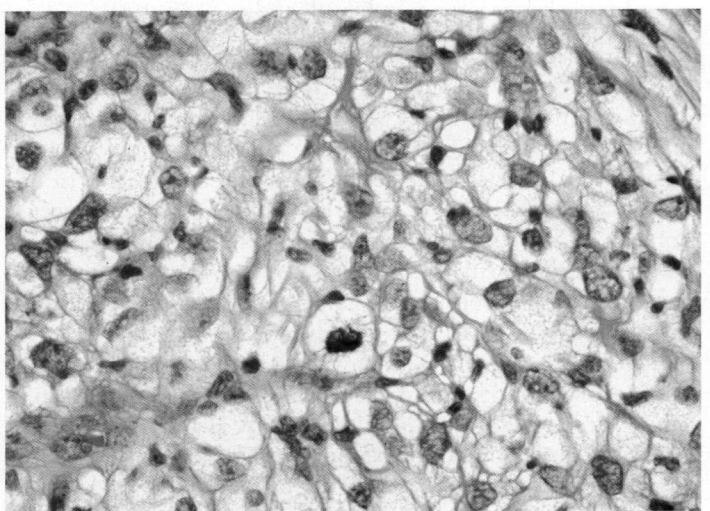

Figure 32-14 Clear-cell atypical fibroxanthoma. The atypical cells exhibit abundant clear cytoplasm in this variant.

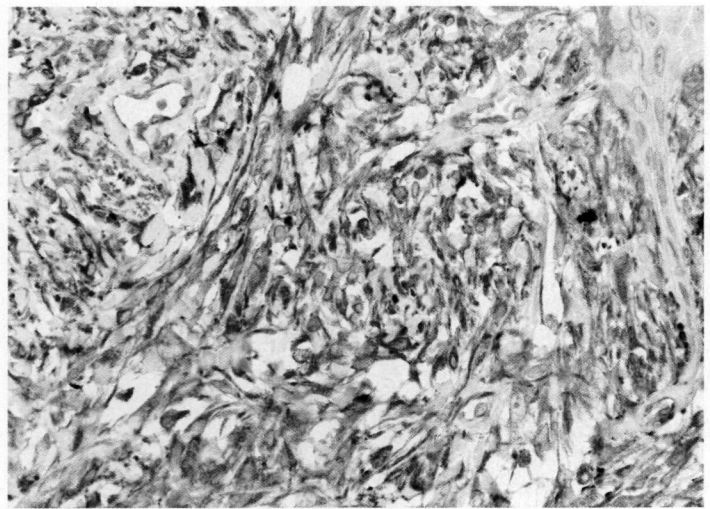

Figure 32-15 Clear-cell atypical fibroxanthoma (AFX). CD68 and CD163 are typically positive in all forms of AFX.

(177,193), the diagnosis of AFX should be carefully reconsidered if CD10 staining is negative or limited. Despite initial hopes, neither CD163 nor CD117 has proven to be of diagnostic value (194,195). The smooth muscle marker h-caldesmon is negative in many AFXs (192), but staining has been reported in over 20% of tumors in one study (196). These differences may be related to the clone employed. h-Caldesmon is typically strongly expressed in leiomyosarcoma (192). CD99 expression is frequent in AFX but not specific (177,197), and it should be noted that some AFXs express EMA (without evidence of other epithelial marker positivity) and CD31 (175).

Principles of Management: Complete local excision should be performed, although recurrences are rare even with incomplete removal (174). Mohs surgery has been reported to be associated with a lower risk of recurrence compared to standard surgery (196).

Pleomorphic Dermal Sarcoma

Clinical Summary. Pleomorphic dermal sarcoma (undifferentiated pleomorphic sarcoma of the skin) appears to be essentially a more advanced or aggressive form of AFX, previously classified as a superficial form of malignant fibrous histiocytoma (MFH) (176). The tumors most often occur in the elderly on severely sun-damaged skin of the head, especially the scalp. An ulcerated nodule or plaque is most commonly present. There is a significant risk of recurrence or metastasis (198). Metastatic disease can be associated with a high mortality.

Histopathology. The pathologic features are those of an AFX, but with the additional presence of features such as large size, necrosis, perineural or lymphovascular invasion, and significant permeation of subcutis or deeper tissues.

Immunohistochemical staining shows a similar profile to AFX (see above) (175). Cytogenetic changes are also like those seen in AFX, with frequent UV-associated mutations. Occasional cytogenetic differences have been identified in some pleomorphic dermal sarcomas compared to AFX (190,191).

Principles of Management: Wide local excision and close follow-up are indicated because of the significant risk of recurrence and potential for metastasis (199). Metastases can involve the skin, lymph nodes, and lung with subsequent death in a number of cases (198). Radiotherapy does not appear to provide any survival benefit (200).

Malignant Fibrohistiocytic Tumors

These are fully malignant tumors, with frequent capacity for metastasis and for causing death.

Malignant Fibrous Histiocytoma

Clinical Summary. The concept of MFH has generally fallen into disrepute because it appears to be neither of histiocytic origin nor a specific entity (1). It is now considered as obsolete in the 2018 WHO Classification of Skin Tumours (3). A large number of theories of histogenesis for these tumors were proposed (201), but using techniques such as immunohistochemistry, cytogenetics, and electron microscopy, most MFHs can be recategorized as other types of sarcoma, melanoma, carcinoma, or even lymphoma (1,202–206). Such tumors usually arise in deep soft tissue, only occasionally reaching the skin by direct growth or metastasis; so, presentation in the skin is uncommon (207,208). CGH of a large series of lesions classified as MFH showed identical cytogenetic changes to many leiomyosarcomas, suggesting that many MFHs are leiomyosarcomas that have become very poorly differentiated to be recognized by most standard techniques (209). Indeed, array-CGH and transcriptome analysis on 160 soft-tissue sarcomas supported the concept that a proportion of MFH-type lesions are leiomyosarcomas (210).

Despite the best techniques available, a small group of MFH-type tumors apparently show no definable line of differentiation (about 20% of lesions in one practice) (201). These are probably best classified for the most part as undifferentiated pleomorphic sarcomas (201,202,204,211). Myxoid MFH is generally considered to be a myxofibrosarcoma, and giant-cell MFH (212,213) probably often represents a form of osteosarcoma or, perhaps, malignant giant-cell tumor of soft tissue (214).

Angiomatoid fibrous histiocytoma was formerly regarded as a subtype of MFH (215) but has been reclassified as a fibrohistiocytic tumor of intermediate grade on the basis of its excellent prognosis (see later) (85,216).

Principles of Management: Complete wide surgical excision is the mainstay of treatment. Radiotherapy and chemotherapy may be used as adjuncts and for palliation. The prognosis is generally poor, especially for incompletely excised and recurrent lesions.

FIBROBLASTIC/MYOFIBROBLASTIC TUMORS

These lesions generally lack the histiocytic differentiation (e.g., presence of giant cells, foam cells, and CD68 reactivity) seen in the so-called fibrohistiocytic tumors described earlier.

Benign Fibroblastic/Myofibroblastic Tumors

These benign lesions may recur locally, but in general, their growth is not destructive and they do not metastasize.

Hypertrophic Scar and Keloid

Clinical Summary. Excessive fibrous tissue deposited in association with scar formation may lead to a hypertrophic scar or keloid.

There are important clinical and pathologic differences between these processes, although it has been suggested that they may form a spectrum of changes (217–219). Keloids may become much more prominent than hypertrophic scars, persist, and can extend beyond the original site of injury, with a high rate of recurrence following surgical treatment. However, contractures are not a feature of keloid scars, tending to occur mostly in postburn hypertrophic scars. Keloids occur mainly on the upper chest and arms, head and neck, and especially on the ear. They are uncommon in the periocular region and on the palms, soles, penis, and scrotum (220,221). Keloids mostly affect people in the second and third decades of life, and they are more common in wounds that have been infected or are under excess tension.

There is frequently a history of prior trauma (such as ear piercing), but some keloids apparently arise spontaneously, especially in the presternal region. Dark-skinned individuals are much more susceptible to keloids, and occasional familial cases have been recorded (221).

Histopathology. Both hypertrophic scars and keloids exhibit excess collagen formation with varying numbers of fibroblastic cells. These tend to form nodular, whorled masses, with vertically aligned vessels in hypertrophic scars and reduced vascularity in keloids (221,222). SMA-positive myofibroblasts are characteristically present in hypertrophic scars and are scant or absent in keloids. In keloids, hypocellular zones of fibrous tissue contain thickened, glassy, eosinophilic collagen bundles, in contrast to the more cellular nodules in hypertrophic scars (Fig. 32-16A, B). In most scars, diffuse moderate-to-strong nuclear beta-catenin immunoexpression was detected in fibroblasts/myofibroblasts, making its utility in the distinction from fibromatoses less useful (223).

Pathogenesis. Keloids have been shown to exhibit abnormal fibroblast activity, with increased hyaluronic acid production and increased levels of transforming growth factor β and other cytokines (224). Decreased apoptosis may also play a role, allowing the keloidal fibroblasts to proliferate and produce more collagen (224). Reduced vascular density in keloids compared to that in hypertrophic scars and normally healing scars suggests that hypoxia may also play an important role (221).

Principles of Management: Simple excision is the principal approach to the treatment of hypertrophic scars (225), and intralesional steroids may enhance resolution. Surgery alone may be problematic in some keloids because this may exacerbate the lesions. Keloid treatments include pressure therapy, a variety of topical and intralesional agents, including corticosteroids injection, interferon, laser therapy, radiotherapy, and cryotherapy (225). These treatments may be combined with surgical debulking.

Dermatomyofibroma

Clinical Summary. Dermatomyofibroma is an uncommon plaque-like proliferation of fibroblasts and myofibroblasts in the dermis, occurring mainly in young females, although any sex and a wide range of ages may be affected (226,227). The lesions are typically small, with a variety of sites involved, although the shoulder region and neck are most commonly affected (226–231).

Histopathology. Uniform spindle cells in elongated and intersecting fascicles are arranged mainly parallel to the epidermis

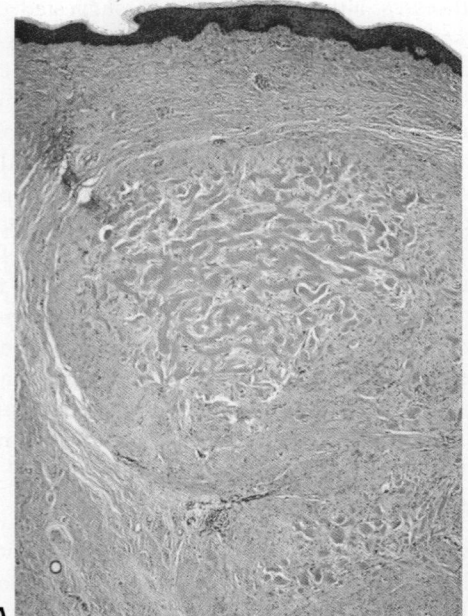
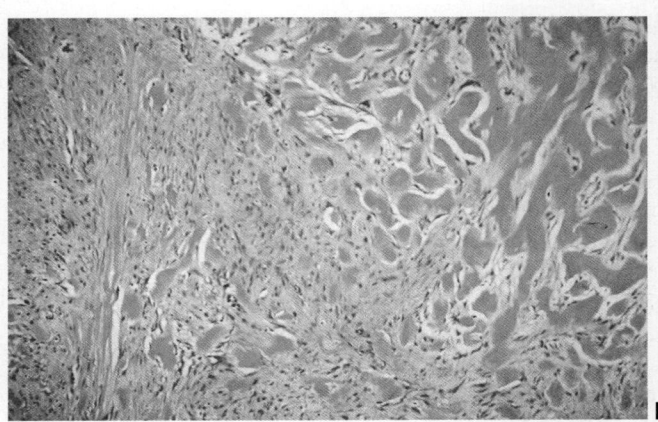

Figure 32-16 Keloid scar. **A:** Nodules of spindle cells with abundant collagen are present in the dermis with prominent hyalinization. **B:** Glassy eosinophilic and hyalinized collagen fibers are interspersed with swathes of fibroblasts.

to form a well-circumscribed plaque. There is occasional involvement of the subcutis, with sparing of adnexa and papillary dermis (Fig. 32-17A, B) (226,228,231). Overlying epidermal hyperplasia and pigmentation may be seen with increased and fragmented elastin within the lesion. Three cases have recently been reported in adult males on the thigh and trunk that showed red blood cell extravasation associated with dilated capillaries and slit-like spaces, giving a resemblance to Kaposi sarcoma (232).

Pathogenesis. Immunohistochemical reactivity for nonspecific muscle actin, variably for α-SMA, and the ultrastructural features suggest myofibroblastic differentiation (228,231,233,234).

Differential Diagnosis. The orientation parallel to the epidermis of monomorphic spindle cells and their location primarily in the reticular dermis are points of distinction from dermatofibroma. Dermatomyofibroma does not express factor XIIIa or

h-caldesmon (231,233). Desmin and S100 are also negative, with only limited CD34 positivity reported (226).

Principles of Management: Conservative local excision is considered adequate treatment, with no recurrence seen in a series of 56 tumors, even when excision was marginal or incomplete (226).

Soft Fibroma (Fibroepithelial Polyp)

Clinical Summary. Soft fibromas, also called fibroepithelial polyps, acrochordons, or skin tags, occur as three types: (a) multiple, 1- to 2-mm, furrowed papules, especially on the neck and axillae; (b) single or multiple filiform, smooth growths in varying locations, up to 5 mm long; and (c) solitary, pedunculated or "bag-like" growths, usually about 10 mm in diameter but occasionally much larger, most often on the lower trunk (235,236).

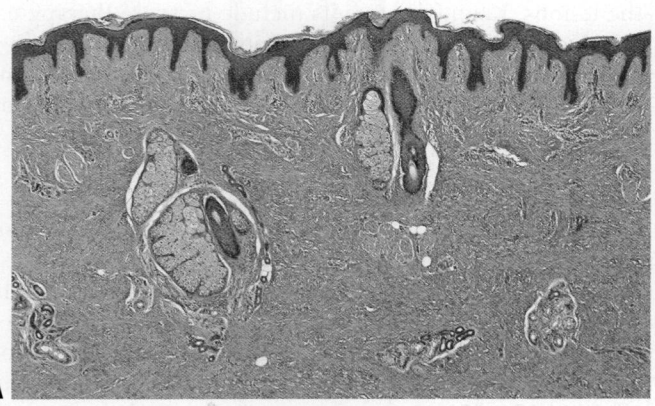
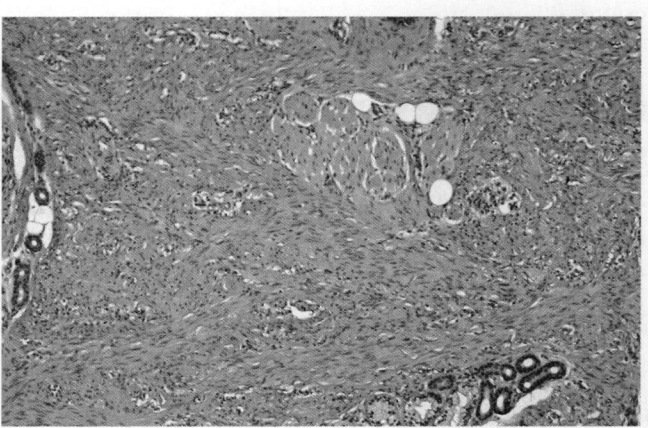

Figure 32-17 Dermatomyofibroma. **A:** The epidermis shows elongated rete ridges overlying a plaque of increased cellularity that surrounds but does not replace appendages. **B:** At higher power, the lesion is composed of uniform spindle cells with eosinophilic cytoplasm that efface the dermis, sparing adnexae.

Several reports have suggested an association between the presence of soft fibroma and colonic polyps (236–239), diabetes (240–242), and acromegaly (243). The association with colonic polyps, however, has not been confirmed by subsequent reports (244–249).

Histopathology. The multiple small furrowed papules usually show papillomatosis, hyperkeratosis, and regular acanthosis. Occasionally, horn cysts are also present, giving a resemblance to a pedunculated seborrheic keratosis. The epidermis of the filiform, smooth growths shows slight-to-moderate acanthosis and, occasionally, mild papillomatosis. The connective tissue stalk is composed of loose collagen fibers and often contains numerous dilated capillaries filled with erythrocytes. Nevus cells are found in as many as 30% of the filiform growths, indicating that some of them represent involuting melanocytic nevi (250). The larger pedunculated growths generally show a flattened epidermis overlying loose collagen fibers and mature fat cells in the center (245). In some instances, the fat is prominent, indicating lipofibroma formation (251), and such lesions may overlap with the morphology of nevus lipomatosus superficialis (see Chapter 34). Malignancy arising in these polyps is an exceedingly rare phenomenon (252) and probably represents a coincidental occurrence rather than indicative of a special propensity for true malignant transformation.

Principles of Management: Lesions are excised for cosmetic purposes.

Pleomorphic Fibroma

Clinical Summary. Pleomorphic fibroma typically presents as a slow-growing exophytic nodule most commonly on the trunk or extremities and rarely at other sites, such as the face and subungual location, of middle-aged to older adults (253–255).

Histopathology. The epidermis is flattened, overlying a circumscribed nodule in the dermis composed of plump mononucleate and multinucleate, spindle-shaped or stellate cells with atypical nuclei and occasional mitoses, distributed sparsely in a fibrous stroma (Fig. 32-18A, B).

Pathogenesis. The tumor cells are variably SMA- and CD34-positive, suggesting either myofibroblastic or dermal dendritic cell origin/differentiation (248,253,254,256).

Differential Diagnosis. Dermatofibromas with monster cells are more cellular, and they have areas with typical histologic features of dermatofibroma and often acanthotic pigmented epidermis overlying the lesion. In contrast to dermatofibroma, pleomorphic fibroma expresses CD34 (256). AFXs present as rapidly growing, highly cellular lesions composed of pleomorphic, spindle-shaped to epithelioid cells with numerous mitotic figures, which may be atypical. Cases with adipocytes may resemble atypical dermal lipomatous tumor. Pleomorphic fibromas, by contrast, are negative for MDM2 by immunohistochemistry with no demonstrable 12q15/MDM2 amplification by fluorescence *in situ* hybridization (257). Diagnosis by cytology is fraught with danger because the pleomorphic cells in this benign lesion may appear malignant (258).

Principles of Management: Excision is curative and recurrences are rare.

Sclerotic Fibroma (Storiform Collagenoma or Plywood Fibroma)

Clinical Summary. This is an uncommon lesion usually occurring as a small, solitary nodule, but occasionally lesions may be as large as 3 cm in diameter (259). Multiple lesions are a marker for Cowden disease (260). A number of cases have been reported in the oral cavity (261).

Histopathology. The tumors are circumscribed and composed of interwoven fascicles of laminated eosinophilic collagen with prominent clefting (Fig. 32-19A, B). Cellularity is low, with inconspicuous nuclei. There can be a resemblance to a Pacinian corpuscle (262) or the late stage of erythema elevatum diutinum (263,264). Occasional cases have been reported containing pleomorphic cells, suggesting a relationship to pleomorphic fibroma (265). Giant cells may be conspicuous in some examples (266). Immunostaining is positive for factor XIIIa, with frequent positivity for CD34 (267,268) and sometimes EMA (268).

Pathogenesis. On the basis of similar fibrotic changes seen in dermatofibroma and in inflammatory lesions (263,264), it has been suggested that sclerotic fibromas may have diverse origins (269,270). Active collagen synthesis, rare recurrence, and detection of proliferative activity with immunohistochemistry have led to the suggestion that the lesions are benign fibroblastic neoplasms (267,271,272).

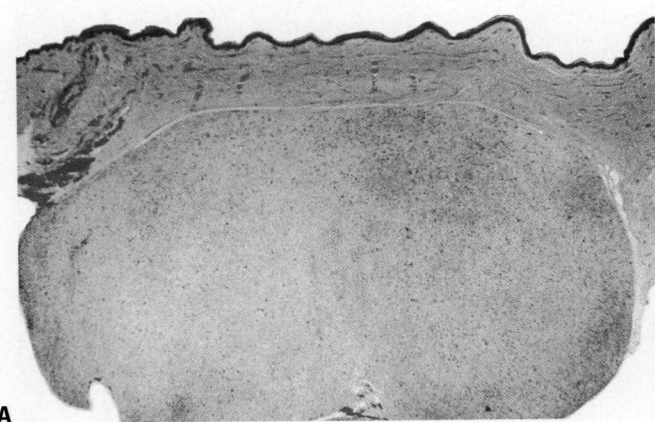
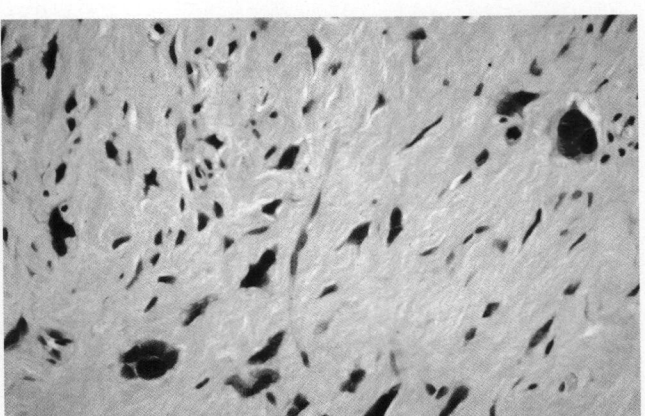

Figure 32-18 Pleomorphic fibroma. **A:** A sharply circumscribed nodule in the dermis and subcutis. **B:** Spindle cells and giant cells with marked nuclear pleomorphism and hyperchromatism in a pale, hyalinized stroma.

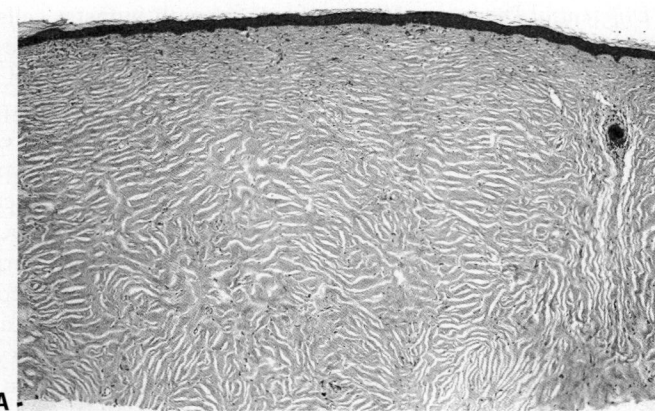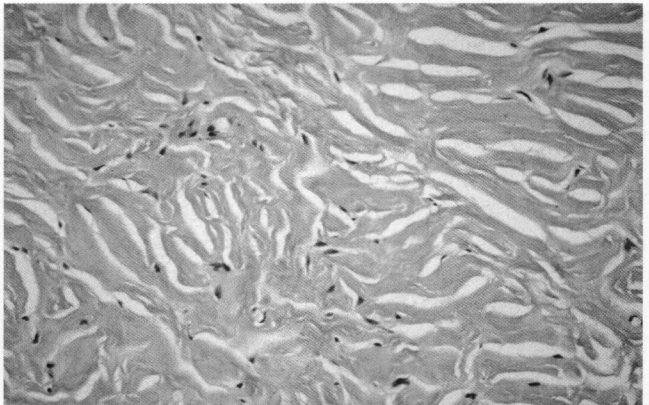

Figure 32-19 Sclerotic fibroma. **A:** A pale, poorly cellular lesion replaces the dermis with some flattening of overlying rete ridges. **B:** Clefts are prominent between lamellated, hyaline, and highly eosinophilic collagen.

Principles of Management: Local excision is typically curative, with recurrence exceptional. Cowden disease should be considered if lesions are multiple (260).

Fibroma of Tendon Sheath

Clinical Summary. Fibroma of tendon sheath presents as a slow-growing nodule near tendinous structures, most frequently in the hands and wrists. Other less common sites include feet, elbows, and knees. It is uncertain whether fibroma of tendon sheath is a neoplasm or a reactive process. A clonal chromosomal abnormality, t(2;11) (q31–32;q12), has been demonstrated (273). The identical translocation has been described in collagenous fibroma, raising the possibility of a genetic link (274). A case of multifocal concurrent fibromas of tendon sheath in the hands and feet (275), as well as intra-articular cases (276), has been reported.

Histopathology. The lesion is characterized by nodules largely composed of interlacing bundles of hyalinized, hypocellular fibrous tissue, with occasional more cellular areas of spindle-shaped, fibroblast-like cells (Fig. 32-20A, B). The more cellular areas may show some degree of pleomorphism, with mitotic figures (277). A characteristic feature is the presence of slit-like vascular channels (278). No foam cells are seen, and multinucleated giant cells are very rare (277).

Pathogenesis. The cells of fibroma of tendon sheath express SMA. Ultrastructural studies show features of myofibroblastic differentiation (279).

Principles of Management: Treatment is by local excision, with a recurrence rate of 24% (280).

Collagenous Fibroma (Desmoplastic Fibroblastoma)

Clinical Summary. Collagenous fibroma is a rare benign tumor mainly affecting men. It typically involves subcutis or skeletal muscle, but occasionally it primarily involves the dermis (281,282). Tumors are usually small (1 to 4 cm in diameter), but lesions up to 20 cm in diameter have been reported (283). Many tumors occur around the shoulder and upper arm or back, although a wide distribution can be seen, with a number of cases recorded, in the oral cavity (284,285).

Histopathology. Tumors are circumscribed, ovoid masses that may be lobulated and are composed of dense, paucicellular collagenous tissue with scattered spindle cells without mitotic activity. These show features of myofibroblasts ultrastructurally

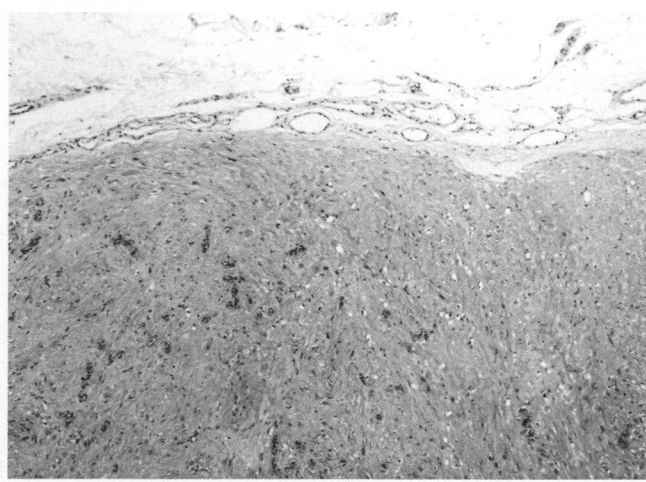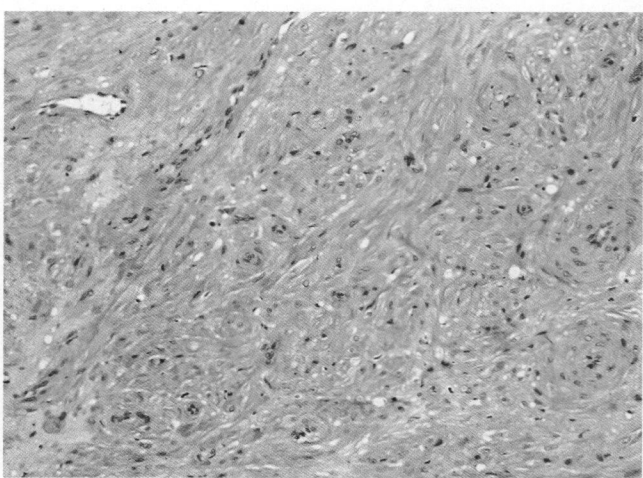

Figure 32-20 Fibroma of tendon sheath. **A:** These lesions are poorly cellular, with ill-defined fascicles of bland, myofibroblast-type cells. **B:** The spindle cells show a smooth muscle–like appearance and are typically actin-positive.

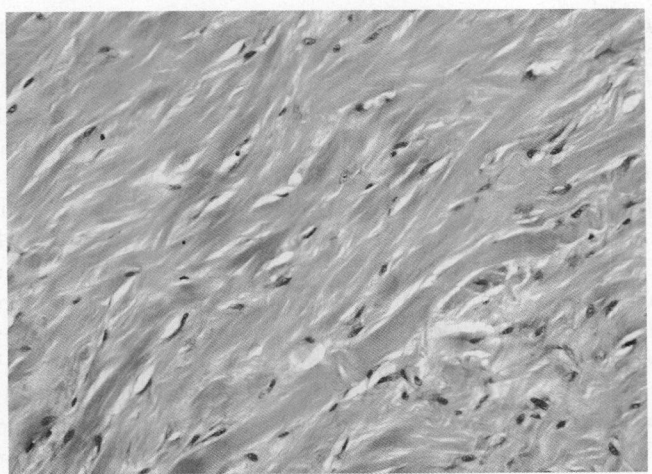

Figure 32-21 Desmoplastic fibroblastoma/collagenous fibroma. Thick bands of hyalinized, eosinophilic collagen are present, giving an appearance resembling a keloid.

(286,287). A fascicular or plexiform growth pattern is absent, and areas reminiscent of a keloid may be seen (Fig. 32-21). Focal myxoid change may be present, with inconspicuous blood vessels (283). The tumor cells variably express α-SMA and are negative for desmin, EMA, S100 protein, and CD34 (283). Strong nuclear immunoreactivity for FOS-like antigen 1 (FOSL1) is seen, which assists in the differentiation from fibroma of tendon sheath and desmoid-type fibromatosis, which are negative (288). Cytogenetic studies have shown a t(2;11) translocation, usually related to 11q12, (281) suggesting a relationship to fibroma of tendon sheath, which has shown similar changes (274,289,290). An 11q12 rearrangement suggesting deregulated expression of *FOSL1* has also been reported (291).

Principles of Management: Excision is curative, with no malignant transformation recorded.

Plexiform Myofibroblastoma

Clinical Summary. In 2020, a series of 36 cases of this novel benign neoplasm was described (292). Patients are usually children or young adults who mostly present with a solitary lesion on the trunk or back, although a wide variety of sites may be affected.

Histopathology. Tumors are composed of bland spindle-shaped cells with pale cytoplasm forming plexiform fascicles in the subcutis and dermis. An infiltrative margin is present, giving a desmoid fibromatosis-like appearance. Keloidal change is seen in a third of cases, with no included osteoclasts-like giant cells or histiocytic areas. Occasional lesions show myxoid or fasciitis-like zones.

Immunohistochemically, SMA is usually demonstrable, with about half of the cases staining with desmin and CD34. S100 and beta-catenin are not features. Only one of seven cases tested showed any abnormality on genetic sequencing.

The tumors can be distinguished from desmoid fibromatoses by their dermal involvement; plexiform architecture; and lack of beta-catenin staining, genetic adenomatous polyposis coli (APC), or CTNNB1 alterations.

Principles of Management: Conservative excision is suggested because no metastases have been recorded and recurrence is exceptional, even after incomplete removal. Occasional cases regress.

Nodular Fasciitis

Clinical Summary. Nodular fasciitis is a rapidly growing benign soft-tissue lesion. It usually presents as a solitary, sometimes tender subcutaneous nodule that reaches its ultimate size of 1 to 5 cm within a few weeks. The lesions tend to regress, even if incompletely excised, usually within a few months (293). Although the arm is the most common site, lesions may occur in any subcutaneous area. Nodular fasciitis occurs in all age groups but is more common in young adults, with an equal sex distribution. The cause is unknown. Although trauma does not seem to play a role, the general view is that nodular fasciitis represents a reactive fibroblastic and vascular proliferation.

Histopathology. Nodular fasciitis occurs usually in the subcutis, less often in muscles, and rarely in the dermis. A prominent feature is the infiltrative growth pattern along fibrous septa of the subcutis, resulting in poor demarcation. The nodule consists of immature spindly myofibroblasts and fibroblasts growing haphazardly in vascular, myxoid stroma, presenting a "tissue culture–like" pattern (Fig. 32-22A, B). The vascular component includes well-formed capillaries and slit-like

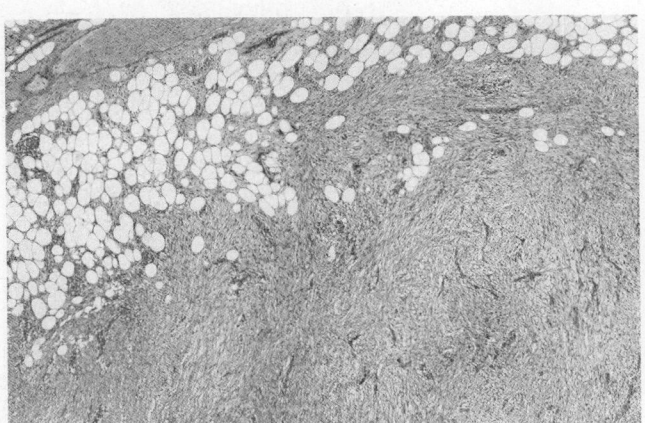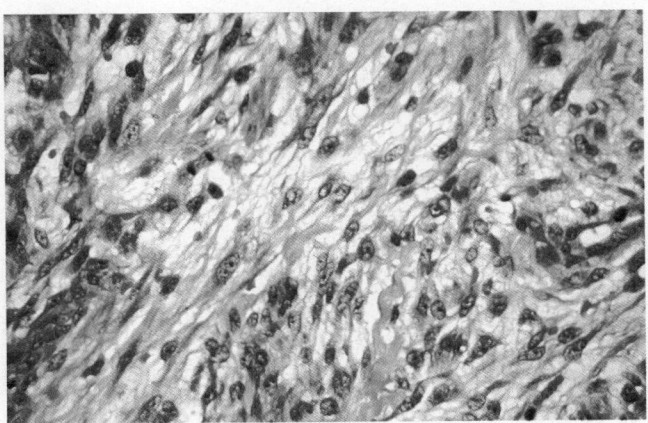

Figure 32-22 Nodular fasciitis. **A:** Plump spindle cells are arranged in varied cellularity in a loosely structured, vascular stroma. **B:** Plump spindle cells with ovoid, vesicular nuclei and scattered mitoses are embedded in the stroma with capillaries and scattered erythrocytes.

spaces with extravasation of red blood cells. The fibroblasts may show numerous mitoses, which are not atypical. Multinucleate, osteoclast-like giant cells are frequently present. In some instances, degenerate muscle fibers simulate multinucleate giant cells (294). A lymphocytic infiltrate is often present, mainly at the periphery of the nodule (295). In older lesions, the fibroblasts appear more mature, showing a more compact arrangement of spindle cells with increased production of collagen (296). It has been reported that *USP6* rearrangements with the formation of the fusion gene *MYH9-USP6* occur in most examples of nodular fasciitis, but *USP6* rearrangements are absent in its histologic mimics in soft tissue, including desmoid-type fibromatosis, fibrosarcoma, and myxofibrosarcoma. Therefore, *USP6* fluorescence *in situ* hybridization (FISH) may be a useful adjunct in the diagnosis of nodular fasciitis (297).

Dermal fasciitis is a rare variant arising within the dermis, usually occurring on the limbs and trunk of young adults (298) and also occurring in the head and neck region (299–303). Only one tumor recurred locally. No lesion metastasized (298). *Postoperative/posttraumatic* spindle-cell *nodule* has also been described as the dermal analog of nodular fasciitis (304). Another variant, *intravascular fasciitis* (305), occurs within vessel walls. *Proliferative fasciitis* appears to be related to nodular fasciitis but includes giant cells resembling ganglion cells, similar to those of proliferative myositis. These show abundant, irregularly outlined, basophilic cytoplasm with one or two large vesicular nuclei and a prominent nucleolus (306,307). Ki67 has not been found to be useful in discriminating the lesion from a sarcoma (308).

Pathogenesis. The spindle cells in nodular fasciitis have the ultrastructural features of myofibroblasts (309). As in other myofibroblastic lesions, the cells are immunoreactive for SMA and muscle-specific actin (MSA) but not for desmin (310). In one study, four of five cases of proliferative fasciitis showed diffuse strong expression of c-FOS, primarily in the epithelioid cells, whereas spindle-cell components were largely negative. Using FISH, all four c-FOS immunopositive tumors also showed *FOS* gene rearrangement in the epithelioid cells (311).

Differential Diagnosis. The presence of numerous large, pleomorphic fibroblasts and the infiltrative type of growth may suggest a malignancy such as sarcoma. In addition to rapid growth and tenderness, however, the combination of fibroblastic and vascular proliferation is the most helpful diagnostic feature of nodular fasciitis. Other findings suggesting the diagnosis are the presence of a mucoid ground substance and an inflammatory infiltrate, especially near the margin of the lesion. Recurrence of a lesion originally diagnosed as nodular fasciitis should spur a careful reappraisal of the clinical and histologic findings (294).

Cranial fasciitis of childhood is considered an unusual variant of nodular fasciitis of uncertain etiology. It occurs in infants and children as a rapidly growing mass in the subcutaneous tissue of the scalp that extends into the underlying cranium. In some cases, the lesion extends through the cranium to involve the dura (312). No recurrence has been reported after excision of the mass with resection or curettage of the underlying bone (312,313). The histologic features closely resemble those of nodular fasciitis. An origin in one of the deep fascial layers of the scalp appears likely (312).

Principles of Management: The lesion follows a benign course, and recurrences are infrequent.

Ischemic Fasciitis

Clinical Summary. This condition is also known as atypical decubital fibroplasia and often occurs at sites of long-standing pressure, typically in the elderly (314). Not all cases are associated with immobility, and some appear trauma-related (315). The limb girdle and sacrum chest are most commonly affected, but a 2016 series of 17 cases identified the arm as a frequent location, in addition (316). The resultant ischemia is believed to induce the formation of a reactive fibroblastic proliferation that may mimic nodular or proliferative fasciitis or even a sarcoma.

Histopathology. Reactive fibroblastic tissue is present associated with foci of necrosis and repair. The process extends through dermis and into subcutis and sometimes underlying tissue, including skeletal muscle, often abutting bony prominences. Atypical reactive fibroblasts are seen with a proliferation of fine vessels, and ulceration may be present (Fig. 32-23A, B). A zonal pattern of growth is helpful in establishing the diagnosis, with central fibrin and hemorrhage bordered by enlarged and atypical fibroblasts and reactive blood vessels (316). A myofibroblastic

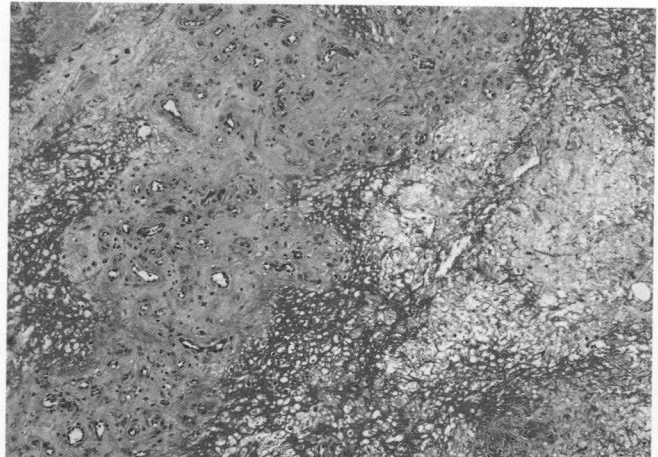
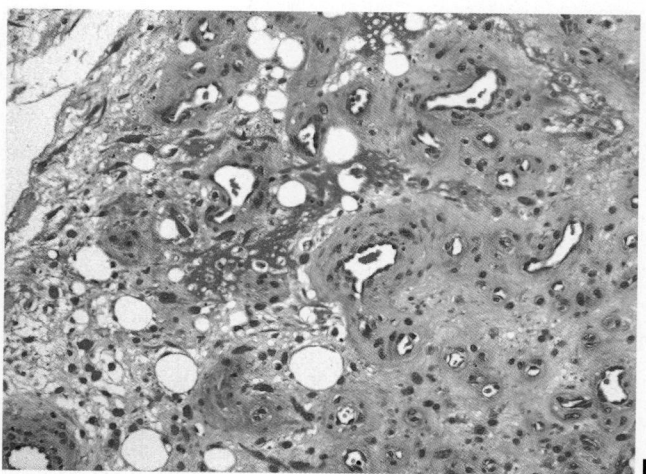

Figure 32-23 Ischemic fasciitis. **A:** Fibrin deposition and granulation tissue are present in this lesion excised from the greater trochanter of an elderly, bedridden man. **B:** Dilated vessels and reactive stromal cells are seen at high power. The degree of atypia may raise the possibility of a sarcoma at times.

origin in at least some of the cells is supported by finding actin and or desmin staining in a number of cases (315). Cytogenetic changes have been identified in one lesion reported in the literature (317).

Principles of Management: Local excision is usually curative if the predisposing factor is removed.

Myofibroma/Myofibromatosis

Clinical Summary. Myofibroma is a benign neoplasm that can present as solitary or multiple lesions. The majority of tumors are solitary, measuring between 0.5 and 7.0 cm in size. The nodules are most commonly confined to the dermis, subcutis, and skeletal muscle of the head, neck, and trunk, but any site may be affected. A recent case was reported in the sole of the foot (316). In *infantile myofibromatosis,* multiple tumors may also develop in bones and viscera in addition to skin involvement, causing death in rare cases (318–320). Death may occur in the first few months of life, usually from cardiopulmonary or gastrointestinal complications, but in survivors and in those with superficial myofibromatosis, spontaneous involution of the lesions usually takes place, often within the first year of life. Involution may be mediated by apoptosis or overgrowth of its own vascular supply (321,322). In adults, the tumors are solitary and superficial, and show no tendency to regress (323,324). Familial cases of infantile myofibromatosis are believed to be inherited in an autosomal dominant manner (325). *Myopericytoma* is a term that has been introduced to describe a spectrum of tumors typified by a hemangiopericytoma-like vascular architecture and features of perivascular myoid (myopericytic) differentiation. The term has been used to describe myofibroma, myopericytoma, and glomangiopericytoma (326) (also see Myopericytoma, Chapter 33).

Histopathology. Most tumors have a characteristic biphasic growth pattern. The lesions consist of nodular dermal aggregates of plump spindle cells resembling smooth muscle cells with pale eosinophilic cytoplasm arranged in short fascicles, sometimes with areas of hyalinization (327) (Fig. 32-24A, B) surrounding a central, hemangiopericytoma-like component where less-differentiated rounded cells with scant cytoplasm are arranged around irregularly shaped, thin-walled blood vessels. There is no atypia or pleomorphism. The stroma may appear mucoid in the less cellular areas (328). Foci of necrosis and calcification may be present centrally. In some cases, the distribution of the two components is reversed; that is, the hemangiopericytoma-like areas are situated peripherally. Other lesions may show a predominance of myoid or hemangiopericytomatous elements.

Pathogenesis. Solitary and multifocal myofibromas stained positively for SMA in 95% and 92% of cases, MSA in 75% and 50% of cases, and desmin in 10% and 14% of cases, respectively, in one large series (329). The cells are believed to be myopericytic in origin (324,330).

Principles of Management: Patients should be evaluated for the possibility of multiple tumors. The treatment of choice is early conservative surgery to minimize functional and/or aesthetic damage. Complete tumor excision is not always possible (331). Most patients in one large study were treated with complete or partial excision. There were no recurrences after treatment (329). A case of facial myofibroma with spontaneous involution has been reported (332).

Fibrous Hamartoma of Infancy

Clinical Summary. Fibrous hamartoma of infancy usually occurs as one or, rarely, two subcutaneous nodules that may be present at birth or develop during the first 2 years of life (333–336). After an initial period of growth, there is no further increase in the size of the nodule. There is a predilection for boys, with male-to-female ratio of up to 2.6:1 (336,337). These lesions

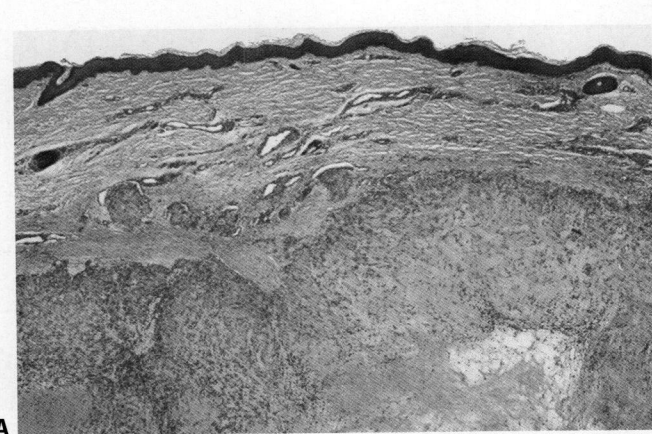
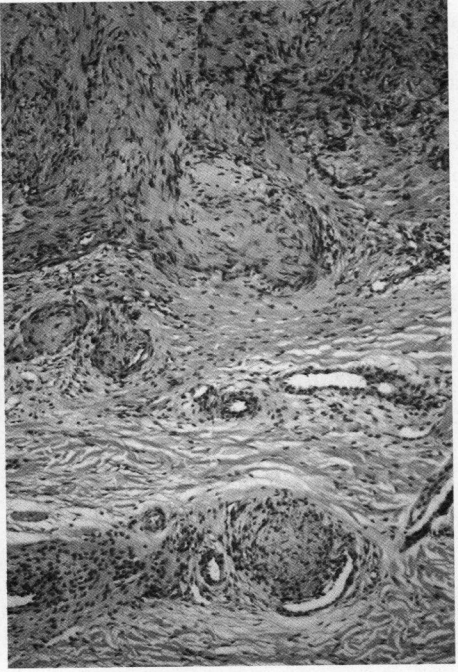

Figure 32-24 Myofibroma. **A:** Circumscribed dermal nodules of varied size, with hyalinization in the center of the largest nodule. **B:** The nodules consist of fascicles of plump spindle cells with pale eosinophilic cytoplasm, some of which indent the walls of blood vessels.

present in a wide range of locations, most commonly the axilla, upper arm, upper trunk, inguinal region, and external genitalia (336). A case with t(2;3) (q31;q21) chromosomal translocation was described (338).

Histopathology. The nodule consists of immature spindly my-ofibroblasts and fibroblasts growing haphazardly in a vascular, myxoid stroma, presenting a "tissue culture–like" pattern (Fig. 32-25A, B) (333,334). The fibrous component varies in cellularity, pattern, and amount and may resemble granulation tissue, deep fibrous histiocytoma, or fibromatosis in some areas (337). The spindle cells in the fibrous trabeculae express actin (336). A pseudoangiomatous pattern has also been reported in up to half of the cases which may mimic giant-cell fibroblastoma (339,340).

In a recent series of 145 cases, 2 tumors showed fibrosarcomatous change with high cellularity, high nuclear grade, and brisk mitotic activity and a focal osteoid-like eosinophilic matrix. Until the natural history of these unusual cases is known, the authors suggest the term "fibrous hamartoma of infancy with sarcomatous morphology" rather than "fibrous hamartoma of infancy with malignant progression." These two tumors showed a hyperdiploid karyotype with loss of heterozygosity of chromosomes 1p and 11p and loss of 10p, chromosome 14, and a large portion of chromosome 22q. One of the cases in an infant required forequarter amputation, but the patient is alive and well (340).

Principles of Management: Complete local excision is usually curative, and the recurrence rate is low (341). Cases with fibrosarcomatous morphology may require more aggressive management (340).

Juvenile Hyaline Fibromatosis

Clinical Summary. Hyaline fibromatosis syndrome is a connective tissue disease with two different clinical manifestations of similar pathophysiology: infantile hyaline fibromatosis and juvenile hyaline fibromatosis (JHF). JHF is a rare autosomal recessive, relatively mild presentation of hyaline fibromatosis syndrome. It starts in early infancy with flexural contractures and innumerable skin papules and nodules that gradually increase in size, with osteolytic bone lesions and gingival hyperplasia. Wart-like papillomatous lesions may occur in the perianal region. The largest nodules are usually seen on the scalp and around the neck. JHF has been reported in association with skull and encephalic abnormalities and in the hand of an adult (342). A mutation of the *CMG2* gene on chromosome 4q21 is hypothesized to result in the abnormal deposition of amorphous hyaline substance in different body tissues (343,344). *Infantile hyaline fibromatosis* (infantile systemic hyalinosis) presents with widespread visceral involvement and an invariably fatal outcome (345).

Histopathology. The nodules are composed of spindle-shaped or round stromal cells and homogeneous, amorphous eosinophilic ground substance to varying degrees. Small, newly developed tumors are more cellular, whereas larger, older tumors contain more ground substance (346,347). The spindle-shaped cells tend to be arranged in interlacing cords, and the ground substance is periodic acid–Schiff-positive and diastase-resistant. In paraffin-embedded, formalin-fixed material, empty spaces are seen around the nuclei of stromal cells, giving these cells a chondroid appearance (348,349).

Pathogenesis. The stromal cells have the ultrastructural features of fibroblasts (349–351). The perinuclear vacuoles are intracytoplasmic, membrane-bound vesicles filled with fibrillogranular material identical in appearance to the ground substance (349). The anthrax toxin receptor 2 (*ANTXR2*) gene has been identified as being responsible for JHF/infantile systemic hyalinosis (352).

Principles of Management: Currently, there is no satisfactory treatment for this stigmatizing, debilitating, and potentially lethal disease. Surgical excision has been considered the main form of treatment for managing both skin and oral lesions but not for joint, bone, and visceral involvement (352).

Infantile Digital Fibromatosis (Inclusion Body Fibromatosis)

Clinical Summary. Infantile digital fibromatosis occurs as single or multiple nodules on the fingers or toes, excluding the great toe and the thumb. Lesions may be present at birth, but they usually appear during the first year of life and occasionally later in childhood. The nodules rarely exceed 2 cm in diameter and involute spontaneously. In about 75% of the cases, recurrences are observed during early childhood (353). A congenital case has been reported and there have been no cases of metastases or death (354).

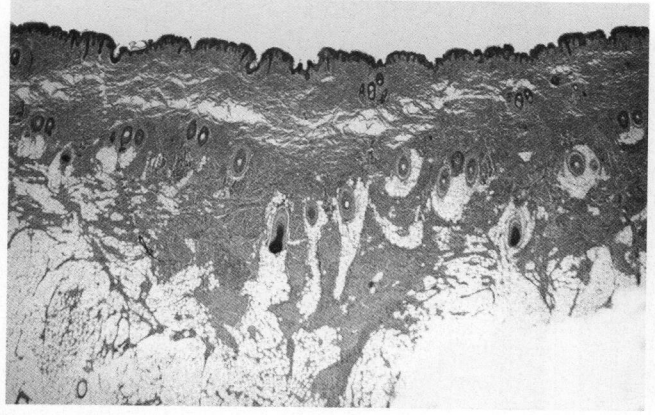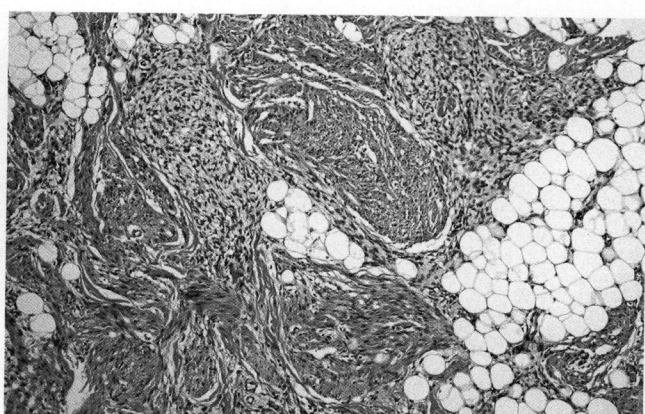

Figure 32-25 Fibrous hamartoma of infancy. **A:** Trabeculae of varied thickness intersect lobules of fat in the subcutis. **B:** The trabeculae are composed of immature spindle cells arranged in loosely structured myxoid areas and more densely collagenous tissue.

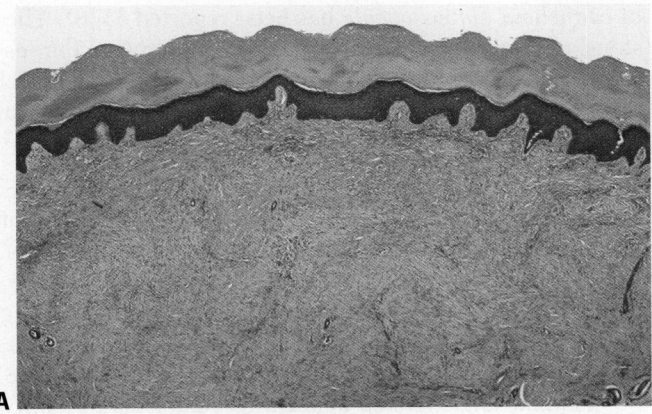
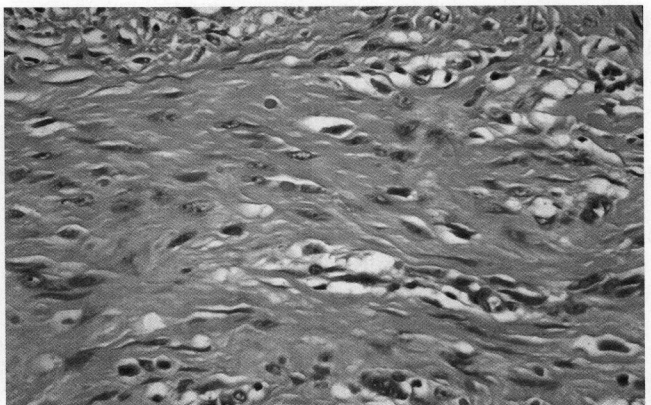

Figure 32-26 Infantile digital fibromatosis. **A:** Intersecting fascicles extend from the papillary dermis into the subcutis. **B:** Fascicles of spindle cells, some of which contain small round, eosinophilic, cytoplasmic inclusions.

Histopathology. The dermis is infiltrated by uniform spindle cells and collagen bundles arranged in interlacing fascicles, extending from just below the epidermis into the subcutis (Fig. 32-26A). A characteristic feature is the presence of eosinophilic cytoplasmic inclusions 3 to 10 μm in diameter resembling erythrocytes, often indenting the nucleus (Fig. 32-26B). These inclusions stain deep red with Masson trichrome and purple with phosphotungstic acid–hematoxylin. They express vimentin and actin (355).

Pathogenesis. Tumor cells are positive for calponin, desmin, α-SMA, and CD99; often positive for CD117; usually negative for heavy caldesmon, nuclear β-catenin, and CD34; and negative for keratins, estrogen/progesterone receptor proteins, and activated caspase 3 (356). Ultrastructurally, the spindle cells show the features of myofibroblasts and contain actin filaments, which extend into, and are continuous with, the granular intracytoplasmic inclusions.

Principles of Management: A management algorithm based on symptomatology has been proposed given the high recurrence rate after surgery and a propensity for cases to spontaneously involute. Treatment options include observation, intralesional steroids or 5-fluorouracil, and surgery as a last resort (356,357).

Elastofibroma (Elastofibroma Dorsi)

Clinical Summary. This condition appears to be a degenerative process that occurs most often in older women beneath the scapula. Lesions form a poorly circumscribed connective tissue mass, which may be as large as 15 cm in diameter. Occasional cases occur away from the scapula, and some lesions are bilateral or multiple (358–362). Many lesions are asymptomatic, but a clunking sensation may be experienced with shoulder movement (361). The behavior is benign, with recurrence exceptionally rare.

Histopathology. Irregular zones of poorly cellular collagen extend into the soft tissues with prominent, abnormally formed elastin bundles (Fig. 32-27). Elastin stains show these to have a globular and beaded morphology. CD34 staining is present in some of the spindle cells in the tumors, and these cells are negative for S100 and actin (363,364).

Pathogenesis. Repeated mild trauma has been suggested as an etiologic factor, with a number of cases reported in baseball

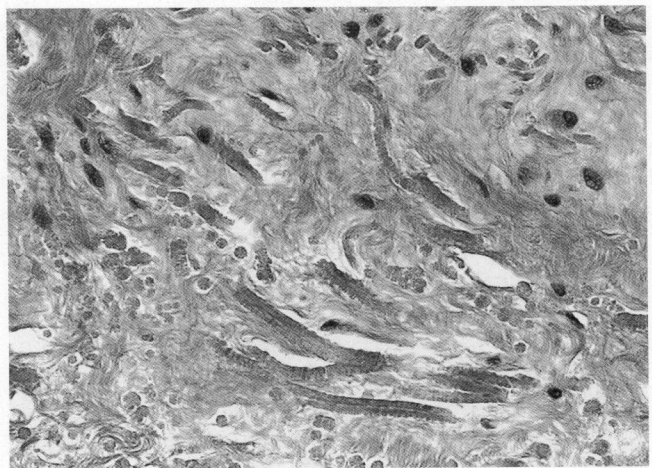

Figure 32-27 Elastofibroma. Coarse elastin fibers are prominent in the lesion, with small globular excrescences. (Courtesy of Dr. E.-.C Jung, University of California, San Francisco, California.)

pitchers (365). Abnormal elastin production is also a possible cause, with various chromosomal changes in lesions in a few patients and some genetic predisposition (366,367).

Differential Diagnosis. The histologic findings may be subtle, but once the presence of abnormal elastin is appreciated, the diagnosis is straightforward. Fibromatoses are more cellular lesions, and nuchal-type fibromas, although occurring in a similar site, typically occur in males and show denser collagen, with only fine elastin bands and, sometimes, a proliferation of fine nerve twigs.

Principles of Management: Local excision is considered adequate treatment, if required, with no reports of malignant transformation. However, conservative treatment is the preferred option (368).

Angiofibromas

Cutaneous angiofibromas occur at various body sites. On the face, they are often referred to as fibrous papules or adenoma sebaceum. On the penis, they are described as pearly penile papules, and under the nail, they are considered by many to be synonymous with periungual fibromas or acral fibrokeratomas (369). Cutaneous angiofibromas may occur in a number of syndromes such as tuberous sclerosis, multiple endocrine neoplasia type 1, and Birt-Hogg-Dube syndrome (370). These tumors appear to be unrelated to nasopharyngeal (juvenile) angiofibromas.

Fibrous Papule of the Face

Clinical Summary. These common lesions typically occur on the nose or adjacent skin of adults. They present as small, firm, dome-shaped papules up to 5 mm in diameter. Although originally believed to represent involuting melanocytic nevi (371,372), they are now established as a discrete entity (373).

Histopathology. The epidermis is raised, overlying a localized area of fibroplasia and fine vascular proliferation in the upper dermis (Fig. 32-28). There are scattered associated enlarged triangulate or stellate cells, which may be multinucleated (372,374). Dendritic CD163-positive macrophages are present, with variable or absent CD10 or CD34 staining (375). Atypia may be evident in these cells, with nuclear hyperchromasia, enlargement, and pleomorphism (Fig. 32-29A, B) as seen in pleomorphic fibromas. In some cases, increased melanocytes are seen at the dermoepidermal junction, sometimes with nuclear enlargement. *Clear-cell fibrous papule* appears to be a variant in which NKI/C3-positive lesional cells show cytoplasmic clearing that is not caused by glycogen (376,377). One series of 10 cases

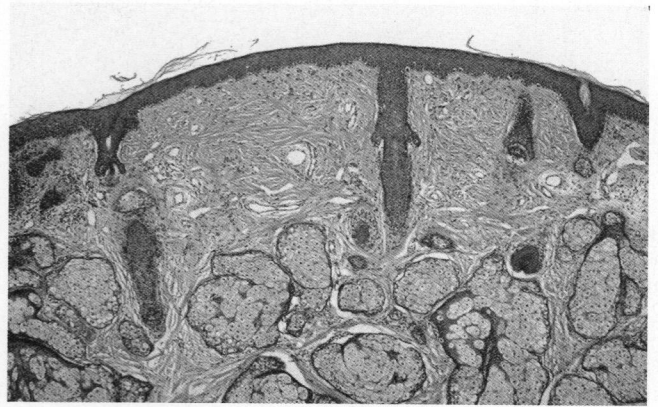

Figure 32-28 Angiofibroma (fibrous papule of the face). The epidermis is elevated over a zone of vascular fibroplasia in the superficial dermis.

of *epithelioid fibrous papule* has been reported (378). These lesions, although possibly related to the more usual fibrous papules, have a markedly contrasting appearance, with cellular nests of epithelioid cells that may closely resemble groups of melanocytes histologically (378).

Pathogenesis. Electron microscopic and immunohistochemical studies indicate that the stromal cells are of fibroblastic or dermal dendrocytic origin rather than of melanocytic (379–381). They express factor XIIIa but not S100 protein (382–386). Tuberous sclerosis-associated angiofibromas are related to germline mutation of the *TSC1* or *TSC2* gene, which activates the mammalian target of the rapamycin (mTOR) pathway (387).

Cellular angiofibroma appears to be a separate entity that occurs almost exclusively on the vulva. It is a condition of superficial soft-tissue origin rather than dermal location and may be related to spindle-cell lipoma and mammary-type myofibroblastoma, which have in common loss of chromosome 13q14 (388,389). Similarly, *giant-cell angiofibroma* appears to be unrelated to dermal angiofibromas, showing features more in common with solitary fibrous tumor (390). The recently described *angiofibroma of soft tissue* is a deeply sited lesion usually of the extremities that appears unrelated to cutaneous angiofibromas (391).

Principles of Management: Conservative excision of angiofibromas may be considered for cosmetic or diagnostic purposes, with no malignant potential recorded. Topical rapamycin appears to be a safe and effective alternative to surgery or laser ablation (392,393).

Pearly Penile Papules

Clinical Summary. These small (1 to 3 mm in diameter), persistent white papules occur mainly on the coronal margin and sulcus of the penis and rarely on the glans in groups or rows. Recent work suggests that they tend to involute with age, with a reported prevalence of 38% in males under 25 years and 11% in those over 50 years (394). They do not appear to be related to human papillomavirus infection (395) and are more common in the uncircumcised (394).

Histopathology. The features are typical of an angiofibroma (with no associated hair follicles owing to the location) (396). A small series of cases suggested that the presence of Ki67

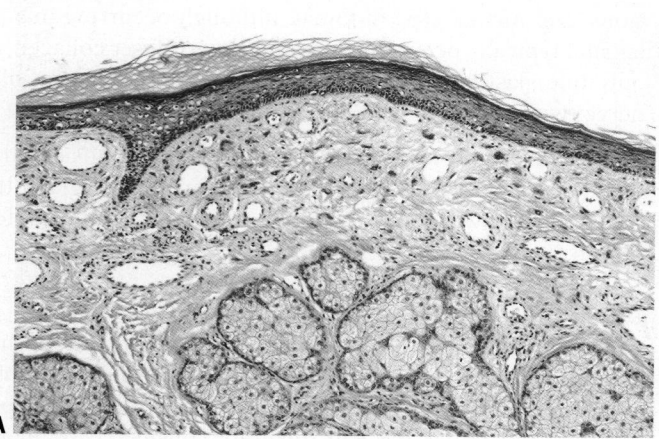

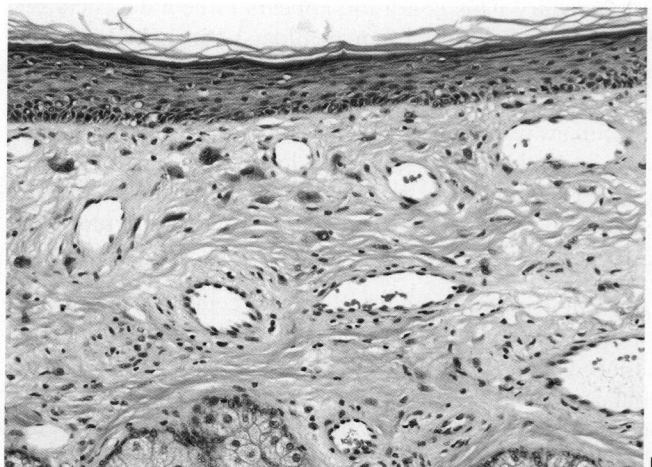

Figure 32-29 A and B: Angiofibroma. This angiofibroma shows prominent atypical stromal cells—a not uncommon finding of no sinister significance.

staining confined to the lower half of the epidermis was of value in differentiating the lesions from viral warts, in which Ki67 staining also occurred in the upper epidermis (397).

Principles of Management: If treatment is desired, cryotherapy and laser ablation have been found to be effective, with laser therapy the preferred approach in a recent literature review (398).

Tuberous Sclerosis

Clinical Summary. Tuberous sclerosis is a rare genetic disorder that may be inherited in an autosomal dominant pattern or more often presents as a new spontaneous mutation (399–401). A variety of cutaneous lesions occur with systemic defects in wide-ranging body systems, including the brain, kidney, eye, and lung (402). Most patients develop multiple facial angiofibromas (previously misleadingly termed adenoma sebaceum). These tumors consist of numerous small, red papules in symmetric distribution over the nose, cheeks, and chin. Soft fibromas may also occur on the face and scalp, with skin tags and subungual or periungual fibromas a frequent finding. Shagreen patches are usually found in the lumbosacral region and consist of slightly raised, yellowish, leathery areas of skin (the term "shagreen" refers to a type of rawhide leather that has a rough pitted surface). Various hypopigmented skin lesions are present in more than half of patients with tuberous sclerosis; significantly, they may be present at birth or appear at an early age and are often the earliest indication of tuberous sclerosis (403).

Genetic studies show linkage to chromosome 9q34 (TSC1) or chromosome 16p31 (TSC 2), which encode for tumor suppressor proteins hamartin and tuberin, respectively (399,400,404–406). These proteins help regulate cell proliferation and survival, and loss of TSC1 or TSC2 function disrupts the mTOR (mechanistic or mammalian target of rapamycin) pathway. Sporadic cases are assumed to result from new mutations, many of which are in TSC 2. TSC 2 patients tend to have more severe disease with greater numbers of hypopigmented lesions (399). Treatment with mTOR inhibitors such as rapamycin may be of great value in the clinical management of tuberous sclerosis (407,408).

Systemic Lesions. Multiple tumors are commonly found in the brain (gliomas, often calcified), retina (gliomas), heart (rhabdomyomas), and kidneys (angiomyolipomas) (409).

Histopathology. The angiofibromas show a fine vascular proliferation in the dermis with associated fibrosis and occasional reactive stromal cells (410). Elastic tissue is absent in these lesions, and compression of adnexa may be seen (Fig. 32-30A, B).

The soft fibromas on the face and scalp show markedly sclerotic collagen arranged in thick, concentric layers around atrophic pilosebaceous follicles. In contrast to the angiofibromas, dilated capillaries are usually absent. Giant angiofibroma (411) and a cluster growth of large nodules (412) have also been reported.

The ungual fibromas show fibrosis, occasionally with capillary dilation. The shagreen patches have the histologic features of connective tissue nevi (collagenomas), with either a dense, sclerotic mass of broad collagen bundles in the dermis, mimicking morphea, or normal collagen bundles interwoven throughout the dermis. The elastic tissue in some instances shows fragmentation and clumping (410) but is generally reduced in amount (413).

The hypopigmented areas show a normal number of melanocytes, with decreased pigmentation. On electron microscopy, the melanosomes within the melanocytes and keratinocytes are smaller and show reduced melanization (403,413).

Differential Diagnosis. The angiofibromas seen in tuberous sclerosis may be histologically identical to solitary angiofibromas (fibrous papules of the face), but their multiplicity, potentially larger size, and at times pedunculated architecture are some distinguishing features.

Principles of Management: Indications for treatment of angiofibromas in patients with tuberous sclerosis can include large size, repeated bleeding, impairment of vision or interference with nasal air flow, and cosmesis. Surgery and laser therapy are potential options, with improvement reported with rapamycin or similar inhibitors of mTOR either topically or orally (407,408,414,415). Consensus guidelines for management of tuberous sclerosis complex have been described (409).

Acral Fibrokeratoma (Acquired Digital Fibrokeratoma, Periungual Fibroma)

Clinical Summary. Acral fibrokeratoma is considered by some authors to fall within the spectrum of angiofibromatous proliferations, although the vascular component may be limited. Lesions

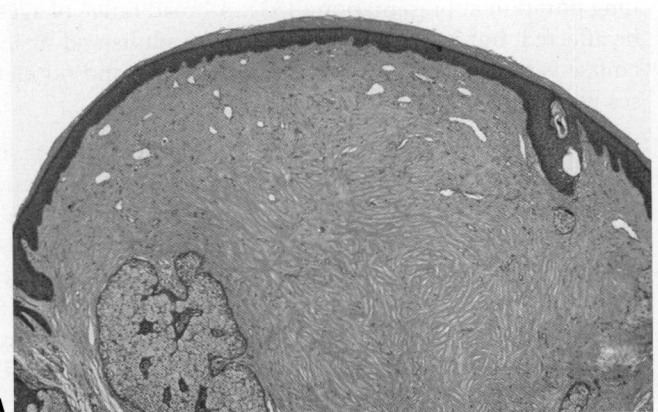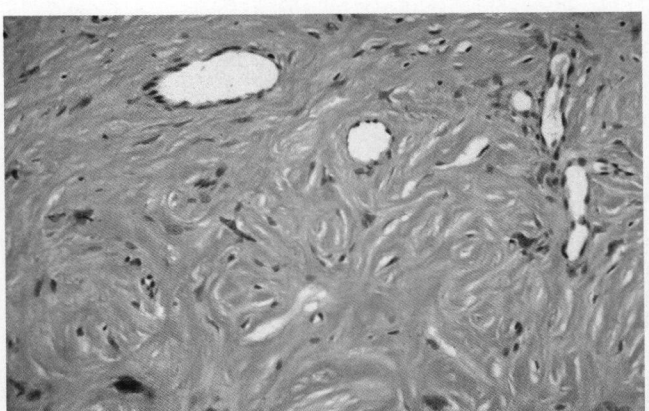

Figure 32-30 Angiofibroma arising in tuberous sclerosis. **A:** The epidermis is raised in a dome-shaped pattern overlying a zone of compact fibroplasia with prominent blood vessels in the upper half. **B:** The typical features of an angiofibroma are seen with sclerotic, hyalinized stroma, with scattered spindle and stellate cells and telangiectatic blood vessels.

normally present as solitary firm, hyperkeratotic projections from the finger or toe but are occasionally sited on the palm or sole (416,417). Some appear to originate from the nail bed (418,419), and there are isolated examples of large size (417). Tumors arise in adults, with rare cases of familial multiple acral mucinous fibrokeratoma and multiple acral fibromas associated with familial retinoblastoma, which may represent cutaneous markers of tumor suppressor gene germline mutation (420,421). Multiple lesions are often associated with tuberous sclerosis.

Histopathology. There is hyperkeratosis and acanthosis with broad, often branching rete ridges. In the core are prominent interwoven collagen bundles mostly vertically oriented (Fig. 32-31). Elastic fibers are present but are normally thin and sparse. Many tumors show abundant fine vessels. A *cellular variant* has been described that has features similar to DFSP, including CD34 positivity (422,423). It has been suggested that this may in fact represent a form of superficial acral fibromyxoma (424,425).

Differential Diagnosis. Rudimentary supernumerary digits may appear similar clinically and histologically. However, rudimentary polydactyly almost always occurs at the base of the fifth finger, is present from birth, and is often bilateral. Histologically, numerous nerve bundles are present, especially at the base of the lesions.

Principles of Management: Complete surgical removal is curative (422).

Nuchal-Type Fibroma (Nuchal Fibroma)

Clinical Summary. Nuchal fibroma is an uncommon lesion typically arising on the posterior neck of adult men (426). Similar changes have also been seen at a number of non-nuchal sites, leading to the designation nuchal-type. A large proportion of patients have diabetes mellitus, and consideration should be given to the possibility of Gardner syndrome (see discussion later) (426). An association with desmoid tumors has been recorded (427,428).

Histopathology. In the dermis and subcutis, there is a poorly circumscribed mass containing haphazardly arranged collagen bundles with sparse, bland, spindle-shaped cells (Fig. 32-32). There is frequent entrapment of fat and a proliferation of fine nerves resembling a traumatic neuroma. Inflammation is not a feature, and elastin fibers may be reduced in number (429).

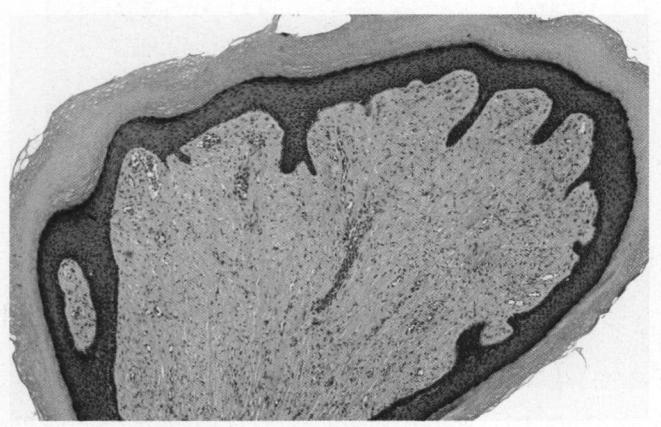

Figure 32-31 Digital fibrokeratoma. A polypoid lesion with acanthotic epidermis overlying dense bundles of collagen in the dermis.

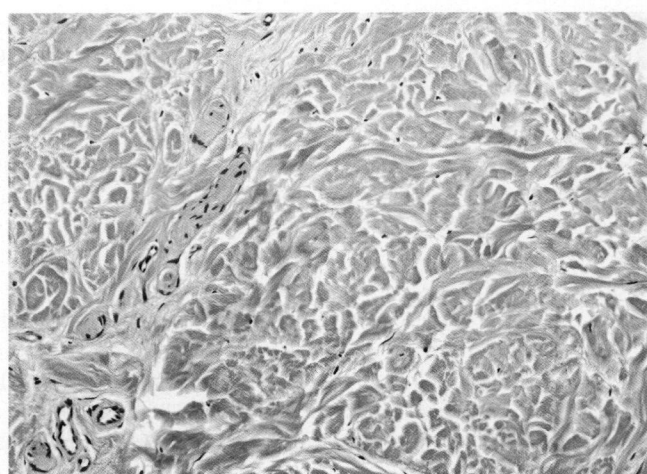

Figure 32-32 Nuchal-type fibroma. The tumor is hyalinized and poorly cellular. Note the small nerve twigs within the lesion.

Pathogenesis. A fibroblastic origin is proposed, with immunohistochemical staining showing CD34 positivity in the spindle cells in some cases (429).

Differential Diagnosis. The *Gardner fibroma* is very similar, if not identical, histologically, but occurs in young people in the context of Gardner syndrome, and most often on the trunk (426–430). It may be the presenting feature of that syndrome, a form of familial APC that may include osteomas, epidermoid cysts, and desmoid tumors (427). There may be subtly different histologic features such as an absence of small nerve fibers (428,430,431). Elastin fibers are decreased in number, in contrast to elastofibroma in which they are markedly increased and abnormal in morphology (429).

Principles of Management: Local excision is considered adequate treatment. Lesions occasionally recur but do not metastasize.

Superficial Acral Fibromyxoma (Digital Fibromyxoma)

Clinical Summary. This uncommon tumor was first described in a series of 37 cases in 2001 (432), with a large series of 124 further cases recently described (433). The lesions are almost always sited on the toes, fingers, or heels, often close to the nail, and average about 2 cm in size (432). A few have been reported on the palm (432), and lesions may be painful or of long duration at presentation (433). A broad range of ages may be affected, but many patients are young adults and male. The course is benign, with occasional recurrences and no metastases recorded (433).

Histopathology. Tumors are sited in the dermis or subcutis and are often poorly circumscribed with a proliferation of spindle-to-stellate cells in loose fascicles. There may be mild nuclear atypia and occasional multinucleated stromal cells, but mitoses are sparse. A myxocollagenous matrix bears fine vessels, with mast cells often conspicuous (Fig. 32-33A, B). Some lesions are more cellular and these are now generally considered to be synonymous with cellular digital fibromas (423–425). Invasion of bone is exceptional (433).

Pathogenesis. The majority of tumors stain prominently with CD34 and some with CD99. Although the presence of EMA positivity was emphasized in early reports, the incidence of

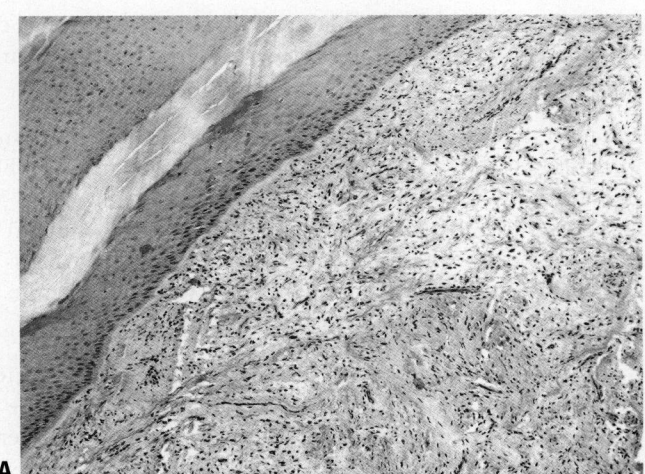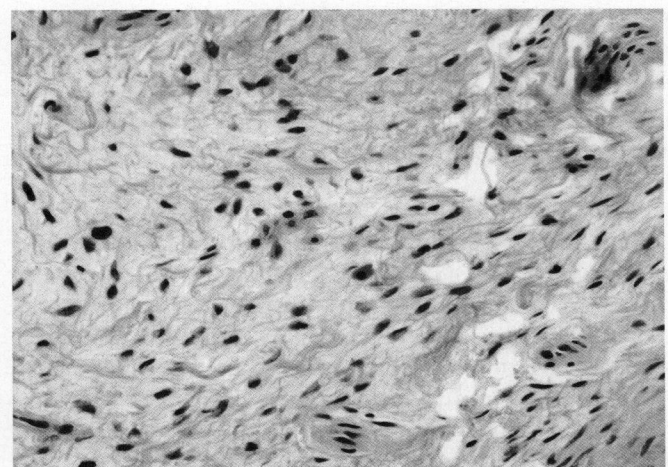

Figure 32-33 Superficial acral fibromyxoma. **A:** This lesion was from under the big toe nail, seen in the upper left of the photograph, a common site of origin. **B:** Myxoid stroma is present with nondescript, bland, spindle-shaped cells. These were CD34- and epithelial membrane antigen–positive on immunohistochemistry.

positive staining is low in some recent series (425,432,433). S100, actin, desmin, keratins, and HMB-45 are typically negative. Some lesions are CD10-positive (434). Nestin is positive (this may also be seen in DFSP) with no staining for MUC4, which helps to exclude the possibility of a low-grade fibromyxoid sarcoma (435).

In a small study, Rb1 loss was found by immunohistochemistry in 90% of the cases (436), indicating a relationship with the RB1-deleted range of tumors that include spindle-cell lipoma, atypical spindle cell/pleomorphic lipoma, pleomorphic liposarcoma, myofibroblastoma, and cellular angiofibroma (437).

Differential Diagnosis. The appearances have features in common with a variety of other connective tissue lesions, especially those with a tendency to become myxoid. However, correlating the clinical setting, histology, and immunostaining pattern should lead to the correct diagnosis.

Principles of Management: Local excision is the treatment of choice, with 24% of incompletely excised lesion recurring in one series (433).

Angiomyofibroblastoma of the Vulva

Clinical Summary. Angiomyofibroblastoma is a benign tumor that occurs mainly in the vulvovaginal region of middle-aged premenopausal women (438) but has also been rarely described in the inguinoscrotal region of males. It presents as a circumscribed tumor 0.5 to 12 cm in size and is often mistaken clinically for a Bartholin gland cyst. The tumors do not recur when treated with local excision (439–441).

Histopathology. Angiomyofibroblastomas are well-circumscribed tumors composed of hypercellular and hypocellular areas. There are plump epithelioid or spindle cells with moderate amounts of eosinophilic cytoplasm arranged singly, in clusters, or forming linear arrays around numerous small to medium-sized dilated capillaries within an edematous stroma. Some of the cells may have eccentric nuclei, imparting a plasmacytoid appearance. Multinucleated cells are not uncommon. There is minimal cytologic atypia, and mitoses are generally difficult to find

(439–443). An adipose tissue component is present in some cases (444).

Pathogenesis. The tumor cells of angiomyofibroblastoma are desmin-positive and actin-negative in most cases. Occasional cases are SMA-positive (439–443). The cells also express estrogen and progesterone receptors (444). No specific or recurrent molecular alterations have been reported.

Differential Diagnosis. In contrast to angiomyofibroblastoma, aggressive angiomyxoma has an infiltrating growth pattern, prominent hyalinized vessels, and mucin within the stroma. The cells of aggressive angiomyxoma are actin-positive and desmin-negative.

Principles of Management: Treatment is surgical.

Fibromatosis Colli

Clinical Summary. Fibromatosis colli presents 2 to 4 weeks after birth as a hard, immobile, fusiform swelling in the mid or lower portions of the sternocleidomastoid muscle, causing the head to tilt toward the side of the affected muscle (445). There is a high associated incidence of preceding breech and forceps delivery. However, the lesion develops *in utero* and not as a consequence of birth trauma as was once believed (446). Some cases are associated with congenital musculoskeletal abnormalities, including congenital dysplasia of the hip and rib cage anomalies (447–449). Most cases respond well to conservative treatment (447). Less than 20% require surgical therapy (445). Fine-needle aspiration cytology has been reported to be a reliable method of diagnosing these tumors (450,451).

Histopathology. There are proliferating fibroblasts of varying cellularity in a collagenous stroma partially replacing the skeletal muscle. There is little or no pleomorphism and a lack of mitotic activity. Atrophic and degenerate skeletal muscle fibers are entrapped with the lesion.

Principles of Management: Most cases respond well to conservative treatment (447). Less than 20% require surgical therapy (445).

Intermediate Biologic Potential (Locally Aggressive Fibroblastic/Myofibroblastic Tumors)

These tumors tend to grow inexorably and cause tissue damage but not to metastasize. Where feasible, complete excision is indicated.

Desmoid-Type Fibromatosis (Aggressive Fibromatosis, Desmoid Tumor, Musculoaponeurotic Fibromatosis)

Clinical Summary. Desmoid-type fibromatoses are benign clonal fibroblastic proliferations that arise as firm, nontender masses from muscular aponeuroses and tend to invade the muscle. This infiltrative growth pattern predisposes to local invasiveness and recurrence, but the lesions do not metastasize. Their rate of growth is slow, but the lesions may attain considerable size, as large as 25 cm in diameter (452). Although usually solitary, they may be multiple (453). Desmoid fibromatoses may occur in children, but they are seen mainly in young adults, particularly in women, the most common type arising from the rectus abdominis muscle after pregnancy. The lesions also occur as extra-abdominal masses in older adults in equal gender distribution (454).

The association of desmoid fibromatoses with familial adenomatous polyposis and Gardner syndrome is well documented. The prevalence in familial adenomatous polyposis is between 10% and 25% (455). APC gene mutation occurs in desmoid-type fibromatosis in patients with familial polyposis and less commonly in sporadic lesions (455–457). Trisomies for chromosomes 8 and 20 have also been demonstrated in some cell subpopulations (458,459). In sporadic cases, there are somatic mutations in the beta-catenin (CTNNB1) gene on 3p21, resulting in immunohistochemically demonstrable overexpression in nuclei. Fibromatosis in patients with familial adenomatous polyposis (FAP) harbors inactivating germline mutations in the desmoid region of the *APC* gene on 5q21-q22 (460).

Histopathology. Desmoid fibromatoses are composed of poorly circumscribed bundles of uniform spindle cells surrounded by abundant collagen with extensive hyalinization, whereas some cases have abundant mucoid matrix. The nuclei are small, regular, and pale staining, with a variable mitotic rate. The lesions frequently infiltrate adjacent striated muscle, entrapping atrophic muscle fibers (Fig. 32-34A, B) (452). A recent study of 165 cases showed seven distinct morphologic patterns, including conventional, hypocellular/hyalinized, staghorn vessel, myxoid,

keloidal, nodular fasciitis-like, and hypercellular. Most cases contained two and some up to five patterns. Intra-abdominal lesions showed the most variations in pattern (461).

Pathogenesis. Ultrastructurally, the spindle cells of desmoid fibromatosis show features of fibroblasts or myofibroblasts (453,462,463). Immunostaining shows variable SMA and MSA positivity (464). Nuclear immunopositivity for β-catenin was detected in 80% of cases of sporadic desmoid fibromatosis and in 67% of tumors in patients with FAP (465). Calretinin was observed in three-fourths of desmoid fibromatosis (466).

Principles of Management: Surgery is still the standard treatment for desmoid fibromatoses, although results can be less than optimal. Chemotherapy, radiotherapy, estrogen therapy, imatinib, and other treatments have shown various degrees of efficacy (467–471). Wide excision with negative margins should be the goal, but not at the expense of function, because fewer than half of the patients with positive margins experienced recurrence in one study (472).

Palmar Fibromatosis (Dupuytren Contracture)

Clinical Summary. Palmar fibromatosis presents as a benign, slow-growing nodule or cordlike thickening on the volar surface of the hands accompanied by flexion contracture of the digits. The incidence rises with increasing age, and bilateral disease is common. There is a higher incidence among patients with epilepsy, diabetes, or alcoholic liver disease and heavy smokers. There is a genetic predisposition, and some studies show an association with manual labor (473–479). *Plantar fibromatosis* is a similar lesion that arises from the plantar aponeurosis and rarely causes flexion contractures of the toes. Palmar and plantar fibromatoses and knuckle pads can develop in the same patient (480,481). Cases of palmar–plantar fibromatoses can occur in children and preadolescents (482).

Histopathology. Early lesions consist of multinodular cellular proliferations of uniform plump, spindle-shaped fibroblastic cells within a collagenous stroma (Fig. 32-35). Mitotic figures may be present but are usually infrequent. Long-standing lesions are less cellular and contain increased amounts of dense collagen.

Pathogenesis. The cells variably express SMA and MSA (483). The cells are often negative for beta-catenin in contrast to

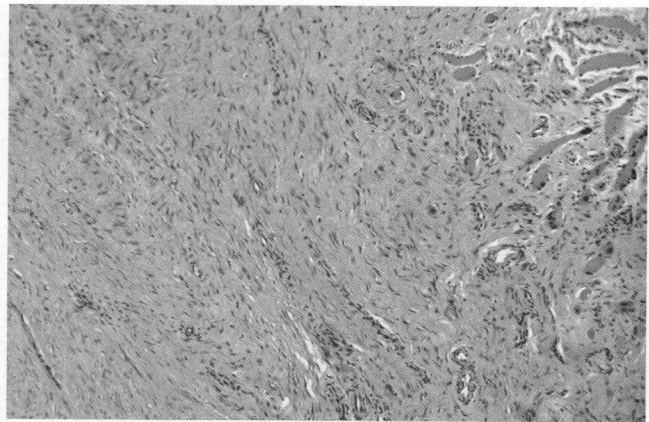
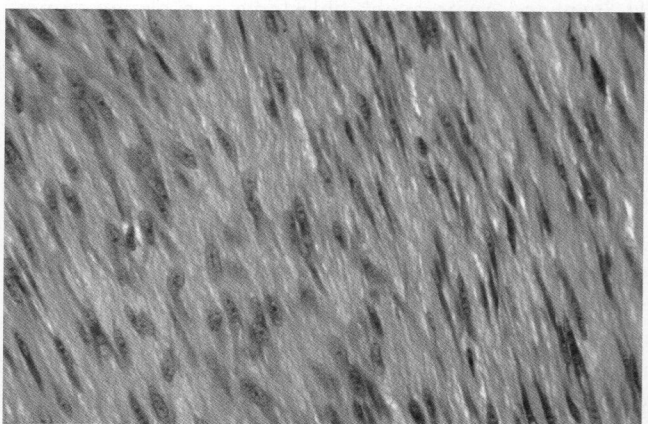

Figure 32-34 Desmoid-type fibromatosis (desmoid tumor). **A:** A mass composed of dense bundles of eosinophilic spindle cells is present within striated muscle (right). **B:** The tumor cells are monomorphic, with regular nuclei and pale eosinophilic cytoplasm.

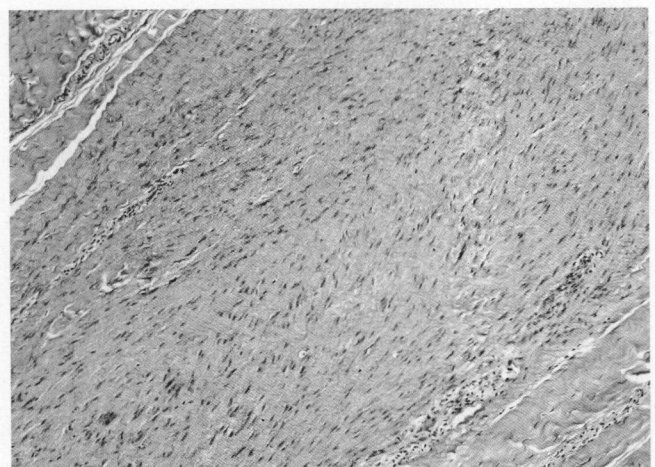

Figure 32-35 Palmar fibromatosis (Dupuytren contracture). There is a proliferation of uniform fibroblastic cells within a collagenous stroma.

desmoid-type fibromatoses (460). Ultrastructural studies show features of fibroblasts and myofibroblasts (484,485).

Principles of Management: Treatment is by surgical excision.

Knuckle Pads

Knuckle pads are uncommon, entirely benign fibroblastic tumors that present as persistent, slow-growing lesions over the extensor surfaces of the proximal interphalangeal and metacarpophalangeal joints (486). The lesions are flesh-colored, flat or dome-shaped, and freely mobile, and they mostly arise in men (486). Some patients have coexisting Dupuytren contractures, and these entities may be related (480).

Histopathology. The histologic features are similar to those of Dupuytren contracture. There is fibroblastic proliferation, with thickened irregular collagen bundles. The overlying epidermis may show hyperkeratosis and acanthosis (486,487).

Principles of Management: Treatment is surgical (488).

Intermediate Biologic Potential (Rarely Metastasizing Fibroblastic/Myofibroblastic Tumors)

These tumors may grow inexorably, causing local tissue damage. Metastases to local or visceral sites are uncommon, and even in the presence of metastases, tumor behavior may be indolent.

Solitary Fibrous Tumor

Clinical Summary. Solitary fibrous tumor is a rare mesenchymal neoplasm that most commonly involves the pleura but has also been reported in numerous extrapleural locations, including rare cases in the skin (489–492). In the skin, lesions present as a circumscribed nodule, mainly on the head and neck (492,493).

Histopathology. The tumors are circumscribed, unencapsulated nodules involving the dermis, subcutis, and fascia. Lesions are typically described as having a "patternless pattern," with hypercellular and hypocellular areas composed of bland spindle cells with pale vesicular nuclei, inconspicuous nucleoli, and indistinct cell borders. The spindle cells form fascicles or storiform patterns similar to DFSP, alternating with a vascular component of ectatic vessels and slit-like staghorn vessels, presenting a hemangiopericytoma-like appearance. Abundant hyalinized collagen makes up the less cellular areas (Fig. 32-36A, B), and mitotic activity is inconspicuous. The cells express CD34 in the majority of cases, CD99 and bcl-2 in some cases, and, focally, factor XIIIa, but they are negative for smooth muscle, neural, and epithelial markers (491,492,494,495). Nuclear expression of STAT6 immunohistochemically distinguishes solitary fibrous tumors from histologic mimics (496).

Principles of Management: Rare metastases from pleural solitary fibrous tumors have been reported, but all documented cutaneous tumors appear to be benign and cured by complete excision, although recurrences can occur, requiring reexcision (489,495).

Inflammatory Pseudotumor

Clinical Summary. Inflammatory pseudotumor encompasses a heterogeneous group of lesions also known as inflammatory myofibroblastic tumor and plasma cell granuloma. The tumor was originally described in the lung but has since been reported in other organs, including rare cases in the skin. The exact pathogenesis of inflammatory pseudotumor is unclear. Some lesions probably represent an exaggerated response to an antigenic stimulus such as an infectious agent, whereas others are true neoplasms (497–500). Although tumors in extracutaneous sites can recur and occasionally metastasize, all cases reported in the skin have behaved in an indolent manner, with no reports of recurrence after complete excision (501).

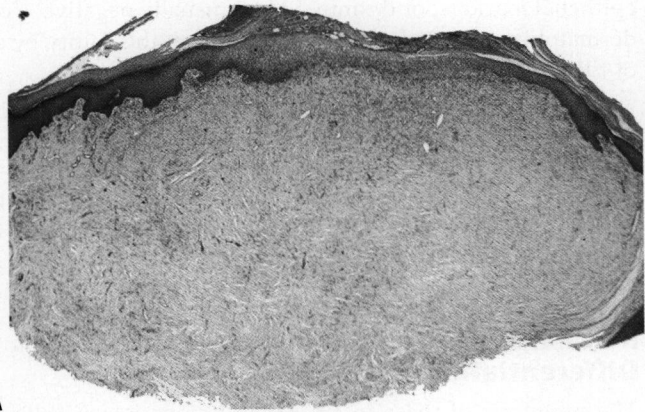

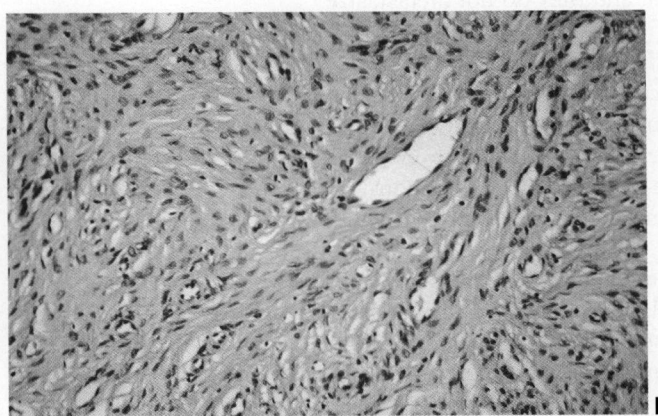

Figure 32-36 Solitary fibrous tumor. A: A circumscribed dermal nodule is present with some overlying reactive epidermal hyperplasia. B: Prominent vascularity is seen extending between bland "patternless" spindle cells.

Histopathology. Inflammatory pseudotumors present as circumscribed, unencapsulated lesions confined to the dermis or involving both dermis and subcutaneous fat. Two histologic patterns have been described in the skin (498–503). The first consists of bland spindle cells arranged in fascicle or storiform pattern admixed with variable numbers of inflammatory cells within myxoid and collagenous stroma. Although mitotic figures are usually present, there is no nuclear pleomorphism. The predominant inflammatory cells are plasma cells and small lymphocytes. Lymphoid follicles with germinal centers, eosinophils, and neutrophils may also be present. The second pattern is characterized by nodules composed of lymphocytes and plasma cells in a background of thick, hyaline collagen bundles arranged in intersecting or onion skin–like pattern without spindle cells. Giant histiocyte-like cells and Reed–Sternberg–like cells were described in one case report (498).

Pathogenesis. The spindle cells are SMA-positive (55,500,501). Ultrastructural studies demonstrate features of myofibroblastic and fibroblastic differentiation (502). Immunoreaction to ALK has been reported in up to 60% of extracutaneous cases, mostly in lesions from the pediatric population and young adults (497,504,505). There have been no reports of ALK in cutaneous lesions. ALK protein is a product of t(2;5) chromosomal translocation, adding support to the belief that some of these tumors are genuine neoplasms of myofibroblasts.

Differential Diagnosis. Nodular fasciitis typically presents as a rapidly developing tumor consisting of plump myofibroblasts within myxoid stroma imparting a "tissue culture" appearance accompanied by a sparse inflammatory infiltrate and red blood cell extravasation. Dermatofibromas are less well circumscribed, are usually associated with epidermal hyperplasia, and lack the prominent lymphoplasmacytic infiltrate.

Principles of Management: Treatment is surgical.

TUMORS OF UNCERTAIN DIFFERENTIATION

This is a heterogeneous group of tumors whose histogenesis is uncertain.

Benign Tumors of Uncertain Differentiation

In general, these lesions do not recur even after incomplete excision, and they do not metastasize.

Multinucleate Cell Angiohistiocytoma

Clinical Summary. Multinucleate cell angiohistiocytoma is an uncommon lesion that presents in middle-aged to elderly women as grouped red-to-brown or violaceous, circumscribed, dome-shaped tumors. Lesions occur in acral regions, most commonly the lower legs, wrists, back of the hands, and on the face. The tumors have a smooth surface and range from 2 to 10 mm in size. Some of the papules may coalesce to form larger annular lesions. They are benign lesions that progress slowly and persist, although spontaneous regression has been reported in some cases (506–511). One case of generalized multinucleated cell angiohistiocytoma was described (512).

Histopathology. The lesions are characterized by fine vessels with prominent endothelium in a fibrous stroma. There are sparse perivascular lymphocytes, with neutrophils and plasma

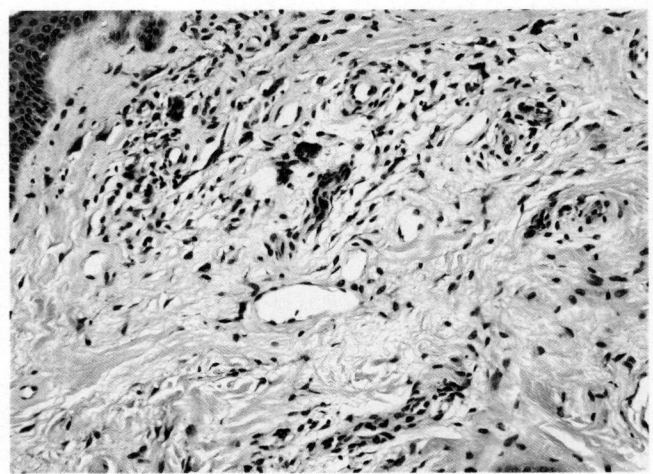

Figure 32-37 Multinucleate cell Angiohistiocytoma. Dilated superficial dermal blood vessels with surrounding multinucleate "histiocytic" cells.

cells present in some cases. Characteristically, there are increased numbers of large, irregular, bizarre mononuclear or multinucleated cells with hyperchromatic nuclei and scalloped basophilic cytoplasm in the interstitium. The epidermis may be hyperplastic (506–511). Increased mast cells have been noted (506) (Fig. 32-37).

Pathogenesis. The pathogenesis of multinucleate cell angiohistiocytoma is uncertain. The mononuclear interstitial cells express lysozyme and factor XIIIa. The multinucleated cells are immunoreactive only for vimentin (506,508,510,511).

Principles of Management: The lesion is benign and does not recur after excision.

EWSR1–SMAD3 Rearranged Fibroblastic Tumor

Clinical Summary. This is a recently described, very rare tumor with a predilection for the extremities of middle-aged women (513,514).

Histopathology. Lesions are usually small (<2 cm in diameter), partly circumscribed, and sited in the dermis or subcutis. Bland spindle-shaped cells are present with a collagenous or myxoid stroma, sometimes with collagen rosettes. Mitotic activity is limited and necrosis is not a feature.

Characteristically, and importantly, there is strong nuclear staining for ERG. No staining is seen for CD34, SOX10, S100, epithelial markers, or desmin. SMA is usually negative. Cellular dermatofibroma can be distinguished from this entity by a lack of ERG staining.

Pathogenesis. All lesions show EWSR1–SMAD3 fusion or rearrangement by FISH or next-generation sequencing.

Principles of Management: The tumors are benign but may occasionally recur. Local excision is, therefore, likely to be curative.

Intermediate Biologic Potential (Rarely Metastasizing Tumors of Uncertain Differentiation)

The prognosis of these intermediate lesions is generally good, with recurrence seen in some cases, primarily related to incomplete excision. Metastases are uncommon and are usually locoregional and/or indolent, but fatalities may occasionally occur.

Angiomatoid Fibrous Histiocytoma

Clinical Summary. This neoplasm occurs most often on the extremities of children and young adults as a fairly small, slowly growing, nodular or cystic mass in the dermis or subcutis (85) and was previously known as "angiomatoid malignant fibrous histiocytoma" (215,216). There may be associated pain and systemic symptoms such as anemia, pyrexia, and weight loss, possibly owing to excess interleukin 6 production (515).

This tumor should not be confused with aneurysmal fibrous histiocytoma, which would be better described as dermatofibroma with aneurysmal change (31) (see earlier discussion).

Histopathology. The tumors show variable appearances and may be challenging to diagnose. Often, hemorrhagic, cystic pseudovascular spaces are present, lined by attenuated tumor cells that are not endothelial. Multinodular sheets of ovoid-to-spindly cells with eosinophilic histiocytoid or myoid appearances are present in varying patterns with an infiltrate of lymphocytes and plasma cells (Fig. 32-38A, B) (516). Mitotic activity and atypia are not usually prominent, but if they are, this is not always predictive of adverse behavior (517). Stromal desmoplasia may efface much of the tumor, and occasional examples have a more solid appearance *solid variant of aneurysmal fibrous histiocytoma*, compounding the difficulty in diagnosis. As would be expected from the hemorrhage, hemosiderin is frequent in tumor cells and macrophages. The overall pattern may suggest a lymph node, with a peripheral lymphoid cuff in 80% of cases, with follicles and germinal centers and a thick pseudocapsule, giving a circumscribed outline (516).

Pathogenesis. The cell of origin is unclear, with varying results using immunohistochemistry (516). Many cases are CD68-positive, with the expression of desmin in about 50% of cases interpreted as evidence of myoid or myofibroblastic differentiation (216). Endothelial markers such as CD31 and CD34 are negative in the tumor cells. It should be noted that myogenin and MyoD1 are negative, in contrast to rhabdomyosarcoma (31). Although MUC4 is usually a fairly specific marker for low-grade fibromyxoid sarcoma, it has been demonstrated in 22% of angiomatoid fibrous histiocytomas (518). Up to 94% of neoplasms are EMA-positive, but cytokeratins are negative (518,519). SOX9 (which is implicated in chondroid differentiation in various neoplasms, possibly regulated by EWS) has been demonstrated by immunostaining in 85% of pediatric tumors (520).

Cytogenetic studies using FISH or RT-PCR show that most tumors have translocations involving EWSR1/ATF, EWSR1/CREB1, or less commonly FUS/ATF1 fusions (521–524). The EWSR1/CREB1 translocation has also been identified in clear-cell sarcoma (523). RT-PCR is the preferred method of ancillary investigation over FISH because it is more sensitive and specific (524).

Principles of Management: Complete surgical excision is indicated. The prognosis is generally good, with recurrence seen in 15% of cases, primarily related to incomplete excision or deep extension into fascia or skeletal muscle (85,514). Metastases arise in up to 5% of patients and are usually confined to local lymph nodes, but fatalities occasionally occur (85,215,216,517,525), sometimes decades later. Although most studies suggest that histology and the specific translocation identified do not affect prognosis, in a 2010 study, two patients who died of disease had tumors with significant pleomorphism and high proliferative activity (517).

Giant-Cell Tumor of Soft Tissue

Clinical Summary. The lesions present as an isolated nodule, often on the limbs, which is painless and slow growing (526). Both children and adults may be affected.

Histopathology. A circumscribed multinodular lesion is seen within the subcutis and sometimes dermis or skeletal muscle. The appearances are akin to a giant-cell tumor of bone (osteoclastoma) with CD68-positive osteoclast-type giant cells among regular mononuclear cells with ovoid nuclei (Fig. 32-39). Mitoses may be prominent and sometimes intravascular impingement may be present within the lesion. Hemorrhage, hemosiderin, and cystic degeneration can occur.

Pathogenesis. Some cases have followed trauma or been associated with Paget disease of the bone. No genetic changes have been identified in a series of 15 tumors, suggesting that they are distinct from giant-cell tumors of bone, in which genetic changes are present in the vast majority of cases (527).

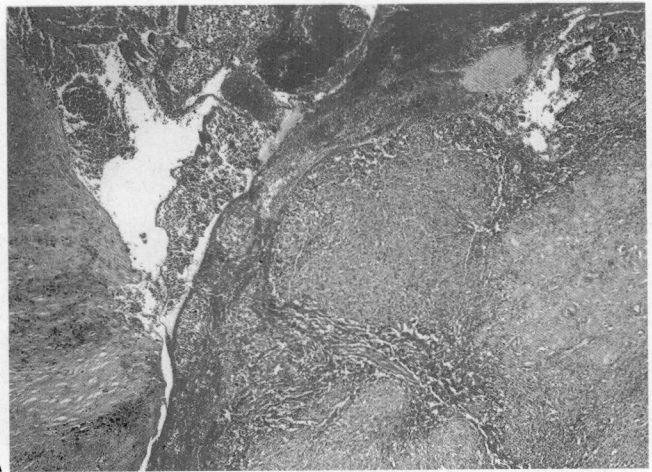
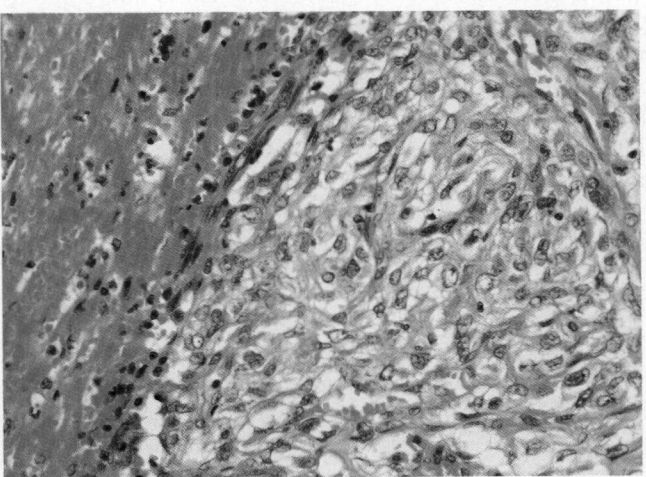

Figure 32-38 Angiomatoid fibrous histiocytoma. **A:** This 20-year-old man had severe anemia associated with this lesion from the shoulder. Blood-filled spaces are prominent, with surrounding pale zones of tissue. **B:** Pale histiocytoid cells are present in the wall of the blood-filled spaces that do not show an endothelial lining.

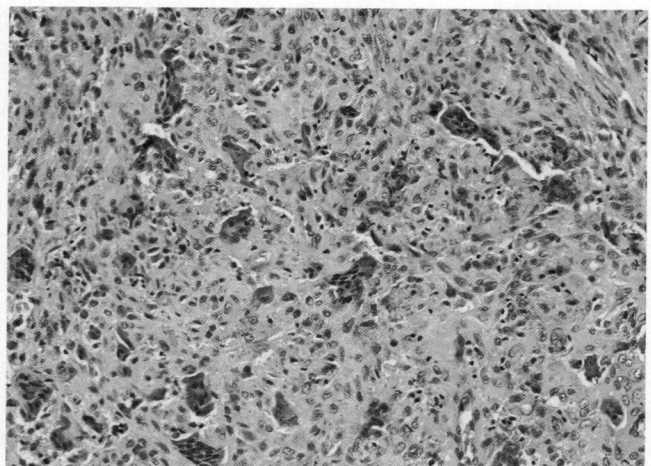

Figure 32-39 Giant-cell tumor of soft tissue. Osteoclast-type giant cells are associated with a background of regular mononuclear cells. The appearances closely resemble an osteoclastoma of bone.

Principles of Management: Complete conservative excision is advisable because of a low risk of recurrence and very rarely lymph node or distant metastases.

Malignant Tumors of Uncertain Differentiation

These are fully malignant neoplasms, which may recur locally even after complete excision, and may metastasize widely and cause death.

Synovial Sarcoma

Clinical Summary. Synovial sarcoma most commonly occurs in the deep connective tissues of the limbs, particularly the thigh, of young and middle-aged adults. Lesions confined to the dermis or subcutis or skin metastases are rare (528–530). The chromosomal translocation t(X;18) has been described in most synovial sarcomas and usually involves fusion of SSX1 or SSX2 with SS18 (previously known as SYT) (531–535).

Histopathology. The tumor typically presents a biphasic pattern, with an epithelioid cell component forming glandular spaces and a uniform small, spindle-cell component resembling fibrosarcoma (Fig. 32-40). Monophasic synovial sarcoma most frequently exhibits solely a spindle-cell element. Purely glandular monophasic synovial sarcoma theoretically exists but, without cytogenetic analysis, would be indistinguishable from adenocarcinoma (536,537). Most tumors express EMA with low- and high-molecular-weight cytokeratins. S100 and CD99 are stainable in some cases (538). TLE1 nuclear immunostaining is highly sensitive for synovial sarcoma (539), but it is not specific, and can be seen in many skin squamous cell carcinomas, basal cell carcinoma, sebaceous tumors, atypical fibroxanthomas, some melanomas, and DFSP (540,541).

Pathogenesis. Immunohistochemical and ultrastructural features indicate that the tumor is not derived from synovium, leading to suggestions of alternative terms such as *connective tissue carcinosarcoma* and *soft-tissue carcinoma* (542,543). The distribution of collagens, fibronectin, laminin, and tenascin in synovial sarcoma suggests similarities with the embryonic development of epithelia from mesenchymal cells, supporting the concept that synovial sarcoma is a soft-tissue carcinosarcoma (544).

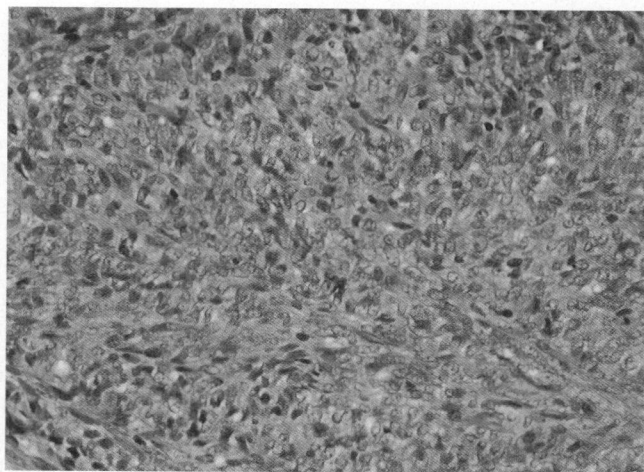

Figure 32-40 Synovial sarcoma. A cellular proliferation of fairly monomorphic, ovoid to spindle-shaped cells is seen in this monophasic tumor. Immunohistochemistry showed cytokeratin positivity in these cells.

Prognostic factors include tumor size, stage, grade, and patient age, with younger patients faring better (545–550). A worse prognosis has also been reported with larger areas of necrosis and increased mitoses (551). The prognostic value of SYT–SSX fusion has been questioned (552), although recent evidence suggests an adverse prognosis in tumors displaying SS18–SSX1, rather than SS18–SSX2 fusion (534). Tumors showing immunohistochemical staining for the cell survival–related factor mTOR may have a worse prognosis (551,553).

Principles of Management: Surgical excision is the mainstay of treatment, with a possible improvement of outlook with associated radiotherapy (548,549). Some improvement of prognosis in metastatic synovial sarcoma has been described using ifosfamide (554).

Epithelioid Sarcoma

Clinical Summary. Epithelioid sarcoma is a rare, highly malignant soft-tissue neoplasm of uncertain histogenesis. It occurs most commonly on the distal limbs of young men as a slowly growing nodule or plaque (Fig. 32-41) (555,556). Other sites of involvement include the head, neck, pelvis, and genital region (557,558). Most lesions are sited in subcutis or soft tissue, but

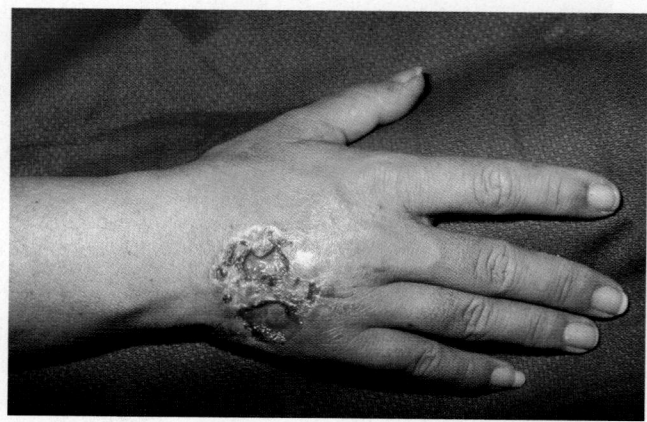

Figure 32-41 Epithelioid sarcoma. Ulcerated nodules on the back of the hand of a 32-year-old. The patient died from systemic metastases 18 months later.

occasional examples present primarily in the dermis and upper subcutis. Recurrence and metastasis are frequent, usually to lymph nodes and lung (556). Prognosis is related to tumor size and may be more favorable in females and those under 16 years of age (559,560). The incidence appears to be rising according to the SEER database in the United States (560).

Histopathology. Tumors are composed of nodules of atypical epithelioid cells with pleomorphic nuclei and variable amounts of eosinophilic cytoplasm. These merge with spindle cells and an associated fibrous stroma, in which there may be hemorrhage, hemosiderin, and mucin deposition with a patchy peripheral lymphocytic infiltrate. On occasions, mucin deposition may be prominent, causing diagnostic difficulty (561). Variable mitotic activity is seen, with frequent vascular and perineural invasion. Necrosis is characteristically present in the center of tumor nodules, contributing to the granulomatous appearance. Foci of calcification and ossification may be present. The lesions are diffusely invasive and may show overlying ulceration (Fig. 32-42A–C).

Positive immunostaining is seen for cytokeratins AE1/AE3, EMA, and vimentin, with more than 50% expressing CD34 and sometimes actin (562). CK7 is negative, in contrast to synovial sarcoma, and negative CK5/6 staining aids distinction from metastatic squamous cell carcinoma. Loss of INI-1 is helpful in differentiating epithelioid sarcoma from pseudomyogenic hemangioendothelioma (epithelioid sarcoma-like hemangioendothelioma) (563). Desmin is negative in both of these tumors. Both *ERG* and D2-40 may be seen in epithelioid sarcoma by immunostaining, although ERG is not present on *ERG* gene rearrangement studies (564).

A spindle-cell (*fibroma-like*) *variant* of epithelioid sarcoma also occurs, in which the spindle-cell pattern predominates without the characteristic epithelioid cells and nodularity (565,566).

Proximal-type epithelioid sarcoma is an aggressive variant occurring predominantly in the pelvis, perineum, and genital tract of older adults. It frequently shows rhabdoid features microscopically, simulating extrarenal rhabdoid tumor (567,568).

Pathogenesis. The histogenesis of epithelioid sarcoma is uncertain, but the ultrastructural features of desmosome-like intercellular junctions, numerous microvilli, and whorled arrangements of intermediate filaments (557,569), allied with immunoreactivity for EMA, cytokeratin, vimentin, and, in many cases, CD34 and actin, suggest an origin from primitive mesenchymal cells with the capacity for epithelial differentiation (562). Inactivation of the *SMARCB1* gene leads to loss of nuclear INI-1 (integrase interactor 1) expression immunohistochemically in more than 90% of cases (570). This is not an entirely specific finding, being also present in malignant rhabdoid tumors and some epithelioid malignant peripheral nerve sheath tumors. INI-1 is a tumor suppressor gene that is constitutively expressed in most normal cells. Cytogenetic studies have shown various chromosomal aberrations, largely related to 22q11 or 12, with inactivation of *SMARCB1*. Abnormalities of chromosomes 8 and 22 have been reported in proximal-type epithelioid sarcoma (571).

Differential Diagnosis. At low power, the features often suggest a granulomatous process such as granuloma annulare or rheumatoid nodule. However, cellular atypia, a general lack

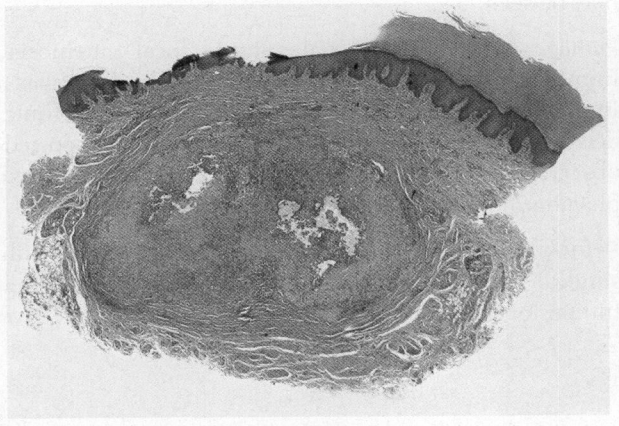

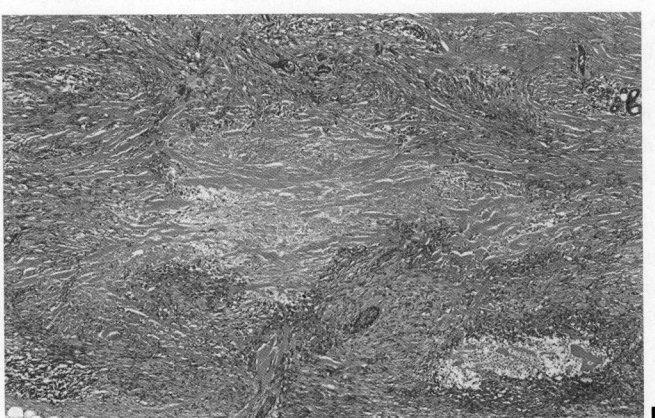

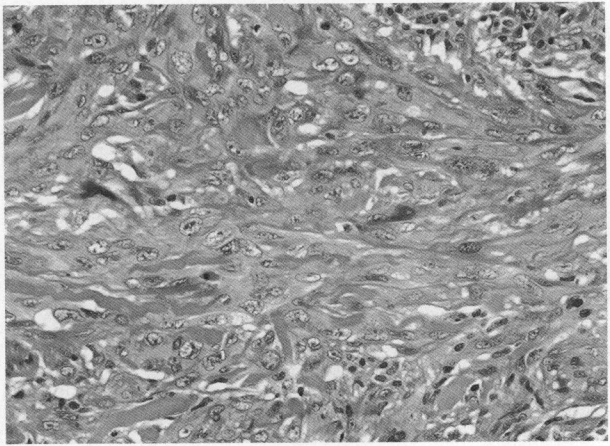

Figure 32-42 Epithelioid sarcoma. **A:** A nodule of tumor is present in the dermis with foci of necrosis. **B:** In this tumor, the pattern of infiltration and necrosis mimics a granulomatous process such as necrobiosis lipoidica. Attention to cellular detail will help avoid such a misdiagnosis. **C:** Enlarged, atypical epithelioid cells are present that stained positively for cytokeratins on immunohistochemistry.

of mucin, and foci of tumor cell necrosis assist in making the correct diagnosis even before immunohistochemical stainings have been performed (569,572). Although epithelioid sarcoma shows both mesenchymal and epithelial differentiation, it lacks the characteristic biphasic pattern of synovial sarcoma, which does not usually express CD34 (536). Epithelioid sarcoma is negative for cytokeratins 5/6 in most cases, which helps to distinguish it from squamous cell carcinoma, which is typically positive (573). Loss of INI-1 staining immunohistochemically can be helpful in supporting a diagnosis of epithelioid sarcoma (see earlier discussions).

Principles of Management: Radical surgical excision is the treatment of choice, with sentinel lymph node biopsy and removal of involved nodes (574,575). The precise role of radiotherapy and cytotoxic therapy is currently unclear (575–577). Research evaluating potential specific targeted therapies is underway (578).

MISCELLANEOUS LESIONS

Cutaneous Myxoma

Clinical Summary. Cutaneous myxomas are sharply demarcated nodules in the dermis or subcutis. They may occur as multiple lesions in association with cardiac and breast myxomas, spotty pigmentation, and endocrine overactivity in Carney complex (579) or as solitary lesions, usually on the head and neck, trunk, or digits (580–583).

Histopathology. Lesions are sharply circumscribed and sparsely cellular, composed of stellate and spindle-shaped fibroblasts, abundant small, thin-walled vessels, and myxoid matrix (Fig. 32-43A, B). An epithelial component is sometimes present, taking the form of linear strands of epithelium with basaloid features, small keratinous cysts, or follicular induction resembling superficial basal cell carcinoma (579,582,584). *Superficial angiomyxoma* describes tumors with a more prominent associated vascular pattern (582).

Differential Diagnosis. Cutaneous myxoma is more sharply circumscribed and more vascular than focal mucinosis (585). The tumor cells in myxomas express vimentin, with variable positivity for CD34 and actin. The cells are usually negative

for S100 protein, which is helpful in the distinction from neuroid tumors such as neurothekeoma and myxoid neurofibroma (586). Neurothekeomas display a multilobular pattern, and the cells in myxoid neurofibromas have wavy nuclei.

Principles of Management: Treatment is surgical with a recurrence rate of 30% to 40% (587).

Digital Mucous Cyst

Clinical Summary. It has been suggested that two types of digital mucous cyst exist (588,589). One type is analogous to focal mucinosis. It differs from focal mucinosis only by its location near the proximal nail fold and by its greater tendency to fluctuation. The other type is located on the dorsum of a finger near the distal interphalangeal joint and is caused by a herniation of the joint lining, thus representing a ganglion (588). Another view is that digital mucous cyst and digital myxoma are identical and that there is no anatomic connection with the interphalangeal joint (589). The lesion can uncommonly occur on the toes.

Histopathology. According to the first concept, digital mucous cyst in its early stage has the same histologic appearance as that seen in focal mucinosis, that is, an ill-defined area of mucinous material. Subsequently, multiple clefts form and then coalesce into one large cystic space containing mucin composed largely of hyaluronic acid, which stains with Alcian blue and colloidal iron (590). The cystic space in early lesions is separated from the epidermis by mucinous stroma, but in older lesions, it is found in a subepidermal location with thinning of the overlying epidermis. The collagen at the periphery of the cyst appears compressed. No lining of the cyst wall is apparent (Fig. 32-44) (590,591). Transepidermal elimination of mucinous material may be seen.

Pathogenesis. The type analogous to focal mucinosis results from overproduction of hyaluronic acid by fibroblasts (590). In the ganglion type of digital mucous cyst, hyaluronic acid is derived from the joint fluid. This concept is supported by the observation that methylene blue injected into the distal interphalangeal joint can be identified in the cyst (591,592).

Principles of Management: Management consists either of a surgical approach, conservative therapy, or simple follow-up. Intralesional steroids have also been shown to be effective (593).

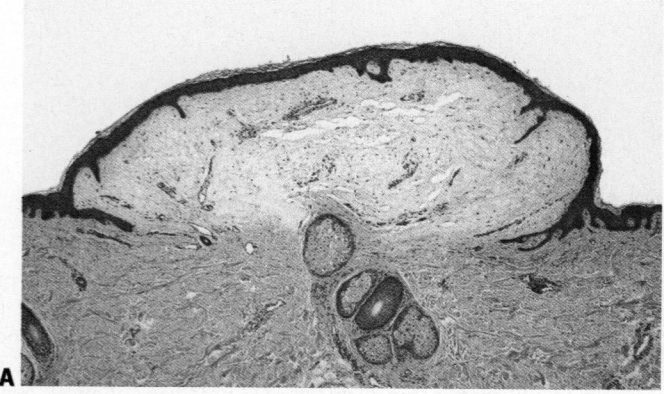
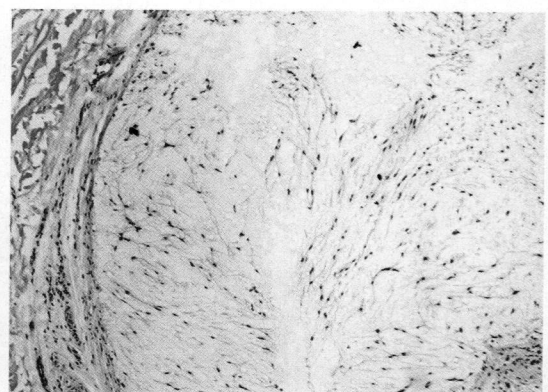

Figure 32-43 A, B: Cutaneous myxoma. The lesion is a sharply circumscribed nodule composed of a vascular mucinous matrix in which spindle cells are scattered.

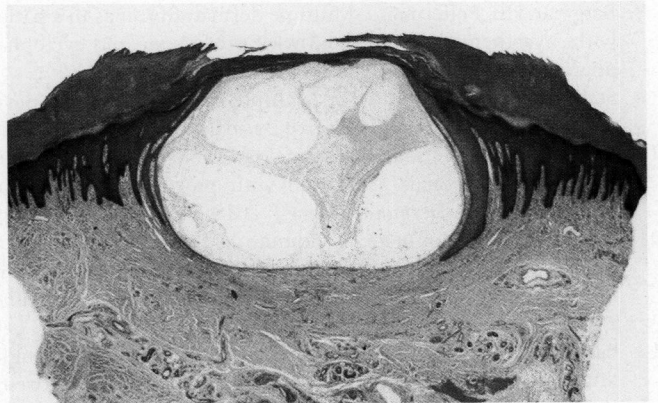

Figure 32-44 Digital mucous cyst. The epidermis is raised and attenuated over a circumscribed mucinous cystic nodule, with an epidermal collarette.

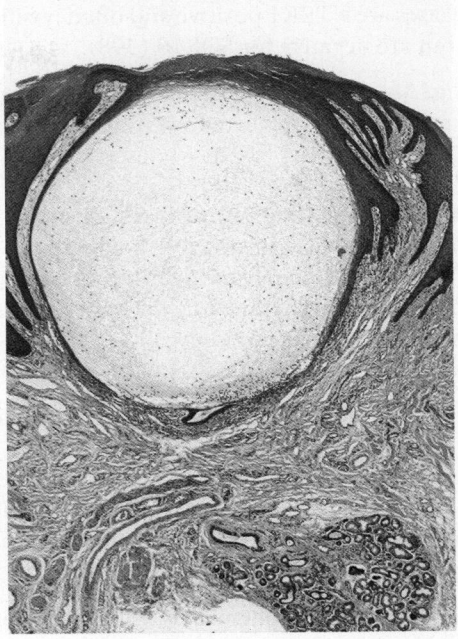

Figure 32-45 Mucous cyst of the oral mucosa. The squamous epithelium is raised and overlies a cyst containing mucin and inflammatory cells. A segment of salivary gland duct opens into the base of the cyst.

Mucous Cyst (Mucocele) of the Oral Mucosa/Mucocele

Clinical Summary. Mucoceles present as solitary asymptomatic lesions, usually on the mucous surface of the lower lip and only rarely elsewhere on the oral mucosa (594). The cysts usually typically measure less than 10 mm in diameter, appear dome-shaped, are translucent, and contain a clear, viscous fluid. Minor trauma causing rupture of a mucous duct appears to initiate the lesion, releasing sialomucin into the tissue. Although most patients with an oral mucous cyst have no preexisting abnormality, mucous cysts of the lower lip may occur in patients with cheilitis glandularis, a condition in which the labial mucous glands and ducts are hyperplastic (595).

Histopathology. Early lesions consist of multiple small spaces filled with sialomucin surrounded by or intermixed with granulation tissue in the submucosa. Older lesions show either a solitary, large cystic space or several large spaces lined by a thick layer of granulation tissue composed of neutrophils, lymphocytes, fibroblasts, muciphages, and capillaries (594). The wall of some cysts shows a ruptured salivary duct opening into the cavity. The sialomucin within the cysts appears as amorphous, slightly eosinophilic material that is periodic acid–Schiff-positive and diastase-resistant and also stains with Alcian blue and colloidal iron. Minor salivary gland ducts in the underlying stroma provide a clue to the diagnosis (Fig. 32-45) (596).

Principles of Management: Treatment is surgical.

Fibroblastic Connective Tissue Nevus

Clinical Summary. This is a rare benign cutaneous mesenchymal lesion (597). Presentation is across a wide age range, although most cases are in children (with a median age of 10 years). Most cases arise on the trunk, head or neck, and limbs. The lesions are solitary, painless, and slow growing, ranging in size from 0.3 to 2.0 cm. No tumor was found to recur, even when excision was incomplete, and no metastases have been recorded.

Histopathology. Histologically, the lesions are poorly circumscribed and unencapsulated, involving the deep dermis/superficial subcutis. Overlying papillomatous epidermis and dermal adipose tissue may be noted. There is a proliferation of bland spindle cells without atypia or mitoses that surround appendages in short fascicles.

Pathogenesis. The tumors are composed of fibroblastic/myofibroblastic cells that are focally positive for SMA and CD34 (weak) and negative for desmin, AE1/3, melan-A, pro-collagen, and S100. Cases can stain for factor XIIIa.

Differential Diagnosis. The main differential diagnoses of fibroblastic connective tissue nevus (FCTN) include plaque-stage DFSP, dermatomyofibroma, pilar leiomyoma, and the fibroblastic-dominant subtype of plexiform fibrohistiocytic tumor. DFSP is classically composed of a uniform proliferation of mildly atypical fibroblasts arranged in a storiform pattern. Strong diffuse CD34 positivity in lesional cells would favor DFSP. Dermatomyofibroma presents in an older age group (with a median age of 30 years) and tends to arise around the shoulder and upper arms. In dermatomyofibroma, fascicles of spindle cells are typically oriented parallel to the overlying epidermis. Pilar leiomyoma usually occurs in an older age group and is often painful, and immunohistochemically, it is consistently desmin-positive.

Plexiform fibrohistiocytic tumor occurs in the dermis and subcutis of children and young adults on the upper extremities, especially the fingers, hand, or wrist. It typically grows as a poorly circumscribed, plexiform proliferation composed of multiple small nodules showing admixed round mononuclear cells and osteoclast-like giant cells and short fibromatosis-like fascicles of fibroblastic/myofibroblastic-appearing spindled cells. Plaque-like CD34-positive dermal fibroma consists of a proliferation of CD34+ fibroblast-like bland cells localized mostly in the upper dermis with rare involvement of subcutis and shows a distinctive orientation to the epidermis, with the superficial elements vertical to it and the deeper cells horizontal. Lipofibromatosis affects the limbs of children and is mostly localized in the fibrous septa of fat and skeletal muscle and has a second component of abundant mature adipose tissue. An emerging entity is the NTRK-rearranged spindle-cell neoplasm that occurs mainly in the first two decades of life and can resemble lipofibromatosis but has a wide morphologic spectrum. Cases are NTRK1 positive and often positive for S100 and CD34 but are negative for SOX10 (598).

Principles of Management: Local surgical excision is considered adequate. No cases recurred even after incomplete excision (599).

Superficial CD34-Positive Fibroblastic Tumor

Clinical Summary. This is a distinctive low-grade neoplasm occurring in adults with equal sex distribution, ranging in size from 1.5 to 10 cm. It is confined to the superficial soft tissues of the limbs or adjacent skin. Only 30 to 40 cases have been reported (600,601).

Histopathology. Histologically, all tumors were characterized by relative circumscription, pleomorphic spindled to polygonal cells with variably enlarged bizarre-appearing cells, intranuclear cytoplasmic pseudoinclusions, and extremely low mitotic activity. The cells showed an abundant granular, fibrillary, or glassy cytoplasm. Necrosis was rarely seen.

Pathogenesis. Immunohistochemically, neoplastic cells showed diffuse and strong expression of CD34 and focal staining with cytokeratin in half of the cases. All tested cases lacked expression of FLI-1, ERG, S100, desmin, and SMA. The tumors showed retained SMARCB1 (INI-1) and lacked TP53 overexpression, with a very low Ki-67-labeling index. Cases tested by FISH for TGFBR3 and/or MGEA5 rearrangements were negative, although three cases have shown PRDM10 rearrangements.

Differential diagnosis. Superficial location, CD34 positivity, and a low mitotic index assist in distinguishing these tumors from histologic mimics.

Principles of Management: Treatment is surgical with the aim of complete excision. An excellent prognosis has been reported, with only one patient developing lymph node metastasis.

REFERENCES

1. Fletcher CDM. The evolving classification of soft tissue tumours: an update based on the new WHO classification. *Histopathology.* 2006;48:3–12.
2. WHO Classification of Tumours Editorial Board. *Soft Tissue and Bone Tumours.* WHO Classification of Tumours Series. Vol 3. 5th ed. International Agency for Research on Cancer; 2020.
3. Elder DE, Massi D, Scolyer RA, Willemze R. *WHO Classification of Skin Tumours.* 4th ed. International Agency for Research on Cancer; 2018.
4. Bedi TR, Pandhi RK, Bhutani LK. Multiple palmoplantar histiocytomas. *Arch Dermatol.* 1976;112:1001–1003.
5. Lehmer LM, Ragsdale BD. Digital dermatofibromas—common lesion, uncommon location: a series of 26 cases and review of the literature. *Dermatol Online J.* 2011;17:2.
6. Mentzel T, Kutzner H, Rutten A, Hügel H. Benign fibrous histiocytoma (dermatofibroma) of the face: clinicopathologic and immunohistochemical study of 34 cases associated with an aggressive clinical course. *Am J Dermatopathol.* 2001;23:419–426.
7. Beatrous SV, Riahi RR, Grisoli SB, Cohen PR. Associated conditions in patients with multiple dermatofibromas: case reports and literature review. *Dermatol Online J.* 2017;23:13030/qt8zv852d8.
8. Bargman HB, Fefferman I. Multiple dermatofibromas in a patient with myasthenia gravis treated with prednisone and cyclophosphamide. *J Am Acad Dermatol.* 1986;14:351–352.
9. Stainforth J, Goodfield MJD. Multiple dermatofibromata developing during pregnancy. *Clin Exp Dermatol.* 1994;19:59–60.
10. Queirós C, Uva L, Soares de Almeida L, Filipe P. Multiple eruptive dermatofibromas associated with pregnancy—a case and literature review. *Dermatol Online J.* 2019;25:13030/qt29d3q6p1.
11. Kanitakis J, Carbonnel E, Delmonte S, Livrozet JM, Faure M, Claudy A. Multiple eruptive dermatofibromas in a patient with HIV infection: case report and literature review. *J Cutan Pathol.* 2000;27:54–56.
12. Bachmeyer C, Cordier F, Blum L, Cazier A, Vérola O, Aractingi S. Multiple eruptive dermatofibromas after highly active antiretroviral therapy. *Br J Dermatol.* 2000;143:1336–1337.
13. Niemi KM. The benign fibrohistiocytic tumours of the skin (review). *Acta Dermatol Venereol (Stockholm).* 1970;50:1–66.
14. Schoenfeld RJ. Epidermal proliferations overlying histiocytomas. *Arch Dermatol.* 1964;90:266–270.
15. Leyva WH, Santa Cruz DJ. Atypical cutaneous fibrous histiocytoma. *Am J Dermatopathol.* 1986;8:467–471.
16. Dalziel K, Marks R. Hair follicle-like changes over histiocytomas. *Am J Dermatopathol.* 1986;8:462–466.
17. Bryant J. Basal cell carcinoma overlying longstanding dermatofibromas. *Arch Dermatol.* 1977;113:1445–1446.
18. Goette DK, Helwig EB. Basal cell carcinomas and basal cell carcinoma–like changes overlying dermatofibroma. *Arch Dermatol.* 1975;111:589–591.
19. Buselmeier TJ, Uecker JH. Invasive basal cell carcinoma with metaplastic bone formation associated with a long-standing dermatofibroma. *J Cutan Pathol.* 1979;6:496–500.
20. Leiphart, P, Chu, C, Helm, K. Two cases of adenodermatofibroma. *J Cutan Pathol.* 2021;48:330–333.
21. Calonje E, Mentzel T, Fletcher CDM. Cellular benign fibrous histiocytoma: clinicopathologic analysis of 74 cases of a distinctive variant of cutaneous fibrous histiocytoma with frequent recurrence. *Am J Surg Pathol.* 1994;18:668–676.
22. Colome-Grimmer MI, Evans HL. Metastasizing cellular dermatofibroma. A report of two cases. *Am J Surg Pathol.* 1996;20:1361–1367.
23. Volpicelli ER, Fletcher CD. Desmin and CD34 positivity in cellular fibrous histiocytoma: an immunohistochemical analysis of 100 cases. *J Cutan Pathol.* 2012;39:747–52.
24. Luzar B, Calonje E. Cutaneous fibrohistiocytic tumours—an update. *Histopathology.* 2010;56:148–65.
25. Colby TV. Metastasizing dermatofibroma. *Am J Surg Pathol.* 1997;21:976.
26. Guillou L, Gebhard S, Salmeron M, Coindre JM. Metastasizing fibrous histiocytoma of the skin: a clinicopathologic and immunohistochemical analysis of three cases. *Mod Pathol.* 2000;13:654–660.
27. Gaufin M, Michaelis T, Duffy K. Cellular dermatofibroma: clinicopathologic review of 218 cases of cellular dermatofibroma to determine the clinical recurrence rate. *Dermatol Surg.* 2019;45:1359–1364.
28. Santa Cruz DJ, Kyriakos M. Aneurysmal ("angiomatoid") fibrous histiocytoma of the skin. *Cancer.* 1981;47:2053–2061.
29. Calonje E, Fletcher CDM. Aneurysmal benign fibrous histiocytoma: a clinicopathological analysis of 40 cases of a tumour frequently misdiagnosed as a vascular neoplasm. *Histopathology.* 1995;26:323–331.
30. Nabatanzi A, Male M, Qu XY, et al. Aneurysmal fibrous histiocytoma: clinicopathology analysis of 30 cases of a rare variant of cutaneous fibrohistiocytoma. *Curr Med Sci.* 2019;39:134–137.

31. Billings SD, Folpe AL. Cutaneous and subcutaneous fibrohistiocytic tumors of intermediate malignancy: an update. *Am J Dermatopathol.* 2004;26:141–155.

32. Botrus G, Sciot R, Debiec-Rycther M. Cutaneous aneurysmal fibrous histiocytoma with a t(12;19)(p12;q13) as the sole cytogenetic anomaly. *Cancer Genet Cytogenet.* 2006;164:155–158.

33. Wood KA, Easson AM, Ghazarian D, Saeed Kamil Z. Metastatic aneurysmal fibrous histiocytoma in a 20-year-old woman: a rare case report with review of the literature and discussion of its genomic features. *J Cutan Pathol.* 2020;47:870–875.

34. Mentzel T, Wiesner T, Cerroni L, et al. Malignant dermatofibroma: clinicopathological, immunohistochemical, and molecular analysis of seven cases. *Mod Pathol.* 2013;26:256–267.

35. Fukamizu H, Oku T, Inoue K, Matsumoto K, Okayama H, Tagami H. Atypical ("pseudocarcinomatous") cutaneous histiocytoma. *J Cutan Pathol.* 1983;10:327–333.

36. Tamada S, Ackerman AB. Dermatofibroma with monster cells. *Am J Dermatopathol.* 1987;9:380–387.

37. Setoyama M, Fukumaru S, Kanzaki T. Case of dermatofibroma with monster cells: a review and an immunohistochemical study. *Am J Dermatopathol.* 1997;19:312–315.

38. Kaddu S, McMenamin ME, Fletcher CDM. Atypical fibrous histiocytoma of the skin: clinicopathologic analysis of 59 cases with evidence of infrequent metastasis. *Am J Surg Pathol.* 2002;26:35–46.

39. Felty CC, Linos K. Epithelioid fibrous histiocytoma: a concise review. *Am J Dermatopathol.* 2019;41:879–883.

40. Dickson BC, Swanson D, Charames GS, Fletcher CD, Hornick JL. Epithelioid fibrous histiocytoma: molecular characterization of ALK fusion partners in 23 cases. *Mod Pathol.* 2018;31:753–762.

41. Kazakov DV, Kyrpychova L, Martinek P, et al. ALK gene fusions in epithelioid fibrous histiocytoma: a study of 14 cases, with new histopathological findings. *Am J Dermatopathol.* 2018;40:805–814.

42. Doyle LA, Mariño-Enriquez A, Fletcher CD, Hornick JL. ALK rearrangement and overexpression in epithelioid fibrous histiocytoma. *Mod Pathol.* 2015;28:904–12.

43. Wilson Jones E, Cerio R, Smith NP. Epithelioid cell histiocytoma: a new entity. *Br J Dermatol.* 1989;120:185–195.

44. Singh Gomez C, Calonje E, Fletcher CDM. Epithelioid benign fibrous histiocytoma of skin: clinico-pathological analysis of 20 cases of a poorly known variant. *Histopathology.* 1994;24:123–129.

45. Glusac EJ, McNiff JM. Epithelioid cell histiocytoma: a simulant of vascular and melanocytic neoplasms. *Am J Dermatopathol.* 1999;21:1–7.

46. Fletcher CD. Benign fibrous histiocytoma of subcutaneous and deep soft tissue. A clinicopathological analysis of 21 cases. *Am J Surg Pathol.* 1990;14:801–809.

47. Coindre JM. Deep benign fibrous histiocytoma. In: Fletcher CDM, Unnik K, Mertens F, eds. *World Health Organisation Classification of Tumours. Pathology and Genetics of Tumours of Soft Tissue and Bone.* IARC Press; 2002:114–115.

48. Frau DV, Erdas E, Caria P, et al. Deep fibrous histiocytoma with a clonal karyotypic alteration: molecular cytogenetic characterization of a t(16;17)(p13.3;q21.3). *Cancer Genet Cytogenet.* 2010;202:17–21.

49. Gleason BC, Fletcher CD. Deep "benign" fibrous histiocytoma: clinicopathologic analysis of 69 cases of a rare tumor indicating occasional metastatic potential. *Am J Surg Pathol.* 2008;32:354–362.

50. Wambacher-Gasser B, Zelger B, Zelger BG, Steiner H. Clear cell dermatofibroma. *Histopathology.* 1997;30:64–69.

51. Zelger BG, Steiner H, Kutzner H, Rütten A, Zelger B. Granular cell dermatofibroma. *Histopathology.* 1997;31:258–262.

52. Iwata J, Fletcher CDM. Lipidized fibrous histiocytoma. Clinicopathologic analysis of 22 cases. *Am J Dermatopathol.* 2000;22:126–134.

53. Zelger BG, Calonje E, Zelger B. Myxoid dermatofibroma. *Histopathology.* 1999;34:357–364.

54. Usmani A, Lal P, Li H, et al. Myofibroblastic differentiation in dermatofibromas [Abstract]. *J Cutan Pathol.* 2000;27:576.

55. Kutchemeshgi M, Barr RJ, Henderson CD. Dermatofibroma with osteoclast-like giant cells. *Am J Dermatopathol.* 1992;14:397–401.

56. Kuo Tt, Hu S, Chan HL. Keloidal dermatofibroma. *Am J Surg Pathol.* 1998;22:564–568.

57. Kiyohara T, Kumakiri M, Kobayashi H, Ohkawara A, Lao LM. Atrophic dermatofibroma. Elastophagocytosis by the tumor cells. *J Cutan Pathol.* 2000;27:312–315.

58. Schwob VS, Santa Cruz DJ. Palisading cutaneous fibrous histiocytoma. *J Cutan Pathol.* 1986;13:403–407.

59. Papalas JA, Balmer NN, Wallace C, Sangüeza OP. Ossifying dermatofibroma with osteoclast-like giant cells: report of a case and literature review. *Am J Dermatopathol.* 2009;31:379–383.

60. Zelger BG, Zelger B. Dermatofibroma (fibrous histiocytoma): an inflammatory or neoplastic disorder? *Histopathology.* 2001;38:379–381.

61. Calonje E. Is cutaneous benign fibrous histiocytoma (dermatofibroma) a reactive inflammatory process or a neoplasm? *Histopathology.* 2000;37:278–280.

62. Chen TC, Kuo Tt, Chan HL. Dermatofibroma is a clonal proliferative disease. *J Cutan Pathol.* 2000;27:36–39.

63. Hui P, Glusac EJ, Sinard JH, Perkins AS. Clonal analysis of cutaneous fibrous histiocytoma (dermatofibroma). *J Cutan Pathol.* 2002;29:385–389.

64. Cheng L, Amini SB, Zaim MT. Follicular basal cell hyperplasia overlying dermatofibroma. *Am J Surg Pathol.* 1997;21:711–718.

65. Morgan MB, Howard HG, Everett MA. Epithelial induction in dermatofibroma: a role for the epidermal growth factor (EGF) receptor. *Am J Dermatopathol.* 1997;19:35–40.

66. Han KH, Huh CH, Cho KH. Proliferation and differentiation of the keratinocytes in hyperplastic epidermis overlying dermatofibroma. Immunohistochemical characterization. *Am J Dermatopathol.* 2001;23:90–98.

67. Calonje E, Fletcher CDM. Cutaneous fibrohistiocytic tumors: an update. *Adv Anat Pathol.* 1994;1:2–15.

68. Cerio R, Spaull J, Wilson Jones E. Histiocytoma cutis: a tumor of dermal dendrocytes (dermal dendrocytoma). *Br J Dermatol.* 1989;120:197–206.

69. Headington JT. The dermal dendrocyte. In: Callen JP, Dahl MV, Golitz LE, eds. *Advances in Dermatology.* Vol 1. Year Book Medical; 1986:159–171.

70. Prieto VG, Reed JA, Shea CR. Immunohistochemistry of dermatofibroma and benign fibrous histiocytomas. *J Cutan Pathol.* 1995;22:336–341.

71. Mihatsch-Konz B, Schaumburg-Lever G, Lever WF. Ultrastructure of dermatofibroma. *Arch Dermatol Forsch.* 1973;246:181–192.

72. Aubock L. Zur ultrastruktur fibroser und histiocytarer hauttumoren. *Virchows Arch A.* 1975;368:253–274.

73. Katenkamp D, Stiller D. Cellular composition of the so-called dermatofibroma (histiocytoma cutis). *Virchows Arch.* 1975;367:325–336.

74. Kindblom LG, Jacobsen GK, Jacobsen M. Immunohistochemical investigations of tumors of supposed fibroblastic-histiocytic origin. *Hum Pathol.* 1982;13:834–840.

75. Kerdel FA, Morgan EW, Holden CA. Demonstration of alpha-1-anti-trypsin and alpha-1-antichymotrypsin in cutaneous histiocytic infiltrates. *J Am Acad Dermatol.* 1982;7:177–182.

76. Burgdorf W, Moreland A, Wasik R. Negative immunoperoxidase staining for lysozyme in nodular subepidermal fibrosis. *Arch Dermatol.* 1982;118:241–243.

77. Kanitakis J, Schmitt D, Thivolet J. Immunohistologic study of cellular populations of histiocytofibromas ("dermatofibromas"). *J Cutan Pathol.* 1984;11:88–94.

78. Zelger B, Sidoroff A, Stanzl U, et al. Deep penetrating dermatofibroma versus dermatofibrosarcoma protuberans. *Am J Surg Pathol.* 1994;18:677–686.

79. Agarwal A, Gopinath A, Tetzlaff MT, Prieto VG. Phosphohistone-H3 and Ki67: useful markers in differentiating dermatofibroma from dermatofibrosarcoma protuberans and atypical fibrohistiocytic lesions. *Am J Dermatopathol.* 2017;39:504–507.

80. Goldblum JR, Tuthill RJ. CD34 and factor XIIIa immunoreactivity in dermatofibrosarcoma protuberans and dermatofibroma. *Am J Dermatopathol.* 1997;19:147–153.

81. Horenstein MG, Prieto VG, Nuckols JD, Burchette JL, Shea CR. Indeterminate fibrohistiocytic lesions of the skin. Is there a spectrum between dermatofibroma and dermatofibrosarcoma protuberans? *Am J Surg Pathol.* 2000;24:996–1003.

82. Franchi A, Santucci M. Tenascin expression in cutaneous fibrohistiocytic tumors. Immunohistochemical investigation of 24 cases. *Am J Dermatopathol.* 1996;18:454–459.

83. Kahn HJ, Fekete E, From L. Tenascin differentiates dermatofibromas from dermatofibrosarcoma protuberans: comparison with CD34 and factor XIIIa. *Hum Pathol.* 2001;32:50–56.

84. Thway K, Fisher C. Angiomatoid fibrous histiocytoma: the current status of pathology and genetics. *Arch Pathol Lab Med.* 2015;139:674–682.

85. Costa MJ, Weiss SW. Angiomatoid malignant fibrous histiocytoma: a follow-up study of 108 cases with evaluation of possible histologic predictors of outcome. *Am J Surg Pathol.* 1990;14:1126–1132.

86. Doyle LA, Fletcher CD. Metastasizing "benign" cutaneous fibrous histiocytoma: a clinicopathologic analysis of 16 cases. *Am J Surg Pathol.* 2013;37:484–495.

87. Lodewick E, Avermaete A, Blom WA, Lelie B, Block R, Keuppens M. Fatal case of metastatic cellular fibrous histiocytoma: case report and review of literature. *Am J Dermatopathol.* 2014;36:e156–162.

88. Tseng YT, Chen KL, Tsai TF. Metastatic cellular fibrous histiocytoma. *Dermatologica sinica.* 2016;34:102–105.

89. Santos-Briz A, García-Gavín J, Pastushenko I, Sayagués JM, Rodríguez-Peralto JL, Requena L. Perineural invasion as a clue to malignant behavior in a dermatofibroma. *Am J Dermatopathol.* 2020;42:533–538.

90. Charli-Joseph Y, Saggini A, Doyle LA, et al. DNA copy number changes in tumors within the spectrum of cellular, atypical, and metastasizing fibrous histiocytoma. *J Am Acad Dermatol.* 2014;71:256–63.

91. Rodríguez-Jurado R, Palacios C, Durán-McKinster C, et al. Medallion-like dermal dendrocyte hamartoma: a new clinically and histopathologically distinct lesion. *J Am Acad Dermatol.* 2004;51:359–363.

92. Kutzner H, Mentzel T, Palmedo G, et al. Plaque-like CD34-positive dermal fibroma ("medallion-like dermal dendrocyte hamartoma"): clinicopathologic, immunohistochemical, and molecular analysis of 5 cases emphasizing its distinction from superficial, plaque-like dermatofibrosarcoma protuberans. *Am J Surg Pathol.* 2010;34:190–201.

93. Marque M, Bessis D, Pedeutour F, Viseux V, Guillot B, Fraitag-Spinner S. Medallion-like dermal dendrocyte hamartoma: the main diagnostic pitfall is congenital atrophic dermatofibrosarcoma. *Br J Dermatol.* 2009;160:190–193.

94. Min HJ, Kim JH, Kim JW, et al. Multiple giant cell tumor of tendon sheath involving both flexor and extensor tendons in a single digit: a case report and review of the literatures. *J Hand Surg Asian Pac.* 2018;23:282–285.

95. King DT, Millman AJ, Gurevitch AW. Giant cell tumor of the tendon sheath involving the skin. *Arch Dermatol.* 1978;114:944–946.

96. Uriburu IJ, Levy VD. Intraosseous growth of giant cell tumors of the tendon sheath (localized nodular tenosynovitis) of the digits: report of 15 cases. *J Hand Surg.* 1998;23:732–736.

97. de St. Aubain Somerhaussen N, Dal Cin P. Giant cell tumour of tendon sheath. In: Fletcher CDM, Unni KK, Mertens F, eds. *World Health Organization Classification of Tumours. Pathology and Genetics of Tumours of Soft Tissue and Bone.* IARC Press; 2002:110–111.

98. Di Grazia S, Succi G, Fragetta F, Perrotta RE. Giant cell tumor of tendon sheath: study of 64 cases and review of literature. *G Chir.* 2013;34:149–52.

99. Reilly KE, Stern PJ, Dale JA. Recurrent giant cell tumors of the tendon sheath. *J Hand Surg.* 1999;24:1298–1302.

100. Vogrincic GS, O'Connell JX, Gilks CB. Giant cell tumor of tendon sheath is a polyclonal cellular proliferation. *Hum Pathol.* 1997;28:815–819.

101. Nakayama S, Nishio J, Nakatani K, Nabeshima K, Yamamoto T. Giant cell tumor of tendon sheath with a t(1;1)(p13;p34) chromosomal translocation. *Anticancer Res.* 2020;40:4373–4377.

102. Ushijima M, Hashimoto H, Tsuneyoshi M. Giant cell tumor of the tendon sheath (nodular tenosynovitis). *Cancer.* 1986;57:875–884.

103. Carstens P. Giant cell tumors of tendon sheath. *Arch Pathol.* 1978;102:99–103.

104. Rao AS, Vigorita VJ. Pigmented villonodular synovitis (giant cell tumor of the tendon sheath and synovial membrane): a review of 81 cases. *J Bone Joint Surg.* 1984;66a:76.

105. Weiss SW, Goldblum JR. Giant cell tumor of tendon sheath. In: *Enzinger and Weiss's Soft Tissue Tumors.* 5th ed. Mosby-Harcourt; 2008:770–777.

106. Alguacil-Garcia A, Unni KK, Goellner JR. Giant cell tumor of tendon sheath and pigmented villonodular synovitis: an ultrastructural study. *Am J Clin Pathol.* 1978;69:6–17.

107. Wood GS, Beckstead JH, Medeiros LJ, Kempson RL, Warnke RA. The cells of giant cell tumor of tendon sheath resemble osteoclasts. *Am J Surg Pathol.* 1988;12:444–452.

108. Medeiros LJ, Beckstead JH, Rosenberg AE, Warnke R, Wood G. Giant cells and mononuclear cells of giant cell tumor of bone resemble histiocytes. *Appl Immunohistochem.* 1993;1:115–122.

109. O'Connell JX, Fanburg JC, Rosenberg AE. Giant cell tumor of tendon sheath and pigmented villonodular synovitis: immunophenotype suggests a synovial cell origin. *Hum Pathol.* 1995;26:771–775.

110. Hao X, Billings SD, Wu F, et al. Dermatofibrosarcoma protuberans: update on the diagnosis and treatment. *J Clin Med.* 2020; 9:1752.

111. Peters CW, Hanke CW, Pasarell HA, Bennett JE. Dermatofibrosarcoma protuberans of the face. *J Dermatol Surg Oncol.* 1982;8:823–826.

112. Gutierrez G, Ospina JE, De Baez NE, de Escorcia EK, Gutiérrez R. Dermatofibrosarcoma protuberans. *Int J Dermatol.* 1984;23:396–401.

113. McKee PH, Fletcher CDM. Dermatofibrosarcoma protuberans presenting in infancy and childhood. *J Cutan Pathol.* 1991; 18:241–246.

114. Martin L, Combemale P, Dupin M, et al. The atrophic variant of dermatofibrosarcoma protuberans in childhood: a report of six cases. *Br J Dermatol.* 1998;139:719–725.

115. Checketts SR, Hamilton TK, Baughman RD. Congenital and childhood dermatofibrosarcoma protuberans: a case report and review of the literature. *J Am Acad Dermatol.* 2000;42:907–913.

116. Kahn LB, Saxe N, Gordon W. Dermatofibrosarcoma protuberans with lymph node and pulmonary metastases. *Arch Dermatol.* 1978;114:599–601.

117. Taylor HB, Helwig EB. Dermatofibrosarcoma protuberans. *Cancer.* 1961;15:717–725.

118. Fletcher CDM, Evans BJ, MacArtney JC, Smith N, Wilson Jones E, McKee PH. Dermatofibrosarcoma protuberans: a clinicopathological and immunohistochemical study with a review of the literature. *Histopathology.* 1985;9:921–938.

119. Bednar F. Storiform neurofibromas of the skin, pigmented and non-pigmented. *Cancer.* 1957;10:368–376.

120. Dupree WB, Langloss JM, Weiss SW. Pigmented dermatofibrosarcoma protuberans (Bednar tumor). A pathologic, ultrastructural, and immunohistochemical study. *Am J Surg Pathol.* 1985;9:630–639.

121. Fletcher CDM, Theaker JM, Flanagan A, Krausz T. Pigmented dermatofibrosarcoma protuberans (Bednar tumour); melanocytic colonization or neuroectodermal differentiation? A clinicopathological and immunohistochemical study. *Histopathology.* 1988;13:631–643.

122. Maire G, Fraitag S, Galmiche L, et al. Clinical, histologic, and molecular study of 9 cases of congenital dermatofibrosarcoma protuberans. *Arch Dermatol.* 2007;143:203–210.

123. Connelly JH, Evans HL. Dermatofibrosarcoma protuberans: a clinicopathologic review with emphasis on fibrosarcomatous areas. *Am J Surg Pathol.* 1992;16:921–925.

124. Diaz-Cascajo C, Weyers W, Borrego L, Iñarrea JB, Borghi S. Dermatofibrosarcoma protuberans with fibrosarcomatous areas: a clinico-pathologic and immunohistochemic study in four cases. *Am J Dermatopathol.* 1997;19:562–567.

125. Goldblum JR, Reith JD, Weiss SW. Sarcomas arising in dermatofibrosarcoma protuberans. A reappraisal of biologic behavior in eighteen cases treated by wide local excision with extended clinical follow up. *Am J Surg Pathol.* 2000;24:1125–1130.

126. Liang CA, Jambusaria-Pahlajani A, Karia PS, et al. A systematic review of outcome data for dermatofibrosarcoma protuberans with and without fibrosarcomatous change. *J Am Acad Dermatol.* 2014;71:781–786.

127. Abbott JJ, Oliveira AM, Nascimento AG. The prognostic significance of fibrosarcomatous transformation in dermatofibrosarcoma protuberans. *Am J Surg Pathol.* 2006;30:436–443.

128. Shmookler BM, Enzinger FM, Weiss SW. Giant cell fibroblastoma: a juvenile form of dermatofibrosarcoma protuberans. *Cancer.* 1989;64:2154–2161.

129. Beham A, Fletcher DC. Dermatofibrosarcoma protuberans with areas resembling giant cell fibroblastoma: report of two cases. *Histopathology.* 1990;17:165–167.

130. Alguacil-Garcia A. Giant cell fibroblastoma recurring as dermatofibrosarcoma protuberans. *Am J Surg Pathol.* 1991;15:798–801.

131. Allen PW, Zwi J. Giant cell fibroblastoma transforming into dermatofibrosarcoma protuberans [Letter]. *Am J Surg Pathol.* 1992;15:1127–1128.

132. Coyne J, Kaftan SM, Craig RD. Dermatofibrosarcoma protuberans recurring as a giant cell fibroblastoma. *Histopathology.* 1992;21:184–187.

133. Michael M, Zamecnik M. Giant cell fibroblastoma with a dermatofibrosarcoma protuberans component. *Am J Dermatopathol.* 1992;14:549–552.

134. Alguacil-Garcia A, Unni KH, Goellner JR. Histogenesis of dermatofibrosarcoma protuberans: an ultrastructural study. *Am J Clin Pathol.* 1978;69:427–434.

135. Zina AM, Bundino S. Dermatofibrosarcoma protuberans: an ultrastructural study of five cases. *J Cutan Pathol.* 1979;6:265–271.

136. Hashimoto K, Brownstein MH, Jacobiec FA. Dermatofibrosarcoma protuberans. *Arch Dermatol.* 1974;110:874–885.

137. Zemecnik M, Michal M, Chlumska A. Composite dermatofibrosarcoma protuberans–giant cell fibroblastoma recurring as Bednar tumor–giant cell fibroblastoma with mucoid lakes and with amputation neuroma. *Cesk Patol.* 2002;38:173–177.

138. Lautier R, Wolff HH, Jones RE. An immunohistochemical study of dermatofibrosarcoma protuberans supports its fibroblastic character and contradicts neuroectodermal or histiocytic components. *Am J Dermatopathol.* 1990;2:25–30.

139. Ma CK, Zarbo RJ, Gown AM. Immunohistochemical characterization of atypical fibroxanthoma and dermatofibrosarcoma protuberans. *Am J Clin Pathol.* 1992;97:478–483.

140. Calonje E, Fletcher CDM. Myoid differentiation in dermatofibrosarcoma protuberans and its fibrosarcomatous variant: clinicopathologic analysis of 5 cases. *J Cutan Pathol.* 1996;23:30–36.

141. Labonte S, Hanna W, Bandarchi-Chamkhaleh B. A study of CD117 expression in dermatofibrosarcoma protuberans and cellular dermatofibroma. *J Cutan Pathol.* 2007;34:857–860.

142. Dal Cin P, Sciot R, De Wever J, et al. Cytogenetic and immunohistochemical evidence that giant cell fibroblastoma is related to dermatofibrosarcoma protuberans. *Genes Chromosomes Cancer.* 1996;15:73–75.

143. McArthur GA. Molecular targeting of dermatofibrosarcoma protuberans: a new approach to a surgical disease. *J Natl Compr Canc Netw.* 2007;5:557–562.

144. Llombart B, Serra-Guillén C, Monteagudo C, López Guerrero JA, Sanmartín O. Dermatofibrosarcoma protuberans: a comprehensive review and update on diagnosis and management. *Semin Diagn Pathol.* 2013;30:13–28.

145. Navarrete-Dechent C, Mori S, Barker CA, Dickson MA, Nehal KS. Imatinib treatment for locally advanced or metastatic dermatofibrosarcoma protuberans: a systematic review. *JAMA Dermatol.* 2019;155:361–369.

146. Weiss SW, Nickoloff BJ. CD-34 is expressed by a distinctive cell population in peripheral nerve, nerve sheath tumors, and related lesions. *Am J Surg Pathol.* 1993;17:1039–1045.

147. Aiba S, Tabata N, Ishil H, Ootani H, Tagami H. Dermatofibrosarcoma protuberans is a unique fibrohistiocytic tumor expressing CD34. *Br J Dermatol.* 1992;127:79–84.

148. Altman DA, Nickoloff BJ, Fivenson DP. Differential expression of factor XIIIa and CD34 in cutaneous mesenchymal tumors. *J Cutan Pathol.* 1993;20:154–158.

149. Calikoglu E, Augsburger E, Chavaz P, Saurat JH, Kaya G. CD44 and hyaluronate in the differential diagnosis of dermatofibroma and dermatofibroma protuberans. *J Cutan Pathol.* 2003;30:185–189.

150. West RB, Harvell J, Linn SC, et al. Apo D in soft tissue tumors: a novel marker for dermatofibrosarcoma protuberans. *Am J Surg Pathol.* 2004;28:1063–1069.

151. Bandarchi B, Ma L, Marginean C, Hafezi S, Zubovits J, Rasty G. D2-40, a novel immunohistochemical marker in differentiating dermatofibroma from dermatofibrosarcoma protuberans. *Mod Pathol.* 2010;23:434–438.

152. Piombino E, Broggi G, Barbareschi M, et al. Wilms' tumor 1 (WT1): immunomarker of dermatofibrosarcoma protuberans-an immunohistochemical study on a series of 114 cases of bland-looking mesenchymal spindle cell lesions of the dermis/subcutaneous tissues. *Cancers (Basel).* 2021;13:252.

153. Mullen JT. Dermatofibrosarcoma protuberans: wide local excision versus mohs micrographic surgery. *Surg Oncol Clin N Am.* 2016;25:827–839.

154. Loghdey MS, Varma S, Rajpara SM, Al-Rawi H, Perks G, Perkins W. Mohs micrographic surgery for dermatofibrosarcoma protuberans (DFSP): a single-centre series of 76 patients treated by frozen-section Mohs micrographic surgery with a review of the literature. *J Plast Reconstr Aesthet Surg.* 2014;67:1315–1321.

155. Jing C, Zhang H, Zhang X, Yu S. Dermatofibrosarcoma protuberans: a clinicopathologic and therapeutic analysis of 254 cases at a single institution. *Dermatol Surg.* 2021;47:e26–e30.

156. Jha P, Moosavi C, Fanburg-Smith JC. Giant cell fibroblastoma: an update and addition of 86 new cases from the Armed Forces Institute of Pathology, in honor of Dr. Franz M. Enzinger. *Ann Diagn Pathol.* 2007;11:81–88.

157. Dymock RB, Allen PW, Stirling JW, Gilbert EF, Thornbery JM. Giant cell fibroblastoma: a distinctive, recurrent tumor of childhood. *Am J Surg Pathol.* 1987;11:263–272.

158. Weiss SW, Goldblum JR. Giant cell fibroblastoma. In: *Enzinger and Weiss's Soft Tissue Tumors.* 5th ed. Mosby-Harcourt; 2008:386–390.

159. Harvell JD, Kilpatrick SE, White WL. Histogenetic relations between giant cell fibroblastoma and dermatofibrosarcoma protuberans. CD34 staining showing the spectrum and a simulator. *Am J Dermatopathol*. 1998;20:339–345.

160. Terrier-Lacombe MJ, Guillou L, Maire G, et al. Dermatofibrosarcoma protuberans, giant cell fibroblastoma, and hybrid lesions in children: clinicopathological comparative analysis of 28 cases with molecular data. *Am J Surg Pathol*. 2003;27:27–39.

161. Enzinger FM, Zhang R. Plexiform fibrohistiocytic tumor presenting in children and young adults. An analysis of 65 cases. *Am J Surg Pathol*. 1988;12:818–826.

162. Leclerc S, Hamel-Teillac D, Oger P, Brousse N, Fraitag S. Plexiform fibrohistiocytic tumor: three unusual cases occurring in infancy. *J Cutan Pathol*. 2005;32(8):572–576.

163. Remstein ED, Arndt CAS, Nascimento AG. Plexiform fibrohistiocytic tumor: clinicopathologic analysis of 22 cases. *Am J Surg Pathol*. 1999;23:662–670.

164. Valiga A, Neidig L, Cusack CA, et al. Plexiform fibrohistiocytic tumor on the chest of a 5-year-old child and review of the literature. *Pediatr Dermatol*. 2019;36:490–496.

165. Salamanca J, Rodríguez-Peralto JL, García de la Torre JP, López-Ríos F. Plexiform fibrohistiocytic tumor without multinucleated giant cells. *Am J Dermatopathol*. 2002;24:399–401.

166. Fisher C. Atypical plexiform fibrohistiocytic tumor. *Histopathology*. 1997;30:271–273.

167. Zelger B, Weinlich G, Steiner H, Zelger BG, Egarter-Vigl E. Dermal and subcutaneous variants of plexiform fibrohistiocytic tumor. *Am J Surg Pathol*. 1997;21:235–241.

168. Hollowood K, Holley MP, Fletcher CDM. Plexiform fibrohistiocytic tumor: clinicopathological, immunohistochemical and ultrastructural analysis in favour of a myofibroblastic lesion. *Histopathology*. 1991;19:503–513.

169. Leclerc-Mercier S, Pedeutour F, Fabas T, Glorion C, Brousse N, Fraitag S. Plexiform fibrohistiocytic tumor with molecular and cytogenetic analysis. *Pediatr Dermatol*. 2011;28:26–29.

170. Jaffer S, Ambrosini-Spaltro A, Mancini AM, Eusebi V, Rosai J. Neurothekeoma and plexiform fibrohistiocytic tumor: mere histologic resemblance or histogenetic relationship? *Am J Surg Pathol*. 2009;33:905–913.

171. Fox MD, Billings SD, Gleason BC, et al. Expression of MiTF may be helpful in differentiating cellular neurothekeoma from plexiform fibrohistiocytic tumor (histiocytoid predominant) in a partial biopsy specimen. *Am J Dermatopathol*. 2012;34:157–160.

172. Moosavi C, Jha P, Fanburg-Smith JC. An update on plexiform fibrohistiocytic tumor and addition of 66 new cases from the Armed Forces Institute of Pathology, in honor of Franz M. Enzinger, MD. *Ann Diagn Pathol*. 2007;11:313–319.

173. Fretzin DFJ, Helwig EB. Atypical fibroxanthoma of the skin. *Cancer*. 1973;31:1541–1552.

174. Beer TW, Drury P, Heenan PJ. Atypical fibroxanthoma: a histological and immunohistochemical review of 171 Cases. *Am J Dermatopathol*. 2010;32:533–540.

175. Luzar B, Calonje E. Morphological and immunohistochemical characteristics of atypical fibroxanthoma with a special emphasis on potential diagnostic pitfalls: a review. *J Cutan Pathol*. 2010;37:301–319.

176. Weiss SW, Enzinger FM. Malignant fibrous histiocytoma: an analysis of 200 cases. *Cancer*. 1978;41:2250–2266.

177. Mirza B, Weedon D. Atypical fibroxanthoma: a clinicopathological study of 89 cases. *Australas J Dermatol*. 2005;46:235–238.

178. Requena L, Sangueza OP, Sánchez Yus E, Furio V. Clear-cell atypical fibroxanthoma: an uncommon histopathologic variant of atypical fibroxanthoma. *J Cutan Pathol*. 1997;24:176–182.

179. Crowson AN, Carlson-Sweet K, MacInnis C, et al. Clear cell atypical fibroxanthoma: a clinicopathologic study. *J Cutan Pathol*. 2002;29:374–381.

180. Diaz-Cascajo C, Borghi S, Bonczkowitz M. Pigmented atypical fibroxanthoma. *Histopathology*. 1998;33:537–541.

181. Orosz Z. Atypical fibroxanthoma with granular cells. *Histopathology*. 1998;33:88–89.

182. Bruecks AK, Medlicott SA, Trotter MJ. Atypical fibroxanthoma with prominent sclerosis. *J Cutan Pathol*. 2003;30:336–339.

183. Offman S, Pasternak S, Walsh N. Keloidal and other collagen patterns in atypical fibroxanthomas. *Am J Dermatopathol*. 2010;32:326–332.

184. Alguacil-Garcia A, Unni KK, Goellner JR, Winkelmann RK. Atypical fibroxanthoma of the skin: an ultrastructural study of two cases. *Cancer*. 1977;40:1471–1480.

185. Barr RJ, Wuerker RB, Graham JH. Ultrastructure of atypical fibroxanthoma. *Cancer*. 1977;40:736–743.

186. Longacre TA, Smoller BR, Rouse RU. Atypical fibroxanthoma: multiple immunohistologic profiles. *Am J Surg Pathol*. 1993;17:1199–1209.

187. Sakamoto A, Oda Y, Yamamoto H, et al. Calponin and h-caldesmon expression in atypical fibroxanthoma and superficial leiomyosarcoma. *Virchows Arch*. 2002;440:404–409.

188. Lai K, Harwood CA, Purdie KJ, et al. Genomic analysis of atypical fibroxanthoma. *PLoS One*. 2017;12:e0188272.

189. Helbig D, Quaas A, Mauch C, et al. Copy number variations in atypical fibroxanthomas and pleomorphic dermal sarcomas. *Oncotarget*. 2017;8:109457–109467.

190. Griewank KG, Wiesner T, Murali R, et al. Atypical fibroxanthoma and pleomorphic dermal sarcoma harbor frequent NOTCH1/2 and FAT1 mutations and similar DNA copy number alteration profiles. *Mod Pathol*. 2018;31:418–428.

191. Thum C, Hollowood K, Birch J, Goodlad JR, Brenn T. Aberrant Melan-A expression in atypical fibroxanthoma and undifferentiated pleomorphic sarcoma of the skin. *J Cutan Pathol*. 2011 Dec;38(12):954–60.

192. Hultgren TL, DiMaio DJ. Immunohistochemical staining of CD10 in atypical fibroxanthomas. *J Cutan Pathol*. 2007;34:415–419.

193. Beer TW. CD163 is not a sensitive marker to identify atypical fibroxanthomas. *J Cutan Pathol*. 2012;39:29–32.

194. Beer TW, Haig D. CD117 is not a useful marker in atypical fibroxanthoma. *Am J Dermatopathol*. 2009;31:649–652.

195. Hartel PH, Jackson J, Ducatman BS, Zhang P. CD99 immunoreactivity in atypical fibroxanthoma and pleomorphic malignant fibrous histiocytoma: a useful diagnostic marker. *J Cutan Pathol*. 2006;33(suppl 2):24–28.

196. Martinez-Ciarpaglini C, Agustí J, Alvarez E, et al. h-caldesmon immunoreactivity in atypical fibroxanthoma: implications for the differential diagnosis. *Pathology*. 2018;50:358–361.

197. Miller K, Goodlad JR, Brenn T. Pleomorphic dermal sarcoma: adverse histologic features predict aggressive behavior and allow distinction from atypical fibroxanthoma. *Am J Surg Pathol*. 2012;36:1317–1326.

198. Tardío JC, Pinedo F, Aramburu JA, et al. Pleomorphic dermal sarcoma: a more aggressive neoplasm than previously estimated. *J Cutan Pathol*. 2016;43:101–112.

199. Winchester D, Lehman J, Tello T, et al. Undifferentiated pleomorphic sarcoma: factors predictive of adverse outcomes. *J Am Acad Dermatol*. 2018;79:853–859.

200. Ibanez MA, Rismiller K, Knackstedt T. Prognostic factors, treatment, and survival in cutaneous pleomorphic sarcoma. *J Am Acad Dermatol*. 2020;83:388–396.

201. Fritchie K, Fisher C, Coindre JM, Lazar AJ, Rubin BP. A brief history and contemporary re-assessment of malignant fibrous histiocytoma: "fact or fancy." *Diagn Histopathol*. 2011;17:340–347.

202. Hollowood K, Fletcher CDM. Malignant fibrous histiocytoma: morphologic pattern or pathologic entity? *Semin Diagn Pathol*. 1995;12:210–220.

203. Fletcher CDM. Pleomorphic malignant fibrous histiocytoma: fact or fiction? A critical reappraisal based on 159 tumors diagnosed as pleomorphic sarcoma. *Am J Surg Pathol.* 1992;16:213–228.

204. Weiss SW, Goldblum JR. Malignant fibrous histiocytoma. In: *Enzinger and Weiss's Soft Tissue Tumors.* 5th ed. Mosby-Harcourt; 2008:406–425.

205. Nakayama R, Nemoto T, Takahashi H, et al. Gene expression analysis of soft tissue sarcomas: characterization and reclassification of malignant fibrous histiocytoma. *Mod Pathol.* 2007;20:749–759.

206. Al-Agha OM, Igbokwe AA. Malignant fibrous histiocytoma: between the past and the present. *Arch Pathol Lab Med.* 2008;132:1030–1035.

207. Fujimura T, Okuyama R, Terui T, et al. Myxofibrosarcoma (myxoid malignant fibrous histiocytoma) showing cutaneous presentation: report of two cases. *J Cutan Pathol.* 2005;32:512–515.

208. Mansoor A, White CR Jr. Myxofibrosarcoma presenting in the skin: clinicopathological features and differential diagnosis with cutaneous myxoid neoplasms. *Am J Dermatopathol.* 2003;25:281–286.

209. Larramendy ML, Gentile M, Soloneski S, Knuutila S, Böhling T. Does comparative genomic hybridization reveal distinct differences in DNA copy number sequence patterns between leiomyosarcoma and malignant fibrous histiocytoma? *Cancer Genet Cytogenet.* 2008;187:1–11.

210. Gibault L, Pérot G, Chibon F, et al. New insights in sarcoma oncogenesis: a comprehensive analysis of a large series of 160 soft tissue sarcomas with complex genomics. *J Pathol.* 2011;223:64–71.

211. Fletcher CDM, van den Berg E, Molenaar WM. Pleomorphic malignant fibrous histiocytoma/undifferentiated high grade pleomorphic sarcoma. In: Fletcher CDM, Unni KK, Mertens F, eds. *World Health Organization Classification of Tumours. Pathology and Genetics of Tumours of Soft Tissue and Bone.* IARC Press; 2002:120–122.

212. Guccion JG, Enzinger FM. Malignant giant cell tumor of soft parts: an analysis of 32 cases. *Cancer.* 1972;29:1518–1529.

213. Fletcher CDM, van den Berg E, Molenaar WM. Myxoid malignant fibrous histiocytoma/undifferentiated high grade pleomorphic sarcoma. In: Fletcher CDM, Unni KK, Mertens F, eds. *World Health Organization Classification of Tumours. Pathology and Genetics of Tumours of Soft Tissue and Bone.* IARC Press; 2002:120–126.

214. Folpe AL, Morris RJ, Weiss SW. Soft tissue giant cell tumor of low malignant potential: a proposal for the reclassification of malignant giant cell tumor of soft parts. *Mod Pathol.* 1999;12:894–902.

215. Enzinger FM. Angiomatoid malignant fibrous histiocytoma: a distinct fibrohistiocytic tumor of children and young adults simulating a vascular neoplasm. *Cancer.* 1979;44:2147–2157.

216. Fanburg-Smith JC, Miettinen M. Angiomatoid "malignant" fibrous histiocytoma: a clinicopathologic study of 158 cases and further exploration of the myoid phenotype. *Hum Pathol.* 1999;30:1336–1343.

217. Al-Attar A, Mess S, Thomassen JM, Kauffman CL, Davison SP. Keloid pathogenesis and treatment. *Plast Reconstr Surg.* 2006;117:286–300.

218. Burd A, Huang L. Hypertrophic response and keloid diathesis: two very different forms of scar. *Plast Reconstr Surg.* 2005;116:150e–157e.

219. Atiyeh BS, Costagliola M, Hayek SN. Keloid or hypertrophic scar: the controversy: review of the literature. *Ann Plast Surg.* 2005;54:676–680.

220. Murray JC, Pollack SV, Pinnel SR. Keloids: a review. *J Am Acad Dermatol.* 1981;4:461–470.

221. Beer TW, Baldwin HC, Goddard JR, Gallagher PJ, Wright DH. Angiogenesis in pathological surgical scars. *Hum Pathol.* 1998;29:1273–1278.

222. Linares HA, Larson DL. Early differential diagnosis between hypertrophic and nonhypertrophic healing. *J Invest Dermatol.* 1974;62:514–516.

223. Goto K, Ishikawa MI, Aizawa D, Muramatsu K, Naka M, Sugino T. Nuclear B-catenin immunoexpression in scars *J Cutan Pathol.* 2021;48:18–23.

224. Shaffer JJ, Taylor SC, Cook-Boldin F. Keloidal scars: a review with a critical look at therapeutic options. *J Am Acad Dermatol.* 2002;46:S63–S97.

225. Wolfram D, Tzankov A, Pülzl P, Piza-Katzer H. Hypertrophic scars and keloids—a review of their pathophysiology, risk factors, and therapeutic management. *Dermatol Surg.* 2009;35:171–181.

226. Mentzel T, Kutzner H. Dermatomyofibroma: clinicopathologic and immunohistochemical analysis of 56 cases and reappraisal of a rare and distinct cutaneous neoplasm. *Am J Dermatopathol.* 2009;31:44–49.

227. Ma JE, Wieland CN, Tollefson MM. Dermatomyofibromas arising in children: report of two new cases and review of the literature. *Pediatr Dermatol.* 2017;34:347–351.

228. Kamino H, Reddy VB, Gero M, Greco MA. Dermatomyofibroma. A benign cutaneous, plaque-like proliferation of fibroblasts and myofibroblasts in young adults. *J Cutan Pathol.* 1992;19:85–93.

229. Hugel H. Plaque-like dermal fibromatosis/dermatomyofibroma. *J Cutan Pathol.* 1993;20:94.

230. Mortimore RJ, Whitehead KJ. Dermatomyofibroma: a report of two cases, one occurring in a child. *Australas J Dermatol.* 2001;42:22–25.

231. Colome MI, Sanchez RL. Dermatomyofibroma: report of two cases. *J Cutan Pathol.* 1994;21:371–376.

232. Mentzel T, Kutzner H. Haemorrhagic dermatomyofibroma (plaque-like dermal fibromatosis): clinicopathological and immunohistochemical analysis of three cases resembling plaque-stage Kaposi's sarcoma. *Histopathology.* 2003;42(6):594–598.

233. Mentzel T, Calonje E, Fletcher CDM. Dermatomyofibroma: additional observations on a distinctive cutaneous myofibroblastic tumour with emphases on differential diagnosis. *Br J Dermatol.* 1993;129:69–73.

234. Ng WK, Cheung MF, Ma L. Dermatomyofibroma: further support of its myofibroblastic nature by electron microscopy. *Histopathology.* 1996;29:181–183.

235. Field LM. A giant pendulous fibrolipoma. *J Dermatol Surg Oncol.* 1982;8:54–55.

236. Chobanian SJ, Van Ness MM, Winters C, Cattau EL Jr. Skin tags as a marker for adenomatous polyps of the colon. *Ann Intern Med.* 1985;103:892–893.

237. Beitler M, Eng A, Kilgour M, Lebwohl M. Association between acrochordons and colonic polyps. *J Am Acad Dermatol.* 1986;14:1042–1049.

238. Chobanian SJ, Van Ness MM, Winters C. Skin tags as a screening marker for colonic neoplasia. *Gastrointest Endosc.* 1986;32:162.

239. Chobanian SJ. Skin tags and colonic polyps: a gastroenterologist's perspective. *J Am Acad Dermatol.* 1987;16:407–409.

240. Margolis J, Margolis LS. Skin tags: a frequent sign of diabetes mellitus. *N Engl J Med.* 1976;294:1184.

241. Kahana M, Grossman E, Feinstein A, Ronnen M, Cohen M, Millet MS. Skin tags: a cutaneous marker for diabetes mellitus. *Acta Dermatol Venereol (Stockholm)* 1987;67:175–177.

242. Agarwal JK, Nigam PK. Acrochordon: a cutaneous sign of carbohydrate intolerance. *Australas J Dermatol.* 1987;28:132–133.

243. Lawrence JH, Tobias CA, Linfoot JA, et al. Successful treatment of acromegaly: metabolic and clinical studies in 145 patients. *J Clin Endocrinol Metab.* 1970;31:180–198.

244. Dalton AD, Coghill SB. No association between skin tags and colorectal adenomas. *Lancet.* 1985;1:1332–1333.

245. Luk GD. Colonic polyps and acrochordons (skin tags) do not correlate in familial colonic polyposis kindreds. *Ann Intern Med.* 1986;104:209–210.

246. Graffeo M, Cesari P, Buffoli F, Mazzola A, Salmi A, Paterlini A. Skin tags: markers for colonic polyps? *J Am Acad Dermatol.* 1989;21:1029–1030.

247. Da La Torre C, Ocampo C, Doval I, Losada A, Cruces MJ. Acrochordons are not a component of Birt-Hogg-Dube syndrome. Does this syndrome exist? Case reports and review of the literature. *Am J Dermatopathol.* 1999;21:369–374.

248. Schulz T, Ebschner U, Hartschuh W. Localised Birt-Hogg-Dube syndrome with localised perivascular fibromas. *Am J Dermatopathol.* 2001;23:149–153.

249. Akhtar AJ, Zhuo J. Non-association between acrochordons and colonic polyps in a minority population. *J Natl Med Assoc.* 2003;95:746–749.

250. Stegmaier OC. Natural regression of the melanocytic nevus. *J Invest Dermatol.* 1959;32:413–419.

251. Huntley AC. Eruptive lipofibromata. *Arch Dermatol.* 1983;119:612–614.

252. Agir H, Sen C, Cek D. Squamous cell carcinoma arising from a fibroepithelial polyp. *Ann Plast Surg.* 2005;55:687–688.

253. Kamino H, Lee JYY, Berke A. Pleomorphic fibroma of the skin: a benign neoplasm with cytologic atypia. A clinicopathologic study of eight cases. *Am J Surg Pathol.* 1989;13:107–113.

254. Hsieh YJ, Lin YC, Wu YH, Su HY, Billings SD, Hood AF. Subungual pleomorphic fibroma. *J Cutan Pathol.* 2003;30:569–571.

255. Hassanein A, Telang G, Benedetto E, Spielvogel R. Subungual myxoid pleomorphic fibroma. *Am J Dermatopathol.* 1998;20:502–505.

256. Rudolph P, Schubert C, Zelger BG, Zelger B, Parwaresch R. Differential expression of CD34 and Ki-Mlp in pleomorphic fibroma and dermatofibroma with monster cells. *Am J Dermatopathol.* 1999;21:414–419.

257. Al-Zaid T, Wang WL, Lopez-Terrada D, et al. Pleomorphic fibroma and dermal atypical lipomatous tumor: are they related? *J Cutan Pathol.* 2013;40:379–384.

258. Yadav YK, Kushwaha R, Sharma U, Gupta K. Cytomorphology of pleomorphic fibroma of skin: a diagnostic enigma. *J Cytol.* 2013;30:71–73.

259. Rapini RP, Golitz LE. Sclerotic fibromas of the skin. *J Am Acad Dermatol.* 1989;20:266–271.

260. Starink TM, Meijer CJLM, Brownstein MH. The cutaneous pathology of Cowden's disease: new findings. *J Cutan Pathol.* 1985;12:83–93.

261. Alawi F, Freedman PD. Sporadic sclerotic fibroma of the oral soft tissues. *Am J Dermatopathol.* 2004;26:182–187.

262. Krivošíková L, Janega P, Babala J, Babál P. Pacinian collagenoma: a distinct form of sclerotic fibroma. *J Cutan Pathol.* 2020;47:291–294.

263. Llamas-Velasco M, Stengel B, Pérez-González YC, Mentzel T. Late-stage erythema elevatum diutinum mimicking a fibroblastic tumor: a potential pitfall. *Am J Dermatopathol.* 2018;40:442–

264. Shi KY, Vandergriff T. Late-stage nodular erythema elevatum diutinum mimicking sclerotic fibroma. *J Cutan Pathol.* 2018;45:94–96.

265. Mahmood MN, Salama ME, Chaffins M, et al. Solitary sclerotic fibroma of the skin: a possible link with pleomorphic fibroma with immunophenotypic expression for O13(CD99) and CD34. *J Cutan Pathol.* 2003;30:631–636.

266. Brito H, Pereira EM, Reis-Filho JS, Maeda SA. Giant cell collagenoma: case report and review of the literature. *J Cutan Pathol.* 2002;29:48–51.

267. Shitaba PK, Crouch EC, Fitzgibbon JF, Swanson PE, Adesokan PN, Wick MR. Cutaneous sclerotic fibroma. Immunohistochemical evidence of a fibroblastic neoplasm with ongoing type 1 collagen synthesis. *Am J Dermatopathol.* 1995;17:339–343.

268. Abdaljaleel MY, North JP. Sclerosing dermatofibrosarcoma protuberans shows significant overlap with sclerotic fibroma in both routine and immunohistochemical analysis: a potential diagnostic pitfall. *Am J Dermatopathol.* 2017;39:83–88.

269. High WA, Stewart D, Essary LR, Kageyama NP, Hoang MP, Cockerell CJ. Sclerotic fibroma–like change in various neoplastic and inflammatory skin lesions: is sclerotic fibroma a distinct entity? *J Cutan Pathol.* 2004;31:373–378.

270. Gonzalez-Vela MC, Val-Bernal JF, Martino M, González-López MA, García-Alberdi E, Hermana S. Sclerotic fibroma–like dermatofibroma: an uncommon distinctive variant of dermatofibroma. *Histol Histopathol.* 2005;20:801–806.

271. Cohen PR, Tschen JA, Abaya-Blas R, Cochran RJ. Recurrent sclerotic fibroma of the skin. *Am J Dermatopathol.* 1999;21:571–574.

272. McCalmont TH. Sclerotic fibroma: a fossil no longer. *J Cutan Pathol.* 1994;21:82–85.

273. Dal Cin P, Sciot R, De Smet L, Van den Berghe H. Translocation 2;11 in a fibroma of tendon sheath. *Histopathology.* 1998;32:433–435.

274. Sciot R, Samson I, van den Berghe H, Van Damme B, Dal Cin P. Collagenous fibroma (desmoplastic fibroblastoma): genetic link with fibroma of tendon sheath? *Mod Pathol.* 1999;12:565–568.

275. Park SY, Jin SP, Yeom B, Kim SW, Cho SY, Lee JH. Multiple fibromas of tendon sheath: unusual presentation. *Ann Dermatol.* 2011;23:S45–S47.

276. Griesser MJ, Wakely PE, Mayerson J. Intraarticular fibroma of tendon sheath. *Indian J Orthop.* 2011;45:276–279.

277. Humphreys S, McKee PH, Fletcher CDM. Fibroma of tendon sheath. *J Cutan Pathol.* 1986;13:331–338.

278. Cooper PH. Fibroma of tendon sheath. *J Am Acad Dermatol.* 1984;11:625–628.

279. Hashimoto H, Tsuneyoshi M, Daimaru Y, Ushijima M, Enjoji M. Fibroma of tendon sheath: a tumor of myofibroblasts. A clinicopathologic study of 18 cases. *Acta Pathol Jpn.* 1985;35:1099–1107.

280. Chung EB, Enzinger FM. Fibroma of tendon sheath. *Cancer.* 1979;44:1945–1954.

281. Nakayama S, Nishio J, Aoki M, Nabeshima K, Yamamoto T. An update on clinicopathological, imaging and genetic features of desmoplastic fibroblastoma (collagenous fibroma). *In Vivo.* 2021;35:69–73.

282. Gong LH, Liu WF, Ding Y, Geng YH, Sun XQ, Huang XY. Diagnosis and differential diagnosis of desmoplastic fibroblastoma by clinical, radiological, and histopathological analyses. *Chin Med J (Engl).* 2018;131:32–36.

283. Miettinen M, Fetsch JF. Collagenous fibroma (desmoplastic fibroblastoma): a clinicopathologic analysis of 63 cases of a distinctive soft tissue lesion with stellate-shaped fibroblasts. *Hum Pathol.* 1998;29:676–682.

284. de Sousa SF, Caldeira PC, Grossmann Sde M, de Aguiar MC, Mesquita RA. Desmoplastic fibroblastoma (collagenous fibroma): a case identified in the buccal mucosa. *Head Neck Pathol.* 2011;5:175–179.

285. Nonaka CF, Carvalho Mde V, de Moraes M, de Medeiros AM, Freitas Rde A. Desmoplastic fibroblastoma (collagenous fibroma) of the tongue. *J Cutan Pathol.* 2010;37:911–914.

286. Alberghini M, Pasquinelli G, Zanella L, Bacchini P, Bertoni F. Desmoplastic fibroblastoma: a light and ultrastructural description of two cases. *Ultrastruct Pathol.* 2004;28:149–157.

287. Huang HY, Sung MT, Eng HL, Huang CC, Huang WT, Chen WJ. Superficial collagenous fibroma: immunohistochemical, ultrastructural, and flow cytometric study of three cases, including one pemphigus vulgaris patient with a dermal mass. *APMIS.* 2002;110:283–289.

288. Kato I, Yoshida A, Ikegami M, et al. FOSL1 immunohistochemistry clarifies the distinction between desmoplastic fibroblastoma and fibroma of tendon sheath. *Histopathology.* 2016;69:1012–1020.

289. Nishio J, Akiho S, Iwasaki H, Naito M. Translocation t(2;11) is characteristic of collagenous fibroma (desmoplastic fibroblastoma). *Cancer Genet.* 2011;204:569–571.

290. Bernal K, Nelson M, Neff JR, Nielsen SM, Bridge JA. Translocation (2;11)(q31;q12) is recurrent in collagenous fibroma (desmoplastic fibroblastoma). *Cancer Genet Cytogenet.* 2004;149:161–163.

291. Macchia G, Trombetta D, Moller E, et al. FOSL1 as a candidate target gene for 11q12 rearrangements in desmoplastic fibroblastoma. *Lab Invest.* 2012;92:735–743.

292. Papke DJ Jr, Al-Ibraheemi A, Fletcher CDM. Plexiform myofibroblastoma: clinicopathologic analysis of 36 cases of a distinctive benign tumor of soft tissue affecting mainly children and young adults. *Am J Surg Pathol.* 2020;44:1469–1478.

293. Hutter RVP, Stewart FW, Foote FW Jr. Fasciitis. *Cancer.* 1962;15:992–1003.

294. Bernstein KE, Lattes R. Nodular (pseudosarcomatous) fasciitis: a nonrecurrent lesion. *Cancer.* 1982;49:1668–1678.

295. Mehregan AH. Nodular fasciitis. *Arch Dermatol.* 1966;93:204–210.

296. Soule EH. Proliferative (nodular) fasciitis. *Arch Pathol.* 1962;73:437–444.

297. Nishio J. Updates on the cytogenetics and molecular cytogenetics of benign and intermediate soft tissue tumors. *Oncol Lett.* 2013;5:12–18.

298. De Feraudy S, Fletcher CD. Intradermal nodular fasciitis: a rare lesion analyzed in a series of 24 cases. *Am J Surg Pathol.* 2010;34:1377–1381.

299. Lai FM-M, Lam WY. Nodular fasciitis of the dermis. *J Cutan Pathol.* 1993;20:66–69.

300. Goodlad JR, Fletcher CDM. Intradermal variant of nodular "fasciitis." *Histopathology.* 1990;17:569–571.

301. Price S, Kahn LB, Saxe N. Dermal and intravascular fasciitis: unusual variants of nodular fasciitis. *Am J Dermatopathol.* 1993;15:539–543.

302. Nishi SPE, Vessels Brey N, Sanchez RL. Dermal nodular fasciitis: three case reports of the head and neck and literature review. *J Cutan Pathol.* 2006;33:378–382.

303. Thompson L, Fanburg-Smith J, Wenig B. Nodular fasciitis of the external ear region: a clinical study of 50 cases. *Ann Diagn Pathol.* 2001;5:191–198.

304. Wick MR, Mills SE, Ritter JH, Lind AC. Postoperative/posttraumatic spindle cell nodule of the skin. The dermal analogue of nodular fasciitis. *Am J Dermatopathol.* 1999;21:220–224.

305. Patchefsky AS, Enzinger FM. Intravascular fasciitis: a report of 17 cases. *Am J Surg Pathol.* 1981;5:29–36.

306. Chung EB, Enzinger FM. Proliferative fasciitis. *Cancer.* 1975;36:1450–1458.

307. Diaz-Flores L, Martin Herrera AI, Garcia Montelongo R, Gutierrez Garcia R. Proliferative fasciitis: ultrastructure and histogenesis. *J Cutan Pathol.* 1989;16:85–92.

308. Lin XY, Wang L, Zhang Y, Dai SD, Wang EH. Variable Ki67 proliferative index in 65 cases of nodular fasciitis, compared with fibrosarcoma and fibromatosis. *Diagn Pathol.* 2013;8:50.

309. Wirman JA. Nodular fasciitis: a lesion of myofibroblasts. *Cancer.* 1976;38:2378–2389.

310. Montgomery EA, Meis JM. Nodular fasciitis: its morphologic spectrum and immunohistochemical profile. *Am J Surg Pathol.* 1991;15:942–948.

311. Makise N, Mori T. Motoi T. Recurrent FOS rearrangement in proliferative fasciitis/proliferative myositis. *Mod Pathol.* 2020;34:942–950.

312. Sarangarajan R, Dehner L. Cranial and extracranial fasciitis of childhood: a clinicopathologic and immunohistochemical study. *Hum Pathol.* 1999;30:87–92.

313. Lauer DH, Enzinger FM. Cranial fasciitis of childhood. *Cancer.* 1980;45:401–406.

314. Perosio PM, Weiss SW. Ischemic fasciitis: a juxta-skeletal fibroblastic proliferation with a predilection for elderly patients. *Mod Pathol.* 1993;6:69–72.

315. Liegl B, Fletcher CD. Ischemic fasciitis: analysis of 44 cases indicating an inconsistent association with immobility or debilitation. *Am J Surg Pathol.* 2008;32:1546–1552.

316. Roh HS, Paek JO, Yu HJ, Kim JS. Solitary cutaneous myofibroma on the sole: an unusual localization. *Ann Dermatol.* 2012;24(2):220–222.

317. Sachak T, Heerema NA, Mayerson J, Payne JE, Parwani A, Iwenofu OH. Novel t(1;2)(p36.1;q23) and t(7;19)(q32;q13.3) chromosomal translocations in ischemic fasciitis: expanding the spectrum of pseudosarcomatous lesions with clonal pathogenetic link. *Diagn Pathol.* 2018;13:18.

318. Venencie PV, Bigel P, Desgruelles C, Lortat-Jacob S, Dufier JL, Saurat JH. Infantile myofibromatosis. *Br J Dermatol.* 1987;117:255–259.

319. Spraker MK, Stack C, Esterly NB. Congenital generalized fibromatosis. *J Am Acad Dermatol.* 1984;10:365–371.

320. Stanford D, Rogers M. Dermatological presentations of infantile myofibromatosis: a review of 27 cases. *Australas J Dermatol.* 2000;41:156–161.

321. Fukasawa Y, Ishikura H, Takada A, et al. Massive apoptosis in infantile myofibromatosis: a putative mechanism of tumor regression. *Am J Pathol.* 1994;144:480–485.

322. Leaute-Labreze C, Labarthe MP, Blanc JF, Sanyas P, Dosquet C, Taïeb A. Self-healing generalized infantile myofibromatosis with elevated urinary bFGF. *Pediatr Dermatol.* 2001;18:305–307.

323. Guitart J, Ritter JH, Wick MR. Solitary cutaneous myofibromas in adults: report of six cases and discussion of differential diagnosis. *J Cutan Pathol.* 1996;23:437–444.

324. Requena L, Kutzner H, Hugel H, Rütten A, Furio V. Cutaneous adult myofibroma: a vascular neoplasm. *J Cutan Pathol.* 1996;23:445–457.

325. Zand DJ, Huff D, Everman D, et al. Autosomal dominant inheritance of infantile myofibromatosis. *Am J Med Genet.* 2004;126A:261–266.

326. Dray M, McCarthy S, Palmer A, et al. Myopericytoma: a unifying term for a spectrum of tumours that show overlapping features with myofibroma. A review of 14 cases. *J Clin Pathol.* 2006;59:67–73.

327. Chung EB, Enzinger FM. Infantile myofibromatosis. *Cancer.* 1981;48:1807–1818.

328. Benjamin SP, Mercer RD, Hawk WA. Myofibroblastic contraction in spontaneous regression of multiple congenital mesenchymal hamartoma. *Cancer.* 1977;40:2343–2352.

329. Oudijk L, den Bakker MA, Hop WC, et al. Solitary, multifocal and generalized myofibromas: clinicopathological and immunohistochemical features of 114 cases. *Histopathology.* 2012;60:E1–E11.

330. Granter SR, Badizadegan K, Fletcher CDM. Myofibromatosis in adults, glomangiopericytoma and myopericytoma. A spectrum of tumors showing perivascular myoid differentiation. *Am J Surg Pathol.* 1998;22:513–525.

331. Gatibelza ME, Vazquez BR, Bereni N, Denis D, Bardot J, Degardin N. Isolated infantile myofibromatosis of the upper eyelid: uncommon localization and long-term results after surgical management. *J Pediatr Surg.* 2012;47:1457–1459.

332. Heath M, Hajar T, Korcheva V, Leitenberger J. Spontaneous involution (regression) of a solitary cutaneous myofibroma in an adult patient. *J Cutan Pathol.* 2018;45:159–161.

333. Enzinger FM. Fibrous hamartoma of infancy. *Cancer.* 1965;18:241–248.

334. Cooper PH. Fibrous proliferations of infancy and childhood. *J Cutan Pathol.* 1992;19:257–267.

335. Scott DM, Peña JR, Omura EF. Fibrous hamartoma of infancy. *J Am Acad Dermatol.* 1999;41:857–859.

336. Dickey GE, Sotelo-Avila C. Fibrous hamartoma of infancy: current review. *Pediatr Dev Pathol.* 1999;2:236–243.

337. Sotelo-Avila C, Bale PM. Subdermal fibrous hamartoma of infancy: pathology of 40 cases and differential diagnosis. *Pediatr Pathol.* 1994;14:39–52.

338. Carretto E, Dall'Igna P, Allagio R, et al. Fibrous hamartoma of infancy: an Italian multi-institutional experience. *J Am Acad Dermatol.* 2006;54:800–803.

339. Saab S, McClain C, Coffin C. Fibrous hamartoma of infancy: a clinicopathologic analysis of 60 cases. *Am J Surg Pathol.* 2014 38(3):394–401.

340. Al-Ibraheemi A, Martinez A, Weiss SW, et al. Fibrous hamartoma of infancy: a clinicopathologic study of 145 cases, including 2 with sarcomatous features. *Mod Pathol.* 2017;30:474–485.

341. Lakshminarayanan R, Konia T, Welborn J. Fibrous hamartoma of infancy: a case report with associated cytogenetic findings. *Arch Pathol Lab Med.* 2005;129:520–522.

342. Hallock GG. Juvenile hyaline fibromatosis of the hand in an adult. *J Hand Surg Am.* 1993;18:614–617.

343. Braizat O, Badran S, Hammouda A. Juvenile hyaline fibromatosis: literature review and a case treated with surgical excision and corticosteroid. *Cureus.* 2020;12(10):e10.

344. Nofal A, Sanad M, Assaf M, et al. Juvenile hyaline fibromatosis and infantile systemic hyalinosis: a unifying term and a proposed grading system. *J Am Acad Dermatol.* 2009;61:695–700.

345. Kan AE, Rogers M. Juvenile hyaline fibromatosis: an expanded clinicopathologic spectrum. *Pediatr Dermatol.* 1989;6:68–75.

346. Kitano Y, Horiki M, Aoki T, Sagami S. Two cases of juvenile hyalin fibromatosis. *Arch Dermatol.* 1972;106:877–883.

347. Mayer-Da-Silva A, Polares-Baptista A, Rodrigo FG, Teresa-Lopes M. Juvenile hyalin fibromatosis. *Arch Pathol.* 1988;112:928–931.

348. Miyake I, Tokumaru H, Sugino H, Tanno M, Yamamoto T. Juvenile hyaline fibromatosis: case report with five years' follow-up. *Am J Dermatopathol.* 1995;17:584–590.

349. Haleem A, Al-Hindi HN, Juboury MA, Husseini HA, Ajlan AA. Juvenile hyaline fibromatosis: morphologic, immunohistochemical, and ultrastructural study of three siblings. *Am J Dermatopathol.* 2002;24:218–224.

350. Winik BC, Boente MC, Asial R. Juvenile hyaline fibromatosis: ultrastructural study. *Am J Dermatopathol.* 1998;20:373–378.

351. Karacal N, Gulcelik N, Yildiz K, Mungan S, Kutlu N. Juvenile hyaline fibromatosis: a case report. *J Cutan Pathol.* 2005;32:438–440.

352. Denadai R, Bertola DR, Stelini RF, Raposo-Amaral CE. Additional thoughts about juvenile hyaline fibromatosis and infantile systemic hyalinosis. *Adv Anat Pathol.* 2012;19:191–192.

353. Santa Cruz DJ, Reiner CB. Recurrent digital fibroma of childhood. *J Cutan Pathol.* 1978;5:339–346.

354. Failla V, Wauters O, Nikkels-Tassoudji N, Carlier A, André J, Nikkels AF. Congenital infantile digital fibromatosis: a case report and review of the literature. *Rare Tumors.* 2009;1:e4.146–147.

355. Choi KC, Hashimoto K, Setoyama M, Kagetsu N, Tronnier M, Sturman S. Infantile digital fibromatosis: immunohistochemical and immunoelectron microscopic studies. *J Cutan Pathol.* 1990;17:225–232.

356. Laskin WB, Miettinen M, Fetsch JF. Infantile digital fibroma/fibromatosis: a clinicopathologic and immunohistochemical study of 69 tumors from 57 patients with long-term follow-up. *Am J Surg Pathol.* 2009;33:1–13.

357. Eyyper EH, Lee JC, Tarasen AJ, Weinberg MH, Adetayo OA. An algorithmic approach to the management of infantile digital fibromatosis: review of literature and a case report. *Eplasty.* 2018;18:167–176.

358. Saint-Paul MC, Musso S, Cardot-Leccia N. Elastofibroma of the stomach. *Pathol Res Pract.* 2003;199:637–639.

359. Shimizu S, Yasui C, Tateno M, et al. Multiple elastofibromas. *J Am Acad Dermatol.* 2004;50:126–129.

360. Montijano HC, Chismol AJ, Pons SA, Seminario EP, Fenollosa GJ. Elastofibroma dorsi. Report of five cases and review of the literature. *Acta Orthop Belg.* 2002;68:417–420.

361. Lococo F, Cesario A, Mattei F, et al. Elastofibroma dorsi: clinicopathological analysis of 71 cases. *Thorac Cardiovasc Surg.* 2013;61:215–222.

362. Deveci MA, Özbarlas HS, Erdoğan KE, Biçer ÖS, Tekin M, Özkan C. Elastofibroma dorsi: clinical evaluation of 61 cases and review of the literature. *Acta Orthop Traumatol Turc.* 2017;51:7–11.

363. Hisaoka M, Hashimoto H. Elastofibroma: clonal fibrous proliferation with predominant CD34-positive cells. *Virchows Arch.* 2006;448:195–199.

364. Kayaselcuk F, Demirhan B, Kayaselcuk U, Ozerdem OR, Tuncer I. Vimentin, smooth muscle actin, desmin, S-100 protein, p53, and estrogen receptor expression in elastofibroma and nodular fasciitis. *Ann Diagn Pathol.* 2002;6:94–99.

365. Hatano H, Morita T, Kawashima H, Ogose A, Hotta T. Symptomatic elastofibroma in young baseball pitchers: report of three cases. *J Shoulder Elbow Surg.* 2010;19:e7–e10.

366. McComb EN, Feely MG, Neff JR, Johansson SL, Nelson M, Bridge JA. Cytogenetic instability, predominantly involving chromosome 1, is characteristic of elastofibroma. *Cancer Genet Cytogenet.* 2001;126:68–72.

367. Nishio JN, Iwasaki H, Ohjimi Y, et al. Gain of Xq detected by comparative genomic hybridization in elastofibroma. *Int J Mol Med.* 2002;10:277–280.

368. Sahin M, Gul VO. Is it necessary to always resect elastofibroma dorsi? *ANZ J Surg.* doi:10.1111/ans.16. Epub ahead of print.

369. Macri A, Kwan E, Tanner LS. Cutaneous angiofibroma. In: *StatPearls [Internet].* StatPearls Publishing; 2022.

370. Sakurai A, Matsumoto K, Ikeo Y, et al. Frequency of facial angiofibromas in Japanese patients with multiple endocrine neoplasia type 1. *Endocr J.* 2000;47:569–573.

371. Graham JH, Saunders JB, Johnson WC, Helwig EB. Fibrous papule of the nose: a clinicopathological study. *J Invest Dermatol.* 1965;45:194–203.

372. Saylan T, Marks R, Wilson Jones E. Fibrous papule of the nose. *Br J Dermatol.* 1971;85:111–118.

373. Meigel WN, Ackerman AB. Fibrous papule of the face. *Am J Dermatopathol.* 1979;1:329–340.

374. McGibbon DH, Wilson Jones E. Fibrous papule of the nose. *Am J Dermatopathol.* 1979;1:345–348.

375. Tokat, F, Sezer, E, Duman, D, Durmaz EÖ, İnce Ü. Histopathological characteristics and CD163 immunostaining pattern in fibrous papule of the face. *J Cutan Pathol.* 2021;482:274–280.

376. Lee AN, Stein SL, Cohen LM. Clear cell fibrous papule with NKI/C3 expression: clinical and histologic features in six cases. *Am J Dermatopathol.* 2005;27:296–300.

377. Bansal C, Stewart D, Li A, Cockerell CJ. Histologic variants of fibrous papule. *J Cutan Pathol.* 2005;32:424–428.

378. Kucher C, McNiff JM. Epithelioid fibrous papule—a new variant. *J Cutan Pathol.* 2007;34:571–575.

379. Ragaz A, Berezowsky V. Fibrous papule of the face: a study of five cases by electron microscopy. *Am J Dermatopathol.* 1979;1:353–355.

380. Kimura S, Yamasaki Y. Ultrastructure of fibrous papule of the nose. *J Dermatol.* 1983;10:571–578.

381. Damman J, Biswas A. Fibrous papule: a histopathologic review. *Am J Dermatopathol.* 2018;40(8):551–560.

382. Spiegel J, Nadji M, Penneys NS. Fibrous papule: an immunohistochemical study with antibody to S100 protein. *J Am Acad Dermatol.* 1983;9:360–362.

383. Nemeth AJ, Penneys NS, Bernstein HB. Fibrous papule: a tumor of fibrohistiocytic cells that contain factor XIIIa. *J Am Acad Dermatol.* 1988;19:1102–1106.

384. Cerio R, Rao BK, Spaull J, Jones EW. An immunohistochemical study of fibrous papule of the nose: 25 cases. *J Cutan Pathol.* 1989;16:194–198.

385. Nemeth AJ, Penneys NS. Factor XIIIa is expressed by fibroblasts in fibrovascular tumors. *J Cutan Pathol.* 1989;16:266–271.

386. Cerio R, Wilson Jones E. Factor XIIIa positivity in fibrous papule. *J Am Acad Dermatol.* 1990;20:138–139.

387. Chan JY, Wang KH, Fang CL, Chen WY. Fibrous papule of the face, similar to tuberous sclerosis complex-associated

angiofibroma, shows activation of the mammalian target of rapamycin pathway: evidence for a novel therapeutic strategy? *PLoS One.* 2014;18(9):e89467.

388. Fletcher CDM. Cellular angiofibroma. In: Fletcher CDM, Unnik K, Mertens F, eds. *World Health Organization Classification of Tumours. Pathology and Genetics of Tumours of Soft Tissue and Bone.* IARC Press; 2002:71–72.

389. Maggiani F, Debiec-Rychter M, Vanbockrijck M, Sciot R. Cellular angiofibroma: another mesenchymal tumour with 13q14 involvement, suggesting a link with spindle cell lipoma and (extra)-mammary myofibroblastoma. *Histopathology.* 2007;51:410–412.

390. Guillou L, Bridge JA. Giant cell angiofibroma. In: Fletcher CDM, Unnik K, Mertens F, eds. *World Health Organization Classification of Tumours. Pathology and Genetics of Tumours of Soft Tissue and Bone.* IARC Press; 2002:79–80.

391. Mariño-Enríquez A, Fletcher CD. Angiofibroma of soft tissue: clinicopathologic characterization of a distinctive benign fibrovascular neoplasm in a series of 37 cases. *Am J Surg Pathol.* 2012;36:500–508.

392. Viswanath V, Thakur P, Pund P. Use of topical rapamycin in facial angiofibromas in Indian skin type. *Indian J Dermatol.* 2016;61:119.

393. Wataya -Kaneda M, Nakamura A, Tanaka M, et al. Efficacy and safety of topical sirolimus therapy for facial angiofibromas in the tuberous sclerosis complex: a randomized clinical trial. *JAMA Dermatol.* 2017;153:39–48.

394. Agha K, Alderson S, Samraj S, et al. Pearly penile papules regress in older patients and with circumcision. *Int J STD AIDS.* 2009;20:768–770.

395. Hogewoning CJ, Bleeker MC, van den Brule AJ, et al. Pearly penile papules: still no reason for uneasiness. *J Am Acad Dermatol.* 2003;49:50–54.

396. Ackerman AB, Kornberg R. Pearly penile papules. Acral angiofibromas. *Arch Dermatol.* 1973;108:673–675.

397. Gardner KM, Crawford RI. Distinction of condylomata acuminata from vulvar vestibular papules or pearly penile papules using Ki-67 immunostaining. *J Cutan Med Surg.* 2019;23:255–257.

398. Honigman AD, Dubin DP, Chu J, Lin MJ. Management of pearly penile papules: a review of the literature. *J Cutan Med Surg.* 2020;24:79–85.

399. Au KS, Williams AT, Roach ES, et al. Genotype/phenotype correlation in 325 individuals referred for a diagnosis of tuberous sclerosis complex in the United States. *Genet Med.* 2007;9:88–100.

400. Leung AK, Robson WL. Tuberous sclerosis complex: a review. *J Pediatr Health Care.* 2007;21:108–114.

401. Schwartz RA, Fernandez G, Kotulska K, Jóźwiak S. Tuberous sclerosis complex: advances in diagnosis, genetics, and management. *J Am Acad Dermatol.* 2007;57:189–202.

402. Rosser T, Panigrahy A, McClintock W. The diverse clinical manifestations of tuberous sclerosis complex: a review. *Semin Pediatr Neurol.* 2006;13:27–36.

403. Fitzpatrick TB, Szabo G, Hori Y, Simone AA, Reed WB, Greenberg MH. White leaf-shaped macules. *Arch Dermatol.* 1968;98:1–6.

404. Kwiatkowski DJ, Short MP. Tuberous sclerosis. *Arch Dermatol.* 1994;130:348–354.

405. Wienecke R, Maize JC Jr, Lowry DR, et al. The tuberous sclerosis gene TSC2 is a tumor suppressor gene whose protein product co-localizes with its putative substrate RAP1 in the cis/medial golgi [Abstract]. *J Invest Dermatol.* 1996;106:811.

406. Napolioni V, Curatolo P. Genetics and molecular biology of tuberous sclerosis complex. *Curr Genomics.* 2008;9:475–487.

407. Leducq S, Giraudeau B, Tavernier E, Maruani A. Topical use of mammalian target of rapamycin inhibitors in dermatology: a systematic review with meta-analysis. *J Am Acad Dermatol.* 2019;80:735–742.

408. Sasongko TH, Ismail NF, Zabidi-Hussin Z. Rapamycin and rapalogs for tuberous sclerosis complex. *Cochrane Database Syst Rev.* 2016;7(7):CD011272.

409. Krueger DA, Northrup H; International Tuberous Sclerosis Complex Consensus Group. Tuberous sclerosis complex surveillance and management: recommendations of the 2012 International Tuberous Sclerosis Complex Consensus Conference. *Pediatr Neurol.* 2013;49(4):255–265.

410. Nickel WR, Reed WB. Tuberous sclerosis: special reference to the microscopic alterations in the cutaneous hamartomas. *Arch Dermatol.* 1962;85:209–226.

411. Willis WF, Garcia RL. Giant angiofibroma in tuberous sclerosis. *Arch Dermatol.* 1978;114:1843–1844.

412. Park YK, Hann SK. Cluster growths in adenoma sebaceum associated with tuberous sclerosis. *J Am Acad Dermatol.* 1989;20:918–920.

413. Kobayasi RT, Wolf-Jurgensen P, Danielsen L. Ultrastructure of shagreen patch. *Acta Dermatol Venereol (Stockholm)* 1973;53:275–278.

414. Leducq S, Giraudeau B, Tavernier E, et al. Topical use of mammalian target of rapamycin inhibitors in dermatology: a systematic review with meta-analysis. *J Am Acad Dermatol.* 2019;80:735–742.

415. Sasongko TH, Ismail NF, Zabidi-Hussin Z. Rapamycin and rapalogs for tuberous sclerosis complex. *Cochrane Database Syst Rev.* 2016;7(7):CD011272.

416. Baykal C, Buyukbabani N, Yazganoglu KD, Saglik E. Acquired digital fibrokeratoma. *Cutis.* 2007;79:129–132.

417. Bron C, Noel B, Panizzon RG. Giant fibrokeratoma of the heel. *Dermatology.* 2004;208(3):271–272.

418. Saito S, Ishikawa K. Acquired periungual fibrokeratoma with accessory germinal matrix. *Dermatology.* 1995;190:169–171.

419. Hashiro M, Fujio Y, Tanaka M, et al. Giant acquired fibrokeratoma of the nail bed. *J Hand Surg Br.* 2002;27:549–555.

420. Dereure O, Savoy D, Doz F, Junien C, Guilhou JJ. Multiple acral fibromas in a patient with familial retinoblastoma: a cutaneous marker of tumour-suppressor gene germline mutation? *Br J Dermatol.* 2000;143:856–859.

421. Moulin G, Balme B, Thomas L. Familial multiple acral mucinous fibrokeratomas. *J Am Acad Dermatol.* 1998;38:999–1001.

422. Ballan A, Zeinaty P, Tomb R, et al. Acquired ungual fibrokeratoma: a systematic review of the literature. *Int J Dermatol.* 2021;60:533–539.

423. McNiff JM, Subtil A, Cowper SE, Lazova R, Glusac EJ. Cellular digital fibromas: distinctive CD34-positive lesions that may mimic dermatofibrosarcoma protuberans. *J Cutan Pathol.* 2005;32:413–418.

424. Guitart J, Ramirez J, Laskin WB. Cellular digital fibromas: what about superficial acral fibromyxoma? *J Cutan Pathol.* 2006;33:762–763.

425. Luzar B, Calonje E. Superficial acral fibromyxoma: clinicopathological study of 14 cases with emphasis on a cellular variant. *Histopathology.* 2009;54:375–377.

426. Michal M, Fetsch JF, Hes O, Miettinen M. Nuchal-type fibroma: a clinicopathologic study of 52 cases. *Cancer.* 1999;85:156–163.

427. Wehrli BM, Weiss SW, Yandow S, Coffin CM. Gardner-associated fibromas (GAF) in young patients: a distinct fibrous lesion that identifies unsuspected Gardner syndrome and risk for fibromatosis. *Am J Surg Pathol.* 2001;25:645–651.

428. Coffin CM, Hornick JL, Zhou H, Fletcher CD. Gardner fibroma: a clinicopathologic and immunohistochemical analysis of 45 patients with 57 fibromas. *Am J Surg Pathol.* 2007;31:410–416.

429. Diwan AH, Graves ED, King JA, Horenstein MG. Nuchal-type fibroma in two related patients with Gardner's syndrome. *Am J Surg Pathol.* 2000;24:1563–1567.

430. Michal M, Boudova L, Mukensnabl P. Gardner's syndrome associated fibromas. *Pathol Int.* 2004;54:523–526.

431. Michal M. Non–nuchal-type fibroma associated with Gardner's syndrome. A hitherto-unreported mesenchymal tumor different from fibromatosis and nuchal-type fibroma. *Pathol Res Pract.* 2000;196:857–860.

432. Fetsch JF, Laskin WB, Miettinen M. Superficial acral fibromyxoma: a clinicopathologic and immunohistochemical analysis of 37 cases of a distinctive soft tissue tumor with a predilection for the fingers and toes. *Hum Pathol.* 2001;32:704–714.

433. Hollmann TJ, Bovée JV, Fletcher CD. Digital fibromyxoma (superficial acral fibromyxoma): a detailed characterization of 124 cases. *Am J Surg Pathol.* 2012;36:789–798.

434. Tardío JC, Butrón M, Martín-Fragueiro LM. Superficial acral fibromyxoma: report of 4 cases with CD10 expression and lipomatous component, two previously underrecognized features. *Am J Dermatopathol.* 2008;30:431–435.

435. Cullen D, Díaz Recuero JL, Cullen R, Rodríguez Peralto JL, Kutzner H, Requena L. Superficial acral fibromyxoma: report of 13 cases with new immunohistochemical findings. *Am J Dermatopathol.* 2017;39:14–22.

436. Agaimy A, Michal M, Giedl J, Hadravsky L, Michal M. Superficial acral fibromyxoma: clinicopathological, immunohistochemical, and molecular study of 11 cases highlighting frequent Rb1 loss/deletions. *Hum Pathol.* 2017;60:192–198.

437. Libbrecht S, Van Dorpe J, Creytens D. The rapidly expanding group of RB1-deleted soft tissue tumors: an updated review. *Diagnostics (Basel).* 2021;11:430.

438. Fletcher CD, Tsang WY, Fisher C, Lee KC, Chan JK. Angiomyofibroblastoma of the vulva: a benign neoplasm distinct from aggressive angiomyxoma. *Am J Surg Pathol.* 1992;16:373–382.

439. Nasu K, Fujisawa K, Takai N, Miyakawa I. Angiomyofibroblastoma of the vulva. *Int J Gynecol Cancer.* 2002;12:228–231.

440. Nucci MR, Fletcher CD. Vulvovaginal soft tissue tumors: update and review. *Histopathology.* 2000;36:97–108.

441. Neilsen GP, Rosenberg AE, Young RH, Dickersin GR, Clement PB, Scully RE. Angiomyofibroblastoma of the vulva and vagina. *Mod Pathol.* 1996;9:284–291.

442. Banerjee K, Datta Gupta S, Mathur SR. Vaginal angiomyofibroblastoma. *Arch Gynecol Obstet.* 2004;270:124–125.

443. Fukunaga M, Nomura K, Matsumoto K, Doi K, Endo Y, Ushigome S. Vulval angiomyofibroblastoma. Clinicopathologic analysis of six cases. *Am J Clin Pathol.* 1997;107:45–51.

444. Laskin WB, Fetsch JF, Tavassoli FA. Angiomyofibroblastoma of the female genital tract: analysis of 17 cases including a lipomatous variant. *Hum Pathol.* 1997;28:1046–1055.

445. Blythe WR, Logan TC, Holmes DK, Drake AF. Fibromatosis colli: a common cause of neonatal torticollis. *Am Fam Physician.* 1996;54;1965–1967.

446. Dunn PM. Congenital sternomastoid torticollis: an intrauterine postural deformity. *J Bone Joint Surg Br.* 1973;55:877.

447. Binder H, Eng GD, Gaiser JF, Koch B. Congenital muscular torticollis: results of conservative management with long-term follow-up in 85 cases. *Arch Phys Med Rehabil.* 1987;68:222–225.

448. Canale ST, Griffin DW, Hubbard CN. Congenital muscular torticollis: a long-term follow-up. *J Bone Joint Surg Am.* 1982;64:810–816.

449. Hummer CD Jr, MacEwen GD. The coexistence of torticollis and congenital dysplasia of the hip. *J Bone Joint Surg Am.* 1972;54:1266–1256.

450. Pereira S, Tani E, Skoog L. Diagnosis of fibromatosis colli by fine needle aspiration (FNA) cytology. *Cytopathology.* 1999;10:25–29.

451. Sharma S, Mishra K, Khanna G. Fibromatosis colli in infants: a cytologic study of eight cases. *Acta Cytol.* 2003;47:359–362.

452. Gonatas K. Extra-abdominal desmoid tumors: report of six cases. *Arch Pathol.* 1961;71:214–221.

453. Goellner JR, Soule EH. Desmoid tumors: an ultrastructural study of eight cases. *Hum Pathol.* 1980;11:43–50.

454. Hayry P, Retamao JJ, Totterman S, Hopfner-Hallikainen D, Sivula A. The desmoid tumor. II. Analysis of factors possibly contributing to the etiology and growth behavior. *Am J Clin Pathol.* 1982;77:674–680.

455. Sturt NJH, Clark SK. Current ideas in desmoids tumours. *Fam Cancer.* 2006;5:275–285.

456. Giarola M, Wells D, Mondini P, et al. Mutations of adenomatous polyposis cell (APC) gene are uncommon in sporadic desmoid tumours. *Br J Cancer.* 1998;78:582–587.

457. Jilong Y, Jian W, Xiaoyan Z, Xiaoqiu L, Xiongzeng Z. Analysis of APC/beta-catenin genes mutations and Wnt signalling pathway in desmoid-type fibromatosis. *Pathology.* 2007;39:319–325.

458. Bridge JA, Swarts SJ, Buresh C, et al. Trisomies 8 and 20 characterize a subgroup of benign fibrous lesions arising in both soft tissue and bone. *Am J Pathol.* 1999;154:729–733.

459. de Wever J, Dal Cin P, Fletcher CD, et al. Cytogenetic, clinical and morphologic correlations in 78 cases of fibromatosis: a report from the CHAMP Study Group. Chromosomes and Morphology. *Mod Pathol.* 2000;13:1080–1085.

460. Fisher C Thway K Aggressive fibromatosis. *Pathology.* 2014 46:135–140.

461. Zreik RT Fritchie KJ. Morphologic spectrum of desmoid-type fibromatosis. *Am J Clin Pathol.* 2016;145:332–340.

462. Stiller D, Katenkamp D. Cellular features in desmoid fibromatosis and well differentiated fibrosarcomas: an electron microscopic study. *Virchows Arch A Pathol Anat.* 1975;369:155–164.

463. Hasegawa T, Hirose T, Kudo E, Abe J, Hizawa K. Cytoskeletal characteristics of myofibroblasts in benign neoplastic and reactive fibroblastic lesions. *Virchows Arch A Pathol Anat.* 1990;416:375–382.

464. Goldblum J, Fletcher JA. Desmoid-type fibromatoses. In: Fletcher CDM, Unni KK, Mertens F, eds. *World Health Organization Classification of Tumours. Pathology and Genetics of Tumours of Soft Tissue and Bone.* IARC Press; 2002:83–84.

465. Carlson JW, Fletcher CD. Immunohistochemistry for beta-catenin in the differential diagnosis of spindle cell lesions: analysis of a series and review of the literature. *Histopathology.* 2007; 51:509–514.

466. Barak S, Wang Z, Miettinen M. Immunoreactivity for calretinin and keratins in desmoid fibromatosis and other myofibroblastic tumors: a diagnostic pitfall. *Am J Surg Pathol.* 2012;36:1404–1409.

467. Bertani E, Testori A, Chiappa A, et al. Recurrence and prognostic factors in patients with aggressive fibromatosis. The role of radical surgery and its limitations. *World J Surg Oncol.* 2012;10:184.

468. Bocale D, Rotelli MT, Cavallini A, Altomare DF. Anti-oestrogen therapy in the treatment of desmoid tumours: a systematic review. *Colorectal Dis.* 2011;13:388–395.

469. Penel N, Le Cesne A, Bui BN, et al. Imatinib for progressive and recurrent aggressive fibromatosis (desmoid tumors): an FNCLCC/French Sarcoma Group phase II trial with a long-term follow-up. *Ann Oncol.* 2011;22:452–457.

470. de Camargo VP, Keohan ML, D'Adamo DR, et al. Clinical outcomes of systemic therapy for patients with deep fibromatoses (desmoid tumors). *Cancer.* 2010;116:2258–2265.

471. Mankin HJ, Hornicek FJ, Springfield DS. Extra-abdominal desmoid tumors: a report of 234 cases. *J Surg Oncol.* 2010;102:380–384.

472. Mullen JT, Delaney TF, Kobayashi WK, et al. Desmoid tumor: analysis of prognostic factors and outcomes in a surgical series. *Ann Surg Oncol.* 2012;19:4028–4035.

473. Geoghegan JM, Forbes J, Clark DI, Smith C, Hubbard R. Dupuytren's disease risk factors. *J Hand Surg Br.* 2004;29:423–426.

474. Godtfredsen NS, Lucht H, Prescott E, Sørensen TI, Grønbaek M. A prospective study linked both alcohol and tobacco to Dupuytren's disease. *J Clin Epidemiol.* 2004;57:858–863.

475. Gudmundsson KG, Arngrímsson R, Sigfússon N, Björnsson A, Jónsson T. Epidemiology of Dupuytren's disease: clinical, serological, and social assessment. The Reykjavik Study. *J Clin Epidemiol.* 2000;53:291–296.

476. Burge P, Hoy G, Regan P, Milne R. Smoking, alcohol and the risk of Dupuytren's contracture. *J Bone Joint Surg Br.* 1997;79:206–210.

477. Arafa M, Noble J, Royle SG, Trail IA, Allen J. Dupuytren's and epilepsy revisited. *J Hand Surg Br.* 1992;17:221–224.

478. Arkkila PE, Kantola IM, Viikari JS. Dupuytren's disease: association with chronic diabetic complications. *J Rheumatol.* 1997;24:153–159.

479. Pojer J, Radivojevic M, Williams TF. Dupuytren's disease: its association with abnormal liver function in alcoholism and epilepsy. *Arch Intern Med.* 1972;129:561–566.

480. Mikklesen OH. Knuckle pads in Dupuytren's disease. *Hand.* 1977;9:301–305.

481. Snyder M. Dupuytren's contracture and plantar fibromatosis: is there more than a causal relationship? *J Am Podiatr Assoc.* 1980;40:410–415.

482. Fetsch JF, Laskin WB, Miettinen M. Palmar-plantar fibromatosis in children and preadolescents: a clinicopathologic study of 56 cases with newly recognized demographics and extended follow-up information. *Am J Surg Pathol.* 2005;29:1095–1105.

483. Goldblum J, Fletcher JA. Superficial fibromatoses. In: Fletcher CDM, Unni KK, Mertens F, eds. *World Health Organization Classification of Tumours. Pathology and Genetics of Tumours of Soft Tissue and Bone.* IARC Press; 2002:81–82.

484. Iwaska H, Muller H, Stutte HJ, Brennscheidt U. Palmar fibromatosis (Dupuytren's contracture). Ultrastructural and enzyme histochemical studies of 43 cases. *Virchows Arch A Pathol Anat Histopathol.* 1984;40:41–53.

485. Meister P, Gokel JM, Remberger K. Palmar fibromatosis "Dupuytren's contracture." A comparison of light, electron and immunofluorescence microscopic findings. *Pathol Res Pract.* 1979;164:402–412.

486. Mackey SL, Cobb MW. Knuckle pads. *Cutis.* 1994;54:159–160.

487. Lagier R, Meinecke R. Pathology of "knuckle pads": study of four cases. *Virchows Arch A Pathol Anat Histopathol.* 1975;365:185–191.

488. Dias JM, Costa MM, Romeu JC, Soares-Almeida L, Filipe P, Pereira da Silva JA. Pachydermodactyly in a 16-year-old adolescent boy. *J Clin Rheumatol.* 2012;18:246–248.

489. Chan JKC. Solitary fibrous tumour—everywhere, and a diagnosis in vogue. *Histopathology.* 1997;31:568–576.

490. Okamura JM, Barr RJ, Battifora H. Solitary fibrous tumor of the skin. *Am J Dermatopathol.* 1997;19:515–518.

491. Cowper SE, Kilpatrick T, Proper S, Morgan MB. Solitary fibrous tumor of the skin. *Am J Dermatopathol.* 1999;21:213–219.

492. Hardisson D, Cuevas-Santos J, Contreras F. Solitary fibrous tumor of the skin. *J Am Acad Dermatol.* 2002;46:S37–S40.

493. Morgan MB, Smoller BR. Solitary fibrous tumors are immunophenotypically distinct from mesothelioma(s). *J Cutan Pathol.* 2000;27:451–454.

494. Suster S, Nascimento AG, Miettinen M, Sickel JZ, Moran CA. Solitary fibrous tumor of soft tissue: a clinicopathologic and immunohistochemical study of 12 cases. *Am J Surg Pathol.* 1995;19:1257–1266.

495. Erdag G, Qureshi HS, Patterson JW, Wick MR. Solitary fibrous tumors of the skin: a clinicopathologic study of 10 cases and review of the literature. *J Cutan Pathol.* 2007;34:844–850.

496. Doyle LA Vivero M, Fletcher CDM Nuclear expression of STAT6 distinguishes solitary fibrous tumor from histologic mimics. *Mod Pathol.* 2014 27(3):390–395.

497. Cook JR, Dehner LP, Collins MH, et al. Anaplastic lymphoma kinase (ALK) expression in inflammatory myofibroblastic tumor: a comparative immunohistochemical study. *Am J Surg Pathol.* 2001;25:1364–1371.

498. Yang M. Cutaneous inflammatory pseudotumor: a case report with immunohistochemical and ultrastructural studies. *Pathology.* 1993;25:405–409.

499. Hurt MA, Santa Cruz DA. Cutaneous inflammatory pseudotumor: lesions resembling "inflammatory pseudotumors" or "plasma cell granuloma" of extracutaneous site. *Am J Surg Pathol.* 1990;14:764–773.

500. Shabrawi-Caelen LE, Kerl K, Cerroni L, Soyer HP, Kerl H. Cutaneous inflammatory pseudotumor—a spectrum of various diseases? *J Cutan Pathol.* 2004;31:605–611.

501. Vadmal MS, Pellegrini AE. Inflammatory myofibroblastic tumor of the skin. *Am J Dermatopathol.* 1999;21:449–453.

502. Nakajima T, Sano S, Itami S, Yoshikawa K. Cutaneous inflammatory pseudotumor (plasma cell granuloma). *Br J Dermatol.* 2001;144:1271–1273.

503. Coffin CM, Fletcher JA. Inflammatory myofibroblastic tumor. In: Fletcher CDM, Unni KK, Mertens F, eds. *World Health Organization Classification of Tumours. Pathology and Genetics of Tumours of Soft Tissue and Bone.* IARC Press; 2002:91–93.

504. Cessna MH, Zhou H, Sanger WG, et al. Expression of ALK1 and p80 in inflammatory myofibroblastic tumor and its mesenchymal mimics: a study of 135 cases. *Mod Pathol.* 2002;15:931–938.

505. Chan JK, Cheuk W, Shimizu M. Anaplastic lymphoma kinase expression in inflammatory pseudotumors. *Am J Surg Pathol.* 2001;25:761–768.

506. Puig L, Fernandez-Figueras MT, Bielsa I, Lloveras B, Alomar A. Multinucleate cell angiohistiocytoma: a fibrohistiocytic proliferation with increased mast cell numbers and vascular hyperplasia. *J Cutan Pathol.* 2002;29:232–237.

507. Shapiro PE, Nova MP, Rosmarin LA, Halperin AJ. Multinucleate cell angiohistiocytoma: a distinct entity diagnosable by clinical and histologic features. *J Am Acad Dermatol.* 1994;30:417–422.

508. Annessi G, Girolomoni G, Giannetti A. Multinucleate cell angiohistiocytoma. *Am J Dermatopathol.* 1992;14:340–344.

509. Sass U, Noel JC, André J, Simonart T. Multinucleate cell angiohistiocytoma: report of two cases with no evidence of human herpesvirus-8 infection. *J Cutan Pathol.* 2000;27:258–261.

510. Pérez LP, Zulaica A, Rodríguez L, et al. Multinucleate cell angiohistiocytoma. Report of five cases. *J Cutan Pathol.* 2006;33:349–352.

511. Blanco Barrios S, Rodríguez Díaz E, Alvarez Cuesta C, et al. Multinucleate cell angiohistiocytoma: a new case report. *J Eur Acad Dermatol Venereol.* 2005;19:208–211.

512. Chang SN, Kim HS, Kim SC, Yang WI. Generalized multinucleate cell angiohistiocytoma. *J Am Acad Dermatol.* 1996;35:320–322.

513. Kao YC, Flucke U, Eijkelenboom A, et al. Novel EWSR1-SMAD3 gene fusions in a group of acral fibroblastic spindle cell neoplasms. *Am J Surg Pathol.* 2018;42:522–528.

514. Habeeb O, Korty KE, Azzato EM, et al. EWSR1-SMAD3 rearranged fibroblastic tumor: case series and review. *J Cutan Pathol.* 2021;48:255–262.

515. Akiyama M, Yamaoka M, Mikami-Terao Y, et al. Paraneoplastic syndrome of angiomatoid fibrous histiocytoma may be caused by EWSR1-CREB1 fusion-induced excessive interleukin-6 production. *J Pediatr Hematol Oncol.* 2015;37:554–559.

516. Thway K, Fisher C. Angiomatoid fibrous histiocytoma: the current status of pathology and genetics. *Arch Pathol Lab Med.* 2015;139:674–682.

517. Matsumura T, Yamaguchi T, Tochigi N, Wada T, Yamashita T, Hasegawa T. Angiomatoid fibrous histiocytoma including cases with pleomorphic features analysed by fluorescence in situ hybridisation. *J Clin Pathol.* 2010;63:124–128.

518. Abrahao-Machado LF, Bacchi LM, Fernandes IL. MUC4 expression in angiomatoid fibrous histiocytoma. *Appl Immunohistochem Mol Morphol.* 2020;28:641–645.

519. Hasegawa T, Seki K, Ono K, Hirohashi S. Angiomatoid (malignant) fibrous histiocytoma: a peculiar low-grade tumor showing

immunophenotypic heterogeneity and ultrastructural variations. *Pathol Int.* 2000;50:731–738.

520. Berklite L, John I, Ranganathan S, Parafioriti A, Alaggio R. SOX9 immunohistochemistry in the distinction of angiomatoid fibrous histiocytoma from histologic mimics: diagnostic utility and pitfalls. *Appl Immunohistochem Mol Morphol.* 2020;28:635–640.

521. Lazar A, Abruzzo LV, Pollock RE, Lee S, Czerniak B. Molecular diagnosis of sarcomas: chromosomal translocations in sarcomas. *Arch Pathol Lab Med.* 2006;130:1199–1207.

522. Demicco EG. Sarcoma diagnosis in the age of molecular pathology. *Adv Anat Pathol.* 2013;20:264–274.

523. Tanas MR, Rubin BP, Montgomery EA, et al. Utility of FISH in the diagnosis of angiomatoid fibrous histiocytoma: a series of 18 cases. *Mod Pathol.* 2010;23:93–97.

524. Thway K, Gonzalez D, Wren D, Dainton M, Swansbury J, Fisher C. Angiomatoid fibrous histiocytoma: comparison of fluorescence in situ hybridization and reverse transcription polymerase chain reaction as adjunct diagnostic modalities. *Ann Diagn Pathol.* 2015;19:137–142.

525. Chow LT, Allen PW, Kumta SM, Griffith J, Li CK, Leung PC. Angiomatoid malignant fibrous histiocytoma: report of an unusual case with highly aggressive clinical course. *J Foot Ankle Surg.* 1998;37:235–238.

526. Mavrogenis AF, Tsukamoto S, Antoniadou T, Righi A, Errani C. Giant cell tumor of soft tissue: a rare entity. *Orthopedics.* 2019;42:e364–e369.

527. Lee JC, Liang CW, Fletcher CD. Giant cell tumor of soft tissue is genetically distinct from its bone counterpart. *Mod Pathol.* 2017;30:728–733.

528. Fletcher CDM, McKee PH. Sarcomas: III. Synovial sarcoma. *Clin Exp Dermatol.* 1985;10:332–349.

529. Li P, Laskin W, Wang WL, Demicco EG, Panse G. Primary superficial synovial sarcoma: clinical and histopathological characteristics in eight cases with molecular confirmation. *J Cutan Pathol.* 2021;48:263–268.

530. Sharma A, Ko JS, Billings SD. Primary cutaneous synovial sarcoma-Sometimes the hoof beats are zebras. *J Cutan Pathol.* 2021;48:281–284.

531. van de Rijn M, Barr FG, Collins MH, Xiong QB, Fisher C. Absence of SYT-SSX fusion products in soft tissue tumors other than synovial sarcoma. *Am J Clin Pathol.* 1999;112:43–49.

532. Guillou L. Contribution of molecular biology and markers to the prognosis and management of patients with soft tissue sarcoma. *Pathol Case Rev.* 2008;13:69–77.

533. Feng X, Huang YL, Zhang Z, et al. The role of SYT-SSX fusion gene in tumorigenesis of synovial sarcoma. *Pathol Res Pract.* 2021;222:153416.

534. Kubo T, Shimose S, Fujimori J, Furuta T, Ochi M. Prognostic value of SS18-SSX fusion type in synovial sarcoma; systematic review and meta-analysis. *Springerplus.* 2015;4:375.

535. Coindre JM, Pelmus M, Hostein I, Lussan C, Bui BN, Guillou L. Should molecular testing be required for diagnosing synovial sarcoma? A prospective study of 204 cases. *Cancer.* 2003;98:2700–2707.

536. Fisher C, de Bruijn DRH, Geurts van Kessel A. Synovial sarcoma. In: Fletcher CDM, Unni KK, Mertens F, eds. *World Health Organization Classification of Tumours. Pathology and Genetics of Tumours of Soft Tissue and Bone.* IARC Press; 2002:203–204.

537. Streich L, Johnson DN, Alexiev BA. Synovial sarcoma with overwhelming glandular (adenocarcinoma-like) component: a case report and review of the literature. *Pathol Res Pract.* 2021;222:153Epub ahead of print.

538. Fos SN, Bosch L. Immunohistochemistry of soft tissue sarcomas. Pathol. *Case Rev.* 2008;13:45–50.

539. El Beaino M, Jupiter DC, Assi T, et al. Diagnostic value of TLE1 in synovial sarcoma: a systematic review and meta-analysis. *Sarcoma.* 2020;2020:7192347.

540. Xiong Y, Dresser K, Cornejo KM. Frequent TLE1 expression in cutaneous neoplasms. *Am J Dermatopathol.* 2019;41:1–6.

541. Pukhalskaya T, Smoller BR. TLE1 expression fails to distinguish between synovial sarcoma, atypical fibroxanthoma, and dermatofibrosarcoma protuberans. *J Cutan Pathol.* 2020;47: 135–138.

542. Miettinen M, Virtanen I. Synovial sarcoma: a misnomer. *Am J Pathol.* 1984;117:18–25.

543. Ghadially FN. Is synovial sarcoma a carcinosarcoma of connective tissue? *Ultrastruct Pathol.* 1987;11:147–151.

544. Guarino M, Christensen L. Immunohistochemical analysis of extracellular matrix components in synovial sarcoma. *J Pathol.* 1994;172:279–286.

545. Bergh P, Meis-Kindblom JM, Gherlinzoni F, et al. Synovial sarcoma: identification of low and high risk groups. *Cancer.* 1999;85:2596–2607.

546. Deshmukh R, Mankin HJ, Singer S. Synovial sarcoma: the importance of size and location for survival. *Clin Orthop Relat Res.* 2004;419:155–161.

547. Thompson RC, Garg A, Goswitz J, Cheng EY, Clohisy DR, Dusenbery K. Synovial sarcoma. Large size predicts poor outcome. *Clin Orthop Relat Res.* 2000;373:18–24.

548. Shi W, Indelicato DJ, Morris CG, Scarborough MT, Gibbs CP, Zlotecki RA. Long-term treatment outcomes for patients with synovial sarcoma: a 40-year experience at the University of Florida. *Am J Clin Oncol.* 2013;36:83–88.

549. Palmerini E, Staals EL, Alberghini M, et al. Synovial sarcoma: retrospective analysis of 250 patients treated at a single institution. *Cancer.* 2009;115:2988–2998.

550. Kyriazoglou A, Timmermans I, De Cock L, et al. Management of synovial sarcoma in a tertiary referral center: a retrospective analysis of 134 patients. *Oncol Res Treat.* 2021;44:232–241.

551. Li YX, Ding SS, Wen WJ, Han L, Wang HQ, Shi HY. Impact of the activation status of the Akt/mtor signalling pathway on the clinical behaviour of synovial sarcoma: retrospective analysis of 174 patients at a single institution. *Cancer Manag Res.* 2020;12:1759–1769.

552. ten Heuvel SE, Hoekstra HJ, Bastiaannet E, Suurmeijer AJ. The classic prognostic factors tumor stage, tumor size, and tumor grade are the strongest predictors of outcome in synovial sarcoma: no role for SSX fusion type or ezrin expression. *Appl Immunohistochem Mol Morphol.* 2009;17:189–195.

553. Setsu N, Kohashi K, Fushimi F, et al. Prognostic impact of the activation status of the Akt/mTOR pathway in synovial sarcoma. *Cancer.* 2013;119(19):3504–3513. doi:10.1002/cncr.28255.

554. Salah S, Yaser S, Salem A, Al Mousa A, Abu Sheikha A, Sultan I. Factors influencing survival in metastatic synovial sarcoma: importance of patterns of metastases and the first-line chemotherapy regimen. *Med Oncol.* 2013;30:639.

555. Enzinger FM. Epithelioid sarcoma: a sarcoma simulating a granuloma or a carcinoma. *Cancer.* 1970;26:1029–1041.

556. Chase DR, Enzinger FM. Epithelioid sarcoma: diagnosis, prognostic indicators and treatment. *Am J Surg Pathol.* 1985;9:241–263.

557. Kodet R, Smelhais V, Newton WA, et al. Epithelioid sarcoma in childhood. *Pediatr Pathol.* 1994;14:433.

558. Schmidt D, Harms D. Epithelioid sarcoma in children and adolescents: an immunohistochemical study. *Virchows Arch A Pathol Anat.* 1987;410:423.

559. Evans HL, Baer SC. Epithelioid sarcoma: a clinicopathologic and prognostic study of 26 cases. *Semin Diagn Pathol.* 1993;10: 286–291.

560. Jawad MU, Extein J, Min ES, Scully SP. Prognostic factors for survival in patients with epithelioid sarcoma: 441 cases from the SEER database. *Clin Orthop Relat Res.* 2009;467:2939–2948.

561. Flucke U, Hulsebos TJ, van Krieken JH, Mentzel T. Myxoid epithelioid sarcoma: a diagnostic challenge. A report on six cases. *Histopathology.* 2010;57:753–759.

562. Miettinen M, Fanburg-Smith JC, Virolainen M, Shmookler BM, Fetsch JF. Epithelioid sarcoma: an immunohistochemical analysis of 112 classical and variant cases and a discussion of the differential diagnosis. *Hum Pathol.* 1999;30:934–942.

563. Caballero GA, Roitman PD. Pseudomyogenic hemangioendothelioma (epithelioid sarcoma-like hemangioendothelioma). *Arch Pathol Lab Med.* 2020;144(4):529–533.

564. Miettinen M, Wang Z, Sarlomo-Rikala M, Abdullaev Z, Pack SD, Fetsch JF. ERG expression in epithelioid sarcoma: a diagnostic pitfall. *Am J Surg Pathol.* 2013;37:1580–1585.

565. Mirra JM, Kessler S, Bhuta S, Eckardt J. The fibroma-like variant of epithelioid sarcoma: a fibrohistiocytic/myoid cell lesion often confused with benign and malignant spindle cell tumors. *Cancer.* 1992;15:1382–1395.

566. Tan SH, Ong BH. Spindle cell variant of epithelioid sarcoma: an easily misdiagnosed tumor. *Australas J Dermatol.* 2001;42:139–141.

567. Guillou L, Wadden C, Coindre JM, Krausz T, Fletcher CD. "Proximal-type" epithelioid sarcoma, a distinctive aggressive neoplasm showing rhabdoid features. *Am J Surg Pathol.* 1997;21:130–146.

568. Hasegawa T, Matsuno Y, Shimoda T, Umeda T, Yokoyama R, Hirohashi S. Proximal-type epithelioid sarcoma: a clinicopathologic study of 20 cases. *Mod Pathol.* 2001;14:655–663.

569. Heenan PJ, Quirk CJ, Papadimitriou JM. Epithelioid sarcoma: a diagnostic problem. *Am J Dermatopathol.* 1986;8:95–104.

570. Hornick JL, Dal Cin P, Fletcher CD. Loss of INI1 expression is characteristic of both conventional and proximal-type epithelioid sarcoma. *Am J Surg Pathol.* 2009;33:542–550.

571. DiCaudo DJ, McCalmont TH, Wick MR. Selected diagnostic problems in neoplastic dermatopathology. *Arch Pathol Lab Med.* 2007;131:434–439.

572. Quezado MM, Middleton LP, Bryant B, Lane K, Weiss SW, Merino MJ. Allelic loss on chromosome 22q in epithelioid sarcomas. *Hum Pathol.* 1998;29:604–608.

573. Lin L, Skacel M, Sigel JE, et al. Epithelioid sarcoma: an immunohistochemical analysis evaluating the utility of cytokeratin 5/6 in distinguishing superficial epithelioid sarcoma from spindled squamous cell carcinoma. *J Cutan Pathol.* 2003;30:114–116.

574. Chbani L, Guillou L, Terrier P, et al. Epithelioid sarcoma: a clinicopathologic and immunohistochemical analysis of 106 cases from the French sarcoma group. *Am J Clin Pathol.* 2009;131:222–1227.

575. de Visscher SA, van Ginkel RJ, Wobbes T, et al. Epithelioid sarcoma: still an only surgically curable disease. *Cancer.* 2006;107:606–612.

576. Maduekwe UN, Hornicek FJ, Springfield DS, et al. Role of sentinel lymph node biopsy in the staging of synovial, epithelioid, and clear cell sarcomas. *Ann Surg Oncol.* 2009;16:1356–1363.

577. PDQ Pediatric Treatment Editorial Board. Childhood soft tissue sarcoma treatment (PDQ®): health professional version. In: *PDQ Cancer Information Summaries [Internet].* National Cancer Institute (US); 2020.

578. Noujaim J, Thway K, Bajwa Z, et al. Epithelioid sarcoma: opportunities for biology-driven targeted therapy. *Front Oncol.* 2015;5:186.

579. Carney JA, Headington JT, Su WPD. Cutaneous myxomas: a major component of the complex of myxomas, spotty pigmentation, and endocrine overactivity. *Arch Dermatol.* 1986;122:790–798.

580. Sanusi ID. Subungual myxoma. *Arch Dermatol.* 1982;118:612–614.

581. Hill TL, Jones BE, Park KH. Myxoma of the skin of a finger. *J Am Acad Dermatol.* 1990;22:343–345.

582. Allen PW, Dymock RB, MacCormac LB. Superficial angiomyxomas with and without epithelial components. *Am J Surg Pathol.* 1988;12:519–530.

583. Allen PW. Myxoma is not a single entity: a review of the concept of myxoma. *Ann Diagn Pathol.* 2000;4:99–123.

584. Mehregan DR, Thomas L, Thomas JE. Epidermal basaloid proliferation in cutaneous myxomas. *J Cutan Pathol.* 2003;30:499–503.

585. Wilk M, Schmoekel C. Cutaneous focal mucinosis: a histopathological and immunohistochemical analysis of 11 cases. *J Cutan Pathol.* 1994;21:446–452.

586. Kempson RL, Fletcher CDM, Evans HL, et al. Tumors of the soft tissues. In: *Atlas of Tumor Pathology.* 3rd Series, Fascicle 30. Armed Forces Institute of Pathology; 2001:425–426.

587. Calonje E, Guerin D, McCormick D, Fletcher CD. Superficial angiomyxoma: clinicopathological analysis of a series of distinctive but poorly recognized cutaneous tumors with a tendency for recurrence. *Am J Surg Pathol.* 1999;23:910–917.

588. Armijo M. Mucoid cysts of the fingers. *J Dermatol Surg Oncol.* 1981;7:317–322.

589. Salasche SJ. Myxoid cysts of the proximal nail fold. *J Dermatol Surg Oncol.* 1984;10:35–39.

590. Johnson WC, Graham JH, Helwig EB. Cutaneous myxoid cyst. *JAMA.* 1965;191:15–20.

591. Goldman JA, Goldman L, Jaffe MS, Richfield DF. Digital mucinous pseudocysts. *Arthritis Rheum.* 1977;20:997–1002.

592. Newmeyer WL, Kilgore ES Jr, Graham WP. Mucous cysts: the dorsal distal interphalangeal joint ganglion. *Plast Reconstr Surg.* 1974;53:313–315.

593. Sechi A, Starace M, Alessandrini A, Caposiena Caro RD, Piraccini BM. Digital myxoid cysts: correlation of initial and long-term response to steroid injections. *Dermatol Surg.* 2021: 47(5): 146–152.

594. Lattanand A, Johnson WC, Graham JH. Mucous cyst (mucocele). *Arch Dermatol.* 1970;101:673–678.

595. Weir TW, Johnson WC. Cheilitis glandularis. *Arch Dermatol.* 1971;103:433–437.

596. Jensen JL. Superficial mucoceles of the oral mucosa. *Am J Dermatopathol.* 1990;12:88–92.

597. De Feraudy S, Fletcher C. Fibroblastic connective tissue naevus. A rare cutaneous lesion analyzed in a series of 25 cases. *Am J Surg Pathol.* 2012;36:1509–1515.

598. Wong D, Vargas A, Bonar F, et al. NTRK-rearranged mesenchymal tumours: diagnostic challenges, morphological patterns and proposed testing algorithm. *Pathology.* 2020;52(4):401–409.

599. Pennacchia I, Kutzner K Kazakov D, Mentzel T. Fibroblastic connective tissue nevus: clinicopathological and Immunohistochemical study of 14 cases. *J Cutan Pathol.* 2017;44:827–834.

600. Carter JM, Weiss SW, Linos K, DiCaudo DJ, Folpe AL. Superficial CD34-positive fibroblastic tumor: report of 18 cases of a distinctive low-grade mesenchymal neoplasm of intermediate (borderline) malignancy. *Mod Pathol.* 2014;27:294–302.

601. Lao W, Yu L Wang J. Superficial CD34-positive fibroblastic tumour: a clinicopathological and immunohistochemical study of an additional series. *Histopathology.* 2017;70(3):394–401.

INTRODUCTION

The classification of vascular lesions and, in particular, benign vascular tumors is far from satisfactory. The division between developmental, reactive, benign (neoplastic), and occasionally malignant vascular tumors is often blurred, and many conditions cannot be neatly classified into a specific category. This often reflects either limited knowledge about the pathogenesis or the presence of overlapping features among different entities. Although advances in knowledge and research have undoubtedly led to the improvement of this situation, the classification of many vascular tumors still remains controversial. A few examples include pyogenic granuloma and angiolymphoid hyperplasia with eosinophilia (reactive vs. neoplastic) and, more importantly, Kaposi sarcoma (neoplastic vs. infectious). The classification of cutaneous vascular tumors proposed in this chapter and in Table 33-1 is partially based on the most recent World Health Organization (WHO) classification of vascular tumors (1) and intends only to provide a framework to define and present different vascular tumors in a coherent manner on the basis of recent developments. It does not intend to be definitive, because future changes in our understanding of vascular tumors will undoubtedly give way to further modifications.

REACTIVE CONDITIONS

Intravascular Papillary Endothelial Hyperplasia (Masson Tumor)

Not an uncommon condition, intravascular papillary endothelial hyperplasia, or Masson tumor, represents an unusual endothelial proliferation in an organizing thrombus that can be misdiagnosed as angiosarcoma (2).

Clinical Summary. Intravascular papillary endothelial hyperplasia arises primarily within a venous channel or secondarily within a preceding angioma or some type of vascular anomaly, including hemorrhoids, as in Masson's original description. Secondary Masson tumor often occurs in deep-seated hemangiomas. Exceptional cases of extravascular location in association with hematoma have been reported (3). The lesions are almost always solitary, arising in the skin, subcutaneous tissue, or even muscle with the head and neck region and the upper extremities. The fingers, especially, are the most common sites. Exceptional instances of multiple lesions of the lower extremities simulating Kaposi sarcoma (4), simultaneous multiple lesions of skin and bone (5), and multiple lesions associated with

interferon beta treatment have also been described (6). All ages can be affected, although there is a slight female predominance (2). Primary lesions are usually tender nodules less than 2 cm in size, whereas secondary lesions occur because some preceding vascular abnormality increases in size.

Histopathology. Often, low-power examination allows recognition of the intravascular nature of the process in a single thin-walled vein (Fig. 33-1) or as part of a preceding angiomatous condition. Extravascular lesions fail to reveal a blood vessel wall despite serial sectioning. The main lesion consists of a mass of anastomosing vascular channels with a variable degree of intraluminal papillary projections (Fig. 33-2). The stroma consists of hyalinized eosinophilic material that may merge with uncanalized thrombus remnants. The infiltrating vascular channels show enlarged and prominent endothelial cells that may be "heaped up" to give rise to intraluminal prominences, but atypia and mitotic activity are slight.

Differential Diagnosis. The occurrence of areas of somewhat atypical endothelial-lined channels apparently showing a "dissection of collagen" appearance can closely simulate a well-differentiated angiosarcoma. However, the stroma is not collagen and is thus not refractile on polarization, and the changes are localized and occur within a preceding vessel or a vascular anomaly. Usually, angiosarcoma shows a much greater degree of nuclear atypia, multilayering, and mitotic activity.

Principles of Management: Simple excision.

Angioendotheliomatosis

For many years, two distinctive forms of angioendotheliomatosis were recognized: an aggressive variant with systemic involvement and poor prognosis and a reactive self-limited form with a benign course usually restricted to the skin. However, the so-called malignant angioendotheliomatosis shows no endothelial differentiation but represents a form of angiotropic lymphoma known as *intravascular lymphomatosis* (see Chapter 31). Rare cases of epithelioid angiosarcoma can present with intravascular lesions in the dermis, particularly when the primary lesion arises in the lumen of a large blood vessel.

Reactive Angioendotheliomatosis

Clinical Summary. Reactive angioendotheliomatosis is an uncommon condition that almost exclusively affects the skin and presents in patients of either gender with a wide anatomic distribution and predilection for the limbs. Clinical presentation varies from erythematous or brown macules to papules and/or

Table 33-1
Classification of Cutaneous Vascular Tumors

Benign Vascular Tumors

Benign Tumors and Tumor-like Conditions

Papillary endothelial hyperplasia (Masson tumor)

Reactive angioendotheliomatosis

Glomeruloid hemangioma

Papillary hemangioma

Bacillary angiomatosis

Vascular ectasias

Nevus flammeus (salmon patch and port-wine stain)

Angiokeratoma

Generalized essential telangiectasia

Cutaneous collagenous vasculopathy

Unilateral nevoid telangiectasia

Angioma serpiginosum

Hereditary hemorrhagic telangiectasia (Osler–Weber–Rendu)

Nevus araneus

Venous lake

Congenital hemangiomas

RICH (rapidly involuting congenital hemangioma)

NICH (noninvoluting congenital hemangioma)

Capillary hemangioma

  Variants:

    Infantile hemangioma

    Cherry angioma

    Tufted angioma (angioblastoma)

    Lobular capillary hemangioma (pyogenic granuloma)

Cavernous hemangioma

  Variant: Sinusoidal hemangioma

Verrucous hemangioma

Microvenular hemangioma

Hobnail hemangioma

Epithelioid hemangioma (angiolymphoid hyperplasia with eosinophilia)

Cutaneous epithelioid angiomatous nodule

Acquired elastotic hemangioma

Poikilodermatous plaque-like hemangioma

Arteriovenous hemangioma

  Variants:

    Superficial (cirsoid aneurysm)

    Deep

Angiomatosis

Spindle cell hemangioma

Symplastic hemangioma

Intermediate Vascular Tumors

Locally Aggressive

Kaposi-like hemangioendothelioma

Giant-cell angioblastoma

Rarely Metastasizing

Kaposi sarcoma

Retiform hemangioendothelioma

Papillary intravascular angioendothelioma (malignant endovascular papillary angioendothelioma, Dabska tumor)

Composite hemangioendothelioma

Pseudomyogenic hemangioendothelioma

Malignant Vascular Tumors

Epithelioid hemangioendothelioma

Angiosarcoma

  Variants:

    Idiopathic (head and neck)

    Associated with chronic lymphedema (Stewart–Treves)

    Postirradiation

    Epithelioid

Tumors of Lymph Vessels

Lymphangioma

  Variants:

    Lymphangioma circumscriptum

    Cavernous lymphangioma/cystic hygroma

    Benign lymphangioendothelioma (acquired progressive lymphangioma)

    Lymphangiomatosis

    Lymphangiomyoma

Multifocal lymphangiomatosis with thrombocytopenia

Atypical vascular proliferation after radiotherapy

Tumors of Perivascular Cells

Glomus tumor

Glomangiomatosis

  Variant: Infiltrating glomus tumor

Glomangiosarcoma

Myopericytoma

RICH, rapidly involuting congenital hemangioma; NICH, noninvoluting congenital hemangioma.

plaques that can be associated with purpura. A livedo-like pattern is sometimes present. In many cases, an association with systemic disease has been documented, including cryoglobulinemia (7); paraproteinemia (8); renal disease; amyloidosis (9); antiphospholipid syndrome (10); rheumatoid arthritis (11); cirrhosis (12); polymyalgia rheumatica (12); sarcoidosis (13); myelodysplastic syndrome (14); and systemic infections, especially tuberculosis and bacterial endocarditis

(15). Localized forms of the disease are less frequent and include a variant associated with peripheral vascular atherosclerotic disease described as *diffuse dermal angiomatosis* (15). The latter presentation has also been described in association with iatrogenic arteriovenous fistulas (16) and in a number of female patients associated with macromastia, obesity, and tobacco use (17,18), occasionally mimicking inflammatory breast carcinoma.

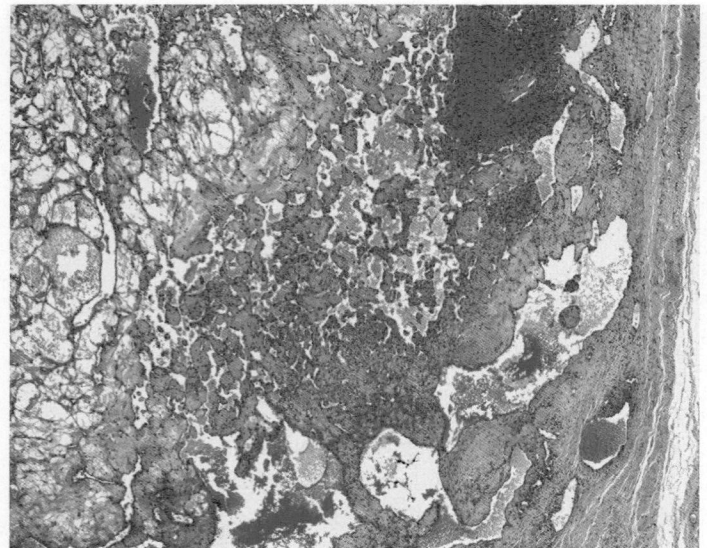

Figure 33-1 Primary intravascular papillary endothelial hyperplasia. Part of a markedly dilated vascular channel with prominent papillary structures intermixed with red blood cells and fibrin.

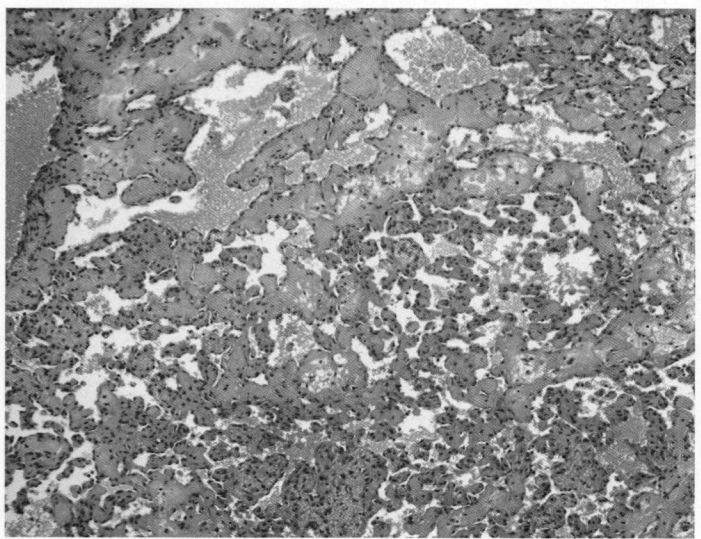

Figure 33-2 Intravascular papillary endothelial hyperplasia. Typical hyaline papillary projections lined by endothelial cells focally mimicking a dissection of collagen pattern.

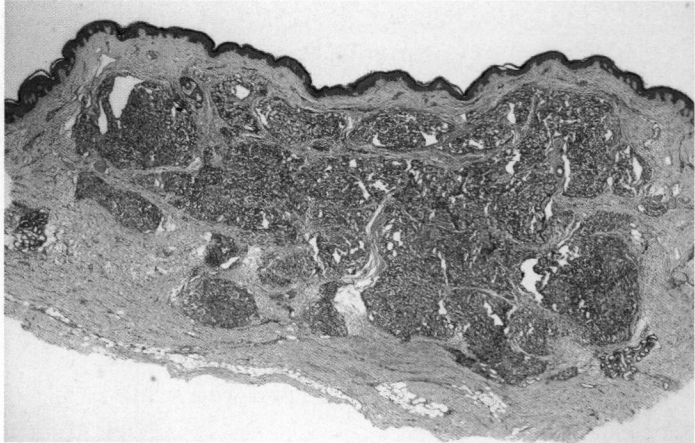

Figure 33-3 Reactive angioendotheliomatosis. Numerous closely packed capillaries within preexisting dilated blood vessels are seen throughout the dermis.

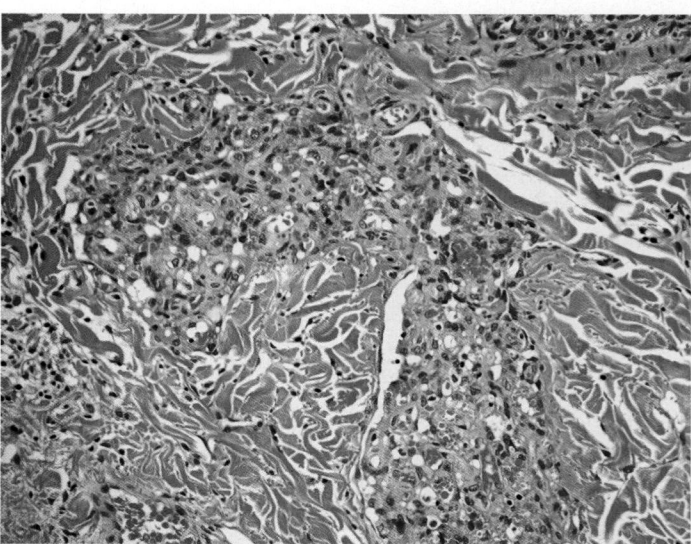

Figure 33-4 Reactive angioendotheliomatosis. Plump endothelial cells and intraluminal eosinophilic globules in a case associated with cryoglobulinemia.

Histopathology. Lesions are predominantly dermal and composed of closely packed, variably dilated vascular spaces (mainly capillaries) (Fig. 33-3) lined by bland but plump endothelial cells surrounded by pericytes. Rare cases display endothelial cells with focal epithelioid change (12). Small lumina might be apparent, some of which are obliterated by endothelial cells or fibrin thrombi. Often, the capillaries appear to proliferate in the lumina of dilated preexisting blood vessels. Hyaline refractile eosinophilic thrombi representing immunoglobulins are present in cases associated with cryoglobulinemia (8) (Fig. 33-4). In diffuse dermal angiomatosis, the proliferating endothelial cells are not present within vascular channels but can be found between dermal collagen fibers.

Histogenesis. Reactive angioendotheliomatosis, in contrast to malignant angioendotheliomatosis, displays universal reactivity for endothelial markers. It has been proposed that the endothelial cell proliferation is induced by a circulating angiogenic

factor or, alternatively, especially in cases associated with cryoglobulinemia or atherosclerotic vascular disease, by occlusion of vascular spaces (9). In many instances, the vascular proliferation is triggered by luminal occlusion, and it is likely that thrombosis plays an important role in pathogenesis.

Differential Diagnosis. The histologic distinction from tufted angioma may be difficult, but the clinical presentation of both entities is different, and tufted angioma shows clusters of capillaries in a typical cannonball distribution throughout the dermis with crescent-like dilated spaces that are probably lymphatic in nature in the periphery of many of the vascular tufts. In intravascular lymphomatosis, thin-walled vascular channels throughout the dermis and subcutis appear distended by atypical lymphoid cells, mainly, but not always, with a B-cell phenotype. Intravascular histiocytosis was originally regarded as the part of the spectrum of angioendotheliomatosis (19). It is, however, now considered a distinctive entity, with lesions most commonly developing close to involved joints of patients with rheumatoid arthritis. Similar features may also be seen as an incidental finding in biopsies performed for other pathologies, including samples from patients with chronic lymphedema. Histologically, collections of histiocytes are present within the lumina of thin-walled blood vessels. These cells are positive for CD68 and CD163 and may be positive for CD31.

Principles of Management: The condition is usually self-limited or improves when the underlying disease is treated.

Glomeruloid Hemangioma

Clinical Summary. Glomeruloid hemangioma is a highly distinctive, rare, reactive vascular proliferation that presents in patients with POEMS syndrome (*P*olyneuropathy, *O*rganomegaly, *E*ndocrinopathy, *M*-protein, and *S*kin changes), usually but not always in association with multicentric Castleman disease (20–23). The skin changes in POEMS syndrome include hypertrichosis, hyperpigmentation, hyperhidrosis, sclerodermoid features, and multiple small, vascular papules on the trunk and limbs. Single or multiple lesions with similar morphology have been described in patients with no evidence of POEMS syndrome (24,25) and in one patient with Erdheim-Chester disease (23). Some single lesions described as such may be examples of the recently described papillary hemangioma (see Papillary Hemangioma section). Hemangiomas with features of capillary hemangioma and glomeruloid hemangioma have been described in an intracranial location in a patient with POEMS syndrome (26).

Histopathology. Most vascular lesions in POEMS syndrome show the features of cherry angiomas, and only a few lesions have the appearance of a glomeruloid hemangioma. Other lesions may display histologic features that do not fit exactly into a definitive diagnostic category. In glomeruloid hemangioma, there are numerous ectatic vascular spaces throughout the dermis that contain in their lumina clusters of small, congested capillaries surrounded by pericytes bearing a striking resemblance to renal glomeruli (Figs. 33-5 and 33-6). Although the endothelial cells are flat, a few scattered cells appear vacuolated and can show periodic acid–Schiff (PAS)-positive hyaline globules. Initially, it

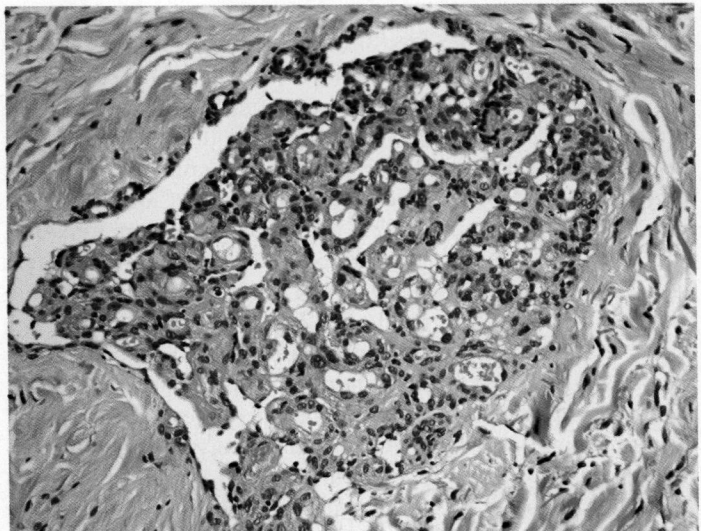

Figure 33-6 Glomeruloid hemangioma. Striking resemblance to a renal glomerulus.

was suggested that the latter correspond to deposition of immunoglobulins. More recently, however, it has been shown that the inclusions represent giant lysosomes with cellular debris and fat vacuoles known as thanatosomes (27). Staining for human herpesvirus 8 (HHV-8) is negative.

Histogenesis. Glomeruloid hemangioma probably represents a variant of reactive angioendotheliomatosis. The cause of the vascular proliferation in POEMS syndrome has not been established, but it may be induced by an angiogenic factor, possibly the abnormal immunoglobulin in the vascular spaces, or vascular endothelial growth factor (VEGF) (23).

Papillary Hemangioma

Clinical Summary. Papillary hemangioma is a recently described variant of hemangioma with a striking predilection for the head and neck of adults with male predominance (28). It presents as a long-standing asymptomatic papule, and local recurrence is exceptional.

Histopathology. Dilated, thin-walled vascular channels occupy the dermis and are characterized by the presence of multiple papillary projections with endothelial cells and pericytes associated with a thick basement membrane–like material. The endothelial cells are bland and contain abundant intracytoplasmic eosinophilic globules.

Histogenesis. The etiology is not known, but it has been suggested that this hemangioma represents a solitary variant of glomeruloid hemangioma. The latter, however, has a distinctive glomeruloid architecture and lacks papillary projections containing basement membrane–like material and pericytes (29).

Principles of Management: Simple excision is the treatment of choice.

VASCULAR ECTASIAS

Nevus Flammeus

Clinical Summary. The term *nevus flammeus* is often used to refer to two different lesions: the *salmon patch* and the *port-wine stain*.

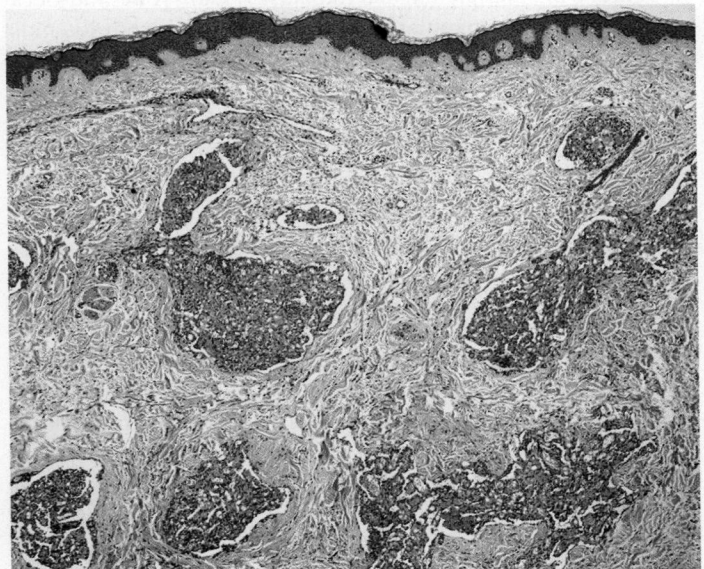

Figure 33-5 Glomeruloid hemangioma. Widely dilated preexisting vascular channels filled with smaller blood vessels. Note the low-power resemblance to reactive angioendotheliomatosis.

Although both lesions are congenital, the former tends to involute in the first few years of life and usually has no association with other types of anomalies, whereas the latter tends to be persistent and is often related to other malformations. The salmon patch is present in up to 50% of newborns of either gender as an ill-defined, red to pale pink macule, mainly in the nape of the neck, the glabella, or the eyelids (30). It was reported to be present in 91.2% of hospitalized neonates (31). The port-wine stain occurs in about 0.3% of newborns as a macular, usually unilateral, red-pink lesion, with a predilection for the face (32). Later in life, the lesion becomes darker and raised. A significant proportion of cases can be associated with accompanying neurological and/or ocular involvement (33). Acquired port-wine stains have rarely been described (Fegeler syndrome) in association with trauma, drugs, and even herpes zoster (34). Familial cases sometimes occur, and they have been attributed to mutations in the RASA1 gene (35,36).

Sturge–Weber syndrome (encephalotrigeminal angiomatosis) is characterized by the presence of a facial port-wine stain, often in the distribution of the trigeminal nerve associated with an ipsilateral leptomeningeal venous malformation, atrophy and calcification of the underlying cerebral cortex, epilepsy, mental retardation, ocular vascular malformations, glaucoma, and contralateral hemiparesis. There is a higher risk of neuro-ocular symptoms when there is involvement of the dermatome V1 by the port-wine stain (33).

In *Klippel–Trenaunay syndrome* (osteohypertrophic nevus flammeus), hypertrophy of the soft tissues and bones of one or several extremities affected with a nevus flammeus is observed. Associated with this are varicosities or arteriovenous fistulas or both and, less commonly, spindle cell hemangioendotheliomas. Cases presenting with arteriovenous fistulas are sometimes known as Parkes–Weber syndrome. Complications of note are cutaneous ulcers and high-output cardiac failure.

In phakomatosis pigmentovascularis, there is a port-wine stain associated with melanocytic lesions, including dermal melanocytosis and nevus spilus (37). Sturge–Weber and Klippel–Trenaunay can also be associated with this condition.

A new clinical syndrome has recently been reported as CLAPO: capillary malformation of the lower lip, lymphatic malformation of the face and neck, asymmetry, and partial/generalized overgrowth (38). Somatic activating *PIK3CA* mutations have been found in most patients (39).

Histopathology. In the *salmon patch*, dilated capillaries are seen in the papillary dermis. In the *port-wine stain*, no telangiectases are apparent histologically until the patient has reached about 10 years of age (40). The capillary ectasias thereafter gradually increase with age. Ultimately, when the lesion is raised or nodular, dilation appears not only in the superficial capillaries but also in some of the blood vessels in the deeper layers of the dermis and in the subcutaneous layer. Many ectatic vessels are filled with red blood cells. Lesions with a deep component can be associated with a cavernous hemangioma or an arteriovenous malformation (40).

Histogenesis. Because no histologic abnormalities are present early in life with a port-wine stain, it appears likely that this malformation is the result of a congenital weakness of the capillary walls (40). Thus, the port-wine stain represents a progressive telangiectasia. Antibodies directed against components of the blood vessel wall, collagenous basement membrane protein

(type IV collagen), fibronectin, and factor VIII–related antigen have an equivalent distribution and intensity in normal skin and nevus flammeus. Although this does not rule out a structural abnormality of these components, it has been suggested that the alteration may be related to the supporting dermal elements rather than to an intrinsic abnormality in the vessel wall. At the molecular level, pathogenesis involves complex interactions within MAPK and PI3K pathways (41) and *GNAQ* mutations (42).

Principles of Management: Salmon patches tend to regress spontaneously, and laser is the treatment of choice for port-wine stains.

Angiokeratoma

Clinical Summary. Four types of angiokeratoma have been described that represent true ectasias of blood vessels of the superficial dermis (43):

1. *Angiokeratoma corporis diffusum.* Patients present with numerous clusters of tiny, red papules in a symmetrical distribution, usually in the "bathing-trunk" area. Although often considered synonymous with Fabry disease, which is an X-linked genetic disorder associated with deficiency of the lysosomal enzyme A-galactosidase, identical clinical appearances have been described in patients with other enzymatic deficiencies, including B-galactosidase, neuraminidase, L-fucosidase, and B-mannosidase (44–46). In exceptional cases, presentation is not associated with detectable biochemical abnormalities, and these cases may be familial (47,48).
2. *Angiokeratoma of Mibelli.* Several dark red papules with a slightly verrucous surface are seen on the dorsa of the fingers and toes. Usually, the lesions appear during childhood or adolescence and measure 3 to 5 mm in diameter (49).
3. *Angiokeratoma of Fordyce.* Multiple vascular papules of 2 to 4 mm in diameter are seen on the scrotum (50). Similar lesions have been described on the vulva (51). They arise in middle or later life. Early lesions are red, soft, and compressible; later, they become blue, keratotic, and noncompressible.
4. *Solitary or multiple angiokeratomas.* Usually one and occasionally several papular lesions arise in young adults, most commonly on the lower extremities. They may be congenital, and when located in a restricted area of the lower limbs the term *angiokeratoma circumscriptum* is used (52). The lesions range from 2 to 10 mm in diameter. Early lesions appear bright red and soft but later become blue to black, firm, and hyperkeratotic. Thrombosed lesions are not uncommonly misdiagnosed clinically as malignant melanomas.

Histopathology. The histologic findings are essentially the same in all the four aforementioned types of angiokeratoma and consist of numerous, dilated, thin-walled, congested capillaries mainly in the papillary dermis underlying an epidermis that shows variable degrees of acanthosis with elongation of the rete ridges and hyperkeratosis (Fig. 33-7). In cutaneous lesions of Fabry disease, cytoplasmic vacuoles representing lipids can sometimes be detected in endothelial cells, fibroblasts, and pericytes.

Principles of Management: In cases of solitary lesions, simple excision is the treatment of choice. Laser therapy is an option in genital angiokeratomas (50). In patients with A-galactosidase

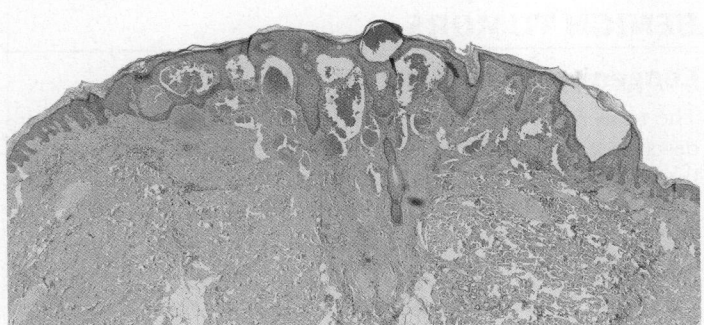

Figure 33-7 Angiokeratoma. Note the ectatic blood vessels in the papillary dermis with overlying epidermal hyperplasia.

deficiency, treatment with the enzyme may result in regression of the lesions (53).

Generalized Essential Telangiectasia

Clinical Summary. Widespread linear telangiectases, mainly on the extremities and sometimes the trunk, may gradually develop in adults, predominantly in women between the third and fourth decades of life (54,55). There is no associated bleeding. Occasional cases are associated with lesions in the conjunctiva and oral mucosa, and, exceptionally, watermelon stomach has been reported (56).

Histopathology. Dilated, often congested, vessels are seen in the papillary dermis. The walls of the vessels are composed only of endothelium. The absence of alkaline phosphatase activity suggests that it is the venous portion of the capillary loop that participates in the disease process (54,55).

Principles of Management: Laser therapy may result in cosmetic improvement (57).

Cutaneous Collagenous Vasculopathy

Clinical Summary. This condition is very rare and presents in adults as asymptomatic, progressive, generalized telangiectasia with no involvement of the oral cavity or nails (58). The clinical appearances are indistinguishable from those seen in essential generalized telangiectasia.

Histopathology. Superficial, small dermal vessels appear dilated, and their walls are thickened by amorphous hyaline material. Rarely, small blood vessels in the reticular dermis are involved (59). This material is positive for PAS and also for colloidal iron. It represents collagen, as demonstrated by electron microscopy; by immunohistochemistry, it is positive for collagen type IV, laminin, and fibronectin. Ultrastructure examination demonstrates that the vessels involved are postcapillary venules.

Principles of Management: Success with pulsed-dye laser has been reported (60).

Unilateral Nevoid Telangiectasia

Clinical Summary. Although unilateral nevoid telangiectasia may be congenital, in most instances, its onset is related to high estrogen levels associated with pregnancy, puberty, and chronic hepatic disease associated with alcoholism and rarely with hepatitis C (61). Neurologic abnormalities may rarely be found (62). It is more common in women, and presentation in children is very rare. The telangiectases, which are largely punctate and stellate rather than linear, follow a dermatomal

distribution, particularly those associated with the trigeminal nerve and cranial nerves III and IV. Exceptional cases are associated with gastric involvement.

Histopathology. Numerous dilated vessels are seen in the upper and middle dermis and, to a lesser extent, in the deeper part of the dermis.

Histogenesis. It has been proposed that the changes seen in this condition are induced by an increase in estrogen receptors in a dermatomal distribution (63). However, this has not been confirmed by immunohistochemistry.

Principles of Management: Some responses can be achieved by the use of pulsed-dye laser.

Angioma Serpiginosum

Clinical Summary. Angioma serpiginosum is a rare acquired vascular lesion that usually presents in the first two decades of life with a predilection for females. Anatomic distribution is wide, but lesions often present on the lower extremities. The disorder is asymptomatic, and slow progression occurs over the years. Focal spontaneous regression rarely occurs. Most cases are sporadic, but inherited cases have been reported (64). A typical lesion is characterized by deep red nonpalpable puncta that are grouped closely together in a macular or netlike pattern. Irregular extension at the periphery of the macules may cause them to have serpiginous borders. The deep red puncta represent dilated capillaries.

Histopathology. Dilated, thin-walled capillaries are seen in some of the dermal papillae and the superficial reticular dermis. Epidermal changes and extravasation of red blood cells do not occur.

Histogenesis. On electron microscopic examination, it is apparent that the thickening of the capillary walls is caused by a heavy precipitate of basement membrane–like material mixed with thin collagen fibers and an increased number of concentrically arranged pericytes. In addition, some of the dilated capillaries show slitlike protrusions of their lumina and endothelial lining into the surrounding thickened vessel walls. These findings indicate that angioma serpiginosum is not just a simple telangiectasia but represents a vascular malformation. It has been reported that the condition is associated with mutations of the gene *PORCN* on chromosome Xp11.3-Xq12 (65). This theory, however, has been disputed (66).

Principles of Management: Lesions may be treated with pulsed-dye laser (64).

Hereditary Hemorrhagic Telangiectasia (Osler–Weber–Rendu Disease)

Clinical Summary. Hereditary hemorrhagic telangiectasia (HHT), or Osler–Weber–Rendu disease, is inherited as an autosomal dominant trait. Up to four variants of the disease have been described, reflecting genetic heterogeneity (see Histogenesis). Although epistaxis may already begin in childhood, the characteristic telangiectases on the mucous membranes do not begin to appear until adolescence, and the cutaneous lesions often appear much later in life, particularly involving the upper part of the body. Typical lesions are small, bright red, nonpulsating papules.

Concomitant involvement of other organs, including the gastrointestinal tract, liver, brain, lungs, spleen, kidneys, and adrenal glands, is common. Associated vascular malformations are often a feature (67). Morbidity and mortality are related mainly to bleeding from internal organs.

Histopathology. Irregularly dilated capillaries and venules lined by flat endothelial cells are seen in the papillary and subpapillary dermis.

Histogenesis. On electron microscopy, the dilated vessels in the skin and oral mucosa are seen to be small postcapillary venules that normally do not possess pericytes. A defect in the perivascular supportive tissue has been found to be responsible for the breakdown of the junctions between endothelial cells and the resultant hemorrhage. A number of genetic abnormalities have been described in the disease. In type 1, HHT is associated with mutations on the *ENG* gene on chromosome 9q34.1 (68). In type 2 HHT, the mutation is located on the *ACVRL1* gene on chromosome 12q13 (69). In other variants of the disease, mutations have been described on chromosome 5 (70) and on gene *SMAD4* located on chromosome 18q21.1 (71). In the latter setting, patients also have juvenile polyposis.

Principles of Management: Management of this systemic condition is complex and involves treatment of acute hemorrhagic complications, as well as screening for significant vascular malformations in visceral organs and preventive treatment (e.g., excision, radiation therapy) if appropriate. Specialized centers exist to provide expert advice and management.

Nevus Araneus (Spider Nevus)

Clinical Summary. Nevus araneus, or spider nevus, considered the most common form of telangiectasia, presents at any age, especially in children, with a predilection for the face and upper limbs (72). It is characterized by a central, slightly elevated, red punctum from which blood vessels radiate. Occasionally, pulsation can be observed. Although spider nevi often arise spontaneously, pregnancy, the use of oral contraceptives, and liver disease are factors predisposing to their appearance (72). Spontaneous regression is common as children grow older and after pregnancy.

Histopathology. In the center of the lesion is an ascending artery that branches and communicates with multiple dilated capillaries.

Principles of Management: Lesions can be treated by electrodesiccation or laser.

Venous Lake

Clinical Summary. Venous lake is a small, dark blue, slightly raised, soft lesion occurring on the exposed skin of elderly persons. It can usually be emptied of most of its blood by using sustained pressure. Usually, several lesions are present. The face, ears, and lips are the most common sites.

Histopathology. Venous lake represents a telangiectasia. In the upper dermis, close to the epidermis, the lesions show either one greatly dilated space or several interconnected dilated spaces filled with erythrocytes and lined by a single layer of flattened endothelial cells and a thin wall of fibrous tissue (73). In some instances, in place of fibrous tissue, there is a thin, irregular, noncontinuous, smooth muscle layer (74).

Principles of Management: Simple excision is the treatment of choice.

BENIGN TUMORS

Congenital Hemangiomas

The term *congenital hemangioma* was first proposed in 1996 to describe a group of hemangiomas that first appear in utero and that are fully developed at birth (75). These lesions were probably classified in the past as infantile hemangiomas (IHs), vascular malformations, and even cavernous hemangiomas. These congenital hemangiomas have been divided into rapidly involuting congenital hemangiomas (RICH) and noninvoluting congenital hemangiomas (NICH). Although they seem to represent distinctive clinicopathologic entities, there is some degree of overlap not only between RICH and NICH but also between RICH and IH (76). This means that accurate diagnosis usually relies on close clinicopathologic correlation. It is still controversial whether these lesions are pathogenetically interconnected, with some lesions described to begin as a RICH but failing to completely involute and persisting as NICH-like lesions (77). Interestingly, RICH and NICH express levels of insulin-like growth factor-2 mRNA at levels that are very similar to those expressed by IHs in children older than 4 years (78). VEGF receptor-1, however, is expressed at increasing levels in both RICH and NICH compared to IH. On a genetic level, congenital hemangiomas are associated with somatic activating mutations in *GNAQ* and *GNA11* (79).

Rapidly Involuting Congenital Hemangioma

Clinical Summary. RICH develops fully before birth and tends to regress during the first year of life. The tumor affects males and females equally and has a wide anatomic distribution with some predilection for the head and limbs (80,81). Some patients with RICH present with thrombocytopenia and coagulopathy early in the neonatal period (82). These alterations are mild, and patients do not progress to true Kasabach–Merritt syndrome.

Histopathology. Lesions are mainly subcutaneous and extend focally into the dermis. The architecture is lobular, and between tumor lobules there are often bands of fibrosis (Figs. 33-8 and 33-9) with focal inflammation, dystrophic calcification, and hemosiderin deposition. Lobules are composed of variably congested

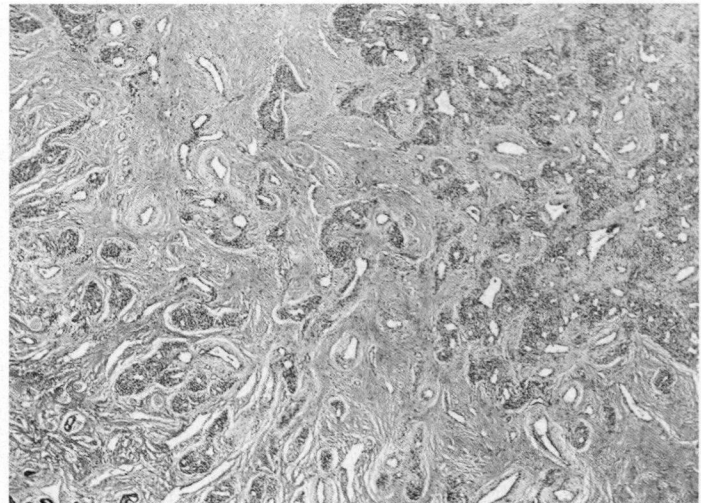

Figure 33-8 Rapidly involuting congenital hemangioma. Fibrous tissue is seen not only within individual tumor lobules but also between different tumor lobules. (Courtesy of H. Kozakevich, MD, Boston, MA.)

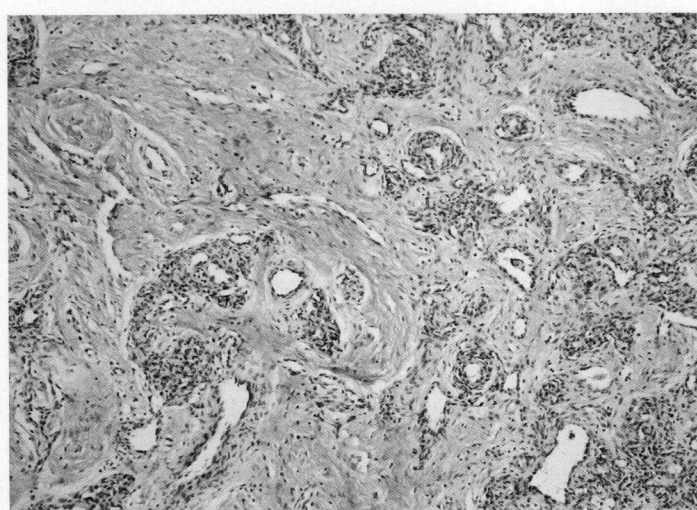

Figure 33-9 Rapidly involuting congenital hemangioma. Individual lobules are identical on high power to those seen in infantile hemangioma, but there is fibrosis with the lobules. (Courtesy of H. Kozakevich, MD, Boston, MA.)

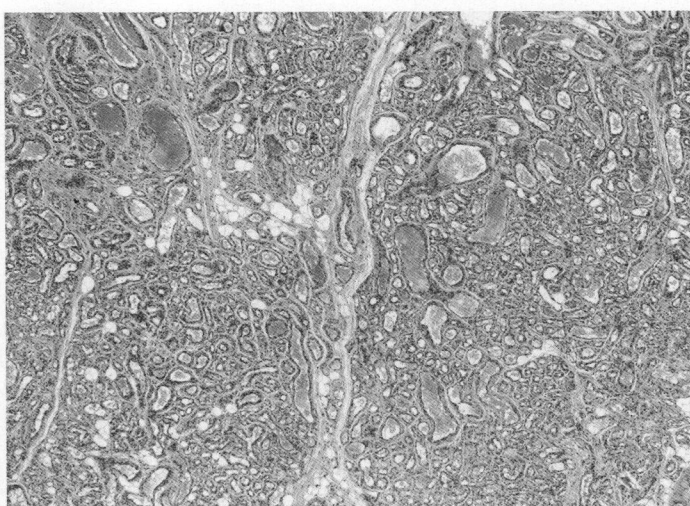

Figure 33-10 Noninvoluting congenital hemangioma. Tumor lobules vary more in size and contain many larger vascular channels.

capillaries, each of which is surrounded by a layer of pericytes. The overlying epidermis and adnexal structures usually appear atrophic. Larger vascular channels may be found in the fibrotic areas. Individual lobules may show variable fibrosis. Extramedullary hemopoiesis may be seen, and perineural extension is absent. GLUT-1 staining is usually negative in tumor lobules. However, in rare cases, focal positivity may be present.

Differential Diagnosis. This is discussed later, under NICH.

Principles of Management: Tumors usually regress spontaneously. In large lesions or those that affect vital organs, various treatment modalities have been attempted, including embolization, surgical excision, and systemic steroids. Propanolol is usually not effective.

Noninvoluting Congenital Hemangioma

Clinical Summary. NICH is fully developed at birth but shows no signs of regression, and it progresses over time (83). There is an equal sex incidence, and although anatomic distribution is wide, there is predilection for the head and limbs.

Histopathology. Vascular lobules tend to be large and are often composed of capillaries and larger, sometimes thicker blood vessels (Fig. 33-10). Draining larger blood vessels are present in tumor lobules. Surrounding the latter, there are areas of fibrosis containing large blood vessels with features of veins and arteries. Arteriovenous fistulas are also identified, and this closely mimics arteriovenous malformations. Histologic distinction can be very difficult, and close clinicopathologic correlation is often necessary. As opposed to vascular malformations, NICH does not tend to recur. GLUT-1 staining is usually negative.

Differential Diagnosis. The main differential diagnosis of RICH and NICH is IH. The latter typically develops shortly after birth, grows rapidly during the first year of life, and tends to involute over a period of several years. The lobules of RICH and IH are often identical, and it has been proposed that distinction between both is based mainly in the presence of bands of fibrosis around tumor lobules, presence of atrophy of adnexal structures and epidermis, and lack of GLUT-1 positivity in the

former. In practice, however, and especially in small biopsies, distinction may be very difficult, and clinicopathologic correlation is paramount. Staining for GLUT-1, the human erythrocyte glucose transporter, is particularly helpful, because IH tends to be diffusely positive for this marker (84), whereas RICH is usually negative, and if positive, the positivity tends to be focal. Distinction between IH and NICH is easier, because the latter tends to display more variability in the size of vascular channels, GLUT-1 staining is usually negative, and arteriovenous fistulas are identified. The main problem with the diagnosis of NICH, RICH, and IH is that there is some degree of overlap between the three entities, as demonstrated by the fact that IH may coexist with either RICH or NICH. The problem is further compounded by the fact that some cases of RICH fail to involute completely and behave more like NICH (so-called PICH). In such cases, the histologic appearances overlap with those of RICH and NICH. At present, the pathogenetic relation between these groups of lesions remains obscure. Distinction between NICH and vascular malformations may be difficult. Radiologic studies are often helpful, and NICH, RICH, and IH are positive for WT1, whereas vascular malformations, particularly those that are arteriovenous in nature, tend to be negative for this marker (85).

Principles of Management: Lesions do not usually respond to medical treatment. Surgery is the treatment of choice but may be difficult in large tumors. Embolization may be used in large tumors involving vital structures.

Capillary Hemangioma Variants

Infantile Hemangioma (Strawberry Nevus, Juvenile Hemangioendothelioma, Juvenile Hemangioma)

Clinical Summary. Infantile capillary hemangioma, mostly represented by strawberry nevus, constitutes the most common vascular tumor of infancy, affecting as many as 1 in every 100 live births. Overall, it comprises between 32% and 42% of all vascular tumors (86). Lesions first appear usually between the third and the fifth weeks of life, increase in size for several months to 1 year, and then start to regress. A typical lesion consists of one or several bright red, soft, lobulated tumors that vary greatly in size and have a wide anatomic distribution with a predilection for the head and neck area. Females are slightly more affected than males. On occasion, lesions can involve deeper soft tissues or even internal organs and can be associated with high morbidity, especially if located near vital structures. Complete spontaneous resolution is common, occurring in about 70% of capillary hemangiomas by the time the patient has reached the age of 7 years.

Contrary to what was believed in the past, capillary hemangiomas are not associated with Kasabach–Merritt syndrome. This syndrome, consisting of thrombocytopenia, microangiopathic hemolytic anemia, and acute or chronic consumption coagulopathy, is seen mainly with kaposiform hemangioendothelioma (usually a subcutaneous lesion, see p. 1237) and less commonly with cavernous hemangiomas (see p. 1232) and tufted angioma (see p. 1229).

Histopathology. All tumors have a lobular architecture (Fig. 33-11), but microscopic features change as the lesion evolves. During their period of growth in early infancy, capillary hemangiomas show considerable proliferation of their endothelial cells. The endothelial cells are large, mitotically active, and aggregated, predominantly in solid strands and masses in which there are only a few small capillary lumina. Not uncommonly, crystalline intracytoplasmic inclusions can be seen in the endothelial cells. The lumina can be highlighted with the use of a reticulin stain. In maturing lesions, the capillary lumina are wider, and the lining endothelial cells then appear flatter (Fig. 33-12). In mature lesions, some of the lumina may be greatly dilated, focally resembling a cavernous hemangioma. In the involuting phase, there is progressive fibrosis with disappearance of the blood vessels. The vascular nature of the tumor may then be difficult to establish. However, the lobular pattern is often preserved. A worrying but entirely benign feature seen in a number of capillary hemangiomas is the presence of perineural invasion (87).

Pathogenesis. Ultrastructural and immunohistochemical studies of capillary hemangiomas have demonstrated that tumors show remarkable cellular heterogeneity. A large proportion of the cells in a given tumor are endothelial cells and pericytes, but fibroblasts and mast cells are also present (88). A complex interaction among these cell populations may modulate

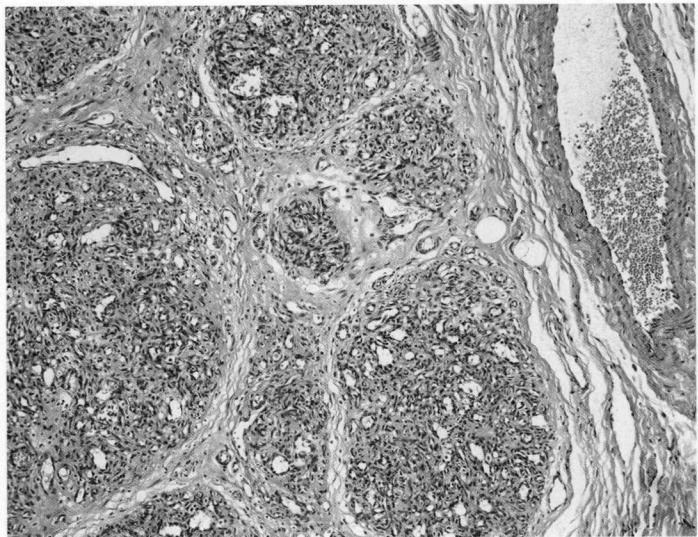

Figure 33-12 Infantile hemangioma. Mature lesion with well-formed canalized capillaries and a neighboring feeding vessel.

the progression and latter evolution of capillary hemangiomas (89). Juvenile hemangiomas share the same unique phenotype with human placenta (89). Immunohistochemical staining for GLUT-1 uniformly stains endothelial cells in IH (84). Gene expression analysis of these tumors has shown that their features are those of a pro-proliferative cell type with altered adhesive properties as compared to endothelial cells of the normal dermal microvasculature (90).

Differential Diagnosis. Distinction between IH and RICH and NICH is discussed in *Differential Diagnosis* in the section Noninvoluting Congenital Hemangioma.

Principles of Management: Oral β-blockers, mainly propranolol, are used in IHs both in the proliferative and in the nonproliferative stages, but they are more successful in the former (91). The effect of β-blockers may be explained by the expression of high levels of $β_2$-adrenoreceptors in these tumors (92). Topical β-blockers have been tried in small and superficial noncomplicated lesions (93).

Cherry Hemangioma (Senile Angioma, Campbell de Morgan Spot)

Clinical Summary. Cherry hemangiomas are bright red lesions varying in size from a hardly visible punctum to a soft, raised, dome-shaped lesion measuring several millimeters in diameter. This very common lesion, often present in large numbers, may start appearing in early adulthood, and the number of lesions increases with age. Cherry hemangiomas may occur anywhere on the skin, but the trunk and the upper limbs are the most common sites.

Histopathology. In the early stage of development, cherry hemangiomas have the appearance of true capillary hemangiomas, being composed of numerous newly formed capillaries with narrow lumina and prominent endothelial cells arranged in a lobular fashion in the subpapillary region. As the lesion ages, the capillaries become dilated. In a fully mature cherry hemangioma, numerous moderately dilated capillaries lined by flattened endothelial cells are observed. The intercapillary stroma shows edema and homogenization of the collagen.

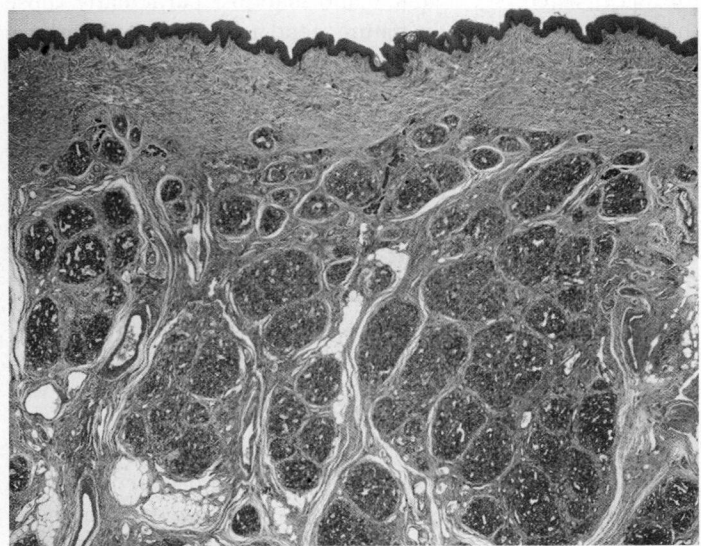

Figure 33-11 Infantile hemangioma. Involvement of the dermis and subcutis by multiple lobules composed of capillaries.

The epidermis is thinned and often surrounds most of the angioma as a collarette.

Pathogenesis. *GNA14/GNAQ/GNA11* mutations are present in most lesions (94).

Differential Diagnosis. In its early stage, cherry hemangioma, like granuloma pyogenicum, shows capillary proliferation; however, endothelial proliferation is much less pronounced than in granuloma pyogenicum, and thus solid aggregates of endothelial cells are not seen.

Principles of Management: Simple excision, if desired.

Tufted Hemangioma (Tufted Angioma, Angioblastoma)

Clinical Summary. Tufted hemangioma is a benign angiomatous condition that can be regarded as identical to the angioblastoma reported by Japanese authors (95) and part of the spectrum of kaposiform hemangioendothelioma. The angiomas affect the genders equally, usually arising between the ages of 1 and 5 years (96–98); occasionally, the lesions are present at birth (99,100), but they may develop in adults or even in old age (101). There are exceptional instances of angiomas arising in pregnancy (102), expressing estrogen and progesterone receptors, with regression after pregnancy, the occurrence in several members of a family (103), and the development of lesions in association with liver disease (105). The most common sites for the angiomatous papules and plaques are the upper trunk, neck, and proximal part of the limbs. Exceptionally, presentation may be in the oral cavity (105). The lesions usually slowly progress for several years and can eventually cover wide segments of the body; some are tender on palpation, and rare lesions regress (106). In rare cases, hypertrichosis may be seen in the skin overlying the lesion. Low-grade coagulopathy and Kasabach–Merritt syndrome are rare associations (107–109).

Histopathology. Circumscribed foci of closely set capillaries are found scattered through the dermis and occasionally reach the subcutis. At lower magnification, these discrete, ovoid angiomatous lobules or tufts have been alluded to as giving rise to a "cannonball" appearance (Fig. 33-13). The vascular nature of the tufts may not be immediately apparent, because vascular lumina are compressed by enlarged endothelial cells and contain few red blood cells. Some of the vascular tufts appear to indent lymphatic-like channels (Figs. 33-14 and 33-15). Mitotic activity and cell atypia are insignificant.

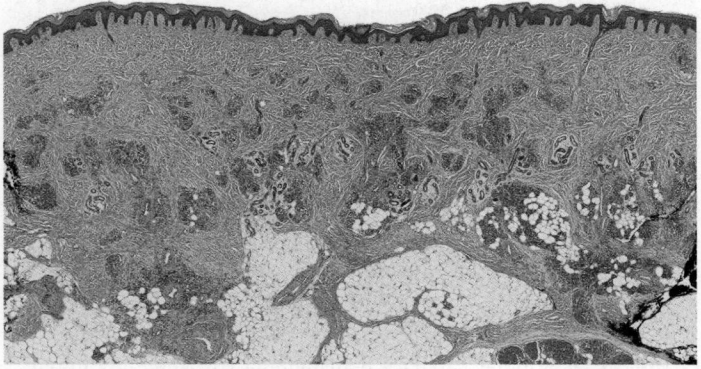

Figure 33-13 Tufted angioma. Scattered, round, or ovoid dermal lobules in a typical "cannonball" distribution.

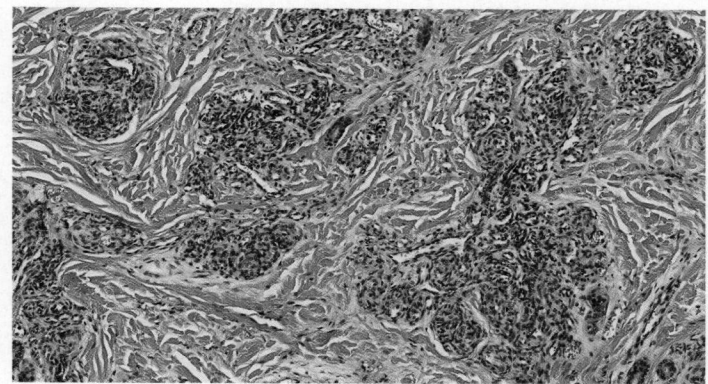

Figure 33-14 Tufted angioma. Lobule composed of bloodless capillaries surrounded by dilated crescent-shaped vascular channels.

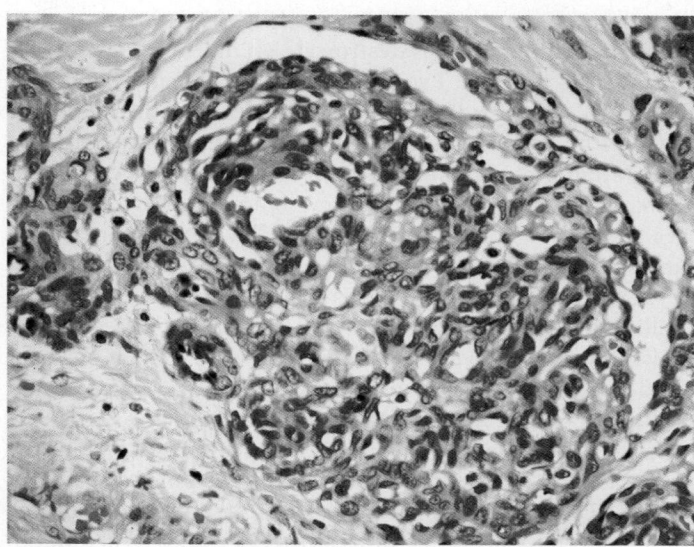

Figure 33-15 Tufted angioma. Often, the capillaries appear poorly canalized, and pericytes are prominent.

The presence of strong labeling for actin indicates a prominent pericytic component among the tumor capillaries.

Pathogenesis. *GNA14* somatic mutation is present in tufted hemangiomas (110).

Differential Diagnosis. The main importance of this uncommon angioma, especially if it develops in adults, is the differential diagnosis from Kaposi sarcoma or, possibly, a low-grade angiosarcoma. Endothelial cells in tufted angioma may show slight spindling but not the elongated spindle cells of Kaposi sarcoma. The discrete focal arrangement of vascular tufts having few red blood cells also differs greatly from the mature lesions of Kaposi sarcoma. The absence of cell atypia is the main distinguishing feature from angiosarcoma.

The hypertrophic cellular appearance of the tufts is similar to the angiomatous tissue in IH, but the vascular aggregates are far more massive in the latter, where they tend to replace wide segments of the dermis and fat.

It is likely that tufted angioma and kaposiform hemangioendothelioma are part of the same spectrum (111). Morphologic overlap is often seen, and their relationship appears to be supported by a similar immunohistochemical profile: the spindle cells in both neoplasms are positive for Prox1, podoplanin,

LYVE-1, CD31, and CD34, whereas the cells within the tufts are negative for Prox1, podoplanin, and LYVE-1 and positive for CD31 and CD34 (112).

Principles of Management: Surgical excision may be performed in small lesions. In cases associated with Kasabach–Merritt syndrome, different treatment modalities have been reported, including vincristine (with or without embolization) (107), systemic steroids, and even propranolol. The latter has shown only very limited response (113).

Pyogenic Granuloma (Lobular Capillary Hemangioma)

Clinical Summary. Pyogenic granuloma, or lobular capillary hemangioma, is a common proliferative lesion that is often related to trauma. Typically, the lesion grows rapidly for a few weeks before stabilizing as an elevated, bright red papule, usually not more than 1 to 2 cm in size (Fig. 33-16); it may then persist indefinitely unless destroyed. Recurrence after surgery or cautery is not rare. Pyogenic granuloma most often affects children or young adults of either gender, but the age range is wide; the hands, fingers, and face, especially the lips and gums, are the most common sites (114,115). Pyogenic granuloma of the gingiva in pregnancy (epulis of pregnancy) is a special subgroup. Lesions may rarely develop within a port-wine stain.

A rare and alarming event is the development of multiple satellite angiomatous lesions at and around the site of a previously destroyed pyogenic granuloma (116,117). This usually occurs following lesions on the shoulder or upper trunk in children. Histologically, lesions that are similar to pyogenic granuloma can occur in the deep dermis, the subcutaneous tissue (118), and even within dilated venous channels (119,120). Widely scattered angiomatous lesions resembling pyogenic granulomas have also been described (121–123), sometimes in association with visceral disease.

Histopathology. The typical lesion presents as a polypoid mass of angiomatous tissue protruding above the surrounding skin. It is often constricted at its base by a collarette of acanthotic epidermis (Fig. 33-17). An intact, flattened epidermis may cover the entire lesion, but surface erosions are common. In ulcerated lesions, a superficial inflammatory cell reaction can give rise to an appearance suggestive of granulation tissue, but inflammation does not appear to be an intrinsic feature. Inflammation is usually slight in the deeper part of the lesion and may be absent when the epidermis is intact. The angiomatous tissue tends to occur in discrete masses or lobules, resembling a capillary hemangioma—hence, the preference by Mills and associates (114) for the term *lobular capillary hemangioma* to describe this condition (Fig. 33-18). The angiomatous tissue is surrounded by myxoid stroma containing scattered spindle- and stellate-shaped connective tissue cells and occasional mast cells. The angiomatous tissue is composed of a variably dilated network of blood-filled capillary vessels and groups of poorly canalized vascular tufts. Mitotic activity varies and can be prominent. Feeding vessels often extend into the adjacent dermis, and rare lesions show a deep component in the reticular dermis. Occasionally, foci of intravascular papillary endothelial hyperplasia occur within the larger deep vessels. Focal epithelioid

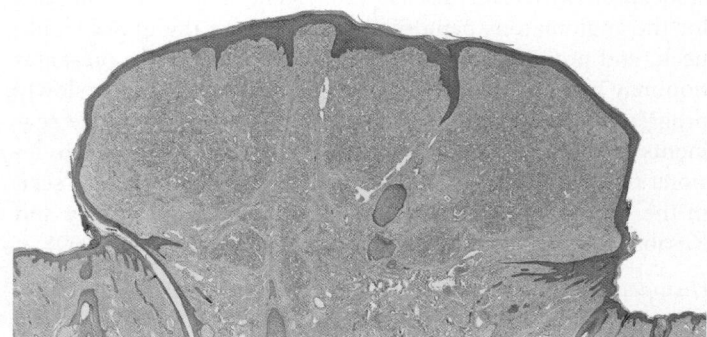

Figure 33-17 Lobular capillary hemangioma (pyogenic granuloma). Early, nonulcerated lesion with the typical epithelial collarette.

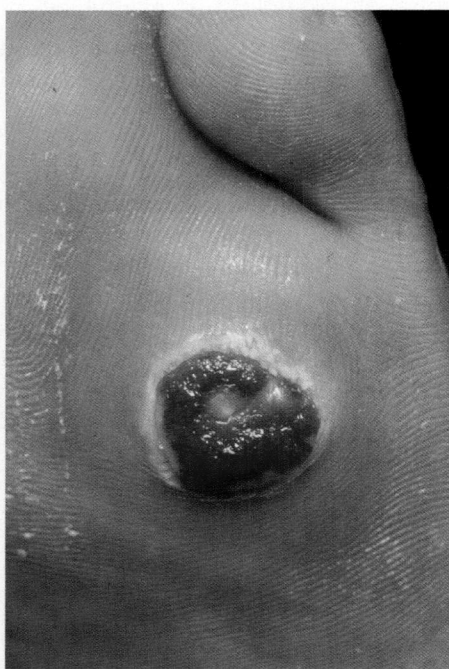

Figure 33-16 Lobular capillary hemangioma (pyogenic granuloma). Ulcerated, polypoid papular lesion.

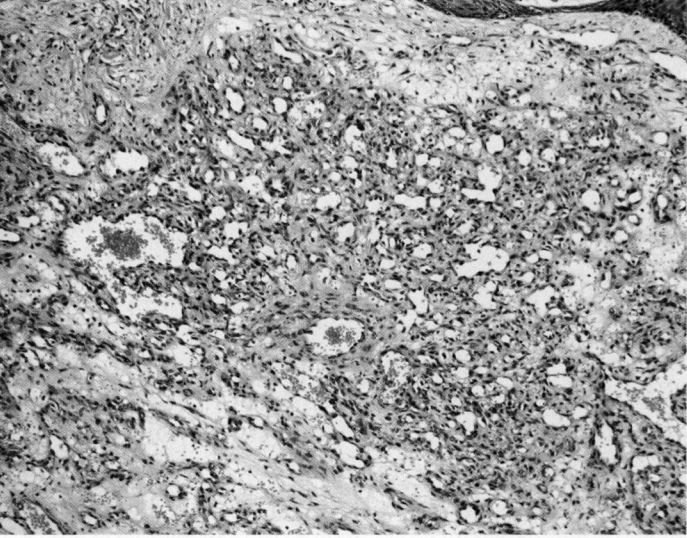

Figure 33-18 Lobular capillary hemangioma (pyogenic granuloma). Distinctive lobules of dilated and congested capillaries in an edematous stroma.

endothelial cells can sometimes be seen. Focal cytologic atypia may be present, particularly in lesions arising in mucosal surfaces such as the mouth (124). The histology of recurrent or satellite lesions is similar, but the angiomatous proliferation can extend more deeply into the dermis. Pyogenic granulomas of the subcutaneous tissue or in veins show similar histologic features but lack an inflammatory component. Intravascular lesions can so distend the veins that the surrounding muscle coat can be thinned and difficult to detect (Fig. 33-19).

Pathogenesis. It was once assumed that granuloma pyogenicum was caused by pyogenic infection. However, the histologic picture of early lesions suggests a capillary hemangioma, and even in eroded lesions that show inflammation, the appearance mimics that of a capillary hemangioma in its deeper portions. Therefore, the term *lobular capillary hemangioma* has been suggested (114). Immunohistochemical studies demonstrate positive labeling of endothelial cells for vascular markers, including CD3 and ERG and also of pericytes for smooth muscle actin. *BRAF* and *RAS* mutations have been identified as a driver of, particularly, secondary pyogenic granuloma (125).

Differential Diagnosis. Both Kaposi sarcoma and angiosarcoma should be considered as part of the differential diagnosis, especially when multiple lesions are present. Elevated polypoid lesions are rare in Kaposi sarcoma; most show obvious spindle cells woven between delicate vascular spaces, unlike in pyogenic granuloma. A much greater degree of cell atypia with intraluminal spreading of malignant cells characterizes well-differentiated angiosarcomas. Focal areas of intravascular papillary endothelial hyperplasia within a pyogenic granuloma can occasionally simulate angiosarcoma, but, even so, nuclear atypia is slight.

A further differential diagnosis of pyogenic granuloma is with bacillary angiomatosis, an infectious, vascular proliferation seen in HIV-infected and immunocompromised patients and caused by *Bartonella henselae* or, less commonly, by *Bartonella quintana*, which are small, gram-negative rods belonging to the family Bartonellaceae (126–128) (see Chapter 21). Bacillary angiomatosis is now rarely seen in the developed countries, because HIV-positive patients are treated with highly active antiretroviral therapy (HAART) and with prophylactic antibiotics. Clinically, and especially histologically, lesions of bacillary angiomatosis can look remarkably similar to a pyogenic granuloma. The low-power architecture in superficial lesions may be almost identical to that seen in pyogenic granuloma (Fig. 33-20). In bacillary angiomatosis, however, the endothelial cells often have abundant pale cytoplasm (Fig. 33-21), and aggregates of neutrophils are present throughout the lesion, often in relation to clumps of granular basophilic material. This basophilic material shows bacilli when stained with Warthin–Starry (Fig. 33-22) or Giemsa stains. The presence of the organism may also be detected by PCR.

Vascular granulomatous lesions mimicking pyogenic granulomas occasionally arise as a complication of retinoid therapy,

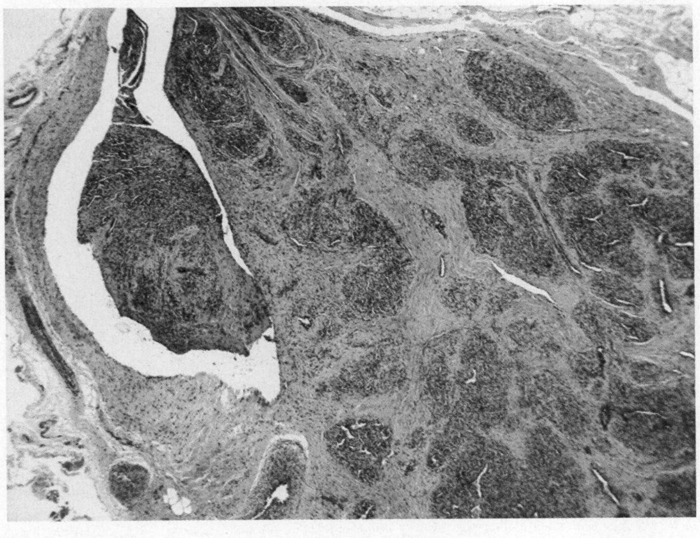

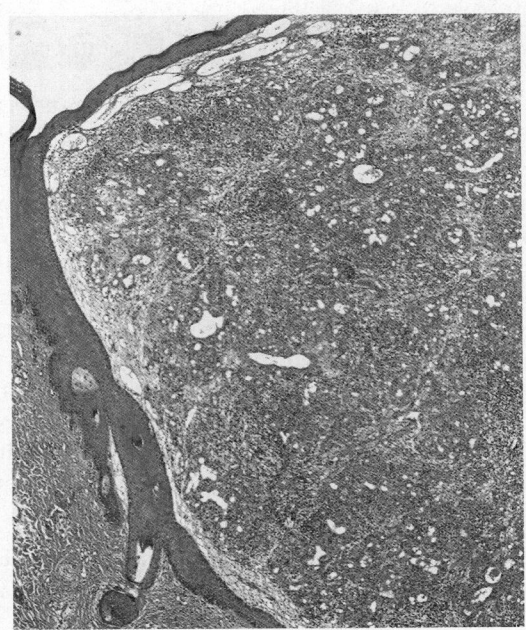

Figure 33-20 Bacillary angiomatosis. Similar low-power architecture to lobular capillary hemangioma, but there is more prominent inflammation in the background.

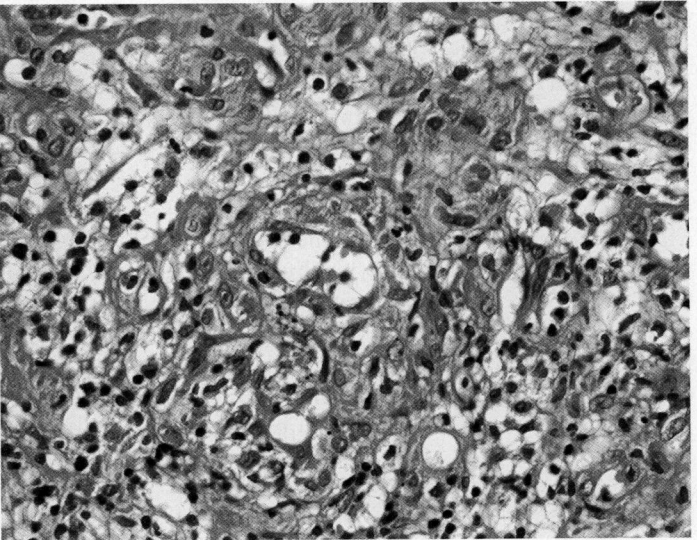

Figure 33-21 Bacillary angiomatosis. The vascular channels are lined by pale epithelioid endothelial cells. Often, neutrophils with nuclear dust are seen in the surrounding stroma.

Figure 33-19 Intravascular lobular capillary hemangioma (pyogenic granuloma). Some cases occur entirely in an intravenous location.

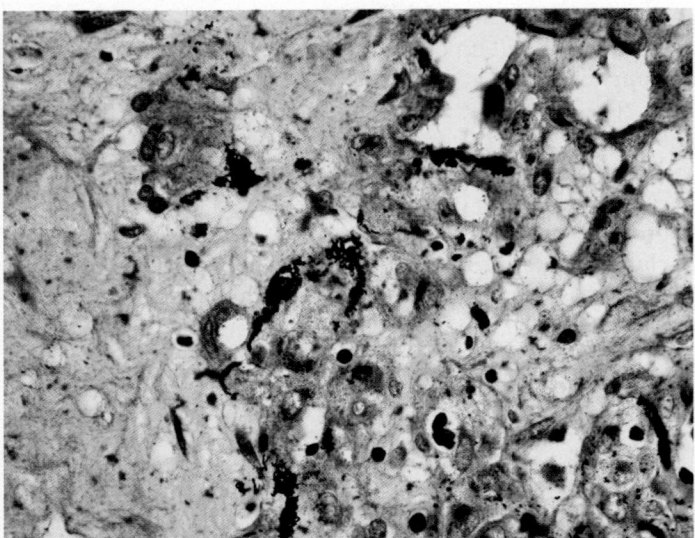

Figure 33-22 Bacillary angiomatosis. Warthin–Starry stain showing numerous clumps of bacilli.

BRAF inhibitors, anti-TNF alpha therapy, and other systemic medications, but the histology is that of nonspecific vascular granulation tissue lacking a lobular architecture (129–132).

Distinction from a nodular lesion of orf or milker's nodule may be difficult, because the low-power architecture may resemble a lobular capillary hemangioma. However, in the former, there is often prominent hyperplasia of the epidermis and the infundibular portion of the hair follicles. The prominent vascular component represents granulation tissue with only a focal lobular architecture, and the keratinocytes often show typical viral inclusions.

Principles of Management: Surgical excision is the treatment of choice. Most lesions are incompletely removed by a shave biopsy, and local recurrence may occur.

Cavernous Hemangioma

Clinical Summary. Sharing with IH the same age, gender, and anatomic distribution, cavernous hemangioma is still less common and tends to be larger, deeper, and less well defined than the former and shows no tendency for spontaneous regression. Rare cavernous hemangiomas may be associated with an overlying capillary hemangioma. There are two rare conditions in which numerous cavernous hemangiomas occur: Maffucci syndrome and the blue rubber bleb nevus.

Maffucci Syndrome

Clinical Summary. The outstanding features of Maffucci syndrome are dyschondroplasia resulting in defects in ossification; fragility of the bones, causing severe deformities; and osteochondromas, which may develop into chondrosarcomas (133). In addition, large, compressible subcutaneous cavernous hemangiomas and spindle cell hemangiomas (SCHs) (see p. 1240) may be present at birth or appear in childhood or early adulthood.

Histopathology. See next section.

Blue Rubber Bleb Nevus

Clinical Summary. In the blue rubber bleb nevus, cavernous hemangiomas are present at birth but may subsequently increase in size and number. The hemangiomas have a distinct appearance, and most of them are protuberant, dark blue, soft, and compressible; some are pedunculated. They vary from a few millimeters to 3 cm in diameter. In addition, subcutaneous hemangiomas are felt on palpation. There are also hemangiomas in the oral mucosa, the gastrointestinal tract, and, less commonly, in other organs (134). Gastrointestinal bleeding from multiple hemangiomas causes severe chronic anemia, which may leave many patients dependent on lifelong blood transfusions. Some blue rubber bleb nevi are probably telangiectatic glomangiomas in which the glomus cells are sparse.

Histopathology. Cavernous hemangiomas appear in the lower dermis and the subcutaneous tissue with large, irregular spaces containing red blood cells and fibrinous material (Fig. 33-23). The spaces are lined by a single layer of bland endothelial cells. Not uncommonly, a capillary component is present, especially in the superficial portion of a tumor. Dystrophic calcification is often present.

Variant of Cavernous Hemangioma: Sinusoidal Hemangioma

Clinical Summary. Sinusoidal hemangioma is a relatively rare variant of cavernous hemangioma (135). The lesion presents as a bluish subcutaneous mass, especially in middle-aged adults, and has a predilection for females. Although the anatomic distribution is wide, tumors often present in the breast, and in this setting, angiosarcoma is considered in the differential diagnosis.

Histopathology. Sinusoidal hemangioma is lobular and focally ill-defined with partial or total replacement of subcutaneous fat lobules. The typical feature is the presence of gaping, markedly dilated and congested, thin-walled, back-to-back vascular spaces in a sievelike or sinusoidal arrangement (Fig. 33-24). Pseudopapillary structures attributable to cross-sectioning of these spaces focally resemble intravascular papillary endothelial hyperplasia (Fig. 33-25). The vascular channels are lined by bland, flat endothelial cells, which can be focally prominent and mildly pleomorphic. Thrombosis, hyalinization, dystrophic calcification, and even areas of infarction can be seen in older

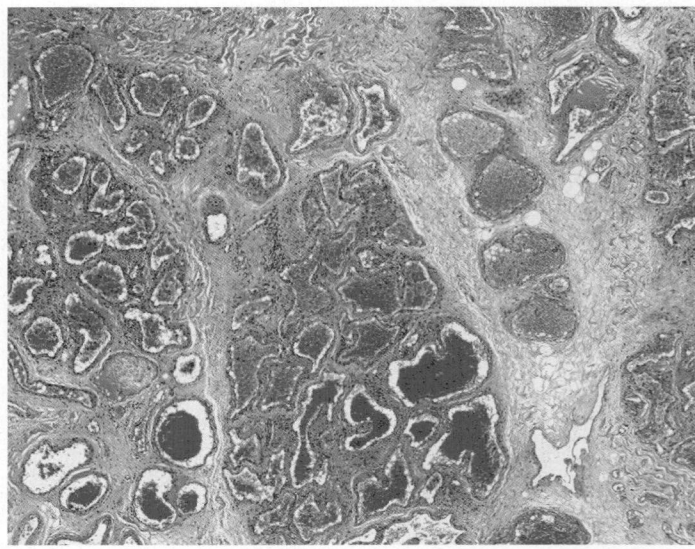

Figure 33-23 Cavernous hemangioma. Markedly dilated and congested vascular spaces.

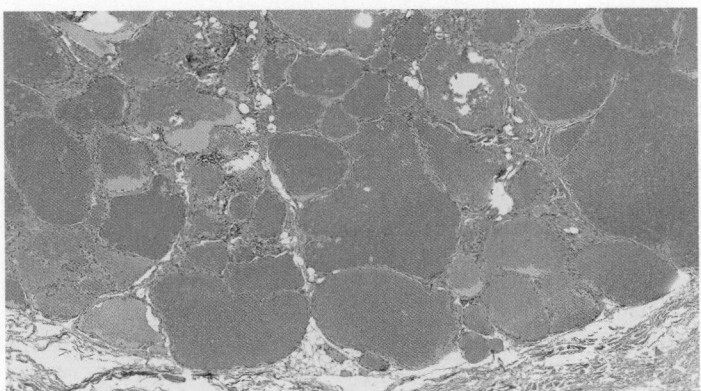

Figure 33-24 Sinusoidal hemangioma. Congested anastomosing vascular channels with a sievelike appearance.

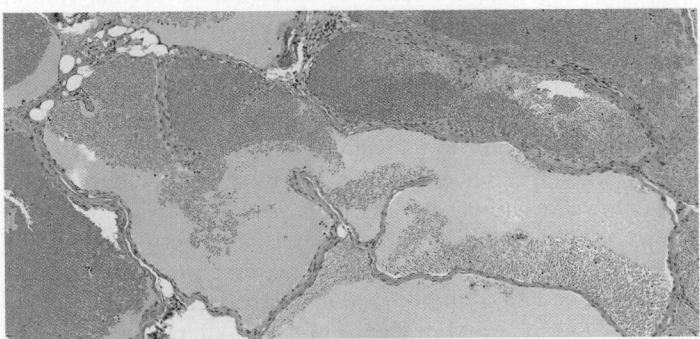

Figure 33-25 Sinusoidal hemangioma. Higher magnification reveals a typical sinusoidal appearance.

lesions. Distinction from a well-differentiated angiosarcoma is based on the presence in the latter of an infiltrative growth pattern, cytologic atypia, and multilayering. In breast lesions, it is worth remembering that mammary angiosarcomas are always intraparenchymal.

Principles of Management: Simple excision is the treatment of choice. Oral sirolimus has been used successfully in the control of blue rubber bleb nevus syndrome (136).

Verrucous Venous Malformation (Verrucous Hemangioma)

Clinical Summary. Verrucous venous malformation is a rare form of vascular malformation that is usually congenital and only rarely presents later in life. Most cases present as wartlike, dark blue papules or nodules, with a special predilection for the distal lower limbs (Fig. 33-26). Although most cases are solitary, an exceptional case with multiple lesions on different parts of the body has been reported (137). Often, cases are confused clinically and histologically with angiokeratomas, but verrucous hemangiomas always have a deep component, and recurrence after incomplete excision occurs in up to one-third of cases (138). A somatic *MAP3K3* mutation is associated with this condition (139).

In *Cobb syndrome*, a lesion identical to a verrucous hemangioma presents on the trunk with a dermatomal distribution and in association with an underlying meningospinal hemangioma (140). Some cases of Cobb syndrome present in association with a port-wine stain.

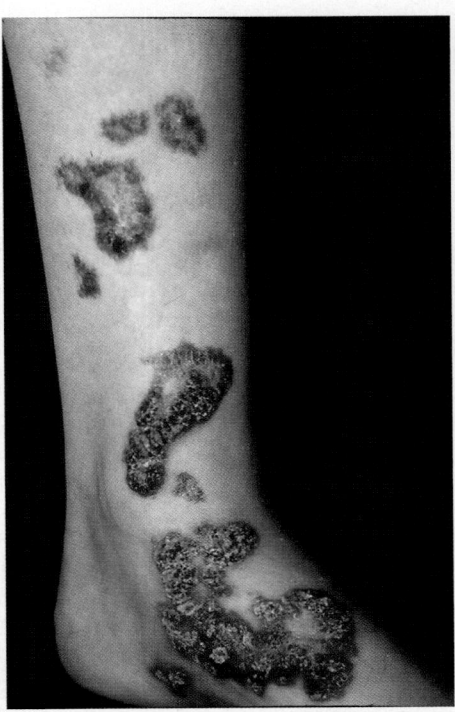

Figure 33-26 Verrucous venous malformation. Verrucous vascular plaques are typically seen.

Histopathology. The superficial portion of a verrucous hemangioma is indistinguishable from an angiokeratoma. However, a combination of congested capillaries and cavernous-like vascular spaces is seen extending into the deep dermis and subcutaneous tissue (Fig. 33-27). These vascular spaces are lined by flattened endothelial cells and are usually surrounded by a layer of pericytes. A lobular growth pattern is often apparent in the deep component.

Principles of Management: Surgical excision is curative only if the deep component is completely removed.

Microvenular Hemangioma

Clinical Summary. This is a relatively rare, acquired vascular lesion that usually arises as a small, reddish lesion in young to middle-aged individuals of either gender (141,142). The arms,

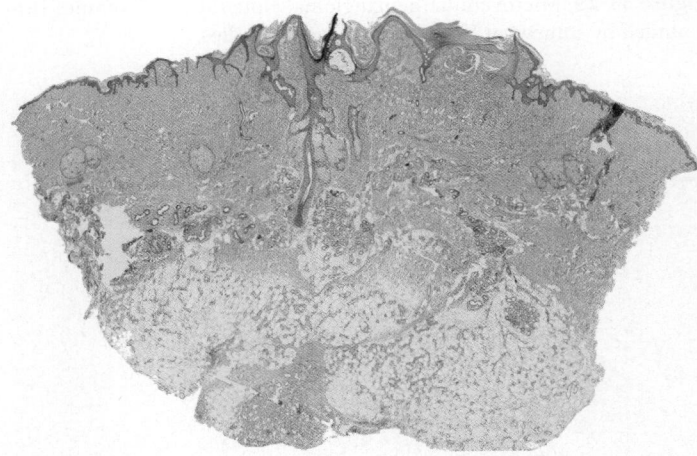

Figure 33-27 Verrucous venous malformation. Note the superficial component similar to angiokeratoma but with a deep component extending to the subcutaneous tissue.

trunk, and legs are favored sites. Multiple lesions are exceptionally seen (143).

Histopathology. Histologically, thin, branching capillaries and small venules with narrow or slightly dilated lumina are found widely throughout the dermis (Fig. 33-28). There is no obvious endothelial cell atypia or accompanying inflammation, but slight dermal sclerosis is often present (Fig. 33-29). The collagen bundles around the vascular channels appear somewhat sclerotic. A fairly constant feature in many cases is the prominent infiltration of arrector pili muscles by the proliferating vascular channels (Fig. 33-30).

Differential Diagnosis. The importance of microvenular hemangioma as an acquired vascular anomaly in young patients lies

in the differential diagnosis from an early or macular lesion of Kaposi sarcoma. The lymphangioma-like channels of Kaposi sarcoma are more delicate, do not contain erythrocytes, show angulated outlines, and tend to wrap around collagen bundles. Furthermore, plasma cells and other inflammatory cells are common in Kaposi sarcoma but not in microvenular hemangioma. HHV-8 is consistently positive in Kaposi sarcoma and negative in microvenular hemangioma. Only a single case of HHV-8-positive microvenular hemangioma in a patient with POEMS syndrome has been reported (144).

Principles of Management: Simple excision is the treatment of choice.

Hobnail Hemangioma (Targetoid Hemosiderotic Hemangioma)

Clinical Summary. Hobnail hemangioma, or targetoid hemosiderotic hemangioma, is a relatively uncommon vascular tumor, likely a superficial lymphatic malformation that usually presents in the trunk or extremities of young or middle-aged adults with a male predominance (145–147). Rare cases occur in the oral mucosa and in children. Multiple lesions are exceptional. The descriptive name initially given to this tumor reflects a typical clinical appearance characterized by a small solitary lesion consisting of a brown to violaceous papule, 2 to 3 mm in diameter, surrounded by a thin, pale area and a peripheral ecchymotic ring. However, these features are present only in a small percentage of cases, and most often the clinical appearance is that of a red-blue or brown papule. The alternative name of *hobnail hemangioma*, which emphasizes a more constant special histologic feature, has therefore been proposed (see text following). Interestingly, some lesions in females change during the menstrual cycle, suggesting that there is a direct hormonal influence (148).

Histopathology. In the superficial reticular dermis, there are thin-walled, dilated, and irregular vascular spaces (Fig. 33-31) often lined by bland endothelial cells with scanty cytoplasm and rounded nuclei that protrude into the lumina and closely resemble hobnails (Figs. 33-32 and 33-33). Intraluminal papillary projections and fibrin thrombi can be seen in the superficial blood vessels (Fig. 33-33). The vascular channels in the deeper dermis become much less conspicuous and eventually

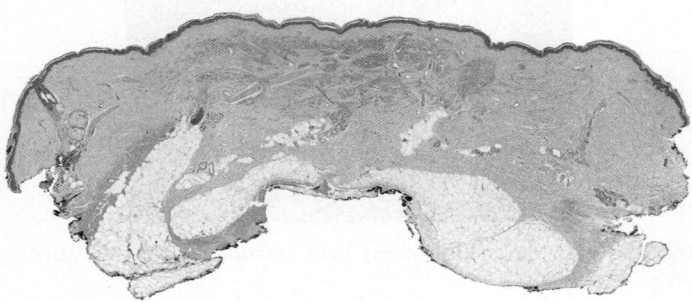

Figure 33-28 Microvenular hemangioma. Irregular, branching, thin-walled venules within the dermis.

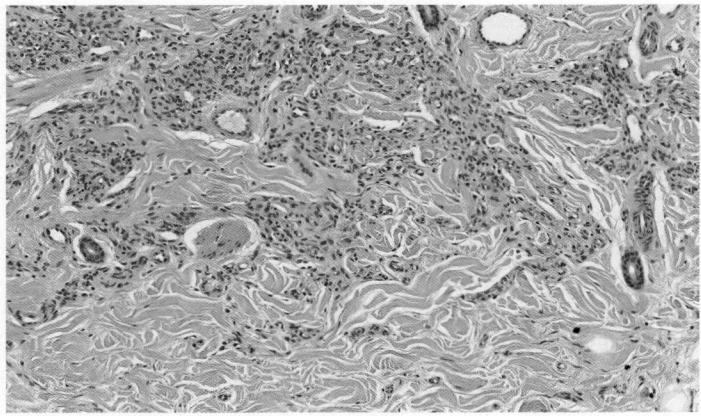

Figure 33-29 Microvenular hemangioma. Note the small venules surrounded by somewhat hyalinized collagen bundles.

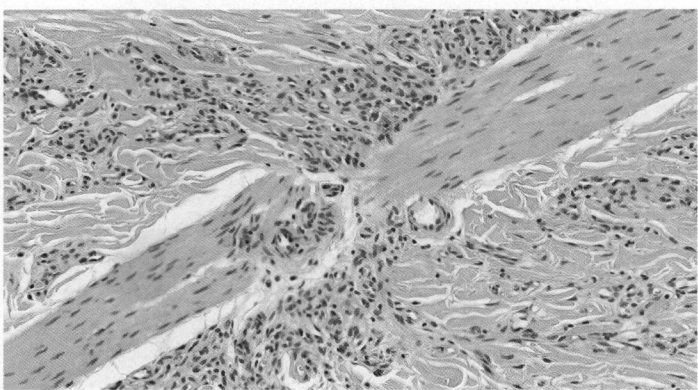

Figure 33-30 Microvenular hemangioma. Prominent infiltration of the arrector pili muscle.

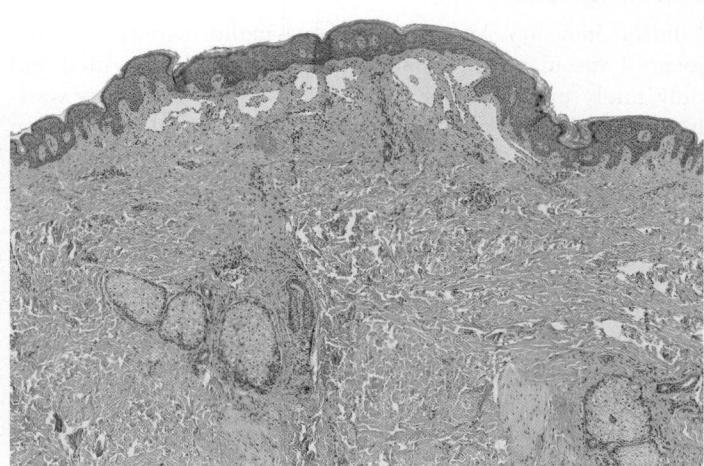

Figure 33-31 Hobnail hemangioma. Typical wedge-shaped architecture with a prominent superficial component.

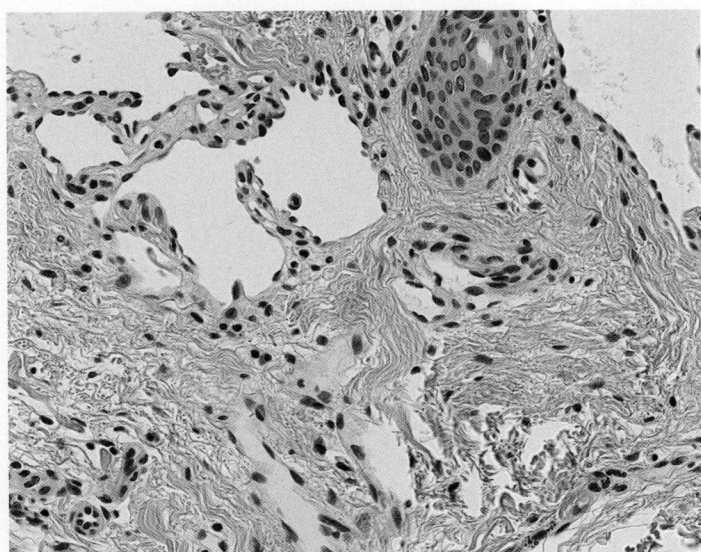

Figure 33-32 Hobnail hemangioma. Irregular congested vascular channels, some of which are lined by hobnail endothelial cells.

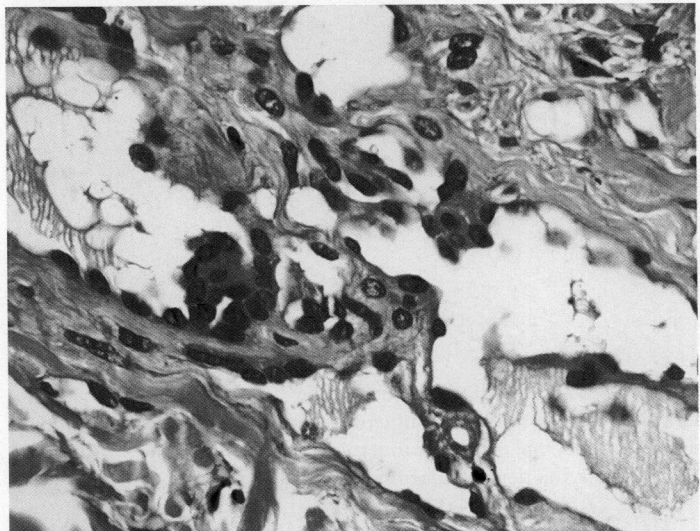

Figure 33-33 Hobnail hemangioma. Hobnail endothelial cells and small papillary projections.

disappear completely. These deeper channels are irregular and angulated, lined by flattened endothelial cells, and dissect between collagen bundles. Extensive red blood cell extravasation and inflammatory aggregates predominantly of lymphocytes are seen. In a later stage, extensive stromal hemosiderin deposition is commonly seen.

Pathogenesis. Because there is a family of vascular tumors characterized by epithelioid endothelial cells, it has been proposed that this tumor represents the benign end of the spectrum of a group of vascular tumors characterized by hobnail endothelial cells that includes *papillary intralymphatic angioendothelioma (PILA, Dabska tumor)* and *retiform hemangioendothelioma* (see p. 1247). The endothelial cells are positive for D2-40 (podoplanin), suggesting a lymphatic line of differentiation (149). These cells are negative for WT1, and on the basis of this finding it has been proposed that the lesion represents a lymphatic malformation (149).

Differential Diagnosis. This includes patch-stage Kaposi sarcoma, retiform hemangioendothelioma, and benign lymphangioendothelioma (see p. 1257).

Principles of Management: Simple excision is the treatment of choice.

Epithelioid Hemangioma (Angiolymphoid Hyperplasia with Eosinophilia)

The terms *epithelioid hemangioma* and *angiolymphoid hyperplasia with eosinophilia* highlight the controversy about whether this entity represents a vascular neoplasm or a reactive process consequent to trauma or some other stimulus. Previously, lesions included within this group were referred to as *histiocytoid hemangiomas*, but this name has been abandoned because, as originally proposed, it included other entities that do not qualify as epithelioid hemangioma (150,151). It was thought that the entity might represent a reactive proliferation secondary to diverse stimuli, but studies have shown a number of gene rearrangements indicating clonal origin (see later) (152). Therefore, the term *epithelioid hemangioma* is generally preferred to encompass vascular lesions at the benign end of the spectrum of conditions characterized by endothelial cells that have an epithelioid morphology.

Clinical Summary. Most lesions arise either superficially in the dermis or in the subcutaneous tissue or deeper tissues, although occasionally both superficial and deep tissues are affected together (153). Blood eosinophilia has been reported in up to 15% of patients (151,153). Local recurrence may be seen in up to 30% of cases.

Superficial Lesions. Young to middle-aged women are mainly affected by the development of pruritic papules (Fig. 33-34) and plaques at or around the external ear. The lesions can be numerous but are limited to one side. Typically, the clinical course is chronic over several years despite excision and other

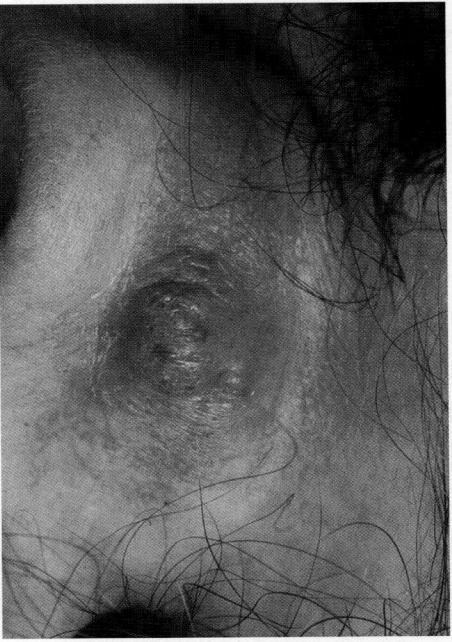

Figure 33-34 Epithelioid hemangioma (angiolymphoid hyperplasia with eosinophilia). Single or multiple vascular papules are often present in the ear.

treatment modalities. Such superficial lesions were originally referred to as *pseudopyogenic granuloma*. Occlusion of the external auditory canal can bring patients to the attention of ear, nose, and throat specialists. Sometimes, other areas in the head and neck region, especially the occipital region and the vicinity of the temporal artery, are affected.

Lesions of Subcutaneous and Deeper Tissues. Adults are mainly affected, and there is no gender predilection. The typical lesion is a solitary, slowly growing, firm, subcutaneous swelling 2 to 10 cm in size in the head and neck region, with some predilection for the pre- or postauricular sites. Sometimes, more than one lesion arises. Most lesions are asymptomatic except for occasional pruritus. Lymphadenopathy is usually not seen. Occasionally, other body sites are affected, such as the arm, hands, axillae, or inguinal region (153–155). Rare cases have been documented in association with a traumatically induced arteriovenous fistula involving the popliteal artery (156). Origin from the radial artery has also been documented (157). The condition can persist for years, but serious complications do not occur.

Epithelioid hemangioma may also rarely occur in the oral cavity (158), tongue (159), lymph node (160), bone (161), and testis (162). A case has also been reported in an ovarian teratoma (163). Epithelioid hemangiomas occurring at sites different from the skin often lack the inflammatory component.

Histopathology. The main components of the pathology include the following:

1. Proliferation of small- to medium-sized blood vessels, often showing a lobular architecture (Fig. 33-35). Many of these vascular channels are lined by greatly enlarged (epithelioid) endothelial cells (Figs. 33-36 and 33-37).
2. A perivascular inflammatory cell infiltrate composed mainly of lymphocytes and eosinophils.
3. Nodular areas of a lymphocytic infiltrate with rare follicle formation.
4. Frequent origin from a small artery or a vein. Rarely, the whole lesion is intravascular (Fig. 33-38) (164).

In superficial lesions, there is a variable degree of vascular hyperplasia, which can include areas in which the proliferation is almost angiomatous. A distinctive feature is the

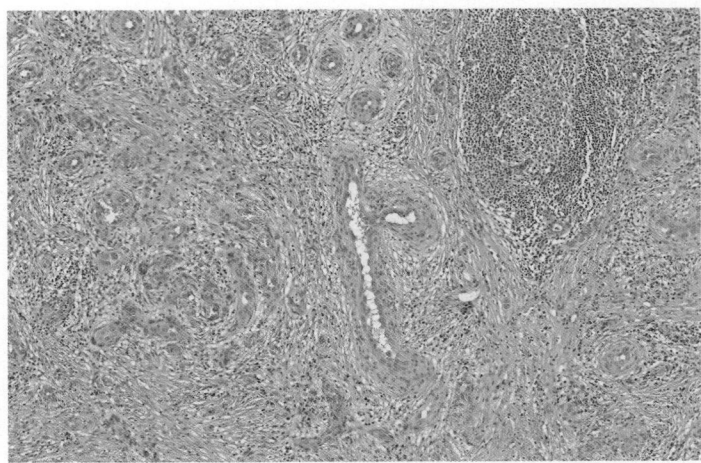

Figure 33-36 Epithelioid hemangioma (angiolymphoid hyperplasia with eosinophilia). Numerous vascular channels lined by prominent large, pink epithelioid endothelial cells and surrounded by inflammation.

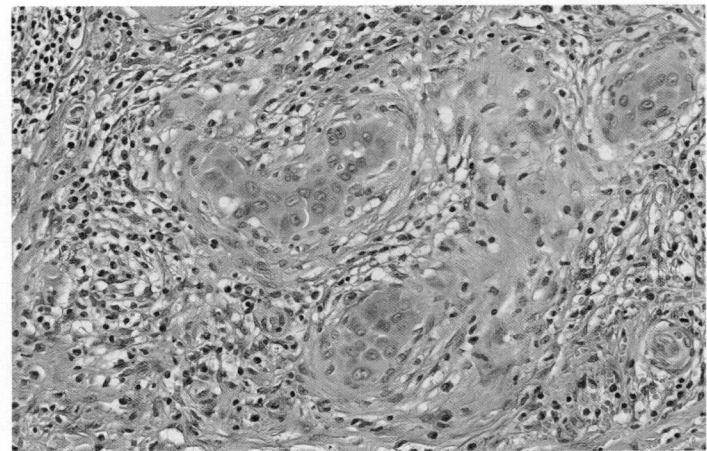

Figure 33-37 Epithelioid hemangioma (angiolymphoid hyperplasia with eosinophilia). Prominent endothelial cells with abundant eosinophilic cytoplasm and numerous eosinophils in the surrounding stroma. Note the perivascular fibrosis.

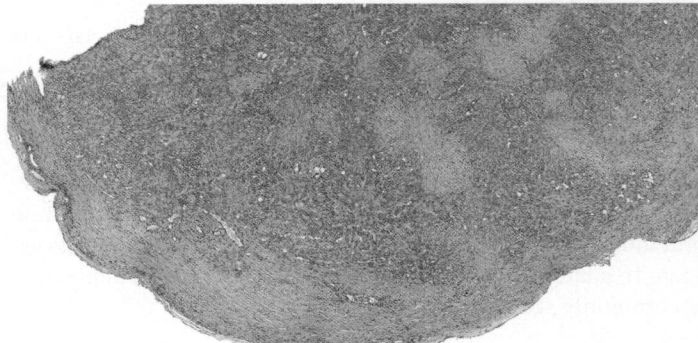

Figure 33-38 Intravascular epithelioid hemangioma (angiolymphoid hyperplasia with eosinophilia). Some cases of epithelioid hemangioma are entirely intravascular.

"cobblestone" appearance of enlarged endothelial cells that project into the lumina of some vessels. The nucleus of these cells is ovoid and orthochromatic without atypia or evidence of mitotic activity. Affected vessels often show endothelial cells with intracytoplasmic vacuoles, which is a prominent feature of diagnostic value (Fig. 33-37). The most abnormal blood vessels

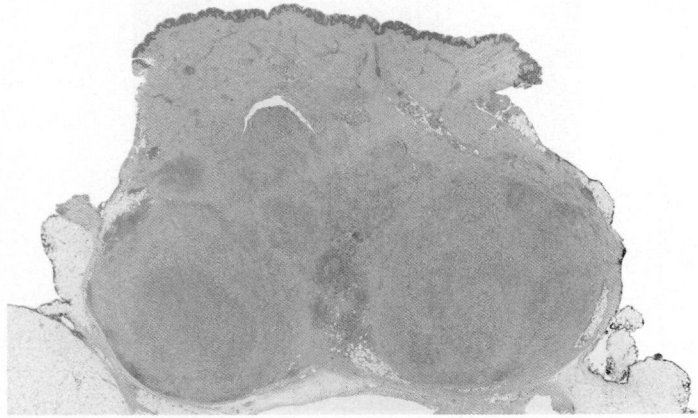

Figure 33-35 Epithelioid hemangioma (angiolymphoid hyperplasia with eosinophilia). Superficial lesion from the ear showing typical lobular architecture and a prominent inflammatory cell infiltrate.

are usually surrounded by stellate and spindle-shaped cells in a mucoid stroma. The associated perivascular inflammatory cell infiltrate is usually loosely scattered around the affected vessel, but it may be almost completely absent in some places. Generally, eosinophils make up 5% to 15% of the cells. Lesions with few inflammatory cells are rarely seen. Inflammatory cells also decrease markedly in late stages when a prominent fibrotic component is often present.

The epidermis above the lesions may show acanthosis or erosions owing to superficial trauma. The skin appendages are usually unaffected except for the occasional finding of follicular mucinosis (165). Intravascular epithelioid hemangioma can represent a serious diagnostic pitfall by mimicking malignant vascular neoplasms with epithelioid morphology. It presents in two morphologic forms, a lobular capillary hemangioma-like proliferation and a solid proliferation (164). Most cases do not express FOSB, but low mitotic activity, and a lack of atypical mitoses, pronounced nuclear atypia, multilayering or tumor necrosis should allow distinction from malignant epithelioid vascular neoplasms (164).

In subcutaneous lesions, the inflammatory cell infiltrate is usually more massive, with a central, poorly circumscribed nodule that replaces the fat. The nodule is composed of confluent sheets of small lymphocytes and eosinophils in which a network of poorly canalized thick-walled capillaries is embedded. Satellite smaller islands of lymphoid cells with lymphoid follicles usually surround the central nodule. Eosinophils can form up to 50% of the cell population.

In about 50% of cases, evidence of involvement of medium- to large-sized arteries can be found. A variable degree of blood vessel damage occurs, with infiltration of the vessel wall by inflammatory cells and occlusion of the lumen. Partial loss of the internal elastic lamina is often seen.

Histogenesis. Occasionally, trauma or external otitis can precede the onset of the disease. Ultrastructural studies have not confirmed that the enlarged endothelial cells are developing histiocytic properties, as has been suggested. Even though transient angiolymphoid hyperplasia with eosinophilia and Kaposi sarcoma have been described after primary infection with HHV-8 in an HIV-positive patient, there is no association with HHV-8 in larger studies (166,167). Human polyomavirus 6 infection has been detected in one case (168). *FOS* and *FOSB* gene rearrangements have been found in approximately one-third of epithelioid hemangiomas, predominantly in deep-seated locations (bone and soft tissue), rarely in cutaneous cases, and in no cases with classic cutaneous presentation and are often referred to as angiolymphoid hyperplasia (152), whereas a smaller subset, mostly in the head and neck region, shows a *GATA6-FOX1* fusion and no expression of FOSB (169). A study focusing on epithelioid hemangioma of bone has found *FOS* or *FOSB* gene rearrangements in all cases tested (170). Most penile cases present with a characteristic fusion involving *FOSB* (171). Interestingly, it has been shown that cutaneous tumors, including ones in the angiolymphoid hyperplasia part of the spectrum, strongly express FOSB regardless of no evident gene rearrangement (172).

Differential Diagnosis. The proliferation of endothelial-lined channels with large irregular cells can be misinterpreted as angiosarcoma. The latter can be accompanied by a lymphocytic infiltrate, but eosinophils are rarely present. The main distinguishing feature is the presence of nuclear atypia with hyperchromatism, mitotic activity, and dissection of collagen pattern in angiosarcoma but not in epithelioid hemangioma. Distinction from the retiform hemangioendothelioma (p. 1247) is easy: Angiolymphoid hyperplasia lacks a retiform growth pattern and does not show tall, narrow endothelial cells with a typical hobnail appearance, as is the case in retiform hemangioendothelioma.

Angiolymphoid hyperplasia can be distinguished from most benign angiomas or ectasias by the absence of an intrinsic inflammatory cell infiltrate in the latter. Greatly enlarged endothelial cells with an eosinophilic cytoplasm rarely feature in benign angiomas, although they can be seen focally in lobular capillary hemangioma (pyogenic granuloma).

Persistent insect bite reactions can show overlapping histologic features with angiolymphoid hyperplasia, but the vascular proliferation is rarely as exuberant. A somewhat similar pathology can also arise as a reaction to injected vaccines (173). The histology is characterized by a deep lymphoid infiltrate with lymphoid follicles, tissue eosinophilia, and fibrosis. Vascular hyperplasia is, however, less marked than in angiolymphoid hyperplasia, and epithelioid endothelial cells are not a feature. A diagnostic feature is the presence of aluminum-containing histiocytes, as demonstrated by solochrome-azurine when aluminum-adsorbed vaccines have been used (173). The presence of aluminum may also be demonstrated by energy-dispersive x-ray microanalysis. Interestingly, a recent study has shown EBER positivity in aluminum-containing histiocytes (174).

When epithelioid hemangioma was first described in Western Europe, similarities to *Kimura disease* as reported in East Asia were noted. Indeed, many authors thought that both conditions might be part of one disease spectrum. However, in later years, most authorities have emphasized differences between the two entities (175,176). Subcutaneous epithelioid hemangioma and Kimura disease occur most commonly in the head and neck region in adults, and both share the histologic features of extensive lymphoid proliferation, tissue eosinophilia, and evidence of vascular hyperplasia. Kimura disease, however, demonstrates a wider age span, with a male predominance and a tendency for more extensive lesions to occur, often with involvement of salivary tissue and lymph nodes and at sites distant from the head and neck region. Authors from East Asia have stressed the histologic differences, the most important of which are the lesser degree of exuberant vascular hyperplasia, lacking prominent eosinophilic endothelial cells, and the absence of uncanalized blood vessels in Kimura disease. Other points of difference are eosinophilic abscesses and marked fibrosis around the lesions in Kimura disease and the absence of lesions centered around damaged arteries. There is an important association between Kimura disease and renal disease, particularly nephrotic syndrome (177).

Principles of Management: Surgery is the treatment of choice. Intralesional steroids may also be used.

Cutaneous Epithelioid Angiomatous Nodule

Clinical Summary. Cutaneous epithelioid angiomatous nodule is a recently described lesion within the spectrum of vascular tumors with epithelioid endothelial cells (178–180). It is rare and presents in adults as a papule or nodule with a predilection for the trunk, followed by the limbs and face. Occasionally, multiple lesions may be seen, and there is no tendency for local recurrence (181,182). An exceptional case has been described in association with a vascular malformation (183).

Histopathology. Scanning magnification shows a superficial, well-circumscribed proliferation (Fig. 33-39) often surrounded by an epidermal collarette. It is composed of sheets of epithelioid endothelial cells with abundant pink cytoplasm, vesicular nuclei, and a single, small nucleolus (Fig. 33-40). A granular cell variant has been described (184). Cytologic atypia is absent, and mitotic figures may be focally seen (Fig. 33-41). There is little tendency for the formation of vascular channels, but individual endothelial cells often contain intracytoplasmic vacuoles. There is very little stroma between tumor cells, and in the background, scattered mononuclear inflammatory cells and eosinophils may be seen.

Differential Diagnosis. Distinction from epithelioid hemangioma is easy, as the clinical setting in the latter is different, and lesions are composed of vascular channels lined by epithelioid endothelial cells and not by solid sheets of epithelioid endothelial cells. Bacillary angiomatosis can be distinguished from epithelioid

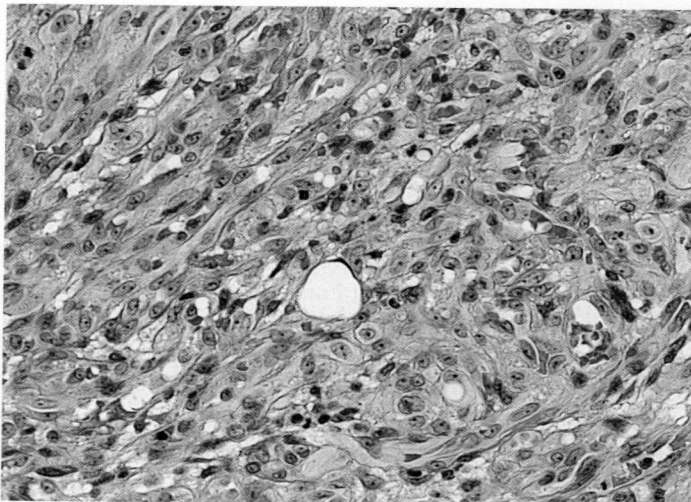

Figure 33-41 Cutaneous epithelioid angiomatous nodule. Cytologic atypia is mild or absent and there are rare mitotic figures.

angiomatous nodule, because lesions in the former are usually multiple, and histologically there is formation of vascular channels lined by pale epithelioid endothelial cells and associated amorphous basophilic aggregates and neutrophils, indicating the areas where the bacteria are located. Distinction from epithelioid angiosarcoma is based on the infiltrative growth pattern, pleomorphism, and mitotic activity in the latter.

Principles of Management: Simple excision is the treatment of choice.

Acquired Elastotic Hemangioma

Clinical Summary. Acquired elastotic hemangioma is a distinctive relatively rare vascular lesion that develops in sun-exposed skin, mainly of the forearms and neck of middle-aged to elderly patients, with predilection for females. The clinical presentation consists of a small, red or blue, circumscribed and asymptomatic plaque (185).

Histopathology. Lesions are well circumscribed and consist of a superficial, bandlike proliferation of capillaries in the background of solar elastosis (Figs. 33-42 and 33-43). Each capillary

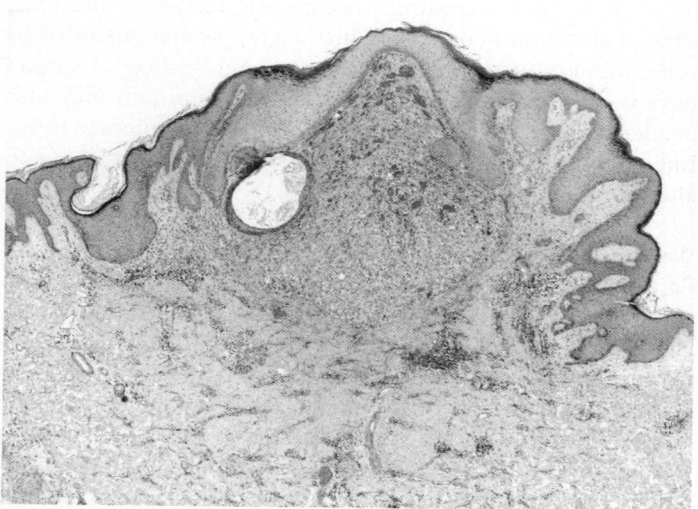

Figure 33-39 Cutaneous epithelioid angiomatous nodule. Superficial, well-defined polypoid lesion.

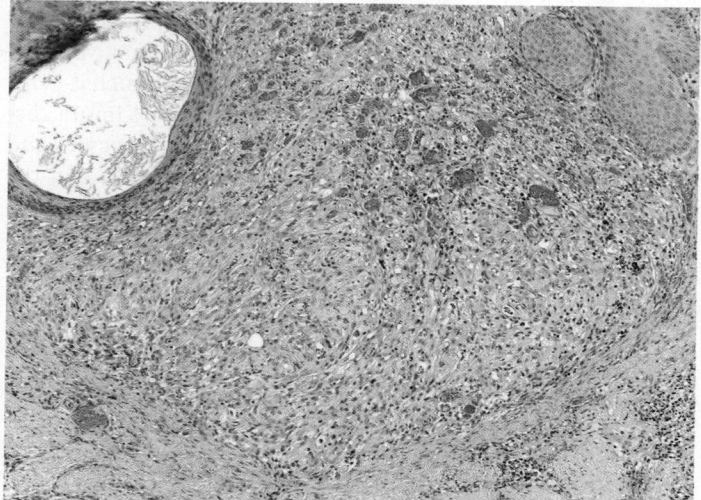

Figure 33-40 Cutaneous epithelioid angiomatous nodule. Sheets of epithelioid endothelial cells with focal intracytoplasmic lumina.

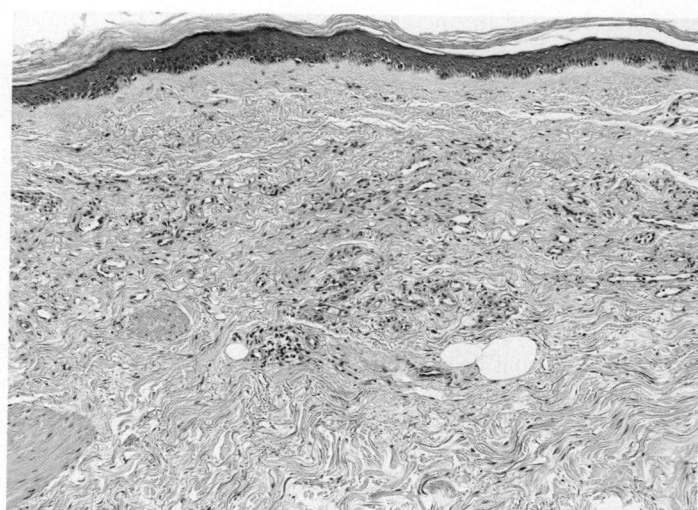

Figure 33-42 Acquired elastotic hemangioma. Superficial plaquelike proliferation of small, round vascular channels. (Courtesy of Dr. T. Mentzel, Friedrichshafen, Germany.)

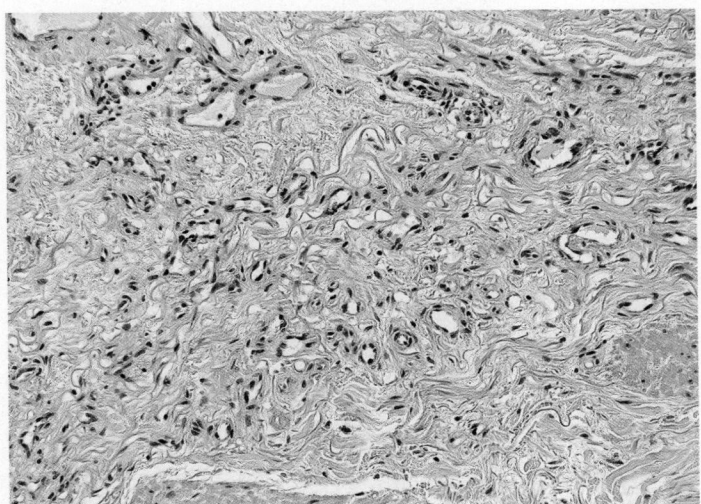

Figure 33-43 Acquired elastotic hemangioma. Note the solar elastosis in the background. (Courtesy of Dr. T. Mentzel, Friedrichshafen, Germany.)

is surrounded by a layer of pericytes. Expression of D2-40 (podoplanin) suggests a lymphatic line of differentiation (186).

Principles of Management: Simple excision is the treatment of choice.

Arteriovenous Malformation (Arteriovenous [Venous] Hemangioma, Cirsoid Aneurysm)

Clinical Summary. Arteriovenous malformation, or cirsoid aneurysm, usually occurs as a solitary dark red papule or nodule on the face (especially the lip) or, less commonly, on the extremities of adults, with equal gender incidence (187,188). Rare cases are present in the oral cavity (189). Most of the lesions measure less than 1 cm in diameter.

Histopathology. Within a circumscribed area, usually restricted to the dermis (Fig. 33-44), densely aggregated, thick-walled, and thin-walled vessels lined by a single layer of endothelial cells are observed (Fig. 33-45). The walls of the thick-walled vessels consist mainly of fibrous tissue but, in most instances, also contain some smooth muscle. Internal elastic lamina is found in very few vessels, indicating that most of the blood

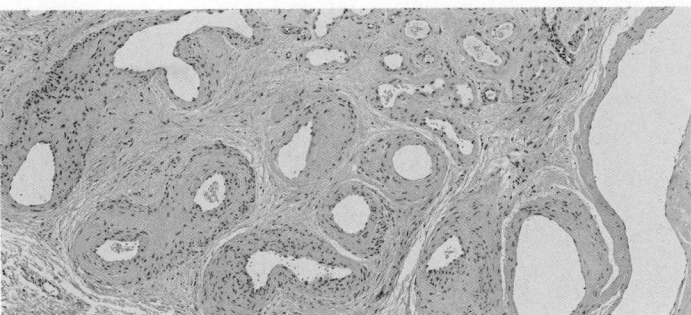

Figure 33-45 Cirsoid aneurysm. A combination of small veins and arteries.

vessels are veins. Many vessels contain red blood cells, and thrombi are occasionally seen (187). Lesions with similar histologic appearances can be seen in the deeper soft tissues of younger patients and can be associated with hemodynamic complications attributable to shunting.

Histogenesis. It seems likely that many of these lesions represent pure venous hemangiomas, some of which have arterialized veins (187). Inherited lesions are associated with germline *RASA1* mutations (36).

Principles of Management: Simple excision is the treatment of choice.

Poikilodermatous Plaque-Like Hemangioma

Clinical Summary. Poikilodermatous plaque–like hemangioma is a recently described (190,191) and rare, mostly solitary vascular lesion in the form of an erythematous or violaceous atrophic plaque with a predilection for the lower limbs and pelvic girdle of elderly males. It clinically resembles patch/plaque mycosis fungoides but follows an indolent course.

Histopathology. Lesion is characterized by a diffuse bandlike proliferation of thin-walled postcapillary venules (Figs. 33-46 and 33-47) within the papillary and superficial reticular dermis, in a background of dermal edema, fibrosis, and diminished or absent elastic fibers. The vessels are lined by a single layer of bland CD31 and ERG-positive endothelial cells without atypia or mitoses. Each vascular channel is surrounded by a layer of pericytes. There may be admixed D2-40 positive dilated lymphatic vessels.

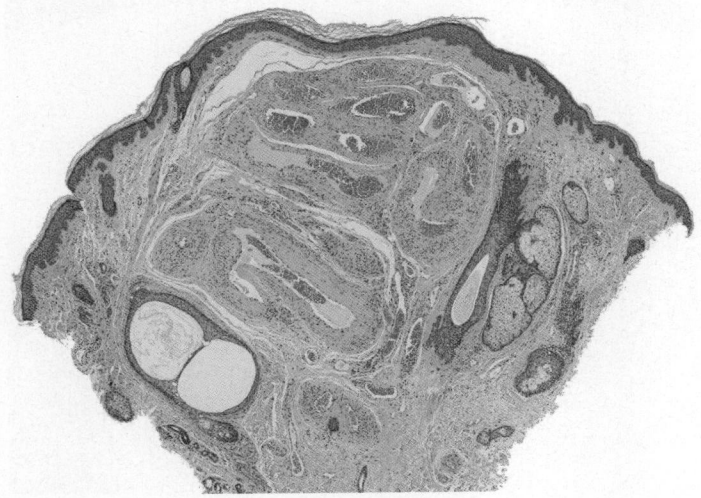

Figure 33-44 Cirsoid aneurysm. Polypoid superficial lesion composed of dilated, thick-walled vascular channels.

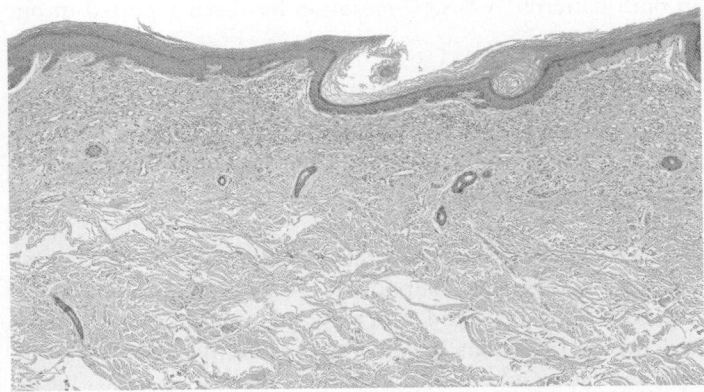

Figure 33-46 Poikilodermatous plaquelike hemangioma. Diffuse bandlike proliferation of small vessels within the papillary and superficial reticular dermis.

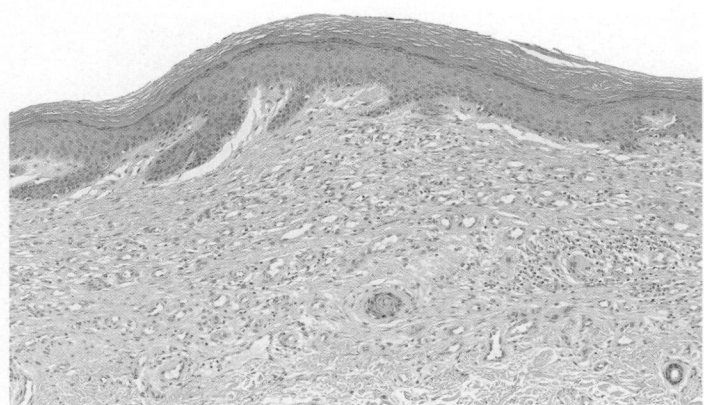

Figure 33-47 Poikilodermatous plaquelike hemangioma. Thin-walled postcapillary venules surrounded by dermal fibrosis.

Pathogenesis. It is not clear whether this distinctive lesion is a true neoplasm or a reactive process secondary to repeated trauma. However, in the original series, no history of sustained trauma could be elicited in any of the patients, and rarely more than one lesion is present.

Principles of Management: Typically, no treatment is needed, but distinction from mycosis fungoides is very important.

Angiomatosis

Clinical Summary. Angiomatosis is an uncommon condition that presents exclusively in children and adolescents and is defined as a diffuse proliferation of blood vessels affecting a large contiguous area of the body (192–194). Anatomic distribution is wide, but there is a preference for limb involvement. A typical case presents with involvement of the skin, underlying soft tissues, and even bones. Associated limb hypertrophy is common. Involvement of parenchymal organs and the central nervous system can be present. Owing to extensive involvement, surgical treatment is difficult, and recurrences are common.

Histopathology. Most tumors are composed of abundant mature fat intermixed with blood vessels in two histologic patterns (193). The most common pattern is a mixture of veins with irregular walls, cavernous vascular spaces, and capillaries. The veins often show an incomplete muscular layer, and smaller blood vessels can be seen in the walls of larger vessels. The second pattern is composed mainly of capillaries with a focal lobular architecture. Perineural invasion can be a feature in both patterns. A *GNAQ* mutation has been reported in one case (194).

Spindle Cell Hemangioma

Clinical Summary. SCH is a tumor that was first described in 1986 (195) as a form of low-grade angiosarcoma. This view was challenged in subsequent publications, and, until very recently, a nonneoplastic process most likely related to a vascular malformation was the dominant theory. However, more recent cytogenetic evidence has supported a benign neoplastic process (see Pathogenesis). Gender incidence is equal, and most lesions arise in the second or third decade of life. It presents as multiple red-blue nodules in the dermis and subcutaneous tissue, most commonly involving the distal aspects of the extremities with a predilection for the hands. Less frequently, lesions are seen on the head and neck. Visceral lesions do not occur, and

involvement of deeper soft tissues and bone is rare (196,197). The clinical course is indolent, with multiple new lesions appearing over the years. Spontaneous regression is exceptional. In approximately 10% of cases, associated anomalies include lymphedema, Maffucci syndrome, Klippel–Trenaunay syndrome, and early-onset varicose veins (198,199).

Histopathology. Tumors tend to be poorly circumscribed and may present totally or partially in an intravascular location, especially involving medium-sized veins. A typical lesion is composed of two elements (Fig. 33-48): (a) irregularly dilated, thin-walled congested cavernous spaces often with organizing thrombi and (b) phleboliths intermixed with more solid areas composed of spindle-shaped cells (Fig. 33-49) generally bland in appearance, although rare cases may show focal degenerative cytologic atypia. Mitotic figures are rare. Commonly, in the solid areas, focal aggregates of epithelioid cells with eosinophilic cytoplasm and bundles of smooth muscle are seen. The epithelioid cells may show vacuolation or intracytoplasmic lumina (Fig. 33-50). Slitlike vascular spaces are common in the solid areas and are accompanied by scattered extravasated red blood cells and hemosiderin-laden macrophages. Focal areas with changes resembling Masson tumor can be a feature. Irregular, thick-walled vascular spaces reminiscent of those seen in vascular malformations are often seen in the periphery of many lesions. Occasionally, cases show combined features of epithelioid hemangioendothelioma and SCH (200). However, these cases are likely to represent examples of composite hemangioendothelioma (see p. 1249).

Pathogenesis. Original classification of this tumor as a form of low-grade angiosarcoma was based on the development of lymph node metastasis in one of the patients reported (201). However, the patient had been treated with radiotherapy, and it is very likely that the metastasis was from a radiation-induced sarcoma. Further case series proposed a reactive condition or a form of vascular malformation. This, however, has been contested as the demonstration of R132C IDH1 mutations identical to those found in Maffucci syndrome and IDH2 mutations in cases of SCH supports a benign neoplastic process (202,203).

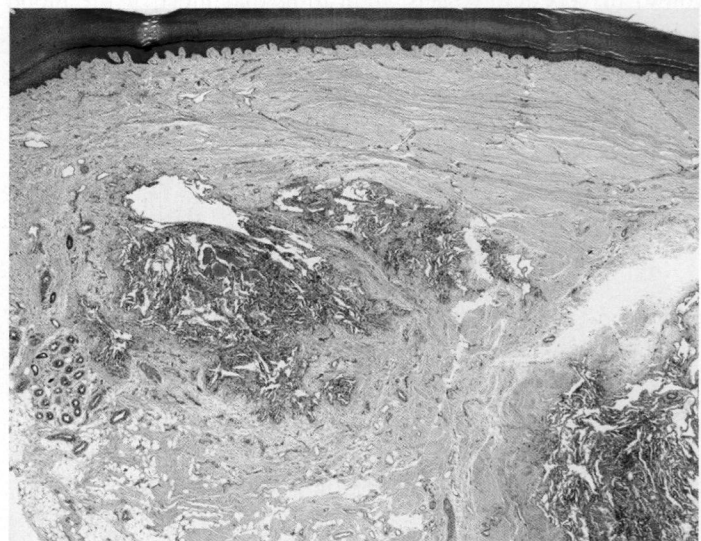

Figure 33-48 Spindle cell hemangioma. Multifocal lesions combining dilated and congested vascular spaces and more cellular areas.

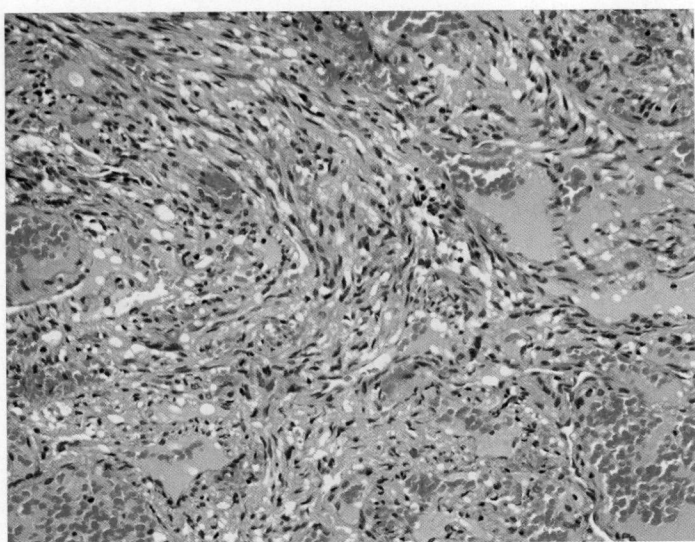

Figure 33-49 Spindle cell hemangioma. Thin-walled, dilated vascular spaces and bland spindle-shaped cells.

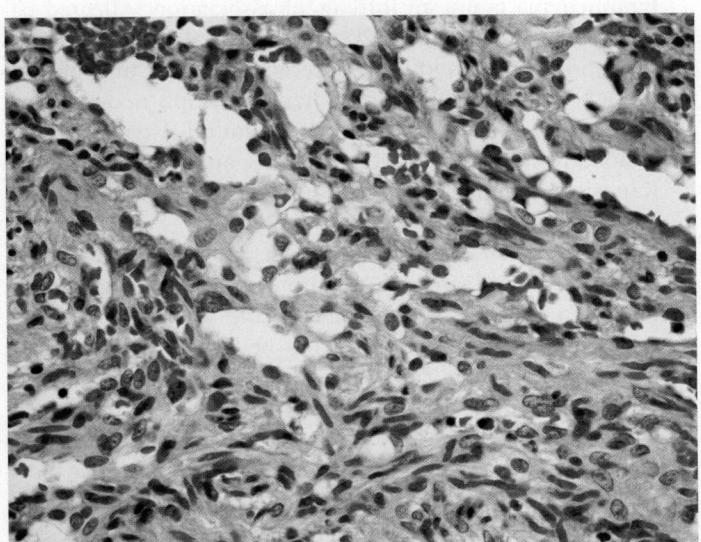

Figure 33-50 Spindle cell hemangioma. Spindle-shaped cells and focal epithelioid pale pink vacuolated cells.

By immunohistochemistry, the endothelial cells lining the vascular spaces and the epithelioid cells in the solid areas stain variably with endothelial markers. The spindle cells stain focally with actin and less commonly with desmin.

Differential Diagnosis. The main differential diagnosis is with nodular-stage Kaposi sarcoma, as discussed later (p. 1245).

Principles of Management: Surgical excision is the treatment of choice.

Symplastic Hemangioma

Clinical Summary. Symplastic hemangioma is not a distinctive variant of hemangioma but rather represents extensive degenerative changes in a preexisting hemangioma, closely mimicking malignancy (204–206). Very few cases have been reported, but from personal experience with a limited number of cases the preexisting hemangioma is often not identifiable, or it represents a cirsoid aneurysm.

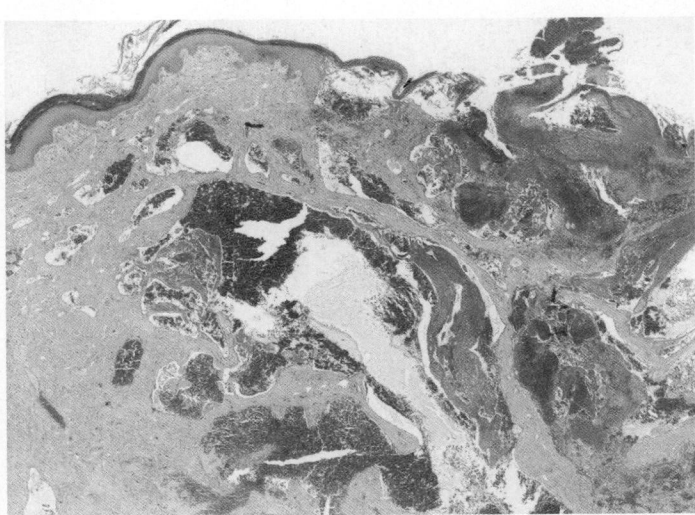

Figure 33-51 Symplastic hemangioma. Lesions are often polypoid, and their vascular nature is apparent at scanning magnification.

Histopathology. Lesions are often polypoid and well circumscribed and do not tend to be ulcerated (Fig. 33-51). Dilated and congested thin- to thick-walled vascular spaces are surrounded by a variable cellular stroma that is often myxoid and hemorrhagic. Stromal cells and smooth muscle cells within the vessel walls display variable cytologic atypia consisting of nuclear enlargement and hyperchromatism (Fig. 33-52). The endothelial cells lining the vascular spaces do not show cytologic atypia (Fig. 33-53). Other cells have a bizarre appearance, and multinucleation is not uncommon. Mitotic figures may be found but are not common. Very occasional atypical mitotic figures may also be seen.

Differential Diagnosis. The main differential diagnosis to consider is angiosarcoma. However, in symplastic angioma, the endothelial cells lining the vascular channels are bland, with no mitotic activity or multilayering. A further differential diagnosis is with pleomorphic hyalinizing angiectatic tumor of soft parts (207). The latter is an infiltrative tumor that occurs mainly in the subcutis or deeper soft tissues and is characterized by thin-walled dilated vascular spaces with prominent

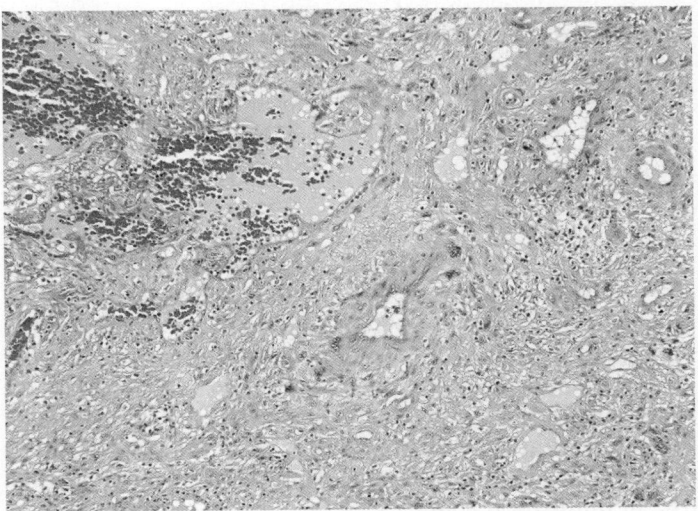

Figure 33-52 Symplastic hemangioma. Atypical cells both within the stroma and in the blood vessel walls.

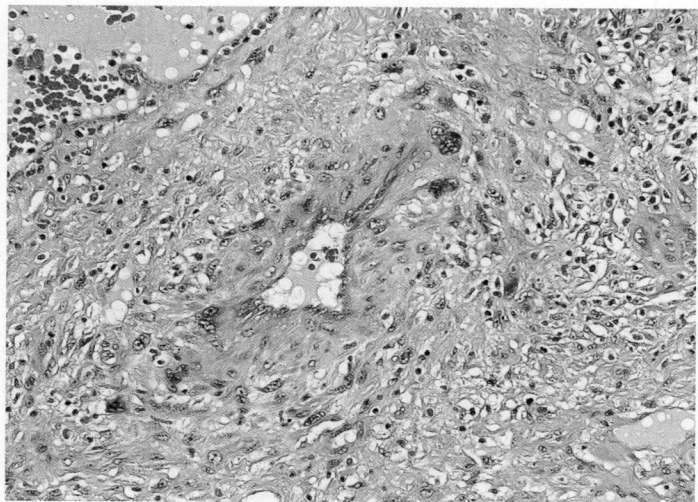

Figure 33-53 Symplastic hemangioma. Endothelial cells show no atypia or mitotic activity.

perivascular hyalinization and pleomorphic stromal cells with low mitotic activity and frequent intranuclear inclusions.

Principles of Management: Simple excision is the treatment of choice.

VASCULAR TUMORS OF INTERMEDIATE MALIGNANCY

Malignant tumors of endothelial cell origin can be broadly divided into intermediate and high-grade malignancy. Strictly used, the term *intermediate malignancy* refers to a tumor that has potential for aggressive local behavior with a tendency for local recurrence and low or negligible potential for metastatic spread. There is a tendency to designate malignant vascular tumors with true potential for metastatic spread as angiosarcomas and low-grade tumors as hemangioendotheliomas. However, some authors use the terms interchangeably, and progress in understanding of some of these tumors has led to certain neoplasms being either upgraded as fully malignant (e.g., epithelioid hemangioendothelioma) or downgraded as benign (e.g., SCH). It must also be remembered that the term *hemangioendothelioma* was used in the past to refer to some benign vascular tumors, especially strawberry nevus in children. The category of vascular tumors of intermediate malignancy also includes lesions like Kaposi sarcoma, a generally indolent process in which a truly neoplastic origin has not clearly been demonstrated.

Kaposi Sarcoma

Introduction. Until the late 1960s, Kaposi sarcoma was described as an uncommon, slowly progressive, multifocal tumor arising mostly in elderly male patients of eastern and southern European descent, a clinical pattern now referred to as the *classic* form of the disease. During the last two decades of the last century, intense interest developed as Kaposi sarcoma became a prime marker of AIDS. Although with the advent of HAART the incidence of Kaposi sarcoma in patients with HIV/AIDS has decreased dramatically in the Western world, the same is not true in third-world countries, particularly in Africa, where access to HAART is still very limited. In addition, Kaposi sarcoma can arise in association with other causes of immunodeficiency,

especially when drug induced, particularly in the setting of organ transplantation and less commonly in different forms of inherited immune deficiency. Despite recent great advances in knowledge regarding the etiology and pathogenesis of Kaposi sarcoma, there remain many unusual facets about the disease that as yet defy adequate scientific explanation. Although it has been demonstrated that all types of Kaposi sarcoma are associated with a novel variant of herpesvirus, HHV-8, it is still controversial whether Kaposi sarcoma is a multifocal reactive process or a neoplastic condition. As such, it is perhaps best viewed as a locally (and potentially systemically) aggressive virus-induced endothelial proliferation.

Clinical Features. Nearly all cases of Kaposi sarcoma can be classified into four groups (208–211):

1. *Classic Kaposi sarcoma.* This arises 10 to 15 times more commonly in men than women, affecting mainly patients of eastern European, Jewish, and Mediterranean origin (212). The disease arises mainly in patients over the age of 50 years with the slow development of angiomatous nodules and plaques on the lower extremities (Fig. 33-54). Chronic lymphedema is not an infrequent association. Affected patients may survive 10 to 20 years; even at late stages with widespread skin nodules, visceral disease is unusual, although asymptomatic involvement of lymph nodes, lungs, or gastrointestinal tract can often be found at necropsy. Occasionally, before the advent of AIDS, an aggressive type of Kaposi sarcoma occurred in young adults or children with early lymph node involvement (213).

2. *Endemic African Kaposi sarcoma.* In the 1960s, it was realized that Kaposi sarcoma was quite common among native blacks in Central Africa, representing the most common tumor in pathology departments in Uganda and parts of what was known as Zaire (now the Democratic Republic of Congo). In South Africa, it has been estimated that Kaposi sarcoma is 10 times more common in blacks than whites (Fig. 33-55). In Africans, the disease can run a similar indolent course as in classic Kaposi sarcoma, but a higher proportion of young people are affected, with a more aggressive disease manifested by widespread tumors, deep infiltrative or elevated fungating lesions, and bone involvement. A distinctive childhood type of Kaposi sarcoma occurs with

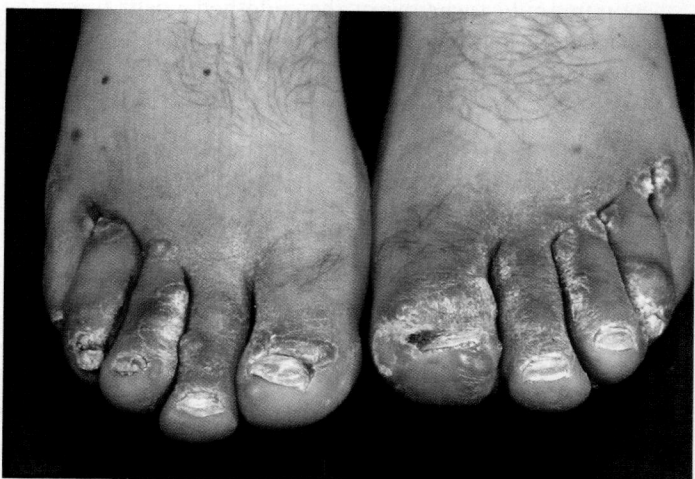

Figure 33-54 Clinical Kaposi sarcoma. Typical endemic case with plaques and nodules on an acral location.

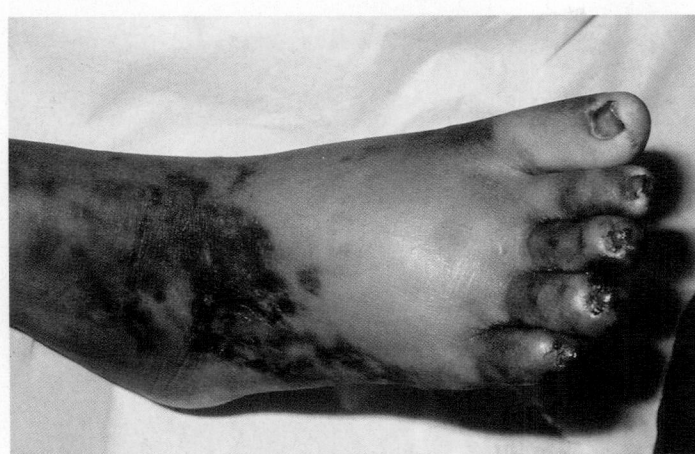

Figure 33-55 Clinical Kaposi sarcoma. In endemic African cases, associated lymphedema is often seen.

massive lymph node involvement and early death. Mucocutaneous lesions are usually a late or minor clinical feature in this lymphadenopathic form (214). The male-to-female ratio in these children is approximately 3:1. Most cases of Kaposi sarcoma that have occurred in sub-Saharan Africa in the last 25 years are in patients with HIV/AIDS (215).

3. *AIDS-associated Kaposi sarcoma*. In the early 1980s, reports of groups of young homosexual males in New York and California who were developing Kaposi sarcoma was one of the keys in establishing the existence of AIDS. Originally, about 40% of patients with AIDS had concomitant Kaposi sarcoma, but this high percentage has gradually and dramatically fallen in the United States and Europe since the advent of HAART (216). Collected data from the Centers for Disease Control and Prevention in the United States have suggested that standardized incidence ratio for Kaposi sarcoma was approximately 500 for AIDS patients compared to the general population (217). The risk of Kaposi sarcoma occurring with AIDS is much greater in active homosexuals than in heterosexual males or females, such as hemophiliacs who receive contaminated blood products or drug abusers who share needles.

The clinical features of AIDS-related Kaposi sarcoma differ from the classic disease in the rapid evolution of the lesions, their atypical distribution affecting the trunk, and the mucosal involvement (218) (Fig. 33-56). Visceral

involvement is very common at autopsy (219,220), but such internal lesions are often unapparent clinically during life. Visceral involvement may be present without any skin lesions. In patients on HAART and according to the degree of restoration of the immune system, lesions may regress, and if they develop during treatment they are usually limited in number and extent.

4. *Kaposi sarcoma and iatrogenic immunosuppression*. Drug-induced immunosuppression to prevent rejection of transplanted organs greatly increases the risk of developing lymphomas and other tumors, including Kaposi sarcoma (221,222). In a large retrospective study over 23 years, Kaposi sarcoma developed in 3.9% of cases of kidney transplant patients (222). A peculiarity of this type of Kaposi sarcoma is the frequent regression or apparent cure on discontinuation of immunosuppressive therapy. The male-dominant gender ratio is much smaller in this group. Kaposi sarcoma can also occur in other causes of immunosuppression, including genetic diseases (223).

Histopathology. The histopathology of fully developed nodules of Kaposi sarcoma in all types of the disease is distinctive and should rarely cause problems for pathologists. The diagnostic pitfalls lie mainly in the early macular lesions, where misinterpretation as banal inflammation or some form of minor angiomatous or lymphatic anomaly is easy to make. Despite the name sarcoma, cytologic atypia is minimal in tumor cells in all stages of evolution of Kaposi sarcoma (except in the rare anaplastic variant).

For descriptive convenience, the histologic spectrum can be divided into stages roughly corresponding to the clinical type of lesion: early and late macules, plaques, nodules, and aggressive late lesions. In reality, there is overlap between stages and multiple biopsies taken at the same time, or even a single biopsy may show features of different histologic stages. There are no differences in the pathology of the disease in the different risk groups.

1. *Macular (patch stage)*. In early macules, there is usually a patchy, sparse, dermal perivascular infiltrate consisting of lymphocytes and plasma cells. Narrow cords of cells, insinuated between collagen bundles, may at first suggest histiocytes or connective tissue cells, but close inspection should reveal evidence of luminal differentiation or connection with discernible small vessels (Fig. 33-57). Usually,

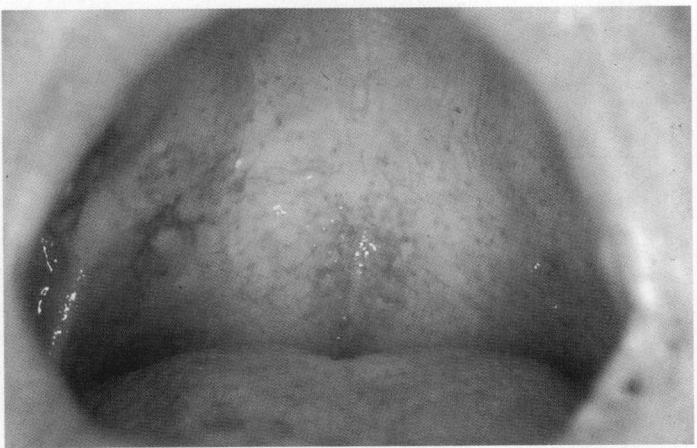

Figure 33-56 Kaposi sarcoma. Oral lesions are often seen in patients with HIV/AIDS, particularly in patients not on HAART.

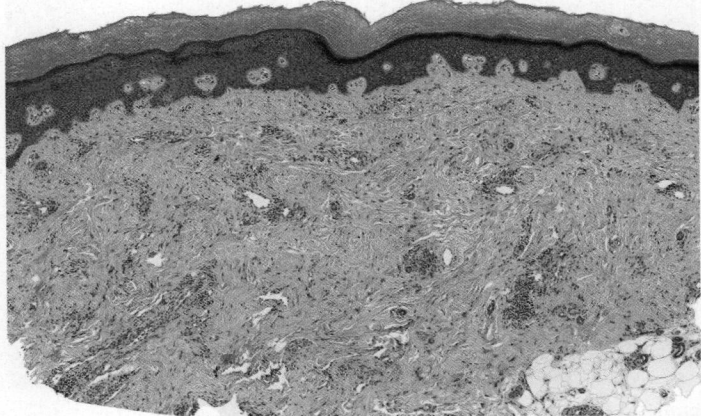

Figure 33-57 Patch-stage Kaposi sarcoma. Numerous slitlike spaces throughout the dermis in the background of hemorrhage.

a few dilated irregular or angulated lymphatic-like spaces lined by delicate, bland endothelial cells are also present. Vessels with "jagged" outlines tending to separate collagen bundles are especially characteristic (Fig. 33-58). Normal adnexal structures and preexisting blood vessels often protrude into newly formed blood vessels (Fig. 33-59). This finding, known as the promontory sign, is commonly present but not specific to Kaposi sarcoma. In late macular lesions, there is a more extensive infiltrate of vessels in the dermis: "jagged" vessels and cords of thicker-walled vessels similar to those in granulation tissue. Some of these vessels may in part be reactive rather than an intrinsic part of the tumor. At this stage, red blood cell extravasation and the presence of siderophages may be encountered. In some lesions, ramifying variably dilated bloodless lymphatic-like spaces dissect out collagen to give an appearance that suggests a well-differentiated angiosarcoma or progressive lymphangioma. This exaggerated lymphangioma-like appearance has led some authors to designate this as a special variant of the disease (224) (Fig. 33-60). Occasional fascicles of spindle-shaped cells may occur independently of blood vessels. In some cases, dilated, congested, thin-walled vascular channels with a sievelike (Fig. 33-61) appearance mimicking a hemangioma are seen.

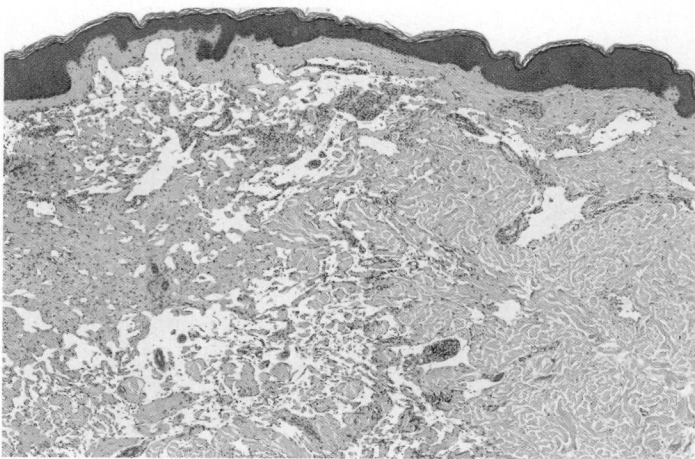

Figure 33-60 Lymphangiomatous Kaposi sarcoma. Numerous, irregular, dilated, bloodless vascular channels with a striking lymphangioma-like appearance.

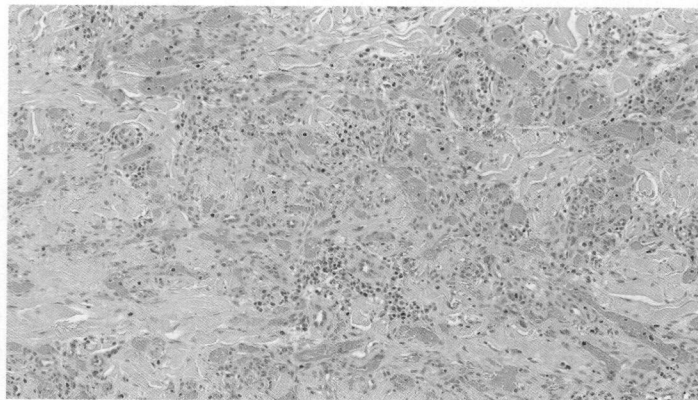

Figure 33-61 Angiomatous Kaposi sarcoma. Congested, small vascular channels in a focal sievelike pattern.

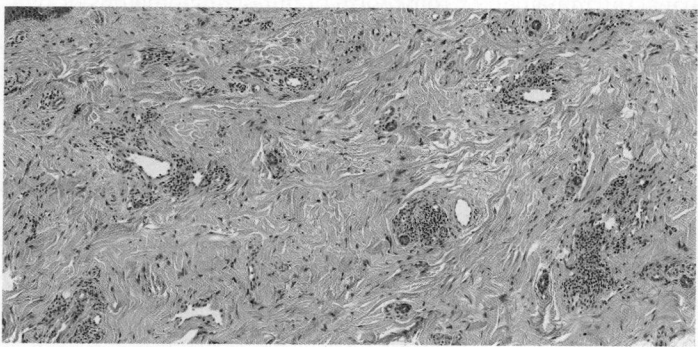

Figure 33-58 Patch-stage Kaposi sarcoma. Irregular, jagged, thin-walled, small vascular channels in association with hemosiderin deposition and focal inflammation.

2. *Plaque stage.* In this stage, a diffuse infiltrate of small blood vessels extends through most parts of the dermis and tends to displace collagen (Fig. 33-62). The vessels show variable morphology, with some occurring as poorly canalized cords, some as blood-containing ovoid vessels, and some showing lymphatic-like features. Loosely distributed spindle cells, arranged in short fascicles, are also encountered (Fig. 33-63). Intracytoplasmic hyaline globules may be found in areas

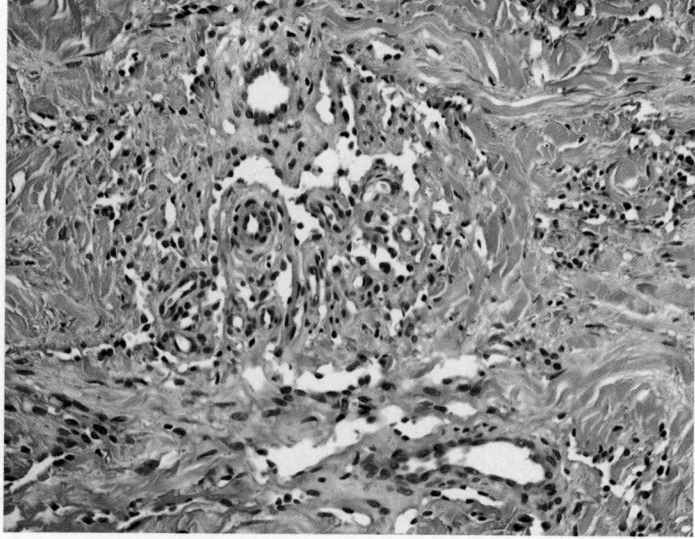

Figure 33-59 Patch-stage Kaposi sarcoma. A normal blood vessel protruding into newly formed blood vessels ("promontory sign") lined by bland endothelial cells.

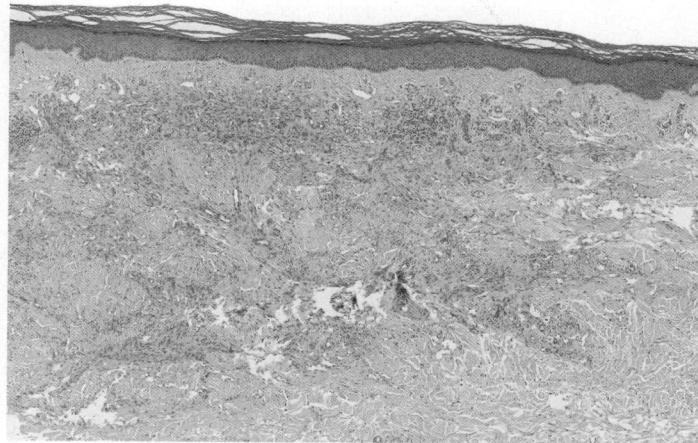

Figure 33-62 Plaque-stage Kaposi sarcoma. A more cellular dermis with extensive hemorrhage.

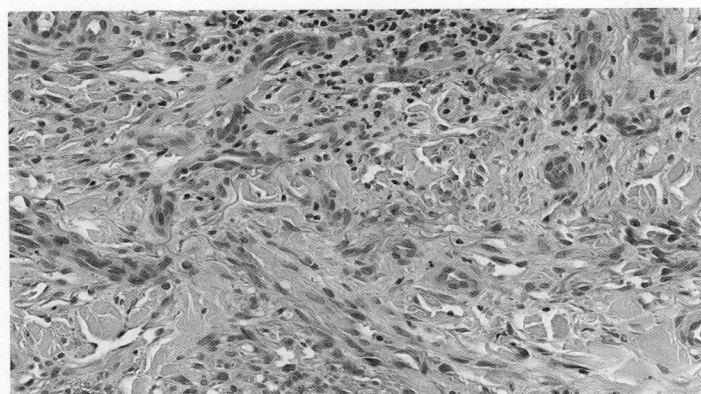

Figure 33-63 Plaque-stage Kaposi sarcoma. Bland spindle-shaped cells with focal formation of cleftlike spaces containing red blood cells.

with a denser infiltrate. These hyaline globules are seen more often in lesions from patients with AIDS.

3. *Nodular stage.* In the tumor stage, well-defined nodules composed of vascular spaces and spindle cells replace dermal collagen (Fig. 33-64). These tumor nodules tend to be compartmentalized by dense bands of fibrocollagenous tissue. Dilated lymphatic spaces can also be seen between tumor aggregates. The characteristic feature is a honeycomb-like network of blood-filled spaces or slits that are closely associated with interweaving spindle cells (Fig. 33-65). Although generally vascular spaces and fascicles of spindle cells are present, either element can focally predominate. The vascular lumina in the angiomatous tissue are so closely set that they lie next to each other in a "back-to-back" arrangement.

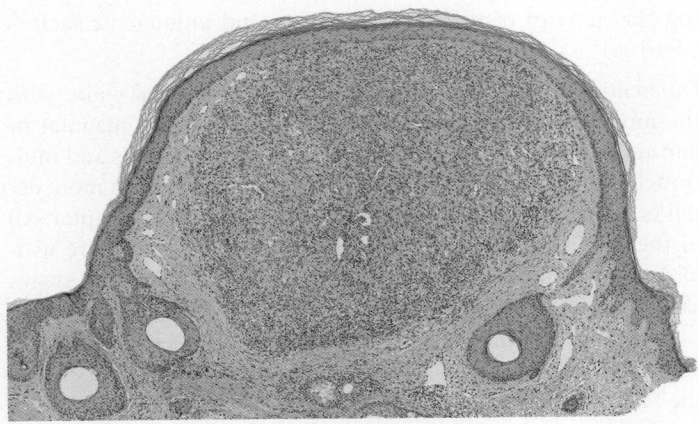

Figure 33-64 Nodular-stage Kaposi sarcoma. Fairly well-circumscribed dermal nodule.

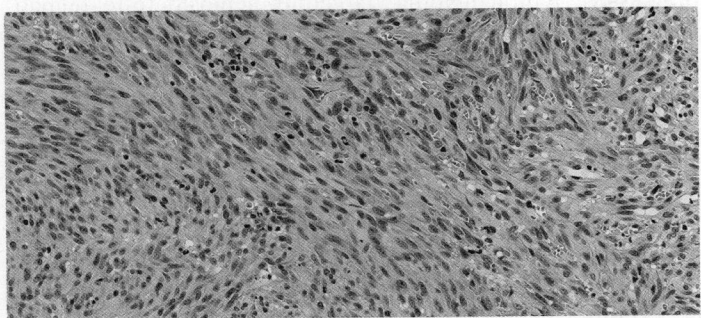

Figure 33-65 Nodular-stage Kaposi sarcoma. Bland spindle cells forming slitlike spaces occupied by red blood cells.

Delicate, flattened endothelial cells lining the vascular clefts are hardly discernible with routine stains but are easily seen with the immunocytochemical markers CD31 and CD34. The vascular slits in the nodules appear to be in direct contact with spindle cells, leading to the suggestion that they are pseudovascular spaces. The presence of a closely set honeycomb-like pattern of vascular spaces is perhaps the single most important diagnostic feature of Kaposi sarcoma. In the vascular spaces of pyogenic granuloma and most angiomas, the endothelial cells of the capillary walls are more prominent, and the vessels are set farther apart by intervening stroma. Around the nodules, varying numbers of thicker-walled vessels are encountered that may represent reactive or "feeder" vessels and are not a basic component of the tumor. Blood pigment–containing macrophages are nearly always prominent adjacent to the nodules, especially in lesions at dependent sites.

The spindle cells in the nodules are elongated and fusiform with a well-defined cytoplasm. The nuclei are ovoid and somewhat flattened with finely granular chromatin in the long axis of the cells. The nucleoli are generally inconspicuous, and nuclear atypia is absent or slight. Mitotic figures are not prominent. Prominent and consistent positivity for CD34 is seen in the spindle cell population.

Intra- and extracellular hyaline globules occur more frequently than in plaque-stage lesions. They present in groups as faintly eosinophilic spheres 1 to 7 μm in size and are PAS-positive and diastase resistant. The globules probably represent partially digested erythrocytes. Usually, the epidermis and skin appendages remain intact.

Lesions of Kaposi sarcoma, particularly in the nodular stage, may be partially or completely intravascular (225). The vessels involved are usually veins.

Distinctive variants of classic Kaposi sarcoma include those with micronodular, lymphangioma-like, lymphangiectatic, ecchymotic, verrucous, keloidal, and pyogenic granuloma–like features (226–229).

HIV-positive patients presenting with Kaposi sarcoma in lymphedematous skin may show focal fibroma-like lesions that may represent an early stage in the evolution of Kaposi sarcoma (230).

4. *Aggressive late-stage lesions.* Mostly in the endemic African setting but sometimes with other types of Kaposi sarcoma, "infiltrating" lesions show a more obviously sarcomatous character with reduction or loss of the vascular component. The spindle cells demonstrate a greater degree of cytologic atypia with regard to size, shape, and nuclear features, with mitosis becoming frequent. In such lesions, phagocytized erythrocytes and the presence of hyaline globules may provide clues about the tumor's origin. Very rarely, angiosarcoma is mimicked by the development of vascular spaces lined by grossly atypical endothelial cells. This variant of Kaposi sarcoma is termed "anaplastic" (Fig. 33-66). It is extremely rare, but case series have been reported in nonendemic settings (231).

A useful diagnostic tool is the demonstration of HHV-8 in samples from patients with all clinical subsets of Kaposi sarcoma. All variants of this tumor are etiologically related to this novel virus. Formerly, demonstration of the virus was possible

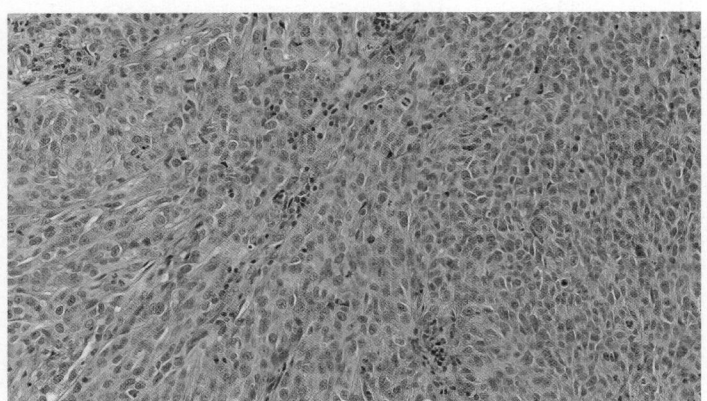

Figure 33-66 Anaplastic Kaposi sarcoma. More pronounced cellular atypia and abundant mitoses.

only by *in situ* hybridization. This has been simplified by the development of a commercially available monoclonal antibody against the latent nuclear antigen (LNA-1) of the virus that can be used in routine practice. Positive cases demonstrate granular nuclear staining (232,233) (Fig. 33-67). Extremely rarely, a negative HHV-8 reaction may be encountered in a tumor with clinical and histologic features of Kaposi sarcoma (234). Such cases should be tested for HHV-8 transcripts by PCR.

The histology of lesions of Kaposi sarcoma that have regressed after chemotherapy or with angiogenesis inhibitors, including Col-3, can be difficult to interpret (235). Regression may be partial or complete. In completely regressed lesions, there is absence of spindle-shaped cells; increase in the number of capillaries in the superficial dermis; a superficial, perivascular lymphohistiocytic inflammatory cell infiltrate; and variable numbers of siderophages. Partially regressed lesions show a prominent decrease in the number of spindle-shaped cells, focal inflammation, and siderophages. The residual spindle-shaped cells tend to be arranged around superficial and mid-dermal capillaries. These changes are correlated with a prominent decrease in the expression of LNA-1.

Pathogenesis. The peculiar epidemiologic aspects of Kaposi sarcoma have stimulated research for many years on whether viruses other than HIV or some other transmissible agent help to induce the disease. Initial studies of the fine structure of tumor cells in Kaposi sarcoma have revealed tuboreticular structures and cylindrical-confronting cisternae, suggestive of a cellular

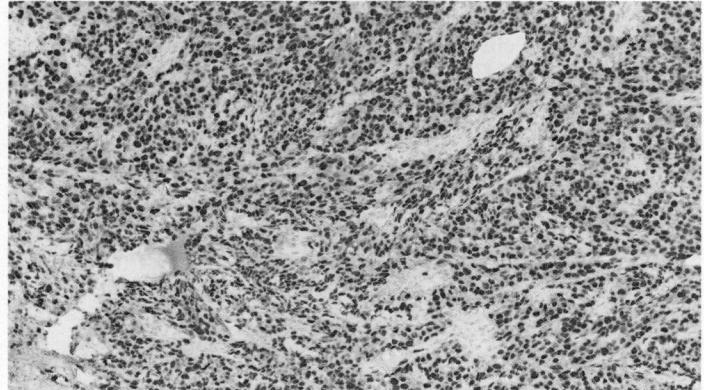

Figure 33-67 Kaposi sarcoma. Staining of the nuclei of tumor cells with an antibody against the LAN-1 of HHV-8 using the ABC (Avidin Biotic Complex) immunohistochemical staining method.

reaction to a viral infection. In the last decade of the 20th century, the riddle of the association between Kaposi sarcoma and a virus was resolved. Chang and colleagues (236) described a new human gammaherpesvirus associated with Kaposi sarcoma. This virus is closely associated with Epstein–Barr virus, has been named *HHV-8*, and it is etiologically associated with Kaposi sarcoma (237–239). DNA sequences of this virus have been detected consistently in all variants of the disease, including AIDS-related Kaposi sarcoma, African endemic Kaposi sarcoma induced by iatrogenic immunosuppression, and Mediterranean Kaposi sarcoma. The virus can be found in the blood of patients before lesions of Kaposi sarcoma develop (240).

For many years, it was suspected that the proliferating cell in Kaposi sarcoma is lymphatic in origin. This has been substantiated by the development of antibodies specific for lymphatic endothelium, including Lyve-1, podoplanin, D2-40, and Prox1 (241,242).

The multifocal development, slow evolution of the classic form of the disease, regression when immunosuppression is reduced or stopped, and histology of inflammation and cells lacking cytologic atypia have led many to suggest that at least initially Kaposi sarcoma is a reactive condition and not a neoplastic process. Initial reports demonstrating the presence of clonality have lent support to the latter (243). However, a number of more recent studies have suggested that the disease starts as a reactive angioproliferative and inflammatory process that progresses to become a monoclonal neoplastic process (244,245). This is a result of close, complex interactions between inflammatory cytokines, angiogenic factors, HHV-8, and, in HIV-positive patients, the HIV virus (246,247). In the latter setting, it has been demonstrated that the HIV-1 transactivating protein Tat-1 promotes the development of lesions by increasing the activity of different cytokines and angiogenic factors (248).

Differential Diagnosis. The differential diagnosis is wide, with the most difficulties encountered with either early macular or late aggressive lesions. Vascular proliferations in stasis and multinucleate cell angiohistiocytoma are discussed here in more detail because they are not described elsewhere in this chapter. All of the different lesions described later in this section are usually negative for HHV-8, whereas Kaposi sarcoma in all stages should be positive for this marker.

In *early macular lesions*, an inflammatory condition or a cell-poor (atrophic) histiocytoma may be suspected because the vascular nature of vessels with collapsed lumina may not be apparent. Appropriate cell markers may clarify the vascular nature of the underlying lesion. In late macular lesions, the differential diagnosis includes a well-differentiated angiosarcoma, progressive lymphangioma, targetoid hemosiderotic hemangioma, and microvenular hemangioma. Angiosarcoma shows not only a "dissection" of collagen infiltrative pattern but also endothelial cell atypia with hyperchromatism and intraluminal shedding of malignant cells. Histologically, progressive lymphangioma is almost indistinguishable from Kaposi sarcoma with prominent lymphangioma-like features, but inflammatory cells, especially plasma cells, tend to be absent in the former. When the clinical features are taken into account, distinction is not difficult. In hobnail hemangioma, lymphangioma-like channels are confined mainly to the upper dermis; in some places, plump "hobnail" endothelial cells invaginate vascular spaces, inflammatory cells are rare, and hemosiderin deposition is prominent, unlike early Kaposi sarcoma. Microvenular hemangioma differs by showing blood-containing vessels, many of which are surrounded by pericytes or smooth muscle cells (positive for smooth muscle actin), suggestive of venular differentiation.

SCH, kaposiform hemangioendothelioma, and moderately differentiated angiosarcomas with spindle cell differentiation are the most important histologic simulants of *nodular Kaposi lesions*.

SCH differs by showing cavernous or widely dilated vascular spaces and collections of epithelioid cells with or without intracytoplasmic lumina.

Kaposiform hemangioendothelioma is mainly a disease of children that usually affects deep soft tissues, although the skin can be affected (249). Histologically, the tumor shows intermediate features of capillary hemangioma and Kaposi sarcoma and has a lobular growth pattern that is absent in Kaposi sarcoma. Furthermore, the capillaries at the periphery of tumor lobules in kaposiform hemangioendothelioma often show focal thrombosis, there may be focal epithelioid endothelial cells, and eosinophilic globules are absent.

Sometimes, spindle cell differentiation is prominent in angiosarcoma, but usually markedly atypical cells are present, allowing differentiation from Kaposi sarcoma.

Other acquired vascular conditions that can cause problems from the clinical and histologic points of view are bacillary angiomatosis and pyogenic granuloma, especially if complicated by satellite lesions, and tufted angioma. Spindle cell fascicles with a bland cytologic appearance do not feature as a prominent component of any of these entities.

Aneurysmal benign fibrous histiocytoma is a nonvascular, highly cellular spindle cell lesion with pseudovascular spaces and hemosiderin deposition that can be confused with nodular Kaposi sarcoma (250). The variability of pathology, the presence of peripheral areas similar to common dermal fibrous histiocytoma, and immunohistochemistry should prevent error in diagnosis.

In *aggressive late-stage lesions*, many malignant spindle cell tumors can come into the differential diagnosis, especially if clinical details are unavailable. The most important differential diagnoses are fibrosarcoma, leiomyosarcoma, monophasic synovial sarcoma, malignant cellular blue nevus with sparse melanin deposition, and desmoplastic malignant melanoma. Accurate diagnosis may be impossible unless reliable immunohistochemistry is available. CD31 and CD34 are particularly helpful in suggesting a vascular derivation, even in poorly differentiated Kaposi lesions.

Hypostasis and high venous pressure give rise to vascular proliferation (pseudo–Kaposi sarcoma and acroangiodermatitis). Angiomatous papules and plaques near the ankles that are secondary to high venous pressure result from incompetent veins and are common causes of Kaposi-like lesions (251). Less commonly, high venous pressure can arise because of congenital or acquired arteriovenous anomalies (252). Histologically, there is an expansion of the whole capillary bed throughout the dermis. In the papillary dermis, there is reduplication and corkscrewing of thick-walled capillaries, which increase in size and become angiomatous in appearance. Similarly, venules and deeper, vertically small veins become hypertrophied and tortuous. Erythrocyte extravasation, fibrosis with horizontally oriented spindle cells, and numerous siderophages are additional features. The angiomatous capillaries appear separated from each other by an edematous matrix, and they do *not* lie "back-to-back" as in Kaposi sarcoma. To complicate matters, hypostatic vascular proliferation can coexist with Kaposi sarcoma. A key difference between Kaposi sarcoma and pseudo–Kaposi sarcoma is that in the latter, vascular hyperplasia results from hyperplasia of the preexisting vasculature, whereas in the former, the vascular proliferation is mainly independent.

Multinucleate cell angiohistiocytoma arises as slowly developing grouped vascular papules usually on the legs (253) but also at other sites including the face and hands (254). Most patients are older women. Histologically, an increased number of capillaries and venules with few inflammatory cells are found throughout the dermis, but the extent of the proliferation does achieve angiomatous proportions. Increased numbers of histiocytes and scattered multinucleate cells are usually found, although not in every biopsy. Blood pigment deposition is generally insignificant.

Immunohistochemical demonstration of HHV-8 is of great help in the histologic differential diagnosis of Kaposi sarcoma, as all of the vascular and nonvascular entities previously discussed are usually not associated with this virus.

Principles of Management: At present no curative treatment exists for Kaposi sarcoma, and the mainstay of treatment is relief of associated symptoms. Surgical excision, external beam radiation, laser treatment, cryotherapy, and photodynamic treatment can be used to control local tumor growth and manage associated discomfort or for cosmetic indications. Systemic chemotherapy is reserved for individual cases with numerous skin lesions, marked involvement of the oral mucosa, symptomatic visceral involvement, and rapidly progressive disease manifestation. Antiretroviral treatment (HAART) has significantly reduced the incidence of HIV-associated Kaposi sarcoma, whereas adjustment of immunosuppressive regimens may be beneficial in cases of iatrogenic Kaposi sarcoma (229).

Retiform Hemangioendothelioma

Clinical Summary. Retiform hemangioendothelioma is a rare variant of low-grade angiosarcoma that is characterized by indolent clinical behavior (255–257). There is a predilection for young adults, and it presents as a slowly growing nondistinct tumor with equal gender incidence and a predilection for the extremities, especially the distal lower limbs. Rare cases can be associated with radiotherapy or chronic lymphedema. A single case with multiple primary tumors has been documented (258). Multiple recurrences are common, but metastasis has so far been reported in only two cases. One case metastasized to a regional lymph node, and a second case presented with a soft tissue metastasis close to the primary tumor (258). Retiform hemangioendothelioma is part of the spectrum of a family of vascular tumors that are characterized by endothelial cells with a distinctive hobnail appearance. This includes a benign tumor originally described as targetoid hemosiderotic hemangioma (hobnail hemangioma) and another low-grade malignant lesion, PILA (p. 1248).

Histopathology. Tumors are ill-defined and involve the reticular dermis with frequent extension into the subcutis. In most cases, there is a striking low-power resemblance to the normal rete testis conferred by the presence of elongated, arborizing blood vessels (Fig. 33-68) lined by monomorphic bland endothelial cells with prominent apical nuclei and scanty cytoplasm. These

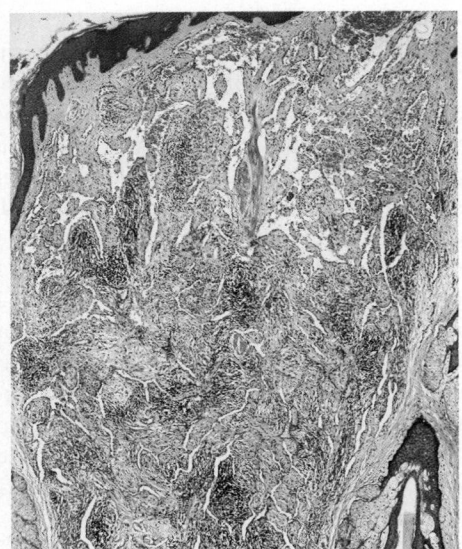

Figure 33-68 Retiform hemangioendothelioma. Branching blood vessels and a prominent lymphocytic inflammatory cell infiltrate.

cells have been described as having a "matchstick" or hobnail appearance (Fig. 33-69). A lymphocytic inflammatory cell infiltrate is frequently seen not only in the stroma but also in the vascular lumina (though not invariably present). The intravascular lymphocytes commonly appear in close contact with the hobnail endothelial cells. Occasional intravascular papillae with hyaline cores can be seen (Fig. 33-69). In most tumors, there are solid areas composed of bland spindle cells or epithelioid cells that stain for endothelial markers. Some lesions present a mini-retiform pattern that may be more difficult to recognize on low-power examination. A sclerotic stroma is seen in some cases.

Pathogenesis. Recurrent *YAP1* and *MAML2* gene rearrangements have been found in retiform hemangioendothelioma (259).

Differential Diagnosis. Retiform hemangioendothelioma shares clinical and histologic features with PILA (Dabska tumor). However, in the latter, cavernous vascular spaces resembling

lymphatics predominate, there is no retiform architecture, and intravascular papillae with collagenous cores are a striking feature. Hobnail hemangioma (targetoid hemosiderotic hemangioma) is more superficial, lacks a retiform architecture, and has hobnail endothelial cells that are seen mainly in vessels near the surface. Angiosarcoma often presents in a different clinical setting and shows cytologic atypia, mitoses, and absence of hobnail endothelial cells.

Principles of Management: Complete surgical excision is the treatment of choice.

Papillary Intralymphatic Angioendothelioma (Malignant Endothelial Papillary Angioendothelioma, Dabska Tumor)

Clinical Summary. PILA is a very rare tumor that was first described in 1969 as malignant endolymphatic angioendothelioma. Until recently, only very few additional cases had been reported in the literature, and there seemed to be a lack of consensus regarding its specific histologic features. However, the largest series of cases published more recently delineated the histologic features of this tumor more accurately, and the alternative name of PILA was proposed (260). Tumors present mainly in infants and children, but around 25% of patients are adults. Males and females are equally affected, and most cases involve the limbs. Clinical presentation is that of a slowly growing, solitary, asymptomatic nodule or plaque. This tumor is classified among tumors with low-grade malignant potential on the basis of reports of local recurrence and rare regional lymph node metastasis in the original series. However, follow-up in 8 of the 12 cases recently reported showed no evidence of either local recurrence or distant spread (260). It is therefore likely that these tumors are benign, although confirmation of these findings is required in larger series with longer follow-up.

Histopathology. Low-power examination reveals a dermal and often subcutaneous tumor composed of markedly dilated, thin-walled vascular channels resembling a cavernous lymphangioma (Fig. 33-70). These vascular channels are lined by bland hobnail endothelial cells with protruding nuclei and very scanty cytoplasm. A prominent intra- and extravascular

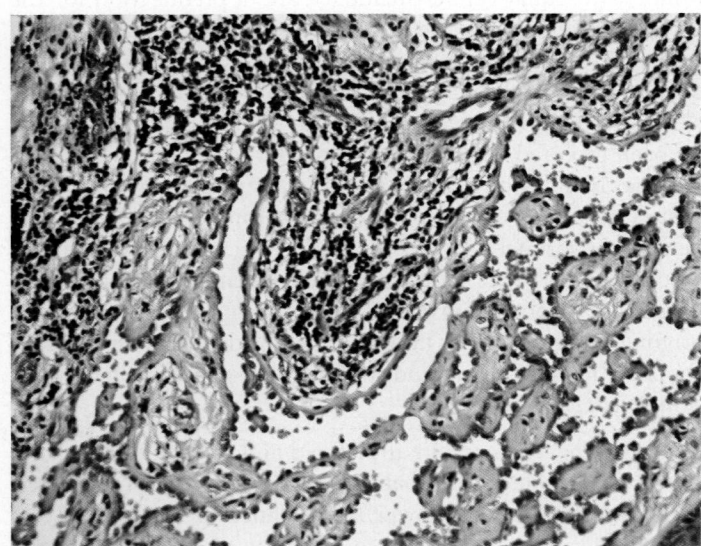

Figure 33-69 Retiform hemangioendothelioma. Typical bland hobnail endothelial cells and focal papillary projections.

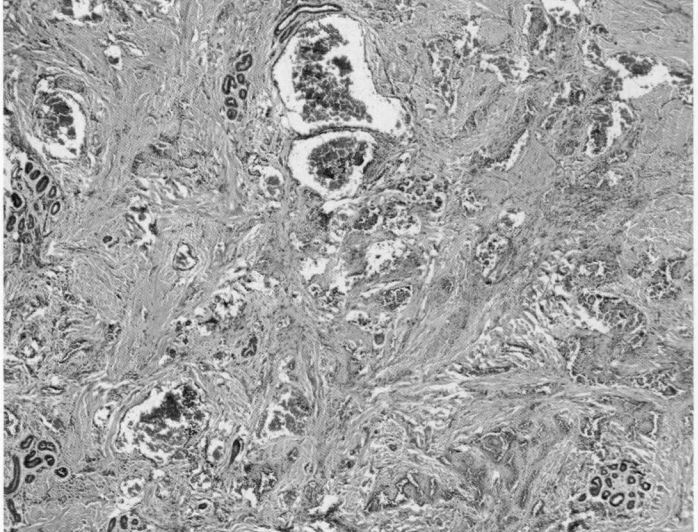

Figure 33-70 Papillary intralymphatic angioendothelioma. Cavernous lymphangioma–like vascular spaces and intravascular papillae.

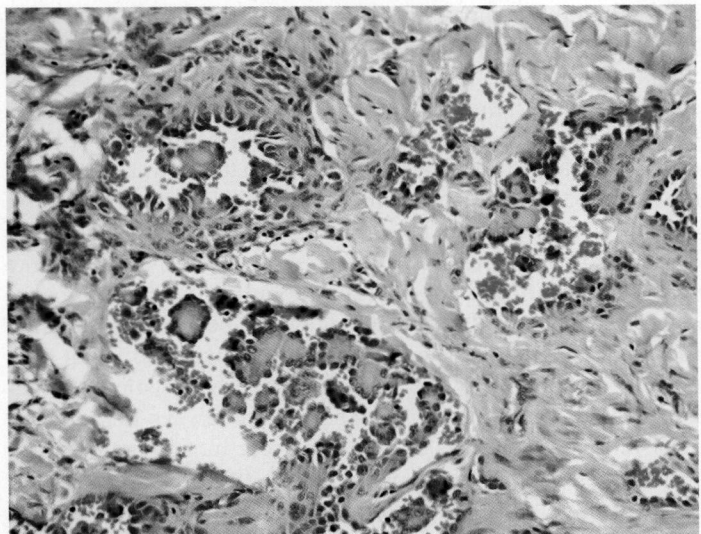

Figure 33-71 Papillary intralymphatic angioendothelioma. Bland hobnail endothelial cells and formation of numerous papillary projections with collagenous cores.

lymphocytic inflammatory cell infiltrate is often present, and intravascular papillae with collagenous cores are a frequent finding (Fig. 33-71). Commonly, the lymphocytes appear to be in close apposition to the endothelial cells.

Pathogenesis. On the basis of the close interaction between lymphocytes and endothelial cells in Dabska tumor, it has been proposed that the hobnail endothelial cells differentiate toward high endothelial cells, which are normally responsible for the selective homing of lymphocytes in lymphoid organs (261). A similar theory can be proposed for retiform hemangioendothelioma, which shares some histologic features with Dabska tumor. The strong expression of vascular endothelial growth factor receptor-3 (VEGFR-3) by tumor cells has led to suggestions that these tumors display lymphatic differentiation (261). However, the specificity of this marker as an indicator of lymphatic differentiation is doubtful.

Differential Diagnosis. Refer to the differential diagnosis for retiform hemangioendothelioma (previous section).

Principles of Management: Local excision is the currently recommended treatment.

Composite Hemangioendothelioma

Clinical Summary. Composite hemangioendothelioma is a low-grade malignant vascular tumor with a tendency for local recurrence but very low metastatic potential. It is defined as a neoplasm containing a mixture of histologic patterns including benign, intermediate, and/or malignant (262–264). It is a very rare tumor presenting mainly in adults. Childhood manifestation is rare, and congenital onset is exceptional (262–266). There is no sex predilection, and most tumors occur in the extremities with a predilection for the hands and feet. In 25% of patients, tumors arise in association with lymphedema. An association with Maffucci syndrome has also been documented. The lesions present as long-standing red-blue nodules or plaques, usually measuring multiple centimeters. The rate of local recurrence is around 50%, and this may occur years after excision of the primary tumor. In conventional composite hemangioendothelioma, there are only rare reported cases with satellites, and metastasis to regional lymph nodes and to the

soft tissues. An exceptional complication is the development of Kasabach–Merritt syndrome. The neuroendocrine variant (see later) is considerably more aggressive, with half of the cases developing distant metastases (267).

Histopathology. Composite hemangioendothelioma is poorly circumscribed, with an infiltrative growth pattern and involvement of the dermis and subcutaneous tissue. The different components vary from tumor to tumor and may include retiform hemangioendothelioma (Fig. 33-72), epithelioid hemangioendothelioma, PILA, SCH, conventional angiosarcoma (low and even high grade), lymphangioma circumscriptum, and areas simulating an arteriovenous malformation. The prognosis is likely to be dictated by the component with the highest histologic grade, but this should be estimated in larger series of cases with adequate follow-up. A subset of cases with more aggressive behavior are positive for neuroendocrine markers (synaptophysin, rarely chromogranin). These tumors usually display retiform and epithelioid components (similar to epithelioid hemangioendothelioma) and hemangioma-like areas in which the vascular channels are lined by hobnail endothelial cells (267). The lesions so far described do not show necrosis or areas with features of angiosarcoma. However, despite the histology being typical of compositive hemangioendothelioma, they have the potential for aggressive behavior with metastatic potential.

Pathogenesis. Composite hemangioendotheliomas exhibit recurrent *YAP1* and *MAML2* gene rearrangements (268).

Principles of Management: Complete excision is the mainstay of treatment.

Kaposiform Infantile Hemangioendothelioma (Kaposi-Like Hemangioendothelioma)

Clinical Summary. Kaposiform infantile hemangioendothelioma, a distinctive vascular neoplasm, was described in the past in individual case reports under different names (249,269–271). It is rare and usually presents in the retroperitoneum or deep soft tissues of infants and neonates. Tufted angioma is likely to be part of the spectrum of this neoplasm, with the former representing an earlier,

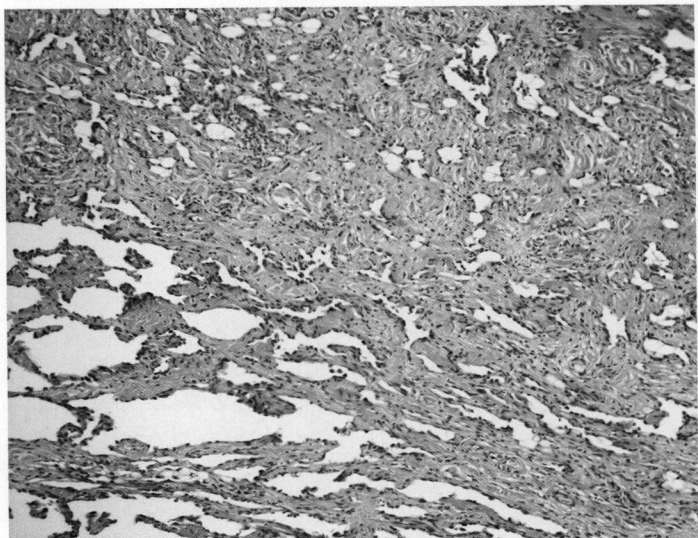

Figure 33-72 Composite hemangioendothelioma. Areas of retiform hemangioendothelioma and well-differentiated angiosarcoma. Elsewhere, the tumor contains areas resembling an epithelioid hemangioendothelioma.

less exuberant variant of the latter with predilection for the skin (see p. 1229). Occasionally, congenital or adult multifocal lesions have been described (272). A high number of cases are associated with Kasabach–Merritt syndrome (up to half of cases or more) or lymphangiomatosis. It is classified as a low-grade malignant vascular tumor because of its locally aggressive growth. Although exceptional regional perinodal soft tissue involvement has been reported, metastases have not been described (269,271). Cutaneous tumors are a common presenting feature but may be entirely absent in one-tenth of patients (272). Lesions with a superficial location tend to behave in a benign fashion except when associated with Kasabach–Merritt syndrome.

Histopathology. Low-power examination shows a tumor with a lobular and focally infiltrative growth pattern (Fig. 33-73). Bands of collagen separate tumor lobules. These lobules are composed of a mixture of congested capillaries surrounded by fascicles of bland spindle-shaped endothelial cells and pericytes (Fig. 33-74). Slitlike vascular spaces are often a feature. Focal

areas with epithelioid cells containing abundant pale pink cytoplasm are often seen. In many areas, the tumor resembles a capillary hemangioma. Toward the periphery of the tumor lobules, small vascular channels frequently show intraluminal thrombi (Fig. 33-75). Hemosiderin deposition and hemorrhage are additional findings. It has been suggested that this tumor consists of vascular and lymphatic components, and there is expression of D2-40 (podoplanin) by endothelial cells (273). The latter is reflected by the presence of dilated, irregular, lymphatic-like spaces in the stroma between tumor lobules. Some tumors have areas resembling tufted angioma. It has been suggested that there is an overlap between both entities, and endothelial cells of both disorders show expression of the lymphatic endothelial cell marker, Prox1 (112). Lesions are always negative for HHV-8. Regression does not tend to occur in patients who survive the Kasabach–Merritt phenomenon (274).

Distinction from Kaposi sarcoma is discussed on page 1247.

Pathogenesis. Although data is limited owing to only a few analyzed cases, somatic activating *GNA14* mutations have been reported (110), and epigenetic analysis shows a shared methylation profile with tufted angioma, distinct from the methylation pattern of vascular malformations (275).

Principles of Management: Treatment is surgical excision. Treatment options for large and deep-seated lesions, not amenable to surgery, include embolization, chemotherapy with vincristine, corticosteroids, sirolimus, and propranolol.

Pseudomyogenic (Epithelioid Sarcoma–Like) Hemangioendothelioma

Clinical Summary. Pseudomyogenic hemangioendothelioma is a rare tumor of low-grade malignant potential with a high risk of local recurrence but only rare metastatic potential. Owing to its clinical and immunohistochemical features, it was initially thought to represent a distinctive variant of epithelioid sarcoma, and it was originally reported in 1992 as the "fibroma-like variant of epithelioid sarcoma" (276). It has subsequently become apparent that the tumor shows endothelial differentiation and it has been referred to as either "epithelioid

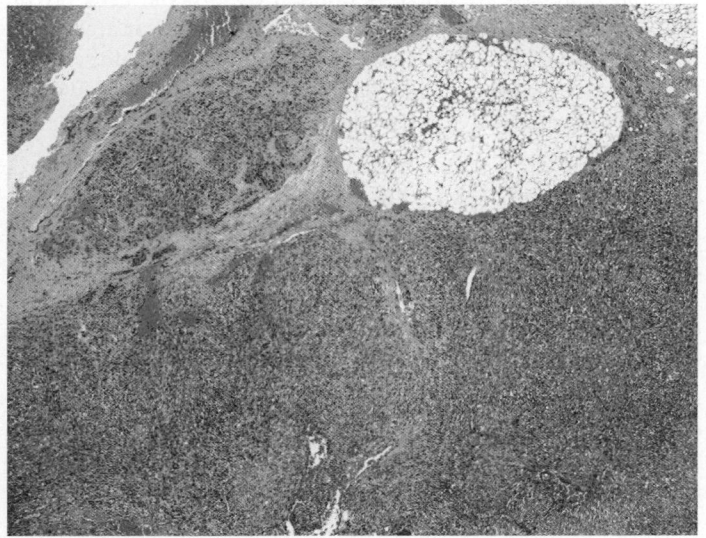

Figure 33-73 Kaposiform hemangioendothelioma. Typical lobular and infiltrative growth pattern with replacement of the subcutaneous tissue.

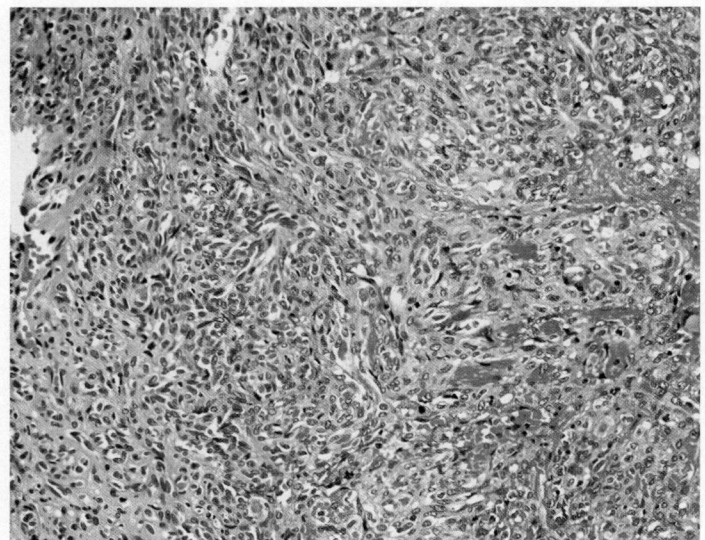

Figure 33-74 Kaposiform hemangioendothelioma. Capillaries intermixed with bland spindle-shaped cells.

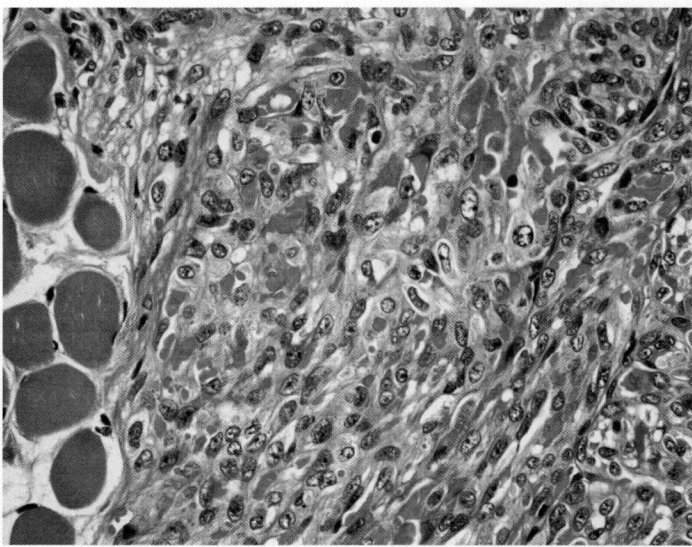

Figure 33-75 Kaposiform hemangioendothelioma. Note the infiltration of skeletal muscle and frequent microthrombi within the capillaries.

sarcoma–like hemangioendothelioma" or, more recently, as "pseudomyogenic hemangioendothelioma" (277,278).

The tumor affects young adults, with a strong male predilection. Although the anatomic distribution is wide, the lower extremities are most commonly involved. The clinical presentation as frequently painful nodules measuring few centimeters is typical, and the disease is multifocal in most cases (279).

The tumors have the potential for local recurrence and development of further lesions. Metastasis to lymph nodes or visceral organs and disease-associated mortality are, however, exceptional (279).

Histopathology. The tumors affect multiple tissue planes and may present within dermis, subcutis, and, less frequently, in skeletal muscle or even bone (Fig. 33-76). The margins are infiltrative, often giving rise to a plexiform growth pattern. The tumor cells are spindled and arranged in loose fascicles and sheets. They contain abundant brightly eosinophilic and occasionally rhabdomyoblast-like cytoplasm and vesicular nuclei with variably sized eosinophilic nucleoli (Fig. 33-77). A minor cellular component with epithelioid differentiation may be admixed. Cytologic atypia is mild. Nuclear pleomorphism is a rare feature, and mitoses are scarce. Tumor necrosis and lymphovascular invasion may be observed, and an intratumoral neutrophil-rich inflammatory cell infiltrate is frequently seen.

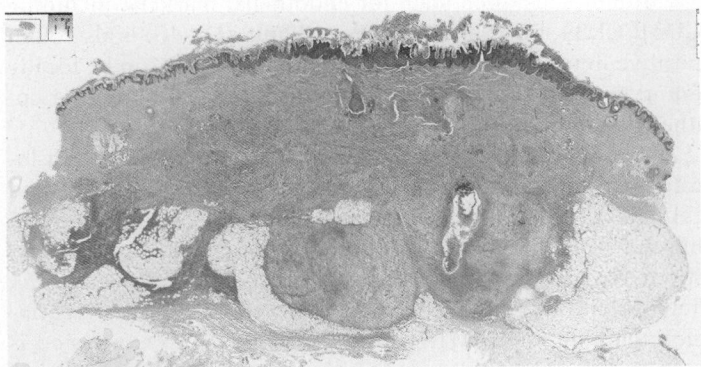

Figure 33-76 Pseudomyogenic hemangioendothelioma. The tumor shows nodular outlines with focally infiltrative growth within skeletal muscle.

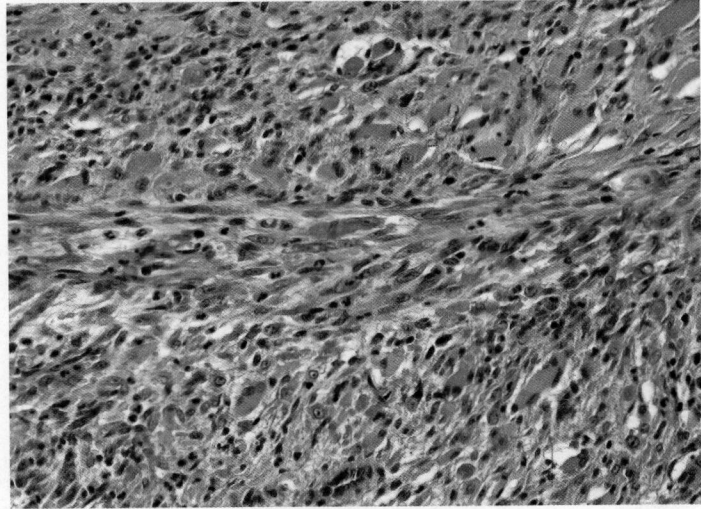

Figure 33-77 Pseudomyogenic hemangioendothelioma. Spindled tumor cells are arranged in fascicles infiltrating skeletal muscle fibers.

By immunohistochemistry, tumor cells consistently express cytokeratin AE1/AE3 in addition to the endothelial markers FLI1 and ERG (277–280). CD31 staining is noted in approximately 50% of cases. Focal expression for cytokeratins CAM5.2 and MNF116, EMA, and SMA may also be observed, but CD34, S-100 protein, and desmin staining are negative, and INI1 expression is intact. Diffuse nuclear immunoreactivity for FOSB in greater than 50% of cells is observed in almost all pseudomyogenic hemangioendotheliomas (281).

Pathogenesis. Various FOSB gene rearrangements have been demonstrated in pseudomyogenic hemangioendothelioma (282,283).

Differential Diagnosis. Pseudomyogenic hemangioendothelioma has a broad differential diagnosis of cutaneous spindle cell tumors. Spindle cell squamous cell carcinoma affects sun-damaged skin, most commonly of the head and neck area of elderly patients. Although it shares the expression of cytokeratins, it is consistently negative for the endothelial cell marker ERG and FOSB. Cellular fibrous histiocytoma lacks the plexiform growth pattern, and its spindle cells are tapered rather than plump and they lack the brightly eosinophilic cytoplasm. The lack of desmin expression excludes leiomyosarcoma. Epithelioid sarcoma is characterized by a multinodular growth pattern composed of sheets of epithelioid cells. In contrast to pseudomyogenic hemangioendothelioma, INI1 expression is consistently lost in epithelioid sarcoma. Spindle cell angiosarcoma has a similar immunohistochemical profile. It is, however, characterized by severe cytologic atypia and nuclear pleomorphism, and vasoformative elements are often present.

Principles of Management: Conservative excision is the treatment of choice.

MALIGNANT TUMORS

Epithelioid Hemangioendothelioma

Clinical Summary. Epithelioid hemangioendothelioma is a neoplasm that was initially described in 1982 as a low-grade tumor of vascular endothelial origin (284). Epithelioid hemangioendothelioma, however, is associated with high morbidity and mortality and should therefore be regarded as a neoplasm with full malignant potential (285). It arises mainly in the superficial and deep soft tissue and muscle of the extremities (286). The tumor can also arise at internal sites and in the viscera (especially the liver, lungs, and bone). Many of such tumors were described previously by different names. Middle-aged patients, with an equal gender distribution, are mainly affected, but the tumor has a wide age distribution. In about half the cases, the tumor apparently arises from a medium-sized vein or, less often, an artery (287,288). Multicentricity is common in visceral lesions, particularly those affecting the lungs, liver, and bones. Skin involvement is uncommon and usually associated with an underlying soft tissue or bone lesion or with multicentric disease (289). Rare cases present with pure cutaneous involvement (290,291). Metastases develop in about 30% of cases involving superficial soft tissues, with a mortality rate of 17% (292). The prognosis is worse for internal sites.

Histopathology. Typically, epithelioid hemangioendothelioma shows an infiltrative growth pattern. However, purely cutaneous tumors often consist of a fairly circumscribed dermal tumor

(Fig. 33-78). Tumor cells are ovoid, cuboidal, or short and spindle shaped with prominent eosinophilic cytoplasm. The nucleus is vesicular, showing variable or no atypia, and the nucleolus lacks prominence (Fig. 33-79). Cells tend to be arranged in short fascicles, small nests, or in a "single file" pattern, often set in a distinctive hyalinized or mucoid stroma rich in sulfated acid mucopolysaccharides. There is often a chondroid appearance. Obvious vascular channels are generally lacking, but intracytoplasmic vacuoles, sometimes containing erythrocytes, are usually present (Fig. 33-79). Infiltration through large-vessel walls and evidence of endothelial origin may be found. A subset of the tumor with a more aggressive clinical course shows prominent cytologic atypia and a high mitotic rate, overlapping histologically with epithelioid angiosarcoma (292) (Fig. 33-80). Rare cases that express synaptophysin seem to pursue an aggressive clinical course (289). Some cases are associated with a prominent osteoclast-like giant-cell reaction (293).

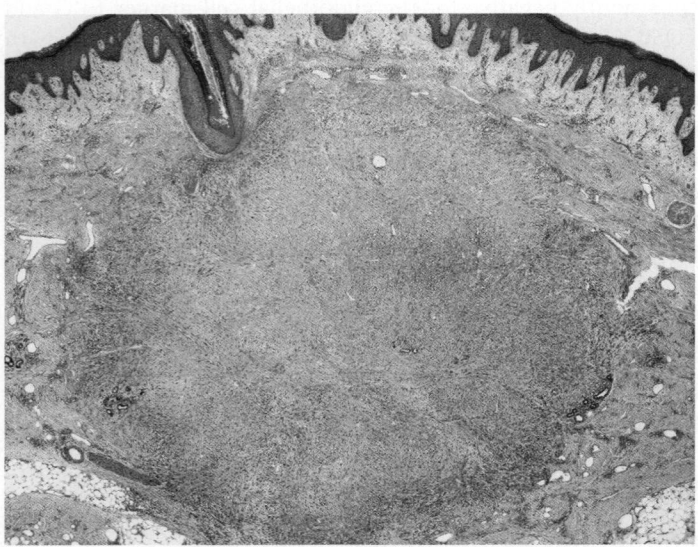

Figure 33-78 Epithelioid hemangioendothelioma. Purely cutaneous tumors often present as a fairly circumscribed nodule with hyalinization or myxoid change.

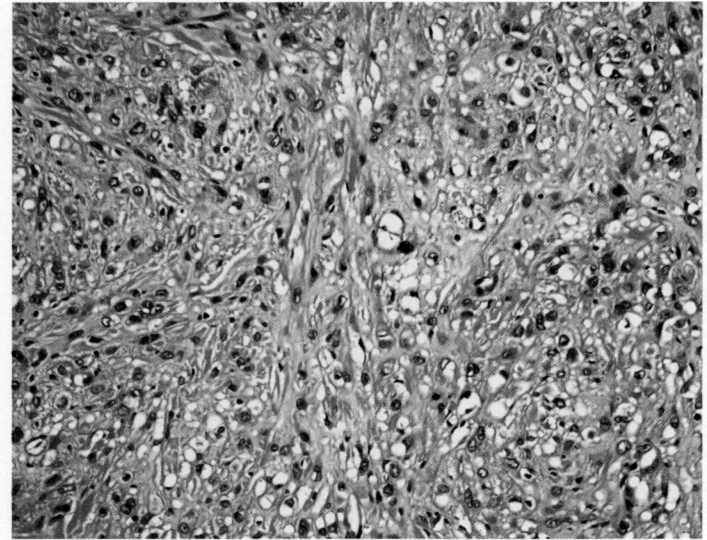

Figure 33-79 Epithelioid hemangioendothelioma. Epithelioid cells with variable atypia organized in short strands or individual units. Notice the formation of intracytoplasmic lumina.

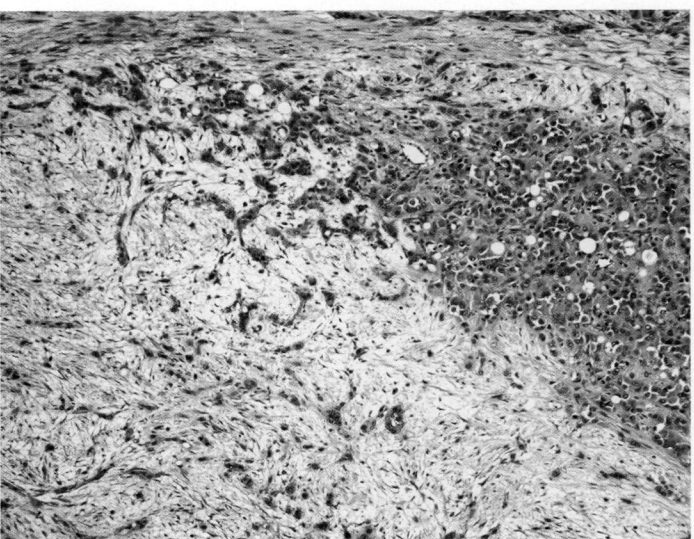

Figure 33-80 Epithelioid hemangioendothelioma. Transition between classic epithelioid hemangioendothelioma and solid, more pleomorphic areas with features of an epithelioid angiosarcoma.

Although lesions with cytologic atypia and mitoses are associated with a poorer prognosis, the behavior of tumors with bland morphology is difficult to predict.

Tumor cells often stain for endothelial markers, including CD31, CD34, FLI1, and ERG. Podoplanin (D2-40) is also often positive in tumor cells. Positivity for pan-keratin can be focally found in up to 20% to 30% of cases (289,292). Staining for epithelial membrane antigen is usually negative.

Cytogenetic analysis revealed a t(1;3) (p36.3;q25) translocation in most cases, resulting in a fusion of the *WWTR1* and *CAMTA1* genes (294–296). More recently, a novel fusion involving the *YAP1* and *TFE3* genes on chromosomes 11 and X, respectively, has been identified in a smaller subset of cases (297). Tumors with *WWTR1-CAMTA1* typically show diffuse strong nuclear staining for CAMTA1 (298), whereas TFE3 expression is seen in *YAP-TFE3* tumors and some of the *WWTR1-CAMTA1* tumors. Interestingly, it has been demonstrated that the fusions are not mutually exclusive and that TFE3-positive cases are characterized by larger solitary tumors with better formed vessels, more substantial nuclear atypia, and hypercellularity (299).

Differential Diagnosis. The differential diagnosis includes epithelioid hemangioma (angiolymphoid hyperplasia with eosinophilia), which often has a lobular architecture, prominent inflammation, and numerous well-formed blood vessels; metastatic adenocarcinoma, which is negative for endothelial markers and positive for mucin stains; myxoid chondrosarcoma, which has a lobular growth pattern, S-100 protein-positive cells, and absence of intracytoplasmic lumina; and myoepithelioma, which usually lacks intracytoplasmic lumina and has cells that are variably positive for keratin, smooth muscle actin, epithelial membrane antigen, glial fibrillary acid protein, and S-100 protein.

Principles of Management: Treatment is surgical excision. Chemotherapy and radiation may be used for tumors not amenable to surgery or for metastatic disease.

Angiosarcoma

Clinical Summary. Most angiosarcomas of the skin arise in the following clinical settings: (a) angiosarcoma of the face and scalp in the elderly, (b) angiosarcoma (lymphangiosarcoma) secondary to chronic lymphedema (Stewart–Treves syndrome), and (c) angiosarcoma as a complication of chronic radiodermatitis or arising from the effects of severe skin trauma or ulceration (300).

An aggressive variant known as *epithelioid angiosarcoma* (301) regarded as distinctive from the variants mentioned before has been described. This tumor is difficult to diagnose histologically without the help of immunohistochemistry because of the exclusive epithelioid morphology and the limited formation of vascular channels (see text following).

Apart from these circumstances, cutaneous angiosarcomas are extremely rare. Exceptional case reports include angiosarcoma arising in preceding benign vascular tumors, including vascular malformations (302), in a large blood vessel (303), in association with a plexiform neurofibroma in neurofibromatosis (304), in a schwannoma (305), in a malignant peripheral nerve sheath tumor (306), in xeroderma pigmentosum (307), in a gouty tophus (308), in association with vinyl chloride exposure (309), in association with immunosuppression in organ transplantation (310), vascular grafts (311), and as the mesenchymal component in a metaplastic carcinoma (312). A case of "cutaneous-type" angiosarcoma has been described arising in a mature teratoma of the ovary (313). Angiosarcoma in children is extremely rare (314). An exceptional case of an angiosarcoma producing granulocyte colony-stimulating factor and inducing a leukemoid reaction has been described (315). With the exception of epithelioid angiosarcoma, the histologic spectrum of angiosarcomas is similar regardless of the clinical setting.

1. *Angiosarcoma of the scalp and face of the elderly.* This is almost invariably a fatal tumor that usually arises innocuously as erythematous or bruiselike lesions on the scalp or middle and upper face with a predilection for men (316–320). Subsequent plaques, nodules, or ulcerations develop (Fig. 33-81); metastasis to nodes or internal organs (mainly lungs, liver, and brain) usually arises as a late complication, with many patients dying as a result of extensive local disease. This sarcoma has only rarely been reported in black patients; the disease affects mainly whites and sometimes Asians (320). Only a very small

percentage of patients, with smaller lesions that are usually less than between 5 and 10 cm in diameter at presentation, can be successfully treated with radical wide field radiotherapy and surgery (316,319). Combined series of idiopathic angiosarcoma of the face and scalp, other cutaneous angiosarcomas, and angiosarcomas occurring in internal organs report 5-year survival rates varying between 24% and 34% (318,319,321,322). The best chance of survival resides in wide surgical excision followed by radiotherapy (323).

2. *Angiosarcoma following lymphedema (postmastectomy lymphangiosarcoma or the Stewart–Treves syndrome).* Typically, the tumor presents in women who have had severe, long-standing lymphedema of the arm following breast surgery (324,325). In most cases, lymphedema is present for about 10 years before the tumor arises, usually in the inner portion of the upper arm. Radiotherapy can usually be excluded as an etiologic factor because the sarcoma nearly always develops beyond the areas of chronic radiodermatitis. Lymphedema-induced angiosarcoma has also been described in men and in a lower extremity (326) from causes other than cancer surgery, including congenital lymphedema (327), tropical lymphedema attributable to filarial infection (328), and massive localized lymphedema of the morbidly obese (329). The prognosis despite radical surgery is extremely poor.

3. *Postirradiation angiosarcoma.* There are many reports of angiosarcoma arising in the skin after radiotherapy for internal cancer. The most common sites are the breast or chest wall (330–335) and the lower abdomen after therapy for breast or gynecologic cancer.

Histopathology. Usually, the tumor extends well beyond the limits of the apparent clinical lesion, and multifocality is frequent. As a rule, the tumor shows varied differentiation in different biopsies, even within different fields in a single biopsy (Fig. 33-82). In well-differentiated areas, irregular anastomosing vascular channels lined by a single layer of somewhat enlarged endothelial cells permeate between collagen bundles (Figs. 33-82 and 33-83). Isolation and enclosure of collagen bundles, figuratively referred to as *dissection of collagen* is a characteristic feature (Fig. 33-84). Nuclear atypia

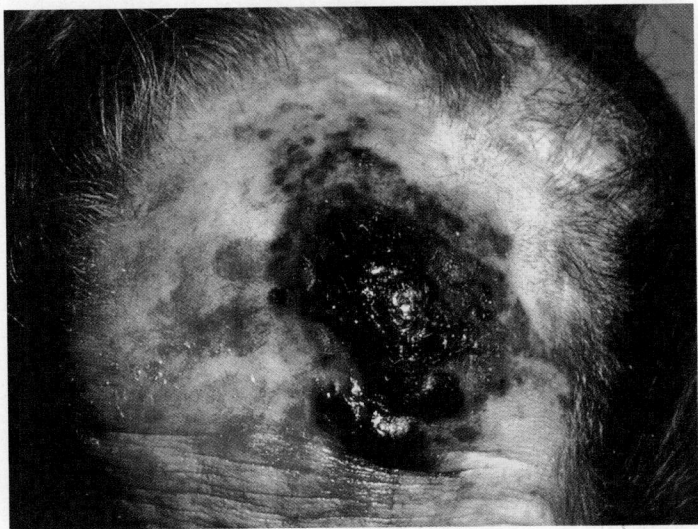

Figure 33-81 Idiopathic angiosarcoma of the face. Hemorrhagic, ulcerated nodule with bruiselike lesions in a multifocal pattern in surrounding skin.

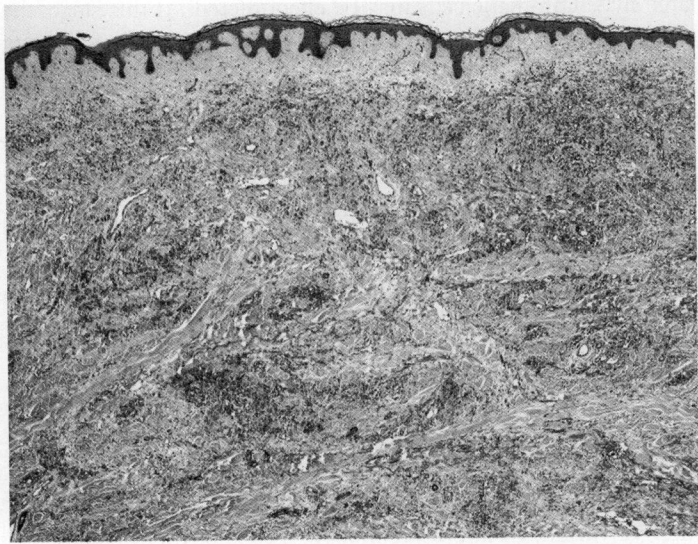

Figure 33-82 Well-differentiated angiosarcoma. Low-power view mimicking plaque-stage Kaposi sarcoma.

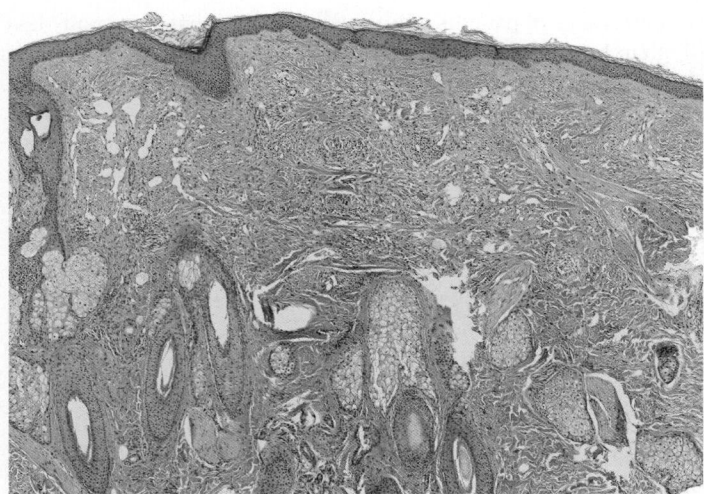

Figure 33-83 Well-differentiated angiosarcoma. Irregular and congested vascular channels infiltrating between collagen bundles.

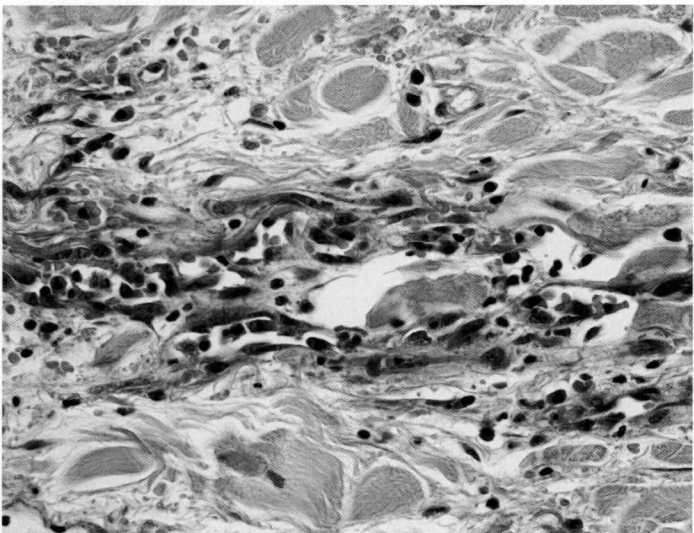

Figure 33-84 Well-differentiated angiosarcoma. Dissection of collagen pattern. Marked cytologic atypia and multilayering.

is always present and may be slight to moderate, but occasional large hyperchromatic cells may be encountered. At this stage, the vascular lumens are generally bloodless but may contain free-lying shed malignant cells. Mitotic figures are invariably present, and it has been suggested that a high mitotic rate correlates with a poor prognosis (336). Other factors that are associated with poor prognosis include depth of invasion and positive tumor margins along with a tumor diameter greater than 5 cm.

In less well-differentiated areas, endothelial cells increase in size and number (Fig. 33-85), forming intraluminal papillary projections where there is enhanced mitotic activity. In poorly differentiated areas, solid sheets of large pleomorphic cells with little or no evidence of luminal differentiation can resemble metastatic carcinoma or melanoma. Focally, areas showing epithelioid cells are not uncommon. The presence of an epithelioid component in the three variants of angiosarcoma described herein should not lead to the classification of a tumor because epithelioid angiosarcoma such as this represents a distinctive variant of angiosarcoma (p. 1255). Other areas of tumors may simulate a poorly differentiated spindle cell sarcoma (Fig. 33-86). Interstitial hemorrhage and widely dilated blood-filled

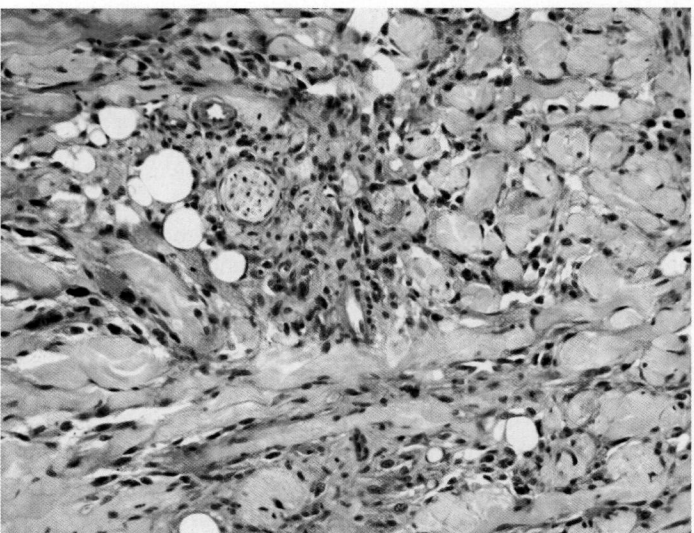

Figure 33-85 Moderately differentiated angiosarcoma. More cellular tumor with less evident vascular differentiation and more cytologic atypia.

spaces may sometimes develop. Rare cases are composed of granular cells, signet ring cells, or foamy cells (337–339). In exceptional cases, tumors may be extensively infiltrated by lymphocytes or macrophages. In the former setting, distinction from a lymphoma may be difficult (340,341).

The histopathology of angiosarcomas secondary to lymphedema and radiotherapy shows a similar range of well-differentiated to poorly differentiated neoplasms as idiopathic angiosarcoma of the face and scalp. There are no reliable histologic differentiating features, although sometimes evidence of chronic lymphedema or chronic radiation dermatitis may be apparent in the tissue adjacent to the sarcoma.

Histogenesis. Sarcomas of probable lymphatic origin cannot be distinguished histologically from those of presumptive vascular endothelial origin; hence, there is a tendency to disregard the term *lymphangiosarcoma* in favor of *angiosarcoma.* For many years, a number of putative specific markers of lymphatic endothelium

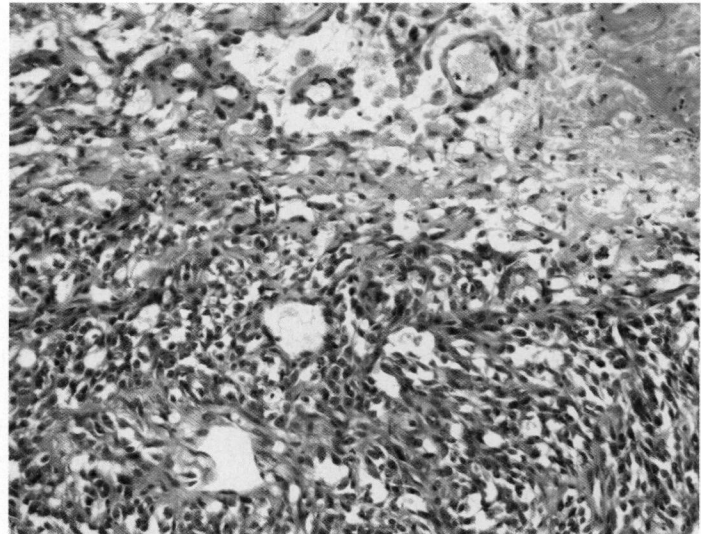

Figure 33-86 Poorly differentiated angiosarcoma. Highly cellular tumor composed of pleomorphic spindle-shaped cells and only focal suggestion of vascular differentiation.

have been described, many of which have been a disappointment. However, a few appear to be specific, and these include LYVE-1, podoplanin, D2-40, and Prox1 (342–345). By using D2-40, it has been shown that a percentage of cases, but by no means all, of angiosarcomas display lymphatic differentiation (346).

CD34 and, especially, the more specific CD31 are much more reliable as sensitive markers of tumors of endothelial cell origin for use in routine biopsies (347). It is important to remember, however, that CD34 is a very poorly specific marker and that CD31 stains macrophages, and this may represent a pitfall in tumors with prominent numbers of macrophages (347). The staining pattern, however, in the latter cells tends to be granular and faint, whereas in endothelial cells the staining is crisp and highlights the cytoplasmic membrane prominently. An antibody against the carboxy terminal of the FLI1 protein, a nuclear transcription factor member of the ETS family of DNA-binding transcription factors, has been shown to be a relatively specific marker of endothelial cells (348,349). More recently, an antibody developed against ERG, another member of the ETS family of DNA-binding transcription factors, appears to show superior specificity and sensitivity (350,351). As opposed to other markers of endothelial cell differentiation, the staining with antibodies against FLI1 and ERG is nuclear. On electron microscopic examination, well-differentiated tumors may show the ovoid laminated organelle-like Weibel–Palade bodies characteristic of vascular endothelial cells, but they are absent in most tumors.

MYC amplification and overexpression can be detected by fluorescence *in situ* hybridization (FISH) and immunohistochemistry in the secondary forms of angiosarcoma (352). In contrast, this appears to be a rare finding in primary cutaneous angiosarcoma (353).

On gene analysis, most cases show complex karyotypes, with upregulation of angiogenesis-related and vascular-specific receptor tyrosine kinase genes (*CIC*, *KDR*, *PTPRB*, and *PLCG*), whereas the epithelioid morphology subset in younger patients is particularly associated with *CIC* alterations (354).

Differential Diagnosis. Well-differentiated angiosarcomas, if cell atypia is slight, may closely resemble early macular lesions of Kaposi sarcoma and benign lymphangioendothelioma, because all of these conditions can demonstrate, to a greater or lesser extent, a "dissection of collagen" pattern. The major differences in clinical presentation of the disorders (absence of mitosis and the bland appearances of the endothelial cells in macular lesions of Kaposi sarcoma and benign lymphangioendothelioma) should prevent any difficulties. Focal dissection of collagen pattern is also mimicked in intravascular papillary endothelial hyperplasia by new vessels invading thrombotic material. In poorly differentiated angiosarcomas, it is usually possible to find evidence of channel formation in peripheral areas that allows diagnosis. However, the use of endothelial markers, especially ERG and CD31, is an important aid in diagnosis. CD31 is the most specific and sensitive marker of endothelial cell differentiation, but it is important to remember that this marker also stains macrophages, and this may represent a diagnostic pitfall. Atypical vascular proliferations that are not uncommonly seen after radiotherapy also need to be distinguished from angiosarcoma, which are discussed on page 1258. Finally, occasionally adenoid squamous carcinomas or sarcomatoid squamous cell carcinoma, with or without intratumoral hemorrhage, can simulate angiosarcoma (355–357). Immunohistochemistry is useful in these cases because only angiosarcomas with epithelioid

morphology are usually positive for cytokeratin, but these also show staining for CD31 and CD34. Angiosarcomas are consistently negative for HHV-8 (358).

Principles of Management: The treatment of cutaneous angiosarcoma is primarily surgical with wide local excision. Adequate surgical margins are often difficult to achieve, and adjuvant radiotherapy may be beneficial. Chemotherapy may be used for advanced disease.

Epithelioid Angiosarcoma

Clinical Summary. Epithelioid angiosarcoma is a rare form of angiosarcoma that usually arises in deep soft tissues (301) but may also occur in the skin and internal organs, including the thyroid and adrenal gland. Personal experience indicates that cutaneous lesions are more common than previously thought, and it is likely that such lesions were diagnosed in the past as epithelial or melanocytic neoplasms. There is a wide anatomic distribution with a predilection for the limbs (359,360). Tumors present in adults without a significant gender predilection. Some examples are multifocal, and it is difficult to establish the source of the primary tumor (346). Epithelioid angiosarcoma occurring in internal organs may rarely metastasize to the skin (361). Rare examples have been associated with radiation therapy (362), an arteriovenous fistula (363), and a foreign body (364). The outlook is extremely poor, although a slow course has been described for some skin tumors (359,360). However, the latter is based on a few cases with short follow-up, and cutaneous tumors appear to be aggressive (360).

Histopathology. Tumors are composed of sheets of pleomorphic large cells with prominent eosinophilic cytoplasm, a large nucleus, and an eosinophilic nucleolus, usually with little evidence of vascular differentiation other than the occasional presence of intracytoplasmic vacuoles sometimes containing red blood cells (Fig. 33-87). This angiosarcoma can easily be mistaken for a carcinoma deposit or even malignant melanoma (Fig. 33-88). Usually, the tumor cells demonstrate consistent positivity for CD34, FLI1, CD31, and ERG (360). However, cytokeratin positivity is present in up to 50% of cases, and rare cases are focally positive for epithelial membrane antigen; this might be a source of confusion with metastatic carcinoma and epithelioid

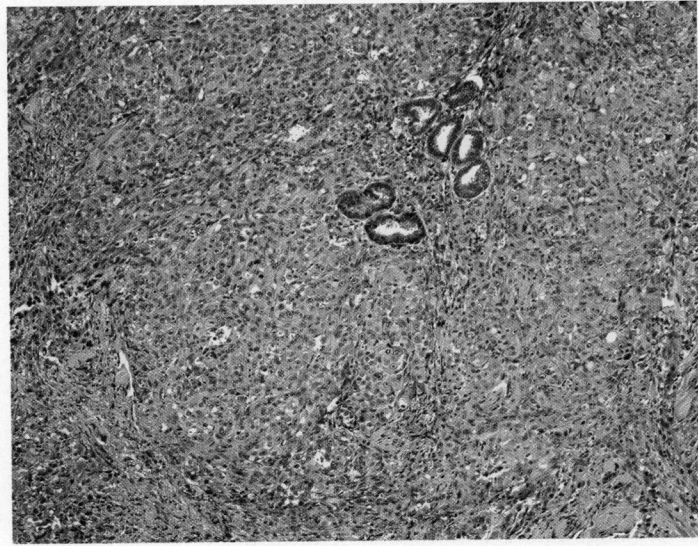

Figure 33-87 Epithelioid angiosarcoma. Solid proliferation of atypical epithelioid cells replacing the dermis.

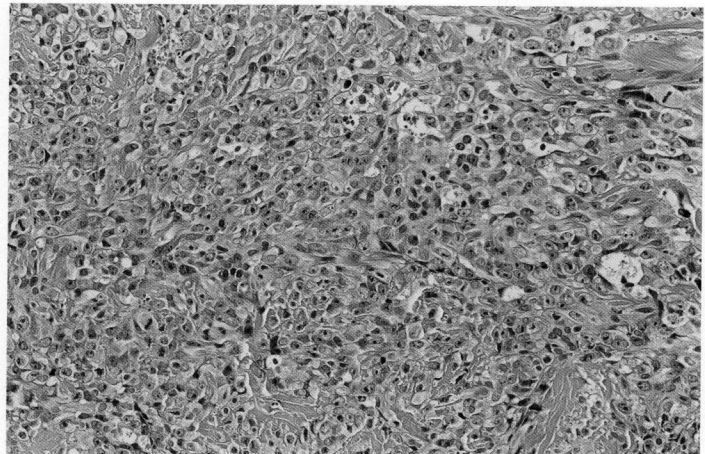

Figure 33-88 Epithelioid angiosarcoma. Large epithelioid cells with abundant pink cytoplasm, vesicular nuclei, and a single prominent eosinophilic nucleolus. Note the resemblance to melanoma cells and the hemorrhage in the background.

sarcoma, which are negative for endothelial markers. However, epithelioid sarcoma is positive for CD34 in up to 60% of cases and negative for INI-1.

Differential Diagnosis. These cases present difficult diagnostic challenges simulating lymphoma, melanoma, lymphoepithelioma-like carcinoma, adnexal carcinoma, neuroendocrine carcinoma, epithelioid sarcoma, and other conditions (359). Awareness of the entity and appropriate immunohistochemical workup are key to establishing the diagnosis.

Principals of Treatment. Wide local excision with or without adjuvant radiation is the treatment of choice. Chemotherapy is reserved for advanced disease.

TUMORS OF LYMPHATIC VESSELS

Lymphangiomas constitute only about 4% of all vascular tumors and about 26% of benign vascular tumors in children (31). They can be classified into four types (365): (a) cavernous lymphangioma, (b) cystic hygroma, (c) lymphangioma circumscriptum, and (d) acquired progressive lymphangioma or benign lymphangioendothelioma (366). In addition, lesions of lymphangiectasia, which are indistinguishable from classic lymphangioma circumscriptum, may occur, although rarely, in association with congenital or acquired lymphedema. Although traditionally cavernous lymphangioma and cystic hygroma have been considered independent entities, it is likely that the latter is an ectatic variant of the former, which arises in areas of loose connective tissue (discussed under the same heading later) (367). The existence of capillary lymphangioma is doubtful and will not be considered further.

Histogenesis. The great majority of tumors of lymphatic vessels are benign, and most of them appear to represent developmental abnormalities rather than true neoplasms. Although in hemangiomas the endothelial cells stain positively for factor VIII–related antigen, the endothelial cells in lymphangiomas are for the most part negative for this marker (368). The presence of fragmented basal lamina and anchoring filaments in hemangiomas is a more reliable ultrastructural feature to use to distinguish lymphatics and blood vessels. However, distinction between angiomas and lymphangiomas is not always clear

even when light microscopy is combined with immunohistochemistry and electron microscopy (369). Somatic mutations in PI3KCA appear to be involved in the pathogenesis of lymphangioma (370).

Cavernous Lymphangioma and Cystic Hygroma

Clinical Summary. Cavernous lymphangioma usually presents at birth or during the first 2 years of life with an equal gender incidence (371,372). The most common locations are the head and neck area (particularly the oral cavity) and, less often, the extremities. It presents as a large, diffuse, subcutaneous, often fluctuant soft mass. Recurrences are common after limited excision.

Cystic hygroma has a similar age and gender distribution, and lesions tend to affect the neck, axillae, and groin (371). Tumors tend to be better circumscribed than cavernous lymphangiomas, but there is also a tendency for local recurrence unless a wide excision is performed. Cystic hygroma of the neck is commonly associated with Turner syndrome (371,373).

Histopathology. Cavernous lymphangioma shows large, irregularly shaped spaces in the dermis and subcutaneous tissue lined by a single layer of bland endothelial cells (Fig. 33-89). The surrounding stroma can be loose or fibrotic and shows a lymphocytic inflammatory cell infiltrate with scattered lymphoid follicles. An incomplete layer of smooth muscle can be seen in the walls of some vessels. The vascular lumina show pink proteinaceous fluid with lymphocytes, but erythrocytes can also be seen. Large cavernous lymphangiomas, particularly in areas of the lip or tongue, may extend between the muscle bundles, separating them from one another (365).

In cystic hygroma, microscopic features are similar to those of cavernous lymphangioma except for the presence of numerous cystically dilated thin-walled lymphatic spaces.

Differential Diagnosis. Distinction from cavernous hemangioma can be impossible because the vascular channels in both

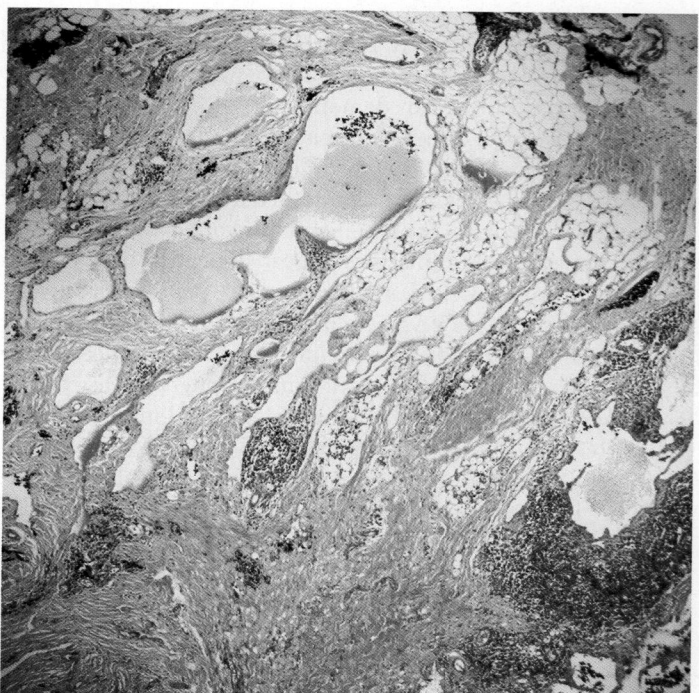

Figure 33-89 Cavernous lymphangioma. Dilated lymphatic channels and aggregates of lymphocytes in the stroma.

conditions can show red blood cells in their lumina. The presence of lymphoid aggregates in the stroma tends to favor the diagnosis of lymphangioma.

Principles of Management: Surgery is the mainstay of treatment. Local recurrences are, however, common following incomplete excision.

Lymphangioma Circumscriptum

Clinical Summary. Lymphangioma circumscriptum is predominantly a developmental malformation of infancy with an equal gender incidence, but it may arise at any age (374,375). Similar acquired lesions arising in adults in relation to chronic lymphedema or radiotherapy are best regarded as *lymphangiectasia.* The anatomic distribution is wide, but the proximal portions of the limbs and limb girdle are most frequently affected. Association with cavernous lymphangioma, cystic hygroma, and even lymphangiomatosis is common. A typical lesion consists of collections of numerous papules with vesicle-like lesions containing clear fluid and, less commonly, blood (Fig. 33-90). Owing to the presence of a deep component (see text following), lesions arising in infancy tend to recur after simple excision.

Histopathology. Lymphangioma circumscriptum is composed of numerous dilated lymphatics in the superficial and papillary dermis (Fig. 33-91). There is clear fluid and, less frequently, red blood cells in their lumina. In the overlying epidermis, there is

some degree of acanthosis and hyperkeratosis. The surrounding stroma shows scattered lymphocytes. Lesions developing in infancy often show a large-caliber, muscular lymphatic space in the subcutaneous tissue, which has to be ligated at the time of excision to avoid recurrence (Fig. 33-92).

Principles of Management: Surgery is the treatment of choice, but local recurrences are common following simple excision.

Progressive Lymphangioma (Benign Lymphangioendothelioma)

Clinical Summary. Progressive lymphangioma (benign lymphangioendothelioma) is a benign rare tumor that has a tendency to present in middle-aged to elderly adults and evolve slowly over years. Males and females are equally affected, and although the anatomic distribution is wide, there is preferential involvement of the limbs (376,377). Clinically, a typical lesion is a solitary well-circumscribed erythematous macule or plaque. Recurrence after simple excision is exceptional, and occasional lesions can show focal or complete spontaneous regression (377).

Histopathology. Most lesions predominantly involve the superficial dermis, but extension into the dermis and subcutis can be present (376,377). Irregular, horizontal, thin-walled vascular channels lined by a single layer of bland endothelial cells are seen dissecting collagen bundles (Fig. 33-93). Endothelial cell atypia and mitotic figures are absent. The vascular channels appear empty or have scanty proteinaceous material and/or a few red blood cells.

Differential Diagnosis. The main differential diagnosis is with well-differentiated angiosarcoma and patch-stage Kaposi sarcoma. Although sharing with angiosarcoma the presence of extensive dissection of collagen bundles, the latter conditions occur in completely different settings, and in angiosarcoma, there is usually, at least focally, cytologic atypia and mitotic figures. Patch-stage Kaposi sarcoma often presents clinically with multiple lesions, and histologically, the abnormal blood vessels tend to cluster around normal preexisting blood vessels. There is hemosiderin deposition with an inflammatory cell infiltrate with lymphocytes and plasma cells.

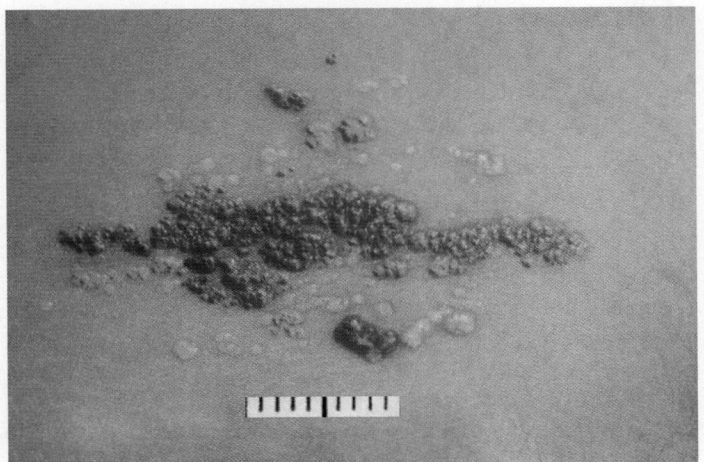

Figure 33-90 Lymphangioma circumscriptum. Localized, plaquelike lesion with multiple slightly warty papules.

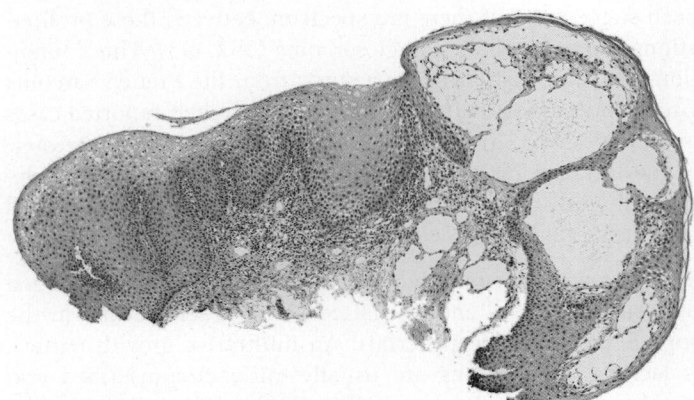

Figure 33-91 Lymphangioma circumscriptum. Numerous dilated lymphatic channels expand the papillary dermis.

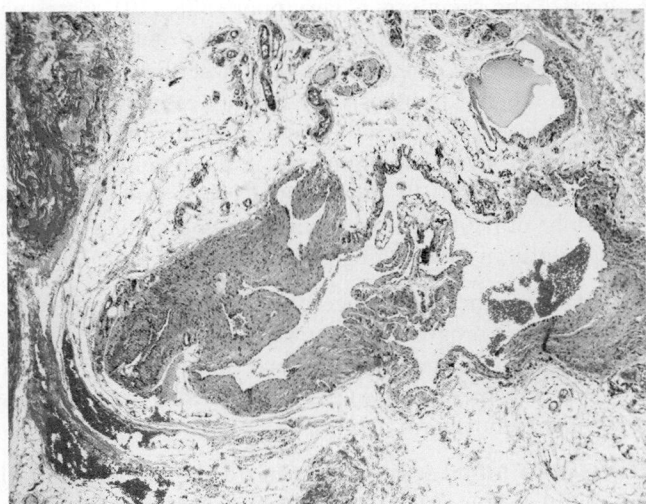

Figure 33-92 Lymphangioma circumscriptum. Deep muscular lymphatic space. If this vessel is not ligated, the lesion will recur.

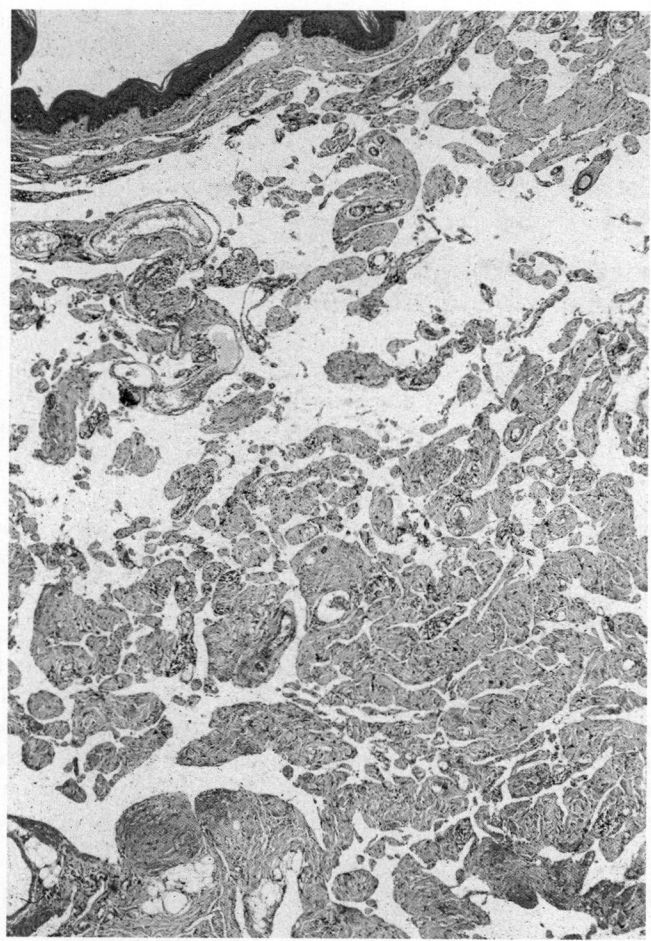

Figure 33-93 Progressive lymphangioma. Extensive dissection of collagen bundles by irregular vascular channels lined by bland, flat endothelial cells.

Principles of Management: Complete excision is curative.

Lymphangiomatosis

Clinical Summary. Lymphangiomatosis is a rare developmental abnormality that affects children with an equal gender incidence. Although most cases appear to be congenital, the disease is often not diagnosed until childhood. Most cases involve soft tissues, skin, bone, and parenchymal organs. When vital organs are affected, the prognosis is very poor (378,379). Cases with involvement limited to skin and soft tissues of a limb (with or without bone involvement) have been described and are associated with a better prognosis (379). Rare cases can present in association with kaposiform hemangioendothelioma of infancy and childhood. Lymphangiomatosis is the lymphatic counterpart of angiomatosis. In some instances, distinction between them can be difficult, although lymphangiographic studies can be very helpful in establishing the difference.

Histopathology. The appearance of lymphangiomatosis is very similar to that of progressive lymphangioma, but the changes in lymphangiomatosis are more extensive and diffuse with the involvement of deeper soft tissues, fibrosis in long-standing cases, and stromal hemosiderin deposition.

Principles of Management: Owing to the extent of the lesion, complete removal is difficult, and local recurrences are common following surgery. Sirolimus has also been used in the treatment of the condition (380).

Multifocal Lymphangioendotheliomatosis with Thrombocytopenia (Cutaneovisceral Angiomatosis with Thrombocytopenia, Infantile Hemorrhagic Angiodysplasia)

Clinical Summary. Multifocal lymphangioendotheliomatosis with thrombocytopenia is a distinctive condition presenting at birth with multiple (sometimes hundreds) red-brown to blue macules, papules, nodules, or plaques (381–384). New lesions appear throughout childhood, and there is often involvement of other sites, including lungs, gastrointestinal tract, liver, spleen, skeletal muscle, bone, synovium, and brain. Thrombocytopenia is a frequently associated finding and tends to be low grade, but some patients die as a result of bleeding, especially in the gastrointestinal tract and brain. An additional complication includes sepsis. In an exceptional case, no thrombocytopenia occurred (385).

Histology. Microscopic examination reveals multiple thin-walled and dilated lymphatic-like vascular channels scattered throughout the dermis and extending into the subcutaneous tissue. These channels are lined by endothelial cells with hobnail morphology. Intraluminal papillary projections may sometimes be seen.

Differential Diagnosis. The main differential diagnosis is with PILA (Dabska tumor), and the histologic findings may be identical in both entities. Distinction is easy, however, as PILA (Dabska tumor) usually presents as a single lesion with no associated thrombocytopenia.

Principles of Management: In cases with more severe thrombocytopenia, systemic steroids may have to be used. In several cases, treatment with bevacizumab, an antibody to VEGF, was successful (386).

Atypical Vascular Proliferation After Radiotherapy

Clinical Summary. Lesions related to atypical vascular proliferation usually develop a few months or years after radiotherapy for breast cancer, but they may also appear in irradiated skin after treatment for ovarian and endometrial carcinoma (387–391). The clinical presentation is not distinctive and varies from skin-colored to red macules, papules, and rarely plaques. The lesions may be multiple at presentation, and further lesions may develop over time. Occasional cases may mimic lymphangioma circumscriptum. The behavior appears to be benign, with occasional local recurrences. However, it has been suggested that there is a spectrum between these proliferations and postradiation angiosarcoma (392,393). This contention has been challenged by a study from the French Sarcoma Group, but, unfortunately, the follow-up in their reported cases is limited (394). In view of the controversy and also because of the fact that histologic diagnosis may be difficult, these lesions should therefore be treated with complete excision, and patients should be followed-up closely.

Histopathology. Irregular lymphatic-like vascular channels lined by a single layer of endothelial cells are present focally in the superficial and/or deep dermis. An infiltrative growth pattern is lacking, and lesions are usually fairly circumscribed and largely confined to the dermis (Fig. 33-94). The cells lining the channels often have a hobnail appearance, and papillary projections may occasionally be seen. There is no cytologic atypia,

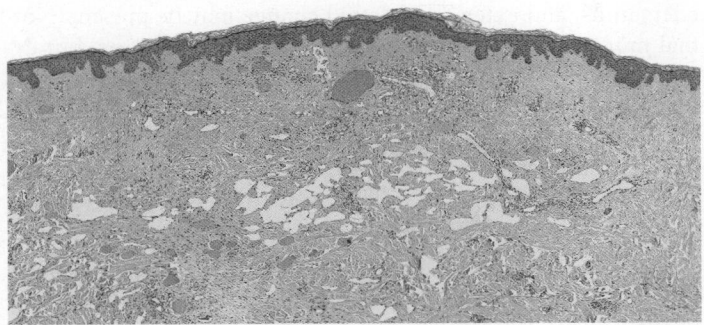

Figure 33-94 Atypical vascular proliferation after radiotherapy. Fairly localized superficial dermal vascular proliferation.

multilayering, or mitotic activity (Fig. 33-95). Interestingly, dermal changes secondary to radiotherapy are not usually seen.

Differential Diagnosis. The differential diagnosis includes well-differentiated angiosarcoma, hobnail hemangioma, and Kaposi sarcoma. As opposed to hobnail hemangioma, the lesion is not symmetrical, and the vascular channels do not have a predominant superficial dermal location. The clinical setting, the absence of inflammation, and the presence of hobnail endothelial cells with focal papillary projections should allow distinction from Kaposi sarcoma. Careful examination of multiple sections is recommended to make sure that there are no mitotic figures and cytologic atypia to distinguish it from a well-differentiated angiosarcoma. This distinction can be very difficult, especially in small biopsies. Studies have identified MYC amplification and overexpression by FISH and immunohistochemistry in radiation-associated angiosarcoma but not in atypical vascular lesions. This can therefore be used as an additional diagnostic tool in this challenging setting (352,395,396).

Principles of Management: Atypical vascular lesions are typically small and should be removed completely to allow for adequate histologic examination and to exclude a more significant underlying disease. This is particularly relevant as cutaneous angiosarcoma not infrequently contains well-differentiated areas closely resembling and often indistinguishable from atypical vascular lesions on partial samples. As patients with atypical vascular lesions are at risk for developing further lesions and even angiosarcoma at the site of previous radiation, careful clinical follow-up is necessary.

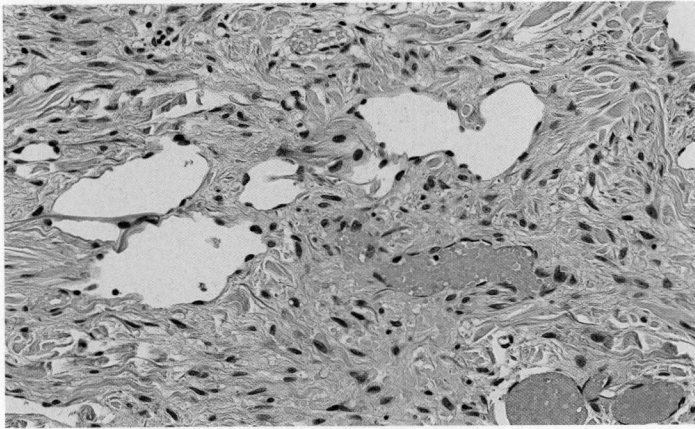

Figure 33-95 Atypical vascular proliferation after radiotherapy. Irregular vascular channels lined by slightly hyperchromatic endothelial cells, some of which have a hobnail appearance.

TUMORS OF PERIVASCULAR CELLS

Glomus Tumor

Clinical Summary. Glomus tumors are relatively rare lesions that usually present in young adults between the third and fourth decades of life with no gender predilection except for subungual tumors, which have a marked female predilection (397). The hand (particularly subungual region and palm) is the most commonly affected site, followed by the foot and forearm. Lesions, however, can occur with a wide anatomic distribution, not only on the skin but also rarely in mucosa and internal organs. Most tumors classically present as solitary, small (<1 cm), blue-red nodules that are characteristically associated with paroxysmal pain often elicited by changes in temperature (especially cold) or pressure. Subungual glomus tumors have been associated with neurofibromatosis type I (398–400).

A very small proportion of glomus tumors are multiple (in up to 10% of patients) (Fig. 33-96). As opposed to solitary glomus tumors, the latter usually arise in children, tend to be asymptomatic, are rarely subungual, and are thought to be inherited in an autosomal dominant fashion (401). The gene for multiple inherited glomangiomas (also known as *glomuvenous malformations*) has been linked to chromosome 1p21-22 (402–405). Clinically, multiple glomangiomas can be confused with lesions of the blue rubber bleb nevus syndrome, and it is likely that cases of this condition reported in the past represented examples of multiple glomangiomas or glomangiomyomas. They can also be confused with venous malformations (406). Histologically, multiple glomus tumors are predominantly glomangiomas (see text following).

The glomus coccygeum is a prominent glomus body measuring up to several millimeters and located near the tip of the coccyx. Awareness of its existence is important because when found incidentally in biopsies it may be confused with a neoplasm (407).

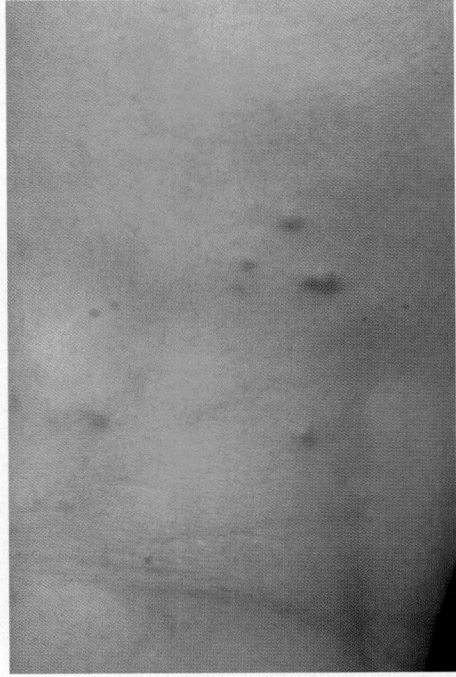

Figure 33-96 Glomangiomas. Multiple bluish dermal lesions.

Local recurrence is uncommon and when seen is usually in deep-seated tumors with an infiltrative growth pattern (so-called infiltrating glomus tumor; see text following) (408). Glomangiomatosis is defined as lesions with clinical features of angiomatosis displaying histologic evidence of glomus cells around the vascular channels (409). Exceptionally, glomus tumors originate within a blood vessel (410,411) or nerve (412). Malignant glomus tumor or glomangiosarcoma is very rare and usually arises in deep soft tissues. It comprises around 1% of all glomus tumors (413) and appears to be an aggressive tumor with a metastasis rate of 40% (413). Exceptionally, a glomangiosarcoma arising in an internal organ may present with metastases to the skin (414).

Histopathology. Glomus tumors show varying proportions of glomus cells, blood vessels, and smooth muscle and are classified accordingly into *solid glomus tumor* (25% of cases), *glomangioma* (60% of cases), and *glomangiomyoma* (15% of cases). Most cases of glomus tumor are well circumscribed, and a classic solid lesion (Fig. 33-97) is composed of sheets of uniform cells with pale or eosinophilic cytoplasm, well-defined cell margins (highlighted distinctively by PAS stain), and round or ovoid punched-out central nuclei (Fig. 33-98). Small blood vessels are uniformly distributed in the tumor but may not be apparent without the use of special stains. The stroma is often

edematous, and extensive myxoid change may be present. Normal mitotic figures may be conspicuous in some cases, but cytologic atypia is usually absent. Numerous stromal nerve fibers may be highlighted with special stains. Exceptional cases show extensive oncocytic change (415). Tumor cells with epithelioid morphology have also been described (416). In glomangioma, there are numerous dilated, cavernous-like, thin-walled vascular spaces surrounded by one or a few layers of glomus cells (Fig. 33-99). In glomangiomyoma, there are a significant number of spindle-shaped smooth muscle cells, which tend to be distributed near the vascular spaces and blend with the adjacent collections of glomus cells (Fig. 33-100).

Infiltrating glomus tumor is a very rare variant that occurs in deep soft tissues and is characterized by solid nests of glomus cells with an infiltrative growth pattern (408). It is associated with a high recurrence rate.

The histologic diagnosis of malignant glomus tumor is difficult because of the few cases reported in the literature

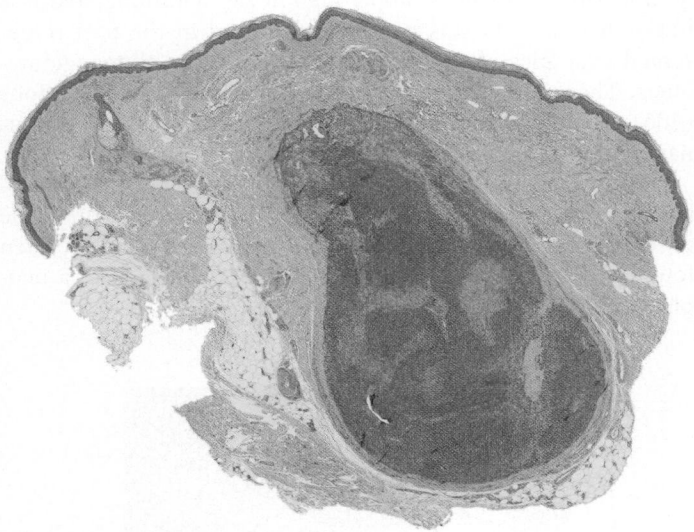

Figure 33-97 Solid glomus tumor. Well-circumscribed dermal nodule.

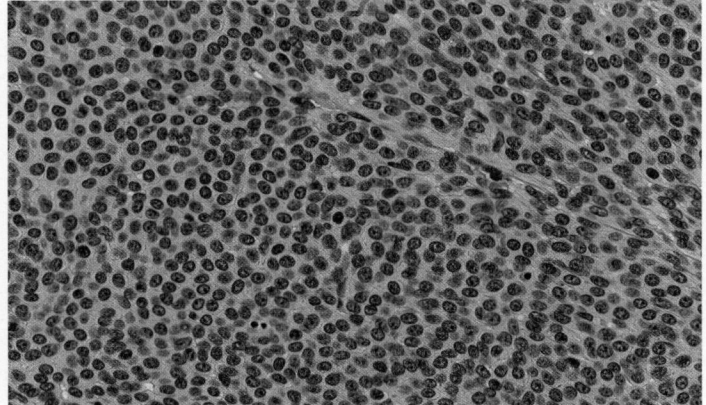

Figure 33-98 Solid glomus tumor. Monomorphic round cells with eosinophilic cytoplasm and central punched-out nuclei.

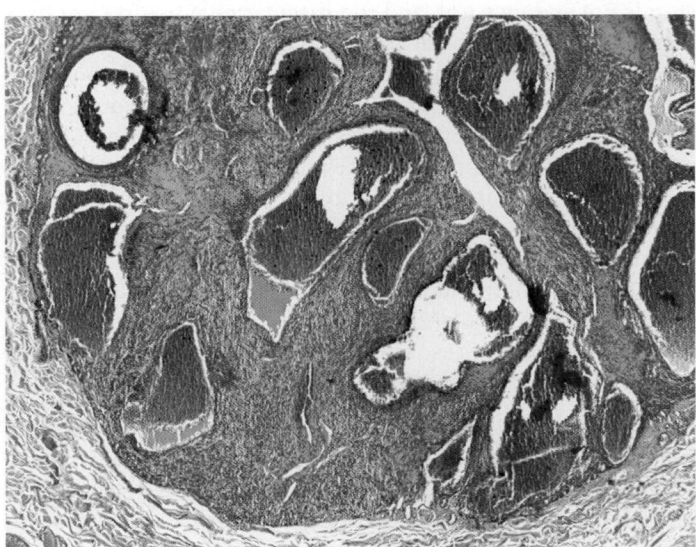

Figure 33-99 Glomangioma. Cavernous vascular spaces surrounded by layers of glomus cells.

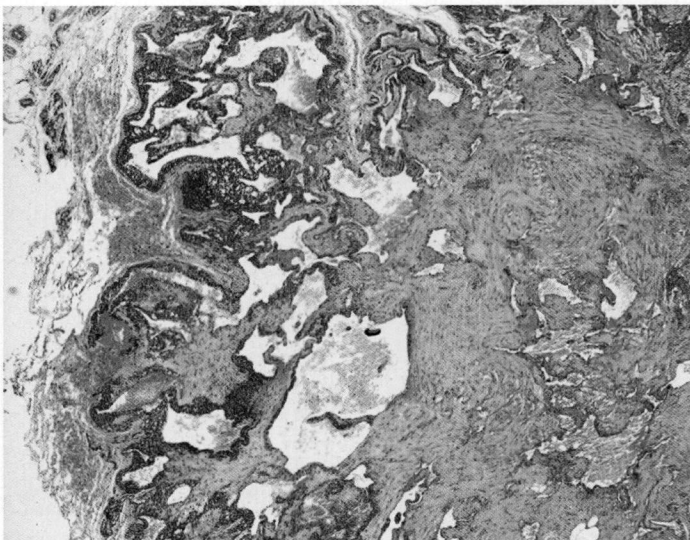

Figure 33-100 Glomangiomyoma. Spindle-shaped cells with pink cytoplasm combined with glomus cells.

(413,417). Criteria for the histologic diagnosis of malignant glomus tumor have been delineated and include (a) size greater than 2 cm and subfascial or visceral location, (b) atypical mitotic figures, or (c) moderate to marked nuclear atypia and five or more mitotic figures per 50 high-power fields (413). A preexisting benign component is common but not invariably present. Tumors arising *de novo* have architectural features resembling a glomus but consist of cells with prominent atypia. In the absence of unequivocal histologic features for glomus tumor, positive immunohistochemical stain for smooth muscle actin and for collagen type IV (in a pericellular distribution) is helpful in both typical and atypical glomus tumors (413). Tumors with focal cytologic atypia but no evidence of other features suggestive of malignancy are classified as symplastic glomus tumors. Glomus tumors of uncertain malignant potential are regarded as those that do not fulfill the criteria for the diagnostics of malignant glomus tumor or symplastic glomus tumor but that have frequent mitotic activity and superficial location only, deep location only, or large size only. Recently, the applicability of these criteria has been evaluated in a cohort of cutaneous glomus tumors, and only tumoral necrosis has been shown to have an association with a higher biological potential (local recurrence) (417). However, it seems that the prognosis of cutaneous malignant glomus tumors is much more favorable than that of their deep-seated counterparts.

Histogenesis. Glomus tumors closely resemble the modified smooth muscle cells of a segment of specialized arteriovenous anastomoses (Sucquet–Hoyer canal) that is involved in the regulation of temperature, the *glomus body*. Glomus bodies are usually found in acral skin, particularly on the hands. However, many glomus tumors arise from sites where glomus bodies are not known to exist. In view of this, it is likely that some glomus tumors arise from the differentiation of pluripotential mesenchymal cells or ordinary smooth muscle cells. On immunohistochemical examination, glomus tumor cells stain for smooth muscle actin, H-caldesmon, muscle-specific actin, and myosin (418). Staining for collagen type IV shows prominent pericellular positivity. Staining for desmin is only occasionally focally positive. CD34 may also be positive in glomus tumors (419). *NOTCH* gene fusions can be seen in approximately half of glomus tumor cases, with a predilection for the extremities of males, even though many of the typical subungual tumors lack the fusion, implying a different pathway (420). A relatively small subset of glomus tumors exhibit BRAF V600E mutation, and they fall within the category of malignant or uncertain malignant potential tumors (421).

Differential Diagnosis. Solid glomus tumor can be distinguished from eccrine spiradenoma by the presence in the latter of two populations of cells, focal ductal differentiation, and positivity for epithelial markers. Occasionally, intradermal nevus with pseudovascular spaces resembles a glomus tumor, but in the former, there is always evidence of nesting, maturation, and positivity of lesional cells for S-100.

Multiple glomus tumors differ from lesions of the blue rubber bleb nevus by the presence of glomus cells in nearly all tumors. It is likely that some, if not all, previously reported cases of blue rubber bleb nevus have actually represented examples of multiple glomangiomas.

Principles of Treatment. Glomus tumors are treated by simple excision.

Myopericytoma

Clinical Summary. Traditionally, tumors thought to differentiate toward perivascular myoid cells or pericytes have been divided into two main categories: infantile hemangiopericytoma and adult hemangiopericytoma. Both variants, however, appear to have very little in common except for the histologic presence of a pericytomatous vascular pattern. Moreover, with the combination of immunohistochemistry and electron microscopy, most tumors classified as adult hemangiopericytoma on light microscopy show other lines of differentiation (422). These include synovial sarcoma, mesenchymal chondrosarcoma, solitary fibrous tumor, and deep benign fibrous histiocytoma. The few cases for which the line of differentiation remains obscure are the "true" adult hemangiopericytomas, but it is likely that they arise from an undifferentiated mesenchymal cell. These rare examples of "true" adult hemangiopericytomas do not usually occur in the skin and will not be discussed further in this chapter.

In recent years, the concept of myopericytoma has been introduced to describe a spectrum of tumors composed of short, oval- to spindle-shaped cells with a myoid appearance and a distinctive concentric perivascular growth (423). These tumors tend to occur mainly in the deep dermis and subcutaneous tissue and include lesions classified in the past as glomangiopericytoma, myopericytoma, myofibroma, and myofibromatosis in adults. Infantile hemangiopericytoma and infantile myofibromatosis represent identical entities, and the only term used now to denote the entity is the latter (424,425).

Infantile myofibroma/myofibromatosis usually presents at birth or in the initial years of life as single or multiple dermal or subcutaneous nodules. Local recurrence is common, and distant spread has been described, but it is likely that the spread represents multicentricity rather than true metastasis (426).

Myopericytoma most commonly occurs in middle-aged adults with a predilection for the limbs, especially the distal lower limb. Lesions are small (<2 cm in diameter), long-standing, usually asymptomatic, and may be single or, less frequently, multiple. Tumors are rarely painful. In the setting of multiple myopericytomas, these often develop simultaneously with a predilection for a single anatomic site. Recurrence is rare and frequently represents either persistence or the development of a new tumor. Very rare malignant examples of myopericytoma have been described (427). Recurrent PDGFRB alterations have been demonstrated in myopericytoma (428).

Histopathology. Infantile myofibroma/myofibromatosis lesions are multinodular and show, at least focally, a biphasic growth pattern (Fig. 33-101). Hemangiopericytomatous areas composed of small, round hyperchromatic cells blend with areas composed of bundles and nodules of more mature spindle-shaped cells with eosinophilic cytoplasm resembling myofibroblasts (Fig. 33-102). This zoning phenomenon is identical to, although less pronounced than, that seen in infantile myofibromatosis (see Chapter 32). Mitosis, necrosis, and vascular invasion are common features.

In infantile hemangiopericytoma, the darker, less mature cells in the pericytomatous areas usually do not stain for any markers, whereas the more mature spindle-shaped cells

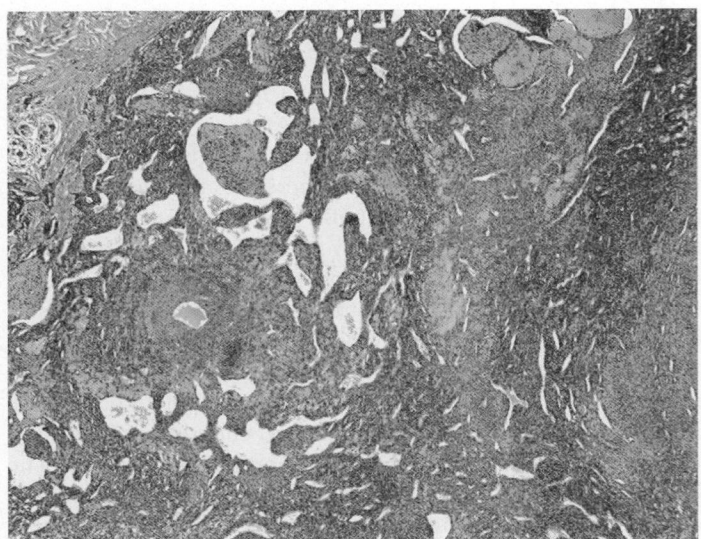

Figure 33-101 Infantile myofibroma. Biphasic tumor with numerous branching blood vessels.

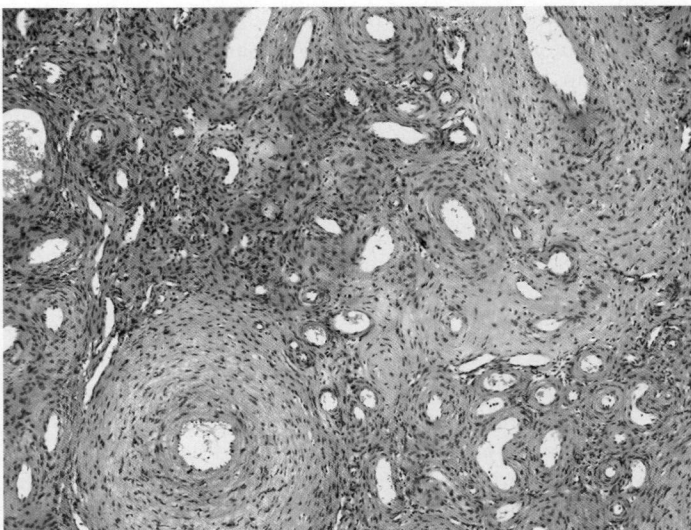

Figure 33-103 Myopericytoma. Biphasic pattern and prominent whirling of tumor cells around blood vessels.

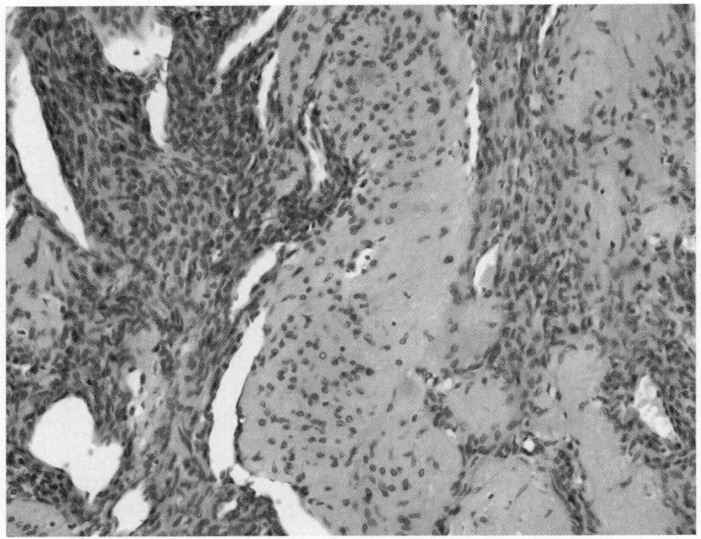

Figure 33-102 Infantile myofibroma. Typical biphasic pattern showing immature round cells with scanty cytoplasm (left) alternating with bundles of spindle cells with a myofibroblastic appearance (right).

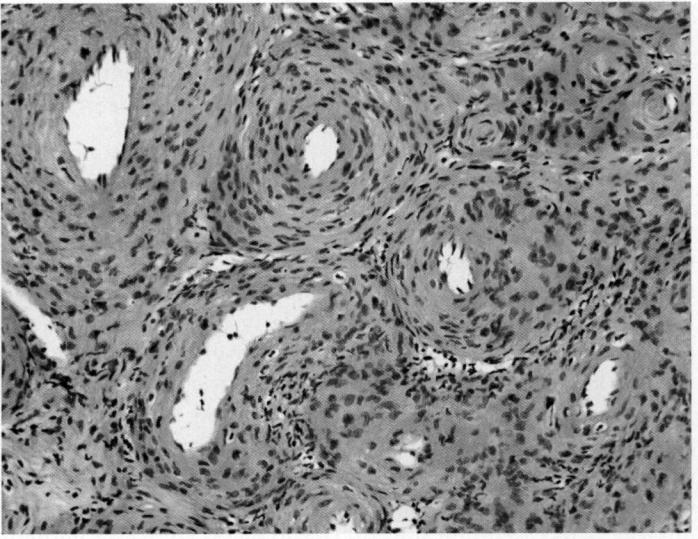

Figure 33-104 Myopericytoma. Bland spindle-shaped pericytes arranged in a concentric manner.

resembling myofibroblasts stain for alpha-smooth muscle actin. Identical features are seen in infantile myofibromatosis, and it is believed that the two entities are part of the same spectrum.

The histologic spectrum of myopericytoma is very wide and varies from lesions that are very similar to myofibromatosis to tumors that closely resemble glomus tumors and even an angioleiomyoma. Tumors are well circumscribed and composed of a mixture of solid cellular areas intermixed with variable numbers of vascular channels (Fig. 33-103). The latter are often elongated and display prominent branching, resulting in a staghorn appearance (hemangiopericytoma-like). The cells in the solid areas are round or short and spindle-shaped with eosinophilic or amphophilic cytoplasm and vesicular nuclei. Cytologic atypia is not usually a feature, and mitotic figures are very rare. A common and striking feature is the presence of concentric layers of tumor cells around vascular channels, resulting in a typical onion ring appearance (Fig. 33-104). Myxoid change may be focally prominent. Occasional findings

include hyalinization, cystic degeneration, and bone formation. Nodules of tumor cells may protrude into the lumina of vascular channels. Rare examples are entirely intravascular (429). In some cases, tumor cells closely resemble glomus cells and are characterized by round punched-out central nuclei and pale eosinophilic cytoplasm. These cases are referred to as *glomangiopericytomas*.

Glomangiopericytoma cells stain diffusely for smooth muscle actin (Fig. 33-105) and are only very rarely focally positive for desmin. Focal staining for CD34 may also be seen.

Differential Diagnosis. Some authors regard angioleiomyoma as part of the spectrum of myopericytoma. Angioleiomyoma, however, is composed of uniform smooth muscle cells, which stain diffusely for both smooth muscle actin and desmin. Furthermore, concentric arrangement of tumor cells around vascular channels is not present.

Principles of Management: Local excision is curative.

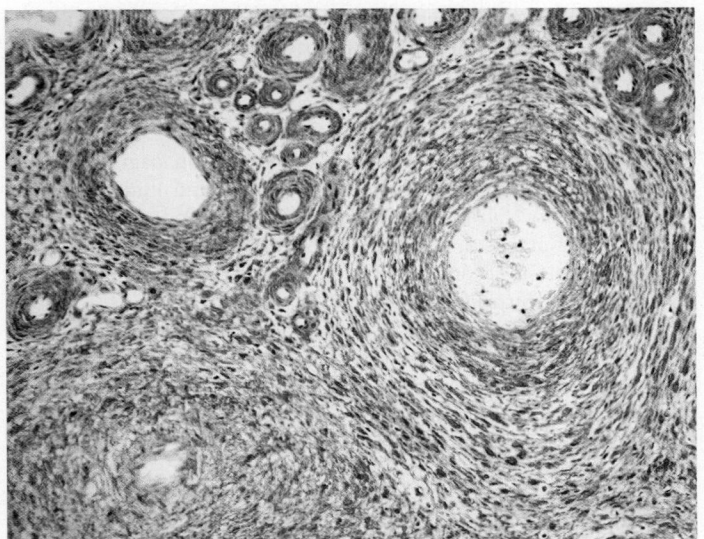

Figure 33-105 Myopericytoma. Diffuse staining of tumor cells with alpha-smooth muscle actin by the ABC method.

REFERENCES

1. WHO Classification of Tumours Editorial Board. *Soft Tissue and Bone Tumours.* 5th ed. WHO; 2020.
2. Hashimoto H, Daimaru Y, Enjoji M. Intravascular papillary endothelial hyperplasia: a clinicopathologic study of 91 cases. *Am J Dermatopathol.* 1983;5:539.
3. Pins MR, Rosenthal DI, Springfield DS, Rosenberg AE. Florid extravascular papillary endothelial hyperplasia (Masson's pseudosarcoma) presenting as a soft tissue sarcoma. *Arch Pathol Lab Med.* 1993;117:259.
4. Reed CN, Cooper PH, Swerlick RA. Intravascular papillary endothelial hyperplasia: multiple lesions simulating Kaposi's sarcoma. *J Am Acad Dermatol.* 1984;10:110.
5. Higashi Y, Uchida Y, Yoshi N, et al. Multiple intravascular papillary endothelial hyperplasia affecting skin and bone. *Clin Exp Dermatol.* 2009;34:740.
6. Durleu C, Bayle-Lebey P, Gadroy A, Loche F, Bazex J. Intravascular papillary endothelial hyperplasia: multiple lesions appearing in the course of treatment with interferon beta [in French]. *Ann Dermatol Venereol.* 2001;128:1336.
7. LeBoit PE, Solomon AR, Santa Cruz DJ, Wick MR. Angiomatosis with luminal cryoprotein deposition. *J Am Acad Dermatol.* 1992;27:969.
8. Di Filippo Y, Cardot-Leccia N, Long-Mira E, et al. Reactive angioendotheliomatosis revealing a glomerulopathy secondary to a monoclonal gammopathy successfully treated with lenalidomide. *J Eur Acad Dermatol Venereol.* 2021;35:e115–e118.
9. Ortonne N, Vignon-Pennamen MD, Majdalani G, Pinquier L, Janin A. Reactive angioendotheliomatosis secondary to dermal amyloid angiopathy. *Am J Dermatopathol.* 2001;23:315.
10. Creamer D, Black MM, Calonje E. Reactive angioendotheliomatosis in association with the antiphospholipid syndrome. *J Am Acad Dermatol.* 2000;45(5, pt 2):903.
11. McMenamin ME, Fletcher CD. Reactive angioendotheliomatosis: a study of 15 cases demonstrating a wide clinicopathologic spectrum. *Am J Surg Pathol.* 2002;26:685.
12. Wick MR, Rocamora A. Reactive and malignant "angioendotheliomatosis": a discriminant clinicopathological study. *J Cutan Pathol.* 1988;15:260.
13. Shyong EQ, Gorevic P, Lebwohl M, Phelps RG. Reactive angioendotheliomatosis and sarcoidosis. *Int J Dermatol.* 2002;41:894.
14. Del Pozo J, Martinez W, Sacristan F, Rodríguez-Lozano J, Fonseca E. Reactive angioendotheliomatosis associated with myelodysplastic syndrome. *Acta Derm Venereol.* 2005;85:269.
15. Kim S, Elenitsas R, James WD. Diffuse dermal angiomatosis: a variant of reactive angioendotheliomatosis associated with peripheral vascular atherosclerosis. *Arch Dermatol.* 2002;138:456.
16. Sommer S, Merchant WJ, Wilson CL. Diffuse dermal angiomatosis due to an iatrogenic arteriovenous fistula. *Acta Derm Venereol.* 2004;84:251–252.
17. Reusche R, Winocour S, Degnim A, Lemaine V. Diffuse dermal angiomatosis of the breast: a series of 22 cases from a single institution. *Gland Surg.* 2015;4:554–560.
18. Hui Y, Elco CP, Heinl NF, Lourenco AP, Wiggins DL, Wang Y. Diffuse dermal angiomatosis mimicking inflammatory breast carcinoma. *Breast J.* 2018;24:196–198.
19. Requena L, El Shabrawi CL, Walsh SN, et al. Intralymphatic histiocytosis: a clinicopathologic study of 16 cases. *Am J Dermatopathol.* 2009;31:140–151.
20. Chan JKC, Fletcher CDM, Hicklin GA, Rosai J. Glomeruloid hemangioma: a distinctive cutaneous lesion of multicentric Castleman's disease associated with POEMS syndrome. *Am J Surg Pathol.* 1990;14:1036.
21. Shinozaki-Ushiku A, Higashihara T, Ikemura M, et al. Glomeruloid hemangioma associated with TAFRO syndrome. *Hum Pathol.* 2018;82:172–176.
22. Tsai CY, Lai CH, Chan HL, Kuo Tt. Glomeruloid hemangioma—a specific cutaneous marker of POEMS syndrome. *Int J Dermatol.* 2001;40:403.
23. Legendre P, Norkowski E, Le Pelletier F, et al. Glomeruloid haemangioma: a possible consequence of elevated VEGF in POEMS and Erdheim-Chester disease. *Eur J Dermatol.* 2018;28:784–789.
24. Pina-Oviedo S, Lopez-Patiño S, Ortiz-Hidalgo C. Glomeruloid hemangiomas localized to the skin of the trunk with no clinical changes of POEMS syndrome. *Int J Dermatol.* 2006;45:1445.
25. Velez D, Delgado-Jimenez Y, Fraga J. Solitary glomeruloid hemangioma without POEMS syndrome. *J Cutan Pathol.* 2005;32:449.
26. Maurer GD, Shittelhelm J, Ernemann U, et al. Intracranial hemangiomas in a patient with POEMS syndrome. *J Neurol.* 2010;287:484.
27. Lee H, Meier FA, Ma CK, Ormsby AH, Lee MW. Eosinophilic globules in 3 cases of glomeruloid hemangioma of the head and neck: a characteristic offering more evidence for the thanatosomes with or without POEMS. *Am J Dermatopathol.* 2008;30:539.
28. Suurmeijer AJ, Fletcher CD. Papillary haemangioma: a distinct cutaneous haemangioma of the head and neck area containing eosinophilic globules. *Histopathology.* 2007;51:638.
29. Suurmeijer AJ. Papillary hemangioma and glomeruloid hemangioma are distinct clinicopathologic entities. *Int J Surg Pathol.* 2010;18:48.
30. Happle R. Capillary malformations: a classification using specific names for specific skin disorders. *J Eur Acad Dermatol Venereol.* 2015;29:2295–2305.
31. Ferahbas A, Utas S, Urkacus M, Gunes T, Mistik S. Prevalence of cutaneous findings in hospitalized neonates: a prospective observational study. *Pediatr Dermatol.* 2009;26:139.
32. Adams B, Lucky AW. Acquired port-wine stains and antecedent trauma: case report and review of the literature. *Arch Dermatol.* 2000;136:897.
33. Ch'ng S, Tan ST. Facial port-wine stains—clinical stratification and risks of neuro-ocular involvement. *J Plast Reconstr Aesthet Surg.* 2008;61:889–893.
34. Freysz M, Cribier B, Lipsker D. Fegelers syndrome, acquired port-wine stain or acquired capillary malformation: three cases and a literature review [in French]. *Ann Dermatol Venereol.* 2013;140:341.
35. Berg JN, Quaba AA, Georgantopoulou A, Porteous ME. A family with hereditary port-wine stain. *J Med Genet.* 2000;37:E12.
36. Eerola I, Boon LM, Mulliken JB, et al. Capillary malformation-arteriovenous malformation, a new clinical and genetic disorder caused by RASA1 mutations. *Am J Hum Genet.* 2003;73:1240–1249.

37. Fernández-Guarino M, Boixeda P, de las Heras E, Aboin S, García-Millán C, Olasolo PJ. Phakomatosis pigmentovascularis: clinical findings in 15 patients and review of the literature. *J Am Acad Dermatol.* 2008;58:88.

38. López-Gutiérrez JC, Lapunzina P. Capillary malformation of the lower lip, lymphatic malformation of the face and neck, asymmetry and partial/generalized overgrowth (CLAPO): report of six cases of a new syndrome/association. *Am J Med Genet A.* 2008;146A:2583.

39. Rodriguez-Laguna L, Ibañez K, Gordo G, et al. CLAPO syndrome: identification of somatic activating PIK3CA mutations and delineation of the natural history and phenotype. *Genet Med.* 2018;20:882–889.

40. Finley JL, Noe JM, Arndt KA, Rosen S. Port-wine stains: morphologic variations and developmental lesions. *Arch Dermatol.* 1984;120:1453.

41. Nguyen V, Hochman M, Mihm MC Jr, Nelson JS, Tan W. The pathogenesis of port wine stain and Sturge Weber syndrome: complex interactions between genetic alterations and aberrant MAPK and PI3K activation. *Int J Mol Sci.* 2019;20:2243.

42. Shirley MD, Tang H, Gallione CJ, et al. Sturge-Weber syndrome and port-wine stains caused by somatic mutation in GNAQ. *N Engl J Med.* 2013;368:1971–1979.

43. Cuestas D, Perafan A, Forero Y, et al. Angiokeratomas, not everything is Fabry disease. *Int J Dermatol.* 2019;58:713–721.

44. Molho-Pessach V, Bargal R, Abramowitz Y, et al. Angiokeratoma corporis diffusum in human beta-mannosidosis: report of a new case and a novel mutation. *J Am Acad Dermatol.* 2007;57:407.

45. Kanitakis J, Allombert C, Doebelin B, et al. Fucosidosis with angiokeratomas: microscopic study of a new case and literature review. *J Cutan Pathol.* 2005;32:506.

46. Germain DP, Moiseev S, Suárez-Obando F, et al. The benefits and challenges of family genetic testing in rare genetic diseases-lessons from Fabry disease. *Mol Genet Genomic Med.* 2021;9:e1666.

47. Kelly B, Kelly E. Angiokeratoma corporis diffusum in a patient with no recognizable enzyme abnormality. *Arch Dermatol.* 2006;142:615.

48. Lipsker D, Kieffer C, Nojavan H, Doray B, Cribier B. Familial ACD with no recognizable enzyme abnormalities. *Arch Dermatol.* 2006;142:1509.

49. Hayes KR, Rebello DJA. Angiokeratoma of Mibelli. *Acta Derm Venereol (Stockh).* 1961;41:56.

50. Cohen PR, Celano NJ. Penile angiokeratomas (PEAKERs) revisited: a comprehensive review. *Dermatol Ther (Heidelb).* 2020;10:551–567.

51. Kontogianni-Katsaros K, Kairi-Vassilatoy E, Grapsa D, Papadias K, Hasiakos D, Kondi-Pafitis A. Angiokeratoma of the vulva: a rare benign tumor mimicking malignancy—case reports. *Eur J Gynaecol Oncol.* 2006;27:632.

52. Ozdemir R, Karaaslan O, Tiftikcioglu YO, et al. Angiokeratoma circumscriptum. *Dermatol Surg.* 2004;30:1364.

53. Fauchais AL, Prev S, Quatara B, Vidal E, Sparsa A. Angiokeratoma regression in a Fabry disease after treatment with agalsidas-beta clinical effectiveness. *J Eur Acad Dermatol Venereol.* 2010;24:737.

54. Blume JE. Generalized essential telangiectasia: a case report and review of the literature. *Cutis.* 2005;75:223.

55. Long D, Marshman G. Generalized essential telangiectasia. *Australas J Dermatol.* 2004;45:67.

56. Tetart F, Lorthioir A, Girszyn N, Lahaxe L, Ducrotté P, Marie I. Watermelon stomach revealing generalized essential telangiectasia. *Intern Med J.* 2009;39:781.

57. Powell E, Markus R, Malone CH. Generalized essential telangiectasia treated with PDL. *J Cosmet Dermatol.* 2021;20:1086–1087.

58. Salama S, Rosenthal D. Cutaneous collagenous vasculopathy with generalized telangiectasia: an immunohistochemical and ultrastructural study. *J Cutan Pathol.* 2000;27:40.

59. Stavrou C, Uthayakumar A, Calonje JE, Bunker CB. Cutaneous collagenous vasculopathy. *BMJ Case Rep.* 2021;14:e241434.

60. Echeverría B, Sanmartín O, Botella-Estrada R, Vitiello M. Cutaneous collagenous vasculopathy successfully treated with pulse dye laser. *Int J Dermatol.* 2012;51:1359.

61. Claudia M, Astrid H, Cozzani E, Cabiddu F, Guadagno A, Parodi A. Unilateral nevoid telangiectasia: a rare and underdiagnosed skin disease. *Eur J Dermatol.* 2020;30:601–602.

62. Akman-Karakas A, Kandemir H, Senol U, et al. Unilateral nevoid telangiectasia accompanied by neurological disorders. *J Eur Acad Dermatol Venereol.* 2011;25:1356.

63. Afsar FS, Ortac R, Diniz G. Unilateral nevoid telangiectasia with no estrogen and progesterone receptors in a pediatric patient. *Indian J Dermatol Venereol Leprol.* 2008;74:163.

64. Ilknur T, Fetil E, Akarsu S, Altiner DD, Ulukuş C, Güneş AT. Angioma serpiginosum: dermoscopy for diagnosis, pulsed dye laser for treatment. *J Dermatol.* 2006;33:252–255.

65. Houge G, Oeffner F, Grzeschik KH. An Xp11.23 deletion containing PORCN may also cause angioma serpiginosum, a cosmetic skin disease associated with extreme skewing of X-inactivation. *Eur J Hum Genet.* 2008;16:1027.

66. Happle R. Angioma serpiginosum is not caused by PORCN mutations. *Eur J Hum Genet.* 2009;17:881.

67. Sharathkumar AA, Shapiro A. Hereditary haemorrhagic telangiectasia. *Haemophilia.* 2008;14:1269–1280.

68. Vincent P, Plauchu H, Hazan J, Fauré S, Weissenbach J, Godet J. A third locus for hereditary haemorrhagic telangiectasia maps to chromosome 12q. *Hum Molec Genet.* 1995;4:945.

69. Berg JN, Gallione CJ, Stenzel TT, et al. The activin receptor-like kinase 1 gene; genomic structure and mutations in hereditary hemorrhagic telangiectasia type 2. *Am J Hum Genet.* 1997;61:60.

70. Cole SG, Begbie E, Wallace GMF, Shovlin CL. A new locus for hereditary hemorrhagic telangiectasia (HHT3) maps to chromosome 5. *J Med Genet.* 2005;42:577–582.

71. Gallione CJ, Repetto GM, Legius E, et al. A combined syndrome of juvenile polyposis and hereditary hemorrhagic telangiectasia associated with mutations in MADH4 (SMAD4). *Lancet.* 2004;363:852.

72. Beard MP, Millington GW. Recent developments in the specific dermatoses of pregnancy. *Clin Exp Dermatol.* 2012;37:1–4.

73. Bean WB, Walsh JR. Venous lakes. *Arch Dermatol.* 1956;74:459.

74. Alcalay J, Sandbank M. The ultrastructure of cutaneous venous lakes. *Int J Dermatol.* 1987;26:645.

75. Boon LM, Enjolras O, Mulliken JB. Congenital hemangioma: evidence for accelerated involution. *J Pediatr.* 1996;128:329.

76. Mulliken JB, Enjolras O. Congenital hemangiomas and infantile hemangioma missing links. *J Am Acad Dermatol.* 2004;50:875.

77. Nasseri E, Piram M, McCuaig CC, Kokta V, Dubois J, Powell J. Partially involuting congenital hemangiomas: a report of 8 cases and review of the literature. *J Am Acad Dermatol.* 2014;70:75–79.

78. Picard A, Boscolo E, Khan ZA, et al. IGF-2 and FLT-1/VEGF-R1 mRNA levels reveal distinctions and similarities between congenital and common infantile hemangioma. *Pediatr Res.* 2008;63:263.

79. Ayturk UM, Couto JA, Hann S, et al. Somatic activating mutations in GNAQ and GNA11 are associated with congenital hemangioma. *Am J Hum Genet.* 2016;98:789–795.

80. North PE, Waner M, James CA, Mizeracki A, Frieden IJ, Mihm MC Jr. Congenital nonprogressive hemangioma: a distinct clinicopathologic entity unlike infantile hemangioma. *Arch Dermatol.* 2002;137:1607.

81. Berenguer B, Mulliken JB, Enjolras O, et al. Rapidly involuting congenital hemangioma: clinical and histopathologic features. *Pediatr Develop Pathol.* 2003;6:495.

82. Baselga E, Cordisco MR, Garzon M, Lee MT, Alomar A, Blei F. Rapidly involuting congenital hemangioma associated with transient thrombocytopenia and coagulopathy: a case series. *Br J Dermatol.* 2008;158:1363.

83. Enjolras O, Mulliken JB, Boon LM, et al. Non-involuting congenital hemangioma: a rare cutaneous vascular anomaly. *Plast Reconstr Surg.* 2001;107:1647.

84. North PE, Waner M, Mizeracki A, Mihm MC Jr. GLUT1: a newly discovered immunohistochemical marker for juvenile hemangiomas. *Hum Pathol.* 2000;31:11.

85. Al Dhaybi R, Powell J, McCuaig C, Kokta V. Differentiation of vascular malformation by expression of Wilms tumor 1 gene: evaluation of 126 cases. *J Am Acad Dermatol.* 2010;63:1052.

86. Léauté-Labrèze C, Harper JI, Hoeger PH. Infantile haemangioma. *Lancet.* 2017;390:85–94.

87. Calonje E, Mentzel T, Fletcher CDM. Pseudosarcomatous neural invasion in capillary hemangiomas. *Histopathology.* 1995;26:159.

88. Johnson EF, Davis DM, Tollefson MM, Fritchie K, Gibson LE. Vascular tumors in infants: case report and review of clinical, histopathologic, and immunohistochemical characteristics of infantile hemangioma, pyogenic granuloma, noninvoluting congenital hemangioma, tufted angioma, and kaposiform hemangioendothelioma. *Am J Dermatopathol.* 2018;40:231–239.

89. North PE, Waner M, Mizeracki A, et al. A unique microvascular phenotype shared by juvenile hemangiomas and human placenta. *Arch Dermatol.* 2001;137:559.

90. Stiles JM, Rowntree RK, Amaya C, et al. Gene expression analysis reveals marked differences in the transcriptome of infantile hemangioma endothelial cells compared to normal dermal microvascular endothelial cells. *Vasc Cell.* 2013;5:6.

91. Léauté-Labrèze C, Hoeger P, Mazereeuw-Hautier J, et al. A randomized, controlled trial of oral propranolol in infantile hemangioma. *N Engl J Med.* 2015;372:735–746.

92. Hadaschik E, Sheiba N, Engster M, Flux K. High levels of B2-adrenoreceptors are expressed in infantile capillary hemangiomas and may mediate the therapeutic effect of propranolol. *J Cutan Pathol.* 2012;39:881.

93. Zheng L, Li Y. Effect of topical timolol on response rate and adverse events in infantile hemangioma: a meta-analysis. *Arch Dermatol Res.* 2018;310:261–269.

94. Liau JY, Lee JC, Tsai JH, Chen CC, Chung YC, Wang YH. High frequency of GNA14, GNAQ, and GNA11 mutations in cherry hemangioma: a histopathological and molecular study of 85 cases indicating GNA14 as the most commonly mutated gene in vascular neoplasms. *Mod Pathol.* 2019;32:1657–1665.

95. Okada E, Tamura A, Ishikawa O, Miyachi Y. Tufted angioma (angioblastoma): case report and review of 41 cases in the Japanese literature. *Clin Exp Dermatol.* 2000;25:627.

96. Wilson Jones E, Orkin M. Tufted angioma (angioblastoma): a benign progressive angioma, not to be confused with Kaposi's sarcoma or low-grade angiosarcoma. *J Am Acad Dermatol.* 1989;20:214.

97. Herron MD, Coffin CM, Vanderhooft SL. Tufted angiomas: variability of clinical morphology. *Pediatr Dermatol.* 2001;19:394.

98. Osio A, Fraitag S, Hadj-Rabia S, Bodemer C, de Prost Y, Hamel-Teillac D. Clinical spectrum of tufted angiomas in childhood: report of 13 cases and a review of the literature. *Arch Dermatol.* 2010;146:758.

99. Browning J, Frieden I, Baselga E, Wagner A, Metry D. Congenital, self-regressing tufted angioma. *Arch Dermatol.* 2006;142:749.

100. Satter EK, Graham BS, Gibbs NF. Congenital tufted angioma. *Pediatr Dermatol.* 2002;19:445.

101. Lee B, Chiu M, Soriano T, Craft N. Adult-onset tufted angioma: a case report and review of the literature. *Cutis.* 2006;78:341.

102. Omori M, Bito T, Nishigori C. Acquired tufted angioma in pregnancy showing expression of estrogen and progesterone receptors. *Eur J Dermatol.* 2013;23:898–899.

103. Tille JC, Morris MA, Brundler MA, Pepper MS. Familial predisposition to tufted angioma: identification of blood and lymphatic vascular components. *Clin Genet.* 2003;53:393.

104. Fernandez AP, Wolfson A, Ahn E, Maldonad JC, Alonso-Llamazares J. Kasabach-Merritt phenomenon in an adult man with a tufted angioma and cirrhosis responding to radiation, bevacizumab, and prednisone. *Int J Dermatol.* 2014;53:1165–1176.

105. Sabharwal A, Aguirre A, Zahid TM, Jean-Charles G, Hatton MN. Acquired tufted angioma of upper lip: case report and review of the literature. *Head Neck Pathol.* 2013;7:291–294.

106. Tomasini C. Cytotoxic-mediated spontaneous regression of eruptive tufted angioma in a teenage girl. *J Eur Acad Dermatol Venereol.* 2017;31:e522–e523.

107. Yesudian PD, Klafowski J, Parslow R, Gould D, Pizer B. Tufted angioma-associated Kasabach-Merritt syndrome treated with embolization and vincristine. *Plast Reconstr Surg.* 2007;119:1392.

108. Brasanac D, Janic D, Boricic I, Jovanovic N, Dokmanovic L. Retroperitoneal kaposiform hemangioendothelioma with tufted angioma-like features in and infant with Kasabach-Merritt syndrome. *Pathol Int.* 2003;53:627.

109. Ramesh R, De Silva B, Atherton DJ. Congenital tufted angioma with persistent low-grade coagulopathy. *Clin Exp Dermatol.* 2009;34:766.

110. Lim YH, Bacchiocchi A, Qiu J, et al. GNA14 somatic mutation causes congenital and sporadic vascular tumors by MAPK activation. *Am J Hum Genet.* 2016;99:443–450.

111. Chu CY, Hsian CH, Chiu HC. Transformation between kaposiform hemangioendothelioma and tufted angioma. *Dermatology.* 2003;206:334.

112. Le Huu AR, Jokinen CH, Rubin BP, et al. Expression of prox1, lymphatic endothelial nuclear transcription factor, in Kaposiform hemangioendothelioma and tufted angioma. *Am J Surg Pathol.* 2010;34:1563–1573.

113. Chiu YE, Drolet BA, Blei F, et al. Variable response to propranolol treatment of kaposiform hemangioendothelioma, tufted angioma and Kasabach-Merritt phenomenon. *Pediatr Blood Cancer.* 2012;59:934.

114. Mills SE, Cooper PH, Fechner RE. Lobular capillary hemangioma: the underlying lesion of pyogenic granuloma: a study of 73 cases from the oral and nasal mucous membranes. *Am J Surg Pathol.* 1980;4:471.

115. Patrice SJ, Wiss K, Mulliken JB. Pyogenic granuloma (lobular capillary hemangioma): a clinicopathologic study of 178 cases. *Pediatr Dermatol.* 1994;8:267.

116. Gupta V, Mridha AR, Sharma VK. Pediatric dermatology photoquiz: multiple erythematous papules on the back. Recurrent pyogenic granulomas with satellitosis. *Pediatr Dermatol.* 2016;33:97–98.

117. Tursen U, Demirkan F, Ikizoglu G. Giant recurrent pyogenic granuloma on the face with satellitosis responsive to systemic steroids. *Clin Exp Dermatol.* 2004;29:40.

118. Fortna RR, Junkins-Hopkins JM. A case of lobular capillary hemangioma (pyogenic granuloma), localized to the subcutaneous tissue and a review of the literature. *Am J Dermatopathol.* 2007;29:408.

119. Gameiro A, Cardoso JC, Calonje E. Intravascular lobular capillary hemangioma in the corpus spongiosum. *Am J Dermatopathol.* 2016;38:e15–e17.

120. Ikeda K, Ichiba T, Seo K, Okazaki Y. Intravenous lobular capillary haemangioma presenting as neck discomfort associated with neck anteflexion. *BMJ Case Rep.* 2021;14:e237529.

121. Lopez-Castillo D, Curto-Barredo L, Sánchez-Schmidt JM, Pujol RM. Multiple eruptive pyogenic granulomas on the proximal nail folds following cast immobilization: a case report with nail unit ultrasound findings. *Acta Derm Venereol.* 2020;100:adv00071.

122. Chae JB, Park JT, Kim BR, Shin JW. Agminated eruptive pyogenic granuloma on chin following redundant needle injections. *J Dermatol.* 2016;43:577–578.

123. Xu Y, Li H, Wang ZX, Yang S. Multiple eruptive pyogenic granulomas occurring in a region of scalded skin. *Pediatr Dermatol.* 2016;33:e27–e28.

124. Dermawan JK, Ko JS, Billings SD. Intravascular lobular capillary hemangioma (intravascular pyogenic granuloma): a

clinicopathologic study of 40 cases. *Am J Surg Pathol.* 2020;44:1515–1521.

125. Groesser L, Peterhof E, Evert M, Landthaler M, Berneburg M, Hafner C. BRAF and RAS mutations in sporadic and secondary pyogenic granuloma. *J Invest Dermatol.* 2016;136:481–486.

126. Chian CA, Arrese JE, Pierard GE. Skin manifestations of *Bartonella* infections. *Int J Dermatol.* 2002;41:461.

127. Plettenberg A, Lorenzen T, Burtsche BT, et al. Bacillary angiomatosis in HIV-infected patients—an epidemiological and clinical study. *Dermatology.* 2000;201:326.

128. Sala M, Font B, Sanfetu I, et al. Bacillary angiomatosis caused by *Bartonella quintana. Ann N Y Acad Sci.* 2005;1063:302.

129. Armstrong K, Weinstein M. Pyogenic granulomas during isotretinoin therapy. *J Dermatol Case Rep.* 2011;5:5–7.

130. Henning B, Stieger P, Kamarachev J, Dummer R, Goldinger SM. Pyogenic granuloma in patients treated with selective BRAF inhibitors: another manifestation of paradoxical pathway activation. *Melanoma Res.* 2016;26:304–307.

131. Patruno C, Balato N, Cirillo T, Napolitano M, Ayala F. Periungual and subungual pyogenic granuloma following anti-TNF-α therapy: is it the first case? *Dermatol Ther.* 2013;26:493–495.

132. Paul LJ, Cohen PR. Paclitaxel-associated subungual pyogenic granuloma: report in a patient with breast cancer receiving paclitaxel and review of drug-induced pyogenic granulomas adjacent to and beneath the nail. *J Drugs Dermatol.* 2012;11:262–268.

133. Amary MF, Damato S, Halai D, et al. Ollier disease and Maffucci syndrome are caused by somatic mosaic mutations of IDH1 and IDH2. *Nat Genet.* 2011;43:1262–1265.

134. Lybecker MB, Stawowy M, Clausen N. Blue rubber bleb naevus syndrome: a rare cause of chronic occult blood loss and iron deficiency anaemia. *BMJ Case Rep.* 2016;2016:bcr2016216963.

135. Calonje E, Fletcher CDM. Sinusoidal hemangioma: a distinctive benign vascular neoplasm within the group of cavernous hemangiomas. *Am J Surg Pathol.* 1991;15:1130.

136. Zhou J, Zhao Z, Sun T, et al. Efficacy and safety of sirolimus for blue rubber bleb nevus syndrome: a prospective study. *Am J Gastroenterol.* 2021;116(5):1044–1052.

137. Singh J, Sharma P, Tandon S, Sinha S. Multiple verrucous hemangiomas: a case report with new therapeutic insight. *Indian Dermatol Online J.* 2017;8:254–256.

138. Chan JKC, Tsang WYW, Calonje E, et al. Verrucous hemangioma: a distinct but neglected variant of cutaneous hemangioma. *Int J Surg Pathol.* 1995;2:171.

139. Couto JA, Vivero MP, Kozakewich HP, et al. A somatic MAP3K3 mutation is associated with verrucous venous malformation. *Am J Hum Genet.* 2015;96:480–486.

140. Ighani M, Aboulafia AJ. Cobb syndrome (cutaneomeningospinal angiomatosis). *BMJ Case Rep.* 2018;2018:bcr2018225208.

141. Hunt SJ, Santa Cruz DJ, Barr RJ. Microvenular hemangioma. *J Cutan Pathol.* 1991;18:235.

142. Napekoski KM, Fernandez AP, Billings SD. Microvenular hemangioma: a clinicopathologic review of 13 cases. *J Cutan Pathol.* 2014;41:816–822.

143. Linos K, Csaposs J, Carlson JA. Microvenular hemangioma presenting with numerous bilateral macules, patches, and plaques: a case report and review of the literature. *Am J Dermatopathol.* 2012;35:98.

144. Hudnall SD, Chen T, Brown K, Angel T, Schwartz MR, Tyring SK. Human herpesvirus-8-positive microvenular hemangioma in POEMS syndrome. *Arch Pathol Lab Med.* 2003;127:1034.

145. Joyce JC, Keith PJ, Szabo S, Holland KE. Superficial hemosiderotic lymphovascular malformation (hobnail hemangioma): a report of six cases. *Pediatr Dermatol.* 2014;31:281–285.

146. Trindade F, Kutzner H, Tellechea Ó, Requena L, Colmenero I. Hobnail hemangioma reclassified as superficial lymphatic malformation: a study of 52 cases. *J Am Acad Dermatol.* 2012;66:112–115.

147. Mentzel T, Partanen TA, Kutzner H. Hobnail hemangioma ("targetoid hemosiderotic hemangioma"): clinicopathologic

148. Ortiz-Rey JA, Gonzalez-Ruiz A, San Miguel P, Alvarez C, Iglesias B, Antón I. Hobnail haemagioma associated with the menstrual cycle. *J Eur Acad Dermatol Venereol.* 2005;19:367.

149. Al Dhaybi R, Lam C, Hatami A, Powell J, McCuaig C, Kokta V. Targetoid hemosiderotic hemangiomas (hobnail hemangiomas) are vascular lymphatic malformations: a study of 12 pediatric cases. *J Am Acad Dermatol.* 2012;66:116–120.

150. Allen PW, Ramakrishna B, MacCormac LB. The histiocytoid hemangiomas and other controversies. *Pathol Ann.* 1992;27:51.

151. Tsang WYW, Chan JKC. The family of epithelioid vascular tumors. *Histol Histopathol.* 1993;8:187.

152. Huang SC, Zhang L, Sung YS, et al. Frequent FOS gene rearrangements in epithelioid hemangioma: a molecular study of 58 cases with morphologic reappraisal. *Am J Surg Pathol.* 2015;39:1313–1321.

153. Olsen TG, Helwig EB. Angiolymphoid hyperplasia with eosinophilia: a clinicopathologic study of 116 patients. *J Am Acad Dermatol.* 1985;12:781.

154. Chan JKC, Hui PK, Ng CS, Yuen NW, Kung IT, Gwi E. Epithelioid hemangioma (angiolymphoid hyperplasia with eosinophilia) and Kimura's disease in Chinese. *Histopathology.* 1989;15:557.

155. Kuo TT, Shih LY, Chan HL. Kimura's disease: involvement of regional lymph nodes and distinction from angiolymphoid hyperplasia with eosinophilia. *Am J Surg Pathol.* 1988;12:843.

156. Moesner J, Pallesen R, Sorensen B. Angiolymphoid hyperplasia with eosinophilia (Kimura's disease): a case with dermal lesions in the knee region and a popliteal arteriovenous fistula. *Arch Dermatol.* 1981;117:650.

157. Sawaimul K, Iqbal B, Kambale T. Kimura's disease embedding radial artery: a very rare presentation. *J Cancer Res Ther.* 2015;11:1031.

158. Saravanam PK, Gajendran A, Dinakaran N, Jayaraman D. Oropharyngeal Kimura's disease: a diagnostic dilemma and therapeutic challenge. *BMJ Case Rep.* 2020;13:e236366.

159. Lin SF, Wei YM, Fan Y, Sun CF. Angiolymphoid hyperplasia with eosinophilia of the tongue with a Sézary syndrome history: evidence for immune mediation of the disease. *Australas J Dermatol.* 2020;61:285–288.

160. Suster S. Nodal angiolymphoid hyperplasia with eosinophilia. *Am J Clin Pathol.* 1987;88:236–239.

161. Xian J, Righi A, Vanel D, Baldini N, Errani C. Epithelioid hemangioma of bone: a unique case with multifocal metachronous bone lesions. *J Clin Orthop Trauma.* 2019;10:1068–1072.

162. Banks ER, Mills SE. Histiocytoid (epithelioid) hemangioma of the testis: the so-called vascular variant of "adenomatoid tumor." *Am J Surg Pathol.* 1990;14:584.

163. Madison JF, Cooper PH. A histiocytoid (epithelioid) vascular tumor of the ovary: occurrence within a benign cystic teratoma. *Mod Pathol.* 1989;2:55.

164. Luzar B, Ieremia E, Antonescu CR, Zhang L, Calonje E. Cutaneous intravascular epithelioid hemangioma. A clinicopathological and molecular study of 21 cases. *Mod Pathol.* 2020;33:1527–1536.

165. Gutte R, Doshi B, Khopkar U. Angiolymphoid hyperplasia with eosinophilia with follicular mucinosis. *Indian J Dermatol.* 2013;58:159.

166. Oksenhendler E, Cazals-Hatem D, Schulz TF, et al. Transient angiolympmhoid hyperplasia and Kaposi's sarcoma after primary infection with human herpesvirus 8 in a patient with human immunodeficiency virus infection. *N Engl J Med.* 1998;338:1585.

167. Bhattacharjee P, Hui P, McNiff J. Human herpesvirus-8 is not associated with angiolymphoid hyperplasia with eosinophilia. *J Cutan Pathol.* 2004;31:612–615.

168. Rascovan N, Monteil Bouchard S, Grob JJ, et al. Human polyomavirus-6 infecting lymph nodes of a patient with an angiolymphoid hyperplasia with eosinophilia or Kimura disease. *Clin Infect Dis.* 2016;62:1419–1421.

and immunohistochemical analysis of 62 cases. *J Cutan Pathol.* 1999;26:279.

169. Antonescu CR, Huang SC, Sung YS, et al. Novel GATA6-FOXO1 fusions in a subset of epithelioid hemangioma. *Mod Pathol.* 2021;34:934–941.

170. Tsuda Y, Suurmeijer AJH, Sung YS, et al. Epithelioid hemangioma of bone harboring FOS and FOSB gene rearrangements: a clinicopathologic and molecular study. *Genes Chromosomes Cancer.* 2021;60:17–25.

171. Antonescu CR, Chen HW, Zhang L, et al. ZFP36-FOSB fusion defines a subset of epithelioid hemangioma with atypical features. *Genes Chromosomes Cancer.* 2014;53:951–959.

172. Ortins-Pina A, Llamas-Velasco M, Turpin S, Soares-de-Almeida L, Filipe P, Kutzner H. FOSB immunoreactivity in endothelia of epithelioid hemangioma (angiolymphoid hyperplasia with eosinophilia). *J Cutan Pathol.* 2018;45:395–402.

173. Chong H, Brady K, Metze, D, Calonje E. Persistent nodule at injection sites (aluminium granuloma)—clinicopathological study of 14 cases with a diverse range of histological reaction patterns. *Histopathology.* 2006;48:182.

174. Frings VG, Roth S, Rosenwald A, Goebeler M, Geissinger E, Wobser M. EBER in situ hybridization in subcutaneous aluminum granulomas/lymphoid hyperplasia: a diagnostic clue to differentiate injection-associated lymphoid hyperplasia from other forms of pseudolymphomas and cutaneous lymphomas. *J Cutan Pathol.* 2021;48:625–631.

175. Abuel-Haija M, Hurford MT. Kimura disease. *Arch Pathol Lab Med.* 2007;131:650.

176. Chen H, Thompson LD, Aguilera NS, Abbondanzo SL. Kimura disease: a clinicopathologic study of 21 cases. *Am J Surg Pathol.* 2004;28:585.

177. Yang S, Wang J, Chen Y, et al. Concurrent kidney glomerular and interstitial lesions associated with Kimura's disease. *Nephron.* 2019;143:92–99.

178. Brenn T, Fletcher CDM. Cutaneous epithelioid angiomatous nodule: a distinct lesion in the morphologic spectrum of epithelioid vascular tumors. *Am J Dermatopathol.* 2004;26:14.

179. Fernandez-Flores A, Montero MG, Renedo G. Cutaneous epithelioid angiomatous nodule of the external ear. *Am J Dermatopathol.* 2005;27:175.

180. Kantrow S, Martin JD, Vnencak-Jones CL, Boyd AS. Cutaneous epithelioid angiomatous nodule: report of a case and absence of microsatellite instability. *J Cutan Pathol.* 2007;34:515.

181. Pavlidakey PG, Burroughs C, Karrs T, Somach SC. Cutaneous epithelioid angomatous nodule: a case with metachronous lesions. *Am J Dermatopathol.* 2011;33:831.

182. Kaushal S, Sharma MC, Ramam M, Kumar U. Multiple cutaneous epithelioid angiomatous nodules of the penis. *J Cutan Pathol.* 2011;38:369.

183. Shiomi T, Kaddu S, Yoshida Y, et al. Cutaneous epithelioid angiomatous nodule arising in capillary malformation. *J Cutan Pathol.* 2011;38:372.

184. Sorrells TC, Winn A, Sulit DJ. Granular cell cutaneous epithelioid angiomatous nodule. *J Cutan Pathol.* 2019;46:864–866.

185. Requena L, Kutzner H, Mentzel T. Acquired elastotic hemangioma: a clinicopathologic variant of hemangioma. *J Am Acad Dermatol.* 2002;47:371.

186. Martorell-Calatayud A, Balmer N, Sanmartin O, Díaz-Recuero JL, Sangueza OP. Definition of the features of acquired elastotic hemangioma reporting the clinical and histopathological characteristics of 14 patients. *J Cutan Pathol.* 2010;37:460.

187. Gurbuz Y, Muezzinoglu B, Apaydin R, Yumbul AZ. Acral arteriovenous tumor (cirsoid aneurysm): clinical and histopathological analysis of 6 cases. *Adv Clin Path.* 2002;6:25–29.

188. Girard C, Graham JH, Johnson WC. Arteriovenous hemangioma (arteriovenous shunt). *J Cutan Pathol.* 1974;1:73.

189. Koutlas IG, Jessurun J. Arteriovenous hemangioma: a clinicopathological and immunohistochemical study. *J Cutan Pathol.* 1994;21:343.

190. Semkova K, Carr R, Grainger M, et al. Poikilodermatous plaque-like hemangioma: case series of a newly defined entity. *J Am Acad Dermatol.* 2019;81:1257–1270.

191. Sullivan M, Hartman R, Mahalingam M. Poikilodermatous plaque-like hemangioma: a benign vasoformative entity with reproducible histopathologic and clinical features. *J Cutan Pathol.* 2020;47:950–953.

192. Aronniemi J, Lohi J, Salminen P, et al. Angiomatosis of soft tissue as an important differential diagnosis for intramuscular venous malformations. *Phlebology.* 2017;32:474–481.

193. Rao VK, Weiss SW. Angiomatosis of soft tissue: an analysis of the histologic features and clinical outcome in 51 cases. *Am J Surg Pathol.* 1992;16:764.

194. Gaeta R, Lessi F, Mazzanti C, et al. Diffuse bone and soft tissue angiomatosis with GNAQ mutation. *Pathol Int.* 2020;70:452–457.

195. Weiss SW, Enzinger FM. Spindle cell hemangioendothelioma: a low-grade angiosarcoma resembling cavernous hemangioma and Kaposi's sarcoma. *Am J Surg Pathol.* 1986;10:521.

196. Ono CM, Mitsunaga MM, Lockett LJ. Intragluteal spindle cell hemangioendothelioma: an unusual presentation of a recently described vascular neoplasm. *Clin Orthop Relat Res.* 1992;281:224–228.

197. Hakozaki M, Tajino T, Watanabe K, et al. Intraosseus spindle cell hemangioma of the calcaneus: a case report and review of the literature. *Ann Diagn Pathol.* 2012;16:369.

198. Cai Y, Wang R, Chen XM, et al. Maffucci syndrome with the spindle cell hemangiomas in the mucosa of the lower lip: a rare case report and literature review. *J Cutan Pathol.* 2013;40:661–666.

199. Fletcher CDM, Beham A, Schmid C. Spindle cell haemangioendothelioma: a clinicopathological and immunohistochemical study indicative of a non-neoplastic lesion. *Histopathology.* 1991;18:291.

200. Tronnier M, Vogelbruch M, Kutzner H. Spindle cell hemangioma and epithelioid hemangioendothelioma arising in an area of lymphedema. *Am J Dermatopathol.* 2006;28:223–227.

201. Perkins P, Weiss SW. Spindle cell hemangioendothelioma: an analysis of 78 cases with reassessment of its pathogenesis and biologic behavior. *Am J Surg Pathol.* 1996;20:1196.

202. Kurek KC, Pansuriya TC, van Ruler MA, et al. R132C IDH1 mutations are found in spindle cell hemangiomas and not in other vascular tumors or malformations. *Am J Pathol.* 2013;183:1494.

203. Ten Broek RW, Bekers EM, de Leng WWJ, et al. Mutational analysis using Sanger and next generation sequencing in sporadic spindle cell hemangiomas: a study of 19 cases. *Genes Chromosomes Cancer.* 2017;56:855–860.

204. Tsang WYW, Chan JKC, Fletcher CDM, et al. Symplastic hemangioma: a distinctive vascular neoplasm featuring bizarre stromal cells. *Int J Surg Pathol.* 1994;1:202.

205. Kutzner H, Winzer M, Mentzel T. Symplastic hemangioma [in German]. *Hautarzt.* 2000;51:327.

206. Goh N, Dayrit J, Calonje E. Symplastic hemangioma: report of two cases. *J Cutan Pathol.* 2006;33:735.

207. Folpe AL, Weiss SW. Pleomorphic hyalinizing angiectatic tumor: analysis of 41 cases supporting evolution from a distinctive precursor lesion. *Am J Surg Pathol.* 2004;28:1417–1425.

208. Beral V, Peterman TA, Berkelman R, Jaffe HW. Kaposi's sarcoma among persons with AIDS: a sexually transmitted infection. *Lancet.* 1990;335:123.

209. Friedman-Kien AE, Saltzman BR. Clinical manifestations of classical, endemic African, and epidemic AIDS-associated Kaposi's sarcoma. *J Am Acad Dermatol.* 1990;22:1237.

210. Tappero JW, Conant MA, Wolfe SF, Berger TG. Kaposi's sarcoma: epidemiology, pathogenesis, histology, clinical spectrum, staging criteria and therapy. *J Am Acad Dermatol.* 1993;28:371.

211. Jessop S. HIV-associated Kaposi's sarcoma. *Dermatol Clin.* 2006; 24:509.

212. Guttman-Yassley E, Bar-Chana M, Yukelson A, et al. Epidemiology of classic Kaposi's sarcoma in the Israeli Jewish population between 1960 and 1998. *Br J Cancer.* 2003;89:1657.

213. Dorfmann RF. Kaposi's sarcoma with special reference to its manifestations in infants and children and to the concepts of Arthur Purdy Stout. *Am J Surg Pathol.* 1986;10(suppl):68.

214. Onunu AN, Okoduwa C, Eze EU, et al. Kaposi's sarcoma in Nigeria. *Int J Dermatol.* 2007;46:204.

215. Mwanda OW, Fu P, Collea R, Whalen C, Remick SC. Kaposi's sarcoma in patients with and without human immunodeficiency virus infection, in a tertiary referral centre in Kenya. *Ann Trop Med Parasitol.* 2005;99:81.

216. Biggar RJ. AIDS-related cancers in the era of highly active antiretroviral therapy. *Oncology (Williston Park).* 2001;15:439.

217. Hernández-Ramírez RU, Shiels MS, Dubrow R, Engels EA. Cancer risk in HIV-infected people in the USA from 1996 to 2012: a population-based, registry-linkage study. *Lancet HIV.* 2017;4:e495–e504.

218. Yarchoan R, Uldrick TS. HIV-associated cancers and related diseases. *N Engl J Med.* 2018;378:1029–1041.

219. Lemlich G, Scham L, Lebwokl M. Kaposi's sarcoma and acquired immunodeficiency syndrome: postmortem findings in twenty-four cases. *J Am Acad Dermatol.* 1987;16:319.

220. McKenzie R, Travis WD, Dolan SA, et al. The causes of death in patients with human immunodeficiency virus infection: a clinical and pathologic study with emphasis on the role of pulmonary diseases. *Medicine (Baltimore).* 1991;70:326.

221. Serraino D, Angeletti C, Carrieri MP, et al. Kaposi's sarcoma in transplant and HIV infected patients: an epidemiologic study in Italy and France. *Transplantation.* 2005;80:1699.

222. Moosa MR. Kaposi's sarcoma in kidney transplant recipients: a 23-year experience. *QJM.* 2005;98:205.

223. Picard C, Mellouli F, Duprez R, et al. Kaposi's sarcoma in a child with Wiskott-Aldrich syndrome. *Eur J Pediatr.* 2006;165:453.

224. Mohanna S, Sanchez J, Ferrufino JC, Bravo F, Gotuzzo E. Lymphangioma-like Kaposi's sarcoma: report of four cases and review. *J Eur Acad Dermatol Venereol.* 2006;20:1010–1011.

225. Luzar B, Antony F, Ramdial PK, et al. Intravascular Kaposi's sarcoma—a hitherto unrecognized phenomenon. *J Cutan Pathol.* 2007;34:861.

226. Kempf W, Cathomas G, Burg G, Trüeb RM. Micronodular Kaposi's sarcoma—a new variant of classic-sporadic Kaposi's sarcoma. *Dermatology.* 2004;208:255.

227. O'Donnell PJ, Pantanowitz L, Grayson W. Unique histologic variants of cutaneous Kaposi sarcoma. *Am J Dermatopathol.* 2010;32:244.

228. Grayson W, Pantanowitz L. Histological variants of cutaneous Kaposi sarcoma. *Diagn Pathol.* 2008;3:31.

229. Radu O, Pantanowitz L. Kaposi sarcoma. *Arch Pathol Lab Med.* 2013;137:289.

230. Ramdial PK, Chetty R, Singh B, Singh R, Aboobaker J. Lymphoedematous HIV-associated KS. *J Cutan Pathol.* 2006;33:474.

231. Tourlaki A, Recalcati S, Boneschi V, et al. Anaplastic Kaposi's sarcoma: a study of eight patients. *Eur J Dermatol.* 2013;23:382–386.

232. Patel RM, Goldblum JR, HsI ED. Immunohistochemical detection of human herpes virus-8 latent nuclear antigen-1 is useful in the diagnosis of Kaposi sarcoma. *Mod Pathol.* 2004;17:456.

233. Cheuk W, Wong KO, Wong CS, Dinkel JE, Ben-Dor D, Chan JK. Immunostaining for human herpesvirus 8 latent nuclear antigen-1 helps distinguish Kaposi's sarcoma from its mimics. *Am J Clin Pathol.* 2004;121:335.

234. Martí N, Monteagudo C, Pinazo I. Negative herpesvirus-8 immunoreactivity does not exclude a diagnosis of Kaposi sarcoma. *Br J Dermatol.* 2011;164:209.

235. Pantanowitz L, Dezube BJ, Pinkus GS, Tahan SR. Histological characterization of regression in acquired immunodeficiency syndrome-related Kaposi's sarcoma. *J Cutan Pathol.* 2004;31:26.

236. Chang Y, Cesarman E, Pessin MS. Identification of herpesvirus-like DNA sequences in AIDS-associated Kaposi's sarcoma. *Science.* 1994;266:1865.

237. Huang YQ, Li JJ, Kaplan MH, et al. Human herpesvirus-like nucleic acid in various forms of Kaposi's sarcoma. *Lancet.* 1995;345:759.

238. Geraminejad P, Memar O, Aronson I, Rady PL, Hengge U, Tyring SK. Kaposi's sarcoma and other manifestations of human herpesvirus 8. *J Am Acad Dermatol.* 2002;47:641.

239. Dupin N, Grandadam M, Calvez V, et al. Herpesvirus-like DNA sequences in patients with Mediterranean Kaposi's sarcoma. *Lancet.* 1995;345:761.

240. Gao SJ, Kinsgley L, Hoover DR, et al. Seroconversion to antibodies against Kaposi's sarcoma-associated herpesvirus-related latent nuclear antigens before the development of Kaposi's sarcoma. *N Engl J Med.* 1996;335:233.

241. Carroll PA, Brazeau E, Lagunoff M. Kaposi's sarcoma-associated herpesvirus infection of blood endothelial cells induces lymphatic differentiation. *Virology.* 2004;328:7.

242. Xu H, Edwards JR, Espinosa O, Banerji S, Jackson DG, Athanasou NA. Expression of a lymphatic endothelial cell marker in benign and malignant vascular tumors. *Hum Pathol.* 2004;35:857.

243. Rabkin CS, Janz S, Lash A, et al. Monoclonal origin of multicentric Kaposi's sarcoma lesions. *N Engl J Med.* 1997;336:988–993.

244. Judde JG, Lacoste V, Brière J, et al. Monoclonality or oligoclonality of human herpesvirus-8 terminal repeat sequences in Kaposi's sarcoma and other diseases. *J Natl Cancer Inst.* 2000;92:677.

245. Duprez R, Lacoste V, Brière J, et al. Evidence for a multiclonal origin of multicentric advanced lesions of Kaposi sarcoma. *J Natl Cancer Inst.* 2007;99:1086.

246. Gessain A, Duprez R. Spindle cells and their role in Kaposi's sarcoma. *Int J Biochem Cell Biol.* 2005;37:2457.

247. Mariggiò G, Koch S, Schulz TF. Kaposi sarcoma herpesvirus pathogenesis. *Philos Trans R Soc Lond B Biol Sci.* 2017;372:20160275.

248. Aoki Y, Tosato G. Interactions between HIV-1 Tat and KSHV. *Curr Top Microbiol Immunol.* 2007;312:309.

249. Schmid I, Klenk AK, Sparber-Sauer M, Koscielniak E, Maxwell R, Häberle B. Kaposiform hemangioendothelioma in children: a benign vascular tumor with multiple treatment options. *World J Pediatr.* 2018;14:322–329.

250. Calonje E, Fletcher CDM. Aneurysmal benign fibrous histiocytoma: clinicopathological analysis of 40 cases of a tumour frequently misdiagnosed as a vascular neoplasm. *Histopathology.* 1995;26:323.

251. Brenner S, Martinez de Morentin E. What's new in pseudo-Kaposi's sarcoma. *J Eur Acad Dermatol Venereol.* 2001;15:382–384.

252. Strutton G, Weedon D. Acro-angiodermatitis: a simulant of Kaposi's sarcoma. *Am J Dermatopathol.* 1987;9:85.

253. Roy SF, Dong D, Myung P, McNiff JM. Multinucleate cell angiohistiocytoma: a clinicopathologic study of 62 cases and proposed diagnostic criteria. *J Cutan Pathol.* 2019;46:563–569.

254. Perez LP, Zuloica A, Rodriguez L, et al. Multinucleate cell angiohistiocytoma: report of 5 cases. *J Cutan Pathol.* 2006;33:349.

255. Calonje E, Fletcher CDM, Wilson Jones E, Rosai J. Retiform hemangioendothelioma: a distinctive form of low-grade angiosarcoma delineated in a series of 15 cases. *Am J Surg Pathol.* 1994;18:115.

256. Fukunaga M, Endo Y, Masui F, et al. Retiform hemangioendothelima. *Virchows Arch.* 1996;428:301.

257. Tan D, Kraybill W, Cheney RT, Khoury T. Retiform hemangioendothelioma: a case report and review of the literature. *J Cutan Pathol.* 2005;32:634.

258. Duke D, Dvorak A, Harris TJ, Cohen LM. Multiple retiform hemangioendotheliomas: a low-grade angiosarcoma. *Am J Dermatopathol.* 1996;18:606.

259. Antonescu CR, Dickson BC, Sung YS, et al. Recurrent YAP1 and MAML2 gene rearrangements in retiform and composite hemangioendothelioma. *Am J Surg Pathol.* 2020;44:1677–1684.

260. Fanburg-Smith JC, Michal M, Partanen TA, Alitalo K, Miettinen M. Papillary intralymphatic angioendothelioma (PILA): a report

of twelve cases of a distinctive vascular tumor with phenotypic features of lymphatic vessels. *Am J Surg Pathol.* 1999;23:1004.

261. Manivel JC, Wick MR, Swanson PE, Patterson K, Dehner LP. Endovascular papillary angioendothelioma of childhood: a vascular lesion possibly characterized by "high" endothelial cell differentiation. *Hum Pathol.* 1986;17:1240.

262. Nayler SJ, Rubin BP, Calonje E, Chan JK, Fletcher CD. Composite hemangioendothelioma: a complex, low-grade vascular lesion mimicking angiosarcoma. *Am J Surg Pathol.* 2000;24:352.

263. Requena L, Luis Díaz J, Manzarbeitia F, Carrillo R, Fernández-Herrera J, Kutzner H. Cutaneous composite hemangioendothelioma with satellitosis and lymph node metastases. *J Cutan Pathol.* 2008;35:225.

264. Fukunaga M, Suzuki K, Saegusa N, Folpe AL. Composite hemangioendothelioma: report of 5 cases including one with associated Maffucci syndrome. *Am J Surg Pathol.* 2007;31:156.

265. Reis-Filho JS, Paiva ME, Lopes JM. Congenital composite hemangioendothelioma: case report and reappraisal of the hemangioendothelioma spectrum. *J Cutan Pathol.* 2002;29:226.

266. Biagioli M, Sbano P, Miracco C, Fimiani M. Composite cutaneous haemangioendothelioma: case report and review of the literature. *Clin Exp Dermatol.* 2005;30:385.

267. Perry KD, Al-Lbraheemi A, Rubin BP, et al. Composite hemangioendothelioma with neuroendocrine marker expression: an aggressive variant. *Mod Pathol.* 2017;30:1589.

268. Antonescu CR, Dickson BC, Sung YS, et al. Recurrent YAP1 and MAML2 gene rearrangements in retiform and composite hemangioendothelioma. *Am J Surg Pathol.* 2020;44(12):1677–1684.

269. Lyons LL, North PE, Mac-Moune Lai F, Stoler MH, Folpe AL, Weiss SW. Kaposiform hemangioendothelioma: a study of 33 cases emphasizing its pathologic, immunophenotypic, and biologic uniqueness from juvenile hemangioma. *Am J Surg Pathol.* 2004;28:559.

270. Alvarez-Mendoza A, Lourdes TS, Ridaura-Sanz C, Ruiz-Maldonado R. Histopathology of vascular lesions found in Kasabach-Merritt syndrome: review based on 13 cases. *Pediatr Dev Pathol.* 2000;3:556.

271. Lai FMM, Choi PCL, Leung PC, et al. Kaposiform hemangioendothelioma: five patients with cutaneous lesions and long follow-up. *Mod Pathol.* 2001;14:1087.

272. Croteau SE, Liang MG, Kozakewich HP, et al. Kaposiform hemangioendothelioma: atypical features and risks of Kasabach-Merritt phenomenon in 107 referrals. *J Pediatr.* 2013;162:142.

273. Debelenko LV, Perez-Atayde AR, Mulliken JB, Liang MG, Archibald TH, Kozakewich HP. D2-40 immunohistochemical analysis of pediatric vascular tumors reveals positivity in kaposiform hemangioendothelioma. *Mod Pathol.* 2005;18:1454.

274. Enjolras O, Mulliken JB, Wassef M, et al. Residual lesions after Kasabach-Merritt phenomenon in 41 patients. *J Am Acad Dermatol.* 2000;42:225.

275. Ten Broek RW, Koelsche C, Eijkelenboom A, et al. Kaposiform hemangioendothelioma and tufted angioma—(epi)genetic analysis including genome-wide methylation profiling. *Ann Diagn Pathol.* 2020;44:151434.

276. Mirra JM, Kessler S, Bhuta S, Eckardt J. The fibroma-like variant of epithelioid sarcoma: a fibrohistiocytic/myoid cell lesion often confused with benign and malignant spindle cell tumors. *Cancer.* 1992;69:1382.

277. Billings SD, Folpe AL, Weiss SW. Epithelioid sarcoma-like hemangioendothelioma. *Am J Surg Pathol.* 2003;27:48.

278. Hornick JL, Fletcher CD. Pseudomyogenic hemangioendothelioma: a distinctive, often multicentric tumor with indolent behavior. *Am J Surg Pathol.* 2011;35:190.

279. Requena L, Santonja C, Martinez-Amo JL, Saus C, Kutzner H. Cutaneous epithelioid sarcomalike (pseudomyogenic)

hemangioendothelioma: a little-known low-grade cutaneous vascular neoplasm. *JAMA Dermatol.* 2013;149:459.

280. Amary MF, O'Donnell P, Berisha F, et al. Pseudomyogenic (epithelioid sarcoma-like) hemangioendothelioma: characterization of five cases. *Skeletal Radiol.* 2013;42:947.

281. Hung YP, Fletcher CD, Hornick JL. FOSB is a useful diagnostic marker for pseudomyogenic hemangioendothelioma. *Am J Surg Pathol.* 2017;41:596–606.

282. Walther C, Tayebwa J, Lilljebjorn H, et al. A novel SERPINE1-FOSB fusion gene results in a transcriptional up-regulation of FOSB in pseudomyogenic haemangioendothelioma. *J Pathol.* 2014;232:534–540.

283. Zhu G, Benayed R, Ho C, et al. Diagnosis of known sarcoma fusions and novel fusion partners by targeted RNA sequencing with identification of a recurrent ACTB-FOSB fusion in pseudomyogenic hemangioendothelioma. *Mod Pathol.* 2019;32:609–620.

284. Weiss SW, Enzinger FM. Epithelioid hemangioendothelioma: a vascular lesion often mistaken for a carcinoma. *Cancer.* 1982;50:970.

285. Mentzel T, Beham A, Calonje E, Katenkamp D, Fletcher CD. Epithelioid hemangioendothelioma of skin and soft tissues: clinicopathologic and immunohistochemical study of 30 cases. *Am J Surg Pathol.* 1997;21:363.

286. Flucke U, Vogels RJ, de Saint Aubain Somerhausen N, et al. Epithelioid hemangioendothelioma: clinicopathologic, immunhistochemical, and molecular genetic analysis of 39 cases. *Diagn Pathol.* 2014;9:131.

287. Ishibashi H, Takasaki C, Akashi T, Okubo K. Successful excision of epithelioid hemangioendothelioma of the superior vena cava. *Ann Thorac Surg.* 2020;109:e271–e273.

288. Alam SI, Nepal P, Sajid S, Al-Bozom I, Salah MM, Muneer A. Epithelioid hemangioendothelioma of the ulnar artery presenting with neuropathy. *Ann Vasc Surg.* 2020;67:563.e13–563.e17.

289. Shibayama T, Makise N, Motoi T, et al. Clinicopathologic characterization of epithelioid hemangioendothelioma in a series of 62 cases: a proposal of risk stratification and identification of a synaptophysin-positive aggressive subset. *Am J Surg Pathol.* 2021;45:616–626.

290. Madura C, Sacchidanand S, Barde NG, Biligi D. Epithelioid hemangioendothelioma in a child. *J Cutan Aesthet Surg.* 2013;6:232–235.

291. Quante M, Patel NK, Hill S, et al. Epithelioid hemangioendothelioma presenting in the skin: a clinicopathologic study of eight cases. *Am J Dermatopathol.* 1998;20:541–546.

292. Deyrup AT, Tighiouart M, Montag AG, Weiss SW. Epithelioid hemangioendothelioma of soft tissue: a proposal for risk stratification based on 49 cases. *Am J Surg Pathol.* 2008;32:924.

293. Williams SB, Bulter CB, Gilkey GW, et al. Epithelioid hemangioendothelioma with osteoclast-like giant cells. *Arch Pathol Lab Med.* 1993;117:315.

294. Mendlick MR, Nelson M, Pickering D, et al. Translocation t(1;3)(p36.3;q25) is a nonrandom aberration in epithelioid hemangioendothelioma. *Am J Surg Pathol.* 2001;25:684.

295. Errani C, Zhang L, Sung YS, et al. A novel WWTR1-CAMTA1 gene fusion is a consistent abnormality in epithelioid hemangioendothelioma of different anatomic sites. *Genes Chromosomes Cancer.* 2011;50:644.

296. Tanas MR, Sboner A, Oliveira AM, et al. Identification of a disease-defining gene fusion in epithelioid hemangioendothelioma. *Sci Transl Med.* 2011;3:98.

297. Antonescu CR, Le Loarer F, Mosquera JM, et al. Novel YAP1-TFE3 fusion defines a distinct subset of epithelioid hemangioendothelioma. *Genes Chromosomes Cancer.* 2013;52:775.

298. Doyle LA, Fletcher CD, Hornick JL. Nuclear expression of CAMTA1 distinguishes epithelioid hemangioendothelioma from histologic mimics. *Am J Surg Pathol.* 2016;40:94–102.

299. Lee SJ, Yang WI, Chung WS, Kim SK. Epithelioid hemangioendotheliomas with TFE3 gene translocations are compossible with CAMTA1 gene rearrangements. *Oncotarget*. 2016;7:7480–7488.

300. Young RJ, Brown NJ, Reed MW, et al. Angiosarcoma. *Lancet Oncol*. 2010;11:983–991.

301. Fletcher CDM, Beham A, Bekir S, Clarke AM, Marley NJ. Epithelioid angiosarcoma of deep soft tissue: a distinctive tumor readily mistaken for an epithelial neoplasm. *Am J Surg Pathol*. 1991;15:915.

302. Rossi S, Fletcher CD. Angiosarcoma arising in hemangioma/vascular malformation: report of four cases and review of the literature. *Am J Surg Pathol*. 2002;26:1319.

303. Al-robaie B, Stephenson M, Evans GH, Sandison AJ. Angiosarcoma mimicking a recurrent carotid artery aneurysm. *Ann Vasc Surg*. 2011;25:19–23.

304. Hasiotou M, Danassi-Afentaki D, Stefanaki K, Sfakianos G, Prodromou N, Moschovi M. Early atypical malignant transformation of a plexiform neurofibroma in a 4-year-old boy with Neurofibromatosis 1. *Pediatr Blood Cancer*. 2005;45:76–77.

305. McMenamin ME, Fletcher CD. Expanding the spectrum of malignant change in schwannomas: epithelioid malignant change, epithelioid malignant peripheral nerve sheath tumor, and epithelioid angiosarcoma: a study of 17 cases. *Am J Surg Pathol*. 2001;25:13–25.

306. Mentzel T, Katencamp D. Intraneural angiosarcoma and angiosarcoma arising in benign and malignant peripheral nerve sheath tumours: clinicopathological and immunohistochemical analysis of four cases. *Histopathology*. 1999;35:114.

307. Marcon I, Collini P, Casanova M, Meazza C, Ferrari A. Cutaneous angiosarcoma in a patient with xeroderma pigmentosum. *Pediatr Hematol Oncol*. 2004;21:23.

308. Folpe AL, Johnston CA, Weiss SW. Cutaneous angiosarcoma arising in a gouty tophus: report of a unique case and a review of foreign material-associated angiosarcoma. *Am J Dermatopathol*. 2000;22:418.

309. Ghandur-Mnaymneh L, Gonzales MS. Angiosarcoma of the penis with hepatic angiomas in a patient with low vinyl chloride exposure. *Cancer*. 1981;47:1318.

310. Kakisis JD, Antonopoulos C, Moulakakis K, et al. Angiosarcoma of a thrombosed arteriovenous fistula in a renal transplant recipient. *Ann Vasc Surg*. 2019;56:357.e1–357.e4.

311. Agaimy A, Ben-Izhak O, Lorey T, Scharpf M, Rubin BP. Angiosarcoma arising in association with vascular Dacron grafts and orthopedic joint prostheses: clinicopathologic, immunohistochemical, and molecular study. *Ann Diagn Pathol*. 2016;21:21–28.

312. Kantrow SM, Boyd AS. Primary cutaneous metaplastic carcinoma: report of a case involving angiosarcoma. *Am J Dermatopathol*. 2007;29:270.

313. Den-Bakker MA, Ansink AC, Ewing-Graham PC. "Cutaneous-type" angiosarcoma arising in a mature cystic teratoma of the ovary. *J Clin Pathol*. 2006;59:658.

314. Bruder E, Perez-Atayde AR, Jundt G, et al. Vascular lesions of bone in children, adolescents, and young adults. A clinicopathologic reappraisal and application of the ISSVA classification. *Virchows Arch*. 2009;454:161–179.

315. Nara T, Hayakawa A, Ikeuchi A, Katoh N, Kishimoto S. Granulocyte colony-stimulating factor-producing cutaneous angiosarcoma with leukaemoid reaction arising on a burn scar. *Br J Dermatol*. 2003;149:1273–1275.

316. Flucke U, Karanian M, Broek RWT, Thway K. Soft tissue special issue: perivascular and vascular tumors of the head and neck. *Head Neck Pathol*. 2020;14:21–32.

317. Cao J, Wang J, He C, Fang M. Angiosarcoma: a review of diagnosis and current treatment. *Am J Cancer Res*. 2019;9:2303–2313.

318. Mark RJ, Pown JC, Tran LM, Fu YS, Juillard GF. Angiosarcoma: a report of 67 patients and a review of the literature. *Cancer*. 1996;77:2400.

319. Morgan MB, Swann M, Somach S, et al. Cutaneous angiosarcoma: a case series with prognostic correlations. *J Am Acad Dermatol*. 2004;50:867.

320. Albores-Saavedra J, Schwartz AM, Henson DE, et al. Cutaneous angiosarcoma: analysis of 434 cases from the surveillance, epidemiology, and end results program, 1973-2007. *Ann Diagn Pathol*. 2011;15:93.

321. Abraham JA, Hamicek FJ, Kaufman AM, et al. Treatment and outcome of 82 patients with angiosarcoma. *Ann Surg Oncol*. 2007;14:1953.

322. Mendenhall WM, Mendenhall CM, Werning JW, et al. Cutaneous angiosarcoma. *Am J Clin Oncol*. 2006;29:524.

323. Pawlik TM, Paulino AF, McGinn CJ, et al. Cutaneous angiosarcoma of the scalp: a multidisciplinary approach. *Cancer*. 2003;98:1716.

324. Milam EC, Rangel LK, Pomeranz MK. Dermatologic sequelae of breast cancer: from disease, surgery, and radiation. *Int J Dermatol*. 2021;60:394–406.

325. Cui L, Zhang J, Zhang X. Angiosarcoma (Stewart-Treves syndrome) in postmastectomy patients: report of 10 cases and review of literature. *Int J Clin Exp Pathol*. 2015;8:11108–11115.

326. Cooper H, Farsi M, Dorton D, et al. Cutaneous angiosarcoma of the leg. *Dermatol Online J*. 2019;25:13030/qt3hq6r0b0.

327. Offori TW, Platt CC, Stephens M, et al. Angiosarcoma in congenital hereditary lymphedema (Milroy's disease): diagnostic beacons and a review of the literature. *Clin Exp Dermatol*. 1993; 18:174.

328. Krishnamoorthy N, Viswanathan S, Rekhi B, et al. Lymphangiosarcoma arising after 33 years within a background of chronic filariasis: a case report with review of literature. *J Cutan Pathol*. 2012;39:52–55.

329. Shon W, Ida CM, Boland-Froemming JM, et al. Cutaneous angiosarcoma arising in massive localized lymphedema of the morbidly obese: a report of five cases and review of the literature. *J Cutan Pathol*. 2011;38:560.

330. Abdou Y, Elkhanany A, Attwood K. Primary and secondary breast angiosarcoma: single center report and a meta-analysis. *Breast Cancer Res Treat*. 2019;178:523–533.

331. Hung J, Hiniker SM, Lucas DR, et al. Sporadic versus radiation-associated angiosarcoma: a comparative clinicopathologic and molecular analysis of 48 Cases. *Sarcoma*. 2013;2013:798403.

332. Sener SF, Milos S, Feldman JL, et al. The spectrum of vascular lesions in the mammary skin, including angiosarcoma after breast conservation treatment for breast cancer. *J Am Coll Surg*. 2001;193:22.

333. Billings SD, McKenney JK, Folpe AL, Hardacre MC, Weiss SW. Cutaneous angiosarcoma following breast-conserving surgery and radiation: an analysis of 27 cases. *Am J Surg Pathol*. 2004;28:781.

334. Cohen-Hallaleh RB, Smith HG, Smith RC, et al. Radiation induced angiosarcoma of the breast: outcomes from a retrospective case series. *Clin Sarcoma Res*. 2017;7:15.

335. Morgan EA, Kozono DE, Wang Q, et al. Cutaneous radiation-associated angiosarcoma of the breast: poor prognosis in a rare secondary malignancy. *Ann Surg Oncol*. 2012;19:3801.

336. Shustef E, Kazlouskaya V, Prieto VG, Ivan D, Aung PP. Cutaneous angiosarcoma: a current update. *J Clin Pathol*. 2017;70:917–925.

337. Hitchcock MG, Hurt MA, Santa Cruz DJ. Cutaneous granular cell angiosarcoma. *J Cutan Pathol*. 1994;21:256.

338. Salviato T, Bacchi CE, Luzar B, Falconieri G. Signet ring cell angiosarcoma: a hitherto unreported pitfall in the diagnosis of epithelioid cutaneous malignancies. *Am J Dermatopathol*. 2013;35:671.

339. Tatsas AD, Keedy VL, Florell SR, et al. Foamy cell angiosarcoma: a rare and deceptively bland variant of cutaneous angiosarcoma. *J Cutan Pathol*. 2010;37:901.

340. Brightman LA, Demierre MF, Byers HR. Macrophage-rich epithelioid angiosarcoma mimicking malignant melanoma. *J Cutan Pathol*. 2006;33:38.

341. Requena L, Santonja C, Stutz N, et al. Pseudolymphomatous cutaneous angiosarcoma: a rare variant of cutaneous angiosarcoma readily mistaken for cutaneous lymphoma. *Am J Dermatopathol.* 2007;29:342.

342. Sleeman JP, Krishnan J, Kirkin V, et al. Markers for the lymphatic endothelium: in search of the Holy Grail? *Microsc Res Tech.* 2001;55:61.

343. Jackson DG. The lymphatic revisited: new perspectives from the hyaluronan receptor LYVE-1. *Trends Cardiovasc Med.* 2003;13:1.

344. Kahn HJ, Bailey D, Marks A. Monoclonal antibody D2-40, a new marker of lymphatic endothelium, reacts with Kaposi's sarcoma and a subset of angiosarcomas. *Mod Pathol.* 2002;15:434.

345. Ordonez NG. Podoplanin: a novel diagnostic immunohistochemical marker. *Adv Anat Pathol.* 2006;13:83.

346. Rao P, Lahat G, Arnold C, et al. Angiosarcoma: a tissue microarray study with diagnostic implications. *Am J Dermatopathol.* 2013;35:432–437.

347. McKenney JK, Weiss SW, Folpe AL. CD31 expression in intratumoral macrophages: a potential diagnostic pitfall. *Am J Surg Pathol.* 2001;25:1167.

348. Folpe AL, Chand EM, Goldblum JR, Weiss SW. Expression of Fli-1, a nuclear transcription factor distinguishes vascular neoplasms from potential mimics. *Am J Surg Pathol.* 2001;25:1061.

349. Ross S, Orvieto E, Furlanetto A, Laurino L, Ninfo V, Dei Tos AP. Utility of immunohistochemical detection of Fli-1 expression in round cell and vascular neoplasms using a monoclonal antibody. *Mod Pathol.* 2004;17:547.

350. McKay KM, Doyle LA, Lazar AJ, Hornick JL. Expression of ERG, an Ets family transcription factor, distinguishes cutaneous angiosarcoma from histological mimics. *Histopathology.* 2012;61:989.

351. Miettinen M, Wang ZF, Paetau A, et al. ERG transcription factor as an immunohistochemical marker for vascular endothelial tumors and prostatic carcinoma. *Am J Surg Pathol.* 2011;35:432.

352. Mentzel T, Schildhaus HU, Palmedo G, Büttner R, Kutzner H. Postradiation cutaneous angiosarcoma after treatment of breast carcinoma is characterized by MYC amplification in contrast to atypical vascular lesions after radiotherapy and control cases: clinicopathological, immunohistochemical and molecular analysis of 66 cases. *Mod Pathol.* 2012;25:75.

353. Shon W, Sukov WR, Jenkins SM, Folpe AL. MYC amplification and overexpression in primary cutaneous angiosarcoma: a fluorescence in-situ hybridization and immunohistochemical study. *Mod Pathol.* 2014;27(4):509–515.

354. Huang SC, Zhang L, Sung YS, et al. Recurrent CIC gene abnormalities in angiosarcomas: a molecular study of 120 cases with concurrent investigation of PLCG1, KDR, MYC, and FLT4 gene alterations. *Am J Surg Pathol.* 2016;40:645–655.

355. Driemel O, Müller-Richter UD, Hakim SG, et al. Oral acantholytic squamous cell carcinoma shares clinical and histological features with angiosarcoma. *Head Face Med.* 2008;4:17.

356. Gu X, Jiang R, Fowler MR. Acantholytic squamous cell carcinoma in upper aerodigestive tract: histopathology, immunohistochemical profile and epithelial mesenchymal transition phenotype change. *Head Neck Pathol.* 2012;6:438–444.

357. Zidar N, Gale N, Zupevc A, Dovsak D. Pseudovascular adenoid squamous-cell carcinoma of the oral cavity—a report of two cases. *J Clin Pathol.* 2006;59:1206–1208.

358. Lasota J, Miettinen M. Absence of Kaposi's sarcoma-associated virus (human herpesvirus-8) sequences in angiosarcoma. *Virchows Arch.* 1999;434:51.

359. Suchak R, Thway K, Zelger B, Fisher C, Calonje E. Primary cutaneous epithelioid angiosarcoma: a clinicopathologic study of 13 cases of a rare neoplasm occurring outside the setting of conventional angiosarcomas and with predilection for the limbs. *Am J Surg Pathol.* 2011;35:60.

360. Bacchi CE, Silva TR, Zambrano E, et al. Epithelioid angiosarcoma of the skin: a study of 18 cases with emphasis on its clinicopathologic spectrum and unusual morphologic features. *Am J Surg Pathol.* 2010;34:1334.

361. Val-Bernal JF, Figols J, Arce FP, et al. Cardiac epithelioid angiosarcoma presenting as cutaneous metastasis. *J Cutan Pathol.* 2001;28:265.

362. Weed BR, Folpe AL. Cutaneous CD30-positive epithelioid angiosarcoma following breast-conserving therapy and irradiation: a potential diagnostic pitfall. *Am J Dermatopathol.* 2008;30:370–372.

363. Aldaabil RA, Alkhunaizi AM, Al-Dawsari NA, Dawamneh MF, Rabah R. Angiosarcoma at the site of nonfunctioning arteriovenous fistula in a kidney transplant recipient. *J Vasc Surg Cases Innov Tech.* 2016;2:53–55.

364. Terrando S, Sambri A, Bianchi G, et al. Angiosarcoma around total hip arthroplasty: case series and review of the literature. *Musculoskelet Surg.* 2018;102:21–27.

365. Goh SG, Calonje E. Cutaneous vascular tumours: an update. *Histopathology.* 2008;52:661–673.

366. Guillou L, Flecher CDM. Benign lymphangioendothelioma (acquired progressive lymphangioma): a lesion not to be confused with well-differentiated angiosarcoma and patch stage Kaposi's sarcoma: clinicopathologic analysis of a series. *Am J Surg Pathol.* 2000;24:1047–1057.

367. Wiegand S, Eivazi B, Barth PJ, et al. Pathogenesis of lymphangiomas. *Virchows Arch.* 2008;453:1–8.

368. Burgdorf WHC, Mukai K, Rosai J. Immunohistochemical identification of factor VIII-related antigen in endothelial cells of cutaneous lesions of alleged vascular nature. *Am J Clin Pathol.* 1981;75:167.

369. Pearson JM, McWilliam LJ. A light microscopical, immunohistochemical, and ultrastructural comparison of hemangiomata and lymphangiomata. *Ultrastruct Pathol.* 1990;14:497.

370. Luks VL, Kamitaki N, Vivero MP, et al. Lymphatic and other vascular malformative/overgrowth disorders are caused by somatic mutations in PIK3CA. *J Pediatr.* 2015;166:1048–1054.

371. Jiao-Ling L, Hai-Ying W, Wei Z, Jin-Rong L, Kun-Shan C, Qian F. Treatment and prognosis of fetal lymphangioma. *Eur J Obstet Gynecol Reprod Biol.* 2018;231:274–279.

372. Alqahtani A, Nguyen LT, Flageole H, Shaw K, Laberge JM. 25 years experience with lymphangiomas in children. *J Pediatr Surg.* 1999;34:1164.

373. Noia G, Maltese PE, Zampino G, et al. Cystic hygroma: a preliminary genetic study and a short review from the literature. *Lymphat Res Biol.* 2019;17:30–39.

374. Vatopoulou A, Anagnostopoulos A, Sujeewa F. Congenital lymphangioma circumscriptum of the vulva. *J Obstet Gynaecol Res.* 2019;45:2137–2138.

375. Chang MB, Newman CC, Davis MD, Lehman JS. Acquired lymphangiectasia (lymphangioma circumscriptum) of the vulva: clinicopathologic study of 11 patients from a single institution and 67 from the literature. *Int J Dermatol.* 2016;55:e482–e487.

376. Yamada S, Yamada Y, Kobayashi M, et al. Post-mastectomy benign lymphangioendothelioma of the skin following chronic lymphedema for breast carcinoma: a teaching case mimicking low-grade angiosarcoma and masquerading as Stewart-Treves syndrome. *Diagn Pathol.* 2014;9:197.

377. Alkhalili E, Ayoubieh H, O'Brien W, Billings SD. Acquired progressive lymphangioma of the nipple. *BMJ Case Rep.* 2014;2014:bcr2014205966.

378. Ramani P, Shah A. Lymphangiomatosis: histologic and immunohistochemical analysis of four cases. *Am J Surg Pathol.* 1993;17:329.

379. Singh GC, Calonje E, Ferrar DW, Browse NL, Fletcher CD. Lymphangiomatosis of the limbs: clinicopathologic analysis of a series. *Am J Surg Pathol.* 1995;19:125.

380. Triana P, Dore M, Cerezo VN. Sirolimus in the treatment of vascular anomalies. *Eur J Pediatr Surg.* 2017;27:86–90.

381. North PE, Kahn T, Cordisco MR, Dadras SS, Detmar M, Frieden IJ. Multifocal lymphangioangiotheliomatosis with thrombocytopenia: a newly recognized clinicopathological entity. *Arch Dermatol.* 2004;140:599.

382. Piggott KD, Riedel PA, Baron HI. Multifocal lymphangioendotheliomatosis with thrombocytopenia: a rare cause of gastrointestinal bleeding in the new born period. *Pediatrics.* 2006; 117:e810.

383. Yeung J, Somers G, Viero S, et al. Multifocal lymphangioendotheliomatosis with thrombocytopenia. *J Am Acad Dermatol.* 2006;54:S214.

384. Maronn M, Katrine K, North P, et al. Expanding the phenotype of multifocal lymphangioendotheliomatosis with thrombocytopenia. *Pediatr Blood Cancer.* 2009;52:531.

385. Khamaysi Z, Bergman R. Multifocal congenital lymphangioendotheliomatosis without gastrointestinal bleeding and/or thrombocytopenia. *Am J Dermatopathol.* 2010;32:804.

386. Kline RM, Buck LM. Bevacizumab treatment in multifocal lymphangioendotheliomatosis with thrombocytopenia. *Pediatr Blood Cancer.* 2009;52:534.

387. Fineberg S, Rosen PP. Cutaneous angiosarcoma and atypical vascular lesion of the skin and breast after radiation therapy for breast carcinoma. *Am J Clin Pathol.* 1994;102:757.

388. Diaz-Cascajo C, Borghi S, Weyers W, Retzlaff H, Requena L, Metze D. Benign lymphangiomatous papules of the skin after radiotherapy: a report of five new cases and review of the literature. *Histopathology.* 1999;35:319.

389. Requena L, Kutzner H, Mentzel T, Durán R, Rodríguez-Peralto JL. Benign vascular proliferations in irradiated skin. *Am J Surg Pathol.* 2002;26:328.

390. Brenn T, Fletcher CD. Radiation-associated cutaneous atypical vascular lesions and angiosarcoma: clinicopathologic analysis of 42 cases. *Am J Surg Pathol.* 2005;29:983.

391. Brenn T, Fletcher CD. Post-radiation vascular proliferation: an increasing problem. *Histopathology.* 2006;48:106.

392. Patton KT, Deyrup AT, Weiss SW. Atypical vascular lesions after surgery and radiation of the breast: a clinicopathologic study of 32 cases analyzing histologic heterogeneity and association with angiosarcoma. *Am J Surg Pathol.* 2008;32:943.

393. Mattoch IW, Robbins JB, Kempson RL, Kohler S. Post-radiotherapy vascular proliferations in mammary skin: a clinicopathologic study of 11 cases. *J Am Acad Dermatol.* 2007;57:126.

394. Gengler C, Coindre JM, Leroux A, et al. Vascular proliferations of the skin after radiation therapy for breast cancer: clinicopathologic analysis of a series in favour of a benign process: a study from the French Sarcoma Group. *Cancer.* 2007;109:1884.

395. Guo T, Zhang L, Chang NE, et al. Consistent MYC and FLT4 gene amplification in radiation-induced angiosarcoma but not in other radiation-associated atypical vascular lesions. *Genes Chromosomes Cancer.* 2011;50:25.

396. Fernandez AP, Sun Y, Tubbs RR, Goldblum JR, Billings SD. FISH for MYC amplification and anti-MYC immunohistochemistry: useful diagnostic tools in the assessment of secondary angiosarcoma and atypical vascular proliferations. *J Cutan Pathol.* 2012;39:234.

397. Schiefer TK, Parker WL, Anakwenze OA, Amadio PC, Inwards CY, Spinner RJ. Extradigital glomus tumor: a 20-year experience. *Mayo Clin Proc.* 2006;81:1337.

398. Schwartz RA, Wilson BN, John AM, Handler MZ. Neurofibromatosis type 1 and subungual glomus tumors: a noteworthy association. *J Am Acad Dermatol.* 2021;84(6):e271.

399. Lipner SR, Scher RK. Subungual glomus tumors: underrecognized clinical findings in neurofibromatosis 1. *J Am Acad Dermatol.* 2021;84(6):e269.

400. Yuen J, Bavan L, Graham A. A rare case of multiple subungual glomus tumours in a neurofibromatosis type 1 patient. *Hand Surg.* 2015;20:159–160.

401. Kromer C, Milani-Nejad N, Chung C, Tyler K. Multiple tender bluish nodules. *JAAD Case Rep.* 2020;6:225–227.

402. Boon LM, Brouillard P, Irrthum A, et al. A gene for inherited cutaneous venous anomalies ("glomangiomas") localizes to chromosome 1p21-22. *Am J Hum Genet.* 1999;65:125.

403. Calvert JT, Burns S, Riney TJ, et al. Additional glomangioma family link to chromosome 1p: no evidence for genetic heterogeneity. *Hum Hered.* 2001;51:180.

404. Brouillard P, Boon LM, Mulliken JB, et al. Mutations in a novel factor, glomulin, are responsible for glomuvenous malformations ("glomangiomas"). *Am J Hum Genet.* 2002;70:866.

405. Brouillard P, Ghassibe M, Penington A, et al. Four common glomulin mutations cause two thirds of glomovenus malformations ("familial glomangioma"): evidence for a founder effect. *J Med Genet.* 2005;42:e13.

406. Boon LM, Mulliken JB, Enjolras O, Vikkula M. Glomuvenous malformation (glomangioma) and venous malformation: distinct clinicopathologic and genetic entities. *Arch Dermatol.* 2004;140:971.

407. Rahemtullah A, Szyfelbein K, Zembowicz A. Glomus coccygeum: report of a case and review of the literature. *Am J Dermatopathol.* 2005;27:428.

408. Skelton HG, Smith KJ. Infiltrative glomus tumor arising from a benign glomus tumor: a distinctive immunohistochemical pattern in the infiltrative component. *Am J Dermatopathol.* 1999;21:562–566.

409. Jalali M, Netscher DT, Connelly JH. Glomangiomatosis. *Ann Diagn Pathol.* 2002;6:326.

410. Beham A, Fletcher CDM. Intravascular glomus tumor: a previously undescribed phenomenon. *Virchows Arch A Pathol Anat Histopathol.* 1991;418:175.

411. Lee SK, Song DG, Choy WS. Intravascular glomus tumor of the forearm causing chronic pain and focal tenderness. *Case Rep Orthop.* 2014;2014:619490.

412. Calonje E, Fletcher CDM. Cutaneous intraneural glomus tumor: report of a case. *Am J Dermatopathol.* 1995;15:395.

413. Folpe Al, Fanburg-Smith JC, Miettinen M, Weiss SW. Atypical and malignant glomus tumors: analysis of 52 cases, with a proposal for reclassification of glomus tumors. *Am J Surg Pathol.* 2001;25:1.

414. Yu DK, Chu KH, Kim YJ, Heo DS. Tracheal glomangiosarcoma with multiple skin metastases. *J Dermatol.* 2004;31:776.

415. Ugras N, Yercİ Ö, Yalçınkaya U, et al. Malignant glomus tumor with oncocytic features: an unusual presentation of dysphagia. *APMIS.* 2015;123:613–617.

416. Pulitzer DR, Martin PC, Reed RJ. Epithelioid glomus tumor. *Hum Pathol.* 1995;26:1022.

417. Luzar B, Martin B, Fisher C, Calonje E. Cutaneous malignant glomus tumours: applicability of currently established malignancy criteria for tumours occurring in the skin. *Pathology.* 2018;50:711–717.

418. Mravic M, LaChaud G, Nguyen A, Scott MA, Dry SM, James AW. Clinical and histopathological diagnosis of glomus tumor: an institutional experience of 138 cases. *Int J Surg Pathol.* 2015;23:181–188.

419. Mentzel T, Hugel H, Kutzner H. CD34-positive glomus tumor: clinicopathologic and immunohistochemical analysis of six cases with myxoid stromal change. *J Cutan Pathol.* 2002;29:426.

420. Agaram NP, Zhang L, Jungbluth AA, Dickson BC, Antonescu CR. A molecular reappraisal of glomus tumors and related pericytic neoplasms with emphasis on NOTCH-gene fusions. *Am J Surg Pathol.* 2020;44:1556–1562.

421. Karamzadeh Dashti N, Bahrami A, Lee SJ, et al. BRAF V600E mutations occur in a subset of glomus tumors, and are associated with malignant histologic characteristics. *Am J Surg Pathol.* 2017;41:1532–1541.

422. Fletcher CD. The evolving classification of soft tissue tumours: an update based on the new WHO classification. *Histopathology.* 2006;48:3–12.

423. Granter SR, Badizadegan K, Fletcher CD. Myofibromatosis in adults, glomangiopericytoma, and myopericytoma: a spectrum

of tumors showing perivascular myoid differentiation. *Am J Surg Pathol*. 1998;22:513.

424. Dray MS, McCarthy SW, Palmer AA, et al. Myopericytoma: a unifying term for a spectrum of tumors that show overlapping features with myofibroma. A review of 14 cases. *J Clin Pathol*. 2006;59:67.

425. Mentzel T, Dei Tos AP, Sapi Z, Kutzner H. Myopericytoma of skin and soft tissues: clinicopathologic and immunohistochemical study of 54 cases. *Am J Surg Pathol*. 2006;30:104.

426. Mentzel T, Calonje E, Nascimiento AG, Fletcher CD. Infantile hemangiopericytoma versus infantile myofibromatosis: a study of a series suggesting a spectrum of infantile myofibroblastic lesions. *Am J Surg Pathol*. 1994;18:922.

427. McMenamin ME, Fletcher CDM. Malignant myopericytoma: expanding the spectrum of tumors with myopericytic differentiation. *Histopathology*. 2002;41:450.

428. Hung YP, Fletcher CDM. Myopericytomatosis: clinicopathologic analysis of 11 cases with molecular identification of recurrent PDGFRB alterations in myopericytomatosis and myopericytoma. *Am J Surg Pathol*. 2017;41:1034–1044.

429. McMenamin ME, Calonje E. Intravascular myopericytoma. *J Cutan Pathol*. 2002;29:557.

Chapter 34

Adipocytic Tumors of the Skin and Subcutis

JORGE TORRES-MORA AND ANDREW L. FOLPE

INTRODUCTION

Normal Fat

Three types of adipocytes are found in the human body: brown, white, and beige. Brown fat, predominantly present in the axillary and subpleural regions in newborns, has a thermogenic function and derives embryonically from cells expressing myogenic nuclear regulatory genes such as *MYOD1* and *MYF5*, thought to represent skeletal muscle precursors (1). Brown fat cells are rich in mitochondria and express high levels of UCP1, the enzyme critical for the uncoupling of oxidative respiration and the generation of heat (2). The characteristic red-brown to tan color of brown fat results from cytochrome pigment in these mitochondria. Almost all "brown fat" in adults represents morphologically identical beige fat. Beige adipocytes are also involved in the regulation of body temperature, but develop after birth either *de novo* or by white-to-brown adipocyte transdifferentiation (so-called browning of white adipose tissue) (2–4). In adults, univacuolated white fat is by far the most common type of adipose tissue and is chiefly responsible for the storage of excess chemical energy as triacylglycerol, in addition to providing mechanical cushioning in areas such as the plantar foot (5).

Pathologic Evaluation of Cutaneous and Subcutaneous Adipocytic Tumors

Careful morphologic evaluation is the keystone to the correct diagnosis of adipocytic tumors of all types, in any anatomic location including the skin. In contrast to many other types of soft tissue tumors, where immunohistochemical evaluation is a standard part of the diagnostic workup, immunohistochemistry plays a very limited role in the evaluation of adipocytic tumors. Although normal white fat cells are invariably S100 protein-positive, S100 protein expression is less common in lipoblasts, and almost never present in the undifferentiated spindled cells seen in pleomorphic or dedifferentiated liposarcomas, or in the primitive round cells of myxoid liposarcoma (6). Nonneoplastic brown fat, beige fat, and tumors showing brown fat differentiation typically show diffuse CD10 expression, a finding that may occasionally be of value in the differential diagnosis of hibernoma (7). As will be discussed at various points in this chapter, immunohistochemistry for CD34 and RB1 protein has some utility in the differential diagnosis of spindle cell and pleomorphic lipomas, but is not necessary in most cases, and may be confusing in some. In contrast, molecular genetic evaluation has become increasingly important in the diagnosis of adipocytic tumors, with specific genetic alterations characterizing various lipomatous lesions (e.g.,

MDM2/CDK4 amplification in atypical lipomatous tumors, *PLAG* rearrangement in lipoblastoma, *DDIT3* rearrangement in myxoid liposarcoma). Table 34-1 summarizes diagnostically useful genetic findings in selected adipocytic tumors of the skin and subcutis.

Fatty tumors of dermatologic interest are common and are generally located in the subcutis, rather than within the skin proper. Aside from nevus lipomatosus, purely *cutaneous* lipogenic tumors are exceptionally rare and have different specific clinicopathologic features in comparison with more deeply located tumors. Thus, when evaluating an adipocytic tumor, the dermatopathologist/pathologist may find it very helpful to discuss with the submitting clinician whether a given tumor is cutaneous, subcutaneous, or more deeply situated and extending up to involve the skin. Review of clinical photographs can also at times be very useful.

General Comments on the Clinical Management of Cutaneous and Subcutaneous Adipocytic Tumors

An extensive discussion of the clinical management of adipocytic tumors involving the skin is beyond the scope of this chapter, but certain general comments can be made. Small tumors confined to the skin or subcutis can generally be primarily excised without prior biopsy, as the risk of malignancy is very low, and re-excision will usually not be challenging from an oncologic perspective. Masses "larger than a golf ball" (~4 cm) (8) involving the subcutis should be studied by magnetic resonance imaging (MRI) scan, with needle biopsy of tumors showing imaging findings worrisome for atypical lipomatous tumor or other sarcomas (9,10). Entirely benign-appearing masses can be excised without needle biopsy, recognizing that there is small but nonzero risk that the specimen will ultimately prove to represent an atypical lipomatous tumor. Simple or even incomplete excision is most often adequate therapy for benign adipocytic tumors of the skin and subcutis. Atypical lipomatous tumors should be excised with histologically negative margins—it is difficult to give a precise figure in millimeters, owing to local anatomic and cosmetic considerations. In cases of atypical lipomatous tumors that undergo clinically complete excision but show microscopically positive margins, it is reasonable to follow the patient closely for local recurrence, rather than performing immediate re-excision, as the risk of local recurrence is low and the risk of malignant progression (dedifferentiation) exceedingly so. Patients having extremely rare fully malignant adipocytic tumors of the skin and subcutis (e.g., pleomorphic liposarcoma, myxoid liposarcoma, dedifferentiated liposarcoma)

Table 34-1

Diagnostically Useful Molecular Genetic and/or "Surrogate" Immunohistochemical Findings in Adipocytic Tumors of the Skin and Subcutis

Tumor Type	Positive Findings	Pertinent Negative Findings	Potential Pitfalls
Typical lipoma	*HMGA2* fusions	Absent *MDM2/CDK4* amplification	MDM2 protein expression in reactive histiocytes
Spindle cell/pleomorphic lipoma	Monoallelic *RB1* deletion and loss of RB1 protein expression	Absent *MDM2/CDK4* amplification Absent *DDIT3* rearrangement Absent STAT6 expression	RB1 protein loss in myxofibrosarcoma infiltrating the skin/subcutis
Chondroid lipoma	*C11orf95-MKL2* fusion	Absent *DDIT3* rearrangement Absent *NR4A3* rearrangement	None
Lipoblastoma	*PLAG1* rearrangements	Absent *DDIT3* rearrangement	None
Lipofibromatosis	Rearrangements involving various tyrosine kinase genes	Absent *NTRK* or *BRAF* rearrangements	Identical *FN1-EGF* fusions in calcifying aponeurotic fibroma
Hemosiderotic fibrolipomatous tumor	*TGFBR3* and/or *OGA* (*MGEA5*) rearrangements	None	None
Atypical lipomatous tumor/ well-differentiated liposarcoma and dedifferentiated liposarcoma	*MDM2/CDK4* amplification	For myxoid tumors, absent *DDIT3* rearrangement	MDM2 protein expression in reactive histiocytes
Myxoid liposarcoma	*DDIT3* rearrangement	For differentiating tumors, *MDM2/CDK4* amplification	*DDIT3* amplification in some myxoid well-differentiated and dedifferentiated liposarcomas

should be evaluated by an experienced multidisciplinary sarcoma team, for planning of surgery and any adjuvant therapy.

BENIGN ADIPOCYTIC AND ADIPOCYTE-RICH TUMORS OF THE SKIN AND SUBCUTIS

Nevus Lipomatosus Superficialis

First described by Hoffman and Zurhelle in 1921, nevus lipomatosus superficialis (NLS) is a relatively rare benign lesion, generally considered to represent a developmental anomaly or hamartomatous growth (11). NLS may be multifocal or solitary and is characterized by the presence of ectopic fat located in the reticular or papillary dermis (12).

Clinical Features. The "classical" (multicentric) form tends to present earlier than the solitary form and can even be present at birth. For unknown reasons, it has a predilection for the pelvic girdle, particularly for the skin of the buttocks and less commonly, the lower back and upper thigh, typically presenting as clusters of soft fleshy papules of variable size, arranged either irregularly or in a bandlike or zosteriform fashion (11).

The solitary form affects older patients with a median age of 43 years and has a slight female predominance. It presents as a sessile, broad-based lesion, lacking the distinctive clinical appearance of the multicentric form, and mimicking a wide variety of other benign skin lesions (Fig. 34-1A). The size of

solitary lesions can vary from a few millimeters to several centimeters (13). The thigh is most often involved, but cases have been reported in essentially any anatomic location (11,14–21).

NLS is not convincingly associated with other clinical anomalies, although a poorly understood association with the syndrome of generalized folded skin ("Michelin baby syndrome") has been reported. This syndrome, inherited in an autosomal dominant fashion, is characterized by mutations in the *MAPRE2* or *TUBB* genes (22).

Pathologic Features
Gross Findings
The lesions in the classical form are dome-shaped papules with the color of the surrounding skin or with a yellow hue. The skin surface is wrinkled and sometimes the lesions coalesce and form cerebriform plaques (12). A rare finding is the presence of multiple comedo-like plugs. The solitary form lacks distinctive features and it is usually thought to represent an accessory nipple, lipoma, neurofibroma, acrochordon, papilloma, or other benign entity (11,21). The cut surface of the lesions is soft with a homogeneous yellow appearance, reflecting the presence of fat.

Microscopic Findings
The characteristic feature is the presence of groups of adipocytes abnormally located in the dermis (Fig. 34-1B, C). The percentage of ectopic fat varies, ranging from cases showing rare clusters of adipocytes present mostly around the subpapillary vessels, to others showing larger amounts of fat arranged

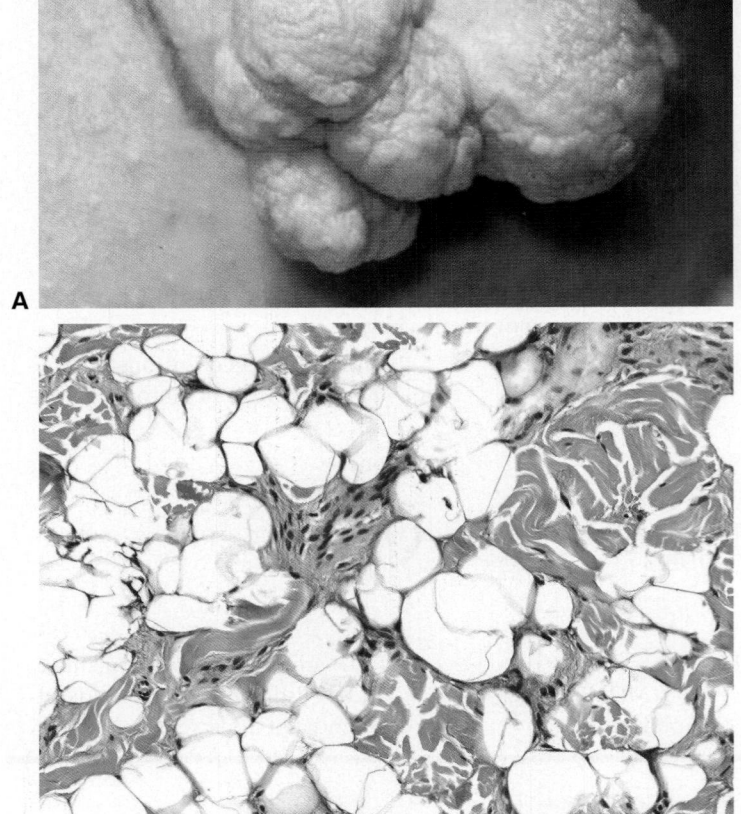

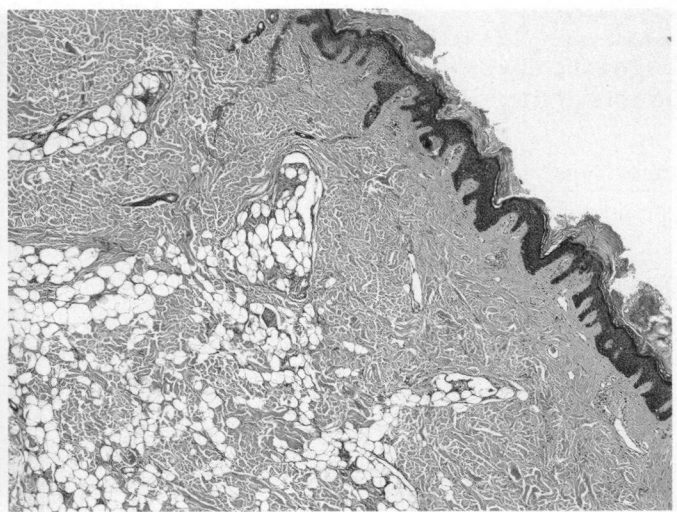

Figure 34-1 Gross photograph of nevus lipomatosis superficialis (NLS), presenting as an inner thigh mass in a 43-year-old woman (**A**). Low-power photomicrograph of NLS involving the skin of the neck in a male infant (**B**). Higher power view, showing mature fat and small aggregates of spindled cells in the same case (**C**).

in irregular lobules and effacing the distinction between the dermis and the subcutaneous tissue. An increased number of vessels in the papillary and subpapillary dermis may be seen, sometimes surrounded by immature adipocytes and spindled cells, resembling an early stage in normal adipogenesis (11,23). The epidermis can show undulation and crypt-like indentations, the latter having irregular epithelial proliferation at the base, reminiscent of abortive follicular structures. Other histologic findings in NLS include disorganized collagen bundles, mild perivascular chronic inflammation, perifollicular fibrosis, and hypertrophy of the pilosebaceous units (21,24,25).

Ancillary Studies
Immunohistochemistry
NLS is a clinical and histologic diagnosis, and immunohistochemistry is not needed.

Genetic/Molecular Studies
A single case of NLS has been shown to harbor a deletion of 2p24-pter, a nonspecific finding (26).

Differential Diagnosis
The differential diagnosis of NLS is limited and includes acrochordons with herniated fat (11), rare primary dermal lipomas, various cutaneous epithelial and mesenchymal tumors with adipocytic metaplasia, and the grossly cerebriform lipomatous proliferation seen in the exceptionally uncommon Proteus syndrome (27). Clinical correlation is generally sufficient for correct classification of the "classical," multicentric form of NLS. Distinction of the solitary form from various mimics generally necessitates identification of specific features of another tumor type (e.g., aggregates of spindled cells in dermal spindle cell lipoma, epithelial cells in adnexal tumors with fatty metaplasia). These distinctions may be rather arbitrary at times and are almost never clinically relevant.

Piezogenic Papules
Piezogenic papules are small nonneoplastic papulonodular lesions, sometimes accompanied with pain and presenting primarily, but not exclusively, in athletes and in patients with Ehlers–Danlos syndrome (28,29). They were first described by Shelley and Rawnsey in 1968, who used the term "piezogenic" to indicate that pressure to the area was the trigger for the fat herniation characteristic of these lesions (30).

Clinical Features
Because most piezogenic papules are asymptomatic, their true incidence is probably underreported but has been estimated to be as high as 76% in the United States (28,29). They typically occur in the posteromedial aspect of the heels and the wrists, and

have no gender, age, ethnic, or other associations. Clinically, the lesions appear as soft compressible skin papules, appearing when pressure is applied to the area and vanishing afterward (28).

Pathologic Features

The pathogenesis of piezogenic papules is felt to be related to the herniation of fat into the dermis. Thus, in Ehlers–Danlos syndrome, piezogenic papules are presumably related to the collagen abnormalities that characterize this syndrome (29), whereas piezogenic papules occurring in athletes, complicating diabetes, peripheral neuropathy, various forms of arthritis, and aging are likely due to ongoing mechanical damage to the interlobular fibrous septa of the fat of the heel pad (31,32). Although most piezogenic papules are not biopsied, those that are typically show changes of ongoing damage and repair to the fat lobules, with loss of fibrous septation, myofibroblastic and vascular proliferation, and nonspecific reactive epidermal changes (Fig. 34-2A, B) (28).

Ancillary Studies

Piezogenic papules is a clinical and to a lesser degree histologic diagnosis, not requiring ancillary studies.

Differential Diagnosis

The differential diagnosis of piezogenic papules includes lesions characterized by intradermal fat, most notably NLS, as well as other tumors characterized by fat, fibroblastic proliferation, and small blood vessels. As noted earlier, the clinical features of piezogenic papules and NLS are wholly dissimilar. The so-called congenital fibrolipomatous hamartoma may represent simply a clinically distinctive form of piezogenic papules (33,34). Appreciation of the normal, hyperseptated appearance of fat from the foot (and the absence of long fascicles of fibroblastic cells, hyperchromatic stromal cells, and abnormal thick-walled vessels, respectively) should allow its confident distinction from plantar fibromatoses, atypical lipomatous tumors, and vascular malformations.

Conventional Lipoma

Lipomas are benign adipocytic neoplasms composed of mature adipose tissue. They are the most common mesenchymal neoplasms encountered by dermatopathologists.

Clinical Features

Lipomas usually present as asymptomatic masses of widely variable size, which come to medical attention only when they impact cosmesis or produce mass effect and discomfort due to large size. Subcutaneous lipomas are far more common than are tumors confined to the dermis. Lipomas may also occur in essentially any other anatomic location (e.g., muscle, bone, joints, viscera). Common locations include the trunk, shoulder, and proximal extremities. Dermal and subcutaneous lipomas usually present in middle-aged adults (40 to 60 years of age), show a male predominance, and appear to be somewhat more common in obese individuals (35). They are usually solitary, but about 5% are multiple and can be associated with Bannayan-Zonana, Cowden, PTEN hamartoma, Legius, Proteus, and Froehlich syndrome (36–38). Rarely, patients can present with a diffuse overgrowth of adipose tissue known as lipomatosis (Fig. 34-3A). Clinically, lipomatosis is subclassified in symmetric, asymmetric, pelvic, and mediastino-abdominal forms.

Pathologic Features
Gross Findings

Subcutaneous lipomas are well circumscribed, surrounded by a thin capsule and generally small, with a median of 3 cm (range 1 to 25 cm) (Fig. 34-3B). The cut surface generally resembles normal, lobulated fat.

Microscopic Findings

The diagnosis of lipomas is typically quite straightforward, as they are comprised of sheets and lobules of mature adipocytes. The distinction of lipomas from simply abundant nonneoplastic fat may be challenging at times, but the presence of a thin fibrous capsule, less well-developed fibrous septa between lobules, and somewhat greater variability in adipocyte size should suggest the diagnosis of lipoma (Fig. 34-3C, D). Lipomas contain a well-developed capillary vasculature, which is typically compressed between adipocytes and inapparent. In thick sections (common in insufficiently fixed fatty tissues), this vasculature may be unusually prominent. The vascularity is well developed but inconspicuous because it is compressed in

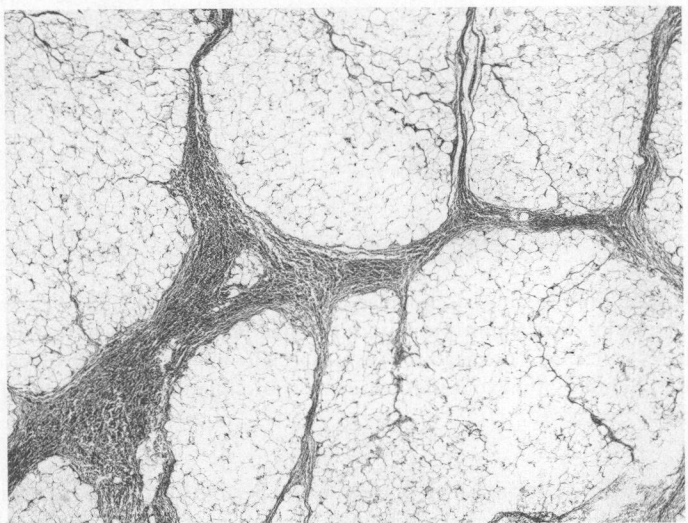
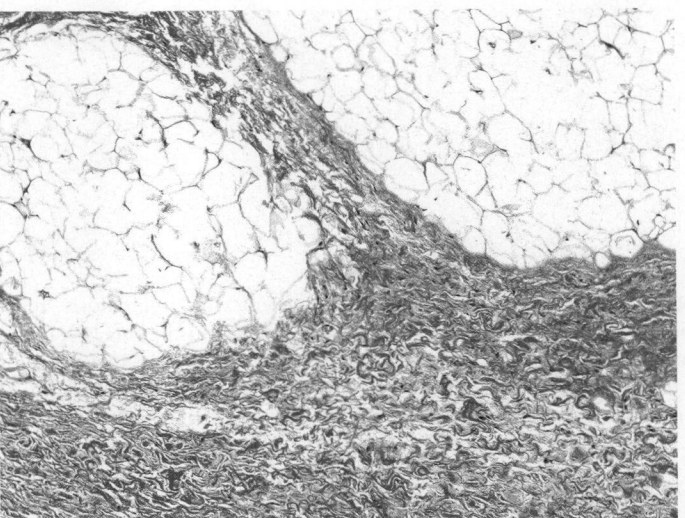

Figure 34-2 So-called piezogenic papules essentially represent herniated fat from the foot and typically show the pronounced lobulation that characterizes fat in this location (**A**). Higher power view of piezogenic papule, with mature fat and fibrous septae with a mildly increased number of reactive fibroblasts (**B**).

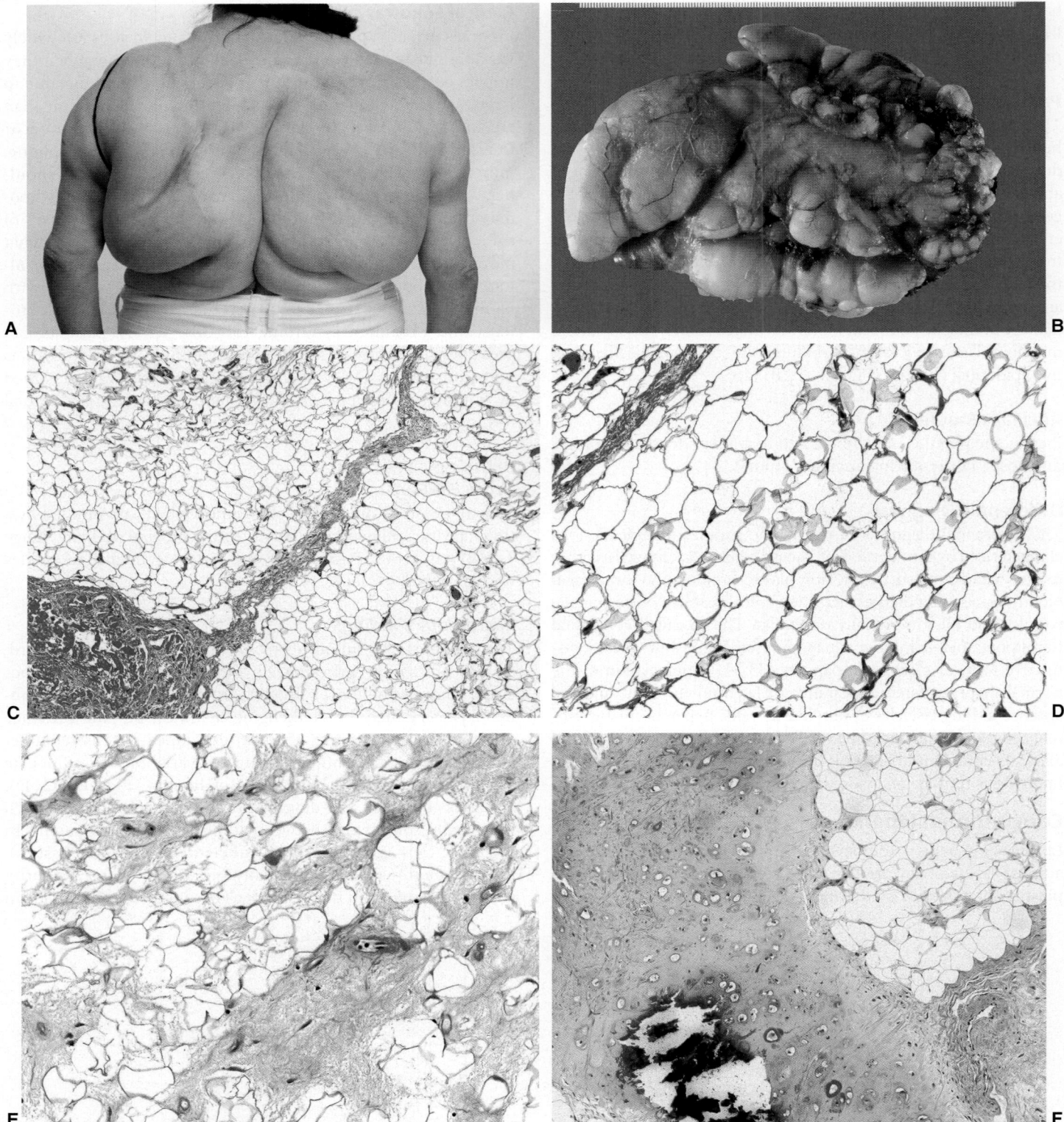

Figure 34-3 Clinical photograph of a patient with lipomatosis, displaying multiple symmetric lipomas (**A**). (Courtesy of Dr. Julia Lehman, Rochester, MN.) Gross photograph of a subcutaneous lipoma (**B**). Lipomas typically show a more pronounced lobular pattern of growth than does nonneoplastic fat (**C**). Ordinary lipomas may show some variation in adipocyte size, and this feature is not especially helpful in the distinction of lipomas from atypical lipomatous tumors (**D**). Lipoma with an increased number of myxoid fibrous septae (fibrolipoma, myxolipoma) (**E**). Chondro-osseous lipoma, containing islands of partially calcified cartilaginous matrix (**F**).

between adipocytes. Lipomas may show stromal myxoid change (myxolipoma) or increased collagenous tissue (fibrolipoma) (Fig. 34-3E). A distinctive subset of lipomas contains relatively mature-appearing cartilage and/or bone (chondro-osseous lipoma) (Fig. 34-3F); such lesions should be distinguished from

chondroid lipoma (see below) (39). Benign tumors containing an admixture of mature fat and benign smooth muscle (myolipoma, lipoleiomyoma), previously discussed in this chapter, are now considered to represent tumors of smooth muscle showing adipocytic metaplasia. Such lesions are unrelated to the distinctive tumor of "myomelanocytic" perivascular epithelioid cells known as "angiomyolipoma," and this term should not be used in the skin.

Lipomas are frequently traumatized, and thus often exhibit a variety of degenerative and reactive changes, including fat necrosis, lipid-laden macrophages, so-called Lochkern cells, and fat atrophy. Because benign adipocytic tumors of the skin and subcutis far outnumber their malignant counterparts, "pseudomalignant" change in lipoma should always be excluded before diagnosing a malignant adipocytic tumor in these locations (see below).

Ancillary Studies
Immunohistochemistry
Immunohistochemistry plays almost no role in the diagnosis of lipomas, although it may be of some value in the differential diagnosis of lipoma and atypical lipomatous tumors. Demonstration of HMGA2 expression, a feature of lipomas but not normal fat, is potentially of some value but is almost never truly necessary. HMGA2 expression is not specific for lipomas, however, and may be seen in a wide variety of other adipocytic and nonadipocytic mesenchymal tumors (40). Immunohistochemistry for MDM2 and CDK4 have been shown in numerous studies to be useful in the distinction of lipomas (negative) from atypical lipomatous tumors (positive) and may be of value. However, the sensitivity and specificity of MDM2/CDK4 immunohistochemistry are lower than those of molecular cytogenetic techniques such as fluorescence *in situ* hybridization (FISH) (41). It is particularly important to appreciate that lipid-laden macrophages in fat necrosis are routinely positive for MDM2 by immunohistochemistry, a potential diagnostic pitfall.

Genetics/Molecular Studies
The majority of lipomas show rearrangements of chromosome bands 12q13-q15, resulting in fusions of the *HMGA2* gene with a variety of gene partners, most commonly *LPP* (42). Less commonly, rearrangements of 6p21 are found, resulting in fusions involving *HMGA1* (43).

Differential Diagnosis
The differential diagnosis of dermal and subcutaneous lipomas includes a variety of benign and malignant lesions. True dermal lipomas are quite rare and can generally be distinguished from NLS on clinical grounds and from fat-rich acrochordons and fibromas by attention to their sessile growth pattern. Benign vascular malformations may contain abundant adipose tissue, simulating lipoma, but are usually ill-defined, extensive lesions with involvement of muscle as well as the subcutis. The distinction of garden-variety subcutaneous lipomas from lipoma variants depends on recognition of variant-specific morphologic features, such as small vessels with fibrin thrombi in angiolipoma, aggregates of spindled cells, wiry collagen and myxoid matrix in spindle cell lipoma, or interspersed multivacuolated brown fat cells in hibernoma. These distinctions are of course of very limited clinical significance.

Much more important is the distinction of benign lipomas with fat necrosis or other degenerative/reactive features from atypical lipomatous tumors. As noted above, lipomas far outnumber atypical lipomatous tumors in the subcutis, and thus the pretest probability that one dealing with a "problematic" (but not strictly atypical) lipoma is quite high. This contrasts

with intramuscular locations, where the relative percentage of atypical lipomatous tumors is greater, or the retroperitoneum, where lipomas are vanishingly rare. Lipomas containing foci of fat necrosis are commonly mistaken for atypical lipomatous tumor (ALT), as such lesions will often show fibrosis (mimicking the irregular fibrous septa of ALT), lipid-laden macrophages (simulating lipoblasts), variation in adipocyte size, and adipocytes with enlarged nuclei, powdery chromatin and intranuclear vacuoles (Lochkern cells), reminiscent of the atypical stromal cells seen in ALT (Fig. 34-4A, B). However, the fibrous septa in lipomas with fat necrosis lack the exceptionally finely fibrillar collagen seen in ALT, and enlarged, hyperchromatic stromal cells are absent. Immunohistochemistry for macrophage markers (e.g., CD163, CD11c, CD68) can sometimes be helpful in establishing the histiocytic lineage of suspected "lipoblasts." It must be remembered that such cells are routinely MDM2-positive by immunohistochemistry (Fig. 34-4C). In difficult cases, FISH for *MDM2/CDK4* may be occasionally needed to confidently exclude ALT. In the subcutis, FISH is indicated for very large tumors occurring in patients older than 50 years, and for recurrent tumors.

Fat atrophy can be seen in lipomas and in nonneoplastic fat and may present as a mass. The adipocytes in fat atrophy may be strikingly shrunken, resembling immature fat, lipoblasts, or even vacuolated endothelial cells (Fig. 34-4D, E). The normal capillary vasculature is relatively accentuated, and in combination with the adipocyte changes, these lesions may resemble ALT, myxoid liposarcoma, or even epithelioid hemangioendothelioma. Attention to the small size of these lesions and their retained lobular architecture are helpful in arriving at the correct diagnosis.

Spindle Cell Lipoma and Pleomorphic Lipoma

Spindle cell lipoma and pleomorphic lipoma (SCL/PL) were described separately and initially considered distinct tumors. However, over time, it has become quite clear that they represent morphologic variants of a single entity, with many cases showing features of both (44,45).

Clinical Features
Most present as subcutaneous lesions, with a striking preference for adult males (45 to 60 years of age). The most common sites include the shoulder and head and neck areas (Fig. 34-5A). SCL/PL may, however, occur in essentially any anatomic location; tumors in less common location more often occur in women. Rare primary SCL/PL of the dermis more often occur in women, with a wide anatomical distribution. SCL/PL are rare in children.

Pathologic Features
Gross Findings
They are usually well circumscribed, except for the intradermal variant, which tends to show poorly defined infiltrative margins (46). The cut surface reflects the proportion of the different components present and can vary from yellowish to white gray and show myxoid foci. They are generally small (3 to 5 cm) but may at times present as rather large masses (>10 cm).

Microscopic Findings
Fundamentally, SCL is composed of well-circumscribed proliferation of mature fat, myxoid matrix, bundles of wiry or "ropy" collagen, blood vessels of varying caliber, and small

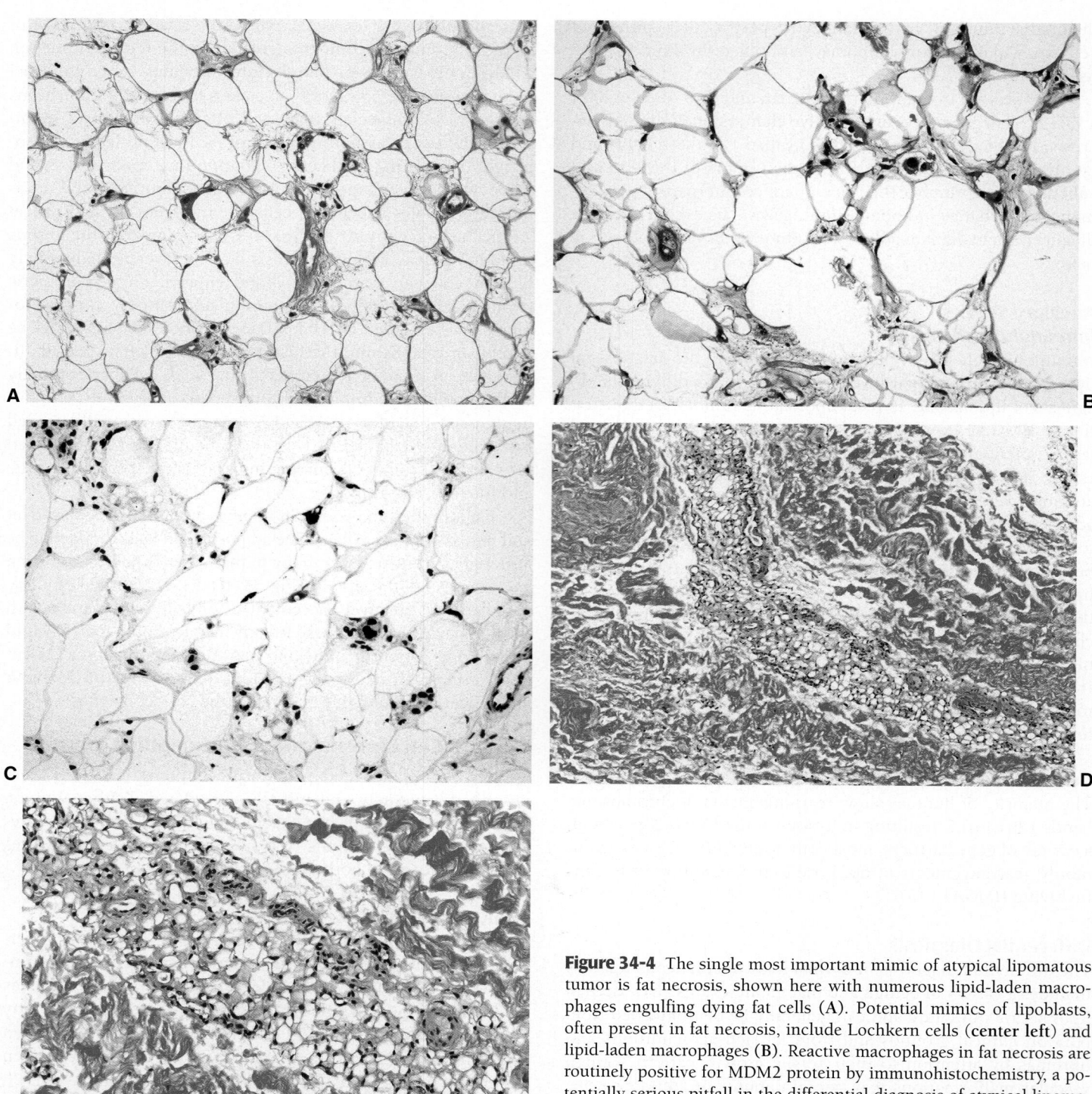

Figure 34-4 The single most important mimic of atypical lipomatous tumor is fat necrosis, shown here with numerous lipid-laden macrophages engulfing dying fat cells (**A**). Potential mimics of lipoblasts, often present in fat necrosis, include Lochkern cells (**center left**) and lipid-laden macrophages (**B**). Reactive macrophages in fat necrosis are routinely positive for MDM2 protein by immunohistochemistry, a potentially serious pitfall in the differential diagnosis of atypical lipomatous tumors (**C**). Atrophic subcutaneous fat, here arising in the site of a prior buttock injection, can present as a mass and mimic a fatty tumor (**D**). Higher power view of fat atrophy, showing atrophic adipocytes, prominent vascularity, and hyalinized stroma (**E**).

aggregates of spindled cells (Fig. 34-5B–F). However, these are exceptionally protean tumors and may consist of any imaginable combination of these elements. Tumors may consist almost entirely of mature fat or be largely devoid of fat ("fat-free" and "low-fat" SCL) (47,48). The spindled cells of SCL are distinctive, having small, ovoid nuclei with one pointed end, and are frequently arranged in small, aligned packets, a growth pattern that has been likened to a "school of fish." Highly cellular SCL are easily confused with other spindle cell tumors

of the subcutis. Myxoid change is almost always present and may at times be so prominent as to mimic other myxoid soft tissue tumors. Highly myxoid SCL may display cracking artifact and pseudovascular change (so-called pseudoangiomatous SCL) (49). A variety of different vascular patterns are seen, including arborizing small capillaries (simulating myxoid liposarcoma) or branching, hyalinized, thick-walled vessels (mimicking solitary fibrous tumor). In addition to showing morphologic features of SCL, pleomorphic lipomas are defined

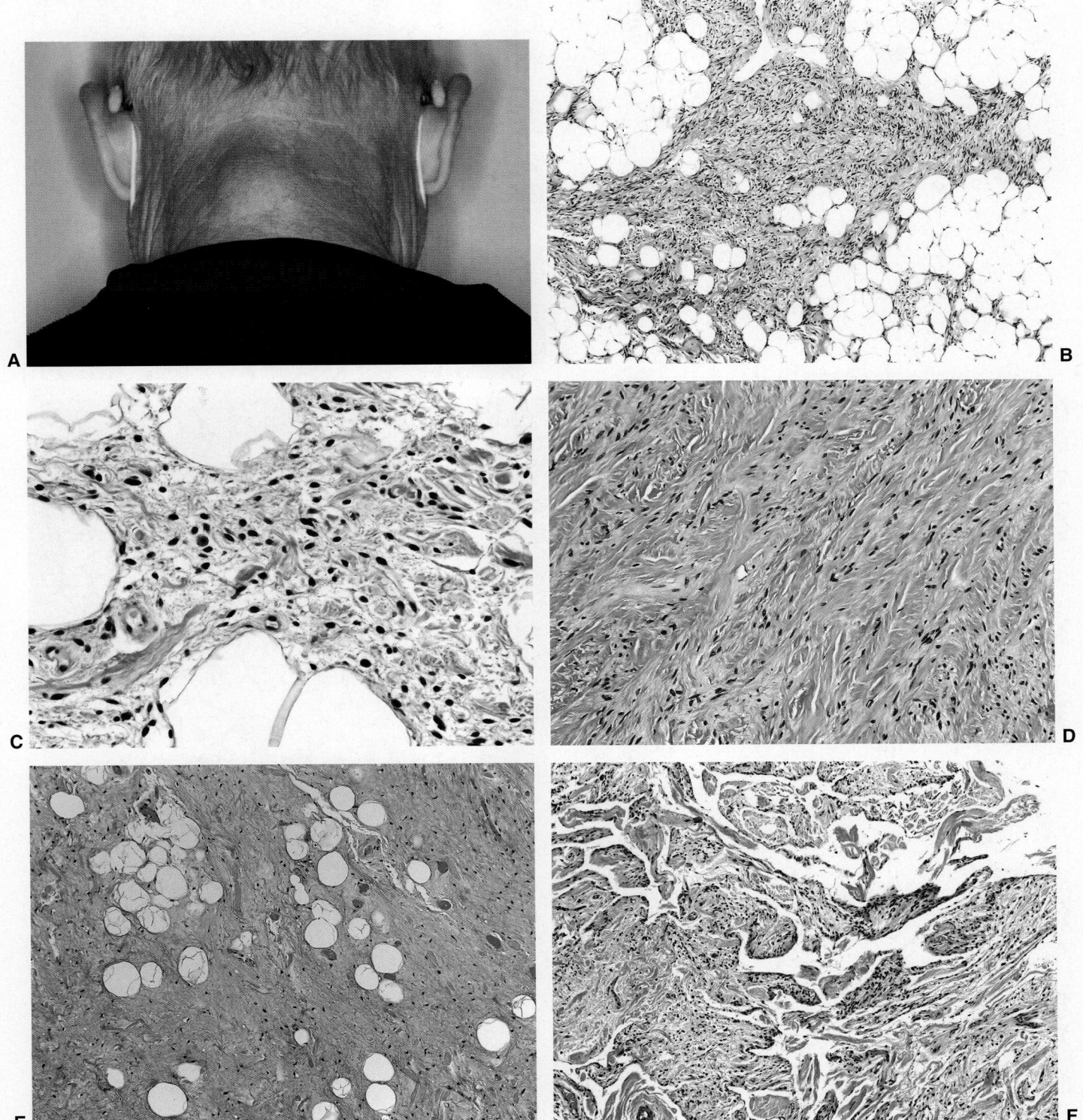

Figure 34-5 Spindle cell lipoma of the neck in an older male, the most common clinical presentation (**A**). (Courtesy of Dr. Julia Lehman, Rochester, MN.) Spindle cell lipomas are composed of small "packets" of aligned, bland spindled cells, wiry collagen, myxoid matrix, and mature fat, in almost any imaginable combination (**B**). Higher power view of typical spindle cell lipoma (**C**). Some spindle cell lipomas contain little or no fat (**D**). Extensively myxoid spindle cell lipoma (**E**). "Pseudoangiomatous" spindle cell lipoma (**F**). Pleomorphic lipomas contain pleomorphic, floret-like giant cells, in addition to areas identical to spindle cell lipoma

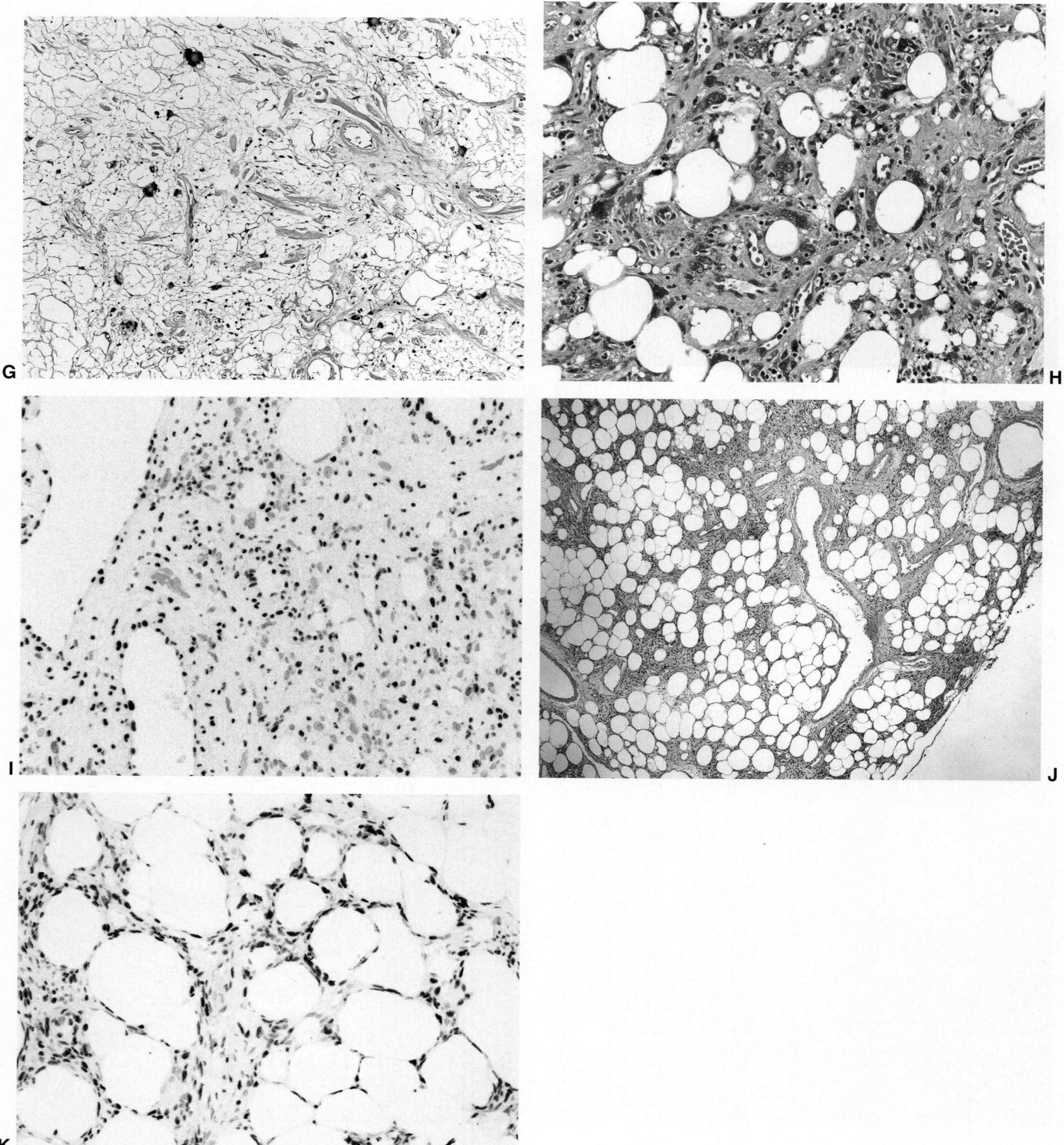

Figure 34-5 (*continued*) (**G**). Some pleomorphic lipomas are highly cellular and contain numerous lipoblast-like cells (atypical pleomorphic lipomatous tumor) (**H**). In such cases, demonstration of lost expression of RB1 protein (shown) and absent *MDM2* amplification (not shown) are reassuring findings (**I**). The closest morphologic mimic of spindle cell lipoma is lipomatous solitary fibrous tumor (**J**). Unlike spindle cell lipomas, solitary fibrous tumors show retained RB1 expression (not shown) and express STAT6 (**K**).

by the presence of a highly variable number of large, multinucleated, hyperchromatic, floret-like neoplastic giant cells. Lipoblast-like cells and occasional mitotic figures may be seen in SCL/PL (Fig. 34-5G).

There also exist rare tumors of the skin and subcutis that show many features of SCL/PL, but display infiltrative growth, greater nuclear atypia, elevated mitotic activity, and more easily identified lipoblasts (Fig. 34-5H, I). Such lesions, previously classified as "spindle cell liposarcoma," are now labeled "atypical spindle cell and pleomorphic lipomatous tumors," reflecting their likely relationship to classical SCL/PL (50,51).

Ancillary Studies
Immunohistochemistry
The spindle cells in SCL/PL express CD34 and androgen receptors (52). S100 protein is negative. Occasional cases show limited desmin expression, and the distinction of these cases from fat-rich mammary-type myofibroblastomas may at times be rather arbitrary. Loss of RB1 protein expression is seen in both SCL and PL, a helpful but nonspecific finding (53).

Genetic/Molecular Studies
SCL/PL is characterized by loss of material from chromosomes 13q and 16q, with monoallelic deletion of *Rb1* on 13q14 (54,55). Identical *Rb1* deletions are also seen in cellular angiofibroma and myofibroblastoma of soft tissue, suggesting common pathogenesis (56,57).

Differential Diagnosis
Although most SCL/PL are readily recognized, their exceptionally broad morphologic spectrum continues to pose challenges for pathologists. Fat-rich SCL can be confused with ordinary lipomas, and although the distinction is not of great clinical significance, attention to the typical clinical setting of SCL and careful search for small aggregates of characteristic spindled cells should allow this distinction. SCL with a minimal adipocytic component may mimic various myxoid soft tissue tumors when extensively myxoid, or other spindle cell lesions when more cellular and collagenized. Myxoid, fat-poor SCL lack the stromal neutrophils and stellate tumor cells of cutaneous angiomyxoma, and have retained expression of PRKAR1A. Cellular, collagenous SCL may closely simulate solitary fibrous tumor, but lack STAT6 expression (Fig. 34-5J and K). SCL of the hands and feet are much better circumscribed than are acral fibromyxomas (cellular digital fibroma), another potential mimic. The distinction of SCL from morphologically similar, RB1-deficient tumors such as mammary-type myofibroblastoma and cellular angiofibroma of the genital region may be extremely difficult, if not wholly subjective. Expression of desmin and estrogen receptors is generally more characteristic of the latter two entities.

Extensively myxoid SCL should be rigorously distinguished from myxoid liposarcoma and myxofibrosarcoma (especially myxofibrosarcoma extending to involve the skin). Unlike the great majority of SCL, myxoid liposarcomas present as deeply situated large masses, most often within the muscles of the thigh. In comparison to myxoid SCL, myxoid liposarcomas have a more prominent, delicately arborizing capillary vasculature, round rather than spindled cells, accentuated peripheral cellularity, and numerous small lipoblasts, often present immediately adjacent to capillaries. In difficult cases, demonstration of *DDIT3* rearrangement is diagnostic of myxoid liposarcoma. Subcutaneous and dermal extension from more deeply situated myxofibrosarcoma may closely mimic SCL/PL and represents a significant pitfall, especially as these lesions may contain relatively bland, CD34-positive spindled cells, ropy collagen, and floret-like giant cells. Most myxofibrosarcomas will contain at least small areas of solid, nonmyxoid growth containing an increased number of mitotically active, pleomorphic tumor cells, a helpful clue. Clinical and radiographic correlation with regard to the size, extent, and delineation of the tumor are often the best ways to avoid misdiagnosis of myxofibrosarcomas involving the skin as SCL/PL. Importantly, nonspecific chromosomal losses involving chromosome 13 may result in RB1 loss in myxofibrosarcoma, and this marker is not helpful here. Finally, SCL/PL with predominantly pleomorphic features may be confused with ALTs and pleomorphic liposarcomas. Careful attention to the presence of areas of classical SCL usually resolves this dilemma without great difficulty. In problematic cases, the absence of MDM2 amplification by FISH points toward SCL/PL. Pleomorphic liposarcomas are usually deeply situated and large, with numerous pleomorphic lipoblasts and areas resembling undifferentiated pleomorphic sarcoma.

Angiolipoma
Angiolipomas are benign neoplasms composed of an admixture of mature fat and branching small vessels containing characteristic fibrin thrombi. Although historically considered an adipocytic tumor, angiolipomas may consist almost entirely of vessels (cellular angiolipoma) and lack the cytogenetic abnormalities seen in essentially all other adipocytic tumors, suggesting they may represent instead vascular tumors with an adipocytic component.

Clinical Features
Angiolipomas are subcutaneous lesions that typically occur in young adults, being rare in children and in adults older than 50 years. The forearm is the single most common site, followed by the trunk and the upper arm (58). Roughly two-thirds of patients with angiolipoma have multiple lesions, which are characteristically tender or painful to manipulation. They are usually sporadic, but a small percentage are familial with an autosomal dominant pattern of inheritance (59). Mammary angiolipomas are frequently identified in patients undergoing various imaging studies for the evaluation of breast disease, where they present as small, well-circumscribed masses (60). Correlation with imaging findings is important to avoid the overdiagnosis of mammary angiolipomas as more aggressive vascular tumors (see below).

Pathologic Features
Gross Findings
Angiolipomas are small ovoid lesions, usually no more than 2 cm in size, relatively well circumscribed, and surrounded by a thin pseudocapsule. The cut surface is fatty and yellow, like lipomas, but they can be firmer and show a variable reddish hue due to the presence of the vascular component.

Microscopic Findings
Angiolipomas are composed of a somewhat haphazard admixture of mature adipose tissue and small blood vessels, often having an elongated, spindled, or "stretched" appearance (Fig. 34-6A–C).

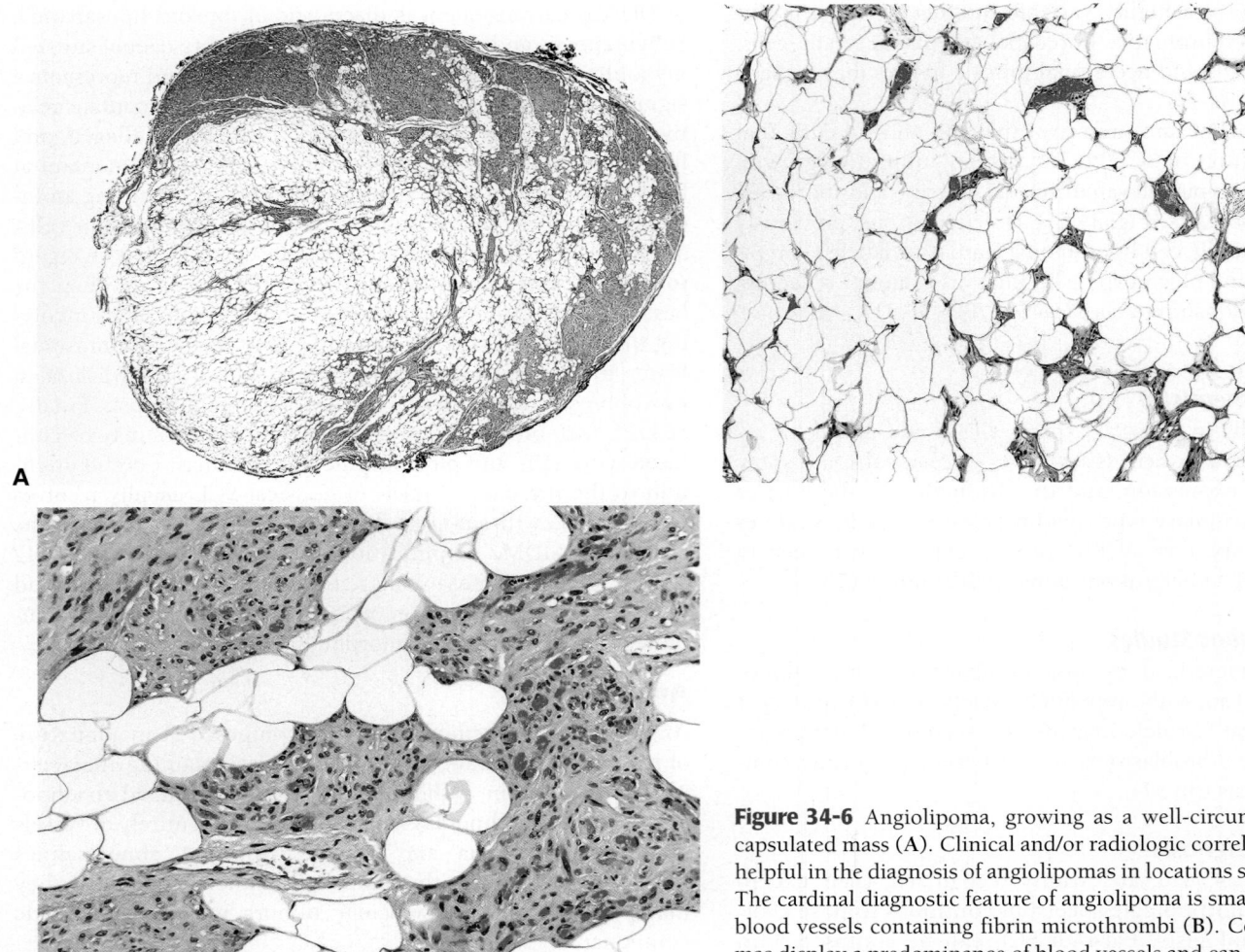

Figure 34-6 Angiolipoma, growing as a well-circumscribed, nonencapsulated mass (**A**). Clinical and/or radiologic correlation can be very helpful in the diagnosis of angiolipomas in locations such as the breast. The cardinal diagnostic feature of angiolipoma is small, capillary-sized blood vessels containing fibrin microthrombi (**B**). Cellular angiolipomas display a predominance of blood vessels and can be confused with a vascular neoplasm infiltrating fat. Note the fibrin microthrombi (**C**).

The relative proportion of fat and vessels is highly variable, with fat-predominant lesions mimicking conventional lipomas and so-called cellular angiolipomas consisting almost entirely of the vascular component and mimicking various benign and malignant vascular tumors (61). The greatest numbers of blood vessels are typically found in a subcapsular location. Perhaps the most characteristic feature of angiolipomas is the presence of small fibrin thrombi, a particularly useful morphologic clue in lesions occurring in locations such as the breast and/or sampled with core needle biopsy.

Ancillary Studies

Immunohistochemistry

Immunohistochemistry plays little or no role in the diagnosis of angiolipoma. As expected, the adipocytes of these tumors express S-100 protein, whereas the endothelial components are positive with various markers of vascular differentiation (e.g., CD31, ERG, and FLI1). HHV8 LANA protein is absent, a pertinent negative finding when the differential diagnosis for cellular angiolipoma includes Kaposi sarcoma.

Genetic Features

Unlike other adipocytic tumors, angiolipomas lack consistent karyotypic alterations (62), although recent studies have highlighted loss or structural rearrangement of chromosome 13 in

some cases (63). At the molecular level, about 80% of cases show low-frequency mutations of the *PRKD2* gene (64).

Differential Diagnosis

The differential diagnosis of angiolipomas varies depending on their relative proportion of fat or vascular components. Fat-predominant angiolipomas may be distinguished from ordinary lipomas by attention to the clinical history of multiple, painful lesions, as well as careful inspection for small, fibrin-filled vessels. Benign vascular malformations may contain a large amount of mature fat in addition to congeries of abnormally configured vessels; in the past, these tumors were sometimes erroneously labeled "infiltrating angiolipoma." Such lesions are much larger than angiolipomas, often involve skeletal muscle, and contain thick-walled vessels lacking fibrin thrombi.

Cellular angiolipomas may be confused with a variety of hemangiomas. Although capillary hemangiomas may contain fat, they grow in a lobular pattern and lack fibrin thrombi. Spindle cell hemangiomas consist of a distinctive admixture of cavernous vascular channels, phleboliths, spindled actin-positive pericytic cells, and vacuolated endothelial cells (65). Although anastomosing hemangiomas may contain both fat and fibrin microthrombi, they involve deep soft tissue and viscera (66).

Among malignant vascular tumors, cellular angiolipomas are most often confused with angiosarcoma, especially when they involve the breast and are sampled with core needle biopsy. This is especially true in previously irradiated patients, where the (dermato)pathologist is anxious about the possibility of postirradiation angiosarcoma. Clinical correlation can be critical in this setting, as angiolipomas of the breast present as small, circumscribed *subcutaneous* masses, whereas postirradiation angiosarcomas involve the mammary skin (60). Mammary parenchymal angiosarcomas typically present as large, poorly circumscribed lesions, with a high clinical index of suspicion for malignancy. In needle biopsies, where the haphazard vascular arrangement of angiolipoma may mimic infiltration of fat by a malignant vascular tumor, close attention to the well-formed nature of the vessels, the absence of endothelial atypia or multilayering, and the presence of fibrin thrombi should allow for this distinction in all instances. Unlike Kaposi sarcoma, predominantly spindled angiolipomas grow in a circumscribed manner within the subcutis, lack prominent chronic inflammation, and are negative for HHV8 LANA protein.

Chondroid Lipoma

Chondroid lipomas are benign lipomatous tumors composed of a distinctive combination of white fat, brown fat, lipoblast-like cells, and vaguely chondroid, myxohyaline matrix (67). Their resemblance to a cartilaginous tumor is underscored by the name under which this entity was first reported: "extraskeletal chondroma with lipoblast-like cells" (68). Despite their unusual appearance, they lack true cartilaginous differentiation (69).

Clinical Features

Chondroid lipomas generally present as slowly growing, asymptomatic masses. Most are deeply situated, involving the superficial muscular fascia or skeletal muscle, but they can also be subcutaneous. The majority are relatively small (median 4 cm), but occasional tumors present as rather large (>10 cm) masses. The most common locations include the proximal extremity and limb girdles, followed by the distal extremities, trunk, and head and neck sites such as the oral cavity (67,70).

Pathologic Features
Gross Findings
The tumors are usually well circumscribed, with a variably lobulated, gelatinous cut surface.

Microscopic Findings
At low-power magnification, chondroid lipomas are well circumscribed, frequently surrounded by a fibrous capsule, and vaguely lobulated (Fig. 34-7A). They are composed of an unusual combination of mature white adipose tissue, multivacuolated cells resembling brown fat, lipoblast-like cells with scalloped nuclei, and eosinophilic, vaguely chondroblast-like cells (67). The cells are surrounded by a hyalinized, myxoid matrix, which may show considerable basophilia, imparting a chondroid appearance (Fig. 34-7B, C). True cartilage with lacunae is not, however, present. The tumors contain a well-developed, thick-walled

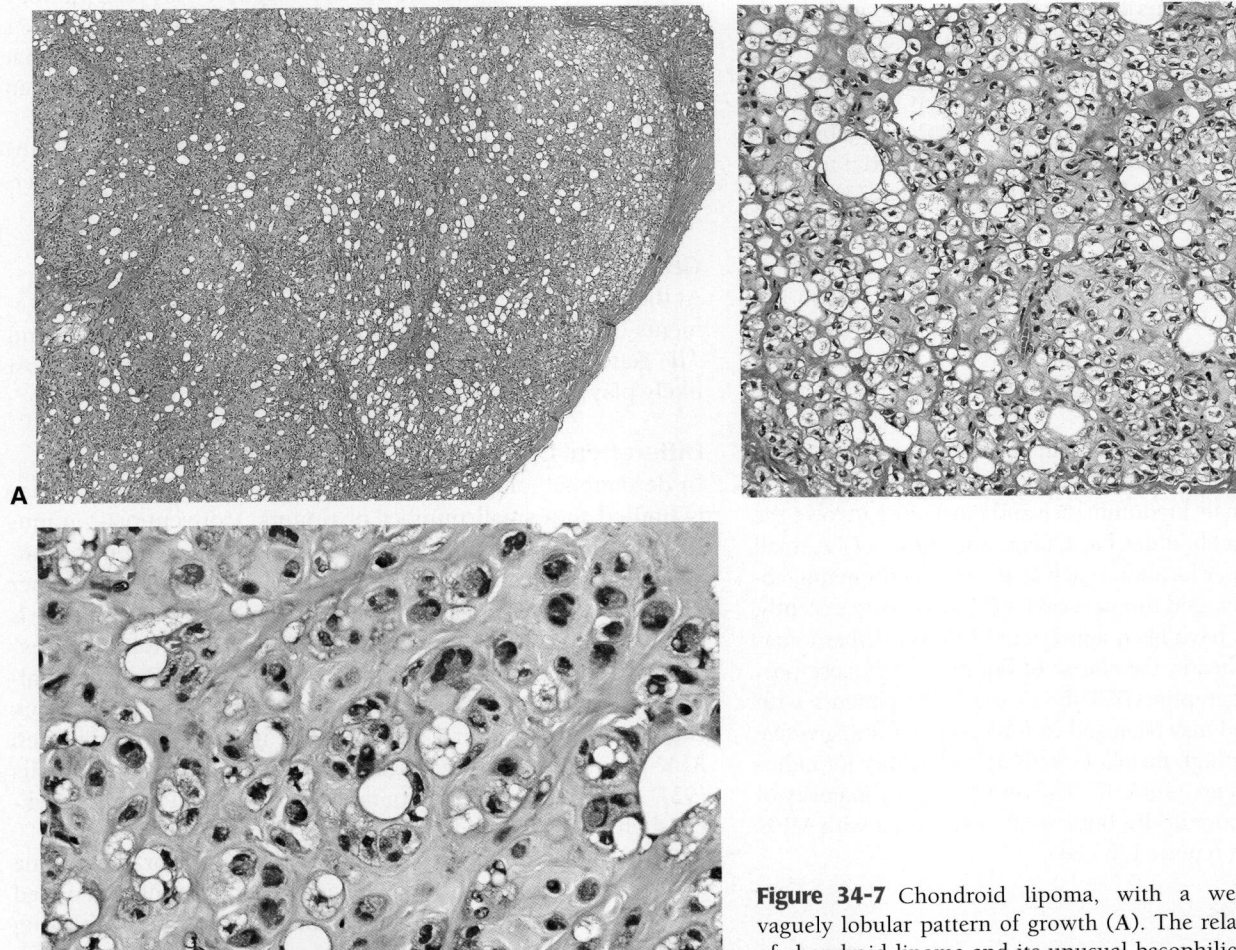

Figure 34-7 Chondroid lipoma, with a well-circumscribed and vaguely lobular pattern of growth (**A**). The relatively high cellularity of chondroid lipoma and its unusual basophilic matrix can suggest a malignant cartilaginous tumor or even myxoid liposarcoma (**B**). Lipoblast-like cells are frequently found in chondroid lipomas (**C**).

vasculature, but lack the arborizing capillary network seen in a potential mimic, myxoid liposarcoma.

Ancillary Studies
Immunohistochemistry
The cells show variable reactivity to S-100 protein and CD68 antibodies and are negative for epithelial membrane antigen.

Genetic Features
Although genetic testing is not necessary for diagnosis, chondroid lipomas harbor a specific t(11;16)(q13;p13) translocation that results in the *C11orf95-MKL2* fusion oncogene (71).

Differential Diagnosis
Because of their unusual appearance, the differential diagnosis of chondroid lipoma includes both adipocytic and cartilaginous tumors. Extraskeletal myxoid chondrosarcomas are typically larger and more deeply situated, frequently contain old and recent hemorrhage, and are notably hypovascular lesions composed of small, eosinophilic cells with clefted nuclei, arranged in cords, chains, and lace-like arrays within a deeply basophilic matrix. Extraskeletal myxoid chondrosarcoma typically lacks S100 protein expression and invariably shows rearrangements of the *NR4A3* gene, detectable by various molecular methods (72,73). Soft tissue chondromas produce true hyaline cartilage, frequently calcify, and often evoke an osteoclast-rich tissue reaction. Although the large numbers of lipoblast-like cells and the myxoid matrix of chondroid lipoma may suggest myxoid liposarcoma, its circumscribed growth pattern and the absence of an elaborately arborizing capillary network should point in the correct direction. In problematic cases, detection of *DDIT3* rearrangements is diagnostic of myxoid liposarcoma (74). Rarely, heavily vacuolated perineurial tumors ("pseudolipoblastic" perineurioma) can mimic chondroid lipoma; expression of perineurial markers (e.g., EMA, claudin-1, GLUT1) may be helpful here (75).

Hibernoma
Hibernomas are rare benign tumors composed of brown fat. The name is derived from the resemblance of these tumors to the brown fat in hibernating animals (76).

Clinical Features
The tumors present more frequently in young adults, with a mean age of 38 years (range 2 to 75 years); roughly 5% occur in children. They show a slight male predominance and most often involve the thigh, followed by the shoulder, back, neck, and chest (77). A small number involve deeper locations such as the retroperitoneum, abdominal cavity, pleura, and thoracic cavity (77–79). More recently, osseous hibernomas have been appreciated (80,81). Hibernomas are frequently identified in the course of fluorodeoxyglucose-positron emission tomography (FGD-PET) scans for patients with metastatic disease and may be mistaken for a potentially aggressive tumor owing to their high metabolic activity and avidity for radionuclide tracer (82) (Fig. 34-8A, B). The overwhelming majority of hibernomas occur sporadically, but a weak association with MEN 1 syndrome has been reported (83,84).

Pathologic Features
Gross Findings
Hibernomas are circumscribed lesions of widely variable size (range 1 to 24 cm). Their cut surface is lobulated and yellow to brown in color, reflecting the proportions of the brown and mature fat present. Occasionally, myxoid change and hemorrhage can be seen.

Microscopic Findings
These distinctive tumors are composed of sheets and lobules of large, polygonal, multivacuolated adipocytes with small, cytologically bland nuclei. The appearance and tinctorial quality of the cytoplasm are variable, with some cells showing abundant granular eosinophilic cytoplasm, vaguely reminiscent of oncocytes or granular cells, whereas others have multivacuolated cytoplasm reminiscent of lipoblasts or univacuolated cytoplasm as in mature adipocytes (Fig. 34-8C, D). The stroma can show varying degrees of myxoid change (85). Based on the relative proportion of eosinophilic and clear cells and the type of stromal change, hibernomas have been subclassified as typical, lipoma-like, myxoid, and spindle cell variants (77). These "variants" have no clinical significance. Interestingly, hibernomas with spindle cell features occur mostly in the head and neck regions of adult males and show CD34 reactivity, suggesting that they represent spindle cell lipomas with brown fat. Some hibernomas may show an increased number of fibrous septae containing somewhat prominent stromal cells, raising concern for an ALT (Fig. 34-8E) (86).

Ancillary Studies
Immunohistochemistry
Almost all hibernomas are readily diagnosed by morphology alone. Immunohistochemistry for uncoupling protein-1 (UCP1 or thermogenin), a mitochondrial protein transporter that uncouples electron transport from ATP production, has been shown to be positive in normal and neoplastic brown fat (87). Much more widely available antibodies to CD10 (neprilysin) have also been shown to be helpful in the distinction of hibernomas from selected morphologic mimics (7).

Genetic Features
At the cytogenetic level, hibernomas show structural rearrangements of 11q13-21, resulting in co-deletions of the *MEN1* and *AIP* genes. Deletions of these tumor suppressor genes most likely play a role in the pathogenesis of hibernomas (88–90).

Differential Diagnosis
In dermatopathology, the differential diagnosis of hibernomas is limited to a small number of tumors. Conventional granular cell tumor may show some similarities to hibernomas composed predominantly of eosinophilic cells; however, the former often shows overlying pseudoepitheliomatous hyperplasia, is composed of cells with distinctive "chunky" granules, and expresses S100 protein, SOX10, and TFE3 (91,92). So-called polypoid non-neural granular cell tumors occur in children, lack expression of peripheral nerve sheath markers, and are often ALK-positive, reflecting underlying *ALK* gene rearrangements (93). Adult-type rhabdomyomas express skeletal muscle markers such as desmin and myogenin.

The most important differential diagnosis for hibernoma is atypical lipomatous tumor, especially when multivacuolated brown fat cells are mistaken for lipoblasts, or in cases displaying stromal sclerosis and myxoid change. Unlike lipoblasts, which contain an enlarged, hyperchromatic nucleus that is displaced to the side of the cell by one or more optically clear vacuoles,

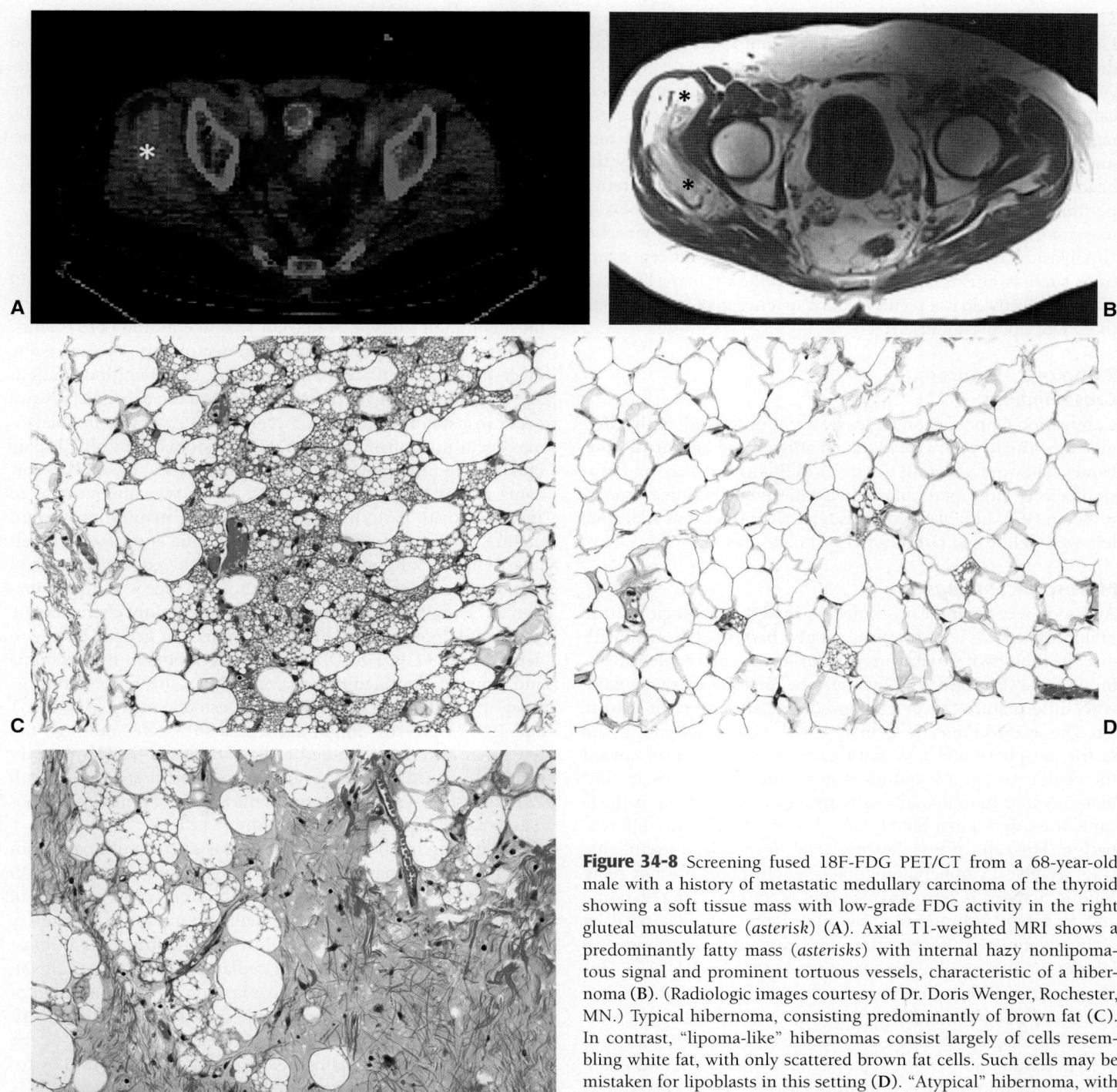

Figure 34-8 Screening fused 18F-FDG PET/CT from a 68-year-old male with a history of metastatic medullary carcinoma of the thyroid showing a soft tissue mass with low-grade FDG activity in the right gluteal musculature (*asterisk*) (**A**). Axial T1-weighted MRI shows a predominantly fatty mass (*asterisks*) with internal hazy nonlipomatous signal and prominent tortuous vessels, characteristic of a hibernoma (**B**). (Radiologic images courtesy of Dr. Doris Wenger, Rochester, MN.) Typical hibernoma, consisting predominantly of brown fat (**C**). In contrast, "lipoma-like" hibernomas consist largely of cells resembling white fat, with only scattered brown fat cells. Such cells may be mistaken for lipoblasts in this setting (**D**). "Atypical" hibernoma, with an increased number of slightly enlarged stromal cells, may also mimic atypical lipomatous tumor (**E**).

brown fat cells have centrally placed, normochromatic nuclei, and a very large number of minute vacuoles. Although stromal cell atypia is obviously subjective, truly enlarged, hyperchromatic stromal cells with smudgy nuclei are not seen in hibernoma. In cases where the dermatopathologist needs only a little reassurance, CD10 immunohistochemistry may be helpful in confirming the diagnosis of hibernoma (7). In more challenging cases, FISH for MDM2 amplification may be required to exclude conventional atypical lipomatous tumors or very rare atypical lipomatous tumors containing brown fat (86).

Lipoblastoma and Lipoblastomatosis

Lipoblastomas are benign tumors composed of immature adipose tissue. Originally described under a variety of other names, such as embryonal lipoma (94), the term "lipoblastoma" was first applied by Vellios and colleagues in their 1958 description of a distinctive tumor of infancy which appeared to recapitulate embryonal fat development (95). The term "lipoblastomatosis" has been used for morphologically similar lesions showing an infiltrative pattern of growth, also known as "infiltrating" or "diffuse" lipoblastoma (96,97).

Clinical Features

Lipoblastoma predominantly affects infants and young children, with the majority of cases appearing before the age of 3 (96–98). However, they may occur in older children, adolescents, and young adults (99,100). Lipoblastomas have a slight male predominance (reported male to female ratio of 1.7), and most often involve the trunk and extremities, followed by the head and neck (101). Unusual tumors have involved the retroperitoneum, pelvis, abdomen, and lung. Ordinary lipoblastomas are usually circumscribed masses of the subcutis, whereas "lipoblastomatosis" is infiltrative and may involve deep structures such as muscle and bone (97). Unlike ordinary lipomas, which typically do not recur, local recurrence may be seen in up to 45% of lipoblastomas (101).

Pathologic Features
Gross Findings

Conventional lipoblastomas are well circumscribed, with a lobulated, white to yellow, myxoid cut surface and delicate fibrous bands. They are generally small (3 to 5 cm) but may on occasion be very large, particularly in locations such as the retroperitoneum (97). Lipoblastomatosis typically presents as multiple, less well-delineated but otherwise similar masses.

Microscopic Findings

At low-power magnification, the cardinal morphologic feature of lipoblastoma is a pronounced lobular pattern of growth, with discrete lobules of variably myxoid fat surrounded by delicate fibrous septa (Fig. 34-9A). Cases may be predominantly myxoid, with little mature fat, or composed almost entirely of mature fat. The lesions typically "zonate," with mature adipose tissue at the periphery and less mature, more myxoid areas toward the center. In the myxoid areas, the tumors may closely simulate myxoid liposarcoma, with arcades of arborizing, delicate capillaries, and small bland cells showing lipoblastic differentiation. The cells of lipoblastoma tend to spindle, a useful clue (Fig. 34-9B). Lymphangioma-like myxoid pools are not seen. Mitotic activity is low, and necrosis is absent. Long-standing and recurrent lesions can show maturation, characterized by almost complete differentiation toward mature fat arranged in lobules divided by fibrous septa (Fig. 34-9C, D) (94,101). This phenomenon is thought to account for misdiagnosis of lipoblastomas as lipomas in older patients. In older adults, lipoblastomas often display "fibroblastic" features, with a predominance of hypocellular fibroblastic septa, within which are found small, partially myxoid nodules of mature fat (Fig. 34-9E) (100). Extremely rare lipoblastomas display atypical features such as nuclear atypia and mitotic activity, requiring molecular genetic testing for definitive diagnosis (102).

Ancillary Studies
Immunohistochemistry

Immunohistochemistry may be of some value in the diagnosis of challenging lipoblastomas or those occurring in older patients. Although the lipoblastic cells have a nonspecific phenotype, with coexpression of S100 protein and CD34 (103), desmin expression is often seen in the spindled cells (104), a peculiar but helpful finding (Fig. 34-9F). Nuclear PLAG1 expression has been reported in up to 80% of lipoblastomas, although this test is not widely available (105).

Genetic Features

Lipoblastomas usually contain extra copies of chromosome 8 and/or structural alterations of 8q11-q13, resulting in rearrangements of the *PLAG1* gene with a variety of partners, including *HAS2*, *COL1A2*, *COL3A1*, *RAB2A*, *BOC*, and *EEF1A1* (106–111). The recently described fibroblastic variant shows *PLAG1* rearrangements with novel partners, including *PCMTD1*, *YWHAZ*, *CTDSP2*, and *PPP2R2A* (100). Unusual cases harbor *HMGA2* gene rearrangements without *PLAG1* alterations (112).

Differential Diagnosis

Extensively myxoid lipoblastomas may closely mimic myxoid liposarcoma, and conversely, myxoid liposarcoma is by far the most common subtype of liposarcoma in children (113). Thus, the distinction of lipoblastoma from myxoid liposarcoma is the most important differential diagnostic consideration. Patient age is helpful, as pediatric myxoid liposarcomas almost always occur in patients older than 5 years of age, whereas lipoblastomas occur in younger children. Lipoblastomas typically display much more pronounced lobulation than does myxoid liposarcoma and is better circumscribed. These two tumors tend to show opposite patterns of zonation, with maturation toward mature fat at the periphery of lipoblastoma and increased cellularity mimicking round cell change at the edge of lobules of myxoid liposarcoma. Extensive myxoid change with the formation of "lymphangioma-like pools" is much more characteristic of myxoid liposarcoma. Ultimately, molecular genetic testing to demonstrate *PLAG1* or *DDIT3* rearrangements in lipoblastoma and myxoid liposarcoma, respectively, is the most definitive assay in challenging cases. Immunohistochemistry for PLAG1 and DDIT3 proteins might serve as a surrogate, although too few cases have been studied to be certain (114). The very recently described "pediatric fibromyxoid soft tissue tumor with *PLAG1* fusion" very likely represents a form of fibroblastic lipoblastoma occurring in young children (115).

Maturing lipoblastomas can be mistaken as ordinary lipomas or "fibrolipomas," a clinically insignificant error. Attention to the pronounced lobularity of lipoblastoma, the presence of small myxoid foci, and occasionally immunohistochemistry for desmin and CD34 should allow these distinctions in most cases. Lipofibromatosis, another pediatric tumor containing fat, grows in a nonlobular, infiltrative fashion and is composed of small, bland fibroblastic cells with multifocal lipoblastic differentiation and a variable amount of mature fat (116). At the genetic level, lipofibromatosis is frequently characterized by fusions involving various tyrosine kinases (117).

Finally, the lipoblastoma-like tumor of the vulva is a rare benign mesenchymal neoplasm of the vulvovaginal region in middle-aged women that shows combined morphologic features of lipoblastoma, myxoid liposarcoma, and spindle cell lipoma (118). At the molecular level, these lesions lack PLAG1, DDIT3, or RB1 alterations, distinguishing them from these other entities (118–120). Extremely rare cases in men have also been reported (121).

Lipofibromatosis

Lipofibromatosis is an unusual neoplasm of infancy and early childhood showing a marked predilection for the hands and feet. Although this entity was formally described in 2000 (116), cases were likely included in older series of infantile and juvenile fibromatosis (122).

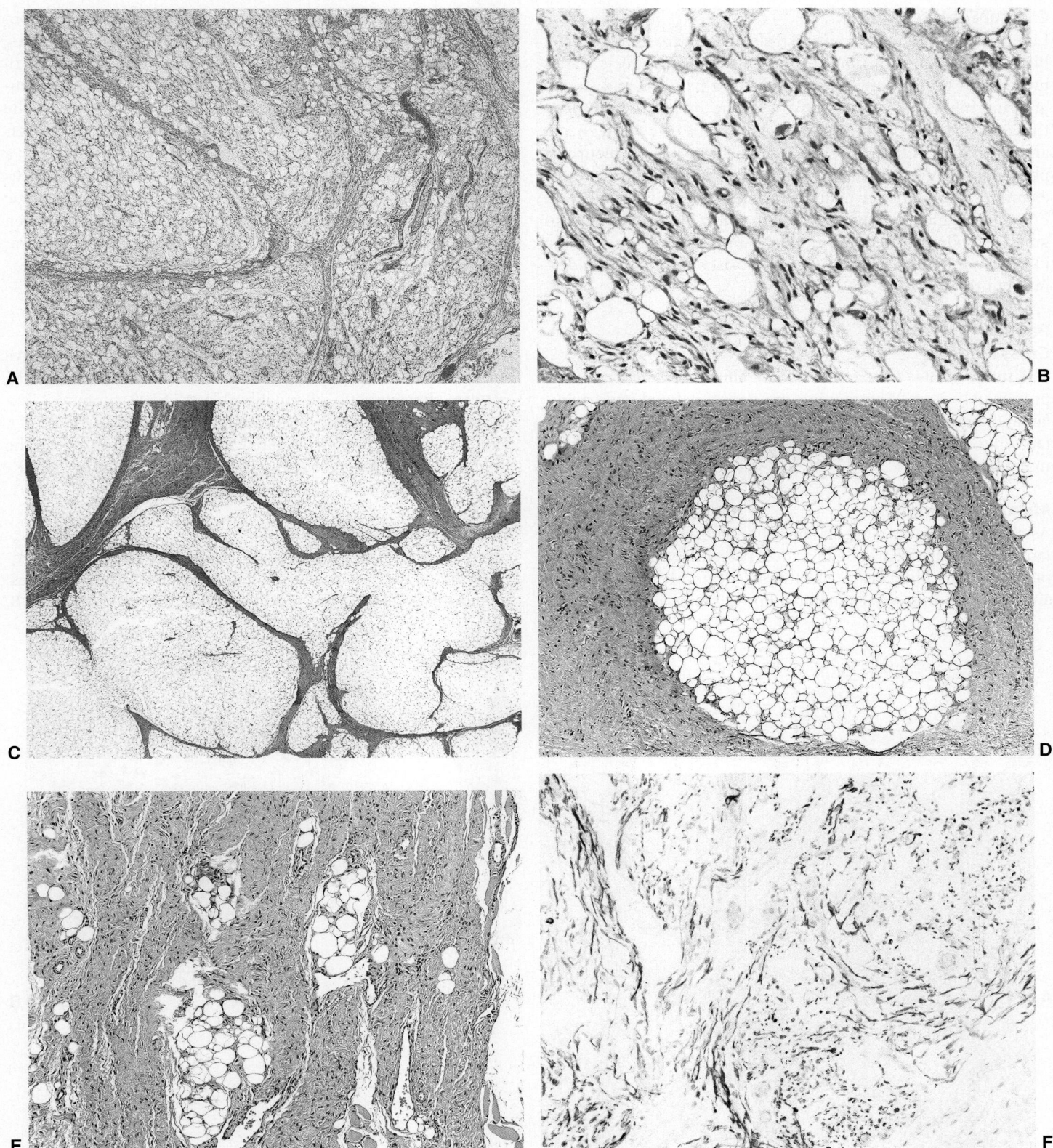

Figure 34-9 Lipoblastoma, showing pronounced lobularity, variable myxoid change, and mature fat (A). Lipoblastomas often display a well-developed capillary vasculature and may mimic myxoid liposarcoma. Cellular spindling is much more characteristic of lipoblastoma (B). Maturing lipoblastoma, consisting largely of mature fat, with only small foci of myxoid matrix (C). Higher power view of a maturing nodule in lipoblastoma (D). Fibroblastic lipoblastoma contains moderately cellular fascicles of fibroblastic cells, in addition to small nodules of variably myxoid fat (E). Desmin expression is common in the stromal cells of lipoblastomas and can be helpful in their distinction from myxoid liposarcomas (F).

Clinical Features

Lipofibromatosis occurs exclusively in children (age range: birth to 14 years; median 1 year of age) and affects males more often than females. It presents as a painless and slowly growing mass, most often involving the hands, followed by the arm, leg, foot, trunk and exceptionally the head, neck, and orbit (116,117,123). The lesions have locally recurring potential but no metastatic risk (116). Exceptional recurrent examples show greater cellularity, stromal calcifications, and *FN1-EGF1* gene fusions, suggesting a close link to a more aggressive pediatric neoplasm, calcifying aponeurotic fibroma (117). Despite its name, lipofibromatosis is not related to desmoid fibromatosis.

Pathologic Features
Gross Findings

The tumors range in size from 1 to 7 cm, with a median of approximately 2 cm. The margins are poorly defined and irregular, and a minority appear vaguely lobulated. The cut surface is tan-white to yellowish, grossly fatty and rubbery, firm or gritty in consistency (116).

Microscopic Findings

As the name would suggest, lipofibromatosis usually consists largely of mature fat, although a small percentage of cases may be predominantly fibroblastic. The tumors are poorly circumscribed and infiltrate into adjacent fibroadipose tissue and sometimes skeletal muscle. The lesions are composed of variably sized lobules of mature fat divided by thickened fibrous septa containing cytologically bland, cuboidal to spindled fibroblastic cells with a small amount of eosinophilic cytoplasm, normochromatic nuclei, and low to absent mitotic activity (Fig. 34-10A, B). At the interface between these fibrous septa and the mature fat, numerous small lipoblast-like cells are present, typically having only a single intracytoplasmic vacuole and a normochromatic nucleus (Fig. 34-10C). These cells appear to represent early adipocytic differentiation by the fibroblastic cells and should not be taken as evidence of "liposarcoma." Myxoid change may be present, particularly in infants, mimicking lipoblastoma.

Ancillary Studies
Immunohistochemistry

The fibroblastic cells of lipofibromatosis are variably positive for CD34 and smooth muscle actin, the latter in a "tram-track" pattern characteristic of myofibroblasts. S100 protein is expressed by mature adipocytes and lipoblast-like cells (116,117). Pan-TRK antibodies are negative, a useful finding when the differential diagnosis of lipofibromatosis includes *NTRK*-rearranged neoplasia (124,125).

Genetic Features

A recent molecular genetic study of lipofibromatosis has identified frequent gene fusions involving tyrosine kinase genes, including *FN1-EGF, EGR1-GRIA1, TPR-ROS1, SPARC-PDGFRB,*

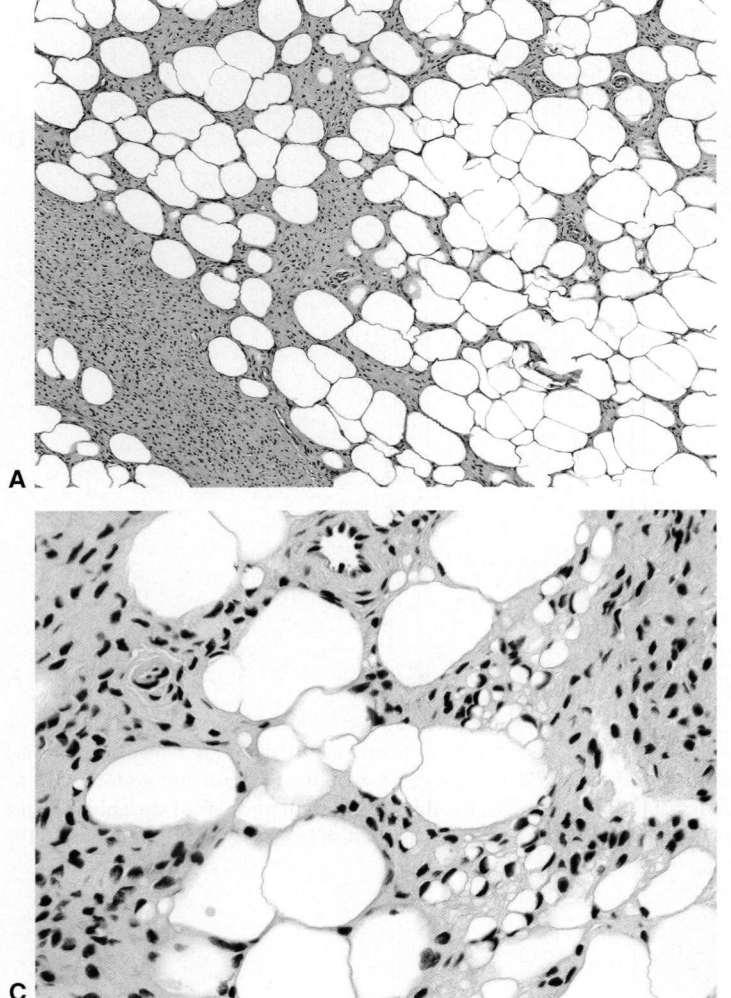

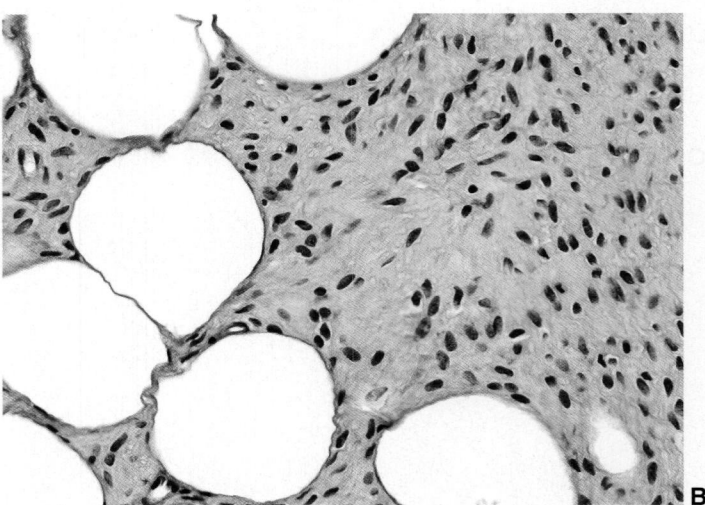

Figure 34-10 Lipofibromatosis typically presents in the distal extremities of infants as a fatty-appearing mass. Microscopically, it consists of mature fat admixed with unusual fibroblastic zones, composed of uniform, small, somewhat cuboidal cells (**A**). Higher power view of fibroblastic areas in lipofibromatosis (**B**). At the interface between the fibroblastic zones and the mature fat numerous lipoblast-like cells are present, suggesting adipocytic differentiation in the fibroblastic cells themselves (**C**).

FN1-TGFA, EGFR-BRAF, VCL-RET, and *HBEGF-RBM27* (117). Identical *FN1-EGF* fusions are seen in calcifying aponeurotic fibroma, suggesting a link between these two pediatric tumors of the distal extremities.

Differential Diagnosis

As the name implies, the closest mimicker of lipofibromatosis is the recently described "lipofibromatosis-like neural tumor" (LFLNT) (126). LFLNT is a member of an ever-growing family of spindle cell neoplasms defined by rearrangements involving the *NTRK* genes, colloquially referred to as "TRKomas" (127). LFLNT occurs in older patients than does lipofibromatosis; shows greater cellularity and nuclear variability; and co-expresses S100 protein, CD34, and TRK protein in the spindle cell component (126). Lipoblastomas usually occur in more proximal locations, show pronounced lobularity, often express desmin and harbor *PLAG1* rearrangements. Fibrous hamartomas of infancy also typically occur in much more proximal locations and show triphasic morphology, with fat, fibromatosis-like fascicles, and nodules of myxoid primitive mesenchyme (128,129).

Hemosiderotic Fibrolipomatous Tumor

Originally described as a reactive process ("hemosiderotic fibrolipomatous lesion"), hemosiderotic fibrolipomatous tumor (HFLT) is an unusual low-grade mesenchymal neoplasm that may recur locally and rarely progress to myxoid sarcoma. Recurrent HFLT commonly show morphologic features of another rare soft tissue tumor, pleomorphic angiectatic tumor of soft parts (PHAT), and close examination of cases of PHAT invariably show foci of HFLT ("early PHAT") (130,131). Identical genetic changes are also seen in HFLT and PHAT, and it is now clear that they represent different manifestations of a single entity (130–133).

Clinical Features

Both HFLT and PHAT typically occur as slowly growing masses in the subcutaneous tissues of the distal extremities, usually the ankles and feet. HFLT is often mistaken clinically for some sort of adipocytic tumor because of its prominent fatty component, whereas PHAT may be mistaken for a hematoma or Kaposi sarcoma because of its vascular appearance.

Although HFLT was originally felt to be reactive in nature, and PHAT to be benign, both have a roughly 50% risk of local recurrence and are considered mesenchymal tumors of borderline malignancy. Extraordinarily rare HFLT and PHAT have progressed to myxoid sarcoma, somewhat resembling myxoinflammatory fibroblastic sarcoma or myxofibrosarcoma (130).

Pathologic Features
Gross Findings

"Pure" HFLT typically appears as infiltrative fatty masses of widely variable size, with areas of hemosiderin staining and myxoid change. Foci of PHAT are better circumscribed, often deeply hemosiderin stained, and may even show grossly visible ectatic blood vessels.

Microscopic Findings

Microscopically, HFLT consists of a partially myxoid proliferation of mature fat, moderately cellular fascicles of hemosiderin-laden spindled cells, chronic inflammatory cells, and macrophages (Fig. 34-11A, B). Areas closely resembling

"miniature" PHAT may be present, with hyalinized vessels, aggregates of damaged small vessels, and scattered hemosiderin-containing tumor cells showing nuclear pleomorphism and intranuclear pseudoinclusions (Fig. 34-11C, D). Mitotic activity is extremely low, and necrosis is absent.

Ancillary Studies
Immunohistochemistry
HFLT are typically CD34 positive and negative for all other markers except vimentin.

Genetic Features
Rearrangements of the *TGFBR3* and/or *OGA* (*MGEA5*) genes are found in substantial subsets of HFLT and in PHAT, supporting their relationship.

Differential Diagnosis

The differential diagnosis of HFLT includes essentially any spindle cell neoplasms infiltrating fat as well as spindle cell lipoma. Perhaps the most distinctive feature of HFLT is the presence of abundant hemosiderin within the spindled cells themselves, sometimes highlighted with Prussian Blue stains for iron. The presence of small aggregates of damaged blood vessels is also extremely characteristic of HFLT and is not generally a feature of other spindle cell tumors involving fat. Spindle cell lipomas may closely resemble HFLT but lack hemosiderin deposition and grow in a well-circumscribed fashion.

MALIGNANT ADIPOCYTIC TUMORS
Atypical Lipomatous Tumor/Well-Differentiated Liposarcoma and Dedifferentiated Liposarcoma

ALT and well-differentiated liposarcoma (WDL) are *synonyms* used in different locations to describe the same locally aggressive, nonmetastasizing adipocytic tumor, harboring in almost all instances of amplifications of a portion of the long arm of chromosome 12, containing (among others) the *MDM2* and *CDK4* genes (134). Dedifferentiated liposarcoma is defined as a (usually) high-grade, nonlipogenic sarcoma arising from a preexisting ALT/WDL, either in direct association or in a local recurrence.

The term "ALT" should be applied to lesions that arise in the superficial and deep soft tissues of the extremities and trunk, whereas the term "WDL" is reserved for tumors arising in the abdomen, mediastinum, retroperitoneum, inguinal and paratesticular area, and viscera (135). This terminology is meant to reflect the very different natural history of these lesions in these different locations, with tumors in the accessible soft tissues having a much lower risk of local recurrence and/or dedifferentiation than their retroperitoneal/visceral counterparts. In the head and neck, tumors arising from the skin and subcutis should be labeled "ALT," with tumors of the upper aerodigestive tract considered "WDL." Tumors of the extremities were previously classified as "atypical lipoma" when suprafascial and "WDL" when subfascial; this classification has been abandoned (6). In practice, almost all tumors of this type seen by dermatopathologists should be labeled "ALT."

Clinical Features

Overall, ALT/WDL is the most common subtype of liposarcoma, presenting most commonly in middle-aged adults with

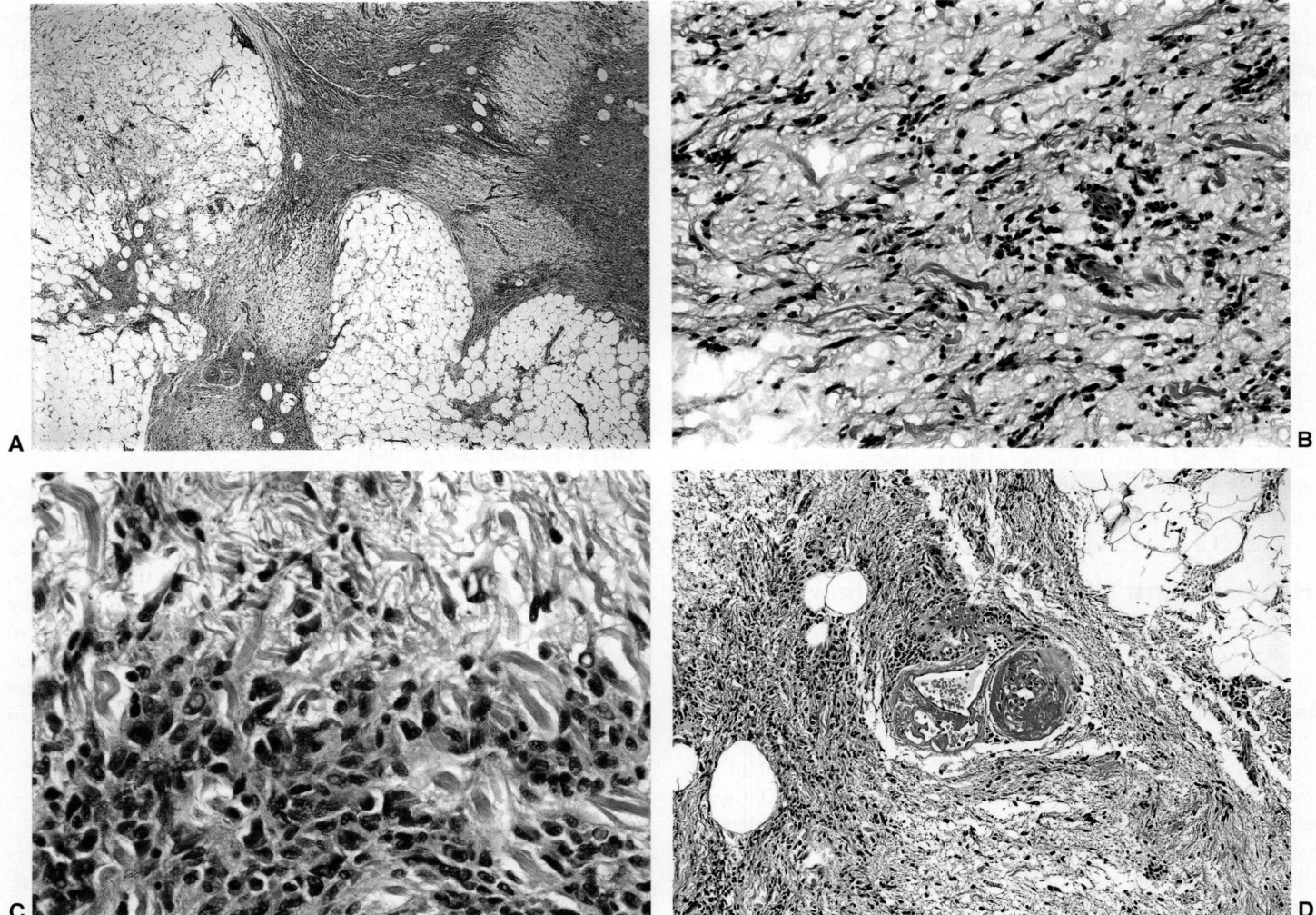

Figure 34-11 Hemosiderotic fibrolipomatous tumor (HFLT) typically contains a large amount of mature fat, in which is found a variably myoid spindle cell proliferation (**A**). Myxoid and spindled area in HFLT, mimicking spindle cell lipoma (**B**). The spindled cells of HFLT contain intracytoplasmic iron pigment and often display nuclear pseudoinclusions, highly characteristic features (**C**). Aggregates of damaged small blood vessels are typically seen, one of the pieces of evidence establishing HFLT as the precursor lesion to the very rare soft tissue tumor known as pleomorphic hyalinizing angiectatic tumor of soft parts (**D**).

a peak incidence between the fourth and fifth decades, with a male predilection (134). Extremely rare pediatric examples are often associated with Li-Fraumeni syndrome (136,137). About 75% occur in the subcutis and muscles of the extremities, 20% in the retroperitoneum, and the remainder in the groin, spermatic cord and a variety of other sites (138,139). Primary ALT of the skin (as opposed to the subcutis) is vanishingly rare and appears most often as a polypoid mass, mimicking a fat-rich acrochordon (140–142). Dedifferentiated liposarcoma is far more common in the retroperitoneum, mediastinum, and paratesticular region than in extremity locations (138,139).

ALT/WDL are nonmetastasizing lesions whose risk for local recurrence and disease-related mortality is location dependent. Local recurrences are seen in roughly 50% of extremity tumors, in contrast to "high-risk" locations such as the retroperitoneum, where the local recurrence rate is essentially 100%. The risk for dedifferentiation appears to be time dependent, rather than site dependent, and has been estimated to be 10% to 15% in high-risk locations dend <5% in the extremities (138,139). Extremely rare cutaneous ALT and small, completely excised tumors confined to the subcutis have an exceedingly low risk for low recurrence and/or dedifferentiation (143).

Pathologic Features

Gross Findings

Reported cases of primary dermal ALT have presented as small (1 to 5 cm) polypoid masses, with an unremarkable, fatty cut surface (140–142). The size of ALT more generally is highly variable, ranging from small subcutaneous tumors resembling ordinary lipomas to massive tumors consisting of fat admixed with areas of fibrosis, hemorrhage, and myxoid change (138,139).

Microscopic Findings

ALT/WDL may be broadly divided into sclerosing, lipoma-like, and inflammatory subtypes (144). However, individual lesions frequently show a mixture of appearances, and the clinical significance of subclassifying these lesions is rather limited.

Fundamentally, ALT/WDL consist of mature adipose tissue transected by irregular, finely fibrillar collagenous septa containing a variable number of enlarged, hyperchromatic stromal cells, often with "smudgy" chromatin. Lipoblasts, defined as cells containing an enlarged, hyperchromatic nucleus indented on more than one side by optical clear vacuoles, may be few or absent and are *not* required for diagnosis. Indeed, as discussed in prior sections of this chapter, the hunt for lipoblasts is a frequent cause for misdiagnosis of various nonneoplastic and benign fatty tumors as "liposarcoma." ALT/WDL may consist largely of fibrous septa with numerous hyperchromatic stromal cells (sclerosing variant) or may be composed almost entirely of mature fat, with only difficult-to-find hyperchromatic cells (lipoma-like variant) (Fig. 34-12A–D). In some cases, enlarged hyperchromatic stromal cells are most easily found within the wall of abnormally configured, thick-walled vessels. A patchy chronic inflammatory cell infiltrate containing lymphocytes and plasma cells is often seen and may be prominent (inflammatory variant). Particularly in the paratestis and retroperitoneum, this chronic inflammatory cell infiltrate may be exceptionally dense, largely obscuring diagnostic hyperchromatic stromal cells, and sometimes resulting in confusion with a sclerosing hematolymphoid malignancy (145,146). Myxoid stromal change may also be seen, and occasionally is so pronounced as to mimic true myxoid liposarcoma (Fig. 34-12E) (147). Variation in adipocyte size has been suggested by some to be a feature of ALT/WDL, but in our experience is neither sensitive nor specific. Primary dermal ALT/WDL may show any combination of these morphologic features (140–142). Very rare ALT/WDL may show heterologous smooth muscle differentiation ("lipoleiomyosarcoma") (148,149), bone formation (150), and hibernoma-like morphology (151).

When present in association with ALT/WDL, the diagnosis of dedifferentiated liposarcoma (DL) is usually very straightforward. The overwhelming majority of DL resemble undifferentiated pleomorphic sarcoma, with high cellularity, overt nuclear atypia, frequent mitotic figures, and foci of necrosis (Fig. 34-12F) (134). Rare cases may appear morphologically low-grade, resembling fibromatosis, low-grade fibromyxoid sarcoma, or a perineurial neoplasm. In these cases, it is the abrupt transition from typical ALT/WDL to "something different" which is the most important clue to the diagnosis of DL (152). Heterologous differentiation in the form of osteosarcoma, chondrosarcoma, rhabdomyosarcoma, leiomyosarcoma, and rarely angiosarcoma may be seen (153). Examples of DL presenting in recurrent lesions, without associated ALT/WDL, usually require clinical correlation with regard to a previously excised mass, although FISH for MDM2 can be helpful in some instances (see below).

Ancillary Studies
Immunohistochemistry
Immunohistochemistry for MDM2 and CDK4 is useful in the distinction of ALT/WDL from potential mimics but is neither entirely sensitive nor specific (154). In particular, MDM2/CDK4-positive cells may be identified in up to 8% of lipomas and perhaps most treacherously in the lipid-laden macrophages of fat necrosis (41). Many spindle cell sarcomas express MDM2, and thus immunohistochemistry is less valuable in the diagnosis of DL than is FISH (see below).

Molecular/Genetic Studies
ALT/WDL and DL are characterized by the presence of supernumerary ring and giant marker chromosomes, which contain amplified sequences from the 12q13-15 region (155,156). MDM2 is thought to be the main driver gene but a variety of other gene co-amplifications in the same segment have been identified, including TSPAN31, CDK4, HMGA2, CPM, and FRS2 (157–159), among others. Rare Li-Fraumeni syndrome–associated tumors

resembling ALT/WDL harbor TP53 mutations, lack MDM2 amplification, and might better be considered a distinct liposarcoma subtype (137). Demonstration of MDM2 amplification in an otherwise undifferentiated-appearing pleomorphic sarcoma is generally considered presumptive evidence of DL, especially in high-risk anatomic locations (160).

Differential Diagnosis
The differential diagnosis in dermal and superficial ALT includes nonneoplastic and neoplastic conditions. Far and away the most common mimic of ALT is fat necrosis, either involving normal fat or lipoma. This is because fat necrosis often shows fibrosis, mimicking the fibrous septa of ALT, may contain an increased number of mildly atypical reactive stromal cells, frequently shows variation in adipocyte size, and contains lipid-laden macrophages and so-called Lochkern cells, mimicking lipoblasts. Lochkern cells are typically seen in somewhat thick sections of fat and represent lipocytes with an enlarged nucleus having powdery chromatin and intranuclear pseudovacuoles. As noted above, immunostains for MDM2 are often positive in lipid-laden macrophages, compounding the problem. Numerous pseudolipoblasts are also very frequently encountered in reactions to exogenous lipids (usually silicone), where they are typically seen in association with potentially helpful clues, such as hyaline fibrosis, chronic inflammation, and foreign-body–type multinucleated giant cells (Fig. 34-12G–I). It is important to keep silicone reaction in mind for masses having "too many lipoblasts," as a history of silicone injection may not always be provided. Massive localized lymphedema, a distinctive pseudosarcoma seen most often in morbidly obese patients, may simulate ALT owing to its large size and the presence of abundant fat with various reactive stromal changes. Attention to the clinical history, the characteristic location in the proximal thigh, and the presence of striking dermal fibrosis, lymphatic proliferation, and lymphangiectasia should allow for its ready distinction from liposarcoma.

Among neoplasms, spindle cell and pleomorphic lipoma of the skin and subcutis is most likely to be mistaken for ALT/WDL, especially in cases containing large numbers of pleomorphic floret-like giant cells and lipoblast-like cells. Clinical correlation with regard to patient age and tumor site is often helpful, as most SCL/PL involve the scalp, neck, or shoulder region in older males, as is attention to the cardinal morphologic features of this tumor type, small aggregates of bland, aligned spindled cells, wiry collagen, and myxoid matrix. In difficult cases, immunohistochemistry for CD34 and RB1 protein and FISH for MDM2 may be very useful (53,161). Fat-forming solitary fibrous tumors (lipomatous solitary fibrous tumor, lipomatous hemangiopericytoma) may contain a large amount of adipose tissue, mimicking liposarcoma, but also show characteristic branching, "staghorn" vessels, and nuclear expression of STAT6 protein (162–164).

The chief differential diagnostic consideration for DL is with other pleomorphic sarcomas infiltrating nonneoplastic fat. Application of strict diagnostic criteria for ALT/WDL is generally the best way to avoid this pitfall. FISH for MDM2 amplification may be helpful in some cases.

Pleomorphic Liposarcoma
Pleomorphic liposarcoma is a rare subtype of liposarcoma characterized by the presence of varying numbers of pleomorphic

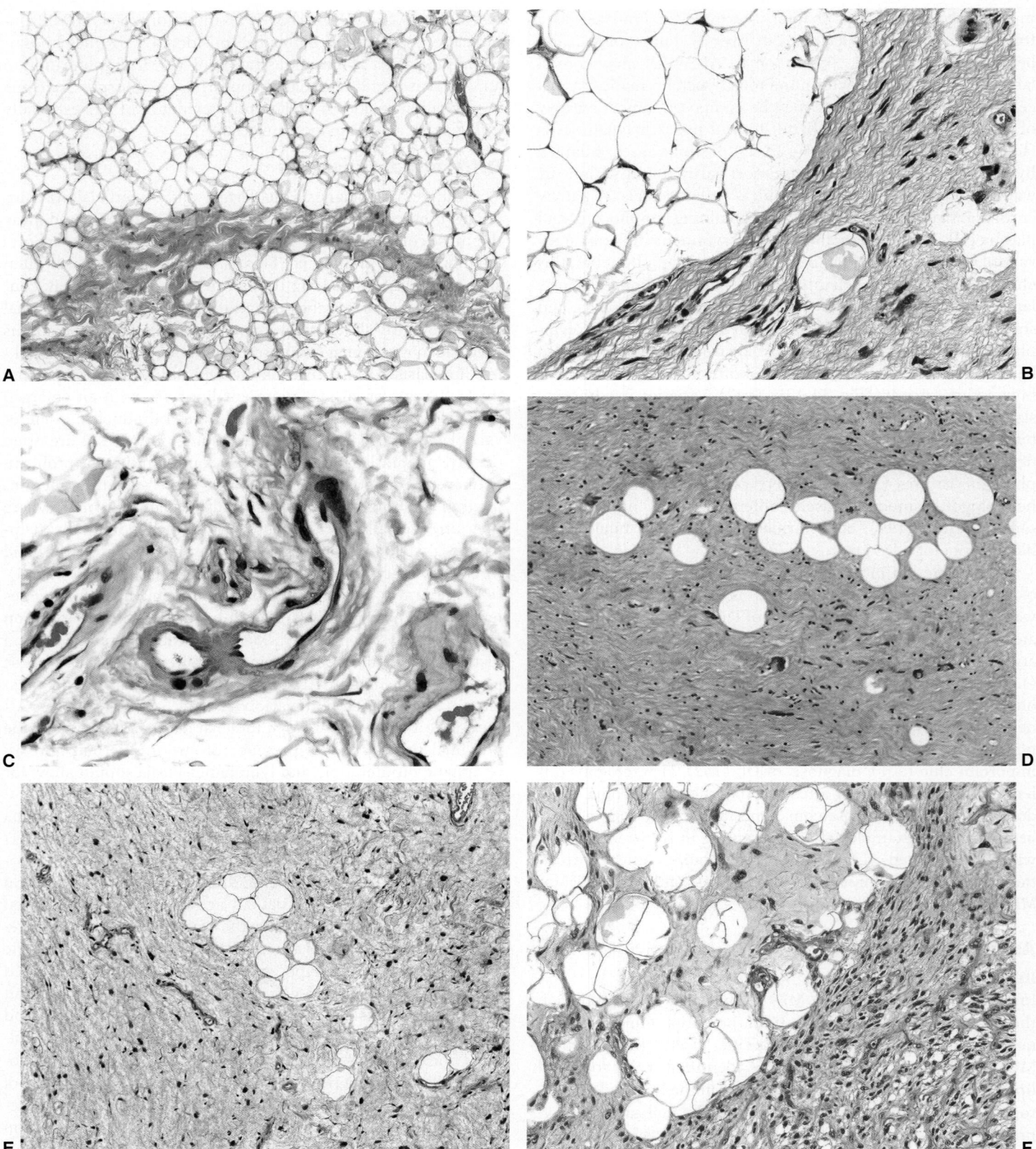

Figure 34-12 "Lipoma-like" atypical lipomatous tumor (ALT) consisting of mature fat transected by irregular fibrous septa, within which are found an increased number of hyperchromatic stromal cells (**A**). Higher power view of hyperchromatic cells in ALT (**B**). In some cases, hyperchromatic stromal cells are most easily identified within blood vessel walls (**C**). Sclerosing ALT, containing a greater amount of collagen and more easily identified hyperchromatic stromal cells (**D**). Myxoid change in ALT can mimic myxoid liposarcoma. However, enlarged hyperchromatic stromal cells are never a feature of true myxoid liposarcoma (**E**). Dedifferentiated liposarcoma, showing an abrupt transition between ALT and undifferentiated spindle cell sarcoma (**F**).

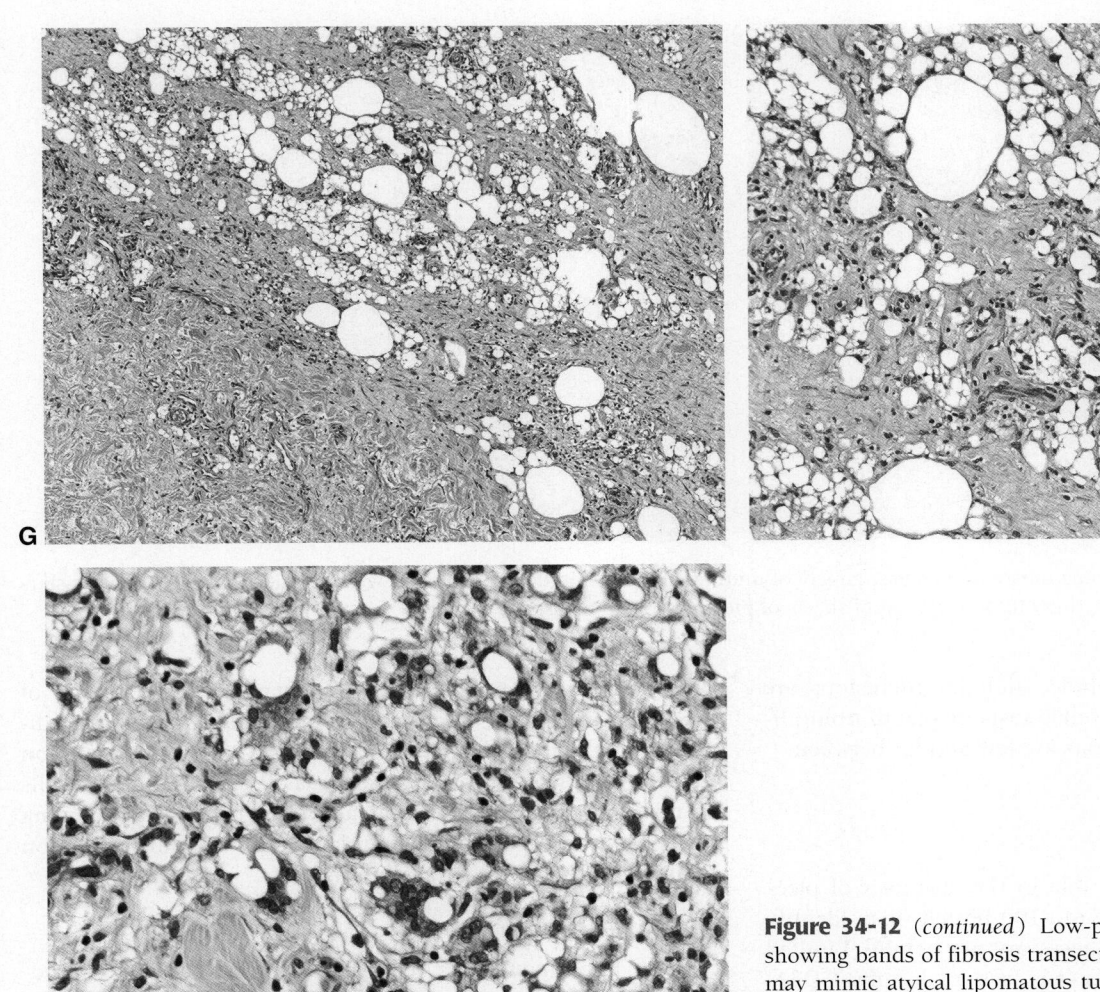

Figure 34-12 (*continued*) Low-power view of a silicone reaction, showing bands of fibrosis transecting adipose tissue. This appearance may mimic atyical lipomatous tumor/well-differentiated liposarcoma (**G**). Higher power view of lipoblast-like cells in silicone reaction (**H**). The presence of multinucleated foreign body giant cells is a useful clue in the distinction of silicone reaction from liposarcoma (**I**).

lipoblasts in a background of pleomorphic spindle cell sarcoma. By definition, they lack molecular and morphologic features diagnostic of other forms of liposarcomas (165–167).

Clinical Features

Pleomorphic liposarcomas almost always occur in deep soft tissue or the subcutis, and purely dermal lesions are vanishingly rare (167). Fewer than 20 primary pleomorphic liposarcomas of the dermis have been reported, some without convincing photomicrographs or appropriate ancillary studies (142,167–172). Based on the provided photomicrographs, we (and others) suspect that at least some reported examples represent instead atypical spindle cell/pleomorphic lipomatous tumors (see above) (173).

In general, pleomorphic liposarcomas occur in adults (median age 54 to 64 years), with the notable exception of the very rare myxoid variant, which occurs in children and has a mediastinal predilection (113,174). They more often involve the lower extremity, with the thigh being the single most commonly affected site, followed by a variety of locations such as the upper extremity and the head and neck area (166,167,175).

Pleomorphic liposarcomas are aggressive tumors having a poor outcome. The local recurrence rate is 25% to 42%, the metastatic rate is between 30% and 50% and the overall 5-year survival rate is as low as 39%. Metastases occur mostly in the lungs and pleura and rarely to the liver, brain, and bone

(166,167,175). The largest series of superficially located pleomorphic liposarcoma reported an excellent prognosis, with only rare local recurrences and no metastasis or death from disease, although as noted above, the classification of these tumors has been questioned (169).

Pathologic Features

Gross Findings

Most are large at the time of diagnosis (8 to 12 cm). The cut surface typically does not appear fatty, resembling instead other high-grade soft tissue sarcomas, with a fleshy, variably hemorrhagic and necrotic appearance (166,167,175).

Microscopic Findings

Pleomorphic liposarcomas are defined by the presence of large, bizarre-appearing pleomorphic lipoblasts. However, such cells are extremely variable in number, with some cases consisting largely of sheets of lipoblasts, and others consisting almost entirely of undifferentiated pleomorphic spindle cell sarcoma (Fig. 34-13A, B). In such cases, careful sampling and close inspection of multiple slides may be necessary for diagnosis. Myxoid change, closely resembling myxofibrosarcoma, may be present. Rare cases consist largely of small, epithelioid cells (epithelioid or small cell variant) (166,167,175). The presence of numerous multinucleated tumor giant cells and pleomorphic

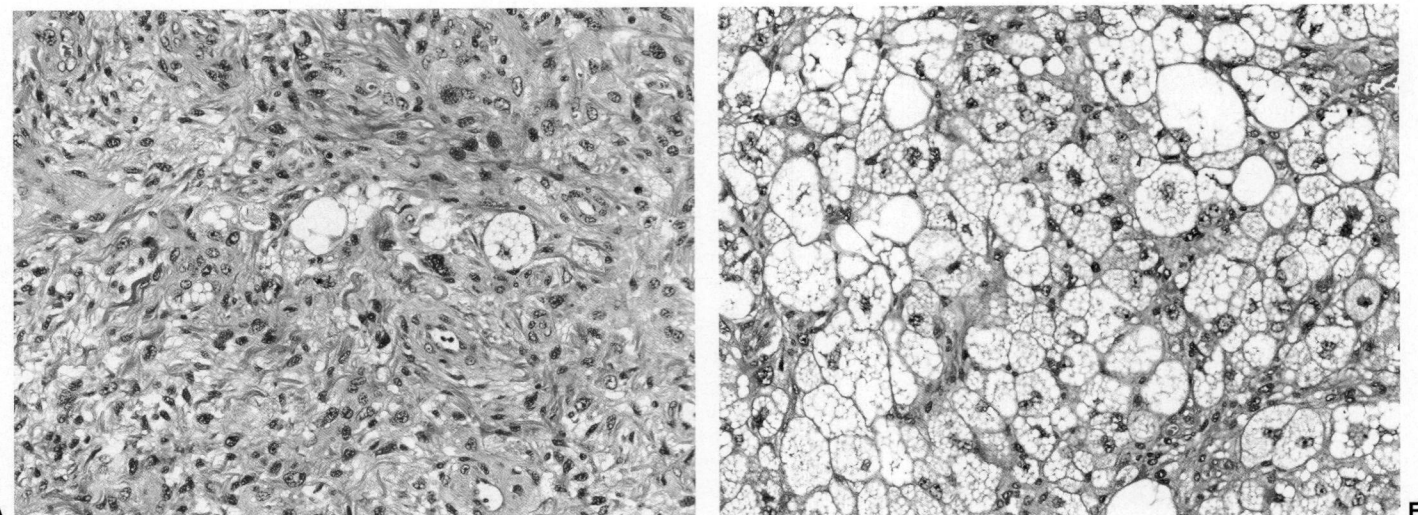

Figure 34-13 Pleomorphic liposarcoma most often consist largely of undifferentiated spindle cell sarcoma, within which is found small clusters of pleomorphic lipoblasts (**A**). Rarely these tumors consist of sheets of pleomorphic lipoblasts (**B**).

tumor cells containing eosinophilic, globular inclusions are useful morphologic clues to the diagnosis of pleomorphic liposarcoma in cases where lipoblasts are few and far between.

Ancillary Studies
Immunohistochemistry
Immunohistochemistry has little role in the diagnosis of pleomorphic liposarcoma. Antibodies to S100 protein may identify lipoblasts but are usually neither necessary nor helpful. Limited expression of a variety of markers (e.g., actins, desmin, CD34) may be present. Keratin expression can be seen in the epithelioid variant, a potentially significant pitfall when the differential diagnosis includes renal cell or adrenocortical carcinoma (167,176).

Genetic Features
Pleomorphic liposarcomas lack a specific genetic alteration, showing instead a complex pattern of chromosomal gains and losses, as in other high-grade pleomorphic sarcomas. Molecular genetic features of other liposarcoma subtypes (e.g., *MDM2* amplification, *DDIT3* rearrangement) are absent. Comparative genomic hybridization shows a higher frequency of chromosomal imbalances than are seen in dedifferentiated liposarcomas, with more chromosomal gains than losses, including gains of 20q13, 5p13-p15, 17p11.2-p12, and 1q21-q22 and 9q22-qter (177). At the molecular level, the most frequent mutations in pleomorphic liposarcoma involve the *NF1* and *TP53* genes (178,179).

Differential Diagnosis
In the skin and subcutis, pleomorphic liposarcomas should be distinguished from spindle cell and pleomorphic lipomas containing large numbers of floret-like giant cells and lipoblast-like cells. This is particularly true for so-called atypical spindle cell and pleomorphic lipomatous tumor, which displays infiltrative growth, elevated mitotic activity, and a relatively large number of lipoblast-like cells (51,180,181). The presence of areas of undifferentiated-appearing spindle cell sarcoma points toward pleomorphic liposarcoma, whereas foci resembling spindle cell lipoma, with small packets of aligned, bland spindled cells in association with wiry collagen obviously suggests the opposite.

Large nodules of lipoblasts are much more characteristic of pleomorphic liposarcoma. Care should be taken also not to diagnose myxofibrosarcoma with pseudolipoblasts (a common finding) as pleomorphic liposarcoma. Pseudolipoblastic cells in myxofibrosarcoma lack optically clear cytoplasm, showing instead intracytoplasmic accumulation of basophilic secretion identical to that seen extracellularly.

Myxoid Liposarcoma
Myxoid liposarcoma is a relatively common subtype of liposarcoma, defined by abundant myxoid matrix, an elaborate capillary vasculature, small, bland cells showing lipoblastic differentiation, and rearrangements of the *DDIT3* locus. Highly cellular, high-grade forms of myxoid liposarcoma were previously classified as "round cell liposarcoma." Essentially all myxoid liposarcomas occur in the deep soft tissue of the extremities, in particular the thigh, and dermal and subcutaneous examples almost always represent metastatic disease. There is only a single report of three genetically confirmed, primary myxoid liposarcomas of the subcutis (182).

Clinical Features
Of the three cases of primary subcutaneous myxoid liposarcoma reported by Buehler and colleagues, two arose in acral locations. Two affected patients were male and one female; all were adults aged 32 to 40 years. Following local excision, these patients were reported to be disease free at 6, 8, and 13 months (182).

Myxoid liposarcomas of deep soft tissue frequently metastasize to unusual locations, with roughly 50% of patients in some series having nonpulmonary metastases, involving peritoneum/pleura, bone, salivary glands, breast, and skin (183,184). Thus, when confronted with a myxoid liposarcoma in the skin or subcutis, the possibility of a previously excised or occult lesion of the extremities should always be excluded. Very late metastases are commonly seen in patients with this disease.

Pathologic Features
Gross Findings
Myxoid liposarcomas appear as gelatinous, usually nonfatty masses of widely variable size.

Microscopic Findings

Myxoid liposarcomas grow in a somewhat circumscribed, vaguely lobular pattern and produce abundant myxoid matrix, within which is found an exceptionally well-developed, arborizing capillary vasculature, often said to resemble chicken wire or crow's feet. The neoplastic cells are small, uniform, and monomorphic and hence the presence of pleomorphic tumor cells should suggest other diagnoses (Fig. 34-14A–C). Lipoblastic differentiation, typically in the form of small, oligovacuolated lipoblasts is typically identified adjacent to the capillaries. Abundantly myxoid tumors may form large acellular pools of myxoid matrix, the so-called pulmonary edema or lymphangioma-like pattern. A variable component of mature fat may be seen. Mitotic activity is usually low, although large areas of necrosis may be present. Accentuated cellularity is typically seen at the periphery of the lobules. High-grade myxoid liposarcomas (round cell) are defined as myxoid liposarcomas showing at least 5% areas displaying high cellularity, with obscuring of the underlying vascular pattern, elevated nuclear grade, and easily identified mitotic figures.

Ancillary Testing

Immunohistochemical Findings

Historically, immunohistochemistry has played no role in the diagnosis of myxoid liposarcoma. However, a very recently developed monoclonal antibody to the DDIT3 protein has shown considerable promise as a surrogate to molecular genetic testing (185). Further study of this antibody is necessary, however, to understand its spectrum of reactivity more fully.

Genetic Findings

Myxoid liposarcoma is characterized in >95% of cases by a t(12;16) that fuses the *DDIT3* gene on 12q13 with the *FUS* gene on 16p11 (186–188). In about 3% of cases, *EWSR1* (22q12) substitutes for *FUS*, generating an *EWSR1-DDIT3* fusion with t(12;22). There are no known clinical or pathologic differences between fusion variants.

Differential Diagnosis

The most important differential diagnostic consideration for myxoid liposarcoma involving the skin or subcutis is with a metastasis from a tumor of deep soft tissue. Such metastases may occur very late in the clinical course, and a careful, detailed clinical history may be needed. Obviously, the presence of synchronous or metachronous multicentric disease should suggest metastases. Extensively myxoid spindle cell lipomas may mimic myxoid liposarcoma but lack an elaborate capillary vasculature and contain small aggregates of bland spindled cells, not a feature of myxoid liposarcoma. Myxoid dermatofibrosarcoma protuberans with extensive fat infiltration may also mimic myxoid

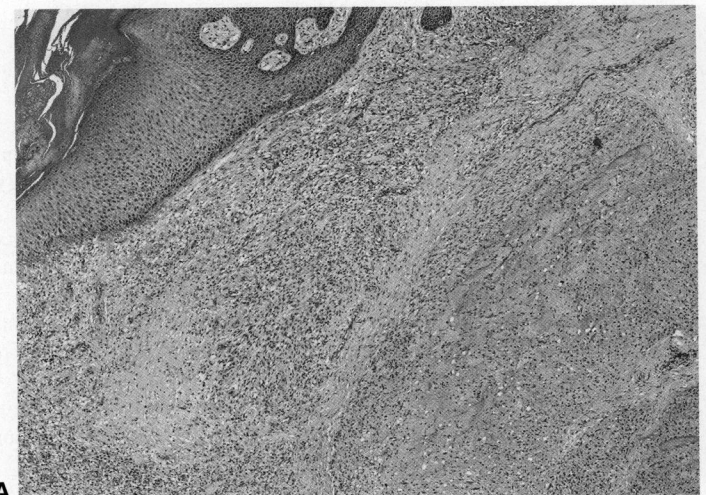

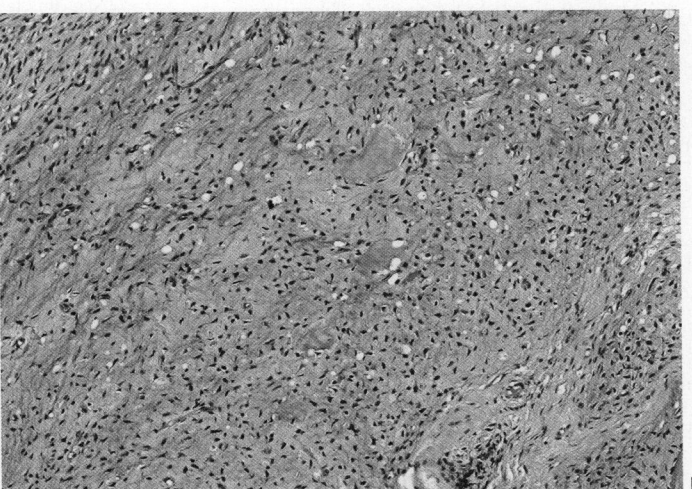

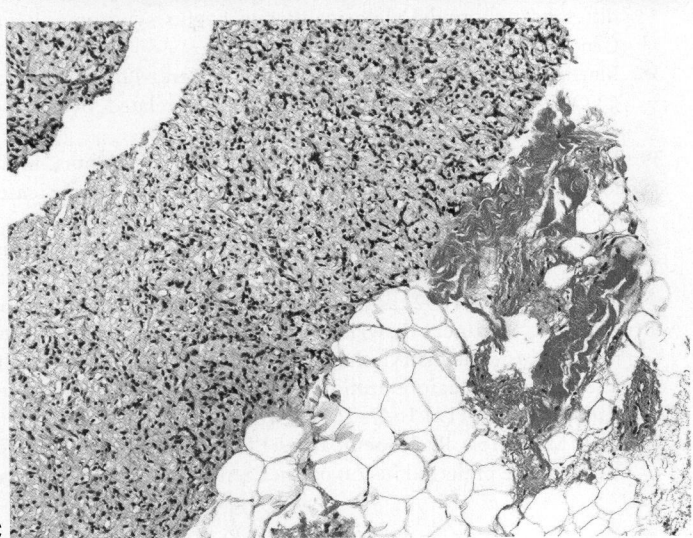

Figure 34-14 An extremely rare case of primary myxoid liposarcoma of the skin (**A**), showing classical morphologic features of this tumor type, including abundant myxoid matrix, an elaborate capillary vasculature, small round cells, and scattered lipoblasts (**B**). (Case courtesy of Dr. Steven Billings, Cleveland, OH.) The overwhelming majority of myxoid liposarcomas seen in the skin or subcutis represent metastases from occult or previously excised deeply seated tumors, as in this axillary subcutaneous metastasis from a myxoid liposarcoma of the thigh in a 30-year-old male (**C**).

liposarcoma. In such cases, identification of less myxoid foci of more conventional dermatofibrosarcoma is typically the best way to resolve this problem, although FISH for *PDGFB* amplification may be helpful in selected cases (189).

REFERENCES

1. Seale P, Bjork B, Yang W, et al. PRDM16 controls a brown fat/skeletal muscle switch. *Nature.* 2008;454(7207):961–967.
2. Wu J, Bostrom P, Sparks LM, et al. Beige adipocytes are a distinct type of thermogenic fat cell in mouse and human. *Cell.* 2012;150(2):366–376.
3. Rui L. Brown and beige adipose tissues in health and disease. *Compr Physiol.* 2017;7(4):1281–1306.
4. Petrovic N, Walden TB, Shabalina IG, Timmons JA, Cannon B, Nedergaard J. Chronic peroxisome proliferator-activated receptor gamma (PPARgamma) activation of epididymally derived white adipocyte cultures reveals a population of thermogenically competent, UCP1-containing adipocytes molecularly distinct from classic brown adipocytes. *J Biol Chem.* 2010;285(10):7153–7164.
5. Maemichi T, Tsutsui T, Matsumoto M, Iizuka S, Torii S, Kumai T. The relationship of heel fat pad thickness with age and physiques in Japanese. *Clin Biomech (Bristol, Avon).* 2020;80:105110.
6. Goldblum JR, Folpe AL, Weiss SW. *Enzinger & Weiss's Soft Tissue Tumors.* 7th ed. Elsevier; 2019.
7. Gjorgova-Gjeorgjievski S, Fritchie K, Folpe AL. CD10 (neprilysin) expression: a potential adjunct in the distinction of hibernoma from morphologic mimics. *Hum Pathol.* 2021;110:12–19.
8. Nandra R, Forsberg J, Grimer R. If your lump is bigger than a golf ball and growing, think Sarcoma. *Eur J Surg Oncol.* 2015;41(10):1400–1405.
9. Mashima E, Sawada Y, Saito-Sasaki N, et al. A retrospective study of superficial type atypical lipomatous tumor. *Front Med (Lausanne).* 2020;7:609515.
10. Thavikulwat AC, Wu JS, Chen X, Anderson ME, Ward A, Kung J. Image-guided core needle biopsy of adipocytic tumors: diagnostic accuracy and concordance with final surgical pathology. *AJR Am J Roentgenol.* 2021;216(4):997–1002.
11. Jones EW, Marks R, Pongsehirun D. Naevus superficialis lipomatosus. A clinicopathological report of twenty cases. *Br J Dermatol.* 1975;93(2):121–133.
12. Lynch FW, Goltz RW. Nevus lipomatosus cutaneus superficialis (Hoffmann-Zurhelle); presentation of a case and review of the literature. *AMA Arch Derm.* 1958;78(4):479–482.
13. Triki S, Mekni A, Haouet S, et al. Nevus lipomatosus cutaneous superficialis: a clinico-pathological study of 13 cases [in French]. *Tunis Med.* 2006;84(12):800–802.
14. Park HJ, Park CJ, Yi JY, Kim TY, Kim CW. Nevus lipomatosus superficialis. *Int J Dermatol.* 1997;36(6):435–437.
15. Saez Rodriguez M, Rodriguez-Martin M, Carnerero A, et al. Naevus lipomatosus cutaneous superficialis on the nose. *J Eur Acad Dermatol Venereol.* 2005;19(6):751–752.
16. Sawada Y. Solitary nevus lipomatosus superficialis on the forehead. *Ann Plast Surg.* 1986;16(4):356–358.
17. Leung AKC, Barankin B. Nevus lipomatosus superficialis on the left proximal arm. *Case Rep Dermatol Med.* 2017;2017:6908750.
18. Abel R, Dougherty JW. Nevus lipomatosus cutaneous superficialis (Hoffman-Zurhelle); report of two cases. *Arch Dermatol.* 1962;85:524–526.
19. Vano-Galvan S, Moreno C, Vano-Galvan E, Arrazola JM, Munoz-Zato E, Jaen P. Solitary naevus lipomatosus cutaneous superficialis on the sole. *Eur J Dermatol.* 2008;18(3):353–354.
20. Hattori R, Kubo T, Yano K, et al. Nevus lipomatosus cutaneous superficialis of the clitoris. *Dermatol Surg.* 2003;29(10):1071–1072.
21. Dudani S, Malik A, Mani NS. Nevus lipomatosis cutaneous superficialis—a clinicopathologic study of the solitary type. *Med J Armed Forces India.* 2016;72(1):67–70.
22. Isrie M, Breuss M, Tian G, et al. Mutations in either TUBB or MAPRE2 cause circumferential skin creases kunze type. *Am J Hum Genet.* 2015;97(6):790–800.
23. Reymond JL, Stoebner P, Amblard P. Nevus lipomatosus cutaneous superficialis. An electron microscopic study of four cases. *J Cutan Pathol.* 1980;7(5):295–301.
24. Inoue M, Ueda K, Hashimoto T. Nevus lipomatosus cutaneus superficialis with follicular papules and hypertrophic pilo-sebaceous units. *Int J Dermatol.* 2002;41(4):241–243.
25. Takashima H, Toyoda M, Ikeda Y, Kagoura M, Morohashi M. Nevus lipomatosus cutaneous superficialis with perifollicular fibrosis. *Eur J Dermatol.* 2003;13(6):584–586.
26. Cardot-Leccia N, Italiano A, Monteil MC, Basc E, Perrin C, Pedeutour F. Naevus lipomatosus superficialis: a case report with a 2p24 deletion. *Br J Dermatol.* 2007;156(2):380–381.
27. Hoey SE, Eastwood D, Monsell F, Kangesu L, Harper JI, Sebire NJ. Histopathological features of Proteus syndrome. *Clin Exp Dermatol.* 2008;33(3):234–238.
28. Laing VB, Fleischer AB Jr. Piezogenic wrist papules: a common and asymptomatic finding. *J Am Acad Dermatol.* 1991;24(3):415–417.
29. Kahana M, Feinstein A, Tabachnic E, Schewach-Millet M, Engelberg S. Painful piezogenic pedal papules in patients with Ehlers-Danlos syndrome. *J Am Acad Dermatol.* 1987;17(2, pt 1):205–209.
30. Shelley WB, Rawnsley HM. Painful feet due to herniation of fat. *JAMA.* 1968;205(5):308–309.
31. Buschmann WR, Jahss MH, Kummer F, Desai P, Gee RO, Ricci JL. Histology and histomorphometric analysis of the normal and atrophic heel fat pad. *Foot Ankle Int.* 1995;16(5):254–258.
32. Espana A, Pujol RM, Idoate MA, Vazquez-Doval J, Romani J. Bilateral congenital adipose plantar nodules. *Br J Dermatol.* 2000;142(6):1262–1264.
33. Semadeni BL, Mainetti C, Itin P, Lautenschlager S. Precalcaneal congenital fibrolipomatous hamartomas: report of 3 additional cases and discussion of the differential diagnosis. *Dermatology.* 2009;218(3):260–264.
34. Jakhar D, Kaur I, Singal A, Sharma S. Precalcaneal congenital fibrolipomatous hamartoma: rare or under-reported? *J Cutan Pathol.* 2019;46(4):277–279.
35. Rydholm A, Berg NO. Size, site and clinical incidence of lipoma. Factors in the differential diagnosis of lipoma and sarcoma. *Acta Orthop Scand.* 1983;54(6):929–934.
36. Wanner M, Celebi JT, Peacocke M. Identification of a PTEN mutation in a family with Cowden syndrome and Bannayan-Zonana syndrome. *J Am Acad Dermatol.* 2001;44(2):183–187.
37. Tucci A, Saletti V, Menni F, et al. The absence that makes the difference: choroidal abnormalities in Legius syndrome. *J Hum Genet.* 2017;62(11):1001–1004.
38. Martinez-Lopez A, Blasco-Morente G, Perez-Lopez I, et al. CLOVES syndrome: review of a PIK3CA-related overgrowth spectrum (PROS). *Clin Genet.* 2017;91(1):14–21.
39. Fritchie KJ, Renner JB, Rao KW, Esther RJ. Osteolipoma: radiological, pathological, and cytogenetic analysis of three cases. *Skeletal Radiol.* 2012;41(2):237–244.
40. Dreux N, Marty M, Chibon F, et al. Value and limitation of immunohistochemical expression of HMGA2 in mesenchymal tumors: about a series of 1052 cases. *Mod Pathol.* 2010;23(12):1657–1666.
41. Clay MR, Martinez AP, Weiss SW, Edgar MA. MDM2 and CDK4 immunohistochemistry: should it be used in problematic differentiated lipomatous tumors?: a new perspective. *Am J Surg Pathol.* 2016;40(12):1647–1652.
42. Petit MM, Mols R, Schoenmakers EF, Mandahl N, Van de Ven WJ. LPP, the preferred fusion partner gene of HMGIC in lipomas,

is a novel member of the LIM protein gene family. *Genomics.* 1996;36(1):118–129.

43. Wang X, Zamolyi RQ, Zhang H, et al. Fusion of HMGA1 to the LPP/TPRG1 intergenic region in a lipoma identified by mapping paraffin-embedded tissues. *Cancer Genet Cytogenet.* 2010;196(1):64–67.

44. Enzinger FM, Harvey DA. Spindle cell lipoma. *Cancer.* 1975;36(5):1852–1859.

45. Shmookler BM, Enzinger FM. Pleomorphic lipoma: a benign tumor simulating liposarcoma. A clinicopathologic analysis of 48 cases. *Cancer.* 1981;47(1):126–133.

46. French CA, Mentzel T, Kutzner H, Fletcher CD. Intradermal spindle cell/pleomorphic lipoma: a distinct subset. *Am J Dermatopathol.* 2000;22(6):496–502.

47. Billings SD, Folpe AL. Diagnostically challenging spindle cell lipomas: a report of 34 "low-fat" and "fat-free" variants. *Am J Dermatopathol.* 2007;29(5):437–442.

48. Sachdeva MP, Goldblum JR, Rubin BP, Billings SD. Low-fat and fat-free pleomorphic lipomas: a diagnostic challenge. *Am J Dermatopathol.* 2009;31(5):423–426.

49. Hawley IC, Krausz T, Evans DJ, Fletcher CD. Spindle cell lipoma—a pseudoangiomatous variant. *Histopathology.* 1994;24(6):565–569.

50. Marino-Enriquez A, Nascimento AF, Ligon AH, Liang C, Fletcher CD. Atypical spindle cell lipomatous tumor: clinicopathologic characterization of 232 cases demonstrating a morphologic spectrum. *Am J Surg Pathol.* 2017;41(2):234–244.

51. Creytens D, Mentzel T, Ferdinande L, et al. "Atypical" pleomorphic lipomatous tumor: a clinicopathologic, immunohistochemical and molecular study of 21 cases, emphasizing its relationship to atypical spindle cell lipomatous tumor and suggesting a morphologic spectrum (atypical spindle cell/pleomorphic lipomatous tumor). *Am J Surg Pathol.* 2017;41(11):1443–1455.

52. Syed S, Martin AM, Haupt H, Podolski V, Brooks JJ. Frequent detection of androgen receptors in spindle cell lipomas: an explanation for this lesion's male predominance? *Arch Pathol Lab Med.* 2008;132(1):81–83.

53. Chen BJ, Marino-Enriquez A, Fletcher CD, Hornick JL. Loss of retinoblastoma protein expression in spindle cell/pleomorphic lipomas and cytogenetically related tumors: an immunohistochemical study with diagnostic implications. *Am J Surg Pathol.* 2012;36(8):1119–1128.

54. Dal Cin P, Sciot R, Polito P, et al. Lesions of 13q may occur independently of deletion of 16q in spindle cell/pleomorphic lipomas. *Histopathology.* 1997;31(3):222–225.

55. Dahlen A, Debiec-Rychter M, Pedeutour F, et al. Clustering of deletions on chromosome 13 in benign and low-malignant lipomatous tumors. *Int J Cancer.* 2003;103(5):616–623.

56. Maggiani F, Debiec-Rychter M, Vanbockrijck M, Sciot R. Cellular angiofibroma: another mesenchymal tumour with 13q14 involvement, suggesting a link with spindle cell lipoma and (extra)-mammary myofibroblastoma. *Histopathology.* 2007;51(3):410–412.

57. Maggiani F, Debiec-Rychter M, Verbeeck G, Sciot R. Extramammary myofibroblastoma is genetically related to spindle cell lipoma. *Virchows Arch.* 2006;449(2):244–247.

58. Howard WR, Helwig EB. Angiolipoma. *Arch Dermatol.* 1960;82:924–931.

59. Garib G, Siegal GP, Andea AA. Autosomal-dominant familial angiolipomatosis. *Cutis.* 2015;95(1):E26–E29.

60. Sebastiano C, Gennaro L, Brogi E, et al. Benign vascular lesions of the breast diagnosed by core needle biopsy do not require excision. *Histopathology.* 2017;71(5):795–804.

61. Hunt SJ, Santa Cruz DJ, Barr RJ. Cellular angiolipoma. *Am J Surg Pathol.* 1990;14(1):75–81.

62. Sciot R, Akerman M, Dal Cin P, et al. Cytogenetic analysis of subcutaneous angiolipoma: further evidence supporting its difference from ordinary pure lipomas: a report of the CHAMP Study Group. *Am J Surg Pathol.* 1997;21(4):441–444.

63. Panagopoulos I, Gorunova L, Andersen K, Lobmaier I, Bjerkehagen B, Heim S. Consistent involvement of chromosome 13 in angiolipoma. *Cancer Genomics Proteomics.* 2018;15(1):61–65.

64. Hofvander J, Arbajian E, Stenkula KG, et al. Frequent low-level mutations of protein kinase D2 in angiolipoma. *J Pathol.* 2017;241(5):578–582.

65. Perkins P, Weiss SW. Spindle cell hemangioendothelioma. An analysis of 78 cases with reassessment of its pathogenesis and biologic behavior. *Am J Surg Pathol.* 1996;20(10):1196–1204.

66. John I, Folpe AL. Anastomosing hemangiomas arising in unusual locations: a clinicopathologic study of 17 soft tissue cases showing a predilection for the paraspinal region. *Am J Surg Pathol.* 2016;40(8):1084–1089.

67. Meis JM, Enzinger FM. Chondroid lipoma. A unique tumor simulating liposarcoma and myxoid chondrosarcoma. *Am J Surg Pathol.* 1993;17(11):1103–1112.

68. Chan JK, Lee KC, Saw D. Extraskeletal chondroma with lipoblast-like cells. *Hum Pathol.* 1986;17(12):1285–1287.

69. Nielsen GP, O'Connell JX, Dickersin GR, Rosenberg AE. Chondroid lipoma, a tumor of white fat cells. A brief report of two cases with ultrastructural analysis. *Am J Surg Pathol.* 1995;19(11):1272–1276.

70. Darling MR, Daley TD. Intraoral chondroid lipoma: a case report and immunohistochemical investigation. *Oral Surg Oral Med Oral Pathol Oral Radiol Endod.* 2005;99(3):331–333.

71. Huang D, Sumegi J, Dal Cin P, et al. C11orf95-MKL2 is the resulting fusion oncogene of t(11;16)(q13;p13) in chondroid lipoma. *Genes Chromosomes Cancer.* 2010;49(9):810–818.

72. Flucke U, Tops BB, Verdijk MA, et al. NR4A3 rearrangement reliably distinguishes between the clinicopathologically overlapping entities myoepithelial carcinoma of soft tissue and cellular extraskeletal myxoid chondrosarcoma. *Virchows Arch.* 2012;460(6):621–628.

73. Flucke U, Mentzel T, Verdijk MA, et al. EWSR1-ATF1 chimeric transcript in a myoepithelial tumor of soft tissue: a case report. *Hum Pathol.* 2012;43(5):764–768.

74. Rao UN, Cieply K, Sherer C, Surti U, Gollin SM. Correlation of classic and molecular cytogenetic alterations in soft-tissue sarcomas: analysis of 46 tumors with emphasis on adipocytic tumors and synovial sarcoma. *Appl Immunohistochem Mol Morphol.* 2017;25(3):168–177.

75. Torres-Mora J, Ud Din N, Ahrens WA, Folpe AL. Pseudolipoblastic perineurioma: an unusual morphological variant of perineurioma that may simulate liposarcoma. *Hum Pathol.* 2016;57:22–27.

76. Gery L. In discussion of MF Bonnel's paper. *Bull Mem Soc Anat (Paris).* 1914;89:111–112.

77. Furlong MA, Fanburg-Smith JC, Miettinen M. The morphologic spectrum of hibernoma: a clinicopathologic study of 170 cases. *Am J Surg Pathol.* 2001;25(6):809–814.

78. Jaroszewski DE, Petris GD. Giant hibernoma of the thoracic pleura and chest wall. *World J Clin Cases.* 2013;1(4):143–145.

79. Hertoghs M, Van Schil P, Rutsaert R, Van Marck E, Vallaeys J. Intrathoracic hibernoma: report of two cases. *Lung Cancer.* 2009;64(3):367–370.

80. Kumar R, Deaver MT, Czerniak BA, Madewell JE. Intraosseous hibernoma. *Skeletal Radiol.* 2011;40(5):641–645.

81. Song B, Ryu HJ, Lee C, Moon KC. Intraosseous hibernoma: a rare and unique intraosseous lesion. *J Pathol Transl Med.* 2017;51(5):499–504.

82. Kim JD, Lee HW. Hibernoma: intense uptake on F18-FDG PET/CT. *Nucl Med Mol Imaging.* 2012;46(3):218–222.

83. Hedayati V, Thway K, Thomas JM, Moskovic E. MEN1 syndrome and hibernoma: an uncommonly recognised association? *Case Rep Med.* 2014;2014:804580.

84. Deguidi G, Mirandola S, Nottegar A, Tsvetkova V, Bianchi B, Pellini F. Axillary hibernoma in woman with lobular breast cancer and MEN1 syndrome: a case report. *Int J Surg Case Rep.* 2020;77:834–838.

85. Chirieac LR, Dekmezian RH, Ayala AG. Characterization of the myxoid variant of hibernoma. *Ann Diagn Pathol.* 2006; 10(2):104–106.

86. Al Hmada Y, Schaefer IM, Fletcher CDM. Hibernoma mimicking atypical lipomatous tumor: 64 cases of a morphologically distinct subset. *Am J Surg Pathol.* 2018;42(7):951–957.

87. Malzahn J, Kastrenopoulou A, Papadimitriou-Olivgeri I, et al. Immunophenotypic expression of UCP1 in hibernoma and other adipose/non adipose soft tissue tumours. *Clin Sarcoma Res.* 2019;9:8.

88. Mertens F, Rydholm A, Brosjo O, Willen H, Mitelman F, Mandahl N. Hibernomas are characterized by rearrangements of chromosome bands 11q13-21. *Int J Cancer.* 1994;58(4):503–505.

89. Nord KH, Magnusson L, Isaksson M, et al. Concomitant deletions of tumor suppressor genes MEN1 and AIP are essential for the pathogenesis of the brown fat tumor hibernoma. *Proc Natl Acad Sci U S A.* 2010;107(49):21122–21127.

90. Gisselsson D, Hoglund M, Mertens F, Dal Cin P, Mandahl N. Hibernomas are characterized by homozygous deletions in the multiple endocrine neoplasia type I region. Metaphase fluorescence in situ hybridization reveals complex rearrangements not detected by conventional cytogenetics. *Am J Pathol.* 1999;155(1):61–66.

91. Karamchandani JR, Nielsen TO, van de Rijn M, West RB. Sox10 and S100 in the diagnosis of soft-tissue neoplasms. *Appl Immunohistochem Mol Morphol.* 2012;20(5):445–450.

92. Schoolmeester JK, Lastra RR. Granular cell tumors overexpress TFE3 without corollary gene rearrangement. *Hum Pathol.* 2015;46(8):1242–1243.

93. Cohen JN, Yeh I, Jordan RC, et al. Cutaneous non-neural granular cell tumors harbor recurrent ALK gene fusions. *Am J Surg Pathol.* 2018;42(9):1133–1142.

94. Van Meurs DP. The transformation of an embryonic lipoma to a common lipoma. *Br J Surg.* 1947;34(135):282–284.

95. Vellios F, Baez J, Shumacker HB. Lipoblastomatosis: a tumor of fetal fat different from hibernoma; report of a case, with observations on the embryogenesis of human adipose tissue. *Am J Pathol.* 1958;34(6):1149–1159.

96. Mentzel T, Calonje E, Fletcher CD. Lipoblastoma and lipoblastomatosis: a clinicopathological study of 14 cases. *Histopathology.* 1993;23(6):527–533.

97. Collins MH, Chatten J. Lipoblastoma/lipoblastomatosis: a clinicopathologic study of 25 tumors. *Am J Surg Pathol.* 1997;21(10): 1131–1137.

98. Chung EB, Enzinger FM. Benign lipoblastomatosis. An analysis of 35 cases. *Cancer.* 1973;32(2):482–492.

99. de Saint Aubain Somerhausen N, Coindre JM, Debiec-Rychter M, Delplace J, Sciot R. Lipoblastoma in adolescents and young adults: report of six cases with FISH analysis. *Histopathology.* 2008;52(3):294–298.

100. Fritchie K, Wang L, Yin Z, et al. Lipoblastomas presenting in older children and adults: analysis of 22 cases with identification of novel PLAG1 fusion partners. *Mod Pathol.* 2021;34(3): 584–591.

101. Coffin CM, Lowichik A, Putnam A. Lipoblastoma (LPB): a clinicopathologic and immunohistochemical analysis of 59 cases. *Am J Surg Pathol.* 2009;33(11):1705–1712.

102. Shinkai T, Masumoto K, Ono K, et al. A case of unusual histology of infantile lipoblastoma confirmed by PLAG1 rearrangement. *Surg Case Rep.* 2015;1(1):42.

103. Abdul-Ghafar J, Ahmad Z, Tariq MU, Kayani N, Uddin N. Lipoblastoma: a clinicopathologic review of 23 cases from a major tertiary care center plus detailed review of literature. *BMC Res Notes.* 2018;11(1):42.

104. Kubota F, Matsuyama A, Shibuya R, Nakamoto M, Hisaoka M. Desmin-positivity in spindle cells: under-recognized immunophenotype of lipoblastoma. *Pathol Int.* 2013;63(7):353–357.

105. Matsuyama A, Hisaoka M, Hashimoto H. PLAG1 expression in mesenchymal tumors: an immunohistochemical study with special emphasis on the pathogenetical distinction between soft tissue myoepithelioma and pleomorphic adenoma of the salivary gland. *Pathol Int.* 2012;62(1):1–7.

106. Chen Z, Coffin CM, Scott S, et al. Evidence by spectral karyotyping that 8q11.2 is nonrandomly involved in lipoblastoma. *J Mol Diagn.* 2000;2(2):73–77.

107. Gisselsson D, Hibbard MK, Dal Cin P, et al. PLAG1 alterations in lipoblastoma: involvement in varied mesenchymal cell types and evidence for alternative oncogenic mechanisms. *Am J Pathol.* 2001;159(3):955–962.

108. Hibbard MK, Kozakewich HP, Dal Cin P, et al. PLAG1 fusion oncogenes in lipoblastoma. *Cancer Res.* 2000;60(17): 4869–4872.

109. Yoshida H, Miyachi M, Ouchi K, et al. Identification of COL3A1 and RAB2A as novel translocation partner genes of PLAG1 in lipoblastoma. *Genes Chromosomes Cancer.* 2014;53(7):606–611.

110. Nitta Y, Miyachi M, Tomida A, et al. Identification of a novel BOC-PLAG1 fusion gene in a case of lipoblastoma. *Biochem Biophys Res Commun.* 2019;512(1):49–52.

111. Giovannoni I, Barresi S, Rossi S, Stracuzzi A, Argentieri MG, Alaggio R. Pediatric lipoblastoma with a novel EEF1A1-PLAG1 fusion. *Genes Chromosomes Cancer.* 2021.

112. Pedeutour F, Deville A, Steyaert H, Ranchere-Vince D, Ambrosetti D, Sirvent N. Rearrangement of HMGA2 in a case of infantile lipoblastoma without Plag1 alteration. *Pediatr Blood Cancer.* 2012;58(5):798–800.

113. Alaggio R, Coffin CM, Weiss SW, et al. Liposarcomas in young patients: a study of 82 cases occurring in patients younger than 22 years of age. *Am J Surg Pathol.* 2009;33(5):645–658.

114. Scapa JV, Cloutier JM, Raghavan SS, Peters-Schulze G, Varma S, Charville GW. DDIT3 immunohistochemistry is a useful tool for the diagnosis of myxoid liposarcoma. *Am J Surg Pathol.* 2021;45(2):230–239.

115. Chung CT, Antonescu CR, Dickson BC, et al. Pediatric fibromyxoid soft tissue tumor with PLAG1 fusion: a novel entity? *Genes Chromosomes Cancer.* 2021;60(4):263–271.

116. Fetsch JF, Miettinen M, Laskin WB, Michal M, Enzinger FM. A clinicopathologic study of 45 pediatric soft tissue tumors with an admixture of adipose tissue and fibroblastic elements, and a proposal for classification as lipofibromatosis. *Am J Surg Pathol.* 2000;24(11):1491–1500.

117. Al-Ibraheemi A, Folpe AL, Perez-Atayde AR, et al. Aberrant receptor tyrosine kinase signaling in lipofibromatosis: a clinicopathological and molecular genetic study of 20 cases. *Mod Pathol.* 2019;32(3):423–434.

118. Lae ME, Pereira PF, Keeney GL, Nascimento AG. Lipoblastoma-like tumour of the vulva: report of three cases of a distinctive mesenchymal neoplasm of adipocytic differentiation. *Histopathology.* 2002;40(6):505–509.

119. Mirkovic J, Fletcher CD. Lipoblastoma-like tumor of the vulva: further characterization in 8 new cases. *Am J Surg Pathol.* 2015; 39(9):1290–1295.

120. Schoolmeester JK, Michal M, Steiner P, Michal M, Folpe AL, Sukov WR. Lipoblastoma-like tumor of the vulva: a clinicopathologic, immunohistochemical, fluorescence in situ hybridization and genomic copy number profiling study of seven cases. *Mod Pathol.* 2018;31(12):1862–1868.

121. Gambarotti M, Erdogan KE, Righi A, et al. Lipoblastoma-like tumor of the spermatic cord: case report and review of the literature. *Virchows Arch.* 2021;478(5):1013–1017.

122. Allen PW. The fibromatoses: a clinicopathologic classification based on 140 cases. *Am J Surg Pathol.* 1977;1(3):255–270.

123. Nuruddin M, Osmani M, Mudhar HS, Fernando M. Orbital lipofibromatosis in a child: a case report. *Orbit.* 2010;29(6):360–362.

124. Agaram NP, Zhang L, Sung YS, et al. NTRK1 associated gene fusions in pediatric fibroblastic/myofibroblastic neoplasms: a molecular study of 58 cases. *Mod Pathol.* 2016;29(suppl 2):12A.

125. Hung YP, Fletcher CDM, Hornick JL. Evaluation of pan-TRK immunohistochemistry in infantile fibrosarcoma, lipofibromatosis-like neural tumour and histological mimics. *Histopathology.* 2018;73(4):634–644.

126. Agaram NP, Zhang L, Sung YS, et al. Recurrent NTRK1 gene fusions define a novel subset of locally aggressive lipofibromatosis-like neural tumors. *Am J Surg Pathol.* 2016;40(10):1407–1416.

127. Ayasun R, Guven DC, Gullu I. A novel agnostic tumor: NTRKoma. *J Oncol Pharm Pract.* 2021;27:802–803.

128. Enzinger FM. Fibrous hamartoma of infancy. *Cancer.* 1965; 18:241–248.

129. Al-Ibraheemi A, Martinez A, Weiss SW, et al. Fibrous hamartoma of infancy: a clinicopathologic study of 145 cases, including 2 with sarcomatous features. *Mod Pathol.* 2017;30(4):474–485.

130. Boland JM, Folpe AL. Hemosiderotic fibrolipomatous tumor, pleomorphic hyalinizing angiectatic tumor, and myxoinflammatory fibroblastic sarcoma: related or not? *Adv Anat Pathol.* 2017;24(5):268–277.

131. Folpe AL, Weiss SW. Pleomorphic hyalinizing angiectatic tumor: analysis of 41 cases supporting evolution from a distinctive precursor lesion. *Am J Surg Pathol.* 2004;28(11):1417–1425.

132. Carter JM, Sukov WR, Montgomery E, et al. TGFBR3 and MGEA5 rearrangements in pleomorphic hyalinizing angiectatic tumors and the spectrum of related neoplasms. *Am J Surg Pathol.* 2014;38(9):1182–1992.

133. Zreik RT, Carter JM, Sukov WR, et al. TGFBR3 and MGEA5 rearrangements are much more common in "hybrid" hemosiderotic fibrolipomatous tumor-myxoinflammatory fibroblastic sarcomas than in classical myxoinflammatory fibroblastic sarcomas: a morphological and fluorescence in situ hybridization study. *Hum Pathol.* 2016;53:14–24.

134. Coindre JM, Pedeutour F, Aurias A. Well-differentiated and dedifferentiated liposarcomas. *Virchows Arch.* 2010;456(2):167–179.

135. WHO Classification of Tumours Editorial Board. *WHO Classification of Tumours of Soft Tissue and Bone.* 5th ed. International Agency for Research of Cancer; 2020.

136. Waters R, Horvai A, Greipp P, et al. Atypical lipomatous tumour/well-differentiated liposarcoma and de-differentiated liposarcoma in patients aged ≤ 40 years: a study of 116 patients. *Histopathology.* 2019;75(6):833–842.

137. Debelenko LV, Perez-Atayde AR, Dubois SG, et al. p53+/mdm2-atypical lipomatous tumor/well-differentiated liposarcoma in young children: an early expression of Li-Fraumeni syndrome. *Pediatr Dev Pathol.* 2010;13(3):218–224.

138. Lucas DR, Nascimento AG, Sanjay BK, Rock MG. Well-differentiated liposarcoma. The Mayo Clinic experience with 58 cases. *Am J Clin Pathol.* 1994;102(5):677–683.

139. Weiss SW, Rao VK. Well-differentiated liposarcoma (atypical lipoma) of deep soft tissue of the extremities, retroperitoneum, and miscellaneous sites. A follow-up study of 92 cases with analysis of the incidence of "dedifferentiation." *Am J Surg Pathol.* 1992;16(11):1051–1058.

140. Mathew R, Morgan MB. Dermal atypical lipomatous tumor/well-differentiated liposarcoma obfuscated by epidermal inclusion cyst: a wolf in sheep's clothing? *Am J Dermatopathol.* 2006;28(4):338–340.

141. Paredes BE, Mentzel T. Atypical lipomatous tumor/"well-differentiated liposarcoma" of the skin clinically presenting as a skin tag: clinicopathologic, immunohistochemical, and molecular analysis of 2 cases. *Am J Dermatopathol.* 2011;33(6):603–607.

142. Dei Tos AP, Mentzel T, Fletcher CD. Primary liposarcoma of the skin: a rare neoplasm with unusual high grade features. *Am J Dermatopathol.* 1998;20(4):332–338.

143. Sirvent N, Coindre JM, Maire G, et al. Detection of MDM2-CDK4 amplification by fluorescence in situ hybridization in 200 paraffin-embedded tumor samples: utility in diagnosing adipocytic lesions and comparison with immunohistochemistry and real-time PCR. *Am J Surg Pathol.* 2007;31(10):1476–1489.

144. Evans HL. Atypical lipomatous tumor, its variants, and its combined forms: a study of 61 cases, with a minimum follow-up of 10 years. *Am J Surg Pathol.* 2007;31(1):1–14.

145. Kraus MD, Guillou L, Fletcher CD. Well-differentiated inflammatory liposarcoma: an uncommon and easily overlooked variant of a common sarcoma. *Am J Surg Pathol.* 1997;21(5):518–527.

146. Argani P, Facchetti F, Inghirami G, Rosai J. Lymphocyte-rich well-differentiated liposarcoma: report of nine cases. *Am J Surg Pathol.* 1997;21(8):884–895.

147. Antonescu CR, Elahi A, Humphrey M, et al. Specificity of TLS-CHOP rearrangement for classic myxoid/round cell liposarcoma: absence in predominantly myxoid well-differentiated liposarcomas. *J Mol Diagn.* 2000;2(3):132–138.

148. Evans HL. Smooth muscle in atypical lipomatous tumors. A report of three cases. *Am J Surg Pathol.* 1990;14(8):714–718.

149. Folpe AL, Weiss SW. Lipoleiomyosarcoma (well-differentiated liposarcoma with leiomyosarcomatous differentiation): a clinicopathologic study of nine cases including one with dedifferentiation. *Am J Surg Pathol.* 2002;26(6):742–749.

150. Yoshida A, Ushiku T, Motoi T, Shibata T, Fukayama M, Tsuda H. Well-differentiated liposarcoma with low-grade osteosarcomatous component: an underrecognized variant. *Am J Surg Pathol.* 2010;34(9):1361–1366.

151. Hallin M, Schneider N, Thway K. Well-differentiated liposarcoma with hibernoma-like morphology. *Int J Surg Pathol.* 2016;24(7):620–622.

152. Henricks WH, Chu YC, Goldblum JR, Weiss SW. Dedifferentiated liposarcoma: a clinicopathological analysis of 155 cases with a proposal for an expanded definition of dedifferentiation. *Am J Surg Pathol.* 1997;21(3):271–281.

153. Evans HL, Khurana KK, Kemp BL, Ayala AG. Heterologous elements in the dedifferentiated component of dedifferentiated liposarcoma. *Am J Surg Pathol.* 1994;18(11):1150–1157.

154. Binh MB, Sastre-Garau X, Guillou L, et al. MDM2 and CDK4 immunostainings are useful adjuncts in diagnosing well-differentiated and dedifferentiated liposarcoma subtypes: a comparative analysis of 559 soft tissue neoplasms with genetic data. *Am J Surg Pathol.* 2005;29(10):1340–1347.

155. Pedeutour F, Forus A, Coindre JM, et al. Structure of the supernumerary ring and giant rod chromosomes in adipose tissue tumors. *Genes Chromosomes Cancer.* 1999;24(1):30–41.

156. Sandberg AA. Updates on the cytogenetics and molecular genetics of bone and soft tissue tumors: liposarcoma. *Cancer Genet Cytogenet.* 2004;155(1):1–24.

157. Macarenco RS, Erickson-Johnson M, Wang X, Jenkins RB, Nascimento AG, Oliveira AM. Cytogenetic and molecular cytogenetic findings in dedifferentiated liposarcoma with neural-like whorling pattern and metaplastic bone formation. *Cancer Genet Cytogenet.* 2007;172(2):147–150.

158. Erickson-Johnson MR, Seys AR, Roth CW, et al. Carboxypeptidase M: a biomarker for the discrimination of well-differentiated liposarcoma from lipoma. *Mod Pathol.* 2009;22(12):1541–1547.

159. Wang X, Asmann YW, Erickson-Johnson MR, et al. High-resolution genomic mapping reveals consistent amplification of the fibroblast

growth factor receptor substrate 2 gene in well-differentiated and dedifferentiated liposarcoma. *Genes Chromosomes Cancer.* 2011;50(11):849–858.

160. Kandel RA, Yao X, Dickson BC, et al. Molecular analyses in the diagnosis and prediction of prognosis in non-GIST soft tissue sarcomas: a systematic review and meta-analysis. *Cancer Treat Rev.* 2018;66:74–81.

161. Weaver J, Downs-Kelly E, Goldblum JR, et al. Fluorescence in situ hybridization for MDM2 gene amplification as a diagnostic tool in lipomatous neoplasms. *Mod Pathol.* 2008;21(8):943–949.

162. Creytens D, Ferdinande L. Diagnostic utility of STAT6 immuno-histochemistry in the diagnosis of fat-forming solitary fibrous tumors. *Appl Immunohistochem Mol Morphol.* 2016;24(2):e12–e13.

163. Guillou L, Gebhard S, Coindre JM. Lipomatous hemangiopericy-toma: a fat-containing variant of solitary fibrous tumor? Clinicopath-ologic, immunohistochemical, and ultrastructural analysis of a series in favor of a unifying concept. *Hum Pathol.* 2000;31(9):1108–1115.

164. Folpe AL, Devaney K, Weiss SW. Lipomatous hemangiopericy-toma: a rare variant of hemangiopericytoma that may be confused with liposarcoma. *Am J Surg Pathol.* 1999;23(10):1201–1207.

165. Rubin BP, Fletcher CD. The cytogenetics of lipomatous tumours. *Histopathology.* 1997;30(6):507–511.

166. Gebhard S, Coindre JM, Michels JJ, et al. Pleomorphic liposar-coma: clinicopathologic, immunohistochemical, and follow-up analysis of 63 cases: a study from the French Federation of Cancer Centers Sarcoma Group. *Am J Surg Pathol.* 2002;26(5):601–616.

167. Hornick JL, Bosenberg MW, Mentzel T, McMenamin ME, Oliveira AM, Fletcher CD. Pleomorphic liposarcoma: clinicopathologic analysis of 57 cases. *Am J Surg Pathol.* 2004;28(10):1257–1267.

168. Val-Bernal JF, Gonzalez-Vela MC, Cuevas J. Primary purely intrader-mal pleomorphic liposarcoma. *J Cutan Pathol.* 2003;30(8):516–520.

169. Gardner JM, Dandekar M, Thomas D, et al. Cutaneous and sub-cutaneous pleomorphic liposarcoma: a clinicopathologic study of 29 cases with evaluation of MDM2 gene amplification in 26. *Am J Surg Pathol.* 2012;36(7):1047–1051.

170. Al-Zaid T, Frieling G, Rosenthal S. Dermal pleomorphic liposar-coma resembling pleomorphic fibroma: report of a case and re-view of the literature. *J Cutan Pathol.* 2013;40(8):734–739.

171. Ramirez-Bellver JL, Lopez J, Macias E, et al. Primary dermal pleo-morphic liposarcoma: utility of adipophilin and MDM2/CDK4 immunostainings. *J Cutan Pathol.* 2017;44(3):283–288.

172. Martelosso A, Bitencourt P, Lima RB, et al. Giant primary pleomor-phic dermal liposarcoma. *J Cutan Pathol.* 2017;44(8):724–725.

173. Berg SH, Massoud CM, Jackson-Cook C, Boikos SA, Smith SC, Mochel MC. A reappraisal of superficial pleomorphic liposar-coma. *Am J Clin Pathol.* 2020;154(3):353–361.

174. Boland JM, Weiss SW, Oliveira AM, Erickson-Johnson ML, Folpe AL. Liposarcomas with mixed well-differentiated and pleomor-phic features: a clinicopathologic study of 12 cases. *Am J Surg Pathol.* 2010;34(6):837–843.

175. Downes KA, Goldblum JR, Montgomery EA, Fisher C. Pleomor-phic liposarcoma: a clinicopathologic analysis of 19 cases. *Mod Pathol.* 2001;14(3):179–184.

176. Miettinen M, Enzinger FM. Epithelioid variant of pleomor-phic liposarcoma: a study of 12 cases of a distinctive variant of high-grade liposarcoma. *Mod Pathol.* 1999;12(7):722–728.

177. Rieker RJ, Joos S, Bartsch C, et al. Distinct chromosomal imbal-ances in pleomorphic and in high-grade dedifferentiated liposar-comas. *Int J Cancer.* 2002;99(1):68–73.

178. Schneider-Stock R, Walter H, Radig K, et al. MDM2 amplification and loss of heterozygosity at Rb and p53 genes: no simultaneous alterations in the oncogenesis of liposarcomas. *J Cancer Res Clin Oncol.* 1998;124(10):532–540.

179. Barretina J, Taylor BS, Banerji S, et al. Subtype-specific genomic alterations define new targets for soft-tissue sarcoma therapy. *Nat Genet.* 2010;42(8):715–721.

180. Creytens D. What's new in adipocytic neoplasia? *Virchows Arch.* 2020;476(1):29–39.

181. Creytens D, van Gorp J, Savola S, Ferdinande L, Mentzel T, Libbrecht L. Atypical spindle cell lipoma: a clinicopathologic, immunohistochemical, and molecular study emphasizing its relationship to classical spindle cell lipoma. *Virchows Arch.* 2014;465(1):97–108.

182. Buehler D, Marburger TB, Billings SD. Primary subcutaneous myxoid liposarcoma: a clinicopathologic review of three cases with molecular confirmation and discussion of the differential diagnosis. *J Cutan Pathol.* 2014;41(12):907–915.

183. Estourgie SH, Nielsen GP, Ott MJ. Metastatic patterns of ex-tremity myxoid liposarcoma and their outcome. *J Surg Oncol.* 2002;80(2):89–93.

184. Smith TA, Easley KA, Goldblum JR. Myxoid/round cell liposar-coma of the extremities. A clinicopathologic study of 29 cases with particular attention to extent of round cell liposarcoma. *Am J Surg Pathol.* 1996;20(2):171–180.

185. Baranov E, Black MA, Fletcher CDM, Charville GW, Hornick JL. Nuclear expression of DDIT3 distinguishes high-grade myx-oid liposarcoma from other round cell sarcomas. *Mod Pathol.* 2021;34:1367–1372.

186. Creytens D. A contemporary review of myxoid adipocytic tu-mors. *Semin Diagn Pathol.* 2019;36(2):129–141.

187. Narendra S, Valente A, Tull J, Zhang S. DDIT3 gene break-apart as a molecular marker for diagnosis of myxoid liposarcoma—assay validation and clinical experience. *Diagn Mol Pathol.* 2011;20(4):218–224.

188. Antonescu CR. The role of genetic testing in soft tissue sarcoma. *Histopathology.* 2006;48(1):13–21.

189. Karanian M, Perot G, Coindre JM, Chibon F, Pedeutour F, Neu-ville A. Fluorescence in situ hybridization analysis is a helpful test for the diagnosis of dermatofibrosarcoma protuberans. *Mod Pathol.* 2015;28(2):230–237.

Tumors with Muscular Differentiation Involving the Skin

Chapter 35

SCOTT C. BRESLER AND RAJIV M. PATEL

TUMORS OF SMOOTH MUSCLE

In contrast to most other soft tissue neoplasms, tumors of smooth muscle are thought to arise from their normal tissue counterparts. In the skin, these structures include arrector pili muscles, mural muscle of blood vessels, and specialized smooth muscle at genital sites, which includes nipple, vulva, and scrotum (dartoic smooth muscle).

Smooth Muscle Hamartoma

Clinical Summary. Smooth muscle hamartoma is typically a congenital lesion that appears as a patch or plaque that is skin colored or slightly pigmented and several centimeters in diameter (1). The most affected anatomic location is the lumbosacral area (1). The extensor surfaces of the lower extremities and other locations on the trunk are also common sites, with occasional cases involving the face or breast region (2). Lesions occur more commonly in males (3). Follicular-based papules may be present throughout, and the lesion can also exist in a linear configuration (4). The pseudo-Darier sign (transient induration, sometimes with vermiculation) can be elicited on rubbing in most (80%) cases, which is a visually similar phenomenon to the true Darier sign observed in mastocytoma (5). Some lesions show hypertrichosis, which tends to diminish over time, as does hyperpigmentation (1). Significant morphologic overlap exists with Becker nevus (an acquired lesion also known as Becker melanosis or pigmented hairy epidermal nevus; see Chapter 28). Becker nevi are typically located on the shoulder of adolescent male patients and show marked hyperpigmentation, hypertrichosis, and often an associated proliferation of smooth muscle (3), suggesting that these lesions occupy the opposite ends of the spectrum, with Becker nevi demonstrating more marked epithelial changes than smooth muscle hamartoma. Rare cases of familial clustering have been observed (2). As opposed to the systemic syndrome often observed in association with Becker nevus [Becker nevus syndrome (6)], systemic manifestations, other than the so-called Michelin tire syndrome, which represents generalized cutaneous involvement (7), have not been reported. Malignant transformation is not a feature of smooth muscle hamartoma.

Histopathology. Numerous fascicles of smooth muscle cells are scattered haphazardly throughout the mid- to deep reticular dermis and extend in various directions (Fig. 35-1). On closer inspection, the fascicles are found to be composed of elongated spindle cells with brightly eosinophilic cytoplasm and

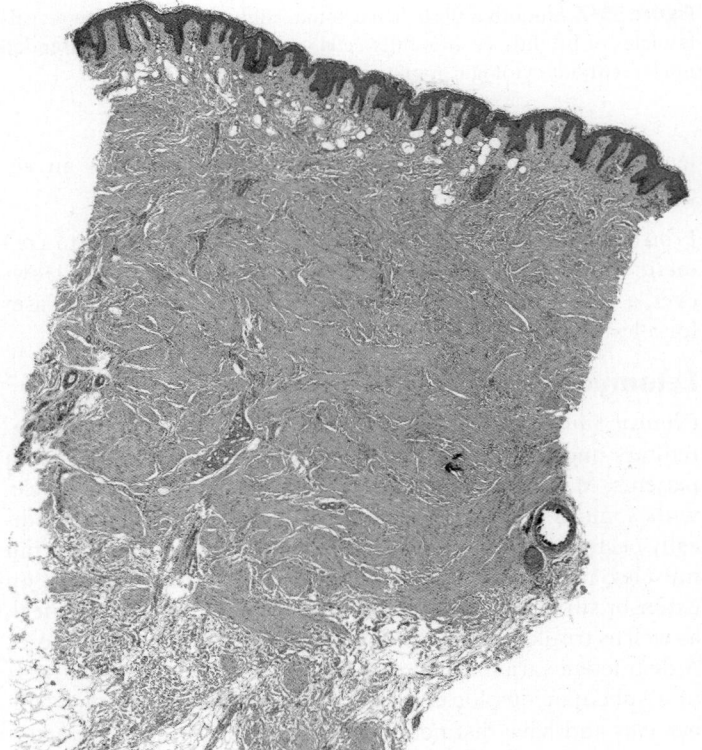

Figure 35-1 Smooth muscle hamartoma. Scanning magnification reveals an ill-defined proliferation of eosinophilic fascicles present throughout the dermis and extending in various directions.

blunt-ended, bland-appearing nuclei lacking hyperchromasia or other atypical features (Fig. 35-2). Some examples show hypertrichosis, which is caused by increased length and shaft diameter of involved hairs rather than by increased density (4,8). Some of the smooth muscle bundles may connect to hair follicles (4).

Pathogenesis. In a recent small study, somatic mutations in *ACTB*, the gene that encodes β actin, have been recently identified in most smooth muscle hamartomas (9). Such mutations have also been found in Becker nevi (10), which is further evidence that these lesions exist along a spectrum.

Differential Diagnosis. To confirm smooth muscle differentiation, immunohistochemical markers for smooth muscle actin (SMA) and/or desmin can be utilized; however, this is rarely necessary in practice. The main differential diagnosis is pilar

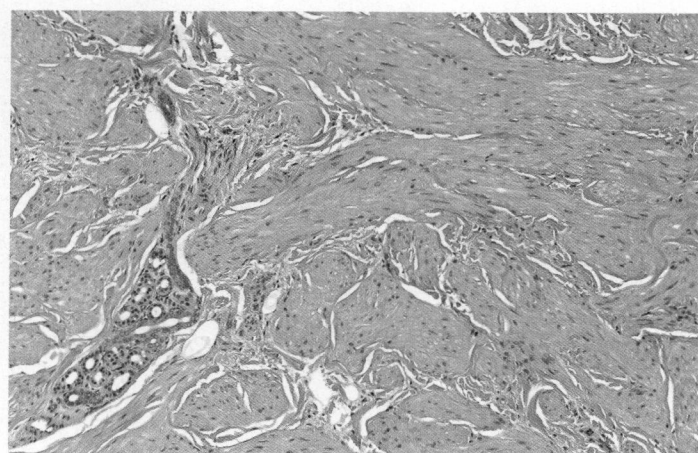

Figure 35-2 Smooth muscle hamartoma. Higher magnification reveals fascicles of brightly eosinophilic cells with cigar-shaped, blunt-ended nuclei without cytologic atypia or appreciable mitotic activity.

leiomyoma, which has better-defined borders and is an acquired lesion.

Principles of Management. If treatment is desired owing to cosmetic concerns, the preferred modality is simple excision. However, a recent case report described the use of pulsed dye laser for a lesion on the face with a good response (11).

Leiomyoma

Clinical Summary. Cutaneous leiomyomas are sporadic or hereditary and most often occur in young to middle-aged adult patients. Males and females appear to have an equal incidence, with some reports of a female predominance (12). Sporadically occurring pilar leiomyomas, which arise from arrector pili muscles, may be solitary or multiple and typically present on extensor surfaces as painful papules or nodules. Head and neck as well as trunk are also commonly affected anatomic locations. A distinctive variant that arises from the walls of blood vessels in a subcutaneous location are typically designated *angioleiomyomas* and have distinctive clinical and histologic characteristics. A third subset of cutaneous leiomyomas, which are the least common, present on genital skin (arising from scrotal or vulvar smooth muscle) or the nipple; tumors arising at these sites tend to be painless. Leiomyomas may occur in combination with additional mesenchymal elements, most commonly adipose tissue (13).

Hereditable leiomyomas that occur as multiple lesions are associated with hereditary leiomyomatosis and renal cell cancer (HLRCC or Reed) syndrome (14). This disorder is inherited in an autosomal dominant fashion and is distinguished by germline mutations in the gene encoding fumarate hydratase (*FH*; 1q42.3-q43) (15–18). Cutaneous leiomyomas are often the presenting feature of this disorder (14). As a significant proportion of affected patients develop an aggressive variant of renal cell carcinoma (RCC), identification at an early age is crucial for the timely implementation of appropriate screening procedures.

Pilar leiomyomas occur as solitary or multiple lesions with no sex predilection (13). These tumors clinically present as firm papules with a pink or red-brown to skin-colored surface, and typically arise on the trunk and extremities (13). Multiple leiomyomas may occur in a linear or agminated distribution or with a zosteriform/segmental distribution, with lesions

numbering in the hundreds (19,20). Approximately half of patients have involvement of more than one area of the body (13). A significant proportion (40% to 50%) of pilar leiomyomas are painful or tender to palpation (13). Lesions tend to gradually increase in size over time, and older lesions tend not to regress (3). On exposure to cold, lesions may become firmer or more protruding or may become painful (20).

The presence of multiple leiomyomas should raise clinical suspicion for HLRCC with a resulting thorough investigation of the patient's clinical and family history. Most affected female patients develop uterine leiomyomas and undergo hysterectomy at a younger age than patients with sporadically occurring uterine leiomyomas (21). Approximately 80% of HLRCC patients will have cutaneous manifestations. HLRCC-associated RCC, a morphologically distinctive variant of RCC (22) previously regarded as type 2 papillary RCC or collecting duct carcinoma, is seen in approximately 20% to 35% of patients with HLRCC (23). However, when selection bias is removed, this proportion is likely lower (14). The high mortality rate of this tumor type, which tends to occur in middle age, necessitates the identification of affected patients in order to begin appropriate surveillance screening. Other neoplasms potentially associated with HLRCC include testicular Leydig cell tumor, pheochromocytoma, adrenal cortical carcinoma, ovarian cystadenoma, and gastrointestinal stromal tumor. Solitary leiomyomas are slightly less common than those occurring as multiple lesions. Solitary leiomyomas are generally somewhat larger, with an average diameter of 6.4 versus 4.8 mm for multiple lesions (13). Giant leiomyomas (>5 cm) have rarely been reported, with larger tumors showing morphologic overlap with smooth muscle hamartoma (24).

Genital leiomyomas differ somewhat from pilar leiomyomas in their clinical presentation. Lesions present as painless, slow-growing masses that typically develop over many years with a mean diameter of approximately 3 to 4 cm (25,26). The labia majora appears to be the most common site for vulvar leiomyomas (25,27), which present at an average age of approximately 40 to 50 years old (27,28). Vulvar leiomyomas have been reported to enlarge during pregnancy (3); however, a minority of tumors cause pruritus or pain (26). Scrotal leiomyomas tend to be slightly larger than vulvar leiomyomas, with a mean diameter of 6 cm (25), and are also generally asymptomatic. Nipple leiomyomas are the least common member of this group and can be painful or can interfere with breastfeeding (29).

Angioleiomyomas, which are currently classified as tumors of pericytic lineage under the current World Health Organization (WHO) classification scheme (30), are typically subcutaneous tumors and only rarely occur in the dermis. Most are slow-growing and less than 2 cm in size (31). The most common site of involvement is the lower extremities (32), and most lesions are painful. Less commonly, angioleiomyomas occur on the trunk, head, or upper extremities. Rare cases of digital and acral tumors have also been described, which have an increased tendency to cause pain (32). An exceptional case of an angioleiomyoma causing bony destruction has also been reported (33). Angioleiomyomas may also occur in the oral cavity (34). Presentation is most common in the fourth to sixth decades with a slight female predominance (31). Rare lesions are congenital (35).

Histopathology. Pilar leiomyomas, whether multiple or solitary, and *nipple leiomyomas* are similar in histologic appearance. They are unencapsulated and tend to be circumscribed but poorly demarcated from the background dermis (Fig. 35-3). Nipple leiomyomas in particular may show an infiltrative appearance (29). Tumors are composed of interlacing bundles of smooth muscle, and background dermal collagen fibers may be intermingled. The smooth muscle cells of leiomyomas contain characteristic blunt-ended nuclei and generally lack cytologic atypia (Fig. 35-4). Approximately 50% of cases show overlying epidermal hyperplasia (Fig. 35-3). Leiomyomas of arrector pili origin may exhibit a low mitotic activity of less than or equal to 1 per 10 high-power field (HPF) (13). Historically, the presence of more than 1 mitosis per 10 HPF has resulted in a diagnosis of cutaneous leiomyosarcoma (atypical intradermal smooth muscle neoplasm). Leiomyomas may have degenerative atypia, and these cases are often referred to as "symplastic leiomyomas" (36), which is a diagnosis that should be made with caution. Interestingly, pilar leiomyomas that are associated with HLRCC tend to have a higher degree of nuclear atypia (though typically

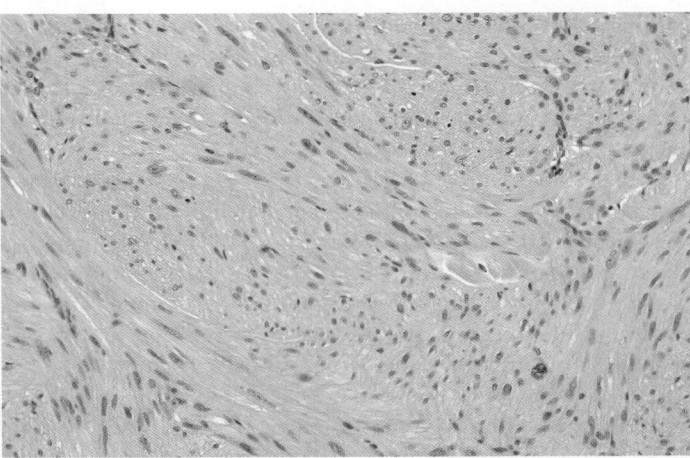

Figure 35-5 Leiomyoma associated with hereditary leiomyomatosis and renal cell cancer syndrome. This example shows mild cytologic atypia that is commonly seen in such lesions.

mild) than sporadically occurring leiomyomas (Fig. 35-5) (37); however, this is not a diagnostically reliable feature, and sporadically occurring lesions cannot be distinguished from those associated with HLRCC by morphologic appearances alone. Although genetic testing is considered the gold standard, loss of FH expression by immunohistochemistry (IHC) is a fairly sensitive (range 70% to 83.3%) and specific (range 75% to 97.6%) indicator for HLRCC (37–39) and can be used for screening purposes (Fig. 35-6). The addition of anti-S-(2-amino)-cystine (2SC) staining by IHC may increase specificity (38).

Vulvar and scrotal leiomyomas, although similar in appearance to pilar and nipple leiomyomas, do show several reliable differences (25,27). Vulvar and scrotal tumors are generally larger and tend to be better circumscribed, although a subset have focally infiltrative margins (25,27). Scrotal tumors are often associated with lymphoid aggregates (25). Additionally, some vulvar leiomyomas exhibit epithelioid cytomorphology, usually in association with typical spindled features (27). Degenerative change in the form of myxoid alteration or hyalinization is present in a significant minority of cases (25,27), the former of which can cause confusion with aggressive

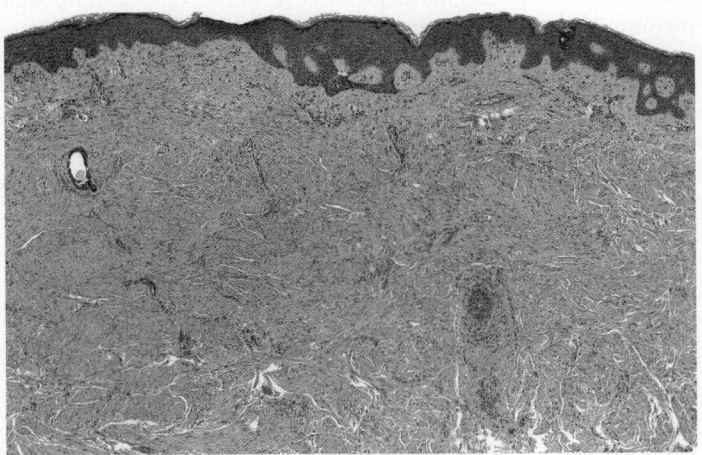

Figure 35-3 Pilar leiomyoma. Low-power image revealing an ill-defined but relatively circumscribed proliferation of smooth muscle present in the dermis. Mild epidermal hyperplasia is seen over the lesion.

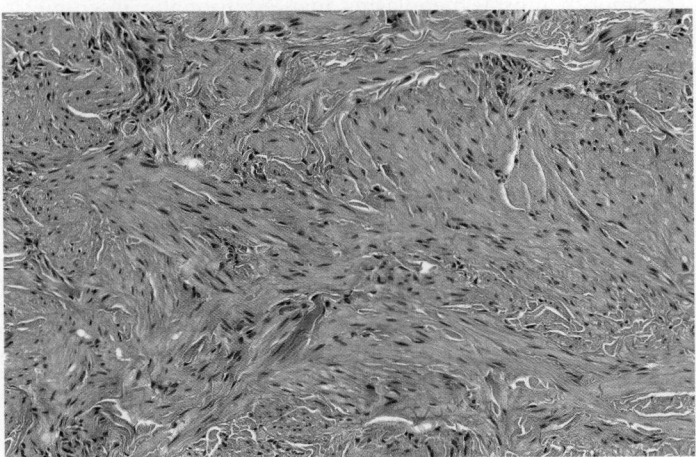

Figure 35-4 Pilar leiomyoma. Higher magnification reveals intersecting smooth muscle fascicles that are composed of spindle cells with brightly eosinophilic cytoplasm containing cigar-shaped, blunt-ended nuclei without significant cytologic atypia.

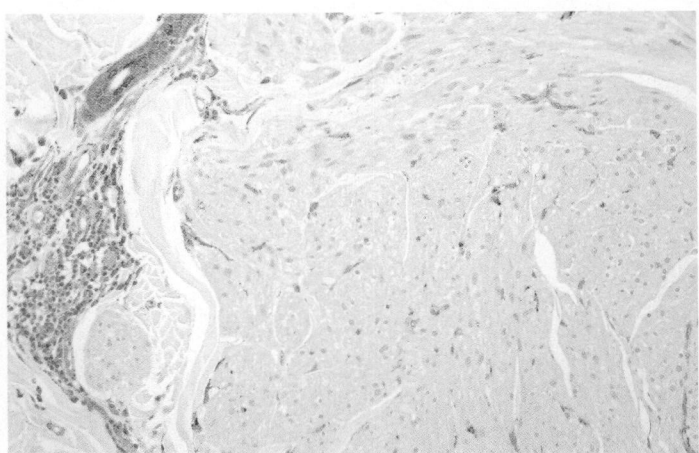

Figure 35-6 Leiomyoma associated with hereditary leiomyomatosis and renal cell cancer syndrome. This example shows loss of fumarate hydratase (FH) staining in tumor cells. Note the positive internal control in background blood vessels, eccrine duct, and inflammatory cells.

angiomyxoma. Vulvar leiomyomas commonly express estrogen and progesterone receptors, unlike pilar tumors (40). Analogously, focal androgen receptor positivity has been reported in scrotal leiomyomas (41). Genital leiomyomas have not been associated with HLRCC to date.

Angioleiomyomas differ from pilar and genital leiomyomas as they are typically located in the subcutaneous tissue, are well circumscribed and encapsulated (Fig. 35-7), and contain numerous blood vessels of varying thickness (Fig. 35-8). The lumina of the blood vessels are usually slit-shaped or stellate. A significant proportion of tumors show myxoid or hyaline change, and thrombosis within tumoral vessels is occasionally encountered (31). Nuclear features of the smooth muscle cells are typically bland; however, rare examples of a pleomorphic variant have been reported that simulate malignancy (42). This pleomorphism is not associated with an increase in proliferative activity, and the atypia is thus likely degenerative rather than neoplastic in nature. Some authors have separated angioleiomyomas into three histologic variants: solid, cavernous, and venous (31). Additionally, a rare intravascular variant has been described (43). Tumoral calcinosis has been seen in association with a subset of acral angioleiomyomas that are posited to arise in the setting of insertional Achilles tendinopathy secondary to tendon neovascularization (44).

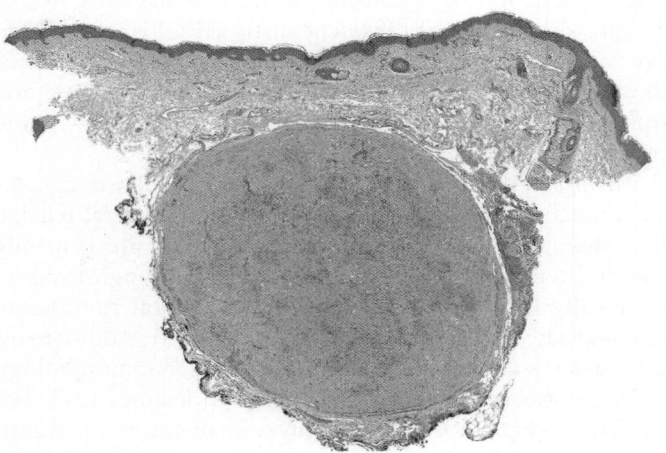

Figure 35-7 Angioleiomyoma. Scanning magnification reveals a sharply circumscribed but unencapsulated subcutaneous mass.

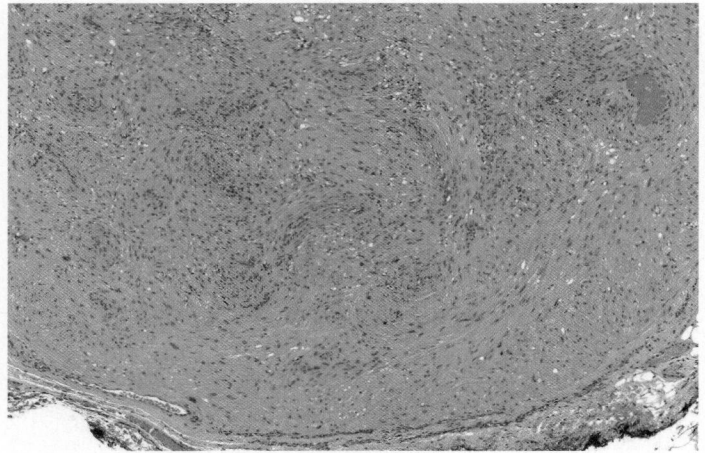

Figure 35-8 Angioleiomyoma. At higher magnification, numerous intratumoral small vessels are seen, intermingled with fascicles of smooth muscle cells without cytologic atypia. Smooth muscle of vessel walls merges without borders into intervening smooth muscle fascicles.

Occasional angioleiomyomas contain adipocytes, which have been referred to in the past as "*angiolipoleiomyoma*"; however, many authors believe that the fat cells in these tumors likely represent divergent adipocytic differentiation (45) or a metaplastic phenomenon and do not warrant distinction as a separate clinicopathologic entity. Other authors have suggested that such lesions represent hamartomas (31). Importantly, these lesions have no relationship to angiomyolipomas of the kidney, do not express HMB-45, and are not associated with tuberous sclerosis (46).

Pathogenesis. As discussed previously, smooth muscle tumors are believed to arise from their normal tissue counterparts, in this case the smooth muscle of subcutaneous blood vessel walls. Angioleiomyomas have been shown to harbor chromosomal imbalances and several nonrecurrent translocations; the most consistent chromosomal aberration is a loss on chromosome 22 (47,48).

Differential Diagnosis. The main differential diagnosis for leiomyoma is cutaneous leiomyosarcoma (atypical intradermal smooth muscle neoplasm). Leiomyosarcomas have greater mitotic activity and a higher degree of cytologic atypia and nuclear pleomorphism than leiomyomas and may also show the presence of necrosis (see later). Dermatomyofibroma may resemble leiomyoma and is comprised of horizontally oriented fascicles of myofibroblasts present within the dermis. Additionally, dermatomyofibromas, although positive for actins, are typically negative for desmin. Vulvar leiomyomas with extensive myxoid degeneration can be confused with aggressive angiomyxoma, which also often expresses SMA and desmin (49). However, epithelioid cell change is not a feature of aggressive angiomyxoma.

Rare variants of leiomyoma show granular (50) or clear cell (51) change, the former of which can cause confusion with granular cell tumor (GCT). S100 protein and SOX-10 can be used as discriminators in this setting because most GCTs strongly and diffusely express these markers. Expression of S100 protein is not observed in leiomyomas with granular cell change (50). A rare architectural pattern of leiomyoma simulating Verocay bodies of schwannoma has also been reported (52), which can be resolved using a panel of immunohistochemical markers, including SMA, desmin, S100 protein, and SOX-10.

Smooth muscle neoplasms may additionally resemble fibroblastic proliferations. However, smooth muscle nuclei are blunt ended and cigar shaped rather than tapered, as seen in fibroblasts. Additionally, collagen tends to have a wavy, buckled appearance, whereas smooth muscle cells are elongated and straight. If in doubt, IHC for markers such as desmin, SMA, calponin, or h-caldesmon, which stain most leiomyomas, can be performed to confirm smooth muscle differentiation.

Large leiomyomas can resemble smooth muscle hamartomas; however, this diagnostic dilemma is easily resolved clinically, because smooth muscle hamartomas are typically congenital lesions that present as patches or plaques, whereas leiomyomas are acquired tumors that present as papules or nodules.

Principles of Management. For a solitary lesion or for leiomyomas that are few in number, simple excision is curative (40). Any significant atypia in a smooth muscle neoplasm, even if a diagnosis of leiomyoma is favored, warrants modest but complete excision. In such cases, a diagnosis of *atypical leiomyoma* is appropriate

(53). In patients with a large number of lesions, surgical excision may not be practical. In such cases, treatment with calcium channel inhibitors may reduce pain in a subset of patients (54). Other medications such as phenoxybenzamine and oral nitroglycerine, have been used with limited success (24).

Epstein–Barr Virus–Associated Smooth Muscle Tumor

Clinical Summary. Epstein–Barr virus (EBV)–associated smooth muscle tumors occur in the setting of immunosuppression, most commonly in young to middle-aged adults who have undergone organ transplantation or have acquired immune deficiency syndrome (AIDS) (55). These tumors also occur in children with human immunodeficiency virus (HIV) infection/AIDS (56). They typically arise in the viscera (most commonly liver), deep soft tissue, or skin in the case of posttransplant-associated tumors, or intra- and extra-axial central nervous system (CNS) in the case of HIV-associated tumors (57). EBV-associated smooth muscle tumors were previously separated into benign and malignant counterparts; however, there appears to be no association between size, degree of cytologic atypia, mitotic rate, or the presence of necrosis with biologic behavior. Rare examples of metastatic tumors have been reported; however, this phenomenon could represent multifocal disease, which is common (55). Multifocal or intracranial tumors appear to be associated with worse overall survival (58).

Histopathology. Typically, these tumors consist of intersecting fascicles of smooth muscle cells exhibiting characteristic cytologic features, such as brightly eosinophilic cytoplasm and elongated, cigar-shaped nuclei (Fig. 35-9). Cytologic atypia can be present, and mitoses may be numerous. Necrosis is seen in a minority of cases (55). Infiltrative growth can be a feature (57). Most cases are positive for SMA; desmin expression is seen in approximately 50% of cases (55). Examples of EBV-associated smooth muscle tumors mimicking angioleiomyomas have been reported (59,60).

Pathogenesis. Given the histopathologic resemblance to angioleiomyoma and in some cases to pilar leiomyoma, EBV-associated smooth muscle tumors likely arise from normal cutaneous

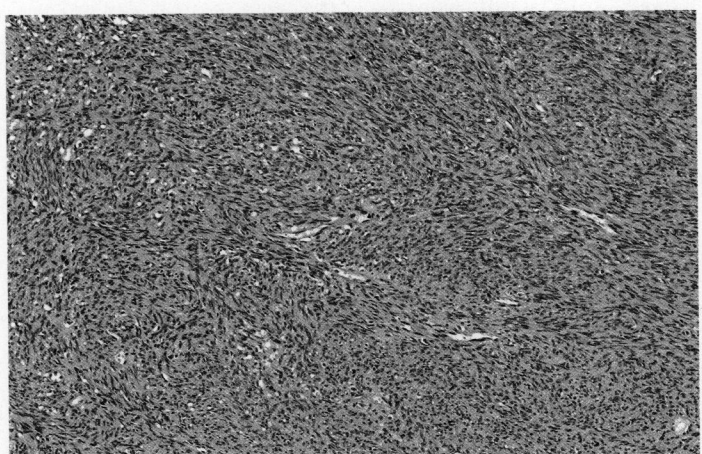

Figure 35-9 Epstein–Barr virus-associated smooth muscle tumor. These tumors most often resemble angioleiomyoma. This example is densely cellular with intersecting fascicles of smooth muscle cells exhibiting bland cytomorphologic features. However, some lesions may show morphologic overlap with leiomyosarcoma.

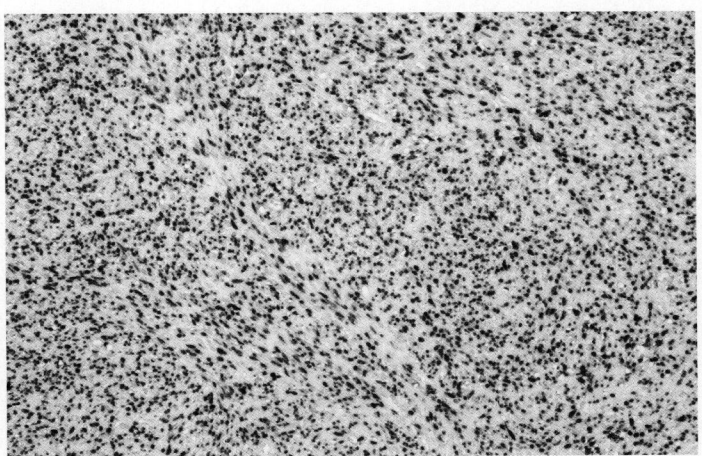

Figure 35-10 Epstein–Barr virus-associated smooth muscle tumor. *In situ* hybridization for Epstein–Barr virus-encoded small RNAs (EBER) can be used to confirm the diagnosis.

smooth muscle found in the walls of blood vessels and arrector pili muscles.

Differential Diagnosis. EBV-associated smooth muscle tumors can resemble angioleiomyoma, pilar leiomyoma, and leiomyosarcoma. *In situ* hybridization for Epstein–Barr virus-encoded small RNAs (EBER) confirms the diagnosis (Fig. 35-10).

Principles of Management. Surgical resection or reduction of immunosuppression is the most commonly pursued treatment modality (58); however, the latter needs to be balanced with maintaining appropriate levels of immune suppression to prevent rejection in organ transplant recipients.

Leiomyosarcoma

Clinical Summary. Superficial leiomyosarcomas, which are less common than those arising in deep soft tissue or the retroperitoneum, can be divided into tumors arising in the subcutis and those arising in the dermis; the latter are termed cutaneous leiomyosarcomas (atypical intradermal smooth muscle neoplasms) and arise from arrector pili muscles. Such tumors present as a nodule and most often arise in the trunk and lower extremities of middle-aged patients in the fifth to seventh decades, with a male preponderance (61,62). Like pilar leiomyomas, these lesions may be painful (61). Cutaneous leiomyosarcomas have a high rate of local recurrence (up to 20% to 50%), particularly if margins are involved in the excision specimen (61,63). Distant metastases are vanishingly rare (64), even when superficial subcutaneous involvement is present, leading some authors to refer to these tumors as "atypical intradermal smooth muscle neoplasms" (61). That being said, distant metastases have been reported in rare cases, particularly those with subcutaneous infiltration (65); therefore, we retain the designation "cutaneous leiomyosarcoma" for these tumors in daily practice to avoid confusion. The term "atypical intradermal smooth muscle neoplasm" theoretically also encompasses atypical (symplastic) leiomyomas. Although we prefer the designation cutaneous leiomyosarcoma for histologically malignant smooth muscle tumors arising in the dermis with only focal superficial subcutaneous involvement, when reporting such cases, we comment on the indolent behavior of most of these tumors and recommend reexcision with adequate follow-up.

Subcutaneous leiomyosarcomas, which arise from vascular smooth muscle and closely resemble deep-seated leiomyosarcomas (66), occur in slightly older patients (aged 50 to 80 years) and appear to affect each sex equally (65). Like cutaneous leiomyosarcomas, they have a predilection for the lower extremity (particularly the thigh) and present as a nodule, which may be painful (62). Subcutaneous tumors have an appreciably higher metastatic rate of up to approximately 50% (62). Common sites of distant metastasis are the lungs and skin (62), whereas lymph node metastases are rare. The 5-year survival rate is approximately 30% to 50%, with tumor size as an independent prognostic indicator (62,66). As with cutaneous leiomyosarcoma, local recurrence is common. Although cases in children are rare, examples have been reported (67).

Like cutaneous leiomyomas, leiomyosarcomas can occur in the context of HLRCC (68,69). An example of cutaneous leiomyosarcoma occurring in the setting of Li-Fraumeni syndrome has also been reported (70).

Although cutaneous metastases of sarcomas are rare, leiomyosarcoma is the most common source (~40% of cases in one large series) of sarcoma metastases to the skin (71).

Histopathology. Cutaneous leiomyosarcomas are typically ill-defined with an infiltrative border. Closer inspection reveals a neoplasm composed of fascicles of eosinophilic spindle cells (Fig. 35-11). Cytologic atypia and mitotic activity are generally readily detected (Fig. 35-12). If graded according to French (FNCLCC) criteria, most tumors confined to the dermis are grade 1. However, as tumor grade does not appear to influence the rate of recurrence, metastasis, or overall survival, we typically do not report histologic grade for cutaneous leiomyosarcomas limited to the dermis. Subcutaneous as well as metastatic leiomyosarcomas tend to be well circumscribed (Fig. 35-13), as opposed to those arising in the dermis but may have focally infiltrative borders. The FNCLCC grade is usually higher (65).

Myxoid stromal change can occur occasionally and may represent greater than 50% of tumor volume in rare cases (72). A subset of cases show epithelioid cytology (67,72). Rare examples of desmoplastic leiomyosarcoma with diffuse involvement presenting clinically as plaques have been reported (73). Such cases are characterized by subtle infiltration of thickened dermal collagen fibers by small bundles or single neoplastic

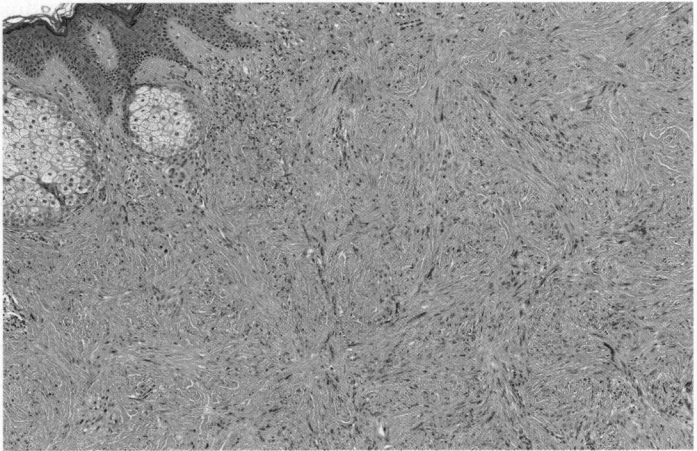

Figure 35-11 Cutaneous leiomyosarcoma. Scanning magnification of a cutaneous leiomyosarcoma showing infiltration of the dermis by intersecting fascicles of eosinophilic spindle cells. Cytologic atypia can be appreciated even at low power in this example.

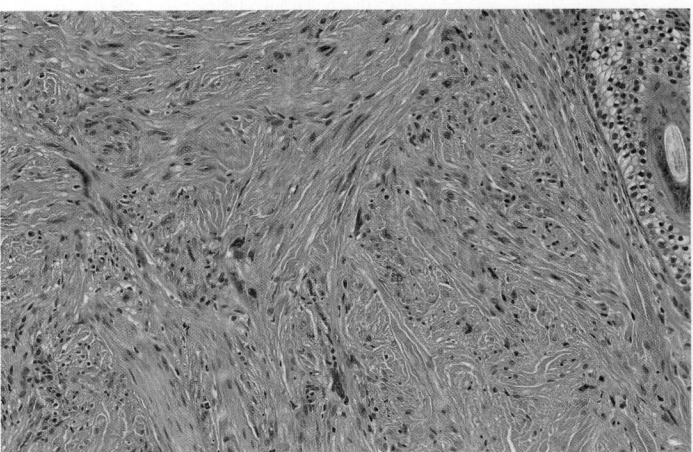

Figure 35-12 Cutaneous leiomyosarcoma. Higher magnification reveals that the tumor cells show nuclear pleomorphism with vesicular to hyperchromatic chromatin. However, occasional nuclei that resemble those of normal smooth muscle cells can occasionally be seen. Additionally, the tumor cells have abundant eosinophilic cytoplasm.

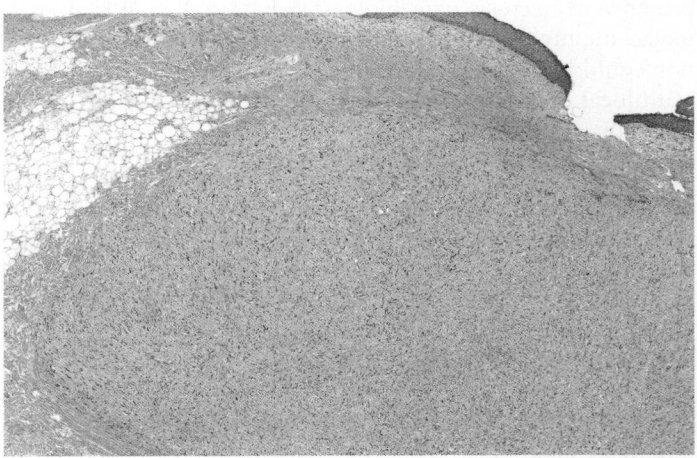

Figure 35-13 Subcutaneous leiomyosarcoma. Scanning magnification showing a relatively circumscribed subcutaneous mass.

smooth muscle cells. As with leiomyomas, mature adipose can be present in leiomyosarcomas (45).

In both cutaneous and subcutaneous leiomyosarcomas, atypical cytologic features include nuclear pleomorphism and hyperchromasia (Fig. 35-14). IHC shows expression of desmin and SMA in most cases, either diffusely or, less commonly, focally. Additional markers such as calponin or h-caldesmon are also often positive. Desmin is more specific than SMA but is not as sensitive. Cytokeratins and epithelial membrane antigen (EMA) are positive in approximately 30% to 40% of cases, which may be focal or extensive (63,67,74), representing an important diagnostic pitfall.

Vulvar and *scrotal leiomyosarcomas* tend to be larger and better circumscribed than cutaneous or subcutaneous leiomyosarcomas arising at other sites (25,28). Several different classifications exist for vulvar leiomyosarcomas. One scheme uses the following criteria to identify vulvar smooth muscle neoplasms with potential for adverse outcome: size greater than or equal to 5 cm in greatest dimension, presence of infiltrative margins, greater than or equal to 5 mitoses per 10 HPF, and the presence of moderate-to-severe cytologic atypia (27). Tumors that fulfill

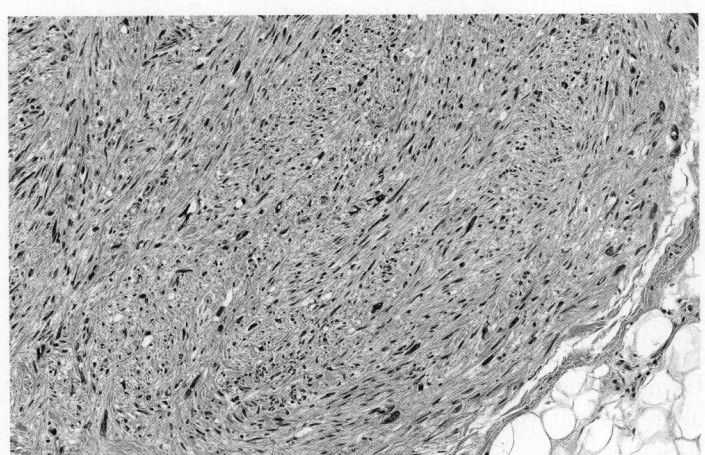

Figure 35-14 Subcutaneous leiomyosarcoma. Higher magnification reveals cytologic atypia with nuclear pleomorphism and hyperchromasia; however, tumor cells are arranged in well-formed fascicles and have brightly eosinophilic cytoplasm. Occasional mitoses are present.

just one of these criteria are classified as leiomyomas, whereas those that fulfill three or more are designated as leiomyosarcoma. Satisfaction of two of the criteria warrants classification as an atypical leiomyoma. Geographic tumor necrosis is not included in this classification scheme, but its presence would increase concern for malignant behavior. Although this classification system is widely used, a more recent small series suggests that vulvar smooth muscle neoplasms are better classified using criteria developed for uterine smooth muscle tumors as outlined in the most recent WHO classification of tumors of female reproductive organs (27,75), which includes assessment for degree of cytologic atypia, presence of necrosis, and mitotic count. Generally, when a tumor fulfills three criteria for malignancy, which include at least moderate cytologic atypia and 10 mitoses/10 HPF, it is classified as malignant (28). This scheme uses the terminology "smooth muscle tumor of uncertain malignant potential" (STUMP) for cases showing borderline histologic features.

Pathogenesis. Like pilar leiomyomas, cutaneous leiomyosarcomas are thought to arise from arrector pili muscles. Similarly, subcutaneous leiomyosarcomas are thought to arise from the walls of blood vessels. Leiomyosarcomas tend to have a complex karyotype (76), the most frequently occurring abnormalities being losses in the 13q4-21 region (77).

Differential Diagnosis. The main differential diagnosis of leiomyosarcoma is leiomyoma, which may contain degenerative atypia. Furthermore, pilar leiomyomas may show an infiltrative growth pattern despite otherwise benign histologic features. Interestingly, in a recent series, a benign diagnosis was rendered on an initial superficial biopsy in 7 of 25 cases, but on repeat biopsy that was deeper or larger, a malignant diagnosis was made, with higher-grade morphology seen in the deeper portions of the tumors (65). These observations further underscore the innumerable pitfalls of superficial biopsies. Leiomyosarcoma has also been reported arising in association with a symplastic leiomyoma (78).

Cellular dermatofibromas, which may show mitotic activity, membranous "tram-track" SMA immunoreactivity, as well as focal desmin positivity (79), typically show collagen entrapment at the periphery of the lesion, display a less uniform fascicular growth pattern, and lack the characteristic cytologic features of smooth muscle neoplasms. Leiomyosarcoma can also be confused for spindle cell melanoma, which typically strongly and diffusely expresses S100 protein and SOX-10. Spindle cell carcinoma is another potential histologic mimic, particularly because a subset of leiomyosarcomas exhibit keratin and/or EMA expression. Atypical fibroxanthoma and pleomorphic dermal sarcoma are common on the head and neck and often show "tram-track" SMA staining but are usually negative for desmin. Metastatic leiomyosarcoma in the dermis is typically well circumscribed with a smooth rounded border; however, clinical correlation is often needed to make the diagnosis.

Tumors with myxoid change may lack prominent fascicular growth, and subcutaneous tumors can thus mimic myxofibrosarcoma, extraskeletal myxoid chondrosarcoma, myxoid liposarcoma, or perhaps even malignant peripheral nerve sheath tumor with myxoid degeneration (72). However, in addition to maintaining cytologic features typical of smooth muscle differentiation, myxoid leiomyosarcomas generally retain expression of SMA, and a subset are reactive for desmin (72). The presence of recurrent translocations such as t(9;22)(q22;q12) *EWSR1-NR34A3* or t(12;16)(q13;p11) *FUS-CHOP* would support a diagnosis of myxoid chondrosarcoma (80) or myxoid liposarcoma (81), respectively. Moreover, additional sampling may reveal areas of more conventional histology (72).

Principles of Management. The mainstay of treatment for superficial leiomyosarcoma is wide local excision. Although seemingly adequate for cutaneous leiomyosarcoma, patients with subcutaneous leiomyosarcoma may benefit from adjuvant radiation treatment (64).

TUMORS OF SKELETAL MUSCLE

Rhabdomyoma

Clinical Summary. Rhabdomyomas are rare benign tumors of striated muscle. Most present in the deep soft tissues or heart. Extracardiac types are subdivided into fetal, adult, and genital types based on clinical and morphologic features. Fetal and adult types tend to arise in the head and neck of infants and young children and adults, respectively, while genital types occur in the genitalia of adults over a wide age range. Typically, these lesions are slow-growing painless masses (82,83). Primary cutaneous lesions are exceedingly rare.

Histopathology. Rhabdomyomas are typically unencapsulated nodular masses. Adult-type lesions are composed of large, polygonal cells with small nuclei and an abundant amount of eosinophilic cytoplasm and typically contain evidence of cross-striations (Fig. 35-15). The fetal type is composed of variable amounts of immature round to spindled rhabdomyoblasts set in a predominantly myxoid stroma. A so-called intermediate (juvenile) type shows greater cellularity, less stroma, differentiating rhabdomyoblasts, and a smooth muscle immunophenotype (Fig. 35-16) (84). Genital rhabdomyomas are small lesions (<2 cm) composed of loose connective tissue containing spindled, polygonal, and straplike rhabdomyoblasts (85). By IHC, constituent cells of rhabdomyoma are positive for desmin, myoblast determination protein 1 (MYOD1), myogenin, and muscle-specific actin. Desmin is typically strong and diffusely positive, whereas myogenin and MYOD1 may be focally so (86).

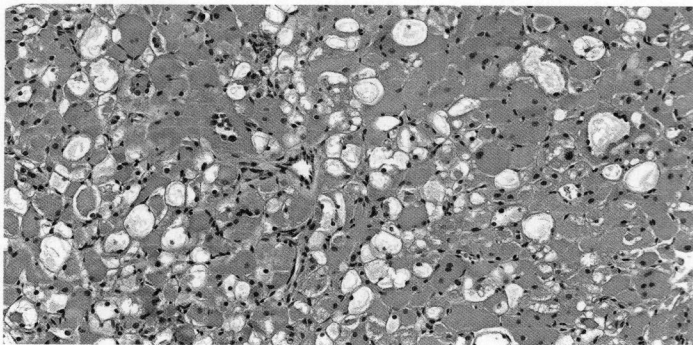

Figure 35-15 Adult rhabdomyoma. Scanning magnification shows large, polygonal cells with small nuclei and an abundant amount of eosinophilic cytoplasm. Evidence of cross-striations is focally seen.

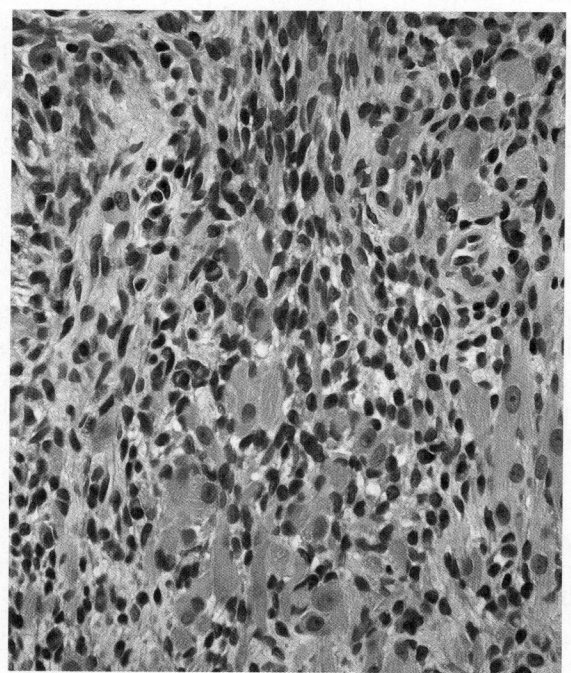

Figure 35-16 Fetal rhabdomyoma. High magnification reveals an example of an intermediate (juvenile) type rhabdomyoma containing cellular bundles of immature spindle cells with features of smooth muscle, a general lack of stroma and differentiated rhabdomyoblasts.

Pathogenesis. Syndromic and nonsyndromic fetal and a subset of adult rhabdomyomas show evidence of activation of the sonic hedgehog pathway by *PTCH1* and non-*PTCH1*–associated mechanisms, respectively (87). This activation has not been found in genital rhabdomyomas.

Differential Diagnosis. Adult and sometimes genital type rhabdomyomas may be confused with GCTs. The granular cytoplasm and S100 protein and SOX10 positivity of the latter allow distinction in difficult cases. Pleomorphic rhabdomyosarcoma has significantly more nuclear atypia and mitotic activity than rhabdomyoma. Nuclear pleomorphism, significant mitotic activity, and a cambium layer distinguish embryonal rhabdomyosarcoma (ERMS) from fetal-type rhabdomyoma.

Principles of Management. Most tumors are cured by simple excision. Recurrence may occur when excision is incomplete. Multifocal lesions may be seen in approximately 3% to 10% of adult rhabdomyoma cases.

Rhabdomyomatous Mesenchymal Hamartoma

Clinical Summary. Rhabdomyomatous mesenchymal hamartoma is an unusual, striated muscle proliferation that typically presents as a polypoid lesion arising in the periorbital and perioral regions of the head and neck of neonates. Cases arising in children and adults have also been reported (88,89). Lesions are typically a few millimeters to 1 to 2 cm in size. It is likely that this lesion is related to other rhabdomyomas. Congenital anomalies such as cleft lip or gum, bilateral sclerocorneas, retinal dysplasia, and amniotic band syndrome may occur in combination with these lesions (88).

Histopathology. Mature skeletal fibers are variably present in the dermis mixed with adipose, fibrous tissue, nerves, and adnexal structures (Fig. 35-17). Calcification or ossification may be seen in some cases.

Pathogenesis. The etiology is unknown, but hypotheses include a yet undiscovered genetic alteration or aberrant embryonic migration.

Differential Diagnosis. Adult-type rhabdomyomas also commonly present in the head and neck; however, they tend to be deeply seated and do not present as superficial polypoid lesions. Adult-type rhabdomyomas have more polygonal cells as well. Cutaneous ERMS is much less differentiated and more atypical.

Principles of Management. This is a benign lesion cured by simple excision.

Rhabdomyosarcoma

Clinical Summary. Primary cutaneous rhabdomyosarcoma is rare. It is important to rule out a metastasis before coming to this diagnosis. Like its deep tissue counterpart, there is a bimodal age distribution with male predominance (90). Alveolar and ERMS tend to affect infants and teenagers. Cutaneous embryonal rhabdomyosarcoma most commonly occurs in the head and neck region, whereas alveolar rhabdomyosarcoma (ARMS) in skin typically arises in the extremities. Pleomorphic rhabdomyosarcoma is the most common subtype in adults and also arises in superficial locations, particularly in the head and neck and extremities; rare cutaneous cases have been reported (91,92). Only very rare cases of epithelioid rhabdomyosarcoma

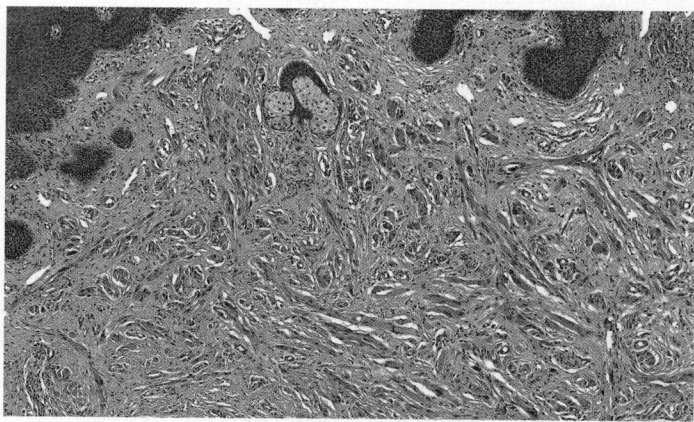

Figure 35-17 Rhabdomyomatous mesenchymal hamartoma. In this scanning photomicrograph, skeletal muscle fibers are variably present in the dermis mixed with fibrous tissue, nerves, and adnexal structures.

have been described in the skin, and these are also more common in the head and neck (93,94). Superficial presentation of epithelioid rhabdomyosarcoma may be more common than in other subtypes (94). The head and neck, followed by the extremities, are the most common sites for spindle cell/sclerosing rhabdomyosarcoma in adults. In children, these tumors arise most often in the paratesticular region, followed by the head and neck and other locations (95). The clinical presentation of rhabdomyosarcoma is not distinctive, apart from botryoid forms of embryonal rhabdomyosarcoma, which have a characteristic polypoid appearance with small clusters of pedunculated nodules abutting the epithelial surface. Most superficial rhabdomyosarcomas present as cutaneous or subcutaneous nodules or masses. In the most recent series of primary cutaneous rhabdomyosarcoma, children presented with embryonal and alveolar histologic subtypes, whereas adults presented with pleomorphic, epithelioid, or not-otherwise-specified (NOS) variants. Tumors ranged in size from 0.7 to 4.4 cm and were found on the head and neck, extremities, or trunk. The prognosis was generally poor; 4 of 11 patients died of disease, with an overall mortality rate of 36%; 6 developed metastases (90). Although they appear to behave aggressively, with metastasis and significant mortality reported for all subtypes, owing to their rarity, it is generally difficult to meaningfully compare the behavior of cutaneous and superficial rhabdomyosarcomas with their deep-seated counterparts. Metastases may also involve superficial sites and are generally a harbinger of poor patient outcome.

Histopathology. Histology is subtype specific. ERMS histology recapitulates cytologic and immunophenotypic features of embryonic skeletal muscle. Primitive cells in various stages of myogenesis are present. Tumors are composed of uniform round to spindled cells with minimal cytoplasm, and alternating cellular and myxoid zones are typically apparent (Fig. 35-18). Rhabdomyoblasts with polygonal to stellate to spindled morphology with abundant eosinophilic cytoplasm may or may not be present in a given tumor. Terminal differentiation in the form of cross-striations may also be seen. Poorly differentiated anaplastic ERMS contain large, markedly atypical cells with

hyperchromatic nuclei and bizarre mitotic figures. Botryoid tumors contain linear aggregates of tumors cells that tightly hug the epithelial surface, forming a "cambium layer." Some cases combine both embryonal and alveolar histology. ERMS are nearly always positive for desmin, but staining may be variable. Muscle-specific markers like myogenin and MYOD1 are essentially always positive, but the extent of staining is also quite variable (Fig. 35-19). Aberrant staining with keratins, S100, and neurofilament may be seen (96).

Alveolar rhabdomyosarcoma (ARMS) is composed of highly cellular sheets of primitive small round blue cells with a high nuclear to cytoplasmic ratio. Aggregates of cells form nodules that are delineated by fibrous septa. Discohesion of cells centrally leads to a "pseudoalveolar" pattern (Fig. 35-20). Multinucleated tumor cells are a common finding. ARMS are immunoreactive for desmin, myogenin, and MYOD1. Nuclear positivity for myogenin is strong and diffuse, unlike in ERMS. MYOD1 may be focal, and there may be expression of other

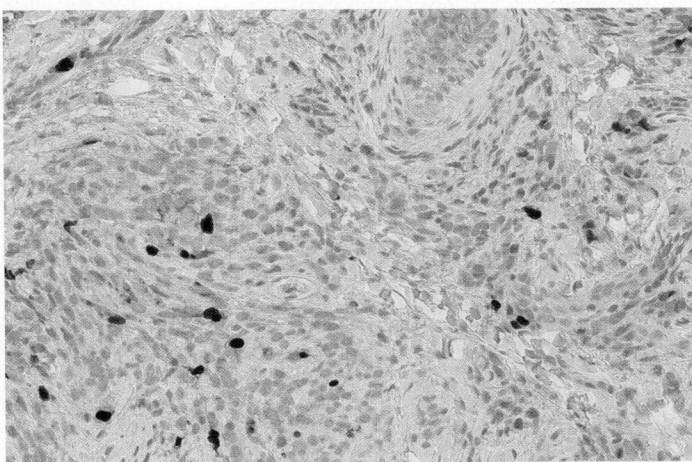

Figure 35-19 Embryonal rhabdomyosarcoma. Muscle-specific markers like MYOD1 are essentially always positive, but the extent of staining is variable and may be focal, as seen here.

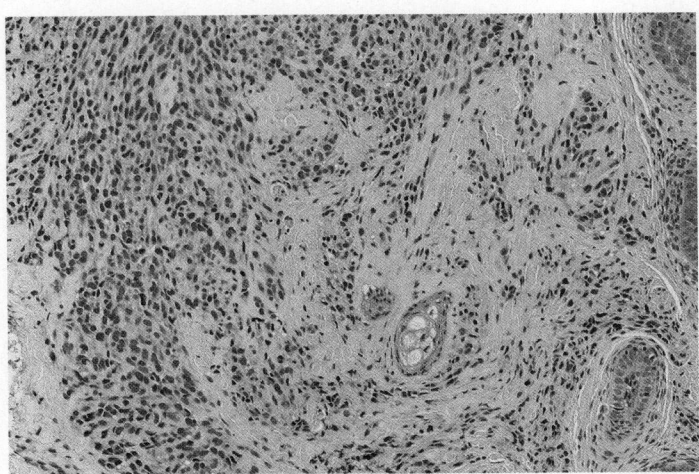

Figure 35-18 Embryonal rhabdomyosarcoma. This high-power view shows tightly packed, uniform round to spindled cells with minimal cytoplasm alternating with less cellular regions. Note the focal myxoid stroma.

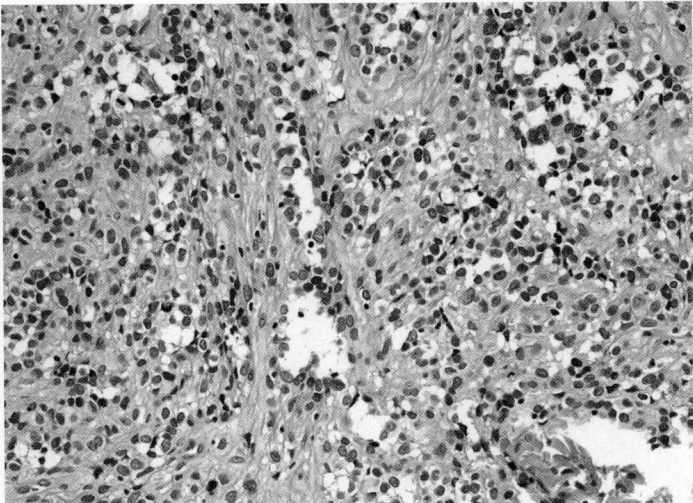

Figure 35-20 Alveolar rhabdomyosarcoma. High-power photomicrograph showing cellular sheets of primitive small round blue cells with high nuclear to cytoplasmic ratio. Nodules of cells are delineated by fibrous septa. Note central cellular discohesion resulting in a "pseudoalveolar" architecture.

markers such as keratin and neuroendocrine markers like synaptophysin, chromogranin, and CD56 (97).

Pleomorphic rhabdomyosarcoma is a high-grade sarcoma composed of sheets of large atypical often multinucleated spindled to rhabdoid cells with abundant eosinophilic cytoplasm (Fig. 35-21). These tumors are desmin positive and show only limited expression of myogenin and MYOD1 (Fig. 35-22) (98).

Epithelioid rhabdomyosarcoma displays sheetlike growth of uniform epithelioid cells with abundant eosinophilic cytoplasm and large vesicular nuclei with prominent nucleoli. There is only focal and at most mild nuclear pleomorphism (93). The histologic features are reminiscent of melanoma or carcinoma (Fig. 35-23). Coexpression of desmin, which is strong and diffuse, with a specific marker of skeletal differentiation, such as myogenin or MYOD1, allows distinction from these morphologic mimics. Similar to other rhabdomyosarcoma subtypes, focal positive staining with cytokeratins is a well-documented pitfall in the differentiation of epithelioid rhabdomyosarcoma from carcinoma (94).

Spindle cell/sclerosing rhabdomyosarcomas show variable histomorphology. Spindle cell rhabdomyosarcoma is composed

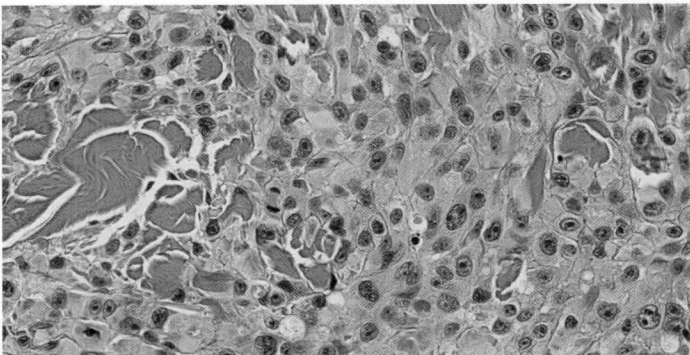

Figure 35-23 Epithelioid rhabdomyosarcoma. High-power view showing uniform epithelioid cells with abundant eosinophilic cytoplasm and large vesicular nuclei with prominent nucleoli. There is at most only focal nuclear pleomorphism. (Image courtesy of Dr. Steven Billings, Cleveland Clinic.)

of intersecting cellular fascicles of spindle cells. Constituent cells have pale eosinophilic cytoplasm with blunted, ovoid nuclei with centrally located small nucleoli (Fig. 35-24). There is significant mitotic activity, and nuclear hyperchromasia and pleomorphism are often seen. Straplike rhabdomyoblasts may be present in some cases. Sclerosing rhabdomyosarcoma has prominent hyalinization that may mimic osteoid seen in osteosarcoma. Tumor cells are arranged in cords, nests, microalveoli, or trabeculae in a pseudovascular growth pattern (Fig. 35-25). Varying combinations of these histologic patterns may be seen in any given tumor. By IHC there is diffuse expression of desmin in all cases and focal expression of myogenin. MYOD1 may be focal or diffuse in the spindle cell component but is usually diffuse in sclerosing areas (99).

Pathogenesis. A t(2;13)(q36;q14) translocation is found in most ARMS, resulting in a *PAX3-FOXO1* fusion, whereas a t(1;13)(p36;q14) translocation resulting in a *PAX7-FOXO1* fusion is seen in a small subset of cases. PAX3 and PAX7 are transcription factors involved in myogenesis (100). Embryonal rhabdomyosarcomas do not result from a single genetic event or driver mutation but from a combination of RAS pathway mutations and copy number alterations (101). Pleomorphic rhabdomyosarcomas have complex karyotypes with numerical and unbalanced structural alterations but no recurrent translocations (102). *TP53* is inactivated in pleomorphic rhabdomyosarcomas (103).

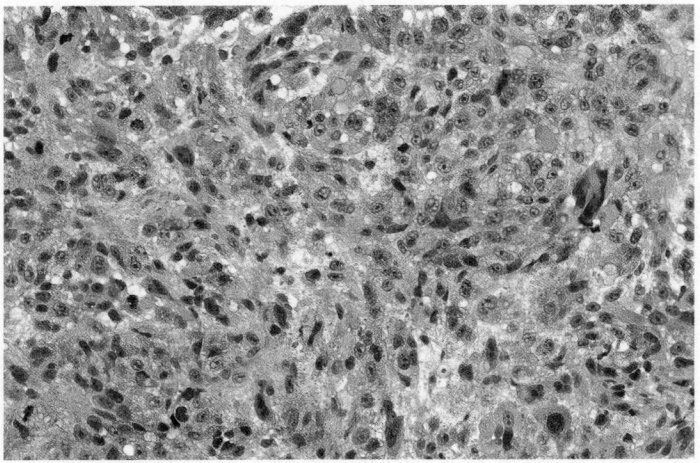

Figure 35-21 Pleomorphic rhabdomyosarcoma. This high-power photomicrograph shows a high-grade sarcoma composed of sheets of large atypical, sometimes multinucleated spindled to rhabdoid cells with abundant eosinophilic cytoplasm.

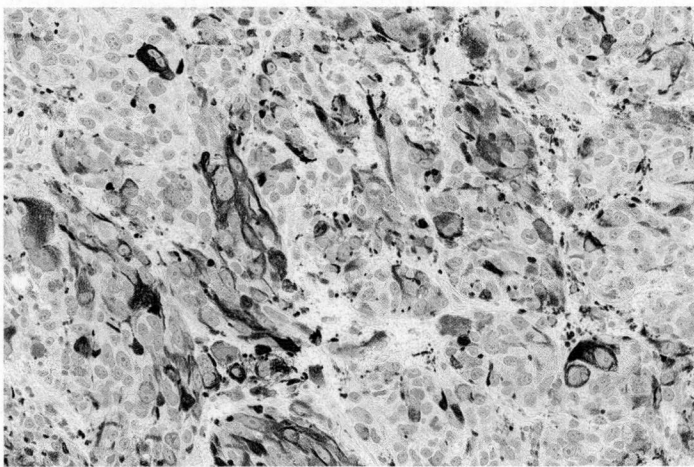

Figure 35-22 Pleomorphic rhabdomyosarcoma. As seen in this high-power view, these tumors are desmin positive. These tumors demonstrate only limited expression of myogenin and MYOD1.

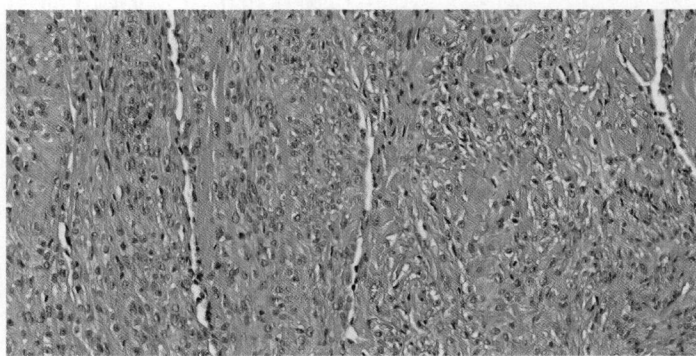

Figure 35-24 Spindle cell/sclerosing rhabdomyosarcoma. Spindle cell rhabdomyosarcoma is composed of intersecting cellular fascicles of spindle cells with pale eosinophilic cytoplasm and blunted, ovoid nuclei with centrally located small nucleoli.

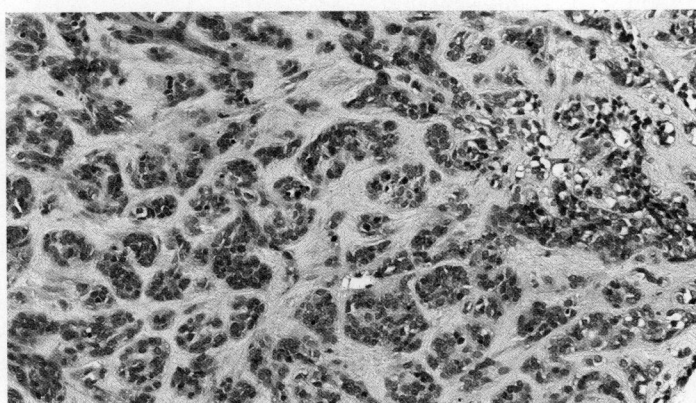

Figure 35-25 Spindle cell/sclerosing rhabdomyosarcoma. High magnification shows a sclerosing rhabdomyosarcoma composed of islands of atypical ovoid tumor cells arranged in cords, nests, microalveoli, and trabeculae in a pseudovascular growth pattern. Note the prominent background hyalinization mimicking the osteoid seen in osteosarcoma.

Epithelioid rhabdomyosarcoma is not currently acknowledged as a distinct subtype of rhabdomyosarcoma (RMS) at the time of this writing, but recent data have demonstrated that a subset of these cases are associated with *TFCP2* fusions, suggesting they may be separated into a distinct subgroup in the future (104).

Genetic abnormalities in spindle cell/sclerosing rhabdomyosarcoma are categorized into three groups. The first is congenital/infantile spindle cell rhabdomyosarcoma with *VGLL2/ NCOA2/CITED2* rearrangements (105). The second group, which comprises most cases of spindle cell/sclerosing RMS in adolescents and young adults as well as a subset in older adults, are characterized by *MYOD1* gene mutation (99). The third group of spindle cell/ sclerosing RMS has no identifiable recurrent genetic alterations.

Differential Diagnosis. The differential diagnosis depends on the subtype under consideration. Embryonal and alveolar RMS need to be differentiated from other small round blue cell tumors such as Ewing sarcoma, lymphoma, and neuroblastoma, among others. Ewing sarcoma is diffusely positive for CD99 in a membranous pattern and is typically negative for desmin. If it is positive for desmin, it is usually focally so. Ewing sarcoma is negative for muscle-specific markers MYOD1 and myogenin and demonstrates *EWSR1* rearrangement detectable by fluorescence *in situ* hybridization (FISH) or polymerase chain reaction (PCR). Depending on the type of lymphoma, there is positivity for CD45 and/or TdT, whereas desmin and other markers of muscular differentiation are negative. Pleomorphic and epithelioid rhabdomyosarcoma need to be distinguished from melanoma and sarcomatoid carcinoma. To complicate matters, rhabdomyosarcomas, in general, may be focally positive for cytokeratins. Addition of desmin to an immunohistochemical screening panel, followed by stains for myogenin or MYOD1, if there is strong desmin positivity, will distinguish pleomorphic rhabdomyosarcoma from sarcomatoid carcinoma. Identifying epithelioid rhabdomyosarcoma can be even more challenging. That being said, any melanoma or carcinoma with cytomorphology resembling epithelioid RMS would be expected to demonstrate strong and diffuse expression of melanocyte markers and cytokeratins, respectively.

Spindle cell rhabdomyosarcoma may resemble leiomyosarcoma or fibrosarcoma. Cutaneous leiomyosarcoma (atypical intradermal smooth muscle neoplasm) is typically composed of long intersecting fascicles of spindle cells with a moderate to extensive amount of eosinophilic cytoplasm and blunt-ended "cigar-shaped" nuclei. Primary cutaneous and metastatic leiomyosarcoma is diffusely positive for actins and variably so for desmin, and negative for more specific markers of skeletal muscle differentiation, such as myogenin and MYOD1. Fibrosarcoma arising in dermatofibrosarcoma protuberans (DFSP) is usually seen in association with classic DFSP. In difficult cases, immunoreactivity for CD34 and molecular demonstration of rearrangement of the *PDGFRB* gene locus is helpful for diagnosis. Fibrosarcomatous DFSP is negative for SMA and desmin. Of note, fibrosarcomatous DFSP may sometimes lose expression of CD34 (106). Infantile fibrosarcoma most commonly arises in infancy. This has a nonspecific immunophenotype with variable expression of actins, desmin, CD34, and S100. These tumors are frequently characterized by an *ETV6-NTRK3* fusion and are often positive with pan-TRK antibodies (107).

Spindle cell/sclerosing RMS with extensive hyalinization may mimic osteosarcoma owing to extensive matrix formation (108). Osteosarcoma lacks a diagnostically specific immunophenotype. SATB2 is a very sensitive marker of osteoblastic differentiation but is nonspecific. Histologic, clinical, and radiologic correlation is essential to differentiating osteosarcoma from its histologic mimics (109). It should be kept in mind that rare cases of true rhabdomyoblastic differentiation have been reported in melanocytic nevi, Merkel cell carcinoma, and other cutaneous carcinomas. A broad immunohistochemical panel should always be employed in order to distinguish rhabdomyosarcoma from its morphologic mimics.

Principles of Management. It is difficult to compare the clinical behavior of cutaneous rhabdomyosarcomas with their deep-seated counterparts owing to the rarity of the former. In general, they appear to behave aggressively, with metastasis and significant mortality reported for most subtypes (90,92,94,110). Congenital/infantile spindle cell/sclerosing rhabdomyosarcoma with gene fusions, however, appear to demonstrate a favorable clinical course (105).

REFERENCES

1. Zvulunov A, Rotem A, Merlob P, Aryeh M. Congenital smooth muscle hamartoma. *Am J Dis Child.* 1990;144(7):782–784.
2. Gualandri L, Cambiaghi S, Ermacora E, Tadini G, Gianotti R, Caputo R. Multiple familial smooth muscle hamartomas. *Pediatr Dermatol.* 2001;18(1):17–20.
3. Holst VA, Junkins-Hopkins JM, Elenitsas R. Cutaneous smooth muscle neoplasms: clinical features, histologic findings, and treatment options. *J Am Acad Dermatol.* 2002;46(4):477–494.
4. Jang HS, Kim MB, Oh CK, Kwon KS, Chung TA. Congenital smooth muscle hamartoma with follicular spotted appearance. *Br J Dermatol.* 2000;142(1):138–142.
5. Kim YJ, Roh MR, Lee JH, Na JI, Ko JY, Jung JM, et al. Clinicopathologic characteristics of early-onset Becker's nevus in Korean children and adolescents. *Int J Dermatol.* 2018;57(1): 55–61.
6. Torchia D. Becker nevus syndrome: a 2020 update. *J Am Acad Dermatol.* 2021;85(2):e101–e103.

7. Glover MT, Malone M, Atherton DJ. Michelin-tire baby syndrome resulting from diffuse smooth muscle hamartoma. *Pediatr Dermatol.* 1989;6(4):329–331.

8. Gagne EJ, Daniel Su WP. Congenital smooth muscle hamartoma of the skin. *Pediatr Dermatol.* 1993;10(2):142–145.

9. Atzmony L, Ugwu N, Zaki TD, Antaya RJ, Choate KA. Post-zygotic ACTB mutations underlie congenital smooth muscle hamartomas. *J Cutan Pathol.* 2020;47(8):681–685.

10. Cai ED, Sun BK, Chiang A, Rogers A, Bernet L, Cheng B, et al. Postzygotic mutations in beta-actin are associated with Becker's nevus and Becker's nevus syndrome. *J Invest Dermatol.* 2017;137(8):1795–1798.

11. Grillo E, Boixeda P, Ballester A, Vano-Galvan S, Gonzalez C, Jaén P. Congenital smooth muscle hamartoma on the face treated using vascular laser. *Pediatr Dermatol.* 2013;30(6):e250–e251.

12. Malik K, Patel P, Chen J, Khachemoune A. Leiomyoma cutis: a focused review on presentation, management, and association with malignancy. *Am J Clin Dermatol.* 2015;16(1):35–46.

13. Raj S, Calonje E, Kraus M, Kavanagh G, Newman PL, Fletcher CDM. Cutaneous pilar leiomyoma: clinicopathologic analysis of 53 lesions in 45 patients. *Am J Dermatopathol.* 1997;19(1):2–9.

14. Alam NA, Olpin S, Leigh IM. Fumarate hydratase mutations and predisposition to cutaneous leiomyomas, uterine leiomyomas and renal cancer. *Br J Dermatol.* 2005;153(1):11–17.

15. Tomlinson IPM, Alam NA, Rowan AJ, et al. Germline mutations in FH predispose to dominantly inherited uterine fibroids, skin leiomyomata and papillary renal cell cancer the multiple leiomyoma consortium. *Nat Genet.* 2002;30(4):406–410.

16. Alam NA, Olpin S, Rowan A, et al. Missense mutations in fumarate hydratase in multiple cutaneous and uterine leiomyomatosis and renal cell cancer. *J Mol Diagn.* 2005;7(4):437–443.

17. Grubb RL, Franks ME, Toro J, et al. Hereditary leiomyomatosis and renal cell cancer: a syndrome associated with an aggressive form of inherited renal cancer. *J Urol.* 2007;177(6):2074–2080.

18. Sanz-Ortega J, Vocke C, Stratton P, Linehan WM, Merino MJ. Morphologic and molecular characteristics of uterine leiomyomas in hereditary leiomyomatosis and renal cancer (HLRCC) syndrome. *Am J Surg Pathol.* 2013;37(1):74–80.

19. Straka BF, Wilson BB. Multiple papules on the leg. *Arch Dermatol.* 1991;127(11):1717, 1720.

20. Kim HJ, Lee M, Lee MG. A twist on piloleiomyoma: segmental cutaneous leiomyomatosis. *J Cutan Pathol.* 2016;43(11):1083–1085.

21. Stewart L, Glenn GM, Stratton P, et al. Association of germline mutations in the fumarate hydratase gene and uterine fibroids in women with hereditary leiomyomatosis and renal cell cancer. *Arch Dermatol.* 2008;144(12):1584–1592.

22. Merino MJ, Torres-Cabala C, Pinto P, Marston Linehan W. The morphologic spectrum of kidney tumors in hereditary leiomyomatosis and renal cell carcinoma (HLRCC) syndrome. *Am J Surg Pathol.* 2007;31(10):1578–1585.

23. Skala SL, Dhanasekaran SM, Mehra R. Hereditary leiomyomatosis and renal cell carcinoma syndrome (HLRCC): a contemporary review and practical discussion of the differential diagnosis for HLRCC-associated renal cell carcinoma. *Arch Pathol Lab Med.* 2018;142(10):1202–1215.

24. Kim GW, Park HJ, Kim HS, et al. Giant piloleiomyoma of the forehead. *Ann Dermatol.* 2011;23(suppl 2):144–146.

25. Newman PL, Fletcher CD. Smooth muscle tumors of the external genitalia: clinicopathological analysis of a series. *Histopathology.* 1991;18(6):523–529.

26. Devereaux KA, Schoolmeester JK. Smooth muscle tumors of the female genital tract. *Surg Pathol Clin.* 2019;12(2):397–455.

27. Nielsen GP, Rosenberg AE, Koerner FC, Young RH, Scully RE. Smooth-muscle tumors of the vulva: a clinicopathological study of 25 cases and review of the literature. *Am J Surg Pathol.* 1996;20(7):779–793.

28. Sayeed S, Xin D, Jenkins S, et al. Criteria for risk stratification of vulvar and vaginal muscle tumors: an evaluation of 71 cases comparing proposed classification systems. *Am J Surg Pathol.* 2018;42(1):84–94.

29. Hammer P, White K, Mengden S, Korcheva V, Raess PW. Nipple leiomyoma: a rare neoplasm with a broad spectrum of histologic appearances. *J Cutan Pathol.* 2019;46(5):343–346.

30. Matsuyama A. Angioleiomyoma. In: *WHO Classification of Tumours: Soft Tissue and Bone Tumours.* 5th ed. International Agency for Research on Cancer; 2020:186–187.

31. Hachisuga T, Hashimoto H, Enjoji M. Angioleiomyoma: a clinicopathologic reappraisal of 562 cases. *Cancer.* 1984;54(1):126–130.

32. Hammond MI, Miner AG, Piliang MP. Acral and digital angioleiomyomata: 14-year experience at the Cleveland Clinic and review of the literature. *J Cutan Pathol.* 2017;44(4):342–345.

33. Park IJ, Kim HM, Lee HJ. Re: Angioleiomyoma in the digit causing bony destruction. *J Hand Surg Eur Vol.* 2009;34(1):131–132.

34. Ishikawa S, Fuyama S, Kobayashi T, Taira Y, Sugano A, Iino M. Angioleiomyoma of the tongue: a case report and review of the literature. *Odontology.* 2016;104(1):119–122.

35. Orozco-Covarrubias L, Carrasco-Daza D, Julian-Gonzalez R, et al. Congenital cutaneous angioleiomyoma. *Pediatr Dermatol.* 2011;28(4):460–462.

36. Matoso A, Chen S, Plaza JA, Osunkoya AO, Epstein JI. Symplastic leiomyomas of the scrotum: a comparative study to usual leiomyomas and leiomyosarcomas. *Am J Surg Pathol.* 2014;38(10):1410–1417.

37. Llamas-Velasco M, Requena L, Kutzner H, et al. Fumarate hydratase immunohistochemical staining may help to identify patients with multiple cutaneous and uterine leiomyomatosis (MCUL) and hereditary leiomyomatosis and renal cell cancer (HLRCC) syndrome. *J Cutan Pathol.* 2014;41(11):859–865.

38. Llamas-Velasco M, Requena L, Adam J, Frizzell N, Hartmann A, Mentzel T. Loss of fumarate hydratase and aberrant protein succination detected with S-(2-succino)-cysteine staining to identify patients with multiple cutaneous and uterine leiomyomatosis and hereditary leiomyomatosis and renal cell cancer syndrome. *Am J Dermatopathol.* 2016;38(12):887–891.

39. Carter CS, Skala SL, Chinnaiyan AM, et al. Immunohistochemical characterization of fumarate cancer syndromes. *Am J Surg Pathol.* 2017;41(6):801–809.

40. McGinley KM, Bryant S, Kattine AA, Fitzgibbon JF, Googe PB. Cutaneous leiomyomas lack estrogen and progesterone receptor immunoreactivity. *J Cutan Pathol.* 1997;24(4):241–245.

41. Suárez-Peñaranda JM, Vieites B, Evgenyeva E, Vázquez-Veiga H, Forteza J. Male genital leiomyomas showing androgen receptor expression. *J Cutan Pathol.* 2007;34(12):946–949.

42. Kawagishi N, Kashiwagi T, Ibe M, et al. Pleomorphic angioleiomyoma: report of two cases with immunohistochemical studies. *Am J Dermatopathol.* 2000;22(3):268–271.

43. Sajben FP, Barnette DJ, Barrett TL. Intravascular angioleiomyoma. *J Cutan Pathol.* 1999;26(3):165–167.

44. Marco VS, Bosch SB, Almeida LV. Acral angioleiomyoma with tumoral calcinosis: a complication of the insertional Achilles tendinopathy. *J Cutan Pathol.* 2017;44(7):661–664.

45. Jones C, Shalin SC, Gardner JM. Incidence of mature adipocytic component within cutaneous smooth muscle neoplasms. *J Cutan Pathol.* 2016;43(10):866–871.

46. Beer TW. Cutaneous angiomyolipomas are HMB45 negative, not associated with tuberous sclerosis, and should be considered as angioleiomyomas with fat. *Am J Dermatopathol.* 2005;27(5):418–421.

47. Nishio J, Iwasaki H, Ohjimi Y, et al. Chromosomal imbalances in angioleiomyomas by comparative genomic hybridization. *Int J Mol Med.* 2004;13(1):13–16.

48. Welborn J, Fenner S, Parks R. Angioleiomyoma: a benign tumor with karyotypic aberrations. *Cancer Genet Cytogenet.* 2010;199(2):147–148.

49. Amezcua CA, Begley SJ, Mata N, Felix JC, Ballard CA. Aggressive angiomyxoma of the female genital tract: a clinicopathologic and immunohistochemical study of 12 cases. *Int J Gynecol Cancer.* 2005;15(1):140–145.

50. Mentzel T, Wadden C, Fletcher CDM. Granular cell change in smooth muscle tumours of skin and soft tissue. *Histopathology.* 1994;24(3):223–231.

51. Dobashi Y, Iwabuchi K, Nakahata J, Yanagimoto K, Kameya T. Combined clear and granular cell leiomyoma of soft tissue: evidence of transformation to a histiocytic phenotype. *Histopathology.* 1999;34(6):526–531.

52. Lespi PJ, Smit R. Verocay body-prominent cutaneous leiomyoma. *Am J Dermatopathol.* 1999;21(1):110–111.

53. Cook DL, Pugliano-Mauro MA, Schultz ZL. Atypical pilar leiomyomatosis: an unusual presentation of multiple atypical cutaneous leiomyomas. *J Cutan Pathol.* 2013;40(6):564–568.

54. Thompson JA. Therapy for painful cutaneous leiomyomas. *J Am Acad Dermatol.* 1985;13(5, pt 2):865–867.

55. Deyrup AT, Lee VK, Hill CE, et al. Epstein-Barr virus-associated smooth muscle tumors are distinctive mesenchymal tumors reflecting multiple infection events: a clinicopathologic and molecular analysis of 29 tumors from 19 patients. *Am J Surg Pathol.* 2006;30(1):75–82.

56. McClain KL, Leach CT, Jenson HB, et al. Association of Epstein-Barr virus with leiomyosarcomas in young people with AIDS. *N Engl J Med.* 1995;332(1):12–18.

57. Matin RN, Ieremia E. Cutaneous Epstein-Barr virus-associated smooth muscle tumor in immunosuppression. *J Cutan Pathol.* 2021;48(2):325–329.

58. Jonigk D, Laenger F, Maegel L, et al. Molecular and clinicopathological analysis of Epstein-Barr virus-associated posttransplant smooth muscle tumors. *Am J Transplant.* 2012;12(7):1908–1917.

59. Chang JYF, Wang CS, Hung CC, Tsai TF, Hsiao CH. Multiple Epstein-Barr virus-associated subcutaneous angioleiomyomas in a patient with acquired immunodeficiency syndrome. *Br J Dermatol.* 2002;147(3):563–567.

60. Petersson F, Huang J. Epstein-barr virus-associated smooth muscle tumor mimicking cutaneous angioleiomyoma. *Am J Dermatopathol.* 2011;33(4):407–409.

61. Kraft S, Fletcher CDM. Atypical intradermal smooth muscle neoplasms: clinicopathologic analysis of 84 cases and a reappraisal of cutaneous "leiomyosarcoma." *Am J Surg Pathol.* 2011;35(4):599–607.

62. Winchester DS, Hocker TL, Brewer JD, et al. Leiomyosarcoma of the skin: clinical, histopathologic, and prognostic factors that influence outcomes. *J Am Acad Dermatol.* 2014;71(5):919–925.

63. Kaddu S, Beham A, Cerroni L, et al. Cutaneous leiomyosarcoma. *Am J Surg Pathol.* 1997;21(9):979–987.

64. Wong GN, Webb A, Gyorki D, et al. Cutaneous leiomyosarcoma: dermal and subcutaneous. *Australas J Dermatol.* 2020;61(3):243–249.

65. Fauth CT, Bruecks AK, Temple W, Arlette JP, Difrancesco LM. Superficial leiomyosarcoma: a clinicopathologic review and update. *J Cutan Pathol.* 2010;37(2):269–276.

66. Jensen ML, Jensen OM, Michalski W, Nielsen OS, Keller J. Intradermal and subcutaneous leiomyosarcoma: a clinicopathological and immunohistochemical study of 41 cases. *J Cutan Pathol.* 1996;23(5):458–463.

67. De Saint Aubain Somerhausen N, Fletcher CDM. Leiomyosarcoma of soft tissue in children: clinicopathologic analysis of 20 cases. *Am J Surg Pathol.* 1999;23(7):755–763.

68. Wang C, Tetzlaff M, Hick R, Duvic M. Reed syndrome presenting with leiomyosarcoma. *JAAD Case Reports.* 2015;1(3):150–152.

69. Badeloe S, van Geest AJ, van Marion AMW, Frank J. Absence of fumarate hydratase mutation in a family with cutaneous leiomyosarcoma and renal cancer. *Int J Dermatol.* 2008;47(suppl 1):18–20.

70. Sabater-Marco V, Ferrando-Roca F, Morera-Faet A, García-García JA, Bosch SB, López-Guerrero JA. Primary cutaneous leiomyosarcoma arising in a patient with Li-Fraumeni syndrome: a neoplasm with unusual histopathologic features and loss of heterozygosity at TP53 Gene. *Am J Dermatopathol.* 2018;40(3):225–227.

71. Wang WL, Bones-Valentin RA, Prieto VG, Pollock RE, Lev DC, Lazar AJ. Sarcoma metastases to the skin: a clinicopathologic study of 65 patients. *Cancer.* 2012;118(11):2900–2904.

72. Rubin BP, Fletcher CDM. Myxoid leiomyosarcoma of soft tissue, an underrecognized variant. *Am J Surg Pathol.* 2000;24(7):927–936.

73. Choy C, Cooper A, Kossard S. Primary cutaneous diffuse leiomyosarcoma with desmoplasia. *Australas J Dermatol.* 2006;47(4):291–295.

74. Iwata J, Fletcher CDM. Immunohistochemical detection of cytokeratin and epithelial membrane antigen in leiomyosarcoma: a systematic study of 100 cases. *Pathol Int.* 2000;50(1):7–14.

75. Kurman RJ, Carcangiu ML, Herrington CS. *WHO Classification of Tumours of Female Reproductive Organs.* IARC Press; 2014.

76. Sreekantaiah C, Davis JR, Sandberg AA. Chromosomal abnormalities in leiomyosarcomas. *Am J Pathol.* 1993;142(1):293–305.

77. Derré J, Lagacé R, Nicolas A, et al. Leiomyosarcomas and most malignant fibrous histiocytomas share very similar comparative genomic hybridization imbalances: an analysis of a series of 27 leiomyosarcomas. *Lab Invest.* 2001;81(2):211–215.

78. Fons ME, Bachhuber T, Plaza JA. Cutaneous leiomyosarcoma originating in a symplastic pilar leiomyoma: a rare occurrence and potential diagnostic pitfall. *J Cutan Pathol.* 2011;38(1):49–53.

79. Volpicelli ER, Fletcher CDM. Desmin and CD34 positivity in cellular fibrous histiocytoma: an immunohistochemical analysis of 100 cases. *J Cutan Pathol.* 2012;39(8):747–752.

80. Hinrichs SH, Jaramillo MA, Gumerlock PH, Gardner MB, Lewis JP, Freeman AE. Myxoid chondrosarcoma with a translocation involving chromosomes 9 and 22. *Cancer Genet Cytogenet.* 1985;14(3–4):219–226.

81. Knight JC, Renwick PJ, Cin PD, Van Den Berghe H, Fletcher CDM. Translocation t(12;16)(q13;p11) in myxoid liposarcoma and round cell liposarcoma: molecular and cytogenetic analysis. *Cancer Res.* 1995;55(1):24–27.

82. Schlittenbauer T, Rieker R, Amann K, et al. Recurrent adult-type rhabdomyoma: a rare differential diagnosis of "swellings in the masticatory muscle." *J Craniofac Surg.* 2013;24(5):e504–e507.

83. De Trey LA, Schmid S, Huber GF. Multifocal adult rhabdomyoma of the head and neck manifestation in 7 locations and review of the literature. *Case Rep Otolaryngol.* 2013;2013:758416.

84. Kapadia SB, Meis JM, Frisman DM, Ellis GL, Heffner DK. Fetal rhabdomyoma of the head and neck: a clinicopathologic and immunophenotypic study of 24 cases. *Hum Pathol.* 1993;24(7):754–765.

85. Schoolmeester JK, Xing D, Keeney GL, Sukov WR. Genital rhabdomyoma of the lower female genital tract: a study of 12 cases with molecular cytogenetic findings. *Int J Gynecol Pathol.* 2018;37(4):349–355.

86. Mccluggage G, Longacre TA, Fisher C. Myogenin expression in vulvovaginal spindle cell lesions: analysis of a series of cases with an emphasis on diagnostic pitfalls. *Histopathology.* 2013;63(4):545–550.

87. Tostar U, Johan Malm C, Meis-Kindblom JM, Kindblom LG, Toftgård R, Birgitte Undén A. Deregulation of the hedgehog signalling pathway: a possible role for the PTCH and SUFU genes in human rhabdomyoma and rhabdomyosarcoma development. *J Pathol.* 2006;208(1):17–25.

88. Rosenberg AS, Kirk J, Morgan MB. Rhabdomyomatous mesenchymal hamartoma: an unusual dermal entity with a report of two cases and a review of the literature. *J Cutan Pathol.* 2002;29(4):238–243.

89. Lee Y-H, Yao X-F, Wu Y-H. Plaque-type variant of acquired rhabdomyomatous mesenchymal hamartoma on the chin. *Am J Dermatopathol.* 2021;43(12):908–912.

90. Marburger TB, Gardner JM, Prieto VG, Billings SD. Primary cutaneous rhabdomyosarcoma: a clinicopathologic review of 11 cases. *J Cutan Pathol.* 2012;39(11):987–995.

91. Kohashi K, Kinoshita I, Oda Y. Soft tissue special issue: skeletal muscle tumors: a clinicopathological review. *Head Neck Pathol.* 2020;14(1):12–20.

92. Watanabe M, Ansai SI, Iwakiri I, Fukumoto T, Murakami M. Case of pleomorphic rhabdomyosarcoma arising on subcutaneous tissue in an adult patient: review of the published works of 13 cases arising on cutaneous or subcutaneous tissue. *J Dermatol.* 2017;44(1):59–63.

93. Jo VY, Mariño-Enríquez A, Fletcher CDM. Epithelioid rhabdomyosarcoma: clinicopathologic analysis of 16 cases of a morphologically distinct variant of rhabdomyosarcoma. *Am J Surg Pathol.* 2011;35(10):1523–1530.

94. Feasel PC, Marburger TB, Billings SD. Primary cutaneous epithelioid rhabdomyosarcoma: a rare, recently described entity with review of the literature. *J Cutan Pathol.* 2014;41(7):588–591.

95. Chen S, Rudzinski ER, Arnold MA. Challenges in the diagnosis of pediatric spindle cell/sclerosing rhabdomyosarcoma. *Surg Pathol Clin.* 2020;13(4):729–738.

96. Morotti RA, Nicol KK, Parham DM, et al. An immunohistochemical algorithm to facilitate diagnosis and subtyping of rhabdomyosarcoma: the children's oncology group experience. *Am J Surg Pathol.* 2006;30(8):962–968.

97. Parham DM, Barr FG. Classification of rhabdomyosarcoma and its molecular basis. *Adv Anat Pathol.* 2013;20(6):387–397.

98. Furlong MA, Mentzel T, Fanburg-Smith JC. Pleomorphic rhabdomyosarcoma in adults: a clinicopathologic study of 38 cases with emphasis on morphologic variants and recent skeletal muscle-specific markers. *Mod Pathol.* 2001;14(6):595–603.

99. Agaram NP, LaQuaglia MP, Alaggio R, et al. MYOD1-mutant spindle cell and sclerosing rhabdomyosarcoma: an aggressive subtype irrespective of age. A reappraisal for molecular classification and risk stratification. *Mod Pathol.* 2019;32(1):27–36.

100. Buckingham M, Relaix F. Seminars in cell & developmental biology PAX3 and PAX7 as upstream regulators of myogenesis. *Semin Cell Dev Biol.* 2015;44:115–125.

101. Bridge JA, Liu J, Weibolt V, et al. Novel genomic imbalances in embryonal rhabdomyosarcoma revealed by comparative genomic hybridization and fluorescence in situ hybridization: an intergroup rhabdomyosarcoma study. *Genes Chromosomes Cancer.* 2000;27(4):337–344.

102. Li G, Ogose A, Kawashima H, et al. Cytogenetic and real-time quantitative reverse-transcriptase polymerase chain reaction analyses in pleomorphic rhabdomyosarcoma. *Cancer Genet Cytogenet.* 2009;192(1):1–9.

103. Hettmer S, Archer NM, Somers GR, et al. Anaplastic rhabdomyosarcoma in TP53 germline mutation carriers. *Cancer.* 2014;120(7):1068–1075.

104. Le Loarer F, Cleven AHG, Bouvier C, et al. A subset of epithelioid and spindle cell rhabdomyosarcomas is associated with TFCP2 fusions and common ALK upregulation. *Mod Pathol.* 2020;33(3):404–419.

105. Alaggio R, Zhang L, Sung YS, et al. A molecular study of pediatric spindle and sclerosing rhabdomyosarcoma identification of novel and recurrent VGLL2-related fusions in infantile cases. *Am J Surg Pathol.* 2016;40(2):224–235.

106. Llombart B, Serra-guillén C, Monteagudo C, Antonio J, Guerrero L, Sanmartín O. Dermatofibrosarcoma protuberans: a comprehensive review and update on diagnosis and management. *Semin Diagn Pathol.* 2013;30(1):13–28.

107. Davis JL, Lockwood CM, Stohr B, et al. Expanding the spectrum of pediatric NTRK-rearranged mesenchymal tumors. *Am J Surg Pathol.* 2019;43(4):435–445.

108. Mentzel T, Katenkamp D. Sclerosing, pseudovascular rhabdomyosarcoma in adults. Clinicopathological and immunohistochemical analysis of three cases. *Virchows Arch.* 2000;436(4):305–311.

109. Hasegawa TSHI, Hirose T, Kudo E. Immunophenotypic heterogeneity in osteosarcomas. *Hum Pathol.* 1991;22(6):583–590.

110. Tsai J-W, ChangChien Y-C, Lee J-C, et al. The expanding morphological and genetic spectrum of MYOD1-mutant spindle cell/sclerosing rhabdomyosarcomas: a clinicopathological and molecular comparison of mutated and non-mutated cases. *Histopathology.* 2019;74(6):933–943.

Tumors with Osseous and/or Cartilaginous Differentiation

Chapter 36

RYAN S. BERRY, STEVEN D. BILLINGS, AND BRUCE D. RAGSDALE

INTRODUCTION

In this chapter, tumors with osseous and/or cartilaginous differentiation are discussed in the context of their relevance to dermatopathology.

DERMATORADIOLOGY

It is axiomatic in dermatopathology that correlation of histopathology with the clinical configuration of skin lesions is the surest route to an accurate and therapeutically relevant diagnosis. Submission of clinical photographs with specimens is easier in the digital age. However, lesions covered in this chapter often appear merely as dome-shaped elevations of otherwise normal skin. For these, the best "clinical photo" is a radiologic study. It will depict depth and location that can narrow a differential diagnosis, identify adjacent structures at risk, size, character of margins that predicts biologic potential and the necessary extent of surgery, and the presence or absence of mineralization. Magnetic resonance imaging (MRI) more specifically predicts composition (fat vs. other soft tissue ± cystic change and necrosis). There are many syndromes with simultaneous skin and bone expression for which radiologic studies are part of the diagnosis. The adequacy of a biopsy can be checked against radiologic studies. Thus, correlation with available radiology can not only assist in the avoidance of misdiagnosis but also contribute to a more accurate diagnosis in dermatopathology (Table 36-1).

DIFFERENTIATION

In tumors, clonality does not always translate into morphologic uniformity. Although most sarcomas exhibit only one line of histologic differentiation, a minority may display a strikingly diverse phenotype. This phenomenon not only presents a diagnostic problem but also raises questions about the commitment of tumor cells toward a specific phenotype. Traditionally, the name of mesenchymal tumors is based on their most differentiated pattern, prognosis on the least differentiated. Even though it may be difficult to explain the pathogenesis of divergent differentiation, the variation illustrates that the phenotype of a tumor cell is not set in stone, but its direction of differentiation can be influenced (modulated) by a number of factors, particularly body location, character of the vascular supply, and signals from surrounding stromal elements.

CUTANEOUS OSSIFICATION

Cutaneous bone formation may be primary or secondary. If it is primary, there is no preceding cutaneous lesion; if it is secondary, bone forms through mesenchymal cell modulation within a preexisting lesion (metaplastic ossification). Primary cutaneous ossification can occur in Albright hereditary osteodystrophy (AHO) and as osteoma cutis. Aggressive, systemic forms of heterotopic ossification exist, generating lesions that often resist surgical treatment and produce a high rate of recurrence. These entities typically manifest during infancy as genetic syndromes such as fibro-osseous ossificans progressiva (FOP) or progressive osseous heteroplasia (POH) (1).

Albright Hereditary Osteodystrophy

Clinical Summary. In AHO (2,3), multiple areas of subcutaneous or intracutaneous ossification are often encountered in infancy and childhood, and their significance should not be overlooked, even in the normocalcemic patient. Early recognition of the skin manifestations of this syndrome and careful follow-up are important to prevent the deleterious effects of hypocalcemia. No definite area of predilection seems to exist; areas of ossification have been described on the trunk, extremities, and scalp. The areas of ossification may be so small as to be hardly perceptible or as large as 5 cm in diameter. Those located in the skin may cause ulceration, and bony spicules may be extruded through the ulcer. In addition to cutaneous and subcutaneous osteomas, bone formation may be observed in some cases along fascial planes.

AHO includes the syndromes of pseudohypoparathyroidism (PHP) and pseudopseudohypoparathyroidism (PPHP). Patients with the former condition have hypocalcemia with resistance to parathyroid hormone (PTH), whereas patients with the latter do not show resistance to PTH and have normal serum calcium levels. The term AHO is used when a specific phenotype is present: short stature, round facies, and multiple skeletal abnormalities. Brachydactyly, described as shortening of II, IV, and V metacarpals and I distal phalanx, is typically the most specific feature of AHO (4). As a result of this shortening, some knuckles are absent when the fists are clenched, and depressions or dimples are apparent there instead (the Albright dimpling sign). Additional manifestations include basal ganglia calcification and mental retardation.

Histopathology. Spicules of bone of various sizes may be found within the dermis or in the subcutaneous tissue. The bone contains numerous osteocytes as well as cement lines that are best

Table 36-1
Utility of Radiologic Studies in Dermatopathology ("Dermatoradiology")

1. Serves as the "clinical photo" for subsurface lesions that are otherwise merely dome-shaped elevations
   - Dermal, subcutaneous, and deeper lesions
2. To unequivocally demonstrate site of origin and extent
   - Subungual exostosis versus fibro-osseous pseudotumor (myositis ossificans) versus osteochondroma in a digit
   - Calvarial osteoma versus mineralized/ossified subcutaneous cyst and others
   - Intracranial extension of occult meningoceles and encephaloceles
   - Scalp hemangioma versus sinus pericranii
3. A cross-check on adequacy of biopsy sampling or removal
   - Diagnostic mineralized portions of soft tissue masses
   - MRI predicts tissue composition and degree of cystic change
4. To detect recurrence
   - Subcutaneous metastasis beneath a surgical site versus hematoma, foreign body, etc.
5. Ancillary evidence for diagnosis
   - Sarcoidosis (chest film), psoriasis (hip arthritis), congenital syphilis (periostitis)
   - Pachydermoperiostosis (thickened cortices), metastatic renal cell carcinoma (kidney tumor)
   - Sterile lytic bone lesions with palmoplantar pustulosis, acne fulminans, and Sweet syndrome
6. To diagnose syndromic associations
   - Maffucci syndrome
   - McCune–Albright syndrome
   - POEMS syndrome
   - Buschke–Ollendorff syndrome
7. An aesthetic dimension and confirmation of early cases
   - Calciphylaxis
   - Dystrophic mineralization in scleroderma

MRI, magnetic resonance imaging; POEMS, polyneuropathy, organomegaly, endocrinopathy, M protein, and skin changes.

revealed with a strong (e.g., Harris) hematoxylin or in polarized light. In addition, osteoblasts are usually aligned along the edges where new bone is being laid down. The osteoblasts that form bone in all forms of primary cutaneous ossification originate in preexisting fibrous connective tissue, and thus their product is termed *intramembranous* rather than *endochondral* bone. Osteoclasts, if present, are cells with multiple large nuclei resembling multinucleated foreign-body giant cells but are distinguished by their attachment to a bone surface. They excavate surface pits called *Howship lacunae* into the bone substance as the initial step in remodeling. Osteons with haversian canals containing blood vessels and connective tissue are produced through internal remodeling and indicate the passage of significant time. The spicules of bone may enclose, either partially or completely, areas of mature fat cells, which represent the maturation of the lesion with the establishment of a medullary cavity. Hematopoietic elements, however, are observed only rarely among the fat cells.

Cutaneous and superficial soft tissue lesions associated with AHO include osteoma, so-called plaque-like osteoma, calcifying aponeurotic fibroma–like lesion, calcinosis circumscripta–like lesion, and osteonevus Nanta–like lesion (5).

Pathogenesis. An autosomal dominant condition, AHO results from heterozygous inactivation of G(s) alpha, encoded by the *GNAS1* locus on the distal long arm of chromosome 20. Small insertions and deletions or point mutations of *GNAS1* are found in approximately 80% of patients with AHO (6). Other cases may be caused by large deletions, broad *GNAS* methylation defects, or isolated loss of methylation (6,7).

The incidence of cutaneous ossification in AHO is fairly high, with studies showing an incidence between 50% and 70% of patients (8,9). Although the conclusion that most cases of primary osteoma cutis are associated with AHO seems somewhat exaggerated, it is apparent that patients with extensive foci of ossification may have AHO.

The reason for the bone formation in AHO is not entirely clear. However, recent studies have suggested that a key role for G(s) alpha in bone is to regulate osteoblast differentiation by maintaining the proper balance between Hedgehog and Wnt signaling pathways (10–12).

Differential Diagnosis. POH is a rare autosomal dominant condition of mesenchymal differentiation in females characterized by dermal ossification during infancy and progressive heterotopic ossification of cutaneous, subcutaneous, and deep connective tissues during childhood (13). Recently, paternally inherited inactivating mutations in the *GNAS1* gene on chromosome 20q13 have been implicated in the pathogenesis, although sporadic cases have also been reported (14). POH can be distinguished from AHO by the progression of heterotopic ossification from skin and subcutaneous tissue into skeletal muscle, by the absence of morphologic features associated with AHO, and by the presence of normal endocrine function (15). The disorder can be distinguished from FOP by the presence of cutaneous ossification, the absence of congenital malformations of the skeleton, the absence of inflammatory tumor-like swellings, the asymmetric mosaic distribution of lesions, and the absence of predictable regional patterns of heterotopic ossification. Also, in FOP, cartilage production precedes ossification of deeper tissues (endochondral ossification), whereas the predominant pathway of bone formation in POH and AHO is intramembranous. Unlike FOP, which is caused by a recurrent activating missense mutation of the gene encoding the bone morphogenetic protein (BMP) type I receptor *ACVR1*, most cases of AOH are caused by alterations of *GNAS* (16).

Principles of Management: Patients with AHO should be referred to an endocrinologist if not already established with one, because calcium imbalances may be life threatening. From the point of view of the dermatologist, osteomas may be removed as medically or cosmetically indicated.

Osteoma Cutis

Clinical Summary. The term *osteoma cutis* is applied to cases of primary cutaneous ossification in which there is no evidence of a preexisting or associated lesion. It can present in a generalized or localized form. The underlying cause can be idiopathic or in the context of a hereditary syndrome.

The four groups of patients with osteoma cutis have osteomas limited in extent in all but the first group: (a) patients with *widespread osteomas* since birth or early life but without evidence of AHO; (b) patients with *single, large, plaquelike or platelike osteomas* present since birth or acquired later in life; (c) patients with *single, small osteomas* arising in later life in various locations; and (d) patients with *multiple miliary osteoma cutis (of the face)*.

Some instances of reported localized or widespread osteomas since birth, as well as familial cases, may represent unrecognized hereditary disorders related to parathyroid hormone (PTH) resistance and PTH signaling pathway impairment, given that many of these articles were published prior to recent molecular characterization and identification of new forms of PTH-related signaling disorders. Inactivating PTH/PTH-related protein signaling disorder (iPPSD) is the new term proposed for this group of disorders (17).

Multiple miliary osteoma cutis (MMOC) is a variant of osteoma cutis that can encompass both primary and secondary ossification, the latter almost always reported as acne sequelae. Most individuals are women with a median age of onset of 51 years. The facial skin is almost always affected (>90%), although extrafacial involvement is reported and appears to be more common in men (18). Germline or somatic mutations in *GNAS* have not been identified in a few individuals with MMOC (19).

Histopathology. The histologic findings in osteoma cutis are the same as those in primary cutaneous ossification occurring in conjunction with hereditary causes (Fig. 36-1). This bone is formed by the activities of flattened osteoblasts that appear to be derived through modulation from dermal fibroblasts. Both intramembranous and endochondral ossification may occur in skin, although the latter method is less common. A minority of the formative cells persist in the osseous product as resident osteocytes. Osteomas undergo a high rate of remodeling (20), enlarging by continued bone application on outer surfaces

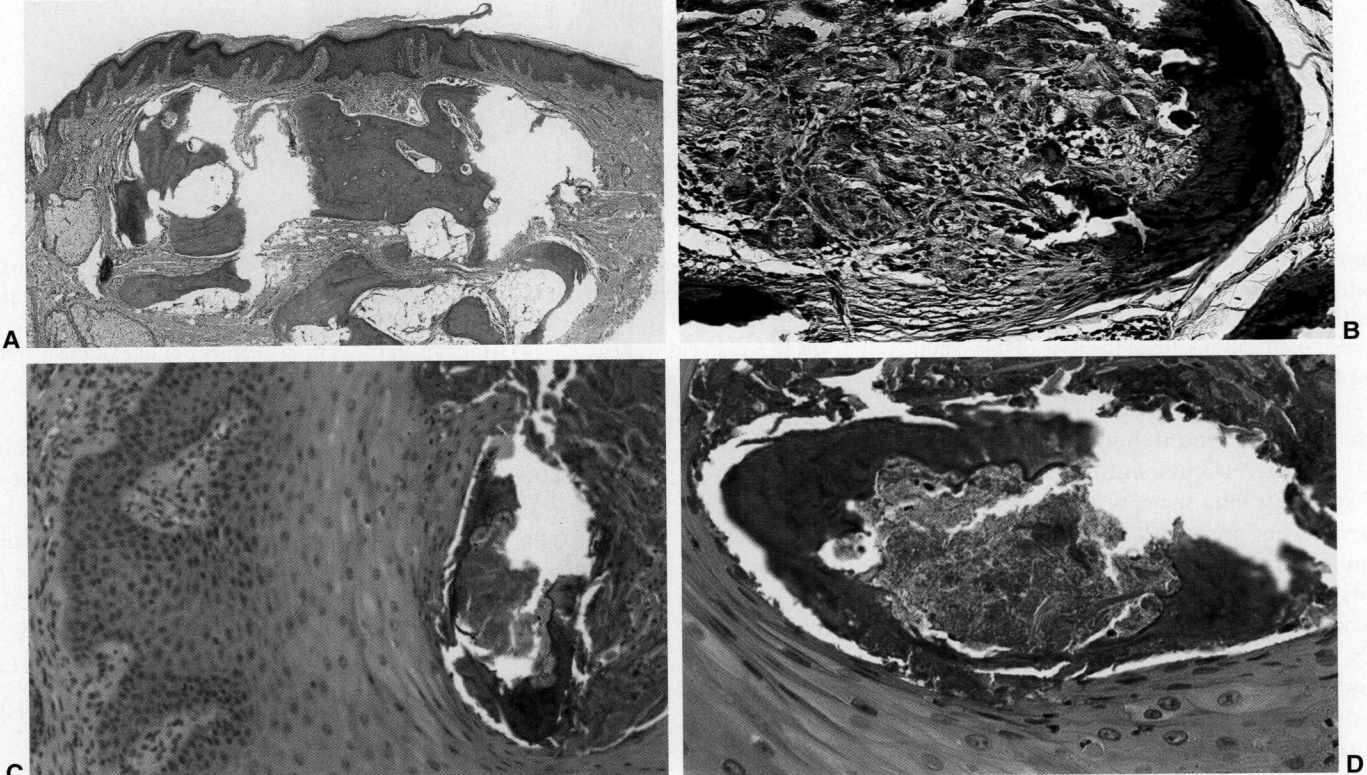

Figure 36-1 Osteoma cutis. **A:** Spicules of bone reside in the superficial dermis in this case. **B:** Exuberant osteoclasia is hollowing out this osteoma that occurred in a nevus (36-year-old woman; face). **C:** An epidermal-lined channel is evacuating a small osteoma, no longer in dermis (74-year-old man; toe). **D:** A high-power view of the osteoma from (**C**) depicts osteoclastic erosions (Howship lacunae).

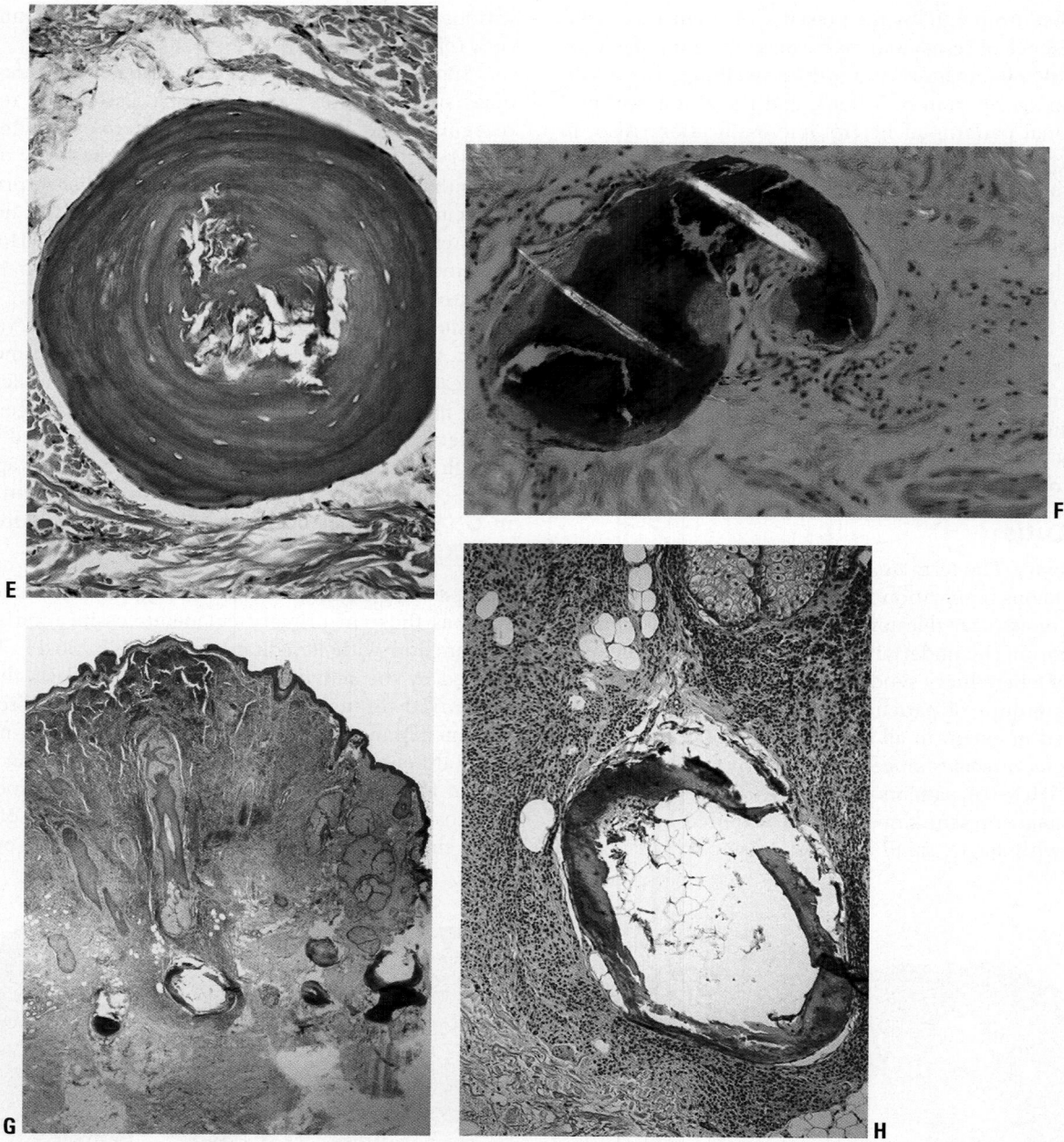

Figure 36-1 (*continued*) **E:** A spherical osteoma cutis has resident osteocytes in oval lacunae of its laminations about a central nidus of mature keratin flakes that were likely extruded from a follicle or cyst (80-year-old woman; shoulder). **F:** A polarized light view highlights two hair shafts crossing an irregular osteoma cutis confirming origin in the mesenchymal reaction following follicle rupture (70-year-old man; midback). **G:** Five rounded ossifications are in the base of this compound nevus (44-year-old woman; cheek). **H:** Fat is in the central chamber of one of the osteomas shown in (G).

with eventual central hollowing out by osteoclastic erosion (Fig. 36-1B). A circular outline is commonly achieved, with central space for fatty marrow and, rarely, trilineage hematopoietic marrow. They are at risk for all the disorders of genuine skeletal members. In cases with transepidermal elimination, some patients show fragments of bone within channels lined by epidermis and leading to the surface (Fig. 36-1C, D), as with a foreign body, and others show such fragments within breaks in the epidermis. When secondarily infected as after overlying ulceration, the differential diagnosis should exclude the possibility of a sinus tract draining an underlying osteomyelitis or septic joint.

Pathogenesis. In the genesis of osteoma cutis, it is posited that stem cells, which reside in all postnatal tissues, including the skin, can commit to an osteogenic lineage (21). BMPs,

hedgehogs, the transcription factor, core-binding factor alpha-1 (Cbfa1) and *GNAS*, play an important role in osteoblast differentiation and bone formation (22–25). Osteoblasts actively deposit type I collagen, forming osteoid, which then becomes mineralized by the deposition of calcium salts to become mature (lamellar) bone. A study analyzing osteoma cutis lesions demonstrated high levels of alkaline phosphatase activity and high expression of osteonectin and type I collagen mRNA (26).

Principles of Management: Osteomas may be removed as medically or cosmetically indicated.

Metaplastic or Secondary Ossification

Clinical Summary. Metaplastic or secondary ossification occurs within a preexisting lesion, such as a response to an inflammatory, neoplastic, or traumatic event. A simple prerequisite seems to be some antecedent relatively rigid substrate. Virtually any process that calcifies may secondarily ossify (27).

Histopathology. The histologic findings in secondary ossification are generally the same as in primary cutaneous ossification. However, there is often a secondary process associated with the ossification. Small, generally spherical spots of ossification within the dermis often start initially against a speck of amorphous mineralization or demonstrably around extravasated keratin debris (Fig. 36-1E), hair shafts (Fig. 36-1F), or in the stroma of another lesion such as a melanocytic nevus (Fig. 36-1G, H).

Metaplastic ossification occurs more commonly in benign neoplasms compared to malignant neoplasms. The most common benign neoplasm to show metaplastic ossification is melanocytic nevi (osteonevus of Nanta), followed by pilomatrixoma (calcifying epithelioma of Malherbe) (28).

In intradermal nevi, ossification usually follows folliculitis. In pilomatricoma, mineralization of shadow cells attracts osteoclastic giant cells. Osteoclastic erosion of mineralized epithelium is followed by ("coupled to") osteoblastic deposition of osteoid against remnants of the shadow cell islands. The process is therefore similar to endochondral ossification, wherein mineralized cartilage is the inducing factor and can lead to a fat-filled cancellous network with thin cortex resembling a normal rib cross section.

Although uncommon, malignant neoplasms of the skin may show secondary ossification. Basal cell carcinomas represent the majority, followed by squamous cell carcinoma and melanoma (28). Ossification takes place usually in the stroma but sometimes around mineralizing keratin microcysts. In some cases of malignant melanoma (29,30), heterotopic bone formed in areas of desmoplastic melanoma with previous procedure site changes, suggests a relationship between desmoplasia, trauma, and bone formation. *Osteogenic melanoma* is the term applied to this rare variant of malignant melanoma, which has a predilection for acral sites (31,32).

The list of secondary lesions associated with metaplastic ossification is continually growing in the medical literature, some of which include scars (especially abdominal wounds) (33), burns (34), venous stasis (Fig. 36-2), nephrogenic systemic fibrosis (35), cutis laxa–like pseudoxanthoma elasticum (36), and in inflammatory processes of the skin such as morphea, systemic scleroderma, dermatomyositis.

Principles of Management: Metaplastic ossification is usually found when the lesion itself is biopsied or removed. Decision-making for complete excision depends on the associated neoplasm.

CUTANEOUS CHONDRO-OSSEOUS LESIONS

Extraskeletal osseous and cartilaginous tumors and tumor-like conditions of the extremities such as subungual exostosis can often be differentiated radiologically; for those that cannot, knowledge of the spectrum of lesions will allow for a suitably ordered differential diagnosis. Of these lesions (myositis ossificans, subungual exostosis, fibro-osseous pseudotumor of the digit, fibrodysplasia [myositis] ossificans progressiva [FOP], and extraskeletal osteosarcoma), all but myositis ossificans and subungual exostosis are relatively rare. Although many of the previously mentioned entities were once considered reactive, recent molecular-genetic evidence has identified recurrent genetic alterations (discussed later), indicating that some of these represent self-limited clonal neoplasms. The differential diagnosis for these extraskeletal osseous and cartilaginous lesions includes soft tissue sarcoma, calcified tophi in gout, melorheostosis, pilomatricoma, and tumoral calcinosis (37).

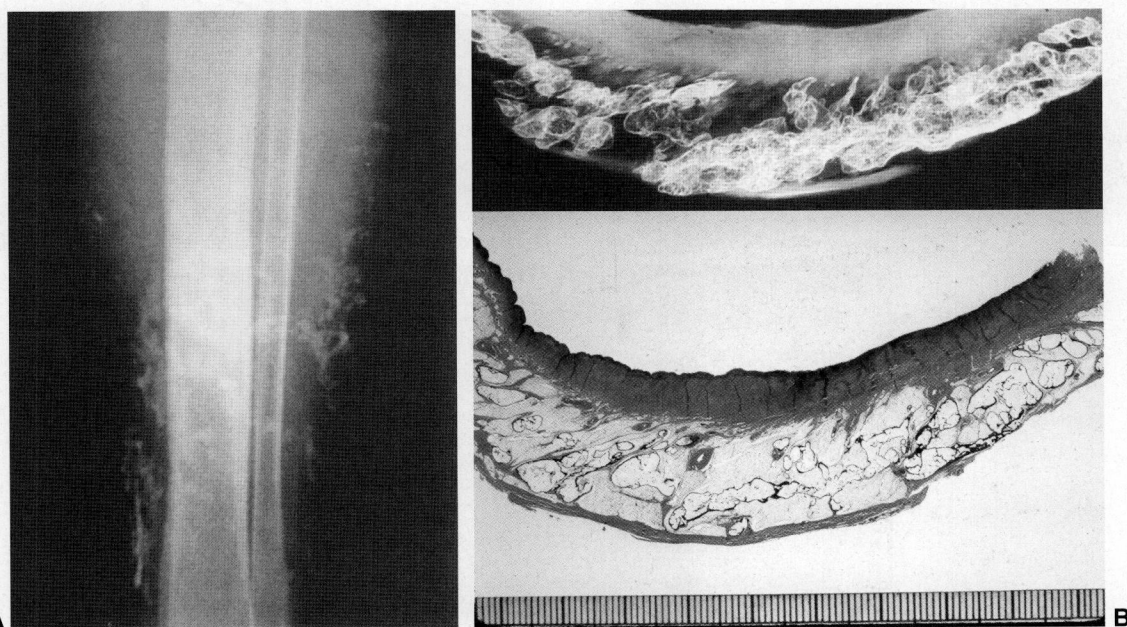

Figure 36-2 Heterotopic subcutaneous ossification associated with chronic venous stasis (60-year-old woman; chronic venous stasis of lower legs). **A:** In this plain film radiograph, irregular bony deposits unrelated to veins occur in the absence of fat necrosis or abnormal serum calcium or phosphorus. **B:** A specimen radiograph (**top**) correlates well with the distribution of irregular lobulated ossific plates in and around subcutaneous fat in the large format histologic section (**bottom**). The ossification has taken place in interlobular septa. In the histologic view, fibrosis markedly thickens dermis. Thick-walled veins of venous incompetency are in subcutaneous fat (e.g., **left of center**).

Myositis Ossificans and Related Entities

Clinical Summary. Myositis ossificans (Fig. 36-3) is a benign, solitary, self-limiting, ossifying soft tissue lesion generally occurring in skeletal muscle but also arising in other tissues such as tendons and subcutaneous adipose (*panniculitis ossificans*). It is generally thought to occur as a posttraumatic event, although a history of trauma is not always present. Young, active adolescent and adult males are most commonly affected (38), whereas it is relatively rare in small children (39). Radiologic findings depend on the modality used and duration of the lesion. In its mature phase (around 6 to 8 weeks) it has a characteristic radiologic appearance of a mass with a peripheral rim of radiodensity, correlating with the more mature bony parts of the lesion, surrounding a relatively radiolucent less well-vascularized cellular center (38,40).

Subungual exostosis (Fig. 36-4) is a common benign bony projection that occurs on a distal phalanx, beneath or beside the nail, often leading to nail deformity (41,42). It has also been reported as *subungual osteochondroma*, a term correctly applied only to the anomalous tumor forming on the surface of metaphyseal portions of long bones in adolescents and young adults (43–45). The great toe is the most common site, but other toes and fingers can also be affected. Although the bony addition usually measures only a few millimeters in diameter, swelling of the entire distal phalanx makes it look larger, possibly with ulceration that is often misdiagnosed as an infected ingrown nail. There is frequently an association with trauma (46). Radiographs reveal a bony projection from the edge of the terminal phalangeal tuft (Fig. 36-4A) and are indispensable in avoiding

assigning an incorrect alternative diagnosis (47). The length and radiologic density are proportional to duration.

Fibro-osseous pseudotumor of the digits (FOPT) is a heterotopic ossification closely related to myositis ossificans. It presents as a painful, localized swelling in the soft tissues of digits, most often the proximal portions of the index or middle finger. The peak incidence is during the third and fourth decades of life (48–50). Radiographs of early lesions show an ill-defined soft tissue mass attached to bone surface with varying amounts of calcification.

Bizarre parosteal osteochondromatous proliferation (BPOP), first described by Nora et al. (51), is an uncommon process involving the small bones of the hands and, less commonly, the long bones (52). There is no significant sex predilection, and patients range from children to elder adults. Radiologically, the lesion is heavily calcified and attached to the underlying cortex by a broad base.

Soft tissue aneurysmal bone cysts (ABC) typically arise in the deep soft tissue of extremities (53) but may also present in skin (54). ABC is a well-circumscribed tumor with blood-filled, cystic spaces with associated fibrous septa that are frequently associated with woven bone. Within the septa are fibroblasts, osteoclasts, and siderophages. ABC is associated with rearrangements of *USP6*, like myositis ossificans.

Button osteomas are benign, slow-growing lesions that present as small, circumscribed growths on calvarial and mandibular surfaces. They are generally biopsied by a dermatologist under a preoperative diagnosis of (palpable) "cyst." They are common in modern (38%) and archaeologic (41%) populations

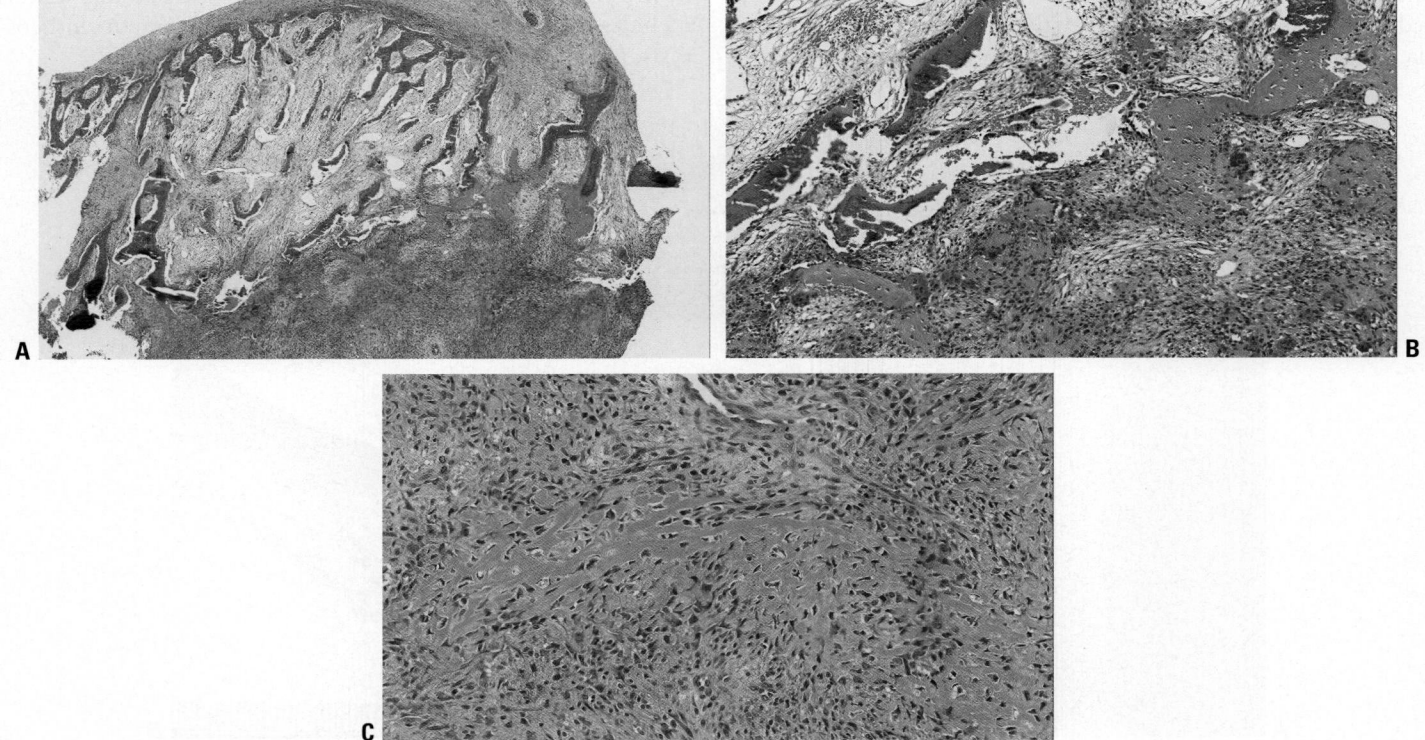

Figure 36-3 Myositis ossificans. **A:** Low-power view showing the zonal pattern characterized by central (**bottom**) immature, fibroblastic/myofibroblastic tissue resembling nodular fasciitis, an intermediate zone where cells are intimately associated with immature bone and osteoid, and peripheral zone (**top**) showing mature lamellar bone. **B:** High-power view of the intermediated zone (**top**) and the central nodular fasciitis–like zone (**bottom**). **C:** Osteoid-like area in the intermediate zone showing a cellular proliferation of cells, which could be mistaken for a malignant process to the undiscerning eye.

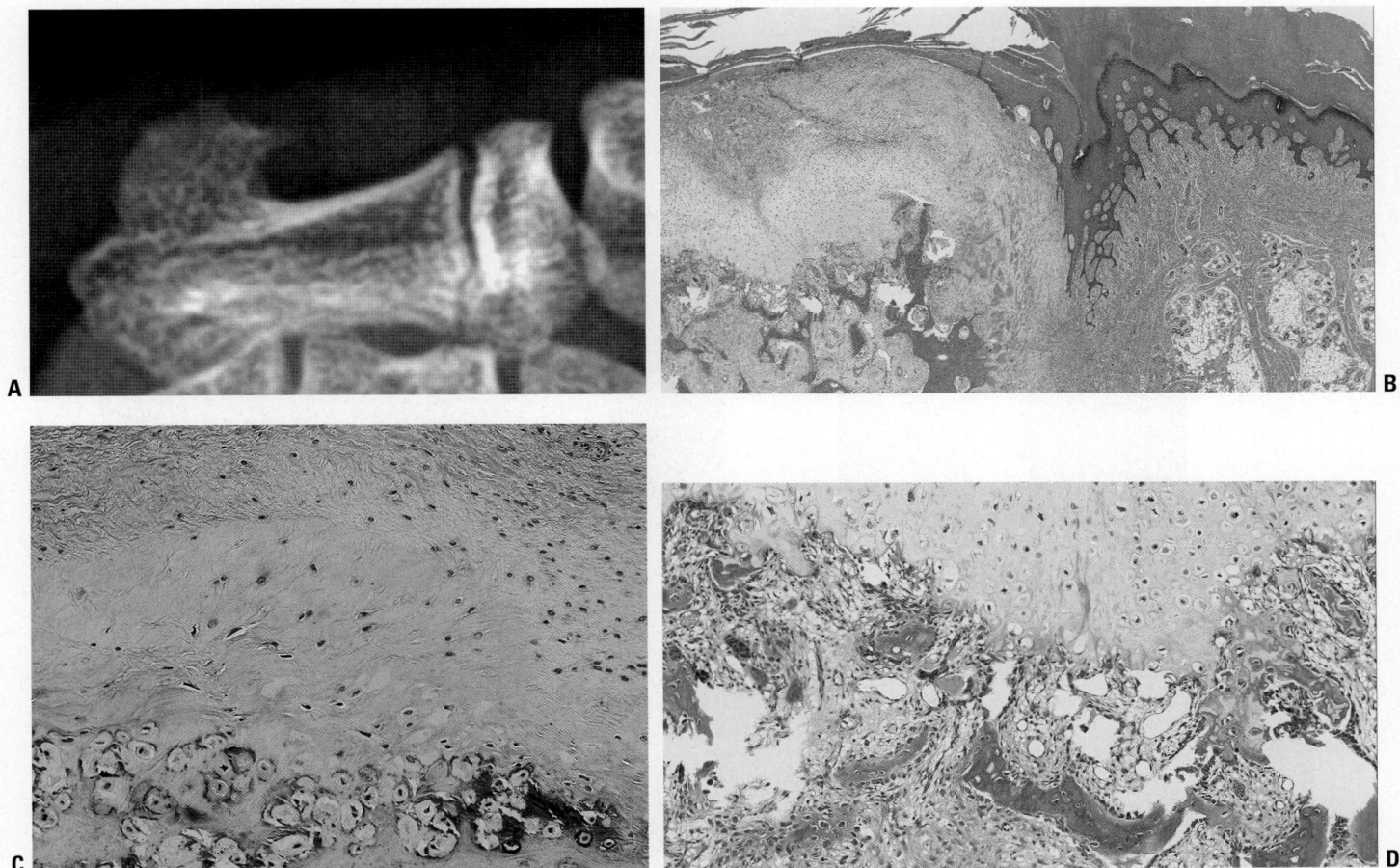

Figure 36-4 Subungual exostosis (12-year-old girl with a painful deformed left hallux nail). **A:** A cancellous stalk in this plain film radiograph extends from intact cortex of the tuft of terminal phalanx beneath the nail. A true osteocartilaginous exostosis (osteochondroma) would attach to the metaphyseal (more proximal) region of the phalanx, not to the tip, and cortex would reflect up its sides, not the picture here. **B:** The excised exostosis was a cartilaginous cap (**top**) overlying the cancellous bony stalk built by enchondral ossification. **C:** The earliest stage in the progressive enlargement of a subungual exostosis is the elaboration of myxoid material between dermal fibroblasts (**top**). With time, the myxoid material assumes the solidity of cartilage, and the intervening cells occupy lacunae within it (**bottom**). **D:** Deletion of cartilage by osteoclastic erosion and substitution of bone follows.

and correlate with age (55). In one-third of cases, there are two or more. Multiple osteomas of this type may be associated with an underlying hereditary condition such as familial adenomatous polyposis (Gardner syndrome) (56).

Histopathology. Myositis ossificans (Fig. 36-3) and its subcutaneous counterpart, *panniculitis ossificans*, portray a cellular, mitotically active spindle cell proliferation in the early growth phase but lack the abnormal mitoses and extreme pleomorphism of malignancy and manifest uniform nuclear chromaticity. Later, greater density and maturity of the bony product in the periphery around the still disturbingly cellular central zones affords less of a diagnostic challenge because it has the reverse architecture of soft tissue osteosarcoma and would not be seen in nodular fasciitis. Rarely, cartilage undergoing endochondral ossification, reminiscent of fracture callus, may be present.

Myositis ossificans can contain areas resembling *ABC* (57), including hemorrhagic cysts lined by fibrous septa containing fibroblasts, osteoclast-like giant cells, and chronic inflammatory cells, as well as foci of woven bone with matrix calcification ("blue bone"). If the entire lesion shows such features, it may be classified as an ABC.

The earliest change in an *exostosis* (Fig. 36-4B) is mucopolysaccharide and osteoid elaboration by periosteum and

modulated fibroblasts in the closely approximated contiguous dermis (Fig. 36-4C), eventuating in a gradational continuum of chondroid (Fig. 36-4D) and osteoid that can be alarmingly cellular. As the cartilage achieves solid qualities, it becomes focally eroded along its deep surface by osteoclastic giant cells, followed immediately by endochondral bone deposition on any chondral remnant. In this way, a cancellous bony stalk is built out from original cortex at the expense of cartilage. The process continues, aggravated perhaps from ongoing irritation by footwear, inducing new fibrocartilaginous cap substance.

Besides position on the bone (terminal tuft vs. proximal metaphyseal portion) as revealed in a plane film radiography, the major difference between subungual exostosis and *subungual osteochondroma* is the composition of the cartilaginous cap. Although both enlarge their bony stalk by endochondral growth, the cartilaginous cap in subungual exostosis is composed of fibrocartilage, whereas the cartilaginous cap of osteochondroma is composed of hyaline cartilage, with a cell configuration similar to that of a normal growing epiphysis. In the center of both entities, endochondral ossification is found as well as trabecular bone with osteocytes, osteoblasts, and occasionally hematopoietic cells (43).

FOPT (Fig. 36-5) closely resembles myositis ossificans histopathologically but may show an irregular multinodular

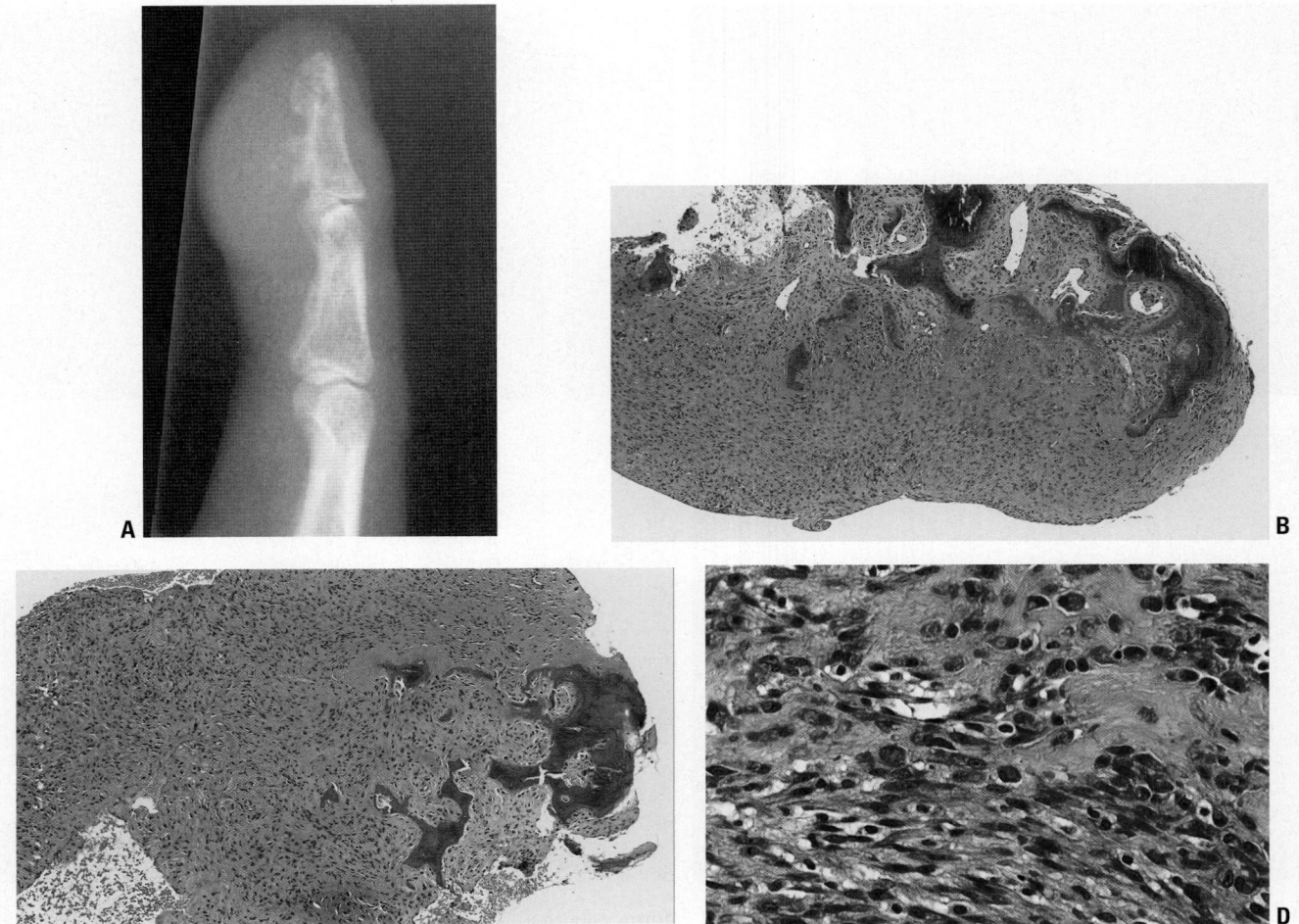

Figure 36-5 Fibro-osseous pseudotumor of digit (42-year-old man; rapidly enlarging fingertip with no recalled history of trauma). **A:** The terminal phalange of the fifth finger in this plain film radiograph has undergone bulbous enlargement and has some internal ossific density that may extend partly from the periosteal surface. **B:** A chaotic pattern of osteoid is emerging in an active spindle cell background. **C:** This highly cellular lesion has basophilic mineralization of part of the osteoid product (**right**). **D:** The cellularity lacks the pleomorphism, hyperchromasia, and abnormal mitoses of osteosarcoma.

growth with a less significant zonal organization (mature woven bone located peripherally and immature woven bone centrally) than seen in myositis ossificans (49,50,58).

BPOP similarly shows overlapping histopathologic features with MO and FOPT. However, the presence of cartilage formation is a prerequisite for the diagnosis of BPOP, which is less commonly present in MO. A zonal architecture is often apparent at low magnification with central or basally located new bone surrounded by a peripheral cap of cartilage. The cartilage often shows areas of hypercellularity, and enlarged, bizarre, and binucleated chondrocytes, which may result in misinterpretation of malignancy. The cartilage undergoes endochondral ossification, producing bone with a characteristic dark blue tinctorial quality (52).

Button osteomas display a macro- and microstructure with parallel lamella of compact bone, sometimes partly haversianized and best appreciated under polarized light (Fig. 36-6).

Pathogenesis. The pathogenesis of *myositis ossificans* and related lesions is still not fully understood. Historically, traumatic injury was believed to be the inciting event resulting in an exuberant, fibroblastic/myofibroblastic proliferation that eventually leads to ossification. However, *USP6* gene rearrangements, first identified in *skeletal aneurysmal bone cyst* (59) and *nodular fasciitis*

(60), have also been detected in *myositis ossificans* (61,62), and *fibro-osseous pseudotumor of digits* (63), suggesting a biologic relationship and clonal neoplastic nature of the entities.

BPOP, similar to MO and related lesions, was thought to represent a reactive process, potentially to prior trauma. However, identification of recurrent chromosomal translocation t(1;17) (q32;q21) or inv(7), supports this representing a self-limited benign neoplasm (64,65).

The demographic characteristics of *button osteomas,* mainly the high frequency among ancient and modern populations, their independence of sex and race, and scarcity in other primates, favor a hamartoma and not a neoplastic osteoma, although posttraumatic exostosis remains an attractive hypothesis.

Differential Diagnosis. A differential diagnosis of these lesions includes extraskeletal osteosarcoma, periosteal and parosteal osteosarcoma, periosteal chondroma, and osteomyelitis. *Myositis ossificans* and its subcutaneous counterpart, *panniculitis ossificans,* in early postinjury stages can mimic a cellular, mitotically active spindle cell sarcoma in its early posttrauma growth but lack the abnormal mitoses and extreme pleomorphism of malignancy manifesting uniform nuclear chromaticity.

Principles of Management: The treatment is surgical.

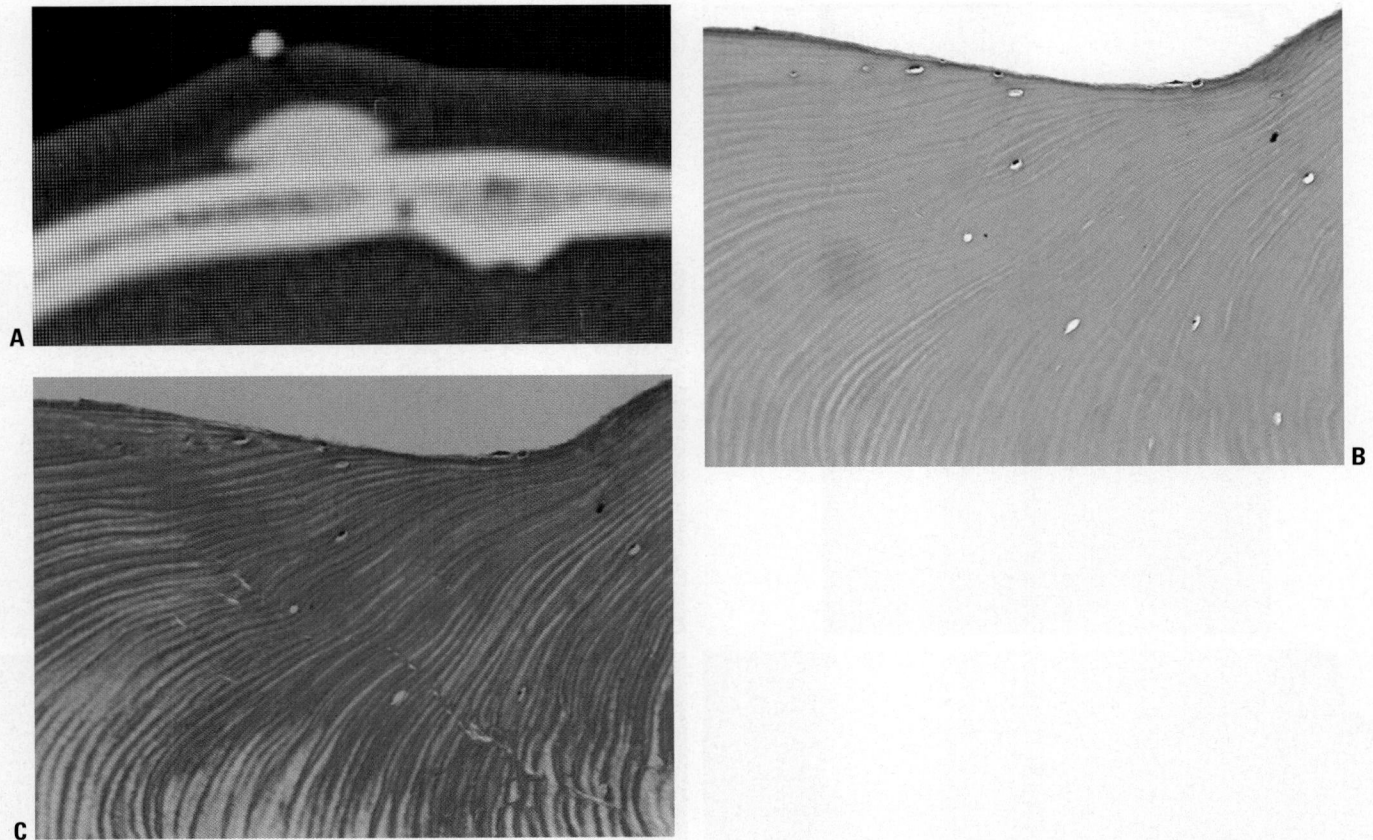

Figure 36-6 Button osteoma. **A:** Radiograph illustrates a bony projection situated on outer skull cortex. **B:** Concentric lamellar pattern of compact bone is sparsely populated by osteocytes. **C:** Polarized light highlights the concentric lamella with alternating collagen fiber direction.

Extraskeletal Osteosarcoma

Clinical Summary. This aggressive tumor, characterized by atypical mesenchymal cells synthesizing osteoid, is extremely rare, especially as a primary cutaneous tumor (66,67). Llamas-Velasco and colleagues characterized 11 reported cases of primary cutaneous osteosarcoma in the literature as of date and reported two additional cases (67). In summary, primary cutaneous extraskeletal osteosarcoma occurs in both men and women with a mean age of 71.3 years, most commonly occurring on the head or extremities. Other extraskeletal sites for primary osteosarcoma that may come to the attention of dermatologists include the penis (68) and tongue (69). Almost half of reported cases presented with metastases or succumbed to disease progression. Extraskeletal osteosarcoma has been reported in the skin with no associated predisposing conditions, adjacent to a basal cell carcinoma, associated with melanoma, in an old burn scar, following radiotherapy, post trauma, and under a previously electrodessicated actinic keratosis (70). There should be no connection to deeper structures and no demonstrable primary bone lesion. Origin in antecedent myositis ossificans has been reported (71,72). When osteosarcoma is concurrent with a distinct carcinoma pattern, such as that found in basal cell carcinoma, the term *carcinosarcoma* should be used. Similarly, when it is associated with melanoma it should be classified as a dedifferentiated/sarcomatous melanoma.

Histopathology. Cutaneous extraskeletal osteosarcoma has the same histologic appearance as primary osteosarcoma of the bone, with malignant mesenchymal cells forming tumor osteoid or fully formed woven bone (Fig. 36-7). Most present as osteoblastic osteosarcoma, others with fibroblastic, chondroblastic, and telangiectatic differentiation. Immunohistochemical reactions are largely used to exclude other malignancies such as malignant melanoma and metaplastic carcinoma (carcinosarcoma) and should therefore be negative for melanocytic markers (Melan-A, HMB45, S100, and Sox10) and pancytokeratin. Special AT-rich sequence-binding protein 2 (SATB2) has been recently described as a novel marker of osteoblastic differentiation in bone and soft tissue tumors (73) and may possibly serve as a useful adjunct in cases of mesenchymal tumors where there is a question of osteoid production versus hyalinized collagen (73,74). However, this marker may not be as specific for osteosarcoma as initially thought (75).

Differential Diagnosis. Metaplastic and reactive ossification may occur in and around various tumors with specific identity such as dermatofibroma (76), atypical fibroxanthoma (77), ossifying fibromyxoid tumor, myositis ossificans and related lesions such as FOPT, mixed tumor of the skin, giant-cell tumor of tendon sheath, all of which by and large lack the cytologic atypia of osteosarcoma. In addition, sarcomatoid (osteogenic) malignant melanoma, undifferentiated pleomorphic sarcoma ("malignant fibrous histiocytoma"), and peripheral nerve sheath tumors (e.g., malignant triton tumor) and Merkel cell carcinoma may demonstrate "divergent" differentiation into bone, cartilage, or myogenous tissue (78). Immunohistochemical panels and molecular studies can assist in detecting these deceptive tumors with differing biologic behaviors.

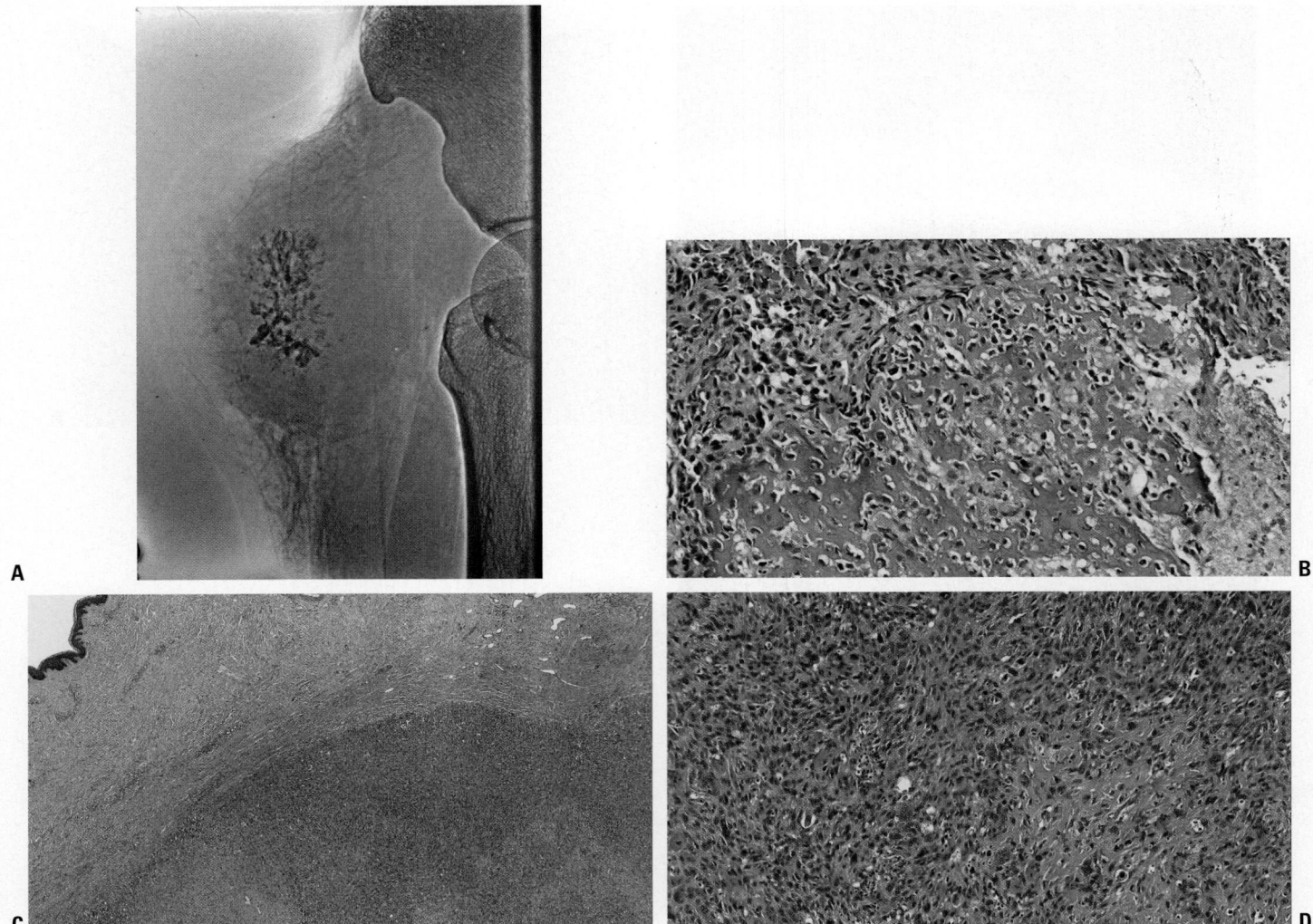

Figure 36-7 Extraskeletal osteosarcoma. **A:** In this plain film, an oval mass lateral to the hip joint has irregular central bony density, unlike the peripheral ossification of myositis ossificans. **B:** Cytologically malignant cells form osteoid. **C:** Another example showing a densely cellular proliferation of hyperchromatic cells deep in the dermis. **D:** High-power view showing focal areas of osteoid formation (**bottom right**) in a background of overtly malignant cells.

A 2011 review of *cutaneous metastasis from osteosarcoma* found only 15 cases with 23 total cutaneous metastases of osteosarcoma and added one that metastasized to the scalp (79).

Principles of Management: Complete surgical excision is the standard treatment. Extraskeletal osteosarcoma is considered poorly responsive to chemotherapy, and the role of adjuvant radiotherapy and chemotherapy, although often used, remains unclear (80,81).

BENIGN CARTILAGINOUS TUMORS OF SKIN AND SOFT TISSUE

Soft Tissue Chondromas

Clinical Summary. The hallmark of all differentiated chondrogenic tumors is neoplastic chondrocytes responsible for the formation of the characteristic cartilaginous tumor matrix. Benign cartilage nodules and masses independent of bone, including cutaneous cartilage tumors, are variously regarded as neoplastic, metaplastic, or anomalous. Generically referred to as *soft*

part or *extraskeletal chondromas* (Fig. 36-8), most of these nodules are located in the hands and feet, especially in the fingers of middle-aged adults (82,83), but may rarely occur at other sites too (e.g., the back) (84) and at different ages, including infancy (85,86). Most extraskeletal chondromas are solitary, but bilateral cases have been reported (87,88). These slowly enlarging nodules are seldom painful or tender and rarely exceed 3 cm in diameter. Local recurrence is uncommon, occurring in up to 10% of individuals. True *cutaneous chondromas*, located primarily in the dermis, are rarely described in the dermatologic literature (89–91) but can be familial (92).

Synovial chondroma (intracapsular and periarticular) and multiple purely cartilaginous (chondromatosis) or chondroosseous (osteochondromatosis) nodules in tenosynovium or joint synovium are thought to represent metaplastic changes of subsynovial fibrous tissue that may create a mass around a joint or along a tendon. When near a joint, intracapsular and para-articular chondromas are to be differentiated from *synovial chondromatosis* (93) (Fig. 36-9). Because of location, these tumors come to the attention of the dermatopathologist only rarely.

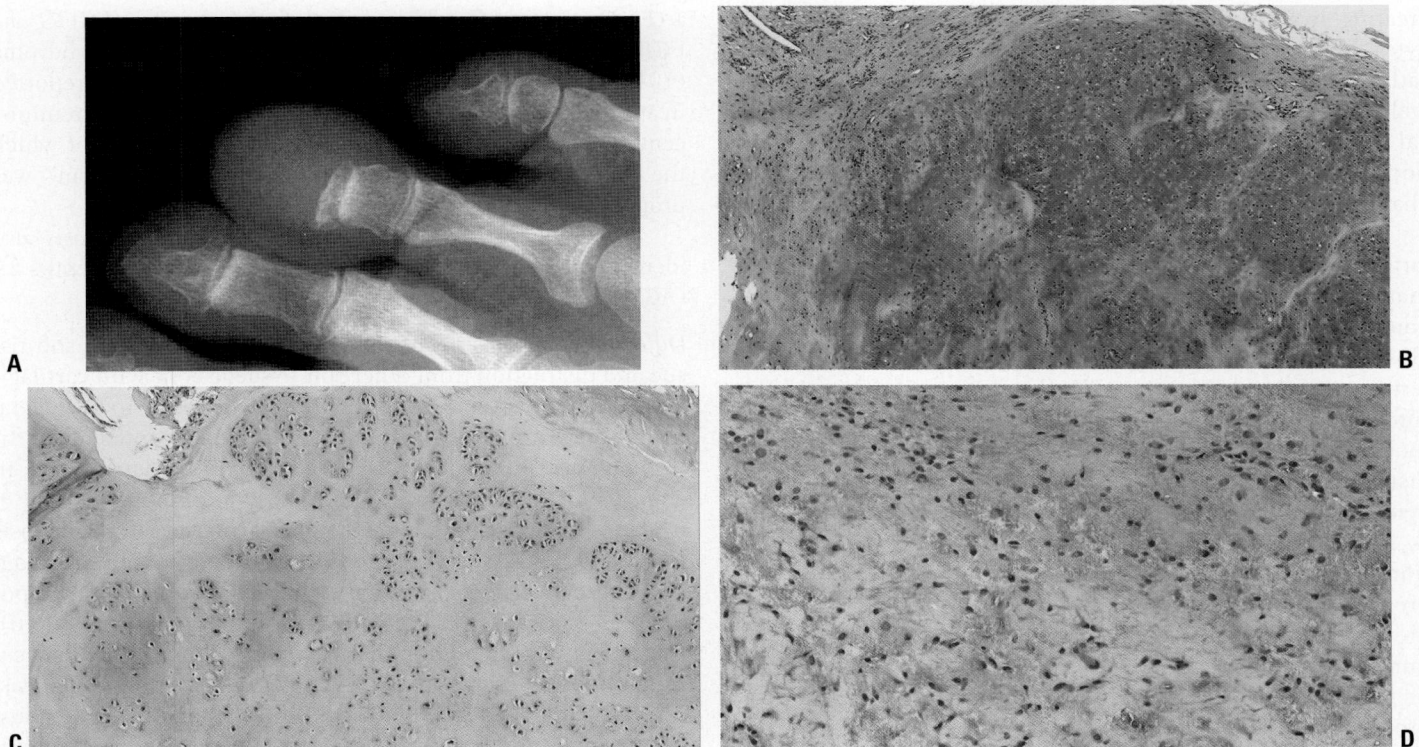

Figure 36-8 Extraskeletal (soft tissue) chondroma (62-year-old man; toe pain and swelling for 18 years). **A:** The plain film radiography shows pressure erosion of all but 2 mm of the proximal end of the distal phalanx, which abuts a 1.4 cm diameter rounded unmineralized soft tissue mass at the tip of the toe. **B:** The tumor consists of a rounded mass of variably cellular, myxoid, and hyaline cartilage. **C:** This example shows lobules of mature hyaline cartilage with less myxoid change. **D:** Chondrocytes often have oblong or reniform nuclei, unlike the round nuclei of synovial and intraosseous chondromas. Nuclear size variation and binucleate cells are commonplace in this benign lesion.

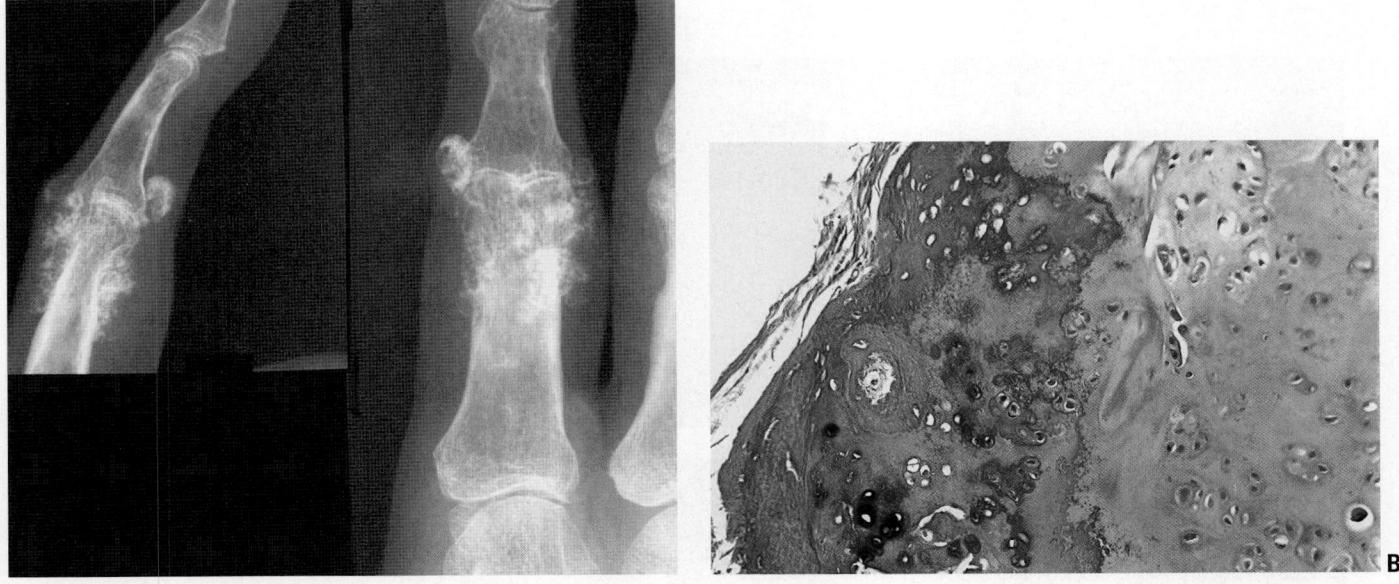

Figure 36-9 Synovial osteochondromatosis (71-year-old man; 5-year history of postinjury finger enlargement). **A:** Multiple lobules of the lesion around a proximal interphalangeal joint have radiodense rims correlating with rims of endochondral bone. **B:** Between radiolucent, moderately cellular, solid-appearing hyaline cartilage (**right**) and the eosinophilic bone that rims in (**left**) is a basophilic zone of mineralized cartilage. (Courtesy of Newton Sampaio.)

Enchondromas are benign intraosseous hyaline cartilage tumors whose location in the distal phalanx (in contrast to more proximal bones) is rare but may be responsible for nail dystrophy (94,95).

Histopathology. Soft tissue chondromas appear to develop and grow at their periphery by the metaplastic enlargement of fibroblasts into plump cells that inflate the preexisting structural fibrous tissue with sulphated mucopolysaccharides, creating hyaline cartilage (Fig. 36-8). The plump chondrocytes frequently have distinctive elongated reniform nuclei rather than the expected round shape in most cartilage. The well-circumscribed, solid-appearing cartilage may exhibit focal or diffuse calcification, focal fibrosis (*fibrochondroma*), endochondral ossification (*soft tissue osteochondroma*), myxoid change (myxochondroma), cystification, and/or hemorrhage.

Hypercellular soft tissue chondromas composed of enlarged chondrocytes within a variable amount of chondroid matrix that often demonstrate delicate calcifications and contain numerous osteoclast-like multinucleated giant cells closely resemble chondroblastoma of bone and have been referred to as *chondroblastoma-like chondroma of soft tissue* (96). Interpretation should ignore substantial atypia in what is radiologically or clinically a small lesion to avoid unnecessarily disfiguring surgery. Plump, immature-appearing chondrocytes that are bi- or multinucleated are not uncommon and, as in bone lesions, do not necessarily connote malignancy. Immunohistochemically, chondrocytes often label with S100 protein. Interestingly, like other chondrogenic tumors, chondromas consistently show nuclear expression of ERG, and this immunohistochemical stain is a useful tool in select diagnostic situations, especially in cases that are negative for S100 protein (97).

Pathogenesis. Cytogenetic analyses of *soft tissue chondroma* report aberrations of chromosomes 2, 3, 6, 11, and 12q13-q15 (98–100). Rearrangements of *HMGA2* have been identified in soft tissue chondroma, with one case harboring an *HMGA2-LPP* fusion (100). More recently, a fusion involving the fibronectin 1 (*FN1*) gene and fibroblast growth factor receptor 1 (*FGFR1 and FGFR2*) was identified in 50% of cases of soft tissue chondroma (101). Additional gene fusion partners with *FN1* were reported in another study of chondroid tumors morphologically reminiscent of chondroblastoma-like soft tissue chondroma, for which the term "calcified chondroid mesenchymal neoplasm" was proposed (102).

Recent molecular studies of *synovial chondromatosis* also identified recurrent alterations of *FN1* and activin receptor 2A (*ACVR2A*) (101,103).

Differential Diagnosis. The diagnosis of chondromas of soft tissue and distinction from other soft tissue lesions with cartilaginous differentiation is not difficult in most cases. Extraskeletal chondromas are to be distinguished from developmental cartilaginous rests of branchial origin usually in the lateral neck in children or infants. A superficial biopsy might retrieve a bit of hyaline cartilage from digital synovial (osteo) chondromatosis (Fig. 36-9). Several soft tissue processes may contain histologically disconcerting cartilage, including mixed tumors (apocrine or eccrine), calcifying aponeurotic fibroma (Fig. 36-10), giant-cell tumor of tendon sheath, metaplastic cartilage in occasional lipoma varieties, (teno)synovial (osteo)chondromatosis, cartilage produced in myositis ossificans and fracture callus, metaplastic cartilage in and around tophaceous pseudogout, chondro-osseous osteophytes from phalanges submitted by hand surgeons, and soft tissue recurrence of a bone tumor (e.g., chondromyxoid fibroma). Heavily calcified chondromas show granular areas with giant-cell reaction resembling tumoral calcinosis or tenosynovial giant-cell tumors. *Tenosynovitis with*

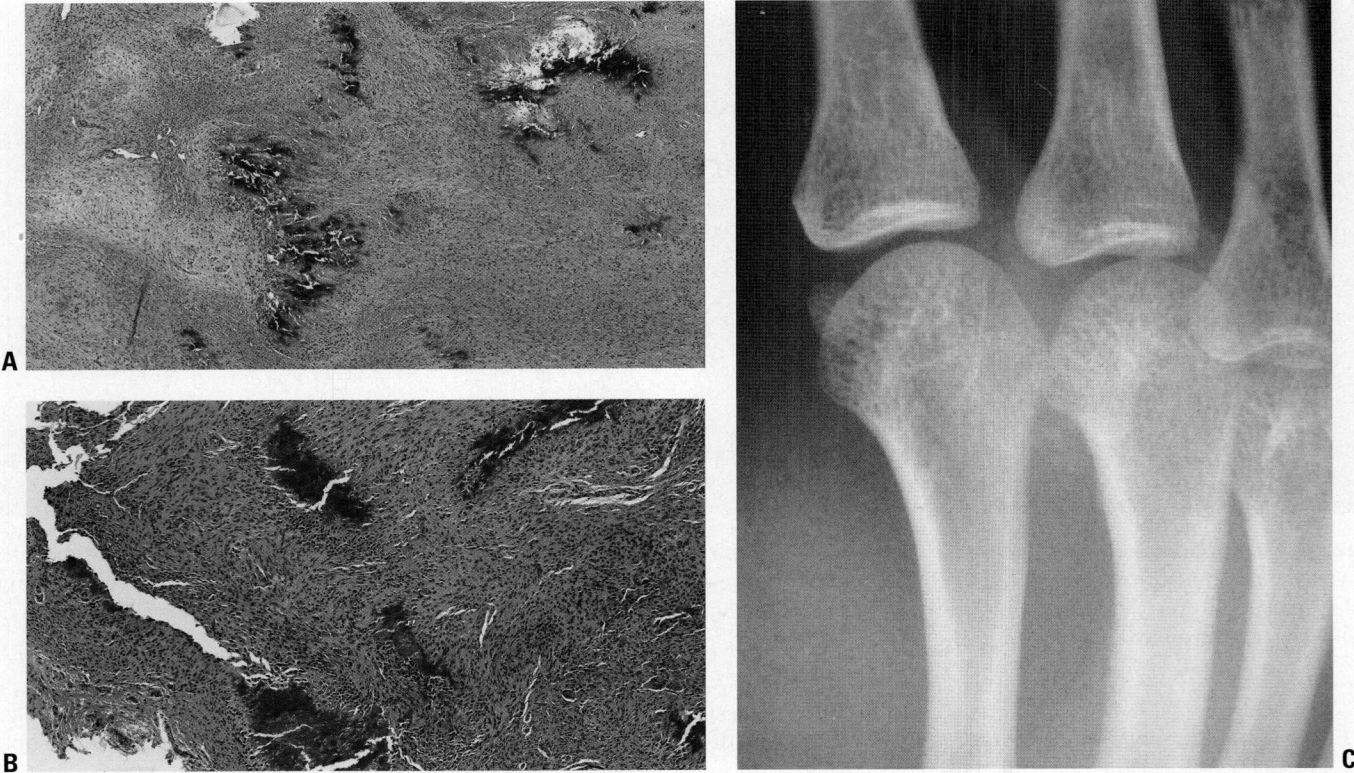

Figure 36-10 Calcifying (juvenile) aponeurotic fibroma (27-year-old man; palm). Cartilage islands with characteristic calcification (**A**) set in a fibromatosis-like background (**B**) explain the speckled densities in the plain film (**C**).

psammomatous calcification could also potentially be confused for a heavily calcified chondroma, but characteristic psammomatous calcification and clinical history should allow accurate classification (104,105).

Radiographs can distinguish tumors extending from bone, such as osteochondroma or subungual exostosis (106). Extraskeletal chondromas with mineralization of the chondroid matrix will show on plain film radiographs (107), and the remainder can be imaged by MRI (108) or sonography (109).

Principles of Management: Chondromas may be observed or conservatively excised if physically or cosmetically bothersome.

Calcifying (Juvenile) Aponeurotic Fibroma

Clinical Summary. Calcifying (juvenile) aponeurotic fibroma (CAF) is a rare benign tumor clinically presenting as a painless, mobile solitary mass with a strong predilection for the distal portion of the hands and feet of children and young adults (110). Uncommonly, it can occur in nonacral sites such as scalp (111), neck (112), lumbosacral (113), back, knee region, thigh, forearm, elbow, and arm (114). Minute calcific foci may be evident grossly and on plain films (Fig. 36-10C). Often adherent to dense fibrous connective tissue (e.g., tendon, fascia, or periosteum), CAFs range from 1 to 5 cm in dimension and are poorly circumscribed with a dense fibrous consistency.

Histopathology. Histologically, at the periphery of each centrally located calcified island, sometimes with cartilage formation, is a palisade of rounded mononuclear and fibroblastic cells reminiscent of chondrocytes (Fig. 36-10A). The intervening fibromatosis-like areas consist of spindle-shaped fibroblastic/myofibroblastic cells that radiate into the surrounding soft tissue via multiple processes (Fig. 36-10B).

Pathogenesis. An *FN1-EGF* gene fusion was identified as a recurrent genetic mutation in a small series of cases and is thought to be the driver mutation in CAF (115).

Differential Diagnosis. Familiarity with this entity should help to avoid confusion with other processes, including infantile and extra-abdominal fibromatoses, chondroma of soft parts, and fibrous hamartoma of infancy.

The recently described *EWSR1-SMAD3-rearranged fibroblastic tumor* shares overlapping histopathologic features with CAF, characterized by a central hyalinized and paucicellular nodular growth surrounded by hypercellular spindle cells arranged in intersecting fascicles (116–118). These lesions are generally found in an older patient population and appear to have a strong female predilection in comparison to CAF. The tumors show consistent strong and diffuse immunoreactivity for ERG, compared to weak-to-moderate labeling in CAF (117). Molecular studies such as fluorescence *in situ* hybridization (FISH) could be used to differentiate these tumors if necessary.

Principles of Management: Surgical management should be conservative for all tumors with the typical appearance of a CAF. In fact, excision and reexcision, if necessary, appear preferable to radical or mutilating surgical procedures to maintain function of the extremity. Fifty percent develop one or more recurrences (114). Rapidity of growth seems to slow down with increasing age. Various references state that no instances of metastasis have been reported, whereas others allude to rare malignant transformation (119,120).

CHONDROSARCOMA

Extraskeletal Myxoid Chondrosarcoma (So-Called)

Clinical Summary. Extraskeletal myxoid chondrosarcoma represents a discrete genetically defined entity that, despite its name, shows no convincing evidence of cartilaginous differentiation and is likely better classified as a tumor of uncertain line of differentiation (121,122). However, it is included in this chapter given its historical consideration as a cartilaginous tumor, and histologically the myxoid matrix has some resemblance to chondroid tumors.

Extraskeletal myxoid chondrosarcoma more commonly affects adult males (male-to-female ratio of ~2:1) with a median age at the time of diagnosis in the fifth decade of life (123–125). Only a small minority have been reported in children (126). The tumor frequently arises in the deep soft tissues, especially of the lower extremity (123). The gradually enlarging mass may or may not be associated with pain. Most extraskeletal myxoid chondrosarcomas are large, ovoid, pseudo-encapsulated, well-circumscribed tumors with a lobular architecture. By MRI, the neoplasm is a nodular, radiolucent mass (Fig. 36-11A). The cut surface is tan, gelatinous, and frequently hemorrhagic (Fig. 36-11B).

Histopathology. Extraskeletal myxoid chondrosarcoma is characterized by a proliferation of ovoid and bipolar cells that are enmeshed in a prominent myxoid matrix (Fig. 36-11C, D). It has a repetitive lobular pattern and chains of neoplastic cells that seem to progress from the periphery toward the center of lobules. Hemorrhage and hemosiderin in the fibrous tissue surrounding the nodules is characteristic. The tumor cells have little-to-moderate amounts of eosinophilic cytoplasm, and the nuclei are uniform rather than pleomorphic. Occasionally, individual tumor cells are surrounded by lacunar spaces; however, the formation of well-developed hyaline cartilage is uncommon. Mitoses are not numerous, and multinucleated giant cells are absent. There may be marked collagenization, spindle-shaped tumor cells, and matrix-poor regions in which the tumor cells grow in solid sheets. The neoplastic cells are variably positive for S-100 protein (17% to 50%), EMA, and neuroendocrine markers such as neuron-specific enolase, synaptophysin, and INSM1 (121,127–129). The tumor does not label with Sox10 (130).

Differential Diagnosis. Myxoid tumors of soft tissue encompass a heterogeneous group of lesions characterized by a marked abundance of extracellular myxoid matrix, with marked differences in biologic potential that generate diagnostic challenges for the clinician and the pathologist alike. The differential diagnosis of extraskeletal myxoid chondrosarcoma is broad and includes many reactive processes and epithelial and mesenchymal neoplasms, chief among them, intramuscular myxoma, juxta-articular myxomas, neural neoplasms, cutaneous and soft tissue myoepitheliomas, myxoid liposarcoma, myxofibrosarcoma, metastatic carcinoma, metastatic melanoma with myxoid stroma, and chordoma. Myxoid chondrosarcoma does not have the vascular pattern typical of myxoid liposarcoma and lacks lipoblasts. FISH testing is proving to be a useful ancillary diagnostic tool in differential diagnosis (131,132). However, selecting the appropriate FISH probe is important given that some entities within the differential (i.e., myoepithelioma) have rearrangements involving *EWRS1*.

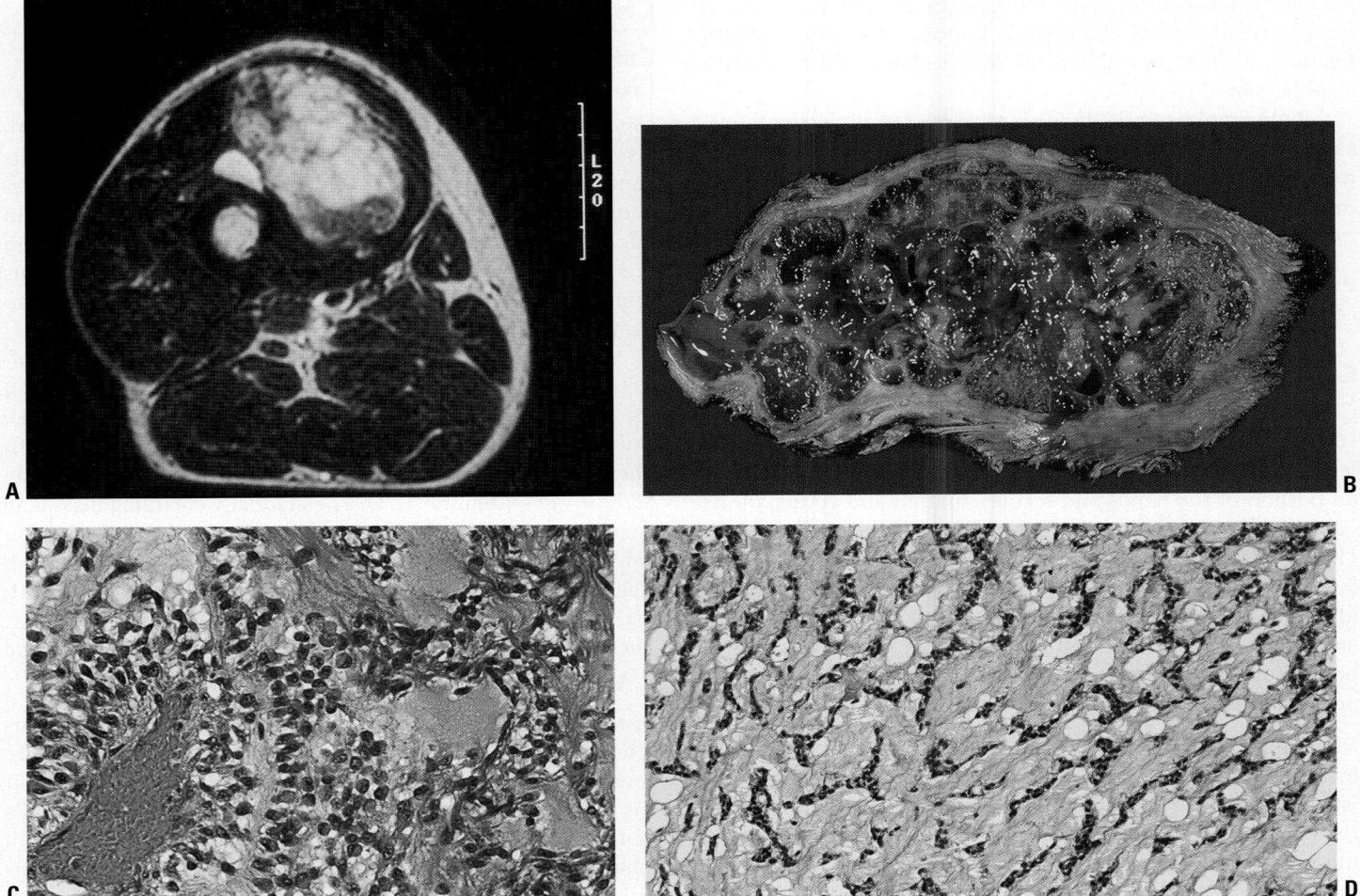

Figure 36-11 Extraskeletal myxoid chondrosarcoma (63-year-old man; 17 × 8 × 8 cm anterior thigh mass; death unrelated to tumor 28 months postoperative.) A: By MRI, this tumor has a high signal intensity because its watery matrix has a high hydrogen content, as does subcutaneous fat. B: The tumor has a glistening myxoid and hemorrhagic cut surface. C, D: Ovoid and stellate tumor cells form perivascular arrays and cords in a basophilic myxoid background.

Pathogenesis. On the basis of the types of collagen synthesized, the cellular phenotype of extraskeletal myxoid chondrosarcoma is not chondrocytic or prechondrocytic but rather is composed of primitive mesenchymal cells with focal, multidirectional differentiation (122). The presence of a fusion gene between the orphan nuclear receptor, *NR4A3* (also known as CHN/NOR1), and, most commonly, *EWSR1*, [t(9;22)(q22;q12)], produces an EWSR1/NR4A3 fusion protein (125,128,132,133). This protein appears to contribute to the overexpression of several genes that may contribute to pathogenesis (134,135). Other less common translocations have also been described.

Principles of Management: Although extraskeletal myxoid chondrosarcoma is considered a low-grade sarcoma with low disease-related mortality, recurrence is common, and definitive initial surgery with careful monitoring for a prolonged period of time is prudent. Adjuvant or palliative radiotherapy may be beneficial, but chemotherapy does not appear to be particularly effective (124,125,136,137).

Extraskeletal Mesenchymal Chondrosarcoma

Clinical Summary. Extraskeletal mesenchymal chondrosarcoma is a high-grade malignant cartilaginous neoplasm primarily affecting adolescents and young adults (138,139). Children may also be affected (140). Although most mesenchymal chondrosarcomas arise in bone, around one-third of cases are extraskeletal. The head and neck region is the principal site involved, followed by the lower extremities. Cutaneous involvement may occur via metastasis from a skeletal or extraskeletal primary location (141).

Histopathology. Chondroid-type flocculent mineralizations and foci of low signal intensity within enhancing lobules reflect its characteristic biphasic histopathologic pattern of differentiated cartilage islands interspersed within highly cellular round-to-spindled undifferentiated mesenchymal cells (Fig. 36-12A) (142). A prominent "hemangiopericytoma-like" vascular pattern may also be a prominent feature (Fig. 36-12B). The cartilaginous areas are S100 protein positive. The mesenchymal component is generally negative for keratin, but around one-third may show focal EMA expression (143). Positivity of small cells for myogenic markers such as desmin, MyoD1, and myogenin may be seen (144); in rare cases, more diffuse rhabdomyoblastic differentiation indicates mesenchymal chondrosarcoma's polyphenotypic potential (145).

Like other undifferentiated small round cell tumors, CD99 immunoreactivity may be found in the immature mesenchymal

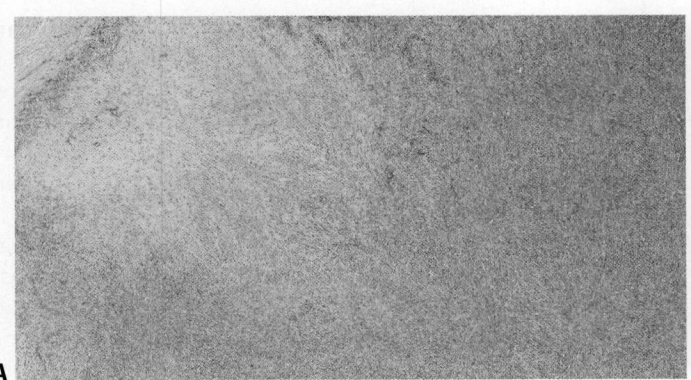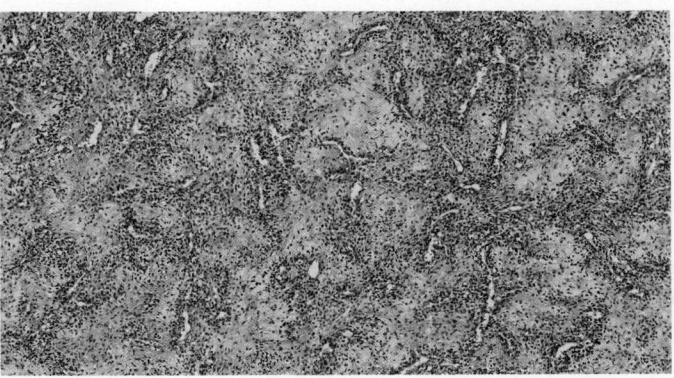

A   B

Figure 36-12 Mesenchymal chondrosarcoma. **A:** Small, round, undifferentiated cells (**right**) might easily be mistaken for Ewing sarcoma or lymphoma were it not for the sporadic islands of cartilage product (**top left**). **B:** Other areas may show a richly vascular pattern with tumor cells arranged in a classic perivascular pattern around sinusoidal vessels.

cells with a distinct membrane pattern of labeling and is therefore not a useful marker to distinguish it from Ewing sarcoma (145,146). NKX2-2, a nuclear marker found to be positive in the majority (up to 93%) of Ewing sarcoma, is also frequently expressed (up to 75%) in extraskeletal mesenchymal chondrosarcoma (147). However, Sox9, a transcription factor thought to be a master regulator of chondrogenesis, appears to be a useful marker to distinguish mesenchymal chondrosarcoma from other small round cell tumors (148,149). NKX3-1, a nuclear marker found to be a highly sensitive and specific marker for prostatic adenocarcinoma (150), may serve as an additional marker to aid in the differential because it was reported to be expressed in 12/12 cases of mesenchymal chondrosarcoma and 9/11 *EWSR1-NFATC2* sarcomas, although negative in histopathologic mimics such as Ewing sarcoma and myoepithelial tumors (151).

Pathogenesis. Few case reports for various chromosomal abnormalities have been reported, but the most common recurrent *HEY1-NCOA2* gene fusion in mesenchymal chondrosarcoma is on chromosome 8. The two genes are only about 10 Mb apart, and for this reason the fusion is thought to occur secondary to a small interstitial deletion del(8)(q13.3a21.1) (152). FISH studies for the detection of the *HEY1-NCOA2* fusion gene are proving to be helpful in confirming the diagnosis (153). More recently, a novel fusion *IRF2BP2-CDX1* was identified in an example of mesenchymal chondrosarcoma with t(1;5) (q42;q32) (154).

Differential Diagnosis. The cellular areas of mesenchymal chondrosarcoma can mimic undifferentiated small round cell tumors such as Ewing sarcoma and other undifferentiated translocation associated sarcomas. Poorly differentiated synovial sarcoma and malignant solitary fibrous tumor may also be mistaken for mesenchymal chondrosarcoma in the absence of overt cartilaginous differentiation. Immunohistochemical and molecular studies should aid in differentiating these neoplasms.

Principles of Management: Complete surgical excision with adjuvant chemotherapy therapy is associated with fewer recurrences in mesenchymal chondrosarcoma (139). Unlike extraskeletal myxoid chondrosarcoma, mesenchymal chondrosarcoma pursues an aggressive clinical course with a high incidence of metastasis (138).

OSSEOUS AND CHONDROID LESIONS, RARER STILL

Embryonic tissue and organ development are initiated from three embryonic germ layers: ectoderm (skin and neuron), mesoderm (blood, bone, muscle, cartilage, and fat), and endoderm (respiratory and digestive tracts). It was formerly believed that cell types in each germ layer were specific and did not cross from one to another throughout life. A new finding is that one tissue lineage can cross to another tissue lineage, and this is termed *transdifferentiation* (155). For example, skin-derived precursor cells (ectoderm) can transdifferentiate to osteoblastic cells (mesoderm); ossification in chondroid syringomas and mixed tumors of the skin employs the enchondral mechanism.

The appearance of cutaneous lesions in a patient with a prior history of chondrosarcoma should alert the clinician to the rare possibility of *metastatic chondrosarcoma* (156). Such metastases preceding the diagnosis of primary chondrosarcoma are anecdotal. These metastases can be either single or multiple, with a slight predilection for the head and neck region (157).

Metaplastic carcinoma (carcinosarcoma, sarcomatoid carcinoma) is a biphasic tumor comprising malignant keratin-positive epithelial component and heterologous keratin-negative mesenchymal elements. Many conclude that the sarcomatous component of the tumor is best regarded as a metaplastic transformation of the carcinomatous component (158). Primary carcinosarcoma of the skin is uncommon, with up to 38 reported cases, according to Tran and coworkers in 2005 (159). Most of these tumors were seen on the head and neck region of older individuals, both male and female. Microscopically, the more common carcinoma component is a squamous cell carcinoma, followed by basal cell carcinoma, whereas the most common sarcomatous component is osteosarcoma.

Cutaneous carcinosarcoma is broadly classified into two distinct groups (159). Epidermal-derived (basal or squamous cell carcinoma epithelial component with a sarcomatous component) carcinosarcomas arise on the sun-damaged skin of the head and neck of elderly males (mean age 72 years) with a 70% 5-year disease-free survival. In contrast, adnexal-derived (spiradenocarcinoma, porocarcinoma, proliferating trichilemmal cystic carcinoma, or matrical carcinoma) carcinosarcomas occur in younger patients (mean age 58 years), present as recent growth in a long-standing nodule, and have a 25% 5-year disease-free survival. Malignant heterologous mesenchymal elements include osteosarcoma, chondrosarcoma, leiomyosarcoma, and rhabdomyosarcoma. In contrast to metaplastic carcinomas arising in visceral sites, those primarily arising in the skin do not appear to behave in a very aggressive manner (159).

Sarcomatoid (metaplastic) carcinoma of the breast, although a well-established aggressive neoplasm, is very uncommon. Its metaplastic elements, derived from carcinomatous elements, span all lines of mesenchymal differentiation. Skin metastasis from such lesions is extremely rare but can be chondrosarcomatous (160).

Malignant melanomas showing foci of divergent differentiation include fibroblastic/myofibroblastic, Schwannian, perineural, smooth muscle, rhabdomyosarcomatous, osteocartilaginous, ganglionic and ganglioneuroblastic, neuroendocrine, and epithelial (161). *Melanomas showing foci of osteocartilaginous differentiation* are extremely rare, but melanoma should be considered in the differential diagnosis of primary cutaneous neoplasms exhibiting osteocartilaginous differentiation (162). Oral mucosal melanomas with osteocartilaginous differentiation are to be distinguished from malignant change in a pleomorphic adenoma, sarcomatoid carcinoma, osteogenic sarcoma, and mesenchymal chondrosarcoma. Primary vaginal melanoma with cartilaginous differentiation must be distinguished from primary malignant mixed Müllerian tumor.

One benign tumor of the tongue that deserves mention is the *ectomesenchymal chondromyxoid tumor (EMT)*, which presents as an asymptomatic nodule of the anterior dorsum (and rarely the ventral aspect) of the tongue in patients in the third to fifth decades of life. Microscopically, unencapsulated lobules are composed of sheets and cords of oval to spindle cells in a variable chondromyxoid background. Rarely, a chondroid component is completely absent, raising the differential diagnosis of a myoepithelioma or extraskeletal myxoid chondrosarcoma. Immunohistochemical reactions for S100 protein, NSE, α-SMA, and GFAP are positive in EMT, whereas myoepithelioma reacts for S100 protein and less strongly for GFAP and is positive for myoepithelial markers and epithelial markers such as p63 and EMA (163).

Atypical fibroxanthoma can contain areas of chondroid differentiation that resemble chondrosarcoma and have S100 positivity (164).

A gastrointestinal carcinoma metastasis to skin with cutaneous osseous metaplasia has been reported (165).

Pseudocyst of the auricle is a benign condition that presents as a fluctuant swelling of the ear, most commonly in young Asian males (166). Histologically, an intracartilaginous cyst will have no epithelial lining and a sparse lymphocytic inflammatory response (Fig. 36-13).

Ossifying fibromyxoid tumor (OFMT) of soft tissue is a rare tumor of uncertain differentiation that typically presents as a subcutaneous mass in the extremities (167–169). It is usually well circumscribed and frequently has an incomplete rim of lamellar bone associated with a dense fibrous pseudocapsule (Fig. 36-14). Bone is found in approximately 75% of histologically typical tumors, compared with approximately 50% of those showing atypical histologic features (170). The tumor cells will variably label with S-100 in approximately 70% of cases (167,168). Recurrent genetic alterations involve the *PHF1* gene (171).

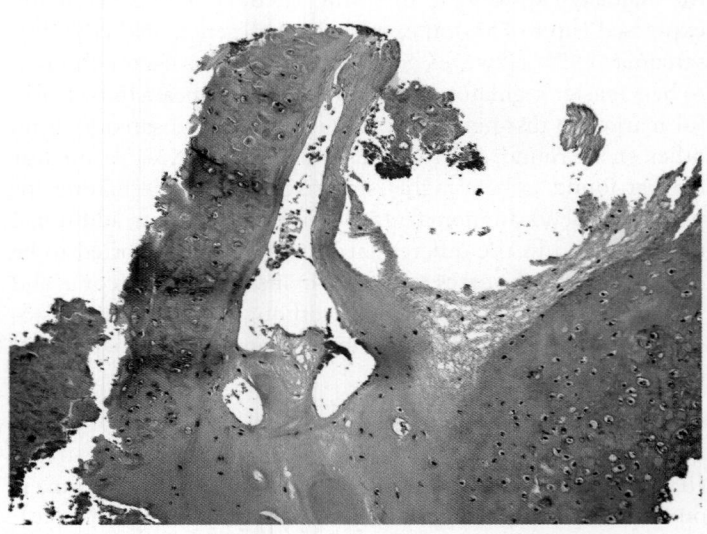

Figure 36-13 Pseudocyst of the auricle. A space in the auricular cartilage is lined by chondroid tissue with a sparse inflammatory response. A pseudocyst has no epithelial lining.

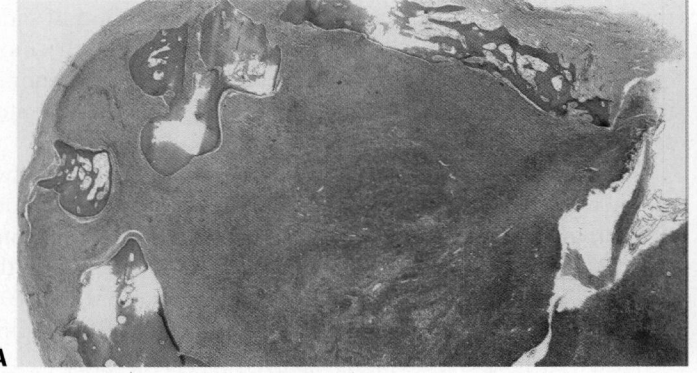
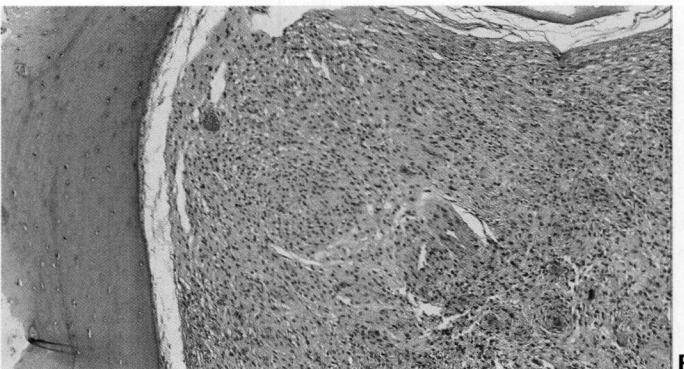

A   **B**

Figure 36-14 Ossifying fibromyxoid tumor. **A:** A well-circumscribed lesion containing an incomplete shell of lamellar bone at the periphery. **B:** Centrally, the tumor is made up of relatively uniform, round-to-ovoid–shaped cells arranged in nests and cords in a fibromyxoid stroma.

REFERENCES

1. Vanden Bossche L, Vanderstraeten G. Heterotopic ossification: a review. *J Rehabil Med.* 2005;37(3):129–136.

2. Albright F, Burnett CH, Smith PH. Pseudo-hypoparathyroidism—an example of "Seabright-Bantam syndrome": report of three cases. *Endocrinology.* 1942;30:922–932.

3. Albright F, Forbes AP, Henneman PH. Pseudo-pseudohypoparathyroidism. *Trans Assoc Am Physicians.* 1952;65:337–350.

4. de Sanctis L, Vai S, Andreo MR, Romagnolo D, Silvestro L, de Sanctis C. Brachydactyly in 14 genetically characterized pseudo-hypoparathyroidism type Ia patients. *J Clin Endocrinol Metab.* 2004;89(4):1650–1655.

5. Kacerovska D, Nemcova J, Pomahacova R, Michal M, Kazakov DV. Cutaneous and superficial soft tissue lesions associated with Albright hereditary osteodystrophy: clinicopathological and molecular genetic study of 4 cases, including a novel mutation of the GNAS gene. *Am J Dermatopathol.* 2008;30(5):417–424.

6. Elli FM, Linglart A, Garin I, et al. The prevalence of GNAS deficiency-related diseases in a large cohort of patients characterized by the EuroPHP Network. *J Clin Endocrinol Metab.* 2016;101(10):3657–3668.

7. Mantovani G, de Sanctis L, Barbieri AM, et al. Pseudohypoparathyroidism and GNAS epigenetic defects: clinical evaluation of Albright hereditary osteodystrophy and molecular analysis in 40 patients. *J Clin Endocrinol Metab.* 2010;95(2):651–658.

8. Salemi P, Skalamera Olson JM, Dickson LE, Germain-Lee EL. Ossifications in Albright hereditary osteodystrophy: role of genotype, inheritance, sex, age, hormonal status, and BMI. *J Clin Endocrinol Metab.* 2018;103(1):158–168.

9. de Sanctis L, Giachero F, Mantovani G, et al. Genetic and epigenetic alterations in the GNAS locus and clinical consequences in pseudohypoparathyroidism: Italian common healthcare pathways adoption. *Ital J Pediatr.* 2016;42(1):101.

10. Regard JB, Malhotra D, Gvozdenovic-Jeremic J, et al. Activation of hedgehog signaling by loss of GNAS causes heterotopic ossification. *Nat Med.* 2013;19(11):1505–1512.

11. Regard JB, Cherman N, Palmer D, et al. Wnt/β-catenin signaling is differentially regulated by Gα proteins and contributes to fibrous dysplasia. *Proc Natl Acad Sci U S A.* 2011;108(50):20101–20106.

12. Wu JY, Aarnisalo P, Bastepe M, Sinha P, et al. Gsα enhances commitment of mesenchymal progenitors to the osteoblast lineage but restrains osteoblast differentiation in mice. *J Clin Invest.* 2011;121(9):3492–3504.

13. Kaplan FS, Craver R, MacEwen GD, et al. Progressive osseous heteroplasia: a distinct developmental disorder of heterotopic ossification. Two new case reports and follow-up of three previously reported cases. *J Bone Joint Surg Am.* 1994;76(3):425–436.

14. Shore EM, Ahn J, Jan de Beur S, et al. Paternally inherited inactivating mutations of the GNAS1 gene in progressive osseous heteroplasia. *N Engl J Med.* 2002;346(2):99–106.

15. Kaplan FS, Shore EM. Progressive osseous heteroplasia. *J Bone Miner Res.* 2000;15(11):2084–2094.

16. Shore EM, Xu M, Feldman GJ, et al. A recurrent mutation in the BMP type I receptor ACVR1 causes inherited and sporadic fibrodysplasia ossificans progressiva. *Nat Genet.* 2006;38(5):525–527.

17. Thiele S, Mantovani G, Barlier A, et al. From pseudohypoparathyroidism to inactivating PTH/PTHrP signalling disorder (iPPSD), a novel classification proposed by the EuroPHP network. *Eur J Endocrinol.* 2016;175(6):P1-P17.

18. Duarte BM, Pinheiro RR, Cabete J. Multiple miliary osteoma cutis: a comprehensive review and update of the literature. *Eur J Dermatol.* 2018;28(4):434–439.

19. Myllylä RM, Haapasaari KM, Palatsi R, et al. Multiple miliary osteoma cutis is a distinct disease entity: four case reports and review of the literature. *Br J Dermatol.* 2011;164(3):544–552.

20. Goldminz D, Greenberg RD. Multiple miliary osteoma cutis. *J Am Acad Dermatol.* 1991;24(5, pt 2):878–881.

21. Elli FM, Boldrin V, Pirelli A, et al. The complex GNAS imprinted locus and mesenchymal stem cells differentiation. *Horm Metab Res.* 2017;49(4):250–258.

22. Pignolo RJ, Xu M, Russell E, et al. Heterozygous inactivation of Gnas in adipose-derived mesenchymal progenitor cells enhances osteoblast differentiation and promotes heterotopic ossification. *J Bone Miner Res.* 2011;26(11):2647–2655.

23. Yamaguchi A, Komori T, Suda T. Regulation of osteoblast differentiation mediated by bone morphogenetic proteins, hedgehogs, and Cbfa1. *Endocr Rev.* 2000;21(4):393–411.

24. Sánchez-Duffhues G, Hiepen C, Knaus P, Ten Dijke P. Bone morphogenetic protein signaling in bone homeostasis. *Bone.* 2015;80:43–59.

25. Kan C, Chen L, Hu Y, et al. Conserved signaling pathways underlying heterotopic ossification. *Bone.* 2018;109:43–48.

26. Oikarinen A, Tuomi ML, Kallionen M, Sandberg M, Väänänen K. A study of bone formation in osteoma cutis employing biochemical, histochemical and in situ hybridization techniques. *Acta Derm Venereol.* 1992;72(3):172–174.

27. Walsh JS, Fairley JA. Calcifying disorders of the skin. *J Am Acad Dermatol.* 1995;33(5, pt 1):693–706; quiz 707–710.

28. Conlin PA, Jimenez-Quintero LP, Rapini RP. Osteomas of the skin revisited: a clinicopathologic review of 74 cases. *Am J Dermatopathol.* 2002;24(6):479–483.

29. Moreno A, Lamarca J, Martinez R, Guix M. Osteoid and bone formation in desmoplastic malignant melanoma. *J Cutan Pathol.* 1986;13(2):128–134.

30. Urmacher C. Unusual stromal patterns in truly recurrent and satellite metastatic lesions of malignant melanoma. *Am J Dermatopathol.* 1984;6(suppl):331–335.

31. Lucas DR, Tazelaar HD, Unni KK, et al. Osteogenic melanoma. A rare variant of malignant melanoma. *Am J Surg Pathol.* 1993;17(4):400–409.

32. Trevisan F, Tregnago AC, Lopes Pinto CA, et al. Osteogenic melanoma with desmin expression. *Am J Dermatopathol.* 2017;39(7):528–533.

33. Marteinsson BT, Musgrove JE. Heterotopic bone formation in abdominal incisions. *Am J Surg.* 1975;130(1):23–25.

34. Kornhaber R, Foster N, Edgar D, et al. The development and impact of heterotopic ossification in burns: a review of four decades of research. *Scars Burn Heal.* 2017;3:2059513117695659.

35. Wiedemeyer K, Kutzner H, Abraham JL, et al. The evolution of osseous metaplasia in localized cutaneous nephrogenic systemic fibrosis: a case report. *Am J Dermatopathol.* 2009;31(7):674–681.

36. Choi GS, Kang DS, Chung JJ, Lee MG. Osteoma cutis coexisting with cutis laxa-like pseudoxanthoma elasticum. *J Am Acad Dermatol.* 2000;43(2, pt 2):337–339.

37. Kransdorf MJ, Meis JM. From the archives of the AFIP. Extraskeletal osseous and cartilaginous tumors of the extremities. *Radiographics.* 1993;13:853–884.

38. Walczak BE, Johnson CN, Howe BM. Myositis ossificans. *J Am Acad Orthop Surg.* 2015;23(10):612–622.

39. Sferopoulos NK, Kotakidou R, Petropoulos AS. Myositis ossificans in children: a review. *Eur J Orthop Surg Traumatol.* 2017;27(4):491–502.

40. Tyler P, Saifuddin A. The imaging of myositis ossificans. *Semin Musculoskelet Radiol.* 2010;14(2):201–216.

41. Landon GC, Johnson KA, Dahlin DC. Subungual exostoses. *J Bone Joint Surg Am.* 1979;61(2):256–259.

42. Miller-Breslow A, Dorfman HD. Dupuytren's (subungual) exostosis. *Am J Surg Pathol.* 1988;12(5):368–378.

43. Lee SK, Jung MS, Lee YH, Gong HS, Kim JK, Baek GH. Two distinctive subungual pathologies: subungual exostosis and subungual osteochondroma. *Foot Ankle Int.* 2007;28(5):595–601.

44. Cates HE, Burgess RC. Incidence of brachydactyly and hand exostosis in hereditary multiple exostosis. *J Hand Surg Am.* 1991; 16(1):127–132.

45. Göktay F, Atış G, Güneş P, Macit B, Çelik NS, Gürdal Kösem E. Subungual exostosis and subungual osteochondromas: a description of 25 cases. *Int J Dermatol.* 2018;57(7):872–881.

46. Davis DA, Cohen PR. Subungual exostosis: case report and review of the literature. *Pediatr Dermatol.* 1996;13(3):212–218.

47. Ragsdale B. Morphologic analysis of skeletal lesions: correlation of imaging studies and pathologic findings. In: Weinstein RS, Graham AR, eds. *Advances in Pathology and Laboratory Medicine.* Mosby-Year Book; 1993:445–490.

48. Spjut HJ, Dorfman HD. Florid reactive periostitis of the tubular bones of the hands and feet. A benign lesion which may simulate osteosarcoma. *Am J Surg Pathol.* 1981;5(5):423–433.

49. Dupree WB, Enzinger FM. Fibro-osseous pseudotumor of the digits. *Cancer.* 1986;58(9):2103–2109.

50. Moosavi CA, Al-Nahar LA, Murphey MD, Fanburg-Smith JC. Fibroosseous [corrected] pseudotumor of the digit: a clinicopathologic study of 43 new cases. *Ann Diagn Pathol.* 2008;12(1): 21–28.

51. Nora FE, Dahlin DC, Beabout JW. Bizarre parosteal osteochondromatous proliferations of the hands and feet. *Am J Surg Pathol.* 1983;7(3):245–250.

52. Meneses MF, Unni KK, Swee RG. Bizarre parosteal osteochondromatous proliferation of bone (Nora's lesion). *Am J Surg Pathol.* 1993;17(7):691–697.

53. Nielsen GP, Fletcher CD, Smith MA, Rybak L, Rosenberg AE. Soft tissue aneurysmal bone cyst: a clinicopathologic study of five cases. *Am J Surg Pathol.* 2002;26(1):64–69.

54. Chung IA, Petelin K, Pižem J, Luzar B. Cutaneous aneurysmal bone cyst—first report of a case and literature review. *J Cutan Pathol.* 2019;46(11):858–863.

55. Eshed V, Latimer B, Greenwald CM, et al. Button osteoma: its etiology and pathophysiology. *Am J Phys Anthropol.* 2002;118(3): 217–230.

56. Dinarvand P, Davaro EP, Doan JV, et al. Familial adenomatous polyposis syndrome: an update and review of extraintestinal manifestations. *Arch Pathol Lab Med.* 2019;143(11): 1382–1398.

57. Zhang L, Hwang S, Benayed R, et al. Myositis ossificans-like soft tissue aneurysmal bone cyst: a clinical, radiological, and pathological study of seven cases with COL1A1-USP6 fusion and a novel ANGPTL2-USP6 fusion. *Mod Pathol.* 2020;33(8):1492–1504.

58. Sleater J, Mullins D, Chun K, Hendricks J. Fibro-osseous pseudotumor of the digit: a comparison to myositis ossificans by light microscopy and immunohistochemical methods. *J Cutan Pathol.* 1996;23(4):373–377.

59. Oliveira AM, Perez-Atayde AR, Inwards CY, et al. USP6 and CDH11 oncogenes identify the neoplastic cell in primary aneurysmal bone cysts and are absent in so-called secondary aneurysmal bone cysts. *Am J Pathol.* 2004;165(5):1773–1780.

60. Erickson-Johnson MR, Chou MM, Evers BR, et al. Nodular fasciitis: a novel model of transient neoplasia induced by MYH9-USP6 gene fusion. *Lab Invest.* 2011;91(10):1427–1433.

61. Sukov WR, Franco MF, Erickson-Johnson M, et al. Frequency of USP6 rearrangements in myositis ossificans, brown tumor, and cherubism: molecular cytogenetic evidence that a subset of "myositis ossificans-like lesions" are the early phases in the formation of soft-tissue aneurysmal bone cyst. *Skeletal Radiol.* 2008;37(4): 321–327.

62. Bekers EM, Eijkelenboom A, Grünberg K, et al. Myositis ossificans—another condition with USP6 rearrangement, providing evidence of a relationship with nodular fasciitis and aneurysmal bone cyst. *Ann Diagn Pathol.* 2018;34:56–59.

63. Flucke U, Shepard SJ, Bekers EM, et al. Fibro-osseous pseudotumor of digits—expanding the spectrum of clonal transient neoplasms harboring USP6 rearrangement. *Ann Diagn Pathol.* 2018;35:53–55.

64. Nilsson M, Domanski HA, Mertens F, Mandahl N. Molecular cytogenetic characterization of recurrent translocation breakpoints in bizarre parosteal osteochondromatous proliferation (Nora's lesion). *Hum Pathol.* 2004;35(9):1063–1069.

65. Broehm CJ, M'Lady G, Bocklage T, Wenceslao S, Chafey D. Bizarre parosteal osteochondromatous proliferation: a new cytogenetic subgroup characterized by inversion of chromosome 7. *Cancer Genet.* 2013;206(11):402–405.

66. Chung EB, Enzinger FM. Extraskeletal osteosarcoma. *Cancer.* 1987;60(5):1132–1142.

67. Llamas-Velasco M, Rütten A, Requena L, Mentzel T. Primary cutaneous osteosarcoma of the skin: a report of 2 cases with emphasis on the differential diagnoses. *Am J Dermatopathol.* 2013;35(6):e106–e113.

68. Sacker AR, Oyama KK, Kessler S. Primary osteosarcoma of the penis. *Am J Dermatopathol.* 1994;16(3):285–287.

69. Dubey SP, Murthy DP, Cooke RA, Chaudhuri D. Primary osteogenic sarcoma of the tongue. *J Laryngol Otol.* 1999;113(4): 376–379.

70. Santos-Juanes J, Galache C, Miralles M, Curto JR, Sánchez del Río J, Soto J. Primary cutaneous extraskeletal osteosarcoma under a previous electrodessicated actinic keratosis. *J Am Acad Dermatol.* 2004;51(5 suppl):S166–S168.

71. Konishi E, Kusuzaki K, Murata H, Tsuchihashi Y, Beabout JW, Unni KK. Extraskeletal osteosarcoma arising in myositis ossificans. *Skeletal Radiol.* 2001;30(1):39–43.

72. Savant D, Kenan S, Kenan S, Kahn L. Extraskeletal osteosarcoma arising in myositis ossificans: a case report and review of the literature. *Skeletal Radiol.* 2017;46(8):1155–1161.

73. Conner JR, Hornick JL. SATB2 is a novel marker of osteoblastic differentiation in bone and soft tissue tumours. *Histopathology.* 2013;63(1):36–49.

74. Falconieri G, Cataldi P, Kavalar R, Štitič V, Luzar B. Cutaneous osteoblastic osteosarcoma: report of 2 new cases integrated with SATB2 immunohistochemistry and review of the literature. *Am J Dermatopathol.* 2016;38(11):824–831.

75. Davis JL, Horvai AE. Special AT-rich sequence-binding protein 2 (SATB2) expression is sensitive but may not be specific for osteosarcoma as compared with other high-grade primary bone sarcomas. *Histopathology.* 2016;69(1):84–90.

76. Papalas JA, Balmer NN, Wallace C, Sangüeza OP. Ossifying dermatofibroma with osteoclast-like giant cells: report of a case and literature review. *Am J Dermatopathol.* 2009;31(4):379–383.

77. Chen KT. Atypical fibroxanthoma of the skin with osteoid production. *Arch Dermatol.* 1980;116(1):113–114.

78. Adhikari LA, McCalmont TH, Folpe AL. Merkel cell carcinoma with heterologous rhabdomyoblastic differentiation: the role of immunohistochemistry for Merkel cell polyomavirus large T-antigen in confirmation. *J Cutan Pathol.* 2012;39(1):47–51.

79. Ragsdale MI, Lehmer LM, Ragsdale BD, Chow WA, Carson RT. Cutaneous metastasis of osteosarcoma in the scalp. *Am J Dermatopathol.* 2011;33(6):e70–e73.

80. Ahmad SA, Patel SR, Ballo MT, et al. Extraosseous osteosarcoma: response to treatment and long-term outcome. *J Clin Oncol.* 2002; 20(2):521–527.

81. Longhi A, Bielack SS, Grimer R, et al. Extraskeletal osteosarcoma: a European Musculoskeletal Oncology Society study on 266 patients. *Eur J Cancer.* 2017;74:9–16.

82. Chung EB, Enzinger FM. Chondroma of soft parts. *Cancer.* 1978;41(4):1414–1424.

83. Dahlin DC, Salvador AH. Cartilaginous tumors of the soft tissues of the hands and feet. *Mayo Clin Proc.* 1974;49(10):721–726.

84. Pollock L, Malone M, Shaw DG. Childhood soft tissue chondroma: a case report. *Pediatr Pathol Lab Med.* 1995;15(3):437–441.

85. Ryu JH, Park EJ, Kim KH, Kim KJ. A case of congenital soft tissue chondroma. *J Dermatol.* 2005;32(3):214–216.

86. Gangopadhyay AN, Khurana SK, Rastogi BL, Kulshrestha S. Soft tissue chondroma in an infant. *J Indian Med Assoc.* 1991;89(11):315.

87. Dellon AL, Weiss SW, Mitch WE. Bilateral extraosseous chondromas of the hand in a patient with chronic renal failure. *J Hand Surg Am.* 1978;3(2):139–141.

88. Temsamani H, Mouhsine A, Benchafai I, Benariba F. Bilateral extraskeletal chondroma of the neck. *Eur Ann Otorhinolaryngol Head Neck Dis.* 2016;133(4):295–296.

89. Hsueh S, Santa Cruz DJ. Cartilaginous lesions of the skin and superficial soft tissue. *J Cutan Pathol.* 1982;9(6):405–416.

90. Ando K, Goto Y, Hirabayashi N, Matsumoto Y, Ohashi M. Cutaneous cartilaginous tumor. *Dermatol Surg.* 1995;21(4):339–341.

91. Batalla A, Suh-Oh HJ, Pardavila R, de la Torre C. True cutaneous chondroma: a case report. *J Cutan Pathol.* 2015;42(9):657–659.

92. Humphreys TR, Herzberg AJ, Elenitsas R, Johnson BL, Goldstein J. Familial occurrence of multiple cutaneous chondromas. *Am J Dermatopathol.* 1994;16(1):56–59.

93. Steiner GC, Meushar N, Norman A, Present D. Intracapsular and paraarticular chondromas. *Clin Orthop Relat Res.* 1994;(303):231–236.

94. Koff AB, Goldberg LH, Ambergel D. Nail dystrophy in a 35-year-old man. Subungual enchondroma. *Arch Dermatol.* 1996;132(2):223, 226.

95. Wilson CA, El-Khayat RH, Somerville J, McKenna K. Digitial endochondroma. *Dermatol Online J.* 2014;21(2):13030/qt9vb4f09s.

96. Cates JM, Rosenberg AE, O'Connell JX, Nielsen GP. Chondroblastoma-like chondroma of soft tissue: an underrecognized variant and its differential diagnosis. *Am J Surg Pathol.* 2001;25(5):661–666.

97. Shon W, Folpe AL, Fritchie KJ. ERG expression in chondrogenic bone and soft tissue tumours. *J Clin Pathol.* 2015;68(2):125–129. doi:10.1136/jclinpath-2014-202601

98. Dal Cin P, Qi H, Sciot R, Van den Berghe H. Involvement of chromosomes 6 and 11 in a soft tissue chondroma. *Cancer Genet Cytogenet.* 1997;93(2):177–178.

99. Sakai Junior N, Abe KT, Formigli LM, et al. Cytogenetic findings in 14 benign cartilaginous neoplasms. *Cancer Genet.* 2011;204(4):180–186.

100. Dahlén A, Mertens F, Rydholm A, et al. Fusion, disruption, and expression of HMGA2 in bone and soft tissue chondromas. *Mod Pathol.* 2003;16(11):1132–1140.

101. Amary F, Perez-Casanova L, Ye H, et al. Synovial chondromatosis and soft tissue chondroma: extraosseous cartilaginous tumor defined by FN1 gene rearrangement. *Mod Pathol.* 2019;32(12):1762–1771.

102. Liu YJ, Wang W, Yeh J, et al. Calcified chondroid mesenchymal neoplasms with FN1-receptor tyrosine kinase gene fusions including FGFR2, FGFR1, MERTK, NTRK1, and TEK: a molecular and clinicopathologic analysis. *Mod Pathol.* 2021;34(7):1373–1383.

103. Agaram NP, Zhang L, Dickson BC, et al. A molecular study of synovial chondromatosis. *Genes Chromosomes Cancer.* 2020;59(3):144–151.

104. Shon W, Folpe AL. Tenosynovitis with psammomatous calcification: a poorly recognized pseudotumor related to repetitive tendinous injury. *Am J Surg Pathol.* 2010;34(6):892–895.

105. Michal M, Agaimy A, Folpe AL, et al. Tenosynovitis with psammomatous calcifications: a distinctive trauma-associated subtype of idiopathic calcifying tenosynovitis with a predilection for the distal extremities of middle-aged women—a report of 23 cases. *Am J Surg Pathol.* 2019;43(2):261–267.

106. Ragsdale BD, Sweet DE, Vinh TN. Radiology as gross pathology in evaluating chondroid lesions. *Hum Pathol.* 1989;20(10):930–951. doi:10.1016/0046-8177(89)90266-9

107. Nakamura R, Ehara S, Nishida J, Shiraishi H, Sato T, Tamakawa Y. Diffuse mineralization of extraskeletal chondroma: a case report. *Radiat Med.* 1997;15(1):51–53.

108. Chandramohan M, Thomas NB, Funk L, Muir LT. MR appearance of mineralized extra skeletal chondroma: a case report and review of literature. *Clin Radiol.* 2002;57(5):421–423.

109. Bianchi S, Zwass A, Abdelwahab IF, Olivieri M, Marinaro E. Sonographic evaluation of soft tissue chondroma. *J Clin Ultrasound.* 1996;24(3):148–150.

110. Allen PW, Enzinger FM. Juvenile aponeurotic fibroma. *Cancer.* 1970;26(4):857–867.

111. Oruç M, Uysal A, Kankaya Y, Yildiz K, Aslan G, Sengül D. A case of calcifying aponeurotic fibroma of the scalp: case report and review of the literature. *Dermatol Surg.* 2007;33(11):1380–1383.

112. Sharma R, Punia RS, Sharma A, Marwah N. Juvenile (calcifying) aponeurotic fibroma of the neck. *Pediatr Surg Int.* 1998;13(4):295–296.

113. Murphy BA, Kilpatrick SE, Panella MJ, White WL. Extra-acral calcifying aponeurotic fibroma: a distinctive case with 23-year follow-up. *J Cutan Pathol.* 1996;23(4):369–372.

114. Fetsch JF, Miettinen M. Calcifying aponeurotic fibroma: a clinicopathologic study of 22 cases arising in uncommon sites. *Hum Pathol.* 1998;29(12):1504–1510.

115. Puls F, Hofvander J, Magnusson L, et al. FN1-EGF gene fusions are recurrent in calcifying aponeurotic fibroma. *J Pathol.* 2016;238(4):502–507.

116. Kao YC, Flucke U, Eijkelenboom A, et al. Novel EWSR1-SMAD3 gene fusions in a group of acral fibroblastic spindle cell neoplasms. *Am J Surg Pathol.* 2018;42(4):522–528.

117. Michal M, Berry RS, Rubin BP, et al. EWSR1-SMAD3-rearranged fibroblastic tumor: an emerging entity in an increasingly more complex group of fibroblastic/myofibroblastic neoplasms. *Am J Surg Pathol.* 2018;42(10):1325–1333.

118. Habeeb O, Korty KE, Azzato EM, et al. EWSR1-SMAD3 rearranged fibroblastic tumor: case series and review. *J Cutan Pathol.* 2021;48(2):255–262.

119. Amaravati R. Rare malignant transformation of a calcifying aponeurotic fibroma. *J Bone Joint Surg Am.* 2002;84(10):1889; author reply 1889.

120. Lafferty KA, Nelson EL, Demuth RJ, Miller SH, Harrison MW. Juvenile aponeurotic fibroma with disseminated fibrosarcoma. *J Hand Surg Am.* 1986;11(5):737–740.

121. Goh YW, Spagnolo DV, Platten M, et al. Extraskeletal myxoid chondrosarcoma: a light microscopic, immunohistochemical, ultrastructural and immuno-ultrastructural study indicating neuroendocrine differentiation. *Histopathology.* 2001;39(5):514–524.

122. Aigner T, Oliveira AM, Nascimento AG. Extraskeletal myxoid chondrosarcomas do not show a chondrocytic phenotype. *Mod Pathol.* 2004;17(2):214–221.

123. Meis-Kindblom JM, Bergh P, Gunterberg B, Kindblom LG. Extraskeletal myxoid chondrosarcoma: a reappraisal of its morphologic spectrum and prognostic factors based on 117 cases. *Am J Surg Pathol.* 1999;23(6):636–650.

124. Drilon AD, Popat S, Bhuchar G, et al. Extraskeletal myxoid chondrosarcoma: a retrospective review from 2 referral centers emphasizing long-term outcomes with surgery and chemotherapy. *Cancer.* 2008;113(12):3364–3371.

125. Paioli A, Stacchiotti S, Campanacci D, et al. Extraskeletal myxoid chondrosarcoma with molecularly confirmed diagnosis: a multicenter retrospective study within the Italian Sarcoma Group. *Ann Surg Oncol.* 2021;28(2):1142–1150.

126. Hachitanda Y, Tsuneyoshi M, Daimaru Y, et al. Extraskeletal myxoid chondrosarcoma in young children. *Cancer.* 1988; 61(12):2521–2526.

127. Oliveira AM, Sebo TJ, McGrory JE, Gaffey TA, Rock MG, Nascimento AG. Extraskeletal myxoid chondrosarcoma: a clinicopathologic, immunohistochemical, and ploidy analysis of 23 cases. *Mod Pathol.* 2000;13(8):900–908.

128. Okamoto S, Hisaoka M, Ishida T, et al. Extraskeletal myxoid chondrosarcoma: a clinicopathologic, immunohistochemical, and molecular analysis of 18 cases. *Hum Pathol.* 2001;32(10): 1116–1124.

129. Karamchandani JR, Nielsen TO, van de Rijn M, West RB. Sox10 and S100 in the diagnosis of soft-tissue neoplasms. *Appl Immunohistochem Mol Morphol.* 2012;20(5):445–450.

130. Yoshida A, Makise N, Wakai S, Kawai A, Hiraoka N. INSM1 expression and its diagnostic significance in extraskeletal myxoid chondrosarcoma. *Mod Pathol.* 2018;31(5):744–752.

131. Wang WL, Mayordomo E, Czerniak BA, et al. Fluorescence in situ hybridization is a useful ancillary diagnostic tool for extraskeletal myxoid chondrosarcoma. *Mod Pathol.* 2008;21(11):1303–1310.

132. Noguchi H, Mitsuhashi T, Seki K, et al. Fluorescence in situ hybridization analysis of extraskeletal myxoid chondrosarcomas using EWSR1 and NR4A3 probes. *Hum Pathol.* 2010;41(3):336–342.

133. Sciot R, Dal Cin P, Fletcher C, et al. t(9;22)(q22-31;q11-12) is a consistent marker of extraskeletal myxoid chondrosarcoma: evaluation of three cases. *Mod Pathol.* 1995;8(7):765–768.

134. Subramanian S, West RB, Marinelli RJ, et al. The gene expression profile of extraskeletal myxoid chondrosarcoma. *J Pathol.* 2005;206(4):433–444.

135. Davis EJ, Wu YM, Robinson D, et al. Next generation sequencing of extraskeletal myxoid chondrosarcoma. *Oncotarget.* 2017;8(13):21770–21777.

136. Chiusole B, Le Cesne A, Rastrelli M, et al. Extraskeletal myxoid chondrosarcoma: clinical and molecular characteristics and outcomes of patients treated at two institutions. *Front Oncol.* 2020;10:828.

137. Kemmerer EJ, Gleeson E, Poli J, Ownbey RT, Brady LW, Bowne WB. Benefit of radiotherapy in extraskeletal myxoid chondrosarcoma: a propensity score weighted population-based analysis of the SEER database. *Am J Clin Oncol.* 2018;41(7):674–680.

138. Nakashima Y, Unni KK, Shives TC, Swee RG, Dahlin DC. Mesenchymal chondrosarcoma of bone and soft tissue. A review of 111 cases. *Cancer.* 1986;57(12):2444–2453.

139. Frezza AM, Cesari M, Baumhoer D, et al. Mesenchymal chondrosarcoma: prognostic factors and outcome in 113 patients. A European Musculoskeletal Oncology Society study. *Eur J Cancer.* 2015;51(3):374–381.

140. Bishop MW, Somerville JM, Bahrami A, et al. Mesenchymal chondrosarcoma in children and young adults: a single institution retrospective review. *Sarcoma.* 2015;2015:608279.

141. Aramburu-González JA, Rodríguez-Justo M, Jiménez-Reyes J, Santonja C. A case of soft tissue mesenchymal chondrosarcoma metastatic to skin, clinically mimicking keratoacanthoma. *Am J Dermatopathol.* 1999;21(4):392–394.

142. Shapeero LG, Vanel D, Couanet D, Contesso G, Ackerman LV. Extraskeletal mesenchymal chondrosarcoma. *Radiology.* 1993;186(3):819–826.

143. Fanburg-Smith JC, Auerbach A, Marwaha JS, et al. Immunoprofile of mesenchymal chondrosarcoma: aberrant desmin and EMA expression, retention of INI1, and negative estrogen receptor in 22 female-predominant central nervous system and musculoskeletal cases. *Ann Diagn Pathol.* 2010;14(1):8–14.

144. Folpe AL, Graham RP, Martinez A, Schembri-Wismayer D, Boland J, Fritchie KJ. Mesenchymal chondrosarcomas showing immunohistochemical evidence of rhabdomyoblastic differentiation: a potential diagnostic pitfall. *Hum Pathol.* 2018;77:28–34.

145. Hoang MP, Suarez PA, Donner LR, et al. Mesenchymal chondrosarcoma: a small cell neoplasm with polyphenotypic differentiation. *Int J Surg Pathol.* 2000;8(4):291–301.

146. Granter SR, Renshaw AA, Fletcher CD, Bhan AK, Rosenberg AE. CD99 reactivity in mesenchymal chondrosarcoma. *Hum Pathol.* 1996;27(12):1273–1276.

147. Hung YP, Fletcher CD, Hornick JL. Evaluation of NKX2-2 expression in round cell sarcomas and other tumors with EWSR1 rearrangement: imperfect specificity for Ewing sarcoma. *Mod Pathol.* 2016;29(4):370–380.

148. Wehrli BM, Huang W, De Crombrugghe B, Ayala AG, Czerniak B. Sox9, a master regulator of chondrogenesis, distinguishes mesenchymal chondrosarcoma from other small blue round cell tumors. *Hum Pathol.* 2003;34(3):263–269.

149. Fanburg-Smith JC, Auerbach A, Marwaha JS, Wang Z, Rushing EJ. Reappraisal of mesenchymal chondrosarcoma: novel morphologic observations of the hyaline cartilage and endochondral ossification and beta-catenin, Sox9, and osteocalcin immunostaining of 22 cases. *Hum Pathol.* 2010;41(5):653–662.

150. Gurel B, Ali TZ, Montgomery EA, et al. NKX3.1 as a marker of prostatic origin in metastatic tumors. *Am J Surg Pathol.* 2010; 34(8):1097–1105.

151. Yoshida KI, Machado I, Motoi T, et al. NKX3-1 is a useful immunohistochemical marker of EWSR1-NFATC2 sarcoma and mesenchymal chondrosarcoma. *Am J Surg Pathol.* 2020;44(6):719–728.

152. Wang L, Motoi T, Khanin R, et al. Identification of a novel, recurrent HEY1-NCOA2 fusion in mesenchymal chondrosarcoma based on a genome-wide screen of exon-level expression data. *Genes Chromosomes Cancer.* 2012;51(2):127–139.

153. Nakayama R, Miura Y, Ogino J, et al. Detection of HEY1-NCOA2 fusion by fluorescence in-situ hybridization in formalin-fixed paraffin-embedded tissues as a possible diagnostic tool for mesenchymal chondrosarcoma. *Pathol Int.* 2012;62(12):823–826.

154. Nyquist KB, Panagopoulos I, Thorsen J, et al. Whole-transcriptome sequencing identifies novel IRF2BP2-CDX1 fusion gene brought about by translocation t(1;5)(q42;q32) in mesenchymal chondrosarcoma. *PLoS One.* 2012;7(11):e49705.

155. Buranasinsup S, Sila-Asna M, Bunyaratvej N, Bunyaratvej A. In vitro osteogenesis from human skin-derived precursor cells. *Dev Growth Differ.* 2006;48(4):263–269.

156. Leal-Khouri SM, Barnhill RL, Baden HP. An unusual cutaneous metastasis of a chondrosarcoma. *J Cutan Pathol.* 1990;17:274–277.

157. Arce FP, Pinto J, Portero I, et al. Cutaneous metastases as initial manifestation of dedifferentiated chondrosarcoma of bone: an autopsy case with review of the literature. *J Cutan Pathol.* 2000;27:262–267.

158. Patel NK, McKee PH, Smith NP, et al. Primary metaplastic carcinoma (carcinosarcoma) of the skin: a clinicopathologic study of four cases and review of the literature. *Am J Dermatopathol.* 1997;19:363–372.

159. Tran TA, Muller S, Chaudahri PJ, et al. Cutaneous carcinosarcoma: adnexal vs. epidermal types define high-and low-risk tumors: results of a meta-analysis. *J Cutan Pathol.* 2005;32:2–11.

160. Sexton CW, White WL. Chondrosarcomatous cutaneous metastasis. A unique manifestation of sarcomatoid (metaplastic) breast carcinoma. *Am J Dermatopathol.* 1996;18:538–542.

161. Banerjee SS, Eyden B. Divergent differentiation in malignant melanomas: a review. *Histopathology.* 2008;52:119–129.

162. Sundersingh S, Majhi U, Murhekar K, et al. Malignant melanoma with osteocartilaginous differentiation. *Indian J Pathol Microbiol.* 2010;53:130–132.

163. Palma Guzman JM, de Andrade BA, Rizo VH, Romañach MJ, León JE, de Almeida OP. Ectomesenchymal chondromyxoid tumor: histopathologic and immunohistochemical study of two cases without a chondroid component. *J Cutan Pathol.* 2012; 39:781–786.

164. Wilson PR, Strutton GM, Stewart MR. Atypical fibroxanthoma: two unusual variants. *J Cutan Pathol.* 1989;16:93–98.

165. Tiemann A, Bosse A, Finke U. Carcinoma metastasis in cutaneous osseous metaplasia. Differential diagnosis of osseous tumor metaplasia [in German]. *Chirurg.* 1992;63:988–989.

166. Lim CM, Ming LC, Goh YH, Lim LH, Lim L. Pseudocyst of the auricle: a histologic perspective. *Laryngoscope.* 2004;114:1281–1284.

167. Folpe AL, Weiss SW. Ossifying fibromyxoid tumor of soft parts: a clinicopathologic study of 70 cases with emphasis on atypical and malignant variants. *Am J Surg Pathol.* 2003;27(4):421–431.

168. Miettinen M, Finnell V, Fetsch JF. Ossifying fibromyxoid tumor of soft parts—a clinicopathologic and immunohistochemical study of 104 cases with long-term follow-up and a critical review of the literature. *Am J Surg Pathol.* 2008;32(7):996–1005.

169. Graham RP, Dry S, Li X, et al. Ossifying fibromyxoid tumor of soft parts: a clinicopathologic, proteomic, and genomic study. *Am J Surg Pathol.* 2011;35(11):1615–1625.

170. Kilpatrick SE, Ward WG, Mozes M, Miettinen M, Fukunaga M, Fletcher CD. Atypical and malignant variants of ossifying fibromyxoid tumor. Clinicopathologic analysis of six cases. *Am J Surg Pathol.* 1995;19(9):1039–1046.

171. Gebre-Medhin S, Nord KH, Möller E, et al. Recurrent rearrangement of the PHF1 gene in ossifying fibromyxoid tumors. *Am J Pathol.* 2012;181(3):1069–1077.

Chapter
37

Tumors of Neural Tissue

VICTOR G. PRIETO

GENERAL ANATOMIC RELATIONSHIPS

Structural Components

A nerve, an anatomic unit, is composed of nerve fibers, endoneurium, and perineurium. Nerve fibers, the functioning element, are aggregated to form axial bundles (parallel arrays of nerve fibers with longitudinal symmetry). Individually, each fiber consists of an axon, or axons, and related Schwann cells (1–4). Axons are cytoplasmic extensions from the perikaryon of neurons in the central nervous system, or ganglion cells in sympathetic ganglia. The peripheral portion of an axon, along its entire length from its origin to terminus, is enclosed by enveloping Schwann cells. Along nonmyelinated nerve fibers, a single Schwann cell encloses segments of several axons in cytoplasmic invaginations. Along myelinated nerve fibers, a single Schwann cell encloses a segment of an axon in concentric layers of its cytoplasmic membrane; a node of Ranvier is formed where neighboring Schwann cells abut end to end. In sympathetic ganglia, each neuron is rimmed by satellite cells; the relationship is reminiscent of that between Schwann cells and axons. Ultrastructurally, axons contain microfilaments, specialized intermediate (neural) filaments, and microtubules. Schwann cells have complex cytoplasmic processes; they are surrounded by continuous basal lamina and contain densely packed intermediate filaments (3).

The *perineurium*, a tubular fibrous sheath, delimits each nerve. It extends from the pia-arachnoid of the central nervous system to the terminus of each nerve or to specialized sensory receptors. Slender bipolar or tripolar cells (*perineurial cells*) are isolated among the concentric fibrous lamellae of the perineurium. Ultrastructurally, discontinuous basal lamina, numerous pinocytotic vesicles, and tight intercellular junctions are characteristics of the perineurial cells (3). The perineurium is a relatively impervious barrier and thus protects the nerves.

The *endoneurium*, a delicate, mucinous matrix, is confined by the perineurium; it provides a cushion for the axial collection of nerve fibers. Components of the endoneurium include fibroblasts (CD34+), mast cells, collagen, a myxoid matrix, and capillaries.

In proximal (axial) locations, several large nerves, in bundles, are encased in a dense fibrous matrix, the *epineurium* (a fibrous sheath that, at the junction of the spinal nerves with the central nervous system, is continuous with

the dura mater). Individual nerves, at some place along their course, leave the bundles to continue without an epineurium. Near the terminus of each nerve, nerve fibers extend beyond an open-ended perineurium into the mesenchyme; naked axons even extend into epithelium. Ensheathed receptors of the skin include mucocutaneous corpuscles, and the corpuscles of Vater-Pacini, Meissner, and Merkel cells. Meissner corpuscles are ovoid structures in which an axon is sinuously enclosed in stacks of distinctive cells. Pacinian corpuscles are spherical structures in soft tissue. In them, concentrically laminated, distinctive cells, and fibrous lamellae are arranged around a centrally located axon (Fig. 37-1). The ultrastructural features of the laminated cells of both Meissner and Pacinian corpuscles are similar to perineurial cells with the exception of the innermost cells that ensheathe the central axon (5).

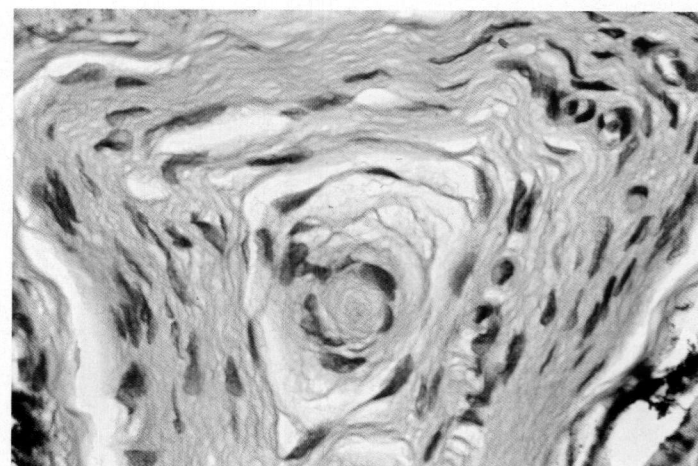

Figure 37-1 Pacinian corpuscle. This pacinian body has a distorted outline. At the periphery, there is a well-formed dense fibrous membrane. Elongated spindle cells are compressed among the compactly arranged collagen fibers. At the center, an acidophilic punctum is representative of a single axon. Cytoplasmic processes of sheath cells are clustered about the axon. There is an intermediate zone in which spindle cells are loosely spaced in a clear matrix. Regardless of the results of immunoreactions, the loosely spaced spindle cells have the morphologic features of perineurial cells. There is a morphologic continuum from periphery to, but not including, axon.

ONTOGENY AND REACTIONS TO INJURY AS RELATED TO THE INTERPRETATION OF PHENOTYPIC EXPRESSIONS OR PATTERNS IN NEOPLASIA

Neurosustentacular cells of peripheral nerves, related cells of the peripheral ganglia, melanocytes, and even cells of some cranial mesenchyme are all of neurocristic origin.

In reactions of peripheral nerves to injury, reserve cells of neural origin proliferate; they subsequently express either schwannian or perineurial phenotypes. Expressions of phenotype are fortuitous; the environs, in which uncommitted reserve cells find themselves, likely influence the final phenotypic expression. The available options probably include a capacity to function facultatively as endoneurial fibroblasts (6).

Histologic morphologies of neural tumors may be classified according to the similarities to either normal structures or to the reactions of normal nerves to injury. Thus, the structure of Meissner corpuscles is recapitulated in the tactile corpuscle–like structures (tactoid bodies) of diffuse (extraneural) neurofibromas (4). Some of the features of neural Wallerian degeneration (Fig. 37-2) are recapitulated in granular cell nerve sheath tumors. The intravaginal hyaline nodules of Renaut (4) may provide a model for the patterns manifested in nerve sheath myxomas. When damaged, axons form multiple, sproutlike extensions (6). In the ensuing reparative process, newly formed Schwann cells accompany newly formed axons (Fig. 37-3). These patterns are very similar to those seen in spontaneous, intraneural neuromas.

PHENOTYPES AND HISTOCHEMICAL AND IMMUNOHISTOCHEMICAL REACTIONS

Neurosustentacular cells, melanocytes, and even some mesenchymal cells, being of neurocristic origin, share a common

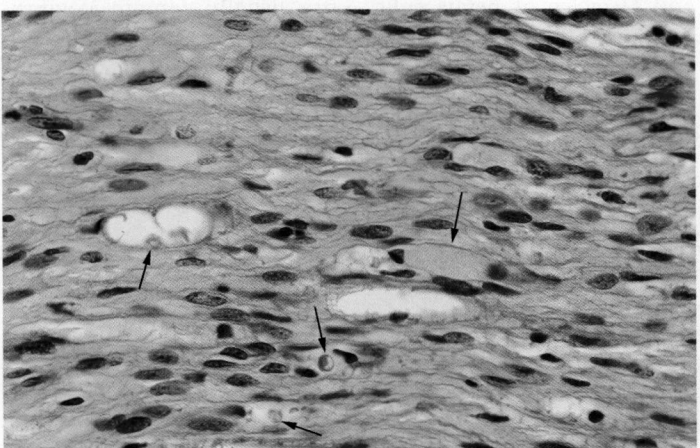

Figure 37-2 Wallerian degeneration. This peripheral nerve, bordering the site of an injury, shows poorly defined myelin sheaths; as a result, reticular fibers (basement membranes) of individual Schwann cells are more closely spaced. Scattered microcystic areas are representative of sites in which myelin sheaths have been disrupted. In some of the defects, there are globular deposits, some of which are concentrically laminated (*black arrows*); these "myelin figures" are collections of lipid membranes. Some of the Schwann cells are swollen and have pale, faintly granular cytoplasm.

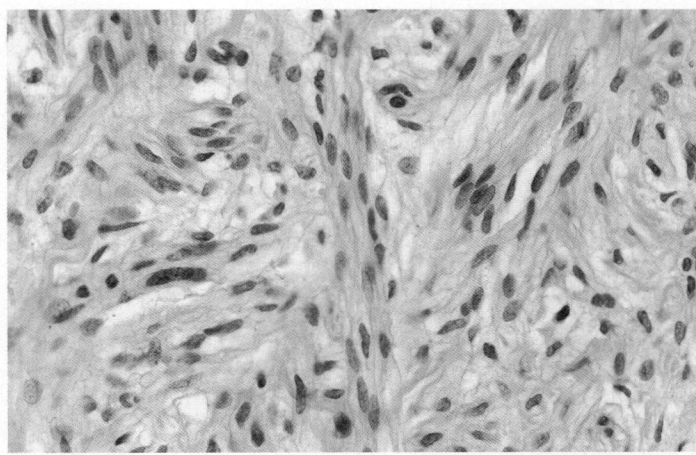

Figure 37-3 Extraneural neuroma. In this extraneural neuroma, Schwann cells cluster to form thin fascicles among collagen bundles of the preexisting soft tissue. Proliferating axons, as they extend in the process of repair into the fibrous tissue, provide a scaffold for proliferating Schwann cells.

progenitor. The cells of tumors of peripheral nerves commonly express the ultrastructural qualities of either Schwann cells or perineurial cells, but there may be conflicting findings; for example, those cells of tactile corpuscles that have the ultrastructural features of perineurial cells mark with antibodies for S-100 protein (as do Schwann cells).

S-100 protein is a lightly acidic, calcium-binding protein of glial cells but is also expressed in the skin in a variety of other cells, including melanocytes, adipocytes, chondrocytes, myoepithelial cells of sweat glands, and Schwann cells. *Neuron-specific enolase* (NSE), neurofilaments, and peripherin are cytoplasmic proteins common to a variety of cells, including neurons and their axons. In addition, peripherin is also expressed by a variety of melanocytes. An immunoreaction for the demonstration of neural filaments or peripherin provides a pure demonstration of the reaction of axons. On a histochemical level, silver impregnation techniques demonstrate axons (Fig. 37-4) but are less sensitive than immunohistochemistry. The luxol-fast blue stain and antibodies for either myelin basic protein (MBP) or CD57 (Leu-7) antigen demonstrate myelin products. An immunoreaction for glial fibrillary acidic protein (GFAP) is positive in glial cells; it is also positive in some of the cells in some

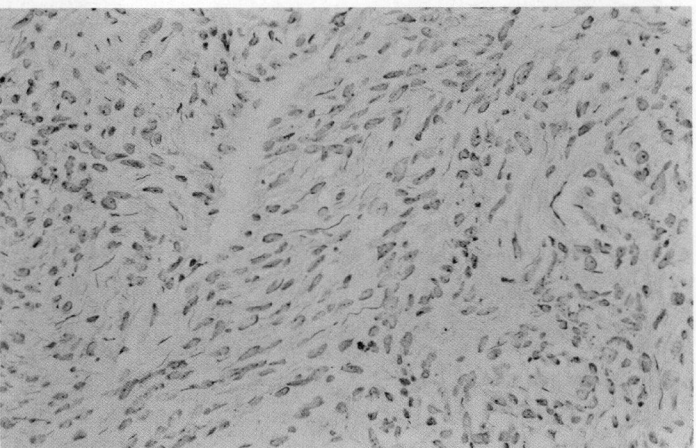

Figure 37-4 Extraneural neuroma (Bodian stain). The loosely spaced, delicate fibers are axons; axons are argyrophilic.

tumors of salivary glands. In some large schwannomas of soft tissue, neoplastic Schwann cells also express GFAP. *Epithelial membrane antigen* (EMA) is a cytoplasmic antigen commonly expressed in a variety of normal and neoplastic tissue, including eccrine/apocrine and sebaceous cells.

NEOPLASMS

Neurofibromas (Hamartomas with Phenotypic Diversity)

Clinical Summary. Cutaneous neurofibromas (CNFs) (the common, sporadic neurofibromas) are soft, polypoid, and skin colored or slightly tan; they are small (rarely larger than a centimeter in diameter) (Fig. 37-5A). They usually arise in adulthood. The identification of CNFs, in the absence of other stigmata, does not establish a diagnosis of neurofibromatosis.

Histopathology. Under low magnification, most examples of CNF are faintly eosinophilic. They are extraneural, small dermal tumors, relatively circumscribed, but not encapsulated (Fig. 37-5B) (3,4). Thin spindle cells with elongated, wavy nuclei are regularly spaced among thin, wavy collagenous strands (Fig. 37-6). The strands are either closely spaced (homogeneous pattern) or loosely spaced in a clear matrix (loose pattern): the two patterns are often intermixed in a single lesion. Rarely are CNFs hypocellular lesions composed of widely spaced spindle and stellate cells in a myxoid matrix. The demonstration of preserved cutaneous adnexa admixed with the cells of a CNF is a combination that qualifies the lesion as hamartomatous (Fig. 37-5B). Small nerves are easily identified around CNFs. On rare occasions, there are tactoid (tactile corpuscle-like) bodies and pigmented, dendritic melanocytes (4,7). Also exceptional is a signet-ring cell–like morphology resembling lipoblasts (8). Traditionally, it has been considered that neurofibromas contain axons, Schwann cells, perineural cells, and fibroblasts. More recently, the term "telocytes" (interstitial Cajal-like cells, endoneurial dendritic cells) has been proposed for those dendritic cells expressing CD34 seen in normal nerve tissue as well as in most peripheral nerve sheath tumors (9,10).

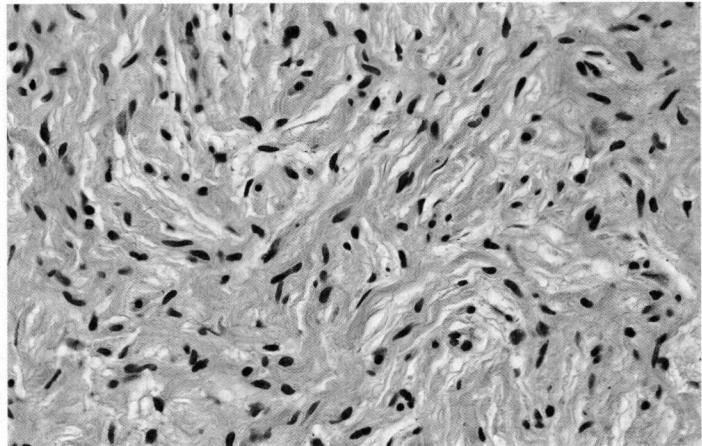

Figure 37-6 Extraneural sporadic cutaneous neurofibroma. Thin spindle cells are associated with thin, wavy collagen bundles. The cells and collagen bundles are loosely spaced in a clear or mucinous matrix.

Histogenesis. Silver impregnations (Bodian or Bielschowsky stain) reveal scattered axons, mostly in small, embedded nerves, throughout the lesion. Immunohistochemically, axons appear more numerous and more uniformly distributed. Antiperipherin and antineurofilaments label the axons in either punctate (when cut perpendicularly) or fiber-like (when cut parallel to their long axis). Anti-NSE labels the axons; the cytoplasm of Schwann cells is faintly, but diffusely, labeled.

Differential Diagnosis. Because schwannomas are intraneural lesions, they are well circumscribed/encapsulated. In contrast to neurofibromas, schwannomas contain very few axons, and they are usually located at the periphery of the lesion, in a subcapsular location between the tumor and the perineurium (tumor capsule). In contrast to neurofibromas, there is no loose intermingling of irregularly dispersed remnants of the axial bundle of the nerve of origin in the tumoral component.

Neurotized nevi show areas indistinguishable from neurofibromas. However, they contain at least a few superficial nests and fascicles of nevus cells. They usually contain Wagner–Meissner corpuscles, which are rare in CNFs.

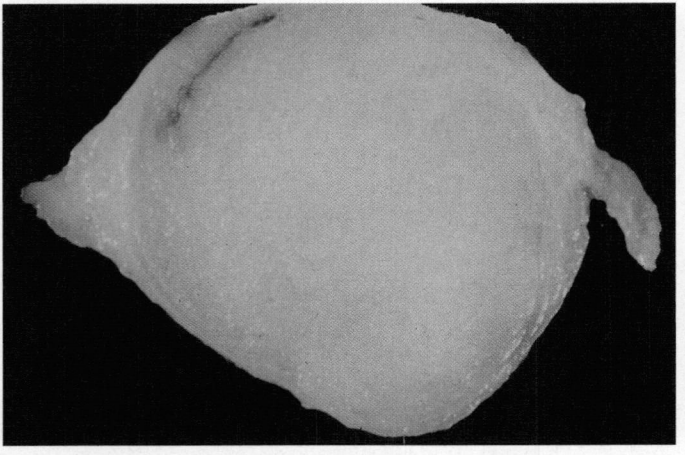

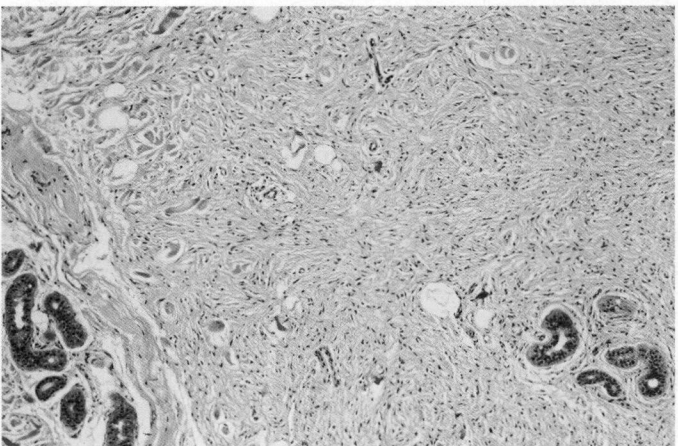

Figure 37-5 **A:** Extraneural sporadic cutaneous neurofibroma. This symmetrically rounded, circumscribed tumor bulges into the subcutaneous fat. The cut surface is white and homogeneous. **B:** Extraneural sporadic cutaneous neurofibroma. A circumscribed, nonencapsulated tumor of the dermis is composed of loosely spaced spindle cells and wavy collagenous strands. Near the margin, collagen bundles of the dermis are entrapped in the lesion. A cluster of sweat glands is also present within the tumor; in this relationship, a defect in dermal mesenchyme has been inlaid with a neurocristic derivative.

Some sporadic neurofibromas, including subcutaneous variants, are confined, at least in part, by the perineurium of the nerve of origin and are thus intraneural and circumscribed. This architecture may thus raise the possibility of plexiform neurofibroma.

Dermatofibromas may also be confused with neurofibromas, particularly those lesions with markedly fibrous stroma. However, dermatofibromas only have rare, scattered dendritic cells expressing S100 protein. Medallion-like dermal dendrocyte hamartoma is another fibrohistiocytic lesion that may be confused with neurofibroma. This is a benign, rare congenital or acquired lesion, comprised of a benign dermal proliferation of fusiform cells, presenting as a well-circumscribed atrophic and wrinkled patch located on the upper trunk or neck. Tumor cells express CD34 and factor XIIIa, but not S100 (11,12); these lesions lack the t(17;22)(q21;q13) characteristic of dermatofibrosarcoma protuberans.

Traumatic neuromas may resemble neurofibroma because of the presence of numerous small nerve twigs (see later).

Principles of Management: Except for malignant transformation (usually associated with rapid growth in a long-standing lesion; see also later), CNF are removed only when they result in cosmetic or functional problems.

NEUROFIBROMATOSIS (NF)

Clinical Summary. Neurofibromatosis is a genetic disease that involves the nervous system. It has three major subtypes: NF1 (the most common subtype, also known as von Recklinghausen disease), NF2, and schwannomatosis.

NF1

Clinical summary: Multiple CNFs are characteristic of most, but not all, examples of NF1. Other important stigmata include plexiform (intraneural), and deep, diffuse (extraneural) neurofibromas; multiple periareolar neurofibromas (Fig. 37-7); intraocular Lisch nodules; and macular, cutaneous hyperpigmentation (e.g., café-au-lait spots and bilateral axillary freckling). These patients may also have neurocognitive delays and skeletal abnormalities (13,14).

Pathogenesis: Neurofibromatosis type I (NF1) may arise as an autosomal dominant condition but is secondary to spontaneous mutation in nearly half of the patients (15). CNFs usually appear first in late childhood or in adolescence; the disease

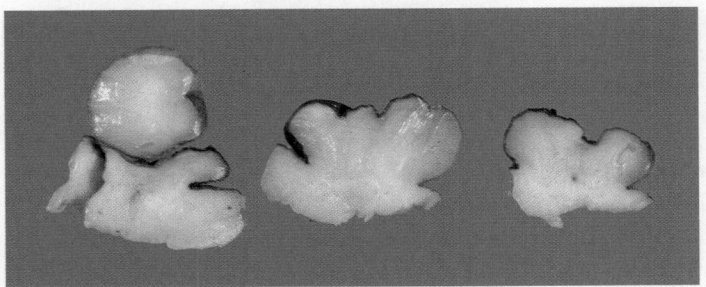

Figure 37-7 Periareolar neurofibroma. The lesion has been breadloafed. Multiple polypoid components project above the skin surface. The cut surface is white and glistening. The lesion diffusely involves the dermis and protrudes irregularly into the subcutaneous fat.

progresses by showing gradual increases in the size and number of neurofibromas.

For NF1, its gene is located in the pericentromeric region of the long arm of chromosome 17 (16). The large gene's size may account for the high incidence of sporadic cases. The gene shows functional and structural homology with the guanosine triphosphatase–activating protein, which controls the *ras* oncogene. As a result, the role of the *ras* oncogene in growth, development, and differentiation may be aberrantly expressed in the NF1 phenotype (16). The protein product of the gene is called neurofibromin (17). This gene may have multiple alterations in NF1, such as point mutations, microdeletions, and exon deletions or duplications; most of them result in premature termination codons and truncated neurofibromin (18). In addition to neurofibromin, there are multiple genetic alterations in some of these tumors, particularly malignant ones, including methylation changes (19).

In NF1, all sorts of nerves may be affected, including superficial peripheral nerves, deep peripheral nerves, nerve roots, and the autonomic nerves of viscera and blood vessels. Large, pendulous plexiform neurofibromas have the flabby texture of a "bag of worms." Deep, diffuse neurofibromas are poorly defined at their limits with the adjacent soft tissue (4). Owing to the diffuse nature of the lesions and their size, the limbs may have an elephantiasic quality. Spinal nerve root tumors may cause compression of the spinal cord (15). Tumors of the central nervous system occur in 5% to 10% of the patients (13). Neurofibromas adjacent to the bone may erode it. Lesions that are variably associated with NF include kyphoscoliosis and an increase in the length of long bones. NF1 may be associated with diffuse intestinal ganglioneuromatosis and multiple endocrine neoplasia (MEN), type 2b (20,21). Gastrointestinal stromal tumors are more common in NF1 than in the general population (22,23), as well as xanthogranulomas and juvenile chronic myelogenous leukemias (23).

In localized or segmental NF, CNFs are few and there is no family history (24–26). Dermoscopy may be helpful for the clinical diagnosis; the lesions tend to show peripheral pigment network, peripheral halo of brown pigmentation, and fingerprint-like structures (18).

NF2

Clinical Summary: NF2 is a rare autosomal dominant disorder (1:200,000 individuals) (27), also called "MISME Syndrome," for "Multiple Inherited Schwannomas, Meningiomas, and Ependymomas." There is a more than 95% penetrance by age 60. Manifestations include hearing loss, café-au-lait spots, neurofibromas, schwannomas, and a variety of intracranial tumors, such as bilateral schwannomas of the acoustic nerve (Fig. 37-8) and meningioangiomatosis. Detection of bilateral acoustic schwannomas is considered diagnostic of the syndrome. The gene locus has been linked to chromosome 22q11-q13. The protein gene product, called *merlin*, is similar to a group of cytoskeleton-linked proteins (17) and appears to work as a tumor suppressor involved in multiple pathways (Ras/Raf/MEK/ERK, PI3K/Akt/mTORC1, NF-kB, and Hippo). Its loss results in de-differentiation and abnormal growth of Schwann cells. Loss of SOX-10 function, a marker present in both neural and melanocytic cells, may contribute to Schwann cell proliferation (28). Interestingly, schwannoma cell lines have receptors for curcumin, which might be useful as a therapeutic tool (29).

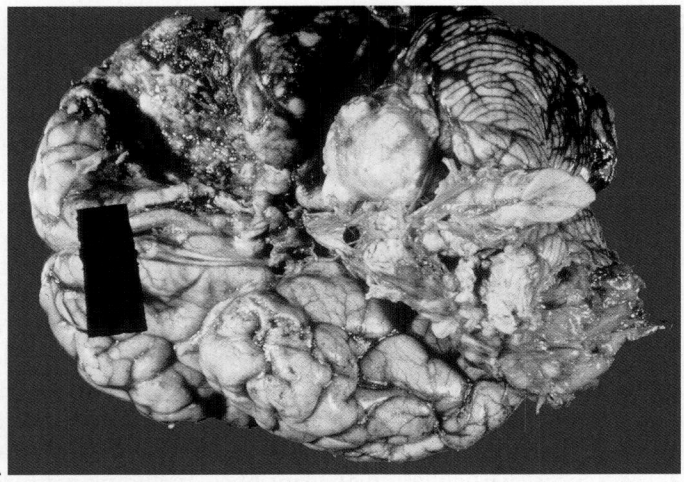
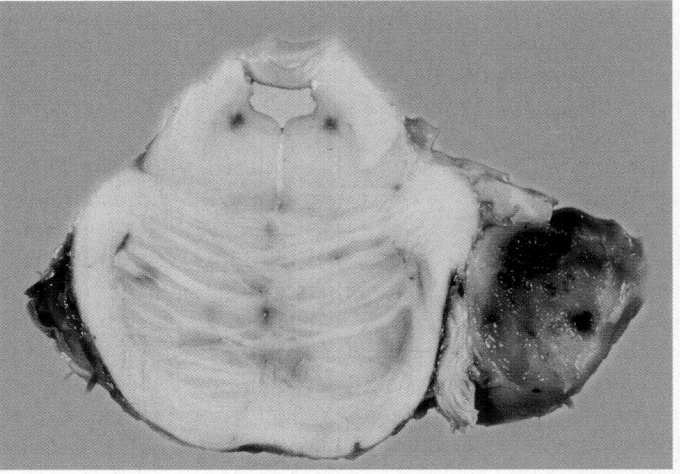

Figure 37-8 **A:** Acoustic neuroma (schwannoma involving the VIII cranial nerve) and meningiomas. The schwannoma is expansile and white. Portions of a meningioma are also represented along the base of the brain; other portions had been surgically removed. The patient had neurofibromatosis. **B:** Acoustic nerve schwannoma (cut surface of brain stem at level of pons). On the right, an acoustic neuroma (schwannoma) involves the VIII cranial nerve. The cut surface is focally hemorrhagic. In other areas, the cut surface is tan, a coloration often seen in association with hemosiderin deposits.

Schwannomatosis

Clinical Summary: **Schwannomatosis** (30) is characterized by multiple and plexiform schwannomas, as a clinical entity distinct from NF2 (31). It accounts for about 15% of patients with NF. Lesions appear in any anatomic location outside the acoustic nerve and are typically associated with significant pain. Mutations of the *SMARCB1* (also known as *INI1* and *BAF47*) tumor suppressor gene occur in 40% to 50% of familial cases and in 8% to 10% of sporadic cases of schwannomatosis (32). Other molecular alterations include mutations in *LZTR1*, somatic mutations in *NF2*, and loss of heterozygosity in chromosome 22q. Furthermore, it has been shown that there are distinct DNA methylation changes (33). This gene is also involved in rhabdoid tumors characterized by the presence of malignant rhabdoid tumors of the kidney, atypical teratoid/rhabdoid tumors, (AT/RT) of CNS, and extrarenal RT that develop in childhood. Café-au-lait spots occur in nearly all patients with NF, and they usually precede cutaneous tumors (14). The presence of more than six spots, each exceeding 1.5 cm in diameter, is indicative of NF (13,15).

Histopathology of lesions in patients with neurofibromatosis. (A complete description of the histologic features of schwannomas appears later.) The histologic spectrum of neurofibromas in NF1 and NF2 is broad. Some CNFs are small; others are large, cutaneous, or deep, circumscribed or plexiform (intraneural) variants (Fig. 37-9), and still others are diffuse (extraneural).

In many deep and circumscribed and in most plexiform neurofibromas, there are axial bundles composed of

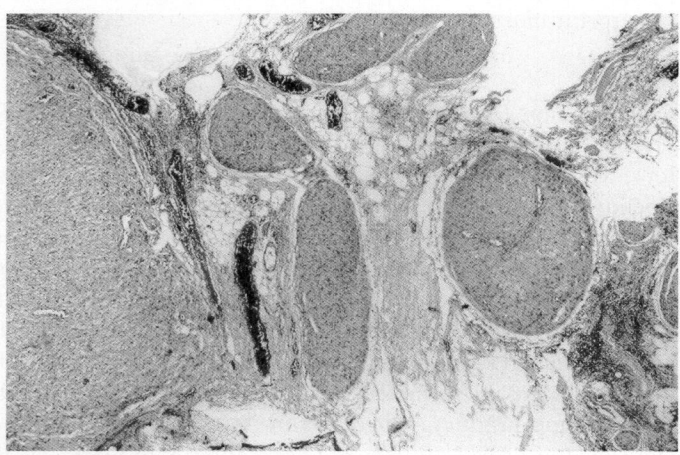
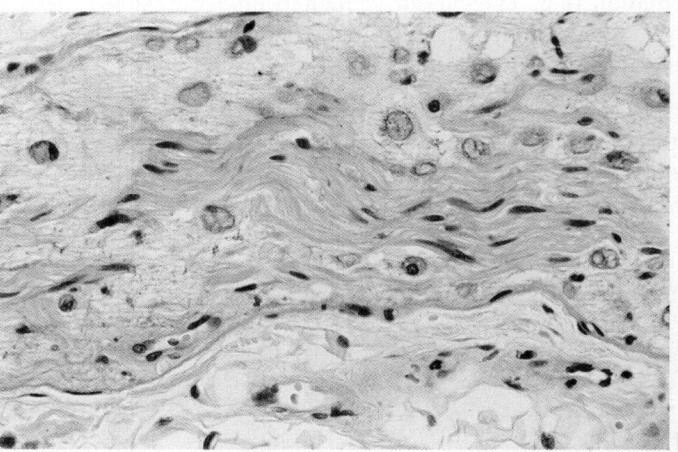

Figure 37-9 **A:** Components of a cutaneous, plexiform, intraneural neurofibroma. For the most part, components of the plexus in this field are cut in cross section. The tumor is intraneural; it sits in fibrofat without an extraneural component. Each component of the plexus is confined by a thickened perineurium. **B:** Plexiform intraneural neurofibroma; mucinous endoneurial type. This small branch of a large, cutaneous, plexiform neurofibroma shows a well-defined, central bundle of Schwann cells (an axial bundle). In this central bundle, Schwann cell fascicles of the pre-existing nerve are symmetrically arranged along the long axis of the nerve. The endoneurial space is widened and mucinous. In it, distinctive, rounded cells (endoneurial mucocytes) are loosely spaced. The expanding mucinous matrix has displaced some of the Schwann fascicles of the axial bundle away from their neighbors. The muciparous cells resemble the "cellules godronné" as seen in the "intravaginal hyaline system" of Renaut. The perineurium is delicate; it is a single layer of flattened cells.

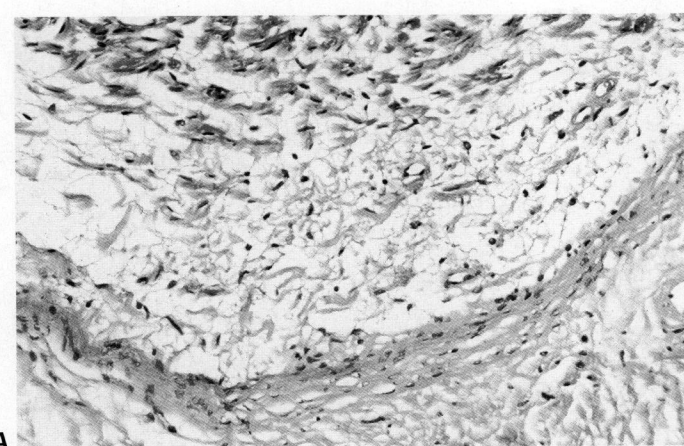
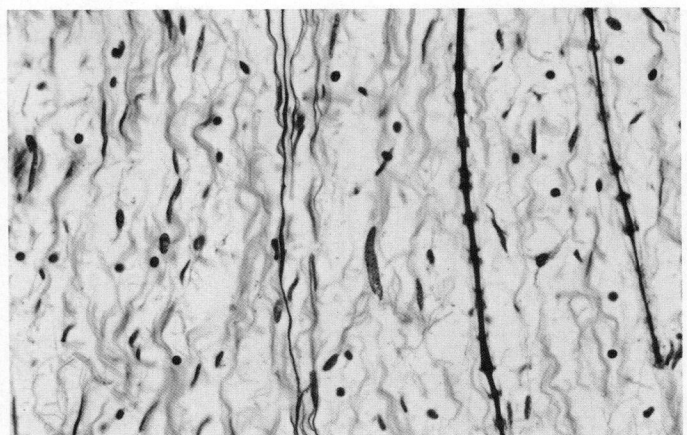

Figure 37-10 **A:** Intraneural neurofibroma; schwannian pattern of differentiation. A thickened perineurium forms a concave band near the bottom of the field; it defines the limits of the tumorous component at the interface with the adjacent soft tissue. At the top of the field, a distorted axial bundle (a remnant of the nerve of origin) is represented. The tumor is represented in the space between the perineurium and the distorted axial bundle; thin, pale collagen bundles are loosely and randomly spaced in a stringy, myxoid matrix. Thin spindle cells with elongated, wavy nuclei are closely associated with some of the collagen bundles. The fibrous component of the lesion is asymmetric in its relationships with both the long axis of the involved nerve and the central axial bundle. **B:** Intraneural neurofibroma; remnant of axial bundle (Bodian stain). Argyrophilic, myelinated, and nonmyelinated axons are parallel; they have axial symmetry and are a remnant of the axial bundle. Wavy collagen bundles of the tumor are more asymmetric in orientation and distribution.

symmetrically arranged nerve fibers, remnants of the axial bundle of the nerve of origin (Figs. 37-9 and 37-10) (3,4,34). Their role in the histogenesis of NF is uncertain. The axial bundle retains its symmetry in a field of distorted and asymmetric patterns (Fig. 37-10). In some axial bundles, Schwann cells are hyperplastic and tightly packed. In areas, these remnants of the nerve of origin focally evolve into micronodules composed of interlacing fascicles of Schwann cells; such micronodules may qualify as *microscopic schwannomatosis* (4). Many of these cellular micronodules may be independent of a true axial bundle, but they might function as growth centers (Fig. 37-11). Cells and collagenous strands stream from their periphery and extend asymmetrically into the expanded, mucinous, endoneurial matrix. In some intraneural variants, there are similar, streaming cells blending with the perineurium and thus suggesting that the perineurium contributes to the tumor. Those cells show features of perineurial cells, such as EMA expression.

The cells of *perineurial variants* are bipolar or tripolar with rigid processes; they are loosely spaced in either a myxoid or fibrous matrix (Figs. 37-12 and 37-13). *Endoneurial (schwannian) variants* are characterized by a thickened perineurium, one or several axial bundles, and isolated cells in an expanded, mucinous endoneurial component (Figs. 37-9 to 37-14). Some of the cells in the mucinous matrix resemble the "cellules godronné" of Renaut (round cells with portions of the mucinous matrix that are either enclosed within the cytoplasm or focally partitioned (encircled and sequestered) by cytoplasmic processes) (Fig. 37-9B) (1,3,4,35). One or several axial bundles may be found among asymmetric collagen bundles of the tumor (Figs. 37-14 and 37-15). In the expanded endoneurial component of both perineurial and endoneurial (schwannian) variants, the matrix is myxoid, rich in hyaluronic acid (4).

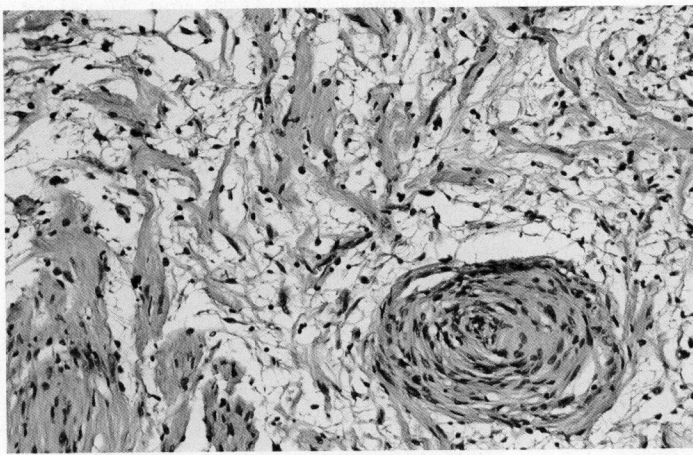

Figure 37-11 Intraneural neurofibroma; focal, microscopic schwannomatosis. Coarse collagen bundles are asymmetrically arranged in a loosely cellular, myxoid matrix. Near the right lower corner, collagen bundles and cells form a whorl; the whorl, as a nidus, is an example of microscopic schwannomatosis.

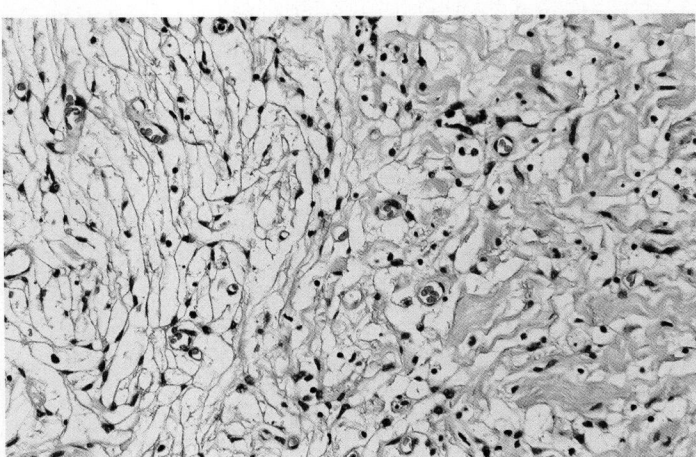

Figure 37-12 Intraneural neurofibroma; biphasic (perineurial and schwannian) patterns. To the right, wavy collagen bundles are loosely spaced; spindle cells are closely associated with the collagen bundles (schwannian pattern). To the left, distinctive, bipolar and tripolar cells are loosely spaced in a clear or myxoid matrix; these distinctive cells have perineurial qualities.

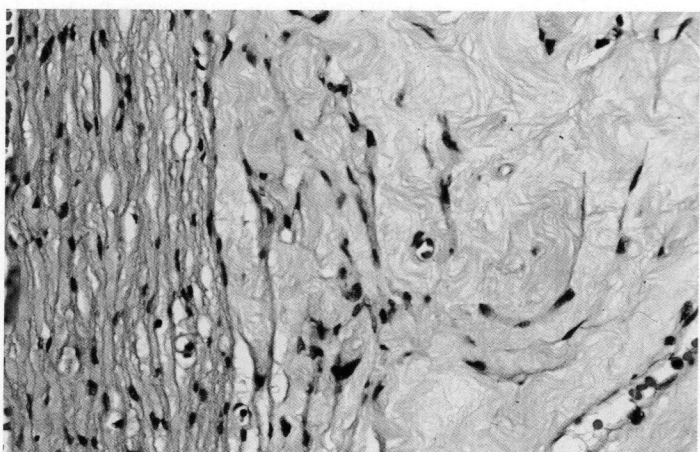

Figure 37-13 Intraneural neurofibroma; perineurial cell differentiation near the capsule of the tumor. The membrane to the left of the field is a thickened perineurium (capsule). In the fibrous matrix to the right of the perineurium, distinctive cells are loosely spaced; some blend with the inner surface of the perineurium. The loosely spaced cells have the morphologic features of perineurial cells.

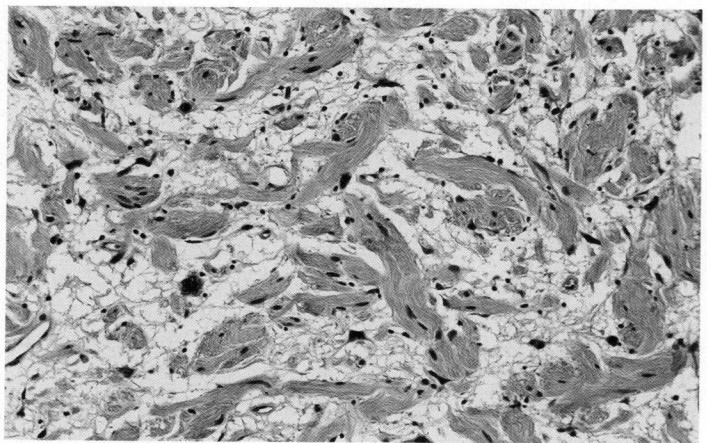

Figure 37-14 Intraneural neurofibroma; cytologic atypia. Coarse collagen bundles are loosely, and randomly, spaced in a myxoid matrix. Spindle cells are closely associated with the collagen bundles. Spindle and stellate cells are present among the collagen bundles in the myxoid matrix. Some of the cells in the myxoid matrix show nuclear atypia; they show variations in nuclear size and outline.

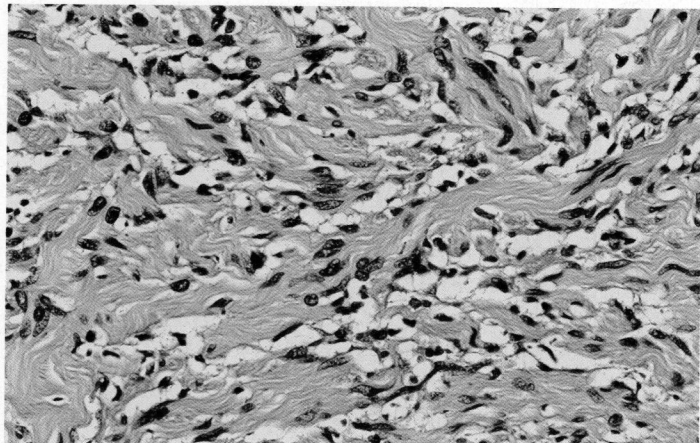

Figure 37-15 Intraneural neurofibroma; cellular pattern. Spindle cells are increased in number among the collagen bundles; focally, they are present within the collagen bundles. The cells have enlarged, wavy nuclei and scanty cytoplasm.

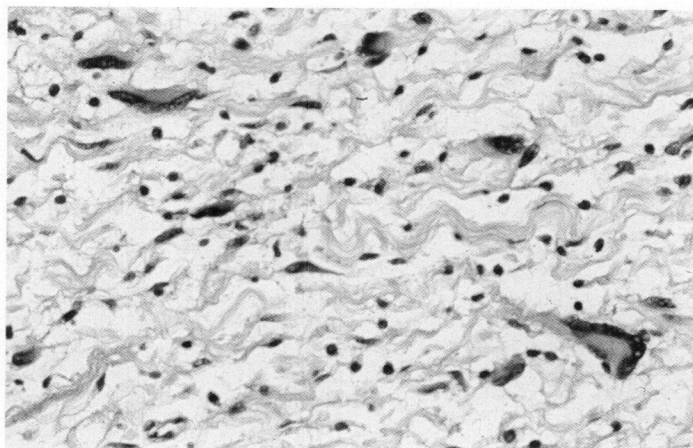

Figure 37-16 Intraneural neurofibroma; cellular atypia. Some of the cells among the collagen bundles are cytologically atypical; some of the atypical cells are multinucleated.

Focal cytologic atypia ("ancient" change), defined as scattered, enlarged, atypical nuclei (Figs. 37-14 and 37-16), is not associated with malignant change, as long as the lesion does not have hypercellularity, necrosis, or mitotic figures (3,4). On a related morphologic variant, the concept of atypical neurofibromatous neoplasms of unknown malignant potential has been proposed for nodular lesions that grow within a preexisting neurofibroma and that could be a precursor for a malignant peripheral nerve sheath tumor (MPNST, please see later) (36). Such lesions seem to have loss of *CDKN2A (arf)*, thus allowing the lesion to escape from senescence (37).

At the peripheral edge of the *extraneural (diffuse) neurofibroma*, margins are poorly defined (Fig. 37-17), typically involving adipocytes (3,38). The matrix of extraneural neurofibroma is either delicately fibrous and faintly acidophilic or more coarsely fibrous and brightly acidophilic. In the absence of plexiform components, nerves within diffuse neurofibromas are usually small, internally symmetric, and hypercellular; perineuria of such nerves are often hyperplastic. In cross section, these nerves resemble Pacinian corpuscles (39). Patterns of both plexiform and diffuse neurofibroma are combined in so-called *paraneurofibroma* (Figs. 37-18 and 37-19) (4).

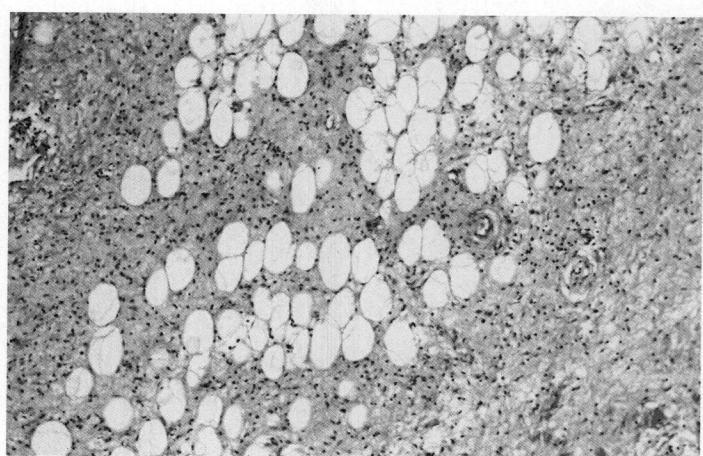

Figure 37-17 Extraneural (diffuse) neurofibroma. A delicately fibrous matrix is loosely cellular. The cells have scanty cytoplasm; they appear as naked nuclei. Adipocytes are entrapped.

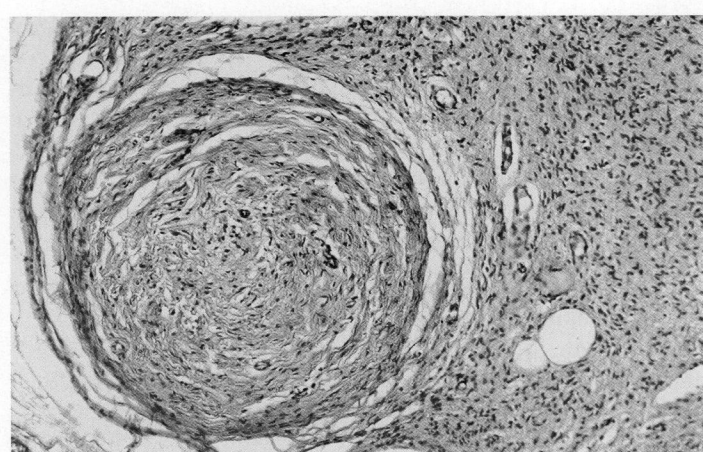

Figure 37-18 Diffuse and plexiform neurofibroma (paraneurofibroma). The round nodule to the left is a portion of an intraneural plexiform neurofibroma; it has been cut in cross section. The delicate fibrous matrix to the right is a portion of a diffuse (extraneural) component.

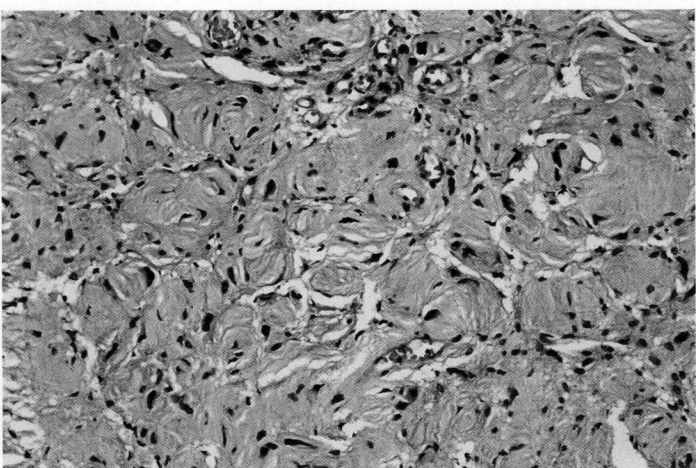

Figure 37-20 Extraneural neurofibroma; tactile corpuscle-like patterns. As a regional variation in this extraneural neurofibroma, spindle cells, in stacked lamellae, form tactile corpuscle-like structures.

Focal collections of structures resembling tactile corpuscles (tactoid bodies) (Fig. 37-20) and pigmented, dendritic melanocytes (a relatively common feature of deep, extraneural [diffuse] neurofibromas) are rare in the intraneural components of plexiform, or circumscribed, intraneural neurofibromas (4,7). Some neurofibromas may have extensive hyalinization (40).

Mucinous and proliferative endarteritis and aneurysms are occasional features in the setting of NF1; they affect mainly muscular renal vessels, but similar changes can be manifested in other sites (4,41,42). Aneurysmal changes have been a prominent feature of muscular vessels in some examples of extraneural neurofibromas of the skin and soft tissue, particularly in the distribution of the trigeminal nerve (4). Such lesions may clinically be mistaken for hemangioma.

Ultrastructurally, the cells of neurofibromas (including those of tactoid bodies) mostly resemble those of perineurial cells (43), but there are also axons and cells with the

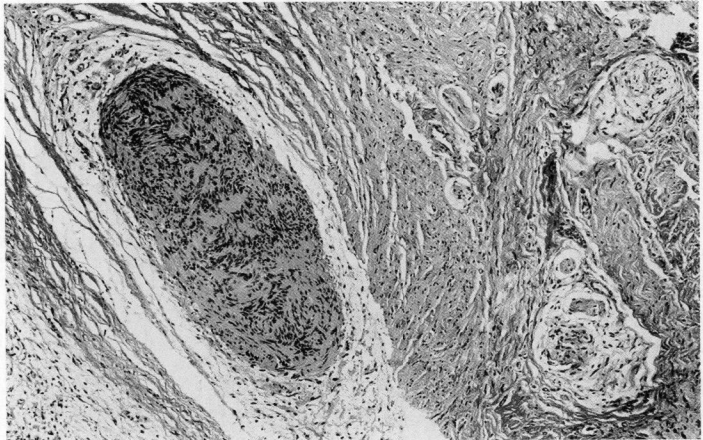

Figure 37-19 Diffuse and plexiform neurofibroma (paraneurofibroma) with focal microscopic schwannomatosis. The intraneural portions are pale, rounded, and faintly basophilic; in these components, wavy collagen bundles are loosely spaced. The extraneural component is a uniformly cellular fibrous matrix. Near the center of the field, a cellular nodule is confined within the intraneural matrix; in this cellular nodule, nuclei are arranged in palisades. The nodule is an example of microscopic schwannomatosis. The patterns of Verocay bodies are represented.

characteristics of Schwann cells and endoneurial fibroblasts (44). Endoneurial fibroblasts, like common mesenchymal fibroblasts, do not have basal lamina. The average diameter of their collagen fibrils lies well below that of dermal collagen fibrils, which is about 100 nm (45).

Histogenesis. The immunohistochemical profile of neurofibroma is as follows: S-100 protein (+), with variable expression of CD57 (Leu-7) antigen (+), and myelin basic protein (+). In extraneural CNFs, axons, as demonstrated with NSE, or with antibodies to neurofilaments or peripherin, are fairly uniform in distribution among collagen bundles. This finding is less consistent in deep, intraneural neurofibromas. Perineural cells express EMA, whereas endoneurial fibroblasts express CD34+ (46). Furthermore, the pattern of CD34 reaction named "fingerprinting" (slender, CD34-positive cells forming whorls around dermal vessels) (47) has been described as being characteristic of neurofibromas and not in melanoma (48), although rare cases of spindle cell melanoma may have similar immunohistochemical features (49).

Immunohistochemical and ultrastructural analysis reveals that Schwann and perineural cells with enclosed axons are variably distributed in CNFs (50,51). Their presence has been interpreted as either being an integral part of the tumor or entrapped nerve fibers (43). Nonplexiform neurofibromas of von Recklinghausen disease contain abundant, peptide-rich nerve fibers (50). Similar associations undoubtedly exist in plexiform variants. Thus, the innervation of neurofibromas of NF1 appears to be much richer than appreciated in the past.

The extraneural distribution of the common dermal neurofibroma may be a manifestation of the extension of tumor through the open-ended terminal of perineurial sheaths or through the thin perineurium of small dermal nerves (34). Deep, extraneural neurofibromas may represent a diffuse, neurocristic dysplasia (52). In this approach, the presence of adipocytes within such a tumor may be evidence of mesenchymal differentiation rather than simple entrapment.

There are hybrid peripheral nerve sheath tumors (53), including neurofibroma-schwannoma (54), schwannoma-perineurioma (55), neurofibroma-perineurioma (56), congenital nevi with features of schwannoma-perineurioma (57), as well as combinations including epithelioid schwannoma (58). That study emphasized histopathologic and immunohistochemical findings with one case having been analyzed ultrastructurally. Furthermore, one case had a point mutation in exon 15 of the NF2 gene (53).

A recent study in mice has suggested that mast cells and macrophages may be important in the maintenance of nerve sheath tumors (59,60). That study has shown that depletion of macrophages with targeted therapy (PLX3397) resulted in cell death and tumor volume regression.

Differential Diagnosis. Plexiform lesions of the skin and subcutaneous tissue include plexiform schwannoma (4), plexiform neuroma (61), neuromas of the mucosal neuroma syndrome (62), nerve sheath myxoma (63), plexiform fibrous histiocytoma (64), and possibly perineurioma (65). Also, some fasciculated melanocytic tumors are described as "plexiform" (66–68). Although most plexiform neurofibromas are associated with NF1, there are rare cases of sporadic lesions without associated syndrome.

Dendritic cell neurofibroma with pseudorosettes is a benign, "plexiform" lesion of the skin (69,70). These lesions have two cell types: large dendritic and small, dark cells. The dark cells tend to cluster in palisades about the large dendritic cells. The tumor cells are immunoreactive for S-100 protein. The large cells are not neurons. In a *Reply to a Letter to the Editor*, Michal et al. (71) showed a tumor that was both diffuse and plexiform. As photographically documented, the dendritic cells were intraneural and sheltered from the small cell component by a complex of cell processes resembling neuropil. The histologic features of the population of small cells can be compared to those of the small cells in some examples of "epithelioid" small cell populations in some variants of schwannoma. Such (34) schwannomas are of the type associated with zones of radial sclerosis. In neither category of nerve sheath tumor do the small cells have the cytologic features of a population of "blast" (immature) cells. To borrow an old designation, but in the process to alter its definition, the patterns of differentiation in the small cell population might qualify as "neuroglial" differentiation. Despite the morphological cellular similarities between dendritic cell neurofibromas and neuroblastomas, we recommend not to use the term "neuroblastoma-like" neurofibroma based upon their markedly distinct clinical behavior.

Subcutaneous, diffuse neurofibromas may be confused with the deep component of *dermatofibrosarcoma protuberans*. Some authors have mislabeled the pigmented form of dermatofibrosarcoma (Bednar tumor) as *pigmented storiform neurofibroma* (39,72).

Fibrous hamartoma (of infancy) has fascicles of spindle cells with a myxoid background, thus resembling diffuse neurofibroma.

The nodular myxoid components of a low-grade *malignant myxoid fibrous histiocytoma* might be misinterpreted as the pattern of a plexiform neurofibroma.

Principles of Management: As mentioned previously, except for malignant transformation (usually associated with rapid growth in a long-standing lesion; see also later), CNF are removed only when they result in cosmetic or functional problems.

TRUE NEOPLASMS OF SCHWANN CELLS: SCHWANNOMAS

Clinical Summary. Schwannomas (neurilemmomas; anaxonal, intraneural, Schwann cell tumors; "peripheral neurogliomas") are benign, circumscribed, expansile neoplasms (1,34,43). The cells of schwannomas mostly have the characteristics of Schwann cells. Schwann cells are specialized sustentacular cells, normally distributed as a single layer about, and along, one or more axons. In a sense, the insulation that they provide along normal nerve fibers favors proper propagation of nerve impulses. In schwannomas, the population of Schwann cells exists independently of a plexus of axons. As solitary, skin-colored tumors along the course of peripheral or cranial nerves, their usual size is between 2 and 4 cm, usually on the head or the flexor aspect of the extremities. Schwannomas are rare in the subcutaneous tissue and even less common in the dermis. In deep soft tissue, they may be large (73). In the central nervous system, the VIII cranial is the favorite site. Internal viscera (74) and bones may be involved. When small, most schwannomas are asymptomatic but may develop pain, localized to the tumor or radiating along the nerve of origin.

Histopathology. Schwannomas, apart from infiltrating, fascicular variants, are intraneural and symmetrically expansile; they are confined by the perineurium of the nerve of origin (Fig. 37-21).

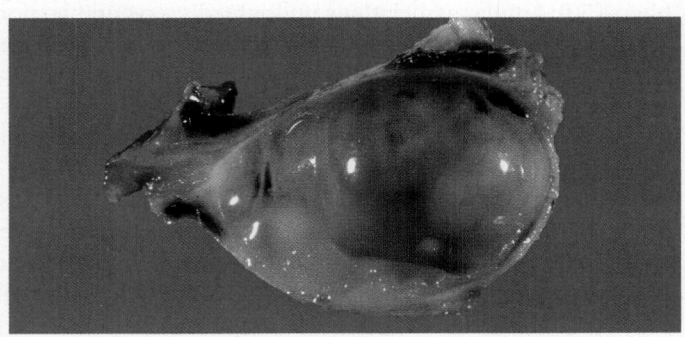

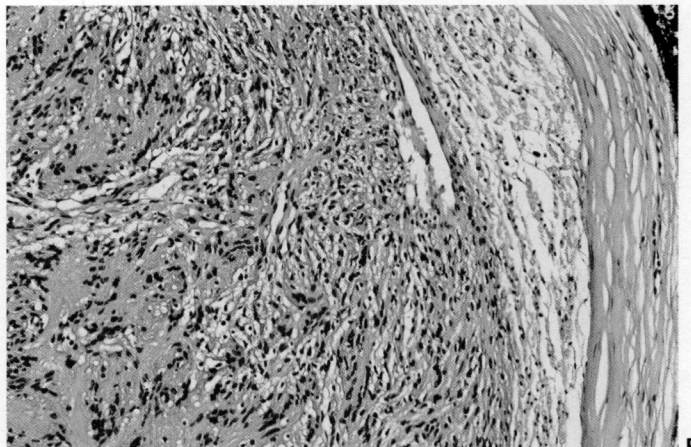

Figure 37-21   A: Schwannoma. The lesion is circumscribed and encapsulated. It bulges over a portion of the cut surface. **B:** Schwannoma and nerve of origin. This schwannoma is uniformly cellular; the Schwann cells focally form nuclear palisades and Verocay bodies. To the right, a thickened perineurium, at its interface with the neighboring soft tissue, defines the limits of the tumor. The loosely cellular zone between the perineurium and the tumor is a compressed nerve of origin; the nerve maintains its identity at the periphery of the tumor; it is not enclosed within the substance of the tumor.

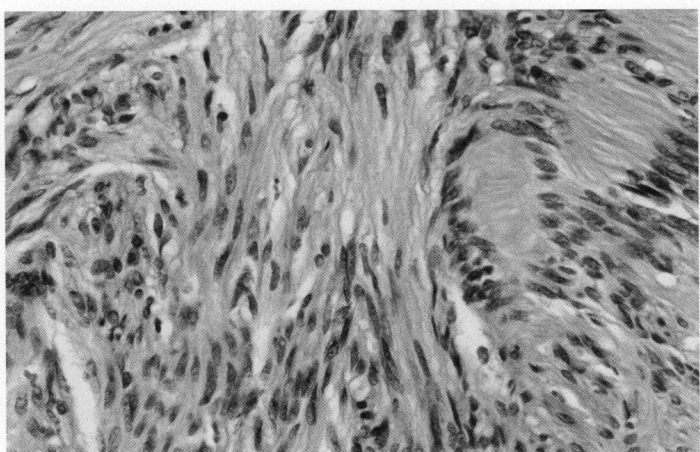

Figure 37-22 Schwannoma; Antoni A patterns. Pale spindle cells with elongated, wavy nuclei are arranged in fascicular patterns. To the right of the field, nuclear palisades are regularly spaced; two nuclear palisades and the enclosed cytoplasmic processes comprise a Verocay body. Cellular components of this type qualify as Antoni A tissue.

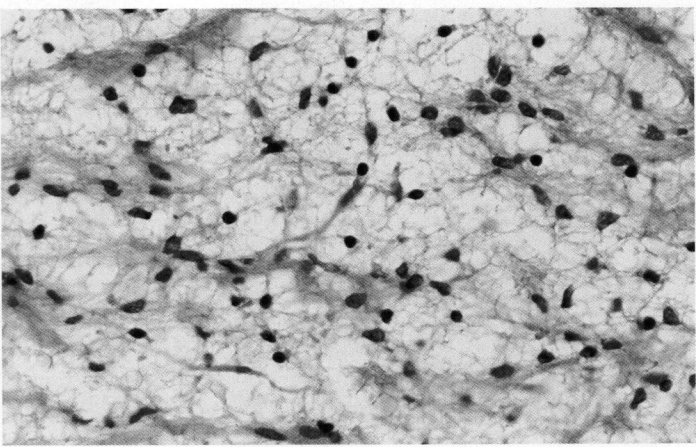

Figure 37-24 Schwannoma; Antoni B patterns. In this example, the cells of an Antoni B component are small with complex, delicate cytoplasmic processes. The cytologic features have a glial cell–like quality.

Most of the symmetrically bundled nerve fibers of the nerve of origin are displaced eccentrically; if identified in a histologic section, they are usually to be found between the tumor and the perineurium (see Fig. 37-21) (4,34). At the interface with the nerve of origin, some of the nerve fibers may extend from the compressed, eccentric axial bundle into the tumor. The observations of Russell and Rubinstein (75) confirm that schwannomas may contain some loosely, and randomly, spaced, nonmyelinated axons, particularly in small peripheral schwannomas, and in small and medium-sized acoustic nerve schwannomas (75).

The tumor cells are arranged in two patterns, *Antoni A* and *Antoni B* (3,74). In the Antoni type A areas, uniform spindle cells are arranged back-to-back (Fig. 37-22); each cell is outlined by delicate, rigid, reticular fibers (basement membranes). The cells tend to cluster in stacks, and the respective nuclei often form palisades. Two neighboring palisades, the intervening cytoplasm of Schwann cells, and associated reticular fibers, all in combination, constitute a *Verocay body* (see Figs. 37-22 and 37-23).

In Antoni type B areas, files of elongated cells, arranged end to end are loosely spaced in a clear, watery, or myxoid matrix (Figs. 37-23 to 37-25) (1); in some examples, the cells somewhat resemble glial cells; in other examples, they resemble perineurial cells. It has been proposed that some of the dendritic cells in these Antoni type B areas are telocytes (9).

Typically, there are clusters of dilated, thick, congested blood vessels (3), occasionally with fibrinoid necrosis or hyalinization, thrombi, or subendothelial collections of foam cells (Fig. 37-26) (76). The vascular changes can be found in both Antoni A and Antoni B tissue. Some lesions may have cystic changes (Fig. 37-27), extravasated erythrocytes, or hemosiderin (4,76). These features are more prominent in ancient schwannomas (see later).

Ultrastructurally, most tumor cells manifest the features of Schwann cells (long cytoplasmic processes and myelin with long-spacing collagen) (43,74).

The patterns in Antoni type B areas are interpreted to be of a "degenerative" nature (76). "Ancient change" characterizes the nuclear atypia as well as the large, thick, dilated vessels with fibrin often seen in some schwannomas (4,76) (see also later).

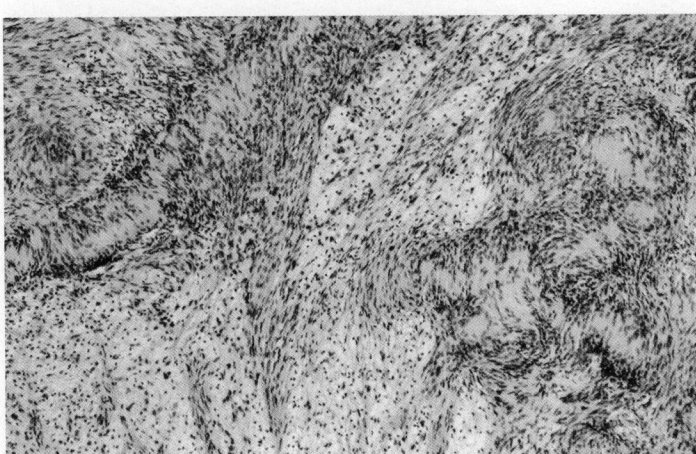

Figure 37-23 Schwannoma; mixed Antoni A and Antoni B patterns. The Antoni A component is cellular; Verocay bodies are a prominent feature. The loosely cellular, pale zones are Antoni B patterns. In the Antoni B component, there is some variation in nuclear size and staining.

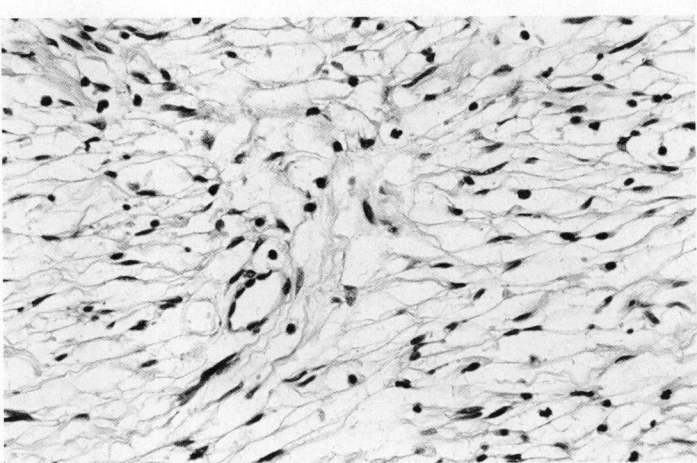

Figure 37-25 Schwannoma; Antoni B Patterns. In this example, the cells of an Antoni B component are bi- or tripolar; the cytoplasmic processes are elongated and straight; the cells cytologically resemble perineurial cells.

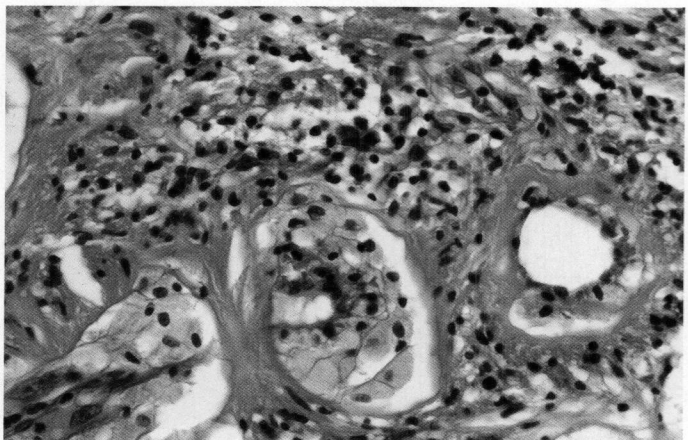

Figure 37-26 Schwannoma; Antoni B component, vascular changes. In this Antoni B component, several vessels are loosely clustered. They have thickened, hyalinized walls. There are prominent, subintimal collections of foam cells. Loose infiltrates of lymphoid cells are adjacent to the vessels and among the foamy histiocytes. In part, the hyalin represents a stage in the organization of fibrinoid; fibrinoid degeneration and thrombosis are common vascular changes in some schwannomas.

Ultrastructurally, tumor cells are widely separated by an electron-lucid, homogeneous matrix containing strands of fibrin and detached segments of the basement membrane. Autophagic lysosomes, some containing myelin figures, are seen in many cells (i.e., a "histiocytic" quality). The cellular changes include extensive loss of basement membrane, disruption of cell membrane, and nuclear degenerative changes (77).

Schwannomas associated with NF2 or schwannomatosis may display prominent myxoid stroma or "mixed" features, resembling a combination of schwannoma, neurofibroma, and perineurioma. Regarding immunohistochemistry, there may be a mosaic pattern of expression of SMARCB1/INI1. Sporadic schwannomas rarely show such a pattern (78).

Histogenesis. The immunohistochemical profile is S-100 protein (+), and two antigens characteristic of basement membrane, collagen type IV and laminin (+). In the capsule, cells are EMA (+). A Bodian stain and an immunoreaction for the demonstration

of neural filaments reveal few or no axons, except in and near the peripherally displaced axial bundle.

Differential Diagnosis. If a nerve sheath tumor involves a significant sensory or motor nerve, the histologic distinction between intraneural neurofibroma and schwannoma becomes an important consideration for a surgeon. The intact, but displaced, symmetric axial bundle (Fig. 37-21) of a schwannoma can often be preserved during surgical dissections. On the other hand, excision of an intraneural neurofibroma requires sacrifice of the nerve of origin. Most neurofibromas are poorly circumscribed and show a "hamartomatous" appearance owing to the combination of Schwann cells, axons, perineural cells, and fibroblasts. Axons are usually distributed through the lesion.

Palisaded and encapsulated neuroma (PEN) (see also later) should be considered in the differential diagnosis of schwannoma. They are mostly located on the face. Although they are circumscribed, as are most schwannomas, they contain numerous axons within the lesion.

Variant Types of Schwannomas

Cellular Schwannoma (CS)

In CS, as defined by Harkin and Reed (3), most cells are arranged with an Antoni A type pattern; Schwann cells are closely aggregated with scanty intercellular matrix. Some scattered cells may have large, hyperchromatic nuclei (Fig. 37-28). Increased cellularity per unit area, a preponderance of type A patterns, and a low mitotic rate are requisites for the diagnosis of "cellular schwannoma" (Fig. 37-29). Other authors have expanded the definition of "cellular schwannoma" (1) to include some features that overlap with MPNST. The dichotomy in the approaches to "cellular" schwannoma is given recognition herein by the definition of two classes: CS1 and CS2 (79).

Clinical Summary. Most examples of CS are large tumors of the retroperitoneum and mediastinum and may show immunoreactivity for GFAP (80,81).

Histopathology: The lesions of CS1 are mostly cellular, with "patternless" areas in which cells form solid sheets, alternating with areas in which intersecting fascicles of spindle cells are seen

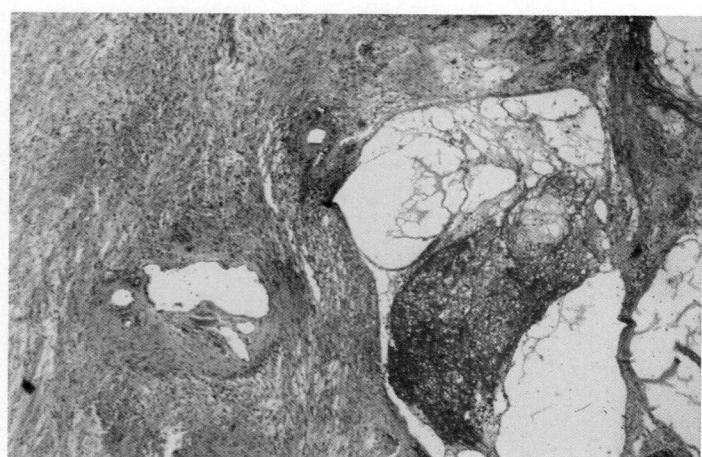

Figure 37-27 Schwannoma; microcystic and vascular changes. With this connective tissue stain, cells have a reddish tinge, and connective tissue is green. Vessels are dilated; their walls are fibrous and irregularly thickened. To the right, multiple, small cysts contain a loose meshwork of fibrin.

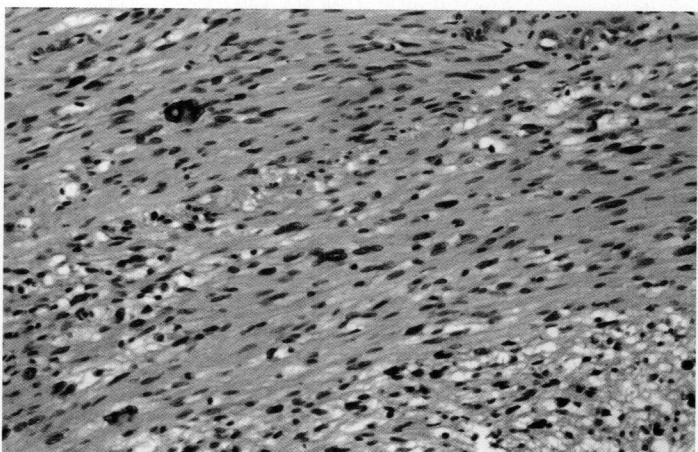

Figure 37-28 Schwannoma; cytologic atypia (ancient change of cytologic type). Spindle cells form interlacing fascicles. The cells show variations in nuclear size, staining, and outlines; in many of the nuclei, chromatin is dense and smudgy. Mitoses are not a feature of "ancient change."

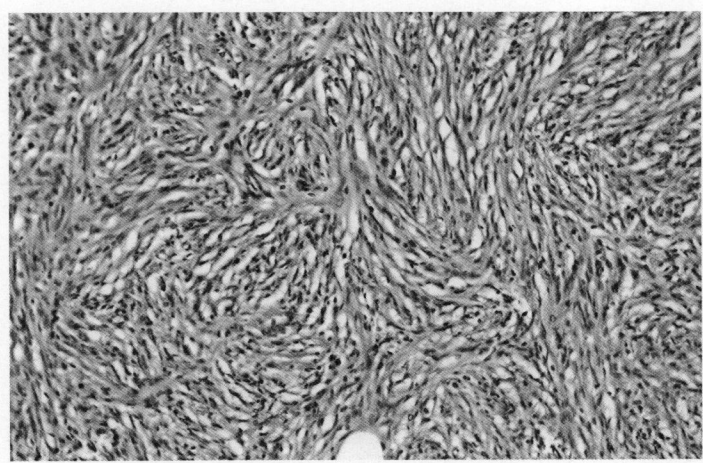

Figure 37-29 Schwannoma; cellular variant (CS1). In this schwannoma, patterns are uniformly cellular (Antoni A type). Uniform spindle cells are arranged in the pattern of interlacing fascicles. In this example, mitotic activity is not a significant feature.

in a storiform pattern (Fig. 37-29). The basic patterns of more classical variants of schwannoma, such as those of a common schwannoma or an epithelioid schwannoma, are preserved, but in some examples, most of the cells are cytologically atypical (Fig. 37-29). In some examples, nuclear atypia is uniform and extensive. By definition, mitotic figures are infrequent (<2/10 hpf). A background population of small lymphocytes may also contribute to the cellularity. Nuclear palisades, Verocay bodies, and Antoni type B components tend to be inconspicuous; there should not be zones of necrosis (3,4).

In CS2 (cellular schwannoma of Woodruff [82]; transformed schwannoma of Reed and Harkin [3]), lesions may have increased cell density, storiform patterns, mitotic figures (up to 20 or more per 10 hpf), necrosis, and focal but frank cytologic atypia (1,81–86). Although histologic features might suggest a transition from benignancy to low-grade malignancy (Fig. 37-30), most of these lesions behave in a benign fashion. Thus, most of these lesions are amenable to local surgery. In making a distinction between these lesions and infiltrating low-grade malignant schwannomas, confinement by the perineurium of the nerve of origin is prognostically and therapeutically important (82).

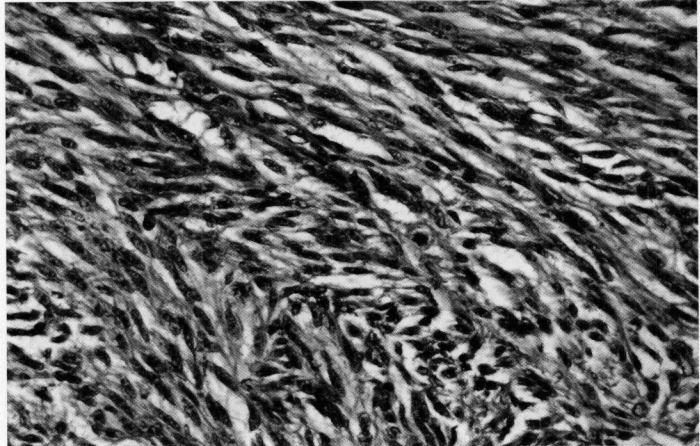

Figure 37-30 Schwannoma; cellular variant with mitotic activity (CS2). In this example of cellular schwannoma, the fascicles are hypercellular; nuclei are enlarged and show hyperchromatism. There are scattered mitotic figures.

Differential Diagnosis. The differential diagnosis of CS1 includes *leiomyoma*, low-grade *leiomyosarcoma*, *gastrointestinal stromal tumor,* and *pleomorphic hyalinizing angioectoid tumor*. Intense and diffuse expression of S100 protein with negative CD34, SMA, and desmin would offer support for a diagnosis of schwannoma. Smooth muscle cells, in turn, react with antibodies to SMA and desmin. In gastrointestinal stromal tumors, divergent phenotypes may be expressed, but CD117 (c-kit) is the commonly expressed antigen. Some pleomorphic hyalinizing angioectoid tumors may express CD34 but definitely lack S100 protein. As mentioned previously, CS2 may be confused with MPNST. Circumscription and strong/diffuse S100 expression are features that support the diagnosis of CS. MPNST may express CD117 (87), p53, and high Ki67 (88,89). Also resembling MPNST, children may develop a plexiform variant of CS (90).

Epithelioid Schwannoma

In the rare *epithelioid schwannoma* (with or without radial sclerosis) (4,91–93) spindle and round cells are clustered in epithelioid patterns. The nuclei are often round (Figs. 37-31 and 37-32) but may be irregular and hyperchromatic. Typically, the cytoplasm is large and eosinophilic. In some cases, cells have round nuclei and scanty cytoplasm, and some of the cells are radially arranged in palisades around distinctive zones of sclerosis (4,94–97). In the zones of sclerosis, fibrous lamellae are radially oriented; they interdigitate with cytoplasmic projections of the surrounding tumor cells (97). Such lesions have been characterized as epithelioid schwannoma with radial sclerosis (4), "collagenous spherulosis" in a schwannoma (96), rosetoid schwannoma (97), and the so-called "neuroblastoma-like" epithelioid schwannoma (94,95). The designation "neuroblastoma-like" schwannoma gives recognition to a lymphocyte-like pattern; the nuclei of the small, blue tumor cells, in size and staining, resemble those of lymphocytes. The small cell component may be extensive or just a focal pattern in what is otherwise a typical schwannoma. The small cells tend to cluster in rosette-like patterns about vessels and spherical zones of radial sclerosis. As with other schwannomas, epithelioid schwannomas may show mitotic figures and cytologic atypia; however, necrosis is not a feature.

In our opinion, owing to the possible confusion with a malignant neoplasm, neither the histology nor the clinical behavior of these lesions justifies a characterization of "neuroblastoma-like." Collagenous spherulosis, as originally defined for breast lesions, is distinct from the patterns of radial sclerosis seen in nerve sheath tumors (98). Some examples of epithelioid schwannoma have been characterized as cellular, and others have a plexiform pattern (see Figs. 37-31 and 37-32).

Epithelioid schwannomas diffusely express S100 and SOX10 and lack melanocytic markers. Approximately 50% of the lesions may show loss of SMARCB1/INI1 (99), and this finding may also be helpful in distinguishing them from melanocytic lesions.

Glandular Schwannoma

Glands, having the features of sweat glands, are occasionally found within subcutaneous schwannomas (100–103). A demonstration of a component of myoepithelial cells has been the basis for positing that the glands are nothing more than entrapped sweat glands. Yoshida and Toot (103) proposed *divergent differentiation* as an alternate explanation for the glandular

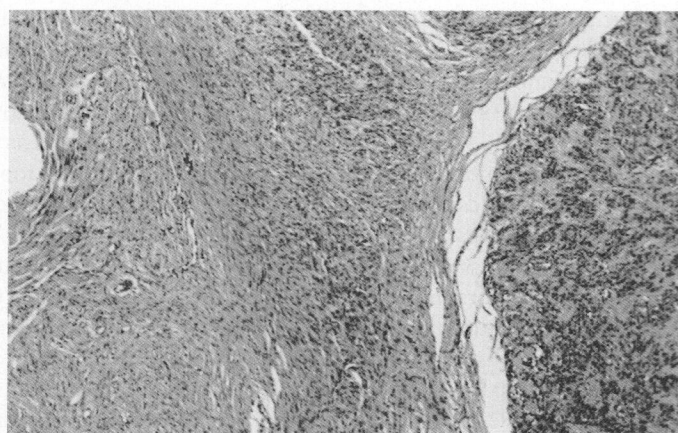
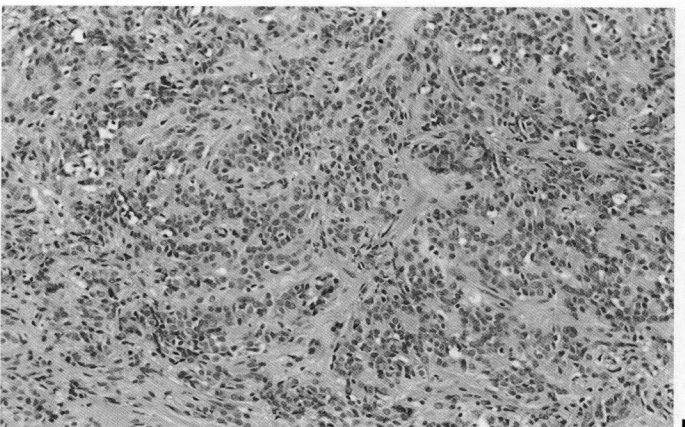

Figure 37-31 A, B: Plexiform epithelioid schwannoma, arising in extraneural neurofibroma. A: To the right, a portion of a plexiform lesion presents a sharp interface with an extraneural (diffuse) neurofibroma. Fascicles of uniform, epithelioid cells are loosely, and regularly, spaced in the plexiform component. B: At higher magnification, the fascicles of uniform, small epithelioid cells are loosely spaced in a fibrous matrix.

inclusions. Glandular differentiation can also be seen in malignant schwannomas and rarely in neurofibromas (102). Some schwannomas may have cysts that contain mucoid material outlined by palisades of Schwann cells; such lesions have been classified as pseudoglandular schwannomas (104).

Plexiform Schwannoma

Clinical Summary. Plexiform schwannomas occur mostly in the subcutaneous tissue and only rarely in the dermis (4,31, 105–111). They may be a feature of the syndrome of *multiple schwannomas* (clinical schwannomatosis or neurilemmomatosis) (108,112), or they may be solitary (109). The same gene is involved in NF2 and multiple schwannomas (30,113).

Histopathology. Plexiform schwannoma is intraneural. Spindle cells, often in solid Antoni A patterns, fill the expanded endoneurial space of a limited segment of a neural plexus; each column and nodule of the tumor is surrounded by perineurium. There may be dilated vascular spaces and Antoni type B tissue. Cystic changes are uncommon. In some examples, fascicles of Schwann cells extend for a short distance beyond the confines of the perineurium

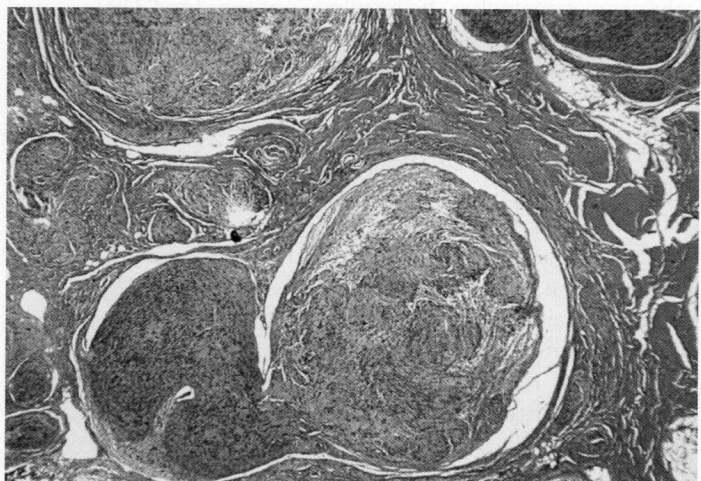

Figure 37-32 Plexiform schwannoma. Components of the plexus are mostly cut in cross section; they are supported by a dense fibrous matrix. Within some of the components, both Antoni A and Antoni B patterns are represented.

into the neighboring mesenchyme. These limited patterns, when encountered in the adjacent soft tissue, resemble those of a small, circumferential, extraneural neuroma (106).

Plexiform schwannomas may be cellular or epithelioid. Those located in the deep soft tissue frequently show histologic features of CS2 (114). In one series, lesions had hypercellularity, pleomorphism, and mitotic figures; tumor necrosis and myxoid change were less common. Females were more commonly affected than males; none of the patients had stigmata of NF. Two of six patients with follow-up had two local recurrences, and one patient had one local recurrence. At the last follow-up, all six patients were free of disease (114).

The category of plexiform schwannoma may be heterogeneous. In a single case, Kao et al. (109) have documented a relationship between neurofibroma and plexiform schwannoma. One of the authors has identified cases of plexiform schwannoma that appear associated with a background of diffuse neurofibroma (79) (Figs. 37-31 and 37-32).

Principles of Management: As mentioned in neurofibromas, schwannomas are removed only when they result in cosmetic or functional problems. The aim then is to excise them while preserving neural function. In the case of CS and melanotic schwannomas, owing to their deep-seated location, they are usually excised to rule out the possibility of a sarcoma.

Schwannoma Arising in Neurofibroma (with Emphasis on Relationships with Intraneural Microscopic Schwannomatosis)

There are reports of schwannomas in continuity with neurofibromas/hybrid peripheral nerve sheath tumors (54,115,116). *Intraneural microscopic schwannomatosis* (see Figs. 37-11 and 37-19) (4), a proliferative change affecting axial bundles of nerve fibers in intraneural neurofibromas, may become a *schwannoma ex neurofibroma* (26). Rarely, remnants of an intraneural neurofibroma are found at the periphery of a CS (CS1).

Borderline Variants

Infiltrating (Extraneural) Fascicular Schwann Cell Tumor (IFSCT) of Infancy and Childhood

Clinical Summary. IFSCT (plexiform peripheral nerve sheath tumor of infancy and childhood) (117); congenital hamartoma of nerve) is a rare Schwann cell neoplasm most often affecting an extremity (118). In contrast to all variants of schwannoma, IFSCT is chiefly extraneural because true plexiform patterns (intraneural by definition) are not a prominent feature. Therefore, IFSCT does not fulfill the criteria of a variant schwannoma. It also lacks the organoid qualities of a hamartoma.

Histopathology. Uniform spindle cells form tortuous, interlacing fascicles varying in size. In some of the thin fascicles, spindle cells tend to cluster in palisades; collections of cytoplasm separate the neighboring palisades. Some cases may show rapid growth, locally aggressive behavior, hypercellularity, and frequent mitotic figures. The lesion infiltrates skin and soft tissue and, in some examples, erodes bone.

Histogenesis. The most characteristic feature of IFSCT is its invasion of soft tissue in a fascicular pattern. Most tumor cells of IFSCT are clearly identifiable as Schwann cells, both immunohistochemically and ultrastructurally.

Principles of Management: In one published collection, four of the six patients with follow-up had local recurrences (117). In addition, one patient, with an invasive lesion of the orbit, died of disease. Woodruff reported six cases (90), ranging in age from 2 to 15 months. There was no association with NF1. Three of the tumors were well circumscribed, but lesions were not encapsulated. Although all tumors recurred locally, children were alive and free of disease at last follow-up.

The documented behavior of reported examples has not convincingly established the nature of the lesion. The histologic patterns, if not the cytologic features, overlap with those of infiltrating and fascicular epithelioid malignant schwannoma (IFEMS); they even share some features with neurotropic melanoma. Their nature is controversial. In our opinion, IFSCT should be characterized as a borderline lesion of indeterminate malignant potential until its nature is better documented.

Psammomatous Melanotic Schwannoma (PMS)
This lesion has a controversial name because many cases do not display the features characteristic of schwannoma (Antoni A and B areas), so there has been a proposal to designate them as malignant melanotic schwannian tumor to highlight the possibility of recurrence and distant metastasis (119,120).

Clinical Summary. This uncommon tumor is typically seen in paraspinal areas, followed by the GI tract, bone, subcutaneous tissue, and other locations. Up to two-thirds of the neoplasms cause symptoms (121). It may be either sporadic or a stigma

of the *Carney complex.* The complex includes some or all of the following: myxomas (including trichogenic and cardiac variants) (122); spotty pigmentation; pigmented adrenal cortical hyperplasia; large-cell calcifying Sertoli cell tumor (123); and endocrine overactivity (including Cushing syndrome) (121,124). Up to 10% of PMS develop metastasis to lungs, liver, and spleen (125), particularly those lesions with very many mitotic figures (>2/10 HPF) (119).

Histologically, there are usually psammoma bodies, and pigmented and dendritic melanocytes (Fig. 37-33). The lesions tend to be heavily pigmented. Most examples of PMS are quite distinctive and only vaguely resembling schwannomas, but a few lesions show nuclear palisades and Verocay bodies as common schwannomas (121,126). Zhang studied 13 cases of nonpsammomatous melanotic schwannomas (125). Positive immunohistochemical markers include S-100, Leu-7, HMB45 antigen, Melan-A, and vimentin. The product, in linear patterns, of immunoreactions for laminin and collagen IV correlates with the Schwann cell nature of the tumor cells. Ultrastructural features also are those of Schwann cells (see later under *Ultrastructure* in MPNST) (125).

The main differential diagnosis is melanoma metastatic to the soft tissue. Such lesions tend to occur in the context of a patient with a prior history of melanoma and tend to have high proliferation (numerous mitotic figures) and monomorphous cells. In the differential diagnosis, we should also consider that standard schwannomas may have psammoma bodies and calcification and thus should not be designated as psammomatous melanocytic schwannomas (127).

These lesions express S100 and SOX10 as well as several melanocytic makers. As with epithelioid blue nevus, these lesions may have loss of PRKAR1A expression (119).

Principles of Management: These lesions are usually excised to rule out malignancy. The main issue is not to confuse this lesion with a metastatic melanoma. Owing to the possibility of recurrence or metastasis, the aim should be complete excision and close follow-up.

Transformed (Borderline) Schwannoma (TBS) (CS2)
This borderline lesion of uncertain malignant potential is, by definition, like its benign counterpart, intraneural (i.e., confined by an expanded perineurium) (4). Its histologic features are reminiscent of those seen in low-grade MPNST of NF (a lesion that is not confined by the perineurium of the nerve of

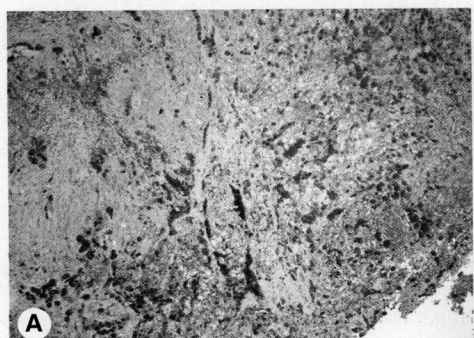
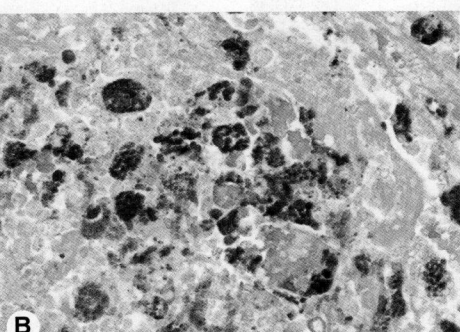
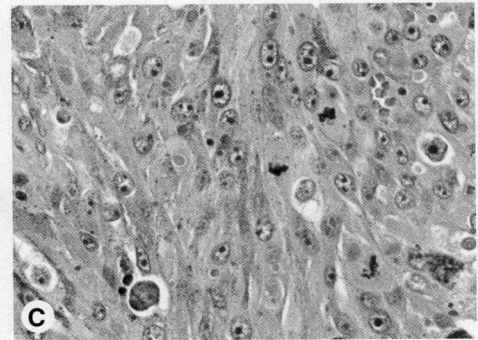

Figure 37-33 A, B: Malignant melanotic schwannian tumor (psammomatous melanotic schwannoma) lesion from the paraspinal region of a young male. A: Low-power view of cellular areas with focal abundant melanin pigment. B: Extensive necrosis. C: Numerous mitotic figures, including atypical forms.

origin). Some examples of CS2 contain scattered globular deposits of melanotic pigment. As defined by Reed and Harkin (4), "transformed" schwannoma shares many features with CS as defined by Woodruff et al. (82), and herein we define this lesion as CS2.

Bona fide malignant transformation of benign schwannoma has been a rarely documented event (128–130). In one report, only histologically "high-grade" variants were represented (131). Such "high-grade" lesions show a marked degree of cellular atypia and pleomorphism and a high mitotic rate. They may show infiltrative growth beyond the confines of the perineurium (131), a quality that excludes CS2.

Principles of Management: As mentioned previously, these lesions are usually removed to rule out sarcoma.

MALIGNANT PERIPHERAL NERVE SHEATH TUMOR OF COMMON TYPE

Clinical Summary. These lesions may be sporadic, associated with a neurofibroma, or appear in the context of NF 1 (Fig. 37-34). Related malignancies may be *de novo* or may be transformations in other neurocristic neoplasms, such as schwannoma or ganglioneuroma (52,132,133). The criteria for the diagnosis of MPNST include some of the following: origin from, or continuity with, a major nerve or neurofibroma; association with classic stigmata of NF; characteristic morphology in histologic patterns of spindled and epithelioid patterns; and demonstration of at least focal expression of S-100; or ultrastructural features of Schwann cells (and/or perineurial cells) (134).

It has been argued that because most "malignant schwannomas" arise in association with neurofibromas of NF, the designation "malignant schwannoma" is best used only for those rare cases of malignant schwannoma ex-schwannoma. On the other hand, it may be argued that the designation "malignant peripheral nerve sheath tumor" provides no distinctions between the common malignancy of NF and an uncommon lesion such as peripheral neuroepithelioma (primitive neuroectodermal tumor). Also, it does not provide distinctions between Schwann cell variants and perineurial variants. Similarly, epithelioid variants and mesenchymal variants are not distinguished in the

concept of MPNST. However, despite all these shortcomings, this designation is the most popular for malignant lesions with features of neurofibromas.

MPNST *(sheath or Schwann cell type: S-100+)* is the common malignant tumor of peripheral nerves (1,3,4,135–141). Its association with NF 1 is established, but, even in this setting, it is uncommon. On the other hand, of the many peripheral stigmata in NF, neurofibromas are the most predisposed to malignant transformations. In a series of 678 patients with NF, an MPNST was observed in only 21 (3.1%) of the patients (138). In only 2 of the 678 patients did an MPNST primarily involve the skin and subcutaneous fat. Allison et al. reviewed the clinicopathologic features of five examples of MPNST involving the skin or subcutaneous tissue (140). Four of the lesions occurred in women. One patient had a diagnosis of type 1 NF. Four of the lesions were associated with a CNF; for the remaining case, the tumor involved a superficial peripheral nerve. Four of the cases were of a common type, whereas the remaining case was an epithelioid variant. There were no local recurrences, but three patients died of metastatic disease.

MPNST usually arise contiguous to a neurofibroma: in turn, they may be intraneural or extraneural. In the deep soft tissue, involvement of a large nerve trunk, such as a femoral, tibial, or intercostal nerve, is characteristic, but in some instances, such a connection is not apparent. MPNST can also arise as sporadic or *de novo* lesions (i.e., not associated with NF) (139). As mentioned previously, there are rare reports of MPNST arising in a schwannoma (131). For many examples of standard MPNST, the patterns are expressive of the patterns of differentiation in embryonic mesenchyme (Fig. 37-35). The expressions can include, singly or in various combinations, fascicles of cells, often alternatingly light and dark (Fig. 37-36A, B); or elements such as chondroid matrix, osteoid (Fig. 37-37A), and rhabdomyoid cells (Fig. 37-37B) (141,142). MPNST of the perineurial type has been promoted as a variant, with the predictable proposal that such a lesion is a malignant perineurioma, but most such cases lack evidence of a relationship between a benign "perineurioma" and an MPNST (143–145). The biologic potential

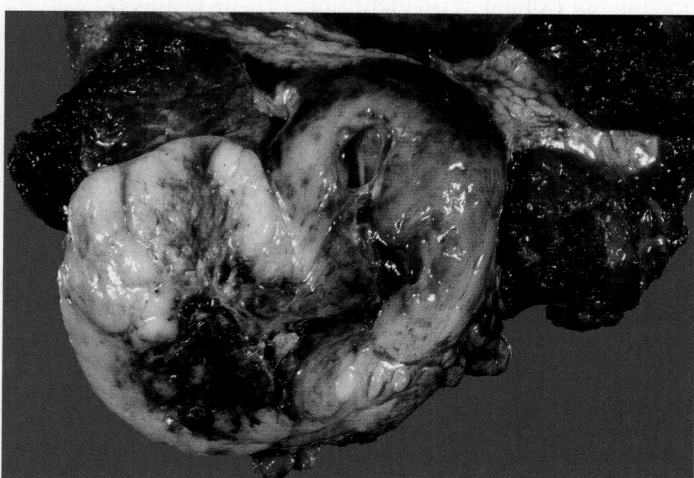

Figure 37-34 Malignant peripheral nerve sheath tumor. The tumor is expansile and circumscribed. The cut surface has a fish-flesh quality. A central, degenerative cyst contains blood clot.

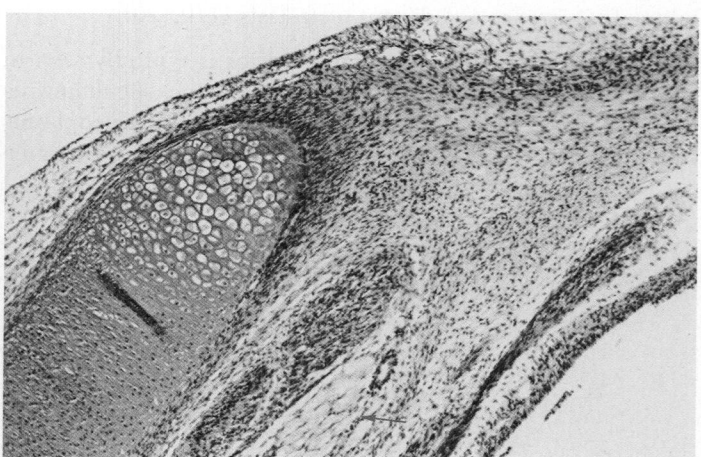

Figure 37-35 Fetal mesenchyme. Fetal mesenchyme shows varying patterns of differentiation. An island of immature cartilage is represented. In the neighboring mesenchyme, there are patterns of alternating light and dark fascicles. One fascicle of developing skeletal muscle fibers (*green arrow*) is represented in the myxoid matrix at the bottom of the field. These patterns are recapitulated, in neoplastic distortions, in many examples of malignant peripheral nerve sheath tumor.

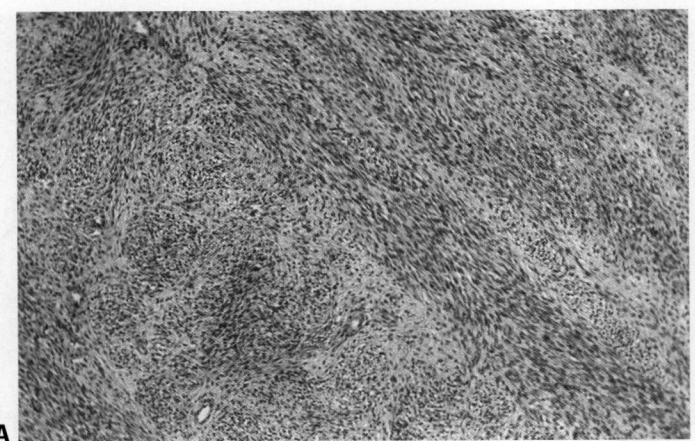
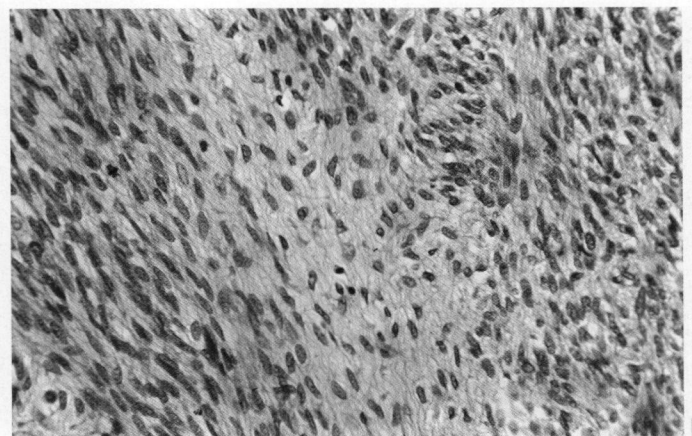

Figure 37-36 A, B: Malignant peripheral nerve sheath tumor; spindle cell variant. A: Atypical spindle cells form intersecting fascicles; the fascicles are alternately light and dark. B: At higher magnification, spindle cells are cytologically atypical, but cytologic features are uniform.

of such perineurial variants has not been adequately defined owing to the limited number of examples.

Histopathology. The variable patterns of differentiation in MPNST include mesenchymal (fibrosarcomatous, osteosarcomatous, and chondrosarcomatous (4); rhabdomyosarcomatous (1,131,141); and liposarcomatous) patterns; glandular (endodermal) patterns (102); epithelioid patterns in which individual spindle and round cells often have acidophilic cytoplasm (4,146,147) and are closely spaced in nests, fascicles, and sheets; and neuroepithelioma-like patterns (148).

Histologically, *mesenchymal patterns* are preponderant in the setting of MPNST that arise in patients with NF (3). Thin, spindle cells are arranged in interlacing fascicles in a fibromyxoid matrix. The fascicles are long and straight. They are alternatingly pale and dark (more intensely stained). Often, the spindle cells are remarkably uniform (Fig. 37-36A, B). Neoplastic cells tend to be concentrically, or radially, arranged about vessels, particularly near areas of necrosis. Endothelial cells may be prominent, resembling the endothelial-proliferation pattern seen in glioblastomas. As mentioned previously, some lesions may show specific patterns of mesenchymal differentiation (Fig. 37-37A, B). When present, such areas are usually spotty in

distribution, and there may be multiple patterns of mesenchymal differentiation in a single lesion. Detection of mitotic figures is very important for a diagnosis of MPNST, although it is not a prime determinant of biologic potential. In the setting of NF, rates may be low (<10/10 hpf) or high (>50/10 hpf), and the outcome for either category may be poor; also important are the size and location of the lesions, and the age of the patient.

Epithelioid patterns are a variant expression of MPNST in the setting of NF (3). *De novo* true malignant schwannomas (139) and "high-grade" MPNST arising in benign schwannomas (*malignant transformed schwannoma*) (131) tend to be predominantly intraneural and show "epithelioid" morphologies (146,147). The study of Hruban et al. does not support this generalization, but we should take into account that it also includes, as *de novo* variants, examples of both neuroepithelioma and MPNST arising in neurofibroma (148).

In these epithelioid variants, plump tumor cells, in nests and sheets, are closely spaced with scanty intercellular matrix (Figs. 37-38 and 37-39). Nuclei are large and often rounded. Giant cells are commonly seen in the pleomorphic variants. In some lesions, cells form nests and cords in a sparsely cellular, myxoid, or hyaline matrix. The "purely epithelioid" (epithelial)

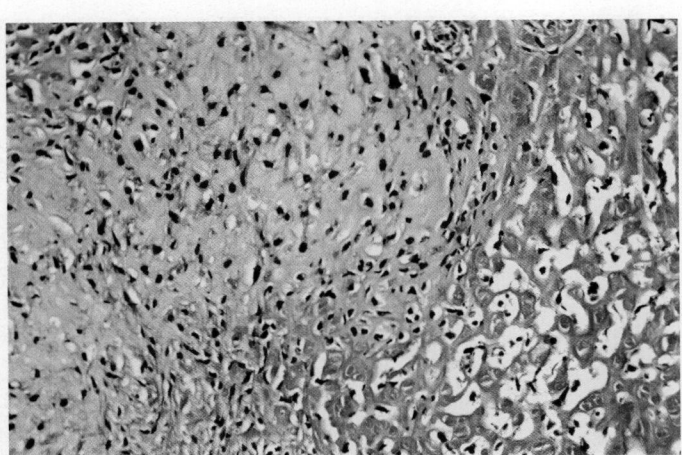
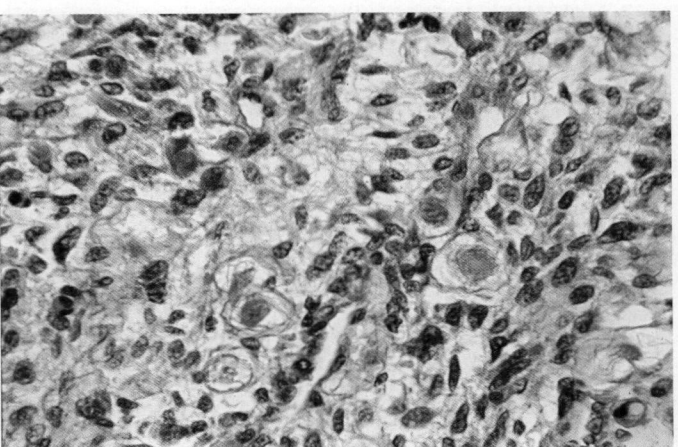

Figure 37-37 A, B: Mesenchymal differentiation in malignant peripheral nerve sheath tumor. A: Chondro-osseous differentiation; Chondroid differentiation is represented to the left of the center of the field; to the right, the patterns are those of neoplastic osteoid. B: Rhabdomyoblastic differentiation. In this field of undifferentiated small cells, there are scattered, rounded cells with plump, round nuclei; these round cells show concentrically arranged cytoplasmic myofibrils.

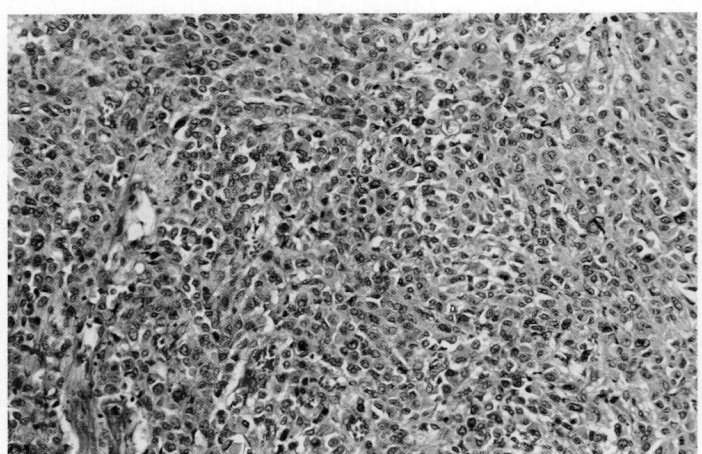

Figure 37-38 Epithelioid malignant peripheral nerve sheath tumor. Plump, atypical, spindle, and epithelioid cells form solid sheets. Intercellular matrix is scanty.

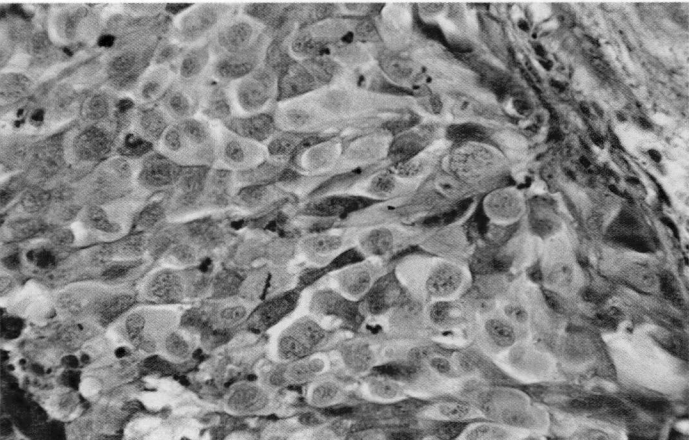

Figure 37-40 Neuroendocrine malignant peripheral nerve sheath tumor (Masson trichrome stain). Large, atypical cells are closely clustered; they form distinct nests in a fibrous matrix. The preponderant cells have pale cytoplasm. Dark cells with dendritic processes are compressed among the pale cells. The dark cells are argyrophilic.

MPNST is rare, representing a lesion without a "sarcomatous" component (149). In some "epithelioid" examples, plump, acidophilic tumor cells manifest a striking cytoplasmic argyrophilia (Fig. 37-40) (4); such examples may represent large-cell neuroendocrine carcinoma.

Some malignant epithelioid peripheral nerve sheath tumors, some of which appear to have had their origin from, and are in continuity with, a peripheral nerve, may manifest extraneural, infiltrating, and fascicular morphologies (39,146); they may qualify as IFEMSs (79). In the skin and subcutis, such a lesion, in recurrences, might be histologically indistinguishable from desmoplastic and neurotropic melanoma (Fig. 37-41).

In both fusiform and epithelioid variants, there may be areas of geographic necrosis with peripheral palisades of tumor cells, reminiscent of patterns in high-grade gliomas of the central nervous system (3).

Regarding possible differences between sporadic and NF 1–associated MPNST, there are no pathognomonic histologic findings, although the latter seem to portray worse prognosis.

Ultrastructure: A light microscopic diagnosis of MPNST of the sheath (Schwann) cell type is supported by a variety of features. Electron microscopy studies reveal features of both

Schwann and perineural cells (43). Slender, overlapping cytoplasmic processes that envelop other processes, or cell bodies, may be connected by intercellular junctions. Granular, flocculent material, preferably along and parallel to the plasma membrane, may occasionally assume the linear form of basal lamina. Fine intracytoplasmic filaments should be absent or relatively scant (134).

Purported histogenesis: In 40% to 80% of cases of MPNST (39,149,150), the tumor cells are immunoreactive for S-100 protein. CD57 can be detected in 30% to 40% of the cases (150). Myelin basic protein is less commonly detected (10%) (151). Laminin and collagen type IV are found in about 25% to 30% of cases. A high Ki67 labeling index (LI) has been correlated with a reduced survival rate; in addition, there seems to be a significant correlation between Ki67 LI and the immunohistochemical expression of p53 or MDM2 (89). It has been suggested that an MPNST that is strongly S-100+ might then be characterized as malignant schwannoma (79).

Immunohistochemistry and ultrastructural analysis have been used to highlight patterns of diverse differentiation (136),

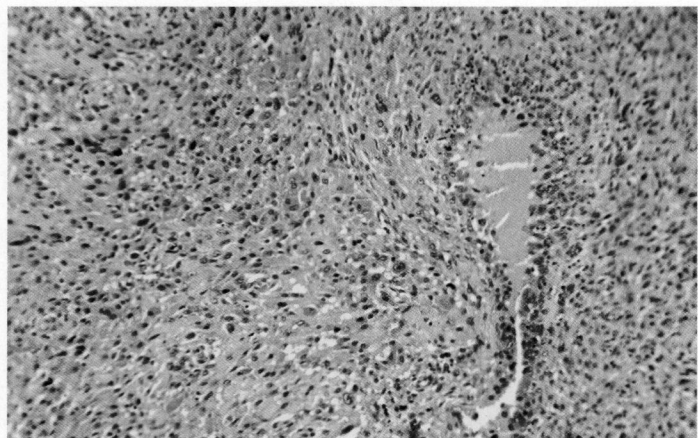

Figure 37-39 Epithelioid malignant peripheral nerve sheath tumor. Plump, rounded cells are arranged in patterns of ill-defined nests. Nuclei show variations in size and staining. A cleft to the right of the center of the field is outlined by palisades of tumor cells.

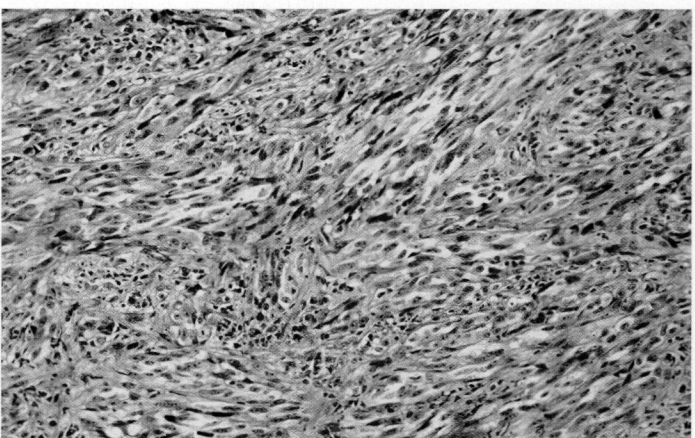

Figure 37-41 Fasciculated, malignant epithelioid peripheral nerve sheath tumor (both melanoma-like and neurotropic). Broad fascicles of atypical spindle cells infiltrate a fibrous matrix; portions of this soft tissue lesion were intraneural.

including schwannian, perineurial and endoneurial, and mesenchymal categories. In that study, some MPNST had a high component of cells immunoreactive for S-100 protein, and without perineurial and mesenchymal features. In a second category, less than 50% of tumor cells were reactive for S-100 protein and, in a third category, the cells did not react for S-100 protein; these latter two groups were interpreted as having patterns of heterologous (mesenchymal) and/or perineurial differentiation. ALDH1 has been recently reported to be expressed in most neural lesions (152).

Differential Diagnosis

A moderate increase in cellularity, focal storiform patterns, mild nuclear atypia, and the presence of mitotic figures (<10/10 hpf) are helpful features that distinguish MPNST from neurofibroma (4,86,88,153). As mentioned previously, the concept of atypical neurofibromatous neoplasms of unknown malignant potential has been proposed for lesions with nodular areas that grow within a preexisting neurofibroma and could be precursors of an MPNS, please see later (36). Such lesions seem to have loss of *CDKN2A* (*arf*), thus allowing the lesion to escape from senescence (37).

Expression of the histone 3 trimethylated in a lysine in position 27 (H3K27me3) may be helpful in distinguishing benign and MPNST, because its expression may be lost in malignant ones (154).

In the absence of discernible stigmata of NF, differentiation of MPNST from fibrosarcoma can be difficult. Patterns of interlacing fascicles that are alternately light and dark are characteristic of MPNST. For those cases of mesenchymal variants of MPNST with patterns of specific differentiation but lacking a history or stigmata of NF, histologic features would be very similar to those of malignant mesenchymomas.

Monophasic synovial sarcoma shares many features with MPNST, namely, the presence of long fascicles of monotonous, spindle cells. In contrast with MPNST, synovial sarcoma has a genetic profile with t(X;18). Common changes are a loss of NF1 locus, and a loss of the band containing gene p53, although such changes are not specific. In 50% of monophasic synovial sarcomas, the cells are focally immunoreactive for cytokeratins and EMA. With the exception of one study, MPNST routinely contains translocations involving chromosomes X and 18: t(X;18) (SYT-SSX) (155).

For deeply located epithelioid variants of MPNST, the main differential diagnosis is melanoma. In general, epithelioid melanocytes tend to express at least other melanocytic markers in addition to S100, e.g., MART1, HMB45 antigen, or MITF.

If confronted with infiltrating and fascicular patterns in a tumor of the skin, a distinction between neurotropic melanoma, desmoplastic melanoma, and cutaneous primary infiltrating and fascicular epithelioid MPNST may be impossible in the absence of lentiginous and junctional, melanocytic patterns in the overlying or adjacent epidermis. For those cases, the intensity and diffuseness of S100 expression may be helpful, because melanomas frequently and strongly express this marker in most tumor cells. Also helpful may be detection of peripherin, because this is a marker that is expressed in many spindle cell melanomas (156) and tends to be absent in MPNST (personal observation).

Infiltrating fascicular Schwann Cell Tumor of infancy (IF-SCT), in its histologic, but not its cytologic features, shows

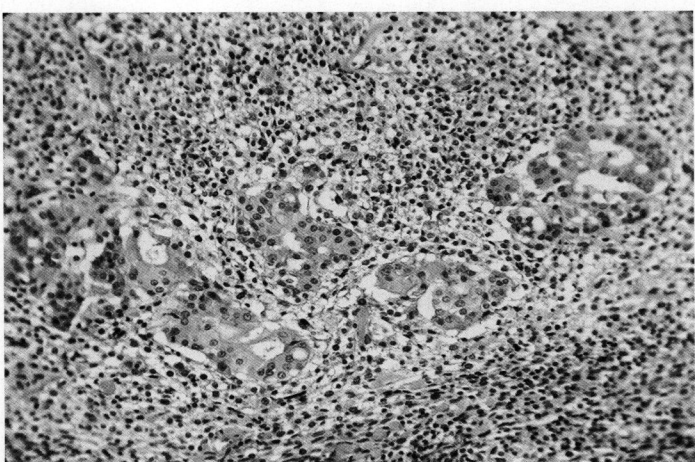

Figure 37-42 Small epithelioid cell malignant peripheral nerve sheath tumor; divergent glandular differentiation. Plump, columnar cells form solid nests and glandular patterns; the cells have small, round nuclei with uniform nuclear characteristics. The glandular spaces contain basophilic mucin. The glandular component is a random manifestation in an epithelioid malignant peripheral nerve sheath tumor.

overlaps with the patterns of both IFEMS and neurotropic melanoma.

Glandular, entoderm-like patterns (Fig. 37-42) may be more commonly associated with epithelioid than with mesenchymal variants of MPNST. When such glandular differentiation is present, the main differential diagnosis is carcinosarcoma. Entoderm-like glandular patterns, in the absence of sarcomatous components, are rarely encountered in the soft tissue in the setting of NF; a lesion showing such patterns may represent a primary neuroendocrine carcinoma/Merkel cell carcinoma (157).

Principles of Management: In the setting of NF, MPNST, in its many guises, generally has a poor prognosis, although a recent meta-analysis indicates that the differences between MPNST associated or not associated with NF1 are decreasing (158). High-grade tumors show high mitotic rates (as many as 50/10 hpf), dense cellularity, scanty stroma, marked nuclear atypia, pleomorphism, and palisaded zones of necrosis. For intraneural, high-grade MPNST ex-schwannoma (confined by the perineurium of the nerve of origin), confinement favorably modifies the significance of the "high grade." In one series of epithelioid MPNST, superficial location (skin and subcutis) and small size were favorable prognostic parameters (146). In general, adverse prognostic factors include large tumor size, age ≥7 years, tumor necrosis ≥25%, and association with von Recklinghausen disease (159,160). A high mitotic rate and the need for resection by amputation have also been cited as factors related to a poor prognosis (148). Aggressive surgical treatment is usually required for high-grade tumors with extensive spread along the involved nerve (161).

TUMORS OF UNCERTAIN NATURE WITH NERVE SHEATH–LIKE FEATURES

Nerve sheath myxoma was originally defined by Reed and Harkin. Gallager and Helwig, under the designation of *neurothekeoma*, described a series of tumors, which they interpreted as nerve sheath tumors; the histologic patterns of neurothekeomas shared some general features with those of nerve sheath myxoma (161). As a result, there has been confusion regarding the relationship between the two categories.

Herein, we use the designation of *nerve sheath myxoma* (*NSM*) to a myxoid and loosely cellular lesion that mostly appears micronodular (3) and is likely related to nerves. A larger group, the neurothekeomas of Gallager and Helwig (cellular *NTK*) (162), includes both a cellular, or epithelioid and fascicular, neurothekeoma, and a variant of neurothekeoma in which epithelioid and myxoid patterns are mixed (163,164). This second group of cellular neurothekeomas is currently included in the group of fibrohistiocytic lesions.

Mature Nerve Sheath Myxoma (NSM)

In 1985, Pulitzer and Reed (165) expanded the concept of NSM. In 2005, Fetsch et al. (166) analyzed their material with emphasis on those cases that would immunohistochemically and clinicopathologically correspond to classic NSM. Their results offer strong support for the neural character of classic NSM. The nature of cellular neurothekeoma is still controversial, although most authors now favor a fibrohistiocytic origin (167).

Clinical Summary. Classic (micronodular) NSM (Pulitzer and Reed) is most common in middle-aged adults with a male–female ratio of approximately 1:2 (3,4,165,166); mean age has been reported as 21.6 to 36 years. Characteristically, it is an asymptomatic, soft, skin-colored, or translucent papule or nodule ranging from 0.5 to 1.0 cm in diameter (63,165). It is typically located on the face and the upper extremities but can occur anywhere on the body; in the material from the American Forces Institute of Pathology (AFIP) acral locations were preponderant (166).

Histopathology. Symmetrically expansile, myxoid micronodules of various sizes are loosely clustered in a fibrous matrix in the reticular dermis. Less frequently, this lesion is located primarily in deep soft tissues. In aggregate, they form a multilobulated mass that is often poorly circumscribed and not always symmetrical (Fig. 37-43). The myxoid matrix is rich in acid mucopolysaccharides (sulfated glycosaminoglycans), with widely and regularly spaced bipolar and tripolar cells (Fig. 37-44). Nuclei are elongated, and often angulated, with inconspicuous nucleoli and uniformly distributed, dense chromatin. Cytoplasms are pale, and cell membranes are sharply defined. Centrally in the micronodules, cells tend to be arranged in loose whorls. Each micronodule is partially or completely outlined, in perineurium-like patterns, by a thin condensation of fibrous tissue. Continuity with adjacent nerves is rarely identified (4,162,165,166). A few of the dendritic cells within or around the nodules are CD34-positive (telocytes) (9).

Ultrastructurally, a continuous basal lamina outlines most cells, but there may be discontinuous basal lamina and pinocytotic vesicles (165,168). Additional features include engulfment of collagen fibers in the manner of Schwann cells as well as fibroblasts and mast cells.

Histogenesis. The most consistent immunohistochemical profile is S-100 protein (+), collagen type IV (+), GFAP (+), and vimentin (+). A smaller number of cells are EMA (+) (167), likely of perineural type.

Principles of Management: These are benign lesions that rarely recur even after incomplete excision.

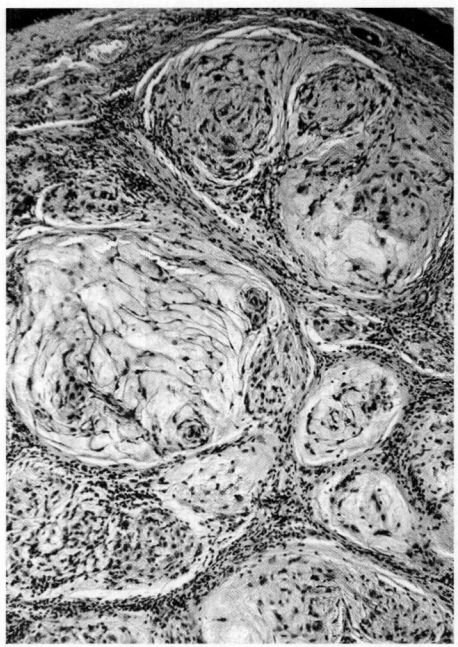

Figure 37-43 Nerve sheath myxoma. The lesion is plexiform; fascicles are represented in both longitudinal and cross sections. Some of the fascicles are outlined by thin sheaths of condensed fibrous tissue. Tumor cells are loosely spaced in a prominent myxoid matrix. Some of the tumor cells have thin polar extensions of cytoplasm; they morphologically resemble perineurial cells. Some are plump and epithelioid. Some of the thin cells form whorls about blood vessels of the fascicles. In this example, lymphoid infiltrates are prominent in the stroma.

Neurothekeoma (NTK)

[Cellular, Epithelioid, and Fascicular (Nerve Sheath Tumor–like) Neurothekeoma, questionably of Nerve Sheath Origin: Cellular Neurothekeoma; NTK]

The lesions of this category should be classified as *neurothekeoma* (*NTK*); the designation *cellular neurothekeoma* was and is, in large part, a political accommodation that may be considered superfluous. The category includes two variants. The classic one shows uniform cellularity arranged with cells arranged in short fascicles. The second variant, sometimes called mixed, fascicles are admixed with myxoid areas, resembling classic NSM.

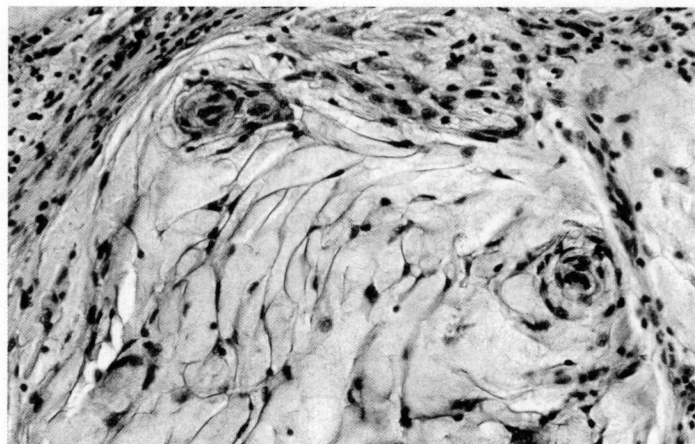

Figure 37-44 Nerve sheath myxoma. At higher magnification, many of the tumor cells have "perineurial cell–like" qualities. Some of the distinctive cells form whorls about vessels.

Clinical Summary. In NTK, the mean age is 24 years, but there are examples in children. The upper body is the favored site. Women are more commonly affected (167). The lesions are firm, pink, red-brown papules or nodules measuring 0.5 to 3.0 cm; some may produce symptoms such as pain or pruritus (168).

Histopathology. In the classic variant, cellular fascicles tend to be rather uniform in diameter, and their margins are poorly defined. They are arranged in infiltrating (dissecting) patterns among collagen bundles of the reticular dermis or are supported by a fibrous matrix (Fig. 37-45A, B); they often extend into the subcutis. Exclusive of the fascicular component, individual tumor cells and small, irregular clusters of tumor cells may infiltrate the reticular dermis; they may even extend into arrector muscles. In the fascicles, the cells are closely spaced; they tend to be polygonal, but in rare examples, they are plump and spindled shaped. Cytoplasm is conspicuous and tends to be acidophilic;

cytoplasmic processes are rigid. The nuclei are plump, rounded or elongated, and somewhat irregular in outline. Nuclear chromatin is stippled, and nuclear membranes are heavy.

In the mixed variant, some of the aggregates become locally expanded to form broad fascicles and nodules with both cellular and myxoid areas (Fig. 37-46). In the myxoid zones, stellate cells are loosely spaced: their cytoplasmic processes are broader and more irregular in diameter than those of the cells of NSM. The myxoid patterns tend to be represented at the periphery of broad fascicles and nodules. Compact whorls of cells are focally prominent in all variations of NTK. Spotty, incomplete condensations of fibrous tissue are observed at the periphery of the broad fascicles and nodules.

In some examples of NTK, the stroma consists of a sclerotic, fibrous matrix without preservation of the interwoven fiber patterns of the reticular dermis (Fig. 37-45A).

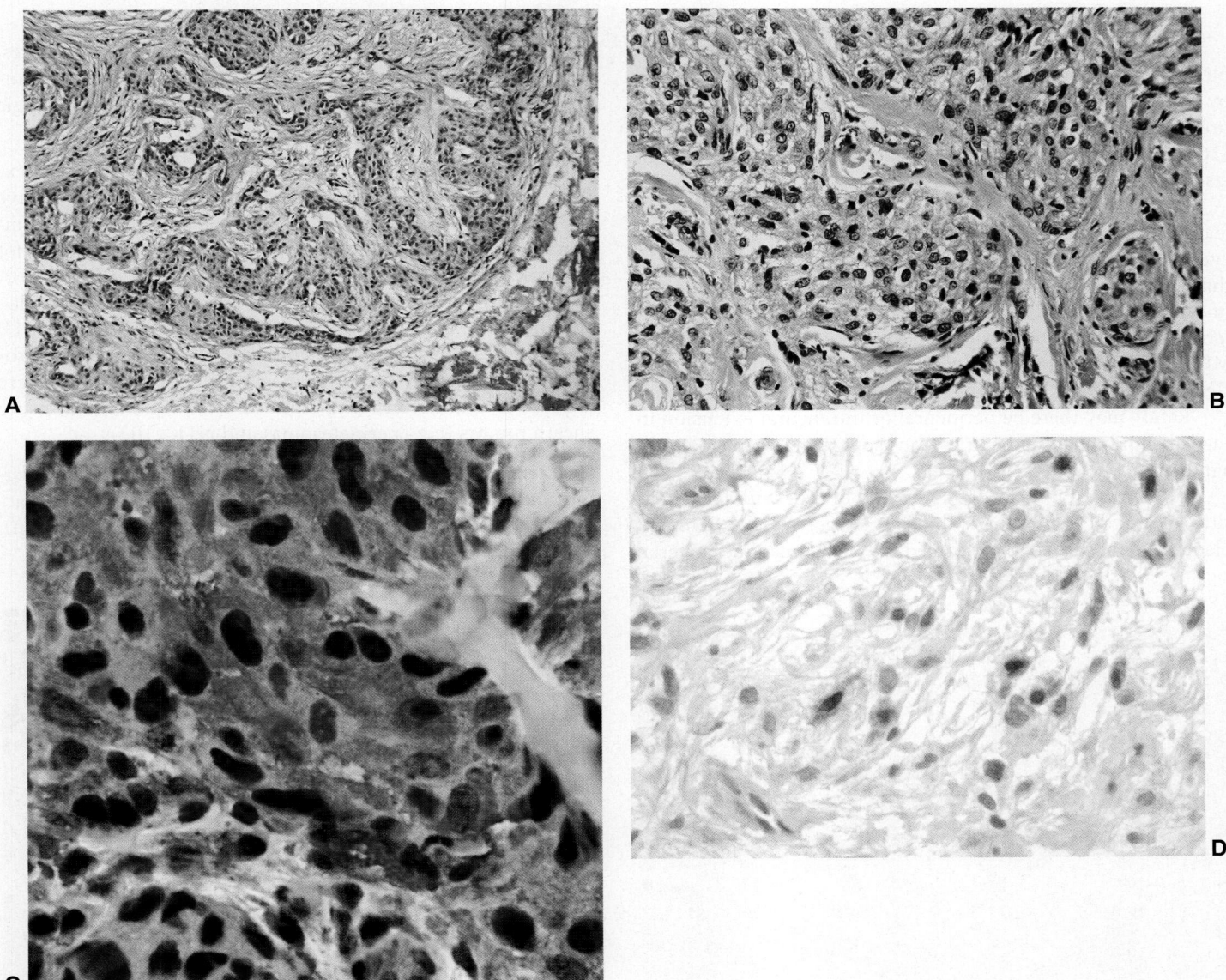

Figure 37-45 A–D: Neurothekeoma. A: Pale, acidophilic epithelioid cells from tortuous, interconnected fascicles in a well-defined fibromyxoid matrix; the lesion is sharply circumscribed. In the fascicles, myxoid matrix is scanty. B: At higher magnification, the epithelioid cells of the fascicles are loosely attached to their neighbors. Defects among the tumor cells contain a mucinous matrix. The tumor cells show regular, round nuclei with well-defined nuclear membranes and stippled chromatin; nuclei are small. C: Expression of S100A6 in a neurothekeoma. D: Expression of MITF1 in a neurothekeoma

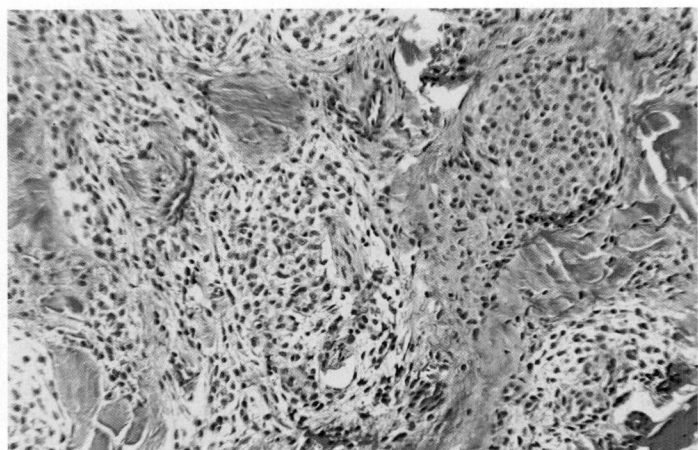

Figure 37-46 Neurothekeoma: myxoid variant. In this example, cellular zones merge with myxoid zones; the lesion is fasciculated; the fascicles extend among collagen bundles of the reticular dermis without inducing a tumor stroma.

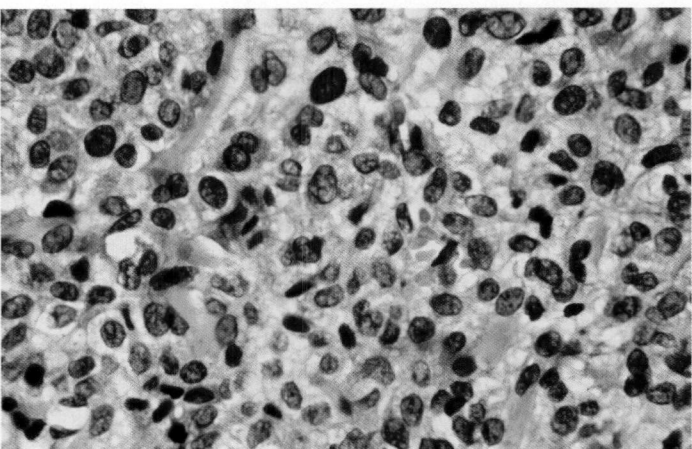

Figure 37-48 Neurothekeoma with atypical features. Cells have scanty cytoplasm. Enlarged, hyperchromatic nuclei vary in size and outline, and some show prominent nucleoli.

Mitotic figures are not a prominent feature in most examples of both variants of NTK. Atypical variants are characterized by nuclear atypia and pleomorphism with scattered mitotic figures (Figs. 37-47 and 37-48), some of which may be atypical (165,169); however, even these cases tend to behave in a benign fashion (see later).

Some examples of NTK contain multinucleated giant cells, a feature that might suggest a diagnosis of plexiform fibrous histiocytoma (Fig. 37-49). Furthermore, some authors have suggested that NTK is the superficial counterpart of plexiform fibrous histiocytoma (170,171), although the immunohistochemical pattern appears to be different, that is, podoplanin, S100A6, and MITF are expressed in the former but not in the latter.(172,173) Gene array analysis offers differences between the two (174).

Rarely may there be perineural or intraneural extension in the surrounding dermal nerves, thus suggesting a malignant diagnosis (175).

Ultrastructurally, NTK is composed of cells with focal densities of the cell membranes, which are suggestive of attachment plaques, and focal, poorly formed, basal lamina–like material

(176). Some of the cells contain phagolysosome-like structures, irregularly arranged microfilaments, and rare microfilament-attached dense bodies (177). Fibroblasts are common. A single case had perineurial cell–like features (168).

Histogenesis. Immunohistochemically, the cells of NTK exhibit a variable and inconsistent phenotype. They are positive for vimentin, CD10 (177), PGP 9.5, podoplanin, MITF (similar to dermatofibroma), and S100A6 (Fig. 37-45) but do not express standard S-100 protein or EMA (167,173,178–180)). There may be weak and variable expression of smooth muscle–specific actin, collagen type IV, NK1/C3, and CD57 (63,181). For these reasons, NTKs are currently classified within fibrohistiocytic lesions. However, it is interesting to note that there are rare hybrid lesions with features of both peripheral nerve sheath tumors (e.g., perineurioma) and NTK (182).

Differential Diagnosis. Intraneural neurofibromas are rare in the dermis, and only slightly more common in the subcutis. Immunoreactive axons (either with silver techniques or with NSE or peripherin), a feature of intraneural neurofibroma, are not detected in NSM.

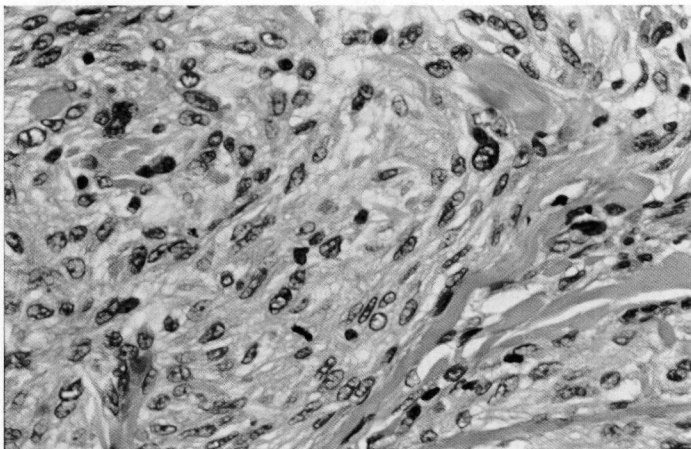

Figure 37-47 Neurothekeoma with atypical features. Tumor cells of this atypical nerve sheath myxoma vary in size and outline; some are hyperchromatic. A mitotic figure is represented to the left and below the center of the field.

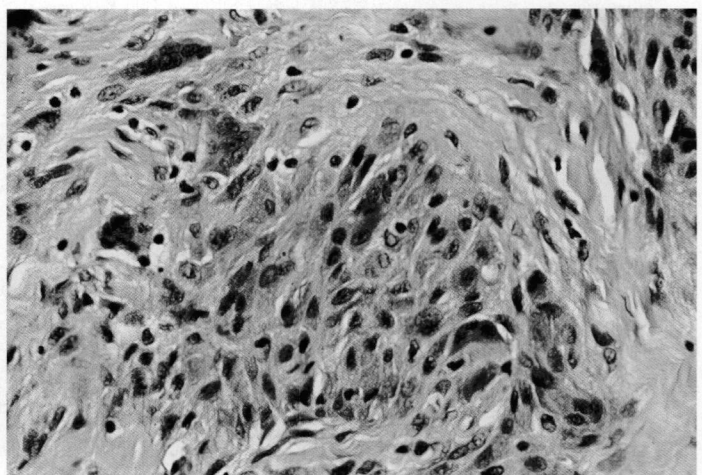

Figure 37-49 Nerve sheath myxoma with multinucleated giant cells. The basic pattern of this "plexiform" lesion suggested a variant of nerve sheath myxoma. Focally, as in this field, the patterns overlap with those of plexiform fibrous histiocytoma.

Cellular myxomas of the skin, including angiomyxomas (183) and trichogenic myxomas (122), are rare lesions. They are solid, uniform lesions, without the micronodular qualities of NSM or the fascicular and nodular qualities of NTK. Cellular myxomas are generally negative for S-100 protein, although there are rare positive examples (63) (personal observation). To complicate the topic, it seems that some examples of cellular myxoma appear to have been reported as NSM. Zelger et al. suggested that some reported examples of NSM are actually perineuriomas (65).

Spindle cell nevus of the Spitz type, particularly dermal variants, might be confused with NTK. A strong and uniform reaction for S-100 protein or MART1 would favor a variant of Spitz nevus or some other variant of nevus, such as a cellular blue nevus with prominent fascicular components. The pigmentation of deep penetrating nevus is not a feature of NTK. HMB45 will usually label the entire lesion in both blue nevi and deep penetrating nevi and the superficial cells in most other nevi (184). Interestingly, NTK may express KBA.62, a marker typically expressed in melanocytic lesions (185).

Spindle cell melanoma with extensive perineural invasion (*neurotropic melanoma*) also mimics NTK. However, the overwhelming majority of spindle cell melanomas are S-100 protein and SOX10 positive (186). Not all desmoplastic and neurotropic melanomas are immunoreactive for HMB45, but a positive reaction would exclude NTK (180,184). Owing to the lack of intraepidermal component, NTK might be mistaken for a metastatic malignant melanoma. As mentioned previously, expression of S-100 protein or MART1 would rule out NTK (180).

Some examples of the myxoid variant of NTK, with involvement of the subcutis, and with multinucleated giant cells, would be difficult to distinguish from plexiform fibrous histiocytoma of children and young adults (Fig. 37-49) (64). In the nodular portions of plexiform fibrous histiocytic tumor, the cells are closely spaced and are often admixed with multinucleated giant cells. Plexiform fibrous histiocytic tumor is a deep lesion and has a close association with fascia. A myxoid matrix is usually not prominent. As mentioned previously, owing to the fascicular ("plexiform") architecture of NTK and the multinucleated giant cells, it has been suggested that NTK and plexiform fibrous histiocytoma might be the same lesion. However, immunohistochemical (172,173) and gene array (174) findings appear to be different.

Sclerosing myofibroblastomas, as well as rare myxoid or epithelioid pilar leiomyomas, of the skin should be considered in the differential diagnosis (187). At least focally myxoid leiomyomas have fascicles of smooth muscle cells with spindle morphology, large nuclei, and perinuclear cytoplasmic vacuoles. Although some NTK may have some cells immunoreactive for smooth muscle actin, unlike leiomyomas, they do not express desmin (63).

Epithelioid fibrous histiocytoma (*EFH*) (epithelioid cell histiocytoma, adventitial cellular myxofibroblastoma) (188,189), a lesion favoring acral sites, tends to be polypoid; it is mostly confined to a widened papillary dermis. Some examples are mostly myxoid. Occasionally, there are large, vacuolated cells with muciparous qualities. Many of the dendritic histiocytes that are found among tumor cells of EFH are reactive for factor XIIIa, and some are reactive for S-100 protein, which may be a diagnostic pitfall. Examples of EFH can be identified in some reports of NSM.

The possible cell of origin in NTK is still unclear. The immunohistochemical distinctions between NSM and NTK provide evidence that "cellular neurothekeoma" might not be a nerve sheath tumor (167). On the other hand, the commonness of many of the histologic patterns in the groups NSM and NTK could be dependent on the degree of differentiation, or the functional status, of Schwann cells. It has been argued that NTK is a variant of dermatofibroma or fibrous histiocytoma (167,190); NK1/C3 positivity is evidence of the "histiocytic" nature of the tumor cells, and thus the lesion could be assigned to the "fibrohistiocytic" category. Positivity for CD10 would also support a "histiocytic" nature of NTK, but this type of positivity has also been observed in myelin sheaths (191) and Wallerian degeneration. Also possibly suggesting a nerve sheath differentiation, there are examples of NTK with features suggesting hybrid morphologies with perineuriomas (192). In summary, NSM and NTK are superficial lesions with multiple morphologies that behave in a benign fashion and have features at least suggesting nerve sheath differentiation.

Principles of Management: NTK behaves in a benign fashion regardless of the degree of atypia (193). However, particularly in those cases with marked cytologic atypia, we recommend complete excision.

Granular Cell Tumors

Granular Cell Tumor (GrCT)

Clinical Summary. Granular cell tumor (granular cell myoblastoma, granular cell schwannoma, granular cell nerve sheath tumor) is usually solitary. However, in about 10% of the cases, lesions are multiple. Forty percent of the cases involve the tongue (Abrikosoff tumor) (194), but the skin and the subcutaneous tissue are also a common site (Fig. 37-50A). Other reported sites include the esophagus, stomach, appendix, larynx, bronchus, pituitary gland, uvea, and skeletal muscle (195).

GrCT of the skin are well circumscribed, raised, firm, and nodular. Some examples are verrucous at the surface. Generally, lesions range from 0.5 to 3.0 cm in diameter. The cut surface is often faintly yellow and homogeneous. Tenderness or pruritus has been an occasional complaint.

Histopathology. Most GrCT are extraneural, but rare examples appear at least focally intraneural. Broad fascicles of tumor cells infiltrate the dermis among collagen bundles (Fig. 37-50B). There is common extension of fascicles of tumor into the subcutis. The tumor cells are large and polygonal (Fig. 37-50B); cell membranes are distinct. Cytoplasms are filled with faintly eosinophilic, uniform, small granules, that are PAS (+) and diastase-resistant, as well as with scattered, laminated, cytoplasmic globules with peripheral halos (residual bodies) (Fig. 37-51). Nuclei are usually small and centrally located. They tend to be round to oval in outline, but, in some examples, they are plump, irregular, and hyperchromatic with a central nucleolus. Mitotic figures are uncommon. Some clusters of tumor cells are surrounded by PAS (+), diastase-resistant membranes, strands of collagen fibers, and occasional flattened, satellite cells (194). Interstitial spindle cells have fibroblast-like qualities (39). Rarely, fascicles of tumor cells are entrapped in a dense fibrous matrix (sclerosing/desmoplastic variant), a possible diagnostic pitfall (196). The overlying epidermis is usually hyperplastic (see Differential Diagnosis).

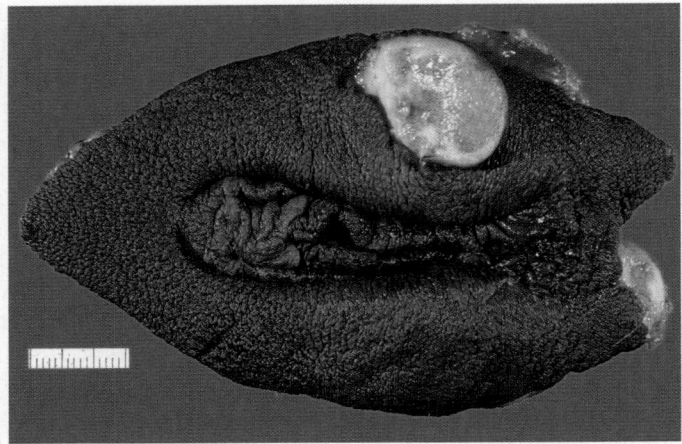
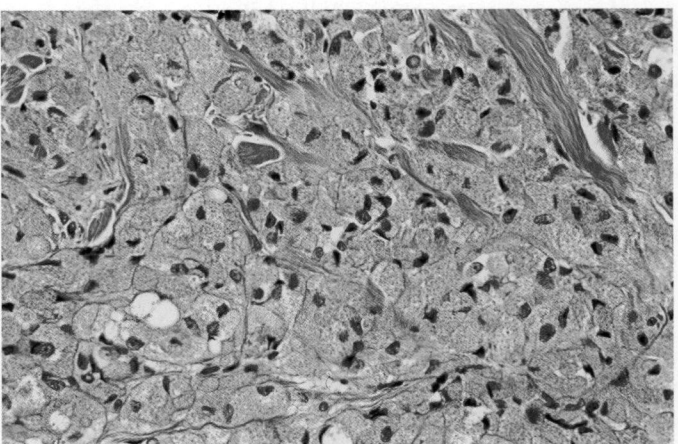

Figure 37-50 A, B: Granular nerve sheath tumor. **A:** This granular cell tumor involves the labia majora of the vulva. The cut surface of the tumor is exposed; it is yellow tan and somewhat granular. The specimen is the product of a vulvectomy. **B:** In this example, the cells are plump and polygonal; fine granules, uniform in size, fill the cytoplasm of each cell. In this category, nuclear characteristics are variable from case to case; in this example, there is some variability in nuclear size and outline. An occasional nucleus contains an inclusion of cytoplasm. Nucleoli are variable in size.

Often, there is neurotropic spread along peripheral nerves both within and at the advancing tumor margins (Fig. 37-51). Rarely, usually in deeply located lesions, there is an intraneural component that expands the involved nerve.

Although most lesions with granular cell features behave in a benign fashion, it may be difficult to predict biologic behavior in GrCT because they may show abundant mitotic figures and infiltrative pattern (197). Because recurrences are common after incomplete excision, GrCT should probably be completely excised. Infiltration of skeletal muscle is a common feature of GrCT involving the squamous mucosae; in such areas, regenerating and degenerating muscle fibers are entrapped among fascicles of tumor cells. *Plexiform GrCT* is characterized by perineurial extensions of tumor along the neural plexus of the dermis in the absence of a discrete mass (198).

Ultrastructurally, tumor cells are outlined by basal lamina (199,200). The preponderant cytoplasmic granules are largely phagolysosomes. They appear as membrane-bound vacuoles measuring 200 to 900 nm in diameter. Some of the larger cytoplasmic bodies have the appearance of residual bodies, or myelin figures (194,199,200). The peripheral satellite cells of the fascicles are outlined by a discontinuous basal lamina (201). Interstitial cells of the tumor contain angulate bodies (39).

Histogenesis. The granular cell category is heterogeneous. Not all examples seem to be nerve sheath tumors (see later); some of the immunohistochemically divergent lesions are also cytologically atypical (202). The classic immunohistochemical profile is S-100 protein, SOX10, peripheral nerve myelin proteins, such as P2 protein and PO protein, Gap43, PGP 9.5, NSE, calretinin, CD68, alpha-inhibin, and TFF-3 (203–205). A protein associated with autophagy, LC3 (microtubule-associated protein 1 light chain 3, a specific marker of autophagy), is expressed in GrCT and also in schwannomas (206).

Differential Diagnosis. Xanthomas are excluded by the identification of cytoplasmic granules (rather than vacuoles) in GrCT. A fascicular arrangement of cells also favors GrCT.

Angulated, elongated columns of bland squamous cells occasionally extend from the epidermis into GrCT among the fascicles of tumor cells (*pseudoepitheliomatous hyperplasia*). On biopsy specimens from tumoral lesions of the tongue, genitalia, or the mucous membranes of the upper respiratory tract, esophagus, or anus, such patterns should be interpreted with caution. If confronted with such patterns on a superficial biopsy specimen, a careful search for a component of granular cells might help avoid a mistaken diagnosis of carcinoma and needless aggressive surgery.

Tumor cells with cytoplasmic granular cell qualities are occasionally a feature of *granular cell lesions of diverse lineage*, such as basal cell carcinoma (207) and dermatofibroma (208). The granules of rare granular squamous cell carcinomas, in contrast to those of other benign and malignant GrCTs, are PAS (–), and desmosomes are seen on electron microscopy (209). In the jawbones, a granular cell variant of ameloblastoma has been described. Granular cell change has been noted in smooth muscle tumors (210).

The *primitive polypoid granular cell tumor* (*dermal nonneural granular cell tumor*) presents as a painless nodule, mainly on the extremities or trunk (207). Lesions are both polypoid and endophytic. The tumor cells are immunoreactive for NKI-C3, and CD68, and are negative for S100 protein, smooth muscle

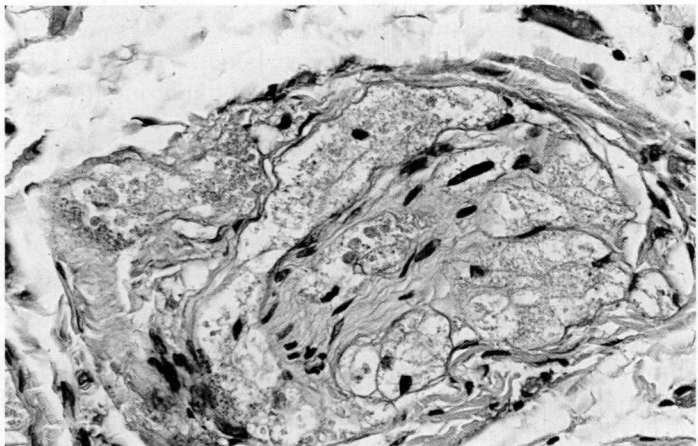

Figure 37-51 Granular cell nerve sheath tumor, neurotropism. Granular cells infiltrate the perineurium and the endoneurial space of this small nerve. In the cytoplasm of some of the cells, in addition to fine, uniform granules, there are larger, rounded, acidophilic bodies that are "residual body–like."

actin, Melan-A, CD34, desmin, and cytokeratin (211). Most reported cases have behaved in a benign fashion (207), although there has been a report of a lymph node metastasis (212).

There have been rare reports of hybrid tumors containing a component of granular cells and perineurioma (213,214). One such lesion had expression of S100 protein in the granular cells and of EMA and GLUT-1 in the perineurioma area. Electron microscopy was reported showing a plethora of lysosomes in the granular cells and of pinocytotic vesicles and tight junctions in perineurial cells (214). One of these hybrid lesions has been shown to be primarily intraneural (213).

Principles of Management: Most GrCT behave in a benign fashion and do not recur after excision.

Granular Cell Epulis of Infancy
Clinical Summary. Granular cell epulis of infancy is a polypoid tumor of the gingiva of the newborn, with a predilection for girls (215). It shares the basic histologic features of *GrCT but* is immunohistochemically distinctive. The immunohistochemical profile is NSE (+), vimentin (+), S-100 protein (–), GFAP (–), CD57 (–), MBP (–), lysozyme (–), alpha1-ACT (–), and laminin (–). Interstitial cells are positive for S-100 protein; they do not contain angulate bodies (216).

Malignant Granular Cell Tumor (MGrCT)
Clinical Summary. MGRCT is uncommon. Most of the reported cases have occurred on the skin or in the subcutaneous tissue (217). As in benign GrCT, a few cases have been reported from other areas, such as the sciatic nerve (218) and the viscera. A variety of malignant tumors may masquerade in granular cell patterns. In all instances, an acceptance of the diagnosis, MGrCT, is predicated on circumspection.

In the skin and subcutaneous tissue, MGrCT, a rapidly growing, poorly defined nodule or mass, may reach a considerable size and undergo ulceration (218).

Histopathology. There are two types of MGrCT (219). In one type, in spite of the clinically malignant course, the histologic appearance of the primary lesion, and even of the metastases, is that of a benign GrCT, except for occasional mitotic figures and mild cellular pleomorphism with nuclei that are slightly larger than those seen in most benign GrCT (219–221). In the general category of GCNST, these cytologic features are too common to provide reliable identification of lesions with the potential for metastasis. In evaluating the malignant potential of histologically benign or indeterminate GrCTs, clinical data, such as large size of the tumor, rapid growth, ulceration, and invasion into adjacent tissue, are of greater diagnostic value than the histologic features (222). The average diameter of "histologically benign, clinically malignant," GrCTs has been found to be 9 cm, as compared with 1.85 cm for the benign variety (219,222,223). In the soft tissues, malignant lesions usually have three or more of the following criteria: necrosis, spindling, vesicular nuclei with large nucleoli, increased mitotic figures (>2/10 high-power fields), high nuclear to cytoplasmic (N:C) ratio, and pleomorphism (224).

In the second type of MGCT, both the primary lesion and the metastases are histologically malignant; they show transitions from typical granular cells through pleomorphic granular cells to pleomorphic, no granular spindle and giant cells with numerous mitotic figures (225,226).

In MGrCT, S-100 protein and NSE may become negative.

Principles of Management: Extensive metastases to viscera, skin, and skeletal musculature occur, either with or without regional lymph node metastases (220). Some lesions, even in the absence of demonstrable metastases, have been characterized as MGrCT (227). Management is complete excision and close follow-up.

Fibrolamellar Nerve Sheath Tumor
Clinical Summary. Fibrolamellar nerve sheath tumor (FNST) is a rare, solitary tumor of the dermis (79,228).

Histopathology. FNST is nonencapsulated, but sharply defined, in the dermis. Coarse, rigid, eosinophilic lamellae are arranged in parallel arrays in stacks of four or more. Neighboring stacks are random in orientation, one to the other, but in some areas, cells are arranged in storiform patterns and abut neighboring stacks. Some examples are mostly myxoid; in them, the fibrous lamellae are more delicate and widely spaced. Tumor cells, each with a small nucleus; scanty perikaryon; and rigid, thin, polar cytoplasmic extensions, resemble perineurial cells. They are isolated in a clear or mucinous matrix among the fibrous lamellae. Rarely, there may be a few loosely clustered, pigmented dendritic cells.

FNST is histologically distinctive but may be simply an exaggeration of perineurial-like patterns that are occasionally manifested in CNFs. Furthermore, in an abstract presentation, it was suggested that sclerotic fibroma is actually an end-stage morphology of some neurofibromas (229).

FNST shares features with *sclerotic fibroma,* as manifested either sporadically or in the setting of *Cowden* disease. A demonstration of immunoreactivity for S-100 protein by some of the tumor cells strongly favors the diagnosis of FNST.

Principles of Management: FNST is a benign lesion. Excision is usually recommended for cosmetic reasons.

TUMORS OF PERINEURIAL CELLS (PERINEURIOMAS)

Storiform Perineurial Cell Fibroma, Soft Tissue type
Clinical Summary. Storiform perineurial cell fibroma, soft tissue type (SPCF; storiform perineurial fibroma; "soft tissue perineurioma"), is a solitary, symmetrically expansile, and well-circumscribed tumor. It most commonly affects the subcutis (4,230–232) but may involve the deep soft tissue and even viscera. In the series reported by Hornick and Fletcher (233), there was a slight preponderance of females. A painless mass in the subcutis was the most common clinical presentation, with the involvement of deep soft tissue in more than 25% of cases. Most of their cases were well circumscribed; 12 cases microscopically showed focal, infiltrative margins.

Histopathology. SPCF may be characterized as a fibroma whose component cells express the phenotype of perineurial cells. This lesion is circumscribed. At its periphery, the interface with soft tissue is defined by a thin capsule consisting of several loosely spaced, delicate fibrous lamellae. Beneath the capsule, thin, collagen fibers form a delicate, fibrous matrix, in which there are loosely spaced cells with plump, angulated nuclei and

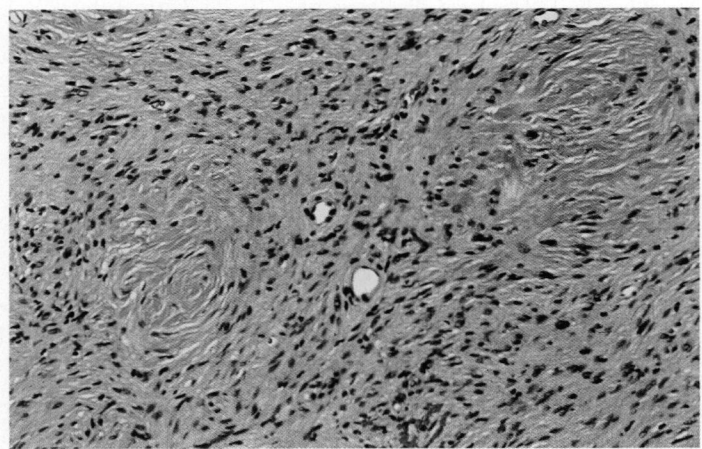

Figure 37-52 Storiform perineurial cell nerve sheath tumor (soft tissue "perineurioma"). Spindle cells are individually isolated in a delicate fibrous matrix. There are two collections of stacked, acidophilic fibrous lamellae.

rigid, polar, cytoplasmic extensions (Fig. 37-52). Some cells are arranged in storiform fascicles. In most examples, small nerves are embedded in, or may be traced into, the tumor. The tumor cells tend to form thin, concentric layers around entrapped small nerves, blood vessels, and collagen bundles. There may be small stacks of hyalinized (skeinoid?) fibrous lamellae, somewhat similar to those of FNST (Fig. 37-52). Fourteen cases were classified as atypical perineuriomas; only two tumors recurred locally, and there were no metastases. This atypical variant of perineurioma does not appear to be a precursor of MPNST of the perineurial type. Rather, MPNST of the perineurial type is grouped in the general category of MPNST (see earlier). Thus, the atypical forms are being promoted as benign lesions in which atypia is dismissed as "degenerative" ("ancient") change. In that series (233), mitotic counts in standard perineuriomas ranged from 1 to >5 mitoses per hpf. Among the atypical perineuriomas, mitotic figures ranged from 0 to 7 per 30 hpf. Therefore, these atypical, mitotically active perineuriomas may be similar to the atypical, mitotically active "cellular schwannomas."

Histogenesis. The cytologic features are perineurial cell–like. In some examples, tumor cells are immunoreactive for vimentin and EMA (231). The latter reaction may be weak or patchy; it is most likely to be best developed in cells in, or near, the capsule. In other examples, scattered aggregates of tumor cells, in more central locations, are reactive for S-100 protein. Claudin-1, a tight junction–associated protein, is commonly expressed (234). An abnormality of chromosome 22 has been reported (235). There is a report of a soft tissue perineurioma in a patient with NF type 2 (236).

Differential Diagnosis. Storiform patterns appear to be variations that are expressed in a variety of nerve sheath tumors. Perhaps variants of both schwannomas and neurofibromas have been included in this category of "perineurioma." This impression is further supported by the reports of hybrid lesions of perineurioma and schwannoma (55,237). Furthermore, there are rare cases of congenital nevi with features of both perineurioma and schwannoma (57) and perineurioma and NTK (see also earlier).

CS may resemble perineurioma; such lesions usually do not express CD34 or EMA.

Fibrous histiocytoma of the subcutaneous fat and dermatofibroma are also considerations in the differential diagnosis. Such lesions, in contrast to perineurioma, contain keloidal collagen and express factor XIIIa and CD163.

Dermatofibrosarcoma protuberans (DFSP), in its nodular, well-differentiated components, might be confused with SPCF. It has been variously classified as a fibroblastic, fibrohistiocytic, or neurocristic tumor. The pigmented variant of DFSP (*Bednar tumor*) has been sometimes considered as a pigmented storiform neurofibroma. The nature of pigmented dermatofibrosarcoma is controversial but, in one study, perineurial cell–like qualities were observed (72). The cells of DFSP, like some cells of nerve sheath tumors, are immunoreactive for CD34 (238). DFSP is described in detail elsewhere (Chapter 32).

Meningiomas also have spindle cells with whirling and express EMA (see also later). In contrast to perineurioma, meningioma lacks GLUT1 or Claudin 1 expression (239).

Principles of Management: Perineuriomas are benign lesion; owing to their circumscribed nature, they are usually excised in the first surgery.

Acral Perineuriomas
Pacinian Neurofibroma
The designation, *Pacinian neurofibroma*, has been assigned to a variety of lesions. It was originally considered to be a neuroma and neurofibroma, but most authors currently include it within the group of perineuriomas. Its name gives recognition to a proliferation of structures resembling Pacinian (Vater-Pacini) corpuscles.

Intraneural Perineurioma
Clinical Summary. Intraneural perineurioma (intraneural symmetrically concentric perineurial cell tumor; hypertrophic interstitial neuritis; hypertrophic mononeuropathy; intraneural PN) is an intraneural, solitary, segmental, and cylindrical enlargement of a nerve, usually accompanied by sensorimotor defects (231,240,241).

Histopathology. In the characterization of this lesion, distinctions are required between onion bulbs and pseudo-onion bulbs. Pseudo-onion bulbs are composed of cells that are immunoreactive for EMA. If the cells of a concentrically arranged cluster are Schwann cells (S-100+), the collection qualifies as an onion bulb pattern; if the concentrically arranged cells are mostly perineurial cells (EMA+), the collection qualifies as a pseudo-onion bulb pattern. In intraneural PN, cells, with both the structural qualities and the immunoreactivity of perineurial cells, form concentric sheaths (pseudo-onion bulbs) around affected nerve fibers (Fig. 37-53), and even around small clusters of pseudo-onion bulbs (231). Collagen bundles and vessels may be similarly embraced. There is usually a specific and concentric orientation of cells about axons, and there usually are demyelination and degeneration of axons; in the center of the clusters, axons may appear enlarged and irregularly shaped.

Histogenesis. In intraneural PN, the concentrically arranged cells express EMA (231) and have the ultrastructural features of perineurial cells.

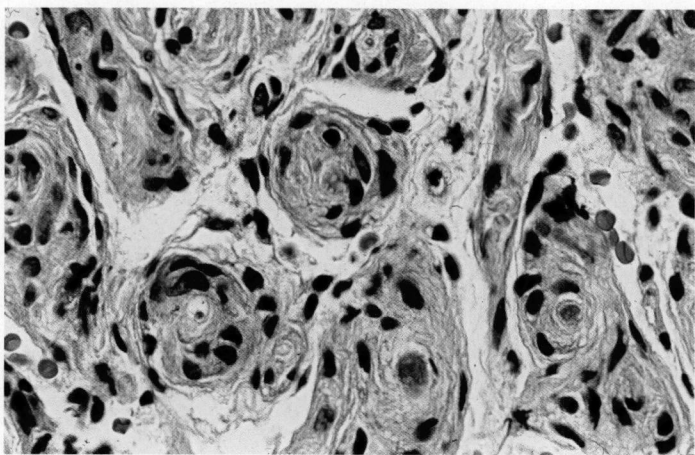

Figure 37-53 Perineurioma, intraneural variant. Axons are surrounded by concentric layers of spindle cells; the spindle cells are layered in onion-skin patterns. The lesion is intraneural; axial symmetry is preserved.

A defect in the integrity of the perineurial barrier has been proposed as the primary alteration. Delamination of the perineurium, and migration of perineurial cells into the endoneurium have been offered as an explanation for the origin of pseudo-onion bulbs (240).

In common with descriptions of the clonal, chromosomal abnormalities in benign and malignant schwannomas, neurofibromas, meningiomas, and gliomas, intraneural PN may also show monosomy of 22q and deletion of 22q11.2-qter; deletion of 22q11 is cited as a finding favoring neoplasia (231).

Differential Diagnosis. The *hereditary degenerative neuropathies* are not localized and segmental (242). In addition, they are characterized by concentric hyperplasia of Schwann cells (onion bulbs) (Fig. 37-54).

Principles of Management: Acral perineurioma is a benign lesion. Excisional surgery may result in further sensorimotor deficit.

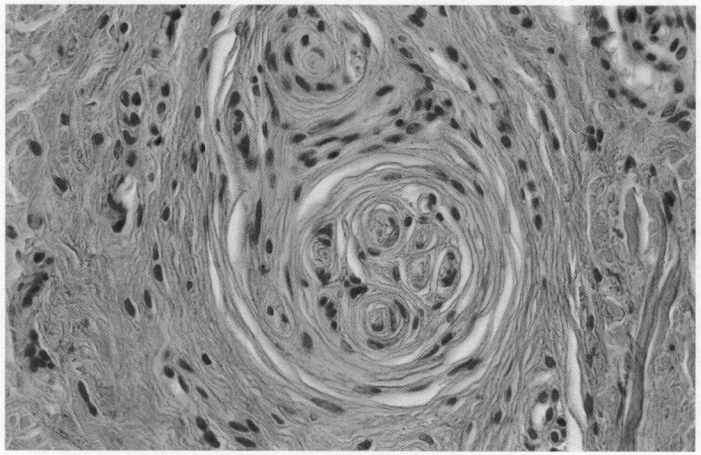

Figure 37-54 Hypertrophic neuropathy. In the center of the field, a small nerve is cut in cross section. The perineurium is thickened. Spindle cells are arranged concentrically about nerve fibers (onion-skin pattern). Some of the spindle cells blend with the thickened perineurium.

Pacinian Perineural Cell Fibroma, Acral Type (Subcutaneous [Sclerosing] or Dermal [Fibrous] Perineurioma, PPCF)

Clinical Summary. An uncommon, small, benign tumor found mainly on the hands has been characterized as either fibrous (dermal) perineurioma (243) or sclerosing (subcutaneous) perineurioma (244,245). It should be noted that most, if not all, of the lesions in this category could, in the past, have been easily accommodated in the category of *Pacinian neuroma* or *neurofibroma.* Such lesions have been also designated as fibrous or sclerosing perineurioma (244).

Histopathology: Whether fibroma, neuroma, neurofibroma, or perineurioma, these small tumors are basically fibrous lesions with focal areas of increased cellularity. They are mostly acral in location and tend to be oval in outline, with the long axis perpendicular to the surface of the skin. The lesions, reported by Skelton et al. had a configuration, at low magnification, that resembled that of a CNF (243). Some of the lesions have ill-defined margins; some are circumscribed, particularly along the deep margin, with cellularity being greatest in the area of circumscription. The cells are spindle shaped or ovoid; they have round nuclei with uniformly distributed chromatin; they have pale or clear cytoplasm. Some of the cells appear to be outlined by a delicate membrane (possible reticulum). In areas, the cells form thin, interconnected ribbons (retiform patterns). In some examples, small spindle and round cells form whorls in patterns strongly suggestive of the arrangement of cells in a Pacinian corpuscle (245). Rarely, there may be extensive areas of adipose tissue (246).

An additional variant of "perineurioma," the *retiform (reticular) perineurioma* (247) is a soft tissue lesion sharing some of the features of the subcutaneous or dermal variants (Fig. 37-55A, B).

These Pacinian lesions show cells immunoreactive for EMA and claudin-1 (234). Some of the tumor cells are immunoreactive for muscle-specific actin and CD 99. Sclerosing perineuriomas express GLUT1, a marker usually detected in hemangiomas (248). The tumor cells show ultrastructural features of perineurial cells.

The differential diagnosis includes glomus tumor. The lack of EMA and claudin-1 expression supports a diagnosis of glomus tumor.

Principles of Management: These are benign lesions that do not require complete excision.

NEUROMAS

Neuromas are hyperplasias of axons and associated nerve sheath cells. In most, but not all, cutaneous neuromas, Schwann cells and axons are arranged in interlacing (tortuous) fascicles. Axons are easily demonstrated with silver impregnation techniques. They are also easily demonstrated with monoclonal antibodies, such as those for neurofilaments, but neither silver impregnation stains nor immune reactions, in themselves, distinguish between the innervated fascicles of a neuroma and those of CNF.

Neuromas can be divided into four types: extraneural (traumatic or acquired); intraneural (isolated and spontaneous, solitary or multiple); intraneural (multiple mucosal), including

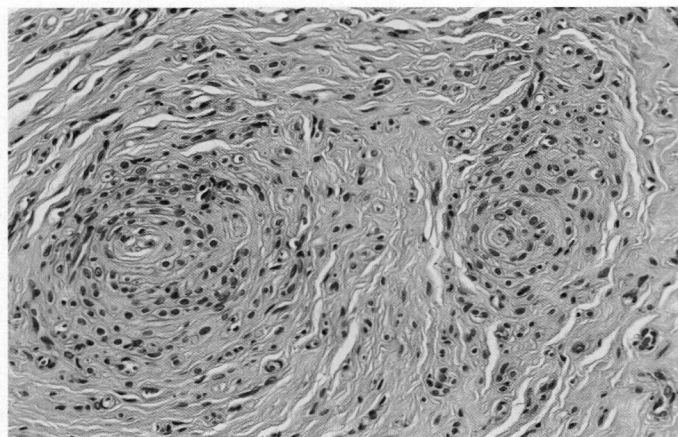
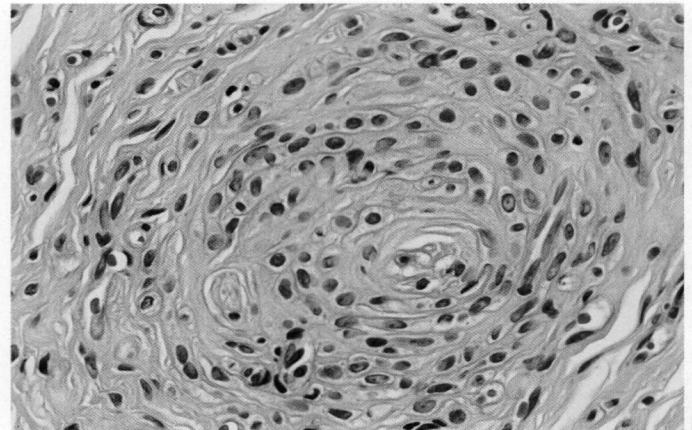

Figure 37-55 **A, B:** Sclerosing perineurial cell nerve sheath tumor (fibrous or sclerosing "perineurioma"). **A:** In two foci, bland, small cells with pale cytoplasm are arranged in whorls among delicate collagen fibers; the cells are round or slightly spindle shaped; some appear to be isolated by basement membranes. The bland cytologic features are reminiscent of glomus cells. The concentric whorls are reminiscent of cellular arrangements in pacinian corpuscles. In the background, the lesion is sclerotic with small spindle cells among collagen bundles. **B:** At higher magnification, the cells form whorls about a central nidus. The cytologic features are more epithelioid than perineurial.

those occurring in MEN, type 2b; and abnormalities of sensory receptors.

Extraneural Neuromas

Acquired (Traumatic) Neuroma

Clinical Summary. Traumatic neuromas are usually solitary, firm papules or nodules at the sites of scars following local trauma (Fig. 37-56A); if they extend to the skin surface, they are skin colored or pink. In mature neuromas, a lancinating type of pain might be elicited in response to local pressure.

Histopathology. Interlacing fascicles of regenerating nerve fibers extend from the proximal end of a damaged nerve; they extend through an acquired defect in the perineurium, and then into the neighboring mesenchyme. They insinuate in asymmetric patterns among collagen bundles (Fig. 37-56B). With maturation, perineuria form around each of the extraneural fascicles. The distal end of a severed nerve does not contribute significantly to the neuroma. In pretumorous stages, nerve fibers of both the proximal and the distal segments of the disrupted nerve show Wallerian degeneration (Fig. 37-2).

Exceptionally, MPNST may arise in a traumatic neuroma (249).

Principles of Management: Traumatic neuromas are reactive lesions that do not require complete excision.

Rudimentary Supernumerary Digits

Clinical Summary. These are usually asymptomatic, smooth, or verrucous papules, usually at the base of the ulnar side of the fifth finger. They are assumed to represent the residua of either autoamputation in utero or postnatal destruction of a supernumerary digit (250).

Histopathology. Much of what comprises a rudimentary digit shows the histologic pattern of an acquired neuroma. Some of the nerve fibers of the neuroma, among those that are located close to the epidermis, terminate in closely spaced Meissner corpuscles (250).

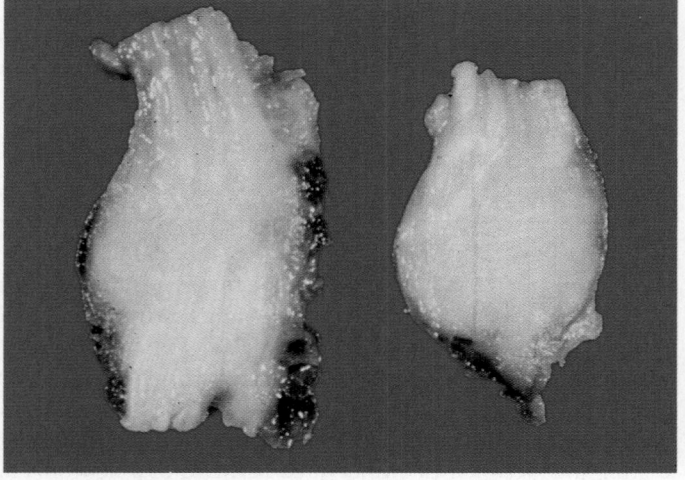
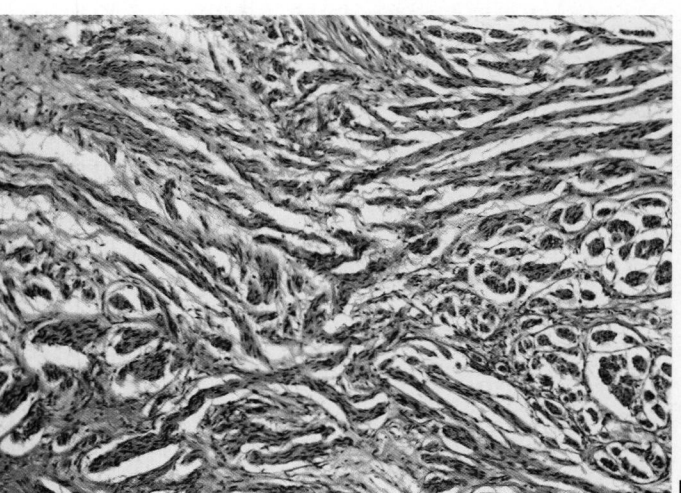

Figure 37-56 **A, B:** Extraneural (traumatic neuroma). **A:** This neuroma has been bisected along the long axis of the specimen. The neuroma is centrally placed; the cut surface in the region of the neuroma is homogeneous and white. Proximal and distal portions of the involved nerve are attached to the tumor. **B:** Fascicles of Schwann cells are arranged haphazardly in a fibrous matrix. A thin perineurium has formed at the periphery of some of the fascicles; the thin perineuria are separated from the respective Schwann cell fascicles by a clear space.

Principles of Management: These are benign lesions. They are usually removed for cosmetic reasons.

Intraneural Neuromas

Palisaded and Encapsulated (Sporadic and Spontaneous) Neuroma (PEN)

Clinical Summary. PEN is a firm, rubbery, skin-colored, or pink papule or nodule (251–254). It commonly affects the "butterfly area" of the face. Solitary examples may arise in either early childhood or adulthood (mean age, 45.5 years). In adulthood, sporadic neuromas can be multiple. Both solitary and multiple cutaneous intraneural neuromas are usually asymptomatic. In neither presentation are the lesions associated with the stigmata of *MEN.* During biopsy, a lesion of PEN is often enucleated from its dermal bed and then submitted to the pathologist with little, if any, surrounding skin.

Histopathology. PEN is a bulbous expansion of a peripheral nerve. Despite its designation of "encapsulated," it lacks a well-formed capsule and appears as a well-circumscribed, ovoid, or rounded nodule in the dermis (Fig. 37-57). Intraneurally, Schwann cells form uniform, broad (often consisting of as many as four or five cell layers), interlacing fascicles that are spaced in a clear or mucinous matrix (Fig. 37-58). Nuclear palisades are ill-defined. Nuclei are uniform and lack mitotic figures. PEN is confined by a thin, expanded perineurial sheath; hence its pseudoencapsulated morphology. This variation might be a consequence of the anatomy of a nerve; the perineurial sheath is open-ended in this site. At some sites along the periphery, it is usually possible to identify, as in-continuity extensions, tumor within the endoneurial space of small neighboring nerves.

The fascicles, with silver stains (Fig. 37-59) (254), and with immunoreactions for NSE (Fig. 37-60), neural filaments, and peripherin, are rich in axons (Fig. 37-59). A weak, sometimes

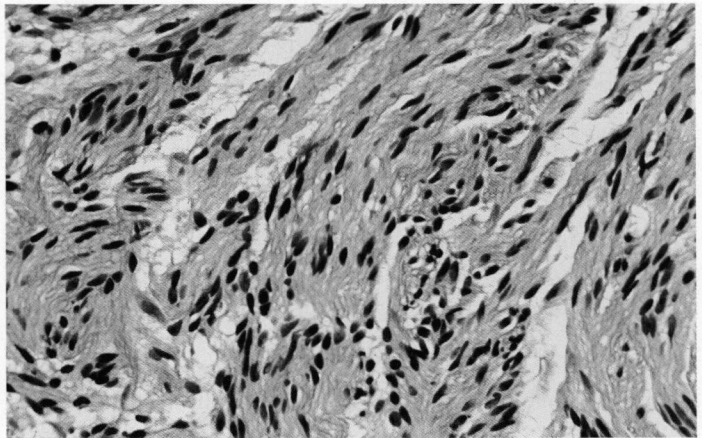

Figure 37-58 Palisaded and encapsulated (intraneural) neuroma. The Schwann cells form broad fascicles that are loosely spaced in a myxoid matrix. There are scattered nuclear palisades. In cross section, the small vacuoles in the cytoplasm of some of the cells are of the type that is produced by nonmyelinated axons. Myelinated fibers are also commonly found in the fascicles.

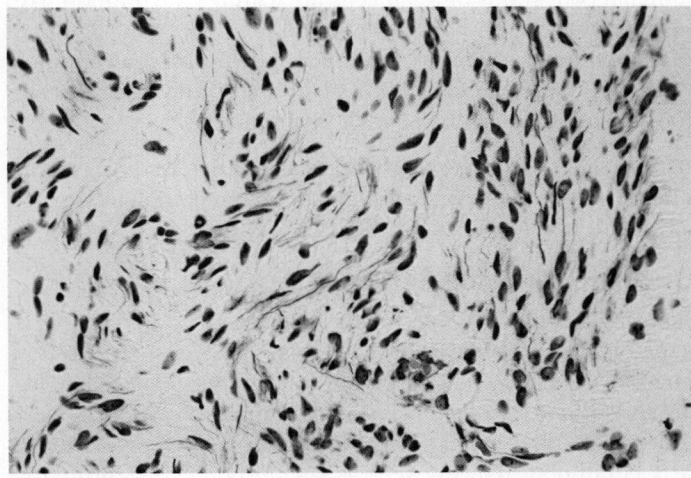

Figure 37-59 Palisaded and encapsulated (intraneural) neuroma (Bodian silver stain). The lesion is axon rich.

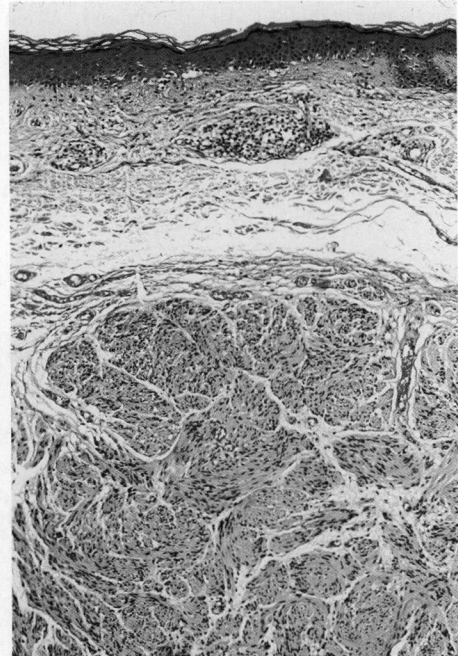

Figure 37-57 Palisaded and encapsulated (intraneural) neuroma. The lesion is encapsulated. Fascicles of Schwann cells are arranged in interlacing patterns; the fascicles are supported by a scanty clear or myxoid matrix. Focally, within some of the fascicles, the nuclei of the Schwann cells form ill-defined palisades.

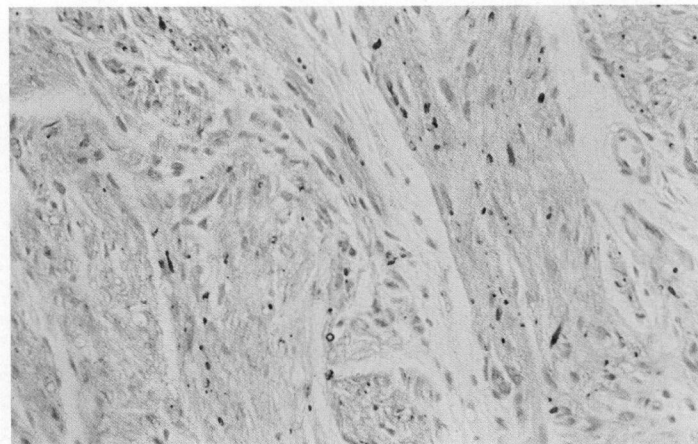

Figure 37-60 Palisaded and encapsulated (intraneural) neuroma (immunohistochemical reaction for neuron-specific enolase). With a reaction for neuron-specific enolase, axons are represented in large part as puncta.

discontinuous, reaction for EMA is a feature in the capsule of PEN (251). The presence of axons sets PEN apart from schwannoma, including all the variants. In PEN, axon representation in the fascicles is variable from lesion to lesion (254). Axon density, as evaluated by an immunoreaction to peripherin, may not be comparable to the relative density of axons with a Bodian stain (255).

Principles of Management: PEN are usually biopsied to differentiate them from basal cell carcinoma or melanocytic lesions. Even after partial excision, they rarely recur.

Intraneural Plexiform Neuroma

Clinical Summary. Plexiform neuroma is an uncommon intraneural tumor of the dermis and subcutis. It has been characterized as a variant of PEN (61), but some examples might represent incipient plexiform schwannoma.

Histopathology. Nodules and broad cords are circumscribed by the perineurium of the involved segment of the nerve. The internal patterns of all the nodules and broad cords are basically those of PEN.

Clustered, dilated vessels with sclerotic walls and subendothelial collections of foam cells are features in common with schwannoma.

In contrast to fully developed plexiform schwannoma, plexiform neuroma, with both silver stains and immunoreactions for neural filaments, is rich in axons.

Principles of Management: These are benign lesions. As with other intraneural tumors, attempts to obtain complete excision may result in a sensorimotor deficit.

Mucosal Neuroma Syndrome

Clinical Summary. MEN, type 2b, first described in 1968 (62), is the only one of three types (i.e., types 1, 2, and 2b) to show mucosal and cutaneous neuromas (*mucosal neuroma syndrome, MNS*). *Multiple (intraneural) neuromas*, many of which are periorificial, are often its earliest manifestation. First appearing in early childhood, they are seen as small nodules, often in large numbers, on the mucosa of the lips, tongue, oral cavity (256), the conjunctiva, and the sclera. Some patients show small, nodular neuromas, usually only in small numbers, on the skin of the face (256). Lesions are occasionally represented in large numbers on and about the nose and eyelids. Quite frequently, the lips are thick, fleshy, and protruding. There may be marfanoid features and skeletal abnormalities (257).

MEN, type 2b, may be inherited as an autosomal dominant trait (257). *Medullary thyroid carcinoma, bilateral pheochromocytoma* (256), and *diffuse alimentary tract ganglioneuromatosis* are associated disorders of variable frequency (258).

Histopathology. The neuromas of the MNS are intraneural and plexiform. Characteristically, the involved nerves are slender. Many are uniform in diameter, but bulbous expansions are also a feature. Within the confines of the perineurium, fascicles, which are uniform in diameter and composed of two or more nerve fibers, are interlaced in asymmetric patterns; they are closely spaced, back-to-back, in a clear or mucinous (endoneurial) matrix. The fascicles of nerve fibers in the mucosal and cutaneous lesions are richly innervated.

Multiple mucocutaneous neuromas may be encountered in the absence of other stigmata of MEN (259,260).

Linear cutaneous neuroma (dermatoneurie en strie), a sporadic variant of an intraneural neuroma, is manifested clinically as a group of raised linearities (261,262). It differs from the MNS in clinical presentation and in the size of the altered nerves in the dermis. It has been proposed that linear cutaneous neuromas are a manifestation of MEN, type 2b (261).

Histologically, nerves of the dermis and subcutis are slightly enlarged and hypercellular (Fig. 37-61A, B). Internally, Schwann cells are increased in number, and nerve fibers are tortuous. This combination of features results in loss of axial symmetry in the affected segments (Fig. 37-61B).

Ensheathed neuroma is a dermal microscopic lesion. Hypercellular nerves of the dermis are ensheathed by benign squamous epithelium (263). This type of reaction is occasionally encountered at the site of a recent biopsy.

Special Stains (Applicable to All Neuromas). With luxol-fast blue stain, some of the fibers in all forms of neuroma may be myelinated.

Electron Microscopy (Applicable to All Neuromas). Ultrastructurally, both extra and intraneural neuromas show fascicles composed of both myelinated and nonmyelinated nerve fibers

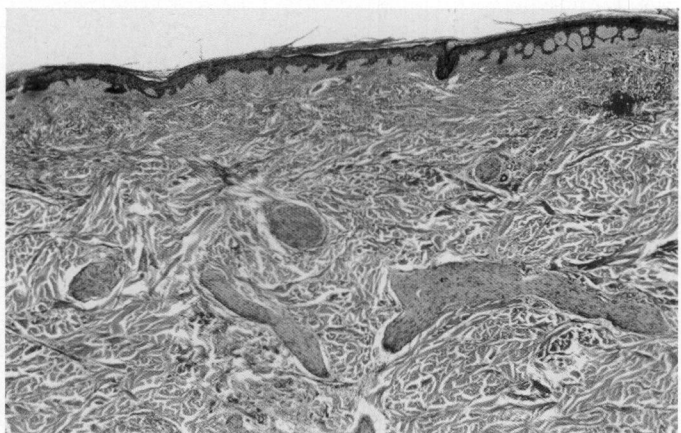
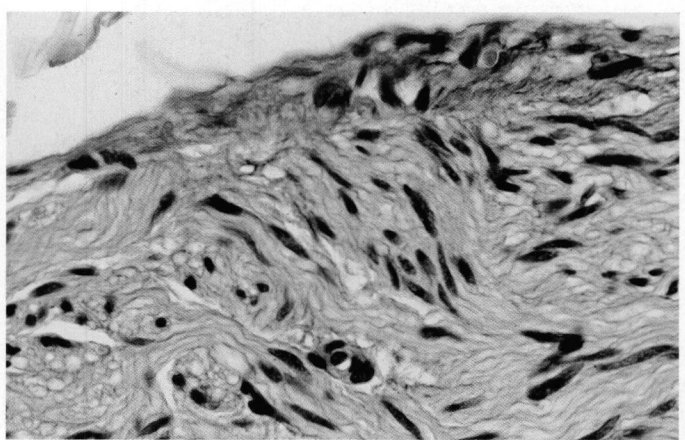

Figure 37-61 A, B: Linear (intraneural) neuroma (hyperneury). A: Nerves of the dermis are enlarged; they show Schwann cell hyperplasia; the cross-sectional diameter is increased. B: At higher magnification, interlacing fascicles of innervated Schwann cells form asymmetric patterns; they are confined by a perineurium.

(262). Those of a mature, extraneural neuroma are ensheathed by multiple lamina of perineurial cells (264). Generally, perineurial cells do not outline the individual, asymmetric fascicles of intraneural neuromas.

Histogenesis (Applicable to All Neuromas). The immunohistochemical profile is S-100 protein (+), collagen type IV (+), vimentin (+), and NSE and neural filaments (+).

In mature traumatic neuroma, most of the individual nerve fascicles are surrounded by cells expressing EMA, thus indicating perineurial differentiation (252). Collagens type I and III are deposited among the fascicles. The nerve fibers of the newly formed fascicles are supported by a matrix rich in acid mucopolysaccharides (252).

Principles of Management: As with other neuromas, these are benign lesions.

Pacinian Neuroma

Clinical Summary. Pacinian neuroma is an occult, painful lesion (265). It is found in the same anatomic sites as Pacinian corpuscles.

Histopathology. Pacinian corpuscles form a localized cluster but are otherwise unremarkable. The corpuscles may vary in size. Some lesions present as multiple nodules, and the term agminated neuroma has been proposed (266).

Principles of Management: As with other neuromas, these are benign lesions. Surgery may be needed for pain control

SMALL BLUE ROUND CELL TUMORS

This category includes *primary, cutaneous, small-cell undifferentiated carcinoma (Merkel cell tumor); primitive neuroectodermal tumors (PNETs),* such as *Ewing sarcoma* and *neuroepithelioma; neuroblastoma; primitive mesenchymal tumors,* such as *small-cell osteosarcoma,* and *embryonal* and *alveolar rhabdomyosarcoma;* rare *melanomas of infancy* that arise in the setting of *giant congenital nevus (melanoblastoma of infancy)* (267); and *melanotic neuroectodermal tumor of infancy* (268). On hematoxylin-eosin–stained sections, the tumor cells of all these lesions have few distinguishing characteristics, other than scanty cytoplasm and closely spaced, "dark" nuclei. The primitive patterns provide a challenge in differential diagnosis; lesions with these characteristics have been grouped as "primitive neuroectodermal tumors." In this category, some of the lesions share certain basic features, but are mostly to be distinguished by patterns of divergent differentiation, as manifested morphologically, or as demonstrated immunohistochemically (269). Small blue round cell tumors are more common in soft tissue or bone (270,271). In the skin, cutaneous small (Merkel) cell undifferentiated carcinoma is most frequent.

Cutaneous Small (Merkel) Cell Undifferentiated/Neuroendocrine Carcinoma

Clinical Summary. Cutaneous small-cell undifferentiated carcinoma (Merkel cell, neuroendocrine, trabecular carcinoma, Carcinoma of Toker cells, MCC) (272–276) is a relatively uncommon tumor. It occurs mostly as a solitary nodule, usually on the head or on the extremities. Multiple lesions have been observed, either localized to one area or widely distributed. The tumors are usually few but are occasionally multiple. MCC have a high rate of recurrence and metastasis (275,277).

The lesions of MCC are firm and red-pink. They are usually nonulcerated and range in size from 0.8 to 4.0 cm in diameter.

Histopathology. Tumor cells, with scanty cytoplasm and round or irregular nuclei, are closely spaced in trabeculae and sheets (Figs. 37-62 and 37-63) (278,279); less commonly, they are arranged in ribbons and festoons, sometimes as pseudorosettes (280). Nuclear chromatin is often dense and uniformly distributed. In some examples, nuclei, focally or uniformly, show margination of chromatin. Nucleoli are generally inconspicuous. Nuclear molding may be a feature, with numerous mitotic figures and nuclear fragments. For some MCC, the nests of cells are supported by scant, delicate, and paucicellular stroma. Lymphoid infiltrates are common, at the margin, and focally in the stroma. In rare cases, there is involvement of the overlying epidermis (pagetoid extension) (281,282). Occasionally, there are areas of squamous and glandular differentiation, including frank squamous cell carcinoma (283–286). Vascular invasion is relatively frequent.

The immunohistochemical profile is NSE (+), protein gene product (+), chromogranin (+), Ber-EP4 (+) (285), and CD57 (+) (287). Insulinoma-associated 1 protein, another neuroendocrine marker, is also expressed in MCC (288). A single punctate zone of cytoplasmic immunoreactivity for cytokeratins, especially CK20, or neurofilaments is most characteristic (289). EMA is expressed in 75% to 80% of MCC (290). CK20 expression is a finding against the diagnosis of metastatic small-cell carcinoma of the lung (290). TTF-1 (thyroid transcription factor-1) is relatively specific for small cell undifferentiated carcinoma of the lung (PSCUC) (291), although the authors have seen rare cases of MCC focally expressing TTF1. MCC can express some clones of Pax8 (292), a marker originally described in renal, Müllerian, and thyroid neoplasms. It has been indicated that MCC expressing bcl-2 or MCPyV may have better prognosis (293), in contrast to p63 expression that would be associated with a worse prognosis (294), although not all authors agree.

Ultrastructurally, cytoplasmic, membrane-bound, round, dense-core granules of neuroendocrine type measure 100 to 200 nm in diameter (274,280). There are perinuclear bundles, or whorls, of intermediate filaments that are 7 to 10 nm wide

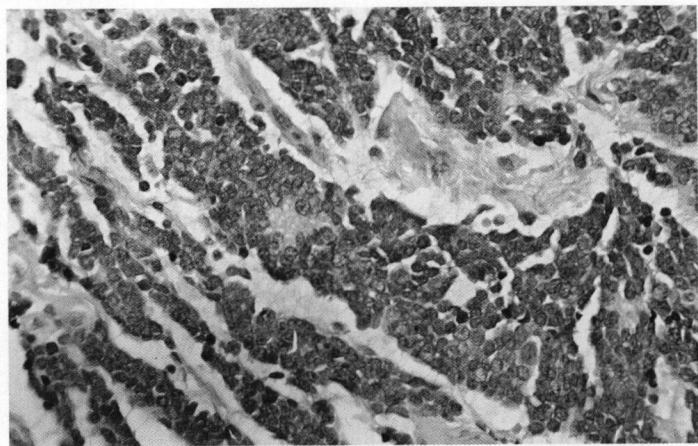

Figure 37-62 Merkel cell tumor. Atypical, but uniform, small blue cells form fascicles that vary in size. The cells have scanty cytoplasm; nuclei are crowded. Chromatin is delicate but uniformly distributed. Nucleoli are inconspicuous. There are scattered pyknotic nuclei. Each fascicle is outlined by a mucinous sheath, which abuts on a fibrous matrix.

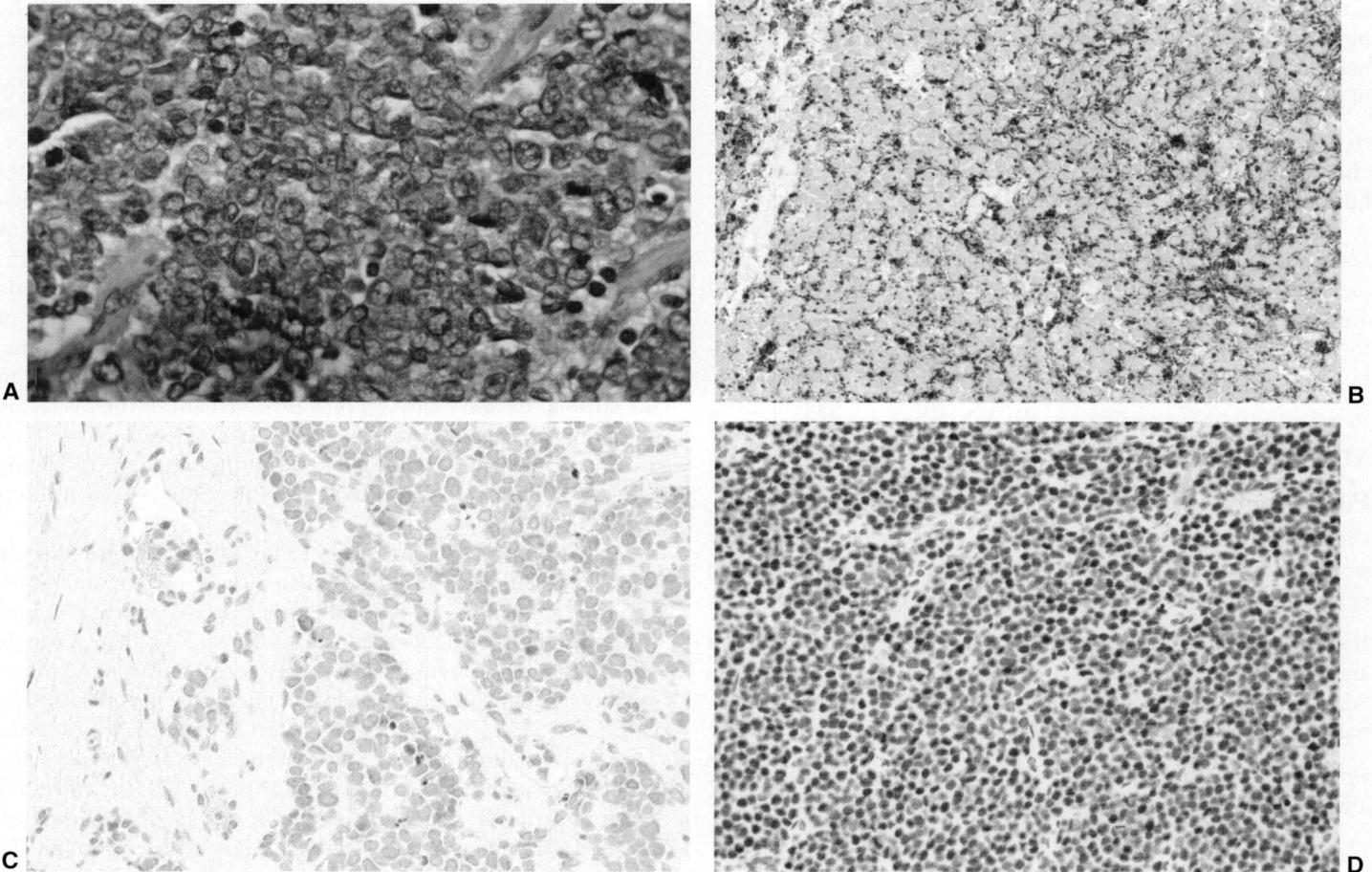

Figure 37-63 A–D: Merkel cell tumor. A: In this field, there is some central clearing of nuclear chromatin. The nuclei contain one or several nucleoli. There are scattered mitotic figures. B: Dot-like expression of CK20. C: Focal and weak expression of TTF1 in the same lesion as (B). D: Expression of the MCC PyV antigen.

(295) and small desmosomes. Tonofilaments attached to the desmosomes have been found only in a few cases (296).

The College of American Pathologists (CAP) has recommended a standard histologic reporting to include the important, prognostically significant histologic features, in particular, size (including thickness in a manner similar to the Breslow method), pattern of infiltration (nodular vs. infiltrative), vascular invasion, amount of lymphocytic infiltrate, presence of adeno/squamous differentiation, and number of mitotic figures (297).

Histogenesis. It is accepted by most authors that MCC derive from Merkel cells, a neuroendocrine cell present in the epithelial structures in the skin, particularly in hair follicles. Divergent differentiation is expressed in neuroendocrine, squamous, adnexal (298,299), and melanocytic phenotypes (300). A majority of MCC contains DNA from a type of Polyoma virus (301), which has been designated Merkel cell virus (MCV). The virus is detected in both standard MCC and MCC with divergent differentiation (squamous and glandular) (302). Because MCV is observed in the skin (and head and neck mucosae [303]) of elderly patients, this finding may explain in part the epidemiology of MCC.

MCC shares genetic changes with tumors of neural crest origin, such as melanoma, pheochromocytoma, and neuroblastoma (304).

Differential Diagnosis. Cutaneous metastases from atypical carcinoids or small-cell undifferentiated carcinoma (oat cell carcinoma) of the lung may be confused with primary MCC (305). Acute leukemia and lymphoma may also enter into the differential diagnosis. Immunohistochemical studies are very helpful. Most lymphomas will express leukocyte common antigen, CD20 or CD-3 (290).

Primary small-cell undifferentiated carcinomas have been observed in most organ systems. They are not peculiar to the skin, but those in the skin often have distinguishing characteristics. Small-cell undifferentiated carcinomas of both the skin and lung are neuroendocrine carcinomas, but the former designation (i.e., small cell undifferentiated carcinoma) has a greater degree of specificity; it gives recognition to basic patterns that are expressed in distinctive primary neoplasms in a variety of organ systems. The nuclei of pulmonary small cell undifferentiated carcinomas (PSCUC) are irregular; they often have a pointed extremity. Squamous and glandular differentiation are variable features of PSCUC. Clinicopathologic correlations are an aid in the differential diagnosis.

Primary basaloid carcinomas and undifferentiated carcinomas of the skin appendages, including lymphoepithelial variants, must also be considered in the differential diagnosis (306). In general, such lesions do not express CK20 and do not show a dot-like pattern of keratin expression.

Tumors that are histologically similar to MCC have been observed as isolated lesions in lymph nodes (307), and it has been suggested that they may correspond to "primary" lesions in the lymph nodes.

Principles of Management: MCC require complete excision with free margins. In a few institutions, patients with primary MCC of the skin are offered sentinel lymph node examination. Radiotherapy and chemotherapy have been used in recurrent/metastatic lesions. Targeted therapies, such as anti-PDL1, are showing promising results (308).

Peripheral Neuroblastoma

Clinical Summary. Neuroblastoma, as a primary soft tissue tumor, is a diagnosis of exclusion. The skin is a most unlikely site. In infancy, the differential diagnosis of undifferentiated, small-cell malignancies of the skin and soft tissue includes metastatic neuroblastoma. A thorough workup is required to rule out a metastasis from an occult site, such as the adrenal gland or paravertebral ganglia. The clinical features of metastatic neuroblastoma in infancy include the patterns of blueberry muffin baby (309) and blanching subcutaneous nodules (310). There are also adult neuroblastomas of the skin (311,312).

Histopathology. Neuroblastomas are undifferentiated, small-cell malignancies. Solid sheets of undifferentiated cells are often the preponderant patterns. Septation, neuropil, differentiation as manifested by variation in cytologic features, and Homer Wright rosettes, if identified, are an aid in diagnosis. Neuroblasts are distinguished by the formation of cell processes. The designation *neuropil* gives recognition to a matrix of cytoplasmic processes, including those of neurons, Schwann cells, and glial cells. It gives recognition to patterns of "matrical" differentiation in neuroectodermal tumors (Fig. 37-64). Larger cells with slightly eccentric, round nuclei, prominent central nucleoli, and marginated chromatin provide evidence of neuronal differentiation (Fig. 37-65); such cells, when identified, are usually sprinkled about among the more primitive cells.

Depending on the degree of differentiation, the immunohistochemical profile is as follows: neural filaments (+), NSE (+), S-100 protein (+), synaptophysin (+). Other neuroendocrine markers may be positive (313). Expression of E2F3 has been associated with impaired prognosis in noncutaneous neuroblastomas (314).

Metastatic neuroblastoma possesses an innate tendency for maturation (differentiation). As a consequence, metastases

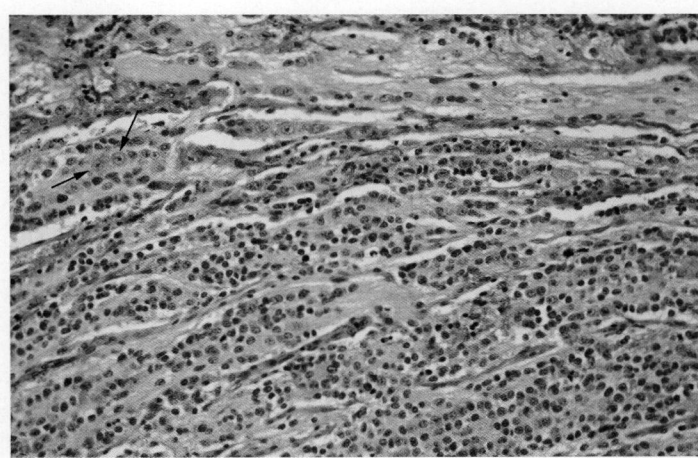

Figure 37-65 Differentiating neuroblastoma. The lesion is partitioned by delicate fibrous septa. Tumor cells are clustered among the septa; the hypocellular, fibrillated matrix among the cells is neuropil. Scattered cells have plump, round nuclei with a central nucleolus (arrow); these distinctive cells are differentiating ganglion cells.

from a neuroblastoma may present as immature or mature ganglioneuroma (315). Problems are complicated by the rare example in which a primary neuroblastoma of the adrenal gland, with distant metastases, undergoes complete regression in the primary site.

Principles of Management: The most important decision is to rule out the possibility of a cutaneous lesion of neuroblastoma being a distant metastasis from an internal location. Neuroblastomas of the skin are highly aggressive lesions. Because there is not much experience with this type of lesions, these patients may be treated usually following protocols for noncutaneous locations.

Ganglioneuroma

Clinical Summary. Ganglioneuroma is exceedingly uncommon in the skin (316,317). Rare examples appear to be in the nature of heterotopias (318). Other examples may represent divergent differentiation of phenotypically pluripotent neurocristic cells. Still other examples may represent metastatic neuroblastoma that has matured into a ganglioneuroma.

Histopathology. The basic pattern of a ganglioneuroma is that of a neuroma in which characteristic ganglion cells are either clustered or individually isolated (318). Small, primary ganglioneuromas of the skin may be characterized by numerous, mature ganglion cells and an inconspicuous background of neurosustentacular cells (319). There is a desmoplastic variant (320).

Histogenesis. Schwann cells express S-100 protein (321). Schwann cell fascicles of a ganglioneuroma, like those of all neuromas, contain axons. Ganglion cells are reactive for NSE and chromogranin. Immaturity, as manifested by foci of small, dark cells, spongy neuropil, and lymphoid infiltrates, signals the need for additional studies to rule out a differentiating metastatic neuroblastoma. In immature ganglioneuroma, the neurons may not be associated with satellite cells.

Principles of Management: Ganglioneuromas are benign lesions that usually require simple excision.

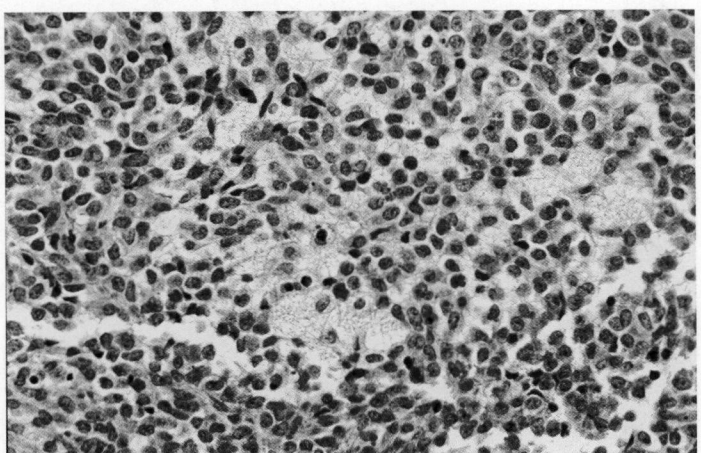

Figure 37-64 Differentiating neuroblastoma. Uniform, atypical, small blue cells form sheets. In areas, the diffuse patterns are interrupted by pale, rounded collections of delicate fibrils (neuropil).

PRIMITIVE NEUROECTODERMAL TUMORS

Ewing Sarcoma (EWS)/Peripheral Neuroepithelioma (PNE)

Originally, the designation *primitive neuroectodermal tumor* served as a taxonomic convenience when confronted with the histologic pattern of a poorly differentiated, small round cell neoplasm showing some evidence of neuroectodermal differentiation. The designation has been attributed to A. P. Stout, but there is no mention of this designation in the commonly cited reference. Currently, the designation has supplanted that of neuroepithelioma, acquiring some degree of specificity.

Ewing sarcoma and peripheral neuroepithelioma are primitive neuroectodermal tumors (PNETs), members of the category of small round cell tumors.

Clinical Summary. EWS, including an atypical variant (322), is a rare malignant neoplasm of bone and soft tissue. *Peripheral neuroepithelioma* (PNE) (the "primitive neuroectodermal tumor") is generally a tumor of the deep soft tissue, with rare examples in bone. It has been reported in internal viscera. *Askin tumor* of the chest wall is also cited as an example of primitive neuroectodermal tumor. Some examples of PNETs have had their origin in a peripheral nerve (323) or have been a component of MPNST (malignant schwannoma) (148). When referring to cutaneous lesions, there is a female predominance, and they tend to occur at a later age, and with a better outcome, than noncutaneous lesions (324).

Histopathology. PNETs are tumors composed of small blue cells (325). In the Ewing category, the cells tend to be glycogen rich. Nuclear characteristics are uniform; chromatin patterns tend to be open (325). In the neuroepithelioma category, the cells focally form pseudorosettes.

Histogenesis. Useful, but variably positive, reactions include NSE, CD57, and synaptophysin. In EWS/PNE, tumor cells are immunoreactive for CD-99 (MIC2) (326,327); the reaction is sensitive but not specific; a positive reaction provides a distinction between PNET (+) and neuroblastoma (-).

Both EWS and PNE are characterized by the presence of chromosomal translocations, usually involving chromosomes 11 and 22 [e.g., t(11;22)(q24;q12)]. The EWS gene has been identified at the breakpoint on chromosome 22 (328). Some small cell sarcomas of the soft tissue may present in "skin" biopsies, including some of the newly described EWS-like lesions, such as CIC-DUX4 (329).

Differential Diagnosis. Neuroepithelioma-like patterns/pseudorosettes may be encountered as a regional variation in MPNST (148) and in the setting of Merkel cell carcinoma (330).

Principles of Management: When primary to the skin, EWS/PNETs are associated with a better prognosis than those in noncutaneous lesions. Furthermore, it has been suggested that these patients with cutaneous lesions should receive a less aggressive treatment (324).

Melanotic Neuroectodermal Tumor of Infancy

Clinical Summary. Melanotic neuroectodermal tumor of infancy affects the tissues of the oral cavity but may also be found in other sites (268,331,332).

Histopathology. This tumor expresses neural and epithelial markers, melanogenesis, and occasional glial and rhabdomyoblastic differentiation. The patterns of melanotic neuroectodermal tumor of infancy have been compared to those of the retina at 5 weeks' gestation (268).

Principles of Management: These are malignant tumors with a high tendency to recur but with a low ability to develop distant metastasis.

HETEROTOPIAS

Clinical Summary. Cephalic brain–like heterotopias (CBHs) (nasal gliomas) are found most commonly in the skin near the root of the nose (333–335), but they may be intranasal (40%) or extranasal (60%). Extranasal CBHs, ranging in size from 1 to 5 cm, are smooth, firm, noncompressible, and skin colored. They do not pulsate or transilluminate. On the external surface of the nose, they are usually not midline. Intranasally, CBHs present as a firm, smooth, red to purple protrusion and usually measure 2 to 3 cm in diameter. They may resemble a hemangioma. Some examples are both intranasal and extranasal, with the two components being connected through a defect in the nasal bone (336). Other common bony defects that are associated with CBH involve the fonticulus frontalis, the cribriform plate, and the space between nasal bone and cartilage. Some examples are connected by a fibrous cord to the dura. Other sites of involvement include the scalp, oropharynx, nasopharynx, tongue, and subcutaneous tissue overlying T-12 (337).

Histopathology. CBHs are not encapsulated. They are disorganized and commonly show admixtures of glial tissue (Fig. 37-66); randomly distributed, mature neurons; increased vascularity; focal calcification; and fibrous tissue (335). Strands of neural tissue and fibrous tissue are interwoven (338). There are fibrillary and gemistocytic astrocytes, activated oligodendrocytes, and giant astrocytes. Astrocytes are the most conspicuous cellular component. In some examples, the astrocytic component may resemble a low-grade astrocytoma. Neurons are usually small; for some examples, they are absent but, for others, they are focally prominent (335). There may also be ependymal and retinal epithelium, and even choroid plexus–like components (339). Focal areas of oligodendroglial differentiation may

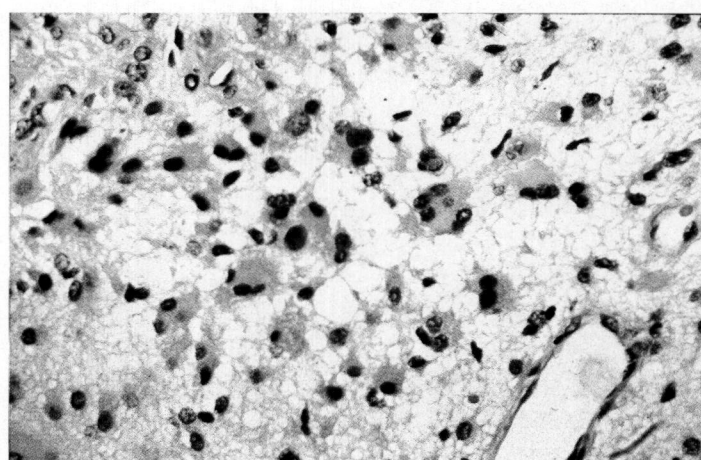

Figure 37-66 Parapharyngeal cephalic brain–like heterotopia. Astrocytes are supported by neuropil.

be prominent; in such areas, the neuropil may be immunoreactive for both NSE and synaptophysin. The degree of differentiation in these heterotopias may reflect the age of the patient at the time of excision. Some examples are remarkable for the diversity of cell types, all of which are representative of neuroectodermal differentiation. There is a report of an oligodendroglioma arising in ectopic brain tissue of the nasopharynx (340).

Immunohistochemically, neurons react for NSE and neural filaments. Astrocytes and ependymal cells are immunoreactive for GFAP, whereas oligodendroglial cells are not. Oligodendroglial cells share some immunoreactions with Schwann cells.

Differential Diagnosis. Encephaloceles (extracranial protrusions of brainlike tissue that are in continuity with the subarachnoid space) may show a high degree of organization (341). CBH and encephaloceles of the same anatomic sites have similar clinical features. A distinction between CBH and encephalocele is not always possible. Because encephaloceles are connected to the subarachnoid space by a sinus tract, such lesions should not be biopsied, because of the possibility of rhinorrhea with leakage of spinal fluid and even septic encephalitis. Thus, computerized tomography (341) and neurosurgical consultation should precede any operative intervention of either CBH or encephalocele.

Principles of Management: These are benign lesions that do not recur with simple excision. The most important element is to rule out the possibility of encephalocele because surgery may result in encephalorrhea and septic encephalitis.

CUTANEOUS MENINGIOMAS AND MENINGOTHELIAL HETEROTOPIAS

Clinical Summary. Cells with the features of meningothelial cells may be encountered in skin and soft tissue (278). They may represent a true neoplasm (and thus be properly characterized as *ectopic* meningioma), or they resemble *meningoceles, meningomyeloceles,* and *meningoencephaloceles* (and thus be properly characterized as heterotopia or dysplasia).

Definitions of various pathways, and an understanding of developmental phenomena, provide an explanation for the presence of meningothelial cells in the skin and soft tissue:

1. Precursors of meningothelial cells may be displaced into the dermis and subcutis during embryogenesis. Such remnants, located mainly in subcutaneous tissue of the scalp, forehead, and paravertebral regions of children and young adults (342–344), may develop into congenital meningeal heterotopias. They are relatively restricted in the distribution along the lines of closure of the developing neural tube. Some of these lesions qualify as acelic meningeal heterotopias (rudimentary meningoceles) (343). For such examples, occult connections with the central nervous system may become apparent only at the time of surgery; a leakage of spinal fluid into the surgical defect will provide the evidence. Histologic patterns include features of those of both the dura and the leptomeninges.
2. True ectopic meningiomas, distributed along the course of cranial nerves of the sensory organs of the face and head, tend to occur in adults; they arise from extensions of arachnoidal lining cells along peripheral nerves (344). Some ectopic meningiomas arise in sites that are far from the axial

skeleton. The histologic patterns of benign ectopic meningiomas recapitulate those of the meningiomas of the central nervous system.

3. Large, intracranial meningiomas may extend in direct continuity through foramina or old operative defects into the neighboring soft tissue; they qualify as *perforating* meningiomas. Their histology corresponds to that of the primary intracranial lesion and, once defined, is predictive of their behavior.
4. *Anaplastic (malignant) meningiomas* (including sarcomatous variants) and *papillary and hemangiopericytomatous variants* may aggressively invade bone, soft tissue, and scalp. They may also be associated with intracranial seeding and with extracranial, mostly pulmonary metastases. Histologically benign meningiomas have rarely seeded the brain surface or metastasized (345).

A related lesion is the hamartomatous meningioma, a lesion occurring on the scalp that may resemble angiosarcoma owing to the presence of slitlike spaces (346).

Histopathology. Heterotopias are not well circumscribed. Cells of such lesions are cytologically bland and loosely attached to their neighbors. They commonly outline thin, angulated clefts, a feature that may be mistaken as evidence of vascular differentiation (Fig. 37-67A) (344,346), particularly in the related lesion, meningothelial hamartoma (Fig. 37-67B). Whorls of cells and psammoma bodies, if identified, are an aid in diagnosis. The supporting fibrous matrix is loosely fissured.

The complexities of the classification of true meningiomas (whether intracranial, ectopic, or metastatic) and the details of the corresponding histopathology preclude a presentation in this section. The basic features include sheets and nests of polygonal or spindle cells; whorls of cells; psammoma bodies (Fig. 37-68); intranuclear inclusions of cytoplasm; immunoreactivity for EMA; and scanty, condensed stroma or thin clefts at the interface between nests.

Anaplastic (malignant) meningiomas are characterized by dense cellularity, nuclear atypia, mitoses, necrosis, and invasion of the brain and even soft tissue (347,348). The basic patterns of common meningiomas are usually preserved, but some examples are frankly sarcomatous.

Ultrastructurally, poorly formed basal lamina; rare desmosomes; abundant mitochondria; and elaborate interdigitating, cytoplasmic processes are all features of meningothelial cells.

Histogenesis. Like intracranial meningiomas, the cells of ectopic meningiomas and meningeal heterotopias react immunohistochemically for vimentin and EMA (349–352). Depending on the histologic subtype, there may also be an expression of cytokeratins and S-100 protein.

Differential Diagnosis. Meningoceles, meningomyeloceles, and meningoencephaloceles, like meningeal heterotopias, present along the lines of closure of the neural tube. Arachnoidal components are associated with both dense, and loosely laminated, vascularized fibrous tissue. If there is an associated encephalocele (or myelocele), then tissue of the central nervous system, other than its coverings, will also be represented.

Ependymal rests may also be found in the sacrococcygeal region. Some are organized in patterns that resemble microscopic myxopapillary ependymomas (353). Such rests may provide an explanation for the origin of rare *ectopic ependymomas* in the sacrococcygeal region (354).

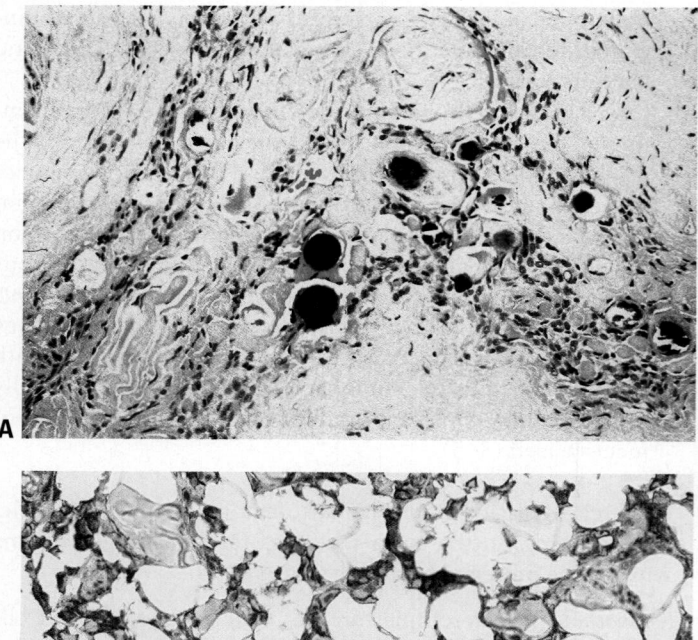

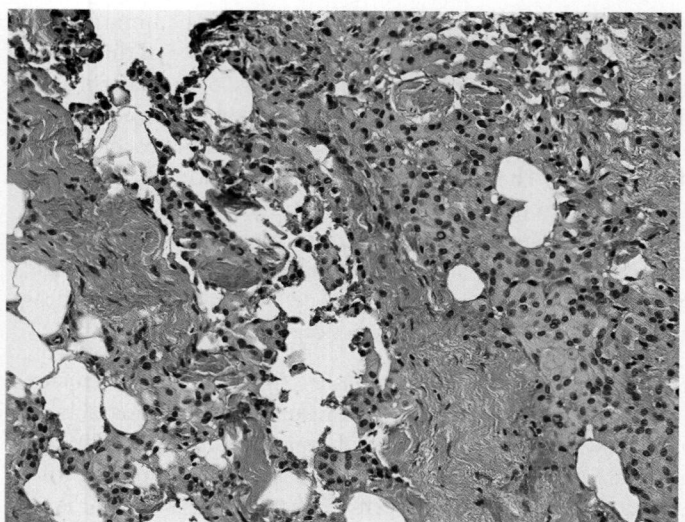

Figure 37-67 A–C: Meningeal heterotopia. A: Spindle cells with angulated, uniform nuclei form traceries among collagen bundles. There are clefts in some of the thin nests of spindle cells. The rounded, basophilic structures are psammoma bodies. B: Meningothelial hamartoma from the scalp shows pseudovascular spaces mimicking angiosarcoma. C: Tumor cells express EMA

The histologic pattern of meningiomas and EMA expression raises the possibility of differential diagnosis with perineuriomas (see later).

The term *meningioma-like tumor of the skin* has been given to lesions expressing CD34 but lacking EMA, MITF1, or NKI-C3 (355). These lesions have dendritic, spindled cells focally arranged in whorled areas resembling those of meningiomas.

Principles of Management: Except for the atypical/malignant cases, meningiomas are benign lesions that do not require wide margins of resection. For the rare malignant cases not amenable to surgery, there have been reports of use of targeted therapies such as vascular endothelial growth factor and platelet-derived growth factor inhibitors (356).

NEURAL TUMORS OF A DEGENERATIVE NATURE

In impingement neurofasciitis (*Morton or interdigital "neuroma"*), the compression of nerves and soft tissue between bony or other hard surfaces may induce degenerative changes. The responses include demyelination and endoneurial fibrosis, mucinous and fibrinous degeneration of soft tissue (fascia), deposition of pre-elastin over the surfaces of elastic fibers (in patterns resembling those seen in lesions of elastofibroma dorsi), and fibrinous bursitis (Fig. 37-69A, B) (357). These lesions have nerves, vessels, soft tissue, and a portion of synovium (Fig. 37-70). All these phenomena, manifested in the interdigital area of the so-called Morton neuroma, have nothing in common with the neuromas. In the altered nerves, localized, oval zones of mucinous or fibrous matrix may focally displace the nerve fibers. In them, spindle and stellate cells are loosely arranged in whorls. Similar epiphenomena,

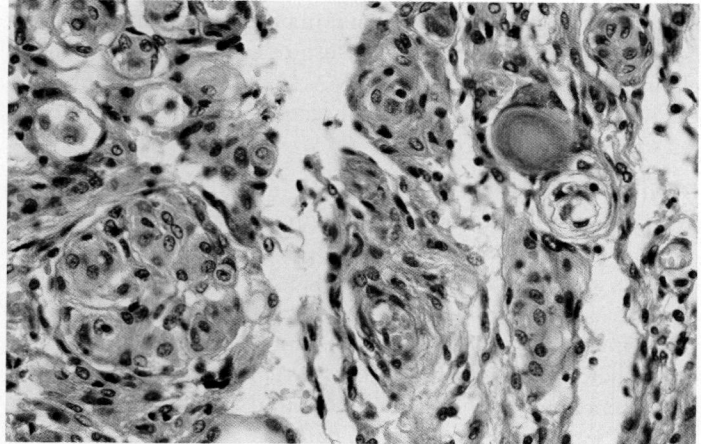

Figure 37-68 Cutaneous meningioma. Small, uniform spindle and epithelioid cells are arranged in nests and whorls; there are clefts among the nests. A psammoma body is represented.

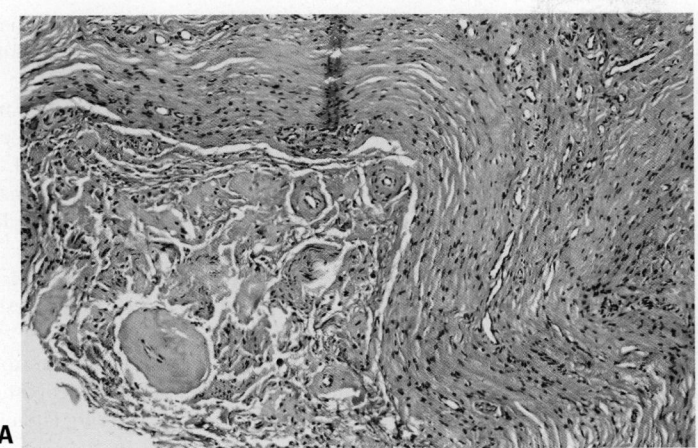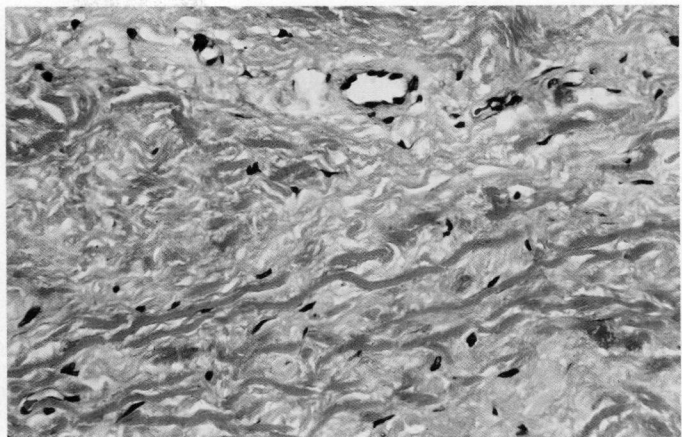

Figure 37-69 A, B: Impingement neuropathy (Morton neuroma). A: To the left and extending to the bottom of the field, a nerve is cut in cross section; the perineurium is thickened and fibrotic. Individual nerve fibers and small clusters of nerve fibers are loosely spaced in a myxoid matrix. There are scattered hyaline deposits in the endoneurial space. Vessels of the endoneurium are cut in cross section; they have thickened, hyalinized walls. B: The connective tissue adjacent to an affected nerve shows hyperelastosis; the elastic fibers are increased in diameter. Often, in Morton neuroma, the changes in the adjacent connective tissue are similar to those of elastofibroma dorsi.

which were characterized by Renaut as an "intravaginal hyaline system," are often encountered as an incidental finding in normal nerves.

Ganglion cyst of nerve is an uncommon tumor of a degenerative nature. In preferential sites, a superficial nerve impinges on a bony protuberance.

Initially, the perineurium and endoneurium are mucinous, expanded, and paucicellular. In one or more sites, cystic changes ensue. The end result is a mucinous cyst that expands the endoneurial space, compresses the axial bundle, and distends the perineurial sheath. A condensation of fibrous tissue forms the wall of the cyst.

Ganglion cyst of nerve is distinguished from periarticular ganglion cyst by location.

NEUROTROPIC GROWTH (GENERAL COMMENTS)

Neurotropic growth of tumor is common in the skin. Generally, the identification of this phenomenon is sufficient to characterize any related primary neoplasm of the skin as aggressive (e.g., neurotropic melanoma [358] and epidermoid carcinoma [359]). Rarely, benign invasion of nerve sheaths by squamous epithelium has been noted in reexcision specimens after a biopsy (360), recently designated as epithelial sheath neuroma (263) (Fig. 37-71), and the cells of benign blue nevi and related lesions, and of congenital nevi, may occasionally be seen within nerves (sometimes designated as perineural "involvement" rather than invasion).

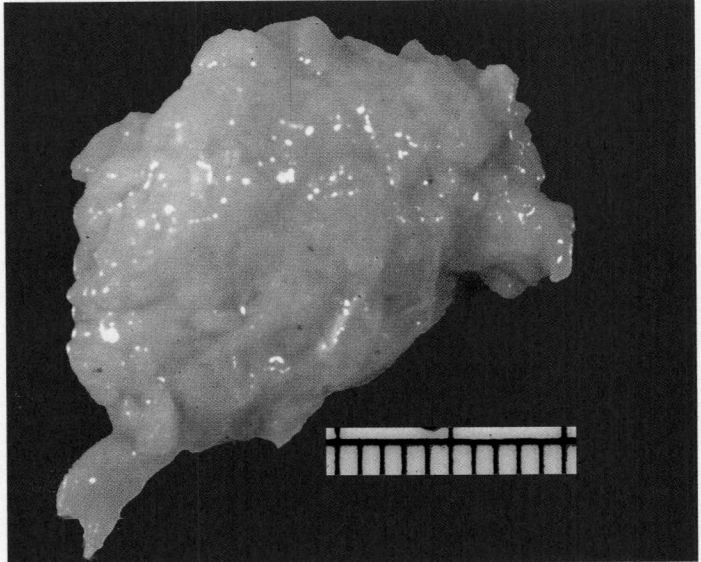

Figure 37-70 Impingement neuropathy (Morton neuroma). A portion of a small nerve enters and exits a tumor. The tumor is not a neoplasm but an inflammatory process. The inflammatory process involves the interdigital nerve, soft tissue, and associated vessels. A portion of inflamed synovium is often included as part of the excised specimen.

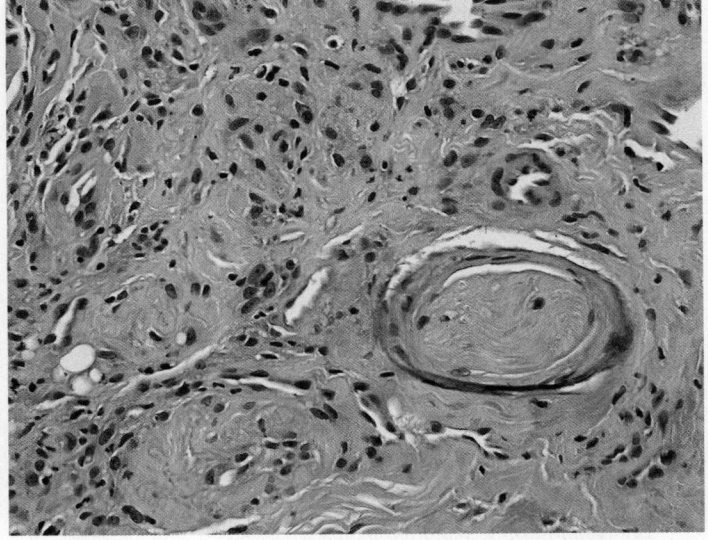

Figure 37-71 Epithelial sheath neuroma. Reexcision specimen for metastatic melanoma. Notice the presence of epithelial cells around a small dermal nerve, mimicking invasive squamous cell carcinoma with perineural invasion.

Primary lymphoma, as a solitary tumor of peripheral nerve, is extremely rare. Misdraji et al. reported a series of four cases (361). The lesions were all diffuse large B-cell lymphomas. The involved sites included sciatic nerve (2 cases), radial nerve (1), and sympathetic chain and T2 spinal nerve. At the time of the report, two of the patients had died of their disease. One patient at autopsy had evidence of neurolymphomatosis. The second patient had evidence of disseminated disease, including lymphomatous meningitis.

ACKNOWLEDGMENT

The author would like to acknowledge the work of Richard J. Reed for his work on this chapter in previous editions.

REFERENCES

1. Scheithauer B, Woodruff JM, Earlandson, R. *Tumors of the Peripheral Nervous System.* Armed Forces Institute of Pathology; 1999.
2. Ortiz-Hidalgo C, Weller R. Peripheral nervous system. In: Sternberg S, ed. *Histology for Pathologists.* Lippincott-Raven Press; 1999:285.
3. Harkin JC, Reed RJ. *Tumors of the Peripheral Nervous System.* Armed Forces Institute of Pathology; 1969.
4. Reed RJ, Harkin JC. *Tumors of the Peripheral Nervous System.* Armed Forces Institute of Pathology; 1983.
5. Weiser G. An electron microscope study of "Pacinian neurofibroma." *Virchows Arch A Pathol Anat Histol.* 1975;366(4):331–340.
6. Morris JH, Hudson AR, Weddell G. A study of degeneration and regeneration in the divided rat sciatic nerve based on electron microscopy. IV. Changes in fascicular microtopography, perineurium and endoneurial fibroblasts. *Z Zellforsch Mikrosk Anat.* 1972;124(2):165–203.
7. Pižem J, Nicholson KM, Mraz J, Prieto VG. Melanocytic differentiation is present in a significant proportion of nonpigmented diffuse neurofibromas: a potential diagnostic pitfall. *Am J Surg Pathol.* 2013;37(8):1182–1191.
8. Vecchio GM, Amico P, Leone G, Salvatorelli L, Magro G. Lipoblast-like signet-ring cells in neurofibroma: a potential diagnostic pitfall of malignancy. *Pathologica.* 2010;102(3):108–111.
9. Díaz-Flores L, Gutiérrez R, García MP, et al. Telocytes in the normal and pathological peripheral nervous system. *Int J Mol Sci.* 2020;21(12):4320.
10. Popescu LM, Faussone-Pellegrini MS. Telocytes—a case of serendipity: the winding way from interstitial cells of Cajal (ICC), via interstitial Cajal-like cells (ICLC) to telocytes. *J Cell Mol Med.* 2010;14(4):729–740.
11. Restano L, Fanoni D, Colonna C, Gelmetti C, Berti E. Medallion-like dermal dendrocyte hamartoma: a case misdiagnosed as neurofibroma. *Pediatr Dermatol.* 2010;27(6):638–642.
12. Rodríguez-Jurado R, Palacios C, Durán-McKinster C, et al. Medallion-like dermal dendrocyte hamartoma: a new clinically and histopathologically distinct lesion. *J Am Acad Dermatol.* 2004;51(3):359–363.
13. Riccardi VM. Von Recklinghausen neurofibromatosis. *N Engl J Med.* 1981;305(27):1617–1627.
14. Crowe FW. Axillary freckling as a diagnostic aid in neurofibromatosis. *Ann Intern Med.* 1964;61:1142–1143.
15. Crowe F, Schull W, Neel J. *Clinical, Pathological, and Genetic Study of Multiple Neurofibromatosis.* Thomas; 1956.
16. Goldberg NS, Collins FS. The hunt for the neurofibromatosis gene. *Arch Dermatol.* 1991;127(11):1705–1707.
17. Zvulunov A, Esterly NB. Neurocutaneous syndromes associated with pigmentary skin lesions. *J Am Acad Dermatol.* 1995;32(6):915–935; quiz 936–937.
18. Wilson BN, John AM, Handler MZ, Schwartz RA. Neurofibromatosis type 1: new developments in genetics and treatment. *J Am Acad Dermatol.* 2020.
19. Lyskjaer I, Lindsay D, Tirabosco R, et al. H3K27me3 expression and methylation status in histological variants of malignant peripheral nerve sheath tumours. *J Pathol.* 2020;252(2):151–164.
20. Shekitka KM, Sobin LH. Ganglioneuromas of the gastrointestinal tract. Relation to Von Recklinghausen disease and other multiple tumor syndromes. *Am J Surg Pathol.* 1994;18(3):250–257.
21. DeLellis RA. Multiple endocrine neoplasia syndromes revisited. Clinical, morphologic, and molecular features. *Lab Invest.* 1995;72(5):494–505.
22. Miettinen M, Fetsch JF, Sobin LH, Lasota J. Gastrointestinal stromal tumors in patients with neurofibromatosis 1: a clinicopathologic and molecular genetic study of 45 cases. *Am J Surg Pathol.* 2006;30(1):90–96.
23. Zvulunov A, Barak Y, Metzker A. Juvenile xanthogranuloma, neurofibromatosis, and juvenile chronic myelogenous leukemia. World statistical analysis. *Arch Dermatol.* 1995;131(8):904–908.
24. Jaakkola S, Muona P, James WD, et al. Segmental neurofibromatosis: immunocytochemical analysis of cutaneous lesions. *J Am Acad Dermatol.* 1990;22(4):617–621.
25. Hager CM, Cohen PR, Tschen JA. Segmental neurofibromatosis: case reports and review. *J Am Acad Dermatol.* 1997;37(5, pt 2):864–869.
26. Schultz ES, Kaufmann D, Tinschert S, Schell H, von den Driesch P, Schuler G. Segmental neurofibromatosis. *Dermatology.* 2002;204(4):296–297.
27. Ren Y, Chari DA, Vasilijic S, Welling DB, Stankovic KM. New developments in neurofibromatosis type 2 and vestibular schwannoma. *Neurooncol Adv.* 2021;3(1):vdaa153.
28. Doddrell RD, Dun XP, Shivane A, et al. Loss of SOX10 function contributes to the phenotype of human Merlin-null schwannoma cells. *Brain.* 2013;136(pt 2):549–563.
29. Angelo LS, Maxwell DS, Wu JY, et al. Binding partners for curcumin in human schwannoma cells: biologic implications. *Bioorg Med Chem.* 2013;21(4):932–939.
30. Honda M, Arai E, Sawada S, Ohta A, Niimura M. Neurofibromatosis 2 and neurilemmomatosis gene are identical. *J Invest Dermatol.* 1995;104(1):74–77.
31. Wolkenstein P, Benchikhi H, Zeller J, Wechsler J, Revuz J. Schwannomatosis: a clinical entity distinct from neurofibromatosis type 2. *Dermatology.* 1997;195(3):228–231.
32. Plotkin SR, Blakeley JO, Evans DG, et al. Update from the 2011 International Schwannomatosis Workshop: from genetics to diagnostic criteria. *Am J Med Genet A,* 2013;161A(3):405–416.
33. Mansouri S, Suppiah S, Mamatjan Y, et al. Epigenomic, genomic, and transcriptomic landscape of schwannomatosis. *Acta Neuropathol.* 2021;141(1):101–116.
34. Masson P. Experimental and spontaneous schwannomas (peripheral gliomas): I. experimental schwannomas. *Am J Pathol.* 1932;8(4):367–388.11.
35. Hattori H. Vacuolated cells in neurofibroma: an immunohistochemical study. *J Cutan Pathol.* 2005;32(2):158–161.
36. Miettinen MM, Antonescu CR, Fletcher CDM, et al. Histopathologic evaluation of atypical neurofibromatous tumors and their transformation into malignant peripheral nerve sheath tumor in patients with neurofibromatosis 1-a consensus overview. *Hum Pathol.* 2017;67:1–10.
37. Rhodes SD, He Y, Smith A, et al. Cdkn2a (Arf) loss drives NF1-associated atypical neurofibroma and malignant transformation. *Hum Mol Genet.* 2019;28(16):2752–2762.
38. Val-Bernal JF, González-Vela MC. Cutaneous lipomatous neurofibroma: characterization and frequency. *J Cutan Pathol.* 2005;32(4):274–279.
39. Enzinger FM, Weiss SW. *Soft Tissue Tumors.* 3rd ed. M.-Y. Book. 1995.

40. McHugh KE, Sturgis CD, Bergfeld WF. Hyalinized neurofibromas: not just rare variants in skin of the female breast. *Am J Dermatopathol.* 2019;41(10):718–721.

41. Greene JF Jr, Fitzwater JE, Burgess J. Arterial lesions associated with neurofibromatosis. *Am J Clin Pathol.* 1974;62(4):481–487.

42. Salyer WR, Salyer DC. The vascular lesions of neurofibromatosis. *Angiology.* 1974;25(8):510–519.

43. Erlandson RA, Woodruff JM. Peripheral nerve sheath tumors: an electron microscopic study of 43 cases. *Cancer.* 1982;49(2):273–287.

44. Friede RL, Bischhausen R. The organization of endoneural collagen in peripheral nerves as revealed with the scanning electron microscope. *J Neurol Sci.* 1978;38(1):83–88.

45. Lassmann H, Jurecka W, Lassmann G, Gebhart W, Matras H, Watzek G. Different types of benign nerve sheath tumors. Light microscopy, electron microscopy and autoradiography. *Virchows Arch A Pathol Anat Histol.* 1977;375(3):197–210.

46. Khalifa MA, Montgomery EA, Ismiil N, Azumi N. What are the CD34+ cells in benign peripheral nerve sheath tumors? Double immunostaining study of CD34 and S-100 protein. *Am J Clin Pathol.* 2000;114(1):123–126.

47. Yeh I, McCalmont TH. Fingerprint CD34 immunopositivity. *J Cutan Pathol.* 2010;37(11):1127–1129.

48. Yeh I, McCalmont TH. Distinguishing neurofibroma from desmoplastic melanoma: the value of the CD34 fingerprint. *J Cutan Pathol.* 2011;38(8):625–630.

49. Yeh I, Vemula SS, Mirza SA, McCalmont TH. Neurofibroma-like spindle cell melanoma: CD34 fingerprint and CGH for diagnosis. *Am J Dermatopathol.* 2012;34(6):668–670.

50. Vaalasti A, Suomalainen H, Kuokkanen K, Rechardt L. Neuropeptides in cutaneous neurofibromas of von Recklinghausen's disease. *J Cutan Pathol.* 1990;17(6):371–373.

51. Weiser G. [Neurofibroma and perineurial cell. Electron microscopic examinations of 9 neurofibromas (author's transl)]. *Virchows Arch A Pathol Anat Histol.* 1978;379(1):73–83.

52. Reed RJ. *The neural crest, its migrants, and cutaneous malignant neoplasms related to neurocristic derivatives.* In: Lynch IH, Fusaro R, eds. *Cancer-Associated Genodermatoses.* Van Nostrand Reinhold; 1982.

53. Kazakov DV, Pitha J, Sima R, et al. Hybrid peripheral nerve sheath tumors: Schwannoma-perineurioma and neurofibroma-perineurioma. A report of three cases in extradigital locations. *Ann Diagn Pathol.* 2005;9(1):16–23.

54. Feany MB, Anthony DC, Fletcher CD. Nerve sheath tumours with hybrid features of neurofibroma and schwannoma: a conceptual challenge. *Histopathology.* 1998;32(5):405–410.

55. Yang X, Zeng Y, Wang J. Hybrid schwannoma/perineurioma: report of 10 Chinese cases supporting a distinctive entity. *Int J Surg Pathol.* 2013;21(1):22–28.

56. Lang SS, Zager EL, Coyne TM, Nangunoori R, Kneeland JB, Nathanson KL. Hybrid peripheral nerve sheath tumor. *J Neurosurg.* 2012;117(5):897–901.

57. Wang L, Wang G, Gao T. Congenital melanocytic nevus with features of hybrid schwannoma/perineurioma. *J Cutan Pathol.* 2013;40(5):497–502.

58. Kacerovska D, Michal M, Kazakov DV. Hybrid epithelioid schwannoma/perineurioma. *Am J Dermatopathol.* 2016;38(7): e90–e92.

59. Staser K, Yang FC, Clapp DW. Pathogenesis of plexiform neurofibroma: tumor-stromal/hematopoietic interactions in tumor progression. *Annu Rev Pathol.* 2012;7:469–495.

60. Prada CE, Jousma E, Rizvi TA, et al. Neurofibroma-associated macrophages play roles in tumor growth and response to pharmacological inhibition. *Acta Neuropathol.* 2013;125(1):159–168.

61. Argenyi ZB, Cooper PH, Santa Cruz D. Plexiform and other unusual variants of palisaded encapsulated neuroma. *J Cutan Pathol.* 1993;20(1):34–39.

62. Gorlin RJ, Sedano HO, Vickers RA, Cervenka J. Multiple mucosal neuromas, pheochromocytoma and medullary carcinoma of the thyroid—a syndrome. *Cancer.* 1968;22(2):293–299 passim.

63. Argenyi ZB, LeBoit PE, Santa Cruz D, Swanson PE, Kutzner H. Nerve sheath myxoma (neurothekeoma) of the skin: light microscopic and immunohistochemical reappraisal of the cellular variant. *J Cutan Pathol.* 1993;20(4):294–303.

64. Enzinger FM, Zhang RY. Plexiform fibrohistiocytic tumor presenting in children and young adults. An analysis of 65 cases. *Am J Surg Pathol.* 1988;12(11):818–826.

65. Zelger B, Weinlich G, Zelger B. Perineuroma. A frequently unrecognized entity with emphasis on a plexiform variant. *Adv Clin Path.* 2000;4(1):25–33.

66. Barnhill RL, Barnhill MA, Berwick M, Mihm MC Jr. The histologic spectrum of pigmented spindle cell nevus: a review of 120 cases with emphasis on atypical variants. *Hum Pathol.* 1991;22(1):52–58.

67. Rose C, Kaddu S, El-Sherif TF, Kerl H. A distinctive type of widespread congenital melanocytic nevus with large nodules. *J Am Acad Dermatol.* 2003;49(4):732–735.

68. Clarke B, Essa A, Chetty R. Plexiform spitz nevus. *Int J Surg Pathol.* 2002;10(1):69–73.

69. Michal M, Fanburg-Smith JC, Mentzel T, et al. Dendritic cell neurofibroma with pseudorosettes: a report of 18 cases of a distinct and hitherto unrecognized neurofibroma variant. *Am J Surg Pathol.* 2001;25(5):587–594.

70. Simpson RH, Seymour MJ. Dendritic cell neurofibroma with pseudorosettes: two tumors in a patient with evidence of neurofibromatosis. *Am J Surg Pathol.* 2001;25(11):1458–1459.

71. Woodruff JM, Busam KJ. Histologically benign cutaneous dendritic cell tumor with pseudorosettes. *Am J Surg Pathol.* 2002;26(12):1644–1648.

72. Dupree WB, Langloss JM, Weiss SW. Pigmented dermatofibrosarcoma protuberans (Bednar tumor). A pathologic, ultrastructural, and immunohistochemical study. *Am J Surg Pathol.* 1985;9(9):630–639.

73. Ackerman LV, Taylor FH. Neurogenous tumors within the thorax; a clinicopathological evaluation of forty-eight cases. *Cancer.* 1951;4(4):669–691.

74. Stout AP. Tumors of the peripheral nervous system. *Mo Med.* 1949;46(4):255–259.

75. Russell D, Rubinstein L. *Pathology of Tumours of the Nervous System.* 5th ed. Williams & Wilkins; 1989.

76. Argenyi ZB, Balogh K, Abraham AA. Degenerative ("ancient") changes in benign cutaneous schwannoma. A light microscopic, histochemical and immunohistochemical study. *J Cutan Pathol.* 1993;20(2):148–153.

77. Sian CS, Ryan SF. The ultrastructure of neurilemoma with emphasis on Antoni B tissue. *Hum Pathol.* 1981;12(2):145–160.

78. Patil S, Perry A, Maccollin M, et al. Immunohistochemical analysis supports a role for INI1/SMARCB1 in hereditary forms of schwannomas, but not in solitary, sporadic schwannomas. *Brain Pathol.* 2008;18(4):517–519.

79. Reed RJ, Pulitzer DR. Tumors of neural tissue. In: Elder DE, ed., *Lever's Histopathology of the Skin.* Lippincott, Williams & Wilkins/Wolters Kluwer; 2009:1107–1150.

80. Kawahara E, Oda Y, Ooi A, Katsuda S, Nakanishi I, Umeda S. Expression of glial fibrillary acidic protein (GFAP) in peripheral nerve sheath tumors. A comparative study of immunoreactivity of GFAP, vimentin, S-100 protein, and neurofilament in 38 schwannomas and 18 neurofibromas. *Am J Surg Pathol.* 1988;12(2):115–120.

81. Lodding P, Kindblom LG, Angervall L, Stenman G. Cellular schwannoma. A clinicopathologic study of 29 cases. *Virchows Arch A Pathol Anat Histopathol.* 1990;416(3):237–248.

82. Woodruff JM, Godwin TA, Erlandson RA, Susin M, Martini N. Cellular schwannoma: a variety of schwannoma sometimes mistaken for a malignant tumor. *Am J Surg Pathol.* 1981;5(8):733–744.

83. Casadei GP, Scheithauer BW, Hirose T, Manfrini M, Van Houton C, Wood MB. Cellular schwannoma. A clinicopathologic, DNA flow cytometric, and proliferation marker study of 70 patients. *Cancer.* 1995;75(5):1109–1119.

84. Fletcher CD, Davies SE, McKee PH. Cellular schwannoma: a distinct pseudosarcomatous entity. *Histopathology*. 1987;11(1):21–35.

85. White W, Shiu MH, Rosenblum MK, Erlandson RA, Woodruff JM. Cellular schwannoma. A clinicopathologic study of 57 patients and 58 tumors. *Cancer*. 1990;66(6):1266–1275.

86. Hajdu SI. Schwannomas. *Mod Pathol*. 1995;8(1):109–115.

87. Leroy X, Aubert S, Leteurtre E, Gosselin B. Expression of CD117 in a malignant peripheral nerve sheath tumour arising in a patient with type 1 neurofibromatosis. *Histopathology*. 2003;42(5):511–513.

88. Lin BT, Weiss LM, Medeiros LJ. Neurofibroma and cellular neurofibroma with atypia: a report of 14 tumors. *Am J Surg Pathol*. 1997;21(12):1443–1449.

89. Watanabe T, Oda Y, Tamiya S, Kinukawa N, Masuda K, Tsuneyoshi M. Malignant peripheral nerve sheath tumours: high Ki67 labelling index is the significant prognostic indicator. *Histopathology*. 2001;39(2):187–197.

90. Woodruff JM, Scheithauer BW, Kurtkaya-Yapicier O, et al. Congenital and childhood plexiform (multinodular) cellular schwannoma: a troublesome mimic of malignant peripheral nerve sheath tumor. *Am J Surg Pathol*. 2003;27(10):1321–1329.

91. Kindblom LG, Meis-Kindblom JM, Havel G, Busch C. Benign epithelioid schwannoma. *Am J Surg Pathol*. 1998;22(6):762–770.

92. Orosz Z. Cutaneous epithelioid schwannoma: an unusual benign neurogenic tumor. *J Cutan Pathol*. 1999;26(4):213–214.

93. Smith K, Mezebish D, Williams JP, et al. Cutaneous epithelioid schwannomas: a rare variant of a benign peripheral nerve sheath tumor. *J Cutan Pathol*. 1998;25(1):50–55.

94. Fisher C, Chappell ME, Weiss SW. Neuroblastoma-like epithelioid schwannoma. *Histopathology*. 1995;26(2):193–194.

95. Goldblum JR, Beals TF, Weiss SW. Neuroblastoma-like neurilemoma. *Am J Surg Pathol*. 1994;18(3):266–273.

96. Skelton HG 3rd, Smith KJ, Lupton GP. Collagenous spherulosis in a schwannoma. *Am J Dermatopathol*. 1994;16(5):549–553.

97. Vélez D, Reina Duran T, Pérez-Gala S, Fernández JF. Rosetoid schwannoma (neuroblastoma-like) in association with an anetoderma. *J Cutan Pathol*. 2006;33(8):573–576.

98. Resetkova E, Albarracin C, Sneige N. Collagenous spherulosis of breast: morphologic study of 59 cases and review of the literature. *Am J Surg Pathol*. 2006;30(1):20–27.

99. Jo VY, Fletcher CDM. SMARCB1/INI1 loss in epithelioid schwannoma: a clinicopathologic and immunohistochemical study of 65 cases. *Am J Surg Pathol*. 2017;41(8):1013–1022.

100. Elston DM, Bergfeld WF, Biscotti CV, McMahon JT. Schwannoma with sweat duct differentiation. *J Cutan Pathol*. 1993;20(3):254–258.

101. Kim YC, Park HJ, Cinn YW, Vandersteen DP. Benign glandular schwannoma. *Br J Dermatol*. 2001;145(5):834–837.

102. Woodruff JM, Christensen WN. Glandular peripheral nerve sheath tumors. *Cancer*. 1993;72(12):3618–3628.

103. Yoshida SO, Toot BV. Benign glandular schwannoma. *Am J Clin Pathol*. 1993;100(2):167–170.

104. Robinson CA, Curry B, Rewcastle NB. Pseudoglandular elements in schwannomas. *Arch Pathol Lab Med*. 2005;129(9):1106–1112.

105. Harkin J, Arrington JH, Reed RJ. Benign plexiform schwannoma: a lesion distinct from plexiform neurofibroma [abstract]. *J Neuropathol Exp Neurol*. 1978;37:622.

106. Iwashita T, Enjoji M. Plexiform neurilemmoma: a clinicopathological and immunohistochemical analysis of 23 tumours from 20 patients. *Virchows Arch A Pathol Anat Histopathol*. 1987;411(4):305–309.

107. Rongioletti F, Drago F, Rebora A. Multiple cutaneous plexiform schwannomas with tumors of the central nervous system. *Arch Dermatol*. 1989;125(3):431–432.

108. Sasaki T, Nakajima H. Congenital neurilemmomatosis. *J Am Acad Dermatol*. 1992;26(5, pt 1):786–787.

109. Kao GF, Laskin WB, Olsen TG. Solitary cutaneous plexiform neurilemmoma (schwannoma): a clinicopathologic,

110. Woodruff JM, Marshall ML, Godwin TA, Funkhouser JW, Thompson NJ, Erlandson RA. Plexiform (multinodular) schwannoma. A tumor simulating the plexiform neurofibroma. *Am J Surg Pathol*. 1983;7(7):691–697.

111. Shishiba T, Niimura M, Ohtsuka F, Tsuru N. Multiple cutaneous neurilemmomas as a skin manifestation of neurilemmomatosis. *J Am Acad Dermatol*. 1984;10(5, pt 1):744–754.

112. Murata Y, Kumano K, Ugai K, Ijichi A, Taomoto K, Tani M. Neurilemmomatosis. *Br J Dermatol*. 1991;125(5):466–468.

113. Rouleau GA, Merel P, Lutchman M, et al. Alteration in a new gene encoding a putative membrane-organizing protein causes neuro-fibromatosis type 2. *Nature*. 1993;363(6429):515–521.

114. Agaram NP, Prakash S, Antonescu CR. Deep-seated plexiform schwannoma: a pathologic study of 16 cases and comparative analysis with the superficial variety. *Am J Surg Pathol*. 2005;29(8):1042–1048.

115. Harder A, Wesemann M, Hagel C, et al. Hybrid neurofibroma/schwannoma is overrepresented among schwannomatosis and neurofibromatosis patients. *Am J Surg Pathol*. 2012;36(5):702–709.

116. Zamecnik M. Hybrid neurofibroma/schwannoma versus schwannoma with Antoni B areas. *Histopathology*. 2000;36(5):473–474.

117. Meis-Kindblom JM, Enzinger FM. Plexiform malignant peripheral nerve sheath tumor of infancy and childhood. *Am J Surg Pathol*. 1994;18(5):479–485.

118. Argenyi ZB, Goodenberger ME, Strauss JS. Congenital neural hamartoma ("fascicular schwannoma"). A light microscopic, immunohistochemical, and ultrastructural study. *Am J Dermatopathol*. 1990;12(3):283–293.

119. Torres-Mora J, Dry S, Li X, Binder S, Amin M, Folpe AL. Malignant melanotic schwannian tumor: a clinicopathologic, immunohistochemical, and gene expression profiling study of 40 cases, with a proposal for the reclassification of "melanotic schwannoma." *Am J Surg Pathol*. 2014;38(1):94–105.

120. Sahay A, Epari S, Gupta P, et al. Melanotic schwannoma, a deceptive misnomer for a tumor with relative aggressive behavior: a series of 7 cranial and spinal cases. *Int J Surg Pathol*. 2020;28(8):850–858.

121. Carney JA. Psammomatous melanotic schwannoma. A distinctive, heritable tumor with special associations, including cardiac myxoma and the Cushing syndrome. *Am J Surg Pathol*. 1990;14(3):206–222.

122. Cohen C, Davis TS. Multiple trichogenic adnexal tumors. *Am J Dermatopathol*. 1986;8(3):241–246.

123. Proppe KH, Scully RE. Large-cell calcifying Sertoli cell tumor of the testis. *Am J Clin Pathol*. 1980;74(5):607–619.

124. Carney JA, Hruska LS, Beauchamp GD, Gordon H. Dominant inheritance of the complex of myxomas, spotty pigmentation, and endocrine overactivity. *Mayo Clin Proc*. 1986;61(3):165–172.

125. Zhang HY, Yang GH, Chen HJ, et al. Clinicopathological, immunohistochemical, and ultrastructural study of 13 cases of melanotic schwannoma. *Chin Med J (Engl)*. 2005;118(17):1451–1461.

126. Foad MS, Kleiner DE, Dugan EM. A case of psammomatous melanotic schwannoma in the setting of the Carney complex. *J Cutan Pathol*. 2000;27:556.

127. Din NU, Fritchie K, Tariq MU, Ahmed A, Ahmad Z. Calcification and ossification in conventional schwannoma: a clinicopathologic study of 32 cases. *Neuropathology*. 2020;40(2):144–151.

128. Carstens PH, Schrodt GR. Malignant transformation of a benign encapsulated neurilemoma. *Am J Clin Pathol*. 1969;51(1):144–149.

129. Nayler SJ, Leiman G, Omar T, Cooper K. Malignant transformation in a schwannoma. *Histopathology*. 1996;29(2):189–192.

130. McMenamin ME, Fletcher CD. Expanding the spectrum of malignant change in schwannomas: epithelioid malignant change, epithelioid malignant peripheral nerve sheath tumor, and

epithelioid angiosarcoma: a study of 17 cases. *Am J Surg Pathol.* 2001;25(1):13–25.

131. Woodruff JM, Selig AM, Crowley K, Allen PW. Schwannoma (neurilemoma) with malignant transformation. A rare, distinctive peripheral nerve tumor. *Am J Surg Pathol.* 1994;18(9):882–895.

132. Ghali VS, Gold JE, Vincent RA, Cosgrove JM. Malignant peripheral nerve sheath tumor arising spontaneously from retroperitoneal ganglioneuroma: a case report, review of the literature, and immunohistochemical study. *Hum Pathol.* 1992;23(1):72–75.

133. Ricci A Jr, Parham DM, Woodruff JM, Callihan T, Green A, Erlandson RA. Malignant peripheral nerve sheath tumors arising from ganglioneuromas. *Am J Surg Pathol.* 1984;8(1):19–29.

134. Taxy JB, Battifora H, Trujillo Y, Dorfman HD. Electron microscopy in the diagnosis of malignant schwannoma. *Cancer.* 1981;48(6):1381–1391.

135. Leroy K, Dumas V, Martin-Garcia N, et al. Malignant peripheral nerve sheath tumors associated with neurofibromatosis type 1: a clinicopathologic and molecular study of 17 patients. *Arch Dermatol.* 2001;137(7):908–913.

136. Takeuchi A, Ushigome S. Diverse differentiation in malignant peripheral nerve sheath tumours associated with neurofibromatosis-1: an immunohistochemical and ultrastructural study. *Histopathology.* 2001;39(3):298–309.

137. Guccion JG, Enzinger FM. Malignant Schwannoma associated with von Recklinghausen's neurofibromatosis. *Virchows Arch A Pathol Anat Histol.* 1979;383(1):43–57.

138. D'Agostino AN, Soule EH, Miller RH. Sarcomas of the peripheral nerves and somatic soft tissues associated with multiple neurofibromatosis (Von Recklinghausen's disease). *Cancer.* 1963;16:1015–1027.

139. D'Agostino AN, Soule EH, Miller RH. Primary malignant neoplasms of nerves (malignant neurilemomas) in patients without manifestations of multiple neurofibromatosis (Von Recklinghausen's disease). *Cancer.* 1963;16:1003–1014.

140. Allison KH, Patel RM, Goldblum JR, Rubin BP. Superficial malignant peripheral nerve sheath tumor: a rare and challenging diagnosis. *Am J Clin Pathol.* 2005;124(5):685–692.

141. Stasik CJ, Tawfik O. Malignant peripheral nerve sheath tumor with rhabdomyosarcomatous differentiation (malignant triton tumor). *Arch Pathol Lab Med.* 2006;130(12):1878–1881.

142. Woodruff JM, Perino G. Non-germ-cell or teratomatous malignant tumors showing additional rhabdomyoblastic differentiation, with emphasis on the malignant Triton tumor. *Semin Diagn Pathol.* 1994;11(1):69–81.

143. Hirose T, Scheithauer BW, Sano T. Perineurial malignant peripheral nerve sheath tumor (MPNST): a clinicopathologic, immunohistochemical, and ultrastructural study of seven cases. *Am J Surg Pathol.* 1998;22(11):1368–1378.

144. Rosenberg AS, Langee CL, Stevens GL, Morgan MB. Malignant peripheral nerve sheath tumor with perineurial differentiation: "malignant perineurioma." *J Cutan Pathol.* 2002;29(6):362–367.

145. Zámecník M, Michal M. Malignant peripheral nerve sheath tumor with perineurial cell differentiation (malignant perineurioma). *Pathol Int.* 1999;49(1):69–73.

146. Laskin WB, Weiss SW, Bratthauer GL. Epithelioid variant of malignant peripheral nerve sheath tumor (malignant epithelioid schwannoma). *Am J Surg Pathol.* 1991;15(12):1136–1145.

147. Lodding P, Kindblom LG, Angervall L. Epithelioid malignant schwannoma. A study of 14 cases. *Virchows Arch A Pathol Anat Histopathol.* 1986;409(4):433–451.

148. Hruban RH, Shiu MH, Senie RT, Woodruff JM. Malignant peripheral nerve sheath tumors of the buttock and lower extremity. A study of 43 cases. *Cancer.* 1990;66(6):1253–1265.

149. DiCarlo EF, Woodruff JM, Bansal M, Erlandson RA. The purely epithelioid malignant peripheral nerve sheath tumor. *Am J Surg Pathol.* 1986;10(7):478–490.

150. Wick MR, Swanson PE, Scheithauer BW, Manivel JC. Malignant peripheral nerve sheath tumor. An immunohistochemical study of 62 cases. *Am J Clin Pathol.* 1987;87(4):425–433.

151. Daimaru Y, Hashimoto H, Enjoji M. Malignant peripheral nerve-sheath tumors (malignant schwannomas). An immunohistochemical study of 29 cases. *Am J Surg Pathol.* 1985;9(6):434–444.

152. Liesche F, Griessmair M, Barz M, Gempt J, Schlegel J. ALDH1—a new immunohistochemical diagnostic marker for Schwann cell-derived tumors. *Clin Neuropathol.* 2019;38(4):168–173.

153. Liapis H, Dehner LP, Gutmann DH. Neurofibroma and cellular neurofibroma with atypia: a report of 14 tumors. *Am J Surg Pathol.* 1999;23(9):1156–1158.

154. Cleven AH, Sannaa GA, Briaire-de Bruijn I, et al. Loss of H3K27 tri-methylation is a diagnostic marker for malignant peripheral nerve sheath tumors and an indicator for an inferior survival. *Mod Pathol.* 2016;29(6):582–590.

155. Coindre JM, Hostein I, Benhattar J, Lussan C, Rivel J, Guillou L. Malignant peripheral nerve sheath tumors are t(X;18)-negative sarcomas. Molecular analysis of 25 cases occurring in neurofibromatosis type 1 patients, using two different RT-PCR-based methods of detection. *Mod Pathol.* 2002;15(6):589–592.

156. Huttenbach Y, Prieto VG, Reed JA. Desmoplastic and spindle cell melanomas express protein markers of the neural crest but not of later committed stages of Schwann cell differentiation. *J Cutan Pathol.* 2002;29(9):562–568.

157. Reed RJ. Case 13. In: Proceedings of the 49th Annual Anatomic Pathology Slide Seminar, American Society of Clinical Pathologists; 1983.

158. Kolberg M, Høland M, Agesen TH, et al. Survival meta-analyses for >1800 malignant peripheral nerve sheath tumor patients with and without neurofibromatosis type 1. *Neuro Oncol.* 2013;15(2):135–147.

159. Meis JM, Enzinger FM, Martz KL, Neal JA. Malignant peripheral nerve sheath tumors (malignant schwannomas) in children. *Am J Surg Pathol.* 1992;16(7):694–707.

160. Wanebo JE, Malik JM, VandenBerg SR, Wanebo HJ, Driesen N, Persing JA. Malignant peripheral nerve sheath tumors. A clinicopathologic study of 28 cases. *Cancer.* 1993;71(4):1247–1253.

161. Sordillo PP, Helson L, Hajdu SI, et al. Malignant schwannoma—clinical characteristics, survival, and response to therapy. *Cancer.* 1981;47(10):2503–2509.

162. Gallager RL, Helwig EB. Neurothekeoma—a benign cutaneous tumor of neural origin. *Am J Clin Pathol.* 1980;74(6):759–764.

163. Barnhill RL, Mihm MC Jr. Cellular neurothekeoma. A distinctive variant of neurothekeoma mimicking nevomelanocytic tumors. *Am J Surg Pathol.* 1990;14(2):113–120.

164. Rosati LA, Fratamico FC, Eusebi V. Cellular neurothekeoma. *Appl Pathol.* 1986;4(3):186–191.

165. Pulitzer DR, Reed RJ. Nerve-sheath myxoma (perineurial myxoma). *Am J Dermatopathol.* 1985;7(5):409–421.

166. Fetsch JF, Laskin WB, Miettinen M. Nerve sheath myxoma: a clinicopathologic and immunohistochemical analysis of 57 morphologically distinctive, S-100 protein-and GFAP-positive, myxoid peripheral nerve sheath tumors with a predilection for the extremities and a high local recurrence rate. *Am J Surg Pathol.* 2005;29(12):1615–1624.

167. Laskin WB, Fetsch JF, Miettinen M. The "neurothekeoma": immunohistochemical analysis distinguishes the true nerve sheath myxoma from its mimics. *Hum Pathol.* 2000;31(10):1230–1241.

168. Barnhill RL, Dickersin GR, Nickeleit V, et al. Studies on the cellular origin of neurothekeoma: clinical, light microscopic, immunohistochemical, and ultrastructural observations. *J Am Acad Dermatol.* 1991;25(1, pt 1):80–88.

169. Busam KJ, Mentzel T, Colpaert C, Barnhill RL, Fletcher CD. Atypical or worrisome features in cellular neurothekeoma: a study of 10 cases. *Am J Surg Pathol.* 1998;22(9):1067–1072.

170. Jaffer S, Ambrosini-Spaltro A, Mancini AM, Eusebi V, Rosai J. Neurothekeoma and plexiform fibrohistiocytic tumor: mere histologic resemblance or histogenetic relationship? *Am J Surg Pathol.* 2009;33(6):905–913.

171. Leclerc-Mercier S, Brousse N, Fraitag S. Is plexiform fibro-histiocytic tumor a deep form of cellular neurothekeoma? *J Cutan Pathol.* 2009;36(10):1123–1125.

172. Fox MD, Billings SD, Gleason BC, et al. Expression of MiTF may be helpful in differentiating cellular neurothekeoma from plexiform fibrohistiocytic tumor (histiocytoid predominant) in a partial biopsy specimen. *Am J Dermatopathol.* 2012;34(2):157–160.

173. Kaddu S, Leinweber B. Podoplanin expression in fibrous histiocytomas and cellular neurothekeomas. *Am J Dermatopathol.* 2009;31(2):137–139.

174. Sheth S, Li X, Binder S, Dry SM. Differential gene expression profiles of neurothekeomas and nerve sheath myxomas by microarray analysis. *Mod Pathol.* 2011;24(3):343–354.

175. Cardoso J, Calonje E. Cellular neurothekeoma with perineural extension: a potential diagnostic pitfall. *J Cutan Pathol.* 2012;39(6):662–664.

176. Argenyi ZB, Kutzner H, Seaba MM. Ultrastructural spectrum of cutaneous nerve sheath myxoma/cellular neurothekeoma. *J Cutan Pathol.* 1995;22(2):137–145.

177. Aronson PJ, Fretzin DF, Potter BS. Neurothekeoma of Gallager and Helwig (dermal nerve sheath myxoma variant): report of a case with electron microscopic and immunohistochemical studies. *J Cutan Pathol.* 1985;12(6):506–519.

178. Misago N, Satoh T, Narisawa Y. Cellular neurothekeoma with histiocytic differentiation. *J Cutan Pathol.* 2004;31(8):568–572.

179. Salama S, Chorneyko K. Neurothekeoma (N.T.): a clinicopathologic study of 13 new cases with emphasis on immunohistochemical and ultrastructural features. *J Cutan Pathol.* 2000;27:571.

180. Plaza JA, Torres-Cabala C, Evans H, Diwan AH, Prieto VG. Immunohistochemical expression of S100A6 in cellular neurothekeoma: clinicopathologic and immunohistochemical analysis of 31 cases. *Am J Dermatopathol.* 2009;31(5):419–422.

181. Page RN, King R, Mihm MC Jr, Googe PB. Microphthalmia transcription factor and NKI/C3 expression in cellular neurothekeoma. *Mod Pathol.* 2004;17(2):230–234.

182. Linos K, Stuart L, Goncharuk V, Edgar M. Benign cutaneous biphasic hybrid tumor of perineurioma and cellular neurothekeoma: a case report expanding the clinical and histopathologic features of a recently described entity. *Am J Dermatopathol.* 2015;37(4):319–322.

183. Allen PW, Dymock RB, MacCormac LB. Superficial angiomyxomas with and without epithelial components. Report of 30 tumors in 28 patients. *Am J Surg Pathol.* 1988;12(7):519–530.

184. Prieto VG, Shea CR. Use of immunohistochemistry in melanocytic lesions. *J Cutan Pathol.* 2008;35(suppl 2):1–10.

185. Suarez A, High W. Immunohistochemical analysis of KBA.62 in eighteen neurothekeomas: a potential marker for differentiating neurothekeoma from melanocytic tumors. *J Cutan Pathol.* 2013.

186. Ramos-Herberth FI, Karamchandani J, Kim J, Dadras SS. SOX10 immunostaining distinguishes desmoplastic melanoma from excision scar. *J Cutan Pathol.* 2010;37(9):944–952.

187. Calonje E, Wilson-Jones E, Smith NP, Fletcher CD. Cellular "neurothekeoma": an epithelioid variant of pilar leiomyoma? Morphological and immunohistochemical analysis of a series. *Histopathology.* 1992;20(5):397–404.

188. Jones EW, Cerio R, Smith NP. Epithelioid cell histiocytoma: a new entity. *Br J Dermatol.* 1989;120(2):185–195.

189. Singh Gomez C, Calonje E, Fletcher CD. Epithelioid benign fibrous histiocytoma of skin: clinico-pathological analysis of 20 cases of a poorly known variant. *Histopathology.* 1994;24(2):123–129.

190. Zelger BG, Zelger B. Cellular "neurothekeoma": an epithelioid variant of dermatofibroma? *Histopathology.* 1998;32(5):414–422.

191. Cadoni A, Mancardi GL, Zaccheo D, et al. Expression of common acute lymphoblastic leukemia antigen (CD 10) by myelinated fibers of the peripheral nervous system. *J Neuroimmunol.* 1993;45(1–2):61–66.

192. Requena L, Sitthinamsuwan P, Fried I, et al. A benign cutaneous plexiform hybrid tumor of perineurioma and cellular neurothekeoma. *Am J Surg Pathol.* 2013;37(6):845–852.

193. Stratton J, Billings SD. Cellular neurothekeoma: analysis of 37 cases emphasizing atypical histologic features. *Mod Pathol.* 2013.

194. Aparicio SR, Lumsden CE. Light-and electron-microscope studies on the granular cell myoblastoma of the tongue. *J Pathol.* 1969;97(2):339–355.

195. Sobel HJ, Marquet E. Granular cells and granular cell lesions. *Pathol Annu.* 1974;9(0):43–79.

196. Fernandes MS, Leitch CS, Al-Qsous W, Biswas A. Desmoplastic stromal changes in cutaneous neural granular cell tumors: an under-recognized histopathologic feature of diagnostic and prognostic importance. *J Cutan Pathol.* 2020;47(5):431–438.

197. Miracco C, Andreassi A, Laurini L, De Santi MM, Taddeucci P, Tosi P. Granular cell tumour with histological signs of malignancy: report of a case and comparison with 10 benign and 4 atypical cases. *Br J Dermatol.* 1999;141(3):573–575.

198. Lee J, Bhawan J, Wax F, Farber J. Plexiform granular cell tumor. A report of two cases. *Am J Dermatopathol.* 1994;16(5):537–541.

199. Ordonez NG. Granular cell tumor: a review and update. *Adv Anat Pathol.* 1999;6(4):186–203.

200. Garancis JC, Komorowski RA, Kuzma JF. Granular cell myoblastoma. *Cancer.* 1970;25(3):542–550.

201. Weiser G. [Granular cell tumor and the phagocytozing form of Schwann cells. Electron microscopic examinations of 3 cases (author's transl)]. *Virchows Arch A Pathol Anat Histol.* 1978;380(1):49–57.

202. Lee MW, Chang SE, Song KY, et al. S-100-negative atypical granular cell tumor: report of a case. *Int J Dermatol.* 2002;41(3):168–170.

203. Ortiz-Hidalgo C, Frias-Soria CL. [The histopathology and immunohistochemistry of granular cell tumour. A study of 12 cases with a brief historical note]. *Rev Esp Patol.* 2019;52(1):11–19.

204. Mukai M. Immunohistochemical localization of S-100 protein and peripheral nerve myelin proteins (P2 protein, P0 protein) in granular cell tumors. *Am J Pathol.* 1983;112(2):139–146.

205. Mahalingam M, LoPiccolo D, Byers HR. Expression of PGP 9.5 in granular cell nerve sheath tumors: an immunohistochemical study of six cases. *J Cutan Pathol.* 2001;28(6):282–286.

206. Shintaku M. Immunohistochemical localization of autophagosomal membrane-associated protein LC3 in granular cell tumor and schwannoma. *Virchows Arch.* 2011;459(3):315–319.

207. LeBoit PE, Barr RJ, Burall S, Metcalf JS, Yen TS, Wick MR. Primitive polypoid granular-cell tumor and other cutaneous granular-cell neoplasms of apparent nonneural origin. *Am J Surg Pathol.* 1991;15(1):48–58.

208. Cheng SD, Usmani AS, DeYoung BR, Ly M, Pellegrini AE. Dermatofibroma-like granular cell tumor. *J Cutan Pathol.* 2001;28(1):49–52.

209. Gilliet F, MacGee W, Stoian M, Delacrétaz J. [Histogenesis of granulated cell tumors]. *Hautarzt.* 1973;24(2):52–57.

210. Mentzel T, Wadden C, Fletcher CD. Granular cell change in smooth muscle tumours of skin and soft tissue. *Histopathology.* 1994;24(3):223–231.

211. Lewin MR, Montgomery EA, Barrett TL. New or unusual dermatopathology tumors: a review. *J Cutan Pathol.* 2011;38(9):689–696.

212. Lazar AJ, Fletcher CD. Primitive nonneural granular cell tumors of skin: clinicopathologic analysis of 13 cases. *Am J Surg Pathol.* 2005;29(7):927–934.

213. Izquierdo FM, Suarez-Vilela D, Honrado E. Intraneural hybrid granular cell tumor-perineurioma. *APMIS.* 2013;121(7):678–680.

214. Matter A, Hewer E, Kappeler A, Fleischmann A, Vajtai I. Plexiform hybrid granular cell tumor/perineurioma: a novel variant of benign peripheral nerve sheath tumor with divergent differentiation. *Pathol Res Pract.* 2012;208(5):310–314.

215. Takahashi H, Fujita S, Satoh H, Okabe H. Immunohistochemical study of congenital gingival granular cell tumor (congenital epulis). *J Oral Pathol Med.* 1990;19(10):492–496.

216. Lack EE, Perez-Atayde AR, McGill TJ, Vawter GF. Gingival granular cell tumor of the newborn (congenital "epulis"): ultrastructural observations relating to histogenesis. *Hum Pathol.* 1982;13(7):686–689.

217. Simsir A, Osborne BM, Greenebaum E. Malignant granular cell tumor: a case report and review of the recent literature. *Hum Pathol.* 1996;27(8):853–858.

218. Shimamura K, Osamura RY, Ueyama Y, et al. Malignant granular cell tumor of the right sciatic nerve. Report of an autopsy case with electron microscopic, immunohistochemical, and enzyme histochemical studies. *Cancer.* 1984;53(3):524–529.

219. Gamboa LG. Malignant granular-cell myoblastoma. *AMA Arch Pathol.* 1955;60(6):663–668.

220. Klima M, Peters J. Malignant granular cell tumor. *Arch Pathol Lab Med.* 1987;111(11):1070–1073.

221. Uzoaru I, Firfer B, Ray V, Hubbard-Shepard M, Rhee H. Malignant granular cell tumor. *Arch Pathol Lab Med.* 1992;116(2):206–208.

222. Strong EW, McDivitt RW, Brasfield RD. Granular cell myoblastoma. *Cancer.* 1970;25(2):415–422.

223. Moten AS, Zhao H, Wu H, Farma JM. Malignant granular cell tumor: clinical features and long-term survival. *J Surg Oncol.* 2018;118(6):891–897.

224. Fanburg-Smith JC, Meis-Kindblom JM, Fante R, Kindblom LG. Malignant granular cell tumor of soft tissue: diagnostic criteria and clinicopathologic correlation. *Am J Surg Pathol.* 1998;22(7):779–794.

225. al-Sarraf M, Loud AV, Vaitkevicius VK. Malignant granular cell tumor. Histochemical and electron microscopic study. *Arch Pathol.* 1971;91(6):550–558.

226. Gartmann H. [Malignant granular cell tumor]. *Hautarzt.* 1977;28(1):40–44.

227. Gokaslan ST, Terzakis JA, Santagada EA. Malignant granular cell tumor. *J Cutan Pathol.* 1994;21(3):263–270.

228. Goo B, Cho SB, Cho YH, et al. Fibrolamellar nerve sheath tumor or sclerotic neurofibroma? *J Cutan Pathol.* 2006;33(11):760–761.

229. Cheshire LB, Stern JB. *Sclerotic neurofibroma (formerly sclerotic fibroma).* In: 32 Annual Meeting of the American Society of Dermatopathology; 1995.

230. Lazarus SS, Trombetta LD. Ultrastructural identification of a benign perineurial cell tumor. *Cancer.* 1978;41(5):1823–1829.

231. Tsang WY, Chan JK, Chow LT, Tse CC. Perineurioma: an uncommon soft tissue neoplasm distinct from localized hypertrophic neuropathy and neurofibroma. *Am J Surg Pathol.* 1992;16(8):756–763.

232. Mentzel T, Dei Tos AP, Fletcher CD. Perineurioma (storiform perineurial fibroma): clinico-pathological analysis of four cases. *Histopathology.* 1994;25(3):261–267.

233. Hornick JL, Fletcher CD. Soft tissue perineurioma: clinicopathologic analysis of 81 cases including those with atypical histologic features. *Am J Surg Pathol.* 2005;29(7):845–858.

234. Folpe AL, Billings SD, McKenney JK, Walsh SV, Nusrat A, Weiss SW. Expression of claudin-1, a recently described tight junction-associated protein, distinguishes soft tissue perineurioma from potential mimics. *Am J Surg Pathol.* 2002;26(12):1620–1626.

235. Giannini C, Scheithauer BW, Jenkins RB, et al. Soft-tissue perineurioma. Evidence for an abnormality of chromosome 22, criteria for diagnosis, and review of the literature. *Am J Surg Pathol.* 1997;21(2):164–173.

236. Pitchford CW, Schwartz HS, Atkinson JB, Cates JM. Soft tissue perineurioma in a patient with neurofibromatosis type 2: a tumor not previously associated with the NF2 syndrome. *Am J Surg Pathol.* 2006;30(12):1624–1629.

237. Hornick JL, Bundock EA, Fletcher CD. Hybrid schwannoma/perineurioma: clinicopathologic analysis of 42 distinctive benign nerve sheath tumors. *Am J Surg Pathol.* 2009;33(10):1554–1561.

238. Weiss SW, Nickoloff BJ. CD-34 is expressed by a distinctive cell population in peripheral nerve, nerve sheath tumors, and related lesions. *Am J Surg Pathol.* 1993;17(10):1039–1045.

239. Dominguez-Malagon HR, Serrano-Arévalo ML, Maldonado J, et al. Perineurioma versus meningioma. A multi-institutional immunohistochemical and ultrastructural study. *Ultrastruct Pathol.* 2021;45(1):71–77.

240. Stanton C, Perentes E, Phillips L, VandenBerg SR. The immunohistochemical demonstration of early perineurial change in the development of localized hypertrophic neuropathy. *Hum Pathol.* 1988;19(12):1455–1457.

241. Mitsumoto H, Wilbourn AJ, Goren H. Perineurioma as the cause of localized hypertrophic neuropathy. *Muscle Nerve.* 1980;3(5):403–412.

242. Kuhlenbaumer G, Young P, Hünermund G, Ringelstein B, Stögbauer F. Clinical features and molecular genetics of hereditary peripheral neuropathies. *J Neurol.* 2002;249(12):1629–1650.

243. Skelton HG, Williams J, Smith KJ. The clinical and histologic spectrum of cutaneous fibrous perineuriomas. *Am J Dermatopathol.* 2001;23(3):190–196.

244. Fetsch JF, Miettinen M. Sclerosing perineurioma: a clinicopathologic study of 19 cases of a distinctive soft tissue lesion with a predilection for the fingers and palms of young adults. *Am J Surg Pathol.* 1997;21(12):1433–1442.

245. Burgues O, Monteagudo C, Noguera R, Revert A, Molina I, Llombart-Bosch A. Cutaneous sclerosing Pacinian-like perineurioma. *Histopathology.* 2001;39(5):498–502.

246. Macarenco AC, Macarenco RS. Cutaneous lipomatous sclerosing perineurioma. *Am J Dermatopathol.* 2008;30(3):291–294.

247. Graadt van Roggen JF, McMenamin ME, Belchis DA, Nielsen GP, Rosenberg AE, Fletcher CD. Reticular perineurioma: a distinctive variant of soft tissue perineurioma. *Am J Surg Pathol.* 2001;25(4):485–493.

248. Yamaguchi U, Hasegawa T, Hirose T, et al. Sclerosing perineurioma: a clinicopathological study of five cases and diagnostic utility of immunohistochemical staining for GLUT1. *Virchows Arch.* 2003;443(2):159–163.

249. Kos Z, Robertson SJ, Purgina BM, Verma S, Gravel DH. Malignant peripheral nerve sheath tumor arising in a traumatic neuroma: a case report. *Hum Pathol.* 2013;44(10):2360–2364.

250. Shapiro L, Juhlin EA, Brownstein MH. "Rudimentary polydactyly": an amputation neuroma. *Arch Dermatol.* 1973;108(2):223–225.

251. Argenyi ZB. Immunohistochemical characterization of palisaded, encapsulated neuroma. *J Cutan Pathol.* 1990;17(6):329–335.

252. Argenyi ZB, Santa Cruz D, Bromley C. Comparative light-microscopic and immunohistochemical study of traumatic and palisaded encapsulated neuromas of the skin. *Am J Dermatopathol.* 1992;14(6):504–510.

253. Fletcher CD. Solitary circumscribed neuroma of the skin (so-called palisaded, encapsulated neuroma). A clinicopathologic and immunohistochemical study. *Am J Surg Pathol.* 1989;13(7):574–580.

254. Reed RJ, Fine RM, Meltzer HD. Palisaded, encapsulated neuromas of the skin. *Arch Dermatol.* 1972;106(6):865–870.

255. Kossard S, Kumar A, Wilkinson B. Neural spectrum: palisaded encapsulated neuroma and verocay body poor dermal schwannoma. *J Cutan Pathol.* 1999;26(1):31–36.

256. Khairi MR, Dexter RN, Burzynski NJ, Johnston CC Jr. Mucosal neuroma, pheochromocytoma and medullary thyroid carcinoma:

multiple endocrine neoplasia type 3. *Medicine (Baltimore)*. 1975;54(2):89–112.

257. Ayala F, De Rosa G, Scippa L, Vecchio P. Multiple endocrine neoplasia, type IIb. Report of a case. *Dermatologica*. 1981;162(4):292–299.

258. Carney JA, Go VL, Sizemore GW, Hayles AB. Alimentary-tract ganglioneuromatosis. A major component of the syndrome of multiple endocrine neoplasia, type 2b. *N Engl J Med*. 1976;295(23):1287–1291.

259. Truchot F, Grézard P, Wolf F, Balme B, Perrot H. Multiple idiopathic mucocutaneous neuromas: a new entity? *Br J Dermatol*. 2001;145(5):826–829.

260. Pujol RM, Matias-Guiu X, Miralles J, Colomer A, de Moragas JM. Multiple idiopathic mucosal neuromas: a minor form of multiple endocrine neoplasia type 2B or a new entity? *J Am Acad Dermatol*. 1997;37(2, pt 2):349–352.

261. Guillet G, Gauthier Y, Tamisier JM, et al. Linear cutaneous neuromas (dermatoneurie en stries): a limited phakomatosis with striated pigmentation corresponding to cutaneous hyperneury (featuring multiple endocrine neoplasia syndrome?). *J Cutan Pathol*. 1987;14(1):43–48.

262. Mason GH, Pitt TE, Tay E. Cutaneous nerve hypertrophy. *Pathology*. 1998;30(4):422–424.

263. Requena L, Grosshans E, Kutzner H, et al. Epithelial sheath neuroma: a new entity. *Am J Surg Pathol*. 2000;24(2):190–196.

264. Waggener JD. Ultrastructure of benign peripheral nerve sheath tumors. *Cancer*. 1966;19(5):699–709.

265. Fletcher CD, Theaker JM. Digital pacinian neuroma: a distinctive hyperplastic lesion. *Histopathology*. 1989;15(3):249–256.

266. Sampath A, Labadie JG, Guitart J. Agminated Pacinian neuroma—immunohistochemical studies and literature review. *J Cutan Pathol*. 2020;47(7):581–583.

267. Reed RJ. Giant congenital nevi: a conceptualization of patterns. *J Invest Dermatol*. 1993;100(3):300S–312S.

268. Pettinato G, Manivel JC, d'Amore ES, Jaszcz W, Gorlin RJ. Melanotic neuroectodermal tumor of infancy. A reexamination of a histogenetic problem based on immunohistochemical, flow cytometric, and ultrastructural study of 10 cases. *Am J Surg Pathol*. 1991;15(3):233–245.

269. Pearson JM, Harris M, Eyden BP, Banerjee SS. Divergent differentiation in small round-cell tumours of the soft tissues with neural features—an analysis of 10 cases. *Histopathology*. 1993;23(1):1–9.

270. Navarro S, Cavazzana AO, Llombart-Bosch A, Triche TJ. Comparison of Ewing's sarcoma of bone and peripheral neuroepithelioma. An immunocytochemical and ultrastructural analysis of two primitive neuroectodermal neoplasms. *Arch Pathol Lab Med*. 1994;118(6):608–615.

271. Kushner BH, Hajdu SI, Gulati SC, Erlandson RA, Exelby PR, Lieberman PH. Extracranial primitive neuroectodermal tumors. The Memorial Sloan-Kettering Cancer Center experience. *Cancer*. 1991;67(7):1825–1829.

272. Gollard R, Weber R, Kosty MP, Greenway HT, Massullo V, Humberson C. Merkel cell carcinoma: review of 22 cases with surgical, pathologic, and therapeutic considerations. *Cancer*. 2000;88(8):1842–1851.

273. Raaf JH, Urmacher C, Knapper WK, Shiu MH, Cheng EW. Trabecular (Merkel cell) carcinoma of the skin. Treatment of primary, recurrent, and metastatic disease. *Cancer*. 1986;57(1):178–182.

274. Ratner D, Nelson BR, Brown MD, Johnson TM. Merkel cell carcinoma. *J Am Acad Dermatol*. 1993;29(2, pt 1):143–156.

275. Skelton HG, Smith KJ, Hitchcock CL, McCarthy WF, Lupton GP, Graham JH. Merkel cell carcinoma: analysis of clinical, histologic, and immunohistologic features of 132 cases with relation to survival. *J Am Acad Dermatol*. 1997;37(5, pt 1):734–739.

276. Toker C. Trabecular carcinoma of the skin. *Arch Dermatol*. 1972;105(1):107–110.

277. Albores-Saavedra J, Batich K, Chable-Montero F, Sagy N, Schwartz AM, Henson DE. Merkel cell carcinoma demographics, morphology, and survival based on 3870 cases: a population based study. *J Cutan Pathol*. 2010;37(1):20–27.

278. Sibley DA, Cooper PH. Rudimentary meningocele: a variant of "primary cutaneous meningioma." *J Cutan Pathol*. 1989;16(2):72–80.

279. Sibley RK, Dehner LP, Rosai J. Primary neuroendocrine (Merkel cell?) carcinoma of the skin. I. A clinicopathologic and ultrastructural study of 43 cases. *Am J Surg Pathol*. 1985;9(2):95–108.

280. Silva EG, Mackay B, Goepfert H, Burgess MA, Fields RS. Endocrine carcinoma of the skin (Merkel cell carcinoma). *Pathol Annu*. 1984;19(pt 2):1–30.

281. LeBoit PE, Crutcher WA, Shapiro PE. Pagetoid intraepidermal spread in Merkel cell (primary neuroendocrine) carcinoma of the skin. *Am J Surg Pathol*. 1992;16(6):584–592.

282. Smith KJ, Skelton HG 3rd, Holland TT, Morgan AM, Lupton GP. Neuroendocrine (Merkel cell) carcinoma with an intraepidermal component. *Am J Dermatopathol*. 1993;15(6):528–533.

283. Foschini MP, Eusebi V. Divergent differentiation in endocrine and nonendocrine tumors of the skin. *Semin Diagn Pathol*. 2000;17(2):162–168.

284. Cerroni L, Kerl H. Primary cutaneous neuroendocrine (Merkel cell) carcinoma in association with squamous-and basal-cell carcinoma. *Am J Dermatopathol*. 1997;19(6):610–613.

285. Traest K, De Vos R, van den Oord JJ. Pagetoid Merkel cell carcinoma: speculations on its origin and the mechanism of epidermal spread. *J Cutan Pathol*. 1999;26(7):362–365.

286. Martin B, Poblet E, Rios JJ, et al. Merkel cell carcinoma with divergent differentiation: histopathological and immunohistochemical study of 15 cases with PCR analysis for Merkel cell polyomavirus. *Histopathology*. 2013;62(5):711–722.

287. Michels S, Swanson PE, Robb JA, Wick MR. Leu-7 in small cell neoplasms. An immunohistochemical study with ultrastructural correlations. *Cancer*. 1987;60(12):2958–2964.

288. Rush PS, Rosenbaum JN, Roy M, Baus RM, Bennett DD, Lloyd RV. Insulinoma-associated 1: a novel nuclear marker in Merkel cell carcinoma (cutaneous neuroendocrine carcinoma). *J Cutan Pathol*. 2018;45(2):129–135.

289. Merot Y, Margolis RJ, Dahl D, Saurat JH, Mihm MC Jr. Coexpression of neurofilament and keratin proteins in cutaneous neuroendocrine carcinoma cells. *J Invest Dermatol*. 1986;86(1):74–77.

290. Wick MR, Kaye VN, Sibley RK, Tyler R, Frizzera G. Primary neuroendocrine carcinoma and small-cell malignant lymphoma of the skin. A discriminant immunohistochemical comparison. *J Cutan Pathol*. 1986;13(5):347–358.

291. Hanly AJ, Elgart GW, Jorda M, Smith J, Nadji M. Analysis of thyroid transcription factor-1 and cytokeratin 20 separates Merkel cell carcinoma from small cell carcinoma of lung. *J Cutan Pathol*. 2000;27(3):118–120.

292. Sangoi AR, Cassarino DS. PAX-8 expression in primary and metastatic Merkel cell carcinoma: an immunohistochemical analysis. *Am J Dermatopathol*. 2013;35(4):448–451.

293. Sahi H, Koljonen V, Kavola H, et al. Bcl-2 expression indicates better prognosis of Merkel cell carcinoma regardless of the presence of Merkel cell polyomavirus. *Virchows Arch*. 2012;461(5):553–559.

294. Asioli S, Righi A, Volante M, Eusebi V, Bussolati G. p63 expression as a new prognostic marker in Merkel cell carcinoma. *Cancer*. 2007;110(3):640–647.

295. van Muijen GN, Ruiter DJ, Warnaar SO. Intermediate filaments in Merkel cell tumors. *Hum Pathol*. 1985;16(6):590–595.

296. Haneke E. Electron microscopy of Merkel cell carcinoma from formalin-fixed tissue. *J Am Acad Dermatol*. 1985;12(3):487–492.

297. Rao P, Balzer BL, Lemos BD, et al. Protocol for the examination of specimens from patients with Merkel cell carcinoma of the skin. *Arch Pathol Lab Med.* 2010;134(3):341–344.

298. Gould E, Albores-Saavedra J, Dubner B, Smith W, Payne CM et al. Eccrine and squamous differentiation in Merkel cell carcinoma. An immunohistochemical study. *Am J Surg Pathol.* 1988;12(10):768–772.

299. Wick MR, Goellner JR, Scheithauer BW, Thomas JR III, Sanchez NP, Schroeter AL. Primary neuroendocrine carcinomas of the skin (Merkel cell tumors). A clinical, histologic, and ultrastructural study of thirteen cases. *Am J Clin Pathol.* 1983; 79(1):6–13.

300. Isimbaldi G, Sironi M, Taccagni G, Declich P, Dell'Antonio A, Galli C. Tripartite differentiation (squamous, glandular, and melanocytic) of a primary cutaneous neuroendocrine carcinoma. An immunocytochemical and ultrastructural study. *Am J Dermatopathol.* 1993;15(3):260–264.

301. Feng H, Shuda M, Chang Y, Moore PS. Clonal integration of a polyomavirus in human Merkel cell carcinoma. *Science.* 2008;319(5866):1096–1100.

302. Iwasaki T, Kodama H, Matsushita M, et al. Merkel cell polyomavirus infection in both components of a combined Merkel cell carcinoma and basal cell carcinoma with ductal differentiation; each component had a similar but different novel Merkel cell polyomavirus large T antigen truncating mutation. *Hum Pathol.* 2013;44(3):442–447.

303. Wu KN, McCue PA, Berger A, Spiegel JR, Wang ZX, Witkiewicz AK. Detection of Merkel cell carcinoma polyomavirus in mucosal Merkel cell carcinoma. *Int J Surg Pathol.* 2010;18(5): 342–346.

304. Vortmeyer AO, Merino MJ, Böni R, Liotta LA, Cavazzana A, Zhuang Z. Genetic changes associated with primary Merkel cell carcinoma. *Am J Clin Pathol.* 1998;109(5):565–570.

305. Wick MR, Millns JL, Sibley RK, Pittelkow MR, Winkelmann RK. Secondary neuroendocrine carcinomas of the skin. An immunohistochemical comparison with primary neuroendocrine carcinoma of the skin ("Merkel cell" carcinoma). *J Am Acad Dermatol.* 1985;13(1):134–142.

306. Rios-Martin JJ, Solorzano-Amoreti A, González-Cámpora R, Galera-Davidson H. Neuroendocrine carcinoma of the skin with a lymphoepithelioma-like histological pattern. *Br J Dermatol.* 2000;143(2):460–462.

307. Eusebi V, Capella C, Cossu A, Rosai J. Neuroendocrine carcinoma within lymph nodes in the absence of a primary tumor, with special reference to Merkel cell carcinoma. *Am J Surg Pathol.* 1992;16(7):658–666.

308. Zelin E, Zalaudek I, Agozzino M, et al. Neoadjuvant therapy for non-melanoma skin cancer: updated therapeutic approaches for basal, squamous, and Merkel cell carcinoma. *Curr Treat Options Oncol.* 2021;22(4):35.

309. Shown TE, Durfee MF. Blueberry muffin baby: neonatal neuroblastoma with subcutaneous metastases. *J Urol.* 1970; 104(1):193–195.

310. Hawthorne HC Jr, Nelson JS, Witzleben CL, Giangiacomo J. Blanching subcutaneous nodules in neonatal neuroblastoma. *J Pediatr.* 1970;77(2):297–300.

311. Aleshire SL, Glick AD, Cruz VE, Bradley CA, Parl FF. Neuroblastoma in adults. Pathologic findings and clinical outcome. *Arch Pathol Lab Med.* 1985;109(4):352–356.

312. Mackay B, Luna MA, Butler JJ, Adult neuroblastoma. Electron microscopic observations in nine cases. *Cancer.* 1976;37(3):1334–1351.

313. Osborn M, Dirk T, Käser H, Weber K, Altmannsberger M. Immunohistochemical localization of neurofilaments and neuron-specific enolase in 29 cases of neuroblastoma. *Am J Pathol.* 1986;122(3):433–442.

314. Parodi S, Ognibene M, Haupt R, Pezzolo A. The over-expression of E2F3 might serve as prognostic marker for neuroblastoma patients with stage 4S disease. *Diagnostics (Basel).* 2020; 10(5):315.

315. Joshi VV, Silverman JF. Pathology of neuroblastic tumors. *Semin Diagn Pathol.* 1994;11(2):107–117.

316. Gambini C, Rongioletti F. Primary congenital cutaneous ganglioneuroma. *J Am Acad Dermatol.* 1996;35(2, pt 2):353–354.

317. Hammond RR, Walton JC. Cutaneous ganglioneuromas: a case report and review of the literature. *Hum Pathol.* 1996;27(7):735–738.

318. Collins JP, Johnson WC, Burgoon Jr CF. Ganglioneuroma of the skin. *Arch Dermatol.* 1972;105(2):256–258.

319. Rios JJ, Diaz-Cano SJ, Rivera-Hueto F, Villar JL. Cutaneous ganglion cell choristoma. Report of a case. *J Cutan Pathol.* 1991;18(6):469–473.

320. Franchi A, Massi D, Santucci M. Desmoplastic cutaneous ganglioneuroma. *Histopathology.* 1999;34(1):82–84.

321. Lee JY, Martinez AJ, Abell E. Ganglioneuromatous tumor of the skin: a combined heterotopia of ganglion cells and hamartomatous neuroma: report of a case. *J Cutan Pathol.* 1988;15(1): 58–61.

322. Hartman KR, Triche TJ, Kinsella TJ, Miser JS. Prognostic value of histopathology in Ewing's sarcoma. Long-term follow-up of distal extremity primary tumors. *Cancer.* 1991;67(1): 163–171.

323. Hashimoto H, Enjoji M, Nakajima T, Kiryu H, Daimaru Y. Malignant neuroepithelioma (peripheral neuroblastoma). A clinicopathologic study of 15 cases. *Am J Surg Pathol.* 1983;7(4):309–318.

324. Delaplace M, Lhommet C, de Pinieux G, Vergier B, de Muret A, Machet L. Primary cutaneous Ewing sarcoma: a systematic review focused on treatment and outcome. *Br J Dermatol.* 2012;166(4):721–726.

325. Banerjee SS, Agbamu DA, Eyden BP, Harris M. Clinicopathological characteristics of peripheral primitive neuroectodermal tumour of skin and subcutaneous tissue. *Histopathology.* 1997;31(4):355–366.

326. Hasegawa SL, Davison JM, Rutten A, Fletcher JA, Fletcher CD. Primary cutaneous Ewing's sarcoma: immunophenotypic and molecular cytogenetic evaluation of five cases. *Am J Surg Pathol.* 1998;22(3):310–318.

327. Fellinger EJ, Garin-Chesa P, Glasser DB, Huvos AG, Rettig WJ. Comparison of cell surface antigen HBA71 (p30/32MIC2), neuron-specific enolase, and vimentin in the immunohistochemical analysis of Ewing's sarcoma of bone. *Am J Surg Pathol.* 1992;16(8):746–755.

328. Ladanyi M, Lewis R, Garin-Chesa P, et al. EWS rearrangement in Ewing's sarcoma and peripheral neuroectodermal tumor. Molecular detection and correlation with cytogenetic analysis and MIC2 expression. *Diagn Mol Pathol.* 1993;2(3):141–146.

329. Brcic I, Brodowicz T, Cerroni L, et al. Undifferentiated round cell sarcomas with CIC-DUX4 gene fusion: expanding the clinical spectrum. *Pathology.* 2020;52(2):236–242.

330. Smith PD, Patterson JW. Merkel cell carcinoma (neuroendocrine carcinoma of the skin). *Am J Clin Pathol.* 2001;115(suppl):S68–S78.

331. Argenyi ZB, Schelper RL, Balogh K. Pigmented neuroectodermal tumor of infancy. A light microscopic and immunohistochemical study. *J Cutan Pathol.* 1991;18(1):40–45.

332. Kapadia SB, Frisman DM, Hitchcock CL, Ellis GL, Popek EJ. Melanotic neuroectodermal tumor of infancy. Clinicopathological, immunohistochemical, and flow cytometric study. *Am J Surg Pathol.* 1993;17(6):566–573.

333. Baran R, Kopf A, Schnitzler L. [Nasal glioma. Apropos of 4 cases, with electron microscopic study of one case]. *Ann Dermatol Syphiligr (Paris).* 1973;100(4):395–407.

334. Christianson HB. Nasal glioma. Report of a case. *Arch Dermatol.* 1966;93(1):68–70.

335. Yeoh GP, Bale PM, de Silva M. Nasal cerebral heterotopia: the so-called nasal glioma or sequestered encephalocele and its variants. *Pediatr Pathol.* 1989;9(5):531–549.

336. Kopf AW, Bart RS. Tumor conference No. 15: nasal glioma. *J Dermatol Surg Oncol.* 1978;4(2):128–130.

337. Skelton HG, Smith KJ. Glial heterotopia in the subcutaneous tissue overlying T-12. *J Cutan Pathol.* 1999;26(10):523–527.

338. Fletcher CD, Carpenter G, McKee PH. Nasal glioma. A rarity. *Am J Dermatopathol.* 1986;8(4):341–346.

339. Mirra SS, Pearl GS, Hoffman JC, Campbell WG Jr. Nasal "glioma" with prominent neuronal component: report of a case. *Arch Pathol Lab Med.* 1981;105(10):540–541.

340. Bossen EH, Hudson WR. Oligodendroglioma arising in heterotopic brain tissue of the soft palate and nasopharynx. *Am J Surg Pathol.* 1987;11(7):571–574.

341. Berry AD III, Patterson JW. Meningoceles, meningomyeloceles, and encephaloceles: a neuro-dermatopathologic study of 132 cases. *J Cutan Pathol.* 1991;18(3):164–177.

342. Chan HH, Fung JW, Lam WM, Choi P. The clinical spectrum of rudimentary meningocele. *Pediatr Dermatol.* 1998;15(5):388–389.

343. El Shabrawi-Caelen L, White WL, Soyer HP, Kim BS, Frieden IJ, McCalmont TH. Rudimentary meningocele: remnant of a neural tube defect? *Arch Dermatol.* 2001;137(1):45–50.

344. Lopez DA, Silvers DN, Helwig EB, Cutaneous meningiomas—a clinicopathologic study. *Cancer.* 1974;34(3):728–744.

345. Laymon CW, Becker FT. Massive metastasizing meningioma involving the scalp. *Arch Derm Syphilol.* 1949;59(6):626–635.

346. Suster S, Rosai J. Hamartoma of the scalp with ectopic meningothelial elements. A distinctive benign soft tissue lesion that may simulate angiosarcoma. *Am J Surg Pathol.* 1990;14(1):1–11.

347. Myong NH, Chi JG. Correlation of histopathologic classification with proliferative activity and DNA ploidy in 120 intracranial meningiomas, with special reference to atypical meningioma. *J Korean Med Sci.* 1997;12(3):221–227.

348. Mackay B, Bruner JM, Luna MA, Guillamondegui OM. Malignant meningioma of the scalp. *Ultrastruct Pathol.* 1994;18(1–2):235–240.

349. Theaker JM, Fleming KA. Meningioma of the scalp: a case report with immunohistological features. *J Cutan Pathol.* 1987;14(1):49–53.

350. Argenyi ZB, Thieberg MD, Hayes CM, Whitaker DC. Primary cutaneous meningioma associated with von Recklinghausen's disease. *J Cutan Pathol.* 1994;21(6):549–556.

351. Theaker JM, Gatter KC, Puddle J. Epithelial membrane antigen expression by the perineurium of peripheral nerve and in peripheral nerve tumours. *Histopathology.* 1988;13(2):171–179.

352. Gelli MC, Pasquinelli G, Martinelli G, Gardini G. Cutaneous meningioma: histochemical, immunohistochemical and ultrastructural investigation. *Histopathology.* 1993;23(6):576–578.

353. Pulitzer DR, Martin PC, Collins PC, Ralph DR. Subcutaneous sacrococcygeal ("myxopapillary") ependymal rests. *Am J Surg Pathol.* 1988;12(9):672–677.

354. Anderson MS. Myxopapillary ependymomas presenting in the soft tissue over the sacrococcygeal region. *Cancer.* 1966;19(4):585–590.

355. Monteagudo C, Jiménez AI, Arnandis A, Barr RJ. Meningioma-like tumor of the skin revisited: a distinct CD34+ dermal tumor with an expanded histologic spectrum. *Am J Surg Pathol.* 2019;43(11):1518–1525.

356. Miedema JR, Zedek D. Cutaneous meningioma. *Arch Pathol Lab Med.* 2012;136(2):208–211.

357. Reed RJ, Bliss BO. Morton's neuroma. Regressive and productive intermetatarsal elastofibrositis. *Arch Pathol.* 1973;95(2):123–129.

358. Reed RJ, Leonard DD. Neurotropic melanoma. A variant of desmoplastic melanoma. *Am J Surg Pathol.* 1979;3(4):301–311.

359. Lawrence N, Cottel WI. Squamous cell carcinoma of skin with perineural invasion. *J Am Acad Dermatol.* 1994;31(1):30–33.

360. Stern JB, Haupt HM. Reexcision perineural invasion. Not a sign of malignancy. *Am J Surg Pathol.* 1990;14(2):183–185.

361. Misdraji J, Ino Y, Louis DN, Rosenberg AE, Chiocca EA, Harris NL. Primary lymphoma of peripheral nerve: report of four cases. *Am J Surg Pathol.* 2000;24(9):1257–1265.

Metastatic Carcinoma of the Skin

PRIYADHARSINI NAGARAJAN AND MICHAEL T. TETZLAFF

Chapter

38

INCIDENCE AND DISSEMINATION

There is a critical need to recognize cutaneous metastases of visceral carcinomas for many reasons. First, they can be an important mimic of primary cutaneous carcinomas. Moreover, their discovery in the skin may be the first presenting indication of underlying disease. Second, the treatment of a tumor producing cutaneous metastasis would be different from that of a primary cutaneous tumor and unique according to the cell of origin. Whereas primary cutaneous carcinoma would be managed with surgical extirpation (and may also include sentinel lymphadenectomy), cutaneous dissemination of an underlying malignancy would more often be managed with systemic therapy, whose efficacy is tailored to the appropriate cell of origin. And, finally, cutaneous involvement by underlying malignancy often heralds advancement of stage and shortened patient survival.

Among patients with visceral malignancy, cutaneous metastases are generally uncommon. In a study of 7,316 patients with internal cancer (including all stages of disease), Lookingbill and colleagues (1) found that 5% (367) developed skin involvement. Among 4,020 patients with underlying malignancy who had known metastatic disease, Lookingbill and associates (2) reported that 10% (420) of these developed skin metastases, and of 7,518 patients with internal cancer who were autopsied at Roswell Park Memorial Institute, 9% had skin metastases (3).

A survey of 1,775 patients who developed cutaneous metastasis (2,4–12) reveals important themes. Overall, there is a relatively equal frequency of men versus women who develop cutaneous metastases (1.1:1), and the average age generally reflects the oncology population with a mean of 68 years (range: 37–90 years). The tumor type is reflected by the general demographics unique to each histology and their relative frequencies in the population. And among over 1,500 patients with cutaneous metastases, the cutaneous lesion was the first indication of underlying malignancy in 34% of the patients reported. The incidence of various tumors that are metastatic to the skin correlates well with the frequency of occurrence of the primary malignant tumor in each gender.

A review of 1,123 patients with cutaneous metastases (excluding melanoma) showed that in women (2,4,7,8,13), among 581 patients with known cutaneous metastases, 76.9% originated from breast carcinomas (447/581), commensurate with the greater frequency of carcinoma of the breast among women. This was followed in relative frequency by colorectal carcinoma (5.5%; 32/581), lung carcinoma (4.0%; 23/581), and ovarian

tumors (3.4%; 20/581). Among cutaneous metastases occurring in 542 men (2,4,7,8,13), the most common organ of origin was lung (27.7%; 150/542), large intestine (21.2%; 115/542), head and neck carcinomas (16.8%; 91/542), and carcinomas arising in the upper gastrointestinal tract (10.3%; 56/542). Metastatic melanoma is covered elsewhere (Chapter 28).

Owing to the relative rarity of carcinomas of the thyroid gland (14,15), pancreas (16), liver, gallbladder, urinary bladder (17), endometrium, prostate (18,19), testes, and neuroendocrine system, cutaneous metastases of these tumors are also relatively rare. A review by Schwartz (20) reported cutaneous metastatic disease as the first sign of internal cancer most commonly seen with cancers of the lung, kidney, and ovary.

Cutaneous metastases most commonly present as multiple, discrete, painless, and freely movable papules or nodules of sudden onset and relatively rapid growth. The nodules vary in size (usually 1 to 3 cm in diameter), although very large lesions have been reported (21). Less common presentations include plaques, rashes, and ulcerative lesions, depending on the extent of lymphatic or hematogenous involvement. A zosteriform pattern of skin metastasis has been reported to occur on the chest wall and abdominal wall, and the most frequent site of the primary was the breast, ovary, lung, prostate, bladder, and stomach (22,23). Dissemination of visceral malignancy may occur through the lymphatics or the bloodstream. Lymphatic spread reflects anatomic proximity to the primary tumor. For example, comparing carcinomas of the breast and oral cavity, because metastases reach the skin largely through lymphatic channels, their distribution in the skin typically reflects their anatomic proximity to those sites: oral cavity lesions most commonly metastasize to the skin of the head and neck, whereas breast carcinomas typically metastasize to the chest wall, abdomen, or breast skin. In contrast, metastatic lesions involving the skin from sites owing to hematogenous dissemination may appear in any area of the skin, although these tend to be enriched in more vascular sites, such as the scalp (head and neck), which accounts for ~5% of all cutaneous metastases (13). Metastasis to the umbilicus is also relatively common, and the underlying primary tumor is usually adenocarcinoma of the stomach, ovaries, endometrium, or breast (18,24).

Distinction of a primary carcinoma of the skin from a metastatic lesion can be a diagnostic challenge, particularly in the setting of a solitary lesion and no known history of an underlying visceral carcinoma. Primary cutaneous carcinomas that are particularly challenging mimics of visceral malignancies include primary mucinous adenocarcinoma of skin (25–27), adenocarcinoma of the mammary-like glands of the vulva (28), cutaneous signet-ring carcinoma (29), primary cutaneous carcinoids (30), and some adnexal carcinomas (31).

Establishing the diagnosis of a primary mucinous carcinoma of the skin involves the presence of a peripheral myoepithelial layer, which if present, is helpful by documenting the presence of an in-situ component (26). Immunoperoxidase positivity with CD15, CK5/6, and 34BE12 (27) might favor a primary lesion. Many have shown that p63 and D2-40 positivity favors a primary adenocarcinoma over a metastatic lesion (31–33). Other markers favoring a primary skin cancer include CK15, D2-40, and nestin (32–34). Except for sebaceous tumors, there is rare reactivity for primary adnexal carcinoma of the skin with CD10 in comparison with metastatic carcinoma, especially metastatic renal cell carcinoma (35). Some immunoperoxidase stains that are helpful in distinguishing primary tumors from metastatic lesions will be discussed in a histology-specific fashion later.

Molecular approaches for identification of tissue can also be used (36–38).

PRINCIPLES OF MANAGEMENT FOR CUTANEOUS METASTASES

The management of cutaneous metastases has been reviewed from a dermatologic perspective (39). A diagnosis of a cutaneous metastasis should prompt an assessment for the extent of metastatic disease and the total tumor burden, which will inform subsequent therapy. Excision of metastases is recommended only when surgically feasible and when this will result in a significant decrease in total tumor burden, such as in patients with oligometastatic disease (rendering the patient without evidence of disease), improved quality of life, or increased functionality.

Therapeutic options for patients with widespread cutaneous and subcutaneous metastases are directed according to the subtype of tumor. Options vary according to the unique biology of a given tumor type but may include radiotherapy, isolated limb perfusion, or interferon alfa injections for skin localized metastases. For patients with more widely disseminated disease, systemic chemotherapy, oncogene-targeted therapy, and immunotherapy are all viable options.

Sometimes, treatment of the primary cancer with an efficacious regimen may induce regression of cutaneous lesions. For example, an "abscopal response" represents an unusual response to radiation therapy in which radiation of a tumor at one location causes untreated distant skin lesions to also dissipate. The abscopal response has been reported with treatment of melanoma, Merkel cell carcinoma, and hematologic, and solid tumors and may be caused by activation of cellular immunity (39).

Novel treatments have had a profound impact on prolonging the survival and improving the quality of life in patients with metastatic cancer. Oncogene-targeted therapy represents a potential revolution, although its benefits so far have been limited for most patients. In general, tumors newly presenting with metastatic disease should be submitted for oncogenic mutation testing, increasingly performed using large gene panels. For instance, appropriate targeted therapy for metastatic melanoma associated with a mutation of the *BRAF* gene results in complete or partial tumor regression in most patients, with an estimated median progression-free survival of more than 7 months,

although recurrence is often inevitable, particularly when single agents are used (39). Current trials emphasize the use of agents targeting more than one oncogene (e.g., BRAF plus MEK inhibitors), in the hope of extending survival.

Even more promising therapy for patients with disseminated metastatic disease is the use of agents that amplify the host antitumor immune response. Examples include the use of immune checkpoint inhibitors, including the anti-CTLA-4 agent, ipilimumab, and monoclonal antibodies directed at the programmed death 1 (PD-1) protein or its ligand, PD-L1, including nivolumab, pembrolizumab, and avelumab. In the near future, use of these agents in various combinations with targeted therapy and other modalities will likely result in improved survival for patients with metastatic melanoma and for other cancers as well.

Carcinoma of the Breast

Cutaneous metastases that occur predominantly by lymphatic dissemination include nodular carcinoma, inflammatory carcinoma, carcinoma en cuirasse, telangiectatic carcinoma, and carcinoma of the inframammary crease. Alopecia neoplastica and mammary carcinoma of the eyelid are probably caused by hematogenous spread (20).

Clinical Summary. Nodular metastatic breast cancer appears as single or multiple firm, variably painful nodules ranging in size from 1 to 3 cm, which are situated in the dermis and/or subcutis and may be ulcerated (40,41). An exophytic nodule may occur in the inframammary crease, resembling a primary squamous cell or basal cell carcinoma, and occurs more frequently in women with large breasts.

Inflammatory breast carcinoma is characterized by an erythematous patch or a plaque with an active spreading border that resembles erysipelas/cellulitis and usually affects the breast and nearby skin (20,42,43). Rarely, inflammatory metastatic carcinoma may arise from primary involvement of other organs (44). The redness and warmth are attributed to capillary congestion.

En cuirasse metastatic carcinoma is characterized by a diffuse morphea-like (scar-like) induration of the skin and rarely involves skin from other primary carcinomas (45,46). It usually begins as scattered papular lesions coalescing into a sclerodermoid plaque without inflammatory changes.

Telangiectatic metastatic breast carcinoma is characterized by violaceous papulovesicles resembling purpura/hemorrhage or also lymphangioma circumscriptum (20,47,48). A violaceous hue, which is often present, is caused by blood in dilated vascular channels.

Alopecia neoplastica occurs as oval plaques or patches of the scalp and may be confused clinically with alopecia areata or a scarring alopecia. Metastatic mammary carcinoma in the eyelid clinically presents as a painless swelling with induration or as a discrete nodule (20). Of 10 metastatic tumors to the eyelids, 4 were breast carcinomas, 2 were renal, and 1 each was thyroid, prostate, lung, and salivary gland (49).

Histopathology. Nodular metastatic breast carcinoma is characterized by a proliferation of neoplastic cells forming expansile or infiltrative nodules in the dermis and/or subcutis (40,41). These nodules consist of variably sized groups of tumor cells arranged as glands, sheets, or cords. There is typically a fibroinflammatory stromal response. Depending on the tumor type (ductal versus lobular) some cells may show a glandular arrangement, which may be quite ill-defined (**Figs. 38-1 to 38-3**).

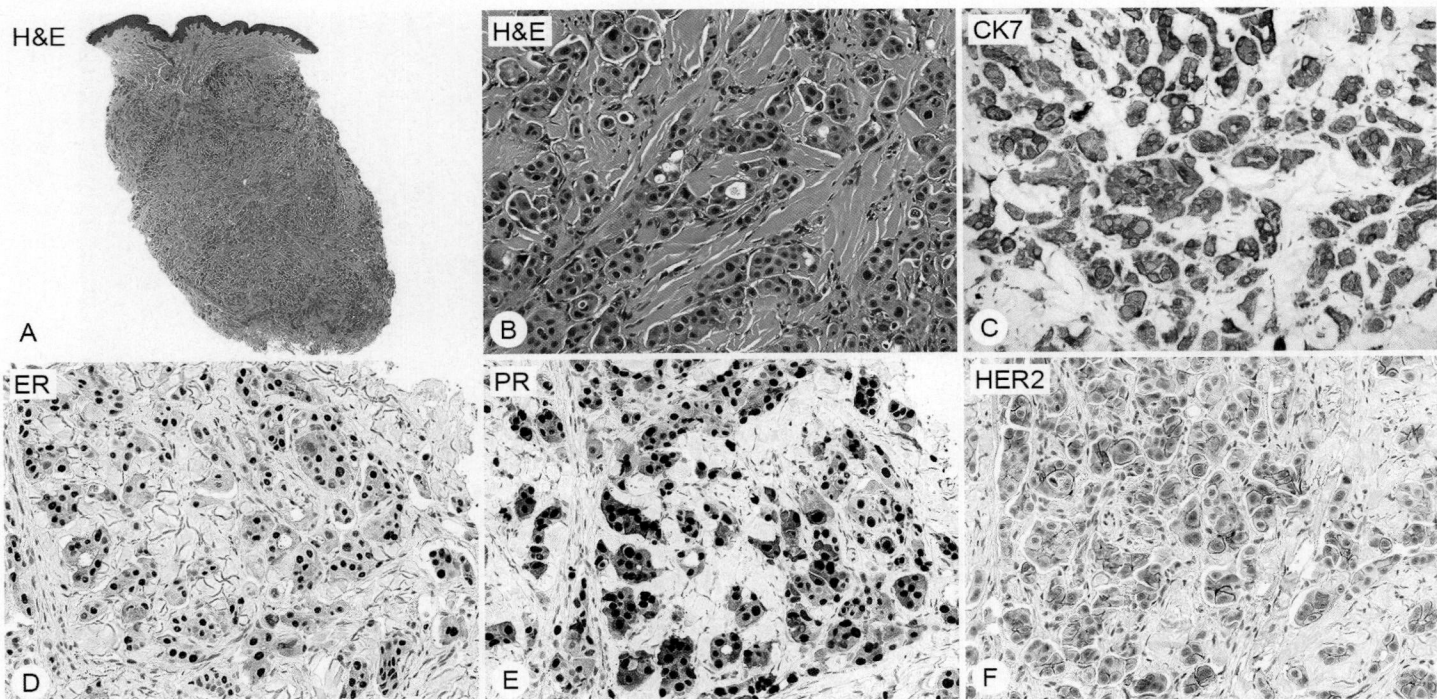

Figure 38-1 Metastatic breast carcinoma involving forehead; hormone-receptor positive, ductal type. A: Nodular tumor in dermis lacking epidermal involvement (hematoxylin and eosin, 20×), (**B**) composed of irregular clusters of epithelioid tumor cells with eosinophilic cytoplasm and round nuclei. Glandular differentiation is also present (hematoxylin and eosin, 200×). Tumor cells are positive for (**C**) cytokeratin 7 (CK7, 200×), (**D**) estrogen receptor (ER, 200×), (**E**) progesterone receptor (PR, 200×), and (**F**) HER2 (200×).

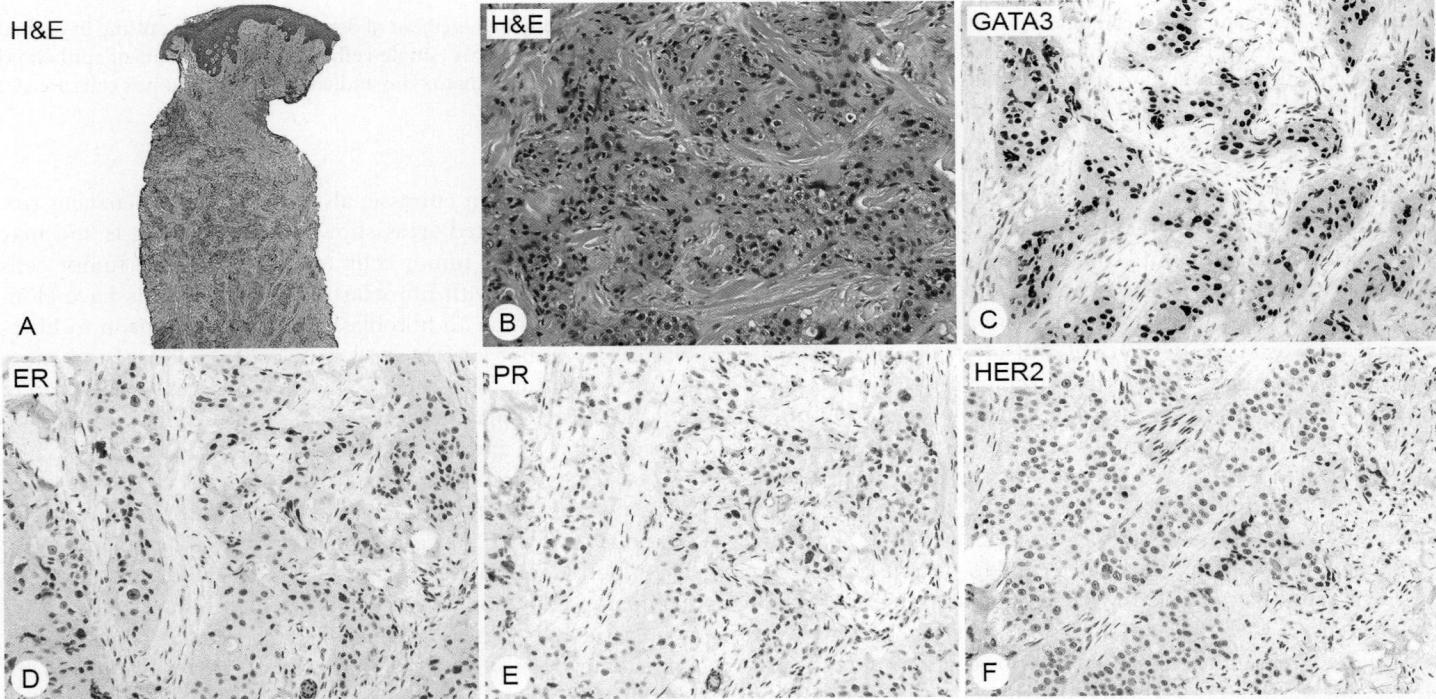

Figure 38-2 Metastatic triple negative breast carcinoma (TNBC) involving epigastric area. A: Nodular tumor in dermis lacking epidermal involvement (hematoxylin and eosin, 20×), (**B**) composed of irregular clusters of epithelioid tumor cells with eosinophilic somewhat granular cytoplasm and round nuclei. Glandular differentiation is not conspicuous (hematoxylin and eosin, 200×). Tumor cells are positive for (**C**) GATA3 (200×), but negative for hormone receptors (**D**) estrogen receptor (ER, 200×), (**E**) progesterone receptor (PR, 200×), (**F**) HER2 (200×).

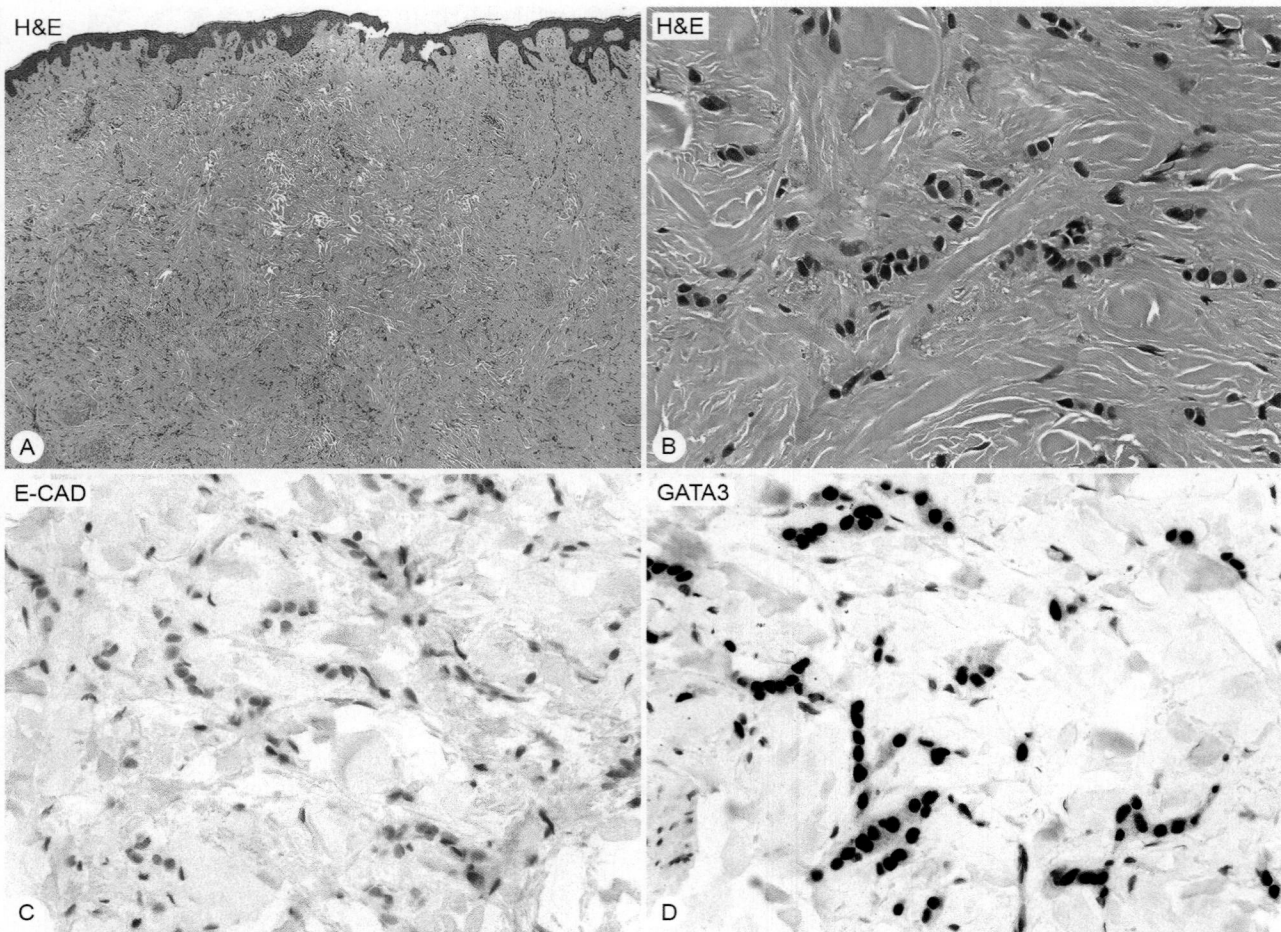

Figure 38-3 Metastatic breast carcinoma, lobular type, involving right upper flank. **A:** Subtle involvement of dermis by tumor, resulting in dermal hypercellularity (busy dermis) (hematoxylin and eosin, 40×). **B:** Tumor is composed of short cords (single-cell files) or single units of epithelioid tumor cells with small amounts of amphophilic cytoplasm and hyperchromatic ovoid nuclei (hematoxylin and eosin, 400×). Tumor cells are **(C)** negative for E-cadherin (E-CAD, 400×) and **(D)** positive for GATA3 (400×).

Sometimes, a nodule may be pigmented and clinically suggestive of a melanoma or pigmented basal cell carcinoma. The pigment results from melanin accumulation within the cytoplasm of neoplastic cells and in the stroma (50).

Inflammatory metastatic breast carcinoma is defined by extensive invasion of the dermal and often the subcutaneous lymphatics by groups and cords of tumor cells (42,43). Many examples of inflammatory carcinoma show restriction of tumor cells to the lymphatics, but there can be variable involvement of the adjacent dermis and subcutis by tumor cells. The morphology of the tumor cells often resembles that of the primary carcinoma and possesses variable amounts of pale eosinophilic cytoplasm and enlarged, overall irregular, often pleomorphic, and hyperchromatic nuclei. Marked capillary congestion—the consequence of tumor emboli—is present together with interstitial edema and underlies the clinical appearance of erythema and warmth (20). There is usually a variable perivascular lymphoid infiltrate. The extensive lymphatic dissemination is thought to be the result of retrograde lymphatic spread into the skin secondary to progressive blockage of the deep lymphatics and lymph nodes. Fibrosis is not a significant feature. Some studies indicate that only 1% to 4% of patients with metastatic breast carcinoma present with the inflammatory or erysipeloid type and that most of these patients have intraductal breast carcinoma (51).

In carcinoma en cuirasse, also referred to as *scirrhous carcinoma*, the indurated areas show hyalinized fibrosis and may contain only a few tumor cells (45,46,52). These tumor cells may be confused with fibroblasts. The tumor cells have elongated nuclei similar to fibroblasts, but in comparison to fibroblasts, the tumor nuclei are larger, more angular, and more deeply basophilic. The tumor cells often lie singly; however, in some areas, they may assemble in small groups or as single rows between fibrotic and thickened collagen bundles.

In telangiectatic carcinoma, the tumor cells tend to be located more superficially in the dermis within dilated lymphatic vessels than those in inflammatory carcinoma (47,48). The blood vessels are congested with red blood cells, as in inflammatory carcinoma, but usually also contain aggregates of neoplastic cells. The presence of many dilated blood vessels immediately beneath the epidermis gives rise to the clinical appearance of hemorrhagic vesicles.

Alopecia neoplastica describes the phenomenon of painless scarring alopecia secondary to metastasis to the heavily vascular skin of the scalp (53). Hematogenous deposition of tumor cells to the scalp skin evokes a fibroinflammatory response that culminates in the destruction of hair follicles and the development of clinical alopecia.

Carcinoma of the inframammary crease has been described as islands of epithelial cells with hyperchromatic nuclei extending contiguously with the epidermis from the dermis (54,55).

Epidermotropic involvement from metastatic breast carcinoma may mimic malignant melanoma and/or Paget disease (56).

The signet-ring cell histologic pattern of breast carcinoma (57) may also be seen in carcinoma of the gastrointestinal tract and urinary bladder (58). This may be confused with a primary cutaneous signet-ring cell carcinoma that occurs most frequently in middle-aged men on the eyelid and less frequently in the axilla (58). A primary mucinous carcinoma of the skin may also require distinction from metastatic lesions from the breast or colon (59). Rarely, a granular cell histologic pattern is seen.

Immunoperoxidase Studies. Cutaneous metastases of mammary carcinoma are positive with most cytokeratins, except for CK20 (59) (**Figs. 38-1 to 38-3**) and are often positive with epithelial membrane antigen (EMA) and carcinoembryonic antigen (CEA), although the latter lack specificity. Metastatic breast carcinomas also typically express GATA3, gross cystic disease fluid protein, estrogen and progesterone receptors, and mammaglobin (60–64). Reactivity with S-100 protein has been reported in cases of primary and metastatic breast carcinoma, particularly those lacking reactivity for hormone receptors, that is, triple negative breast cancers (**Fig. 38-2**) (65). The presence of melanin granules and melanosomes within tumor cells that give a positive HMB-45 is rare and probably occurs secondarily to phagocytosis or melanocyte colonization of the tumor cells (32). In lesions in which there are cells positive with S-100 or SOX10, strong, diffuse reactivity for keratins, EMA, and/or CEA would make melanoma less likely. Primary signet-ring carcinoma of the skin has been reported to be positive with CK7 and CK20, and this would aid in distinction from the breast, which is usually negative with CK20 (58). Most breast carcinomas are negative with D2-40, nestin, and CK15, but a subset showed 5% positive with CK15 (34,66).

Carcinoma of the Lung

Metastasis to the skin is more common in men, but the incidence of lung carcinoma in women is increasing (2,4,7,8,13). Cutaneous involvement from lung carcinoma is thought to occur early in the course of disease. Of 56 patients reported with skin metastasis from an underlying lung carcinoma, 7% had cutaneous involvement prior to the diagnosis of the primary tumor, whereas 16% had developed skin involvement concurrently with their primary lung cancer (67). In over half of the patients with cutaneous metastasis, the skin was the first extranodal site (1).

Clinical Summary. Metastases may occur on any cutaneous surface, but the most common sites are the chest wall and posterior abdomen (20,68–70). Small cell neuroendocrine carcinoma shows predilection for the skin of the back (2). Most lesions present as a localized cluster of cutaneous papules or nodules or as a solitary nodule with a red-purple color, occasionally mistaken for vascular lesions.

Histopathology. Cutaneous metastases from an underlying lung carcinoma (**Figs. 38-4 to 38-6**) showed an undifferentiated histopathologic pattern in approximately 40% of cases, whereas the remaining 60% of cases showed either frank adenocarcinoma or squamous cell carcinoma (4,68–70). The undifferentiated tumors were often of the small cell type with hyperchromatic nuclei and scant cytoplasm, typical of small cell carcinoma (formerly known as *oat cell carcinoma*) (4,68–70). Well-differentiated neuroendocrine tumors (carcinoid tumors) of the lung are derived from the bronchus and consist of solid islands and nests of uniform cells. Other sources include the stomach, small and large intestines, and primarily the skin. The closely packed tumor cells may suggest a malignant lymphoma. Immunoperoxidase studies are extremely helpful in making this distinction (71–74).

Squamous cell carcinomas metastatic to skin are usually poorly or moderately differentiated (**Fig. 38-4**) (4,75). They can usually be distinguished from primary squamous cell carcinoma by the absence of connection to or emanation from the surface epidermis and seldom show an orderly pattern of differentiation. They may show occasional whorls of squamoid cells with imperfect keratinization and individually keratinized cells and sometimes have large, bizarre forms with frequent mitotic figures and even acantholysis (76). In larger tumors, areas of central necrosis are often present. Most cutaneous metastatic squamous cell carcinomas arise in the lung, oral cavity, or esophagus. Tumors from the oral cavity tend to be more differentiated and nearly always appear on the head or neck. Squamous carcinoma metastatic from the esophagus shows essentially similar features to that from the lung.

Adenocarcinomas metastatic to the skin from the lung are often moderately differentiated, but some show well-formed, mucin-secreting, glandular structures (**Fig. 38-5**). Individual tumor cells sometimes contain abundant cytoplasmic mucin but

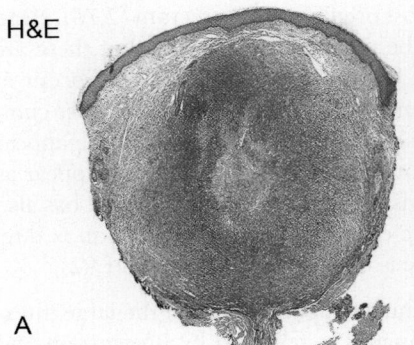
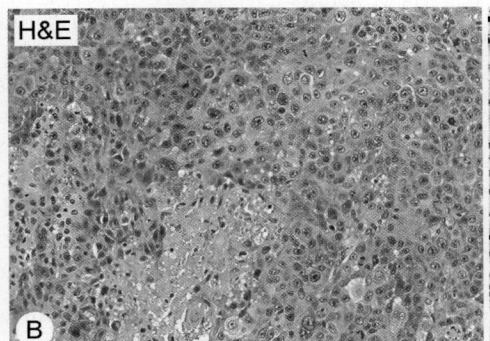
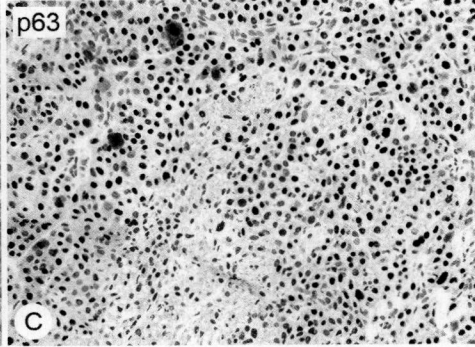

Figure 38-4 Metastatic squamous cell carcinoma from lung involving left lateral back. **A:** Nodular tumor involving dermis (hematoxylin and eosin, 20×), (**B**) composed of sheets of epithelioid cells with eosinophilic cytoplasm, ovoid nuclei, vesicular chromatin and prominent nucleoli, focally necrotic (lower center) (hematoxylin and eosin, 200×). **C:** Tumor cells are diffusely positive for p63 (200×).

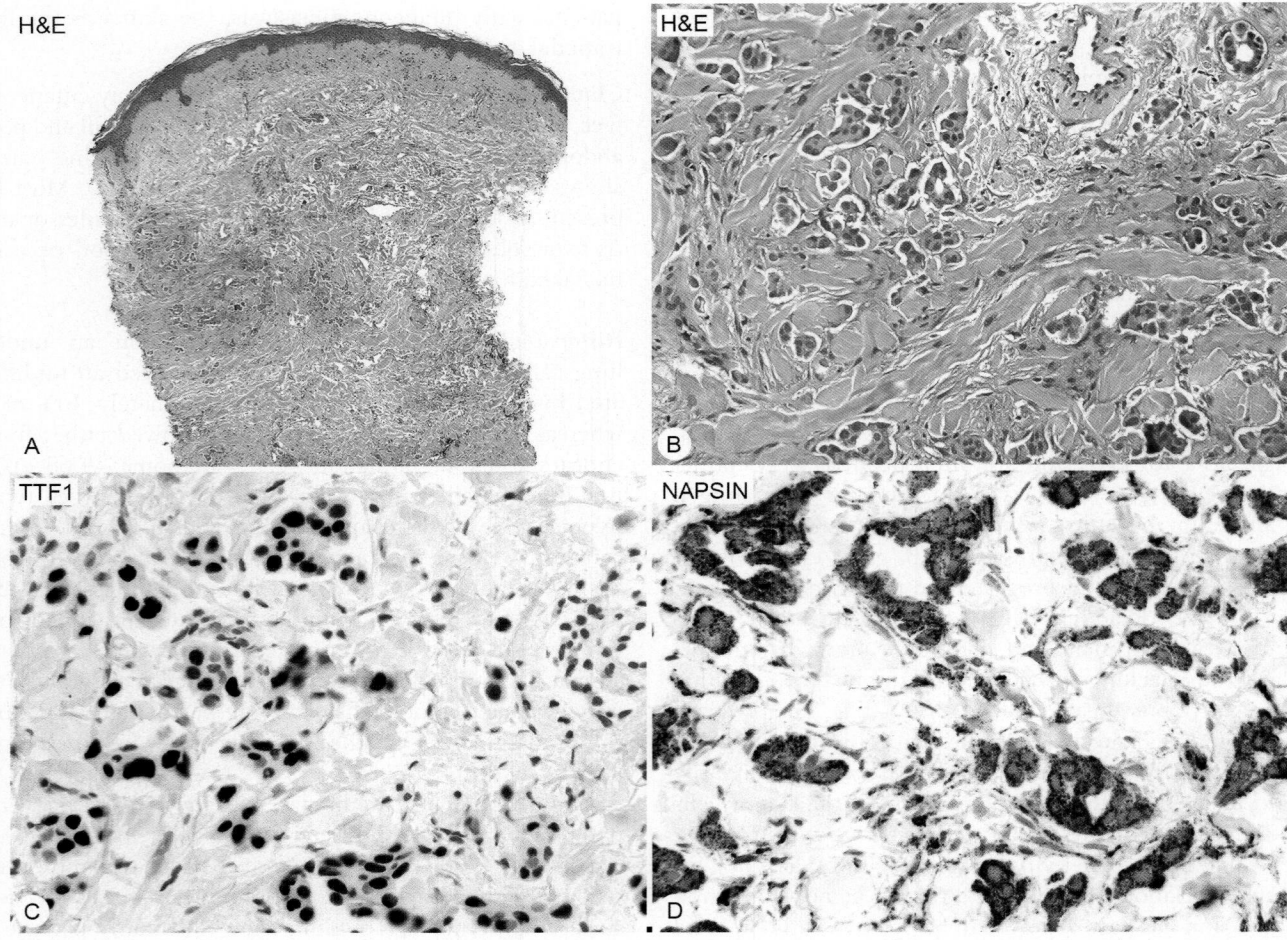

Figure 38-5 Metastatic adenocarcinoma from lung involving sternal notch. **A:** Infiltrative tumor involving dermis (hematoxylin and eosin, 40×), **(B)** composed of irregular nests of epithelioid cells with glandular differentiation. Tumor cells are positive for **(C)** TTF1 (400×) and **(D)** Napsin (400×).

usually lack large pools of mucin, which is more characteristically seen from gastrointestinal metastatic adenocarcinomas (4).

Immunoperoxidase Studies. The immunophenotype of pulmonary metastases to the skin varies according to the histopathologic subtype (**Figs. 38-4 to 38-6**). Undifferentiated small cell carcinoma expresses TTF-1 and Cam5.2 but is negative for CK20 and up to 50% positive for CK7 (**Fig. 38-6**) (77). The latter is critical to distinguishing this from primary cutaneous Merkel cell carcinoma, which usually expresses CK20, NF-1 and, in ~80% of cases, Merkel cell carcinoma polyomavirus T antigen (78–80). Merkel cell carcinomas usually show a CK20, perinuclear dot, and/or diffuse positivity, and this is rarely seen in metastatic neuroendocrine carcinomas (81). Both small cell carcinomas and Merkel cell carcinomas show reactivity to one or more of the following neuroendocrine markers: chromogranin-A, CD56 antigen (Leu-7), synaptophysin, and INSM1 (82,83). Negative reactions with lymphocyte common antigen (LCA) and other lymphoid markers (CD3 and CD20) are most helpful in ruling out malignant lymphomas (79, 80). Thyroid transcription factor 1 (TTF-1) is positive in thyroid carcinoma and small cell lung carcinoma and is negative in most cases of Merkel cell carcinoma (81,84,85). Achaete–scute complex-like 1 (MASH1, ASCL1) is usually positive in small cell carcinoma of the lung dend negative in Merkel cell carcinoma (86).

Although keratins are positive in most metastatic carcinomas, metastatic pulmonary adenocarcinomas are positive for CK7, TTF-1, and napsin as well as EMA and CEA

(60,78,87–89). Metastatic squamous cell carcinoma of the lung expresses CK5/6, p63, and p40 (identical to squamous cell carcinomas from other sites) (87,88).

Gastrointestinal Carcinoma

Carcinoma of the colon and rectum is the second most common type of primary cancer in men and women (2,4,6,8,10,13,20).

Clinical Summary. Cutaneous lesions usually appear after the primary tumor has been recognized and occur more commonly on the skin of the abdomen or perineal areas, reflecting not only their anatomic proximity but also their predilection for previous scar sites (90), because most originate in the rectum (2,70). Head and neck areas may also be the site of metastasis, but these are less common. Metastases from gastric carcinoma may occur at any distant site, but the umbilical region is perhaps most common (the "Sister Mary Joseph nodule"). Clinically, these appear as solitary or multiple grouped nodules but may also appear as plaques or ulcerated lesions. Subcutaneous involvement has also been described. Pancreatic cancer metastatic to the skin is rare, and the most common site is the umbilical area (20,91,92).

Histopathology. Most cutaneous metastases from the large intestine and all from the stomach, as reported by Brownstein and Helwig (4,93), were adenocarcinomas (**Fig. 38-7**). Colorectal carcinomas most commonly colonize the dermis or subcutis with sparing of the epidermis, although epidermotropism has

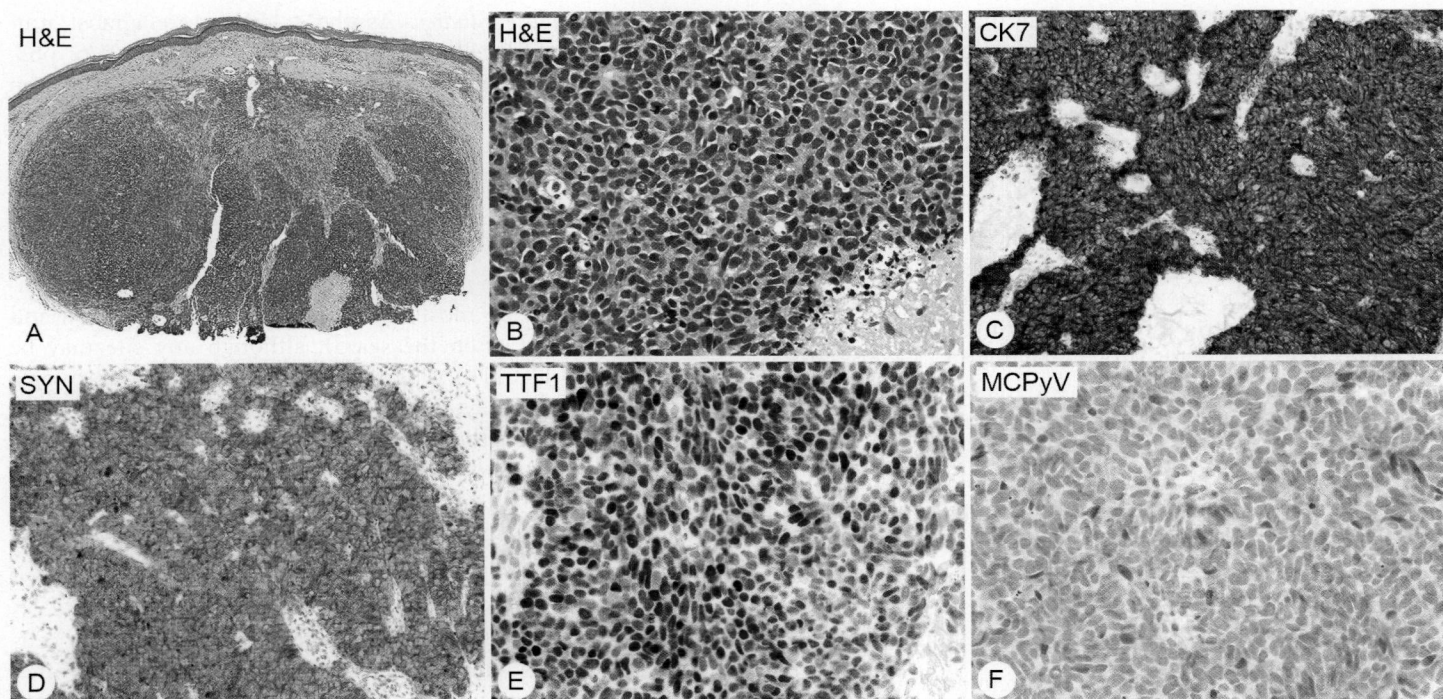

Figure 38-6 Metastatic small cell carcinoma from lung involving right infraclavicular area. **A:** Nodular tumor in dermis lacking epidermal involvement (hematoxylin and eosin, 20×), **(B)** composed of tightly packed sheets of epithelioid cells with minimal eosinophilic cytoplasm, hyperchromatic angulated nuclei (hematoxylin and eosin, 400×). Tumor cell necrosis involving single cells is noted throughout the neoplasm, whereas there is also geographic necrosis (right lower corner). The tumor cells are positive for **(C)** cytokeratin 7 (CK7, 200×), **(D)** synaptophysin (SYN, 200×), and **(E)** TTF1 (400×) but are **(F)** negative for Merkel cell polyomavirus (MCPyV, 400×).

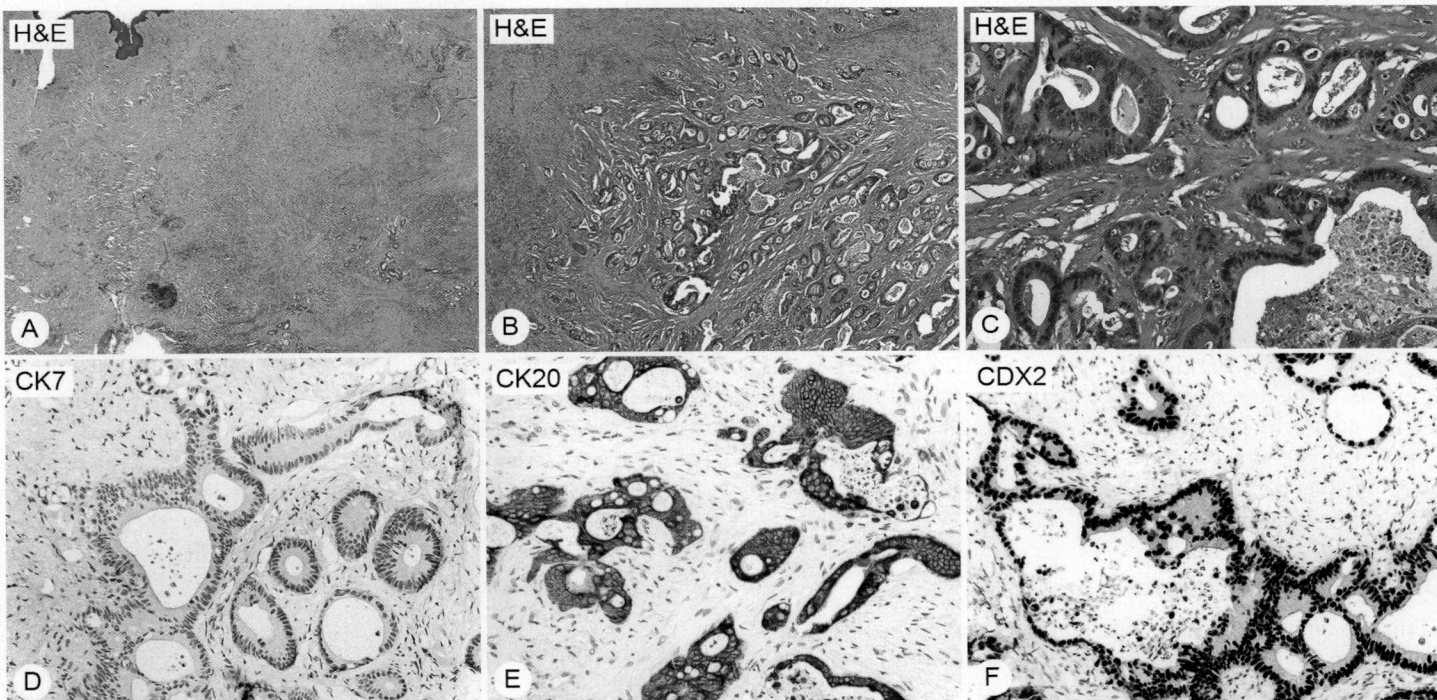

Figure 38-7 Metastatic carcinoma from the colon involving midabdomen (periumbilical area). **A:** Infiltrating glandular cells involving deep dermis and subcutis in a background of dense fibrosis (hematoxylin and eosin, 20×). **B:** The tumor is composed of irregular glandular structures and cords of tumor cells (hematoxylin and eosin, 40×), **(C)** lined by columnar cells with hyperchromatic nuclei (hematoxylin and eosin, 200×). Characteristic dirty necrosis is noted in the right lower corner. The tumor cells are **(D)** negative for cytokeratin 7 (CK7, 200×) and positive for **(E)** cytokeratin 20 (CK20, 200×), and **(F)** CDX2 (200×).

been described (94). Occasionally, the tumor cells closely approximate the epidermis so as to mimic a primary adenocarcinoma. The tumor cells range from well to poorly differentiated glands. A typical feature of colorectal adenocarcinoma is the presence of central necrosis with clusters of admixed neutrophils (so-called dirty necrosis). A mucinous carcinoma pattern with small groups of tumor cells that lie in large pools of mucin is common in lesions from the large intestine. Signet-ring cell differentiation is not usually seen in lesions from the large intestine but may be present in lesions from the stomach (4). Metastases from gastric carcinomas are usually anaplastic, infiltrating carcinomas with variable cellularity, a loose stroma, and varying proportions of signet-ring cells. The mucin present in metastatic carcinoma from the gastrointestinal tract as well as in mucinous carcinomas from the breast and lung is a non-sulfated, hyaluronidase-resistant, sialic acid–type of mucosubstance (95–97). Metastases from underlying pancreatic adenocarcinomas usually present as an adenocarcinoma with similar morphology to that of the primary tumor. The differential diagnosis for metastatic carcinoma includes carcinomas of cutaneous adnexa such as sweat gland carcinomas.

Immunoperoxidase Studies. Colorectal carcinomas typically show positivity for CK20 and CDX2 but negativity for CK7 (**Fig.** 38-7) (60,98–102). CK20 can also be positive in Merkel cell carcinoma (80), pancreatic carcinoma (62%) (103), gastric carcinoma (50%) (104), cholangiocarcinomas (43%) (105), and transitional cell carcinomas (29%) (106,107), and this marker was nearly absent in carcinomas from other organ systems and in malignant mesotheliomas. Mucinous carcinoma of the skin, which is generally thought to derive from the sweat glands, is positive with numerous cytokeratins but is negative with CK20. This would allow distinction from a metastatic mucinous adenocarcinoma of the colon, which would be positive with CK20 (108).

CDX2 expression is seen in most tumors of the intestinal tract and urothelial carcinoma and is thought to be useful in identifying extragenital Paget disease with involvement of the colon (99,109). Gastric carcinomas are typically positive for CK7, CDX2, and CK20 (60,98). Pancreatic carcinomas usually express CK7, CK8, CK18, and CK19, so cytokeratin cocktails containing these can be sensitive markers but lack specificity. Immunoperoxidase with a carbohydrate antigen (CA19-9) may be positive (16,60,92). Finally, loss of SMAD4 (DPC4) expression has been described in approximately 50% of pancreatic ductal adenocarcinomas, 25% of cholangiocarcinomas, and 15% of colorectal carcinomas and can be helpful in delineating possible sites of origin for adenocarcinoma involving the skin (110,111).

Oral Cavity Carcinoma

Clinical Summary. Most lesions metastasizing from carcinomas of the oral cavity are spread by lymphatic invasion and are located on the face or neck (4). They usually appear as multiple or solitary nodules and are sometimes ulcerated.

Histopathology. The lesions are almost always squamous cell in type and are usually moderately or well differentiated (4). They are located usually in the deeper dermis and subcutaneous tissue with sparing of the superficial cutis. In examples with ulceration and involvement of the upper corium, distinction from primary squamous cell carcinoma of skin may not be possible (4).

Immunoperoxidase Studies. As these lesions are almost uniformly squamous cell carcinomas, they express CK5/6, p63, and p40. Depending on the site of involvement, the detection of high-risk human papillomavirus (HPV) and p16 may also be useful in distinguishing an oral cavity metastasis from a primary cutaneous squamous cell carcinoma (1,112).

Renal Cell Carcinoma

Clinical Summary. In metastatic renal cell carcinoma (RCC), cutaneous tumors are most commonly located in the head and neck area (most often the scalp), although any site may be involved (20,113,114). They typically present as solitary or a few nodules and may be skin colored, reddish, or violaceous. They may occur as the first sign of internal cancer or as late as 10 years after diagnosis of the primary. They occur more commonly in men.

Histopathology. The histologic features are usually those of a heavily vascularized clear cell adenocarcinoma. They are often localized, well-circumscribed intradermal nodules and may extend to the overlying epidermis (4) (**Fig.** 38-8). The tumor cells show oval nuclei with abundant, clear cytoplasm and are often in a glandular configuration. Importantly, the cytoplasmic lipid in clear cell RCC does not impact the contours of the nuclear membrane, as seen in tumors with sebaceous differentiation. The stroma is heavily vascularized, and extravasated red blood cells are frequent. Intracytoplasmic glycogen is uniformly present, and can be demonstrated by staining with periodic acid–Schiff (PAS) and diastase-labile intracytoplasmic material. Frozen sections stained with oil red O show the presence of lipid droplets in many tumor cells (113). The histologic differential diagnosis includes adnexal tumors and, especially, nodular hidradenoma. In contrast to the usual unilobular and hemorrhagic RCC, the eccrine acrospiroma tends to be multilobular and nonhemorrhagic, and often distinct ductal structures are present, and a dense hyaline stroma. Sebaceous cell tumors may also be considered, but the markedly vascular stroma and hemorrhagic nature of RCCs is fairly distinctive, whereas in sebaceous tumors, the cytoplasmic clearing is caused by vacuoles, which often impinge or indent the nucleus.

Immunoperoxidase Studies. In most cases, the tumor cells stain positively with pan-cytokeratin, cytokeratin AE1/AE3, CAM5.2, EMA, and CD10 (35,115,116). They are usually negative with CK7 and CK20, and about 60% in one study were positive with vimentin (117–119). Renal cell carcinoma marker (RCC-Ma) is positive (119). Additional stains that are of help in recognizing renal cell metastatic lesions include PAX2 (21,116,120–125), PAX 8, carbonic anhydrase-IX (CA-IX) (**Fig.** 38-8C, **D**), and CD10.

Carcinoma of the Ovary

Clinical Summary. Metastatic carcinoma of the ovary most frequently involves the skin of the abdomen, including the umbilicus, vulva, or back (20,126), reflecting their anatomic proximity to the ovaries. Lesions of the abdomen may involve the scar sites from surgery or diagnostic procedures (2).

Histopathology. These tumors reflect the primary tumor and are most commonly those of a moderately or well-differentiated adenocarcinoma, often having a papillary configuration and

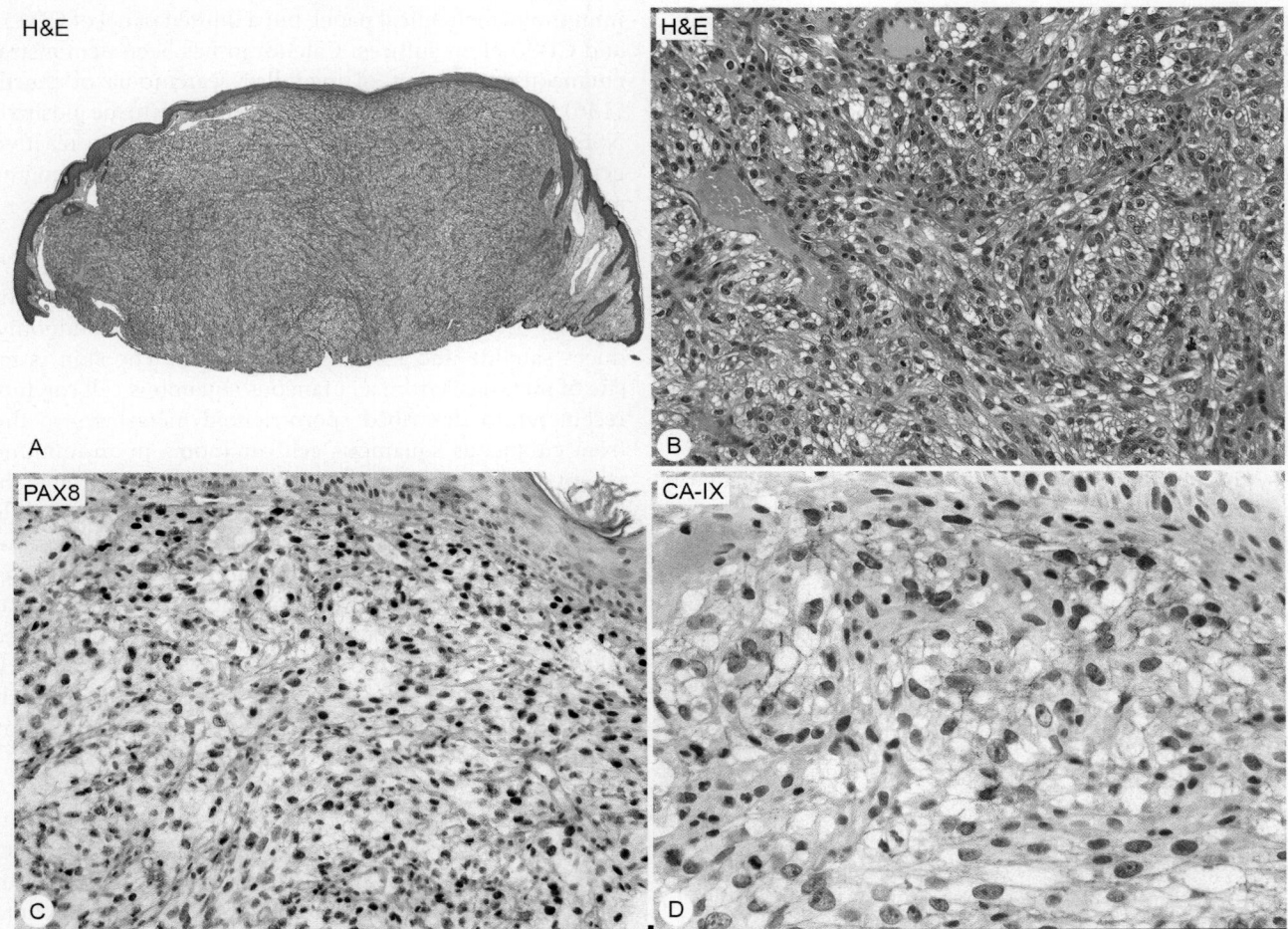

Figure 38-8 Metastatic clear cell renal cell carcinoma involving left postauricular neck. (**A**) Nodular, polypoid tumor in dermis abutting the epidermis (hematoxylin and eosin, 20×). **B:** The tumor is composed of sheets of epithelioid cells with abundant clear and pale amphophilic cytoplasm (hematoxylin and eosin, 200×). The tumor cells are positive for (**C**) PAX8 (200×), and (**D**) carbonic anhydrase-IX (CA-IX, 400×).

sometimes containing psammoma bodies, or with mucinous features. In 724 patients studied by Brownstein and Helwig (4), psammoma bodies in cutaneous masses were found only in metastases from the ovary (but might also be seen in papillary carcinomas from other sites, including, e.g., the thyroid).

Immunoperoxidase Studies. Papillary ovarian tumors are typically strongly and diffusely positive for CK7 and CA125 but negative for CK20 (127). Mucinous ovarian carcinomas (**Fig. 38-9**) were CK7 positive, and a few were CK20 negative

(66). PAX 8 discriminates ovarian metastases from adrenal and other cutaneous metastases but may be positive in renal, thyroid, and endometrial tumors (122,128,129). WT1 is also frequently positive in ovarian carcinomas (130).

Neuroendocrine Carcinomas

Clinical Summary. Lesions appear as solitary or multiple cutaneous papules or nodules and may occur at any site. Primary well-differentiated neuroendocrine tumors (previously

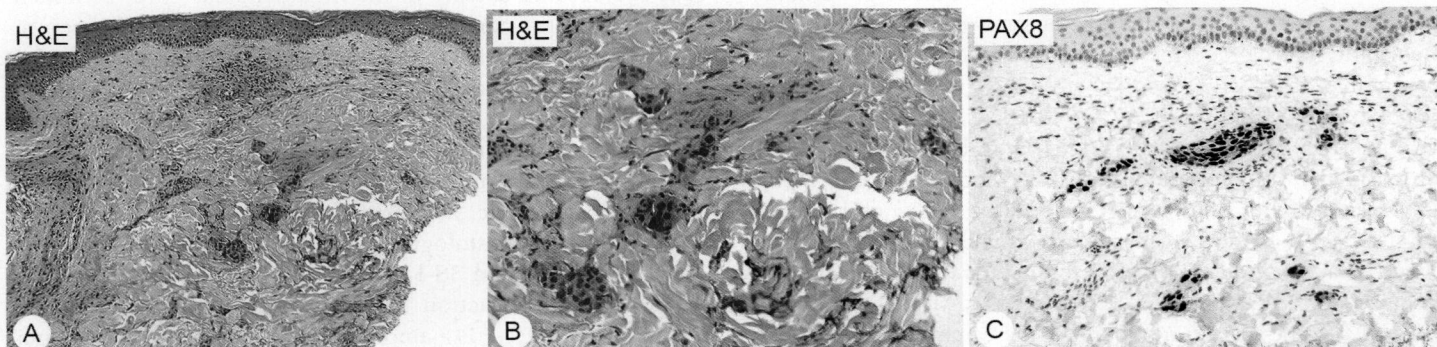

Figure 38-9 Metastatic ovarian serous carcinoma involving left breast skin. **A:** Small clusters of tumor cells in dermis and occasionally also within capillaries (hematoxylin and eosin, 100×), (**B**) composed of epithelioid cells with high nuclear to cytoplasmic ratio (hematoxylin and eosin, 200×). **C:** The tumor cells are positive for PAX8 (200×).

referred to as carcinoids) giving rise to cutaneous metastases (**Fig. 38-6**) occur most frequently in the bronchi but have been reported from various sites containing neuroendocrine cells, including the small intestine, sigmoid colon, pancreas, stomach, thymus, and thyroid (74). In addition, cutaneous metastases from neuroendocrine carcinomas of a variety of sites, including the uterus, vulva, gallbladder, and fallopian tubes, have been reported (20,131). Neuroblastoma, which is the most common cancer among newborns, has been reported to metastasize to the subcutaneous tissue in 32% of patients with congenital neuroblastoma (20,126,132). Clinically, these lesions exhibit a fairly specific appearance, which has been described as a "blueberry muffin." This term has also been used to describe some cases of congenital leukemia and extramedullary hematopoiesis. Cutaneous neuroblastoma is very rare in adults, and it is impossible to distinguish between primary and metastatic lesions except for finding an internal primary tumor (133).

Histopathology. Well-differentiated neuroendocrine (carcinoid) tumor metastases in the skin and subcutaneous tissue consist of solid islands, nests, and cords of tumor cells (**Fig. 38-6**). As a rule, the cells appear quite uniform in size and shape; have small, rounded nuclei; and abundant, clear, or eosinophilic cytoplasm occasionally containing numerous eosinophilic granules (74). However, in some instances, the nuclei are hyperchromatic, and there may be areas in which the nuclei show anaplasia by being irregularly shaped, large, and hyperchromatic. The histologic differential diagnosis may include sweat gland carcinoma or glomus tumor because of the arrangement of cells in well-defined islands, as well as metastases from other neuroendocrine tumors, and primary Merkel cell carcinoma. The latter usually show more immature cells or greater cellular atypia, a greater number of mitotic figures, and a "trabecular" pattern. Involvement of the deep dermis and multiple skin sites favor a metastatic lesion (131). Primary or metastatic neuroblastomas (peripheral neuroectodermal tumor) show identical features of undifferentiated, small, hyperchromatic cells with frequent rosettes of the Homer-Wright type and numerous mitoses (133). Some examples of undifferentiated lesions may not show rosettes. The histologic differential diagnosis includes other small cell carcinomas that sometimes show rosette-like structures, extraskeletal Ewing sarcoma, lymphoma, and leukemia.

Immunoperoxidase and Electron Microscopic Studies. Immunoperoxidase studies are of great value in distinguishing a primary neuroendocrine (Merkel cell) carcinoma of the skin from a metastatic neuroendocrine carcinoma (**Fig. 38-6**). Merkel cell carcinomas are usually positive with CK20 (79,80,134) but are negative with TTF-1 and CK7 (79–81,85). If the lesion is positive for CEA in non-ductal or non-glandular sites, this would strongly favor a metastatic lesion (83). The presence of a positive reaction with neuron specific enolase (NSE) and EMA is not necessarily helpful, because these can be reactive in primary or secondary neuroendocrine carcinomas as well as sweat gland carcinomas. Reactivity with CK20 favors a Merkel cell tumor but may also be seen in neuroendocrine carcinomas of salivary origin (135). If the tumor is positive with S-100, this favors an eccrine sweat gland carcinoma, metastatic breast carcinoma, or malignant melanoma. Exclusion of cutaneous involvement by lymphoma (systemic or primary cutaneous) requires a broad immunohistochemical panel, but a limited panel of CD45, CD3, and CD20 often suffices. Calcitonin has been demonstrated in cutaneous metastasis of medullary carcinoma of the thyroid (136). Neuroblastoma has been reported to be positive with NSE but is often negative with other commonly reactive antigens of neuroendocrine tumors such as EMA, chromogranin-A, and synaptophysin (133).

Carcinoma of the Skin

Metastases can occur from primary skin cancers to other cutaneous sites. Malignant melanoma not uncommonly produces satellite and in-transit metastases. The skin is rarely a site of metastasis from a cutaneous squamous cell carcinoma. A recent report described sporotrichoid metastases to the skin from cutaneous squamous cell carcinoma in an immunocompetent patient (137). In another example illustrated here, a lesion was clinically described as a subcutaneous nodule, and histopathology shows an atypical squamous proliferation without a connection to the overlying epidermis. In such a case, the possibility of metastasis from another site, such as head and neck or lung, should be considered by immunohistochemistry and clinically. The tumor cells were positive with CKAE1/AE3, p63, D2-40, and CK15 (**Fig. 38-10**). Review of records showed that a squamous cell carcinoma had been excised from a nearby skin site a month before.

Miscellaneous Carcinomas

In metastatic hepatocellular carcinoma from the liver, the arrangement of malignant hepatocytes in irregular columns is fairly distinctive, and if there are acinar structures containing bile, the diagnosis is definite (138). The tumor cells express polyclonal CEA (in a canalicular pattern similar to that seen in primary hepatocellular carcinoma), alpha-fetoprotein (AFP), and alpha-1-antitrypsin.

In choriocarcinoma, the cutaneous metastases show the two types of cells that arise from the fetal trophoblast: cytotrophoblasts and syncytiotrophoblasts. The cytotrophoblasts usually grow in clusters, and the cells appear cuboidal with large, vesicular nuclei and a pale cytoplasm. The syncytiotrophoblasts, which have large and irregular nuclei and a basophilic cytoplasm, grow around the clusters of cytotrophoblasts in a plexiform pattern resembling chorionic villi (77,139). The syncytiotrophoblasts have been reported to be strongly positive for human chorionic gonadotropin (HCG) antigen (140).

Metastatic carcinoma of the prostate to the skin is rare, and if it occurs, it is usually in the inguinal area, lower abdomen, or thighs, but distant sites of the scalp and face have been reported (20). Reactivity with prostate-specific antigen (PSA) and/or prostatic acid phosphatase (PAP) helps to establish the diagnosis (141).

Cutaneous metastases from thyroid carcinoma tend to involve the abdominal skin or the head area (20). Papillary, follicular, anaplastic, and medullary thyroid carcinomas typically retain their histologic patterns in the cutaneous metastases (**Figs. 38-11 and 38-12**). Immunoperoxidase studies often show a positive reaction to CK7, antithyroglobulin antibody (142), and TTF1 (34) among papillary and follicular carcinomas, whereas PAX8 also highlights papillary, follicular, and anaplastic carcinomas. Medullary carcinoma of the thyroid is positive for calcitonin but, in contrast to the other subtypes, lacks reactivity for PAX8.

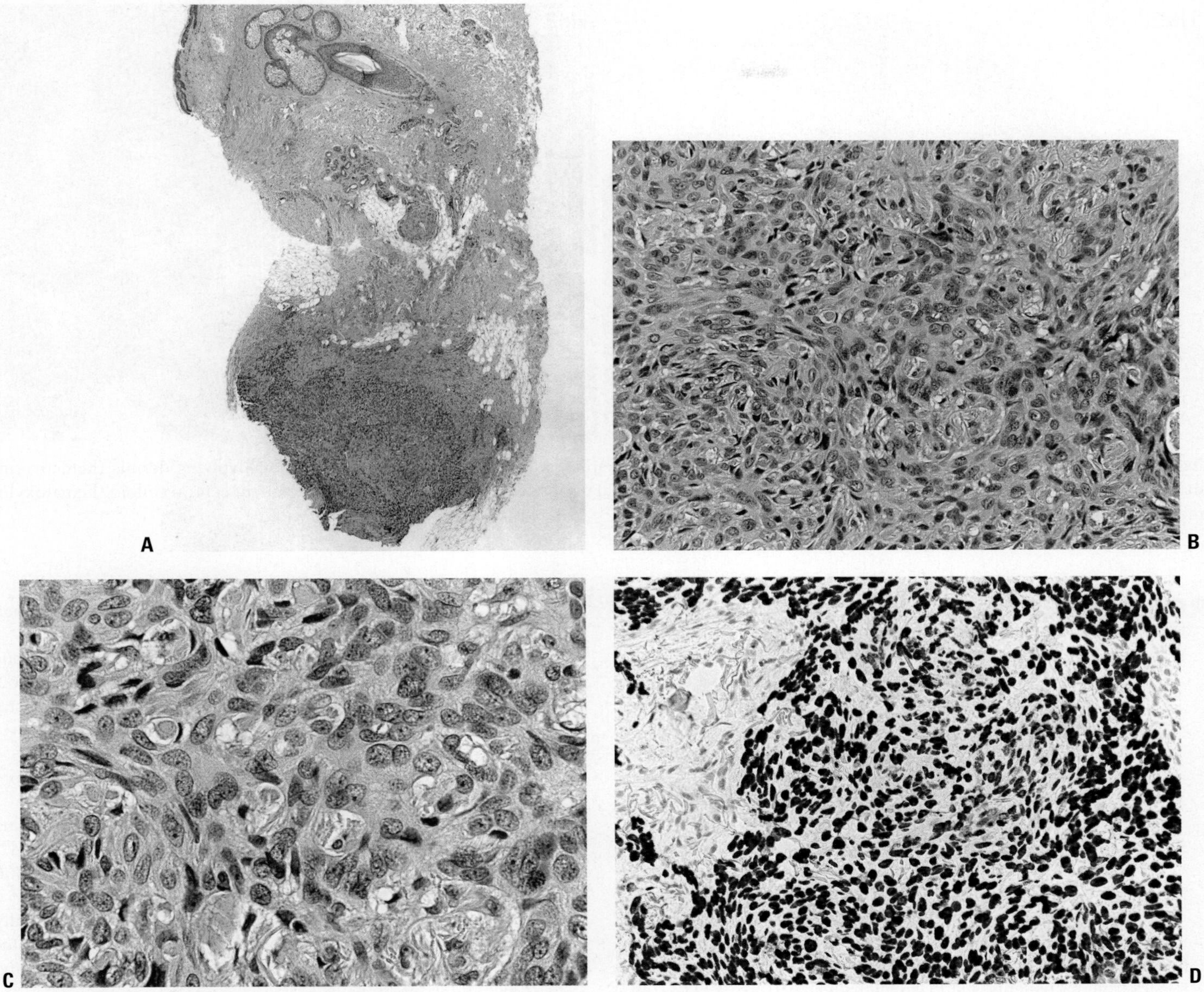

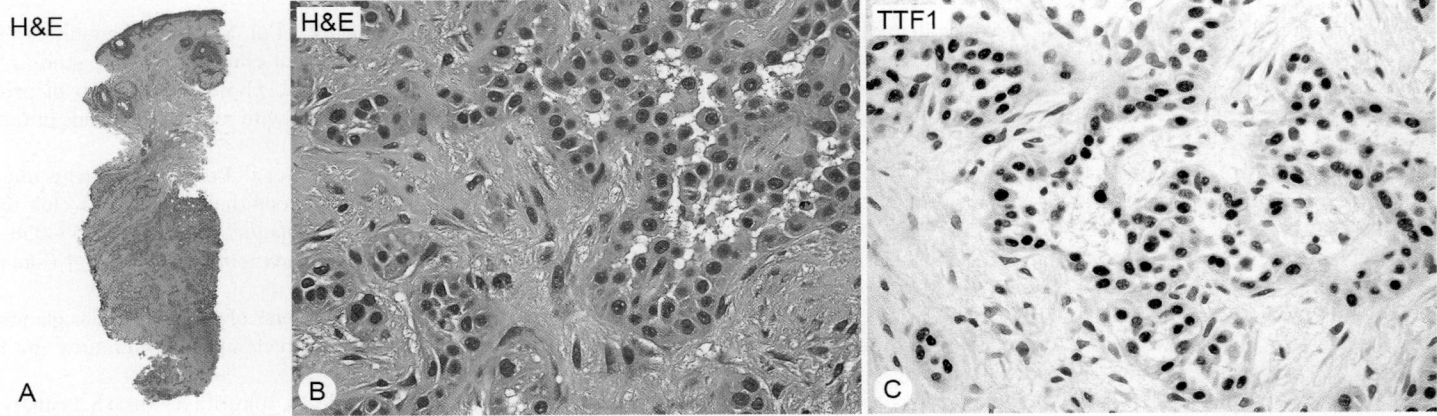

Figure 38-10 **Metastatic squamous cell carcinoma, skin primary.** Squamous cell carcinoma metastatic to the skin. A: hematoxylin and eosin, 20×. B: hematoxylin and eosin, 200×. C: hematoxylin and eosin, 400×. D: p63, 200×.

Figure 38-11 Metastatic poorly differentiated papillary thyroid carcinoma involving vertex of scalp. A: Deep dermal-subcutaneous nodular tumor (hematoxylin and eosin, 20×), (**B**) composed of irregular nests of epithelioid cells with acantholysis (hematoxylin and eosin, 400×), (**C**) positive for TTF1 (400×).

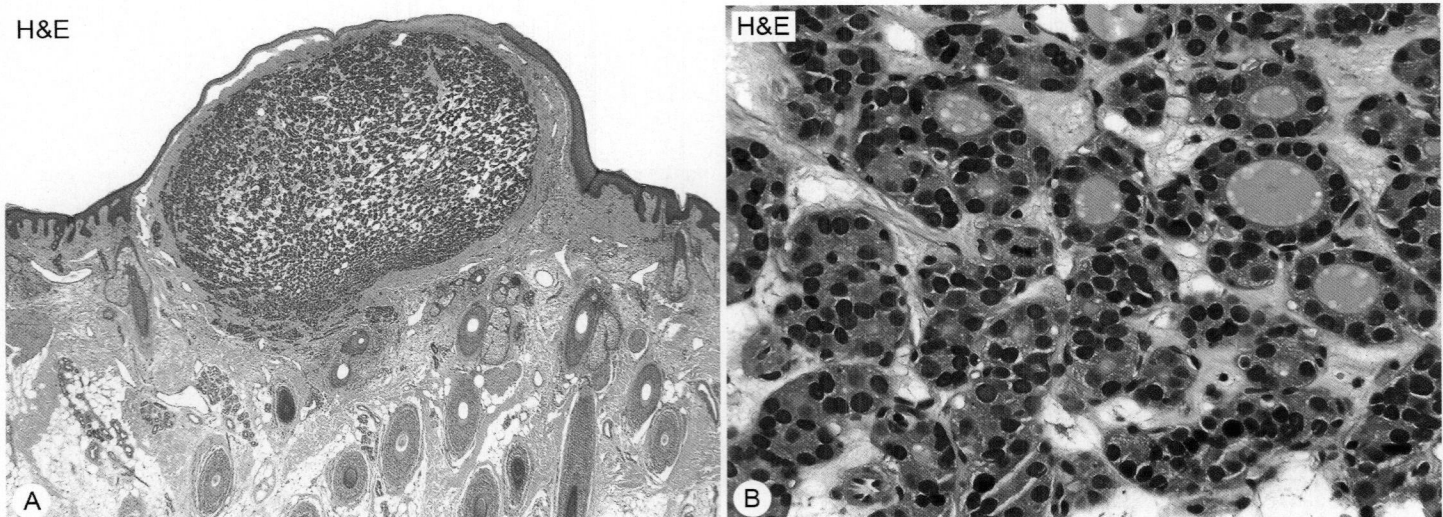

Figure 38-12 Metastatic follicular thyroid carcinoma involving left occipital scalp. **A:** Nodular, polypoid tumor involving dermis (hematoxylin and eosin, 20×), (**B**) composed of variably sized circular nests of cuboidal tumor cells with ovoid nuclei, and frequent central colloid (hematoxylin and eosin, 400×).

REFERENCES

1. Lookingbill DP, Spangler N, Sexton FM. Skin involvement as the presenting sign of internal carcinoma. A retrospective study of 7316 cancer patients. *J Am Acad Dermatol.* 1990;22(1):19–26.

2. Lookingbill DP, Spangler N, Helm KF. Cutaneous metastases in patients with metastatic carcinoma: a retrospective study of 4020 patients. *J Am Acad Dermatol.* 1993;29(2, pt 1):228–236.

3. Spencer PS, Helm TN. Skin metastases in cancer patients. *Cutis.* 1987;39(2):119–121.

4. Brownstein MH, Helwig EB. Metastatic tumors of the skin. *Cancer.* 1972;29(5):1298–1307.

5. Chopra R, Chhabra S, Samra SG, Thami GP, Punia RP, Mohan H. Cutaneous metastases of internal malignancies: a clinicopathologic study. *Indian J Dermatol Venereol Leprol.* 2010;76(2):125–131.

6. Fernandez-Flores A. Cutaneous metastases: a study of 78 biopsies from 69 patients. *Am J Dermatopathol.* 2010;32(3):222–239.

7. Gan EY, Chio MT, Tan WP. A retrospective review of cutaneous metastases at the National Skin Centre Singapore. *Australas J Dermatol.* 2015;56(1):1–6.

8. Hu SC, Chen GS, Lu YW, Wu CS, Lan CC. Cutaneous metastases from different internal malignancies: a clinical and prognostic appraisal. *J Eur Acad Dermatol Venereol.* 2008;22(6):735–740.

9. Itin P, Tomaschett S. Cutaneous metastases from malignancies which do not originate from the skin. An epidemiological study [in German]. *Internist (Berl).* 2009;50(2):179–186.

10. Saeed S, Keehn CA, Morgan MB. Cutaneous metastasis: a clinical, pathological, and immunohistochemical appraisal. *J Cutan Pathol.* 2004;31(6):419–430.

11. Sariya D, Ruth K, Adams-McDonnell R, et al. Clinicopathologic correlation of cutaneous metastases: experience from a cancer center. *Arch Dermatol.* 2007;143(5):613–620.

12. Schoenlaub P, Sarraux A, Grosshans E, Heid E, Cribier B. Survival after cutaneous metastasis: a study of 200 cases [in French]. *Ann Dermatol Venereol.* 2001;128(12):1310–1315.

13. Brownstein MH, Helwig EB. Patterns of cutaneous metastasis. *Arch Dermatol.* 1972;105(6):862–868.

14. Junik R, Kłubo-Gwieździńska J, Zuchora Z, Zmyslowski W. Papillary thyroid cancer with metastasis to the skin. *Clin Nucl Med.* 2006;31(7):435–436.

15. Quinn TR, Duncan LM, Zembowicz A, Faquin WC. Cutaneous metastases of follicular thyroid carcinoma: a report of four cases and a review of the literature. *Am J Dermatopathol.* 2005;27(4):306–312.

16. Ambro CM, Humphreys TR, Lee JB. Epidermotropically metastatic pancreatic adenocarcinoma. *Am J Dermatopathol.* 2006;28(1):60–62.

17. Block CA, Dahmoush L, Konety BR. Cutaneous metastases from transitional cell carcinoma of the bladder. *Urology.* 2006;67(4):846.e15–e17.

18. Fukuda H, Saito R. A case of Sister Mary Josephs nodule from prostatic cancer. *J Dermatol.* 2006;33(1):46–51.

19. Sharma R, Chandra M. Cutaneous metastases from carcinoma of the prostate: a case report. *Dermatol Online J.* 2005;11(1):24.

20. Schwartz RA. Cutaneous metastatic disease. *J Am Acad Dermatol.* 1995;33(2, pt 1):161–182; quiz 183–186.

21. Lee JH, Lee PK, Ahn ST, Oh DY, Rhie JW, Han KT. Unusually huge metastatic cutaneous renal cell carcinoma to the right buttock: case report and review of the literature. *Dermatol Surg.* 2006;32(1):159–160.

22. Ahmed I, Holley KJ, Charles-Holmes R. Zosteriform metastasis of colonic carcinoma. *Br J Dermatol.* 2000;142(1):182–183.

23. Kikuchi Y, Matsuyama A, Nomura K. Zosteriform metastatic skin cancer: report of three cases and review of the literature. *Dermatology.* 2001;202(4):336–338.

24. Steck WD, Helwig EB. Tumors of the umbilicus. *Cancer.* 1965;18:907–915.

25. Kazakov DV, Suster S, LeBoit PE, et al. Mucinous carcinoma of the skin, primary, and secondary: a clinicopathologic study of 63 cases with emphasis on the morphologic spectrum of primary cutaneous forms: homologies with mucinous lesions in the breast. *Am J Surg Pathol.* 2005;29(6):764–782.

26. Qureshi HS, Salama ME, Chitale D, et al. Primary cutaneous mucinous carcinoma: presence of myoepithelial cells as a clue to the cutaneous origin. *Am J Dermatopathol.* 2004;26(5):353–358.

27. Vodovnik A. Primary mucinous carcinoma of the skin. *J Cutan Pathol.* 2006;33(1):61–62.

28. Abbott JJ, Ahmed I. Adenocarcinoma of mammary-like glands of the vulva: report of a case and review of the literature. *Am J Dermatopathol.* 2006;28(2):127–133.

29. Kiyohara T, Kumakiri M, Kouraba S, Tokuriki A, Ansai S. Primary cutaneous signet ring cell carcinoma expressing cytokeratin 20 immunoreactivity. *J Am Acad Dermatol.* 2006;54(3):532–536.

30. Cokonis CD, Green JJ, Manders SM. Primary carcinoid tumor of the skin. *J Am Acad Dermatol.* 2004;51(5 suppl):S146–S148.

31. Ivan D, Nash JW, Prieto VG, et al. Use of p63 expression in distinguishing primary and metastatic cutaneous adnexal neoplasms from metastatic adenocarcinoma to skin. *J Cutan Pathol.* 2007;34(6):474–480.

32. Mahalingam M, Nguyen LP, Richards JE, Muzikansky A, Hoang MP. The diagnostic utility of immunohistochemistry in distinguishing primary skin adnexal carcinomas from metastatic adenocarcinoma to skin: an immunohistochemical reappraisal using cytokeratin 15, nestin, p63, D2-40, and calretinin. *Mod Pathol.* 2010;23(5):713–719.

33. Plaza JA, Ortega PF, Stockman DL, Suster S. Value of p63 and podoplanin (D2-40) immunoreactivity in the distinction between primary cutaneous tumors and adenocarcinomas metastatic to the skin: a clinicopathologic and immunohistochemical study of 79 cases. *J Cutan Pathol.* 2010;37(4):403–410.

34. Celis JE, Gromova I, Cabezón T, et al. Identification of a subset of breast carcinomas characterized by expression of cytokeratin 15: relationship between CK15+ progenitor/amplified cells and pre-malignant lesions and invasive disease. *Mol Oncol.* 2007;1(3):321–349.

35. Bahrami S, Malone JC, Lear S, Martin AW. CD10 expression in cutaneous adnexal neoplasms and a potential role for differentiating cutaneous metastatic renal cell carcinoma. *Arch Pathol Lab Med.* 2006;130(9):1315–1319.

36. Igbokwe A, Lopez-Terrada DH. Molecular testing of solid tumors. *Arch Pathol Lab Med.* 2011;135(1):67–82.

37. Monzon FA, Koen TJ. Diagnosis of metastatic neoplasms: molecular approaches for identification of tissue of origin. *Arch Pathol Lab Med.* 2010;134(2):216–224.

38. Monzon FA, Medeiros F, Lyons-Weiler M, Henner WD. Identification of tissue of origin in carcinoma of unknown primary with a microarray-based gene expression test. *Diagn Pathol.* 2010;5:3.

39. Wong CY, Helm MA, Kalb RE, Helm TN, Zeitouni NC. The presentation, pathology, and current management strategies of cutaneous metastasis. *N Am J Med Sci.* 2013;5(9):499–504.

40. Whitaker-Worth DL, Carlone V, Susser WS, Phelan N, Grant-Kels JM. Dermatologic diseases of the breast and nipple. *J Am Acad Dermatol.* 2000;43(5, pt 1):733–751; quiz 752–754.

41. Pipkin CA, Lio PA. Cutaneous manifestations of internal malignancies: an overview. *Dermatol Clin.* 2008;26(1):1–15, vii.

42. De Giorgi V, Grazzini M, Alfaioli B, et al. Cutaneous manifestations of breast carcinoma. *Dermatol Ther.* 2010;23(6):581–589.

43. Marneros AG, Blanco F, Husain S, Silvers DN, Grossman ME. Classification of cutaneous intravascular breast cancer metastases based on immunolabeling for blood and lymph vessels. *J Am Acad Dermatol.* 2009;60(4):633–638.

44. Panse G, Bossuyt V, Ko CJ. Metastatic serous carcinoma presenting as inflammatory carcinoma over the breast—report of two cases and literature review. *J Cutan Pathol.* 2018;45(3):234-239.

45. Salemis NS, Christofyllakis C, Spiliopoulos K. Primary breast carcinoma en cuirasse. A rare presentation of an aggressive malignancy and review of the literature. *Breast Dis.* 2020;39(3–4):155–159.

46. Ben Hamouda M, Aounallah A, Tlili T, et al. Morphea-like carcinoma en cuirasse revealing a bilateral breast cancer. *Am J Med.* 2021;134(6):e394–e395.

47. Dobson CM, Tagor V, Myint AS, Memon A. Telangiectatic metastatic breast carcinoma in face and scalp mimicking cutaneous angiosarcoma. *J Am Acad Dermatol.* 2003;48(4):635–636.

48. Shiraishi K, Sayama K. Atypical case of telangiectatic metastatic breast carcinoma presenting as purpura. *JAAD Case Rep.* 2017;3(4):316–318.

49. Bianciotto C, Demirci H, Shields CL, Eagle RC Jr, Shields JA. Metastatic tumors to the eyelid: report of 20 cases and review of the literature. *Arch Ophthalmol.* 2009;127(8):999–1005.

50. Shamai-Lubovitz O, Rothem A, Ben-David E, Sandbank M, Hauben D. Cutaneous metastatic carcinoma of the breast mimicking malignant melanoma, clinically and histologically. *J Am Acad Dermatol.* 1994;31(6):1058–1060.

51. Cox SE, Cruz PD Jr. A spectrum of inflammatory metastasis to skin via lymphatics: three cases of carcinoma erysipeloides. *J Am Acad Dermatol.* 1994;30(2, pt 2):304–307.

52. Mullinax K, Cohen JB. Carcinoma en cuirasse presenting as keloids of the chest. *Dermatol Surg.* 2004;30(2, pt 1):226–228.

53. Paolino G, Pampena R, Grassi S, et al. Alopecia neoplastica as a sign of visceral malignancies: a systematic review. *J Eur Acad Dermatol Venereol.* 2019;33(6):1020–1028.

54. Sanki A, Spillane A. Diagnostic and treatment challenges of inframammary crease breast carcinomas. *ANZ J Surg.* 2006;76(4):230–233.

55. Waisman M. Carcinoma of the inframammary crease. *Arch Dermatol.* 1978;114(10):1520–1521.

56. Requena L, Sánchez Yus E, Núñez C, White CR Jr, Sangueza OP. Epidermotropically metastatic breast carcinomas. Rare histopathologic variants mimicking melanoma and Paget's disease. *Am J Dermatopathol.* 1996;18(4):385–395.

57. Hui Y, Wang Y, Nam G, et al. Differentiating breast carcinoma with signet ring features from gastrointestinal signet ring carcinoma: assessment of immunohistochemical markers. *Hum Pathol.* 2018;77:11–19.

58. Gonzalez-Lois C, Rodríguez-Peralto JL, Serrano-Pardo R, Martínez-González MA, López-Ríos F. Cutaneous signet ring cell carcinoma: a report of a case and review of the literature. *Am J Dermatopathol.* 2001;23(4):325–328.

59. Wesche WA, Khare VK, Chesney TM, Jenkins JJ. Non-hematopoietic cutaneous metastases in children and adolescents: thirty years experience at St. Jude Children's Research Hospital. *J Cutan Pathol.* 2000;27(10):485–492.

60. Chu P, Wu E, Weiss LM. Cytokeratin 7 and cytokeratin 20 expression in epithelial neoplasms: a survey of 435 cases. *Mod Pathol.* 2000;13(9):962–972.

61. Fernandez-Flores A. Cutaneous metastases from breast carcinoma: calretinin expression and estrogen, progesterone and Her2/neu status of the metastases, compared to primary cutaneous apocrine tumors. *Rom J Morphol Embryol.* 2013;54(3 suppl):695–699.

62. Ni YB, Tsang JY, Chan SK, Tse GM. GATA-binding protein 3, gross cystic disease fluid protein-15 and mammaglobin have distinct prognostic implications in different invasive breast carcinoma subgroups. *Histopathology.* 2015;67(1):96–105.

63. Yang Y, Lu S, Zeng W, Xie S, Xiao S. GATA3 expression in clinically useful groups of breast carcinoma: a comparison with GCDFP15 and mammaglobin for identifying paired primary and metastatic tumors. *Ann Diagn Pathol.* 2017;26:1–5.

64. Peng Y, Butt YM, Chen B, Zhang X, Tang P. Update on immunohistochemical analysis in breast lesions. *Arch Pathol Lab Med.* 2017;141(8):1033–1051.

65. Stroup RM, Pinkus GS. S-100 immunoreactivity in primary and metastatic carcinoma of the breast: a potential source of error in immunodiagnosis. *Hum Pathol.* 1988;19(8):949–953.

66. Bayer-Garner IB, Smoller B. Androgen receptors: a marker to increase sensitivity for identifying breast cancer in skin metastasis of unknown primary site. *Mod Pathol.* 2000;13(2):119–122.

67. Brady LW, O'Neill EA, Farber SH. Unusual sites of metastases. *Semin Oncol.* 1977;4(1):59–64.

68. Ferreira L, Luis F, Cabral F. Lung cancer and cutaneous metastasis [in Portuguese]. *Rev Port Pneumol.* 2004;10(6):475–484.

69. Nashan D, Meiss F, Braun-Falco M, Reichenberger S. Cutaneous metastases from internal malignancies. *Dermatol Ther.* 2010;23(6):567–580.

70. Hussein MR. Skin metastasis: a pathologist's perspective. *J Cutan Pathol.* 2010;37(9):e1–e20.

71. Courville P, Joly P, Thomine E, et al. Primary cutaneous carcinoid tumour. *Histopathology.* 2000;36(6):566–567.

72. Donati, P, Panetta C, Cota C, Paolino G, Muscardin L. Carcinoid metastasis of the skin appearing as painful tumor. *J Dermatol.* 2013;40(5):415–417.

73. Falto-Aizpurua L, Seyfer S, Krishnan B, Orengo I. Cutaneous metastasis of a pulmonary carcinoid tumor. *Cutis.* 2017;99(5):E13–E15.

74. Rodriguez G, Villamizar R. Carcinoid tumor with skin metastasis. *Am J Dermatopathol.* 1992;14(3):263–269.

75. Babacan NA, Kiliçkap S, Sene S. A case of multifocal skin metastases from lung cancer presenting with vasculitic-type cutaneous nodule. *Indian J Dermatol.* 2015;60(2):213.

76. Yorita K, Tsuji K, Takano Y, et al. Acantholytic squamous cell carcinoma of the lung with marked lymphogenous metastases and high titers of myeloperoxidase-antineutrophil cytoplasmic antibodies: a case report. *BMC Cancer.* 2018;18(1):300.

77. Travis WD. Update on small cell carcinoma and its differentiation from squamous cell carcinoma and other non-small cell carcinomas. *Mod Pathol.* 2012;25(suppl 1):S18–S30.

78. Yang DT, Holden JA, Florell SR. CD117, CK20, TTF-1, and DNA topoisomerase II-alpha antigen expression in small cell tumors. *J Cutan Pathol.* 2004;31(3):254–261.

79. Tetzlaff MT, Nagarajan P. Update on Merkel cell carcinoma. *Head Neck Pathol.* 2018;12(1):31–43.

80. Tetzlaff MT, Harms PW. Danger is only skin deep: aggressive epidermal carcinomas. An overview of the diagnosis, demographics, molecular-genetics, staging, prognostic biomarkers, and therapeutic advances in Merkel cell carcinoma. *Mod Pathol.* 2020;33(suppl 1):42–55.

81. Byrd-Gloster AL, Khoor A, Glass LF, et al. Differential expression of thyroid transcription factor 1 in small cell lung carcinoma and Merkel cell tumor. *Hum Pathol.* 2000;31(1):58–62.

82. Lilo MT, Chen Y, LeBlanc RE. INSM1 is more sensitive and interpretable than conventional immunohistochemical stains used to diagnose Merkel cell carcinoma. *Am J Surg Pathol.* 2018;42(11):1541–1548.

83. Wick MR, Swanson PE, Ritter JH, Fitzgibbon JF. The immunohistology of cutaneous neoplasia: a practical perspective. *J Cutan Pathol.* 1993;20(6):481–497.

84. Guinee DG Jr, Fishback NF, Koss MN, Abbondanzo SL, Travis WD. The spectrum of immunohistochemical staining of small-cell lung carcinoma in specimens from transbronchial and open-lung biopsies. *Am J Clin Pathol.* 1994;102(4):406–414.

85. Tot T. The value of cytokeratins 20 and 7 in discriminating metastatic adenocarcinomas from pleural mesotheliomas. *Cancer.* 2001;92(10):2727–2732.

86. Ralston J, Chiriboga L, Nonaka D. MASH1: a useful marker in differentiating pulmonary small cell carcinoma from Merkel cell carcinoma. *Mod Pathol.* 2008;21(11):1357–1362.

87. Jagirdar J. Application of immunohistochemistry to the diagnosis of primary and metastatic carcinoma to the lung. *Arch Pathol Lab Med.* 2008;132(3):384–396.

88. Ordonez NG. Napsin A expression in lung and kidney neoplasia: a review and update. *Adv Anat Pathol.* 2012;19(1):66–73.

89. El-Maqsoud NM, Tawfiek ER, Abdelmeged A, Rahman MF, Moustafa AA. The diagnostic utility of the triple markers Napsin A, TTF-1, and PAX8 in differentiating between primary and metastatic lung carcinomas. *Tumour Biol.* 2016;37(3):3123–3134.

90. Greenberg HL, Lopez L, Butler DF. Peristomal metastatic adenocarcinoma of the rectum. *Arch Dermatol.* 2006;142(10):1372–1373.

91. Grossi U, Petracca Ciavarella L, Fuso P, Crucitti A. Sister Mary Joseph's nodule and colorectal cancer: an aggressive treatment for an aggressive disease. *ANZ J Surg.* 2020;90(7–8):1504–1505.

92. Taniguchi S, Hisa T, Hamada T. Cutaneous metastases of pancreatic carcinoma with unusual clinical features. *J Am Acad Dermatol.* 1994;31(5, pt 2):877–880.

93. Brownstein MH, Helwig EB. Spread of tumors to the skin. *Arch Dermatol.* 1973;107(1):80–86.

94. Oku T, Nakayama F, Takigawa M. A peculiar form of epidermotropism in cutaneous metastatic carcinoma. *J Dermatol.* 1990;17(1):59–61.

95. Johnson WC, Helwig EB. Histochemistry of primary. *Ann N Y Acad Sci.* 1963;106:794–803.

96. Johnson WC, Helwig EB. Histochemistry of the acid mucopolysaccharides of skin in normal and in certain pathologic conditions. *Am J Clin Pathol.* 1963;40:123–131.

97. Werner I. Studies on glycoproteins from mucous epithelium and epithelial secretions. *Acta Soc Med Ups.* 1953;58(1–2):1–55.

98. Park SY, Kim HS, Hong EK, Kim WH. Expression of cytokeratins 7 and 20 in primary carcinomas of the stomach and colorectum and their value in the differential diagnosis of metastatic carcinomas to the ovary. *Hum Pathol.* 2002;33(11):1078–1085.

99. Werling RW, Yaziji H, Bacchi CE, Gown AM. CDX2, a highly sensitive and specific marker of adenocarcinomas of intestinal origin: an immunohistochemical survey of 476 primary and metastatic carcinomas. *Am J Surg Pathol.* 2003. 27(3):303–310.

100. Azoulay S, Adem C, Pelletier FL, Barete S, Francès C, Capron F. Skin metastases from unknown origin: role of immunohistochemistry in the evaluation of cutaneous metastases of carcinoma of unknown origin. *J Cutan Pathol.* 2005;32(8):561–566.

101. Saad RS, Silverman JF, Khalifa MA, Rowsell C. CDX2, cytokeratins 7 and 20 immunoreactivity in rectal adenocarcinoma. *Appl Immunohistochem Mol Morphol.* 2009;17(3):196–201.

102. Park JH, Kim JH. Pathologic differential diagnosis of metastatic carcinoma in the liver. *Clin Mol Hepatol.* 2019;25(1):12–20.

103. Perysinakis I, Minaidou E, Leontara V, et al. Differential expression of beta-Catenin, EGFR, CK7, CK20, MUC1, MUC2, and CDX2 in intestinal and pancreatobiliary-type ampullary carcinomas. *Int J Surg Pathol.* 2017;25(1):31–40.

104. Altree-Tacha D, Tyrrell J, Haas T. CDH17 is a more sensitive marker for gastric adenocarcinoma than CK20 and CDX2. *Arch Pathol Lab Med.* 2017;141(1):144–150.

105. Kim DH, Joo JE, Kim EK, Lee HJ, Lee WM. The expressions of cytokeratin 7 and 20 in epithelial tumors: a survey of 91 cases. *Cancer Res Treat.* 2003;35(4):355–363.

106. Jung S, Wu C, Eslami Z, et al. The role of immunohistochemistry in the diagnosis of flat urothelial lesions: a study using CK20, CK5/6, P53, Cd138, and Her2/Neu. *Ann Diagn Pathol.* 2014;18(1):27–32.

107. Parker DC, Folpe AL, Bell J, et al. Potential utility of uroplakin III, thrombomodulin, high molecular weight cytokeratin, and cytokeratin 20 in noninvasive, invasive, and metastatic urothelial (transitional cell) carcinomas. *Am J Surg Pathol.* 2003;27(1):1–10.

108. Ohnishi T, Takizawa H, Watanabe S. Immunohistochemical analysis of cytokeratin and human milk fat globulin expression in mucinous carcinoma of the skin. *J Cutan Pathol.* 2002;29(1):38–43.

109. Lora V, Kanitakis J. CDX2 expression in cutaneous metastatic carcinomas and extramammary Paget's disease. *Anticancer Res.* 2009;29(12):5033–5037.

110. Yan P, Klingbiel D, Saridaki Z, et al. Reduced expression of SMAD4 is associated with poor survival in colon cancer. *Clin Cancer Res.* 2016;22(12):3037–3047.

111. Ritterhouse LL, Wu EY, Kim WG, et al. Loss of SMAD4 protein expression in gastrointestinal and extra-gastrointestinal carcinomas. *Histopathology.* 2019;75(4):546–551.

112. Pereira TC, Share SM, Magalhães AV, Silverman JF. Can we tell the site of origin of metastatic squamous cell carcinoma? An immunohistochemical tissue microarray study of 194 cases. *Appl Immunohistochem Mol Morphol.* 2011;19(1):10–14.

113. Connor DH, Taylor HB, Helwig EB. Cutaneous metastasis of renal cell carcinoma. *Arch Pathol.* 1963;76:339–346.

114. Corgna E, Betti M, Gatta G, Roila F, De Mulder PH. Renal cancer. *Crit Rev Oncol Hematol.* 2007;64(3):247–262.

115. Heatley MK. Keratin expression in human tissues and neoplasms. *Histopathology.* 2002;41(4):365–366.

116. Barr ML, Jilaveanu LB, Camp RL, Adeniran AJ, Kluger HM, Shuch B. PAX-8 expression in renal tumours and distant sites: a useful marker of primary and metastatic renal cell carcinoma? *J Clin Pathol.* 2015;68(1):12–17.

117. Chu P, Arber DA. Paraffin-section detection of CD10 in 505 nonhematopoietic neoplasms. Frequent expression in renal cell carcinoma and endometrial stromal sarcoma. *Am J Clin Pathol.* 2000;113(3):374–382.

118. Laury AR, Perets R, Piao H, et al. A comprehensive analysis of PAX8 expression in human epithelial tumors. *Am J Surg Pathol.* 2011;35(6):816–826.

119. Perna AG, Ostler DA, Ivan D, et al. Renal cell carcinoma marker (RCC-Ma) is specific for cutaneous metastasis of renal cell carcinoma. *J Cutan Pathol.* 2007;34(5):381–385.

120. Tong GX, Memeo L, Colarossi C, et al. PAX8 and PAX2 immunostaining facilitates the diagnosis of primary epithelial neoplasms of the male genital tract. *Am J Surg Pathol.* 2011;35(10):1473–1483.

121. Hu Y, Hartmann A, Stoehr C, et al. PAX8 is expressed in the majority of renal epithelial neoplasms: an immunohistochemical study of 223 cases using a mouse monoclonal antibody. *J Clin Pathol.* 2012;65(3):254–256.

122. Tacha D, Qi W, Zhou D, Bremer R, Cheng L. PAX8 mouse monoclonal antibody [BC12] recognizes a restricted epitope and is highly sensitive in renal cell and ovarian cancers but does not cross-react with b cells and tumors of pancreatic origin. *Appl Immunohistochem Mol Morphol.* 2013;21(1):59–63.

123. Ozcan A, de la Roza G, Ro JY, Shen SS, Truong LD. PAX2 and PAX8 expression in primary and metastatic renal tumors: a comprehensive comparison. *Arch Pathol Lab Med.* 2012;136(12):1541–1551.

124. Mentrikoski MJ, Wendroth SM, Wick MR. Immunohistochemical distinction of renal cell carcinoma from other carcinomas with clear-cell histomorphology: utility of CD10 and CA-125 in addition to PAX-2, PAX-8, RCCma, and adipophilin. *Appl Immunohistochem Mol Morphol.* 2014;22(9):635–641.

125. Costantino C, Thomas GV, Ryan C, Coakley FV, Troxell ML. Metastatic renal cell carcinoma without evidence of a renal primary. *Int Urol Nephrol.* 2016;48(1):73–77.

126. Schwartz RA. Histopathologic aspects of cutaneous metastatic disease. *J Am Acad Dermatol.* 1995;33(4):649–657.

127. Baker PM, Oliva E. Immunohistochemistry as a tool in the differential diagnosis of ovarian tumors: an update. *Int J Gynecol Pathol.* 2005;24(1):39–55.

128. Fujiwara M, Taube J, Sharma M, McCalmont TH, Kim J. PAX8 discriminates ovarian metastases from adnexal tumors and other cutaneous metastases. *J Cutan Pathol.* 2010;37(9):938–943.

129. Xiang L, Kong B. PAX8 is a novel marker for differentiating between various types of tumor, particularly ovarian epithelial carcinomas. *Oncol Lett.* 2013;5(3):735–738.

130. Zhao L, Guo M, Sneige N, Gong Y. Value of PAX8 and WT1 immunostaining in confirming the ovarian origin of metastatic carcinoma in serous effusion specimens. *Am J Clin Pathol.* 2012;137(2):304–309.

131. Fogaca MF, Fedorciw BJ, Tahan SR, Johnson R, Federman M. Cutaneous metastasis of neuroendocrine carcinoma of uterine origin. *J Cutan Pathol.* 1993;20(5):455–458.

132. Isaacs H Jr. Cutaneous metastases in neonates: a review. *Pediatr Dermatol.* 2011;28(2):85–93.

133. Van Nguyen A, Argenyi ZB. Cutaneous neuroblastoma. Peripheral neuroblastoma. *Am J Dermatopathol.* 1993;15(1):7–14.

134. Scott MP, Helm KF. Cytokeratin 20: a marker for diagnosing Merkel cell carcinoma. *Am J Dermatopathol.* 1999;21(1):16–20.

135. Chan JK, Suster S, Wenig BM, et al. Cytokeratin 20 immunoreactivity distinguishes Merkel cell (primary cutaneous neuroendocrine) carcinomas and salivary gland small cell carcinomas from small cell carcinomas of various sites. *Am J Surg Pathol.* 1997;21(2):226–234.

136. Ordonez NG, Samaan NA. Medullary carcinoma of the thyroid metastatic to the skin: report of two cases. *J Cutan Pathol.* 1987;14(4):251–254.

137. Ciocca O, Vassallo C, Brazzelli V, Fiandrino G, Rosso R, Borroni G. Sporotrichoid metastases to the skin from cutaneous squamous cell carcinoma in an immunocompetent patient. *Am J Dermatopathol.* 2010;32(4):395–397.

138. Kahn JA, Sinhamohapatra SB, Schneider AF. Hepatoma presenting as a skin metastasis. *Arch Dermatol.* 1971;104(3):299–300.

139. Cosnow I, Fretzin DF. Choriocarcinoma metastatic to skin. *Arch Dermatol.* 1974;109(4):551–553.

140. Chhieng DC, Jennings TA, Slominski A, Mihm MC Jr. Choriocarcinoma presenting as a cutaneous metastasis. *J Cutan Pathol.* 1995;22(4):374–377.

141. Segal R, Penneys NS, Nahass G. Metastatic prostatic carcinoma histologically mimicking malignant melanoma. *J Cutan Pathol.* 1994;21(3):280–282.

142. Brody HJ, Stallings WP, Fine RM, Someren A. Carcinoid in an umbilical nodule. *Arch Dermatol.* 1978;114(4):570–572.

Index

Note: Page number followed by "*f*" indicate figure; those followed by "*t*" indicate table.

Drug(s) (*continued*)
  biological agents, reaction to, 399–400
  bleomycin pigmentation, 394, 394*f*
  bullous disorders, 388–390
  chemotherapeutic agents, reactions to,
      396–397, 396–397*f*
  chrysiasis, 395
  clofazimine-induced pigmentation,
      393–394
  coma blister, 388–389, 388*f*
  diltiazem pigmentation, 394
  drug-induced bullous pemphigoid, 390
  drug-induced fibrosing disorders,
      387–388, 388*f*
  drug-induced pemphigus, 389–390, 390*f*
  dysmaturation, 396, 396*f*
  elastosis perforans serpiginosa,
      penicillamine induced, 401–402
  erythema multiforme, 382, 382*f*
  exanthematous drug eruptions, 391, 391*f*
  exanthemic drug eruptions, 391
  fixed drug eruption, 383, 384*f*
  halogen eruptions, 387, 387*f*
  halogenodermas, 387
  HCV, antiretroviral therapy for, 400–401, 401*f*
  HIV, antiretroviral therapy for, 401
  hydroxyurea pigmentation, 394
  interface dermatitis, 381–385
  krokodil, 403
  levamisole, 402–403, 403*f*
  lichenoid drug eruption, 383, 383*f*
  linear IgA bullous dermatosis, 390
  lupus erythematosus, 384–385, 384*f*
  mercury pigmentation, 395, 396*f*
  minocycline pigmentation, 393, 393*f*
  nephrogenic systemic fibrosis, 388, 388*f*
  neutrophilic drug eruptions, 385–388
  neutrophilic eccrine hidradenitis,
      396–397, 397*f*
  noninterface lymphocytic drug eruptions,
      385, 385*f*
  penicillamine-induced dermatoses,
      401–403, 402*f*
  photoallergic drug eruption, 391, 391*f*
  photodistributed hyperpigmentation,
      392–393, 392*f*
  phototoxic drug eruption, 392, 392*f*
  pigmentary disorders, 393–395
  pseudolymphoma syndrome, 385, 385*f*
  pseudoporphyria, 389
  scleroderma-like conditions, 388
  Sweet syndrome, 387–388, 387*f*
  systemic lupus erythematosus and, 357*t*
  TEN and SJS, 382–383, 383*f*
  toxic acral erythema, 397
  toxic epidermal necrolysis and, 333
DSAP. *See* Disseminated superficial actinic
      porokeratosis
Ductal cells, of eccrine hidrocystoma, 1052
Ductal eccrine carcinoma, malignant eccrine
      poroma and, 1056
Dupuytren contracture (palmar fibromatosis),
      1198–1199
Dwarfism, mucopolysaccharidosis and, 530
Dysbetalipoproteinemia, 806
Dyschromatosis symmetrica hereditaria. *See*
      Acropigmentation symmetrica of Dohi
Dyschromia, radiation dermatitis and, 425

Dyshidrotic dermatitis, 291–292, 291*f*
  clinical summary of, 291
  histopathology of, 113, 291–292, 291*f*
  principles of management, 292
Dyskeratosis. *See also* Focal acantholytic
      dyskeratosis
  acantholysis with, 959
  in acantholytic squamous cell carcinoma, 987
  PAMS and, 311
  transient acantholytic dermatosis with, 337
Dyskeratosis congenita (DKC), 158–159, 819
  clinical summary of, 158
  differential diagnosis of, 159
  histopathology of, 158
  pathogenesis of, 159
  poikiloderma atrophicans vasculare and, 365
  principles of management, 159
Dyskeratotic acanthoma, 959
Dyskeratotic keratinocytes
  acute ultraviolet burn, 422*f*
  of Bowenoid papulosis of genitalia, 783
  in verrucous lupus erythematosus, 353
Dyskerin gene, 159, 819
Dysmaturation, 396
  clinical summary of, 396
  histopathology of, 396
  ultraviolet recall and, 422
Dyspareunia, necrolytic migratory erythema, 489
Dysplastic nevus, 855–858, 856–527*f*
  differential diagnosis of, 861–863, 863*f*
  histopathology of, 110
  as intermediate lesions of tumor
      progression, 860–861
  melanocytic dysplasia, grading of, 858–859,
      858–859*t*
  as melanoma precursors, 859
  principles of management of, 863
  radial growth phase melanoma v., 861*t*
  as risk markers, 859–860
  significance of, 859
Dysplastic nevus syndrome, 855
Dystrophic calcinosis cutis, 520, 520*f*
  with burn scars, 422
  clinical summary of, 520
  histopathology of, 520
  principles of management, 520
Dystrophic epidermolysis bullosa
  milia and, 968
  with nail unit, 603

EAC. *See* Erythema annulare centrifugum
Early spongiotic dermatitis, histopathology
      of, 117
Ears
  discoid lupus erythematosus and, 351
  relapsing polychondritis and, 583
  vellus hairs, 57
Ear skin nevi, 849
EB. *See* Epidermolysis bullosa
EBA. *See* Epidermolysis bullosa acquisita
EBV. *See* Epstein–Barr virus
EBV-positive mucocutaneous ulcer (MCU),
      1103–1105, 1104*f*
  clinical features of, 1103
  differential diagnosis of, 1105
  histogenesis of, 1105
  histopathology of, 1103
  principles of management of, 1105

Eccrine acrospiroma, 1059
Eccrine adenocarcinoma, histopathology of, 126
Eccrine angiomatous hamartoma, 131, 1051,
      1052*f*
Eccrine glands, 11*t*, 33–38
  carcinomas of, 1066–1070
    adenoid cystic carcinoma, 1068–1069, 1068*f*
    classic type of, 1067
    digital papillary adenocarcinoma, 1068,
        1068*f*
    endocrine mucin-secreting sweat gland
        carcinoma, 1066–1067
    microcystic adnexal carcinoma, 1066*f*,
        1067–1069
    mucinous eccrine carcinoma, 1067, 1067*f*
    mucoepidermoid carcinoma, 1068
    syringoid eccrine carcinoma, 1067–1068*f*
  chilblains and, 430–431*f*, 432
  collagen fibers and, 50
  coma blisters and, 336
  in dermoid cyst, 970
  discoid lupus erythematosus and, 352
  embryology of, 33–34
  histopathology of, 104, 104*f*, 130–131
  inflammatory processes of, 90
  morphea and, 367, 367*f*
  neutrophilic eccrine hidradenitis, 581–582*f*
  normal microanatomy of, 34–35, 35*f*
  Paget disease and, 1007
  porokeratotic eccrine ostial and dermal duct
      nevus of, 959
  regional variation of, 35–36, 37*f*
  specialized structure and function of, 36–37
  special stains for, 36–38*f*, 37–38
  S100 protein in, 79–80
  tumors of, 103, 103*f*, 126, 1051–1064
    eccrine hidrocystoma, 1051, 1052*f*
    eccrine nevus, 1051, 1051*f*
    eccrine poroma, 1054–1055, 1054–1055*f*
    eccrine syringofibroadenoma, 1056, 1056*f*
    hidradenocarcinoma, 1060–1061, 1061*f*
    malignant eccrine poroma, 1051–1056*f*,
        1055–1056
    malignant mixed tumor, 1065–1063*f*,
        1065–1066
    mixed tumor of the skin, 1061–1062*f*,
        1061–1063
    mucinous syringometaplasia, 1057
    nodular hidradenoma, 1059–1060,
        1059–1060*f*
    papillary eccrine adenoma, 1059, 1059*f*
    spiradenocarcinoma, 1058–1059, 1059*f*
    spiradenoma, 1057–1058, 1057–1058*f*
    syringoma, 1052–1054, 1053*f*
Eccrine glandular ridges, Merkel cells at, 21
Eccrine hidrocystoma, 1051
  additional studies of, 1051
  apocrine hidrocystoma v., 1046
  clinical summary of, 1051
  differential diagnosis of, 1052
  histopathology of, 104, 104*f*, 130, 1052,
      1052*f*
  principles of management, 1052
Eccrine nevus, 1051, 1051*f*
  clinical summary of, 1051
  histopathology of, 105, 105*f*, 126, 131,
      1051, 1051*f*
  principles of management, 1051